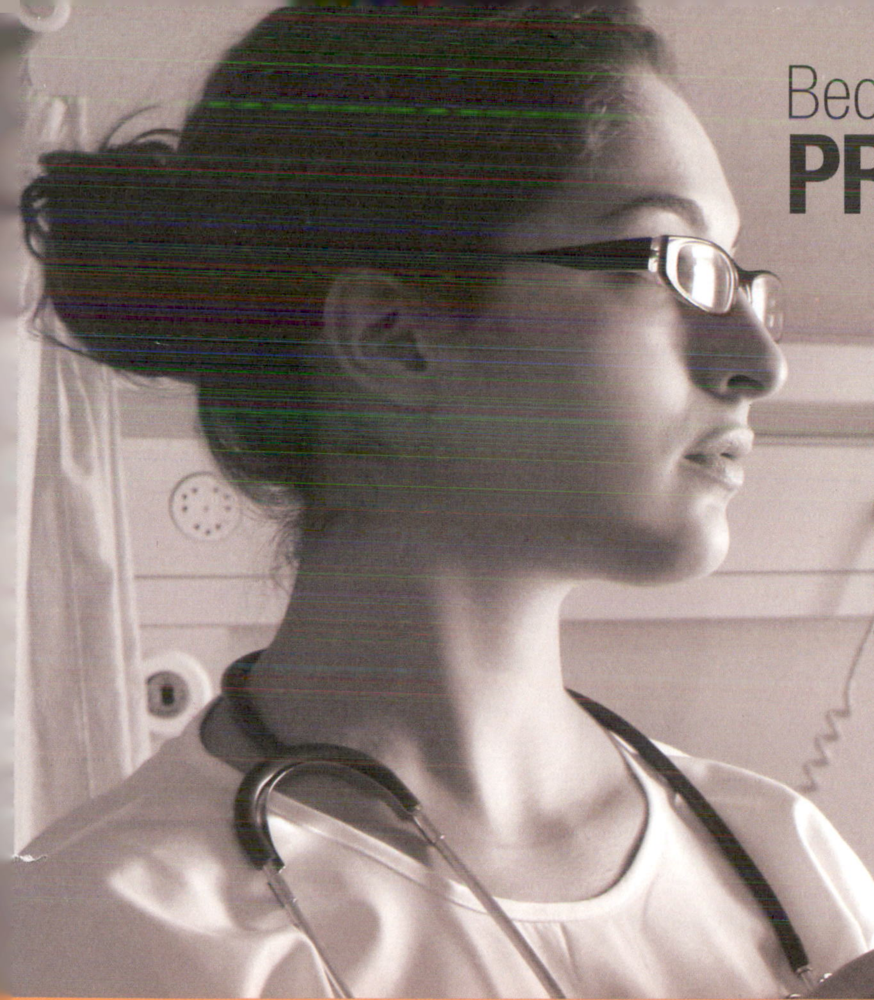

Become
PRACTICE-READY
using your
PEARSON
RESOURCES

Simplify your study time by using the resources included with this textbook at **http://nursing.pearsonhighered.com.**

This book includes the following materials for you to use:

- Learning Outcomes
- NCLEX® Review Questions
- Critical Thinking Activities
- Case Studies
- Care Plans
- Media Links
- and More.

Enhance your SUCCESS with the additional resources be... For more information and purchasing options visit **www.mypearsonstore.com.**

D0145880

For Your Classroom Success
MyNursingLab®

MyNursingLab provides a guided learning path that is proven to help students synthesize vast amounts of information, guiding them from memorization to true understanding through application.

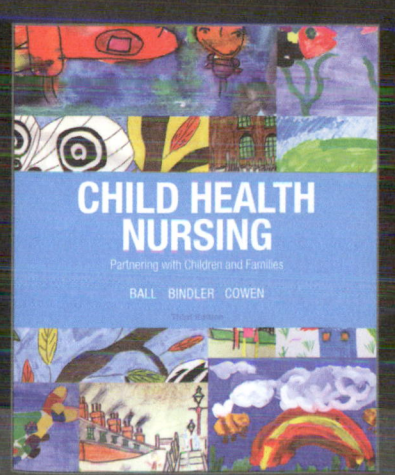

For Your Clinical Success
MyNursingApp™

Clinical references across the nursing curriculum available!

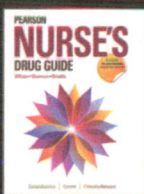

Pearson's Nurse's Drug Guide

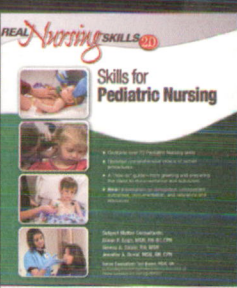

visit:
www.realnursingskills.com

For Your NCLEX-RN® Success

MaryAnn Hogan, MSN, RN provides clear, concentrated, and current review of "need to know" information for effective classroom and NCLEX-RN® preparation.

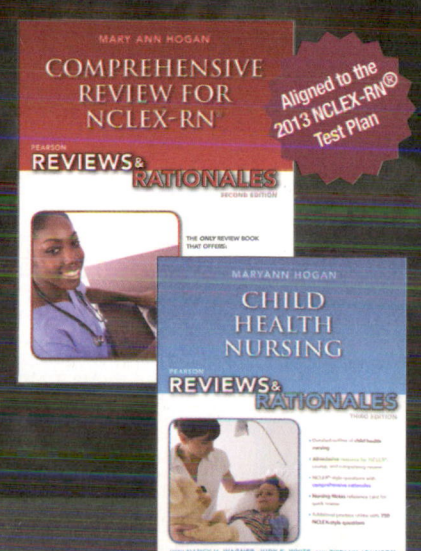

Aligned to the 2013 NCLEX-RN® Test Plan

ALWAYS LEARNING

PEARSON

MyNursingLab®

www.mynursingapp.com

Learn more about and purchase
access to MyNursingLab.

MyNursingApp™

www.mynursinglab.com

MyNursingApp puts all the information
you need in the palm of your hand.

myPEARSONstore.com

Find your textbook and everything
that goes with it.

ALWAYS LEARNING

PEARSON

CHILD HEALTH NURSING
Partnering with Children and Families

Third Edition

Jane W. Ball, RN, CPNP, DRPH
Consultant, Trauma Systems Evaluation and Planning Committee
American College of Surgeons
Gaithersburg, Maryland

Ruth C. Bindler, RNC, PhD
Professor Emeritus
Washington State University College of Nursing
Spokane, Washington

Kay J. Cowen, RN-BC, MSN
Clinical Professor
University of North Carolina at Greensboro School of Nursing
Greensboro, North Carolina

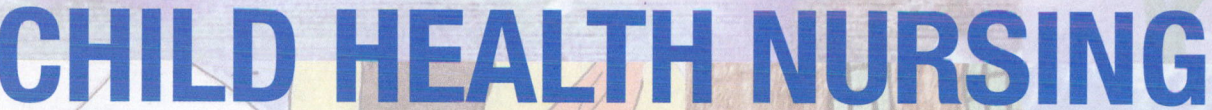

PEARSON

Boston   Columbus   Indianapolis   New York   San Francisco   Upper Saddle River
Amsterdam   Cape Town   Dubai   London   Madrid   Munich   Paris   Montréal   Toronto
Delhi   Mexico City   São Paulo   Sydney   Hong Kong   Seoul   Singapore   Taipei   Tokyo

Publisher: Julie Levin Alexander
Publisher's Assistant: Regina Bruno
Executive Acquisitions Editor: Kim Norbuta
Editorial Assistant: Erin Rafferty
Development Editor: Kim Wyatt
Managing Editor, Production: Patrick Walsh
Production Liaison: Maria Reyes
Production Editor: Lynn Steines, S4Carlisle Publishing Services
Manufacturing Manager: Lisa McDowell
Art Director: Mary Siener
Interior Designer: Mary Siener
Cover Design: Jodi Notowitz
Cover Image: Shutterstock
Director of Marketing: David Gesell
Marketing Manager: Phoenix Harvey
Marketing Specialist: Michael Sirinides
Media Project Managers: Leslie Brado/Michael Dobson
Composition: S4Carlisle Publishing Services
Printer/Binder: Courier/Kendallville
Cover Printer: LeHigh Phoenix Color/Hagerstown
Cover/Interior Illustrations: Jelena Voronova/Shutterstock;
Tumarkin Igor/ITPS, Shutterstock; Viktoriya Field/Shutterstock;
Aleksandar Mijatovic/Shutterstock; Brian J. Abela/Shutterstock

Notice: Care has been taken to confirm the accuracy of information presented in this book. The authors, editors, and the publisher, however, cannot accept any responsibility for errors or omissions or for consequences from application of the information in this book and make no warranty, express or implied, with respect to its contents.

The authors and publisher have exerted every effort to ensure that drug selections and dosages set forth in this text are in accord with current recommendations and practice at time of publication. However, in view of ongoing research, changes in government regulations, and the constant flow of information relating to drug therapy and drug reactions, the reader is urged to check the package inserts of all drugs or the hospital formulary for any change in indications of dosage and for added warnings and precautions. This is particularly important when the recommended agent is a new and/or infrequently employed drug.

Copyright © 2014, 2010, 2006 by Pearson Education, Inc. All rights reserved. Manufactured in the United States of America. This publication is protected by Copyright and permission should be obtained from the publisher prior to any prohibited reproduction, storage in a retrieval system, or transmission in any form or by any means, electronic, mechanical, photocopying, recording, or likewise. To obtain permission(s) to use material from this work, please submit a written request to Pearson Education, Inc., Permissions Department, One Lake Street, Upper Saddle River, New Jersey 07458 or you may fax your request to 201-236-3290.

Many of the designations by manufacturers and seller to distinguish their products are claimed as trademarks. Where those designations appear in this book, and the publisher was aware of a trademark claim, the designations have been printed in initial caps or all caps.

Library of Congress Cataloging-in-Publication Data
Ball, Jane (Jane W.)
  Child health nursing: partnering with children and families / Jane W. Ball, Ruth C. Bindler, Kay J. Cowen. — 3rd ed.
     p.; cm.
  Includes bibliographical references and index.
  ISBN-13: 978-0-13-284007-1
  ISBN-10: 0-13-284007-3
  I. Bindler, Ruth McGillis II. Cowen, Kay J. III. Title.
    [DNLM: 1. Pediatric Nursing. WY 159]
    LC Classification not assigned
    618.92'00231—dc23
    2012026325

10 9 8 7 6 5 4 3 2 1

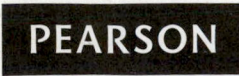

www.pearsonhighered.com

ISBN-13: 978-0-13-284007-1
ISBN-10: 0-13-284007-3

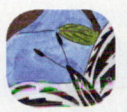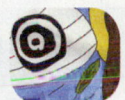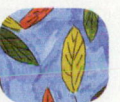

Jane W. Ball

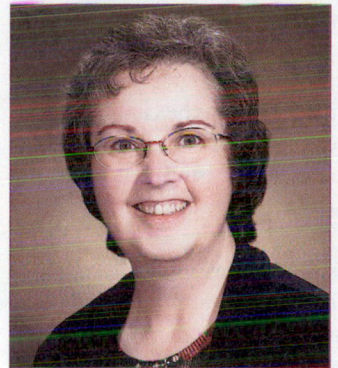

Jane W. Ball graduated from the Johns Hopkins Hospital School of Nursing, and subsequently received a BS from the Johns Hopkins University. She worked in the surgical, emergency, and outpatient units of the Johns Hopkins Children's Medical and Surgical Center, first as a staff nurse and then as a pediatric nurse practitioner, beginning her career as a pediatric nurse and advocate for children's health needs. Jane obtained both a master of public health and a doctor of public health degree from the Johns Hopkins University Bloomberg School of Public Health with a focus on maternal and child health. After graduation she became the chief of child health services for the Commonwealth of Pennsylvania Department of Health. In this capacity she oversaw the state-funded well-child clinics and explored ways to improve education for the state's community health nurses. After relocating to Texas, she joined the faculty at the University of Texas at Arlington School of Nursing to teach community pediatrics to registered nurses returning to school for a BSN. During this time she became involved in writing her first textbook, *Mosby's Guide to Physical Examination*, which is currently in its seventh edition. After relocating to the Washington, DC, area, she joined Children's National Medical Center to manage a federal project to teach instructors of emergency medical technicians from all states about the special care children need during an emergency. Exposure to the shortcomings of the emergency medical services system in the late 1980s with regard to pediatric care was a career-changing event. With federal funding, she developed educational curricula for emergency medical technicians and emergency nurses to help them provide improved care for children. A textbook entitled *Pediatric Emergencies, A Manual for Prehospital Providers* was developed from these educational ventures. For 15 years she managed the federally funded Emergency Medical Services for Children's National Resource Center. As executive director, Dr. Ball directed the provision of consultation and resource development for state health agencies, health professionals, families, and advocates about successful methods to improve the health care system so that children get optimal emergency care in all health care settings. Having left that position, she devotes more time to writing and serves as a consultant to the American College of Surgeons, supporting state trauma system development. In 2010, Dr. Ball received the Distinguished Alumna Award from the Johns Hopkins University.

Ruth C. Bindler

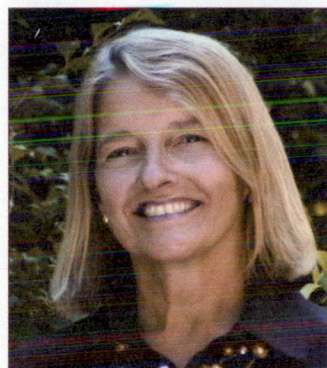

Ruth C. McGillis Bindler received her BSN from Cornell University—New York Hospital School of Nursing. She worked in oncology nursing at Memorial-Sloan Kettering Cancer Center in New York, and then moved to Wisconsin and became a public health nurse in Dane County, Wisconsin. Thus began her commitment to work with children as she visited children and their families at home, and served as a school nurse for several elementary, middle, and high schools. Due to this interest in child health care needs, she earned her MS in child development from the University of Wisconsin. A move to Washington State was accompanied by a new job as a faculty member at the Intercollegiate Center for Nursing Education in Spokane. Dr. Bindler has been fortunate to be involved for over 35 years in the growth of this nursing education consortium, which is a combination of public and private universities and colleges and is now the Washington State University (WSU) College of Nursing. Ruth obtained a PhD in human nutrition at WSU. She has taught theory and clinical courses in child health nursing, cultural diversity and health, graduate research, pharmacology, and assessment, as well as serving as lead faculty for child health nursing and Associate Dean for Graduate Programs. She is now a professor emeritus at Washington State University. Her first professional book, *Pediatric Medications*, was published in 1981, and she has continued to publish articles and books in the areas of pediatric medications and pediatric health. Research efforts are focused in the area of childhood obesity, type 2 diabetes, metabolic syndrome, and cardiometabolic risk factors in children. Ethnic diversity and interprofessional collaboration have been additional themes in her work. Dr. Bindler believes that her role as a faculty member has enabled her to continually, foster the development of students in nursing, mentor junior faculty into the teaching role, and particip the profession of nursing. In addition to teaching, rese tion, and leadership, she enhances her life by profes munity service, and by activities with her family.

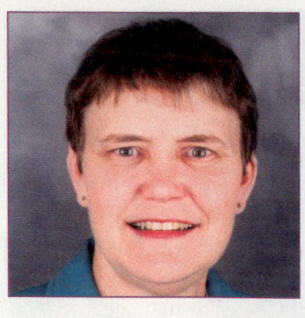

Kay J. Cowen

Kay J. Cowen received her BSN from East Carolina University in Greenville, North Carolina, and began her career as a staff nurse on the pediatric unit of North Carolina Baptist Hospital in Winston-Salem. She developed a special interest in the psychosocial needs of hospitalized children and preparing them for hospitalization. This led to the focus of her master's thesis at the University of North Carolina at Greensboro (UNCG) where she received a master of science in nursing education degree with a focus in maternal child nursing.

Mrs. Cowen began her teaching career in 1984 at UNCG where she continues today as clinical professor in the Parent Child Department. Her primary responsibilities include coordinating the pediatric nursing course, teaching classroom content, and supervising a clinical group of students. Mrs. Cowen shared her passion for the psychosocial care of children and the needs of their families through her first experience as an author in the chapter "Hospital Care for Children" in Jackson & Saunders' *Child Health Nursing: A*

Comprehensive Approach to the Care of Children and Their Families published in 1993.

In the classroom, Mrs. Cowen realized that students learn through a variety of teaching strategies and became especially interested in the strategy of gaming. She led a research study to evaluate the effectiveness of gaming in the classroom and subsequently continues to incorporate gaming in her teaching. In the clinical setting, Mrs. Cowen teaches her students the skills needed to care for patients and the importance of family-centered care, focusing on not only the physical needs of the child but also the psychosocial needs of the child and family.

During her teaching career, Mrs. Cowen has continued to work part time as a staff nurse: first on the pediatric unit of Moses Cone Hospital in Greensboro and then at Brenner Children's Hospital in Winston-Salem. In 2006 she became the part-time pediatric nurse educator in Brenner's Family Resource Center. Through this role she is able to extend her love of teaching to children and families.

Through her role as an author, Mrs. Cowen is able to extend her dedication to pediatric nursing and nursing education. She is married and the mother of twin sons.

We dedicate this book to our partners:
~our families for their unwavering support
~colleagues who have grown and learned with us, and continue to help expand our thinking
~families and children with whom we work, for teaching us the essentials of child health nursing
~students who are our collaborators now and in their future careers as nurses

Thank You

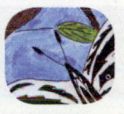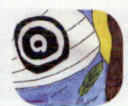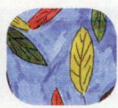

We would like to express our deep gratitude to our colleagues from schools and hospitals across the country for their time over the past 3 years. These individuals assisted us in the revision of this book by contributing and reviewing manuscript chapters and contributing to the supplements that accompany this title. **Child Health Nursing: Partnering with Children & Families** has benefited immeasurably from your efforts, insights, and willingness to share your expertise as teachers and nurses.

CONTRIBUTOR

Chapter 4: Genetics and Genomics Influence

Linda D. Ward, MN, ARNP
Clinical Assistant Professor
Washington State University College of Nursing
Spokane, Washington

SUPPLEMENTAL CONTRIBUTORS

Jane Brown, MSN, RN
Associate Professor
Walters State Community College
Morristown, Tennessee

Laura L. Brown, RN, MSN, CPN
Nursing Instructor
Asheville Buncombe Technical Community College
Asheville, North Carolina

Pamela P. DiNapoli, PhD, RN
Associate Professor
University of New Hampshire
Durham, New Hampshire

Donna Eberly, RN, MSN
Instructor
Western Iowa Tech Community College
Sioux City, Iowa

Sharon Koval Falkenstern, PhD, CRNP, PNP-C, CNE
Assistant Professor, Coordinator of NP Option
The Pennsylvania State University
University Park, Pennsylvania

Leslie Holmes, RN, BSN, MSN
Instructor, Family and Community Nursing
Nell Hodgson Woodruff SON Emory University
Atlanta, Georgia

Mary Jo Konkloski, RN, MSN, ANP
Coordinator, RN Program
Finger Lakes Health College of Nursing
Geneva, New York

Patricia Kuster, PhD, RN, CPNP
Assistant Professor
Samuel Merritt College School of Nursing
Sacramento, California

Brenda Lykins, RNC-NIC, BSN
Neonatal Outreach Coordinator
MultiCare Regional Perinatal Outreach Program
Tacoma, Washington

Adelaide R. McCulloch

Brenda Millet, MSN, RN-BC
Staff Development Specialist
Children's National Medical Center
Washington, DC

Cheryl Shaffer, RN, MS, PNP, ANP, PhD(c)
Associate Professor
Suffolk County Community College
Selden, New York

Lisa D. South, RN, DSN
Assistant Professor
The University of Alabama at Birmingham
Birmingham, Alabama

Jane K. Walker, BBA, RN, CLNC, PhD(c)
Associate Professor of Nursing
Walters State Community College
Morristown, Tennessee

Jeannie Weston, MS, CNS, BSN
Assistant Clinical Instructor
Emory University
Atlanta, Georgia

REVIEWERS

Mike Aldridge, Concordia University Texas
Kim Amer, DePaul University
Janice Bidwell, San Diego State University
Patricia Bobbitt, Wake Forest University School of Medicine
Sally Brooks, The University of Louisiana at Monroe
Michael Brown, The University of Texas Health Science Center at Houston
Karyn Casey, The University of Tennessee
Teresa Chase, University of Kentucky
Jennifer Compere, Brenner Children's Hospital
Joseph De Santis, University of Miami
Linda Esposito, Wake Forest Baptist Medical Center
Melissa Ethington, The University of Texas Health Science Center at Houston
Niki Fogg, Texas Woman's University
Betty Freund, Kent State University
Julie Garcia, The University of Texas Health Science Center at San Antonio
Carol Hall Grantham, Georgia State University
Debbie Hancock, The University of North Carolina at Greensboro
Kristen Harrison, Wake Forest Baptist Medical Center
Amy Zlomek Hedden, California State University, Bakersfield
Michelle Howell, Wake Forest Baptist Medical Center
Kim Hutchinson, Wake Forest Baptist Medical Center
Arlene Johnson, Clemson University
Eleanor Kehoe, College of Staten Island
Mary Kishman, College of Mount St. Joseph
Julie Kordsmeier, The University of North Carolina at Greensboro
Heidi Krowchuk, The University of North Carolina at Greensboro
Laura Kubin, Texas Woman's University

Sarah Kulinski, Lenoir-Rhyne University
Patricia Kuster, Samuel Merritt University
Lin Lin, The University of Texas Health Science Center at Houston
Antoinette McCray, Norfolk State University
Cheryl Mele, Drexel University
Mary Ellen Mitchell-Rosen, Nova Southeastern University
Heidi Monroe, Seattle Pacific University
Brenda Pavill, University of North Carolina Wilmington
Sue Perkins, Washington State University
Kathleen Peterson, The College at Brockport
Janice Pitman, Brenner Children's Hospital
Kari Crawford Plant, Levine Children's Hospital
Deborah Roberts, Sonoma State University
T. Kim Rodehorst-Weber, University of Nebraska Medical Center
Carol Rossman, Calvin College
Michele Shaw, Washington State University
Anita Smith, Wake Forest University School of Medicine
Daphnee Stewart, Mercer University
Phyllis Thatcher, Wake Forest Baptist Medical Center
Debra Thomson, Wake Forest Baptist Medical Center
Maureen Tippen, University of Michigan-Flint
Theresa Turick-Gibson, Hartwick College
Diane Van Os, Westminster College
Darla Vogelpohl, University of Toledo
Beverly Bockstruck West, University of Memphis
Melissa Williams, Augusta State University
Cecilia Wilson, Texas Woman's University

Preface

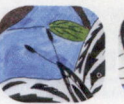 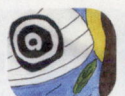 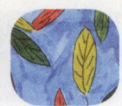

The world children grow up in today is vastly different from the world we experienced in our early years. Our evolving social environment has resulted in diverse family structures and roles. Multiple racial and ethnic groups now commonly share communities, work environments, and recreation. A variety of technology applications are part of children's daily routines. Nutritional patterns have changed due to the complexity of daily lives and food marketing, and the environment is identified as an increasing influence on child and adolescent health. The geospatial design elements of communities, including schools, modes of transportation, and safety in neighborhoods, have altered daily behaviors. Life in complex societies offers new challenges to mental health, and homes provide diverse risk and protective factors in managing the health and illness of child family members. New ways of treating diseases, from applications of genomics to a current generation of medications, influence youth health. Healthcare reform, electronic health records, new approaches to chronic and acute condition management, and a focus on prevention have contributed to changes in the information that nurses and other healthcare providers need. We draw heavily upon *Healthy People 2020* in this text to guide our suggested interventions and evaluation of goals for health conditions.

In addition to an evolution of influences on child health, there have been incredible achievements in nursing education. The American Association of Colleges of Nursing (AACN) published the *Essentials of Baccalaureate Education for Professional Nursing Practice* in 2008. While we know that many Associate Degree Nursing programs use our books, we also are aware that a number of those programs also use "the Baccalaureate Essentials" in establishing their curricula. We have therefore applied the Essentials throughout the book and cite them in a new feature (see a description later in this preface). In 2009, the "Carnegie Report" on *Educating Nurses: A Call for Radical Transformation* was published. This long-awaited study emphasized the importance of connecting classroom and clinical learning, focusing on clinical reasoning when working with students, and fostering career ladders and lifelong learning. These recommendations inform our clinical judgment and clinical reasoning features. Finally, in 2010, the Institute of Medicine (IOM) released *The Future of Nursing: Leading Change, Advancing Health*. The IOM recommended that nurses function to the full extent of their education and training, achieve higher levels of education, be full partners with physicians and other healthcare professionals in the redesign of health care, and work to plan policies that ensure data collection and information infrastructure.

Child Health Nursing: Partnering with Children & Families is a contemporary pediatric nursing textbook. Excellence in pediatric nursing care, whether it is in the acute care setting or in the community, is a challenge and the major objective guiding today's pediatric nurse. You, as a student, will be challenged to synthesize previous information with new knowledge, apply evidence-based findings, collaborate with other healthcare professionals and families, and integrate current knowledge to use clinical reasoning skills in planning pediatric nursing care. You will be challenged to lead, examining ways in which you can positively influence the health care of children and their families in the challenging times of healthcare reform.

The third edition of *Child Health Nursing* builds upon the strong foundation and planning of the first two editions and addresses the need for fresh approaches to child and adolescent health care and nursing education in several ways. Themes in this book include:

- Partnering with Children and Their Families
- The Roles and Essential Functions of the Nurse
- Health Promotion and Health Maintenance
- Collaboration with Families and Healthcare Providers
- Evidence-Based Practice
- Clinical Reasoning

The subtitle, *Partnering with Children & Families*, reflects the core value of our textbook—emphasizing family-centered care, recognition of the family as the central influence in each child's life, and respect for families from all cultures. Families are viewed as case managers, as partners with healthcare providers, and as integral participants in care in all pediatric nursing settings. Partnership and interprofessional collaboration are other key concepts of our textbook. In the past, we introduced the *Bindler-Ball Child Healthcare Model* as a paradigm with which to view health care of children. This model illustrates an important core value—that all children need health promotion and maintenance interventions, no matter where they seek care or what health conditions they may be experiencing. Families may visit offices or other community settings, specifically to obtain health supervision care; or nurses may integrate health promotion and maintenance into the care for children with acute and chronic illness in a variety of inpatient and outpatient settings. The Bindler-Ball Healthcare Model places health promotion and maintenance at the foundation of a pyramid to demonstrate the need to apply these concepts with all children. See Chapter 1 for an introduction to this model.

WHAT'S NEW IN THIS EDITION

- Baccalaureate Essentials Boxes highlight the nine essentials of nursing education identified by the American Association of Colleges of Nursing.
- NANDA-I 2012-2014 nursing diagnoses for multiple conditions.
- Updated *Healthy People 2020* goals for the pediatric population.
- More Evidence-Based Practice features emphasize nursing research and offer a critical thinking element.
- Clinical Judgment speed bumps to encourage critical thinking.
- Clinical Reasoning section at the end of chapter to help with application of concepts and synthesis.
- New statistics, and integration of current health care implications and environmental considerations.

ORGANIZATION

The six units in this textbook have a unifying theme. The first unit, *Nurses, Children, and Families,* lays the foundation for a thorough understanding of pediatric nursing in today's world. It discusses the nurse's roles in caring for children in the hospital, community, and home, as well as the concepts of family-centered care and cultural considerations.

The second unit focuses on *Child Concepts and Application,* melding theory with application so that concepts can be applied to pediatric nursing care in a variety of settings. Genetics and genomics are current concepts that will be increasingly employed in future health care. We describe concepts of growth and development and child/family communication in separate chapters, and examine applications to pediatric nursing. The pediatric assessment chapter provides basic and detailed information that will be applied in all pediatric healthcare settings.

The third unit focuses on *Health Promotion and Maintenance Through Childhood.* The first chapter introduces basic concepts, and each of the remaining five chapters applies health promotion and maintenance concepts with specific approaches for children at each developmental stage from newborn through adolescence. Nurses assess children thoroughly, establish goals in partnership with the family, intervene to promote and maintain health and foster development, and evaluate the outcomes of care. This unique approach minimizes repetition throughout the book, and underscores the need for all children to receive routine health promotion and health maintenance to achieve optimal health.

The fourth unit, *Child Healthcare Settings and Considerations,* explores the various settings in which care occurs. In addition to the hospital, nurses and nursing students are likely to provide care in community settings, such as health centers, schools, and homes, where health promotion and maintenance activities predominate. Special considerations for the care of children during disasters are also discussed. Shorter hospitalizations have become the norm, thereby increasing the need for more comprehensive care in community settings, such as specialty outpatient centers where nurses coordinate care for children with various health conditions. Children need special attention when they have chronic health conditions, when they have life-threatening illnesses or injuries, or when they need end-of-life care.

The fifth unit discusses *Nursing Care for Common Health Conditions.* The unit begins with a chapter on infant, child, and adolescent nutrition, which discusses both nutritional requirements for health and some common nutritional disruptions. A chapter on social and environmental influences addresses topics pertinent to children and

their families in today's world, such as violence and substance use. A chapter on pediatric pain assessment and management provides general nursing care concepts that are woven through the remainder of the book. Another chapter focuses on the prevention and treatment of infectious and communicable diseases, a significant role in pediatric nursing care.

The sixth unit consists of 14 chapters that address *Nursing Care of Specific Health Conditions.* Information about health conditions, including both illnesses and injuries, is grouped by body systems, eliminating the need for duplication at various places in the text. This streamlined approach builds on previous concepts rather than repeating them, integrating a developmental approach with pertinent conditions affecting all age groups from newborn to adolescent.

The chapters fully describe diseases and injuries beginning with an anatomic and physiologic overview, pediatric differences, and system-specific assessment guidelines. This is followed by a discussion of the etiology, pathophysiology, clinical manifestations, and **collaborative care**, including diagnostics and clinical therapy sections for each of the major conditions. **Nursing management** of major conditions contains detailed sections on assessment and diagnosis, planning and intervention, and evaluation of care. The book is readable and understandable, taking the student from present knowledge level to mastery of new material. The many features further enhance the readability of the material for students coming from various backgrounds and nursing programs and curricula.

Sample nursing care plans will assist you in applying developmental, psychosocial, and physiologic concepts to the care of children with specific conditions. North American Nursing Diagnosis Association (NANDA International) diagnoses are used, as well as the current Nursing Intervention Classifications (NIC) and Nursing Outcomes Classifications (NOC).

Visuals That Teach

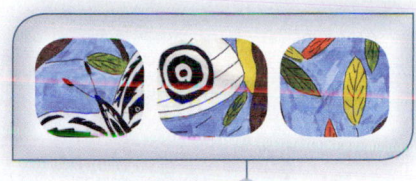

The art program of this book continues to use a thoroughly integrated approach, beginning with the cover and carried through the interior of the textbook. The cover of *Child Health Nursing* features hand-painted tiles from Rydal Elementary School in Abington, Pennsylvania. Art is both a method of expression and a healing modality, and the feelings, design, and colors of the tiles integrated throughout this book will help you identify with children and their families, and understand their experiences.

A Day in the Life of a Nurse helps identify the roles and focus of nursing care in each of three settings: the hospital, the healthcare center, and the school setting.

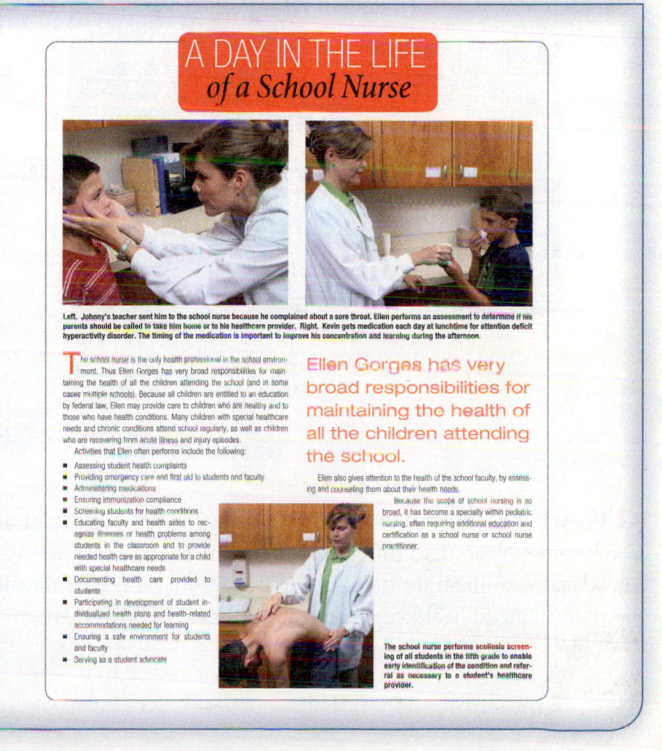

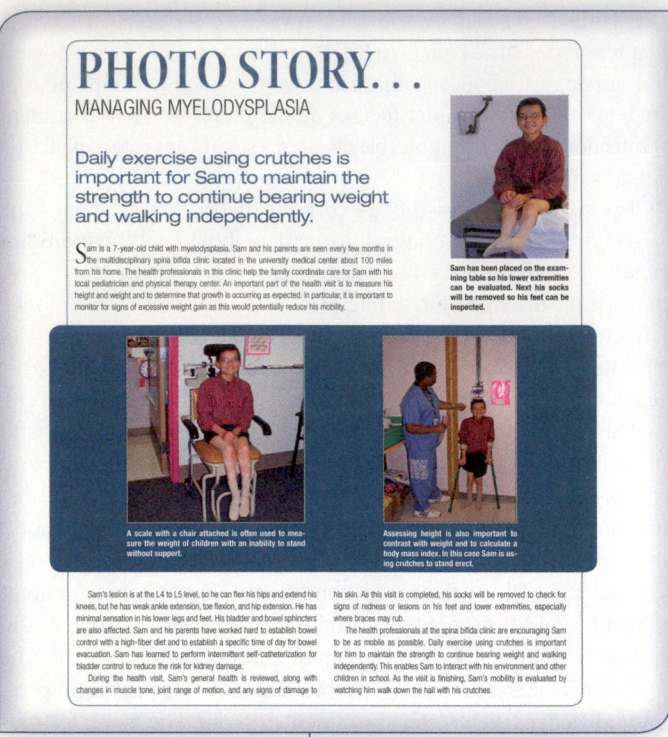

PHOTO STORY...
MANAGING MYELODYSPLASIA

Daily exercise using crutches is important for Sam to maintain the strength to continue bearing weight and walking independently.

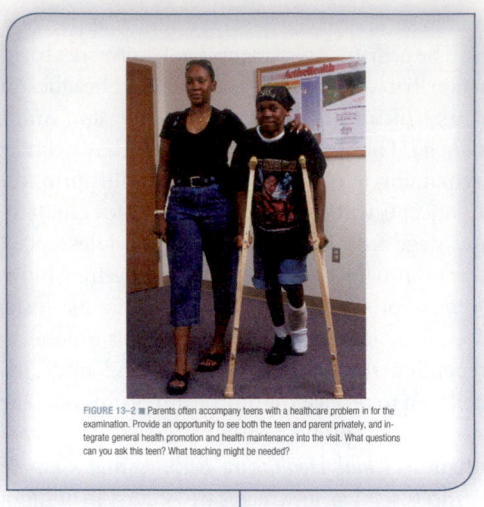

FIGURE 13–2 ■ Parents often accompany teens with a healthcare problem in for the examination. Provide an opportunity to see both the teen and parent privately, and integrate general health promotion and health maintenance into the visit. What questions can you ask this teen? What teaching might be needed?

The photographs and drawings throughout the textbook do more than illustrate concepts and examples. You will find critical thinking opportunities among the figure captions. These unique highlights, also appearing in the text itself, encourage you to apply information and analyze the nursing implications needed to provide care for children and their families, thus adding true learning value to the visuals.

Photo Stories help bring information and concepts "alive" to develop a deeper understanding about the effect of a specific condition on the child and family. These stories include photographs of a child or situation to demonstrate the challenges a child and family may face in managing the condition.

The text explains in-depth pathophysiology of pediatric conditions, and accompanying **Pathophysiology Illustrated** figures allow you to see into the body to visualize the causes and effects of conditions on children. These elaborate drawings illustrate conditions on a cellular or organ level, and may also portray the step-by-step process of a disease. Drawings or photos with artistic overlays relate disease to its anatomic location and action.

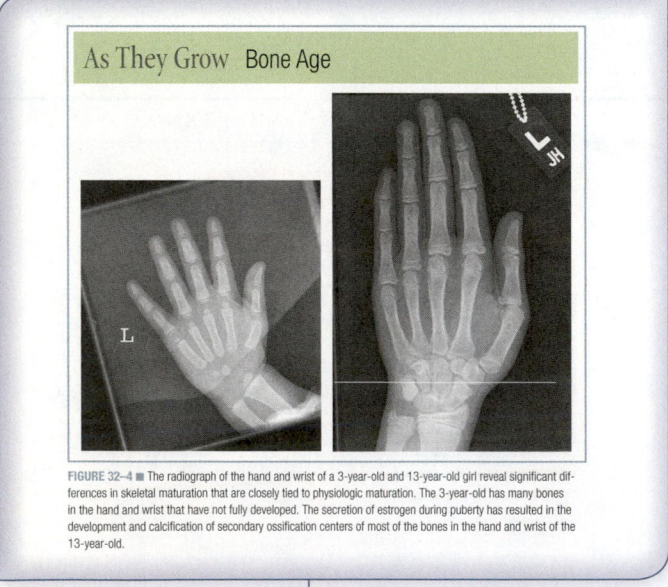

As They Grow   Bone Age

FIGURE 32–4 ■ The radiograph of the hand and wrist of a 3-year-old and 13-year-old girl reveal significant differences in skeletal maturation that are closely tied to physiologic maturation. The 3-year-old has many bones in the hand and wrist that have not fully developed. The secretion of estrogen during puberty has resulted in the development and calcification of secondary ossification centers of most of the bones in the hand and wrist of the 13-year-old.

As They Grow illustrations help you visualize the important anatomic and physiologic differences between a child and an adult. These features illustrate the important ways that a child's development influences healthcare needs and how the child progresses through developmental stages.

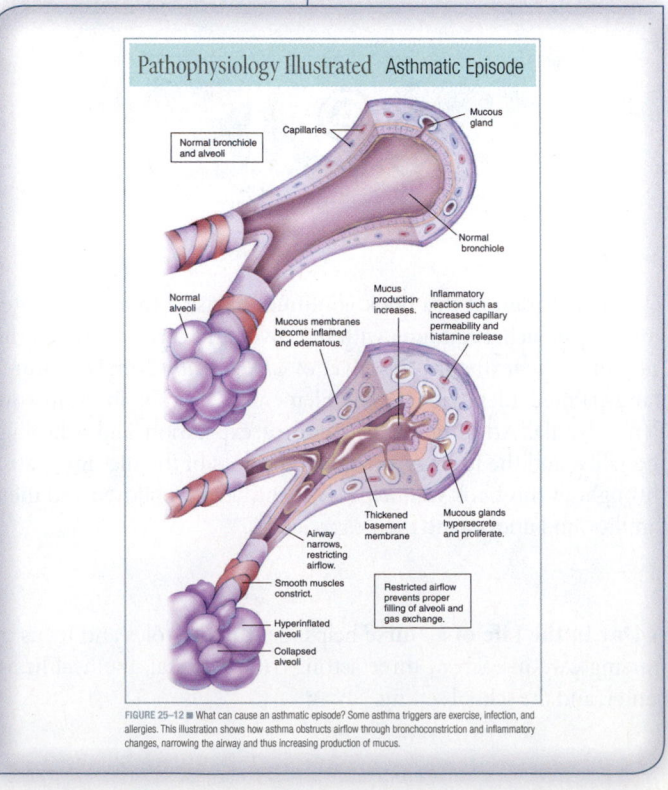

Pathophysiology Illustrated   Asthmatic Episode

FIGURE 25–12 ■ What can cause an asthmatic episode? Some asthma triggers are exercise, infection, and allergies. This illustration shows how asthma obstructs airflow through bronchoconstriction and inflammatory changes, narrowing the airway and thus increasing production of mucus.

Features That Help You Use This Book Successfully

Nursing students face challenges in their education—managing demands on their time, applying research findings, evaluating components of evidence-based practice, and developing their critical thinking skills. Thus instructors and students alike value the in-text learning aids that we include in our textbooks to meet the challenges of pediatric nursing in today's world. We developed a textbook that is easy to learn from and easy to use as a professional reference. The following guide will help you use the features and resources from *Child Health Nursing* to succeed in the classroom, in the clinical setting, on the NCLEX-RN® examination, and in nursing practice.

Assessment Guidelines for the Child tables in each of the systems chapters provide an overview of the key aspects of an integrated assessment for conditions within the body system.

TABLE 33–3	Assessment Guidelines for the Child with a Neurologic Condition
ASSESSMENT FOCUS	**ASSESSMENT GUIDELINES**
Level of consciousness	■ Is the infant or child difficult to arouse?
	■ Is the infant or child irritable or difficult to calm or console?
	■ Is the child oriented? Can the child tell the examiner his or her name and age?
	■ What is the child's ability to concentrate? Can the young child name pictures of animals? Can the older child answer simple math questions or spell words?
	■ The Glasgow Coma Scale provides a numeric score for future comparison. See Table 33–5.
Cranial nerves	■ Assess the cranial nerves. See Table 7–18 ⏺. See Table 33–6 for methods to indirectly assess cranial nerves in the unconscious child.
Fontanels and sutures	■ Palpate fontanels and suture lines on the infant's scalp.
Cognitive function	■ Are the child's verbal skills developmentally appropriate for age?
	■ Does the child follow directions and respond appropriately?
Pupils	■ Check the pupils for size and reaction to light and accommodation. See Figure 33–4 on page 1154.
Vital signs	■ Assess heart rate, respiratory rate, and blood pressure.
	■ Monitor for an increased systolic blood pressure, a widened pulse pressure, bradycardia, and irregular respirations (late signs of increased intracranial pressure).
Posture and movement	■ Inspect the infant's posture and movement by using the primitive reflexes. See Table 7–19 ⏺.
	■ Observe the child's play or other spontaneous activity to assess strength as well as symmetry and smoothness of movements.
	■ Are the child's motor skills developmentally appropriate for age? Were motor skills acquired at the appropriate age? Has the child lost a previously acquired skill?
	■ Evaluate muscle strength and tone, comparing side to side. Is any weakness present?
	■ Test the child's coordination for smoothness and symmetry of response.

Practice Alert

When the child has a chronic respiratory or neuromuscular condition, development of respiratory failure may be gradual as muscles associated with breathing may be weakened. Signs will be subtle. Be particularly alert to behavior changes in addition to respiratory signs. Pulse oximetry and serial blood gases may be needed to monitor the child.

Practice Alerts warn you of safety precautions and other nursing alerts to consider in providing safe care.

Clinical Tip

Insulin binds to IV tubing. Run 50 to 100 mL of insulin through the new IV tubing to saturate all the binding sites. This ensures that the full dose of insulin reaches the child from the outset.

Clinical Tips are "pearls" from clinical nursing experts embedded throughout the textbook.

Clinical Judgment

Some signs of the intact neurologic status of an infant (newborn to 2 months of age) are a cry with a loud and energetic quality, a strong suck, and suck-swallowing coordination. What is one additional sign?

NEW! Clinical Judgment speed bumps appear when an opportunity for critical thinking arises.

Case Scenarios and photos at the beginning of the chapter engage you with a child's real-life experience with a specific health challenge. Additional information about the child and family appears throughout the chapter to illustrate application of nursing care. Use the questions embedded in each scenario to apply pathophysiologic, psychosocial, family, culture, developmental, or nursing process considerations. At the end of the chapter, a detailed **Clinical Reasoning in Action** exercise picks up the opening scenario and asks you to apply what you have read.

> **"Why do they need to take my tonsils out? They're fine where they are!"**
> —*Tiona, age 5*

Five-year-old Tiona Lewallen has a history of frequent tonsillitis and is scheduled for a tonsillectomy and adenoidectomy in the morning. Her mother has brought her in today for preoperative evaluation and instruction. Tiona has no other health problems. Her experience with health care is limited to well-child checkups and immunizations as well as several visits to the otolaryngologist in the past year. She has no prior hospitalizations. Tiona will return at 6:30 a.m. for surgery. She will be admitted to the pediatric day short-stay unit for a few hours following surgery and will then be discharged home as long as she is able to drink fluids and take oral pain medication. How should the nurse assess what Tiona knows about her surgery? What techniques should be used to teach Tiona about the surgery? What instructions should Tiona's

Clinical Reasoning in Action

INTRODUCTION
Recall Tiona, the child described in the beginning of the chapter. She is a 5-year-old girl who was admitted to the hospital for a tonsillectomy and adenoidectomy (T&A).

DESCRIPTION
Following Tiona's operation, she refused to drink liquids because it hurt when she swallowed. After receiving intravenous pain medication, Tiona realized that she could swallow without too much pain and began to eat Popsicles and drink liquids. She was then switched to oral pain medication. Later in the day, Tiona was drinking liquids well enough to be discharged home.

DISCUSSION
1. What information should the nurse include in the discharge teaching plan for Tiona's mother?

2. As Tiona and her mother are preparing to leave the hospital, Tiona says, "I am going to be good so I do not have to come to the hospital anymore!" How should the nurse respond?

3. Tiona's mother states that she is worried that her daughter will not drink enough at home. What can the nurse suggest to Tiona's mother to encourage her to drink fluids? What are the symptoms of dehydration that Tiona's mother should watch for over the next few days?

4. Children Tiona's age have many fears and stressors related to hospitalization and surgery. How can her mother assist Tiona to express her feelings about the hospital experience once she is home?

Tables of **Diagnostic Procedures and Laboratory Tests** pertinent to the specific systems assist you in clinical when you need the information.

TABLE 32–3	Diagnostic Procedures and Laboratory Tests for the Endocrine System*	
DIAGNOSTIC PROCEDURES	**LABORATORY TESTS**
ACTH stimulation test	Fasting plasma glucose
Adrenal (ACTH) suppression test	Hemoglobin A_{1c}
Bone age	Hormone levels
Computed tomography (CT)	Insulin-like growth factor (IGF-1) and Insulin-like growth factor-binding protein 3 IGFBP-3
Fluid deprivation test	
Karyotype	
Magnetic resonance imaging (MRI)	Newborn metabolic screening
Thyroid radioactive iodine uptake (RAIU) scan	Provocative growth hormone testing
	Thyroid antibodies

Note: *See Appendixes D and E 🔴 for information about these diagnostic procedures and for expected laboratory tests values.

Complementary Therapy
Muscular Dystrophy

Many families who have a child with muscular dystrophy use different types of complementary care. The nurse always assesses for such approaches, provides information as needed by the family, makes recommendations for complementary therapies that may be helpful, and cautions against those that could be harmful due to interactions with medications or other problems. Common complementary care used in muscular dystrophy includes dietary enhancement. This enhancement includes vitamins A, C, E, D, and B-complex; minerals such as calcium, magnesium, zinc, and selenium; probiotic supplement; omega-3 fatty acids; herbal remedies such as green and rhodiola rosea teas; muscular and immunologic enzymes such as coenzyme Q10, N-acetyl cysteine, acetyl-L-carnitine, creatine, and L-theanine; melatonin to promote sleep; and massage to assist with reduction of muscle spasms (University of Maryland Medical Center, 2011).

Complementary Therapy boxes present approaches other than traditional medical prescriptions that may be used by children and families to maintain health or treat diseases. These boxes discuss research when it is present to support or refute the efficacy of these modalities. At other times, they alert you about information to gather from the family and to consider when planning care.

Developing Cultural Competence
Growth Grids

The growth grids now in use were standardized using a cross section of the U.S. population and are generally reflective of most children. However, children from some other countries or cultures may fall outside these curves. For example, new immigrants or adoptees may be in lower percentiles, and catch up over several months or years. Children of immigrants from developing countries tend to be larger than their parents. Even when small, children should follow normal growth patterns. For example, a child may remain at the 10th or 25th percentile for height, but continue to slowly grow and not fall to a lower percentile.

Developing Cultural Competence boxes challenge you to explore differences among racial, ethnic, and social groups, and to plan nursing care that addresses the issues of health disparity.

Legal and Ethical Considerations
Child Nutrition Reauthorization Act

The Child Nutrition Reauthorization Act of 2010, titled the Healthy, Hunger-Free Kids Act of 2010, continues the federal school meal programs (breakfast, lunch, after-school snack, and summer food service) for low-income children and increases access to nutritional foods. The program also has goals for nutrition education and physical activity in an effort to address childhood obesity. School nurses may work with food service personnel in the nutrition programs for healthy eating and in creating a nutrition education program for students (Sherry, 2008). See Chapter 19.

Legal and Ethical Considerations boxes identify laws and ethical issues pertinent to pediatric nursing topics.

Medications Used to Treat boxes list the actions, indications, and important nursing implications for medications.

Medications Used to Treat Asthma

QUICK-RELIEF MEDICATION	ACTION/INDICATION	NURSING MANAGEMENT
Short-Acting Beta₂-Agonists (SABA) Albuterol Levalbuterol Pirbuterol: *Metered dose inhaler (MDI) or nebulizer*	Relaxes smooth muscle in airway leading to rapid bronchodilation (within 5–10 minutes) and mucus clearing Drug of choice for acute therapy and for prevention of exercise-induced bronchospasm	■ Use this rescue medication before inhaled steroid, wait 1–2 minutes between puffs, wait 15 minutes to give inhaled steroid. Child should hold breath 10 seconds after inspiring. Then rinse mouth and avoid swallowing medication. Use a spacer. ■ Differences in potency exist, but all products are comparable on a per puff basis. ■ Some dose-related side effects include tachycardia, nervousness, nausea and vomiting, and headaches. ■ Regular use more than 2 days a week for symptom control indicates a loss of control and need for additional therapy.
Corticosteroids Methylprednisolone Prednisone Prednisolone: *Oral*	Diminishes airway inflammation, secretions, and obstruction, enhances bronchodilating effect of beta₂-agonists Used for acute asthma episodes that are not completely responsive to beta₂-agonists; helps reduce rate of hospitalization	■ Short-term therapy should continue until child achieves 80% peak expiratory flow rate personal best or symptoms resolve. ■ Give with food to reduce gastric irritation. ■ Give oral dose in early morning to mimic normal peak corticosteroid blood level. ■ Assess for potential adverse effects of long-term therapy: decreased growth, unstable blood sugar, and immunosuppression.
Anticholinergic Ipratropium: *Metered dose inhaler (MDI) or nebulizer*	Inhibits bronchoconstriction and decreases mucus production with an onset of action in 30–90 minutes	■ Do not use for primary emergency treatment because of delayed onset. ■ Rinse mouth afterward to get rid of bitter taste. ■ Side effects include increased wheezing, cough, nervousness, dry mouth, tachycardia, dizziness, headache, and palpitations. ■ Prevent medication contact with eyes.
DAILY CONTROL MEDICATIONS	ACTION/INDICATION	NURSING MANAGEMENT

Evidence-Based Practice boxes further enhance the approach to research. We describe a particular nursing problem and investigate the evidence from several studies that explore solutions to the problem. We emphasize nursing research, provide an interpretation explaining the implications of the studies, and then invite you to apply critical thinking skills to further identify nursing care approaches.

Evidence-Based Practice   Care Coordination for Children with Special Healthcare Needs

PROBLEM
Children with special healthcare needs require assistance from a variety of programs and services to maximize their potential. Fragmentation of care may result in the child's needs being unmet.

EVIDENCE
Data were analyzed from the 2005–2006 National Survey of Children with Special Healthcare Needs to determine the association between receiving adequate care coordination, family–provider relations, and outcomes in the child and family. Data indicated that 68.2% of the families reported receiving some type of assistance with care coordination. Of these, 59.2% indicated they received adequate help, and 40.8% indicated the assistance was inadequate. Adequate care coordination was associated with family-centered care, satisfaction with care received, and a partnership with healthcare professionals. Families who reported receiving adequate care coordination were less likely to have problems with specialty referrals, family financial burden, and reduction in work hours. These families also had less out-of-pocket expenses, fewer visits to the emergency department per month, and fewer missed days of school for the CSHCN than families who reported receiving inadequate assistance with care coordination (Turchi, Berhane, Botholi, et al., 2009).

A descriptive study of six pediatric primary care practices was conducted to

coordination by nurses as an integral aspect of each visit decreased the number of visits to the primary care provider and to the emergency department (Antonelli, Stille, & Antonelli, 2008).

A longitudinal study compared the use of pediatric practice-based care coordination to an agency-based model of care coordination. Six pediatric practices participated in the study. Three of the practices continued agency-based care coordination (comparison group) while three practices had a nurse care coordinator placed onsite, who received training and quality improvement (intervention group). Children and youth with special healthcare needs were identified. At baseline, 262 of these families/children were interviewed. At 18 months, 76 families/children in the intervention group and 68 in the comparison group were interviewed. Results of the study indicated that families who received practice-based care coordination reported a higher level of satisfaction with care coordination, were more likely to report that their experience with care coordination had improved, reported fewer barriers to healthcare services, and were treated better by the staff in the office (Wood et al., 2009).

IMPLICATIONS
Practice-based care coordination in which the nurse works with families to facilitate coordination of services is effective and leads to greater satisfaction with

Baccalaureate Essential II
Basic Organizational and Systems Leadership for Quality Care and Patient Safety

Quality improvement and safety is a priority for healthcare organizations. Nurses at the bedside have a major influence on the quality of care provided and the safety of the patient; however, it is the responsibility of the organization's leadership to provide the staffing and resources so that safe and quality care can be provided (Disch, Dreher, Davidson, et al., 2011). Healthcare providers must advocate for best practices that focus on risks unique to children. Children in the healthcare setting are at risk for harm related to misidentification, adverse effects from high-alert medications, and healthcare-acquired or associated infection (Steering Committee on Quality Improvement and Management & Committee on Hospital Care, 2011). Young children are especially vulnerable to injury because of their developmental immaturity, including the inability to recognize safety risks. It is essential that the hospital environment be free of hazards that pose risks for children.

NEW! Baccalaureate Essentials boxes focus on the nine essentials of nursing education identified by the American Association of Colleges of Nursing.

BOX 32–6	Research: Communication Between Adolescents with Type 1 Diabetes and Their Parents

Transcripts of interactions between adolescents ages 11 to 15 years with type 1 diabetes and their parents were analyzed. Participation in the study required that the adolescent had been diagnosed with type 1 diabetes for at least a year and have no other chronic illness, psychologic problems, or learning disability. Transcripts were based on a 10-minute interaction between the adolescent and his or her parents in which a diabetes management task, identified by the teen as a source of disagreement, was discussed.

Five themes were identified from the transcripts: fear, frustration, discounting, normalizing, and trusting. Parents demonstrated frustration, fear, and difficulty in trusting the child with the daily management of diabetes. Parents were also fearful of long-term complications. Adolescents demonstrated frustration because they did not feel their parents recognized their successes in their diabetes management. Discounting was noted in statements by parents that showed a lack of respect for the adolescents' opinions and failure to include the adolescents in decisions related to their care. These statements further added to the child's frustration. The theme of normalizing was noted in only a few families and included statements indicating that the family was attempting to view diabetes as a normal aspect of the adolescent's life. The other themes of fear, frustration, trust, and discounting were cited as barriers to achieving the goal of normalcy.

The study concluded that effective communication between parents and adolescents with type 1 diabetes is essential and that nurses should work with families to facilitate communication related to diabetes management (Ivey, Wright, & Dashiff, 2009).

RESEARCH boxes focus on relevant research studies to give students additional information and background information.

 ## Partnering with Families

Helping the Infant Sleep

Helping an infant to self-regulate and be able to sleep for longer periods is often a stressful challenge for families. Parents need to have substantial sleep periods themselves to be refreshed and able to deal with daily life. When up several times during the night with a baby, parents may become irritable and fatigued. Question the family about the baby's sleep routine. The infant passes into light sleep several times at night and may awaken; self-regulation will assist in helping the infant get back to sleep. Suggestions helpful for the family are as follows:

- Place the baby to sleep in a quiet and darkened room, a "sleep friendly" environment.
- Establish a consistent sleep routine and time; the routine may involve some cuddling and rocking time but should not be vigorous, stimulating play.
- Provide a consistent transitional object, such as a favorite blanket each night.
- Put the baby to bed while still awake but drowsy rather than after falling asleep, so the infant learns self-soothing skills.
- Do not try to awaken the baby in non-rapid eye movement (NREM or quiet) sleep.
- For the baby who has trouble going to sleep, remain in the room for a few minutes but do not establish eye contact; place a hand on the abdomen or chest or gently hold flailing arms and legs.

Source: *Data from National Sleep Foundation. (2011). Sleep, infants, and parents. Retrieved from http://www.sleepfoundation.org/articles/ask-the-expert/sleep-infants-and-parents*

Partnering with Families boxes help you to apply the concepts of family-centered nursing care by providing approaches and teaching in a format directly applicable when you work with families.

Clinical Manifestations   Acute Otitis Media and Otitis Media with Effusion

ETIOLOGY	CLINICAL MANIFESTATIONS	CLINICAL THERAPY
Acute otitis media—bacterial infection in the middle ear from pathogens transferred from the nasopharynx; most common infectious agents are *S. pneumoniae, H. influenzae, M. catarrhalis.*	*Behavioral*—ear pain, pulling at ear, rapid onset, irritability, malaise, poor feeding. *Examination*—bulging tympanic membrane, air or fluid bubbles present behind tympanic membrane; immobile or poorly mobile tympanic membrane, red (or other color change such as white, gray, or yellow as long as bulging is present) tympanic membrane, reduced visibility of tympanic membrane landmarks with displaced light reflex.	Treat ear pain with anesthetic eardrops, herbal pain products instilled into the auditory canal, or systemic acetaminophen or ibuprofen. Verify that the tympanic membrane is intact before inserting eardrops. Observe the child's condition for 48–72 hours and if not improved, treat with course of antibiotics.
Otitis media with effusion—collection of fluid in the middle ear behind the tympanic membrane which is not infected with bacteria.	*Behavioral*—difficulty hearing or responding as expected to sounds. *Examination*—signs of acute inflammation are NOT present; tympanic membrane is retracted or neutral; immobile or partly mobile tympanic membrane; yellow or gray tympanic membrane; opaque or thickened tympanic membrane with visibility of landmarks reduced.	Provide symptomatic treatment of pain. Carefully assess hearing acuity over several months. Assess speech if loss of hearing acuity occurs. Assess development.

Clinical Manifestations boxes link etiology, clinical manifestations, and clinical therapy for specific conditions.

Nursing Care Plans are present in every chapter dealing with health conditions. They illustrate the conceptual approach that nurses need in caring for children, including assessment, NANDA nursing diagnoses, goals, plans, interventions (with NIC), and evaluation (with NOC).

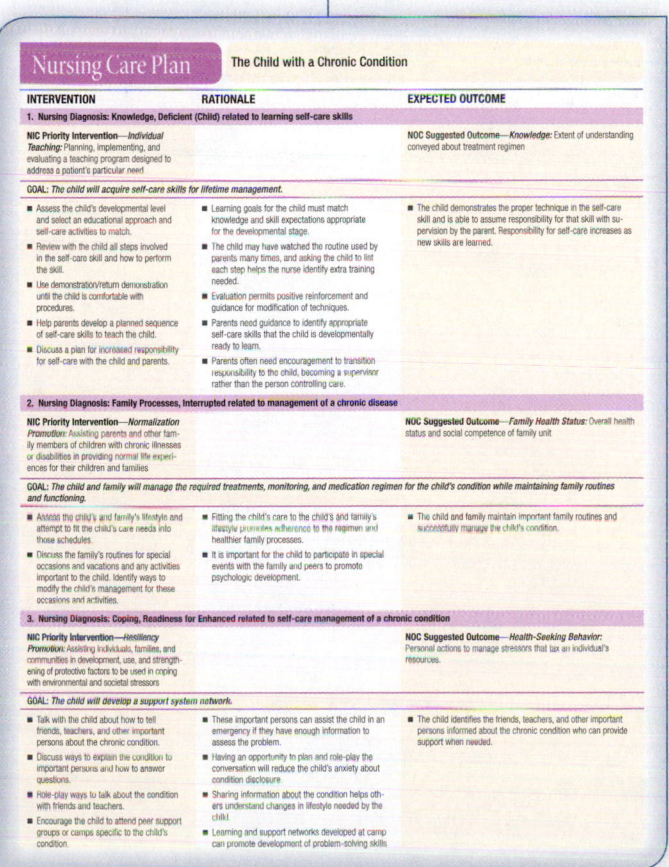

Nursing Care Plan   The Child with a Chronic Condition

INTERVENTION	RATIONALE	EXPECTED OUTCOME
1. Nursing Diagnosis: Knowledge, Deficient (Child) related to learning self-care skills		
NIC Priority Intervention—*Individual Teaching:* Planning, implementing, and evaluating a teaching program designed to address a patient's particular need		**NOC Suggested Outcome**—*Knowledge:* Extent of understanding conveyed about treatment regimen
GOAL: *The child will acquire self-care skills for lifetime management.*		
▪ Assess the child's developmental level and select an educational approach and self-care activities to match. ▪ Review with the child all steps involved in the self-care skill and how to perform the skill. ▪ Use demonstration/return demonstration until the child is comfortable with procedures. ▪ Help parents develop a planned sequence of self-care skills to teach the child. ▪ Discuss a plan for increased responsibility for self-care with the child and parents.	▪ Learning goals for the child must match knowledge and skill expectations appropriate for the developmental stage. ▪ The child may have watched the routine used by parents many times, and asking the child to list each step helps the nurse identify extra training needed. ▪ Evaluation permits positive reinforcement and guidance for modification of techniques. ▪ Parents need guidance to identify appropriate self-care skills that the child is developmentally ready to learn. ▪ Parents often need encouragement to transition responsibility to the child, becoming a supervisor rather than the person controlling care.	▪ The child demonstrates the proper technique in the self-care skill and is able to assume responsibility for that skill with supervision by the parent. Responsibility for self-care increases as new skills are learned.
2. Nursing Diagnosis: Family Processes, Interrupted related to management of a chronic disease		
NIC Priority Intervention—*Normalization Promotion:* Assisting parents and other family members of children with chronic illnesses or disabilities in providing normal life experiences for their children and families		**NOC Suggested Outcome**—*Family Health Status:* Overall health status and social competence of family unit
GOAL: *The child and family will manage the required treatments, monitoring, and medication regimen for the child's condition while maintaining family routines and functioning.*		
▪ Assess the child's and family's lifestyle and attempt to fit the child's care needs into those schedules. ▪ Discuss the family's routines for special occasions and vacations and any activities important to the child. Identify ways to modify the child's management for these occasions and activities.	▪ Fitting the child's care to the child's and family's lifestyle promotes adherence to the regimen and healthier family processes. ▪ It is important for the child to participate in special events with the family and peers to promote psychologic development.	▪ The child and family maintain important family routines and successfully manage the child's condition.
3. Nursing Diagnosis: Coping, Readiness for Enhanced related to self-care management of a chronic condition		
NIC Priority Intervention—*Resiliency Promotion:* Assisting individuals, families, and communities in development, use, and strengthening of protective factors to be used in coping with environmental and societal stressors		**NOC Suggested Outcome**—*Health-Seeking Behavior:* Personal actions to manage stressors that tax an individual's resources.
GOAL: *The child will develop a support system network.*		
▪ Talk with the child about how to tell friends, teachers, and other important persons about the chronic condition. ▪ Discuss ways to explain the condition to important persons and how to answer questions. ▪ Role-play ways to talk about the condition with friends and teachers. ▪ Encourage the child to attend peer support groups or camps specific to the child's condition.	▪ These important persons can assist the child in an emergency if they have enough information to assess the problem. ▪ Having an opportunity to plan and role-play the conversation will reduce the child's anxiety about condition disclosure. ▪ Sharing information about the condition helps others understand changes in lifestyle needed by the child. ▪ Learning and support networks developed at camp can promote development of problem-solving skills.	▪ The child identifies the friends, teachers, and other important persons informed about the chronic condition who can provide support when needed.

Health Promotion & Maintenance Overview   The Child Receiving Cancer Treatment

Cancer treatment often extends for several years, so the child needs to continue health promotion and health maintenance visits.

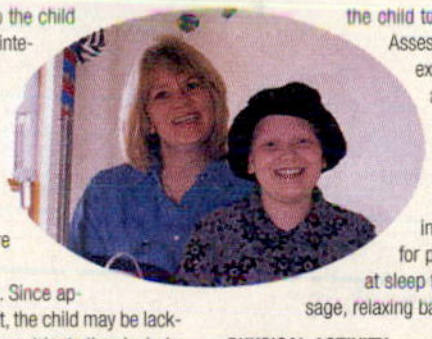

GROWTH AND DEVELOPMENT SURVEILLANCE
▪ The child is assessed for height, weight, and body mass index. This provides information about growth patterns which may be altered by cancer treatment. If indicated, 24-hour diet recalls and other nutritional assessments are performed.
▪ Teaching is provided about age-appropriate foods. Since appetite may be impaired during periods of treatment, the child may be lacking fruits, vegetables, or other foods, as well as the nutrients they include. Encourage parents to be sure the child has a well-balanced diet during periods of remission.
▪ Perform developmental screening of young children. Provide suggestions for parents about the stimulation that is appropriate for the child's age. Include quiet activities that can be used when the child is fatigued or receiving therapy. These might include reading books, listening to music, and working on a computer. Have the parent plan for those activities on days that the child goes for chemotherapy or other treatment.
▪ Ask about the school-age child's progress in school. Performance may be altered due to neurologic effects of treatment as well as missing school. Plan for the family to partner with the school personnel for provision of tutors, computer programs, or other needed assistance.
▪ Encourage continued social contact with peers when blood counts are adequate to prevent infection.

PHYSICAL ASSESSMENT AND SCREENING
▪ Careful physical assessments are performed to identify any abnormalities that may result from cancer or its treatment. Be alert for signs of anemia, neutropenia, and thrombocytopenia; refer for treatment and suggest preventive measures such as infection control for neutropenia. Cardiopulmonary and neuromuscular assessments are particularly important. Vision and hearing should be assessed prior to treatment and periodically throughout. Include measurements of fine and gross motor activity.

ELIMINATION
▪ Toddlers may have an interruption in toilet training during periods when they do not feel well. Help parents to understand this regression, and encourage them to start again when the child is feeling better.
▪ Some medications cause diarrhea or constipation, so evaluate bowel patterns and provide guidance as needed. Skin care instruction may be needed if the child has diarrhea and is relatively immobile. Increasing fluids and fiber foods may be needed for constipation.
▪ Evaluate urinary output since many medications have effects on kidney function. Encourage adequate fluids for age to ensure elimination of medications.

SLEEP AND FATIGUE
▪ Children undergoing treatment often have disturbed sleep patterns. Parents of young children may become exhausted working all day, getting the child to treatments, and having disturbed sleep at night. Assess both the child's sleep patterns and the family's experiences. Encourage plans for respite care to enable rest periods. Provide cots, rocking chairs, and other comfortable settings for the child and family members during treatments.
▪ Both the child and parents may not expect or understand the profound fatigue that occurs during cancer treatment. They can be helped to plan for providing quiet times, eliminating electronic media at sleep time, and replenishing energy through naps, massage, relaxing baths, and spending time with family.

PHYSICAL ACTIVITY
▪ Since the child has periods of fatigue, patterns of physical activity may decrease. Emphasize the importance of integrating physical activity when the child feels well, since it is needed for learning gross motor skills, facilitating blood flow, improving mental status, and setting patterns for the future.

DISEASE AND INJURY PREVENTION STRATEGIES
▪ The child with cancer has the same safety hazards as other children of the same age, and such topics as car safety seats, fire prevention, water safety, and violence prevention should be addressed.
▪ An important hazard for children with cancer is infection due to decreased immune response and neutropenic episodes. Keep records of immunization status. Follow the recommendations of the CDC and AAP for other immunizations. Teach the hazards of exposure to large groups and those with infections when the child's immune system is compromised and neutropenia is present. Teach care of central lines and other potential sources of infection. Have families report signs of infection and exposure to known illnesses promptly.

MENTAL AND SPIRITUAL HEALTH
▪ Evaluate the child and family for signs of anxiety and depression. Ask how they are managing the cancer treatment and what poses the greatest challenges. Refer to other families with similar circumstances for support.
▪ Ensure that the child has contact with friends through childcare or school, or via phone, letters, and computer.
▪ Find out the impact of the child's cancer on the parents' jobs. Ask how the siblings have been coping, what changes there are in school performance, and whether teachers and others are aware of the stress the sibling may be experiencing.

TRANSITIONAL CARE
▪ As the child's treatment ends, instruct them about needed periodic follow-up with the oncologist. Continue to perform neurologic examinations and ascertain school performance. Be alert for signs of secondary tumors.
▪ Ask about worries regarding the future. As teens grow older, have them take over more responsibility for informing care providers of their cancer history and assist them to transition to adult healthcare providers.

Health Promotion & Maintenance Overviews summarize the needs of children with specific chronic conditions, such as asthma or diabetes. These overviews teach you to look at the child who has a chronic illness like any other child, with health maintenance needs for prevention, education, and basic care.

End-of-Chapter Review

Chapter Highlights summarize key points of the chapter.

Clinical Reasoning in Action refers back to the chapter-opening scenario and asks critical thinking questions to help students apply knowledge to real patient care.

NCLEX-RN® Review prepares students for course exams on chapter content and gives exposure to all formats of NCLEX®-style questions.

Detailed **References** provide the basis for evidence-based nursing care and support the currency and accuracy of the textbook.

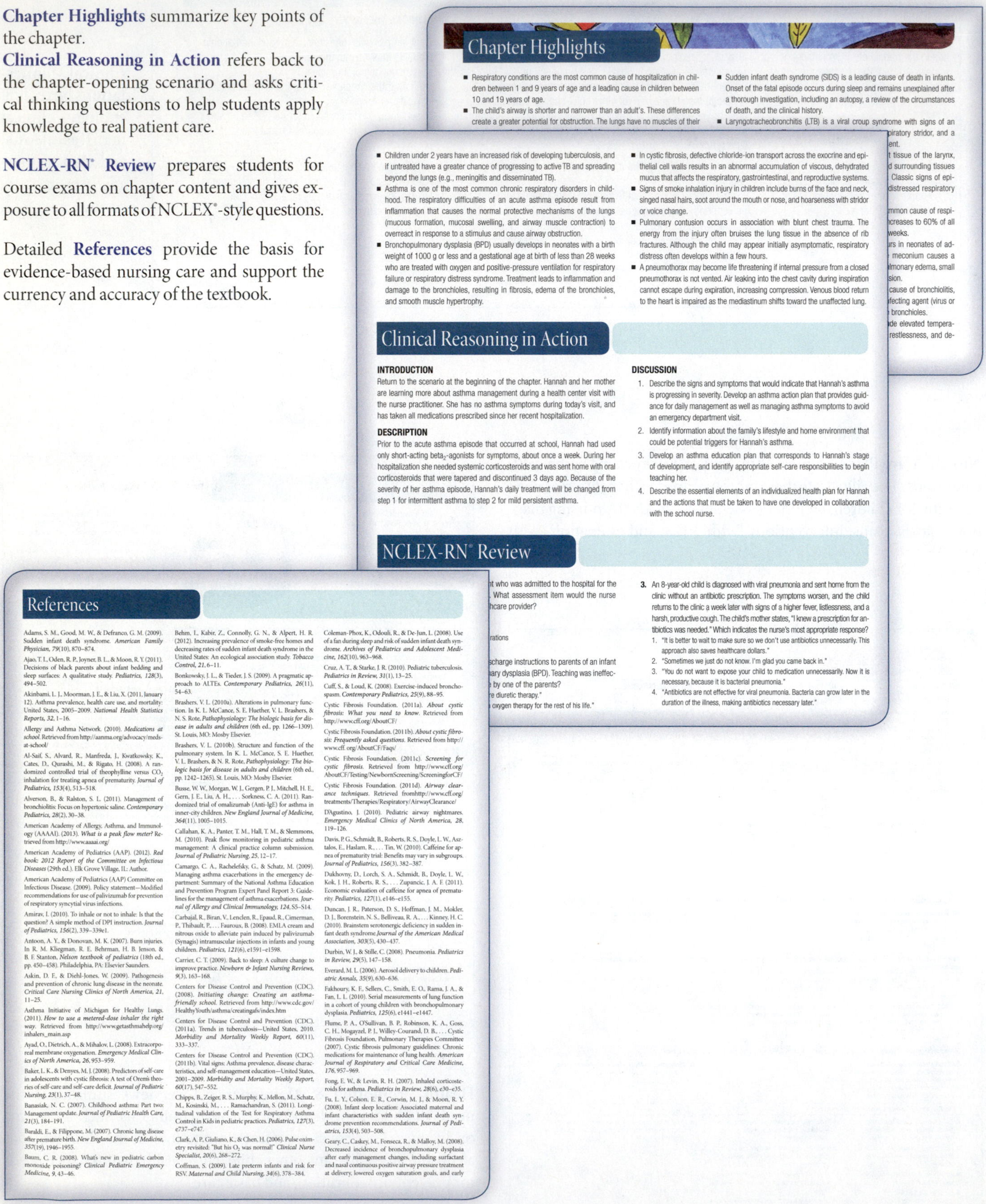

Chapter Highlights

- Respiratory conditions are the most common cause of hospitalization in children between 1 and 9 years of age and a leading cause in children between 10 and 19 years of age.
- The child's airway is shorter and narrower than an adult's. These differences create a greater potential for obstruction. The lungs have no muscles of their
- Children under 2 years have an increased risk of developing tuberculosis, and if untreated have a greater chance of progressing to active TB and spreading beyond the lungs (e.g., meningitis and disseminated TB).
- Asthma is one of the most common chronic respiratory disorders in childhood. The respiratory difficulties of an acute asthma episode result from inflammation that causes the normal protective mechanisms of the lungs (mucous formation, mucosal swelling, and airway muscle contraction) to overreact in response to a stimulus and cause airway obstruction.
- Bronchopulmonary dysplasia (BPD) usually develops in neonates with a birth weight of 1000 g or less and a gestational age at birth of less than 28 weeks who are treated with oxygen and positive-pressure ventilation for respiratory failure or respiratory distress syndrome. Treatment leads to inflammation and damage to the bronchioles, resulting in fibrosis, edema of the bronchioles, and smooth muscle hypertrophy.

- Sudden infant death syndrome (SIDS) is a leading cause of death in infants. Onset of the fatal episode occurs during sleep and remains unexplained after a thorough investigation, including an autopsy, a review of the circumstances of death, and the clinical history.
- Laryngotracheobronchitis (LTB) is a viral croup syndrome with signs of an
- In cystic fibrosis, defective chloride-ion transport across the exocrine and epithelial cell walls results in an abnormal accumulation of viscous, dehydrated mucus that affects the respiratory, gastrointestinal, and reproductive systems.
- Signs of smoke inhalation injury in children include burns of the face and neck, singed nasal hairs, soot around the mouth or nose, and hoarseness with stridor or voice change.
- Pulmonary contusion occurs in association with blunt chest trauma. The energy from the injury often bruises the lung tissue in the absence of rib fractures. Although the child may appear initially asymptomatic, respiratory distress often develops within a few hours.
- A pneumothorax may become life threatening if internal pressure from a closed pneumothorax is not vented. Air leaking into the chest cavity during inspiration cannot escape during expiration, increasing compression. Venous blood return to the heart is impaired as the mediastinum shifts toward the unaffected lung.

Clinical Reasoning in Action

INTRODUCTION
Return to the scenario at the beginning of the chapter. Hannah and her mother are learning more about asthma management during a health center visit with the nurse practitioner. She has no asthma symptoms during today's visit, and has taken all medications prescribed since her recent hospitalization.

DESCRIPTION
Prior to the acute asthma episode that occurred at school, Hannah had used only short-acting beta₂-agonists for symptoms, about once a week. During her hospitalization she needed systemic corticosteroids and was sent home with oral corticosteroids that were tapered and discontinued 3 days ago. Because of the severity of her asthma episode, Hannah's daily treatment will be changed from step 1 for intermittent asthma to step 2 for mild persistent asthma.

DISCUSSION
1. Describe the signs and symptoms that would indicate that Hannah's asthma is progressing in severity. Develop an asthma action plan that provides guidance for daily management as well as managing asthma symptoms to avoid an emergency department visit.
2. Identify information about the family's lifestyle and home environment that could be potential triggers for Hannah's asthma.
3. Develop an asthma education plan that corresponds to Hannah's stage of development, and identify appropriate self-care responsibilities to begin teaching her.
4. Describe the essential elements of an individualized health plan for Hannah and the actions that must be taken to have one developed in collaboration with the school nurse.

NCLEX-RN® Review

who was admitted to the hospital for the
. What assessment item would the nurse
thcare provider?

rations

scharge instructions to parents of an infant
ary dysplasia (BPD). Teaching was ineffec-
e by one of the parents?
re diuretic therapy."
oxygen therapy for the rest of his life."

3. An 8-year-old child is diagnosed with viral pneumonia and sent home from the clinic without an antibiotic prescription. The symptoms worsen, and the child returns to the clinic a week later with signs of a higher fever, listlessness, and a harsh, productive cough. The child's mother states, "I knew a prescription for antibiotics was needed." Which indicates the nurse's most appropriate response?
   1. "It is better to wait to make sure so we don't use antibiotics unnecessarily. This approach also saves healthcare dollars."
   2. "Sometimes we just do not know. I'm glad you came back in."
   3. "You do not want to expose your child to medication unnecessarily. Now it is necessary, because it is bacterial pneumonia."
   4. "Antibiotics are not effective for viral pneumonia. Bacteria can grow later in the duration of the illness, making antibiotics necessary later."

References

Adams, S. M., Good, M. W., & Defranco, G. M. (2009). Sudden infant death syndrome. *American Family Physician, 79*(10), 870–874.

Ajao, T. I., Oden, R. P., Joyner, B. L., & Moon, R. Y. (2011). Decisions of black parents about infant bedding and sleep surfaces: A qualitative study. *Pediatrics, 128*(3), 494–502.

Akinbami, L. J., Moorman, J. E., & Liu, X. (2011, January 12). Asthma prevalence, health care use, and mortality: United States, 2005–2009. *National Health Statistics Reports, 32*, 1–16.

Allergy and Asthma Network. (2010). *Medications at school.* Retrieved from http://aanma.org/advocacy/meds-at-school/

Al-Saif, S., Alvard, R., Manfreda, J., Kwatkowsky, K., Cates, D., Qurashi, M., & Rigato, H. (2008). A randomized controlled trial of theophylline versus CO₂ inhalation for treating apnea of prematurity. *Journal of Pediatrics, 153*(4), 513–518.

Alverson, B., & Ralston, S. L. (2011). Management of bronchiolitis: Focus on hypertonic saline. *Contemporary Pediatrics, 28*(2), 30–38.

American Academy of Allergy, Asthma, and Immunology (AAAAI). (2013). *What is a peak flow meter?* Retrieved from http://www.aaaai.org/

American Academy of Pediatrics (AAP). (2012). *Red book: 2012 Report of the Committee on Infectious Diseases* (29th ed.). Elk Grove Village, IL: Author.

American Academy of Pediatrics (AAP) Committee on Infectious Disease. (2009). Policy statement—Modified recommendations for use of palivizumab for prevention of respiratory syncytial virus infections.

Amirav, I. (2010). To inhale or not to inhale: Is that the question? A simple method of DPI instruction. *Journal of Pediatrics, 156*(3), 339–339e1.

Antoon, A. Y., & Donovan, M. K. (2007). Burn injuries. In R. M. Kliegman, R. E. Behrman, H. B. Jenson, & B. F. Stanton, *Nelson textbook of pediatrics* (18th ed., pp. 450–458). Philadelphia, PA: Elsevier Saunders.

Askin, D. F., & Diehl-Jones, W. (2009). Pathogenesis and prevention of chronic lung disease in the neonate. *Critical Care Nursing Clinics of North America, 21*, 11–25.

Asthma Initiative of Michigan for Healthy Lungs. (2011). *How to use a metered-dose inhaler the right way.* Retrieved from www.getasthmahelp.org/inhalers_main.asp

Ayad, O., Dietrich, A., & Mihalov, L. (2008). Extracorporeal membrane oxygenation. *Emergency Medical Clinics of North America, 26*, 953–959.

Baker, L. K., & Denyes, M. J. (2008). Predictors of self-care in adolescents with cystic fibrosis: A test of Orem's theories of self-care and self-care deficit. *Journal of Pediatric Nursing, 23*(1), 37–48.

Banasiak, N. C. (2007). Childhood asthma: Part two: Management update. *Journal of Pediatric Health Care, 21*(3), 184–191.

Baraldi, E. & Filippone, M. (2007). Chronic lung disease after premature birth. *New England Journal of Medicine, 357*(19), 1946–1955.

Baum, C. R. (2008). What's new in pediatric carbon monoxide poisoning? *Clinical Pediatric Emergency Medicine, 9*, 43–46.

Behm, L., Kabir, Z., Connolly, G. N., & Alpert, H. R. (2012). Increasing prevalence of smoke-free homes and decreasing rates of sudden infant death syndrome in the United States: An ecological association study. *Tobacco Control, 21*, 6–11.

Bonkowsky, J. L., & Tieder, J. S. (2009). A pragmatic approach to ALTEs. *Contemporary Pediatrics, 26*(11), 54–63.

Brashers, V. L. (2010a). Alterations in pulmonary function. In K. L. McCance, S. E. Huether, V. L. Brashers, & N. S. Rote, *Pathophysiology: The biologic basis for disease in adults and children* (6th ed., pp. 1266–1309). St. Louis, MO: Mosby Elsevier.

Brashers, V. L. (2010b). Structure and function of the pulmonary system. In K. L. McCance, S. E. Huether, V. L. Brashers, & N. R. Rote, *Pathophysiology: The biologic basis for disease in adults and children* (6th ed., pp. 1242–1265). St. Louis, MO: Mosby Elsevier.

Busse, W. W., Morgan, W. J., Gergen, P. J., Mitchell, H. E., Gern, J. E., Liu, A. H., . . . Sorkness, C. A. (2011). Randomized trial of omalizumab (Anti-IgE) for asthma in inner-city children. *New England Journal of Medicine, 364*(11), 1005–1015.

Callahan, K. A., Panter, T. M., Hall, T. M., & Slemmons, M. (2010). Peak flow monitoring in pediatric asthma management: A clinical practice column submission. *Journal of Pediatric Nursing, 25*, 12–17.

Camargo, C. A., Rachelefsky, G., & Schatz, M. (2009). Managing asthma exacerbations in the emergency department: Summary of the National Asthma Education and Prevention Program Expert Panel Report 3: Guidelines for the management of asthma exacerbations. *Journal of Allergy and Clinical Immunology, 124*, S5–S14.

Carbajal, R., Biran, V., Lenclen, R., Epaud, R., Cimerman, P., Thibault, P., . . . Fauroux, B. (2008). EMLA cream and nitrous oxide to alleviate pain induced by palivizumab (Synagis) intramuscular injections in infants and young children. *Pediatrics, 121*(6), e1591–e1598.

Carrier, C. T. (2009). Back to sleep: A culture change to improve practice. *Newborn & Infant Nursing Reviews, 9*(3), 163–168.

Centers for Disease Control and Prevention (CDC). (2008). *Initiating change: Creating an asthma-friendly school.* Retrieved from http://www.cdc.gov/HealthyYouth/asthma/creatingafs/index.htm

Centers for Disease Control and Prevention (CDC). (2011a). Trends in tuberculosis—United States, 2010. *Morbidity and Mortality Weekly Report, 60*(11), 333–337.

Centers for Disease Control and Prevention (CDC). (2011b). Vital signs: Asthma prevalence, disease characteristics, and self-management education—United States, 2001–2009. *Morbidity and Mortality Weekly Report, 60*(17), 547–552.

Chipps, B., Zeiger, R. S., Murphy, K., Mellon, M., Schatz, M., Kosinski, M., . . . Ramachandran, S. (2011). Longitudinal validation of the Test for Respiratory Asthma Control in Kids in pediatric practices. *Pediatrics, 127*(3), e737–e747.

Clark, A. P., Giuliano, K., & Chen, H. (2006). Pulse oximetry revisited: "But his O₂ was normal!" *Clinical Nurse Specialist, 20*(6), 268–272.

Coffman, S. (2009). Late preterm infants and risk for RSV. *Maternal and Child Nursing, 34*(6), 378–384.

Coleman-Phox, K., Odouli, R., & De-Jun, L. (2008). Use of a fan during sleep and risk of sudden infant death syndrome. *Archives of Pediatrics and Adolescent Medicine, 162*(10), 963–968.

Cruz, A. T., & Starke, J. R. (2010). Pediatric tuberculosis. *Pediatrics in Review, 31*(1), 13–25.

Cuff, S., & Loud, K. (2008). Exercise-induced bronchospasm. *Contemporary Pediatrics, 25*(9), 88–95.

Cystic Fibrosis Foundation. (2011a). *About cystic fibrosis: What you need to know.* Retrieved from http://www.cff.org/AboutCF/

Cystic Fibrosis Foundation. (2011b). *About cystic fibrosis: Frequently asked questions.* Retrieved from http://www.cff.org/AboutCF/Faqs/

Cystic Fibrosis Foundation. (2011c). *Screening for cystic fibrosis.* Retrieved from http://www.cff.org/AboutCF/Testing/NewbornScreening/ScreeningforCF/

Cystic Fibrosis Foundation. (2011d). *Airway clearance techniques.* Retrieved from http://www.cff.org/treatments/Therapies/Respiratory/AirwayClearance/

D'Agustino, J. (2010). Pediatric airway nightmares. *Emergency Medical Clinics of North America, 28*, 119–126.

Davis, P. G., Schmidt, B., Roberts, R. S., Doyle, L. W., Asztalos, E., Haslam, R., . . . Tin, W. (2010). Caffeine for apnea of prematurity trial: Benefits may vary in subgroups. *Journal of Pediatrics, 156*(3), 382–387.

Dukhovny, D., Lorch, S. A., Schmidt, B., Doyle, L. W., Kok, J. H., Roberts, R. S., . . . Zupancic, J. A. F. (2011). Economic evaluation of caffeine for apnea of prematurity. *Pediatrics, 127*(1), e146–e155.

Duncan, J. R., Paterson, D. S., Hoffman, J. M., Mokler, D. J., Borenstein, N. S., Belliveau, R. A., . . . Kinney, H. C. (2010). Brainstem serotonergic deficiency in sudden infant death syndrome. *Journal of the American Medical Association, 303*(5), 430–437.

Durbin, W. J., & Stille, C. (2008). Pneumonia. *Pediatrics in Review, 29*(5), 147–158.

Everard, M. L. (2006). Aerosol delivery to children. *Pediatric Annals, 35*(9), 630–636.

Fakhoury, K. F., Sellers, C., Smith, E. O., Rama, J. A., & Fan, L. L. (2010). Serial measurements of lung function in a cohort of young children with bronchopulmonary dysplasia. *Pediatrics, 125*(6), e1441–e1447.

Flume, P. A., O'Sullivan, B. P., Robinson, K. A., Goss, C. H., Mogayzel, P. J., Willey-Courand, D. B., . . . Cystic Fibrosis Foundation, Pulmonary Therapies Committee (2007). Cystic fibrosis pulmonary guidelines: Chronic medications for maintenance of lung health. *American Journal of Respiratory and Critical Care Medicine, 176*, 957–969.

Fong, E. W., & Levin, R. H. (2007). Inhaled corticosteroids for asthma. *Pediatrics in Review, 28*(6), e30–e35.

Fu, L. Y., Colson, E. R., Corwin, M. J., & Moon, R. Y. (2008). Infant sleep location: Associated maternal and infant characteristics with sudden infant death syndrome prevention recommendations. *Journal of Pediatrics, 153*(4), 503–508.

Geary, C., Caskey, M., Fonseca, R., & Malloy, M. (2008). Decreased incidence of bronchopulmonary dysplasia after early management changes, including surfactant and nasal continuous positive airway pressure treatment at delivery, lowered oxygen saturation goals, and early

Acknowledgments

It is both challenging and a significant responsibility to write a pediatric textbook. Pediatric nursing is constantly changing due to new knowledge and technologies. It is inspiring to observe this evolution of pediatric nursing practice and to have the opportunity to share with nursing students much of our enthusiasm for working with children and their families. We appreciate the opportunity to contribute to the education of a new generation of nurses.

This edition of the textbook used the strong foundation of the first edition and integrated some new features. The production of a textbook requires a team that is fully committed to the vision from the beginning of the revision through the final production process. We were fortunate to have a close collaborative relationship with our publishing company, Pearson. Kim Norbuta, our nursing editor, infused new ideas and approaches into the textbook and accompanying learning aids. We are excited about the coming application of simulations as methods of expanding understanding of pediatric nursing for the student. Julie Alexander, vice president and publisher, has once again enthusiastically supported this venture on behalf of Pearson.

Our developmental editor, Kim Wyatt, has worked with us for several books; she is a cheerleader and a friend, and she has an exquisite eye for detail. She worked side by side with a new editor, Mary Cook, to ensure the quality and timeliness of the present edition. Mary was essential in cultivating our relationship with reviewers—her pleasant and competent manner was outstanding. We thank Maria Reyes, production editor; Patrick Walsh, production managing editor; and editorial assistant Erin Rafferty, for their expertise and valuable contributions. Our thanks also go to Mary Siener for

the textbook design. At S4Carlisle Publishing Services, we thank Lynn Steines for coordinating production, and Joan Lyon for her copyediting skills.

George Dodson took many of the photos in this book. We sincerely thank the children, families, and nurses who allowed us to illustrate development, pediatric healthcare conditions, and nursing care of children in hospital, home, and community settings.

One chapter in the book was written by an expert in a specialized field. We particularly thank Linda Ward for her contributions on genetics and genomics. She is a participant in the National Institutes of Health Summer Genetics Institute and a researcher in education of nurses on these important topics, and we could have no better contributor. We would also like to acknowledge the academic- and clinical-based pediatric nurses who served as reviewers and consultants. Their valuable feedback enabled us to more appropriately focus our chapters for today's student nurses and the practice of pediatric nursing.

This book emphasizes partnering with families to provide comprehensive care for children. Our own families are also critically important to our lives. Without them we could not reach our own personal and professional goals, and we depend on them every day for support, love, and caring. We thank them for their enduring partnerships and contributions that made this book a reality.

Jane W. Ball
Ruth C. Bindler
Kay J. Cowen

Contents

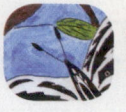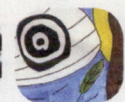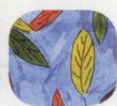

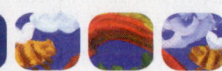

UNIT II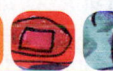

Child Concepts and Application 77

UNIT III

Health Promotion and Maintenance Through Childhood 228

Chapter 8
Concepts of Health Promotion and Maintenance 229

Chapter 9
Health Promotion and Maintenance of the Newborn 252

Chapter 10
Health Promotion and Maintenance of the Infant 275

Chapter 11
Health Promotion and Maintenance of the Toddler and Preschooler 295

UNIT IV
Child Healthcare Settings and Considerations 358

UNIT V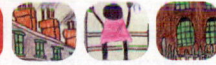

Nursing Care for Common Health Conditions 481

Chapter 19
Infant, Child, and Adolescent Nutrition 482

UNIT VI

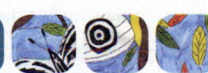

Nursing Care of Specific Health Conditions 649

Chapter 23
Alterations in Fluid, Electrolyte, and Acid–Base Balance 650

Chapter 24
Alterations in Eye, Ear, Nose, and Throat Function 694

Chapter 27
Alterations in Immune Function 864

Chapter 30
Alterations in Gastrointestinal Function 989

Chapter 31
Alterations in Genitourinary Function 1046

Chapter 32
Alterations in Endocrine and Metabolic Function **1097**

Chapter 33
Alterations in Neurologic Function 1148

Chapter 34
Alterations in Mental Health and Cognition   1214

Nurses, Children, and Families

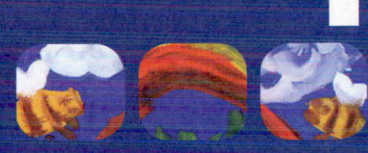

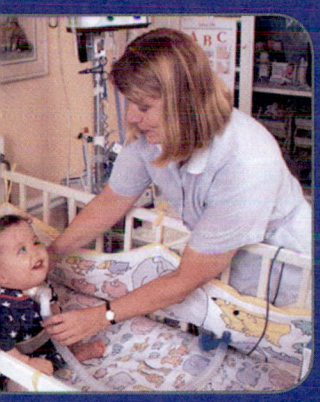
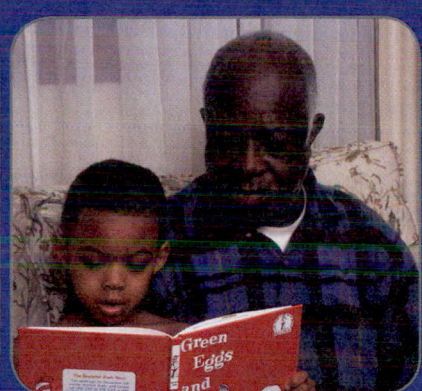
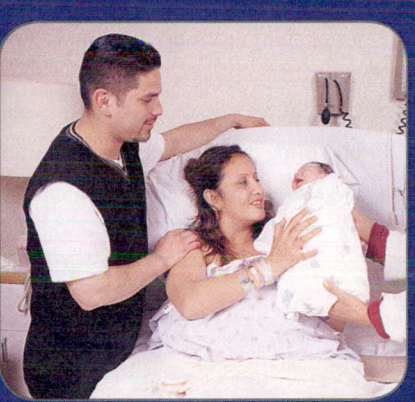
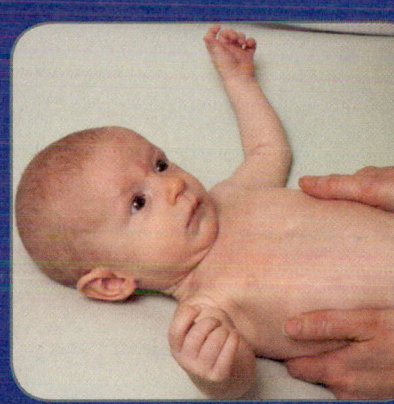

Pediatric nurses care for children and their families in many different settings, including the hospital, healthcare centers, physicians' offices, specialty care centers, the home, schools, and elsewhere in the community, such as homeless shelters and disaster shelters. Pediatric nurses develop partnerships with children and their families to address the child's acute or chronic health condition, to prevent disease, or to promote the child's health, growth, and development. The partnerships formed enable the pediatric nurse to learn about the family's culture and belief system, potential genetic or hereditary influences, family strengths and resources, and preferences for care. This information provides the foundation for the nursing care plan, developed in collaboration with the child and family. Pediatric nurses implement the nursing care plan by providing direct care and education. In some cases, the pediatric nurse functions as the advocate for the child and family in the healthcare system and serves as case manager for children with complex health conditions.

Child Health Nursing: Concepts, Roles, and Issues

 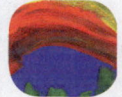 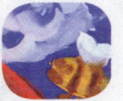

Learning Outcomes

After completing this chapter, you will be able to:

1. Differentiate between the general nurse and advanced practice nurse roles in child health nursing.

2. Examine the historical and current societal influences on pediatric health care and nursing practice.

3. Analyze the current causes of child morbidity and mortality and identify opportunities for nursing intervention.

4. Plan strategies to improve pediatric patient safety in the healthcare setting.

5. Contrast the policies for obtaining informed consent of minors with policies for adults.

6. Identify unique pediatric legal and ethical issues in pediatric nursing practice.

> *"Drew's seizure was scary, so I called Mom. He was shaking all over and wouldn't wake up. He even wet his pants, and he has not done that for a long time."*
>
> —Kevin, age 8

Drew Santo is a 3-year-old boy who has a seizure disorder that until a week ago was fairly well controlled by medication. He and his family receive health care at the center serviced by their health plan. A pediatric nurse and pediatrician collaborate in providing Drew's health care and monitoring his developmental progress.

Drew had a seizure in the last week. His phenytoin blood level, taken the day of the seizure, was slightly lower than the therapeutic range. Because of the recent seizure, an electroencephalogram (EEG) is ordered to identify any change in the electrical pattern in the brain. Other laboratory tests are also ordered, following the guidelines of the health center's clinical pathway for children with seizure disorders.

Over the past 2 years, Drew's family and the pediatric nurse have worked in partnership to ensure that Drew is treated as a healthy child with a chronic condition. The nurse has helped his parents to obtain information about his condition, to understand the action of his medication, and to take appropriate measures when he has a seizure. Drew's parents are upset that he has again had a seizure, especially when they have done everything they could to keep the seizures under control. They have been able to think of him as a healthy boy because he had not had a seizure for a long time. Now they wonder if they will be able to keep treating him that way. In how many different settings could you find nurses providing care to children with this condition? Does the type of nursing care provided to children differ among these settings?

OVERVIEW OF PEDIATRIC HEALTH CARE

Nurses provide care to healthy children, as well as to those with illnesses, injuries, and chronic conditions, in a wide variety of settings. Fortunately, most children in the United States are healthy, experiencing only occasional short-term health problems, and nurses have the opportunity to partner with them to prevent disease and promote a healthy lifestyle. However, children with special healthcare needs require frequent contact with the healthcare system to achieve and maintain their optimal level of health.

In all cases, nurses working with children have the pleasure of watching children grow, achieve milestones in development, and adapt to and manage their health conditions. Nurses find reward in knowing they made a contribution to the health and welfare of these children.

Nurses who choose to specialize in pediatrics need all of the foundational knowledge provided during nursing education such as:

- The nursing process
- Anatomy and physiology
- Physical assessment
- Pathophysiology and healthcare condition recognition and management
- Communication skills and clinical nursing skills

Building upon the principles, knowledge, and skills already learned, pediatric nurses integrate additional competencies related to the care of children and their families into their practice. The special knowledge and skills that nurses caring for children must acquire and apply are listed in Box 1–1.

BOX 1–1	Expected Competencies of the Pediatric Nurse

The Society of Pediatric Nurses has described these concepts and competencies for the beginning generalist pediatric nurse:

- An understanding of the unique anatomical, physiological, and developmental differences among neonates, infants, children, adolescents, and young adults in transition;
- The ability to care for children in the context of their families;
- Sensitivity to cultural issues, especially those related to how the family and healthcare providers tend to children's healthcare needs;
- The ability to communicate effectively with children, families, and other healthcare providers and appropriate educational agency staff;
- The provision of safety assurance and injury prevention to children and their families;
- The ability to promote children's health in the context of their families;
- The assessment of the unique growth and development needs of children who have chronic conditions and of their families;
- The provision for the exceptional needs of children with episodic injuries and illnesses;
- An understanding of the economic, social, and political influences outside the family that have an impact on children's health and development and family functioning; and
- An understanding of the ethical, moral, and legal dilemmas involving children, families, and healthcare professionals.

Source: *From American Nurses Association, National Association of Pediatric Nurse Practitioners, and Society of Pediatric Nurses. (2008). Pediatric nursing: Scope and standards of practice* (p. 17). Silver Spring, MD: Nursesbooks.org.

Pediatric health care occurs along a continuum that reflects not only care to the child as he or she ages, but also a continuum of various healthcare settings used by some individual children who have complex health conditions. For example, all children need health promotion and health maintenance services, but some children will need care for chronic conditions, acute illnesses and injuries, and even end-of-life care. See Figure 1–1 ■ for the model of pediatric health care upon which this text is based.

The range of healthcare services provided by nurses specializing in pediatrics leads to many exciting professional opportunities in a wide variety of clinical settings. The array of settings where pediatric nurses work includes the following:

- Hospitals, such as the pediatric unit, intensive care unit, newborn nursery, emergency department, radiology, and specialty clinics
- Physicians' offices, clinics, and healthcare centers
- Home of the child
- Rehabilitation centers and residential treatment centers
- Schools, childcare centers, and camps

Nurses play a significant role in the provision of health care for children, with varied responsibilities in different settings. Regardless of the settings in which nurses work, assessment, nursing care interventions, education, and advocacy are universal roles.

ROLE OF THE NURSE IN THE CARE OF CHILDREN

Pediatric nursing uses a family-centered care approach; focuses on protecting newborns, infants, children, and adolescents from illness and injury; promotes child health; and assists children to attain optimal levels of health, regardless of health problems, and rehabilitation. This also involves the alleviation of suffering through the diagnosis and treatment of the child's responses, and advocacy in the care of children and their families (American Nurses Association, National Association of Pediatric Nurse Practitioners, & Society of Pediatric Nurses, 2008). The predominant nursing roles in caring for children and their families include direct care, education, advocacy, and case management.

Direct Care Provider

The primary role of pediatric nurses is to provide direct nursing care to children and their families in hospitals and various community settings such as health centers, schools, and the home. The nursing process provides the framework for delivery of direct pediatric nursing care. The nurse assesses the child and identifies the nursing diagnoses that describe the responses of the child and family to the health promotion and health maintenance plan and to any illness or injury experienced. The nurse then implements and evaluates nursing care.

Pediatric nursing care is designed to meet the child's physical and emotional needs. It is offered in a manner sensitive to and compatible with the child's and family's cultural beliefs (see Chapter 3 🔴). It is tailored to the child's developmental stage, giving the child additional responsibility for self-care with increasing age, and ultimately assisting the adolescent with transition to adult health care. This care is also provided in partnership with the family, embracing the principles of family-centered care (see Chapter 2 🔴).

Nurses play an important role in minimizing the psychologic and physical distress experienced by children and their families. Providing support to children and their families is one important aspect of

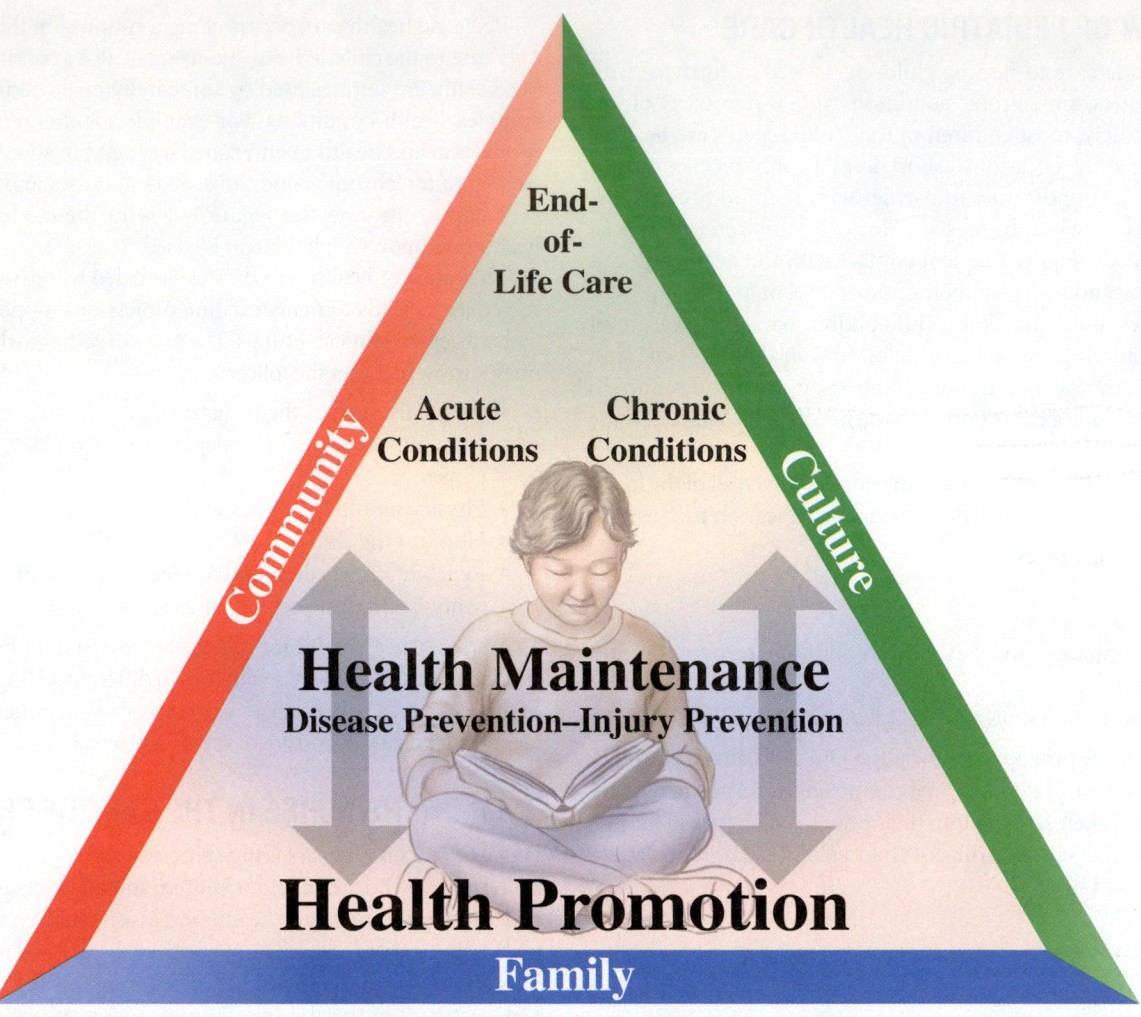

FIGURE 1–1 ■ **The Bindler-Ball Continuum of Pediatric Health Care for Children and Their Families**

The outer bars represent the family, cultural, and community influences on the care that the child receives, either through the services sought by the family or the services provided in the community. Cultural influences include the family's decision to seek health care and follow recommendations, as well as the healthcare provider's cultural competence in caring for a child and family.

The inner categories represent the different types of health care needed by children. All children need health promotion and health maintenance services, represented by the base of the triangle. Notice the arrows representing the upward and downward movement between the levels of care as the child's condition changes.

Children may be healthy with episodic acute illnesses and injuries. Some children develop a chronic condition for which specialized health care is needed. A child's chronic condition may be well controlled, but acute episodes (such as with asthma) or other illnesses and injuries may occur, and the child also needs health promotion and health maintenance services to continue. Some children develop a life-threatening illness and ultimately need end-of-life care. A healthy child can also experience a catastrophic injury that causes death, and the family needs supportive end-of-life care (Bindler & Ball, 2007).

direct nursing care. This often involves listening to the concerns of children and parents, being present during stressful or emotional experiences, and implementing strategies to help children and family members cope. Nurses can help families by suggesting ways to support their children in the hospital, in out-of-hospital settings, and in the home. Nurses can also support families with informational resources, support groups, referrals for healthcare services, and in some cases respite care.

As a member of the child's healthcare team, the nurse is responsible for collaborating with other health professionals and ensuring that the nursing care is coordinated with that of other professionals. Experienced pediatric nurses or those with graduate-level education often assume a leadership role in coordinating the collaboration of an interprofessional (interdisciplinary) team of healthcare providers. In some cases the nurse recognizes that the child and family need care that is outside the nurse's scope of practice or

specific skill level, so a referral must be initiated. In other cases an interprofessional team will meet to jointly develop a care plan for a child with a chronic condition. See the case management information on page 6.

Nurses continually expand the range of direct care they provide. After developing experience and a comfort level in the care of children typically seen in one setting, the pediatric nurse is often ready to move to a different setting or specialty area or to accept a leadership position. In some cases the experienced nurse may be given supervisory responsibility for nursing care provided by other members of the nursing care team.

Other nursing professionals you will find in pediatric settings include advanced practice nurses (e.g., clinical nurse specialists and pediatric nurse practitioners) who have a graduate-level nursing education and are prepared to practice in a specialty area or at a higher level of responsibility.

- Clinical nurse specialists serve as educators and role models, members of the clinical research team, consultants to the healthcare team, and change agents within the healthcare system. They often have a nursing practice with a specialty focus such as respiratory, cardiovascular, or oncology.
- Pediatric nurse practitioners, in collaboration with physicians and other healthcare team members, perform assessment, diagnosis, and management of health conditions in office settings, schools, and hospitals. Nurse practitioners are now assuming a larger role within hospital settings in the management of children with acute illnesses or the exacerbation of chronic health problems.

Experienced pediatric nurses and advanced practice nurses who enjoy teaching may choose to become nurse educators. Experienced pediatric nurses can be mentors to new nurses, serving as role models, supporting their professional development, and promoting their clinical skills development. Advanced practice nurses may join a school of nursing faculty to teach pediatrics or support the nursing education programs provided within clinical health settings.

Patient Educator

The education of children and their families or caregivers improves treatment results. For example, education can be direct teaching to the child and family members about the medications needed to treat a specific health condition as well as other therapies that will be needed once the child is discharged. In pediatric nursing, patient education is especially challenging, because nurses must be prepared to work with children at various levels of understanding. More than providing simple facts, the goal of the education is to help the child and family make informed choices about health and healthy behavior. Depending on the needs of the child and family at any particular time, education can focus on health promotion, health maintenance, self-care, and management of a health condition.

As patient educators, nurses help children adapt to the hospital setting and prepare them for procedures (Figure 1–2 ■). Most hospitals encourage a parent to stay with the child and to provide much of the direct and supportive care. Nurses teach parents to watch for important signs and responses to therapies, to increase the child's comfort, and even to provide advanced care. Taking an active role prepares and empowers the parent to assume total responsibility for care after the child leaves the hospital.

Planning and preparation, as well as an understanding of the child's developmental level, are needed to effectively educate children and parents. The nurse needs to become fully informed about the condition and information to be taught, and then think about strategies and resources that will help the child and family learn to manage the health condition. An assessment of the child's and family's knowledge about the condition or health practices, their past experiences, their attitudes and beliefs, and health literacy is a starting point for education. An understanding of the child's developmental capabilities is also important. See Developing Cultural Competence: Health Literacy. See Box 1–2 for suggestions to lower the reading level of patient education materials.

Developing Cultural Competence
Health Literacy

Among U.S. adults, 20% read at a fifth-grade level or below, and 90 million people have difficulty using and understanding health information (Hawkins, Kantayya, & Sharkey-Asner, 2010). **Health literacy** is the degree to which individuals have the capacity to obtain and understand basic health information needed to make appropriate health decisions (Ferguson & Pawlak, 2011). It involves the ability to read as well as to listen and analyze information. Health literacy also involves the ability to make decisions and apply information. Individuals at higher risk for low health literacy include those who did not graduate from high school, nonnative English speakers, various racial and ethnic minority groups, and those below the poverty level.

BOX 1–2	**Adapting the Reading Level of Patient Education Materials**

Understanding written information in patient care instructions, education materials, and even prescription labels is important to promote **adherence** (the extent to which a patient or parent acts consistently with regard to recommended care). Printed materials to educate children and families about a health condition might be readily available, but they often are written at too high a reading level. Educational materials should be written at a fifth- or sixth-grade reading level (Hawkins, Kantayya, & Sharkey-Asner, 2010). Just because printed material may be available in the primary language of the patient and family, do not assume the family members have reading skills in that language.

Some tips to developing patient education material with a lower reading level include:

- Use short, familiar words with one or two syllables and short sentences.
- Substitute simple language that defines a medical term rather than using the term.
- Use pictures or graphics to give directions when possible.
- Use active voice rather than passive voice.
- Use "must" to express a requirement.
- Use lists and tables to simplify content.
- Divide the content into small sections and use headers.
- Color code information to help readers know it is important.
- Use a computer program to evaluate the reading level of materials you develop.

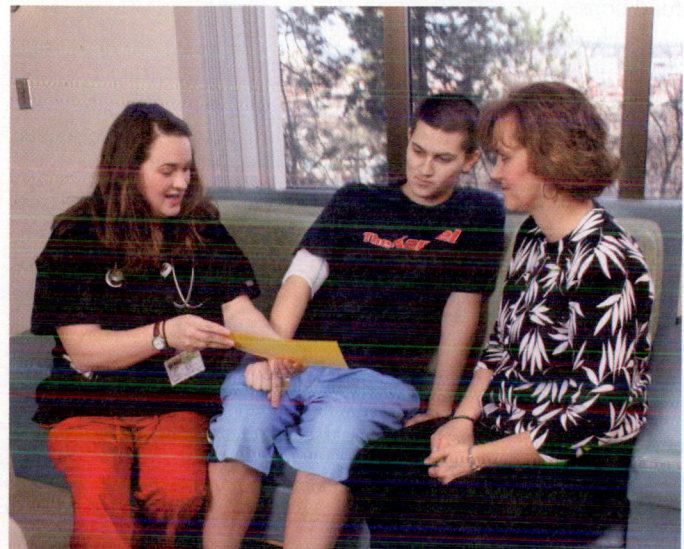

FIGURE 1–2 ■ Explaining procedures can reduce the patient's and family's fears and anxieties about what to expect and how to cooperate during the procedure.

Weblink | Tips for Writing Simple Information Sheets

Weblink | Tool Kit for Literacy

Establishing rapport with the child and family makes it easier for the nurse to provide education. Family members and the child will be more comfortable asking questions. During educational sessions, the nurse can also provide support for the emotional needs of the child and family. Children and families should be encouraged to express their feelings and thoughts about the impact of the health condition, which may result in the exploration of potential strategies that could improve the psychologic aspects of living with the condition. Outcomes of education can be evaluated during future visits, particularly for children receiving ongoing health promotion and health maintenance care and for those with a chronic condition that requires home management.

Advanced practice nurses and experienced pediatric nurses often have responsibility for providing education and counseling that is directed toward helping the child or family solve a problem or deal with an acute crisis.

Patient Advocacy

Advocacy—acting to safeguard and advance the interests of another—is directed at enabling the child and family to adjust to the changes in the child's health in their own way. To be an effective advocate, the nurse must be aware of the child's and the family's needs, the family's resources, and the healthcare services available in the hospital and the community. The nurse can then assist the family and the child to make informed choices about these services and to act in the child's best interests. For example, a nurse works to make sure the family member and child (to his or her level of understanding) have adequate information about treatment options to make an informed decision. The nurse must also protect the child and family by taking appropriate actions related to any potential or actual incidents of incompetent, unethical, or illegal practices by any member of the healthcare team.

As advocates, nurses also work to ensure that the policies and resources of healthcare agencies meet the psychosocial needs of children and their families. This often requires nurses to become active participants on committees that develop policies or guidelines for nursing and medical care or modernizing the healthcare facility design. In each case, the knowledge that the pediatric nurse contributes about the developmental and psychosocial needs of children is important in ensuring that the needs of children are appropriately addressed in their healthcare facility.

According to the United Nations Convention on the Rights of the Child, every child has a right to enjoy the highest attainable standard of health and access to healthcare facilities, and governments should take appropriate measures to help children achieve these rights (Todres, 2010). Pediatric nurses should become active at the community level, advocating for legislative and regulatory changes that improve the health of children. Nurses also advocate for improved health through community education about important health measures, such as universal health insurance for children or immunizations. Some pediatric nurses choose to obtain advanced education to specialize in ethics or public policy, or to become an attorney. In these roles, the nurse then takes a leadership position to promote and implement ethical practices and policy changes that benefit children and their families.

Case Manager

When a child has a significant health problem or disabling condition, physicians, nurses, social workers, physical and occupational therapists, and other specialists come together to create an interdisciplinary plan to address the child's medical, nursing, developmental, educational, and psychosocial needs. Because nurses spend large amounts of time providing nursing care for the child and family, they often know more than other healthcare professionals about the family's wishes and resources. As a member of the interprofessional (interdisciplinary) care plan team, one important role for the nurse as the family's advocate is to ensure that the care plan considers the family's wishes and contains appropriate services. An experienced pediatric nurse or advanced practice nurse often becomes the child's case manager, coordinating the implementation of the plan of care. Sometimes the parent or a social worker becomes the case manager.

Case management is a process of coordinating the delivery of healthcare services in a manner that focuses on timely access to health services, patient safety, quality, and cost-effectiveness (Campagna & Stanton, 2010). This is often a collaborative practice with other healthcare providers that helps optimize the patient's self-care abilities, promotes continuity of care (an interprofessional process facilitating a patient's transition between and among settings based on changing needs and available resources), and encourages effective utilization of healthcare resources. The family is included in the planning and decision-making process, adhering to the family-centered care philosophy described in Chapter 2 🔗. This approach involves regular interaction between the case manager and the child and family to develop an individualized care plan in collaboration with the healthcare team. The case manager is also responsible for communication with all health team members for care coordination and advocating for the child and family.

The nurse case manager often has a role in carefully matching healthcare resources appropriate for the patient's condition and links the child and family to these services. These may include community medical resources, home care agencies qualified to care for children, healthcare services offered in the school setting, educational interventions, and services reimbursed by the child's health plan. The goal is to help the child and family have the best healthcare outcome and decrease fragmentation of care, while controlling the cost of healthcare services. Case management may be used for care of the patient when hospitalized as well as for long-term care of chronic conditions.

Discharge planning is a form of case management. Good discharge planning promotes a smooth, rapid, and safe transition into the community and improves the results of treatment begun in the hospital. To be a discharge planner, the nurse must have obtained information from the family about their capabilities and resources for caring for the child after an emergency department visit or hospitalization. The nurse then analyzes the care needs and begins to educate the family about care to provide at home, signs of a deteriorating or worsening condition, and who and when to call for assistance. Appropriate Internet sites and community resources may be recommended. In some cases, healthcare providers use telehealth to connect the family to some services.

Research

Research is conducted on pediatric healthcare issues to advance the science associated with pediatric nursing care and to increase the integration of an evidence-based nursing practice (Sawin, Gralton, Harrison, et al., 2010). Research can focus on evaluating innovations in care to determine if practice is improved.

Pediatric nurses need to become consumers of new pediatric research, reading and analyzing the research findings and applying those findings to practice. Such findings may potentially improve healthcare outcomes, improve comfort, or even reduce the cost of care. This research is also used in developing specific healthcare facility evidence-based practice guidelines. For example, pediatric nurses may identify issues in patient care processes that involve clinical practice, education, ethical issues, and specific needs of particular populations of children. In collaboration with advanced practice nurse researchers or other health professionals, pediatric nurses can help identify research questions, assist with the design of research studies, and collect data. With advanced education the pediatric nurse can become a nurse researcher. See pages 19–20 for issues related to consent and assent.

HISTORY OF CHILD HEALTH CARE

By examining the roots of pediatric nursing and how certain nursing roles have evolved, we may better understand the historical context of current child health issues and pediatric nursing practice.

The Beginnings of Child Health Nursing

During the 18th and 19th centuries, and much of the 20th century, infectious disease caused the majority of deaths in children, along with falls, burns, and poisoning. In 1900 to 1902, more than 12% of infants listed in the Census Bureau's Death Registration Area died before reaching 1 year of age, often due to gastrointestinal and respiratory disorders (Golden, 2011).

Significant efforts to address child health were initiated in 1880 to improve the infant mortality rate. Lack of refrigeration or milk from sick cows often resulted in infantile diarrhea and tuberculosis. Regulations to improve the sanitation of milk, provision of pasteurized milk to infants in poor families in milk stations, and the development of artificial infant formulas all occurred during this period. Milk stations became infant welfare stations, providing the model for future well-baby examinations (Golden, 2011). Social welfare reformers began addressing principles of hygiene, plumbing, housing, and social reform (Fairchild, Rosner, Colgrove, et al., 2010).

In 1895, Lillian Wald, the pioneer of home visiting nursing, recognized the need for health promotion and disease prevention among New York City's poor immigrant population, and she, along with Mary Maud Brewster, organized nursing services to children and their families at the Henry Street Settlement (Berman, 2010). Although the nurses in these settings could not help their patients overcome poverty, they did actively seek improvements in social conditions affecting their health. The nurses made home visits, taught parents about nutrition and hygiene, and made arrangements for sick children to see a physician at a dispensary or hospital (Figure 1–3 ■). In the early 1900s, some hospitals had pediatric dedicated wards.

Improving the health conditions for children attending public schools became a focus in the 1890s and early 20th century. Many children were absent or sent home from school because of illness. Physicians inspected schools and examined students in New York, Boston, Chicago, and Philadelphia to identify infectious disease and to quarantine students as necessary. In 1902, Lillian Wald assigned nurse Lina Rogers to a school for a 1-month experimental project at the request of the New York City Board of Education and the city's health commissioner. The project was so successful in reducing absenteeism from schools that more school nurses were hired

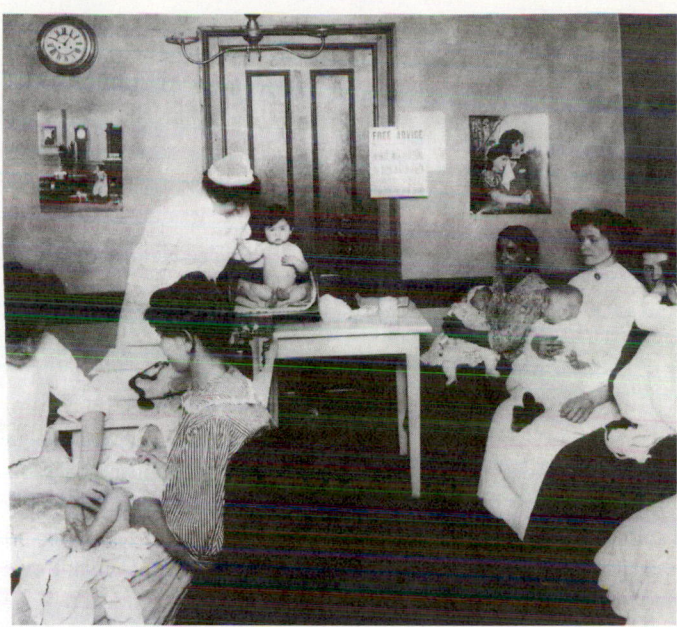

FIGURE 1–3 ■ A well-baby clinic for recently immigrated mothers and their babies, circa 1912.

Source: *Photo courtesy of the National Archives, photo no. 90-G-5-1.*

(Hawkins & Watson, 2010). School nursing was thus initiated in New York City, and the model soon spread to other cities in the United States and Canada. Children and their parents were educated about personal hygiene and disease prevention in these school health programs, and school nurses also visited homes during the summer to meet and educate new mothers. See Figure 1–4 ■. Nurses were

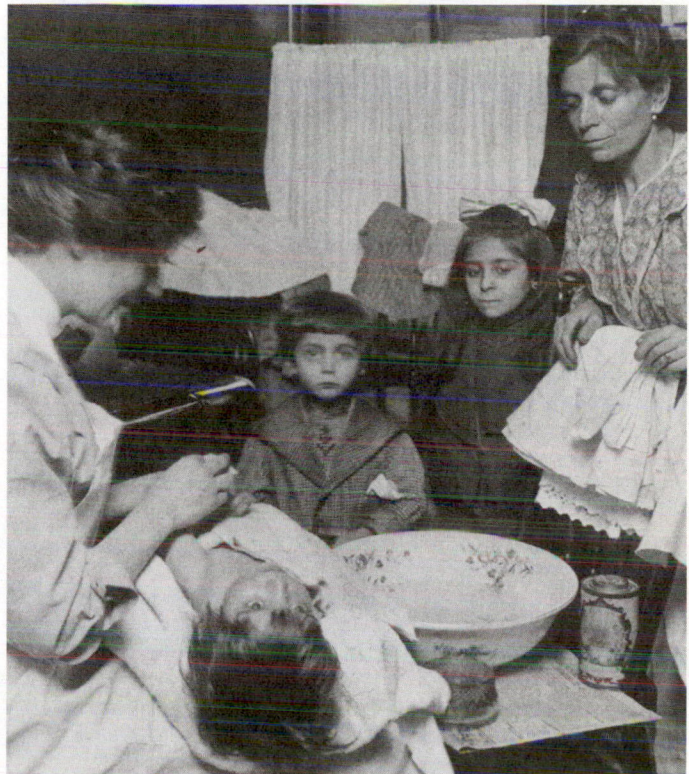

FIGURE 1–4 ■ A community health nurse visits children who are not attending school due to a communicable disease outbreak.

Source: *Photo courtesy of the Visiting Nurses Association of Boston.*

additionally active in educating and encouraging parents to permit their children to receive the first vaccines for smallpox and diphtheria (Colgrove, 2007).

Efforts by physicians, nurses, and other social activists during the first decade of the 20th century increased the awareness of child health and welfare issues at the federal level. The first White House Conference on Children was held in 1909, and it addressed the care of dependent children and working conditions of children. In 1912, the Children's Bureau, the first U.S. agency devoted to the condition and welfare of children, was formed (Theerman, 2010).

Historic Legislation

The first U.S. program supporting health services to mothers and infants was the Sheppard-Towner Child Welfare Act, enacted in 1920. It provided matching funds to states to establish programs promoting infant and child health such as visiting nurses, preventive health clinics to improve health services for all classes of children and their families, and education about proper methods of infant care and feeding (Theerman, 2010). Despite a significant reduction in the infant mortality rate, Congress did not reauthorize the program. See Box 1–3 for a timeline of other significant federal legislation that has benefited children.

BOX 1–3	**Significant Federal Legislation Affecting Child Health**

- 1920—The Sheppard-Towner Act supported services to mothers and infants.
- 1935—The Social Security Act included two important programs for children: Aid to Families with Dependent Children (AFDC), now called Temporary Assistance to Needy Families (TANF), and Title V of this act, which initiated programs to improve the health of mothers and children.
- 1946—The National School Lunch Act created the modern school lunch program.
- 1965—Medicaid, under Title XIX of the Social Security Act, enabled indigent pregnant women and children to have access to health care.
- 1966—The Child Nutrition Act initiated the school breakfast program.
- 1970—The Poisoning Prevention Packaging Act required that dangerous medications were to have childproof caps.
- 1972—The Women, Infants, and Children (WIC) program began providing supplemental food for low-income pregnant women, infants, and children.
- 1973—The Rehabilitation Act required that accommodations be made for children with disabilities to have access to schools and other public programs.
- 1974—The Child Abuse Prevention and Treatment Act provided funding for recognition of child abuse and development of child protection teams. This law also specified that every baby, regardless of disabilities, should receive nutrition, hydration, and medication.
- 1975—The Education for All Handicapped Children Act mandated that children with disabilities receive a free and appropriate education in the least restrictive environment. This act was reauthorized as the Individuals with Disabilities Education Act (IDEA) in 1997 and 2004, and children with disabilities were provided with educational opportunities and benefits equivalent to their peers without disabilities.
- 1984—The Emergency Medical Services for Children program was created to improve the quality of and access to emergency care for children with acute illnesses and injuries.
- 1997—State Children's Health Insurance Program (SCHIP) legislation expanded health coverage to children through 19 years of age in families with an income too high to qualify for Medicaid.

In 1935, as part of the Social Security Act, child welfare was addressed through the establishment of the Aid to Families with Dependent Children program to support needy children without fathers. Title V of the Social Security Act focused on promoting and improving the health of mothers and children nationwide. The Title V program has supported many landmark projects over the past 70 years to improve the health of pregnant women and children (Health Resources and Services Administration, Maternal and Child Health Bureau, 2010):

- Through maternal and child health grants to states and territories, states established agencies to address the needs of pregnant women and children.
- Over the next six decades, special programs were developed to address emerging issues such as infant mortality, children with intellectual disabilities, and newborn hearing screening.
- National guidelines were developed for child health supervision from infancy through adolescence, and safety standards for out-of-home childcare facilities were developed.
- Nutrition care during pregnancy and lactation has been enhanced through the Women, Infants, and Children's (WIC) supplemental nutrition program.
- Successful strategies for childhood injury prevention were identified. See pages 13–14 to understand why injury prevention became a major focus for maternal and child health programs.

Other Advances in Child Health Care

Other significant advances in society have had a major impact on the health of children:

- The development of antibiotics and vaccines beginning in the 1940s and 1950s has saved innumerable children who would have died of infectious diseases.
- Technologic advances have enabled new treatments for children with conditions that would have proven fatal, such as the heart-lung machine in the 1950s that made possible new surgical treatments for children with congenital heart defects.
- The National Aeronautic Space Administration (NASA) engineered miniaturized equipment that could be carried into space to monitor the astronauts. That equipment was then modified for use in health care. Much of the portable equipment used for pediatric health care is based on this research and engineering.
- Access to health information by computers (publications, patient data, and scientific studies) has enabled health professionals to collect, contrast, and analyze information about the care of children with specific conditions in different settings. Significant advances in the treatment and outcomes of children with many conditions are constantly being made.

Nurses have been instrumental in the development of pediatric health care and the specialty of pediatric nursing. They continue to help the specialty develop and to make sure that the needs of children are addressed in all settings. Exciting contributions are being made by pediatric nurses today, including:

- Conducting research to improve the care of children in areas such as self-management of health conditions, palliative care, and end-of-life care
- Identifying strategies to provide health services to homeless children

- Promoting healthy behaviors and lifestyles for children to address obesity and reduce their risk of chronic diseases as adults
- Developing strategies to reduce medication errors and improve patient safety
- Improving emergency medical systems to ensure access to appropriate and high-quality care

NURSING PROCESS IN PEDIATRIC CARE

The systematic framework for practice provided by the nursing process is the same for pediatric patients as for other patients. Consider how the five steps of the nursing process relate to children:

- *Assessment* involves collecting patient and family data and performing physical examinations during community-based health services, at admission, periodically during the child's hospitalization, and when home care services are provided. The nurse analyzes and synthesizes data to make a judgment about the patient's problems.
- *Nursing diagnoses* describe the health promotion and health patterns that nurses observe in the child and family and for which specific nursing actions can be planned, implemented, and evaluated. The North American Nursing Diagnosis Association (NANDA) has responsibility for endorsing the standard language for these nursing diagnoses to describe the health promotion and health patterns that nurses can independently manage.
- *Nursing care plans* are based on goals that will improve the child's or family's health and health conditions. Specific expected outcomes should be realistic. Nursing care plans have nursing interventions classifications (NICs) and nursing outcomes classifications (NOCs). NIC provides a standard language for general nursing actions that are specific for a nursing diagnosis. NOC provides a standard language for patient states or behaviors that should be monitored in children and families with a specific nursing diagnosis.

  Standard care plans for specific diagnoses are often used in the pediatric unit of the hospital and by home health agencies. The nurse is responsible for individualizing standard care plans based on data collected from the child's assessment, the cultural values of the child and family, and evaluation of the child's response to care. The family (and the child, when old enough) and the nurse should collaborate in the planning and agree upon the care plan goals. Individualized nursing action plans provide directions for nursing care.

- *Implementation* is the carrying out of interventions outlined in the nursing care plan. Interventions may be modified, depending on outcomes and the child's responses.
- *Evaluation* is the use of specific objective and subjective measures (often called outcome measures or criteria) to assess the progress of the child and family in reaching the goals defined in the nursing care plan. Following the evaluation of their progress toward the goals, the nursing care plan may be modified. For example, as the child's condition improves and goals are attained, new goals and nursing action plans should be defined.

In several chapters throughout this textbook, specific examples of the nursing process used in nursing care plans are provided for

health promotion activities and for the management of a child with a specific condition.

Clinical Reasoning

Clinical reasoning is "the process by which nurses collect cues, process the information, come to an understanding of a patient problem or situation, plan and implement interventions, evaluate outcomes, and reflect on and learn from the process" (Lapkin, Levett-Jones, Bellchambers, et al., 2010, p. e209). Clinical reasoning skills develop when the nurse builds upon previously acquired knowledge and past experience while learning to solve problems associated with a patient's health status or health condition. It involves assessment, planning, implementation of care, and evaluation of outcomes. **Critical thinking** is an individualized, creative thinking or reasoning process that the nurse uses to solve problems. Critical thinking and clinical reasoning are terms sometimes used interchangeably. As with clinical reasoning, the process of critical thinking involves several skills including the following (Jones, 2010):

- Analyzing data from the history, physical examination, and laboratory tests
- Applying standards of care
- Discriminating between signs, therapies, or appropriate nursing actions
- Seeking additional information or evidence regarding appropriate care to provide
- Using logical reasoning when developing a plan of care
- Predicting outcomes associated with the plan of care
- Transforming knowledge through the evaluation of care
- Evaluating new clinical practice guidelines

Clinical reasoning and critical thinking skills are essential for nurses because nursing and health care are dynamic. The patient's condition can change dramatically during a hospitalization, requiring the recognition of subtle cues that need attention to prevent the patient's deterioration. Research and new knowledge change the manner in which nursing care is provided. The healthcare system is under great pressure to improve the quality of care within an environment of fiscal constraints.

Evidence-Based Practice

Evidence-based practice is a problem-solving approach that combines the best evidence from well-designed studies with an individual's clinical expertise and the patient's circumstances and values or preferences (Gallagher-Ford, Fineout-Overholt, Melnyk, et al., 2011). It provides a bridge between research and practice by using a systematic search for the most relevant evidence and a critical review of that evidence to answer a clinical question. This is one strategy to keep nursing practice current and to promote positive healthcare outcomes for children and their families. It has also become an important strategy for healthcare institutions focusing on patient safety and quality of care. The Institute of Medicine has set a goal that by 2020, 90% of all healthcare decisions will be evidence based (Melnyk, Fineout-Overholt, Stillwell, et al., 2009).

The process of evidence-based practice involves several steps (Melnyk, Fineout-Overholt, Stillwell, et al., 2010):

1. Clearly identify the specific clinical question to be investigated.
2. Collect the most relevant and best evidence.
3. Critically review and synthesize the evidence.

4. Apply the evidence to practice by integrating it with one's clinical experience and patient preferences and values, leading to a practice decision or change.
5. Evaluate the practice decision or change.
6. Disseminate the results of the evidence-based practice process.

The PICOT acronym describes a method for refining the clinical question and identifying the search terms for a literature search (Melnyk et al., 2010):

- **P**—defining the patient *population* (e.g., by age, sex, ethnicity, and health problem)
- **I**—*identifying* the health condition or current nursing actions of interest
- **C**—identifying the *comparison* intervention or patient population
- **O**—identifying the effectiveness of the intervention on the patient population's clinical *outcomes*
- **T**—defining a *time* interval for the question

To integrate the best research evidence, the health professional must analyze and evaluate all clinical studies related to a specific health condition or clinical problem. However, clinical judgment is needed to determine if the research findings fit the population of care served by the health professional or by the healthcare setting. As partners in the healthcare process, the child's and family's preferences must be considered in any care provided.

The new evidence may result in a proposed change in the process of care, such as a revised clinical practice guideline, if the analysis reveals that the children have a better outcome or the cost of care is reduced with a new procedure or treatment. In some cases, the care change is implemented in a nursing unit or healthcare setting as a pilot project. Data are collected to evaluate the changed practice to see if the outcomes occur as predicted by the evidence. If the changed practice does result in improved outcomes, then the new practice is adopted more broadly. It is the responsibility of the nurses involved in the project to publish the results so that findings are more widely disseminated.

In some cases, multiple disciplines collaborate in an evidence-based practice process to answer a clinical question that leads to the development of a clinical practice guideline. For example, the international Cochrane Collaboration conducts systematic reviews of health care and health policy research and publishes evidence-based healthcare recommendations in the *Cochrane Reviews* (Cochrane Collaboration, 2011). A **clinical practice guideline** (sometimes called a clinical pathway) is a consensus of evidence-based and expert opinion statements about the care for a specific diagnosis used to assist healthcare providers to make decisions about the appropriate care of a child with that condition (Harbaugh, 2009; Kavanagh, Adams, & Wang, 2009). These clinical practice guidelines are often developed by a national professional organization, government agency, or expert panel for a specific condition. They serve as an interface between research and practice, encouraging practice changes that improve quality and are more cost-effective. Practice guidelines promote uniformity in care so that patient outcomes and health professional performance can be measured. For an example, see the asthma guidelines developed by the National Asthma Education Program of the National Institutes of Health in Chapter 25 .

Assessing Quality of Health Care

Quality of care is defined by the Institute of Medicine as "the degree to which healthcare services for individuals and populations increase the likelihood of desired health outcomes and are consistent with current professional knowledge" (Kavanagh et al., 2009, p. 458). To determine if care provided is of high quality, it must be measured. For this reason, measurable healthcare indicators (also known as performance indicators and review criteria) that can be used to assess the appropriateness of healthcare decisions, services, and outcomes are the focus of several organizations and federal agencies. Indicators can focus on the structure or environment where care is delivered, the process of care, or patient outcomes. Examples of pediatric indicators that have been developed include the following (Kavanagh et al., 2009):

- The Agency for Healthcare Research and Quality (AHRQ) has 18 indicators for pediatric inpatient care. Most of these indicators are associated with complications of care, such as accidental puncture or laceration, postoperative hemorrhage and hematoma, postoperative sepsis, postoperative respiratory failure, and transfusion reaction (McDonald, 2009).
- The Joint Commission has indicators for inpatient pediatric asthma care and for care in the pediatric intensive care unit.
- The Cystic Fibrosis Foundation has quality indicators to improve care provided in its sponsored care centers.
- The Rand Corporation has developed a comprehensive set of inpatient indicators for children and adolescents, and for the follow-up care of very low-birth-weight infants.

Electronic patient records make it possible to evaluate the quality of care provided to all children with the specific health status or health condition of interest. When the child's record of care reveals an indicator of an unexpected outcome, it is then possible to fully investigate the circumstances of the care to identify opportunities for improvements. When a pattern of variations from the expected process of care is found, education can be provided to all healthcare providers to improve compliance with the process of care. Nurses have a role in assessing the quality of care by participating on performance improvement committees. Quality indicators will become increasingly more important in healthcare settings as the Centers for Medicare and Medicaid Services plan to use quality measures to guide reimbursement (Scanlon, Harris, Levy, et al., 2008). See Box 1–4 for research conducted on pediatric healthcare quality.

BOX 1–4	Research: Quality of Pediatric Health Care

Through a consensus-based process, nine measures of inpatient asthma care that were considered appropriate and reliable were identified. The measures were then tested using a retrospective chart review of 252 children admitted to a tertiary care hospital who were cared for by 109 different physician providers. The compliance with these measures of asthma care was variable. A documented assessment of asthma severity on admission was found in 39% of cases. Systemic corticosteroids were used in 98% of cases, but only 87% had oral (versus intravenous) corticosteroids. Only 20% of children over 5 years of age had albuterol administered by metered dose inhaler versus nebulizer. Several measures identified potential roles for nurses; for example, 33% of cases had parental participation in an asthma education class, 5% of cases had a written asthma action plan, and 22% of cases had a follow-up appointment with a primary care provider at the time of discharge. This project demonstrates the importance of interprofessional collaboration in the improvement of care quality (Nkoy, Fassl, Simon, et al., 2008).

CONTEMPORARY CLIMATE FOR PEDIATRIC NURSING CARE

As of the 2010 national census, an estimated 83.3 million children and youth under 20 years of age live in the United States, and they account for approximately 27% of the population. (See Figure 1–5 ■ for a distribution of the population by age group.) The percentage of children and youth within the U.S. population continues to decline as the elderly live longer. The median age of the population has increased from 35.3 years in 2000 to 37.6 years in 2010 (U.S. Census Bureau, 2011).

Partnering with Families: Family-Centered Care

To develop a trusting partnership with families, healthcare providers must recognize that the family is a constant influence and support in the child's life. A **partnership** is a relationship in which participants join together to ensure health care is delivered in a way that recognizes the critical roles and contributions of each partner in promoting health, preventing illness, and managing healthcare conditions. The family is the principal caregiver and center of strength and support for the child (Figure 1–6 ■). Partnerships with families are important in all healthcare settings because of the vital role that families play in meeting the emotional, social, and developmental needs of their children and in ensuring their health and well-being. **Family-centered care** is a dynamic, deliberate approach to building collaborative relationships between health professionals and families that is respectful of their diversity and beliefs about the nature of the child's condition and ways to manage it. See Chapter 2 ☻ for methods of implementing family-centered care and building partnerships with families.

All children need a **medical home** or **healthcare home**—a continuous, comprehensive, family-centered, and compassionate source of health care provided throughout the child's developmental years. Criteria for a medical or healthcare home include the following: being well known by a physician or nurse who provides the usual source of sick care, having access to specialty care and other services or therapies, spending adequate time communicating clearly with the family, providing help with care coordination when needed, respecting the family's values and partnering with the family in the child's care, and providing interpreters when necessary.

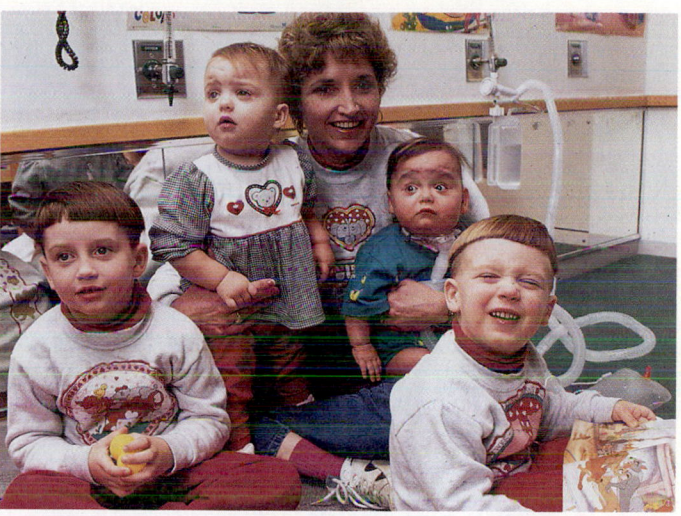

FIGURE 1–6 ■ Many facilities now encourage family visitation for children with health problems that require long-term hospitalization. Extended family visits enable parents to learn about the child's care, and provide siblings with opportunities to interact with the hospitalized child.

An estimated 57.5% of children have a healthcare home that meets these criteria (Health Resources and Services Administration, 2009, p. 25). See Chapter 8 ☻ for additional information about the healthcare home.

When a family has an established relationship with a care provider, a partnership between the parent and healthcare provider enables the child to receive health services based on the family's risks and protective factors. See Chapters 8 and 14 ☻ for more information about the role of nurses in the medical or healthcare home model of care.

Culturally Competent Care

The U.S. population has a varied mix of cultural groups, with ever-increasing diversity. Approximately 46% of all children less than 18 years of age are from families of minority populations (Federal Interagency Forum on Child and Family Statistics, 2011). Consider the current issues:

- In 2010, 23% of children in the United States lived with at least one parent who was foreign born.
- In 2009, 21% of school-age children in the United States spoke another language other than English, and 5% had difficulty speaking English.
- In 2009, about 6% of school-age children spoke a language other than English at home and lived in a home in which a language other than English was spoken and no person over 14 years spoke English "very well."

The 2010 U.S. population illustrates the diversity of children under 18 years of age: 54% of U.S. children were non-Hispanic White, 23% Hispanic, 14% Black, 4% Asian, and 5% all other races. The racial and ethnic diversity is expected to increase significantly over the next few decades as 39% of U.S. children are projected to be Hispanic by 2050 (Federal Interagency Forum on Child and Family Statistics, 2011). It is also important to recognize the diversity among the non-Hispanic White population as they represent many cultural groups, such as immigrants from former Soviet bloc countries in Eastern Europe.

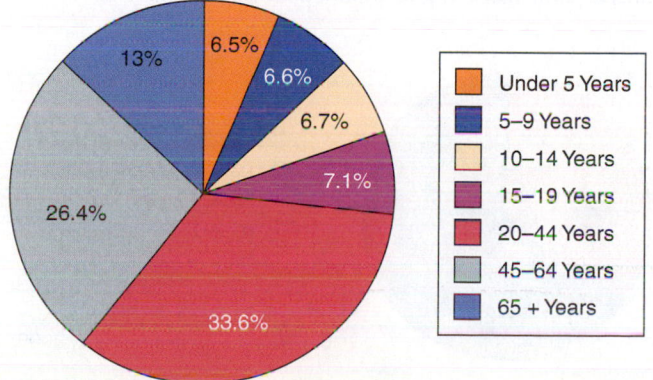

🟧	Under 5 Years
🟦	5–9 Years
🟨	10–14 Years
🟥	15–19 Years
🟥	20–44 Years
⬜	45–64 Years
🟦	65 + Years

FIGURE 1–5 ■ United States Population by Age Group, 2010
In 2010, children from birth to 19 years of age accounted for approximately 27% of the total population in the United States.

Source: *U.S. Census Bureau. (2011). Age and sex composition: 2010. 2010 Census Briefs. Retrieved from http:// www.census.gov/prod/cen2010/briefs/c2010br-03.pdf*

Weblink

Federal Interagency Forum on Child Health

Developing Cultural Competence
Integrating Tradition

Conflicts can occur within a family when traditional rituals and practices of the family's elders do not conform to current healthcare practices. Nurses need to be sensitive to the potential implications for the child's health care, especially when the child is being cared for in the home. Specific cultural groups often practice complementary and alternative therapies. Information about these practices needs to be obtained during the history. Although some complementary therapies are beneficial or cause no harm, other therapies may interact with prescribed medications and cause harm. See Chapter 3 🔵 for more information about complementary and alternative therapies.

When cultural values are not included as part of the nursing care plan, parents may be forced to decide whether the family's beliefs and values should take priority over the healthcare professional's guidance. Make an effort to understand traditional health practices and to integrate them into the care plan. When the family's cultural values are incorporated into the care plan, the family is more likely to accept and adhere to the needed care, especially in the home care setting. Avoid imposing your personal cultural values on the children and families in your care. By learning about the values of the different ethnic groups in the community—religious beliefs that have an impact on healthcare practices, beliefs about common illnesses, and their specific healing practices—you can develop an individualized nursing care plan for each child and family. See Chapter 3 🔵 for guidelines in developing a culturally competent practice in pediatric nursing.

Culture involves the knowledge, beliefs, and behaviors that define an individual's personal identification, language, thoughts, communications, actions, customs, and values (U.S. Department of Health and Human Services, National Institutes of Health, 2010). It develops from socially learned beliefs, lifestyles, values, and integrated patterns of behavior that are characteristic of the family, religious faith, ethnic or racial group, and geographic area. The cultural background and values of children and their parents are often quite different from those of the nurse. This lack of knowledge about the family's cultural values may lead to practices that either inadvertently offend the family or result in less than optimal outcomes of care. Awareness of differences in cultural values is the first step in developing cultural competence. See Developing Cultural Competence: Integrating Tradition for initial steps in integrating culture into nursing care plans.

Pediatric Health Statistics

Infant Mortality

The U.S. infant mortality rate was 6.42 per 1,000 live births in 2009 (Kochanek, Xu, Murphy, et al., 2011). The leading causes of infant mortality (death occurring during the first year of life) vary according to the age and race of the infant. For example, the infant mortality rate in the United States during 2009 was 5.27 per 1,000 live births for non-Hispanic Whites, 12.71 for Blacks, and 5.44 for Hispanic infants (Kochanek, et al., 2011). See Figure 1–7 ■ for the 10 most common causes of infant mortality in 2008.

Approximately 65% of infant deaths in 2009 occurred within the first 28 days of life. See Figure 1–8 ■ for a comparison of the neonatal and postneonatal mortality rates. Infants have different causes of mortality in the first 28 days of life than in the remaining 11 months of the first year of life. Leading causes of neonatal mortality include prematurity and low birth weight, congenital malformations, and conditions originating in the perinatal period, such as maternal complications related to pregnancy or birth-related complications.

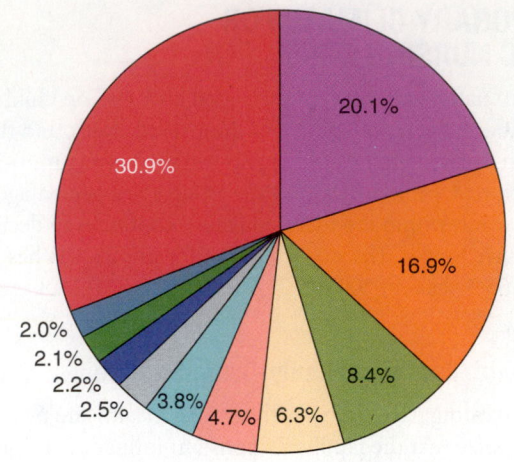

Legend:
- Congenital Malformations
- Low Birth Weight
- Sudden Infant Death Syndrome
- Complications of Pregnancy
- Unintentional Injuries
- Newborn Affected by Complications of Placenta, Cord, and Membranes
- Bacterial Sepsis of Newborn
- Respiratory Distress of Newborn
- Diseases of Circulatory System
- Neonatal Hemorrhage
- All Others

FIGURE 1–7 ■ Leading causes of infant mortality (birth to 1 year of age) in the United States in 2008.

Source: Data from Miniño, A. M., Murphy, S. M., Xu, J., & Kochanek, K. D. (2011). Deaths: Final data for 2008. National Vital Statistics Reports, 59(10), 1–157.

Leading causes of postneonatal mortality include sudden infant death syndrome (SIDS), congenital malformations, and unintentional injuries (U.S. Department of Health and Human Services, 2011a).

Sudden infant death syndrome (SIDS) accounts for nearly 8% of deaths to infants and usually occurs during the postneonatal period (between 1 and 12 months of age). Compared to non-Hispanic White infants, mortality rates due to SIDS were 2.4 times higher in American Indian and Alaska Native infants and 1.9 times higher in non-Hispanic Black infants (Mathews & MacDorman, 2011). What

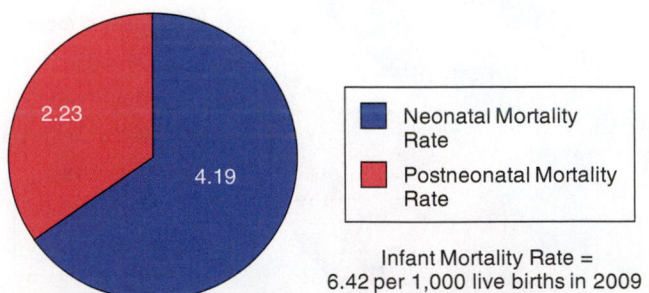

Legend:
- Neonatal Mortality Rate
- Postneonatal Mortality Rate

Infant Mortality Rate = 6.42 per 1,000 live births in 2009

FIGURE 1–8 ■ Comparison of Neonatal and Postneonatal Mortality Rates, 2009
Neonatal mortality refers to all deaths that occur in an infant 28 days of life and younger. Postneonatal mortality refers to infants between 29 days and 1 year of age. Mortality rates are calculated as the number of deaths per 1,000 live births.

Source: Kochanek, K. D., Xu, J., Murphy, S. L., Miniño, A. M., & Kung, H. (2011). Deaths: Preliminary data for 2009, National Vital Statistics Reports, 59(4), 1–51.

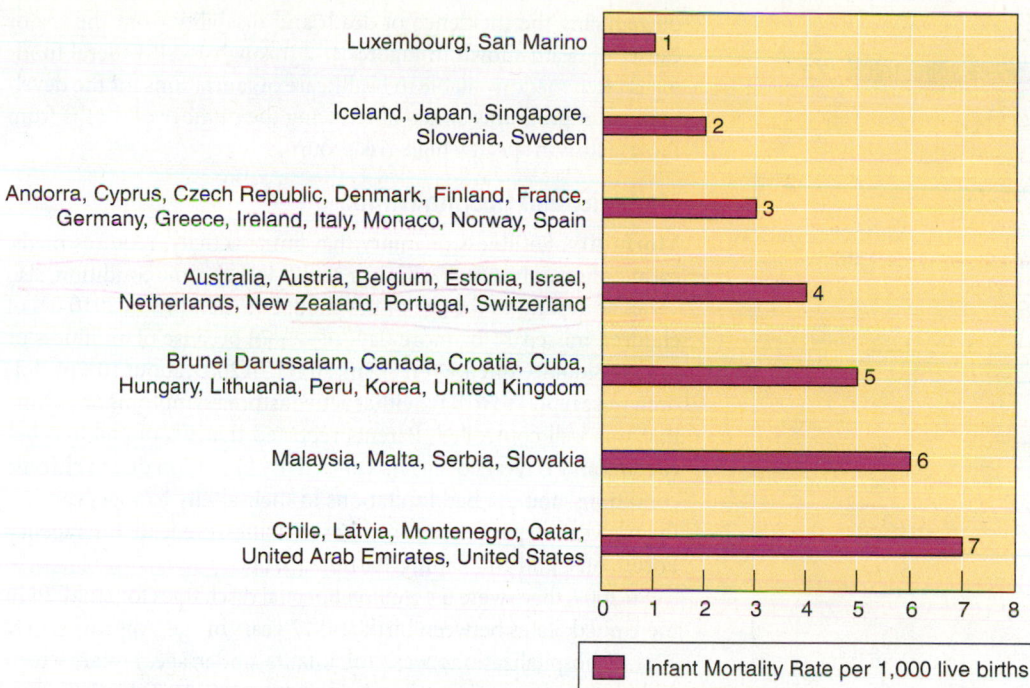

could potentially account for the higher risk of SIDS in these infants? See Chapter 25 🔗 for an answer. What do you think are the leading causes of injury deaths in infants? See Table 1–1 for an answer.

Despite the historical success in reducing the infant mortality rate over many decades, the United States does not compare well to the infant mortality rates found in other industrialized or developed countries with a population of at least 1 million. In 2009, the United States ranked 45th behind such developed nations as Singapore, Iceland, Sweden, Japan, France, and Germany (World Health Organization, 2011). See Figure 1–9 ■ for the comparison of infant mortality rates by nations with the lowest infant mortality rates in 2009. Several factors may account for the higher rate of infant mortality

FIGURE 1–9 ■ 2009 Infant Mortality Rates in Selected World Nations

Ranking of the nations with the lowest infant mortality rates in the world in 2009. Note the 47 nations that have a lower infant mortality rate than the United States. What could account for the United States' poorer ranking?

Source: *Data from World Health Organization Global Health Observatory Data Repository. (2011).* Child mortality data, 2009. *Retrieved from* http://apps.who.int/ghodata/?vid=1320

in the United States, such as a high rate of prematurity, aggressive treatment to save very low-birth-weight infants, health disparities in different populations, and different methods of reporting fetal and infant deaths. Research and perinatal care programs for high-risk pregnant women and infants are directed at reducing the infant mortality rate.

Child Mortality

Children have different healthcare problems than adults, and the problems may depend on age and development. The most common cause of death in 2009 for U.S. children between 1 and 19 years of age was unintentional injury. Congenital anomalies, cancer, homicide, and diseases of the heart are the other major causes of death in children between 1 and 9 years of age. See Figure 1–10 ■. The major causes of death to children in this age group are similar to those in the last decade, and progress has been made in lowering the rates of mortality for most of these leading causes of death. Dramatic reductions in the causes of death by type of injury have also occurred over the past decade. In older children and adolescents between 10 and 19 years of age, the leading causes of mortality include cancer, homicide, suicide, congenital anomalies, and diseases of the heart, in addition to unintentional injuries. See Figure 1–11 ■.

Unintentional injury is a leading cause of death in all pediatric age groups, except neonates. The rate of death for causes such as motor vehicle crashes, drowning, falls, and burns has been decreasing over the last 20 years. It is alarming that intentional injury (homicide and suicide) has become a leading cause of death in children. See Table 1–1 for the leading causes of injury death by age group. Injury prevention became a major focus of many national organizations and the federal maternal and child health programs in the United States beginning in the 1980s. What specific injury prevention interventions do you think contributed to reduced deaths due to these mechanisms of injury? See Chapters 9 to 13 🔗 for answers.

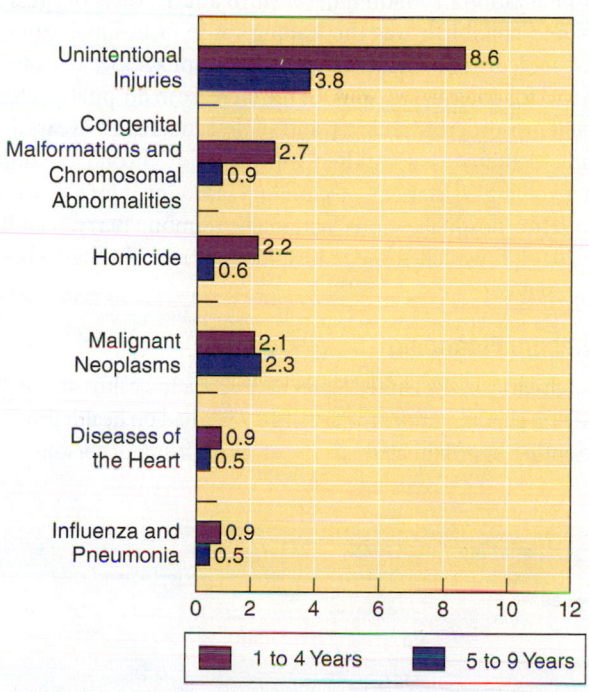

FIGURE 1–10 ■ Age-specific mortality rate per 100,000 children in the United States in 2009 for the six leading causes of death in children 1 to 4 years of age and 5 to 9 years of age. Unintentional injuries (potentially preventable deaths) are the leading cause of mortality in these age groups. Why would the rate of unintentional injury be higher in the 1 to 4 year old age group? Which types of injuries cause the most deaths? See Table 1–1. See Chapters 10–12 🔗 for more information.

Source: *Centers for Disease Control and Prevention, National Center for Health Statistics. (2012).* Underlying Cause of Death 1999–2009 on CDC WONDER Online Database, released 2012. *Retrieved from* http://wonder.cdc.gov/ucd-icd10.html

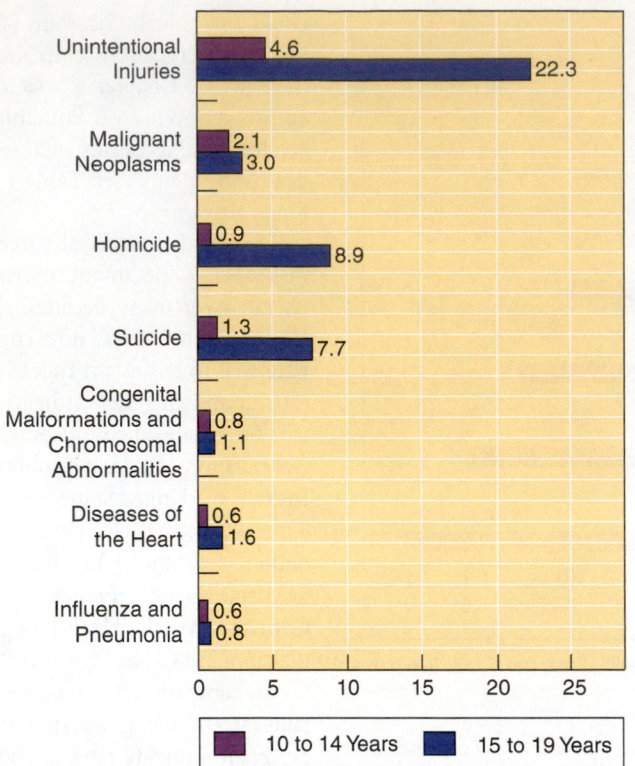

FIGURE 1–11 ■ Age-specific mortality rate per 100,000 children in the United States in 2009 for children 10 to 14 years of age and 15 to 19 years of age. The leading cause of mortality in children and adolescents in 2009 was unintentional injury. Why do you think the rate is higher in the 15 to 19 year age group? Which type of injury causes the most deaths? Drowning? Fires and burns? Motor vehicle crashes? See Table 1–1 for the answer.

Source: *Centers for Disease Control and Prevention, National Center for Health Statistics. (2012).* Underlying Cause of Death 1999–2009 on CDC WONDER Online Database, released 2012. *Retrieved from* http://wonder.cdc.gov/ucd-icd10.html

Healthy People 2020

The U.S. government set objectives to improve the health of all citizens, including children and young adults, by the year 2020 in the report entitled *Healthy People 2020* (U.S. Department of Health and Human Services, 2011b). This national effort strives to identify nationwide priorities for health improvement and provides goals and measurable objectives for improving health status at the local, state, and national level. See Chapter 14 🔗 for a listing of national health goals and some objectives that relate to children. Additional objectives are highlighted in many other chapters. These objectives focus

on reducing the incidence of death and disability from the major causes of death shown in Figures 1–7 through 1–11. Federal funding is often made available to healthcare organizations for the development of programs aimed at reducing the number of deaths from these factors in specific high-risk groups.

Morbidity and Hospitalization

Morbidity, an illness or injury that limits activity, requires medical attention or hospitalization, or results in a chronic condition, also varies according to the age of the child. For example, in 2010 6% of children missed 11 or more days of school because of an illness or injury (Bloom, Cohen, & Freeman, 2011). In 2009, about 10% of children were reported to have either active asthma symptoms or asthma that was well controlled. Parents reported that 9% of children between 5 and 17 years of age had an activity limitation due to chronic conditions, and 2% had limitations in their ability to walk, care for themselves, or participate in other activities (Federal Interagency Forum on Child and Family Statistics, 2011).

In 2009, there were 6.4 million hospital discharges for children in the United States between birth and 17 years of age. Approximately 72% of hospitalizations were for infants under age 1 year, which includes newborns (Yu, Wier, & Elixhauser, 2011). Table 1–2 illustrates the leading causes of hospitalization of children by age group in 2009. Respiratory diseases are a leading cause of hospitalization in children of all ages. Injury and poisoning are also a leading cause of hospitalization. Examine the leading causes of injury mortality; what specific injuries in each age group might be represented in these hospitalizations? Mental disorders were the leading cause of hospitalization in children between 10 and 17 years of age. Pregnancy and childbirth was the leading cause of hospitalization for adolescent females between 15 and 17 years of age. See Chapters 20 and 34 🔗 for potential reasons for the increase in hospital discharges for mental disorders in children and adolescents 10 to 17 years. It was recently identified that children with complex chronic conditions, often involving assistance by technology, accounted for about 10.1% of pediatric hospitalizations nationally (Simon, Berry, Feudtner, et al., 2010). In which cause of hospitalization might these children be represented?

Healthcare Financing

Not all children in the United States have access to health care. In 2009, 9.5 million children under the age of 18 years had no health insurance, representing approximately 16.2% of all uninsured persons in the

TABLE 1–1	Five Leading Causes of Injury Death by Age Group Highlighting Unintentional Injuries, 2009*				
	Ranking of Injury Mortality Causes				
AGE GROUP	**1st**	**2nd**	**3rd**	**4th**	**5th**
0 to 12 months	Suffocation	Motor vehicle, traffic	Drowning	Fire, burns	Poisoning
1 to 4 years	Drowning	Homicide	Motor vehicle, traffic	Fire, burns	Suffocation
5 to 9 years	Motor vehicle, traffic	Drowning	Fire, burns	Homicide	Motor vehicle, other land transport
10 to 14 years	Motor vehicle, traffic	Suicide	Homicide	Drowning	Motor vehicle, other land transport
15 to 19 years	Motor vehicle, traffic	Homicide	Suicide	Poisoning	Drowning

*Shaded boxes indicate unintentional injuries.

Source: *Data from National Center for Health Statistics, National Vital Statistics System. (2012).* Leading causes of injury deaths by age group highlighting unintentional injury deaths, United States—2009. *Retrieved from http://webappa.cdc.gov/cgi-bin/broker.exe*

TABLE 1–2	Leading Causes of Hospitalization for Children and Number of Hospital Discharges for Each Cause in 2009				
	Ranking of Causes				
AGE GROUP	**1st**	**2nd**	**3rd**	**4th**	**5th**
Infants less than 1 year	Diseases of the respiratory system 170,352	Congenital anomalies and chromosomal abnormalities 52,368	Infectious and parasitic diseases 32,164	Diseases of the digestive system 29,298	Diseases of the genitourinary system 22,869
1 to 4 years	Diseases of the respiratory system 220,804	Injury and poisoning 50,943	Endocrine, nutrition, metabolic, and immune disorders 48,286	Disorders of the skin and subcutaneous tissues 33,206	Diseases of the digestive system 30,520
5 to 9 years	Diseases of the respiratory system 100,634	Diseases of the digestive system 42,861	Injury and poisoning 39,950	Endocrine, nutrition, metabolic, and immune disorders 22,557	Diseases of the nervous system and sense organs 21,210
10 to 14 years	Diseases of the digestive system 56,415	Mental disorders 55,699	Injury and poisoning 48,652	Diseases of the respiratory system 47,463	Endocrine, nutrition, metabolic, and immune disorders 22,603
15 to 17 years	Complications of pregnancy, childbirth, and puerperium 148,293	Mental disorders 74,477	Injury and poisoning 60,568	Diseases of the digestive system 48,901	Diseases of the respiratory system 27,738

Source: *Data from Agency for Healthcare Research and Quality, HCUP Kids' Inpatient Database, 2009. (2011).* Patient and hospital characteristics for ICD-9-CM principal diagnosis code. *Retrieved from* http://hcupnet.ahrq.gov

United States (Fox, 2010). Nationally, approximately one third of children with special healthcare needs are uninsured (Kogan, Newacheck, Blumberg, et al., 2010). More than two thirds of uninsured children are eligible for public insurance programs such as Medicaid or the Children's Health Insurance Program (CHIP). See Legal and Ethical Considerations: Children's Health Insurance Program. *Medicaid* provides coverage to children and individuals with disabilities who meet income level qualifications set by the state. Children covered under the Temporary Assistance to Needy Families (TANF) are usually eligible.

Not all eligible children are enrolled in Medicaid or CHIP, potentially because of difficulties in getting enrolled or limitations in state funding. Hispanic children (14%) are more than twice as likely as non-Hispanic White (6%) or Black (6%) children to be uninsured for health care (Leininger & Meurer, 2011). Low-income immigrant children are more likely to be uninsured than other children from low-income families, and public policy makes many immigrant children ineligible for CHIP (Yu, Huang, & Kogan, 2008).

Clinical Tip

The federal poverty rate is used to determine eligibility for many health and welfare services. The rate is a sliding scale based on the number of persons in the family, and it is updated annually. For example, the poverty rate for a family of four in 2011 was $22,350 (Centers for Medicare and Medicaid Services, 2011a).

Of children who do have healthcare coverage, more than 20% experience breaks in public and private health insurance coverage that jeopardize consistent care for chronic conditions and preventive health services (Cassedy, Fairbrother, & Newacheck, 2008). Uninsured children often do not have a usual source of health care and have difficulty obtaining basic preventive health care, including immunizations or care for chronic conditions. When children were enrolled in CHIP, their health care improved with a significantly increased access to care and their families experienced fewer financial burdens (Smith-Campbell & Pile, 2010).

Legal and Ethical Considerations
Children's Health Insurance Program

Congress created the Children's Health Insurance Program (CHIP) in 1997 and reauthorized it in 2009 through 42 USC 1305 Public Law 111–3. This program provides health insurance for children when their family's income is too high to qualify for Medicaid but too low to pay for private insurance.

Despite the availability of CHIP, many eligible children are not enrolled. Reasons families have not enrolled their eligible children may include the following (Leininger & Meurer, 2011):

- They may not know their child is eligible.
- The enrollment requirements and income verification tests are barriers.
- Some state plans require a monthly premium or co-payment for healthcare visits, and even a minimal co-pay reduces enrollment and use of health services.

Nurses can play an important role in encouraging families to investigate their eligibility for the program. Obtain current guidelines in your state about eligibility requirements and coverage benefits.

Health Benefits

Children enrolled in CHIP must be provided with health benefits coverage that is substantially equal to the benefits coverage in the federal or state employee health benefits plan or the plan of the largest health maintenance organization in the state. In 2010, 7.7 million children were enrolled in CHIP at some time during the year (Centers for Medicare and Medicaid Services, 2011b). Approximately 34.4 million children were enrolled in Medicaid in 2010 (Centers for Medicare and Medicaid Services, 2011c). Children enrolled in Medicaid are provided services through the Early Periodic Screening, Diagnostic, and Treatment (EPSDT) service. This is

Medicaid Early Periodic Screening and Diagnostic Treatment Benefits

Weblink

BOX 1–5	Preventive Health Services Covered Under Medicaid's Early Periodic Screening, Diagnostic, and Treatment Service

- Comprehensive health and developmental history
- Comprehensive unclothed physical examination
- Appropriate immunizations
- Laboratory tests (statewide screening requirements and lead toxicity screening)
- Health education
- Vision services—screening, treatment for defects in vision, including eyeglasses
- Dental services—dental screening, relief of pain and infection, restoration of teeth, and maintenance of dental health by a dentist
- Hearing services—diagnosis and treatment of hearing defects, including hearing aids
- Other necessary health care—to correct or ameliorate defects, physical and mental illnesses, and conditions discovered by the screening process

Source: *From Centers for Medicare and Medicaid Services. (2011). Early periodic screening diagnosis & treatment. Retrieved from http://www.medicaid.gov/Medicaid-CHIP-Program-Information/By-Topics/Benefits/Early-Periodic-Screening-Diagnosis-and-Treatment.html*

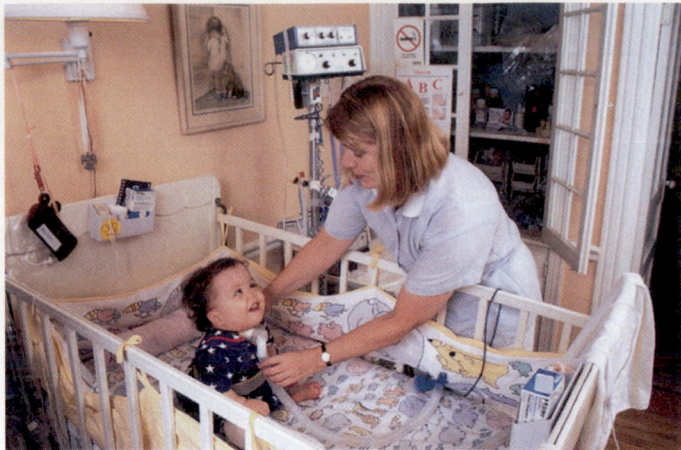

FIGURE 1–12 ■ It is often desirable from a family and cost perspective to provide health care in the home, and technologic advances have made this possible. But is it really less costly to provide care in the home for a child with technology assistance? How does one factor in parents' out-of-pocket expenses for medical supplies that are not reimbursed, lost time from work or the need for a parent to discontinue employment to care for the child, and the emotional strain on families who care for their child 24 hours a day, 7 days a week? What support is needed by these families to continue providing this level of care at home? See Chapters 14 and 16.

a comprehensive and preventive child health program for individuals under 21 years. See Box 1–5 for a list of covered services.

Managed care is a health delivery system that focuses on the delivery of specified healthcare services while attempting to control the costs of such services. Depending on the managed care plan, certain essential elements include contracting with clinicians for provision of services at a predetermined fee, use of clinical standards of care such as clinical practice guidelines, care coordination of children with chronic conditions, and quality improvement programs to evaluate the services provided. Many state Medicaid programs have converted to a managed care process. Children with special healthcare needs utilize significantly more healthcare services than other children, and managed care programs for these children must take into consideration the lifelong needs for services such as technology support and home care.

Healthcare Technology

Research and technology have enabled many children with congenital anomalies and low birth weights to survive, with and without chronic conditions. Lifesaving technology has also created such burdens as high healthcare costs and stresses on the functioning of the child's family. Technologic advances have resulted in the design of portable medical and infusion therapy equipment for home care. Many children are dependent upon or assisted by technology for physiologic functions. For example, approximately 11% of children with special healthcare needs use medical equipment such as ventilators, feeding tubes, and intravenous or central lines along with their associated pumps, cardiorespiratory monitors, peritoneal dialysis, and pacemakers (Health Resources and Services Administration, Maternal and Child Health Bureau, 2008). The number of children assisted by technology continues to increase as scientific and technologic advances grow. Generators are often used in cases of power outages in the home. Some families have regained control over their lives by creating intensive care units in their homes (Figure 1–12 ■). Children who 15 to 25 years ago would have died from respiratory, neurologic, or other medical conditions are thriving with home care and are participating in family, community, and school life.

LEGAL AND ETHICAL CONCEPTS AND RESPONSIBILITIES

Regulation of Nursing Practice

Because nurses are accountable for their professional actions, each state regulates nursing practice with a nurse practice act. A state's nurse practice act defines the legal roles and responsibilities of nurses. Become familiar with this act in your state. As professionals, nurses set standards for education and practice that conform to state regulations, and these standards are modified as the science of nursing advances.

Standards of clinical nursing practice developed by the American Nurses Association, the Society of Pediatric Nurses, and the National Association of Pediatric Nurse Practitioners in 2008 define standards for both nursing care and performance. Standards of care describe the competent level of nursing care using the nursing process and form the foundation of clinical decision making. Standards of performance describe the expectations for patient care and professional performance. See Box 1–6.

Accountability and Risk Management

Accountability

The family entrusts the child's care to the healthcare team. Family members expect this team to provide good medical and nursing care and to avoid mistakes that cause harm. Nurses are personally accountable for:

- Expanding their knowledge base
- Staying current regarding changes in medical and nursing practice for specific conditions
- Recognizing important changes in the child's condition that require intervention
- Taking action as necessary to protect the child

Patient Safety

Patient safety is defined as the freedom from unintentional injury caused by medical care; it includes freedom from harm by

BOX 1–6	Professional Practice Standards for Pediatric Nursing Practice

STANDARDS OF CARE

- Collection of comprehensive data pertinent to the patient's health or situation
- Analysis of the assessment data to determine diagnoses or healthcare issues
- Identification of expected outcomes for a plan of care individualized to the child, family, or situation
- Development of a plan of care that prescribes strategies and alternatives to attain expected outcomes
- Implementation of the identified plan of care
- Evaluation of progress toward attainment of outcomes

STANDARDS OF PERFORMANCE

- Systematic enhancement of the quality and effectiveness of nursing care
- Evaluation of own nursing practice in relation to professional practice standards and guidelines, relevant statutes, rules, and regulations
- Attainment of knowledge and competency that reflects current nursing practice
- Interaction with and contribution to the professional development of peers and colleagues
- Collaboration with the child, family, and others in the conduct of nursing practice
- Integration of ethical considerations and processes in all areas of practice
- Integration of research findings into practice, and where appropriate, participation in the generation of new knowledge
- Consideration of factors related to safety, effectiveness, cost, and impact on practice in planning and delivering patient care
- Provision of leadership in the professional practice setting and the profession
- Advocacy for the pediatric client and family

Source: *American Nurses Association, National Association of Pediatric Nurse Practitioners, and Society of Pediatric Nurses. (2008). Pediatric nursing: Scope and standards of practice. Silver Spring, MD: Nursesbooks.org.*

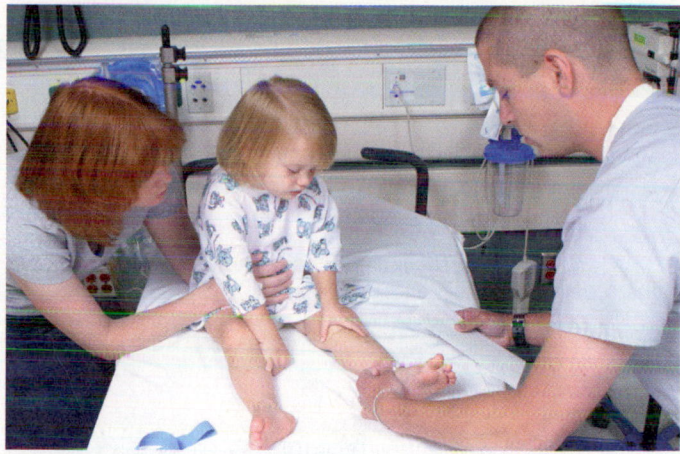

FIGURE 1–13 ■ An important patient safety action is to verify the identity of the child prior to performing any procedure or administering medication. The nurse needs two forms of identification. In this case the child's identification bracelet is compared to the name and birth date on the laboratory test form, and the parent also confirms the child's identity.

medication errors within hospitals are "systems" errors, such as incorrect transcription of physician orders, malfunctioning equipment used for administering medications, interruptions during medication administration, and delayed medication delivery by the pharmacy, rather than an error by a single individual. Reduction of medication errors is one focus of patient safety since children have been found to experience medication errors at a rate 3 times greater than adults (American Academy of Pediatrics, 2011b). Incorrect dosing is the most commonly reported medication error, and reasons for this increased risk among children include the following (Gonzales, 2010):

- Medication dosage is based on weight or body surface area, often making dosage calculations more complex. This means the optimal dose is based on mg/kg and divided by number of doses to be given a day. An additional problem is that children often need suspensions or liquid preparations, adding to the dosage calculation complexity. Not only must the correct dose be calculated, but also the amount of liquid preparation with that dose. Some medications are in concentrations that require dilution, further complicating the accurate medication dosage calculation. See Chapter 15 and the Skills Manual for more information about medication administration to children.
- The misplacement of a decimal in the medication dosage calculation can result in an overdose that can cause harm to the child or even death. Critically ill or injured children do not have the reserves to deal with an overdose of medication like a healthy child.
- Some medications (e.g., acetaminophen) have different dosage forms (drops, liquids, tablets).
- Medications are sometimes prescribed that are not yet approved by the Food and Drug Administration for use in children, and pediatric standard dosage guidelines have not been established.
- Young children cannot communicate well if they are having a reaction to the medication.

Another cause of potential medical error involves family members with limited English proficiency who must read and interpret administration instructions at home. Communication challenges

death-related or adverse drug events, misidentification of the patient, and healthcare-associated infections (American Academy of Pediatrics, 2011b). Correct patient identification is essential prior to all procedures and medication administration (Figure 1–13 ■). Improving communication at the change of shift is important to ensure that the child receives all needed care in a continuous manner. Hand hygiene practices and other processes (e.g., standardizing central line dressings) are used to reduce infections. The Joint Commission has National Patient Safety Goals (NPSGs) that healthcare facilities must meet for accreditation. The 2011 NPSGs focus on the correct identification of patients, improved staff communication, safe medication administration, infection control, identification of patients at risk for suicide, and prevention of mistakes in surgery (Joint Commission, 2011).

Clinical Tip

Parents need to be actively engaged as a member of the child's healthcare team and know it is important to keep their child safe in the hospital or other healthcare setting. Parents should be encouraged to ask questions, challenge decisions they do not agree with or understand, and speak up until they are satisfied that they understand or agree with the outcome (Sandlin-Leming, 2010).

Children are at a higher risk for medical errors than other patients. They also may be more vulnerable to harm from errors made because of their immature physiology, which may affect their ability to metabolize and excrete medications (Gonzales, 2010). Many

Weblink | American Nurses Association

Evidence-Based Practice | Medication Errors and Institutional Culture

PROBLEM

Medication errors are a serious problem in pediatric nursing because children are at higher risk for severe adverse effects. Dosages are calculated by the weight of the child, and an error in decimal placement results in a potential serious overdose or underdose.

A systems approach to medication errors encourages nurses and other healthcare providers to report their mistakes without pointing fingers so that the system can be improved. Nurses need to be accountable when they make a mistake, but how can nurses be encouraged to report errors? Is the hospital culture part of the answer?

EVIDENCE

A study, involving 279 nursing units in 146 U.S. acute care hospitals, investigated the antecedents of severe and nonsevere medication errors over a 6-month period. Medical errors were defined as the wrong dose, wrong patient, wrong time, wrong drug, wrong route, or omission. Severe errors were defined as those needing increased nursing observation or technical monitoring, laboratory or radiologic testing, medical intervention, or transfer to another unit. Nonsevere errors did not need increased attention or interventions. Antecedents investigated included work dynamics, percentage of RNs among nursing staff, communication with physicians, nursing expertise, education level, experience, medication-related support services, and patient characteristics. Study findings revealed that as the percentage of nurses with a bachelor's degree (BSN) increased, severe medication errors decreased; nursing units with more experienced nurses reported more nonsevere medication errors; and medication-support services were positively related to nonsevere errors. Results indicate that severe and nonsevere medication errors might have different antecedents, and thus different approaches may be needed to prevent or reduce severe and nonsevere medication errors (Chang & Mark, 2009).

A systematic review was conducted of 12 studies evaluating the implementation of computerized physician order entry with a focus on adult and pediatric/neonatal critical care settings. Although the use of this system did reduce medication prescription errors, the benefits of this system in preventing potential and actual adverse drug events and mortality were not consistently found (van Rosse, Maat, Rademaker, et al., 2009).

Anonymous adverse event recording in a large children's hospital was used to evaluate medication errors and to identify strategies to prevent medication errors; however, it was believed that events were underreported. Initially RNs were surveyed to identify situations in which they would report a safety event or near miss (an error intercepted before it reached the patient) and reasons why reports were not filed. Reasons for not reporting events included not enough time and not being aware of a need to report events that did not cause harm or near misses. Education was provided to help nurses recognize events to report and tips to decrease the time needed to report events. Trends in reported data were provided to help nurses see the value of reporting (e.g., incorrect intravenous fluid use was a common problem, and better storage supply bin labeling and separation of similarly named fluids helped address this problem). Efforts resulted in an increased reporting of events, and events reported decreased the severity of consequences. While improvement in event reporting occurred, nurses still reported inadequate time to submit reports (Hession-Laband & Mantell, 2011).

IMPLICATIONS

Medication errors resulting from multiple dosage calculations associated with different dosage forms (different concentrations) or decimal placement can lead to potential overdose or underdose, and may cause serious adverse effects. Special system approaches are needed to prevent pediatric medication error, especially when nurses are in settings where children are not the only patient population, such as family practice settings and emergency departments. Increased reporting by nurses, physicians, and pharmacists would help identify the extent of medication errors along with important system information that could be used to identify prevention strategies. Studies on the culture of healthcare institutions that successfully encourage reporting of medication errors and near misses are needed. Nurses need to learn about the system problems contributing to medication error, so they can help identify solutions to reduce the risk for error.

CRITICAL THINKING APPLICATION

Identify the medication error reporting guidelines and strategies used to reduce medical errors in your clinical healthcare setting. What medication safety practices have resulted from a review of error reports? Identify any potential strategies to improve medication safety in these settings.

---

between the health professional and the family member, such as failure to obtain information about a drug allergy, may lead to serious adverse effects. See Chapters 3 and 6 🔗 . When using a hospital interpreter, it is essential to communicate instructions on dose, route, frequency, and duration of medications to reduce the chance of medical error. See Evidence-Based Practice: Medication Errors and Institutional Culture.

Risk Management

Healthcare institutions make every effort to promote optimal patient care and reduce liability by various activities. **Risk management** is a process established by a healthcare institution to identify, evaluate, and reduce the risk of injury to patients, staff, and visitors, and thus reduce the institution's liability. This involves studying the causes of unintentional injury (e.g., infection, medical errors, patient falls, technology failure, and poor communication) within a healthcare institution and implementing system changes to prevent future errors. See Box 1–7 for strategies to reduce medication errors. Policy and procedure manuals should be current and provide guidance on patient care and the use of technology specifically related to potentially serious situations.

Quality improvement is the continuous study and improvement of the processes and outcomes of providing healthcare services

---

| BOX 1–7 | Strategies to Reduce Pediatric Medication Error |

- Do not rely on memory; verify medication dosages and their calculations.
- Medications with a sound-alike medication should be reviewed to make sure the correct medication has been prescribed for the patient's condition.
- Every prescription should include the child's weight and age as well as the calculated dose and mg/kg dose. The dosage form (vial, tablet, or ampule) should not be used on the prescription, as medication preparations and concentrations may vary by pharmaceutical company.
- Handwritten prescription information should be written in legible printed letters to prevent confusion with other drugs having similar names.
- Abbreviations for medications and frequency of administration should not be used.
- The administration rate for all intravenous (IV) medications should be specified.
- A zero should not be used after a whole number (e.g., 5.0 could be misread as 50 which can potentially result in a 10-fold dosage increase).
- A computerized physician order system with clinical decision support can reduce errors from poor handwriting and check for potential drug interactions and allergies.
- Bar coding for medications and timers and alarms should be used to remind nurses to administer medications.
- Unit dose dispensing systems should be used.
- Nurses should have time protected from interruption for medication preparation and administration.

BOX 1–8

Baccalaureate Essential II: Basic Organizational and Systems Leadership for Quality Care and Patient Safety

Knowledge and skills in leadership, quality improvement, and patient safety are necessary to provide high-quality health care.

A recent study of interruptions that pediatric nurses experience in daily care of patients and the related systems issues was conducted to identify potential negative consequences. Findings revealed that 33% of interruptions occurred when nurses were engaged in patient care or procedures, 25% occurred during documentation, and 9.3% occurred while preparing or administering medications. Interruptions reduce focus and concentration related to the work being performed and sometimes result in an increased risk for error (Hall, Pedersen, Hubley, et al., 2010). Nurses should be involved in analyzing interruptions and identifying solutions that could increase the time available for patient assessment and communication with family members.

to meet the needs of patients, by examining the systems and processes of how care and services are delivered (Box 1–8). Nurses caring for children participate in the development of institutional policies and standards of pediatric nursing practice. Hospitals and home health agencies encourage the development of diagnosis-specific nursing care plans or interprofessional clinical practice guidelines that serve as minimal institutional standards of care.

The facility's healthcare quality committee identifies indicators of effective care by pediatric nurses and other providers during the development of institutional standards of care. These indicators may measure either the process of care, the institution's systems, or the expected outcome of care for a specific patient condition. Patient records are regularly reviewed by risk management nurses to identify deviations from the institutional standards or clinical practice guidelines. When deviations from expected processes and outcomes are identified, the facility explores opportunities to improve the system or processes of care provision with all care providers. Recommendations for the revision of institutional standards to further improve care by pediatric nurses and other health providers in the institution often result.

Documentation of nursing care is an essential part of risk management and quality assurance. The patient's record is a legal document that is admissible evidence in court. If a patient record is subpoenaed, documented care is considered the only care provided, regardless of the quality of undocumented care. Nurses must also report any untoward incidents that could inhibit the patient's recovery.

Practice Alert

Information in the patient's record must be legibly written in objective terms or appropriately recorded in the computerized medical record. Nurses must accurately and sequentially document the patient assessment, the nursing care plan, and the child's responses to medical therapies and nursing care, including the regularly scheduled evaluation of the patient's progress toward nursing goals. When recording a patient's response to therapy, the nurse must include physiologic responses and exact quotes. The date, time, and nurse's signature and title are required.

Legal and Ethical Issues in Pediatric Care

Numerous legal and ethical dilemmas develop when caring for children. Examples include informed consent, the child's participation in healthcare decisions, the child's rights versus the parents' rights, confidentiality, withholding or withdrawing medical treatment, genetic testing, and organ transplantation issues.

Legal and Ethical Considerations
Informed Consent

Information that must be provided to obtain informed consent includes an explanation of the condition, a detailed description of the treatment (such as surgical procedures, blood products, sedation, anesthesia, and certain diagnostic procedures), possible benefits and significant risks associated with the proposed treatments, possible alternative treatments, answers to questions, and notification of a parent's or guardian's right to refuse treatment on behalf of the child.

Informed Consent

Informed consent is a formal preauthorization by the child's parent or guardian for an invasive procedure or participation in research. See Legal and Ethical Considerations: Informed Consent. Informed consent was originally a principle to ensure the disclosure of information, but now informed consent also focuses on the comprehension by the patient or parents of the disclosed information. Informed consent also allows persons to disagree with treatment. The physician is legally responsible for obtaining informed consent. In the case of research, the investigative researcher may formally designate a person to obtain informed consent. The nurse's role is to verify that informed consent has been obtained prior to any procedure or research participation, alert physicians to the need for informed consent, serve as a witness for informed consent, and respond to questions asked by parents and children.

Consent must be given voluntarily and prior to the procedure or research. Because children are not considered competent to make informed healthcare decisions, parents, as the legal custodians of minor children, are customarily requested to give informed consent on behalf of a child. Both children and parents must understand that they have the right to refuse treatment at any time. In an emergency, the doctrine of implied consent provides exception to informed consent. Initial medical examination and treatment of the child's condition needed to preserve life or prevent permanent disability or harm can be performed while attempting to locate a parent and obtain informed consent (American Academy of Pediatrics, 2011a).

When parents are divorced, some states limit the parental rights to give informed consent to the parent with custody. When parents have joint custody, in most cases either may give consent. Many children live in homes with a parent and other adult (stepparent, cohabiting unmarried adult, or grandparent) who does not have legal authority to sign consent. In such cases, the child should have a medical screening examination to ensure that an emergency condition does not exist. Non-urgent treatment should not be provided until the parent or guardian with legal authority can be reached (even if by telephone) (American Academy of Pediatrics, 2011a). Obtain information about your state law regarding custody and who can provide informed consent for healthcare procedures and treatments. Obtain legal advice from the agency's designated legal experts for complex family issues related to guardianship, divorced parents who disagree about the child's treatment, or a caregiver who is not the legal guardian.

Research issues Children are vulnerable subjects who cannot provide truly informed consent and as such require additional protections. Risk needs to be minimized as much as possible while maintaining the child's confidentiality and a sound research design. Harm

BOX 1–9	Growth & Development

By 7 to 8 years of age, a child is able to understand concrete explanations about assent for research participation. By age 11 years, a child's abstract reasoning and logic are advanced. By age 14 years, an adolescent can usually weigh options and make decisions regarding consent as capably as an adult.

must be considered from the perspective of the child (such as pain, anxiety, or distress related to procedures, or any physical or psychologic harm) and minimized as much as possible (National Association of Pediatric Nurse Practitioners, 2010).

Assent is the voluntary agreement to participate in a research project or to choose not to participate (dissent). Without the opportunity to dissent, seeking assent is meaningless. Assent requires children to have a basic understanding of cause and effect, some ability to weigh risks, and recognition of benefits of participation. See Box 1–9. With regard to participation in research, federal guidelines state that children 7 years of age and older must receive information about a research project with developmentally appropriate methods and with terms that are appropriate to the child's comprehension. Children should be given adequate time to ask questions and be told that they have the right to refuse to participate in the study. The child is then asked if he or she wishes to participate. If the child assents, parents then provide signed permission for the child to participate in the research project.

Child Participation in Healthcare Decisions

Children are considered to have the cognitive capacity to make medical decisions when they can understand that a decision must be made, they are able to receive and process information about the decision to be made, they are able to state an opinion using the presented information, and they recognize the consequences of the decision (Van Norman, 2008; Sinclair, 2009). Children under 18 or 21 years of age (the age of majority), depending on state law, are considered minors, and consent from the parent or guardian is required to perform a medical or surgical procedure or treatment. Each state has a minor consent statute, but they vary in which situations or conditions a mature minor may give consent independently. In some states minors can legally give informed consent in the following circumstances (American Academy of Pediatrics, 2011a):

- The minor is a parent or pregnant.
- The adolescent is a legally **emancipated minor** (self-supporting adolescent under 18 years of age not living at home, married, or on active duty in the military, or granted emancipation by the court). In some cases, the minor must convince a judge that he or she is mature enough to make an independent judgment about consent for treatment.
- **Mature minors** (adolescents between 14 and 18 years able to understand treatment risks) may give independent consent to receive or refuse treatment for some limited conditions such as testing and treatment for sexually transmitted infections, family planning, drug and alcohol abuse, blood donation, and mental health care (American Academy of Pediatrics, 2008).

Learn about the facility's policies and procedures on the rights of minors in the informed consent process.

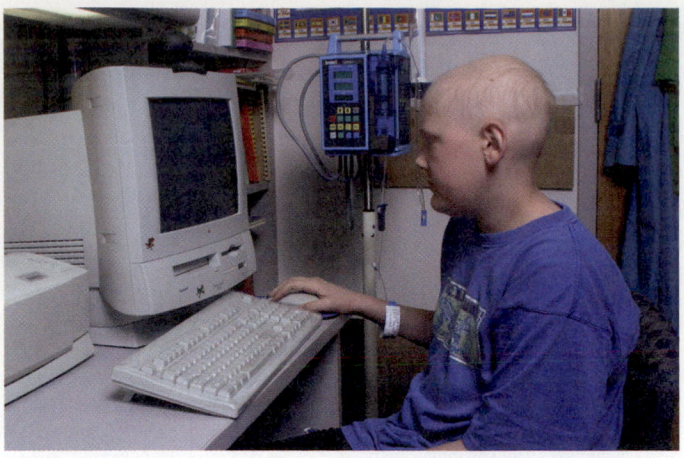

FIGURE 1–14 ■ Marvin, a 15-year-old boy with acute myelocytic leukemia, has come out of his second remission with an acute onset of fever, joint pain, and petechiae. A bone marrow transplant is one of the few remaining therapeutic options. Although Marvin has agreed to a transplant if a suitable donor is found, he does not want to be resuscitated and placed on life support equipment should he have a cardiac arrest. He has talked extensively with the hospital chaplain and social worker and feels comfortable with his decision. His parents want an all-out effort to sustain his life until a donor is located. At what age can children make an informed decision about whether to accept or refuse treatment? What happens when the parents and children have conflicting opinions about treatment? How are ethical decisions made?

Children should become more actively involved in decision making about treatment procedures as their reasoning skills develop. Each child's developmental level needs to be evaluated individually to determine how extensive a role he or she should have in the decision-making process. Assuming a larger role in the decision-making process with increasing age helps the child develop into a self-determining person. Adolescents are increasingly able to use abstract thought processes, reason, consider possible outcomes and consequences, and evaluate facts from different perspectives—the adult way of thinking (Sinclair, 2009). Research is needed to develop valid and reliable tools to assist health professionals in identifying those children with more advanced problem-solving skills who should have a larger role in making decisions about their own care.

Child's Rights Versus Parents' Rights

As adolescents develop more mature thinking skills, their opinions about consenting for medical or surgical procedures for serious health conditions may conflict with their parents (Figure 1–14 ■). Parents have the legal authority to make choices about their child's health care except in the following cases:

- When the parents' choice of treatment does not permit lifesaving treatment for the child (see Developing Cultural Competence: Religion and Blood Products for information about religious beliefs and emergency treatment)
- When there is a potential conflict of interest between the child and parents, such as with suspected child abuse or neglect

If adolescents and parents or guardians disagree about a major treatment intervention (e.g., bone marrow transplant, heart transplant), adolescents must convince their parents to refuse treatment on their behalf, seek designation as an emancipated minor, or back down and agree to treatment (Sinclair, 2009). Healthcare providers may try to use negotiation and compromise as a first step to help the adolescent and parents reach agreement about interventions

Developing Cultural Competence
Religion and Blood Products

Jehovah's Witnesses oppose blood transfusions for themselves and their children because they believe transfusions are equivalent to the oral intake of blood, which is morally and spiritually wrong according to their interpretation of the Bible (Leviticus 17:13–14). A Jehovah's Witness who receives a transfusion believes he or she has committed a sin and may have forfeited everlasting life. Transfusions of any blood products, including plasma and the patient's own blood, are forbidden. Most healthcare institutions have developed policies to address the care of these children when blood products are needed. Every effort is made to avoid the use of blood products with alternative therapies, except when a blood product will be lifesaving. Then, the child may need to be placed in protective custody, and healthcare providers are authorized to provide lifesaving treatment by the state's child protective service agency (American Academy of Pediatrics, 2011a).

so that the adolescent's voice and opinion are considered. Medical consultation may be sought to identify other treatment options that might be acceptable to both the adolescent and parents. The facility's ethics committee (often composed of health professionals, clergy, consumer representatives, and an ethics expert) usually becomes involved to help resolve the issue. In some cases, the adolescent may feel the only recourse is to seek emancipated minor status.

Confidentiality

The Health Insurance Portability and Accountability Act (HIPAA), Public Law 104-191, enacted by Congress in 1996, requires the confidential management of patient medical record data. One goal of the law is to protect the **privacy** (the ability of an individual to maintain information in a protected manner) of citizens by establishing standards for management of confidential medical information. Healthcare organizations have developed policies to prevent the inappropriate disclosure of protected health information. Patients have the right to determine who can have access to their health information. Violating confidentiality guidelines puts the nurse at risk for liability and legal action (U.S. Department of Health and Human Services, 2009).

Confidentiality is an agreement between a patient and a provider that information discussed during the healthcare encounter will not be shared without the permission of the patient. Adolescents' concerns about confidentiality influence if and when they seek health care because they do not want their parents informed about sensitive health conditions (Shapiro, 2010). State laws vary, and if the state law does not require the consent of the parent for the adolescent's condition, the consenting minor controls the healthcare decisions as well as the parent's access to the health information related to that care. However, the issue of minors giving consent is complicated by the healthcare system that holds the parents responsible for the financial costs of the healthcare services sought in confidence. Parents may learn about the adolescent's healthcare visit if the health insurer sends a statement of fees paid or owed. See Partnering with Families: Adolescents and Confidentiality.

Breaching confidentiality is a potential problem for adolescents, who are just learning whom they can trust in the healthcare system. Make sure you openly discuss the limits of confidentiality for topics, such as mandatory reporting requirements, with the patient and family. Inadvertent disclosure of personal information may lead to psychologic, social, or physical harm in some patients.

Practice Alert

If the adolescent has a reportable disease, such as a sexually transmitted infection, confidentiality may create a public health hazard. In such cases, the healthcare professional is obligated to report the disease to the appropriate state or county agency. Suspected cases of child abuse must be reported to the appropriate agency specified by state law.

Patient Self-Determination Act

The federal Patient Self-Determination Act directs healthcare institutions to inform hospitalized patients about their rights, which include expressing a preference for treatment options and making **advance directives** (writing a living will or authorizing a durable power of attorney for healthcare decisions on the patient's behalf). Nurses often discuss these issues with patients and their families. Minor children and their parents should also be informed of their rights. An adolescent with a serious or life-limiting condition, such as the child in Figure 1–14, has a strong and legitimate interest in expressing an opinion about aggressive therapy. The adolescent and parents should be encouraged to talk and reach a joint therapy decision. If the parents and adolescent are unable to agree, the legal issues

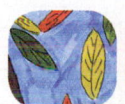

Partnering with Families

Adolescents and Confidentiality

Adolescents need a safe and confidential environment to discuss healthcare issues so that they seek health care when needed. Ways to promote confidentiality include the following actions:

- Ensure that adolescents and parents talk separately to the healthcare provider about their concerns.
- Ensure privacy when collecting an adolescent's medical history or discussing sensitive issues. Create a comfortable atmosphere and environment for adolescents to discuss private concerns regarding their health.
- Display and offer educational materials on confidentiality to adolescents and parents.

- Explain how confidentiality is protected between the healthcare professional and the adolescent, as well as his or her parents, at the beginning of the healthcare visit. Discuss situations in which there are limits to the confidentiality that can be provided.
- Obtain a phone number or other contact information to enable the health professional to contact the adolescent.
- Make sure clinic literature is small enough to fit discreetly into a purse or wallet.

become complex, as described in the Child's Rights Versus Parents' Rights section on page 20. Adolescent decisions to forgo life-prolonging treatment have been upheld in some courts of law (American Academy of Pediatrics, 2008).

Do-not-attempt-resuscitation (or allow natural death) orders have become more common for children with terminal illnesses in which no further aggressive treatments are available or desired. In many cases, these children are cared for at home or in a hospice program, but some still attend school. Implementation of do-not-attempt-resuscitation orders for such children then becomes a community issue to ensure that no resuscitation measures are initiated by any emergency care provider when the child has a life-threatening event. State health policies must be developed so children with these signed orders are easily identified and appropriate documentation of the orders is on file. See Chapter 18 ⊘ for issues related to end-of-life care.

Ethical Concepts and Issues

Ethics is the philosophic study of morality, and the analysis of moral problems and moral judgments. It is an inquiry into the justification of particular actions. Major advances in medical technology, such as the ability to save the lives of newborns with severe impairments, the ability to extend the lives of children who are chronically ill or seriously injured, genetic testing, and gene therapy, have led to challenges for healthcare professionals and parents to make the best decision for the child's condition. For example, dying used to be a natural process, but dying in the pediatric intensive care unit may be managed for severely ill children by limiting or withdrawing life-sustaining treatment (Kodish & Weise, 2011). Healthcare professionals have a moral obligation to deliver care with compassion and respect for the worth and uniqueness of each individual; they must understand and respect religious and cultural differences that affect parental decisions about requesting or refusing a treatment.

Ethical issues may arise from a **moral dilemma,** a conflict involving individual beliefs, social values, and ethical principles. Problems may develop because physicians, nurses, and parents have differing opinions about treatments for an infant or child with a serious or terminal condition. Each side of the conflict may support different courses of action (e.g., performing or refraining from performing a therapy). Emotions play a significant role in the development of ethical dilemmas. Parents want to protect the child, and they have their vision of what is good for the child. Healthcare professionals have different values than families because of their culture and life experiences. Value differences may also exist between members of the healthcare team caring for the child. Regardless, all health professionals want the child to benefit from the care provided.

An ethical theory or framework for decision making is often used in healthcare institutions to guide family members and healthcare professionals to determine an appropriate action. Theories focus on different outcomes, such as the consequences of the decision, the greatest good, the avoidance of suffering, or utilitarianism (a comparison of consequences or burdens with the benefits resulting from the action). The four general ethical principles used in the development of a decision-making framework include (Twomey, 2011):

- **Beneficence**—a care provider's obligation to act or to make a decision that benefits the patient, promoting the child's and family's well-being

- Respect for the patient's **autonomy**—right for self-determination or decision making, to protect the informed choices (consent and refusal) of patients capable of decision making
- **Nonmaleficence**—to reduce the risk for harm, and to use interventions with the most beneficial risk-benefit ratio
- **Justice**—to treat all patients with fairness and respect, and to use scarce resources wisely to avoid waste in ineffective treatments

Nurses face many ethical dilemmas when providing pediatric care. They witness parents struggling to decide among treatment options. Pediatric nurses have a responsibility to become knowledgeable about the moral and legal rights of their patients and families and to protect and support those rights. Professional integrity with regard to telling the truth and keeping promises is also important. To avoid conflicts in medical decision making for a child's care, the physicians, nurses, parents, and the adolescent (or child when appropriate) should jointly discuss all relevant information, consider the risks and benefits of all treatment options, and reach a shared decision (Cummings & Mercurio, 2010).

Work with parents to form a therapeutic alliance and attempt to prevent conflicts when the family's values and the health professionals' values do not match. Make sure that families understand the uncertainty regarding their child's condition without giving a perception that a decision has been made, and find out what is important to them in the care of their child. They may be able to describe what they wish to avoid having happen to their child, and this may be a starting point for discussion and negotiation about their child's care.

Healthcare institutions have ethics committees to resolve conflicts about treatment decisions. Ethics committees may employ the following functions (Kodish & Weise, 2011):

- Perform individual case consultations to resolve a conflict between health professionals and the child and family
- Resolve a dispute between health professionals about the care to provide to a child
- Create and review healthcare facility policies on ethical issues such as genetic testing, do-not-attempt-resuscitation orders, or withdrawing life-sustaining therapies
- Educate health professionals, patients, and families about ethical issues in health care

Withholding or Withdrawing Medical Treatment

Due to technologic advances that sustain life, parents must sometimes face difficult decisions, such as when an infant or child has a life-limiting condition or serious disability. See Figure 1–15 ■. Decisions are made with regard to what is in the best interest of the child, using analysis of the expected burdens and benefits of an intervention. In some cases, the benefits, risks, and burdens to the family are considered.

How do federal regulations for care of infants with severe defects affect current healthcare practice? The Child Abuse and Treatment Act of 1984, also known as the Baby Doe regulations, defines withholding of medically indicated treatment as child abuse, except when care is futile (Curtin, 2008). This act was enacted to protect the rights of infants with severe defects. **Futility** is a situation in which treatments do not provide a clear clinical benefit. Physicians are not obligated to offer interventions that cause extreme pain and suffering

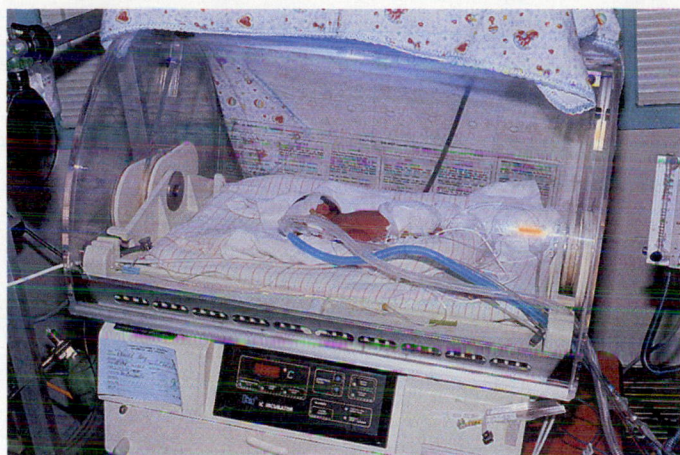

FIGURE 1–15 ■ Infant John, at 5 days of age, has a birth weight of 1200 g, acute respiratory distress, and a severe intraventricular hemorrhage. His physicians are seeking his parents' consent for surgical placement of a ventriculoperitoneal shunt. Regardless of intensive medical care and planned surgical intervention, the infant is expected to have a severe disability. The infant's condition is critical, and it is not certain how well he will respond to surgery. The parents, after much consideration and discussions with their family and pastor, have requested that comfort measures only be provided. They want life-sustaining treatment to be withheld, because they believe the additional procedures will cause excessive suffering for the infant, especially when the outcome is uncertain. How do federal regulations protecting newborns with severe disabilities affect current healthcare practice? How is the best interest of this infant with a severe disability determined?

Source: *Courtesy of Carol Harrigan, RNC, MSN, NNP.*

BOX 1–10	Steps in Ethical Problem Solving

- Recognize that a potential or actual ethical dilemma exists.
- Collect as much information as possible:
  - About the medical facts and the physician's goals
  - About the child's and family's wishes or preferences
  - About your values and beliefs
- Identify if surrogate decision makers exist (e.g., a court-appointed guardian).
- State the dilemma as clearly as possible.
- Seek consultation on all possible courses of action or inaction.
- Identify the strengths and weaknesses of each therapeutic action.
- Identify the realistic expectations, benefits, and burdens of each potential therapeutic action or inaction.
- Set goals and establish a decision-making process, and implement a plan of action.
- Evaluate the results.

---

when there is no or little benefit. Treatments that only prolong life without improving quality of life are often considered to represent a misuse of expensive healthcare resources.

Parents are the recognized decision makers for infants and they are entitled to full information about the risks and benefits of a procedure or treatment, as well as the child's long-term prognosis. Factors important to parents in making their decision include clear information on the seriousness of the child's condition and prognosis, the child's potential quality of life, degree of pain and suffering, a trusting relationship with the physician, and physician recommendations (Kendall & Guo, 2008; Racine & Shevell, 2009). Often the parents have time to consult with family members and faith leaders, and seek second or third opinions before making a decision (Diekema, Botkin, & Committee on Bioethics, 2009). Conflict sometimes arises when parents choose to withhold therapy or request aggressive therapy on behalf of their child and the healthcare provider recommendations differ.

To address such a case, an ethics consultation may be requested by healthcare providers or by the family. A common question brought before ethics committees is whether to withhold or withdraw life-sustaining treatment. The ethics committee often recommends treatment decisions using the process of data collection and evaluation outlined in Box 1–10. In some cases, a compromise is reached that does not totally satisfy the parents or the healthcare providers. Courts should make ethical decisions only when healthcare professionals and parents are unable to agree about providing or withholding treatment.

Genetic Testing of Children

With advances in genetics research, it is now possible to conduct genetic testing and screen infants for the presence of disease carrier status. It is also possible to conduct presymptomatic detection of a specific condition, such as Huntington disease or Duchenne muscular dystrophy. In some cases, testing can be performed to determine a child's predisposition to develop a condition, such as breast cancer or colon cancer (Twomey, Bove, & Cassidy, 2008). Genetic screening of newborns, such as for inborn errors of metabolism, cystic fibrosis, sickle cell disease, and other conditions, routinely occurs. In this case, the early identification of the genetic condition will have a clear benefit to the child, a system is in place to confirm the diagnosis, and treatment and follow-up are available to affected newborns. See Chapter 4 🔗 for more information about ethical issues regarding genetic testing. See Chapter 32 🔗 for more information on newborn screening.

Organ Transplantation Issues

In 2010, 1,827 children less than 18 years of age received an organ transplant. In 2011, approximately 1,933 children less than 18 years of age were on the list waiting for a transplant. Children between 11 and 17 years of age account for nearly 45% of all children waiting for a transplant (Health Resources and Services Administration, 2011). The death of a child can benefit another child through organ transplantation, and organ transplantation has become an accepted therapeutic option for some life-threatening conditions.

The limited supply of organs has created numerous ethical issues. See Legal and Ethical Considerations: The Children's Health Act. Which patients on the waiting list should receive the organs available? Should a patient with multiple congenital anomalies or abnormal chromosomes be eligible for a transplant? Should families be permitted to pay donor families for organs? Should the family's ability to pay for an organ transplant give a child higher priority for an organ? Should a patient receive a second organ transplant, replacing an organ deteriorating because of rejection? Should parents conceive another child hoping that the new baby is a potential stem cell donor for a child with an illness? If so, what pressures does this knowledge place on each child as they grow older? Each institution performing organ transplants develops guidelines for ethical decision making regarding these questions. See Chapter 27 🔗 for more information on organ transplants.

Legal and Ethical Considerations
The Children's Health Act

The Children's Health Act, Public Law §106-310 passed in 2000, directed the development of specific criteria, policies, and procedures to address the specific needs of children regarding priorities for organ allocation. Guidelines for the allocation of hearts, lungs, livers, and kidneys for children have been developed that give preference to children based on factors in addition to time on the waiting list (American Academy of Pediatrics, 2010).

PARTNERING WITH CHILDREN AND THEIR FAMILIES

As illustrated throughout this chapter, partnering with parents and children is the foundation for our interactions with families for all pediatric nursing care. Developing relationships is challenging, exciting, and ultimately gratifying for nurses who choose to specialize in pediatrics. Partnering is essential every step of the way:

- Obtaining informed consent and assent
- Respecting that the parent is the expert with regard to the child's care
- Acknowledging and supporting cultural values in the provision of care
- Preparing parents to assume ongoing complex healthcare responsibilities for their child

Use the information in Partnering with Families boxes provided in other chapters to enhance your relationships with families and to provide appropriate care in a supportive environment that promotes the family unit and the child's development.

Chapter Highlights

- Roles of nurses in caring for children include providing direct care (health promotion, health maintenance, and nursing care for health conditions), patient education, patient advocacy, and case management, and minimizing the psychologic and physical distress experienced by children and their families.
- Nurses care for children in many different settings: various units within the hospital and outpatient clinics, schools, childcare centers, physician offices, community health centers, rehabilitation centers, and the home.
- Family-centered care is a method designed to meet the emotional, social, and developmental needs of children and families needing health care.
- Nurses must identify culturally relevant facts about their patients to provide appropriate and competent care to an increasingly diverse population.
- Unintentional injury is the leading cause of death for children between 1 and 19 years of age.
- Efforts to increase the number of low-income children with access to health care include expansion of the Children's Health Insurance Program (CHIP) nationwide.
- Documentation of nursing care is essential for risk management and quality improvement. Documentation must include the patient assessment, the nursing care plan, the child's responses to medical therapies and nursing care, and regular evaluation of the child's progress toward nursing goals.

- Informed consent is the formal preauthorization for an invasive procedure or participation in research. Parents typically give informed consent for children under 18 years of age unless the child is an emancipated minor, a self-supporting adolescent not subject to parental control.
- Children need to become more actively involved in decisions about their care as their decision-making abilities develop. Even though they cannot provide informed consent, federal guidelines mandate that children as young as 7 years of age receive information about treatment procedures and research project participation and give their assent.
- Because adolescents fear disclosure of confidential information, they may avoid seeking health care. When adolescents have a reportable disease, it is important to inform them that confidentiality cannot be maintained, as a report must be made to a public health agency.
- Adolescents at a higher risk of death due to a life-limiting or chronic condition should be encouraged to talk with their parents and jointly prepare advance directives.
- Federal regulations require a formalized ethical decision-making process to assist healthcare providers and families in making important decisions about withholding, withdrawing, or limiting a child's therapy.

Clinical Reasoning in Action

INTRODUCTION

Return to the scenario about Drew at the beginning of the chapter. Despite his seizure disorder Drew has been developing normally, meeting expected developmental milestones as evaluated by the Denver II (see Chapter 10 🔗).

DESCRIPTION

The pediatric nurse has worked closely with the family to ensure that all of Drew's healthcare needs are addressed during health promotion and health maintenance visits. Prior to the most recent seizure, the nurse had been helping the parents to ensure that all healthcare requirements were met for Drew to attend a new childcare center. The pediatric nurse will now modify the nursing care plan to integrate the needed diagnostic procedures and treatment for Drew's seizure disorder and to help the parents manage their increased concerns about his seizure disorder.

DISCUSSION

1. Identify all the roles of Drew's nurse in working with this child and his family. What other roles could nurses have within this healthcare center and in other settings to support the nursing care provided to Drew and his family? Consider the roles of a nurse manager in the healthcare setting, a nurse consultant to the childcare center, and a nurse in the emergency department.

2. Informed consent is needed before diagnostic procedures are performed and prior to releasing healthcare information. What is the process for obtaining informed consent in your healthcare setting? What is the nurse's role in the process? What needs to happen before health information is released to the childcare center? How does this healthcare facility ensure compliance with HIPAA?

3. The healthcare setting where Drew receives care has an evidence-based clinical practice guideline for the management of children with seizures. Identify a clinical practice guideline that has been developed for a pediatric healthcare condition in your healthcare setting. How is the clinical practice guideline used and how does this process differ from implementation of a nursing care plan?

4. Describe the nursing interventions to be added to Drew's modified nursing care plan for diagnostic procedures, treatment, and family concerns.

NCLEX-RN® Review

1. A new registered nurse (RN) is preparing to care for a group of pediatric patients. The nurse is unable to participate in which of the following activities?
   1. Patient advocacy
   2. Family education
   3. Case management
   4. Prescription of medication

2. In which situations are children at risk of injury? Choose all that apply.
   1. An infant is crawling on the floor while older children are playing nearby.
   2. An adolescent is learning how to become a safe baby-sitter.
   3. A toddler is playing on the playground while at preschool.
   4. A school-age child likes to imitate her older sibling's movements while on her bike.
   5. An adolescent is attending a gathering of school friends after a dance.

3. In planning an educational session for parents of toddlers concentrating on primary prevention, which indicates the most appropriate topic on which the nurse should concentrate?
   1. Unintentional injury prevention
   2. Seizure management
   3. Child abuse prevention
   4. Sudden infant death prevention

4. A child and his grandfather arrive in the emergency department after a car collision. The grandfather does not have custody of the child. What should be the nurse's next action?
   1. Obtain the custodial parent's telephone number for permission.
   2. Provide emergency care to both under implied consent.
   3. Register and provide care to the grandfather but transfer the child.
   4. Ensure permission to treat is obtained prior to registering them.

See Appendix I ⊘ for answers.

References

American Academy of Pediatrics, Levetown, M., & Committee on Bioethics. (2008). Communicating with children and families: From everyday interactions to skill in conveying distressing information. *Pediatrics, 121*(5), 21441–21442.

American Academy of Pediatrics, Committee on Hospital Care, Section on Surgery, & Section on Critical Care. (2010). Policy statement—Pediatric organ donation and transplantation. *Pediatrics, 125*(4), 822–828.

American Academy of Pediatrics, Committee on Pediatric Emergency Medicine, & Committee on Bioethics. (2011a). Policy statement—Consent for emergency medical services for children and adolescents. *Pediatrics, 128*(2), 427–433.

American Academy of Pediatrics, Steering Committee on Quality Improvement and Management, & Committee on Hospital Care. (2011b). Policy statement—Principles of pediatric patient safety: Reducing harm due to medical care. *Pediatrics, 127*(6), 1199–1210.

American Nurses Association, National Association of Pediatric Nurse Practitioners, & Society of Pediatric Nurses. (2008). *Pediatric nursing: Scope and standards of practice*. Silver Spring, MD: Nursesbooks.org.

Berman, P. (2010). Mary Maud Brewster: A closer look at a long-neglected public health pioneer. *American Journal of Nursing, 110*(8), 62–63.

Bindler, R. C., & Ball, J. W. (2007). The Bindler-Ball healthcare model: A new paradigm for health promotion. *Pediatric Nursing, 33*(2), 121–126.

Bloom, B., Cohen, R. A., & Freeman, G. (2011). Summary health statistics for U.S. children: National health interview survey, 2010, Publication No. (PHS)-2012-1578. *Vital and Health Statistics, 10*(250), 1–146.

Campagna, V., & Stanton, M. P. (2010). Case managers can improve hospital resource management. *Nurse Leader, 8*(5), 40–43.

Cassedy, A., Fairbrother, G., & Newacheck, P. (2008). The impact of insurance instability on children's access, utilization, and satisfaction with health care. *Ambulatory Pediatrics, 8*(5), 321–328.

Centers for Medicare and Medicaid Services. (2011). *Early periodic screening diagnosis & treatment*. Retrieved from http://www.medicaid.gov/Medicaid-CHIP-Program-Information/By-Topics/Benefits/Early-Periodic-Screening-Diagnosis-and-Treatment.html

Centers for Medicare and Medicaid Services. (2011a). *2011 poverty level guidelines*. Retrieved from http://www.cms.gov/MedicaidEligibility/downloads/POV11Combo.pdf

Centers for Medicare and Medicaid Services. (2011b). *FY 2010 number of children ever enrolled in year—CHIP by program type*. Retrieved from http://www.medicaid.gov/Medicaid-CHIP-Program-Information/By-Topics/Childrens-Health-Insurance-Program-CHIP/Downloads/CHIPEverEnrolledYearGraph.pdf

Centers for Medicare and Medicaid Services. (2011c). *FY 2010 number of children ever enrolled in year—Medicaid.*

Retrieved from http://www.cms.gov/NationalCHIPPolicy/downloads/FY2010StateXIXTotalTable020111FINAL.pdf

Chang, Y., & Mark, B. A. (2009). Antecedents of severe and nonsevere medication errors. *Journal of Nursing Scholarship, 41*(1), 70–78.

Cochrane Collaboration. (2011). *Cochrane reviews.* Retrieved from http://www.cochrane.org/cochrane-reviews

Colgrove, J. (2007). Foot soldiers against infectious diseases: Nurses, families, and immunization in the twentieth century. *Pediatric Nursing, 33*(5), 449–451.

Cummings, C. L., & Mercurio, M. R. (2010). Autonomy, beneficence, and rights. *Pediatrics in Review, 31*(6), 252–255.

Curtin, L. (2008). The Babies Doe: Finding middle ground. *American Nurse Today, 3*(1), 7–10.

Diekema, D. S., Botkin, J. R., & Committee on Bioethics. (2009). Clinical report—Forgoing medically provided nutrition and hydration in children. *Pediatrics, 124*(2), 813–822.

Fairchild, A. L., Rosner, D., Colgrove, J., Bayer, M., & Fried, L. P. (2010). The exodus of public health: What history can tell us about the future. *American Journal of Public Health, 100*(1), 54–63.

Federal Interagency Forum on Child and Family Statistics. (2011). *America's children: Key indicators of well-being, 2011.* Retrieved from http://www.childstats.gov/americaschildren

Ferguson, L. A., & Pawlak, R. (2011). Health literacy: The road to improved health outcomes. *Journal for Nurse Practitioners, 7*(2), 123–129.

Fox, J. B. (2010). Vital signs: Health insurance coverage and health care utilization—United States, 2006–2009 and January–March 2010. *Morbidity and Mortality Weekly Report, 59* (November 9), 1–7.

Gallagher-Ford, L., Fineout-Overholt, E., Melnyk, B. M., & Stillwell, S. B. (2011). Implementing an evidence-based practice change. *American Journal of Nursing, 111*(3), 54–60.

Golden, J. (2011). Pediatrics, public health, and infant mortality in the early 20th century. *Archives of Pediatrics and Adolescent Medicine, 165*(2), 102–103.

Gonzales, K. (2010). Medication administration errors and the pediatric population: A systematic search of the literature. *Journal of Pediatric Nursing, 25*, 555–565.

Hall, L. M., Pedersen, C., Hubley, P., Ptack, E., Hemingway, A., Watson, C., & Keatings, M. (2010). Interruptions and pediatric patient safety. *Journal of Pediatric Nursing, 25*, 167–175.

Harbaugh, N. (2009). Pay for performance: Quality and value-based reimbursement. *Pediatric Clinics of North America, 56*, 997–1007.

Hawkins, A. O., Kantayya, V. S., & Sharkey-Asner, C. (2010). Health literacy: A potential barrier in caring for underserved populations. *Disease-a-Month, 56*, 734–740.

Hawkins, J. W., & Watson, J. C. (2010). School nursing on the Iron Range in a public health nursing model. *Public Health Nursing, 27*(6), 571–578.

Health Resources and Services Administration, Maternal and Child Health Bureau. (2008). *The national survey of children with special health care needs chart book 2005–2006.* Retrieved from http://mchb.hrsa.gov/cshcn05/

Health Resources and Services Administration, Maternal and Child Health Bureau. (2009). *The National Survey of Children's Health 2007.* Rockville, MD: U.S. Department of Health and Human Services. Retrieved from http://www.mchb.hrsa.gov/nsch/07emohealth/index.html

Health Resources and Services Administration, Maternal and Child Health Bureau. (2010). *About Title V History.* Retrieved from https://perfdata.hrsa.gov/mchb/tvisreports/LearnMore/TitleVHistory.aspx

Health Resources and Services Administration, Organ Procurement and Transplant Network. (2011). *Transplants in the U.S. by recipient age, and current U.S. waiting list by age.* Retrieved from http://www.optn.transplant.hrsa.gov/latestData/rptData.asp

Hession-Laband, E., & Mantell, P. (2011). Lessons learned: Use of event reporting by nurses to improve patient safety and quality. *Journal of Pediatric Nursing, 26*(2), 149–155.

Joint Commission. (2011). *Hospital: 2011 National Patient Safety Goals.* Retrieved from http://www.jointcommission.org/hap_2011_npsgs/

Jones, J. H. (2010). Developing critical thinking in the perioperative environment. *AORN Journal, 91*(2), 248–256.

Kavanagh, P. L., Adams, W. G., & Wang, C. J. (2009). Quality indicators and quality assessment in child health. *Archives of Diseases in Childhood, 94*, 458–463.

Kendall, A., & Guo, W. (2008). Evidence-based neonatal bereavement care. *Newborn & Infant Nursing Reviews, 8*(3), 131–135.

Kochanek, K. D., Xu, J., Murphy, S. L., Miniño, A. M., & Kung, H. (2011). Deaths: Preliminary data for 2009, *National Vital Statistics Reports, 59*(4), 1–51.

Kodish, E., & Weise, K. (2011). Ethics in pediatric care. In R. M. Kliegman, B. F. Stanton, J. W. St. Geme, N. F. Schor, & R. E. Behrman, *Nelson textbook of pediatrics* (19th ed.). Philadelphia: Elsevier Saunders. Retrieved from http://www.expertconsultbook.com

Kogan, M. D., Newacheck, P. W., Blumberg, S. J., Heyman, K. M., Strickland, B. B., Singh, G. K., & Zeni, M. B. (2010). State variation in underinsurance among children with special healthcare needs in the United States. *Pediatrics, 125*(4), 673–680.

Lapkin, S., Levett-Jones, T., Bellchambers, B., & Fernandez, R. (2010). Effectiveness of patient simulation manikins in teaching clinical reasoning skills to undergraduate nursing students: A systematic review. *Clinical Simulation in Nursing, 6*(6), e207–e222.

Leininger, L. J., & Meurer, J. (2011). Access to care for children: Recent progress, remaining challenges. *Pediatric Annals, 40*(3), 161–168.

Mathews, T. J., & MacDorman, M. F. (2011). Infant mortality statistics from the 2007 period linked birth/infant death data set. *National Vital Statistics Reports, 59*(6), 1–47.

McDonald, K. M. (2009). Approach to improving quality: The role of quality measurement and a case study of the Agency for Healthcare Research and Quality pediatric quality indicators. *Pediatric Clinics of North America, 56*, 815–829.

Melnyk, B. M., Fineout-Overholt, E., Stillwell, S. B., & Williamson, K. M. (2009). Igniting a spirit of inquiry: An essential foundation for evidence-based practice. *American Journal of Nursing, 109*(11), 49–52.

Melnyk, B. M., Fineout-Overholt, E., Stillwell, S. B., & Williamson, K. M. (2010). The seven steps of evidence-based practice. *American Journal of Nursing, 110*(1), 51–53.

Miniño, A. M., Murphy, S. M., Xu, J., & Kochanek, K. D. (2011). Deaths: Final data for 2008. *National Vital Statistics Reports, 59*(10), 1–157.

National Association of Pediatric Nurse Practitioners. (2010). NAPNAP position statement on protection of children involved in research studies. *Journal of Pediatric Health Care, 24*(1), 17A–18A.

National Center for Health Statistics & National Vital Statistics System. (2011). *Fatal injury reports, 2008.* Retrieved from http://webapppa.cdc.gov/cgi-bin/broker.exe

Nkoy, F. L., Fassl, B. A., Simon, T. D., Stone, B. L., Srivastava, R., Gesteland, P. H., . . . Maloney, C. G. (2008). Quality of care for children hospitalized with asthma. *Pediatrics, 122*(5), 1055–1063.

Racine, E., & Shevell, M. I. (2009). Ethics in neonatal neurology: When is enough enough? *Pediatric Neurology, 40*(3), 147–155.

Sandlin-Leming, D. (2010). Pediatric patient safety: Educating parents. *Journal of PeriAnesthesia Nursing, 25*(2), 116–118.

Sawin, K. J., Gralton, K. S., Harrison, T. M., Malin, S., Balchunas, M. K., Brock, L. A., . . . Schiffman, R. F. (2010). Nurse researchers in children's hospitals. *Journal of Pediatric Nursing, 25*, 408–417.

Scanlon, M. C., Harris, J. M., Levy, F., & Sedman, A. (2008). Evaluation of the Agency for Healthcare Research and Quality pediatric quality indicators. *Pediatrics, 121*(6), e1723–e1731.

Shapiro, N. A. (2010). Confidentiality and access to adolescent health care services. *Journal of Pediatric Health Care, 24*(2), 133–136.

Simon, T. D., Berry, J., Feudtner, C., Stone, B. L., Sheng, X., Bratton, S. L., . . . Srivastava, R. (2010). Children with complex chronic conditions in inpatient hospital settings in the United States. *Pediatrics, 126*(4), 647–655.

Sinclair, S. J. (2009). Involvement of adolescents in decision making for heart transplants. *Maternal and Child Nursing, 34*(5), 276–281.

Smith-Campbell, B., & Pile, D. (2010). Children's Health Insurance Program and pediatric nurses. *Journal of Pediatric Nursing, 25*, 138–141.

Theerman, P. (2010). Julia Lathrop and the Children's Bureau. *American Journal of Public Health, 100*(9), 1589–1590.

Todres, J. (2010). Children's health in the United States: Assessing the potential impact of the Convention on the Rights of the Child. *Child Welfare, 89*(5), 37–56.

Twomey, J. (2011). Ethical, legal, psychosocial, and cultural implications of genomics for oncology nurses. *Seminars in Oncology Nursing, 27*(1), 54–63.

Twomey, J. G., Bove, C., & Cassidy, D. (2008). Presymptomatic genetic testing in children for neurofibromatosis 2. *Journal of Pediatric Nursing, 23*(3), 183–194.

U.S. Census Bureau. (2011). *Age and sex composition: 2010.* 2010 Census Briefs. Retrieved from http://www.census.gov/prod/cen2010/briefs/c2010br-o3.pdf

U.S. Department of Health and Human Services. (2009). *Health information privacy.* Retrieved from http://www.hhs.gov/ocr/privacy/

U.S. Department of Health and Human Services, National Institutes of Health. (2010). *Cultural competency.* Retrieved from http://www.nih.gov/clearcommunication/culturalcompetency.htm

U.S. Department of Health and Human Services, Health Resources and Services Administration, Maternal and

Child Health Bureau. (2011a). *Child Health USA 2011.* Rockville, MD: Author. Retrieved from www.mchb .hrsa.gov

U.S. Department of Health and Human Services. (2011b). *Healthy People 2020.* Washington, DC: Author. Retrieved from http://www.healthypeople.gov/2020/about/default.aspx

Van Norman, G. A. (2008). Ethical issues in informed consent. *Perioperative Nursing Clinics, 3,* 213–221.

Van Rosse, F., Maat, B., Rademaker, C. M. A., van Vught, A. J., Egberts, A. C. G., & Bollen, C. W. (2009). The effect of computerized physician order entry on medication prescription errors and clinical outcome in pediatric and intensive care: A systematic review. *Pediatrics, 123*(4), 1184–1190.

World Health Organization. (2011). *Child health indicators.* Retrieved from http://apps.who.int/ghodata/?vid=160

Yu, H., Wier, L. M., & Elixhauser, A. (2011). *Hospital stays for children, 2009.* HCUP Statistical Brief No. 118. Rockville, MD: Agency for Healthcare Research and Quality. Retrieved from http://www.hcup-us.ahrq.gov/reports/statbriefs/sb118.pdf

Yu, S. M., Huang, Z. J., & Kogan, M. D. (2008). State-level healthcare access and use among children in U.S. immigrant families. *American Journal of Public Health, 98*(11), 1996–2003.

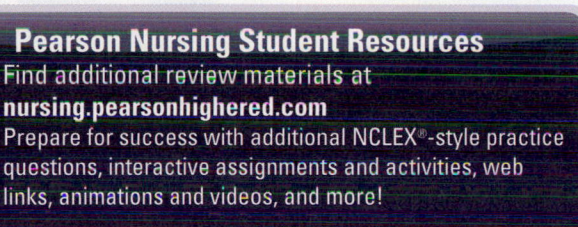

Pearson Nursing Student Resources
Find additional review materials at
nursing.pearsonhighered.com
Prepare for success with additional NCLEX®-style practice questions, interactive assignments and activities, web links, animations and videos, and more!

Family-Centered Care: Theory and Application

 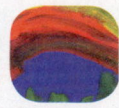 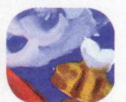

Learning Outcomes

After completing this chapter, you will be able to:

1. Design a nursing care plan for the child and family that integrates key concepts of family-centered care.

2. Compare the characteristics of different types of families.

3. Analyze the impact of each of the four different parenting styles on child personality development.

4. Contrast the categories of family strengths that help families cope with stressors.

5. Explain the effect of major family changes on children, including divorce, gaining a stepparent, being placed in foster care, and adoption.

6. Review various family theories and apply them to the nursing process.

7. Summarize the advantages of using a family assessment tool.

8. Assemble a list of family support services that might be available in a community.

> **"Mom and Dad are so worried about Casey. They were scared he was going to die, and now they wonder if he'll ever be normal again. We've been talking about how to take care of him when he comes home and how we'll all have to help out more around the house."**
>
> —*Casey's sister Teresa, 16 years old*

Casey DeProspero, a 14-year-old, is recuperating from injuries sustained in a motor vehicle crash in which he was the passenger. He was not wearing a seat belt and experienced a brain injury after striking the windshield. His cognitive and motor functions are impaired. Following a 7-day acute care hospital stay, he was moved to the inpatient rehabilitation hospital where he has been for the past 5 days. He is much more responsive to stimuli and to family members 12 days after his injury. Physical therapy is provided twice a day to promote range of motion and muscle tone and to prevent contractures. Plans are being made to discharge him home with outpatient rehabilitation care within the next 5 days. A case manager will be assigned to coordinate his healthcare services.

Casey lives with his mother, sister, two half-brothers (10 and 6 years old), and stepfather. Both his mother and stepfather are employed full time and are trying to determine how to manage care for Casey once he returns home. Casey's father has not been actively involved in his life since the divorce 12 years ago. Casey's grandparents reside in the same town and may provide some support to the family.

What family support will Casey need as he continues his rehabilitation from the brain injury? What family assessment information is needed to effectively plan nursing care for this adolescent and his family? Does this family have strengths and coping strategies that will help them adapt to Casey's disability?

Video
Defining Family

FAMILY ROLES

The U.S. Census Bureau defines a **family** as two or more individuals who are joined together by marriage, birth, or adoption and live together (U.S. Census Bureau, 2010a). More broadly, however, a family may be a self-identified group of two or more persons joined together by sharing resources and emotional closeness. Family members can also include "honorary relatives" of the family, whether or not they are related by blood, marriage, or adoption, or even live in the same household. The family as defined by its members is likely to be dynamic, because membership often changes over time. For example, second marriages often integrate children into a newly formed family. Spouses of married children are integrated into an existing family, and the newly married couple begins a new family. In today's world, it is even more likely that families will live in different cities, states, or even countries than their extended families. So, there is no *typical* family.

Generally, family members depend on each other for emotional, physical, and economic support. Families are guided by a common set of values or beliefs about the worth and importance of certain ideas and traditions. These values often bind family members together, and these values are greatly influenced by external factors, including cultural background, social norms, education, environmental influences, socioeconomic status, and beliefs held by peers, coworkers, political and community leaders, and other individuals outside the family unit. Because of the influence of these external factors, a family's values may change considerably over the years, or members within a family may hold values that conflict with those of other family members.

A family is generally understood to be a safe haven for its members as they learn group values, norms, and acceptable behaviors. However, child abuse and neglect are significant problems and can occur within any family configuration (see Chapter 20 🔴). Individual family members take on certain social and gender roles and hold a designated status within the family. Parental roles are usually learned through a socialization process during childhood and adolescence. Roles of the family are listed in Box 2–1.

Parents have important roles that involve childrearing and the long-term care of children until they reach adulthood. Depending on their other roles in society, parents work to successfully nurture and rear children, helping them to meet role expectations. Parents must also meet the needs of the family unit and provide economic support for the family. Children also learn specific roles through a socialization process. Parents set expectations of behavior with discipline and modeling of appropriate behavior.

Ideally the family is a child's source of strength and support, the major constant in the child's life. Families are intimately involved in their children's physical and psychologic well-being, and they play a vital role in the health promotion and health maintenance of their children. By respecting the family's role, strengths, and experiences with the healthcare system, nurses have an opportunity to develop an effective partnership with the child and family as they make healthcare decisions that promote the child's health. This partnership between nurses and families is known as family-centered care.

FAMILY-CENTERED CARE

Family-centered care is a philosophy of health care in which a mutually beneficial partnership develops between the family and the nurse, and also other health professionals. In this way the priorities and needs of the family are addressed when the family seeks health care for the child. Each party respects the knowledge, skills, and experience that the other brings to the healthcare encounter. This is in contrast to family-focused care in which the role of health professionals is that of an expert who directs care, tells the family what to do, and intervenes on behalf of the family.

History of Family-Centered Care

Family-centered care became integral to the nursing care of children when it was recognized that families had a significant role in promoting the psychosocial and developmental needs of children in the hospital. When parents were initially allowed to stay with hospitalized children, nurses and other health professionals noticed that children were quieter, happier, and recovering sooner. Family-centered care promotes the presence of support systems during hospitalization and during invasive and painful procedures. Allowing parental involvement in the plan of care is beneficial to both the hospitalized child and the family (Pruitt, Johnson, Elliott, et al., 2008) (Box 2–2).

Nurses have long embraced the family-centered care philosophy. This philosophy is becoming more widely accepted by other health professionals. Parents are now recognized as partners in their child's care, not as visitors in the healthcare setting as patient- and family-centered care has become the standard of care in the pediatric setting (Moretz, 2010) (Figure 2–1 ■). The Society of Pediatric Nurses and the American Nurses Association have developed nursing practice guidelines for family-centered care (Table 2–1). See Chapter 16 🔴 for additional information related to the hospitalized child.

BOX 2–1	Roles of the Family

- Caring, nurturing, and educating children
- Maintaining the continuity of society by transmitting its knowledge, customs, values, and beliefs to children
- Receiving and giving love
- Preparing children to become productive members of society
- Meeting the needs of its members
- Serving as a buffer between its members and environmental and societal demands while addressing the interests and needs of the individual family members

---

BOX 2–2	Research: Parental Presence During Procedures

Increasingly, parents are permitted to be present during medical procedures performed on their children. Resistance to parental presence has been based on the fear that parents would delay the procedure, interfere with the procedure, distract or increase the anxiety of the health professionals performing the procedure, and increase parental anxiety. Studies have investigated parental presence in various situations involving medical procedures, such as venipuncture, lumbar puncture, laceration repair, resuscitation, and induction of anesthesia (Arai, Ito, Kandatsu, et al., 2007; Jones, Qazi, & Young, 2007; Maxton, 2008). In most cases, parents are less anxious and the ability of health professionals to perform procedures is not affected (Dingeman, Mitchell, Meyer, et al., 2007; O'Malley, Brown, Krug, et al., 2008).

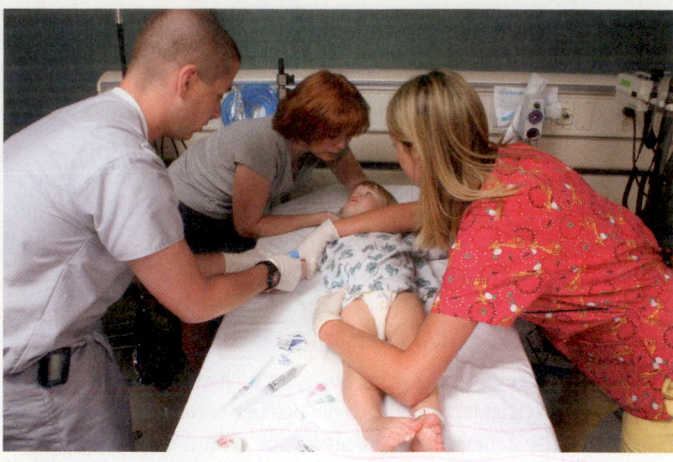

FIGURE 2–1 ■ A health facility policy that permits parents to be present during a procedure performed on their child is an example of a family-centered care policy. The parent is providing security and comfort to this child who is having blood drawn.

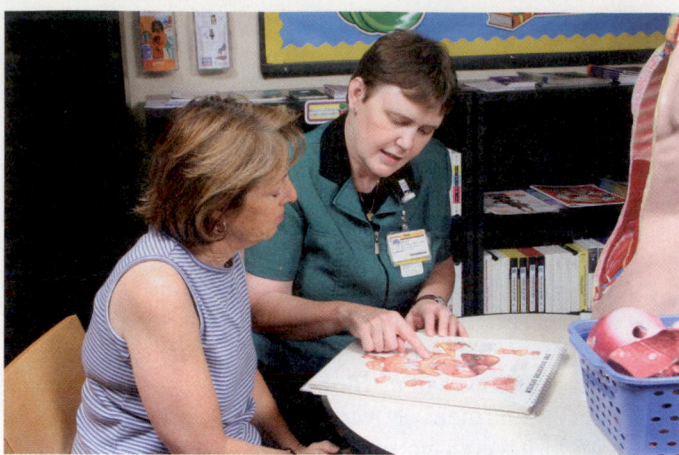

FIGURE 2–2 ■ The family resource center provides an opportunity for family members to obtain more information about their child's illness from the pediatric nurse educator. This nurse uses pictures from a chart to explain a child's illness to the parent.

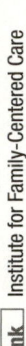

Weblink | Institute for Family-Centered Care

Promoting Family-Centered Care

Partnering with families in the provision of health care is essential to promote the best outcome when caring for children. Families have important knowledge to share about their child, their child's health condition, and how their child responds to various actions and events. They also need access to information that will make it possible for them to fully participate in planning and decision making.

Some healthcare facilities are developing patient and family resource centers to provide information and support. In most cases, the resource center is a consumer-oriented health library with staffing, but peer support services may also be coordinated through the center (Institute for Patient- and Family-Centered Care, 2011). Families can be supported to access useful print or online information that helps them to become informed participants in decision making about their child's care. Resources can often be provided in the preferred language and appropriate reading level. Models and anatomically correct dolls may be available that provide hands-on learning for both parents and children. In addition, the family resource center may serve as a place for family members to read, rest, and reflect (Institute for Patient- and Family-Centered Care, 2011). See Figure 2–2 ■.

Clinical Tip

It is important to consider how a healthcare setting's written policies, procedures, and literature for families refer to families and what attitudes these materials convey. Words like *policies*, *allowed*, and *not permitted* imply that hospital personnel have authority over families in matters concerning their children. Words like *guidelines*, *working together*, and *welcome* communicate an openness and appreciation for families in the care of their children.

Parents want to participate in decisions about their child's care. Cultural beliefs must be taken into consideration when working with the family to plan care for the child. See Developing Cultural Competence: Family-Centered Care.

In almost all cases, the child leaves the healthcare setting and the family assumes responsibility for provision of needed care in the home. The family caregivers must not feel alienated from a healthcare system they need for continuing assistance. (See Partnering with Families: Guidelines for Effective Partnership.) At the same time,

however, parents need to consider their own limitations. Before planning how to add more caregiving responsibilities to their routines, parents should assess their strengths in managing their ongoing family and caregiving responsibilities.

Beyond the provision of nursing care itself, children and parents can participate in the development of policies and guidelines for family-centered care in all types of healthcare settings. Their experiences while receiving care in the healthcare setting may reveal valuable insights. Considering parents' perspectives can be critical for staff and hospital administrators to provide quality patient care and achieve successful patient satisfaction. Parents who exhibit leadership qualities can be empowered to serve on advisory boards or councils, representing the family and community perspective. Parental roles may include:

- Assisting in the design and evaluation of programs and systems
- Assessing a healthcare setting for its family-centered policies and care practices, as well as its cultural appropriateness

Developing Cultural Competence
Family-Centered Care

When planning and providing care for children, it is essential that the nurse includes concerns and cultural beliefs of members of the child's family (Giger & Davidhizar, 2008). A collaborative relationship among the family and the healthcare team that addresses cultural values and diversity is essential in providing optimal culturally and linguistically competent family-centered care (Goode, Haywood, Wells, et al., 2009).

The nurse should also consider the possibility that an extended family member may need to be consulted regarding the treatment plan for the child, especially if the child spends a lot of time with extended family members. For example, in African American culture, grandmothers are a key member of the family. They are frequently relied upon to help care for the child, including care of the child who is ill (Purnell & Paulanka, 2008). Native Americans may consult tribal elders (considered part of the extended family) before agreeing to health care for their child. In some Hispanic cultures, major decisions for the child's health care include input from grandparents and other extended family members. It is important for the nurse to use the nursing process to incorporate beliefs and concerns of family members into the plan of care for the child (Giger & Davidhizar, 2008).

TABLE 2–1 Elements of Family-Centered Care and Recommendations for Nursing Practice

ELEMENTS	NURSING PRACTICE RECOMMENDATIONS
The Family at the Center Incorporate into policy and practice the recognition that the family is the constant in a child's life, while the service systems and support personnel within those systems fluctuate, and that the illness or injury of a child affects all members of the family system.	■ Establish a therapeutic relationship with the family. ■ Perform a comprehensive family assessment in collaboration with the family, identifying both strengths and needs. ■ Use the family assessment when working with the family to plan, implement, and evaluate care, considering the impact of the child's illness or injury on the entire family, with special attention to the siblings. ■ Provide siblings with information about their sibling's illness/injury at an appropriate developmental level and answer questions honestly. ■ Promote sibling visitation in hospital settings and participation in home care activities. ■ Identify extended family members who should receive information and be included in the educational process.
Family-Professional Collaboration Facilitate family-professional collaboration at all levels of hospital, home, and community care for: ■ Care of an individual child ■ Program development, implementation, evaluation, and evolution ■ Policy formation	■ Develop provider–family relationships that are guided by goals and expectations of both the family and the provider. ■ Ensure that parents are integral and critical collaborators in the decision-making process about their child's care. Involve children and adolescents in the decision-making process as appropriate for their cognitive and emotional development. ■ Assure that parents have 24-hour access to their children, and facilitate their participation in the child's care. ■ Provide parents with the option to stay with their child during procedures and tests, and provide ways for the parent to support the child during the procedure. ■ Provide comfort and hygiene facilities for families who spend long hours at the facility or travel great distances. ■ Promote the development of expertise in the special care of the child, fostering family independence and empowerment. ■ Incorporate parents and children into the quality assessment/improvement process. ■ Integrate family members into institutional and community advisory groups and in policy development.
Family-Professional Communication Exchange complete and unbiased information between families and professionals in a supportive manner at all times.	■ Provide information about the child's problem, prognosis, and needs in a manner that respects the child and family as individuals and promotes two-way dialogue. ■ Encourage the family to share information about the child and the illness/injury so that care planning and decisions are made in the most informed and collaborative manner.
Cultural Diversity of Families Incorporate into policy and practice the recognition and honoring of cultural diversity, strengths, and individuality within and across all families, including ethnic, racial, spiritual, social, economic, educational, and geographic diversity.	■ Practice family-centered care in a culturally competent manner with respect and sensitivity for the wide range of families with diverse values and beliefs. ■ Seek to understand the family's beliefs and practices related to race, culture, and ethnicity when developing relationships and collaborating in the child's health care. ■ Seek to understand and respect the family's religious/spiritual beliefs and practices and integrate these into the child's care, as the family desires. ■ Work with the family to address issues in care related to socioeconomic status, geographic considerations, access to health care, and insurance status. ■ Integrate training programs on diversity, cultural understanding, and culturally competent care into staff development programs.
Coping Differences and Support Recognize and respect different methods of coping, and implement comprehensive policies and programs that provide families with the developmental, educational, emotional, spiritual, environmental, and financial supports needed to meet their diverse needs.	■ Assess the strengths and weaknesses of the family's coping strategies and their resiliency factors and characteristics. Identify maladaptive coping mechanisms and assist the family to augment their coping efforts. ■ Assess the family's needs and desires for support, and assist the family in accessing and accepting assistance from support networks as needed or desired.
Family-Centered Peer Support Encourage and facilitate family-to-family support and networking.	■ Educate parents about parent-to-parent and family support resources and assist them to access such resources in the institution and community. ■ Provide access to psychoeducational groups that might be useful to parents, siblings, or ill/injured children.
Specialized Service and Support Systems Ensure that hospital, home, and community service and support systems for children needing specialized health and developmental care and their families are flexible, accessible, and comprehensive in responding to diverse family-identified needs.	■ Provide collaborative, flexible, accessible, comprehensive, and coordinated services to children and their families. ■ Provide comprehensive case management/care coordination for children and families with ongoing care needs. ■ Along with families, take an active role in advocating for the needs of ill and injured children.
Holistic Perspective of Family-Centered Care Appreciate families as families and children as children, recognizing that they possess a wider range of strengths, concerns, emotions, and aspirations beyond their need for specialized health and developmental services and support.	■ Encourage attention to the normal developmental needs and developmental tasks of the entire family unit and individual family members. ■ Encourage and facilitate the development of individual and family identities beyond a focus on illness or injury. ■ Facilitate "normalization" as valued and desired by the family.

Source: Adapted with permission from Lewandowski, L. A., & Tesler, M. D. (Eds.). (2003). Family-centered care: Putting it into action. The SPN/ANA guide to family-centered care. Washington, DC: American Nurses Association.

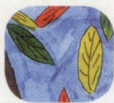

Partnering with Families

Guidelines for Effective Partnership

Parents have a role in developing an effective collaborative relationship with nurses and other health professionals. Parents often become experts in their child's health condition and learn to advocate for their child. They also must learn to communicate effectively with the health professionals caring for their child, and in the process develop a trusting relationship.

Guidelines for improved parental communication include encouraging parents to (Bright Futures, 2008a):

- Realize that strong communication with healthcare professionals develops over time.
- Share information about the child.
- Bring a list of questions to each visit and take notes during the visit.

- Ask questions related to the child's expected development.
- Get information about the child's health and safety including brochures, lists of resources, and appropriate websites.
- Ask how and when to contact the healthcare professional between visits.

Tips for nurses include:

- Provide information and honestly discuss issues of concern to both the family and healthcare providers.
- Demonstrate respect for the family's choices and methods for providing needed care.
- Continue to collaborate with the child and family and be willing to continue problem solving as new issues arise.

- Participating in the renovation or construction of healthcare facilities
- Recommending changes that will ultimately improve the quality of care
- Educating health professionals about working effectively with families as partners in the child's care

Parents can also serve a valuable role in family-to-family support networks by mentoring families entering the healthcare system for a new chronic condition. Parents may also help raise awareness about specific healthcare issues, serve as advocates for public policy issues, and assist with fund-raising activities.

Guidelines for working with families as advisors and tools for assessing the family-centered policies in various healthcare settings are available from the Institute for Family-Centered Care.

Clinical Judgment

When providing care to children, recall that the family is central to all healthcare interventions, with parents and children as the partners in care. Families need to sense that the nurse cares about them and respects them as an integral part of the child's life. What are some actions by the nurse that indicate a sense of caring for both the child and the family?

FAMILY COMPOSITION

Families are diverse in structure, roles, and relationships. Various types of families—both those considered traditional and nontraditional—exist in contemporary American society. This section identifies common types of family structure.

Nuclear Family

In the nuclear family, children live with both biological parents, and no other relatives or persons live in the household. One parent may stay home to rear the children while one parent works, but more commonly, both parents are employed by choice or necessity. Two-income families must address important issues such as childcare arrangements, household chores, and how to ensure quality family time. Dual-career/dual-earner families are now considered the norm in modern society. In cases of excessive job demands and lack of

control over the job, parental stress can have a negative impact on the family. These families often find it difficult to meet family and individual child needs as well as career demands. Important nursing considerations include:

- Respecting a parent who stays home to rear the children while appreciating the value of childrearing
- Helping parents to develop strategies to ensure that the child's health promotion needs are met, such as a nutritious diet with appropriate calories and adequate physical exercise

Blended or Reconstituted Family

The blended or reconstituted nuclear family includes two parents with biological children from a previous marriage or relationship who marry or cohabit. This family structure has become increasingly common due to high rates of divorce and remarriage. Potential advantages to the children may include better financial support and a new supportive role model. Stressors that can cause challenges in forming a cohesive family unit may include:

- Lack of a clear role for the stepparent
- Lack of acceptance of the stepparent
- Financial stresses when two families must be supported by stepparents
- Communication problems

Parents in the blended family may have difficulties overcoming differences in parenting styles, discipline, and values. Important nursing considerations include directing families to resources that may help reduce the potential conflicts associated with different parenting styles, discipline, and manipulative behaviors by children that can develop with the blended family. See the discussion on page 39 regarding stepparenting.

Another type of blended family includes two parents with adopted or foster children, sometimes including biological children. Many parents choose adoption because of infertility. In other cases, a couple or single adult chooses to adopt a child or take in foster children for personal, religious, or family reasons. The adoptive or foster parent may be a relative of the child. See the discussion beginning on page 40 regarding foster care and adoption.

Extended Family

Extended families exist when one parent or a couple shares expenses as well as household and childrearing responsibilities with grandparents, the sibling of a parent, or other relatives. For example, in multigenerational family living, three generations share the same household. See Box 2–3. Families may reside together to share housing expenses and childcare responsibilities. However, in many cases, the child may reside with the grandparent and one parent because of issues associated with unemployment, parental separation, parental death, or parental substance abuse. Grandparents may raise children due to the inability of parents to care for children. Grandparents endure emotional, physical, and financial stresses when taking on the childrearing role of one or more grandchildren (Figure 2–3 ■).

Also in the extended relative network family, two nuclear families of primary relatives or unmarried relatives live in close proximity to each other. The families share a social support network in which chores, goods, and services are exchanged. This type of family model may be common in the Latino community.

Single-Parent Family

The family of a single parent is formed when the mother or father is widowed, divorced, abandoned, or separated. According to 2007 data, 25% of children under 18 years of age lived in single-parent families (Kreider & Elliott, 2009). Although the majority of children who live with a single parent reside with their mother, the number of children residing with their father has increased significantly over the past several years (Clark, 2008). Reasons for the increasing rate of single-parent families include high rates of divorce and an increase in the number of births to never-married mothers (Shore & Shore, 2009).

Single-parent families often face difficulties because the sole parent may lack social and emotional support, need assistance with childrearing issues, and face financial strain. Single-parent families experience higher rates of poverty. In 2007, 9% of children living with their married parents lived at the poverty level, compared to 43% who lived with only their mother (Childstats.gov, 2009). Depending on social support and family resources, the single parent may be stressed from working to support the family, managing household responsibilities, serving as both mother and father, and attempting

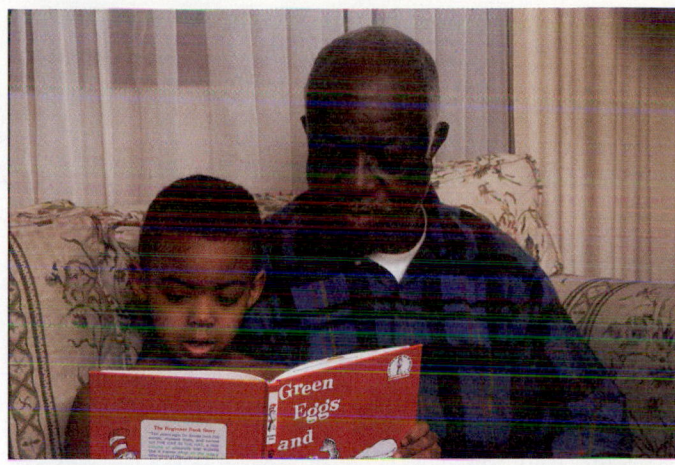

FIGURE 2–3 ■ This child lives with his mother and grandparents following the divorce of his parents. The special attention provided by his grandfather is helping him to adapt to the change in his family, and it enables the mother to work feeling confident that her son is safely cared for before and after school.

to have a personal life. Single mothers are often impoverished due to lack of child support, inequitable pay for work performed, work skill deficiencies, and cutbacks in social welfare programs. An important nursing consideration for working with single parents is to assess their strengths and needs in providing care to the child, such as after-school and backup childcare arrangements that enable the parent to fulfill work commitments (Figure 2–4 ■). Determine if the child has access to all resources available to support growth and development, such as school breakfast and lunch programs that provide nutritional support.

Binuclear Family

In a postdivorce family the biological children can be members of two nuclear households, with parenting shared by the father and the mother. The children alternate between the two homes, spending varying amounts of time with both parents in a situation called co-parenting, usually involving joint custody. **Joint custody** is a legal situation in which both parents have equal responsibility and legal rights, regardless of where the children live. The binuclear family is

BOX 2–3	**Community Care: Grandparents Raising Grandchildren**

The percentage of children under the age of 18 years living with a grandparent increased from 8% to 10% between 2001 and 2010. Statistics show that 7.5 million children lived with a grandparent in 2010, and 22% of these children did not have a parent present (U.S. Census Bureau, 2010b).

There are many reasons why children live with their grandparents, including death of a parent, parental substance abuse, teenage childbearing, and incarceration of the parents. In addition to the financial strain that is often present in homes where children live with a grandparent, caring for grandchildren can be stressful. Grandparents and other relatives who care for children are at risk for depression and other mental health problems (Linsk, Mason, Fendrich, et al., 2009).

Assess grandparents' knowledge related to developmental needs of children of different ages and teach them any special considerations in the care of the child. Grandparents are frequently older adults who may have alterations in senses and their own health concerns. Adapt communication and teaching to meet the needs of the grandparent if indicated (Barba, Tesh, Cowen, et al., 2010).

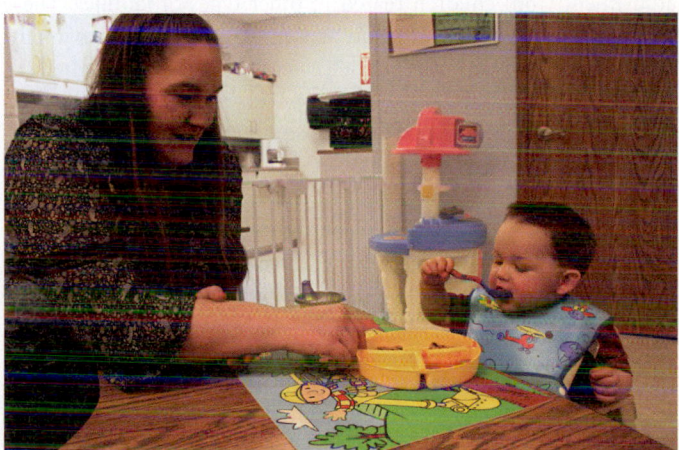

FIGURE 2–4 ■ Adolescents who become single parents often have challenges with balancing school, personal time, and care of the infant.

a model for effective communication. It enables both biological parents to be involved in a child's upbringing and provides additional support and role models from extended family members. Special nursing considerations in this family type involve ensuring that health promotion guidance and education for care of the child with an acute or chronic condition are communicated effectively to both biological parents.

Heterosexual Cohabiting Family

In this family type, a heterosexual couple who may or may not have children lives together outside of marriage. This may include never-married individuals as well as divorced or widowed persons. Biological children may result from the relationship, or in some cases children of one parent are present and help form a blended type of cohabiting family. In 2008, 6% of all children in the United States lived with a cohabiting parent or parents (Childstats.gov, 2009). Special concerns exist regarding the increased likelihood of economic hardship and child abuse (Kalil & Ryan, 2010; Clark, 2008). An important nursing consideration for children who live in informal stepfamilies is that the nonbiological parent has no legal authority to seek emergency medical care for the child. However, in the case of a true emergency—one that could result in loss of life or diminished functioning—health professionals are obligated to provide care and obtain consent as soon as possible afterward. The nonbiological parent also may not have knowledge of the child's medical history.

Gay and Lesbian Family

A gay or lesbian family involves two adults of the same sex who live together as domestic partners with or without children, or a gay or lesbian single parent rearing a child. Children in these families may be from a previous heterosexual union, or be born to or adopted by one or both member(s) of the same-sex couple. A biological child may be born to one of the partners through artificial insemination or through a surrogate mother. In the United States, 96% of all counties have at least one gay or lesbian couple living in the county. Approximately 30% of lesbian couples and 20% of gay couples are raising a child (Bowen, 2008).

Children who are adopted or born into lesbian and gay families are highly valued, as with heterosexual families (Figure 2–5 ■). Small studies that have evaluated children reared by same-sex couples found no significant differences in childrearing or in the children's adjustment from children reared in other types of families. These children have been found to do as well emotionally, behaviorally, and socially as those born into heterosexual families (Chamberlain, Miller, & Bornstein, 2008).

Children in homosexual families sometimes have only one biological or adoptive legal parent. The other partner is the co-parent and has no legal parental status in the majority of states. Several states do allow second-parent adoption for same-sex couples (Evan B. Donaldson Adoption Institute, 2008). Co-parent adoption would help maintain the child's rights to a continuing relationship if the legal parent dies or becomes incapacitated, or if the parents separate. Either parent could then provide consent for health care and make other important decisions on behalf of the child. Financial support of the child is more ensured if one parent dies or parents separate. Nursing considerations in this type of family involve respect for the relationship between partners and recognition of the nurturing capacity in these families.

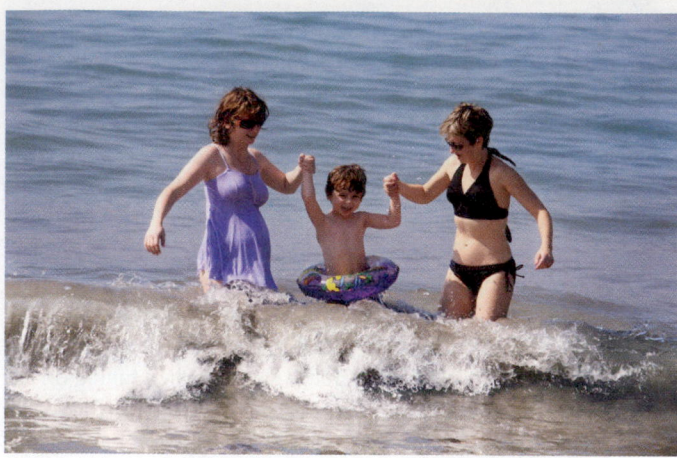

FIGURE 2–5 ■ Children raised in a homosexual family have been found to do as well emotionally, behaviorally, and socially as those born into heterosexual families (Chamberlain, Miller, & Bornstein, 2008). These parents are as dedicated as heterosexual parents to promoting the growth and development of their children.
Source: Galina Barskaya/Fotolia.

Practice Alert
It is important to identify the biological or adoptive parent, or a caregiver's legal documentation proving the right to medical decision making, when obtaining consent for the child's health care.

FAMILY FUNCTIONING
Transition to Parenthood

Choosing to become a parent is a major life change for adults. Couples experience significant family and cultural pressure to have a child. Mothers may be eager to have a child, but be concerned about fulfilling all the expectations of others (the father, the baby, other children, her parents, close friends, and her employer). Fathers anticipate increased responsibility and may be concerned about their ability to provide adequate support for the family. See Legal and Ethical Considerations: Family and Medical Leave Act.

At the time of birth the parents experience stresses and challenges along with feelings of pride and excitement. Mothers and fathers both make adjustments to their lifestyles to give priority to parenting. The baby is dependent for total care 24 hours a day, and this often results in sleep deprivation, irritability, less personal time, and less time for the couple's relationship. In addition the family often experiences a change in financial status.

Several factors influence how well the parents adjust to their new role. Social support provided to the mother, especially by the father, is important for the mother's adjustment. Marital happiness during

Legal and Ethical Considerations
Family and Medical Leave Act

Eligible parents of newborns and adopted children are entitled to 12 weeks of unpaid leave during any 12-month period, initially authorized under the federal Family and Medical Leave Act of 1993. Vacation or sick leave may often be used to pay for time away from work. This act also applies if a child, spouse, or parent of the employee develops a serious health condition. The employee is entitled to return to the previous position or an equivalent position with all the same pay, benefits, and other conditions (U.S. Department of Labor, 2009).

pregnancy is an important adjustment factor for both parents. Infants with significant health conditions or those with difficult temperaments can cause extra stress for the parents and affect their adjustment to the parenting role.

With the birth of the first child, mothers and fathers both have challenges related to renegotiating their employment to accommodate family and childcare time. Fathers are sometimes additionally challenged to develop closeness with the infant and to learn how to care for the infant, especially when they may not have had role models or any childcare experience. Most parents find that caring for infants and children takes more time than anticipated.

Nurses can help parents through this important transition by listening to the challenges they describe during the infant's first health visits. Encourage fathers and mothers to attend and participate in health promotion visits with the healthcare provider so that positive parenting can be supported. Answer questions and offer ideas to address described problems that the parents may be too tired to solve on their own. Help them recognize that frustrations and feelings they have regarding the challenges of infant care are normal and expected. Encourage both parents to become active in caring for the infant and to gain comfort in that care. Help each parent find activities that they enjoy with regard to infant care to encourage interaction and bonding with the infant.

Parental Influences on the Child

The qualities of family relationships and family behaviors are important aspects of family strengths and family functioning. Positive family relationships are characterized by parent–child warmth and supportiveness. Warm parent–child relationships can buffer children from stress and promote positive cognitive and social outcomes. Parents who are warm and place high demands on their children for appropriate behavior have children who tend to be content, self-reliant, self-controlled, and open to learning in school.

Mothers and fathers each contribute to the psychologic, emotional, and social health and development of their children. Both parents provide affection, nurturing, and comfort. They teach children life skills and healthy lifestyles. Although focus is frequently on the role of the mother, research has demonstrated that fathers too are important in the child's development (Bright Futures, 2008b).

Family Size

The size of the family influences the amount of attention given to children. In small families, parents often have more time to give attention to the children, to encourage achievement, and to support involvement in community activities. Children in larger families are encouraged to be cooperative so that the family group functions well. The child usually receives less personal attention from the parents and must often turn to others in the family for support. Family finances may be more limited. Children may adopt a specialized family role to gain family recognition, such as the "responsible one," "the clown," or "the black sheep."

Sibling Relationships

Siblings are the first peers of a child and often have a lifelong relationship lasting up to 70 or more years. Siblings, especially those of the same gender who are closer in age, tend to have a closer relationship because they often share many common experiences through childhood and adolescence. In general, for children who are more widely spaced in age, the parents have greater influence than siblings. However, the older sibling may be a very strong role model for younger siblings.

Sibling rivalry exists between children at times in all families. Children learn to share, compete, and compromise with their siblings. Some siblings take on other roles such as protector, problem solver, friend, and supporter for dealing with issues in the family and in the environment. Some siblings learn to work well together to maintain privacy or to form a coalition for negotiating with the parents. An older sibling helps reinforce rules and roles in the family by prompting and inhibiting certain patterns of behavior in the younger siblings. However, one sibling may test the waters by breaking a previously implicit rule to determine what rule flexibility is allowed in the family.

Children develop different personalities because of the need to establish a distinct identity for themselves and to be seen as unique in the family. Siblings may share some experiences, but they are often exposed to different environmental experiences that also help shape their personalities. Few if any personality differences tend to result solely from the birth order of the child. First-born children on average have slightly higher IQs and greater achievement in school and in their careers. This may be related to the fact that first-born children receive all of the attention from their parents until a sibling is born. Their intellectual development may also be enhanced through experiences of teaching their younger siblings (Craig & Dunn, 2010).

PARENTING

The family is an important component in the lives of all children, and it plays an essential role in fostering the development of infants, children, and youth. A significant concept in families is that of parenting. **Parenting** is a leadership role in the family in which children are guided to learn acceptable behaviors, beliefs, morals, and rituals of the family and to become socially responsible, contributing members of society. The manner in which children are parented, in combination with their individual personality traits and characteristics, influences their developmental outcomes.

Parents have responsibility for providing stability to children with a nurturing, safe, and structured environment. The child needs to have physical and emotional space to grow and develop. This space enables the child to personally find the relationship balance between closeness and distance, as well as safety and risk. Parents also enculturate their children with the values, beliefs, rituals, and behaviors learned and transmitted across family generations. See Developing Cultural Competence: Culture and Family Structure. To be successful in parenting, parents must have a certain flexibility that enables the family to adapt and adjust to family changes with time and other significant stressors and challenges (Figure 2–6 ■).

Parents should practice reasonable **limit setting** (established rules or guidelines for behavior) on children's autonomy, encouraging them to learn values and self-control. Yet at the same time, parents need to foster the child's curiosity, initiative, and sense of competence. Styles of parenting may differ, but they can be evaluated by examining two factors that are important in the development of children: parental warmth and parental control. Parental warmth refers to the amount of affection and approval parents display. Parental control refers to how restrictive the parents are. See Table 2–2 for the characteristics associated with parental warmth and control.

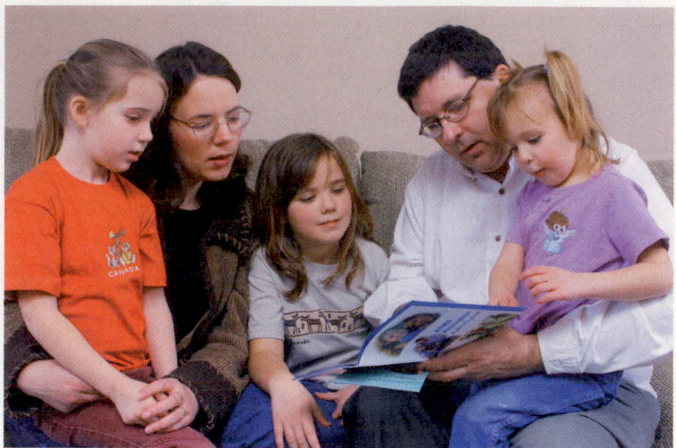

FIGURE 2–6 ■ Family time is important, especially during those times when all members of the family need to work together toward a common goal. In this family, everyone is learning more about the condition of one child and what each can do to help.

TABLE 2–2	**Characteristics of Significant Parenting Attributes**	
PARENTING ATTRIBUTE	**PARENTAL WARMTH**	**PARENTAL CONTROL**
High level	Warm, nurturing	Restrictive control of behavior
	Express affection and smile at children frequently	Survey and enforce compliance with rules
	Limit criticism, punishment	Encourage children to fulfill their responsibilities
	Express approval of child	May limit freedom of expression
Low level	Cool, hostile	Permissive, minimally controlling
	Quick to criticize or punish	Make fewer demands
	Ignore children	Fewer restrictions on behavior or expression of emotion
	Rarely express affection or approval	Permit freedom in exploring environment
	Rejection may be seen	

Developing Cultural Competence
Culture and Family Structure

A family's structure and roles are largely dependent upon cultural influence. For example, culture may determine who has authority (head of household) and is the primary decision maker for other members of the family. Sometimes the decision maker role varies by the type of decisions to be made. In some cultures, such as Hispanic, decisions regarding the health care of children are primarily the responsibility of the female, while other decisions are male dominated. Family dominance patterns may be *patriarchal*, as seen in some Appalachian cultures; *matriarchal*, as seen in some African American cultures; or more *egalitarian*, as seen in some European American cultures.

Diana Baumrind identified three parenting styles (*authoritarian, authoritative, permissive*) and described the influences each style has on children. This proposed classification is still useful in identifying parenting behavior (Baumrind, 2005). Another parenting style, called *indifferent*, exists in some families (Craig & Dunn, 2010). Although families will generally exhibit one style, it may vary in certain situations. See Table 2–3 for characteristics of parenting styles by levels of warmth and control.

Authoritarian Parents

Authoritarian parents tend to be punitive and adhere to rigid rules or be more dictatorial. Parents who use this style might say, "Because I'm your parent, that's why," "A rule is a rule," or "Just do what I say." This style sets firm limits, and those limits or rules are not negotiable or open to any discussion. Parents expect family beliefs and principles to be accepted without question. Children have no opportunity to participate in the family decision-making process. Children with authoritarian parents do not develop the skills to examine why a certain behavior is desirable or how their actions might influence others.

Authoritative Parents

Authoritative parents use firm control to set limits, but they establish an atmosphere with open discussion or are more democratic. Limits for behavior are clear and reasonable, but the child is encouraged to talk about why certain behaviors occurred and how the situations might be handled differently another time. Parents provide explanations about inappropriate behaviors at the child's level of understanding. Children are allowed to express their opinions and objections, and some flexibility is permitted when appropriate. However, parents make it clear that they are the ultimate authority for decisions. Children with authoritative parents develop a sense of social responsibility since they converse about their responsibilities and approaches.

Permissive Parents

Permissive parents show a great deal of warmth, but set few controls or restraints on the child's behavior. Parents are so intent on showing unconditional love that they fail to perform some important parenting functions. Children are allowed to regulate their own behavior. Discipline is inconsistent and parents may threaten punishment but not follow through. Both extremes result in excessive permissiveness, and the child does not learn socially acceptable limits of behavior. As the parent does not impose any controls on the child, the child ends up controlling the parents.

Indifferent Parents

Indifferent parents display little interest in their children or in their roles as parents. They do not demonstrate affection or approval of the children, and they do not set limits or controls on the children. This may occur because of disinterest or because their lives are busy and stress filled, leaving little time or energy for their children. Children who experience this style of parenting often have the worst outcomes, such as destructive impulses and delinquent behavior. If the parents are also hostile, the child often develops delinquent behavior (Craig & Dunn, 2010).

Parent Adaptability

Parents who are able to adapt their behavior to meet the needs of children at different developmental stages are also more effective. Eleanor Maccoby (1980) expanded upon Diana Baumrind's perspectives on parenting style by examining how parents and children interact during the parenting process. Parenting styles may change

TABLE 2–3	Parenting Styles by Level of Warmth and Control		
PARENTING STYLE	**WARMTH/CONTROL**	**BEHAVIOR OF PARENTS**	**CHILD OUTCOMES**
Authoritarian	High control Low warmth	Highly controlling, issue commands and expect them to be obeyed Little communication with children Inflexible rules Permit little independence	No negotiation skills No ability to direct and initiate own activities Frustrated in efforts to achieve autonomy May become fearful, withdrawn, and unassertive Girls often passive and dependent during adolescence Boys often rebellious and aggressive
Authoritative	Moderately high control High warmth	Set reasonable limits on behavior Accept and encourage growing autonomy of children Open communication with children Flexible rules	More willingly accept restrictions Tend to be more self-reliant, self-controlled, and socially competent Higher self-esteem Better school performance
Permissive	Low control High warmth	Few or no restraints Unconditional love Communication flows from child to parent Much freedom and little guidance No limit setting	May become rebellious, aggressive, or socially inept, self-indulgent, or impulsive May be creative, active, and outgoing
Indifferent	Low control Low warmth	No limit setting Lack affection for children Parents focused on stress in own lives Parents may show hostility or neglect	May show a high expression of destructive impulses and delinquent behavior

Source: *Adapted from Craig, G. J., & Dunn, W. L. (2010). Understanding human development (2nd ed., p. 191). Reprinted and electronically reproduced by permission of Pearson Education, Inc., Upper Saddle River, New Jersey.*

as the child grows older. For example, parents may use negotiation to help the child develop problem-solving skills and to learn how to compromise, which is necessary to get along with others. This enables the child to have more self-control and self-responsibility over time. Parents and some children can develop shared goals and jointly participate in decision making, whereas other children require constant negotiation for decision making. See Partnering with Families: Guidelines for Promoting Acceptable Behavior in Children.

Assessing Parenting Styles

Nurses can assess parenting styles by asking families how they handle different situations that require limit setting. The nurse, in all settings, is often in a position to discuss parenting styles and to offer suggestions for managing certain types of child behaviors that are frustrating to the family. Keep in mind that children all differ, and parents often must vary their parenting styles for different children in the family. For example, the child's temperament is often tied to

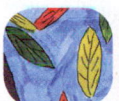

Partnering with Families

Guidelines for Promoting Acceptable Behavior in Children

- Set realistic expectations and directions for behavior based on the child's age and understanding; enforce the expected directions and behaviors consistently.
- Focus on promoting appropriate and desirable behaviors in the child.
  - Model or suggest appropriate behavior.
  - Review expected behavior for special situations, such as a family party, going to the movies, or other social events.
  - Help the child distinguish between inside and outside voice and behaviors.
  - Praise or reward the child using appropriate behaviors.
- Tell the child about his or her inappropriate behavior as soon as it begins and offer guidelines for behavior change or provide a distraction.
- When reprimanding the child, focus on the behavior rather than stating that the child is bad. Explain how the behavior is inappropriate and how

it makes you as the parent and any other person involved feel. Avoid ridicule or accusation that can take the form of shame or criticism. These actions can have an impact on the child's self-esteem if repeated often enough.
- Be alert for situations when the child could potentially misbehave, such as when tired or overexcited. Use a distraction to control or calm the child.
- Help children gain self-control with friendly reminders (count to three, as soon as the clothes are on the doll, as soon as you finish the game) regarding the timing for transition to the next event of the day, such as bedtime, putting the toys away, or washing hands before dinner.
- Discuss reasons and social rules for expected behaviors when the child is old enough to understand.

Developing Cultural Competence
Cultural Influences on Parenting

Some cultural influences on parenting are associated with a chosen lifestyle. For example, living in a predominantly ethnic neighborhood makes it possible to participate in special ethnic events that help teach the child about the culture. Parents use the community for social contacts that help to reinforce patterns of parenting and to establish behavioral expectations of their children. Frequent contact or living with the extended family helps the child learn family and ethnic traditions, behaviors, and values. Children may be sent to religious or parochial schools that foster values important to the family.

behavioral style. One child may need clear limits set with discussion and reinforcement needed, whereas a sibling may immediately respond to the parents' limit setting without a need for discussion. See Chapter 5 🔗 for more information on the temperaments of children from infancy through adolescence. Also see Developing Cultural Competence: Cultural Influences on Parenting.

Discipline and Limit Setting

Discipline is a method for teaching the rules that govern behavior or conduct. **Punishment** is the action taken to enforce the rules when the child misbehaves. Parenting styles play an important role

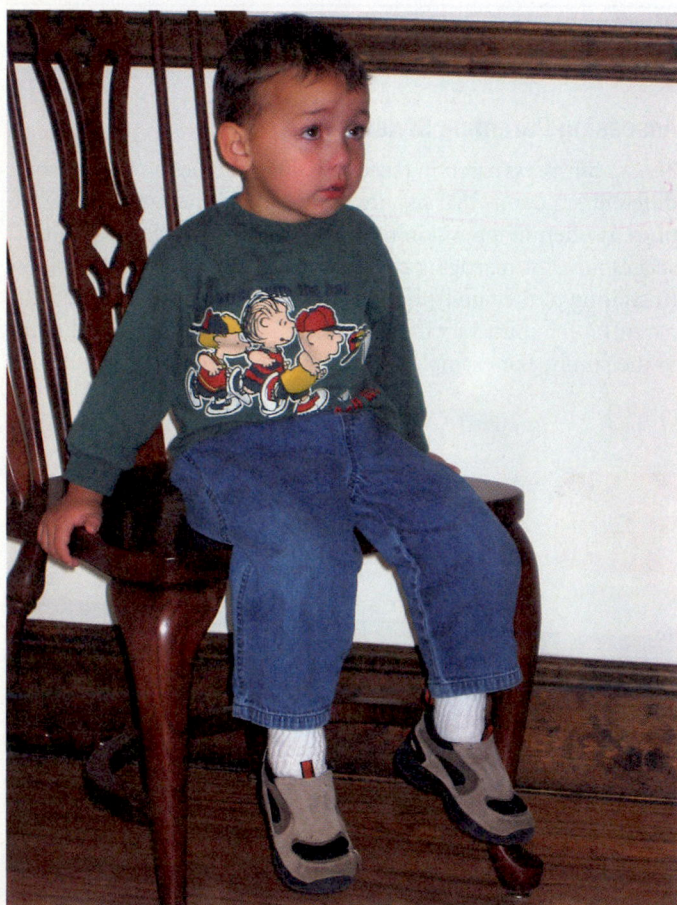

FIGURE 2–7 ■ One effective discipline method is to remove the child to an isolated area where no interaction with children and adults can occur and no toys are present. This is used to demonstrate that there is a consequence to misbehavior. For older children, consider the loss of phone, computer, or other privileges.
Source: Conor Murcar.

in the type of discipline used with children. When clear limits are set and consistently maintained, as with authoritative parenting, punishment may be needed less often. Limit setting and firm control of those limits are important for children to learn to what extent they can safely and independently operate within the environment. Firm limits also help children to feel secure because they are reassured by consistency and the sense of protection perceived by the limits. Punishment helps children learn that there are consequences for misbehavior and that other individuals may be affected by the behavior. This helps children develop a sense of responsibility for their behavior.

Parents use various strategies for discipline and punishment. Factors that affect what type of discipline is used are related to sex of the child, education level and age of the parents, family income, and race. In addition, the type of misbehavior and the location in which it occurs affect the type of discipline used (Socolar, Savage, & Evans, 2007).

Discipline strategies used with children include (Gershoff, Lansford, Zelli, et al., 2010; Hicks-Pass, 2009; Socolar et al., 2007):

- **Reasoning**—explaining why a behavior or action is inappropriate or describing how limit setting is important. By reasoning, parents can help the child to understand why certain behaviors are wrong. Similarly, parents can share personal stories and fables to help children understand social and moral values or to better understand acceptable behavior.
- **Behavior modification**—giving positive rewards (such as treats or privileges) or reinforcement for good behavior or consistently ignoring inappropriate behavior to minimize the behavior. This encourages children to behave in specified ways.
- **Experiencing consequences**—allowing the child to learn important lessons associated with misbehavior, such as taking away a toy, using a time-out, withdrawing privileges, or providing no dessert if the child misses dinner or does not eat nutritious foods (Figure 2–7 ■).
- **Corporal punishment**—spanking or inflicting pain with a paddle, whip, or other object. While some parents report using this type of discipline every day, many report never or rarely using it. Recent research indicates that corporal punishment is one of the three least common methods used to discipline preschoolers (Gershoff et al., 2010).
- **Scolding or yelling**—using harsh language directed at the child. Both spanking and scolding or yelling have been associated with more aggression in children (Gershoff et al., 2010).

See Chapters 11 through 13 🔗 for age-specific discipline strategies.

Clinical Tip
Time-out is a punishment method of placing the child in a location away from toys and attention as a consequence of misbehavior. The general rule for the length of time-out is 1 minute per age.

Clinical Tip
Nurses have an important educational role in helping parents to identify an appropriate discipline method and to take an authoritative role with their children. Encourage and educate parents about the need to be in charge, to set the rules, and to stand by them so that children learn how to behave.

SPECIAL FAMILY CONSIDERATIONS
Divorce and Its Effects on Children

The divorce rate in the United States is estimated to be around 50% of all marriages. Each year, an additional 1 million children are affected by divorce (Portnoy, 2008). Children are affected in many ways when the family breaks apart due to divorce, even if the divorce was preceded by many periods of stress and tension in the home.

Many children believe they are at fault for the separation and divorce, that they said or did something to make the parent leave. When one parent leaves, the children may feel abandoned and divorced by that parent. They may fear being abandoned by the remaining parent. Also, children may become engaged in the disputes of parents and experience conflicts of loyalty when parents fight for their affection.

In divorces involving a lot of conflict and hostility, the children may have increased problems with adjustment. When children must make a lot of changes in their lives in addition to the parents' separation (new home, different school), their adjustment is made more difficult as their sense of order is upset. Predictable routines have changed, and children may test limits to see if they still apply. The more changes they must make in the period immediately after the divorce, the more challenging is their adjustment. The disruption associated with divorce is also linked to academic and behavior problems among children (Portnoy, 2008). See Table 2–4 for potential effects of divorce on children of different ages.

Sometimes parents are so stressed that their customary parenting styles become inconsistent. They may be unable to provide the warmth, affection, and support that the children need during this time. Battles over custody, child support, property division, and visitation rights all cause more distress for the children.

Nurses can assist families experiencing divorce by inquiring about the circumstances and changes that the child is experiencing. Talk with parents about the child's fears of abandonment and concerns, reminding them that even infants and toddlers can sense tensions in the home. Remind parents about the need to keep children out of the middle of confrontations and to maintain limits of acceptable behavior. Encourage parents to avoid saying negative statements about the other parent, and encourage them to make every effort to maintain their relationship with the children. And most important, help parents recognize their children's needs for love and security during this difficult period.

The quality of the relationship between the divorced parents has an important impact on the future relationships their children have with them as adults. Children do better when both parents remain involved with their children and cooperate with each other after divorce (American Academy of Child and Adolescent Psychiatry, 2008).

Fathers who do not live with their children but live nearby are more likely to have involvement with their children if they have a good relationship with the child's mother, financial resources, and work experience. The relationship between father and child may be improved when the father can interact with the child in a conflict-free environment. See Partnering with Families: Promoting Relationships with Parents Following Separation and Divorce.

Stepparenting

When divorced or widowed parents remarry, the child may respond with ambivalence, divided loyalty, anger, or uncertainty. Parents should anticipate how the child and the entire family will respond to

TABLE 2–4	Potential Effects of Divorce on Children of Different Ages
AGE (YEARS)	**BEHAVIOR***
3–5	Fear, anxiety, worry Sorrow and grief Anger Regression Searching and questioning Temper tantrums Increased crankiness and aggression Self-blame Loneliness, unhappiness, depression
6–8	Worry, anxiety, depression Sadness Insecurity Fantasy Guilt Self-blame Inability to concentrate on schoolwork Regression Confusion Grief Anger and aggression Resentment Behavioral problems at school and home
9–10	Anger Anxiety and depression Grief Manipulation of parents Withdrawal from friends and activities Resentment Behavioral problems at school and home Loneliness Fear
11–13	Panic Fear Depression Guilt Risk taking Fear of loneliness and abandonment Denial Anger
14–17	Struggle with morality Loneliness Sadness Anger Fear Depression Guilt Aggressiveness Truancy, use of drugs and alcohol Sexual acting out

*This table lists some of the behaviors that could potentially be seen with different age groups and is not all inclusive. There are many other behaviors that could be present as well, depending on the individual child.

Source: *Data from Wallerstein, J. S., & Blakeslee, S. (2004). What about the kids? Raising your children before, during, and after divorce. New York: Hyperion; Douglas, E. (2006). The effects of divorce on children. University of New Hampshire Cooperative Extension. Retrieved from http://ceinfo .unh.edu; Craig, G. J., & Dunn, W. L. (2010). Understanding human development (2nd ed.). Upper Saddle River, NJ: Pearson/Prentice Hall; Portnoy, S. M. (2008). The psychology of divorce: A lawyer's primer, Part 2: The effects of divorce on children. American Journal of Family Law, 21(4), 126–134; Weston, F. (2009). Effects of divorce or parental separation on children. British Journal of School Nursing, 4(5), 237–243.*

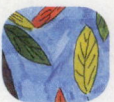

Partnering with Families

Promoting Relationships with Parents Following Separation and Divorce

Guidelines that may help reduce conflict and foster maintenance of a close relationship between the child and each parent include the following:

- Develop a way to stay in touch with the child even when apart, such as phone calls, faxes, or e-mail.
- Encourage a liberal visitation schedule so that each parent has time to be a normal parent. Overnight stays rather than a few hours at a time allow for more normal interactions.

- When parents have difficulty minimizing conflict in front of the child, transition the child to the other parent after school or childcare, or from a friend's home. This keeps the child from feeling responsible for the conflict.

changes in lifestyles, routines, and interaction patterns and address them early in the formation of the new family relationship. When a stepparent joins a ready-made family, opportunities for improved emotional and financial support of the child can result, but the development of a new cohesive family requires many adjustments on the part of all family members. Although relationships between the child and the stepparent may be tense in the beginning, close relationships that promote the child's development and emotional well-being often develop (Amato, 2007).

Blending of two families often results in the need to identify or negotiate new customs, traditions, rituals, and routines for the family. Children may lose or fear losing a close relationship with the noncustodial parent, neighborhood friends (if a move was required), contact with grandparents, and family traditions. Discussions with children about their feelings may help the new family develop plans that ease the transition.

Stepparents must adjust to the habits and personality of the child and then work to gain trust and acceptance. If the child has not accepted the divorce or loss of a biological parent, the stepparent faces more challenges in developing a trusting, affectionate, and respectful relationship. Sharing in childrearing decisions and responsibilities is an important task for stepparents, but their roles and the role of the joint or noncustodial parent need to be discussed and negotiated.

Stepparents are additional parents, not replacement parents. The child and the stepparent need to adjust to each other. The stepparent should try to establish a position in the child's life that is different from that of the missing biological parent, rather than competing with the biological parent. Stepmothers often have more challenges than stepfathers adjusting to their new role. This may be because they spend more time with the children.

In most stepparent families, discipline is a challenge. Family members must agree upon standards of behavior, as well as when, how, and by whom discipline is used, and those guidelines need to be consistently maintained. Discipline by a stepparent is difficult until a bond develops between the stepparent and stepchild. The development of this bond cannot be forced. Time and honest communication are needed to gain the child's trust.

Contact with the biological parent often continues through custody arrangements, financial support, and visitation. Children may actually move between two households, adding to the complexity and stressors in their lives. Children may have divided loyalties between the two sets of parents (Dupuis, 2010). Power conflicts may emerge if the biological parents do not make efforts to cooperate in parenting decisions. Children benefit when their parents maintain a cooperative co-parenting relationship. Parents must agree to work together for the child's benefit. Making sure that children maintain frequent contact with their nonresidential parent is essential to positive relationships with that parent. Children have fewer emotional and behavioral problems when the nonresident parent is involved in the child's life (Amato, 2007).

FOSTER CARE

Foster care is the provision of protection and shelter for a child in an approved living situation away from the family of origin. It is legally coordinated by the state's child welfare system. The goal of foster care is to ensure the safety and well-being of vulnerable children. On September 30, 2008, approximately 463,000 children were in foster care. Of these children, 40% were White non-Hispanic, 31% were Black non-Hispanic, 20% were Hispanic, and 10% were other races or multiracial (U.S. Department of Health and Human Services, 2010a).

During 2008, 273,000 children entered foster care and 285,000 exited. Of those children exiting foster care, 52% were united with their parent or primary caregiver, 19% were adopted, 15% were placed with a relative or guardian, 10% were emancipated, and 3% had other outcomes (U.S. Department of Health and Human Services, 2010a).

Children enter the foster care system for many reasons. The primary reason is child abuse and neglect. Other reasons, but to a much lesser extent, include a parent's inability to care for the child because of drug addiction or health issues (Whenan, Oxlad, & Lushington, 2009). Each state has guidelines regarding qualifications and standards for foster care parents and the process for becoming a foster parent. In an effort to ensure that the child is placed in a safe and nurturing environment, the state guidelines used to investigate the home often include an interview with the interested adults to check for readiness to be a foster parent, health of all family members, legal background checks, and safety of the residence. Foster parents are also required to have initial training and annual continuing education.

Foster care parents may be relatives (kinship care) or unrelated families with whom the child has a strong emotional bond. However, many children needing foster care are placed in extended families because there are fewer suitable nonkinship family foster homes. Although there are psychologic benefits in keeping the child within the extended family, especially for helping the child learn and understand cultural and family values, the kinship foster parents have more challenges than other foster parents. They may be older or in poorer health, have less income, and have less education. Kinship foster parents may receive less funding than licensed foster care parents. In addition, they tend to receive less supervision and family service support than in nonkinship foster care (Raphel, 2008).

Foster Parenting

Foster parenting is very demanding. Foster parents must provide for the daily needs of children, support them emotionally, and provide appropriate responses to their behaviors; however, they may not feel they are prepared to do so (Whenan et al., 2009). Foster parents provide transportation to medical and mental health counseling appointments, coordinate visits with birth parents and caseworkers, and advocate for the child in school settings. When the child has complex problems or needs, the challenge of caring for the foster child is even greater. Foster parents receive some funding to care for children, but it is often inadequate for the child's needs, so the family subsidizes the child's care from their own funds. Low reimbursement rates, inadequate respite care, and the increasing complexity of problems in foster children contribute to a foster parent's decision to leave the foster care system (Lauver, 2008). Foster parents may feel like they are the only ones available to support the child, and they may become frustrated with the system or burn out. Strategies must be developed to include foster parents in decision making and educate them regarding their role in the child welfare system and legal system to increase retention of foster parents (Marcellus, 2010). When the child must be moved to a different foster family, this may further exacerbate the ongoing stress that the individual child experiences in the foster care system.

Much of the child's adjustment rests with the stability of the family and available resources. Even though foster care is intended to be a temporary short placement—until the child can be returned home or an adoptive home is found—placed children may actually reside with the foster family for a lengthy time, sometimes for years. For the child who has come from an unstable, abusive, or neglectful environment, the foster care home can be supportive to the child's health status, development, and academic achievement.

Children in foster care are more likely to have compromised growth and development and mental health disorders (Bruskas, 2008). Many of the problems are related to the reason foster care was sought, such as physical or sexual abuse, neglect, or abandonment. For the optimal psychologic outcome of children placed in foster care, caregivers should seek permanent placement as rapidly as possible, so the child perceives a sense of belonging and develops psychologic ties.

Foster parents caring for children need to provide continuity, consistency, and predictability. It is essential that foster parents provide a nurturing environment for these children and show love and affection toward them. Developmentally appropriate activities are essential to foster the child's long-term physical and emotional development.

Health Status of Foster Children

Children placed in foster care often have complex health problems and chronic illness. They are also more likely to have developmental delays, behavioral and psychiatric disorders, and academic difficulty (Whenan et al., 2009). Efforts to ensure that children receive appropriate health care while in foster care are challenged by various barriers such as lack of coordination between healthcare providers and social workers. Lack of preventive care for foster children may result because of fragmentation in caregiving systems, loss of medical records, and foster parents who simply do not know how to obtain the services the foster child needs (Schneiderman, 2006).

Every child entering foster care should receive an initial health screening, followed by a more comprehensive health assessment within a month. Findings and recommendations from the health assessment and additional health evaluations should be incorporated into the child's social service case plan. Nurses can play an important role in partnering with foster parents to arrange for and obtain the services needed by the child. Foster parents need to be supported in their efforts to be the caring adult for these children, helping them to develop self-esteem and resilience.

Transition to Permanent Placement

Foster care is not intended to be a long-term solution for a safe and secure home for the child. Although many children are reunited with birth parents, other children are not. The Adoption and Safe Families Act of 1997 (PL 105-89) led to significant changes in child placement (Strijker, Knorth, & Knot-Dickscheit, 2008):

- A process was developed to evaluate the performance of care providers.
- Timelines were shortened for decision making about permanent placement of children.
- Incentives were established for states to encourage adoption.
- States were given guidelines regarding when reasonable efforts to reunite children with birth parents are no longer necessary. Actions are required in certain circumstances to terminate parental rights.
- Finally, kinship foster care was formally recognized.

The Fostering Connections to Success and Increasing Adoptions Act of 2008 was enacted to amend portions of the Social Security Act. Purposes of the legislation include support of caregivers who are relatives of the child in foster care, improved outcomes of children in foster care, and improved incentives for adoption (U.S. Department of Health and Human Services, 2008a). See Legal and Ethical Considerations: Foster Care Independence Act.

Legal guardianship (a permanent placement option for the child, often with relatives, in which parental rights are not terminated) was established as an alternative to **adoption** (a legal relationship between the child and parents not related by birth in which the adoptive parents assume all legal and financial responsibility for the child). Long-term foster care was eliminated as a permanent

---

Legal and Ethical Considerations
Foster Care Independence Act

The Foster Care Independence Act of 1999 (PL 106-169) requires states to provide youth 18 to 21 years of age with services to help them make the transition to self-sufficiency—training and education with services to help them gain employment, mentors for personal and emotional support, as well as financial, housing, counseling, and other supports and services (U.S. Department of Health and Human Services, 2010b).

Weblink   National Adoption Information Clearinghouse

placement option in nonkinship care, but it could continue for kinship foster care to promote stability for the involved children (Adoption.com, 2010).

For those children with kinship foster care, adoption is often not perceived as the best option. Legal guardianship enables the child to retain legal connections with the birth family and a relationship with the extended family. The guardian assumes limited financial liability for the child's care. Legal guardianship can be reversed at a future point in time if the birth parents petition the court.

ADOPTION

Motivations for adoption of a child vary with the families seeking adoption. In some cases, couples have fertility problems and are unable to have a biological child. In a family that already has biological children, the reasons may include:

- A desire to provide a home to a child who needs one or to have a larger family without additional biological children
- Fertility issues requiring invasive medical procedures that are too extensive, expensive, or psychologically too overwhelming for a subsequent pregnancy
- Adoption of a foster child with whom the family has established strong bonds
- Adoption by a family relative or stepparent

The supply of healthy infants available for adoption is much smaller than the number of families who want to adopt. Most children in the United States available for adoption are older children, often of minority populations or of mixed races, and those with special healthcare needs. In 2008, the number of children waiting to be adopted was 130,000, down from 134,000 in 2002 (U.S. Department of Health and Human Services, 2008b). Because most families choosing to adopt children prefer to have an infant, many children have been adopted from foreign nations. In 2007, the nations that provided the largest number of orphans for adoption in the United States were China, Guatemala, Russia, Ethiopia, South Korea, Vietnam, Ukraine, and Kazakhstan (Howard & John, 2009). Adopted children account for approximately 2% of all children in the United States (U.S. Department of Health and Human Services, 2009).

Legal Aspects of Adoption

Controlled by individual state law, adoption may be arranged through an authorized agency, such as a licensed social service agency. Some adoptions are arranged through independent agencies in collaboration with physicians, lawyers, nurses, and members of the clergy. State laws require any family who wants to adopt a child to undergo a home study, a process in which parents are interviewed about a large number of topics and issues and are provided education and guidelines to prepare for the adoption. The National Adoption Information Clearinghouse provides information about state adoption laws.

Birth mothers and birth fathers are each required to relinquish legal rights to a child before an adoption can occur. The legal period between the child's birth and when the birth mother relinquishes legal rights varies by state. Efforts are made to ensure that the birth mother is not coerced into relinquishing legal rights to the child immediately after birth. In an open adoption, the birth

mother and adoptive parents often have contact with each other prior to the birth and have jointly planned potential future contacts between the child and biological mother. In some adoptions, birth mothers write a letter that is given to the child at an appropriate age.

Preparation for Adoption

Parents often benefit from preadoption counseling, which may help provide the support and reassurance about parenting and the adoptive process, and help adopting parents make connections with support groups or other families with adopted children. Parents may wonder about their ability to love and parent the child. They may have concerns about the responses of relatives, other children, and friends, especially if the child is from a different ethnic or racial group. Children already present in the family need to be reassured that they will not be displaced by the new child. Families need information about the child's understanding of what adoption means and guidance to help inform the child about being adopted (Box 2–4). See Partnering with Families: Informing the Child About Adoption.

Children who are older when adopted must also make the commitment to the family relationship. They often have a memory of parents and other caregivers, so developing a close relationship with the adoptive parents takes more time. It may also be more challenging for parents to develop a close emotional bond to the adopted older child than to an adopted infant. Even when a serious commitment has been made to adopt an older child, adjustment of the family and child may be difficult for everyone. Counseling may be helpful to some families during the transition process.

BOX 2–4	Understanding of and Responses to Adoption by Children at Various Ages

- Children under 3 years of age do not recognize a difference between being adopted into a family versus being a biological child in the family.
- Starting at about 3 years of age, children like to hear more about their adoption story and they begin to ask what adoption means. Children adopted at this age may experience the separation from their other family and relatives. They are aware of physical differences between themselves and the adoptive family when they are of a different race or ethnic group. They may also be fearful of abandonment by the adoptive family.
- By 5 years of age adopted children begin to recognize they are different from most of their peers who were not adopted. Some children develop a feeling of responsibility for their biological parents' decision not to keep them.
- School-age children may fantasize about their biological family and what their life might have been like if they were not adopted. Their self-esteem may be affected as they think there was a flaw in them that led their biological parents to give them up for adoption.
- Adolescents may continue to fantasize about the "ideal" biological family and try out identities similar to what they know or imagine about their biological parents. They may also become angry that their own life experience is different from societal norms. They may choose to seek information about their biological family through a reunion registry.

Source: *Data from Borchers, D., & Committee on Early Childhood, Adoption, and Dependent Care, American Academy of Pediatrics. (2003). Families and adoption: The pediatrician's role in supporting communication. Pediatrics, 112(6), 1437–1441.*

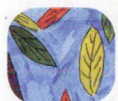

Partnering with Families

Informing the Child About Adoption

Most parents have anxiety about when and how to tell the child that he or she is adopted. There is no perfect age to tell the child about the adoption, so consider the child's age and developmental stage when sharing information.

- Some authorities believe the child should be told at such a young age that the child will always know that he or she is adopted. This may be especially important when the child is of a different ethnic or racial group, or has very different physical characteristics than the parents.
- The terms *adoption*, *adopted*, *birth family*, or *biological family* should be part of the family's natural conversation (Borchers & Committee on Early Childhood, Adoption, and Dependent Care, 2003).
- Decide when you and the child are most ready to introduce the topic of adoption—such as when a discussion of babies and where they come from occurs. However, avoid waiting for "just the right moment" because children may wonder what other information has not yet been shared.
- Make sure the child is told before a third party is likely to say something. The chances of this happening increase as the child enters school.
- Tell the child in a matter-of-fact manner about the adoption. Let the child know how much he or she was wanted and that some personal qualities of the child made the selection special. Avoid phrases such as "given up" for adoption. A more positive phrase to use is that the biological family made an adoption plan in the best interest of the child's future.

- Share the adoption story that includes the child's birth. Then the story can continue with the adoptive family's desire to adopt a child and that the adopted child was specifically chosen.
- Make sure the child understands that his or her place in the family is permanent. The adoptive family's commitment to the child should be repeated frequently.
- Maintain honesty and an open opportunity for discussion about adoption with the child. Be willing to discuss the child's biological family and the adoption process so the child feels comfortable asking questions. This helps make the adoption a positive process. More discussion about adoption will be needed as the child grows older, especially when the child begins to ask at about 5 to 6 years of age why he or she was not wanted by the biological parents. Anticipate that the child will grieve the loss of the birth parents.
- As the child grows older and asks for more information about the birth parents, provide what information is known and try to help the child deal with information that is difficult to hear. If requested information is not available, be honest and admit it. Help the child decide what information to share with strangers, friends, and extended family members.
- Recognize that the adolescent may fantasize about the birth parents and want to find them. Listening to the adolescent's concerns and providing support during this challenging time of development is important.

International Adoptions

Approximately 21,449 children from other countries are adopted yearly by families from the United States (Howard & John, 2009). These children are likely to need healthcare services. Many of them have spent time in orphanages and are at increased risk for developmental delay and emotional problems. Health problems can potentially exist, including infectious diseases (tuberculosis, hepatitis B and C) and parasites. Nurses work with families that have adopted children from other countries to provide a comprehensive evaluation of the child to detect developmental, vision, and hearing delays as well as infectious diseases as soon as the child is brought into the country (Smit, 2010).

Emotional and psychologic problems, such as inconsistency in interpersonal development and delayed developmental milestones, may be the result of long-term institutionalization in an orphanage. The child and family may need counseling and support to help the child adjust to being part of a family. The initial response of the child who has been in an orphanage to the new parents may be crying or turning away. Children need a transition period of several months to adjust to a different daily routine and to bond with the parents. Exposing the child to large numbers of family members or to busy environments may be stressful for the child. The nurse may become involved in providing counseling to the family trying to integrate the adopted child into the family's life and routine. As the child grows, efforts to help the child understand the cultural birth heritage are also important (Figure 2–8 ■). See Developing Cultural Competence: Adopting a Child from a Different Heritage.

FAMILY THEORIES

Families must be understood in their own context. It is important to understand each family's strengths and unique qualities and how the family and its members respond to the complex and often conflicting demands for time and attention.

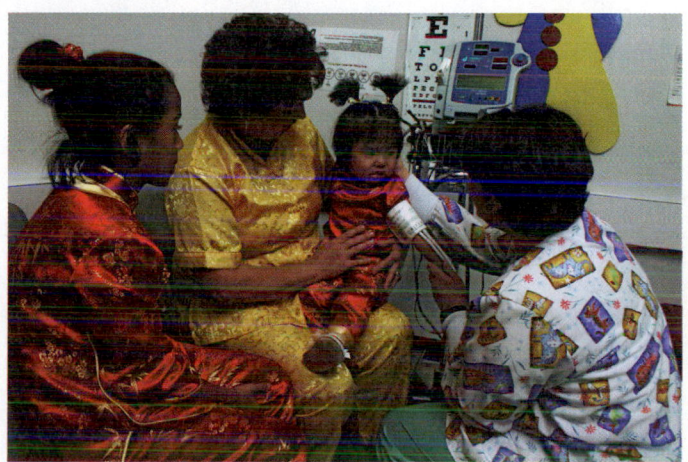

FIGURE 2–8 ■ Adopted children who are of mixed race or a different ethnic group than the parents may cause a few additional challenges for the adoptive parents. Family members may be less supportive of the adoption initially. Because the child may have different physical characteristics, the family may capture more attention than it wishes. The family needs to learn to appreciate the different cultures represented in the newly formed family.

Developing Cultural Competence
Adopting a Child from a Different Heritage

Families adopting a child of another race or culture often want to learn about the traditions of the child's birth culture so they can show respect for and promote an understanding of that culture in the child. This information helps promote the child's development of identity and self-esteem. It is also the responsibility of the parents to involve the adopted child in cultural socialization (Vonk, Lee, & Crolley-Simic, 2010). Strategies to learn and foster an understanding of the child's culture of origin include the following:

- Interact with people of the child's heritage or race—join a cultural association or church and make friends.
- Identify successful professionals from the child's culture who can be role models. Discuss ways to help the child develop an identity within the culture and to interact effectively with members of the culture.
- Live in a multicultural neighborhood. Enroll the child in a school with diversity of students and faculty.
- Learn about the culture through books, magazines, and movies targeted to the cultural group. Identify Internet sites with information and discussions to understand important issues.
- Celebrate special holidays of the cultural group.
- Take family field trips to learn about historical events important to the culture and encourage cultural pride. Help all members of the family develop a bicultural view.

TABLE 2–5	Eight-Stage Family Life Cycle
STAGES	**CHARACTERISTICS**
Stage I	Beginning family, newly married couples*
Stage II	Childbearing family (oldest child is an infant through 30 months of age)
Stage III	Families with preschool children (oldest child is between 2.5 and 6 years of age)
Stage IV	Families with school-age children (oldest child is between 6 and 13 years of age)
Stage V	Families with teenagers (oldest child is between 13 and 20 years of age)
Stage VI	Families launching young adults (all children leave home)
Stage VII	Middle-aged parents (empty nest through retirement)
Stage VIII	Family in retirement and old age (retirement to death of both spouses)

*Keep in mind that this was the norm at the time the model was developed, but today families form through many different types of relationships.

Source: *Adapted from Duvall, E. M. (1977). Marriage and family development (5th ed.). Philadelphia: Lippincott; Duvall, E. M., & Miller, B. C. (1985). Marriage and family development (6th ed.). New York: Harper Row; Friedman, M. M., Bowden, V. R., & Jones, E. G. (2003). Family nursing: Research, theory, and practice (5th ed.). Upper Saddle River, NJ: Prentice Hall; Gedaly-Duff, V., Nielsen, A., Heims, M. L., & Pate, M. D. (2010). Family child health nursing. In J. R. Kaakinen, V. Gedaly-Duff, D. P. Coehlo, & S. M. H. Hanson, Family health care nursing: Theory, practice, and research (4th ed., pp. 332–378). Philadelphia: F. A. Davis.*

Family social system theories are helpful in understanding family functioning, environment–family interchange, family changes over time, and family response to health and illness. A brief review of family theories provides a context about family functioning that can assist with planning nursing care and developing future partnerships with families and their children.

Each family has a structure and functions to help it maintain stability while responding continuously to various stresses and strains, within the family and in the family's interactions and functioning within the community. Families develop and modify their responses and functioning over time to adapt or be tolerant of family, community, and environmental changes. Family processes include the behaviors and strategies that help to regulate space, time, energy, and other aspects of family functioning to promote family stability, growth, and control.

Family Development Theory

Family development theories use a framework to categorize a family's progression over time according to specific, typical stages in family life. These are predictable stages in the life cycle of every family, but they follow no rigid pattern. Duvall's (1977) eight stages in the family life cycle of a traditional nuclear family have been used as the foundation for contemporary models of the family life cycle that describe the developmental processes and role expectations for different family types. Table 2–5 lists Duvall's eight stages to illustrate important developmental transitions that occur at some point in most families.

Life cycle stages have been developed for the more contemporary blended families, dual-career families, and others. Although each family is unique, the members experience fairly predictable, similar, and consistent changes (Friedman, Bowden, & Jones, 2003).

Developmental tasks, goals, or challenging issues for the family in each stage have been defined for different family types.

Nurses can assess families by their development stage, how well they are fulfilling the tasks of that stage, and the availability of resources to accomplish developmental tasks. The stages provide a method for anticipating transitions and potential stressors with family role changes that occur at different points along the developmental continuum for different family types. By understanding the family's developmental stage, the nurse can analyze the family growth and health promotion needs and identify developmental transitions and potential stressors. This enables the nurse to identify the types of teaching and anticipatory guidance that might be needed.

Family Systems Theory

Family systems theory, in which there is interaction between the components (family members) of the system (family) and between the system and the environment, was developed by Murray Bowen in the mid-1970s (Friedman et al., 2003). A family is a living social system, consisting of a small group of individuals who are closely interrelated and interdependent while collaborating to attain family functions and goals. In short, the family is more than the sum of its members (Clark, 2008; Kaakinen & Hanson, 2010). In family systems theory, due to the amount of interrelationship and interdependence in the family, any change or stressor experienced by one or more family members affects the entire family and causes disruption. Families are adaptable, and they can change interactions and behaviors associated with the disruption in response to positive feedback.

From a systems perspective, the family may or may not exchange materials, energy, and information with its physical, social, and cultural environments. An *open family* seeks information and resources, and actively interacts with the community to solve problems. A *closed family* views change and offered support as a threat, and resistance to outside influences is a strategy the family uses to maintain control. These attributes have an effect on the capacity of the family to adapt—to modify behavior and change as the situation demands (Clark, 2008; Kaakinen & Hanson, 2010).

Family systems theory encourages nurses to see the child and parents as participating members of a whole family (Kaakinen & Hanson, 2010). It encourages looking at the processes within the family and the relationships between subsystems (spouse, parent, child, and siblings) and suprasystems (the community within which it is embedded). Stress and crises motivate the family to mobilize its resources and to begin problem solving.

Using this perspective, the nurse can assess the effects of illness or injury on the entire family system and the reciprocal effects of the family on the illness or injury. Assessing how open or closed the family is to information and resources is important in planning nursing care. Open families will be more receptive to referrals and interventions from health professionals. The nurse will need to work with the closed family to establish trust and acceptance before the family is receptive to ideas and interventions proposed.

Family Stress Theory

Family stress theory focuses on the family's response to unexpected or unplanned events. These events are generally stressful and can be very disruptive for the family (Kaakinen & Hanson, 2010). Most families have developed coping strategies to deal with routine stressors (completion of household chores, homework, etc.). Nonroutine stressors (such as surgery or the birth of a child) and unexpected events (accidents or emergency department visits) are often more stressful because the family has not had time to review resources and prepare a response.

Families experience many stressors as an inevitable part of life. Some stressors are positive, such as the birth of a child. Other stressors are unexpected and not considered positive, such as learning that a child has a serious health condition. Many families live in a stressed state due to inadequate finances, healthcare concerns, relationship challenges, and other pressures.

No one theory is sufficient for viewing the needs and behaviors of all families. The theories described here continue to evolve as researchers identify new or broadened explanations for behaviors, so it is difficult to attach one specific theorist to each family theory. When assessing families, you may also find it useful to consider more than one of these theories for particular families to help you understand the full set of behaviors associated with individual families and to plan effective nursing interventions.

FAMILY ASSESSMENT

Nurses need to assess family strengths and support mechanisms, identify strategies for **coping** (the use of learned behavioral and cognitive strategies to manage or relieve perceived stress), and determine when families have overextended their resources and need additional support. In some cases, nurses can provide the additional support needed. At other times, referral to other health professionals is appropriate to address the family's needs.

Children and families live their lives within a variety of settings and interact with those settings in ways that directly or indirectly influence behaviors and learning. Because of these environmental influences on the family, it is important to consider the relationship of the family with the social networks within the community.

Family Stressors

A child's illness or injury affects every member of the family. Such a stressor demands a response from the family members that can change the way they interact with each other and with other people. Nurses need to identify and assess how families respond to the stress of illness or injury of a child, or other family members, because of the potential hardships it causes the entire family.

Clinical Tip

Identify the parent who can legally provide consent for medical treatment when there has been a divorce and potentially a remarriage. In some states, the noncustodial parent cannot give consent. The stepparent cannot give consent unless the custodial parent grants written permission. Stepparents or other family members may also not know the child's medical history. Identify the legal framework for informed consent with regard to these children so that care is provided in an appropriate and responsible manner.

Family Strengths

Family strengths are the positive relationships and processes that support and protect families and family members during times of adversity and change. Nurses can use family strengths as an effective tool in problem solving within the family (Wright & Leahey, 2009).

An important focus for family assessment prior to planning nursing interventions is to identify the family's **resilience,** its capacity to develop strengths and abilities, to "bounce back" from the stress and challenges. When a family can control and deal with events satisfactorily, its members gain a sense of competence, making them more resilient, in contrast to families who are overwhelmed by traumatic experiences. Characteristics of a resilient family include (Benard, 2007):

- Social competence, involving cultural flexibility, empathy, and caring
- Developing competence in communication skills
- Problem solving that involves planning, help seeking, and critical and creative thinking that enables them to make decisions
- Maintaining family flexibility and adapting to changing circumstances, while maintaining a commitment to the family as a unit
- Having a sense of purpose and belief in a positive outcome (can set goals, have optimism and faith)
- Connectedness and maintenance of supportive relationships outside the family

Most families have the capacity for resilience. However, they often need nursing support to help family members learn new skills, make adaptations, and gain confidence in their abilities to manage new challenges. Potential resources to foster resilience include religious faith, finances, social support, physical health, family flexibility, and family coping mechanisms. Families with diminished resources will be more susceptible to disruption because of a healthcare crisis or event. Nurses need to help families identify their strengths, as well as areas for improvement that will lead to increased resiliency.

Functional families use their strengths and a variety of coping strategies to successfully reduce stress. Coping strategies of

TABLE 2–6	Coping Strategies Used by Functional Families and Dysfunctional Families

FUNCTIONAL FAMILY COPING STRATEGIES	DYSFUNCTIONAL FAMILY COPING STRATEGIES
■ Family relationships—increased structure and organization within the home and family, strengthening family cohesion, and increased role flexibility of family members	■ Denial of family problems
■ Gathering information and knowledge, family joint problem solving	■ Exploitation of family members such as by scapegoating (negatively labeling and stigmatizing a family member, often a child) to avoid examining the real problem in the family
■ **Normalization**—the process of family management that involves acknowledging a life-changing situation, such as a child having a chronic health problem, but making an effort to lead a normal life (Family life is normal because the impact of the condition on the family functioning is minimized as demonstrated by behaviors, rituals, and routines that show others that the family is normal.)	■ Use of threat or withdrawal of affection and support to keep family members together at the expense of the emotional health of its members
■ Passive acceptance about an event or situation about which little or nothing can be done and determining that it will take care of itself over time	■ Myths or images the family has of itself that obscure reality and enable the family to deny some of its problems
■ Direct, open, honest, and clear communication	■ Extreme dominance and submission patterns
■ Use of humor and laughter	■ Family addictions (drug or alcohol)
■ Maintaining active linkages with the community and using social support networks	■ Domestic violence (partner, child, sibling to sibling, and elder abuse)
■ Spiritual supports	

Source: *Data from Friedman, M. M., Bowden, V. R., & Jones, E. G. (2003).* Family nursing: Research, theory, and practice *(5th ed., pp. 476–494). Upper Saddle River, NJ: Prentice Hall.*

dysfunctional families are defensive and do not effectively manage the stress. See Table 2–6 for coping strategies used by functional and dysfunctional families.

Nurses can use recognition of family strengths to develop rapport with the family. One approach is to help family members recognize that the strengths they have used in prior life experiences can apply to the current healthcare experience. Focus on family competence and acknowledge and validate family members' emotions. See Box 2–5 for types of family strengths. The more a family recognizes its strengths in managing the child's healthcare problem, the more likely that family will become an effective partner in the process.

Collecting Data for Family Assessment

To obtain an accurate and concise family assessment, establish a trusting relationship with the child and family. Identify the parent's and the child's greatest concern, and expect these concerns to be different. It is important to acknowledge these multiple concerns and demonstrate respect for the diversity of the family. The goal is to obtain family information that will be helpful in planning nursing interventions designed to help the family care for the child and improve the child's outcomes while valuing each person within the family.

During the healthcare process, information about the family is collected continuously through interviews, observations of the family interactions, reports from other healthcare providers or agencies working with the family, and a family assessment tool. See Box 2–6 for family assessment information to collect. (See Chapter 7 🔗 for suggested psychosocial history data collection and Box 7–3, Daily Living Patterns, as family assessment information is also obtained during the child's health history.) Observation of the home and family members is recommended in some cases to obtain valuable information about family functioning.

Family Assessment Tools

Family assessment tools help us to gather additional information about the family's functioning, with particular focus on family stresses, coping strategies, and family strengths. Nurses collect information about the way the family functions—in nurturing its

BOX 2–5	Family Strengths Helpful in Managing Stressors

- **Communication skills.** The ability of family members to listen and to discuss their concerns
- **Shared family values and beliefs.** The family's common perceptions of reality and willingness to have hope and to appreciate that change is possible
- **Intrafamily support.** The provision of support and reinforcement by extended family members, as well as establishing an atmosphere of belonging
- **Self-care abilities.** The family's ability to take responsibility for health problems and the demonstrated willingness of individual members to take good care of themselves
- **Problem-solving skill.** The family's use of negotiation in problem solving, using everyday experiences as resources, and focusing on the present rather than past events or disappointments

BOX 2–6	Family Assessment Information to Collect

- Name, age, sex, and family relationship of all people residing in the household
- Family type, structure, roles, and values
- Cultural associations, including cultural norms and customs related to childrearing and infant feeding
- Faith-based affiliations
- Support systems network, including extended family, friends, and faith-based and community associations
- Communication patterns, including language barriers
- Environmental data—place of residence, condition of housing, number of persons living in the residence, sleeping arrangements, play areas, and neighborhood characteristics

members, problem solving, and communicating—to help identify strategies that are potentially more effective for management of the child's health care. These tools enable the nurse to work more effectively with the family, such as collaborating with the family in planning for health maintenance and health promotion strategies.

Genogram

Information about family structure can be illustrated on a **genogram** (a pedigree that incorporates information about the family members' significant life events, health, and illness status over at least three generations). See Figure 4–12 on page 96 ⊘. A genogram is used most often to focus on the health history of a family, although additional identifying features such as social class, occupation, place of residence, religion, and ethnicity may be added for the family assessment process.

Family Ecomap

By illustrating the family's relationships and interactions with social networks in the community, an **ecomap** enables nurses and other healthcare providers to visualize the family's social network. Family participation in the preparation of the ecomap may reveal information about how the family perceives or receives social support, as well as the strength of family relationships with significant other persons and organizations. The ecomap provides an opportunity to identify the community resources being used by the family and to highlight any potential community resources that may help promote the family's health. Figure 2–9 ■ shows a sample ecomap for Casey's family.

Family APGAR

The **family APGAR** is a quick five-item questionnaire measuring family adaptability, partnership, growth, affection, and resolve. Used as an initial screening tool for family assessment (Table 2–7), the questionnaire can be administered quickly to family members over 10 years of age (Smilkstein, Ashworth, & Montano, 1982). Ask all family members to complete a separate copy of the questionnaire to gain a picture of the family's perspective on family functioning. Be more concerned if the majority of responses fall in the "hardly ever" category or responses vary widely among family members. This may indicate a family that needs much more support to cope with the demands of daily life and management of the child's condition. This tool continues to be used to assess family functioning (Preechawong, Zauszniewki, Heinzer, et al., 2007).

Home Observation for Measurement of the Environment

The Home Observation for Measurement of the Environment (HOME) is an assessment tool developed to measure the quality and quantity of stimulation and support available to the child in the home environment (Caldwell & Bradley, 1984). The tool is also used to identify relationships between the home environment and the child's development (Totsika & Sylva, 2004). Four age-specific scales are available: birth to 3 years, 3 to 6 years, 6 to 10 years, and 10 to 15 years. Each age-specific scale includes subscales, such as parental responsivity, acceptance of child, the physical environment, learning materials, variety in experience, and parental involvement. Data are collected during an informal, low-stress interview and observation

Ecomap of Casey's Family

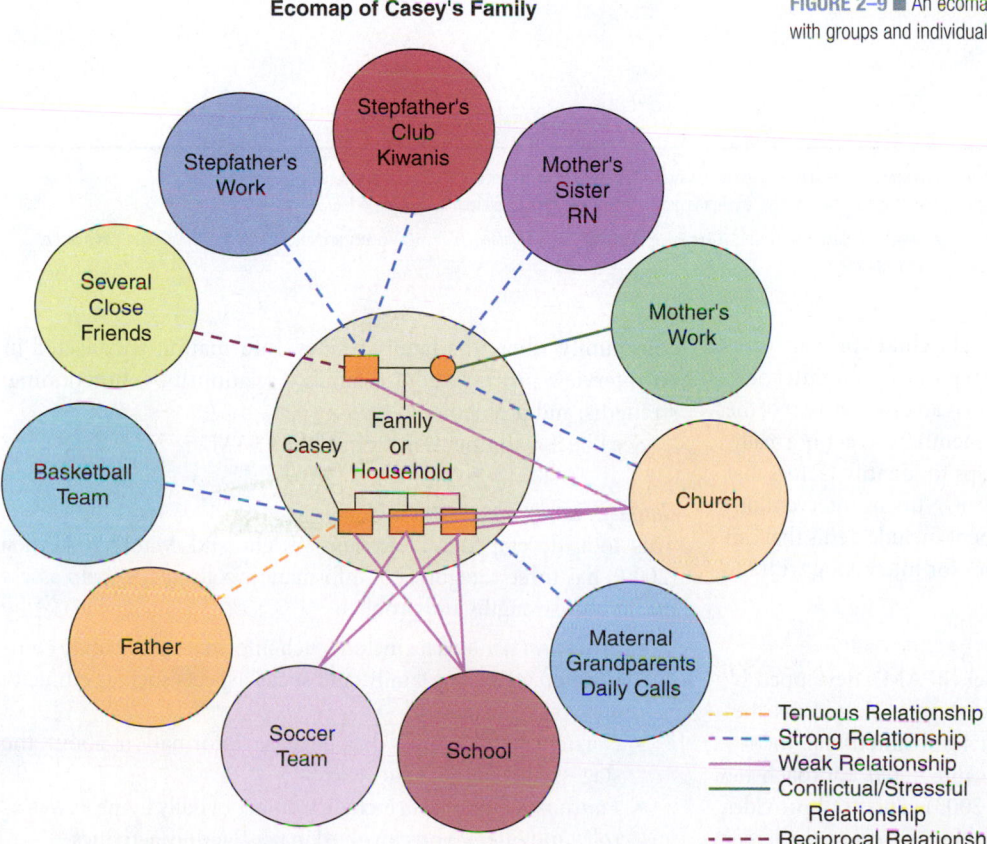

FIGURE 2–9 ■ An ecomap illustrates the family's relationships and interactions with groups and individuals in the immediate external environment.

TABLE 2–7	The Family APGAR Questionnaire

Directions

The following questions have been designed to help us better understand you and your family. You should feel free to ask questions about any item in the questionnaire.

Comment space should be used if you wish to give additional information or if you wish to discuss the way the question is applied to your family. Please try to answer all questions. *Family* is defined as the individual(s) with whom you usually live. If you live alone, your family consists of persons with whom you now have the strongest emotional ties.

For each question, check only one box.

	ALMOST ALWAYS 2	SOME OF THE TIME 1	HARDLY EVER 0
I am satisfied that I can turn to my family for help when something is troubling me. Comments:			
I am satisfied with the way my family talks over things with me and shares problems with me. Comments:			
I am satisfied that my family accepts and supports my wishes to take on new activities or directions. Comments:			
I am satisfied with the way my family expresses affection and responds to my emotions, such as anger, sorrow, and love. Comments:			
I am satisfied with the way my family and I share time together. Comments:			

According to which member of the family is being interviewed, the interviewer may substitute for the word family *either* spouse, significant other, parents, *or* children.

Responses are scored (2, 1, or 0) and added. The total score ranges from 0 to 10. The larger the score, the greater amount of satisfaction with family functioning.

Source: *Directions and scoring information adapted from and chart reprinted with permission from Smilkstein, G., Ashworth, C., & Montano, D. (1982). Validity and reliability of the family APGAR as a test of family function.* Journal of Family Practice, 15*(2), 303–311; Dowden Health Media.*

over 45 to 90 minutes in the home setting. The child's primary caregiver and child must be present and awake during the interview. Observation of the parent–child interaction is an essential part of the assessment. The intent is to allow family members to act normally. Assessment of the home environment helps to identify factors that promote the child's growth and development. Nursing interventions that could result from the HOME assessment include items that can be used in the home for toys and strategies for interacting with the child to promote learning.

Friedman Family Assessment Model

The Friedman Family Assessment Model (FFAM), developed by Marilyn Friedman, comprises elements of general systems theory, family developmental theory, structural-functional theory, and cross-cultural theory to provide an integrated approach for assessment of families (Friedman et al., 2003). This tool provides a method to examine the whole family in the context of the larger

community where the family resides. Information is collected in an interview process about a family's relationships, functioning, strengths, and problems.

See Box 2–7 for the short form of the FFAM.

Calgary Family Assessment Model

This tool, developed by Lorraine Wright and Maureen Leahey (2009), has three categories of information collected to help assess the family's strengths and problems.

- *Structural* family data include such information as family composition, extended family, and social aspects such as ethnicity and spirituality.
- *Developmental* family data include information about the stages of the family's life cycle.
- *Functional* family data include routines of daily living as well as roles and interactions involved in usual family activities.

BOX 2–7	The Friedman Family Assessment Model (Short Form)

The following form is shortened for ease in assessing a family. If you are not sure what data should be covered in each of the assessment areas below, please refer to the original reference where more detailed questions/areas are presented.

Before using the following guidelines in completing family assessments, note that not all areas included below will be germane for each of the families visited. The guidelines are comprehensive and allow depth when probing is necessary. Do not feel that every subarea needs to be covered when the broad area of inquiry poses no problems to the family or concern to the health worker. Second, by virtue of the interdependence of the family system, one will find unavoidable redundancy. The assessor should try not to repeat data, but to refer the reader back to sections where this information has already been described.

IDENTIFYING DATA

1. Family Name
2. Address and Phone
3. Family Composition: The Family Genogram
4. Type of Family Form
5. Cultural (Ethnic) Background
6. Religious Identification
7. Social Class Status
8. Social Class Mobility

DEVELOPMENTAL STAGE AND HISTORY OF FAMILY

9. Family's Present Developmental Stage
10. Extent of Family Developmental Tasks Fulfillment
11. Nuclear Family History
12. History of Family of Origin of Both Parents

ENVIRONMENTAL DATA

13. Characteristics of Home
14. Characteristics of Neighborhood and Larger Community
15. Family's Geographical Mobility
16. Family's Associations and Transactions with Community

FAMILY STRUCTURE

17. Communication Patterns
    Extent of Functional and Dysfunctional Communication (types of recurring patterns)
    Extent of Emotional (Affective) Messages and How Expressed
    Characteristics of Communication Within Family Subsystems
    Extent of Congruent and Incongruent Messages
    Types of Dysfunctional Communication Processes Seen in Family
    Areas of Closed Communication
    Familial and Contextual Variables Affecting Communication

18. Power Structure
    Power Outcomes
    Decision-making Process
    Power Bases
    Variables Affecting Family Power
    Overall Family System and Subsystem Power (Family Power Continuum Placement)

19. Role Structure
    Formal Role Structure
    Informal Role Structure
    Analysis of Role Models (optional)
    Variables Affecting Role Structure

20. Family Values
    Compare the Family to American Core Values or Family's Reference Group Values and/or Identify Important Family Values and Their Importance (priority) in Family.

Congruence Between the Family's Values and the Family's Reference Group or Wider Community
Disparity in Value Systems
Presence of Value Conflicts in Family
Effect of the Above Values and Value Conflicts on Health
Status of Family

FAMILY FUNCTIONS

21. Affective Function
    Mutual Nurturance, Closeness, and Identification
    Separateness and Connectedness
    Family's Need–Response Patterns

22. Socialization Function
    Family Child-rearing Practices
    Adaptability of Child-rearing Practices for Family Form and Family's Situation
    Who Is (Are) Socializing Agent(s) for Child(ren)?
    Value of Children in Family
    Cultural Beliefs That Influence Family's Child-rearing Patterns
    Social Class Influence on Child-rearing Patterns
    Estimation About Whether Family Is at Risk for Child-rearing Problems and If So, Indication of High-Risk Factors
    Adequacy of Home Environment for Children's Needs to Play

23. Health Care Function
    Family's Health Beliefs, Values, and Behavior
    Family's Definitions of Health–Illness and Its Level of Knowledge
    Family's Perceived Health Status and Illness Susceptibility
    Family's Dietary Practices
    Adequacy of Family Diet (recommended 3-day food history record)
    Function of Mealtimes and Attitudes toward Food and Mealtimes
    Shopping (and its planning) Practices
    Person(s) Responsible for Planning, Shopping, and Preparation of Meals
    Sleep and Rest Habits
    Physical Activity and Recreation Practices
    Family's Therapeutic and Recreational Drug, Alcohol, and Tobacco Practices
    Family's Role in Self-care Practices
    Medically Based Preventive Measures (physicals, eye and hearing tests, immunizations, dental care)
    Complementary and Alternative Therapies
    Family Health History (both general and specific diseases— environmentally and genetically related)
    Health Care Services Received
    Feelings and Perceptions Regarding Health Services
    Emergency Health Services
    Source of Payments for Health and Other Services
    Logistics of Receiving Care

FAMILY STRESS, COPING, AND ADAPTATION

24. Family Stressors, Strengths, and Perceptions
    Stressors Family Is Experiencing
    Strengths That Counterbalance Stressors
    Family's Definition of the Situation

25. Family Coping Strategies
    How the Family Is Reacting to the Stressors
    Extent of Family's Use of Internal Coping Strategies (past/present)
    Extent of Family's Use of External Coping Strategies (past/present)
    Dysfunctional Coping Strategies Utilized (past/present; extent of use)

26. Family Adaptation
    Overall Family Adaptation
    Estimation of Whether Family Is in Crisis

27. Tracking Stressors, Coping, and Adaptation Over Time

Source: *From Friedman, M. M., Bowden, V. R., & Jones, E. G. (2003).* Family nursing: Research, theory, and practice *(5th ed., pp. 593–594). Reprinted and electronically reproduced by permission of Pearson Education, Inc., Upper Saddle River, N.J: Prentice Hall.*

The model enables assessment of extensive information about the family, but the originators of the model encourage focusing on specific data collection that matches the challenges that exist in the family, such as transitions of a child through adolescence or problems in managing a treatment plan within the family's routines. A family genogram or ecomap is also considered helpful in completing the assessment and ultimately in promoting a positive working relationship with the family (Wright & Leahey, 2009).

FAMILY SUPPORT SERVICES

Family support services exist in all communities with a purpose of supporting families in the rearing of healthy children. Contemporary lifestyles stress families trying to provide for their children's needs because of many factors, including divorced or single parents, both parents being in the workforce, more time each day that parents and children are separated, and families separated from extended families and natural support systems. Families may also be stressed by economic factors, poor living conditions, or even homelessness. Many communities have worked to develop social support programs to support the health and development of children and to promote positive family relationships. Examples of these family support services include the following:

- Head Start and Early Head Start
- Before- and after-school programs for children of working parents
- School-based health and counseling services
- Play groups for preschool children
- Peer support groups
- Social service programs offered by the faith community
- Home visiting programs for high-risk children and parents
- Job skills training, adult education, and literacy programs
- Crisis care and respite care programs
- Funding for military family support programs

Many of these family support services work to promote positive family relationships, parental competencies, and behaviors that contribute to the health and development of the children and family. Most programs are designed with the premise that no family is entirely self-sufficient and most can benefit from some external support.

Think about the formal and informal family support services in your community. Nurses play an important role in linking families to community support services after performing a family assessment and collaborating with families to identify and seek assistance most beneficial to their needs.

Nursing Management

The goal of family-centered nursing management is to assess and help families recognize their strengths and resiliency. This information can be used in collaboratively planning the nursing care with the child and family members.

Nursing Assessment and Diagnoses

The presence of a newly acquired disability, as occurred in Casey's family, adds a dimension of developmental risk. The child and family members may respond with either psychologic or behavioral problems, or they may respond in a more positive manner.

Collect the psychosocial history and daily living patterns data from the family and child. Assessment of the culturally diverse child and family additionally includes determining the family's healthcare practices such as health traditions, health beliefs, health-seeking behaviors, healthcare practitioner, and religion or spirituality.

Select the appropriate family assessment tool to collect information that can help evaluate the family's strengths and resources. Analyze the information collected and focus on key information that will help develop a plan of care for the child and family. Follow these steps:

- Determine how this condition influences family functioning.
- Identify how all of the family members have responded to the child's acute condition and disability.
- Obtain information about how the family is considering management of the child's care at home.
- Determine if other family issues or stressors must be integrated into the plan of care.
- Identify the family's expectations of different health professionals and facilities to help manage the child's care.
- Prepare an ecomap and genogram.

Examples of nursing diagnoses that may result from the family and home assessment include:

- Coping: Family, Compromised related to multiple simultaneous stressors
- Family Processes, Interrupted related to child with a significant disability requiring alteration in family functioning
- Caregiver Role Strain, Risk for related to child with a newly acquired disability and the associated financial burden
- Social Interaction, Impaired (parents and child) related to lack of family or respite support
- Parenting, Readiness for Enhanced related to well child care

NANDA-I © 2012

Planning and Implementation

Like all families, Casey's family needs support to increase resources and coping behaviors so they can successfully manage the multiple stressors of daily living along with a child's chronic condition.

Establishing a therapeutic relationship with the family is an important intervention. This relationship should be characterized by empathy and trust, as well as the development of mutually identified goals for the child's care. To help families develop resiliency, focus on family competence and strengths. Acknowledge and validate their emotions. Provide information in a clear, timely, and sensitive manner. Ask questions that help direct the family's thinking rather than providing them with all of the answers. Work with families by teaching them to identify solutions until they are able to solve problems without assistance. It may be helpful for them to meet other families who have faced similar situations.

Assist the family to begin planning for ongoing care using family-centered principles:

- Identify the primary decision maker for the child's health care.
- Discuss the family's goals for managing the child's health care in the home setting.
- Consider how the family's strengths and previous family problem-solving experiences can be integrated into the intervention.

- Consider the family's ethnic and religious background in developing intervention recommendations. Partner with the child and family to assist them in determining how they can incorporate prescribed therapies with their religious or cultural practices. Ensure that the child and family understand the child's illness, treatment, or health promotion. Apply culturally sensitive techniques when dispelling any cultural myths. (See Developing Cultural Competence: Healthcare Providers.)

- Offer the family one or more potential interventions rather than trying to force one intervention. Be open to modifying the intervention or devising an alternative intervention to better match the family's lifestyle preferences.

- Identify what type of support or assistance the family would like to have.

- Identify potential resources in the community that match the child's and the family's needs for support. Collaborate with the family to discuss those resources and to select those that are acceptable to the family.

- Make sure the family has a care coordinator, especially when a family member seems to be unable to assume the case management role initially. Assist families in obtaining resources through such actions as role rehearsal, providing instructions and support when making an initial call, or connecting with

---

Developing Cultural Competence
Healthcare Providers

When appropriate, collaborate with the family to determine the role traditional healthcare providers and other practitioners, such as folk healers, curanderos or curanderas, and spiritualists, will have in the care of the child. Encourage collaboration and communication between practitioners to ensure continuity of care.

---

another family support person who can help with resource linkage.

- Refer families with moderate or severe dysfunction to community resources for social support and counseling as appropriate.

Evaluation

Expected outcomes of nursing care include:

- Collaboration of the child and family with an assigned case manager
- Implementations of interventions as recommended by the nurse and healthcare team
- Appropriate care provided by the family to the child with an acquired disability

---

Chapter Highlights

- A family is composed of individuals who are joined together by marriage, blood, adoption, or residence in the same household, sharing resources and emotional closeness. Family membership often changes over time.

- Family-centered care is the development of a mutually beneficial partnership between families and the nurse, and also other health professionals. Each party respects the knowledge, skills, and experience that the other brings to the healthcare encounter. Partnering with families in the provision of health care is essential to promote the best outcome when caring for children.

- Various family composition models are common in today's society, including nuclear families, extended families, blended or reconstituted families, single-parent families, binuclear families, heterosexual cohabiting families, and gay and lesbian families.

- Health-related events may cause unexpected stresses for the parents, such as changed relationships with their parents, changes regarding employment, and lifestyle changes.

- Positive family relationships are characterized by parent–child warmth and supportiveness, and these traits help buffer children from stress while promoting positive social and cognitive outcomes.

- Parenting is a leadership role in the family in which children are guided to learn acceptable behaviors, beliefs, morals, and rituals of the family, and to become socially responsible contributing members of society.

- Discipline is a method for teaching the rules that govern behavior or conduct. Punishment is the action taken to enforce the rules when a child misbehaves.

- The quality of the relationship between the divorced parents has an important impact on their future relationships with their children. Better maintenance of

family and kinship ties results when divorced parents are able to minimize the conflict and continue sharing parenting.

- Stepparenting that involves the blending of two families leads to the need to identify and renegotiate new customs, traditions, rituals, and routines for the family. A child must adjust to the stepparent, and the stepparent to the child.

- The goal of foster care is to ensure the safety and well-being of vulnerable children by placing them in an approved living situation away from the family of origin that is legally coordinated by the state's child welfare system.

- Adoption is a legal relationship between a child and parents not related by birth in which the parents assume legal and financial responsibility for the child. Many children are adopted from foreign nations.

- Family social systems theories help in understanding the family functioning, environment–family interchange, family changes over time, and family response to health and illness.

- Resilience is the family's capacity to develop strengths and abilities to bounce back from the stresses and challenges faced, and to eliminate or minimize negative outcomes.

- Family strengths are the relationships and processes that support and protect families and family members during times of adversity and change. These strengths enable families to develop, adapt to change, and cope with challenges.

- Family assessment tools are used to gather information about the family's functioning with regard to characteristics such as nurturing its members, problem solving, and communication. Information gathered helps the nurse work more effectively with the family in meeting the child's healthcare needs.

Clinical Reasoning in Action

INTRODUCTION

Reflect back to the scenario about Casey and his family at the beginning of the chapter, and review the ecomap on page 47. Casey's family is coping with his initial survival of a serious brain injury, and facing a long rehabilitation process. Family members are just now recognizing that life as they have known it is changing.

DESCRIPTION

Casey is totally dependent on others for care including bathing, toileting, feeding, and mobilizing. Although he is expected to regain self-care abilities, the impact of the injury on his cognitive ability and future functioning is unknown.

Casey's extended family has provided support to the family during the past 12 days, but the level of support in the future weeks will decrease because of other family obligations. Casey's aunt, a nurse, has been especially helpful to his family during the initial crisis. Casey's mother has already initiated a leave of absence from work so she can care for him when he returns home; however, this will mean the family has reduced income during that time. Casey's sister, Teresa, will try to earn more money baby-sitting to help the family out. Casey's younger brothers have been able to visit him, but they are very anxious because

Casey cannot talk with them. They have been trying to avoid bothering their mother and father during this time, but they wonder when life will be more normal and they can again participate in their usual after-school activities.

DISCUSSION

1. What information about family strengths, needs, and resilience can be identified from the scenario, the information on page 45, the ecomap on page 47, and the information above?

2. What additional information would be helpful to know about family strengths and needs prior to developing a nursing care plan?

3. Based on your assessment of the family and challenges facing them, list at least one nursing diagnosis (in addition to those listed on page 50) that addresses an issue important for planning nursing care for Casey and his family.

4. Describe the use of family-centered care principles in planning Casey's nursing care in collaboration with the family.

5. What potential parenting issues could this family anticipate for Casey and his brothers?

NCLEX-RN® Review

1. A mother who uses time-out as a method of discipline for her 5-year-old child is asking the nurse what type of parenting this exemplifies. What response would be the most appropriate?
   1. Indifferent
   2. Authoritative
   3. Authoritarian
   4. Permissive

2. A 16-year-old male begins to act out in school, and his teacher observes a sudden drop in his grades. Knowing this adolescent was adopted 10 years ago, which indicates what might be causing these behavioral changes?
   1. Industry versus inferiority
   2. Trust versus mistrust
   3. Identity versus role confusion
   4. Intimacy versus isolation

3. A nurse is caring for a 4-year-old child in a pediatric clinic. The child's parents both work and have mentioned they are having financial difficulties and can no longer afford a private babysitter. Which support service would be the most appropriate for the nurse to recommend to this family?
   1. School-based counseling services
   2. Play groups
   3. Head Start or Early Head Start
   4. Home visiting programs

4. The father of a 9-year-old Orthodox Jewish patient has requested a kosher diet for his son during his hospitalization. Which statement by the nurse indicates that she is sensitive to the cultural needs of this family?
   1. "I will call the kitchen and see if they can provide a kosher meal."
   2. "Just make sure your child does not eat anything not kosher."
   3. "I will place the order for a kosher diet. I will check with you when his meal comes to make sure he received the appropriate foods."
   4. "The physician ordered a regular diet and that is what I must enter into the computer."

See Appendix I 🔗 for answers.

References

Adoption.com. (2010). *Summary of the Adoption and Safe Families Act of 1997*. Retrieved from http://library.adoption.com/articles/summary-of-the-adoption-and-safe-families-act-of-1997.html

Amato, P. R. (2007). The impact of family formation change on the cognitive, social, and emotional well-being of the next generation. *International Child and*

Youth Care Network: CYC-Online, Issue 102. Retrieved from http://www.cyc-net.org/cyc-online/cycol-0707-amato.html

American Academy of Child and Adolescent Psychiatry. (2008). *Children and divorce*. Retrieved from http://www.aacap.org/cs/root/facts_for_families/children_and_divorce

Arai, Y.-C. P., Ito, H., Kandatsu, N., Kurokawa, S., Kinugasa, S., & Komatsu, T. (2007). Parental presence during induction enhances the effect of oral midazolam on emergence behavior of children undergoing general anesthesia. *Acta Anaesthesiologica Scandinavica, 51*, 858–861.

Barba, B. E., Tesh, A. S., Cowen, K., & Hancock, D. (2010). Older adults: What every pediatric nurse should know. *Childcare in Practice, 16*(3), 275–286.

Baumrind, D. (2005). Patterns of parental authority and adolescent autonomy. *New Directions for Child and Adolescent Development, 108*, 61–69.

Benard, B. (2007). *The foundations of the resiliency framework: From research to practice.* Retrieved from http://www.resiliency.com/htm/research.htm

Borchers, D., & Committee on Early Childhood, Adoption, and Dependent Care, American Academy of Pediatrics. (2003). Families and adoption: The pediatrician's role in supporting communication. *Pediatrics, 112*(6), 1437–1441.

Bowen, D. M. (2008). The parent trap: Differential familial power in same-sex families. *William and Mary Journal of Women and the Law, 15*(1), 1–49.

Bright Futures. (2008a). Families + health-care professionals = Partners for healthy children. Retrieved from http://brightfutures.aap.org/pdfs/familypartnership.pdf

Bright Futures. (2008b). Promoting family support. *Bright Futures: Guidelines for health supervision of infants, children and adolescents.* Retrieved from http://brightfutures.aap.org/pdfs/Guidelines_PDF/2-BF_Promoting_Family_Support.pdf

Bruskas, D. (2008). Children in foster care: A vulnerable population. *Journal of Child and Adolescent Psychiatric Nursing, 21*(2), 70–77.

Caldwell, B. M., & Bradley, R. H. (1984). *The home observation for measurement of the environment.* Little Rock: University of Arkansas.

Chamberlain, J., Miller, M. K., & Bornstein, B. H. (2008). The rights and responsibilities of gay and lesbian parents: Legal developments, psychological research, and policy implications. *Society for the Psychological Study of Social Issues, 2*(1), 103–126.

Childstats.gov. (2009). *America's children: Key national indicators of well-being, 2009.* Retrieved from http://www.childstats.gov/americaschildren/famsoc1.asp

Clark, M. J. (2008). Care of families. In M. J. Clark, *Community health nursing: Advocacy for population health* (5th ed., pp. 317–348). Upper Saddle River, NJ: Pearson Prentice Hall.

Craig, G. J., & Dunn, W. L. (2010). *Understanding human development* (2nd ed.). Upper Saddle River, NJ: Pearson Prentice Hall.

Dingeman, R. S., Mitchell, E. A., Meyer, E. C., & Curley, M. A. Q. (2007). Parent presence during complex invasive procedures and cardiopulmonary resuscitation: A systematic review of the literature. *Pediatrics, 120*, 842–854.

Douglas, E. (2006). *The effects of divorce on children.* University of New Hampshire Cooperative Extension. Retrieved from http://ceinfo.unh.edu

Dupuis, S. (2010). Examining the blended family: The application of systems theory toward an understanding of the blended family system. *Journal of Couple and Relationship Therapy, 9*, 239–251.

Duvall, E. M. (1977). *Marriage and family development* (5th ed.). New York: Harper & Row.

Duvall, E. M., & Miller, B. L. (1985). *Marriage and family development* (6th ed.). New York: Harper & Row.

Evan B. Donaldson Adoption Institute. (2008). *Expanding resources for waiting children II: Eliminating legal and practice barriers to gay and lesbian adoption from foster care. Policy & practice perspective.* Retrieved from http://www.adoptioninstitute.org/publications/2008_09_Expanding_Resources_Legal.pdf

Friedman, M. M., Bowden, V. R., & Jones, E. G. (2003). *Family nursing: Research, theory, and practice* (5th ed.). Upper Saddle River, NJ: Prentice Hall.

Gedaly-Duff, V., Heims, M. L., & Nielsen, A. E. (2010). Family child health nursing. In J. R. Kaakinen, V. Gedaly-Duff, D. P. Coehlo, & S. M. H. Hanson, *Family health care nursing: Theory, practice, and research* (4th ed., pp. 332–378). Philadelphia: F. A. Davis.

Gershoff, E. T., Lansford, J. E., Zelli, A., Grogan-Kaylor, A., Chang, L., Deater-Deckard, K., & Dodge, K. A. (2010). Parent discipline practices in an international sample: Association with child behaviors and moderation by perceived normativeness. *Child Development, 81*(2), 487–502.

Giger, J. N., & Davidhizar, R. E. (2008). *Transcultural nursing: Assessment & intervention* (5th ed.). St. Louis, MO: Mosby Elsevier.

Goode, T. D., Haywood, S. H., Wells, N., & Rhee, K. (2009). Family-centered, culturally, and linguistically competent care: Essential components of the medical home. *Pediatric Annals, 38*(9), 505–512.

Hicks-Pass, S. (2009). Corporal punishment in America today: Spare the rod, spoil the child? Systematic review of the literature. *Best Practices in Mental Health, 5*(2), 71–88.

Howard, C. R., & John, C. C. (2009). International adoptions. *Travelers Health-Yellow Book.* Retrieved from http://www.nc.cdc.gov/travel/yellowbook/2010/chapter-7/international-adoptions.aspx

Institute for Patient- and Family-Centered Care. (2011). *Patient and family resource centers.* Retrieved from http://www.ipfcc.org/advance/topics/pafam-resource.html

Jones, M., Qazi, M., & Young, K. D. (2007). Ethnic differences in parent preference to be present for painful medical procedures. *Pediatrics, 116*(2), 191–197.

Kaakinen, J. R., & Hanson, S. M. H. (2010). Theoretical foundations for the nursing of families. In J. R. Kaakinen, V. Gedaly-Duff, D. P. Coehlo, & S. M. H. Hanson (Eds.), *Family health care nursing: Theory, practice and research* (4th ed., pp. 63–102). Philadelphia: F. A. Davis.

Kalil, A., & Ryan, R. M. (2010). Mothers' economic conditions and sources of support in fragile families. *Future of Children, 2*(2), 39–61.

Kreider, R. M., & Elliott, D. B. (2009). America's families and living arrangements: 2007. *Current Population Reports.* Washington, DC: U.S. Census Bureau.

Lauver, L. S. (2008). Parenting foster children with chronic illness and complex medical needs. *Journal of Family Nursing, 14*(1), 74–96.

Lewandowski, L. A., & Tesler, M. D. (Eds.). (2003). *Family-centered care: Putting it into action. The SPN/ANA guide to family-centered care.* Washington, DC: American Nurses Association.

Linsk, N., Mason, S., Fendrich, M., Bass, M., Prubhughate, P., & Brown, A. (2009). "No matter what I do they still want their family": Stressors for African American grandparents and other relatives. *Journal of Family Social Work, 12*, 25–43.

Maccoby, E. E. (1980). *Social development: Psychological growth and the parent-child relationship.* New York: Harcourt Brace Jovanovich.

Marcellus, L. (2010). Supporting resilience in foster families: A model for program design that supports recruitment, retention, and satisfaction of foster families who care for infants with prenatal substance exposure. *Child Welfare, 89*(1), 7–29.

Maxton, F. J. C. (2008). Parental presence during resuscitation in the PICU: the parents' experience. Sharing and surviving the resuscitation: a phenomenological study. *Journal of Clinical Nursing, 17*, 3168–3176.

Moretz, J. G. (2010). Strengthening patient- and family-centered care: Learning through webinars. *Pediatric Nursing, 36*(3), 168–170.

O'Malley, P. J., Brown, K., & Krug, S. E. and the Committee on Pediatric Emergency Medicine. (2008). Patient- and family-centered care of children in the emergency department. *Pediatrics, 122*(2), e511–e521.

Portnoy, S. M. (2008). The psychology of divorce: A lawyer's primer, Part 2: The effects of divorce on children. *American Journal of Family Law, 21*(4), 126–134.

Preechawong, S., Zauszniewski, J. A., Heinzer, M. M. V., Musil, C. M., Kercsmar, C., & Aswinanonh, R. (2007). Relationships of family functioning, self-esteem, and resourceful coping of Thai adolescents with asthma. *Issues in Mental Health Nursing, 28*, 21–36.

Pruitt, L. M., Johnson, A., Elliott, J. C., & Polley, K. (2008). Parental presence during invasive procedures. *Journal of Pediatric Health Care, 22*(2), 120–127.

Purnell, L. D., & Paulanka, B. J. (2008). *Transcultural health care: A culturally competent approach* (3rd ed.). Philadelphia: F. A. Davis.

Raphel, S. (2008). Kinship care and the situation for grandparents. *Journal of Child and Adolescent Psychiatric Nursing, 21*(2), 118–120.

Schneiderman, J. U. (2006). Innovative pediatric nursing role: Public health nurses in child welfare. *Pediatric Nursing, 32*(4), 317–321.

Shore, R., & Shore, B. (2009). Increasing the percentage of children living in two-parent families. *Annie E. Casey Foundation Kids Count Indicator Brief Online.* Retrieved from http://www.aecf.org/~/media/Pubs/Initiatives/KIDS%20COUNT/K/KIDSCOUNTIndicatorBriefIncreasingthePercentage/Two%20Parent%20Families.pdf

Smilkstein, G., Ashworth, C., & Montano, D. (1982). Validity and reliability of the family APGAR as a test of family function. *Journal of Family Practice, 15*(2), 303–311.

Smit, E. M. (2010). International adoption families: A unique health care journey. *Pediatric Nursing, 36*(5), 253–258.

Socolar, R. R. S., Savage, E., & Evans, H. (2007). A longitudinal study of parental discipline of young children. *Southern Medical Journal, 100*(5), 472–477.

Strijker, J., Knorth, E. J., & Knot-Dickscheit, J. (2008). Placement history of foster children: A study of placement history and outcomes in long-term family foster care. *Child Welfare, 87*(5), 107–124.

Totsika, V., & Sylva, K. (2004). The home observation for measurement of the environment revisited. *Child Psychology and Psychiatry, 9*(1), 25–35.

U.S. Census Bureau. (2010a). *Current Population Survey (CPS)—Definitions and explanations.* Retrieved from http://www.census.gov/population/www/cps/cpsdef.html

U.S. Census Bureau. (2010b). *U.S. Census Bureau reports men and women wait longer to marry.* Retrieved from http://www.census.gov/newsroom/releases/archives/families_households/cb10-174.html

U.S. Department of Health and Human Services. (2008a). *Fostering Connections to Success and Increasing Adoptions Act of 2008 P.L. 110-351.* Retrieved from http://

www.childwelfare.gov/systemwide/laws_policies/federal/index.cfm?event=federalLegislation.viewLegis&id=121

U.S. Department of Health and Human Services. (2008b). *Trends in foster care and adoption—FY2002–FY2007*. Retrieved from http://www.acf.hhs.gov/programs/cb/stats_research/afcars/trends_02-07.pdf

U.S. Department of Health and Human Services. (2009). *Adoption USA: A chartbook based on the 2007 national survey of adoptive parents*. Retrieved from http://aspe.hhs.gov/hsp/09/NSAP/chartbook/chartbook.cfm?id=1

U.S. Department of Health and Human Services. (2010a). *Foster care statistics*. Retrieved from http://www.childwelfare.gov/pubs/factsheets/foster.cfm#child

U.S. Department of Health and Human Services. (2010b). *Foster Care Independence Act of 1999*. Retrieved from http://www.acf.hhs.gov/programs/cb/laws_policies/cblaws/public_law/pl106_169/pl106_169.htm

U.S. Department of Labor. (2009). *Fact Sheet No. 28: The Family and Medical Leave Act of 1993*. Retrieved from http://www.dol.gov/esa/whd/regs/compliance/whdfs28.pdf

Vonk, M. E., Lee, J., & Crolley-Simic, J. (2010). Cultural socialization practices in domestic and international transracial adoption. *Adoption Quarterly, 13*, 227–247.

Wallerstein, J. S., & Blakeslee, S. (2004). *What about the kids? Raising your children before, during, and after divorce*. New York: Hyperion.

Weston, F. (2009). Effects of divorce or parental separation on children. *British Journal of School Nursing, 4*(5), 237–243.

Whenan, R., Oxlad, M., & Lushington, K. (2009). Factors associated with foster carer well-being, satisfaction, and intention to continue providing out-of-home care. *Children and Youth Services Review, 31*, 752–760.

Wright, L., & Leahey, M. (2009). *Nurses and families: A guide to family assessment and intervention* (5th ed.). Philadelphia: F. A. Davis.

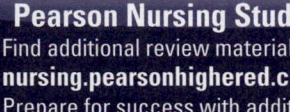
Pearson Nursing Student Resources
Find additional review materials at
nursing.pearsonhighered.com
Prepare for success with additional NCLEX®-style practice questions, interactive assignments and activities, web links, animations and videos, and more!

Cultural Influences

 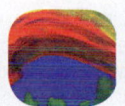 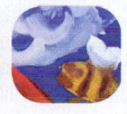

Learning Outcomes

After completing this chapter, you will be able to:

1. Discuss specific concepts related to culture such as diversity, race, ethnicity, and assimilation.

2. Describe cultural influences on the family's beliefs about health, illness, and treatments.

3. Identify cultural disparities in health care and barriers to health care for the child and family.

4. Analyze the various uses of complementary and alternative medicine in child health care.

5. Examine the role of the nurse in promoting cultural competence.

6. Apply strategies for nurses to achieve cultural competence when providing care to the child and family.

7. Compare nursing assessment strategies for various components of culture.

8. Summarize nursing interventions for providing culturally sensitive and competent care to the child and family.

"I don't want to talk to her . . . I want Mimi, she makes me feel better."
—Raven, age 4

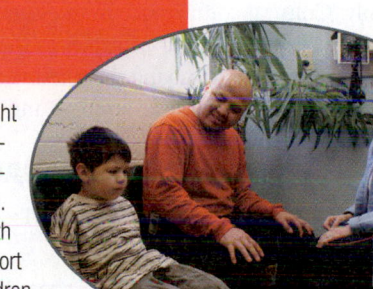

Raven Roanhorse is a 4-year-old Native American male brought to the health clinic by his father, Alex. Growing up on a reservation, Raven is one of four children in the family who recently began to go to the clinic in a nearby town for health care. The nurse there, Carol, has formed a positive relationship with Raven's family. Alex appreciates Carol's concern and rapport with the family and asks to see her when he brings in his children.

The purpose for the visit to the clinic is to evaluate Raven due to complaints of an earache. Alex also requests that Raven receive a thorough health examination and asks the nurse to identify and provide intervention for any health concerns. Alex acknowledges that the family has never taken Raven to a conventional healthcare facility and that his care has always been given by the family or tribal healer, Mimi. Some immunizations have been administered at a tribal clinic on the reservation. Raven has never experienced any major illnesses, but he has been treated routinely by the tribal healer for "usual childhood illnesses" such as colds, fever, and stomachaches. What questions should the nurse ask the father specific to Raven's current complaints of an earache? What additional information should the nurse gather related to Raven's past medical history and immunizations status?

The United States is undergoing demographic shifts, resulting in increasingly varied ethnic and cultural groups. Some of the reasons for immigration include improved access to transportation, sponsorship of individuals and families from countries with limited opportunities for work or with dangerous political situations, and assistance from family members already in North America. Nurses will come into contact with families of diverse backgrounds who seek health care for their children. Children reflect the cultures of both parents in their own specific adaptation and manifestation. As children mature, they may also become strongly influenced by school peers and the greater society, sometimes conflicting with the cultural values of the family. In response, nurses must continually strive to provide culturally competent care to children and their families. Although it is impossible to know all of the mores (customs) and values of each culture, the nurse who possesses an understanding of the cultural factors that influence the child and family can accurately assess those factors and incorporate them into an individualized plan to deliver culturally competent, family-centered care to individual children.

Culture is not strictly defined by race, ethnicity, and geography. Culture is far broader. Many groups form customs, ways of viewing the world, and patterns of behavior that can be described as cultures. Examples of these groups might include individuals with hearing impairments, gays and lesbians, the homeless, people in the military, and professional groups such as nurses. See Chapter 2 for a discussion on gay and lesbian families and Chapter 20 🔴 for a discussion on the homeless and military families.

This chapter provides an overview of culture and related concepts and the associated influences on health and health care for the child and family. Cultural competence is an essential element of nursing care, and we provide specific examples in the nursing management section to assist you in applying the nursing process when working with culturally diverse children, families, and populations.

CULTURE—DEFINITIONS AND BASIC CONCEPTS

Culture has many definitions and is described as the following:

The combination of a body of knowledge, a body of belief, and a body of behavior. It involves a number of elements, including personal identification, language, thoughts, communications, actions, customs, beliefs, values, and institutions that are often specific to ethnic, racial, religious, geographic, or social groups (U.S. Department of Health and Human Services, National Institutes of Health, 2010).

Table 3–1 provides an overview of definitions of culture according to several common theories. As nurses, we should study culture since it determines how people perceive health and health care. Specifically, culture informs us about how to view the body, mind, and spirit; what to do to maintain health; and what is acceptable as healthcare treatment. The child's concept of health is formed while growing up in a culture with its unique approaches and belief systems.

Culture and Nurse Theorists

Although numerous theories about culture may provide a framework for understanding and assessment, we will focus on four theories developed by and directly applicable to nursing. These theories offer threads that, when woven together, create a foundation nurses can utilize to understand and integrate culture into nursing care of

TABLE 3–1	Definitions of Culture
THEORIST	**DEFINITION**
Giger & Davidhizar (2008)	"A patterned behavioral response that develops over time as a result of imprinting the mind through social and religious structures and intellectual and artistic manifestations" (p. 2)
Leininger (2006)	"The learned, shared, and transmitted values, beliefs, norms, and lifeways of a particular culture that guides thinking, decisions, and actions in patterned ways and often intergenerationally" (p.13)
Purnell (2009)	"The totality of socially transmitted behavioral patterns, arts, beliefs, values, customs, and lifeways, and all other products of human work and thought characteristics of a population that guide their worldview and decision making" (p. 1)
Spector (2009)	"Nonphysical traits, such as values, beliefs, practices, habits, attitudes, and customs, that are shared by a group of people and passed from one generation to the next" (p. 348)

Source: Giger & Davidhizar (2008); Leininger (2006); Purnell (2008); Spector (2009).

children and families. All of these theories involve partnering and collaborating with families and sometimes community leaders to include cultural approaches in planned interventions.

One important theory is *culture care diversity and universality*, developed by nurse anthropologist Dr. Madeleine Leininger. In the 1950s, Leininger predicted that nurses in the future would need to understand more about culture to provide nursing care and that care was foundational to nursing but would change in the next decades. She developed her visionary concepts by travel and work with various cultural groups; many of her views were formed by caring for children in different cultures. Leininger views care as an essential part of nursing and believes that all care must be culturally based to contribute to the well-being, healing, growth, and survival of healthcare recipients (Leininger, 2006). Leininger (2006, pp. 24–25) describes her "sunrise enabler" as a guide that can be used to examine a variety of influences on care and culture. Its components are cultural values and lifeways, political and legal factors, economic factors, educational factors, kinship and social factors, religious and philosophical factors, and technological factors.

Dr. Larry Purnell, another nurse theorist, has developed a useful approach to assessing and planning culturally based nursing care. Purnell's *model for cultural competence* describes important components of the individual, family, and community within the larger global society (Purnell, 2008). He identified 12 major concepts that are common to all cultures and can be assessed to provide important information about an individual child and family (Purnell, 2008, p. 22). They are:

- Overview and heritage
- Communications
- Family roles and organization
- Workforce issues
- Biocultural ecology
- High-risk health behaviors
- Nutrition
- Pregnancy and child-bearing practices
- Death rituals

- Spirituality
- Healthcare practices
- Healthcare practitioners

You may choose to use these categories to focus your questions during assessments of children. For a family recently immigrated to this country, you might ask about the life history: "What places have you lived in? What did those countries or geographic areas look like? Were you in a temporary shelter or a family home? How did you travel here? What do you miss about your native land?" Consider the area of family roles. When caring for a child recently diagnosed with type 1 diabetes, what questions about family roles are important to plan teaching that fits within the family's cultural patterns?

Dr. Joyce Newman Giger and Dr. Ruth Davidhizar are nurse theorists who have examined **transcultural** (across cultures) nursing. Giger and Davidhizar (2008) developed the *transcultural assessment model* in direct response to student need for a framework that would provide structure for assessments of clients. In this framework, the client is the center of care and culturally unique. Knowledge of the cultural heritage, beliefs, attitudes, and behaviors of the client is required to provide culturally competent care. This model is based on six phenomena that nurses must assess (Giger & Davidhizar, 2008, p. 7):

- Communication
- Space
- Social organization
- Time
- Environmental control
- Biological variations

For example, the concept of space involves information about the distance or proximity that is comfortable for persons during interactions with others, information about visual and auditory perception, and body movements or positions. The nurse is alert for the child's eye contact patterns, ability to hear and see, positioning in the bed or chair, and response to touch. Such observations, combined with data from the health record and responses of the child and family members, will help the nurse to structure the space to best support healing in the child. What do you know about differences in eye contact among cultural groups? Look back to Raven in the opening scenario. Many Native American groups are uncomfortable with prolonged eye contact and will look away even while speaking or listening to someone. How will you adapt your care when dealing with a child who does not return eye contact? What are your own cultural patterns regarding eye contact, proximity to other people, and touch?

An additional view of health is provided by Dr. Rachel Spector, a nurse whose work has focused on cultural diversity and its relationship to health and illness beliefs and practices. According to Spector (2009), HEALTH (written in this manner to indicate the model) reflects the balance of the person—physical, mental, and spiritual—in the outside world. The *HEALTH traditions model* is predicated on the concept of holistic health and describes practices that can be used to maintain, protect, and restore health (Table 3–2). Spector states health is a complex, interrelated, and balanced state of the physical, mental, and spiritual (2009). These facets of health are as follows:

- *Physical*—all physical aspects, such as anatomical organs, gender, age, nutrition, genetic inheritance, body chemistry, and physical condition
- *Mental*—cognitive processes, such as memories, thoughts, and knowledge of such emotional processes as feelings, self-esteem, and defenses
- *Spiritual*—both positive and negative learned spiritual practices and teachings, dreams, stories, and symbols; protecting forces; and metaphysical or innate forces

Nurses must also consider contexts, such as the person's family, culture, work, community, history, and environment. The person must be in a state of balance within all personal and contextual parts. Illness occurs as a result of imbalance of one or all parts of the person (mind, body, spirit). When applying this theory, the pediatric nurse assesses the child's physical, cognitive, and spiritual states and examines all of the contexts in which the child has experiences. This theory directly relates to activities that are described in the unit on health promotion (which Spector calls health protection) and health maintenance later in this text. See Chapter 8 for further description of health promotion and health maintenance.

TABLE 3–2	Spector's Facets of Health (Physical, Mental, and Spiritual) and Personal Methods of Maintaining, Protecting, and Restoring Health		
	PHYSICAL	**MENTAL**	**SPIRITUAL**
Maintain Health	Proper clothing	Concentration	Religious worship
	Proper diet	Social and family support systems	Prayer
	Exercise/rest	Hobbies	Meditation
Protect Health	Special foods and food combinations	Avoid certain people who can cause illness	Religious customs
	Symbolic clothing	Family activities	Superstitions
			Wearing amulets and other symbolic objects to protect from the "evil eye" or defray other sources of harm
Restore Health	Homeopathic remedies, liniments	Relaxation	Religious rituals, special prayers
	Herbal teas	Exorcism	Meditation
	Special foods	Curanderos and other traditional healers	Traditional healings
	Massage	Nerve teas	Exorcism
	Acupuncture/moxibustion		

Source: *From Spector, R. (2009). Cultural diversity in health and illness (p. 78). Upper Saddle River, NJ: Pearson.*

Application of Cultural Theories

You may apply elements of these four frameworks as you assess cultural influences while working with children and families. Although their descriptions of culture differ, key elements are common to many of the theories. For example:

- *Culture is based on shared values and beliefs*—Each culture identifies and articulates its shared values and beliefs. Expected behaviors and roles emerge that are consistent with those values and beliefs. A belief system suggests what preventive health measures and treatment for diseases are sought and accepted. It may also state the importance of children, the family, other individuals, and the collective group, all of which can influence the choices people in the culture make regarding health. In short, a person's worldview may determine his or her actions related to health care.

- *Culture is learned and dynamic*—A child born into a culture starts learning the beliefs and practices of the group from birth. Children who are members of two cultural groups, such as African and immigrant, learn about both groups as they grow and develop. Immigrants may face challenges when integrating the rules of the dominant culture. Children who have family members from two or more cultural groups integrate parts of the worldview from each group. Therefore, although culture is connected with groups, each individual's manifestation of his or her own cultural background will be unique. Culture is therefore dynamic and constantly changing. It evolves and adapts as new members are born into or join the group and as the surrounding social and physical environments change. For example, as first-generation immigrants enter a new country they generally closely follow the cultural patterns of their native lands. As their children grow, the youth maintain some of the family cultural patterns but begin to incorporate some of the new culture.

- *Culture is integrated into life and uses symbols*—Culture is integrated through social institutions such as schools, houses of worship, friendships, families, and occupations (Figure 3–1 ■). This provides a variety of opportunities for learning about one's culture. The sense of integration may be disrupted or harder to maintain as individuals move frequently and as cultures intertwine. Symbols are an important way that many cultures communicate with each other and with the outside world. Language, dress, music, tools, and nonverbal gestures are symbols a culture uses to display and transmit the culture.

Definitions Related to Culture

Nurses should be aware of the distinctions between several aspects of culture. We assume that you already have some personal and academic experience with culture, so we will define terms briefly and focus on their relevance to pediatric nursing.

- **Race** refers to a group of people who share biological similarities such as skin color, bone structure, and genetic traits. Examples of races include White (sometimes called Caucasian or European American), Black, Hispanic, Natives (such as Native Americans, Alaskan Natives, Hawaiian Natives, and First Nation people of Canada), and Asian.

- **Ethnicity** describes a "cultural group's sense of identification associated with the group's common social and cultural heritage" (Spector, 2009, p. 349). Examples of ethnic groups

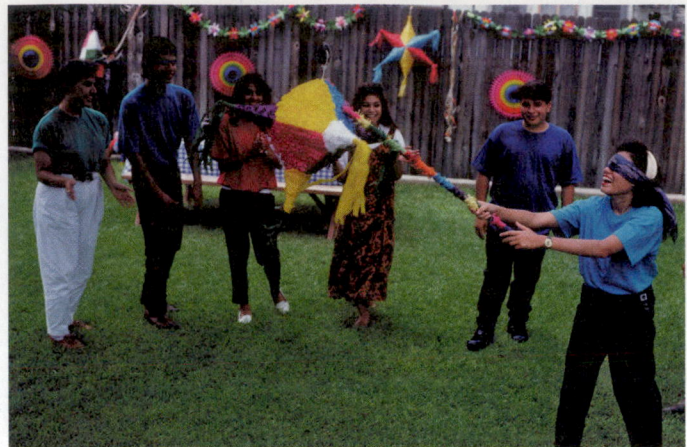

FIGURE 3–1 ■ These children are engaged in a cultural birthday tradition of breaking the piñata. Maintaining cultural traditions is one way families can continue their cultural heritage. Can you think of other common cultural traditions related to special occasions?

include African Americans, Hmong, Jewish, and Irish Americans. Ethnicity is the group's identity, or perception, of itself. It may be demonstrated when a group's members feel different from other groups; come from a common ancestry, country, or region; enjoy certain foods; speak a distinct language; practice a certain religious faith; have dances, music, or other pastimes; dress in a distinct way; or share other practices and background with group members. Even the mainstream or majority groups usually identify with some ethnic group. How would you describe your own ethnic identity? Is it based on your race, the country of origin of your parents, or the place where you live? How does your ethnic group determine your views of health and the type of health care you seek?

Think of some of the children you are working with in clinical settings. What are predominant ethnic groups in your area? What languages are spoken? Do children and their parents speak the same languages? What countries are represented? Are certain holidays commonly celebrated? Is there a common faith-based practice? Are certain ethnic groups more receptive in general to healthcare teaching and other interventions? Do some practice herbal medicine or other approaches? Some of these practices will be discussed later in the chapter.

- **Stereotyping** is assuming that all members of a group have the same characteristics. When caring for a Hispanic child, a nurse who stereotypes would assume that the child speaks Spanish or that the parents are migrant farm workers. A nurse must individually assess each situation to see which characteristics common to a group are possessed by a particular child rather than ascribing all traits to the child.

- **Prejudice** is a negative stereotype about a certain group that is applied to all individuals within the group.

- **Bias** refers to a preference for a certain set of ideas. Cultural bias generally refers to preference for one's own cultural values.

- All people at times demonstrate **ethnocentrism,** or believing that one's own ethnic perspective and way of thinking is best. This belief necessarily affects all relationships with others. Think about how you treat a cold, what food you think is best to eat if you have an upset stomach, or how you think a child should be toilet trained. How can you work with children and families in a way that honors their beliefs and health practices rather than simply presenting the practices that are common in your ethnic group?

- **Acculturation** refers to modifying one's culture to fit within the new or dominant culture.
- **Assimilation** is related to acculturation and is described as adopting and incorporating characteristics of the new culture within one's practices (Spector, 2009).

Awareness of these cultural concepts will enhance your ability to learn about diverse cultural groups, understand their concepts of health, work with individuals in the culture to evaluate their particular health practices, and become effective in planning nursing care for children of many racial and ethnic backgrounds.

DEMOGRAPHICS AND CULTURAL DIVERSITY IN THE UNITED STATES

According to the latest data from the U.S. Census Bureau (2011), the White non-Hispanic population increased from 194.6 million to 196.8 million between 2000 and 2010. However, White non-Hispanics comprised 64% of the population in 2010, a decrease from 69% of the population in 2000. Considering current data, we can see that minority groups now represent approximately 36% of the population and are steadily growing.

The United States continues to experience an influx of millions of immigrants and refugees. **Immigrants** are individuals who are foreign born (anyone who is not born a U.S. citizen) and are admitted as permanent residents to the United States to live and work. **Refugees** are those who leave their country based on fear of persecution due to race, religion, nationality, social group membership, or political opinion (U.S. Citizenship and Immigration Services, 2011). The foreign-born population of the United States grew from 11.1% in 2000 to 12.5% in 2009 (Grieco & Trevelyan, 2010).

All nurses must have an understanding of the major cultural groups found in their regions and be able to perform culturally sensitive assessments and plan interventions that are appropriate for the children and families in clinical settings. For that reason, nurses should be familiar with community and world demographics. Immigrants may have different healthcare needs related to understanding of the majority healthcare system, variations in immunizations given to children in native countries, and mental health issues related to integration within a new country. See Developing Cultural Competence: Culture Shock.

Although over one third of the U.S. population consists of minority and ethnic groups (U.S. Census Bureau, 2011), the percentage of registered nurses (RNs) in the country from minority groups is much lower. Results of a 2004 survey estimated that 81.8% of RNs were White non-Hispanic, and 10.6% were from another race or ethnic group. Approximately 7.5% did not indicate their racial or ethnic background (American Nurses Association, 2007). Of the physicians in the United States whose racial or ethnic background is known, approximately 22% belong to a minority group (American Medical Association, 2008). This general lack of diversity among healthcare providers has contributed to a lack of adequate health care for some minority groups, resulting in health disparities.

The nursing shortage is a great concern of all people providing health care; however, the shortage of minority nurses is critical as well and affects the provision of culturally competent patient care (Xu, 2008). Nurses from the majority cultural group may not fully understand the views of health and the healthcare practices of other groups. Nurses who are members of minority groups offer distinct skills by being able to understand and interpret both healthcare institutions and the healthcare needs of certain minority groups. It is therefore important for all nurses to increase their knowledge about groups in their communities in order to provide culturally competent care. Do you work with student peers from various ethnic and racial groups? How can you learn from them and how can you share your cultural knowledge with others? All nurses have the responsibility to increase diversity of the profession and augment diverse knowledge of healthcare providers. Go to your state, provincial, and local websites to find information about the cultural groups in your community; focus your learning and research on these groups as you continue to read this chapter.

CULTURAL COMPETENCE IN NURSING

Cultural competence refers to the ability of the nurse to understand and effectively respond to the needs of patients and families from different cultural backgrounds (Spector, 2009) (Figure 3–2 ■). It involves identifying and integrating the family's health beliefs, practices, and cultural and linguistic needs into patient care (U.S. Department of Health and Human Services, National Institutes of Health, 2010). Cultural competence also requires that nurses become aware

Developing Cultural Competence
Culture Shock

The experience that a person has in attempting to understand or adapt to a culture that is fundamentally different from his or her own culture is known as **culture shock.** The person may experience feelings of discomfort, powerlessness, anxiety, and disorientation. Immigrants to the United States may experience culture shock when differences or conflicts arise between their own values, beliefs, and customs and the ways of their new surroundings. The nurse should assess children and their families who have recently immigrated for indications of culture shock. Referring the family to counseling and/or support from representatives of their own culture, or a community group, may be helpful.

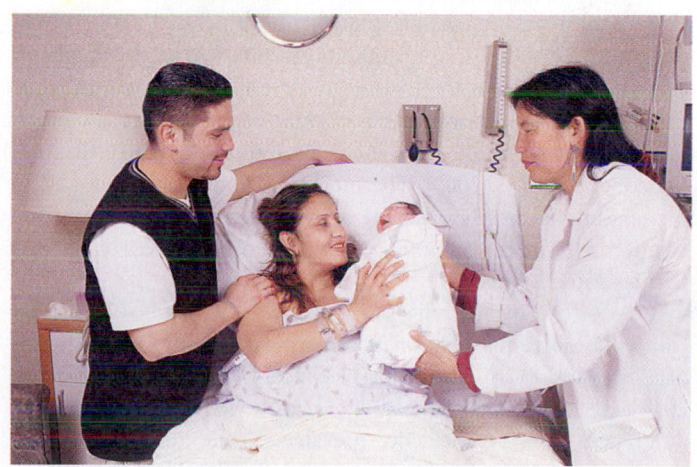

FIGURE 3–2 ■ Nurses increasingly have opportunities to provide culturally competent care as demographics continue to evolve; however, there continues to be disparity among ethnicity of nurses and the populations they serve. Nurses, such as this nurse providing care to the family of a newborn, must develop an understanding of the cultural beliefs and practices of the population. How can nurses improve their understanding of the individuals representing various cultures?

Weblink National Center for Cultural Competence

of themselves and their environment without letting these factors influence the care they provide to patients and families. Nurses must become culturally competent in order to deliver effective nursing care (Tuck, Moon, & Allocca, 2010). Cultural competence must include knowledge of cultural groups, attitudes that honor various cultures and seek to increase competence, and skills to ensure appropriate assessments and interventions. The Office of Minority Affairs of the U.S. Department of Health and Human Services and the Agency for Healthcare Research and Quality have been primary agencies in investigating issues regarding cultural competence and setting standards for healthcare providers. See Table 3–3 for the Office of Minority Health Standards and examples of application to pediatric nursing.

You may be wondering how you can increase your cultural competence. What are your responsibilities? What are the steps you can take to achieve competence? The first essential step to developing cultural competence is for you, the nurse, to examine your own perceptions, stereotypes, and prejudices regarding various cultures. You can begin to identify individual beliefs that are ethnocentric, biased, or prejudiced through an examination of your own personal heritage and values. Complete a cultural assessment on yourself. Describe heritage, beliefs and values, language, and exposure to diverse cultures. Examine your childhood and the practices and beliefs of your family. Through this understanding of your own background, you establish a foundation for the appreciation of the values and beliefs of others. Additionally, this examination assists you in identifying similarities and differences of cultures other than your own.

HEALTH CARE AND CULTURE

Culture influences concepts of health and health care in many ways. The worldview of people in the family determines how health is viewed. Is an illness seen as fate or punishment for actions? Is preventive care viewed as important and an essential part of life? The family and cultural views influence the child, who gradually takes on parts of the culture during development. Let's explore some of the important ways in which culture and health care interact.

Disparities in Health and Barriers to Health Care

Research indicates that racial and ethnic minorities in the United States continue to receive lower quality health care than the White population (Kaiser Family Foundation, 2008). African Americans, Hispanics, and Asians are less likely to have a regular healthcare provider than Whites. Individuals from minority groups are also much less likely to have health insurance than Caucasians (Lillie-Blanton, Maleque, & Miller, 2008). The morbidity and mortality for these populations is disproportionate as compared to Caucasians (see Chapter 1 🔗). See Developing Cultural Competence: Health Disparities and Hispanics.

One of the overarching goals of *Healthy People 2020* is to "achieve health equity, eliminate disparities, and improve the health of all groups" (U.S. Department of Health and Human Services, 2010). Health disparity populations are those groups with significant differences in disease incidence, prevalence, morbidity, mortality, or survival rates as compared to the general populations. Disparities in relation to gender, race, ethnic group, education, income, disability, geographic location, and sexual orientation are common. For example, while 20.7% of all children were living in poverty in 2009, the numbers were much higher in Black (35.4%) and Hispanic (33.1%) children (U.S. Census Bureau, 2010a). African Americans, Hispanic

Developing Cultural Competence
Health Disparities and Hispanics

There are 50.5 million Hispanics in the United States, comprising 16% of the population. This number represents a 43% growth since 2000 (U.S. Census Bureau, 2011). This large group experiences many ethnic disparities such as lack of health insurance, low immunization rates, limited prenatal care, and high rates of obesity. Certain diseases such as diabetes, human immunodeficiency virus (HIV), and cancer of the cervix are more common in Hispanics (U.S. Census Bureau, 2010b). Many of these problems affect children.

When working with Hispanic groups, perform accurate weight and height measurements and plot on growth grids. Include additional nutritional assessment and guidance if overweight is evident. Ask about access to health insurance and health care. Investigate the immunization record for all children and update as needed. At the same time, recognize that healthcare needs may vary according to location and group. Look at each person and your area individually.

Americans, American Indians, Asian Americans, Native Hawaiians, and other Pacific Islanders have higher rates of infant mortality, low birth weight, cancer, diabetes, heart disease, stroke, and substance abuse and a shorter life expectancy (U.S. Department of Health and Human Services, National Institutes of Health, 2011). These conditions have direct relevance to pediatric nurses. Infant mortality is directly related, while some other conditions such as heart disease and diabetes have their roots in youth due to a high rate of overweight among several minority youth groups.

Clinical Tip

Obesity and conditions related to it such as diabetes are prevalent among persons who are poor. Children who have Medicaid coverage are 6 times more likely to be obese than those children who are covered by a private insurance policy. Latino children ages 2 to 18 years are most at risk for being overweight, followed by Black children (National Institute for Health Care Management, 2007). Well-child visits with a focus on weight monitoring, evaluating community resources for availability of access to nutritious foods and physical activity, and education related to diet and activity are essential with these children to prevent complications such as diabetes and heart disease.

Why do disparities exist? Let's examine some of the many reasons.

Access and Barriers

One reason disparities exist among cultural groups relates to access and barriers to care. Access ensures that children of all races, ethnic groups, and income levels can obtain preventive care and treatment for illness or injury. Barriers delay or prevent health care for the child and may be related to the following factors (Nield, 2008; Schneiderman, McDaniel, Xie, et al., 2010):

- Lack of health insurance among low-income families
- Communication difficulties such as those experienced when families do not speak English
- Lack of knowledge about cultural approaches to health care on the part of care providers
- Transportation problems

See Evidence-Based Practice: Investigating Culture and Healthcare Barriers.

Lack of health coverage is a major barrier for children in many groups. Those in immigrant families are at particular risk, and the number of immigrants is increasing in the United States. In 2009, 10% of all children in the United States (or 7.5 million) under 18 years of

TABLE 3–3 · National Standards for Culturally and Linguistically Appropriate Services in Health Care

STANDARD	NURSING IMPLICATIONS FOR CHILD HEALTH
1. Healthcare organizations should ensure that patients/consumers receive from all staff members effective, understandable, and respectful care that is provided in a manner compatible with their cultural health beliefs and practices, and preferred language.	Ask about cultural health beliefs of the family and child. Inquire about desired language. Integrate these assessment areas into all care for the child.
2. Healthcare organizations should implement strategies to recruit, retain, and promote at all levels of the organization a diverse staff and leadership representative of the demographic characteristics of the service area.	Turn to diverse staff members for guidance in working with members of their groups. Collaborate with family and community members to plan care for children. Decide on location, types, and timing of services.
3. Healthcare organizations should ensure that staff at all levels and across all disciplines receive ongoing education and training in culturally and linguistically appropriate service delivery.	Request training in cultural approaches for groups in your area. Invite community members to participate in training for cultural competence. Partner with your agency and families to enhance care for children.
4. Healthcare organizations must offer and provide language assistance services, including bilingual staff and interpreter services, at no cost to each patient/consumer with limited English proficiency at all points of contact, in a timely manner during all hours of operation.	Investigate agency resources. Collaborate to assemble lists of qualified interpreters and translators and other resources. Arrange to have brochures and other health materials translated and available for children and families.
5. Healthcare organizations must provide to patients/consumers in their preferred language both verbal offers and written notices informing them of their right to receive language assistance services.	Post signs in the common languages used at health clinics, vans, hospitals, and other settings where children receive care to describe language services provided. Include resources for patients and their families who are not literate in their native language.
6. Healthcare organizations must ensure the competence of language assistance provided to patients/consumers with limited English proficiency by interpreters and bilingual staff. Family and friends should not be used to provide interpretation services (except on request by the patient/consumer).	Consider taking language classes to increase proficiency with children and families. Do not use children as translators for other family members.
7. Healthcare organizations must make available easily understood patient-related materials and post signage in the languages of the commonly encountered groups and/or groups represented in the service area.	Materials essential in care must be translated and available for families, including consent forms, health histories, and treatment instructions.
8. Healthcare organizations should develop, implement, and promote a written strategic plan that outlines clear goals, policies, operational plans, and management accountability/oversight mechanisms to provide culturally and linguistically appropriate services.	Ask in your clinical settings about services that are available for culturally diverse populations and what goals the agencies have for dealing with children and families from diverse groups.
9. Healthcare organizations should conduct initial and ongoing organizational self-assessments of activities and are encouraged to integrate cultural and linguistic competence-related measures into their internal audits, performance improvement programs, patient satisfaction assessments, and outcomes-based evaluations.	Ask questions of each child and family to evaluate their satisfaction with the services that they have received. Were their expectations for service met?
10. Healthcare organizations should ensure that data on the individual patient's/consumer's race, ethnicity, and spoken and written language are collected in health records, integrated in the organization's management information systems, and periodically updated.	Collect data on written health histories and verbal questions about the child's race, ethnicity, and languages. Record the information and note its application within care for the individual child.
11. Healthcare organizations should maintain a current demographic, cultural, and epidemiological profile of the community as well as a needs assessment to accurately plan for and implement services that respond to the cultural and linguistic characteristics of the service area.	Consult your national, state, provincial, and regional websites and documents to learn what childhood health conditions and healthcare needs are present in your communities. Integrate your knowledge of these needs as you approach children and parents; partner with them to plan care to meet healthcare needs.
12. Healthcare organizations should develop participatory, collaborative partnerships with communities and utilize a variety of formal and informal mechanisms to facilitate community and patient/consumer involvement in designing and implementing CLAS*-related activities.	Invite parents to participate in health teaching and screening programs at schools. Suggest that members of the community could assist with design of waiting areas in clinics and hospitals. Engage children and parents in projects that involve translation of signs.
13. Healthcare organizations should ensure that conflict and grievance resolution processes are culturally and linguistically sensitive and capable of identifying, preventing, and resolving cross-cultural conflicts or complaints by patients/consumers.	Ask children and parents to review care received. Refer them to appropriate sources for follow-up as needed. Be sensitive to situations when people are concerned that you were not aware of cultural concerns of a family; openness to one's biases and methods of interaction is the first step in increased sensitivity.
14. Healthcare organizations are encouraged to regularly make available to the public information about their progress and successful innovations in implementing the CLAS standards and to provide public notice in their communities about the availability of this information.	Post information about new cultural services available to families. Consider the use of community flyers, radio, or other approaches to inform families about culturally sensitive services in your facility.

*CLAS = Culturally and Linguistically Appropriate Services

Source: *Standards from U.S. Department of Health and Human Services, Office of Minority Health. (2007).* National standards for culturally and linguistically appropriate services in health care. Washington, DC: Author.

Evidence-Based Practice

Investigating Culture and Healthcare Barriers

PROBLEM

Health disparities exist among various cultural groups. Although examination of factors in adults has identified some barriers to care, there has been little research about barriers that exist among families with children. An understanding of the factors that improve healthcare access and those that act as barriers is needed to provide accessible care for children from minority ethnic groups.

EVIDENCE

A study of the child healthcare decision making and practices of 12 immigrant women from the Caribbean revealed concerns related to communication and trust with healthcare providers. The women shared feelings that they were not valued in the healthcare setting. Their use of herbs and folk practices was also frequently misunderstood or frowned upon, often resulting in a failure to disclose this information. The women also felt that they did not have the abilities to effectively navigate the healthcare system (Yearwood, 2007).

Baker, Dang, Ly, et al. (2010) examined barriers to immunizations for Hmong children in California. Responses from 417 parents were analyzed to determine what factors contributed to perceived barriers. Parents of Hmong children who used traditional Hmong health care, such as the herbalists and shamans, and were of lower socioeconomic status had higher perceived barriers to immunizations.

Schneiderman, McDaniel, Xie, et al. (2010) examined the perceptions of 237 parents at a child welfare pediatric medical clinic related to healthcare access barriers and pediatric healthcare use. Difficulty understanding the explanations given by physicians was identified as the greatest healthcare access barrier and could affect compliance with recommended health care among this population.

NURSING IMPLICATIONS

A theme in two of the previous studies is socioeconomic status. Nurses need to refer families to sources for healthcare services and then follow up to be sure the families were able to access care. Referrals to community health centers and instructions for transportation to the health setting are important for many families. A need for understandable information is another theme among most groups. Explaining why an immunization is needed as well as providing information about the child's condition are important nursing roles. Referring the family to others from the same ethnic or racial group and assisting them in navigating complex systems such as school and social services may also be necessary. Cultural differences and practices were also cited as a barrier to health care. It is essential that healthcare providers become familiar with other cultures and be accepting of practices that are safe for the child. By being open to practices of other cultures, healthcare providers will find families more willing to share openly about how they treat their children. This may lead to an opportunity for education related to unsafe practices.

CRITICAL THINKING APPLICATION

What is the process that immigrant families in your state or province must follow to secure health care for their children? How would you help to guide someone through this process?

What cultural groups are common in your community? Do you speak their language? If not, what measures should you take to ensure that they understand the teaching offered in clinical settings? What type of support groups will be helpful for families when they have a child with special healthcare needs?

---

age were uninsured. Of children living in poverty, 15.1% were uninsured. The percentage of children who were uninsured varied greatly depending on race. While 7% of non-Hispanic White children were uninsured, 11.5% of Black children, 16.8% of Hispanic children, and 10% of Asian children were without insurance (DeNavas-Walt, Proctor, & Smith, 2010). Recall the discussion in Chapter 1 🔗 that encouraged all families with children to seek a "home" that they can turn to for care and questions. Identification of a pediatric healthcare home makes it more likely that preventive care is received, that early diagnosis of healthcare problems can occur, and that prompt treatment or referral takes place.

Families need access to healthcare services in their own communities, and they must have means of transportation to the services. Working parents need services available at times that do not require them to miss work. Obtaining even basic or emergency services for children in rural areas may be difficult due to the lack of providers. Service hours must meet the needs of the population served. Language translators should be readily available. A welcoming atmosphere, pleasant surroundings, and reasonable wait time will all enhance use of health care. Pediatric nurses are instrumental in surveying families and planning approaches that welcome them to healthcare settings. See Developing Cultural Competence: Use of Cultural Brokers in the Healthcare Setting.

Lack of trust of healthcare providers can also be a barrier to care. Historically, groups such as Blacks and Native Americans were the recipients of inferior care and even unethical research studies. Members of these groups may continue to distrust healthcare providers. If inadequate care was received at some time or if care providers appear rude or noncaring, some families may prefer to treat children at home and seek care only in emergency situations. Trust can be enhanced when children and families of all races, ethnic groups, religious groups, and

Developing Cultural Competence
Use of Cultural Brokers in the Healthcare Setting

Use of a **cultural broker,** one who serves as a go-between, negotiator, or advocate for people from different cultural backgrounds, can help maximize the family's understanding of and access to health care (Andrews & Boyle, 2008; Moore, 2010; Purnell, 2009). Communication between the healthcare provider and the family is enhanced as well as the family's understanding of the child's plan of care. Families may be more motivated to utilize services available to them and to encourage others to do so as well. The role of a cultural broker can be fulfilled by a nurse, physician, interpreter, teacher, family member, or anyone who is interested in helping provide a cultural connection for families (National Center for Cultural Competence, 2004).

other populations are treated fairly and with respect. Collaborate with families to learn their healthcare goals and provide relationships with a stable group of health professionals when possible.

Biological Differences

Genetic and physical differences occur among cultural groups (Figure 3–3 ■) and can lead to disparity in needs and care. Differences include blood type, body build, skin color, drug metabolism, and susceptibility to certain diseases. Other disparities occur because of fundamental differences between genders, ages, and races. For example, male children are more likely to manifest pyloric stenosis and attention deficit disorder, whereas female children more often have congenital hip dysplasia and systemic lupus erythematosus. Age provides another biological variation as infants are more likely to manifest the cancer neuroblastoma, whereas adolescents have a higher incidence of Hodgkin disease. Race is also connected with certain disease processes. Blacks are more likely to experience diabetes and

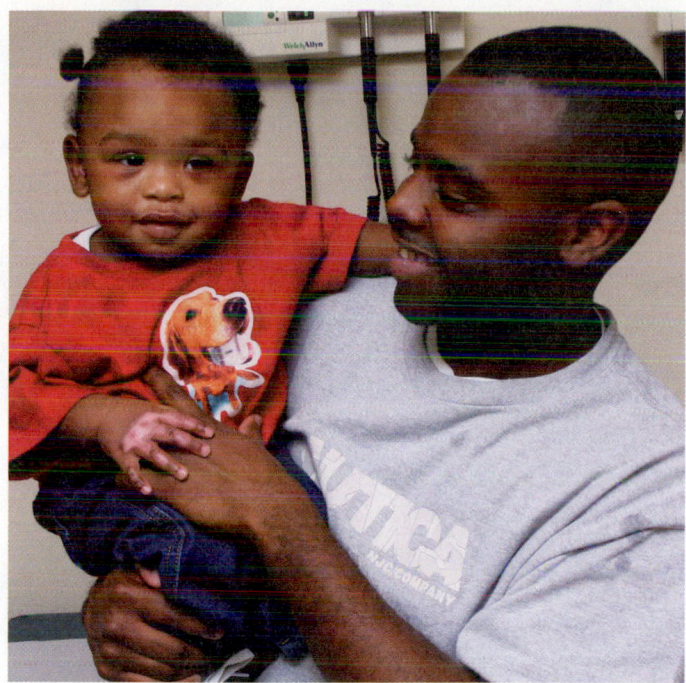

FIGURE 3–3 ■ Children manifest physical characteristics related to their ethnic groups. How will you integrate this knowledge into developmental assessments of children?

sickle cell anemia (see chapters throughout this text for a discussion of these conditions). Thalassemia, another type of anemia, is most common in Mediterranean people. Whites from certain geographic origins are more likely to manifest cystic fibrosis, celiac disease, and Crohn disease. Hispanics have high rates of diabetes and lactose intolerance. Asians and Native Americans often do not metabolize alcohol readily and are more prone to injury after alcohol ingestion or to alcohol abuse (Giger & Davidhizar, 2008).

Clinical Tip
Although certain conditions are more common in various racial or ethnic groups, it is best to approach each family individually. For example, there are marked differences in rates of diabetes among Native American tribes (Giger & Davidhizar, 2008). Thus, knowing the most common conditions for a race in general may not be directly applicable to the specific location and group in your area.

Nurses must understand other genetic characteristics in order to perform culturally competent nursing assessments and interventions. Differences in skin color and tones may make cyanosis, pallor, and jaundice difficult to recognize and describe. Mongolian spots are darkened skin on the lower back and buttocks of some babies with dark skin tones. Variations in texture of hair require different approaches to hygiene among various racial groups. See Chapters 4 and 7 🔗 for more detail about biological variations and implications for assessment.

Clinical Tip
When assessing patients with darker skin, pallor is exhibited by yellow-brown skin in a brown-skinned person and ashen gray skin in a black-skinned person. Cyanosis is noted by inspection of the conjunctiva, lips, soles of the feet, and palms of the hands.

Environmental Differences
Some conditions are clearly genetic in origin, such as sickle cell anemia, whereas others are linked to environmental conditions,

especially socioeconomic status. (See Chapter 20 🔗.) For example, mortality rates in Native Americans have increased secondary to rising rates of suicide, homicide, and accidental injury (Andrews & Boyle, 2008). These injuries may be directly related to the high unemployment rate common on some reservations, which leads to poor self-esteem and promotes depression. Families with inadequate finances are more likely to live in crowded conditions and experience more infectious disease. Conditions in their neighborhoods may be unsafe and result in injury to children. Falls, fires, and other hazards may be common. Peeling paint may result in conditions such as lead poisoning. Lack of knowledge about transmission, poor access to treatment, and use of intravenous drugs can increase incidence of HIV in populations with high rates of poverty.

Some conditions may result from interrelated biological and environmental factors, which are often hard to separate. Lack of access to health care, lower rates of immunization, poor nutritional status, and lack of transportation may all interact with biological factors to promote high incidence of certain disease states. Native Americans or Hispanics who eat traditional diets have low rates of obesity and diabetes, but those who eat the "typical American diet," which is high in fat and low in fruits and vegetables, have high rates of these conditions. Likewise, medication metabolism differences are sometimes further altered by exposure to environmental pollution, alcohol, and diet. In many cases, these biological and environmental factors interact to create certain healthcare risks.

Cultural Practices That Influence Health Care
Family Roles and Organization
A family's organization and the roles played by individual family members are largely dependent upon cultural influence. For example, culture may determine who has authority (head of household) and is the primary decision maker for other members of the family. Additionally, the role of decision maker may change according to specific decisions. In some cultures, decisions regarding the health care of children are primarily the responsibility of the female, whereas other decisions are male dominated. Family dominance patterns may be patriarchal, as seen in some Appalachian cultures; matriarchal, as seen in some African American cultures; or more egalitarian, as seen in some European American cultures. Nurses should be alert for roles and functions in families since teaching may need to be directed to those responsible for decision making to effectively promote child health.

Culture also defines gender roles, as well as the roles of the elderly and of extended family. For example, Native Americans may consult tribal elders (considered part of the extended family) before agreeing to medical care for their child. In some cultures, major decisions for the family, including a child's health care, involve input from grandparents and other extended family members (Figure 3–4 ■). Grandparents may even assume responsibility for care of the children in the family (see Chapter 2 🔗). In these cases, nurses must direct teaching for health promotion and demonstration for treatment procedures to the grandparent.

Family goals are also determined by cultural values and practices, as are family member roles and childrearing practices and beliefs. In some families, children are expected to take on responsibilities early and may be expected to take on tasks such as management of their own chronic disease and nutritional intake. In other families, children are given long periods to grow up and are not expected to

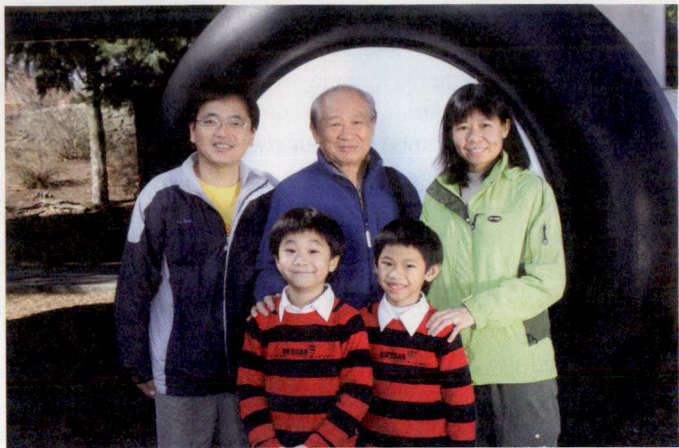

FIGURE 3–4 ■ Many cultures value the input of grandparents and other elders in the family or group. For example, in this multigenerational family, the grandfather's guidance is highly valued and significantly influences the family's childrearing practices.

manage healthcare needs. Direct teaching to a child with diabetes in the latter family type may not be appropriate. Nurses often provide information and ask about developmental milestones for children; however, there may be variations in family goals and it is not unusual that families accomplish these tasks with children at younger or older ages. For example, it is commonly expected that children are weaned by 1 year of age and toilet trained at about 2 years of age, but this is not always the case. Ask about the norms in the family and whether the child is developing according to the parents' expectations. As long as the child is progressing in motor, language, and social tasks, some variation is expected due to cultural norms. Views about alternative lifestyles such as sexual orientation and single parenting are also established by the family's values and beliefs. Understanding such values assists the nurse in providing sensitive care. Examples of childrearing practices common to particular cultures are listed in Table 3–4. Realize that the practices listed are common in these cultures, but not necessarily practiced by all members of that culture. (See Chapter 2 🔗 for further discussion of family structures.)

Communication

Communication is the method by which members of cultural groups share information and preserve their beliefs, values, norms, and practices. Information is transmitted through both verbal and nonverbal methods. Verbal communication consists of spoken or written words, including tone and level of voice, language, verbal style and dialect, and written material.

Obviously, verbal communication is improved when a healthcare provider speaks the same language as the patient and family. Recall the national standards related to language assistance services (see Table 3–3). Children are most likely to speak both the language of the parents and the healthcare providers and may appear to be likely interpreters. However, it is recommended that children never be used to interpret in healthcare situations due to the confidentiality needs of both parent and child. Additionally, if children are used as interpreters, it can create an imbalance in power that could adversely affect parental authority. Interpreters should be culturally competent and have training in both health literacy and medical interpretation (Singleton & Krause, 2009). Signs, posted literature, and brochures should also be available in the languages of the children and families served. Even when children speak the language of the healthcare

TABLE 3–4	Childrearing Practices of Selected Cultures
CULTURE	**CHILDREARING PRACTICES**
African American	Grandmothers play an important role in the care of children.
	Children are expected to demonstrate respectfulness, conformity to rules, obedience, and good behavior.
	Extended family is very important.
Amish	There is an average of seven children per family.
	Childrearing is regarded as the highest priority for parents.
	Grandparents often provide care to children.
	Children are expected to continue with the Amish tradition.
	Children are expected to follow the rules as prescribed by the church district.
Appalachian	Large families are common.
	Strict parenting practices and physical punishment are common.
	Grandparents frequently provide care to children.
Arab	The father is typically the disciplinarian.
	The child's character is considered a reflection of the family's influence.
	Children are expected to respect their elders and to have good behavior.
	Adolescents are expected to do well in their studies.
	Discipline may include physical punishment and shaming.
Chinese	The family may lavish resources on the child.
	Children typically depend on the family for all needs and may not be expected to earn their own money as adolescents.
	Male children are often more valued than female children.
	Children may be taught to avoid displaying their emotions/feelings.
	Children are expected to assist parents in the home (chores).
	High educational achievement is expected.
Mexican	Children are closely protected and are not encouraged to leave the home.
	Extended family members frequently live close by.
	Children are expected to demonstrate respect for parents and elder family members.
	Discipline may include physical punishment.
	Education is a priority.
Navajo Indian	Large families are important.
	Infants may be kept in a cradleboard to protect them.
	Grandmothers are important decision makers in the family.
	Children are allowed to make decisions about their care.

Source: *Data from Purnell, L. D., & Paulanka, B. J. (2008). Transcultural health care: A culturally competent approach (3rd ed.). Philadelphia: F. A. Davis; Purnell, L. D. (2009). Guide to culturally competent health care (2nd ed.). Philadelphia: F. A. Davis.*

providers, written material must be provided at a level that the family can read and understand.

Clinical Judgment

The nurse is providing care to a 10-year-old Hispanic male who speaks both English and Spanish fluently. His parents know very little English. The nurse is preparing to teach the mother how to do a sterile dressing change. Is it appropriate for the nurse to use the patient to interpret the instructions for the procedure to the mother?

Clinical Tip

Speaking and reading may not occur in the same language. For example, an immigrant may read and speak fluently in a primary language and speak but not read the language of the new country. The immigrant's child may read and speak the language of the present country and speak but not read the native language of the family. Always ask about both reading and speaking preferences.

Language can also affect health literacy skills, as a large number of instructions are given in writing, including prescriptions and directions on medication bottles, signs hanging in health facilities, consent forms for procedures and surgery, insurance forms, directions for techniques or procedures, future appointment dates, and health promotion materials. Verify what the child and family can read and whether alternative methods should be used. Nurses can verbally give the information and provide paper and pencil so that the family can take notes in their own language. Translation services should be available in all healthcare settings, including the pharmacy, the appointment desk, and for phone calls, to ensure access to services for all patients served.

Variations in communication among cultures are reflected in word meaning, voice inflection and quality, and verbal styles. Culture influences not only affect the manner in which feelings are expressed, but also which verbal and nonverbal expressions of communication are considered appropriate. An individual's willingness to discuss certain topics or to express or conceal certain thoughts and feelings is also influenced by the cultural norms. Some groups may be expected to remain quiet when experiencing pain, whereas other cultures may loudly and dramatically express pain. Watch for the cues that family members give to children in pain, such as "Oh, you're all right—be a big boy," or "You go ahead and cry. How can you take that pain?" Remember that culture is constantly evolving, so children commonly exhibit communication patterns seen in their parents as well as reflecting the patterns of the majority culture and of childhood peers.

Use of first names and surnames varies among cultural groups, so nurses should make no assumptions, as the use of a person's first name may be considered disrespectful. Always ask upon admission to any facility what the child wishes to be called. Address family members respectfully, usually using terms such as Mr., Mrs., and Ms. If the person has a title such as doctor, judge, or senator, it should be used. Ask what the person prefers to be called and record this in the health record for future reference. In the Korean, Cambodian, and Filipino cultures, the first name used is actually the family name. Asking for the "family name" rather than the "last name" may clarify this practice.

Nonverbal communication refers to body language such as posture, gestures, facial expressions, eye contact, and touch, as well as the use of silence. The nurse's use of nonverbal communication may hinder or help communication. Gestures and body language may be misunderstood or misinterpreted. For example, eye contact has different meanings among cultures. Silence is considered a sign of respect in

some cultures. Among those groups, offering an immediate response to a question may be viewed as being disrespectful because an instant reply could indicate that no thought was given to the matter. Watch for patterns in various cultures and alter your own approach to be more congruent. For example, many nurses commonly nod and say "yes" or "oh, I see" when a patient is speaking. This may seem disruptive to some cultures. If you note that the listener is silent and does not use such patterns of agreement, alter your own response to match more closely the acceptable method of communication for the child or family.

Touch is another form of nonverbal communication. The appropriateness of touch varies by culture. For example, an Asian may consider touching an unfamiliar person of the opposite gender to be inappropriate, while a person of another culture believes touch between men and women is appropriate. Adults commonly feel that it is acceptable to touch children of all ages, but this may not be accurate. Look for responses from the child and family to touch. Does the parent touch the child, stroke the crying baby, or put an arm around a school-age child? What is the response as the nurse touches the child to take a blood pressure or pulse? If you think it might be reassuring to stroke an arm during a painful procedure and are unsure of the child's response, ask if it would be helpful to do that. As nurses, we must touch children to weigh them, take blood pressures, and give immunizations. This does not mean that close touch is appropriate at all times. Tell all children when you will touch them for procedures so they understand what is happening. Refer to Chapter 6 for further information on communication.

An individual's sense of personal space also differs by culture. Space refers to the physical distance and relationships between the individual and other persons and objects in the environment. Cultures may have specific spatial preferences, such as personal distance and social distance. Some cultures tend to prefer close contact with less space since they use touch as a form of communication (Box 3–1). Be alert for how close a child comes to you and other individuals. Try to maintain this space in your interactions. Realize that nursing procedures often cause the space barrier to be broken.

Time Orientation

Cultures have specific values and meanings regarding time orientation. Cultural groups may place emphasis on the events of the past, those events that occur in the present, or those that will occur in the

---

BOX 3–1 Zones of Personal Space

Four "zones" of personal space to consider during communication are as follows:

- The *intimate zone* is within 18 inches of the body. This zone is for close personal contact and is generally reserved for those who have a close relationship. Nurses often bridge this zone for weighing, taking blood pressure, and performing other procedures.
- The *personal zone* is 18 inches to 4 feet from the body. This zone is used when talking to the family and child during interviews and history assessment. Be alert that some people have closer or more remote distances for personal interactions. Try to maintain the comfort zone of the child and family.
- The *social zone* is 4 to 12 feet from the body. This zone is used for impersonal communication and is usually the first zone nurses use before entering the personal zone, such as when calling someone in from a waiting room.
- The *public zone* is greater than 12 feet from the body. This zone is used when giving speeches or lectures to a group of people.

Source: Data from Spector, R. E. (2009). Cultural diversity in health and illness (7th ed.). Upper Saddle River, NJ: Pearson Prentice Hall.

future. Children reflect the time orientation of their families and of the cultures in which they live. Time is also influenced by development so that young children sometimes do not understand the use of clocks, the importance ascribed to being "on time," or other time orientations.

Cultures that are oriented predominantly to the past may want to begin healthcare encounters with lengthy descriptions of past health-care treatments, family history of diseases, or individual past experiences with health. There may be little interest in learning methods of adapting to or maintaining a new plan of care.

For cultures that are oriented predominantly to the present, little consideration may be given to either the past or the future. For example, adolescents commonly focus on the present and may not engage in preventive health practices for long-term health. Therefore, short-term goals often provide more incentive to adolescents.

Cultures that are oriented predominantly to the future, such as European Americans, may not focus on what is important at the present time. For example, the family focusing on the future may dream of a child's education or sports performance and have trouble setting present goals for treatment of a disease such as juvenile arthritis. One commonly hears that it was a big adjustment to learn to "take one day at a time." Not living up to the family's expectation for future success may be difficult for a child who has developed an illness that has a chronic course.

Time also refers to punctuality regarding schedules and appointments. In the United States, the predominant culture respects being on time and considers time valuable and not to be wasted. Other cultures may not emphasize the concern for time. This may be manifested by a family's inability to follow timed medication schedules or treatments, or to show up as scheduled for an appointment. In these cases, it is not intended as a sign of disrespect.

Nutrition

Nutritional practices begin even before birth as many cultural groups have beliefs that determine foods that are healthy to eat or should be avoided during pregnancy. Nutritional habits and patterns vary among cultures and are related to both religious practices and health beliefs. Certain cultures and religions have restrictions on or prescriptions about specific foods and preparation methods. Ritualistic behaviors involving eating and drinking, for example on special occasions and holidays, are observed by most cultures (Figure 3–5 ■). Many religions recommend fasts during specific holiday seasons, such as Lent for Roman Catholics, Yom Kippur for Jews, and Ramadan for Muslims; however, in most cases, small children, pregnant women, and sick individuals are not required to fast.

Additionally, some cultures value large size or may associate a healthy child with being "large." Other cultures value slimness and look down upon overweight individuals. Both of these views influence family eating patterns and expectations for the child; the child's self-esteem can therefore be influenced. The U.S. culture honors being slim in the media but reinforces eating and large size by the availability of fast food and the positive image of large sports stars such as some football players, which can result in confusion about health and body image.

Nutrition may also be essential to the culture's practices for health promotion and care during illness. Specific food preferences are identified in Table 3–5. Health problems associated with specific cultures, which may require dietary changes, are also identified. Recognize that nutrition may be closely related to environmental situations. Families with few resources may not be able to obtain or eat cultural foods due to access or financial issues. Nutrition plays a

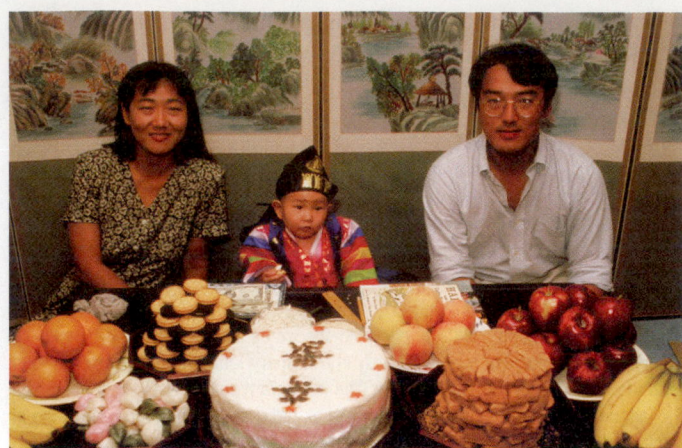

FIGURE 3–5 ■ Food traditions are common in many cultures and are often associated with rituals and celebrations. This family is celebrating the child's birthday with traditional foods.

Source: *Robert Brenner/PhotoEdit.*

powerful role in maintaining health so resources for nutritious and desired foods may be needed.

Health Beliefs, Approaches, and Practices

Health beliefs and practices have a profound impact on the health of a child. Those beliefs influence the family's healing approaches and practices. They determine what the family perceives as the cause of the child's illness, the purpose of illness, and how illness should be treated. Moreover, because beliefs and practices vary, not all families will seek traditional Western medical care for their children.

Health Beliefs

Three views of health beliefs described by Andrews and Boyle (2008) are magico-religious, scientific, and holistic. In reality, many people ascribe to a view that combines more than one of these belief systems, but it is helpful to examine them separately. In the **magico-religious paradigm,** health and illness are determined by supernatural forces such as God, gods, magic, spirits, or fate. Illness of a child may be perceived as a punishment for actions. Children of preschool age usually have this view of illness; some adults also believe that higher or supernatural powers determine health and illness. It is wise to ask both children and their families what they think caused an illness or how they believe they can stay well. People who believe in this paradigm may gain comfort from prayer, healing rituals, and faith healing. Young children who believe that they have caused their own illness because of their developmental level (usually preschool and early school age) can be expressly told that it was not something they did that caused the illness in order to decrease their feelings of guilt.

Balance and harmony of the body and nature are important concepts in the **holistic health paradigm.** It is believed that the child's illness results when the natural balance or harmony is disturbed. Infection and other illness gain entry into the body when it is not in balance. This health belief is most common in North American Indian and Asian cultures (Andrews & Boyle, 2008). Increasingly, the ideas of holism are being integrated into Western health care and combined with other approaches. An example of integration of approaches is use of a medication or radiation for illness in combination with adequate rest and a diet that is designed to increase immune function. An associated holistic health belief is the hot and cold theory of disease, which subscribes to the thought that illnesses and

TABLE 3–5	Food Preferences of Selected Cultures	
CULTURE	**FOOD PREFERENCES**	**HEALTH CONDITIONS THAT MAY REQUIRE MODIFIED DIETARY HABITS**
African American	Collard greens	Anemia
	Cornbread	Coronary heart disease
	Fried foods, such as fat-back (pork fat) and chicken wings	Obesity
		Hypertension
	Grits	Lactose intolerance
	Pork	
Hispanic/ Latin American	Rice	Coronary heart disease
	Beans	Diabetes
	Tortillas	Obesity
	Cheese	
	Chili	
	Fried foods	
	Carbonated beverages	
Native American	Blue cornmeal	Diabetes
	Corn, squash, beans	Hypertension
	Carbonated beverages	Malnutrition
	Fish and game	
	Fruits, such as berries	
	Snack foods, such as chips and prepackaged pastries	
Asian American	Raw fish	Coronary heart disease
	Rice	Liver disease
	Soy sauce	Ulcers

Source: Data from Andrews, M. M., & Boyle, J. S. (2008). Transcultural concepts in nursing care (5th ed.). Philadelphia: Lippincott Williams & Wilkins; Giger, J. N., & Davidhizar, R. E. (2008). Transcultural nursing: Assessment and intervention (5th ed.). St. Louis, MO: Mosby-Elsevier; Purnell, L. D. (2009). Guide to culturally competent health care (2nd ed.). Philadelphia: F. A. Davis.

diseases are a result of disruption in the hot and cold balance of the body. Therefore, consuming foods of the opposite variety can cure or prevent specific hot and cold illnesses. Hot and cold therapies related to healing are practiced in some African American, Asian, Latino, Arab, Muslim, and Caribbean cultures (Andrews & Boyle, 2008). See page 70 for further information.

The **scientific or biomedical health paradigm** assumes that physiology explains all illness and life itself (Andrews & Boyle, 2008). Biochemical reactions and the genomic code are used to explain all health states, and a child's illness is always caused by viruses, bacteria, or damage to the body. This approach is often called Western medicine. Families who hold this view expect a traditional Western medical intervention, such as medication, treatment, or surgery, to treat the child's health problems. Parents may be dissatisfied with care if they are told that the child is to rest, drink fluids, and use comfort measures; they feel a medication is most likely to help. Within this belief system it is difficult to understand certain health conditions. Families may struggle to "explain" an illness by wondering if the child was exposed to something harmful during fetal life, or has an environmental exposure; a reason for the condition is needed to understand it. Most physicians, nurses, and other healthcare professionals adhere primarily to biomedical or scientific theories to explain and

treat illnesses. However, certain therapies such as therapeutic touch, biofeedback, and other nontraditional methods that are more common in a holistic health paradigm are gaining popularity within these professions. For the family with scientific or biomedical health beliefs, health professionals sometimes need to emphasize that certain conditions have no known cause, and to suggest treatments other than traditional Western medicine if other approaches may be helpful.

Health Approaches and Practices

The family's health beliefs influence their approaches and practices regarding health and illness. The young child has a view of health and illness connected with developmental understanding and gradually takes on the family's cultural view while growing older. Additionally, some families, when faced with a life-threatening illness of their child, may seek alternative health practices that are not considered part of their cultural heritage. This is especially true if the family becomes frustrated with traditional biomedical treatments that are unable to cure their child. See Table 3–6 for examples of health practices common to specific cultures.

Healthcare practitioners The family seeking care for the child may choose one or a combination of magico-religious, holistic, or biomedical healthcare providers. Recall Raven in the opening scenario. His family has used a combination of a native healer and Western care. Nurses and other healthcare professionals seek to learn about the family's belief system and to integrate all types of care that the family wishes as long as there is no danger offered to the child.

Practice Alert

Families often combine treatments from more than one healthcare approach, both in seeking practitioners and in applying treatments such as medicines. Most often that is helpful to them and to the child. Nurses must be alert, however, to any practices that would be unsafe for the child. For example, the child with type 1 diabetes must be treated with insulin, and to rely only on a folk healer or herbs places the child in a life-threatening situation. Certain herbs may be harmful to children with some conditions (e.g., renal disorders) or in interaction with prescribed medication, and should not be used. In cases when the family's cultural practice is placing the child in a hazardous situation, civil courts may intervene to provide care for the child, for example, mandating a life-preserving chemotherapy for a child even when the family is opposed to treatment. Support families in their beliefs and healthcare practices but remain alert for any care that could be harmful to the child and report it promptly.

The use of **folk healers** varies according to the culture. Although the healer's role and position in the community differ among cultures, healers do share commonalities. Healers speak the language of the cultural group, use common methods of communication for the culture, and live in the same community. Several types of healers are specific to certain groups. Mexican American and some Hispanic cultures may seek healing by a **curandero** (male healer) or **curandera** (female healer), who deals with all levels of illness, from minor colds to cancer (Spector, 2009). The curandero's holistic treatment may include use of herbs, laying on of hands, massaging the afflicted area, cleansing the body with herbs, preparing an amulet to be worn, burning a candle with a specific prayer printed on the candle jar, or calling the spirit of a saint to bless the patient. Essential to the curandero/a and patient relationship is the faith the child and family have in his or her abilities. Families may combine curanderismo (Hispanic medical system) with a Western approach for some conditions. For example, a child with seizures may be given medications for the disorder obtained from Western care and may be fed a tea that the healer believes will treat the condition.

Puerto Ricans may use an **espiritista,** a healer who communicates with spirits for the physical and emotional development of the patient (Purnell, 2009). Mexican Americans may use this type of healer when the ailment is thought to be caused by witchcraft. However, use of an espiritista is frowned upon in some Hispanic cultures. **Sobadores,** individuals who use massage and manipulation to treat patients with joint and muscle problems, are another type of healer who might be used by Mexican Americans (Zoucha & Zamarripa, 2008).

Native Americans may seek healing from a **shaman,** "a woman or man who enters an altered state of consciousness, at will, to contact and utilize another type of reality to acquire knowledge and power and to help other people" (Fontaine, 2011, p. 355). Similar to the healing tradition of shamanism, Native Americans may also use a

healer, or medicine man or woman. Because Native Americans generally believe in the balance of nature and a state of harmony, they seek advice to identify what they have done to disrupt their body harmony. The healer then prescribes the required treatment for restoration of balance and harmony. Teas, other herbal products, smudges, meditation, and other approaches are common. Returning to one's family, home, and roots may produce a sense of balance. See Developing Cultural Competence: Smudging. Children who are ill and hospitalized may be surrounded and cared for by family members and tribal elders.

African Americans often combine Western and traditional beliefs about illness. Some believe in spirits as causes of illness and may use powders, oils, and ceremony to maintain health. Other healers that might be used by individuals from different cultures are listed in Table 3–6.

TABLE 3–6	Health Practices of Selected Cultures		
CULTURE	**HEALTH PRACTICES**	**CULTURE**	**HEALTH PRACTICES**
African American	Religious healing (laying on of hands)	Hispanic or Latin American	Hot and cold foods
	Talismans (amulets or lucky charms)		Herbs
	Herbal remedies/oils		Massage
	Use of healers:		Prayers
	"Old woman" healers		Religious medals
	Voodoo healers		Use of healers:
	Shamans		Curanderos/curanderas
	Spiritualists		Yerberos or jerberos (herbalists)
	Root doctors		Brujos/brujas (witches)
Asian American	Acupuncture/acupressure		Espiritistas (spiritualists)
	Coin rubbing		Sobadores
	Cupping	Native American	Ceremony
	Herbs		Counseling
	Hot and cold foods		Herbs and plants
	Massage		Healing touch/acupressure
	Meditation		Medicine bundle
	Moxibustion (heat therapy)		Singing
	Qi gong (combines meditation, movement, and regulation of breathing)		Pipe ceremony
	Restoring energy between yin and yang		Drumming and chanting (prayer)
	Tai chi		Smudging
	Tiger balm		Sun dance
	Use of healers:		Sweat lodge (purification ceremony)
	Physicians		Vision quest (a powerful ceremony)
	Herbalists		Use of healers:
	Acupuncturists		Medicine men or women
European American	Amulets		Shamans
	Healing rituals		
	Dietary modifications		
	Exercise		
	Traditional medicine		
	Use of healers:		
	Traditional healthcare providers: physicians, nurses, and nurse practitioners		

Source: Data from Andrews, M. M., & Boyle, J. S. (2008). Transcultural concepts in nursing care (5th ed.). Philadelphia: Lippincott Williams & Wilkins; Giger, J. N., & Davidhizar, R. E. (2008). Transcultural nursing: Assessment & intervention (5th ed.). St. Louis, MO: Mosby Elsevier; Fontaine, K. L. (2011). Complementary & alternative therapies for nursing practices (3rd ed.). Upper Saddle River, NJ: Prentice Hall; Spector, R. E. (2009). Cultural diversity in health and illness (7th ed.). Upper Saddle River, NJ: Pearson Prentice Hall.

Developing Cultural Competence
Smudging

Smudging is a process used by Native Americans and some religious groups during healing ceremonies. Sacred herbs such as sage, cedar, or tobacco are burned and the smoke is used to smudge people and sacred objects so that healing can begin. The smoke is believed to clear negativity, cause purification, and serve as a prayer to the creator (Fontaine, 2011).

Faith-based belief and spirituality Faith-based belief and practice is an integral part of culture for some families. Views of religion and spirituality can shape their approaches and responses to a child's illness and guide practices to maintain health. Religious beliefs may influence the family's explanation of the cause of a child's illness, their perception of the severity of the illness, and choices of treatments for the illness, and can offer solace to the family and child. For these reasons, it is important to determine the influence of religion and spirituality within the family.

Faith and spirituality can be a source of great comfort and support for children who are ill and their families. Conversely, conflicts may arise between the family's religion or spirituality and biomedical care for the child. For example, the family's pursuit of specific religious therapies can serve as a barrier to biomedical care, because some parents may believe that their spiritual practices can substitute for medical treatment of the child. **Religion,** commonly referred to as **faith-based belief,** is an organized system of shared beliefs regarding the significance of the nature, cause, and purpose of life and of the universe. Religion is usually centered on the belief in or the worshipping of a supernatural or supreme being (such as God or Allah). **Spirituality** refers to the individual's experience and own interpretation of his or her relationship with a supreme being. Children are spiritual beings and generally express their spirituality through behavior such as imaginative play, art, dance, and song (Mueller, 2010). Prayer, one of the most common expressions of religious faith, is a frequently used therapy in which many children and families engage (Grossoehme, VanDyke, Jacobson, et al., 2010; Lambert, Fincham, & Graham, 2011).

Although spirituality and faith-based beliefs are generally positive means of support for children and families in maintaining and restoring health, at times they can have potentially negative effects for children. Certain groups may blame individuals for their own illnesses, and children may develop guilt as a result. If prejudice against other groups occurs, unhealthy responses may interfere with the child's psychosocial development. Abuse may result from parental religious beliefs regarding corporal punishment and discipline. If a religious group denies lifesaving treatments, courts may intervene to ensure care for the child.

Christianity is overwhelmingly the most common faith tradition in the United States. In 2008, 76% of U.S. adults identified themselves as Christian, 3.9% identified themselves as belonging to a non-Christian group, 15% did not specify a religious affiliation, 4.1% refused to answer the question, and 0.9% did not know their religious identification (Kosmin & Keysar, 2009) (Figure 3–6 ■). Although adherence to a religious tradition is predominant in the United States, it should not be assumed that all individuals believe in or practice organized religion. Always ask family members if

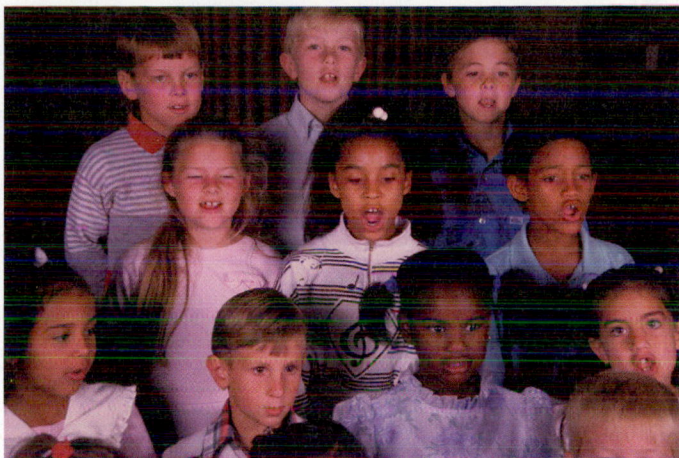

FIGURE 3–6 ■ No longer are communities limited to one culture. The children in this multicultural choir are representative of the changes in demographics in the United States. Even though they may differ in cultural background, a common thread is found in their religious preference. Can you identify other ways in which multicultural groups interact?

Source: Myrleen Pearson/PhotoEdit.

they follow a faith and would like a representative from that faith to visit when in the hospital. Adolescents may follow different faith traditions than their parents and should be asked the question individually.

Collaboration between the healthcare team and family is essential to providing care congruent with the child's and family's expectations. Although spirituality is important for many families, it is often overlooked as a healing strategy. Illness and injury may cause the family to turn to spiritual guidance as a method of understanding and coping. Assessment of the family and child's spiritual needs is an important aspect of nursing care (Mueller, 2010). At all times, the nurse must respect the family's view and avoid being judgmental toward their beliefs. Partner with the child and family to incorporate their traditional practices and beliefs with prescribed therapies to ensure the delivery of safe and effective care for the child.

Healing approaches Most health professionals in the United States practice traditional Western medicine; however, some families prefer healers. There are multiple approaches, and some families and practitioners will choose alternative treatments. Several other medical approaches are described here and further explored in the section on complementary and alternative modalities later in the chapter. One way to treat illness is by *homeopathy,* or treating a person with small doses of medicines that would cause illness when given to someone who is healthy. Traditional Western (or *allopathic*) medicine generally gives medicine or treatments that suppress symptoms. Analgesics for pain or antibiotics for infection are examples of such treatments. In homeopathy, the symptoms are viewed as the body's method of healing and small doses of medications are given to enhance the symptoms. For example, medications are chosen to promote fever and inflammation since they are thought to be healing forces (Fontaine, 2011; Spector, 2009).

Another approach to treatment is that of *osteopathic medicine,* which integrates many of the approaches of Western medicine with a belief that many of the body's disorders can be treated by mechanical correction of body imbalances. Several osteopathic medical schools are based in the United States. A doctor of osteopathy

TABLE 3–7	Hot and Cold Conditions and Foods		
HOT CONDITIONS	**COLD FOODS USED TO TREAT HOT CONDITIONS**	**COLD CONDITIONS**	**HOT FOODS USED TO TREAT COLD CONDITIONS**
Diarrhea	Barley water	Cancer	Beef
Fever	Chicken	Earaches	Cheese
Constipation	Dairy products	Headaches	Eggs
Infection	Raisins	Musculoskeletal conditions	Grains
Kidney problems	Fish	Pneumonia	Liquor
Sore throats	Fresh fruits	Malaria	Onions
	Fresh vegetables		Spicy foods
	Goat meat		Chocolate

Source: Data from *Giger, J. N., & Davidhizar, R. E. (2008). Transcultural nursing: Assessment & intervention (5th ed.). St. Louis, MO: Mosby Elsevier; Purnell, L. D. (2009). Guide to culturally competent health care (2nd ed.). Philadelphia: F. A. Davis; Purnell, L. D., & Paulanka, B. J. (2008). Transcultural health care: A culturally competent approach (3rd ed.). Philadelphia: F. A. Davis; Spector, R. E. (2009). Cultural diversity in health and illness (7th ed.). Upper Saddle River, NJ: Pearson Prentice Hall.*

(DO) may practice in the same health facilities as other physicians (Spector, 2009).

Naturopathy is a form of medicine that ascribes to the healing forces of nature. Naturopathic physicians focus on the restoration of health. They utilize opportunities to educate families about healthy lifestyles. A variety of interventions may be used including herbs, nutrition, acupuncture, and stress management. Counseling is also a commonly used approach as it focuses on the holistic needs of the individual, including mental, spiritual, and emotional factors (Fontaine, 2011).

Chiropractic medicine focuses on the relationship between body structure (primarily that of the spine) and function, and how that relationship affects the preservation and restoration of health. Chiropractors use manipulative therapy as an integral treatment tool (Fontaine, 2011).

Nutrition is another healing approach used by nearly all cultural groups. A common statement repeated in some groups is "Feed a cold, starve a fever." Some ascribe to certain foods for illness and health promotion while other foods may be withheld in certain situations. Recall the description of the need for balanced nutrition to treat disease in many cultures. Hot and cold conditions and foods and their links to culture are explained on page 70. Table 3–7 lists examples of hot and cold conditions and foods used to treat these conditions. Dietary intake and food patterns are integrally connected to culture and so it is logical that food is used to maintain health, restore balance, and treat illness. As children become older, they often practice a combination of food patterns that derive from their cultural group and the larger society in which they live. Diet recalls, food frequencies, and questions about what foods are recommended for certain conditions are good approaches to learn about nutritional intake. (See Chapter 7 🖉 for examples of assessment techniques.) As long as a child is receiving fluids needed and no part of intake is contraindicated for the illness, cultural patterns should be honored.

Complementary and alternative modalities   Complementary and alternative modalities (CAM) are defined as a "group of diverse medical and healthcare systems, practices, and products that are not presently considered to be part of conventional Western medicine"

(National Center for Complementary and Alternative Medicine [NCCAM], 2010a, p. 1). For the purposes of this text we refer to CAM as complementary and alternative modalities, recognizing that not all are medical approaches and most are not applied by traditional medical doctors. A wide array of practitioners use CAM techniques; several types of CAM have already been discussed in this chapter, such as homeopathy and nutrition. The use of CAM therapies in the United States is widespread and is observed in some manner within all cultures (Figure 3–7 ■). An estimated 38.3% of adults and 11.8% of children in the United States use CAM (Nahin, Barnes, Stussman, et al., 2009).

Although the terms *complementary* and *alternative* are often used interchangeably, they have different meanings and applications. **Complementary medicine** is used in combination with conventional medicine (NCCAM, 2010a). An example of a complementary therapy is the use of massage therapy in conjunction with biomedical therapy, such as narcotic analgesics, for a child with cancer pain.

Alternative medicine is used in place of conventional medicine (NCCAM, 2010a). An example of an alternative therapy is the use of herbal medicines instead of traditional Western medical care for a

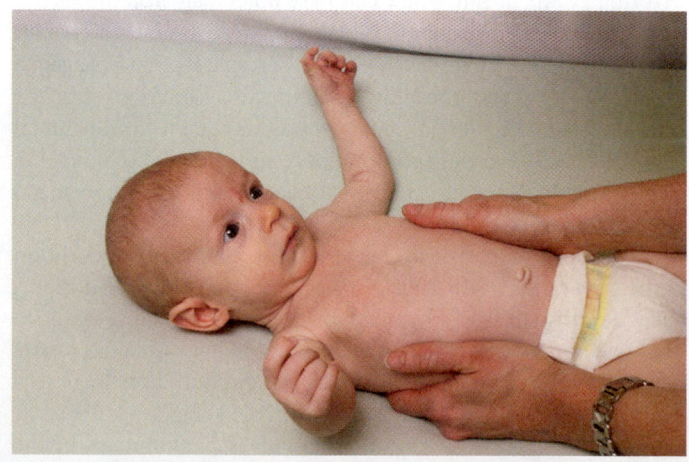

FIGURE 3–7 ■ Infant massage can be used to soothe infants. See Chapter 5, 🔗.

TABLE 3–8	Categories of Complementary and Alternative Medicine	
NATURAL PRODUCTS	**MIND–BODY MEDICINE**	**MANIPULATIVE AND BODY-BASED PRACTICES**
Natural products include herbal medicines, dietary supplements, vitamins, and minerals used to improve health.	Mind–body medicine uses a variety of techniques designed to enhance the mind's capacity to affect body function and symptoms.	Manipulative and body-based practices in CAM are based on manipulation and/or movement of one or more parts of the body.
Probiotics (live microorganisms similar to those found in the digestive tract) are also included in this category and are available in yogurt and dietary supplements.	Mind–body techniques include meditation, yoga, acupuncture, deep-breathing exercises, guided imagery, hypnotherapy, progressive relaxation, qi gong, and tai chi.	Examples include chiropractic or osteopathic spinal manipulation and massage therapy.

Source: *Data from National Center for Complementary and Alternative Medicine. (2010a). What is complementary and alternative medicine? Retrieved from http://nccam.nih.gov/health/whatiscam/D347.pdf*

child's health condition, such as surgery, radiation, prescribed medications, or other medical interventions.

The NCCAM (2010a) classifies CAM into three broad categories: natural products, mind–body medicine, and manipulative and body-based practices. Table 3–8 provides an overview of these three categories. Some CAM practices may fit into more than one category. In addition to these broad categories, other examples of CAM include movement therapies, traditional healers, and energy therapies such as Reiki and healing touch. Whole medical systems, based on theory and practice, may also be considered CAM and have evolved apart from the Western medical approach; whole medical systems include naturopathy and homeopathy. See page 70 for further explanations of these types of medicine. Some examples of CAM used in children are provided in Table 3–9.

Safety issues concerning CAM therapies   The use of CAM in the care of children must be addressed because of the limited research with this age group and developmental variations that may influence efficacy and safety. Although many CAM therapies may have been proven effective in adults, they may have little effect on children, or even be harmful. The National Institutes of Health and the Agency for Healthcare Research and Quality have set research agendas to investigate the effectiveness of CAM therapies for treatment.

CAM practices must be assessed for safety, including positive and negative benefits, cost, efficacy, and clinical usefulness. The use of herbs and natural products raises many issues, such as standards of products, misleading claims, safety related to megadoses of some products, and standardization of natural products. Determine the family's use of complementary and/or alternative medicine such as the type of remedies and healthcare practices used. Also determine the side effects, risks, and other implications to the child receiving this type of therapy. Partner with the family to ensure safe practices with the use of complementary and/or alternative modalities. See Partnering with Families: CAM Therapies.

Practice Alert

Several professional organizations, including the Society of Pediatric Nurses and the American Academy of Pediatrics, have affirmed that children and families should be educated about the benefits and risks of CAM, while being respectful of the family's desires to use these therapies. All healthcare providers must become knowledgeable about the broad range of CAM therapies to help families understand potential benefits and risks to the child (Asher, 2007; Kemper, Vohra, Walls, et al., 2008).

Nursing Management

The focus of nursing care is assessment of cultural influences on the child's health. The nurse providing culturally competent care to the child and family considers all facets of their culture. Identification of cultural influences as well as cultural barriers will enable the nurse to provide culturally competent nursing care in the management and support of the culturally diverse child and family.

Nursing Assessment

Assessment of the child and family includes determining the family's cultural healthcare beliefs and practices.

Questions may include:

- What is your child's condition?
- What do you think caused the child's illness?
- How do you think the child could best be treated?
- Has your child had this condition before and how was it treated?
- What are the most important results you hope to achieve for your child?

When the family is new to the healthcare facility, ask about former healthcare providers and if cultural healers are used. Ask family members how they would like to partner with other healing practices and the goals they have for their interaction with you as the nurse.

Determine barriers to the child's health care:

- Do the child and family speak a language different from the healthcare providers?
- Is there adequate transportation to healthcare facilities?
- Is the living situation supportive of treatment and prevention of illness and injury?
- Do the child and family have adequate funds or coverage for health care?

Faith-based practice and spirituality may influence a child's health. Identify any religious or spiritual practices the child and family use, as well as the significance of religion and spirituality on health promotion and during the child's illness.

- Do the child and family have any religious or spiritual beliefs?
- How important are those beliefs in the child's life and health and other family members' life and health?
- Do the child and family belong to a religious/spiritual community (e.g., church, synagogue, mosque)?

TABLE 3–9	Selected Types of Complementary and Alternative Medicines		
THERAPY	**DESCRIPTION**	**POTENTIAL USE IN CHILDREN**	**NURSING IMPLICATIONS**
Aromatherapy	Essential oils (extracts or essences) from flowers, herbs, and trees provide strong pleasant odors to promote relaxation, health, and well-being.	The family may use candles or oils to promote a child's pain relief or to encourage the child's relaxation. Use of aromatherapy in the hospital may reduce nausea due to hospital odors.	Few side effects when used as directed; however, allergies to oils may worsen symptoms in a child with asthma and other pulmonary disorders. Caution families to avoid aromatherapy.
Dietary supplements	A product (other than tobacco) is taken by mouth that contains an ingredient intended to supplement the diet, such as vitamins, minerals, herbs or other botanicals, amino acids, and substances such as enzymes, organ tissues, and metabolites. Dietary supplements come in many forms, such as extracts, tablets, capsules, liquids, and powders. They have special labeling requirements.	Many parents administer daily multiple vitamins to their children. Adolescents may use creatine to improve body image or athletic performance (Kemper et al., 2008). Echinacea is an herb that is frequently used to treat a cold.	Assess the family's use of dietary supplements for the child. Determine potential interactions between supplements and prescribed medications. Teach parents about safe dosages and safe storage of vitamins and other dietary supplements for children.
Massage	Therapists press, rub, and manipulate muscle and soft tissues to enhance function of those tissues and promote relaxation, well-being, and relief from pain.	Massage has been found to be beneficial for reducing the symptoms of asthma, insomnia, colic, cystic fibrosis, and juvenile arthritis. It is used in neonatal intensive care units (NICUs) to promote growth of preterm infants (Kemper et al., 2008).	Assess the child for benefits of massage. Potential contraindications to massage therapy may include bleeding disorders, fractures, and an open or healing wound.
Therapeutic touch	In therapeutic touch, the healing force of the therapist affects the patient's recovery. Healing is promoted when the body's energies are in balance. By passing their hands over the patient without touching the patient, healers can identify energy imbalances.	The family may enlist a spiritualist or other practitioner to perform therapeutic touch on the child to promote pain relief or a quicker recovery.	Assess the benefits of therapeutic touch on the child (e.g., pain relief). Partner with the family to establish other methods of pain relief if therapeutic touch is not effective.
Faith-based therapies	Spiritual healing, including prayer, is the most prevalent complementary therapy in the United States (Kemper et al., 2008). Other faith-based therapies include faith healing, laying on of hands, meditation, and anointing.	Families may include a variety of faith-based therapies, depending on the child's condition. Spiritual health may help improve quality of care, decrease anxiety, and increase positive feelings, such as hope, optimism, and freedom from regret.	Provide the child and family a private environment for faith-based practices. Assess for benefits of the therapies. Partner with the family to determine alternative methods of therapy if needed.

Source: *Data from National Center for Complementary and Alternative Medicine. (2010a). What is complementary and alternative medicine (CAM)? Retrieved from http://nccam.nih.gov/health/whatiscam/ D347.pdf. National Cancer Institute (2011). Spirituality in Cancer Care. Retrieved from http://www.cancer.gov/cancertopics/pdq/supportivecare/spirituality/Patient/; Kemper, K. J., Vohra, S., Walls, R., & the Task Force on Complementary and Alternative Medicine, the Provisional Section on Complementary, Holistic, and Integrative Medicine. (2008). The use of complementary and alternative medicine in pediatrics. Pediatrics, 122(6), 1374–1386.*

- How do the child's and family's religious/spiritual beliefs affect their practices for health and illness?
- What religious/spiritual healing rituals and practices are performed? By whom?
- Are any healthcare interventions forbidden by religious or spiritual beliefs?
- In what general religious practices (e.g., prayer, church attendance, meditation) does the family participate?

Identifying the roles of family members and who is responsible for healthcare decisions is an integral role of the nurse during the initial assessment interview. Determine the following:

- What is the family's structure (e.g., nuclear, extended)?
- Is the family patriarchal, matriarchal, or egalitarian?
- Who is the primary decision maker for the child's health care?
- Are the family roles clearly delineated?
- Who does the child depend on for comfort and support?

To communicate effectively, the nurse assesses the communication patterns and needs of the child and family:

- What language(s) does the child speak?
- What language(s) do the parents speak?
- What language does the child read?

- What language do the parents read?
- What is the family's literacy level either in English or in their native language?
- Is an interpreter necessary or helpful?
- What language would the child and family prefer healthcare providers use to communicate with them?
- Who is doing the majority of the talking and answering of questions?
- What gestures, facial expressions, and body language are used?
- Are there specific ways of demonstrating respect or disrespect for the culture?
- How does the child learn best (e.g., demonstration, reading, hearing)?
- How do the parents learn best (e.g., demonstration, reading, hearing)?

To avoid misinterpretation of a child's or family member's behavior, the nurse observes cues from the family to determine the appropriate spatial zone. Determine the following:

- What are the cultural preferences or restrictions related to spatial distancing, eye contact, touching, and other verbal and nonverbal forms of communication?

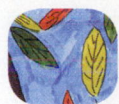

Partnering with Families

CAM Therapies

Once the nurse has been informed about CAM therapies used, potential side effects and risks can be considered, such as interactions between an herb and a prescribed medication. Partner with the family to promote and inform parents of the following safe practices for CAM use (NCCAM, 2010b):

- Ensure that your child has received an accurate diagnosis from a licensed healthcare provider and that CAM use does not replace or delay conventional medical care.

- If you decide to use CAM for your child, do not increase the dose or length of treatment beyond what is recommended. More is not necessarily better.
- If your child experiences an effect from a CAM therapy that concerns you, contact your child's healthcare provider.
- Store herbal and other dietary supplements out of the sight and reach of children.

- Does the family plan for the future?
- Is being on time considered important to the family?
- How do the parent and other family members prefer to be addressed?
- How does the child prefer to be addressed (e.g., nicknames)?
- Explore the meaning of food to the child and family. Identify the following:
  - Acceptable foods and preparation practices
  - Foods that are prohibited or taboo
  - Specific food rituals (e.g., holidays, fasting)
  - Dietary practices used in promoting the child's health and in treating the child's illnesses
  - Foods the child typically likes to eat
  - Foods the child dislikes
  - The family's usual mealtimes
  - The child's height, weight, and other developmental indicators of nutritional health

Refer to Chapter 19 🔗 for further discussion of nutrition assessment.

Assess the child's biological features for variations of physical characteristics of an ethnic or cultural group (e.g., bone structure, skin color). Assess the child's parental history for the existence of diseases such as hypertension, diabetes, and blood disorders. Determine if the child has been screened for ethnic or culturally specific diseases, for example, sickle cell disease.

For the dying child or child who has died, determine culturally specific rituals. Determine the family's cultural beliefs regarding death and practices for care of the body. For a comprehensive discussion of end-of-life issues, including cultural considerations, refer to Chapter 18 🔗.

Nursing Diagnoses

The use of NANDA nursing diagnoses to describe situations specifically related to culture may be in itself culturally biased since the focuses of these diagnoses are based on Western cultural beliefs. Diagnoses such as Impaired Verbal Communication or Deficient Knowledge should not be used solely because a person does not speak English. Is someone who speaks a different language "impaired" in communication?

Specific nursing diagnoses are dependent upon the reason the family seeks contact with healthcare professionals, ranging from the child's health promotion and health maintenance

(e.g., immunizations) to the care of a child who is chronically or terminally ill. Examples include:

- Therapeutic Regimen Management: Family, Ineffective related to mistrust of healthcare personnel
- Fear related to separation from support system in stressful situation such as hospitalization
- Spiritual Distress related to discrepancy between spiritual beliefs and prescribed treatment
- Family Processes, Interrupted related to shift in family roles due to illness

NANDA-I © 2012

Planning and Implementation

The planning and implementation of nursing care for the culturally diverse child and family depends specifically on the findings of the previous assessments. Partner with the child and family to establish a safe, effective, and desirable plan of care. Establish access to an interpreter if needed and evaluate if the match with a particular interpreter is appropriate for the child and family. See Table 3–3 and Chapter 6 🔗 for further guidelines for interpreters.

Recognizing the influence of culture on one's own beliefs, values, and healthcare practices is essential for the nurse to deliver culturally competent care. Nurses demonstrate appropriate strategies to delivering culturally sensitive care when they develop techniques in assessing the influence of culture on the child and family and incorporate that information into an individualized plan of care. As a nurse, you will also collaborate with a multidisciplinary team, including social workers and language specialists, to help the family in receiving assistance to overcome barriers to care such as transportation, financial issues, remote access, and others.

Partner with the child and family in determining how they can incorporate prescribed therapies with their healthcare practices. Recognize the predominant decision maker of the child's health care. If culturally appropriate, encourage all family members to participate in the child's care. Ensure that the child and family understand the child's illness, treatment, or health promotion activities. If discrepancies are noted, be particularly sensitive if attempting to dispel any cultural myths. Recognize that cultural beliefs are deeply rooted, and the most sensitive explanation may not have the desired impact.

Partner with the family to determine the role traditional healthcare providers and other practitioners, such as folk healers, curanderos or curanderas, and spiritualists, will have in the care of the child.

Encourage collaboration and communication between practitioners to ensure continuity of care. Collaborate with the child and family to meet specific spiritual needs. This involves showing respect and allowing time and privacy for religious rituals. Offer to have a religious advisor visit and arrange for inclusion of the child's religious symbols such as displaying a cross in the room, wearing a medicine bag around the neck or wrist, and wearing prayer shawls.

Ensure that the child's nutritional preferences are available. Provide nutritional guidance for the child and family if necessary. Provide education to the family regarding high-risk dietary practices. Partner with the family to establish a well-balanced meal plan for the child. Incorporate cultural preferences in the diet plan. Refer the family to a nutritionist if necessary.

Encourage screening for the child and other family members for disorders associated with specific ethnic groups (e.g., sickle cell disease in African Americans, Tay-Sachs disease in Jews) if they have not been screened. Provide education regarding specific diseases of high incidence in specific populations. Determine the family's awareness of those specific diseases. Encourage early preventive care in children at risk for culturally specific diseases.

Evaluation

A desired outcome for the nurse is an awareness and understanding of the cultural influences on the health promotion and illness care of the child, and integration of this understanding into care for all children. Expected outcomes of nursing care that demonstrate culturally sensitive care for the child and family include:

- Inclusion of cultural influences in the plan of care
- Collaboration of the child and family with the nurse related to cultural needs and issues of the family
- Integration of cultural influences into health promotion/health maintenance visits
- Integration of cultural influences into illness/injury care

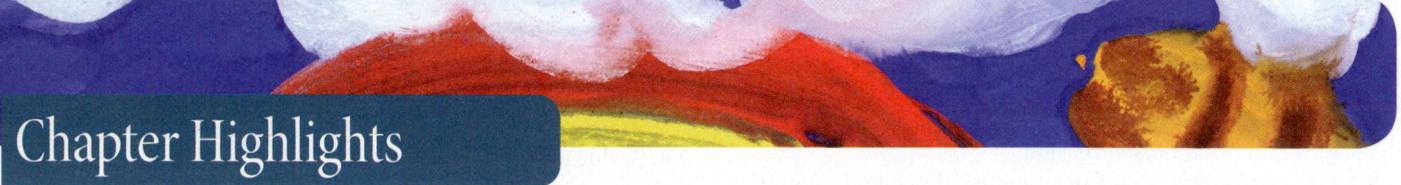

Chapter Highlights

- Culture is a significant determinant of an individual's beliefs, behavior, and response to health and illness. Parental beliefs and behaviors can either promote the child's health care or impede preventive care, delay or complicate medical care, or result in the use of ineffective or harmful remedies.
- The morbidity and mortality rate for some racial and ethnic populations is disproportionate as compared to the White population.
- Cultural barriers to health care include lack of cultural awareness and sensitivity in healthcare providers, health-seeking behaviors, perceptions of health and illness, how health information is communicated, socioeconomic factors, and inadequate access.
- Cultural competence refers to the ability of the nurse to understand and respond effectively to the cultural needs of the child and family.

- The development of cultural competence is an enduring process. Strategies include a self-assessment of one's own beliefs, changes in nursing school curriculum to reflect the diverse nature of the population, increasing diversity of the nursing workforce, and increasing understanding through nursing research.
- Health beliefs of the family inform and determine its use of healthcare practitioners and therapies. A combination of Western and alternative practitioners and therapies is commonly used.
- Complementary and alternative modalities (CAM) are defined as diverse medical and healthcare systems, practices, and products that are not presently considered to be part of conventional medicine.

Clinical Reasoning in Action

INTRODUCTION

Recall Raven, the 4-year-old boy brought to the clinic for complaints of an earache. His father requests a health and physical examination to determine if any healthcare interventions are necessary. Raven does not seem to understand the purpose of the visit and indicates that he has no desire to talk to the nurse.

DESCRIPTION

As the nurse in this situation, you will implement developmentally and culturally appropriate interventions to communicate with Raven. You discuss Raven's living arrangements, education, and nutritional habits with his father, allowing Raven time to adjust to the surroundings of the examination room. Additional information collected relates to care provided for Raven's fever and pain, such as teas and herbs, prior to this visit to the clinic. Raven is observant of your communication with his father.

DISCUSSION

1. What are the most appropriate interventions for communicating with Raven?
2. What approach will you take to assess Raven?
3. How will you examine your cultural values in an effort to provide culturally competent care?
4. How will you demonstrate the role of the nurse to Raven, since his major experience with health care has been through his healer?
5. What short-term and long-term collaborative plans should you establish with this family?

NCLEX-RN® Review

1. The nurse is asked to care for a child whose family is from a culture different from the nurse's culture. Which is the most effective strategy for this nurse to quickly learn how to care for this family?
   1. Listen to the family's preferences.
   2. Complete an Internet search about the culture.
   3. Ask other nurses who have cared for the child.
   4. Involve other disciplines in the child's care.

2. When working with cultural differences, which of the following areas may differ from one culture to another? Select all that apply.
   1. Religious beliefs
   2. Alternative therapies
   3. Time orientation
   4. Nutrition
   5. Hand signals

3. The nurse manager is teaching new graduates that it is important to assess culture when caring for a child. Which of the following questions is not particular to a cultural assessment?
   1. "What do you usually do when your child has a fever?"
   2. "Who is responsible for caring for the children in your family?"
   3. "How do you know when your child is sick?"
   4. "Is there a spiritual counselor you would like me to call?"

4. In learning cultural competence, which statement best exemplifies a cultural perspective to avoid?
   1. "I don't know of any other way that is better than mine."
   2. "I think immigrants are required to have a green card."
   3. "I think different kinds of people make life interesting."
   4. "I hope to understand how different people view medicine."

See Appendix I 🔁 for answers.

References

American Medical Association. (2008). *Physician characteristics and distribution in the US, 2008 edition.* Retrieved from http://www.ama-assn.org/ama/pub/about-ama/our-people/member-groups-sections/minority-affairs-consortium/physician-statistics/total-physicians-raceethnicity-2006.shtml

American Nurses Association. (2007). *Nursing facts: Today's registered nurses: Numbers and demographics.* Retrieved from http://www.ana.org/readroom/fsdemogr2.htm

Andrews, M. M., & Boyle, J. S. (2008). *Transcultural concepts in nursing care* (5th ed.). Philadelphia: Lippincott Williams & Wilkins.

Asher, C. (2007). Position statement on complementary and alternative medicine in pediatrics. *Journal of Pediatric Nursing, 22*(2) 159–161.

Baker, D. L., Dang, M. T., Ly, M. Y., & Diaz, R. (2010). Perception of barriers to immunization among parents of Hmong origin in California. *American Journal of Public Health, 100*(5), 839–845.

DeNavas-Walt, C., Proctor, B. D., & Smith, J. C. (2010). *Income, poverty, and health insurance coverage in the United States: 2009.* Retrieved from http://www.census.gov/prod/2010pubs/p60-238.pdf

Fontaine, K. L. (2011). *Complementary & alternative therapies for nursing practice* (3rd ed.). Upper Saddle River, NJ: Pearson.

Giger, J. N., & Davidhizar, R. E. (2008). *Transcultural nursing: Assessment & intervention* (5th ed.). St. Louis, MO: Mosby-Elsevier.

Grieco, E. M., & Trevelyan, E. N. (2010). *Place of birth of the foreign-born population: 2009 American community survey briefs.* U.S. Census Bureau. Retrieved from http://www.census.gov/prod/2010pubs/acsbr09-15.pdf

Grossoehme, D. H., VanDyke, R., Jacobson, C. J., Cotton, S., Ragsdale, J. R., & Seid, M. (2010). Written prayers in a pediatric hospital: Linguistic analysis. *Psychology of Religion and Spirituality, 2*(4), 227–233.

Kaiser Family Foundation. (2008). *Eliminating racial/ethnic disparities in health care: What are the options?* Retrieved from http://www.kff.org/minority-health/h08_7830.cfm

Kemper, K. J., Vohra, S., Walls, R., and the Task Force on Complementary and Alternative Medicine, the Provisional Section on Complementary, Holistic, and Integrative Medicine. (2008). The use of complementary and alternative medicine in pediatrics. *Pediatrics, 122*(6), 1374–1386.

Kosmin, B. A., & Keysar, A. (2009). *American Religious Identification Survey (ARIS 2008) summary report.* Retrieved from http://www.americanreligionsurvey-aris.org/reports/ARIS_Report_2008.pdf

Lambert, N. M., Fincham, F. D., & Graham, S. M. (2011). Understanding the layperson's perception of prayer: A prototype analysis of prayer. *Psychology of Religion and Spirituality, 3*(1), 55–65.

Leininger, M. (2006). Culture care diversity and universality theory and evolution of the ethno-nursing method. In M. M. Leininger & M. R. McFarland (Eds.), *Culture care diversity and universality: A worldwide nursing theory* (2nd ed., pp. 1–41). Boston: Jones and Bartlett.

Lillie-Blanton, M., Maleque, S., & Miller, W. (2008). Reducing racial, ethnic, and socio-economic disparities in health care: Opportunities in National Health Reform. *Journal of Law, Medicine and Ethics, 36*(4), 693–702.

Moore, J. (2010). Cultural brokers in health care. *American Diversity Report.* Retrieved from http://www.americandiversityreport.com/index.php?option=com_content&view=article&id=19:cultural-brokers-in-health-care&catid=1:us-diversity&Itemid=2

Mueller, C. R. (2010). Spirituality in children: Understanding and developing interventions. *Pediatric Nursing, 36*(4), 197–203, 208.

Nahin, R. L., Barnes, P. M., Stussman, B. J., & Bloom, B. (2009). Costs of complementary and alternative medicine (CAM) and frequency of visits to CAM practitioners: United States, 2007.

National Cancer Institute (2011). Spirituality in Cancer Care. *Retrieved from* http://www.cancer.gov/cancertopics/pdq/supportivecare/spirituality/Patient/

National Center for Complementary and Alternative Medicine (NCCAM). (2010a). *What is complementary and alternative medicine?* Retrieved from http://nccam.nih.gov/health/whatiscam/D347.pdf

National Center for Complementary and Alternative Medicine (NCCAM). (2010b). *Complementary and alternative medicine use in children.* Retrieved from http://nccam.nih.gov/health/children/#discuss

National Center for Cultural Competence. (2004, Spring/Summer). *Bridging the cultural divide in healthcare settings: The essential role of cultural broker programs.* Georgetown University Center for Child and Human Development, Georgetown University Medical Center. Retrieved from http://www.culturalbroker.info/11_contents/index.html

National Health Statistics Report, 18. Retrieved from http://nccam.nih.gov/news/camstats/costs/nhsrn18.pdf

National Institute for Health Care Management. (2007). *Reducing health disparities among children: Strategies and programs for health plans.* Retrieved from http://www.nihcm.org/pdf/HealthDisparitiesFinal.pdf

Nield, L. S. (2008). Improving cultural competence in the pediatric clinic. *Pediatric Annals, 37*(12), 830–835.

Purnell, L. D. (2009). *Guide to culturally competent health care* (2nd ed.). Philadelphia: F. A. Davis.

Purnell, L. D. (2008). The Purnell model for cultural competence. In L. D. Purnell & B. J. Paulanka, *Transcultural health care: A culturally competent approach* (3rd ed., pp. 19–55). Philadelphia: F. A. Davis.

Purnell, L. D., & Paulanka, B. J. (2008). *Transcultural health care: A culturally competent approach* (3rd ed.). Philadelphia: F. A. Davis.

Schneiderman, J. U., McDaniel, D. D., Xie, B., Cabassa, L. J., & Suh, J. (2010). Child welfare caregivers of differing English-language use: Perceptions of pediatric health care access barriers. *Journal of Ethnic & Cultural Diversity in Social Work, 19,* 18–33.

Singleton, K., & Krause, E. M. S. (2009). Understanding cultural and linguistic barriers to health literacy. *Online Journal of Issues in Nursing, 14*(3), Manuscript 4.

Spector, R. E. (2009). *Cultural diversity in health and illness* (7th ed.). Upper Saddle River, NJ: Pearson Prentice Hall.

Tuck, I., Moon, M. W., & Allocca, P. N. (2010). An integrative approach to cultural competence education for advanced practice nurses. *Journal of Transcultural Nursing, 21*(4), 402–409.

U.S. Census Bureau. (2010a). *Income, poverty, and health insurance coverage in the United States: 2009: Current Population Reports*. Retrieved from http://www.census.gov/prod/2010pubs/p60-238.pdf

U.S. Census Bureau. (2010b). *Highlights in minority health & health disparities September/October, 2010*. Retrieved from http://www.cdc.gov/omhd/Highlights/2010/HSeptOct10.html

U.S. Census Bureau. (2011). *Overview of race and Hispanic origin: 2010*. Retrieved from http://www.census.gov/prod/cen2010/briefs/c2010br-02.pdf

U.S. Citizenship and Immigration Services. (2011). *Refugee questions and answers*. Retrieved from http://www.uscis.gov

U.S. Department of Health and Human Services. (2010). *Healthy People 2020*. Retrieved from http://www.healthypeople.gov/2020/TopicsObjectives2020/pdfs/HP2020_brochure.pdf

U.S. Department of Health and Human Services, National Institutes of Health. (2010). *Cultural competency*. Retrieved from http://www.nih.gov/clearcommunication/culturalcompetency.htm

U.S. Department of Health and Human Services, National Institutes of Health. (2011). *Health disparities*. Retrieved from http://report.nih.gov/nihfactsheets/ViewFactSheet.aspx?csid=124&key=H

U.S. Department of Health and Human Services, Office of Minority Health. (2007). *National standards for culturally and linguistically appropriate services in health care*. Retrieved from http://minorityhealth.hhs.gov/templates/browse.aspx?lvl=2&lvlID=15

Xu, Y. (2008). Mentoring and career development of minority nurses and faculty. *Home Health Care Management and Practice, 20*(6), 503–505.

Yearwood, E. L. (2007). Child health care decision making and experiences of Caribbean women. *Journal of Pediatric Health Care, 21*(2), 89–98.

Zoucha, R., & Zamarripa, C. A. (2008). People of Mexican heritage. In L. D. Purnell & B. J. Paulanka, *Transcultural health care: A culturally competent approach* (3rd ed., pp. 309–324). Philadelphia: F. A. Davis.

Pearson Nursing Student Resources

Find additional review materials at
nursing.pearsonhighered.com
Prepare for success with additional NCLEX®-style practice questions, interactive assignments and activities, web links, animations and videos, and more!

Child Concepts and Application

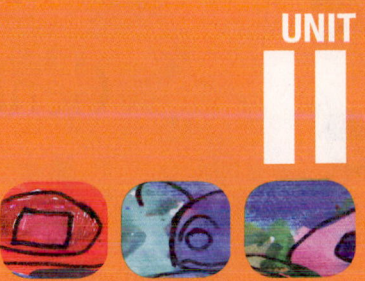

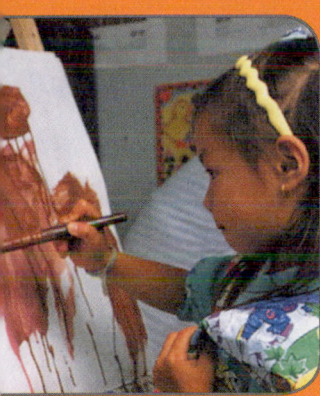 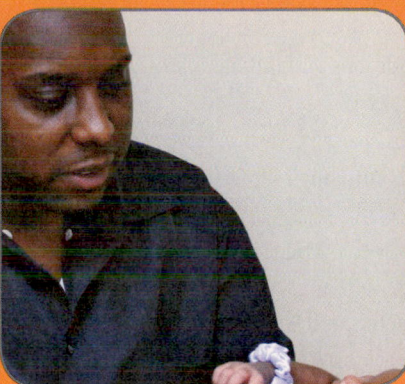 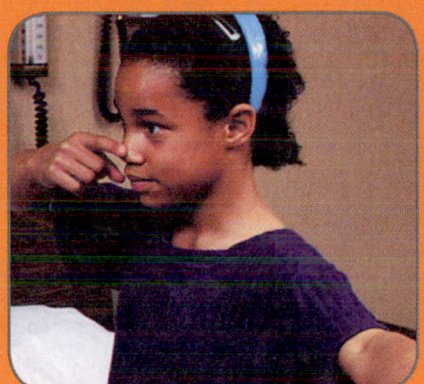 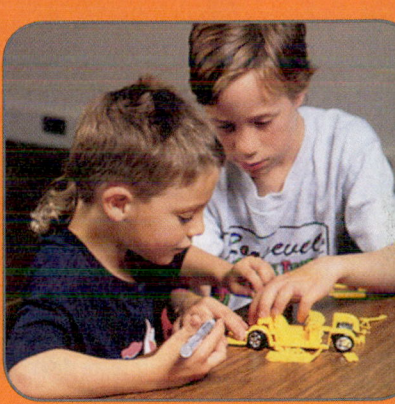

Pediatric nurses rely on a thorough knowledge base to formulate appropriate nursing interventions. Understanding the child's physical, cognitive, and psychosocial developmental stages is essential to providing care. The nurse applies communication principles when working with both children and their family members. The nurse applies knowledge of growth and development, as well as communication, during physical assessment of young children. Descriptions of findings and identification of abnormalities and risk factors are crucial to providing effective nursing care.

Genetic and Genomic Influences

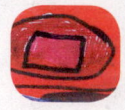 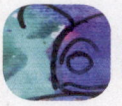 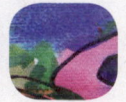

Learning Outcomes

After completing this chapter, you will be able to:

1. Apply genetic concepts to health promotion and health maintenance.

2. Integrate basic genetic concepts into child and family education and the reinforcement of information provided to patients by genetic professionals.

3. Incorporate genetic physical assessment and a family history pedigree into the delivery of nursing care.

4. Identify children or families with actual or potential genetic conditions and initiate referrals to a genetics professional.

5. Prepare children and their families for a genetic evaluation.

6. Recognize the significance of delivering genetic education and counseling follow-up in a professional manner.

7. Explain the implications of genetic advances on the role of nurses with particular attention to spiritual, cultural, ethical, legal, and social issues.

8. Summarize the significance of recent advances in human genetics and the impact on healthcare delivery.

> **"If I know whether I have the gene alteration that causes Huntington disease, then I will be able to be honest with myself and plan my life with more straightforward choices."**
> —*Sarah, age 17*

Sarah Hart is a mature 17-year-old who arrives alone at the clinic for a sports physical. Sarah was raised by her mother, Diane, and does not know her father. Sarah appears anxious and tells the nurse about her concerns. Sarah has memories of her mother's father dying from Huntington disease when she was 8 years old, and she has recently begun researching information. She knows that Huntington disease is inherited in an autosomal dominant inheritance pattern with symptoms often manifesting by age 40 years, but it often presents earlier as it is inherited from generation to generation. Sarah also knows there is no treatment or cure for Huntington disease. Diane will not discuss her father's death or the inheritance issues with Sarah even though they have a very close relationship. Sarah states that her mother is a free spirit and always "lives in the moment." Sarah, on the other hand, has told the nurse that she is concerned about whether she should save money, attend college, pursue a career, get married, and have children, or just live in the moment herself, travel, and take on no responsibilities. Sarah would like to be tested to see if she has the altered gene and will have Huntington disease, but her mother strongly objects. Diane is not interested in knowing if she has the altered gene. If Sarah were found to have the dominant gene that causes Huntington disease, it would be inferred that her mother also has the gene.

Does the nurse have enough knowledge about genetics to evaluate Sarah's knowledge and also to provide reinforcement of information and guidance to Sarah? Is Sarah able to give informed consent for genetic testing or is she too young to make a decision? Where can the nurse refer Sarah to find the answers to her questions in order to make an informed decision? How might Sarah's test result, positive or negative, affect her self-identity and life planning? Her relationship with her mother?

PARTNERING WITH FAMILIES: MEETING THE STANDARD OF GENETIC NURSING CARE DELIVERY

Completion of the Human Genome Project in 2003 heralded the dawn of the genomic era of health care (Box 4–1). It has long been known that some diseases occur due to specific gene defects and therefore are often inherited. **Genetic diseases** have traditionally been thought of as inherited diseases involving dysfunction of a single gene. Although these "typical" genetic diseases have enormous health consequences for affected individuals and families, they have relatively little public health impact. Research associated with the Human Genome Project has revealed a genetic component to virtually all diseases; together, genetic and environmental forces contribute to health and illness. The human **genome** is the entire deoxyribonucleic acid (DNA) sequence of an individual, and the study of **genomics** takes a holistic view of gene function. Human genomics is the study of all the DNA in the human genome, including gene interactions with other genes and with environmental, psychosocial, and cultural factors. While essentially all diseases and conditions have both genetic and environmental components, the genetic contribution to various diseases varies widely (Figure 4–1 ■).

DNA is central to our state of health because each individual's DNA sequence directs the formation of the hundreds of thousands of proteins available to carry out cellular functions (Figure 4–2 ■). Proteins include enzymes, cell receptors, ion channels, structural molecules, antibodies, transport molecules, and many other molecules necessary for biological function. Protein structure is dictated by the DNA sequence within the encoding gene, while gene function is affected by all manner of environmental and **epigenetic** effects. Good health is dependent on both normal gene structure and normal gene function. Genetic abnormalities may cause too much or too little of a specific protein, or perhaps a dysfunctional protein, to be formed. This can result in increased risk for disease. Both traditional genetic disorders and common complex diseases such as heart disease, stroke, diabetes, and cancer are now known to be related to gene structure and function. Research has uncovered many genetic and environmental factors that increase risk for disease, resulting in treatments that range in scope from promoting healthy lifestyles to specific genetic therapies. Knowledge gained from human genome research is changing all aspects of health care, including health promotion, disease prevention, screening, treatment, and monitoring of treatment effectiveness.

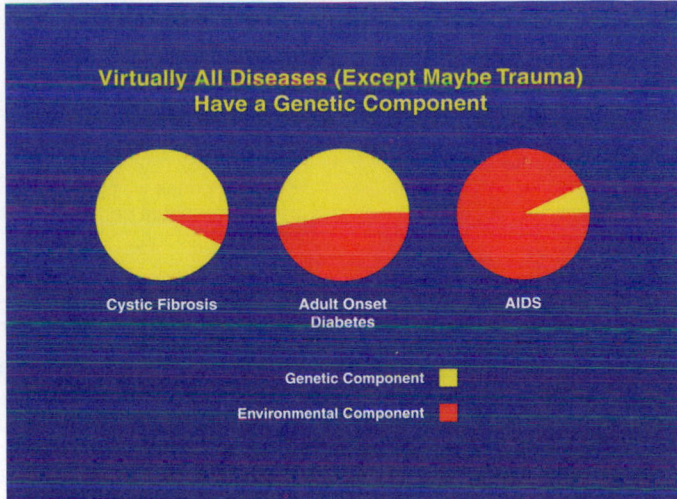

FIGURE 4–1 ■ Although the causes for nearly all diseases and health conditions have both genetic and environmental components, the relative contribution of genetic and environmental influences varies widely. At one end of the spectrum lie "traditional" genetic diseases such as cystic fibrosis (CF). Although CF is caused by a gene alteration, its morbidity and mortality vary according to environmental effects such as medical management. On the other hand, AIDS is an infectious disease that will not occur without environmental exposure to the HIV virus. Still, there are genetic alterations that cause some people to be resistant to HIV infection. In type 2 diabetes, the genetic and environmental contributions are fairly equivalent.

Source: *Reprinted with permission of Francis Collins, M.D., Ph.D., Director, National Human Genome Research Institute, National Institutes of Health.*

The translation of genetic and genomic knowledge to clinical care requires nurses to be prepared to deliver genetically competent care in all healthcare settings to individuals, families, communities, and populations. Nurses in newborn nurseries and mother-baby units may be the first to suspect a newborn has a genetic condition. Pediatric nurses often care for children with genetic conditions, who may require frequent hospitalization. Nurses in general and specialty clinics must be prepared to help asymptomatic individuals and families who are increasingly seeking information about their risk for an inherited disease or condition. Nurses must achieve genetic and genomic literacy to deliver competent care in the genomic era.

An expectation for nurses to acquire proficiency in genetics and genomics was formally established in 2007 by the American Nurses Association (ANA) and the International Society of Nurses in Genetics (ISONG) in a joint statement, *Genetics/Genomics Nursing: Scope and Standards of Practice.* This document outlines the levels of genetic knowledge required of all registered nurses, including basic and advanced practice nurses in general practice, as well as those who specialize in genetics nursing (Box 4–2). In addition, a set of essential competencies in genetics and genomics has been defined and endorsed by nearly 50 nursing organizations. These competencies represent the minimal level of genetic and genomic competency expected of every registered nurse across all practice settings (Consensus Panel, 2009) (Box 4–3). In response to advances in science and technology, genetic and genomic concepts now represent core knowledge for nurses (American Association of Colleges of Nursing, 2008).

Nurses must have basic genetic and genomic knowledge to care for the needs of patients and their families with known or suspected

BOX 4–1	Human Genome Project

In 1990, the U.S. Department of Energy joined with the National Institutes of Health to develop the Human Genome Project (HGP), a 15-year endeavor to sequence the entire human genome and identify all human genes. The project's completion was announced in April 2003, two years earlier than anticipated. The sequence of the 3.1 billion nucleotide bases that make up human DNA is available to all in a public database. New knowledge and technology associated with the HGP have led to a greater understanding about the biological basis for human variation and the identification of genes associated with both rare and common human disease. With the HGP completed, a new set of goals was put forth, including learning more about gene function and human genetic variation, understanding the genetic contribution to disease, and translating genetic knowledge into health benefits.

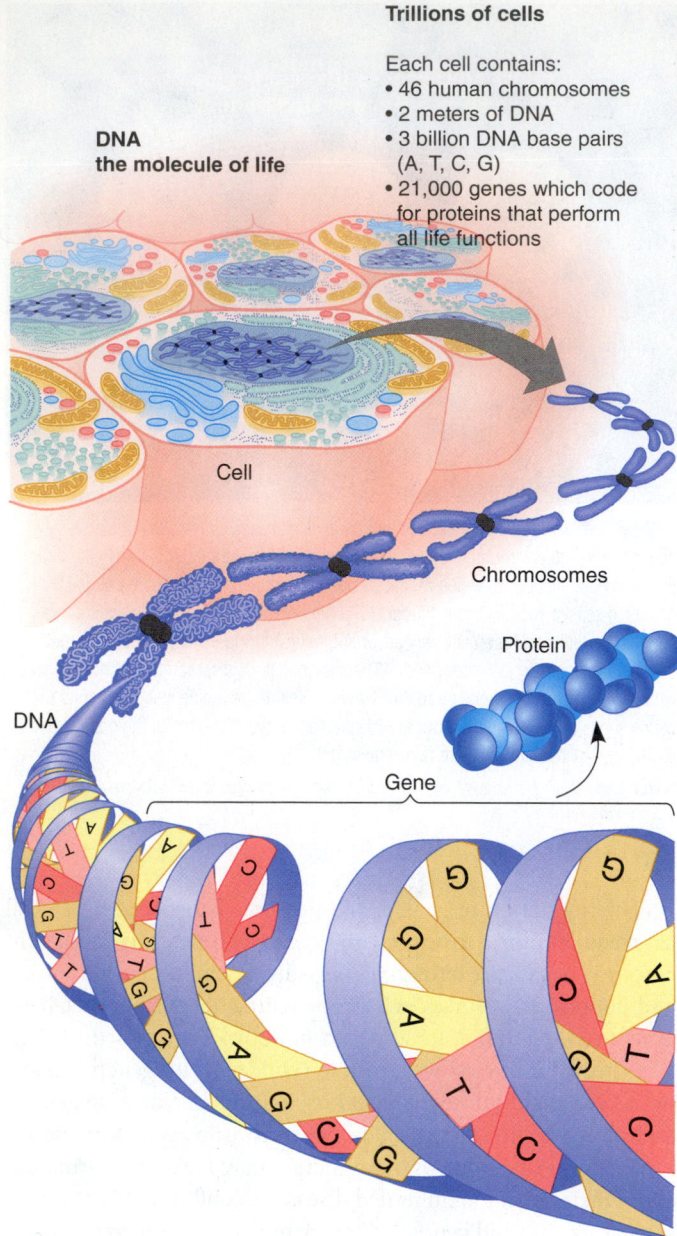

DNA
the molecule of life

Cell

Chromosomes

Protein

Gene

DNA

Trillions of cells

Each cell contains:
- 46 human chromosomes
- 2 meters of DNA
- 3 billion DNA base pairs (A, T, C, G)
- 21,000 genes which code for proteins that perform all life functions

FIGURE 4–2 ■ Each cell nucleus throughout the body contains DNA, which makes up the genes and chromosomes that represent the majority of an individual's genome. The remaining portion of the human genome is contained in a small amount of DNA in the mitochondria.

genetic disease. Examples of nursing activities that reflect application of genetic competence include:

- Identifying disease risk by collecting a family history and drawing a three-generation pedigree
- Providing nondirective counseling to assist families who have questions or concerns about their reproductive risks
- Helping individuals and families to identify credible sources of genetic information
- Helping individuals and families to understand the implications and limitations of genetic testing
- Anticipating variable responses among individuals to "standard" medication doses, due to pharmacogenetic effects

BOX 4–2   **ANA/ISONG Scope and Standards of Genetics/ Genomics Nursing**

The ANA/ISONG statement on the scope and standards of genetics and genomic nursing practice is as follows:

All licensed registered nurses, regardless of their practice setting, have a role in the delivery of genetics services and the management of genetic information. Nurses require genetics and genomics knowledge to identify, refer, support, and care for persons affected by, or at risk for manifesting or transmitting conditions or diseases with a genetic component. As the public becomes more aware of the genetic contribution to health and disease, nurses in all areas of practice are being asked to address basic genetics- and genomics-related questions and service needs.

Source: *Used with permission from American Nurses Association and International Society of Nurses in Genetics. Copyright 2007, p. 17. Silver Spring, MD: Nursesbooks.org*

- Recognizing dysmorphic features that may indicate a genetic condition in a newborn
- Applying concepts of health promotion and health maintenance to assist children and families at increased risk to develop common chronic conditions, such as heart disease, to make informed lifestyle choices
- Partnering with families affected by genetic conditions, including providing advocacy, supporting the child's and family's decisions, teaching, making appropriate referrals, clarifying information, and providing further information about available resources and services
- Partnering with the community to educate the public and supporting legislation that protects genetic information and those with genetic conditions from discrimination
- Ensuring the delivery of genetically competent care for the child and family
- Applying knowledge of the ethical, legal, and social implications of genetic information

By integrating fundamental genetic concepts into practice, nurses can significantly improve the nursing care provided to children and their families. In fact, an understanding and application of genetic concepts is an essential part of child and family nursing.

Impact of Genetic Advances on Health Promotion and Health Maintenance

Health promotion and health maintenance for children and their families are foundational for all nursing care. (See Chapter 8 🔗.) The genome era offers a promise of personalized healthcare based on an individual's or a population's risk for disease, which varies according to the set of genes they inherited and a multitude of environmental factors. However, most individuals do not know details of their genetic makeup. While some people may be aware that they carry an altered gene associated with a specific disease, the majority do not know with certainty how their genetic inheritance influences their future health. This is particularly true for common conditions such as heart disease and diabetes, where risk varies with inheritance of a number of gene variations and is modified by lifestyle factors such as diet and physical activity. Having specific knowledge about one's genetic makeup and associated risk for disease provides a basis for health screening and may provide motivation for people to maintain a healthy lifestyle. Imagine, then, if people knew their statistical risks for inheriting or developing disease, based on their specific genotype.

BOX 4–3	**Essential Nursing Competencies for Genetics and Genomics**

In a national effort to establish the minimum basis by which to prepare nurses to deliver competent genetic- and genomic-focused nursing care, a consensus panel composed of nursing leaders from clinical, research, and academic settings developed the following essential competencies. These competencies are applicable to the practice of all registered nurses, regardless of academic preparation, practice setting, role, or specialty. The competencies are related to professionalism, clinical practice, and client education and support.

PROFESSIONAL RESPONSIBILITIES

All registered nurses are expected to:

- Recognize when one's own attitudes and values related to genetic and genomic science may affect care provided to clients.
- Advocate for clients' access to desired genetic/genomic services and/or resources including support groups.
- Examine competency of practice on a regular basis, identifying areas of strength, as well as areas in which professional development related to genetics and genomics would be beneficial.
- Incorporate genetic and genomic technologies and information into registered nurse practice.
- Demonstrate in practice the importance of tailoring genetic and genomic information and services to clients based on their culture, religion, knowledge level, literacy, and preferred language.
- Advocate for the rights of all clients for autonomous, informed genetic- and genomic-related decision making and voluntary action.

PROFESSIONAL PRACTICE

The registered nurse:

- Demonstrates an understanding of the relationship of genetics and genomics to health, prevention, screening, diagnostics, prognostics, selection of treatment, and monitoring of treatment effectiveness.
- Demonstrates ability to elicit a minimum of three-generation family health history information.
- Constructs a pedigree from collected family history information using standardized symbols and terminology.
- Collects personal, health, and developmental histories that consider genetic, environmental, and genomic influences and risks.
- Conducts comprehensive health and physical assessments which incorporate knowledge about genetic, environmental, and genomic influences and risk factors.
- Critically analyzes the history and physical assessment findings for genetic, environmental, and genomic influences and risk factors.

- Assesses clients' knowledge, perceptions, and responses to genetic and genomic information.
- Develops a plan of care that incorporates genetic and genomic assessment information.
- Identifies clients who may benefit from specific genetic and genomic information and/or services based on assessment data.
- Identifies credible, accurate, appropriate, and current genetic and genomic information, resources, services, and/or technologies specific to given clients.
- Identifies ethical, ethnic/ancestral, cultural, religious, legal, fiscal, and societal issues related to genetic and genomic information and technologies.
- Defines issues that undermine the rights of all clients for autonomous, informed genetic- and genomic-related decision making and voluntary action.
- Facilitates referrals for specialized genetic and genomic services for clients as needed.

EDUCATION, CARE, AND SUPPORT

The registered nurse:

- Provides clients with interpretation of selective genetic and genomic information or services.
- Provides clients with credible, accurate, appropriate, and current genetic and genomic information, resources, services, and/or technologies that facilitate decision making.
- Uses health promotion/disease prevention practices that consider genetic and genomic influences on personal and environmental risk factors and incorporate knowledge of genetic and/or genomic risk factors (e.g., a client with a genetic predisposition for high cholesterol who can benefit from a change in lifestyle that will decrease the likelihood that the genetic risk will be expressed).
- Uses genetic- and genomic-based interventions and information to improve clients' outcomes.
- Collaborates with healthcare providers in providing genetic and genomic health care.
- Collaborates with insurance providers/payers to facilitate reimbursement for genetic and genomic healthcare services.
- Performs interventions/treatments appropriate to clients' genetic and genomic healthcare needs.
- Evaluates impact and effectiveness of genetic and genomic technology, information, interventions, and treatments on clients' outcome.

Source: *From Consensus Panel on Genetic/Genomic Nursing Competencies. (2009). Essentials of genetic and genomic nursing: Competencies, curricula guidelines, and outcome indicators (2nd ed.). Silver Spring, MD: American Nurses Association.*

Health promotion and health maintenance teaching and nursing interventions could be targeted to individuals according to their disease risk. Children and families may experience increased motivation to adhere to lifestyle choices and health screenings that are personalized according to their disease risk. Individualized health care is a major goal in the genomic era.

With knowledge of genetic conditions, the pediatric nurse can implement health teaching and promote early detection of complications from genetic conditions with emphasis on primary and secondary care interventions. For example:

- Nurses should ensure informed consent for newborn screening and provide teaching and support to families whose infants have positive screens.
- Nurses should stress to all teenage girls the importance of folic acid (see Chapter 19 🔗) whether they are sexually active or not. Folic acid supplementation around the time of conception is demonstrated to significantly reduce the incidence of neural tube defects, a relatively common birth defect.

- A child who screens positive for scoliosis (see Chapter 7 🔗) should be assessed for axillary freckling and café au lait spots, due to the relationship between scoliosis and neurofibromatosis.
- Screening for Marfan syndrome (see Chapter 35 🔗) should be a part of all sports physicals, due to the lethal cardiovascular complication of aortic dilation. This can be accomplished by assessing for common characteristics such as myopia, scoliosis, tall stature, long fingers and thumbs, a hollow chest, and an arm span greater than the height.
- Nurses should both teach and support families regarding any specific interventions necessary to avoid complications in children with genetic conditions. Examples are the importance for children with phenylketonuria (PKU) to maintain a phenylalanine-free diet for life, and the need to maintain children with sickle cell disease (see Chapter 28 🔗) on penicillin.
- When caring for the child with Down syndrome (see Chapter 34 🔗), the pediatric nurse can help the parents shift from the more expected and traditional focus of disease

BOX 4–4	**Using the People-First Approach**

The nurse should incorporate a person-first philosophy and use genetic terminology that is sensitive to the maintenance of an individual's positive self-image. When communicating genetic concerns to children, families, other healthcare providers, or the public, take care to use words that do not reflect value.

Name the diagnosis rather than apply the label. For example, newborn Sammy, who exhibits Down syndrome, should not be identified as the "Down baby" but as Sammy who has Down syndrome. Describe Sally as having (a diagnosis of) autism, not as being autistic.

Also, the term *developmental disability* is preferred (rather than "mental retardation").

Use the term **wild type gene** or *expected gene* or *unaltered gene*, rather than "normal" gene. Use *altered gene* or *disease-producing gene*, rather than "mutated" or "abnormal" gene.

Source: *Adapted from Snow, K. (2010).* People First Language *at http://www.disabilityisnatural.com*

management to health promotion and protection, by teaching parents about the established guidelines for exams and screenings specific to children with Down syndrome.

- With late-onset diseases such as Huntington, the pediatric nurse should be aware of the child's struggle to maintain a healthy lifestyle and meet society's expectations while struggling with the knowledge of potentially having a lethal gene alteration.

Early diagnosis and early intervention with health-promoting care that is specific to the genetic diagnosis allows children affected with genetic alterations to achieve maximal function, better health, and improved quality of life. The pediatric nurse must be able to identify available community-based and genetic-based resources to assist the child or adolescent and the family with strategies to support health promotion and health maintenance activities. See Box 4–4.

GENETIC BASICS

A basic knowledge of cell structure, function, and division, and of the structure and function of genetic material within cells is essential to deliver the genetic standard of care to children, adolescents, and their families.

The **cell** is the basic unit of life and the working unit of all living systems. Life starts as a single cell, but the developed human body is made up of trillions of cells. These cells share common features such as a nucleus that contains 46 chromosomes, and **organelles** such as mitochondria. Cells are specialized in appearance and function, according to their location. For example, pancreatic cells are much different than nerve cells.

All human cells, except mature red blood cells, contain in their nucleus a complete set of DNA molecules. DNA molecules consist of long sequences of nucleotides or bases represented by the letters A, T, C, and G. The order, or sequence, of these bases provides instructions for protein building. The entire DNA in a human cell is referred to as the **human genome** and represents the complete set of inheritance for an individual. Most of the DNA is organized into chromosomes, which are contained in the cell nucleus. A small amount of DNA is found in the mitochondria, which will be discussed later in this section. Each person's genome is unique, with the exception of monozygotic twins who are derived from the same fertilized ovum and share identical DNA.

Each cell nucleus contains about 6 feet of DNA that is tightly wound and packaged into 23 pairs of chromosomes, making a complete set of 46 chromosomes. The set includes 22 pairs of **autosomes,** which are by tradition numbered according to size, with chromosome 1 being the largest and chromosome 22 the smallest. There are two copies of each autosome—one inherited from the mother and the other from the father. Members of a chromosome pair are called **homologous chromosomes.** The 23rd chromosome pair, the **sex chromosomes,** determine an individual's gender. A female has two copies of the X chromosome (one copy inherited from each parent), and a male has one X chromosome (inherited from his mother) and one Y chromosome (inherited from his father). The structure and number of chromosomes can be shown by a **karyotype,** which is a picture of an individual's chromosomes (Figure 4–3 ■). The sperm and ova represent exceptions to the 23-pair rule, containing only a single chromosome from each homologous pair.

Cell Division

Mitosis and meiosis are the two types of cell division in human cells (Figure 4–4 ■). **Mitosis** takes place in somatic or tissue cells of the

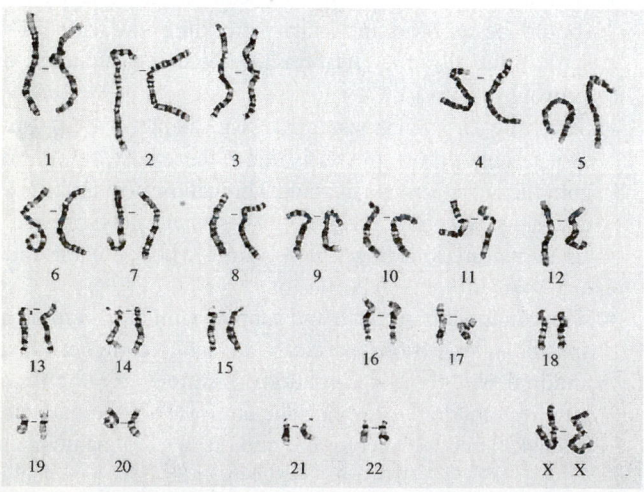

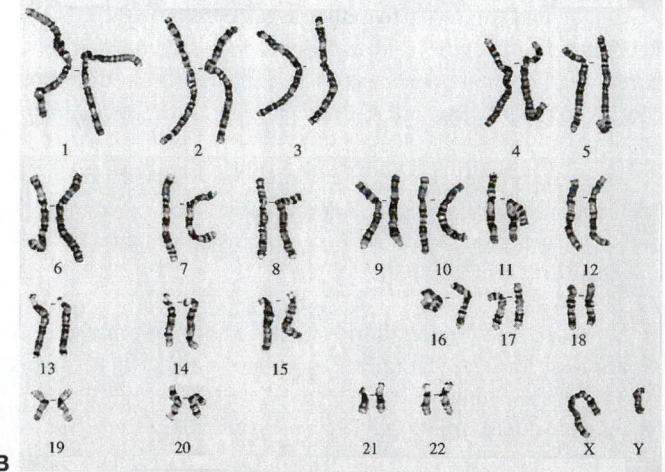

FIGURE 4–3 ■ A karyotype is a picture of an individual's chromosomes. It depicts the number and structure of the 22 pairs of autosomes and the sex chromosomes. *A,* Female. *B,* Male.

Source: *Courtesy of the Greenwood Genetic Center, Greenwood, SC.*

FIGURE 4–4 ■ Comparison of mitosis and meiosis. Two pairs of homologous chromosomes are shown. Mitosis results in two diploid daughter cells that are replicas of the original cell. But in meiosis, crossing over during Meiosis I results in variable distribution of genetic material to the resulting four haploid cells.

Source: *From Klug, William S.; Cummings, Michael R., Concepts of Genetics, 6th Ed. © 2000. Reprinted and electronically reproduced by permission of Pearson Education, Inc., Upper Saddle River, New Jersey.*

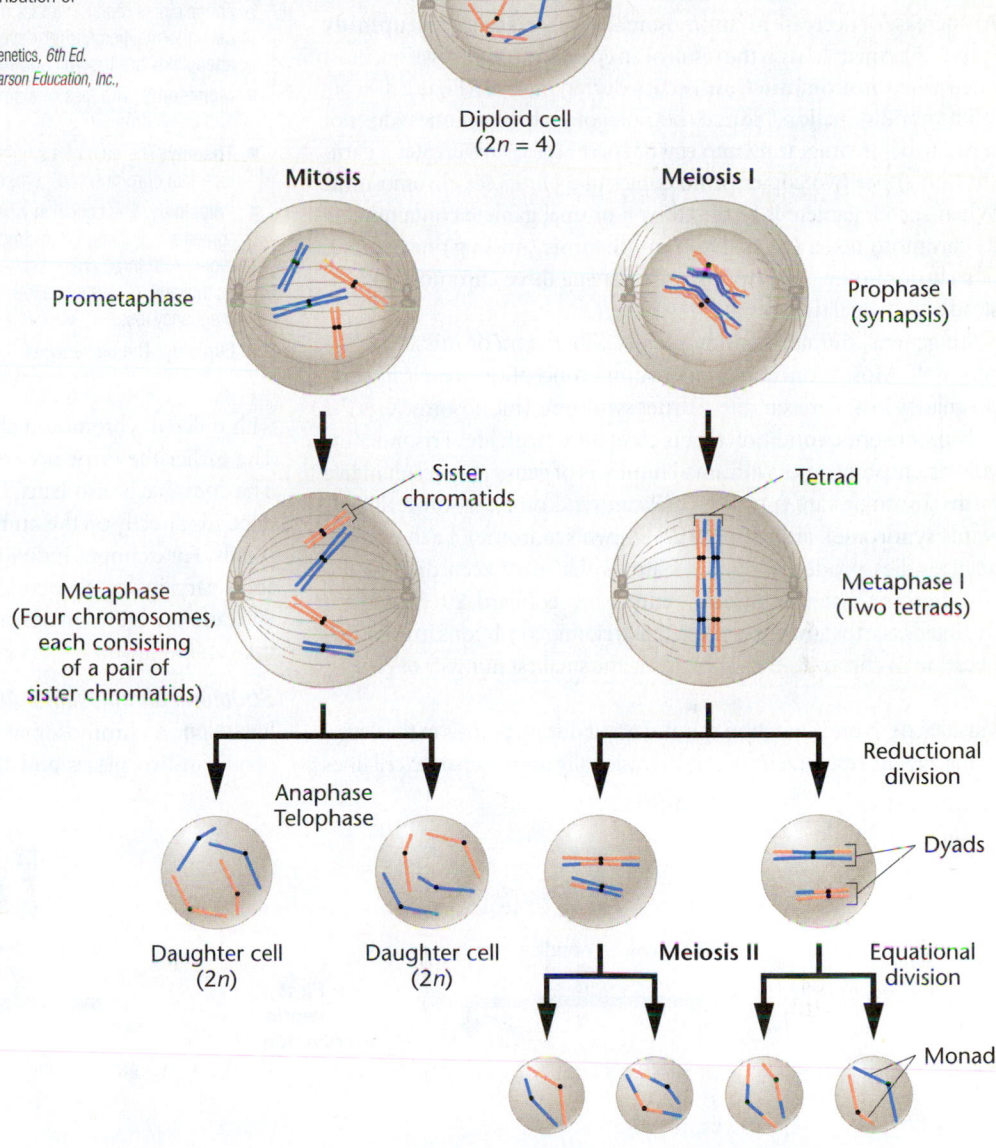

body and represents how the body makes new cells. Cell division through mitosis results in two cells called daughter cells that are genetically identical to the original cell and to each other. Mitosis is responsible for rapid human growth in early life. The mitotic activity of a **zygote** (fertilized ovum) and its daughter cells is the foundation for human growth and development. A zygote undergoes mitosis to form a multicellular embryo, then a fetus, then an infant. Mitosis also replaces cells lost daily from skin surfaces and the lining of gastrointestinal and respiratory tracts.

Meiosis is also known as reduction division of the cell. Meiosis occurs only in the reproductive cells of the testes and ovaries and results in the formation of sperm and oocytes (**gametes**). Meiosis is similar to mitosis in that it is a form of cell division; however, through a series of complex mechanisms, the amount of genetic material is reduced to half. Each gamete contains a single copy of each of the 22 autosomes, plus a single sex chromosome. This is critical to ensure that when the two gametes combine during fertilization,

the correct total number of chromosomes (46) is present in the offspring's cells. The other purpose of meiosis is to make new combinations of genetic material through processes of crossing over and independent assortment. New combinations are necessary to promote diversity in the human population. **Crossing over** results from an exchange or reshuffling of material between homologous chromosomes during gamete formation. This exchange results in new intact chromosomes that represent a patchwork of maternal and paternal genetic material. **Independent assortment** means that each chromosome pair segregates randomly into one or another gamete, further enhancing the genetic diversity that is possible at fertilization.

Chromosomal Alterations

Alterations in chromosomes often occur during cell division (meiosis or mitosis) and are classified as either structural alterations or alterations in the number of chromosomes. The clinical consequences of both types of alterations vary according to the amount of DNA affected by the alterations.

Alterations in Chromosome Number

An increase or decrease in chromosomal number is called **aneuploidy** (Box 4–5). Aneuploidy is the result of an error during cell division, most often when **nondisjunction** occurs during meiosis (Figure 4–5 ■). With nondisjunction, paired homologous chromosomes do not separate before migrating into egg or sperm cells. This creates a gamete with either two copies or no copies of a particular chromosome. When such a gamete is fertilized by a normal gamete containing all 23 chromosomes, a zygote that is **monosomic** (missing one member of a chromosome pair) or **trisomic** (having three chromosomes instead of the usual two) results.

In general, humans do not tolerate either extra or missing DNA very well. Most monosomic or trisomic conceptions result in early pregnancy loss. For example, Turner syndrome (monosomy X) is the only monosomic condition that is compatible with life. Trisomies involving chromosomes with small numbers of genes may result in live births. Examples are trisomy 13 (Patau syndrome), trisomy 18 (Edwards syndrome), and trisomy 21 (Down syndrome). Each of these aneuploidies produces clinical features that vary according to the chromosome that is duplicated (Turnpenny & Ellard, 2012). It is not a coincidence that the three nonlethal trisomic conditions involve duplication of chromosomes containing the smallest number of genes.

Mosaicism Nondisjunction can also occur during mitosis in the developing zygote, resulting in two, or occasionally more, separate cell lines

---

BOX 4–5   **Variations in Chromosomal Number**

- **Aneuploidy.** The condition of having extra or missing chromosomes. Most aneuploidies result in lethal mutations, but if the individual lives, physical abnormalities and/or developmental delay often occur. Examples of aneuploidy are trisomy and monosomy conditions.
- **Monosomy.** The loss of a single chromosome from a pair, for example, Turner syndrome (45, X).
- **Trisomy.** The gain of a single chromosome, making a total of three copies of a certain chromosome (e.g., trisomy 21, which is Down syndrome).
- **Polyploidy.** The condition when more than two complete sets of chromosomes are present. For example, nondisjunction during meiosis can result in a zygote with three entire sets, or 69 chromosomes. This genotype, known as triploidy, represents a lethal mutation and is a significant cause of early pregnancy loss.
- **Euploidy.** The presence of the normal number of 46 chromosomes.

---

with different chromosomal makeup. This is known as **mosaicism.** The earlier the error occurs, the more cells that will be abnormal. The converse is also true. The degree to which a person is affected depends directly on the number or percentage of cells with the aneuploidy. For example, individuals with mosaic Turner syndrome may show varying degrees of infertility or short stature, and an individual with mosaic Down syndrome may have a higher intelligence level than children whose every cell has three copies of chromosome 21.

Structural Chromosomal Alterations

Inversion A chromosomal **inversion** occurs when a chromosome breaks in two places and the piece between the breaks turns end

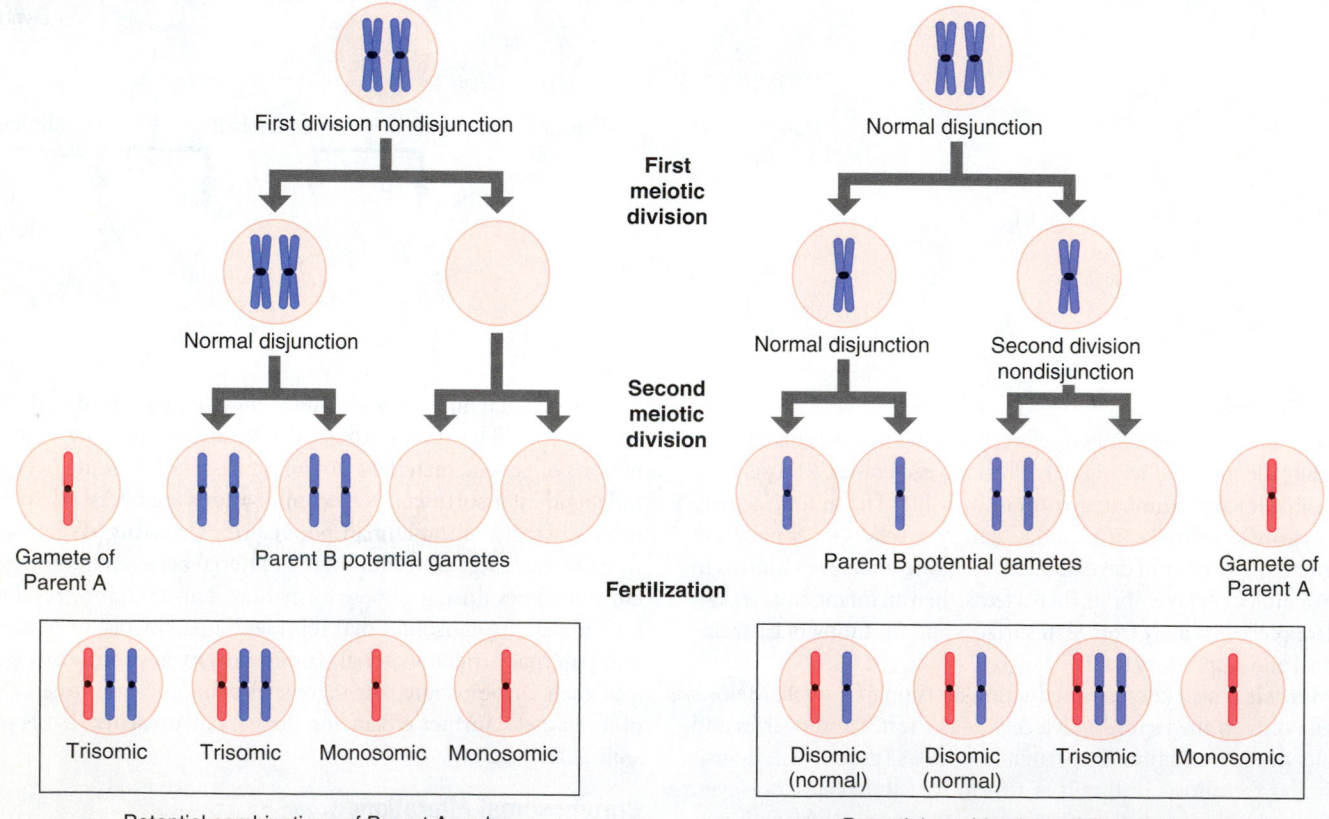

FIGURE 4–5 ■ Examples of nondisjunction—a random error that occurs when a chromosome pair fails to separate during cell division. Nondisjunction results in more (e.g., trisomy) or less (e.g., monosomy) than the expected number of chromosomes present in the new cell. Nondisjunction is the most common cause of trisomy 21 (Down syndrome).

for end and reattaches within the same chromosome. An inversion changes the DNA sequence for that portion of the chromosome. Inversions result in *balanced* rearrangements, because the amount of DNA in the chromosome remains normal. The clinical consequences of an inversion depend on how much chromosomal material is involved and where the inversion occurs. An inversion within the gene that codes for factor VIII, a clotting factor, is an important cause of hemophilia A.

Deletion and duplication Chromosomal alterations sometimes occur when unequal crossing over or abnormal segregation causes a chromosome to have a missing segment (deletion) or an additional segment (duplication) of genetic material. These are called *unbalanced* rearrangements. Large deletions or duplications may be visible microscopically, whereas smaller alterations are detectable only with high-resolution genetic tests. Conditions associated with unbalanced rearrangements may be incompatible with life or cause altered physical and/or mental development. An example is cri du chat syndrome (with developmental delays, a cry sounding like a cat mewing, and low-set ears) from a large deletion on chromosome 5 (Turnpenny & Ellard, 2012).

Translocation Translocation occurs when two, usually nonhomologous, chromosomes exchange segments of DNA. A translocation that results in a correct amount of chromosomal material but a new arrangement is a *balanced translocation*. The individual who has a balanced rearrangement has all of the chromosomal material present and therefore does not usually have any physical or mental disabilities. However, individuals with a balanced translocation are at high risk to produce gametes with unbalanced rearrangements. This leads to increased risk of pregnancy loss or having children with mental and/or physical disabilities due to missing or extra genetic material. A common *unbalanced translocation* between chromosomes 14 and 21 is responsible for about 3% of children diagnosed with Down syndrome (Ranweiler, 2009). See Figure 4–6 ■. When

a child with Down syndrome is born, it is important to conduct a chromosome study to determine if the cause is nondisjunction or translocation. Translocation, while unrelated to maternal age, carries a significantly greater recurrence risk with subsequent pregnancies (Ranweiler, 2009).

Genes

In addition to understanding chromosomal alterations, the nurse must also have knowledge of genes—what they are, their function, and the consequences of gene alterations. The nurse must understand the inheritance of gene alterations in order to provide correct information to the child, adolescent, and family affected by or at risk for a known genetic condition. As the genetic contribution to common chronic disease is better understood, knowledge of the function and inheritance of genes has become increasingly relevant in designing health promotion and health maintenance activities.

A **gene** is a segment of a chromosome that can be identified with a particular function, most commonly production of one or more proteins. Each chromosome contains numerous genes arranged in a linear order. The number of genes present on each chromosome varies. Chromosome 1 is the largest chromosome with the largest number of protein-encoding genes, over 3,000, whereas the Y chromosome has the smallest number of genes, about 200 (Chromosome Map, n. d.). Genes that reside on autosomes (chromosomes 1 through 22) are present in pairs, with one copy on each homologous chromosome. Because each gene copy is inherited from a different parent, differences in their nucleotide sequence likely exist; these different forms or versions of genes are called **alleles.** An individual who has two functionally identical alleles of a gene is said to be **homozygous** (*homo* = same) for that gene. An individual who has two different alleles of the gene is said to be **heterozygous** (*hetero* = different). See Figure 4–7 ■.

Genes have a specific location on a certain chromosome; this is called the *genetic locus*. Gene mapping has documented the locus

FIGURE 4–6 ■ *A*, Example of translocation which occurs when a segment of a chromosome transfers (moves and attaches itself to another chromosome). When meiosis occurs in the balanced carrier parent (B), an ovum or sperm has the potential to have one single copy of chromosome 21 plus the copy of chromosome 21 that is attached to chromosome 14, making a total of two copies of chromosome 21. When combined with the other parent's chromosome 21, the offspring then has three copies of chromosome 21. *B*, Chromosomal translocation is responsible for 3% to 4% of all Down syndrome occurrences.

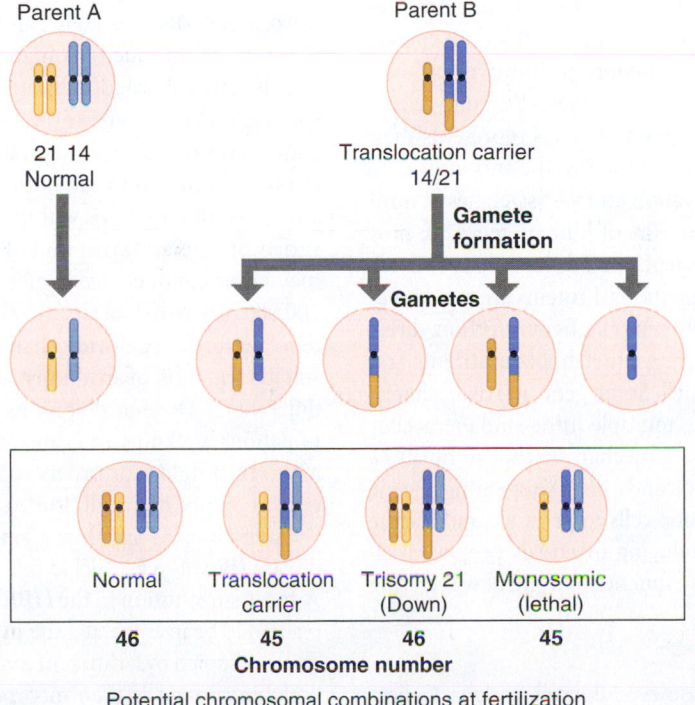

Parent A

21 14
Normal

Parent B

Translocation carrier
14/21

Gamete formation

Gametes

Normal	Translocation carrier	Trisomy 21 (Down)	Monosomic (lethal)
46	45	46	45

Chromosome number

Potential chromosomal combinations at fertilization

A

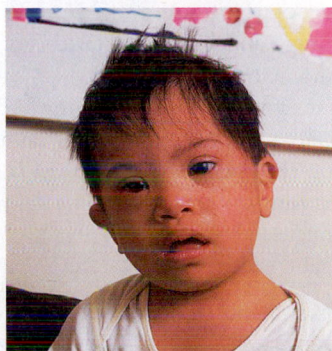

B

Genotype is most often represented as:

- Homozygous
  – *RR* or *rr*
- Heterozygous
  – *Rr*

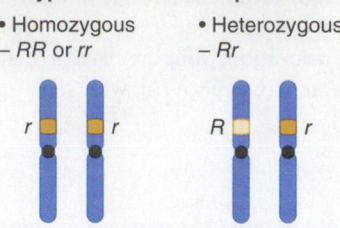

FIGURE 4–7 ■ Sample homozygous (two identical alleles of a gene) and heterozygous (two different alleles of a gene) genotypes. A capital letter is used to represent the dominant form of the gene (the dominant allele), and a small letter represents the recessive allele.

for most human genes. For example, it is known that the Huntington gene is located at the tip of chromosome 4 and that one of several genes for eye color is located at a specific site on chromosome 19.

Genes are described as *altered* or *mutated* when a change has taken place in the nucleotide sequence of the gene. When the gene is *expressed,* or actively making protein, the alteration may or may not cause the protein product to be defective. A gene alteration that does not change the protein product is called a **polymorphism** or silent mutation. Other changes in nucleotide sequence, perhaps at a locus some distance from the gene itself, may affect **gene expression,** or a gene's activity in making protein. Smaller, non-DNA molecules are also involved in gene expression; these **epigenetic effects** can cause genes to be overexpressed (making more protein product than expected), underexpressed (making less than expected), or expressed at a time in development when the gene is normally inactive.

The observable, outward expression of an individual's entire physical, biochemical, and physiologic makeup, as determined by the person's genotype and environmental factors, is referred to as **phenotype.** Phenotype may be apparent as a trait, such as curly or straight hair, or as signs or symptoms of a disease.

Distribution and Function of Genes

It is believed that less than 2% of the human genome is actually represented by genes. The vast majority of human DNA does not encode proteins and, in fact, has unknown function. In humans, protein-coding DNA is organized into about 21,000 genes (Ensembl release 63, 2011); each individual's particular set of genes represents their **genotype.** Genes are distributed unevenly across the chromosomes, with random areas of gene concentration and vast stretches of non-coding DNA. The functions of over 90% of human genes are now known. Collectively, 21,000 human genes encode hundreds of thousands of proteins that carry out all functions. Proteins are highly specialized. They transmit messages between cells, fight infection, direct genes to turn on or off, form structures, metabolize nutrients and drugs, and sense light, taste, and smell. Some gene activities change moment to moment, in response to multiple intra- and extracellular signals. An example is the feedback mechanism that stimulates a cell to produce insulin after eating a candy bar. After eating, a gene on chromosome 11 directs pancreatic cells to produce and secrete insulin. Although the gene for producing insulin is present in all nucleated cells of the body, it is only functional in insulin-secreting pancreatic cells.

Mitochondrial Genes

Nearly all genes reside on chromosomes in the cell nucleus. Collectively these genes represent the nuclear genome; however, DNA is

also present in cell cytoplasm. Mitochondria (organelles involved in energy metabolism, or the "powerhouse" of the cell) contain a small amount of DNA identified as mitochondrial DNA (mtDNA). There are 37 genes in mitochondrial DNA; these genes have a higher mutation rate than nuclear DNA (Turnpenny & Ellard, 2012). Clinical manifestations occurring as a result of mitochondrial gene alterations primarily affect high-energy tissues such as brain, skeletal muscle, and heart muscle. Because ova have many mitochondria and the mitochondria of the sperm are located in the tail of the sperm that detaches at fertilization, mtDNA is inherited only from the mother in a *matrilineal* pattern. This creates a unique pattern of inheritance. A female with a mutation of a mitochondrial gene will pass that mutation to all of her children, whereas an affected male will not pass the mtDNA mutation to any of his children (Jorde, Carey, & Bamshad, 2010).

Gene Alterations and Disease

An alteration in the DNA sequence of a gene may cause a defective protein to be formed, which may directly cause or increase risk for a health condition or disease. Gene alterations can be inherited or they can be acquired. Mutations inherited from one or both parents (hereditary mutations) are also known as germline mutations, because the mutation exists in the reproductive cells, the parental sperm or ovum. Consequently, the DNA in every cell of that offspring will have the gene alteration, which can then be transmitted to following generations. Single-gene alterations are responsible for approximately 6,000 hereditary diseases such as cystic fibrosis, Duchenne muscular dystrophy, and phenylketonuria. Each of these disorders is relatively rare, although collectively they affect 1 of every 300 newborns (Centers for Disease Control and Prevention [CDC], n.d.). While they are of enormous consequence to affected families, they constitute a relatively small portion of the total public health burden.

Gene alterations can also occur in an individual's DNA at any time throughout a lifetime. They result from errors during cell division (mitosis) or from environmental influences such as radiation or toxins. These acquired mutations are also called sporadic or *de novo* mutations. See Figure 4–8A and B ■. Most cases of cancer, for example, are due to somatic mutations. Somatic mutations are not directly inherited, although some conditions associated with somatic mutations are known to aggregate in families. Genes vary enormously in size, from several hundred to more than a million nucleotides. A mutation can occur anywhere along the gene sequence, and different mutations within a particular gene can result in a wide variety of signs and symptoms. For example, the cystic fibrosis transmembrane conductance regulator (CFTR) gene is a large gene (over 200,000 base pairs) located on chromosome 7. CFTR encodes a protein that forms a chloride channel, and mutations in CFTR can result in formation of an abnormal chloride channel. More than 1,700 different CFTR gene alterations have been identified. Some of those mutations are known to cause cystic fibrosis, while others result in a variety of milder disorders such as absence of the vas deferens, or even no symptoms at all (Jorde et al., 2010).

Alterations as small as a single nucleotide are known to cause disease (Box 4–6 ■). Sickle cell anemia is such a disorder. A single A-for-T substitution in the *HBB* gene causes an incorrect amino acid (valine) to be inserted at a site in the protein product (β-globin) normally occupied by a different amino acid (glutamic acid). The altered β-globin protein is then incorporated into hemoglobin molecules. Under conditions of low oxygen tension, the altered β-globin causes

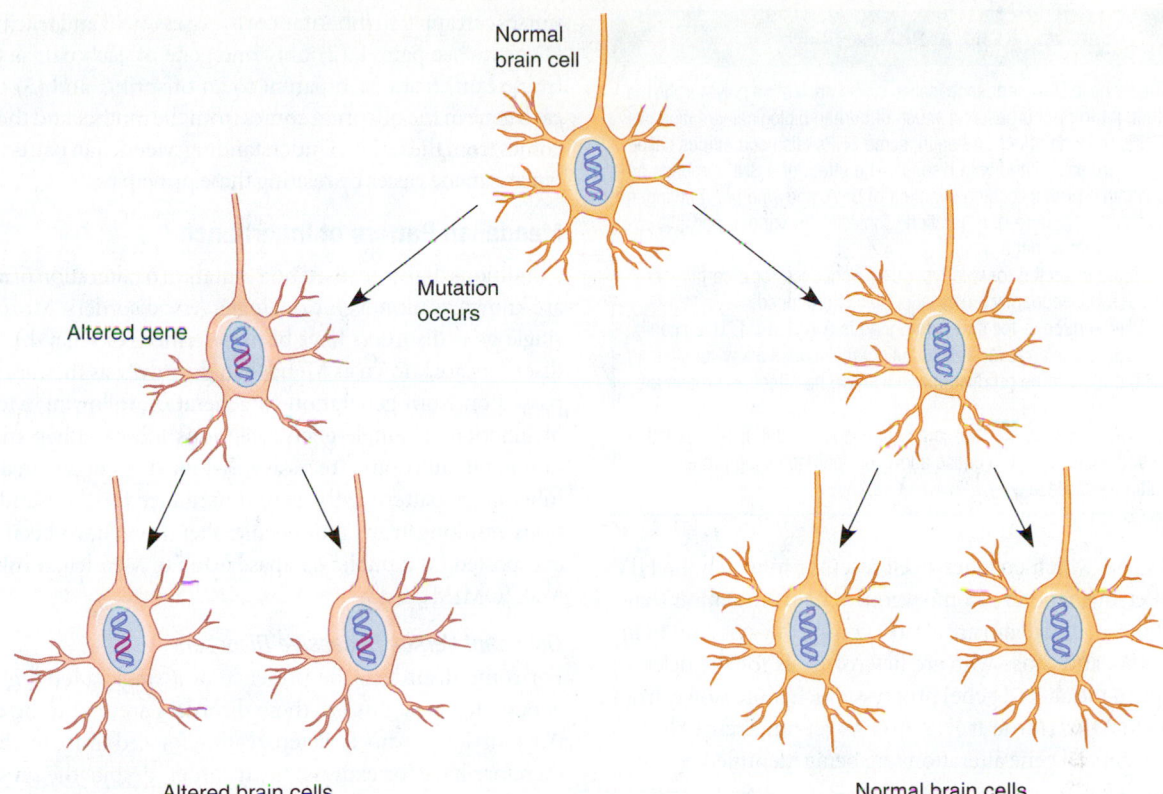

Normal
brain cell

Mutation
occurs

Altered gene

Altered brain cells

Normal brain cells

FIGURE 4–8A ■ Acquired DNA mutations occur in the body's tissue (somatic) cells throughout an individual's lifetime. Consequently, all new cells resulting from cell division of the cell with the DNA mutation will have the same DNA alteration (mutation) in that tissue, but these mutations are not inheritable. Most cancers result from acquired DNA alterations.

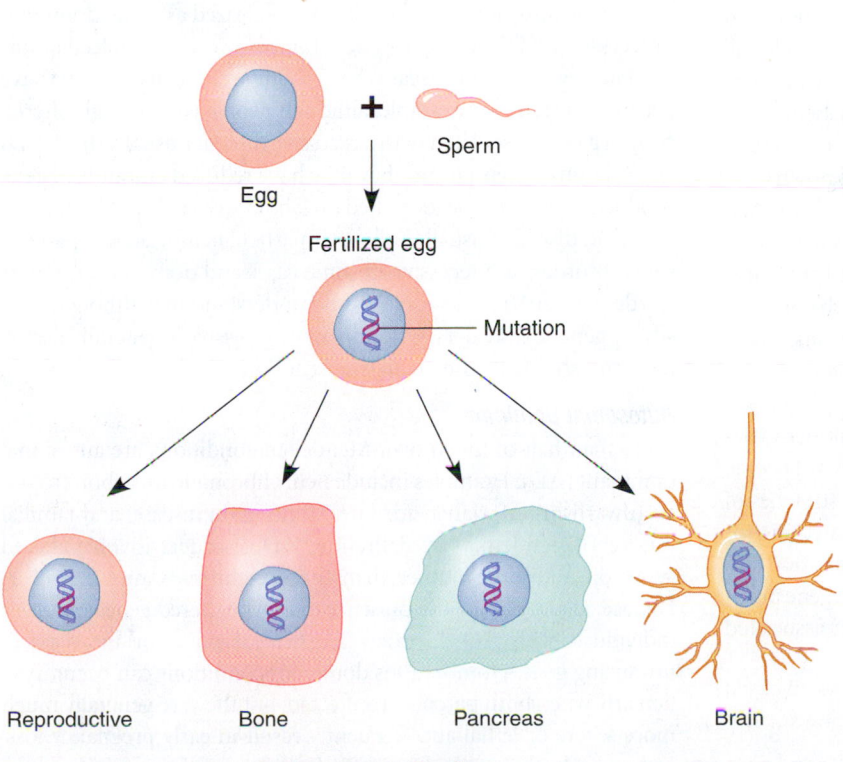

Sperm

Egg

Fertilized egg

Mutation

Reproductive   Bone   Pancreas   Brain

Body cells of offspring

FIGURE 4–8B ■ A germline mutation can occur in the egg, sperm, or single-cell zygote (fertilized egg). The resulting individual will carry that mutation in all of his or her body cells and may pass the altered gene on to his or her offspring.

red blood cells to assume an abnormal, sickle-like shape. This leads to vascular occlusion and hemolytic anemia (Steinberg, 2008). In other situations, multiple gene alterations combine with environmental factors and lead to a health condition or disease. These conditions are referred to as **multifactorial.** Most common chronic disorders, including hypertension, heart disease, type 2 diabetes, and cancer, are multifactorial. Alterations in regulatory genes may also occur. Regulatory elements are stretches of DNA located away from a gene which control gene expression. They include gene promoters, enhancers, silencers, and other control mechanisms and are important in maintaining homeostasis (Turnpenny & Ellard, 2012). Mutation of a regulatory gene might lead to the loss of expression of a gene, unexpected expression in a tissue in which it is usually silent, or a change in the time when a gene is usually expressed. Epigenetic factors also affect gene function and are of great interest in genetics research.

Gene Alterations That Decrease Risk of Disease

Although gene mutations are commonly associated with disease, it is important to remember that gene mutations can also be helpful and decrease the risk of disease. One example is the protective value of a single copy of some genes known to cause autosomal recessive disorders. Sickle cell disease (SCD) is one example; individuals with a single altered SCD gene have protection against malaria. Another protective gene alteration involves a deletion in the DNA sequence

| BOX 4–6 | Genes and Health or Disease |

Single-letter variations in DNA sequence (called single nucleotide polymorphisms or SNPs) are thought to be the basis for much of human biological variation. Although most SNPs have no effect on health, some SNPs (also sometimes called "point mutations") are associated with disease. The effect of a SNP depends on whether it lies within a protein-coding segment of DNA, and whether it changes the resulting protein's structure and function. Consider the various possible results when a SNP occurs within a gene:

Person 1 has the expected, or wild type, DNA sequence for a certain gene, which is A A **A T** T T. Consequently a normal protein is produced.

Person 2's DNA sequence for that same gene is A A **A A** T T. This specific variation in DNA sequence (an A-for-T substitution) may cause a low-functioning or nonfunctioning protein to be produced, or may have no effect on protein production at all.

Person 3's DNA sequence for that same gene is A A **C T** T T. This variation (a C-for-A substitution) is known to cause a low- or nonfunctioning protein to be produced, resulting in disease.

in the *CCR5* gene, which encodes a cell receptor to which the HIV virus binds. Persons who are homozygous for this mutation (have two copies of the altered gene) are almost completely resistant to infection with HIV, and those who are heterozygous for the deletion (have one copy of the altered gene) progress much more slowly from HIV infection to AIDS (Jorde et al., 2010). As genomic research continues, more beneficial gene alterations are being identified.

Genetic Variation: Single Nucleotide Polymorphisms and Copy Number Variants

Humans are remarkably similar to each other at the DNA level, with 99.5% of the nucleotide sequence being identical between individuals. Much genetic variation in humans is attributed to single-nucleotide (or "single-letter") changes in DNA sequence, which are known as **single nucleotide polymorphisms** (SNPs, pronounced "snips"). On average, the DNA sequence of two unrelated people will vary at roughly one of each thousand nucleotides; each site of variation represents a SNP (Jorde et al., 2010). Most SNPs are benign, although collectively they account for most phenotypic variation such as appearance and risk for disease. By convention, SNPs known to be associated with disease are considered to be mutations and are often called point mutations, indicating the single nucleotide cause.

Scientists have mapped SNPs all over the genome and are working to identify the multiple gene variations associated with common diseases that cannot be explained by single-gene alterations. These complex diseases include hypertension, cancer, cardiovascular disease, and diabetes.

In recent years, DNA research has identified copy number variation as an additional source of human genetic variation. Most people have two copies of each gene, but in some individuals, stretches of DNA of variable size (up to 3 million bases) are replicated one or more times. These DNA segments appear to be fairly common and can contain entire genes, resulting in more than expected gene product. In some cases, **copy number variants** have been associated with disease (Zhang, Gu, Hurles, et al., 2009).

PRINCIPLES OF INHERITANCE

Knowledge of inheritance allows the nurse not only to offer and reinforce genetic information to children, adolescents, and their families but also to assist them in managing their care and in making reproductive decisions. The basic underlying principles of inheritance that

nurses can apply to inheritance risk assessment and teaching include: (1) genes are paired, (2) only one gene of each pair is transmitted (passed on) from each parent to an offspring, and (3) one copy of each gene in the offspring comes from the mother and the other copy comes from the father. Understanding Mendelian patterns of inheritance is made easier by relating these principles.

Mendelian Pattern of Inheritance

Conditions that are caused by a mutation or alteration of a single gene are known as monogenic or single-gene disorders. More than 6,000 single-gene disorders have been described (CDC, n.d.). Single-gene disorders are known as Mendelian disorders, as they are predictably passed on from generation to generation following Mendel's laws of inheritance. Single-gene mutations follow either an autosomal dominant, autosomal recessive, X-linked, or occasionally Y-linked inheritance pattern. Modes of inheritance for thousands of conditions resulting from monogenic alterations have been catalogued and posted on a public database (Online Mendelian Inheritance in Man [OMIM], n.d.).

Dominant Versus Recessive Disorders

For some disorders, the presence of a single altered gene allele is enough to cause disease; these disorders are said to be **dominant.** An individual who is heterozygous for a dominant disorder will therefore have (or express) the disorder, despite the presence of the one functioning allele. Other disorders occur only when both alleles of a gene pair are altered. In these **recessive** disorders, the gene product produced from a single unaltered gene is enough to perform the expected function and maintain homeostasis. Because most human genes reside on autosomes, the most common inheritance patterns are autosomal dominant and autosomal recessive.

Genetic disorders have long been categorized as being dominant or recessive as if the categories were rigid; however, as molecular understanding of genetic diseases has progressed, the distinctions have become blurred. For example, although people with a single altered copy of a gene associated with a recessive disorder usually display no clinical signs or symptoms, they may have reduced amounts of gene product, which may be identified on laboratory analysis. Also, while a genetic disorder usually follows a particular inheritance pattern, some disorders are recessive in some cases and dominant in others (Jorde et al., 2010). The nurse should understand that although classifying genetic disorders as dominant or recessive is generally useful, the terms should be used with some caution.

Autosomal Dominant

More than half of the known Mendelian conditions are autosomal dominant (AD). Examples include neurofibromatosis, achondroplasia (dwarfism), Marfan syndrome, Huntington disease, and familial hypercholesterolemia. By definition, AD disorders involve altered genes on autosomes rather than the sex chromosomes X and Y. Disease occurs despite the presence of one unaltered gene, and most individuals with AD disorders are heterozygous for the disease-producing gene. Homozygous dominant conditions can occur, particularly when both parents are affected, but they are generally much more severe or lethal and frequently result in early pregnancy loss. For example, the child who is born homozygous for achondroplasia (a form of dwarfism) is much more severely affected than a child who is heterozygous and usually will not survive early infancy. Huntington disease is a notable exception to this rule, however. Individuals who

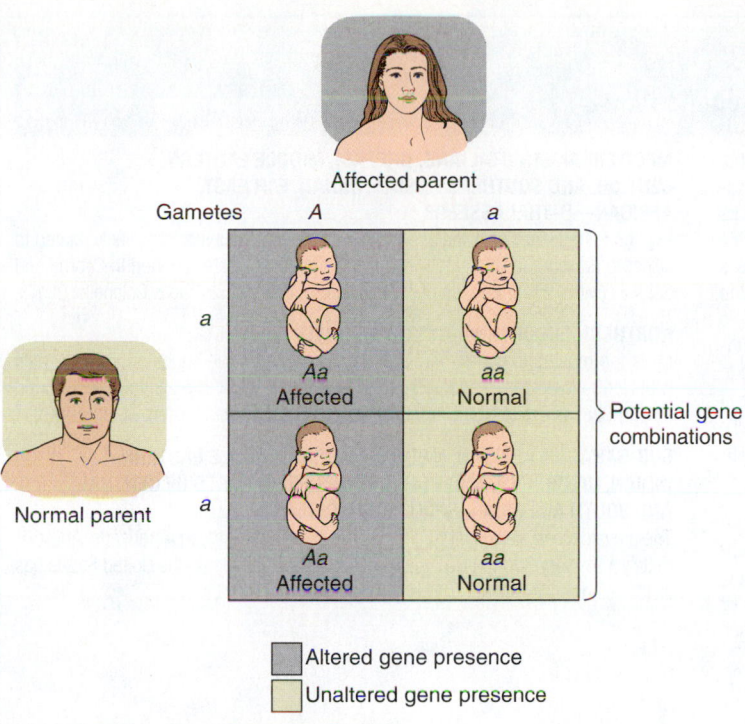

Affected parent

Gametes

FIGURE 4–9 ■ Autosomal Dominant Inheritance

This Punnett square shows potential gene combinations (genotypes) and resulting phenotypes of children who have one parent with an autosomal dominant altered gene. Phenotypes are expressed (resulting in an affected offspring, male or female) when a single copy of the altered gene is inherited. Possible genotypes and phenotypes for each pregnancy are shown.

have two copies of the altered Huntington gene do not have earlier onset of symptoms, although the disease may progress more rapidly than in heterozygous individuals (Warby, Graham, & Hayden, 2010). In general, the nurse should expect an individual exhibiting an AD condition to be heterozygous.

Inheritance risk in autosomal dominant conditions Because the gene alteration in AD conditions occurs on an autosome rather than a sex chromosome, both males and females have an equal chance of being affected. There is a 50% chance that an affected parent will pass the altered disease-producing gene on to a child (Figure 4–9 ■). Nurses must remember and teach families that each pregnancy is an independent event with a 50% chance of an affected child, no matter how many of a couple's previous children have inherited the altered gene. Family histories will often reflect this 50% inheritance rate as well as both males and females being affected. An affected child always has an affected parent, who in turn also has an affected parent.

BOX 4–7	**Autosomal Dominant Mendelian Inheritance Characteristics**

When gathering a family history, the nurse should assess for the following characteristics of autosomal dominant inheritance:

1. Both males and females are affected.
2. Males and females are usually affected in equal numbers.
3. An affected child will have an affected parent and/or all generations will have an affected individual (appearing as a vertical pattern of affected individuals on the family pedigree).
4. Unaffected children of an affected parent will have unaffected offspring.
5. A significant proportion of isolated cases are due to a new mutation.

See Box 4–7. Exceptions to this inheritance pattern occur when the condition is due to a spontaneous new mutation.

Autosomal Recessive

Autosomal recessive (AR) conditions occur when both copies of the same gene in an individual are altered. Generally, AR conditions are more severe and have an earlier onset than conditions with other patterns of inheritance. Examples of AR conditions include cystic fibrosis, PKU, sickle cell anemia, and most inborn errors of metabolism. Like autosomal dominant disorders, AR conditions involve genes on one of the 22 autosomes. A condition is called *recessive* when two altered gene copies are needed to express the condition. A child born with a recessive condition has therefore inherited one altered gene from each parent. Most often, both parents are **carriers** of the condition, with one altered and one unaltered gene copy. Carriers usually exhibit no signs or symptoms. There are, however, exceptions to this general rule: Sickle cell disease (SCD) is an example. An individual with a single copy of the altered sickle cell gene is usually asymptomatic; however, symptoms can occur in situations of extremely low oxygenation such as high altitudes. These individuals are said to have sickle cell trait. Carrier status for a number of AR conditions has an evolutionary benefit; for example, a single copy of the SCD gene affords increased resistance to malaria. Individuals whose ancestors are from malaria-endemic areas are therefore more likely to carry the altered sickle cell gene. See Developing Cultural Competence: Ethnic or Population Groups and Autosomal Recessive Inheritance. Because carrier status usually confers no symptoms, parents are often unaware of their carrier status until they have an affected child (Figure 4–10 ■).

Inheritance risk in autosomal recessive conditions Because AR conditions do not involve genetic material on the sex chromosomes, males and females have an equal chance of inheriting the altered gene and exhibiting the condition. When both parents are carriers of an autosomal recessive gene alteration, each pregnancy presents the same inheritance risks. Each child born to carrier parents has a 25% chance of inheriting two copies of the altered disease-producing gene, a 50% chance of being a carrier with only one copy of the altered gene, and a 25% chance of inheriting both unaltered genes and being neither affected nor a carrier. Remembering that each pregnancy is an independent event, these probability percentages remain constant with each pregnancy, no matter how many affected or unaffected children a family already has. This is often a difficult concept for parents to grasp, and the nurse should carefully evaluate their level of understanding of this important detail about inheritance. See Box 4–8.

The transmission percentages stated previously apply when both parents are carriers of an autosomal recessive condition. Percentages will change if only one parent is a carrier, or if a parent is homozygous for the condition. The nurse must be able to teach a parent about these simple inheritance percentages. Drawing a Punnett square, as in Figures 4–9 and 4–10, is a useful method of illustrating inheritance patterns for families.

X-Linked

X-linked conditions are the result of an altered gene on the X chromosome. Examples include hemophilia A and Duchenne muscular dystrophy. Most X-linked disorders are caused by recessive genes;

Developing Cultural Competence
Ethnic or Population Groups and Autosomal Recessive Inheritance

Because the prevalence of autosomal recessive conditions varies around the globe, certain recessive genetic conditions are more prevalent in particular ethnic populations. Nurses should ask about the country of origin of an individual's ancestors when collecting a family history. In populations where individuals tend to marry within their own community, autosomal recessive conditions are especially common. This is known as the "founder effect." Population-based screening has been implemented in many countries for certain severe recessive disorders. Most screening programs are voluntary, although some are mandated by law or religious authority. A voluntary program in the United States offers carrier screening for Tay-Sachs disease to Ashkenazi Jewish individuals. Since the program began in 1970, the incidence of Tay-Sachs disease in that population has been reduced by 90% (Zlotogora, 2009).

Common examples of disorders that occur more commonly in specific populations are as follows.

ASHKENAZI JEWISH—TAY-SACHS DISEASE, GAUCHER DISEASE
Tay-Sachs disease is rare in non-Jewish populations, but has a carrier rate of approximately 1 in 30 among individuals of Ashkenazi Jewish (central-eastern Europe) ancestry (Jorde et al., 2010). The carrier rate for Gaucher disease is as high as 1 in 18 in the Ashkenazi Jewish population, compared to 1 in 100 in the general population (Pastores & Hughes, 2011).

TURKISH, IRISH, EAST ASIAN POPULATIONS, PENNSYLVANIA AMISH—PHENYLKETONURIA (PKU)
PKU carrier rates as high as 1 in 26 have been found in Turkish populations. The PKU gene is especially rare in African and Ashkenazi Jewish populations (Mitchell & Scriver, 2010).

MEDITERRANEAN (ITALIANS, GREEKS), MIDDLE EASTERN, CENTRAL AND SOUTHEAST ASIAN, INDIAN, FAR EAST, AFRICAN—β-THALASSEMIA
High gene frequency of β-thalassemias in these populations is most likely related to selective pressure from malaria. The highest incidences are reported in Cyprus and Sardinia (with 12% to 14% carrier rates) and southeast Asia (Cao & Galanello, 2010).

NORTHERN EUROPEAN—CYSTIC FIBROSIS (CF)
CF is the most common life-limiting autosomal recessive condition in individuals with Northern European ancestors. Carrier rates of about 1 in 28 have been found among Caucasians in North America (Moskowitz, Chmiel, Sternen, et al., 2008).

SUB-SAHARAN AFRICAN, MEDITERRANEAN, MIDDLE EASTERN, INDIAN, CARIBBEAN, AND POPULATIONS FROM PARTS OF CENTRAL AND SOUTH AMERICA—SICKLE CELL DISEASE
The prevalence of sickle cell trait is 8% to 10% among African Americans. Approximately 1 in every 300 to 500 African American infants born in the United States has sickle cell disease (Bender & Hobbs, 2009).

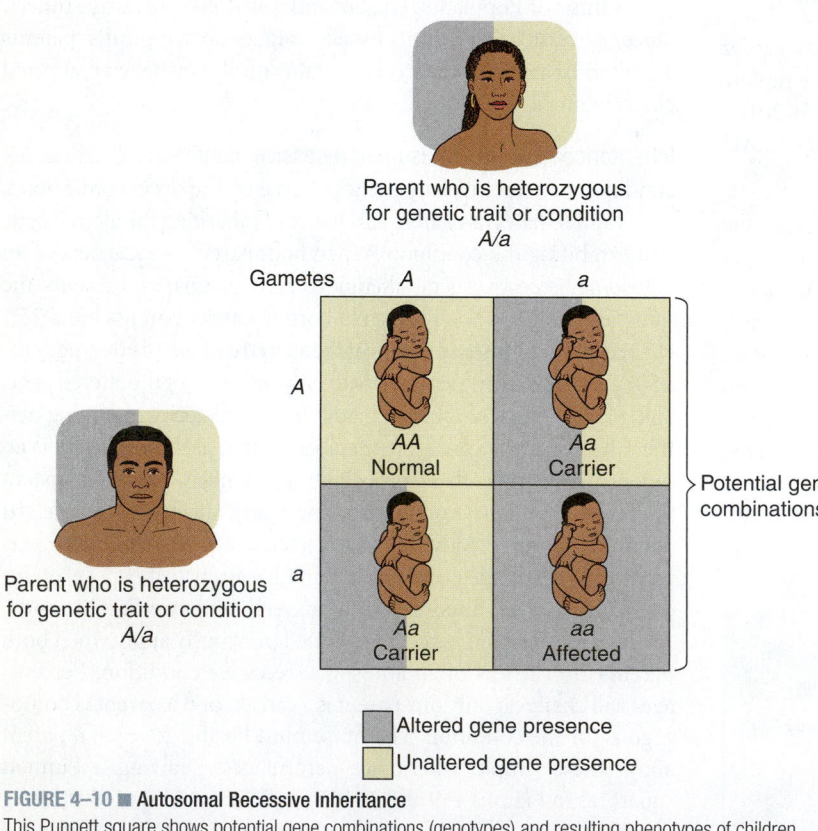

FIGURE 4–10 ■ Autosomal Recessive Inheritance
This Punnett square shows potential gene combinations (genotypes) and resulting phenotypes of children whose parents each have a single copy of an autosomal recessive altered gene. Phenotypes are expressed (resulting in an affected offspring, male or female) only when two copies of the altered gene are inherited. Possible genotypes and phenotypes for each pregnancy are shown.

although X-linked dominant conditions can occur, they are rare and will not be discussed here. Recall that the sex chromosomes are unevenly represented in males and females. Males, with their single X chromosome, have just a single copy of each of the approximately 1,600 genes that reside on the X chromosome. Any altered X gene will consequently be expressed in males, because an unaltered allele is not present for "backup." Females, on the other hand, have two copies of each X gene, and an unaltered gene generally compensates for an altered allele, making the female a carrier.

Inheritance risk in X-linked conditions In families with X-linked disorders, a pattern of maternal transmission is seen. Females who are carriers of X-linked conditions have a 50% chance of passing the altered gene to their offspring. Any daughter who receives the altered gene is likely to receive an unaltered X chromosome from her father and therefore be a carrier like her mother. Sons of carrier mothers, however, have no backup X chromosome, having inherited a Y chromosome from their father. Therefore, a son who inherits the altered X will display the condition and go on to pass that altered X to each of his daughters, who will then be carriers of the altered gene (Figure 4–11 ■). A male can never transmit an altered gene on the X chromosome to his sons because males transmit only the Y chromosome to sons. Because of these transmission patterns, the most common occurring transmission of an X-linked condition is through a female who is a carrier of an altered gene. See Box 4–9.

BOX 4–8	Autosomal Recessive Mendelian Inheritance Characteristics

When gathering a family history, the nurse should assess for the following characteristics of autosomal recessive inheritance:

1. Both males and females are affected.
2. Males and females are usually affected in equal numbers.
3. An affected child will usually have an unaffected parent but may have affected siblings (appearing as a horizontal pattern of affected individuals on the family pedigree).
4. The condition may appear to skip a generation.
5. The parents of the affected child may be consanguineous (close blood relatives).
6. The family may be descendants of an ethnic group that is known to have a more frequent occurrence of a certain genetic condition.

X Inactivation

Early in embryonic life, one of the X chromosomes inherited by females is inactivated. This process is believed to be completed by the end of the first week of development and results in equalizing the expression of X-linked genes in the two sexes. Each female receives one X chromosome from her mother (maternal X) and one from her father (paternal X). The inactivation of either the maternal or paternal X chromosome is random. However, once an X has been inactivated in any given cell, all of the cell's descendants (through mitosis) contain the same inactive X chromosome. This process results in females being mosaic for X-linked genes; some cells will express genes from the maternal X

chromosome, while other cells will express genes from the paternal X. Females who inherit an altered gene on an X chromosome therefore show variable expression, because the gene alteration will be present in only some cells. Expression of symptoms can vary from extremely mild to a full manifestation of the condition. For example, female carriers of the X-linked recessive conditions hemophilia A or Duchenne muscular dystrophy may exhibit mild symptoms of those disorders.

Most X-linked conditions are considered to be recessive, because the presence of an unaltered X masks the effects of the altered X. While X-linked dominant conditions do exist, they are rare. An example is vitamin D–resistant rickets. If a male is affected, the condition is severe and often lethal. A family history of multiple male miscarriages may be a sign of an X-linked dominant condition.

Y-Linked Disorders

Because the Y chromosome has very few genes, alterations on the Y chromosome are not often associated with health problems. Several genes involved in sperm formation are carried on the Y chromosome, and alterations in these genes may be associated with male infertility. Y-linked disorders are transmitted only from father to son.

Variability in Classic Mendelian Patterns of Inheritance

In addition to classic Mendelian inheritance patterns, nurses must be prepared to help families understand several other concepts that affect risk for inheriting a genetic disorder. Such concepts include the following variations in traditional Mendelian patterns of inheritance.

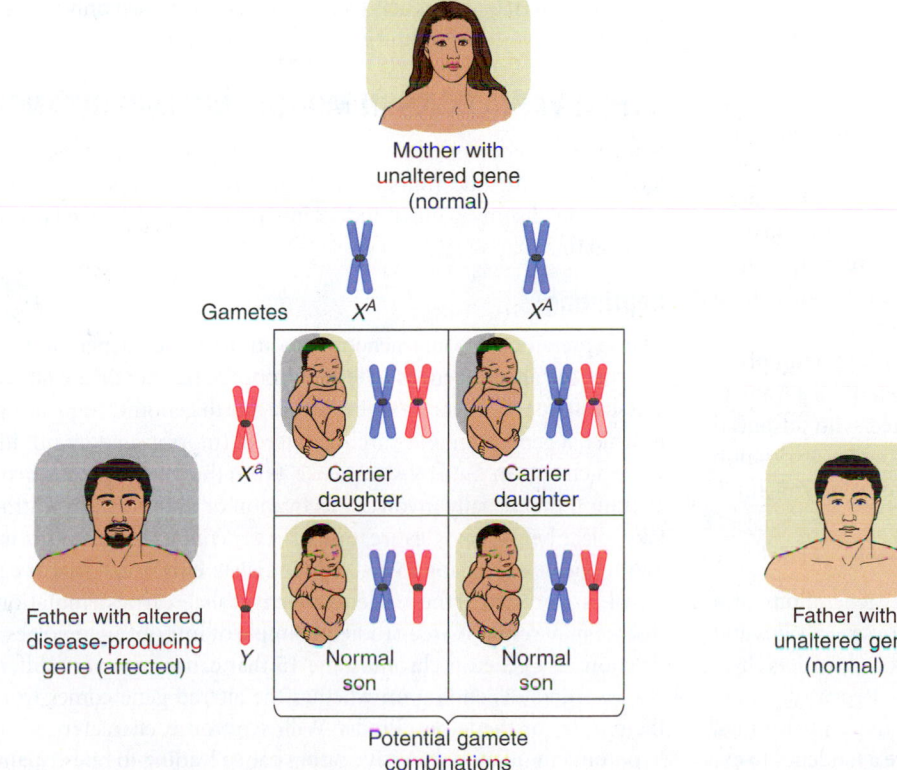

FIGURE 4–11 ■ X-Linked Inheritance

These Punnett squares show potential gene combinations (genotypes) and resulting phenotypes of children whose parents have different genotypes involving an X-linked gene alteration. Male offspring who inherit a copy of the altered gene will be affected, and female offspring who inherit a copy of the altered gene will be carriers for the disorder. Possible genotypes and phenotypes for each pregnancy are shown.

BOX 4–9	X-Linked Mendelian Inheritance Characteristics

When gathering a family history, the nurse should assess for the following characteristics of X-linked inheritance:

1. More males will be affected than females; females are rarely affected.
2. An affected male will have all carrier daughters.
3. There is no male-to-male inheritance.
4. Affected males are related by carrier females.
5. Female carriers may report milder symptoms of the condition.
6. A sporadic case could occur due to a new mutation.

Penetrance

Some individuals will inherit an altered gene associated with a disorder, and may even transmit the disorder to their offspring, without ever exhibiting the disorder themselves. This "skipping" of a generation is due to reduced penetrance, which is associated with certain genetic conditions. **Penetrance** is the probability that a gene will be expressed phenotypically. It is an "all or none" concept in that a gene is considered to be penetrant if it is expressed to any degree. Penetrance can be measured in the following way. In a certain group of individuals with the same genotype, what percentage of them will exhibit at least some signs and/or symptoms of the condition? If the number is less than 100%, then that condition is said to show *reduced penetrance*. Reduced penetrance is thought to be caused by modifying effects of genes other than the altered gene. Reduced penetrance is a feature of some autosomal dominant disorders. Others (for example, achondroplasia and Huntington disease) exhibit 100% penetrance, and all individuals with one copy of the gene alteration will exhibit signs and symptoms of the disease.

New Mutation

When there is no previous family history of a condition, the disease may be caused by a spontaneous new mutation. A new mutation is said to be sporadic or *de novo.* New mutations of a gene are most frequently seen in autosomal dominant and X-linked conditions because one copy of an altered gene is all that is necessary to alter health. Mutation rates for inherited disorders vary over a thousand-fold due to a number of factors, only some of which are understood (Nussbaum, McInnes, & Willard, 2007). Diseases in which new mutations are common include neurofibromatosis, achondroplasia (dwarfism), Duchenne muscular dystrophy, and hemophilia A and B. A number of new mutations have been associated with advanced parental age, both maternal (consider the well-known association between aneuploidies and maternal age) and paternal (Arnheim & Calabrese, 2009).

Anticipation

Anticipation is said to occur when successive generations of a family exhibit earlier onset of symptoms and more severe signs and symptoms of certain diseases. Anticipation occurs in disorders characterized by expansion of unstable repeat units. Repeat units are DNA sequences with repeating units of three or more nucleotides, for example CAGCAG . . . CAG. Repeat units have a tendency to expand, or accumulate repeats, during meiosis, especially during spermatogenesis. As a result, the number of repeats tends to increase in successive generations. Individuals with greater numbers of repeats have earlier onset of symptoms, more severe symptoms, or both.

More than a dozen diseases, usually neurologic in nature, result from unstable repeat expansions. These include Huntington disease, fragile X syndrome, and myotonic dystrophy.

Variable Expressivity

Expressivity describes the degree to which a phenotype is expressed. When people with the same genetic makeup (genotype) exhibit signs and/or symptoms with varying degrees of severity, the phenotype is described as showing *variable expression.* Variable expression is common in the autosomal dominant condition neurofibromatosis type 1. Although neurofibromatosis has 100% penetrance, members of the same affected family often exhibit variation in degree of signs and/or symptoms.

Sex-Limited Traits

Sex-limited traits are autosomal traits that are expressed in either males or females but not both. In these traits, gene expression is linked to an individual's hormonal environment, especially estrogen and testosterone levels. It is important to note that although one gender does not express the trait, the gene is present in the individual's genome and can be passed on to offspring. An example is ambiguous genitalia in female infants caused by congenital adrenal hyperplasia (CAH). CAH is an autosomal recessive disorder in which cortisol and aldosterone formation are blocked, resulting in overproduction of androgen and virilization of female external genitalia (Turnpenny & Ellard, 2012).

Sex-Influenced Traits

Sex-influenced traits are those that act differently in males and females. Pattern baldness acts as an autosomal dominant trait in males and requires only one copy to be expressed. In females, however, the gene for pattern baldness acts recessive and is expressed only when a woman has two copies of the gene (Jorde et al., 2010).

OTHER VARIATIONS IN MONOGENIC INHERITANCE

Some single-gene disorders follow unique types of inheritance patterns. These include mitochondrial inheritance, imprinting, and uniparental disomy. Mitochondrial inheritance was discussed previously in this chapter.

Imprinting

The expression of some genetic conditions varies depending on whether the altered gene is inherited from the mother or the father. These differences in gene expression are due to genomic imprinting, in which a gene from one parent is altered. Imprinting does not involve a change in the DNA sequence, but rather an epigenetic gene alteration that usually involves inactivation of the gene. Imprinting takes place before gametes are formed. After conception, the imprint controls gene expression so that only one allele, either maternal or paternal, is expressed. If the unsilenced (active) allele carries a mutation, disease may result. A well-studied example of imprinting involves a deletion in a gene on chromosome 15 that causes two very different disorders depending on whether the altered gene comes from the mother or the father. Prader-Willi syndrome, characterized by hypotonia in infancy, excessive eating habits leading to obesity, and mild-to-moderate developmental delay, is due to a deletion on chromosome 15 that is inherited from the father. Angelman syndrome is due to a similar deletion in the same gene on chromosome 15, but it is inherited from the mother. The clinical presentation is very different. Individuals with Angelman syndrome have severe developmental delay, a jerky gait, seizures, and a happy, sociable disposition (Gurrieri & Accadia, 2009).

Uniparental Disomy

In cases of uniparental disomy, the child inherits both copies of a chromosome pair (or homologous parts of a chromosome pair) from the same parent instead of one copy from each parent. If there are no altered genes on these chromosomes, the child may not be affected by this event. However, if the chromosome contains an altered gene for an autosomal recessive disease, the child will receive two copies of the altered gene and express the disease. For instance, if a child inherits two copies of chromosome 7 carrying an altered cystic fibrosis gene from a mother who is a carrier, the child will exhibit signs and symptoms of cystic fibrosis. Interestingly, about 25% of individuals with Prader-Willi syndrome and 3% to 5% of individuals with Angelman syndrome inherit their disorders due to uniparental disomy for chromosome 15 (Gurrieri & Accadia, 2009).

POLYGENIC AND MULTIFACTORIAL INHERITANCE

Most inheritable traits are polygenic. That is, they occur as a result of variations on several genes. Polygenic traits include fingerprint patterns, eye color, height, and skin color. Most diseases and health conditions are caused by more than one gene, and the expression of those genes is often modified by environmental influences. These conditions are called multifactorial and include many birth defects such as cleft lip and palate, pediatric conditions such as autism and asthma, and adult-onset conditions such as cancer and heart disease. Because the term *polygenic* does not infer the influence of the environment, the term *multifactorial* is preferred. The relative contribution of genetic and environmental influences varies across disorders.

Multifactorial conditions accumulate in families but do not follow characteristic Mendelian inheritance patterns. Recurrence risk predicts whether a condition will occur again in subsequent pregnancies. Recurrence risk varies among multifactorial conditions but is usually less than that of Mendelian disorders. Calculation of recurrence risk is complex, and for some disorders recurrence risk is not easily predicted. Calculations are based on population studies and expressed as a percentage. Risk of recurrence is higher when more than one family member is affected, when the affected family member has severe expression of the disease, and when the affected family member is closely related (Jorde et al., 2010).

Neural Tube Defects

A neural tube defect (NTD) is a condition that occurs early during fetal development with incomplete closure of the neural tube. Severity of the disorder varies, depending on which part of the tube does not close. Anencephaly, meningomyelocele, and spina bifida are examples of NTD. Recurrence risk for NTD is increased in families with an affected child, but that risk can be reduced by maternal dietary folic acid supplementation (Jorde et al., 2010).

Congenital Heart Defects

Most congenital heart defects are thought to be of multifactorial cause. Chromosomal disorders such as deletions or trisomy conditions, alterations in genes involved in the complex process of heart development, and maternal disease and drug exposure have all been associated with cardiac deformities. Often a specific genetic disorder cannot be identified. Recurrence risk varies widely with the condition and the number and degree of relationship of affected family members (Oyen, Poulsen, Boyd, et al., 2009; Sadowski, 2009).

Cleft Lip and Palate

Cleft lip and/or palate (CL/P) occur due to failure of bony fusion at about day 35 of gestation. While rare gene mutations can cause CL/P, in most cases the disorder is thought to be multifactorial. Maternal smoking and a number of gene variations have been associated with CL/P. Recurrence risk for families increases with the severity of the clefting in the affected child (Turnpenny & Ellard, 2012).

Autism Spectrum Disorder

While the etiology of autism spectrum disorder remains poorly understood, most experts believe it to be multifactorial. Twin studies suggest a strong genetic component, with 60% to 92% concordance between identical twins. A number of environmental influences have been suspected to influence the development of autism, as well (Inglese & Elder, 2009).

Collaborative Care

Many health professionals work together in screening, diagnosis, identification, and treatment of genetic disorders. The goals of collaborative care are early diagnosis through assessment and testing, development of an effective treatment plan combined with psychosocial support to enhance coping, and referral to a genetic specialist when needed.

Diagnostic Procedures

Genetic testing Genetic testing is available for both chromosomal and gene-based alterations, and the field of genetic testing is advancing rapidly. New methodologies and broader applications of older techniques have greatly expanded the number of conditions for which genetic testing is available. Increasingly, genetic testing is offered directly to consumers, with limited counseling to explain test results. Patients and families may use unreliable sources for information about genetic testing. They can easily form misconceptions about the types of genetic tests available and what information the tests are able and not able to provide. For example, a test for cystic fibrosis may be reported as negative, but the significance of that finding relies on how many of the multiple CFTR mutations associated with CF were included in the test. The pediatric nurse needs knowledge of available genetic tests and understanding of implications related to genetic testing in order to assist patients and their families as they weigh choices regarding genetic testing. See Box 4–10.

BOX 4–10	**What Is a Genetic Test?**

A genetic test involves the analysis of chromosomes, DNA, RNA, genes, or gene products (e.g., enzymes and other proteins) to detect heritable or somatic variations related to disease or health. Whether a laboratory method is considered a genetic test also depends on the intended use, claim, or purpose of a test. For example, amino acid analysis to detect a metabolic disorder such as PKU is considered a genetic test, but the use of this same analysis to monitor general nutritional status is not (U.S. Department of Health and Human Services, 2008).

Recommendations for genetic testing Genetic tests are useful to diagnose disease, predict risk of future disease, inform reproductive decision making, and manage patient care. Guidelines regarding who should be tested and when to test are available for some genetic conditions. However, new knowledge accumulates rapidly, and recommendations for practice often lag behind research findings by several years.

Categories of genetic tests Genetic tests have been used for some time to detect heritable conditions that are passed from generation to generation. There are several categories of genetic testing, each with a unique purpose. See Table 4–1. Genetic testing utilizes a variety of methods and may analyze DNA, products of DNA, or other substances that indicate a genetic defect. DNA can be analyzed on a number of levels, from karyotyping an entire set of chromosomes to examining a specific gene for a mutation. Tests of DNA products (RNA or proteins) are sometimes done to measure gene function or expression, which vary from one tissue to another. Some genetic tests measure metabolites that accumulate when individuals lack a specific enzyme due to a gene mutation.

In pediatrics, the most common types of genetic testing are diagnostic tests, prenatal tests, and newborn screening. It is especially important for the pediatric nurse to understand the difference between screening tests and diagnostic tests. Screening tests are used in populations to find individuals at risk for a disorder, while diagnostic tests are used to establish a specific diagnosis in an individual. Screening tests provide a cost-effective means of identifying people at high risk to have a disease, so that more expensive diagnostic testing can be targeted to those at greatest risk. Diagnostic tests may be ordered when a child is suspected of having a specific disorder based on clinical presentation or screening test results. Diagnostic testing may be carried out prenatally to identify genetic disease such as an aneuploidy in a fetus.

Newborn screening is carried out on most newborns in developed countries and provides a means to identify children who may have a genetic disease such as PKU, sickle cell disease, or congenital hypothyroidism. In recent years, a laboratory technique called tandem mass spectroscopy has allowed greatly expanded newborn screening with little increase in laboratory cost. However, even the most specific of screening tests will result in false-positive results, and every positive screening test must be followed by a diagnostic test. In fact, a positive newborn screen is more likely to represent a false positive than to lead to clinical diagnosis (Wilfond & Ross, 2009). The cost to follow up positive screening tests is significant both in terms of parental anxiety and financial burden, and expanded newborn screening has raised a number of ethical, legal, and social concerns (Bailey, Skinner, Davis, et al., 2008). Criteria for conditions included in newborn screening programs include demonstrated benefit of early detection and the availability of disease-altering treatment. Cost-effectiveness is also a concern, as many of the disorders included in expanded newborn screening are rare. See Chapter 10 ⏺ for further description of newborn screening.

Another category of genetic testing that pediatric nurses should be aware of is preimplantation genetic diagnosis. This involves the detection of disease-causing gene alterations in human embryos just after in vitro fertilization and before implantation

TABLE 4–1	Types of Genetic Tests
TYPE OF TEST	**DESCRIPTION**
Diagnostic testing	Used to establish a diagnosis of a genetic disorder in an individual who is symptomatic or has had a positive screening test.
Prenatal testing	Testing to identify a fetus with a genetic disease or condition. Testing is usually initiated due to family history or maternal factors. Some prenatal testing is offered routinely.
Newborn screening	Testing of newborn to identify the presence of a condition that requires immediate initiation of treatment to prevent death or disability.
Preimplantation testing	Following in vitro fertilization, testing is performed on embryos to identify embryos with a particular genetic condition.
Carrier testing	Testing in an asymptomatic individual to identify carrier status for a genetic condition.
Predictive testing	Offered usually to asymptomatic individuals to detect genetic conditions that occur later in life. May be presymptomatic or predispositional.
	Presymptomatic testing detects mutations that, if present, are likely or certain to eventually cause symptoms (an example is Huntington disease).
	Predispositional testing detects mutations that increase the likelihood that symptoms will develop (such as BRCA 1 and 2).

of the embryo in the uterus, thus providing an opportunity for preselection of unaffected embryos for implantation. Couples at risk to pass on a genetic disease such as Tay-Sachs commonly use preimplantation genetic diagnosis and preselection of unaffected embryos.

Still another purpose of genetic testing is for carrier screening. This involves the identification of an individual who is asymptomatic but may be a carrier for an autosomal or X-linked recessive genetic disease. Carrier screening is often utilized by potential parents who want to make informed reproductive decisions, both in families with known conditions such as Tay-Sachs or cystic fibrosis, but also more commonly by couples without a family history of genetic conditions. Since 2001, the American College of Obstetricians and Gynecologists (ACOG) has recommended that cystic fibrosis carrier screening be made available to all couples, with the decision whether to have the test to be based on personal choice (ACOG Committee on Genetics, 2011).

Predictive testing involves testing an asymptomatic individual for the presence of a late-onset genetic disease. The hope with predictive testing is that by identifying individuals at risk for a specific condition early in their lives, targeted prevention, surveillance, and/or treatment may ultimately reduce morbidity and mortality. An example is testing for genes associated with adult-onset cancers, such as breast or medullary thyroid cancer. Prediction is tempered, however, by the fact that many late-onset genetic conditions are multifactorial, influenced by both genetic and environmental factors. Consequently, even a positive test documenting the presence of a gene alteration may be unable to predict with certainty whether signs and symptoms will appear, when they may occur, or how severe those signs and symptoms might be. An exception to this general rule occurs when an autosomal dominant gene has complete penetrance; the most common example is Huntington disease. A positive Huntington test virtually guarantees that the individual will develop the disease. Predictive testing is complicated further by the ability to detect altered genes when there is no preventive treatment for the disease. Examples are Alzheimer disease and Huntington disease. The issue of predictive testing among children and adolescents, in particular, has been the focus of considerable concern. (See the following section on the role of the nurse in genetic testing.) Consider the opening scenario, in which 17-year-old Sarah considers the personal implications around testing for the Huntington gene. Although there is no preventive treatment for Huntington disease, Sarah is exploring the possibility of gene testing so that she can make informed life decisions.

Diagnosing chromosomal alterations **Cytogenetics,** or the study of chromosomes, describes the microscopic examination of chromosomes to reveal alterations such as additions, deletions, and chromosomal breaks with rearrangements or rejoinings (translocations). Prenatally, amniocentesis and chorionic villi sampling (CVS) can be undertaken to provide specimens for cytogenetic examination. After a child is born, chromosomal diagnostic examination can be accomplished with a blood, skin, or buccal cell sample.

Both amniocentesis and CVS provide fetal cells from which a karyotype can be prepared to examine chromosome number and structure. Cells sloughed off by the fetus and containing the genome of the fetus are present in amniotic fluid. With CVS, fetal cells are obtained directly from the chorionic villi. These cells also contain the genome of the developing fetus. Whether the cells come from amniocentesis, CVS, or blood, a karyotype can be completed in a cytogenetics laboratory. Chromosomes can be identified by their size and unique light and dark banding patterns. The pairs of autosomal chromosomes are arranged from 1 to 22 according to each chromosome's size, unique banding patterns, and centromere position. The sex chromosomes complete the picture, with the X chromosome(s) first, then the Y chromosome (if present). The karyotype shows all of the chromosome pairs lined up, allowing for visual analysis (Figure 4–3). The final report contains numeric data reporting the total number of chromosomes present. If there is an additional or deleted chromosome, it is identified with a plus ($+$) or minus ($-$) symbol. For example, a male individual with a genotype of 47, XY, $+18$ has 47 chromosomes (instead of the expected 46), with an additional copy of chromosome 18 (trisomy 18).

Fluorescence in situ hybridization (FISH) is another way to screen cells for chromosomal changes. FISH analyzes chromosomes from amniotic fluid or other sources by adding DNA probes that attach to specific chromosomes, chromosomal regions, or genes. A fluorescent signal attached to the probe is visible through a microscope, allowing rapid diagnosis of an abnormal chromosome number or particular chromosomal rearrangement. FISH does not require growth of cells in an incubator, so results can be obtained faster than with karyotyping. Cells can be analyzed within hours after the DNA probes are added. FISH analysis is particularly useful to identify trisomy of chromosomes 13, 18, 21, X, and Y (the only nonlethal trisomies) but is capable of detecting smaller chromosomal

alterations, such as the deletions associated with Prader-Willi and Angelman syndromes as well (Jorde et al., 2010). It cannot, however, detect gene alterations that involve very short nucleotide sequences. For gene testing of high resolution, molecular methods of DNA testing are required.

Diagnosing gene alterations Recent advances in molecular genetic technology along with the mapping of the human genome have resulted in tremendous expansion of available genetic testing. Genetic testing is currently available for more than 2,200 diseases, with more being added each day (GeneTests, 2011). DNA-based tests involve new, sophisticated technology that permits examination of the DNA sequence itself, so that even single-nucleotide variations can be detected. DNA-based testing can be performed on blood, bone marrow, amniotic fluid, fibroblast cells of the skin, or buccal cells from the mouth. Tests commonly require several days to weeks to complete, and occasionally several months are required before results are reported.

Genes are made up of many nucleotides, or base pairs. For example, the CFTR gene on chromosome 7, which in an altered form causes cystic fibrosis, is over 200,000 base pairs long. It is reasonable, then, that alterations at various sites on the CFTR gene may affect its function and lead to expression of the disease. Indeed, more than 1,700 mutations of the CFTR gene leading to cystic fibrosis have been identified (ACOG, 2011). Most of these mutations are rare; the most common alteration, named delta F508, causes about 70% of cystic fibrosis. It is not feasible to test for all possible alterations, however, and current clinical guidelines recommend testing for 25 mutations (ACOG, 2011; Moskowitz et al., 2008). Therefore, a negative test does not eliminate all chance of carrying a gene alteration associated with cystic fibrosis. This is just one of the limitations of genetic testing that nurses must understand to provide genetically competent care. See The Role of the Nurse in Genetic Testing later in this chapter.

Other genetic tests examine gene products, rather than the makeup of the gene itself. These include biochemical-based methods that examine protein products of genes or their substrates. An example of a biochemical test is the PKU test. Although PKU is caused by a deficiency of the enzyme phenylalanine hydroxylase (PAH), the PKU test actually measures phenylalanine levels, which are markedly elevated in individuals with PAH deficiency. Many of these biochemical tests have been in use for years.

Tests of gene expression are available as well. For example, **microarray analysis** can detect levels of messenger RNA in cells, which indicates which genes are "turned on" or being expressed. Microarray analysis is especially useful to examine tumor cells (Jorde et al., 2010).

Quality and accuracy of genetic tests Genetic nurses express concern that genetic tests are becoming available too quickly without regulation of the companies offering them. The quality, accuracy, and reliability of genetic test results are not measured against any common standard. Of particular concern is the growing popularity of direct-to-consumer genetic testing, which is increasingly accessible and affordable and allows individuals to order genetic tests without consulting a healthcare provider. In many cases minimal or no education is provided for the individual undergoing testing, nor is counseling or follow-up uniformly provided. Individuals may

Legal and Ethical Considerations
Implications of Genetic Testing

Since its inception, the National Human Genome Research Institute has designated a percent of its budget to examine the ethical, legal, and social implications (ELSI) of genetic and genomic information. Genetic testing raises many questions that have been addressed by ELSI. Genetic exceptionalism, the idea that genetic information should be treated differently from other health information, continues to be a subject of great interest and little consensus. Proponents of genetic exceptionalism point out that genetic information is unique and deserving of special consideration and protection because it is predictive, is potentially stigmatizing, and may reveal information about family members other than the patient undergoing testing. The contrasting view points out that other information is also predictive (consider blood cholesterol and risk for cardiovascular disease) and stigmatizing (for example, information about sexually transmitted infections).

Federal health privacy protection, as mandated under the federal Health Insurance Portability and Accountability Act (HIPAA) privacy rule, does not afford special protection to genetic information, treating it as being no more sensitive than other health-related information. However, the majority of states have enacted legislation that takes the exceptionalist view, providing protection against discrimination based on genetic information and penalties for violating genetic privacy (U.S. Department of Health and Human Services, 2008). Federal legislation to prohibit discrimination based on genetic information in health insurance and employment (the Genetic Information Nondiscrimination Act, or GINA) was enacted in 2008.

make hard and irrevocable life-altering decisions after receiving test results, so accuracy and reliability, along with professional counseling, are essential. See Legal and Ethical Considerations: Implications of Genetic Testing.

Nursing Management

By integrating into practice the genetic aspects of assessment, observation, and history gathering, the pediatric nurse can improve the standard of care delivered and have a positive impact on the child and family. The pediatric nurse does not need to be a genetic expert, but with heightened awareness, appropriate inquiries and referrals to genetic specialists can be completed.

Family Risk Assessment

Genetic Family History
While gathering a family history, the nurse must assess the information that is provided by the family, looking for significant information that might indicate the need for a follow-up or a referral to a genetic specialist. Multiple pregnancy losses, developmental delay, congenital conditions, or birth defects are some of the conditions that may be identified when collecting a family history and would indicate the family may benefit from a genetic referral.

Pedigrees
Pediatric nurses should know how to collect a three-generation family history, record the history in a pedigree, and think "genetic." A **pedigree** is a pictorial representation or diagram of the medical history of a family (Figure 4–12 ■). A pedigree is constructed around a designated "index" patient, called the **proband** (if he or she is affected with the genetic disorder of interest) or **consultand** (if he or she seeks genetic counseling without being known to have the disorder). Multiple symbols (Figure 4–13 ■) are utilized to present this picture, and the finished pedigree presents a family's medical data and biological relationship information at a glance. A pedigree provides a clear, visual representation of relationships of affected individuals to the immediate and extended family. It can identify other individuals in the family who might benefit from a genetic consultation. A pedigree can also indicate a Mendelian or multifactorial pattern of inheritance. On the basis of the pedigree, genetic referral and/or reproductive risk teaching for the individual and family can occur. The visual nature of a pedigree enhances a family's learning and can be used to clarify any inheritance misunderstandings or misconceptions. If completed correctly and comprehensively, a pedigree permits all healthcare professionals working with the child or family to quickly see what history and background information has been collected (Box 4–11).

It is important to gather a three-generation family pedigree even if the nurse believes this is a first occasion of the condition within a

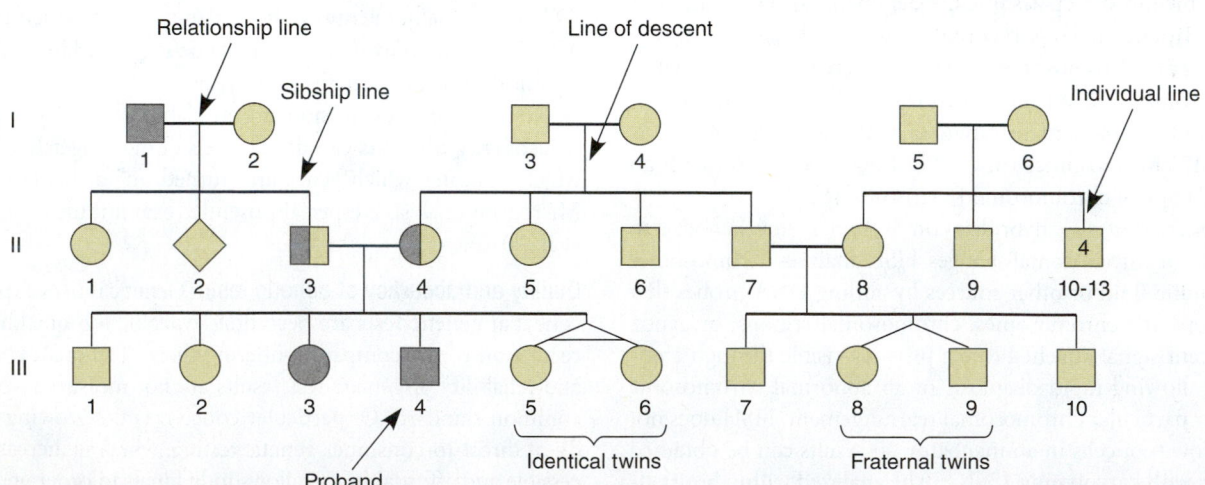

A representative pedigree for a single characteristic or genetic condition through three generations.

FIGURE 4–12 ■ Sample three-generation pedigree.

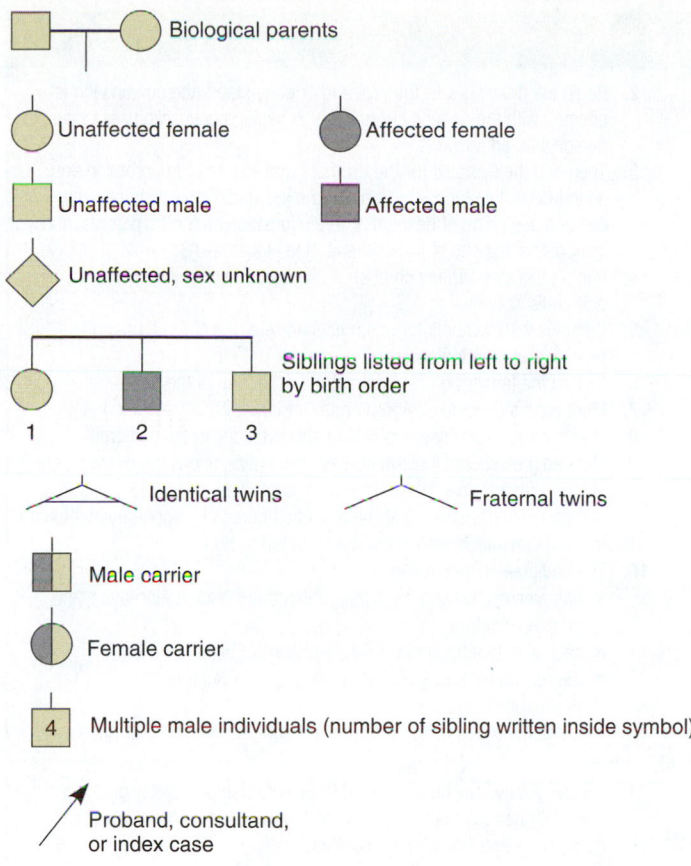

FIGURE 4–13 ■ Selected standardized symbols for use in drawing a pedigree.

family. A condition without any identifiable inheritance pattern on the pedigree may be due to a new mutation or variable expressivity. Throughout the process of gathering family history data, the nurse must remember family confidentiality at all times. All information related to a pedigree is confidential information. The history may reveal sensitive details that include infertility problems, elective termination of pregnancy, or nonpaternity. This information may not even be known by a current partner or other family members. Other sensitive issues include pregnancies conceived by technology, a history of suicides, drug or alcohol abuse, and same-sex relationships. See Box 4–12.

Challenges inherent in recalling the family history include the parents' inability to remember conditions that may have been surgically repaired and then forgotten, or reporting conditions that may have been attributed incorrectly to other causes. Also, the family history may contain information previously unknown to extended family members. Reproductive decisions may have been made that were against the family's religious or cultural beliefs. Both immediate and extended family members may be unaware of these "family skeletons" and the parent may be reluctant to reveal this information (Bennett, 2010).

Genetic Physical Assessment

The pediatric nurse in any healthcare setting should incorporate genetic aspects into the comprehensive assessment (see Chapter 8 🔗). An early finding by the nurse provides the child and the family with an opportunity for a genetic referral and more comprehensive health care.

Major and Minor Anomalies

Dysmorphology refers to the study of human congenital defects or abnormalities of body structure that begin before birth. Traditionally, congenital anomalies have been included under the umbrella of genetic disorders whether they occur due to a gene alteration or another cause of abnormal embryonic or fetal development. Dysmorphic anomalies can occur anywhere in the body, but are perhaps most often associated with facial features. As a routine part of patient assessment, the nurse should complete a screening for minor anomalies or malformations. A **minor anomaly** or malformation is an unusual morphologic feature that in itself is of no serious medical or cosmetic concern to the individual or family. Some minor anomalies are merely family traits or are present in certain ethnic groups. Minor anomalies include such traits as wide-set eyes, single palmar creases, café au lait patches, low anterior hairline, preauricular (in front of the ears) pits and tags, broad face, or mild proportionate short stature. Examples of variations associated with ethnic origin include upward-slanting eyes or prominent epicanthal folds among individuals of Asian descent. The presence of a single minor anomaly is relatively common and is usually of no consequence. However, minor anomalies may be important diagnostic clues, especially if several are found in the same individual. For example, a newborn with a short, broad head, a single palmar crease, and up-slanting eyes that do not resemble his parents' eyes should be evaluated for Down syndrome (Ranweiler, 2009). Infants with three or more minor anomalies often have a major anomaly as well, or an underlying genetic syndrome (Askin, 2009). Therefore, the nurse who notes three or more minor anomalies in a newborn or child should consider the possibility of a major anomaly or an underlying genetic condition and advocate for a genetic referral.

About 3% of all children have a **major anomaly,** defined as a serious structural defect present at birth that may have severe medical or cosmetic consequences, interfere with normal functioning of body systems, lead to a lifelong disability, or even cause an early death. Congenital heart defects, cleft lip and/or palate, neural tube defects, duodenal atresia, and craniosynostosis are considered major anomalies (Bennett, 2010). Some major anomalies are present at birth but are not apparent, such as deafness, various skeletal dysplasias, and some types of congenital heart defects.

A **syndrome** is a collection of multiple anomalies, major or minor, that occur in a consistent pattern and have a common cause. For example, Down syndrome is the cause of a variety of anomalies that can appear in multiple body systems, including the eyes, ears, hair, mouth and tongue, heart, and brain. An **association** is a group of abnormalities of unknown cause that occur together more often than is expected by chance (Turnpenny & Ellard, 2012).

The nurse can identify clues to genetic problems by inspecting the child, the parents, and other family members (Table 4–2). Nurses may even ask to look at family photographs and examine them for common dysmorphic features and family traits. Several standardized craniofacial measurements have been defined, and tables are available displaying normal values according to age, so that dysmorphic

BOX 4–11　Steps in Drawing a Pedigree

I. How to
  1. Work in pencil (because family historians often remember additional relatives and details only after questioning is almost completed).

II. Organization
  1. Begin recording data in the middle of the sheet of paper (to allow enough room for both the maternal and paternal sides of the family).
  2. Use only standard pedigree symbols (see Figure 4–13).
  3. Place the male individual in a couple on the left of the relationship line; the paternal side of the family also goes on the left side of the paper.

III. Determining Family Relationships
  1. Determine relationships within the family by asking questions such as:
    ■ Do you have a partner or are you married?
    ■ How many biological brothers and sisters do you have?
    ■ How many children do you have?
    ■ Do all the children have the same biological father?
    ■ Do all the children share the same mother and father?
  2. Referral to "the baby's father or mother" can be helpful until the relationship between parents is established.
  3. Referral to a "union" if marriage does not exist can also help communication.

IV. Who Should or Should Not Be Included
  1. To ensure accuracy, the pedigree should include the parents, offspring, siblings, aunts, uncles, grandparents, and first cousins of the individual seeking counseling.
  2. Detailed information about the spouses of the proband's family can be omitted unless there is a history of some kind of disorder or condition.
  3. Eliminating persons or information that does not contribute any valuable information can help keep the pedigree small and more manageable.

V. Recording the Family History
  1. Determine the approximate size of the family (to plan spacing on the paper).

  2. Begin the drawing with the proband or consultand (the person who is affected with the genetic condition or is seeking counseling). Mark that person with an arrow.
  3. Then add the symbols for the brothers and sisters of the proband and an individual line for each. Connect the individual lines with a sibship line and add a line of descent, the relationship line for the parents, and symbols for parents of the proband. See Figure 4–13.
  4. Repeat this step for any children of the proband or children of the proband's siblings.
  5. Continue with symbols for all immediate relatives of the proband's parents and grandparents.
  6. Record the family's ethnic background at the top of the page.
  7. Mark each symbol to designate relevant information (see Box 4–13).
  8. Create a key to clarify symbols and abbreviations in the pedigree.
  9. The pedigree should include at least three generations. Mark each generation with a Roman numeral along the left side of the paper, with the first generation marker (I) at the top. Each person in a generation should follow an imaginary horizontal line from left to right.
  10. The pedigree should include
    ■ half-siblings, pregnancy losses, stillbirths, previous marriages, and adopted children
    ■ causes of death, age at death, and current health problems
    ■ the reason for taking the pedigree (e.g., developmental delay, dysmorphology, etc.)
    ■ the name of the family historian (person relaying the information)

VI. Other
  1. Consanguinity may be suspected if the historian repeatedly gives the same last name on both sides of the family. Ask if any relatives in the family have ever had a child together.

VII. Completing the Pedigree
  1. When completed, the pedigree should be dated and signed with the name, credentials, and position of the person drawing it.

Source: *Data from Bennett, R. L. (2010). The practical guide to the genetic family history (2nd ed.). New York: John Wiley & Sons. Reproduced with permission of John Wiley & Sons, Inc.*

BOX 4–12　Specific Facts and Health Information to Include in a Pedigree

■ Age/birth date or year of birth
■ Age of death (year, if known)
■ Cause of death
■ Full siblings versus half or stepsiblings
■ Relevant health information (including medical conditions and age at diagnosis)
■ Affected/unaffected status for familial conditions—define shading of symbols in a legend key
■ Pregnancy with gestational age (LMP) or estimated date of delivery (EDD)
■ Pregnancy complications with gestational ages noted (e.g., 6 wk, 32 wk): miscarriage/spontaneous abortion (SAB), stillbirth (SB), pregnancy termination (TOP), ectopic (ECT)

■ Infertility versus no children by choice
■ Ethnic background (country of origin for each grandparent)
■ Consanguinity
■ First names (if appropriate—be cautious of privacy)
■ Date pedigree taken or updated
■ Reason pedigree taken
■ Name of person who took pedigree and credentials
■ Key or legend (symbols or acronyms used on the chart)

Source: *Bennett, R. L. (2010). The practical guide to the genetic family history (2nd ed.). New York: John Wiley & Sons. Reproduced with permission of John Wiley & Sons, Inc.*

facial features are more easily identified (Figure 4–14 ■). By making a genetic referral, the pediatric nurse can make a difference in the child's state of health.

The Role of the Nurse in Genetic Testing

Many people have misconceptions about genetic testing, and nurses play an important role in helping parents and children understand the implications and limitations of genetic tests. Communication

with the child and family should include a discussion regarding the reason the test is being considered, as well as potential positive and negative outcomes of the test. Are there existing treatments for the condition being tested? What are the potential psychologic issues associated with a positive or negative test? Who will be affected by the test results? Will the test results be shared with extended family members? When helping families to make decisions about genetic testing, nurses should focus on determining whether the test is in

TABLE 4–2	Selected Dysmorphic Physical Assessment Findings*		
Skull	Asymmetric head/face	**Eyes**	Blue sclera
	Brachycephaly (short, broad head shape) (See Figure 33–17.)		Different colored eyes
	Flattened or prominent occiput		Down-slanting eyes
	Fontanels too large or small		Epicanthal folds (See Figure 7–16.)
	Frontal bossing (prominent central forehead)		Extreme hyperopia (farsightedness)
	Micrognathia (small jaw)		Extreme myopia (nearsightedness)
	Prognathism (projection of jaw beyond that of the forehead)		Hypertelorism (widely spaced eyes)
			Hypotelorism (closely spaced eyes)
Extremities	Abnormally positioned feet		Short palpebral fissures (distance between inner and outer canthus of eyes)
	Arachnodactyly (long fingers or toes)		Up-slanting eyes (See Figure 7–17.)
	Brachydactyly (short fingers or toes)	**Skin**	Axillary freckling (See Figure 33–18.)
	Camptodactyly (permanent flexion of fingers or toes)		Café au lait spots (See Figure 33–18.)
	Clinodactyly (curved fingers or toes, most often the fifth finger)		Excessive skin
	Extremely long, thin extremities		Extremely loose skin
	Hypoplastic (very small) or absent nails		Hyperelastic skin
	Loose joints		Leaf-shaped white markings
	Single transverse palmar crease		Syndactyly (webbing between fingers and toes)
	Polydactyly (extra fingers and/or toes)	**Mouth**	Cleft lip with or without cleft palate (See Figure 30–3.)
	Rocker bottom feet		Large or small tongue
	Syndactyly (webbing between fingers and toes)		Misshapen, missing, or extra teeth
	Unusually tall or short stature		Early loss of teeth
Ears	Ear tags or pits		Late eruption of teeth
	Ears that are posteriorly rotated		Smooth or abnormal philtrum
	Hearing loss		Thin upper lip
	Low-set ears	**Other**	Catlike mewing cry
	Malformed ears		Hoarse, weak cry
Hair	Excessive body hair		Hypogonadism
	Abnormal hairline or hair distribution		Obesity
	Large section of white hair in otherwise pigmented hair		Short, webbed neck
	Sparse or brittle hair		Multiple fractures

*This list is not all-inclusive, but is meant to increase the nurse's awareness of assessment findings that may be significant and require a referral to genetic specialists.

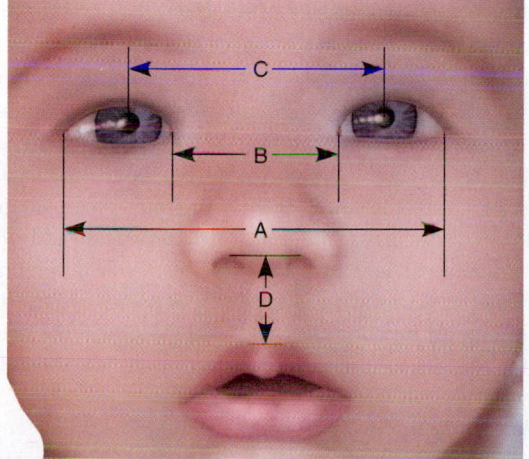

FIGURE 4–14 ■ Classic facial measurements for assessment with a genetic focus on faces/eyes, e.g., hypertelorism, hypotelorism, as described in Table 4–2. *A*, Outer intercanthal distance. *B*, Intercanthal distance. *C*, Interpupillary distance. *D*, Philtrum length.

the child's best interests, ensuring informed consent, promoting the child's autonomy, considering the family perspective, and addressing psychosocial issues. Often, the role of the nurse is to initiate a genetic referral.

Reasons for genetic testing in minors   The primary purpose of genetic testing in children should be to promote the child's well-being. The nurse must therefore help families to understand the purpose of a specific genetic test.

In general, there are four reasons to consider testing minors for genetic alterations. The first is if the testing offers an immediate medical benefit for the child in terms of diagnosis, disease prevention, or early treatment. Examples include studies to establish a diagnosis in a child with features of a genetic syndrome or to test a child for familial adenomatous polyposis (a genetic disease in which removal of the colon during adolescence is often required to prevent colon cancer). Another example is testing for familial hypercholesterolemia, an inherited condition that results in early death from extremely high cholesterol levels if left untreated. In all these conditions, diagnosis and treatment at a young age guide health management and improve health outcomes.

A second kind of situation occurs when an adolescent is facing a reproductive decision of his or her own. If an adolescent has a family history of a genetic condition, he or she may be interested in genetic testing that offers no specific medical benefit to that adolescent other than family planning. Recall Sarah, the young woman in the opening scenario who wanted to be tested for Huntington disease. Might genetic testing affect her reproductive decisions?

A third situation occurs when a parent or child requests genetic testing for a condition for future planning in the absence of any immediate benefit. This situation may arise with carrier testing or predictive testing for adult-onset inherited disorders. For example, an older child related to an individual affected with familial (early-onset) Alzheimer disease may wish confirmation of whether he or she carries the altered gene, in order to plan for a life career or to make relationship decisions such as marriage. Parents, as well, sometimes request predictive or carrier testing for their children who are well below reproductive age. More research is needed to better understand ethical concerns around genetic testing in children (Wilfond & Ross, 2009); however, most medical ethicists and professional organizations recommend that carrier testing and predictive genetic testing for adult-onset diseases usually be deferred until a child reaches adulthood (Borry, Evers-Kiebooms, Cornel, et al., 2009). Exceptions may occur when there is sufficient medical concern for the child (Lwiwski, Greenberg, & Mhanni, 2008).

Finally, a family member may request genetic testing for a child when the test results are entirely for the benefit of another family member, with no direct benefit to the child. This may occur during DNA linkage studies, in which multiple blood samples from both affected and unaffected individuals within a family must be analyzed and compared to produce a recognized DNA pattern for diagnosing a genetic condition in that particular family.

The pediatric nurse must be aware of these potential situations and know that decisions to perform genetic tests on children and adolescents are not made easily. The primary focus of genetic testing in children should be to promote the well-being of the child. In order to justify a genetic test on minors, the potential benefits must outweigh the potential harms. Otherwise genetic testing should be postponed until the child is capable of making an informed decision. That time often comes when an adolescent is making reproductive decisions.

Ensuring informed consent for genetic testing The pediatric nurse is responsible for alerting children and their families of their right to make an informed decision prior to *any* genetic testing with consideration of the special circumstances arising from the family, culture, and community life. All genetic testing should be voluntary, and it is the nurse's responsibility to ensure that the consent process includes discussion of the risks and benefits of the test, including any physical harm as well as potential psychologic and societal injury by stigmatization, discrimination, or emotional stress.

Promoting autonomy in genetic testing To the degree possible, children and adolescents should participate in decision making about genetic testing (Borry et al., 2009). The nurse should

therefore advocate for the child, considering the child's decision-making ability. Is the child's cognitive and emotional development sufficient to make a decision about genetic testing? Children of the same age have varying levels of development, and the complexity of genetic testing is variable; therefore, participation of children and adolescents in decisions about genetic testing should be considered on a case-by-case basis (Borry et al., 2009). As the child grows, his or her own genetic knowledge may exceed the parents' knowledge level. Older children and adolescents may be better prepared to participate in decision making and may disagree with their parents. The pediatric nurse can help facilitate understanding on both sides of the issue or refer the family to experienced professionals.

Considering the family perspective Recognizing that genetic testing affects families and not just individuals, the nurse should use a family perspective when assisting parents and children who are making decisions about genetic testing. Each family member's decisions should be respected, whether it is to participate in genetic testing or to decline. Not all people want to know their genetic risks. For example, if Sarah, the young woman in the opening scenario, has a positive Huntington test, the implication is that her mother (who does not wish to know her Huntington status) also carries the altered gene. A nondirective approach is critical; nurses must take care to avoid imposing their own values or personal opinions onto patients and families.

Ensuring confidentiality and privacy for genetic testing Although confidentiality and privacy are an integral part of delivery of care for all nurses, this issue is of greater concern as it relates to genetic information. Results of genetic tests can be far reaching. Although federal law offers some protections against genetic discrimination, risks persist. What effect will a genetic diagnosis have on the availability and affordability of life insurance? Can genetic information be released to the courts, military, schools, or adoption agencies? Would a child with a known gene alteration for Huntington disease be offered a college scholarship for the best law school? The technology that has made genetic testing possible has far outpaced the ability of health policy makers and legislators to put in place systems to protect genetic information.

Addressing psychosocial issues Pediatric nurses must be prepared to assist children and families to manage anxiety around genetic testing. Uncertainty and stress associated with making a decision to undertake genetic testing may extend into weeks or even months before results are available. That stress may be increased or relieved once test results are known. Although receiving favorable test results may decrease anxiety for the family or the individual, potential problems do occur, and the pediatric nurse must be prepared to address them. Concerns about carrier status may interfere with development of interpersonal relationships and intimacy. A positive test result may lead to feelings of unworthiness and self-image disturbance. Survivor guilt may affect children with negative results if their siblings are positive. Younger children may blame themselves, thinking they did or said something to cause the gene alteration. The adolescent carrying a gene alteration for a late-onset disease may have an increased tendency for risky behaviors. The adolescent who has inherited an altered disease-producing gene may foster resentment toward the parent who carries the altered gene. Parental guilt may exist for passing the altered gene to the child. Finally, parent–child bonds may be altered if parents become either overprotective or overly permissive. The parent and other family members may unconsciously form lowered expectations for the child or adolescent. Nurses must use counseling interventions to assist patients to process, adjust to, and utilize genetic information.

The nurse should also be aware that health insurance policies may not cover genetic testing, which is often very expensive. Even if the insurance benefit will cover the test, many individuals are fearful of discrimination based on genetic test results that are included in their medical record. The pediatric nurse should inform the child and the family of their right to know who will have access to the genetic test results.

Planning and Implementation

The pediatric nurse is responsible for comprehensively delivering the standard of care to children and families, while at the same time being aware of the limitations of his or her own knowledge and expertise. In addition to the continuous integration of genetic aspects into the nurse's assessment of family history and physical assessment, the nurse is also responsible for carrying out interventions that include initiating referrals to genetic specialists and delivering care to the individual or family in any of the following ways (Consensus Panel, 2009).

Genetic Referrals and Counseling

After gathering assessment data that incorporate genetic concepts, the pediatric nurse is able to partner with children and their families by initiating a referral to a genetic specialist if there are indicators for a genetic referral (Box 4–13). The nurse should provide the family with information about the advantages of a referral to genetic specialists, and the disadvantages of not following through with the referral. The nurse should inform the child and family that a genetic referral can provide information and answer many questions they may have concerning genetic health. Families should be encouraged to address all their concerns with the genetic specialist, who will be able to answer questions regarding genetic conditions, inheritance, availability of treatment, and future implications, as well as economic or insurance questions.

Those who are concerned about genetic disease may benefit from a genetic consultation whether or not genetic testing is available for that condition. Many people seek information and coping strategies as much as they do test results. Referral of a child with a suspected genetic problem to a geneticist, genetic nurse specialist, or genetic clinic is an expected nursing responsibility in the same way as referral to a dietitian or a social worker. When in doubt, the pediatric nurse should contact the advanced practice genetic clinical nurse, genetic counselor, or geneticist to discuss concerns.

Family Preparation for Genetic Referrals and Genetic Counseling

Not knowing what to expect from a genetic referral is common, and the fear of the unknown may cause anxiety for both the child and family. In order to facilitate the referral to genetic specialists, the pediatric nurse should educate the patient and family so that they know what to expect during as well as after a genetic evaluation. See Partnering with Families: Ethical Implications of Genetic Information.

Usually before the first genetic evaluation visit, the parent(s) will be contacted to provide a detailed medical and family history and to

---

BOX 4–13	Child or Family Indicators for a Referral to a Genetic Specialist

PRENATAL HISTORY INDICATORS FOR A GENETIC REFERRAL

- Infertility
- Repeated spontaneous abortions (usually 2–3 or more)
- Stillbirths or infant deaths due to unknown or genetic causes
- Females exposed to radiation, infectious disease, toxic agents, or certain drugs immediately before or during pregnancy
- Males exposed to radiation, toxic agents, or certain drugs who are contemplating *immediate* paternity (e.g., received chemotherapy in childhood)

OTHER INDICATORS FOR A PRENATAL GENETIC REFERRAL

- Unexpected drug or anesthesia reactions
- If the child or family reports a known or "believed" genetic condition in the family
- Any anomaly affecting more than one member of a family
- Single or multiple congenital anomalies
- Familial occurrence of neoplasms
- The early onset of common complex disorders such as coronary heart disease or cancer
- Consideration of marriage to a blood relative (**consanguinity**)
- Women who are 35 years and older and are considering pregnancy or are already pregnant
- Men who are 45 years and older and are considering paternity
- Members of ethnic groups in which certain genetic disorders are frequent and screening, testing, or prenatal diagnosis is available

- History of heritable conditions such as bleeding disorders, sickle cell disease, cystic fibrosis, thalassemia, or childhood cancers
- Any other situation where suspicious signs and/or symptoms might suggest genetic disease and the nurse feels further evaluation may be needed

POSTNATAL DEVELOPMENTAL INDICATORS FOR A GENETIC REFERRAL

- Delayed or abnormal development
- Developmental regression
- Mental retardation
- Speech problems
- Learning disability

POSTNATAL PHYSICAL INDICATORS FOR A GENETIC REFERRAL

- Failure to thrive in an infant or child
- Delays in physical growth, unusual body proportions, or low muscle tone
- Abnormal or delayed development of secondary sex characteristics or sex organs
- Short or extremely tall stature
- Blindness, cataracts in infants or children
- Deafness
- Hypotonia in an infant or child
- Seizures in newborns or infants
- Skin lesions such as café au lait spots

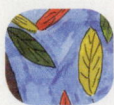

Partnering with Families

Ethical Implications of Genetic Information

The nurse must consider the enormity of the ethical issues facing all families who have knowledge of their genetic makeup. The ethical issues a nurse may have to discuss with the child and family are numerous. A few of the issues are listed here.

ACCESS TO INFORMATION

- Who should have access to personal genetic information, and how will it be used?
- Do insurers, employers, courts, law enforcement, schools, universities, adoption agencies, and the military have a right to access this information?

SELF-PERCEPTION

- How does personal genetic information affect an individual's perception of self?
- How does personal genetic information affect society's perceptions of that individual?
- How does personal genetic information affect an individual's cultural identity?
- How are self-identity and self-worth affected by a confirmed genetic risk or condition?

FAMILY ROLES AND RELATIONSHIPS

- Should an individual be tested for an autosomal dominant condition if the siblings or parents are opposed to knowing if they, themselves, have the altered gene?
- Should potential mates have genetic information?
- Should two people with increased genetic risk be prohibited from having children?
- Should a child be tested?
- Should the father be told if genetic testing and/or genetic counseling reveals nonpaternity?
- Should adoption records contain a complete genetic history of the biological parents?

- Is there an obligation to tell other family members if an altered gene that demands a change in lifestyle (nutrition, exercise, smoking, etc.) is diagnosed?
- Is there an obligation to tell other family members if an altered gene that causes early debilitation and/or death is diagnosed?

INFORMED CONSENT

- Are all individuals undergoing genetic testing giving true informed consent? Do they understand all of the consequences of agreeing to even a simple blood test in the doctor's office that may reveal a diagnosis or increased risk for a genetic condition?

HEALTH AND LIFE INSURANCE

- Should insurance companies have access to genetic test results?
- Should medical insurance costs be higher for persons with a gene alteration known to produce disease? For a gene alteration known to increase disease risk?
- Should medical insurance costs be higher for persons with known increased risk for disease because of any gene alteration if they make unhealthy lifestyle choices and do nothing to lower their risk?
- Should individuals be required to have a large life insurance policy to financially protect their families?

FINANCIAL

- Should a child with a life-limiting genetic condition be eligible for government grants or scholarship money?
- Should society be expected to financially support such children through government programs or private insurance?
- What is the motivation for children with life-limiting conditions to save money for the future?

EMPLOYMENT

- Should an employer have access to an individual's genetic profile?
- Will the individual's productivity be affected by the genetic condition?

make an appointment for genetic consultation. The parents should be prepared to give as exact a family history as possible so that a detailed three-generation pedigree can be constructed. The parents should be informed that a genetic consultation usually lasts several hours. During the appointment, a genetic clinical nurse, genetic counselor, and/or physician will interview the parents and their child to collect information about the family history and the child's medical history. A geneticist will examine the child and possibly the parents to establish an accurate diagnosis. Photos may be taken, and tests may be ordered. These may include chromosome analysis, DNA-based testing, radiographs, biopsy, biochemical tests, developmental testing, and/or linkage studies. After the exam and the completion of any applicable testing, the geneticist and/or genetic counselor will discuss the findings with the parents and/or child and make recommendations. Information will be provided about the likelihood of a genetic condition; or, if a diagnosis is made, information about the specific condition will be shared. The discussion will include the natural history of the condition, inheritance patterns, current preventive or treatment options, and risks to the child and/or family. The visit will also include opportunities for questions and answers as well as the assessment and evaluation of the family's understanding (Pediatric

Genetic Evaluations, n.d.). It is typical for the information retention of a family facing a new genetic diagnosis to be very low. This makes it imperative for the nurse to take advantage of opportunities to reinforce genetic concepts at a later time when the individual or family is ready.

As the visit concludes, the child and parents can expect appropriate referrals to be made, discussion of available services, and a follow-up visit may be scheduled. A summary of the information is usually sent to the family. The child's healthcare provider will receive a report if requested by the individual or parents.

Genetic healthcare providers present the individual and the family with information to promote informed decisions. They should recognize the importance of protecting the individual's autonomy. A challenge during any visit to a genetic specialist is to provide nondirective counseling. Families should be permitted to make decisions that are not influenced by biases or values from the nurse, counselor, or geneticist. Many families are accustomed to practitioners and nurses providing direction and guidance in their decision making, and families may be uncomfortable with the nondirectional approach. They may believe that the nurse or healthcare provider is withholding very bad news. The nurse should discuss the positives and negatives of each decision and present as many options as possible through the use of therapeutic listening and communication skills.

Family Teaching

The pediatric nurse must be aware of available genetic resources and participate in the education of genetic disorders as well as health promotion and prevention. Informing children and their families of what to expect from a genetic referral as well as clarifying and/or reinforcing information obtained during a genetic referral or genetic test results are also important.

Cultural and religious beliefs and values of the individual and family must be assessed by the nurse prior to teaching. Are the gene alterations viewed as uncontrollable and believed to be occurring secondary to cultural beliefs such as a stranger looking at the infant? Or, are the gene alterations considered a "punishment"? A family's readiness to learn can be influenced by cultural or religious beliefs and values. Obtaining educational materials in the primary language of the child or family will also help facilitate the teaching-learning experience.

The nurse must be aware of common inheritance misconceptions such as a parent's belief that with a 25% recurrence risk, after one child is affected the next three children will be unaffected, or with a 50% recurrence risk every other child will be affected. The recurrence risk *for each pregnancy* should be continually stressed by the nurse. Families often believe that a family member has inherited a genetic condition because they look like or "take after" a relative with a genetic condition. When new gene alterations or mutations are discussed, families will often exhibit surprise because no one else in the family has the condition so they perceive that the trait or condition cannot possibly be inherited (Bennett, 2010). Helping families to understand these genetic concepts is fundamental to delivering competent genetic nursing care.

Psychosocial Care

In order to meet the psychosocial needs of the child and family, the nurse should identify their expectations and needs as well as their cultural, spiritual, value, and belief systems. From where does the individual or family receive strength? Denial of the genetic diagnosis is common, and nurses must be aware of the family's state of acceptance. Individuals and families often will not believe that a genetic condition exists. Nurses must also provide care to help alleviate any anxiety or guilt in the child or family. Anxiety related to uncertainty while awaiting diagnosis or test results is common, but individuals also experience anxiety from not understanding the future implications of a confirmed genetic disease. Guilt may be associated with knowledge of the existence of a genetic condition in the family. The nurse must support families as they contemplate telling extended family members, friends, and neighbors about a confirmed diagnosis. Immediate family members often do not want to tell extended family members until they are ready. It is important for the nurse to reassure parents that the genetic condition is not the result of something they did or did not do during pregnancy. The nurse should encourage open discussions and the expression of fears and concerns. Guilt and shame are common as a family deals with the loss of the expectation and dream of a healthy child, grandchild, niece, or nephew. Reinforce to parents that genetic alterations are caused by changes within a gene and not by superstitions related to sin or other

cultural beliefs. It is important to remember that everyone has superstitions or beliefs. The pediatric nurse must remain nonjudgmental. As mothers, fathers, and extended family members provide continuous care for the individual with a genetic condition, depression can result. Depression also can occur in the individual with the chronic condition. The nurse must maintain awareness of the possibility of depression and be proactive in obtaining support for the individual or family. See Chapter 34 🔗.

The nurse also is responsible for assessing the family's coping mechanisms (see Chapter 2 🔗) as well as available family, spiritual, cultural, and community support systems. Genetic conditions can cause a permanent strain on family dynamics and relationships (Lehmann, Speight, & Kerzin-Storrar, 2011). The pediatric nurse may need to help the child and family reaffirm self-worth and value. Parents and children may feel they are part of a "production line" even though they are present for a very private problem. Nurses must be sensitive to these perceptions, provide open communication, and encourage discussion of feelings. Growth and development can be altered by actual or potential genetic disorders. Especially unique is the potential or actual inheritance of a late-onset condition such as Huntington disease, as discussed in the chapter-opening scenario. Like Sarah, the adolescent with this altered gene may not meet any of the developmental tasks in moving toward adulthood. Should the adolescent attend college or worry about the future? The pediatric nurse must identify the impact of genetic knowledge on activities of daily living but also movement through developmental milestones. Both individual and family strengths need to be identified. See Chapter 5 🔗.

The nurse can refer the individual or family to a support group. However, it is important to have permission from the child or family if the nurse is providing a support group with the patient's name and contact information. Electronic sources of genetic information abound and are unregulated; many of them are proprietary, offering expensive genetic testing or products that may have little scientific basis. Nurses should help families to both select and evaluate credible websites and online discussion groups.

Another key role for the nurse is to help families with the often difficult task of communicating genetic information such as inheritance patterns to extended family members. Cultural values of autonomy and privacy are affected when a person must consider whether to communicate genetic information to extended family members who may also carry the altered gene. The genetic alteration, in a form that causes disease or does not, may be extensive within a family, affecting multiple family members. Family members often have difficulty understanding that some genetic conditions have variable expressivity. Members of the extended family often are shocked and feel a profound sense of guilt that they carry the gene alteration that has caused their loved one to have a genetic condition.

Managing Care Through Advocacy

Careful self-assessment of feelings is essential for the nurse. The pediatric nurse must continually advocate for the child and family and support their decisions even if the decisions contradict the nurse's own ideals and morals. Coping with genetic revelations and making genetic-related treatment decisions are difficult activities for everyone. The nurse must remember that families will need resources and support, and also help in gathering information about reproductive options.

BOX 4–14 **Research: Genomics**

By deciphering the human DNA sequence and making it available to all researchers, the Human Genome Project represents basic research predicted to have a profound impact on health care. Now that the basic human genome sequence is known, researchers are identifying genetic variations that are associated with disease or have other health implications. Examples of genomic research include:

- **Pharmacogenomics,** determining how an individual's genome affects his or her response to medications. For example, children with leukemia are screened for a genetic variation that limits metabolism of mercaptopurine, a drug used in maintenance therapy. Prior to the availability of this genetic test, children with the altered gene were at risk to develop mercaptopurine toxicity and potentially fatal bone marrow suppression.

- The study of epigenetics, or how non-DNA molecules regulate gene expression. Environmental factors influence gene expression without changing the actual DNA sequence through epigenetic processes. For example, children whose mothers had inadequate nutrition during pregnancy appear to have increased risk to develop type 2 diabetes in later life. This increased risk is thought to be due to epigenetic influences on genes regulating sugar absorption and metabolism.

- **Proteomics,** research around the total "collection" of proteins an individual has available to carry out cellular functions. Just as an individual's genome is unique, so is his or her proteome.

- Examining the human microbiome, or the genomes of the microbes that inhabit humans. Adults have 10 times more microbial cells than human cells, and proteins made by those microbes contribute to an individual's proteome, influencing human metabolism, disease susceptibility, and drug response.

- The International HapMap project, which explored DNA sequence variation of individuals around the globe. HapMap data provide a baseline view of human genetic variation and underpin research to identify DNA sequence variations that contribute to disease risk.

- The Cancer Genome Atlas Project, a pilot study to identify specific DNA alterations that cause cells to become cancerous. The gene alterations associated with specific cancers can then be treated as genetic targets in cancer prevention, diagnosis, and treatment.

- Genome-wide association studies, in which the entire genomes of individuals known to have a specific disease are sequenced and compared to the genomes of individuals without the disease. Type 1 diabetes and attention deficit hyperactivity disorder are among the diseases included in genome-wide association studies.

Evaluation

Expected outcomes of delivering nursing care with a genetic focus include:

- The child and family will make informed and voluntary decisions related to genetic health issues.
- The child and family will accurately identify:
  - Basic genetic concepts and simple inheritance risk probabilities
  - What to expect from a genetic referral
  - The influence of genetic factors in health promotion and health maintenance
  - Social, legal, and ethical issues related to genetic testing

VISIONS FOR THE FUTURE

Nurses are often the primary caregivers that children and their families turn to for information, guidance, and clarification of ideas. This nursing role is essential not only in providing direct nursing care but also as a member of the community. As more information about the genomic revolution is available to consumers—in areas such as pharmacogenomics, gene transfer, ethics, genetic engineering, and stem cell research—the role of nurses grows enormously. Nurses should remain educated, informed, knowledgeable, and ready to discuss trends and changes with children, adolescents, and their families (Box 4–14).

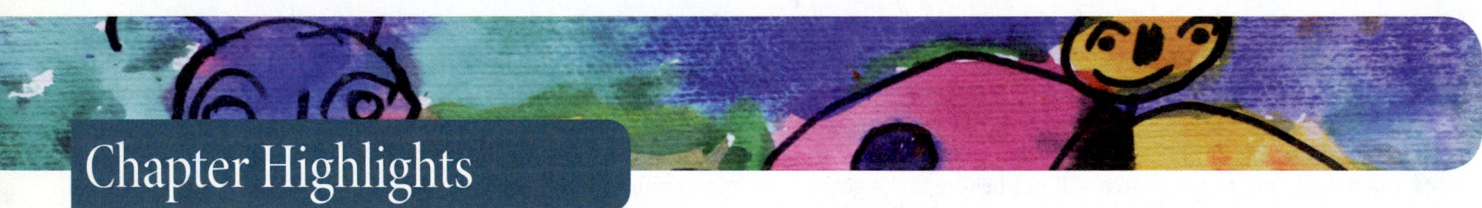

Chapter Highlights

- Nurses are responsible for basic genetic knowledge and delivering the expected standard of genetic nursing care.
- Genetic concepts can be applied to health promotion and health maintenance.
- When cell division does not occur as expected, chromosomal alterations on the autosomes or sex chromosomes can result.
- Mosaicism will present varied clinical manifestations of chromosomal alterations.
- Chromosomal alterations can be seen in a human karyotype.
- Protein-encoding genes are important to life and physiologic function, because proteins perform a variety of functions within the cell.
- Different forms of a gene that occupy the same place on a pair of chromosomes are alleles.
- An individual may be identified as heterozygous or homozygous for a single gene.
- Some gene alterations cause disease, and some protect individuals from disease.
- Mitochondrial gene alterations are inherited from the mother and primarily affect high-energy organs such as skeletal and cardiac muscle and brain.

- Knowledge of the principles of inheritance allows the nurse not only to offer and reinforce genetic information to children, adolescents, and their families but also to assist them in managing their care and in making reproductive decisions.
- Multifactorial inheritance does not follow Mendelian inheritance patterns.
- Basic genetic nursing care involves family risk assessment through a detailed family history, drawing a three-generation pedigree, and integrating genetic concepts into physical assessment.
- Basic genetic nursing involves initiating a referral to genetic specialists.
- Genetic healthcare providers present the individual and the family with information to promote informed decisions.
- There are several types of genetic tests available, all with special considerations related to the genetic testing of minors.
- The nurse must be aware of the social, ethical, cultural, and spiritual issues related to the delivery of genetic nursing care.

Clinical Reasoning in Action

INTRODUCTION

Recall 17-year-old Sarah from the chapter-opening scenario. While at the sports clinic for a routine physical, she questions the nurse about the likelihood that she will acquire Huntington disease. Huntington disease is a progressive disorder of motor, cognitive, and psychiatric disturbances. Symptoms typically present between age 35 and 44 years, with a median survival time of 15 to 18 years after onset.

Huntington disease is inherited in autosomal dominant fashion and displays virtually 100% penetrance. Anticipation is a common feature of Huntington disease. In about two thirds of affected individuals, the first symptoms are neurologic, including changes in eye movements and coordination, minor involuntary movements, and difficulty in mental planning. Other individuals experience psychiatric changes as the first symptoms, developing a depressed or irritable mood (Warby, Graham, & Hayden, 2010).

DESCRIPTION

Sarah's mother, Diane, is of western European Caucasian descent. Sarah's knowledge about her father is limited. She knows that he is a third-generation Filipino American but has no medical information on him or his extended family.

Sarah's grandmother on her mother's side has three sisters and two brothers. The two brothers died of myocardial infarctions at the ages of 37 and 55 years, respectively. Sarah's maternal grandfather had no brothers but two sisters. Her maternal grandfather died at age 62 years of Huntington disease. The sisters are alive and well and have no medical problems.

Diane has two brothers and two sisters. She is the youngest of the siblings. Her oldest brother, Ken, was diagnosed 10 years ago with Huntington disease at age 41 years. Ken has two daughters ages 21 and 25 years. Sarah is very close to these cousins and she knows that they have no medical problems beyond seasonal allergies and migraine headaches. Diane's other brother, Brian (age 38 years), has recently had bouts of depression and has noticed slight difficulties in coordination and involuntary movements. Brian and his wife Sally adopted a son,

Dave, with Down syndrome, and he is 19 years old. All of Brian's other children (ages 10, 6, and 3 years) are alive and well. Diane's sister Marion has had two pregnancy losses at 22 weeks and 10 weeks gestation. Marion also has two children, ages 3 and 12 years, who are alive and well. She has informed the family that she has had genetic testing for the Huntington gene alteration with a negative result. Sarah's maternal aunt Kathy has a daughter from a previous relationship and two sons from her current marriage. Her daughter was born with a cleft lip and palate. Sarah's brother is age 12 years and does not have any medical problems.

DISCUSSION

1. What further data would you gather from Sarah before referring her to a genetic specialist?
2. Search websites and other literature to learn more about Huntington disease. What are the signs and symptoms? The prognosis? Is it linked to any ethnic group?
3. Create a family pedigree for Sarah based on the family information she has provided. What does the pedigree reveal, and what nursing actions would you plan for Sarah?
4. Based on a summary of Sarah's risk and protective factors (see Chapter 5 🔗), list three nursing diagnoses that encompass both physical and psychosocial health.
5. Should Sarah be tested at this time? Give a rationale for your answer.
6. How might Sarah's identity be affected by a positive or negative genetic testing result?
7. What key points should the nurse consider when developing a teaching plan for Sarah?

NCLEX-RN® Review

1. Which statement indicates correct information has been given to the parents of a child having genetic screening? Autosomal recessive characteristics:
   1. Affect males greater than females.
   2. Mean an affected male can have only carrier daughters.
   3. Mean an affected child will have an affected parent.
   4. Affect males and females equally.

2. In discussing concerns with a pregnant woman, which information is crucial for the nurse to collect to ensure the most accurate genetic information is available? Choose all that apply.
   1. A family medical history for the three previous generations
   2. Relationships between any affected family members
   3. The birth history for any siblings of the baby
   4. A medical history for both the mother and father
   5. The estimated date of birth

3. The nurse is caring for a child who is hospitalized for hyponatremia. The health care provider is considering a genetic referral based upon the nurses developmental assessment. Which developmental indicators would support this referral?
   1. Deafness
   2. Speech problems
   3. Short stature
   4. Skin lesions

4. Which will best facilitate gathering genetic information from a child?
   1. Implement developmentally appropriate assessment skills.
   2. Ask the adults to leave the room to allow for privacy.
   3. Allow the parent to answer the questions for the child.
   4. Include a detailed explanation of the process prior to beginning.

See Appendix I 🔗 for answers.

References

American Association of Colleges of Nursing (AACN). (2008). *The essentials of baccalaureate education for professional nursing practice.* Washington, DC: Author.

American College of Obstetricians and Gynecologists (ACOG). (2011). Update on carrier screening for cystic fibrosis. *Obstetrics & Gynecology, 117*(4), 1028–1031.

American Nurses Association (ANA) & International Society of Nurses in Genetics (ISONG). (2007). *Genetics/genomics nursing: Scope and standards of practice.* Silver Spring, MD: Nursesbooks.org

Arnheim, N., & Calabrese, P. (2009). Understanding what determines the frequency and pattern of human germline mutations. *Nature Reviews: Genetics, 10,* 478–488.

Askin, D. F. (2009). Physical assessment of the newborn. *Nursing for Women's Health, 13*(2), 140–149.

Bailey, D. B., Skinner, D., Davis, A. M., Whitmarsh, I., & Powell, C. (2008). Ethical, legal, and social concerns about expanded newborn screening: Fragile X syndrome as a prototype for emerging issues. *Pediatrics, 121*(3), 693–704.

Bender, M. A., & Hobbs, W. (2009). Sickle cell disease. In *GeneReviews* at GeneTests: Medical Genetic Information Resource. Retrieved from http://www.ncbi.nlm.nih.gov/books/NBK1377/

Bennett, R. L. (2010). *The practical guide to the genetic family history* (2nd ed.). Hoboken, NJ: John Wiley & Sons.

Borry, P., Evers-Kiebooms, G., Cornel, M. C., Clarke, A., & Dierickx, K. (2009). Genetic testing in asymptomatic minors. *European Journal of Human Genetics, 17,* 711–719.

Cao, A., & Galanello, R. (2010). Beta-thalassemia. In *GeneReviews* at GeneTests: Medical Genetic Information Resource. Retrieved from http://www.ncbi.nlm.nih.gov/books/NBK1426/

Centers for Disease Control and Prevention (CDC). (n.d.). *Single gene disorders and disability (SGDD).* Retrieved from http://www.cdc.gov/ncbddd/single_gene/default.htm

Chromosome Map. (n.d.). Retrieved from http://www.ncbi.nlm.nih.gov/books/NBK22266/#A296

Consensus Panel on Genetic/Genomic Nursing Competencies. (2009). *Essentials of genetic and genomic nursing: Competencies, curricula guidelines, and outcome indicators* (2nd ed.). Silver Spring, MD: American Nurses Association.

Ensembl release 63. (2011). *Genome statistics.* Retrieved from http://www.ensembl.org/Homo_sapiens/Info/StatsTable?db=core

GeneTests: Medical Genetics Information Resource. (2011). Copyright, University of Washington, Seattle. 1993–2011. Retrieved from http://www.ncbi.nlm.nih.gov/sites/GeneTests/

Gurrieri, F., & Accadia, M. (2009). Genetic imprinting: The paradigm of Prader-Willi and Angelman syndromes. *Endocrine Development, 14,* 20–28.

Inglese, M. D., & Elder, J. H. (2009). Caring for children with autism spectrum disorder. Part 1: prevalence, etiology and core features. *Journal of Pediatric Nursing, 1,* 41–48.

Jorde, L. B., Carey, J. C., & Bamshad, M. J. (2010). *Medical genetics.* Philadelphia: Mosby Elsevier.

Lehmann, A., Speight, B. S., & Kerzin-Storrar, L. (2011). Extended family impact of genetic testing: The experiences of X-linked carrier grandmothers. *Journal of Genetic Counseling, 20,* 365–373.

Lwiwski, N., Greenberg, C. R., & Mhanni, A. A. (2008). Genetic testing of a child at risk for adult onset conditions: When is testing indicated? *Journal of Genetic Counseling, 17,* 523–525.

Mitchell, J. J., & Scriver, C. (2010). Phenylalanine hydroxylase deficiency (2007). In *GeneReviews* at GeneTests: Medical Genetic Information Resource. Retrieved from http://www.ncbi.nlm.nih.gov/books/NBK1504/

Moskowitz, S. M., Chmiel, J. F., Sternen, D. L., Cheng, E., & Cutting, G. R. (2008). CFTR-related disorders. In *GeneReviews* at GeneTests: Medical Genetic Information Resource. Retrieved from http://www.ncbi.nlm.nih.gov/books/NBK1250/

Nussbaum, R. L., McInnes, R. R., & Willard, H. F. (2007). *Thompson & Thompson genetics in medicine* (7th ed.). Philadelphia: Saunders.

Online Mendelian Inheritance in Man, OMIM (TM). (n.d.). Baltimore: McKusick-Nathans Institute for Genetics Medicine, Johns Hopkins University; Bethesda, MD: National Center for Biotechnology Information Library of Medicine. Retrieved from http://www.ncbi.nlm.nih.gov/omim

Oyen, N., Poulsen, G., Boyd, H. A., Wohlfahrt, J., Jensen, P. K. A., & Melbye, M. (2009). Recurrence of congenital heart defects in families. *Circulation, 120,* 295–301.

Pastores, G. M., & Hughes, D. A. (2011). Gaucher disease. In *GeneReviews* at GeneTests: Medical Genetic Information Resource. Retrieved from http://www.ncbi.nlm.nih.gov/books/NBK1269/

Pediatric genetic evaluations. (n.d.). Retrieved from http://louisville.edu/childevaluation/clinical-genetic-services-1/medical-genetics-evaluation.html

Ranweiler, R. (2009). Assessment and care of the newborn with Down syndrome. *Advances in Neonatal Care, 9*(1), 17–24.

Sadowski, S. L. (2009). Congenital cardiac disease in the newborn infant: Past, present, and future. *Critical Care Nursing Clinics of North America, 21,* 37–48.

Snow, K. (2010). *People first language.* Retrieved from http://www.disabilityisnatural.com/images/PDF/pfl09.pdf

Steinberg, H. H. (2008). Sickle cell anemia, the first molecular disease: Overview of molecular etiology, pathophysiology, and therapeutic approaches. *Scientific World Journal, 8,* 1295–1324.

Turnpenny, P., & Ellard, S. (2012). *Emery's elements of medical genetics* (14th ed.). Philadelphia: Elsevier.

U.S. Department of Health & Human Services. (2008). *United States system of oversight of genetic testing: A response to the charge of the secretary of Health and Human Services. Report of the Secretary's Advisory Committee on Genetics, Health, and Society (SACGHS).* Retrieved from http://oba.od.nih.gov/oba/SACGHS/reports/SACGHS_oversight_report.pdf

Warby, S. C., Graham, R. K., & Hayden, M. R. (2010). *Huntington disease.* In *GeneReviews* at GeneTests: Medical Genetic Information Resource. Retrieved from http://www.ncbi.nlm.nih.gov/books/NBK1305/

Wilfond, G., & Ross, L. R. (2009). From genetics to genomics: Ethics, policy, and parental decision making. *Journal of Pediatric Psychology, 34*(6), 639–647.

Zhang, F., Gu, W., Hurles, M. E., & Lupski, J. R. (2009). Copy number variation in human health, disease, and evolution. *Annual Review of Genomics and Human Genetics, 10,* 451–481.

Zlotogora, J. (2009). Population programs for the detection of couples at risk for severe monogenic genetic diseases. *Human Genetics, 126,* 247–253.

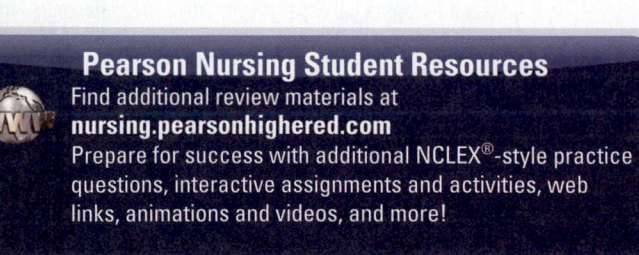

Pearson Nursing Student Resources

Find additional review materials at **nursing.pearsonhighered.com**

Prepare for success with additional NCLEX®-style practice questions, interactive assignments and activities, web links, animations and videos, and more!

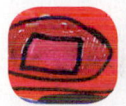 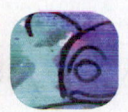 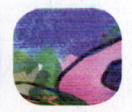

Concepts of Growth and Development

KEY TERMS

Learning Outcomes

After completing this chapter, you will be able to:

1. Describe the major psychologic theories of development as formulated by Freud, Erikson, Piaget, Kohlberg, social learning theorists, and behaviorists.

2. Explain contemporary developmental approaches such as temperament theory, ecologic theory, and the resilience framework.

3. Recognize major developmental milestones for infants, toddlers, preschoolers, school-age children, and adolescents.

4. Synthesize information from several theoretic approaches to plan assessments of the child's growth and developmental milestones.

5. Plan nursing interventions that are appropriate for the child's developmental state and that apply developmental theories and frameworks.

6. Recognize risks to normal developmental progression, and plan assessments of the child's development.

7. Use data collected during developmental assessments to plan appropriate nursing interventions that promote development of children and adolescents.

"We were so worried when Sergio was born prematurely. I had tried to do everything right during pregnancy, but I felt responsible somehow when I went into labor early. We're so happy to have Sergio home now and I spend every moment I can with him."

—*Yolanda, mother of Sergio, who was born prematurely*

Yolanda and Pepe Gomez are the parents of Sergio, who was born at 29 weeks' gestation. Sergio is their first child, and all appeared to be going well in the pregnancy until Yolanda went into labor. The family had no significant history of congenital conditions or premature births. Sergio was born after a short labor and weighed 1250 grams (2.75 pounds). Although he did well initially, Sergio soon developed respiratory distress syndrome and was placed on a ventilator in the neonatal intensive care unit. He required parenteral feedings but as he grew and improved, he was able to start gavage feedings of his mother's breast milk, and finally learned to breast-feed. Sergio was discharged from the hospital in stable condition at 2 months of age. He is now 6 months, and other than two respiratory illnesses, he has continued to grow and develop without additional health problems. The nurse in the pediatric healthcare home monitors Sergio monthly, performing developmental assessments, monitoring his visual and hearing responses, and providing ideas for his parents about how to best promote his development.

How can the nurse best facilitate Sergio's continued developmental progression? What do the parents need to know about prematurity and how to best support their son?

Children develop as they interact with their surroundings. They learn skills at different ages, but the order in which they learn them is universal. Development is affected by factors such as nutrition and cultural practices, as well as the social situation in the country or neighborhood. Although Sergio will develop in a unique manner influenced by his prematurity, environmental factors, and the interaction between these factors, certain principles of development can assist his parents and the nurse in fostering positive adaptations for him.

This chapter covers general principles of growth and development and several theories related to childhood development, as well as their nursing applications. We discuss each age group, from infancy through adolescence, and examine developmental milestones, physical and cognitive characteristics, psychosocial concerns, and communication strategies. This basic information will help you to assess accurately and to plan developmentally appropriate care for children in each age group. We mention conditions that interfere with usual developmental progression, such as prematurity, adoption, and genetic influences. You can apply appropriate nursing assessments and interventions to these special situations, such as the one described in the opening scenario. The nurse's role in developmental screening, as well as descriptions of developmental tests appropriate at various ages, can be found in the Health Promotion and Health Maintenance chapters for each age group (Chapters 9 through 14 ⊘).

PRINCIPLES OF GROWTH AND DEVELOPMENT

Nurses who work with children must not only understand the pathophysiology of disease practices and the health promotion and health maintenance needs, but also integrate knowledge of development into each encounter with a child. The child's age and organ maturity influence the pathophysiologic process, metabolism of medications, and healing process. The child's age and developmental stage determine health promotion needs regarding topics such as safety measures and immunizations. Nurses also must consider developmental factors for therapeutic communication to occur, using appropriate language, providing explanations for procedures, and integrating approaches such as stories and pictures.

Growth refers to an increase in physical size. Growth represents quantitative changes such as height, weight, blood pressure, and number of words in the child's vocabulary. **Development** refers to an increase in capability or function. Developmental skills, such as the ability to sit without support or to throw a ball overhand, unfold in a complex manner as the child's innate capabilities interact with the stimuli and support provided in the environment. The quantitative and qualitative changes in body organ functioning, ability to communicate, and performance of motor skills unfold over time and are key considerations for nurses planning pediatric health care.

Each child displays a unique maturational pattern during the process of development. Although the exact age at which skills emerge differs, the sequence or order of skill performance is uniform among children. Skill development proceeds according to two processes: from the head down and from the center of the body out to the extremities. Development that proceeds from the head downward through the body and toward the feet is called **cephalocaudal development** (Figure 5–1 ■). For example, at birth, an infant's head is much larger proportionately than the trunk or extremities.

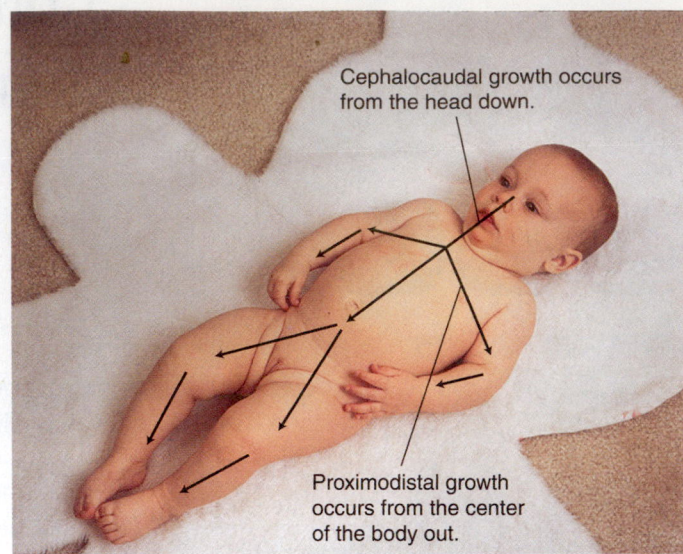

Cephalocaudal growth occurs from the head down.

Proximodistal growth occurs from the center of the body out.

FIGURE 5–1 ■ In normal cephalocaudal growth, the child gains control of the head and neck before the trunk and limbs. In normal proximodistal growth, the child controls arm movements before hand movements. For example, the child reaches for objects before being able to grasp them. Children gain control of their hands before their fingers; that is, they can hold things with the entire hand before they can pick something up with just their fingers.

Similarly, infants learn to hold up their heads before sitting, and to sit before standing. Skills such as walking that involve the legs and feet develop last in infancy. Development that proceeds from the center of the body outward to the extremities is called **proximodistal development** (see Figure 5–1). For example, infants are first able to control the trunk, then the arms; only later are fine motor movements of the fingers possible. Pediatric nurses use these concepts of predictable and sequential developmental direction to analyze the infant's or child's present state and to partner with families to encourage and support emerging developmental abilities.

During the childhood years, extraordinary changes occur in all aspects of development. Physical size, motor skills, cognitive ability, language, sensory ability, and psychosocial patterns all undergo major transformations. Nurses study normal patterns of development to identify and assess children who demonstrate slow or abnormal growth development. These assessments can guide the nurse in planning interventions for the child and family, such as referring the child for a diagnostic evaluation or rehabilitation, or teaching the parents how to provide adequate stimulation for the child. The nurse caring for Sergio in the opening scenario needed to possess this skill and knowledge. When development is proceeding normally, the nurse uses the knowledge of usual patterns to plan teaching approaches based on the child's cognitive and language ability, to offer appropriate toys and activities during illness, and to respond therapeutically during interactions with the child. The information discussed in this chapter will lead you directly to Chapters 8 through 13 ⊘ where growth and development knowledge is applied to planning health promotion and maintenance visits with newborns, children, and adolescents.

MAJOR THEORIES OF DEVELOPMENT

Child development is a complex process. Many theorists have attempted to organize their observations of behavior into a description of principles or a set of stages. Each theory focuses on a particular facet of development, but no one theory provides all necessary information, and stages are not absolute. That is, rates of progression differ among children and stages overlap, even for a specific child. Most developmental theorists separate children into age groups by common characteristics. Some commonly used groupings include:

- *Prenatal period*—Includes the time from conception to birth; influenced by the genetics of the baby and the health of parents, particularly the mother.
- *Newborn*—From birth to 1 month of life. Although part of infancy, the first month is marked by the need for adaptation to extrauterine life and requires special support and care. The infant who is born before 37 weeks' gestation is called a preterm and has unique developmental challenges.
- *Infancy*—From 1 to 12 months. Includes infants up to 1 year of age; they require a high level of care in daily activities.
- *Toddlerhood*—From 1 to 3 years. Characterized by increased motor ability and independent behavior.
- *Preschool*—From 3 to 6 years. The preschooler refines gross and fine motor ability and language skills and often participates in a preschool learning program.
- *School age*—From 6 to 12 years. Begins with entry into a school system and is characterized by growing intellectual skills, physical ability, and independence.
- *Adolescence*—From 12 to 18 years. Begins with entry into the teen years. Mature cognitive thought, formation of identity, and influence of peers are important characteristics.

Freud's Theory of Psychosexual Development

Theoretic Framework

The psychoanalytic techniques used by Sigmund Freud (Table 5–1) led him to believe that early childhood experiences form the unconscious motivation for actions in later life. He developed a theory that sexual energy is centered in specific parts of the body at certain ages. Unresolved conflict and unmet needs at a certain stage lead to a fixation of development at that stage (Craig & Dunn, 2010).

Freud viewed the personality as a structure with three parts: the **id,** the basic sexual energy that is present at birth and drives the individual to seek pleasure; the **ego,** the realistic part of the person, which develops during infancy and searches for acceptable methods of meeting impulses; and the **superego,** the moral and ethical system, which develops in childhood and contains a set of values and a conscience (Craig & Dunn, 2010). He viewed all of these forces as largely out of conscious awareness.

Development and behaviors then unfold as the ego balances the tension between the two opposing forces of id and superego. The ego diverts impulses of the id and protects itself from excess anxiety created by the superego by use of **defense mechanisms.** These unconscious techniques distort reality to guide actions and prevent painful challenges to the personality. Defense mechanisms used by children can include regression to earlier stages of development, and repression of painful experiences such as child abuse. See Table 5–2 for more examples.

Stages

Oral (birth to 1 year) The infant derives pleasure largely from the mouth, with sucking, eating, chewing, and mouthing objects as primary desires. These oral behaviors also release tension for the infant and play an important part in formation of the ego.

Anal (1 to 3 years) The young child's pleasure is centered in the anal area, with control over body secretions as a prime force in behavior.

Phallic (3 to 6 years) Sexual energy becomes centered in the genitalia, and children explore touching their sexual organs. Freud also viewed this period as the time when the child works out relationships with parents of the same and opposite sexes. He believed that children love the parent of the opposite sex and want to take the place of the parent of their same sex. The child needs to accept the presence of both parents and begin to identify with the parent of the same sex.

Latency (6 to 12 years) Sexual energy is at rest in the passage between earlier stages and adolescence. Freud believed that the child focuses on other activities related to social and cognitive growth during this stage.

Genital (12 years to adulthood) Mature sexuality is achieved as physical growth is completed, sexual pleasure reemerges, and relationships develop with others outside the family.

Nursing Application

Freud emphasized the importance of meeting the needs of each stage in order to move successfully into future developmental stages. His work has been criticized for several reasons (Thornton, 2010):

- He developed a theory of childhood by his work with adults, primarily women, who sought help in dealing with emotional issues.
- He viewed males as dominant because of their possession of a penis.
- He ignored the effects of culture and other external experiences.

However, some aspects of his theory appear to be supported by more current research and can be applied in nursing. Both the normal developmental progression of children and disruptions that occur in illness are pertinent nursing considerations.

The preschooler's concern about sexuality guides the nurse to provide privacy and clear explanations during any procedures involving the genital area. It may be necessary to teach parents that masturbation by the young child is normal and to help parents deal with it through distraction or refocusing. The adolescent's focus on relationships suggests that the nurse should include questions about significant friends during history taking. Table 5–3 summarizes techniques the nurse can use to apply these theoretic concepts to the care of children.

Illness can interfere with normal developmental processes and add challenges for the nurse who is striving to meet an ill child's needs. For example, the importance of sucking in infancy guides the nurse to provide a pacifier for the infant who cannot have oral fluids. Recall Sergio from the opening scenario. He did not have the ability or strength to suck after birth and was fed parenterally and by gavage. However, as soon as he was able, he was assisted to breastfeed in order to foster his oral musculature and his ability to gain comfort from sucking.

Erikson's Theory of Psychosocial Development

Theoretic Framework

Erikson's theory establishes psychosocial stages during eight periods of human life. For each stage, Erikson identified a crisis, that is, a particular challenge that exists for healthy personality development to occur (Erikson, 1963, 1968). The word *crisis* in this context refers

TABLE 5–1	Major Developmental Theorists	
THEORIST	**YEARS OF LIFE**	**BACKGROUND**
Sigmund Freud	1856–1939	Freud was a physician in Vienna, Austria. His work with adults who were experiencing a variety of nervous disorders led Freud to develop the approach called psychoanalysis, which explored the driving forces of the unconscious mind.
Erik Erikson	1902–1994	Erikson studied Freud's theory of psychoanalysis under Freud's daughter, Anna, but later established his own developmental theory emphasizing the psychosocial nature of individuals. Erikson's theory is one of the few that addresses development over the entire life span.
Jean Piaget	1896–1980	Piaget was a 20th-century Swiss scientist who watched his own three children carefully and wrote detailed journals of their behaviors and verbalizations. He studied the intellectual abilities of children, focusing on child psychology and its application to education.
Lawrence Kohlberg	1927–1987	Kohlberg used Piaget's cognitive stage theory as the basis for his theory of moral development. He worked with children in his native Germany and in many other countries, including Kenya, Taiwan, and Mexico.
Albert Bandura	b. 1925	Bandura is a Canadian who has conducted psychologic research at Stanford University for many years. He believes that children learn from their social environment, particularly by modeling the observed behaviors of others.
John Watson	1878–1958	Watson was an American scientist who applied the work of animal behaviorists, such as Ivan Pavlov and B. F. Skinner, to children.
Urie Bronfenbrenner	1917–2005	Bronfenbrenner established the ecologic theory of development and served as a professor at Cornell University. He viewed the child as interacting with the environment at different levels, or systems. This revolutionary approach emphasizes the series of mutual interactions between the child and the various systems.
Stella Chess and Alexander Thomas	Chess, 1914–2007; Thomas, 1914–2003	Chess and Thomas were psychiatrists who began the New York Longitudinal Study in 1956 with 141 children, which they expanded in 1961 with 95 additional children. Most of these individuals are still being assessed periodically as adults. Their research identified characteristics of personality and provides a basis for the ongoing study of temperament (Chess & Thomas, 1995).

TABLE 5–2	Common Defense Mechanisms Used by Children	
DEFENSE MECHANISM	**DEFINITION**	**EXAMPLE**
Regression	Return to an earlier behavior	A previously toilet-trained child becomes incontinent when separated from parents during a hospitalization.
Repression	Involuntary forgetting of uncomfortable situations	An abused child cannot consciously recall episodes of abuse.
Rationalization	An attempt to make unacceptable feelings acceptable	A child explains hitting another because "he took my toy."
Fantasy	A creation of the mind to help deal with unacceptable fear	A hospitalized child who is weak pretends to be Superman.

to normal maturational social needs rather than to a single critical event. Each developmental crisis has two possible outcomes:

1. When needs are met, the consequence is healthy and the individual moves on to future stages with particular strengths.
2. When needs are not met, an unhealthy outcome occurs that will influence future social relationships.

Stages

Trust versus mistrust (birth to 1 year) The task of the first year of life is to establish trust in the people providing care. Trust is fostered by provision of food, clean clothing, touch, and comfort. If basic needs are not met, the infant will eventually learn to mistrust others. Developing a sense of trust leads the child, as he or she matures into an adult, to have confidence that the world is a good place and to approach life with a general sense of optimism. However, a balance between trust and mistrust is important. If a child is too trusting, child abuse or other poor outcomes may occur. The sense of trust must predominate, but individuals need mistrust at times for healthy development.

Autonomy versus shame and doubt (1 to 3 Years) The toddler's sense of autonomy or independence is shown by controlling body excretions, saying no when asked to do something, and directing motor activity. Children who are consistently criticized for expressions of autonomy or for lack of control—for example, during toilet training—will develop a sense of shame about themselves and doubt in their abilities. Developing a healthy sense of autonomy results in a person who can function with independence and self-direction. It is also important for the toddler to recognize feelings and needs of others, as excessive autonomy could lead to disregard and inability to work with others (Figure 5–2A ■).

Initiative versus guilt (3 to 6 Years) The young child is exposed to more people outside of the family and therefore initiates new activities and considers new ideas. This interest in exploring the world creates a child who is involved and busy. The child learns to assume new responsibilities and becomes aware of guiding principles for actions. Constant criticism for the child's activities, on the other hand, leads to feelings of guilt and a lack of purpose. Preschoolers' sense of initiative leads to the ability to start projects but they may not always

TABLE 5–3	Nursing Applications of Theories of Freud, Erikson, and Piaget	
AGE GROUP	**DEVELOPMENTAL STAGES**	**NURSING APPLICATIONS**
Infant (birth to 1 year)	Oral stage (Freud): The baby obtains pleasure and comfort through the mouth.	When a baby is to be offered nothing by mouth (NPO), offer a pacifier if not contraindicated. After painful procedures, offer a baby a bottle or pacifier or have the mother breastfeed.
	Trust versus mistrust stage (Erikson): The baby establishes a sense of trust when basic needs are met.	Hold the hospitalized baby often. **(1)** Offer comfort after painful procedures. Meet the baby's needs for food and hygiene.
		Encourage parents to room in.
		Manage pain effectively with use of pain medications and other measures.
	Sensorimotor stage (Piaget): The baby learns from movement and sensory input.	Use crib mobiles, manipulative toys, wall murals, and bright colors to provide interesting stimuli and comfort.
		Use toys to distract the baby during procedures and assessments.
Toddler (1–3 years)	Anal stage (Freud): The child derives gratification from control over body excretions.	Ask about toilet training and the child's rituals and words for elimination during the admission history.
		Continue the child's normal patterns of elimination in the hospital.
		Do not begin toilet training during illness or hospitalization.
		Accept regression in toileting during illness or hospitalization.
		Have potty chairs available in the hospital and childcare centers.
	Autonomy versus shame and doubt stage (Erikson): The child is increasingly independent in many spheres of life.	Allow self-feeding opportunities.
		Encourage the child to remove and put on own clothes, brush teeth, or assist with hygiene. **(2)**
		If restraint for a procedure is necessary, proceed quickly, providing explanations and comfort.
	Sensorimotor stage (end); preoperational stage (beginning) (Piaget): The child shows increasing curiosity and explorative behavior. Language skills improve.	Ensure safe surroundings to allow opportunities to manipulate objects.
		Name objects and give simple explanations.
Preschooler (3–6 years)	Phallic stage (Freud): The child initially identifies with the parent of the opposite sex but by the end of this stage has identified with the same-sex parent.	Be alert for children who appear more comfortable with male or female nurses, and attempt to accommodate them.
		Encourage parental involvement in care.
		Plan for playtime and offer a variety of materials from which to choose.
	Initiative versus guilt stage (Erikson): The child likes to initiate play activities.	Offer medical equipment for play to lessen anxiety about strange objects. **(3)**
		Assess children's concerns as expressed through their drawings.
		Accept the child's choices and expressions of feelings.
	Preoperational stage (Piaget): The child is increasingly verbal but has some limitations in thought processes. Causality is often confused, so the child may feel responsible for causing an illness.	Offer explanations about all procedures and treatments.
		Clearly explain that the child is not responsible for causing the illness.

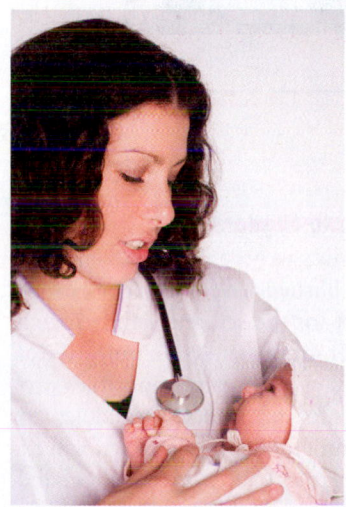

(1) Comfort baby often

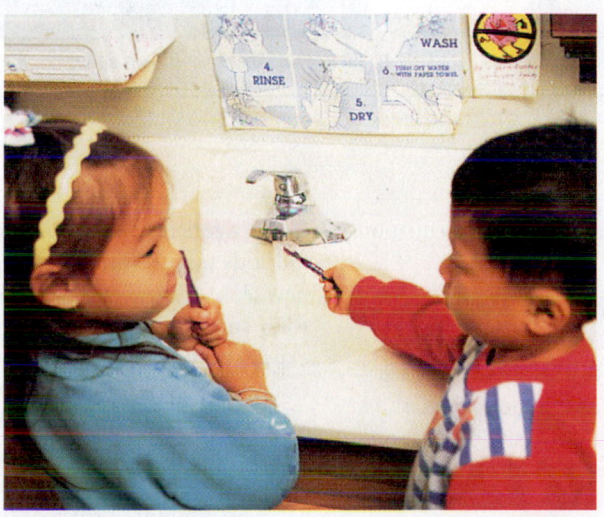

(2) Encourage hygiene

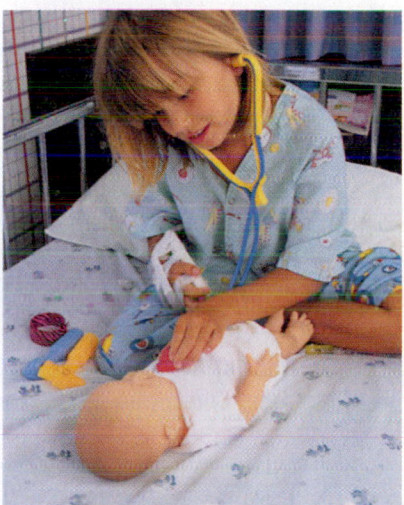

(3) Use toys to lessen anxiety

Source: aletia2011/Fotolia.

(Continued)

TABLE 5–3	Nursing Applications of Theories of Freud, Erikson, and Piaget (*Continued*)	
AGE GROUP	**DEVELOPMENTAL STAGES**	**NURSING APPLICATIONS**
School age (6–12 years)	Latency stage (Freud): The child places importance on privacy and understanding the body.	Provide gowns, covers, and underwear. Knock on door before entering. Explain treatments and procedures.
	Industry versus inferiority stage (Erikson): The child gains a sense of self-worth from involvement in activities.	Encourage the child to continue schoolwork while hospitalized. Encourage the child to bring favorite pastimes to the hospital. **(4)** Help the child adjust to limitations on favorite activities.
	Concrete operational stage (Piaget): The child is capable of mature thought when allowed to manipulate and see objects.	Give clear instructions about details of treatment. Show the child equipment that will be used in treatment.
Adolescent (12–18 years)	Genital stage (Freud): The adolescent's focus is on genital function and relationships.	Ensure access to gynecologic care for adolescent females and education for testicular examination for males. Provide information on sexuality. Ensure privacy during health care. Have brochures and videos available for teaching about sexuality.
	Identity versus role confusion stage (Erikson): The adolescent's search for self-identity leads to independence from parents and reliance on peers.	Provide a separate recreation room for teens who are hospitalized. **(5)** Take the health history and perform examinations without parents present. Introduce the adolescent to other teens with the same health problem.
	Formal operational stage (Piaget): The adolescent is capable of mature, abstract thought.	Give clear and complete information about health care and treatments. Offer both written and verbal instructions. Continue to provide education about the disease to the adolescent with a chronic illness, as mature thought now leads to greater understanding.

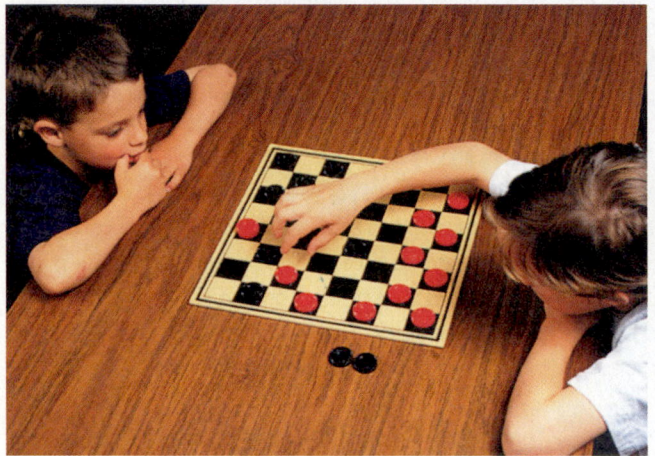

(4) Encourage favorite pastimes

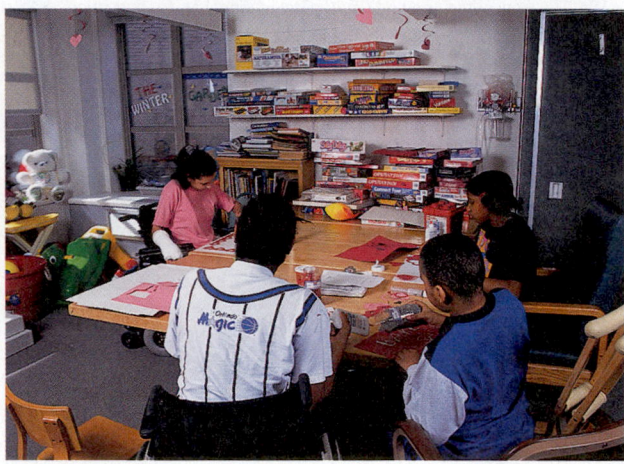

(5) Provide teens their own space

see the value in completing them, a potentially frustrating situation for parents (Figure 5–2B ■).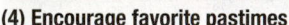

Industry versus inferiority (6 to 12 years) The middle years of childhood are characterized by development of new interests and by a focus on intellectual or cognitive pursuits. The child takes pride in accomplishments in sports, school, home, and community. Developing a sense of industry provides the child with purpose and confidence in his or her ability to be successful. If the child cannot accomplish what is expected, however, the result will be a sense of inferiority. The child's sense of industry must be balanced by a realistic perspective gained over time, that there is always more to learn and that one cannot be the "best" at every activity (Figure 5–2C ■).

Identity versus role confusion (12 to 18 years) In adolescence, as the body matures and thought processes become more complex, a new sense of identity or self is established. The adolescent tries out roles and examines what fits best for the self and family/society expectations. The self, family, peer group, and community are all examined and redefined. Identifying with values and roles provides guidance as the adolescent enters adulthood. The adolescent who is unable to establish a meaningful definition of self will experience confusion in one or more roles of life. On the other hand, a certain amount of role confusion is desirable as it is the impetus for self-examination and provides the basis for establishment of identity.

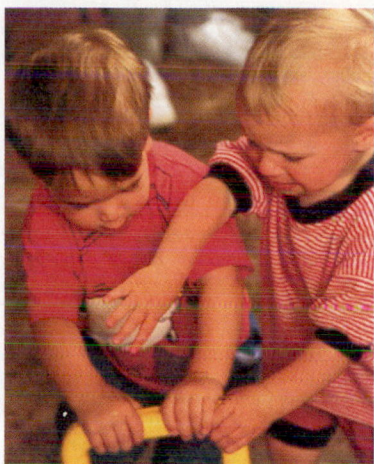

A

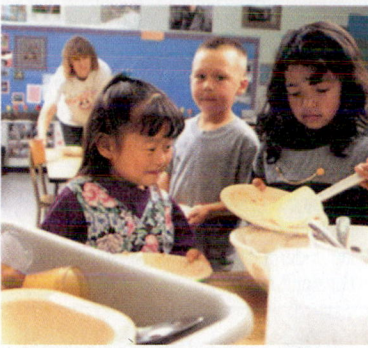

B

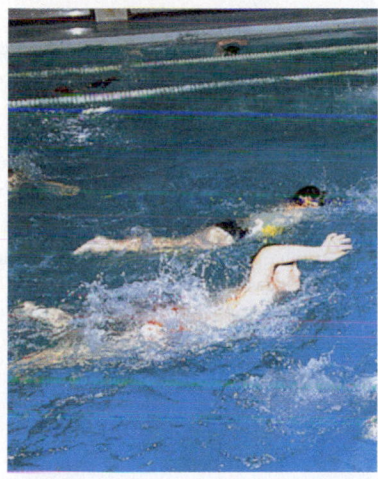

C

FIGURE 5–2 ■ Erikson's psychosocial stages.

A, The toddler shows *autonomy* by exerting control over toys and activities.

B, Preschoolers demonstrate *initiative* by planning and carrying out activities.

C, School-age children excel at *industry* by participating in activities such as sports.

Nursing Application

Erikson's theory is directly applicable to the nursing care of children. Health promotion and health maintenance visits in the community provide opportunities for helping caregivers to meet children's needs. The nurse asks for examples of the child's social interactions and self-concept. The child's behaviors can be explained within the perspective of developmental stages. Parents benefit from learning what the child's developmental tasks are at each stage and from discussing ideas about how to encourage healthy psychosocial development. Such discussions also may highlight parental concerns and provide a forum for reassurance about normal developmental characteristics, such as a preschooler who does not follow through on each activity, or an adolescent who tries different hairstyles each month.

The child's usual support from family, peers, and others is interrupted by hospitalization. The challenge of hospitalization also adds a situational crisis to the normal developmental crisis a child is experiencing. Although the nurse may meet many of the hospitalized child's needs, continued parental involvement is necessary both during and after hospitalization to ensure progression through expected developmental stages (see Table 5–3). Asking parents about the child's developmental progression provides clues to activities and provides information about what the child needs in the hospital. (See Chapter 15 🔗.)

Piaget's Theory of Cognitive Development

Theoretic Framework

Based on his observations and work with children, Jean Piaget formulated a theory of cognitive, or intellectual, development. He believed that the child's view of the world is influenced largely by age, experience, and maturational ability. Given nurturing experiences, the child's ability to think matures naturally (Ginsberg & Opper, 1988; Piaget, 1972). The child incorporates new experiences via **assimilation** and changes to deal with these experiences by the process of **accommodation.** The child is an active participant in this cognitive building process. For example, an infant first sucks and grasps by reflex. As feedback occurs—some actions produce more satisfaction than others—the infant learns to change behaviors by sucking a breast, bottle, or fingers. Similarly, an infant learns to grasp a rattle, to shake it to create sound, to bring it close to the face to examine, or to let go to watch it fall. In these examples, can you describe which parts of the behaviors represent assimilation and which represent accommodation?

Some earlier theories viewed children as being totally formed and shaped by adults around them. John Locke, a 17th-century theorist, formulated the theory of *tabula rasa*, or blank slate, to explain children. He believed that they entered the world with nothing but genetic potential and the way they developed was a result of experiences provided. Although this theory is similar to Piaget's in recognizing the importance of experiences in building cognitive processes, Piaget believed that children were active participants in the unfolding of their inborn cognitive structures, taking in information and modifying behavior as a result.

Another important characteristic of Piaget's theory is that each stage he described is qualitatively different. A child does not simply learn by having *more* experiences. Instead, the child's mind unfolds so that the processes used to understand reality at different ages are unlike those of earlier stages. Piaget identified the characteristics of thought that are found at various stages. Examine Table 5–4 as you read about the following stages.

Stages

Sensorimotor (birth to 2 years) Infants learn about the world by input obtained through the senses and by their motor activity. Six substages are characteristic of this stage.

TABLE 5–4	Characteristics of Thought Identified by Piaget		
CHARACTERISTIC	**DEFINITION**	**DEVELOPMENT STAGE**	**NURSING IMPLICATIONS**
Object permanence	Ability to understand that when something is out of sight it still exists	Sensorimotor period, especially in coordination of secondary schemes substage from 8–12 months	Before development of object permanence, babies will not look for toys or other objects out of sight; as the concept is developing they are concerned when a parent leaves since they are not certain the parent will return.
Egocentrism	Ability to see things only from one's own point of view	Preoperational thought	Peers or others who have gone through an experience will not impress the preschooler; teaching should focus on what an experience will be like to the child.
Transductive reasoning	Connecting two events in a cause-and-effect relationship simply because they occur together in time	Preoperational thought	Ask the child what he or she thinks caused an occurrence; ask how the two events are connected; correct misconceptions to lessen the child's guilt.
Centration	Focusing only on one particular aspect of a situation	Preoperational thought	Listen to the child's comments and deal with concerns in order to present new concepts to the child.
Animism	Giving lifelike qualities to nonliving things	Preoperational thought	Ask preschool children to describe how a machine works, or how the trees move. Provide opportunities to learn about machines that may move and make noises (intravenous pumps, magnetic resonance imaging) to decrease fears.
Magical thinking	The belief that events occur because of one's thoughts or actions	Preoperational thought	Ask young children how they became ill, or what caused a parent's or sibling's illness. Correct misconceptions when the child blames self for causing problems by wishing someone ill or having bad behavior.
Conservation	Knowledge that matter is not changed when its form is altered	Concrete operational thought	Before conservation of thought is reached, the child may think that gender can be changed when hair is cut or that the leg under a cast is broken in separate pieces. Ask perceptions and clarify misconceptions.

Use of reflexes (birth to 1 month) The infant begins life with a set of reflexes such as sucking, rooting, and grasping. By using these reflexes, the infant receives stimulation via touch, sound, smell, and vision. The reflexes thus pave the way for the first learning to occur.

Primary circular reactions (1 to 4 months) Once the infant responds reflexively, the pleasure gained from that response causes repetition of the behavior. For example, if a toy grasped reflexively makes noise and is interesting to watch, the infant will grasp it again (see Figure 5–3A ■).

Secondary circular reactions (4 to 8 months) Awareness of the environment grows as the infant begins to connect cause and effect. The sounds of bottle preparation will lead to excited behavior. If an object is partially hidden, the infant will attempt to uncover and retrieve it.

Coordination of secondary schemes (8 to 12 months) Infants exhibit intentional behavior, using learned behavior to obtain objects, create sounds, or engage in other pleasurable activity. **Object permanence** (the knowledge that something continues to exist even

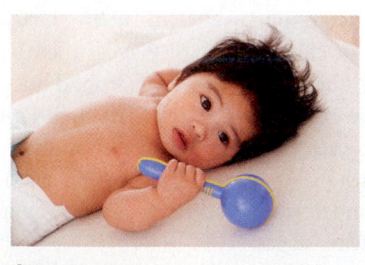
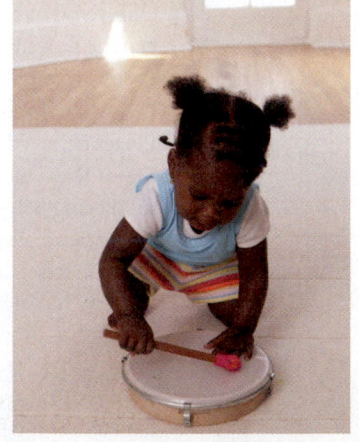
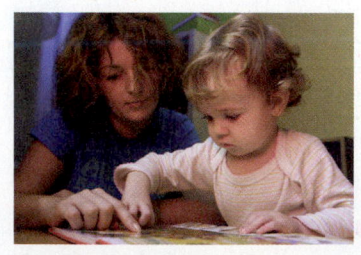

A   B   C

FIGURE 5–3 ■ Piaget's cognitive stages.
A, A young infant displays *primary circular reactions* when a reflexive response, such as shaking a rattle, results in pleasure and is repeated.
B, As the infant becomes a toddler, *tertiary circular reactions* are demonstrated when the child experiments with objects by turning them, placing them in the mouth, and banging them.
C, Toddlers and preschoolers demonstrate *mental combinations* as they increasingly use language to describe and understand their worlds.

Source: *A,* Ruth Jenkinson © Dorling Kindersley; *B,* Vanessa Davies © Dorling Kindersley; *C,* Artyom Yefimov/Fotolia.

when out of sight) begins when the infant remembers where a hidden object is likely to be found; it is no longer "out of sight, out of mind."

The concept of object permanence is not fully developed, however. The infant knows the parent well, objects to new people, and seems very worried when the parent leaves. Other caretakers may be rejected because the infant does not understand that the parent will return. This phase of "stranger anxiety" is quite common and heralds the infant's growing recognition of and desire to be cared for by the parent.

Tertiary circular reactions (12 to 18 Months) Curiosity, experimentation, and exploration predominate as the toddler tries out actions to learn results. Objects are turned in every direction, placed in the mouth, used for banging, and inserted in containers as their qualities and uses are explored (Figure 5–3B ■).

Mental combinations (18 to 24 months) Language provides a new tool for the toddler to use in understanding the world. Language enables the child to think about events and objects before or after they occur. Object permanence is now fully developed as the child actively searches for objects in various locations and out of view. The child who has had successful separations from the parents followed by return, such as hours spent in another's home or a childcare center, begins to understand that the missing parent will return (Figure 5–3C ■).

Preoperational (2 to 7 years) The young child thinks by using words as symbols, but logic is not well developed. During the preconceptual substage (2 to 4 years), vocabulary and comprehension increase greatly, but the child shows **egocentrism** (an inability to see things from the perspective of another). In the intuitive substage (4 to 7 years), the child relies on **transductive reasoning** (drawing conclusions from one general fact to another). For example, when a child disobeys a parent and then falls and breaks an arm that day, the child may ascribe the broken arm to bad behavior. Cause-and-effect relationships are often unrealistic or a result of **magical thinking** (the belief that events occur because of thoughts or wishes). Additional characteristics noted in the thought of preschoolers include **centration,** or the ability to consider only one aspect of a situation at a time, and **animism,** or giving life to inanimate objects because they move, make noise, or have certain other qualities.

Concrete operational (7 to 11 years) Transductive reasoning has given way to a more accurate understanding of cause and effect. The child can reason quite well if concrete objects are used in teaching or experimentation. The concept of conservation (that matter does not change when its form is altered) is learned at this age.

Formal operational (11 years to adulthood) Fully mature intellectual thought has now been attained. The adolescent can think abstractly about objects or concepts and consider different alternatives or outcomes. A certain amount of idealism, however, is characteristic at this stage.

Nursing Application

Piaget's theory is essential to pediatric nursing. The nurse must understand a child's thought processes in order to design stimulating activities and meaningful, appropriate teaching plans. Presence of the parent, as much as possible, is important for the infant experiencing stranger anxiety, while links to peers may be important to the teen (Box 5–1).

BOX 5–1	Research: Cognitive Theories

All developmental theories are simply that—theories. A theory is developed to explain a collection of observations or facts and to predict future occurrences. No theory can explain all of reality, and all have some strengths and some weaknesses. Although Piaget's theory of cognitive development provides a useful framework to examine and understand the thought process of young children, it is not perfect. He developed the theory mainly by observation of his own three children. It may lack some applicability in cross-cultural contexts, and it does not explain the importance of social contexts in learning. Two other important cognitive theories help to expand the work of Piaget and may provide assistance for nurses planning to teach young children:

1. Lev Vygotsky (1896–1934) agreed with Piaget's theory of child cognition. However, he believed that children are embedded in social contexts that influence learning. As parents and others guide and assist children, they learn tasks that were impossible for them to master alone. He also viewed the social structure of language as essential to development of thought (Santrock, 2011; Vygotsky, 1962).

2. Information processing is another theory about cognitive development that views attention and memory as the most important parts of learning, rather than the structures described by Piaget. Infants tend to habituate or become bored with the same stimuli. They are more attentive to, and learn from, new stimuli. Both long-term and short-term memory are important to learning. The older child actively engages in strategies to assist with memorization, thereby playing an active part in learning (Mundy & Jarrold, 2010; Santrock, 2011).

Nurses use their understanding of cognitive stages to tailor health teaching. For example, the teaching that a 6-year-old needs about newly diagnosed diabetes would focus on very different topics than the teaching provided for a 16-year-old with the same diagnosis. The nurse would apply knowledge of the young child's magical thinking and egocentrism by asking about possible causes of the disease and planning teaching that focuses on the child's experiences. The adolescent would receive teaching with others of the same age or teaching by teens who are managing the disease. With adolescents, the nurse can address causation and possible outcomes.

Nurses in community settings apply knowledge of development when planning interventions in clinics, schools, and homes. For example, fire prevention and actions to take during fires is a part of teaching for young children (do not play with matches, know how to notify someone of an emergency), as well as older children (learn fire-starting safety for outdoor activities, ask family to practice a home fire drill). Nurses in preschools teach about poisons and have children label harmful substances in the home with "Mr. Yuk."

By understanding a child's concept of time, the nurse can plan how far in advance to prepare that child for procedures. Similarly, the nurse's decision to offer manipulative toys, read stories, draw pictures, or give the child reading material to explain healthcare measures depends on the child's cognitive stage of development (see Table 5–3).

Kohlberg's Theory of Moral Development

Theoretic Framework

Lawrence Kohlberg's focus was on a particular type of cognitive development concerned with moral decisions. He presented stories involving moral dilemmas to children and adults and asked them to solve the dilemmas. In one story, a woman was very ill and the drug that would help her was too expensive for her family. The scientist who made that drug would not sell it for less money, so the woman's husband broke in to the store to steal the drug. Kohlberg asked a series of questions about whether it was right or wrong to steal the drug, and to charge a high price for it. Kohlberg then analyzed the motives people expressed when making decisions about the best course to take. Based on the explanations given, Kohlberg established three levels of moral reasoning. Although he provided age guidelines, he stated that they are approximate and that many people never reach the highest (postconventional) stage of development (Santrock, 2011).

Kohlberg's work has been criticized for insensitivity to cultural differences in moral reasoning, lack of consideration of the family in moral development, an emphasis on moral reasoning rather than actual actions, and sexual bias (Santrock, 2011). However, it remains a useful framework for some to help understand moral decision making.

Stages

Preconventional (4 to 7 years) Decisions are based on the desire to please others and to avoid punishment.

Conventional (7 to 11 years) Conscience or an internal set of standards becomes important, but these standards are based on the beliefs and teachings of others such as parents. Rules are important and must be followed to please other people and "be good."

Postconventional (12 years and older) The individual has internalized ethical standards on which to base decisions, and uses awareness of the common good and ethical principles rather than relying on the standards of others. Social responsibility is recognized. The value in each of two differing moral approaches can be considered and a decision made.

Nursing Application

Decision making is required in many areas of health care. Children can be assisted to make decisions about health care and to consider alternatives when available. The nurse should keep in mind that young children may agree to participate in research simply because they want to comply with adults and appear cooperative. Guidelines for child participation in research are available (see Chapter 1 🔗).

Provide parents with information so that they can assist their children in moral judgments. Encourage talking with a child or adolescent about how a given decision was made. Parents can then add information and help the child learn to integrate more factors into decision making. Talking about the process is important in helping children progress to higher moral development stages. Focusing on the feelings of others, using positive discipline techniques, and clearly identifying positive and negative behaviors are important. See Chapters 11 through 13 🔗 for positive discipline techniques at each age.

Social Learning Theory

Theoretic Framework

Albert Bandura, a contemporary psychologist, believes that children learn attitudes, beliefs, customs, and values through their social contacts with adults and other children. Children imitate (or model) the behavior they see; if the behavior is positively reinforced, they tend to repeat it. However, Bandura also believes that people can consciously choose how to act, such as deciding to handle problems by talking rather than hitting or yelling, even when some role models engage in the latter approach. The external environment (the behavior of others) and the child's internal processes and characteristics are thus

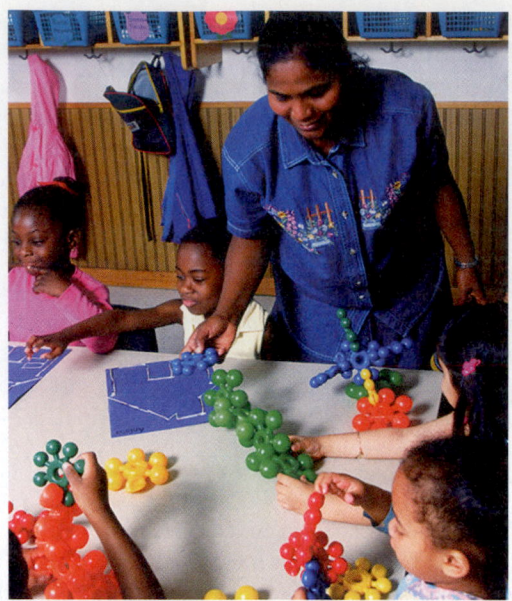

FIGURE 5–4 ■ Children exposed to pleasant stimulation and who receive positive feedback from an adult for engaging in activities will develop and refine their skills faster, demonstrating the importance of a nurturing environment. Group activities provide an opportunity for motor skill and psychosocial development. Which skills are being developed by children in this photograph?

both key elements in the behaviors a child manifests (Bandura, 1986, 1997a).

Bandura believes that an important determinant of behavior is **self-efficacy,** or the expectation that someone can produce a desired outcome. For example, if adolescents believe they can avoid use of drugs or alcohol, they are more likely to do so. A child who has confidence in his or her ability to exercise regularly or lose weight has a greater chance of success with these behavior changes. Parents who have confidence in their ability to care adequately for their infants are more likely to do so (Bandura, 1997b).

Nursing Application

The importance of modeling behavior can readily be applied in health care. Children are more likely to cooperate if they see adults or other children performing a task willingly. A frightened child may watch another child perform vision screening or have blood drawn and overcome fear of a procedure. Contact with positive role models is useful when teaching children and adolescents self-care for chronic diseases such as diabetes. Positive reinforcement should be given for desired performance (Figure 5–4 ■).

Nurses can use the concept of self-efficacy to increase the chance of success with lifestyle behavior changes. For example, methods of fostering self-efficacy include encouraging youth who are trying to quit smoking, providing role models for parents and youth, and encouraging parents by pointing out their successes with their children. See Evidence-Based Practice: Self-Efficacy.

Behaviorism

Theoretic Framework

John Watson studied the research of Pavlov and Skinner, who both demonstrated that one's actions are determined by the responses one receives from the environment. Pavlov and, later, Skinner worked with animals, presenting a stimulus such as food and pairing it with

Evidence-Based Practice   Self-Efficacy

PROBLEM

Nurses often provide information for parents and children that will encourage them to adopt healthy lifestyles. Providing information may not be enough; many of us know about healthy behaviors but do not consistently apply them. The concept of self-efficacy helps to explain why some people take on healthy behaviors whereas others do not. People who are convinced they can make a positive change are more likely to do so. In fact, research has demonstrated that lower physical activity and dietary self-efficacy scores in early adolescents were significantly related to higher waist circumference and skinfold thickness (Steele, Daratha, Bindler, et al., 2011). A number of research projects test and apply self-efficacy in teaching about health. Four examples follow.

EVIDENCE

- Parental self-efficacy is the belief that parents can manage a range of tasks and situations in caring for their children. Parents with higher self-efficacy scores were significantly more likely to manage conduct problems of their adolescents successfully, and their adolescents displayed fewer behavioral problems than adolescents of parents with lower parental self-efficacy. This study was carried out with Mexican American families, demonstrating the cross-cultural applicability of the concept of self-efficacy (Dumka, Gonzales, Wheeler, et al., 2010).

- Mothers who have a greater degree of self-efficacy about ability to breastfeed are significantly more likely to begin and to continue breastfeeding. A Breastfeeding Self-Efficacy Scale has been developed by nurses to identify risk and protective factors that influence the self-efficacy of new mothers. A network of support for breastfeeding is important, and evaluating breastfeeding

self-efficacy can identify women at risk for early discontinuation of breastfeeding (McCarter-Spaulding & Dennis, 2010).

- A program that was designed using self-efficacy theory to create opportunities for personal empowerment among adolescents resulted in improved health lifestyle choices and lower depression and anxiety scores (Melnyk, Jacobsen, Kelly, et al., 2009).

- An intervention with over 1,000 students in grades 5 and 6 was effective in increasing self-efficacy regarding television viewing time and decreasing television viewing time (Salmon, Jorna, Hume, et al., 2011).

IMPLICATIONS

In addition to providing information about health behaviors, nurses need to integrate methods to increase self-efficacy in teaching projects with families, children, and adolescents. Assessments should be designed to identify self-efficacy of parents and children around health topics of interest. Interventions can then be planned to enhance the self-efficacy of family members.

CRITICAL THINKING

Nurses can apply the concept of self-efficacy in teaching children and families. Plan a teaching project for school-age children to foster healthy eating. Include expected outcomes for the children and interventions. Could your outcome be improved if you focus not just on getting the content across, but also on increasing the belief and confidence that the children will be able to integrate the new behaviors into their lives? What activities could your teaching plan include that would be likely to improve the self-efficacy of these school-age children?

---

another stimulus such as a ringing bell. Eventually the animal being fed began to salivate when the bell rang. As Skinner and then Watson began to apply these concepts to children, they showed that behaviors can be elicited by positive reinforcement, such as a food treat, or extinguished by negative reinforcement, such as by scolding or withdrawal of attention. Watson believed that he could make a child into anyone he desired—from a professional to a thief or beggar—simply by reinforcing behavior in certain ways (Santrock, 2011).

Nursing Application

Behaviorism has been criticized for its simplicity and its denial of the inherent capability of persons to respond willfully to events in the environment. This theory does, however, have some use in health care. When particular behaviors are desired, healthcare providers can establish positive reinforcement to encourage these behaviors. Using behavioral techniques, nurses may alter behavior of children who misbehave or teach skills to children who are physically challenged. Parents often use reinforcement in toilet training. Indeed, combining behaviorism with social learning theory can be beneficial. For example, children might have desired activities, such as toothbrushing, modeled by an adult or older child (social learning theory) and be rewarded (behaviorism) for carrying out the activity on a regular basis.

Ecologic Theory

Theoretic Framework

You may have noticed that theorists disagree over the relative importance of heredity versus environment—or nature versus nurture—in human development. **Nature** refers to the genetic or hereditary capability of an individual. **Nurture** refers to the effects of the environment on a person's performance. Piaget believed in the importance

of internal cognitive structures that unfold at appointed times, given any environment that provides basic opportunities. He emphasized the strength of nature. The behaviorist John Watson, on the other hand, believed that behaviors are primarily shaped by environmental responses; he thus stressed the predominance of nurture. Contemporary developmental theorists increasingly recognize the interaction of nature and nurture in determining the child's development.

Clinical Judgment

Does nature or nurture have primary importance in the theories of Freud, Erikson, Kohlberg, Piaget, social learning, and behaviorism? Think about whether each of the theories emphasizes the role of heredity (nature) or the role of the environment (nurture) in influencing the development of children. Contrast these theories with the ecologic theory of Bronfenbrenner. What is a key difference? How does the ecologic theory view the roles of nature and nurture?

The ecologic theory of development was formulated by Urie Bronfenbrenner to explain the unique relationship of the child to all of life's settings, from close to remote (Bronfenbrenner, 1986; Bronfenbrenner, McClelland, Ceci, et al., 1996; Bronfenbrenner, 2005). **Ecologic theory** emphasizes the presence of mutual interactions between the child and these various settings. Neither nature nor nurture is considered of more importance. Bronfenbrenner believed that each child brings a unique set of genes—and specific attributes such as age, gender, health, and other characteristics—to his or her interactions with the environment. The child then interacts in many settings at different levels or systems (Figure 5–5 ■).

Levels or Systems

Microsystem The microsystem level is defined as the daily, consistent, close relationships such as home, childcare center, school,

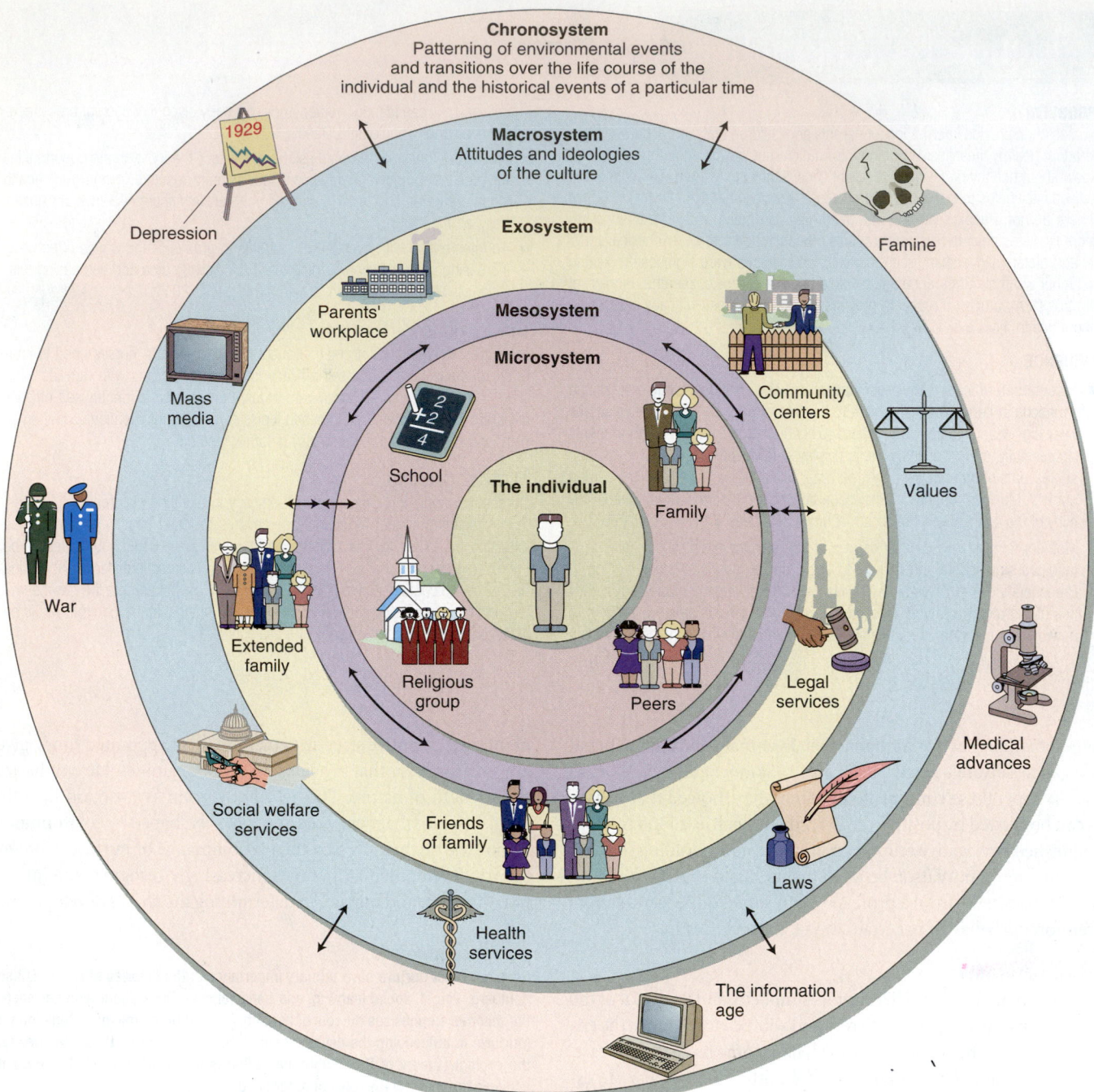

FIGURE 5–5 ■ Bronfenbrenner's ecologic theory of development views the individual as interacting within five levels or systems.

Source: *Redrawn from Santrock, J. W. (2005).* Life span development. *Madison, WI: Brown & Benchmark. Based on Bronfenbrenner's (1979, 1986) works in Contexts of child rearing: Problems and prospects.* American Psychologist, 34, *844–850; Ecology of the family as a context for human development: Research perspectives.* Developmental Psychology, 22, *723–742.*

friends, and neighbors. For the child with a chronic illness requiring regular care, the healthcare providers may even be part of the microsystem. Consider Sergio, the baby born prematurely who is described in the opening scenario. The family provides essential care for him, and the nurse provides regular assessments and teaching for the parents. Both the family and the nurse in the healthcare setting constitute important parts of Sergio's microsystem. In the ecologic model, the child influences each of the settings in the microsystem in addition to being influenced by them, in a series of reciprocal interactions.

Mesosystem The mesosystem level includes relationships of microsystems with one another. For example, two microsystems for most children are the home and the school. The relationships between these microsystems are shown by parents' involvement in their children's school. This involvement, in turn, influences the effects of the home and school settings on the children.

Exosystem The exosystem level is composed of those settings that influence the child even though the child is not in close daily contact with them. One exosystem may be the workplaces of parents

TABLE 5–5	Assessment of Ecologic Systems in Childhood—Bronfenbrenner			
MICROSYSTEMS	**MESOSYSTEMS**	**EXOSYSTEMS**	**MACROSYSTEMS**	**CHRONOSYSTEMS**
Parents	Parents' involvement in childcare or school	Community centers	Cultural group membership	Child's age
Significant others in close contact		Local political influences	Beliefs and values of group	Parents' ages
Childcare arrangements	Parents' involvement in community	Parents' work	Political structure	
School	Parents' relationships with significant others (e.g., grandparents, care providers)	Parents' friends and activities		
Neighborhood contacts		Social services		
Clubs		Health care		
Friends, peers	Influences of religious community (e.g., church, synagogue, mosque) or parents and school	Libraries		
Religious community (e.g., church, synagogue, mosque)				

or caregivers. Although children may rarely visit such settings, they can be influenced by policies related to health care, sick leave, inflexible work hours, overtime, or travel, or even by the mood of the boss (through its impact on the parent). The child's needs may influence a parent to give up a certain job or to work harder to obtain money for the child's education. How could having a premature baby, such as Sergio, influence the work plans of parents?

Macrosystem The macrosystem level includes the beliefs, values, and behaviors expressed in the child's environment. Culture is a powerful influence in the macrosystem, as are the political system and faith-based beliefs.

Chronosystem The outer level, the chronosystem, brings the perspective of time to the previous settings. The time period during which the child grows up influences views of health and illness. For example, the experiences of children with influenza in the 19th versus 20th centuries were quite different.

Nursing Application

Nurses use ecologic theory when they assess the child's settings to identify influences on development. Table 5–5 provides an assessment tool based on this theory. Interventions are planned to enhance the strengths of the child's settings and to improve on areas that are not supportive.

Temperament Theory

Theoretic Framework

In contrast to behaviorists such as Watson or maturational theorists such as Piaget, Stella Chess and Alexander Thomas recognize the innate qualities of personality that each individual brings to the events of daily life. They, like Bronfenbrenner, believe the child is an individual who both influences and is influenced by the environment. However, Chess and Thomas focus on one specific aspect of development—the wide spectrum of behaviors possible in children, identifying nine parameters of response to daily events (Table 5–6). Infants generally display clusters of responses, which Chess and Thomas have classified into three major personality types (Box 5–2). Although most children do not demonstrate all behaviors described for a particular type, they usually show a grouping indicative of one personality type (Chess & Thomas, 1995, 1996).

Current research demonstrates that personality characteristics displayed during infancy are often consistent with those seen later in life. They do not, however, predict future characteristics due to the complex and dynamic interaction of personality traits and environmental reactions.

Many other researchers have expanded the work of Chess and Thomas, developing assessment tools for temperament types. The concept of "goodness of fit" is an outgrowth of this theory.

TABLE 5–6	Nine Parameters of Personality—Chess and Thomas	
PARAMETER	**DESCRIPTION**	**SCORING**
Activity level	Degree of motion during eating, playing, sleeping, bathing	High, medium, or low
Rhythmicity	Regularity of schedule maintained for sleep, hunger, elimination	Regular, variable, or irregular
Approach or withdrawal	Response to a new stimulus such as a food, activity, or person	Approachable, variable, or withdrawn
Adaptability	Degree of adaptation to new situations	Adaptive, variable, or nonadaptive
Threshold of responsiveness	Intensity of stimulation needed to elicit a response to sensory input, objects in the environment, or people	High, medium, or low
Intensity of reaction	Degree of response to situations	Positive, variable, or negative
Quality of mood	Predominant mood during daily activity and in response to stimuli	Positive, variable, or negative
Distractibility	Ability of environmental stimuli to interfere with the child's activity	Distractible, variable, or nondistractible
Attention span and persistence	Amount of time devoted to activities (compared with other children of the same age) and the degree of ability to stick with an activity in spite of obstacles	Persistent, variable, or nonpersistent

Source: *Data from Chess, S., & Thomas, A. (1996).* Temperament: Theory and practice. *Philadelphia: Brunner/Mazel Publishers.*

BOX 5–2 **Patterns of Temperament—Chess and Thomas**

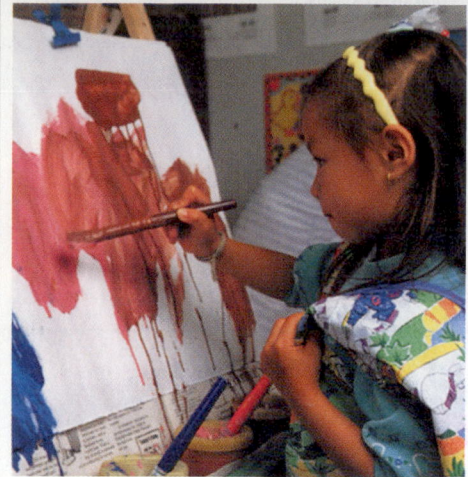
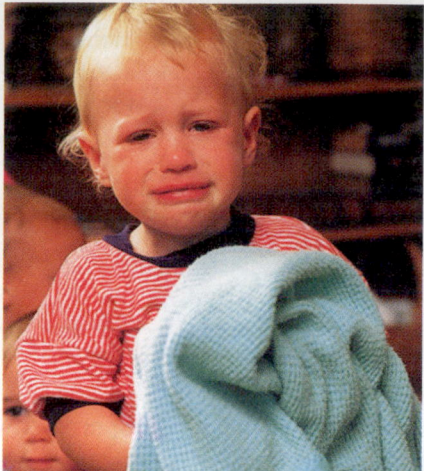
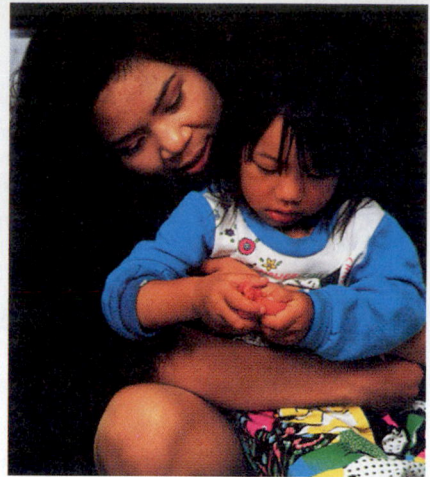

The **"easy" child** is generally moderate in activity; shows regularity in patterns of eating, sleeping, and elimination; and is usually positive in mood and when subjected to new stimuli. The easy child adapts to new situations and is able to accept rules and work well with others. About 40% of children in the New York Longitudinal Study displayed this personality type.

The **"difficult" child** displays irregular schedules for eating, sleeping, and elimination; adapts slowly to new situations and persons; and displays a predominantly negative mood. Intense reactions to the environment are common. About 10% of children in the New York Longitudinal Study displayed this personality type.

The **"slow-to-warm-up" child** has reactions of mild intensity and slow adaptability to new situations. The child displays initial withdrawal followed by gradual, quiet, and slow interaction with the environment. About 15% of children in the New York Longitudinal Study displayed this personality type. The remaining 35% of children studied showed some characteristics of each personality type.

Source: *Data from Chess, S., & Thomas, A. (1996).* Temperament: Theory and practice. *Philadelphia: Brunner/Mazel Publishers.*

Goodness of fit refers to whether parents' expectations of their child's behavior are consistent with the child's temperament type. A "good fit" exists when the properties of the environment are in accord with the child's capabilities, characteristics, and style of behavior (Burney & Leerkes, 2010; Chess & Thomas, 1999). As an example of lack of good fit, an active infant who reacts strongly to verbal stimuli may be unable to sleep when placed in a room with older siblings. When parents understand a child's temperament characteristics, they are better able to shape the environment to meet the child's needs. The active infant described previously should be put to sleep in a quiet room.

Nursing Application

The concept of personality type or temperament is a useful one for nurses. Nurses can assess the temperament of young children and alter the environment to meet their needs. This may involve moving a hospitalized child to a single room to ensure adequate rest if the child is easily stimulated, or allowing a shy child time to become accustomed to new surroundings and equipment before beginning procedures or treatments.

Parents are often relieved to learn about temperament characteristics. They learn to appreciate their children's qualities and to adapt the environment to meet the children's needs. A burden of guilt can also be lifted from parents who feel that they are responsible for their child's actions. The nurse can teach parents ways of enhancing goodness of fit between the child's personality and the environment (Table 5–7). See further suggestions for helping parents understand temperament during health promotion and health maintenance visits in Chapters 9 through 13 ⓔ.

TABLE 5–7	Ways to Improve Goodness of Fit Between Parent and Child
CHILD'S BEHAVIOR	**PARENT'S ACTIVITY**
Extremely active	Plan periods of active play several times in a day. Have restful periods before bedtime to foster sleep.
Shy	Allow time to adapt at own pace to new people and situations.
Easily stimulated	Have a quiet room for sleeping as an infant. Have a quiet room for homework for the school-age child.
Short attention span	Provide projects that can be completed in a short period.
	Gradually encourage longer periods at activities.

Resiliency Theory

Theoretic Framework

Why do some children coming from similar backgrounds have such different behavioral outcomes? The resiliency model is a theory that examines both the individual's characteristics and the interaction of these characteristics with the environment. **Resilience** is the ability to function with healthy responses, even with significant stress and adversity (Henderson, Benard, & Sharp-Light, 2007). In this model, the individual or family members experience a crisis that provides a source of stress, and the family interprets or deals with the crisis based on resources available. Families and individuals have **protective factors** that provide strength and assistance in dealing with crises, and **risk factors** that promote or contribute to their challenges

TABLE 5–8	Components of Resiliency Model
COMPONENT	**EXAMPLE**
Internal risk/protective factors	Health
	Developmental level
	Genetic traits
	Temperament
	Coping ability
External risk/protective factors	Family members
	Quality of relationships
	Knowledge level
	Environmental characteristics
	Community services
Interventions	Enhance knowledge
	Minimize risk factors
	Enhance protective factors
	Enhance supportive resources
	Strengthen family and community resources

Source: *Data from Daly, B. P., Shin, R. Q., Thakral, C., Selders, M., & Vera, E. (2009). School engagement among urban adolescents of color: Does perception of social support and neighborhood safety really matter?* Journal of Youth and Adolescence, 38(1), 63–74.

TABLE 5–9	Assessment Questions to Determine Resilience Capability

Questions to Determine Risk Factors

- What has this event been like for your family?
- What other stressors do you have in your family right now?
- Are there financial worries?
- Are there things you think and worry about late at night?
- How would you describe your job? Your friends?
- What do you do on a typical day?
- What is your neighborhood like?
- Do you have friends or other people to call in emergencies?

Questions to Determine Protective Factors

- What gives you strength?
- How do you deal with this stress?
- What do you think you do well in your family?
- Who do you call when you need help?
- Do you have a computer? Internet access?
- Are you religious? Spiritual?
- Do you exercise regularly?
- How do you spend free time?

(Daly, Shin, Thakral, et al., 2009; Henderson et al., 2007). Risk and protective factors can be identified in children, in their families, and in their communities (see Chapter 20 ⊘ for further description of the interplay of social and environmental factors with individual characteristics). Children and their families undergo stresses and experience crises throughout life. For example, a crisis for a young child might be a transfer to a new childcare provider. Protective factors could involve past positive experiences with new people, an "easy" temperament, and awareness of the new childcare provider about adaptation needs of young children to new experiences. Risk factors for a similar child might be repeated moves to new care providers, limited close relationships with adults, and a "slow-to-warm-up" temperament.

Once confronted by a stress or crisis, the child and family adjust and adapt to the situation based on the particular risk and protective factors involved. Adaptation may lead to increasing resilience as the child and family learn about new resources and inner strengths and develop the ability to deal more effectively with future crises. Examples of risk and protective factors are listed in Table 5–8.

Nursing Application

Nurses gather information about the individual characteristics, prior life experiences, and environmental factors that act as protective and risk factors for children. Table 5–9 lists questions that can be helpful as the nurse gathers information from a child or family members. Nurses then use concepts of resiliency theory in planning interventions for children and families. Nursing strategies can target risk factors. For example, in families with firearms, the nurse can encourage family behaviors to ensure gun safety by teaching about use of gun trigger locks and locked gun cabinets. In addition, nurses can emphasize protective factors, such as encouraging holding and verbalization to parents of infants to provide an environment that meets needs for trust establishment and speech development.

INFLUENCES ON DEVELOPMENT

Development is a complex process that involves the interplay of inherited genetic traits and the social experiences of the child. For example, genetic traits common in certain ethnic or cultural groups may predispose children to be at the upper or lower ranges of growth and may influence other physical characteristics. Certain groups are more prone to develop specific diseases due to genetic variations (see Chapter 4 ⊘ for a thorough discussion of genetic factors). Genetic traits interact in a mutually influential way with the child's health status, as well as social and environmental factors. These factors include prematurity, adoption and parenting, cultural influences, and more.

The normal pregnancy lasts for 40 weeks. A preterm infant is one born before 37 weeks' gestation. About 1 in every 8 infants born in the United States (over 500,000 annually) are premature, and the number has risen 20% in the last two decades (Centers for Disease Control and Prevention [CDC], 2010). The reasons for the increase in prematurity rates are not clear. A growing number of multiple births (resulting from fertility treatment) and increasing maternal age at birth may be potential contributors. Inadequate nutrition, tobacco use, substance use, lack of prenatal care, maternal diseases such as diabetes, and psychologic influences may also play a part (CDC, 2010). Infants who are premature have immature body systems, requiring medical support in the newborn period. In spite of treatment, infants may experience episodes that adversely affect development, such as (CDC, 2010):

- Inadequate respiratory function, leading to infection and poor perfusion of the brain and other organs
- Inability to suck and to adequately metabolize food intake
- Inadequate kidney function, complicating the administration of drugs and the ability of the infant to manage fluid and electrolyte variations
- Lowered immune protection against pathogens

- Variations in neurologic maturity leading to decreased responses and to complications such as intraventricular hemorrhage
- Neurologic conditions such as cerebral palsy

Premature infants are thus at risk for a number of conditions that can compromise normal developmental progression. They need support early in life to ensure careful monitoring and stimulation to encourage development. See the description of Sergio in the opening scenario for a glimpse of the parental challenges and the nursing role with premature infants.

As we have seen, both nature and nurture are important in determining individual patterns of development. These two forces interact in distinctive ways in each individual, explaining differences in time frames for acquisition of developmental skills among children, personality variations between identical twins, and other unique characteristics of individuals. An environmental factor that is extremely important in the development of children is the profile of family characteristics. The family is an important component in the lives of all children, and it plays an essential role in fostering the development of youth. A significant concept in families is that of parenting. How children are parented interacts with their individual characteristics to influence risk and protective factors, personality characteristics, and developmental outcomes. Chapter 2 🕐 discusses types of families, frameworks used to understand families, the roles of families in fostering the development of children, and types of parenting styles.

The families into which children are born influence them profoundly. Early bonding, institutionalization followed by adoption, multiple foster homes—all interact with the child's inherited characteristics to influence the rate of development and the characteristics that the child manifests. Children are supported in different ways and acquire various worldviews depending on such factors as whether they have one or two parents or stepparents, whether one or both parents work outside the home, how many siblings are present, and whether an extended family is close. Note should be made of variations in family structure such as single parent, homosexual parents, extended family, and stepparents. In addition, factors such as nutritional support, early childcare, stress among family members, access to physical activity, presence of environmental hazards such as radon or lead, and reading/playing with the child influence the child's growth and development.

Another factor that influences child development is that of culture, through traditional practices among some ethnic groups. The traditional customs of the many cultural groups represented in North America influence the growth and development of the children in these groups. Nutritional practices of various ethnic groups may influence the rate of growth for infants. In addition, development may be influenced by childrearing practices. For example, the Native American practice of carrying infants on boards often delays walking when it is measured against the norm for walking on some developmental tests. These infants begin walking later than other babies, but achieve other gross motor skills on schedule. Children who are carried by straddling the mother's hips or back for extended periods have a low incidence of developmental dysplasia of the hip, since the practice keeps their hips in an abducted position. It is important for nurses to take cultural practices into account when performing developmental screening; some tests may not be culturally sensitive and can inaccurately label a child as delayed when the pattern of development is simply different in the group, perhaps due to childrearing practices in the family. In these cases there is no lasting delay in any milestone but variation in acquiring skills may occur.

All cultural groups have rules regarding patterns of social interaction. Schedules of language acquisition are determined by the number of languages spoken and the amount of speech in the home. The particular social roles assumed by men and women in the culture affect school activities and ultimately career choices. Attitudes toward touching and other methods of encouraging developmental skills vary among cultures. Chapter 20 🕐 includes further description of other factors that influence child development such as school and childcare, community services, environmental hazards, and additional community and family factors. In addition, Chapters 9 through 13 🕐 describe assessment of development at each age.

GROWTH AND DEVELOPMENT BY AGE GROUP

Nurses use information about developmental milestones to assess children, to identify those with delays, and to plan interventions that will foster development. To do so requires a comprehensive understanding of expected physical growth and development, cognitive abilities, and psychosocial characteristics (Commonwealth Fund, 2011). Potential risks—such as prematurity, international adoption, and presence of health problems—necessitate a more frequent and in-depth assessment of observed milestones. Nurses compare the expected findings with assessment results, make referrals for further evaluation when appropriate, and use the results to plan nursing interventions. Chapters 9 through 13 🕐 examine further details about analyzing developmental results. See the Photo Story for an example of developmental findings in a child who was adopted from Romania.

NEWBORN (UP TO 1 MONTH)
Physical Growth and Development and Prenatal Influences

Some Asian cultures calculate age from the time of conception. This practice acknowledges the profound influence of the prenatal period. Nurses work closely with pregnant women to encourage safe health practices during pregnancy.

The mother's nutrition and general state of health play a part in pregnancy outcome. During pregnancy, mothers should seek early prenatal care, eat well, exercise regularly, and avoid harmful exposure to substances. Early prenatal care provides an opportunity to evaluate the health of the mother and the development of the fetus, to intervene when possible to eliminate fetal risks, and to teach the mother healthy lifestyles that positively influence pregnancy outcome. Teaching focuses on health habits that directly affect the unborn child; deleterious habits are discouraged and programs are offered to decrease risky behaviors. Maternal smoking is associated with low-birth-weight infants. Ingestion of alcoholic beverages, including beer and wine, during pregnancy may lead to fetal alcohol syndrome (see Chapter 32 🕐 for further description). Substance abuse by the mother may result in neonatal addiction, convulsions, hyperirritability, poor social responsiveness, and other neurologic disturbances of the infant, as well as changes in neurobehavioral and cognitive function of children (Murphy-Oikonen, Montelpare, Southon, et al., 2010). See Chapter 32 🕐 for a discussion of neonatal withdrawal syndrome.

PHOTO STORY...

DEVELOPMENTAL OBSERVATIONS OF A YOUNG CHILD

Two-year-old Irena was adopted from Romania several months ago by U.S. parents Michael and Alyssa. Irena was left at an orphanage by her mother when she was about 7 months old; the mother stated that the pregnancy and delivery were normal. She gave up the child because she had two older children to care for and her husband had left home nearly a year before and had not been heard from since. Irena appears small for her age, but is thriving in her new environment. She is learning a few English words and is responding appropriately to care and interactions. Follow Irena as she goes about her daily activities.

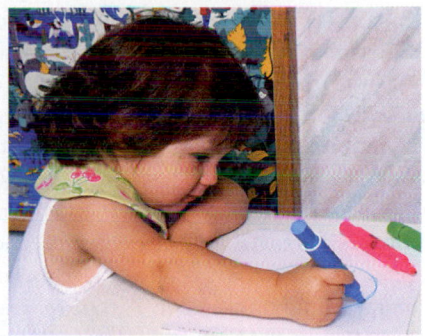

Irena shows fine motor skills as she begins to scribble and color in a circle provided by a parent.

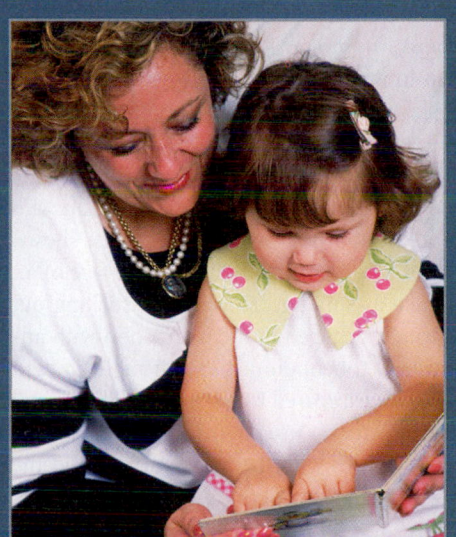
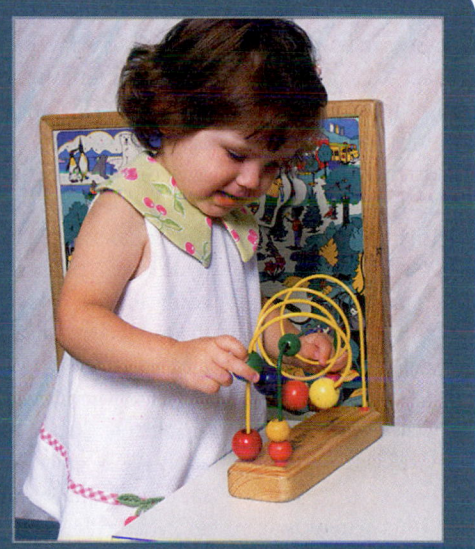

Left. Alyssa reads with Irena and provides positive reinforcement for activities. Right. Cognitive development is enhanced as toddlers manipulate objects. What is Irena learning about color, texture, and spatial relationships?

PSYCHOSOCIAL DEVELOPMENT
Play

Irena is observed playing with toys and making sounds with her dolls. This is expected behavior, as toddlers often engage in solitary play. Toddlers also begin to enjoy the presence of other children, even though they do not yet play cooperatively with them. Irena's parents can encourage the emergence of parallel play commonly seen in toddlers by arranging to have Irena play with other children. The parents can be available at first so that Irena feels secure; once she shows comfort with other children, her parents can gradually increase their absence during these playtimes.

PHYSICAL GROWTH AND DEVELOPMENT

Although many international adoptees are small for their age, Irena appears well nourished. (See Chapter 19 🔗 for a discussion of nutritional needs during toddlerhood.) Her gross motor skills, including walking up steps, running, and kicking a ball, are well developed. Fine motor skills are evident in her ability to brush teeth and dress with help, scribble on paper, and build a tower of cubes. As her physical abilities continue to develop, her family needs to integrate injury prevention to keep her safe from falls, car crashes, and other injuries.

COGNITIVE DEVELOPMENT

Cognitive development relates to intellectual or thinking processes. It is hard to identify Irena's cognitive stage at this time, as she knows only a few English words and is shy during interactions with strangers. As she adapts to her new home, frequent assessments of her cognitive development will be necessary.

Personality and Temperament

Irena has been demonstrating what experts term an "easy" temperament; that is, she has readily acquired a regular schedule for eating and sleeping, her mood is generally pleasant, and she is easily comforted when upset. These temperamental characteristics will form a critical link to communication with family, teachers, and friends.

Communication

Irena has only learned a few words. This is abnormal for a toddler, since most know several hundred words. However, it is expected that Irena will learn language quickly as she adapts. Michael and Alyssa should speak with Irena often, pointing out names of people and objects. Positive reinforcement for Irena's attempts at speech can involve smiles, phrases such as "that's right," and further elaboration such as "Yes, that is a bus; it's a big, yellow bus." *What else can you suggest to her parents as activities that will enhance speech development?*

Good nutrition is particularly important during pregnancy, and therefore is a focus of prenatal teaching. Poor nutrition can lead to low-birth-weight infants and infants with compromised neurologic performance, slow development, or impaired immune status with resultant high disease rates. Low maternal stores of iron can result in anemia in the infant (American Academy of Pediatrics, 2009). Exercise has regular health benefits. It encourages blood flow that can improve circulation to the fetus. Mothers often report an improved sense of well-being from regular exercise. Although new and vigorous or risky exercise should not be started in pregnancy, women can usually continue established exercise regimens; walking is nearly always safe.

Many other prenatal influences have been identified. Even prescription drugs may adversely affect the fetus. For example, the drug thalidomide, commonly used in Europe to treat nausea during the 1950s, resulted in the birth of infants with limb abnormalities to women who used the drug during pregnancy. Differences in physiology related to gastric emptying, renal clearance, drug distribution, and other factors contribute to variations in pharmacokinetics during pregnancy. Drugs can cause **teratogenesis** (abnormal development of the fetus) or **mutagenesis** (permanent changes in the fetus's genetic material) (van Gelder, van Rooij, Miller, et al., 2010). Certain drugs can cause bleeding, stained teeth, impaired hearing, or other defects in the infant. The U.S. Food and Drug Administration (FDA) has established risk categories for drugs in pregnancy. Category A indicates drugs with no known risk. Categories B, C, and D indicate increasing risk, and Category X indicates drugs with known danger of fetal risk (U.S. Food and Drug Administration, 2011).

Some maternal illnesses are harmful to the developing fetus, such as rubella (German measles), which is rarely a serious disease for adults but can cause deafness, vision defects, heart defects, and mental retardation in the fetus if it is acquired by a pregnant woman. A fetus can also acquire diseases, such as acquired immunodeficiency syndrome (AIDS) and human immunodeficiency virus (HIV) infection or hepatitis B, from the mother.

Paternal influence may be important as well. Either parent may have been exposed to toxic chemicals during war, toxins in the workplace, steroids, or street drugs. Radiation, chemicals, and other environmental hazards may adversely affect a fetus when the parent has been exposed to these influences. The best outcomes for infants occur when both parents have had minimal exposure to environmental toxins, have enjoyed general good health, and have refrained from use of drugs, excessive alcohol, and tobacco.

Among a newborn's physical characteristics, its reflexes (see Chapter 7 ✪ for a description) help it receive input, nourishment, and comfort from the environment. For example, the infant's sucking reflex provides food, physical contact with the mother, and a way to comfort the self. This food enables the baby to grow and perform a gradually expanding array of motor skills. Nurses closely monitor developmental progression during the baby's first month of life, as the transition of all body systems to extrauterine life occurs.

Cognitive Development

Piaget's theory of cognitive development recognized the importance of the newborn reflexes in determining the newborn's cognitive development. Reflexes are not just a way to obtain food or maintain safety, but are the tools that help the newborn transition from the uterus to the external world. The baby uses reflexes and learns through them. Grasping opens the world to many objects that the baby will gradually learn to manipulate. When comfort needs are met, the baby learns from the experiences of eating and being clothed and held. The foundations of thought have been laid.

Psychosocial Development

Many people believe that the newborn is incapable of anything but eating and sleeping. However, some observant care providers and researchers, such as Dr. T. Berry Brazelton and Dr. Kathryn Barnard, have noted that the newborn is particularly attuned to people in the environment, especially the parents. Relationships begin and will continue to develop throughout infancy. **Attachment** is a strong emotional bond between people, and it can begin in the newborn period. When women hold their babies directly after birth, they tend to progress from touching them by fingertip, to full palm, and then enfolding them in hands and arms. Newborns are often alert after birth and follow the mother's face carefully with their eyes. This first interaction fosters attachment between the mother and baby. For many families, the process also involves attachment with the father, and sometimes siblings. The newborn learns quickly in the first month about safety and security, comfort, and food. If fed when hungry, held and comforted when in pain or distress, and played with several times daily, the baby learns that the parents and other caretakers can be trusted to meet its basic needs. Once the infant learns to trust that people will provide care, it is free to move on to explore the environment more actively. T. Berry Brazelton, a pediatrician who has worked extensively with newborns and their parents, has shown that even in the first days of life infants can focus on the face of an adult; imitate behaviors such as smiling, frowning, or sticking out the tongue; and become totally engaged in the interaction with another person. He has identified "touchpoints" or predictable times in early life when young children are geared to learn new skills (Lester & Sparrow, 2010). The term *en face* is used to indicate the baby and adult gazing into each other's faces with their faces oriented in the same positions (Figure 5–6 ■). There are periods in the day when the

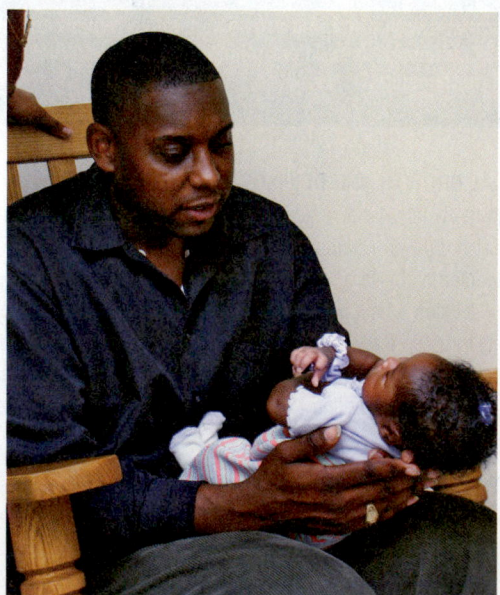

FIGURE 5–6 ■ Note that the parent's and infant's faces are in the same plane. This "en face" position enables both to examine each other's faces and establish eye contact, fostering attachment between parent and child.

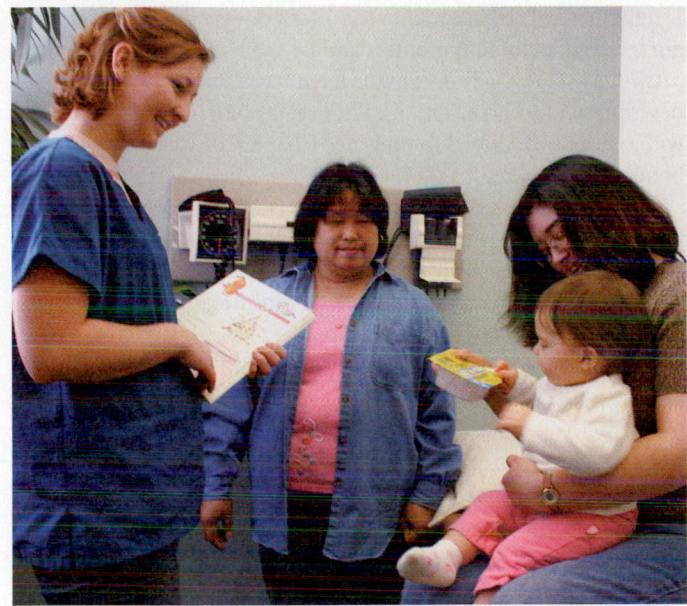

FIGURE 5–7 ■ Nurses in many settings with young children are applying the attachment facilitation techniques suggested by Dr. T. Berry Brazelton. Health professionals can teach parents to recognize the nonverbal cues of their infants and toddlers. The nurse can also model and positively reinforce the mother's interactions with her infant.

baby's level of alertness supports the ability to focus on faces of caretakers and to learn positive aspects of the interpersonal relationship. Nurses support parents to recognize these times (or touchpoints) and use them to interact with the baby when possible (Figure 5–7 ■). See Table 5–10 for a description of infant states of alertness and suggested parental responses.

Nurses play an important role in helping new parents to learn about their babies' communication ability and to respond appropriately (Box 5–3). Some parents may need ongoing help for a period of time to foster attachment with the child, such as parents who are very young or have limited experience with babies, parents with mental health problems, or the parents of a premature newborn. Reflect back on Sergio, described in the chapter beginning. His parents are

---

BOX 5–3   **Research: Nursing Assessment**

One of the first nurses to apply information about development, attachment, and infant/child behaviors was Dr. Kathryn Barnard. She sought to understand the impact of the first years of life on later health and founded Nursing Child Assessment Satellite Training (NCAST), a program to teach nurses and other healthcare providers how to evaluate the parent–child interaction. Her work continues through an active program that provides training and tools for parent–child interaction, promoting early relationships, understanding babies' cues, promoting maternal mental health during pregnancy, assessing the child's environment, and assessing sleep (NCAST, 2011).

very motivated and spend much time with him. However, they remain anxious about his condition, and his mother experiences guilt about his premature birth. Challenges for parents of a high-risk infant include:

- Guilt and grieving about the child's condition
- Worry upon hospital discharge about whether skills are present to be competent in care of the baby
- Concern about future development
- Constant adaptation to changes as the child grows and develops

Nursing interventions that can promote positive attachment with the high-risk infant include:

- Encouraging frequent visits to the baby in the newborn care unit
- Promoting holding of the baby
- Providing for skin-to-skin contact of the baby and parent
- Pointing out the baby's attributes and responses to voice or touch
- Involving parents in care of and decisions about the baby
- Advocating for healthcare agency policies that are supportive of attachment between the infant and parents
- Giving information and repeating as needed; letting parents have a telephone number they can call at any time to get information about the baby or talk with a supportive person
- Arranging for ongoing developmental assessments on a regular basis once the infant is discharged from the hospital

---

TABLE 5–10	Infant States of Alertness	
STATE	**DESCRIPTION**	**RECOMMENDED PARENTAL RESPONSES**
Drowsiness or dozing	The baby's eyes are open or closed but there is not concentration on surroundings; the eyelids flutter, extremities move slowly, and occasional startles occur. The baby transitions to either deeper sleep or wakefulness.	Parents can provide a quiet place for sleep or encourage wakefulness if that is desired.
Quiet alert (or wide awake)	The baby is wide awake and follows objects, sounds, and faces; there is minimal motor movement. The infant is learning from the environment and will look away every few seconds and then look back at the face or object of interest.	Parents can talk and sing to the baby, assume the en face position, or provide objects for the baby to look at.
Active alert (or active awake)	The baby is very active with movements of extremities and head. The baby responds to all stimuli with movement.	Parents may swaddle or quiet the infant if desired or allow the baby to move about, understanding that either crying or settling into quiet alert will likely occur next.
Crying	The baby cries and has movements of extremities.	Parents can look for reasons for the crying and intervene to provide comfort. The baby may be tired and need swaddling, or the baby may be hungry, have gastric distress, or be wet or cold. Sometimes the source of crying is not known and an episode of crying, while annoying to parents, may continue to occur.

Source: *Adapted from London, M. L., Ladewig, P. W., Ball, J. W., et al. (2011). Maternal & child nursing care (3rd ed.). Upper Saddle River, NJ: Prentice Hall Health.*

INFANT (1 MONTH TO 1 YEAR)

Can you imagine tripling your present weight in a single year? Or becoming proficient in understanding fundamental words in a new language and even speaking a few? These and many more accomplishments take place in the first year of life. Starting the year as a mainly reflexive creature, the infant can walk and communicate by the year's end. Never again in life is development so swift (Figure 5–8 ■).

Video Understanding Growth and Development

The first year of life is one of rapid change for the infant. The birth weight usually doubles by about 5 months and triples by the end of the first year. Body proportions begin to change (Figure 5–9 ■).

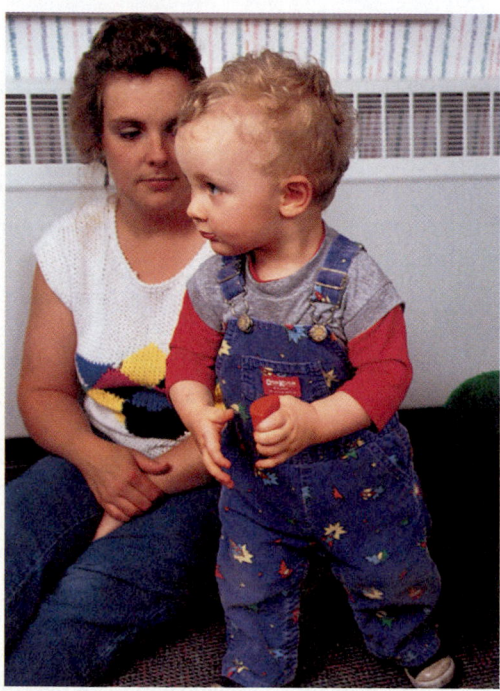

FIGURE 5–8 ■ A 12-month-old child has tripled his birth weight, is learning to walk, and is beginning to talk.

Height increases by approximately 1 foot during this year. Teeth begin to erupt at about 6 months, and by the end of the first year the infant has six to eight deciduous teeth (see Chapter 7 ⊘ for a full description of tooth eruption). Physical growth is closely associated with type and quality of feeding. See Chapter 19 ⊘ for a discussion of nutrition in infancy.

Body organs and systems, although not fully mature at 1 year of age, function differently than they did at birth. Kidney and liver maturation helps the 1-year-old excrete drugs or other toxic substances (such as those acquired from environmental exposure) more readily than in the first weeks of life. The changing body proportions mirror changes in developing internal organs. Maturation of the nervous system is demonstrated by increased control over body movements, enabling the infant to sit, stand, and walk. Some infants take a few steps by 1 year of age, while others walk easily by then. Generally sometime between 12 and 18 months, walking is mastered. Sensory function also increases as the infant begins to discriminate visual images, sounds, and tastes (Table 5–11). See Table 10–1 in Chapter 10 ⊘ for a detailed list of the developmental milestones of the infant that are observed during health promotion visits.

Cognitive Development

The brain continues to increase in complexity during the first year. Most of the growth involves maturation of cells, with only a small increase in cell number. This growth of the brain is accompanied by development of its functions. One has only to compare the behavior of an infant shortly after birth with that of a 1-year-old to understand the incredible maturation of brain function. The newborn's eyes widen in response to sound; the 1-year-old turns to the sound and recognizes its significance. The 2-month-old cries and coos; the 1-year-old says a few words and understands many more. The 6-week-old grasps a rattle for the first time; the 1-year-old reaches for toys and self-feeds.

The infant's behaviors provide clues about thought processes. Piaget's work outlines the infant's actions in a set of rapidly progressing changes in the first year of life. The infant receives stimulation through sight, sound, and feeling, which the maturing brain interprets. This input from the environment interacts with internal cognitive abilities to enhance cognitive functioning.

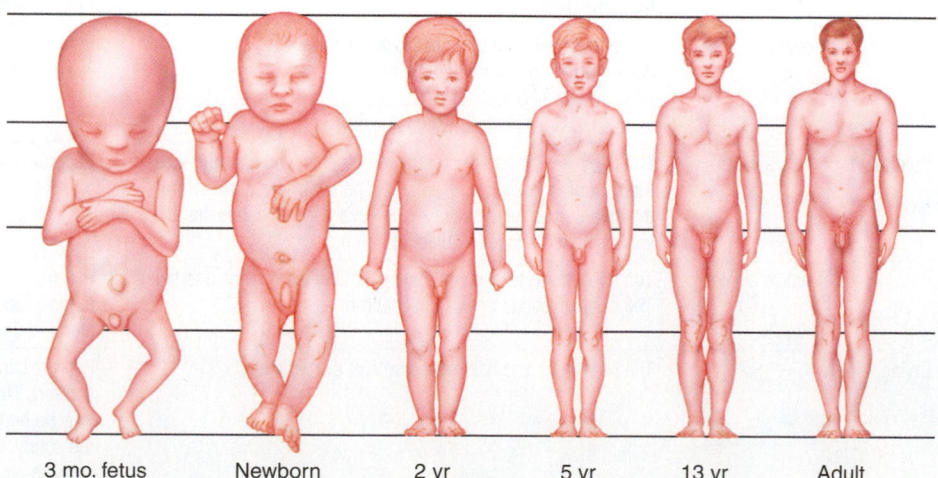

FIGURE 5–9 ■ Body proportions at various ages.

3 mo. fetus   Newborn   2 yr   5 yr   13 yr   Adult

TABLE 5–11	Physical Growth and Development Milestones During Infancy			
AGE	**PHYSICAL GROWTH**	**FINE MOTOR ABILITY**	**GROSS MOTOR ABILITY**	**SENSORY ABILITY**
Birth to 1 month	Gains 5–7 oz (140–200 g)/week Grows 1.5 cm (1/2 in.) in first month Head circumference increases 1.5 cm (1/2 in.)/month	Holds hand in fist **(1)** Draws arms and legs to body when crying	Inborn reflexes such as startle and rooting are predominant activity May lift head briefly if prone **(2)** Alerts to high-pitched voices Comforts with touch **(3)**	Prefers to look at faces and black-and-white geometric designs Follows objects in line of vision **(4)**

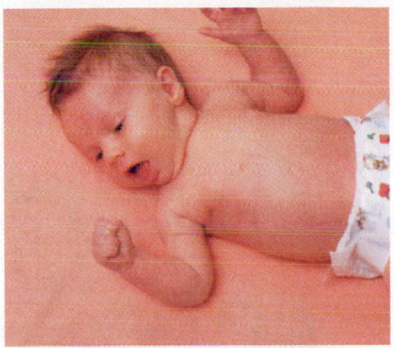

(1) Holds hand in fist

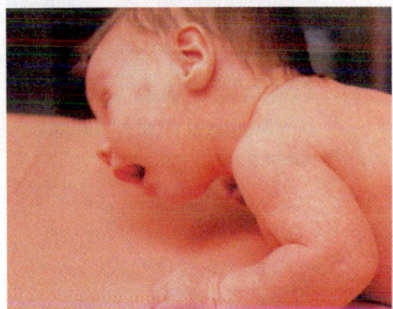

(2) May lift head

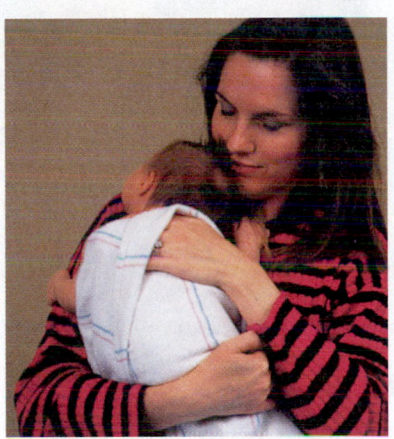

(3) Comforts with touch

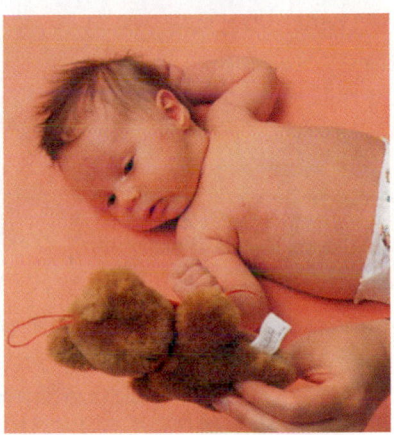

(4) Follows objects

| 2–4 months | Gains 5–7 oz (140–200 g)/week
Grows 1.5 cm (1/2 in.)/month
Head circumference increases 1.5 cm (1/2 in.)/month
Posterior fontanel closes
Ingests 120 mL/kg/24 hr (2 oz/lb/24 hr) | Holds rattle when placed in hand **(5)**
Looks at and plays with own fingers
Brings hands to midline | Moro reflex fading in strength
Can turn from side to back and then return **(6)**
Decrease in head lag when pulled to sitting; sits with head held in midline with some bobbing
When prone, holds head up and supports weight on forearms **(7)** | Follows objects 180 degrees
Turns head to look for voices and sounds |

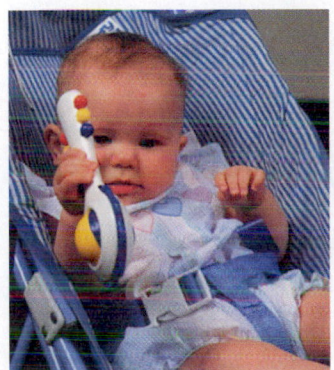

(5) Holds rattle

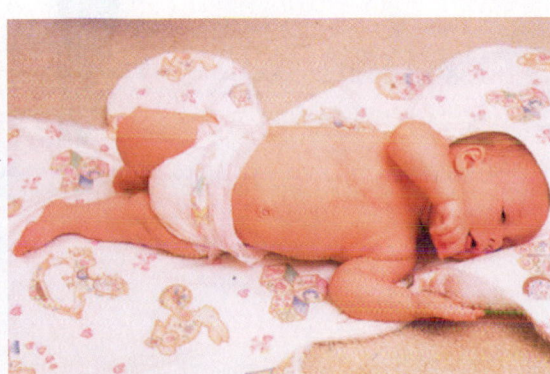

(6) Can turn from side to back

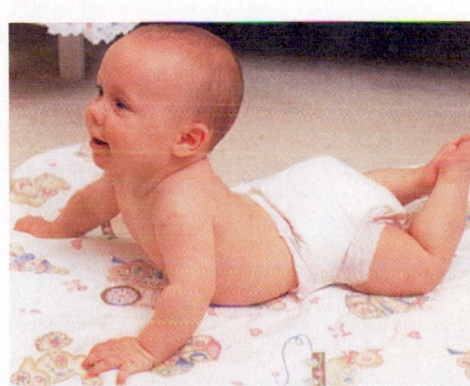

(7) Holds head up and supports weight with arms

(Continued)

TABLE 5-11	Physical Growth and Development Milestones During Infancy (*Continued*)			
AGE	**PHYSICAL GROWTH**	**FINE MOTOR ABILITY**	**GROSS MOTOR ABILITY**	**SENSORY ABILITY**
4–6 months	Gains 5–7 oz (140–200 g)/week Doubles birth weight at 5–6 months Grows 1.5 cm (1/2 in.)/month Head circumference increases 1.5 cm (1/2 in.)/month Teeth may begin erupting by 6 months Ingests 100 mL/kg/24 hr (1 1/2 oz/lb/24 hr)	Grasps rattles and other objects at will; drops them to pick up another offered object **(8)** Mouths objects Holds feet and pulls to mouth Holds bottle Grasps with whole hand (palmar grasp) Manipulates objects **(9)**	Head held steady when sitting No head lag when pulled to sitting Turns from abdomen to back by 4 months and then back to abdomen by 6 months When held standing, supports much of own weight **(10)**	Examines complex visual images Watches the course of a falling object Responds readily to sounds

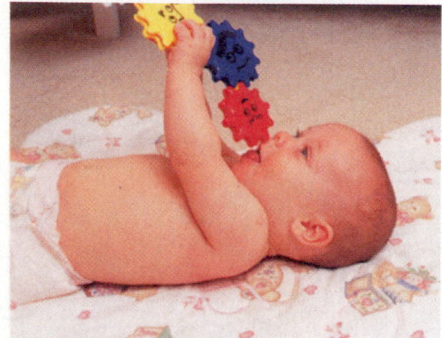

(8) Grasps objects at will

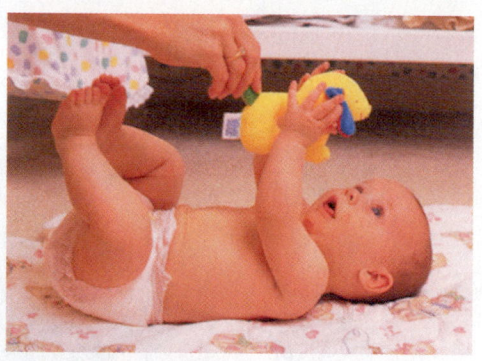

(9) Manipulates objects

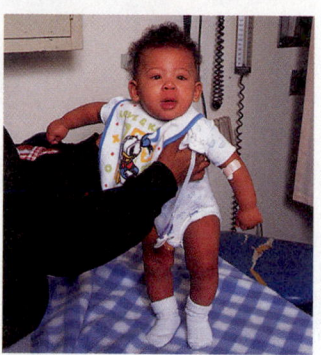

(10) Supports most of weight when held standing

6–8 months	Gains 3–5 oz (85–140 g)/week Grows 1 cm (3/8 in.)/month Growth rate slower than first 6 months	Bangs objects held in hands Transfers objects from one hand to the other Beginning pincer grasp at times	Most inborn reflexes extinguished Sits alone steadily without support by 8 months **(11)** Likes to bounce on legs when held in standing position	Recognizes own name and responds by looking and smiling Enjoys small and complex objects at play

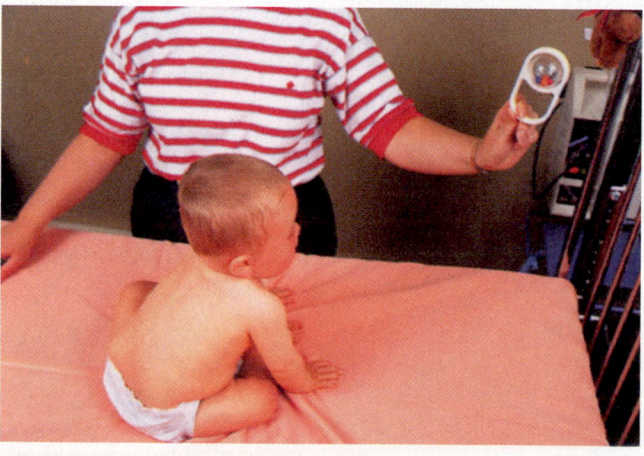

(11) Sits alone without support

TABLE 5–11	Physical Growth and Development Milestones During Infancy (*Continued*)			
AGE	**PHYSICAL GROWTH**	**FINE MOTOR ABILITY**	**GROSS MOTOR ABILITY**	**SENSORY ABILITY**
8–10 months	Gains 3–5 oz (85–140 g)/week Grows 1 cm (3/8 in.)/month	Picks up small objects **(12)** Uses pincer grasp well **(14)**	Crawls or pulls whole body along floor by arms **(13)** Creeps by using hands and knees to keep trunk off floor Pulls self to standing and sitting by 10 months Recovers balance when sitting	Understands words such as "no" and "cracker" May say one word in addition to "mama" and "dada" Recognizes sound without difficulty

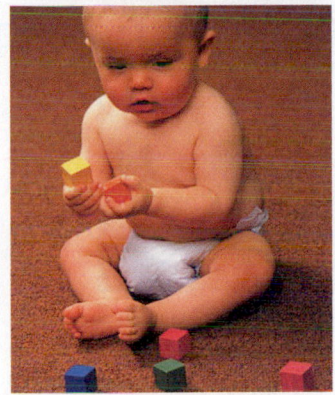

(12) Picks up small objects

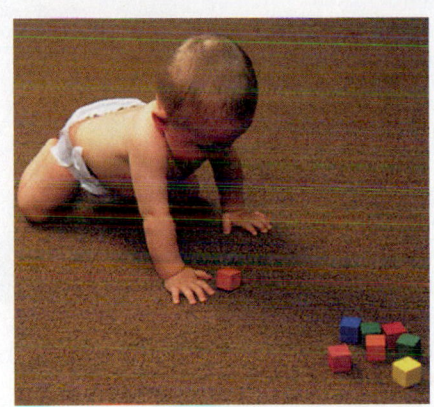

(13) Crawls or pulls body by arms

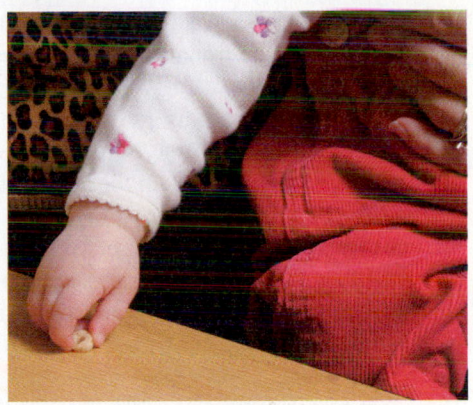

(14) Uses pincer grasp well

10–12 months	Gains 3–5 oz (85–140 g)/week Grows 1 cm (3/8 in.)/month Head circumference equals chest circumference Triples birth weight by 1 year	May hold crayon or pencil and make mark on paper Places objects into containers through holes **(15)**	Stands alone **(16)** Walks holding onto furniture Sits down from standing **(17)**	Plays peek-a-boo and patty cake

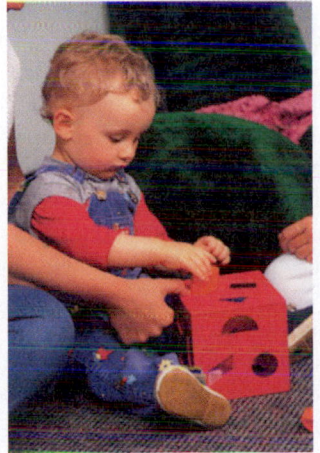

(15) Places objects in container through holes

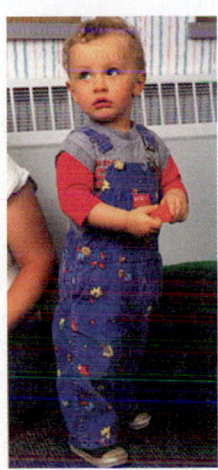

(16) Stands alone

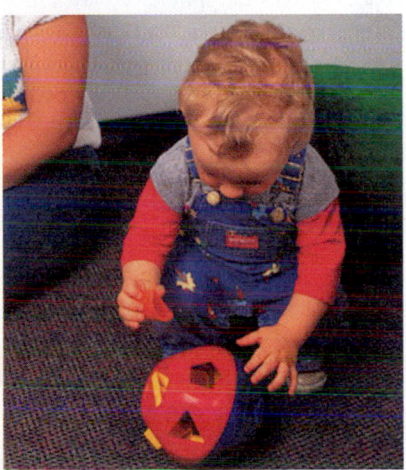

(17) Sits down from standing

Psychosocial Development

Video Stages of Play

An 8-month-old infant is sitting on the floor, grasping blocks and banging them on the floor. Infants spend much of their time engaging in **solitary play,** or playing by themselves. However, when a parent walks by, the infant laughs and waves hands and feet wildly, showing that periodic interactions with others are pleasurable (Figure 5–10 ■). Physical capabilities enable the infant to move toward and reach for objects of interest. Cognitive ability is reflected in manipulation of the blocks to create different sounds. Social interaction enhances play. The presence of a parent or other person increases interest in surroundings and teaches the infant different ways to play.

The play of infants begins in a reflexive manner. When infants move extremities or grasp objects, they experience the foundations of play. They gain pleasure from the feel and sound of these activities, and gradually perform them purposefully. For example, when a parent places a rattle in the hand of a 6-week-old infant, the infant grasps it reflexively. As the hands move randomly, the rattle makes an enjoyable sound. The infant learns to move the rattle to create the sound and then finally to grasp the toy at will to play with it. The next phase of infant play focuses on manipulative behavior. The infant examines toys closely, looking at them, touching them, and placing them in the mouth. The infant learns a great deal about texture, qualities of objects, and all aspects of the surroundings. At the same time, interaction with others becomes an important part of play. The social nature of play is obvious as the infant plays with other children and adults.

Toward the end of the first year, the infant's ability to move in space enlarges the sphere of play. Once infants crawl or walk, they can get to new places, find new toys, discover forgotten objects, or seek out other people for interaction. Play is a reflection of every aspect of development, fostering psychosocial skills and enhancing learning and maturation (Table 5–12).

Personality and Temperament

Why does one infant frequently awaken at night crying whereas another sleeps for 8 to 10 hours undisturbed? Why does one infant smile much of the time and react positively to interactions while another is withdrawn around unfamiliar people and frequently frowns and cries? Such differences in responses to the environment are believed to be inborn characteristics of temperament. Infants are born with a tendency to react in certain ways to noise and to interact differently with people. They may display varying degrees of regularity in activities such as eating and sleeping, and manifest a capacity for concentrating on tasks for different amounts of time.

Nursing assessment identifies personality characteristics of the infant that the nurse can share with the parents. With this information, the parents can appreciate more fully the uniqueness of their infant and design experiences to meet the infant's needs. Parents can learn to modify the environment to promote adaptation. For example, an infant who does not adapt easily to new situations may cry, withdraw, or develop another way of coping when adjusting to new people or places. Parents might be advised to use one or two babysitters rather than engaging new sitters frequently. If the infant is easily distracted when eating, parents can feed the infant in a quiet setting to encourage a focus on eating. Although the infant's temperament is unchanged, the ability to fit with the environment is

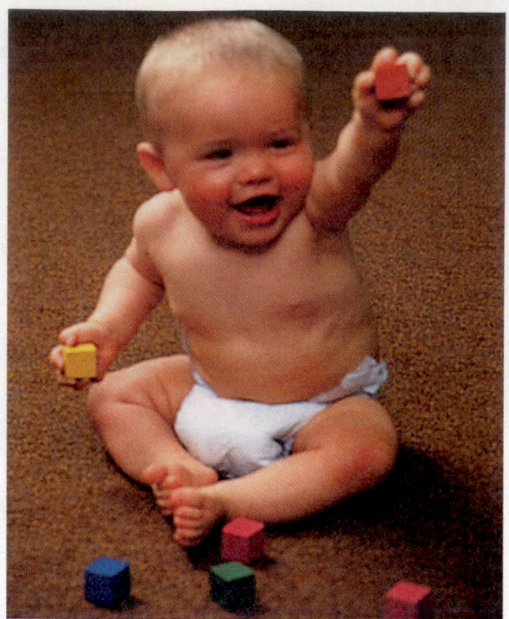

FIGURE 5–10 ■ Garrett shows us that an 8-month-old child can play with blocks, demonstrating physical, cognitive, and social capabilities.

enhanced. See Chapter 10 ⏺ for further ideas about how nurses apply information on infant temperament to health promotion and health maintenance visits.

Communication

Even at a few weeks of age, infants communicate and engage in two-way interaction, and express comfort by soft sounds, cuddling, and eye contact. Newborns respond best to a high-pitched voice, something that most parents inherently seem to know. Even fathers raise their voice to a higher pitch when talking with a young infant. The infant displays discomfort by thrashing the extremities, arching the back, and crying vigorously. From these rudimentary skills, communication ability continues to develop until the infant speaks several words at the end of the first year of life (see Table 5–12).

Nurses assess the infant's communication to identify possible abnormalities or developmental delays. Language ability may be assessed with the Denver II Developmental Test and other specialized language screening tools (see Chapter 8 ⏺). Infants and toddlers understand (**receptive speech**) more words than they can speak (**expressive speech**). Abnormalities may be caused by a hearing deficit, developmental delay, or lack of verbal stimulation from caretakers. Further assessment may be required to pinpoint the cause of an abnormality.

Nursing interventions focus on providing a stimulating and loving environment. Parents are encouraged to speak and sing to infants frequently and teach words. Descriptive verbalizations encourage the infant's speech. For example, when a 1-year-old says "bottle," the parent can say, "Oh you want your warm bottle of milk now? This is your blue bottle." Hospital nurses should include the infant's known words when providing care, and talk to infants using comforting and descriptive terminology. To encourage feelings of security, care providers can hold the infant for feedings, cuddle and play gently often during the day, and swaddle and hold the young infant securely during crying episodes. Parents may enjoy receiving information about how to swaddle the infant or perform infant massage. (See Complementary Therapy: Infant Massage.)

TABLE 5–12	**Psychosocial Development During Infancy**	
AGE	**PLAY AND TOYS**	**COMMUNICATION**
Birth–3 months	Prefers visual stimuli of mobiles, black-and-white patterns, mirrors	Coos
	Auditory stimuli are music boxes, tape players, soft voices	Babbles
	Responds to rocking and cuddling	Cries
	Moves legs and arms while adult sings and talks	
	Likes varying stimuli—different rooms, sounds, visual images	
3–6 months	Prefers noisemaking objects that are easily grasped like rattles	Vocalizes during play and with familiar people
	Enjoys stuffed animals and soft toys with contrasting colors	Laughs
		Cries less
		Squeals and makes pleasure sounds
		Babbles multisyllabically (mamamamama)
6–9 months	Likes teething toys	Increases vowel and consonant sounds
	Increasingly desires social interaction with adults and other children	Links syllables together
	Soft toys that can be manipulated and mouthed are favorites	Uses speechlike rhythm when vocalizing with others
9–12 months	Enjoys large blocks, toys that pop apart and go back together, nesting cups, and other objects	Understands "no" and other simple commands
	Laughs at surprise toys like jack-in-the-box	Says "dada" and "mama" to identify parents
	Plays interactive games like peek-a-boo	Learns one or two other words
	Uses push-and-pull toys	Receptive speech surpasses expressive speech

Complementary Therapy Infant Massage

Infant massage is a technique for communicating with and soothing infants. It has been used in many cultures throughout history, but it is not traditional within most families in the United States and Canada. It has many benefits both for infants and parents and can be taught to families who are interested. Premature infants are particularly benefited from this intervention. Some of the benefits for babies include improved sleep, soothability, decreased stress hormones, improved respiratory and gastrointestinal function, and positive parent–child interaction. Preterm infants have improved weight gain, gastric motility, and bone density with shorter hospital stays (Field, Diego, & Hernandez-Reif, 2010). Massage periods of 10 to 15 minutes daily can be encouraged and facilitated to enhance bonding and attachment between parents and infant. Several books and massage classes are available for the nurse or parent desiring to learn more about this technique.

TODDLER (1 TO 3 YEARS)

Toddlerhood is sometimes called the first adolescence. An infant only months before, the child from 1 to 3 years displays independence and negativism. Pride in newfound accomplishments emerges.

Physical Growth and Development

The rate of growth slows during the second year of life. Parents may become concerned because the child has a limited intake and may need reassurance that this is normal. See Chapter 19 🖉 for further discussion of nutrition in toddlerhood. By age 2 years, the birth weight has usually quadrupled and the child is about one half of the adult height. Body proportions begin to change, with legs longer and head smaller in proportion to body size than during infancy (see Figure 5–9). The toddler has a pot-bellied appearance and stands with feet apart to provide a wide base of support. By approximately 33 months, eruption of deciduous teeth is complete, with 20 teeth present.

Gross motor activity develops rapidly (Table 5–13), as the toddler progresses from walking to running, kicking, and riding a tricycle (Figure 5–11 ■). As physical maturation occurs, the toddler develops the ability to control elimination patterns. See Chapter 11 🖉 for a discussion of the nurse's role in assisting parents in the process of toilet training toddlers, and Developing Cultural Competence: Toilet Training. See Table 11–1 in Chapter 11 for a detailed list of the developmental milestones of toddlerhood.

Cognitive Development

During the toddler years, the child moves from the sensorimotor to the preoperational stage of development. The early use of language awakens in the 1-year-old the ability to think about objects or people when they are absent. Object permanence is well developed.

At about 2 years of age, the increasing use of words as symbols enables the toddler to use preoperational thought. Rudimentary problem solving, creative thought, and an understanding of cause-and-effect relationships are now possible.

TABLE 5–13	Physical Growth and Development Milestones During Toddlerhood			
AGE	PHYSICAL GROWTH	FINE MOTOR ABILITY	GROSS MOTOR ABILITY	SENSORY ABILITY
1–2 years	Gains 8 oz (227 g) or more per month Grows 3.5–5 in. (9–12 cm) during this year Anterior fontanel closes	By end of second year, builds a tower of four blocks **(1)** Scribbles on paper **(2)** Can undress self **(3)** Throws a ball	Runs Shows growing ability to walk, and finally walks with ease Walks up and down stairs a few months after learning to walk with ease **(5)** Likes push-and-pull toys	Visual acuity 20/50
2–3 years	Gains 1.4–2.3 kg (3–5 lb)/year Grows 5–6.5 cm (2–2.5 in.)/year	Draws a circle and other rudimentary forms Learns to pour Learning to dress self **(4)**	Jumps Kicks ball Throws ball overhand	

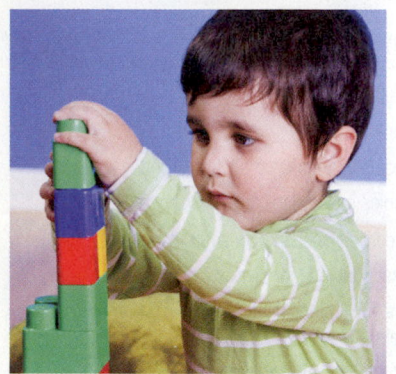

(1) Builds tower of four blocks

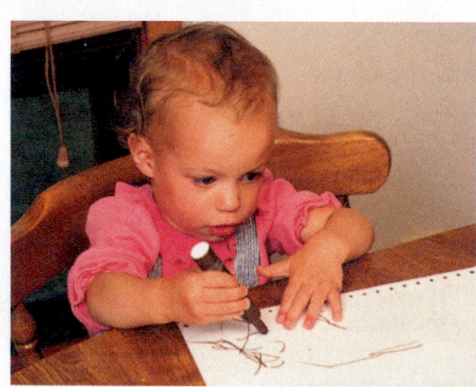

(2) Scribbles on paper

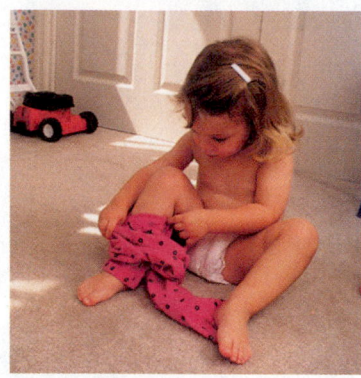

(3) Can undress self

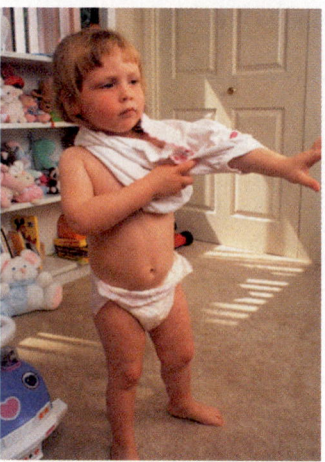

(4) Learning to dress self

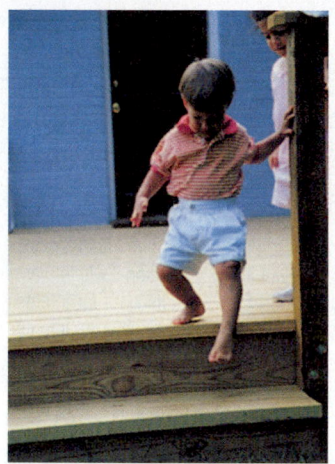

(5) Walks up and down stairs

Source: (1) Fernando Cortes/Shutterstock.

Psychosocial Development

Play

Many changes in play patterns occur between infancy and toddlerhood. Developing motor skills enable toddlers to bang pegs into a pounding board with a hammer. The social nature of toddler play is also readily seen. Toddlers find the company of other children pleasurable, even though socially interactive play may not occur. Two toddlers tend to play with similar objects side by side, occasionally trading toys and words. This is called **parallel play.** This playtime with other children assists toddlers to develop social skills. Toddlers engage in play activities they have seen at home, such as talking on the phone. This imitative behavior teaches new actions and skills (Figure 5–12 ■).

Physical skills are manifested in play as toddlers push and pull objects, climb in and out and up and down, run, ride a tricycle with big wheels, turn the pages of books, and scribble with a pen. Both gross motor and fine motor abilities are enhanced during this age period.

Cognitive understanding enables the toddler to manipulate objects and learn about their qualities. Stacking blocks and placing rings on a building tower teach spatial relationships and other lessons that provide a foundation for future learning. Various kinds of play objects should be provided for the toddler to meet play needs.

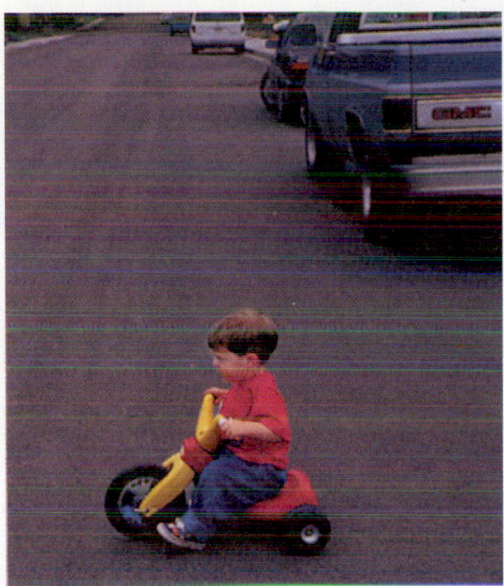

FIGURE 5–11 ■ This toddler has learned to ride a Big Wheel tricycle, which he is doing right into the street. Toddlers must be closely watched to prevent injury.

Developing Cultural Competence
Toilet Training

In traditional Native American families, children are allowed to unfold and develop naturally at their own pace. Children thus wean and toilet train themselves with little interference or pressure from parents. In other groups, toilet training is accomplished at an early age. Nurses should honor the beliefs and practices of families rather than suggesting that one approach, for example, a single age for toilet training, is right for all families and situations.

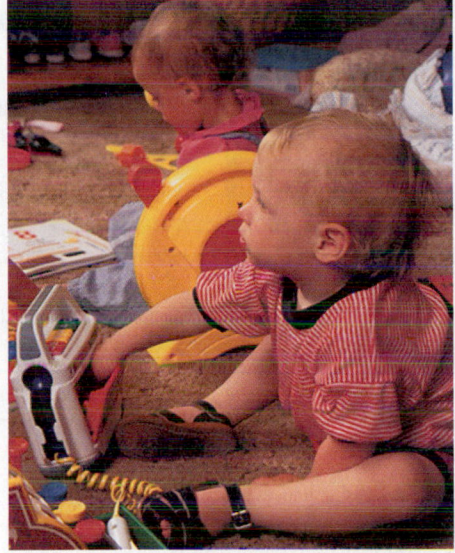

A

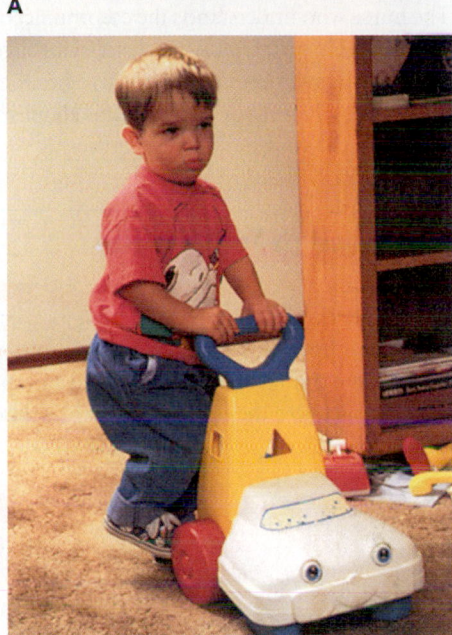

B

FIGURE 5–12 ■ *A,* Two children are displaying typical parallel play since they enjoy playing near other children, but are not engaging in social interactions with each other. Which cognitive and motor skills are these children developing? *B,* Imitative play such as pushing and pulling a vacuum allows this toddler to develop gross and fine motor skills.

These play needs can easily be met whether the child is hospitalized or at home (Table 5–14).

Personality and Temperament

The toddler retains most of the temperamental characteristics identified during infancy, but may demonstrate some changes. The normal developmental progression of toddlerhood also plays a part in responses. For example, the infant who previously responded positively to stimuli, such as a new baby-sitter, may appear more negative in toddlerhood. The increasing independence characteristic of this age is shown by the toddler's use of the word *no.* The parent and child constantly adapt their responses to each other and learn anew how to communicate with each other.

Communication

Because of the phenomenal growth of language skills during the toddler period, adults should communicate frequently with children in this age group. Toddlers imitate words and speech intonations, as well as the social interactions they observe.

At the beginning of toddlerhood, the child may use four to six words in addition to "mama" and "dada." Receptive speech (the ability to understand words) far outpaces expressive speech. By the end of toddlerhood, however, the 3-year-old has a vocabulary of almost 1,000 words and uses short sentences.

Communication occurs in many ways, some of which are nonverbal. Toddler communication includes pointing, pulling an adult over to a room or object, and speaking in **expressive jargon** (using unintelligible words with normal speech intonations as if truly communicating in words). Another communication method occurs when the toddler cries, pounds feet, displays a temper tantrum, or uses other means to illustrate dismay. These powerful communication methods can upset parents, who often need suggestions for handling them. It is best to verbalize the feelings shown by the toddler, for example, by saying, "You must be very upset that you cannot have that candy. When you stop crying you can come out of your room," and then to ignore further negative behavior. The toddler's search for autonomy and independence creates a need for such behavior. Sometimes an upset toddler responds well to holding, rocking, and stroking.

TABLE 5–14	**Psychosocial Development During Toddlerhood**	
AGE	**PLAY AND TOYS**	**COMMUNICATION**
1–3 years 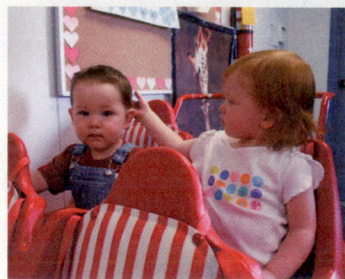	Refines fine motor skills by use of cloth books, large pencil and paper, wooden puzzles Facilitates imitative behavior by playing kitchen, grocery shopping, toy telephone Learns gross motor activities by riding tricycle with big wheels, playing with soft ball and bat, molding water and sand, tossing ball or beanbag Develops cognitive skills through educational television shows, music, stories, and books	Increasingly enjoys talking Exponential growth of vocabulary especially when spoken and read to regularly Needs to release stress by pounding board, frequent gross motor activities, and occasional temper tantrums Likes contact with other children and learns interpersonal skills

The toddler from a bilingual home is at an optimal age to learn two languages. If the parents do not speak English, the toddler will benefit from a childcare experience because both languages can then be learned. The nurse who understands the communication skills of toddlers is able to assess expressive and receptive language and communicate effectively, thereby promoting positive healthcare experiences for these children. Parents often need ideas about strategies for communication with the young child. See Partnering with Families: Communicating with a Toddler.

PRESCHOOL CHILD (3 TO 6 YEARS)

The preschool years are a time of new initiative and independence. Most children are in a childcare center or school for part of the day and learn a great deal from this social contact. Language skills are well developed, and the child is able to understand and speak clearly. Endless projects characterize the world of busy preschoolers. They may work with play dough to form animals, then cut out and paste paper, then draw and color (Figure 5–13 ■).

Physical Growth and Development

Preschoolers grow slowly and steadily, with most growth taking place in long bones of the arms and legs. The short, chubby toddler gradually gives way to a slender, long-legged preschooler (Table 5–15).

Physical skills continue to develop (Figure 5–14 ■). The preschooler runs with ease, holds a bat, and throws balls of various types. Writing ability increases, and the preschooler enjoys drawing and learning to write a few letters. The preschooler becomes interested in the body and its function. The nurse can teach hand washing, general hygiene, dental care, and other health promotion topics to both parents and child. See Chapter 11 🔗 for further information about partnering with families to promote and maintain health of preschoolers.

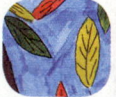 # Partnering with Families

Communicating with a Toddler

Procedures such as drawing blood, getting immunizations, or even having ears checked can be frightening for a toddler. Parents and nurses can partner to provide effective communication that minimizes the trauma caused by such procedures. Nurses should give the following suggestions to parents when their toddler needs a healthcare procedure:

- Avoid telling toddlers about the procedure too far in advance. They do not have an understanding of time and can become quite anxious. Telling them just before the procedure begins is most appropriate.
- Use simple terminology: "We need to get a little blood from your arm. It will help us to find out if you are getting better." If the parent is willing to hold the child, he or she can say, "I will hold your arm still so the nurse can do it quickly." Approach positively and confidently.
- Give short, clear instructions. Do not give choices if none exist. Offer a choice of two alternatives when possible. "Would you like apple or grape juice after you drink this medicine?"
- Tell the toddler what is being done; name objects. For example, "The nurse can hear your heart through that stethoscope. Let's listen. . . ."
- Allow the toddler to cry. Acknowledge that it must be frightening and that you understand. Allow the child to cry out during a procedure or other frightening event.

- If in a hospital or clinic, ask if frightening or painful procedures can be performed in a treatment room so that the toddler's room and the clinic examination room are both safe havens.
- Be sure the toddler is restrained, with the joints above and below the procedure immobilized so the procedure can be quickly accomplished with the least trauma. The nurse should ask the parent if he or she wishes to hold the child, and if so, explain how to position the child safely and securely.
- Use a Band-Aid to cover the site and to reassure the toddler that the body is still intact.
- Allow the toddler to choose a reward such as a sticker after the procedure. Bring the child to a special place like the library or a playroom, and do an activity together if possible.
- Praise the toddler for cooperation, and acknowledge that you know this was difficult.
- Comfort the toddler by rocking, offering a favorite drink, playing music, and holding. Parents are the best comfort a child has when undergoing stressful procedures.

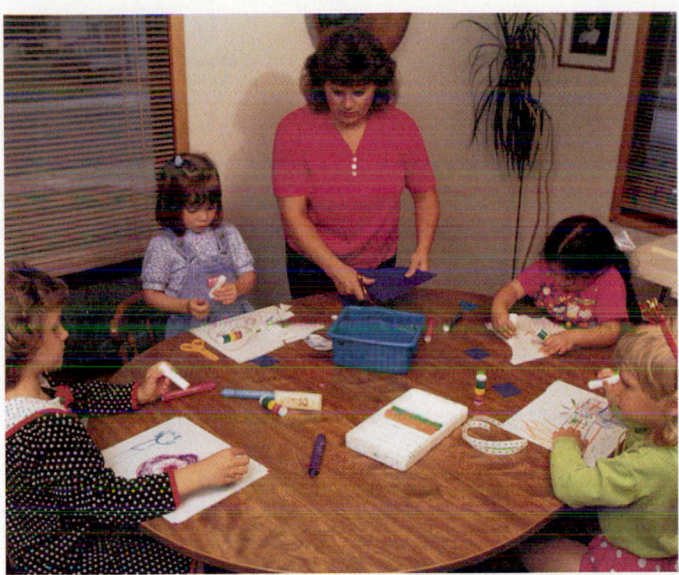

FIGURE 5–13 ■ Preschoolers have well-developed language, motor, and social skills, and they can work creatively together on an art project, as this group is doing at an in-home childcare center.

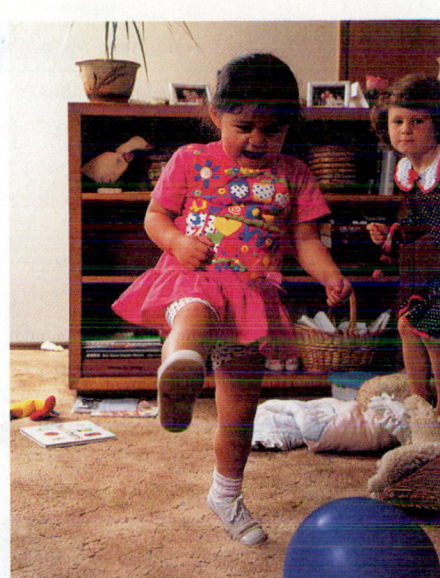

FIGURE 5–14 ■ Preschoolers continue to develop more advanced motor skills, such as kicking a ball without falling down.

Cognitive Development

The preschooler exhibits characteristics of preoperational thought. Symbols or words are used to represent objects and people, enabling the young child to think about them. This is a milestone in intellectual development; however, the preschooler still has some limitations in thought (Table 5–16). According to Piaget, the young child does not have "less thought" than adults, but the thought is qualitatively different. Understanding the child's thought will help you to explain procedures, conduct health teaching, and communicate more effectively with the preschooler. For example, as you plan to teach about how hand washing can prevent colds, what connections will you need to make for the preschooler? Consider the transductive reasoning of the child and formulate an effective teaching approach.

Psychosocial Development

Play

The preschooler has begun to play in a new way. Toddlers simply play side by side with friends, each engaging in his or her own activities; but preschoolers interact with others during play. One child cuts out colored paper while her friend glues it on paper in a design. This new type of interaction is called **associative play,** and it is characterized by children interacting in groups and participating in similar activities (Figure 5–15A ■). The child life therapist in hospital settings recognizes the therapeutic value of play in planning activities for children that enable them to work through feelings about procedures and separation, as well as facilitating the normal developmental need for interaction with other children. The role of the child life therapist is further discussed in Chapter 15 🕑.

In addition to this social dimension of play, other aspects of play also differ. The preschooler enjoys large motor activities such as swinging, riding a tricycle, and throwing a ball. Increasing manual dexterity is demonstrated in greater complexity of drawings and manipulation of blocks and modeling. These changes necessitate

planning of playtime to include appropriate activities. Preschool programs and child life departments in hospitals help meet this important need.

Materials provided for play can be simple but should guide activities in which the child engages. Because fine motor activities are popular, paper, pens, scissors, glue, and a variety of other such objects should be available. The child can use them to create important images such as pictures of people, hospital beds, or friends. A collection of dolls, furniture, and clothing can be manipulated to represent parents and children, nurses and physicians, teachers, or other significant people. Because fantasy life is so powerful at this age, the preschooler readily uses props to engage in **dramatic play,** that is, living out the drama of human life (Figure 5–15B ■).

The nurse can use playtime to assess the preschooler's developmental level, knowledge about health care, and emotions related to healthcare experiences. Observations about objects chosen for play, content of dramatic play, and pictures drawn can provide important assessment data. The nurse can also use play periods to teach the child about healthcare procedures and offer an outlet for expression of emotions (see Table 5–16). See Chapter 15 🕑 for further information about use of play with hospitalized children, and Chapter 33 🕑 for a description of play therapy with children who have psychiatric and mental health needs.

Personality and Temperament

Characteristics of personality observed in infancy tend to persist over time. The preschooler may need assistance as these characteristics are expressed in the new situations of preschool or nursery school. An excessively active child, for example, will need gentle, consistent handling to adjust to the structure of a classroom. Encourage parents to visit preschool programs to choose one that would best foster growth in their child. Some preschoolers enjoy the structured learning of a program that focuses on cognitive skills, whereas others are happier and more open to learning in a small group that provides much time for free play. Nurses can help parents to identify their

TABLE 5–15	Physical Growth and Development Milestones During the Preschool Years		
PHYSICAL GROWTH	**FINE MOTOR ABILITY**	**GROSS MOTOR ABILITY**	**SENSORY ABILITY**
Gains 1.5–2.5 kg (3–5 lb)/year	Uses scissors **(1)**	Throws a ball overhand	Visual acuity continues to improve
Grows 4–6 cm (1 1/2–2 1/2 in.)/year	Draws circle, square, cross **(2)**	Climbs well **(6)**	Can focus on and learn letters and numbers **(8)**
	Draws at least a six-part person	Rides tricycle **(7)**	
	Enjoys art projects such as pasting, stringing beads, using clay		
	Learns to tie shoes at end of preschool years **(3)**		
	Buttons **(4)**		
	Brushes teeth **(5)**		
	Uses spoon, fork, knife		

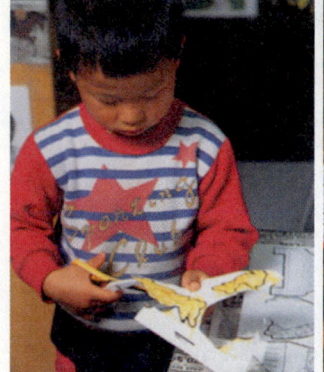

(1) Uses scissors

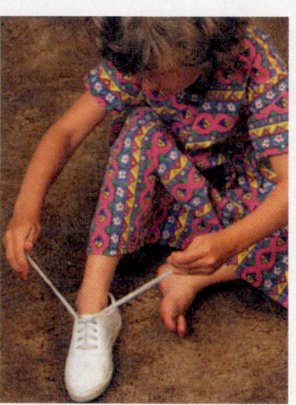

(2) Draws circle, square, cross

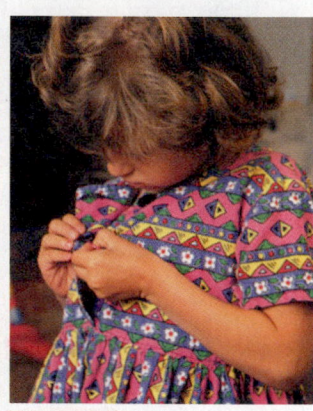

(3) Ties shoes

(4) Buttons clothes

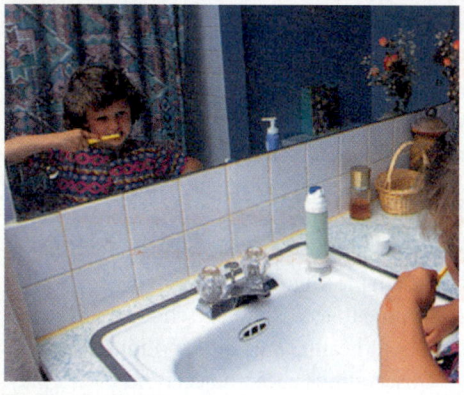

(5) Brushes teeth

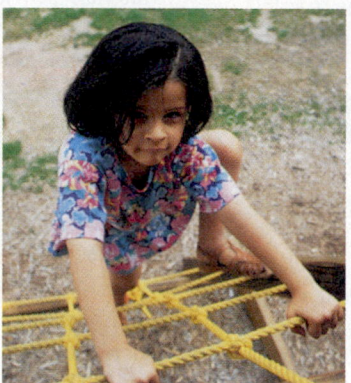

(6) Climbs well

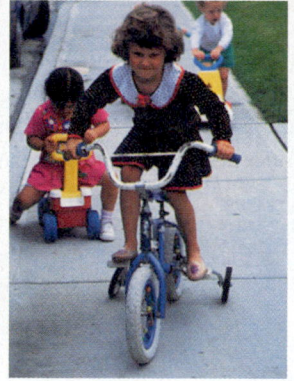

(7) Rides tricycle or bicycle with training wheels

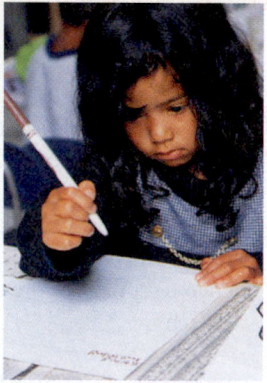

(8) Learns letters and numbers

TABLE 5–16	Psychosocial Development During Preschool Years	
AGE	**PLAY AND TOYS**	**COMMUNICATION**
3–6 years	Associative play is facilitated by simple games, puzzles, nursery rhymes, and songs.	All parts of speech are developed and used, occasionally incorrectly.
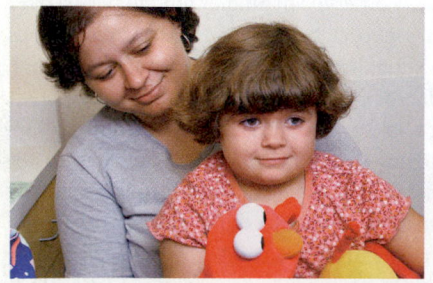	Dramatic play is fostered by dolls and doll clothes, play houses and hospitals, dress-up clothes, and puppets.	The child communicates with a widening array of people.
	Stress is relieved by pens, paper, glue, and scissors.	Play with other children is a favorite activity.
	Cognitive growth is fostered by educational television shows, music, stories, and books.	Health professionals can:
		■ Verbalize and explain procedures to children.
		■ Use drawings and stories to explain care.
		■ Use accurate names for body functions.
		■ Allow the child to talk, ask questions, and make choices.

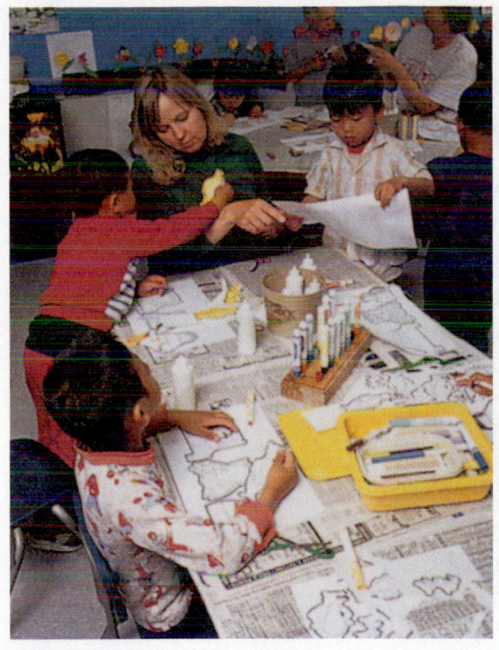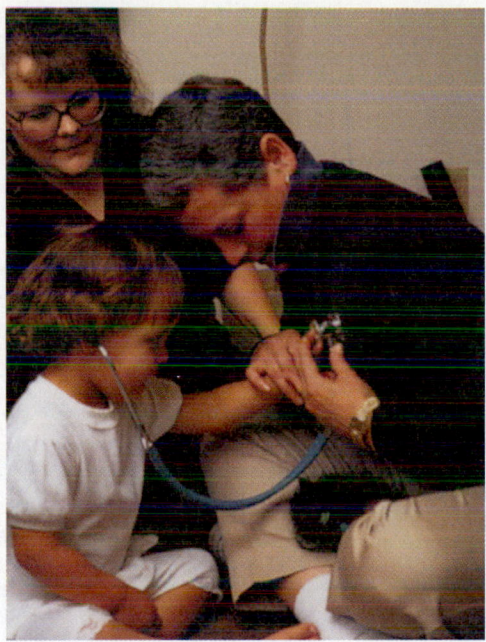

A

B

FIGURE 5–15 ■ *A*, These preschoolers are participating in associative play, which means that they can interact with each other. One child is cutting out shapes, and the other is gluing them in place. *B*, Jasmine is participating in dramatic play with a nurse while her mother looks on. In dramatic play, the child uses props to play out the drama of life. It can be an excellent way for a nurse to assess the developmental level of children while talking to them. Notice that the child and the nurse are on the floor at the same level and that the atmosphere is informal. Why is it important to be at the same level as the child?

child's personality or temperament characteristics and to find the best environment for growth.

Communication

Language skills blossom during the preschool years. The vocabulary grows to over 2,000 words, and children speak in complete sentences of several words and use all parts of speech. They practice these new-found language skills by endlessly talking and asking questions.

The sophisticated speech of preschoolers mirrors the development occurring in their minds and helps them to learn about the world around them. However, this speech can be quite deceptive. Although preschoolers use many words, their grasp of meaning is usually literal and may not match that of adults. These literal interpretations have important implications for healthcare providers:

- The preschooler who is told she will be "put to sleep" for surgery may think of a pet recently euthanized.
- The child who is told that a dye will be injected for a diagnostic test may think he is going to die.
- Mention of "a little stick" in the arm can cause images of tree branches rather than of a simple immunization.
- The nurse's explanation that a shot is "like a mosquito bite" may signal the idea of buzzing and itching for a child.

The child may also have difficulty focusing on the content of a conversation. The preschooler is unable to consider the perspective of another and may be unable to move from individual thoughts to those the nurse is proposing, as the following conversation illustrates:

Nurse: I'd like to tell you about the operation that you will have tomorrow.

Sharisse: OK. Did you know my brother just got a new squirt gun?

Nurse: That's nice. Now, first thing in the morning you will wake up early and your foot will be scrubbed with a special soap.

Sharisse: The gun can spurt for about 40 feet—you have to pump it up.

Nurse: We'll talk about that later. Let me tell you about your operation now. After your foot is scrubbed, the nurse will measure your blood pressure and temperature and feel the pulse in your arm. Do you remember me doing those things today?

Sharisse: Yes. And I got a sticker when I came into the hospital today, too. Do you know that my Mom is going to stay here tonight?

During this interchange, Sharisse engages in **collective monologue,** in which separate conversations occur even though each person waits for the other to speak. Though waiting for the nurse to speak, Sharisse is not generally responding to the nurse's content but is instead focusing on content from her own mind. She exhibits centration or a focus on just one aspect of a situation (the squirt gun). The nurse needs to respond to Sharisse's content and then reinsert more facts about the preparations for surgery.

Concrete visual aids such as pictures of a child undergoing the same procedure or a book to read together enhance teaching by meeting the child's developmental needs. Handling medical equipment such as intravenous bags and stethoscopes increases interest and helps the child to focus. Teaching may have to be done in several short sessions rather than one long session. Use short, directive approaches: "I know this hurts; it will feel like a pinch. It will be over soon. Hold your mom's hand and let's count while we give you this medicine. One, two, three, four, oh it's over!"

SCHOOL-AGE CHILD (6 TO 12 YEARS)

Errol, 10 years old, arrives home from school shortly after 3 p.m. each day. He immediately calls his friends and goes to visit one of them. They are building models of cars and collecting baseball cards. Hours are spent on these projects and on discussions of events at school that day (Figure 5–16 ■).

Nine-year-old Karen practices soccer two afternoons a week and plays in games each weekend. She also is learning to play the flut

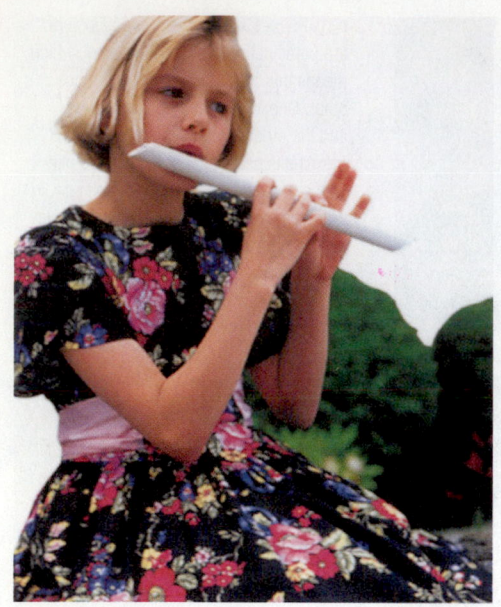

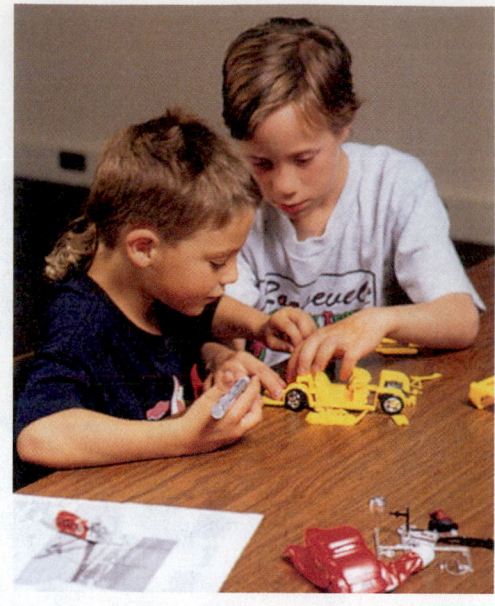

A   **B**

FIGURE 5–16 ■ *A,* School-age children may take part in activities that require practice. This is a consideration when children are hospitalized and unable to practice or perform. Why? *B,* School-age children enjoy spending time with others the same age on projects and discussing the activities of the day. This is an important consideration when they are in an acute care setting. When you are in the clinical setting, look for examples of this type of interaction taking place.

and spends her free time at home practicing. Although practice time is not her favorite part of music, Karen enjoys the performances and wants to play well in front of her friends and teacher. Her parents now allow her to ride her bike unaccompanied to the store or to a friend's house.

These two school-age children demonstrate common characteristics of their age group. They are in a stage of industry in which it is important to the child to perform useful work. Meaningful activities take on great importance and are usually carried out in the company of peers. A sense of achievement in these activities is important to develop self-esteem and to prevent a sense of inferiority or poor self-worth.

Physical Growth and Development

School age is the last period in which girls and boys are close in size and body proportions. As the long bones continue to grow, leg length increases (see Figure 5–9). Fat gives way to muscle, and the child appears leaner. Jaw proportions change as the first deciduous tooth is lost at 6 years and permanent teeth begin to erupt. Body organs and the immune system mature, resulting in fewer illnesses among school-age children. Medications are less likely to cause serious side effects, because they can be metabolized more easily. The urinary system can adjust to changes in fluid status. Physical skills are also refined as children begin to play sports, and fine motor skills are well developed through school activities (Table 5–17).

TABLE 5–17	Physical Growth and Development Milestones During the School-Age Years		
PHYSICAL GROWTH	**FINE MOTOR ABILITY**	**GROSS MOTOR ABILITY**	**SENSORY ABILITY**
Gains 1.4–2.2 kg (3–5 lb)/year	Enjoys craft projects	Rides two-wheeler **(1)**	Can read
Grows 4–6 cm (1 1/2–2 1/2 in.)/year	Plays card and board games	Jumps rope **(2)**	Able to concentrate for longer periods on activities by filtering out surrounding sounds **(3)**
		Roller skates or ice skates	

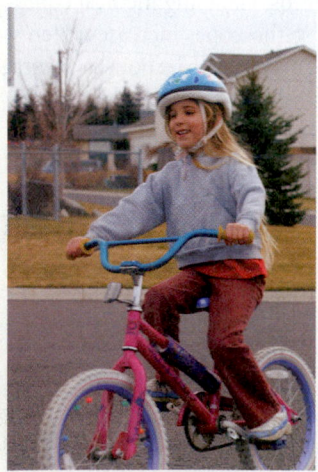

(1) Rides two-wheeler

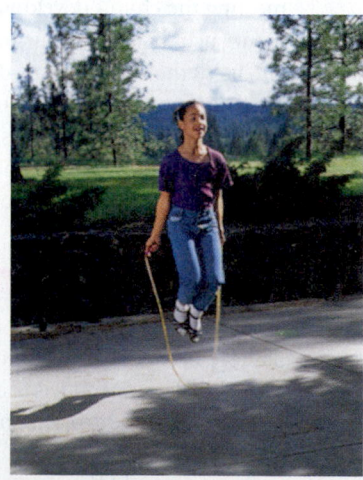

(2) Jumps rope

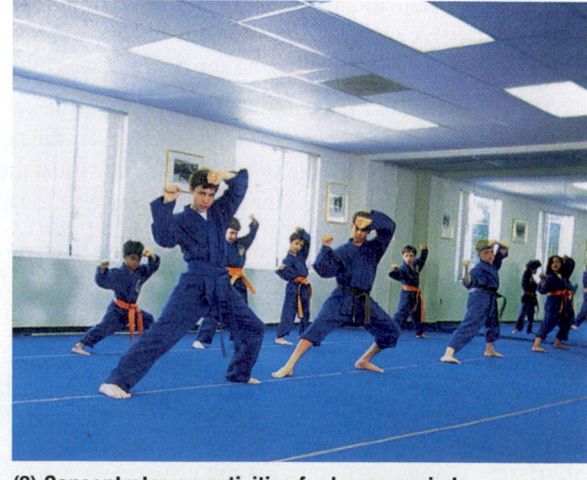

(3) Concentrates on activities for longer periods

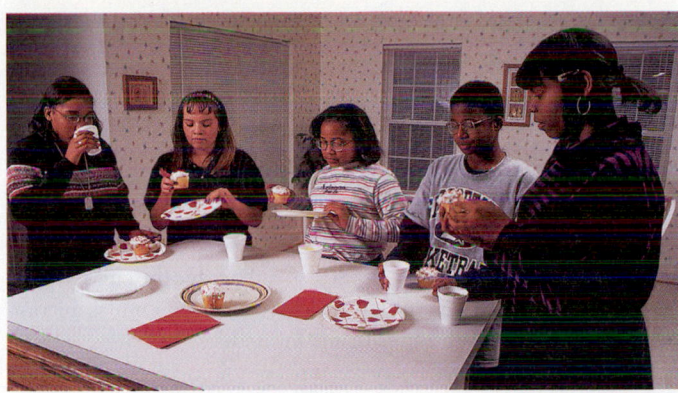

FIGURE 5–17 ■ Because girls have a growth spurt earlier than boys, girls often are taller than boys of the same age. Remember what it was like at your first dance?

Although it is commonly believed that the start of adolescence (age 12 years) heralds a growth spurt, the rapid increases in size commonly occur during school age. Girls may begin a growth spurt by 9 or 10 years and boys a year or so later (Figure 5–17 ■). Nutritional needs increase dramatically with this spurt.

The loss of the first deciduous teeth and the eruption of permanent teeth usually occur at about age 6 years, or at the beginning of the school-age period. Of the 32 permanent teeth, 22 to 26 erupt by age 12 years and the remaining molars follow during the teenage years. The school-age child should be closely monitored to ensure that brushing and flossing are adequate, that fluoride is taken if the water supply is not fluoridated, that dental care is obtained to provide for examination of teeth and alignment, and that loose teeth are identified before surgery or other events that may lead to loss of a tooth.

Cognitive Development

The child enters the stage of concrete operational thought at about 7 years. This stage enables school-age children to consider alternative solutions and solve problems. However, school-age children continue to rely on concrete experiences and materials to form their thought content.

During the school-age years, the child learns the concept of **conservation** (that matter is not changed when its form is altered). At earlier ages, a child believes that when water is poured from a short, wide glass into a tall, thin glass, there is more water in the taller glass. The school-age child recognizes that although it may look like the taller glass holds more water, the quantity is the same. The concept of conservation is helpful when the nurse explains medical treatments. The school-age child understands that an incision will heal, that a cast will be removed, and that an arm will look the same as before once the intravenous infusion is removed.

Psychosocial Development

Play

When a preschool teacher tries to organize a game of baseball, both the teacher and the children become frustrated. Not only are the children physically unable to hold a bat and hit a ball, but they also seem to have no understanding of the rules of the game and do not want to wait for their turn at bat. By 6 years of age, however, children have acquired the physical ability to hold the bat properly and may occasionally hit the ball. School-age children also understand that everyone has a role—the pitcher, the catcher, the batter, the outfielders. They cooperate with one another to form a team, are eager to learn the rules of the game, and want to ensure that these rules are followed exactly (Table 5–18).

The characteristics of play exhibited by the school-age child are cooperation with others and the ability to play a part in order to contribute to a unified whole. This type of play is called **cooperative play.** The concrete nature of cognitive thought leads to a reliance on rules to provide structure and security. Children have an increasing desire to spend much of playtime with friends, which demonstrates the social component of play. Play is an extremely important method of learning and living for the school-age child. Active physical play has decreased in recent years as television viewing and playing of computer games have increased, leading to poor nutritional status and other health risks in children. See Chapter 19 🔗 for further discussion of nutrition and physical activity in children.

When a child is hospitalized, the separation from playmates can lead to feelings of sadness and purposelessness. School-age children often feel better when placed in multibed units with other children. Games can be devised even when children are using wheelchairs (Figure 5–18 ■). Normal, rewarding parts of play should be integrated into care. Friends should be encouraged to visit or call a hospitalized child. Discharge planning for the child who has had a cast

TABLE 5–18	Psychosocial Development During the School-Age Years	
AGE	**ACTIVITIES**	**COMMUNICATION**
6–12 years	Gross motor development is fostered by ball sports, skating, dance lessons, water and snow skiing/boarding, and biking.	Mature use of language
	A sense of industry is fostered by playing a musical instrument, gathering collections, starting hobbies, and playing board and video games.	Ability to converse and discuss topics for increasing lengths of time
	Cognitive growth is facilitated by reading, crafts, word puzzles, and schoolwork.	Spends many hours at school and with friends in sports or other activities
		Health professionals can:
		■ Assess the child's knowledge before teaching
		■ Allow the child to select rewards following procedures
		■ Teach techniques such as counting or visualization to manage difficult situations
		■ Include both parent and child in healthcare decisions

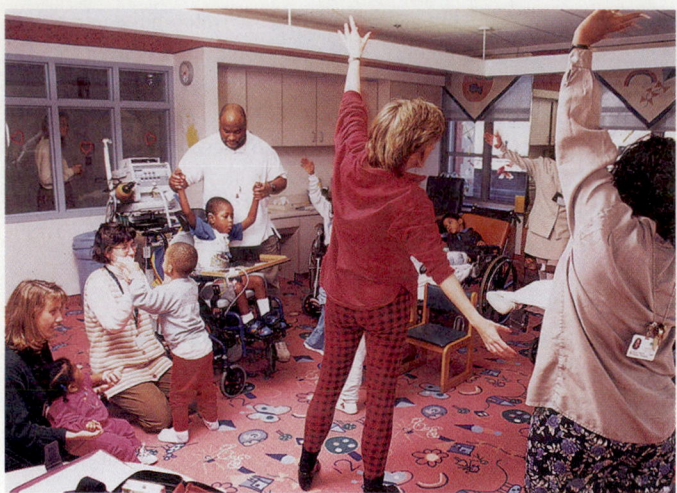

FIGURE 5–18 ■ The nurse can help the child and family accept and adjust to new circumstances. Encouraging the child who uses a wheelchair to participate in group activities can help build confidence in physical skills. Good self-esteem, goal attainment, personal satisfaction, and general health are the continued benefits.

or brace applied should address the activities in which the child can participate and those the child must avoid. Reinforce the importance of playing games with friends.

Personality and Temperament

The enduring aspects of temperament continue to be manifested during the school years. The child classified as "difficult" at an earlier age may now have trouble in the classroom. Advise parents to provide a quiet setting for homework and to reward the child for concentration. For example, after homework is completed, the child may play a game with the parent. Creative efforts and alternative methods of learning should be valued. Encourage parents to see their children as individuals who may not all learn in the same way. The "slow-to-warm-up" child may need encouragement to try new activities and to share experiences with others, whereas the "easy" child will readily adapt to new schools, people, and experiences.

Communication

During the school-age years, the child should learn how to correct any lingering pronunciation or grammatical errors. Vocabulary increases, and the child learns about parts of speech in school. School-age children enjoy writing and can be encouraged to keep a journal of their experiences while in the hospital as a method of dealing with anxiety. The literal translation of words characteristic of preschoolers is uncommon among school-age children; they understand the meaning of phrases such as being "put to sleep" or "getting a little stick in the arm."

Sexuality

Although children become aware of sexual differences between genders during preschool years, they deal much more consciously with sexuality during school age. As children mature physically, they need information about their body changes so that they can develop a healthy self-image and an understanding of the relationships between their bodies and sexuality. Children become interested in sexual issues and are often exposed to erroneous information on television shows, in magazines, or from friends and siblings. Schools and families need to use opportunities to teach school-age children

factual information about sex and to foster healthy concepts of self and others. It is advisable to ask occasional questions about sexual issues to learn how much the child knows and to provide correct information when answers demonstrate confusion. Appropriate and inappropriate touch should be discussed, with lists of trusted people who can be approached (teachers, clergy, school counselors, family members, neighbors) to discuss any episodes with which the child feels uncomfortable. Recognize that even these trusted people can be implicated in inappropriate episodes, so encourage the child to go to more than one person, an important approach if the child is uncomfortable about a relationship with any individual.

ADOLESCENT (12 TO 18 YEARS)

Adolescence is a time of passage, signaling the end of childhood and the beginning of adulthood. Although adolescents differ in behaviors and accomplishments, they are in a period of identity formation. If a healthy identity and sense of self-worth are not developed in this period, role confusion and purposeless struggling will ensue. The adolescents in your care will represent various degrees of identity formation, and each will offer unique challenges.

Physical Growth and Development

The physical changes ending in **puberty,** or sexual maturity, begin near the end of the school-age period. The prepubescent period is marked by a growth spurt at an average age of 10 years for girls and 13 years for boys. The increase in height and weight is generally remarkable and is completed in 2 to 3 years (Table 5–19). The growth spurt in girls is accompanied by an increase in breast size and growth of pubic hair. Menstruation occurs last and signals achievement of puberty. In boys, the growth spurt is accompanied by growth in size of the penis and testes and by growth of pubic hair. Deepening of the voice and growth of facial hair occur later, at the time of puberty. See Chapter 7 ⊘ for a description of the pubertal stages.

During adolescence children grow stronger and more muscular and establish characteristic male and female patterns of fat distribution. The apocrine and eccrine glands mature, leading to increased sweating and a distinct odor to perspiration. All body organs are now fully mature, enabling the adolescent to take adult doses of medications.

The adolescent must adapt to a rapidly changing body for several years. Height, weight, and body proportions increase. Such changes occur with great variability so an adolescent may be at different points of maturation than peers. These physical changes, hormonal variations, and differences in timing offer challenges to identity formation. The adolescent must incorporate the new body and its functions, and retain a healthy sense of self in relationship to peers. The formation of self-identity is a psychologic process but is necessarily closely connected with the body changes occurring.

Cognitive Development

Adolescence marks the beginning of Piaget's last stage of cognitive development, the stage of formal operational thought. The adolescent no longer depends on concrete experiences as the basis of thought but develops the ability to reason abstractly. Concepts such as justice, truth, beauty, and power can be understood. The adolescent revels in this newfound ability and spends a great deal of time thinking, reading, and talking about abstract concepts.

TABLE 5–19	Physical Growth and Development Milestones During Adolescence			
PHYSICAL GROWTH		**FINE MOTOR ABILITY**	**GROSS MOTOR ABILITY**	**SENSORY ABILITY**
Variation in age of growth spurt During growth spurt, girls gain 7–25 kg (15–55 lb) and grow 2.5–20 cm (2–8 in.); boys gain approximately 7–29.5 kg (15–65 lb) and grow 11–30 cm (4 1/2–12 in.)		Skills are well developed **(1)**	New sports activities are attempted and muscle development continues **(2)** Some lack of coordination common during growth spurt	Fully developed

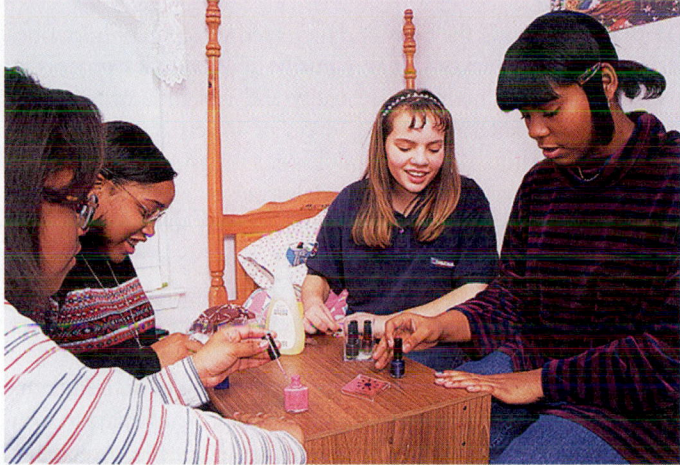

(1) Motor skills are well developed

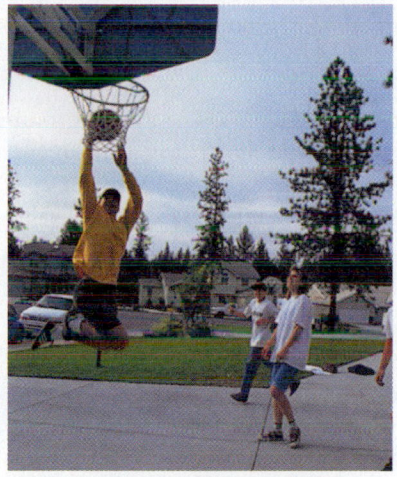

(2) New sports activities attempted

The ability to think and act independently leads many adolescents to rebel against parental authority. Through these actions, adolescents seek to establish their own identity and values.

Psychosocial Development

Activities

Maturity leads to new activities. Adolescents may drive, ride buses, or bike independently. They are less dependent on parents for transportation and spend more time with friends. Activities include participation in sports and extracurricular school activities, as well as "hanging out" and attending movies or concerts with friends (Table 5–20). The peer group becomes the focus of activities, regardless of the teen's interests. Peers are important in establishing identity and providing meaning. Although same-sex interactions predominate, boy–girl relationships are more common than at earlier stages. Adolescents thus participate in and learn from social interactions fundamental to adult relationships (Arnett, 2007).

TABLE 5–20	Psychosocial Development During Adolescence		
AGE		**ACTIVITIES**	**COMMUNICATION**
12–18 years 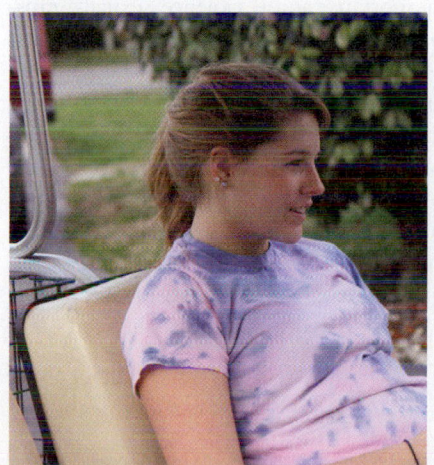		Sports—ball games, gymnastics, water and snow skiing/boarding, swimming, school sports School activities—drama, yearbook, class office, club participation Quiet activities—reading, schoolwork, television, computer, video games, music	Increasing communication and time with peer group—movies, dances, driving, eating out, attending sports events Applying abstract thought and analysis in conversations at home and school

Personality and Temperament

Characteristics of temperament manifested during childhood usually remain stable in the teenage years. For instance, the adolescent who was a calm, scheduled infant and child often demonstrates initiative to regulate study times and other routines. Similarly, the adolescent who was an easily stimulated infant may now have a messy room, a harried schedule with assignments always completed late, and an interest in many activities. It is also common for an adolescent who was an easy child to become more difficult due to the psychologic changes of adolescence and the need to assert independence.

Similar to the child's earlier ages, the nurse's role may be to inform parents of different personality types and to help them support the teen's uniqueness while providing necessary structure and feedback. Nurses can help parents to understand their teen's personality type and to work with the adolescent to meet expectations of teachers and others in authority.

Communication

All parts of speech are used and understood by the adolescent. Colloquialisms and slang are commonly used with the peer group. The adolescent often studies a foreign language in school, having the ability to understand and analyze grammar and sentence structure.

The adolescent increasingly leaves the home base and establishes close ties with peers. These relationships become the basis for identity formation. There is generally a period of stress or crisis before a strong identity can emerge. The adolescent may try out new roles by learning a new sport or other skills, experimenting with drugs or alcohol, wearing different styles of clothing, or trying other activities. It is important to provide positive role models and a variety of experiences to help the adolescent make wise choices.

The adolescent also has a need to leave the past, to be different, and to change from former patterns to establish a self-identity. Rules that are repeated constantly and dogmatically will probably be broken in the adolescent's quest for self-awareness. This poses difficulties when the adolescent has a health problem, such as diabetes or a heart defect that requires ongoing care. Introducing the adolescent to other teens who manage the same problem appropriately is usually more successful than telling the adolescent what to do.

Privacy should be ensured during the taking of health histories or interventions with teens. Even if a parent is present for part of a history or examination, the adolescent should be given the opportunity to relay information or ask questions alone with the healthcare provider. The adolescent should be given a choice of whether to have a parent present during an examination or while care is provided. Most information shared by an adolescent is confidential. Some states mandate disclosure of certain information to parents such as an adolescent's desire for an abortion. In these cases, the adolescent should be informed of what will be disclosed to the parent. (See Chapter 1 for further discussion.)

Setting up teen rooms (recreation rooms for use only by adolescents) or separate adolescent units in hospitals can provide necessary peer support during hospitalization. Most adolescents are not pleased when placed on a unit or in a room with young children. Choices should be allowed when possible, and include preference for evening or morning bathing, the type of clothes to wear while hospitalized, timing of treatments, and visitation guidelines. Use of negotiation and agreements with adolescents may increase compliance. Firmness, gentleness, choices, and respect must be balanced during care of adolescent patients.

Sexuality

With maturation of the body and increased secretion of hormones, the adolescent achieves sexual maturity. This complex process involves a growing interest in sexuality and romantic or sexual relationships, an interplay of the forces of society and family, and identity formation. The early adolescent progresses from dances and other social events to the late adolescent who is mature sexually and may have regular sexual encounters. About 46% of high school students in the United States have had intercourse, and over 34% are currently sexually active; nearly 39% of sexually active youth did not use a condom at their last sexual encounter (Eaton, Kann, Kinchen, et al., 2010).

Teenagers need information about their bodies and emerging sexuality. To make informed decisions about their behavior, teenagers should understand the interests and forces they experience. Including sex education in school classes and healthcare encounters is important. Information on methods to prevent sexually transmitted diseases is given, with most school districts now providing some teaching on AIDS. Far more common risks to teens, however, are diseases such as gonorrhea, herpes, and hepatitis. Health histories should include questions on sexual activity, sexually transmitted diseases, and birth control use and understanding. Most hospitals routinely perform pregnancy screening on adolescent girls before elective procedures.

Adolescents will benefit from clear information about sexuality, an opportunity to develop relationships with adolescents in various settings, an open atmosphere at home and school where problems and issues can be discussed, and previous experience in problem solving and self decision making. Sexual issues should be among topics that adolescents can discuss openly in a variety of settings. Alternatives and support for their decisions should be available.

Some adolescents identify with a sexual minority group such as lesbian, gay, bisexual, or transgendered, or they may be questioning their own sexual orientation. Some studies identify a higher than normal rate of depression, substance abuse, violence, sexually transmitted infections, and homelessness in these adolescents (Dowshen & Garofalo, 2009). Nurses are instrumental in helping these youth by establishing a welcome atmosphere in healthcare facilities, providing information for them and their parents, integrating sexual minority content into sexual education curricula, and providing referrals for health and social care when needed. Nurses must examine their own beliefs and communication styles to provide culturally competent care. They can promote trust and acceptance among youth and in the general school community. See Chapter 13 for further information about the health issues related to homosexuality and other sexual minority practices.

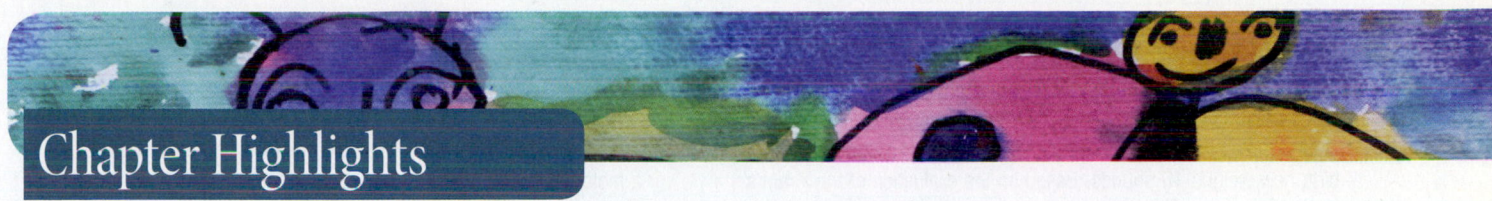

Chapter Highlights

- Development unfolds in a predictable pattern, but at different rates dependent on the particular characteristics and experiences of each child.
- Major theories of development encompass the psychosexual (Freud), psychosocial (Erikson), cognitive (Piaget), moral (Kohlberg), social learning (Bandura), and behavioral (Skinner and Watson) components of individuals.
- The ecologic theory of Bronfenbrenner and the temperament theory of Chess and Thomas emphasize the interactions of the individual within the environment.
- Resiliency theory examines risk and protective factors that hinder or help children and families when dealing with developmental and life crises.
- Influences on the developmental process include one's genetic potential and a series of environmental influences unique to each family and individual.
- The newborn period begins at birth and ends at about 1 month, and is characterized by adaptation to extrauterine life, establishing periods of varying alertness, and specific physical findings.
- Infancy spans the time from 1 month to 1 year, and is marked by rapid physical growth, mastery of basic fine and gross motor skills, and beginning cognitive and language skills.
- Toddlers range in age from 1 to 3 years, and become increasingly mobile and communicative. They master control over excretion and are known for exerting their own opinions and wishes to parents. Injury prevention and toilet training are specific parental teaching needs.
- Preschool years range from 3 to 6 and are marked by increasing social skills. Most preschool children attend childcare programs and learn to play with other children. Continued mastery of physical coordination and language occurs.
- School age spans the years from 6 to 12, when children mature in many areas. They show slow, steady growth until reaching puberty between 9 and 12 years, when a growth spurt marks increased height and weight, as well as sexual maturation. School-age children play cooperatively with other children and participate in various school and community activities.
- Adolescence occurs from about 12 years of age through the teen years. Adolescents establish their own identities distinct from parents and other adults. They are mature physically and cognitively. The peer group exerts the major influence at this age.
- The nurse is involved in assessing development at each stage, and in providing anticipatory guidance to families to foster optimal development.

Clinical Reasoning in Action

INTRODUCTION

Consider Sergio, who was introduced in the chapter-opening scenario. He is now 6 months of age and growing well. His mother has altered her work schedule to stay with him each day; she works for a few hours in the evening when her husband is home. One pair of grandparents lives about 30 miles away and visits frequently. The family has medical insurance but has had to budget carefully to pay household bills since Yolanda is working less and they have expenses connected with Sergio's care.

DESCRIPTION

Since they have no other children and have limited experience with children, Pepe and Yolanda, Sergio's parents, have all the needs of new parents. Due to prematurity, Sergio has additional needs for developmental surveillance and parental education.

Sergio is 24.5 inches (62 cm) long and weighs 15 lb (6.8 kg). Some developmental milestones that the nurse observes include:

- Personal social—smiles, watches his own hand
- Fine motor—hands meet at midline, regards and watches small objects, and has begun to grasp a rattle
- Language—turns to sounds and voices, squeals and makes a variety of other sounds

- Gross motor—holds head steady when in sitting position; holds head and chest up using arms when prone

DISCUSSION

1. Sergio and his parents have many challenges and yet possess many strengths. Using the theory of resilience, list the infant's and family's risks and protective factors.

2. Calculate Sergio's height and weight percentiles. Consult the growth grids in Appendix A 🔗 and the Skills Manual for correct analysis. Since he is steadily growing, what summary can you provide for Sergio's parents? What nutritional advice should you provide for them?

3. Analyze Sergio's developmental milestones. Consult the list of expected milestones in this chapter and on the Denver II Developmental Test in Chapter 8 🔗. What skills will Sergio learn next? What specific suggestions do you have for his parents as they seek to encourage his development?

4. Assume that you are the nurse in the clinic where Sergio receives health care. Briefly outline the physical measurements, developmental observations, and family assessments that you will complete at each visit.

NCLEX-RN® Review

1. The nurse notes that a 6-month-old infant boy who weighed 7 pounds at birth now weighs 15 pounds. Based on the evaluation of the infant's current weight, what is the nurse's next action?
   1. Ask the parent why the child does not eat enough.
   2. Immediately inform the physician.
   3. Chart the assessment.
   4. Teach how not to overfeed the baby.

2. When planning nursing care for a hospitalized 9-year-old child, which intervention is most developmentally appropriate?
   1. Encourage the child to continue schoolwork.
   2. Provide a separate recreation room for activities.
   3. Encourage the child to brush teeth twice a day.
   4. Offer medical equipment for play.

3. The nurse is caring for an 8-year-old child who is hospitalized following a motor vehicle accident. Based upon what the nurse knows about this child's development what is the most appropriate nursing intervention?
   1. Using toys for distraction from painful medical procedures
   2. Offering medical equipment for play to decrease anxiety
   3. Knocking on the door before entering the room
   4. Providing information on sexuality

4. During a developmental assessment, a parent complains that she has a "difficult" toddler. What advice would the nurse offer to the parent?
   1. "Toddlers are flexible. Accepting new rules will occur quickly."
   2. "Do not expect the child to adapt quickly to new situations."
   3. "Encourage associative play and this will get better."
   4. "Spanking your child will make the difficult behavior improve."

See Appendix I ⓔ for answers.

References

American Academy of Pediatrics. (2009). *Pediatric nutrition handbook* (6th ed.). Elk Grove Village, IL: Author.

Arnett, J. J. (2007). *Adolescence and emerging adulthood* (3rd ed.). Upper Saddle River, NJ: Pearson Prentice Hall.

Bandura, A. (1986). *Social foundations of thought and actions: A social cognitive theory*. Englewood Cliffs, NJ: Prentice Hall.

Bandura, A. (1997a). *Self-efficacy: The exercise of control*. New York: W. H. Freeman.

Bandura, A. (1997b). *Self-efficacy in changing societies*. New York: Cambridge University Press.

Bronfenbrenner, U. (1986). Ecology of the family as a context for human development: Research perspectives. *Developmental Psychology, 22*, 723–742.

Bronfenbrenner, U., McClelland, P. D., Ceci, S. J., Moen, P., & Wethington, E. (1996). *The state of Americans*. New York: Free Press.

Bronfenbrenner, U. (Ed.). (2005). *Making human beings human*. Thousand Oaks, CA: Sage Publications.

Burney, R. V., & Leerkes, E. M. (2010). Links between mothers' and fathers' perceptions of infant temperament and coparenting. *Infant Behavior and Development, 33*(2), 125–135.

Centers for Disease Control and Prevention (CDC). (2010). *Premature birth*. Retrieved from http://www.cdc.gov/Features/Prematurebirth/

Chess, S., & Thomas, A. (1995). *Temperament in clinical practice*. New York: Guilford Press.

Chess, S., & Thomas, A. (1996). *Temperament: Theory and practice*. Philadelphia: Brunner/Mazel.

Chess, S., & Thomas, A. (1999). *Goodness of fit: Clinical applications from infancy through adult life*. Philadelphia: Brunner/Mazel.

Commonwealth Fund. (2011). *Child development and preventive care*. Retrieved from http://www.commonwealthfund.org/content/Program-Areas/Archived-Programs/Child-Development-and-Preventive-Care.aspx

Craig, G. J., & Dunn, W. L. (2010). *Understanding human development* (2nd ed.). Upper Saddle River, NJ: Pearson Prentice Hall.

Daly, B. P., Shin, R. Q., Thakral, C., Selders, M., & Vera, E. (2009). School engagement among urban adolescents of color: Does perception of social support and neighborhood safety really matter? *Journal of Youth and Adolescence, 38*(1), 63–74.

Dowshen, N., & Garofalo, R. (2009). Optimizing primary care for LGBTQ youth. *Contemporary Pediatrics, 26*(10), 58–66.

Dumka, L. E., Gonzales, N. A., Wheeler, L. A., & Millsay, R. E. (2010). Parenting self-efficacy and parenting practices over time in Mexican American families. *Journal of Family Psychology, 24*(5), 522–531.

Eaton, D. K., Kann, L., Kinchen, S., Shanklin, S., Ross, J., Hawkins, J., . . . Wechsler, H. (2010). Youth risk behavior surveillance—United States, 2009. *Morbidity and Mortality Weekly Report, 59*(SS-5), 1–146.

Erikson, E. (1963). *Childhood and society*. New York: W.W. Norton.

Erikson, E. (1968). *Identity: Youth and crisis*. New York: W.W. Norton.

Field, T., Diego, M., & Hernandez-Reif, M. (2010). Preterm infant massage therapy research: A review. *Infant Behavior and Development, 33*, 115–124.

Ginsberg, H., & Opper, S. (1988). *Piaget's theory of intellectual development* (3rd ed.). Paramus, NJ: Prentice Hall.

Henderson, N., Benard, B., & Sharp-Light, M. (2007). *Resiliency in action*. Ojai, CA: Resiliency in Action.

Lester, B. M., & Sparrow, J. D. (2010). *Nurturing children and families: Building on the legacy of T. Berry Brazelton*. Hoboken, NJ: Wiley-Blackwell.

London, M. L., Ladewig, P. W., Ball, J. W., & Bindler, R. C. (2011). *Maternal & child nursing care* (3rd ed.). Upper Saddle River, NJ: Prentice Hall Health.

McCarter-Spaulding, D. E., & Dennis, C. L. (2010). Psychometric testing of the Breastfeeding Self-Efficacy Scale-Short Form in a sample of Black women in the United States. *Research in Nursing and Health, 33*(2), 111–119.

Melnyk, B. M., Jacobsen, D., Kelly, S., O'Haver, J., Small, L., & Mays, M. Z. (2009). Improving the mental health, healthy lifestyle, and physical health of Hispanic adolescents: Random controlled pilot study. *Journal of School Health, 79*(12), 575–584.

Mundy, P., & Jarrold, W. (2010). Infant joint attention, neural networks and social cognition. *Neural Network, 23*(8–9), 985–997.

Murphy-Oikonen, J., Montelpare, W. J., Southon, S., Bertoldo, L., & Persichino, N. (2010). Identifying infants at risk for neonatal abstinence syndrome: A retrospective cohort comparison study of 3 screening approaches. *Journal of Perinatal and Neonatal Nursing, 24*(4), 366–372.

NCAST. (2011). *NCAST programs*. Retrieved from http://www.ncast.org/

Piaget, J. (1972). *The child's conception of the world*. Totowa, NJ: Littlefield, Adams.

Rew, L., Whittaker, T. A., Taylor-Seehafer, M. A., & Smith, L. R. (2005). Sexual health risks and protective resources in gay, lesbian, bisexual, and heterosexual homeless youth. *Journal of Specialists in Pediatric Nursing, 10*, 11–19.

Salmon, J., Jorna, M., Hume, C., Arundell, L., Dhahine, J., Tienstra, J., & Crawford, C. (2011). A translational research intervention to reduce screen behaviours and promote physical activity among children: Switch-2-Activity. *Health Promotion International, 26,* 311–321.

Santrock, J. (2011). *Child development* (13th ed.). Boston: McGraw-Hill.

Steele, M. M., Daratha, K. B., Bindler, R. C., & Power, T. G. (2011). The relationship between self-efficacy for behaviors that promote healthy weight and clinical indicators of adiposity in a sample of early adolescents. *Health Education & Behavior, 38,* 596–602.

Thornton, S. P. (2010). *Sigmund Freud.* Retrieved from Internet Encyclopedia of Philosophy at http://www.iep.utm.edu/freud/#H7

U.S. Food and Drug Administration. (2011). *Pregnancy and lactation labeling.* Retrieved from http://www.fda.gov/Drugs/DevelopmentApprovalProcess/DevelopmentResources/Labeling/ucm093307.htm

van Gelder, M. M., van Rooij, I. A., Miller, R. K., Zielhuis, G. A., de Jong-van den Berg, L. T., & Roeleveld,

N. (2010). Teratogenic mechanisms of medical drugs. *Human Reproductive Update, 16*(4), 378–394.

Vygotsky, L. (1962). *Thought and language.* Cambridge, MA: MIT Press.

Yancy, A. K., Grant, D., Kurosky, S., Kravitz-Wirtz, N., & Mistry, R. (2011). Role modeling, risk, and resilience in California adolescents. *Journal of Adolescent Health, 48*(1), 36–43.

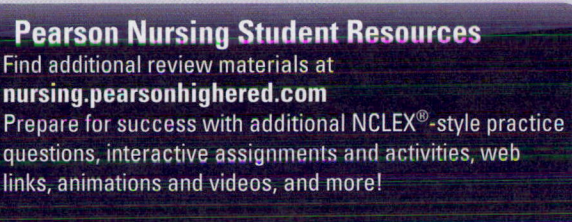

Pearson Nursing Student Resources
Find additional review materials at
nursing.pearsonhighered.com
Prepare for success with additional NCLEX®-style practice questions, interactive assignments and activities, web links, animations and videos, and more!

CHAPTER 6

Child and Family Communication

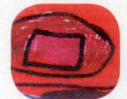 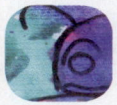 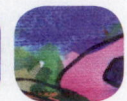

Learning Outcomes

After completing this chapter, you will be able to:

1. Describe the major components of the communication process as they apply to nursing care of children and their families.

2. Identify forms of communication and their related concepts.

3. Analyze factors influencing the communication process.

4. Apply concepts of communication to the developmental levels of childhood.

5. Give examples of barriers and challenges to communication with the child and family.

6. Integrate the nursing process to promote effective communication and establish a therapeutic nurse–child–family relationship.

7. Communicate with patients and families with special needs, including those with low literacy levels, alterations in sensory perception, and language barriers.

8. Collaborate with other members of the healthcare team to provide optimal communication to patients and families.

"I'm so glad the nurse came to our house and talked to Brittney and Madeline about my arthritis. I think it helped my mom and dad, too."

—Madison, age 7

Madison Clarke has been discharged from the hospital after a workup and diagnosis of juvenile arthritis, a chronic condition. The nurse has worked with Madison and her family in the hospital, and now the focus shifts to meeting with the siblings, Brittney, age 9, and Madeline, age 4. The nurse is in their home to explain the disease process, the treatment regimen, how their lives might be affected, and how they can be involved in Madison's care.

The nurse tells Brittney and Madeline that on some days Madison's knees may hurt more than on other days and she may not be able to play. She tells the girls that a physical therapist will come to the house to help Madison with some exercises for her legs and will show them how to gently move Madison's knees to help her stay active. The nurse provides guidance in communications with family members to assist them in developing coping mechanisms for the changes in routine. Effective communication can also assist Madison and her family to identify creative hobbies or activities to further her sense of self-worth.

What communication skills are required to explain the disease and treatment to children at various developmental stages? What factors influence communication? What are potential barriers to communication?

Communication, the exchange of information, thoughts, and feelings, is an essential component of human interaction, as it provides the means by which individuals, from birth through adulthood, learn about the physical and social world. Two theoretical frameworks describe the communication process. In the linear model, the message includes a sender and a receiver. The message is sent using one of the five senses. In the circular or transactional model, communication is viewed as continuous. This framework takes into account the context in which the communication occurred and includes how the characteristics of both the sender and the receiver influence communication (Bach & Grant, 2009).

The nurse–child–family relationship is dependent on effective communication. The nurse's communication with the child and family serves as a key connection between the family and the healthcare system. Establishing a therapeutic relationship with the child and family is essential to promote the health of the child. However, effective communication is a learned process. Pediatric nurses must understand and apply techniques of effective communication, including listening, interpreting the various forms of communication, and being aware of factors that can positively or negatively influence the process. Ongoing evaluation will help nurses identify strategies to modify their communication techniques for children at different ages and developmental stages.

In this chapter, we will survey the communication process and examine factors that influence communication with the child and family. Then, we will address developmental considerations for communication and approaches for special pediatric populations. The remainder of the chapter focuses on nursing management of communication with the child and family. Refer to Chapter 5 for information related to language acquisition.

COMMUNICATION AND THE NURSE–CHILD–FAMILY RELATIONSHIP

Communication is an ongoing cyclical process in which people constantly connect, either consciously or unconsciously, through verbal and nonverbal techniques. Major components of the communication process are the *sender, message, channel, receiver,* and *response* (Figure 6–1 ■).

Communication begins when the child and family enter the healthcare setting. Effective communication with the child and the family leads to the development of trust in the healthcare professional and helps facilitate the family's management of their child's illness. As the child and family interact with the nurse, anxiety may be reduced as they become aware of the nurse's interest and caring. This feeling of trust and security can generate open communication where families feel free to discuss their concerns.

Parents need accurate information and assurance from someone they can trust, as they may be relinquishing the care of their child to strangers. The nurse is the healthcare professional who will experience the majority of the interaction with the child and family. Therefore, the nurse is challenged to also meet the parent's psychologic and educational needs.

Effective communication helps ensure that families receive the information they need to adhere to the prescribed plan of care. Children who receive adequate developmentally appropriate patient education are also more likely to follow the prescribed regimen (Chilman-Blair, 2010). The overall goal of the nurse is to establish

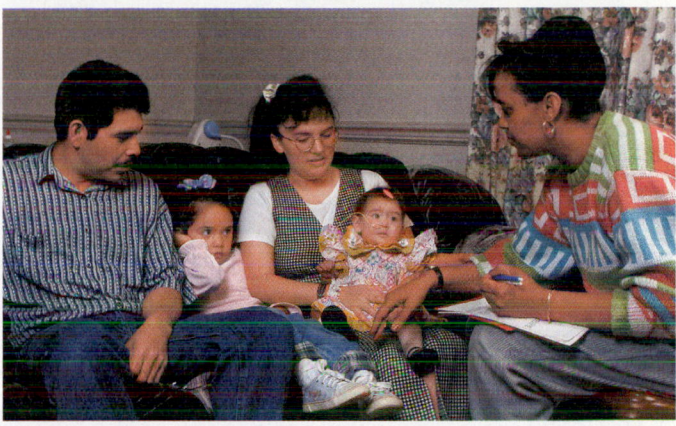

FIGURE 6–1 ■ The nurse is sending a message to the older child, the receiver. Notice the nonverbal communication expressed by the young girl. What message is she communicating? How should the nurse respond?

rapport with the child and family to assist them in identifying mutual goals and to facilitate positive health outcomes, as in this chapter's opening scenario. What indications are present to suggest that the nurse is establishing a therapeutic relationship with positive rapport?

FORMS OF COMMUNICATION

Communication can be categorized into three forms: verbal, nonverbal, and abstract. **Verbal communication** is the use of spoken language, written language, or vocalizations, such as laughter or crying, to convey messages. **Nonverbal communication** is the use of body language, including gestures, facial expressions, posture, touch, and reactions. **Abstract communication** is displayed through play, visual images, and even the selection of clothing. While the younger child may choose to communicate through play, the adolescent may select specific clothes to "send the message."

Verbal Communication

The use of language—as well as nonverbal communication—is crucial to the nurse's assessment and interaction. However, the way the nurse frames the interaction verbally is of great importance to how the message is understood. For example, if the nurse states, "I will be back in a few minutes and we will draw your blood," the young child may think that the nurse will return with paper and crayons and together the two of them will "draw blood" on the paper. A nurse's understanding and application of the developmental and cognitive stages of children is essential to ensure clear communication.

A child's vocabulary and means of expression depend not only on developmental level and cognitive stage, but also on the patterns of language usage in a child's family and individual differences among children. Recall that expressive and receptive language can be different (see Chapter 5), as children may understand more (**receptive language**) than they verbalize (**expressive language**).

In every healthcare encounter, pay attention to tone of voice, inflection, and volume. Consider cultural influences as well. If you encounter a communication barrier, allow adequate time or seek an interpreter to enable the child and parents to express their thoughts.

Nonverbal Communication

Nonverbal communication patterns provide meaningful clues to the intended messages, especially when you are working with a pediatric population. Nonverbal communication can include facial expressions, body language, eye contact, touch, and physical appearance. Children communicate by *what* they do and *how* they do it. Children naturally express themselves nonverbally. They may cling to a parent when frightened, cry when hungry or tired, or moan when attempting to communicate desires. A child's silence may indicate fear, shyness, or anger. Aggressive nonverbal behaviors include biting, kicking, banging fists, and hitting; they may signify anger, frustration, or fear. Table 6–1 gives examples of how the nurse might communicate nonverbally. Look back to the picture in the opening scenario. What nonverbal cues are the parents and children displaying?

Interpretation of nonverbal communication may be ambiguous depending on the culture and the context of the situation (Table 6–2). For example, a child may not understand the meaning of certain gestures in the nurse's culture and thus misinterpret them. Likewise, it is essential for nurses to be familiar with the cultures

in their community and understand the communication patterns. (See Developing Cultural Competence: Periods of Silence During Communication.)

What happens when a patient perceives that a verbal message conflicts with a nonverbal one? The receiver may interpret the nonverbal message rather than the verbal. For example, if a nurse smiles while preparing to change a painful dressing, the child may interpret that to mean the nurse enjoys causing pain.

Paralanguage, another essential aspect of nonverbal communication, includes the tone and pitch of the voice; speed, pace, and volume; and other vocalizations such as laughing, sobbing, and snorting (Fontaine, 2009). Paralanguage has as much, if not more, significance to the receiver as verbal messages do, especially with young children. From infancy, children understand paralanguage long before they know the meaning of the words. They sense anger and stress by the volume, pitch, and rate of the spoken word. Paying attention to the

TABLE 6–1	Forms of Nonverbal Communication	
BEHAVIOR	**POSSIBLE MEANING**	**NURSING IMPLICATION**
Standing		
At the beginning or end of interaction	Initiation/termination of interaction	The nurse may choose to stand if the parent or child stands during an interaction.
Over other person while talking	Intimidation or domination	The nurse can invite (with open hands) the patient or family member to sit while conversing.
Sitting		
Face to face	Interest	The nurse can encourage further communication by a caring and calming voice and facial expression.
Side by side	Neutrality	
Turned away	Termination of the interaction	
At the edge of the chair	Anxiety or eagerness	
Body Posture		
Relaxed	Friendliness, warmth	Constant awareness of body language by the nurse can result in enhanced communication.
Rigid or tense	Fear or anger	
Leaning back	Withdrawal, distance	
Leaning forward	Interest, friendliness	
Arms and/or legs tightly crossed	Self-protection, withdrawal	
Shrinking in	Depression, low self-esteem	
Turned away	Distance, withdrawal	
Gestures		
Leg or foot shaking, finger tapping	Anxiety, frustration, anger	The nurse can display an empathetic and caring attitude to help patients and families relax during stressful events. Listening is an effective tool for exhibiting support.
Fidgety, restless movements	Anxiety, embarrassment	
Finger shaking, hands on hips	Authority, intimidation	
Hiding hands	Shyness, insecurity	
Fist clenching	Anger, frustration	
Wringing hands	Hopelessness, helplessness	
Eyes		
Frequent eye contact	Interest, honesty	The type of eye contact can display positive as well as negative feelings from the patient/family.
Minimal eye contact	Low self-esteem, shyness, boredom	
Rapidly shifting eye contact	Confusion	
Frequent blinking	Anxiety	
Touch		
Touching arm or hand	Interest and concern	The nurse should be aware of how touch might be interpreted. May need to ask permission, depending on the situation.

Source: *Adapted from Fontaine, K. L. (2009). Illness management: Communication and psychoeducation. In* Mental health nursing *(6th ed., p. 128). Upper Saddle River, NJ: Pearson/Prentice Hall.*

TABLE 6–2	Nonverbal Communication Patterns in Major Cultural Groups
CULTURAL GROUP	**NONVERBAL COMMUNICATION PATTERNS***
African American	Close personal space is typical.
	Touch is common with family members and close friends.
	Eye contact is generally acceptable.
Hispanic	Close personal space is typical.
	Touch is common and generally viewed as supportive and sincere.
	Eye contact is acceptable.
	A handshake is important.
Asian	Distant personal space is typical.
	Touch may be viewed as intrusive.
	Direct eye contact may be considered disrespectful.
	A handshake is acceptable.
Native American	Direct eye contact may be considered disrespectful.
	A firm handshake may be viewed as aggressive.
	Touch is not acceptable unless the person knows the other very well.

*Behavioral patterns of nonverbal behavior vary within groups, so avoid stereotyping any one group with these communication characteristics.

Source: *Data from Antai-Otong, D. (2007). Nurse-client communication. Sudbury, MA: Jones and Bartlett; Giger, J. N., & Davidhizar, R. E. (2008).* Transcultural nursing: Assessment and intervention *(5th ed.). St. Louis, MO: Mosby Elsevier; Purnell, L. D. (2009). Guide to culturally competent health care (2nd ed.). Philadelphia: F. A. Davis Company.*

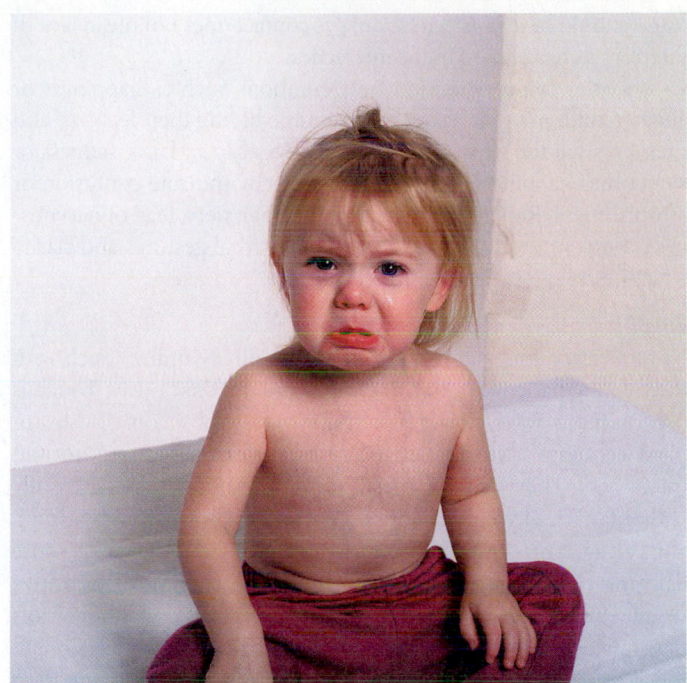

FIGURE 6–2 ■ Facial expressions are a powerful means of communication. What does this child's facial expression convey? What actions can the nurse take to reduce her distress?

Developing Cultural Competence
Periods of Silence During Communication

Certain cultures, such as Asians and Native Americans, are generally comfortable with silence. The nurse should respect this silence and allow the person time to think, reflect, and formulate a response (Giger & Davidhizar, 2008; Purnell, 2009). Nursing care is enhanced when the nurse understands the meaning of silence among patients and families from other cultures (Giger & Davidhizar, 2008).

---

rate of speech is imperative when speaking to children, especially toddlers and preschoolers. The nurse who speaks hurriedly while instructing or informing the child likely will not capture the full attention or the cooperation that he or she would if speech were slower and more distinct.

Facial Expressions

The facial expressions of the nurse and child convey nonverbal messages more than any other body language (Figure 6–2 ■). Facial expressions include smiling, frowning, raising or lowering of eyebrows, and wrinkling of forehead. A child may be observed pouting or with lips quivering, suggesting impending crying.

Children with limited verbal expression are masters at using facial expression, eye contact, and gestures to send powerful messages about themselves, their feelings, and their needs. This method of communication can help guide the nurse when providing care. For example, while changing a dressing, a nurse can observe a child's facial expressions for signs of pain and proceed accordingly. Nonverbal communication offers a much wider context than verbal expression,

which is often less precise in expressing emotion. When aware of nonverbal cues, a nurse can make comprehensive assessment, which enhances the care of the child.

Body Language

Body language includes both gestures and posture. Senders often use gestures to add emphasis to their verbal messages. Gestures can include nodding or shaking one's head, shrugging one's shoulders, waving one's hands, tapping one's foot, or other repetitive movements of the feet or hands. How the patient responds to communication may be conveyed in a gesture. Therefore, be aware of how a patient responds to a gesture and remember that the response may vary, depending on the patient's cultural background. Refer to Table 6–2. The nurse can demonstrate a caring presence through gestures such as nodding and smiling.

The nurse's posture can convey a positive or negative feeling to the child or parents. By sitting in a chair at the child's eye level and leaning forward, a nurse can indicate interest and a desire for open communication. By standing, or leaning back in a chair, with arms crossed, a nurse can indicate disinterest or an unwillingness to communicate. An erect posture generally indicates self-assuredness, whereas a slouched posture can indicate a low self-esteem or not feeling well.

Eye Contact

The importance of maintaining eye contact varies according to cultural influences. For European Americans, maintaining eye contact during communication is essential to establishing trust and conveying interest. In other cultures, such as Native American and some Asian cultures, sustained eye contact may be considered rude or disrespectful. Children in these cultures are taught from an early age to avert their gaze and to look downward when being addressed. The nurse should be aware that lack of eye contact does not mean lack of interest or engagement in the interaction.

The eyes can also demonstrate emotions such as happiness or anger. Children often have a difficult time hiding their feelings, and their eyes tell the story. Tearing of the eyes can indicate sadness or sometimes happiness. Raising eyebrows may indicate confusion or astonishment. Rapid blinking may indicate anxiety, fear, or nervousness. Nurses need to recognize these nonverbal gestures and clarify what the child is experiencing at that time.

Touch

Nurses caring for infants and children routinely utilize touch with their young patients, both consciously and unconsciously. Touch is used in many ways, however, and may not involve consciously applied techniques. Nurses use touch while performing procedures and treatments. They also use social, communicative touch, especially with infants and young children. Touch conveys trust, compassion, and caring. It can be calming to a parent and child. Touch may cause discomfort as a child grows older, and the nurse must be sensitive to the child's and adolescent's response. In addition, although often considered a demonstration of caring by nursing professionals, touch may be culturally inappropriate for some children and their families. Depending on the circumstances, touch can be considered a method of personalizing communication or a violation of personal space. Various factors modify how, when, and even if touch should be utilized. These factors include the patient's age and physiologic and psychologic status, the setting, a variety of sociocultural factors, and the child's previous experience with touch (for example, if the child has experienced abuse or neglect).

Pediatric nurses should inform the parents and the child prior to touch, for example, when listening to the heart rate. Constant observations of the child's response to touch will help the nurse modify the approach or technique. If a child is in pain, the nurse can ask if it is all right to rub the child's back or stroke a hand. Be sensitive to responses and whether the child settles with touch or pulls away.

Therapeutic touch is a noninvasive technique that utilizes hand movements to balance and equalize energy fields (Jackson, Kelley, McNeil, et al., 2008). Healing touch is a biofield therapy and is closely related to and derived from therapeutic touch. It is a specific type of touch that involves hand placement in a specific sequence and requires certification. Healing touch is thought to be useful in alleviating pain, facilitating recovery from surgery, and reducing anxiety and stress (Johnston, 2009; Tang, Tegeler, Larrimore, et al., 2010).

Physical Appearance

The physical appearance of the child and family members can convey significant nonverbal messages to the nurse. Clothing style, grooming, tattoos, and jewelry items such as religious artifacts can provide insight to the child's care and cultural beliefs. Children's clothing can often represent their values—what is important to them as represented by current fashion statements. The nurse should avoid making judgments based on how the child or family is dressed.

Similarly, the nurse's physical appearance communicates nonverbal messages to the child and family. The nurse in the pediatric setting frequently wears colorful uniforms depicting children's favorite cartoon characters (Figure 6–3 ■). White uniforms are often avoided since children sometimes associate a white uniform with medical procedures, which may instill fear and block therapeutic communication.

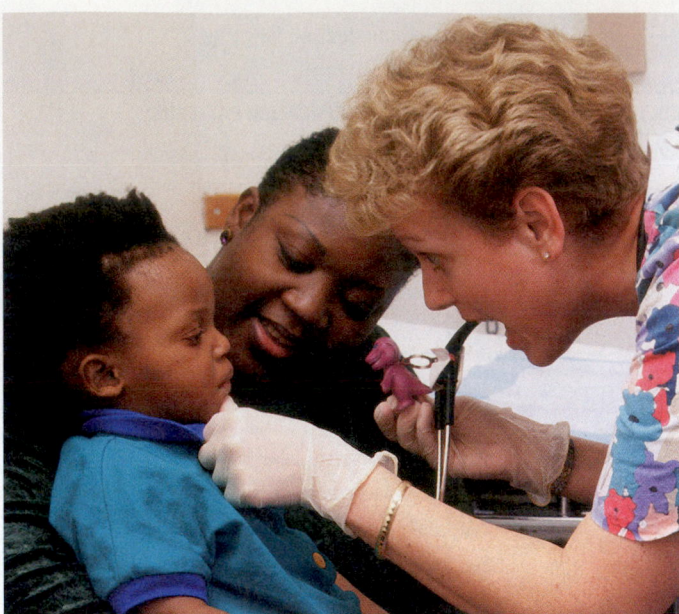

FIGURE 6–3 ■ Notice the nurse's brightly colored uniform and her attempts to allay the child's fears. She is showing a toy and is ready to quickly examine the mouth if the boy smiles.

FACTORS INFLUENCING COMMUNICATION WITH CHILDREN AND THEIR FAMILIES

Essentially every aspect of children's lives affects how they communicate. From an infant crying to a teenager slamming a door, the child's style of communication is influenced by his or her environment, spatial distancing, time, and culture (Table 6–3).

The nurse needs to consider factors unique to each family and situation that can block effective communication, whether these barriers are physical or psychosocial. Physical factors include:

- Language used (such as medical jargon)
- Gender
- Environment
- Linguistic barriers

Psychosocial barriers include:

- Child's health status
- Parents' emotions related to their child's health status
- Culture
- Spatial distancing patterns

Medical Jargon

People who work in health care use certain language that is unique to the profession. The technical language associated with health care is called **medical jargon.** When a nurse is discussing information with a child and family, the use of medical jargon can create major barriers in communication.

Because the child and family members may have no prior experience with medical terminology, they may get confused or feel powerless when faced with unfamiliar language in an unfamiliar environment. Older adolescents and adults may feel embarrassed or offended because they are unable to understand the meaning of medical terminology and may even feel the offense was intentional. By translating jargon into more accessible terms, a nurse can foster understanding.

TABLE 6–3	Factors Influencing Communication

FACTOR	NURSING IMPLICATIONS
Environmental Factors Surroundings and sensory stimuli affect the communication process.	■ The physical environment should include a quiet, private room at a comfortable temperature and with adequate lighting. ■ Move any chairs or equipment that separates the child and family from the nurse or other health team member. ■ Adequate seating for the child and immediate family members should be readily available, with chairs facing each other to promote communication. ■ Remove any unnecessary medical equipment that may be frightening to the small child. ■ Provide privacy and comfort for difficult conversations; the child's and family's privacy are maintained at all times.
Spatial Distancing Patterns The distance between the participants in communication is often referred to as "personal space." Each person defines his or her own personal space zone, and cultural influence is a key determinant in establishing this zone of comfort. The zone may also vary according to the specific situation and with whom the space is shared. (See Chapter 3 🔗 for further discussion of spatial distancing patterns.)	■ Determine the appropriate spatial distancing pattern preference prior to the session. ■ Assess for nonverbal cues in level of comfort with personal closeness and contact.
Time Ample time is needed to communicate with the child and family. The appearance of being rushed may be perceived negatively.	■ The nurse may have difficulty with balancing response to questions and provision of information within the time available. ■ Focus on the family and child for the time available, and avoid giving signals concerning the need to move on to other tasks during that dedicated time.
Culture Culture influences the child's and family's communication patterns. Linguistic barriers associated with culturally diverse populations provide a unique opportunity for the nurse to employ a variety of communication techniques.	■ Assess the impact that culture has on communication to determine the best methods for communication. ■ The use of interpreters, translators, foreign language dictionaries, and symbols or pictures from the family's native language can help to decrease a language barrier. ■ An interpreter or translator may not be available at all times; however, be aware of when to have one available for significant conversations and consent for treatment. ■ Prior to the session, discuss with the interpreter the plan of care for the child and a list of possible questions from the nurse.

Source: *Data from Arnold, E. C., & Boggs, K. U. (2011).* Interpersonal relationships: Professional communication skills for nurses *(6th ed.). St. Louis, MO: Saunders; Spector, R. E. (2009). Cultural diversity in health and illness (7th ed.). Upper Saddle River, NJ: Prentice Hall.*

Gender

Gender is an important consideration in establishing effective communication. A child may respond more positively to females than males if the child associates caring and nurturing with women. Furthermore, if the child associates negative experiences with a particular gender, such as a male physician who performed a bone marrow biopsy in which the child experienced pain, the child may also withdraw from other healthcare professionals who appear similar (e.g., a male wearing a white jacket).

In addition, some cultures place less value on the female's authority. Others do not consider females to be experts or have authority, including the female nurse discussing health-related issues. The child that has been taught that the female has no authority may not cooperate with the female nurse or follow instructions.

Child's Health Status

The family dealing with a child's illness and hospitalization may be experiencing stress, anxiety, confusion, or shock. Parental emotions regarding their child's illness may range from overt exhibition of anger to complete withdrawal. When the family is preoccupied with their child's condition, they may be unable to communicate effectively and may even be unable to understand simple messages.

However, families who have confidence in and trust the nurse caring for their child exhibit decreased anxiety. Nurses can decrease parental stress by providing parents with information and education in a nonjudgmental and helpful manner. Communication with the distraught family requires skill, patience, compassion, and the use of therapeutic techniques described later in the chapter.

Nursing Attitudes

The nurse's attitude transcends all actions and is extremely important in establishing open lines of communication. Children and families can readily identify the nurse who is caring, empathetic, and family centered, versus the nurse who is indifferent or concerned with interests related only to nursing tasks. When the nurse's communication techniques are individualized according to developmental stage and abilities, the child and family may be comforted and reassured.

Caring refers to the nurse's emotional investment in the child and family. The caring nurse evokes feelings of security and comfort in the child and family by perceiving the child's needs and concerns, displaying behaviors that indicate the child is valued, comforting, and offering presence of self. A caring environment provides the child and family the atmosphere needed for open communication.

Empathy is the ability to perceive another person's experience from that person's point of view, in other words, imagining "oneself in another's shoes." Empathy differs from sympathy, which means generally to share in the feelings of another. A sympathizing nurse associates with the feelings of the child, while an empathizing nurse can understand them. Sympathy is not always therapeutic in caring for a child as it can lead nurses to emotional overinvolvement and, possibly, professional burnout. Although some nurses are naturally empathetic, others can learn empathy by focusing on the child's developmental parameters and verbal and nonverbal language.

DEVELOPMENTAL AND COGNITIVE CONSIDERATIONS FOR COMMUNICATION WITH CHILDREN

By virtue of their developmental stages, children process information differently than adults. Children may not necessarily comprehend what they hear, despite indicating that they do understand. Children also express themselves through nonverbal messages more frequently than adults, since by adulthood more control is exercised over nonverbal forms of communication. The nurse must consider the developmental and cognitive levels of the child for whom communication is intended.

Newborn

The primary mode of communication for the newborn is through nonverbal methods and crying. Newborns have no comprehension of words; however, they are attentive to human voice and presence. The newborn responds to touch through patting, stroking, rocking, and comforting. Touch has been shown to be a significant positive factor in the development of newborns and infants. "Kangaroo care," or wrapping a baby to the mother's chest, has proven to be a positive influence on the infant's physiologic outcomes. Early skin-to-skin contact between infant and mother is accomplished by putting the baby on the mother's chest soon after birth. Research has demonstrated that kangaroo care reduces pain during heel stick procedures and intramuscular injection of vitamin K in term infants (Kashaninia, Sajedi, Rahgozar, et al., 2008). Kangaroo care is also frequently used with preterm infants. See Evidence-Based Practice: Preterm Infants and Touch. Nurses can encourage infant touch by parents, can teach techniques of infant massage, and can use touch to comfort babies in healthcare encounters. See Chapter 5, Complementary Therapy: Infant Massage, and Figure 3–7 🔴.

Infant

Like the newborn, young infants have no comprehension of words, although they are also attentive to human voice and presence. The infant continues to respond to touch through patting, stroking, rocking, and comforting. Other stimuli such as singing and developmentally appropriate toys, such as rattles, elicit responses in the infant.

Evidence-Based Practice | Preterm Infants and Touch

PROBLEM
Preterm infants are neurologically immature and therefore are commonly more difficult to soothe and comfort. Their frequent crying may tire both the infant and the parents and interfere with attachment and bonding.

EVIDENCE
Researchers attempt to find ways to simulate the womb and to provide comforting touch and surroundings for preterm babies. One technique that is used is "kangaroo care," or holding the infant in a way that facilitates skin-to-skin contact. This type of care was developed in treatment of premature infants. It involves clothing the baby in only a diaper and placing the infant in an upright position against the skin of the parent's chest (Kearvell & Grant, 2010; Tessier, Charpak, Giron, et al., 2009). Kangaroo care may be provided for one to several hours daily or 24/7 (Nyqvist, Anderson, Bergman, et al., 2010).

Kangaroo care promotes physiologic stability, in addition to facilitating the relationship between the infant and the parent. A study of 194 families in the Kangaroo Mother Care (KMC) group and 144 families in a traditional care group examined the effects of keeping infants in the kangaroo position continually. Infants in the traditional group were kept in the incubator until they could maintain their temperature and were generally not discharged until they had reached a weight of about 1,700 grams. Infants in the KMC group were discharged from the hospital, regardless of weight, once they had adapted to extrauterine life and were able to breastfeed. These infants were maintained in the kangaroo position 24/7 until around 37 to 38 weeks gestational age. Fathers and other caregivers were also allowed to provide the kangaroo position. Infants were monitored closely for weight gain. The Home Observation for Measurement of the Environment (HOME) (Chapter 2 🔴) tool showed that kangaroo care provided a developmentally oriented caregiving environment, especially with neurologically at-risk infants and male infants. There was a positive correlation between an environment of kangaroo care and the father's involvement. There was also a strong correlation

between the infants' HOME score and their developmental quotient, suggesting that infants benefit from this positive environment (Tessier et al., 2009).

A study by Leonard and Mayers (2008) examined the experiences of six parents who provided continuous kangaroo care to their preterm infants in the neonatal nursery of a tertiary care center. In-depth interviews conducted with the parents demonstrated that providing kangaroo care empowered them, improved communication with staff, and increased the connection with their infants.

An additional study investigated the effects of music therapy combined with kangaroo care (dual therapy) on premature infants as compared to the effects of kangaroo care alone. Sixty-one infants born between 24 and 36 weeks' gestation were included in the study. Results showed that kangaroo care alone and kangaroo therapy combined with music therapy decreased the infants' pulse, respiration, and blood pressure, and increased the oxygen saturation levels. Dual therapy was more effective in decreasing the infants' blood pressure than kangaroo care alone, suggesting that combination therapy might be beneficial on the physiologic responses of premature infants (Teckenberg-Jansson, Huotilainen, Polkki, et al., 2011).

IMPLICATIONS
Nurses who care for preterm infants need to integrate knowledge of touch, positioning, and other modalities that provide neurologic comfort for babies and enhance the parents' feelings of connection to the newborn. It is important for the nurse to promote attachment between the mother and the infant through breastfeeding, kangaroo care, and encouragement of participation in care of the infant (Kearvell & Grant, 2010). Fathers should also be encouraged to participate in care of the infant.

CRITICAL THINKING APPLICATION
How will you integrate this information in the neonatal intensive care unit and with babies who have left the hospital and are at home with parents? How will your practice and the teaching you provide to parents be altered?

Infants initially communicate through nonverbal methods and crying. Facial expressions, quivering, and thrashing arms and legs may indicate distress or pain. Cooing, leg kicking, and arm waving may mean contentment and interest in engaging in interaction.

Over time, infants learn to communicate through touch, hearing, and sight. Verbal communication is demonstrated by cooing and crying. Infants communicate hunger, pain, and other discomforts through crying. Infants develop a bonding relationship with parents, siblings, other family members, and caregivers through touch, as touch can convey safety and love. Nurses can facilitate the communication between an infant and parent, as well as model positive communication techniques.

The following may help to promote communication with the newborn or infant and family:

- Allow the parents to be in the infant's view whenever possible during care and nursing procedures.
- Remove the infant from the parent's arms only if necessary.
- Speak in a higher pitched, soft tone.
- Establish eye contact with the baby, but be sensitive that when the baby turns away a period of relaxation is needed.
- Avoid leaning over the infant's face and talking in a forceful tone.
- Use swaddling, rubbing, patting, cuddling, or rocking to quiet a crying baby.
- Communicate through play, such as peek-a-boo.
- Be aware that stranger anxiety may occur in infants age 6 to 12 months.

Toddler and Preschooler   1-3 / 3-6

Toddlers and preschoolers need the opportunity to express their thoughts without being interrupted. These children must learn to recognize nonverbal cues that indicate it is okay for them to talk. Ask parents questions initially and then direct questions to the child once they are comfortable with the setting.

The toddler and preschooler are egocentric, meaning they often have difficulty in understanding another person's point of view. They expect those around them to understand what they are thinking or feeling without the prerequisite exchange of information. In other words, they assume that another's experiences are the same as their own, so others should understand how they feel.

The toddler is developing a sense of self and asserts independence. Allowing the toddler choices when possible promotes communication.

The preschooler is concrete and literal. The child may misinterpret words or phrases that have more than one meaning (Boggs, 2011a). Avoid using expressions and vocabulary that are likely to be misunderstood by the child. For example, the nurse may say, "We will put *dye* in your arm," and the child may interpret this statement as "the arm will *die*." Instead, the nurse might state, "We will put some warm medicine into your arm." See Table 6–4.

Preschoolers also have short attention spans and limited memory of recent events, so asking them what they did yesterday would likely not reveal an accurate recounting. At about 3 years of age, preschoolers can state their name and address if they are taught this information. They can describe the names of toys and family members, but they may not be able to give details of an event unless it had special significance, such as a situation that caused them to feel happy or sad, or was painful.

TABLE 6–4	Language Alternatives When Communicating with Children
POTENTIALLY CONFUSING OR AMBIGUOUS WORDS OR STATEMENTS	**ALTERNATIVE COMMUNICATION CHOICE**
"We will give you some dye in your arm."	"We will put some warm medicine into your arm."
"I will give you a shot."	"I will give you some medicine through a small needle."
"This will hurt or burn."	"It might feel sore or very warm."
"The doctor will make a small cut/incision."	"The doctor will make a small opening."
"You are going to have some anesthesia."	"You will get some medicine that you breathe or get through your arm to make you sleep."
"The medicine tastes bad."	"Some children say the medicine tastes different to them."
"I'm going to take your blood pressure."	"I'm going to measure how hard your heart is working."

Preschoolers ask numerous questions, and they should be given ample opportunity to ask more questions if they desire. For the child to comprehend the information, the responses to these questions should be brief and honest.

Preschoolers engage in magical thinking and believe that inanimate objects, such as the blood pressure cuff, may come alive and harm them. The sounds of electronic equipment may seem to give the machine life as a "monster." The child can act out feelings and thoughts through dramatic play, puppets, and drawings (Boggs, 2011a).

To promote communication with the toddler or preschooler:

- Acknowledge the child, but interact with parents before communicating with the child. This allows the child the opportunity to become accustomed to the nurse's presence.
- Communicate with the child at his or her eye level.
- Communicate using simple language and short sentences.
- Be honest in responses to the child.
- Avoid discussing frightening matters in front of the child.
- Encourage the child to engage in imaginative play with dolls, drawings, or puppets to allow the child to act out feelings and thoughts.
- Encourage toddlers to engage in parallel play.
- Encourage preschoolers to engage in dramatic and associative play (see Chapter 5 🔗 for further description of play in childhood).
- Allow the child the opportunity to ask questions.
- Allow additional time for the child to express thoughts without interruption.
- Offer the toddler choices when possible, such as "Do you want ice cream or a Popsicle?" This helps the child assert his or her independence.

Clinical Judgment

The nurse needs to provide preprocedure teaching to a 5-year-old who will have a procedure that involves the infusion of contrast or radiographic material. How can the nurse best explain this procedure to this age child? What words should be avoided?

School-Age Child (6-12 yrs)

The school-age child is able to use logic and understand certain events. School-age children also begin to comprehend the viewpoints of others, making them capable of empathy. School-age children begin to know body parts and organs, which allows them the opportunity to better understand hospitalization and illness. The nurse must assess the child's cognitive level of understanding and then give explanations accordingly. This assessment, prior to teaching, should decrease chances that the child will misinterpret the information. Medical terminology can be used when appropriate with an opportunity for the child to ask questions (Boggs, 2011a). Doll models with removable body parts that give the child a chance to find the body parts, remove them, and put them back in the appropriate place are valuable teaching tools when accompanied by explanations. In addition, showing diagrams of the body to school-age children or giving them an opportunity to express themselves through art, poems, or stories can enhance the learning experience (Boggs, 2011a).

School-age children possess a large vocabulary and are capable of verbally expressing their feelings. Also, because they are capable of making some decisions, it is important to involve them in discussions about their illness and in the planning of their care. When nurses do this, fears are diminished and the child generally remembers information for a longer period of time (Boggs, 2011a).

The following approaches may help to promote communication with the school-age child:

- Explain all procedures, techniques, and events.
- Speak directly to the child.
- Be honest in responses to the child's questions.
- Encourage the child to express thoughts and feelings through drawing, writing, or painting.
- Provide the school-age child with third-person conversation prompts, such as "Sometimes kids have told me that they are afraid of having surgery." This may encourage the child to admit fears or learn about the situation by asking about the other children.

Adolescent

Adolescents pose a particular communication challenge because they wish to be viewed as adults, even though they have not yet achieved adult cognitive abilities. Adolescents have adequate cognitive capacity to understand and employ abstractions in communication, but their ability to **decode** or interpret medical terminology is limited to their past healthcare experiences.

Adolescents have a need for independence from their parents and respect from the healthcare provider. The adolescent needs to be empowered and involved in his or her care (Rutherford, Pitetti, Zuckerbraun, et al., 2010). To build an effective communication relationship with an adolescent, the nurse must allow time to build rapport and establish trust.

The following approaches may help to promote communication with the adolescent:

- Provide the adolescent the opportunity to interact with the nurse in private, without the parents present.
- Explain the purpose of the interaction in a straightforward manner.
- Encourage the adolescent's participation by initiating a topic unrelated to health, such as "Tell me about your favorite music."

- Reassure the adolescent that he or she does not have to talk about anything until ready.
- Avoid comments or expressions that convey disapproval or surprise.
- Be aware of laws and limits regarding confidentiality. Inform the adolescent that anything affecting his or her immediate safety (such as suicidal ideation) must be communicated to the parent. Issues such as birth control vary from state to state, so clarify guidelines in the jurisdiction where the teen is seen for health care. (See Chapter 1 🔴 for more on confidentiality and consent.)
- Listen to what the teen is saying.
- Answer all questions honestly and directly.
- Offer the adolescent choices when possible (e.g., procedure times, lunch times).
- Do not assume that the adolescent has the same cognitive understanding as adults regarding health care and procedures; verify understanding and provide opportunities for questions.

See Table 15–6 in Chapter 15 🔴 for guidelines on preparing a child for procedures according to developmental level.

The Child with Special Needs

Effective communication is reciprocal. Children who are unable to communicate verbally due to physical, developmental, or acquired disabilities such as autism, cerebral palsy, brain injuries, or intubation may experience anxiety and frustration. See Chapter 34 🔴 for information about communicating with the child with autism. Children who have alterations in visual and hearing perception and those who do not speak English also have special needs related to communication; see page 155. (See Box 6–1.)

Feelings of helplessness may be exacerbated in young children, who are at a developmental disadvantage because they are frightened by the unfamiliar sights and sounds of the hospital and, at the same time, powerless to communicate to the people in charge of caring for them. Other family members may also become anxious due to the child's frustration with his or her communication impairment.

Positive communication strategies with the nonverbal child include signs or gestures, picture cards, or writing tablets. For the child who may be neurologically impaired, the nurse must be sensitive to nonverbal cues such as facial expressions, eye gaze, and body language. To help decrease the child's anxiety, try using direct eye contact, repeating the child's name, and speaking in a calm voice. To elicit responses from the child, a system such as head nods or eye blinks for "yes" or "no" can be established.

When the child is intubated, the tube blocks the vocal cords and speech is prohibited. Children experiencing oral surgery, dental surgery, oral trauma, or facial trauma may also not be able to verbally communicate. The nurse can decrease the child's anxiety by thoroughly explaining that he or she will be able to speak when the tube is removed. Alternative means of communication such as a writing board, alphabet board, keyboard, or symbol cards are essential for the child's physical and psychologic well-being.

Communicating with the Child with an Alteration in Visual Perception

Children who have visual impairment are challenged when removed from their familiar environment, especially during hospitalization.

| BOX 6–1 | Baccalaureate Essential VI: Interprofessional Communication and Collaboration for Improving Patient Health Outcomes |

Nurses and healthcare professionals have the responsibility to communicate effectively with patients and families regardless of the language, reading skills, and any hearing or speech challenges. Effective communication is essential to understanding the diagnosis and plan of care. Adherence to the treatment plan is dependent on the patient's and family's full understanding of the plan. Interprofessional collaboration improves quality of care and patient safety (Rose, 2011; Wagner, Liston, & Miller, 2011). Nurses must collaborate and effectively communicate with other healthcare professionals to maximize outcomes for all patients and families. Examples of interprofessional communication and collaboration include:

- Interdisciplinary rounds to discuss patients with complex healthcare needs
- Care coordination that integrates healthcare services among a variety of healthcare providers (see Chapter 16 🔗)

- Collaboration with the patient education department to develop easy-to-read education materials
- Working with developmental specialists to determine the most effective ways to communicate with children with special needs (see Chapter 16 🔗)
- Calling interpretation services to provide interpreters in different languages as needed
- Collaboration with pharmacists to establish plans for education of patients and families regarding prescribed and OTC medications
- Utilizing the speech and hearing department to provide guidance regarding communication with patients and families with auditory impairment

---

As the nurse, you can enhance communication with the child by using the following approaches:

- Identify yourself when entering the room; encourage others to do so.
- Orient the ambulating child to the objects in the room.
- Speak with a calm, slow voice—do not shout.
- Explain procedures before touching the child.
- Allow the child to handle the equipment when appropriate.
- Explain any unfamiliar sounds the child may hear.
- Encourage parents to stay with young children.
- Continually observe the child's facial expressions.
- Announce your departure before exiting the room.

See Chapter 24 🔗 for additional information related to visual impairment.

Communicating with the Child with an Alteration in Hearing Perception

Children with hearing deficits may be challenged in healthcare settings because they do not hear healthcare personnel or equipment; this can result in increased anxiety and stress. Nurses can enhance communication with a child who has a hearing impairment by using the following approaches:

- Always enter the child's room slowly—sudden images may startle the child.
- Face the child when speaking—to get his or her attention.
- Assess the degree of the hearing impairment and method of communication—to consider the necessity of using a registered interpreter and interpretation skill needed (e.g., specific sign language used, lip reading).
- Clarify the roles of the nurse and the interpreter—the nurse's awareness of how to use an interpreter will increase his or her credibility from the child's viewpoint.
- Inform the child that the interpreter is bound to confidentiality.

See Chapter 24 🔗 for additional information related to hearing impairment.

If the child is both hearing and visually impaired, only a few of the techniques listed previously will be useful. Special reading devices that convert letters in print into vibration may be used (Boggs, 2011b).

Communicating with the Child Who Does Not Speak English

Given the variety of cultures in the United States and the number of immigrants from other countries, most nurses will come in contact with a child and family who do not speak English. (See Chapter 3 🔗 for a discussion of culture.)

Children who are hospitalized and do not understand English are examined by people they do not know, and they see and hear things that may make no sense to them because they cannot benefit from the nurse's explanation. Therefore, when the nurse is interacting with a child who speaks another language, the goal is to minimize the possible negative outcomes related to the circumstances surrounding the child's treatment regimen. Any attempts to communicate with the child through picture cards, gestures, or just a few words in the child's language lessen the communication barrier and help promote trust. See Developing Cultural Competence: Suggested Guidelines for Communicating Using an Interpreter.

Clinical Tip

Family members who speak English as a second language may still need an interpreter in complex and stressful situations. Evaluate the need for an interpreter when teaching is needed related to administration of medications, in socially or psychologically complex situations such as with mental health issues, in patient safety situations such as concern for abuse or self-harm, and when informed consent is needed (Phillips, 2010).

Some additional tips for communicating with a child or family who do not speak English include:

- Speak to the child in a normal tone of voice.
- Use a communication board with pictures and names of basic needs or requests printed in both languages (e.g., bathroom, water, food, pain, hot, cold).
- Learn commonly used words in the child's language when possible.
- Allow all family members the opportunity to express their feelings.
- Encourage parents and other family members to participate in the child's care.
- Develop a plan of care that includes acknowledgment of and respect for the child's culture.
- Offer the family appropriate reassurance.
- Acknowledge effective parenting.

Nursing Management

The goal of nursing management is to collaborate with the child and family in establishing effective communication in order to plan and provide nursing care.

Developing Cultural Competence
Suggested Guidelines for Communicating Using an Interpreter

Nurses sometimes provide care to children and families with whom they cannot directly communicate. The family members may speak a language with which the nurse is not proficient, or the child may be deaf and might use sign language to communicate. Whatever the reason, certain guidelines can foster positive communication with the child and family, such as when the nurse can speak at least a few words in the child's language or is able to sign to introduce self. Other general guidelines are as follows:

- Obtain a skilled interpreter who is adept at both languages or systems of communication.
- Arrange seating so that the nurse and child or family face each other and both can readily see the interpreter. Speak to the child and family, rather than to the interpreter (Figure 6–4 ■).
- Ensure a situation that fosters communication such as soft and appropriate lighting, quiet environment, and comfort for all present.
- Ensure that all information is transmitted. If preliminary introductions occur with the translator, ask him or her to tell the child and family what was said. If the

family has much to say to the interpreter but the interpreter relays only a few words to the nurse, ask for further explanation of content.

- Have the family evaluate the interpreter services at a later time so they can state positive and negative parts of the experience. Another interpreter may be needed to successfully accomplish this evaluation. Adjust use of interpreters as needed to meet the family's needs, considering their preference for gender, age, and other characteristics.
- Avoid using children as interpreters for family members because the family may not feel comfortable sharing all healthcare issues with the child, and it can be a burden for the child to translate for the family. Confidentiality is also an issue.
- Be sensitive to issues that are confidential such as child abuse, alcoholism, pregnancy, and others. Watch for nonverbal communication that shows discomfort with the discussions occurring.

Note: *Further guidelines can be found in Standards from U.S. Department of Health and Human Services, Office of Minority Health. (2007). National standards for culturally and linguistically appropriate services in health care. Washington, DC: Author.*

Nursing Assessment and Diagnosis

A thorough assessment of the child's mental, physical, developmental, and cognitive abilities is necessary to identify the most effective method of communication with the child. Assess the child's developmental level, communication abilities, factors influencing communication, and potential barriers to communication. In addition, assess the language, communication skills, and level of understanding of the parent. (See Chapter 7 🔗 for assessment and interviewing techniques.)

Nursing diagnoses related to communication that may apply to the child and family include:

- Communication: Verbal, Impaired related to language development (toddler)
- Coping: Readiness for Enhanced related to communication about planned diagnostic procedures

- Social Interaction, Impaired related to verbal communication disability
- Communication, Readiness for Enhanced related to availability of a medical interpreter or translator

NANDA-I © 2012

Planning and Implementation

The focus of nursing interventions is facilitation of effective therapeutic communication with the child and family, and the resulting establishment of an effective nurse–child–family relationship (Table 6–5). The nurse accomplishes these tasks through the use of specific techniques, attitudes, and skills tailored to the needs of the child and family (Figure 6–5 ■). See Partnering with Families: Establishing Rapport with Children. Providing an appropriate

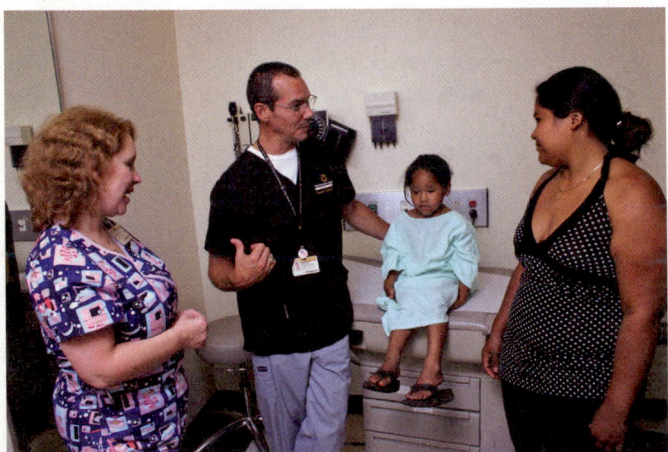

FIGURE 6–4 ■ Most hospitals have designated interpreters that you should use. If not available, find a professional interpreter whom you have identified beforehand and who knows medical terms and the cultural norms of the family. The interpreter should be positioned to improve communication. Maintain eye contact with the parent or patient, not the interpreter. To ensure confidentiality of information for parents, avoid using a family member for history taking.

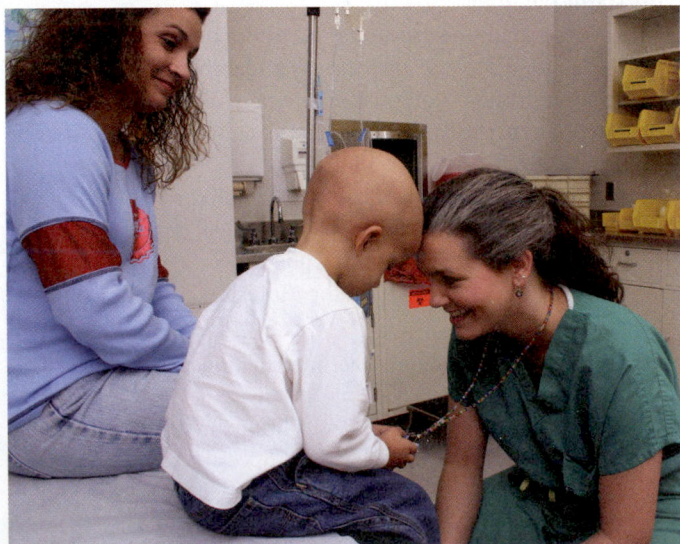

FIGURE 6–5 ■ Taking time to listen to the family members and child is important to the establishment of trust and developing a rapport with the child and family.

TABLE 6–5	Using Therapeutic Communication Techniques with Children	
COMMUNICATION TECHNIQUE	**EXAMPLE**	**NURSING IMPLICATIONS**
Accepting	"It is okay to cry. I know that this hurts."	The nurse should empathize with the child's thoughts and feelings. Conveying acceptance includes respecting the child's emotions by allowing the child to cry when in pain or letting the child know that crying is okay.
Active listening	Pay attention to what the child says, acknowledge the child's feelings, and avoid interruption.	Involve children in the discussion and encourage them to relay their points of view.
		Face the child and parents when talking to let the child and family know that the nurse is listening and understands what is being communicated.
Broad openings	"Tell me about school."	Use open-ended questions to allow the child to choose the discussion topic.
Clarifying	*Child:* "Whenever the doctor tells me I have to stay in the hospital longer, I get so mad." *Nurse:* "It sounds like you are very angry. What does that feel like?"	Communicate understanding by asking the child to clarify or elaborate on the thoughts expressed.
Collaborating	"Perhaps we can work together and figure out the best way to go about handling this."	Assist the child and family through the problem-solving process. The nurse first suggests collaboration with the child and/or family, and then assists them to work through each step of the problem-solving process.
Exploring	"Can you tell me more about how you feel after you receive your chemotherapy?"	Exploring helps the child to organize thoughts and focus on particular issues. It also encourages the child to freely discuss issues in more detail.
Focusing	"I do want to hear about your dog in a little while, but right now could you tell me about your stomachache?"	Utilize focusing to guide the direction of the conversation. This is useful for small children who often wish to discuss a variety of topics rather than focus on one topic. Focusing allows the nurse to explore the child's concern further.
Giving recognition	"That is a very colorful picture you are drawing."	Identify observed behaviors or cues of the child. This indicates an interest in the child.
Observations	"You tell me you aren't hurting, but your fists are clenched and your mouth is quivering." "You seem sad today."	Pay close attention to the behavioral aspect of communication. The nurse acknowledges behaviors that indicate the child's thoughts and feelings.
Offering self	"I will stay with you while your mother goes to the cafeteria to eat lunch."	The nurse is available to listen and be with the child.
Placing the event in time or sequence	"Which happened first . . .?" "When did you first start feeling . . .?"	Assist the child to determine what happened and in what order. The goal is to help the child and nurse understand the progression of events.
Reflection	*Adolescent:* "I keep thinking about what my friends are doing while I am in the hospital, and if they miss me." *Nurse:* "It is hard not being with your friends."	Repeat a phrase or sentence the child just said. By reflection, the nurse indicates an interest in the discussion and validates the child's concerns.
Restatement or paraphrasing	*Child:* "I think I should tell my mother that I have been smoking." *Nurse:* "You want to tell your mother about your smoking?"	The nurse repeats what the child has said using different words. By restating, the nurse acknowledges to the child that he or she is listening. It also provides a means to validate the interpretation of the child's statement.
Summarizing	"The two things that you are most concerned about are. . . ."	Highlight the key facts obtained in the conversation by condensing the information the child related. Summarizing provides the child and nurse an opportunity to consider further direction of the discussion or to give the discussion closure. The nurse can summarize at various points during the conversation; it is not necessary to wait until the discussion is nearing completion.
Validating perceptions	"It sounds like you are sad about being sick. Is that correct?"	The nurse shares the conclusions drawn from the discussion with the child. Validating perceptions provides an opportunity for the child to confirm or deny the nurse's interpretation of the meaning of their communication.

Source: *Data from Antai-Otong, D. (2007). Therapeutic communication techniques. In Nurse-client communication (pp. 53–97). Sudbury, MA: Jones and Bartlett; Arnold, E. C. (2011). Developing therapeutic communication skills. In E. C. Arnold & K. U. Boggs (Eds.), Interpersonal relationships: Professional communication skills for nurses (6th ed., pp. 175–196). St. Louis, MO: Saunders; Fontaine, K. L. (2009). Illness management: Communication and psychoeducation. In Mental health nursing (6th ed., pp. 122–145). Upper Saddle River, NJ: Pearson/Prentice Hall.*

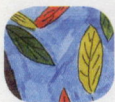

Partnering with Families

Establishing Rapport with Children

A child will be more responsive to the nurse when efforts are made to help the child feel like he or she is an important person in the interaction. By following these guidelines, nurses can help establish rapport with the child and encourage the child to share personal information and feelings.

- Sit or otherwise lower yourself so that you are at the child's eye level. *Sitting at eye level suggests that the nurse cares.*
- Note what the child is playing with or reading; ask about this or perhaps his favorite cartoon character. *Interest displayed by the nurse encourages the child's feeling of security.*
- Agree with the child when appropriate and share your feelings: "I don't like the taste of that medicine either, but sometimes I have to take it when I am sick—but then I have juice." *This statement offers encouragement to the child and family.*
- Compliment a physical feature or activity performed by the child: "You are really strong" or "You picked really nice colors for that picture." *This observational statement may reduce anxiety and imparts status for the child.*

- Use a calm tone of voice, with developmentally appropriate language. *Children want to talk and share information on their level of comprehension.*
- Pace the discussion or procedure in a nonhurried manner. *Trying to rush the child will only add to his or her anxiety.*
- Preschoolers have a limited concept of time. Explain concepts in terms they understand: "Your mother will be back after lunch." *This type of response provides them with a concrete time frame.*
- Include the adolescent in discussion about his or her care. *They have the cognitive ability to employ abstract communication and comprehend scientific terminology.*
- Listen more than you talk, and avoid distractions. *This attentive behavior of the nurse conveys an attitude of interest in the child.*
- Be truthful with the child. *They will respect your honesty.*

Source: *Data from Boggs, K. U. (2011a). Communicating with children. In E. C. Arnold & K. U. Boggs, Interpersonal relationships: Professional communication skills for nurses (6th ed., pp. 349–368). St. Louis, MO: Saunders; Chilman-Blair, K. (2010). Communicating with children about their illness. Practice Nursing, 21(12), 631–633.*

---

environment will foster effective nurse–child–family communication. Remember to provide privacy to ensure confidentiality.

Establish Trust

Trust plays a critical role for an effective nurse–child–family relationship. To establish an atmosphere of trust, the nurse should do the following:

- Follow through with promises to the child and family—this ensures secure feelings for the family.
- Respect confidentiality—this promotes protection of the family.
- Be truthful with the child and family—they will respect the nurse, even if the truth is not what they want to hear.

If a child asks whether a procedure is painful, answer truthfully, but follow with positive words. For example, if a child asks if his "shot" is going to hurt, you might reply, "Yes, but it will only hurt for a moment, and then it will be over. Your mother can hold your hand while I give you the medicine, if that will make you feel better."

Maintain Confidentiality

Essential to the development of trust between the nurse, child, and family is an understanding of the confidentiality of shared information, especially when it is of a sensitive nature. To foster trust, assure the child and family that information is shared only with those directly involved in the child's care. Offer the older child and adolescent the opportunity to discuss matters privately, without the presence of their parents. Explain any exceptions to confidentiality to the child or adolescent. Exceptions to confidentiality include situations such as the child potentially posing a danger to self or others, for example, with suicidal ideation or homicidal thoughts.

Practitioners are increasingly concerned about losing the trust of their patient if they disclose information gained in confidence. However, if the child has consented, either verbally or in writing, that the information may be shared, there is no breach of confidentiality. In

other cases, the child needs to be informed that confidential information must be shared because of state reporting requirements for infectious disease or safety concerns for the child. The nurse should take the time to explain the rationale for sharing confidential information in an effort to gain the child's assent and maintain trust.

Convey Respect

Nursing behaviors that demonstrate respect for the child and family include:

- Knocking before entering the room to denote a respectful attitude
- Addressing the child by first name and parents by "Mr." or "Ms."
- Looking at the child when asking questions to encourage response from the child
- Considering the family's values, culture, and feelings, such as spatial distancing and eye contact, to enhance communication
- Explaining needed procedures before beginning assessments or interventions
- Encouraging their participation in discussions with the multidisciplinary team

Implement Appropriate Communication Strategies

Implement appropriate verbal and nonverbal communication strategies. Be aware of nontherapeutic communication techniques that can lead to communication barriers, as they are often based in bias or judgment. It is essential for the nurse to recognize his or her own feelings and separate those from the child and family. Table 6–6 provides examples of ineffective communication techniques and nursing implications.

Encourage Communication Through Alternative Techniques

Children have the ability to communicate thoughts and feelings in ways other than verbal expression. Play, drawing, journaling, storytelling, bibliotherapy, and humor are effective methods to encourage the child's communication.

TABLE 6–6	Ineffective Communication Techniques	
INEFFECTIVE COMMUNICATION TECHNIQUE	**EXAMPLE**	**NURSING IMPLICATIONS**
Advising (nurse tells the child what to do)	"If I were you, I would tell your parents that you've been drinking with your friends."	Advising prevents the child (and family) from problem solving and makes the nurse rather than the family responsible for the outcome.
Belittling expressed feelings (nurse may be ignoring the importance of the child's problems and not listening carefully)	"Don't you know that big boys don't cry?"	Common expressions may cause the child to "feel like a baby."
Challenging (arguing with the child indicates that his or her perceptions are not genuine or legitimate)	"Was that a good reason to become angry?"	Arguing or challenging the child or family may imply judgment. It is not productive to the progress of the communication.
Changing the topic (introduction of an unrelated topic to the child's discussion)	*Child:* "I wish that I would just die so I wouldn't have to go through this pain anymore." *Nurse:* "Has your mom been in to see you yet today?"	The child may believe that his or her thoughts are not important. It interrupts the child's thought pattern and spontaneity. The nurse should allow the child to discuss feelings and encourage further discussion.
Disagreeing (opposing the child's or parent's thoughts and emotions denies self-respect)	*Child's mother:* "That doctor doesn't know what he is doing—our child is sicker now than when he first came to the hospital." *Nurse:* "Your child's doctor is an expert in his field and he is a highly respected pediatrician. Your child is getting the best care around."	Disagreeing with the child or family limits the opportunity to establish rapport or to increase the child's or parent's self-understanding. The nurse should encourage the child and family to express their thoughts.
False reassurance (telling the child how to feel ignores his or her real feelings of distress)	"You're going to be just fine." "You don't have anything to worry about."	This minimizes the child's situation and increases anxiety. The nurse should be caring and honest in responses to questions.
Imposing values (nurse applies own biases and prejudices to impose values, judgments, and morals)	*Nurse to parent:* "You should let your child have that vaccine!" *Nurse to child:* "You were bad to refuse your medicine." Terms imposing values are *should, good, bad, wrong, right.*	Biases and prejudices can impede open communication and cause the child or family to mistrust the nurse.
Multiple questions (asking more than one question at a time)	"When did you first start feeling bad? How did you feel when you first got sick? How do you feel now?"	Expecting a young child to answer multiple questions results in the child's frustration and limits his or her participation. Also, the nurse will not know which question was answered.
Parroting (repeating the child's words)	*Child:* "I'm so tired." *Nurse:* "You're so tired."	No further expectations of the child are required. The child often misunderstands meaning and ceases to respond. The nurse should rephrase the child's statement or ask questions for clarification.
Probing (failure of nurse to respect the child's or family's decisions and privacy)	"Tell me what secrets you keep from your parents." "I won't be able to help you unless you tell me everything."	This approach implies secrecy or blame of one family member to another. The nurse should demonstrate respect for the child's and family's decisions—unless the decision may cause harm to the child or delay his or her recovery.
Requesting an explanation (similar to challenging and begins with "why?")	"Why can't you just take your medicine like you are supposed to?"	The child interprets "why" as misbehavior. This also implies devaluation of his or her feelings and thoughts. The nurse should ask questions such as "Can you tell me the reason that you don't want to take your medication?"
Stereotypical comments or idiomatic expressions (an indication to the child and family that the nurse may have little concern about their experiences; often references from folklore and proverbs, which means they may be culture specific)	"It's all water under the bridge." "That's the way the ball bounces."	The nurse should avoid expressions that children from different backgrounds may not understand.

Source: *Adapted from Fontaine, K. L. (2009). Illness management: Communication and psychoeducation. In* Mental health nursing *(6th ed., p. 136). Upper Saddle River, NJ: Pearson/Prentice Hall.*

Play

Play promotes growth and development and is crucial for the mental health of children. It has been described as the "work" of children in that it confirms what children know about their world and allows them to explore the rest. Play has been further described as the "language" of childhood; it is the talk, and the toys are its words.

Children have limited experience with stressful events; therefore, when illness or hospitalization occurs, their fears and anxieties rise. Where hospitalization forces a passive role on children, play allows them to take an active role, thus allowing them to gain an increased sense of independence. Role or fantasy play using puppets, dolls, stuffed animals, skits, and visits from cartoon characters offers children an opportunity to learn about health issues affecting them as well as providing an opportunity to communicate their feelings. Allowing children to play with unfamiliar equipment (that has been thoroughly inspected to ensure the child's safety) is another effective means of play. Handling and pretending to use the equipment, such as giving the doll a "shot," helps the child to understand what will happen and further allows expression of fears and concerns. For children engaged in magical thinking, playing with the equipment diminishes some of its influence as a frightening object as the child determines that the equipment is not "alive" (Figure 6–6 ■).

Expressive Play—Painting, Drawing

Younger children have developed fine motor ability to draw with crayons, markers, chalk, and colored pencils. While drawings are used as an assessment tool to determine a child's developmental level, they are also a therapeutic activity for children to put into pictures what they may not be able to put into words. By expressing themselves through forms of art, such as paintings, clay, textiles, or embroidery, children can communicate their feelings about being in the hospital. Additionally, expressive arts such as make-believe, dramatic sketches, and skits help children to cope with the stress of hospitalization (Basso, 2010).

Although the stress of hospitalization and illness can easily be interpreted, other drawings, such as those related to abuse and trauma, should be interpreted by a certified play therapist, someone specially trained in interpretation of children's drawings. Provide the child with opportunities and necessary equipment to draw or paint. Ask if the child would prefer to draw or paint, though both approaches may be used. See Chapter 15 🔗 for further description of communication techniques with hospitalized children.

Journaling

Older children and adolescents may find journaling a good method to express their thoughts and feelings as well as to vent frustrations, fears, and the effects of their illness and treatments (Figure 6–7 ■). Provide the child or adolescent with a journal or notebook in which to write thoughts. Assure the child or adolescent that the journal is his or her property and assist in determining a safe place for the journal when not in use.

Storytelling

Storytelling is an effective means to communicate with the child. The child can engage in storytelling verbally, or by writing and drawing, providing an opportunity for self-expression. The nurse can begin a story by saying, "Once upon a time, there was a little girl named (child's name or a fictitious name) and she had to go to the hospital. . . ." Then ask the child to tell what happens next or to finish the story. Another method is to have the child complete a sentence. For example, begin a sentence such as "What hurts me the most is . . ." and have the child complete the sentence.

Bibliotherapy

Bibliotherapy describes the use of books related to topics and events the child is experiencing or will experience. Reading materials are selected based on the individualized needs of the patient and are of therapeutic value (Chamberlin, Heaps, & Robert, 2008; Fanner & Urquhart, 2008). Through books, the child can learn about life events such as illness, hospitalization, and the birth of a sibling. Children can be encouraged to draw and write their own stories. Many developmentally appropriate books are available to explain a variety of illnesses, treatments, and other concepts such as those related to death and tragedy.

In collaboration with the family, the nurse determines the appropriate materials specific to the child's needs. The nurse assists the family in obtaining these resources either through the institution's sources or by other means such as websites, bookstores, and support groups.

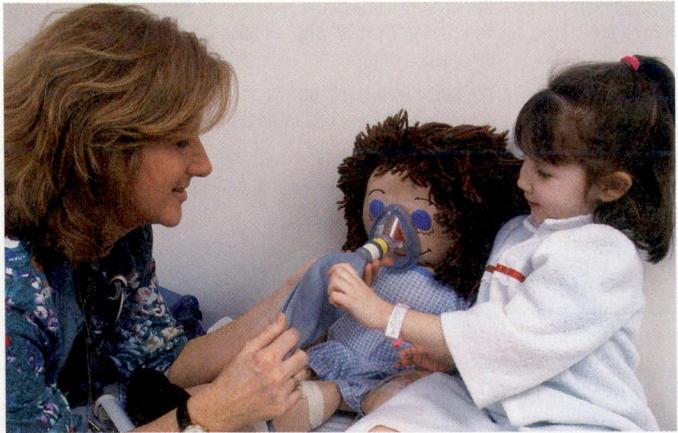

FIGURE 6–6 ■ Putting a mask on her doll gives this child some mastery over her coming surgical experience. It is important for children to see and touch medical equipment in order to allay fears of the unknown.

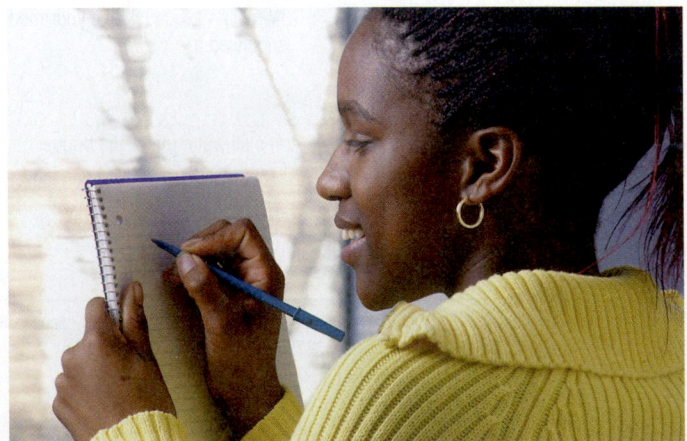

FIGURE 6–7 ■ Most teens are happy to keep a journal of important events and feelings. Ensure them confidentiality.

Humor

The use of humor to communicate in the pediatric setting can serve to bridge communication gaps. It can help to reduce a child's fear of illness, injury, and hospitalization. Children age 3 to 4 years take great delight in distorting familiar concepts. Many children enjoy the verbal expressions of humor in stories like *The Cat in the Hat* (Seuss, 1957), *The Stinky Cheese Man* (Scieszka & Smith, 1992), and *Where the Sidewalk Ends* (Silverstein, 1974). Children age 7 to 8 years try to understand the incongruous nature of humor by responding seriously to riddles and telling jokes without a punch line. Using funny books to help the child relax and laugh can lessen anxiety and enhance relaxation in healthcare settings.

Knowing when to use humor is important. Although humor can facilitate healing, it may not always be appropriate. Prior to using humor with a patient, establishing a therapeutic relationship is essential. The nurse should then take cues from the patient. Timing is essential. If the patient or family members are using humor, then it is probably okay. The nurse should realize that patients from different cultures respond to humor in different ways (Fontaine, 2009).

Laughter has many therapeutic benefits including muscle relaxation, pain reduction, exercise for the heart, decreased stress, and improved mood (Mora-Ripoll, 2010). Nurses can look for that particular time when laughter is appropriate for the child. Engaging in a familiar activity or task in an unfamiliar way, such as wearing a lab or scrub jacket backwards, can offer a coping strategy to a stressed child. Acting silly, such as dancing around to the music the child is listening to or joining the child in playing with a favorite toy, can provide a light moment for both the child and the family.

Evaluation

Evaluation is dependent on assessment findings and specific interventions. General anticipated outcomes for the child and family include:

- Validation of the child's and family's feelings and thoughts
- Establishment of a therapeutic nurse–child–family relationship
- Ability of the family to ask questions and communicate needs

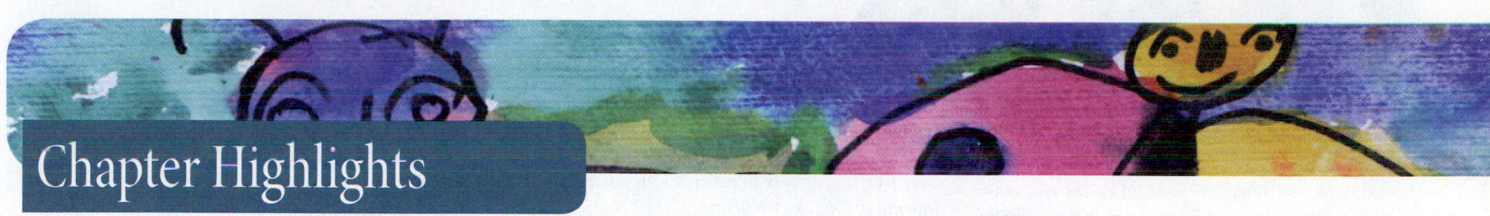

Chapter Highlights

- The nurse–child–family relationship is dependent on effective communication. The nurse's communication with the child and family serves as the connection between the family and the healthcare system.
- Communication is the exchange of information, thoughts, and feelings. It is an ongoing, cyclic process. Individuals are constantly communicating, either consciously or unconsciously, through verbal and nonverbal techniques.
- The two primary modes of communication are verbal and nonverbal communication.
- A child's communication ability and the variety of techniques used to communicate directly correspond with his or her developmental and cognitive levels.

- The challenge of communication with the child is compounded when the child has a sensory or other neurologic impairment.
- Nursing care focuses on identifying communication patterns and needs of the child and family. A thorough assessment of the child's mental, physical, developmental, and cognitive abilities is necessary to determine the most effective method of communication with the child and family.
- Nursing techniques and skills in communication include establishing an appropriate environment, establishing rapport and trust, conveying respect, maintaining professional boundaries, maintaining confidentiality, and implementing appropriate verbal and nonverbal communication techniques.

Clinical Reasoning in Action

INTRODUCTION

Recall the family in the opening vignette. Madison, age 7, was recently hospitalized and diagnosed with juvenile arthritis. A nurse is visiting the home to explain Madison's condition to her siblings, Brittney and Madeline, and to further develop a plan of care with Madison and her parents.

DESCRIPTION

The nurse will collaborate with the clinic's multidisciplinary team and the family to establish a plan of care for Madison. The nurse's first priority is to establish a therapeutic relationship with the family, and the home visit provides an opportunity to discuss Madison's condition with her siblings.

DISCUSSION

1. What developmental considerations will the nurse address when communicating with Madison?

2. What information do the parents need regarding Madison's understanding of the disease process based on her developmental level?

3. How will the nurse present information to Madison's 4-year-old sibling? What therapeutic communication techniques will the nurse implement? How do these techniques differ from techniques used with school-age Madison?

4. How will the nurse present information to Madison's 9-year-old sibling? What therapeutic communication techniques will the nurse implement? How would that differ from presenting information to her 4-year-old sibling?

5. How will the nurse evaluate the effectiveness of teaching to Madison, her parents, and her siblings?

6. What are the benefits of involving the siblings in Madison's care? In what ways can they assist and participate?

NCLEX-RN® Review

1. In speaking with an adolescent, which exemplifies an appropriate method of communication?
   1. "I need to discuss your medical history with you. Should your dad leave or stay?"
   2. "I am not sure that is behavior appropriate for a child your age. Tell me more."
   3. "Lunch will be up at 11:30 and you can play video games until then."
   4. "I really need you to tell me everything so we can get this over with."

2. The nurse is caring for a 4-year-old preschooler who has just had an IV placed. The child is upset and crying. The nurse tells the patient, "It is okay to cry, I know that it hurt." What therapeutic communication technique is this nurse using?
   1. Accepting
   2. Collaborating
   3. Giving recognition
   4. Offering self

3. Which action indicates that a student nurse understands how to promote effective communication through a therapeutic nurse–child–family relationship? The student:
   1. Gets the family whatever they need as promised.
   2. Gives the family reassurance that everything will be OK.
   3. Listens and observes the family interactions.
   4. Steers discussions away from worrisome topics.

4. Which is the most important nursing intervention to facilitate communication with a hospitalized preschool-age child?
   1. Provide detailed explanations of procedures to the child.
   2. Encourage the child to engage in play with dolls, puppets, or safe medical equipment.
   3. Ask the child to write a story about the hospitalization.
   4. Keep visitors to a minimum.

See Appendix I ✏ *for answers.*

References

Antai-Otong, D. (2007). *Nurse-client communication.* Sudbury, MA: Jones and Bartlett.

Arnold, E. C., & Boggs, K. U. (2011). *Interpersonal relationships: Professional communication skills for nurses* (6th ed.). St. Louis, MO: Saunders

Arnold, E. C. (2011). Developing therapeutic communication skills. In E. C. Arnold & K. U. Boggs (Eds.), *Interpersonal relationships: Professional communication skills for nurses* (6th ed., pp. 175–196). St. Louis, MO: Saunders.

Bach, S., & Grant, A. (2009). *Communication & interpersonal skills for nurses.* Exeter, United Kingdom: Learning Matters Ltd.

Basso, R. (2010). Expressive arts in pediatric orientation groups. *Journal of Pediatric Nursing, 25*(6), 482–489.

Boggs, K. U. (2011a). Communicating with children. In E. C. Arnold & K. U. Boggs (Eds.), *Interpersonal relationships: Professional communication skills for nurses* (6th ed., pp. 349–368). St. Louis, MO: Saunders.

Boggs, K. U. (2011b). Communicating with clients with communication disabilities In E. C. Arnold & K. U. Boggs (Eds.), *Interpersonal relationships: Professional communication skills for nurses* (6th ed., pp. 337–347). St. Louis, MO: Saunders.

Chamberlin, D., Heaps, D., & Robert, I. (2008). Bibliotherapy and information prescriptions: A summary of the published evidence-base and recommendations from past and ongoing Books on Prescription projects. *Journal of Psychiatric and Mental Health Nursing, 15,* 24–36.

Chilman-Blair, K. (2010). Communicating with children about illness. *Practice Nursing, 21*(12), 631–633.

Fanner, D., & Urquhart, C. (2008). Bibliotherapy for mental health service users Part 1: A systematic review. *Health Information and Libraries Journal, 25,* 237–252.

Fontaine, K. L. (2009). Illness management: Communication and psychoeducation. In *Mental health nursing* (6th ed., pp. 122–145). Upper Saddle River, NJ: Pearson/Prentice Hall.

Giger, J. N., & Davidhizar, R. E. (2008). *Transcultural nursing: Assessment and intervention* (5th ed.). St. Louis, MO: Mosby Elsevier.

Jackson, E., Kelley, M., McNeil, P., Meyer, E., Schlegel, L., & Eaton, M. (2008). Does therapeutic touch help reduce pain and anxiety in patients with cancer? *Clinical Journal of Oncology Nursing, 12*(1), 113–120.

Johnston, S. L. (2009, December). Healing touch and SCI. *Paraplegia News,* 19–23.

Kashaninia, Z., Sajedi, F., Rahgozar, M., & Noghabi, F. A. (2008). The effect of kangaroo care on behavioral responses to pain of an intramuscular injection in neonates. *Journal for Specialists in Pediatric Nursing, 13*(4), 275–280.

Kearvell, H., & Grant, J. (2010). Getting connected: How nurses can support mother/infant attachment in the neonatal intensive care unit. *Australian Journal of Advanced Nursing, 27*(3), 75–82.

Leonard, A., & Mayers, P. (2008). Parents' lived experience of providing kangaroo care to their preterm infants. *Health SA Gesondheid* (13)4, 16–28.

Mora-Ripoll, R. (2010). The therapeutic value of laughter in medicine. *Alternative Therapies in Health and Medicine, 16*(6), 56–64.

Nyqvist, K. H., Anderson, G. C., Bergman, N., Cattaneo, A., Charpak, N., Davanzo, R., . . . Widström, A. M. (2010). State of the art and recommendations. Kangaroo mother care: Application in a high-tech environment. *Breastfeeding Review, 18*(3), 21–28.

Phillips, C. (2010). Using interpreters: A guide for GPs. *Australian Family Physician, 39*(4), 188–195.

Purnell, L. D. (2009). *Guide to culturally competent health care* (2nd ed.). Philadelphia: F. A. Davis.

Rose, L. (2011). Interprofessional collaboration in the ICU: How to define? *Nursing in Critical Care, 16*(1), 5–10.

Rutherford, K. A., Pitetti, R. D., Zuckerbraun, N. S., Smola, S., & Gold, M. A. (2010). Adolescents' perceptions of interpersonal communication, respect, and concern for privacy in an urban tertiary-care pediatric emergency department. *Pediatric Emergency Care, 26*(4), 257–263.

Spector, R. E. (2009). *Cultural diversity in health and illness* (7th ed.). Upper Saddle River, NJ: Prentice Hall.

Tang, R., Tegeler, C., Larrimore, D., Cowgill, S., & Kemper, K. J. (2010). Improving the well-being of nursing leaders through healing touch training. *Journal of Alternative and Complementary Medicine, 16*(8), 837–841.

Teckenberg-Jansson, P., Huotilainen, M., Polkki, T., Lipsanen, J., & Jarvenpaa, A. (2011). Rapid effects of neonatal music therapy combined with kangaroo care on prematurely-born infants. *Nordic Journal of Music Therapy, 20*(1), 22–42.

Tessier, R., Charpak, N., Giron, M., Cristo, M., de Calume, Z. F., & Ruiz-Peláez, J. G. (2009). Kangaroo mother care, home environment and father involvement in the first year of life: A randomized controlled study. *Acta Paediatrica, 98,* 1444–1450.

Wagner, J., Liston, B., & Miller, J. (2011). Developing interprofessional communication skills. *Teaching and Learning in Nursing, 6,* 97–101.

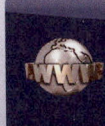

Pearson Nursing Student Resources
Find additional review materials at
nursing.pearsonhighered.com
Prepare for success with additional NCLEX®-style practice questions, interactive assignments and activities, web links, animations and videos, and more!

Pediatric and Newborn Assessment

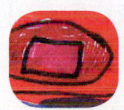 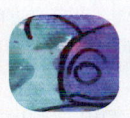 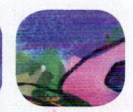

KEY TERMS

Learning Outcomes

After completing this chapter, you will be able to:

1. Discuss the elements of a health history appropriate for an infant and child at different ages.

2. Demonstrate strategies to gain cooperation of a young child for assessment.

3. List five normal variations in pediatric physical findings (such as a Mongolian spot in an infant) observed during a physical assessment.

4. Demonstrate the differences in sequence of the physical assessment for infants, children, and adolescents.

5. Modify physical assessment techniques according to the age and developmental stage of the child.

6. Determine the sexual maturity rating of males and females based upon physical signs of secondary sexual characteristics present.

7. Analyze findings from the assessment of multiple systems and identify signs indicating the presence of a health condition.

8. Distinguish between the assessment procedures used for newborns and older infants.

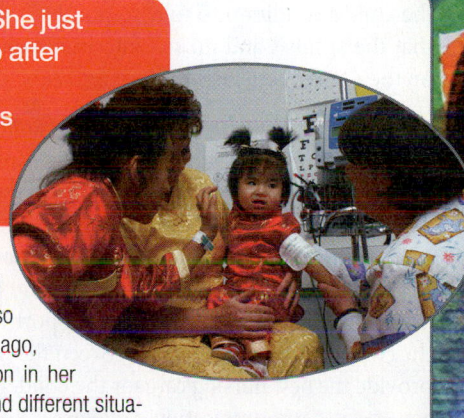

"Jasmine is really afraid of all these people. She just started playing with me a couple of days ago after getting to know me. I know she doesn't feel good, because she wouldn't play with me this morning."

—*Monique, Jasmine's 6-year-old sister*

Jasmine, 27 months old, was recently adopted into the Porter family. She is visiting the health clinic for internationally adopted children with her new mother and sister Monique, who was also adopted, for a comprehensive health assessment. Until 3 weeks ago, Jasmine was living in a center for children eligible for adoption in her native China. She speaks no English and is very fearful of new and different situations. Mrs. Porter is trying to reduce Jasmine's anxiety and assist her adaptation by wearing clothing familiar to her.

Mrs. Porter is anxious to have Jasmine evaluated to identify any health promotion or special healthcare issues that need to be addressed, such as development, growth, nutrition, immunizations, and health conditions. Jasmine had many immunizations before leaving China, and she has never had a major illness or injury. Limited information is available about her biological parents and their health.

Mrs. Porter thinks Jasmine seems small for her age, and she is also concerned that she may have an ear infection. Jasmine's appetite has not been good for the past day, and she has been irritable. Mrs. Porter also thinks she has a slight fever.

Do examination techniques need to vary for children of different ages? How does the nurse gain cooperation for the examination from infants and toddlers? This chapter answers these questions and provides an overview of pediatric assessment, including communication and history taking followed by examination techniques geared to the unique needs of newborns and pediatric patients.

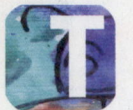

The patient history and physical examination provide a structure and a sequence for collecting and analyzing relevant assessment data. The initial physical examination findings provide the baseline for monitoring a child's future growth and development and his or her response to care for any previously identified health problems. Strategies for obtaining the child's history will be presented first. The remainder of the chapter describes a systematic process for physical examination of the infant, child, and adolescent. A separate section at the end of the chapter addresses newborn assessment. The data obtained from an accurate and complete assessment are the foundation for:

- The nursing process and development of nursing diagnoses
- Development of a plan of care
- Implementation and evaluation of nursing interventions

OBTAINING THE CHILD'S HISTORY
Communication Strategies

What makes communication effective? What does it mean when a parent or caretaker will not look you in the eye when speaking with you? What types of cues indicate that a parent may be withholding historical information?

The health history interview is a personal conversation between a nurse and a parent, caretaker, or adolescent. It takes place in many different healthcare settings—hospital, school, clinic, office setting, or home—but regardless of setting, the privacy of information must be maintained (Box 7–1). Try to ensure that this exchange of information between you and the parent or child is clearly understood by both parties. Effective communication is difficult to accomplish for many reasons: Parents and children may not correctly interpret what the nurse says, the nurse may not understand completely what the parent or child says, or parents may be too stressed with life events or the child's condition to fully respond to questions. Also remember that the family's and nurse's interpretation of information is based on their life experiences, culture, and education.

Strategies to Build Rapport with the Family and Child

As you begin taking the history, make sure the parents understand the purpose of the interview and assure them that the information will be used appropriately. To develop rapport, demonstrate your interest in and concern for the child and family by actively listening to the information shared. Communicate as a nonjudgmental and noncontrolling professional. This rapport forms the foundation for the collaborative relationship between the nurse and parent that will provide the best nursing care for the child. Refer to Chapter 6 for age-specific communication strategies. The following strategies help to establish rapport with the child's family during the nursing history:

- **Introduce yourself** (your name, your title or position, and your role in caring for the child). To demonstrate respect, ask all family members present what name they would prefer you to use when talking with them.
- **Explain the purpose of the interview** and why the nursing history is different from the information collected from other health professionals. For example, "The nurses will use this information to plan nursing care best suited for your child."
- **Provide privacy** and remove as many distractions as possible during the interview. If the patient's room does not offer privacy, attempt to find a vacant patient room or lounge.

BOX 7–1	Health Insurance Portability and Accountability Act (HIPAA)

Assure the parents and child that the information provided during the assessment is protected under the Health Insurance Portability and Accountability Act (HIPAA), a federal law that established guidelines for the electronic transmission of patient information. See Chapter 1 for more information about HIPAA.

- **Direct the focus of the interview** with open-ended questions. Use close-ended questions or directing statements to clarify information. Open-ended questions are useful to initiate the interview, develop a rapport, and understand the parent's perceptions of the child's problem; for example, "What problems led to Roberto's admission to the hospital?" Close-ended questions are used to obtain detailed information; for example, "How high was Tommy's fever this morning?"
- **Ask one question at a time** so that the parent or child understands what piece of information you want and so that you know which question is being answered. "Does any member of your family have diabetes, heart disease, or sickle cell anemia?" is a multiple question. Ask about each disease separately to ensure the most accurate response. See Developing Cultural Competence: Questioning.
- **Use nonverbal behavior** such as nodding, smiling, and eye contact at appropriate times to communicate that you are hearing the information shared. See Chapter 6. Paraphrasing or providing a brief summary of the information shared often helps assure you and the parent and child that you have heard the information correctly.
- **Observe the parent–child interaction and behavior** during the interview and try to sense their feelings. Be alert for the emotional tone of the family and child during the interview. If two or more adults are present, consider who does the talking (mother or father, parent or grandparent, parent or child) and note areas of agreement or disagreement. Direct questions to the child when appropriate, and look to the child for verification of responses from the accompanying adult.
- **Be honest** with the child when answering questions or when giving information about what will happen. Children need to learn that they can trust you.
- **Choose the language style that is best understood** by the parent and child. Commonly used phrases can have different meanings to persons in various regions of the country or to different ethnic groups. Parents may have previously heard clinical terms and use them to describe the child's condition. Parents may not have a full understanding about the condition the terms describe, but think these terms match the signs noted in their child. To improve communication, clarify the parents' understanding

Developing Cultural Competence
Questioning

Some cultural groups, particularly Asians, try to anticipate the answers you want to hear, or they say yes even if they do not understand the question. This practice is done in an effort to please you or as an expression of politeness. Remember to phrase your questions in a neutral manner. It is also important to assess the family's understanding of English or the language used for history taking.

of clinical terms or request frequent feedback from the parents or child to ensure you understand their meaning. For example, "You used the term hyperactivity. I think I know what you mean, but would you explain the behavior a bit more for me?"

- **Use an interpreter** to improve communication when you are not fluent in the family's primary language. Look at and direct questions to the family members rather than to the interpreter. This helps the family see themselves as the focus of care. (See Chapter 6 🔵.)

Subtle nonverbal and verbal cues often indicate that the parent has not provided complete information about the child's problem. Observe for behaviors such as avoidance of eye contact, change in voice pitch, or hesitation when responding to a question. Being supportive and asking clarifying questions encourage further description or the expression of information that is difficult for the parent or child to share; for example, "It sounds like that was a very difficult experience. How did Jasmine react?" See Table 6–2 in Chapter 6 🔵 for nonverbal communication patterns in cultural groups. Encourage parents to share information, even if it is private or sensitive, especially when it influences nursing care planning. Often parents avoid sharing some information because they want to make a good impression, or they do not understand the value of the missing information. If you detect a hesitation to share information, briefly explain why the question was asked, for example, to make their child's hospital experience more pleasant or to begin planning for the child's discharge and home care. Silence is common in some Asian and Native American groups as they attempt to form responses to questions.

In some cases, the parent becomes too agitated, upset, or angry to continue responding to questions. When the information is not needed immediately, move on to another portion of the history to determine whether the parent is able to respond to other questions. Depending on the emotional state of the parent, it may be more appropriate to collect the remaining historical data at a later time.

Data to Be Collected

Nurses collect and organize health, medical, and personal-social history to plan a child's nursing care. In addition, health status, psychosocial, and developmental data are organized to help develop the nursing diagnoses and the nursing care plan (Figure 7–1 ■).

Patient Information

Obtain the child's name and nickname, age, sex, and ethnic origin. The child's birth date, race, religion, address, phone number, and cell phone number can be obtained from the admission form. Ask the parent for an emergency contact address and phone number, as well as a work phone number. Record the name of the person providing the patient history and that person's relationship to the patient. If the historian is not a parent, determine if this individual has authority to consent for the child's medical care.

Physiologic Data

Information about the child's health problems and diseases is collected chronologically in a format similar to the traditional medical history.

Chief complaint The chief complaint is the child's primary problem or reason for hospital admission or visit to a healthcare setting, stated in the parent's or child's exact words.

History of present illness or injury The history of the present illness or injury is a detailed description of each current health problem. This includes the onset and sequence of events, characteristics

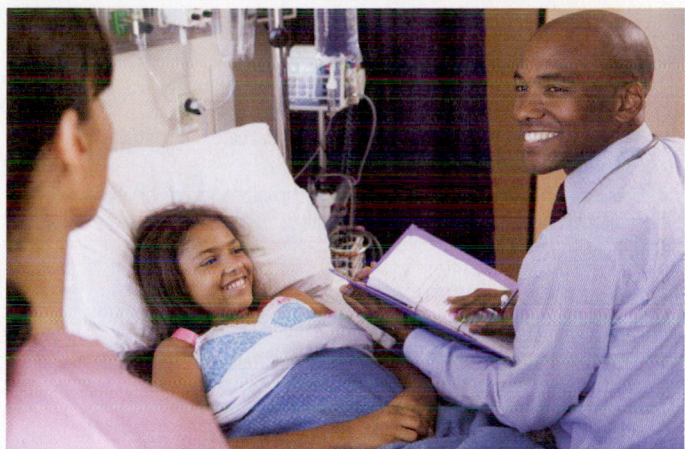

FIGURE 7–1 ■ Observe the behavior of children and family members while you are collecting historical and physiologic data.
Source: *Monkey Business / Fotolia.*

of and changes in symptoms over time, influencing factors, and the current status of the problem. Each problem is described separately. See Table 7–1.

Past history The past history is a more detailed description of the child's prior health status, including all major past illnesses and injuries. A detailed and complete birth history is obtained for a newborn or when the young child's present problem may be related to the birth history. Use the guidelines provided in Box 7–2 to obtain a birth history. Document the child's age at the time of each illness, injury, surgery, or hospitalization. Obtain information about each specific diagnosis, treatment, outcome, complication, or residual problem, and the child's reaction to the event.

Collect information about the child's past history and the child's age at each occurrence. Identify all major illnesses including common communicable diseases. Identify major injuries, their cause or mechanism, and their severity. For past surgeries, obtain information

TABLE 7–1	Characteristics for Illness or Injury Data Collection
CHARACTERISTIC	**DEFINING VARIABLES**
Onset	Sudden or gradual, previous episodes, date and time began
Type of symptom	Pain, itching, cough, vomiting, runny nose, diarrhea, rash, for example
Location	Generalized or localized—anatomically precise
Duration	Continuous or episodic, length of episodes
Severity	Effect on daily activities (e.g., interrupted sleep, decreased appetite, unable to attend school)
Influencing factors	What relieves or worsens symptoms, what precipitated the problem, recent exposure to infection or allergen
Past evaluation for the problem	Laboratory studies, physician's office or hospital where performed, results of past examinations
Previous and current therapies	Prescribed and over-the-counter drugs used, alternative and complementary therapies, other treatment measures tried (e.g., heat, ice, rest), response to treatments

BOX 7–2	Obtaining a Birth History

PRENATAL CONDITION

- Mother's age, health during pregnancy, prenatal care, weight gained, special diet, expected date of delivery
- Details of illnesses, radiograph findings, hospitalizations, medications, complications, and timing during pregnancy
- Prior obstetric history

INTRAPARTUM—DESCRIPTION OF DELIVERY

- Site of delivery (hospital, home, birthing center)
- Labor length, induced or spontaneous, time of rupture of membranes
- Medications or anesthesia used during labor/birth
- Quantity and appearance of amniotic fluid
- Vaginal or cesarean birth, forceps or suction used, vertex or breech position
- Single or multiple birth, gestational age at birth

CONDITION OF BABY AT BIRTH

- Weight, Apgar score, immediate cry
- Need for incubator, oxygen, suctioning, ventilator
- Any abnormalities detected, meconium staining

POSTNATAL CONDITION

- Difficulties in the nursery—feeding, respiratory problems, jaundice, cyanosis, rashes
- Length of hospital stay, special nursery, home with mother
- Breastfed or formula fed, weight lost/gained in hospital
- Medical care needed in first week—readmission to hospital

about the specific type and if the surgery required overnight hospitalization. For all hospitalizations, record the reason and length of hospitalization. If any transfusions (blood or blood products) have been given in the past, identify the circumstances, type and date of transfusion, and reactions to the transfusion.

Current health status Obtain a detailed description of the child's typical health status. Obtain information about allergies, current medications, immunization status, activities and exercise, sleep patterns, nutrition, safety measures used, and health maintenance care as follows:

Health promotion and health maintenance Identify when the last visit was made to the child's primary care provider, dentist, and other healthcare providers (such as specialty physicians, emergency department, or urgent care clinic). Identify the name of each provider.

Medications Provide names of prescribed and over-the-counter medications (such as acetaminophen, cough medications, vitamins, ointments, creams) taken daily or frequently, their purpose, and their effectiveness. If the child is being assessed for an episodic illness or injury, inquire about the medications used for home management of conditions such as fever, colds, coughs, cuts, and rashes. Ask about the use of plants, herbs, teas, or other complementary therapies and their purpose and effectiveness.

Allergies List the child's allergies to food, medication, animals, insect bites, or environmental exposure, and the type of reaction (e.g., respiratory difficulty, rash, hives, or itching).

Immunizations Review the child's record for vaccines and dates received. Ask about any unexpected reactions. Identify any immunizations still needed. See Chapter 22 🔗.

Safety measures used Determine if age-appropriate safety measures are used, such as a car safety seat, window guards, medication storage, bicycle helmet and other sports protective gear, smoke detectors, and storage of household chemicals and firearms.

Activities and exercise Identify the child's play and/or sports activities; identify any physical mobility problem, limitations, and adaptive equipment used.

Nutrition For infants, determine if the baby is formula fed or breastfed, and if ever breastfed, for how long. Determine the type and amount of formula and other liquid intake each day. Identify when solid foods were introduced, which ones, and the amounts eaten each day. Inquire about enrollment in the special nutrition program for Women, Infants, and Children (WIC). Contrast food intake to the appropriate intake for age and weight as described in Chapter 19 🔗.

For children, determine the amount of foods and milk consumed each day. Identify eating and snacking habits, the variety of foods consumed, "junk foods" eaten, and appetite. Inquire about the family eating patterns such as meals eaten together, food consumption in the childcare center or school, and foods eaten during other social events.

Sleep Identify the length and timing of naps and nighttime sleep, presence of nightmares or night terrors or other sleep disturbances, where the child sleeps, and bedtime rituals.

Family history Obtaining a family history is important to identify any major familial and hereditary diseases that could potentially affect the child. Examples of specific diseases the nurse may inquire about are listed in Table 7–2. Information is collected for three

TABLE 7–2	Genetic or Hereditary Diseases
CATEGORY OF DISEASES	**EXAMPLES**
Infectious diseases	Tuberculosis, HIV, hepatitis, varicella, herpes
Cardiac disorders	Heart defects, hypertension, dyslipidemia, sudden childhood deaths
Allergic disorders	Atopic eczema, hay fever, asthma
Eye disorders	Glaucoma, cataracts, vision loss
Ear disorders	Hearing loss
Respiratory disorders	Cystic fibrosis, asthma
Hematologic disorders	Sickle cell disease, thalassemia, G6PD deficiency, hemophilia
Cancer	Retinoblastoma, cancer with early age of onset
Endocrine disorders	Type 1 or type 2 diabetes, hypothyroidism, hyperthyroidism, Turner syndrome
Kidney disorders	Polycystic kidneys
Neurologic disorders	Epilepsy, spina bifida, anencephaly
Musculoskeletal disorders	Muscular dystrophy, achondroplasia, scoliosis, arthritis
Gastrointestinal disorders	Pyloric stenosis, ulcers, colitis, celiac disease
Skin disorders	Neurofibromatosis
Metabolic disorders	Phenylketonuria, galactosemia, maple syrup urine disease, Tay-Sachs disease
Learning problems	Attention deficit disorder, Down syndrome, fragile X syndrome, intellectual disability (mental retardation)
Problem pregnancies	Repeated miscarriages, stillbirths

TABLE 7–3	Data Collection Guidelines for Review of Systems
BODY SYSTEM	**EXAMPLES OF PROBLEMS TO IDENTIFY**
General	General growth pattern, overall health status, ability to keep up with other children or tires easily with feeding or activity, fever, sleep patterns
	Allergies, type of reaction (hives, rash, respiratory difficulty, swelling, nausea), seasonal or with each exposure
Skin and lymph	Rashes, dry skin, itching, changes in skin color or texture, tendency for bruising, swollen or tender lymph glands
Hair and nails	Hair loss, changes in color or texture, use of dye or chemicals on hair
	Abnormalities of nail growth or color
Head	Headaches, concern about size of head
Eyes	Vision problems, squinting, crossed eyes, "lazy eye," wears glasses
	Eye infections, redness, tearing, burning, rubbing, swelling eyelids
Ears	Ear infections, frequent discharge from ears, tubes in ears or myringotomy
	Hearing loss (no response to loud noises or questions, inattentiveness, date of last hearing test), hearing aids or cochlear implants
Nose and sinuses	Nosebleeds, nasal congestion, colds with runny nose, sinus pain or infections
	Nasal obstruction, difficulty breathing, snoring at night
Mouth and throat	Mouth breathing, difficulty swallowing, sore throats, strep infections, mouth odor
	Tooth eruption, cavities, braces
	Voice change, hoarseness, speech problems
Cardiac and hematologic	Heart murmur, anemia, high blood pressure, cyanosis, edema, rheumatic fever, chest pain, easily bruises
Chest and respiratory	Trouble breathing, choking episodes, cough, wheezing, cyanosis, exposure to tuberculosis, other infections
Gastrointestinal	Bowel movements, frequency, color, regularity, consistency, discomfort, constipation or diarrhea, abdominal pain, bleeding from rectum, flatulence
	Usual appetite, nausea or vomiting
Urinary	Frequency, urgency, dysuria, dribbling, strength of urinary stream, foul-smelling urine, blood in urine, past urinary tract infections, genitourinary defects (e.g., undescended testicles)
	Toilet trained—age when day and night dryness was attained, enuresis
Reproductive	For pubescent children:
Female	Menses onset, amount, duration, frequency, discomfort, problems; vaginal discharge; breast development
Male	Puberty onset, emissions, erections, pain or discharge from penis, swelling or pain in testicles
Both	Sexual activity, use of contraception, sexually transmitted diseases
Musculoskeletal	Weakness, clumsiness, poor coordination, balance, tremors, abnormal gait
	Painful muscles or joints, swelling or redness of joints, fractures, scoliosis
Neurologic	Seizures, fainting spells, dizziness, numbness, brain injuries or concussions
	Number of words spoken appropriate for age, problems with articulation
	Concentration, attention span, hyperactivity, memory or learning problems

generations of family members, including the parents, grandparents, aunts, uncles, cousins, child, and siblings. Collect information about the health status of each parent. If there is the potential for a genetic disorder, a family pedigree (genogram) will likely be constructed. See Chapter 4 🔗 for information about constructing a pedigree and important questions used in data collection.

Review of systems The review of systems provides a comprehensive overview of the child's health. This is an opportunity to identify additional signs and symptoms associated with the child's health or hospital admission problem. The review of systems may identify other problems not directly related to the child's current health problem, but these problems could complicate nursing care or home care. For example, asking about allergies may reveal that a child has a latex allergy. The nurse would then need to ensure that the child is not exposed to latex and be prepared for allergic reactions. For each problem, obtain the treatment, outcomes, residual problems, and age at time of onset. Data collection guidelines for review of systems are given in Table 7–3.

Psychosocial Data

Obtain information about family composition to establish a socioeconomic and sociologic context within which to plan care for the newborn or child in the hospital and at home. (See Chapter 20 🔗 to review societal and environmental issues that should be considered in data collection, such as food insecurity.) Include the following:

- **Family composition**—family members living in the home, their relationship to the child, marital status of parents or other family structure, and persons helping to care for the child
- **Financial resources**—household members employed, family income, healthcare resources (e.g., private health insurance, Medicaid, Children's Health Insurance Program [CHIP]), and other resources (e.g., food stamps, Temporary Assistance for Needy Families [TANF], or WIC)
- **Home environment**—housing description (condition, safe play area, pets, child's sleeping area); environmental

atmosphere (emotional stresses, family activities); city or well water; and availability of electricity, heat, and refrigeration

- **Community environment**—neighborhood description, safety, playgrounds, transportation, lighting, sidewalks, and access to shopping; school or childcare arrangements
- **Family or lifestyle changes**—for example, unemployment, relocations, divorce; how the child and family members have coped with the changes

Newborns and infants The psychosocial history for parents of newborns should focus on readiness to care for the infant at home. Inquire about support for the parent in the initial postpartum period, safe transport, and a home environment that provides heat, refrigeration, and safe water supplies. Determine if referral for WIC or TANF is needed to ensure adequate nutrition and financial support for the mother and newborn. See Chapters 9 and 10 🕮 for more information on newborn and infant health promotion.

Children Information about the child's daily routines, psychosocial information, and other living patterns should focus on issues that may have an impact on the quality of daily living (Box 7–3). See Chapters 11 and 12 🕮 for more information on health promotion in toddlers, preschoolers, and school-age children.

Adolescents The psychosocial history for adolescents should focus on critical areas in their lives that may contribute to a less than optimal environment for normal growth and development. See the companion website for questions that should be asked about key topics that are included in the HEEADSSS screening tool (Brown, 2011):

- Home environment
- Education/employment, Eating
- Activities
- Drugs (substance abuse)
- Sexuality, Suicidal thoughts, Safety from injury and violence

Developmental Data

Information about the child's motor, cognitive, language, and social development will help when planning nursing care. Some information is gained by observation of the child during the history and physical examination. Ask the parent about the child's milestones and current fine and gross motor skills. Obtain the age at which the child first used words appropriately, and the child's current words or language ability. Actual assessment of the child with the Denver II Developmental Test or a parent questionnaire may also be used to collect this information (see Chapter 8 🕮). For children in school, ask about academic performance to assess cognitive development. Ask the parent about the child's behavior and manner of interaction with other children, family members, and strangers (see Chapter 12 🕮). For adolescents, ask about activities indicating development of independence and autonomy (see Chapter 13 🕮).

The developmental data will help the nurse plan care that is appropriate for the child. Guidelines for a nursing assessment of development can be found in Chapter 5 🕮.

DEVELOPMENTAL APPROACH TO THE EXAMINATION

The sequence and approach to the examination varies by age, but the techniques are the same for all ages (Box 7–4). Provide a comfortable atmosphere for the examination with privacy so that the patient's modesty is respected. Explain the procedures as you begin to perform them. In young children, a foot-to-head sequence is often used so that the least distressing parts of the examination are completed first. In older cooperative children, the head-to-toe approach is generally used. The sequence is often varied by experienced examiners, such as by auscultating the lungs, heart, and abdomen when an infant or toddler is asleep or quiet.

Standard precautions are used during the physical examination. Good hand hygiene should be performed before contact with the

---

BOX 7–3	Daily Living Patterns

ROLE RELATIONSHIPS

- Family relationships/alterations in family process
- Social and peer relationships and interactions: child care, preschool, school, sports, groups

SELF-PERCEPTION/SELF-CONCEPT

- Personal identity and role identity
- Self-esteem, body image, presence of a nonvisible disorder such as brain injury

COPING/STRESS TOLERANCE

- Temperament
- Coping behaviors
- Discipline
- Any substance abuse

VALUES AND BELIEFS

- Part of a spiritual group or faith community
- Any foods, drinks, or medical interventions prohibited according to spiritual beliefs, special food preparation
- Personal values/beliefs

HOME CARE PROVIDED FOR CHILD'S CONDITION

- Resources needed/available, availability of respite care
- Knowledge and skills of parents, other family members

SENSORY/PERCEPTUAL PROBLEMS

- Any sensory loss (vision, hearing, cognitive, or motor) and adaptations made

---

BOX 7–4	Examination Techniques

- **Inspection**—purposeful observation of the child's physical features and behaviors performed during the entire physical examination. Physical feature characteristics include size, shape, color, movement, position, and location. Adequate lighting is essential. Detection of odors is also a part of inspection.
- **Palpation**—use of touch to identify characteristics of the skin, internal organs, and masses. Characteristics include texture, moistness, tenderness, temperature, position, shape, consistency, and mobility of masses and organs. The palmar surface of the fingers and fingertip pads are used for determining position, size, consistency, and masses. The ulnar surface of the hand is best for detecting vibrations.
- **Auscultation**—listening to sounds produced by the airway, lungs, stomach, heart, and blood vessels to identify their characteristics. Auscultation is usually performed with a stethoscope to enhance the sounds heard in the chest and abdomen. Speech is also assessed during auscultation.
- **Percussion**—striking the surface of the body, either directly or indirectly, to set up vibrations that reveal the density of underlying tissues and borders of internal organs in the chest and abdomen. As the density of the tissue increases, the percussion tone becomes quieter. The tone over air is the loudest, and the tone over solid areas is soft.

child. Gloves should be worn for any contact with mucous membranes and body fluids.

Newborns and Infants Under 6 Months of Age

Infants are among the easiest children to examine, as they do not resist the examination procedure. Keep the parent present to provide comfort and security to the infant. The young infant can be placed on the examining table as long as safety is ensured. When needed, provide physical comfort during the examination by feeding, using a pacifier, cuddling, or changing the diaper to keep the infant calm and quiet. Distraction, such as rocking or clicking noises, may help when the infant begins to get distressed. Observe the infant for general level of activity, overall mood, and responsiveness to handling.

Make sure your hands and stethoscope are warmed and your motions are gentle. Be flexible with the sequence of the examination to take advantage of times the infant is quiet or asleep to auscultate the lungs, heart, and abdomen. If the infant continues to be quiet or can be quieted with a pacifier, palpate the abdomen while the muscles are relaxed. Then proceed to palpate the femoral pulses. The remainder of the examination can proceed in a head-to-toe sequence. Portions of the examination that will disturb the infant, such as examination of the hips, should be performed at the end.

Infants over 6 Months of Age

Because of developing separation and stranger anxiety, the older infant often resists portions of the physical examination. For this reason, it is often best to keep the older infant with the parent. The infant and toddler can be examined on the parent's lap and then held against the parent's chest for some steps, such as the ear examination. See the Photo Story on page 170. If the infant must be placed on the examining table for any procedure, keep the parent close. The infant will not object to having clothing removed, but make sure the room is warm for the infant's comfort. Observe the infant's general level of activity, mood, and responsiveness to handling by the parent.

Toddlers

Toddlers may be active, curious, shy, cautious, or slow to warm up. Because of stranger anxiety, keep toddlers with their parents. One can often examine a toddler on the parent's lap. Let the child hold a security object if it helps. Attempt to reduce the child's anxiety about the examination instruments by demonstrating their use on the parent or letting the parent hold the instrument first. Perform the cranial nerve assessment or developmental assessment as a method to gain cooperation for other procedures.

Avoid asking the child if you can perform a part of the examination as the typical response will be "no." Tell the child what you will do at each step of the examination, using a confident voice that expects cooperation. When a choice is possible, let the child have some control by selecting which part of the examination to do next, such as touching the chest or the abdomen or letting the child choose to stand or sit for a certain part of the examination. Begin the examination by touching the feet and then moving gradually toward the body and head. Instruments to examine the ears, eyes, and mouth are usually viewed as the most fearful and should be used at the end of the examination.

Much of the examination can be performed with the child sitting. Create a flat surface for the abdominal and genital examination by placing the knees of the parent and nurse together. For examination

of the ears, eyes, and mouth, the parent can hold the child closely to the chest with legs between the parent's legs. (See Figure 7–19.) Much of the neurologic and musculoskeletal assessment can be conducted by observing the child play and walk around in the examining room.

Preschoolers

Assess the willingness of the child to be separated from the parent. Younger children will often prefer to be examined on the parent's lap, whereas older children will be comfortable on the examining table. They are usually willing to undress, but leave the underpants on until conducting the genital examination. Most preschoolers are cooperative during the physical examination; however, consider which examination sequence is best for the child. Some children prefer to have the head, eyes, ears, and mouth examined first; others prefer to postpone them to the end of the examination.

Allow the child to touch and play with the equipment. Use games to reduce anxiety about the examination, such as listening to and looking in the ears of the child's stuffed animal first. Give simple explanations about assessment procedures, and, when possible, offer choice during the examination, such as which ear to look into first. Use distraction to gain cooperation during the examination, such as asking the child to count, name colors, or talk about a favorite activity. Give positive feedback when the child cooperates.

School-Age Children

School-age children are willing to cooperate and want to be helpful during the physical examination, so have the child sit on the examining table. Provide guidance about what they can do at each step to help during the examination. Anticipate the development of modesty in school-age children and offer a patient gown to cover the underwear. Let the older school-age child determine if the examination will be conducted in privacy or with the parent or siblings present.

A head-to-toe sequence is usually well accepted by school-age children. Demonstrate how the instruments are used and offer to let the child handle them. As you perform the examination, explain what you are doing and why. Offer as many choices as possible to help the child feel empowered. The examination is a good opportunity to teach the child about how the body works, such as letting the child listen to heart and breath sounds.

Adolescents

Protect the adolescent's modesty by providing a private place to undress and put on the patient gown, and then during the examination by covering the parts of the body not being assessed. Examine the adolescent in a head-to-toe sequence as used for adults. Perform the examination in private without parent or siblings unless the adolescent specifically requests the parent's presence. Provide a chaperone (preferably the same sex as the patient) during the examination when the parent or accompanying adult does not stay in the room.

Adolescents often have concerns regarding their developing bodies. When appropriate provide reassurance about the normal progression of secondary sexual characteristic development and what further changes to expect.

Anatomic and Physiologic Characteristics of Infants and Children

Infants and children have significant differences in physiology than adults. By knowing pediatric anatomic and physiologic differences,

PHOTO STORY...

EXAMINING AN INFANT OR TODDLER

The behaviors of older infants and toddlers sometimes make the physical examination a challenging experience. These children are often fearful of strangers and resist the close contact the nurse needs for the examination. Despite this challenge, it is essential to perform good assessments to identify any health problems the child may have.

Rhenda is flexible in her approach to examining infants and toddlers. She knows that separating the infant or toddler from the parent will often increase the child's distress and make the examination even more difficult. She chooses to examine Benny on his parent's lap to improve the infant's comfort and to enhance the assessment process. Rhenda is also aware that, for toddlers, conducting some of the examination on the floor may be helpful. Additionally, being flexible with regard to the sequence of the examination is important to take advantage of opportunities for assessment of certain body systems.

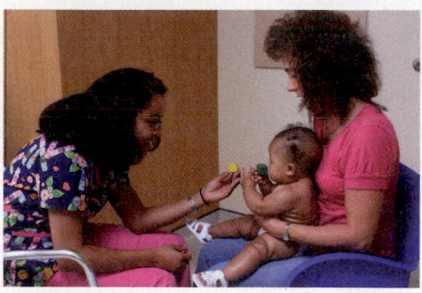

Use a toy to assess Benny's development and motor skills, such as reaching for and grasping a block.

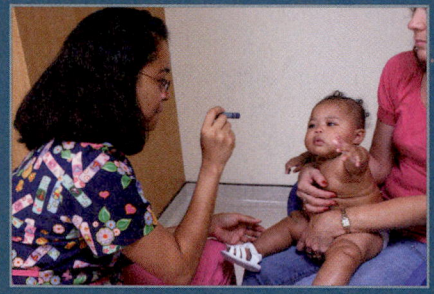

A penlight is an effective tool to assess Benny's level of alertness, as well as his ability to track an object with the eyes. Movement of the head and neck may also be assessed with this maneuver.

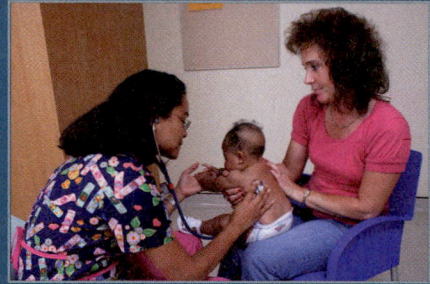

When Benny is comfortable with Rhenda, and feeling secure on his parent's lap, he is less likely to resist having his chest auscultated.

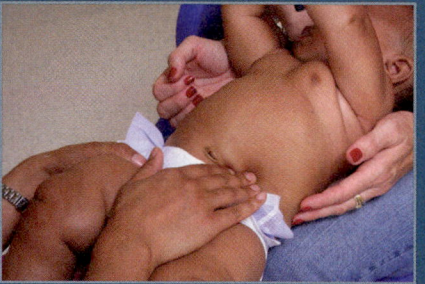

Rhenda places her knees against the mother's to create a flat surface for the abdominal and genital examination.

For example, Rhenda tries to auscultate the heart, lungs, and abdomen when the child is quiet or asleep.

Rhenda smiles and talks soothingly to Benny during the examination. A pacifier or bottle may be used to quiet him when necessary. Because Benny may be fearful when touched by a stranger, Rhenda begins with Benny's feet and hands before moving to the trunk. She uses toys to distract Benny and to assess development, range of motion, and reflexes.

As They Grow Anatomic and Physiologic Characteristics of Children

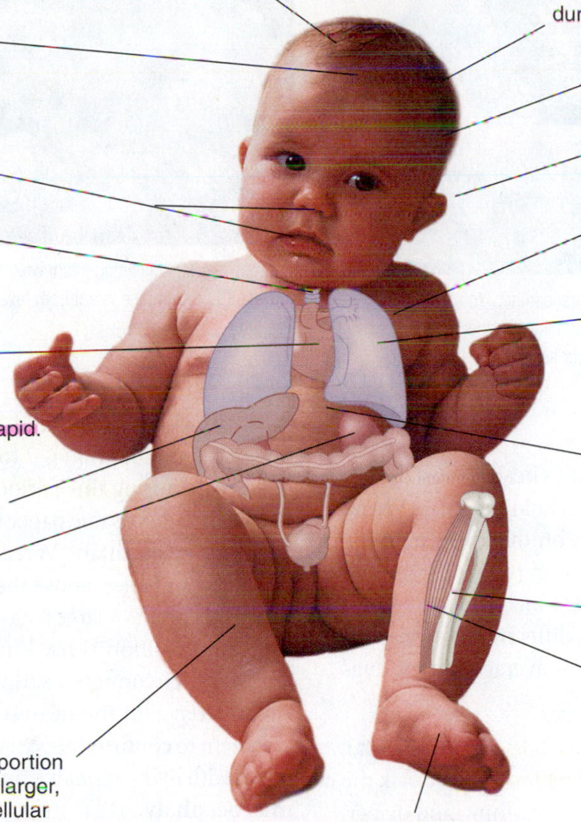

Body surface area large for weight, making infants susceptible to hypothermia.

Anterior fontanel and open sutures palpable up to about 18 months. Posterior fontanel closes between 2 and 3 months.

Tongue large relative to small nasal and oral airway passages.

Short, narrow trachea in children under 5 years makes them susceptible to foreign body obstruction.

Until late school age and adolescence, cardiac output is rate dependent not stroke volume dependent, making heart rate more rapid.

Abdomen offers poor protection for the liver and spleen, making them susceptible to trauma.

Until 12 to 18 months of age, kidneys do not concentrate urine effectively and do not exert optimal control over electrolyte secretion and absorption.

Until later school age, proportion of body weight in water is larger, with more water in extracellular spaces. Daily water exchange rate is much higher.

All brain cells present at birth; myelinization and further development of nerve fibers occur during first year.

Head proportionately larger, making child susceptible to head injury.

Higher metabolic rate, higher oxygen needs, higher caloric needs.

Until puberty, percentage of cartilage in ribs is higher, making them more flexible and compliant.

Until about 10 years, there is a faster respiratory rate, fewer and smaller alveoli, and less lung volume. Tidal volume is proportional to weight (7 to 10 mL/kg).

Up to about 4 or 5 years, diaphragm is primary breathing muscle. CO_2 is not effectively expired when child is distressed, making child susceptible to metabolic acidosis.

Until puberty, bones are soft and more easily bent and fractured.

Muscles lack tone, power, and coordination during infancy. Muscles are 25% of weight in infants versus 40% in adults.

Blood volume is weight dependent: 80 mL/kg.

FIGURE 7–2 ■ Children are not just small adults. There are important anatomic and physiologic differences between children and adults that will change based on a child's growth and development. Can you identify which of these differences are of greatest concern for the hospitalized child and why?

you will recognize normal variations found during the physical examination, and you will better understand the different physiologic responses children have to illness and injury. Figure 7–2 ■ provides an overview of important anatomic and physiologic differences between children and adults.

GENERAL APPRAISAL

The examination begins when you first meet the child in any setting (Figure 7–3 ■). Observe the child's general appearance and behavior. The child should appear well nourished and well developed, as Jasmine appeared during her visit to the health clinic at the beginning of the chapter. Infants and young children are often fearful and seek reassurance from their parents. The child may resist interacting with you until rapport is established.

Observe the behavior and tone of voice used by the parent when he or she is talking to the child. Is the child encouraged to speak? Is the child appropriately reassured or supported by the parent? The child should feel secure with the parent and perceive permission to interact with the nurse.

Anthropometric Measurements

Measure the child's weight, length or height, and head circumference, if appropriate. Accurate assessment of growth throughout childhood is important for several reasons: to ensure health, to identify the impact of disease on the child, and for medication dosage calculation. Plot the height, weight, and head circumference measurements on appropriate growth charts for the child's age and sex to compare with prior measurements and to assess trends in growth. See Appendix A 🔗.

Clinical Tip
See the companion website for links to special growth curves for children with Down syndrome, children with Turner syndrome, and children adopted from other countries.

Infants and Toddlers

Length Measure the length of all children under age 2 years in the supine position, even when they are able to stand independently. Growth charts for children under age 2 years are based on length rather than height. A difference in length and standing height measurement for a child does exist. If height is plotted on a length-based growth chart, assessment of the child's growth over time will be inaccurate.

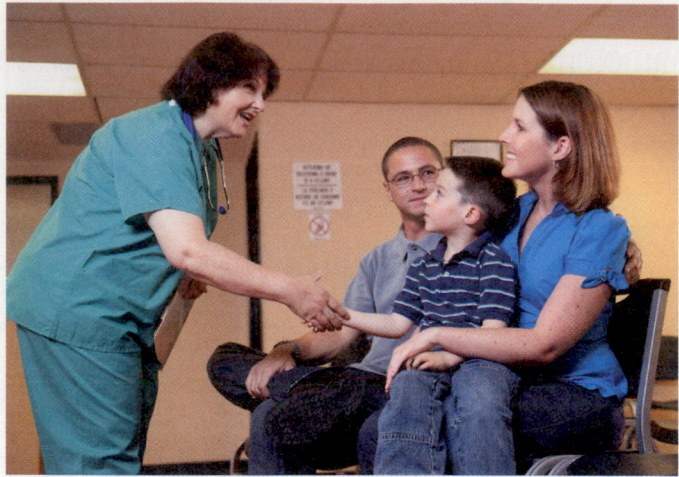

FIGURE 7–3 ■ Examination of the child begins from the first contact. You should observe the behavior of the child and parent by using visual cues to make a proper assessment. Does the child appear well nourished? Does the child appear secure with the parent?

Source: *Getty / Yellow Dog Productions.*

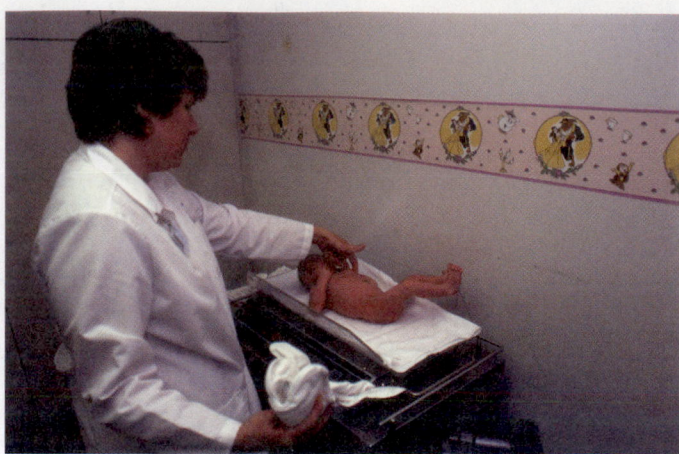

FIGURE 7–5 ■ Measuring infant weight. Place a hand close to the chest without touching the infant to prevent the infant from falling. Record the weight to the nearest 10 g or 1/2 oz.

Source: *Michael Newman / PhotoEdit.*

Use a measuring board and place the infant's head against the top of the board. Ask the parent or an assistant to hold the infant's head in the midline while you gently push down on the knees until the legs are straight. Position the heels of the feet on the footboard and record the length to the nearest 0.5 cm or 1/4 inch (Figure 7–4 ■). Repeat the measurement for accuracy. If a difference between the two readings is found, take a third reading or average the readings for documentation.

Weight Infants are weighed on a platform scale (Figure 7–5 ■), either in a supine or sitting position, depending on their age. Ask the parent or assistant to remove all of the infant's clothing and diaper. Keep a diaper close at hand in case the baby voids while unclothed. Keep the room warm for comfort. Check the balance of the scale before placing the infant on it, and put a paper cover on the scale. Distract the infant, and take the reading when the infant stops moving. Take care to ensure the infant's safety by placing a hand close to the chest without touching the infant to prevent falls. Record the weight to the nearest 10 g or 1/2 oz.

Head circumference Head circumference is measured at regular intervals until the child is 2 to 3 years old because the brain is growing rapidly during this period, achieving 80% of adult size by age 2 years. Use a disposable paper tape, but take care to prevent the paper from cutting the infant. Wrap the tape around the head at the supraorbital prominence, above the ears, and around the occipital prominence, the point of largest circumference of the head (Figure 7–6 ■). The same position is used in newborns, although this may not be the largest circumference due to molding or swelling. Record the circumference to the nearest 0.5 cm or 1/4 inch. Repeat the measurement to confirm the reading. A larger-than-normal head is associated with hydrocephalus, and a smaller-than-normal head suggests **microcephaly.**

Preschoolers and School-Age Children

Height After the age of 2 to 3 years, a **stadiometer,** a height-measuring device attached to the wall, is used to improve the accuracy of the height measurement (Figure 7–7 ■). Have the child

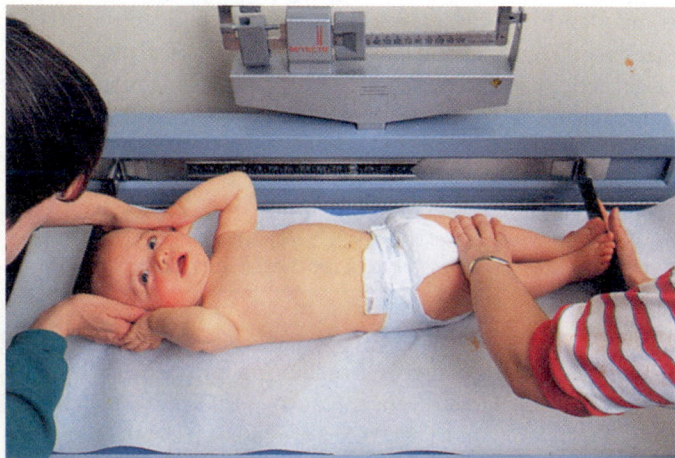

FIGURE 7–4 ■ Measuring infant length. Have an assistant hold the infant's head in the midline while you gently push down on the knees until the legs are straight. Position the heels of the feet on the footboard, and record the length to the nearest 0.5 cm or 1/4 inch.

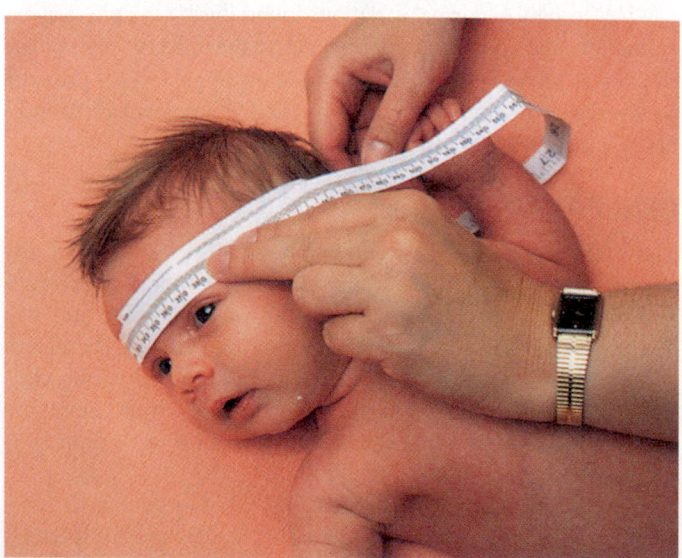

FIGURE 7–6 ■ Measuring head circumference. Wrap the tape around the head at the supraorbital prominence, above the ears, and around the occipital prominence, the point of largest circumference of the head.

stand straight with shoes removed and the back to the wall. The head should be held erect and in the midline position. The shoulders, buttocks, and heels should touch the wall. The canthi of the eyes should be on the same horizontal plane as the stadiometer headpiece. Move the headpiece down to touch the crown. Measure the height reading to the nearest 0.5 cm or 1/4 inch.

Weight Measure the child's weight on a standing scale. Check the balance of the scale before use. Weigh young children in their underclothes. Weigh older children in their street clothes with coats, other heavy clothing, and shoes removed. Record the weight to the nearest 0.1 kg or 1/4 lb. Provide privacy for the older child and adolescent.

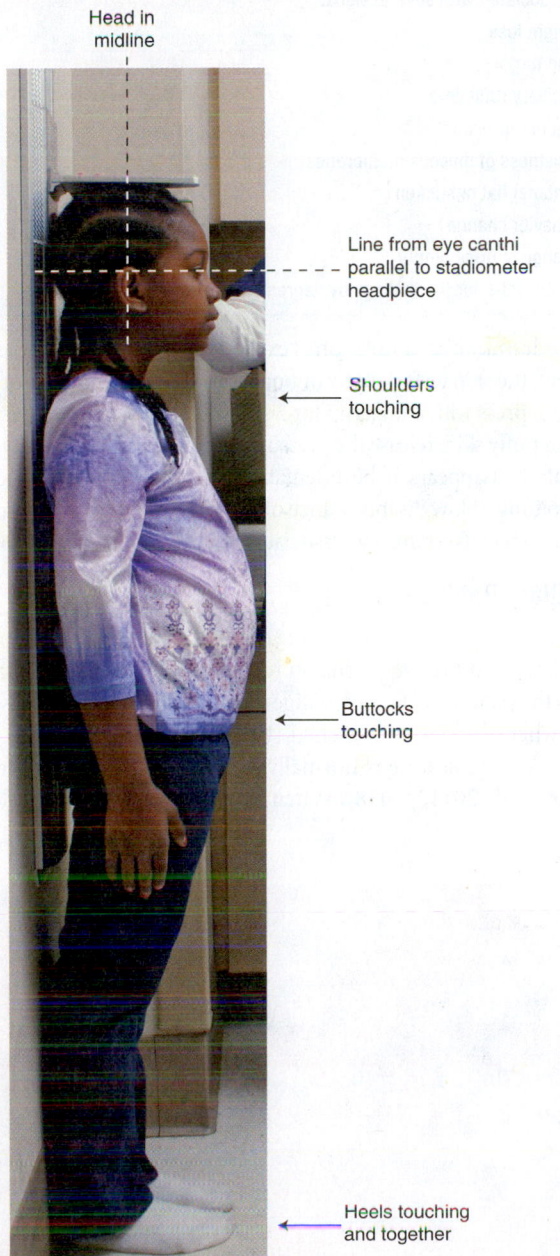

Head in midline

Line from eye canthi parallel to stadiometer headpiece

Shoulders touching

Buttocks touching

Heels touching and together

FIGURE 7–7 ■ Standing height measurements are taken routinely using a stadiometer at each well-child visit beginning at 2 to 3 years to assess the child's rate of growth. Position the head in an erect and midline position while the shoulders, buttocks, and heels touch the wall. Move the headpiece down to touch the crown. Measure the height reading to the nearest 0.5 cm or 1/4 inch.

Clinical Judgment

Jasmine, currently 27 months in age, weighed 10.2 kg and measured 81 cm in height at her visit to the health clinic. Her head circumference measured 47 cm. At what percentiles are her weight, height, head circumference, and body mass index? No prior growth measurements are available. How would you explain these findings to Mrs. Porter?

Body mass index The body mass index (BMI) is a formula (weight in kilograms divided by meters² of height) used to assess total body fat and nutritional status, using the child's height and weight. See Box 19–8 in Chapter 19 for the formula for the BMI calculation, or visit the Centers for Disease Control and Prevention (CDC) website for the automatic calculation of BMI using the child's height and weight. Interpretation of the BMI for children is as follows:

- BMI for age less than 5th percentile—underweight
- BMI for age greater than 85th percentile—overweight
- BMI for age greater than 95th percentile—obesity

Older Children and Adolescents

Height, weight, and BMI Measure the height using a stadiometer attached to the wall or with a stature-measuring device attached to a platform scale. Have the child stand erect with the back to the scale. Move the stature-measuring device to the top of the head. Have the child step off the scale, and read the height in centimeters or inches. Then measure the weight as described for school-age children. Calculate the child's BMI and plot it on the growth curve.

ASSESSING SKIN AND HAIR

What is indicated when the child's skin is not uniform in color or when it feels spongy to the touch? What are each of the primary skin lesions called, and what characteristics are used to describe them? How can cyanosis and jaundice be detected in children with darker skin? Why is skin turgor assessed?

Inspection of the Skin

Use gloves to inspect the child's skin for color and the presence of imperfections, elevations, variations, or lesions. Examination of the skin requires good lighting to detect variations in skin color and to identify lesions. Natural daylight is preferred when available. Rather than inspecting the entire skin surface of the child at one time, examine the skin simultaneously with other body systems as each region of the body is exposed.

Skin Color

Expect the color of the child's skin to be evenly distributed. Look for color variations—such as increased or decreased pigmentation, pallor, mottling, bruises, erythema, cyanosis, or jaundice—that may be associated with health conditions. The palms of the hands and soles of the feet are often lighter than the rest of the skin surface in darker-skinned children. In addition, their lips may appear slightly bluish. Some variations in skin color are common and normal, such as freckles found in the White population and hyperpigmented macules (Mongolian spots) found on infants with dark skin (Figure 7–8 ■). Mongolian spots usually fade during the first few years of life and disappear by puberty. Note any hemangiomas or other birthmarks.

Ecchymosis or small bruises are common over bony prominences (the knees, shins, forehead, and scalp) and the front of the body because children stumble and fall. Bruises are uncommon in

Weblink | *BMI Calculator*

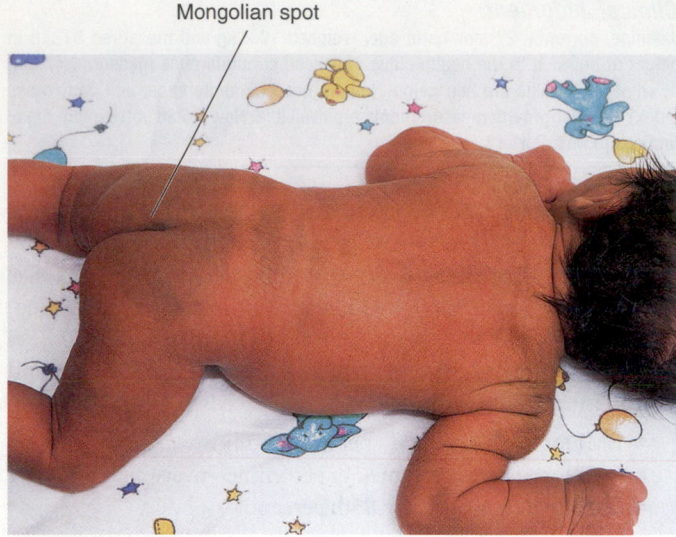

Mongolian spot

FIGURE 7–8 ■ Hyperpigmented macules (Mongolian spots) are large patches of bluish skin often seen on the buttocks. They are a normal occurrence in a large majority of American Indian, Asian, Black, and Hispanic infants, but are sometimes mistaken for bruises.

infants under 9 months of age without known medical conditions (Harris, 2010). Bruises on other parts of the body, especially in various stages of healing, should raise a suspicion of child abuse (see Chapter 20 ✍). Bruises often go through several skin color changes (red, purple, black, blue, yellow, green, and brown) as the body breaks down hemoglobin and blood cells over several days before returning to normal skin color. Note any tattoos or body piercings.

When a skin color abnormality is suspected, the buccal mucosa and tongue should be inspected to confirm the color change. This is especially important in children of darker skin because the mucous membranes are usually pink, regardless of skin color. The gums are pressed lightly for 1 to 2 seconds. Any residual color, such as jaundice or cyanosis, is more easily detected in blanched skin. Jaundice may also be noticed in the sclerae of the eyes. Generalized cyanosis is associated with respiratory and cardiac disorders. Jaundice is associated with liver disorders. Infants who eat a lot of carrots may have a yellow or orange tint to the skin.

Palpation of the Skin

Lightly touch or stroke the skin's surface to evaluate the following characteristics. Follow standard precautions by wearing gloves when palpating mucous membranes, open wounds, and lesions.

Temperature

The child's skin normally feels warm to the touch when placing the wrist or dorsum of the hand against the child's skin. Excessively warm skin may indicate the presence of fever or inflammation, whereas abnormally cool skin may be a sign of shock or cold exposure.

Texture

Children have soft, smooth skin over the entire body. Identify any areas of roughness, thickening, or **induration** (an area of extra firmness with a distinct border). Abnormalities in texture are associated with endocrine disorders, chronic irritation, and inflammation.

Moistness

The child's skin is normally dry to the touch. The skin may feel slightly damp when the child has been exercising or crying. Excessive

sweating without exertion may be associated with a fever, bronchopulmonary dysplasia, or an uncorrected congenital heart defect.

Resilience (Turgor)

The child's skin is elastic and mobile because of the balanced distribution of intracellular and extracellular fluids. To evaluate skin turgor, pinch a small amount of skin on the abdomen, release the skin, and watch the speed of recoil (Figure 7–9 ■). Skin with good turgor immediately returns to its previous contour. Skin with poor turgor tents or takes longer to return to its original contour. Poor skin turgor is commonly associated with dehydration.

Clinical Tip

The degree of dehydration can be estimated by considering the assessment findings associated with several signs:

  Weight loss
  Skin turgor
  Capillary refill time
  Amount of tears
  Moistness of mucous membranes
  Fontanel flat or sunken
  Behavior change
  Change in urine output

See Table 23-5 for the findings by degree of dehydration.

If **edema,** an accumulation of excess fluid in the interstitial spaces, is present, the skin feels doughy or boggy. To test for the degree of edema present, press with a fingertip for 5 seconds against a bone beneath the area of puffy skin, release the pressure, and observe how rapidly the indentation disappears. If the indentation disappears rapidly, the edema is "nonpitting." Slow disappearance of the indentation indicates "pitting" edema, which is commonly associated with kidney or heart disorders.

Capillary Refill Time

Capillary refill time is a technique used to determine the adequacy of circulation and tissue perfusion (oxygen circulating to the tissues). Press the palmar surface of a fingertip and immediately release pressure when the skin is blanched (Figure 7–10 ■). The color return or capillary refill time is normally less than 2 seconds (Seidel, Ball, Dains, et al., 2011, p. 438). When capillary refill time is prolonged,

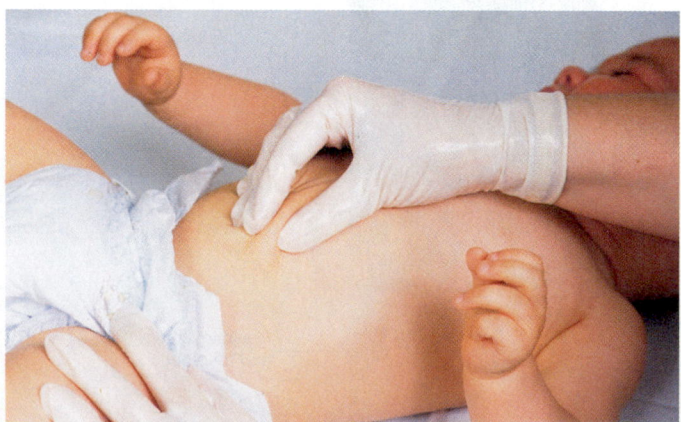

FIGURE 7–9 ■ Testing skin turgor. Pinch a small amount of skin on the abdomen between the thumb and forefinger. Release the skin, and watch the speed of recoil. Skin with normal turgor will quickly return to its usual contour. Tenting of the skin is associated with poor skin turgor.

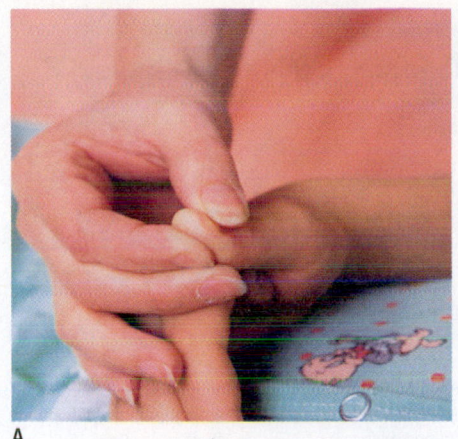

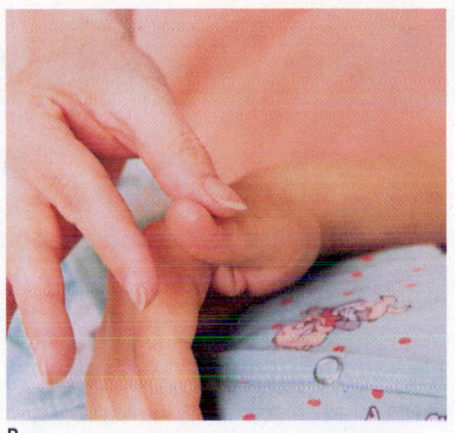

A   B

FIGURE 7–10 ■ Capillary refill technique: *A*, Press the palmar tip of a finger with the arm held at heart level until the skin is blanched. *B*, Quickly release the finger and watch the blood return to the finger. Less than 2 seconds for the color to return (capillary refill time) is expected. Best results occur when the child is in a warm environment. Prolonged capillary refill time can be related to shock or tissue constriction due to a tight bandage or cast.

immediately assess the child for a condition with decreased circulation (e.g., dehydration or shock) or a physical constriction such as a cast or bandage that is too tight.

Skin Lesions

Skin lesions usually indicate an abnormal skin condition. Characteristics, such as location, size, type of lesion, pattern, and discharge, if present provide clues about the cause of the condition. Inspect and palpate the skin color abnormalities, elevations, lesions, or injuries to describe all characteristics present.

Primary lesions (such as macules, papules, and vesicles) are often the skin's initial response to injury or infection. Hyperpigmented macules (freckles and Mongolian spots) are normal findings also classified as primary lesions. Figure 7–11 ■ describes common primary lesions. See Table 36–1 in Chapter 36 🖋 for the characteristics of some common secondary lesions such as scars, ulcers, and fissures.

Primary lesions often appear in common patterns that help distinguish between lesions:

- **Linear**—in a row or stripe (e.g., poison ivy).
- **Annular**—ring-shaped with a central clearing (e.g., ringworm). Annular lesions running together are polycyclic.
- **Herpetiform**—grouped or clustered (e.g., herpes, chickenpox).
- **Reticulated**—networked or lacelike (e.g., parvovirus B19).

Inspection of the Hair

Inspect the scalp hair for color, distribution, and cleanliness. The hair shafts should be evenly colored, shiny, and either curly or straight. Variation in hair color not caused by bleaching or coloring can be associated with a nutritional deficiency. Investigate areas of hair loss. Hair loss in a child may result from tight braids or skin lesions such as ringworm (see Chapter 36 🖋). Notice any unusual hair growth patterns. An unusually low hairline on the neck or forehead may be associated with a congenital disorder such as hypothyroidism.

Children are frequently exposed to head lice. Inspect the individual hair shafts for small nits (lice eggs) that adhere to the hair. None should be present. See Chapter 36 🖋 for more information about head lice.

Observe the distribution of body hair as other skin surfaces are exposed during examination. Fine hair covers most areas of the body. The presence of body hair in unexpected places should be noted. For example, a tuft of hair at the base of the spine often indicates a pilonidal cyst.

Pubic hair begins to develop in children between 8 and 12 years of age, and axillary hair usually develops about 6 months later (see page 201).

Facial hair is noted in boys shortly after axillary hair develops. Note the age at which pubic and axillary hair develop in the child. Development at an unusually young age is associated with precocious puberty.

Palpation of the Hair

Palpate the hair shafts for texture. Hair should feel soft or silky with fine or thick shafts. See Developing Cultural Competence: Hair Characteristics. Endocrine conditions such as hypothyroidism may result in coarse, brittle hair. Part the hair in various spots over the head to inspect and palpate the scalp for crusting or other lesions. If lesions are present, describe them using the characteristics in Figure 7–11.

ASSESSING THE HEAD AND FACE

What can cause a child's head or face to be asymmetric? How does a normal fontanel feel? What does an unusually large or small head suggest in an infant?

Inspection of the Head and Face

During early childhood, the skull's sutures permit expansion for brain growth. See page 172 for the measurement of head circumference. Infants and young children normally have a rounded skull with a prominent occipital area. See Figure 7–12 ■. The shape of the head changes during childhood, and the occipital area becomes less prominent. An abnormal skull shape can result from premature closure of the sutures.

Clinical Tip

Children who were low-birth-weight infants often have a flat, elongated skull because the soft skull bones were flattened by the weight of the head early in infancy. Head flattening is also associated with the recommended sleeping position for infants—on their back. See Chapter 33 🖋.

Inspect the child's face for symmetry when the child is resting, smiling, talking, and crying (Figure 7–13 ■). Significant asymmetry

---

Developing Cultural Competence
Hair Characteristics

Hair varies by genetic origin. Children of African origin often have hair that can appear curly, wavy, or coiled, and this hair more easily breaks. Children of Asian origin have hair that is coarse and straight. Children of Caucasian origin have hair with fine to medium coarseness that is straight or wavy.

Pathophysiology Illustrated   Common Primary Skin Lesions and Associated Conditions

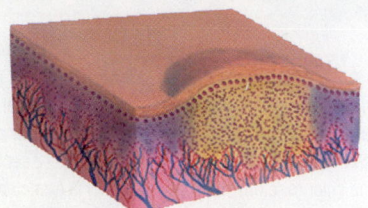

Lesion Name: Papule
Description: Elevated, firm, diameter less than 1 cm (1/2 in.)
Example: Warts, pigmented nevi

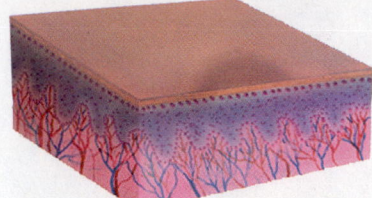

Lesion Name: Macule
Description: Flat, nonpalpable, diameter less than 1 cm (1/2 in.)
Example: Freckle, rubella, rubeola, petechiae

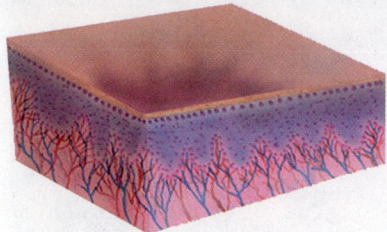

Lesion Name: Patch
Description: Macule diameter greater than 1 cm (1/2 in.)
Example: Vitiligo, Mongolian spot

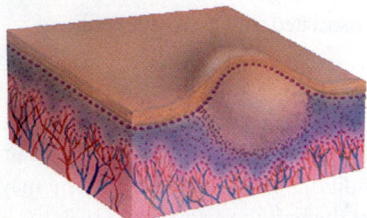

Lesion Name: Pustule
Description: Vesicle filled with purulent fluid
Example: Impetigo, acne

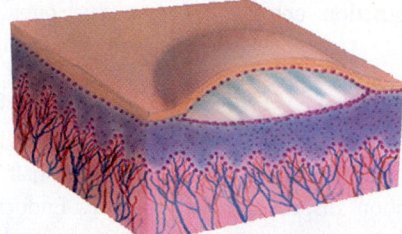

Lesion Name: Vesicle
Description: Elevated, filled with fluid, diameter less than 1 cm (1/2 in.)
Example: Early chickenpox, herpes simplex

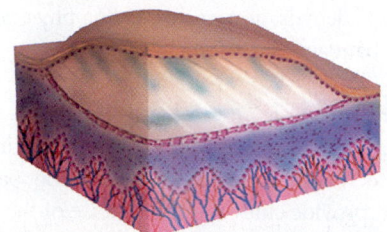

Lesion Name: Bulla
Description: Vesicle diameter greater than 1 cm (1/2 in.)
Example: Burn blister

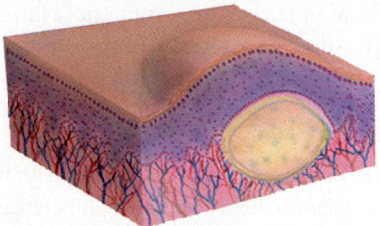

Lesion Name: Nodule
Description: Elevated, firm, deeper in dermis than papule, diameter 1–2 cm (1/2 in.–1 in.)
Example: Erythema nodosum

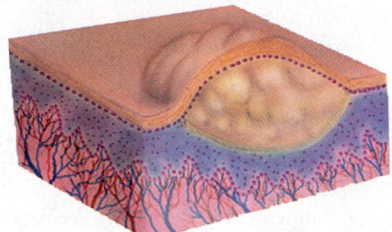

Lesion Name: Tumor
Description: Elevated, solid, diameter greater than 2 cm (1 in.)
Example: Neoplasm, hemangioma

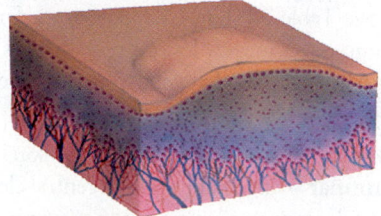

Lesion Name: Wheal
Description: Irregular elevated solid area of edematous skin
Example: Urticaria, insect bite

FIGURE 7–11 ■ Skin lesions usually indicate abnormal skin conditions. Identifying characteristics of these lesions can provide clues about the cause of the condition.

may result from paralysis of trigeminal or facial nerves (cranial nerves V or VII), in utero positioning, and swelling from infection, allergy, or trauma.

Next inspect the face for unusual facial features such as coarseness, wide eye spacing, or disproportionate size. Tremors, tics, and twitching of facial muscles are often associated with seizures.

Palpation of the Skull

Palpate the skull in infants and young children to assess the sutures and fontanels and to detect soft bones. (See Developing Cultural Competence: Touching the Head.)

Sutures

Use your fingertip pads to palpate each suture line. The edge of each bone in the suture line is felt, but normally there is no separation of the two bones. If additional bone edges are felt, it may indicate a skull fracture.

Developing Cultural Competence
Touching the Head

The head is a sacred part of the body to some Southeast Asians. Ask for permission before touching the infant's head to palpate the sutures and fontanels (Purnell, 2009, p. 383). When a Hispanic child is examined, however, not touching the head is considered bad luck by many families.

Fontanels

At the intersection of the sutures, palpate the anterior and posterior fontanels. The fontanel should feel flat and firm inside the bony edges. The anterior fontanel is normally diamond shaped and smaller than 5 cm (2 in.) in diameter at 6 months of age. The anterior fontanel then becomes progressively smaller and closes between

As They Grow Sutures and Fontanels of the Skull

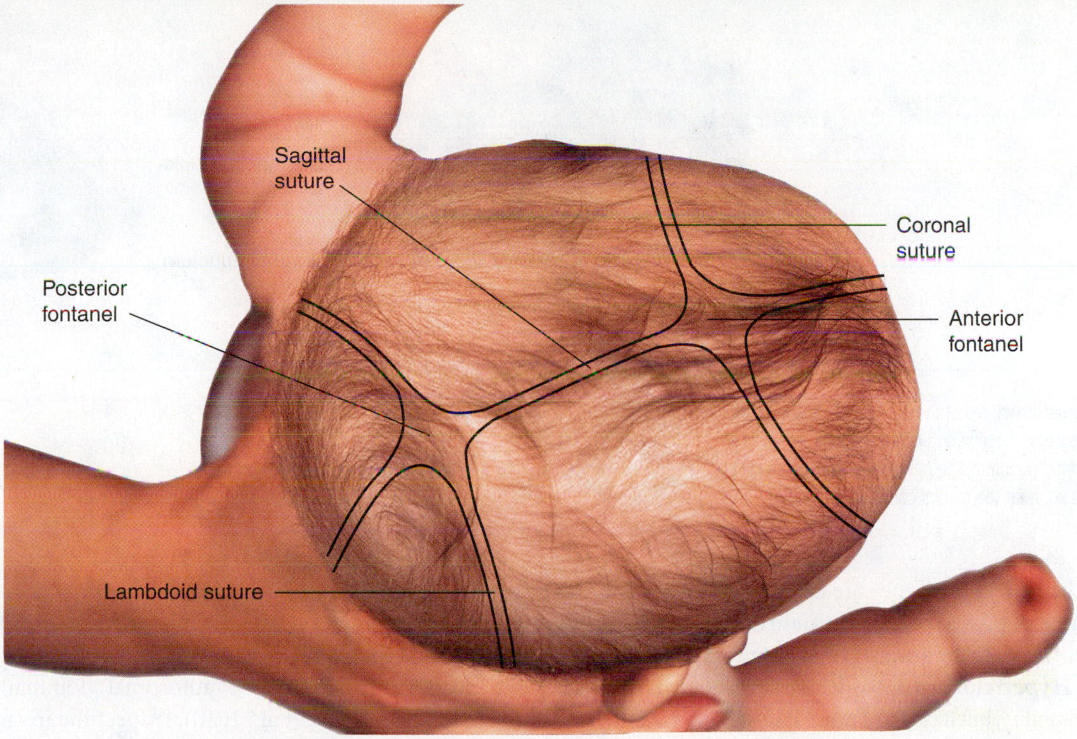

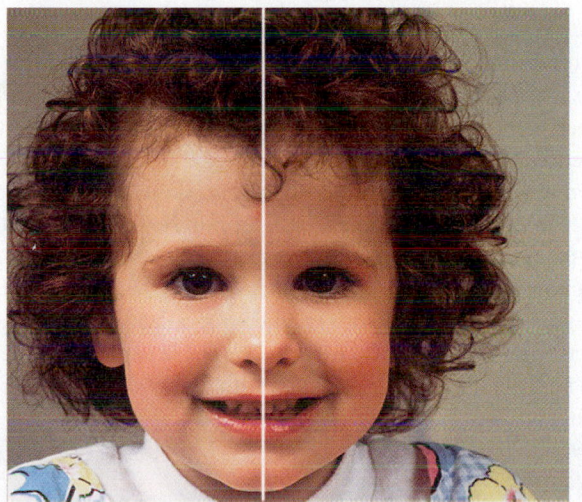

FIGURE 7–12 ■ The **sutures** are fibrous connections between the bones of the skull that have not yet ossified. The fontanels are formed at the intersection of these sutures where bone has not yet formed. Fontanels are covered by tough membranous tissue that protects the brain. The posterior fontanel closes between 2 and 3 months after birth. The anterior fontanel and sutures are palpable up to the age of 18 months. The suture lines of the skull are seldom palpated after 2 years of age. After that time, the sutures rarely separate.

FIGURE 7–13 ■ When inspecting the face, draw an imaginary line down the middle of the face over the nose and compare the features side to side. Significant asymmetry may be caused by paralysis of cranial nerve V or VII, in utero positioning, or swelling from infection, allergy, or trauma.

12 and 18 months of age. The posterior fontanel closes between 2 and 3 months of age. The suture lines of the skull are seldom palpated after 2 years of age. After that time the sutures rarely split.

A tense fontanel, bulging above the margin of the skull, is an indication of increased intracranial pressure. If you suspect that the fontanel is tense, palpate while the child is quietly sitting to determine if the brain tissues bulge above the skull opening and feel tense. A soft fontanel, sunken below the margin of the skull with prominent margins of the skull, is associated with dehydration.

ASSESSING EYES AND VISION

What is the red reflex and what does it indicate? How is eye muscle balance tested? Is it normal for a child's visual acuity to be different at certain ages?

Inspection of the External Eye Structures

The function of the external and internal eye structures and related cranial nerves makes vision possible. Inspect the external eye structures, including the eyeballs, eyelids, and eye muscles (Figure 7–14 ■). Test the function of cranial nerves II, III, IV, and VI, which innervate the eye structures (see page 209). Equipment needed for this examination includes an ophthalmoscope or small flashlight, a vision chart, a penlight, a small toy, and an index card or paper cup.

Eye Size and Spacing

Inspect the eyes and surrounding tissues simultaneously when examining facial features. The eyes should be the same size but not unusually large or small. Observe for a sunken appearance or eye bulging, which can be identified by retracted eyelids. Bulging may be associated with a tumor, and a sunken appearance may reflect dehydration. Note the characteristics of the eyebrows.

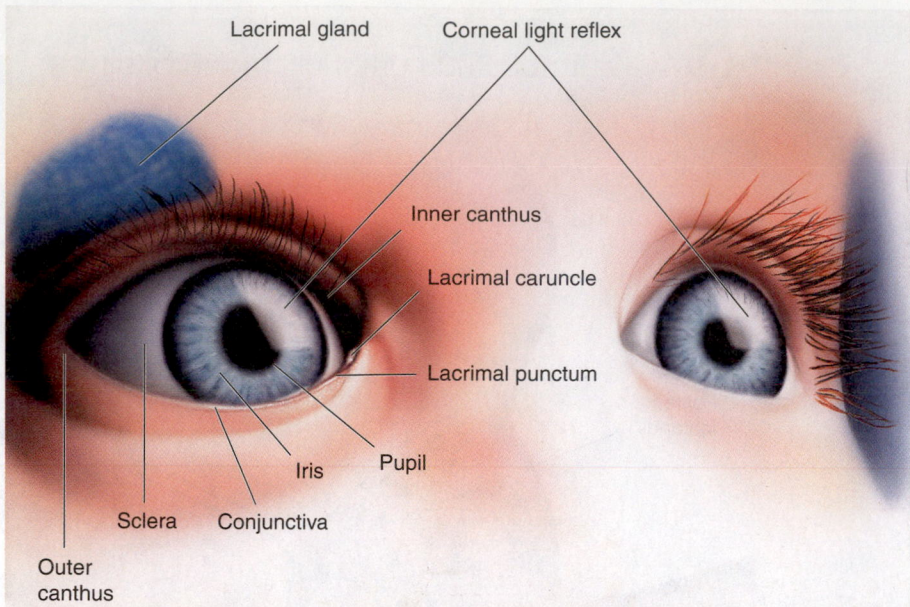

FIGURE 7–14 ■ External structures of the eye. Notice that the light reflex is at the same location on each eye. Note the location of the lacrimal punctum, the opening for the lacrimal gland on each lid, near the medial canthus.

Next inspect the eyes to see if they are appropriately spaced from each other. The distance between the inner canthi of the eyes should be equal to the distance between the inner and outer canthi of the child's eye (Hummel, 2011). **Hypertelorism,** or widely spaced eyes, is associated with intellectual disability, but it can be a normal variation in children.

Eyelids and Eyelashes

Inspect the eyelids for color, size, position, mobility, and condition of the eyelashes. Eyelids should be the same color as surrounding facial skin and free of swelling or inflammation along the edges. Sebaceous glands that look like yellow striations are often present near the hair follicles. Eyelashes curl away from the eye to prevent irritation of the conjunctivae.

Inspect the conjunctivae lining the eyelids by pulling down the lower lid and then everting the upper lid. The conjunctivae should be pink and glossy. No excess tearing should be present.

When the eyes are open, inspect the level at which the upper and lower lids cross the eye. Each lid normally covers part of the iris but not any portion of the pupil. The lids should also close completely over the iris and cornea. **Ptosis,** drooping of the lid over the pupil, is often associated with injury to the oculomotor nerve, cranial nerve III. *Sunset sign*, in which the sclera is seen between the upper lid and the iris, may indicate retracted eyelids or hydrocephalus.

Inspect the eyes for the palpebral slant (Figure 7–15A ■). The eyelids of most children open horizontally. An upward slant is a normal finding in Asian children; however, children with Down syndrome also often have an upward slant (Figure 7–15B ■). A downward slant is seen in some children as a normal variation. Children of Asian descent often have an **epicanthal fold,** an extra layer of skin covering all or part of the medial canthus of the eye.

Eye Color

Inspect the color of each sclera, iris, and bulbar conjunctiva. The sclera is normally white or ivory in children with darker skin. Sclerae of another color may suggest the presence of an underlying disease. For example, yellow sclerae indicate jaundice. An excessive blue tinge to the sclerae may be associated with some types of osteogenesis imperfecta. Typically, the iris is blue or light colored at birth and becomes pigmented within 6 months. Rarely the irises are different colors due to autosomal dominance inheritance (Tuli, Kockler, Kelly, et al., 2010). Inspect the iris for the presence of *Brushfield spots*, white specks in a linear pattern around the iris circumference, which are often associated with Down syndrome. The bulbar conjunctivae, which cover the sclera to the edge of the cornea, are normally clear. Redness can indicate eyestrain, infection, allergies, or irritation.

Pupils

Inspect the pupils for size and shape. Normally the pupils are round, clear, and equal in size. Some children have a **coloboma,** a keyhole-shaped pupil caused by a notch in the iris. This sign can indicate the presence of other congenital anomalies.

To test the pupillary response to light, shine a bright light into one eye. A brisk constriction of both the pupil exposed to direct light and the other pupil (consensual response) is a normal finding. To test pupillary response to accommodation, ask the child to look first at a near object (such as a toy) and then at a distant object (such as a picture on the wall). The expected response is pupil constriction with near objects and pupil dilation with distant objects. These procedures test the optic nerve, cranial nerve II.

Clinical Tip
Some infants resist having their eyes examined by keeping them closed. Often they will open their eyes if held in an upright position over the parent's shoulder. The examiner can then walk around behind the parent and use the ophthalmoscope or a penlight to assess pupil size, shape, and responsiveness to light as well as the corneal light reflex and red reflex.

Inspection of the Eye Muscles

A common pediatric eye disorder is **strabismus,** a muscle imbalance causing the eyes to look crossed. This condition is important to detect because, if uncorrected, it can cause vision impairment.

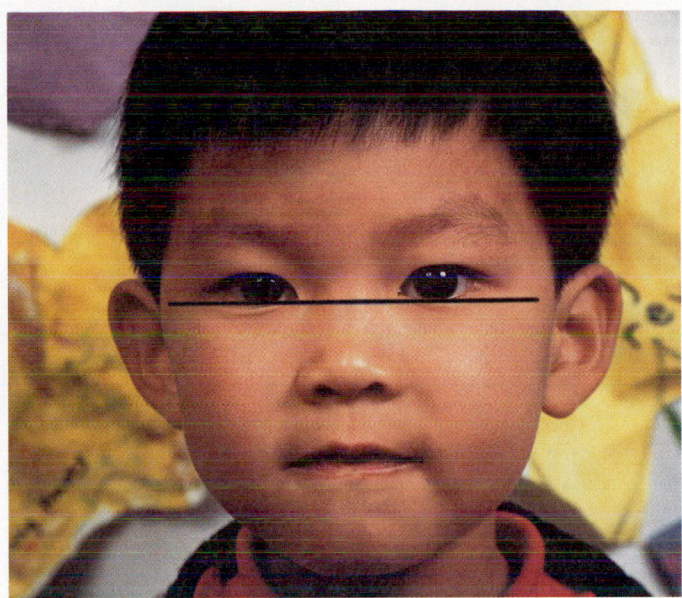

A

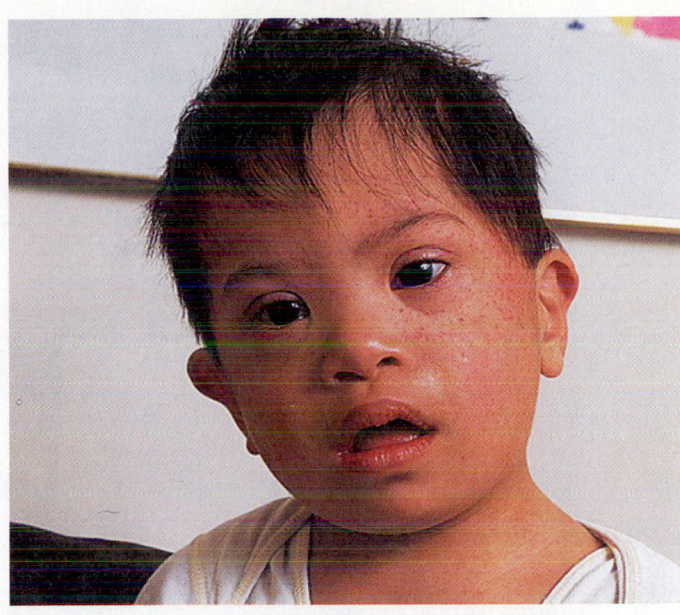

B

FIGURE 7–15 ■ Assessment of the palpebral slant. *A,* Draw an imaginary line across the medial canthi and extend it to each side of the face to identify the slant of the palpebral fissures. When the line crosses the lateral canthi, the palpebral fissures are horizontal and no slant is present. When the lateral canthi fall above the imaginary line, the eyes have an upward slant. A downward slant is present when the lateral canthi fall below the imaginary line. What type of slant does this child have? Are epicanthal folds present? *B,* The eyes of this boy with Down syndrome show an upward slant.

Several tests are used to detect the presence of a muscle imbalance, including the evaluation of extraocular movements, the corneal light reflex, and the cover–uncover test.

Extraocular Movements

For children of 3 years or older, seat the child at your eye level to evaluate the extraocular movements. Hold a toy or penlight 30 cm (12 in.) from the child's eyes and move it through the six cardinal fields of gaze illustrated in Figure 7–16 ■. You may need to hold the young child's head still until fine motor eye movement develops. Both eyes should move together, tracking the object in all directions. This procedure tests the oculomotor, trochlear, and abducens nerves (cranial nerves III, IV, and VI).

Corneal Light Reflex

Shine a light on the infant's or child's nose, midway between the eyes to identify where the light is reflected on the cornea of each eye. The light reflection is normally symmetric, at the same spot on each cornea (see Figure 7–14). An asymmetric corneal light reflex after 6 months of age indicates a muscle imbalance.

Cover–Uncover Test

The cover–uncover test can be used only for older, cooperative children. While standing slightly to one side, but in a position from which you are still able to see the child's eyes, ask the child to look at a picture on the wall or have the parent hold a toy for the child to look at. See Figure 7–17 ■ for the technique. Repeat the procedure with the other eye. Because the eyes work together, no obvious movement of either eye is expected. Eye movement indicates a muscle imbalance.

Inspection of the Internal Eye Structures

The funduscopic examination with an ophthalmoscope allows the structures of the internal eye—the retina, optic disc, arteries and veins, and macula—to be examined. This examination is usually performed by experienced examiners. To assist the examiner, darken the room so the child's pupils dilate. Explain the procedure to the child to gain full cooperation. Have a picture on the wall or hold a toy for the child to stare at so that the child's eye will not have to be held open forcibly.

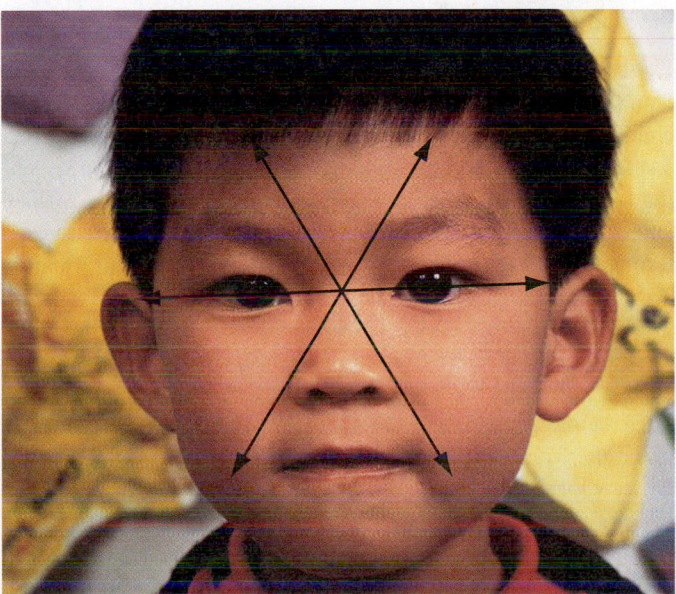

FIGURE 7–16 ■ Inspection of the extraocular movements. Have the child sit at your eye level. Hold a toy or penlight about 30 cm (12 in.) from the child's eyes and move it in all six directions indicated. Both eyes should move together, tracking the object.

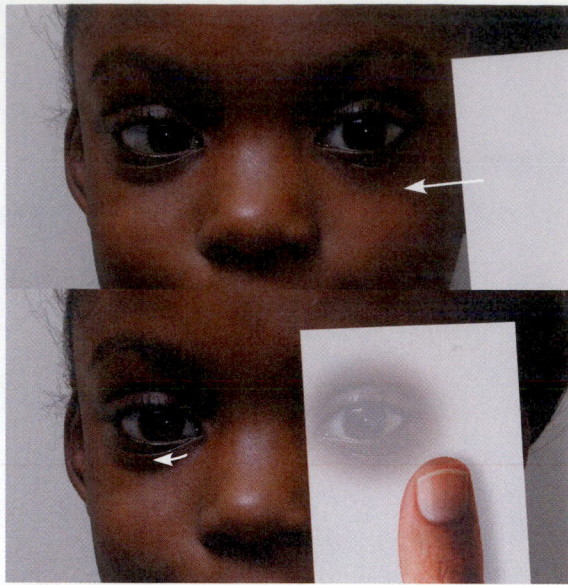

A Right, uncovered eye is weaker

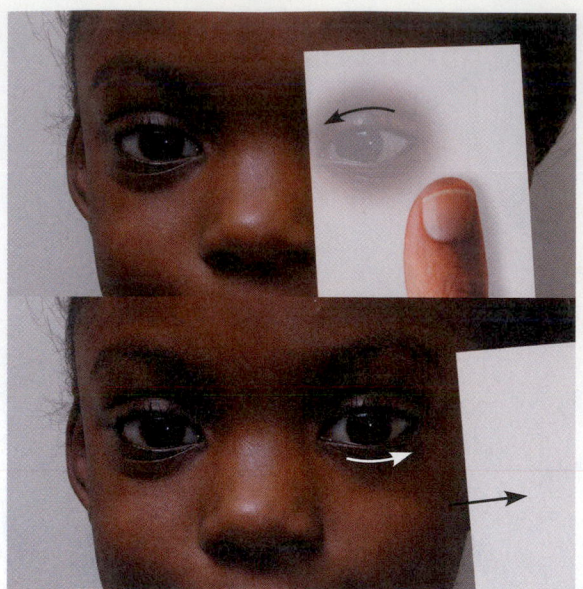

B Left, covered eye is weaker

FIGURE 7–17 ■ Cover–uncover test. With the child at your eye level, ask the child to look at a picture on the wall. *A,* As you cover one eye with an index card or paper cup, observe for any movement of the uncovered eye. If it jumps to fixate on the picture, the uncovered eye has a muscle weakness. *B,* As you remove the cover from the eye, observe the covered eye for any movement to fixate on the picture. If an eye has a muscle weakness, it will drift to a relaxed position when covered.

Red Reflex

A penlight or the light of the ophthalmoscope can be used to assess the **red reflex,** the orange-red glow of the vascular retina as the light travels through the cornea, aqueous humor, lens, and vitreous humor to the retina. Shine light at both eyes from a distance of 45 cm (18 in.). The red reflex of each eye should be symmetric and uniform in shape and color (American Academy of Pediatrics Section on Ophthalmology, 2008). Black spots or opacities within the red reflex are abnormal and may indicate congenital cataracts, hemorrhage, or corneal scars. A white reflex is associated with a tumor or retinoblastoma. See Chapter 24 🔗.

Vision Assessment

Because vision is such an important sense for learning, assessment is essential to detect any serious problems. Vision is evaluated using an age-appropriate vision test, but no simple method exists. It is possible to assess the presence of vision in infants and children by observing their behavior in response to certain maneuvers and during play. Visual assessment techniques focus on light perception, visual acuity, ability of eyes to fixate on and follow an object, and color perception.

Infants and Toddlers

When the infant's eyes are open, test the blink reflex by moving your hand quickly toward the infant's eyes. A quick blink is the normal response. Absence of the blink reflex can indicate that the infant is blind.

To test an infant's ability to visually track an object, hold a light or toy about 15 cm (6 in.) from the infant's eyes. When the infant has fixated on or is staring at the object, move it slowly to each side. The infant should move the head and follow the object with the eyes.

Once an infant has developed skills to reach for and then pick up objects, observe play behavior to evaluate vision. The ability to easily find and pick up small toys is a good indicator of vision in children under 3 years of age. See Table 24–4 in Chapter 24 🔗 for screening questions to identify vision problems in children. Photo screening or an autorefractor may be used to assess vision in some preschool and school-age children.

Visual Fields

Peripheral vision is evaluated by a confrontation test in children over 3 years of age. Have the child look at your nose or chin, and keep the head still. Move both hands beyond your field of vision and slowly move the hands with fingers wiggling toward the space between your head and the child's head. Ask the child to tell you when the moving fingers are seen. The child should see the fingers at the same time as the examiner. Observe for eye or head movement by the young child to indicate when the fingers are seen, rather than depend only upon the child's verbal report.

Standardized Vision Charts

Standardized vision charts cannot be used to test vision until the child can understand directions and cooperate, usually at about 3 years of age. For preschool children, several types of vision screening tools can be used before the alphabet is mastered. The Snellen letter chart and several variations are used for standardized vision testing in children and adolescents. See Table 7–4 for information about vision screening tools.

For all screening tools used to test far vision, make sure the child is the appropriate distance from the chart, usually 10 or 20 feet. Cover one eye with a paper cup or index card, so each eye is evaluated separately before testing them together. Preschool children should be tested after a practice session to ensure that directions are understood. Observe for squinting, moving the head forward, excessive blinking, or tearing. If the child wears glasses or contact lenses, test the child without corrective lenses before testing with lenses. If the child correctly reads the letters on the line designated "20 feet" while standing 20 feet away, vision is "20/20." If, however, the child can only read the line labeled "40 feet" while standing 20 feet away, vision is "20/40." See the Practice Alert for referral indications. See Chapter 24 🔗 for information about vision problems.

TABLE 7–4	Standardized Vision Testing for Children and Adolescents

TEST	DESCRIPTION
Snellen Letter Chart For children who know the alphabet	This alphabet chart consists of lines of letters in decreasing size. The child is asked to read all letters across an indicated line. Designed for reading from a distance of 10 or 20 ft.
HOTV Chart For children who may not know the alphabet or speak English	This chart uses the letters *H, O, T,* and *V* on lines in decreasing size. The child is given a paper with the four letters on it. During the screening, point to a letter and ask the child to select the letter on the paper. Designed for testing from a distance of 10 or 20 ft.
Snellen E Chart For children who do not know the alphabet or speak English	This chart consists of capital Es shown facing in different directions in lines of decreasing size. The child is asked to point in the direction of the "legs" of the E that the examiner indicates. Or, give the child a paper with an E on it and ask the child to turn it in the direction the E is pointing on the chart. Designed for testing from a distance of 10 or 20 ft.
Blackbird Vision Screening For children who do not know the alphabet	In this variation of the Snellen E chart, blackbirds fly in a shape similar to an E. Ask the child to identify in which direction the bird is flying. Designed for testing from a distance of 10 or 20 ft.
The Picture Chart For children who may not know the alphabet	This chart uses commonly identified silhouettes (e.g., house, apple, umbrella) placed on lines in decreasing size. Ask the child to identify the pictures either by naming them or by pointing to each one on a piece of paper. Designed for testing from a distance of 10 or 20 ft.
Allen Cards For children who may not know the alphabet	These cards contain seven familiar pictures: birthday cake, teddy bear, tree, house, car, telephone, and horse with rider. Show the pictures to the child to be sure that the child can recognize them during the test. The child should be able to name objects on three of seven cards within three to five trials. Designed for testing from a distance of 15 ft.
Stereograms (Titmus Stereograms or Random Dot E Game) For children as young as 4 years who can follow instructions	For testing *stereoacuity,* the ability of the eyes to work together for depth perception, in older children. The child wears stereoscopic glasses and is asked to distinguish between cards that are blank, have a raised E, and have a recessed E. The child should consistently be able to identify the cards with Es. Designed for testing at a distance of 16 in. from the face.
Jaeger or Rosenbaum Chart For children who have mastered the alphabet	This standardized card with graduated letters is used to test near vision. Designed for reading at a distance of 12 to 14 in. from the face.
Ishihara Chart For boys as young as 4 years	This chart is used for testing color vision to identify X-linked color blindness. A series of polychromatic cards includes a pattern of dots printed against a background of many colored dots. Ask the child to identify the pattern. The boy who is color blind cannot identify the letter within the colored field. Designed for testing at a distance of 12 to 14 in. from the face.

Practice Alert

Criteria for referral for further vision evaluation include:

- Age 3 to 12 months—failure to fix on an object and follow
- Age 3 to 4 years—20/50 or worse
- Age 5 years—20/40 or worse
- Age 6 years and older—20/30 or worse
- A difference in vision between the eyes of two lines or more on the Snellen eye chart; for example, 20/20 in one eye and 20/40 in the other eye, even though one eye is within the expected range
- Any problems with ocular alignment
- Any other indication of vision impairment, regardless of acuity

Source: *Data from American Academy of Ophthalmology Pediatric Ophthalmology/Strabismus Panel. (2007). Preferred Practice Pattern® Guidelines. Pediatric eye evaluations. San Francisco, CA: Author.* Retrieved from http://www.aao.org/ppp

ASSESSING THE EARS AND HEARING

How do you identify proper ear placement on the head? What is the significance of low-set ears? What play activities can be used to test hearing in young children?

Inspection of the External Ear Structures

As a continuation of the head and eye examination, inspect the position and characteristics of the pinna, the external ear. Equipment needed for this assessment includes an otoscope, noisemakers (bell, rattle, tissue paper), and a tuning fork of 500 to 1000 Hz.

The pinna is considered "low set" when the junction of the upper pinna lies below an imaginary line drawn through the medial and lateral canthi of the eye toward the ear (Figure 7–18 ■). Low-set ears are often associated with congenital renal disorders.

Inspect the pinna for any malformation. The pinna should be completely formed, with an open auditory canal. Next, inspect the tissue around the pinna for abnormalities. A pit or hole in front of the pinna may indicate the presence of a sinus. If the pinna protrudes outward, there may be swelling behind the ear, a sign of infection in the mastoid process of the temporal bone of the skull.

Inspect the external auditory canal for any discharge. A foul-smelling, purulent discharge may indicate the presence of a foreign body or an infection in the external canal. Clear fluid or a blood-tinged discharge may indicate a cerebrospinal fluid leak caused by a basilar skull fracture.

Inspection of the Tympanic Membrane

Examination of the tympanic membrane is important in infants and young children because they are prone to otitis media, a middle ear infection. To examine the internal auditory canal and tympanic membrane, use an otoscope, an instrument with a magnifying lens, bright light, and speculum. The largest ear speculum that fits into the auditory canal is used to form a seal for testing the movement of the tympanic membrane and to reduce the chance of injury to the auditory canal if the child moves suddenly.

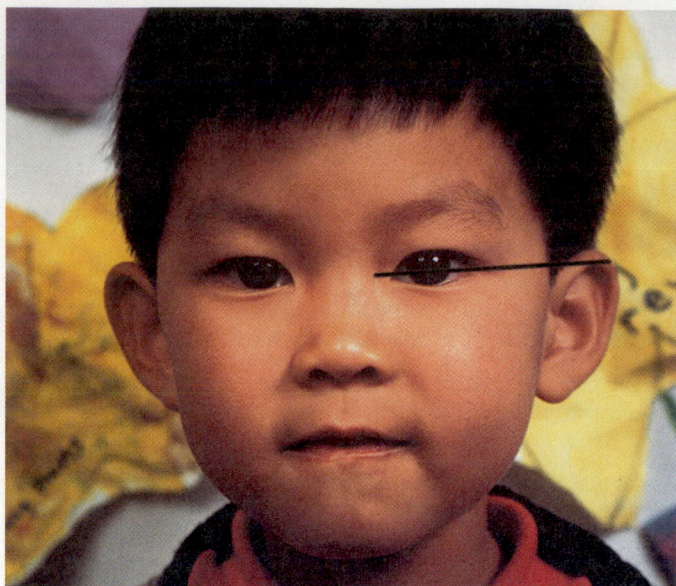

FIGURE 7–18 ■ To detect the correct placement of the external ears, draw an imaginary line through the medial and lateral canthi of the eye toward the ear. This line normally passes through the upper portion of the pinna. The pinna is considered "low set" when the top lies completely below the imaginary line. Low-set ears are often associated with renal disorders. Does this child have normal ear placement? (Yes, he does.)

Toddlers and young children often resist the otoscope examination because of past painful experiences, so postpone it until the end for this age group. Use simple explanations to prepare the child. Let the child play with the otoscope or demonstrate how it is used on the parent or a doll. Figure 7–19 ■ illustrates one method of human restraint for an uncooperative toddler or preschool child.

Hold the handle of the otoscope in the palm of your hand that is closest to the child's face. If a pneumatic squeeze bulb is used, hold it between the index finger and the handle. When the child is cooperative, rest the back of your hand against the child's head to stabilize it. Use your other hand to pull the pinna toward the back of the head either up or down, whichever position straightens the auditory canal and provides the best view for inspecting the tympanic membrane (Figure 7–20 ■).

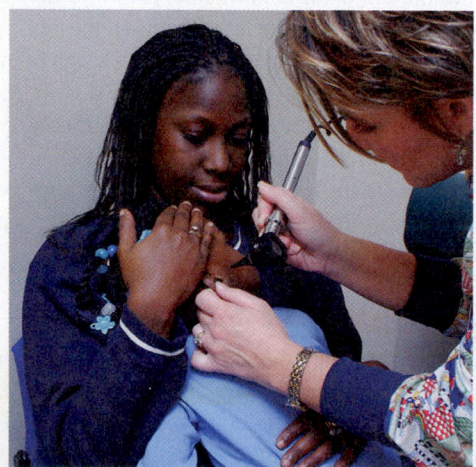

FIGURE 7–19 ■ Human restraint for the otoscopic examination. Place the uncooperative toddler on the parent's lap with legs held between the parent's legs. One of the parent's arms holds the child's head to the chest and the other arm holds the child's arms and upper torso against the chest.

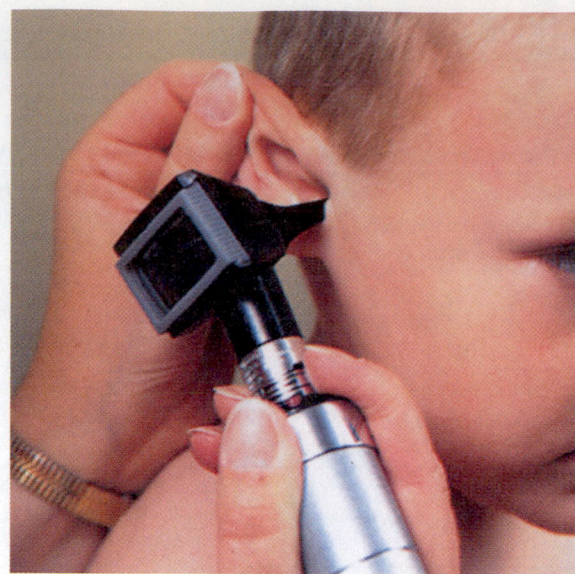

FIGURE 7–20 ■ To examine the tympanic membrane with an otoscope, straighten the auditory canal by pulling the pinna back and up for children over 3 years of age or pulling the pinna down and back for children under 3 years of age.

Slowly insert the speculum into the auditory canal, inspecting the walls for signs of irritation, discharge, or a foreign body. The walls of the auditory canal are normally pink, with some cerumen present. Children often put beads, peas, or other small objects into their ears. If cerumen or a foreign body obstructs the auditory canal, warm water irrigation can be used to clean the canal. Refer to the Skills Manual ⬭ for procedures.

Practice Alert

Never irrigate the ear canal if any discharge is present, as the tympanic membrane may be ruptured. Irrigation would allow the water to enter the middle ear and potentially worsen the infection.

The tympanic membrane, which separates the outer ear from the middle ear, is usually pearly gray and translucent. It reflects light, and the bones (ossicles) in the middle ear are normally visible (Figure 7–21 ■). When the auditory canal is sealed and the pneumatic attachment is squeezed, the tympanic membrane normally moves in and out in response to the positive and negative pressure applied. Table 7–5 lists the unexpected findings of a tympanic membrane examination and their associated conditions. See Figure 24–7 and Figure 24–8 ⬭ for the tympanic membrane appearance with otitis media.

Clinical Judgment

Jasmine's right tympanic membrane is red and has no light reflex. It has no visible landmarks, and it does not move to positive or negative pressure. Jasmine also has a temperature of 38°C (100.4°F). What health condition is most likely present?

Hearing Assessment

Hearing is essential for normal speech development and learning. Hearing loss may occur at any time during early childhood as the result of birth trauma, frequent otitis media, meningitis, or antibiotics that damage cranial nerve VIII. Hearing loss may be associated with other congenital anomalies and genetic syndromes. The hearing of newborns is evaluated at birth (see Chapter 24 ⬭), and hearing is evaluated throughout childhood.

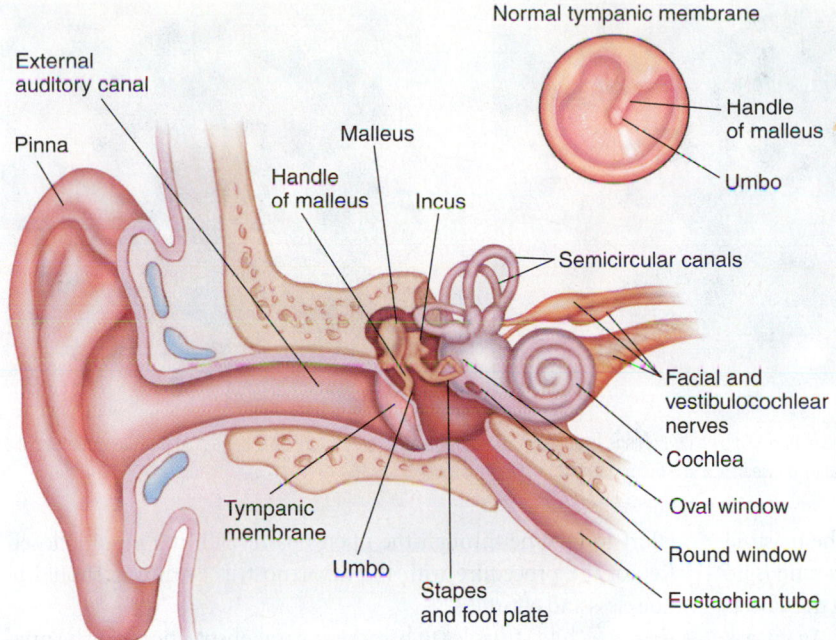

External
auditory canal
Pinna
Malleus
Handle
of malleus   Incus
Normal tympanic membrane
Handle
of malleus
Umbo
Semicircular canals
Facial and
vestibulocochlear
nerves
Cochlea
Oval window
Round window
Eustachian tube
Tympanic
membrane
Umbo
Stapes
and foot plate

FIGURE 7–21 ■ Anatomy of the ear. The tympanic membrane separates the outer ear from the middle and inner ear. It normally has a triangular light reflex pointing toward the center with the base on the nasal side. The bony landmarks, the umbo and handle of malleus, are seen through the tympanic membrane.

CHARACTERISTICS OF TYMPANIC MEMBRANE	UNEXPECTED FINDINGS	ASSOCIATED CONDITIONS
Color	Redness	Infection in middle ear
	Slight redness	Prolonged crying
	Amber	Serous fluid in middle ear
	Deep red or blue	Blood in middle ear
Light reflex	Absent	Bulging tympanic membrane, infection in middle ear
	Distorted, loss of triangular shape	Retracted tympanic membrane, serous fluid in middle ear
Bony landmarks	Extra prominent	Retracted tympanic membrane, serous fluid in middle ear
Movement	No motility	Infection or fluid in middle ear
	Excess motility	Healed perforation

TABLE 7–5 Unexpected Findings on Examination of the Tympanic Membrane and Their Associated Conditions

Evaluate hearing by observing the child's responses to various auditory stimuli using age-appropriate methods. Use hearing and speech articulation milestones as an initial hearing screen. Select an age-appropriate method to screen hearing. When a hearing deficiency is suspected as a result of screening, the child is referred for audiometry or tympanometry to obtain the most accurate evaluation of hearing. **Audiometry** is a screening procedure using air conduction that measures hearing for pure-tone frequencies and loudness. The high- and low-pitched sounds are presented through earphones testing different sound frequencies and the loudness needed to hear each sound. Hearing loss is determined when the child needs higher decibels (louder sound) to hear a tone. **Tympanometry** is a test to estimate the pressure in the middle ear and an indirect measure of tympanic membrane

movement. See Chapter 24 for more information. Refer to the Clinical Skills Manual.

Infants and Toddlers

Select noisemakers with different frequencies, such as a rattle, bell, and tissue paper that will attract the young child's attention. Ask the parent or an assistant to entertain the infant with a quiet toy, such as a teddy bear. Stand behind the infant, about 60 cm (2 ft) away from the infant's ear but outside the infant's field of peripheral vision, and make a soft sound with the noisemaker. Make sure that no air movement provides a clue to the child to turn the head. Have the parent or an assistant observe the child for any of the following responses when the noisemaker is used: widening the eyes, briefly stopping all activity to listen, or turning the head toward the sound. Repeat the test in the other ear and with the other noisemakers. See Table 7–6 for indicators of hearing loss in infants and young children.

Preschool and Older Children

Whispered words are used to evaluate the hearing of children over 3 years of age. Position your head about 30 cm (12 in.) away from the child's ear, but out of the child's range of vision so your lips cannot be read. Use words easily recognized by the child, such as *Mickey Mouse, hot dog,* and *Popsicle,* and ask the child to repeat the words. Repeat the test with different words in the opposite ear. The child should correctly repeat the whispered words.

When the child will not repeat the whispered words, try an alternative procedure. As you whisper directions, ask the child to point to different body parts such as an eye, ear, and hand. Remember to stay out of the child's range of vision so the child cannot read your lips. The child should point to the correct body part each time.

Bone and Air Conduction of Sound

A tuning fork is used to evaluate the hearing of school-age children who can follow directions. Stroke the tines of the tuning fork to begin the vibration. Avoid touching the vibrating tines, which will dampen the sound. Bone conduction is tested when the handle of the tuning fork is placed on the child's skull. Air conduction is tested when the vibrating tines are held close to the child's ear (Figure 7–22 ■).

Weber test   Place the vibrating tuning fork on top of the child's skull in the midline. Ask the child to tell you where the sound is heard the best, either in both ears equally or in one ear. The sound should be heard equally in both ears.

AGE OF CHILD	INDICATORS
Infant	■ No startle reaction to loud noises ■ Does not turn toward sounds by 4 months of age ■ Babbles as a young infant, but does not keep babbling or develop speech sounds after 6 months of age
Young Child	■ No speech by 2 years of age ■ Inability to follow age-appropriate directions, such as "bring me the block" ■ Speech sounds are not distinct as expected at appropriate ages

TABLE 7–6 Indicators of Hearing Loss

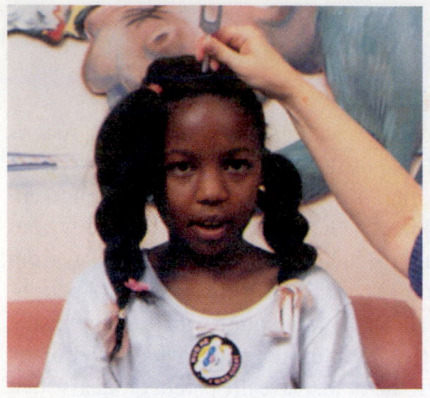 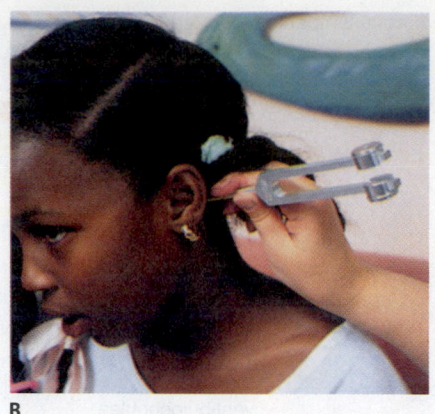 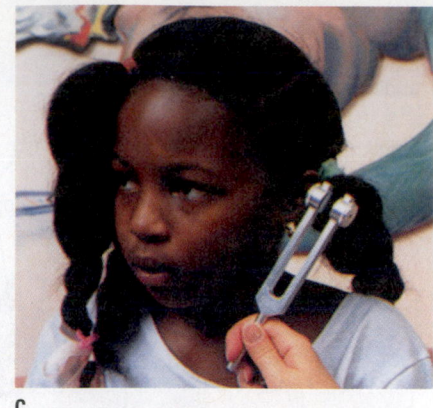

A   B   C

FIGURE 7–22 ■ *A*, Weber test. Place a vibrating tuning fork on the midline of the child's head. *B*, Rinne test, step 1. Place a vibrating tuning fork on the mastoid process until the child no longer hears the sound. *C*, Rinne test, step 2. Reposition still-vibrating tines between 2.5 and 5 cm (1 and 2 in.) from the ear.

Rinne test Place the vibrating tuning fork handle on the mastoid process behind an ear. Ask the child to tell you when the sound is no longer heard. Immediately move the tuning fork, holding the vibrating tines about 2.5 to 5 cm (1 to 2 in.) from the same ear. Again, ask the child to indicate when the sound is no longer heard. The child normally hears the air-conducted sound twice as long as the bone-conducted sound. Repeat the Rinne test on the other ear.

When the sound is heard longer by bone conduction than air conduction, the affected ear may have a conductive hearing loss. When sound is heard longer by air conduction than by bone conduction, but less than twice as long, the affected ear may have a sensorineural hearing loss.

ASSESSING THE NOSE AND SINUSES

What is the most common cause of a nasal obstruction in children? What does nasal flaring indicate? What signs indicate that a foreign body might be lodged in the nose?

Inspection of the External Nose

The external nose characteristics and placement on the face are examined simultaneously with the facial features. Inspect the external nose for size, shape, symmetry, midline placement on the face, and any unusual characteristics. For example, a crease across the nose between the cartilage and bone is often caused by the allergic child's wiping an itchy nose upward with a hand. **Nasal flaring,** widening of the nares with breathing, is a sign of respiratory distress and should not be present.

The nose should be proportional in size to other facial features and positioned in the middle of the face. A flattened nasal bridge is the expected finding in Asian and Black children but may also be seen in children with Down syndrome. A saddle-shaped nose is associated with congenital defects such as cleft palate. The nasolabial folds are normally symmetric. Asymmetry of these folds may be associated with injury to the facial nerve (cranial nerve VII).

Palpation of the External Nose

When a deformity is noted, gently palpate the nose to detect any pain or break in contour. No tenderness or masses are expected. Pain and a contour deviation are usually the result of trauma.

Nasal Patency

The child's airway must be patent to ensure adequate oxygenation. To test for nasal patency, occlude one nostril and observe the child's effort to breathe through the open nostril with the mouth closed. Repeat the procedure with the other nostril. Breathing should be noiseless and effortless.

If the child struggles to breathe, a nasal obstruction may be present. Young infants under 6 months of age will not automatically open the mouth to breathe when the nose is occluded, such as by mucus. Nasal obstruction may be caused by a foreign body, congenital defect, dry mucus, discharge, polyp, or trauma. Young children commonly place objects up their noses, and unilateral nasal flaring is a sign of such an obstruction.

Assessment of Smell

The olfactory nerve (cranial nerve I) is rarely tested in preschool children, but it can be tested in school-age children and adolescents. When testing smell, choose scents the child will easily recognize such as orange, chocolate, peanut butter, and mint. When the child's eyes are closed, occlude one nostril and hold the scent under the nose. Ask the child to take a deep sniff and identify the scent. Alternate odors between the nares. The child can normally identify common scents.

Inspection of the Internal Nose

Inspect the internal nose for color of the mucous membranes and the presence of any discharge, swelling, lesions, or other abnormalities. Use a bright light, such as an otoscope light or penlight. For infants and young children, push the tip of the nose upward and shine the light at the end of the nose (Figure 7–23 ■). The nasal speculum for the otoscope can be used in older children. Avoid touching the septum of the nose with the speculum to prevent injury.

Mucous Membranes

The mucous membranes should be dark pink and glistening. A film of clear discharge may be present. Turbinates, if visible, should be the same color as the mucous membranes and have a firm consistency. When the turbinates are pale or bluish gray, the child may have allergies. A *polyp*, a rounded mass projecting from the turbinate, is also associated with allergies.

Nasal Septum

Inspect the nasal septum for alignment, perforations, bleeding, or crusting. The septum should be straight. Crusting will be noted over the site of a nosebleed.

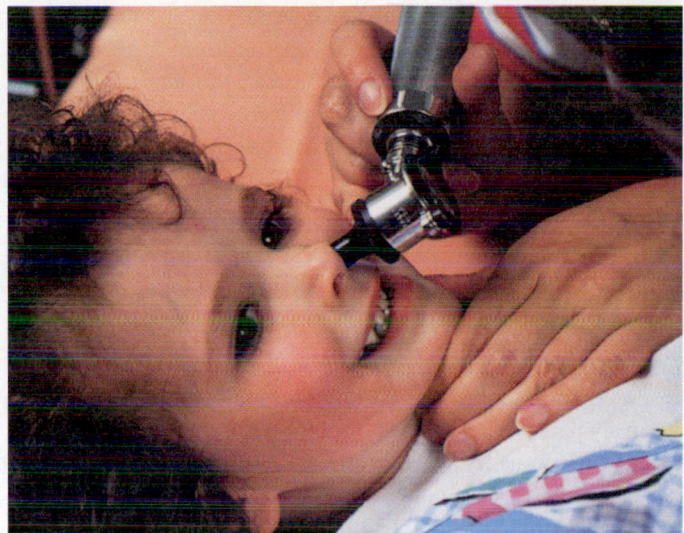

FIGURE 7–23 ■ Technique for examining the nose of a child.

TABLE 7–7	Nasal Discharge Characteristics and Associated Conditions	
DISCHARGE DESCRIPTION	**ASSOCIATED CONDITIONS**
Watery	
Clear, bilateral	Allergy
Serous, unilateral	Spinal fluid from fracture of cribriform plate
Mucoid or purulent	
Bilateral	Upper respiratory infection
Unilateral	Foreign body
Bloody	Nosebleed, trauma

Discharge

Observe for the presence of nasal discharge, noting if the drainage is from one or both nares. Nasal discharge is not a normal finding unless the child is crying. Discharge may be watery, mucoid, purulent, or bloody. A foul-smelling discharge in only one nostril is often associated with a foreign body. Table 7–7 lists conditions associated with nasal discharge.

Inspection of the Sinuses

The maxillary and ethmoid sinuses are present at birth, and all sinuses are fully developed by adolescence (Brook, 2007) (Figure 7–24 ■). Sinus infections can occasionally occur in young children. Suspect a sinus problem when the child has a headache or pain and swelling around one or both eyes.

Inspect the face for any puffiness around one or both eyes; normally neither is present. To palpate over the maxillary sinuses, press up under both zygomatic arches with the thumbs. To palpate the ethmoid sinuses, press against the bone above both eyes with the thumbs. No swelling or tenderness is expected. Tenderness may be an indication of sinusitis.

ASSESSING THE MOUTH AND THROAT

What is the best site to evaluate cyanosis in children? What is the expected sequence of tooth eruption? How is it determined that the tongue has adequate movement for all speech sounds? How can the throat be inspected without causing the child to gag?

Inspection of the Mouth

Young children often need coaxing and simple explanations before they will cooperate with the mouth and throat examination. Most children readily show their teeth. If the child resists by clenching the teeth, the teeth can be gently separated with a tongue blade. Equipment needed for examination of the mouth includes a tongue blade and penlight. Wear gloves when examining the mouth because of contact with mucous membranes. See Figure 7–25 ■ for structures of the mouth.

Practice Alert

Avoid examining the mouth if there are signs of respiratory distress, high fever, drooling, and intense apprehension. These may be signs of epiglottitis. Inspecting the mouth may trigger a total airway obstruction. See Chapter 25 🔗 for more information.

Lips

Inspect the lips for color, shape, symmetry, moisture, and lesions. The lips are normally symmetric without drying, cracking, or other lesions. Lip color is normally pink in White children and more bluish in children with darker skin. Pale, cyanotic, or cherry red lips are indicators of poor tissue perfusion caused by various conditions, such as anemia, respiratory distress, and carbon monoxide poisoning. Note any clefts or edema.

Teeth

Inspect and count the child's teeth. The timing of tooth eruption is often genetically determined, but it

As They Grow Sinus Development

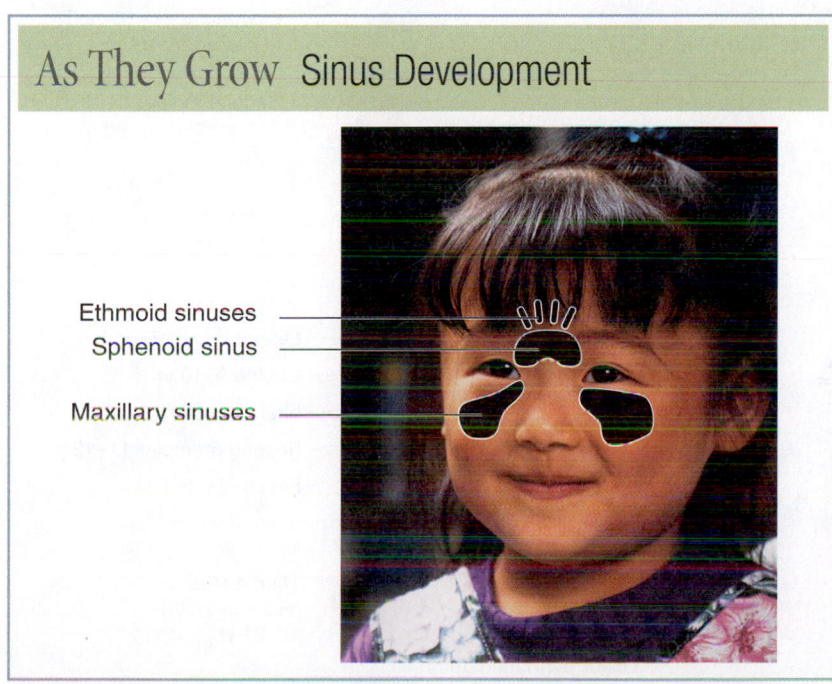

Ethmoid sinuses
Sphenoid sinus
Maxillary sinuses

FIGURE 7–24 ■ The ethmoid and maxillary sinuses form during gestation and are fully formed at birth. Sphenoid sinuses begin developing by 3 years and are fully formed by 7 to 8 years of age. The frontal sinuses form from 5 to 8 years of age but are not complete until adolescence (Taylor, 2006).

Animation Mouth and Throat Examination

Hard palate
Soft palate
Palatoglossal arch
Palatopharyngeal arch
Palatine tonsil
Uvula
Tongue
Oropharynx

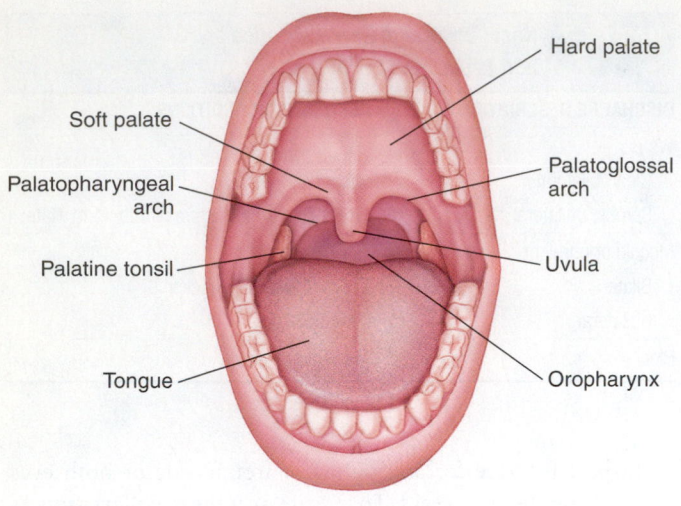

FIGURE 7–25 ■ The structures of the mouth.

involves a regular sequence. Figure 7–26 ■ presents the typical sequence of tooth eruption for both deciduous and permanent teeth.

Inspect the condition of the teeth, look for loose teeth, and note any spaces where teeth are missing. Compare empty tooth spaces with the child's developmental stage of tooth eruption. Once the permanent teeth have erupted, none should be missing. Teeth are normally white, without a flattened, mottled, or pitted appearance. Discoloration on the crown of a tooth may indicate caries. Discoloration of the tooth surface may be associated with some medications and fluorosis. See Chapter 24. Dentin erosion may be associated with chronic vomiting with bulimia nervosa. See Chapter 19.

Mouth Odors

During inspection of the teeth, be alert to any abnormal odors that may indicate problems such as diabetic ketoacidosis, infection, or poor hygiene. In older children be alert for odors of alcohol that could indicate substance use.

Gums and Buccal Mucosa

Inspect the gums for color and adherence to the teeth. The gums are normally pink, with a stippled or dotted appearance. Use a tongue blade to help visualize the gums around the upper and lower molars. No raised or receding gum areas should be apparent around the teeth. When inflammation, swelling, or bleeding is observed, palpate the gums to detect tenderness. Inflammation and tenderness are associated with infection and poor nutrition. Hyperplasia may be associated with some medications, such as phenytoin.

Inspect the mucous membrane lining the cheeks for color and moisture. The mucous membrane is usually pink, but patches of hyperpigmentation are commonly seen in children with darker skin. The *Stensen duct*, the parotid gland opening, is opposite the upper second molar bilaterally. Normally pink, the duct opening becomes red when the child is infected with mumps. Small pink sucking pads

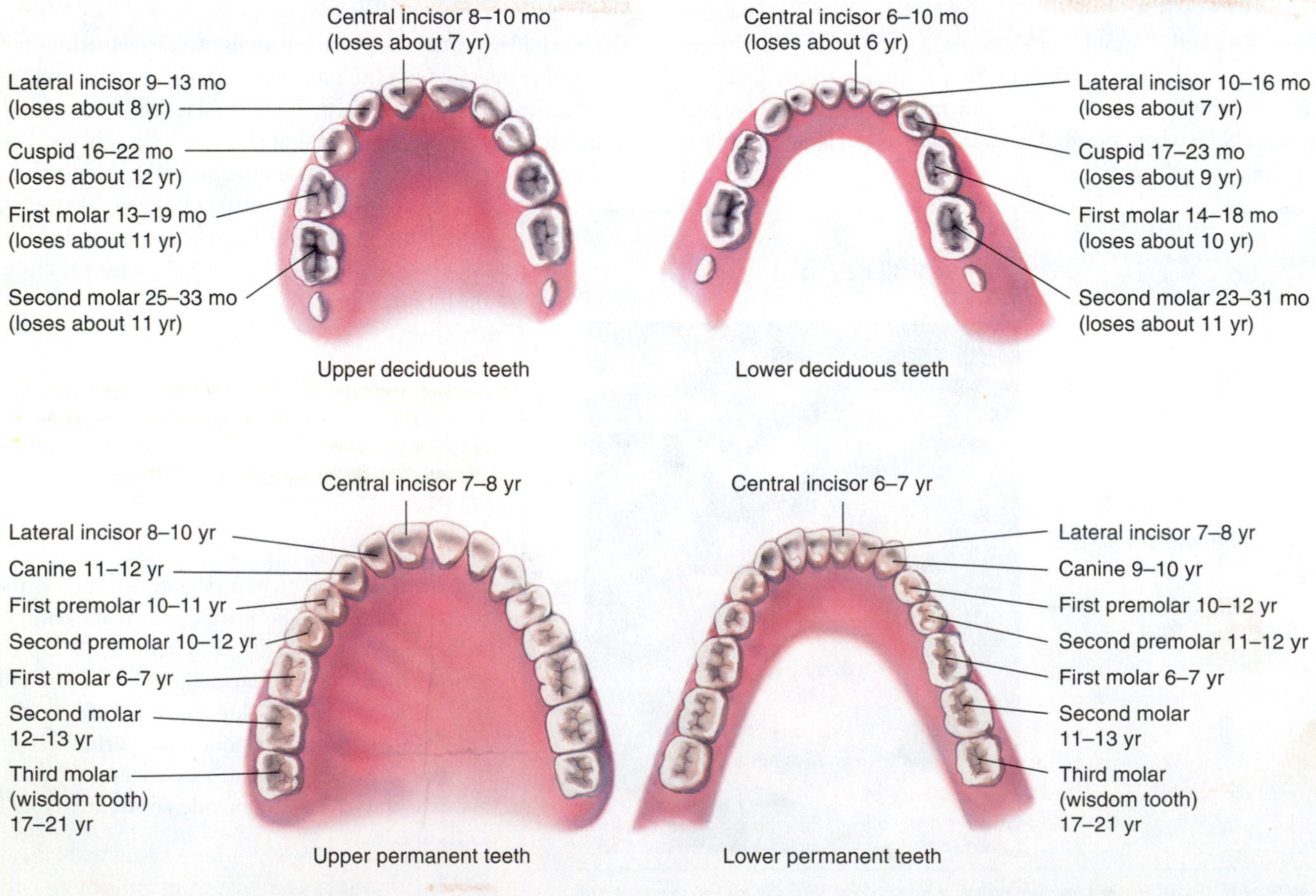

Central incisor 8–10 mo
(loses about 7 yr)
Lateral incisor 9–13 mo
(loses about 8 yr)
Cuspid 16–22 mo
(loses about 12 yr)
First molar 13–19 mo
(loses about 11 yr)
Second molar 25–33 mo
(loses about 11 yr)
Upper deciduous teeth
Central incisor 6–10 mo
(loses about 6 yr)
Lateral incisor 10–16 mo
(loses about 7 yr)
Cuspid 17–23 mo
(loses about 9 yr)
First molar 14–18 mo
(loses about 10 yr)
Second molar 23–31 mo
(loses about 11 yr)
Lower deciduous teeth
Central incisor 7–8 yr
Lateral incisor 8–10 yr
Canine 11–12 yr
First premolar 10–11 yr
Second premolar 10–12 yr
First molar 6–7 yr
Second molar
12–13 yr
Third molar
(wisdom tooth)
17–21 yr
Upper permanent teeth
Central incisor 6–7 yr
Lateral incisor 7–8 yr
Canine 9–10 yr
First premolar 10–12 yr
Second premolar 11–12 yr
First molar 6–7 yr
Second molar
11–13 yr
Third molar
(wisdom tooth)
17–21 yr
Lower permanent teeth

FIGURE 7–26 ■ Typical sequence of tooth eruption for both deciduous and permanent teeth. Notice that bottom teeth come in first for each kind of tooth: incisors, cuspids, and molars. They are lost in the same pattern.

can be present in infants. No areas of redness, swelling, or ulcerative lesions should be present.

Tongue

Inspect the tongue for color, moistness, size, tremors, and lesions, and inspect the floor of the mouth. The child's tongue is normally pink and moist, without a coating, and it fits easily into the mouth. A protuberant tongue is associated with various genetic conditions, such as Down syndrome. A pattern of gray, irregular borders that form a design (geographic tongue) is often normal, but it may be associated with fever, allergies, or drug reactions. Tremors are abnormal. A white adherent coating on an infant's tongue and extending to the buccal mucosa may be caused by thrush, a *Candida* infection.

Observe the mobility of the tongue to assess the frenulum. The child should be able to touch the gums above the upper teeth with the tongue. This tongue movement is adequate to enunciate all speech sounds clearly. Ask the child to stick out the tongue and lift it so the underside of the tongue and the floor of the mouth can be inspected for distended veins.

Palate

Inspect the hard and soft palate to detect any clefts, masses, or an unusually high arch. The palate is normally pink, with a dome-shaped arch and no cleft. The uvula hangs freely from the soft palate. Newborns often have Epstein pearls, white papules in the midline of the palate that disappear in a few weeks. A high-arched palate can be associated with sucking difficulties in young infants.

Palpation of the Mouth Structures

Using a gloved finger, palpate any masses seen in the mouth to determine their characteristics, such as size, shape, firmness, and tenderness. No masses should be found.

Assess the tongue's strength while simultaneously testing the hypoglossal nerve (cranial nerve XII). Place an index finger against the child's cheek and ask the child to push against your finger with the tongue. Normally, some pressure against the finger is felt.

The palate of an infant is palpated by inserting the gloved little finger, with the fingerpad upward, into the mouth. While the infant sucks against your finger, palpate the entire palate. This procedure also tests the strength of the sucking reflex, innervated by the hypoglossal nerve (cranial nerve XII). No clefts should be palpated.

Inspection of the Throat

Inspect the throat for color, swelling, lesions, and the condition of the tonsils. Ask the child to open the mouth wide and stick out the tongue. Use a flashlight to illuminate the throat. A tongue blade can be used, if needed, to visualize the posterior pharynx. Moistening the tongue blade may decrease the child's tendency to gag. The throat is normally pink without lesions, drainage, or swelling. The epiglottis lies behind the tongue and is normally pink like the rest of the buccal mucosa. Swelling or bulging in the posterior pharynx may be associated with a peritonsillar abscess (see Chapter 24 🕮). The gag reflex is not commonly tested in children (see Table 7–18).

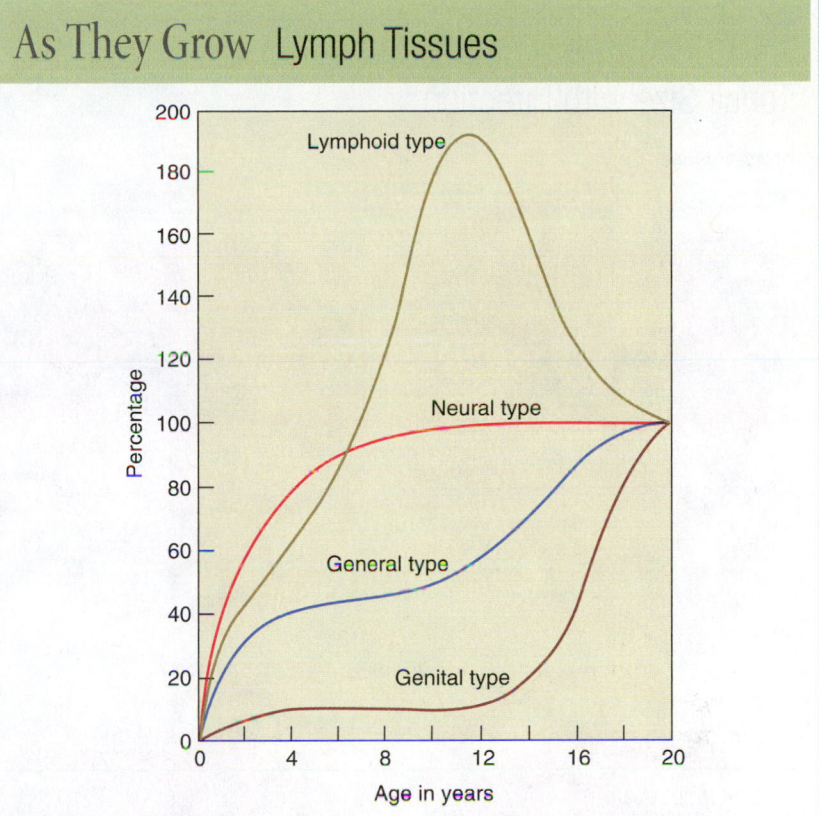

As They Grow Lymph Tissues

FIGURE 7–27 ■ The lymph tissues are well developed at birth and grow rapidly to reach adult dimensions by 6 years of age. They continue growing until 10 to 12 years when they reach their peak in size, and then decrease in size until adult size is achieved during late adolescence. Only the neurologic tissues grow faster than lymph tissue during early childhood. In contrast, the genital and other body organs reach their peak in development during adolescence.

During childhood the tonsils are large in proportion to the size of the pharynx because lymphoid tissue grows fastest in early childhood. See Figure 7–27 ■. The tonsils should be pink without exudate, but crypts (fissures) may be present as a result of prior infections. Significantly enlarged tonsils can cause respiratory distress. The size of tonsils can be graded as indicated in Figure 7–28 ■.

ASSESSING THE NECK

What does it mean when a child's head is tilted to one side? By what age should an infant be able to control his or her head? What does an enlarged lymph node feel like?

Inspection of the Neck

Inspect the neck for size, symmetry, swelling, and any abnormalities. A short neck with skinfolds is normal for infants. The neck is normally symmetric without swelling. Swelling may be caused by local infections such as mumps or a congenital defect. The neck lengthens between 3 and 4 years of age.

Inspect the child's neck for any webbing, an extra skinfold on each side of the neck. Webbing is commonly associated with Turner syndrome. See Chapter 32 🕮.

Infants develop head control by 2 months of age. By this age, an infant can lift the head up and look around when lying on the stomach. A lack of head control can result from neurologic injury, such as an anoxic episode.

Pathophysiology Illustrated
Tonsil Size with Infection

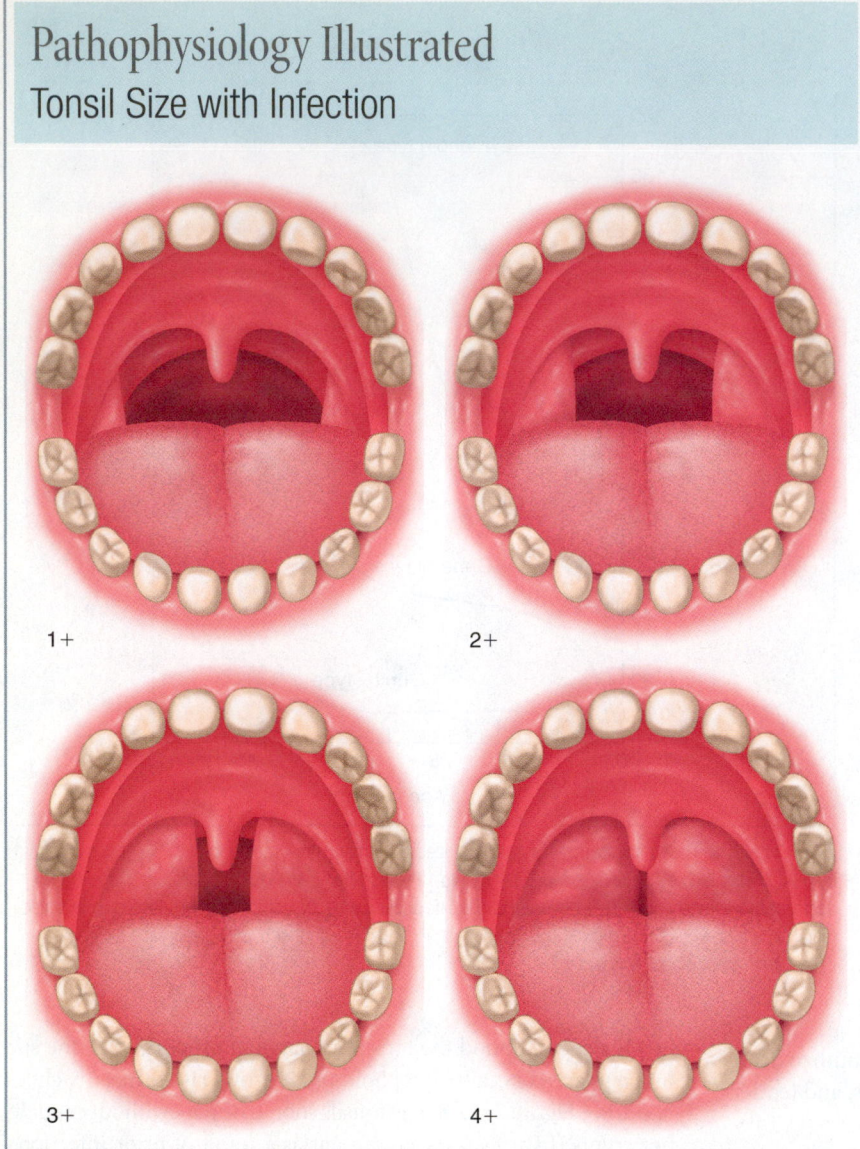

1+

2+

3+

4+

FIGURE 7–28 ■ Tonsil size can be graded from 1+ to 4+ in relation to how much of the airway is obstructed. Tonsil size of 1+ or 2+ is normal. Tonsil size of 3+ is common with infections such as strep throat. Tonsils that "kiss" or nearly touch each other (4+) significantly reduce the size of the airway.

Palpation of the Neck

Face the child and use the fingerpads to simultaneously palpate both sides of the neck for lymph nodes, as well as the trachea and thyroid.

Lymph Nodes

To palpate the lymph nodes, slide your fingertip pads gently over the lymph node chains in the head and neck. The sequence for lymph node palpation is as follows: around the ears, under the jaw, in the occipital area, and in the cervical chain of the neck (Figure 7–29 ■). Firm, clearly defined, nontender, movable lymph nodes up to 1 cm (1/2 in.) in diameter are common in young children. When a lymph node is palpated, a gentle circular motion helps define its characteristics. Enlarged, firm, warm, tender lymph nodes indicate the presence of local infection. Enlarged, nontender, nonmovable lymph nodes can be associated with lymphoma.

Trachea

To palpate the trachea, place your thumb and forefinger on each side of the trachea near the chin and slowly slide down the trachea to determine its position and the presence of any masses. The trachea is normally in the midline of the neck. It is difficult to palpate in children less than 3 years of age because of their short necks. Any shift to the right or left of midline may indicate a tumor or a collapsed lung.

Thyroid

As the fingers slide over the trachea in the lower neck, attempt to feel the isthmus of the thyroid, a band of glandular tissue crossing over the trachea. The lobes of the thyroid wrap behind the trachea and are normally covered by the sternocleidomastoid muscle. Because of the anatomic position of the thyroid, the lobes of the thyroid are not usually palpable in the child unless they are enlarged.

Range of Motion Assessment

To test the neck's range of motion, ask the child to touch the chin to each shoulder and to the chest and then to look at the ceiling. Move a light or toy in all four directions when assessing infants. Children should freely move the neck and head in all four directions without pain.

When the child is unable to move the head voluntarily in all directions, passively move the child's neck through the expected range of motion. Limited horizontal range of motion may be a sign of torticollis, persistent head tilting. Torticollis results from a birth injury to the sternocleidomastoid muscle or from unilateral vision or hearing impairment. Pain with flexion of the neck toward the chest (Brudzinski sign) may indicate meningitis. See Chapter 33 🔗.

ASSESSING THE CHEST

What terms are used to describe the location of specific sounds heard when auscultating the chest? What are retractions and what do they indicate? How can normal and adventitious breath sounds be distinguished when auscultating the lungs?

Examination of the anterior and posterior chest includes the following procedures: inspecting the size and shape of the chest, palpating chest movement that occurs during respiration, observing the effort of breathing, and auscultating breath sounds. A stethoscope is needed for the chest examination.

Topographic Landmarks of the Chest

The chest skeleton provides most of the landmarks used to describe the location of findings during examination of the chest, lungs, and heart. The intercostal spaces are the horizontal markers. The sternum and spine are the vertical landmarks. When both a horizontal and a vertical landmark are used, the location of findings can be precisely described (Figures 7–30 ■ and 7–31 ■). Be sure to indicate

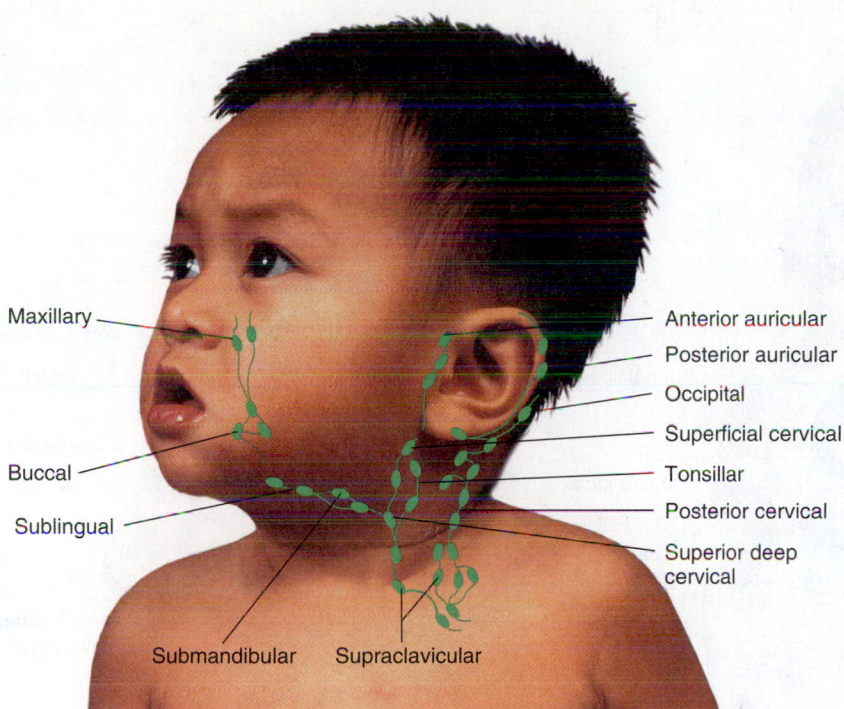

Maxillary

Buccal

Sublingual

Submandibular   Supraclavicular

Anterior auricular

Posterior auricular

Occipital

Superficial cervical

Tonsillar

Posterior cervical

Superior deep cervical

FIGURE 7–29 ■ The neck is palpated for enlarged lymph nodes around the ears, under the jaw, in the occipital area, and in the cervical chains of the neck.

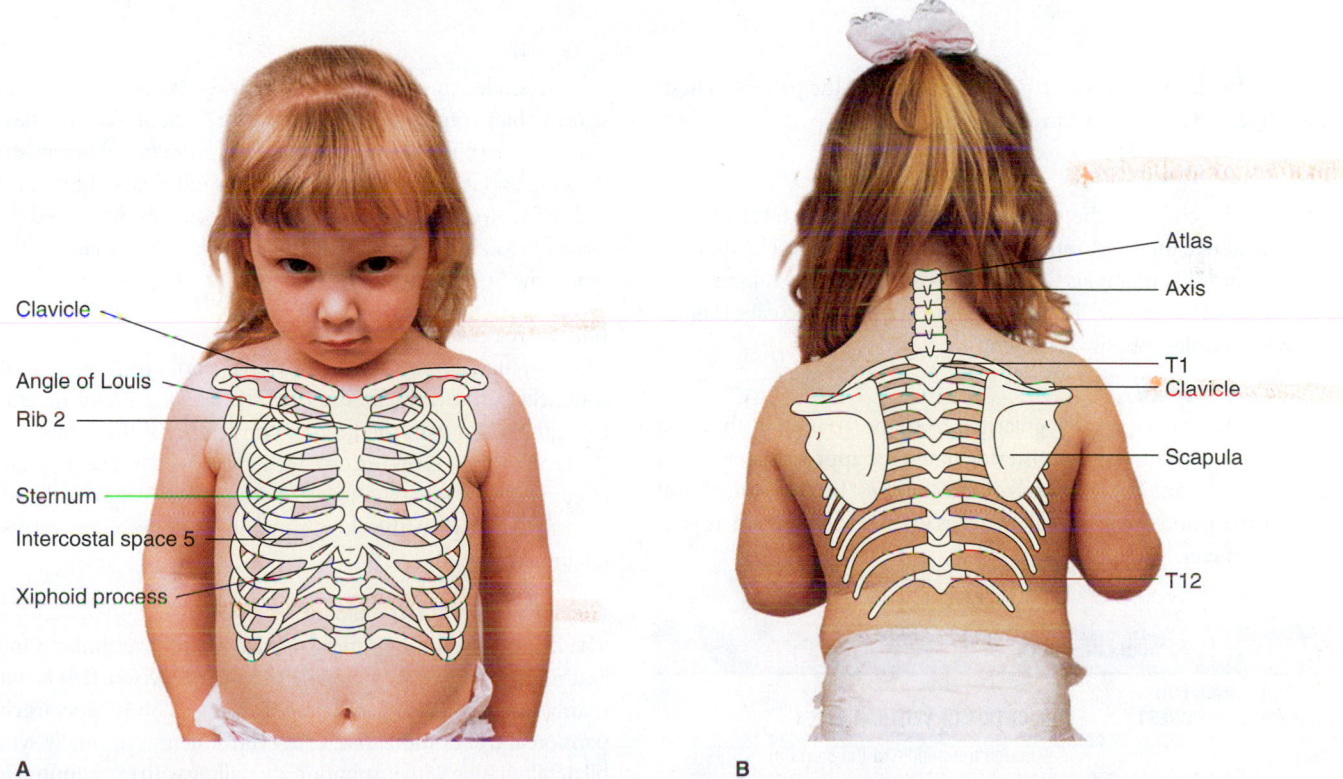

Clavicle

Angle of Louis

Rib 2

Sternum

Intercostal space 5

Xiphoid process

Atlas

Axis

T1

Clavicle

Scapula

T12

A

B

FIGURE 7–30 ■ Intercostal spaces and ribs are numbered to describe the location of findings. *A,* To determine the rib number on the anterior chest, palpate down from the top of the sternum until a horizontal ridge, the angle of Louis, is felt. Directly to the right and left of that ridge is the second rib, and the second intercostal space is immediately below it. Ribs 3 to 12 and the corresponding intercostal spaces can be counted as the fingers move toward the abdomen. *B,* To determine the rib number on the posterior chest, find the protruding spinal process of the seventh cervical vertebra at the shoulder level. The next spinal process belongs to the first thoracic vertebra, which attaches to the first rib.

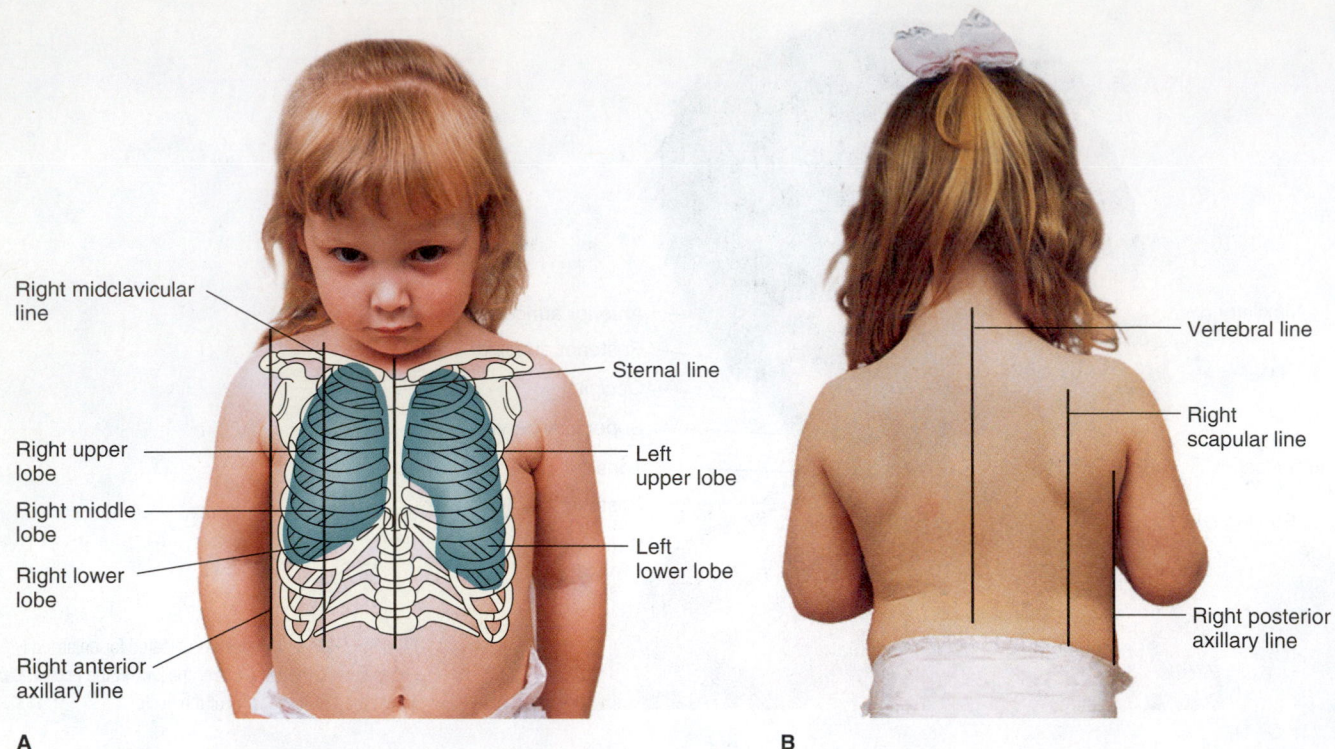

A

B

FIGURE 7–31 ■ The sternum and spine are the vertical landmarks used to describe the anatomic location of findings. The distance between the finding and the center of the sternum (sternal line) or the vertebral line can be measured with a ruler. Imaginary vertical lines, parallel to the sternal and vertebral lines, such as the midclavicular and scapular lines are used to further describe the location of the findings.

whether the finding is on the right or left side of the patient's chest. See Table 7–8 for vertical landmarks of the chest.

Inspection of the Chest

Position the child on the parent's lap or examining table with all clothing above the waist removed to inspect the chest. The thoracic muscles and subcutaneous tissue are less developed in children than in adults, so the chest wall is thinner. As a result, the rib cage is more prominent unless obesity is present.

Shape of the Chest

Inspect the chest for any irregularities in shape. In infants, the chest is rounded with the anteroposterior diameter approximately equal to the lateral diameter. By 2 years of age, the chest becomes more oval with growth, and the lateral diameter is greater than the anteroposterior diameter.

TABLE 7–8	Vertical Landmarks of the Chest
VERTICAL LINES FOR ASSESSING THE CHEST	**LOCATION OF VERTICAL LINES**
Sternal	Through the middle of the sternum
Midclavicular	From the middle of the clavicle
Anterior axillary	From the anterior axillary fold
Midaxillary	From the middle of the axilla
Posterior axillary	From the posterior axillary fold
Spinal	Through the spinous processes of the vertebrae
Scapular	Through the bottom angle of the scapula

If a rounded chest is found in a child over 2 years of age, a chronic obstructive lung condition such as asthma or cystic fibrosis may be present. An abnormal chest shape may also result from two different structural deformities (Figure 7–32 ■). Scoliosis, curvature of the spine, causes a lateral deviation of the chest (see Chapter 35 🔗). A shield-shaped chest, unusually broad with widely spaced nipples, may be associated with Turner syndrome. See Chapter 32 🔗.

Chest Circumference

Chest circumference may be measured until age 1 year, but it is not routinely performed. Chest circumference is a useful measurement for comparison with the head circumference if the growth of either the head or chest is of concern. See Figure 7–33 ■. The head and chest circumferences are expected to be approximately equal until after 1 year of age, when the chest circumference begins to surpass head circumference.

Chest Movement and Respiratory Effort

The diaphragm is the primary muscle used for respiration in infants and young children. As the thoracic muscles develop, they become primarily responsible for ventilation. Inspect for simultaneous chest expansion and abdominal rise. Chest movement is normally symmetric bilaterally, rising with inspiration and falling with expiration. The chest movement of infants and young children is less pronounced than the abdominal movement. Asymmetric chest rise is associated with a collapsed lung.

The thoracic muscles serve as accessory respiratory muscles in infants and young children. When the child has a condition, such as an airway obstruction, the accessory muscles are used for inspiration and retractions are seen. **Retractions,** visible depressions of tissue

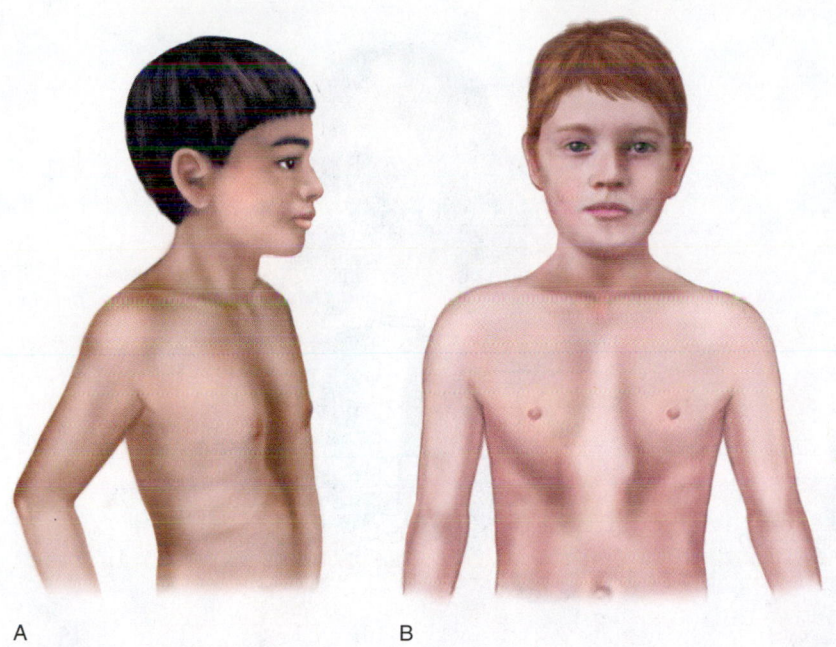

TABLE 7–9	Normal Respiratory Rate Ranges for Each Age Group
AGE	**RESPIRATORY RATE PER MINUTE**
Newborn	30–55
1 year	25–40
3 years	20–30
6 years	16–22
10 years	16–20
17 years	12–18

FIGURE 7–32 ■ Two types of abnormal chest shape. *A,* Pectus excavatum (funnel chest), the sternum protrudes, increasing the anteroposterior diameter. *B,* Pectus carinatum (pigeon chest), the lower portion of the sternum is depressed, decreasing the anteroposterior diameter.

Infants and children have a faster respiratory rate than adults because of their higher metabolic rate and resulting oxygen requirement. **Tachypnea,** an elevated respiratory rate, occurs in response to excitement, fear, respiratory distress, fever, and other conditions that increase oxygen needs. A sustained respiratory rate higher than normal for age is an important sign of respiratory distress. The child is at risk for developing hypoxemia if treatment is not started.

Palpation of the Chest

Palpation is used to evaluate chest movement, respiratory effort, deformities of the chest wall, and tactile fremitus.

Chest Wall

To palpate the chest motion with respiration, place your hands with thumbs together and fingers spread on each side of the child's chest. Confirm the bilateral symmetry of chest motion. Use your fingerpads to palpate any depressions, bulges, or unusual chest wall shape that might indicate abnormal findings such as tenderness, cysts, other growths, crepitus, or fractures. None should be found. **Crepitus,** a crinkly sensation palpated on the chest surface, is caused by air escaping into the subcutaneous tissues. It often indicates a serious injury to the upper or lower airway.

Tactile Fremitus

To palpate **tactile fremitus,** vibrations produced by crying and talking, place the palms of your hands on each side of the chest to evaluate the quality and distribution of these vibrations. Ask the child to repeat a series of words or numbers, such as Cinderella, Donald Duck, or ice cream flavors while you compare the quality of findings side to side over the anterior and posterior chest. The vibration or tingling sensation is normally palpated over the entire chest. Decreased sensations indicate that air is trapped in the lungs, as occurs with asthma. Increased sensations indicate lung consolidation, as occurs with pneumonia.

Auscultation of the Chest

Auscultate the chest with a stethoscope to assess the quality and characteristics of breath sounds, to identify abnormal breath sounds, and to evaluate vocal resonance. Use an infant or pediatric stethoscope when available to help you localize any unexpected breath sounds. Use the stethoscope diaphragm because it transmits the high-pitched breath sounds more clearly.

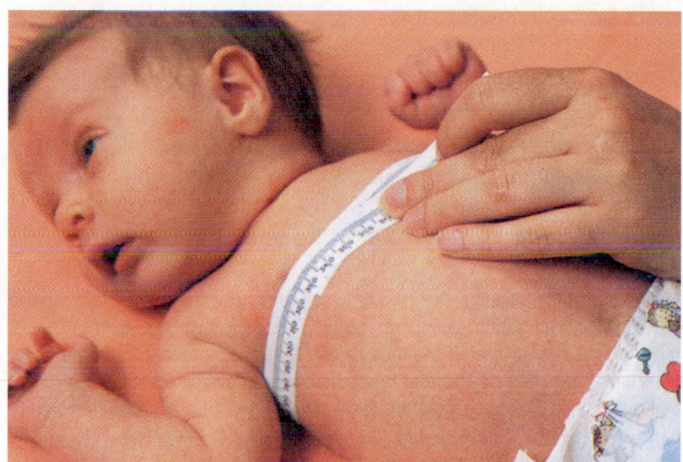

FIGURE 7–33 ■ Measuring chest circumference. Place a tape measure just under the axilla and at the nipple line and record the chest circumference to the nearest 0.5 cm or 1/4 inch.

between the ribs of the chest wall with each inspiration, indicate an increased work of breathing and often respiratory distress (see Figure 25–4 in Chapter 25 🔗).

Respiratory rate Because infants and young children use the diaphragm as the primary breathing muscle, observe or feel the rise and fall of the abdomen to count the respiratory rate in children under age 6 years. Table 7–9 gives the normal respiratory rates for each age group.

Clinical Tip

To get the most accurate reading of a newborn's and young infant's respiratory rate, wait until the baby is sleeping or quietly resting. Place your hand on the abdomen or auscultate the chest. Count the number of breaths for an entire minute because newborns and young infants may have irregular respirations.

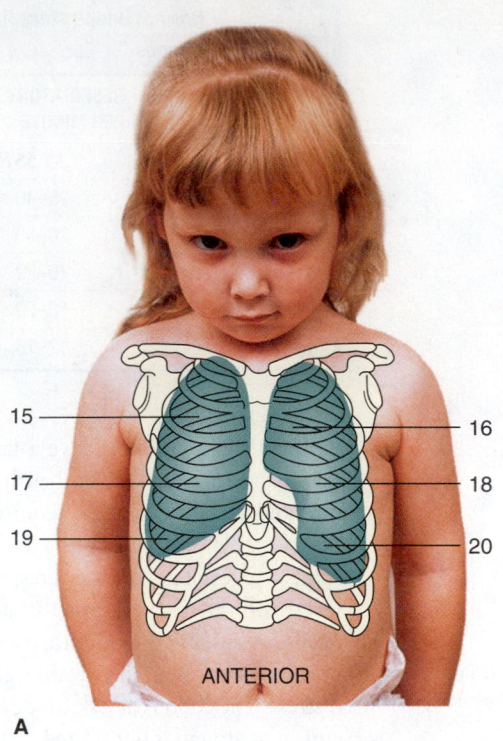

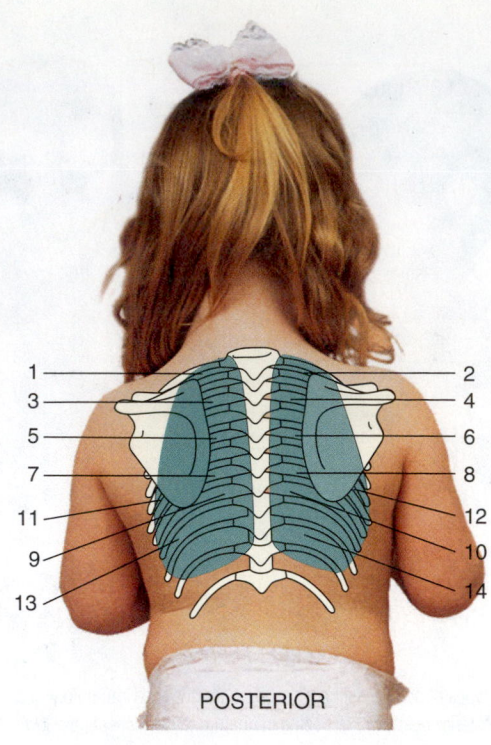

FIGURE 7–34 ■ One example of a sequence for auscultation of the chest.

Breath Sounds

Evaluate the quality and characteristics of breath sounds over the entire chest, comparing sounds between the sides. Select a routine sequence for auscultating the anterior and posterior chest so you will consistently assess all lobes of the lungs. See Figure 7–34 ■ for one suggested chest sequence. Listen to an entire inspiratory and expiratory phase at each site on the chest before moving to the next site.

Clinical Tip

Auscultation of breath sounds is difficult when an infant is crying. If the infant continues to cry after given a pacifier, bottle, or toy, all is not lost. At the end of each cry the infant takes a deep breath, which you can use to assess breath sounds, vocal resonance, and tactile fremitus.

Encourage toddlers and preschoolers to take slow, deep breaths by blowing a pinwheel or piece of tissue off your hand. This may enhance auscultation of subtle wheezes that occur at the end of expiration.

When encouraging the child to breathe normally while auscultating the chest, use suggestive language to increase cooperation: "You certainly are good at breathing slowly. Have you been practicing?" The child will often deepen and slow the breathing pattern as you praise the effort.

Three types of normal breath sounds are usually heard when the chest is auscultated:

1. *Vesicular breath sounds* are low-pitched, swishing, soft, short expiratory sounds. They are usually heard in older children but not in infants and young children.
2. *Bronchovesicular breath sounds* are medium-pitched, hollow, blowing sounds heard equally on inspiration and expiration in all age groups. The location of these sounds on the chest is related to the child's developmental status.
3. *Bronchial/tracheal breath sounds* are hollow and higher pitched than vesicular breath sounds.

Breath sounds normally have equal intensity, pitch, and rhythm bilaterally. Absent or diminished breath sounds generally indicate a partial or total obstruction, such as from a foreign body or mucus that does not permit airflow.

Practice Alert

Infants and young children have a thin chest wall because of immature muscle development. The breath sounds of one lung are heard over the entire chest. It takes practice to accurately identify absent or diminished breath sounds in infants and young children. Because the distance is greatest between the apices and midaxillary areas in young children, these sites are best for identifying absent or diminished breath sounds in a lung. Carefully auscultate, comparing the quality of breath sounds heard bilaterally.

Vocal Resonance

Auscultate the chest to evaluate how well voice sounds are transmitted. Have the child count or repeat a series of words, such as "apple," "banana," and "Cheerios." Use the stethoscope to auscultate the chest, comparing the quality of sounds from side to side and over the entire chest. Voice sounds, with words and syllables muffled and indistinct, are normally heard throughout the chest.

If voice sounds are absent or more muffled than usual, an airway obstruction such as asthma may be present. When a lung consolidation condition such as pneumonia is present, the vocal resonance quality changes in characteristic ways. These abnormal characteristics are:

- **Whispered pectoriloquy:** Syllables are heard distinctly in a whisper.
- **Bronchophony:** Sounds are increased in intensity and clarity while the words remain indistinct.
- **Egophony:** The "eee" sound is transmitted as a nasal "ay" sound.

TABLE 7–10 | **Description of Adventitious Sounds Heard When Auscultating the Chest**

TYPE	DESCRIPTION	CAUSE
Fine crackles	High-pitched, discrete, noncontinuous sound heard at end of inspiration; does not clear with coughing *(Rub pieces of hair together beside your ear to duplicate the sound.)*	Air passing through watery secretions in the smaller airways (alveoli and bronchioles)
Wheezing	Musical, squeaking, or hissing noise usually heard continuously during inspiration or expiration, but generally louder on expiration; does not clear with coughing	Air passing through mucus or fluids in a narrowed lower airway (bronchioles), as with asthma
Sonorous rhonchi	Coarse, low-pitched sound like a snore, heard during inspiration or expiration; may clear with coughing	Air passing through thick secretions that partially obstruct the larger bronchi and trachea

Abnormal Breath Sounds

Abnormal breath sounds, also called *adventitious sounds*, generally indicate the presence of a disease process. Examples of abnormal breath sounds are crackles, rhonchi, and **wheezing** (a noise resulting from the passage of air through mucus or fluids in a narrowed lower airway). To further assess abnormal breath sounds, identify the following:

- Location, for example, side of body and lung lobe(s)
- Presence during part or entire phase of inspiration or expiration
- Change in character or disappearance when the child coughs or shifts position

To routinely identify these adventitious sounds takes practice. Absent or diminished breath sounds may indicate a pneumothorax or airway obstruction. Table 7–10 describes adventitious sounds.

Abnormal Voice Sounds

Observing the quality of the voice and other audible sounds is also important during an examination of the lungs. These sounds include the following:

- **Stridor,** a high-pitched crowing sound often associated with croup, results from air moving through a narrowed trachea and larynx.
- A cough, the reflexive clearing of the airway, is associated with a respiratory infection.
- *Hoarseness,* a change in vocal quality, may be associated with inflammation of the larynx.

Percussion of the Chest

Percussion is a method sometimes used to assess the resonance of the lungs and the density of underlying organs, such as the heart and liver. Today, however, radiograph examination is used more commonly for these evaluations. Percussion of the lungs may be performed by an experienced examiner.

ASSESSING THE BREASTS

What does breast tissue feel like? Do boys have breast development during puberty?

Inspection

The nipples of prepubertal boys and girls are symmetrically located near the midclavicular line at the fourth to sixth ribs. The areola is normally round and more darkly pigmented than the surrounding skin. Inspect the anterior chest for other dark spots that may be **supernumerary nipples,** which are extra small, undeveloped nipples and areolae that may be mistaken for moles. Supernumerary nipples can occur anywhere along the mammary line, from the neck to the pubic area, but they are typically below a normal breast or on the abdomen. Their presence may be associated with congenital renal or cardiac anomalies.

See pages 201–203 for the assessment of pubertal development.

Palpation

Prepubertal boys and girls have no palpable breast tissue. The developing breasts of adolescent females are palpated for abnormal masses or hard nodules. While the adolescent is lying down with one arm behind the neck, palpate the breast and axilla on that side. Palpate in a concentric pattern or vertical strip pattern covering all areas of the breast including the axilla, areola, and nipple. Gently squeeze the nipple to assess for discharge. The fingers should move in small concentric circles in each position. Repeat the procedure on the opposite breast. Breast tissue normally feels dense, firm, and elastic. Any masses need further investigation, but are usually not malignancies. The physical examination is a good opportunity to teach adolescent females how to perform breast self-examination.

The majority of boys have unilateral or bilateral breast enlargement during adolescence (gynecomastia), generally most noticeable around 14 years of age. The breast tissue generally regresses by the time of full sexual maturity. Palpate the tissue to differentiate actual breast tissue from fatty tissue in the pectoral area, and to detect any masses.

ASSESSING THE HEART

What is the point of maximum intensity and where is it located? Where are the pulse points to assess pulse quality? What is the normal heart rate of infants and children? What is the difference between heart sounds and murmurs? Equipment needed for the heart examination includes a stethoscope and sphygmomanometer.

Inspection of the Precordium

Begin the heart examination by inspecting the *precordium*, or anterior chest. Place the child in a reclining or semi-Fowler position, either on the parent's lap or on the examining table. Inspect the shape and symmetry of the anterior chest from the front and side views. Bulging of the left side of the chest wall may indicate an enlarged heart. Observe for any chest movement associated with the heart's contraction. A **heave,** an obvious lifting of the chest wall during contraction, may indicate an enlarged heart.

Palpation of the Precordium

Place the entire palmar surface of your fingers together lightly on the chest wall to palpate the precordium. Systematically palpate the entire precordium to detect any pulsations, heaves, or vibrations.

Apical Impulse

The **apical impulse,** or point of maximum intensity, is the point at which the heart is closest to the anterior chest wall. The apical impulse is sometimes seen on the anterior chest wall of thin children, but it is normally felt as a slight tap against one fingertip. Use the topographic landmarks of the chest to describe its location (see Figures 7–30 and 7–31). See Figure 7–35 ■ to visualize the expected location of the apical impulse in infants and children. Any other sensation palpated is usually abnormal.

Abnormal Sensations

A *lift* is the sensation of the heart lifting up against the chest wall. It may be associated with an enlarged heart or a heart contracting with extra force. A *thrill* is a rushing vibration that feels like a cat's purr. It is caused by turbulent blood flow from a defective heart valve and a heart murmur. If present, the thrill is palpated in the right or left second intercostal space. To describe a thrill's location, use the topographic landmarks of the chest (see Figures 7–30 and 7–31) and estimate the diameter of the thrill palpated.

Percussion of the Heart Borders

Percussion of the heart borders is rarely performed during physical examination, as they are better identified by radiograph examination. Percussion of the heart may be performed by an experienced examiner.

Auscultation of the Heart

Auscultation is used to count the apical pulse, to assess the characteristics of the heart sounds, and to detect abnormal heart sounds. Use the bell of the stethoscope to detect lower pitched sounds.

To assess heart sounds completely, auscultate the heart with the child in both sitting and reclining positions. Differences in heart sounds caused by a change in the child's position or by a change in the position of the heart near the chest wall can then be detected. If differences in heart sounds are detected with a position change, then place the child in the left lateral recumbent position and auscultate again.

Heart Rate and Rhythm

The apical heart rate can be counted at the site of the apical impulse, either by palpation or by auscultation. Count the apical rate for 1 minute in infants and in children who have an irregular rhythm. The brachial or radial pulse rate should be the same as the auscultated apical heart rate. Table 7–11 gives normal heart rates in children of different ages.

Clinical Tip

The child's heart rate varies with age, decreasing as the child grows older. The heart rate also increases in response to exercise, excitement, anxiety, and fever. Such stresses increase the child's metabolic rate, creating a simultaneous need for more oxygen. Children respond to the need for more oxygen by increasing their heart rate, a response called sinus tachycardia.

Listen carefully to the heart rate rhythm. Children often have a normal cycle of irregular rhythm associated with respiration called *sinus arrhythmia*. With sinus arrhythmia, the child's heart rate is

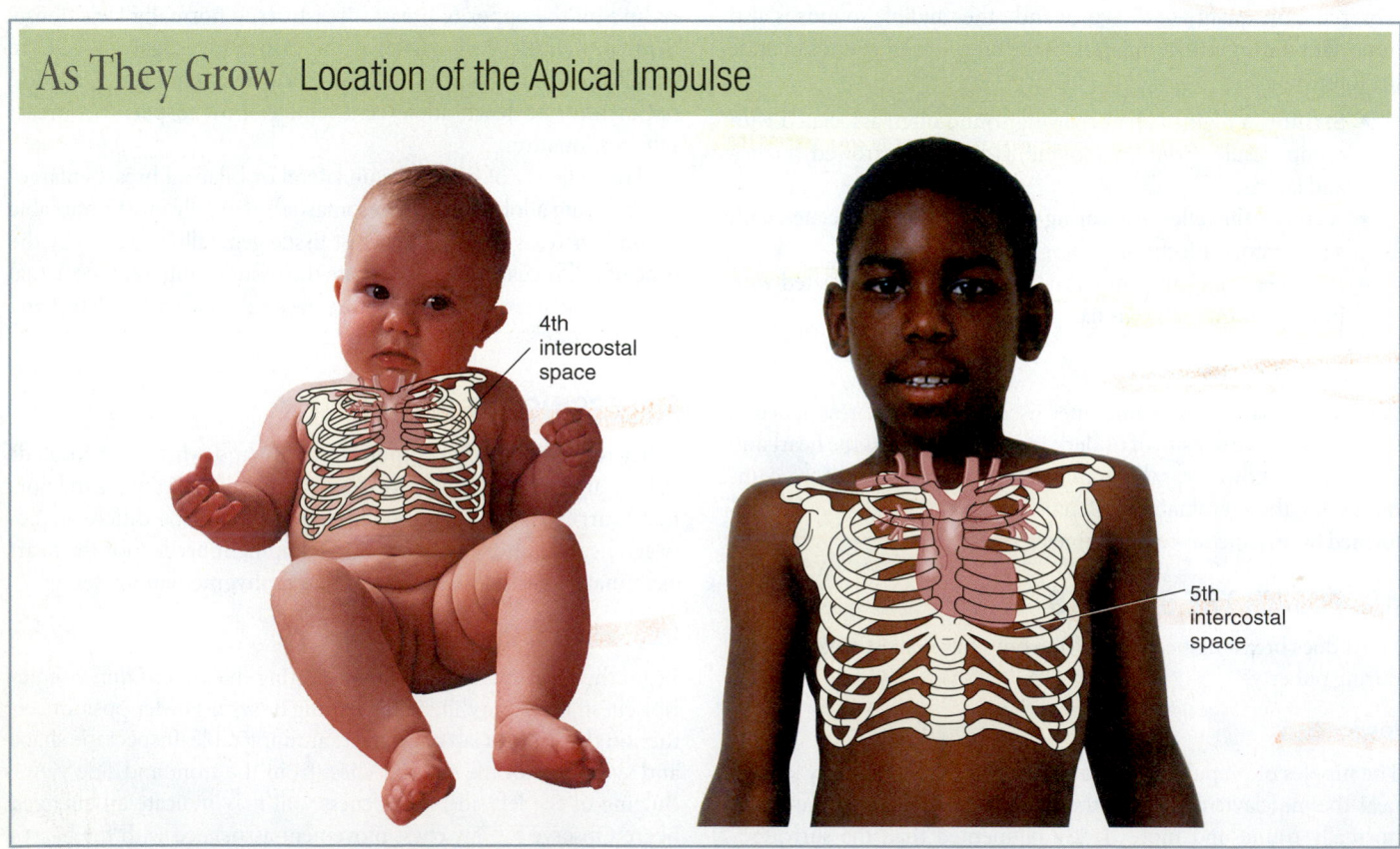

As They Grow Location of the Apical Impulse

4th intercostal space

5th intercostal space

FIGURE 7–35 ■ The location of the apical impulse changes as the child's rib cage grows. In children under 7 years, it is located in the fourth intercostal space just medial to the left midclavicular line. In children over 7 years, it is located in the fifth intercostal space at the left midclavicular line.

TABLE 7–11	Normal Heart Rates for Children of Different Ages	
AGE	**HEART RATE RANGE (BEATS/MINUTE)**	**AVERAGE HEART RATE (BEATS/MINUTE)**
Newborns	100–170	120
Infants to 2 years	80–130	110
2–6 years	70–120	100
6–10 years	70–110	90
10–16 years	60–100	85

faster on inspiration and slower on expiration. When any rhythm irregularity is detected, ask the child to take a breath and hold it while you listen to the heart rate. The rhythm should become regular during inspiration and expiration. Other rhythm irregularities are abnormal. See Chapter 26 ⊘.

Differentiation of Heart Sounds

Heart sounds are due to the closure of the valves and the vibration or turbulence of blood produced by that valve closure. Two primary sounds, S_1 and S_2, are heard when the chest is auscultated.

S_1, the first heart sound, is produced by closure of the tricuspid and mitral valves when the ventricular contraction begins. The two valves close almost simultaneously, so only one sound is normally auscultated.

S_2, the second heart sound, is produced by the closure of the aortic and pulmonic valves. Once blood has reached the pulmonic and aortic arteries, the valves close to prevent blood leakage to the ventricles during diastole. The closure of these valves varies with respirations. Sometimes S_2 is heard as a single sound and at other times as a split sound, that is, two sounds heard a fraction of a second apart.

Clinical Tip

To distinguish between S_1 and S_2 heart sounds in each listening area, palpate the carotid pulse when auscultating the heart. The heart sound heard simultaneously with the carotid pulsation is S_1.

Sound is easily transmitted in liquid, and it travels best in the direction of blood flow. Auscultate heart sounds at specific areas on the chest wall in the direction of blood flow, just beyond the valve (Figure 7–36 ■). The sounds produced by the heart valves or blood turbulence are heard throughout the chest in thin infants and children. Both S_1 and S_2 can be heard in all listening areas.

Auscultate heart sounds for quality (distinct versus muffled) and intensity (loud versus weak). Heart sounds are usually distinct and crisp in children because of their thin chest wall. Muffling or indistinct sounds may indicate a heart defect or congestive heart failure. Document the area where heart sounds are heard most clearly. Table 7–12 and Figure 7–36 review the location where each sound is normally heard most clearly for assessment of quality and intensity. In a child with a potential murmur, auscultate the heart sounds when the child is in the sitting, reclining, and left lateral recumbent positions.

Splitting of the Heart Sounds

After distinguishing the first and second heart sounds, try to detect *physiologic splitting*, the split second heart sound heard more often after a deep breath. More blood returns to the right ventricle, causing the pulmonic valve to close a fraction of a second later than the aortic valve. To detect physiologic splitting, auscultate over the pulmonic area while the child breathes normally and then while the child takes a deep breath. Splitting is normally more easily detected after a deep breath. The splitting returns to a single sound with regular breathing. If splitting does not vary with normal and deep inspiration, it is called *fixed splitting*, an abnormal finding associated with an atrial septal defect.

TABLE 7–12	Listening Sites for Heart Sound Auscultation	
HEART SOUND	**SITES WHERE BEST HEARD**	**SITES WHERE HEARD SOFTLY**
S_1	Apex of the heart	Base of the heart
	Tricuspid area	Aortic area
	Mitral area	Pulmonic area
S_2	Base of the heart	Apex of the heart
	Aortic area	Tricuspid area
	Pulmonic area	Mitral area
Physiologic splitting	Pulmonic area	
S_3	Mitral area	

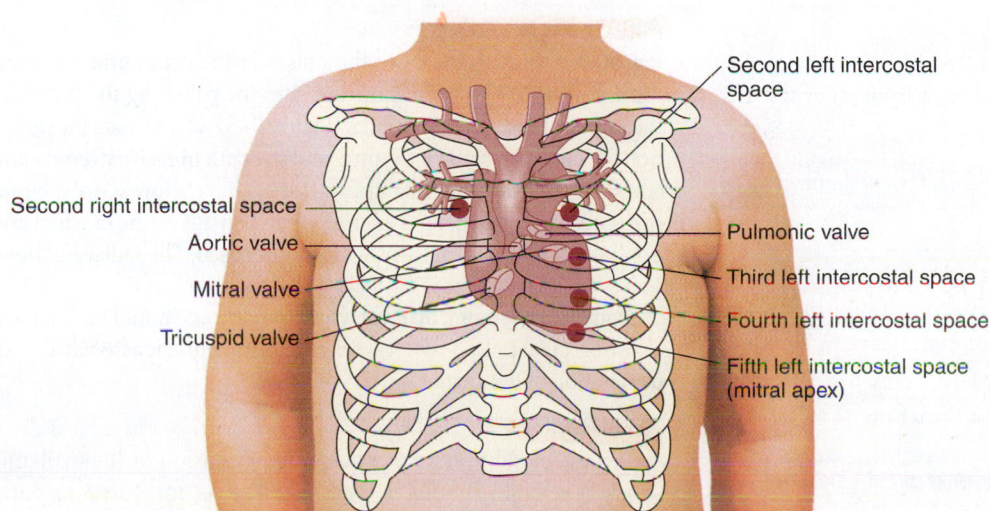

Second left intercostal space

Second right intercostal space
Aortic valve
Mitral valve
Tricuspid valve

Pulmonic valve
Third left intercostal space
Fourth left intercostal space
Fifth left intercostal space (mitral apex)

FIGURE 7–36 ■ Sound travels in the direction of blood flow. Listen for heart sounds caused by valve closure at specific areas on the chest wall away from the valve itself. These areas are named for the valve producing the sound.

- *Aortic:* Second right intercostal space near the sternum.
- *Pulmonic:* Second left intercostal space near the sternum.
- *Tricuspid:* Fifth right or left intercostal space near the sternum.
- *Mitral (apical):* In infants—third or fourth intercostal space, just left of the left midclavicular line; in children—fifth intercostal space at the left midclavicular line.

Third Heart Sound

A third heart sound, S_3, is occasionally heard in children and well-trained athletes as a normal finding. S_3 is a low-frequency sound that occurs when blood rushes through the mitral valve and splashes into the left ventricle. It is heard in diastole, just after S_2. It is distinguished from a split S_2 because it is louder in the mitral area than in the pulmonic area.

Murmurs

Occasionally abnormal heart sounds are auscultated. These sounds are produced by blood passing through a defective valve, great vessel, or other heart structure. Some murmurs are benign or innocent whereas others may indicate a congenital heart defect. Consult an experienced examiner to distinguish between murmurs.

It takes practice to hear murmurs in children. Often murmurs must be very loud to be detected. For softer murmurs, normal heart sounds must be distinguished before an extra sound is recognized. Once a murmur is detected, define the characteristics of the extra sound. Murmurs are classified by the following characteristics.

- **Intensity**—How loud is it? Can a thrill also be palpated? See Table 7–13 for grades of murmur intensity.
- **Location**—Where is the murmur the loudest? Identify the listening area and precise topographic landmarks. Is the child sitting or lying down? Do the characteristics of the child's murmur change when the child changes position?
- **Radiation or transmission**—Is the sound transmitted over a larger area of the chest, to the axilla, or to the back?
- **Timing**—Is the murmur heard best after S_1 or S_2? Is it heard during the entire phase between S_1 and S_2?
- **Quality**—What does the murmur sound like? For example, is it machinelike, musical, or blowing?

Venous Hum

A venous hum is a continuous low-pitched hum heard throughout the cardiac cycle caused by turbulent blood flow in the internal jugular veins. Auscultate for a venous hum over the supraclavicular fossa above the middle of the clavicle or over the upper anterior chest with the bell of the stethoscope. It is heard louder during diastole or when the child stands, and it does not change with respiration. A venous hum may be quieted when the child turns the neck or lies down, or when the jugular vein is occluded. A venous hum may be associated with anemia, but it has no pathologic significance.

Completing the Heart Examination

The complete heart assessment includes palpating the pulses, measuring blood pressure, and evaluating signs from other systems.

TABLE 7–13	Guidelines for Grading the Intensity of a Murmur
INTENSITY	**DESCRIPTION**
Grade I	Barely heard in a quiet room
Grade II	Quiet, but clearly heard
Grade III	Moderately loud, no thrill palpated
Grade IV	Louder, a thrill is usually palpated
Grade V	Very loud, heard when the stethoscope is barely on the chest wall, a thrill is easily palpated
Grade VI	Heard without the stethoscope in direct contact with the chest wall, a thrill is palpated

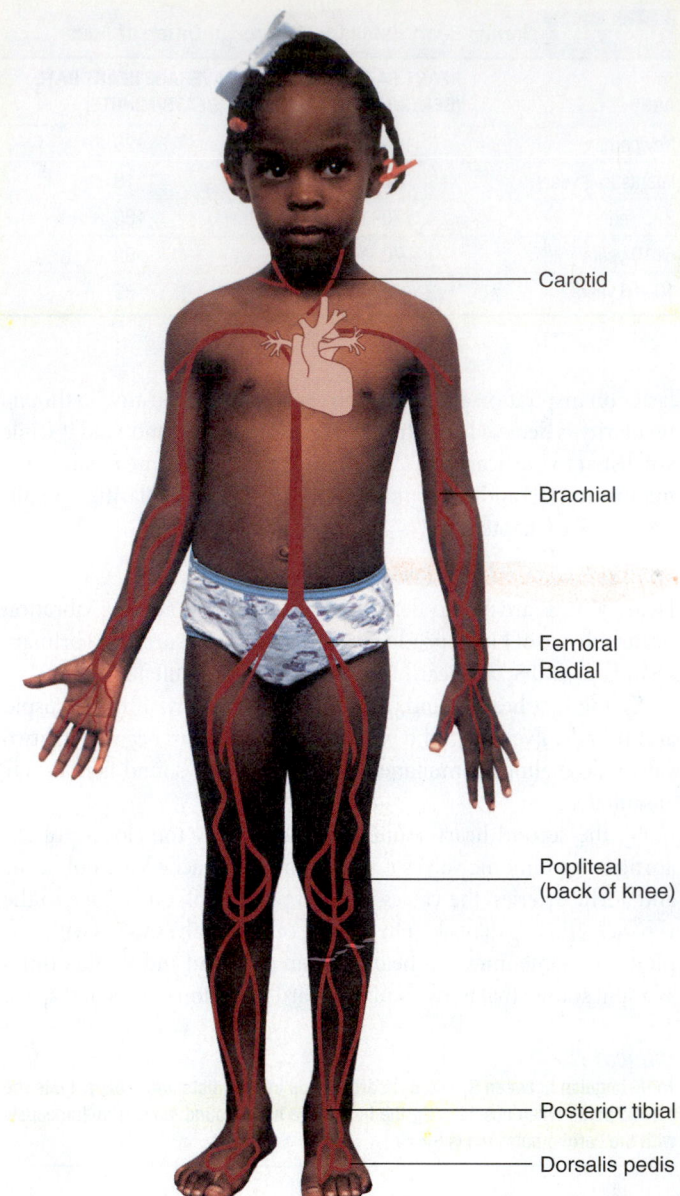

FIGURE 7–37 ■ The sites used to assess pulses in children.

Palpation of the Pulses

Palpate the characteristics of the pulses in the extremities to assess the circulation. The technique and sites for palpating the pulse are the same as those used for adults (Figure 7–37 ■). Evaluate the pulsation for rate, regularity of rhythm, and strength in each extremity and compare your findings bilaterally. Infants have a low systolic blood pressure, making distal pulses difficult to palpate, so the brachial and popliteal or femoral arteries are most often used. The radial and tibial pulses are palpated more easily in older children.

Palpate the femoral arteries whose pulsations should be as strong as the brachial pulsations. A weaker femoral pulse is associated with coarctation of the aorta.

Blood Pressure

Assess the blood pressure to detect hypertension or hypovolemic shock. The child should be seated and quiet for 3 to 5 minutes before blood pressure measurement. To obtain the most accurate

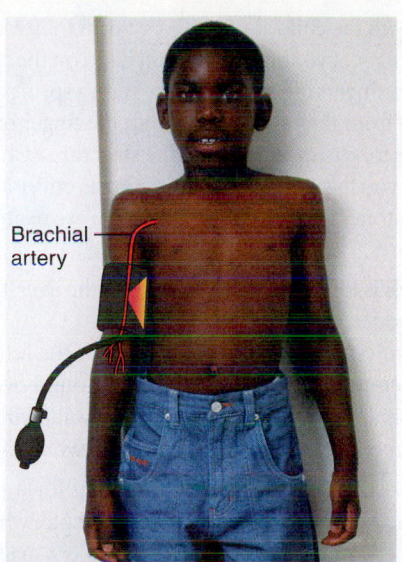

FIGURE 7–38 ■ Choose a cuff with a bladder width that is approximately 40% of the circumference of the upper arm or extremity used. When the cuff is wrapped around the upper arm, the bladder length usually covers 80% to 100% of the arm's circumference and 50% to 75% of the length of the arm (axilla to antecubital fossa).

reading, select an appropriately sized cuff for the extremity used (Figure 7–38 ■).

The recommended method of blood pressure determination is by auscultation. Use the right arm consistently as this arm is used for development of blood pressure standards. With the cuff snugly wrapped around the arm, hold the arm with the antecubital fossa at the level of the heart. See the Clinical Skills Manual ⬭ for the technique.

Use the bell of the stethoscope to hear softer Korotkoff sounds. The systolic reading is the onset of Korotkoff sounds. The diastolic reading is the fourth Korotkoff sound in children up to age 12 years, and the fifth Korotkoff sound in adolescents (Park, 2008, p. 19).

Measure the blood pressure twice and average the two readings. Compare the systolic and diastolic blood pressure reading with the table of age, gender, and height-percentile blood pressure values in Appendix B ⬭. A blood pressure value at the 50th percentile is considered the midpoint of the normal range. A reading at or above the 95th percentile indicates hypertension. To confirm hypertension repeat the readings on several visits.

Oscillometric devices are commonly used to measure a child's blood pressure. These devices measure the systolic blood pressure and the mean arterial blood pressure and calculate the diastolic blood pressure from these two values.

For any child in which there is a concern about a heart condition, obtain an additional blood pressure reading from both an arm and a leg when the child is supine or prone, and then compare the readings. The blood pressure in the leg should be the same or up to 10 mmHg higher than the arm reading (Park, 2008, p. 22). If the reading in the leg is lower than the arm, coarctation of the aorta may be present.

Other Signs

To assess the heart and tissue perfusion, assess other signs including skin color, respiratory distress, and capillary refill (see page 174). The mucous membranes are usually pink. Cyanosis is most commonly associated with a congenital heart defect in children. Signs of respiratory distress, such as tachypnea, nasal flaring, and retractions, may be associated with the child's attempts to compensate for hypoxemia caused by a congenital heart defect.

ASSESSING THE ABDOMEN

What does a sunken abdomen indicate? What do bowel sounds normally sound like? How frequently should bowel sounds be heard in children? What do the various percussion tones indicate? What does a rigid abdomen indicate?

Topographic Landmarks of the Abdomen

The location of underlying organs and structures of the abdomen must be visualized upon examination. The abdomen is commonly divided by imaginary lines into quadrants for the purpose of identifying underlying structures (Figure 7–39 ■). A stethoscope is needed to examine the abdomen.

Clinical Tip

Perform the inspection and auscultation before palpation and percussion, because touching the abdomen may change the characteristics of the bowel sounds.

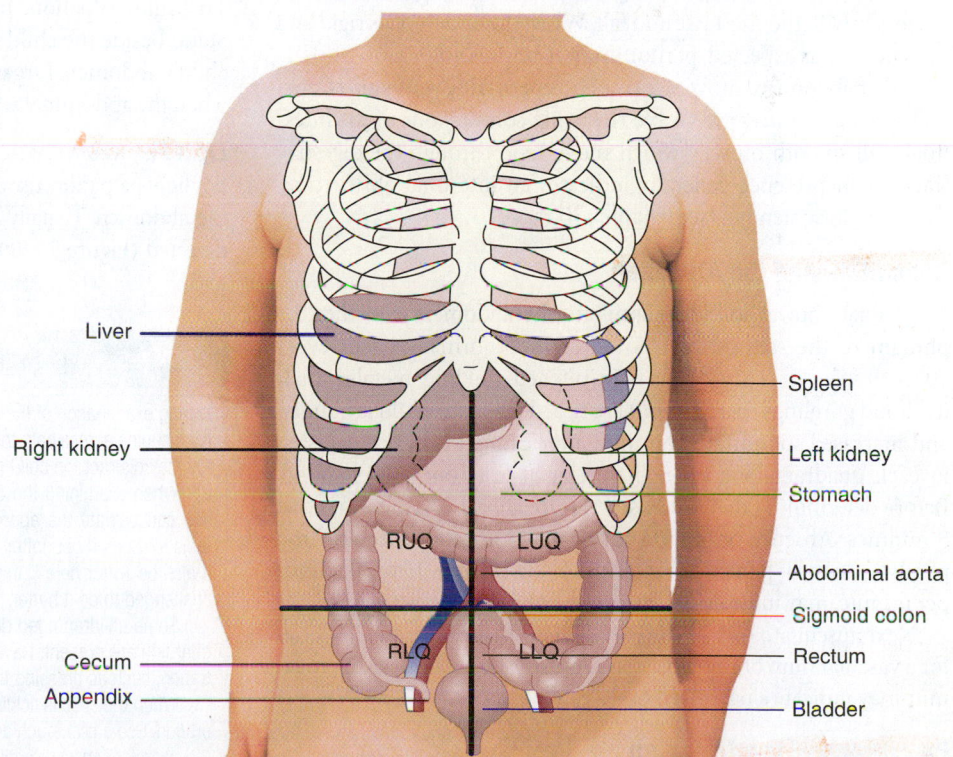

FIGURE 7–39 ■ Topographic landmarks of the abdomen. The abdomen is commonly divided by imaginary lines into quadrants for the purpose of identifying underlying structures.

Inspection of the Abdomen

Begin the examination of the abdomen by inspecting its shape and contour, condition of the umbilicus and rectus muscle, and abdominal movement. Inspect the child's abdomen from the front and side with good lighting. Note any creases, striae, or scars.

Shape

Inspect the shape of the abdomen to identify an abnormal contour. The child's abdomen is normally symmetric and rounded or flat when the child is supine. A scaphoid or sunken abdomen is abnormal and may indicate dehydration or a diaphragmatic hernia (see Chapter 30 🔗) in a newborn.

Umbilicus

The umbilical stump of a newborn normally falls off between 7 and 14 days after birth. After the stump falls off, inspect the umbilicus for complete healing. Continued drainage may indicate an infection or a granuloma. Inspect the umbilicus in infants and toddlers as these children may have an umbilical hernia, a protrusion of abdominal contents through an open umbilical muscle ring. See page 224 for the assessment of the newborn's umbilicus.

Rectus Muscle

Inspect the abdominal wall for any depression or bulging at midline above or below the umbilicus, indicating separation of the rectus abdominis muscles. The depression may be up to 5 cm (2 in.) wide. Measure the width of the separation to monitor change over time. As abdominal muscle strength develops, the separation usually becomes less prominent. However, the splitting may persist if congenital muscle weakness is present.

Abdominal Movement

Infants and children up to 6 years of age breathe with the diaphragm. The abdomen rises with inspiration and falls with expiration, simultaneously with the chest rise and fall. When the abdomen is rigid and does not rise as expected, peritonitis may be present.

Other abdominal movements such as peristaltic waves are abnormal. *Peristaltic waves* are visible rhythmic contractions of the intestinal wall smooth muscle, which move food through the digestive tract. Their presence generally indicates an intestinal obstruction, such as pyloric stenosis (see Chapter 30 🔗).

Auscultation of the Abdomen

To evaluate bowel sounds, auscultate the abdomen with the diaphragm of the stethoscope. Bowel sounds normally occur every 10 to 30 seconds. They have a high-pitched, tinkling, metallic quality. Loud gurglings (*borborygmi*) are heard when the child is hungry, and increased sounds are common after eating or drinking. Listen in each quadrant long enough to hear at least one bowel sound. Before determining that bowel sounds are absent, auscultate at least 5 minutes. Absence of bowel sounds may indicate peritonitis or a paralytic ileus. Hyperactive bowel sounds, as many as 15 to 30 sounds per minute, may indicate gastroenteritis or a bowel obstruction.

Next auscultate over the abdominal aorta and the renal arteries for a vascular hum or murmur. No murmur should be heard. A murmur may indicate a narrowed or defective artery.

Percussion of the Abdomen

Indirect percussion is often used by experienced examiners to evaluate borders and sizes of abdominal organs and masses. Percussion is performed with the child supine. To perform indirect percussion, lay the middle finger of your nondominant hand on the child's abdomen, keeping other fingers off the abdomen. With a spring-like motion, use the fingertip from the other hand to tap the finger on the abdomen. Listen for the tone to detect underlying structures. Choose a sequence that permits you to systematically percuss the entire abdomen.

Different tones heard during percussion are related to the underlying structures.

- *Dullness* is found over organs such as the liver, the spleen, and a full bladder.
- *Tympany* is found over the stomach or the intestines when an obstruction is present. It may also be found over areas beyond the stomach in infants because of air swallowing.
- *Resonance* may be heard over other areas.

Organ size can be identified by listening for a percussion tone change at the border of an organ. For example, when you percuss down the chest, the upper edge of the liver is usually detected by a tone change from resonant to dull near the fifth intercostal space at the right midclavicular line. The lower liver edge is usually detected 2 to 3 cm (about 1 in.) below the right costal margin in infants and toddlers, but closer to the costal margin in older children.

Palpation of the Abdomen

Both light and deep palpation are used to examine the abdomen's organs and to detect any masses. *Light palpation* is used to evaluate the tenseness of the abdomen (how soft or hard it is), the liver, the presence of any tenderness or masses, and any defects in the abdominal wall. *Deep palpation* is used to detect masses, define their shape and consistency, and identify tenderness in the abdomen.

To make the most accurate interpretation, perform the abdominal examination when the child is calm and cooperative (Box 7–5). To begin palpation, position the child supine with knees flexed. Stand beside the child and place your warmed fingertips across the child's abdomen. Organs and other masses are more easily palpated when the abdominal wall is relaxed.

Light Palpation

For light palpation, use a superficial, gentle touch that slightly depresses the abdomen. Usually the abdomen feels soft and no tenderness is detected (Figure 7–40 ■). Palpate any bulging along the abdominal

---

BOX 7–5	Growth & Development: Abdominal Examinations

During examination of the abdomen, infants and toddlers often feel more secure lying supine across both the parent's and the examiner's laps. A bottle, pacifier, or toy may distract the child and improve cooperation for the examination.

When examining the child, use suggestive words to help the child relax so you can palpate the abdomen. "How soft will your tummy get when my hand feels it? Does it get softer than this? Yes. See, it softens as you breathe out. Will it also be softer here?" In this way, the child learns to relax the abdomen and is challenged to do it better.

Some children need distraction, especially when abdominal tenderness and guarding are present. Have the child perform a task that requires some concentration, such as pressing the hands together or pulling locked hands apart.

When the child is ticklish, some special approaches are needed to gain cooperation. Use a firm touch and do not pretend to tickle the child at any point during the examination. Alternatively, put the child's hand on the abdomen and place your hand over the child's. Let your fingertips slide over to touch the abdomen. The child has a sense of being in control, and you may be able to palpate directly.

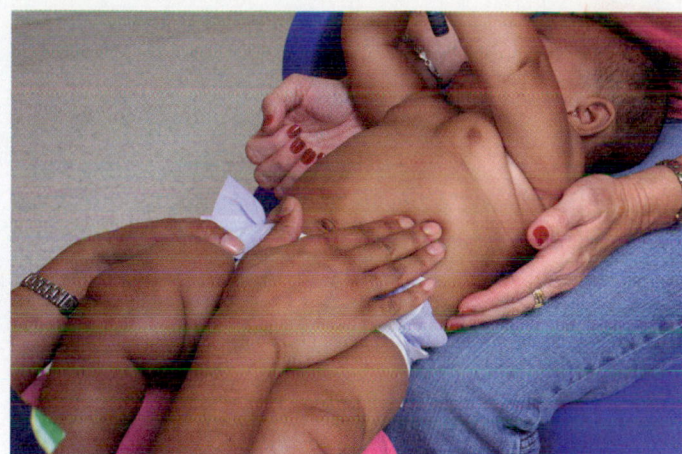

FIGURE 7–40 ■ To palpate the abdomen, use the edge of your fingers, not just your fingerpads, and palpate in a sequence to examine the entire abdomen. Watch the child's face as you palpate for a grimace or constriction of the pupils, which indicates the presence of pain.

Source: *George Dodson.*

wall, especially along the rectus muscle and umbilical ring, which could indicate the presence of a hernia. Measure the diameter of the umbilical muscle ring, rather than the protrusion, to monitor change over time; it normally becomes smaller and closes by 4 years of age.

Locate and lightly palpate the lower liver edge. Place the fingers in the right midclavicular line at the level of the umbilicus and gently move them toward the costal margin during expiration. As the liver edge descends with inspiration, a flat, narrow ridge is usually felt. Measure the distance of the liver edge from the right costal margin at the right midclavicular line. The liver edge is normally palpated 2 to 3 cm (approximately 1 in.) below the right costal margin in infants and toddlers. It may not be palpable in older children. The liver is enlarged when the edge is more than 3 cm (1.25 in.) below the right costal margin. An enlarged liver may be associated with congestive heart failure or hepatic disease.

Deep Palpation

To perform deep palpation, press the fingers of one hand (for small children) or two hands (for older children) more deeply into the abdomen. Because the abdominal muscles are most relaxed when the child takes a deep breath, ask the child to take regular deep breaths when each area of the abdomen is palpated.

The spleen tip may be felt at the left costal margin in the midclavicular line when the child takes a deep breath. The spleen is enlarged when it can be easily palpated below the left costal margin. The kidneys are in a deep layer of abdominal muscles and intestines, and they are rarely palpated except in newborns. If a kidney is actually palpated, an abnormal mass may be present.

Practice Alert

If an enlarged kidney or mass is detected during abdominal palpation, do not continue to palpate the kidney. Notify the primary care provider immediately. The mass could be a Wilms tumor.

Other Masses

Occasionally other masses, both normal and abnormal, can be palpated in the abdomen. A tubular mass commonly palpated in the lower left or right quadrant is often an intestine filled with feces. A distended bladder is often palpated as a firm, central, dome-shaped mass above the symphysis pubis in young children. Any fixed mass that moves laterally, pulsates, or is located along the vertebral column may be a neoplasm.

Assessment of the Inguinal Area

The inguinal area is inspected and palpated during the abdominal examination to detect enlarged lymph nodes or masses. The femoral pulse, a part of the heart examination, may be assessed simultaneously with this examination.

Inspection

Inspect the inguinal area for any change in contour, comparing sides. A small bulging noted over the inguinal area in girls may be associated with a femoral hernia. A bulging in the inguinal area in boys may be associated with an inguinal hernia.

Palpation

Palpate the inguinal area for lymph nodes and other masses. Small lymph nodes, less than 1 cm (0.5 in.) in diameter, are often present in the inguinal area because of minor injuries on the legs. Any tenderness, heat, or inflammation in these palpated lymph nodes could be associated with a local infection.

ASSESSING THE GENITALIA AND PERINEUM

What can a vaginal discharge indicate in a preadolescent girl? Is swelling in a newborn's scrotum normal? Where is the proper location of the urethral meatus on the penis?

Nurses may perform an external genital examination or assist another healthcare provider. Gloves, lubricant, and a penlight are needed for the examination.

Preparation of Children for the Examination

Examination of the genitalia and perineal area can cause stress in children because they sense their privacy has been invaded. To make young children feel more secure, position them on the parent's lap with their legs spread apart. Children can also be positioned on the examining table with their knees flexed and the legs spread apart like a frog. In young children the genital and perineal examination is performed immediately after assessment of the abdomen. The genitals and perineum may be examined last in older children and adolescents.

Clinical Tip

Preschool-age children are often taught that strangers are not permitted to touch their "private parts." When a child this age actively resists examination of the genital area, ask the parent to tell the child that the nurse or doctor has permission to look at and touch these parts of the body. You may wish to reinforce the teaching by saying the nurse or doctor can look only when the parent is in the room.

Some children develop modesty during the preschool period. Briefly explain what you need to examine and why. Then calmly and efficiently examine the child.

Females

Inspection of the External Genitalia

The external genitalia of girls are inspected for color, size, and symmetry of the mons pubis, labia, urethra, and vaginal opening (Figure 7–41 ■). See page 224 for a description of the newborn's genitalia. Simultaneously look for any abnormal findings such as swelling, inflammation, masses, lacerations, or discharge.

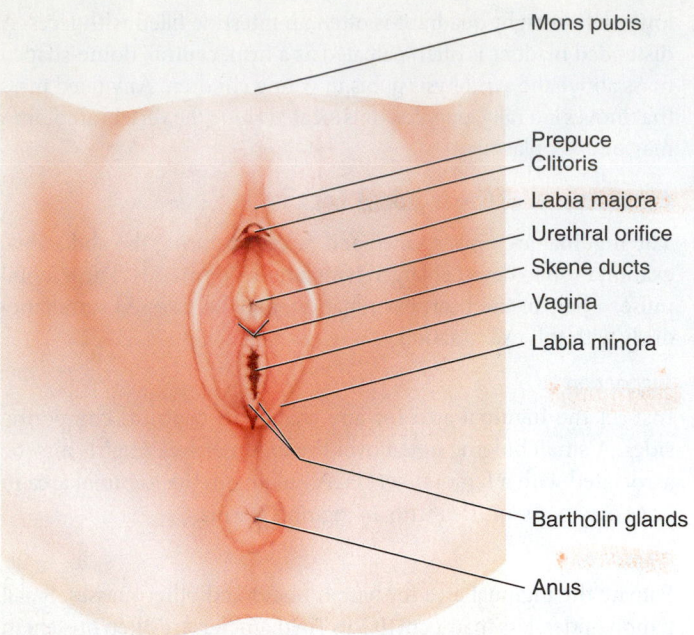

Mons pubis

Prepuce
Clitoris

Labia majora

Urethral orifice

Skene ducts

Vagina

Labia minora

Bartholin glands

Anus

FIGURE 7–41 ■ Anatomic structures of the female genital and perineal area.

Inspect the mons pubis for the presence of pubic hair and its characteristics. See pages 201–203 for guidelines to assess the stage of pubic hair development.

The labia minora are usually thin and pale in preadolescent girls but become dark pink and moist after puberty. In young infants, the labia minora may be fused and cover the structures in the vestibule. These adhesions may need to be separated.

Use the thumb and forefinger of one hand to separate the labia minora for viewing structures in the vestibule. The hymen is just inside the vaginal opening. In preadolescents it is usually a thin membrane with a crescent-shaped opening. The vaginal opening is usually about 1 cm (0.5 in.) in adolescents when the hymen is intact. Sexually active adolescents may have a vaginal opening with irregular edges.

Inspect the vestibule for lesions. No lesions or signs of inflammation are expected around the urethral or vaginal opening. Redness and excoriation are often associated with an irritant such as bubble bath or pinworms.

Preadolescent girls do not normally have a vaginal discharge. Adolescents often have a clear discharge without a foul odor. Menses generally begin approximately 2 years after breast bud development. A foul-smelling discharge in preschool-age children may be associated with a foreign body. Various organisms may cause a vaginal infection in older children.

Practice Alert

Signs of sexual abuse in young children include bruising or swelling of the vulva, foul-smelling vaginal discharge, enlarged opening of the vagina, and a rash or lesions in the perineal area. See Chapter 20 ⊘.

An internal vaginal examination is indicated when abnormal findings such as a vaginal discharge or trauma to the external structures are noted. Only an experienced examiner should perform the vaginal examination of the child. Refer to other assessment texts for guidelines in performing this examination.

Palpation

Palpate the vaginal opening with a finger of your free hand. The Bartholin and Skene glands are not usually palpable. If these glands are palpated in preadolescent children, this indicates enlargement because of an infection such as gonorrhea.

Males

Inspection of the External Genitalia

The male genitalia are inspected for the structural and pubertal development of the penis, scrotum, and testicles. Have boys sit with their legs crossed in front of them. This position puts pressure on the abdominal wall to push the testicles into the scrotum. Note the presence and characteristics of pubic hair. See pages 202–203 for guidelines to assess the staging of pubic hair and external genital development.

Penis Inspect the penis for size, foreskin, hygiene, and position of the urethral meatus. The length of the nonerect penis in the newborn is normally 2 to 3 cm (1 in.). The penis enlarges in length and breadth during childhood and at puberty. The penis is normally straight. A downward bowing of the penis may be caused by a *chordee*, a fibrous band of tissue associated with hypospadias. Note any bruising, swelling, or rashes.

When the penis is circumcised, the glans penis is exposed. The glans penis is normally clean and smooth without inflammation or ulceration. The urethral meatus is a slit-shaped opening near the tip of the glans. No discharge should be present. If the boy is not circumcised, a foreskin opening large enough for a good urinary stream is normal, even when the foreskin does not fully retract, a common finding in boys between 3 and 6 years of age. To inspect the glans penis of an uncircumcised boy, the foreskin is gently retracted by the child, parent, or examiner. Avoid forcible retraction of the foreskin to prevent damage to the tissues and the formation of adhesions between the foreskin and glans. Evaluate the degree of foreskin retraction and the meatal location and size. It is usually possible to visualize the meatus.

Location of the urethral meatus at another site on the penis is abnormal, indicating *hypospadias* (meatus is located on the ventral or undersurface of the penile shaft between the perineum and tip of the glans) or *epispadias* (meatus is located on the dorsal surface of the penile shaft). A round, pinpoint urethral meatus may indicate meatal stenosis. Phimosis is the presence of an abnormal ring of tissue distal to the glans that prevents retraction of the foreskin to allow visualization of the meatus. Erythema and edema of the glans (*balanitis*) may result from an infection or trauma.

Inspect the urinary stream. The stream is normally strong and straight without dribbling.

Scrotum Inspect the scrotum for size, symmetry, presence of the testicles, and any abnormalities. The scrotum is normally loose and pendulous with rugae, or wrinkles. The scrotum of infants often appears large in comparison to the penis. A small, undeveloped scrotum that has no rugae indicates that the testicles are undescended. Enlargement or swelling of the scrotum is abnormal and may indicate an inguinal hernia or hydrocele. To distinguish between a hydrocele and an incarcerated hernia, place a bright penlight under the scrotum and look for a red glow or transillumination through the scrotum. A hydrocele transilluminates; a hernia does not. In older children, scrotal enlargement may be associated with torsion of the spermatic

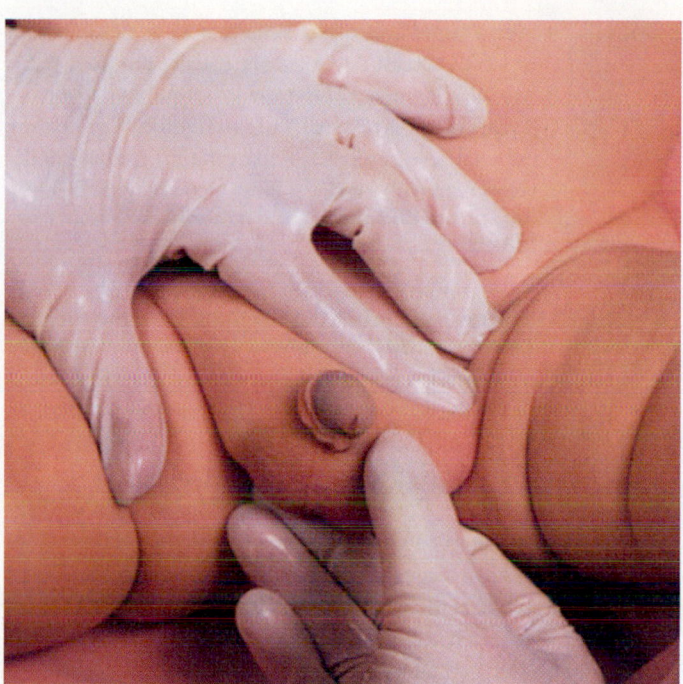

FIGURE 7–42 ■ Palpating the scrotum for descended testicles and spermatic cords.

cord or testicular inflammation. See Chapter 31 🔗. A deep cleft in the scrotum may indicate ambiguous genitalia.

Palpation

Make sure your hands are warm and have the boy sit with legs crossed to prevent stimulation of the cremasteric reflex that causes the testicles to retract.

Penis Palpate the shaft of the penis for nodules and masses. None should be present.

Testicles Palpate the scrotum for the presence of the testicles. Place your index finger and thumb over the inguinal canals located in the groin on each side of the penis. This keeps the testicles from retracting into the abdomen (Figure 7–42 ■).

Gently palpate each testicle with only enough pressure to identify the shape and size. The testicles are normally smooth and equal in size. They are approximately 1 to 1.5 cm (0.5 in.) in diameter until puberty, when they increase in size. A hard, enlarged, painless testicle may indicate a tumor.

If a testicle is not palpated in the scrotum, the examiner palpates the inguinal canal for a soft mass. When the testicle is found in the inguinal canal, an experienced examiner should try to move it to the scrotum to palpate the size and shape. The testicle is descendible when it can be moved into the scrotum. An undescended testicle is one that does not descend into the scrotum or cannot be palpated in the inguinal canal.

Scrotum Palpate the length of the spermatic cord between the thumb and forefinger from the testicle to the inguinal canal. It normally feels solid and smooth. No tenderness is expected.

When bulging or swelling of the scrotum is present, palpate the scrotum to identify the characteristics of the mass. Try to determine whether the mass is unilateral or bilateral. An experienced examiner may attempt to reduce the mass by pushing it back through the external inguinal ring. A mass that decreases may indicate an inguinal hernia. A mass that does not decrease may indicate a hydrocele or an incarcerated hernia.

Inspection of the Anus and Rectum

With the child in a supine or prone position, inspect the anus for sphincter control and any abnormal findings such as inflammation, fissures, or lesions. The external sphincter is usually closed. Inflammation and scratch marks around the anus may be associated with pinworms. A protrusion from the rectum may be associated with a rectal wall prolapse or a hemorrhoid.

Palpation of the Anus and Rectum

Lightly touching the anal opening should stimulate an anal contraction or "wink." Absence of a contraction may indicate the presence of a lower spinal cord lesion.

A rectal examination is not routinely performed on children. It is indicated for symptoms of intra-abdominal, rectal, bowel, or stool abnormalities. The rectal examination should be performed only by an experienced examiner. To reduce anxiety associated with this examination, distract the child with an age-appropriate toy or discussion when assisting with this procedure. Let the child know that the lubricant might feel cold. As the examiner's finger is positioned, help the child to relax the sphincter by telling the child to "push out the poop."

ASSESSMENT OF PUBERTAL DEVELOPMENT AND SEXUAL MATURATION

What is the first stage of breast development in girls? What is the first stage of pubertal development in boys? How is the stage of pubertal development determined in girls and boys?

The age of onset of secondary sexual characteristics can vary with race and ethnicity, environmental conditions, geographic location, and nutrition. For example, in the United States, Black females and males have an earlier onset of secondary sexual characteristics than White females and males (Susman, Houts, Steinberg, et al., 2010). A higher body mass index appears to contribute to earlier development of puberty in females, but not in males (Walvoord, 2010).

Females

Breast development in females usually precedes other pubertal changes. See Figure 7–43 ■ for Tanner stages of breast development. *Thelarche*, or breast budding, is the first stage of pubertal development in the majority of girls, indicating breast Tanner stage II. Breast tissue is seen and palpated below a slightly enlarging areola (1 cm in diameter of palpable glandular tissue) (Hermann-Giddens, Bourdony, Dowshen, et al., 2011). Although stage II breast budding normally occurs between 9 and 14 years of age, it begins as early as 7 years in some girls (Biro, Galvez, Greenspan, et al., 2010).

Inspect the adolescent's breasts while she is sitting to determine the stage of development. A girl's breasts may develop at different rates and appear asymmetric.

Next observe the development of pubic hair. Preadolescent girls have no pubic hair. Initial pubic hair is lightly pigmented, sparse, and straight, along the labia majora. Pubic hair develops in consistent stages for all girls. The hair then becomes coarse and curly and extends

As They Grow   Tanner Stages of Breast Development

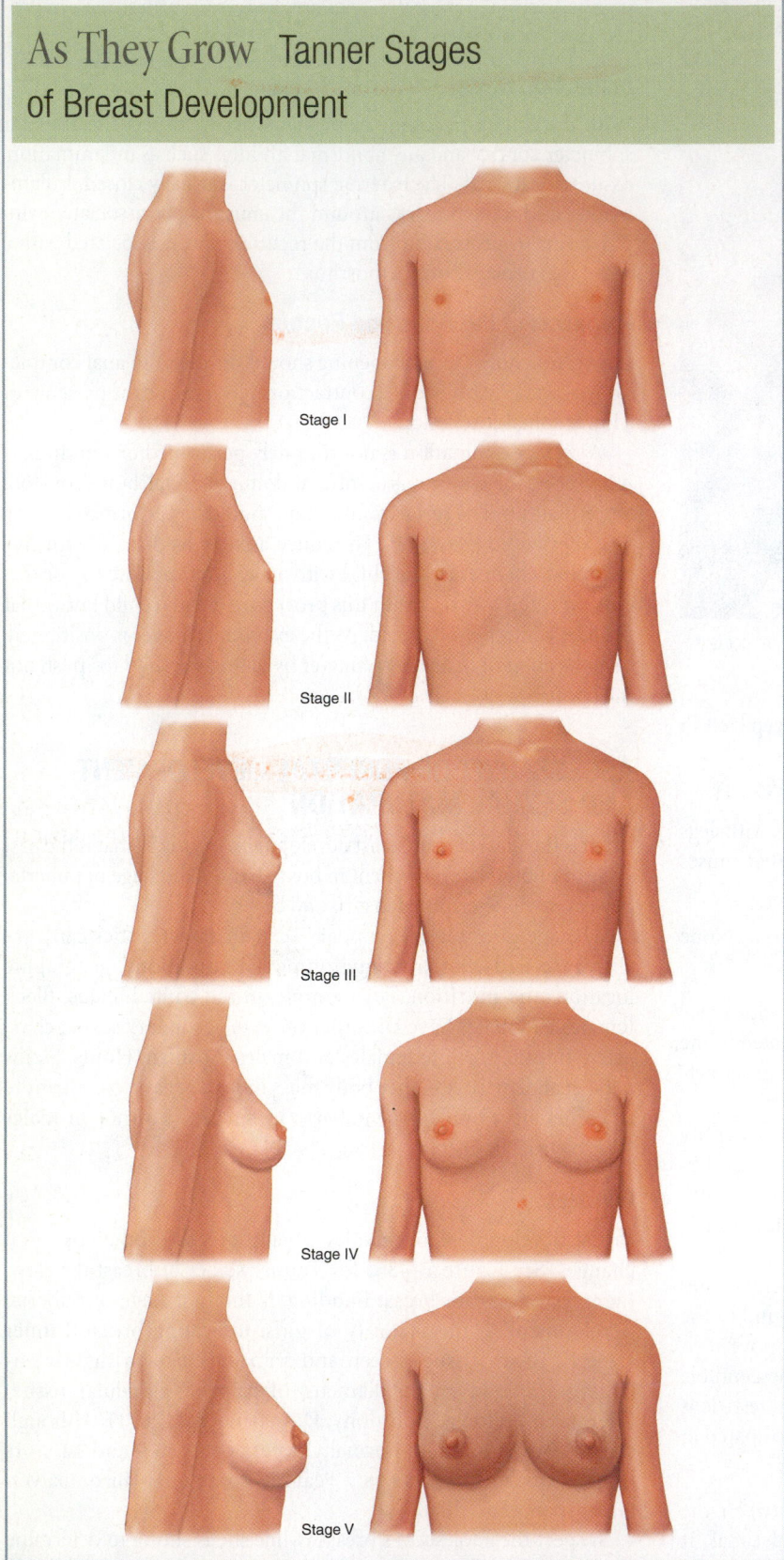

Stage I

Stage II

Stage III

Stage IV

Stage V

FIGURE 7–43 ■ Tanner stages of breast development. *I*, Preadolescent. Only the nipple is raised above the level of the breast, as in the child. *II*, Budding stage. Areola increased in diameter and surrounding area slightly elevated. *III*, Breast and areola enlarged. No contour separation. *IV*, Areola forms a secondary elevation above that of the breast in half of girls. *V*, Areola is usually part of the general breast contour and is strongly pigmented. Nipple usually projects.

over a larger area of the labia majora as development proceeds. Breast development usually precedes pubic hair development. The presence of pubic hair before 8 years of age is unusual and could indicate premature pubertal development. Compare the girl's pubic hair development with the stages illustrated in Figure 7–44 ■.

Males

Initial signs of pubertal development in males are enlargement of the testicles and thinning of the scrotum. This is followed by pubic hair development about 6 months later. Straight, downy pubic hair first develops at the base of the penis. The hair becomes darker, dense, and curly, extending over the pubic area in a diamond pattern by the completion of puberty. The presence of pubic hair before 9 years of age is uncommon and could indicate premature pubertal development. Delayed onset of testicular enlargement after 14 years of age needs evaluation. Penile enlargement generally follows testicular enlargement about 1 year later, genitalia Tanner stage III. Tanner stages of genital growth and pubic hair development follow a standard pattern, as illustrated in Figure 7–45 ■.

Sexual Maturity Rating

The **sexual maturity rating** (SMR) is an average of the breast and pubic hair Tanner stages in females and of the genital and pubic hair Tanner stages in boys. The rating is a number between 2 and 5, as stage 1 is prepubertal. The sexual maturity rating is then related to other physiologic events that happen during puberty. Compare the stage of the child's secondary sexual characteristics with information in Figure 7–46 ■ to identify the timing of other pubertal changes.

In females, menarche generally occurs in SMR 4 or breast stage III to IV. While the mean age of stage II breast development has lowered for females over time, the age at menarche has remained fairly constant, between 12 and 13 years (Walvoord, 2010). The peak height velocity usually occurs before menarche at a mean age of 11.5 years. Identifying the stage of pubertal development provides an opportunity to educate the girl about her body and when to anticipate menarche.

In males, ejaculation usually occurs at SMR 3, with semen noted between SMR 3 and 4. The peak height velocity usually occurs in SMR 4 or genital development stage IV to V, at about 13.5 years of age.

ASSESSING THE MUSCULOSKELETAL SYSTEM

What do extra skinfolds on an arm or leg indicate? What condition does a rib hump indicate? At what age is it normal for children to be knock-kneed and bowlegged?

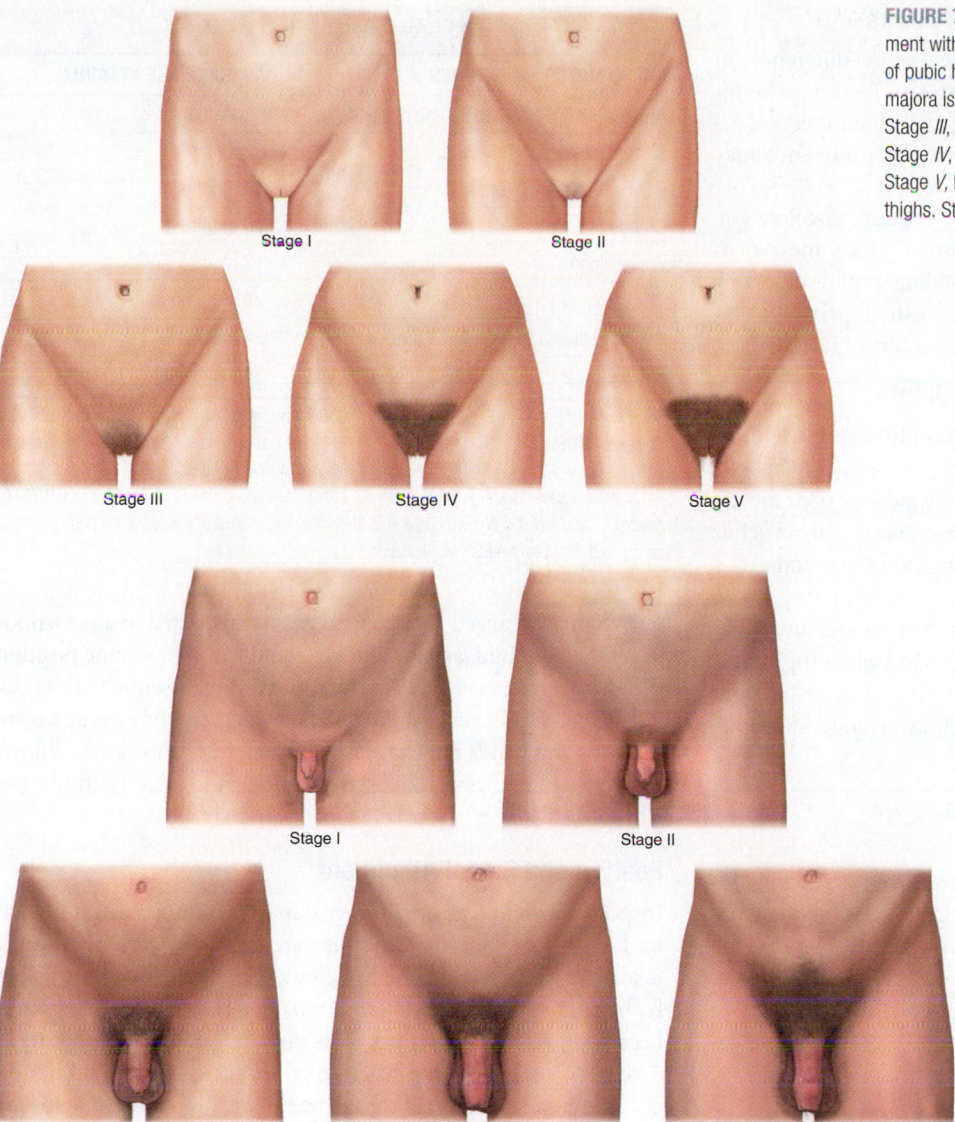

FIGURE 7–44 ■ The Tanner stages of female pubic hair development with sexual maturation. Stage *I*, Preadolescent, no growth of pubic hair. Stage *II*, Soft downy straight hair along the labia majora is an indication that sexual maturation is beginning. Stage *III*, Sparse, dark, visibly pigmented curly pubic hair on labia. Stage *IV*, Hair coarse and curly, abundant but less than adults. Stage *V*, Lateral spreading in triangle shape to medial surface of thighs. Stage *VI*, Further extension laterally and upward.

FIGURE 7–45 ■ The Tanner stages of male pubic hair and external genital development with sexual maturation. Stage *I*, Preadolescent, hair present is no different than that on the abdomen. Testes, scrotum, and penis are the same size and shape as in a young child. Stage *II*, Pubic hair slightly pigmented, longer, straight hair, often still downy, usually at base of penis, sometimes on scrotum; enlargement of scrotum and testes. Stage *III*, Pubic hair dark, definitely pigmented, curly pubic hair around base of penis; enlargement of penis, especially in length, further enlargement of testes, descent of scrotum. Stage *IV*, Pubic hair definitely adult in type but not in extent, spread no further than inguinal fold. Continued enlargement of penis and sculpturing of glans, increased pigmentation of scrotum. Stage *V*, Hair spread to medial surface of thighs in adult distribution. Adult stage, scrotum ample, penis reaching nearly to bottom of scrotum.

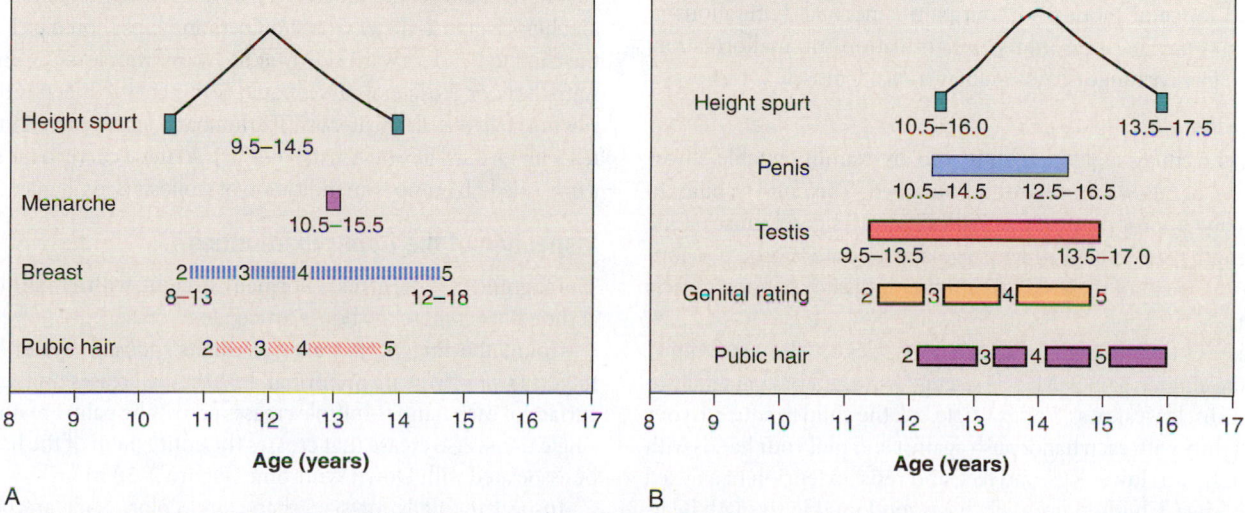

FIGURE 7–46 ■ Sexual maturity rating. Use the Tanner figures to determine the stage of breast and pubic hair development for females or the stage of genital and pubic hair development in males with the numbers (2, 3, 4, 5) corresponding to the child's age and stages listed on the sexual maturity rating figures. The sexual maturity rating figures can then provide information about where the child is in regard to other pubertal changes such as the height spurt and menarche. *A*, Females. *B*, Males.

Source: A, *Redrawn from Marshall, W. A., & Tanner, J. M. (1969). Variations in pattern of pubertal changes in girls. Archives of Disease in Childhood, 44, 291.* B, *Marshall, W. A., & Tanner, J. M. (1970). Variations in pattern of pubertal changes in boys. Archives of Disease in Childhood, 45, 13.*

Inspection of the Bones, Muscles, and Joints

Inspect and compare the arms and then the legs for differences in alignment, contour, skinfolds, length, and deformities. The extremities normally have equal length, circumference, and number of skinfolds bilaterally. Extra skinfolds and a larger circumference may indicate a shorter extremity.

Inspect and compare the joints bilaterally for size, discoloration, and ease of voluntary movement. Joints are normally the same color as surrounding skin, with no sign of swelling. Children should voluntarily flex and extend joints during normal activities without pain. Redness, swelling, and pain with movement may indicate injury or infection.

Palpation of the Bones, Muscles, and Joints

Palpate the bones and muscles in each extremity for muscle tone, masses, or tenderness. Muscles normally feel firm, and bony masses are not normally present. Doughy muscles may indicate poor muscle tone. Rigid muscles, or hypertonia, may be associated with an active seizure or cerebral palsy. A mass over a long bone may indicate a recent fracture or a bone tumor.

Palpate each joint and surrounding muscles to detect any swelling, masses, heat, or tenderness. None is expected when the joint is palpated. Tenderness, heat, swelling, and redness can result from injury or a chronic joint inflammation such as juvenile idiopathic arthritis (see Chapter 27 🔗).

Range of Motion and Muscle Strength

Active Range of Motion

Observe the child during typical play activities, such as reaching for objects, climbing, and walking, to assess range of motion of all major joints. Children spontaneously move their joints through the full normal range of motion with play activities when no pain is present. Limited range of motion may indicate injury, inflammation of a joint, or a muscle abnormality.

Passive Range of Motion

When a joint is suspected of having limited active range of motion, perform passive range of motion. Flex and extend, abduct and adduct, or rotate the affected joint cautiously to avoid causing extra pain. Full range of motion without pain is normal. Limitations in movement may indicate injury, inflammation, or malformation. Increased passive range of motion may indicate muscle weakness.

Muscle Strength

Observe the child's ability to climb onto an examining table, throw a ball, clap hands, or move around on a bed. The child's ability to perform age-appropriate play activities indicates good muscle tone and strength. See Table 7–14 for age-appropriate motor development. Attainment of these skills is another indicator of good muscle strength.

To assess the strength of specific muscles in the extremities, engage the child in games. Muscle strength is compared bilaterally to identify muscle weakness. For example, ask the child to squeeze your fingers tightly with each hand; push against and pull your hands with his or her hands, lower legs, and feet; and resist extension of a flexed elbow or knee. Children normally have good muscle strength bilaterally. Unilateral muscle weakness may be associated with a nerve injury. Bilateral muscle weakness may result from hypoxemia or a congenital disorder such as Down syndrome. Asymmetric weakness may be associated with conditions such as cerebral palsy.

TABLE 7–14	Selected Gross Motor Milestones for Age
GROSS MOTOR MILESTONES	**AVERAGE AGE ATTAINED**
Rolls over from prone to supine position	7 months
Sits without support	6 months
Pulls self to standing position	10 months
Creeps or crawls	10 months
Walks alone	12 months
Climbs on furniture	24 months
Walks up stairs, one step at a time	24 months
Rides tricycle	36 months

Source: *Data from Zitelli, B. J., & Davis, H. W. (2007). Atlas of pediatric physical diagnosis (5th ed.). St. Louis, MO: Elsevier Mosby; Feigelman, S. (2011). The first year. In R. M. Kliegman, B. F. Stanton, J. W. St Geme, N. F. Schor, & R. E. Behrman, Nelson textbook of pediatrics (19th ed., pp. 26–31). Philadelphia: Elsevier Saunders; Feigelman, S. (2011). The second year. In R. M. Kliegman, B. F. Stanton, J. W. St Geme, N. F. Schor, & R. E. Behrman, Nelson textbook of pediatrics (18th ed., pp. 31–33). Philadelphia: Elsevier Saunders.*

When generalized muscle weakness is suspected in a preschool- or school-age child, ask the child to stand from the supine position. Children are normally able to rise to a standing position without using their arms as levers. Children who push their body upright using the arms and hands may have generalized muscle weakness, known as a positive Gowers sign. This may indicate muscular dystrophy (see Chapter 35 🔗).

Posture and Spinal Alignment

Inspect the child's posture when standing from a front, side, and back view. The shoulders and hips are normally level. The head is held erect without a tilt, and the shoulder contour is symmetric. After beginning to walk, young children often have a pot-bellied stance because of a lumbar lordosis. This posture generally disappears by 5 years of age. The spine has normal thoracic convex and lumbar concave curves after 6 years of age. See Figure 7–47 ■ for the expected developmental sequence of posture and spinal curves by age.

Assess the school-age child and adolescent for *scoliosis*, a lateral spine curvature. Stand behind the child, observing the height of the shoulders and hips (Figure 7–48 ■). The shoulders and hips should be level. Ask the child to bend forward slowly at the waist, with arms extended toward the floor. No lateral curve should be present in either position. The ribs normally stay flat bilaterally. The lumbar concave curve should flatten with forward flexion (Figure 7–49 ■). A lateral curve to the spine or a one-sided rib hump is an indication of scoliosis (see Chapter 35 🔗).

Inspection of the Upper Extremities

The alignment of the arms is normally straight, with a minimal angle at the elbows, where the bones articulate.

Count the fingers. Extra finger digits (*polydactyly*) or webbed fingers (*syndactyly*) are abnormal. Inspect the creases on the palmar surface of each hand. Multiple creases across the palm are normal. A single transverse crease that crosses the entire palm of the hand may be associated with Down syndrome (Figure 7–50 ■).

Inspect the nails for size, shape, and color. Nails are normally convex, smooth, and pink. **Clubbing,** widening of the nail bed with an increased angle between the proximal nail fold and nail, is abnormal. Clubbing is associated with chronic respiratory and cardiac conditions.

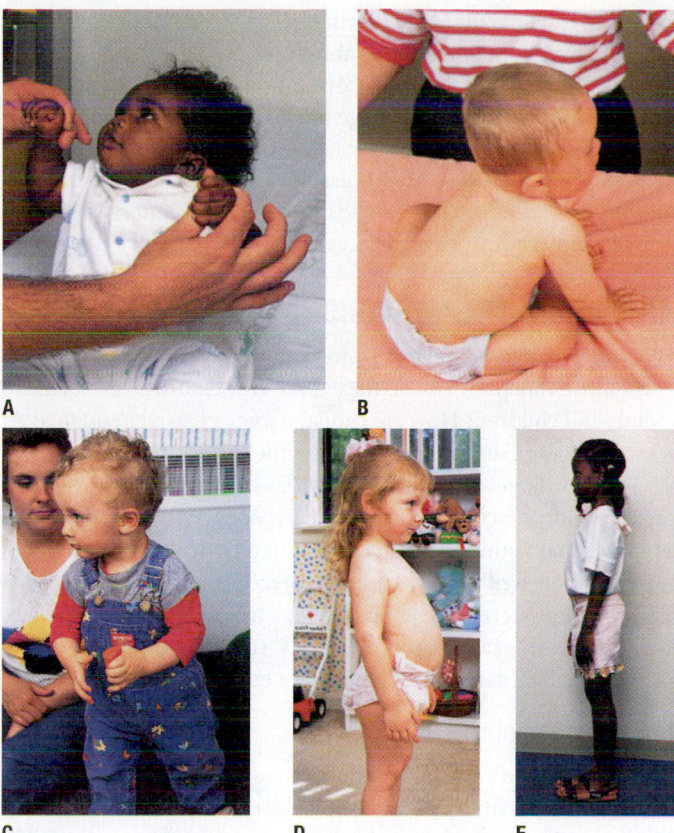

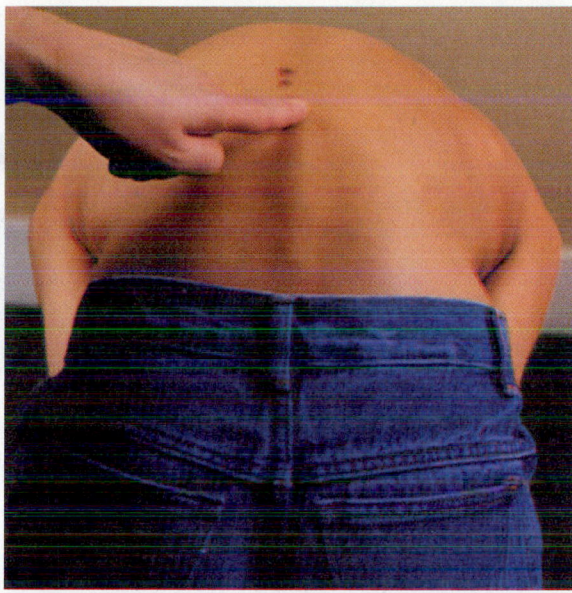

FIGURE 7–49 ■ Inspection of the spine for scoliosis. Ask the child to slowly bend forward at the waist, with arms extended toward the floor. Run your forefinger down the spinal processes, palpating each vertebra for a change in alignment. A lateral curve to the spine or a one-sided rib hump is an indication of scoliosis.

FIGURE 7–47 ■ Normal development of posture and spinal curves. *A,* Infant 2 to 3 months—Holds head erect when held upright; thoracic kyphosis when sitting. *B,* 6 to 8 months—Sits without support; spine is straight. *C,* 10 to 15 months—Walks independently; straight spine. *D,* Toddler—Protruding abdomen; lumbar lordosis. *E,* School-age child—Height of shoulders and hips is level; balanced thoracic convex and lumbar concave curves.

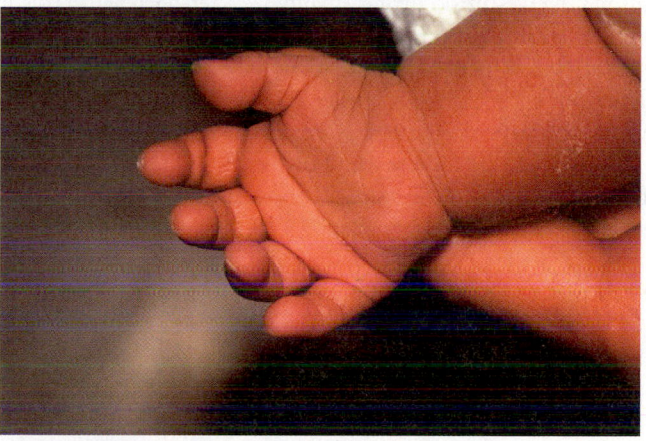

FIGURE 7–50 ■ Transverse crease on palmal surface of the hand is associated with Down syndrome.

Source: *NMSB / Custom Medical Stock Photo, Inc.*

Inspection of the Lower Extremities

Hips

Assess the hips of young infants for dislocation or subluxation. The skinfolds on the upper legs are inspected first. The same number of skinfolds should be present on each leg. Uneven skinfolds may indicate a hip dislocation or difference in leg length. Check for a difference in knee height symmetry (Allis sign, also known as Galeazzi sign). See Figure 7–51 ■ for a description of the technique. The Ortolani-Barlow maneuver is used to assess an infant's hips for dislocation or subluxation. See Figure 7–52 ■ for a description of this assessment maneuver. The Ortolani-Barlow maneuver should be performed by a trained healthcare practitioner.

The child who can stand is asked to stand first on one leg and then the other. The iliac crest height should stay level. If the iliac crest on the lifted leg appears lower, the hip abductor muscles on the weight-bearing side are weak, known as Trendelenburg sign.

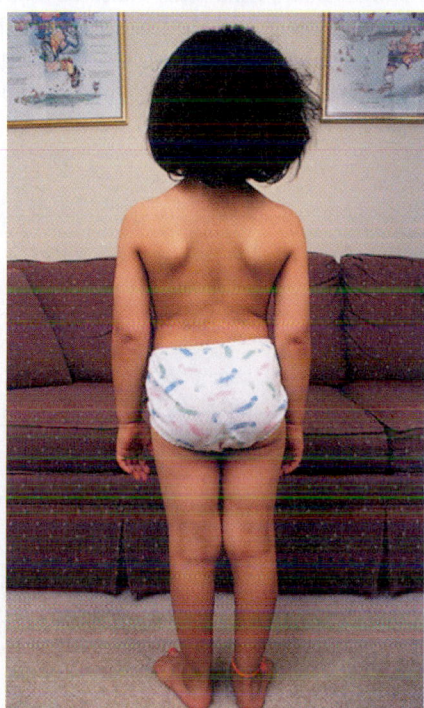

FIGURE 7–48 ■ Does this child have legs of different lengths or scoliosis? Look at the level of the iliac crests and shoulders to see if they are level. See the more prominent crease at the waist on the right side? The right shoulder appears lower than the left. This child could have scoliosis.

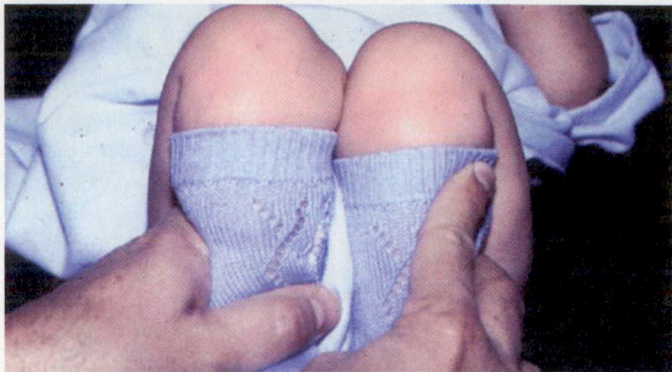

FIGURE 7–51 ■ Flex the infant's hips and knees so the heels are as close to the buttocks as possible. Place the feet flat on the examining table. The knees are usually the same height. A difference in knee height (Allis or Galeazzi sign) is an indicator of hip dislocation (see also Chapter 35 🔗).

Source: *Used with permission International Hip Dysplasia Institute.*

Legs

Inspect the alignment of the legs with the child standing. After a child is 4 years of age, the alignment of the long bones is straight, with minimal angle at the knees and feet where the bones articulate. Assess alignment of the lower extremities in infants and toddlers to ensure that normal changes are occurring. Infants are often born with a twisting of the tibia caused by positioning in utero (tibial torsion). The infant's toes turn in as a result of the tibial torsion. Toddlers go through a skeletal alignment sequence of bowlegs (genu varum) and knock-knees (genu valgum) before the legs assume a straight alignment.

To evaluate the toddler with bowlegs, have the child stand on a firm surface. Measure the distance between the knees when the child's ankles are together. No more than 3.5 cm (1.5 in.) between the knees is normal. See Figure 7–53 ■ for the technique to assess knock-knees.

Inspect the feet for alignment, the presence of all toes, and any deformities. The weight-bearing line of the feet is usually in alignment with the legs. Many newborns have a flexible forefoot

inversion (metatarsus adductus) that results from uterine positioning. Any fixed foot deformity is abnormal. See Chapter 35 🔗.

Inspect the feet for the presence of an arch when the child is standing. Children up to 3 years of age normally have a fat pad over the arch, giving the appearance of flat feet. Older children normally have a longitudinal arch. The arch is usually seen when the child stands on tiptoe or is sitting. If no arch is present, pes planus (flat foot) is present. Inspect the nails on the feet in the same manner as the hands.

ASSESSING THE NERVOUS SYSTEM

What aspects of developmental information are useful for assessment of cognitive function? How is the level of consciousness evaluated in infants and children? How are cranial nerves assessed in infants? At what age does a Babinski response become abnormal?

The neurologic examination provides an opportunity to develop rapport with the child. Many of the procedures can be presented as games that young children enjoy. Cognitive function can be assessed by how well the child follows directions for the game. As the assessment proceeds, the child develops trust and is more likely to cooperate with examination of other systems. Equipment needed includes a reflex hammer, cotton balls, penlight, and tongue blades.

Cognitive Function

Observe the child's behavior, facial expressions, gestures, communication skills, activity level, and level of consciousness to assess cognitive functioning. Match the neurologic examination to the child's stage of development. For example, cognitive function is evaluated much differently in infants than in older children because infants cannot use words to communicate.

Behavior

The alertness of infants and children is indicated by their behavior during the assessment. Infants and toddlers are curious, but they seek the security of the parent, either by clinging or by making frequent eye contact. Older children are often anxious and watch the examiner's

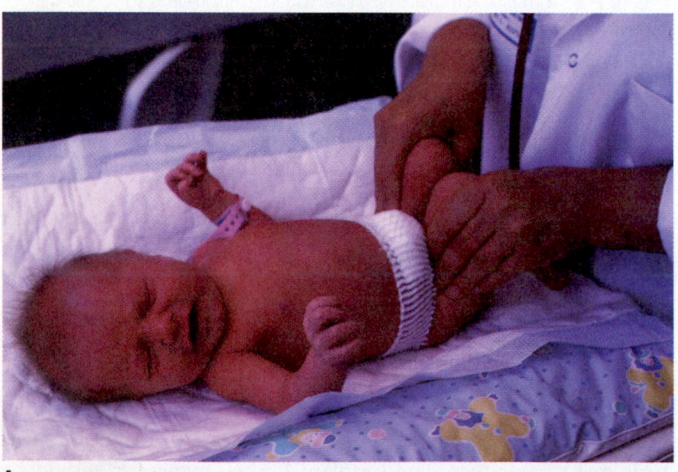

A

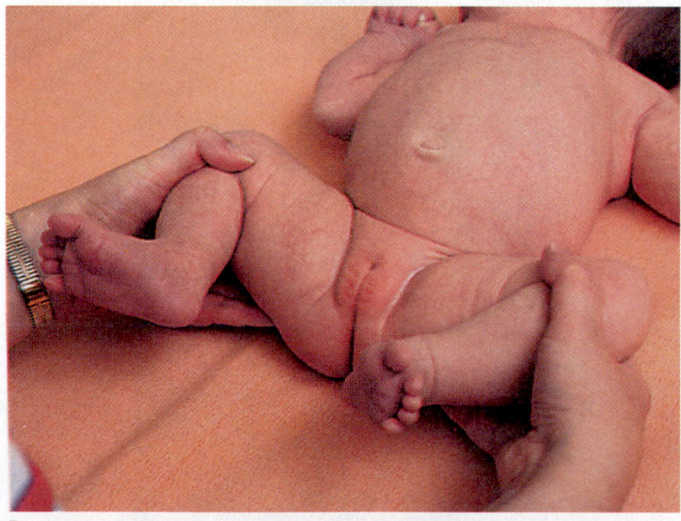

B

FIGURE 7–52 ■ Ortolani-Barlow maneuver. *A,* Place the infant on his or her back and flex the hips and knees at a 90-degree angle. Place a hand over each knee with the thumb over the inner thigh, and the first two fingers over the upper margin of the femur. Move the infant's knees together until they touch, and then put downward pressure on one femur at a time to see if the hips easily slip out of their joints or dislocate. *B,* Slowly abduct the hips, moving each knee toward the examining table. Keep pressure on the hip joints with the fingers in a lever-type motion. Equal hip abduction, with the knees nearly touching the examining table, is normal. Any resistance to abduction or a clunk felt on palpation can be an indication of a congenital hip dislocation.

Source: *A,* © ASTIER—www.agefotostock.com

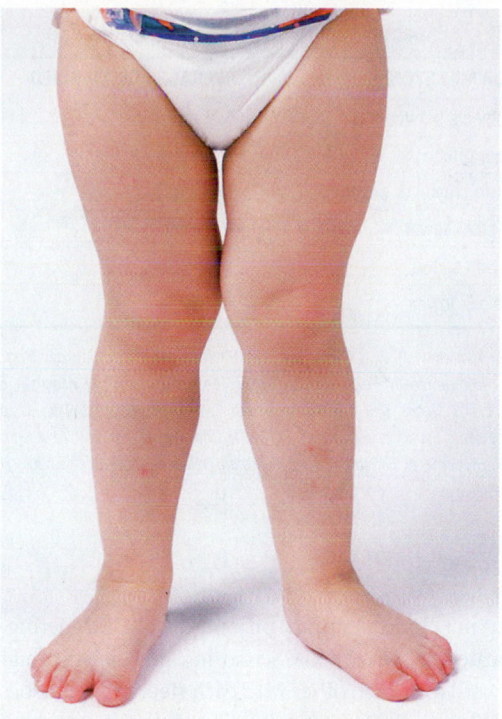

FIGURE 7–53 ■ To evaluate the child with knock-knees, have the child stand on a firm surface. Measure the distance between the ankles when the child stands with the knees together. The normal distance is not more than 5 cm (2 in.) between the ankles.

actions. Lack of interest in assessment or treatment procedures may indicate a serious illness. Excessive activity or an unusually short attention span may be associated with attention deficit hyperactivity disorder.

Communication Skills

Speech, language development, and social skills provide clues to cognitive functioning. Listen to speech articulation and words used, comparing the child's performance with standards of social development and expected language development for age (Table 7–15). Toddlers can normally follow simple directions such as "Show me your mouth." By 3 years of age, the child's speech should be easily understood. Delay in language and social skill development may be

associated with intellectual disability (mental retardation) or hearing loss.

Memory

Immediate, recent, and remote memory can be tested in children starting at approximately 4 years of age. Immediate memory can be tested by asking the child to repeat a series of words or numbers, such as the names of favorite characters from a book, television show, or movie. Children can remember more words or numbers with age:

- Age 4 years—three words or numbers
- Age 5 years—four words or numbers
- Age 6 years—five words or numbers

To evaluate recent memory, ask the child to remember a special name or object. Then 5 to 10 minutes later during the examination have the child recall the name or object. To evaluate remote memory, ask the child to repeat his or her address or birth date or a nursery rhyme. By 5 or 6 years of age, children are normally able to recall this information without difficulty.

Level of Consciousness

When approaching the infant or child, observe his or her level of consciousness and activity, including facial expressions, gestures, and interaction. Children are normally alert, and sleeping children arouse easily. The child who cannot be awakened is unconscious. A lowered level of consciousness may be associated with a number of neurologic conditions such as a brain injury, seizure, infection, or brain tumor. See Chapter 33 .

Cerebellar Function

Observe the young child at play to assess coordination and balance. Development of fine motor skills in infants and preschool children provides clues to cerebellar function.

Balance

Observe the child's balance during play activities such as walking, standing on one foot, and hopping. See Table 7–16 for expected balance development for age. The Romberg procedure can also be used to test balance in children over 3 years of age (Figure 7–54 ■). Once balance and other motor skills are attained, children do not normally stumble or fall when tested. Poor balance may indicate cerebellar dysfunction or an inner ear disturbance.

Coordination

Tests of coordination assess the smoothness and accuracy of movement. Development of fine motor skills can be used to assess coordination in young children. See Table 7–17 for expected fine motor development for age. After 6 years of age, the tests for adults

TABLE 7–15 Expected Language Development for Age

LANGUAGE MILESTONES	AGE ATTAINED
Babbles speechlike sounds, including *p, b,* and *m*	4–6 months
Has 1–2 words like "mama," "dada," "bye-bye"	12 months
Increases words each month, 2-word combinations (e.g., "Where baby?" and "Want cookie")	1–2 years
Uses 2- to 3-word sentences to ask for things or talk about things, large vocabulary, speech understood by family members	2–3 years
Sentences may have 4 or more words, speech understood by most people	3–4 years
Says most sounds correctly except a few like *l, s, r, v, z, ch, sh,* and *th*. Tells stories and uses same grammar as rest of family	4–5 years

Source: *Data from American Speech and Language Association. (2011). How does your child hear and talk?* Retrieved from http://www.asha.org/public/speech/development/chart.htm

TABLE 7–16 Expected Balance Development for Age

BALANCE MILESTONES	AGE ATTAINED
Stands without support briefly	12 months
Walks alone well	15 months
Walks backwards	2 years
Balances on one foot for 5 seconds	4 years
Hops on one foot, heel-toe walking	5 years
Heel-toe walking backwards	6 years

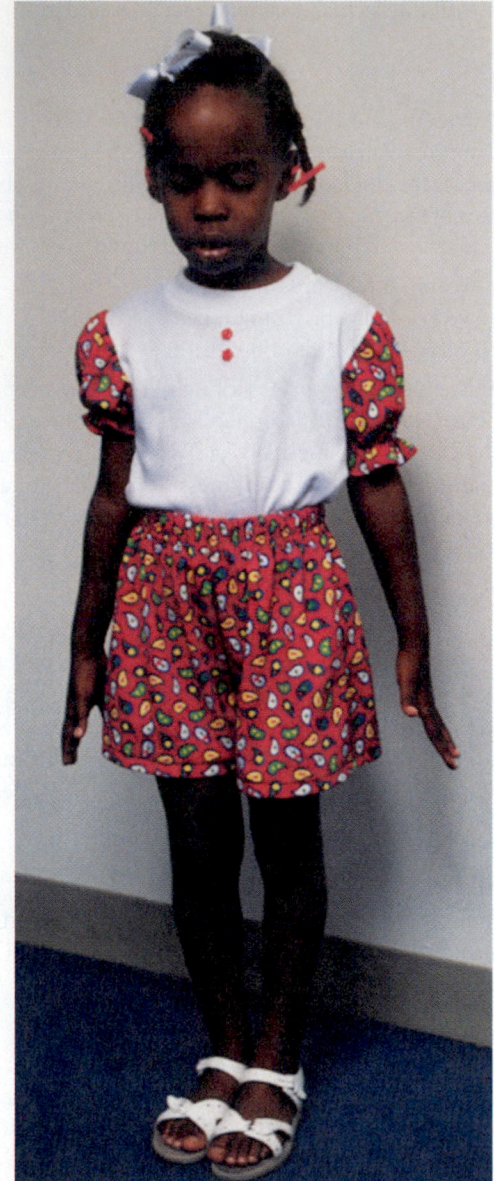

FIGURE 7–54 ■ Romberg procedure. Ask the child to stand with feet together and eyes closed. Protect the child from falling by standing close. Preschool children may extend their arms to maintain balance, but older children can normally stand with arms at their sides. Leaning or falling to one side is abnormal and indicates poor balance.
Source: *George Dodson / Pearson.*

TABLE 7–17	Expected Fine Motor Development for Age
FINE MOTOR MILESTONES	**AVERAGE AGE ATTAINED**
Transfers objects between hands	5–6 months
Thumb finger grasp	8 months
Scribbles with crayon or pencil	13 months
Builds two-block tower	15 months
Feeds self with spoon	18 months
Builds six-block tower	22 months

Source: *Data from Zitelli, B. J., & Davis, H. W. (2007). Atlas of pediatric physical diagnosis (5th ed.). St. Louis, MO: Elsevier Mosby; Feigelman, S. (2011). The first year. In R. M. Kliegman, B. F. Stanton, J. W. St. Geme, N. F. Schor, & R. E. Behrman, Nelson textbook of pediatrics (19th ed., pp. 26–31). Philadelphia: Elsevier Saunders; Feigelman, S. (2011). The second year. In R. M. Kliegman, B. F. Stanton, J. W. St. Geme, N. F. Schor, & R. E. Behrman, Nelson textbook of pediatrics (18th ed., pp. 31–33). Philadelphia: Elsevier Saunders.*

(finger-to-nose, finger-to-finger, heel-to-shin, and alternating motion tests) can be used (Figure 7–55 ■). The child usually responds enthusiastically when these tests are presented as games. Jerky movements or inaccurate pointing (past pointing) indicates poor coordination, which can be associated with delayed development or a cerebellar lesion.

Gait

A normal gait requires intact bones and joints, muscle strength, coordination, and balance. Inspect the child when walking from both a front and a rear view. The iliac crests are normally level during walking, and no limp is expected. Gait stance is related to the motor development of the child. Toddlers beginning to walk have a wide-based gait and limited balance. With practice, the toddler's balance improves and the gait develops a narrower base.

A limp may indicate injury or joint disease. Staggering or falling may indicate cerebellar ataxia. Scissoring, in which the thighs tend to cross forward over each other with each step, may be associated with cerebral palsy or other spastic conditions. Persistent walking on the toes may indicate a possible neurologic dysfunction.

Sensory Function

To assess sensory function, compare the responses of both sides of the body to various types of stimulation. Equal responses bilaterally are normal. Loss of sensation may indicate a brain or spinal cord lesion. An infant's sensory function is not routinely assessed. Withdrawal responses to painful procedures indicate normal sensory function.

Superficial Tactile Sensation

Stroke the skin on the lower leg or arm with a cotton ball or a finger while the child's eyes are closed. Cooperative children over 2 years of age can normally point to the location touched.

Superficial Pain Sensation

Break a tongue blade to get a sharp point. After asking the child to close the eyes, touch the child in various places on each arm and leg, alternating the sharp and rounded ends of the tongue blade. Children over 4 years of age can normally distinguish between a sharp and dull sensation each time. To improve the child's accuracy with the test, let the child practice telling you the difference between the sharp and dull stimulation.

An inability to identify superficial touch and pain sensation may indicate sensory loss. Identify the extent of sensory loss, such as all areas below the knee. Other sensory function tests (temperature, vibratory, deep pressure pain, and position sense) are performed when sensory loss is found. Refer to other texts for description of these procedures.

Cranial Nerve Function

Cranial nerves are assessed in cooperative children much as they are for adults; however, the assessment is modified for infants and toddlers. See Table 7–18 for cranial nerve assessment guidelines. Abnormalities of cranial nerves may be associated with compression of an individual nerve, brain injury, or infection.

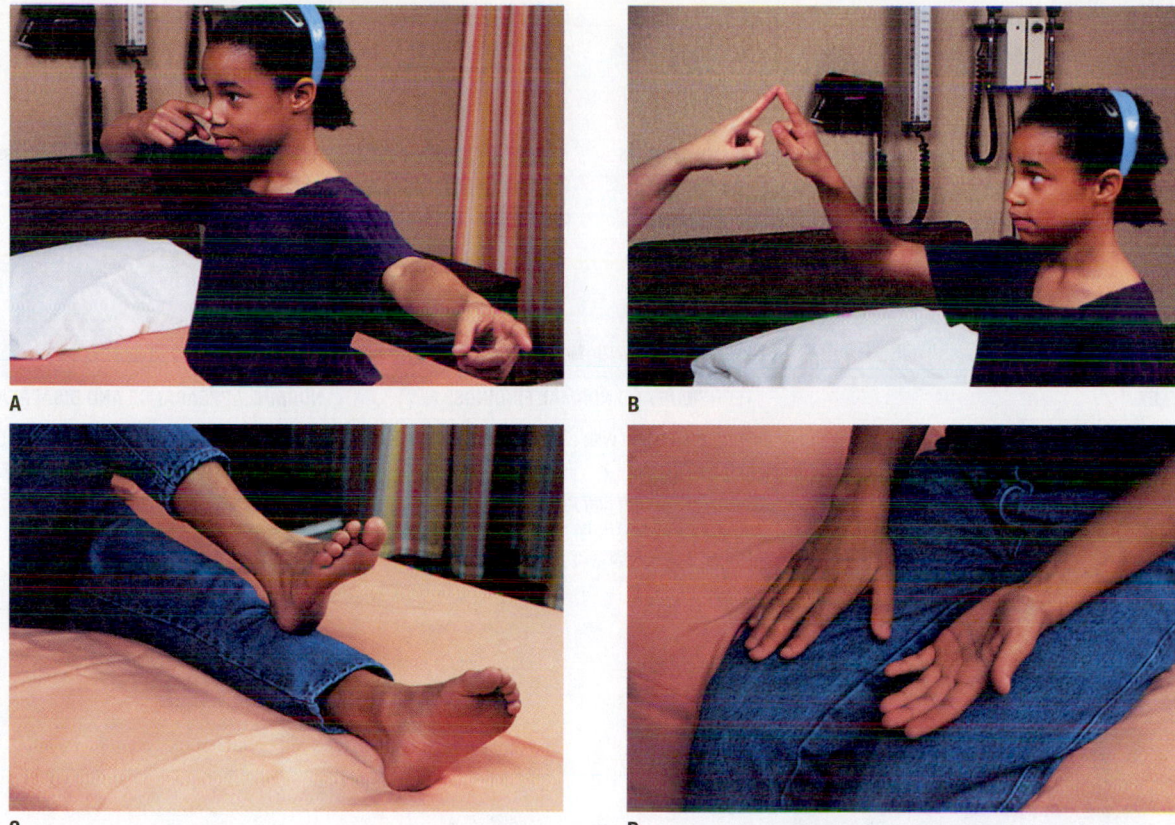

FIGURE 7–55 ■ Tests of coordination. *A, Finger-to-nose test.* Ask the child to close the eyes and touch his or her nose, alternating the index fingers of the hands. *B, Finger-to-finger test.* Ask the child to alternately touch his or her nose and your index finger with his or her index finger. Move your hand to several positions within the child's reach to test pointing accuracy. Repeat the test with the child's other hand. *C, Heel-to-shin test.* Ask the child to rub his or her leg from the knee to the ankle with the heel of the other foot. Repeat the test with the other foot. This test is normally performed without hesitation or inappropriate placement of the foot. *D, Rapid alternating motion test.* Ask the child to rapidly rotate his or her wrist so the palm and dorsum of the hand alternately pat the thigh. Repeat the test with the other hand. Hesitating movements are abnormal. Mirroring movements of the hand not being tested indicate a delay in coordination skill refinement.

TABLE 7–18	Cranial Nerve Assessment in Infants and Children
CRANIAL NERVE[a]	**ASSESSMENT PROCEDURE AND NORMAL FINDINGS**[b]
I Olfactory	Infant: Not tested.
	Child: Not routinely tested. Give familiar odors to child to smell, one naris at a time. *Identifies odors such as orange, peanut butter, and chocolate.*
II Optic	Infant: Shine a bright light in eyes. *A quick blink reflex and dorsal head flexion indicate light perception.*
	Child: Test vision and visual fields if cooperative. *Visual acuity appropriate for age.*
III Oculomotor	Infant: Shine a penlight at the eyes and move it side to side. *Focuses on and tracks the light to each side.*
IV Trochlear	Child: Move an object through the six cardinal points of gaze. *Tracks objects through all fields of gaze.*
VI Abducens	All ages: Inspect eyelids for drooping. Inspect pupillary response to light. *Eyelids do not droop, and pupils are equal sized and briskly respond to light.*
V Trigeminal	Infant: Stimulate the rooting and sucking reflex. *Turns head toward stimulation at side of mouth, and sucking has good strength and pattern.*
	Child: Observe the child chewing a cracker. Touch forehead and cheeks with cotton ball when eyes are closed. *Bilateral jaw strength is good. Child pushes cotton ball away.*
VII Facial	All ages: Observe facial expressions when crying, smiling, frowning, etc. *Facial features stay symmetric bilaterally.*
VIII Acoustic	Infant: Produce a loud sound near the head. *Blinks in response to sound, moves head toward sound, or freezes position.*
	Child: Use a noisemaker near each ear or whisper words to be repeated. *Turns head toward sound and repeats words correctly.*
IX Glossopharyngeal	Infant: Observe swallowing during feeding. *Good swallowing pattern.*
X Vagus	All ages: Elicit gag reflex (not routinely tested). *Gags with stimulation.*
XI Spinal accessory	Infant: Not tested.
	Child: Ask child to raise the shoulders and turn the head side to side against resistance. *Good strength in neck and shoulders.*
XII Hypoglossal	Infant: Observe feeding. *Sucking and swallowing are coordinated.*
	Child: Tell the child to stick out the tongue. Listen to speech. *Tongue is midline with no tremors. Words are clearly articulated.*

[a]Bracketed nerves are tested together.

[b]Italics indicate normal findings.

Infant Primitive Reflexes

Use the guidelines in Table 7–19 to evaluate the movement and posture of newborns and young infants by the Moro, palmar grasp, plantar grasp, placing, stepping, and tonic neck primitive reflexes. These reflexes appear and disappear at expected intervals in the first few months of life as the central nervous system develops. Movements are normally equal bilaterally. An asymmetric response may indicate a serious neurologic problem on the less responsive side.

Superficial and Deep Tendon Reflexes

Evaluate the superficial and deep tendon reflexes to assess the function of specific segments of the spine. The best response to deep tendon reflex testing is achieved when the child is relaxed or distracted.

TABLE 7–19	Techniques for Assessing Selected Primitive Reflexes, with Normal Findings and Their Expected Age of Occurrence	
PRIMITIVE REFLEX	**TECHNIQUE AND NORMAL FINDINGS**[a]	**NORMAL APPEARANCE AND DISAPPEARANCE**
Moro 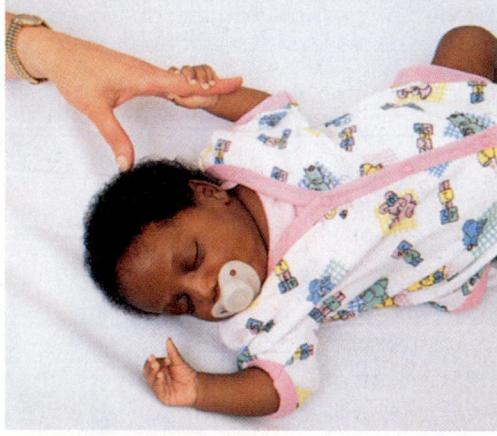	Startle the infant with a sudden noise or change in position. *The arms extend and the fingers form a **C** as they spread. The arms slowly move together as in a hug. The legs may make a similar motion.*	Present at birth. Decreases in strength by 4 months of age. Disappears by 6 months of age.
Palmar grasp 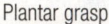	Place a finger across the infant's palm and avoid touching the thumb. *A strong grip around the finger is normal.*	Present at birth. Disappears by 3 months of age.
Plantar grasp 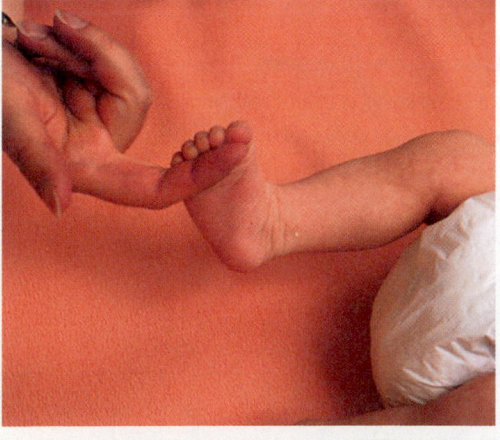	Place a finger across the foot at the base of the toes. *The toes normally curl as if gripping a finger.*	Present at birth. Disappears at about 8 months of age.

TABLE 7–19 Techniques for Assessing Selected Primitive Reflexes, with Normal Findings and Their Expected Age of Occurrence (*continued*)

PRIMITIVE REFLEX	TECHNIQUE AND NORMAL FINDINGS[a]	NORMAL APPEARANCE AND DISAPPEARANCE
Placing 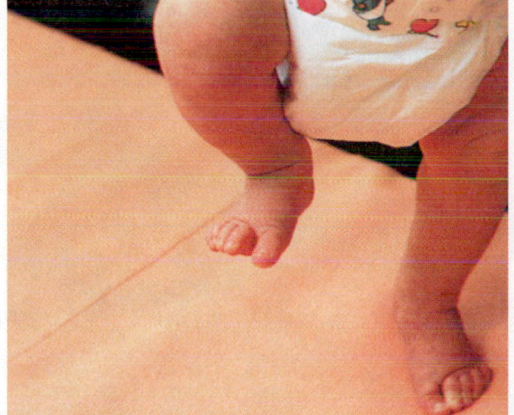	Hold the infant erect and touch the top of one foot with the edge of the table or chair. *The infant normally lifts the foot as if to step up onto the surface.*	Present within days of birth. Disappears at various times.
Stepping 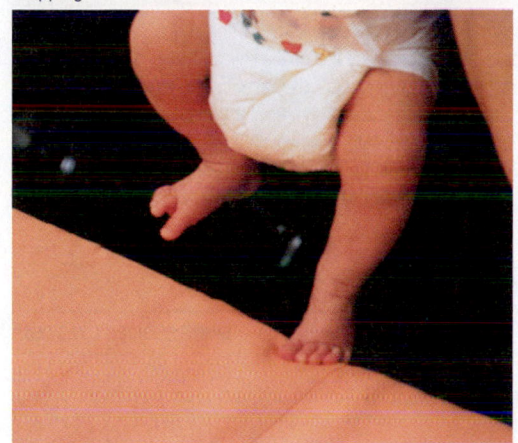	Hold the infant erect and touch the bottom of one foot on the surface of a table or chair. *The feet lift in an alternating pattern as if to walk.*	Present at birth. Disappears between 4 and 8 weeks of age.
Tonic neck 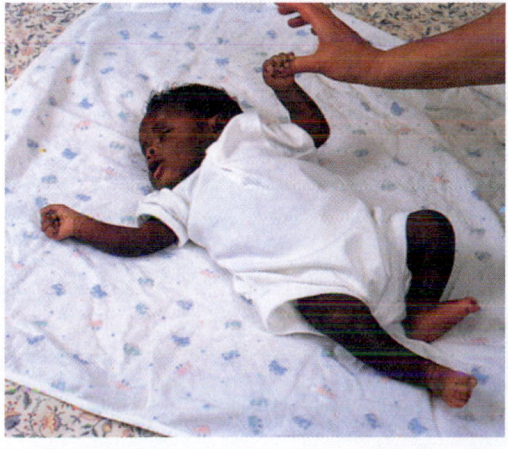	Place the infant in a supine position and, when relaxed, turn the head to one side. Repeat by turning the head to the opposite side. *The arm and leg on the side to which the face is turned normally extend; the opposite arm and leg flex, as if to assume a fencing position.*	Appears about 2 months of age. Decreases by 4 months of age. Disappears no later than 6 months of age. This reflex must disappear before the infant can turn over.

[a] Italics indicate expected findings.

Children often anticipate the knee jerk and either tighten up or exaggerate the response. Making the child focus on another set of muscles may provide a more accurate response. When testing the reflexes on the lower legs, have the child press his or her hands together or try to pull them apart when gripped together.

Superficial Reflexes

Assess superficial reflexes by stroking a specific area of the body. The plantar reflex, testing spine levels L4 through S2, is routinely evaluated in children (Figure 7–56 ■). To assess the cremasteric reflex in boys, stroke the inner thigh of each leg, testing spine levels T12, L1, and L2. The testicle and scrotum on the stroked side normally rise.

Deep Tendon Reflexes

To assess the deep tendon reflexes, tap a tendon near specific joints with a reflex hammer (or with the index finger for infants), comparing responses bilaterally. The biceps, triceps, brachioradialis, patellar, and Achilles tendons are usually evaluated in children. See Table 7–20 for guidelines for assessment of deep tendon reflexes. Inspect for movement in the associated joint, and palpate the strength of the expected muscle contraction. Table 7–21 outlines the numeric scoring of deep tendon reflexes. Responses are normally symmetric bilaterally. The absence of a response is associated with decreased muscle tone and strength. Hyperactive responses are associated with muscle spasticity.

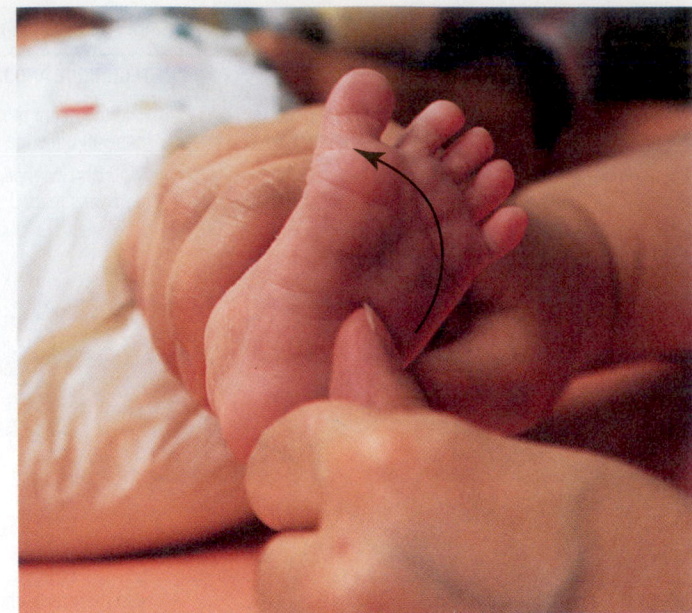

FIGURE 7–56 ■ To assess the plantar reflex, stroke the bottom of the infant's or child's foot from the heel, along the lateral sole, and across the ball. Watch the toes for plantar flexion or the Babinski response, fanning and dorsiflexion of the big toe. The Babinski response is normal in children under 2 years of age. Plantar flexion of the toes (absent Babinski sign) is the normal response in older children. A Babinski sign present in children over 2 years of age can indicate neurologic disease.

TABLE 7–20	Assessment of Deep Tendon Reflexes and the Spinal Segment Tested with Each	
DEEP TENDON REFLEX	**TECHNIQUE AND NORMAL FINDINGS**[a]	**SPINE SEGMENT TESTED**
Biceps 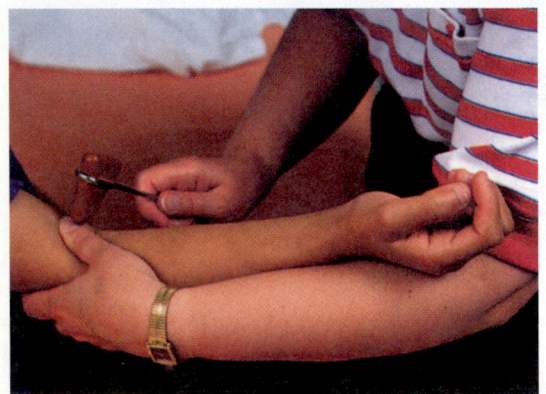	Flex the child's arm at the elbow, and place your thumb over the biceps tendon in the antecubital fossa. Tap your thumb. *Elbow flexes as the biceps muscle contracts.*	C5 and C6
Triceps 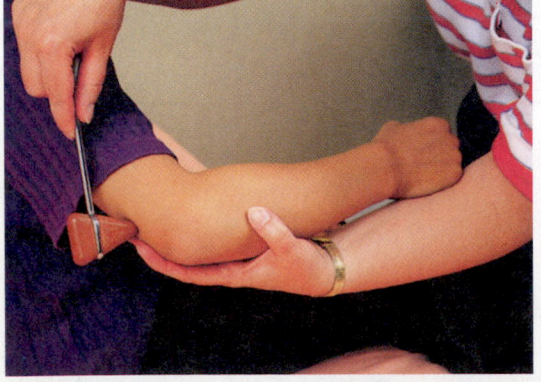	With the child's arm flexed, tap the triceps tendon above the elbow. *Elbow extends as the triceps muscle contracts.*	C6, C7, and C8

TABLE 7–20 | Assessment of Deep Tendon Reflexes and the Spinal Segment Tested with Each (*continued*)

DEEP TENDON REFLEX	TECHNIQUE AND NORMAL FINDINGS[a]	SPINE SEGMENT TESTED
Brachioradialis 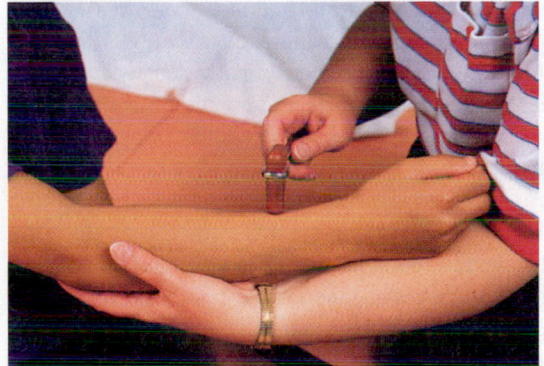	Lay the child's arm with the thumb upright over your arm. Tap the brachioradial tendon 2.5 cm (1 in.) above the wrist. *Forearm pronates (palm facing downward) and elbow flexes.*	C5 and C6
Patellar 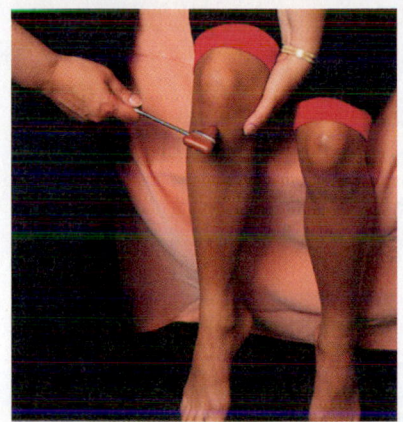	Flex the child's knees, and when the legs are relaxed, tap the patellar tendon just below the knee. *Knee extends (knee jerk) as the quadriceps muscle contracts.*	L2, L3, and L4
Achilles 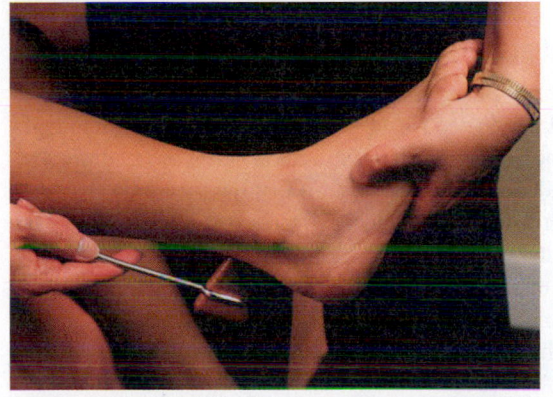	While the child's legs are flexed, support the foot and tap the Achilles tendon. *Plantar flexion (ankle jerk) as the gastrocnemius muscle contracts.*	S1 and S2

[a] Italics indicate normal findings.

TABLE 7–21 | Numeric Scoring of Deep Tendon Reflex Responses

GRADE	RESPONSE INTERPRETATION
0	No response
1+	Slow, minimal response
2+	Expected response, active
3+	More active or pronounced than expected
4+	Hyperactive, clonus may be present

ANALYZING DATA FROM THE PHYSICAL EXAMINATION

Once the physical examination has been completed, legibly record the findings in the child's medical record in the detail and format expected by the facility. Review all abnormal findings, group them together, and contrast them with expected findings. Use clinical reasoning to identify common patterns of signs and physiologic responses that could be associated with health conditions. Individual abnormal physiologic responses are also the basis of many nursing diagnoses.

NEWBORN ASSESSMENT

The newborn is examined at specific intervals while in the birthing facility due to the rapid transitions occurring from intrauterine to extrauterine life. It is important to know that the newborn is adapting to extrauterine life before discharge home. The primary changes that the newborn experiences are noted in the cardiovascular and respiratory systems, and these changes are triggered by the birthing process, exposure to the environment, and cutting the umbilical cord.

Newborn Transition

Prior to birth, a fetus is oxygenated by blood transferred from the placenta. At birth, an infant must initiate respirations. A series of mechanical, chemical, thermal, and sensory stimuli lead to the initiation of breathing.

- **Mechanical**—Pressure on the thorax as the newborn passes through the birth canal forces some of the fluid out of the lungs. When the chest and lungs recoil, air begins replacing the fluid. As the newborn cries and exhales, the air remaining in the lungs is distributed through the alveoli. With each succeeding breath the lungs continue to expand.
- **Chemical**—The aortic and carotid chemoreceptors are stimulated by the falling PO_2 level and rising PCO_2 level after the umbilical cord is clamped. This triggers the respiratory center to initiate breathing.
- **Thermal**—The change in temperature between the uterine and external environments stimulates nerve endings that lead to rhythmic respirations.
- **Sensory**—Various tactile, auditory, and visual stimuli also support the initiation of breathing.

The cardiovascular system begins transitioning after breathing has been initiated.

- The PO_2 rises in the alveoli after air enters the lungs, allowing blood to flow to the lungs as the pulmonary arteries relax and pulmonary vascular resistance falls.
- Blood flow to the extremities through the patent ductus arteriosus and foramen ovale is reduced as systemic vascular resistance increases. The ductus arteriosus and foramen ovale close within hours of birth. See Chapter 26 🗗 for more details of hemodynamic changes at birth.

Assessment at Birth

The initial newborn assessment focuses on the need for resuscitation. The Apgar score is used to determine the newborn's adaptation to extrauterine life at 1 and 5 minutes after birth. The heart rate, respiratory effort, muscle tone, grimace or irritability, and color are evaluated. The score for each physiologic response is 0, 1, or 2 according to criteria listed in Table 7–22. If the 1-minute score is low, health professionals implement aggressive resuscitation without waiting for a 5-minute score. Newborns with a 5-minute Apgar score less than 7 are at greater risk for morbidity and ongoing organ system dysfunction.

After the newborn is stable, a brief examination is conducted to identify the general condition of the cardiovascular, respiratory, neurologic, and gastrointestinal systems, as well as any congenital anomalies. With the newborn on a warming table, auscultate the heart and lungs and obtain the initial vital signs (temperature, heart rate, respiratory rate). Palpate the abdomen and examine the umbilical cord for the presence of three vessels. Inspect the head, face, oral cavity, extremities, genitalia, and perineum for the presence of any visible defects. Assess reactivity; the newborn's behavioral responses immediately after birth should be active and alert. The infant may appear hungry and have a strong sucking reflex. Bursts of random diffuse movements alternating with no movement may also be noted.

Practice Alert

Newborns have a large skin surface area and lose body heat quickly. They lose body heat in four ways:

- **Evaporation**—Water or liquid on the newborn's skin is converted to vapor and cools the newborn.
- **Convection**—Movement of cool air currents across the newborn's skin removes heat.
- **Radiation**—Body heat transfers to a cooler surface not in contact with the skin.
- **Conduction**—Body heat transfers to a cooler surface in contact with the skin.

Special care is provided to help the newborn conserve body heat. Immediately drying the infant after birth and moving the newborn to the mother's abdomen or a radiant warmer helps reduce heat loss at the time of birth. What measures are used to conserve the newborn's body temperature in the newborn nursery?

Assessment of the Newborn

A comprehensive newborn assessment, including a gestational age assessment, is conducted within the first few hours of birth to make sure the newborn's transition to extrauterine life is proceeding as expected or to identify specific problems that put the newborn at risk. The newborn assessment is repeated prior to discharge from the birthing facility. Most physical assessment techniques used for the newborn are the same as used for infants and children. Their application to the newborn, additional special procedures, and newborn findings are the focus of this section.

TABLE 7–22	The Apgar Scoring System		
	SCORE		
SIGN	**0**	**1**	**2**
Heart rate	Absent	Slow; less than 100 beats/min	Greater than 100 beats/min
Respiration	Absent	Slow, irregular	Good breathing with crying
Muscle tone	Flaccid	Some flexion of extremities	Active movement of extremities
Reflex irritability	Absent	Grimace; noticeable facial movement	Vigorous cry; coughs; sneezes; pulls away when touched
Skin color	Pale or blue	Pink body, blue extremities	Pink body and extremities

Source: Data from Apgar, V. (1966). *The newborn (Apgar) scoring system, reflections and advice.* http://profiles.nlm.nih.gov/ps/access/CPBBJY.pdf

Gestational Age Assessment

Gestational age assessment is performed on all newborns to assess the stage of newborn maturity and to determine the risk for conditions associated with prematurity or postmaturity. Knowledge of the birth weight and gestational age helps determine if a newborn had adequate growth in utero. Newborns found to be small (weight less than the 10th percentile) or large (weight greater than the 90th percentile) for gestational age are at risk for greater morbidity. For example, preterm infants may be large for gestational age but still experience the problems of prematurity, such as respiratory distress syndrome, temperature instability, and feeding problems. A higher birth weight is not always associated with increased maturity of the newborn. Conversely, a term or postterm newborn with a low birth weight may be at increased risk for respiratory distress, hypoglycemia, infection, and temperature instability. The preterm newborn's gestational age is also used to evaluate the infant's developmental progress during future health promotion visits.

Gestational age can be calculated counting the number of completed weeks between the first day of the mother's last menstrual period and the date of birth, if the mother's menstrual history is reliable. Prenatal ultrasound is also used to estimate gestational age. The Ballard Gestational Age Assessment provides an estimate of the newborn's gestational age after birth. Gestational ages of 37 to 41 completed weeks are considered to be full term. Infants born before 37 weeks of gestation are preterm. Infants born after 41 completed weeks of gestation are postterm.

The Ballard assessment evaluates six physical and six neuromuscular characteristics of newborn maturity, and it includes extreme preterm newborn characteristics. See Table 7–23 with Figures 7–57 through 7–69 ■ for the assessment guidelines and images of these

(Text continued on p. 218)

| TABLE 7–23 | Ballard Gestational Age Assessment Guidelines for Preterm Physical and Neuromuscular Characteristics |

CHARACTERISTICS AND ASSESSMENT GUIDELINES	EXAMPLES
Physical Characteristics	
Skin—Assess for thickness, transparency, and texture. The preterm infant's skin is thin and smooth, and has visible blood vessels. The extremely preterm infant has sticky, transparent skin. The term infant has thick skin that may have a flaky texture, and blood vessels are difficult to see.	See Figure 7–57 ■.
Lanugo—Assess for the quantity of **lanugo**, the fine, soft hair covering the fetus during intrauterine development. This hair begins to appear at approximately 19 to 20 weeks' gestation and is most prominent at 27 to 28 weeks' gestation. It is mostly shed by 37 weeks' gestation. It first begins to thin over the lower back, and then disappears last from the shoulders.	See Figure 7–58 ■.
Plantar surfaces—Assess the number of deep folds and creases over the sole of the foot. One to two creases appear at approximately 32 weeks' gestation. By 36 weeks' gestation, creases cover the anterior two thirds of the foot. At term, creases cover the entire foot. For extremely preterm infants, a measurement of the foot length from the tip of the great toe to the back of the heel is taken.	See Figure 7–59A and B ■.
Breast—Assess the chest for visibility of the nipple and areola. Then assess the size of the breast bud when grasped between the thumb and forefinger. The extremely preterm infant has no visible nipple and areola. The nipple and areola become more defined and raised by 34 weeks' gestation. A small breast bud appears by 36 weeks' gestation, and grows to 5 to 10 mm in term infants.	See Figure 7–60A and B ■.
Eye/ear—Assess eye opening and the formation of the ear cartilage and curving of the pinna. At earlier gestational ages the lack of cartilage allows the ear to fold easily and retain the fold. As gestational age increases, the resistance of the ear to folding increases and recoil is seen. In extremely preterm infants the pinnae are flat. Incurving proceeds from the top down toward the lobes with advancing gestational age. In extremely preterm infants the eyelids are examined with gentle flexion to determine the amount of fusion. Eye opening begins at 22 weeks, and lids are completely unfused by 28 weeks.	See Figure 7–61A and B ■.
Genitals (male)—Assess whether testicles are in the scrotum and presence of scrotal rugae. The testicles are in the inguinal canal around 28 weeks' gestation and scrotal rugae are becoming visible. By 36 weeks, the testicles are in the upper scrotum and rugae cover the anterior third of the scrotum. At term, rugae cover the scrotum, and at postterm the testicles are pendulous.	See Figure 7–62A and B ■.
Genitals (female)—Assess labial development. The clitoris is initially prominent and the labia minora are flat. By 36 weeks, the labia majora are larger and the clitoris is nearly covered.	See Figure 7–63A and B ■.
Neuromuscular Characteristics	
Posture—Assess the position the supine infant assumes at rest. The extremely preterm infant will lie with arms and legs extended or in any posture placed. With advancing gestational age, the infant has more flexion in the arms and legs. At term the infant lies with arms flexed to the chest, hands fisted, and legs flexed toward the abdomen.	See Figure 7–64A and B ■.
Square window—Assess the angle of the wrist when the palm is flexed toward the forearm. The preterm infant has poor flexion and is unable to flex the arm at the elbow more than 90 degrees. The extremely preterm infant has no flexor tone and cannot achieve a 90-degree angle. The term infant can achieve complete flexion against the forearm.	See Figure 7–65A and B ■.
Arm recoil—Assess the amount of elbow flexion as illustrated. Term infants resist extension and briskly return their arms to the flexed position. Very preterm infants do not resist extension. They respond with weak and delayed flexion in a small arc.	See Figure 7–66A and B ■.
Popliteal angle—Assess the angle of the knee in the supine infant, holding the pelvis flat as illustrated. Estimate the angle of the knee. The infant with more advanced gestational age has greater flexion.	See Figure 7–67 ■.
Scarf sign—Assess the infant's resistance to pulling the arm across the chest toward the opposite shoulder when in supine position. The term infant's elbow will not cross the midline of the chest. The infant's elbow moves closer to the opposite shoulder with decreasing gestational age.	See Figure 7–68A and B ■.
Heel-to-ear extension—Assess the amount of resistance to extension of the leg toward the ear without holding the knee or thigh in place. The infant's heel comes closer to the head with decreasing gestational age.	See Figure 7–69 ■.

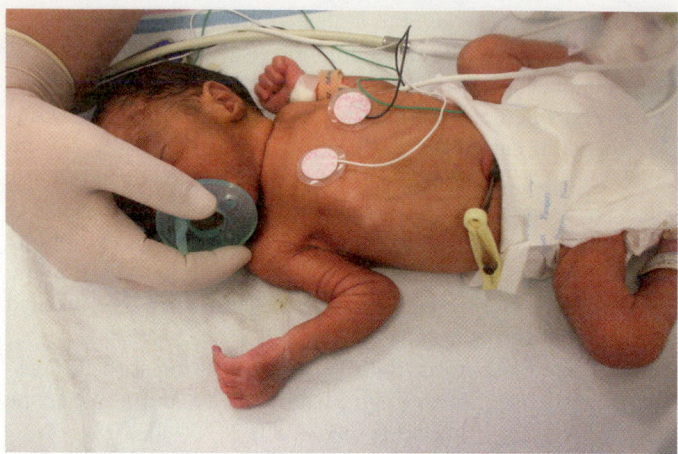

FIGURE 7–57 ■ Transparent skin with visible blood vessels on abdomen of a preterm infant.

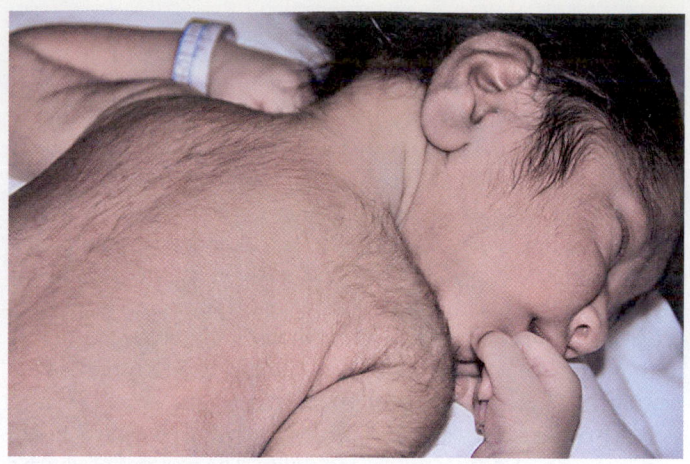

FIGURE 7–58 ■ Lanugo or fine body hair in a preterm infant.
Source: *Vanessa L. Howell, RNC, MSN.*

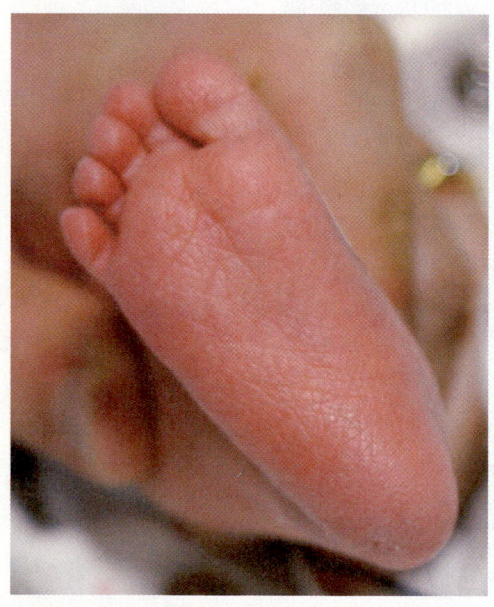

A

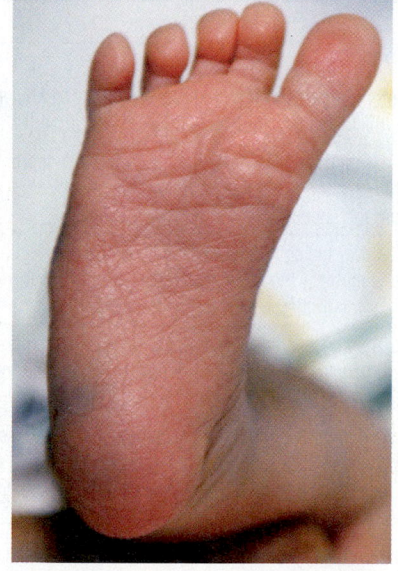

B

FIGURE 7–59 ■ Sole creases. *A,* At a gestational age of approximately 35 weeks, the newborn has few sole creases only on the anterior portion of the foot. *B,* At term, the newborn has deep creases down to and including the heel as the skin loses fluid and dries after birth.

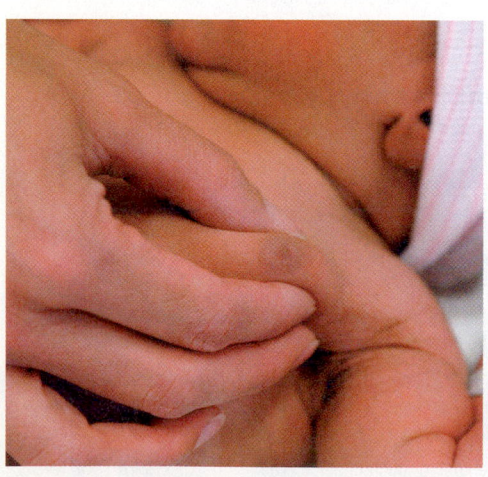

A

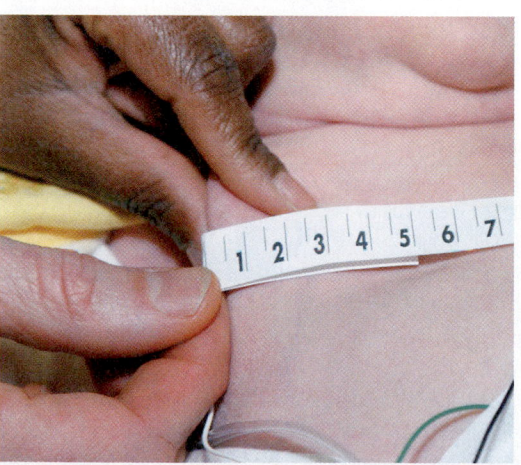

B

FIGURE 7–60 ■ Breast tissue. To assess breast tissue, gently compress the tissue between the middle and index fingers and measure the tissue in millimeters. *A,* At a gestational age of 38 weeks, the newborn has a visible raised area that is 4 mm in diameter on palpation. *B,* At a gestational age of 40 to 44 weeks, the newborn has 10 mm breast tissue.

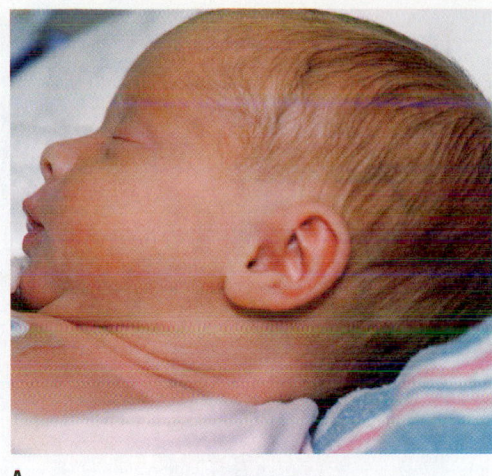
A

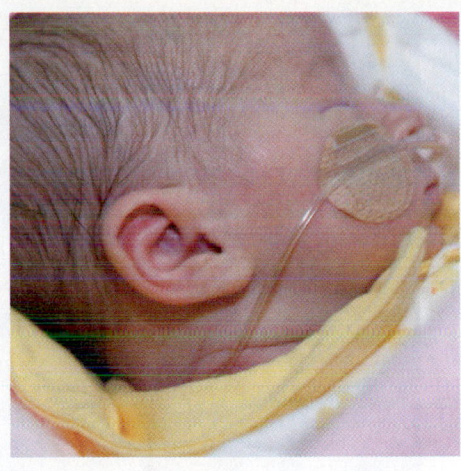
B

FIGURE 7–61 ■ Ear form and cartilage. Press the pinna over to see how quickly it returns to its original position. If it stays in the pressed position or returns slowly to the original position, the gestational age is usually less than 38 weeks. *A,* At a gestational age of approximately 36 weeks, the ear of the infant shows incurving of the upper two thirds of the pinna. *B,* At term, the ear of the infant shows well-defined incurving of the entire pinna.

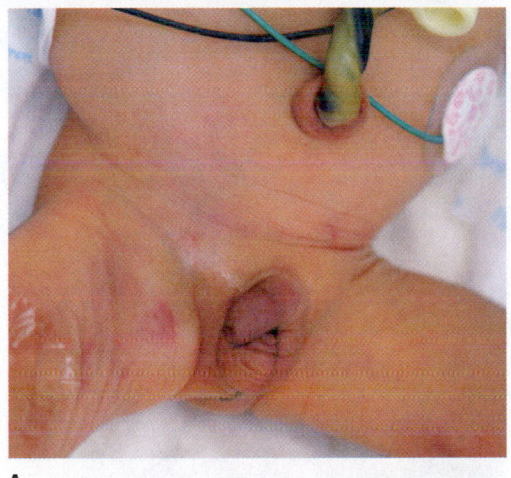
A

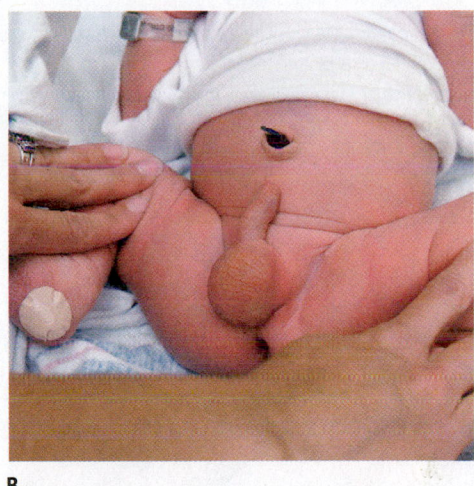
B

FIGURE 7–62 ■ Male genitals. *A,* Note the absence of the testicles in the scrotum, and a scrotum with few rugae in the preterm newborn. *B,* In the term newborn, the testicles are usually descended into the scrotum, and the scrotum is covered by rugae.

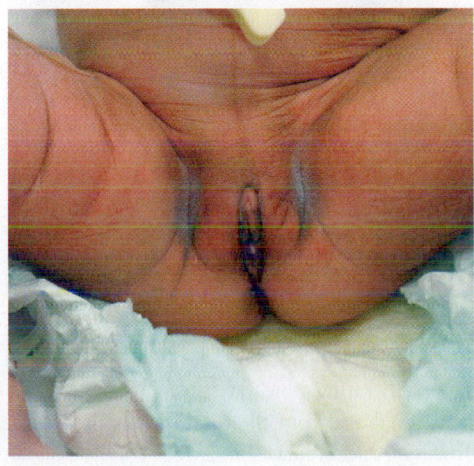
A

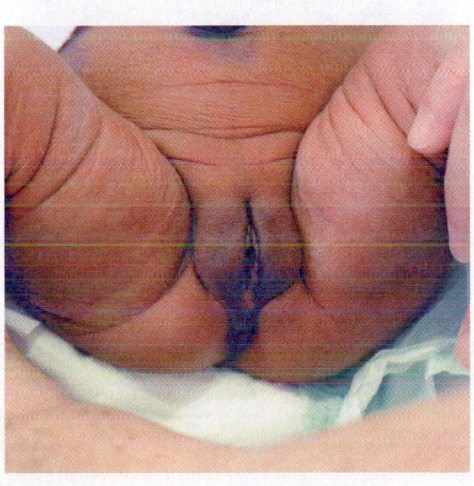
B

FIGURE 7–63 ■ Female genitals. *A,* At a gestational age of 30 to 36 weeks, the newborn has a prominent clitoris, widely separated labia majora, and labia minora protruding beyond the labia majora (when viewed laterally). *B,* At term, the labia majora are well developed and cover both the clitoris and labia minora.

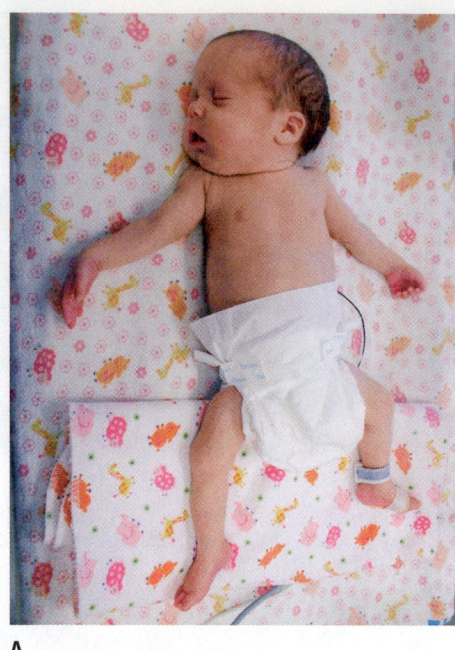
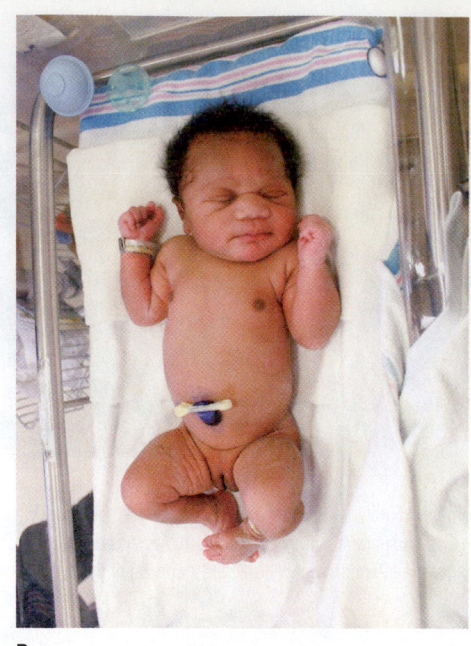

A   **B**

FIGURE 7–64 ■ Resting posture. *A,* At a gestational age of approximately 31 weeks, there is extension of the upper extremities and beginning flexion of the thighs. *B,* At term, the newborn exhibits hypertonic flexion of all extremities.

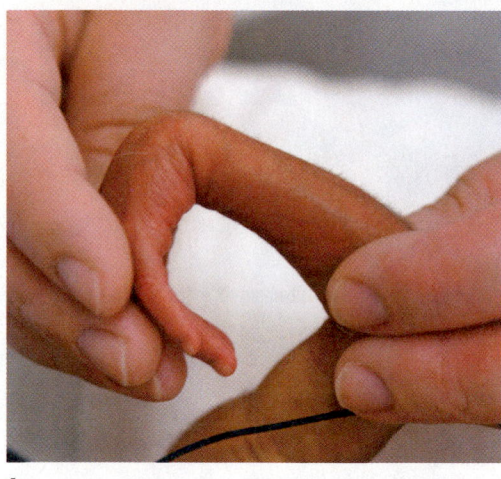
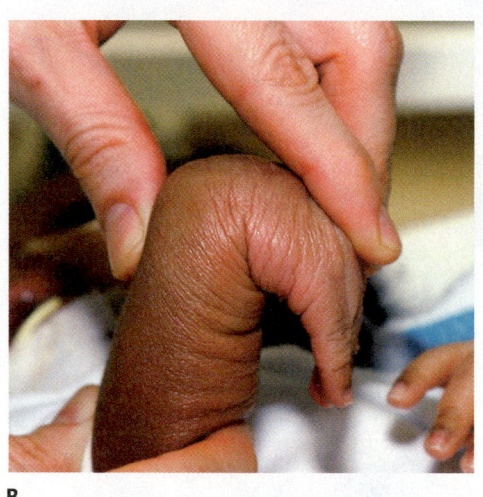

A   **B**

FIGURE 7–65 ■ Square window sign. *A,* At approximately 28 to 32 weeks' gestation, the angle is 90 degrees. *B,* At a gestational age of approximately 39 to 40 weeks, the angle is commonly 30 degrees.

Weblink | Ballard Assessment Tool

physical and neuromuscular characteristics. The score for each of the 6 physical and 6 neuromuscular characteristic ranges from –1 to 4 or 5. Newborns do not necessarily have consistent scores for each characteristic as maturity of different characteristics may vary in that newborn. Once the scoring for each characteristic is completed, the scores are added together. The minimum score with this tool is –10, corresponding to a gestational age of 20 weeks. The maximum score is 50, corresponding to a gestational age of 44 weeks. The Ballard tool has a maturity rating table that is used to identify the newborn's estimated gestational age from the total score. The findings of the assessment process are accurate within 2 weeks of the assigned gestational age. The Ballard assessment is usually performed within the first 48 hours of life.

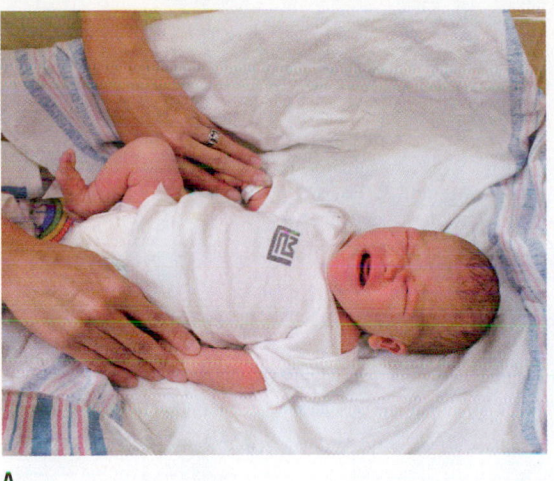
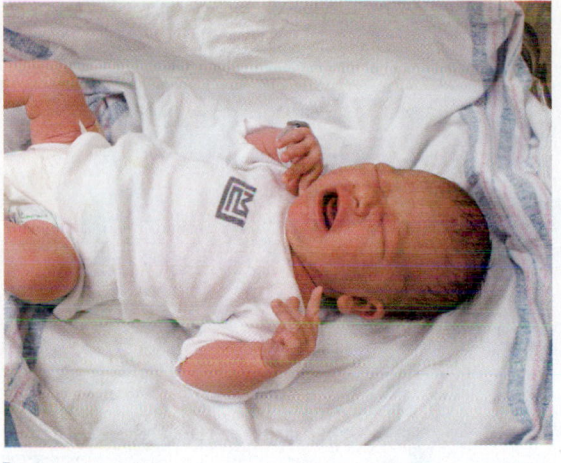

A   **B**

FIGURE 7–66 ■ Elicit the arm recoil by flexing the arms at the elbows to the chest for 5 seconds. *A*, Then extend the arms at the elbows. *B*, Release the arms to see the amount of recoil. In healthy newborns, the angle of flexion is usually less than 90 degrees followed by rapid recoil to the flexed position.

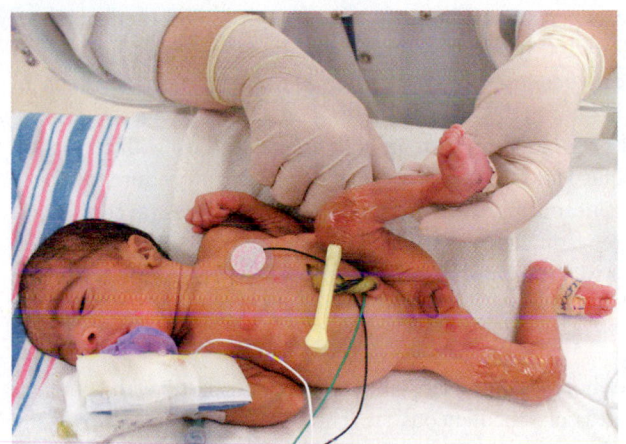

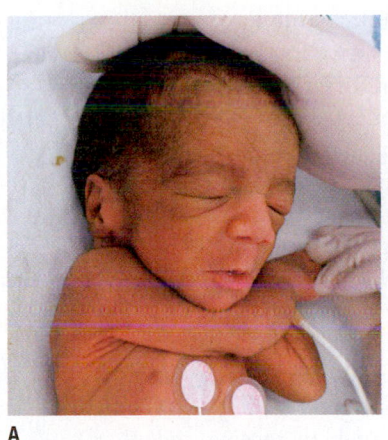
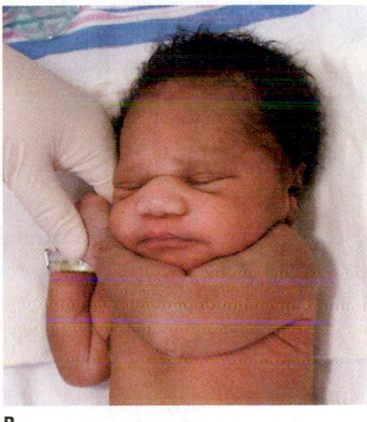

A   **B**

FIGURE 7–67 ■ To assess the popliteal angle, flex and hold the thigh to the abdomen while extending the leg at the knee.

FIGURE 7–68 ■ Scarf sign. *A*, Until approximately 30 weeks' gestation, the elbow moves past midline with no resistance. *B*, The elbow will not reach midline after 40 weeks' gestation.

Size for Gestational Age

Once the gestational age is assessed, a standardized intrauterine growth curve is used to plot the newborn's anthropometric measurements (birth weight) for the gestational age. See Appendix A, Figure A–1 ⊘. Small-for-gestational-age infants fall below the 10th percentile. Appropriate-for-gestational-age infants fall between the 10th and 90th percentiles. Large-for-gestational-age infants fall above the 90th percentile. See Appendix A ⊘, Figure A–2 for a growth curve for preterm infants.

Length is also measured, but it is difficult to obtain a reliable measurement because of the natural flexion of the newborn and molding of the head. One method of length measurement is to place the infant on his or her back with the legs extended as far as possible. Place the top of the measuring tape at the top of the head and stretch the tape to the heel of the foot as shown in Figure 7–70 ■. Each facility establishes guidelines for a consistent length measurement technique to increase the reliability between examiners. Verify the accuracy of the length with a second measurement. Plot the newborn's length on the gestational age growth curve in Appendix A ⊘.

Head circumference is measured as described on page 172 and is contrasted to the chest circumference. The head circumference is generally 2 cm larger than the chest circumference. Plot the head circumference on the gestational age growth curve in Appendix A ⊘.

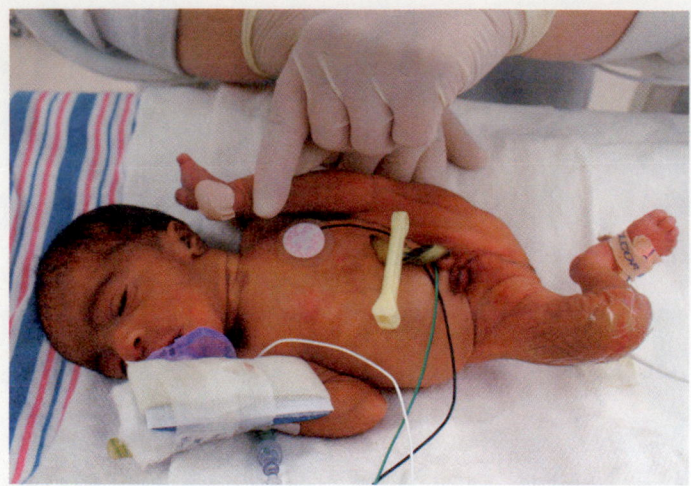

FIGURE 7–69 ■ Heel-to-ear scoring. Move the infant's foot as near to the head or ear as possible and determine the distance between the heel and head.

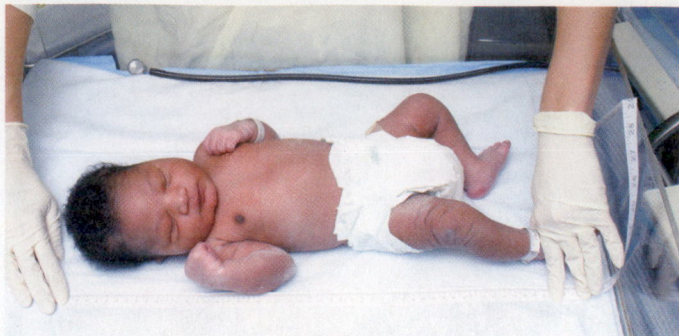

FIGURE 7–70 ■ Measuring the length of the newborn.

General Appearance

Observe the newborn's general appearance, body proportions, posture, and movements. The newborn's head is about one fourth of the total body size. The body appears long with short extremities due to their flexed position. Full-term newborns generally lie in a symmetric position with the limbs semiflexed similar to their position in utero. The legs are partially abducted at the hip. The chest appears rounded and the abdomen appears prominent. The head is slightly flexed and positioned in midline or turned to one side. The hands are held in a tight fist, but fingers may occasionally be extended. Infants of breech birth have the legs and head extended. In frank breech, the legs are abducted and externally rotated, and the feet may be dorsiflexed.

The newborn typically has a second phase of reactivity lasting 4 to 6 hours that occurs following a short sleep phase. The newborn is awake and alert, making this a good time to assess motor and neurologic responses such as sucking, rooting, and other primitive reflexes. Spontaneous motor activity with flexion and extension alternating between the arms and legs is common. Tremors of the arms, legs, and body may be seen with vigorous crying or at rest for the first 48 hours. Be alert for asymmetric movements as they may indicate birth injuries, congenital anomalies, or a neurologic problem.

Listen to the quality of the newborn's cry; it should be strong, lusty, and of medium pitch. A high-pitched cry with a shrill quality may indicate hypoglycemia or a neurologic condition. **Grunting,** a sound produced by the rapid release of air at the end of expiration, with respirations indicates respiratory distress.

Vital Signs

Regular temperature measurements are important because newborns are at risk for heat loss and are unable to stabilize their temperature in the first few hours after birth. Temperature is taken by an axillary thermometer or thermal skin sensor. Axillary temperatures range from 36.4° to 37.2°C (97.5° to 99.0°F).

Count the respiratory rate for a full minute when the newborn is sleeping or resting quietly. Use a stethoscope on the chest or place your hand over the abdomen. The respiratory rate may range between 30 and 55 breaths per minute. *Periodic breathing*, vigorous breathing followed by apnea lasting less than 20 seconds, is common in term infants for a few days after birth. No skin color or heart rate changes should accompany these episodes.

Count the heart rate with the stethoscope over the apical impulse for a full minute. The heart rate may range between 100 and 180 beats per minute immediately after birth, and then stabilizes to 120 to 160 beats per minute. The heart rate may increase to 180 beats per minute with crying. Wider variations are seen in preterm infants.

Take the blood pressure in both an arm and leg with a Doppler technique. Hold the extremity used during the procedure to reduce movement and improve the accuracy of the reading. An average blood pressure reading is 60/40 to 80/45 mmHg at birth for a term infant. Alternatively, the mean arterial pressure (MAP) is reported from the Doppler machine.

Skin

The newborn's skin is thin, smooth, soft, and elastic with some defined areas of subcutaneous fat. The baby's skin dimples over the joints. The feet and hands may have peeling. Lanugo may be seen, depending on the newborn's gestational age. *Vernix*, the greasy yellow or white substance produced from sebaceous gland secretions, lanugo, and shed skin cells, is often found in the skinfolds. Leathery skin with deep creases is seen in postterm newborns.

Assess the newborn for signs of skin disruptions related to the birth process such as forceps marks, site where the internal fetal monitor was attached, or lacerations sustained during the birth process.

The newborn's skin has a ruddy flush for the first 24 hours due to vasomotor instability. It gradually fades to its normal color. Black newborns initially have lighter toned skin than their parents because the pigment function is not yet in full production. The full melanotic color is seen in the nail cuticles and scrotal folds. Bruising over the buttocks of a breech presentation or over the eyes and forehead of a facial presentation may be seen. Identify and record the color, location, and size of all birthmarks, including the hyperpigmented macule (Mongolian spot). See Table 7–24 for common transient skin color changes in newborns that rarely indicate a pathologic condition.

TABLE 7–24	Transient Color Variations in Newborns

COLOR CHANGE	DESCRIPTION
Harlequin	A unilateral erythema on the dependent half of the body and pallor on the other half with a distinct demarcation line down the middle when the newborn is in a side-lying position. The transient color change occurs in up to 10% of newborns and has no pathologic significance (O'Connor, McLaughlin, & Ham, 2008).
Acrocyanosis	A bluish color around the lips, hands, fingernails, feet, and toenails may occur, lasting a few hours and disappearing without warning.
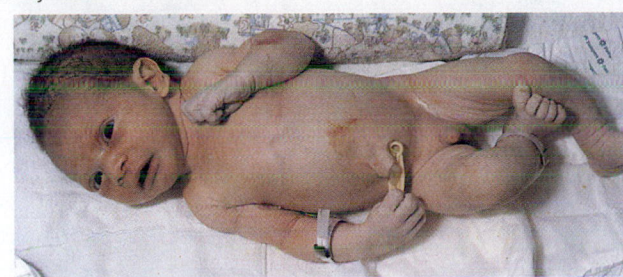	
Cutis marmorata (mottling)	Transient mottling that surrounds the trunk and extremities in response to cooler room temperatures. It persists or is more pronounced in preterm infants.
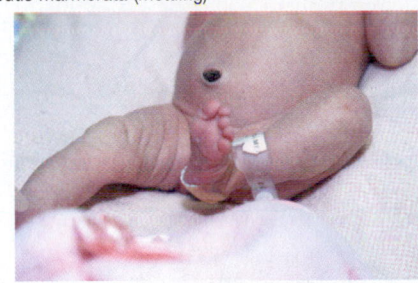	

The following color changes in the newborn are unexpected and cause for concern:

- **Jaundice**—press the tip of the nose, forehead, or sternum to blanch the skin. A yellowish color of the blanched skin indicates the presence of jaundice. Jaundice appearing within 24 hours of birth may indicate hemolytic disease due to blood incompatibility. Jaundice may also be associated with the hemolysis of red blood cells from hematomas, bruises from forceps, or immature liver function. Jaundice appearing after 2 weeks of age may indicate biliary tract obstruction.
- **Meconium staining**—green-brown discoloration of the skin, nails, and cord may indicate fetal distress.
- **Cyanosis or pallor**—may indicate a respiratory or cardiac problem, cold stress, central nervous system damage, loss of blood volume, or infection.

Skin alterations that may be seen in newborns include the following:

- Milia, tiny white papules on the face, are due to occlusion of the hair follicles by sebum (Figure 7–71A ■).
- Erythema toxicum is a common rash (tiny red macules and papules on the cheeks, trunk, back, and buttocks) that appears in the first 3 to 4 days of life (Figure 7–71B ■).
- Storkbite or salmon patch, a vascular marking or common birthmark, is a flat irregularly shaped red or pink patch found on the back of the neck, forehead, eyelid, or upper lip. The mark fades by about 1 year of age.
- Hemangiomas include nevus flammeus (port-wine stain), nevus vasculosus (strawberry hemangioma), and cavernous hemangioma. See Chapter 36 🔗.
- Petechiae on the head and neck may be associated with a breech presentation or a cord around the neck.

Head

Inspect the contour of the head from all angles. A **caput succedaneum,** an edematous swelling and ecchymosis over the presenting part of the head, may be noted in newborns with vaginal delivery (Figure 7–72 ■). It feels soft and may extend across suture lines. It resolves over the first few days of life without treatment. A **cephalhematoma** is a subperiosteal hemorrhage resulting from birth trauma. It may take months to resolve. It is a soft, fluctuant elevation without discoloration that is well defined over one cranial bone (Figure 7–73 ■). **Molding,** an overriding of the cranial bones to accommodate the head's passage through the vaginal canal, may be noted in newborns with vaginal delivery and in those who experienced a long labor prior to cesarean birth. Molding resolves after a few days.

Palpate the head for suture lines. Suture lines may feel more like ridges and be more prominent if molding has occurred. Palpate the fontanels. The anterior fontanel is generally diamond shaped and 3 to 4 cm long by 2 to 3 cm wide. The posterior fontanel is 1 to 2 cm

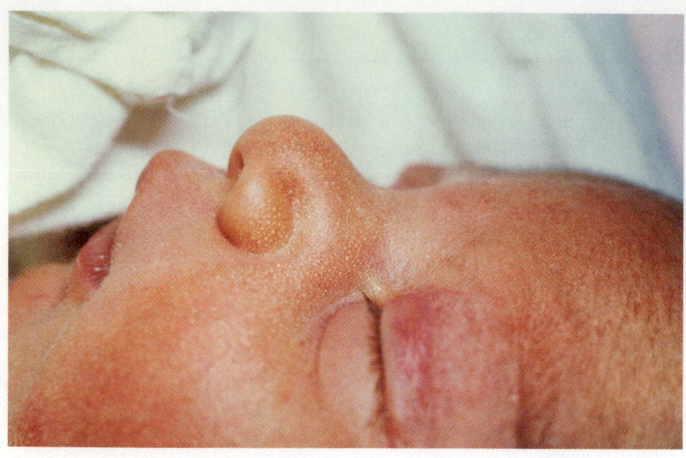

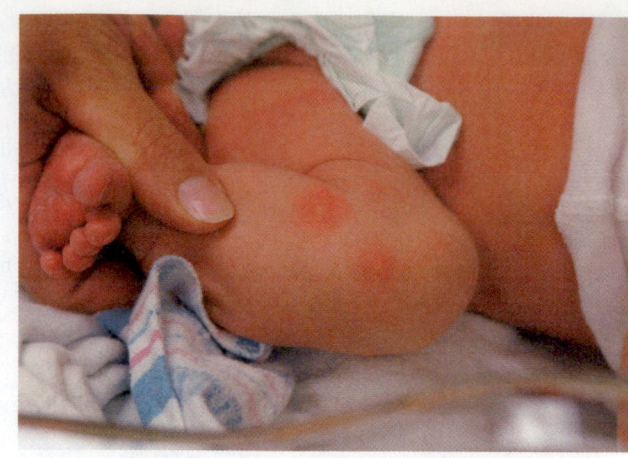

A   **B**

FIGURE 7–71 ■ *A*, Milia. *B*, Erythema toxicum.

Source: *Biophoto Associates/Science Source. B, Saiman, L. (2009). Endocarditis and intravascular infections. In S. S. Long, L. K. Pickering, & C. G. Prober, Principles and practice of pediatric infectious diseases (3rd ed., pp. 269-277), New York: Elsevier Churchill Livingstone; McDonald, J. R. (2009). Acute infectious endocarditis, Infectious Disease Clinics of North America, 23, 642-664; American Heart Association, Baddour, L. M., Wilson, W. R., Bayer, A. S., Fowler, V. G., Bolger, A. F., et al. (2005). Infective endocarditis: Diagnosis, antimicrobial therapy, and management of complications. Circulation, 111, e394-e433.*

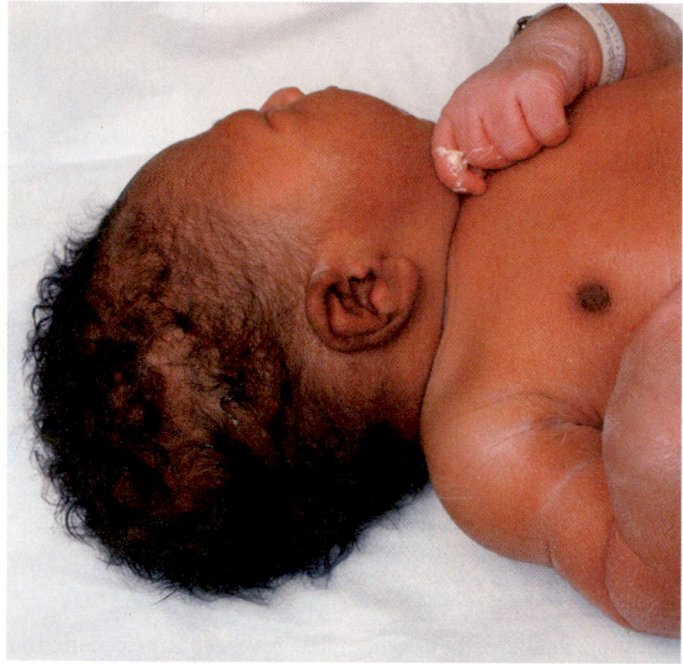

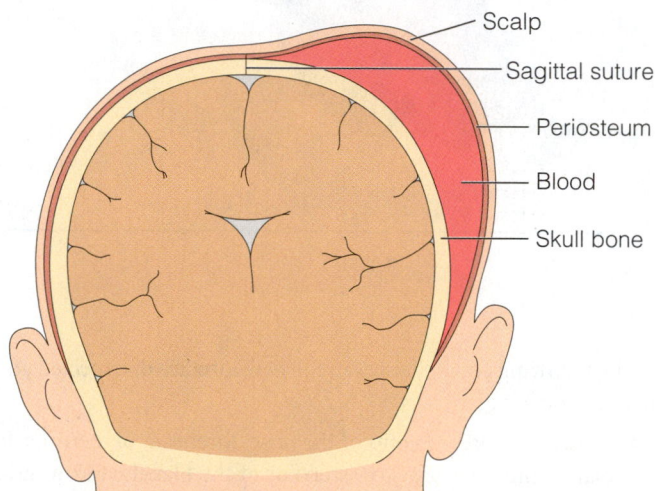

FIGURE 7–72 ■ Caput succedaneum. Following vaginal birth, some newborns develop swelling and a collection of serous fluid in the scalp due to birth trauma. The swelling often crosses the suture lines.

and triangular. A mild pulsation may be palpated over the anterior fontanel. Note the quality and distribution of hair.

Note the features of the face for spacing and symmetry of facial expression at rest and when crying. Asymmetry of facial features may indicate injury to the fifth cranial nerve.

Eyes

The eyes should be clear and have no swelling or discharge. The eyes may be irritated by the prophylactic antibiotics used to prevent ophthalmia neonatorum, but no discharge should be present. A purulent discharge may be due to a bacterial or viral infection acquired during birth.

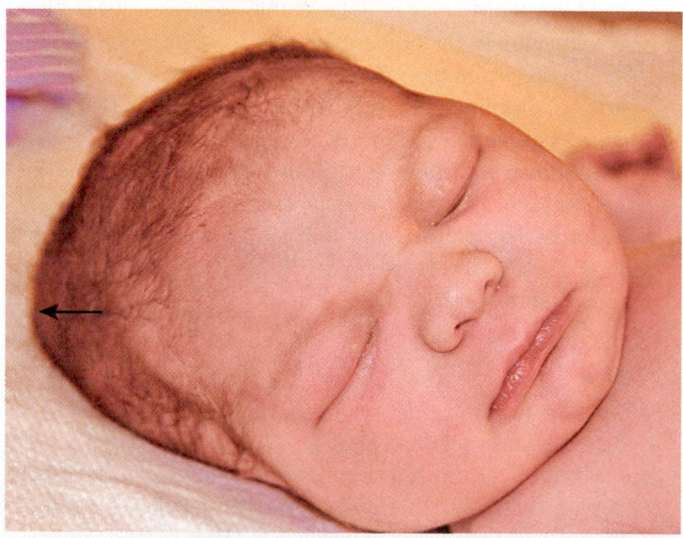

FIGURE 7–73 ■ Cephalhematoma. Following vaginal birth, some newborns develop a collection of blood between the surface of the cranial bone and the periosteal membrane due to birth trauma. The swelling is usually confined to one cranial bone and does not cross the suture lines.

Source: *Vanessa L. Howell, RNC, MSN.*

Use the ophthalmoscope to check for a red reflex or lens opacities bilaterally. The newborn's response to bright light should be a blink reflex. Dim the lights or rock the newborn from upright to horizontal position so that the infant opens the eyes, and then check the pupillary response to light.

The iris of the eyes should be evenly colored. The sclerae should appear white and clear, but they may have a slight bluish tint due to their thinness. Subconjunctival hemorrhage may be present. No tears are generally seen when the newborn cries.

Vision is present and can be noted by the newborn's fixation on high-contrast geometric shapes or a face that is held 8 to 12 inches from the eyes. Term newborn vision is 20/200. The eyes should track a moving object to the midline; however, a slight nystagmus may be seen.

A doll's eye phenomenon is an expected response within the first 10 days after birth. Hold the infant upright and as the head is moved from left to right, the eyes move in the opposite direction. This response disappears as head–eye coordination develops.

Ears

Inspect the pinna for position and any lesions. Note any preauricular skin tags. Inspect the ears for the presence of an auditory canal. Otoscopic examination is rarely performed because the canals are filled with vernix and other substances. Hearing is present after mucus from the middle ear is absorbed and the eustachian tube is aerated. For a gross hearing assessment, note whether the infant awakens to loud noises or responds to sudden sounds with the Moro reflex.

Nose

Inspect the external nose that may appear flattened during the birth process. To assess for nasal patency, gently close the newborn's mouth. Occlude one naris at a time and observe the baby's chest rise with inspiration. Newborns who become distressed with an occluded naris may have choanal atresia, an obstructed nasal passage. The presence of choanal atresia is confirmed by the inability to insert a small feeding tube from the naris into the hypopharynx. Choanal atresia may be unilateral or bilateral.

Observe for any flaring of the nares with respiration, a sign of respiratory distress. The newborn can smell after the nose is cleared of mucus and amniotic fluid, as noted by the search for milk.

Mouth

Inspect the mouth for any defects. The hard palate should be dome shaped and the uvula should be midline. Sucking pads should be present. The tongue should move freely and be proportionately sized for the mouth. Observe the newborn for coordinated sucking and swallowing. Using a gloved finger, palpate the hard and soft palate to detect any clefts.

Findings noted in the mouth include *Epstein pearls*, small white cysts containing keratin that feel hard to the touch. Occasionally a tooth may be noted. Inclusion cysts, gray-white lesions on the gums, may look like teeth.

Neck

Note the position of the head. The head should be positioned midline. The neck is generally short and creased with skinfolds. The neck is not strong enough at birth to fully support the head. Generally, the newborn can raise the head slightly when in the prone position, but head lag is seen when the newborn is raised from supine to sitting position.

Move the newborn's head through a full range of motion. Limitation in movement may be associated with torticollis or a wry neck, resulting from injury to the sternocleidomastoid muscle during birth or due to a congenital defect. Palpate the neck to verify that the trachea is in the midline position. Assess the thyroid for any enlargement, and palpate the neck for masses. Note any webbing or extra folds of skin on the posterior neck that could be associated with Turner syndrome.

Palpate the entire length of the clavicles to detect any sign of a fracture, such as a ridge or mass over a clavicle or crepitus. If a fracture is present, the newborn will have limited range of motion of the arm on that side.

Chest and Lungs

The newborn has a rounded thorax with equal anteroposterior-to-transverse chest diameter. The xiphoid cartilage may appear to protrude because of the thinness of the tissue covering the chest. Observe for any unexpected shapes in the chest such as protrusion or depression of the sternum. The newborn's chest circumference ranges between 30 and 36 cm and is 2 cm smaller than the head circumference.

Breasts may be enlarged and visible in both males and females because of exposure to maternal hormones crossing the placenta. For a few days after birth, the breasts may also secrete a clear or white fluid, known as "witch's milk."

Observe the newborn's chest for respiratory effort. Chest movement should be symmetric and no retractions should be present. During rapid eye movement sleep, periods of apnea lasting less than 20 seconds are common. In cases of respiratory distress, retractions are an indication of accessory muscle use to inflate stiff, noncompliant lungs. If retractions are noted, determine if they are minimal (subcostal) or marked (suprasternal and intercostal). Paradoxical or seesaw respirations, when the chest flattens as the abdomen bulges on inspiration, are a sign of respiratory distress.

Auscultate the anterior and posterior chest for breath sounds with an infant stethoscope. Breath sounds may be louder than in older children, and they are transmitted over the entire chest wall due to thin chest tissue. Localizing breath sounds will be difficult, but auscultated adventitious sounds should be further evaluated. Grunting is a mechanism used by newborns in respiratory distress to prevent atelectasis. The newborn exhales against a closed glottis to increase transpulmonary pressure, producing the sound. Indicate if grunting is heard with or without a stethoscope. Audible grunting without a stethoscope is indicative of greater respiratory distress.

Heart

Locate the apical impulse to identify the placement of the heart in the chest. It should be located in the left side with the point of maximum intensity in the fourth intercostal space along the left midaxillary line a few hours after birth. Listen to the heart tones to ensure their appropriate location in the chest. Sounds heard nearer to the mediastinum or in the right side of the chest may indicate dextrocardia, diaphragmatic hernia, or a pneumothorax.

The transition from fetal to pulmonic circulation occurs in the immediate newborn period. See Chapter 26 🔗 for illustrations and explanation. Fetal shunts (ductus arteriosus and atrial septal defect) normally close within 10 to 15 hours, but may take up to 48 hours. Assess the heart sounds several times during the first 48 to 72 hours of life. Soft systolic murmurs (grade 1 to 2), such as the low-pitched, continuous flow musical murmur of the patent ductus arteriosus, are relatively common in the first 2 to 3 days with the closure of the fetal shunts. Other significant murmurs may also be heard and need further evaluation. See pages 193–196 for characteristics of murmurs and the assessment of the cardiovascular system in infants.

Palpate the peripheral pulses at the brachial, femoral, and pedal sites. Compare the strength and quality of the brachial pulses with the femoral pulses. Weak femoral pulses may indicate coarctation of the aorta. Note other unusual characteristics with regard to pulsations and quality.

Abdomen

Observe the abdomen while the newborn is quiet. Abdominal movement is synchronous with chest movement. The abdomen should appear rounded and slightly protruding. The abdominal muscles may appear relaxed. Note diastasis recti or the presence of an umbilical hernia. Few if any blood vessels should be seen. If distention is present or develops, be suspicious of a gastrointestinal congenital anomaly. If the abdomen is scaphoid or hollow, be concerned about the presence of a diaphragmatic hernia when the abdominal contents are located in the chest cavity.

Auscultate the abdomen for bowel sounds that are present shortly after birth. Absent bowel sounds may indicate a bowel obstruction.

The umbilical cord should be clamped. Inspect the umbilical cord for the presence of two arteries and one vein. At birth these blood vessels are surrounded by mucoid connective tissue called Wharton's jelly. The stump dries quickly and is shriveled and blackened by the third day. See the Clinical Manifestations table for various findings associated with the umbilical cord.

Palpate the abdomen for softness, tenderness, and the presence of masses. Feel the liver edge, the spleen tip, both kidneys, and the bladder.

Genitalia and Anus

In females, inspect the external genitalia and compare to expected size for the newborn's gestational age. A thick white mucoid or blood-tinged vaginal discharge is commonly observed because of the withdrawal of maternal hormones. A hymenal tag is noted in some female newborns.

In males, inspect the penis and palpate the scrotum for the presence of the testes as described on page 201. Note the size of the penis and the location of the urethral meatus. Carefully inspect the external genitalia for signs of ambiguous genitalia. The urine stream should be forceful and straight.

Inspect the anus to ensure that it is patent and that no fissures are present. Observe stool passage to make sure the anus is patent and that the stool passed through the anal opening. Passage of greenish black meconium, the newborn's first stool, should occur within the first 24 hours. When passage of meconium is delayed, a lubricated catheter may be inserted 1 cm (0.5 in.) into the anus. Resistance in passage of the catheter may indicate an obstruction. The stool transitions by the fourth day to a more yellow to yellow-brown pasty or firm consistency.

Lightly stroke the anal area to elicit the anal wink reflex. Constriction of the sphincter indicates good muscle strength.

Extremities

Inspect the arms and legs for any deformities in shape or position. Compare the length and skinfolds of arms and legs to detect differences that could indicate a potential problem. Inspect the hands and feet for extra digits (polydactyly), webbing (syndactyly), and creases. The hands are typically held in fisted position, but will open periodically.

Many newborns have a flexible forefoot inversion (metatarsus adductus) that results from uterine positioning. Any fixed deformity is abnormal. Move the feet toward midline position to identify any

---

Clinical Manifestations Findings Associated with the Umbilical Cord

CLINICAL MANIFESTATION	ETIOLOGY	CLINICAL THERAPY
Bleeding from the cord	Cord clamp is loose or the cord has been pulled	Control bleeding with pressure and tighten or replace the cord clamp.
One artery (two-vessel cord)	Associated with congenital anomalies	Carefully examine the newborn for congenital anomalies such as trisomy 18.
Redness surrounding the cord and spreading to the abdomen; discharge and odor	Infection	Administer antibiotic therapy and monitor for signs of worsening infection.
Draining urine or moistness at the base of the cord	Patent urachus, abnormal connection between the bladder and the umbilicus	Surgery to remove the fistula. Monitor for urinary tract infection.
Serous or serosanguineous drainage after the cord falls off	Granuloma	Clean with alcohol several times a day. Cauterize granuloma with silver nitrate.

positional deformities such as clubfoot or metatarsus adductus. See Chapter 35 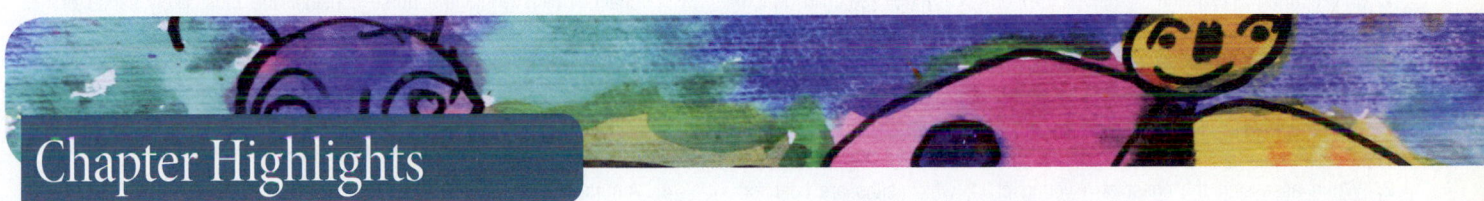.

Note any problems with movement of the extremities. Paralysis of the arm may be associated with a difficult birth and injury to the brachial plexus (Erb-Duchenne paralysis or Erb's palsy).

Note any asymmetry in skin creases on the legs. Check the hips for dislocation with the Ortolani-Barlow maneuver as described on page 206.

Inspect the spine for a dimple, cyst, mass, hemangioma, or tuft of hair in the midline that might indicate an underlying condition such as spina bifida, meningocele, or a dermoid sinus. A hemangioma in the midline lumbosacral area of 2.5 cm (1 in.) in diameter is associated with a spinal abnormality (Drolet, Chamlin, Garzon, et al., 2010). Palpate each vertebra of the spine to assess uniformity in shape. Assess the range of motion of the spine.

Assess muscle tone by observing the resting posture. The position is generally a symmetric flexed posture with extremities folded inward, hips slightly abducted, and fists flexed. Move all the extremities to determine the range of motion and resistance to extending the knee and elbow joints. The newborn should be slightly hypertonic and resist full extension of the legs and arms at the knees and elbows. See Table 7–25 for abnormal postures of the newborn. Limpness or flaccidity is abnormal in a full-term newborn and may indicate a central nervous system disorder.

Assess head control and upper body strength by pulling the supine newborn a few inches off the mattress by holding the arms. Hold the arms carefully so the newborn does not fall back suddenly. The newborn holds the head in the same plane as the body with minimal head lag. When the baby is held in a prone position with one hand under the chest, the newborn holds the head at an angle of 45 degrees or less from horizontal when the back is straight or slightly flexed. Lower body strength can be tested with the stepping primitive reflex (see page 211).

Neurologic System

The newborn should appear alert with eyes open after swelling subsides. A strong suck and coordinated swallow should be noted.

Occasional spontaneous, brief jerky or twitching tremors are common. Prolonged or repeated tremors may be caused by hypoglycemia, hypocalcemia, nicotine withdrawal, or opiate withdrawal.

TABLE 7–25	Abnormal Postures of the Newborn
POSTURE	**DESCRIPTION**
Frog position	Hips abducted and externally rotated, nearly flat against the table; seen after a breech delivery
Opisthotonos	Head arched back, stiff neck, arms and legs extended; seen with meningeal or brainstem irritation and kernicterus
Extended limbs	Intracranial hemorrhage
Continuous asymmetry	Brachial plexus palsy of upper extremity

Signs of seizures may be subtle, such as chewing or swallowing movements, lip smacking, deviations of the eyes, rigidity or flaccidity, or bicycling movement of the legs.

Clinical Tip
To help distinguish between a seizure and a tremor, gently hold the newborn's extremity in your hand. If the held extremity stops moving, the baby is jittery. If the extremity continues to shake, the newborn is more likely to be having a seizure.

Newborns have protective reflexes that may be observed during the assessment: blink, yawn, sucking, cough, sneeze, and withdrawal from pain. Yawns often indicate the newborn has been overstimulated. Sneezing helps clear nasal passages. Assessment of the central nervous system can be performed with the following steps:

- Insert a gloved finger in the mouth to elicit the sucking reflex.
- When the newborn is sucking vigorously, note a change in sucking when exposed to a light, rattle, and voice. A brief cessation of sucking is followed by continuous sucking with repetitious stimulation (Ladewig, London, & Davidson, 2010, p. 615).

Primitive reflexes are also used to assess the neurologic development of the newborn. See Table 7–19 for techniques to assess primitive reflexes and the expected findings.

At the conclusion of the assessment, carefully review the findings to determine if any cluster of findings indicates a particular health condition or to determine if the newborn is adapting as expected to extrauterine life.

Chapter Highlights

- Establish a rapport with the family and use careful listening techniques to collect historical information about the child's health status.
- Collection of historical data includes the chief complaint, history of the present illness or injury, past history, current health status, review of systems, and family history. In addition, psychosocial and developmental data are collected.

- The physical examination sequence includes assessment of the following:
  - Skin and hair
  - Head, eyes, ears, nose, and mouth structures and function
  - Neck
  - Chest and lungs
  - Breasts

- Heart and pulses
- Abdomen
- Inguinal area
- Genitalia and perineal areas
- Musculoskeletal system
- Nervous system
- Assessment sequences vary by the age of the child and the child's cooperation with the procedures.
- Clinical judgment is used to identify common patterns of physiologic responses associated with medical conditions.

- The physiologic responses and family and child responses to health conditions become the basis for many nursing diagnoses.
- The initial newborn assessment at the time of birth includes the Apgar score to identify the need for immediate resuscitation.
- The comprehensive newborn assessment, including a gestational age assessment, is conducted within the first days of birth to make sure the newborn's transition to extrauterine life is proceeding as expected and to identify any specific problems that put the newborn at risk.
- Knowledge of the birth weight and gestational age helps to determine if newborns are large, appropriate, or small for gestational age and potentially at risk for morbidity.

Clinical Reasoning in Action

INTRODUCTION

Return to the opening scenario involving Jasmine, who is 27 months old and has been adopted by the Porter family. She appears well nourished. Her weight is 10.2 kg, her height is 81 cm, and her head circumference is 47 cm.

DESCRIPTION

Jasmine has been with the Porter family for the past 3 weeks and has slowly been developing a relationship with family members. She seems to enjoy playing with her 6-year-old sister Monique. She has exhibited clinging behavior to Mrs. Porter since she left the adoption center in China. She eats small portions of food 4 to 5 times a day, generally feeding herself using her fingers, and she is able to walk and climb without difficulty. Jasmine has learned a few single words of English, mostly names and some foods.

DISCUSSION

When Jasmine was seen in the international adoption clinic, a complete physical assessment was performed. Jasmine sat quietly on Mrs. Porter's lap during the history taking. When the nurse attempted to interest Jasmine in a toy, she refused to take the toy and moved closer to Mrs. Porter. The nurse continued to work to gain Jasmine's trust. She demonstrated the use of some of the equipment on Monique. During the examination Jasmine cried frequently. After about 5 minutes Jasmine stopped crying and cooperated with some portions of the examination. A thorough physical assessment of Jasmine has revealed fever and signs of an acute otitis media.

1. What behaviors would you look for that might indicate that Jasmine is beginning to develop a relationship with Mrs. Porter and Monique?

2. What actions could you take during the physical examination to develop a rapport with Jasmine and to reduce her anxiety?

3. List the information that should be collected during a history of the present illness related to Mrs. Porter's concern about an ear infection.

4. What are the physical findings of an ear infection? How would you determine if Jasmine has an ear infection since she cried during the examination?

5. What is your interpretation of Jasmine's current growth status?

6. Complete the nursing assessment and develop two nursing diagnoses related to her physical condition.

NCLEX-RN® Review

1. In preparing to examine the genital area of a preschool-age child, which action by the nurse will most likely result in the best outcome?
   1. Position the child on the parent's lap with his or her legs apart.
   2. Position the child on the examination table.
   3. Examine the genital area first.
   4. Examine the genital area last.

2. When assessing the chest of a young child, which sites are best for auscultation?
   1. At the bases and midaxillary areas
   2. At the apices and midaxillary areas
   3. Just below the clavicles
   4. Just above the clavicles

3. During an assessment of the neck of a 2-year-old child, the nurse notes firm, nontender, movable lymph nodes 1 cm in diameter in the cervical chain. Which would the nurse consider the most likely cause of this finding?
   1. Abnormal and indicative of illness requiring antibiotic treatment
   2. Abnormal and probably related to minor upper respiratory infection
   3. Normal finding in a child at this age
   4. Abnormal and potentially indicative of a serious health problem

4. A nurse is assessing a 2-year-old boy with the following vital signs: temperature 97.8°F axillary, apical pulse 100, respirations 28 breaths per minute, blood pressure 125/80. Which action by the nurse would be most appropriate?
   1. Reevaluate the child's temperature in 1 hour.
   2. Report the blood pressure to the physician.
   3. Assess for additional signs of respiratory distress in the child.
   4. Determine why the child has tachycardia.

See Appendix I 🔗 *for answers.*

References

American Academy of Ophthalmology Pediatric Ophthalmology/Strabismus Panel. (2007). *Preferred Practice Pattern® Guidelines. Pediatric eye evaluations.* San Francisco, CA: Author. Retrieved from http://www.aao.org/ppp

American Academy of Pediatrics Section on Ophthalmology, American Association of Pediatric Ophthalmology and Strabismus, American Academy of Ophthalmology, and American Association of Certified Orthoptists. (2008). Red reflex examination of neonates, infants, and children. *Pediatrics, 122*(6), 1401–1404.

American Speech and Language Association. (2011). *How does your child hear and talk?* Retrieved from http://www.asha.org/public/speech/development/chart.htm

Biro, F. M., Galvez, M. P., Greenspan, L. C., Succop, P. A., Vangeepuram, N., Pinney, S. M., . . . Wolff, M. S. (2010). Pubertal assessment method and baseline characteristics in a mixed longitudinal study of girls. *Pediatrics, 126*(3), e583–e590.

Brook, I. (2007). Acute and chronic sinusitis. *Infectious Disease Clinics of North America, 21,* 421–448.

Brown, N. (2011). Adolescent medicine. In M. M. Tschudy & K. M. Arcara, *The Harriet Lane handbook* (19th ed., pp. 118–135). St. Louis, MO: Elsevier.

Drolet, B. A., Chamlin, S. L., Garzon, M. C., Adams, D., Baselga, E., Haggstrom, A., . . . Frieden, I. J. (2010). Prospective study of spinal anomalies in children with infantile hemangiomas of the lumbosacral skin. *Journal of Pediatrics, 157*(5), 789–794.

Feigelman, S. (2011). The first year. In R. M. Kliegman, B. F. Stanton, J. W. St. Geme, N. F. Schor, & R. E. Behrman, *Nelson textbook of pediatrics* (19th ed., pp. 26–31). Philadelphia: Elsevier Saunders.

Feigelman, S. (2011). The second year. In R. M. Kliegman, B. F. Stanton, J. W. St. Geme, N. F. Schor, & R. E. Behrman, *Nelson textbook of pediatrics* (19th ed., pp. 31–33). Philadelphia: Elsevier Saunders.

Harris, T. S. (2010). Bruises in children: Normal or child abuse? *Journal of Pediatric Health Care, 24*(4), 216–221.

Hermann-Giddens, M. E., Bourdony, C. J., Dowshen, S. A., & Reiter, E. O. (2011). *Assessment of sexual maturity stages in girls and boys.* Elk Grove Village, IL: American Academy of Pediatrics.

Hummel, P. (2011). Newborn assessment. In E. M. Chiocca, *Advanced pediatric assessment* (pp. 199–229). Philadelphia: Wolters Kluwer Lippincott Williams & Wilkins.

Ladewig, P. W., London, M. L., & Davidson, M. R. (2010). *Contemporary maternal-newborn nursing care* (7th ed.). Upper Saddle River, NJ: Pearson.

O'Connor, N. R., McLaughlin, M. R., & Ham, P. (2008). Newborn skin: Part I. Common rashes. *American Family Physician, 77*(1), 47–52.

Park, M. K. (2008). *Pediatric cardiology for practitioners* (5th ed.). Philadelphia: Mosby Elsevier.

Purnell, L. D. (2009). *Guide to culturally competent care* (2nd ed.). Philadelphia: F. A. Davis.

Seidel, H. M., Ball, J. W., Dains, J., Flynn, J. A., Solomon, B. S., & Stewart, R. W. (2011). *Mosby's guide to physical examination* (7th ed.). St. Louis, MO: Mosby Elsevier.

Susman, E. J., Houts, R. M., Steinberg, L., Belsky, J., Cauffman, E., De Hart, G., . . . Eunice Kennedy Shriver NICHD Early Child Care Research Network. (2010). Longitudinal development of secondary sexual characteristics in girls and boys between ages 9 1/2 and 15 1/2 years. *Archives of Pediatrics and Adolescent Medicine, 164*(2), 166–173.

Tuli, S. S., Kockler, V., Kelly, M. N., & Tuli, S. Y. (2010). What's your diagnosis? Heterochromia iridis. *Consultant for Pediatricians, 9*(11), 405–406.

Walvoord, E. C. (2010). The timing of puberty: Is it changing? Does it matter? *Journal of Adolescent Health, 47*(5), 433–439.

Zitelli, B. J., & Davis, H. W. (2007). *Atlas of pediatric physical diagnosis* (5th ed.). St. Louis, MO: Elsevier Mosby.

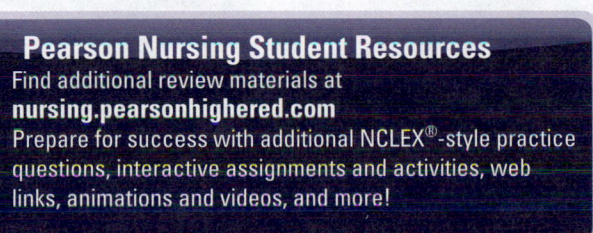

Pearson Nursing Student Resources

Find additional review materials at **nursing.pearsonhighered.com**

Prepare for success with additional NCLEX®-style practice questions, interactive assignments and activities, web links, animations and videos, and more!

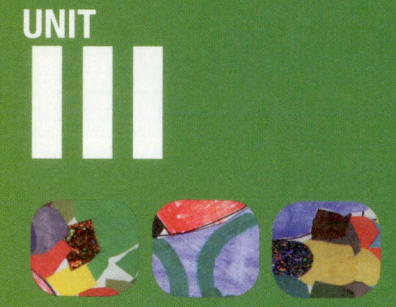

Health Promotion and Maintenance Through Childhood

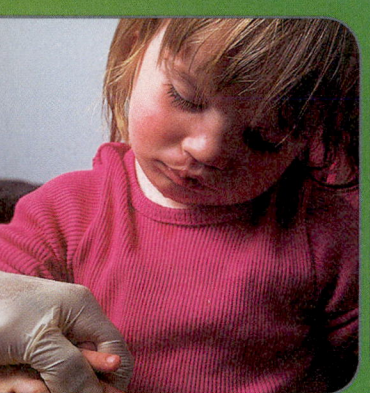
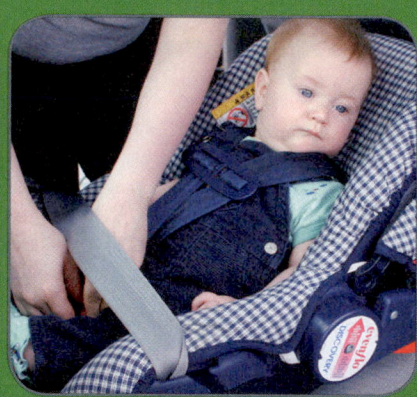
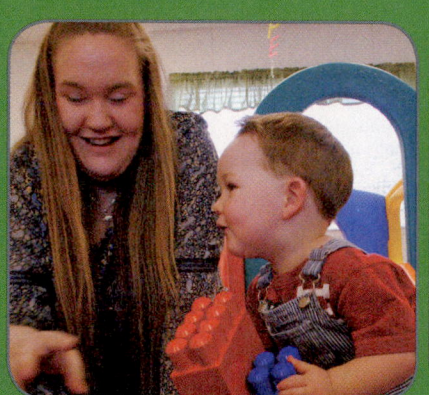
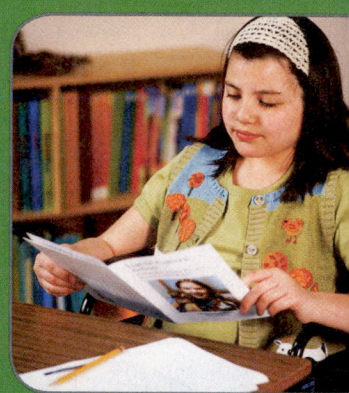

The concepts of health promotion and health maintenance are critical components of pediatric health care. During healthcare encounters, the nurse applies knowledge of development, ecologic theory, and resilience theory to accurately assess growth and development, nutrition, physical activity, oral health, mental and spiritual status, and relationships with families and other people. Pediatric nurses partner with other health professionals to provide health promotion and health maintenance for children from the newborn through adolescent age groups. The nurse plans interventions to enhance the child's health status. Disease and injury prevention strategies are applied during interactions that occur in well-child visits, schools, hospitalizations, and other encounters with children.

Concepts of Health Promotion and Maintenance

CHAPTER 8

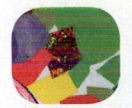 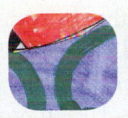 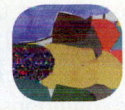

Learning Outcomes

After completing this chapter, you will be able to:

1. Define health promotion and health maintenance.

2. Examine the importance of a medical home, also known as a pediatric healthcare home.

3. Integrate concepts of health promotion and health maintenance in partnership with families during health supervision visits.

4. Describe the components of a health supervision visit.

5. Analyze the nurse's role in providing health promotion and health maintenance for children of different ages in a variety of settings.

6. Perform general observations of children and their families as they come to the pediatric healthcare home for health supervision visits.

7. Synthesize the areas of assessment and intervention for health supervision visits—growth and developmental surveillance, nutrition, physical activity, oral health, mental and spiritual health, family and social relationships, disease prevention strategies, and injury prevention strategies.

8. Apply the nursing process to assess, diagnose, establish goals, intervene, and evaluate care related to health promotion and health maintenance of children and adolescents in a variety of settings.

> "It's kind of fun to come to the van. We've never been to the dentist before. We just moved from Lithuania and my parents don't speak English very well. I like the nurses here. They're always nice to me and my brother."
>
> —*Tony, age 7*

Mr. and Mrs. Yevteshenko have brought their two young sons to a mobile van for care. Tony and Ilya are 7 and 5 years of age. The nurse has arranged to have an interpreter present to assist in history taking, explaining procedures, and family education. The family came from Lithuania about 9 months ago, sponsored by a local ministry. The mother is caring for the children at home, although she worked in an office in her native country. Mr. Yevteshenko had a job in the computer industry, but now he works as a custodian. The parents are devoted to the health and well-being of their children and are eager to learn more English so they can understand the clinic personnel. The school nurse recommended that the family consider using the van, which is locally managed by nurse practitioners. In addition to offering health promotion and health maintenance visits, a dentist and dental hygienists come weekly to the van to provide dental care. Nurses and dental personnel partner with the family to provide care and perform necessary teaching.

The nurse focuses not only on health screening and immunization, but also on the stress of adaptation to life in a new country for each family member. Links are made to community resources that can help the family with basic necessities and educational needs. These resources may also provide a sense of belonging.

How will the needs of the family change as they spend more time in the country? (See Chapter 6 for information about translation of health messages and accurate communication.) What are the major health promotion and health maintenance needs for each child? How can nurses in various settings such as schools and mobile healthcare facilities partner with each other to promote health of families in the community?

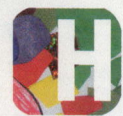

Video

Healthy People 2020

ealthy People 2020 established important goals to meet the vision of a society in which all people live long, healthy lives. The overarching goals are:

- Attain high-quality, longer lives free of preventable disease, disability, injury, and premature death.
- Achieve health equity, eliminate disparities, and improve the health of all groups.
- Create social and physical environments that promote good health for all.
- Promote quality of life, healthy development, and healthy behaviors across all life stages (*Healthy People 2020*, 2011).

The concepts of health promotion and health maintenance provide a framework for nursing interventions that contributes to meeting these goals. Many students in health professions begin their studies with a strong interest in the care of ill individuals. However, as time progresses, they learn that "well" people need care also. They need teaching to improve diet, reduce stress, and obtain immunizations. They may seek information about how to exercise properly or ensure safe environments for their children. These examples of care and teaching are components of health promotion and health maintenance.

Nursing is a holistic profession that examines and works with all aspects of the lives of individuals and has a strong focus on family and community as well. Nurses therefore are uniquely positioned to provide health promotion and health maintenance activities, and indeed these activities should be a part of each encounter with families.

The pediatric nurse applies health promotion and health maintenance in all settings in which children and adolescents are served—well-child clinics, schools, mobile vans, physician and nurse practitioner offices, and hospitals. The nurse must possess a comprehensive background in all aspects of child health care and a solid understanding of child growth and development (see Chapter 5 🔗). The family's role in children's health is critical (see Chapter 2 🔗). The impact of contemporary influences on children provides an essential context to realistic nursing care planning (see Chapter 20 🔗). Finally, a thorough understanding of the healthcare conditions that affect children is needed so that health promotion and health maintenance can be integrated within the framework of comprehensive health care. Both acute and chronic healthcare needs are integrated into the provision of health promotion and health maintenance.

What is the difference between health promotion and health maintenance? When should nurses engage in activities that focus on health? How are these activities integrated into health supervision visits? How do nurses partner with other healthcare professionals to offer comprehensive health services in settings accessible to parents and children? How can nurses help children and their families to maximize length and quality of life? We will consider these and other questions in this chapter and discuss specific activities for certain age groups in the next five chapters.

DEFINITIONS OF HEALTH PROMOTION AND MAINTENANCE

To understand health promotion and health maintenance, we should first agree on a definition of health. The World Health Organization defines **health** as a "state of complete physical, mental, and social well-being and not merely the absence of disease and infirmity" (World Health Organization, 2010). Others view the quality of "complete well-being" as impossible to attain and therefore have further developed

the concept to apply to persons with health challenges as well as those who are "healthy." Health in this expanded view is dynamic, changing, and unfolding; it is the realization of a state of actualization or potential (Pender, Murdaugh, & Parsons, 2011). The basic human right of health is necessary for development of societies (Box 8–1).

Health promotion refers to activities that increase well-being and enhance wellness or health (Pender et al., 2011). These activities lead to actualization of positive health potential for all individuals, even those with chronic or acute conditions. Health promotion activities include providing information and resources to:

- Enhance nutrition at each developmental stage
- Integrate physical activity into the child's daily events
- Provide adequate housing
- Promote oral health
- Foster positive personality development

Health promotion emerged in nursing literature following a Canadian document known as the *Lalonde Report* (Lalonde, 1974). The concept has subsequently been developed by the World Health Organization through conferences and statements about health promotion. Conferences were held in Canada, Australia, Sweden, Indonesia, Mexico, Thailand, and Kenya from 1986 to 2009. Health promotion is viewed as an integrated, cost-effective, essential strategy to safeguard and improve the health of populations (World Health Organization, 2011a). In the United States, health promotion is strongly integrated into the *Healthy People 2020* program, the Bright Futures publications, and the HealthierUS initiative. Many other countries have embraced and developed the concept of health promotion, and the International Union for Health Promotion and Education seeks to link policy, practice, and research to examine and improve health promotion at a global level (International Union for Health Promotion and Education, 2009).

Health promotion assists people to have increased control over their health, make healthy choices, and improve health. Improved health requires positive health policy, supportive environments, strong communities, improved health services, and personal skills that promote health (World Health Organization, 2009). Nurses have important roles in influencing policies, laws, and the cultural milieu that encourages health promotion. They engage directly in health promotion by partnering with children and families to promote family strengths in the areas of lifestyles, social development, coping, and family interactions. You will provide **anticipatory guidance** for families when you understand the child's upcoming developmental stages and teach families how to provide an environment to assist in meeting

---

BOX 8–1	**Prerequisites for Health**

The World Health Organization has established fundamental social conditions that are needed for health: peace, shelter, education, food, income, stable ecosystem, sustainable resources, social justice, and equity. When nurses work with families who cannot meet one of these fundamental resources, activities should first be directed at security for the absent condition, and then other health activities will be more successful. This view is consistent with Maslow's hierarchy of needs, which established that basic physiologic needs must be met before the person can focus on higher needs such as safety, belongingness and love, or self-actualization activities. For example, assisting a family to identify resources for adequate food if they are hungry will increase the family's ability to respond to teaching about safety or immunizations.

the milestones of the stages. The concept of anticipatory guidance is a cornerstone for health promotion and is explored later in this chapter.

Health maintenance (or **health protection**) refers to activities that preserve an individual's present state of health and that prevent disease or injury occurrence, such as when a nurse performs developmental screening or surveillance to identify early deviations from normal development, provides immunizations to prevent illnesses, and teaches about common childhood safety hazards (see A Day in the Life of the Clinic Nurse on page 232). **Screening** is a procedure to detect the possible presence of a health condition before symptoms are apparent. **Surveillance** is a continuous process in which skilled observations are carried out in collaboration with families, specialists, childcare providers, and other professionals; it may include growth surveillance, developmental surveillance, or other components (American Academy of Pediatrics, 2010). Health maintenance activities are commonly preventive in nature and presented in layman's terms to explain the levels and aims of preventive actions. Prevention levels are identified as **primary prevention**, **secondary prevention**, and **tertiary prevention** (Table 8–1).

Although health promotion and health maintenance activities are closely linked and often overlap, we should note how they differ:

- Health *maintenance* focuses on known potential health risks and seeks to prevent them or to identify them early so that intervention can occur.
- Health *promotion* examines the strengths and goals of individuals, families, and populations, and seeks to use them to assist in reaching higher levels of wellness. It involves partnerships with the family as health goals are set, and with other health professionals and resources to provide for meeting the goals.

The nurse must apply both health promotion and health maintenance concepts when providing health care, recognizing that the concepts overlap. See Figure 8–1 ■ for examples of the application of each concept and how they relate to each other.

Health promotion and health maintenance are integrated into healthcare visits for children, with the care provider applying knowledge of health maintenance concepts and adding information the family has identified that will assist in increasing health or wellness (health promotion). These activities commonly take place at well-child or health supervision visits. Ideally, the child has a consistent healthcare provider known as a healthcare home. (See detailed descriptions of health supervision and the pediatric healthcare home later in this chapter.)

Consider the scenario that opened this chapter. Tony and his brother have come to a mobile van that is parked near their school.

The nurse identifies a need for immunizations and connection to resources to assist the newly relocated family. At the same setting, dental care is provided and teaching is performed for these children who have never had a dental visit before. What nursing activities represent health promotion? Which represent health maintenance? With what other professionals must the nurse partner to provide culturally competent care for the family?

APPLICATION OF RESILIENCE AND ECOLOGIC THEORIES

In Chapter 5 ⟳, we discussed two theories that provide useful approaches to children and families: resilience and the ecologic theory. Both of these theories can be linked to concepts of health promotion and health maintenance.

The concept of resilience focuses on the ability of children to use their protective factors or strengths to overcome risks and emerge as healthy and strong individuals. Nurses assess both the protective factors and the risk factors of individual children and their families, and use this information in planning appropriate health-related activities. For example, the nurse may identify the following protective factors for a toddler:

- Both parents are present in the home and share in childcare activities.
- Parents express interest in learning how to limit television time and plan alternative activities for the child.
- The toddler has been weaned from a bottle, is eating family table foods, and has a body mass index in the 50th percentile.

The nurse may also have identified the following risks:

- The grandmother who cares for the toddler three times weekly smokes in her home.
- The family has recently moved and expresses concern that their new jobs do not provide adequate healthcare insurance.
- The toddler has recently been biting and hitting the parents when frustrated.

The nurse uses the information gathered to plan the following health promotion and health maintenance activities:

- Information is provided about the effects of environmental tobacco smoke, and ideas are discussed with the parents about ways to suggest that the grandmother not smoke when the toddler is present (*health maintenance*).
- The nurse finds low-cost but comprehensive healthcare resources and presents them to the family (health maintenance).

TABLE 8–1	Levels of Preventive Health Maintenance Activities	
LEVEL	**DESCRIPTION**	**NURSING ACTIONS**
Primary prevention	Activities that decrease opportunity for illness or injury	Giving immunizations Teaching about car safety seats
Secondary prevention	Early diagnosis and treatment of a condition to lessen its severity	Developmental screening Vision and hearing screening
Tertiary prevention	Restoration to optimal function	Rehabilitation activities for child after a car crash

Source: Adapted from Murray, R. B., Zentner, J. P., & Yakimo, R. (2009). *Health promotion strategies through the life span* (8th ed.). Upper Saddle River, NJ: Prentice Hall Health.

A DAY IN THE LIFE
of the Clinic Nurse

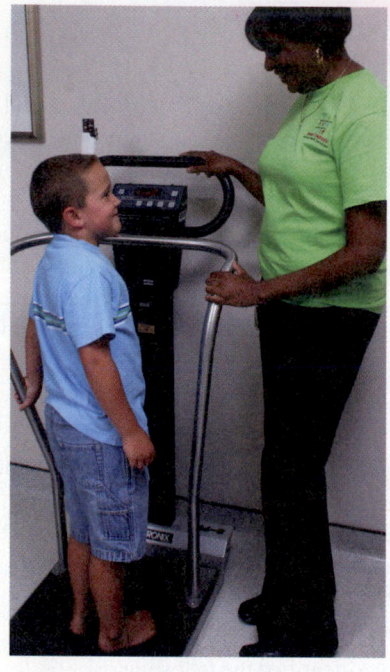

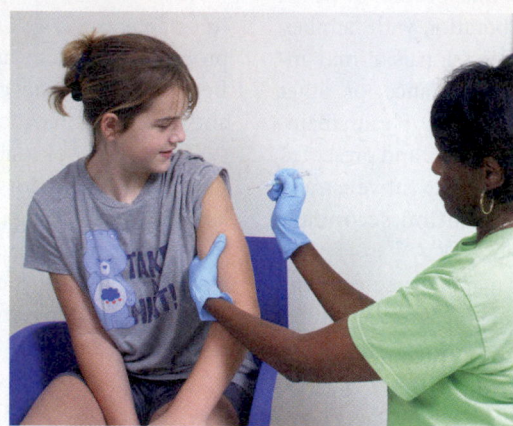

Above. Shalene administers a hepatitis B injection to this teen who did not receive the recommended immunization at a younger age. What other immunizations are commonly needed in the early adolescent years?

Left. As Shalene weighs this young boy, she takes the opportunity to interact with him to assess language and social skills.

Health promotion and health maintenance begin at birth and are a part of every healthcare visit throughout childhood. The nurse is instrumental in performing thorough assessments, integrating teaching, and performing interventions that help to promote health and to prevent disease or injury. Shalene Wilson is a nurse at a clinic that performs well-child assessments and sees children for minor illnesses and injuries.

Health visits often begin with growth measurement, which provides the opportunity for the nurse to introduce herself to the child in a nonthreatening way and to begin the interaction. When reporting growth patterns to the child and parent, the nurse inserts information about diet intake and

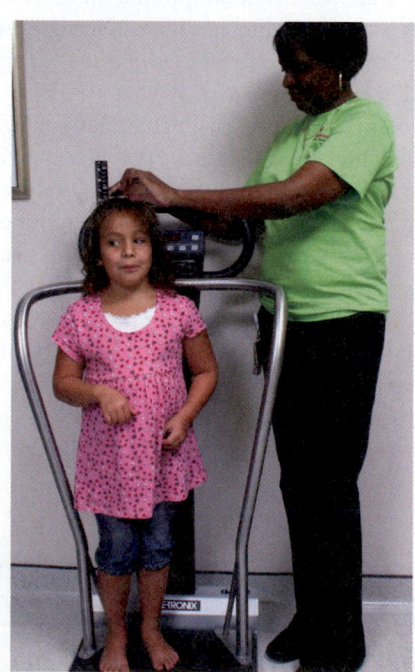

Previous experiences at the clinic have been positive for this young girl. She is complaining of an earache, and Shalene performs body measurements since some medications that might be prescribed require an accurate weight for establishment of dose.

> "What I like best about being a clinic nurse is that every day is different. The challenges are exciting and I am constantly learning."

seeks additional information about nutrition and physical activity. Assessment and teaching are thus integrated into the nurse's interactions with the family during the clinic visit.

Health visits are adapted for older children and adolescents to meet their developmental needs. The adolescent is often seen alone, and Shalene offers teaching regarding nutrition and safety during the physical and psychosocial assessment. She integrates current knowledge of topics such as immunization recommendations into her practice by assessing immunization records and using the opportunity to catch the teen up with any that have not yet been administered.

The clinic nurse is often called upon to participate in community activities. Shalene has attended a bicycle rally to encourage safe riding practices and physical activity. She integrates health promotion activities (such as encouraging vigorous physical activity) with health maintenance activities (safety practices to prevent injury). Shalene has also participated in Head Start screening, food and nutrition events, programs to prepare young children for a new sibling, and other health promotion and health maintenance activities.

Shalene enjoys the variety in her job as the nurse in a community clinic. In a typical day she sees infants and young parents, conducts health supervision for children of all ages, and sees children with minor illnesses. She integrates safety teaching, anticipatory guidance, and guidance for healthy lifestyles into every visit. Her job requires a firm foundation in growth and development; communication skills for varying ages; a knowledge of epidemiology of common conditions and disease; and recommendations for healthcare screenings, immunizations, and other interventions. Shalene's clinic has a list of suggested health maintenance topics that can be addressed at each visit. The list, and the results of her assessment of individual children and families, guides Shalene in addressing topics to promote health and to prevent injury and disease. See Chapters 9 through 13 for specific topics for health promotion and health maintenance at various ages.

- Information is provided on setting limits for common toddler behaviors, and a local support group for parents of toddlers is recommended; ideas for activities appropriate for the age group are discussed, and the parents choose their favorites (*health promotion*).
- The parents are praised for their management of the child's weight; teaching to enhance health nutritional knowledge is integrated into the visit (*health promotion*).

The nurse uses the list of protective factors and risk factors to plan topics for the visit. Information is provided that parents need to keep the child safe and prevent injury (health maintenance). Goals that the family has set are recognized, and resources are provided that will help the family to meet these goals (health promotion). The family and the nurse establish a health partnership to maintain and promote the health of the young toddler in the family.

Using ecologic theory, the nurse also assesses the child and then progresses on to assess several systems in the child's life:

1. The *microsystem* involves those settings in which the child has close contact. These involve the parents and the grandmother for the toddler described previously.
2. The *mesosystem* involves relationships between the microsystems. At this point, the nurse can seek additional information about the relationship between the parents and the grandmother that will provide clues to methods of dealing with the issue of smoking near the child.
3. The *exosystem* is outside the child's daily contacts but influences the child indirectly. It is reflected in the family's concern about lack of healthcare resources due to a recent move and job change.
4. The child is part of a *macrosystem* or society that provides ready access to television and other media, necessitating health teaching about wise use of media and planning for alternative activities.

The ecologic theory provides guidance that is particularly useful in health promotion activities. Several components of health promotion relate to the systems of ecologic theory, as shown in Table 8–2.

Use resilience theory, ecologic theory, or both to assist you in the assessment of children and families, and to point you toward other data to gather. Using the information obtained, you can plan appropriate health promotion and health maintenance activities. Remember that guidelines for topics at various ages are just guidelines; using your assessment data wisely will help you to individualize the specific information needed by a particular family.

Health Promotion and Health Maintenance Overlap

Health Promotion	Overlap	Health Maintenance
• Nutrition to meet all RDAs and enhance health and well-being, with emphasis on whole grains, fruits, vegetables.	• Nutrition that provides for growth and energy needs also helps prevent chronic diseases.	• Nutrition to prevent obesity or growth retardation.
• Activities to promote self-concept formation including body image and decision-making skills.	• Integrating positive activities will both promote self-image and decrease potential for injury.	• Limiting television viewing to decrease exposure to violence which may lead to disturbed sleep and aggressive behaviors.

FIGURE 8–1 ■ While the focus and goals for health promotion and health maintenance differ, there is often overlap in nursing activities and expected outcomes, as demonstrated in these examples.

TABLE 8–2	Socioecologic Approach to Health Promotion Objectives	
HEALTH PROMOTION OBJECTIVES	**SYSTEMS OF ECOLOGIC THEORY**
Develop personal skills	Individual in microsystems
■ Enhance life skills	
■ Provide information	
Strengthen community action and capacity building	Mesosystems
■ Enable resources to work together	
■ Enhance systems for public participation	
■ Improve self-help and social support	
Create supportive environments	Exosystems
■ Assess health impacts of rapidly changing environments	
■ Protect natural and built environments	
Reorient health services	Macrosystems
■ Embrace an expanded role to address health promotion as well as disease treatment	
■ Enhance health research and training for health promotion	
Build healthy public policy through networking	Macrosystems
■ Inform policy makers of health consequences of decisions and policies	
■ Foster equity and eliminate disparities among diverse groups	
■ Identify obstacles to health public policy	

Source: *Data from Health Promotion Objectives from the Ottawa Charter for Health Promotion (World Health Organization, 2005); Health promotion (World Health Organization, 2011b); Ecologic Theory from Bronfenbrenner (2005).*

HEALTH SUPERVISION IN THE PEDIATRIC HEALTHCARE HOME

Health supervision is the provision of services that focus on health promotion, growth and developmental surveillance, and disease and injury prevention (health maintenance) at key intervals during the

BOX 8–2	National Guidelines for Health Promotion

- *Bright Futures*, American Academy of Pediatrics (original editions by Maternal and Child Health Bureau, Health Resources and Services Administration, DHHS)
- *Put Prevention into Practice*, Agency for Healthcare Quality and Research
- *The Guide to Clinical Preventive Services*, U.S. Preventive Services Task Force
- *Guidelines for Adolescent Preventive Services*, American Medical Association

child's life. What health promotion and health maintenance activities are parts of health supervision visits? How can these activities be integrated into all settings where care is provided for children? What are the recommended times for health visits to occur, and what care is provided at certain times? How can you organize a health supervision visit to accomplish goals of the family and health professionals? We will address these and other questions here and in the nursing management section.

All children need a medical home where accessible, continuous, and coordinated health supervision is provided during the developmental years. *Accessibility* refers to both financial and geographic access; *continuous* indicates that the care is ongoing with consistent care providers; *coordination* refers to the need for communication among health professionals to provide for the needs of the child. A medical home or **pediatric healthcare home** is therefore the site of comprehensive health care by a pediatric healthcare professional to ensure optimal health (National Association of Pediatric Nurse Practitioners [NAPNAP], 2009). See Chapter 1 🔗 for additional descriptions of the medical home or pediatric healthcare home. When a family has an established partnership with a care provider, comprehensive, family-centered health services can be provided based on the family's risks and protective factors. These services may be provided in physician offices, community health clinics, the family's home, schools, childcare centers, shelters, or mobile vans (Figure 8–2 ■). National guidelines for preventive health services have been developed for infants, children, and adolescents by the U.S. Department of Health and Human Services (DHHS), the American Academy of Pediatrics (AAP), and the American Medical Association (Box 8–2). NAPNAP supports the list of comprehensive services identified by the AAP (Box 8–3). The guidelines are important references for the

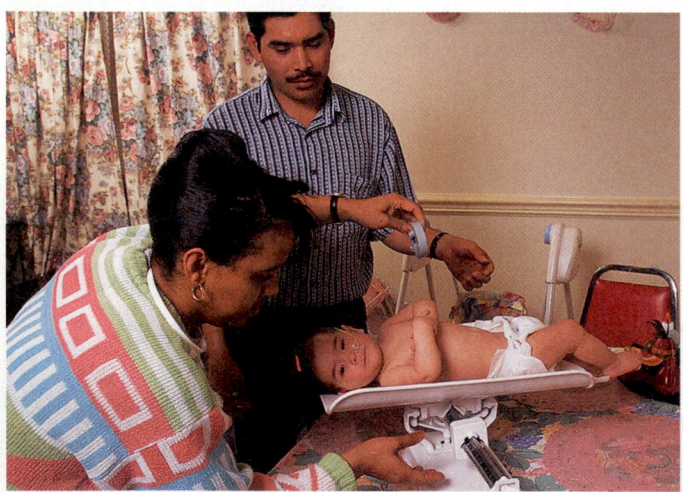

A

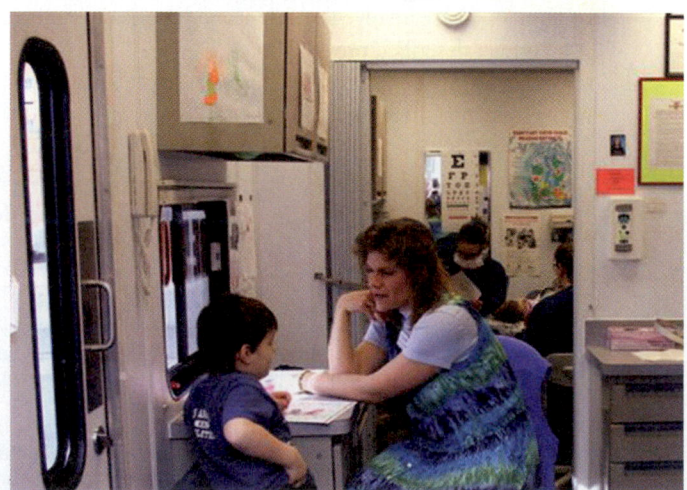

B

FIGURE 8–2 ■ *A*, The nurse is providing a health supervision visit in the child's home after discharge from the hospital for an acute illness. *B*, A nurse is providing information to a child visiting a mobile healthcare van.

BOX 8–3 Elements of a Pediatric Healthcare Home

The AAP and NAPNAP concur that a pediatric healthcare home should offer:

- Family-centered care and trusting partnership
- Sharing of unbiased and clear information
- Provision of primary care to include acute and chronic care; breastfeeding promotion; immunizations; growth and development screenings; healthcare supervision; and counseling about health, nutrition, safety, parenting, and psychosocial issues
- Continuously accessible care with transition from pediatric to adult care
- Continuity of care
- Provision of compassionate, developmentally appropriate, and culturally competent care
- Referral to early intervention and childcare
- Coordination of services and collaboration of professionals
- Maintenance of a comprehensive central record
- Referral to specialists as needed

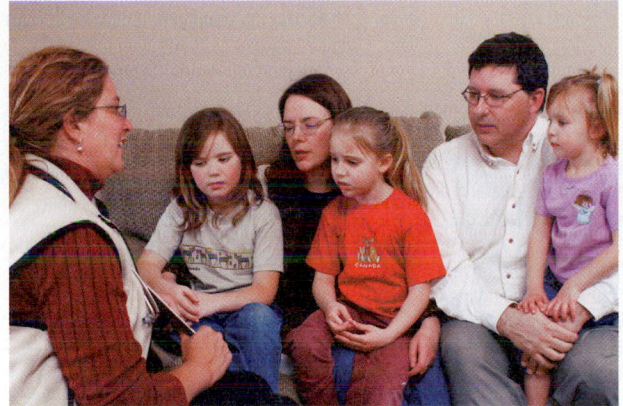

Source: *Data from American Academy of Pediatrics. (2008).* The National Center for Medical Home Initiatives for Children with Special Needs. *Retrieved from http://www .medicalhomeinfo.org/training/index.html; National Association of Pediatric Nurse Practitioners (NAPNAP). (2009). NAPNAP position statement on the pediatric health care/medical home.* Journal of Pediatric Health Care, 23*(3), 23A–24A.*

pediatric nurse; they apply an evidence base to recommend care components for children and adolescents.

The health supervision visit is individualized to the family and child. Standardized screenings and examinations are included, but time is provided for the family's specific concerns and questions about the child's health. Nurses play an integral part in these comprehensive visits, and they partner with other healthcare providers to accomplish health supervision.

An information management tracking system in the pediatric healthcare home site helps to identify appropriate health supervision activities for each child at every visit; electronic health records list appropriate topics for visits at specific ages. If a child misses a visit, the family can be contacted by phone, email, or other preferred electronic media, and encouraged to come in for the recommended care. A family may be contacted if the young child is lacking immunizations. Because not all families get into the healthcare home for each visit, every health visit, including an episodic illness visit or care for a chronic illness, may provide an opportunity for nurses to complete health promotion and health maintenance activities. For example, if the child has missed a prior health supervision visit, immunizations may be given during a visit for an acute condition such as otitis media. When caring for children in hospitals, emergency rooms, or other settings, nurses should ask about their pediatric healthcare home and when the last visit occurred. Identify children who need basic health supervision services and provide them, or refer the children to other settings to meet these needs at another time (Bindler & Ball, 2007).

Nurses play an important role in managing health supervision visits (Figure 8–3 ■). Depending on the setting, the nurse may provide all services or support other care providers by obtaining an updated health history, screening for diseases and other conditions, conducting a developmental assessment, and providing immunizations, anticipatory guidance, and health education. Nurses in all settings are instrumental in identifying children who need health supervision and are not obtaining recommended care.

Although health supervision visits can address many health-related topics, there is generally a limited time in which to engage a child or family. The nurse needs to direct the encounters and have ideas for pertinent agendas. *Bright Futures*, an initiative of the U.S. Maternal and Child Health Bureau, promotes the foundational belief that each child deserves to be healthy and that the community, health professional, family, and child must partner

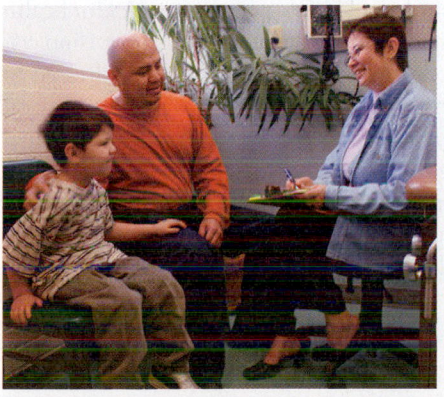

A

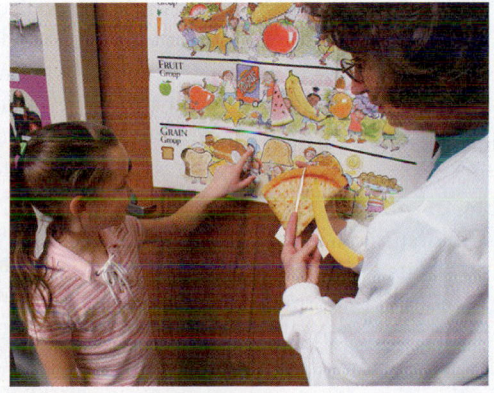

B

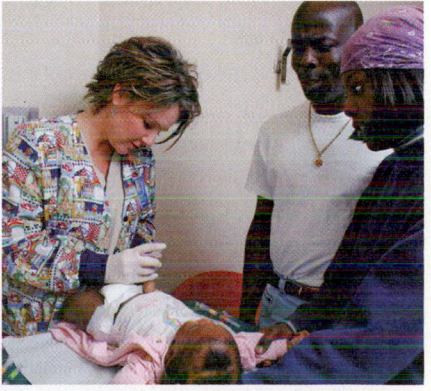

C

FIGURE 8–3 ■ The nurse plays many roles in providing health promotion and health maintenance for children. *A,* Data are collected from the time a nurse calls the child and family to the examination room and during the history-taking phase. The nurse asks questions while observing the child's behaviors and the relationship between parent and child. The nurse also performs screening tests, including blood pressure, tuberculosis, vision and hearing, and developmental screening. *B,* Interventions that include teaching may take place. *C,* A nurse may administer immunizations as parents watch and assist by holding the child. Nurses also play important roles in teaching families information to enhance health.

together to achieve this goal. A series of *Bright Futures* booklets on health supervision, nutrition, physical activity, and mental health provide guidance about how the nurse can manage health supervision visits. These publications are available through the AAP and are referred to throughout Chapters 9 to 13 🔗.

The following six concepts should be integrated into care for children to promote health and prevent disease and injury:

1. **Build effective partnerships with families. A partnership** is a relationship in which participants join together to ensure healthcare delivery in a way that recognizes the critical roles and contributions of each partner in promoting health and preventing illness. The partners in child health include the child, family, health professional, and community. Strategies the nurse can use to build partnerships include:
   - Modeling and encouraging open, supportive communication
   - Recognizing and respecting family strengths
   - Using open-ended questions to identify health issues
   - Mutually identifying goals for the health encounter
   - Mutually establishing a plan of action to meet goals
   - Sustaining the partnership and evaluating the goals

2. **Foster family-centered communication.** The nurse fosters family-centered communication by:
   - Showing interest in the family and their concerns
   - Conveying understanding and empathy
   - Clarifying information as needed

   (*See Chapter 6 🔗 for a thorough discussion of communication with children and families.*)

3. **Address health promotion and health maintenance needs.** The nurse *focuses on health promotion and health maintenance topics during visits*, recognizing that families may not initiate these discussions. Topics include developmental progression, sleep, nutrition, social interactions, physical activity, and other areas pertinent to the family and age of the child.

4. **Manage time to provide for health promotion during routine healthcare visits.** This may involve:
   - Preparing for the visit by reviewing the child's health record and selecting discussion topics appropriate for the child's age
   - Clarifying key health promotion topics for the family
   - Planning together to meet goals not accomplished in the visit due to lack of time or the need to focus only on certain high-priority concerns

5. **Educate in the family's teachable moments.** Large teaching plans are not always needed. Children and families often learn best when presented with small bits of information. The family may not need a large amount of information on preschool nutrition but may benefit from knowing the recommendations for limiting fruit juice intake (see Chapter 19 🔗). These bits of information are geared to a specific question or topic the family has brought up or an observation you have made during the history or other conversation.

TABLE 8–3	Advocating for Children and Families
HEALTH NEED EXAMPLE	**NURSE ADVOCACY ACTIONS**
Members of the community need to learn about places to obtain immunizations.	■ Make a list of agencies that provide immunizations, including those with low-cost immunizations through the Vaccines for Children program (see Chapter 22 🔗). ■ Obtain financial assistance from a local foundation to print your findings. ■ Make copies available in childcare centers and other community agencies.
A local homeless shelter has little in the way of self-image amenities for the residents.	■ Obtain donations of hotel lotions, soaps, and shampoos from classmates and faculty that can be given to the shelter. ■ Visit several local hotels and ask if they will each donate a box of small toiletries for the residents. ■ Encourage volunteers to provide haircuts and styling, or obtain donations to provide this service.
Your state has a law protecting the rights of any woman to bring her unwanted newborn baby to certain sites and give the child up without legal recriminations. Many women do not know about the law, and babies are abandoned in unsafe locations.	■ Find a local newspaper reporter who is willing to write an article about the law. ■ Run off copies of the article to distribute. ■ Make posters with necessary information for several community sites.

6. **Advocate for children and their families.** When an issue arises as you care for a child, seek additional data from various sources. Talk with others and strategize how the problem could be solved. Obtain the support you need and begin to advocate on the issue (see Table 8–3 for examples of nursing advocacy).

COMPONENTS OF HEALTH PROMOTION AND MAINTENANCE VISITS

As a nurse, you will identify and isolate pertinent topics for health promotion and health maintenance during health supervision visits. Apply your knowledge of areas that need to be addressed to a particular age and developmental stage, and then make general observations of the child and family to guide you to additional topics. Although categories to consider vary depending on the age of the child, the family's particular needs, and community resources, common topics generally require attention. Start with the areas described below, integrate general observations as you progress with the visit, and add topics pertinent to promote health in particular situations. Concepts central to health promotion and health maintenance include:

- Contacts with the family
- General observations
- Growth and developmental surveillance
- Nutrition

- Physical activity
- Oral health
- Mental and spiritual health
- Relationships
- Disease prevention strategies
- Injury prevention (safety) strategies

What local child healthcare issues could benefit from advocacy in your community?

Contacts with the Family

Healthcare providers work with families in diverse settings and must adapt approaches and interventions dependent on the needs of these families (see Chapter 2 🖉 for further information on family assessment). Prospective parents sometimes interview potential healthcare providers while pregnant with a child to choose the pediatric healthcare home that will best meet their needs and approaches to child health. In other situations, parents choose the most convenient setting or a facility that is included in their health insurance coverage. Some families remain with one care provider for years, whereas others have multiple providers.

Whatever the individual situation, the nurse recognizes that all contacts with family members are a vital link to the child. Contacts are a time to learn about the child's development, to observe interactions among family members, and to implement effective nursing interventions. Telephone calls, face-to-face meetings, email communication, and brief encounters all serve to provide a mutual interaction with the goal of ensuring child health. Consider the Yevteshenko family described in the opening scenario. They needed dental care and therefore visited a mobile van with that service. How can the nurse interact with them to improve the general health of the children?

General Observations

As a pediatric nurse, you will make general observations of children and their families whenever you encounter them. Be observant during the health supervision visit, and you will have many opportunities to assess the family. These general observations begin as you call the family in and welcome them to the facility. They continue as you weigh and measure the child, and throughout the visit. Key observations include the following:

- Do the child and care provider have close physical contact, eye contact, and vocalization frequently during the visit?
- Do the parents appear relaxed or stressed?
- What are the child's behaviors? Are they what you would expect?
- If a sibling is present, can the parent attend to both children appropriately?
- What responses are you able to elicit in the baby related to eye contact, interest in voice, and motor movements?
- What verbal and nonverbal behaviors do you see in the child or adolescent? Are they within expected norms?

Use your general observations to guide questions. Include additional examination if you have concerns about your observations. For example, if a 2-month-old sleeps for most of the visit, ask questions about the baby's amount of sleep and usual state of alertness. If a mother seems impatient with a crying infant, ask how she usually calms the baby at home. Her answer may reveal that she needs information about how to comfort an infant. If a father is nervously trying to quiet an active child, ask if the child's behavior is typical in new settings. Inquire about how the family sets limits, how much physical activity the child gets daily, and what concerns the father has about the child's behavior. As you progress in your child health nursing experiences, you will become more skilled at integrating your knowledge of development into observations during the visit. Practice these skills and check your observations with more experienced nurses.

Growth and Developmental Surveillance

Growth and developmental surveillance provides important clues about the child's condition and environment. At each health supervision visit, measure the child's height and weight, calculate body mass index, and place each visit's results on percentile charts (see Chapters 7 and 19 🖉). Give parents the information in written form and have it interpreted for them if needed. Adequate growth suggests good nutrition and positive relationships with parents or other care providers. Poor growth could indicate lack of food, lack of a supportive environment, or an underlying child illness.

Perform a physical assessment to ensure that the child is growing as expected and has no abnormal or unexplained physical findings (see Chapter 7 🖉). Health maintenance activities focus on disease prevention and might involve teaching adolescent athletes or an infant's parents proper methods for avoiding fluid imbalance in either of these two vulnerable groups. Health promotion activities related to growth include encouraging at least five servings of fruits and vegetables daily and switching to low-fat dairy products at about 2 years of age.

Developmental surveillance is a flexible, continuous process of skilled observations that also provides data about the child's capabilities, allows for early identification of any neurologic problems, and helps to verify that the home environment is stimulating. Early development is important to later health, and it must be evaluated consistently and systematically during healthcare visits (American Academy of Pediatrics, 2010). Information may be collected from several sources, such as a questionnaire that the parent completes, questions asked during the interview, or observation of the child during the visit. Parents can also be interviewed separately to identify any developmental concerns they may have about the child or adolescent.

When talking with parents, review physical, social, and communication milestones for infants, young children, older children, or adolescents. Detailed milestones for each age group are found in Chapter 5 🖉, and specific examples of questions to ask at particular ages are provided in Chapters 9 through 13 🖉. Be aware that parents' recall of past developmental milestones is often imperfect. The child may be reported to have achieved milestones at ages earlier than actually occurred. When accuracy of developmental milestones is critical, ask to see the child's baby diary or review the past health history at ages closer to the milestone achievement. The parents' report of current skills and achievements is usually accurate. Parents are key participants in their child's developmental screening. They often recognize problems not observed in brief healthcare encounters. Enable them to ask questions and state their observations of the

TABLE 8–4	Developmental Surveillance Questionnaires
QUESTIONNAIRE	**GUIDELINES FOR ADMINISTRATION**
Parents' Evaluation of Developmental Status[a] (birth to 8 years)	Consists of 10 questions for parents to answer in interview; based on research on parents' concerns.
	Requires less than 5 minutes to complete.
	English and Spanish forms are available.
Prescreening Development Questionnaire (PDQ and Revised-PDQ)[b] (birth to 6 years)	Parents complete age-specific forms. Helps identify children who need Denver II assessment.
	Requires less than 10 minutes to complete.
	PDQ is available in English, Spanish, and French versions; R-PDQ in English only.
Ages and Stages Questionnaire[c] (4–48 months)	Questionnaires for 11 specific ages, with 10–15 items each in areas of fine motor, gross motor, communication, adaptive, personal, and social skills. Parents try each activity with the child.
	Requires less than 10 minutes to complete.
	English and Spanish versions are available.
Child Development Inventories[d] (3–72 months)	Consists of 60 yes-no descriptions for three separate instruments to identify children with developmental difficulties.
	Requires about 10 minutes to complete.
Modified Checklist for Autism in Toddlers (M-CHAT)[e]	Consists of 23 yes-no questions for parents of toddlers from 16 to 30 months of age to identify children with possible autism spectrum disorders (see Chapter 34 🔗).
	Requires 5 minutes to administer and 2 minutes to score.

[a]Frances P. Glascoe, Ellsworth & Vandermeer Press Ltd., P.O. Box 68164, Nashville, TN 37206.
[b]Denver Developmental Material, Inc., P.O. Box 371075, Denver, CO 80237-5075.
[c]Brookes Publishing Co., P.O. Box 10624, Baltimore, MD 21285-0625.
[d]Behavior Science Systems, Box 580274, Minneapolis, MN 55458.
[e]Dr. Diana Robins, University of Michigan, 1241 E Catherine St SPC 5618, Ann Arbor, MI 48109. Tool available from www.firstsigns.org or from http://www2.gsu.edu/~wwwpsy/faculty/robins.htm

child, provide them with information, and encourage them to write down observations to bring to the next healthcare visit.

Review school performance for older children and adolescents, including report cards, school achievement records, and any performance on psychoeducational tests when indicated. Inquire about the child's participation in sports and other activities, as well as noted abilities.

Development is a fragile process determined by both innate conditions and environmental influences. Developmental screening of all children requires the use of a regular and organized approach, since about 12% to 13% of children have some type of developmental or behavioral disability (Lipkin, 2011). Standardized developmental questionnaires are effective for developmental surveillance of most children, especially when time for health supervision visits is limited. These questionnaires are easy to administer, do not require the child's cooperation, and can be completed by parents in the waiting area. Screening tests should be administered at the 9-, 18-, and 24- or 30-month visits or at additional times when the parent or healthcare provider has concerns (Lipkin, 2011). Children in need of more extensive developmental surveillance can be identified during these screenings. See Table 8–4 for a list of commonly used developmental screening questionnaires that have been tested for validity and reliability (Box 8–4).

If a developmental delay or abnormality is suspected, a developmental screening test is needed, and a detailed developmental and medical evaluation should be performed (Lipkin, 2011). See Table 8–5 for a list of commonly used developmental screening tests. A frequently administered test is the Denver II (Figures 8–4 ■ page 240 and 8–5 ■ on pages 242–243). Keep in mind that developmental screening tests are not diagnostic tests. They simply help to confirm that most children are progressing along an age-appropriate

BOX 8–4	Research: Validity and Reliability

Validity of a test or tool refers to its ability to measure the characteristics it is intended to measure. For example, a valid test for language measures both understanding and communication of language; it has enough items to measure language abilities, and scores correlate with findings on other language tests. **Reliability** of a test or tool indicates its consistent ability to achieve similar results over time or when administered by various examiners (Polit & Beck, 2008).

norm, and they help document suspicions or patterns of developmental problems. Each test addresses a unique combination of **domains**, which are categories or foci of developmental progression. Some common domains tested include fine motor skills, gross motor skills, language, self-help skills, social skills, and reading.

Clinical Tip

A series of developmental screening tests are available to evaluate the interactions between caregiver and child. Developed by a nurse, Dr. Kathryn Barnard, the Nursing Child Assessment Satellite Training (NCAST) initiated scales to evaluate feeding and teaching interactions between parent and young child; these tools are now part of the Parent-Child Interaction (PCI) program. The Department of Family-Child Nursing and the Center for Human Development and Disability at the University of Washington currently offer training in these important developmental scales, as well as other resources for child health, communication, and environment.

To perform developmental screening with any of the standardized screening tools, make sure all directions are followed:

- Choose the proper test for the child's age and desired information.
- Read directions thoroughly or utilize specific training tools available.

TABLE 8–5	Developmental Screening Tests for Infants and Young Children
SCREENING TEST	**GUIDELINES FOR ADMINISTRATION**
Denver II[a] (birth to 6 years)	Consists of observation of the child in four domains: personal social, fine motor-adaptive, language, and gross motor. Requires 30 minutes to complete. A training video is available.
Bayley Infant Neurodevelopmental Screener (BINS)[b] (3–24 months)	Consists of observation of the child with 10–13 items for each of six age-specific scales to assess neurologic processes, neurodevelopmental skills, and developmental accomplishments. Requires 10–15 minutes to complete.
McCarthy Scales of Children's Abilities[b] (2.5–8.5 years)	Consists of observation of the child in domains of motor, verbal, perceptual-performance, quantitative, general cognition, and memory. Requires 45 minutes to complete.
Denver Articulation Screening Exam (DASE)[a] (2.5–6 years)	Consists of observation of the child's articulation of 30 sound elements and intelligibility. Requires 5 minutes to complete.
Early Language Milestone Scale—2 (ELM)[c] (birth to 36 months)	Consists of observation of the child to assess auditory expressive, auditory receptive, and visual components of speech.
Parent-Child Interactions (PCI) Program[d]	The healthcare provider observes and evaluates a parent-child interaction while the parent feeds the child, and another when the child is taught a new task. Characteristics are provided about the strengths and weaknesses of the parent-child interaction that assist the healthcare provider in improving recognition of cues between parent and child.

[a]Denver Developmental Materials, Inc., P.O. Box 371075, Denver, CO 80237-5075.
[b]Harcourt Assessment: The Psychological Corporation, 19500 Bulverde Rd., San Antonio, TX 78259.
[c]PRO-ED, Inc., 8700 Shoal Creek Blvd., Austin, TX 78758-6897.
[d]NCAST-AVENUW, University of Washington, Box 357920, Seattle, WA 98195-07920.

- Practice as needed until proficient with the test.
- Calculate the infant's or child's age correctly, especially if premature.
- Attempt to develop rapport with the infant or child to get the best performance.
- In some cases, parents can be asked if a child demonstrates specific skills at home, especially if the child is not cooperative.
- Note the behavior and cooperativeness of the child during the screening process.
- Analyze the findings using the test instructions to make the correct interpretation.

Failure to perform an item in a single domain does not mean the child has failed the test (see Developing Cultural Competence: Developmental Testing). The child should be reevaluated at a future visit. Schedule the appointment at a time of day when the child is awake and rested. Provide parents with guidance on specific methods for stimulating the child. Failure of multiple items within one domain or across multiple domains is of greatest concern. When delayed development patterns in one or more domains are revealed, referral for diagnostic developmental assessment is needed.

Both health promotion and health maintenance activities relate to developmental surveillance. Health promotion during a health supervision visit could involve teaching about the next milestones the child will be learning and how to provide an environment where that can occur. This type of anticipatory guidance helps to foster the child's developmental progression. Health maintenance seeks to prevent developmental delay, and activities are focused on deficits found during the visit. For example, if a preschool-age child does not attend school or daycare and the parents have arranged no playmates, the child is likely to have problems with language and social

Developing Cultural Competence
Developmental Testing

Children who have recently come from other countries, and even some born in this country who live in families from minority ethnic groups, may have difficulty with some items on developmental tests. For example, children who are not skilled in the English language may not understand some instructions or be able to answer questions about definitions of words. If an item such as "wave good-bye" or "plays patty-cake" represents a practice not common in another culture, the child may not have had exposure to the skill. In various geographic areas different terms may be used, and children may be confused by certain elements of standardized testing. Be alert for cultural variations, allow the child time to learn a developmental skill, and retest at a later time.

interaction skills. To avoid these health problems, the nurse suggests ways to add social interactions to the child's experience.

Nutrition

Nutrition evaluation is a vital part of each health supervision visit and is closely linked to both health promotion and health maintenance. Good nutrition makes important contributions to general health and fosters growth and development. Eating the proper foods for age and activity level ensures that children have the energy for proper growth, physical activity, cognition, and immune function. Enhancing one's diet with more fruits and vegetables can lead to a stronger immune system and sense of well-being, thus promoting health. It can also contribute to health maintenance by preventing problems such as obesity and some cancers.

For infants, monitoring weight gain, and type and amounts of feedings is essential. Food introduction, infant ability to eat, and

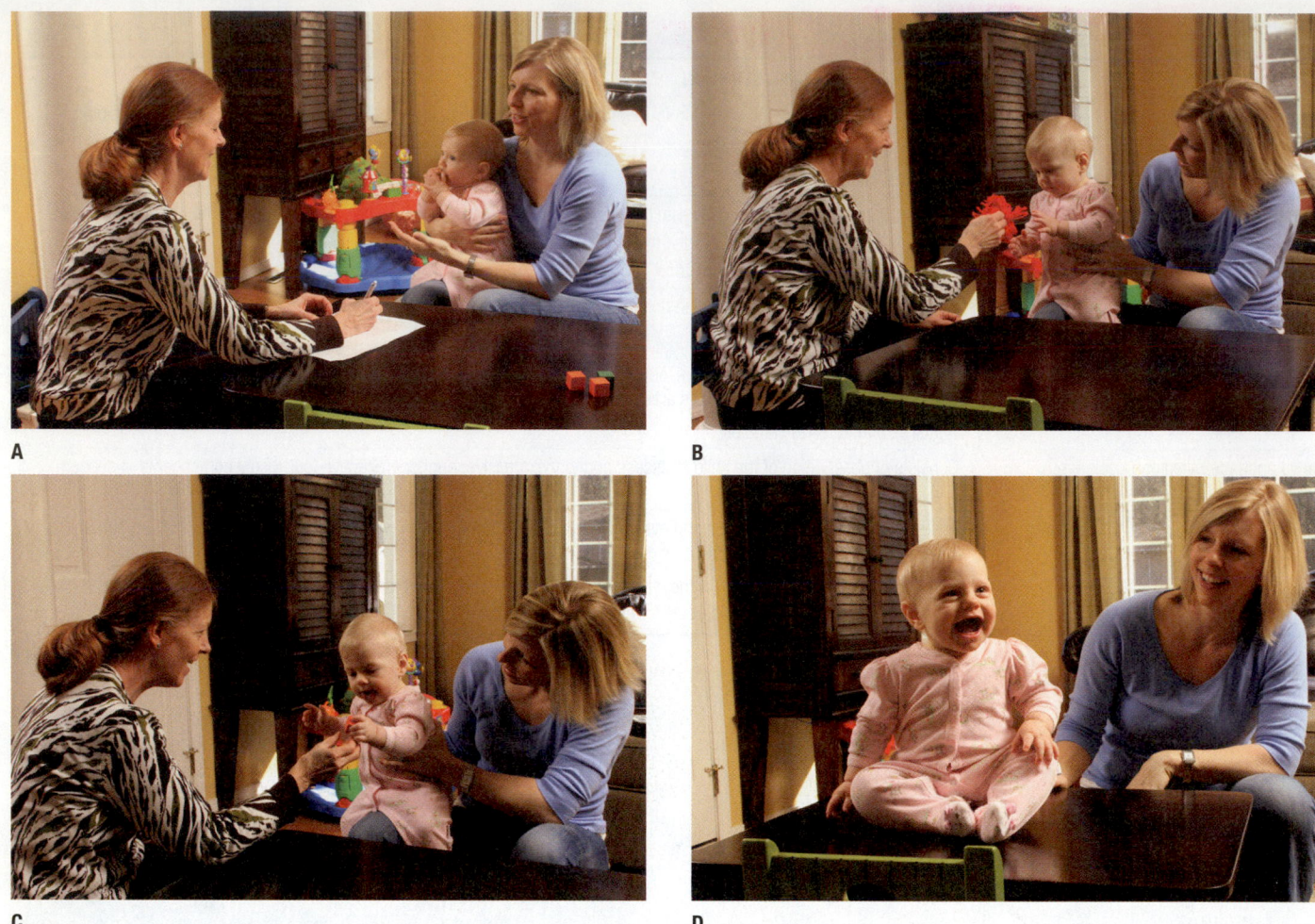

FIGURE 8–4 ■ Follow all directions for performing the Denver II assessment and for interpreting responses. Use the kit provided with the test to ensure accuracy of results. For example, yarn is provided to test the infant's ability to follow an object, a block of a uniform size tests fine motor coordination, and pictures on the score sheet are used to test language abilities. Develop rapport with the child and approach the assessment as fun. This often helps the child participate more actively during the entire Denver II screening. *A,* The nurse making a home visit asks the mother about personal-social tasks the child has accomplished, such as feeding self and waving bye-bye. The girl, who is 6 months of age, is tested for performance of the following age-appropriate behaviors: *B,* Looking for yarn and following 180 degrees. *C,* Banging two cubes. *D,* Sitting without support.

integration of food intake and developmental skills are important to ascertain. Good nutrition requires balance and should be woven into all aspects of daily life. As the baby grows, food patterns of the family become important. Consider childcare settings as well. School-age children and adolescents are establishing food patterns that are most likely to remain with them for life. Ask if the child or adolescent eats breakfast or lunch at school. Inquire about vending machines in the school and how much the child uses them. How often does the family or the adolescent eat at fast-food restaurants? Analyze growth patterns carefully and ask sensitive questions. Find out if the child or adolescent or parents have any concerns about weight or nutrition.

See Chapter 19 🔗 for detailed nutritional assessment recommendations, and Chapters 9 through 13 🔗 for specific nutritional questions to ask for each age group. Include observations and screening relevant to nutritional intake at each health supervision visit. Determine what questions parents have about feeding their children. Integrate the special nutritional needs of children with chronic conditions. Use the information gathered to provide both health promotion and health maintenance interventions. In the area of nutrition, health promotion and health maintenance are closely linked—information provided is likely to both promote a general state of health and prevent disease in the future.

Physical Activity

Physical activity provides many physical and psychologic health benefits. However, there is growing disparity between recommendations and reality among most children. Research by the Centers for Disease Control and Prevention (CDC) has identified that about 23% of children from 9 to 13 years report no free-time physical activity. When schools do not offer daily physical education, many children have no regular activity. About 23% of youth have had no vigorous or moderate physical activity in the last 7 days, only 37% had at least 60 minutes of exercise five days of the previous week, and only 18% had daily activity as recommended (Centers for Disease Control and Prevention, 2010a). Participation in physical activity declines as youth get older, and females are considerably less active than males. For example, while 46% of teen boys have 60 minutes of exercise 5 out of 7 days, only 28% of girls get that amount of activity (Centers for Disease Control and Prevention, 2010a).

The physical activity of infants and young children gives clues to gross motor development status. Observe the infant for symmetric movement, flexion and extension of extremities when excited, and ability to engage with objects and play. Important developmental milestones include sitting, walking, and throwing a ball. Ask what activities the child prefers and amount of time that is spent in activity during the day. As the child grows older, ask questions about sedentary activities such as number of hours spent watching television, playing video games, searching the Internet, or engaging in activities such as social web networking. Determine if the child plays sports at school or in the community. Ask about activities in a typical day to measure amount of activity. Are parents satisfied with the child's activity level, or do they have questions about sports, athletics, other physical activity, and sedentary behaviors? Do the child's weight or body mass index percentile and reported activity level correspond?

Once the nurse gathers data about physical activity, interventions are implemented with the parent and child to enhance activity patterns. Examples of health promotion include suggestions for allowing safe infant crawling and other gross motor activities for periods each day, recommending places to provide sports for a child interested in soccer or hockey, or encouraging a teen to register for a local fun run. These activities will lead the child to a higher state of wellness. The purpose of health maintenance activities is to prevent disease and injury. Include provision of information about safety gear for sports and safe practices such as warm-ups and adequate fluid to prevent injury. Adequate physical activity will contribute to prevention of obesity and its related diseases.

Oral Health

Although oral health may seem to require the knowledge of a specialist, many implications of oral health relate to general health care. Oral health is important because teeth assist in language development, impacted or infected teeth lead to systemic illness, and teeth are related to positive self-image formation. **Dental caries** (cavities, tooth decay, decalcification of enamel and dentin) is the most common chronic disease of children. Many youth in the United States are affected by tooth decay and pain that interfere with activities of daily living such as eating, sleeping, attending school, and speaking. From 41% to 75% (depending on their state of residence) of third graders have had caries, and from 12% to 43% (again depending on state of residence) have untreated tooth decay (Centers for Disease Control and Prevention, 2011). By the teen years, even more youth have caries and untreated decay. In addition, puberty marks the beginning of gingivitis and periodontal disease for some youth; in those with eating disorders, erosion of tooth enamel may occur (American Academy of Periodontology, 2011). The increased use of sealants (38% of youth have obtained these) has improved the oral health of children whose families receive regular dental care (Dye, Tan, Smith, et al., 2007).

When families have financial challenges, dental care is often not obtained. Low-income children account for 80% of all childhood dental decay, the reason for the disparity in caries across states. When decay has already occurred, care is more costly and difficult for the child. Rampant caries, or multiple lesions in the same child, is a complicated and costly condition to manage. Nurses address oral health issues by performing oral assessments during school screenings and health supervision visits, asking about dental care access, and referring families to resources as needed (see Developing Cultural Competence: Dental Care Resources).

Clearly, health promotion is needed for dental health. Nurses assess for risk factors such as intake of sweetened beverages and food, teach

---

Developing Cultural Competence
Dental Care Resources

Over one half of all children from homes with low incomes have not received dental care in the last year; twice as many of them have unmet dental needs as children in families with adequate finances (Child Trends, 2011). Hispanic children, children with disabilities, and children with parents who are poor, have low educational level, or lack health insurance are also more likely to have unmet dental needs (Child Trends, 2011; Tanski, Garfunkel, Duncan, et al., 2010). Since children in homes with low incomes are especially prone to poor dental health, efforts are being extended to help families receive care. Many of the State Children's Health Insurance Programs (SCHIPs) offer dental services, although some have been decreased in the financial crisis of the last few years. All children in the Medicaid program are eligible for dental coverage in the Early and Periodic Screening, Diagnostic, and Treatment (EPSDT) services. See Chapter 1 for further description of programs mentioned here. Private and public clinics in many communities provide low-cost or free care for families with limited financial resources. Recall the family in the opening scenario and their need for dental care. Note that the nurse referred them for further healthcare resources. Many families do not realize their children could receive dental care services. Find out what resources are available in your state and community, and refer families as needed. Be particularly attentive to families who live in poverty, have a child with disabilities, are from an ethnic minority, or have low parental educational levels.

---

about oral care, and ensure access to dental visits. Health maintenance activities relate to prevention of caries and illness related to dental disease. Use of fluoride and sealants to strengthen teeth and referral for care when poor dental care is apparent are examples of these activities.

Mental and Spiritual Health

Mental and spiritual health are important concepts to address in health promotion and health maintenance visits. Families usually are accustomed to questions about physical status of the child but may be unprepared to discuss mental health. Encourage parents to keep a record of mental health issues to bring to health supervision visits. This helps them understand that the healthcare professional is willing to partner with them to assist in dealing with mental health. Suggest topics such as child and parental mood, child temperament, stresses and ways that family members manage stress, or sleep patterns. Make notes in the record as a reminder of questions to ask at the next visit. The healthcare professional addresses mental health issues in relation to prevention, risk assessment, and diagnosis of conditions (Hagan, Shaw, & Duncan, 2008).

The nurse establishes both health promotion and maintenance goals related to child and family mental health. Health promotion goals relate to adequate resources to meet family challenges, as well as protective factors like involvement in extended family and the community. For example, the sleep-deprived child needs help to establish healthy sleep patterns to prevent psychologic and physical problems. It can be helpful to teach stress reduction techniques such as meditation, relaxation, and imagery to the child, as well as providing resources for yoga classes to the family. See Chapter 3 for further discussion. For health maintenance goals related to the prevention of mental health problems, nurses may act by providing resources when domestic violence occurs, or referring cases of suspected child abuse or neglect. Observe the child and family for appropriateness of affect and mood. Be alert for signs of depression, stress, or anxiety (see Chapter 33 for more detail). Note any signs of abuse, neglect, or domestic violence.

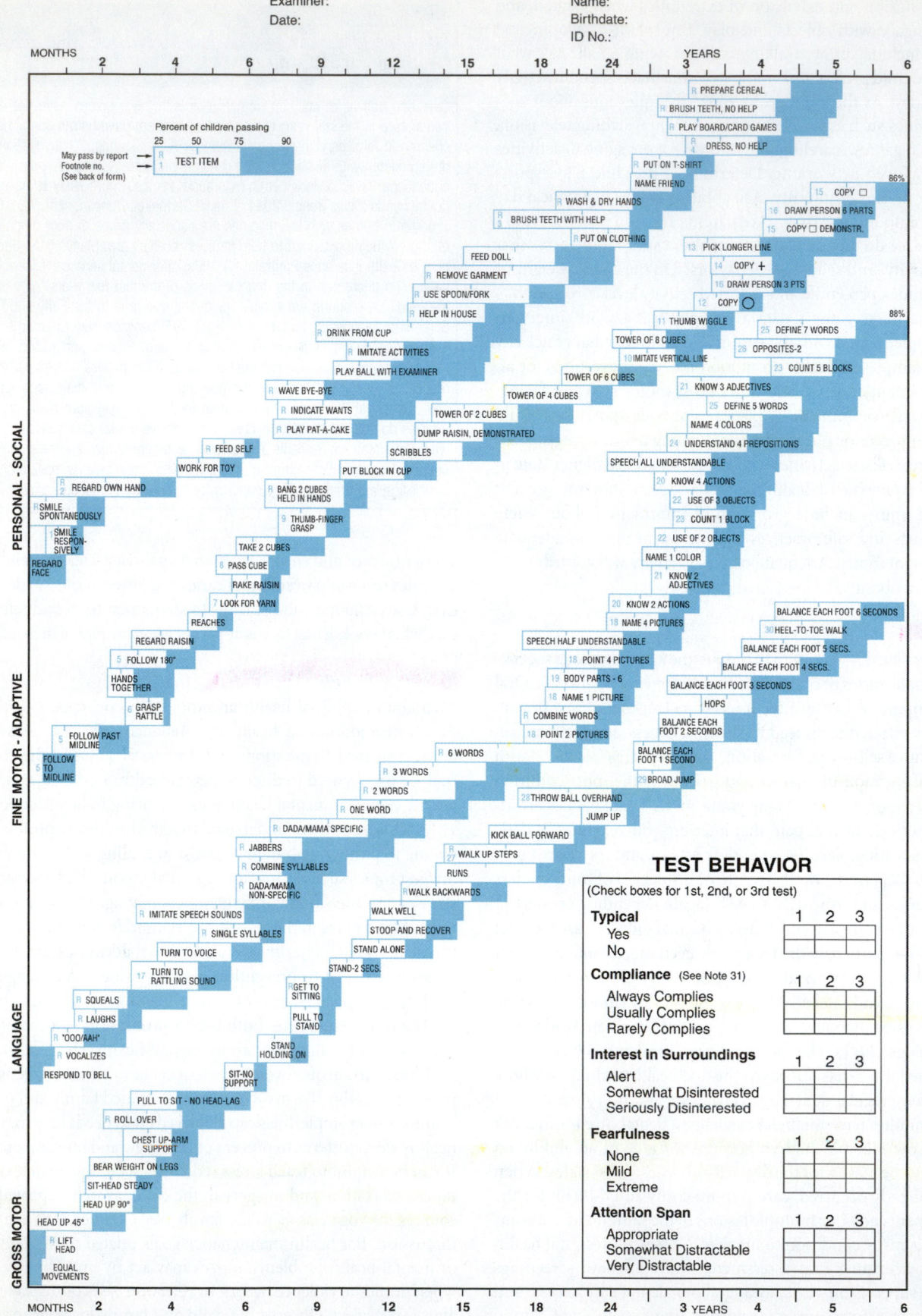

FIGURE 8–5 ■ Denver II.

Source: From W. K. Frankenburg, Denver Developmental Materials, Inc., PO Box 371075, Denver, CO 80237-5075, 1-800-419-4729, www.denverii.com. © 1969, 1989, 1990 W. K. Frankenburg and J. B. Dodds. © 1978 W. K. Frankenburg. © 2009 Wilhelmine R. Frankenburg. Reproduced with permission.

DIRECTIONS FOR ADMINISTRATION

1. Try to get child to smile by smiling, talking or waving. Do not touch him/her.
2. Child must stare at hand several seconds.
3. Parent may help guide toothbrush and put toothpaste on brush.
4. Child does not have to be able to tie shoes or button/zip in the back.
5. Move yarn slowly in an arc from one side to the other, about 8" above child's face.
6. Pass if child grasps rattle when it is touched to the backs or tips of fingers.
7. Pass if child tries to see where yarn went. Yarn should be dropped quickly from sight from tester's hand without arm movement.
8. Child must transfer cube from hand to hand without help of body, mouth, or table.
9. Pass if child picks up raisin with any part of thumb and finger.
10. Line can vary only 30 degrees or less from tester's line.
11. Make a fist with thumb pointing upward and wiggle only the thumb. Pass if child imitates and does not move any fingers other than the thumb.

  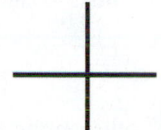 

12. Pass any enclosed form. Fail continuous round motions.
13. Which line is longer? (Not bigger.) Turn paper upside down and repeat. (pass 3 of 3 or 5 of 6)
14. Pass any lines crossing near midpoint.
15. Have child copy first. If failed, demonstrate.

When giving items 12, 14, and 15, do not name the forms. Do not demonstrate 12 and 14.

16. When scoring, each pair (2 arms, 2 legs, etc.) counts as one part.
17. Place one cube in cup and shake gently near child's ear, but out of sight. Repeat for other ear.
18. Point to picture and have child name it. (No credit is given for sounds only.)
    If less than 4 pictures are named correctly, have child point to picture as each is named by tester.

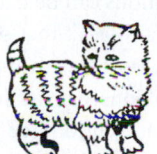 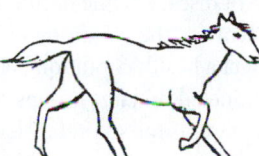 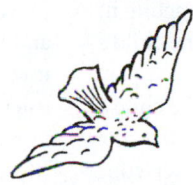 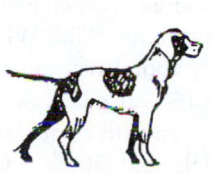 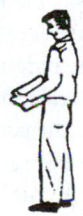

19. Using doll, tell child: Show me the nose, eyes, ears, mouth, hands, feet, tummy, hair. Pass 6 of 8.
20. Using pictures, ask child: Which one flies?...says meow?...talks?...barks?...gallops? Pass 2 of 5, 4 of 5.
21. Ask child: What do you do when you are cold?...tired?...hungry? Pass 2 of 3, 3 of 3.
22. Ask child: What do you do with a cup? What is a chair used for? What is a pencil used for?
    Action words must be included in answers.
23. Pass if child correctly places _and_ says how many blocks are on paper. (1,5).
24. Tell child: Put block **on** table; **under** table; **in front of** me, **behind** me. Pass 4 of 4.
    (Do not help child by pointing, moving head or eyes.)
25. Ask child: What is a ball?...lake?...desk?...house?...banana?...curtain?...fence?...ceiling? Pass if defined in terms
    of use, shape, what it is made of, or general category (such as banana is fruit, not just yellow). Pass 5 of 8, 7 of 8.
26. Ask child: If a horse is big, a mouse is ___? If fire is hot, ice is ___? If the sun shines during the day, the moon shines
    during the ___? Pass 2 of 3.
27. Child may use wall or rail only, not person. May not crawl.
28. Child must throw ball overhand 3 feet to within arm's reach of tester.
29. Child must perform standing broad jump over width of test sheet (8 1/2 inches).
30. Tell child to walk forward, ⟿ heel within 1 inch of toe. Tester may demonstrate.
    Child must walk 4 consecutive steps.
31. In the second year, half of normal children are non-compliant.

OBSERVATIONS:

FIGURE 8–5 ■ *(Continued)* Directions for administration of Denver II.

Source: *From W. K. Frankenburg, Denver Developmental Materials, Inc., PO Box 371075, Denver, CO 80237-5075, 1-800-419-4729, www.denverii.com. © 1969, 1989, 1990 W. K. Frankenburg and J. B. Dodds. © 1978
W. K. Frankenburg. © 2009 Wilhelmine R. Frankenburg. Reproduced with permission.*

Weblink | Centers for Disease Control and Prevention

BOX 8–5	Spiritual Dimension

The **spiritual dimension** is a connection with a power greater than that in the self, and guides a person to strive for inspiration, respect, meaning, and purpose in life (Murray, Zentner, & Yakimo, 2009). Some individuals develop and reinforce the spiritual dimension through membership in a religious group, whereas others study or honor positive human and moral qualities.

BOX 8–6	Mental and Spiritual Health Components

There are many components to mental health. Some areas that can be focused upon during health supervision visits include:

- Mood, especially evidence in any family member of depression, anxiety, or anger
- Sleep patterns, especially of the child
- Presence of domestic violence
- Presence of substance abuse
- Family support system
- Family stresses such as illness, incarceration, financial concerns, marital discord, deaths, recent moves, or job loss
- Spiritual health and meaning in life
- Participation in faith-based groups

Apply resilience theory by asking about both risk and protective factors. What are the mental health issues and how do family members handle them? One family may have financial concerns but has the resources to face and solve problems, whereas another family resorts to fighting and other behaviors that influence the child's environment.

Spiritual health is seen in the larger context of entities that provide meaning in life. For some, this may be membership in a faith-based group; for others, it may be feeling part of a society with a purpose of greater good, or setting goals for the future (Boxes 8–5 and 8–6). Ask about the family's meaningful activities. Provide links to faith-based groups as needed.

Relationships

The relationships that a child establishes with others begin at birth. The first and most important set of relationships develops within the family. The mother, father, siblings, and perhaps extended family are the contexts in which the baby learns to relate with others. As the child grows, the world widens to encompass other children, friends of the family, peers, school, and the larger community network. Analyzing the child's relationships at all ages provides important clues to social interactions.

From the moment the family is called in from a waiting area, be alert for clues to family relationships. Who brought the child to the visit? What was the family doing when you called them from the waiting room? Were they reading to the child or interacting in some way? Do the parents talk with the child? What is the child's response? Are developmentally appropriate interactions apparent? For example, the parent of a 5-year-old might hold the child's hand, but this would rarely be seen with an adolescent. Does the parent of an older child or adolescent let the child answer your questions?

Likewise, other social interactions are important to evaluate. Does the young infant interact in an age-appropriate manner with the healthcare provider or other children in the area? See Chapter 5 for social milestones at various ages.

Ask the parents questions about family and social interactions. What is easy and difficult in caring for the infant? What kind of temperament does the child have? **Temperament** is the characteristic behavioral style of the infant. Babies' temperaments represent inborn characteristics about responses to the environment, such as regularity of sleeping and eating, and to new people and situations. See Chapter 5 for a detailed description of temperament. Does the older child have playmates? What are they like? What activities do the children do together? Ask older children to describe their best friends and how they spend time. Common tools to assess temperament during health supervision visits are Carey Infant and Child Questionnaires (see Chapter 5).

Once you have completed the assessment, establish goals and interventions related to family and social relationships. Health promotion issues include anticipatory guidance for parents of young children about needs for socialization of the child with others, as well as discipline techniques to be used at various ages. Health promotion for the older child may involve teaching related to how to show friends you care and how to solve disputes in a

positive manner. Health maintenance activities are aimed at preventing family and social interaction problems. Provide information to children about bullying in schools and dealing with conflict at home. Specific examples for different age groups can be found in Chapters 9 through 13 .

Disease Prevention Strategies

Disease prevention strategies focus mainly on health maintenance, or prevention of disease. Some health disruptions can be detected early and treatment for the condition can begin. Recall that screening is used to detect a health condition before symptoms are apparent; it is usually conducted on large groups of individuals at risk for a condition and represents the secondary level of prevention (see Table 8–1). Most screening tests are not strictly diagnostic but are followed by further diagnostic tests if the screening result is positive. Once a screening test identifies the existence of a health condition, early intervention can begin, with the goal of reducing the severity or complications of the condition. For example, all newborns are screened within 1 week of birth for at least two genetic diseases: congenital hypothyroidism and phenylketonuria. Appropriate interventions (medication or diet therapy) reduce the chances or severity of mental retardation if either of these conditions is present. (See Chapters 4, 9, and 35 for more information about newborn screening.) Infants are commonly screened for diseases and for growth parameters, young children for growth and disorders such as anemia, and school-age children for growth, blood pressure, hearing, and vision. In addition, adolescents may be screened for scoliosis, substance abuse, and sexually transmitted infections.

Screening tests are administered at times when children are most likely to develop a condition, or to identify the greatest number of children at highest risk for the condition. Screening tests are also expected to correctly identify children who do have the condition. Some children are at greater risk of contracting certain conditions due to their environment. For example, young children living in housing built before 1960 are screened more frequently for lead poisoning than children who live in newer houses where only lead-free paints have been used (see Chapter 20 for a discussion of lead poisoning). Tables 8–6 and 8–7 outline the recommended screening

TABLE 8–6 **Recommendations for Preventive Pediatric Health Care, Committee on Practice and Ambulatory Medicine, American Academy of Pediatrics, United States**

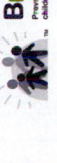

American Academy of Pediatrics
DEDICATED TO THE HEALTH OF ALL CHILDREN™

Recommendations for Preventive Pediatric Health Care

Bright Futures™
Prevention and health promotion for infants, children, adolescents, and their families™

Each child and family is unique; therefore, these **Recommendations for Preventive Pediatric Health Care** are designed for the care of children who are receiving competent parenting, have no manifestations of any important health problems, and are growing and developing in satisfactory fashion. **Additional visits may become necessary** if circumstances suggest variations from normal.

Developmental, psychosocial, and chronic disease issues for children and adolescents may require frequent counseling and treatment visits separate from preventive care visits.

These guidelines represent a consensus by the American Academy of Pediatrics (AAP) and Bright Futures. The AAP continues to emphasize the great importance of **continuity of care** in comprehensive health supervision and the need to avoid **fragmentation of care.**

The recommendations in this statement do not indicate an exclusive course of treatment or standard of medical care. Variations, taking into account individual circumstances, may be appropriate.

Copyright © 2008 by the American Academy of Pediatrics.

No part of this statement may be reproduced in any form or by any means without prior written permission from the American Academy of Pediatrics except for one copy for personal use.

	INFANCY								EARLY CHILDHOOD						
Age[a]	Prenatal[b]	Newborn[c]	3–5 d[d]	By 1 mo	2 mo	4 mo	6 mo	9 mo	12 m	15 mo	18 mo	24 mo	30 mo	3 y	4 y
HISTORY															
Initial/interval	•	•	•	•	•	•	•	•	•	•	•	•	•	•	•
MEASUREMENTS															
Length/height and weight		•	•	•	•	•	•	•	•	•	•	•	•	•	•
Head circumference		•	•	•	•	•	•	•	•	•	•	•			
Weight for length		•	•	•	•	•	•	•	•	•	•				
Body mass index												•	•	•	•
Blood pressure[e]		★	★	★	★	★	★	★	★	★	★	★	★	•	•
SENSORY SCREENING															
Vision		★	★	★	★	★	★	★	★	★	★	★	★	•[f]	•
Hearing		•[g]	★	★	★	★	★	★	★	★	★	★	★	★	•
DEVELOPMENTAL/BEHAVIORAL ASSESSMENT															
Developmental screening[h]								•			•		•		
Autism screening[i]											•	•			
Developmental surveillance[h]		•	•	•	•	•	•		•	•		•		•	•
Psychosocial/behavioral assessment		•	•	•	•	•	•	•	•	•	•	•	•	•	•
Alcohol and drug use assessment															
PHYSICAL EXAMINATION[j]		•	•	•	•	•	•	•	•	•	•	•	•	•	•
PROCEDURES[k]															
Newborn metabolic/hemoglobin screening[l]		←	•	—	→										
Immunization[m]		•	•	•	•	•	•	•	•	•	•	•	•	•	•
Hematocrit or hemoglobin[n]						★			•		★	★		★	★
Lead screening[o]							★	★	• or ★[p]		★	• or ★[p]		★	★
Tuberculin test[q]				★			★		★		★	★		★	★
Dyslipidemia screening[r]												★			★
STI screening[s]															
Cervical dysplasia screening[t]															
ORAL HEALTH[u]							★	★	• or ★[u]		• or ★[u]	• or ★[u]	• or ★[u]	•[v]	
ANTICIPATORY GUIDANCE[w]	•	•	•	•	•	•	•	•	•	•	•	•	•	•	•

	MIDDLE CHILDHOOD						ADOLESCENCE										
Age[a]	5 y	6 y	7 y	8 y	9 y	10 y	11 y	12 y	13 y	14 y	15 y	16 y	17 y	18 y	19 y	20 y	21 y
HISTORY																	
Initial/interval	•	•	•	•	•	•	•	•	•	•	•	•	•	•	•	•	•
MEASUREMENTS																	
Length/height and weight	•	•	•	•	•	•	•	•	•	•	•	•	•	•	•	•	•
Head circumference																	
Weight for length																	
Body mass index	•	•	•	•	•	•	•	•	•	•	•	•	•	•	•	•	•
Blood pressure[e]	•	•	•	•	•	•	•	•	•	•	•	•	•	•	•	•	•
SENSORY SCREENING																	
Vision	•	•	★	•	★	•	★	•	★	★	•	★	★	•	★	★	★
Hearing	•	•	★	•	★	•	★	★	★	★	★	★	★	★	★	★	★
DEVELOPMENTAL/BEHAVIORAL ASSESSMENT																	
Developmental screening[h]																	
Autism screening[i]																	
Developmental surveillance[h]	•	•	•	•	•	•	•	•	•	•	•	•	•	•	•	•	•
Psychosocial/behavioral assessment	•	•	•	•	•	•	•	•	•	•	•	•	•	•	•	•	•
Alcohol and drug use assessment							★	★	★	★	★	★	★	★	★	★	★
PHYSICAL EXAMINATION[j]	•	•	•	•	•	•	•	•	•	•	•	•	•	•	•	•	•
PROCEDURES[k]																	
Newborn metabolic/hemoglobin screening[l]																	
Immunization[m]	•	•	•	•	•	•	•	•	•	•	•	•	•	•	•	•	•
Hematocrit or hemoglobin[n]	★	★	★	★	★	★	★	★	★	★	★	★	★	★	★	★	★
Lead screening[o]	★	★															
Tuberculin test[q]	★	★	★	★	★	★	★	★	★	★	★	★	★	★	★	★	★
Dyslipidemia screening[r]		★		★		★	★	★	★	★	★	★	★	←	—	•	→
STI screening[s]							★	★	★	★	★	★	★	★	★	★	★
Cervical dysplasia screening[t]							★	★	★	★	★	★	★	★	★	★	★
ORAL HEALTH[u]		•[v]															
ANTICIPATORY GUIDANCE[w]	•	•	•	•	•	•	•	•	•	•	•	•	•	•	•	•	•

a If a child comes under care for the first time at any point on the schedule, or if any items are not accomplished at the suggested age, the schedule should be brought up to date at the earliest possible time.

b A prenatal visit is recommended for parents who are at high risk, for first-time parents, and for those who request a conference. The prenatal visit should include anticipatory guidance, pertinent medical history, and a discussion of benefits of breastfeeding and planned method of feeding per AAP statement "The Prenatal Visit" (2001) [URL: http://aappolicy.aappublications.org/cgi/content/full/pediatrics;107/6/1456].

c Every infant should have a newborn evaluation after birth, breastfeeding encouraged, and instruction and support offered.

d Every infant should have an evaluation within 3 to 5 days of birth and within 48 to 72 hours after discharge from the hospital, to include evaluation for feeding and jaundice. Breastfeeding infants should receive formal breastfeeding evaluation, encouragement, and instruction as recommended in AAP statement "Breastfeeding and the Use of Human Milk" (2005) [URL: http://aappolicy.aappublications.org/cgi/content/full/pediatrics;115/2/496]. For newborns discharged in less than 48 hours after delivery, the infant must be examined within 48 hours of discharge per AAP statement "Hospital Stay for Healthy Term Newborns" (2004) [URL: http://aappolicy.aappublications.org/cgi/content/full/pediatrics;113/5/1434].

e Blood pressure measurement in infants and children with specific risk conditions should be performed at visits before age 3 years.

f If the patient is uncooperative, rescreen within 6 months per AAP statement "Eye Examination and Vision Screening in Infants, Children, and Young Adults" (1996) [URL: http://aappolicy.aappublications.org/cgi/reprint/pediatrics;98/1/153.pdf].

g All newborns should be screened per AAP statement "Year 2000 Position Statement: Principles and Guidelines for Early Hearing Detection and Intervention Programs" (2000) [URL: http://aappolicy.aappublications.org/cgi/content/full/pediatrics;106/4/798]. Joint Committee on Infant Hearing. Year 2007 position statement: principles and guidelines for early hearing detection and intervention programs. *Pediatrics.* 2007;120:898–921.

h AAP Council on Children With Disabilities, AAP Section on Developmental Behavioral Pediatrics, AAP Bright Futures Steering Committee, AAP Medical Home Initiatives for Children With Special Needs Project Advisory Committee. Identifying infants and young children with developmental disorders in the medical home: an algorithm for developmental surveillance and screening. *Pediatrics.* 2006;118:405–420 [URL: http://aappolicy.aappublications.org/cgi/content/full/pediatrics;118/1/405].

i Gupta VB, Hyman SL, Johnson CP, et al. Identifying children with autism early? *Pediatrics.* 2007;119:152–153 [URL: http://pediatrics.aappublications.org/cgi/content/full/119/1/152].

j At each visit, age-appropriate physical examination is essential, with infant totally unclothed, older child undressed and suitably draped.

k These may be modified, depending on entry point into schedule and individual need.

l Newborn metabolic and hemoglobinopathy screening should be done according to state law. Results should be reviewed at visits and appropriate retesting or referral done as needed.

m Schedules per the Committee on Infectious Diseases, published annually in the January issue of *Pediatrics*. Every visit should be an opportunity to update and complete a child's immunizations.

n See AAP *Pediatric Nutrition Handbook*, 5th Edition (2003) for a discussion of universal and selective screening options. See also Recommendations to prevent and control iron deficiency in the United States. *MMWR Recomm Rep.* 1998;47(RR-3):1–36.

o For children at risk of lead exposure, consult the AAP statement "Lead Exposure in Children: Prevention, Detection, and Management" (2005) [URL: http://aappolicy.aappublications.org/cgi/content/full/pediatrics;116/4/1036]. Additionally, screening should be done in accordance with state law where applicable.

p Perform risk assessments or screens as appropriate, based on universal screening requirements for patients with Medicaid or high prevalence areas.

q Tuberculosis testing per recommendations of the Committee on Infectious Diseases, published in the current edition of *Red Book: Report of the Committee on Infectious Diseases*. Testing should be done on recognition of high-risk factors.

r "Third Report of the National Cholesterol Education Program (NCEP) Expert Panel on Detection, Evaluation, and Treatment of High Blood Cholesterol in Adults (Adult Treatment Panel III) Final Report" (2002) [URL: http://circ.ahajournals.org/cgi/content/full/106/25/3143] and "The Expert Committee Recommendations on the Assessment, Prevention, and Treatment of Child and Adolescent Overweight and Obesity." Supplement to *Pediatrics*. In press.

s All sexually active patients should be screened for sexually transmitted infections (STIs).

t All sexually active girls should have screening for cervical dysplasia as part of a pelvic examination beginning within 3 years of onset of sexual activity or age 21 (whichever comes first).

u Referral to dental home, if available. Otherwise, administer oral health risk assessment. If the primary water source is deficient in fluoride, consider oral fluoride supplementation.

v At the visits for 3 years and 6 years of age, it should be determined whether the patient has a dental home. If the patient does not have a dental home, a referral should be made to one. If the primary water source is deficient in fluoride, consider oral fluoride supplementation.

w Refer to the specific guidance by age as listed in Bright Futures Guidelines. (Hagan JF, Shaw JS, Duncan PM, eds. *Bright Futures: Guidelines for Health Supervision of Infants, Children, and Adolescents*. 3rd ed. Elk Grove Village, IL: American Academy of Pediatrics; 2008.)

• = to be performed ★ = risk assessment to be performed, with appropriate action to follow, if positive ←—•—→ = range during which a service may be provided, with the symbol indicating the preferred age

Source: *Reproduced with permission from* Pediatrics, *120, 1376. Copyright ©2007 by the American Academy of Pediatrics. No part of this statement may be reproduced in any form or by any means without prior written permission from the American Academy of Pediatrics except for one copy for personal use.*

TABLE 8–7	Components of Well-Child Assessments at Various Ages, Pediatric Clinical Practice Guidelines for Nurses in Primary Care, Health Canada
HEALTH PARAMETER	**MOST IMPORTANT AGES FOR ASSESSMENT**
Height, weight	Every visit from birth to 16 years of age
Head circumference	Every visit in the first 2 years of life
Growth chart plotting	Every visit
Blood pressure	Once in the first 2 years, once at 4–6 years, during school-age years only if there is a risk or concern about high blood pressure, and every second year during adolescence
Eye assessment	Every visit in the first year of life
Strabismus assessment	Every visit in the first year of life
Visual acuity testing	Initial screening (e.g., Snellen chart) at 3–5 years of age; every 2 years between 6 and 10 years of age, then every 3 years until 18 years of age
Dental assessment	Every visit
Speech assessment	Every visit
Developmental assessment	Every visit
Sexual development	Every visit
School adjustment	Every visit after child reaches school age
Chemical abuse	Consider during assessments of children older than 8 years of age
Immunizations	According to schedule: at 2, 4, 6, 12, and 18 months and at 4–6 and 14–16 years
Hemoglobin	Screen at 6–12 months
Safety counseling	Every visit
Nutrition counseling	From birth to 5 years, and for teenagers
Parenting counseling	Every visit

Source: Pediatric Clinical Practice Guidelines for Nurses in Primary Care. Health Canada, 2008. Reproduced with permission from the Minister of Health, 2012.

tests by age for infants, children, and adolescents. Box 8–7 discusses interpretation of screening tests.

Another way to prevent diseases is to immunize children against common communicable diseases. See Chapter 22 🔗 for the complete list of childhood immunizations and schedules for administration. Refer to the Centers for Disease Control and Prevention website and Chapters 9 through 13 🔗 for usual immunization needs at specific ages. The nurse who administers immunizations is performing a health maintenance activity. However, even health promotion activities can occur when a parent expresses interest in learning more about certain immunizations, how they act, and the risks and benefits of immunizations and corresponding diseases. Meeting the parent's goal to understand more and make intelligent choices and healthcare decisions is an example of a health promotion activity.

Injury Prevention (Safety) Strategies

Most childhood mortality and hospitalization is related to injury (see Chapter 1 🔗). Unintentional injury is the leading cause of death among individuals from 1 to 19 years of age (Centers for Disease Control and Prevention, 2010b). Therefore, it is important for the nurse to integrate injury prevention strategies in all health supervision visits. These strategies represent health maintenance activities because they recognize injury risks and aim to prevent potential injuries.

The family is constantly challenged to maintain a safe environment as the child grows older, reaches more advanced developmental levels, is exposed to a widening world outside the family, and has less supervision. Asking parents to bring their questions about

BOX 8–7	Screening Test Interpretation

Sensitivity is the ability of the test to accurately identify those with the condition. High sensitivity is seen in a test that is able to detect the condition when only a small amount of the indicator is present, or early in the disease process. Some children who test positive for a condition do not actually have it; they are classified as false positives.

Specificity is the ability of the test to exclude those who do not have the condition. Some children who test negative may actually have the disease; they are classified as false negatives. The best screening tests have both high sensitivity and high specificity. In addition to this accuracy, other considerations include cost, ease of administration, and acceptability.

Source: Adapted from Clark (2008).

safety to each visit can be a good starting point for discussion. Safety teaching should be integrated with developmental progression. For example, as the child begins to crawl, the family needs to be aware of hazards on the floor of the house, such as electrical outlets and stairs. When the school-age child is riding a bicycle to school, traffic patterns and helmet use should be discussed. Ask the teen driver about drinking patterns of self and friends.

The nurse considers knowledge about the age of the child and information from the health supervision visit to plan health maintenance interventions related to injury. Teaching is performed, resources are made available, and parents and children who have experienced injury are invited to present their experiences. Some common universal injury prevention topics include car safety, pedestrian safety, sport injury prevention, poison prevention, and child abuse prevention. What other activities and approaches would you plan to prevent injuries at specific ages?

Additional Topics

Many other topics might be discussed during health supervision visits. They may relate to either health maintenance activities designed to preserve health, or health promotion activities intended to enhance or improve the state of wellness. They include topics such as extended family members and their role in the child's life, cultural variations or inclusion, or development of moral values and ethical behaviors. The nurse should be alert for clues to potential areas for discussion and should invite the family several times during a visit to ask any questions that they might have. See Developing Cultural Competence: Culture and Disease.

Nursing Management

Nursing Assessment and Diagnosis

During health supervision visits, a portrait of the child and family will emerge. The nurse applies knowledge of populations and development to tailor assessment gathering and planned interventions (Box 8–8). Observe the parent–child interaction in the waiting room and throughout the examination. If siblings are present, watch for interactions among all family members. Observe affect and mood of the child and parents. Nursing assessment of the child and family at each visit for health supervision then focuses on the following:

- Interviewing the family and child to update the health history, to ask about the child's developmental or educational progress, and to identify dietary habits, physical activity, and safety practices
- Eliciting questions and concerns that the parent or child may have
- Conducting developmental surveillance assessments, including review of questionnaires completed by the parent in the waiting room

Developing Cultural Competence
Culture and Disease

Culture and health are intimately linked. Some ethnic groups may have a greater incidence of certain diseases, and screening for these diseases should be more commonly performed (see Chapter 3 🔗). For example, type 2 diabetes is common in African Americans and Native Americans, while ischemic heart disease is at low risk in Chinese Americans. Fair-skinned people are more likely to get skin melanoma.

Significant differences in injury rates are observed in various ethnic groups. High rates of motor vehicle death and drowning occur in American Indian/Alaska Native youth. Blacks have high rates of unintentional suffocation, homicide, and fires. In general, the highest rates of injury-related death occur in American Indian/Alaska Natives, followed by Blacks. Hispanics and Whites have nearly the same rates, and Asian/Pacific Islanders have the lowest rates (Centers for Disease Control and Prevention, 2010b).

At other times the perception of health or illness may differ among cultures. Certain Asian cultures may view illness as an imbalance in the body and will need to have certain ceremonies or other procedures done to restore balance. Bad dreams are believed to be responsible for mental illness in some cultural groups. There is varying acceptance of screening tests such as blood work among various groups. Health takes on different meanings for various people—it may be the absence of disease, the ability to be active in spite of illness, or a state of complete balance.

Be familiar both with common diseases and injuries in the groups you see in clinical settings and with the beliefs about health and illness within the groups. Teach prevention techniques that respond to the greatest proportion of injuries. Honor the beliefs of others and learn from them, as you share your knowledge in a respectful manner.

BOX 8–8 **Baccalaureate Essential VII: Clinical Prevention and Population Health**

An important part of the nursing role is to understand the health of population groups, such as children, adolescents, and families. Epidemiology, or the study of health-related conditions and determinants in certain population groups, form the basis for the nurse's planned interventions related to health promotion and maintenance. Statistics appear about certain conditions throughout this chapter and the entire book text, so that you can understand the prevalence, contributing factors, and protective factors for those conditions. This assists the nurse in planning for interventions that promote health and prevent disease or injury in a population. Some factors that can protect or create risks for population health include genetics, lifestyle behaviors, and environmental conditions. Thus, the nurse examines ethnic and racial characteristics; nutrition, activity, and substance use patterns; genetic history; and emergency preparedness of populations. Populations can be viewed widely such as childhood or adolescence, or in a more specialized approach such as migrant workers, those experiencing homelessness, or families that have no health insurance. *Name a population group that you work with in your pediatric clinical setting, and list the particular risks and protective factors that guide your health promotion and maintenance plans for that population.*

- Performing age-appropriate screening tests (Figure 8–6 ■)
- Performing a physical assessment

Following a thorough assessment, the nurse derives nursing diagnoses that are pertinent to the health status of the child and that consider the family's needs. Nursing diagnoses are developed jointly with the family as an essential component of the partnership between nurse and family. Examples of nursing diagnoses for an 18-month-old child who is brought by parents for regular health supervision and immunizations may include the following:

- Nutrition, Imbalanced: More than Body Requirements related to lack of basic nutritional knowledge
- Poisoning, Risk for related to lack of proper precautions with increased mobility to reach and climb
- Health Behavior, Risk-Prone related to needed immunizations
- Caregiver Role Strain, Risk for related to mother's plans to return to full-time work

NANDA-I © 2012

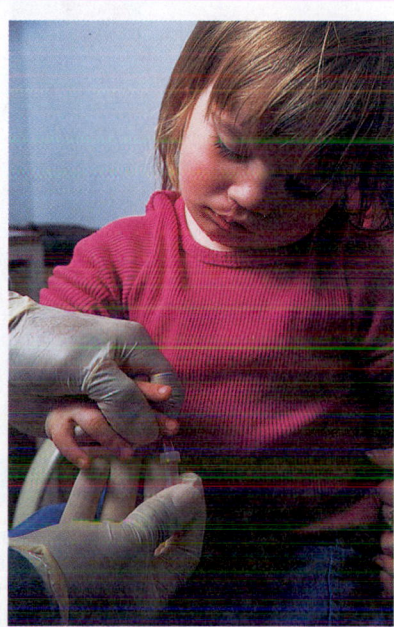

FIGURE 8–6 ■ This 18-month-old toddler is having a blood screening test to detect iron deficiency anemia. Children are often screened for adequate levels of iron in later infancy and during toddlerhood.

Planning and Implementation

Nursing management for health supervision visits begins with collaborative planning with family members. They share their concerns and questions, and the nurse also lists procedures and discussion topics to be addressed. These may include providing immunizations, offering anticipatory guidance about discipline, educating parents and children about healthy behaviors, addressing health promotion regarding nutrition, suggesting ways to prevent disease and injury, and providing referrals for follow-up care. For more information about the recommended schedule for immunizations and the nurse's role in ensuring full immunization status for children, refer to Chapter 22 🖉.

Most parents want to know how to contribute to their child's growth and development. Discussions at the conclusion of the health supervision assessments should focus on building family strengths by promoting the development of competence, confidence, and self-esteem in the growing child. By offering examples of health promotion activities such as these, the nurse can provide a positive ending for the visit.

Although health supervision most likely takes place in an office or clinic setting, nursing management for health supervision can occur in any setting. The nurse recognizes that health promotion and health maintenance activities are key to any nurse–family relationship. For example, if the child is seen in an emergency department for treatment of a fracture, the nurse should ask about immunization status and safety issues. A child with a chronic disorder such as cerebral palsy may obtain most health promotion and health maintenance services in the outpatient clinic at an orthopedic hospital. A child hospitalized for an acute respiratory illness often has a parent present, and the nurse should explore the health promotion questions that parent has and perform some teaching about developmental findings. Indeed, health promotion is a constant and foundational aspect of all pediatric care. Viewing it as essential ensures that this part of health care, which most closely reflects a partnership with families, will be part of every healthcare encounter. Health maintenance information should be included in all healthcare encounters to lessen disease and injury risk. See Figure 8–7 ■. Also see Box 8–9 for information about evidence-based nursing.

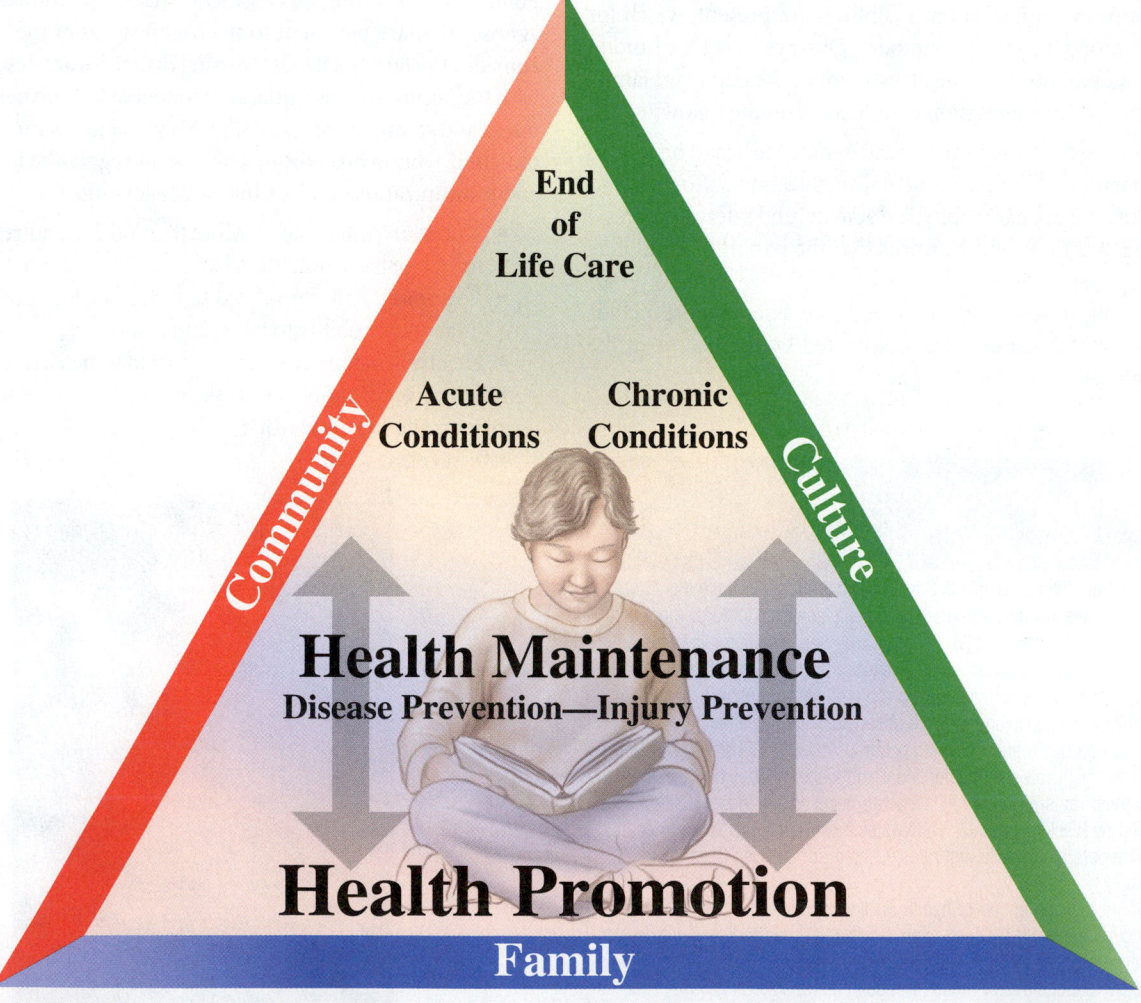

FIGURE 8–7 ■ The Bindler-Ball Continuum of Pediatric Healthcare for Children and Their Families. Health promotion is foundational to all care in pediatric nursing. Health promotion and health maintenance activities take place at health supervision visits and provide the strong foundation for health as the infant grows into childhood and adolescence. The influences from these activities are carried forward as the child experiences any chronic or acute conditions. Likewise, health promotion and maintenance activities can take place at any health encounter. Health promotion goals of balance and spiritual peace may even be met at the end of life. Notice that the family is the strong foundation upon which the child's health encounters rest. The family is an integral part of the child's health and has a strong influence upon it. The community and culture must also be examined to understand their ramifications regarding the child's health status.

BOX 8–9	Research: Evidence-Based Nursing Activities

Nurses are instrumental in providing and analyzing health care in a variety of settings. In one project, a school nurse and physical education teacher partnered to establish an evidence-based guideline to provide strategies to increase physical activity in kindergarten through eighth grade. The extensive guideline provides tools for monitoring children, observing play, evaluating student knowledge, and structuring physical education (Bagby & Adams, 2007). Another example of nurse activity is the construction of an evaluation tool for use with teens at a nurse-managed health center (Benkert, George, Tanner, et al., 2007). Adolescent ratings of care necessarily can influence their acceptance of care provided, so ratings of student perception are important to consider when evaluating outcomes of health centers.

Provide Anticipatory Guidance

Anticipatory guidance involves prediction of the upcoming developmental tasks or needs of a child and gears teaching to those needs. It provides the family with information on what to expect during the child's current and next stage of development. Topics for each visit should include age-appropriate information about healthy habits, prevention of illness and injury, prevention of poisoning, nutrition, oral health, and sexuality. Use health promotional guidance to help the child and family develop strategies that support and enhance social development, family relationships, parental health, community interactions, self-responsibility, and school or vocational achievement.

Because the time for each visit is limited, build upon the parents' current knowledge and care practices, and start with a topic about which they expressed interest. Time can be used to focus on anticipatory guidance to introduce new information, to reinforce what the family is doing well, and to clear up any poorly understood concepts.

Take advantage of other sources of information in the community to enhance the guidance provided. For example, state and local SAFE KIDS Coalitions help inform families about injury prevention strategies. School health programs such as the National Fire Prevention Association's "Risk Watch" may educate children about injury prevention, and other school programs may educate students about smoking and drug avoidance. Keep informed about the types of health education provided in different community settings so it is easier to reinforce the concepts already being taught.

Encourage Health Promotion Activities

Families often need health education and counseling to promote healthy behaviors in their own children, such as information about environmental control to limit sedentary behaviors, dietary changes to increase fruit and vegetable intake, and switching to low-fat dairy products. Partner with the parents to learn what concerns they have and how they want to improve their parenting.

Patient education and counseling are most effective when the family understands the relationship between a behavior change and the resulting health outcome. The parents and child can then work in partnership with the nurse or healthcare provider and make a commitment to the change needed. The health belief model (Pender et al., 2011; Polit & Beck, 2008) helps to explain how people decide whether to participate in programs or activities to prevent disease or enhance health (Table 8–8). They consider whether the health problem is serious and whether they are likely to get the condition. For example, in a family with several members with diabetes, a father is more likely to believe his overweight child will develop diabetes. He is aware of the seriousness of the disease from direct observation. He may weigh the benefits of his teenage daughter's weight loss and activity increase (disease prevention) against the barriers (child fighting with him over food, difficulty managing teen's intake). Then, several modifying factors may influence the situation. The family may have health care so that she can get screened and enter a weight loss program, media announcements may have been made about diabetes, and the teen's motivation to change and confidence in her ability to alter her diet may affect decision making. When finding a family that would benefit from a change in health behavior, consider their perceptions, modifying factors, barriers, and benefits, and plan interventions to enhance the possibility for change.

Perform Health Supervision Interventions

After you collect and analyze all of the information from the interviews, physical assessment, and screening tests, summarize specific health and developmental achievements for the parents and child. Immunizations are provided as appropriate. Offer anticipatory guidance at various points during the health supervision visit.

When a child is found to be at risk for a health condition, integrate health maintenance interventions to lessen the possibility of disease or injury. If an actual health problem is detected, follow-up

Weblink

safekids.org

TABLE 8–8	Health Belief Model			
INDIVIDUAL PERCEPTION OF HEALTH THREAT	**INFLUENCES ON MOTIVATION TO TAKE ACTION**	**MODIFYING FACTORS**	**LIKELIHOOD OF ACTION**
Susceptible to disease or condition	Benefits (e.g., prevent pain and maintain activity)	Social, psychologic, community factors (e.g., age, social class, media, knowledge, previous experiences with condition)	Perceived benefits minus perceived barriers
Disease or condition is serious	Barriers (e.g., time or change required for new behavior)	**Self-efficacy** (e.g., confidence in one's own ability to make change)	

How might the child's self-efficacy (confidence in ability to change) affect the likelihood that the child will adapt to increased physical activity? How can you decrease barriers to health behavior changes?

Source: Adapted from Pender, Murdaugh, & Parsons. (2011).

care must be arranged. The child may need to return for another visit to the primary care provider for further evaluation, or referral to another provider may be needed. Learn about all of the available community resources to make appropriate referrals. The range of such services may include:

- Hospital- and community-based healthcare specialists from a variety of disciplines (dentists, physicians, physical therapists, speech therapists, nutritionists, social workers)
- Community-based programs (childcare centers, developmental stimulation programs, home visitor programs, early intervention programs, mental health centers, diagnostic and evaluation centers, schools, family support centers, food and nutrition referral centers, public health clinics, churches, and other organizations that support families and children)

Evaluation

Expected outcomes of nursing care include the following:

- The child and family collaborate in a partnership with the healthcare provider in joint problem solving and decision making regarding management of the child's healthcare needs after appropriate education and counseling.
- The child and family prepare for future health supervision visits by identifying questions or concerns they want to discuss.

Chapter Highlights

- Health is a dynamic state of physical, mental, and social well-being and is the objective of health promotion and health maintenance activities.
- Theories of resilience and ecology provide guidance in health promotion and health maintenance activities.
- Health supervision visits are healthcare encounters designed to provide assessment, screening, developmental surveillance, immunizations, and health information.
- Partners in providing health supervision are the child, family, health professional, and community.
- Families are best educated in "teachable moments" with small bits of information.
- Developmental surveillance is an essential part of health supervision that provides for observations of children's fine and gross motor skills, language, and psychosocial behavior milestones.

- Nutrition, physical activity, and oral health are essential topics during health supervision visits.
- Mental health, spiritual status, and the relationships of the child within the family and larger community are assessed at each health supervision visit.
- The nurse establishes diagnoses based on a thorough assessment of the child and family during healthcare visits.
- The nurse establishes goals for visits collaboratively with families, and plans interventions to meet goals.
- Health promotion and health maintenance interventions are essential components of all child health care, even during periods of acute or chronic illness.

Clinical Reasoning in Action

INTRODUCTION

Recall the Yevteshenko family in the opening scenario. Tony is receiving dental care for the first time as a 7-year-old, and his 5-year-old brother is waiting his turn. The family recently emigrated from Lithuania and is adjusting to life in this country.

DESCRIPTION

The nurse in the mobile van finds that Tony has well-developed English skills and often acts as interpreter when his parents do not understand questions. He states that he and his brother Ilya like school and that the school nurse is nice to them. She had referred the family to the mobile van for health and oral care. The boys had medical visits and immunizations in Lithuania but never had been to a dentist. They are excited about this visit and interact positively with all staff members. The children and parents appear well nourished and state that they live in a comfortable home, have adequate clothing, and are able to find foods they like to eat.

DISCUSSION

1. With the father's limited employment, what health and dental care insurance needs might the family have? Are there programs in your community or state to which a family such as the Yevteshenkos could be referred?

2. The family has several protective factors such as their willingness to make an appointment and come to the van for care. What other protective factors can you identify? What risk factors?

3. Relationships are an important part of development for school-age children. How would you assess the relationships that Tony and Ilya have at school with peers? How could you as the nurse in the mobile van partner with the school nurse to provide comprehensive health promotion and health maintenance for these boys?

4. Consider that the visit to the mobile van provides a "teachable moment" when the family is focused on dental care. Plan a teaching session to include Tony and Ilya that demonstrates toothbrushing and flossing and allows for return demonstration. How could you and the dental hygienist partner with the family to be sure oral care at home is adequate, and access to professional dental care occurs on a regular basis?

NCLEX-RN® Review

1. The parents of an 8-year-old are at the pediatric healthcare home for a health supervision visit. The child has a history of dental caries. What part of the family history puts him at risk for poor dental care?
   1. The family grows their own vegetables in a garden.
   2. The family is vegetarian.
   3. The family has moved frequently due to the father's employment.
   4. The family does not have health insurance.

2. Which is the priority nursing diagnosis related to child health promotion and maintenance for a family with a first-born child?
   1. Potential for Deficient Knowledge related to inexperience as a parent
   2. Impaired Parenting related to poor cognition
   3. Risk for Impaired Communication related to difference in spoken language between family and nurse
   4. Self-Care Deficit related to activities of daily living

3. Which is true about health maintenance and promotion?
   1. It can take place in any healthcare setting.
   2. It should only occur during annual health supervision visits.
   3. It should be accomplished primarily by the physician.
   4. Health promotion can only be a focus after other healthcare needs are met.

4. Which is the priority intervention for an adolescent who complains to the nurse about changing schools and having no friends?
   1. Discuss why the adolescent had to change schools.
   2. Explore with the teen ways the adolescent might forge new friendships.
   3. Ask the parents why the adolescent has no friends.
   4. Tell the adolescent that he or she must be a friend to have friends.

See Appendix I 🔥 for answers.

References

American Academy of Periodontology. (2011). Protecting children's oral health. Retrieved from http://www.perio.org/consumer/children.htm

American Academy of Pediatrics. (2008). The National Center for Medical Home Initiatives for Children with Special Needs. Retrieved from http://www.medicalhomeinfo.org/training/index.html

American Academy of Pediatrics. (2010). Integrating surveillance and screening with the medical home. Retrieved from http://www.medicalhomeinfo.org/downloads/pdfs/Integsurveil.pdf

Bagby, K., & Adams, S. (2007). Evidence-based practice guideline: Increasing physical activity in schools—Kindergarten through 8th grade. Journal of School Nursing, 23, 137–143.

Benkert, R., George, N., Tanner, C., Barkauskas, V. H., Pohl, J. M., & Marszalek, A. (2007). Satisfaction with a school-based teen health center: A report card on care. Pediatric Nursing, 33, 103–109.

Bindler, R. C., & Ball, J. W. (2007). The Bindler-Ball Healthcare Model: A new paradigm for health promotion. Pediatric Nursing, 33, 121–126.

Bronfenbrenner, U. (2005). Making human beings human: Bioecological perspectives on human development. Thousand Oaks, CA: Sage Publications.

Centers for Disease Control and Prevention. (2010a). Youth Risk Behavior Surveillance—United States, 2009. Morbidity and Mortality Weekly Report, 59(SS-5), 1–148.

Centers for Disease Control and Prevention. (2010b). Causes of death by age group. Retrieved from http://www.cdc.gov/injury/wisaars/leadingcauses.html

Centers for Disease Control and Prevention. (2011). Caries experience and untreated tooth decay. Retrieved from http://apps.nccd.cdc.gov/nohss/IndicatorV.asp?Indicator=2,3

Child Trends. (2011). Unmet dental needs. Retrieved from http://www.childtrendsdatabank.org/?q=node/77

Clark, M. J. (2008). Community health nursing: Advocacy for population health (5th ed.). Upper Saddle River, NJ: Prentice Hall Health.

Dye, B. A., Tan, S., Smith, V., Lewis, B. G., Barker, L. K., Thornton-Evans, G., . . . Li, C. H. (2007). Trends in oral health status: United States, 1988–1994 and 1999–2004. U.S. Department of Health and Human Services, National Center for Health Statistics. Vital and Health Statistics, 11(248), 1–104.

Hagan, J. F., Shaw, J. S., & Duncan, P. M. (2008). Bright futures: Guidelines for health supervision of infants, children, and adolescents (3rd ed.). Elk Grove Village, IL: American Academy of Pediatrics.

Healthy People 2020. (2011). The vision, mission, and goals of Healthy People 2020. Retrieved from http://www.healthypeople.gov/2020/Consortium/HP2020Framework.pdf

International Union for Health Promotion and Education. (2009). Making a difference to global health. Retrieved from http://www.iuhpe.org/index.html?page=5&lang=en

Lalonde, M. (1974). A new perspective on the health of Canadians. Ottawa: Health and Welfare Canada.

Lipkin, P. H. (2011). Developmental and behavioral surveillance and screening within the medical home. In R. G. Voight, Developmental and behavioral pediatrics (pp. 69–92). Elk Grove Village, IL: American Academy of Pediatrics.

Murray, R. B., Zentner, J. P., & Yakimo, R. (2009). Health promotion strategies through the life span (8th ed.). Upper Saddle River, NJ: Prentice Hall Health.

National Association of Pediatric Nurse Practitioners (NAPNAP). (2009). NAPNAP position statement on

the pediatric health care/medical home. Journal of Pediatric Health Care, 23(3), 23A–24A.

Pender, N. J., Murdaugh, C. L., & Parsons, M. A. (2011). Health promotion in nursing practice (6th ed.). Upper Saddle River, NJ: Prentice Hall.

Polit, D. F., & Beck, C. T. (2008). Nursing research: Generating and assessing evidence for nursing practice (8th ed.). Philadelphia: Lippincott Williams & Wilkins.

Tanski, S., Garfunkel, L. C., Duncan, P. M., & Weitzman, M. (2010). Performing preventive services: A Bright Futures book. Elk Grove Village, IL: American Academy of Pediatrics.

World Health Organization. (2005). Global health promotion scaling up for 2015—A brief review of major impacts and developments over the past 20 years and challenges for 2015. Retrieved from http://www.who.int

World Health Organization. (2009). Social determinants of health. Retrieved from http://www.who.int/chp/en/

World Health Organization. (2010). Health promotion. Retrieved from http://www.who.int/topics/health_promotion/en/

World Health Organization. (2011a). Health promotion: 7th global conference on health promotion. Retrieved from http://www.who.int/healthpromotion/conferences/7gchp/en/

World Health Organization. (2011b). Health promotion: Areas of work. Retrieved from http://www.who.int/healthpromotion/areas/en/

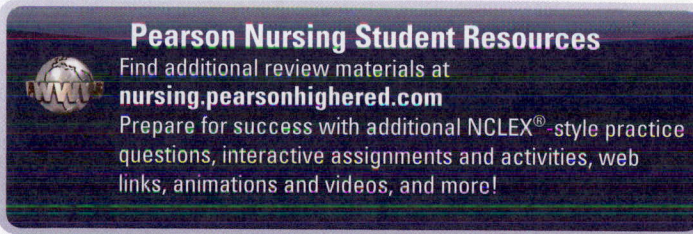

Pearson Nursing Student Resources
Find additional review materials at
nursing.pearsonhighered.com
Prepare for success with additional NCLEX®-style practice questions, interactive assignments and activities, web links, animations and videos, and more!

Health Promotion and Maintenance of the Newborn

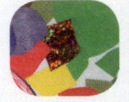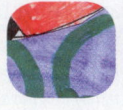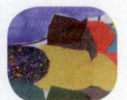

Learning Outcomes

After completing this chapter, you will be able to:

1. Analyze the important link between prenatal care and health promotion and maintenance of the family and newborn.

2. Identify the major health concerns of the newborn.

3. Describe physical and developmental milestones expected during the newborn period.

4. Apply assessment skills to gather data regarding nutrition, physical activity, mental health status, and growth and development of newborns.

5. Integrate therapeutic communication skills with the newborn and family during health supervision visits.

6. Diagnose and plan interventions with newborns and their families to integrate health promotion and maintenance behaviors.

7. Synthesize data from the history and examination of the newborn and family to plan approaches useful with the family during health supervision encounters.

8. Confirm for families the advantages of breastfeeding, and promote breastfeeding whenever possible.

> **"I'm a big sister! Mommy says she's excited, but she takes naps a lot. She says new babies are mixed up about sleeping. Rhonda sleeps in the daytime and the nighttime."**
>
> —*Denise, 5 years old*

Shannon Regis comes to the pediatric clinic with her 10-day-old daughter, Rhonda. Shannon is a 22-year-old single mother who lives with her 5-year-old daughter and boyfriend of 2 years. Shannon had an uncomplicated pregnancy and birth. Rhonda was born at 37 weeks' gestation. She required phototherapy for newborn jaundice and had initial difficulties breastfeeding. Rhonda was discharged at 5 days of age in good health. The nurse weighs and measures Rhonda and notices that she weighs just 1 oz more than her birth weight. Shannon voices concerns that Rhonda sleeps very little, cries a lot at night, and makes sleep difficult for her boyfriend, who has to get up early for work. The nurse asks Shannon how she knows when Rhonda is ready to feed. Shannon recognizes only Rhonda's crying as a feeding cue. The nurse gives Shannon information on newborn states and cues, and encourages Shannon to notice more subtle feeding cues. The nurse calls the lactation consultant, and together they assess the effectiveness of Rhonda's breastfeeding. The lactation consultant works with Shannon on a feeding plan to ensure that Rhonda is getting enough milk to gain weight. The pediatric nurse then partners with Shannon to strategize how to help Rhonda sleep for longer periods, recognizing that newborns often do not settle into a schedule until well into the second month.

What ongoing assessment will Rhonda and her parents need? How can the nurse encourage shared parenting between Shannon and her boyfriend? What coordinated follow-up is required between the pediatric nurse and the lactation consultant?

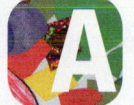 healthy pregnancy usually results in the birth of a healthy newborn. The expectant mother and her partner focus on the pregnancy and the major event of labor and birth. Often the expectant mother is so focused on her pregnancy and anticipated labor experience that the responsibilities and demands of parenthood pose challenges that require support after the birth period.

For a healthy woman, prenatal care, labor, and birth may be her first experience of an ongoing relationship with healthcare professionals. The quality of that experience is key to ensuring a continuing partnership between her and her child's healthcare providers.

The month following delivery is a time of transition for the new mother and her family. Not only is the mother coping with hormonal shifts and a **postpartum** (after giving birth) body, but roles and relationships are also changing. The nurse then assesses knowledge about self-care and newborn care, teaches health promotion and maintenance activities, promotes parental confidence in newborn caregiving, and facilitates a partnership among healthcare professionals and the family.

EARLY CONTACTS WITH THE FAMILY
Prenatal

The nurse who sees the expectant mother during **prenatal care** (healthcare supervision during pregnancy) has the unique opportunity to help parents prepare for their new roles. The nurse listens attentively and provides information and support. During prenatal visits, parents learn to value health supervision and an active partnership with healthcare professionals.

Prenatal Assessment of Risk and Protective Factors

The nurse who interacts with the family in the prenatal period assesses risk and protective factors. A pregnant woman is more likely to change risky health behaviors during pregnancy than at any other time in her life (World Health Organization, 2011). The motivation to give birth to a healthy newborn is usually strong, and the nurse can use maternal readiness for change to promote behaviors that improve maternal and newborn health.

Risk factors should be assessed during the prenatal visit. The nurse begins with the questions that demonstrate interest in the woman's health and well-being. The more sensitive questions, such as use of drugs and alcohol and **domestic violence,** a pattern of assaultive or coercive behaviors within a family, are asked after the nurse establishes rapport with the woman. Questions to assess risk factors include (Hagan, Shaw, & Duncan, 2008):

- "Is this a good time for you to be pregnant?"
- "How does your family feel about having a new baby?"
- "How has your pregnancy been for you so far? Have you had any physical or emotional problems?"
- "What is the most exciting part of becoming parents? The most worrisome part?"
- "How do you think a baby will change your lives?"
- "How were you raised? Will you raise your baby the same way, or what things would you change?"
- "Who will help you with caring for the baby in the first few weeks?"
- "Do you plan to breastfeed or formula feed? How did you make that decision? Do you need more information?"
- "Do you have concerns about labor and giving birth? What are they?"
- "If your newborn is a boy, are you considering circumcision?" (See Developing Cultural Competence: Circumcision.)
- "Are you considering umbilical cord blood collection?" (See Box 9–1.)
- "Are you ready at home for your baby? Do you have clothing, diapers, a crib, and a car safety seat that is intended for a newborn? Do you know how to use your newborn's car safety seat?"
- "Do you have financial worries? Do you worry about being able to pay your rent or obtaining food or baby supplies?"
- "Do you have a gun at home? Is the gun unloaded and locked up? Where is the ammunition stored? Would you consider getting rid of the gun because of the danger to children and other family members?"
- "Are you safe in your relationships? Does your partner ever kick, slap, shove, hit, or yell at you?" (Ask this question to the

---

| **BOX 9–1** | **Umbilical Cord Blood Collection** |

Umbilical cord blood is a rich source of stem cells, unspecialized blood cells that produce all other blood cells. In some cases, cord blood is an alternative to bone marrow transplant and has been used to treat a number of oncologic, hematologic, and immunologic disorders (American Academy of Pediatrics [AAP] Committee on Bioethics, 2010).

Public umbilical cord blood banks receive blood from donor families when infants are born, and the donation can be accessed by healthcare professionals to treat ill persons needing stem cells. Private banks are those where families pay to store their own child's cord blood over time, in case it is needed in the future. Parents may be influenced by the emotional appeal to collect umbilical cord blood for future healthcare usage in their families. Who should consider umbilical cord blood banking?

The American Academy of Pediatrics acknowledges that it is difficult to estimate the likelihood of a family needing cord blood cells for transplantation. Umbilical cord blood banking should be considered if the family has a child with a genetic disorder that is potentially treatable with stem cell transplantation. Private cord blood banking comes at a price: an initial fee of $1,700 to $2,000 and an annual storage fee of about $125 (March of Dimes, 2010). Therefore, private

storage of cord blood as "biological insurance" is not recommended for most families at this time.

Public cord blood donation provides the option of donating cord blood at no cost to a public bank, which makes the cord blood available to any appropriately matched individual in need of a stem cell transplant. The National Marrow Donor Program provides a complete list of participating hospitals. Parents should be aware that with public donation, testing will be done for genetic and infectious disease and if abnormalities are identified, they will be notified. Parents should also be aware that the cord blood banked in a public program may not be accessible for future private use (AAP, 2010).

Arrangements for umbilical cord blood collection must be made well before labor and birth. Consent for the procedure should be obtained during a prenatal visit (AAP, 2010). The parents are responsible for making arrangements with the umbilical cord blood bank of their choosing. A member of the delivery room staff attempts to collect approximately 3 to 5 oz of cord blood immediately after delivery using a collection kit provided by the cord blood storage agency. The cord blood is then shipped to the designated laboratory, processed, and stored for potential future use (March of Dimes, 2010).

Developing Cultural Competence
Circumcision

Circumcision is uncommon in Asia, South and Central America, and most of Europe. It is commonly performed at puberty in some African countries. A majority of newborn males in the United States are circumcised; however, the rate of circumcision varies by region, religion, and socioeconomic status (Lipson & Dibble, 2008). Growing evidence that male circumcision reduces risk of heterosexually acquired HIV infection in men by 60% is increasing the prevalence in some African countries (World Health Organization, 2010). Nurses can encourage discussion during the prenatal period to ascertain cultural and religious practices of a given family about circumcision and provide information as the family desires.

woman when she is alone, never when her partner is in the room with her.)

- "How many cigarettes do you smoke in a day? Did you use alcohol before you knew you were pregnant? How many drinks do you drink in a day (or in a week) now? Tell me about any street drugs or prescription drugs that you take now. Does your partner use any street drugs?"

Most obstetric care providers encourage the expectant mother to choose her newborn's care provider prior to the baby's birth. Pediatric care providers usually welcome a short office visit, sometimes at no charge, to allow the expectant mother and care provider to assess their compatibility prior to initiating the care provider relationship (see Partnering with Families: Prenatal Visit to the Pediatric Care Provider). Many pediatric care providers have written information

for expectant parents, explaining their professional philosophy of care as well as information about services.

At Birth

The hospital length of stay for a healthy mother and newborn is short, approximately 48 hours for a vaginal birth and 72 to 96 hours for an uncomplicated cesarean birth. Early discharge of mother and baby should only occur after term delivery, appropriate growth, and normal physical examination, which generally requires 48 hours after delivery. There should be time to identify any problems and to make certain that the family can care for the infant at home, and ideally the mother and infant should be discharged together (AAP, 2010, 2011a). During the hospital stay, the nurse provides ongoing physical assessment of the mother and newborn and psychosocial assessment of the mother, while providing education and anticipatory guidance to prepare the mother to care for herself and her newborn following hospital discharge.

The birth experience and first few postpartum days can be busy and distracting for new mothers, making it difficult for them to focus on self-care and newborn care instructions. Most hospitals offer discharge instructions in a variety of formats in the hope that parents will retain the most essential information. To facilitate learning for parents with different learning styles and literacy levels, nurses use bedside teaching, return demonstration, and written pamphlets for parent education. Many hospitals and birthing centers have a series of videotapes, DVDs, or closed-circuit TV channels with information for new families. Parents can watch when it is convenient, and the nurse can discuss their questions and thoughts after they view. In

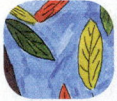

Partnering with Families

Prenatal Visit to the Pediatric Care Provider

Encourage parents to visit the pediatric healthcare home before the baby is born. This will help the parents decide if the healthcare provider offers the type of care they want for their infant. Assist parents to prepare questions and make an appointment to visit the provider they are interested in interviewing. Questions they can ask the provider include:

- How soon after birth will the baby be seen? Can parents be present during the initial physical examination? Will you speak with us again before hospital discharge?
- What is your view about male circumcision? Do you perform circumcision? If not, who does this procedure? Is circumcision performed in the hospital before discharge or in the office later?
- What if our baby needs intensive care? Under what circumstances would our baby need to be transported to a different hospital?
- When is our newborn's first office visit? Do we call for that appointment or is it made for us while we are in the hospital?
- What can I expect from you as our baby's provider? What is your most important job? What do you enjoy most about your work? What are the most important things you offer to new families like us?
- What do you expect from us as the parents of a new baby? What is our most important job?
- What are the costs of care? Do you accept my method of payment/insurance/assistance? How much time is usually spent on office visits? Do we have time to ask questions?

- What are your office hours? What number do we call if we have a question or if the baby is sick outside of office hours?
- Who covers your office when you are unavailable? Do you have partners in the office or colleagues in the community who cover for you when you are out? May I have a list of their names and phone numbers?
- Who else answers our questions about routine baby and child care? What is that person's training? Do you have resources to support breastfeeding mothers? Working mothers?
- If our child needs hospitalization, what hospital do you prefer to use? Would you be our child's doctor in the hospital, or would you refer the hospital care to someone else? Why?

After the interview, parents can ask themselves the following questions:
- Was I comfortable talking with this person? Did this person listen to me?
- Did I get clear answers to my questions?
- Do I feel that I can trust this provider with my child's care?
- Was I comfortable in the office? Did I feel welcome? Were staff members friendly, helpful, and competent?
- Will this provider be a good "fit" for my family?

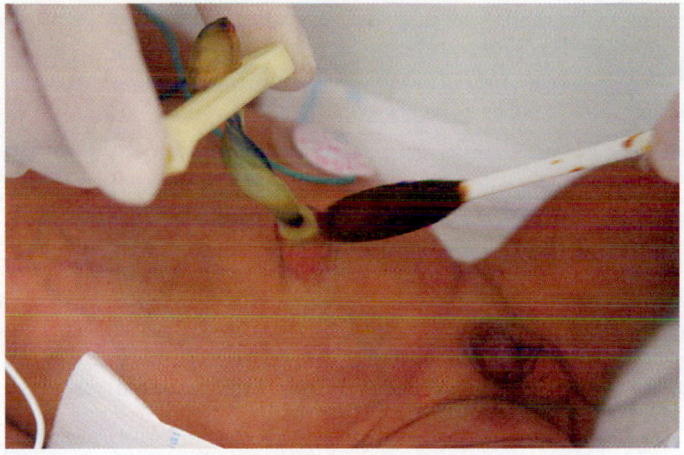 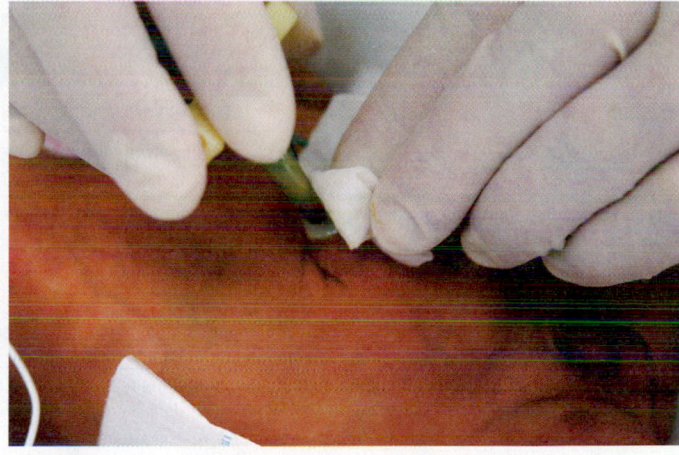

FIGURE 9–1 ■ Two different methods for cord care: *A,* Betadine cleaning and *B,* alcohol cleaning.

addition, some hospitals send parents home with a video or DVD of postpartum and baby care instructions, and some hospitals have a social networking platform for ongoing support.

Although challenging, the nurse incorporates many newborn health promotion and maintenance activities into this short stay. Starting at the moment of birth, the newborn is continuously assessed and procedures are performed to ensure newborn health. For the healthy newborn, basic activities usually include:

- First bath (to remove blood and amniotic fluid from the newborn's skin and prevent transmission of microorganisms to others)
- Umbilical cord care (Figure 9–1 ■ and Box 9–2)
- Vitamin K injection to prevent vitamin K deficiency bleeding (VKDB) (see the Medications table on page 256)
- Eye prophylaxis (administration of ophthalmic antibiotic ointment to prevent gonococcal ophthalmia neonatorum) within 1 hour of birth
- Newborn physical assessment (see Chapter 7 🔗)
- Newborn feeding assessment (see Chapter 19 🔗)
- Newborn screening (see Chapter 32 🔗)
- Hepatitis B vaccination (see Chapter 22 🔗)
- Hearing screening (see Chapter 24 🔗)
- Maternal diseases and assessment reviewed for risk factors
- Other screening tests obtained dependent on history and state regulations
- Assessment of parental ability to adequately care for the newborn and to recognize and report signs of illness

---

BOX 9–2	Umbilical Cord Care

Umbilical cord care practices vary according to region and are often based on institutional tradition. Evidence demonstrates that objectives of cord care are to prevent infection and promote cord separation, accomplished by keeping the cord clean and dry (AAP, 2011b). Cord care practices include no care; sterile water cleansing; application of triple dye; and application of povidone-iodine, isopropyl alcohol, or antimicrobial ointments (AAP & American College of Obstetricians and Gynecologists [ACOG], 2007). Parents are instructed to fold the diaper under the stump to prevent rubbing and to report oozing, bleeding (more than a drop on the diaper), and red or other abnormal appearance of the cord stump.

Clinical Tip

Administration of medications can be stressful for the newborn and parents.

- Provide an opportunity for the newborn and parent(s) to see each other and bond after birth before administering ophthalmic eye treatment.
- Administer eye antibiotic ointment before, or at a different time than, the vitamin K injection. The newborn may cry after the vitamin K injection, making it difficult to administer ophthalmic ointment.
- Administer eye prophylaxis when the newborn is calm. Do not attempt to pry the newborn's eyes open when the newborn is crying, or supine and facing bright overhead lights. Dim the room, swaddle or contain the newborn's limbs, and hold the newborn semi-upright. If the newborn is awake or drowsy, the eyes will usually open, allowing easier administration of the ophthalmic ointment.
- The newborn is less likely to cry during the vitamin K injection if the nurse lays the newborn on a firm surface and the parent gently holds the newborn's arms across the newborn's chest during the injection. This "containment" helps the newborn stay calm during the procedure.

Assessment of Risk and Protective Factors

During this short period of hospitalization, the nurse must establish rapport with the mother and family to accurately assess not only physical recovery and well-being but also psychosocial status and preparation for parenthood. Risk and protective factors are assessed and appropriate referrals are made if necessary. Discussion includes the following:

- "How are you feeling?"
- "Was labor and birth what you had expected? What was different?"
- "What do you think of your new baby? Are you surprised by anything about her?"
- "Does your baby seem easy to comfort? What seems to calm the baby when she is crying?"
- "Are you ready to take your baby home? What supplies do you have for baby care (diapers, blankets, and clothing)? Do you have a car safety seat? Will the person who brings you home have the seat in the car today?"
- "Do you have help at home? Who will answer your questions?"
- "Who will you call if you have concerns about yourself or your new baby?"
- "How is feeding your baby going so far? Do you have questions about feeding your baby? Who will you call for breastfeeding

Medications   Used to Treat Newborns

MEDICATION	PROPHYLACTIC ACTION/IMPLICATION	NURSING MANAGEMENT
Vitamin K (phytonadione)	To prevent vitamin K–dependent hemorrhagic disease of the newborn	1 mg intramuscular (IM) within 6 hours of birth
Sterile ophthalmic ointment containing tetracycline (1%) or erythromycin (0.5%) or one of a variety of topical agents, including ophthalmic solution of povidone-iodine (2.5%)	As prophylaxis against gonococcal ophthalmia neonatorum	1–2 cm ribbon along the conjunctival sac of each eye within 1 hour of birth, taking care that the agent reaches all areas of the conjunctival sac
Hepatitis B virus (HBV) immunoprophylaxis	■ All women should be screened for hepatitis B as part of routine prenatal care. Review the mother's record of hepatitis screening so the infant can be treated as recommended. ■ The first hepatitis B vaccination (HBV) for the newborn is received prior to hospital discharge.	■ For babies of HBsAg-negative women, the first dose of HBV vaccine is administered during the newborn period (recommended time) or by age 2 months, second dose 1–2 months later, and third dose by age 6–18 months. (See Chapter 22 🔗.) ■ Babies of HBsAg-positive women must receive HBV within 12 hours of birth AND receive one dose of hepatitis B immune globulin (HBIG) within 12 hours of birth at a second IM site (opposite thigh). Continue HBV series at 1–2 months of age. (See Chapter 22 🔗.)

Source: *Duncan, P. M. (Eds.). (2008). Bright futures: Guidelines for health supervision of infants, children, and adolescents (3rd ed.). Elk Grove Village, IL: American Academy of Pediatrics.*

questions?" or "What formula will you use? How will you prepare the bottles, nipples, and formula?"

■ "Do you have concerns about going home today?"

Discharge teaching is provided at every available moment. See Partnering with Families: Discharge Teaching for New Parents.

The nurse works closely with both the mother's and newborn's healthcare providers to coordinate services. For many families, few referrals are necessary and may be routine; for example, all first-time breastfeeding mothers may receive a referral to a lactation consultant, or for a follow-up visit in a hospital-sponsored postpartum/newborn clinic. For families with complex needs, a multidisciplinary team of nurses, physicians, social workers, mental health professionals, and staff from community agencies may be involved in providing comprehensive and coordinated services.

When the nurse assesses a need for referral, the assessment information should be discussed with the primary care provider and documented in the mother's and/or newborn's chart. The nurse's scope of responsibilities for making referrals varies with hospital policy and state regulations. Some referrals require a written order from the mother's primary healthcare provider.

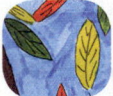

Partnering with Families

Discharge Teaching for New Parents

Parents should receive newborn teaching prior to hospital discharge. They should also have access at home to educational resources to help ensure adequate care of the newborn and instructions regarding how to access healthcare providers for consultation.

Discharge teaching includes:

■ Breastfeeding technique (position, latch, adequacy of urine and stool output, lactation referral and resources) or formula-feeding technique (formula type, preparation, safety, feeding)

■ Umbilical cord care

■ Bathing and skin care

■ Diapering and dressing a newborn

■ Temperature assessment using a thermometer

■ Signs of newborn illness

  ■ Axillary temperature higher than 100.4°F for babies less than 3 months old

  ■ Abdominal swelling, especially if accompanied by no bowel movement for 1 or 2 days and/or vomiting

  ■ Blue skin coloring, especially of the face, lips, or tongue (blue hands and feet are normal in the newborn)

■ Persistent coughing or choking during feedings

■ Unusually long period of crying that will not stop despite comfort measures

■ Jaundice (yellow coloring of the skin) that appears over the whole body

■ Sleeping through feedings, baby seems tired or uninterested in eating

■ Drainage or redness of the umbilical cord stump

■ No movement unless stimulated

■ Respiratory difficulty

  ■ Fast breathing (more than 60 breaths/minute)

  ■ Retractions (muscles between ribs suck in with each breath)

  ■ Flaring of nose

  ■ Grunting while breathing

  ■ Persistent blue skin color

■ Newborn safety

  ■ Infant car seat use

  ■ Supine sleeping position

Source: *Adapted from the American Academy of Pediatrics & American College of Obstetricians and Gynecologists. (2007). Guidelines for perinatal care (6th ed.). Elk Grove Village, IL: AAP.*

To help ensure that the mother follows through with the referral, the nurse or primary care provider should involve the mother in decision making, discuss the purpose of the referral, and state how the mother or newborn will benefit from the service.

Newborn Visit Following Hospital Discharge

The first follow-up visit of a newborn should occur by 5 days of age. The purpose of this visit is to ensure that the newborn is continuing to progress normally and that no previously undiscovered problems have surfaced.

The nurse who assesses the newborn in the clinic or home setting reviews the prenatal and birth history and continues the assessment of the newborn and of ongoing maternal recovery and postpartum adjustment. The nurse weighs the newborn and calculates weight loss; assesses general health, feeding, voiding, and stooling patterns; and observes mother–infant interaction. This is also an important opportunity to assess the degree of newborn jaundice to prevent the occurrence of newborn kernicterus (Box 9–3).

At this initial contact, the nurse promotes maternal confidence in caregiving and offers education and anticipatory guidance. Following hospital discharge, most new mothers are extremely open to learning about infant care (bathing, diapering, soothing) and breastfeeding. The nurse ensures that the parent knows how to contact the obstetric and pediatric care provider for questions and confirms follow-up appointments. The nurse communicates any concerns about the newborn to the primary care provider on the same day as the visit, and interventions are agreed upon (such as an immediate clinic appointment) or referrals are made (for example, to a lactation specialist).

Routine Health Supervision Visits

The schedule for routine infant health supervision visits varies somewhat; however, an assessment by a physician, nurse practitioner, or nurse is recommended at 3 to 5 days of age and within 48 to 72 hours after hospital discharge, with subsequent follow-up visits for newborns at risk for hyperbilirubinemia or feeding problems (AAP & ACOG, 2007; Hagan et al., 2008). An additional health supervision visit should then occur at 1 month of age. These first pediatric office visits set the stage for the partnership among the baby's family members and office staff that is essential to ensuring a **continuum of care,** an ongoing relationship between the healthcare provider and family.

The parent must believe that health supervision and surveillance are important to the child's health in order to keep appointments and follow through with suggested health promotion and maintenance activities. Clear communication with parents in a culturally competent setting helps establish trust and impart the value of frequent interactions with providers in the pediatric healthcare home.

The first outpatient visits influence the tone and effectiveness of future visits (Hagan et al., 2008). The office staff should welcome the baby and family to the office in an unhurried and genuine manner. It is important to convey that the family's and baby's needs are a high priority for the entire staff. The nurse should take time to comment on the baby and validate good parenting ("I like the way you talk to your baby when he makes noises. He really responds to your voice"). The nurse models nurturing behavior by handling the baby gently and respectfully, and responding to any distress appropriately. Parents should be involved in decreasing the newborn's stress, such as holding and comforting the baby during immunizations. Clinical findings, such as the baby's current weight and growth percentile, should be explained to parents. Provide pamphlets and reading materials to reinforce information and discussion. Include parents in decision making when possible, such as discussing the need for referrals and making follow-up appointments.

GENERAL OBSERVATIONS

At the first health promotion visit, the nursing assessment begins with general observations of the newborn and family (Figure 9–2 ■). This often occurs as the family is called in from the waiting area. See Table 9–1.

Welcome the family to the facility and comment on the newborn. Ask how the family is adjusting. In the first month of the newborn's life, parents are frequently exhausted and experiencing stressful adjustments in their relationship with each other. The nurse gathers information to assess the needs of the family, to invite discussion, to validate positive parenting efforts, and to promote partnership between the family and the healthcare team. Questions for new parents may include (Hagan et al., 2008):

- "How are you feeling these days?"
- "How is your baby doing? What do you enjoy most about your baby?"

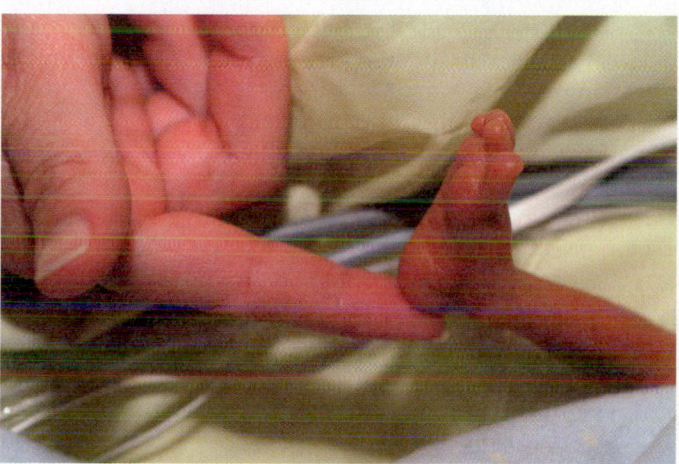

FIGURE 9–2 ■ Assess the mother's interaction with the newborn, including touch and stroking in an intentional and caring manner, indicating progress in bonding with the newborn. This mother of a preterm infant carefully strokes her child's skin.

Source: *Wake Forest Baptist Health (WFBH) Photography.*

BOX 9–3	Prevention of Kernicterus

Kernicterus is a lifelong neurologic syndrome caused by severe and untreated hyperbilirubinemia (jaundice) during the neonatal period. Kernicterus may result in cerebral palsy, mental retardation, hearing loss, and motor and developmental abnormalities. Because hyperbilirubinemia can be treated with phototherapy and exchange transfusions, kernicterus is a preventable condition. (See Chapter 30 🐾 for more information about newborn hyperbilirubinemia.)

All birth settings should provide information for parents about newborn jaundice and when to call their pediatric provider. Be certain that all infants are assessed for jaundice before hospital discharge and again at 3 to 7 days of age. The pediatric nurse must be alert to parents' reports of signs indicating hyperbilirubinemia in the newborn's first few weeks of life and facilitate immediate medical evaluation. Signs of hyperbilirubinemia in the newborn include yellowing of skin and eyes, listlessness, poor feeding, and high-pitched cry (Mayo Clinic, 2011a).

TABLE 9–1	General Observations and Implications for Newborn and Family During Health Promotion and Maintenance Visits	
ASSESSMENT PARAMETER	**NORMAL FINDING**	**OBSERVATION THAT REQUIRES FURTHER ASSESSMENT**
Who brings the baby in for care?	Mother and/or father or partner, baby's grandparent(s), and siblings are in attendance.	Baby's mother is absent.
Is the parent on time (or nearly on time) for the appointment? Does the parent have adequate transportation? Does the parent share the care provider's philosophy of the importance of timeliness or do cultural differences make timeliness less important to the family than to the care providers?	Parent is on time or nearly on time. Parent calls to say she will be late or reschedules appointment if necessary. Parent may be late if common in culture.	Parent misses appointment and does not reschedule.
Are family members, including the newborn, dressed appropriately for weather conditions?	Family members and the newborn are dressed appropriately for current weather conditions.	Baby, siblings, or parent are overdressed or underdressed.
Is interaction among parents and siblings relaxed and appropriate for the setting?	Parent is attentive to the child's needs. Parent speaks to the newborn in a soothing voice. Parent makes appropriate comments to the infant, such as "You're such a good baby!" or "Let's see how much you weigh today."	Parent ignores the child's needs or requests for attention. Parent is verbally or physically abusive. Parent makes abusive comments to the baby or sibling(s) such as "You always want something!" or "You're as stupid as your father!"
Is the parent's behavior appropriate?	Parent is engaged in the activity, alert, and interactive with the newborn and office staff.	Parent is apathetic, lethargic, depressed, hallucinating, belligerent, or aggressive; has alcohol on breath, slurred speech, frantic behavior, uncontrollable crying, or suicidal ideology.
Does the baby appear healthy, well nourished, and cared for?	Baby appears to be in good health with no respiratory distress, little or no evidence of newborn jaundice, flexed with good muscle tone, responsive to the environment and parent's efforts to calm baby. Baby is clean and appropriately dressed. Parent holds the baby protectively and supports the baby's head.	Baby is limp, lethargic, or crying excessively. Baby is working hard to breathe or has central cyanosis. Baby is markedly jaundiced. Baby is not appropriately dressed or cleaned. Parent places the baby in unsafe situations, such as leaving the baby unattended on a chair or exam table. Parent does not hold the newborn in a supportive manner. Baby has injuries or bruises unrelated to birth.

Source: *Data from Hagan, J. F., Shaw, J. S., & Duncan, P. M. (2008).* Bright futures: Guidelines for health supervision of infants, children, and adolescents *(3rd ed.). Elk Grove Village, IL: American Academy of Pediatrics.*

- "How can you tell when your baby wants to eat? To sleep? What calms your baby when she's crying?"
- "How is breastfeeding going? How often does your baby breastfeed? How long are feedings? What questions or concerns do you have?"

Or, if formula feeding:

- "How much formula does your baby drink at a feeding? How often? What questions or concerns do you have about feeding?"
- "Do you have an infant car safety seat? What questions do you have about using the car seat?"
- "How do you position your baby for sleep?"
- "How are your other children doing?"
- "Do you have a pet? If so, has the pet appeared jealous of the newborn?"
- "How do you and your partner manage some time for yourselves?"
- "Have you been feeling sad? All the time or for short periods? What seems to help?"
- "This first month can be really stressful. What do you do when problems really get to you? Who do you turn to for help?"
- "Describe your transportation situation. Tell me about your living situation."
- "What is the most helpful thing we can do for you today?"

Through these questions the nurse assesses development of **attachment behaviors** (behaviors that demonstrate an emotional connection between newborn and caregiver), parental perception of infant **temperament** (characteristic style of activity, mood, and reaction), feeding status, safety, family integration, parental mental health, and parental coping mechanisms. The nurse may determine that further assessment is required, for example, if the parent states that breastfeeding is so painful she wants to switch to formula, she is continuously depressed, she has started smoking again, or she cannot calm her crying baby. The nurse in the pediatric setting is aware that the baby's health is closely connected to the health of the entire family. Many concerns require referral for parents outside the pediatric care setting; therefore, the office or clinic should have a system in place and ready access to referrals and resources for parents in need.

GROWTH AND DEVELOPMENTAL SURVEILLANCE

At Birth

Assessment of growth and development begins at birth (Figure 9–3 ■). An experienced neonatal or labor nurse can accurately assess many parameters of newborn health within a few moments of the infant's birth. The nurse notes posture, flexion, reflexes, and a battery of physical attributes that help the nurse assess appropriate development for gestation. The nurse determines, by physical assessment findings and prenatal history, if the newborn is **preterm** (born prior to 37 weeks' gestation), **term** (born between 37 completed weeks and 42 weeks), or **postterm** (born after 42 weeks' gestation). See Figure 9–4 ■. In addition, the nurse

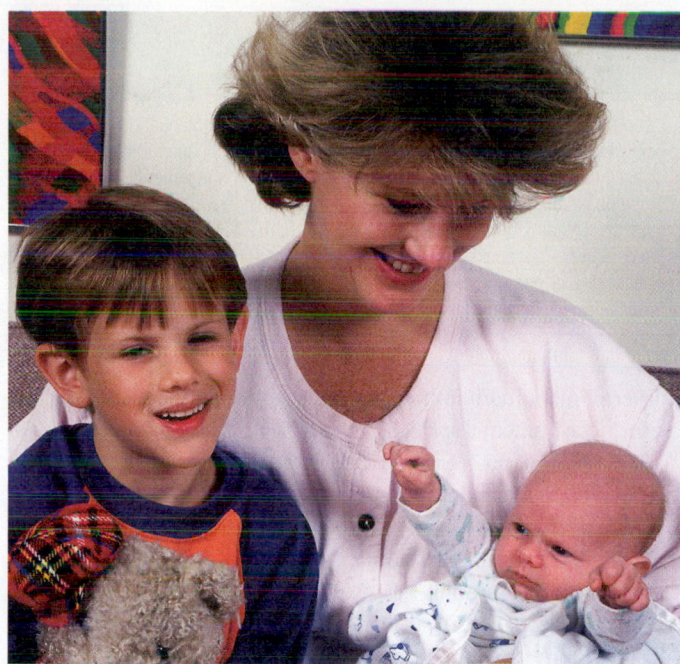

FIGURE 9–3 ■ Observation of the newborn and family begins at first contact during the health supervision and maintenance visit.

determines if the newborn is the expected size and weight for the time spent in utero. See Chapter 7 🔵 for further assessment information. This is done by plotting the baby's weight and measurements on a standard intrauterine growth chart to determine if the newborn is:

- **Appropriate for gestational age (AGA)**—a newborn whose weight, length, and head circumference fall between the 10th and 90th percentiles when plotted on a standard intra-uterine growth/gestational age chart
- **Small for gestational age (SGA)**—a newborn whose weight (and possibly length and head circumference) falls below the 10th percentile when plotted on a standard intrauterine growth/gestational age chart
- **Large for gestational age (LGA)**—a newborn whose weight (and possibly length and head circumference) falls above

the 90th percentile when plotted on a standard intrauterine growth/gestational age chart

The combination of head circumference, body length, and weight, in relation to the length of pregnancy, is an important factor in newborn health and development. The healthy newborn is the product of an uncomplicated pregnancy and birth, is term, and is appropriate for gestational age. Newborns who are not term or not appropriately grown require careful nursing and medical management to prevent or manage complications such as respiratory distress, infection, hypoglycemia, hyperbilirubinemia, feeding problems, and temperature instability. (See Chapters 19, 22, 25, and 30 for specific conditions and Appendix A 🔵 for a preterm infant growth chart.)

Assessing Growth and Development in the Outpatient Setting

The first outpatient visit usually occurs 3 to 5 days following the birth of a healthy term newborn who was discharged more than 48 hours after vaginal birth or one week after discharge following cesarean section or other condition (Hagan et al., 2008). At this visit, the baby's current weight, length, and head circumference are measured and plotted on a growth chart (see Appendix A 🔵), and a basic physical examination is performed (see Chapter 7 🔵).

In the first week of life, most babies lose about one tenth of their birth weight. For example, a baby weighing 3500 g (7 lb, 12 oz) could lose up to 350 g (nearly 12 oz). Growth spurts are evident at around 7 to 10 days and again between 3 and 6 weeks of age. By day 10, most babies are back to their original birth weight and gaining about 2/3 oz or 20 grams per day. Length increases by 1 to 1.5 inches or 2 to 4 cm in the first month, and head circumference increases about 1 inch or 2.5 cm (AAP Committee on Nutrition, 2009). Additional milestones are listed in Table 9–2.

Developmental surveillance includes assessment of the baby's ability to calm when being held or spoken to, and response to sounds by blinking, crying, quieting, or startling. The baby should be able to fixate on a human face and follow it with his or her eyes. The baby should be able to lift his or her head momentarily when placed prone, demonstrate a flexed position, and move all extremities. Most babies will sleep for 3 or 4 hours at a time and stay awake for an hour or longer (Hagan et al., 2008). See Box 9–4.

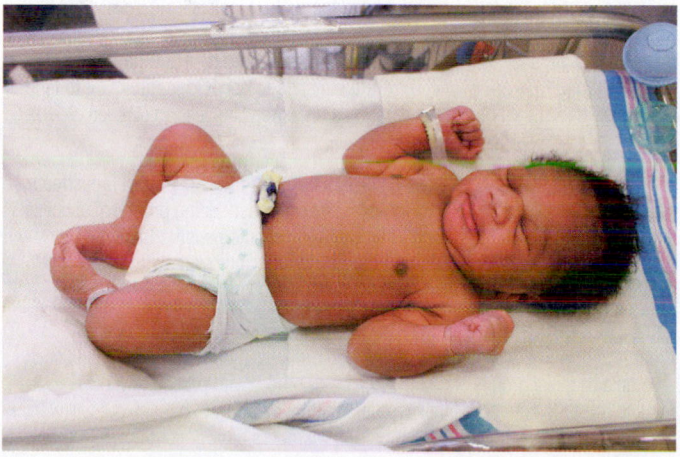

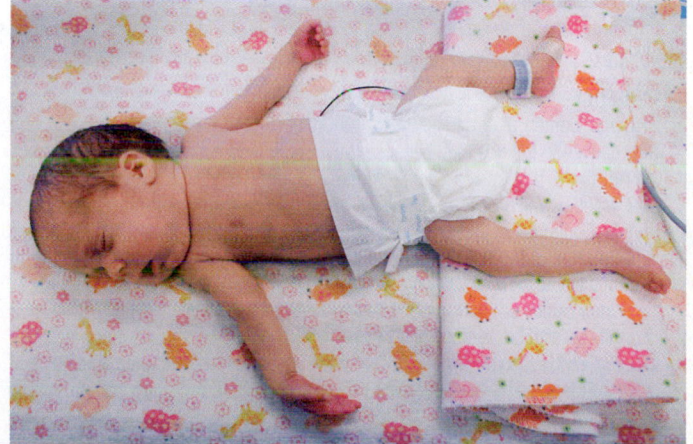

A

B

FIGURE 9–4 ■ The pediatric nurse can determine from the initial observation of position and muscle tone that one baby is *A*, term, and the other is *B*, preterm.

TABLE 9–2	Newborn Growth and Developmental Milestones Observed in Health Promotion and Maintenance Visits
Growth	■ Weight: baby may lose up to one tenth of birth weight in the first week; birth weight should be regained by day 10; weight gain is about 2/3 oz (20 g) per day thereafter. ■ Feeding is vigorous and occurs every 2–4 hours. ■ Infant has 6–8 wet diapers and 2 or more stools daily.
Vision	■ Focuses 8 to 12 inches away. ■ Eyes wander and may cross. ■ Prefers black and white or high-contrast patterns. ■ Prefers the human face to all other patterns.
Hearing	■ May turn toward familiar sounds and voices. Responds to sounds with increased movement, quieting, or calming.

Clinical Tip

Preterm infants do not reach developmental milestones at the same chronologic age as their full-term counterparts. A baby born at 32 weeks' gestation (8 weeks early) may reach developmental milestones approximately 8 weeks later than if he or she had been born full term. For example, a 4-week-old, full-term baby should be able to move the head from side to side while lying prone. A baby born at 32 weeks' gestation should not be expected to meet this milestone until about 12 weeks of age. This baby is said to have a corrected age of 4 weeks at 12 weeks of age. **Corrected age** is a term used to describe children up to 3 years of age who were born preterm. It is calculated by subtracting the number of weeks born before 40 weeks' gestation from the chronologic age.

It is normal for parents to compare their newborn's developmental skills with others of the same age. Every baby develops according to his or her own timetable; however, when a baby falls far behind, fails to reach a developmental milestone, or loses a previously acquired skill, the baby requires further evaluation. In the first month of life, signs of **developmental delay**—a delay in mastering functions, such as motor coordination and behavioral skills—in a

BOX 9–4	Growth & Development: Signs of Developmental Delay

During the second, third, or fourth week of life, signs of potential developmental delay require a complete medical and developmental evaluation to determine if a disability exists and to plan interventions and future management. The pediatric nurse observes the newborn for these signs and may have an opportunity to assess for problems through discussing the newborn's abilities and behaviors with the caregiver. Poor sucking, no response to light or sound, asymmetric movement or flaccidity, or parental concern that something is wrong should be investigated further (Tanski, Garfunkel, Duncan, et al., 2010).

full-term infant merit immediate investigation by a pediatrician, pediatric developmental specialist, pediatric neurologist, or a multidisciplinary team of professionals. Parents require additional emotional support, clear and honest communication, and resources to cope with the stress of this situation (see Chapter 16 🔗).

Table 9–2 summarizes some growth and developmental milestones that can commonly be observed in the first month of life.

NUTRITION

Breastfeeding

Breastfeeding is a valuable contributor to infant health. Breast milk is the perfect food for infants, and breastfeeding offers lifelong benefits for both mother and baby. The American Academy of Pediatrics recommends exclusive breastfeeding (no water, juice, or other foods) for the first 6 months of life. Solid foods may be introduced in the second half of the first year to complement the breast milk diet, with breastfeeding continuing at least until the infant's first birthday, and beyond if mutually desired (AAP Committee on Nutrition, 2009).

Advantages of breastfeeding for the infant include decreased incidence or severity of ear infections (otitis media), allergies, diarrhea, vomiting, respiratory tract infection, meningitis, and other infections. Breastfeeding may also provide the infant protection against

Evidence-Based Practice — Nursing Influence on Breastfeeding Behaviors

PROBLEM

The prevalence of breastfeeding has increased in the United States in the last decade but still lags behind goals set by *Healthy People 2020* and maternal-newborn organizations. Strategies are needed to increase breastfeeding rates, particularly among populations with a traditionally low prevalence of breastfeeding.

EVIDENCE

Hispanic women who immigrate to the United States become acculturated and may choose to formula feed because that appears more mainstream. Breastfeeding rates in acculturated Hispanic women are only about 33%. Breastfeeding support groups, which have materials available in Spanish, plan breastfeeding into mothers' schedules, and use "fotonovelas" or photographic booklets with stories to deliver health promotion messages, are suggested to increase breastfeeding in Hispanic women (Faraz, 2010).

When babies are born prematurely, mothers may believe that they cannot successfully breastfeed. A study of 114 nurses and 18 mothers found that a neonatal intensive care unit provided information and support for mothers, breast pumps and locations for pumping, and available lactation specialists. Deficiencies in support were noted when not all nurses had the degree of education and training that allowed them to work with and support the breastfeeding mother. Training of all staff members and consistency of approach were identified as needs for unit nurses (Cricco-Lizza, 2009).

Another study with late preterm births, or those close to term delivery, found that these infants and mothers were often discharged within the first two days after birth. In this case, the infant may not have the maturity to suck vigorously and has a higher risk of health problems in the neonatal period. Nurses should ensure that these infants are seen in the office at 3 to 5 days of age, or 1 to 2 days after hospital discharge. Mothers will need extra assistance to encourage the infant to feed adequately and should be observed during a breastfeeding session (Ahmed, 2010).

IMPLICATIONS

The nurse plays a key role in teaching all families about the benefits of breastfeeding and in identifying risk factors for low rates of breastfeeding or lack of success with the process. Nurses working with newborns should become trained as lactation specialists and maintain a role in teaching other nurses how to best provide lactation information.

CRITICAL THINKING APPLICATION

What is the rate of breastfeeding in your community? Are there populations such as ethnic or racial groups, working women, or others with particularly low breastfeeding rates? What approaches (verbal, written, video, group teaching) will work best for encouraging breastfeeding among members of your community with low rates of breastfeeding?

the following: **sudden infant death syndrome (SIDS)**, insulin-dependent (type 1) and non-insulin-dependent (type 2) diabetes mellitus, obesity and overweight, asthma, and lymphoma and leukemia (AAP Committee on Nutrition, 2009).

Despite obvious health and developmental advantages of breastfeeding, efforts are needed to promote breastfeeding in the United States. Education of both parents before and after delivery of the infant is an essential component of successful breastfeeding. Barriers to breastfeeding include insufficient prenatal breastfeeding education, disruptive hospital practices, media portrayal of bottle feeding as normative and advertising of infant formula, lack of lactation consultation, nonsupportive work environment for breastfeeding, and lack of routine follow-up and home visits (AAP Committee on Nutrition, 2009).

The decision about whether to breastfeed or formula feed the newborn is usually made prior to birth. Expectant mothers pondering this decision are influenced by previous experience with breastfeeding, support (or lack of support) from friends and family members, cultural norms, and current knowledge regarding differences between breastfeeding and formula feeding.

Healthcare providers in the prenatal setting play a vital role in educating expectant mothers about the health benefits of breastfeeding and providing anticipatory guidance prior to childbirth. The nurse in the birth setting promotes breastfeeding by facilitating nursing in the first 30 to 60 minutes following birth and by providing supportive guidance as the mother begins to develop this skill prior to discharge. Continued assessment, encouragement, and support of breastfeeding are vital to the success of breastfeeding mothers; reasons cited for early cessation are amenable to nursing interventions. See Partnering with Families: The Nurse's Role in Breastfeeding Promotion, and see Evidence-Based Practice: Nursing Influence on Breastfeeding Behaviors.

There are very few contraindications to breastfeeding. Mothers who should not breastfeed are usually aware, prior to giving birth, of the reasons formula feeding is a safer choice for them than breastfeeding. Communication should be clear and coordinated between prenatal care providers and pediatric care providers to ensure that the mother visiting the pediatric care provider is not asked how breastfeeding is going, counseled about the benefits of breastfeeding versus formula feeding, or repeatedly asked about her decision to formula feed instead of breastfeed. (See Chapter 19 for further information about support of mothers during both breastfeeding and formula feeding.)

Practice Alert

For some women, formula feeding is a safer choice than breastfeeding. Nursing is contraindicated in women who (AAP & ACOG, 2007, p. 238; Murray, Zentner, & Yakimo, 2009):

- Use illegal or addictive drugs
- Have an infant with galactosemia
- Are positive for human T-cell lymphotropic virus type I or II
- Are infected with HIV
- Take certain medications (cytotoxic drugs, some psychotropic drugs)
- Have untreated active tuberculosis (her milk can be expressed and given to the infant)
- Are receiving or have exposure to radioactive isotopes, toxic chemicals, or pesticides
- Are receiving antimetabolites or chemotherapeutic agents
- Have active herpes simplex lesions on a breast

The decision to breastfeed or formula feed may be influenced more by economic and social factors than health information. Despite evidence that breastfeeding reduces healthcare costs and

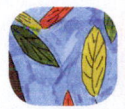

Partnering with Families

The Nurse's Role in Breastfeeding Promotion

Because breastfeeding offers many health benefits for both mother and newborn, the nurse promotes and supports the practice of breastfeeding in the prenatal period, at birth, and in the outpatient setting.

AT BIRTH

- Encourage initial breastfeeding in the first 30 to 60 minutes after delivery unless medically contraindicated or not desired by the mother.
- Discourage separation of mother and infant (baby should room in with mother at all times).
- Teach infant feeding cues to breastfeeding mothers and promote breastfeeding on demand.
- Observe at least one breastfeeding period to assess technique and offer teaching.
- Discourage use of artificial nipples and pacifiers until breastfeeding is well established.
- Avoid distribution of discharge packages that contain formula.
- Provide referral to a lactation support group or lactation specialist as necessary.
- Schedule early follow-up after discharge.

IN THE OUTPATIENT SETTING

- Provide anticipatory guidance about breastfeeding at every infant health screening visit.

- Educate all staff on aspects of breastfeeding support and management of common breastfeeding problems.
- Use visual images and slogans in the office that depict breastfeeding as normative behavior by women and families of diverse backgrounds.
- Post signs in waiting and examination rooms encouraging mothers to breastfeed; the signs should explain the locations of breastfeeding rooms. Provide a private place for breastfeeding in offices.
- Use culturally appropriate educational resources. Meet literacy and language needs of mothers.
- Remove commercial logos and other indirect formula endorsement (e.g., notepads, pens, calendars) and store formula out of view.
- Encourage staff members to become lactation specialists.
- Identify community resources to support breastfeeding and establish office referral guidelines.
- Coordinate with hospital maternity units to promote consistent information and resources.
- Commend breastfeeding mothers at every visit for continuing to breastfeed.

Source: *American Academy of Pediatrics Committee on Nutrition. (2009). Pediatric nutrition handbook (6th ed.). Elk Grove Village, IL: Author.*

BOX 9–5   *Healthy People 2020* National Goals for Breastfeeding

Breastfeeding offers important long-term health benefits for both mother and baby. *Healthy People 2020*, a national public health initiative, has set the following goals for breastfeeding initiation and duration:

- Increase the proportion of women who initiate breastfeeding to 82%.
- Increase the proportion of women who continue breastfeeding their babies until 6 months of age to 61%.
- Increase the proportion of women who breastfeed their babies until 1 year of age to 34%.

Source: *From U.S. Department of Health and Human Services, Office of Disease Prevention and Promotion. (2011).* Healthy People 2020. *Retrieved from http://www.healthypeople.gov/*

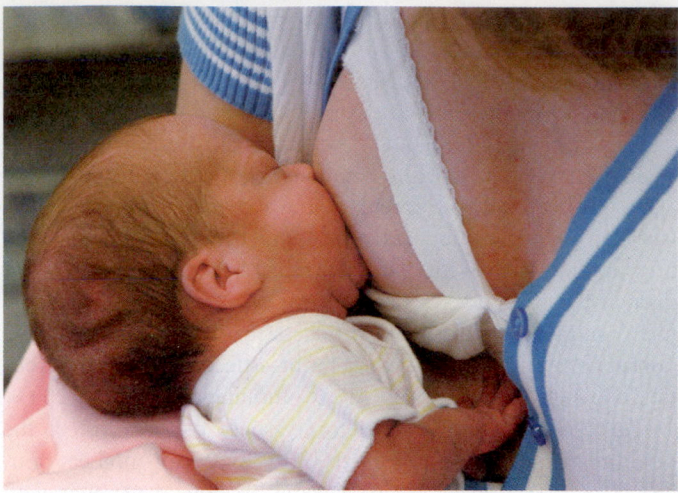

FIGURE 9–5 ■ Breastfeeding has lifelong benefits for the mother and child and should be promoted prenatally, in the hospital, and through the first year of health supervision visits.

employee absenteeism due to infant illness, few states have laws that promote accommodating breastfeeding mothers in the workplace. Pediatric care providers can promote breastfeeding through partnering with employers in the community, educating them about the economic benefits of supporting breastfeeding mothers, and supporting their efforts to do so.

Although breastfeeding initiation rates vary among states, the overall baseline rate of breastfeeding initiation for all women is 75%; by 4 weeks 63% of mothers are breastfeeding, and by 6 months just 43% are breastfeeding (Centers for Disease Control and Prevention, 2008; U.S. Department of Health and Human Services, 2011). See Box 9–5 for *Healthy People 2020* goals for breastfeeding. Many states have passed laws to support breastfeeding, allowing women to breastfeed in public and exempting breastfeeding from public indecency laws. A handful of states have also funded or supported breastfeeding awareness and education campaigns.

Nurses play a vital role in assisting and supporting breastfeeding mothers. The nurse who encounters breastfeeding mothers should understand the basics of breastfeeding management (Figure 9–5 ■). See Partnering with Families: Breastfeeding Basics. Ideally, the pediatric setting has a lactation specialist or resource person who can assess breastfeeding and problem solve with the mother. Referrals to a community lactation specialist or support group may be necessary. See Chapter 19 🖉 for more information.

Formula Feeding

Formula is not the same as breast milk. Breast milk specifically meets the needs of the human infant and provides ideal nutrition for brain growth in the first 12 months of life. Breast milk, in contrast to formula, has elements available from the mother's bloodstream that are immediately available for infant nutrition. Breast milk contains elements that work together to enhance absorption; formula is a mix of isolated single nutrients that do not guarantee the same nutritional benefits of breast milk. Breast milk also contains substances called antibodies that help protect a baby from many illnesses.

In some cases, formula feeding is a safer choice than breastfeeding, or the mother and family may prefer to feed with infant formula. Mothers who use infant formula should feed iron-fortified formula (containing between 4 and 12 mg/L of iron) from birth to 12 months (AAP Committee on Nutrition, 2009). This helps ensure adequate iron stores and very low rates of iron deficiency between 6 and 18 months of age. (See Chapter 19 🖉 for more information about formulas.)

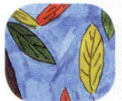

Partnering with Families

Breastfeeding Basics

The pediatric nurse in the outpatient setting receives numerous questions about breastfeeding, especially from new mothers in the first month of their breastfeeding experience. Responsibilities for counseling and referring breastfeeding mothers to lactation resources vary according to office protocols; however, the new mother may simply need reassurance and basic information.

SIGNS THAT YOUR BABY IS WELL FED INCLUDE WHEN YOUR BABY

- Is alert and active
- Is happy and satisfied after breastfeeding
- Breastfeeds at least 8 times in every 24 hours
- Has 3–4 stools daily, with color gradually changing from black to yellow in the first week
- Has 6–8 wet diapers daily

OTHER QUESTIONS FOR THE MOTHER

- Does your baby open his/her mouth and grasp onto the nipple readily?
- Does your baby suck enough to elicit letdown of milk and continue to feed in a rhythmic manner?
- Are your nipples comfortable and without redness or discomfort?
- What other questions do you have? How can we help to improve your breastfeeding experience?

Source: *Adapted from London, M. L., Ladewig, P. W., Ball, J. W., Bindler, R. C., & Cowen, K. C. (2011).* Maternal & child nursing care *(3rd ed.). Upper Saddle River, NJ: Pearson Prentice Hall.*

PHYSICAL ACTIVITY

Muscle development begins early in fetal life. Buoyed by amniotic fluid and contained within the uterus, fetal movements are usually smooth and limited in range. After birth, however, gravity exerts a strong effect and newborn movements are often weak and jerky (Blackburn, 2007). Even so, strong muscle tone is evident in the term newborn. The flexed position of the newborn demonstrates development of the flexor muscles and relaxation of the extensor muscles. This flexed position protects the newborn, conserves energy by reducing movement, and reduces heat loss (Blackburn, 2007).

Parents may need to be reminded that a preterm infant will develop according to his or her "corrected age." If the baby was born 8 weeks premature, at 32 weeks' gestation, parents can expect their otherwise healthy preterm baby to reach developmental milestones about 8 weeks later than if the baby had been born at term. During the first month of life, the newborn gradually "unfolds" and the body straightens. Movements begin to change from reflexive to purposeful. By the end of the first month, the newborn should be able to do the following:

- Bring hands to eyes and mouth
- Move head side to side when lying on abdomen
- Attempt to lift head when prone

In addition, the newborn's hands are kept in tight fists and primitive reflexes are strong (see Chapter 7).

Health promotion teaching for the family includes the following activities:

- Position the baby on the stomach for supervised play periods. This allows the newborn to lift the head and turn it from side to side, make crawling motions, and push up on the arms. Allowing supervised "tummy time" is also important for prevention of flat spots on the back of the baby's head caused by constant supine positioning (Koren, Reece, Kahn-D'angelo, et al., 2010). Be sure to place the baby in a supine position when tiring and starting to fall asleep.
- Beginning at birth, prevent flat spots on the newborn's head from supine positioning by nightly alternating the head position from left to right during sleep and moving the position of the crib daily so the baby has to move the head in different directions to look at the door.
- Encourage switching positions when bottle feeding. It may be most comfortable for the mother to hold the baby in a cradle position with the bottle in her right hand (or left hand if left-handed); however, switching arms encourages newborn muscle development and control on each side of the baby's body. Breastfeeding babies automatically feed from both sides. Parents who bottle feed may need to be reminded to promote this skill in their newborn.
- Allow the baby free movement of arms and hands. If the baby is swaddled, allow the hands to be outside the blanket and positioned in midline. This allows flexion and extension of arms, brings hands into line of vision, and brings hands to mouth.
- Encourage appropriate toys such as a mobile with contrasting colors and patterns; a plastic mirror; music boxes and exposure to soft music on the radio, tape recorder, or CD player; and soft toys with colors, patterns, and gentle sounds.

ORAL HEALTH

Ideally, pediatric oral health begins with prenatal oral health counseling for parents. Promotion of healthy oral hygiene practices and routine preventive dental care for parents establishes a foundation for a lifetime of good oral health for their children.

Protective factors for good oral health include good general health and regular use of dental care in an established **dental home,** a specialized primary dental care provider who manages and facilitates all aspects of oral health care.

Risk factors include infant's siblings with **dental caries** (cavities, or tooth decay) in the past 12 months, active caries present in the mother, suboptimal fluoride exposure, frequent between-meal exposure of family members to simple sugars, low socioeconomic status, no usual source of dental care, and children with special healthcare needs (Centers for Disease Control and Prevention, 2011).

Parents can help prevent decay in their new baby by practicing good oral health habits from birth, even before the teeth erupt. In the first month of life, parents should be warned against propping the bottle in the baby's mouth while the baby falls asleep. Babies who sleep with their teeth exposed to juice, formula, or breast milk can develop early childhood caries, formerly known as "baby bottle tooth decay," in primary teeth, even before they emerge. (See Chapter 19 .)

Oral disease may be prevented if strategies are applied early enough in the child's life. The nurse plays an important role in assessing risk factors for dental disease, promoting oral hygiene beginning in infancy, and providing anticipatory guidance to help parents ensure good oral health for their children.

MENTAL AND SPIRITUAL HEALTH

The first 3 years of a child's life are critically important to the child's development of skills that allow for learning, thinking, responding, and solving problems. The environment that parents create for their baby and young child influences the way the child develops and how nearly the child achieves his or her full potential. A "child-centered" environment provides for basic needs such as adequate nutrition, loving family members and caregivers, a feeling of safety and predictability, opportunities for play, positive reinforcement, exchange of ideas through conversation, exposure to books and music, and a balance of freedom and limits.

An infant's mental health—the developing capacity of the child to experience emotions, form attachments, and learn—is also affected by physical health, temperament, and resiliency. Through a combination of genetic attributes and the environment provided by the newborn's parents, the baby develops personality, strategies for **self-regulation** (the ability to maintain state and self-console), attachments to the family, and cognitive abilities (Hagan et al., 2008).

In the first year of life, infants form emotional attachments and learn to trust caregivers to meet their needs (Figure 9–6). Newborns begin to meet these goals by making their needs known through verbal and nonverbal **cues** (see Partnering with Families: Newborn Engagement and Disengagement Cues). The parent who can interpret these signals and respond to the newborn's needs in a timely and appropriate manner strengthens attachment and promotes optimal infant mental health. In addition, the parent benefits from understanding infant sleep-wake states and the activities most appropriate to the newborn's level of attention (Table 9–3). **Infant state** refers to a group of characteristics that regularly occur together: body activity, eye movements,

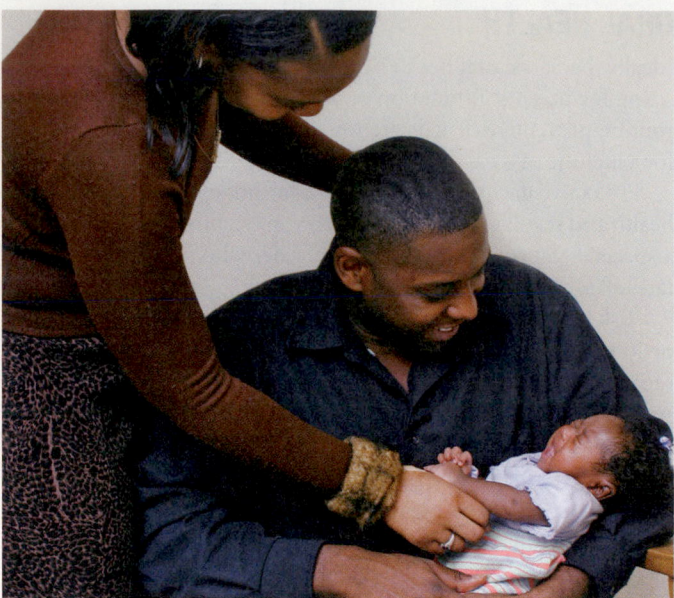

FIGURE 9–6 ■ A healthy parent forms strong attachments to the newborn and is motivated to ensure physical and mental health for the child.

facial movements, breathing pattern, and level of response to external stimuli (e.g., handling) and internal stimuli (e.g., hunger).

The mature newborn will transition smoothly from one state to another, and a parent who knows the behavioral implications of each state is able to respond appropriately to the baby's cues and elicit responses that make the parent feel successful in meeting the baby's needs. A newborn with developmental problems may demonstrate difficulty with state control and move unpredictably from one state to another. These babies can be more difficult to parent, and the family is at risk for impaired parent–infant attachment.

The nurse assesses signs of a growing secure attachment between parent and child in the first month of life by making the following observations:

- Parent looks at the newborn frequently.
- Parent has specific questions and observations about the individual characteristics of the newborn.
- Parent touches, massages, or gently rubs the newborn.
- Parent attempts to soothe the newborn when the newborn is upset, and the newborn responds to the parent's soothing efforts.

- Newborn looks content.
- Newborn signals needs.
- Newborn feeds well.

The newborn's mental health and development is highly dependent on the mental and spiritual health of the primary caregiver, usually the mother. The mother who is emotionally whole and fully present in her newborn's life is best able to provide the nurturing environment necessary for optimal growth and development (Hagan et al., 2008).

Promoting Maternal Mental Health

Bringing a newborn home can be an overwhelming emotional experience for the mother, her partner, and other family members. An immediate shift in roles and responsibilities must occur within the family. In addition to meeting the needs of the newborn, the new mother must also deal with meeting other family members' needs, rapidly shifting emotions, and her postpartum body.

The nurse in the pediatric care setting may be the first healthcare provider encountered by the postpartum woman. Because the mother's and newborn's health are so closely intertwined, the nurse should be alert to signs and symptoms of marked maternal psychosocial stress and mood disorders.

Most women experience **postpartum "blues"** or temporary sadness in the first week after delivery due to hormonal shifts and sleep deprivation. This usually resolves without intervention after a few hours to several days without interfering with the woman's ability to function. **Postpartum depression** is a more serious, persistent, and debilitating **postpartum mood disorder (PPMD)** that usually occurs 2 to 3 months after delivery. Counseling and medication originating from the mother's primary care provider may be necessary interventions. **Postpartum psychosis** is a serious condition that occurs within the first 2 weeks after delivery and is considered a psychiatric emergency (Tanski et al., 2010). See Table 9–4.

Promoting Newborn Mental Health

Beginning at birth, parents can take advantage of the newborn's short periods of wakefulness to communicate and play together. Following are suggestions for parents to promote newborn mental health:

- Encourage your newborn to look at your face while feeding. Imitate the baby's soft sounds and accommodate his or her movements.

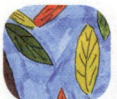 ## Partnering with Families

Newborn Engagement and Disengagement Cues

Newborns use verbal and nonverbal cues to communicate with caregivers. When a newborn is interested in eliciting care and attention, he or she demonstrates engagement cues:
- Turns toward caregiver
- Reaches toward caregiver
- Opens eyes and gazes at caregiver

When the newborn needs to stop interaction, he or she demonstrates disengagement cues:
- Turns head away
- Begins to hiccup or drool
- Falls asleep
- Begins to cry

Source: *Adapted from Hagan, J. F., Shaw, J. S., & Duncan, P. M. (Eds.). (2008). Bright futures: Guidelines for health supervision of infants, children, and adolescents (3rd ed.). Elk Grove Village, IL: American Academy of Pediatrics.*

TABLE 9–3	Infant Sleep and Awake States				
STATE	**BODY ACTIVITY**	**EYE AND FACIAL MOVEMENTS**	**BREATHING PATTERN**	**LEVEL OF RESPONSE**	**IMPLICATIONS FOR CAREGIVING**
Sleep States					
Quiet Sleep (also called deep sleep)	Nearly still, except for occasional startle	No eye movements No facial movements, except for occasional sucking movement at regular intervals	Smooth and regular	The infant is difficult to arouse.	Quiet sleep is restorative and promotes growth. Caregivers trying to feed an unresponsive infant in quiet sleep will find the experience frustrating. Feeding will be more pleasant if nurses and parents respect the infant's needs by waiting until the infant moves to a higher, more responsive state. Even if caregivers use disturbing stimuli, chances are the infant will arouse only briefly, then return to quiet sleep.
Active sleep (rapid eye movement [REM] sleep)	Some body movements	Rapid eye movements (REM); fluttering of eyes beneath closed eyelids May smile and make brief fussy or crying sounds	Irregular	The infant can arouse and then return to sleep.	Active sleep is associated with processing and storing of information and has been linked to learning. It accounts for the highest proportion of newborn sleep and usually precedes wakening. There are brief fussy or crying sounds, but when left undisturbed the infant will quiet.
Awake States					
Drowsy	Increasing body movements	Eyes occasionally open and close, are heavy-lidded or slitlike	Irregular	Infants react to sensory stimuli, although their responses are delayed. A change to alert, active alert, or crying after stimulation is frequently noted.	To awaken infants, caregivers can provide stimulation or feeding. If infants are left alone without stimuli, they may return to a sleep state.
Alert	Minimal	Eyes brighten and search surroundings Attentive appearance	Regular	During this state, infants are attentive to the environment.	Immediately after birth, many new-borns experience intense alertness before a long sleeping period. As infants become older, they spend more time in this state. Providing interaction through talking, maintaining eye contact, or feeding may prolong the state of alertness. Infants in this state provide pleasure and positive feedback to caregivers.
Active alert	Variable activity level with mild startles interspersed	Eyes are open, with dull, glazed appearance May have some facial movements; often none, and face appears still	Irregular	Infants react to sensory stimuli. The infant may change to quiet alert or crying.	Infants may fuss and become increasingly sensitive to disturbing stimuli (hunger, fatigue, noise, excessive handling). If needs are not attended to, the infant will begin to cry. Fatigue or caregiver interventions often interrupt this state, allowing infants to progress to a drowsy or sleep state.
Crying	Increased motor activity Skin color darkens or changes to red or ruddy	Eyes may be tightly closed or open Grimaces	More irregular than in other states	Infants are sensitive to any stimuli and increase crying behavior in response to noise or continued discomfort.	An infant cries in response to unpleasant stimuli. Care by adults decreases crying.

Source: From Hagan, J. F., Shaw, J. S., & Duncan, P. M. (2008). Bright futures: Guidelines for health supervision of infants, children, and adolescents (3rd ed.). Elk Grove Village, IL: American Academy of Pediatrics.

TABLE 9–4	Postpartum Mood Disorders	
DISORDER	**SYMPTOMS**	**ONSET**
Postpartum blues	Predominantly positive mood punctuated by: ■ Labile and intense episodes of tearfulness, irritability, sadness, reactivity to slights ■ Exaggerated sense of empathy	Begins during first few weeks after delivery
Postpartum depression	Five or more of the following symptoms present for at least 2 weeks: ■ Consistently depressed mood ■ Loss of pleasure/interest ■ Poor concentration or indecisiveness ■ Feelings of worthlessness or guilt ■ Recurrent thoughts of death ■ Psychomotor agitation or retardation ■ Fatigue or loss of energy ■ Insomnia or hypersomnia* ■ Significant decrease or increase in appetite*	Can be insidious, but starts within the first 2–3 months after delivery
Postpartum psychosis	Early signs typically include: ■ Restlessness ■ Irritability ■ Insomnia ■ Rapidly evolving or shifting depressed or elated mood ■ Disorganized behavior, with confusion and disorientation ■ Hallucinations or delusions (frequently focused on the infant)	Usually starts within 2–4 weeks of delivery, but can start as early as 2–3 days after delivery; onset can be dramatic and abrupt

*Symptoms are often difficult to assess in the postpartum period.

Source: Data from Tanski, S., Garfunkel, L. C., Duncan, P. M., & Weitzman, M. (2010). Performing preventive service. Elk Grove Village, IL: American Academy of Pediatrics.

■ Respond quickly to your baby's feeding cues and avoid rigid feeding schedules. Hunger and feeding times are unpredictable, especially in the first few months.

■ Identify ways to soothe your crying newborn. Babies cry for reasons other than hunger. (See Partnering with Families: Responding to Your Baby's Cry.)

■ Learn infant massage. For healthy infants, massage reportedly facilitates bonding, helps induce sleep in the baby, and makes parents feel good while massaging their baby. (See Chapter 5 🔗).

■ Allow your baby to suck fingers and hands or a pacifier. (See Box 9–6 and Partnering with Families: Making the Pacifier Decision.)

■ Make eye contact with your baby, hold and rock the baby frequently, and read and sing to your baby. If you cannot think of what to say, tell the baby about your day, or talk about what is happening, for example, "Are you hungry now?" "Is that milk nice and warm?" "Do you hear that dog barking outside?" "You are very alert. I like it when you look at me that way."

■ Be consistent and predictable in the way you respond to the newborn's needs.

During the health supervision visit, the nurse models behavior for parents that promotes positive infant mental health, such as handling the newborn gently, speaking in a soft voice, noticing attributes ("Look how you hold your head up today! You're really getting strong!"), and noticing likes and dislikes. The nurse strengthens parental confidence by asking the parent what the baby likes,

BOX 9–6   Research: Pacifiers, SIDS Reduction, and Breastfeeding

A meta-analysis (overall review of existing research) was done in 2005 of nine studies to review the effect of pacifier use and SIDS reduction (Hauck, Omojokun, & Siadaty, 2005). The published article concluded that the studies demonstrated a significantly reduced risk of SIDS with pacifier use, particularly when used while sleeping. The study recommended that pacifiers can be used for infants over 1 month and up to 1 year old, should be offered at sleep, and can be introduced after breastfeeding has been well established for infants who are nursing. Subsequent studies have verified these findings and recommendations (Adams, Good, & DeFranco, 2009).

Many factors influence breastfeeding duration, such as cultural practices, prenatal education, hospital practices, and postpartum support; therefore, it is unclear whether pacifier use should be discouraged due to a negative effect on breastfeeding. Until more conclusive research is available on any positive link between pacifier use and SIDS prevention, expectant and postpartum mothers should be educated about methods to calm an infant other than pacifier use, the importance of frequent feeding to establish and maintain milk supply, and the benefits of full breastfeeding in the first 6 months of life with addition of appropriate foods to complement the breast milk diet in the second 6 months of life.

such as, "How does he like to be carried, in your arms or up on your shoulder?" and then following the parent's advice. The nurse also promotes nurturing behavior by parents during procedures, such as allowing the parent to hold and comfort the baby while the nurse administers immunizations or draws blood.

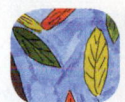

Partnering with Families

Responding to Your Baby's Cry

Babies cannot be spoiled by having their cries answered each time during the newborn period and in the first 6 months of life. Babies cry for multiple reasons; they may be tired, hungry, hot, cold, uncomfortable, overexcited, bored, lonely, or sick. The parent can try several approaches to calm the crying infant. As the baby progresses through infancy, techniques to enhance self-regulation should also be integrated (see Chapter 10).

In response to their newborn's cries, parents should:

- **Answer the cry quickly and consistently.** Answering a cry each time it occurs teaches newborns that their needs will be met and decreases the amount of crying.
- **Answer the cry with touch and verbalization.** When the parent responds to the cry, the parent should be within the newborn's visual field (10 to 13 inches from the face), speak to the newborn in a reassuring tone, and use gentle but firm touch. If the newborn does not stop crying, the parent should hold the newborn chest to chest with knees flexed, providing containment and flexion.

- Try one thing at a time to calm a crying newborn, such as changing the diaper, feeding the newborn, and adding or removing a layer of clothing.
- Gently pat or stroke the newborn's back or bottom in a rhythmic pattern.
- Wrap the newborn in a blanket to keep arms and legs close to the body.
- Rock the newborn forward and backward, as if in a swing.
- Lay the baby's bare skin against your bare skin.
- Dim the lights and rock the baby in a quiet room.
- Give the baby a warm bath.

Crying can be a sign of illness. If a baby continues to cry despite all efforts to calm him, contact the baby's healthcare provider. If you feel frustrated with the baby and need help, contact your healthcare provider immediately.

Source: *London, M. L., Ladewig, P. W., Ball, J. W., Bindler, R. C., & Cowen, K. C. (2011). Maternal & child nursing care (3rd ed.). Upper Saddle River, NJ: Pearson Prentice Hall.*

RELATIONSHIPS

Family adaptation to a new baby begins in pregnancy, and evidence of initial family adaptation to pregnancy may be predictive of future parental coping (Hagan et al., 2008). In the prenatal period, the nurse has the opportunity to gather information about the family and their concerns, educate the family about newborn care and characteristics, provide support and strategies for the immediate postpartum period, and begin to develop a trusting relationship between the family and healthcare professionals.

After the newborn has spent some time with the parent at home, the nurse assesses current protective factors and risks (Table 9–5). A healthy newborn with normal behavior and mature engaged parents has fewer risks than a newborn with special needs and family dysfunction. Based on assessment of the newborn and family, the pediatric nurse may need to coordinate services and resources for a

family at risk, or work with resources already in place, such as those begun prior to discharge from the neonatal intensive care nursery. (See Chapter 2 for more discussion about family assessment and interventions.)

New parents may need assistance in identifying activities that promote family health and positive parent–newborn interaction. Activities could include the following:

- Share newborn care activities. Recognize that you may do things differently than your partner, such as the way you change a diaper or give a bath, but if the baby is cared for, safe, and secure, these differences in technique do not matter.
- Compliment one another on newborn caregiving strengths, such as the mother's ability to breastfeed and the partner's ability to calm the crying baby.
- Attend health supervision visits together as much as possible.

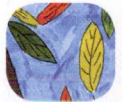

Partnering with Families

Making the Pacifier Decision

In the preterm infant, pacifiers are used for nonnutritive sucking, which means the baby sucks for reasons other than to provide nutrition. In the preterm infant, pacifier use facilitates self-consolation and self-regulation and provides positive oral stimulation in preparation for nutritive sucking and feeding. However, the benefits and potential risks of pacifier use in the healthy full-term infant are unknown. Some facts to share with parents include:

- Pacifiers do not cause medical or psychologic harm.
- Sucking on a pacifier can satisfy a baby's need to suck beyond breastfeeding or bottle feeding.
- Pacifier use during sleep during the first year of life has been shown to reduce the risk of sudden infant death syndrome (Moon, Tanabe, Yang, et al., 2012).

- Parents may incorrectly use a pacifier to soothe a newborn who is actually hungry and needs to feed. For example, the newborn who grows accustomed to falling asleep with a pacifier may awaken and cry frequently when it falls from the mouth.
- A meta-analysis showed that use of a pacifier had no significant effect on the number of infants breastfed at 3 and 4 months of age (Jaafar, Jahanfar, Angolkar, et al., 2011).
- Parents should purchase a one-piece pacifier with ventilation holes and never use a homemade pacifier from a bottle nipple that could come loose and choke the newborn.

TABLE 9–5	Risk and Protective Factors in Newborn and Family Relationships	

NEWBORN PROTECTIVE FACTORS	NEWBORN RISK FACTORS
■ Good health	■ Preterm birth, congenital disabilities, chronic illness
■ Normal eating, bowel, and sleep patterns	■ Feeding and sleep problems
■ Positive temperament	■ Fussing, crying, irritability, difficulty consoling
■ Responds to parents' attention	■ Diminished social interactions and responsiveness
■ Normal growth and development	■ Undernutrition, developmental delay

PARENTAL PROTECTIVE FACTORS	PARENTAL RISK FACTORS
■ Welcome baby at birth	■ Baby unplanned and unwanted at birth; potential for neglect or rejection
■ Meet newborn's basic needs for food, shelter, clothing, and health care	■ Financial insecurity, homelessness, lack of knowledge about how to care for newborn
■ Provide a strong nurturing environment	■ Cannot promote strong nurturing environment due to serious problems such as abusive behavior, depression, mental illness, or substance abuse
■ Parents have a strong relationship with one another, share care of newborn	■ Severe marital problems, absent parent, or frequent change of partners
■ Strong self-esteem, developmental maturity, developing knowledge of infant development	■ Lack of parenting skills, lack of parenting self-esteem, inability to cope with multiple roles, inappropriate coping strategies
■ No history of maltreatment as a child	■ History of maltreatment as a child (risk increases with positive history)

Source: *Data from Hagan, J. F., Shaw, J. S., & Duncan, P. M. (2008).* Bright futures: Guidelines for health supervision of infants, children, and adolescents *(3rd ed.). Elk Grove Village, IL: American Academy of Pediatrics.*

■ Be sensitive to when your partner is overstressed and overtired. Ask how you can help and then follow through with suggested activities. Sometimes listening is the most helpful thing you can do.

■ Rest and take time for yourself. Make decisions about what must be done (paying bills, laundry, grocery shopping) and what could wait (traveling to visit grandparents, painting the house, cleaning closets). Accept help from family and friends.

■ Discuss how you will raise your baby in a loving, supportive, and respectful environment.

■ Discuss how you were raised and what you would like to be different in your new family. Learn about parenting strategies and try out what feels comfortable for you.

■ Keep in contact with family and friends. Maintain community ties that are important to you, such as social, religious, cultural, or recreational organizations or programs.

■ Leave the baby with a trusted friend or family member and take time to be alone occasionally. Talk about something other than the baby.

■ Prepare siblings for the new baby prior to the baby's arrival. Allow siblings to "help" care for the new baby in age-appropriate ways. Praise siblings for positive attention they give to the baby, and allow siblings to express their feelings about the new baby and changes in the family.

■ Support one another in seeking and using community resources to strengthen parenting skills, such as classes and parenting groups.

■ Cuddle, hold, and rock the baby as much as possible. Babies cannot be spoiled by too much attention.

■ Take advantage of the baby's awake time to play with the baby. Singing, reading, and simply talking to the baby about what is happening provide developmental stimulation.

Family assessment should include screening for domestic violence, substance abuse, and child neglect or abuse (Box 9–7). See Chapter 20 *e*. Problems with parental bonding and attachment may also be apparent and require further assessment and interventions. The nurse should seek consultation and coordination of services

BOX 9–7	Screening for Domestic Violence

Domestic violence is a pattern of assaultive and coercive behaviors, including physical, sexual, and psychologic attacks, as well as economic coercion, that adults or adolescents use against their intimate partners to gain or maintain power and control. Domestic violence occurs in heterosexual, gay, lesbian, bisexual, and transgender intimate relationships and crosses all socioeconomic, religious, racial, ethnic, cultural, disability status, class, and age groups. However, domestic violence is primarily a crime against women. Women in abusive relationships may be motivated to disclose domestic violence during pregnancy and postpartum. This may be due to an increase in abuse during pregnancy or postpartum, or they may seek help for the sake of the baby. Women abused before or during pregnancy are at increased risk of abuse after the baby is born. The newborn is then at risk for child abuse and the long-term effects of violence and anger in the child's future relationships (Mayo Clinic, 2011b).

HOW TO ASK ABOUT ABUSE

Asking the question is in and of itself an intervention. The nurse's role is to identify abuse and assist women who are pregnant or have babies and young children to obtain the help they need to remain safe and keep the children safe. Questions about violence should be a part of each prenatal and newborn care visit. Verbal or written surveys may be used (Kataoka, Yaju, Eto, et al., 2010). Nursing implications include:

■ Ask about domestic violence. ("Have you ever been scared or hurt by your partner?")

■ Acknowledge the woman's response and validate her experience. ("I'm so sorry this is happening. It must be hard for you.")

■ Assess the immediate physical safety of the mother and children. ("Is it safe for you to go home today?")

■ Refer to a local domestic violence program for a safety plan and support.

■ Ensure medical follow-up and support.

■ Document findings in the chart.

■ Report to appropriate agencies when the safety of a child is at risk (see Chapter 20 *e* for further discussion of domestic violence and child abuse).

Conversations should be respectful, private, and confidential:

■ Children should not be present.

■ Use an interpreter when necessary.

■ Never use children to interpret.

■ Never ask about domestic violence in front of the woman's partner.

Source: *From Washington State Department of Health. (2008).* Domestic violence and pregnancy: Guidelines for screening and referral. *Retrieved from http://www.doh.wa.gov/cfh/mch/documents/DVFactsheet2008.pdf*

National Newborn Screening and Genetics Resource Center

Weblink

BOX 9–8 | **Newborn Screening**

The purpose of newborn screening is to identify those newborns who require further diagnostic testing for an array of genetic diseases and metabolic disorders. The test involves a small amount of blood, usually taken by heelstick sample, which is then analyzed for indicators of specific disorders. The baby's healthcare provider is notified of the screening results and should be alert to these results at the newborn's first outpatient visit. The department of health in each state regulates newborn screening, including the timing of the test, the need for repeat testing, and which tests are included in the screen. See Chapter 32 ✪. See further information at the National Newborn Screening and Genetics Resource Center website.

---

when encountering serious problems with family dynamics. For instances in which the children are in immediate jeopardy, the nurse needs to be aware of reporting mandates and protocols for child protective services and how to access assistance with interventions.

The setting in which the family seeks care should be aware of resources and how to refer family members in a timely and culturally appropriate fashion. For example, an interpreter from the family's community may know the family, causing mutual discomfort between the family members and the interpreter when discussing culturally sensitive or intensely private matters, such as domestic violence or substance abuse.

DISEASE PREVENTION STRATEGIES

Most babies born in the United States (about 71%) are discharged from the hospital without clinical problems or complicating diagnoses. The most common neonatal conditions that require extension of the newborn hospital stay or return to the hospital are associated with bilirubin metabolism, prematurity (including respiratory distress), respiratory problems, infections, and birth defects.

Disease prevention in the first month includes the following health maintenance activities:

- **Newborn screening**—all states require screening for congenital newborn diseases such as phenylketonuria (PKU) (see Figure 9–7 ■, Box 9–8, and Chapter 32 ✪)

BOX 9–9 | **Newborn Hearing Screening**

Hearing loss occurs in 1 to 2 of every 1,000 healthy newborns and 20 to 40 of every 1,000 newborns requiring intensive care. Universal hearing screening (all newborns tested regardless of risk factors) prior to hospital discharge is now the recommended standard of care (AAP & ACOG, 2007; National Institute on Deafness and Other Communication Disorders [NIDCD], 2011). The percentage of infants screened annually in the United States increased from 38% to 95% between 2000 and 2007 (AAP, 2007).

Newborn hearing screening is not diagnostic, but it can assist in early detection of possible hearing loss. A baby who "fails" the initial screen may be retested prior to hospital discharge. Parents should be advised that a "failed" screen is only an indication for referral to an audiologist for more conclusive testing. The evaluation should occur as soon as possible but no later than 3 months of age. If treatment is delayed for longer than 6 months in an infant with hearing loss, permanent developmental delays can occur in an otherwise healthy infant (AAP & ACOG, 2007; NIDCD, 2011). Early detection and intervention can contribute to an optimized outcome for the infant. Encourage parents to return for follow-up screening, and provide suggestions about observing for infant hearing loss.

- Hearing screening (see Box 9–9 and Chapter 24 ✪)
- Eye examination
- Immunizations (see Chapter 22 ✪)
- Prevention of secondhand smoke exposure
- Sudden infant death syndrome (SIDS) risk reduction (see Figure 9–8 ■ and Chapter 25 ✪)
- Formula safety (see Chapter 19 ✪)
- Hand washing is the key to preventing illness in the newborn and family members. Parents and family members should be taught about the importance of washing hands with soap and warm water:
  - After diaper changes
  - Before feeding the newborn
  - After using the bathroom or assisting someone to use the bathroom
  - Before preparing food or eating
  - When returning home after being out in the community (e.g., at work, day care, church, playing with friends, the mall)
  - After handling pets
  - After blowing nose or sneezing

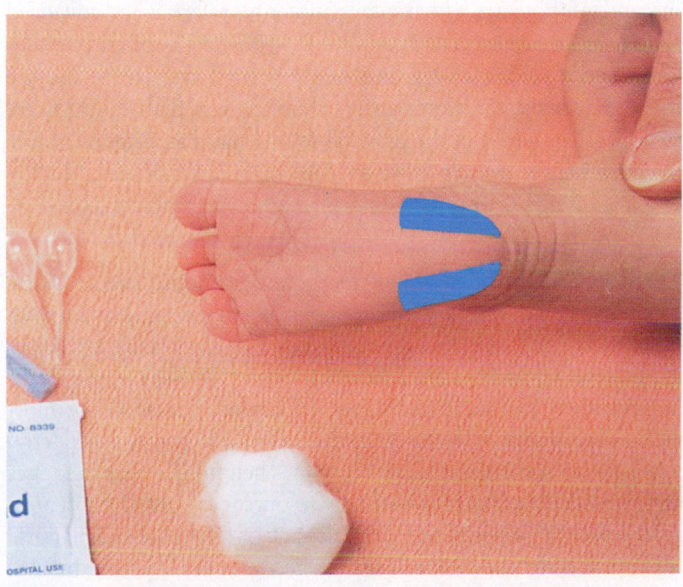

FIGURE 9–7 ■ Heel sites for capillary puncture.

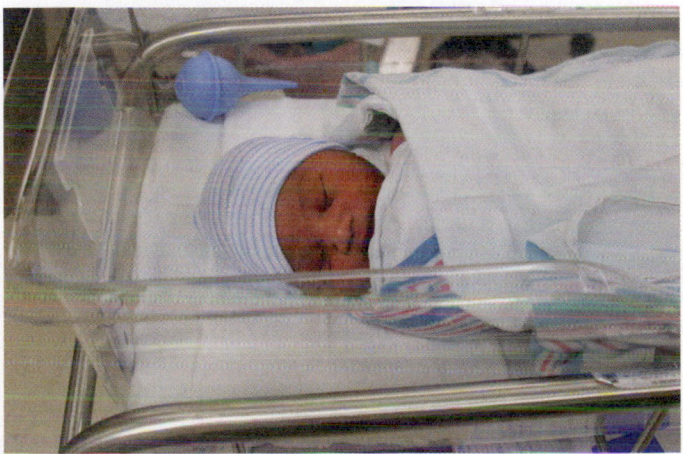

FIGURE 9–8 ■ Parents are more likely to place their newborn in the back-sleeping position when they see it used in the hospital.

■ Minimizing the newborn's exposure to disease by avoiding infant exposure to large crowds, especially in cold and flu season; covering coughs and sneezes and using good hand washing technique especially if parent/caregiver is ill; alerting the baby's caregiver if newborn is exposed to varicella, pertussis, or other serious communicable disease

INJURY PREVENTION STRATEGIES

New parents are sometimes unaware of sources of potential injury for the newborn. Some aspects of injury prevention are pertinent to the newborn's immediate care. Other topics promote discussion and provide opportunities for anticipatory guidance. In the immediate newborn period, the nurse should assess the parents' knowledge of injury prevention strategies and promote healthy and safe habits. Injury prevention strategies include proper and consistent use of an infant car seat, and strategies to prevent falls, burns, choking, drowning, and suffocation (see Box 9–10 and Table 9–6).

Newborn safety awareness begins in the birth setting. Parents should be cautioned to lay the baby in a bassinet or crib rather than on the mother's bed. Teach the parents to use the bulb syringe in the event that the baby spits up a large amount of fluid, and to position the baby for sleep on the back rather than side-lying or prone. Parents should also be oriented to procedures in place to prevent newborn abduction and to their critical role in ensuring newborn safety and security.

Following hospital discharge, the nurse promotes safety by encouraging parents to think about the hazards that the newborn could encounter and how to eliminate them. In the newborn period, the parent or caregiver is uniquely responsible for ensuring that the newborn is not placed in a dangerous situation. The newborn cannot turn on a hot water faucet or run with a sharp object, but it is possible for the parent to inadvertently place the newborn in danger. The newborn is capable of twisting and rolling off any surface higher than the floor, falling out of an infant carrier seat, or drowning while left unattended for a moment in a bathtub filled with only an inch or two of water.

Parents might find it helpful to be aware that most pediatric injuries occur when the parents are under stress; for example, when a parent is hungry and tired (the hour before dinner), during pregnancy, during illness or death in the family, when there is tension between parents, and during changes in the environment, such as a change in the child's caregiver or the family's living environment. At these times, the parent should be particularly vigilant and supervise children closely.

| BOX 9–10 | Car Seat Assistance and Education |

Nurses should help hospitals to develop discharge guidelines for newborns related to car safety seats. They are responsible for referring parents to a local trained child passenger safety technician for assistance. Call 1-877-366-8154 to find a car seat inspection location. You can also refer parents to the AAP car seat guide.

Source: *From* Child restraints for newborn infants: A health care provider's guide. *(2008).* Edmonds, WA: Safe Ride News Publications; American Academy of Pediatrics. *(2011c).* Car safety seats. *Retrieved from http://www.healthychildren.org/English/safety-prevention/ on-the-go/pages/Car-Safety-Seats-Information-for-Families.aspx*

Car Seat Safety

Weblink

Nursing Management

Nursing Assessment and Diagnosis

An essential skill for the nurse in the hospital, clinic, or community setting is the ability to assess the family and newborn and identify potential health promotion and health maintenance activities. Many health promotion and health maintenance activities are pertinent to prenatal health as well as the postpartum period. If maternal and pediatric care providers are located at different agencies, nurses must coordinate and integrate services so that the new mother and family benefit from a seamless continuum of care.

Based on nursing assessments, the nursing diagnoses form the basis for subsequent interventions. Possible nursing diagnoses for the family and newborn in the first month following birth might include:

■ Anxiety (parent) related to change in role status
■ Risk for Impaired Attachment, Parent/Infant related to postpartum depression
■ Attachment, Risk for Impaired related to parental exhaustion or lack of knowledge of infant cues
■ Parenting, Impaired related to premature birth
■ Breastfeeding, Readiness for Enhanced related to infant needs
■ Breastfeeding, Ineffective related to inadequate sucking by infant
■ Parenting, Readiness for Enhanced related to desire to bond with infant

NANDA-I © 2012

Planning and Implementation

Newborn health maintenance and promotion begins in the prenatal period. In most cases, the expectant mother is highly motivated to engage in activities that result in a healthy newborn, and the healthcare team has a unique window of opportunity to promote maternal and newborn health.

In the prenatal period, the nurse's goal is to promote an optimal outcome for both mother and newborn. Comprehensive quality prenatal care is outside the scope of this text; however, important health maintenance and health promotion activities include interventions to help ensure healthy diet and exercise; avoidance of alcohol, tobacco, and drugs; and establishment or maintenance of a dental home. The nurse may assess the need for assistance with food, clothing, and safe housing, which entails numerous referrals and advanced skills to ensure coordinated community services. The nurse provides anticipatory guidance regarding newborn care and safety, and the nurse may assist the woman with choosing a pediatric healthcare provider. The nurse in the prenatal setting plays an important role in educating the woman about the lifelong benefits of breastfeeding and in guiding her toward an informed infant feeding decision.

Hospital-Based Care

The hospital length of stay is short for the healthy mother and newborn. The nurse in the birth setting is responsible for assessing and implementing nursing care during a time of dramatic physiologic changes in both mother and newborn, as well as helping the new parents learn basic newborn care skills. Consistent and accurate breastfeeding information is essential to ensure continued efforts at home, and referral to a lactation specialist or support group is helpful. The nurse assesses and refers the mother to community resources as needed for depression; domestic violence; and drug, alcohol, or tobacco use. The nurse may coordinate interventions such as access to the Women, Infants, and Children (WIC) nutrition program to help ensure adequate food and nutritional support, and refer the mother to parenting classes or

TABLE 9–6	Injury Prevention Topics for Parents of Newborns
TOPIC	**INJURY PREVENTION TEACHING TOPICS**
Motor vehicle safety	■ Choose an infant-only seat or a convertible seat suitable for an infant. ■ The infant rides rear-facing until at least 2 years of age or until the child has reached the highest height and weight of the seat manufacturer. ■ The safest place for all children to ride is in the back seat. Never place a rear-facing car safety seat in the front seat with an active passenger air bag. ■ Use a car safety seat every time the infant is in the car. ■ Read and follow the manufacturer's instructions for the car safety seat and the vehicle owner's manual for installation information. ■ Dress the infant in clothes that allow the straps to go between the legs. Never place blankets under the baby or under the belts. Buckle the baby into the seat, and place blankets over the baby. ■ To make sure the car safety seat is installed correctly and the baby is positioned correctly, go to a car seat inspection station. A certified child passenger safety (CPS) technician will assist you. Find a list of certified CPS technicians and safety seat inspection stations by state or zip code on the National Highway Traffic Safety Administration website or call 1-888-327-4236 or 1-866-732-8243 (SEAT-CHECK) (AAP, 2011c).
Shaken baby syndrome	Never shake a baby. Recognize that sometimes you will not be able to console your baby. Shaking a baby, even for only a few seconds, can cause serious brain damage and death. One of four shaken babies dies. There are materials available for parents and professionals at http://www.dontshake.com
Crib	Use a safety approved crib. Slats should be no more than 2 3/8 inches apart. The mattress should be firm and fit snugly into the crib. Affix the crib rails so they are not able to drop down.
Bed-sharing	The American Academy of Pediatrics discourages bed-sharing by infant and parent due to an increased risk of SIDS and the danger of suffocation associated with this practice. Sleep with the baby nearby, but not in the parental bed. If the parent must sleep with the baby, ensure that the infant is supine, separated from any soft surfaces such as pillows; ensure that no blankets will cover the infant's head; beware of spaces between the mattress and the wall, headboard, or footboard; and do not sleep with the baby when under the influence of drugs or alcohol. The infant should never sleep in the same bed with siblings due to the high risk of suffocation (AAP Task Force on Sudden Infant Death Syndrome, 2011).
Baby toys	Use age-appropriate baby toys. Check toys for sharp edges or loose parts. Keep older siblings' toys out of the baby's reach. Do not use toys with loops or string cords.
Drowning	Never leave a baby alone in the bathtub. If you must turn your back on the baby or leave the room, take the baby out of the tub.
Suffocation	Keep plastic bags and wrappings away from the baby (take the plastic bag off the crib mattress). Shake baby powder into your hand first, then apply it so the baby does not inhale it. Do not allow a baby or sibling to play with a latex balloon. Keep small objects (such as safety pins, coins, small toys) out of the baby's reach. Do not attach pacifiers, medals, or other objects to the crib or to the baby's body with a string or cord. Do not put the crib near blinds, curtains, or anything with a hanging cord. Do not let the baby wear clothing with strings near the neck (such as a sweatshirt hood that ties with a cord) or a headband that could slip down and wrap around the baby's neck. Use a tight-fitting crib sheet that does not come loose when the corner is pulled.
Burns	Set the hot water heater thermostat to 120°F (49°C). Do not smoke or drink hot liquids while holding the baby. Do not microwave bottles of formula or breast milk due to uneven heating. Do not expose the baby to direct sunlight.
Falls	Keep a hand on the baby while dressing or changing the diaper on a surface other than the floor. Never leave the baby unsupervised on any high surface such as a bed, changing table, or sofa. Always keep one hand on the baby.
Pet safety	Keep some distance between the newborn and the pet until the pet's initial reaction to the new baby is assessed. Never leave the baby unsupervised with the family dog or cat, or any animal capable of harming the newborn.
Sibling supervision	Never leave the baby alone with a young sibling. When young children hold the baby, seat the child on a large soft surface, such as the couch, and supervise closely. Watch siblings for aggressive behavior toward the newborn, such as hitting or biting. Siblings may take on a caregiving role and imitate adults; watch for "feeding" of nonfood items or choking hazards.
Fire safety	Install working smoke detectors on every floor of the house and in every sleeping area. Have a fire escape plan from the house and practice it.
Poisoning	Post the universal phone number for the poison control center near your telephone and program it into your cell phone: 1-888-222-1222.
Gun safety	Keep the household guns unloaded and locked up. Keep the ammunition locked up separately from the gun. Consider not keeping a gun in the household due to safety hazards for family members.
In case of emergency	■ Know when and how to call the pediatric care provider. ■ Know when it is appropriate to go to the emergency department. ■ Take a first-aid class and learn CPR for children and adults.

Source: *Data from Hagan, J. F., Shaw, J. S., & Duncan, P. M. (Eds.). (2008).* Bright futures: Guidelines for health supervision of infants, children, and adolescents *(3rd ed.). Elk Grove Village, IL: American Academy of Pediatrics; Murray, R. B., Zentner, J. P., & Yakimo, R. (2009).* Health promotion strategies through the life span *(8th ed.). Upper Saddle River, NJ: Pearson Prentice Hall.*

support groups. Through listening to the family's concerns, providing nurturing responses, respecting cultural differences, and validating parental efforts to learn parenting skills, the nurse further develops the partnership between the family and the healthcare providers.

Prior to discharge the newborn has blood taken for newborn screening, should have initial hearing screening, and may receive the first hepatitis B vaccination. Follow-up after these interventions requires communication among multiple community agencies and the pediatric care provider to ensure that the newborn receives appropriate continuing care.

Care in the Community

In the outpatient setting, the goal of the pediatric healthcare team is to assist the family to develop the knowledge and confidence to safely care for their infant and to incorporate the infant into the family unit. In the first month of the newborn's life, health promotion and maintenance activities may include teaching the parents how to interact with their baby to promote attachment, provide a safe sleeping environment, ensure motor vehicle safety, and prevent accidents or exposure to toxins. The nurse will provide information about baby care practices, especially breastfeeding, and help parents begin to learn about the newborn's temperament in order to respond to needs and thereby promote infant mental health.

The relationship between the family and pediatric healthcare team must be nurtured. Time should be allowed for parents' questions. Cultural differences in perspectives must be considered. Results of screening and testing should be explained. When the nurse involves the parents in healthcare activities of the infant in these ways, it is more likely that they will be cooperative and interested in promoting and maintaining their child's health.

Evaluation

Expected outcomes for the family and healthy newborn by the end of the first month are as follows:

- The newborn makes a successful transition from intrauterine to extrauterine life.
- Risk factors are identified in the prenatal and newborn period, and nursing assessment coordinates with medical intervention to prevent or manage complications.
- The newborn achieves expected physical and developmental milestones.
- Breastfeeding is established and the mother has identified sources of support to continue breastfeeding.
- The family begins successful integration of the newborn into the family.
- Parents demonstrate newborn care skills and beginnings of healthy attachment behaviors.
- Parents recognize the importance of health promotion and health maintenance activities and partner with healthcare professionals to promote and maintain the physical and mental health of the newborn and family.

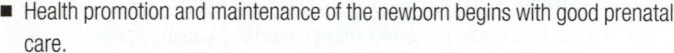 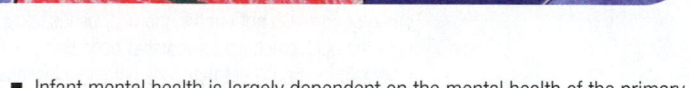

Chapter Highlights

- Health promotion and maintenance of the newborn begins with good prenatal care.
- The expectant mother is encouraged to choose her baby's care provider prior to the baby's birth.
- Family partnership is promoted when the family has warm and supportive interactions with healthcare professionals who respect the parent's ability to learn about and participate in decisions related to the child's pediatric health care.
- The initial pediatric visits focus on infant growth and development, identification of problems not discovered at birth, parent teaching and support, and assessment of family–infant interaction.
- Breastfeeding advocacy is one of the most important health promotion activities that occurs during prenatal care and the first year of life.
- Infant mental health is promoted by parents who create a "child-centered" environment that allows the infant to develop a full set of skills for learning, thinking, responding, and solving problems.

- Infant mental health is largely dependent on the mental health of the primary caregiver, usually the infant's mother.
- Infant mental health and parent–infant attachment are promoted by such activities as responding quickly to the infant's expressed needs; holding, rocking, singing, and talking to the baby; and providing consistent and predictable responses to the baby's needs.
- Disease prevention strategies include immunizations, back sleeping position, preventing secondhand smoke exposure, hand washing, screening, and minimizing newborn exposure to disease.
- Injury prevention strategies include proper and consistent use of an infant car seat, and strategies to prevent falls, burns, choking, drowning, and suffocation.

Clinical Reasoning in Action

INTRODUCTION

Recall 22-year-old Shannon who was described at the beginning of the chapter. She is a single mother with two daughters, 5-year-old Denise and 10-day-old Rhonda. Shannon lives with her boyfriend of the past 2 years. Rhonda was born at 37 weeks' gestation, weighed 2800 g (6 lb, 3 oz) at birth, required phototherapy for newborn jaundice, and had initial difficulties breastfeeding. She was discharged from the nursery at 5 days of age.

DESCRIPTION

Rhonda is an active and fussy baby who reacts strongly to everything that happens around her. Shannon carries her into the exam room in her car seat. Rhonda is dressed appropriately for the weather and appears clean and well cared for. As the nurse undresses Rhonda, the baby arches and screams. Her diaper is dry. Shannon strokes her head and speaks quietly to her. Rhonda now weighs 2830 g (6 lb, 4 oz). The nurse swaddles Rhonda in a blanket. She quiets, and the nurse places her in Shannon's arms. The nurse learns that Rhonda sleeps for only an hour or two at a time, then fusses. Shannon tries to feed her each time she stirs, but sometimes she has short drowsy feedings and does not seem hungry. Rhonda has about four wet diapers and two stools per day. Shannon's boyfriend is increasingly irritable as Rhonda is keeping him awake at night. Shannon states that Rhonda is a much more difficult baby than Denise was. She is exhausted, and feels like a bad mother and partner.

DISCUSSION

1. Shannon is an experienced mother, yet this newborn poses unexpected challenges. List the risk factors in the family, as well as the protective factors.

2. Based on the risk and protective factors, list three or four nursing diagnoses related to the family. What interventions will assist the family to better integrate Rhonda into their lives?

3. Lack of sleep is a major issue for Shannon's family. Describe infant states and determine what sleep state Rhonda is in when she stirs and fusses and makes crying sounds. How could Shannon extend the time between feedings so that Rhonda is more awake and interested in breastfeeding well 8 to 10 times per day? What other strategies could Shannon use to calm her sensitive newborn?

4. What questions would the pediatric nurse and lactation consultant ask Shannon to assess the adequacy of breastfeeding at this time? Calculate the percentage of Rhonda's weight loss since birth. Is this concerning? What other factors should be assessed at this visit?

5. Shannon feels sad and discouraged about her life at this point. What factors could be influencing her mood? What questions should be asked to assess Shannon's coping strategies? What interventions might be suggested? What positive aspects of Shannon's parenting could be noted and validated?

NCLEX-RN® Review

1. Which is an indication of positive parent–newborn attachment during a health supervision visit?
   1. The parent denies having questions about the care, nutrition, or behavior of the newborn.
   2. The parent allows the newborn to self-comfort as he or she starts to cry with the assessment.
   3. The parent touches, massages, and gently rubs the infant in an attempt to soothe.
   4. The father is the primary comforter and nurturer at the visit while the mother observes.

2. The home health nurse is providing education to the parents of a newborn infant. In order to promote health and health maintenance needs, what topics are appropriate for this nurse to include during the home visit? (Select all that apply.)
   1. Developmental progressions
   2. Newborn sleep patterns
   3. Dietary needs
   4. Establishing a plan of action for further care
   5. Clarifying information

3. The nurse notices a mother failing to support a newborn's neck while moving the infant to the exam table. Which is the nurse's most appropriate action?
   1. Document the observation in the notes to discuss later.
   2. Ask to hold the baby while discussing safer holding techniques.
   3. Take the infant from the mother while explaining the weak neck muscles.
   4. Encourage the mother to quickly put the infant on the exam table.

4. The nurse is assessing a small-for-gestational-age newborn who had an older sibling who died of sudden infant death syndrome. Knowing this, the nurse must include which in the plan of care for the newborn?
   1. Encourage the parent(s) to place the infant on his or her abdomen to sleep.
   2. Place the infant in a crib with a tight-fitting, firm mattress.
   3. Place the infant in a crib with a soft mattress with extra blankets.
   4. Encourage the parent(s) to sleep with the infant for close observation.

See Appendix I 🔵 for answers.

References

Adams, S. M., Good, M. W., & DeFranco, G. M. (2009). Sudden infant death syndrome. *American Family Physician, 79,* 870–874.

Ahmed, A. H. (2010). Role of the pediatric nurse practitioner in promoting breastfeeding for late preterm infants in primary care settings. *Journal of Pediatric Health Care, 24*(2), 116–122.

American Academy of Pediatrics (AAP). (2007). Year 2007 position statement: Principles and guidelines for early hearing detection and intervention programs. *Pediatrics, 120*(4), 898–921.

American Academy of Pediatrics (AAP). (2010). Policy statement: Hospital stay for healthy term newborns. *Pediatrics, 125*(2), 405–409. doi:10.1542/peds.2009-3119

American Academy of Pediatrics (AAP). (2011a). *Where we stand: Newborn discharge from hospital.* Retrieved from http://www.healthychildren.org/English/ages-stages/prenatal/delivery-beyond/pages/

American Academy of Pediatrics (AAP). (2011b). *Umbilical cord care.* Retrieved from http://www.healthychildren.org/English/ages-stages/baby/bathing-skin-care/pages/Umbilical-Cord-Care.aspx

American Academy of Pediatrics (AAP). (2011c). *Car safety seats: A guide for families.* Elk Grove Village, IL: Author.

American Academy of Pediatrics (AAP) Committee on Bioethics. (2010). Children as hematopoietic stem cell donors. *Pediatrics, 125,* 392–404. doi:10.1542/peds.2009-3078

American Academy of Pediatrics (AAP) Committee on Nutrition. (2009). *Pediatric nutrition handbook* (6th ed.). Elk Grove Village, IL: Author.

American Academy of Pediatrics (AAP) Task Force on Sudden Infant Death Syndrome. (2011). SIDS and other sleep-related infant deaths: Expansion of recommendations for a safe infant sleeping environment. *Pediatrics, 128,* e1341–e1367.

American Academy of Pediatrics (AAP) & American College of Obstetricians and Gynecologists (ACOG). (2007). *Guidelines for perinatal care* (6th ed.). Elk Grove Village, IL: Author.

Blackburn, S. T. (2007). *Maternal, fetal, and neonatal physiology: A clinical perspective.* St. Louis, MO: Saunders.

Centers for Disease Control and Prevention. (2008). *New CDC study finds gaps in breastfeeding support in U.S. hospitals and birth centers.* Retrieved from http://www.cdc.gov/media/pressrel/2008/r080612.htm

Centers for Disease Control and Prevention. (2011). *Oral health.* Retrieved from http://www.cdc.gov/chronicdisease/resources/publications/AAG/doh.htm

Cricco-Lizza, R. (2009). Rooting for the breast: Breastfeeding promotion in the NICU. *MCN: American Journal of Maternal Child Nursing, 34*(6), 356–364.

Faraz, A. (2010). Clinical recommendations for promoting breastfeeding among Hispanic women. *Journal of the American Academy of Nurse Practitioners, 22,* 292–299.

Hagan, J. F., Shaw, J. S., & Duncan, P. M. (Eds.). (2008). *Bright futures: Guidelines for health supervision of infants, children, and adolescents* (3rd ed.). Elk Grove Village, IL: American Academy of Pediatrics.

Hauck, F. R., Omojokun, O. O., & Siadaty, M. S. (2005). Do pacifiers reduce the risk of sudden infant death syndrome? A meta-analysis. *Pediatrics, 116,* e716–e723.

Jaafar, S. H., Jahanfar, S., Angolkar, M., & Ho, J. J. (2011). Pacifier use versus no pacifier use in breastfeeding term infants for increasing duration of breastfeeding.

Cochrane Library Issue 3, Art. No. CD007202. doi:10.1002/14651858.CD007202.pub2

Kataoka, Y., Yaju, Y., Eto, H., & Horiuchi, S. (2010). Self-administered questionnaire versus interview as a screening method for intimate partner violence in the prenatal setting in Japan: A randomized controlled trial. *BMC: Pregnancy & Childbirth, 10,* 84.

Koren, A., Reece, S. M., Kahn-D'angelo, L., & Medeiros, D. (2010). Parental information and provider practices related to tummy time and back to sleep. *Journal of Pediatric Health Care, 24*(4), 222–230. doi:10.1016/j.pedhc.2009.05.002

Lipson, J. G., & Dibble, S. L. (2008). *Culture and clinical care.* San Francisco: UCSF Nursing Press.

March of Dimes. (2010). *Umbilical cord blood.* Retrieved from http://www.marchofdimes.com/pregnancy/labor_umbilical.html

Mayo Clinic. (2011a). *Infant jaundice.* Retrieved from http://www.mayoclinic.com/health/infant-jaundice/DS00107/DSECTION=symptoms

Mayo Clinic. (2011b). *Domestic violence against women: Recognize patterns, seek help.* Retrieved from http://www.mayoclinic.com/health/domestic-violence/WO00044

Moon, R. Y., Tanabe, K. O., Yang, D. C., Young, Y. A., & Hauck, F. R. (2012). Pacifier use and SIDS: Evidence for a consistently reduced risk. *Maternal Child Health Journal, 16,* 609–614. doi: 10:1007/s10995-011-0793-x

Murray, R. B., Zentner, J. P., & Yakimo, R. (2009). *Health promotion strategies through the life span* (8th ed.). Upper Saddle River, NJ: Pearson Prentice Hall.

National Institute on Deafness and Other Communication Disorders (NIDCD). (2011). *It's important to have your baby's hearing screened.* Retrieved from http://www.nidcd.nih.gov/health/hearing/pages/screened.aspx

Tanski, S., Garfunkel, L. C., Duncan, P. M., & Weitzman, M. (2010). *Performing preventive services.* Elk Grove Village, IL: American Academy of Pediatrics.

U.S. Department of Health and Human Services. (2011). *Healthy People 2020.* Washington, DC: U.S. Government Printing Office.

World Health Organization. (2010). *Male circumcision for HIV prevention.* Retrieved from http://www.who.int/hiv/topics/malecircumcision/en/index.html

World Health Organization. (2011). *Health promotion.* Retrieved from http://www.who.int/healthpromotion.areas/en/

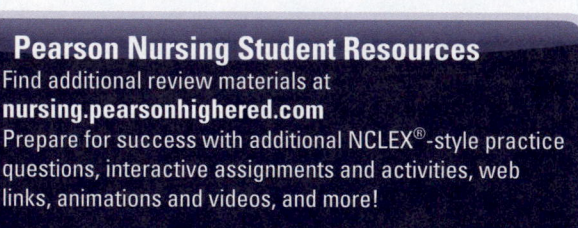

Pearson Nursing Student Resources

Find additional review materials at
nursing.pearsonhighered.com
Prepare for success with additional NCLEX®-style practice questions, interactive assignments and activities, web links, animations and videos, and more!

Health Promotion and Maintenance of the Infant

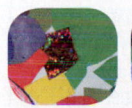 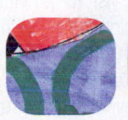 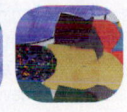

Learning Outcomes

After completing this chapter, you will be able to:

1. Describe the general observations made of infants and their families as they come to the pediatric healthcare home for health supervision visits.

2. Identify the major health promotion and health maintenance needs during infancy.

3. Assess nutrition, physical activity, mental health status, and growth and development of infants.

4. Apply therapeutic communication skills with the infant and family during health supervision visits in infancy.

5. Prioritize interventions for infants and their families to promote health and prevent disease and injury.

6. Synthesize data from the history and examination of the infant and family with knowledge of infant development to plan approaches useful with the family during health supervision encounters.

> "Mommy was really glad to go see the nurse today. She brought our baby, and Grandma said that they would give us a card that would help us buy food. Mommy said we could get some milk and juice."
>
> *—Melody, age 4*

Colleen Agamata arrives at the Women, Infants, and Children (WIC) clinic with her 7-month-old infant Amanda. Colleen works full time, so her mother accompanies her to take Amanda home by bus after the examination by the nurse and a meeting with the dietitian.

It has been hard for Colleen to manage with Amanda and her 4-year-old daughter Melody, but she is determined to support them. She was recently referred to the WIC program to receive screening and examination of her infant, and teaching related to nutrition. The eligibility card enables her to purchase food for herself and her children. She has had several episodes of food insecurity (see Chapter 19 🔗 for a description of food insecurity) when she did not have enough money to buy food for herself or Melody. Now, with a new infant, the challenges are even more difficult to meet. Colleen's mother helps as much as possible, but she has impaired vision and also needs assistance with some tasks.

The nurse screens Amanda for iron intake, obtains a hematocrit, and weighs and measures her so that growth can be monitored. The nurse and dietitian collaborate to teach Colleen health promotion information related to the benefits of nutritious intake, and health maintenance data about ways that food intake can help to prevent such diseases as iron deficiency anemia. They make an appointment to have Colleen bring in both Melody and Amanda for a visit in 2 months.

What ongoing assessments will Melody and Amanda need? How can the nurse in the WIC clinic work with Colleen and the rest of her family to ensure food security and food intake that will both promote healthy growth and prevent disease? What additional health promotion and health maintenance topics are important for this family?

nfancy is a major life transition for the infant and parents. The infant accomplishes phenomenal physical growth and many developmental milestones while the family adapts to the addition of a new member and establishes new goals for each of its existing members. Infant health supervision visits are important to support the health of the infant and the family unit. These visits begin after the newborn period, at about 1 month of age. This is the time when parents establish an ongoing partnership with a primary healthcare provider. A "medical home" or "pediatric healthcare home" is identified to serve the infant's health needs. (See Chapters 1 and 8 ✏ for further description of the medical or pediatric healthcare home.) The goals of health supervision visits are to identify and address the health promotion and health maintenance (or health protection) needs of the infant.

Health promotion activities focus on promoting the highest level of wellness possible for the infant. These activities include facilitating breastfeeding, helping parents to understand their infant's temperament, and employing strategies to ensure adequate sleep by the infant and parents. In contrast, health maintenance activities focus on disease and injury prevention, such as administering immunizations and teaching about infant car seats. Both health promotion and health maintenance interventions are integrated into each health supervision visit.

Recall the Bindler-Ball Continuum of Pediatric Health Care from Chapters 1 and 8. All children require health promotion and maintenance activities, even if they have frequent acute health conditions or chronic health diagnoses. Care in the healthcare home should be coordinated with other resources to provide referral as needed, consistent and continuous in services rendered, and family centered. A true partnership should exist with the care providers and family (Voigt, Macias, & Myers, 2010).

Establishment of the relationship with a healthcare provider and agency is important so that trust develops and the family feels comfortable turning to professionals for information and guidance as the infant grows. Nurses play a vital role in welcoming new families into office and clinic settings, establishing rapport, and applying principles of communication so that trust and positive partnerships develop between providers and families. Infancy is a time when the child grows in physical, psychologic, and cognitive ways; health supervision visits play a key role in fostering healthy growth and development. When should the infant be seen for health supervision visits? What are key components of these visits? How can the nurse best assess and intervene to ensure the infant's health and safety? We will address these and other questions in this chapter.

EARLY CONTACTS WITH THE FAMILY

Health promotion and maintenance occur in a series of health supervision visits during the first year of life. Schedules vary among facilities, but a common pattern includes visits at about 1 month, 2 months, 4 months, 6 months, 9 months, and 1 year of age. In addition, most children have some episodic illnesses such as gastrointestinal illness or otitis media and visit the facility at other times for treatment of these illnesses. A few children have chronic or serious healthcare problems during the first year and have extensive contact with the healthcare home and other services. See Developing Cultural Competence: First Visit for Infant Health Care.

Since the family relies on the healthcare provider for support and interventions during infancy, the family has preferably established

Developing Cultural Competence
First Visit for Infant Health Care

In the United States and Canada, the first healthcare visit for an infant commonly takes place in an office setting, with the parents bringing the infant in for examination. In many other countries, such as Australia, England, and Sweden, community-based maternal and child health nurses (sometimes called "visitors") may be the family's first contact with health professionals. In developing countries with high infant mortality rates, such as Bangladesh, India, and Pakistan, home visits for infants can decrease infant deaths by 30% to 60% (World Health Organization [WHO] & United Nations Children's Fund [UNICEF], 2009). What advantages can you identify for systems that partner nurses and physicians to deliver health promotion and health maintenance visits? What are the roles of nurses, physicians, and other healthcare professionals in the health supervision visits in your clinical agencies?

contact with the provider before the infant is born. If the family has not chosen a care provider during pregnancy and the newborn period, they can visit potential agencies when the baby is an infant and ask questions related to the services, personnel, and other components of care. (See Chapter 9 ✏ for questions the parents can ask at this visit and for clues about how to evaluate their fit with the care provider.) At whatever time it occurs, the purpose of the visit is to ensure that the family understands the services offered and the policies related to provision of care, and feels comfortable with the personality of the providers. Sometimes parents visit two or more providers and choose the best fit for the family.

Chapter 9 ✏ discusses the first health supervision visits that occur in the immediate newborn period and up to 1 month of life. At about 1 month, the visits of infancy begin. During these first visits, assess the family for protective factors and risks. Protective factors might include parental knowledge level of infant needs, support from family and friends, and the mother's good health and nutritional state during pregnancy. Risk factors could include limited financial resources, lack of preparation for the infant, and illness or other stress among family members. Ask about how the family traveled to the visit and if convenient times and transportation are available. Lack of access during times the family is not at work and other health system barriers sometimes interfere with attendance at health supervision visits. Knowledge of these factors will shape the nursing interventions in health supervision in infancy. The nurse applies health promotion principles by building on strengths and fosters health maintenance by intervening to minimize risks. Many examples of these activities follow throughout this chapter.

GENERAL OBSERVATIONS

When the family comes to the clinic or office for care with an infant, general observation should begin at first contact (Figure 10–1 ■). This often occurs as the family is called in from the waiting area. The nurse can observe factors such as:

- Who is bringing the infant in for care?
- What are interactions like between the adults present, other siblings, and the infant?
- Is the infant awake or sleeping?
- If awake, is the infant's body posture and alertness appropriate for age and developmental level?
- Does the infant look well nourished and cared for?

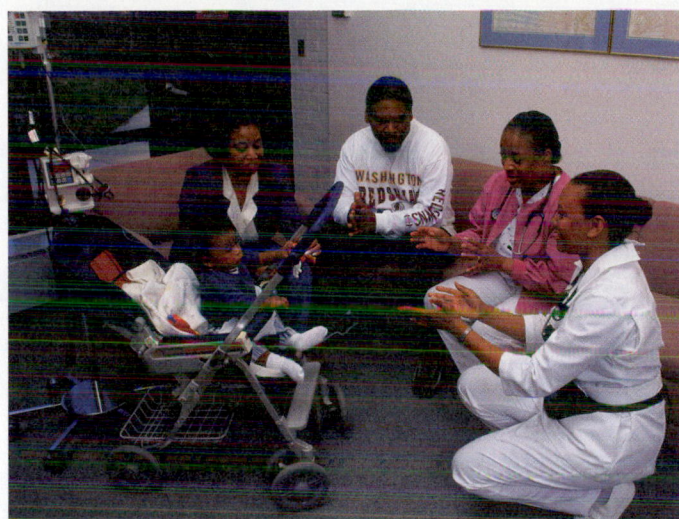

FIGURE 10–1 ■ The nurse begins assessment of the infant's family when they are seen in the waiting room and called in for care. What observations can you make of the infant's general appearance? Developmental accomplishments? Interaction of parents with the baby?

Welcome each member of the family warmly to the facility and comment on the infant. Make special note of the family members present, such as a grandparent. Recall the grandmother who attended the visit in the opening scenario and her central role in the family. Increasing numbers of fathers attend well-child visits. By attending these visits, they exhibit the support of their children, an ability to ask questions and express concerns, and a desire to gather information (Hagan, Shaw, & Duncan, 2008).

Ask how the family is doing with the baby and how the adjustment is going. Inquire about developmental skills and what questions the family would like to ask. Be alert for signs of fatigue or depression in the parents, as these can occur when caring for an infant and can interfere with bonding and positive transition (Box 10–1). Postpartum blues and postpartum depression are two specific types of mood disorders sometimes observed in new mothers; postpartum psychosis is more serious and less common. We will refer to these conditions later in this chapter; Chapter 9 ✪ discusses them in greater detail.

Upon entering the examination room, it is helpful to explain the plans for the visit, such as "I will weigh and measure Sarah now and show you how she is growing. Then I'll ask a few questions about her eating, sleeping, and other things. Then the nurse practitioner will be in to do Sarah's physical examination. Do you have any

---

BOX 10–1	Signs of Sleep Deprivation in Parents

- Confusion and disorientation
- Forgetfulness
- Lack of alertness, judgment, and coordination
- Fatigue
- Increased injuries
- Anxiety
- Decreased motivation
- Disturbed appetite

Source: Data from Murray, R. B., Zentner, J. P., & Yakimo, R. (2009). Health promotion strategies through the life span (8th ed.). Upper Saddle River, NJ: Prentice Hall Health.

---

questions as we start? Will you undress Sarah now so we can weigh her accurately?"

GROWTH AND DEVELOPMENTAL SURVEILLANCE

Physical growth and developmental milestones provide important information about infants. The infant is measured for accurate length, weight, and head circumference (see the Skills Manual ⊂⊃ and Chapter 7 ✪). The measurements should be placed on growth grids and interpreted. (See Appendix A ✪.) Parents enjoy seeing how the infant is progressing and are usually eager to learn about the child's weight gain and growth percentiles (Figure 10–2 ■). Be alert for an infant who demonstrates a change in percentile range. For example, if the infant was in the 75th percentile for length and weight at birth but has fallen to below the 50th percentile for weight, additional assessment will be needed about the infant's feedings. Likewise, if the head circumference is much lower or higher than the length and weight percentiles, further neurologic and developmental assessment should be done. See Partnering with Families: Percentile Measurements.

Practice Alert

If an infant is observed to fail to meet an expected developmental milestone during a healthcare visit, inquire about the milestone and related tasks with the parents. Investigate if the infant was born prematurely because this may delay milestones. Do not alarm them during this data-gathering stage. Examine the results of any developmental questionnaire the parents may have completed. Plan to administer the Denver II or other developmental test to obtain further information. Observe the infant carefully. For example, if a 4-month-old baby fails to hold the head erect when sitting or prone, ask the parents if the baby has ever done so. Inquire about how the baby is positioned at home. Have the baby follow an object to see if the eyes can track. Observe the infant in the prone position and observe how far the head is held and whether the body is supported on the hands. Use the observation time to point out to the parents the skills the infant is accomplishing. For example, hand the infant a block and comment to the parents about how the infant transfers it to the other hand or carries it to the mouth. Discuss the developmental findings with the primary care provider, and create a collaborative plan to foster development of the infant.

In some settings, other growth measurements may be taken, such as chest circumference. If the infant was premature or has specific healthcare needs, particular attention must be paid to physical growth measurements.

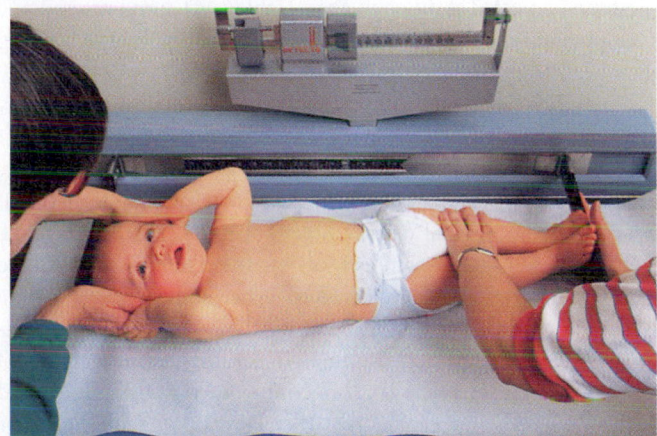

FIGURE 10–2 ■ Weighing and measuring length during health supervision visits provides important information about the child's nutrition and general development. This young infant was measured and then, while the parents dressed the child, the nurse placed the findings on the growth grid.

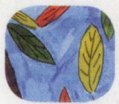

Partnering with Families

Percentile Measurements

Parents commonly do not understand what the term *percentile* means. When you tell them that their infant is in the 50th percentile for length, it is good to add, "If there were 10 babies of the same age, about half would be longer than your baby and about half would be shorter." Then explain that each baby has individual characteristics and that percentile measurements help to see if the infant is staying in approximately the same percentile range over time and growing at the expected rate. Show them the grid on which the percentile ranking is placed.

Growth measurement is followed by a physical assessment. The nurse may complete parts of the assessment, with the remainder performed by the physician, nurse practitioner, or other primary care provider. The assessment evaluates each body system, with particular attention paid to heart, skin, musculoskeletal system, abdomen, and neurologic status. See Chapter 7 🔗 for a thorough discussion of physical assessment.

During the assessment, ask about care of the infant, observing areas where the family appears comfortable and those where the family needs assistance.

- Ask about the infant's bath routine and general skin and nail care. If the infant is a boy, do the parents have questions about care for the circumcised or uncircumcised penis?
- Find out about bowel patterns and if the family has questions about normal bowel movements for infants. (See Chapter 30 🔗 for a description of bowel movements in infants.) Although breastfed babies rarely become constipated, they may not have daily bowel movements.
- Was the infant wrapped appropriately for the temperature? Some parents wrap babies in many layers of clothing even in very hot weather.
- Does the parent have a nonmercury thermometer and know how to take the baby's temperature? Ask the parent to demonstrate the technique used at home.

Developmental surveillance is integrated into each visit from birth to 3 years of age (see Chapter 8 🔗). Begin by observing developmental milestones in the infant (see Chapter 5 🔗 for a summary of milestones expected at different ages). Table 10–1 summarizes some developmental milestones that can commonly be observed during infant healthcare visits.

When there is no opportunity to observe a skill directly, ask parents about whether the infant performs the skill. In addition to direct observation at every health supervision visit, parents are usually requested to fill in a paper or electronic form that asks questions about common developmental tasks. (Table 8–4 in Chapter 8 lists some commonly used questionnaires.) Review the results and determine if additional questions should be asked. When some milestones have not been met, make an appointment for the infant to have a developmental test by a certified examiner. In addition, administration of a developmental screening test is recommended at the 9-, 18-, and 30-month visits (Voigt et al., 2010). (See Developing Cultural Competence: Developmental Milestones. Tests commonly used with young children are listed in Table 8–5.) If you are convinced that the infant is behind on developmental tasks, refer your entire developmental findings to a physician or other pediatric specialist.

TABLE 10–1	Developmental Milestones Observed in Health Promotion and Maintenance Visits
AGE	**DEVELOPMENTAL MILESTONES**
1 month	■ Responds to sound by startle or increased alertness ■ Follows objects and human face with eyes ■ Has periods of alertness and restfulness ■ Is comforted by touch or feeding by parent ■ Has symmetric movements and generally has arms and legs flexed ■ Lifts head momentarily when prone
2 months	■ Has above characteristics ■ Makes noises such as cooing in response to interaction with adult ■ Smiles ■ Lifts head, neck, upper chest when prone ■ Has increasing head control when held in sitting position
4 months	■ Increases cooing and babbling ■ Smiles, laughs, makes other noises during interactions ■ Supports self on hands when prone ■ Rolls front to back ■ Touches objects and grasps rattle placed near hand
6 months	■ Uses sounds in repeated speech such as "bababa, dadadada" ■ Shows interest in surroundings and toys ■ Has no head lag when pulled to sitting ■ Sits with support ■ Grasps objects easily and places in mouth ■ Transfers objects from one hand to other ■ Bears weight on legs when held in standing position
9 months	■ Understands simple words and uses more sounds in babbling ■ Responds to name ■ Enjoys interactive games with parent ■ Moves when placed on floor by crawling, creeping, or rolling repeatedly ■ Sits without support ■ Stands holding on to support ■ Plays with toys ■ Feeds self readily with fingers and tries to use cup
12 months	■ Has one or more words ■ Imitates sounds readily ■ Shows increasing interactions and interest in surroundings ■ Follows directions such as saying "bye-bye" or waving goodbye ■ Pulls to standing, walks a few steps holding on ■ Has well-developed pincer grasp ■ Is able to drink from cup

Developing Cultural Competence
Developmental Milestones

Be alert for differences in cultural practices and beliefs that may influence developmental milestones. For example, if a child is kept on a cradleboard for much of the time, the infant may be slow in learning to crawl. This infant may progress directly to standing by furniture without demonstrating as much creeping or crawling as other infants. In addition, when parents do not have English as a primary language and the examiner uses English, common terms might be misinterpreted. Parents might not understand what is meant if you ask, "Does your baby have a mobile over the crib at home?" or "Is she starting to be afraid of strangers?" How can you be alert for language differences and become sensitive to miscommunication? Refer to Chapter 3 for additional examples of cultural influences and Chapter 6 ⓔ for communication principles.

Practice Alert
When inquiring about a child's performance of a skill, begin with open-ended questions. Parents want their children to perform well, so they may answer that the child can do any skill about which the nurse inquires. Open-ended questions can help avoid this problem. For example, rather than asking "Does Jeremiah reach for a rattle with his hand?" it is better to say "Describe what Jeremiah does if you hold a rattle in front of him."

The nurse establishes health promotion and health maintenance interventions related to growth and development assessment data. Anticipatory guidance related to development is a major component of health promotion. The nurse anticipates the next milestones the infant will be meeting, and recommends ways for the parents to support the infant in progression. Health promotion activities include the following:

- Teaching about food introduction that will foster growth
- Encouraging toys and activities that will assist in meeting the next developmental milestones
- Demonstrating gross and fine motor skills that the infant has achieved
- Demonstrating to parents how the child will focus on their faces and mimic their vocal sounds

Other interventions are focused on health maintenance or disease and injury prevention. For example, some characteristics make certain accidents more likely to occur, as when a 6-month-old is reaching for objects, readily places things in the mouth, and is able to move around on the floor. Ask if the parents are providing the infant with any finger foods. Suggest foods that would be appropriate and discuss foods that commonly cause choking and should be avoided (see Chapter 19 ⓔ). Likewise, since the infant is becoming more mobile, parents should get onto the floor and look for hazards at the infant's eye level. Safety hazards and ways to avoid them are discussed, and parents are given brochures, website addresses, or DVDs to enhance injury prevention information. Can you outline additional health promotion and health maintenance interventions that relate to the infant's growth and development?

NUTRITION

The importance of nutrition during the first year of life cannot be overestimated. The infant will triple in birth weight by 1 year of age and has a need for nutritional balance. From the first sips of breast milk or formula as a newborn, to eating the family meal at 1 year of age, the fast

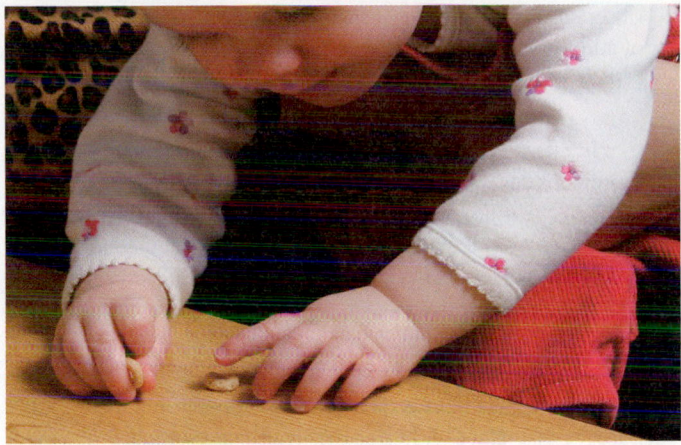

FIGURE 10–3 ■ During the first year of life, nutritional intake patterns reflect the developmental progression of the infant. The baby first receives all nutrition from human milk or formula, and closely bonds with the parent during feeding. As the infant becomes able to take in and metabolize other foods, parents begin to feed soft foods. When the infant can sit, reach for objects, and place them in the mouth, finger foods are introduced. The baby in this picture has developed the pincer grasp and is able to feed foods to self using this ability. Choices should include nutritionally sound food that helps to meet the baby's recommended allowances. By the first birthday, the child has developed the social and motor ability to eat most of the food commonly consumed in the family. Eating has been a mirror of social, metabolic, and developmental progression throughout the first year.

progression of nutritional intake patterns is obvious (Figure 10–3 ■). See Chapter 19 ⓔ for a thorough description of nutritional needs during infancy and further information about breastfeeding.

During each visit, the nurse seeks to learn what the infant is eating and whether the family has any questions or concerns related to intake. Once again, open-ended questions are a good way to begin, with more specific questions inserted after the parent's perceptions are known. For the parents or caregivers of a breastfeeding infant named Kara, the nurse might ask:

- How is Kara's breastfeeding going?
- How do you know when Kara is hungry? Satisfied?
- How often does Kara eat and for how long?
- Do you think she eats enough? Too much?
- Is there anything you would change about the eating patterns?
- What does Kara do when you hold her on your lap and are eating?
- Which foods are more likely to cause a baby to choke?
- Describe your diet, weight, and energy level.
- What questions and concerns do you have related to your breastfeeding?
- Does your family always have access to adequate foods? Are you ever hungry or worried about having enough food for yourself or your family? Do you ever go without food so your children have enough to eat?
- What is the source of your drinking water? Describe how and when you give fluoride to your baby.

Once the infant is in the second half of the first year, food patterns of the family become more important. Consider childcare settings as well. Questions could include:

- Kara goes to an infant care center each day. Do you know what they feed her there?
- What unusual reactions has your baby shown to foods? Are there foods she dislikes?

Observations from other portions of the visit can provide clues about additional observations the nurse can make.

- If an infant has not gained weight as expected and has fallen into a lower channel of weight percentile, more specific analysis of intake is needed. Ask for a recall of the infant's intake in the previous day.
- When the infant does not meet developmental milestones on schedule or is lethargic, intake may be inadequate for age. In these cases support may be needed to ensure adequate intake; a thorough description of feeding may be the first step in analyzing the problem and planning interventions.
- When the child's ability to take in nutrients or the parent's ability to feed the infant is questioned, an observation of a feeding might take place, either at the healthcare setting or during a home visit.
- For the infant who has gained more weight than expected, it is important to ask how often the child is eating and what types of foods are consumed. The family may need information about the recommended number of feedings and types of foods appropriate for the child.

Nurses can use many tools to evaluate the feeding interactions of infants and their parents, including the Feeding Scale, which is part of the Nursing Child Assessment Satellite Training (NCAST) program described in Chapter 8 ⊘. Such tools require training and provide the nurse with a method to make reliable observations about the child's feeding patterns and the corresponding interaction with the parent.

Infants with health conditions such as a congenital heart defect often have difficulty eating and may need additional support. Other health conditions can create the need for increased intake of certain nutrients. For example, a premature infant might need milk enhancers for breast milk or preterm formulas during infancy. Whatever the health condition, the principles of health promotion and health maintenance visits are still followed, with addition of approaches specific for the child's health needs.

As the infant grows, the nurse asks questions about the types of foods the infant has been offered. Parents are invited to describe feedings and any concerns they have. Other family members may have provided information about how to feed infants, and the parents need an opportunity to ask about the family's recommendations. Ask about fluid intake of the infant and assess the parent's knowledge of signs of dehydration (see Chapter 23 ⊘). Integrate your knowledge of infant nutritional needs (see Chapter 19 ⊘) to develop a set of questions specific to each health supervision visit.

Clinical Judgment

How will nutritional needs of the 9-month-old infant differ from those of the 4-month-old infant? When should transition to cow milk occur for the infant fed with formula? Describe the history taken at each age and the teaching performed with the parent.

Additional nutritional assessment measures are used at certain points in the first year. A hematocrit or hemoglobin test is generally performed between 9 and 12 months of age. Lead screening may be needed in certain population groups (see Chapter 20 ⊘). Screening for food security, or the family's access at all times to adequate food, can be used when appropriate (see Chapter 19).

Each visit includes nutritional teaching about important items. The topics for discussion vary according to age group. See Table 10–2

for suggested teaching topics at specific ages. Can you identify which topics are mainly health promotion and which are mainly health maintenance? Most of the activities listed are related to health promotion; however, a few relate to health maintenance as they are directed at disease prevention. Offering adequate fluids helps to prevent dehydration. Using only cups for juice limits amounts, thereby helping to prevent obesity, and limits the exposure, thus preventing dental caries in newly erupting teeth. Do you see any other health maintenance interventions for nutrition teaching in Table 10–2?

Desired outcomes for nutrition in infancy include adequate growth, normal nutritional assessment findings, and knowledge by parents of the nutritional needs of the infant.

PHYSICAL ACTIVITY

Infants need physical activity for optimum development of fine and gross motor skills. Unlike other times of life, the focus is on providing only the opportunities for activity, without a need to focus on motivation. As long as infants are meeting developmental milestones and have a stimulating environment that provides opportunity for fine and gross motor activity, they will use their motor skills, thus enhancing their performance. Time should be provided each day for the infant to reach for objects, exercise legs and arms freely, and increasingly use head control. Playing with parents or others and being surrounded by toys and other stimulating items will encourage motor behavior in all body parts. Ask the parents for a description of the infant's typical day and listen for these types of play periods. Observe the physical skills of the infant (see Chapter 5 ⊘ for motor developmental norms), ask questions about play periods provided, and compose a list of the family protective factors and risk factors in this area. Table 10–3 lists risk and protective factors related to physical activity during infancy.

When the child has a special health or developmental condition, such as mental retardation or neuromuscular disease, it is important for the nurse to evaluate the child's physical activity. General guidelines for the child with a disability include the following:

- Focus on assessment of usual routines and skills needed to accomplish daily tasks such as eating and moving the head to follow objects.
- Consider assessing the child in the natural environment of home or childcare to ensure validity.
- Search out and use tools designed to measure physical performance of infants with developmental delay.
- Include the family in the assessment process.

Based on the results of assessment and using the concept of anticipatory guidance, the nurse plans appropriate teaching for the family. Health promotion teaching related to physical activity includes the following:

- Frequent and supervised play opportunities are needed. Encourage parents to play with their infants daily.
- Holding the infant in various positions, helping the older infant to stand, and providing positive feedback for the infant's accomplishments are encouraged.
- Toys should be placed to encourage movement.
- Participation in parent–infant play groups provides stimulation for the child and social interaction with other infants, and increases the parent's knowledge of the child's abilities.
- The next expected fine and gross motor skills are anticipated, and opportunities for their development are provided.

TABLE 10–2	Nutrition Teaching for Health Promotion and Maintenance Visits

AGE	NUTRITION TEACHING
1 month	Support breastfeeding efforts.
	Teach correct formula types and preparation if used.
	Teach burping and rate of feeding information.
	Encourage families to view feedings as social interactions; emphasize importance of holding the infant and not propping bottles.
2 months	Continue teaching factors listed above.
	Review fluid needs of infants.
	Suggest water during hot weather or if family wants to use a bottle at baby's bedtime.
	Reinforce food safety for partially used bottles of breast milk or formula.
	Use warm water for heating bottles rather than microwave to avoid hot spots due to uneven heating, thereby burning the infant.
	Warn against feeding honey in the first year of life due to the threat of botulism.
	Begin cleaning of infant gums daily.
	Provide information about any supplements needed (e.g., iron for premature infant, vitamin D for babies not exposed to adequate sunlight).
4 months	Continue teaching factors listed above.
	Discuss introduction of first foods between 4 and 6 months, and surveillance for symptoms of allergy or intolerance.
	Recommend that fruit juice not be used until 6 months of age, be fed only by cup, and be limited to 4–6 ounces (120–180 mL) per day (American Academy of Pediatrics, 2011a).
	Discuss changing food patterns such as increasing amounts and decreasing numbers of daily milk feedings.
6 months	Continue teaching factors listed above.
	Reinforce proper introduction of new foods, to include rice cereal, fruits, and vegetables.
	Discuss any unusual food reactions observed.
	Introduce cup for drinking.
	Introduce soft finger foods.
	Serve juice only in a cup and limit to no more than 6 ounces daily.
	Caution about common foods and items that can cause choking.
	Provide information about fluoride supplements if water supply is not fluoridated.
9 months	Continue teaching factors listed above.
	If mother does not continue to breastfeed, teach family to use iron-fortified formula for the first year of life.
	Encourage self-feeding of finger foods, integrating common foods for the family.
	Introduce source of protein such as tofu, cheese, mashed beans, and slivers of meat.
12 months	Continue teaching factors listed above.
	Support the mother who wishes to continue breastfeeding beyond 1 year of age.
	Encourage cups for all feedings other than breast.
	For the formula-fed infant, discuss introduction of cow milk at this age, avoiding skim or 1% milk, which do not have a high enough fat content. (See Chapter 19 for a detailed discussion of nutritional needs and teaching topics.)

TABLE 10–3	Risk and Protective Factors Regarding Physical Activity in Infancy

RISK FACTORS	PROTECTIVE FACTORS
■ Premature birth	■ Meets developmental milestones at expected ages
■ Delayed developmental milestones	■ Has contact with parents, siblings, and others for significant time each day
■ Limited stimulation by family or other care providers	■ A supportive environment with room to play safely, stimulating surroundings
■ Lack of knowledge by family about infant's physical activity needs	■ Physically active family
■ Limited community resources for families with infants	■ Family knowledge about infant's physical activity needs
	■ Community programs that promote physical activity in infants and information for families

Source: *Data from Hagan, J. F., Shaw, J. S., & Duncan, P. M. (2008).* Bright futures: Guidelines for health supervision of infants, children, and adolescents *(3rd ed.). Elk Grove Village, IL: American Academy of Pediatrics.*

Clinical Tip

Parents remember healthcare teaching best when a limited number of topics or facts are discussed. Plan your teaching so that you include important topics and supplement with brochures, web addresses, and other resources the family can take home and review later.

Health maintenance deals with prevention of physical development delays. When an infant is developing more slowly than expected, was premature, or has a diagnosed condition such as a cardiac defect, additional support may be needed. Explain physical activities that the child will be learning next. Make specific suggestions to foster stimulation, ensure adequate range of motion, and maximize developmental progression. The nurse may partner with a physical therapist or other specialist during the health supervision visit to enhance the physical activity of the infant. Referral for developmental screening or to infant programs that work with infants who are developmentally delayed should be considered. The Zero-to-Three Project: National Center for Infants, Toddlers, and Families works to promote the healthy development of infants and toddlers by supporting and strengthening families, communities, and those who work on their behalf. How would you go about locating this resource or other services in your community to assist with health maintenance of infants with physical delays?

The nurse evaluates success of interventions by the child's progression in physical activity milestones at the next health supervision visit. Adequate parental understanding of the importance of physical activity and the means of supporting the child's activities is an important outcome of care.

ORAL HEALTH

The first teeth begin to erupt about midway during infancy. Two front teeth are common at about 6 months of age. However, even before this, parents lay the foundation for good oral health. The mother's intake during pregnancy and breastfeeding is essential to ensuring adequate availability of calcium and other nutrients that will be used as the infant's teeth develop. The nurse in child health supervision settings ensures that the infant has adequate intake of these nutrients via breastfeeding and other foods. A dietary recall of the mother's and

Weblink | The Zero-to-Three Project

infant's intake is one way of assessing for nutrients. When the water supply is not fluoridated, inquire about use of fluoride drops. When there is naturally occurring fluoride in the water, consult the city or town water analysis to be certain it is in the range recommended for optimum oral health and is not too high (when a filter should be used) or too low (when a supplement is needed).

Practice Alert

Be sure that parents do not give the child excessive fluoride since it can permanently discolor the teeth. For example, parents may administer fluoride drops each morning if their water supply has no fluoride, but then have the child at a childcare center several days each week where the water supply is fluoridated. This could cause an overdosage of fluoride. Clarify both the fluoride content of water used in each setting and the use of all fluoride supplements.

Help the family to establish healthy dental habits. The parents should wipe the infant's gums with soft moist gauze once or twice daily. This helps to clean residues of food from the gums and gets the infant accustomed to having something wiping the gums, a practice that may assist when toothbrushing begins. Families are also cautioned to avoid having the infant nurse when sleeping, to avoid use of bottles in bed, and not to allow the infant to drink at will from a bottle during the day. These practices are linked to early childhood caries (see Chapter 8 🕮) and can lead to tooth decay. Although some parents are convinced that this involves "baby teeth" that will be lost, teach that these teeth are needed for healthy food intake, for maintaining proper spaces for permanent teeth eruption, and for speech development.

Nurses assess for the presence of teeth and whether patterns are similar to those expected (see Chapter 7 🕮, Figure 7–26). It is wise to ask if the infant has had any difficulty with teeth eruption. Many babies have increased crying, and parents have disrupted sleeping during these periods. Suggest comfort measures such as offering cool beverages and safe "teething toys" for the baby. Although infancy may seem early for a dental visit, an oral examination is recommended within 6 months of the eruption of the first tooth and no later than 12 months of age (American Academy of Pediatric Dentistry, 2010). Partner with parents to identify a dental care facility for their use. Refer families to resources such as Medicaid, State Children's Health Insurance Programs, and local resources for dental care.

A good deal of overlap exists in health promotion and health maintenance activities related to oral health. Many interventions are designed to prevent caries and infections, which relate to health maintenance. At the same time, they contribute to health promotion by improving dentition, language development, appearance, and self-image. Desired outcomes of care include the eruption of a set of healthy teeth and regular oral health examination.

MENTAL AND SPIRITUAL HEALTH

How do you assess the mental health of an infant? What characteristics indicate that an infant is developing the resources needed for future mental health? The infant's mental health is related to early experiences, inborn characteristics such as temperament and resilience, and relationships with caregivers. The first year of life provides many opportunities for the infant to develop positive mental health; interventions during this important period can enhance the child's future mental status.

One way to evaluate mental health is to look carefully at growth and developmental surveillance data, as described earlier. Children who feel secure and have nurturing environments usually grow as expected and perform milestones at usual times. Slow growth and delayed development are sometimes related to feeding disorders of infancy and early childhood (see Chapter 19 🕮). In these cases, a disturbed relationship with the primary caregiver influences the psychologic state of the infant and results in decreased food intake. Growth is slowed, energy is not available for activity, and development is therefore delayed.

Another way to assess mental health is to observe the child and parent interacting. Does the parent hold the infant securely and does the child cuddle and settle into the parent's arms (Figure 10–4 ■)? Is there eye contact between parent and child? Does the parent appear comfortable in holding and comforting the infant? These interactions indicate bonding or positive attachment (see Chapter 9 🕮 for further discussion of these topics).

During the first year, the infant learns to identify parents; beginning at about 6 months of age, infants may cry or protest when another person holds them. This so-called **stranger anxiety** indicates expected attachment to parents. Similarly, in the second half of the first year of life, infants may exhibit **separation anxiety** by inconsolable crying and other signs of distress when parents are not present. Recognize that these behaviors are normal, demonstrate healthy attachment to primary caregivers, and indicate good mental health. Help parents to recognize them as expected occurrences. Provide them ideas of how to deal with this behavior. Parents can remain in sight and talk to the infant during health supervision examinations. They should be encouraged to hold and comfort the infant after painful procedures such as immunizations. Further techniques for dealing with separation during hospitalization can be found in Chapter 15 🕮. Once the

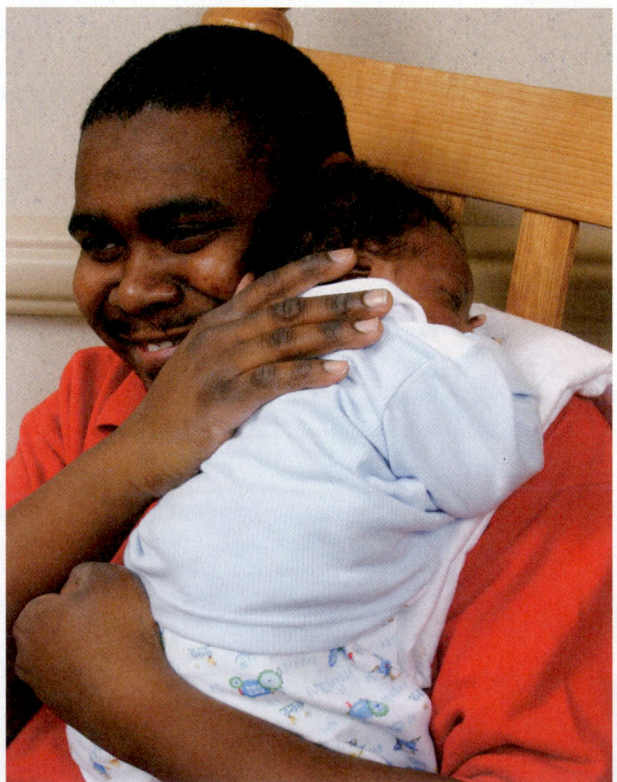

FIGURE 10–4 ■ Interactions between the parent and infant provide clues to mental health. Do the adult and child appear comfortable with each other? Is eye contact and vocalization present? Are their bodies soft and relaxed or tense?

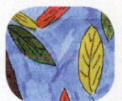

Partnering with Families

Comforting the Distressed Infant

Teen parents and those with little prior experience with babies need help to develop a repertoire of interventions to try when a baby is crying. Ask about how they comfort the baby. Suggest the following interventions if the parent does not state them:

- Offer a breast or bottle feeding, especially if the last feeding was more than 2 hours ago.
- If feeding was recent, hold the baby in a sitting position and rub or pat the back to help expel gastric gas.
- Change the diaper if wet or dirty.
- Place a hand on the abdomen and feel for movement. If movement or passing gas is present, hold the baby against the chest, walk slowly, and pat the back.

- Swaddle the baby securely in a blanket and hold horizontally while rocking.
- Hold the baby on your lap, secure the hands in yours, and talk softly.
- Stroke the infant's skin; rock and sing to the baby.
- Never shake or throw the baby, no matter how long the crying. Call your healthcare provider for suggestions if you feel like nothing works and you are very frustrated. *See Chapter 9 ⊘ for further details about responding to the cries of newborns and young infants. See Chapter 19 ⊘ for a discussion of infant colic, or the "period of purple crying."*

---

infant has experienced that the parent leaves and returns, security in the care of others can emerge.

The infant provides a series of cues about feelings and needs. These include a different type of cry when hungry, wet, or in pain; clearly seeking the nipple when hungry; and readily establishing eye contact when desiring interaction. Parents who are aware of these cues respond to them and meet the infant's needs for contact and comfort, thus increasing trust and a positive state of mental balance. Watch to see how parents respond when an infant cries, falls asleep, or appears hungry. Parents who have a selection of options promote their infant's health. That is, they are most likely to promote infant mental health if they attempt to rock an infant who continues to cry, then change to swaddling and holding securely, or perhaps try feeding or changing the infant. If you notice that the parent is not responding to the infant, point out your observations of the infant's cues. "Look at how your son is watching your face. That usually means that a baby is eager to be talked to and looked at directly." "Your son seems really unhappy right now. Let's try to wrap him securely in the blanket and see if that helps. This is something you can try at home when he is unable to calm himself." See Partnering with Families: Comforting the Distressed Infant.

Another important indication of infant mental health is the ability to comfort oneself. **Self-regulation** is the process of dealing with feelings, learning to soothe oneself, and focusing on activities for increasing periods of time. Infants learn early how to comfort and calm themselves. Ask parents if the child sucks a finger, softly rocks, or otherwise comforts self when distressed. Some babies prefer to be alone and quiet when tired or distressed; others calm better when held, rocked, or placed in an infant swing. Help the parents to identify and reinforce the infant's methods of self-soothing. Teach swaddling and rocking techniques.

Practice Alert

Many infants are assisted in soothing themselves when they are swaddled or tightly wrapped (see the Skills Manual ▭▭▭). Start by placing the baby on a blanket on a flat surface. Securely take the bottom edge of the blanket and pull it tightly over the feet and up to the chest. Wrap the sides of the blanket around the baby so the arms are secured. Many babies will immediately quiet once swaddled, and will either sleep or become quietly alert. However, be aware that some babies find this position uncomfortable. If they fight the blanket and try to free themselves, this may not be an approach that works for quieting those particular babies.

The important function of sleep needs to be assessed at each health visit. Circadian rhythms emerge by 1 to 3 months of age, and the infant has longer sleep times at night, with increasing wakefulness during the day (Murray, Zentner, & Yakimo, 2009). Self-regulation is needed by the infant when learning to go to sleep while tired and agitated. Most parents have periods when an infant is not sleeping well, and some infants regularly stay awake for long periods at night. When this occurs, parents consequently become sleep deprived and have little energy left to deal with the challenges and responsibilities of the family. Nurses use health promotion principles to teach about sleep patterns in infants, and implement health maintenance when partnering with families to deal with problem sleep behaviors that lead to infant and parent fatigue (Box 10–2). (See Table 9–3 in Chapter 9 ⊘ for further information about infant sleep.) See Partnering with Families: Helping the Infant Sleep, and Evidence-Based Practice: Infant Sleep.

The infant is born into a family with spiritual strengths and limitations. The nurse assesses the family and provides additional resources when needed. The infant is not mature enough to understand the family's spiritual framework, but it can sense the atmosphere in the family that relates to nurturing, valuing children, providing a safe and secure environment, and recognizing mental balance. The infant's social

---

BOX 10–2	Infant Sleep Patterns

BIRTH–3 MONTHS

12–16 hours of sleep daily in about five sleep periods of 30 minutes to 4 hours

Sleep spans both day and night hours

3–6 MONTHS

13 hours of sleep daily with a longer sleep at night plus two or three naps daily

6–12 MONTHS

12–14 hours of sleep daily with a longer sleep at night plus one or two naps daily

Source: *Data from Hagan, J. F., Shaw, J. S., & Duncan, P. M. (2008).* Bright futures: Guidelines for health supervision of infants, children, and adolescents *(3rd ed.). Elk Grove Village, IL: American Academy of Pediatrics.*

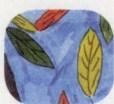

Partnering with Families

Helping the Infant Sleep

Helping an infant to self-regulate and be able to sleep for longer periods is often a stressful challenge for families. Parents need to have substantial sleep periods themselves to be refreshed and able to deal with daily life. When up several times during the night with a baby, parents may become irritable and fatigued. Question the family about the baby's sleep routine. The infant passes into light sleep several times at night and may awaken; self-regulation will assist in helping the infant get back to sleep. Suggestions helpful for the family are as follows:

- Place the baby to sleep in a quiet and darkened room, a "sleep friendly" environment.
- Establish a consistent sleep routine and time; the routine may involve some cuddling and rocking time but should not be vigorous, stimulating play.

- Provide a consistent transitional object, such as a favorite blanket each night.
- Put the baby to bed while still awake but drowsy rather than after falling asleep, so the infant learns self-soothing skills.
- Do not try to awaken the baby in non-rapid eye movement (NREM or quiet) sleep.
- For the baby who has trouble going to sleep, remain in the room for a few minutes but do not establish eye contact; place a hand on the abdomen or chest or gently hold flailing arms and legs.

Source: *Data from National Sleep Foundation. (2011).* Sleep, infants, and parents. *Retrieved from http://www.sleepfoundation.org/articles/ask-the-expert/sleep-infants-and-parents*

and psychologic health are closely related to these factors. For many parents, membership in a faith-based congregation provides spiritual sustenance and an important sense of belonging. This group may also provide food, clothing, and care for the new infant. Sometimes parents who have not attended institutionalized services will choose to do so to offer a significant spiritual home for their new child. Services such as christening and blessing an infant welcome the child formally into the family and provide meaning to parents and extended family members. Having a baby often helps parents to feel that they have an important meaning and purpose in life, regardless of a faith-based membership. An atmosphere where the infant is valued and offers meaning to the lives of the adults present is a positive atmosphere for emotional growth. Assess the family's meaningful activities, practices, and engagement in faith-based rituals. Ask about needs or desires for referrals in the community such as to an organized religious group or other meaningful activities.

While there are risks to mental health there are also protective factors. The partnership that is developing between the health professional and the parents is an important resource. It leads to increased knowledge, support, and parenting skills. The family knowledge and skills lead them to face challenges with courage and resilience. When mental health topics related to the infant and parents are included in each visit, parents are more likely to share with professionals the stresses and challenges that inevitably emerge. Acknowledge in a nonjudgmental manner the parent's feelings of fatigue and frustration with an infant who does not sleep well. Help parents identify the strengths and resources they have to meet their challenges. Assure them that their child will learn from them a positive sense of self and the feeling that a positive outcome is possible.

Many of the nurse's interventions are aimed at positive mental health development in the infant. Health promotion activities focus on teaching parents the needs of infants for security and interaction. Suggest healthy sleep patterns and how they can be achieved. Teach self-regulation skills so that the parents can help the child become quiet and calm.

Health maintenance seeks to identify babies with disruptions in mental health status, often manifested by growth or interaction abnormalities. When the infant has disturbed sleep patterns or difficulty calming self when upset, or the parents do not interpret infant cues related to hunger or discomfort, the nurse plans interventions to help prevent further problems. Teaching, demonstrations, and acknowledging parent success are all health maintenance actions. An expected outcome for these activities is the reestablishment of expected growth and development, and age-appropriate interactions of the infant with others.

RELATIONSHIPS

Family

The infant's social interactions, both within and outside the family, display enormous growth in the first year. The family is the primary unit where the infant learns to interact with other people. Therefore, nurses should examine family dynamics during health supervision visits. Strengths and needs of the family are identified during psychosocial screening. See Chapter 2 🔗 for more discussion about the role of the family in child health, and techniques of family assessment. Identify strengths of the family and positively reinforce them, including the following:

- Playing with the infant each day
- Vocalizing frequently to the infant
- Reading to the infant (provide books so parents are encouraged to do this)
- Avoiding use of television and other media until after 2 years of age
- Providing for basic physical and emotional needs of the infant and other family members
- Sharing infant care among parents and other family and friends
- Encouraging positive relationships among parents and other children
- Knowing infant needs
- Accessing adequate community services and resources

On the other hand, certain risk factors in every family affect family interaction patterns. Questions that may help to identify risk include:

- What do you do when you are frustrated? Do you ever get away together (parents) and can you maintain your own special relationship?

Evidence-Based Practice   Infant Sleep

PROBLEM

Many babies have limited sleeping periods during the night, and their night awakenings disturb parents' sleep. Parents may have busy days and be unable to nap for adequate sleep to perform at a safe and productive level during the day. Parental stress and depression are associated with frequent child awakenings.

EVIDENCE

Sleep of the infant is an important concern for many parents, but there is little research-based evidence about how to help parents understand infant sleep. Several studies enlighten the problem of infant sleep. A study of 314 twin pairs found that most sleep disturbances in early childhood are linked to environmental factors, and thus behavioral interventions with parents are suggested for altering infant sleep patterns (Brescianini, Volzone, Fagnani, et al., 2011). Consistent with these findings, a study evaluating 170 parents for knowledge of child sleep found that most parents could not answer the majority of questions correctly. The researchers suggested that evaluating parental knowledge and teaching about developmental progression of sleep patterns should occur in health visits (Schreck & Richdale, 2011). A cross-cultural study found that parents from predominantly

Asian countries were more likely to identify sleep disturbance in their children than those from countries with a majority of White parents. These findings suggest that information is needed about cultural differences in sleep expectations of parents (Sadeh, Mindell, & Rivera, 2011).

IMPLICATIONS

The evidence provides implications for nursing care. Ask parents of young newborns to record the infant sleep patterns, and inquire about their expectations of infant sleep. As the infant nears 3 to 4 months, patterns should demonstrate few night awakenings and feedings. Teach parents how to minimize stimulation and interaction at night. Provide opportunities to review results at future health supervision visits, or offer telephone or other support to parents.

CRITICAL THINKING

What information do parents of infants need about infant sleep patterns? What questions will assist you to learn what parents know about infant sleep and how they are coping with these sleep patterns?

- (For a teen parent) Are you able to do things with your friends each week? Do friends maintain contact and visit?
- All parents experience fatigue related to childrearing. Is there a resource to provide help when you need it? Can you sleep through the night occasionally while someone else bottle-feeds the infant for a night feeding? Can you nap during the day while the infant sleeps?
- Babies each have a unique temperament (see Chapter 5 🔗). What are the challenges and the positive aspects of your baby's temperament?

Evaluate if the parents are able to laugh about the infant who is very social and wants to be part of everything happening in the house. Be alert to learn if parents have developed mechanisms to quiet the infant's environment so the baby can rest and parents can get a break from care, or if everyone in the family is chronically fatigued.

Factors in the mental health of the parents directly affect the atmosphere in the home and the resulting health of the infant. Depression in parents or other family members has the potential to influence the infant's health. Interactions with parents who are depressed will be altered; caretaking, both physical and emotional, may be impaired. See Chapter 9 🔗 for further discussion of postpartum blues and postpartum depression.

Depression in the mother or other caretaker can have serious implications for the infant. The baby may not get the physical care that is needed, leading to poor nutrition, an inadequate state of cleanliness and health, or neglect of other basic needs (see Chapter 20 🔗 for a description of child neglect). These infants may appear in unkempt conditions to healthcare providers and may cry and appear uncomfortable. In addition, the social interactions may be disrupted and the infant may show decreased vocalization, may display lack of interest in the environment or in people, and may be fussy and irritable or withdrawn and nonengaging. Without positive interactions with caretakers, infants may develop a feeding disorder and fail to gain adequate weight (see Chapter 19 🔗 for a description of feeding disorders of infancy and childhood).

The nurse's role in depression for families with young children relates to health maintenance goals and involves recognizing the condition and referring for care. The safety and well-being of the infant is important, so resources for childcare may be needed while the parent obtains treatment. Other family members can assist by caring for the infant until the parent is able to do so. Be alert for parents who are sad, cry readily, fail to interact during the visit, and show little emotion in caring for the infant. Likewise, as described in the section on the infant's mental health, identify infants who do not establish eye contact or interactions with adults, are withdrawn or seem sad, or are unkempt. See Chapter 34 🔗 for further information about depression.

Intimate partner violence (physical, sexual, or emotional abuse or threat) presents another challenge to the mental health of families and infants. (See Chapter 9 🔗.) Men most commonly commit acts of violence toward their female companions (85% of the cases of intimate partner violence), but women also are sometimes violent toward men. Approximately 4.8 million women are assaulted annually by male partners. Over 2,000 deaths occur annually in the home related to intimate partner violence. Children are often present in the home and are exposed to the violence (Centers for Disease Control and Prevention, 2011; Tanski, Garfunkel, Duncan, et al., 2010).

Women who are abused may be reluctant to tell about such violence either out of fear for safety or reluctance to deal with the psychologic distress entailed. Be alert for women who appear with bruises, black eyes, or other conditions common with violence. Routine screening for domestic violence should be part of clinic and hospital questionnaires and history forms. Ask questions with the woman alone at each health supervision visit, such as:

- What happens in your family if you and the baby's father disagree about something?
- Has your partner ever threatened you or made you feel afraid for your safety?
- I see you have a black eye. Sometimes people are hurt in their family. Can you tell me how it happened?

Intimate partner violence makes it difficult for the mother to provide loving and secure care, and as the infant gets older, witnessing such episodes can be harmful. Children exposed to domestic violence experience more common social, emotional, and cognitive problems. Can you list the names of shelters and other resources that provide services for domestic violence victims in your community? As a nurse, you will need to provide resources to parents as needed. Recognize that these situations are reportable by law and must be referred to departments of social and health services for investigation.

Another risk that occurs in some families with infants is child abuse or maltreatment. This problem is a serious issue that causes disturbed mental status in the infant. See Chapter 20 🔗 for a detailed description of child abuse and its effect on infants and older children. Suspected child abuse must be reported to legal authorities.

Social Interactions

The infant's social interactions both within and outside the family display remarkable growth in the first year. See Chapter 5 🔗 for a full description of social milestones. The newborn tracks with eyes over part of the visual field, focuses on the human face, and even mimics facial movements of adults. By 6 weeks of age, the infant smiles responsively and soon after that coos in response to parental vocalizations. By 4 months, the infant babbles and laughs, gets excited about toys in the environment, and recognizes the parent's voice. By 6 months, the infant imitates sounds, is aware of and shows anxiety about strangers, and has definite personality characteristics. In the remainder of the first year, the infant continues to develop some words, with the first words usually representing people ("mama" or "dada"); builds strong relationships with siblings in the family; and has a well-established temperament. An environment is needed to support the infant in establishment of positive social skills during the first year.

One aspect of the child's personality that influences social interactions, both within and outside the family, is temperament. See Chapter 5 🔗 for detailed descriptions of temperament. Help the parents to identify if the infant's temperament is primarily:

- Easy (moderate activity, easy to console, regular sleep and eating patterns)
- Slow to warm up (slow adaptation to new events and people or to changes in environment and schedule)
- Difficult (high activity, difficult to console, irregular sleep and eating patterns)

Point out the positive aspects of the child's temperament: "Your daughter has already established the ability to sleep through the night. That shows she is able to comfort herself." "Your son does have difficulty sleeping, but he is so interactive and learns a lot from everyone around him." Evaluate the "goodness of fit" between the child's temperament characteristics and the parents' expectations and lifestyle (see Chapter 5). Parents who are on flexible schedules and available much of the day may not find it difficult to care for an infant with irregular sleeping and eating habits, whereas other families have trouble adapting to the infant's patterns. When the fit is not good, parents will need more support and suggestions as they and the infant adapt to each other.

The role of the nurse related to infant social interactions in health supervision visits is to evaluate the social skills of the infant, learn what parents have noticed about the infant's temperament and how it fits with their lives, and make suggestions for positive social development.

These are primarily health promotion activities since they aim to enhance the infant's developing social skills. Be aware of health maintenance needs also if any signs of abnormal social interactions are noted. Questions to help identify problems early might include:

- What happens when you are close to your baby's face and smile? What happens if you coo and make sounds?
- What sounds has your infant made so far?
- Describe how your baby goes to sleep each night. Is the pattern stable or does the schedule vary?
- How do your other children respond to your new baby? Describe what the infant is like around your children and other people.
- You say that you are interested in getting your daughter into an infant center. What experience has she had so far with other infants and children? How do you think she might respond when you first leave her? Has she shown any anxiety or crying so far when she meets new people?

Remember that social skills are closely linked with both physical capabilities and mental health status. For example, an infant who is not smiling responsively may have a visual impairment or may have parents who are not interacting appropriately with him. An infant who is not babbling may have a hearing impairment or might have a lack of vocal stimulation from care providers. Gather as much information as possible in order to complete a thorough assessment that provides clues to possible risk factors.

Clearly, family and other social interactions play an important role in development in the first year of life. Concepts related to these interactions must be inserted in every health supervision visit through promotion activities such as:

- Encouraging parents to hold, read to, and talk to babies. The nurse should positively reinforce these behaviors when observed.
- Pointing out the infant's abilities to respond to faces and voices, to smile and laugh, and to reflect the mood of adults in the home.
- Reviewing sleep patterns and making recommendations for methods to plan bedtime routines.
- Being sure that parents have resources to turn to when needing assistance with infant care or other household responsibilities.

Health maintenance activities, designed to prevent disturbed mental health in the infant, include:

- Reporting suspected child abuse immediately.
- Providing resources in cases of domestic violence.
- Referring infants for further diagnostic workup who do not appear to respond to sound, do not follow objects with their eyes, or do not have normal vocalization.

Desired outcomes for the infant include establishment of close relationships with parents and other family members, a stimulating home environment that is responsive to the infant's temperament, and developmental progression in social interactions.

DISEASE PREVENTION STRATEGIES

Infants are prone to many infectious diseases, especially once passive immunity from the mother wanes at about 6 months of age (see Chapters 22 and 27 🔗). Recommended immunizations are administered on schedule to provide protection from some diseases. Recommended immunizations for infancy are listed in Table 10–4. Further details on immunizations can be found in Chapter 22, including

TABLE 10–4	Routine Immunizations Recommended During Infancy
IMMUNIZATION	**AGE RECOMMENDED**
Hepatitis B	After birth up to 2 months (#1)
	1–4 months (#2)
	6–18 months (#3)
Diphtheria, tetanus, acellular pertussis	2, 4, and 6 months (3 doses)
Haemophilus influenzae type b	2, 4, and 6 months (3 doses; last dose is not needed if PRP-OMP [Pedvax HIB or ComVax] is used for primary series)
Inactivated poliovirus	2, 4, and 6–18 months (3 doses)
Pneumococcal	2, 4, and 6 months (3 doses)
Influenza	Annually from 6 months of age
Rotavirus	2, 4 months (2 doses) or 2, 4, and 6 months (3 doses), dependent on vaccine used

recommended immunization schedules, Figures 22–4 and 22–5. Instruct parents about upcoming immunizations and when the infant should be seen again. Be sure the parent understands the risks and benefits of each immunization. Answer their questions truthfully and have resources on hand such as brochures and DVDs for interested parents.

Infants may have other conditions that have not yet been identified, so screening is helpful for these conditions. During each health supervision visit, the nurse performs screenings recommended by the American Academy of Pediatrics and other child health organizations, and counsels the parents about why such screening is important. Vision and hearing screenings are consistently performed. Screenings for anemia and lead poisoning are added at particular times or with certain groups. Families with certain genetic diseases may choose to have screening for the infant so that supportive care could begin early if the child has the disease (see Chapter 4 for further information about genetic diseases) (Table 10–5).

Parents benefit from teaching about common diseases and conditions of young children and measures for their prevention (Box 10–3). Ask about environmental tobacco smoke (ETS) and encourage smoking parents to quit smoking. This will lower the chance of sudden infant death syndrome, tooth decay, and asthma (see Chapter 25). Teach parents to put infants to sleep on their backs to lower the risk of sudden infant death syndrome. Have them instruct daycare providers about this recommended sleep position.

When an infant is in a childcare setting or has siblings at home, nurses may discuss common infectious diseases such as otitis media (ear infection), gastroenteritis, and skin infection. Provide parents

TABLE 10–5	Screening During Health Promotion and Health Maintenance Visits
AGE	**RECOMMENDED SCREENING TESTS**
1 month	Vision (follow objects, red reflex, opacities)
	Hearing (response to sound; screening by machine if not completed in the hospital)
	Physical examination with special attention to skin problems, hip dysplasia, foot position and range of motion, mouth, abdomen, cardiac abnormality, tearing of eyes, neurologic (including child abuse), anthropometric measurements
	Developmental milestones
	Dietary screening and stool/urine pattern assessment
	Review immunization record
2 months	Include those noted above
4 months	Include those noted above
	Vision (add cover–uncover test for strabismus); ocular mobility for lateral gaze
6 months	Include those noted above
	Vision (add ability to follow object bilaterally, corneal light reflex for eye alignment)
	Physical examination with special attention to muscle tone, extremities, appearance of first teeth, tympanic membrane, testicle descent for males
9 months	Include those noted above
	Lead levels if exposure is possible
	Anemia (earlier if the mother was anemic in pregnancy or the infant has health risks)
	Physical examination with special attention to symmetry of movement
12 months	Include those noted above
	Tuberculosis test if exposed to the disease
	Physical examination with special attention to condition of teeth

Source: *Data from Hagan, J. G., Shaw, J. S., & Duncan, P. M. (Eds.). (2008). Bright futures: Guidelines for health supervision of infants, children, and adolescents (3rd ed.). Elk Grove Village, IL: American Academy of Pediatrics.*

with needed information about prevention and treatment of conditions. Be sure they have a phone number to call when they have questions; provide information about when they should call or see the healthcare provider (Box 10–4).

BOX 10–4	When to Contact a Healthcare Provider

Instruct parents to contact a provider if the infant has:

- Temperature of 100.4°F (38.0°C) or above
- Seizure
- Skin rash, purplish spots, petechiae; change in skin color
- Change in activity or behavior that makes the parent uncomfortable
- Unusual irritability, lethargy, prolonged or unusual cry
- Failure to eat or drink
- Vomiting
- Diarrhea
- Decreased urine
- Respiratory infection that concerns the parent

BOX 10–3	Common Health Conditions of Infants

- Otitis media (see Chapter 24)
- Respiratory infection (see Chapter 25)
- Gastrointestinal infection (see Chapter 30)
- Skin conditions (see Chapter 36)

If the infant has had a health condition, evaluate with the parents how they managed the situation. Did they have the resources needed? Could they call and get needed information? Was a thermometer available? Did they have access to fluid and electrolyte solution, medication, or transportation to get care for the child? Did they have insurance or other coverage for bills? Did the childcare center provide necessary information about a child at the center who had an infectious disease? What situations need to be altered for more successful management of health threats in the future?

Disease prevention strategies focus on health maintenance. These activities are designed to identify diseases in early stages (such as vision impairment or cystic fibrosis) so that they can be managed effectively. This prevents complications and additional health issues. This is a type of secondary prevention (see Table 8–1 in Chapter 8 🔴). In addition, teaching regarding topics such as immunizations and management of communicable diseases prevents serious diseases from occurring.

Desired outcomes for disease prevention strategies include adequate management of health problems, integration of immunization and other preventive measures into care of the infant, and family understanding of preventive measures recommended for infants.

INJURY PREVENTION STRATEGIES

During the first year of life, injury becomes an increasingly common cause of mortality. Strategies must be included in each health supervision visit to lower the risk of injury. Nurses should never assume that parents understand how to insert an infant car seat correctly or what types of toys and foods can lead to choking. Know the most common hazards at each age and teach parents methods of avoiding them (Tables 10–6 and 10–7). Review at each visit the recommendation to place infants to sleep on their backs to lower the risk of sudden infant death syndrome (see Chapter 25 🔴).

Begin the conversation by asking parents what safety hazards they are aware of in the child's environment. Use this information as the starting point for discussion. Give positive feedback for their awareness of hazards and measures they have taken to prevent them. Consider using a home assessment survey that assists parents in identifying hazards that may be present in their homes. When infants visit friends, relatives, or neighbors, they may be exposed to other hazardous situations. Grandparents may not have a home that

is "babyproofed" and the infant could have access to electrical cords, machinery, medicines, or other hazards. Help the parents to evaluate the childcare home or center. Are babies adequately supervised? Do older children have toys that could be harmful to the babies present? Do infants have access to cooking areas, hot water, or heaters? Can they crawl into bathrooms where there is access to toilets or other water sources?

Focus on car safety, as this is a frequent cause of injury for infants. Provide brochures and other types of information about recommendations. Become a certified car seat examiner if possible and ask to view the infant's car seat. If this is not possible, locate examination centers in your community (frequently fire or police stations) and refer every family for a car seat examination. Provide resources for car seats if the family is not able to afford one. Discuss other possible safety hazards such as extensions on the parent bicycle and use of infant strollers in areas where cars are present. See the Photo Story on page 292 and Partnering with Families: Car Seats for Infants.

Injury prevention assessment and teaching strategies are examples of health maintenance activities. They are designed to minimize the exposure to hazardous environmental materials and practices. Consult materials from the Safe Kids Campaign (national and worldwide) for specific helpful tips. Be certain that all care providers, including baby-sitters and family members, have emergency numbers readily available.

Nursing Management

Nursing Assessment and Diagnosis

The nurse working in clinics, offices, and other settings that offer primary care for infants should be skillful in assessing health promotion and health maintenance. The infant's growth, developmental level, general physical health, and mental/social health are assessed. Family interactions and other settings where the infant spends time are evaluated for risks and protective factors that influence the child's development. Assess the health of siblings and patterns of integrating the infant into the rest of the family. Direct particular attention at assessment of risk for diseases and injuries. The data-gathering phase always provides parents with the opportunity to ask questions and relay concerns. Further assessment may need to be directed at these areas.

Based on the assessment data, the nurse establishes nursing diagnoses that become the basis for nursing interventions. Areas of

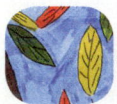

Partnering with Families

Car Seats for Infants

Review the family's routines for transporting an infant by car at every health supervision visit. Recommendations for infants from birth to 2 years:

- Infant-only seats can be used up to a weight of 22–35 pounds, depending on manufacturer directions.
- Rear-facing convertible seats can be used up to a weight of 30–40 pounds and will convert later to toddler seats.
- The seat is always placed in the back seat in the rear-facing position.
- Harness straps should be at or below shoulder level, and the seat should be tightly installed.

- Be sure to follow guidelines for every trip, no matter how short.
- Have the car seat and car checked by a certified child passenger safety technician (locate an inspection station at 866-732-8243).
- If the car seat is changed between two or more cars, it should be checked for proper installation in each car.

Source: *Data from National Highway Traffic Safety Administration (NHTSA). (2011). Traffic safety. Retrieved from http://www.nhtsa.gov/DOT/NHTSA/Traffic%20Injury%20Control/Articles/ Associated%20Files/4StepsFlyer.pdf; American Academy of Pediatrics. (2011). Car safety seats: A guide for families for 2011. Retrieved from http://www.healthychildren.org/English/ safety-prevention/on-the-go/Pages/Car-Safety-Seats-Information-for-Families.aspx*

Weblink | Car Seat Safety

TABLE 10–6	Injury Prevention in Infancy	
HAZARD	**DEVELOPMENTAL CHARACTERISTICS**	**PREVENTIVE MEASURES**
Falls	Mobility increases in first year of life, progressing from squirming movements to crawling, rolling, and standing.	Do not leave infant unsecured in infant seat, even in newborn period. Do not place on high surfaces such as tables, hood of car, or beds unless holding child. **(1)** Once mobile by crawling, keep doors to stairways closed or use gates. Standing walkers have led to many injuries and are not recommended.
Burns	Infant is dependent on caretakers for environmental control. The second half of the first year is marked by crawling and increased mobility. Objects are explored by touching and placing in mouth.	Check temperature of bath water and food/liquids for drinking. Do not hold infant while drinking hot beverages. Cover electrical outlets. Supervise infant so that play with electrical cords cannot occur.
Motor vehicle crashes	Infant is dependent on caretakers for placement in car. On impact with another motor vehicle, an infant held on a lap acts as a torpedo.	Use only approved restraint systems (according to federal Motor Vehicle Safety Standards). The seat must be used for every trip, even if very short. The seat must be properly buckled to the car's lap belt system. **(2)**
Drowning	Infant cannot swim and is unable to lift head.	Never leave infant alone in a bath of even 2.5 cm (1 in.) of water. Supervise when in water even when a life preserver is worn. Flotation devices such as arm inflatables are not certified life preservers.
Poisoning	Infant is dependent on caretakers to keep harmful substances out of reach.	Keep medicines out of reach. Teach proper dosage and administration of medicines to parents. Cleaning products and other harmful substances should not be stored where the infant can reach them. Remove plants from play areas. Have poison control center number by telephone and programmed into cell phones.
Choking	The second half of infancy is marked by exploratory reaching and mouthing objects. Infant explores objects by placing them in the mouth. **(3)**	Avoid foods that commonly cause choking. Keep small toys and all items with small parts away from infants, especially toys labeled "not intended for use by those under 3 years."
Suffocation	Young infant has minimal head control and may be unable to move if vomiting or having difficulty breathing.	Position infant on back for sleep. **(4)** Do not place pillows, stuffed toys, or other objects near head. Do not use plastic in crib. Avoid latex balloons.
Strangulation	Infant is able to get head into railings or crib slats but cannot remove it. Curtain or blinds cords can strangulate the crawling or reaching infant.	Be sure older cribs have slats spaced 6 cm (2 3/8 in.) or less apart. The mattress must fit tightly against the crib rails.

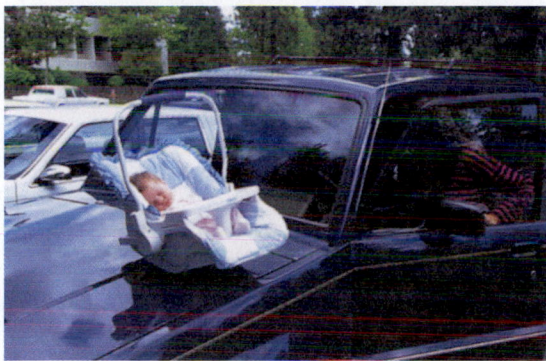

(1) Never leave an infant unsecured or on a high surface.

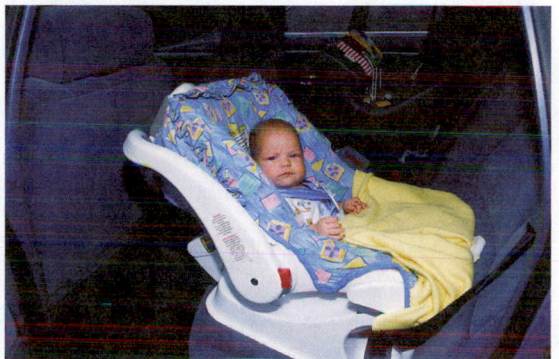

(2) Always use an approved restraint system. Place the infant in a rear-facing seat in the back seat of the car.

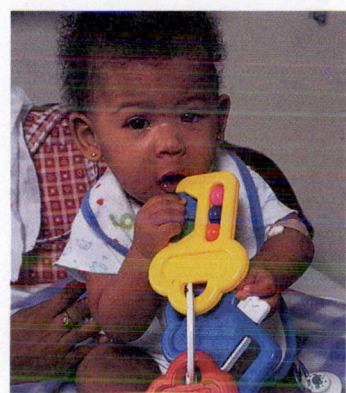

(3) The infant explores objects with his mouth.

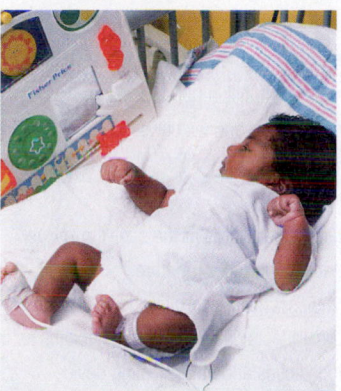

(4) Place the infant on the back for sleeping, and keep toys clear.

TABLE 10–7	Injury Prevention Topics by Age
AGE	INJURY PREVENTION TEACHING TOPICS
1 month	Follow infant car safety guidelines.
	Put the baby to sleep on back.
	Avoid loose bedding and toys in crib; do not have bracelets, necklaces, string toys, or cords near the infant.
	Avoid tobacco use in the environment.
	Provide adult supervision of the baby at all times by trusted individuals.
	Test bath water temperature and never leave the baby alone in bath.
	Never place the baby on a high object such as a counter, table, or bed; always keep one hand on the baby during such activities as diaper changes to prevent falling.
	Wash hands correctly and often.
	Avoid contact with persons with communicable diseases.
	Have smoke alarms and avoid fire hazards.
	Learn infant CPR and airway obstruction removal.
	Never shake the baby.
	Have plans for emergency care.
2 months	Include topics above.
	Use only recommended playpens or cribs and keep sides up.
	Avoid moldy environments.
	Keep baby toys clean.
	Avoid direct sunlight for the baby.
	Keep sharp and small objects out of the baby's environment.
	Keep the hot water heater lower than 120°F.
	Review emergency plan with all care providers.
4 months	Include topics above.
	Get all poisonous substances out of the baby's view and reach; install locks to keep them inaccessible.
	Do not use latex balloons or plastic bags near the baby.
	Never use infant walkers.
	Be sure tap water is no hotter than 120°F.
6 months	Include topics above.
	If an infant-only car seat was used, switch to a rear-facing convertible safety seat (intended for babies up to 40 lb) when the baby is 20–30 lb or 26 inches.
	Empty containers of water immediately after use; be sure pools or other bodies of water are locked and not accessible to the baby.
	Use sunscreen, hat, and long sleeves when the baby is in the sun.
	Keep heavy and sharp objects out of reach; check that all poisons are locked away, including in homes visited; keep pet food and cosmetics out of reach.
	Do not drink hot liquids or eat soup while holding the baby.
	Have the poison control number by phones and programmed into cell phones.
	Be alert for dangers of hot curling irons and other appliances.
	Have electrical cords out of reach and not hanging down.
	Have the home and environment checked for lead hazards.
	Lower the infant crib mattress if still in upper position.
	Install gates and guards on stairs and windows.
	Never use an infant walker.
9 months	Include topics above.
	Crawl on the floor and look for hazards at the baby's eye level.
	Pad sharp corners on tables and other furniture.
	Be alert for and move tables, chairs, and other devices the baby may use for climbing to unsafe places.
	Do not leave heavy or hot objects on tables with tablecloths as the infant may pull the cloth.
	Use barriers around woodstoves and other heating devices.
	Do not allow siblings or other children to have the responsibility to watch the infant in the yard, house, or bath.

TABLE 10–7	Injury Prevention Topics by Age (*Continued*)
AGE	**INJURY PREVENTION TEACHING TOPICS**
12 months	Include topics above.
	Continue to use a rear-facing car safety seat until 2 years of age or until the child is the highest weight or height allowed for the car seat; never place the seat in the front seat with a passenger air bag but use in the back seat of the car. Have the installation rechecked by a certified car seat examiner.
	Start showing the child how to wash hands frequently.
	Provide own personal items such as clothing and blankets to childcare providers; wash often.
	Change batteries in home smoke alarms and check the system.
	Turn handles to back of the stove; use back rather than front burners; keep away from hot liquids.
	Check the care provider setting for safety hazards.
	Remember that responsible adults should always supervise your infant, not other children.
	Peruse the home once again for hazards now that the child is more active, climbing, and walking.
	Do not allow guns in the area where the young child plays or lives; guns must be unloaded, locked securely away, with ammunition locked in a separate location.

Source: Data from Hagan, J. G., Shaw, J. S., & Duncan, P. M. (Eds.). (2008). *Bright futures: Guidelines for health supervision of infants, children, and adolescents* (*3rd ed.*). *Elk Grove Village, IL: American Academy of Pediatrics.*

both strength and need are included; often the family's strengths can be used to further promote health. Possible nursing diagnoses established during a health supervision visit of an infant are as follows:

- Breastfeeding, Ineffective related to the mother's resumption of employment outside the home
- Coping: Family, Compromised related to recent role changes
- Attachment, Risk for Impaired related to anxiety of parents associated with new roles
- Sleep Pattern, Disturbed related to frequently changing sleep cycles and needs
- Skin Integrity, Impaired related to developmental immaturity
- Infection, Risk for related to immature acquired immunity
- Injury, Risk for related to environmental hazards
- Growth and Development, Delayed related to lack of parental interaction with infant

NANDA-I © 2012

Planning and Implementation

The nurse plays a vital role in successful health promotion and health maintenance activities. Explain to the parents what procedures are being performed and their purpose. Encourage them to ask questions and share their perceptions of the infant's personality, development, and other traits. This will enhance their understanding that health care involves a partnership between them and the care providers. It will lead to trust that promotes their ability to share concerns honestly. Recognize that the first year of the infant's life is a key time for establishing a trusting relationship with health professionals.

Much of the visit is spent in teaching parents about topics such as safety measures, providing anticipatory guidance related to development, assisting with integration of the new infant into the family, and relaying resources for support of the family in the community, on the Internet, or elsewhere. Common parental needs include parenting classes, childcare facilities, and family planning resources.

Perform recommended physical and developmental assessments, administer screening tests, and give immunizations. Recognize the importance of data provided by simple assessments such as length and weight. Analyze all findings to learn if the child is developing

as expected. Be sure parents understand the need for tests and treatments, and relay the results of tests to them.

Nurses who work in hospitals, emergency services, and other facilities are also an important link in health supervision. Ask where and how often the child is seen for care. Check immunization schedules to be sure they are up to date. When the child is not being seen regularly, find out if the family does not understand the importance of these visits or lacks resources to obtain the necessary care. Refer them to resources as needed so they can identify a pediatric healthcare home. Agencies that provide health supervision sometimes perform home visits on a regular basis or in case of special need. When nurses make regular home visits to families with risk factors, health outcomes are improved. Seeing the family in the natural setting enables the nurse to tailor interventions to the specific situation. Nutrition, safety, and other teaching is more effective when it is delivered in a format appropriate for the family and matches the family's needs. For example, showing how to set up a stimulating environment with safe materials, even if toys are limited, is an effective nursing strategy. Ensure that home visits are performed when appropriate and available, either through the pediatric healthcare home or through another community agency. Utilize teaching strategies that are effective for the family (see Baccalaureate Essentials box).

Baccalaureate Essential IV
Information Management and Application of Patient Care Technology

Healthcare providers continue exploring strategies to determine which ones families will accept for receiving health information. A project called Baby LifeCheck targets parents of infants from 5 to 8 months and provides information about topics such as diet, sleep, and safety (Wood, 2010). Internet use may include questionnaire administration, kiosks, home monitoring of health practices, referrals, and prescription information (Kind, 2009). Implementing tested and evidence-based strategies for developmental screening and anticipatory guidance is helpful for both the infant and the family (Piotrowski, Talavera, & Mayer, 2009).

Nurses can perform screening, establish anticipatory guidance teaching outcomes, explore with families the best ways to distribute information in specific settings, and measure the satisfaction and effectiveness of strategies. Consider the Internet, kiosks, home monitoring through phone calls, and other creative teaching strategies.

PHOTO STORY...

PLACEMENT OF INFANT IN A CAR SAFETY SEAT

"I thought I had the seat in correctly, but wanted to check. They showed me that it was not attached right, so it could actually have allowed Sammie to be thrown and injured in a crash. I'm so glad it got checked. We've changed where and how I put the seat in the car."

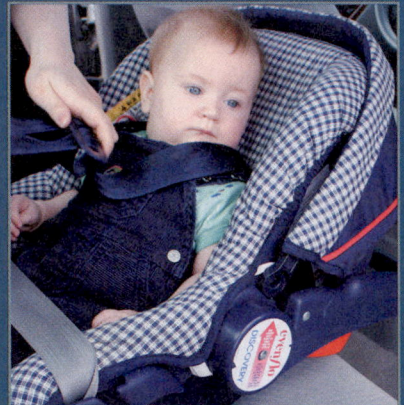

The child must be rear facing and securely harnessed.

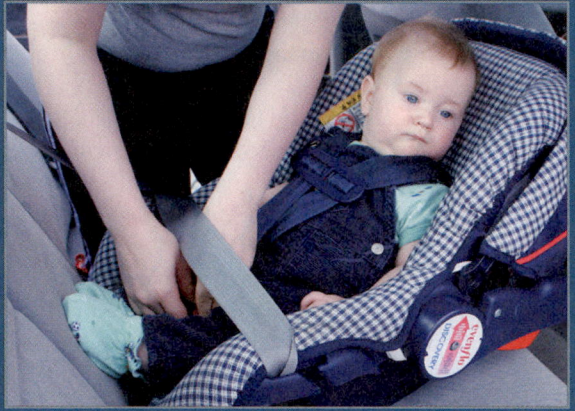

To ensure a proper fit, slide hand under harness and secure belt tightly.

This mother attends a high school alternative program that offers child-care for her infant son. The local police station was invited to send the car seat examiner to the program to evaluate car safety seats for the children. This mother learned to place the seat securely in the back seat, facing to the rear of the car. She also learned how to lift her child in, adjust the harness to fit him properly, and fasten the belt. Many parents do not correctly install and use car seats. Intentions are good, but seats may be old and not meet current standards, instructions for installation in cars may be hard to follow, and the care needed may not be taken. Young parents, such as the teen mother whose baby is shown here, are at particular risk. They may not be able to afford a seat, may rely on "hand me downs" from friends, and may not realize the importance of securing the child in a manner that meets current standards. What are the benefits of having someone come to an alternative school to teach and evaluate car safety? What programs are available in your community for providing car seats for parents who have difficulty affording them?

Before the family leaves the facility, be sure they have the next appointment scheduled. Summarize content of the present visit, emphasizing the family's strengths and the infant's newly acquired developmental skills. Sensitively list any areas that require work in the coming weeks, such as "babyproofing" the home or encouraging the infant to reach for objects. Provide a journal or notebook in which the parents can record the infant's development and write down questions to ask in future visits. Suggest possible topics for the parents to think about, and provide books, brochures, and other printed material.

Evaluation

Expected outcomes of nursing care for the infant and family in health promotion and health maintenance are as follows:

- The infant demonstrates normal patterns of growth and progression in developmental milestones.

- The infant is well adjusted, showing positive response to the environment and interactions with significant others.
- The infant remains free of disease and injury.
- Parents state common safety hazards at the child's present and upcoming ages.

Chapter Highlights

- The first contact between the infant's primary healthcare provider and the parents should occur prior to birth.
- A trusting relationship between the family and the care provider fosters a partnership that is influential in promoting the development of the infant.
- Health supervision visits begin with careful observations of the infant and parent–child interactions.
- Surveillance of growth and development provides important clues to the infant's well-being.
- Nutrition assessment and teaching are important to provide for the challenging nutritional needs of the first year of life.

- The mental health of parents influences the atmosphere in the home and the development of the infant.
- Patterns of interaction between parent and child as well as relationships with other adults and children provide the infant with strong emotional bonds that are essential to normal development.
- Disease and injury prevention strategies are integrated into each infant healthcare supervision visit.

Clinical Reasoning in Action

INTRODUCTION

Recall the chapter-opening scenario. Colleen has come to the WIC clinic with her 7-month-old daughter Amanda. A nutritional assessment is performed, teaching begins, and an appointment is made for a follow-up visit in 2 months for both Amanda and her 4-year-old sister Melody. The children's grandmother is a support person for Colleen, who is a single mother; however, the grandmother's impaired vision limits her somewhat in interactions with the children.

DESCRIPTION

Upon examination, Amanda appears adequately nourished. Her skin is well hydrated and in good condition. She is alert and shows expected developmental progression. Her hematocrit is 33%, weight is 17 lb 8 oz, and length is 26.5 in. Colleen drives Amanda and Melody to childcare each morning on her way to work; they spend afternoons with their grandmother. Colleen is motivated to provide safe and stimulating care for the children and has a supportive group of neighbors and friends.

DISCUSSION

Colleen clearly has many strengths or protective factors to draw from as she cares for her family. The nurse can address several areas of Amanda's development to enhance the family's strengths.

1. Evaluate Amanda's physical findings. Is the hematocrit within expected norms? What percentiles are her height and weight? What foods are recommended at her age?

2. What questions will you ask and what suggestions will you make to ensure that Amanda is safely transported to childcare each day in Colleen's car? How will you ensure a safe environment for Amanda at the grandmother's home when she provides childcare for the children?

3. Suggest several toys and activities that are appropriate for Amanda at her age. What developmental milestones do you expect to observe in areas of language, fine motor, gross motor, and social interactions?

NCLEX-RN® Review

1. Which observation during a healthcare visit alerts the nurse to the need for further developmental assessment in an infant?
   1. A 4-month-old has just started to roll from front to back.
   2. A 9-month-old now stands while holding on to furniture.
   3. A 9-month-old is able to sit with support from pillows on each side.
   4. A 12-month-old says two words, "dog" and "bottle."

2. Which observation in a health supervision visit leads the nurse to be concerned about an infant's mental health?
   1. When the nurse reaches for a 9-month-old, the infant grabs her mother and cries.
   2. The parent swaddles her 1-month-old who is crying after an immunization.
   3. A 10-month-old reportedly sleeps about 12 hours total per day.
   4. A 9-month-old avoids eye contact with parents and the nurse.

3. While at a health supervision visit, the nurse learns the parents are using a "hand-me-down" crib for their infant. Which action is the nurse's priority?

1. Discuss that the crib should have a soft, tight-fitting mattress.
2. Ask the parents what the distance is between slats on the side of the crib and whether the sides drop down.
3. Chart the information. No other action is necessary.
4. Immediately inform the healthcare provider.

4. Which growth pattern discovered at a health supervision visit necessitates a further inquiry into the infant's nutritional intake?

1. A 6-month-old infant whose birth weight was at the 50th percentile and current weight is just above the 25th percentile
2. A 4-month-old infant whose length was at the 25th percentile at 2 months of age and is still at the 25th percentile at 4 months of age
3. A 6-month-old infant whose head circumference was at the 75th percentile at 4 months and remains at the 75th percentile at 6 months
4. An infant whose weight was at the 25th percentile at 6 months and is above the 50th percentile at 9 months

See Appendix I 🔗 for answers.

References

American Academy of Pediatric Dentistry. (2010). *Get it done in Year One.* Retrieved from http://www.aapd.org/parents.pdf

American Academy of Pediatrics. (2011a). *Where we stand: Fruit juice.* Retrieved from http://www.healthychildren.org/English/healthy-living/nutrition/Pages/Where-We-Stand-Fruit-Juice.aspx

American Academy of Pediatrics. (2011b). *Car safety seats: A guide for families for 2011.* Retrieved from http://www.healthychildren.org/English/safety-prevention/on-the-go/Pages/Car-Safety-Seats-Information-for-Families.aspx

Brescianini, S., Volzone, A., Fagnani, C., Patriarca, B., Grimaldi, V., Lanni, R., . . . Stazi, J. A. (2011). Genetic and environmental factors shape infant sleep patterns: A study of 18-month-old twins. *Pediatrics, 127,* e1296. doi:10.1542/peds.2010-0858

Centers for Disease Control and Prevention. (2011). *Understanding intimate partner violence.* Retrieved from http://www.cdc.gov/violenceprevention/pdf/IPV_factsheet-a.pdf

Hagan, J. G., Shaw, J. S., & Duncan, P. M. (2008). *Bright futures: Guidelines for health supervision of infants, children, and adolescents* (3rd ed.). Elk Grove Village, IL: American Academy of Pediatrics.

Kind, T. (2009). The Internet as an adjunct for pediatric primary care. *Current Opinions in Pediatrics, 21,* 806–810.

Murray, R. B., Zentner, J. P., & Yakimo, R. (2009). *Health promotion strategies through the life span* (8th ed.). Upper Saddle River, NJ: Prentice Hall Health.

National Highway Traffic Safety Administration. (2011). *Traffic safety.* Retrieved from http://www.nhtsa.gov/DOT/NHTSA/Traffic%20Injury%20Control/Articles/Associated%20Files/4StepsFlyer.pdf

National Sleep Foundation. (2011). *Sleep, infants, and parents.* http://www.sleepfoundation.org/article/ask-the-expert/sleep-infants-and-parents

Piotrowski, C. C., Talavera, G. A., & Mayer, J. A. (2009). Health steps: A systematic review of a preventive practice-based model of pediatric care. *Journal of Developmental and Behavioral Pediatrics, 30,* 91–103.

Sadeh, A., Mindell, J., & Rivera, L. (2011). "My child has a sleep problem": A cross-cultural comparison of parental definitions. *Sleep Medicine, 12*(5), 478–482.

Schreck, K. A., & Richdale, A. L. (2011). Knowledge of childhood sleep: A possible variable in under or misdiagnosis of childhood sleep problems. *Journal of Sleep Research, 20,* 589–597. doi:10.1111/j.1365-2869.2011.00922.x

Tanski, S., Garfunkel, L. C., Duncan, P. M., & Weitzman, M. (2010). *Performing preventive services.* Elk Grove Village, IL: American Academy of Pediatrics.

Voigt, R. G., Macias, M. M., & Myers, S. M. (eds.) (2010). *AAP Developmental and behavioral pediatrics.* Elk Grove Village, IL: American Academy of Pediatrics.

World Health Organization (WHO) & United Nations Children's Fund (UNICEF). (2009). *Home visits for the newborn child: A strategy to improve survival.* Retrieved from http://www.who.int/maternal_child_adolescent/documents/who_fch_cah_09_02/en/

Wood, A. (2010). Baby LifeCheck—Is it a public health initiative? *Journal of Family Health Care, 20*(1), 9–10.

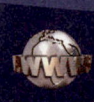
Pearson Nursing Student Resources
Find additional review materials at
nursing.pearsonhighered.com
Prepare for success with additional NCLEX®-style practice questions, interactive assignments and activities, web links, animations and videos, and more!

Health Promotion and Maintenance of the Toddler and Preschooler

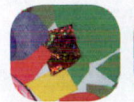 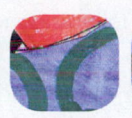 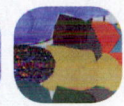

KEY TERMS

Learning Outcomes

After completing this chapter, you will be able to:

1. Describe the general observations made of toddlers/preschoolers and their families as they come to the pediatric healthcare home for health supervision visits.

2. Identify the major health concerns of toddlers and preschoolers.

3. Apply assessment skills to gather data regarding nutrition, physical activity, mental health status, and growth and development of toddlers and preschoolers.

4. Apply therapeutic communication skills with the toddler/preschooler and family during health supervision visits in toddlerhood/preschool.

5. Prioritize interventions to promote health and to prevent disease and injury for toddlers/preschoolers and their families.

6. Synthesize data from the history and examination of the toddler/preschooler and family with knowledge of toddler/preschooler development to plan approaches useful with the family during health supervision encounters.

> "Clarence is so busy! I babysit for all my cousins and he is the hardest one. He's always moving and does not stay interested in anything for very long."
> —*Clarence's cousin Miranda, age 14*

Clarence Kaufman has been brought in for his 15-month-old health supervision visit by his parents, Ben and Karie. Clarence is a healthy toddler, but his parents have questions about his development. They are concerned about his high activity level and need for constant supervision. As both parents work while Clarence is at childcare, they are busy in the evening trying to spend time with him and meet other family obligations. You notice on the record that Clarence missed his 12-month health supervision visit and was last seen when he was 9 months old.

What health promotion activities will be appropriate for this visit? How will you integrate his parents' questions about Clarence's activity level into the visit? Since Clarence has not been seen in health care for some time, what are some likely health maintenance needs? How can you partner with his parents to ensure his visits to the healthcare home?

The years following infancy are challenging for parents as the child grows and acquires new developmental skills. The child progresses from the first tentative steps and words at a year of age, through the "terrible twos" of toddlerhood (about 1 through 2 years of age), and into preschool age (about 3 to 5 or 6 years) when most children attend some type of educational program, have well-developed verbal communication, and acquire many gross and fine motor skills. Toddler and preschool ages are often grouped as "young childhood," as the family remains the primary system within which the child interacts, and caregivers deal with many common concerns such as nutrition, sleep, and growing independence. Facing consistent changes in development, parents rely on the pediatric healthcare home (medical home) for advice and information (see Chapter 8 🖉 for a detailed description of the pediatric healthcare home). Nurses apply concepts of anticipatory guidance during visits for health promotion and health maintenance to assist parents in the transitions they face.

What are some of the unique concerns of the family with a toddler or preschooler? How can the nurse facilitate healthy growth and development during these stages? What resources can parents use to provide support in their task of raising a young child and providing experiences to ready the child for school entry? These are some of the topics that will be addressed in this chapter.

GENERAL OBSERVATIONS

A collaborative relationship between the family and the healthcare providers should already be established. If, however, the family is new to this healthcare home, reach out to welcome them warmly and express interest in them as individuals and parents. As families often feel uncomfortable in healthcare settings, establish positive rapport so they will be able to ask questions and bring up concerns about the child.

As you prepare to call a toddler in from the waiting room, remember to watch for developmental advances, such as an 18-month-old child's desire for independence or signs of continuing reliance on the parent. Does the child strike out independently or cling to the parent once a stranger is seen? Make note of this temperament characteristic, comment about it to the family, and learn how they describe the child's temperament (see Chapter 5 🖉 for a description of child temperament). In addition, observe mobility. Does the child walk independently? What other means are used for locomotion? Again, verify your observations of mobility with the parents during the visit.

Health supervision visits are adapted for older toddlers and preschoolers to include observations of parental discipline and interaction style. Does the parent respond to the child's questions? Were age-appropriate toys or activities brought to the visit to help occupy the child while waiting? Is the child alert and observant of the environment? By preschool age, the child is walking skillfully and usually engages in conversations easily. The nurse welcomes the child warmly and assesses social skills and motor activities. Direct greetings or questions to the child can evaluate stranger anxiety and the ability to understand simple commands or questions. What verbal skills are observed? The parent usually allows the child some independence in answering questions and provides support for the child who is quiet and appears apprehensive. Watch for these interactions.

Recall Ben and Karie, described in the chapter-opening scenario. They are concerned about the impact of their son's activity level and their busy lives on his development. Since the family has not been at the facility for some time, they will need to be welcomed and shown that the healthcare providers are eager to work with them in a partnership to provide care to benefit their child. How can you put them at ease?

Most parents enjoy talking about their children, so asking questions and commenting positively about a child's traits will encourage them to share thoughts about the child. The following questions promote opportunities to educate:

- "Your son is really able to walk so well now, isn't he?"
- "Your daughter has grown so much and she is talking a lot. What is she interested in?"

Once they answer, respond appropriately and ask for additional specific information pertinent to the visit:

- "Yes, it is a challenge now that your son can walk and climb. We'll talk about some safety precautions that are advised at this age."
- "Preschoolers who are outgoing like your daughter are a real pleasure. At the same time, it is sometimes hard to keep them occupied. What do you do to keep her busy?"

What questions could you ask Clarence's parents, described in the opening scenario, about their son? Remember that he is 15 months old; include your knowledge of development in the questions.

The mental health of the parents and the social environment of the home influence the environment in which the child is growing and learning (Halfon, Larson, & Russ, 2010). It is therefore important to ask questions about the parent who comes with the child and the family in general. Inquire about how the family is adjusting to the growing child. If there are other children, ask about their health and the challenges they bring to the family. Were there recent job or insurance changes, or has the family moved? Are there parental concerns about the neighborhood or resources for the child? Does the parent want to talk about any personal problems such as depression, substance use, illness, or stress? (We will explore these topics later in this chapter.)

Health supervision of young children includes:

1. *Assessments,* such as screening tests, evaluations, and observations
2. *Education* that includes anticipatory guidance about coming developmental tasks
3. *Intervention,* including parent counseling, home visits when appropriate, and scheduling further visits
4. *Care coordination* among resources serving the family and community

Nurses establish partnerships with families by demonstrating respect, positive communication, and a receptive attitude. See Chapter 1 🖉 for further description of the partnership between nurses and families.

Consult the record to see when the child was last seen. Parents of toddlers and preschoolers need to know the ages when children should be examined for health promotion and health maintenance. List these ages, and at each visit, make the next appointment or provide written information about where and when to call for the next visit. Encourage families who speak languages other than English to bring an interpreter or arrange for one to be present in the visit. Be sure they understand the information provided about future visits. Keep in mind that some parents may benefit from additional visits or referrals to other community resources, especially during the preschool years when annual healthcare visits become the norm. Be alert during the visit for families that may benefit from such approaches. The recommended ages for care during the toddler and preschool years are 12, 15, and 19 months; from 2 to 3 years; from 3 to 4 years; and from 4 to 5 years.

See Table 11–6 later in this chapter for recommended screening tests at each of these visits.

GROWTH AND DEVELOPMENTAL SURVEILLANCE

An essential assessment skill in the visit is measurement of growth. Weight and length measurement are described in Chapter 7 ✪ and in the Skills Manual ⊂⊃, and expected patterns of growth are discussed in Chapter 5 ✪. Once the child can stand to be measured, sometime between 2 to 3 years of age, use charts for standing height rather than recumbent length. Body mass index (BMI) is first calculated at 2 years of age and provides information about the relationship of height and weight (see Chapter 19 ✪). Head circumference is usually measured until up to 2 years of age. Consult growth charts in Appendix A ✪. Growth continues to be a primary way of evaluating the child's nutritional status. It may also provide clues about conditions that have not yet been identified or evaluated (Box 11–1). Depending on the results of growth measurement, the nurse may need to gather additional data. For a child under the 5th percentile for weight or BMI, detailed nutritional intake records should begin. Laboratory studies such as hematocrit and hemoglobin can be performed. Patterns of family growth can be examined. Ask if the child has had any illness or hospitalization. Observe the body proportions. The toddler has short legs and a wide stance, whereas the preschooler begins to develop longer legs and increased physical skills. Gross motor skills such as standing, walking, running, and riding a tricycle should be described. Fine motor skills can be observed by giving the child a marker and paper to draw upon while asking the parent questions.

The physical assessment is performed, with some parts conducted by the nurse and others by the primary care provider such as a physician or nurse practitioner. See Chapter 7 ✪ for a thorough discussion of physical examination and suggested sequence for different ages. The order of the examination and the approaches to the child are particularly important at this age. Leave intrusive procedures,

BOX 11–1	Health Conditions Related to Growth in Young Children

GROWTH PATTERN	POSSIBLE CONDITIONS
Low percentile for weight, height, and BMI, especially decreasing percentile or growth channels	■ Cardiac defect ■ Cystic fibrosis ■ Gastrointestinal anomaly or parasites ■ Malabsorption ■ Cerebral palsy ■ Endocrine disorder ■ Eating disorder of infancy and childhood (failure to thrive)
High percentile for weight and BMI, especially increasing percentile channels	■ Excess caloric intake ■ Low physical activity ■ Endocrine disorder

such as ear and eye exam for toddlers and visualization of genitalia for preschoolers, until the end of the exam. Integrate techniques such as allowing the child to play with the stethoscope or to "blow out" the light from the otoscope, or make a game of pushing the legs against the examiner to measure symmetry of strength (Figure 11–1 ■). Preschoolers are generally interested in their bodies, and teaching about parts of the examination is helpful. Ideas include comments such as:

- "Do you know what your heart sounds like? Do you want to listen to it?"
- "When you take a deep breath, where does the air go?"
- "This is your tummy. Your food goes here when you eat, then into your blood, and all around your body to make it strong."

During the physical examination, ask the parents pertinent questions. Consider the young child's expected developmental milestones (see Chapter 5) and ask questions related to them. Important questions might include:

- "What are Clarence's sleep patterns like now?"
- "How often does Cassandra have a bowel movement? Are you concerned that they are too frequent or not often enough?

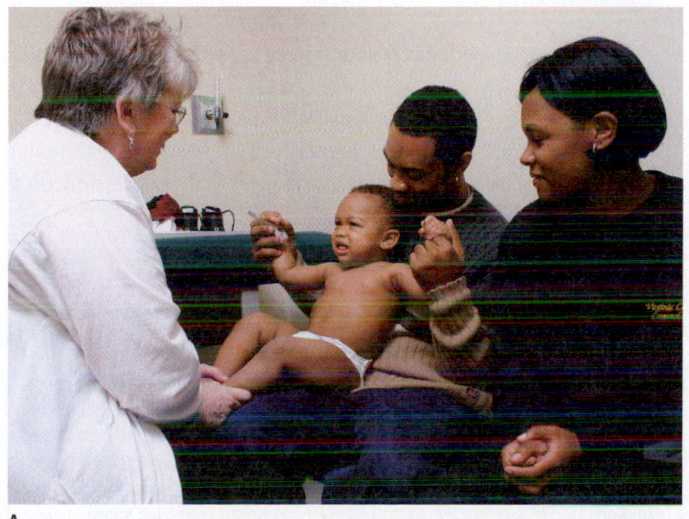

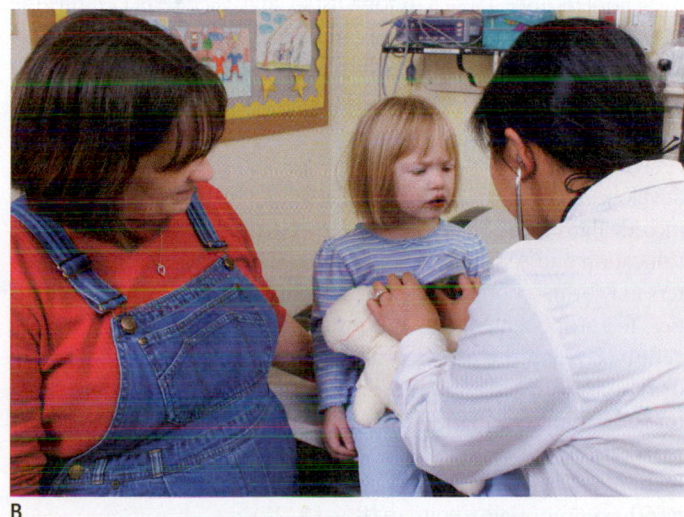

A

B

FIGURE 11–1 ■ The approach to examination of the toddler or preschooler is important to elicit cooperation. A, The toddler may accept parts of the examination best when seated on the parent's lap such as shown in this photo of Clarence. B, The preschooler likes the opportunity to touch and become comfortable with equipment used. In this instance, the preschooler holds a doll that receives the same examinations as the child.

Does she ever appear constipated? What are the symptoms she displays?"

■ "You mentioned that Jim is in a Head Start program. How often does he go? Has he had any illnesses that have kept him home?"

■ "Do you have a thermometer at home? What type is it? Have you used it to take a temperature on your child?"

Remember that some parents understand child growth and development, and your questions give them an opportunity to discuss observations or concerns, as well as help the child to see that the parents trust and have positive rapport with the examiner. When parents answer questions readily and bring up concerns, move into a discussion of these topics during the examination. This encourages the child to relax and also establishes trust.

Development is the key organizing principle of early childhood health care. Developmental screening and services should be integrated within healthcare, childcare, and school settings, to include the multiple sites common for young children (Halfon, DuPlessis, & Inkelas, 2007; Halfon, Stanley, & DuPlessis, 2010). Developmental surveillance is integrated throughout the well-child visit, and developmental screening and testing are performed. See Table 11–1 for developmental milestones commonly observed during health promotion and health maintenance visits of toddlers and preschoolers. Ask if the child has had developmental testing done at a childcare agency or another site. Although health promotion and health maintenance visits commonly address issues such as immunizations, nutrition, and sleep positions, pediatricians in the United States may be less likely to address topics such as child communication, reading, parental stress, or other issues related to developmental progression. Sharing well-child care among professionals such as nurses and other care providers would increase the quality and comprehensiveness of services (Halfon et al., 2010). Nurses generally have in-depth knowledge of child development, through growth and development courses and pediatric nursing curricula, and are thus well positioned to address parental concerns related to child development (Table 11–2). Watch for the inclusion of development in child health visits, identify deficits in your agency, and take steps to meet the needs of parents and children.

Developmental screening and testing are addressed in Chapters 8 through 10 🔗, and the principles continue here for toddlers and preschoolers. (See Table 8–5 for a list of suggested tests.) During the early childhood years, common areas addressed on developmental screening tests include social skills, continuing gross and fine motor activity, and language skills.

Many children, especially by preschool age, attend a childcare center. Ask about the family's experience with the center and whether developmental skills are a focus of activity. Governmental programs include Early Head Start and Head Start (federal) or Early Childhood Education and Assistance Program (ECEAP) (state); nonprofit centers may be in schools, YMCA or YWCA, or related to religious entities; for-profit centers may be run by individuals or as cooperative ventures. Ask if the parent is pleased with the childcare experience or requires further resources. Payment for care can be problematic for some families and should be explored. Resources to assist families with promotion of the social, intellectual, and emotional development of young children are available. Refer families to Zero to Three or other appropriate resources (Box 11–2).

Health promotion growth and development issues for toddlers and preschoolers are addressed at each visit. Examples include:

TABLE 11–1	Developmental Milestones Observed During Health Promotion and Maintenance Visits of Toddlers and Preschoolers
AGE	**DEVELOPMENTAL MILESTONES**
12 months	■ Walks alone or with help
	■ Enjoys social games and interactions
	■ Speaks 1–3 words and understands simple commands
	■ Drinks from cup and feeds self
15 months	■ Walks by self, crawls or walks up stairs
	■ Stacks two blocks
	■ Points to one or more body parts
	■ Is increasingly interactive
	■ Explores environment
18 months	■ Walks with ease
	■ Pushes or pulls toy
	■ Stacks three or more blocks
	■ Uses spoon to eat, spilling often
	■ Follows directions and uses 15–20 words
2–3 years	■ Goes up and down steps
	■ Kicks ball
	■ Scribbles and draws lines on paper
	■ Imitates words and actions of adults
3–4 years	■ Jumps
	■ Rides tricycle
	■ Draws precise lines on paper; attempts to imitate circle, line, and cross
	■ Always feeds self
	■ Dresses self though sometimes clothes are backwards
	■ Has friends and plays with others
4–5 years	■ Recites rhymes and songs
	■ States name
	■ Draws a rudimentary person
	■ Builds tower of blocks and bridges with blocks
	■ Throws ball overhand

■ Explaining growth patterns and what is expected in the months ahead

■ Providing toys that encourage development of the coming developmental milestones (see Chapter 5 🔗 for specific suggestions)

■ Showing parents the child's developmental progression on a screening tool

BOX 11–2	Zero to Three

Zero to Three is a national organization that seeks to promote the healthy development of the nation's infants, toddlers, and their families, by informing, educating, supporting, and strengthening families, communities, and those who work on their behalf. The results of research are used to establish policies and practices that integrate the latest research into practice. Zero to Three works closely with Early Head Start centers, trains program employees, provides information to parents and health professionals, and publishes results in professional and lay journals. Find out how Zero to Three activities influence your community.

TABLE 11–2	Sample Questions and Teaching Topics Pertinent to Early Childhood Visits	
TOPIC	**QUESTIONS**	**TEACHING**
Sleep	How long does Cassandra sleep at night? Does she take naps? Does Jim ever wake at night crying? Do you have trouble consoling him? Is your daughter able to concentrate on preschool and stay alert during the hours she is there? What concerns do you have about your son's sleep patterns?	■ Normal amounts of sleep at various ages ■ Establishment of consistent sleep routines ■ Types of sleep disruptions and their treatment
Discipline	Does Cassandra ever misbehave? When it happens, what does she typically do? How do you respond to her behavior? Have you tried using time-out when she seems out of control? How does the childcare center deal with inappropriate behavior? Do you agree with the center's techniques?	■ Consistency and limit setting ■ Appropriate consequences for behaviors ■ Evaluating methods of discipline ■ Adapting methods to individual children
Toilet training	Have you thought about beginning to toilet train your toddler? How do you think you will do it? What signs have you seen that he might be ready soon? You mentioned that Cassandra has occasional accidents. How often are they, and are you concerned about them? What rewards do you use when your son is successful in using the toilet? Do you have a small toilet for him to use?	■ Readiness cues for toilet training (see Chapter 5 🔗) ■ Introducing toilet training ■ Positive reinforcement for children ■ Transitions to childcare and other settings away from home
Learning/reading	Describe the things that Jim is learning now. Is he progressing as you would expect or like? How often do you read to Jim? How does he like reading with you? Have you been able to get books to keep for him at home? Do you ever visit the library together? Does your library have a story time for young children?	■ Providing stimulating environments for learning ■ Importance of reading to children ■ Importance of providing books for children to look at during playtime ■ Pointing out letters to preschool children
Communication	What is Cassandra's language like now? Are you concerned or particularly pleased about any of her ways of communicating? How does she get along with other children in Head Start? What has she been learning about getting along with other children?	■ Expected language skills ■ Social interaction with adults and other children ■ Childcare resources and evaluation
Parental issues	How is your life going right now? Do you or does anyone else in your family drink more than two drinks per day, smoke, or take street drugs? How is your general mood? Are you often tired, sad, or depressed? Who helps out when you need something? Are there friends or family close to call upon? What resources that you do not have would be helpful to you (e.g., more food, counseling, other parents)?	■ Effects of parental substance abuse on children ■ Need for healthy mental status to meet child's developmental needs ■ Referrals to needed community resources to meet basic mental status needs

Likewise, health maintenance activities are included in health supervision visits, with the primary purpose being prevention of disease and injury. Specific examples are included throughout the chapter, but general areas addressed are as follows:

■ Connecting developmental skills with risks for injury such as drowning, poisoning, and falls

■ Recognizing the possibility of infectious diseases as the child begins a childcare experience and addressing recognition and treatments for common diseases

Expected outcomes for the child include normal growth and development patterns for motor, language, and social skills; parental knowledge of stimulating activities for the child; awareness of the family about risks to growth and development; and healthy body systems for the child.

NUTRITION

The child's nutritional status continues to play an important part in promoting health and preventing health disruptions during toddler and preschooler years. Good nutrition fosters normal growth patterns, promotes developmental progression, and helps prevent disorders such as anemia, tooth decay, and immune dysfunction. In addition, intake of food takes on an increasingly social dimension during early childhood as children interact more with adults and other children at mealtimes.

As with infants, the measurements of weight and height form the basis of the nutritional assessment. Once the child is 2 years of age, the height and weight proportion are used to calculate BMI percentile. See Chapter 19 🔗 for further explanation about evaluation of these percentiles and Appendix A 🔗 for the percentile grids. Children usually stay within the same percentile range over time, even though rates of growth vary somewhat from child to child. For example, if an infant is consistently between the 25th and 50th percentiles for length and weight, the percentiles generally remain about the same as the child gets older. When children change percentile ranges, or when the BMI percentile increases or decreases, additional nutritional data will be collected. The child may be consuming too many calories for activity if the height stays in the same range and the weight increases. Other physical assessment data that provide information about nutrition include energy level of the child; condition of hair, nails, and skin; and meeting developmental milestones.

Practice Alert

When you examine growth grids (in Appendix A 🔗), you will find that the percentiles can be grouped along the lines presented. The ranges described are:

- Below 5th percentile (needs nutritional assessment)
- 5th–10th percentile
- 10th–25th percentile
- 25th–50th percentile
- 50th–75th percentile
- 75th–95th percentile (above 85th percentile needs nutritional assessment)
- Above 95th percentile (needs nutritional assessment)

A child who generally falls between the 25th and 50th percentile may have weight closer to the 25th percentile at one visit and closer to the 50th percentile on the next, which simply reflects normal patterns of fluctuation. On the other hand, a child going from the 25th–50th weight percentile range on one visit to the 75th–95th percentile range on a visit a few months later may have nutritional problems. Weigh the child a second time to verify your findings, add dietary questions to the health supervision visit, collect additional nutritional data, and refer to the physician or nurse practitioner in the facility. See Chapter 19 🔗 for further information about nutritional assessment. What nutritional problems do you think are most common for toddlers and preschoolers?

For toddlers, questions for the family focus on introduction of foods, the child's eating patterns, and transition from breast or bottle to other liquids. The toddler often consumes small amounts of foods, and parents consequently worry about the change in appetite. Showing them that the child is growing normally can help allay their anxiety about this common developmental variation.

Preschoolers increasingly interact with others during food preparation and meal consumption. Questions focus on the child's likes and dislikes for particular foods, behavior at the table, and establishment of healthy family eating patterns. Ask how often the family eats out, especially at fast-food restaurants. Excess intake of fat and salty foods, as well as large portion sizes, is associated with eating out frequently. See Chapter 19 🔗 for further discussion of the issues related to fast foods.

When parents are busy and older siblings are in activities, both toddlers and preschoolers may be eating foods such as french fries or milk shakes several times weekly. Suggest alternative approaches to the busy lifestyle, such as bringing fresh fruit slices along when an older sibling is at a sporting event, keeping a cooler in the car to maintain cool items, and limiting fast-food meals to no more than one or two each week. Obtain nutritional information about common fast-food options in your community and share these with parents. Assist them to make healthy choices when eating out. Encourage the family to establish times to eat together, even if only a few times weekly. If children help with preparations for this family meal and then eat together, nutritional knowledge and intake can be positively enhanced. When the child is in a childcare center, encourage the parents to find out what food is provided in that setting. If the parents would prefer to send food or have particular food requests, assist them in dealing with the childcare personnel.

Questions that provide information to be used as the basis for nutritional teaching include:

- "What type of milk is Jim drinking now? How much does he drink each day? How much juice does he drink each day?"
- "Does your son like to eat with the family at the table? What foods does he like? Dislike?"
- "What types of foods are served at Cassandra's childcare center? Do children eat together at tables there?"

- "What kinds of things does Cassandra like to do with you in the kitchen? How often do you prepare meals at home each week? Which meals do you most commonly prepare? How often does your family eat together? How often do you eat at fast-food restaurants? What are the major times when it is hard to feed your family the foods you would like to or that are good for them? Does your family eat breakfast each day? What do you eat for breakfast?"
- "Are you giving your children any vitamins? Fluoride?"
- "What questions do you have about your child's food needs and patterns?"
- "What access do you have to fresh fruits and vegetables at your local market or farmer's market? Are they affordable? Do you know how to prepare the foods that are healthy to offer your children?"

During the toddler and preschool years, children are gaining much more independence about food choices and patterns of eating. At the same time, their eating patterns depend mainly on the family and so assessment should involve the entire family unit. See Developing Cultural Competence: Family Nutrition.

Parents can benefit from receiving information about nutrition in young children (Table 11–3). Health promotion interventions are designed to focus on leading the child and family to a higher state of wellness and may include actions such as supporting breastfeeding for young toddlers and being sure preschoolers have a role in selecting foods for healthy snacks. Parental education is influential in shaping the young child's diet and should be integrated into all visits (Holt, Wooldridge, Story, et al., 2011). Teach the amounts of food that should be offered and frequency of meals. Encourage parents to make food preparation and meals a pleasant experience. For example, important health promotion teaching to include with every family is the need to include "5 a day," or five servings of fruits and vegetables in the daily diet. (See Chapter 12 🔗 for further description of the 5-a-day program.) Inclusion of adequate fruits and vegetables promotes health by boosting the immune system, providing for regular elimination patterns, and leading to healthy hair and nails. Likewise, "3 a day of dairy" encourages families to provide at least three servings of dairy for children every day. See Chapter 19 for additional information about the nutritional needs of young children. Nurses and parents partner to ensure that the young child establishes healthy eating habits at home and in other daily settings.

Developing Cultural Competence
Family Nutrition

Families integrate their own cultural backgrounds and past experiences into food preparation and choices. Ask what foods are common in the child's cultural group, and help the family learn when to introduce each food. For example, rice may be a first food for an Asian baby, rather than rice cereal. Simply be sure the child also takes in adequate iron sources in the first foods offered. Tofu or bean paste may be a common protein source in some diets. A Native American child may eat fish or wild game, along with berries and roots. Ask and learn about each family's cultural patterns. Learn what you can about cultural groups in your community. Encourage the family to offer the young child their usual foods, as long as they meet needs for requirements, are prepared with minimal salt and seasoning, and are soft enough to avoid choking. Perform diet recalls and analyses to identify specific teaching needs in all families.

TABLE 11–3	Nutrition Teaching for Health Promotion and Health Maintenance Visits
AGE	**NUTRITION TEACHING**
1 year	Support the mother who continues to breastfeed.
	Wean the child from the bottle by substituting a cup.
	If beginning to use cow milk, use whole milk.
	Limit juice to 4–6 oz daily; offer water several times daily.
	Encourage safety measures—use a high chair with a strap, secure the child and use caution in grocery carts, and do not allow foods to be eaten in the car.
	Provide information on choking and airway obstruction removal training.
	Provide food and water safety guidelines (see Chapter 19 🔗).
	Be sure all major food groups have been introduced.
	Limit high-fat and high-sugar foods.
	Review amounts of food commonly consumed and frequency of feedings.
	Review use of fluoride if the water supply is not fluoridated.
2 years	Ask if the mother is still breastfeeding, and support the decision to continue or to wean the child.
	Encourage total removal of a bottle if still in use.
	Ensure that all foods common to the family have been offered.
	Offer child-size eating utensils.
	The child can change to low-fat or skim milk if the family desires.
	Limit milk to two to three servings daily and fruit juice to no more than 4–6 ounces (120–180 mL) daily.
	Teach parents methods for dealing with temper tantrums over food—make food available at meal and snack times only, do not force intake, and offer a variety of foods.
	Teach that the child may have days of very low intake due to slowing growth rate.
3 years	Most children are weaned from breastfeeding and drinking 1% or 2% milk.
	Teach normal intake and decreasing number of snacks.
	Engage the child in food preparation and pouring liquids from a small pitcher.
	Recognize that **food jags** (periods when only one or two foods are eaten) are common.
	Recognize the importance of the social nature of eating; expect the child to sit for a short period at meals with the family.
	Meals and snacks should not be eaten while watching television.
4 years	Encourage involving the child in snack selection and preparation.
	Start to teach food groups and the importance of nutrition for the body.
	Alter intake as appropriate depending on weight and BMI.
	Dairy products consumed should all be low or reduced fat.

Health maintenance activities focus primarily on disease and injury prevention. Examples include feeding practices that avoid common choking foods, and limiting daily fruit juice intake to prevent dental caries (see Chapter 8 🔗) and excessive caloric intake.

Desired outcomes related to nutrition include meeting normal growth and development milestones, maintaining recommended weight, increasing understanding of healthy food patterns, and preventing nutrition-related disorders.

PHYSICAL ACTIVITY

Both children and adults are commonly overweight and sedentary in today's society, so emphasis on physical activity should be a part of each health supervision visit. Nurses and parents are partners in planning activities for the young child; patterns set in motion at this early age will continue throughout childhood and into adulthood.

The toddler and preschooler consistently show gains in fine and gross motor abilities. They move around independently and have more physical activity away from the home base. They commonly visit parks, swim, attend childcare centers, and help with some household tasks. These activities are important, both because they assist the child to continue to develop motor skills and because they limit the amount of time spent in sedentary behavior. The toddler and preschool years are an important time for setting the habits for physical activity during all of childhood.

The caregiver's main emphasis should be on providing experiences that encourage further motor development. The child needs to walk, run, hop, push and pull objects, and throw balls. Motor activity is a major component in all playtimes, and activities should engage the child's large and small muscle groups. The National Association for Sport and Physical Education (NASPE) has established recommendations for toddlers and preschoolers: a minimum of 60 minutes per day of unstructured physical activity, a minimum of 60 minutes per day of structured physical activity, and a maximum of 60 minutes of sedentary behavior at any one time exclusive of sleep (Beets, Bornstein, Dowda, et al., 2011; Centers for Disease Control and Prevention, 2010).

By the preschool years, coordination becomes increasingly important (Figure 11–2 ■). Physical activity is important for all children,

Weblink

NASPE

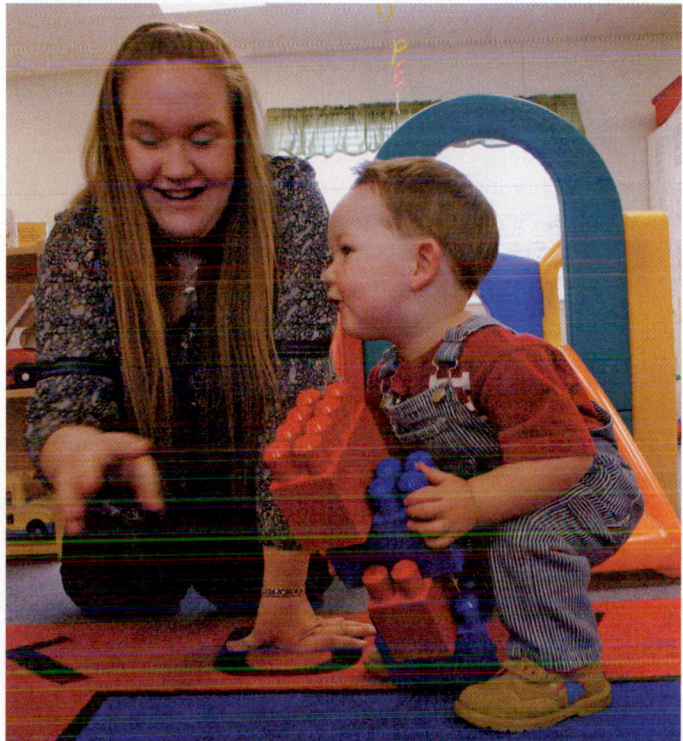

FIGURE 11–2 ■ This toddler enjoys motor activity that uses large muscle groups. The preschooler begins to spend increasing amounts of time in coordination of both small and large muscle mass. List several physical activities you can suggest for the parents of children in each of these age groups.

TABLE 11–4	Risk and Protective Factors Regarding Physical Activity in Toddlerhood and Preschool
RISK FACTORS	**PROTECTIVE FACTORS**
■ Developmental delay ■ Slow development of social skills	■ Expected developmental progression
■ Limited stimulation by family or other care providers ■ Limited social time with other children ■ Long work hours by parents	■ Easily engaged socially with others ■ Daily contact with other young children
■ Reluctance to try new physical activity ■ Limited access to balls, slides, balance beams, tricycles, and other materials that foster physical activity ■ Lack of adequate safety gear for activities	■ Eagerness to try new physical activity ■ Access to balls, slides, balance beams, tricycles, and other materials that foster physical activity ■ Adequate safety gear that properly fits child
■ Parents who have little physical activity on a daily basis ■ Lack of knowledge by family about child physical activity needs	■ Daily physical activity engaged in by all family members, 2 hours of physical activity with child daily ■ Family understanding of motor developmental milestones and importance of physical activity in childhood
■ More than 2 hours daily engaged in television or other screen activities ■ Limited community resources for childcare and physical activity ■ Unsafe neighborhood and lack of lawns, parks, and other facilities	■ Television and other screen activities limited to no more than 2 hours daily ■ Access to childcare that integrates physical activity ■ Safe neighborhood, with lawns, parks, and other facilities

including those with developmental disabilities. The preschooler learns to balance, balance and hop on one foot, skip, and throw and catch with greater accuracy. **Kinesthesia,** or the sense of one's body position and movement, develops during these years. Eye-hand coordination improves at the same time that visual acuity matures. The social component plays an important role as children learn to engage in games and activities cooperatively with others.

The nurse applies the concept of *resilience* by identifying both risk and protective factors related to physical activity (Table 11–4). The concept of resilience is explored in Chapter 5 ⊘. This assessment becomes the basis for nursing interventions, both to reinforce positive physical activity and to make recommendations for changes where needed. When the family has many responsibilities or lives in an unsafe neighborhood, suggest methods to integrate physical activity into daily life. Nurses working in inner-city settings help teachers to add physical activity to childcare center activities, and seek to keep schools open for toddler and preschool programs in early mornings and late afternoons and evenings. Soft beach balls and other items can be provided to assist the family in designing activities that foster the young child's physical capacities. Safety is always a concern. Nurses teach about safety gear, safe playground construction, and emergency care in case of injury. Encourage families to limit television and other "screen" activities like computers and video games to a total of no more than 2 hours daily. As these sedentary behaviors decrease, physical activity will naturally increase.

Children who have special healthcare needs often have particular physical activity limitations or requirements. The toddler or preschooler with diabetes may require glucose monitoring and insulin adjustment during activity (see Chapter 32 ⊘). The child with cystic fibrosis or asthma may need respiratory support or monitoring during exercise (see Chapter 25 ⊘). The child with a musculoskeletal abnormality may require special shoes or other devices to promote activity (see Chapter 35 ⊘ and Figure 11–3 ■). The nurse partners with the family to plan for the child's special health needs while engaging in physical activity.

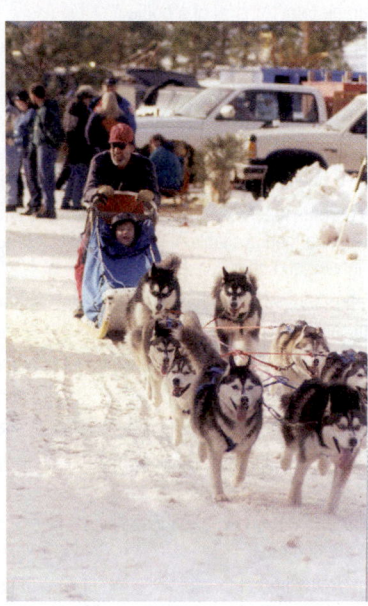

FIGURE 11–3 ■ Special events such as this dog sled ride for children with disabilities ensure that children experience movement and learn to enjoy physical activity.

Health promotion teaching imparts to parents the benefits of activity, such as healthy immune and cardiovascular systems, positive self-concept of the child, and the child's learning of important motor skills. Health maintenance teaching focuses on disease prevention, such as avoidance of overweight, and injury prevention, with use of protective gear for sports. Suggestions for the family may include setting guidelines to limit television and other screen activities to a maximum of 2 hours daily to facilitate adequate physical activity time. Children should not have television and computers in their bedrooms. Parents need encouragement to be active with their children and ideas for activities they can engage in together.

Expected outcomes of health promotion and health supervision related to physical activity are daily inclusion of at least 60 minutes of activity into life patterns, normal developmental progression of the musculoskeletal system, growth in coordination, and appropriate balance between dietary intake and physical activity so that normal weight is maintained.

ORAL HEALTH

The early childhood years play an important part in the child's future oral health, and yet dental care remains one of the most preventable and common unmet healthcare needs for children in developed countries. Dental caries have increased in the 2- to 5-year-old age group from 19% in the 1988–1994 National Health and Nutrition Examination Survey (NHANES) to 24% in the most recent survey (Centers for Disease Control and Prevention, 2009). **Early childhood caries (ECC)** is defined as one or more decayed, missing (due to caries), or filled tooth surfaces in a child less than 6 years of age (National Maternal & Child Oral Health Resource Center, 2010; Wagner & Oskouian, 2008). Former terms for this condition included "bottle mouth syndrome" or "baby bottle tooth decay." Caries occur when bacteria (often *Streptococcus mutans*) in the mouth metabolize food carbohydrates and produce acid. Acids promote loss of tooth minerals, leading to tooth deterioration. This condition is caused by inadequate preventive care, which can include diet, brushing, feeding habits, and lack of dental care. ECC is serious because young children with the condition are more likely to have continuing dental problems that can influence speech, cause pain, and delay development. Teaching prevention at an early age is key to preventing the problem. See Chapter 19 🔗 for further information about this condition (Box 11–3).

By 1 year of age the child should have made a first visit to the dentist. By about 2 years of age, the toddler has a full set of 20 teeth. Evaluate these teeth for condition and number. They help to maintain space for the permanent teeth, foster positive eating habits, and are needed for language development. Inquire about how the family cleans the teeth, and ask them to demonstrate if the child has any dental decay. At the end of preschool, the first of these **deciduous teeth** (primary teeth) are lost, an important developmental event for most children. (See Figure 7–26 in Chapter 7 🔗.)

By 2 to 4 years of age, young children should be discontinuing pacifiers and thumb sucking. These habits are harmful when

| BOX 11–3 | Research: Dental Care Needs |

While dental care has generally improved for the U.S. population, specific groups have more profound dental care needs. Trends demonstrate that dental sealant use has increased and caries have decreased in most children. However, caries in primary teeth of children 2 to 5 years are present in 25% of children. Much higher rates of decay are present in families with low income; two thirds of children from these families have caries and one quarter have untreated caries (Centers for Disease Control and Prevention, 2011). Hispanic families report much lower access to oral health resources and poorer oral health for their young children than Black or White families (Dietrich, Culler, Garcia, et al., 2008). Another group at risk of poor oral health is children with special healthcare needs; these children often experience unmet preventive and restorative care, and their major unmet need is oral care (Lewis, 2009).

In many community settings, nurses are influential in identifying families who may need dental care. Identification of resources for care, education about the importance of dental visits, and demonstration of home care are all needed. Such teaching should occur in all settings—homes, clinics, childcare settings, and schools. Of particular focus are children in homes with low incomes, ethnic minorities, and those with special healthcare needs.

permanent teeth begin erupting around 6 years of age. Parents should be instructed to gradually remove the pacifier by 1 to 2 years of age. Many young children continue to thumb suck, which is a comforting and reassuring habit. Usually the child who is 2 to 4 years is ready to discontinue thumb sucking, and parents can promote this process by praising the child for not sucking, helping the child to find alternative sources of comfort such as rubbing a blanket, putting a sock on the hand at nap or nighttime to serve as a reminder, and working with the preschooler to identify the reward when no thumb sucking is seen for a week or more (American Dental Association, 2011).

The nurse assists the family to ensure oral health for the young child. Some questions during the health promotion visit elicit important information:

- "How many teeth does your toddler have? Did they all come in without problems? What comfort measures have helped when he is teething? Do you have any concerns about his teeth?"
- "What is the source of your drinking water? Do you know if it is fluoridated? If not, does your child take fluoride? How much? How often?"
- "Describe how Cassandra's teeth get brushed and how often. Do you use toothpaste? What type? How much? Is it hard for you to afford toothbrushes?"
- "Are there any loose teeth?"
- "How much juice or sweetened drinks does Jim have each day? How does he drink these (bottle, cup)? How many sweet foods such as candy, gum, cookies, cake, and doughnuts are eaten daily?"
- "Has Jim been to the dentist? When was the last time? Do you have dental insurance? If not, do you have a resource for dental care or are financial concerns limiting dental visits?"

Based on the results of the assessment of the child's teeth, observation of language skills, and answers to questions directed at parents, plan interventions that will foster maintenance of oral health, thus preventing dental disease. (See Chapter 24 🔗 for emergency treatment of dental injury.) These may include referral to low-cost dental clinics, provision of a toothbrush and toothpaste, demonstration to the parents and young child about proper brushing technique, and teaching about limiting sweet snacks and drinks. Remember to positively reinforce health promotion practices such as good oral hygiene for toddlers and preschoolers who brush, visit the dentist, and are careful to limit intake of sweets. See Partnering with Families: Oral Care.

Desired outcomes for oral health are eruption of a normal set of deciduous teeth, regular dental care, nutrition and hygiene practices that foster dental health, and knowledge of child and parent about oral health.

MENTAL AND SPIRITUAL HEALTH

In Chapter 10 🔗, we examined the relationship between normal growth and development and the child's mental health. This relationship continues into the toddler and preschool years, since young children with a sense of security and self-worth generally grow and develop as expected. During the toddler and preschool years, the child develops a conscious sense of self through interactions with others and in play activities. Be sure the office or clinic setting is set up to provide space and activities for young children to promote a positive sense of self.

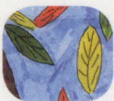

Partnering with Families

Oral Care

Ask parents to describe their child's oral hygiene practices, and enhance with teaching as needed. Recommendations of the American Dental Association include the following:

- Help the child to brush twice daily with a pea-sized amount of fluoride toothpaste, using a small, soft children's brush. Brush for the time it takes to think about the words to a favorite song such as the ABC song. The toddler and preschooler need help to brush for the proper time and to use the right amount of toothpaste. Be sure the child spits out the toothpaste to avoid ingesting too much fluoride which can discolor the teeth. Until about age 2 years, the child may not be able to spit out the toothpaste without swallowing it, in which case toothpaste without fluoride should be used.
- Once the child has two teeth together that are nearly touching, use dental floss once daily.
- Limit sweet snacks and drinks to once daily, followed by brushing.

Practice Alert

While toddlers and preschoolers are waiting for a health supervision visit, they should be in a pleasant setting with age-appropriate activities. As you visit various clinics and offices, evaluate the setting:

- Are the colors bright and yet restful?
- Are there books for young children, child-sized chairs and tables, crayons, paper, and other activities provided?
- Can parents sit and observe the child in play activities?
- Is the setting safe, without hazards such as glass that can be pulled down and break, sharp corners, or access to the street or other unsafe places?
- Are there stimulating surroundings that include a variety of items to look at and things to do?
- Can surfaces and toys be easily cleaned to discourage transfer of microorganisms?

The family is key in fostering a positive self-image and setting the stage for the child's mental health. As the family is called in for the visit, begin your assessment of the family's methods of influencing mental health.

- Do parents communicate readily with the child?
- Are interactions generally warm, caring, and loving, or are there constant criticisms of behavior?
- Do the parents seem willing to point out the child's accomplishments, or do they have trouble making any positive statements about the child?
- Does the child appear at ease with the parents? Is the child at ease in the healthcare setting? Toddlers often still have some stranger anxiety and may show discomfort, whereas preschoolers are more often eager and excited to meet you.

Next ask for a description of a typical day or what the child has recently begun to do. The child's sense of self and mental status are related to new accomplishments. Inquire about toilet training, toothbrushing, choosing clothes and getting dressed, using crayons, or other developmental tasks. See the Denver II Developmental Test in Chapter 8 and a list of tasks in Chapter 5 . Direct questions or comments to the child. If the toddler or preschooler appears nervous or shy, return to questioning the parent and quietly offer a toy or book to the child. Once the nurse appears to be trusted by the parent, rapport can often be established with the child.

Toddlers and preschoolers use self-regulation (the ability to soothe and comfort the self) to control anger, excessive desires for objects or foods, and other nonsocial behaviors. To assist the child in developing the ability to control and regulate self, parents often use discipline techniques. Ask about how the parent responds to the child who is having a temper tantrum or showing other undesirable behaviors. Reinforce positive ways of helping the child set limits for self, and make suggestions when parents need assistance. Spanking or other physical forms of discipline are not more effective than less physical methods and can have negative outcomes, such as increased child aggression and anger (American Academy of Pediatrics [AAP], 2011a). Share principles that can be used for positive limit setting, such as time-out, logical consequences of behavior, and withholding privileges (AAP, 2011a). Model positive limit setting when the child is in the office. "Oh, here's a book you can look at. This instrument on the wall is just for the nurse to use." (See Partnering with Families: Positive Discipline, and Evidence-Based Practice: Discipline.) The goal of discipline is to help the child develop a sense of right and wrong and to learn acceptable ways of dealing with other people. Help parents of the toddler with temper tantrums to learn specific management techniques for these behaviors. (See Partnering with Families: Handling Temper Tantrums.) Continued and extremely disruptive behavior should be referred to a mental health specialist, as there may be underlying causes such as disturbed family issues or childhood depression (Belden, Thomson, & Luby, 2008; Degnan, Calkins, Keane, et al., 2008).

Adequate sleep and rest are needed for children to master self-regulation. Most toddlers and preschoolers have established regular sleeping patterns with occasional night awakenings. They sleep about 8 to 12 hours at night with one or two daytime naps; naps decrease with movement into the preschool years (Hagan, Shaw, & Duncan, 2008; Murray, Zentner, & Yakimo, 2009). Some quiet playtime in the afternoon can be beneficial, even for the preschooler who does not nap. Parents have usually learned to establish clear sleep routines such as reading a story, rubbing a back, and then leaving the child alone. Occasionally parents who work during the day may feel guilty about putting the child to bed early in the evening. Encourage them to spend quality time with the child after arriving home, and then to establish clear sleeping expectations. Transitional objects such as blankets or toys are important for the toddler and can be used during childcare experiences to provide comfort and help maintain normal routines. Some parents prefer to have children sleep in the bed with them. If this is the parents' decision, be sure they are aware of safety hazards such as suffocation in excessive bedding, injury related to falling between headboard and frame, parental smoking that could lead to fire, or parental deep sleeping or alcohol and drug use, which can lead to being so soundly asleep that rolling onto and suffocating the young child is possible.

During early childhood years, some children develop awakenings at night and may need some assistance in falling back to sleep.

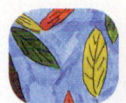

Partnering with Families

Positive Discipline

TO PROVIDE STRUCTURE THAT ENHANCES THE POSSIBILITY OF DESIRABLE BEHAVIORS:

- Limit rules to those that are essential. It is easier to enforce a few important rules than many that are nonessential.
- Provide an environment where the child is mainly free to explore safely in order to avoid constant cautions. For example, have adequate play space for toddlers with limited fragile glassware in the usual daily environment. It is easier for the toddler to learn not to touch a few objects when adequate objects are provided for play.
- Spend time interacting with the child several times each day. Praise positive behaviors frequently. Preschoolers often like to have charts with stars to record picking up toys, helping a parent, and performing other positive behaviors. Once preschoolers obtain a certain number of stars, they earn a reward such as stickers or an outing with the parent.

WHEN THE CHILD SHOWS UNDESIRABLE BEHAVIORS:

- Use distraction as the first approach and praise the child for selecting the new activity suggested by the parent.
- Tell the child one time that the behavior is unsatisfactory and what will happen if the behavior persists.

- Separate the child from a setting in which behavior is undesirable. Place the child in "time-out," a separate place that is safe. Toddlers can be placed in a playpen or crib, while preschoolers are told to sit on a chair. One minute of time-out per year of age is a good length of time. Once time-out is over, provide a positive activity and move the child directly toward the activity.

WHEN UNDESIRABLE BEHAVIORS INCLUDE OTHER PEOPLE, SUCH AS BITING OR HITTING:

- Tell the child clearly that it is not appropriate to hurt another person.
- Separate the child immediately from the situation and use time-out.
- If there are repeated episodes, be sure the child is getting adequate sleep and food, has opportunities for active play that releases energy, and has positive attention from many people in the environment. Be sensitive to stresses such as a recent trauma or a new sibling.
- Encourage children to "use words" instead of hitting or biting. Until able to do so on their own, parents can model this behavior. "You feel like saying 'I am really upset that you took my toy away.' Let's use words instead of hitting so your sister knows that."

Nightmares are frightening dreams that awaken the child who is often crying and upset. Parents can reassure the child, rub the child's back, provide some repeat of a bedtime routine such as reading a story, and then allow the child to settle into sleep again. It is not advisable to bring the child to the parental bed because the child may start to awaken at night to continue this practice. **Night terrors** are characterized by a child who cries out, appears frightened, and has tachycardia and tachypnea. However, in contrast to nightmares, the child having a night terror is not fully awake and may appear disoriented (Murray et al., 2009). Parents should quietly talk to and comfort the child, allowing the child to return to sleep. There is no recollection of these events the next morning.

The toddler gains more independence in many aspects of life such as mobility and speech. Control over toileting is another milestone that signals greater independence and can lead to a sense of self-control. Ask parents if the toddler has shown interest in toilet training and how they intend to work with the child to attain control over bowel and bladder. See Partnering with Families: Toilet Training, and refer to Chapter 5 🔗 for further discussion of readiness for toilet training.

Preschoolers are generally well trained for bowel and bladder with only occasional accidents. These should be treated with understanding rather than blame in order for healthy self-concept to develop. Preschoolers are increasingly aware of gender and sexuality issues. They may ask questions about kissing, love, or their

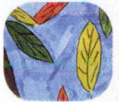

Partnering with Families

Handling Temper Tantrums

Temper tantrums are common in toddlers and are manifested as episodes of screaming, crying, pounding objects, kicking, and otherwise showing anger. Toddlers may be expressing frustration with something that has occurred. They have learned that they are independent individuals and have an effect by showing their dismay. Temper tantrums should gradually decrease in number as the child grows into the preschool years. Parents can learn that although tantrums are normal, techniques exist that can assist in handling them successfully. The approaches are similar to those used when the child bites or hits. Some specific suggestions for tantrums include:

- Learn the signals that a tantrum is about to occur. Most toddlers become increasingly agitated and upset. Touching, holding, and distracting them at that point may help avoid a tantrum.
- Do not respond to minor anger that includes crying and screaming.

- Separate the child from others with a time-out equivalent to 1 minute/year of child's age.
- Leave public places to return home or to a quiet setting.
- Be sure the child is safe and not throwing self against objects that could cause injury.
- Remain calm, holding the child firmly still if needed.
- Talk calmly to the child, verbalizing his or her feelings and what the child needs to do to calm down. Firmly state that "no hitting" or other harmful behavior is allowed.
- Reward the child briefly after control is gained. "It was really good that you could calm down and say you were sorry. Now let's go back to the living room."

Source: *Adapted from American Academy of Pediatrics. (2011b). What should I do when my child has a temper tantrum? Retrieved from http://healthychildren.org*

Evidence-Based Practice   Discipline

PROBLEM

All parents have to discipline their children. Although physical measures such as spanking are not recommended, many parents believe that is the best technique to use. Immigrant families bring both their cultural influences and present challenges to their parenting repertoire, and nurses may be unaware of how to assess or work with such families.

EVIDENCE

In a nursing study of the relationship between Korean immigrant family discipline techniques and children's behavior, harsh discipline by fathers was associated with behavior problems in their children (Kim, Guo, Koh, et al., 2010). In a study of Turkish immigrant families, toddlers with challenging temperament characteristics, such as high activity and difficulty in soothing, were adversely affected by harsh parenting techniques (Yaman, Mesman, van IJzendoorn, et al., 2010). A study of Chinese immigrant families showed that parental belief in the importance of control over the child and cultural distress in adapting to a new life in the United States were associated with more physical discipline (Lau, 2010).

IMPLICATIONS

The American Academy of Pediatrics classifies discipline as *positive* when hugging and praising are used for desired behaviors; *appropriate* when distraction,

time-out, or ignoring are used for undesirable behaviors; and *harsh* when physical discipline and loud verbalizations and harsh criticisms are used (Kim et al., 2010). Parents need assistance to learn positive and appropriate techniques. Ask them what things the child does well and help them select rewards such as special attention at those times. Suggest that they praise the child for desirable behaviors, such as "I really like it when you pick up your toys. Great job." Have them devise a chart with the preschool-age child and place a star whenever a desired behavior, such as kindness to a sibling or friend, is displayed. The child and parent agree that a certain number of stars will result in a reward, such as watching a movie together or going to a favorite restaurant. Parents who use or have used corporal punishment need information about the potential for injury to the child and fostering of violence in the child; they will need many suggestions for positive ways to discipline the child.

CRITICAL THINKING

What questions can you ask to determine the discipline techniques a family uses? How can you provide information about the recommended use of positive and appropriate discipline?

---

genitals. These questions should be truthfully answered, leaving the child with a positive sense of sexuality. Exploration of genitals can occur, and children should be told simply that it is something that should take place in private; offer other activities to engage them when with other people.

For some toddlers or preschoolers, extraordinary stresses can cause challenges to mental health. Traumatic events such as witnessing or being involved in a car crash or losing a parent to death have profound effects on young children. If it is learned during a health supervision visit that a toddler or preschooler has experienced a severe trauma or has

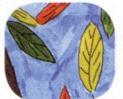

Partnering with Families

Toilet Training

When are children ready to learn toileting? Are parents responsible for the differences in ages at which toilet training is accomplished? Does toilet training provide clues to a child's intellectual ability?

Most children are ready to begin toilet training from 2 to $2\frac{1}{2}$ years of age. We know that children are not ready for toilet training until several developmental capabilities exist: to stand and walk well, to pull pants up and down, and to recognize the need to eliminate and then be able to wait until in the bathroom. The child stays dry for more than 2 hours, follows simple instructions, and displays interest in toileting activities. Once this readiness is apparent, parents can start preparation for toileting. At about 18 months of age, words for elimination (such as "pee" or "potty") are introduced to the child. Then a few months later, the child can be given a small potty chair and the procedure can be explained. Suggest the parent or caregiver read books or watch videos with the child that explain toileting. Having the child select new "big boy" or "big girl" underwear can be an incentive.

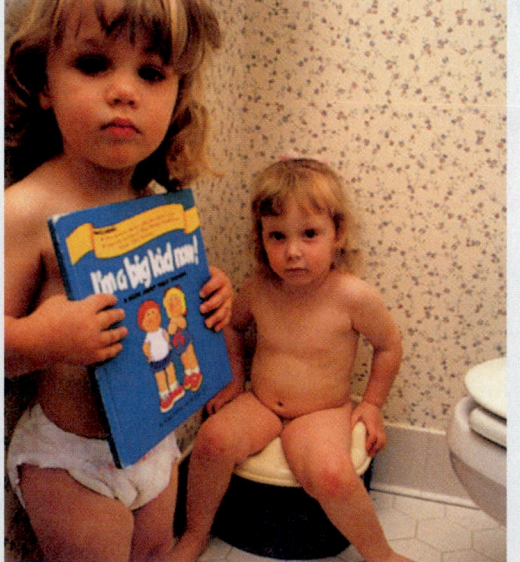

Children often prefer their own chair on the floor to using the large toilet. The child should be placed on the chair at regular intervals for a few moments and can be given a reward or praise for successes. If the child seems not to understand or does not wish to cooperate, it is best to wait a few weeks and then try again. Watching other children using the potty chair or toilet can assist. Just as all of development is subject to individual timetables, toilet training occurs with considerable variability from one child to another. Identify for parents the developmental characteristics of their child and encourage them to appreciate without anxiety the unfolding of skills. These timetables are not predictive of future development.

The child who is ill or hospitalized or has other stress often regresses in toilet-training activities. It is best to quietly reinstitute attempts at training after the trauma. Potty chairs should be available on pediatric units and toileting habits identified during initial assessment so that regular routines can be followed and the child's usual words for elimination can be used.

ongoing stress, refer the family to specialized services such as psychiatric and mental health experts for care. See Chapter 34 🔗 for further descriptions of these challenges to mental health.

In all families, toddlers and preschoolers are learning about moral codes, what is right and wrong, and the rules that guide behaviors. (See Chapter 5 🔗 for further description of moral development in young children.) The family's spiritual orientation takes on additional meaning for the toddler and preschooler. They can participate in the family's faith-based practices, which enlarge their microsystem influences to include that of the religious group, thus reinforcing the child's learning about right and wrong. The nurse assesses the family's faith-based or spiritual beliefs and provides support for the family's approach, whether it occurs in established religious organizations or in the family's other meaningful activities.

Identify strengths and risks in the mental and spiritual health of toddlers and preschoolers. Examples of strengths include:

- The child has adapted positively to both family and childcare routines.
- The toddler is generally able to quiet within a few moments after a temper tantrum.
- The preschooler is showing increasing ability to identify undesirable behavior and readily goes to time-out when needed.
- Family patterns have established a sleep routine that is working well and providing adequate rest for the child.
- Parents have time each day to spend individually with their children, and they provide much positive feedback for desirable behaviors.
- The family attends regular faith-based or spiritual activities meaningful to them.

Risk factors that may indicate the need for more teaching and problem solving with the family include:

- Parents express frustration that the toddler is often not able to sleep through the night.
- The preschooler frequently awakens with night terrors.
- The child was recently in a car accident.
- The preschooler is having several episodes daily at the childcare center of biting or hitting other children.
- Parents commonly spank the child for undesirable behaviors but report that the behaviors are increasing.
- Parents express interest in having others help the child learn right from wrong but do not have ideas about how to access such assistance.

Health promotion activities focus on development of a healthy self-concept in the toddler and young child by helping parents to set up successful play experiences, to praise the child for successes, to use effective limit-setting techniques, and to realize and appreciate the child's unique characteristics. Health maintenance seeks to avoid poor self-image that can occur with constant criticism or expectations not in alignment with the toddler or preschooler developmental capabilities. Further examples of family interactions that can influence the child's self-concept are provided in the following section on relationships.

Desired outcomes for the child related to mental and spiritual health include emergence of a positive self-esteem, ability to self-regulate behaviors, emergence of methods to handle daily stressors, and normal developmental progression in tasks such as toilet training and sleep.

RELATIONSHIPS

As described by Bronfenbrenner's ecologic theory (see Chapter 5 🔗), family members are part of the microsystem for the toddler and preschooler. They form a vital part of the child's environment. Families with members who handle stress well and have healthy lifestyle patterns offer security for the young child. As described in Chapter 10 🔗, when parents are stressed or depressed, the mental status of all family members can be affected. Ask how things are going for the family in general. Inquire about siblings and whether there are any issues of concern that might influence the toddler or preschooler. Illness or behavior problems in a sibling can decrease the parent's ability to deal with other children. The focus on a sibling in need can be confusing to a toddler or preschooler. See Chapter 15 🔗 for further information about concerns of children who have a sibling hospitalized.

Ask about the ages of siblings and the relationships among siblings in the family. Parents may have questions about sibling rivalry, as young children may not always interact positively with brothers and sisters. Sibling rivalry may occur when there is a sense of competition among children, particularly when they are close in age. Rivalry is more common during stressful times, when a child is sick or tired, or when one child gets special privileges. Parents can set an example about fairness and methods to work out issues. Guidelines about unacceptable behavior (physical violence, name-calling, or loud noise) should be clear. Negotiation and other talking skills can be modeled. Parents should also provide quiet time to be alone with each child and should avoid comparing children to each other (AAP, 2011c, 2011d). Preparing the young child with pictures and activities that teach about a coming baby can facilitate the introduction of a new baby into the family (Murray et al., 2009).

Young children often have difficulty distinguishing between reality and their own thinking, making lying or dishonesty possible. They may respond "No" or "I don't know" to questions about whether they did something wrong, in order to avoid punishment or displeasing the parent. Parents should talk about honesty and praise the child for telling the truth, even when they admit to doing wrong. Teach them that there is a penalty for lying such as being in "time out" or not participating in a desired activity.

Mental health issues, discussed in the preceding section, often relate directly to family members. As you inquire about discipline techniques and whether there has been violence in the family or neighborhood, realize that these family-related events can have a profound influence on the child. Be alert for signs of child abuse and for substance abuse in family members. See Chapter 20 🔗 for further discussion of both child abuse and substance abuse. Have the parents become separated or divorced? Is there a new stepparent?

Clinical Tip

Children may experience stress, sadness, and loss when parents become separated or divorced. Identify both the risk and protective factors when a family experiences separation or divorce. Ask parents to identify things that are stressful for the child, such as changes in living situation or being present during fighting. Ask also what positive outcomes there are for the family, such as increased time with the custodial parent, decreased parental stress, and no fighting. Parents who can cooperate in planning for the children are able to surround the children with more support from parents, grandparents, stepparents, and siblings. Assist parents to access resources that will enhance their ability to ensure strong parenting and family relationships for their children (Yu, Pettit, Lansford, et al., 2010).

During questions and observations, the nurse identifies family risks and protective factors. Reinforce strengths and provide services and referrals to deal with risks. Strengths include:

- The family spends time together each day.
- Parents are proud of the child's accomplishments and knowledgeable about developmental progression.
- Childcare center personnel and family members interact regularly to plan consistent approaches for the toddler and preschooler.
- The teen mother of a toddler is enrolled in a high school continuation program with a childcare component.

Examples of risks to mental health include:

- A parent is diagnosed with depression.
- A relative in the home uses street drugs.
- The child awakens with night terrors.

- The teen mother is estranged from her own family and has few goals and resources.

Temperament of the toddler and preschooler plays an important part in how they respond to people and events, and how others perceive them. Remember that the child is usually classified as primarily easy, difficult, or slow to warm up (see Box 5–2: Patterns of Temperament on page 120 🔗). The concept of goodness of fit with the environment still warrants consideration. If there was a good fit between the infant and expectations of those in the surroundings, the fit may change as the child grows older. For example, most people appreciate "easy" infants because they are generally positive, adaptable, and regular in routines. However, in some families there may be a value on independent behaviors as children grow into toddlerhood and preschool age. Parents who were pleased with the infant's temperament may not value the same characteristics in the preschooler; they might prefer the child to be more outgoing and

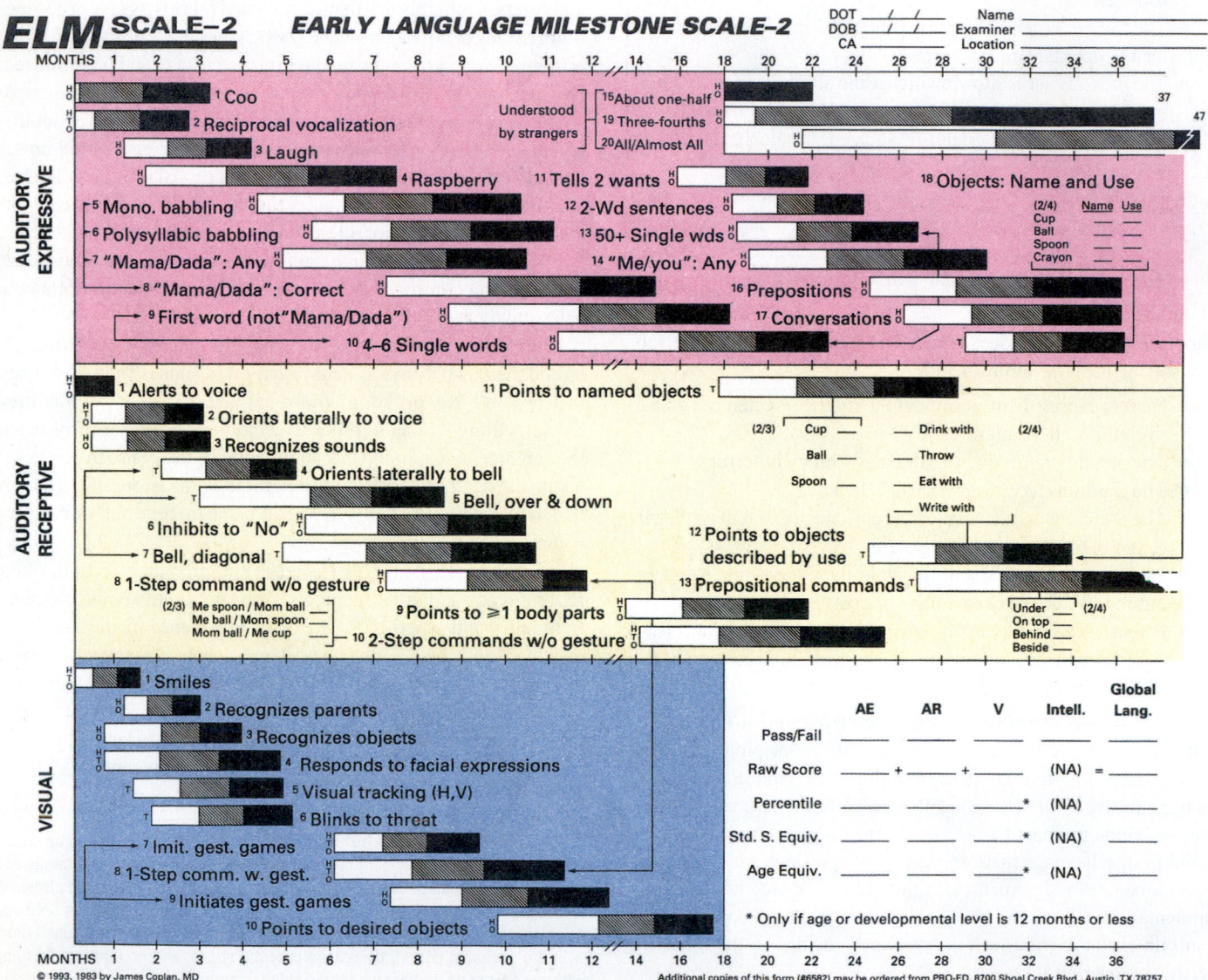

FIGURE 11–4 ■ The Early Language Milestone (ELM) Scale is one method of evaluating speech in young children. It differentiates receptive from expressive speech, recognizing that children may understand some language even though they do not speak to their level of understanding. Examine this tool to see what receptive and expressive language you would expect to see in 15-month-old Clarence in the opening scenario.

Source: *Used with permission from Slossen Educational Publications, Inc.* The Early Language Milestone (ELM) Scale.

less accepting of changes in others. Assist parents in identifying their child's characteristic temperament and learning to appreciate it. They may need help to structure the difficult child's environment to establish routines to facilitate more regular schedules, or the slow-to-warm-up child's environment to provide more time to adapt to new settings and care providers.

Toddlers continue to grow in social abilities, while preschoolers demonstrate large strides in socializing with others. Expect that most toddlers will enjoy playing with other children, although they play "side by side" and not cooperatively. They also engage in play with adults for short periods, such as throwing a ball. On the other hand, preschoolers begin to engage in activities that involve other children directly. They play "house," with one child playing the mother or father, and another the child. They engage in simple games where each plays a separate role. Their interactions with adults display similar maturity as they take on tasks such as setting the table for dinner or picking up books from the floor. Social skills involve getting along with others. Ask the parents how this child does with siblings or other children. Although a few arguments are common, a growing ability to share toys and communicate with others is expected. Ask parents about the child's favorite activities with other children. Preschoolers are usually able to name their best friend and what they like to play together. See Chapter 5 🔾 for a thorough description of the developmental social activity of toddlers and preschoolers.

Young children exhibit increasing skill in language development, a primary medium for social exchange. Recall that the child has both receptive and expressive communication skills. In the receptive domain, the 1-year-old can follow a simple command, the 2-year-old follows a two-step command, and the 3-year-old can understand and follow conversations. In the expressive domain, from just a few words at 1 year, the child has progressed to two-word statements at 2 years, and to stating three-word sentences by 3 years of age. Although all parts of speech are not in place, preschool children certainly have the ability to make needs and thoughts known. Assessment of language skills provides a mirror into this important means of socializing. One example of a language screening tool is the Early Language Milestone Scale (Figure 11–4 ■). The Denver II Developmental Screening Test

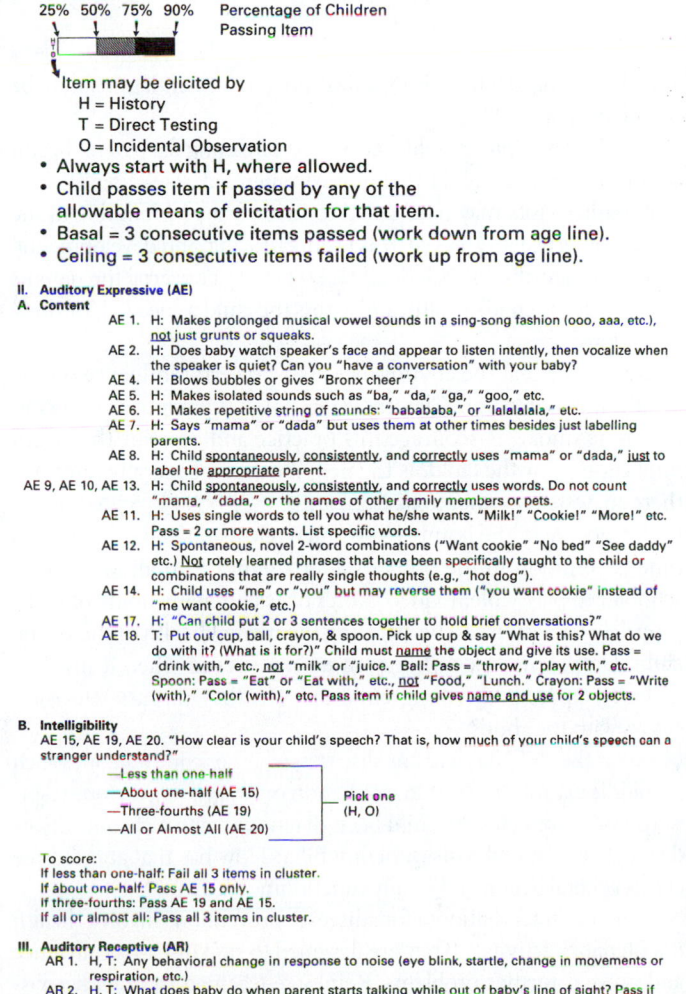

FIGURE 11–4 ■ (Continued) The Early Language Milestone (ELM) Scale.

BOX 11–4	Stuttering

All children have some episodes of **dysfluency,** or a disruption in the smooth transition between sounds, syllables, and words. Examples include repeating a word or phrase or inserting sounds such as "um" in sentences. This "developmental stuttering" generally abates gradually in the early years. Occasionally it persists and becomes accompanied by other behaviors such as frowning, blinking, or squeezing the eyes. The child with persistent or worsening stuttering or associated behaviors should be referred to a speech and language pathologist, who can best perform assessment and effective interventions. Intervention at an early age (before 4 years) is most effective in decreasing stuttering behaviors (Prasse & Kikano, 2008).

TABLE 11–5 Routine Immunizations Recommended During Toddlerhood and Preschool Age

IMMUNIZATION	AGE RECOMMENDED
Hepatitis B	6–18 months: Administer #3 if series not completed during infancy
Hepatitis A	Series of 2 doses with first at 12 months and second at least 6 months later
Diphtheria, tetanus, pertussis	15–18 months (#4)
	4–6 years (#5)
Haemophilus influenzae type b	12–15 months (#4 or will be #3 for PRP-OMP type that requires only 3 doses for whole series)
Inactivated poliovirus	4–6 years (#4)
Measles, mumps, rubella	12–15 months (#1)
Varicella	12–18 months (#1)
	4–6 years (#2)
Pneumococcal	12–15 months (#4)
Influenza	Annually from 6–23 months

Note: Schedule may need to be adapted if child did not receive all recommended immunizations during infancy. See the Centers for Disease Control and Prevention and the American Academy of Pediatrics websites for recommended catch-up schedules. Also see Chapter 22 for further information about immunization schedules.

described in Chapter 8 🖉 also has a language component. As the child nears school entry, communication skills should be assessed again. By that time, the child should be easy to understand, use plurals appropriately, answer questions with ease, and interact readily with others. These skills are necessary for success in kindergarten classrooms. School readiness tools include language components as parts of their testing. Recognize that children who speak a different language at home from that in the dominant culture may need extra time to learn language skills. (See Chapter 6 🖉 for detailed information about working with families when they have a primary language other than English.) When children display slow language development or problems such as stuttering they should be referred to a language specialist (Box 11–4).

Successful social skills involve separating from the parent at times. During toddlerhood, most children spend some time away from parents. Initially, they may be fearful and display crying, but gradually they learn to adapt to the new person and place. Preschoolers need to begin developing relationships with other adults and children in order to adapt to the school setting at about 5 years of age. Ask how many people the child has contact with each week and how the child manages separation from the parent. Encourage parents to see separation as a skill the child is learning rather than something that is guilt-producing for them. When they leave the child in a secure setting, they should hug, provide a favorite object, and leave. Short periods initially will teach the child that the parent can be trusted to return.

Expected outcomes of health promotion and health maintenance activities with young children include increasing social skills with parents, siblings, and other children and adults; successfully managing temperament characteristics; adjusting to time away from the home; and improving language/communication skills.

DISEASE PREVENTION STRATEGIES

Toddlers remain prone to many infectious diseases due to immature immune systems and limited previous exposure to a variety of infections. By the preschool age, immune defenses are more mature and communicable diseases are less common. Some immunizations are given during this age period to complete the basic series. For the child who has not had all immunizations, extra visits to catch up to recommended levels may be needed. At the end of the preschool period, the child has a complete review of the immunization record so any needed injections are given before school entry. See Table 11–5 for immunizations recommended during toddlerhood

and preschool; detailed immunization recommendations can be found in Chapter 22 🖉.

Toddlers and preschoolers also need screening for several health conditions. See Table 11–6 for recommended screening at each visit. Earlier visits may have failed to identify a problem due to the child's young age, so areas such as vision, hearing, and developmental milestones are always included. Ascertain any concerns the parents have about the child's health, and assess the child as needed for these conditions.

Recognize that the environment is a powerful influence on the health of children (see Chapter 20 🖉). Ask if parents or others in the home smoke. Discourage this practice and describe the health implications for the child. Is the neighborhood generally safe? Are there air, water, or other toxic exposures? (See Box 11–5.) Ask about lead exposure in the home. How much television and other screen time is common in the home? Older siblings who allow the preschooler to play violent video games or watch many hours of inappropriate television can be affecting the mental health of the young child. Do parents watch the evening news, even when it involves violence, in front of young children? Do they discuss television shows with the child?

Ask if the child has had any diseases, whether common ones such as middle ear infection, or less common ones such as a serious respiratory infection. Has the child been diagnosed with a chronic disorder such as cystic fibrosis or hemophilia? How has that affected the child's general health and family functioning?

Nursing interventions for disease prevention involve health maintenance activities. They are designed to stop disease occurrence and prevent further problems. Reinforce teaching from earlier visits about recognition of infectious disease, particularly if the child

TABLE 11–6	Screening During Health Promotion and Health Maintenance Visits
AGE	**RECOMMENDED SCREENING TESTS**
15 months	Vision
	Hearing
	Anemia (if not previously done)
	Tuberculosis (if at risk)
	Teeth present and condition
	Physical examination with special attention to skin, gait, bruising, and other signs of possible abuse
	Developmental milestones
	Dietary screening
	Review immunization record
18 months	Continue screening listed above
2–3 years	Continue screening listed above
	Language development
	Lead exposure risk
	Hyperlipidemia risk
3–4 years	Continue screening listed above
	Blood pressure
	Behavioral abnormalities
4–5 years	Continue screening listed above
	Dental malocclusion problems

Source: *Adapted from Hagan, J. F., Shaw, J. S., & Duncan, P. M. (Eds.). (2008).* Bright futures: Guidelines for health supervision of infants, children, and adolescents *(3rd ed.). Elk Grove Village, IL: American Academy of Pediatrics.*

is in a new setting for childcare or other activities. Provide sources for clean water and information about food safety if these seem to be areas of concern. Draw blood for lead screening if the child is exposed to lead sources. Give the immunizations recommended for the age of the child. If parents smoke, review the possible problematic effects on young children such as increased incidence of otitis media and asthma. Refer parents who wish to quit smoking to resources for cessation. Recommend that children not be exposed to more than 2 hours of television or other screen activities each day. Teach parents

BOX 11–5	Research: The Children's Health Study

The Children's Health Study is a large longitudinal study of children across the United States, designed to identify long-term effects of environmental factors on child growth, development, and health. The study began in 1992 with a focus on air pollution effects on California children. Reduced lung development in children exposed to high amounts of particulate contaminants was observed, although children improved if they moved to other communities. A wide range of natural and human-caused environmental conditions such as air, water, diet, sound, family dynamics, community, cultural influences, and genetics are being studied (Children's Health Study, 2011). Nurses should understand the environmental influences in the areas where they work and tailor teaching in healthcare visits to minimize them. Are there days with unsafe air in your community? What is the rate of radon, lead, or other hazardous substances in homes? What are the positive community influences?

to avoid violent shows and video games, to watch television with the child, and to discuss programs together. Emphasize the importance of not installing television, computer, or game machines in the young child's bedroom.

The results of the examination should be summarized for parents. They need to know the normal findings and whether there are concerns that will need further evaluation. Provide time for parents to ask questions about health conditions. Verify that they have financial resources and transportation to continue obtaining health care for the child. Now that visits are further apart, write down the next recommended appointment date, arrange for a telephone reminder, and provide the phone and contact information for questions or emergencies that may occur in the interim.

Desired outcomes for disease prevention include integration of prevention methods into the family's daily lives, prompt treatment of acute conditions, and individualization of all health supervision topics for the child with a chronic condition or special healthcare need.

INJURY PREVENTION STRATEGIES

Injuries remain a common healthcare problem for children during the toddler and preschooler years. The child's mobility, physical skills, and lack of understanding about the presence of hazards put the child at particular risk. In addition, children are sometimes left to play alone for short periods, and toddlers and preschoolers can quickly get into dangerous situations. Every healthcare visit needs to include an assessment of risks and teaching to prevent injuries. Tables 11–7 and 11–8 list injury hazards during these age periods.

Ask parents to name the most common hazards for the age of their child, and add other hazards to their awareness. Reinforce car safety, as the types of seats change when the child reaches 20 lb and then 40 lb. Be certain that parents provide children from 20 to 40 lb the following:

- A convertible forward-facing seat that has been placed in the back seat
- Harness straps at or above the shoulders

Toddlers and preschoolers should be in an appropriate seat for their size:

- In the back seat
- That uses both lap and shoulder belts
- With the lap belt low and tight across the lap/upper thigh area and shoulder belt snug across the chest and shoulder

Recommend that parents have their car seat checked by a childcare inspector. Give them the addresses of the closest inspection stations, which you can locate through the National Highway Traffic Safety Administration. Check your particular state laws regulating car safety seats for children (Figure 11–5 ■).

Other common and serious safety hazards are falls and drowning. In addition to providing general guidelines about safety, these most common injuries should be directly addressed. Children often fall down stairs, from counters where they have been placed or crawled, and from grocery carts. Drowning episodes occur when toddlers and preschoolers are not watched every moment while in the bathtub,

TABLE 11–7   **Injury Prevention in Toddlerhood**

	HAZARD	DEVELOPMENTAL CHARACTERISTICS	PREVENTIVE MEASURES
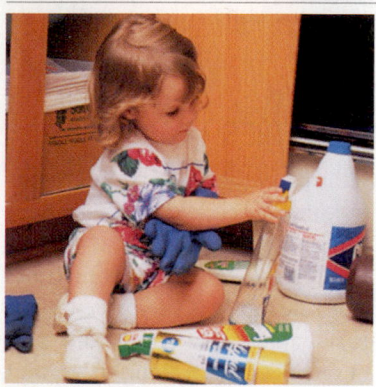	Falls	Gross motor skills improve. Toddler is able to move chairs to counters and can climb up ladders.	Supervise toddler closely. Provide safe climbing toys. Begin to teach acceptable places for climbing.
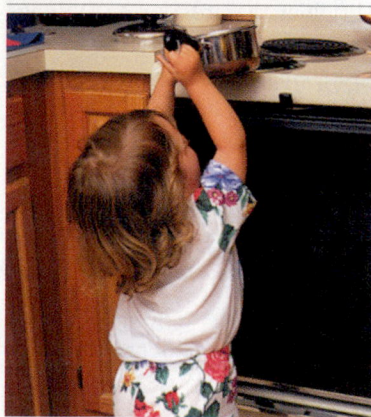	Poisoning	Gross motor skills enable toddler to climb onto chairs and then cabinets. Medicines, cosmetics, and other poisonous substances are easily reached. Some chemical substances that are poisonous can look like sports drinks to young children.	Keep medicines and other poisonous material locked away. Use child-resistant containers and cupboard closures. Post the poison control center number (1-800-222-1222) by every telephone and program it into cell phones. (See Chapter 20 for comprehensive information about poisons.)
	Burns	Toddler is tall enough to reach stove top. Toddler can walk to fireplace and may reach into fire.	Keep pot handles turned inward on stove. Do not burn fires without close supervision. Use a fire screen.
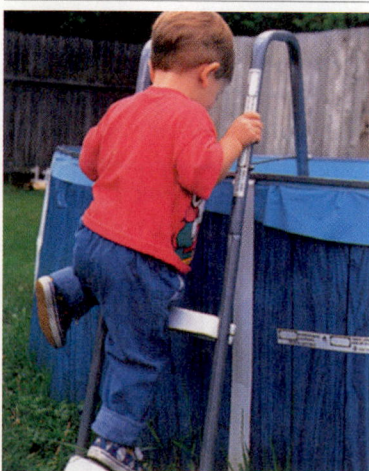	Drowning	Toddler can walk onto docks or pool decks. Toddler may stand on or climb seats on boat. Toddler may fall into buckets, toilets, and fish tanks and be unable to get top of body out.	Supervise any child near water. Swimming classes do not protect a toddler from drowning. Use child-resistant pool and spa covers. Use approved child life jackets near water and on boats. Empty buckets when not in use.
	Motor vehicle crashes	Toddler may be able to undo seat belt, may resist using car seat, demonstrating characteristic negativism and autonomy.	Insist on car safety seat use for all trips. Use approved safety seat only. Keep the child in a rear-facing seat until 2 years of age or until achieving the highest weight or height recommended for the seat by the manufacturer.

TABLE 11–8 Injury Prevention in the Preschool Years

	HAZARDS	DEVELOPMENTAL CHARACTERISTICS	PREVENTIVE MEASURES
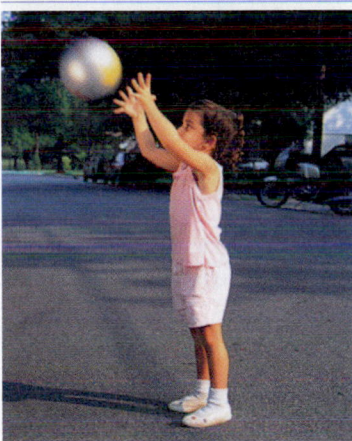	Motor vehicle crashes	Older preschooler independently gets into car and puts on seat belt. Child may forget to belt up or may do so incorrectly.	Verify that the child is belted in properly before starting car. Car seats and booster seats should be placed in the back seat. Child restraint systems must be used until the child is 57 inches tall (8–12 years of age) and can safely use regular car safety belts.
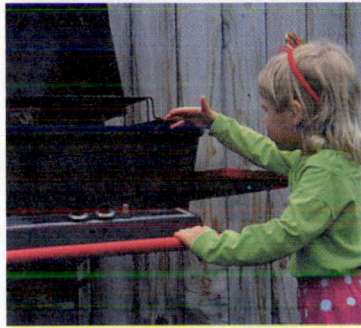	Motor vehicle and pedestrian accidents	Preschooler increasingly plays outside alone or with friends. Preschooler is unable to judge speed of moving car and assumes driver knows that he or she is present.	Teach the child never to go into the road. A safe, preferably enclosed, play yard is recommended. The child should be supervised at all times.
	Drowning	Preschooler who has had swimming lessons may choose to go into a lake or pool.	Teach the child never to go into water without an adult. Provide supervision whenever the child is near water.
	Burns	Preschooler can understand the hazards of fire. Children often find matches and lighters fascinating.	Instruct the child in the dangers of matches, lighters, and similar items. Teach the child to stop, drop, and roll if clothes are on fire. Practice escapes from home are useful. A visit to a fire station can reinforce learning. Teach the child how to call 911.
	Needlesticks in hospital	Preschooler can ambulate and is interested in new objects.	Keep needles out of reach. Remove from unit immediately after use.
	Electrical injury in hospital	Preschooler is mobile and may trip over cords and equipment or may choose to examine them.	Avoid use of electrical cords if possible. Keep equipment out of major traffic areas. Cover any electrical outlets not being used for equipment. Monitor the child closely.

near a pool or spa, at a lake or ocean, or when they fall from boats without personal flotation devices on. Although all young children should begin to take swimming lessons, this does not guarantee their safety around water. Children play with balls and may follow them as they roll or are thrown into the street. Fenced yards and constant supervision are needed.

Geographic areas should be considered. Urban dwelling may increase the chance of exposure to air pollutants. Rural life may be accompanied by exposure to insecticides or by activities with machinery that lead to injuries. Ask about a typical day for the child to identify potential hazards in the environment. Nursing interventions concentrate on relaying to parents the severity of the risk of falls, environmental exposures, drowning, and other hazards for children.

Teach parents to be aware of the dangers and to avoid them, both at home and in other settings. Refer them to classes on first aid and cardiopulmonary resuscitation.

Clinical Tip

A number of young children die each year when they are left confined in parked vehicles. Occasionally children gain access to a vehicle and accidentally lock themselves inside. However, in most cases a parent leaves a child unattended, either forgetting the child is in the car, or remembering but underestimating the danger of heat effects. Nurses can be effective in instructing families to keep cars locked so young children cannot gain access and to never leave a child in a parked car, either in or out of a car seat, even for a few moments, no matter what the outside temperature (Safe Kids, 2011c).

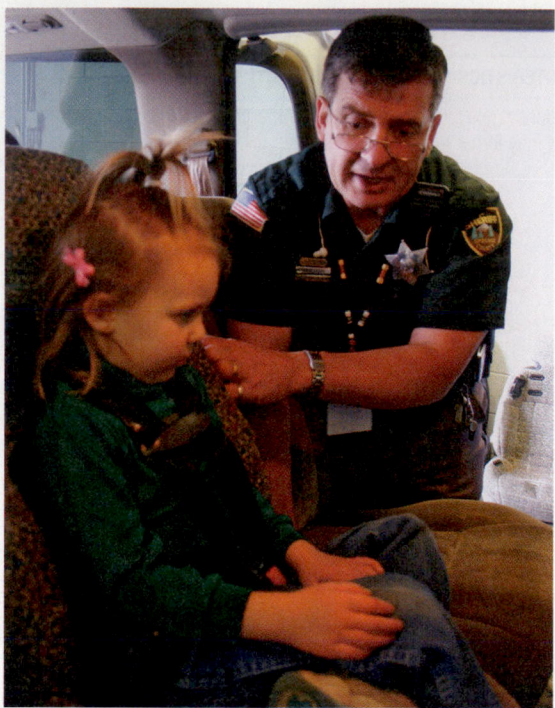

FIGURE 11–5 ■ The officer at this police station is certified to examine car seats for children and make recommendations for parents. He is examining a preschooler in a booster seat for proper fit and alignment. Many car seats are improperly installed or not the proper type for a specific age of child, so centers that check seats provide an important service.

The child spends increasing time away from the parent. Childcare situations should provide the same supervision the child receives at home. Help parents to ask questions and feel confident in safety at other settings. For example, while parents may be cautious about gun safety at home, few of them inquire if a home the child is visiting has guns and how they are stored.

Preschoolers are generally interested in health and their bodies. This is a time when teaching can become directed at both the parents and the child. Preschoolers are receptive to practicing street crossing and tricycle/bicycle riding skills. It may be helpful to have a place in the clinic or office where they can be taught basic skills such as hand washing or street crossing. Consider the time of year, climate, and geographic location and teach appropriately. Spring is often a good time to teach bicycle and water safety. Winter hazards may include woodstoves or other heating devices. See Table 11–9 for additional listings of toddler and preschooler hazards and safety teaching needed. Injury prevention efforts represent health maintenance activities since they are aimed at preventing injuries from occurring.

Nursing Management

Nursing Assessment and Diagnosis

Nurses partner with other healthcare professionals, including physicians, nurse practitioners, and speech therapists, to assess health promotion and health maintenance status of young children. The toddler and preschool years are characterized by much developmental progression, and strategies need to be constantly adapted to meet the particular needs of the child and family.

Parents are partners in the care of the child, and every health supervision visit should address their questions and concerns. Their observations of the child are an invaluable part of the process. As preschoolers become more verbal, they also become partners with the healthcare team. Ask preschoolers what they want to learn, what they want to know about staying well, and other pertinent questions.

Toddlers and preschoolers are examined for growth, physical health status, and mental/social characteristics. Development is an area that many pediatricians feel ill-prepared to address, but which parents commonly want addressed. Additionally, developmental surveillance must occur at every healthcare visit, with standardized screening at least at 9, 18, and 24 to 30 months (Drotar, Stancin, & Dworkin, 2008). Nurses are adept at describing normal developmental milestones, evaluating the progression of children, and using anticipatory guidance to address parental developmental concerns.

Based on a thorough assessment, you will establish nursing diagnoses that are appropriate for the young child and family. Potential nursing diagnoses established during a health supervision visit of a toddler or preschooler might include:

- Anxiety related to change of environment (new care provider)
- Parenting, Impaired related to lack of support from significant others
- Growth and Development, Delayed related to lead exposure
- Health Maintenance, Impaired related to lack of safety knowledge by parent
- Skin Integrity, Impaired related to hyperthermia (sunburn)

NANDA-I © 2012

Planning and Implementation

Based on the nursing diagnoses, the nurse works with others to plan strategies to meet the needs of the family. Explain that assessment questions are asked to provide a picture of the child that can be helpful in partnering with parents to plan health care. Reinforce the importance of the family coming to health supervision visits with their own list of issues. Work with other healthcare professionals to ensure all needs of a particular child and family are addressed.

Clinical Judgment
Teaching for the family takes place as the examination occurs. How can you explain weight and height measurements? Dietary intake? Immunizations?

If the family has been reluctant to ask questions, reflect on the child's development. "Many children have trouble sleeping through the night; is that the case for Cassandra? What helps her to sleep? What is it like at her bedtime?" Developmental areas such as sleep, discipline, toilet training, and expected developmental milestones should be addressed. If the parents were given a journal in an earlier visit to record observations and questions, ask if they have brought it with them.

Health promotion activities should be emphasized during the visit. Health promotion related to physical activity includes teaching about toys that encourage activity, such as balls, musical toys, push toys, and tricycles. See Partnering with

TABLE 11-9	Disease and Injury Prevention Topics by Age
AGE	**INJURY PREVENTION TEACHING TOPICS**
15 months	Wash adult's hands and child's hands frequently.
	Clean toys with soap and water regularly.
	Provide child's own bedding for childcare setting and wash weekly.
	Use forward-facing car safety seat if child is 20 lb; install correctly and have installation checked; place in back seat and never in front seat with a passenger air bag.
	Empty containers of water immediately after use; be sure pools or other bodies of water are locked and not accessible.
	Use sunscreen, hat, and long sleeves in the sun.
	Keep heavy and sharp objects out of reach; check that all poisons are locked away, including in homes visited; keep pet food and cosmetics out of reach.
	Have poison control number by phones and programmed into cell phones.
	Be alert for dangers of hot curling irons and other appliances.
	Have electrical cords out of reach and not hanging down.
	Keep water temperature no higher than 120°F to 125°F.
	Have home environment checked for lead hazards.
	Secure the child in shopping carts.
	Do not let the child have access to alcoholic drinks.
	Remember that responsible adults should always supervise children; other children should not be asked to supervise young children.
	Know CPR, airway obstruction removal, and other first aid.
18 months	As above.
	Bolt heavy objects (such as bookcases and televisions that might be pulled down) securely to the wall.
	Be cautious of the toddler near machinery in the yard (e.g., lawn mowers, farm equipment).
	Use a helmet on the child when on the back of a bicycle.
	Check batteries in home smoke alarms and carbon monoxide or radon monitors; check system monthly; change batteries on a scheduled basis as recommended by manufacturer.
	Ask care providers about discipline methods; do not allow corporal punishment.
2-3 years	As above.
	Use a child seat as directed by manufacturer in the back seat of the car.
	Teach hand washing after toileting and other activities.
	Clean potty chair thoroughly.
	Keep guns unloaded and locked away in a different locked place than ammunition; have trigger locks installed.
	Teach how to cross streets.
	Provide a helmet for riding tricycles.
	Check playgrounds for safety hazards and ensure cushioned surfaces under equipment.
3-4 years	As above.
	Do not let the child play unsupervised.
	Know CPR, airway obstruction removal, and other first aid for the child who has become a preschooler.
4-5 years	As above.
	Continue teaching safety skills to the child.
	Continue supervising when near streets and water sources.
	Teach safety around strangers (never go with a stranger; find a trusted person such as a parent or police officer).

Source: *Adapted from Hagan, J. F., Shaw, J. S., & Duncan, P. M. (Eds.). (2008). Bright futures: Guidelines for health supervision of infants, children, and adolescents (3rd ed.). Elk Grove Village, IL: American Academy of Pediatrics.*

Families: Toy and Playground Safety. Review nutritional intake and encourage introduction of new foods, healthy snack and meal choices, and positive eating for busy families. Emphasize the importance of play to healthy child development. Young children need free playtime each day. Additionally, encourage parents to engage in play with the child every day. This fosters the parent–child relationship, assists the parent in recognizing the child's strengths and needs, and ensures physical activity for both parent and child.

It is essential to apply concepts of anticipatory guidance as you address the child's approaching developmental progression. If the child will soon be toilet trained, provide information about possible

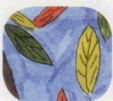

Partnering with Families

Toy and Playground Safety

Play is essential to the physical and cognitive growth of toddlers and preschoolers. However, toys can present hazards for young children. Parents need to receive guidelines to follow in selecting toys. These include (Safe Kids, 2011a):

- Select toys intended for the age of your child. Some toys have small parts or can break into small parts and should not be given to children under 3 years. They should not be too heavy for the child to manipulate them appropriately. Toys with strings, straps, or cords longer than 7 inches pose strangulation hazards.
- Assemble toys as directed and check them frequently for breakage; remove all packing materials before providing toys for the child.
- Do not use older repainted toys unless certain that paint used contained no lead.
- Select cloth toys that are nonflammable, flame resistant, or flame retardant. Avoid electrical and battery-powered toys in children under 8 years.
- Do not allow latex balloons and especially noninflated balloons to be used as toys.

Playgrounds provide a location for healthy development of children, but they can also be responsible for child injuries. Home playgrounds are the site of most playground injuries. Falls, strangulation, and head impacts are examples of frequent playground injuries. Some tips can be provided for parents (Safe Kids, 2011b):

- Surfaces should be composed of soft and loose material such as mulch, shredded rubber, or fine sand. The surface should be 12 inches deep and extend 6 feet around equipment.
- Equipment should not allow the child to be more than 5 feet off the surface.
- Strangulation is a high risk so be sure to remove ties, ribbons, drawstrings, and other hanging items from clothing and play areas.
- Ensure that the equipment is intended for the age of the child. Separate playgrounds for young and older children are recommended.
- Consult the U.S. Consumer Product Safety Commission for playground equipment standards. Inspect equipment regularly.
- Always supervise the young child on a playground at all times.

approaches. If the child is learning to swim or has access to water, reinforce safety precautions near water. For the child going to a new childcare center, provide the parents with a list of questions they can ask the care provider and tips to assist in the transition to a new setting (see Chapter 5 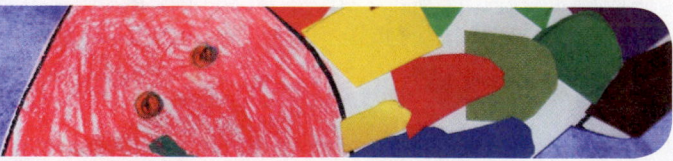). Consider aspects of your climate and geographic location, and teach appropriately for the upcoming season.

Health maintenance activities are added to the visit as you give immunizations and screen for tuberculosis, lead exposure, and problems with language, vision, or hearing. The focus of these activities is to prevent disease or to find it early before there are serious consequences. When you find information that may indicate a problem, be sure to refer the child to the primary care provider, such as a physician or nurse practitioner. You may even recommend that another specialist, such as a speech pathologist or dentist, see the child. Other health maintenance activities that must be part of each visit with a toddler or preschooler involve teaching about common hazards and how to avoid them. Include toy safety teaching in every visit. Emergency care in case of injury is also helpful information for parents, so first aid classes can be recommended.

Conclude the visit with some words of praise about the parent and child accomplishments. Provide the date for the next visit. List any resources helpful to the family, including the clinic/office contact information and emergency services.

Evaluation

Parents should be asked occasionally to evaluate the care they are receiving at the health promotion and health maintenance site. Use these comments to monitor and adjust procedures as needed. The expected outcomes for nursing care of the toddler and preschooler include the following:

- The child demonstrates normal patterns of growth and progression in developmental milestones.
- The child remains free of disease and injury.
- Parents relay satisfaction with the pediatric healthcare home.
- The child manifests positive physical, social, and emotional adjustment.

Chapter Highlights

- General observations of physical ability and social interactions are made as the toddler and preschooler are called back for the healthcare visit.
- Questions about growth and information related to physical health are integrated during the physical examination.

- The approaches and order of the physical examination should be adapted to minimize threats to the young child.
- Developmental surveillance is integrated within each health promotion/health maintenance visit.

- Toddlers and preschoolers gradually take on mature eating patterns; assessment of nutritional status involves growth, food eaten, and family food patterns.
- Physical ability progresses steadily in young children. Opportunities for daily active periods are necessary for healthy growth.
- By 2 years of age a full set of primary teeth is present; they will be kept until the first one is lost at about 6 years.

- Early years are essential to development of a positive sense of self, positive social interactions with others, and healthy lifestyle behaviors.
- Screening for common diseases is performed during routine care. Immunizations are administered to prevent infectious diseases.
- Safety hazards for toddlers and preschoolers are addressed at each visit, with suggestions given to parents to provide safe environments.

Clinical Reasoning in Action

INTRODUCTION

Recall the parents of 15-month-old Clarence. They are working parents who are overwhelmed by the activity level of their son. They express concern about how to spend time with and ensure safety for Clarence, while having some time to spend with each other.

DESCRIPTION

During the examination of Clarence, he is constantly moving and squirming. However, he is a pleasant and happy child who interacts appropriately with adults. His parents are loving and patient with him but express that they are often tired and wonder how to manage such an active child. They recognize that some children are normally active. They request information about how to handle his activity and particularly how to keep their home a safe place for him. Clarence naps at the childcare center each day and does not go to sleep until 10 p.m. each evening. Since the parents are up early, they get him ready to leave at about 6 a.m. The parents have only lived in this city for 2 years. Extended family visit occasionally, but the parents socialize mainly with other employees at work. As you examine the record you find that Clarence has had three doses of DTaP, three doses of hepatitis B, three doses of *Haemophilus influenzae* type b, and two doses of pneumococcal vaccine.

DISCUSSION

1. Clarence's mother and father show many strengths as parents. List the protective factors that you identify in their parenting.
2. How would you classify Clarence's temperament? Consult Chapter 5 🕑 for a description of the different types of temperament in children.
3. What techniques can the nurse use in examining Clarence that will contribute to his cooperation?
4. As you review the safety hazards that the parents have identified for Clarence, what injury prevention is essential to address?
5. How much should Clarence be sleeping at night? What questions will you ask his parents about the sleeping situation, and what recommendations might you suggest to enhance sleep patterns?
6. What immunizations should Clarence receive today? What history questions will you ask and what teaching will you perform related to immunizations? (Consult this chapter and Chapter 22 🕑 for information about immunizations.)

NCLEX-RN® Review

1. When performing a developmental assessment of a 4-year-old child, the nurse notes the child can stack two blocks, roll a ball, scribble on paper, and identify two body parts. What do these milestones indicate?
   1. Normal development for a 4-year-old child
   2. Developmental delay for a 4-year-old child
   3. The presence of a developmental disability
   4. The need for a complete developmental evaluation

2. The nurse knows that the teaching about car seat safety to the parents of a 4-year-old girl has been effective when which statement is made?
   1. "Now that our child is 4 years old we will still need to use a car seat with a harness until she reaches the top height or weight limit that is allowed by the car seat's manufacturer."
   2. "Now that our child is 4 years old, she can sit in the regular car seat and use the seat belt and shoulder belt like adults."
   3. "Now that our child is 4 years old, she can sit in her booster seat in the front seat."
   4. "Our 4-year-old must stay in her forward-facing car seat until she is 6 years old."

3. Which is the best advice the nurse can give to parents asking for help in handling their toddler's temper tantrums?
   1. "I think you should start using time-outs when he throws a temper tantrum."
   2. "Reward him for good behavior, and the temper tantrums will decrease."
   3. "There is nothing to be done. They are a symptom of emotional instability."
   4. "Temper tantrums will increase in number through the preschool years."

4. The nurse teaches the parents of 3-year-old Jim about the "5-a-day" program. What does this mean?
   1. The child should have five glasses of milk daily.
   2. The child should have a food from each of the five food groups at each meal.
   3. The parents should offer five snacks to the child each day.
   4. The child should eat five servings of fruits and vegetables each day.

See Appendix I 🕑 *for answers.*

References

American Academy of Pediatrics (AAP). (2011a). *Disciplining your child*. Retrieved from http://www.healthychildren.org/English/family-life/family-dynamics/communication-discipline/Pages/Disciplining-Your-Child.aspx

American Academy of Pediatrics (AAP). (2011b). Temper Tantrums. Retrieved from http://www.healthychildren.org/English/family-life/family-dynamics/communication-discipline/Pages/Temper-Tantrums.aspx

American Academy of Pediatrics (AAP). (2011c). *Dealing with sibling rivalry*. Retrieved from http://www.healthychildren.org/English/family-life/family-dynamics/Pages/Dealing-with-Sibling-Rivalry.aspx

American Academy of Pediatrics (AAP). (2011d). *Sibling rivalry*. Retrieved from http://www.healthychildren.org/English/family-life/family-dynamics/pages/Sibling-Rivalry.aspx

American Dental Association. (2011). *Thumbsucking*. Retrieved from http://www.ada.org/2977.aspx

Beets, M. W., Bornstein, D., Dowda, M., & Pate, R. R. (2011). Compliance with national guidelines for physical activity in U.S. preschoolers: Measurement and interpretation. *Pediatrics, 127*(4), 658–664.

Belden, A. C., Thomson, N. R., & Luby, J. L. (2008). Temper tantrums in healthy versus depressed and disruptive preschoolers: Defining tantrum behaviors associated with clinical problems. *Journal of Pediatrics, 152*(1), 117–122.

Centers for Disease Control and Prevention. (2009). Quick stats: Percentage of children ages 2–4 years who ever had caries in primary teeth, by race/ethnicity and sex—National Health and Nutrition Examination Survey, United States, 1988–1994 and 1999–2004. *Morbidity and Mortality Weekly Report, 58*(2), 34.

Centers for Disease Control and Prevention. (2010). *Physical activity guidelines for Americans: Children and adolescents*. Retrieved from http://www.cdc.gov/HealthyYouth/physicalactivity/guidelines.htm

Centers for Disease Control and Prevention. (2011). *Oral health program: Strategic Plan 2011–2014*. Washington, DC: Author.

Children's Health Study. (2011). *What is the National Children's Study?* Retrieved from http://www.nationalchildrensstudy.gov/Pages/default.aspx

Degnan, K. A., Calkins, S. D., Keane, S. P., & Hill-Soderlund, A. L. (2008). Profiles of disruptive behavior across early childhood: Contributions of frustration reactivity, physiological regulation and maternal behavior. *Child Development, 79*(5), 1357–1376.

Dietrich, T., Culler, C., Garcia, R. I., & Henshaw, M. M. (2008). Racial and ethnic disparities in children's oral health. *Journal of the American Dental Association, 139*(11), 1507–1517.

Drotar, D., Stancin, T., & Dworkin, P. (2008). *Pediatric developmental screening: Understanding and selecting screening instruments*. Washington, DC: Commonwealth Fund.

Hagan, J. F., Shaw, J. S., & Duncan, P. M. (2008). *Bright futures: Guidelines for health supervision of infants, children, and adolescents*. Elk Grove Village, IL: American Academy of Pediatrics.

Halfon, N., DuPlessis, H., & Inkelas, M. (2007). Transforming the U.S. child health system. *Health Affairs, 26*, 315–330.

Halfon, N., Larson, K., & Russ, S. (2010). Why social determinants? *Healthcare Quarterly, 14*, 8–20.

Halfon, N., Stanley, L., & DuPlessis, H. (2010). Measuring the quality of developmental services for young children: A new approach. *Issue Brief (Commonwealth Fund), 84*, 1–14.

Holt, K., Wooldridge, N., Story, M., & Sofka, D. (2011). *Bright futures: Nutrition* (3rd ed.). Elk Grove Village, IL: American Academy of Pediatrics.

Kim, E., Guo, Y., Koh, C., & Cain, K. C. (2010). Korean immigrant discipline and children's social competence and behavior problems. *Journal of Pediatric Nursing, 25*, 490–499.

Lau, A. S. (2010). Physical discipline in Chinese American immigrant families: An adaptive culture perspective. *Cultural Diversity and Ethnic Minority Psychology, 16*(3), 313–322.

Lewis, C. W. (2009). Dental care and children with special health care needs: A population-based perspective. *Academic Pediatrics, 9*(6), 420–426.

Murray, R. B., Zentner, J. P., & Yakimo, R. (2009). *Health promotion strategies through the lifespan*. (8th ed.). Upper Saddle River, NJ: Prentice Hall Health.

National Maternal & Child Oral Health Resource Center. (2010). *Resource highlights: Focus on early childhood caries*. Retrieved from http://www.mchoralhealth.org/highlights/ecc.html

Prasse, J. E., & Kikano, G. E. (2008). Stuttering: An overview. *American Family Physician, 77*(9), 1271–1276.

Safe Kids. (2011a). *Preventing injuries: At home, at play, and on the way*. Retrieved from http://www.safekids.org/our-work/research/fact-sheets/toy-safety-fact-sheet.html

Safe Kids. (2011b). *Playground safety fact sheet*. Retrieved from http://www.safekids.org/our-work/research/fact-sheets/playground-safety-fact-sheet.html

Safe Kids. (2011c). *Never leave your child alone in a car*. Retrieved from http://www.safekids.org/safety-basics/safety-guide/kids-in-and-around-cars.html

Wagner, R., & Oskouian, R. (2008). Are you missing the diagnosis of the most common chronic disease of childhood? *Contemporary Pediatrics, 25*(9), 60–79.

Yaman, A., Mesman, J., van IJzendoorn, M. H., & Bakermans-Kranenburg, M. J. (2010). Parenting and toddler aggression in second-generation immigrant families: The moderating role of child temperament. *Journal of Family Psychology, 24*(2), 208–211.

Yu, T., Pettit, G. S., Lansford, J. E., Dodge, K. A., & Bates, J. E. (2010). The interactive effects of marital conflict and divorce on parent–adult children's relationships. *Journal of Marriage and the Family, 72*(2), 282–292.

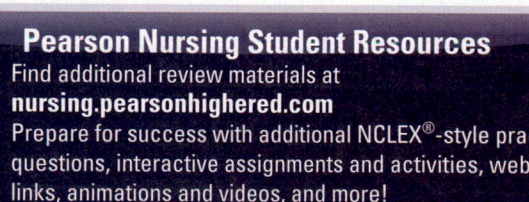

Pearson Nursing Student Resources

Find additional review materials at
nursing.pearsonhighered.com
Prepare for success with additional NCLEX®-style practice questions, interactive assignments and activities, web links, animations and videos, and more!

Health Promotion and Maintenance of the School-Age Child

CHAPTER

12

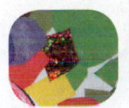 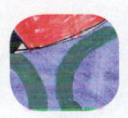 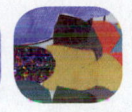

KEY TERMS

Learning Outcomes

After completing this chapter, you will be able to:

1. Describe the general observations made of school-age children and their families as they come to the pediatric healthcare home for health supervision visits.

2. Plan interventions that address the major health concerns of school-age children.

3. Assess nutrition, physical activity, oral health, mental health status, and growth and development of school-age children.

4. Apply therapeutic communication skills with the school-age child and family during health supervision visits.

5. Intervene with school-age children and their families to integrate activities to promote health and to prevent disease and injury.

6. Synthesize data from the history and examination of the school-age child and family.

7. Plan developmentally appropriate approaches for the school-age child and family during health supervision encounters.

> "Our school nurse is really great. She answers our questions about diabetes without making us feel like we're different from other kids. We can keep equipment like syringes in her office and she helps us program our insulin pumps."
>
> *—Jessalyn, age 12*

Jessalyn McIntyre is 12 years old and in sixth grade. She and her friend Kelly Gutierrez both have type 1 diabetes and need to test their blood glucose each day during school. They also both use insulin pumps. When they started using the pumps, the school nurse met with their parents and talked with the endocrinologist in order to help them manage in school. Their careful management of diabetes has enabled Jessalyn and Kelly to participate in sports and other school activities. The school nurse performs many of the girls' health supervision activities, such as nutrition assessment, growth monitoring, physical assessment, and fostering relationships with other children. She partners with other healthcare providers to plan comprehensive care for Jessalyn and Kelly.

Youth such as Jessalyn and Kelly require the same health promotion and health maintenance activities as all school-age children. They need teaching about nutrition and physical activity. Their immunization records should be reviewed, and safety needs addressed. Due to their chronic disease they need additional growth monitoring, teaching regarding dietary management, and assistance in monitoring and managing their insulin needs. The chronic disease may also cause mental health challenges due to differences from peers. What health promotion interventions will you plan for students such as Jessalyn and Kelly? How will you adapt usual needs of school-age children when a chronic disease is being managed? What adaptations will parents have to make as a child with diabetes grows older and begins to manage the disease independently?

School age spans the time from when most children enter kindergarten (around age 5) through the beginning of adolescence (12 to 13 years). Health promotion and health maintenance needs continue during this time, but less frequent visits to the pediatric healthcare home are recommended. In addition, most children are relatively healthy and need few immunizations, which may lead to only sporadic visits for care. When school-age children are seen in health care, even for illness or emergency care, ask for the date of the last well-child or health supervision visit, and encourage the parents to make an appointment if the child is due for a visit. The frequency of health promotion visits decreases during the school-age years, so parents need information about the recommended ages for such visits and a reminder at each visit about when the next one should be scheduled. The American Academy of Pediatrics and the U.S. Department of Health and Human Services recommend annual visits from 5 to 12 years of age.

Visits during the school-age years will focus on:

- Establishing good health habits related to issues such as nutrition, physical activity, and mental health
- Monitoring physical and developmental changes
- Learning the importance of avoiding tobacco, alcohol, and drugs
- Ensuring success in school, family, and extracurricular activities
- Fostering good decision-making and problem-solving skills

Health supervision concepts are applied to children with special healthcare needs, such as Jessalyn and Kelly, described in the opening scenario. See other chapters in this text for information specific to conditions that may affect school-age children such as asthma (Chapter 25), eating disorders (Chapter 19), and diabetes (Chapter 32). What are common sites for health promotion visits for school-age children? What resources are available for working with parents and children? How can nurses assist young children in establishing positive health practices? What special challenges do children face today that readily affect health? These are some of the questions that we will discuss in this chapter.

GENERAL OBSERVATIONS

The first school-age visit usually occurs just before entry into kindergarten. During this visit, the child receives a thorough examination to be certain that physical development is normal, developmental milestones have been met for fine and gross motor skills, school readiness is displayed in social skills and language, and final sets of basic immunizations are completed (see the immunization schedules in Chapter 22 and the Disease Prevention Strategies section later in this chapter). Often, the child is excited about the visit, because it is associated with beginning school. The child may feel some anxiety, as it may be the first time he or she is aware of getting "shots." As with earlier visits, your observations begin as the child is called in for the visit. Speak to the child first, introducing yourself and welcoming the child and parents to the office or clinic. Many children of this age actively participate in conversations, making teaching and gathering data easy (Figure 12–1). For children who are quiet or look to the parents, allow more time for them to get to know the personnel, directing most initial questions to parents. This may be the first visit where the child is old enough to be a partner in the healthcare visit. Establishing positive rapport with the child will enhance health teaching efforts. At the same time, recognize the importance of family-centered care, or a partnership to include decision making jointly by the family and the healthcare provider (Kuo, Houtrow, Arango, et al., 2012).

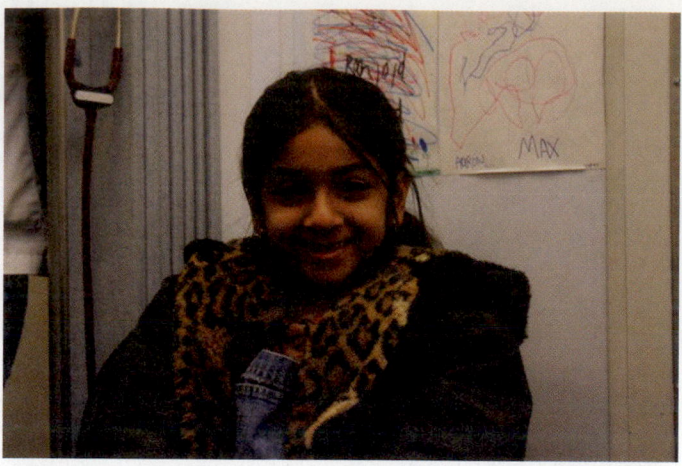

FIGURE 12–1 ■ Children generally interact readily with healthcare providers and appear at ease when welcomed and engaged in interactions. Notice the pleasant setting with child art posted on the wall.

Observe the interaction between the parents and the child. What types of speech tones are used? Is there mutual respect or are parents and child ignoring each other or having disagreements? The child should walk showing symmetry and ease of movement, follow instructions about where to go and taking off shoes for weighing, and demonstrate clear language skills with parents or healthcare personnel.

By the time children come for health visits at 6, 7, 8, and later years, they are expected to be increasingly active in sports, school activities, music, or other interests. Look for clues about their interests as they arrive, and comment upon them during the visit. Did they bring books or an iPod/iPad? What are the book topics or favorite types of music? Ask what they are doing during the summer, or what their two favorite after-school activities entail. What two subjects do they like best in school? Which do they not like? Have they learned to swim? What activities would they like to do that they have not been able to engage in yet? Who are their best friends? How would they describe their best friends? Do they have brothers and sisters? What are the best things and worst things about having siblings? Have them describe a typical day. The questions serve both to put the child at ease and to learn about the child's interests and activities. Compare the child's answers with your understanding of school-age development (see Chapter 5). If you have concerns about an answer, follow it up later in the visit. For example, if the child does not know how to swim, suggest to the parent that this is an important skill and offer resources for swim classes.

Some children do not commonly come to clinics, offices, or other settings for health supervision visits. Therefore, school nurses or nurse practitioners in school-based clinics sometimes offer health promotion and health maintenance activities in the school setting. Children with special healthcare needs, such as Jessalyn and Kelly, may need more frequent monitoring of health, which can be performed in the school setting. A major focus of school nurses is making the environment conducive to health for groups of children (see Chapter 14 for further discussion of the role of the school nurse). School nurses may offer specific examinations to individual children, such as growth and developmental surveillance and health screening for vision, hearing, or scoliosis; they may work with food service personnel and administration to improve meal and snack quality and minimize unhealthy choices in vending machines; and they may work with teachers to integrate concepts such as physical activity and self-esteem into classroom activities.

School-based health clinics and school nurses offer healthcare services that are often integral to children's health status. The nurse often links children with healthcare needs to other community services. Although not a substitute for health supervision visits, such health approaches can be important to provide both health promotion and maintenance services to children. Parents are generally proud of their children. During health supervision visits, watch the parents' responses as children answer questions. Be alert for the parent who interrupts the child or constantly "corrects" what is said. Comments by the parent should involve praise of the child or looking to the child for opinions on certain topics. This indicates that a partnership is developing in the family and that family members work together and value each other. Direct some questions to the parents. Ask if they came with specific concerns that should be addressed. If the child has an individualized education or health plan (see Chapter 16 🔗), ask if the parent brought a copy, if the plan is still appropriate, or if it needs updating. Allow the parent an opportunity to meet with the physician, nurse practitioner, or other professional in a private place and without the child present if desired. Be alert for family dynamics that can influence mental health status. Ask if there have been any important changes in the family and how they have influenced the child. During conversations, be alert for reports of separation, divorce, remarriages, ill siblings or grandparents, recent or upcoming moves, parent job changes, substance abuse, incarceration of family members in jail, custody disputes, or other issues. Such topics can be followed up with further questions, as described later in the mental health section, to learn how they influence the child.

GROWTH AND DEVELOPMENTAL SURVEILLANCE

As the child comes into the health supervision site, height and weight are measured. Be sure to have the child remove shoes and coat. Ask the child and parents if they know the child's current height and weight, and if they have any questions. Plot the percentiles for these measurements, calculate body mass index (BMI) and its percentile, and explain the meaning of these findings later in the visit. See Partnering with Families: Percentile Measurements in Chapter 10 🔗 for an example of how to explain this concept to parents. Watch for children who have changed channels on a growth grid. For example, if the child was in the 25th percentile for height in earlier visits and is presently in the 50th percentile, a growth spurt might be occurring. Most children do not grow uniformly; they have periods of slow growth followed by fast spurts. School age is a time when overweight can begin to be a problem, so look for significant differences in weight and height percentiles, as reflected in a high BMI percentile, and gather additional data as needed (see Chapter 19 🔗 for nutritional assessment approaches). Health promotion and maintenance needs regarding growth are addressed further in the nutrition section of this chapter.

School-age children have logical thought processes and are learning about their bodies. They should be active participants in the physical examination. Explain what you are doing and why. "I'm listening to your heart with this stethoscope and counting how many times it beats in a minute. Have you heard your heart? When have you noticed it beating hard?" Ask if they are nervous about any part of the examination. Verbalizing this anxiety allows you to explain what will be done and why it is important. Most children understand the purpose of the examination; a few will be very nervous, possibly related to a negative experience in health care at a younger age. They can be helped to verbalize their concerns and will often work through the feelings of insecurity or worry by talking about the prior experience. Young children generally want parents present during the examination, whereas children of 9 to 10 years may choose to have a parent wait outside. Allow children to choose what is comfortable, and meet with parents to relay the findings from the examination.

A head-to-toe examination is carried out, with particular attention to systems and skills that influence success in school, such as vision, hearing, muscular strength, and coordination. See Chapter 7 🔗 for detailed information about the physical examination. Remember to provide feedback about the findings; families appreciate knowing that the child's vision is normal and strength is well developed. They should be told what is normal as well as areas that may need more assessment or intervention. Inquire about the child's sleep patterns. During the examination, ask for a description of any illnesses the child has had. Children of school age are generally healthy, with only a few upper respiratory infections or other minor illnesses annually. Some children complain of growing pains, and all complaints are reviewed thoroughly. Unusual complaints may indicate a need for further testing; examples will be discussed in the Disease Prevention Strategies section later in this chapter.

Clinical Tip

The growing skeleton sometimes causes growing pains or osteochondrosis. The most common areas of discomfort are the legs, but arms, elbows, feet, and other body parts may be involved. Growing pains are thought to result from inflammation along the areas of ossification or growth plates, although the etiology is not well described. Consistent sports inflammation or injury may exacerbate growing pains (Atanda, Shah, & O'Brien, 2011). Most growing pain is alleviated by massage, short-term rest, and mild analgesics (Pavone, Lionetti, Gargano, et al., 2011). Growing pains should always be differentiated from musculoskeletal disorders such as Osgood-Schlatter disease and Perthes disease (see Chapter 35 🔗 for a description of these conditions).

School-age children frequently have minor injuries. These might include falls from a bicycle, skin rashes from exposure to plants on a hiking trip, bruises from a ball sport, and other minor mishaps. Be alert for more serious problems that may indicate a need for additional detailed data gathering and teaching. We will discuss examples in the Injury Prevention Strategies section later in the chapter.

Developmental surveillance continues to be an important part of the examination for school-age children. Some milestones can be observed during the visit, while other information is obtained by report of the parent and child. Provide an opportunity for both the parent and child to be alone with the healthcare provider for a few moments to encourage open communication about any sensitive issues. This information is combined with reports about school and other activities to establish that the child is developing as desired. You can ask parents:

- "Does your daughter seem like most 8-year-olds to you? Tell me about her school performance. Do you have any questions or concerns about her behavior or school performance?"
- "Describe your son's best friends and what they like to do."
- "What are the ways that he has been growing up this year?"

Although milestones for development are quite different than at earlier ages, it is still important to evaluate progression (Hamilton & Glascoe, 2010). Direct observations, history questions, and questionnaires that parents complete are possible methods for development data collection. See Table 12–1 for developmental milestones of school-age children. Consider use of questionnaires such as the Ages and Stages Questionnaire or Parents' Evaluation of Developmental Status (PEDS).

TABLE 12–1	Developmental Milestones Observed During Health Promotion and Maintenance Visits of School-Age Children
AGE	**DEVELOPMENTAL MILESTONES**
5 years	■ Is independent in bathroom and dressing activities ■ Ties shoes, buttons ■ Runs well, jumps, may skip, balances on one foot for 10 seconds ■ Pours fluids well, uses hands to catch ball ■ Prints some letters, first name ■ Draws triangle, square, 3- to 5-part person ■ Knows full name, address, phone
6–8 years	■ Is skilled in physical activities such as running, skipping, jumping, hopping ■ Learns to ride bicycle ■ Can cut, paste, write all letters ■ Reads
8–10 years	■ Has increasingly longer periods of concentration for both physical activity and school or other quiet activity ■ Can throw objects far and with accurate aim ■ Shows increased coordination ■ Develops hobbies such as model building, playing a musical instrument, video production, building with wood, needlework
10–12 years	■ Has fine and gross motor skills similar to adult in ability ■ Writes well, adept at computer use ■ May develop some clumsiness as prepubertal growth spurt begins

Once children attend school, parents may need to alter childcare arrangements. Ask whether the child comes home after school on a school bus, takes public transportation, rides in a car, or walks. Is someone at home to supervise the young child? Do the parents feel that the child's after-school activities are safe? If the child goes to a childcare center, are parents satisfied with the program offered? Provide resources as needed to after-school programs that may be available in the school and at other childcare providers. Search your community resource directories to learn about local sites. Help the parent to decide when the child is able to stay alone for a period of time after school. (See Partnering with Families: After-School Self-Care.)

Desired outcomes for growth and developmental surveillance include normal progression with developmental tasks, absence of physical and psychosocial abnormalities or trauma, and integration of safe practices into daily life.

NUTRITION

Key concepts related to nutrition in school-age children are independence and formation of habits that influence the future. Children are increasingly independent in food choices. They usually have strong likes and dislikes of certain foods. They may come home alone and prepare snacks. During school, they choose what to eat from the school lunch or the sack lunch sent by the family. They may even have access to vending machines or sales of snacks during school hours. While independence in food choices is growing, the child is greatly influenced in those choices by friends and the media. Foods that may be rejected often include fresh vegetables and fruits, since they get little media attention, and friends may not prefer them.

At a time when the child chooses many of the foods in the daily diet, habits are being formed that will affect nutrition and health in the years to come. Good choices will help to promote health, maintain weight at a recommended level, provide nutrients for adequate growth and activity, and prevent onset of some chronic diseases. On the other hand, poor choices can lead to overweight and its accompanying problems, lack of adequate calcium and resultant osteoporosis, eating disorders, or lack of energy for brain growth and optimal performance in school. The patterns established during this period are influential in later nutritional status. Knowledge about foods, family participation in good nutritional practices, eating as a family several times weekly, and access to healthy foods can all be enhanced by nursing intervention during this critical formative period.

The first nutritional status assessment includes height and weight measurement, BMI calculation, and examination of percentiles for each measurement on growth grids (see Chapter 19 and Appendix A 🔗). See the discussion of measurement in the previous Growth and Developmental Surveillance section. Slow, steady growth is the norm during the early school-age years; it will be followed by a growth spurt when the child nears puberty.

During the visit, observations provide information about nutritional status. What is the condition of the nails, skin, and hair? What is the energy level and reported physical activity? Does the child look lean or overweight? As the child nears puberty, there may be an increase in fat stores as a preparation for the pubertal growth spurt. Integrate questions for the parent and child into the visit that provide clues about diet:

- "Do you eat school lunch or pack a lunch from home?"
- "Do you eat breakfast? What do you usually eat in the morning?"
- "You mentioned that you are without a car now, Mrs. Jennings. How are you able to get your groceries?"
- "What did you have to eat so far today?"
- "Do you ever worry that you do not have enough food to feed your family?"
- "Do you use WIC (Women, Infants, and Children Nutrition Program), food banks, farmers' markets, or other resources?"
- "Do you have a garden? Would you like to?"
- "What is your favorite grocery store? Why?"
- "You mentioned that all of your children are in activities after school. How do you usually fit in an evening meal for everyone? How often do you eat fast food? How often does the whole family eat together?"
- "How do you feel about your weight and the way you look?"

As you observe the child and family and ask dietary questions, list risks and protective factors related to nutrition. Perhaps protective factors relate to adequate access to nutritious foods, a family garden, and weight and height within normal limits. Reinforce the positive practices of the family and inform the child of how food choices relate to energy level, school performance, and general health. Risk factors become the basis for teaching and planning with the family for necessary change. It is difficult to tackle several nutritional changes at one time, so concentrate on those most needing attention and on those the family agrees are important. Provide information about healthy snacks to keep at home, ways to improve calcium intake, limitation of soda pop to one can daily, and the importance of family meals (Box 12–1). Nutrition teaching can take

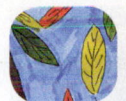

Partnering with Families

After-School Self-Care

Children who come home to an empty house after school are called **latchkey children.** About 15% of children from 5 to 12 years of age spend time in self-care on a regular basis, with an average of 5 to 6 hours weekly. Inquire about self-care practices for youth in the family, and suggest types of care as needed by the parents, such as school-based programs, family members, and center care (Latchkey-Kids, 2011; Safe Kids, 2010). The age at which children are ready for the responsibility of self-care varies, although 12 to 13 years is a usual guideline. Parents need help to decide when the child can come home and stay alone, and then plan for safety precautions for the child. Characteristics that indicate a child may be ready to stay alone for 1 to 3 hours include the following:

- The child has had opportunities to stay alone for shorter periods and has successfully planned appropriate activities and felt secure.
- The child has several activities and interests that can be pursued at home after school (e.g., music, model building, reading).
- The neighborhood and the route home are considered safe.
- The child understands major safety hazards such as not taking rides and not talking on the phone to strangers.
- The child understands fire, firearm, water, and other safety hazards and what to do in emergencies.
- Someone is always directly available by phone.
- A neighbor or other close resource is available.

Provide guidelines that a parent can use to help prepare the child for self-care. These include the following:

- Teach the child where to keep a key so that it is not available to others, such as pinned inside a backpack. Alternatively, a touch pad key code may be used; be sure the child does not give the code to anyone, even friends. Have alternative plans of a place the child is to go in case the child loses a key, the power is off, or door is ajar indicating possible breakin.
- Teach the child to never get in a car with a stranger, open the door of the home to someone the parent has not said will arrive and can enter; do not leave windows or doors unlocked.

- Review the amount of time that can be spent on television, computer, or games. Place a child control on the computer and television to limit access to adult viewing.
- Tell the child that other children are not to come home and stay while an adult is not present.
- Review fire safety, such as avoiding use of matches, open flames, or small appliances. Microwave ovens may be safest for preparing snacks.
- Be sure firearms are locked, with guns unloaded and ammunition in a separate place. The child should not have access to the key to firearm cabinets; remember that children know the house and often are successful in finding the parent's hiding places.
- Review first aid for scratches or minor incidents.
- Review use of 911 and other resources. Keep these numbers by the phones.
- Be sure the child makes good decisions about what to do in case of fire, someone seeking entry to the house, power outage, or severe weather. Provide scenarios and ask the child what should be done. Reinforce teaching as needed.
- Arrange for friends, family members, or neighbors who the child can call if lonely, scared, in need of help, or in danger. Be sure the child knows that it is all right to feel afraid sometimes. Some communities have phone services that help with homework or talk to children who are home alone. Find out if such a service is available in your community.
- Call the child every hour or so during the first few months of staying alone. Consider getting a cell phone so the child can use that phone and does not need to answer the family phone. If the home phone is answered, the child should tell callers that the parents are busy, rather than not at home.
- Never leave a child alone for extended periods or overnight.

Source: *Adapted from Murray, R. B., Zentner, J. P., & Yakimo, R. (2009). Health promotion strategies through the life span (8th ed.). Upper Saddle River, NJ: Prentice Hall Health.*

BOX 12–1	The 5-a-Day Program and 3-a-Day of Dairy

The 5-a-day program is a comprehensive, coordinated national nutrition program designed to increase the consumption of fruits and vegetables to at least five servings daily. The National Cancer Institute and the Produce for Better Health Foundation joined together to launch the program; now many states and local areas have initiatives to raise awareness of the benefits of fruits and vegetables for health.

Most children do not consume this ideal, so concentrating on this topic may help families. Explain that fruits and vegetables contain vitamins necessary for good health and have been associated with lower rates of several cancers, diabetes, and obesity. Ask what vegetables and fruits are available and which they like. Apples, oranges, and bananas comprise the most commonly selected fruits, and carrots, potatoes (most in the form of fries), and tomatoes are common vegetables. Recognize that likes may relate to cultural group. Compose a list, including both common fruits and vegetables like beans, corn, and pears, and less commonly eaten items such as beets, mangoes, pineapple, kiwi, cantaloupe, berries, and other seasonal or geographically related foods. Ask families to choose two or three fruits and two or three vegetables that everyone in the family likes, and teach them to purchase those foods weekly. Recommend that fresh fruits and vegetables always be cut and readily available in the refrigerator; this encourages their consumption when a child comes home alone and is hungry. Add berries and other fruits to cereals.

Make shakes with nonfat frozen yogurt and added fruit. Recognize that frozen and canned fruits and vegetables are a good way to get these food groups. See if local food programs like WIC provide vouchers to obtain foods in local farmers' markets; this is often a good resource for produce in low-income families. Are there field gleaning programs if you live in an agricultural area? (Gleaning describes the process of a farmer allowing people to come into a field that has been harvested to collect any remaining foods.) Set the goal with a family of increasing by one to two servings daily the intake of fruits and vegetables. Ask them to keep a log, and invite them to call and tell you how they are doing. Health promotion programs in schools can offer incentives and prizes to children who eat five servings a day. Work with school nurses to facilitate these programs.

Similarly, we know that most individuals consume only about half the recommended amount of calcium daily. Three servings a day of dairy products such as milk, cheese, and yogurt are recommended for everyone. Dairy products provide intake of calcium, phosphorus, potassium, riboflavin, niacin, and vitamins A, D, and B_{12}. Review the intake of dairy products for children and recommend ways to increase dairy product intake if needed. Consult the National Dairy Council and your state's Dairy Council for more information and for helpful teaching aids.

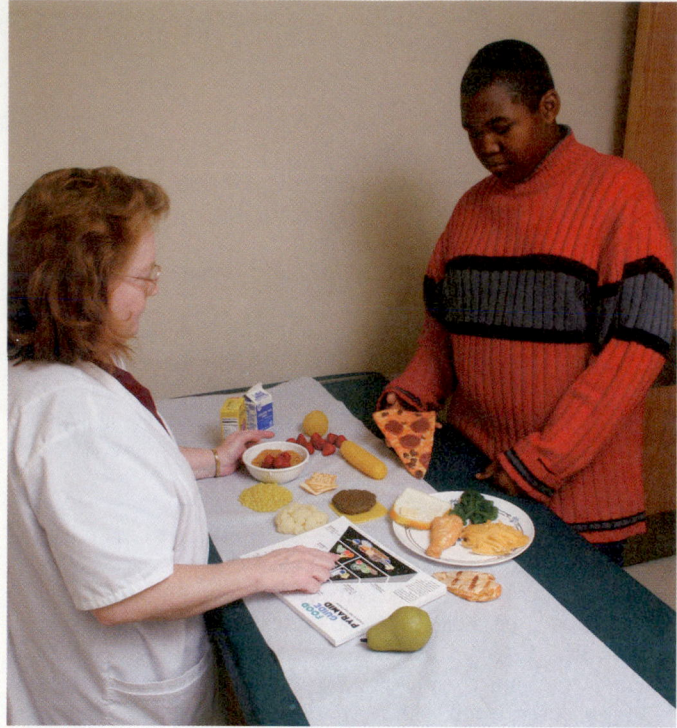

FIGURE 12–2 ■ This school-age child is receiving teaching from the nurse about food choices. What benefit do the food models provide in this situation? What other teaching techniques can you suggest?

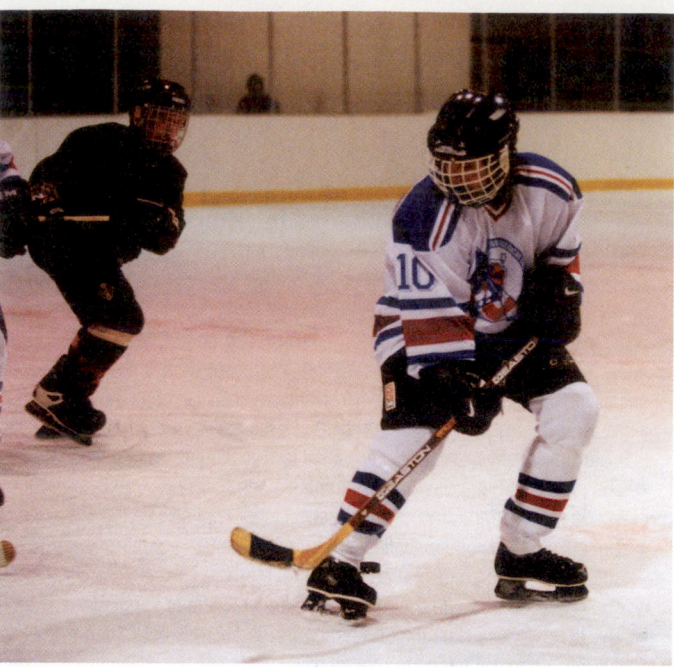

FIGURE 12–3 ■ Everyone needs to be physically active. Some children participate in school sports. Others, such as these boys playing hockey, choose a sport that is available in the community. Other children prefer to walk, ride a bike, or engage in other more solitary activities. Determine what is enjoyable for a particular child and provide assistance in integrating desirable exercise into daily routines.

place during visits, at schools, and in other settings with school-age youth (Figure 12–2 ■).

Clearly, teaching about nutrition can promote health of children. Desired outcomes for health maintenance include absence of overweight and future chronic disease, adequate intake of all nutrients, and increasing child and family knowledge about nutrition.

PHYSICAL ACTIVITY

Just as food choices during the school-age years are likely to influence the child's future nutrition, physical activity during these years is often crucial to development of lifelong exercise. During these years, the child who is physically active continues to refine skills such as eye-hand coordination, muscular strength, agility, and speed. Some children become skilled at ball sports such as basketball, football, soccer, or baseball. Others focus on gymnastics, wrestling, horseback riding, or hockey (Figure 12–3 ■). Some do not like team or organized sports but choose skateboarding, skiing, or biking. Whatever the interest, it is important that children identify some physical activity and continue to develop motor skills. The benefits include socialization, positive sense of accomplishment and self-esteem, weight control, and increasing physical ability (Figure 12–4 ■). Children who do not have an activity of importance often fall behind their peers in agility and skill, making future attempts at an activity very difficult and less likely to be successful.

The nurse should ask about the total amount of time spent daily on screen activities, such as computers, video games, and cell phones. These sedentary activities provide direct competition to time spent in physical activity, reading, and other more healthy pursuits. While no more than 2 hours of daily screen activity is recommended, many youth spend much more time using such media. See Chapter 20 🔋

for further discussion of the effects of media and ways to encourage alternative choices.

Similar to earlier periods in life, the nurse lists risk and protective factors related to school-age physical activity (Table 12–2). Families are often significant in promoting physical activity for children. Find out what the parents do for physical activity and how often. Do they attend a sports club after work, or does the child see them engaging in exercise? Most families can include some walking, yard work, or other activity that is done together to engage the

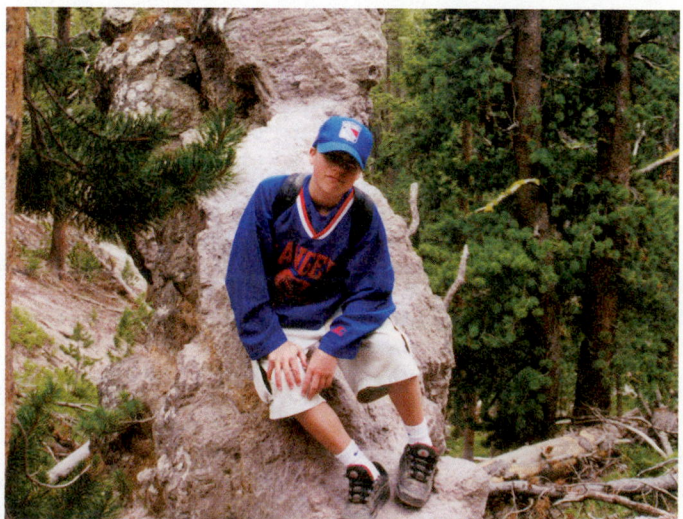

FIGURE 12–4 ■ School-age children often enjoy hikes with family, clubs, or other groups. How many physical and mental health benefits of this physical activity can you list?

TABLE 12–2	**Risk and Protective Factors Regarding Physical Activity in School-Age Children**
RISK FACTORS	**PROTECTIVE FACTORS**
■ Developmental delay and special needs	■ Expected developmental skill level
■ Limited role modeling of daily physical activity by parents and other family members	■ Parents exercise daily and exercise with the child some of this time in settings the child can see ■ Parents set expectations that everyone in the family will choose a physical activity and engage in it regularly
■ Limited facilities in the neighborhood to encourage activity, such as parks, skateboard facilities, rinks, ball courts/fields	■ Neighborhood provides access to parks, skateboard facilities, rinks, ball courts, and other facilities
■ Inadequate financial resources to join clubs or pay for organized sports	■ Family has adequate financial resources to pay for health club or organized sports
■ Lack of safety gear for activities chosen due to cost, or reluctance to use the gear	■ Recommended safety gear that properly fits child is available ■ Child understands importance of safety gear and accepts using such equipment
■ School cuts to physical education programs and recess	■ Schools provide physical education each day with a variety of offerings; student gets to choose and set goals for some activities ■ Schools schedule recess or physical activity breaks twice daily
■ School tryouts for sports that eliminate all but the best players in certain sports	■ Sports teams are leveled so that all students desiring to play a particular sport, such as soccer, are able to do so
■ Reluctance to try new activity	■ Willing to try new activities
■ Worry about competence and physical appearance	■ Feels self-confident in ability and physical appearance ■ Sets goals for learning physical skills
■ Television viewing or other screen activities for more than 2 hours daily	■ Television viewing and other screen activities limited to no more than 2 hours daily

child. Do they walk to a neighbor's house or a nearby store rather than driving? Do they take elevators or choose the stairs in buildings? What is the activity level of siblings? When older siblings are involved in sports, the younger child often is encouraged to develop skills in the same sport.

The child spends much of the day in school; therefore, this setting is important to consider. In an effort to conserve financial resources, some schools have decreased physical education (PE) programs. Children may not have regular PE classes, and there may be few standards of performance. In addition, many states and provinces have established tests and standards for performance in certain cognitive areas. In an attempt to increase teaching time to meet these standards, some schools have cut recess and other breaks. Schools are sometimes located in unsafe areas, and outside recreation is not advisable. However, it is unrealistic to expect children to sit for long periods without physical activity, and such practice reinforces the poor habits of inadequate exercise among children. Schools that offer a variety of activities, including intramural (rather than only organized competitive) sports, are more likely to encourage a greater number of children to be active. At least 30 of the recommended 60 minutes of daily vigorous physical activity should be provided in school, along with an adequate amount of unstructured playtime during recess (Centers for Disease Control and Prevention, 2011). Nurses are influential members of school committees and can encourage the integration of activity in the school day. You may be able to serve on a school or community committee, educating other committee members of the benefits of exercise to enhance cognitive performance and general health. Teachers and school administrators can be supplied with models of successful school activity programs.

Some elementary schools offer sports programs in after-school settings. Children report that it is difficult to begin participating in a sport that was not started early in life since so many accomplished athletes have played for years. When these organized sports have tryouts and eliminations, the children who most need activity may be those eliminated. The child who has a pubertal growth spurt early (see Chapter 5 🔗) is often better at certain organized sports and has many more opportunities to engage in them. Eliminating smaller children or those less adept at sports means that they are unable to learn the skills necessary to play the sport. However, some of them may actually become better at the sport as they grow older and bigger. It is best if different levels are available so that all interested children can play and learn the physical skills needed to improve. Again, school finances make this difficult, so nurses can often be influential in finding community volunteers to work with teams of students. Student nurses, physical education students, senior citizens, and others are often able to help young children play baseball, tennis, or soccer. Other volunteers may teach stretching or warm-up activities. Community partners such as businesses may provide protective gear or uniforms for school sports, especially if the business name can be displayed. In addition, schools can offer alternative activities that some children might prefer to traditional organized sports. Nurses can work with school personnel to encourage physical education and fitness offerings that maximize the numbers of children involved. Can the school obtain a climbing wall? Is there a skate park near the school? Will a local ski resort sponsor a weekly or monthly bus of children from the school? Is swimming available at a nearby city or YMCA/YWCA pool? What can you do in your local community schools to ensure equal access to sports for all children? How can you help parents to become influential in the community to improve options for their children?

It is essential to consider physical activity for the child who has special healthcare needs (Kuo, Frick, & Minkovitz, 2011). It may be difficult for schools to plan an activity for the child with cerebral palsy, visual impairment, or developmental delay. Search for other community resources and help the family to access them. There may be programs for children to ride horses, swim, ski, and engage in other physical activities. Search out the Special Olympics programs in your area. Imagine the thrill that awaits a child who has rarely moved quickly when he or she has the chance to ride a sled or slide on skis.

In summary, the nurse plays an important role in meeting desired outcomes of health promotion by suggesting activities that families can do together, becoming active in physical education programs in schools, acting as a positive role model, and helping interested children to partner with community resources for activity. Health maintenance outcomes include use of safety gear and correct techniques to prevent injury from sport participation.

ORAL HEALTH

Many changes occur in the mouth during the school-age years, necessitating periodic examination. At about 6 years of age, most children lose a tooth, usually in the front. Following that, all 20 of the deciduous or primary teeth will be lost, and the permanent teeth will simultaneously begin to erupt. See Figure 7–26 in Chapter 7 for the schedule of tooth loss of deciduous teeth and tooth eruption of permanent teeth. (See Developing Cultural Competence: Tooth Loss.) In addition, the jaw line elongates and teeth move into new positions. Periodic dental visits focus on both the placement of teeth and oral hygiene.

During the health promotion visit, examine the teeth. Look to see how many deciduous and permanent teeth are present. Describe the child's oral hygiene. Ask how often the child brushes, flosses, and visits the dentist. The child should have learned how to brush and floss during preschool years but is now performing the skills independently. If caries or poor oral hygiene is apparent, ask the child to demonstrate brushing and flossing. Reinforce the need for brushing twice daily and flossing once daily. Provide toothpaste and toothbrushes as gifts during health supervision visits. Local dentists will often provide these supplies so that you can encourage oral hygiene.

Dental visits are recommended every 6 months, so if the child is not visiting on that schedule, ask if finances or transportation are issues, if the family needs a referral to a dentist, or if there is some other reason. If caries or malocclusion is present, stress the need for a dental

appointment. Inquire about use of fluoride if the water supply is not fluoridated. Ask if the child has had sealants applied to the permanent teeth; these will help to prevent future caries. During school age some children are referred to an orthodontist for occlusion and other dental issues. Offer to help the parents locate resources to assist with this additional recommendation for care.

Many children have a high intake of sugared foods and snacks. If this is apparent from the nutritional assessment, discuss the importance of limiting these foods and brushing after their consumption. Frequent brushing is needed when the child has braces. Ask how they are caring for them and what the orthodontist has recommended.

The nurse's health promotion activities include positive reinforcement of good hygiene habits. Health maintenance involves teaching about the need for improved care and limiting food that furthers the formation of caries. Desired outcomes include good oral hygiene, attendance at recommended dental visits, and absence of dental caries.

MENTAL AND SPIRITUAL HEALTH

The school-age years are marked by the emergence of new cognitive skills, the ability to interact cooperatively with others, and a feeling of accomplishment in achievements. The child's self-concept and mental health are linked to these important developmental tasks (see Table 5–3 in Chapter 5 for nursing applications of theories of Freud, Erikson, and Piaget).

Self-Concept

School age is an important period in the development of self-esteem and one's self-concept. **Self-esteem** reflects feelings of self-worth or value. **Self-concept** refers to evaluations of the self in certain specific areas, such as those related to academic achievement, athletic ability, physical appearance, and social interactions (Santrock, 2011). A child with a positive self-concept feels competent, is able to meet challenges, and applies lessons from successes and failures. Specific facets of self-concept include **body image,** the idea that one forms about one's body, and **sexuality,** the person's view of self as a sexual being. Together, self-concept and self-esteem include all of the cognitive, spiritual, sexual, and physical aspects of the individual.

The nurse's aim is to establish a high sense of self-esteem, even in the face of adversity and challenge. The child who believes in his or her ability to face good times and bad has a lowered chance of mental illness such as depression, eating disorder, and anxiety. Parents are encouraged to evaluate and help to build the child's sense of self-esteem (see Partnering with Families: Evaluating and Fostering Self-Esteem).

Many of the areas we have discussed so far in this chapter provide clues to the child's self-concept. Does the child engage in sports or other physical activities? The child may then reflect a positive self-concept and body image. On the other hand, if the child is forced to do these sports by parents and feels inadequate in performance, he or she may reflect a negative self-concept and body image. Be sure to ask about the child's activities and the child's feelings about them. Does the child enjoy them? How does the child rate his or her performance? Inquire about school performance and best friends. Is there an increasing independence and responsibility for self? Success in

---

Developing Cultural Competence
Tooth Loss

In the mainstream U.S. and Canadian cultures, lost teeth signal growing up and are celebrated events. It is common for the tooth lost at school or in the hospital to be sent home to the parents with a note about when it was lost. Many children place the lost tooth under the pillow at night and expect the "tooth fairy" to leave a small gift. Parents remove the tooth while the child sleeps and place a gift. Ask about how tooth loss is handled in the family.

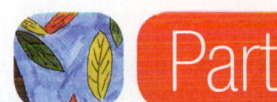

Partnering with Families

Evaluating and Fostering Self-Esteem

Parents play an important part in fostering the child's self-esteem. The nurse can ask parents to evaluate the child and provide suggestions about positive actions.

EVALUATION QUESTIONS	POSITIVE ACTIONS
What does your child do well?	■ Build on the child's strengths and talents. ■ Affectionately point out the child's abilities.
How does your child respond to failure?	■ Assist the child to assess performance. ■ Help the child see that mistakes are expected and have lessons to teach.
Does your child have close friends?	■ Arrange structured playtimes such as going to a movie or cooking with a friend.
How does your child respond to new challenges?	■ Give the child responsibilities at home; encourage your child to try new experiences. ■ Help the child feel a sense of control over outcomes.
How does your own personality compare to your child's?	■ Recognize differences in style. ■ Appreciate the unique qualities of the child. ■ Tailor expectations to the child and not to self or other children.
Are you setting reasonable and attainable expectations for your child?	■ Be a positive role model. ■ Establish goals for behaviors together.

Source: *Adapted from Kids Health. (2011). Developing your child's self-esteem. Retrieved from http://kidshealth.org/parent/emotions/feelings/self_esteem.html*

achieving developmental milestones leads to a positive sense of self-esteem in the child.

A low sense of self-esteem is noted when the child states a disinterest in exercise, school clubs, and family activities. This can lead to loneliness, depression, and mental health problems such as eating disorders. When these feelings are noted during a health supervision visit, the nurse should recommend that the child see a counselor at school or another setting, and should recommend that parents be included in the sessions so that they can best help the child.

It is obvious that the family plays a critical part in the child's developing self-esteem and mental health. To understand the child, it is necessary to ask questions about and explore dynamics in the family. Several protective factors have been identified for families (U.S. Department of Health and Human Services, 2011):

- Nurturing bonds and attachment are formed.
- Parents have knowledge about parenting skills and child development.
- Parents demonstrate resilience by recognizing their own stress and enhancing their problem-solving abilities.
- Parents have a wide array of support systems to provide social connections.
- Caregivers are available that provide resources to meet basic needs, such as finances, housing, and food.

Reinforce these positive factors when they are present, and make suggestions about protective factors for parents who need to broaden their support for the child. Ask about and observe the family's relationships when you are with them. Evaluate the effect of family interactions on the child. Model respectful interchanges by listening carefully to the child, as well as the parent. Gently recognize children if parents answer for them or seem to put them down. You might say, "Jared seems to have something to say and I'd like to hear his opinion.

What were you saying, Jared, about what you do not enjoy at school?" Provide brochures and examples of ways to show children their importance. Encourage both parents to come to child healthcare visits, and support the involvement of both parents in childrearing. Ask about family stressors such as job changes, financial concerns, illness, substance abuse, and domestic violence. About one half of marriages end in divorce, so be prepared to offer suggestions to deal with this situation (see Chapter 2 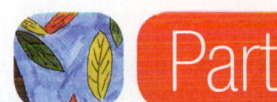). Likewise, when parents remarry and the child is in a blended or growing family again, the new roles and family dynamics may provide both challenges and strengths. Ask about risk factors and protective factors. Remember that resilience is the ability to use strengths to help deal with adversity (see Chapter 5 for a detailed description of resilience theory). Look for risk and protective factors in the family and suggest ways to use protective factors to foster resilience. The child's strengths are used to assist the family functioning and will, in turn, give the child a sense of accomplishment. Examples include the following:

- A child who is able to act independently can be given responsibility for parts of the home or family function, such as planning the menu for dinner two evenings weekly.
- A creative child can be given the task of planning books and other activities for a younger sibling.
- A child with a talent for artistic design can be asked to set the table for dinner guests.

School-age children continue to develop their abilities to self-regulate activities and responses to situations. At this age, the abilities to solve problems and assume more responsibility for self are important. Encourage parents to discuss issues with the child and to seek solutions together when appropriate. For example, the parent may tell the child that there is enough money to sign up for one summer camp and let the child help to choose which one it should be. If the child is having difficulty in getting homework done, he or she can be included in a discussion about possible solutions. If the child suggests doing homework when first coming home, or limiting television time on weeknights, it is more likely that the solution will work. The child assumes more responsibility for assisting with meal preparation and home chores, coming home alone after school, and caring for younger siblings. Encourage the parents to praise the child for assuming more family responsibilities and recognize that the child will need some guidance when taking on new tasks.

Sexuality

The school-age child is developing a sense of body image and sexuality. Look at the child's appearance and dress. Some children may have poor posture, display a sense of insecurity, and seem uncomfortable with themselves. Others may dress as if they were much older, seem sophisticated, and are clearly assuming the role identification with their gender group. Ask the parents in a private setting what observations they have about the child's body image and sexuality. Inquire about friends in whom the child seems romantically or sexually interested, and whether the parent has concerns about this interest.

Questions related to sexuality will emerge during school years. They should be answered truthfully and fully. Even children who do not ask questions usually need information related to sexuality education. They may receive information in school beginning in approximately fourth grade but often have misconceptions about the bodies of men and women, sexual intercourse, how babies are born, and other topics. Suggest that parents read books with their children that deal with these issues at an appropriate developmental level. If books are available at home, children will be likely to look at them and ask questions. Provide titles and lists in offices so that parents can view and choose from resources. Many young girls have body changes as early as 9 or 10 years of age (see Chapter 5 🕮), and reading material can put both parent and child at ease and open the door to discussion. Parents should be advised to talk with teachers to learn what is presented in school and be able to supplement and clarify this information. Having discussions at a young age will encourage further discussion as the child gets older. Nurses often perform sexuality education in schools or work with school districts in establishing policies regarding sexuality education plans.

Computers and other media provide information that can confuse children. Encourage parents to watch movies with their children, to have frank discussions related to sexuality observed, and to answer questions truthfully. Children generally learn about topics such as sexual intercourse, sexual orientation, and childbirth from school discussions and the media. A few moments alone with parents and the child separately at healthcare visits may help to identify the concerns of each related to sexuality.

By approximately grades 4 to 6, most girls have started to have prepubertal body changes and may begin to menstruate. This is another opening to discussions about mature bodies of men and women and the transformation from childhood to greater maturity. Boys mature about 2 years later than girls, and without an event such as menstruation, parents may be less likely to start discussions with male children. Suggest that parents consciously begin conversations with boys periodically to explain changes they see in themselves and their peers. See Chapters 5 and 7 🕮 for further discussion of the body changes seen in the prepubertal period and during puberty.

Sleep

Sleep is important for children to have the energy to perform well in school and other activities. They generally take charge of bedtime routines with reminders about the time to go to sleep, and they sleep through the night. Sleep time varies from 8 to 12 hours, depending on the child and activity level. Busy schedules may interrupt this pattern, leading to irritability, lack of concentration, or even hyperactive behavior. Help children and families plan for healthy practices of **sleep hygiene,** or behaviors that foster a regular and sufficient sleep pattern, as well as daytime alertness (Mayo Clinic, 2009; Mindell, Meltzer, Carskadon, et al., 2009).

Practice Alert

Nurses should inquire about the sleep patterns and amount of sleep that children receive. Ask if they are frequently tired or have trouble sleeping. Some simple behaviors help to promote sleep and are referred to as sleep hygiene. They include (Mayo Clinic, 2009; Mindell et al., 2009):

- Go to bed and get up at approximately the same time each day, including weekends.
- Follow a bedtime routine to prepare for sleep.
- Recognize that we do not "make up" sleep that is "lost" by sleeping in.
- Avoid caffeine, including tea, coffee, and carbonated beverages, for several hours before sleep.
- Gradually slow down activity about an hour or two before bedtime.
- Do not watch television, play games, text on the phone, or conduct other activities in the sleep location.
- Avoid naps in the late afternoon or evening.
- Darken the room for sleep.

Sleepwalking and sleep talking sometimes occur at this age but usually decrease as the child nears adolescence. Children who have stress at home, such as parental fighting, ill family members, or inadequate food or shelter, may not get enough sleep and fall asleep at school. Ask the child if he or she falls asleep in class, and seek additional information about family stressors. This can lead to interventions such as recommending family counseling or referring to resources to obtain better housing or more stable food sources. Children with obesity or large tonsils and adenoids are prone to sleep apnea. They often snore and have otherwise noisy sleep. In such cases, weight loss or adenoidectomy may improve sleep (Bonuck, Chervin, Cole, et al., 2011). (See Chapter 25 🕮 for a thorough discussion of sleep apnea.)

School

Along with family and peers, school is a major microsystem influence in the lives of children, and plays a role in self-concept and mental health formation. Parents may need guidance when the young child is of school age. Ask if they have decided what year the child will begin kindergarten and what school the child will attend. Become familiar with the local schools and whether they perform school readiness testing. The child is usually ready for kindergarten when communication and cognitive skills are sufficient to support learning, the child can successfully separate from parents, experiences with other children show ability to make friends and regulate own behavior, and the child can follow rules and directions (Hagan, Shaw, & Duncan, 2008). Help parents to learn the ways they can facilitate a healthy transition to school, such as ensuring good sleep and eating routines, reading with the child, showing interest in school activities, and finding a space in the home for the child's school-related work.

For the child who is attending school, ask for a description of a best friend; if the child is unable to describe a best friend, isolation may be occurring. Inquire about what the three best and three worst things are about school. Children with low self-concept often have trouble talking about and evaluating school. Find out where the child attends school, if the area is generally safe, and how the child gets to school. Are there clubs, after-school sports, or school performances for parents on occasion? What are the child's grades like? Do the parents and child feel that the child is challenged intellectually but not unduly stressed? Encourage the parents to meet the child's teachers, to become active in school activities, and to be available to solve problems with school personnel when needed. Partner with the parents and child when interventions are needed. An office nurse may contact a school nurse when the child needs support in the school environment. This may occur if the child has become ill and missed school, has family stressors, does not get along well with a teacher, or has a condition such as attention deficit disorder. Identify the risk and protective factors in the school environment and plan interventions to support the child when risks are present. See the following section in this chapter and Chapters 20 and 34 🔗 for more information about attention deficit disorder, bullying, and other issues in the school environment.

Mental Health Disorders

Certain mental health disorders are common during the school years, including anxiety problems that result in worries, fears, physical symptoms, stress, and sleep disorders. These problems may occur without significantly impairing daily functioning, but anxiety disorders affect functioning and have more striking characteristics such as clinging, abdominal pain and headache, fear of embarrassment, and refusal to attend school (Kodish, Rockhill, Ryan, et al., 2011; Ramsawh, Chavira, & Stein, 2010). Posttraumatic stress syndrome and depression may also be seen. See Chapter 34 🔗 for further description of these disorders. Anxiety disorder, posttraumatic stress, and depression should be referred to a mental health specialist for treatment. However, all children worry at times, and learning coping skills and relaxation techniques can help this type of anxiety.

Spiritual Health

Spiritual health is the ability to develop a spiritual nature, including awareness of a life purpose or meaning, a sustaining power during times of stress, a feeling of harmony with the universe, and a sense of fulfillment (Murray, Zentner, & Yakimo, 2009; Pender, Murdaugh, & Parsons, 2011). School age is a time when children learn more about the people and the world around them and begin to find their place in that world. Connection with faith-based groups assists some children and families in defining the purpose of life, while others may do so through social activity or a strong moral sense of responsibility. Ask children what brings happiness, how they help other people, or if they are members of a church, synagogue, or mosque. If families seem to have little purpose, parents are withdrawn or depressed, or the child has difficulty answering questions about meaningful activities, suggest methods of engagement in the community. These might include providing contacts at local religious events, posting flyers about community events designed to bring unity to various cultural groups, or suggesting services needing volunteers in the community. Families who spend time together and find meaning in supporting each other nurture the spiritual health of their members. Suggest that every family plan a "family night" weekly when they play games, talk, eat, or engage in other activities together.

Nursing Role

The nurse has an important role in fostering the mental and spiritual health of school-age children. Health promotion fosters strengths of families and children, leading to healthy self-concept and positive self-esteem. Some strengths to consider in health promotion include:

- The family spends time together in activities several times weekly.
- The child is able to verbalize school and home activities that are important and meaningful.
- The family is engaged in religious or community activities on a regular basis.
- There are adequate resources for housing, food, and other basic necessities.

Health maintenance seeks to prevent mental health disruptions. Be alert for risk factors in families since they represent the need for intervention. Some examples include:

- Family schedules are chaotic with little chance for interaction among family members.
- The family is isolated and feels little connection to the community.
- Basic necessities are often not met, whether for food, housing, or health care.
- The child has no school or community activities such as sports or clubs.

Expected outcomes for health promotion and health maintenance activities with school-age children include formation of a positive sense of self-esteem and healthy body image, use of coping skills to deal with stress, sleep patterns that meet needs for rest, and a growing purpose and meaning in life.

RELATIONSHIPS

While the school-age child is gradually moving away from the family as the center of life, the family remains an important anchor. As we discussed in the preceding section, parents foster a child's development related to several health issues. Ask also about siblings, grandparents, and other extended family members. Sometimes these persons assist in the child's formation of a self-concept. Peers are increasingly important to the school-age child's self-identity. School age is a time of cooperative engagement with others (see Chapter 5 🔗). All children need to learn how to make and maintain friendships and work with others on projects and in recreation.

Inquire about the child's best friends at school, and ask parents if they are comfortable with the child's selection of friends. Find out if the parents facilitate friendships by allowing other children to come to the home and providing transportation as needed. When the child experiences a risk factor such as a move to a new town or school, role-play how to meet new children and how to make friends. If the child feels like an outcast or outsider among peers at school, explore how the family can create a safe and secure place for the child in extracurricular activities with children who have similar interests. When children are homeschooled, the family may need to plan social events and contacts after usual school hours.

Since peers are important at this stage, the school-age child begins to feel pressure to appear like others, to fit in, and to do what others encourage. Although such pressures are often associated with teen years, they usually begin earlier, at least by 8 or 9 years of age. Ask children what things friends try to get them to do that they know they should not do, or if friends have tried to get them to smoke. Middle school years are the most common age for smoking to begin, so always ask if the child has tried smoking. The child may tell you about activities when parents are not in the room, such as playing with guns, trying alcohol or other substances, or partaking in other risky behavior. It is best to ask what the child does in these situations, what the child wants to do, and to whom the child can turn to talk about these events. Offer information about the risks connected with behaviors that are described, and suggest people such as parents, teachers, counselors, or clergy who are possible resources. If the child's health is at risk, be sure to report the activity to the physician or other healthcare provider so that it can be pursued and the child's safety can be ensured. Activities such as playing with firearms or visiting a friend whose parents are making methamphetamine, for example, place children in extreme danger.

Parents often need guidance to help them in setting limits for their school-age children. The child is becoming more independent, but unacceptable behaviors must still be managed by successful discipline techniques. Some guidelines that can help families include (American Academy of Pediatrics, 2011a; Knox, 2010):

- *Talking calmly*—Express the behavior observed, why it is not acceptable, and its effects on others. If appropriate, the child can help decide what should be done to change the behavior (i.e., removing a privilege or other solution).
- *Using natural or logical consequences*—For example, if the child breaks in anger an item he or she owns, the item should not be replaced. If the broken item belongs to someone else, the child should be expected to earn the money to replace the item.
- *Withholding privileges*—Be consistent in privileges withheld and be certain that they are privileges (such as attending a movie with friends) rather than essential (a meal).
- *Using time-out to separate the child from others*—This technique can be helpful when the child needs time to redirect a temper or other such behavior. It is not helpful as a frequent technique for all undesirable behavior, especially when sent to the bedroom that may have a television, cell phone, and other technologic devices.
- *Applying distraction*—The child who is frustrated may learn to handle the stress if the parent suggests a brisk walk or other physical outlet.
- *Avoiding spanking and yelling*—These techniques are not generally helpful and fail to teach the child positive substitutions for undesirable behavior.

School age is often a time when children first experience violence in relationships with others. Some children are bullied, while others are the bullies. Anger and aggression can occur, and children get in fights with each other. Ask children to describe when they last had a disagreement with someone and how the problem was solved. Have they ever been hit, been called names, or had fights? How did it make them feel? What did they do about it? Suggest people who can help, such as school nurses, teachers, and counselors, and be sure that children feel safe in schools, neighborhoods, and homes. Ask parents how they resolve arguments between children at home and what help they need to teach children problem-solving skills. Find

out what policies the schools have in your community to assist in decreasing harassment of and by children. As you progress in your career, become active on school committees that help children learn how to solve problems peacefully and how to respond to episodes of violence. See Chapter 20 🔗 for further discussion of violence in children and a detailed discussion of bullying.

The child's temperament still plays a part in response to situations and the ability to self-regulate (see Chapter 5 🔗 for a discussion of patterns of temperament in children). The "difficult" child may have trouble getting to sleep or being quiet in the classroom. Have parents plan more physical activity for this child. Teach the child that bedtime routines are helpful and that sitting near the front of the class can help with concentration. The "slow to warm up" child may need ideas about what to say when meeting new people. Parents can help this child prepare for a new school by visiting the school with the child, talking about it, and meeting with the teacher so that a warm welcome can occur. The "easy" child is usually adaptable in most situations and is regular in activities. However, this child may object when other children interrupt in conversation, fail to take turns, or otherwise "break the rules" of behavior. Children may need help to understand differences in temperament in order to be more tolerant of classmates and their behaviors. Often nurses in schools address the issue of individual differences by speaking with classes or small groups of children.

Once again, the nurse promotes the child's health by anticipating developmental issues and preparing the parents and child to deal with them. Health maintenance outcomes include preventing problems in interactions with others.

DISEASE PREVENTION STRATEGIES

School-age children are generally healthy. The immune system is mature (see Chapter 27 🔗), personal hygiene practices are more mature than at earlier ages, and immunizations are usually complete. Engage school-age children in active pursuit of their own health. Teach strategies that can enhance the prevention of diseases. Nurses in offices and schools can teach children how to wash hands effectively, how respiratory infections are transmitted, and what can cause gastrointestinal illness. Ask children in your settings what topics are of most interest to them, and be prepared to suggest common areas of concern. Children are interested in their bodies and can understand the connection between eating well and avoiding illness, maintaining normal weight and preventing type 2 diabetes, avoiding smoking to prevent cancer and other respiratory diseases, maintaining oral hygiene to promote oral health, and exercising to prevent hypertension. Include safety teaching in all interactions, provide information about skin care and how to deal with common skin problems, and teach about drug use.

Clinical Judgment

Recall Jessalyn who was described in the chapter-opening scenario. How will you integrate exercise, nutrition knowledge, and management of her diabetes to prevent related diseases such as high blood pressure, retinal damage, renal damage, or cardiovascular disease? See Figure 12–5 ■.

School-age children are in the concrete stage of intellectual development, according to Piaget's theory (see Chapter 5 🔗). This means that teaching is most effective when opportunities are provided to touch, feel, and otherwise become actively engaged in learning. When teaching about smoking, provide models of lungs and have

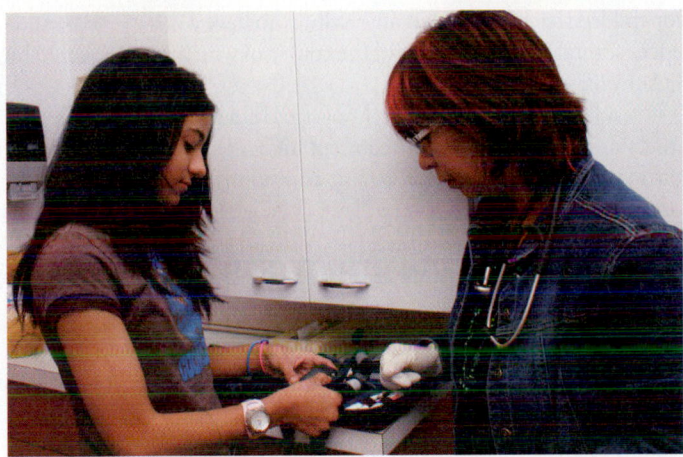

FIGURE 12–5 ■ Jessalyn is showing the school nurse how she programs her insulin pump. The nurse has partnered with nurses in the endocrinologist's office to learn about the type of pump Jessalyn is using. Such collaboration enhances the chances that diabetes will be well monitored and managed.

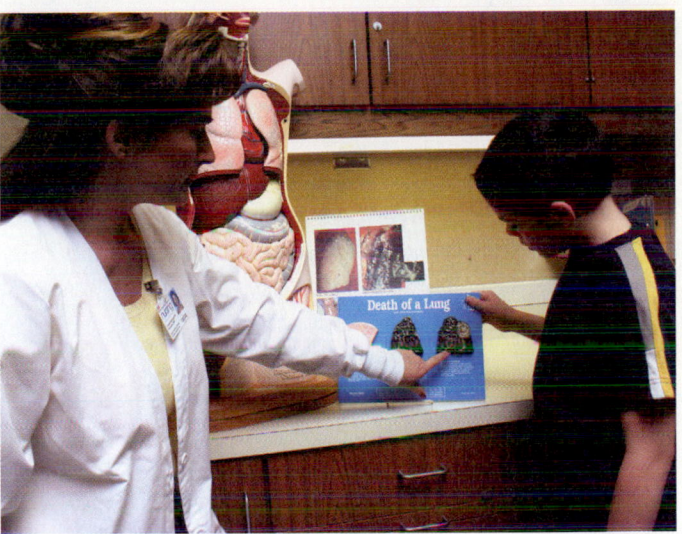

FIGURE 12–6 ■ This boy is learning about the effects of smoking on the body through the concrete experience of examining a model of the lungs. Why does this type of hands-on technique help school-age children to learn concepts?

students breathe through a straw to demonstrate the effects of airway narrowing. These concrete activities will teach them concepts better than simple lecture or reading (Figure 12–6 ■). Concepts of health promotion tend to be abstract since they deal with supporting one's highest potential for wellness. Thus it becomes even more important to provide concrete methods of learning.

Immunizations are generally up to date for school-age children. However, some children may have missed earlier doses due to illness or missed healthcare visits (see Chapter 22 🔗). Evaluate the immunization record to be sure it meets all recommendations. The most common immunization needs at this time are as follows:

- Hepatitis B (whole series or a missed third dose)
- Hepatitis A (two doses if not previously administered)
- Polio and measles-mumps-rubella (if booster doses of each were not given prior to school entry)
- Tetanus and diphtheria and acellular pertussis (Tdap) at the 11-year visit or after
- Varicella if not given earlier and the child has not had the disease
- Human papillomavirus (HPV) three-dose series at 9 years or older
- Meningococcal conjugate vaccine at 11 years with booster at 16 years
- Influenza vaccine annually
- Certain vaccines for children at high risk, such as pneumococcal (see Chapter 22 🔗 for further information on immunizations)

Screening for health risks should occur during the visit (Table 12–3). Unusual complaints such as the following may indicate a need for further testing:

- Pain other than brief discomfort after an injury
- Headaches
- Bruising
- Lack of coordination
- Repeated infections
- Decreasing vision or hearing
- Problems or changes in school performance or behavior

Children who have an identified health problem or developmental disability may have additional needs for screening and for interventions to assist with health maintenance. For example, the child with cystic fibrosis will need information to lessen the risk of respiratory infection, and the child with diabetes may need additional blood studies. The child who has difficulty reading will need alternative approaches to teaching correct hand washing; demonstration with explanation may be the best approach. A family history of diseases increases the child's risk and necessitates testing. For example, if a parent has had early cardiovascular disease (before age 55 years), a lipid profile should be performed on the child.

Inquire about any medications the child takes, including vitamins and fluoride. Ask how often over-the-counter medications are used, which ones, and at what dosages. Both parents and school-age children should understand the correct use and dosages of medications, as well as how to observe for side effects. Some families use complementary therapy for common conditions such as respiratory infections or gastrointestinal complaints. Complementary and alternative medicine (CAM) therapy is quite common in families where children have chronic conditions such as attention deficit hyperactivity disorder (ADHD), autism, or skin conditions (Ben-Arye, Traube, Schachter, et al., 2011; Sibinga & Kemper, 2010). (See Chapter 34 🔗 for a description of CAM for autism and ADHD.) Consult references and websites to find current information about any products used, and insert this teaching into health visits.

Parents should receive explanations about the screening tests performed and the results obtained. Inform them about vision and hearing results. Send home or call in results of blood tests when available. Be sure they understand the findings and have resources to assist in preventing or treating the specific disease in their children. Encourage parents to call with questions about health problems the child develops, and provide information about lowering risks of diseases. Be sure that families know when to keep children home from school (elevated temperature, active vomiting or diarrhea, coughing up brown or green mucus). Assist schools in setting guidelines for

TABLE 12–3	Screening During Health Promotion and Health Maintenance Visits
AGE	**RECOMMENDED SCREENING TESTS**
5 years and 6 years	Vision
	Hearing
	Lead exposure risk (and lead screening if at risk)
	Hematocrit or hemoglobin if at risk of anemia
	Cholesterol if at risk of hyperlipidemia (at 6 years)
	Height and weight (and BMI)
	Blood pressure
	Urinalysis
	Tuberculin test (if at risk)
	Psychosocial/behavioral health
7 and 8 years	Vision
	Hearing
	Hematocrit or hemoglobin if at risk of anemia
	Cholesterol if at risk of hyperlipidemia (at 8 years)
	Height and weight (and BMI)
	Blood pressure
	Oral health
	Tuberculin test (if at risk)
	Psychosocial/behavioral health
9 and 10 years	Vision
	Hearing
	Hematocrit or hemoglobin if at risk of anemia
	Cholesterol if at risk of hyperlipidemia (at 10 years)
	Height and weight (and BMI)
	Blood pressure
	Tuberculin test (if at risk)
	Psychosocial/behavioral health
11 and 12 years	Vision
	Hearing
	Hematocrit or hemoglobin if at risk of anemia
	Cholesterol if at risk of hyperlipidemia
	Sexually transmitted infection (STI) screening if at risk
	Cervical dysplasia screening if at risk
	Height and weight (and BMI)
	Blood pressure
	Tuberculin test (if at risk)
	Psychosocial/behavioral health

Source: Adapted from American Academy of Pediatrics, Committee on Practice and Ambulatory Medicine. (2008). Recommendations for preventive pediatric health care. In J. F. Hagan, J. S. Shaw, & P. M. Duncan, Bright Futures. Elk Grove Village, IL: American Academy of Pediatrics.

management of infectious diseases in that setting. Contact your local county and state health department for infectious disease guidelines for schools; consult Chapter 22 ⊘ for further ideas.

Many disease prevention strategies are designed as health maintenance activities, since their objectives are to prevent health problems. Some health promotion is also integrated when teaching to children emphasizes how their bodies work and how they can best promote their own health. Health promotion activities are important

for children such as Jessalyn and Kelly, who have a disease that influences several body systems and the course of which can be altered by healthy lifestyles.

Desired outcomes for the school-age child include prevention of infectious diseases, prompt treatment for acute infections, and careful management of existing health conditions to maximize health potential.

INJURY PREVENTION STRATEGIES

Injuries are a common cause of morbidity and mortality among school-age children, and each health maintenance encounter should include injury prevention strategies. Children at this age are increasingly independent and may be harmed by activities they engage in without adults, such as playing with fire or firearms. They participate in many sports and other physical activities and may suffer related injuries. In addition, some children unfortunately suffer harm due to physical abuse. See Chapter 20 ⊘ for further discussion of violence prevention.

Many common injuries are preventable by using protective gear and following safety guidelines. About 10% of youth rarely or never wear seat belts in automobiles (Centers for Disease Control and Prevention, 2010a). Many children ride bicycles, but 85% never wear a protective helmet, contributing to 23,000 bicycle-related head injuries annually. Bike helmets could prevent up to 88% of serious brain injuries from bicycle crashes (Centers for Disease Control and Prevention, 2010a). Certain groups of children are more at risk than others of not taking protective measures (see Developing Cultural Competence: Use of Safety Protection). Strategies to make helmet use more attractive and to ensure correct wearing of helmets are needed (see Evidence-Based Practice: Bicycle Helmet Effectiveness and Use). Other risky behaviors that require protective gear include:

- Rollerblading
- Skateboarding
- Roller hockey
- Ice hockey
- Football
- Baseball
- Soccer
- Scooters
- Skiing or snowboarding
- Snowmobiling
- Motorcycle and all-terrain vehicle riding

Developing Cultural Competence
Use of Safety Protection

There are marked differences in behaviors that influence unintentional injuries. Although only about 11% of children rarely or never wear a seat belt in the car, males are most at risk; almost 14% of Black males, 14% of Hispanic males, and 13% of White males do not use seat belts (Centers for Disease Control and Prevention, 2008). Approximately 93% of Black youth, 89% of Hispanic youth, and 82% of White youth do not wear bicycle helmets (Centers for Disease Control and Prevention, 2010a). How will you inquire about seat belt and bicycle helmet use in an open-ended manner during health promotion visits? Consider asking these questions: Where do you usually ride in the car? Who do you usually ride with? Are there seat belts? How often do you use them? Plan strategies to include for all children and families, especially those at high risk of not using seat belts.

Evidence-Based Practice   Bicycle Helmet Effectiveness and Use

PROBLEM

Approximately 90 children die of bicycle-related injuries annually in the United States, and many more are injured. Children ages 5 to 14 years have a high rate of bicycle injuries (Bicycle Helmet Safety Institute, 2011). Although helmets can reduce injury, many times they are not worn or are worn incorrectly.

EVIDENCE

Wearing bicycle helmets is associated with higher household incomes, living in a state with a bicycle helmet law, younger ages, and having health insurance (Dellinger & Kresnow, 2010; Devoe, Tillotson, Wallace, et al., 2012). Many children wear a helmet incorrectly, most often positioning it too far back on the head (Hagel, Lee, Karkhaneh, et al., 2010). A meta-analysis of research on helmet use found that community-based interventions, particularly those providing free helmets, and school-based interventions were effective in increasing helmet use; interventions were most effective with younger children (Owen, Kendrick, Mulvaney et al., 2011).

IMPLICATIONS

Interventions can significantly increase parental and child knowledge about benefits of helmets and their correct use. Interventions to increase helmet use can be integrated into schools and, perhaps more importantly, into community presentations. Providing free or low-cost helmets directly relates to helmet use, so strategies to fund such programs are important. Nurses should not assume that reports of safety precautions such as wearing helmets or seat belts mean that children use these measures correctly. Teach about the benefits of helmets at each health supervision visit. Ask for demonstrations and provide suggestions to improve technique as needed. Common injury causes such as car and bicycle crashes necessitate including at least these evaluations as part of health maintenance activities.

CRITICAL THINKING APPLICATION

Where will you find information about helmet safety? What educational programs are available in your schools and communities? Are helmets made available for families that might not be able to afford their purchase? How do you determine if a child is wearing a helmet correctly? Plan educational materials and programs for children who bicycle.

Identify youth engaging in these activities and teach them safe practices. Partner with schools and community groups to establish education programs. Provide information about adequate conditioning for sports to decrease the chance of overuse injury.

Each visit should contain basic history questions related to injury prevention and then pursue topics that appear to indicate problems. The following questions are appropriate:

- "How often does your daughter wear a seat belt in the car?" (If less than "always" this issue must be addressed.)
- "What sports or other physical activities do you like, Kelly?"
- "Who would you go to if someone was touching you inappropriately or if you felt uncomfortable with anyone?"
- "Do you have firearms, Mr. Bonci? Describe how you store them in the house."
- "You say you come home after school now. How long do you spend at home before your parents or big brother gets home? What do you do during that time?"
- "I see you're playing video games today. How long do you play at home each day? What are your favorite games? Do your parents have any rules about the types of games you can play?"

Once information is collected during the visit, plan two or three health maintenance topics that seem most important for injury prevention in this family. To address the questions raised in the preceding list, plan the following related interventions:

- Emphasize the importance of wearing a shoulder and lap belt for every car trip. Evaluate by demonstration whether the child wears the belts properly. Review Partnering with Families: Car Safety for the School-Age Child for recommendations.
- Teach about protective gear necessary for any sport in which the child participates. Provide resources for financial assistance for such gear. Bike shops often provide discounts on helmets for low-income families, health fairs may provide gear, and local community groups will often make contributions.
- Teach all children safe resources such as teachers, school counselors, and police. If they do not feel safe with one person, even if in these groups, encourage them to contact someone else. Further information on child abuse is found in Chapter 20 ✪
- Be sure parents store firearms locked, with ammunition locked in a separate place. Remind them that most school-age children

---

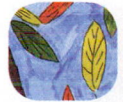 # Partnering with Families

Car Safety for the School-Age Child

Even though parents may have been diligent about car seat and seat belt use when children were younger, guidelines change and parents need teaching about requirements for the school-age child. Recommendations include:

- For children who have grown too large for the child restraint seat used during earlier years, use a booster seat in the back seat. Always use both lap and shoulder belts. Make sure the lap belt fits low and tight across the lap/upper thigh area and the shoulder belt is snug across the chest and shoulder to avoid abdominal injuries.

- Children 4′ 9″ and taller can sit in a regular car seat restrained with lap and shoulder belt that are snug and correctly located across the lap and chest. The back seat is preferred for all children and should be the only location used for children 13 years and younger (American Academy of Pediatrics, 2011b).

can find keys that are stored in desks, drawers, and other locations at home. Have them get the keys out of accessible household locations and install trigger locks if they are not already in place as an additional safeguard.

- Suggest activities for the child at home alone, and provide resources for the child. See Partnering with Families: After-School Self-Care on page 323 for further suggestions.

- Encourage parents to limit television and video game time to less than 2 hours daily. They should avoid violent television shows and games, and look at ratings on boxes to learn about violence and sexual content. Encourage children to begin self-monitoring to limit screen time and avoid violence.

When you have identified a history of injury in the child, partner with the family to plan ways to avoid repeated harm. Examples that indicate a need for specific discussion are:

- Firearm injury
- Fractures
- Known or suspected child abuse
- Dirt bike, all-terrain vehicle, or motorcycle injury
- Burns from setting fires

See Table 12–4 for common injury hazards during the school years. See Table 12–5 for injury prevention teaching.

Nursing Management

Nursing Assessment and Diagnosis

Assessment of health promotion and health maintenance topics occurs in many settings with school-age children. They may be seen in offices or clinics, or in other settings designed to provide such care. They may come for episodic care for a fracture or infection, and health promotion and health maintenance can be easily integrated. They may be seen in the home or neighborhood center and are frequently encountered by nurses in schools. Take advantage of opportunities for assessment and intervention when they occur. The individual child is examined, and the family, friends, school, and community are addressed. These visits provide an opportunity to identify early and intervene in health-related problems that emerge or become apparent during school age, including:

- Anxiety
- Mood disorders
- Attention deficit hyperactivity disorder
- Child abuse
- Domestic violence
- Eating disorders
- Learning problems
- Intellectual disability and developmental disabilities
- Aggression and violence
- Substance abuse
- Parental depression and other mental disorders

Hagan et al., 2008

Inquire about any medications the child uses, and perform teaching about these as needed. Use of complementary therapy is common, and healthcare providers should question all families about use of these therapies. For example, ask about use of vitamins, minerals, herbal supplements, massage, and other therapies. See Complementary Therapy: Use in Children.

Complementary Therapy Use in Children

Recent research shows that many families use complementary and alternative therapy in treatment of children. A survey of 278 military families showed that 23% used complementary therapy with their children (Huillet, Erdie-Lalena, Norvell, et al., 2011). Most common therapies included special diets (often with herbs or high doses of vitamins/minerals), melatonin, and massage. Such high rates of complementary therapy necessitate healthcare provider knowledge and assessment skills (Gilmour, Harrison, Cohen, et al., 2011). Ask questions related to complementary therapy use and outcomes, become knowledgeable about the therapies described by the family, and adapt assessment to identify both desired and unfavorable outcomes from the therapy. Provide education about the products and practices to assist families with their decisions.

Assessment can be considered on two levels with school-age children. Individual children may be assessed for height and weight, for immunization status, and for use of protective gear during sports. Populations of children may also be assessed since school age is the first time that large numbers of children are together in certain settings. The findings from such assessments will become the basis of an **individualized approach** or a **population-based approach** to health promotion and health maintenance. For example, nurses commonly measure height and weight and calculate BMI for individual children seen in a clinic. The results are shared with the family, and appropriate teaching about weight control and nutritious intake can be addressed. In other settings, nurses may measure a classroom of children and use the collective data to plan appropriate interventions. If 40% of children in a school are classified as overweight by BMI percentile, much emphasis should be placed on teaching about dietary intake, physical activity, and the relationship of recommended weight levels to chronic disease risk. However, if only a small number of children are overweight, interventions may not be as extensive.

Assessment techniques with groups of children consider the contexts or systems of a group of children and integrate them into care. Recall the theory of ecology of human development (see Chapter 5 🔗); see Table 12–6 for examples of how the ecologic theory application leads to assessments for specific populations of children. Another example of a data-gathering tool for populations of children is the Youth Risk Behavior Surveillance. See Chapter 20 🔗 for further description of this tool, which is administered by the Centers for Disease Control and Prevention.

Data can be analyzed geographically, by ethnic group, by age categories, or by other criteria to describe the risks of groups of children. Nurses look to these national data and to regional surveys to provide profiles of children in the populations they serve. These collective data can suggest areas that can be applied with groups of children in the local community, as well as with individual children. Many states, cities, and counties provide collective data about health of youth on their websites. Can you find such data for your geographic location on the Internet? How will you use these data to assist in planning assessment of groups of school-age children or individual children?

Nurses perform growth assessment in school-age children, look for achievement of developmental tasks, assess physical and mental health, and note social characteristics. Based on the assessment of an individual or populations of children, nursing diagnoses for children

TABLE 12–4   **Injury Hazards in the School-Age Years**

	HAZARD	DEVELOPMENTAL CHARACTERISTICS	PREVENTIVE MEASURES
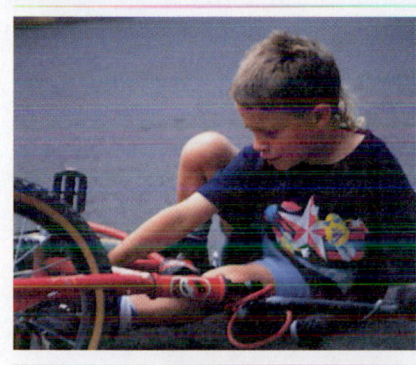	Motor vehicle/ pedestrian/ biking crashes	Child plays outside; may follow ball into road; rides two-wheeler. Child may not know safe street-crossing behaviors.	■ Teach child safe outside play, especially near streets. ■ Reinforce use of bike helmet. ■ Teach biking safety rules and provide safe places for riding. ■ Teach safe street-crossing behaviors.
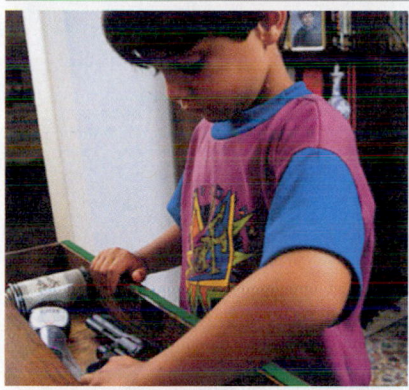	Firearms	Child may have been shown location of guns; is interested in showing them to friends.	■ Teach child never to touch guns without parent present. ■ Guns should be kept unloaded and locked away. Guns and ammunition should be stored in different locations. ■ Be sure guns have trigger locks.
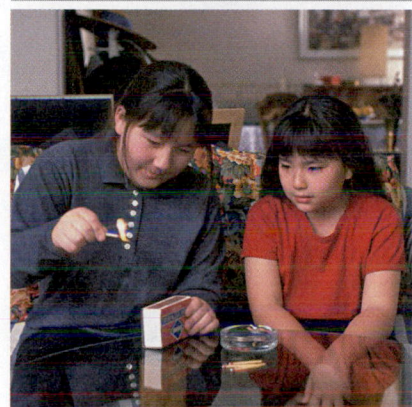	Burns	Child may perform experiments with flames or toxic substances.	■ Teach child what to do in case of fire or if toxic substances touch skin or eyes. ■ Reinforce teaching about 911.
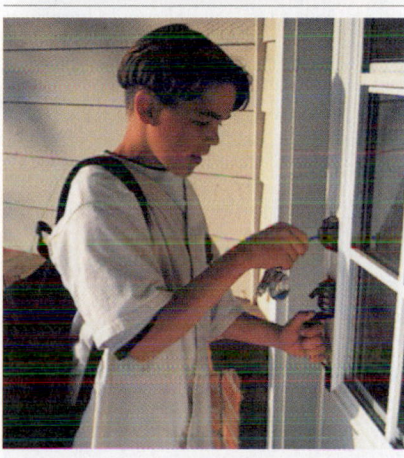	Assault	Child may be left alone after school and may walk, bike, or take public transportation alone.	■ Provide telephone numbers of people to contact in case of an emergency or if child feels lonely. ■ Leave child alone for brief periods initially, and evaluate child's success in managing time. ■ Teach child not to accept rides from or talk to or open doors to strangers. ■ Teach child how to answer the phone.

TABLE 12–5	Injury Prevention Topics by Age
AGE	**INJURY PREVENTION TEACHING**
5–8 years	*Car safety:*
	Use an approved child restraint system, properly positioned in the back seat of the car; use lap and shoulder belts as directed.
	Once large enough for the vehicle seat belt alone, use both lap and shoulder belts.
	All children younger than 13 years should be restrained in the rear seat.
	Never place the child in a front car seat with a passenger air bag.
	Activities:
	Be sure the child knows how to swim and works on this skill regularly.
	Provide protective gear for bicycling and other activities and insist that it be worn.
	Teach safety precautions for bicycling and other activities.
	Home safety:
	Have an escape plan in case of fire in the home.
	Keep poisons, electrical appliances, and fire starters locked.
	Limit screen time to 2 hours daily; do not allow violent games, videos, or television programs.
	Safety outside the home:
	Teach safety with strangers.
	Review behavior with strangers regularly such as not getting in cars and not engaging in phone or Internet conversations.
	Provide a list of people a child can approach if feeling threatened by touch or other experience.
	Choose care providers carefully; occasionally pick up the child earlier than expected; ask policies about discipline and do not leave the child with someone who uses corporal punishment.
	Be sure the child knows emergency numbers, names, and plans.
	Review carefully any hazardous event that has occurred with the child and summarize what was done correctly and how response could be improved.
8–10 years	Use a car booster seat until the child sits upright against back seat with bent knees over edge of seat; insist on use of lap and shoulder belts.
	Do not place the child in front seat of car with a passenger air bag.
	Do not allow a child to operate power tools or machinery.
	Continue to reinforce other teaching described above, including the child more fully and enlarging the child's responsibility with increasing age.
10–12 years	Continue to reinforce teaching described above.
	Parents and child should attend class on cardiopulmonary resuscitation (CPR) and airway obstruction removal.
	Avoid high noise levels such as when listening to music through earphones.

Source: Adapted from Hagan, J. F., Shaw, J. S., & Duncan, P. M. (Eds.). (2008). Bright futures: Guidelines for health supervision of infants, children, and adolescents (3rd ed.). Elk Grove Village, IL: American Academy of Pediatrics.

TABLE 12–6	Application of Ecology of Development to Assessment of Child Populations*
SYSTEM	**ASSESSMENT EXAMPLES**
Microsystem	■ Types of common injuries in the community
	■ Neighborhood services for swimming, bicycle safety
	■ School curriculum offerings about abuse issues
	■ Peer activities available in school and neighborhood
Exosystem	■ School board policies related to teaching health promotion and maintenance activities; school policies related to physical education
	■ Parks department offerings for youth
	■ Amount of involvement of adult volunteers and local businesses in area schools
Macrosystem	■ State grants for smoking prevention and cessation among youth
	■ Insurance reimbursement for health promotion teaching
	■ Availability of results of Youth Risk Behavior Surveillance and other studies to local communities

Note: *See Chapter 5 ⊘ for information about Bronfenbrenner's ecologic theory of development.

and families are established. Possible nursing diagnoses include the following:

- Growth and Development, Delayed, related to abuse
- Parenting, Risk for Impaired, related to lack of knowledge about child health maintenance
- Sleep Deprivation related to sleep terrors
- Violence: Other-Directed, Risk for, related to history of witnessing family violence
- Loneliness, Risk for, related to long periods alone after school
- Health: Community, Deficient, related to locating swimming classes

NANDA-I © 2012

Planning and Implementation

The nurse is instrumental in planning interventions to promote and maintain health in school-age children. You will use a variety of information sources to plan the best interventions to use with families in your community.

When working with individuals, summarize the strengths and needs that you have identified during the visit, and ask the child and family if they concur. Plan together to provide the needed information for topics you have identified as a group. Be sure to emphasize those areas where the family excels. For example, positively reinforce use of car seat belts, use of protective sports gear, and being current with immunizations. Summarize the next expected developmental tasks, such as increasing independence and growing self-responsibility for choosing snacks and television shows. Provide anticipatory guidance to assist with the child's growing independence and how that may affect relationships with parents, siblings, and other family members. As peers are becoming more important, focus discussion on maintaining healthy social relationships through school and faith-based or community events. Most families welcome a combination of discussion and reading material or pertinent websites for later exploration. Provide telephone numbers of resources for questions and community contacts. Inform the parents of the next health promotion/health maintenance visit recommendation. If you come in contact with schoolchildren for episodic care, ask when the last health maintenance visit occurred. If a child is seen for health care after a bicycle crash, the family may be receptive to teaching about safety precautions. When exposed to injuries to the skin, a review of the last tetanus booster may reveal health maintenance needs.

Use every opportunity to work with individual children and insert appropriate health promotion and health maintenance topics. When working with groups of children, health promotion should focus on known needs, interests, and risk areas. Sometimes a combined approach is necessary. For example, stress reduction teaching should be provided on group and individual levels. Nurses can teach or assist in development of progressive relaxation, deep breathing, biofeedback, yoga, or meditation, and can help families to find relaxing activities rather than overscheduling children in multiple activities. See Chapter 3 🕮 for an overview of stress reduction techniques.

In school settings, nurses have used a variety of creative approaches to promote the health of youth. Nurses in this setting can establish programs to train students in health topics; these students then become coaches or health advocates who can work with other students, especially those of younger ages. Nurses may also evaluate the components of school health programs and offer recommendations for additions as needed (Box 12–2).

A nurse might also develop a newsletter to inform school-age children and/or parents about health topics. Bulletin boards, community newspapers, television, and community group membership may each be as effective as teaching in school classrooms. Interventions will be most effective if they begin with an understanding of the population served. What is important to the families of children in your community or school? What are the values, beliefs, and

BOX 12–2   Coordinated School Health

The Centers for Disease Control and Prevention (2010b) recommends the use of coordinated school health as a strategy to improve health and learning. They propose that planning and coordination of school health include the following components:

- Health education
- Physical education
- Health services
- Mental health and social services
- Food services
- Healthy and safe environment
- Family and community involvement
- Staff wellness

See Chapter 14 for further information about health objectives in schools.

motivation needed for children to make changes that will enhance health? See Chapter 14 🕮 for further analysis of the community that will help you to plan population-based interventions for health promotion and health maintenance.

Evaluation

Seek evaluation from parents during visits for care. Were their questions answered? Do they know where to turn for advice? Do they know when the child should be seen again for health promotion and health maintenance?

The expected outcomes for nursing care of individual school-age children include:

- The child demonstrates normal patterns of growth and development.
- The family and community provide a supportive and nurturing environment for the child.
- The child shows growing independence in directing own health promotion activities.

Expected outcomes of nursing care for groups of children include:

- Children identify lifestyle decisions that influence their health status.
- The school and community offer resources that help to lessen risk factors related to health and disease/injury prevention.

Chapter Highlights

- School-age health promotion and health maintenance visits begin with a pre-kindergarten examination.
- Health promotion should take place in any setting where the child is seen, even for episodic or emergency care.
- Growth measurement and developmental surveillance provide the basis for establishing risk and protective factors for an individual child.

- Schoolchildren have increasing independence in making food choices; teaching is needed for the child and family to promote healthy choices.
- Physical activity should be included in the home and school setting for every child.
- Establishment of self-esteem is an important mental health task of the school-age child.

- Peer relationships play an important role in the lives of school-age children, even though they still depend on families for support and nurturing.
- Injury prevention efforts focus on common causes of morbidity and mortality in young children, such as firearms, abuse, motor vehicle crashes, and sports-related injuries.
- The nurse integrates population-based health promotion activities into all settings where groups of children are seen; individualized approaches are used primarily in clinics and offices and focus on the particular needs of a given child.

Clinical Reasoning in Action

INTRODUCTION

Recall the chapter-opening scenario involving two sixth graders with type 1 diabetes. The school nurse meets with Jessalyn and Kelly regularly to monitor their management of diabetes and use of insulin pumps. The nurse is in close contact with the endocrinologist who treats the girls and with the parents of each of them.

DESCRIPTION

Jessalyn has had diabetes for 2 years and is still learning about the disease. She attended a summer camp for children with diabetes last year, which gave her the confidence to try the insulin pump for constant infusion of insulin this academic year. Her parents were surprised about the diagnosis and are now worried about their younger son and whether he will develop the disease. There is no other diabetes history in their family. Jessalyn's recent blood lipid studies indicate a total cholesterol of 180 mg/dL, low-density lipoprotein (LDL) of 120 mg/dL, and high-density lipoprotein (HDL) of 32 mg/dL. Her most recent hemoglobin A_{1c} was 7%.

Kelly has an uncle and grandmother with type 1 diabetes, and she has had the diagnosis for 7 years. For the last 4 years, she has been using an insulin pump. She has recently started to ask whether inhaled insulin would be appropriate for her. Kelly's major issues with management of the disease are difficulty maintaining blood glucose at proper levels during a recent growth spurt, and integration of her basketball and volleyball activities into diabetes management.

DISCUSSION

1. Strengths for both Jessalyn and Kelly are their interest in disease management, access to a school nurse, and supportive families. What other protective factors can you identify?

2. What support and information would be helpful for the parents of Jessalyn and Kelly? How do their needs for information differ? How do these differences relate to the specific situations in the microsystems of their families?

3. Jessalyn and Kelly are in a transition stage between school age and adolescence. Consult Chapter 5 🔗 to examine their expected cognitive stages. How would you approach teaching based on their developmental level?

4. How might the physical growth patterns of 12-year-old girls affect management of diabetes?

5. Consider the psychosocial stages of Jessalyn and Kelly. Are there diabetes management issues that could be related to expected social interactions during older school age? What are the benefits of summer camp attendance for school-age children with a health problem?

6. Examine Jessalyn's lipid levels. Consult Chapter 26 🔗 and the laboratory values in Appendix D 🔗 to evaluate these findings. Review your knowledge of pathophysiology to describe why lipid levels should be measured in children with diabetes.

7. What does hemoglobin A_{1c} measure? What is your evaluation of Jessalyn's level? Consult Chapter 32 🔗 to learn more about hemoglobin A_{1c} and its meaning in diabetes.

8. Outline health promotion related to nutrition and physical activity that you will plan for Jessalyn and Kelly.

NCLEX-RN® Review

1. In working with children who have health alterations that involve body changes, such as loss of hair, the nurse would be most concerned about which age group?
   1. 3–5 years
   2. 6–8 years
   3. 9–11 years
   4. 12–14 years

2. A nurse is planning to teach a first-grade child about good hand hygiene. Which method of teaching would be best suited for this age group?
   1. Use a special black light solution to show the child how effectively she washed her hands.
   2. Demonstrate good hand washing techniques so all children can see and understand.
   3. Give the child a handout that includes a step-by-step guide to hand washing with coloring pages.
   4. Show the child a video and then ask if the child has any questions afterwards.

3. The school nurse is planning to teach fourth-grade students regarding prepubescent body changes. In order for the program to be successful, what should be the nurse's initial action?
   1. Before announcing the program, discuss the content with the parents.
   2. Invite parents to be present during the presentation.
   3. Talk to all the fourth-grade students at one time.
   4. Plan the program for after school.

4. The nurse is planning guidance for the parents of a 9-year-old child during a health supervision visit. He is at the 50th percentile for height and greater than the 95th percentile for weight. Which are appropriate suggestions for the family?
   1. Increase access to play equipment.
   2. Use whole milk and limit servings to two per day.
   3. Increase contact with other children for stimulation.
   4. Limit all screen viewing time to a maximum of 2 hours per day.

See Appendix I 🔗 for answers.

References

American Academy of Pediatrics. (2007a). *Healthy children: Back to school.* Retrieved from http://www.aap.org

American Academy of Pediatrics. (2011a). *Discipline.* Retrieved from http://www.healthychildren.org

American Academy of Pediatrics. (2011b). *Car safety seats.* Retrieved from http://www.healthychildren.org

Atanda, A., Shah, S. A., & O'Biren, K. (2011). Osteochondrosis: Common causes of pain in growing bones. *American Family Physician, 83,* 286–291.

Ben-Arye, E., Traube, Z., Schachter, L., Jaimi, M., Levy, M., Schiff, E., & Lev, E. (2011). Integrative pediatric care: Parents' attitudes toward communication of physicians and CAM practitioners. *Pediatrics, 127*(1), 384–395.

Bicycle Helmet Safety Institute. (2011). *Helmet related statistics.* Retrieved from http://www.bhsi/stats.htm

Bonuck, K. A., Chervin, R. D., Cole, T. J., Emond, A., Henderson, J., Xu, L., & Freeman, K. (2011). Prevalence and persistence of sleep disordered breathing symptoms in young children: A 6-year population-based cohort study. *Sleep, 34,* 875–884.

Centers for Disease Control and Prevention. (2008). Youth risk behavior surveillance—2007. *Morbidity and Mortality Weekly Report, 57*(SS-4), 1–136.

Centers for Disease Control and Prevention. (2010a). Youth risk behavior surveillance—United States, 2009. *Morbidity and Mortality Weekly Report, 59*(SS-5), 1–148.

Centers for Disease Control and Prevention. (2010b). *Coordinated school health.* Retrieved from http://www.cdc.gov/HealthyYouth/CSHP/

Centers for Disease Control and Prevention. (2011). *How much physical activity do children need?* Retrieved from http://www.cdc.gov/physicalactivity/everyone/guidelines/children/html

Dellinger, A. M., & Kresnow, M. J. (2010). Bicycle helmet use among children in the United States: The effects of legislation, personal and household factors. *Journal of Safety Research, 41,* 375–380.

Devoe, J. E., Tillotson, C. J., Wallace, L. S., Lesko, S. E., & Pandhi, H. (2012). Is health insurance enough? A usual source of care may be more important to ensure a child receives preventive health counseling. *Maternal and Child Health Journal, 16*(2), 306–315.

Gilmour, J., Harrison, C., Cohen, M. H., & Vohra, S. (2011). Pediatric use of complementary and alternative medicine: Legal, ethical, and clinical issues in decision-making. *Pediatrics, 128,* S149–S154.

Hagan, J. F., Shaw, J. S., & Duncan, P. M. (2008). *Bright futures: Guidelines for health supervision of infants, children, and adolescents* (3rd ed.). Elk Grove Village, IL: American Academy of Pediatrics.

Hagel, B. E., Lee, R. S., Karkhaneh, M., Voaklander, D., & Rowe, B. H. (2010). Factors associated with incorrect bicycle helmet use. *Injury Prevention, 16*(3), 178–184.

Hamilton, S. S., & Glascoe, F. P. (2010). Making developmental-behavioral screening work for school-aged kids. *Contemporary Pediatrics, 27*(9), 63–87.

Huillet, A., Erdie-Lalena, C., Norvell, D., & Davis, B. E. (2011). Complementary and alternative medicine used by children in military pediatric clinics. *Journal of Alternative and Complementary Medicine, 17,* 531–537.

KidsHealth. (2011). *Developing your child's self-esteem.* Retrieved from http://kidshealth.org/parent/emotions/feelings/self_esteem.html

Knox, M. (2010). On hitting children: A review of corporal punishment in the United States. *Journal of Pediatric Health Care, 24*(2), 103–107.

Kodish, I., Rockhill, C., Ryan, S., & Varley, C. (2011). Pharmacotherapy for anxiety disorders in children and adolescents. *Pediatric Clinics of North America, 58*(1), 56–72.

Kuo, D. Z., Frick, K. D., & Minkovitz, C. S. (2011). Association of family-centered care with improved anticipatory guidance delivery and reduced unmet needs in child health care. *Maternal Child Health Journal, 15,* 1228–1237. doi:10.10076/s10995-010-0702-8

Kuo, D. Z., Houtrow, A. J., Arango, P., Kuhlthau, K. A., Simmons, J. M., & Neff, J. M. (2012). Family-centered care: Current applications and future directions in pediatric health care. *Maternal Child Health Journal, 16,* 297–305. doi:10.1007/s10995-011-0751-7

Latchkey-Kids. (2011). *Age restrictions for latchkey kids.* Retrieved from http://www.latchkey-kids.com/latchkey-kids-age-limits.htm

Mayo Clinic. (2009). *Teen sleep: Why is your teen so tired?* Retrieved from http://www.mayoclinic.com/health/teens-health

Mindell, J. A., Meltzer, L. J., Carskadon, M. A., & Chervin, R. D. (2009). Developmental aspects of sleep hygiene: Findings from the 2004 National Sleep Foundation Sleep in America Poll. *Sleep Medicine, 10*(7), 771–779.

Murray, R. B., Zentner, J. P., & Yakimo, R. (2009). *Health promotion strategies through the life span* (8th ed.). Upper Saddle River, NJ: Prentice Hall Health.

Owen, R., Kendrick, D., Mulvaney, C., Coleman, T., & Royal, S. (2011). Non-legislative interventions for the promotion of cycle helmet wearing by children. *Cochrane Database Systematic Review, 11:* CD003985

Pavone, V., Lionetti, E., Gargano, V., Evola, F. R., Costarella, L., & Sessa, G. (2011). Growing pains: A study of 30 cases and a review of the literature. *Journal of Pediatric Orthopedics, 31,* 606–609.

Pender, N. J., Murdaugh, C. L., & Parsons, M. A. (2011). *Health promotion in nursing practice* (6th ed.). Upper Saddle River, NJ: Prentice Hall.

Ramsawh, H. J., Chavira, D. A., & Stein, M. B. (2010). Burden of anxiety disorders in pediatric medical settings: Prevalence, phenomenology, and a research agenda. *Archives of Pediatrics and Adolescent Medicine, 164*(10), 965–972.

Safe Kids. (2010). *Preventing injuries: At home, at play, and on the way.* Retrieved from http://www.safekids.org/who-we-are/contact.html

Santrock, J. W. (2011). *Child development* (13th ed.). Boston: McGraw-Hill.

Sibinga, E. M., & Kemper, K. J. (2010). Complementary, holistic, and integrative medicine: Meditation practices for pediatric health. *Pediatric Reviews, 31*(12), e91–e103.

U.S. Department of Health and Human Services. (2011). *Strengthening families and communities.* Washington, DC: Author.

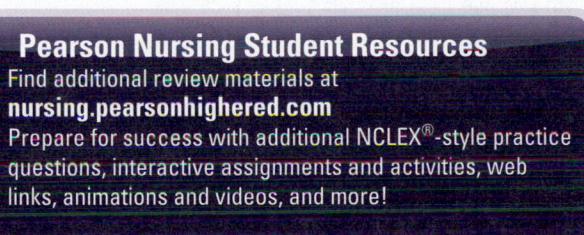

Pearson Nursing Student Resources

Find additional review materials at
nursing.pearsonhighered.com
Prepare for success with additional NCLEX®-style practice questions, interactive assignments and activities, web links, animations and videos, and more!

13 Health Promotion and Maintenance of the Adolescent

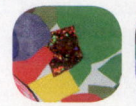 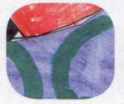 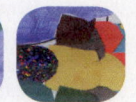

Learning Outcomes

After completing this chapter, you will be able to:

1. Describe the general observations made of adolescents and their families during health supervision visits to the pediatric healthcare home.

2. Identify the major health concerns of adolescents.

3. Apply assessment skills to gather data regarding nutrition, physical activity, mental health status, and growth and development of adolescents.

4. Synthesize data from history and examination of the adolescent and family.

5. Demonstrate therapeutic communication skills with the adolescent and family during health supervision visits.

6. Partner with the adolescent to prioritize health goals and desired interventions.

7. Intervene with adolescents and their families to integrate activities to promote health and to prevent disease and injury.

8. Evaluate care provided for adolescents and families and revise goals and plans as needed.

KEY TERMS

modeling	342
outcome expectancy	342
self-efficacy	342

"I've never really liked going to see the doctor or nurse. But now that I need some birth control, I have to do it. They're actually pretty nice here and have helped me with a lot of things. It doesn't even seem like a doctor's office. It feels like I can ask questions and they won't just lecture me about what to do."

—*Kim, age 16*

Kim Patterson is a sexually active 16-year-old female who has come to the clinic to obtain birth control pills. The nurse takes Kim's history and performs a physical examination. Kim is found to be anemic upon examination of her hematocrit level. Kim states that she has trouble talking with her parents about her boyfriend and other important things; she wishes she could talk with them more freely. The nurse teaches Kim about the risks of sexually transmitted infections, helps Kim examine what makes it difficult to talk with her parents, and helps her identify where she can go to get support and discuss issues that she does not want to explore with her parents. The room offers a casual sofa for seating as the nurse collects the history before the examination and for performing teaching afterward; teens feel comfortable with this approach.

What should the nurse do for follow-up during the next visit with Kim? Which immunizations does Kim need for disease prevention? What special skills are needed to partner with an adolescent in health supervision visits? Consider these questions as you read this chapter.

Even though visits are recommended annually, adolescents are often seen only sporadically for health care. They are usually healthy, may not need immunizations, and consequently do not often come for health care. If adolescents do visit for a minor illness, birth control, a chronic condition requiring periodic assessments, or a sports examination, the visit should be viewed as a health supervision opportunity. Youth with a disability may primarily seek care related to that condition; health promotion should be inserted into those healthcare visits (Figure 13–1 ■). If time is limited, the nurse has to decide which topics to address during a healthcare visit. It is advisable to start with the topic of most interest to the adolescent and then to include injury prevention teaching, since injury is the greatest risk to teens. (See Chapter 1 🔴.) Health promotion topics such as dietary and exercise habits could be discussed if time permits.

Lifestyle behaviors are responsible for most of the preventable diseases in adults, and all typically have their origin in the adolescent years, including sedentary lifestyle, unhealthy diet, tobacco and other substance use, and risk taking that leads to injuries. Assess for these behaviors at all visits and include teaching in the form of verbal information, brochures, videos, DVDs, or social media that can be watched in the healthcare facility. These behaviors directly relate to health promotion topics such as dietary and exercise habits, which should be integrated into health encounters. Mental health assessment and teaching are other areas of prime importance. Of course, if the adolescent suggests he or she is at immediate risk, such as considering suicide in response to depression, this must be dealt with immediately by collaborating with a mental health specialist.

What general principles can guide programs to promote health in adolescents? Researchers have analyzed theory application and approaches of programs, and others have suggested key elements of programs (Box 13–1). Programs assist adolescents in taking on health promotion behaviors by fostering a sense of competence, promoting decision making by the youth, and increasing motivation for change toward healthy behaviors (Murray, Zentner, & Yakimo, 2009). When establishing youth programs, whether with individual adolescents or with groups, the nurse includes evaluation of the effectiveness of the plan and methods to expand and sustain successful approaches.

Clinical Tip

Many teenagers come in for care only sporadically. However, it is recommended that health supervision visits occur annually from 12 to 19 years, since many health topics are important to address.

When you see adolescents who come in for an illness or injury, or in a school or other setting, find out when they were last seen for a health supervision visit. Ask if they have a pediatric healthcare home, and reinforce the need to make an appointment. If an agency relationship is not established, suggest a resource in the community.

How does the nurse interact with the adolescent in order to be effective in health promotion and health maintenance activities? What are the major health supervision needs of adolescents? How does the nurse recognize the independence of the teen but yet include parents as partners in the youth's healthcare team? These are some of the questions that will be addressed in this chapter.

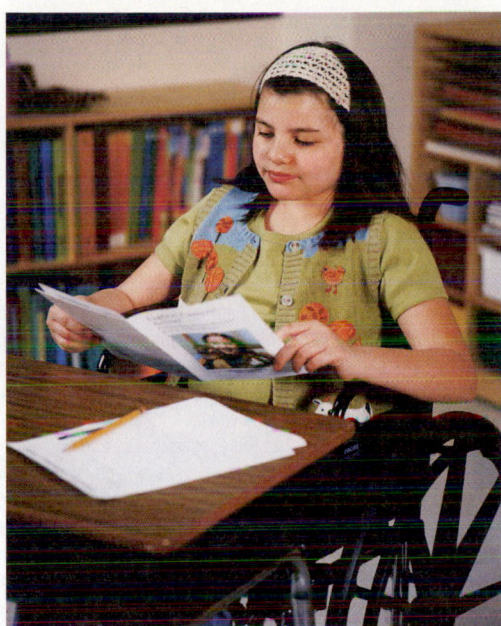

FIGURE 13–1 ■ This teen, who uses a wheelchair, does well in school and has many friends and activities. When she comes for periodic healthcare visits, health promotion and health maintenance activities should be integrated into the examinations.

GENERAL OBSERVATIONS

The beginning of the visit with an adolescent can be an important time to gather information, just as it is with younger children. However, the observations you make will relate to the adolescent's more advanced stage of development.

Ideally, the facility has a waiting area that is designed for adolescents. Teens may not want to wait for health care with either young children or older adults. Teen waiting areas are popular because they provide a special place, thereby relaying that the adolescent is important. Video kiosks and other contemporary methods can be used to impart health information while the teen waits.

As you call the adolescent in for care, observe if parents or friends are present, or if the teen is alone. Young adolescents often come with parents to the facility, and parents may wait in the waiting room during the examination (Figure 13–2 ■). If the teen comes in for a specific problem such as a skin lesion or other health concern, the parent may accompany the adolescent into the examination room. If someone does come with the teen, be aware that you may need to provide private time by asking the other person to wait outside for a moment. Reassure parents that you will talk with them about any of their concerns and questions, and provide them with an opportunity to ask questions and obtain information.

The adolescent is able to respond to questions and requests, and to state the reason for the visit. Be alert for teens who cannot perform these basic skills, and examine them carefully as described later in this chapter. Observe interactions with parents and others who accompany the adolescent to the visit. Some teens are comfortable in healthcare settings and actively engage in conversation, whereas others are nervous and will need more explanations and reassurance as you progress with the first steps of measurement and blood pressure.

BOX 13–1   **Research: Theories Used in Health Promotion Programs for Adolescents**

Several theories guide healthcare specialists in establishing health promotion programs for adolescents. Why are these theories important? They provide an organized approach to planning and suggest the strategies that will be most successful, based on the person's motivation and developmental age (Murray et al., 2009). Some of the major theories used include:

1. **Social Cognitive Theory.** The key components of this theory (Bandura, 1986, 1995, 1997), which is frequently applied in research and health interventions with youth (Bricker, Liu, Comstock, et al., 2010; Connor, George, Gullo, et al., 2011; Hortz & Petosa, 2008), involve **self-efficacy** (the person's belief in his or her ability to perform a behavior) and **outcome expectancy** (what the person expects to get from performing a certain behavior). Learning a new behavior occurs through **modeling,** or imitation of the behavior of someone else. Individuals make decisions about health behaviors based on thought about the consequences and outcomes of those behaviors. The *person's characteristics*, such as self-efficacy and outcome expectancy, interact with the external *environment* and the *behavioral choices* available. All of these components interact to determine health behaviors, and all can be influenced to promote health. If you were seeking to promote physical activity behaviors in youth, some essential components would be:

   - Encourage youth to believe they could perform the activity (self-efficacy).
   - Point out the positive aspects of the behavior (outcome expectancy).
   - Show youth how to do the activity (modeling).
   - Provide a physical setting and opportunity for performing the behavior (environment).
   - Allow trial and error, and choice in time and extent of activity (behavioral choices).

2. **Health Belief Model.** This theory attempts to explain why some individuals take actions to prevent disease or promote health while others do not. Factors that influence the likelihood of taking on preventive behaviors include the *perceived susceptibility to disease, seriousness of the disease, perceived benefits of preventive action*, and *barriers to preventive action*. Modifying factors include knowledge, personality, and peer influence. Cues such as media or reminders by a healthcare professional also influence perception of the condition and therefore influence action (Pender, Murdaugh, & Parsons, 2011). When using this theory to encourage physical activity in youth, the program would include information about the following:

   - Necessity of exercise to prevent problems such as obesity, diabetes, and cardiovascular disease
   - Prevalence of serious diseases in those with low levels of activity
   - Benefits of physical activity to weight control, health, and sense of well-being
   - Common reasons people do not exercise, along with methods to dispel these reasons

3. **Transtheoretical Stages of Change Model.** This model suggests that individuals engage in stages prior to taking any actions that lead to change in health behaviors. The five stages are *precontemplation, contemplation, preparation, action*, and *maintenance* (Erol & Erdogan, 2008). Those in early stages are unlikely to begin behavioral change before about 6 months, while the action phase includes immediate readiness to change. Understanding the adolescent's stage of change can guide the nurse to approach teaching and motivation activities in a more realistic manner. If you were planning an intervention with adolescents who smoke, some strategies could include the following:

   - Ask if the teen is ready to take steps now to stop smoking, or would like to do it in the future.
   - Assist the adolescent to move from precontemplation and contemplation phases to the action phase by providing information and resources about smoking dangers and cessation programs.
   - Assist the adolescent in the action phase with strategies to remain smoke-free.
   - If the individual has recently quit smoking, ask about times when tempted to smoke and strategize to increase the potential for maintenance.

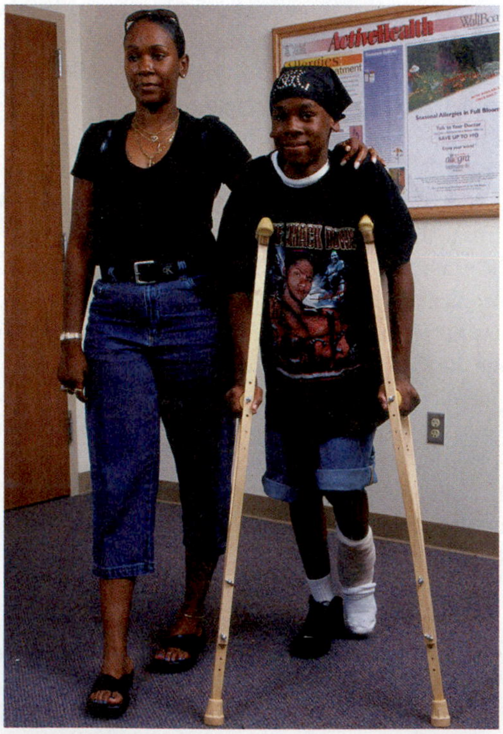

FIGURE 13–2 ■ Parents often accompany teens with a healthcare problem in for the examination. Provide an opportunity to see both the teen and parent privately, and integrate general health promotion and health maintenance into the visit. What questions can you ask this teen? What teaching might be needed?

Initial observations will guide some of the interactions with the teen. For example, if a teen is overweight, provide a quiet and private location while taking the weight, and do not announce the weight aloud. Being alert, quiet, and sensitive are all important qualities of the nurse working with adolescents.

In the discussion of health promotion and health maintenance of the school-age child (see Chapter 12 🔗), it was noted that the healthcare partnership grew from one with parents to one encompassing the child as a partner as well. By adolescence, children should be assuming more of a partnership role in their own health care. As the visit begins, greet adolescents warmly, ask about their concerns and questions, and ask for their opinions and reactions throughout the visit. This will demonstrate that their thoughts are valued and that they play an important role in guiding the healthcare visit. When adolescents are visiting the same office or clinic that they came to during childhood, they usually know and feel comfortable with the care providers. If the setting is new to them, explain procedures and introduce personnel so they feel more at ease.

GROWTH AND DEVELOPMENTAL SURVEILLANCE

Adolescence spans several years, and growth and developmental issues vary throughout the period. For young adolescents, those from about 12 to 13 years of age, growth measurement remains important. Many youth are still growing, and use of percentile grids continues to be an important part of care. Growth should remain in the same percentile channel as during childhood (see description of growth percentile ranges in Chapter 11 ⊘), with girls reaching nearly adult height at this age, and boys still continuing to grow. Be alert, as always, for youth who have either increased or decreased percentiles, or are above the 85th percentile or below the 5th percentile for body mass index (BMI). They will need additional assessment of nutritional intake and physical activity (see Chapter 19 ⊘).

By middle and late adolescence, adult growth is nearly achieved, earlier for girls than boys. While measurement continues to be performed, nurses assess the BMI more carefully to be sure the height and weight indicate appropriate intake and exercise. Overweight at this age is likely to continue into adulthood, particularly if parents are overweight, so early intervention will be needed to decrease this potential. Other youth may have eating disorders and should be referred to a specialist for care. Children from homes without sufficient financial resources may be hungry and lack adequate food of high quality (known as food insecurity). Parents who were eligible for the Women, Infants, and Children (WIC) Nutrition Program services when children were younger may not receive them once the child is an adolescent, so the increasing dietary intake needs of their teens cannot be met. If an adolescent is thin and has little energy, consider this possibility; administer the food security questionnaire found in Chapter 19 ⊘. Even the child who is overweight may live in a family with insufficient resources since foods with high fat and caloric content are often less expensive than those with greater nutrient value. For example, a "dollar menu" at a fast-food restaurant meets hunger needs faster and with less expense than a home-prepared meal of fresh fruits, vegetables, and grains. Additionally, persons who have experienced periods of hunger from inadequate food resources may overeat when food is available, a pattern that promotes weight gain (Smith & Richards, 2008).

Few options exist for measuring the developmental competence of adolescents, but observations and questions during care provide information about meeting developmental milestones. Key tasks for adolescents involve separating from the parents and establishing positive relationships with peers. The young teen may come to an appointment with a parent and rely on that parent to answer some questions during the examination. However, the middle and late teen should be increasingly able to come alone, answer questions, and assume responsibility for healthcare decisions. Offer older teens the option of coming into the room alone, stating, "Your mom can wait here and we can come and get her later. Does that sound all right?" During your time with an adolescent, ask questions such as the following to learn about peer interactions and activities:

- "How would you describe your two best friends?"
- "What are the two things you like best about school? What do you not like?"
- "How do you generally spend Friday and Saturday nights?"
- "Describe what you do before and after school."
- "What do you like about the way your parents treat you? What do you not like?"
- "What are your plans for (the summer, the vacation coming up, after high school)?"

The adolescent receives a physical examination, often by the nurse practitioner or physician. See Chapter 7 ⊘ for components of the examination. Particular parts of the examination for teens include:

- Scoliosis screening
- Sexual maturity rating (Tanner stages)
- Breast exam
- Testicular exam
- Testing for sexually transmitted infections (among those sexually active)
- Pelvic exam and Pap smear (for sexually active females)
- Hematocrit for anemia annually in menstruating adolescents
- Hearing screening at 12, 15, and 18 years
- Vision screening annually
- Blood pressure annually
- Lipid screening for those with a family history of early heart disease or other risk factors
- Tuberculosis for those in high-risk areas

Most adolescents do not want parents present during the examination but occasionally will want a parent for a first pelvic examination or a blood draw. Ask them their preference in a confidential setting so they can freely make the choice. They also may choose to have a healthcare provider of the same gender complete the genitourinary examination. A chaperone (another healthcare provider) should always be present for genital examinations.

During all parts of the admission and measurement process, and during the physical examination, the nurse remains aware of the teen's developmental progression. Teaching is applied throughout the entire visit. Details about essential components are discussed throughout this chapter. Table 13–1 provides a list of topics that should be addressed, along with questions to ask the adolescent and teaching to include. Health promotion approaches are used when the teaching emphasizes common teen issues and provides ideas for the adolescent and parent to deal with these concerns. Health maintenance issues are those designed to keep the youth healthy by avoiding disease and preventing injury.

Expected outcomes of care include screening and early identification for common health problems, normal patterns of growth, and meeting of developmental milestones.

NUTRITION

The young adolescent needs a well-balanced diet to support the growth of this period, and the late adolescent requires intake that supports physical activity and provides nutrients for metabolism and to promote the immune system. Although nutritional intake is important, teens often do not eat well. They may be busy and do not want to plan meals. They like to eat foods that are popular with other teens, so high fat and sugar intake can be common. Or, they may be dieting to achieve weight loss. Some adolescents do not have enough financial resources for purchasing proper foods.

Questions that can guide data gathering include:

- "You mentioned while you were being weighed that you are trying to lose weight. What are you doing to lose the weight? Have you lost any weight yet? How much would you like to weigh? Describe how you exercise."
- "What is your favorite meal? What foods do you dislike or avoid? What do you eat for snacks? Do you drink milk? Do you ever eat cheese or ice cream or yogurt? How often?"
- "Do you take vitamins? Fluoride? Do you take any dietary supplements because of your weight lifting? Do you have to cut back on foods to get into your weight category in wrestling?"
- "Do you bring a lunch to school or eat school lunch? How often does your family eat together?"

TABLE 13–1	Sample Questions and Teaching Topics Pertinent to Adolescence	
TOPIC	**QUESTIONS**	**TEACHING**
Sleep	"What time do you generally go to bed on school nights? On weekends? Do you feel rested when you get up? Do you have trouble getting to sleep?"	Importance of adequate sleep and rest to school performance, alertness, and safety Recommended hours of sleep Allowing time for bedtime routines and limiting caffeine intake, especially in the afternoon and evening Turning off screen equipment (television, computer, cell phone) and making them inaccessible during sleep
School performance	"Describe how school is going for you. Are you getting the grades you expected? What is most difficult for you? Are your teachers available for help when you need it?"	Study habits including adequate time and a quiet setting Resources for getting assistance such as meeting teachers before or after school
Peer interactions	"Describe your best friend. What do you like to do together? Do you usually hang out with one or two friends or in groups? Do you have dates? What do you do on them? Do you have a boyfriend/girlfriend?"	Importance of friends Influence of friends on decisions regarding studying, risky behaviors Sexuality education including decision making about close relationships with others Showing respect and concern for self and friends
Discipline	"What happens when you do something that your parents do not approve of, Carrie? Is it hard for you to set limits for yourself or to do things different than your friends?" (For parents): "How often do you have to discipline Carrie? What kinds of things does she do to get into trouble? How do you feel about your ability to handle discipline for Carrie?"	Establishing limits for self and still feeling accepted by friends (For parents): Deciding appropriate discipline methods such as withdrawing privileges like driving Limiting rules to those necessary and then consistently enforcing them
Injury prevention	"What sports do you enjoy? What protective gear do you wear for this sport? Have you been hurt doing the sport?" "You have had your driver's license about a year now, Franco. Have you had any tickets? Any accidents? Do you ever drive after drinking? Do you ride with friends who have been drinking?" "So you have been helping with the harvest this year. What part of that is your job?"	Protective gear and practices that decrease sports injury Bicycle and automobile safety Importance of avoiding drinking and driving or operating any machinery Farm and environmental safety measures
Planning for future	"You're a junior this year, Franco? Have you started to think about what you will do after graduation? What skills will you need to get that type of job?" "It looks like you have managed well with your baby, Carrie. You will have your GED soon. Do you know what you will do then, and how you'll continue to care for your baby?"	Resources for future planning, such as school counselors, parents, and the Internet Suggesting a visit to potential job sites or colleges to get a realistic view Resources and realistic planning for the teen parent

Combine the information from measurement of the adolescent with the answers to questions about diet to identify possible areas for intervention. Determine any questions the teen has about foods, diet, maintaining desired weight, and topics like vegetarianism or supplements to enhance athletic performance. (See Chapter 19 🔗 for further detail about these special nutritional topics.) Health promotion plans focus on practices that lead to healthy growth and development, including topics such as:

- Consuming five fruits and vegetables daily
- Including whole grain products to replace refined products when possible
- Eating three meals each day, including breakfast and lunch
- Eating together as a family several times weekly
- Planning menus and preparing foods for balanced intake

Health maintenance plans center on those practices that prevent disease, including:

- Limiting refined sugar and high fat intake (such as soft drinks and fried foods) in order to maintain weight at the recommended level

- Including two to three servings of dairy products daily to enhance bone formation and decrease chance of osteoporosis as an adult
- Using resources for treatment of eating disorders if they are identified (see Chapter 19 🔗)

While much of nutrition teaching should be aimed directly at the adolescent, parents are also included. They can be effective contributors to healthy intake by providing plenty of fruits and vegetables for snacks, having foods attractively prepared and ready for consumption when the teen is hungry, planning several meals together as a family each week, encouraging milk or other forms of calcium intake, and setting a good example for food intake. Nurses can help parents to identify youth with an eating disorder and provide resources for intervention in these cases (see Chapter 19 for a full discussion of eating disorders).

Consider as well the teen mother. The adolescent who is pregnant or breastfeeding has increased needs for nutritional teaching and may require financial resources to access sufficient food. How will you combine the growth and developmental needs of an adolescent with those of her infant when planning teaching? See the Photo Story on the next page.

PHOTO STORY...
CHARISSE AND JEREMY AT SCHOOL

Charisse is the 17-year-old mother of Jeremy. She is enrolled in a "choice" (alternative) high school that supports teens in their education by providing childcare in a stimulating environment. The teens take child development courses as part of the curriculum and spend time each day in the childcare center. Charisse's baby Jeremy is an active, alert toddler who attends the childcare center at the high school, and both he and Charisse enjoy the time they spend together during the day. Charisse is often too busy with school and childcare to fix nutritious meals for herself and her son, and she lacks knowledge of how to plan a diet. She wants to feed her baby well, but needs to learn that she influences her child's nutrition by her own example. At the center, she has learned to prepare nutritious food and to join her son in eating so that he learns healthy eating patterns. Teachers work in the childcare center with the teens to enhance knowledge of child development. The teachers use discussion, show the teens how to find valuable information in books and magazines, help them analyze websites for accuracy, and have many guests and speakers from the community so that the teens learn about local resources. In addition, the teachers act as resources to connect the teens to each other in order to enhance their own developmental need of socializing with peers. The adolescents often have complex social and family situations that require much support and a variety of resources. Develop a plan for the

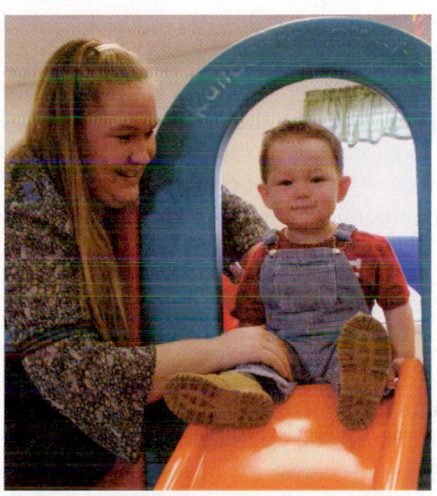

Charisse and Jeremy take time to play together at the school's childcare center.

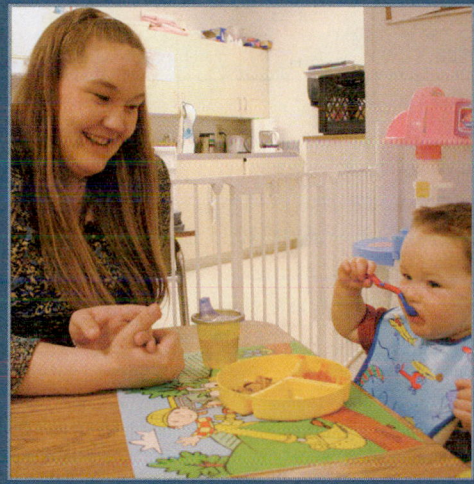

Learning good nutritional practices at school will help Charisse plan better meals at home. She has learned to sit with Jeremy while he eats.

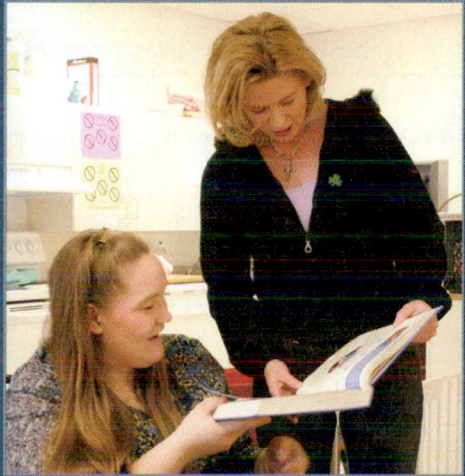

The child development teacher discusses anticipatory guidance with Charisse, who has questions about Jeremy's growth.

ways in which the school nurse can partner with teachers and others to support young teens and their infants in a setting such as this.

Jeremy is just over 1 year of age and has begun to walk. Charisse was unfamiliar with safety hazards for 1-year-olds and has benefited from demonstrations in the childcare center about hazardous toys, furniture, wall plugs, and other parts of the environment. A teacher and the school nurse visit each teen's home every month. *What environmental assessment would you plan for Charisse's home to ensure a safe environment for Jeremy? What teaching is important to avoid some of the most common injuries of toddlers?* (See the

section on injury prevention later in this chapter for ideas to integrate into the teaching plan.)

Plan a nutritious daily menu for Jeremy. Consult Chapter 19 🔗 for details about the recommended daily intake of nutrients and the types and amounts of food needed at Jeremy's age. *What common foods that teens like could be part of Jeremy's diet? Which foods that Charisse likes for herself might not be good choices for Jeremy?* In addition to nutrition, Jeremy's health depends on physical activity. Notice some of the large climbing toys at the child center. *Which gross and fine motor skills are expected at his age?* See Chapter 5 🔗.

PHYSICAL ACTIVITY

Many adolescents suffer from the effects of inadequate physical activity. As children grow and enter the teenage years, physical activity decreases, particularly in girls. Although 60 minutes daily of moderate or vigorous activity is recommended for teens, 23% do not get this level of exercise even one day a week (Eaton, Kann, Kinchen, et al., 2010). Only about 37% of adolescents report daily vigorous activity for 5 days a week. The percentage is lower among certain groups, with only 28% of females reporting that level of activity. The incidence of exercise decreases to about 31% of teens in 12th grade (Eaton et al., 2010). At a time when teens are not very active as a group, physical education requirements in school are also decreasing. Only 23% of 12th-grade students regularly attend a physical education class (Centers for Disease Control and Prevention, 2008). The lack of intramural or noncompetitive school sports can be problematic; students who have played a sport since early childhood make the school team, while those with lower skill levels who cannot make the team are left with no other options for playing a sport. Thus, some adolescents may be active daily, while others become increasingly inactive. Nurses can work with schools, neighborhoods, and other community groups to establish safe, fun, and noncompetitive activities that include all youth.

Physical activity levels must be assessed at each health supervision visit or in other contacts with adolescents. Apply resilience theory and assess youth, families, and the community for risk and protective factors regarding physical activity (Table 13–2).

Some youth have established regular physical activity programs, and this behavior should be encouraged (Figure 13–3 ■). Parents who have regular physical activity are important in influencing children, so encourage parental exercise at pediatric healthcare visits. Be alert for adolescents who exercise but have other health problems. Some athletes try to eat very little to remain a certain weight for wrestling, running, or other sports. Integrate nutritional teaching that includes the importance of adequate intake for sports performance. Other athletes use nutritional supplements or hormones to enhance performance (see Chapter 19 🔗 for a list of some popular products). Although most are not harmful, few have proven benefits and their cost is not warranted.

Other youth have very little physical activity and feel incompetent in performing many sports. Work with them to find at least one thing they can do on a daily basis—walking their dog in the neighborhood, riding a bike to the store, using stairs instead of elevators when possible, parking on the far side of the school lot and walking farther, swimming at a club their parents belong to or at a local YMCA or YWCA, or saving money to take lessons for horseback riding or golf. Form interest groups at schools and community centers that provide an outlet for adolescents who cannot "make the team" for school sports. Encourage parents and adolescents to set goals together to integrate some physical activity daily.

The nurse's activities for health promotion concentrate on teaching the health and mental benefits of physical activity such as increased energy, weight control, and a feeling of control and success. Health maintenance focuses on viewing physical activity as a method to prevent disease such as cardiovascular disease and diabetes. Youth who have

TABLE 13–2 Risk and Protective Factors Regarding Physical Activity in Adolescence	
RISK FACTORS	**PROTECTIVE FACTORS**
■ Lives in rural or other isolated setting with little opportunity for contact with other teens	■ Has opportunities for participation in physical activity at home, at school, and in the community
■ Lives in urban area that is unsafe or provides little opportunity for outside physical activity	■ School provides daily physical education classes
■ Presence of neighborhood hazards and unsafe areas	■ Neighborhood and community provide physical activity options
■ Lack of neighborhood programs for physical activity promotion	■ Has many friends living close who participate in physical activity
	■ Public policies maintain parks, green spaces, biking trails, playgrounds
■ Has a developmental disability that impairs physical movement	■ Programs are available for adolescents with developmental disabilities or other healthcare needs
■ Does not like physical activity	■ Likes physical activity
■ Has a pattern and history of low activity levels	■ Has exercised during all of childhood, often with parents
■ Is overweight	
■ Does not feel competent in most sports	
■ Limited financial resources to pay registration fees or buy protective gear for sports	■ Availability of financial and other resources for sports gear and protective equipment
■ Family members who have little physical activity	■ Parents participate in regular physical activity and encourage the adolescent to do so also
■ Parents who are not active in school sports and committees	
■ Parents who do not like physical activity and have had low levels while their teen was growing up	■ Youth and parents agree to a limit of 2 hours daily of screen time
■ Parents who have little time or facilities for exercise or always exercise at a club—out of view of their family	
■ Lack of youth and parent knowledge about physical activity needs and benefits	■ Knowledgeable about benefits of activity; committed to maintaining exercise patterns
What risk and protective factors for physical activity are present in the local communities you serve?	

Source: *Adapted from Hagan, J. F., Shaw, J. S., & Duncan, P. M. (2008). Bright futures: Guidelines for health supervision of infants, children, and adolescents (3rd ed.). Elk Grove Village, IL: American Academy of Pediatrics.*

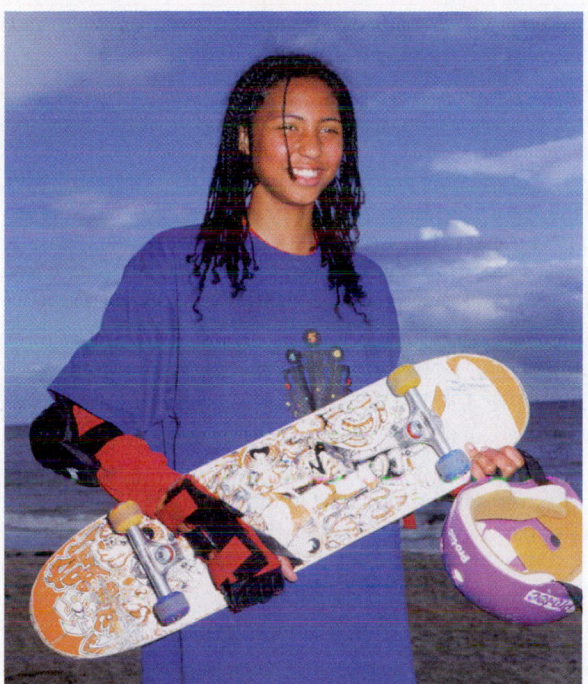

FIGURE 13–3 ■ This teen girl is an avid "boarder." How can you encourage and praise her for the activity? What clues do you have that she is using adequate safety measures?

Developing Cultural Competence
Dental Care

Analysis of several national surveys such as the National Center for Health Statistics and the National Health Interview Survey shows marked disparity in oral health. The major factor in disparity of dental care is lack of dental insurance. While 49% of youth from families without insurance did not have a dental visit in the previous year and 27% of them had unmet dental needs, only 17% of youth from families with insurance lacked a previous year visit and only 4% had unmet dental needs. People without dental insurance commonly are poor. In these families, 21% of children have unmet dental needs in contrast with 4% in families living above the poverty level. Hispanic youth are most at risk; 11% have unmet dental needs (Child Trends, 2010).

When you work with adolescent populations from groups at high risk for lack of dental coverage or high incidence of caries, be certain to include dental assessment in health supervision visits and have resources for care readily available.

family members with these diseases or meet adults who have them are more likely to understand the importance of their own activity.

Desired outcomes include maintenance of weight within recommended level, daily exercise of 60 minutes, and establishment of lifetime exercise routines.

ORAL HEALTH

Continued dental care during the adolescent years can ensure oral health. The recommendations remain the same as those for young children. The adolescent should floss daily, brush twice daily with a small amount of fluoridated toothpaste, and visit a dental provider every 6 months. By about 14 years of age, those who do not have fluoridated water and have been taking fluoride can stop this supplement. Even the molars have been formed by that age, so fluoride tablets are no longer needed. Continue to examine the condition of the teeth and the number of erupted permanent teeth present. Be alert for any unusual growths and ulcers in the mouth and refer for care as needed. Certain activities influence the condition of the teeth and mouth. Examples include self-induced vomiting such as in anorexia or bulimia, which may harm normal teeth enamel; use of certain drugs that might cause ulcers or destroy enamel; or sexually transmitted infections acquired by oral sex.

The availability of dental insurance for the adolescent is a potential concern. The teen whose family does not have dental insurance needs referrals for care to affordable resources. Dental specialists clean off plaque that has formed, apply sealants to erupting molars, examine the teeth for caries, and perform restorative care. Certain groups are more at risk for inadequate dental care; see Developing Cultural Competence: Dental Care. When working with these populations, nurses can question access to care and make recommendations that foster regular checkups. Some teens may wish to whiten their teeth or get orthodontia to improve appearance. The nurse helps the youth and parents to find resources for needed care.

Evaluate risk factors for threats to oral health such as tobacco use (see Chapter 20 ☞ for further information). For example, chewing tobacco is fairly prevalent among certain groups and can lead to nicotine addiction, oral ulcers, cancers, and other problems. Smokeless tobacco is often not considered by health professionals as a risk factor for youth. However, statistics tell us that some groups are at significant risk for this form of tobacco use. About 9% of youth admit to using chew within the previous 30 days. Males have much higher incidence (15%) than females (2%). The ethnic group with the highest rate of usage is Whites, with 20% of males and 2% of females using chew. About 8% of Hispanic males and 4% of Hispanic females use chew, while only 5% of Black males and 1% of Black females use chew (Eaton et al., 2010). Among certain groups, such as hockey or baseball players, using chew can bring acceptance into the peer group. What youth in the community might be using chewing tobacco? What resources are available for them to quit?

Another threat to oral health, similar to earlier ages, is engagement in certain sports. Ask about physical activity. If the youth engages in hockey, football, and similar sports, a mouth guard should be worn during sport activities.

Expected outcomes for oral health include dental visits twice annually, daily positive oral health habits, absence of risk factors for poor oral health, and obtaining recommended follow-up care for problems.

MENTAL AND SPIRITUAL HEALTH

Adolescents have many challenges to their mental health and need support to emerge from adolescence with mental and spiritual strengths. Mental health topics must be addressed at each health supervision opportunity to promote mental health among teens. Mental health is closely linked to developmental tasks such as growing independence, formation of close relationships with peers, becoming confident in accomplishments, becoming part of a social group, and setting goals for the future (Figure 13–4 ■).

Self-Concept

As during other developmental stages, self-concept continues to evolve, influencing how the adolescent reacts to the environment. Academic accomplishments, athletics, and social interactions are examples of factors that influence self-concept. Self-regulation—making decisions to govern oneself—becomes critically important

Video | Teen Mental and Spiritual Health

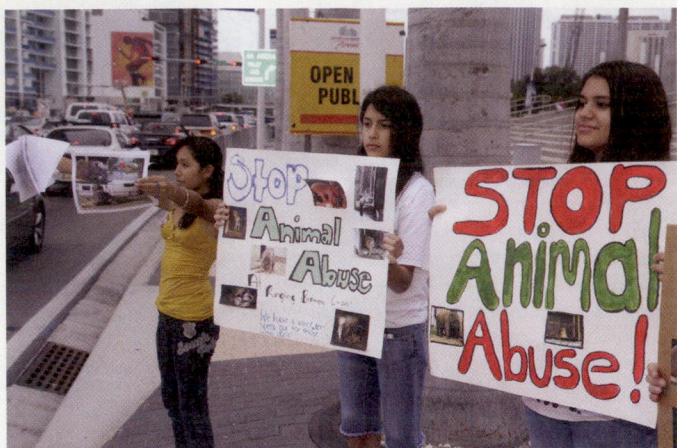

FIGURE 13–4 ■ Teens often become associated with causes. This helps them to feel part of a social group and also provides them with opportunities to examine belief systems and make decisions about meaningful activities.

Source: *Jeff Greenberg/Alamy.*

during adolescence. Self-esteem, or a positive feeling about the self, is key to meeting life's challenges. Questions that provide information about self-esteem include:

- "What things have you accomplished that make you feel proud?"
- "What are some of your major disappointments? How have you dealt with them?"

Ask parents how the adolescent generally feels about him- or herself. Provide resources to deal with disappointments, and give praise for the teen's accomplishments.

The adolescent's self-esteem is often tied to perceptions of body image (see Chapter 12 🔗 for a thorough discussion of self-concept and self-esteem). Factors such as early or late maturation, overweight or underweight, or the role of the media can influence the teen's body image. A healthy image includes the realization that the body has positive and less positive attributes and that the individual can influence the body by healthy eating and physical activity. Be alert for the teen whose wish for a different body leads to eating disorders and excessive exercise or intake of nutritional supplements (see Chapter 19 🔗).

Sexuality

Sexuality involves both body changes that signal mature sexual development and the mental concept of oneself as a sexual being. See Figures 7–43, 7–44, and 7–45 in Chapter 7 🔗 for stages of body change during adolescence. Body changes and mental concepts do not necessarily mature at the same time, and adolescents may not be ready for sexual maturity and the decisions about sexual behavior simply due to achieving sexual maturation. Most young adolescent girls have begun menstruating, and by early to middle adolescence, boys are having nocturnal emissions and ejaculations. Ask teens if they have received information about puberty, body changes, and sexuality. Inform young adolescents that most teens have questions and that you will talk with them about any areas of interest, including contraception and sexually transmitted infections. Ask older adolescents directly if they have had sexual intercourse and, if so, what they are doing to protect against pregnancy and sexually transmitted infections. Provide support for the adolescent who has decided not to have sexual intercourse; reinforce that sexual feelings are normal, but that decisions about sexual intercourse are their right and privilege.

Ask if the teen has confusion about sexuality. If teens identify as gay, lesbian, or bisexual, let them know they are welcome at the healthcare agency and ask about decisions regarding sexual practices, reinforcing the need for protection against sexually transmitted infections. Provide community resources to support gay, lesbian, or bisexual teens so that they can develop a social group in which they feel comfortable. Ask if the adolescent has ever experienced unwanted pressure for intercourse and if there has been help and support to deal with the situation. Intimate partner violence, date rape, and other trauma signals a need for referral to a mental health specialist. See Chapter 20 🔗 for further information on these topics.

Some adolescents are seen for health care at the time they become sexually active. Use this opportunity to reinforce and correct prior knowledge about the body and protection against pregnancy and sexually transmitted infections. Recall Kim in the opening scenario. How will you ensure that she gets the information she needs for safe sex? Since she has come for health care, what other information and interventions does she need? Has she received a tetanus booster in the last 10 years? Has she ever had hepatitis B vaccine? Has she heard about the human papillomavirus vaccine? Kim is having trouble talking openly with her parents. What topics would she like to address? What resources might be available in her school or community to assist her?

Practice Alert

The nurse who works with adolescents dealing with sexuality issues may find that the values of some teens are very different from the nurse's personal values. How do you react when a teen decides to have sexual intercourse or has become pregnant? Can you help teens to make wise decisions without telling them what they should do? It is important for adolescents to learn the importance of sexual intercourse and the meaning of close relationships. Teaching them early about this will enable them to respect others at the time they do have intimate relations. Nurses should also treat teens with respect, expecting them to consider options and make wise decisions. Nurses who cannot work with certain groups of teens due to differences in moral values have the obligation to refer the teens for care to resources where they can receive the information and services they are requesting.

Sleep

Sleep is necessary for anyone to function safely and at a level of one's potential. Unfortunately, many youth do not get the sleep needed for healthy functioning. Teens have an increased need for sleep due to their growth rates and activity levels. At the same time, their internal clocks change, making it more difficult to get to sleep at the usual time. It is thought that a decrease in secretion of melatonin occurs, so the teen does not feel tired in the late evening. However, they often have not received the number of hours of sleep needed by the time they wake up for school or work. The problem may be worsened if the student participates in sports or other activities. They may need to get to school early for music, sports, or other activities, or perhaps stay late into the evening for practices. Some adolescents work on weekends or evenings as well. Of course, social activities usually fill much of their time.

While about 9 hours of sleep are needed, most adolescents get about 6 hours (Mayo Clinic, 2009). The effects of sleep deprivation can be serious. Teens cannot perform to their potential in school or at work. Many parents state that adolescents are moody and difficult to communicate with when they are tired. There may be a connection between lack of sleep and substance abuse, and teens commonly use caffeinated beverages to stay awake. Some people tend to eat more when they are tired, and get less physical activity. Perhaps one of the most serious consequences deals with the danger of driving while sleepy; this is a common cause of accidents. Ask adolescents what time they go to bed and when they awake. Inquire about whether the teen is frequently tired. Suggestions that may help include:

- Try to keep to similar hours for sleeping so the body becomes accustomed to a schedule.
- Avoid caffeine in the late afternoon and evening.
- Do homework early, and relax a bit before going to bed.
- Make screen technology (television, computer, cell phone texting) unavailable during sleep time.
- Plan a day each weekend to simply relax and have few demands.

School

School plays an increasingly important role in adolescent mental health. School provides peer support, meaningful activities, and a forum for learning time management and other skills. At the same time, some youth feel much stress because of inability to fit in, worry about grades and their future, and violent or unsupportive school situations. Choice schools and even online completion of high school are available in some locations to offer alternatives from the mainstream schools. Discuss the elements of school that adolescents like and those they do not like. Evaluate presence of support in the schools such as teachers and counselors. Ask the adolescent about future plans and how those are influencing choices for courses and friends in school at present.

Mental Health Disorders

While most teenagers have many protective factors that can be identified and fostered, a few have risks that can harm mental health. It is important to identify the risks and to use health maintenance techniques to lessen the risk factors. Depression and substance use are two common risks to mental health. Depression is discussed in Chapter 34 and substance use in Chapter 20. See Table 13–3 to help in identification of these problems during health supervision visits.

Spiritual Health

Spirituality offers comfort and support for the adolescent. Being a member of a teen group in a faith-based home can offer a peer group with similar values and bring meaning to life. Some adolescents reject the faith of their parents and seek a different group. Others seek to leave religious practices totally, whereas others become more committed to them. Ask teens if they have the resources they need to bring meaning to their lives, and provide referrals if needed. In addition to faith-based practices, participation in community food kitchens, raising money for causes, and other activities can provide meaning for many adolescents.

Nursing Role

The nurse actively promotes the mental health of youth by understanding their developmental needs, partnering with youth to establish healthcare goals of importance to them, and providing information and resources. Gentle guidance and active partnership with youth help to ensure healthy self-concept, sexuality, and personality development. Although health promotion and health maintenance activities commonly occur in office or clinic settings, there are many other settings where nurses work with adolescents; mental health activities are often integrated into these settings. Consider offering health promotion and health maintenance wherever you might see students.

| TABLE 13–3 | Signs of Depression and Substance Abuse |
DEPRESSION	SUBSTANCE ABUSE
■ Changes in behavior, school performance, sleep, and appetite	■ Changes in behavior, school performance, sleep, and appetite
■ Physical complaints	■ Multiple accidents
■ Loss of interest and pleasure in usual activities	■ Lack of responsibility
■ Difficulty in motivating self; low energy	■ Labile (changeable) mood, attitude, and behavior
■ Sadness, irritability, poor concentration	■ Inability to set goals
■ Change in friends	■ Hopelessness
■ Feelings of worthlessness	■ Feelings of ambivalence
■ Thoughts of death or suicide	■ A variety of physical changes, depending on substances used

Source: Adapted from Tanski, S., Garfunkel, L. C., Duncan, P. M., & Weitzman, M. (2011). *Performing preventive services. Elk Grove Village, IL: American Academy of Pediatrics.*

Some nontraditional settings include correctional facilities, school-based health centers, and programs for pregnant teens. Adolescents in these facilities can benefit from services to improve diet, physical activity, and lifestyle behaviors that influence mental health (Box 13–2).

The desired outcomes for mental and spiritual health promotion and maintenance include meaningful activities in the adolescent's life, emerging independence, good choices about lifestyle behaviors, and development of successful coping skills.

RELATIONSHIPS

Adolescents form stronger bonds with friends than at any time earlier in development; at the same time they need their parents for guidance and reassurance as they become more independent. However, as teenagers strive for independence they frequently strike out at parents, test limits, and engage in conflicts. Interactions in the family provide consistent and important ties at the same time that social interactions outside the family become a central part of life (Figure 13–5 ■). Health promotion helps teens to form strong friendships with peers and to continue to value and participate in the family, and helps parents to understand developmental needs and their role in establishing a new type of relationship with the emerging young adult in the family. Partnerships with care providers are important to help families work together to achieve these outcomes.

When adolescents are seen for healthcare visits, assess relationships with others. Provide time alone with both the adolescent and the parents (if they are present) so that everyone has time to freely talk and ask questions. Some areas already discussed, such as school performance and activities, provide information about the adolescent's friends and how time is spent. Ask teens to describe their best friends and what they do together. Ask parents their opinions of the youth's friends.

Temperament or personality type characteristics continue into adolescence, but they generally do not change from earlier years. For example, the active infant and young child is usually an active teenager. The slow-to-warm-up baby may be the adolescent who needs more time to adjust to a new school or teachers. If the adolescent or parent has trouble with personality characteristics, it may be helpful to talk about these traits, help them to establish a positive sense about the attributes, and discuss ways to adapt the environment as

---

BOX 13–2 | **Community Care: Health Promotion and Maintenance in Nontraditional Settings**

Nurses offer health promotion and health maintenance to adolescents in a variety of settings in addition to offices and clinics in the community. Examples include:

1. **Youth correctional facilities.** Although the American Academy of Pediatrics has recommended that juvenile justice facilities provide care for incarcerated youth, only a very small number of facilities in the United States have received accreditation for care provided. Incarcerated youth arrive with a high probability of preexisting acute conditions such as sexually transmitted diseases, substance use, and mental illness; additional acute problems emerge from the arrest or conditions in the facility (National Commission on Correctional Health Care, 2011). Nurses often provide care in correctional facilities and are instrumental in improving the level of care. Risk assessment of incarcerated youth, health education programs, and intervention services such as immunizations are needed. Gynecologic care and obstetric services for females are essential services.

2. **School-based health centers.** There has been a growth of school-based health care, and the National Assembly on School-Based Health Care (NASBHC) has performance evaluation standards for such care (National Assembly on School-Based Health Care, 2010). Many of these centers are nurse-managed, with a variety of nurse practitioners and registered nurses providing care. Services provided include physical assessment and treatment, mental health assessment and intervention, medication management, and oral health screening and treatment. Integrating services into school settings improves access, increases referrals, fosters collaboration among professionals, and provides screening of populations to find youth with health needs. Personnel in the health centers are viewed by students as part of the school and are therefore often accepted more readily by the adolescents than are professionals in offices or other settings. (See Chapter 14 🔗 for further discussion of school health.)

3. **Pregnancy care.** Nurses often provide care for adolescents who are pregnant in offices, clinics, and schools. When providing services to these teens, nurses can focus on many health promotion and health maintenance topics. Youth are commonly interested in these topics since they realize that their behaviors may influence the fetus. For example, a program that addresses smoking cessation for pregnant teenagers can be instituted, providing information about effects of smoking on the fetus, infants, and children. Pregnancy is also a time when adolescents may be receptive to learning about dietary needs and improved intake. Sleep, child development, and other pertinent topics can be integrated into care in many settings with pregnant youth. Peers and social support are essential for the pregnant teen, and positive support systems can be enhanced by nursing care.

4. **Homeless shelters.** Adolescents may live in homeless shelters or on the street, either with other family members or on their own. These youth often experience health problems such as poor nutrition, interrupted access to dental care and preventive health services, injury from exposure to climate and other hazards, and mental health disruptions (National Coalition for the Homeless, 2009). Nurses in homeless shelters often coordinate mental and physical health services, provide resources for needed care, and facilitate movement into more stable housing in the community.

What clinical settings are used in your nursing program to provide interactions with adolescents? How can you integrate health promotion and health maintenance interventions within these settings, whether they are in the hospital, clinics, offices, schools, homes, or other settings?

---

needed. For example, parents should not expect a slow-to-warm-up teen to be interested in running for a class office. An adolescent with irregular sleep and eating habits will find it difficult to have a job at a set time and will need to set alarms and other reminders.

Inquire about the youth's roles in the family. Does the teen have jobs and responsibilities? What freedom is allowed? What are

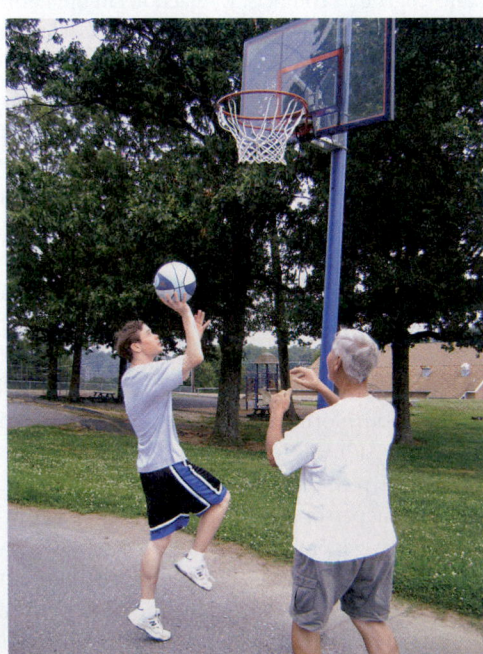

FIGURE 13–5 ▪ This father and son have an opportunity to talk, share a common athletic interest, and enjoy a bonding experience that can last for many years. The teen can transfer the relationship skills he has learned to many future interactions.

relationships like with siblings and extended family members such as grandparents and cousins? What activities are done together as a family? Are there differences in the teen's and the parents' answers to these questions? What are the risk and protective factors in the teen–parent relationship?

Most adolescents require discipline or guidance from parents at certain times. However, constant battles over daily events are counterproductive. Instead, it is best if parents respect the teenager's need for a level of autonomy and enact a few rules on important issues, so that parents have to enforce them only rarely. Guidelines that can help parents include the following:

- Gradually increase the teen's independence. If there is success with growing responsibility, the teen may be ready for more. If the teen misuses independence (perhaps by staying out too late, having a party at home without parents present, lying about location on an evening out), there should be clear limits and loss of privileges.
- Be willing to talk with and hear the teen's story. On the other hand, do not be talked out of consequences for the teen's bad decisions.
- Recognize that driving a car, staying out late, and other activities are not a given. They are privileges for responsibility displayed.
- Comment on a teen's behavior rather than making belittling comments about him or her as a person.
- Realize that the teen is establishing independence and that the relationship will change. Be consistent and loving as the adolescent tries out and learns about limits and the self.

Provide an opportunity alone with the teen to talk about issues such as domestic violence. Is the youth abused, or is there violence between adults in the family? Are there stressors such as lack of sufficient finances, an ill parent, or a lost job? How have these occurrences affected the adolescent? Minor adjustments can be helped by discussion, but some major problems will need referral to mental health specialists (see Chapter 34 🔗 for discussion of mental health problems and approaches).

Help families realize that the roles of all members change when a teenager is present. The following information may be useful for parents:

- It is common to feel rejected as the teen becomes more independent and critical of parents; talk about this with other parents; recognize that a new and positive relationship will likely emerge.
- Provide opportunities for the teen to talk, but do not force the conversation.
- Use open-ended questions. Say, "Tell me something good that happened today" rather than "How was your day?"
- Recognize that it will take time for the teen to take on responsible mature behaviors and that guidance is needed throughout the teen years.
- Provide discipline by talking about the unacceptable behavior, rather than belittling the teen.
- Provide plenty of positive feedback for good grades, participation in activities, help at home, or other behaviors.
- Insist on a few rules; important rules are to give respect to family members and other people and to avoid risky behaviors such as drinking and driving.

Some helpful tips for adolescents include:

- Most teens get frustrated with their parents at times; list some things you like and some you don't like about your family.
- Be sure to focus complaints on specific issues like wanting a later curfew rather than telling parents they don't know anything.
- Most parents, like kids, want to know what they do right; occasionally tell your parents things that are going well or things that you appreciate.
- Talk to your parents; if you don't feel you can, find another adult you respect, like an older sibling, a teacher, a counselor, or a member of the clergy.

In their relationships with peers, adolescents often have many of the same issues that emerge with parents. They may have disagreements with friends or feel hurt by things that are said or done. Ask teens about how things are going with friends and what problems they have. Talk about negotiating, joining groups to form new friendships, and the importance of respecting and not making fun of others. Give them strategies for living up to their own standards even when friends are enticing them to do other things. Say, "Most teenagers have trouble saying no when friends ask them to drink and drive, or smoke, or sneak into the house late. When has it been difficult for you to say no to friends?" Suggest that having friends one can trust and who have the same ideals can be very supportive in adolescent years.

Expected outcomes are the formation of strong relationships both within and outside the family, along with independence in decision making.

DISEASE PREVENTION STRATEGIES

Teenagers typically do not have many diseases, and most are minor illnesses such as respiratory and gastrointestinal illness. However, there are some diseases that occur and health professionals must be aware of signs of potential disease. Common adolescent health issues that are described throughout this book 🔗 include:

- Acne and skin infections (Chapter 36)
- Body piercing and tattooing (Chapter 20)
- Sports overuse injuries (Chapter 35)
- Constipation and diarrhea (Chapter 30)

Other observations may signal more serious health concerns and need to be referred for further evaluation 🔗. Examples include:

- Scoliosis (Chapter 35)
- Anemia (Chapter 28)
- Excessive tiredness (fatigue) (Chapter 29)
- Bruising (Chapter 29)
- Sexually transmitted infections (Chapter 31)
- Eating disorders (Chapter 19)
- Abuse or severe bullying (Chapter 20)

Several screening tests should be performed during health supervision visits with adolescents. Physical examination is combined with mental health screening as described in the previous sections to provide a complete picture of the child's risks for diseases. See Table 13–4.

Screening tests with abnormal results require follow-up and intervention. For example, if the adolescent is anemic, iron tablets may be needed and teaching about high-iron foods should be performed (see Chapter 19 🔗). Vision impairment requires referral to an eye specialist. Presence of sexually transmitted infections requires teaching and medication treatment. History of sexual activity will guide you to tests that should be included in the examination.

Practice Alert

Sexually active teens should be screened annually for:

- Chlamydia
- Gonorrhea
- Trichomoniasis
- Human papillomavirus
- Herpes simplex virus
- Bacterial vaginosis
- Human immunodeficiency virus

Individuals should be screened for syphilis if they request testing or meet any of these criteria:

- History of STIs
- More than one sexual partner in past 6 months
- Intravenous drug use
- Sexual intercourse with a partner at risk
- Sex in exchange for drugs or money
- Homelessness
- Males—sex with other males
- Residence in areas where syphilis is prevalent

Source: *From Hagan, J. F., Shaw, J. S., & Duncan, P. M. (2008). Bright futures: Guidelines for health supervision of infants, children, and adolescents (3rd ed.). Elk Grove Village, IL: American Academy of Pediatrics; Tanski, S., Garfunkel, L. C., Duncan, P. M., & Weitzman, M. (2011). Performing preventive services. Elk Grove Village, IL: American Academy of Pediatrics.*

The adolescent should receive extensive information about ways to protect health and prevent disease. The hazardous outcomes of tobacco are discussed, and smoking/tobacco cessation programs are encouraged for smokers. Unprotected sexual activity is presented as a serious health threat. Use of sunscreens to prevent burns and future skin cancer is encouraged. Females are taught breast self-exam, and males are taught

TABLE 13–4	Screening During Health Promotion and Health Maintenance Visits of Adolescents	
AGE	RECOMMENDED MENTAL HEALTH/BEHAVIORAL SCREENING	RECOMMENDED PHYSICAL HEALTH SCREENING TESTS
11–14 years	Use of tobacco and alcohol	Vision
	History of abuse	Hearing
	Unsatisfactory school performance	Anemia
	History of depression or other mental health problems	Lipids
	History of violence or risk taking	Blood pressure
	History of multiple personal or family stresses	Urinalysis
	Loneliness or lack of friends	Tuberculosis (if at risk)
		Pap smear (for sexually active females)
		Breast exam
		Sexually transmitted disease risks
15–17 years	As above	As above
18–21 years	As above	As above
	Difficulty with job	Offer pelvic exam for all females even if not sexually active

Source: *Adapted from Hagan, J. F., Shaw, J. S., & Duncan, P. M. (2008).* Bright futures: Guidelines for health supervision of infants, children, and adolescents *(3rd ed.). Elk Grove Village, IL: American Academy of Pediatrics.*

testicular exam. For youth who are overweight and sedentary, involve teaching about the possible outcomes such as type 2 diabetes and cardiovascular disease (see Health Belief Model discussion on page 342). Although it is not advisable to threaten or frighten an adolescent with descriptions of diseases, an understanding of the potential serious outcomes of tobacco use or diabetes can be motivators for behavior change.

In addition to teaching disease prevention, the nurse also administers any needed immunizations. Many adolescents have not had immunizations since school entry; therefore, their record should be carefully reviewed. Common immunizations needed by adolescents are as follows:

- Last tetanus-diphtheria (TD) booster—recommended every 10 years if no wounds have required an update in the interim, so if the child received it at age 5 years, a booster is needed at 15 years. A Tdap (tetanus-diphtheria and acellular pertussis) booster is given, with the preferred age from 11 to 12 years. If a dose of TD was given during adolescence, wait at least 5 years, and administer one dose of Tdap.
- Second measles-mumps-rubella—a second dose may not have been routine when teens were younger so they may need it now.
- If hepatitis A is common in the state where you as a nurse provide care, the teen needs to receive the vaccine.
- Hepatitis B vaccine—important for all youth, and some may not have received it as infants.
- Varicella vaccine—required in absence of a documented history of varicella disease.
- Meningococcal vaccine—recommended.
- Human papillomavirus vaccine (three-dose series)—recommended for females and males.
- Annual influenza vaccine—now recommended for all children and adolescents. See Chapter 22 ✪ for further discussion of immunizations.

The results of health screening are shared with the teen and with the parent as appropriate. Teaching and other interventions for disease prevention are examples of health maintenance activities. Expected outcomes are increasing knowledge of common diseases and

methods of prevention among the teen and parents, use of screening tests by the healthcare provider, and use of the healthcare home by the adolescent for treatment of diseases.

INJURY PREVENTION STRATEGIES

Injury is the greatest health hazard for adolescents; therefore, injury prevention must be integrated into every health contact with youth. The major hazard is automobile crashes (see Chapter 1 ✪). Many teens learn to drive and have a license by 16 years of age (Figure 13–6 ■). They often transport friends, get distracted by social interactions in the car, have little experience with actions to take if a car slides or has mechanical problems, may drink and drive, and are often tired when driving. Most states have instituted graduated driver licensing to help decrease some risks. Driving should always be presented as a privilege and a responsibility. Serious consequences

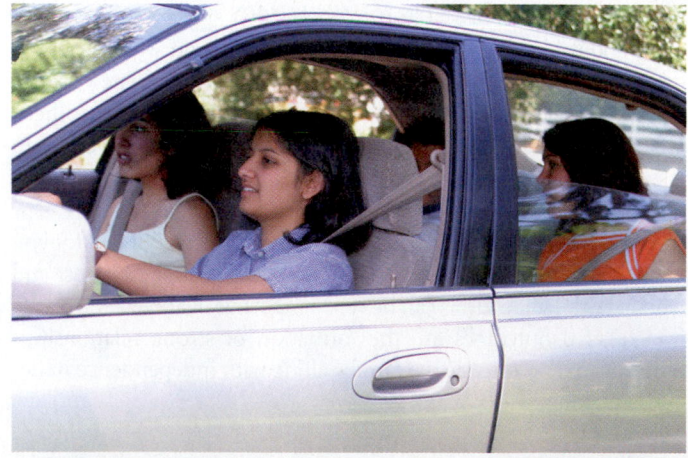

FIGURE 13–6 ■ Adolescents often drive motorized vehicles and may be at risk for injury if not properly prepared or protected. What teaching and experience do these youth need for safe enjoyment of the experience of driving and riding with friends? Do schools in your area offer driver education classes? What are the state requirements for driver licensure?

Source: © Michael Newman/PhotoEdit.

| BOX 13–3 | Research: Parent Restrictions and Teen Driving |

Major risk factors for teen drivers include inexperience (the especially vulnerable time is in the first 6 months of driving), transporting other teens, night driving, non-use of a seat belt, and distractions such as texting and playing music. Graduated driver licensing is an approach used to decrease motor vehicle crashes among novice teen drivers. The Centers for Disease Control and Prevention recommends that no learners' permits be allowed before 16 years of age, that permits must be held for at least 6 months, that driving from 10 p.m. to 5 a.m. not be allowed except with an adult chaperone, that other youth not be transported, and that regular licenses (without youth restrictions) not be allowed until 18 years of age. Zero-tolerance policies for drinking, texting or cell phone use, and nonuse of seat belts should be enforced (Centers for Disease Control and Prevention, 2010). How can nurses be active in political discussions to promote graduated driver licensing and support for parents of novice teen drivers?

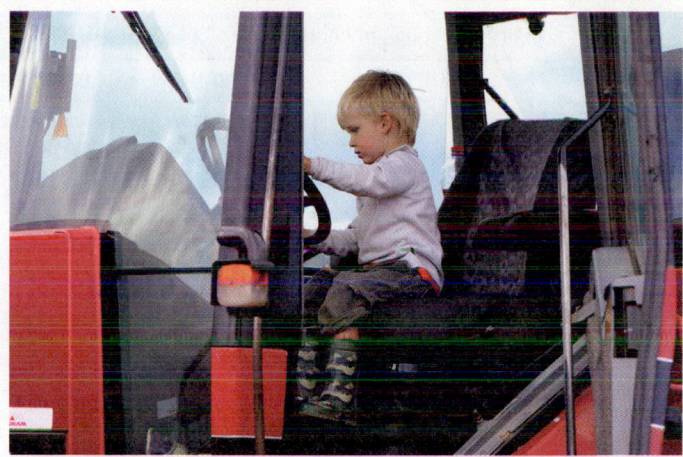

FIGURE 13–7 ■ What items would you include on a checklist for parents of children on a farm? How might pesticides or other chemicals used on a farm injure youth who work near them? What injuries from animals or equipment are common?

Source: *Petr Bonek/Alamy.*

such as losing the ability to drive for a time after any infraction can be suggested to parents. Because of the great risk of injury and death from car crashes, ask at each health visit if the teen drives or rides with other teens, what rules parents have established about driving, and whether the teen ever drinks and drives or rides with someone who does. Know the graduated driver license laws in the state where you work as a nurse. Reinforce the law's mandates, importance of lap and shoulder belt use at all times, and absolute rules to never drink and drive (Box 13–3).

Youth are at risk for injury with other motorized vehicles. Motorcycles, four-wheelers (all-terrain vehicles or ATVs), boats, jet skis, farm machinery, and tools are other sources of injury. Ask about the youth's exposure, teach about avoiding alcohol and drug use, and encourage safety gear and precautions to be used. See Evidence-Based Practice: Farm Injury and Hazards.

Every health visit should also include other questions that help to identify injury hazards:

- "You mentioned that you like target practice. What type of gun do you have? Describe how you store it. Are there other guns in your home?"

- "What is your favorite summer activity? Oh, you jump from the cliffs. How often? Do you jump or dive? How do you know how deep the water is there? How would you describe your swimming skills? Do you ever go alone? Do your parents know you are jumping from the cliffs?"

- "People are sometimes hurt or abused by others. Has that happened to you, either at home or somewhere else?"

- "Do you know what date rape is? Has that ever happened to you?"

Once you have asked about common causes of injury, be sure to discuss and provide written material to perform injury prevention teaching. Such measures are important health maintenance activities. See Tables 13–5 and 13–6 for injury prevention topics

Evidence-Based Practice Farm Injury and Hazards

PROBLEM

Injury is common in communities where children live and work on farms. More than 23,000 farm-related injuries occur annually in the United States among youth, and over 100 die (Zaloshnja, Miller, & Lee, 2011). Most injuries occur on weekends during the spring or summer. Before lunch and late afternoon are common times of the day for injury.

EVIDENCE

Farms contain a number of hazards and commonly employ youth. Machinery is a major cause of injury; other examples of hazards include electric currents, bodies of water, grain storage, and actions of large animals. Nearly half of the injuries occur on beef cattle farms (Centers for Disease Control and Prevention, 2011; Zaloshnja et al., 2011). Exposure to pesticides and other environmental elements also influence youth. Approximately 9% of youth from 16 to 19 years working on farms have been diagnosed with asthma, and 8% have had an asthma attack in the last year; nearly 10% of those who drive tractors have had a recent asthma attack (Syamlal & Mazurek, 2008). Most farms are in rural areas located far from emergency medical facilities. One study found that training high school students on farms in first aid and safety was one effective strategy to lower injury rates and provide emergency care (Carruth, Pryor, Cormier, et al., 2010).

IMPLICATIONS

Nurses should work with families from rural areas to help them promote safety for children on the farm (Figure 13–7 ■). Many rural families seek health care in urban areas so even if you are working in a city, you may have rural families in the agency. Encourage parents to consult the North American Guidelines for Children's Agricultural Tasks to match the child's physical and mental abilities with the tasks on a farm. Then suggest that parents supervise children in farm tasks, know first aid to follow for injuries, realize that serious accidents can occur, have a cell phone to call for help, and know what facilities are available for phone advice and for emergency rescue. Help families plan ahead to keep rural children safe. www.cdc.gov/niosh

CRITICAL THINKING APPLICATION

What items would you include on a checklist for parents of children on a farm? How might pesticides or other chemicals used on a farm injure youth who work near them? Plan educational materials and programs for families that live on farms.

TABLE 13–5 Injury Prevention in Adolescence

	HAZARD	DEVELOPMENTAL CHARACTERISTICS	PREVENTIVE MEASURES
	Motor vehicle crashes	Adolescents learn to drive, enjoy new independence, and often feel invulnerable.	■ Insist on driver's education classes and graduated license law adherence. ■ Enforce rules about safe driving. ■ Use seat belts for every trip. ■ Take license away from youth who drink and drive, even once.
	Sporting injuries	Adolescents may participate in physically challenging sports such as soccer, gymnastics, or football. They may be allowed to drive motorboats.	■ Encourage use of protective sporting gear. ■ Teach safe boating practices. ■ Perform teaching related to hazards of drug and alcohol use, especially when using motorized equipment.
	Drowning	Adolescents overestimate endurance when swimming. They take risks diving.	■ Encourage swimming only with friends. ■ Reinforce rules and teach about risks.

and interventions. Desired outcomes for nursing care include absence of serious injury, the ability to state sources of risk for injury, and emergency plans for assistance when engaging in any risky activities.

Nursing Management

Nursing Assessment and Diagnosis

Nurses assess adolescents in a variety of settings, including offices, clinics, schools, homes, correctional facilities, extended care facilities, sports-related endeavors, and family planning clinics. A wide array of health concerns should be included in these assessments. They include measurement of growth; presence of any unusual findings on physical examination; lifestyle choices related to dietary intake, physical activity, and oral hygiene; assessment of mental status, family interactions, and social connections with peers; and any risky behaviors the adolescent engages in such as smoking, unprotected sexual relations, alcohol or drug use, or unsafe driving practices. The people and organizations around the adolescent such as family, school, and neighborhood are all assessed, using Bronfenbrenner's theory of the ecology of development (Table 13–7). Remember to list both risks and protective factors. The protective factors can be used during implementation to enhance the youth's resilience.

Based on a thorough assessment, the nurse partners with the adolescent to establish nursing diagnoses that are appropriate for the adolescent and family. Possible nursing diagnoses include:

- Rape-Trauma Syndrome related to date rape
- Dentition, Impaired, related to ineffective oral hygiene
- Nutrition, Imbalanced: More than Body Requirements related to lack of basic nutritional knowledge and obesity in both parents
- Nutrition, Readiness for Enhanced, related to increasing interest in nutritional knowledge
- Sleep Pattern, Disturbed, related to frequently changing sleep/wake schedule
- Self-Esteem, Situational Low, related to crisis of friends making fun of adolescent related to situational crisis of friends making fun of adolescent
- Family Processes, Readiness for Enhanced, related to emerging maturity in patterns of communication

NANDA-I © 2012

Planning and Implementation

Whatever the setting, the nurse partners with the adolescent, the parents, teachers, and school counselors to plan appropriate goals and related interventions. Nurses work with individual adolescents in offices, schools, and other settings, and often work with groups of adolescents to perform teaching. Apply communication skills effective

TABLE 13–6	Injury Prevention Topics for Adolescents
TOPIC	**TEACHING**
Driving	Always wear seat and shoulder belts.
	Do not drink and drive or ride with others who do.
	Do not talk or text on a cell phone while you drive.
	Do not drive when you are tired.
	Drive with parents or other adults for several months in winter driving conditions if you live where there is snow, ice, or heavy rains.
	Keep cars in good repair.
Sun	Wear sunscreen.
	Limit time outside especially early in summer.
Machinery	Learn how to use power tools correctly.
	Always have someone near when you use tools or machinery.
	Wear ear and eye protection.
Emergency care	Learn first aid, CPR, and airway obstruction removal.
Water safety	Learn to swim well.
	If you supervise younger children near water, never leave them alone, even for a minute.
Fires	Do not play with fire.
	Follow guidelines to avoid igniting gasoline.
	Test smoke alarms in the house every 6 months and change batteries annually.
Firearms	Know and follow rules to keep firearms locked, with ammunition locked in a separate place.
	Never take out a gun to show a friend unless a parent is also present.
	Take firearm safety classes if you hunt or target shoot.
Hearing	Avoid loud music especially for long periods and through earphones.
Sports	Wear protective gear recommended for sports.
Abuse	Report any abuse to an adult you trust.
	Date with other couples when possible and report date rape.
	Do not drink or take drugs.

Source: *Adapted from Hagan, J. F., Shaw, J. S., & Duncan, P. M. (2008).* Bright futures: Guidelines for health supervision of infants, children, and adolescents *(3rd ed.). Elk Grove Village, IL: American Academy of Pediatrics.*

with teens (see Chapter 6 🔗) such as listening to concerns, allowing for discussion, and bringing peers with similar experiences together for discussion.

Healthy People 2020 recommends policies and programs to target major disruptions to adolescent health. Many interventions involve teaching, so it is wise to develop a number of resources for working with teens. Visit agencies in the community to gather appropriate materials. Teaching topics will be directed both at health promotion (providing information to enhance the adolescent's state of health) and at health maintenance (sharing tips about how to avoid disease and injury). A good starting point is to have the adolescent identify a personal health goal and begin teaching there.

Clinical Tip

Healthy People 2020 recognizes the importance of programs for graduated driver licensing; teen pregnancy, violence, and delinquency prevention; substance abuse treatment; mental health; and HIV prevention (U.S. Department of Health and Human Services, 2011). Identify the local rules and resources.

Clinical Judgment

Recall Kim from the chapter opener. She wants help in talking with her parents and information about birth control. How will you provide the information she requests and insert additional topics such as protection from sexually transmitted infections, immunization needs, and general health screening?

One challenge during health supervision for adolescents is including the right mix of teen and parent decision making and involvement. You will again apply communication skills by tactfully allowing time for both parent and adolescent to be seen alone. Realize that you are supporting and providing information for parents, such as useful discipline techniques, recognition of common parental feelings about teens, and the need for growing independence by their youth. When you provide teaching to groups of teens in schools, there may be policies about what needs to be sent home to parents. Some schools require that an outline of topics such as sexually transmitted infections or substance use be sent home for parents to read. Parents may call you with questions about content and approach, or some may choose to attend and sit in on the presentation. This obviously requires that you partner with the school administration, teachers, parents, and others to be effective in your presentation. Collaboration with many individuals and agencies is an important skill.

TABLE 13–7	Application of Ecology of Development to Assessment of Adolescent Populations*	
MICROSYSTEM	**EXOSYSTEM**	**MACROSYSTEM**
■ Incidence of adolescent injury for common problems like teen driving, boating, farm injury, firearms, drowning	■ School board policies related to sexuality teaching, HIV education, and other risks for teens	■ State grants for tobacco use prevention and cessation among youth
■ Neighborhood agencies that offer services to adolescents such as driver education, firearm training	■ Community agencies providing jobs and other services for youth	■ Insurance reimbursement for health promotion teaching
■ School curricula related to substance use and sexual behaviors	■ Availability of healthcare services that youth can access	■ Availability of results of Youth Risk Behavior Surveillance and other studies to local communities
■ Student and family behaviors related to nutrition and physical activity	■ Integration of health promotion and health maintenance into community services	
	■ Amount of involvement of adult volunteers and local businesses in area schools	

*See Chapter 5 🔗 for information about Bronfenbrenner's ecologic theory of development.

Whether you see adolescents in offices or other private settings, or in schools, correction facilities, or other places with groups present, leave information about how you or another nurse or care provider can be contacted. Provide brochures, referral numbers, names, and email addresses related to the topics discussed. Encourage annual health supervision visits and suggest a variety of places to obtain this care. For example, if a youth will soon graduate from high school, find out if he or she will be working or attending college and provide links to health insurance or care providers in the new location. Partner with other healthcare professionals to improve the environments of adolescents and help meet adolescents' health goals.

Evaluation

Inquire about the care received by teens and their families. They should feel comfortable with care providers and settings and believe that healthcare concerns are well addressed.

Some expected outcomes for care of adolescents and their families include:

- Normal growth patterns and maintenance of healthy weight are manifested.
- Physical activity of 30 to 60 minutes daily is reported.
- There is absence of debris and plaque on dental surfaces.
- The adolescent shows evidence of a positive self-concept.
- The adolescent achieves amount and pattern of sleep needed for mental and physical rejuvenation.
- Positive relationships are demonstrated with peers, family members, teachers, and others.
- The adolescent practices healthy lifestyle habits that promote disease and injury prevention.

Chapter Highlights

- Health promotion and maintenance of adolescents takes place in settings with individual youth as well as in facilities with groups of adolescents.
- Observations of youth and their parents provide valuable clues that assist the nurse in deciding which health issues need most attention during a given interaction.
- Growth measurement provides useful clues about the nutrition status of teenagers. Further nutritional assessment provides information about the teen's food choices, knowledge, and nutritional intake.
- Physical activity is important for youth, but large numbers do not get adequate amounts of exercise.

- The adolescent has many mental health challenges to meet in order to emerge with a positive self-concept and body image.
- Adolescents often have conflicts with parents as they grow to become more independent individuals. Parents must learn that family roles are changing during the teenage years.
- Peers form a primary source of companionship, self-worth, and influence for the adolescent.
- Since they are not seen often for health care, adolescents have needs for disease and injury prevention that must be met at any healthcare encounter.

Clinical Reasoning in Action

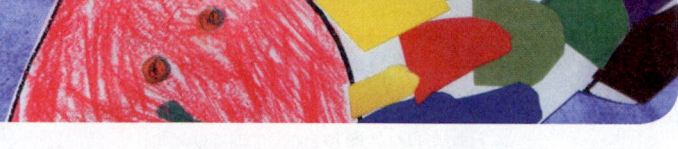

INTRODUCTION

Recall 16-year-old Kim who was described in the opening scenario. She has come to a health clinic for birth control. It is common to see adolescents for health care only when they come for a specific need. Nurses will maximize the opportunity by providing needed health care during this health encounter.

DESCRIPTION

When talking with Kim, you learn that she talks with her parents about most other health concerns and problems but does not feel comfortable talking about her sexual activity. She feels that they will be disappointed in her. She also thinks they do not approve of her boyfriend because he is 2 years older and has dropped out of high school. Kim's partner has been using a condom and will continue to do so; she wants birth control pills to be sure she avoids pregnancy. Her tests for sexually transmitted infections are all negative. Her hematocrit today is 30%.

DISCUSSION

1. What is Kim's psychosocial stage according to Piaget? Review these stages in Chapter 5 🖉 if necessary. How does her difficulty in telling her parents about her sexual activity relate to her development? How does it relate to her role in the family, and her parents' role? What suggestions might be helpful to enhance Kim's communication with her parents?
2. What protective factors do you identify in Kim's sexual behaviors?
3. What nursing diagnoses can you develop based on the history given in the scenario and the previous description?
4. Examine again the photograph in the opening scenario. How can the setting influence the receptivity of an adolescent to care? What do you see in this setting that would help to make the teen comfortable?
5. Plan the information that Kim needs about disease and injury prevention at her developmental stage. How can such information best be transmitted?
6. Kim is found to be anemic. What common dietary patterns of adolescents could contribute to this problem? What nutritional assessment will you perform? What interventions are appropriate?
7. List the immunizations that Kim might need. Which ones directly protect against a sexually transmitted infection?

NCLEX-RN® Review

1. When assessing an early adolescent's nutritional status, what should be included in the assessment?
   1. Anthropometric measurements, 24-hour dietary recall, and activity information
   2. Blood pressure screening, activity information, and lipid screening
   3. Lipid screening and screening for scoliosis
   4. Activity information, blood pressure screening, and lipid screening

2. A 16-year-old female complaining of abdominal pain is waiting in the exam room with her mother. It is important the nurse assess whether the girl is sexually active. What action should the nurse take to gather this information?
   1. Suggest to the mother that she can join her daughter after the exam to discuss findings and have questions answered.
   2. Let the physician ask the question, so the girl does not have to discuss her sexual history twice.
   3. Ask the girl if she is sexually active, as the mother needs to know and be involved with her daughter's care.
   4. Ask the mother to leave the room when sexual history questions will be asked to protect the girl's privacy.

3. The high school principal asks the school nurse to provide injury prevention information to the students. What does the nurse identify as a priority for the majority of students?
   1. Driving and substance abuse
   2. CPR and emergency care
   3. Sports injuries
   4. Driving patterns

4. Which statement best illustrates the concept of self-efficacy?
   1. "I will avoid smoking because I know it leads to cancer."
   2. "I am inspired by my aunt who recently stopped smoking."
   3. "I have the knowledge, support, and strength to achieve my goal to quit smoking."
   4. "I have heard that I should stop smoking but cannot imagine how to accomplish that."

See Appendix I 🔴 *for answers.*

References

Bandura, A. (1986). *Social foundations of thought and actions: A social cognitive theory*. Englewood Cliffs, NJ: Prentice Hall.

Bandura, A. (1995). *Self-efficacy in changing societies*. New York: Cambridge University.

Bandura, A. (1997). *Self-efficacy: The exercise of control*. New York: W. H. Freeman.

Bricker, J. B., Liu, J., Comstock, B. A., Peterson, A. V., Kealey, K. A., & Marek, P. M. (2010). Social cognitive mediators of adolescent smoking cessation: Results from a large randomized intervention trial. *Psychology of Addictive Behaviors, 24*(3), 436–445.

Carruth, A. K., Pryor, S., Cormier, C., Bateman, A., Matzke, B., & Gilmore, K. (2010). Evaluation of a school-based train-the-trainer intervention program to teach first aid and risk reduction among high school students. *Journal of School Health, 80*(9), 453–460.

Centers for Disease Control and Prevention. (2008). Youth Risk Behavior Surveillance—2007. *Morbidity and Mortality Weekly Report, 57*(SS-4), 1–136.

Centers for Disease Control and Prevention. (2010). *Policy impact—teen driver safety*. Retrieved from http://www.cdc.gov/motorvehiclesafety/teenbrief/

Centers for Disease Control and Prevention. (2011). *Agricultural safety*. Retrieved from http://www.cdc.gov/niosh/topics/aginjury/

Child Trends. (2010). *Unmet dental needs*. Retrieved from http://www.childtrendsdatabank.org/?q=node/282

Connor, J. P., George, S. M., Gullo, M. J., Kelly, A. B., & Young, R. M. (2011). A prospective study of alcohol expectancies and self-efficacy as predictors of young adolescent alcohol misuse. *Alcohol and Alcoholism, 46*(2), 161–169.

Eaton, D. K., Kann, L., Kinchen, S., Shanklin, S., Ross, J., Hawkins, J., . . . Wechsler, H. (2010). Youth Risk Behavior Surveillance—United States, 2009. *Morbidity and Mortality Weekly Report, 59*(SS-5), 1–146.

Erol, S., & Erdogan, S. (2008). Application of a stage based motivational interviewing approach to adolescent smoking cessation: The transtheoretical model-based study. *Patient Education and Counseling, 72*(1), 42–48.

Hagan, J. F., Shaw, J. S., & Duncan, P. M. (Eds.). (2008). *Bright futures: Guidelines for health supervision of infants, children, and adolescents* (3rd ed.). Elk Grove Village, IL: American Academy of Pediatrics.

Hortz, B., & Petosa, R. L. (2008). Social cognitive theory variables mediation of moderate exercise. *American Journal of Health Behavior, 32*, 305–314.

Mayo Clinic. (2009). *Teen sleep: Why is your teen so tired?* Retrieved from http://www.mayoclinic.com/health/teens-health

Murray, R. B., Zentner, J. P., & Yakimo, R. (2009). *Health promotion strategies through the life span* (8th ed.). Upper Saddle River, NJ: Prentice Hall Health.

National Assembly on School-Based Health Care. (2010). *School-based health centers play increasingly important role in children's health*. Retrieved from http://www.nasbhc.org

National Coalition for the Homeless. (2009). *Health care and homelessness*. Retrieved from http://nationalhomeless.org/factsheets/health.html

National Commission on Correctional Health Care. (2011). *Standards for health services in juvenile detention and confinement facilities*. Retrieved from http://www.ncchc.org

Pender, N., Murdaugh, C., & Parsons, M. A. (2011). *Health promotion in nursing practice* (6th ed.). Upper Saddle River, NJ: Pearson.

Smith, C., & Richards, R. (2008). Dietary intake, overweight status, and perceptions of food insecurity among homeless Minnesotan youth. *American Journal of Human Biology, 20*(5), 550–563.

Syamlal, G., & Mazurek, J. M. (2008). Prevalence of asthma among youth on Hispanic-operated farms in the United States. *Journal of Agromedicine, 13*(3), 155–160.

Tanski, S., Garfunkel, L. C., Duncan, P. M., & Weitzman, M. (2011). *Performing preventive services*. Elk Grove Village, IL: American Academy of Pediatrics.

U.S. Department of Health and Human Services. (2011). *Healthy People 2020*. Retrieved from http://www.healthypeople.gov/2020

Zaloshnja, E., Miller, T. R., & Lee, B. C. (2011). Incidence and cost of nonfatal farm injuries, United States, 2001–2006. *Journal of Agromedicine, 16*(1), 6–18.

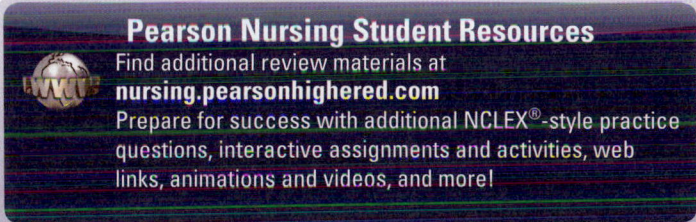

Pearson Nursing Student Resources

Find additional review materials at
nursing.pearsonhighered.com
Prepare for success with additional NCLEX®-style practice questions, interactive assignments and activities, web links, animations and videos, and more!

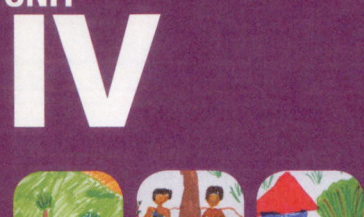

Child Healthcare Settings and Considerations

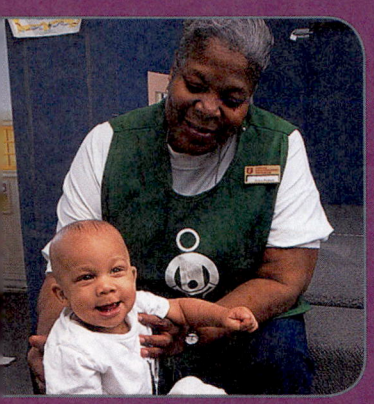
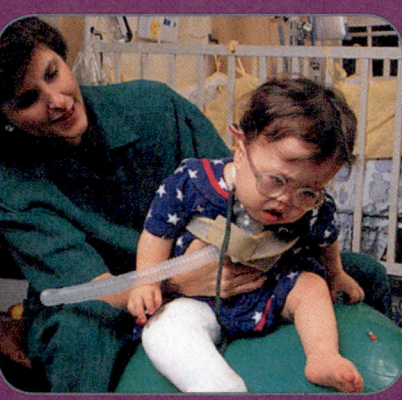
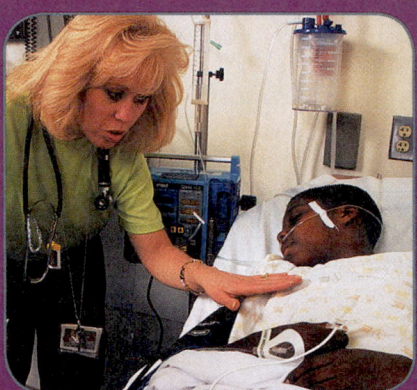
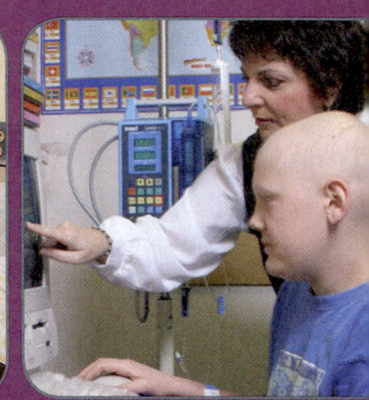

Because children receive the majority of their health care in community settings, pediatric nurses have an important role in promoting the child's health and partnering with families to plan care for the child with episodic or chronic health conditions. In many cases, pediatric nurses develop long-term relationships with the children and families who return for continued care in a particular healthcare setting, such as a health center, physician's office, or school. When working with the hospitalized child and family, pediatric nurses additionally develop individualized nursing care plans that promote coping strategies to deal with the stressors of hospitalization and support the child's optimal growth and development. Pediatric nurses also have an important role in care and support for the child and family when the child has a life-threatening illness or injury or a terminal condition.

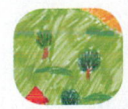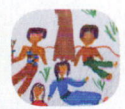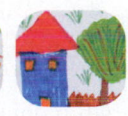

Nursing Care of the Child in the Community

CHAPTER

14

KEY TERMS

Learning Outcomes

After completing this chapter, you will be able to:

1. Discuss the types of community healthcare settings where nurses provide health services to children.

2. Compare the roles of the nurse in each identified community healthcare setting.

3. Plan a family-centered assessment for the child and family in a community setting.

4. Develop a nursing care plan that promotes the health of the child in the community.

5. Summarize the potential roles of the pediatric nurse or school nurse in supporting a community assessment process.

6. Examine the special needs of children that should be considered in disaster preparedness.

> "The baby sure takes a lot of Mom's time. If she cries someone has to figure out what she needs. I try to help by playing with her sometimes, but I am in school most of the day."
>
> —*Nathan, age 7*

Four-month-old Torrey Lowell has been brought by her parents and 7-year-old brother Nathan to the health center for her checkup and next immunizations. Several pediatricians provide care to children in the health center, and nurse practitioners and registered nurses have an active role in providing health promotion services. Torrey's parents have selected a primary care provider in the center for their children's ongoing healthcare services.

Torrey is a healthy baby who is growing at an appropriate rate, and she has not yet had any illnesses. Her parents have experienced much pleasure over the past 4 months watching her grow and gain new developmental skills. The pediatrician talked with the parents and assessed Torrey, and now the nurse is giving her immunizations and providing additional guidance regarding Torrey's next stages of growth and development. The focus of the nurse's discussion is nutrition, the next developmental skills that will emerge, methods to promote Torrey's development, and how the family and Nathan have adapted to the baby in the family. Torrey's mother plans to return to work in the next month, so an important discussion involves selecting a childcare provider and what to observe and ask about when visiting potential childcare centers. Because the hurricane season is beginning, the nurse also reminds the parents of supplies to have on hand in case a disaster is declared.

What is the role of the nurse in community health settings? What information should be shared with parents about selecting a childcare center or any special care needed for a child in the school setting? What information should the nurse share with the parents regarding family preparedness for a natural disaster and the additional supplies needed for an infant?

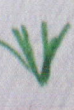

COMMUNITY-BASED HEALTH CARE

The majority of pediatric health care occurs in community settings, as most children are healthy and need health promotion, health maintenance, and episodic acute care. Every child should have a healthcare home or medical home (see Chapter 8 🔗). The healthcare providers in the healthcare home or medical home assume responsibility for coordinating the health care needed by the child. In some cases the primary care provider is a school nurse, community health nurse, or nurse practitioner working alone or in partnership with a physician. In other cases, the nurse collaborates with the physician or other healthcare providers in provision of care.

Health care for children has been rapidly shifting from the hospital to the community setting over the past 15 years. Health plans and healthcare providers continue to explore options to provide safe, high-quality care with fewer hospitalizations or shorter stays when hospitalization is needed. Patterns of healthcare delivery are changing due to technology developments and efforts to reduce healthcare costs, as these examples illustrate:

- Day surgery and invasive diagnostic procedures can be performed in outpatient surgical settings.
- Full-term newborns are usually discharged after 24 to 48 hours.
- Short-stay units associated with emergency departments have reduced the number of hospital admissions.
- Long-term intravenous antibiotics can be provided in the home with the support of home care nursing services.
- Pediatric hospice and palliative care is offered in the home setting more frequently as services specific to children and their families have emerged.

The trend in out-of-hospital care is particularly seen among children with chronic health conditions and advanced disease states. Families are often willing to care for their child who is **medically fragile** (having significant health conditions that require skilled nursing, with or without medical equipment, to support vital functions) in the home because of their desire to have the child integrated into the family and community. Technologic advances, such as portable medical equipment, now make it possible to provide complex healthcare services in the home and other community settings. The healthcare system has supported the family preferences because care in the community is less costly. Home care services and other support services have been developed to support these families.

Characteristics of Community-Based Health Care

Pediatric health care in the community occurs along a continuum that covers the entire child healthcare system. This continuum is reflected in the Bindler-Ball Continuum of Pediatric Health including health promotion and health maintenance services; care for chronic conditions, acute illnesses, and injuries; and end-of-life care (see Chapter 1 🔗). Depending upon the community, its healthcare resources, and the age of the child, this care may be provided in a variety of settings, some of which offer a limited or extensive range of services.

- A healthcare center or a physician's office is often the site of a child's healthcare home (medical home) where the full range of health services are provided, including health promotion, health maintenance, episodic acute care, and health maintenance care for children with chronic conditions. See Chapters 9 through 13 🔗 for age-specific health promotion and health maintenance guidelines. Many children have a chronic health condition that needs ongoing nursing and medical management that is also often offered in these settings.
- A public health clinic may provide only health promotion and health maintenance services. A homeless shelter may also have the capacity to offer such services.
- A hospital outpatient center may provide specialized services to children with chronic conditions or a full range of services similar to a health center.
- Schools usually provide health promotion and health maintenance services at a minimum, plus first aid and emergency care as needed. School-based health centers may additionally provide counseling, health education, and care for acute conditions. Some school settings offer other services, such as preschool and after-school childcare services.
- Childcare centers provide first aid for emergencies and some health promotion services.
- Camp settings, particularly for children with specific health conditions, offer health promotion and education to promote self-care of the chronic condition.
- The home is a site for acute care of minor conditions and for chronic condition management, rehabilitation, and end-of-life care. Children with acute illnesses and complex health conditions, including those with advanced disease states assisted by technology, can be cared for at home when their families are supported by home health services.

Other settings for community-based pediatric health care include:

- **Community events**—Many health education and injury prevention activities occur in the community, sponsored by hospitals, voluntary organizations, and the health department. Bike rodeos, for example, teach children about the need for bicycle helmets and bicycle riding safety. Health fairs offer opportunities to demonstrate correct car safety seat installation.
- **Urgent care centers, walk-in clinics, and emergency departments**—Care for acute illnesses and injuries is provided in these settings when other sources of acute health care are closed or unavailable.
- **Emergency medical services (EMS) system**—Children with a serious injury or illness may need to receive immediate care and transport to the hospital emergency department.
- **Disaster shelters**—Children and their families need food and safe shelter, health promotion, and occasionally acute care services within the community during a natural or man-made disaster. Children dependent on medical technology will need access to shelters with power and healthcare providers.
- **Respite facilities**—Families with a child who has a special healthcare need (disability or chronic illness) often need **respite care,** a family support service that provides periodic breaks from the constant stress of caring for the child (see Legal & Ethical Considerations: Children's Disabilities Temporary Care Reauthorization Act). Respite care, matched to the family's and child's specific needs, can be provided in the home or in out-of-home respite facilities. For example, a crisis nursery allows the family of an infant with special healthcare needs to have a break from providing constant care, and offers counseling and linkage with other community services. Other respite services may be provided in a childcare or after-school program. The goal is to support families so the child can remain in the home. See Chapter 16 🔗.

Legal and Ethical Considerations
Children's Disabilities Temporary Care Reauthorization Act

The Children's Disabilities Temporary Care Reauthorization Act (PL 101-127) authorizes federal funding to the states to develop and implement affordable respite care services and crisis nurseries. Families may be charged a fee for the respite services.

ROLES OF NURSES IN COMMUNITY SETTINGS

An individual child may receive care in all the above settings, or only a few. The nurse in any of these settings has an important role in promoting the health and safety of the child, being a leader in setting policies in the center, as well as using the five steps of the nursing process (as defined in Chapter 1 🔗) to help families meet the healthcare needs of their children.

Health care for individual children is improved when there is continuity of care and communication between settings in this continuum, such as between a health center and the child's school. The pediatric nurse working with families in a community setting is more successful when using knowledge of how the larger environment influences the child's health and development and the family's activities. (See Chapter 20 🔗.) That knowledge needs to be integrated into the nursing care plan.

Nurses act in a variety of positions within these settings, from pediatric nurse in an office setting to school nurse to home health nurse. The nurse may assume the role of direct care provider, educator, advocate, or planner in any of these positions. To work effectively in the community, the nurse needs to gain experience and skills in the following areas:

1. Partnering with families to conduct a child and family assessment and to plan individualized healthcare strategies, as well as implementing and evaluating nursing care strategies to match the family's economic, cultural, and social situation, and available resources
2. Assisting community agencies or voluntary organizations (e.g., schools, churches, and Safe Kids coalitions) to conduct a community assessment and then to plan, implement, and evaluate approaches addressing the healthcare needs of the community's children

Role of the Pediatric Nurse in an Office or Health Center Setting

Nurses use the nursing process when providing care for children in the primary care setting. The range of assessment responsibilities may vary by setting, as well as the preparation and experience of the nurse (Figure 14–1 ■). Specific functions of the pediatric nurse in primary care include the following:

- Collecting health history data
- Performing nursing assessments including vital signs, growth and development, nutritional status, immunization status, and family strengths and challenges
- Conducting physical examinations
- Performing age-appropriate screening tests to detect health problems such as vision or hearing loss, anemia, and lead

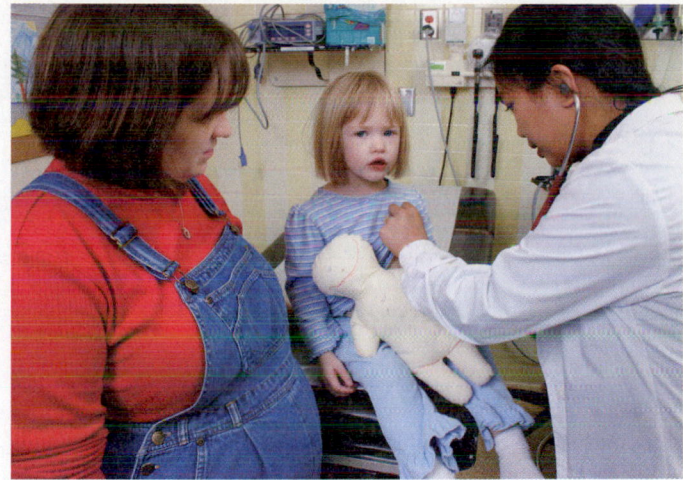

FIGURE 14–1 ■ Nurses carefully assess children in the office setting who present with an acute care illness. It is important to identify how serious the child's illness is and to monitor the child for progression of symptoms during the visit. This is also a time to gather information about the child's illness and to identify health information that will be needed for the family to care for the child at home.

poisoning to ensure that the child has access to all needed health services (see Chapters 9 to 13 🔗)
- Developing nursing diagnoses and implementing a plan of care
- Assisting with health examinations and performing diagnostic tests
- Providing immunizations
- Providing information about procedures and offering reassurance
- Providing patient education for health promotion or management of the health condition
- Linking families with community resources
- Ensuring a safe environment and that infection control guidelines are followed
- Participating in the health center's performance improvement program to identify ways to enhance services provided to children and their families

An important goal for nurses in the office or healthcare setting is to develop a positive partnership with the child and family so that optimal health care is provided. The relationship with the family grows over the months and years of providing care to the child and family. (See Partnering with Families: The First Interaction.)

Identifying Severely Ill and Injured Children

Children with serious illnesses often present at a health center or physician office and require emergency care. Children with episodic illnesses and injuries must be assessed on arrival to determine the urgency of care that will be needed. A rapid assessment for changes in mental status, airway patency, breathing, and circulation is used to identify the child who needs immediate medical attention (see Appendix F 🔗). The child with an urgent condition must be monitored frequently to detect any worsening of the condition and need for emergency care.

The nurse collaborates with the physician and office manager to develop an emergency response plan for the health setting. The nurse is often responsible for teaching the office receptionist to identify a child who needs immediate assessment by the nurse (e.g., extremely labored breathing, cyanosis, wheezing or stridor, seizure, altered

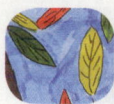

Partnering with Families

The First Interaction

Developing a relationship with the child and family in a community setting is equally as important as in the hospital. In many cases, the initial interaction sets the stage for the long-term relationship with the family that returns to the healthcare environment over many years. Remember to put aside the stressors you may be feeling before you approach the child and family. Take a few moments to play with the infant or child and to comment on a positive attribute of the child to the parents. The parents', and perhaps the child's, stress level will also be reduced. This helps set the stage for a long-term partnership with the child and family.

---

consciousness, vomiting after a head injury, uncontrolled bleeding, or parent agitation) (American Academy of Pediatrics Committee on Pediatric Emergency Medicine, 2007). The nurse should also frequently scan the waiting room for the child with a serious illness needing rapid care. The nurse often assumes a leadership role in promoting basic life support training of office personnel and in coordinating mock drills with all staff in the healthcare setting so that all employees know and perform their designated role when a true emergency occurs. Developing a relationship with the local emergency medical services agency is also important in preparation for the child with a true emergency needing ambulance transport to the hospital.

Practice Alert

Nurses have an important role in ensuring that a health center is prepared to manage a child with an emergency. The steps that should be taken to prepare for a patient emergency include the following:

- Review the most common types of pediatric emergencies that have occurred in the office and how often they have occurred. Determine how close the office is to an emergency department. Determine how long the response time is by the local emergency rescue squad (American Academy of Pediatrics Committee on Pediatric Emergency Medicine, 2007).

- Take responsibility for ordering resuscitation equipment and medications (Box 14–1). Check and restock expired and used supplies and medications at least weekly or after each emergency and record this activity on a log.

- Collaborate with the physician to develop guidelines for **triage** (the rapid assessment to sort patients by the urgency of their condition) and standing orders for management of common pediatric emergencies, such as respiratory distress or anaphylaxis.

- Collaborate with the physician and office manager to plan a role for all staff members in responding to the emergency. Ensure that each staff member knows the location of emergency equipment. Coordinate mock drills to practice the emergency response.

- Post on all appropriate phones the number for calling the local emergency medical services to transport the child to the emergency department.

- Post the poison control number on all phones.

Telephone Advice

Some nurses in the office or healthcare setting perform **telephone triage,** talking with a family member by telephone to address concerns about the child, analyze the child's symptoms, and determine if or how quickly the child needs to be seen by the healthcare provider (Box 14–2). Nurses performing telephone triage and providing telephone advice to parents and caregivers need extensive knowledge of pediatrics and excellent skills in teaching and communicating with the caller. They must be good listeners and able to interpret the information given by the parent to identify the most appropriate information to provide or action to take. Nurses use protocols or published

BOX 14–1	Emergency Equipment in an Office Setting

Essential equipment for managing an emergency in an office setting includes the following in various pediatric sizes as appropriate (American Academy of Pediatrics Committee on Pediatric Emergency Medicine, 2007):

- Oxygen delivery system, including bag-valve masks in 450- and 1000-mL sizes, clear oxygen masks (both breather and nonrebreather masks with a reservoir)

- Airway management equipment, including oral and nasopharyngeal airways, suction devices, laryngoscope handle and blades, endotracheal tubes and stylet, end-tidal CO_2 detector, nasogastric tubes

- Pulse oximeter, peak flow meter, a nebulizer or metered dose inhaler with a spacer/mask

- Intravenous and intraosseous needles, intravenous tubing, and IV solution such as normal saline or lactated Ringer's

- A length-based resuscitation tape or preprinted drug dosage chart needed to quickly identify equipment sizes and drug dosages for the child's weight

- Drugs (epinephrine 1:1000, albuterol for inhalation, racemic epinephrine, activated charcoal, naloxone, 25% dextrose, atropine, dexamethasone, lorazepam, lidocaine, and many others for specific emergencies) (Hegenbarth & the Committee on Drugs, 2010).

Locate the emergency equipment in every clinical setting where you have assignments so you can quickly take the child to it or bring the equipment to the site of an emergency if needed.

---

manuals approved by the health facility to guide the questions to ask about the child's condition and advice to give parents. The call information is then documented in the child's medical record. Telephone advice nursing has become a specialty practice with established competencies and a national certification exam.

Educating the Child and Family

An important nursing role in the healthcare or medical home is to provide patient education regarding injury prevention, growth and development, nutrition, healthy lifestyles, and the home care of episodic illnesses and injuries. The nurse may be responsible for selecting patient education materials that are provided in the waiting area and those specifically used for management of various conditions. Knowledge of community health problems and of the characteristics of the pediatric population served enables the nurse to select culturally and linguistically appropriate education materials.

Nurses teach families to provide the condition-specific care for the child at home, and they assess the need for repeated or additional education (Figure 14–2 ■). This information may include:

- Signs that the condition is not improving as expected, and when to return to the physician

| BOX 14–2 | Telephone Triage Principles |

Parents and caregivers placing telephone calls to the healthcare provider need assistance with determining the extent of the child's illness or injury, the urgency of a needed visit with the healthcare provider, and ideas for home care management. Before any advice can be given, the nurse must collect the following essential health information about the child and ensure that it gets recorded:

- Child's name, age, significant past medical history (chronic conditions, allergies, medications, treatments, recent immunizations)
- Reason for the call—chief complaint
- Present illness or injury—symptoms, duration, severity, pain, appetite, fever
- Review of systems related to the present illness

Once the information is collected and analyzed, the nurse may consult with the physician or follow specific written guidelines for telephone advice that matches the child's condition. Parents will be directed to call 911 or the local emergency phone number if an emergency condition exists. An appointment may be made to see the healthcare provider, or guidelines for care at home are provided. Parents are routinely provided with information about signs of a worsening condition or when to call back if signs have not improved.

- How and when to administer prescribed medications and their potential side effects
- Modification to diet and activity
- Other supportive care for the child's condition (e.g., ice or heat on an injury, wound care)
- Education to help the child and family recognize the need to initiate care for a new episode of a chronic condition (e.g., asthma, sickle cell anemia, or hemophilia) that may prevent the need for a healthcare visit or reduce the severity of the episode

Identifying Community Resources

Nurses in the healthcare home are often involved in identifying community resources that are needed by the child and family to help promote the child's health. Because of the range of issues that can present in the healthcare setting, the nurse's knowledge of health-related resources in the community is important. Compiling a manual of community resources and regularly updating names and phone numbers of contacts will make it easier to provide information

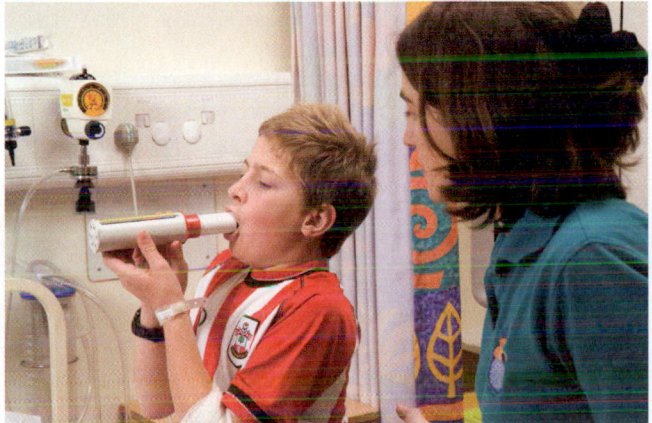

FIGURE 14–2 ■ Nurses provide patient education to help families learn to recognize the early stages of an asthma episode by using a peak flow meter. The child learns the proper method for taking a deep breath and blowing into the peak flow meter so the best reading is obtained.

Source: Copyright 2012 Science Photo Library-Custom Medical Stock Photo, All Rights Reserved.

efficiently. For example, knowledge of how to access the community's early intervention programs for infants and toddlers ensures that families of children with developmental disabilities have educational services under the Individuals with Disabilities Education Improvement Act of 2004 (PL 108-446). Other community resources that might be included are support groups, language and translation services, food banks, lead paint abatement services, social services, and mental health services.

The nurse may also be responsible for coordinating referrals for diagnostic or therapeutic services such as physical therapy, nutritionist consultation, or diagnostic testing. Because the child usually returns to the primary care provider after the consultant visit, the nurse may have the opportunity to review the consultant's recommendation with the family and ensure that the family understands the results of diagnostic testing or recommended care. Reinforcing care recommendations may well improve the family's adherence to them and the child's outcome.

Ensuring a Safe Environment for Children

Another responsibility of the nurse in the healthcare setting is to ensure a safe environment for the child. The healthcare center and office settings have many potential hazards such as equipment, cleaning supplies, sharps, medications, and laboratory chemicals and supplies from which the child needs to be protected. The child must be attended at all times when in the examination area. Guidelines for infection control must be developed and implemented to reduce the transmission of infectious diseases between child patients and between the healthcare providers and children.

Role of the Pediatric Nurse in a Hospital Outpatient Setting

Pediatric nurses provide care for children with acute and chronic conditions within hospital outpatient or ambulatory settings. With experience, pediatric nurses working in a hospital ambulatory setting develop specialized knowledge and skills to meet the specific needs of the population of children they care for in that setting. Many hospital-supported clinics provide health promotion, health maintenance, and episodic illness care, and the roles for nurses are similar to those described for office and health center settings.

Specialty Care Ambulatory Clinics

Many children are referred to pediatric specialists based in specialty care ambulatory clinics for diagnostic workups and the long-term management of their chronic conditions. Nurses in these settings often collect health history data and perform nursing assessments that include vital signs, growth and development, nutritional status, immunization status, and family strengths and challenges. Advanced practice nurses and nurse practitioners assume a larger role in patient assessment, implementing a care plan for the health condition, educating the child and family to manage the condition at home, and linking the child and family with community resources. For example, diabetes nurse educators teach parents and children with newly diagnosed diabetes how to manage their disease. See Figure 14–3 ■ . See Chapter 25 for the Nursing Care Plan for the child with asthma in the community setting. Some advanced practice nurses work as case managers of children with specific health conditions such as spina bifida, promoting coordination of care between all providers (including primary care), helping families get appropriately linked to community resources, and educating them about treatment options.

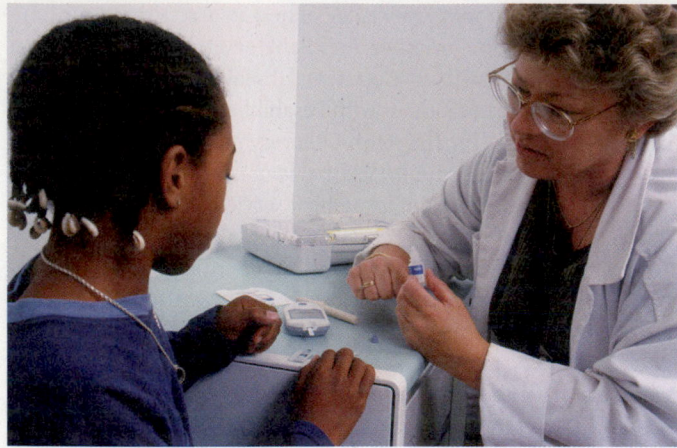

FIGURE 14–3 ■ Nurses often assume a larger role in working with children and families with a chronic health condition in the hospital ambulatory setting. Developing a care plan and educating the family to manage type 1 diabetes is an important role of this pediatric nurse, who is also a certified diabetes educator.

Urgent Care or Emergency Department Settings

Children with acute illnesses may be seen by nurses in the emergency department or in an urgent care setting. Nurses working in an emergency department or urgent care setting need advanced skills in assessment to identify subtle changes in physiologic status while these children receive treatment during the emergency department visit or in a short-stay observation unit. Some of the nurses most experienced in care of children perform the initial triage assessment to identify those children most seriously ill and injured needing immediate care. Other important roles of nurses in emergency departments and urgent care settings include:

- Keeping the emergency department or urgent care center resuscitation area in a state of readiness for care of children with life-threatening emergencies
- Frequently monitoring each child's health status and ensuring the child's safety during the visit
- Assisting with diagnostic procedures
- Collaborating with various health professionals providing treatments, such as respiratory therapists providing nebulizer treatments to children with asthma
- Educating the child and family about the diagnostic procedures and emergency department treatments implemented
- Providing emotional support because children and families are usually stressed by the urgency of the child's condition (see Chapter 17 🔗)
- Identifying and coordinating the child's need for follow-up health care and treatment for the emergent condition

Role of the Nurse in a School Setting

School nursing is a specialized practice of professional nursing in the education setting that advances the well-being, academic success, and lifelong achievement of students. School nurses address a wide range of physical and mental health challenges among the students. They advocate for the children by becoming active in policies developed that affect the school community. They are proactive in health promotion and health maintenance

and serve as a safety net for children (Robert Wood Johnson Foundation, 2010).

Many societal changes have expanded the need for more health services in the school setting, and new morbidities, such as obesity, have expanded opportunities for school nurses to engage in health promotion. Parents who are employed may depend on the school nurse to provide initial health assessments to determine if a healthcare visit (and time away from work) is really needed. An estimated 50 million children and adolescents attend public schools in the United States, and 15% have one or more known medical conditions (Lear, Barnwell, & Behrens, 2008). The Individuals with Disabilities Education Act (PL 94-142) entitles all children with developmental, physical, psychosocial, and behavioral conditions to an education (see Chapter 16 🔗). As a result many children dependent on medical technology, such as peritoneal dialysis, tracheostomies, and ventilators, need nursing and other healthcare services in the school setting (Raymond, 2009). Other children have special healthcare needs such as medication administration for their chronic health conditions (e.g., asthma, diabetes, and seizures). The breadth of school health issues addressed by school nurses is illustrated in national health objectives published in *Healthy People 2020* (Box 14–3).

BOX 14–3	*Healthy People 2020* Objectives That Relate to School Health Issues

- Increase the proportion of elementary, middle, and senior high schools that provide comprehensive school health education to prevent health problems in the following areas: unintentional injury; violence; suicide; tobacco use and addiction; alcohol or other drug use; unintended pregnancy, HIV/AIDS, and STD infection; unhealthy dietary patterns; and inadequate physical activity.
- Increase the proportion of elementary, middle, and senior high schools that have a nurse-to-student ratio of at least 1:750.
- Increase the proportion of elementary, middle, and senior high schools that have health education goals or objectives that address the knowledge and skills articulated in the National Health Education Standards (high school, middle, elementary).
- Increase the proportion of public and private schools that require students to wear appropriate protective gear when engaged in school-sponsored physical activities.
- Reduce weapon carrying by adolescents on school property.
- Increase the percentage of schools with a school breakfast program.
- Increase the percentage of schools that offer nutritious foods and beverages outside of school meals.
- Increase the proportion of school-based health centers with an oral health component.
- Increase the proportion of states and school districts that require regularly scheduled elementary school recess.
- Increase the proportion of public and private schools that require daily physical education for all students.
- Increase the proportion of adolescents who spend at least 50% of school physical education class time being physically active.
- Increase the proportion of children and youth with disabilities who spend at least 80% of their time in regular education programs.

Source: *Data from U.S. Department of Health and Human Services, Office of Disease Prevention and Health Promotion. (2010). Healthy People. Washington, DC: Author. Retrieved from http://www.healthypeople.gov/Default.htm*

Weblink | National Association of School Nurses

The school nurse practices independently as the only licensed healthcare provider in the setting. The National Association of School Nurses and many other national organizations, including *Healthy People 2020*, recommend a ratio of nurse to students in the general school population of 1 to 750, and only 45.1% of all schools are staffed at this ratio (Maughan, 2009a). Schools with fewer students per nurse often have an increased number of children with complex medical conditions in the school (Maughan, 2009b). Depending on the school system, some school nurses may be responsible for providing health promotion and health supervision to children in one or several schools. In a few states they serve more than 3,000 to 5,000 children (Maughan, 2009a). Health aides or licensed practical nurses (LPNs) may be present in the school setting and need training and supervision by the school nurse. Healthcare needs of faculty and staff are also addressed. Many school nurses have obtained certification or advanced education to become a school nurse practitioner, enabling them to better manage this independent practice.

The role of school nurses has changed over the past decade as the population of children attending school has changed. School nurses work to remove or minimize the health barriers to learning so students can perform academically (Figure 14–4A and B ▪). School nurses are also in a position to refer families to community resources to support their children's development and health (see Legal & Ethical Considerations: Child Nutrition Reauthorization Act). Approximately 4% to 6% of children are administered daily medication at school (Clay, Farris, McCarthy, et al., 2008). Even though the school administrator, secretary, or health aide may give the medications in the absence of a school nurse, the nurse is responsible for training and ensuring competence of the person delegated to give medications and for establishing safe medication storage, administration, and record-keeping guidelines (Resha, 2010). See Box 14-4 and A Day in the Life of a School Nurse.

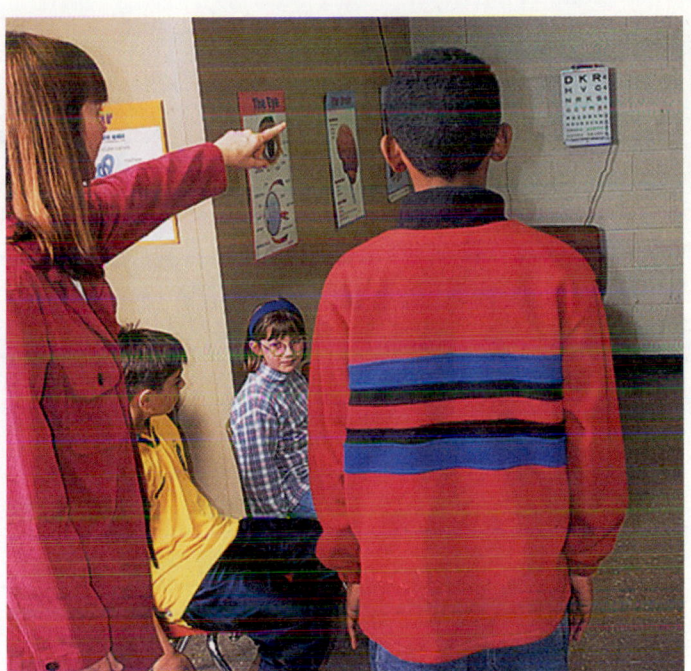

A

B

FIGURE 14–4 ▪ *A,* The school is often the setting for screening tests of large groups of students at risk for a problem. Screening tests are often organized so all children in a particular grade are assessed, as in this test to detect vision problems. State laws mandate grades for screening and selected children who must be screened for conditions such as visual or hearing problems, and scoliosis screening in public schools. *B,* The school nurse treats this child with a nebulizer to determine if the asthma episode can be controlled before calling the parent to come and pick up the child and seek care from the primary care provider. The parent should be informed of nebulizer treatment provided in case the child's asthma episode continues and additional treatment is needed.

BOX 14–4	Roles of a School Nurse

- Provides direct care to children with acute illnesses and injuries, providing first aid and handling life-threatening allergy and asthma events
- Screens students for conditions that impair learning, such as poor vision and hearing, and refers them for further evaluation
- Promotes a healthy school environment by ensuring immunization compliance, monitoring playground equipment safety, promoting infection control, and implementing programs for bullying and violence prevention
- Educates students about healthy lifestyles, good nutrition, exercise, oral health, smoking cessation, sexually transmitted infections, and pregnancy prevention
- Manages students with chronic conditions, administers medications, and participates in the development of individualized health plans (IHPs) and individualized education plans (IEPs) for those with disabilities
- Refers students' families to healthcare providers and insurance programs and connects students with needed services (e.g., for substance abuse treatment, behavioral and mental health, and reproductive health)
- Serves as a leader in the preparation of policies for school-wide emergencies, school health programs, mental health intervention, and student and faculty health emergencies
- Identifies and reports clusters of symptoms that may indicate an epidemic

Source: *Data from American Academy of Pediatrics Council on School Health. (2008). Role of the school nurse in providing school health services. Pediatrics, 121(5), 1052–1056; Robert Wood Johnson Foundation. (2010). Unlocking the potential of school nursing: Keeping children healthy, in school, and ready to learn. Retrieved from http://www.rwjf.org/files/research/cnf14.pdf*

Legal and Ethical Considerations
Child Nutrition Reauthorization Act

The Child Nutrition Reauthorization Act of 2010, titled the Healthy, Hunger-Free Kids Act of 2010, continues the federal school meal programs (breakfast, lunch, after-school snack, and summer food service) for low-income children and increases access to nutritional foods. The program also has goals for nutrition education and physical activity in an effort to address childhood obesity. School nurses may work with food service personnel in the nutrition programs for healthy eating and in creating a nutrition education program for students (Sherry, 2008). See Chapter 19 🔴.

A DAY IN THE LIFE
of a School Nurse

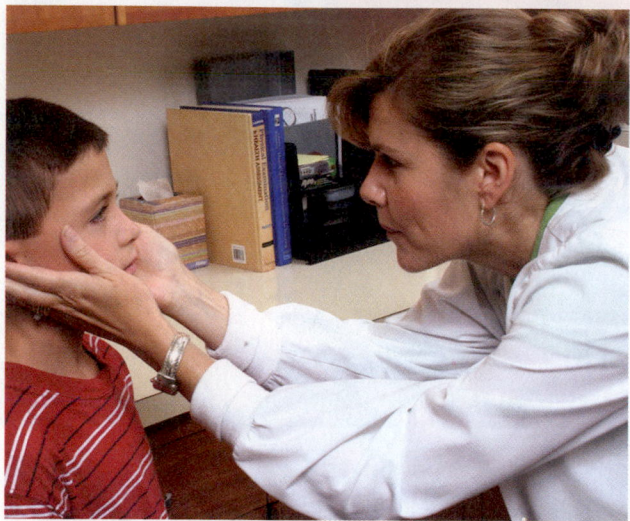
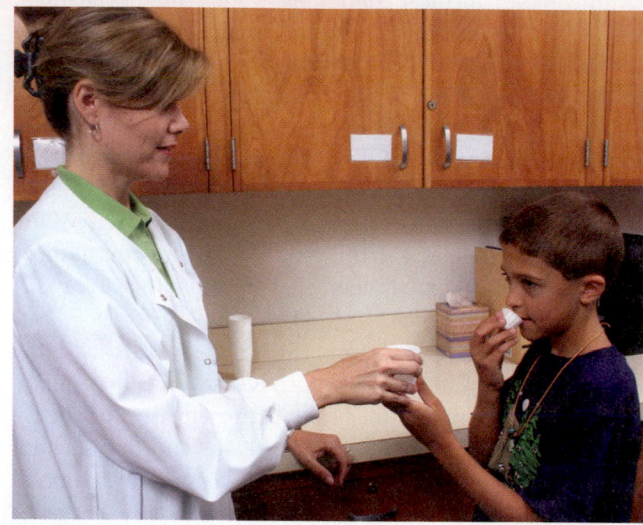

Left. Johnny's teacher sent him to the school nurse because he complained about a sore throat. Ellen performs an assessment to determine if his parents should be called to take him home or to his healthcare provider. **Right.** Kevin gets medication each day at lunchtime for attention deficit hyperactivity disorder. The timing of the medication is important to improve his concentration and learning during the afternoon.

The school nurse is the only health professional in the school environment. Thus Ellen Gorges has very broad responsibilities for maintaining the health of all the children attending the school (and in some cases multiple schools). Because all children are entitled to an education by federal law, Ellen may provide care to children who are healthy and to those who have health conditions. Many children with special healthcare needs and chronic conditions attend school regularly, as well as children who are recovering from acute illness and injury episodes.

Activities that Ellen often performs include the following:

- Assessing student health complaints
- Providing emergency care and first aid to students and faculty
- Administering medications
- Ensuring immunization compliance
- Screening students for health conditions
- Educating faculty and health aides to recognize illnesses or health problems among students in the classroom and to provide needed health care as appropriate for a child with special healthcare needs
- Documenting health care provided to students
- Participating in development of student individualized health plans and health-related accommodations needed for learning
- Ensuring a safe environment for students and faculty
- Serving as a student advocate

Ellen Gorges has very broad responsibilities for maintaining the health of all the children attending the school.

Ellen also gives attention to the health of the school faculty, by assessing and counseling them about their health needs.

Because the scope of school nursing is so broad, it has become a specialty within pediatric nursing, often requiring additional education and certification as a school nurse or school nurse practitioner.

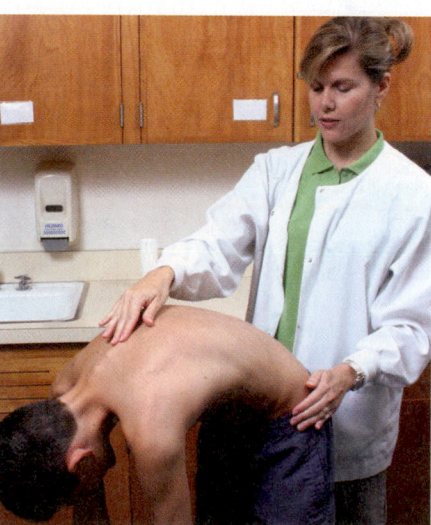

The school nurse performs scoliosis screening of all students in the fifth grade to enable early identification of the condition and referral as necessary to a student's healthcare provider.

Health and Safety Guidelines for Schools

Weblink

BOX 14–5   Standards of Professional School Nursing Practice

1. The school nurse collects comprehensive data pertinent to the healthcare consumer's health and/or the situation.

2. The school nurse analyzes the assessment data to determine the diagnoses or issues.

3. The school nurse identifies expected outcomes for a plan individualized to the healthcare consumer or the situation.

4. The school nurse develops a plan that prescribes strategies and alternatives to attain expected outcomes.

5. The school nurse implements the identified plan by coordinating care delivery; using strategies to promote a healthy and safe environment, especially regarding health education; and providing consultation to influence the identified plan, enhance the abilities of others, and effect change.

6. The school nurse evaluates progress toward attainment of outcomes.

7. The school nurse practices ethically.

8. The school nurse attains knowledge and competency that reflect current nursing practice.

9. The school nurse integrates evidence and research findings into practice.

10. The school nurse contributes to quality nursing practice.

11. The school nurse communicates effectively in a variety of formats in all areas of nursing practice.

12. The school nurse demonstrates leadership in the professional practice setting and the profession.

13. The school nurse collaborates with the healthcare consumer, family, and others in conduct of nursing practice.

14. The school nurse evaluates one's own nursing practice in relation to professional practice standards and guidelines, relevant statutes, rules, and regulations.

15. The school nurse utilizes appropriate resources to plan and provide nursing services that are safe, effective, and financially responsible.

16. The school nurse practices in an environmentally safe and healthy manner.

17. The school nurse manages school health services.

Source: *Reprinted with permission from American Nurses Association and National Association of School Nurses, School Nursing: Scope and Standards of Practice (2nd ed., pp. 12–14),* ©2011 Nursebooks.org, Silver Spring, MD.

Pediatric nurses interested in school nursing usually have a strong interest in community health and seek continuing education to learn more about nursing in a school environment. See Box 14–5 for the standards of professional school nursing.

Community Health Focus

The school nurse also plans, develops, manages, and evaluates healthcare services to all children in the educational setting. In many cases, the nurse works with families of the students to ensure that needed care is provided. Collaboration with other health professionals in the community is becoming increasingly important to promote health in the school setting, as the following examples illustrate:

- Partnering with the physician consultant to discuss and update standing orders for the care of children. These standing orders usually address urgent and emergency care potentially needed by students as well as the variety of healthcare problems present in the population of students.

- Working with the parent-teacher association and other community organizations to organize health fairs and injury prevention programs for students.

- Communicating with the primary healthcare provider or with the pediatric specialist about children with specific health conditions that need to be effectively managed in the school setting. See Evidence-Based Practice: Improving Asthma Management at School. It is essential to have the parent's permission and follow confidentiality requirements. Because the school nurse has regular opportunities to monitor the health status of these children, the information shared helps primary healthcare providers with their ongoing management.

School-Based Health Centers

Approximately 1,500 school-based health centers exist in 44 states (Schlitt, Juszczak, & Eichner, 2008). These are often individually incorporated health centers funded by multiple sources and not formally part of the district's education system. Comprehensive physical, dental, reproductive, and mental health services plus health education are often provided by a multidisciplinary team of nurse practitioners, physicians, physician assistants, mental health providers, and other supporting staff. The availability of school-based health centers increases the access of children and adolescents who have difficulty obtaining health care, such as those who are uninsured or underinsured (Soleimanpour, Geierstanger, Kaller, et al., 2010). School-based health centers encourage students to actively participate in age-appropriate decisions regarding their health care, and they integrate prevention activities with clinical care.

Services provided include physical examinations, acute and chronic illness management, immunizations, mental health, and referrals to other care providers. Access to care is increased, since it is provided in a setting easily accessible to the child. Children may also miss less school time for their appointments. School-based health centers have a documented impact on the health of middle school and high school students, such as increased physical activity and eating healthier food (McNall, Lichty, & Mavis, 2010). Education provided at the center about a condition, like asthma or diabetes, may help students more easily begin the transition to self-manage the condition.

Mental health counseling is a leading reason for student visits to school-based health centers. Students can be assessed for depression, substance abuse, eating disorders, mood or anxiety disorders, or risk factors for suicide. Depending upon the center, the student may receive or be referred for comprehensive evaluations, case management, individual counseling, crisis management, substance abuse treatment, or support groups. Other potential problems addressed may include family conflicts, peer relationships, anger management, and bereavement. Individual therapy is often offered (Soleimanpour et al., 2010).

School nurses who effectively collaborate will find that the school-based health center supplements their role, rather than competing with it. School nurses should develop communication channels with the school-based health center to facilitate collaboration.

Preparation for Emergencies

Because children spend so much of their day in school, this setting is a common location of injury. In addition, acute illnesses occur frequently during school hours. Every school needs a plan to ensure effective emergency care and transport for an acutely ill or injured child. To develop the plan for managing the emergency care of students, the school nurse often works with the school administrators, the physician consultant, and the local EMS agency. The plan developed should also include actions to take when children are on school-sponsored field

Evidence-Based Practice   Improving Asthma Management at School

PROBLEM

Many children with asthma attend school, and some struggle because of frequent absences. They often need help managing their illnesses to participate in the school setting. What are some strategies for assisting children with asthma to improve their school performance?

EVIDENCE

Children with persistent asthma from 36 schools (n = 240) with a mean age of 11 years participated in a randomized controlled trial to determine if school-based supervised asthma therapy would increase adherence to inhaled steroid therapy compared to parent-supervised asthma therapy. Poor asthma control, an outcome measure, was defined as one or more absences from school due to respiratory illness or asthma each month, average use of a rescue inhaler more than 2 times a week (excluding use for pre-exercise treatment), or one or more peak expiratory flow meter (PEFM) readings in the red or yellow zone. Children in the school-based treatment group were supervised by study staff when taking dry-powder inhaler medication, and education was provided if the technique was incorrect. Data were collected regarding daily PEFM readings, use of rescue medications, and school absences. Children in both groups had the same likelihood of poor asthma control episodes at the beginning of the study. Study findings revealed improved asthma control in the school-based treatment group (Gerald, McClure, Mangan, et al., 2009).

A second study recruited 530 children with persistent asthma, 3 to 10 years of age, from 67 schools for a randomized control trial with school-based observed daily therapy compared to parent-administered therapy. Families of all children received a diary to track the child's symptoms, which were retrieved by a monthly telephone interview. Children in the school-based treatment group had more symptom-free days, significantly fewer nights with symptoms, fewer days with activity limitations, and fewer days of school absence than children in the control group. Children in the school-based treatment group were also less likely to have an asthma episode requiring prednisone treatment (Halterman, Szilagyi, Fisher, et al., 2011).

The Asthma Inventory for Children (measuring asthma self-management behaviors) and the Asthma Belief Survey (measuring asthma self-efficacy) were tools used to evaluate the perceptions of 81 African American children, 7 to 12 years of age, to self-manage their asthma. Findings revealed that the children who scored higher on the self-efficacy scale also scored high on the asthma self-management scale. This means that the children who believed they could manage their asthma well also reported using more self-management behaviors to control their asthma (Kaul, 2011).

IMPLICATIONS

It is important to find effective strategies to reduce the number of acute asthma episodes, such as supervised medication administration and teaching children about asthma, daily management, and management of episodes. Education that teaches asthma self-management may help children develop confidence in their ability to manage their asthma. Past research has revealed a relationship between how well the child self-manages his or her asthma and the child's asthma symptoms and morbidity (Kaul, 2011).

CRITICAL THINKING APPLICATION

When in a school for clinical placement, identify the estimated numbers of children with asthma and how many children report to the school nurse with asthma episodes in a month.

What strategies has the school nurse used to reduce the number of asthma episodes in children with persistent asthma? Do these strategies include educating students on self-management of asthma, educating teachers to identify children with asthma, providing daily inhaler medication at school, or seeking an asthma action plan for the student? What evidence exists that the strategy is effective in reducing the number of asthma episodes or reducing the severity of episodes in individual children?

---

trips. Because the school nurse may not be employed at a school full time, other school personnel need to learn how to provide emergency care until the EMS providers arrive at the scene. Therefore, school personnel (administrators, secretaries, and health aides) need training to distinguish between a true emergency that requires activation of the local EMS system and an urgent problem that parents can be called to manage. See Box 14–6 for elements of an emergency response plan.

Additionally, because other potential emergencies can impinge upon the school setting—such as natural and man-made disasters, and behavioral crises—each school needs an **emergency preparedness** plan, a community-based coordinated response plan for the incident. For example, a plan to evacuate students with disabilities is needed. Schools may serve as disaster shelters, but the disaster could occur during the school day. Children may need to be maintained on site for hours or potentially days. Plans for protecting the health and supervision of children should be developed. Adequate supplies of food and water should be stockpiled for the number of days recommended by local disaster planning experts. See page 380 for more information.

Children with Special Healthcare Needs

Children with complex healthcare conditions Previously homebound children who are medically fragile now attend school. Classifications of children who are medically fragile include those with prolonged dependence on a medical device that is required to sustain life (mechanical ventilators, intravenous nutrition or drugs, tracheostomy, suctioning, oxygen, or tube feedings) or to compensate for vital body functions, such as a child with diabetes who uses an insulin pump.

As these children attend school, they must be provided with complex healthcare services. Some of these children have an assigned nurse or skilled health aide because of the need for care and monitoring during the school day. The school nurse must be prepared to provide acute, episodic, chronic, and emergency care to medically fragile children, including such procedures as suctioning and tracheostomy care, IV medications, and gastrostomy feedings. See the Skills Manual ⊂⊃ for these procedures. The school nurse has a vital role in facilitating the **individualized health plan (IHP)** (a formal mechanism to ensure that the child's health needs are effectively managed in the school setting) so that a child is integrated successfully into the classroom while receiving appropriate health care. See Chapter 16 ⊘ for a discussion of individualized health plans and individualized education plans.

BOX 14–6   Elements of a School Emergency Response Plan

- An emergency response plan developed by the school nurse, school or team physicians, athletic trainers, school administrators, and the local EMS agency
- A communication system between all locations within the school campus and the central office personnel who call 911
- Designated persons to direct the EMS providers to the location of the child needing care and transport to the emergency department
- School nurse and other designated school personnel trained to recognize a child needing emergency care and to provide that initial emergency care
- Mock drills to practice the emergency response and to make improvements
- Emergency equipment available to trained school personnel

BOX 14–7	Research: Case Management

A study of school-nurse case management of 114 children (5 to 9 years of age) with chronic conditions such as diabetes, asthma, severe allergies, seizures, and sickle cell anemia evaluated the impact of services on academic health and quality-of-life outcomes over a school year. Selected children had needs that were ongoing and interfering with their school performance. Case managers worked with children and families on a regular basis to help control symptoms and to prevent problems. Children who were case managed had an improved quality of life, better skills, knowledge to manage their health condition, and greater participation in extracurricular activities (Engelke, Guttu, Warren, et al., 2008).

Children with chronic health conditions Children with chronic conditions, such as asthma or diabetes, also need attention from the school nurse. These children may develop acute illnesses or become injured while at school and need nursing care. Some of these children need special accommodations in the school setting to fully participate in the learning environment (Box 14–7). An IHP is developed collaboratively by the parent, child, school nurse, school administrator, and teachers (Figure 14–5 ■).

The IHP is used when the student has a relatively chronic health condition, such as diabetes or cystic fibrosis, or when a need for modification of the school environment exists due to the child's health condition. For example, when the child has a lower extremity fracture and uses crutches, more time is allowed to change classes, and use of the elevator is arranged if classes occur above the ground floor. The IHP should include the health history, baseline health status, medications and procedures required during school, equipment and transportation needs, the nursing care plan, and an emergency action plan (Raymond, 2009). This information is used to maximize the student's participation in the educational program. The parent provides medications, supplies, and equipment along with the physician's written instructions for care at school, on the school bus, on field trips, or during extracurricular activities.

The nursing process provides the format for development of the IHP. In many cases the health plan is integrated into the child's individualized education plan or individual family service plan. See Chapter 16 🔗. Treat the information in this plan as confidential, but

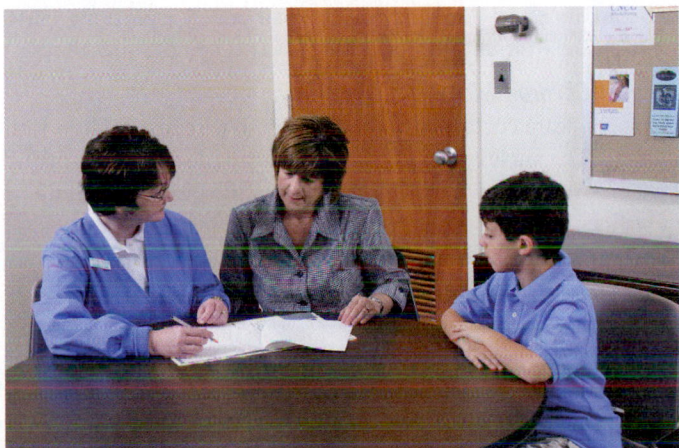

FIGURE 14–5 ■ Because some children need medications or other therapies during school hours, the parents, child, and school nurse often discuss what is needed to manage a child's condition. This is in preparation for a meeting with the teacher and school administrators to develop the child's individualized health plan.

make sure it is stored in an easily accessible area for personnel who must provide emergency care. Train the school personnel to care for the child who needs medications or has special equipment, including special precautions to use when providing care.

Facilitating the Child's Return to School

The school nurse also helps transition the child back into the classroom following an acute illness or injury. Examples include making environmental adaptations, creating an IHP when a new health condition is diagnosed, or revising the IHP when a significant change in the status of the child's chronic condition has occurred. This transition is greatly assisted when the pediatric nurse in the hospital or community setting or the child's primary care provider contacts the school nurse to coordinate the child's return to school. Educational materials about the child's condition sent to the school also assist with this transition. The school nurse then begins to work with the family to prepare teachers and school administrators for the child's special needs. The child's teacher and classmates can be prepared for the child's physical changes if appropriate. Sometimes the teacher's expectations of the child need to be modified, as in the case of a child with a mild brain injury who may have decreased ability to concentrate for several weeks during recovery.

Clinical Judgment

A child has returned to school after fracturing his tibia. He has a cast and must use crutches for the next 4 to 6 weeks. Identify key elements to include in an IHP to facilitate this child's return to school.

Because the nurse has continuing contact with the child throughout the school year, it is possible to evaluate the effectiveness of the IHP, the nursing care provided, and the administration's policies regarding school health care. Evaluation of the IHP and emergency plans leads to future improvements in the school health program.

Outcomes of school nursing care may include the following:

- Completing screening assessments of children and making appropriate referrals for children who need further medical, dental, vision, or hearing assessment
- Protecting students from harm, such as ensuring a safe playground
- Finding resources for children without insurance to receive needed health assessments and resources
- Providing first aid, emergency care, and services for acute healthcare needs
- Meeting healthcare needs of students with chronic conditions and providing needed nursing interventions (e.g., medications and procedures)
- Decreasing absences from school
- Ensuring a safe learning environment

Nursing in Childcare Settings

An estimated 12 million children under 6 years receive care in out-of-home childcare settings while parents are at work (Crowley & Kulikowich, 2009). Many different types of childcare arrangements are available, including these most common settings:

- In-home care by a family member, baby-sitter, or nanny
- A licensed childcare family home setting for up to five children, cared for by a single childcare provider
- A licensed childcare center that cares for six or more children

National Resource Center for Health and Safety in Child Care

Weblink

| BOX 14–8 | Growth & Development: Childcare Outcomes |

When low-income children receive quality childcare that addresses their health and developmental needs and provides support to parents, numerous benefits have been noted in research (e.g., improved behavioral outcomes in school-age children, improved school readiness, and improved academic outcomes). Other long-term studies of quality childcare outcomes for low-income children have found decreased juvenile arrests, enhanced academic achievement, and delayed average age of childbearing (Rosenthal, Crowley, & Curry, 2009).

States establish minimum licensure requirements and guidelines for the safe operation of childcare settings that include the qualifications of staff, staff-to-child ratio, staff training requirements, safe food handling, safe health practices, and environmental safety. The goal is to promote the health and safety, as well as growth and development, of the children served (Box 14–8). Guidelines for the safe operation of childcare centers are available through the National Resource Center for Health and Safety in Child Care.

Although nurses are not often employed in childcare centers, they can provide consultation for the health and safety of the center (Box 14–9). Nurses can assume an important role in establishing the childcare center's policies for health practices, teaching staff about safe health practices, and monitoring health practices in the setting. The nurse consultant can also teach staff to identify children with illnesses and to provide first aid for injured children. In some cases, especially in childcare centers for ill children, nurses provide health screening and direct nursing care.

Reducing Disease Transmission

The nurse works with the childcare center administrators to develop guidelines and to assess childcare practices to identify opportunities for reducing infectious disease transmission among the staff and children. This is crucial because children are close together in large numbers, they put things in their mouths, they may be contagious before symptoms occur, and they are susceptible to most infectious agents. The nurse can educate the childcare center manager and staff to reduce disease transmission in the following ways (Mink & Yeh, 2009):

- Teach staff when and how to perform hand hygiene, manage a child's secretions, sanitize toys and surfaces, and manage a child's cuts and scrapes.
- Monitor the immunization status of children and encourage parents to get their child immunized according to the most current vaccine schedule.
- Develop guidelines for the exclusion of unimmunized children when a vaccine-preventable disease occurs in a child attending the facility as well as guidelines for the exclusion and return of children with various infectious conditions. See Chapter 22 🪀.

| BOX 14–9 | Research: Nurse Consultant Effectiveness |

A study was designed to evaluate the effectiveness of nurse consultants in 111 licensed childcare centers in five California counties. The 73 childcare centers with nurse consultants were found to have a greater number and higher quality of written health and safety policies consistent with national standards in contrast to 38 comparison centers. The centers with nurse consultants also improved many health and safety practices, such as emergency preparedness and hand washing (Alkon, Bernzweig, To, et al., 2009).

- Conduct a daily health check of each child, looking for behavior changes, rashes, fever, complaints of not feeling well, and other signs and symptoms, such as vomiting, diarrhea, or eye drainage, that indicate an acute illness. The child can be isolated, which may help reduce exposure of other children to the infection until the child returns home.
- Develop guidelines for diapering infants and toddlers to reduce the transmission of diseases. For example, use a specific diaper-changing area, dispose of diapers properly, and follow guidelines to reduce contact of urine and feces with various surfaces and staff clothing. Hand hygiene and sanitizing the diaper-changing surface are also necessary.
- Develop and follow guidelines for safe food preparation and handling.

Health Promotion

Health promotion activities within a childcare center encourage the child's highest level of functioning and development, such as having activities that stimulate physical, emotional, and cognitive development, and nutritious food to foster growth. Physical activity guidelines should include structured periods of active play and outdoor play to develop motor skills. It is also important to arrange rest periods and naps for young children. Health maintenance activities, such as immunization monitoring, infection control, and placing infants on their backs to sleep (see Chapter 25 🪀), help prevent injury and disease.

The nurse promotes healthy behaviors by designing and offering health education programs for the children. For example, teach proper oral hygiene, blowing the nose into a tissue, sneezing or coughing into the elbow, and hand washing after toileting and before eating. If childcare providers encourage these practices, they will become habits that the children use routinely.

Environmental Safety

Ensure that the childcare center maintains a current list of which family members may take a child from the facility and has guidelines for verifying identity when necessary. These guidelines are important to prevent child abduction.

The nurse should inspect the childcare environment to identify hazards that could cause injury to the children. Be sure that cleaning supplies and other toxins are stored in a locked cabinet to prevent exposure. Toys used by children should be inspected to ensure that there are no sharp edges or points, small parts, or pinching parts. Check the playground equipment for safety (Figure 14–6 ■).

Care for Children with Illnesses

Some childcare centers have the capacity to care for children with illnesses. The nurse can work as a consultant to develop plans to care for and manage children with communicable diseases. Additional guidelines for infection control are needed to prevent the spread of infection to other children in the center.

Emergency Care Planning

As in the school setting, guidelines for assessing and identifying the child with an emergency health condition are essential. An emergency care plan should be developed to care for an acutely ill or injured child until transported to the emergency department. This plan should include the following elements:

- Giving first aid
- Calling 911 for emergency medical response to transport the child to the emergency department

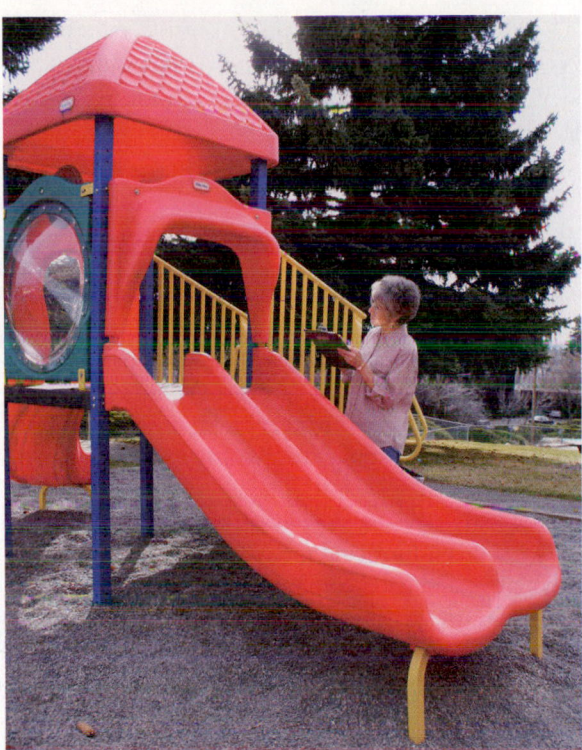

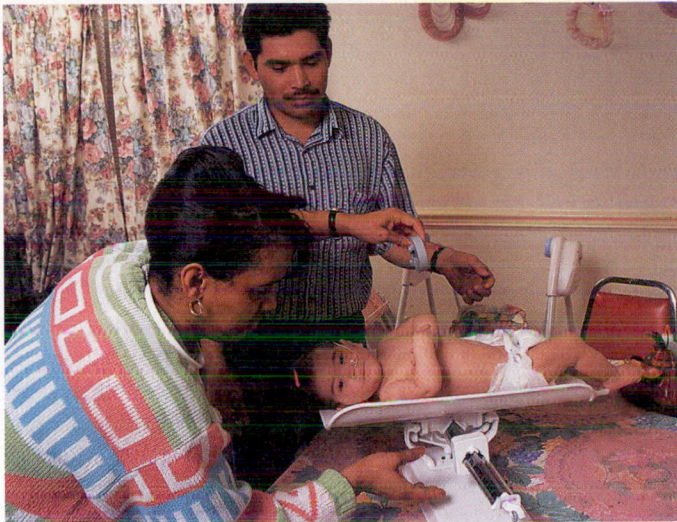

FIGURE 14–7 ■ Nurses provide both short-term and long-term services to families in the home setting. In some cases, families need support for a short time after the child is discharged from the hospital following an acute illness. In other cases, families need assistance with complex nursing care for the child dependent on technology for survival.

FIGURE 14–6 ■ Assess the childcare center's environment for safety hazards. Check the area around playground equipment, making sure that there are wood chips or cushioned tiles under the equipment. Inspect the playground equipment for protruding screws, loose nuts and bolts, and instability at least monthly.

- Calling the parent or emergency contact person to notify someone about the child's condition
- Accompanying the child to the emergency department to stay with the child until the parent arrives

Other Community Settings

In many other community settings, the nurse's role may be similar to that in a school setting. Promoting health, preventing disease, and preventing injury are equally important in childcare centers, camps, health department clinics, and disaster or homeless shelters. For example, nurses may work with homeless shelter administrators to address infection control issues and to assess the safety of the children's environment. See Chapter 20 🌐.

Role of the Nurse in Camp Settings

Nurses care for approximately 10 million children who attend summer camp each year. At residential camps, the nurse is responsible for the health of the camp staff and children for 24 hours a day (Broussard & Meaux, 2007). The majority of camps focus on the needs of healthy children. Nurses in these settings assess and improve the safety of the children's environment, provide nursing care to children with acute and chronic illnesses and injuries, administer medications, and plan activities to promote health. Some special camps for children with chronic conditions must have trained personnel to provide needed medical and nursing care while children are participating in recreational activities. Nurses working at camps for children with special needs should be familiar with treatments and medications of the children attending.

Home Healthcare Nursing

Home health care is a component of the continuum of comprehensive health care provided to children and families. Children with episodic or long-term health conditions can benefit from home health services, including health promotion, health maintenance, and health restorative care, to promote their optimal function and participation in the family. Home health services include the care provided to children with complex health conditions, short-term acute care conditions, and even terminal conditions (Figure 14–7 ■). See Chapter 18 🌐 for more information about palliative and hospice care in the home setting.

Pediatric in-home services for children with complex healthcare conditions have increased for many reasons, including the increased survival of preterm infants, infants with complex congenital conditions, children with severe trauma, and children with life-limiting or life-threatening conditions (Cervasio, 2010). Advances in medical technology and development of portable medical equipment make it possible to sustain children's lives outside the hospital. The home environment is believed to be optimal for the long-term care of these children, allowing them to be integrated into the family and to have their growth and development promoted. Many families prefer to care for their child in the home, rather than in hospital settings, to gain some control over their lives. Some families feel that they have no choice about assuming responsibility for the ongoing nursing and technologic care of their child (Boroughs & Dougherty, 2009). These families live with significant social, psychologic, and physical burdens related to their child's constant care requirements. Home healthcare nurses are essential to provide the intense level of assistance and supervision trained family caregivers require for medically fragile children.

Home health care is costly, but it is considered a cost-effective alternative to hospital inpatient care. Health insurers pay many of the costs associated with home care, but because they cap the total amount of care covered, state Medicaid programs are often the primary payer for these services (Sender, 2011). However, the family ends up paying some costs out of pocket—such as some medications, supplies, and transportation—and incurs a financial burden. In some cases, a parent gives up employment to provide care to the child and to qualify for Medicaid. Challenges in the provision of home health care exist because of the limited number of home health nurses with pediatric expertise. Another challenge involves healthcare payers who offer low reimbursement rates or set restrictions or limitations on home-based services that will be reimbursed (McKenzie, 2011).

Characteristics of Children in Home Care Services

Many of the children needing home health care are medically fragile. Parents and other care providers without backgrounds in health care are given tremendous responsibilities to provide technology-assisted health care to their child. Technology-assisted care in the home may include any of the following: ventilators, tracheostomies, suctioning, cardiorespiratory monitors, nutritional support (enteral, intravenous, or gastrostomy feedings) and feeding pumps, peritoneal dialysis, intravenous fluids with pumps, and medication administration by gastrostomy tube or IV. In some cases, families have created mini intensive care units in the home. Examples of some serious chronic conditions requiring technology-assisted care include congenital heart defects before corrective surgery, bronchopulmonary dysplasia, renal failure, and cancer in its terminal stage.

Only a small number of these children have chronic conditions serious enough to need continuous (daily, or up to 24 hours a day) private-duty care in the home. Nurses or home health aides may remain in the home for an 8- to 12-hour period providing direct nursing care to the child. Healthcare systems (healthcare providers and insurers) are challenged to simultaneously plan and provide services that address the child's long-term health condition and developmental needs. Families also need support so they and their children do well in their environments. For example, the parent needs adequate sleep to provide ongoing daily care for the child. In many cases other healthcare professionals provide needed services, such as physical and occupational therapists, social workers, nutritionists, and personal care aides.

The family also needs help to support the growing child, particularly when of preschool and school age. Options for interaction with children the same age are also important. The federal mandate for the education of children with disabilities provides an avenue to ensure education in the preschool and school setting (see Chapter 16). The school system is mandated to provide appropriate health services for the child's condition.

Most children receive intermittent skilled nursing visits to assess the child and to see how family members are managing the child's healthcare needs. Intermittent home healthcare services (one to several visits a week) may be provided to help families during the child's acute recovery, such as a child with osteomyelitis receiving home antibiotic infusion therapy.

Role of the Pediatric Nurse in Home Care

Home care nursing is focused on assisting a family to gain a greater ability to more independently manage the care of a child with a chronic condition or an acute condition following hospital discharge. There are two major goals of working with families in the home care setting:

- Promoting or restoring health while attempting to minimize the effects of the disability and illness, including palliative care for an illness that is ultimately terminal, such as muscular dystrophy

- Promoting child or family self-care capacity in the home

Nurses develop strategies to support and partner with families who provide care to their children in the home. To work in the home care setting, nurses need a variety of skills:

- Knowledge and experience in pediatric care, pediatric assessment skills for children with various complex health conditions, and acute care practice with various medical technologies (These skills enable nurses to provide direct care, teach the family and child self-care practices, and monitor the child's progress.)
- The ability to be adaptable, creative, and prepared to deal with the unexpected, such as equipment malfunctions
- Skill in collaboration with other healthcare team members
- Skill in educating family members to assess and manage the child's care
- Community assessment skills; an understanding of community resources, financing mechanisms, and multiagency collaboration; and good communication skills (This knowledge helps the nurse better assist families to find the most supportive services to match the child's and family's needs.)
- An understanding of the cultural diversity in the community and the specific cultural values of the families served

Nursing Management

Nursing Assessment and Diagnosis

For most children, home health care is initiated after an acute hospitalization. The hospital nurse, discharge planner, or case manager usually has responsibility for coordinating the child's and family's transition from hospital to home care in collaboration with the home health agency and an assigned home health nurse. The home health nurse works in collaboration with hospital nurses by assessing caregiver readiness to care for the child at home, available resources, and safety of the environment for the child's care (Figure 14–8 ■).

Home Assessment

The following aspects of the home are assessed:

- Home readiness (safe sleeping arrangements, adequate supplies, ability to meet nutritional and fluid needs, telephone

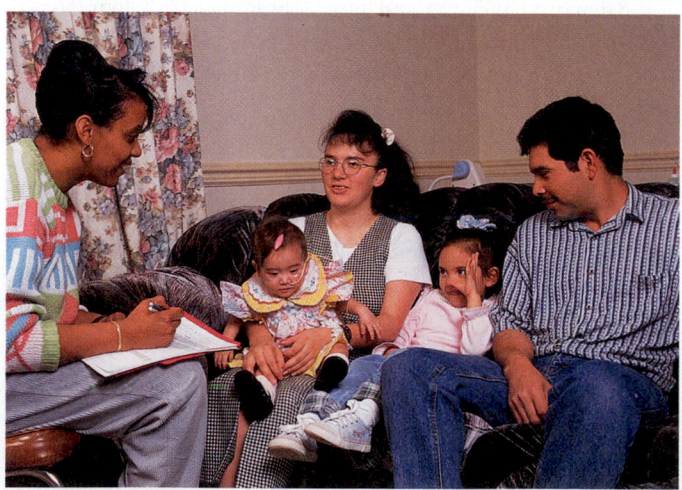

FIGURE 14–8 ■ A visit to the home when all family members are present provides the best information for assessing caregiver readiness to care for the child being discharged from the hospital with a complex health condition.

access, heat, electricity, refrigeration, and lack of any communicable diseases in the home). Sometimes modification in the home is needed to provide access, such as a ramp for a stretcher or wheelchair or additional electric outlets for medical equipment. In many cases a backup generator for power is important.

- Potential hazards related to the child's age, condition, and requirements for technology-assisted care (if extension cords are needed to reach electrical outlets, the equipment may lose power if someone trips over the cord and disconnects it by mistake).
- Features in the home environment that could cause an acute illness, such as family members who smoke tobacco or use of a woodstove or fireplace for heating that could cause respiratory distress. Renovation of a house built before 1978 or renovated in the last 6 months could expose the child to lead dust or other chemicals.

Child and Family Assessment

Assessment of the child is focused on the current health status, growth, developmental progress, and social interaction with family members and healthcare providers. Observation of the potential for abuse and neglect is an important ongoing assessment for these children.

The family is assessed for parenting skills, as well as their abilities in providing the child's needed medical procedures, accurately administering medications, and detecting significant signs that the child's condition has changed. Family strengths and coping abilities are evaluated using the family assessment guidelines in Chapter 2 ⊘. The presence of siblings, their developmental and physical status, and their needs should also be assessed. See Developing Cultural Competence: Respecting Family Preferences.

Examples of nursing diagnoses that could apply to the family as the child transitions from the hospital to home setting include the following:

- Home Maintenance, Impaired related to insufficient family organization and planning
- Caregiver Role Strain related to multiple stressors in caring for a child with a complex health condition in the home
- Therapeutic Regimen Management: Family, Ineffective related to complexity of medical interventions and misinterpreted information
- Social Interaction, Impaired related to therapeutic isolation

NANDA-I © 2012

Developing Cultural Competence
Respecting Family Preferences

When assessing the child and family in the home, recognize that there are potential conflicts between recommended medical care and the family's preferences. Identify which family member is most influential in decisions about care provided for the child. Use open-ended questions to talk with families and understand the health problem from their point of view. Ask the family to identify the issue, why it is a concern, and its impact on the lives of family members. Information gained can then be used to educate the family and to develop a nursing care plan that integrates the family's preferences for the child's care. For example, families from many cultures hang an amulet on a string around an infant's neck to protect health or to protect against the evil eye. Consider making recommendations for a safer way for the child to wear the charm or amulet, such as pinning it to clothing.

Planning and Implementation

Nursing care should focus on promoting an environment within the home for the child to develop, learn social skills, and gain a sense of identity based on family values. Nurses help families in the home setting in the following ways:

- Ensuring that the child will be safe at home
- Providing competent nursing care to the child
- Educating family members about the child's condition and physical signs and symptoms that may indicate a change in health status
- Educating family members to safely administer medications, feedings, and medical procedures
- Demonstrating methods and encouraging family members to promote the child's development and integration into the family
- Linking the family to community resources, including support groups, respite care, and therapeutic recreation
- Assisting families in time management skills and patient care management
- Advocating for increased health insurance coverage or locating other sources of financial assistance

Partnering with the Family

The nurse and family work in partnership in the home to promote the health of the child and of the family as a unit. The nurse must develop a respectful and trusting relationship with the family, remembering that control belongs to the family in the home care setting. The parents are the employer with the ability to hire and fire. Open communication is essential so the nurse can learn what is important to the child and family, and then modify the nursing care plan when appropriate.

Role expectations of the nurse, especially when in the home for extended hours, must be clearly understood to reduce stress in the family. House rules for such things as parking, private areas in the home, door to use, where to store belongings, and routines need to be negotiated, but then rules need to be followed. The success of home care is also based on effective cultural communication. For example, some Jewish families follow strict dietary guidelines that do not permit milk and meat to be served together in the same dishes. The nurse needs to abide by the dietary guidelines and observe the family's food preparation practices.

The range of nursing care activities that may be included in a child's care plan in the home setting include sensory stimulation, routines of daily living, positioning and skin care with gentle handling, respiratory care, nutrition and elimination, medications, and other supportive therapies. Other providers, such as physical therapists, speech-language therapists, occupational therapists, and social workers, may provide other healthcare services in collaboration with the home health nurse.

When nurses provide home care, it is important for a parent to be present and work in partnership with the nurse. Informed consent is needed for invasive treatments and decisions for provision of emergency care to avoid serious risk to life and limb. A plan for communication of key patient-care information and meetings with family members at set intervals are important for the family and nurse to share information and help family members evaluate how well the nurse meets their expectations for care of the child.

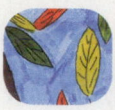

Partnering with Families

Developing a Fire Escape Plan

Developing a fire escape plan is important when the family has one or more children with special healthcare needs. Important steps for families to take in developing the plan include the following:

- Have working smoke and carbon monoxide detectors in the home and teach children what the alarm means. Make sure batteries are changed at least twice a year.
- Draw a diagram of your house. Mark all windows and doors. Plan two routes out of every room. Think about an escape plan if the fire starts in the kitchen, bedroom, or basement.
- Figure out the best way to get infants and young children out of the house. Will you carry them? Is there more than one small child, and if so how will you get them out if you are the only adult?

- Teach preschool and school-age children to follow the escape plan by crawling, touching doors, and going to the window if the door is hot. Show children how to cover the nose and mouth to reduce smoke inhalation.
- Prepare an alternative fire escape plan in case you are alone with the child when the fire begins.
- Keep home exits clear of toys and debris.
- Select a safe meeting place outside the home. Teach children not to go back inside the burning home.

Weblink   Checklist for Pediatric Emergency Preparation   Weblink   AAP Emergency Family Form

Emergency Preparedness

Families need to work with the home health nurse to develop an emergency care plan for any child whose condition could worsen rapidly and become life threatening (e.g., severe congenital heart defect, tracheostomy, or apnea), or be beyond the care that the parents or home health nurse can provide. The emergency care plan should provide guidance as to when to call 911. The local ambulance company needs to be notified that a child dependent on technology is cared for at home. The emergency care plan should include a brief medical history that gives the emergency care providers enough information to understand the child's health condition, to prevent delays in disease-specific treatment, and to minimize unnecessary interventions until the child's personal physician can be consulted. See the American Academy of Pediatrics recommended emergency information form in English and Spanish.

Families should also develop an emergency plan for the safe evacuation of the home in case of fire or other emergency. This is even more challenging when the child cannot mobilize independently and requires equipment for continued survival or quality of life. See Partnering with Families: Developing a Fire Escape Plan for information to help families plan for safe evacuation.

When the child is dependent upon technology, the family should notify the power company so that high priority can be given to getting resources to the child when needed. Backup generators may be needed if electric power for life-sustaining equipment is essential. The child should also be registered for a disaster shelter that can accommodate the healthcare needs of the child and at least one caregiver.

Evaluation

Expected outcomes of nursing care include the following:

- The child's medical needs are integrated into the family's routines when possible.
- An emergency response plan is developed for family use for the child in the event of a disaster, a weather emergency, or a sudden worsening of the child's condition.
- The home health nurse partners with the family to promote the child's health, growth, and development.

Community Health Nursing

Public health promotes the health of the **population** (the collection of individuals that make up a community) rather than the care of individuals, with an emphasis on health promotion and disease prevention. (Emergency medical services and disaster preparedness are addressed in a later section.)

Depending upon the manner in which healthcare services are organized in a community, community health nurses may provide care to children in a variety of settings, such as the following:

- **Public health clinics**—providing well-child care, immunizations, and care for other populations such as adolescents seeking family planning services or treatment for sexually transmitted diseases
- **Schools**—serving as school nurses or consultants on school health issues
- **Childcare settings**—serving as consultants for the health and safety of enrolled children
- **Home**—providing skilled nursing care through a visiting nurse's service, or by assisting high-risk families with the transition of a newborn into the family
- **Homeless shelters**—providing health promotion, health maintenance, and episodic illness care

Community health nurses help the population obtain health services through assessing community needs and resources, advocating for needed resources and services, and then developing health programs to address the needs of children and their families.

Assessment of Community Needs and Resources
Community Assessment

Community assessment is a process of compiling data about a community's health status and resources to develop a public health plan to address the needs of a target population within that community. For example, the target population could be all children, a specific age group such as adolescents, or even a special group of children (such as those with a chronic condition). The community assessment process involves community partners, but follows the nursing process format. Information gained about the number of individuals with the health need and knowledge of existing resources help health professionals determine if additional programs or resources are needed. An overview of the community assessment process is described here, but additional resources such as a community health nursing textbook are needed to complete a full assessment.

Community assessments may be conducted for the following reasons:

- A request is made by interested community advocates or the local health department.
- Justification is needed to fund a new or expanded healthcare program.
- Evaluation of responses to healthcare programs or interventions (such as immunizations, injury prevention program, or services targeted to new immigrants in the community) may provide the data to determine if the children with greatest needs have been appropriately targeted and are benefiting equally from the intervention.

The focus of a community assessment is on the target population. For example, a community assessment might involve ensuring that all children in the community, including those in all racial and ethnic groups, have access to care or specific interventions such as injury prevention programs, immunizations, school health services, or suicide prevention programs.

A community assessment is often initiated because one or more individuals (e.g., parents, school nurse, or community leader) are concerned about a health or social issue, such as a child who is severely injured in a pedestrian crossing on the way to school. The concerned individuals partner with other **stakeholders** (all community residents, policy makers, health providers, and funders concerned with the outcome of the assessment) to investigate if this is an isolated event or if similar incidents have happened at other locations and to identify ways to protect other children. Community partners for this investigation may include nurses, family members, local organizations (e.g., Kiwanis, Safe Kids, parent-teacher association), faith communities, local trauma centers, epidemiologists, elected officials, and health department representatives.

Family members, a pediatric nurse, and a school nurse are important members of the group when pediatric health issues are being addressed. See Developing Cultural Competence: Integrating Cultural Groups into Community Assessments.

The first step in beginning a community assessment is to clearly define its purpose and scope, so the process is focused. The purpose is often associated with a specific problem that an advocate or community leader would like to have addressed by the community. Example issues could be one of the following:

- Several child pedestrians and bicyclists have been injured or killed by motor vehicles over the past 3 months in the same neighborhood.
- Two children drowned at the local lake in a boating incident.
- Three teens from a local high school have committed suicide in the past 2 months.
- The number of children who are fully immunized upon school entry has decreased in the last year.

Once the purpose and scope of the assessment is determined, various factors that influence the health of a community should

Developing Cultural Competence
Integrating Cultural Groups into Community Assessments

Community assessment leaders should invite community members representing different cultural groups to participate in the community assessment process. They help provide an important perspective of the community's needs and help identify culturally appropriate and culturally acceptable strategies to address the health problem.

be considered when collecting assessment data (Clark, 2008, pp. 351–356):

- Demographic characteristics such as age composition of the community, birth statistics, age-specific and cause-specific mortality rates, racial composition, and **morbidity** (incidence and prevalence of certain diseases), as well as the immunization status of children
- Community prospects for continuing growth or economic challenges; cohesion of the community in dealing with past health problems or crises; existing tensions between various community groups; adequacy of personal safety services; communication networks; stresses in the community; and incidence of crime, homicide, and suicide
- Type of community (rural, urban, suburban), size, climate, topographic features, housing adequacy, water supply, waste disposal, and potential hazards that could lead to a disaster
- Sociocultural characteristics such as local government and community leadership, transportation, income and education levels, employment rates, occupations, family composition, faith communities, cultural groups represented, language barriers to health care, number of homeless families and children, recreation, shopping, and social service agencies
- Behavioral characteristics such as nutrition, specific dietary patterns, and use of harmful substances; exercise and recreational opportunities; population use of safety practices
- Health services available to children in the community covered by health insurance, Medicaid, or the State Children's Health Insurance Program (SCHIP); uninsured children; and barriers to healthcare access

Stakeholders next make plans for data collection (types of data to be gathered, sources of data, and methods for obtaining the data) and data analysis. Some of the best data to use are those calculated as rates. See Box 14–10 for commonly used rates. National, neighboring state, and state data can be compared with community data using rates to determine how similar or different the community statistics are for the health problem.

Data may be collected from many sources. See Table 14–1 for suggested sources of community data. Focus groups or interviews with key community representatives may provide information on perceptions of health needs (Clark, 2008). An **epidemiologist,** a specialist with training in the study of patterns of diseases or health risks in a population, is often responsible for analyzing the data. Data trends are analyzed over several years to determine if the identified problem is a cluster of events that is part of a larger significant pattern. For example, the timing and clustering of events, such as the

BOX 14–10	Common Health Statistics Examples

The data for health statistics (e.g., births and deaths) can be obtained from the National Center for Health Statistics with different rates already calculated for the nation, region, state, county, and often large cities. Data are most often calculated for a year, but other time periods may be selected. Census data are often used as the denominator for rates. The common health statistics are calculated with the following formulas:

$$\text{Birth rate} = \frac{\text{number of births in a county in 2011}}{\text{total county population in 2011}} \times 1{,}000$$

$$\text{Mortality rate} = \frac{\text{number of deaths in a state in 2010}}{\text{total state population in 2010}} \times 100{,}000$$

$$\text{Age-specific mortality rate} = \frac{\text{number of deaths in children aged 1–4 years in a city in 2010}}{\text{total population of children aged 1–4 years in the city in 2010}} \times 100{,}000$$

$$\text{Cause-specific mortality rate} = \frac{\text{number of deaths due to a specific injury or illness in the U.S. in 2011}}{\text{total U.S. population in 2011}} \times 100{,}000$$

$$\text{Incidence rate} = \frac{\text{number of new cases of a condition (e.g., type 2 diabetes) in the U.S. in a specific time period}}{\text{U.S. population at risk for the condition in the time period}} \times 100$$

$$\text{Prevalence rate} = \frac{\text{number of new and existing cases of a condition (e.g., asthma) in a state in a specific time period}}{\text{state population during the same time period}} \times 100$$

TABLE 14–1	Sources of Data for a Community Assessment

SOURCE OF COMMUNITY DATA	EXAMPLES
State vital records	Birth rate, age-specific death rate
Census, state population estimates	Age and racial/ethnic composition of the population
Local health agencies	Hospital trauma registry for number of injured children admitted to hospital, child abuse incidents from child protective services, number of infants receiving WIC services, number of children with type 1 diabetes, immunization registry for rate of complete immunizations
Local chapters of voluntary organizations	Volunteers to assist with community assessment and program implementation
Faith-based community	Number of refugee families sponsored, number of children in the families
Community surveys	Frequency of health services used, such as public health clinic for immunizations
Asset map	Geographic map of the community that identifies the location of specific community resources (e.g., education and health centers)
Telephone book	Numbers and types of healthcare providers, faith communities
Law enforcement agencies	Motor vehicle crash reports, crime, homicides, potentially using geographic information systems (GIS) to display their location
Observation	Physical characteristics of the community (e.g., number of schools, recreational facilities)
Focus groups or interviews with key informants	Perception of personal/child health needs, perception of community health needs

Source: *Adapted from Clark, M. J. (2008).* Community health nursing *(5th ed., pp. 357–363). Upper Saddle River, NJ: Prentice Hall Health.*

number of child pedestrians and bicyclists killed or injured, provide a clue to explore recent changes in the community. Have traffic patterns changed because of construction? Does this happen every year as school sessions begin? Is it related to children enjoying spring weather after school? Once the data are collected and analyzed, the community group can then develop a plan to address the problem and have baseline data for evaluation of the planned community intervention.

Key community assets should also be identified during the data collection stage. A **windshield survey,** a walking or driving tour around a neighborhood or community for the purpose of identifying resources and characteristics of the community, often provides important information needed to plan interventions. For example, to address obesity a windshield survey may look at the location of grocery stores, fast-food restaurants, recreation facilities, parks, sidewalks, and safety of play areas. A community assets map can also be developed.

School nurses and community health nurses may use the data collected and analyzed to develop community or target group nursing diagnoses. Examples may include:

- Injury, Risk for related to lack of safe bicycle paths in high traffic areas
- Coping: Community, Readiness for Enhanced related to development of disaster plans and drills to evaluate their effectiveness
- Health: Community, Deficient related to lack of community programs for childhood obesity prevention
- Health Maintenance, Impaired related to refusal of many community families to permit their children to receive immunizations for philosophical reasons

NANDA-I © 2012

Planning and Evaluation

An intervention is planned and implemented after the collected data have been analyzed and the community health problem has been clearly described. The collaborative planning effort involves all the stakeholders who as a group contribute ideas, develop strategies, and consider funding sources. Ultimately the intervention plan is promoted and advertised in the community. The collaboration often has persons with different talents who can assume leadership roles for specific tasks associated with the intervention. The planning group's knowledge of the community's cultural beliefs, primary languages, income levels, reading levels, sources of community health education, and potential community partners is valuable in designing the intervention. Knowledge about potential community funding resources or barriers helps in determining strategies that may be approved and endorsed by community decision makers.

Community Plan and Intervention Example

In trying to improve the safety of children riding their bicycles to school, a grassroots organization determined that constructing new bike paths in the high-traffic areas was not possible unless state funding could be obtained. Funding for such a project could not be obtained without legislative action, so an alternative plan was needed. The nurse, working with other community leaders, identified a number of alternative routes with less traffic for children to use when bicycling to school and other important destinations. Approval was obtained from the community government to mark and advertise these routes. Potential actions to promote the use of the new bike routes include the following:

- Increase awareness of the alternative bike routes through the local media (radio, television, and newspapers in all languages), church bulletins, and flyers sent home from school.
- Encourage use of the alternative routes by working with local businesses to provide incentives to children (e.g., an ice cream cone) to use the alternative bike paths, especially to those wearing a bike helmet and riding safely. Local firefighters and police officers could give reward coupons to children riding the alternative routes.
- Partner with local voluntary organizations to sponsor a bike rodeo to teach new riders safe biking skills and the rules of riding.

Community leaders can then work with the community government to develop the state transportation proposal for constructing bike paths in the high-traffic areas.

Evaluation

The plan and intervention for the health problem needs to be evaluated. Data collected before the intervention can serve as one comparison for the evaluation. Evaluation should also focus on the intervention and how well the target population accepted it, as well as the outcome, such as reduced injuries and deaths.

In the case of the bike routes, community leaders can monitor the use of the recommended bike routes versus the more dangerous routes. An increase in numbers of children using the recommended bike routes should be seen and sustained over an extended period. Nurses can monitor the newspapers, and local hospital emergency departments may be able to provide data on the number of children with bicycle-related injuries in the high-traffic areas and the alternative bike routes. Actual comparison of bicycle-related injuries and deaths should be made between the preintervention phase and at annual intervals to determine if the intervention was associated with the desired outcome.

EMERGENCY CARE PLANNING
Emergency Medical Services for Children

The emergency medical services (EMS) system is the organized community-based public health response to ensure that adults and children with acute illnesses and injuries receive emergency care and timely transport to the hospital emergency department. The EMS system at the local community level is composed of an agency with ambulances and trained emergency medical personnel who respond to emergencies. In some communities this EMS agency is part of the fire department, and in others it is a separate organization. Regardless, each local EMS agency has a medical director who establishes the protocols used by emergency medical personnel when caring for ill and injured individuals. The public accesses the EMS system by placing a call to 911. A dispatcher directs the ambulance unit to respond, takes information, and provides information to the caller about how to manage the ill or injured person until the emergency personnel arrive. State EMS offices set the guidelines for training and certification of emergency medical personnel, equipment to be carried on ambulances, data collection about the patient care provided, and communication systems used. In addition, the state EMS office works closely with hospital emergency departments and trauma centers to coordinate emergency care of patients transported by the EMS system. Children have special needs during emergency care that have been integrated into the overall EMS system. See Legal & Ethical Considerations: Emergency Medical Services for Children.

Important Pediatric Physiologic Differences

Children have different physiologic responses to emergencies because of their smaller anatomy and developing organ systems (see Appendix F 🔗). Small children cannot communicate and describe their health problems, and they are dependent upon family members for security and recognition of the emergency. Due to differences in anatomy, pediatric-size equipment and supplies are essential. EMS providers need education to assess the child and recognize the signs that the child's condition is a true emergency, and then to provide the appropriate medical intervention before and during transport to the hospital.

Hospitals and their emergency departments are also part of the EMS system, and these emergency departments must be prepared to treat children as well as adults. Emergency departments need to have appropriately sized resuscitation equipment for children of all ages and well-trained emergency department physicians and nurses. Educational programs like Pediatric Advanced Life Support provide opportunities for nurses and physicians to work together effectively

Video | EMS for Children

Legal and Ethical Considerations
Emergency Medical Services for Children

Federal legislation was first passed in 1984 to ensure that children's needs were addressed by the EMS system. This program has been renewed and is now authorized in the Public Health Service Act, Section 1910, as of January 2011. States receive funding to improve their systems of emergency care so that all children with severe injuries or critical illnesses have access to optimal emergency care.

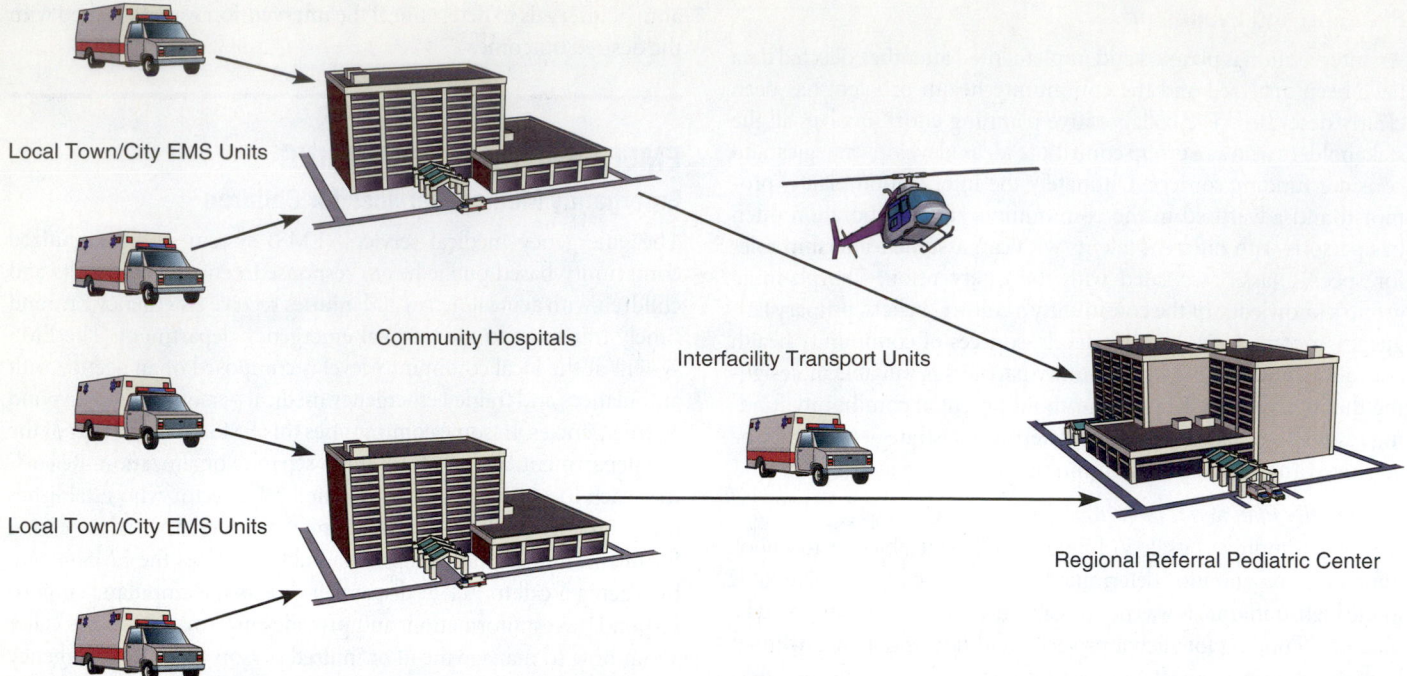

Local Town/City EMS Units

Community Hospitals

Interfacility Transport Units

Local Town/City EMS Units

Regional Referral Pediatric Center

FIGURE 14–9 ■ The emergency medical services (EMS) system is a carefully linked set of resources in the community and region that enable children with serious illnesses and injuries to get the care needed in the most appropriate hospital. The continuum of emergency care includes the caregiver of the child at the scene, the communications center taking the call for help, the EMS personnel responding to the scene who provide immediate emergency care and transport the child to the emergency department, and the hospital emergency department. If the child is transported to a community emergency department but needs more complex care, transfer to a larger hospital or trauma center is then coordinated. A team of specially trained pediatric emergency care providers often manages the transfer between hospitals in an ambulance, helicopter, or small plane. The goal is to get the child to the medical and specialty care resources needed to have the best chance of survival and optimal functional outcome.

to resuscitate a child who is critically ill or injured. In addition, clinical guidelines for a well-orchestrated response for serious trauma and medical emergencies are developed and rehearsed. Urgent care centers and smaller emergency departments need to have agreements with major medical centers or trauma centers to ensure that children with life-threatening injuries or illnesses can be quickly transferred and transported to a more advanced level of care.

Nurses sometimes work as volunteer EMS providers in their communities. Nurses also work as interfacility transport team members, providing care to critically ill children who need to be transferred by ground or air ambulance from a community hospital to a hospital with more advanced care. Figure 14–9 ■ shows the interconnection between the EMS system, community hospitals, and major referral hospitals for provision of emergency services.

Disaster Preparedness

Disasters are serious and massive events that often occur suddenly and cause extensive damage, hardship, deaths, injuries, and psychologic trauma. The amount of destruction and number of people impacted often mean that a community is unable to manage the recovery process without assistance. Many types of disasters occur each year in the United States. Natural disasters may occur suddenly and include floods, mudslides, ice storms, hurricanes, earthquakes, volcanic eruptions, tornados, and fires. Other types of disasters can occur when trains or trucks carrying toxic chemicals and nuclear waste crash or explode. Concerns of terrorism with infectious organisms, toxic chemicals, or radioactive agents have elevated the need for disaster and emergency preparedness. See Chapter 22 ✇ for information about infectious organisms used for terrorism.

State and federal agencies, hospitals, and health professionals are developing community **disaster preparedness** plans for response to natural and man-made disasters that involve multiple casualties. Special planning for the needs of infants, children, and adolescents must be integrated in these efforts, especially since children are often clustered in schools and childcare centers, separated from their family during the day. Health services are needed to treat injuries and potential illnesses caused by contaminated water or other exposures.

Children have special vulnerabilities during a disaster (Box 14–11). Disasters are very traumatic for children involved, and there may be immediate and delayed responses. Fear and panic are among the most common behaviors exhibited when families are not prepared (Murray, 2010). Children may lose their homes and personal possessions. Children may be separated from their family. Friends, pets, and family members may be injured or dead. They have problems expressing their feelings about the disaster.

BOX 14–11   Growth & Development: Disaster Planning

Developmental stages must be considered during disaster planning, since young children may be unable to do the following (American Academy of Pediatrics, 2008):

- Understand what is happening or efforts to reduce the consequences of the disaster
- Figure out how to flee or take evasive action to escape danger
- Follow the instructions given to adults regarding evacuation or safe actions
- Tell others they need help
- Distinguish between reality and fantasy

Video Disaster Preparedness

As They Grow Response to Toxic Chemicals and Terrorism Agents

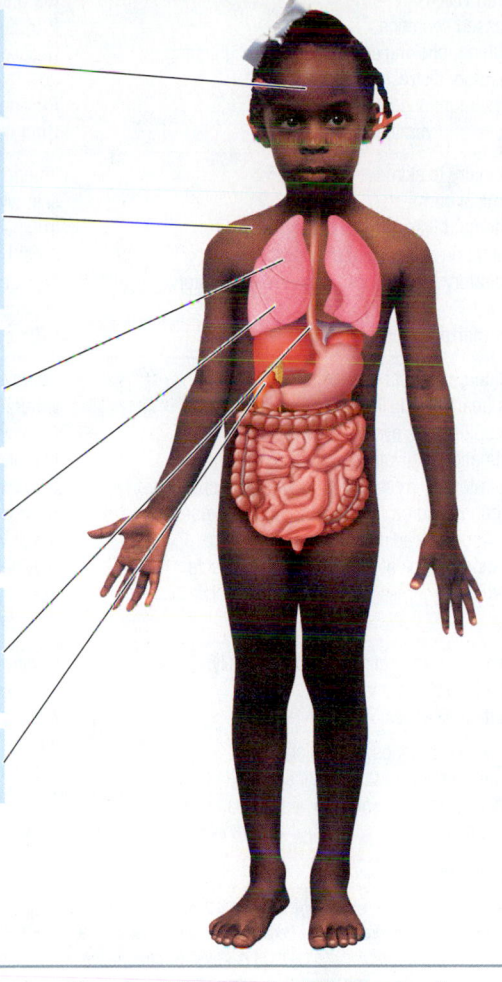

Children's developmental abilities and cognitive levels may interfere with their ability to escape danger.

Children's skin is thinner, so toxic agents falling on the skin can be absorbed more rapidly. Their increased body surface area means greater exposure to toxic agents falling on the skin.

Children breathe faster and inhale more air per weight than adults, meaning a greater exposure to aerosol toxins.

Children are shorter and have greater exposure to heavier aerosol agents that fall to the ground.

Children drink more fluids per kilogram than adults, so there is greater exposure to contaminants in water or other fluids such as milk.

Children also differ in their ability to detoxify and excrete toxic substances.

FIGURE 14–10 ■ Children have different physiologic and cognitive vulnerabilities than adults in response to various chemical toxins or radiologic agents.

Children's size and physiology also make them vulnerable when exposed to toxic chemicals or radiologic agents used by terrorists or released during another type of exposure, such as a train wreck (Figure 14–10 ■).

Clinical Manifestations

Some common initial responses to a disaster, whether it is natural or man-made, include fear, anxiety, sadness, and confusion. The responses of children may be even greater if parents are also anxious or overwhelmed. Developmental stage, prior life experience, and the ability of the primary caregiver to meet needs of safety and security will determine a child's response to disaster. Responses by age group and initial support interventions include the following (Murray, 2010):

- Infants may respond with changes in sleeping and eating patterns, crying and irritability, exaggerated startle response, or apathy. Support involves providing a consistent caregiver and maintaining routines as close to normal as possible.

- Toddlers may respond with changes in appetite, disrupted sleep, nightmares, clinging behaviors, withdrawal, temper tantrums, and helplessness. Support involves providing a routine mealtime, play, bedtime routine, comfort item, and storytelling.

- Preschoolers may respond with regressive behaviors such as bed-wetting, thumb sucking, fear of the dark, alterations in eating and sleeping patterns, feelings of guilt, anxiety, and complaints of stomachaches or headaches. Support involves letting children know they are not responsible, allowing regression during stress, and promoting play and storytelling to express feelings.

- School-age children may respond with preoccupation with the disaster, fear for themselves and their family, withdrawal from friends, decreased interest in daily activities, changes in temperament, and acting out. Support involves restricting media exposure, explanations of the event in age-appropriate terms, opportunities to express their feelings, and play therapies.

- Adolescents may respond with anxiety, acting out, anger, changes in mood, stomachaches, headaches, and risk-taking behaviors. Other adolescents may cope by helping in disaster response efforts. Support involves engaging adolescents in disaster response efforts when it is safe, encouraging them to talk with peers about their feelings, relaxation techniques, exercise, and journal writing.

Because disasters cause disruption for extended periods, such as the 2011 tornados in Alabama and Mississippi that destroyed homes and schools, the child has prolonged periods of emotional distress. These factors place the child at risk for acute stress and posttraumatic stress reactions (Murray, 2010). See Chapter 34 🔗 for more information on posttraumatic stress disorder (PTSD).

See the Clinical Manifestations table for initial clinical therapy for various chemical and radiologic exposures.

Clinical Therapy

The initial response to the scene of any disaster is to get the victims to safety and fresh air, and then to quickly identify the level of injury or illness severity of all individuals. Emergency care and transportation to facilities that can provide needed care for injuries and illnesses is initiated. If the child was exposed to a chemical or radiologic agent, clinical therapy focuses on determining the type of exposure and providing immediate care to reduce the agent's effects, such as decontamination.

Decontamination, the removal of chemicals and nerve agents from the skin, should be performed as soon as possible (Box 14–12). Clothing is removed and the child is washed with soap and water.

Clinical Manifestations Chemical and Radiologic Exposure

TYPE OF EXPOSURE, POTENTIAL AGENTS	POTENTIAL CLINICAL MANIFESTATION	INITIAL CLINICAL THERAPY
Chemical inhalation exposure (pulmonary agents such as chlorine and phosgene)	Burning sensation in nose, throat, and eyes Blurred vision Increased secretions Coughing, choking sensation, chest tightening, respiratory distress, bronchospasm, and pulmonary edema Nausea and vomiting	Get the child to fresh air. Decontaminate the child with water. Provide supplemental oxygen. Secure the airway with an endotracheal tube and assist ventilations if needed. Provide bronchodilators and corticosteroids. Offer symptomatic care.
Chemical skin and eye exposure (cryogenic liquids, acids, alkalis, corrosives, mustard gas, nitrogen mustard)	Cold injury to skin Chemical burns Erythema, blistering Eye inflammation, pain, blindness Respiratory tract inflammation and respiratory distress Bone marrow suppression with leukopenia	Immediately decontaminate; remove clothing and wash skin with soap and water. Irrigate the eyes. Treat burns (see Chapter 36 🔗). Provide fluid resuscitation. Provide analgesia. Offer symptomatic care.
Nerve agents (tabun, sarin, soman, VX, organophosphates)	Cholinergic effects include: Eyes (tearing, pupillary constriction, red conjunctiva, eye pain, blurry vision) Lacrimation, salivation, sweating, runny nose Respiratory distress due to increased respiratory secretions and bronchospasm, cough, wheezing, and dyspnea leading to respiratory failure Neurologic signs of seizures, coma, muscle weakness progressing to flaccid paralysis	Remove clothing and wash skin and hair with soap and water. Administer atropine or pralidoxime as an antidote IV or IM. Give benzodiazepines for seizures. Secure the airway with an endotracheal tube and assist ventilation as needed. Give supplemental oxygen. Keep the child hydrated. Provide analgesia.
Radiation	May be few signs and symptoms initially; nausea, vomiting, malaise Radiation sickness ■ Intense immunosuppression ■ Diarrhea and gastrointestinal infection ■ Disorientation, confusion, loss of balance, and seizures Radiation burns	Remove clothing and decontaminate the child. Administer potassium iodide. Assess airway, breathing, and circulation if a blast injury. Provide fluid resuscitation and treatment for infection. Treat burns.

Source: *Data from Henretig, F. M. (2009). Preparation for terrorist threats: Biologic and chemical agents. Clinical Pediatric Emergency Medicine, 10(3), 130–135; Scalzo, A. J., Lehman-Huskamp, K. L., Sinks, G. A., & Keenan, W. J. (2008). Disaster preparedness and toxic exposures in children. Clinical Pediatric Emergency Medicine, 9, 47–60; Siegel, D. (2009). Preparation for terrorist threats: Radiation injury. Clinical Pediatric Emergency Medicine, 10 (3), 136–139; Tracy, M. A. (2008). Kids and chemicals: A pediatric disaster. Journal of Emergency Nursing, 34(3), 266–267.*

Eye irrigation may be needed to reduce pain and eye damage. Decontamination removes the chemical from the child's skin and reduces the child's absorption of the chemical. It also helps to protect medical personnel who will care for the child.

Other specific antidotes and medications, as well as supportive care, are provided for specific chemical and radiologic exposures. See the Clinical Manifestations table for more information.

Nursing Management

Nurses have an important role in disaster preparedness planning and as first responders to disasters. They also provide continuing care for individuals and families as a community emerges from the initial trauma. A primary role of nurses is to prevent disasters when possible and to assist communities with emergency preparedness for disasters. Nurses work with schools and community agencies to identify potential hazards and prevent them from causing harm.

Disaster Preparation

Pediatric nurses in schools and other community settings play a significant role in preparing families for a disaster. They can help families use developmentally appropriate information to talk with their

BOX 14–12	Growth & Development: Decontamination

Decontamination is a challenge with small children. Fortunately taking off the clothing removes 85% of the exposure. If it will take a prolonged time to get the child into a shower because of the number of victims, remove the child's clothing and provide a clean privacy cover. When possible, put the child in a 5- to 6-minute shower with lukewarm water (98° F) to prevent hypothermia in the child. The water pressure should be adequate but not cause pain. The shower should have a handheld sprayer to use on infants and young children to make sure their airway is protected. The infant or young child should be placed on a stretcher or container with holes for water drainage, so the caregiver can be adequately decontaminated while assisting the infant or young child. Group older children by sex for the shower when there are multiple casualties (Heon & Foltin, 2009).

children about disaster planning and convey information about disasters when they occur. Families who have discussions with health professionals about disaster planning are more likely to comply with disaster preparedness recommendations, and children may cope better if they are involved in the family's disaster planning (Kelly, 2010). Children need to know what to do in case of a disaster and that police officers, firefighters, and emergency medical personnel are available to help them. They should be taught how to call for help, how to shut off the power and gas, when to use the emergency number, and how to contact the family members when separated (American Academy of Pediatrics, 2010).

Nurses can help the family develop a disaster plan for staying at home or for evacuation. Families must prepare to manage on their own at home for at least 72 hours following a major disaster or epidemic. This means the family should have a 3-day supply of nonperishable food and bottled water, flashlights and batteries, a battery-powered radio, over-the-counter medications, and many other resources. Remember to have formula, diapers, bottles, powdered milk, moist towelettes, and diaper rash ointment for infants and children if needed. A plan for family pets should also be made. Refer to the Federal Emergency Management Agency (FEMA) website for the most current recommendations for family supplies to have on hand.

Parents should also carry phone numbers of out-of-town contacts, schools, and neighbors at all times. Developing a list of each family member's medications, clothing, food, water, and other essentials is important so the family can quickly pack and respond to an evacuation order.

Clinical Tip

Resources needed for infants and children in disaster shelters include diapers, baby wipes, formula, baby food, and oral hydrating fluids. Toys and games are also valuable to provide recreation for older children who may be staying in a shelter for several days. If an emergency and evacuation continues for more than a couple of days, nurses may be effective in planning developmentally appropriate activities for children in shelters. They can plan for and obtain supplies and volunteers to facilitate drawing activities and games, and give parents a respite.

Disaster Response

When a disaster occurs, nurses are often on the front line, providing emergency health care, first aid, and general public health interventions (e.g., vaccines, sanitation, food, and water). Nurses can use their knowledge of child and adolescent development to meet the needs of youth during a disaster.

The child's response to psychologic trauma must be addressed. Because parents will be stressed, encourage them to take care of their personal needs for emotional support so they can care for themselves as well as their children. The child's ability to cope is often influenced by the parent's coping with the disaster stress.

Psychologic first aid for families and children involves responding to families in a compassionate and supportive manner, comforting and consoling children, providing information, protecting them from further threat or distress, providing some guidelines for positive coping, recognizing when more psychologic help is needed, and getting the child access to that additional help (Schonfeld & Gurwitch, 2009). Nurses can provide a safe place for children, away

from media and unfolding traumatic events, such as the rescue of dead and injured. Do not leave children unattended or permit them to leave a scene without a responsible adult. Assess for panic reactions, unexpected behaviors, and changing conditions.

Once the initial disaster is managed and children return to home or other settings, they may need extra time with their parents. Parents should attempt to reestablish daily routines for school, meals, play, and rest as soon as possible.

Encourage parents to listen and answer the child's questions about the disaster honestly and in language the child can understand. If they cannot answer a question, it is better to be honest and say so, but also reassure the child that they are trying to do everything to keep the child safe. Let young children know that a lot of adults are working hard to protect everyone. Avoid saying everything will be fine, as this does not always address a child's specific concerns. Encourage older children and adolescents to discuss the disaster with family members and peers if desired.

Allow children to express their feelings about the disaster, and reassure them that it is normal to be upset. Use *play therapy* (e.g., art, playing with action figures or dolls, and storytelling) to allow young children to express their feelings, develop a sense of mastery, and reduce their anxiety. Giving older children special tasks lets them feel that they are helping and gives them a sense of control.

Help schools and other community agencies arrange for mental health specialists to assist children in exploring their feelings in safe settings. Provide grief counseling for youth who have lost peers, family members, or pets. Nurses must remain vigilant for children and families who develop posttraumatic stress disorder (PTSD) (see Chapter 34 🔗). Refer individuals and families for mental health services when anxiety levels remain high or they have difficulty performing normal life tasks.

Because children may be separated from family members in childcare and school settings for many hours a day, the family should provide a phone number for an out-of-state family contact that can be used if the family is unable to get to the child. This would enable the care provider to call and report the child's location and safety. Telephone (cell and landline) communication outages in the disaster area may limit the communication between family members. Make sure the children know what to do in case of an emergency. Family members should choose two meeting locations: one at home and the other outside the neighborhood. All children should have a method for contacting family members by phone or email. All children and family members should memorize the family contact information and planned meeting location address so that reunification is possible if separated (Nager, 2009).

Advance planning is needed to ensure that medically fragile children who need technology for survival or have the potential for life-threatening episodes have the resources needed in the event of a disaster. The designated shelter for such children with health professionals and electric power for the needed equipment should be identified and known to the family. In the meantime, battery packs for power backup should be available at all times. Additionally, parents need to arrange for durable power of attorney so that consent for emergency medical care can be available as needed. The child and parents may become separated during the disaster, or the parents may become injured and unable to care for the child.

Weblink — Federal Emergency Management Agency

Weblink — Disaster Resources for Child Victims

Chapter Highlights

- Pediatric care in the community occurs in the following settings: physician offices and healthcare centers, public health clinics, schools and childcare centers, urgent care centers, outpatient departments, homes, homeless shelters, and disaster shelters.

- Working with the child and family in the community setting requires an understanding of how the larger environment influences the child's health and development and integration of that knowledge into the nursing care plan.

- Nurses working in many office or healthcare settings develop a relationship with the child and family over time. A positive partnership with the child and family is important so that optimal health care is provided.

- During episodic care for illnesses and injuries, the nurse collects health information, assesses the child, assists the primary care provider with diagnostic or therapeutic procedures, and educates the child and family about care of the child at home.

- Pediatric nurses in hospital outpatient clinics assist with diagnostic workups and management of children with chronic health problems, including patient assessment, health education, health promotion, and linking families with community resources.

- School nursing focuses on removing or minimizing health barriers to learning so children can perform academically. Services include prevention, health promotion, health education, emergency care, and managing chronic health problems.

- An individualized health plan describes the school-based care of the child with a chronic condition for optimal participation in school and class activities.

- Nurse consultants to childcare settings assist the administrators in establishing the childcare center's policies for health practices, teach staff about safe health practices, and monitor health practices. They may also assist caregivers to identify and minimize hazards that could injure children.

- Nurses in camps assess and improve the safety of the children's environment, provide nursing care to children with acute and chronic illnesses and injuries, administer medications, and plan activities to promote health.

- Home care nursing goals include promoting or restoring the health of the child while attempting to minimize the effects of the disability and illness as well as promoting child or family self-care capacity in the home.

- Community health nurses help the population obtain health services through assessing community needs and resources, advocating for needed resources and services, and then developing health programs to address the needs of children and their families.

- A community assessment is a process of compiling data about a community's health status and resources for the purpose of public health planning to address a population's health needs.

- The emergency medical services (EMS) system is the organized community-based public health response to ensure that children and adults with acute illnesses and injuries receive emergency care and timely transport to the hospital emergency department.

- Pediatric nurses have a significant role in working with families in preparing for a disaster. They can help families develop a disaster plan, use developmentally appropriate information to talk with children about what to do when disasters occur, and provide direct care in a disaster shelter.

Clinical Reasoning in Action

INTRODUCTION

Return to the scenario at the beginning of the chapter. Four-month-old Torrey, her brother Nathan, and their parents have come to the health center for Torrey's health assessment and immunizations. Torrey is growing and developing well. Nathan seems to have adapted to having a baby sister, and his parents have described their strategy to make him feel secure within the family.

DESCRIPTION

Torrey's parents have been responsive to health promotion and health maintenance recommendations provided by the nurse, as well as suggestions related to childcare arrangements for when the mother returns to work. However, as hurricane season is beginning and the family lives in a town near the coast of the Gulf of Mexico, the nurse spends a little extra time discussing the resources needed for sheltering at home during a disaster as well as preparing for evacuation if necessary.

DISCUSSION

1. Describe the nursing interventions that should be provided to Torrey and her family in the health center serving as Torrey's healthcare home.

2. What preparation should the health center have in case Torrey has a rare serious allergic reaction to a given vaccine? What information is provided to the parents to prepare them for common vaccine reactions?

3. Discuss important aspects of childcare that the parents should consider before selecting a childcare provider for Torrey.

4. List the supplies and resources that Torrey's parents should have on hand to be prepared for a natural disaster.

NCLEX-RN® Review

1. The school nurse has been notified that an 8-year-old who has had a tracheostomy for 2 years will be attending one of the schools to which the nurse is assigned. Which best describes the nurse's role in this situation?
   1. Inform parents they will need to hire a registered nurse to stay with the child at school.
   2. Notify administration that a child with a tracheostomy is not safe attending the school.
   3. Provide training for teachers and health aides to provide appropriate care for the child.
   4. Ask that the nurse only have responsibility for the school the child will be attending.

2. After a chemical explosion, the community nurse arrives at the local shelter to assess pediatric displaced victims. What is the nurse's main concern?
   1. Whether the children were actively exposed to any chemical agents
   2. The existence of posttraumatic stress syndrome in the displaced children
   3. The fear the children have experienced both during and after the explosion
   4. The requests for video games and board games from the children

3. The nurse is preparing a disaster education plan for school-age children to discuss fire prevention and fire evacuation planning. What information is priority in the plan?
   1. It is essential for the child to stay with the family at the time of the fire.
   2. The child and family need to have a definite evacuation plan in place.
   3. The child should stay indoors in the event of a fire.
   4. It is important the child remember to drink more water than usual after a fire.

4. A school nurse is packing a portable emergency bag for a potential disaster. Which indicates the need for further education in disaster preparedness?
   1. A list of staff and students and their location
   2. A blueprint of the school and its grounds
   3. Handheld portable radios with batteries
   4. A portable automatic external defibrillator

See Appendix I ⊘ for answers.

References

Alkon, A., Bernzweig, J., To, K., Wolff, M., & Mackie, J. F. (2009). Child care health consultation improves health and safety policies and practices. *Academic Pediatrics, 9*(5), 366–370.

American Academy of Pediatrics. (2008). *The youngest victims: Disaster preparedness to meet children's needs.* Retrieved from http://www.aap.org/disasters/pdf/Youngest-Victims-Final.pdf

American Academy of Pediatrics. (2010). *Safety and prevention: Getting your family prepared for disasters.* Retrieved from http://www.healthychildren.org/English/safety-prevention/at-home/pages/Getting-Your-Family-Prepared-for-a-Disaster.aspx?nfstatus=401&nftoken=00000000-0000-0000-0000-0000-00000000&nfstatusdescription=ERROR%3a+No+local+token

American Academy of Pediatrics Committee on Pediatric Emergency Medicine. (2007). Preparation for emergencies in the offices of pediatricians and pediatric primary care providers. *Pediatrics, 120*(1), 200–212.

American Academy of Pediatrics Council on School Health. (2008). Role of the school nurse in providing school health services. *Pediatrics, 121*(5), 1052–1056.

American Nurses Association & National Association of School Nurses. (2011). *School nursing: Scope and standards of professional school nursing practice* (2nd ed., pp. 12–14). Silver Spring, MD: nursesbooks.org.

Boroughs, D., & Dougherty, J. A. (2009). Technology-dependent children in the home. *Home Healthcare Nurse, 27*(1), 37–42.

Broussard, L., & Meaux, J. (2007). Camp nursing: Rewards and challenges. *Pediatric Nursing, 33*(3), 238–242.

Cervasio, K. (2010). The role of the pediatric home health care nurse. *Home Healthcare Nurse, 28*(7), 424–431.

Clark, M. J. (2008). *Community health nursing* (5th ed.). Upper Saddle River, NJ: Prentice Hall.

Clay, D., Farris, K., McCarthy, A. M., Kelly, M. W., & Howarth, R. (2008). Family perceptions of medication administration at school: Errors, risk factors, and consequences. *Journal of School Nursing, 24*(2), 95–102.

Crowley, A. A., & Kulikowich, J. M. (2009). Impact of training on child care health consultant knowledge and practice. *Pediatric Nursing, 35*(2), 93–100.

Engelke, M. K., Guttu, M., Warren, M. B., & Swanson, M. (2008). School nurse case management for children with chronic illness: Health, academic, and quality of life outcomes. *Journal of School Nursing, 24*(4), 205–214.

Gerald, L. B., McClure, L. A., Mangan, J. M., Harrington, K. F., Gibson, L., Erwin, S., . . . Grad, R. (2009). Increasing adherence to inhaled steroid therapy among schoolchildren: Randomized, controlled trial of school-based supervised asthma therapy. *Pediatrics, 123*(2), 466–474.

Halterman, J. S., Szilagyi, P. G., Fisher, S. G., Fagnano, M., Tremblay, P., Conn, K. M., . . . Borrelli, B. (2011). Randomized controlled trial to improve care for urban children with asthma. *Archives of Pediatrics and Adolescent Medicine, 165*(3), 262–268.

Hegenbarth, M. A., & the Committee on Drugs. (2010). Preparing for pediatric emergencies: Drugs to consider. *Pediatrics, 121*(2), 433–443.

Henretig, F. M. (2009). Preparation for terrorist threats: Biologic and chemical agents. *Clinical Pediatric Emergency Medicine, 10*(3), 130–135.

Heon, D., & Foltin, G. L. (2009). Principles of pediatric decontamination. *Clinical Pediatric Emergency Medicine, 10*(3), 186–194.

Kaul, T. (2011). Helping African American children self-manage asthma: The importance of self-efficacy. *Journal of School Health, 81*(1), 29–33.

Kelly, F. (2010). Keeping PEDIATRICS in pediatric disaster management: Before, during, and in the aftermath of complex emergencies. *Critical Care Nursing Clinics of America, 22*, 465–480.

Lear, J. G., Barnwell, E. A., & Behrens, D. (2008). Healthcare reform and school-based health care. *Public Health Reports, 123*, 704–708.

Maughan, E. (2009a). Part I—Factors associated with school nurse ratios: An analysis of state data. *Journal of School Nursing, 25*(3), 214–221.

Maughan, E. (2009b). Part II—Factors associated with school nurse ratios: Key state informants' perceptions. *Journal of School Nursing, 25*(4), 292–301.

McKenzie, H. (2011). Children's health insurance programs: Do they provide the coverage that is needed? *Home Healthcare Nurse, 29*(2), 124–125.

McNall, M. A., Lichty, L. F., & Mavis, B. (2010). The impact of school-based health centers on the health outcomes of middle school and high school students. *American Journal of Public Health, 100*(9), 1604–1610.

Mink, C. M., & Yeh, S. (2009). Infections in childcare facilities and schools. *Pediatrics in Review, 30*(7), 259–268.

Murray, J. S. (2010). Responding to the psychosocial needs of children and families in disasters. *Critical Care Nursing Clinics of North America, 22*, 481–491.

Nager, A. L. (2009). Family reunification—Concepts and challenges. *Clinical Pediatric Emergency Medicine, 10*(3), 195–207.

Raymond, J. A. (2009). The integration of children dependent on medical technology into public schools. *Journal of School Nursing, 25*(3), 186–194.

Resha, C. (2010). Delegation in the school setting: Is it a safe practice? *Online Journal of Issues in Nursing, 15*(2). doi:10.3912/OJIN.Vol15No02Man05

Robert Wood Johnson Foundation. (2010). *Unlocking the potential of school nursing: Keeping children healthy, in school, and ready to learn.* Retrieved from http://www.rwjf.org/files/research/cnf14.pdf

Rosenthal, M. S., Crowley, A. A., & Curry, L. (2009). Promoting child development and behavioral health: Family child care providers' perspectives. *Journal of Pediatric Health Care, 23*(5), 289–297.

Scalzo, A. J., Lehman-Huskamp, K. L., Sinks, G. A., & Keenan, W. J. (2008). Disaster preparedness and toxic exposures in children. *Clinical Pediatric Emergency Medicine, 9*, 47–60.

Schlitt, J. J., Juszczak, L. J., & Eichner, N. H. (2008). Current status of state policies that support school-based health centers. *Public Health Reports, 123*, 731–738.

Schonfeld, D. J., & Gurwitch, R. H. (2009). Addressing disaster mental health needs of children: Practical guidance for pediatric emergency health care providers. *Clinical Pediatric Emergency Medicine, 10*(3), 208–215.

Sender, S. (2011). Pediatric home care: The best-kept secret. *Home Healthcare Nurse, 29*(2), 63.

Sherry, J. S. (2008). An evaluation of elementary school nutrition practices and policies in a Southern Illinois county. *Journal of School Nursing, 24*(4), 222–228.

Siegel, D. (2009). Preparation for terrorist threats: Radiation injury. *Clinical Pediatric Emergency Medicine, 10*(3), 136–139.

Soleimanpour, S., Geierstanger, S. P., Kaller, S., McCarter, V., & Brindis, C. D. (2010). The role of school health centers in health care access and client outcomes. *American Journal of Public Health, 100*(9), 1597–1603.

Tracy, M. A. (2008). Kids and chemicals: A pediatric disaster. *Journal of Emergency Nursing, 34*(3), 266–267.

U.S. Department of Health and Human Services, Office of Disease Prevention and Health Promotion. (2010). *Healthy People.* Washington, DC: Author. Retrieved from http://www.healthypeople.gov/Default.htm

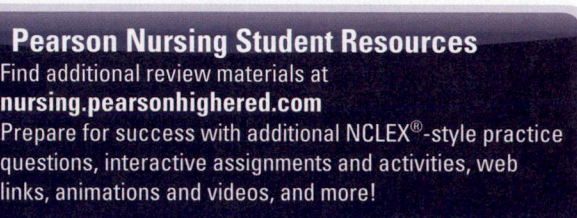

Pearson Nursing Student Resources

Find additional review materials at
nursing.pearsonhighered.com
Prepare for success with additional NCLEX®-style practice questions, interactive assignments and activities, web links, animations and videos, and more!

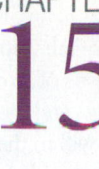

Nursing Care of the Hospitalized Child

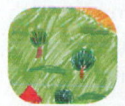 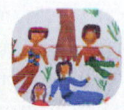 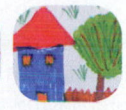

Learning Outcomes

After completing this chapter, you will be able to:

1. Compare and contrast the child's understanding of health and illness according to the child's developmental level.

2. Explain the effects of and response to illness and hospitalization on children and their families.

3. Describe the child's and family's adaptation to hospitalization.

4. Apply family-centered care principles to the hospital setting.

5. Identify nursing strategies to minimize the stressors related to hospitalization.

6. Integrate the concept of family presence during procedures and nursing strategies to prepare the family.

7. Summarize strategies for preparing children and families for discharge from the hospital setting.

8. Evaluate the effectiveness of teaching strategies used with the hospitalized child and his or her family.

> "Why do they need to take my tonsils out? They're fine where they are!"
>
> —*Tiona, age 5*

Five-year-old Tiona Lewallen has a history of frequent tonsillitis and is scheduled for a tonsillectomy and adenoidectomy in the morning. Her mother has brought her in today for pre-operative evaluation and instruction. Tiona has no other health problems. Her experience with health care is limited to well-child checkups and immunizations as well as several visits to the otolaryngologist in the past year. She has no prior hospitalizations. Tiona will return at 6:30 a.m. for surgery. She will be admitted to the pediatric day short-stay unit for a few hours following surgery and will then be discharged home as long as she is able to drink fluids and take oral pain medication. How should the nurse assess what Tiona knows about her surgery? What techniques should be used to teach Tiona about the surgery? What instructions should Tiona's mother receive from the nurse in the preoperative clinic related to care prior to surgery?

Hospitalization, whether it is elective, planned in advance, or the result of an emergency or trauma, is stressful for children of all ages and their families. Because most pediatric conditions can be managed within the home and community setting, hospitalization is not always required to manage the child with an illness. However, those children who are hospitalized usually have a high level of illness acuity as the complexity of hospitalized children has increased over the past several years (Stubenrauch, 2010). (See Table 1–2 in Chapter 1 🔗 for the most common reasons for hospitalization in children.)

Hospitalized children experience a variety of emotions as they are in an unknown environment, surrounded by strangers, unfamiliar equipment, and frightening sights and sounds. These children are subjected to unfamiliar procedures, some of which are invasive or painful and may even require surgery. For both children and families, routines are disrupted and normal coping strategies are tested.

Nurses today are challenged to provide individualized care for the hospitalized child with complex medical conditions, acute illnesses, or injury. As a key aspect of that role, nurses must address the psychosocial and developmental concerns that accompany hospitalization. To minimize the stress of hospitalization, nurses provide support and education to children and their families before, during, and after hospitalization.

During hospitalization, nurses use a family-centered approach and work collaboratively with parents to implement various strategies that promote coping and adaptation and to prepare children for necessary procedures. Nurses also collaborate with members of a multidisciplinary team and partner with families to prepare them for discharge home or transfer to a long-term care or rehabilitation facility.

EFFECTS OF HOSPITALIZATION ON CHILDREN AND THEIR FAMILIES

Children's Understanding of Health and Illness

Can you remember as a child thinking that yelling at your mother caused your strep throat? Young children have limited knowledge about the body and its relation to health and illness. They do not understand what causes them to get sick. Their understanding is based primarily on their cognitive ability at various developmental stages and on previous experiences with healthcare professionals. As children become older, their concept of illness becomes more sophisticated and they demonstrate an understanding of the cause of illness (Drahota & Malcarne, 2008). For example, perhaps as an adolescent you believed that you would never become ill or have an accident. Or, maybe you feared being in a car crash like that of a friend. Table 15–1 provides a discussion of children's understanding of health and illness according to their developmental level.

Hospitalization and the accompanying medical procedures are stressful for children, especially very young children such as toddlers and preschoolers. The child's attempts to deal with these stressors affect both the psychologic and physiologic well-being of the child. Infants, toddlers, and preschoolers lack the cognitive skills to understand hospitalization and are the most likely age groups to exhibit regressive behaviors. Young children have fears and anxieties related to things such as the dark, strangers, and monsters. A hospital's unfamiliar environment can exacerbate those anxieties. Significant stressors for hospitalized children of all ages include:

- Separation from parents, the primary caretaker, or peers
- Loss of self-control, autonomy, and privacy
- Painful or invasive procedures
- Fear of bodily injury and disfigurement

Table 15–2 highlights key stressors of hospitalization for children at each developmental stage. See Evidence-Based Practice: Fears in Children Related to Hospitalization.

Nursing care of the hospitalized child focuses on minimizing the child's fears, anxieties, and disruption of the usual routine, and supporting the family through the stressful experience. Strategies include minimizing separation anxiety, loss of control, pain related to procedures, and fear. See Partnering with Families: Stress Reduction Techniques.

Newborn

Newborns requiring hospitalization are generally admitted to the neonatal intensive care unit (NICU). In some circumstances, an infant that is a few days old may be admitted to the general pediatric unit because of jaundice or concerns about sepsis. At a time when

TABLE 15–1	Children's Understanding of Health and Illness According to Developmental Level		
INFANT	**TODDLER AND PRESCHOOLER**	**SCHOOL-AGE CHILD**	**ADOLESCENT**
By approximately 6 months of age, infants have developed an awareness of themselves as separate from their mother or father.	Toddlers and preschoolers are beginning to understand illness, but not its cause.	School-age children understand how germs are spread.	Adolescents are increasingly aware of the physiologic, psychologic, and behavioral causes of illness and injury.
They are unaware of the effects of illness.	Preschoolers have a beginning understanding of germs but not how they spread.	Older school-age children have a more realistic understanding of the reasons for illness and are able to understand more about disease and how body organs are affected.	They understand that the disease may involve several causes and effects and that multiple organs or body parts may be involved.
They feel anxious when approached by strangers.	The child's concept of the body usually is limited to names and locations of some body parts.	The school-age child's concept of body parts and function is maturing.	The adolescent understands how symptoms can be related to certain organ functions in the body.
	The child's concept of internal organs and body functions is vague.		Adolescents are concerned with appearance and perceive an illness or injury in terms of its effect on their body image.
	They may view illness as a form of punishment for bad behavior or something magical.		
	Events that occur just before the onset of the illness may be mistakenly associated with the illness.		

Source: Data from Drahota, A., & Malcarne, V. L. (2008). Concepts of illness in children: A comparison between children with and without intellectual disability. Intellectual and Developmental Disabilities, 46(1), 44–53; Myant, K. A., & Williams, J. M. (2008). What do children learn about biology from factual information? A comparison of interventions to improve understanding of contagious illnesses. British Journal of Educational Psychology, 78, 223–244; Myant, K. A., & Williams, J. M. (2005). Children's concepts of health and illness: Understanding of contagious illnesses, non-contagious illnesses and injuries. Journal of Health Psychology, 10(6), 805–819; Piko, B. F., & Bak, J. (2006). Children's perception of health and illness: Images and lay concepts in preadolescence. Health Education Research: Theory & Practice, 21(5), 643–653.

TABLE 15–2 Stressors of Hospitalization for Children at Various Developmental Stages

DEVELOPMENTAL STAGES AND STRESSORS	RESPONSES	NURSING MANAGEMENT
Infant		
Separation anxiety	Sleep–awake cycle disrupted	■ Encourage parental presence.
Stranger anxiety	Feeding routines disrupted	■ Adhere to the infant's home routine as much as possible.
Painful, invasive procedures	Displays excessive irritability	■ Utilize topical anesthetics or preprocedural sedation as prescribed.
Immobilization		
Sleep deprivation, sensory overload		■ Promote a quiet environment and reduce excess stimuli.
Toddler		
Separation anxiety	Cries if parents leave the bedside	■ Encourage parental presence.
Loss of self-control	Is frightened if forced to lie supine	■ Allow parents to hold the child in their lap for examinations and procedures when possible.
Immobilization	Wonders why parents don't come to the rescue	■ Allow choices when possible.
Painful, invasive procedures	Associates pain with punishment	■ Utilize topical anesthetics or preprocedural sedation as prescribed.
Bodily injury or mutilation		■ Explain all procedures using simple developmentally appropriate language.
Fear of the dark		■ Provide a night-light.
Preschooler		
Separation anxiety and fear of abandonment	Displays difficulty separating reality from fantasy	■ Encourage parental presence.
Loss of self-control	Fears ghosts and monsters	■ Allow choices when possible.
Bodily injury or mutilation	Fears body parts will leak out when skin is not intact	■ Utilize topical anesthetics or preprocedural sedation as prescribed.
Painful, invasive procedures	Fears that tubes are permanent	■ Explain all procedures.
Fear of the dark and monsters	Demonstrates withdrawal, projection, aggression, regression	■ Provide a night-light or flashlight.
School-Age Child		
Loss of control	Displays increased sensitivity to the environment	■ Encourage parental participation.
Loss of privacy and control over body functions	Demonstrates detailed recall of events to self and other patients	■ Allow the child choices when possible.
Bodily injury		■ Explain all procedures and offer reassurance.
Separation from family and friends		■ Utilize topical anesthetics or preprocedural sedation as prescribed.
Painful, invasive procedures		■ Encourage peer interaction via the Internet, phone calls, and other methods of communication.
Fear of death		
Adolescent		
Loss of control	Displays denial, regression, withdrawal, intellectualization, projection, displacement	■ Include the adolescent in the plan of care.
Fear of altered body image, disfigurement, disability, and death		■ Encourage discussion of fears and anxieties.
Separation from peer group		■ Explain all procedures.
Loss of privacy and identity		■ Ask the adolescent his or her desire for parental involvement.
		■ Encourage peer interaction.

newborns are usually being held and comforted by parents in the safety of their own home, these newborns are instead exposed to a busy, high-technology area and multiple healthcare professionals.

The NICU environment often adds to the anxiety of parents who are already dealing with the fear of losing their child. Depending on the neonate's condition, the presence of ventilatory support and other technical equipment—and even the parent's own fears—may interfere with the parent–newborn attachment phase. As a result, hospitalized neonates may have less physical contact and nurturing than the newborn at home. Because failure to form parental–newborn attachment can have lifelong negative effects on the neonate, nurses should assist parents in establishing physical contact with the newborn. Nursing care to support the parents and newborn involves:

■ Explaining and emphasizing the importance of parent–newborn attachment and bonding to the parents

■ Demonstrating how to touch, hold, feed, and stimulate the newborn

■ Explaining the purpose of all equipment and procedures to the parents

Even neonates with numerous monitoring and supportive lines and tubes can be gently stroked, verbally stimulated, and held when possible. Be sure to incorporate quiet times into the newborn's schedule to allow for periods of rest. Encourage the family to remain with and be active participants in care of the hospitalized child. If parents are unable to remain at the hospital, encourage them to visit the newborn as often as possible.

Infant

By about 6 months of age, infants have developed an awareness of themselves as separate from their mother or father. They are able to identify primary caretakers and may feel anxious when in contact with

Evidence-Based Practice — Fears in Children Related to Hospitalization

PROBLEM

Children experience many fears related to hospitalization and medical care. These fears vary depending on the child's developmental age and experience with the healthcare system.

EVIDENCE

In the past several years, many research studies have focused on the child's response to procedures and hospitalization and how best to prepare children of different ages. Recent studies have focused specifically on the child's view of hospitalization, the impact of this event, and specific stressors and fears related to this experience.

Wilson, Megel, Enenbach, et al. (2010) explored the views of 93 children ages 5 to 9 years related to hospitalization. Both hospitalized and never-hospitalized children were included in the study. The Barton Hospital Picture Test, a tool consisting of eight drawings related to situations that occur in the hospital, was shown to the children. The children were asked to tell a story about the pictures. The main theme that emerged from the stories was fear of being alone. Other feelings included being scared, mad, sad, bored, and lonely. The stories also indicated that the children wanted to be protected from uncertainty and scary things, and they wanted companions because they were not at home.

A study by Salmela, Salanterä, and Aronen (2009) examined fears related to the hospital in 90 children ages 4 to 6 years. The children were interviewed in either a kindergarten classroom or a hospital setting. Interviews were semistructured and accompanied by pictures of sick children, doctors, nurses, and medical equipment. An average of 6.48 fears were expressed by hospitalized children while an average of 4.2 fears were expressed by the children in kindergarten. The largest category of fears (29%) was those related to nursing interventions such as shots, sample taking, and tests. Fears related to being a patient comprised 28% and were primarily related to pain, staying in the hospital, being admitted to the hospital, and having symptoms of an illness. Fears related to the developmental stage of the child accounted for 14% and were related primarily to being left alone, imagination, and loss of autonomy.

A smaller study by Forsner, Jansson, and Söderberg (2009) examined the meaning of being afraid of medical care in nine children ages 7 to 11 years.

Children included in the study were identified by their parent as being afraid of visiting a doctor or a nurse. Experience with health care ranged from office visits for immunizations to frequent contact with health care due to chronic conditions. Children were asked to tell about an experience in which they were afraid of a doctor or nurse and were videotaped in either an actual appointment with the doctor or in a play session of a scary experience. A reflective conversation with the children in which the video was discussed was the final aspect of the study. This study found that children were afraid of medical "stuff" and staff, and it was likened to being threatened by a monster. The children felt unsafe around doctors and nurses and felt like the medical equipment was designed to hurt them. They felt that although they were afraid, the adults (doctors and nurses) ignored them and performed the procedure anyway. The children felt overpowered, and they were hoping to be rescued. While the children in this study were afraid of health care, other themes that emerged included hoping for good (trusting they would not be hurt), being received (caring staff made them feel safe), receiving liberating aid (being consoled or reassured), and facing the feared (playing with equipment).

IMPLICATIONS

Research demonstrates that children have fears related to health care and hospitalization. These fears vary among preschool and school-age children, and those in well settings versus the hospital setting. Children fear medical staff, equipment, pain, and procedures, and they fear being left alone. Policies that provide open visitation for parents and include them in the care of the child will decrease fears related to being alone. Therapeutic nursing interventions that provide developmentally psychosocial care and education to hospitalized children are essential to decrease fear and anxiety related to staff and procedures.

CRITICAL THINKING APPLICATION

How can children in school settings be prepared for future encounters with health care? Describe policies that promote parental presence for hospitalized children. How can fears related to medical staff, equipment, pain, and procedures be reduced in hospitalized preschool and school-age children?

---

strangers. Hospitalization can be a traumatic time for an infant, particularly if the parents are not staying with the child. Infants can sense the anxiety their parents are experiencing during a hospitalization.

Clinical Tip

Parents often feel guilty for leaving their infant, especially if he or she protests adamantly or cries upon their return. Reassure the parents that this protest is a normal behavior that illustrates a healthy parent–infant attachment. Support them as they leave and provide information when they return about the child's activities during their absence.

Common stressors to the infant include painful procedures, immobilization of extremities, and the sleep deprivation caused by the disruption of the infant's normal sleep patterns and routines. However, the most common stressor of hospitalization for the infant is separation from parents, which is manifested by **separation anxiety.** Bowlby identified three phases of separation anxiety exhibited in young children who were separated from their mothers for long periods. This theory remains an essential component of family-centered nursing care and must be incorporated as policies related to family presence are formulated (Jolley & Shields, 2009). Characteristic behaviors of children in the three phases of separation anxiety are listed in Table 15–3. Infants as well as toddlers between the ages of 6 and 18 months who are hospitalized often display some of these behaviors, particularly if parents are unable to remain with the child.

In addition to separation anxiety, children between 6 and 18 months of age may display **stranger anxiety** (wariness of strangers) when confronted with unfamiliar healthcare professionals.

Just like parent–newborn attachment, parent–infant attachment is critical to the infant's developmental achievements (see Chapter 5 🔗). Encourage family members to be active participants in the care of the hospitalized infant through touch, sight, and sound. Infants get satisfaction from meeting their oral needs, so the parents and nurses

TABLE 15–3	Stages of Separation Anxiety	
PROTEST	**DESPAIR**	**DENIAL (DETACHMENT)**
Screaming, crying	Sadness	Lack of protest when parents leave
Clinging to parents	Quiet, appear to have "settled in"	Appearance of being happy and content with everyone
May resist attempts by other adults to comfort them	Withdrawal or compliant behavior	Show interest in surroundings
	Crying when parents return	Close relationships not established

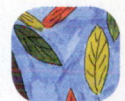

Partnering with Families

Stress Reduction Techniques

Strategies the nurse and family can implement to reduce the hospitalized child's stress include:

1. Encouraging recreation and physical activity (if appropriate for the child and not restricted due to condition)
2. Ensuring that the child obtains sufficient rest
3. Ensuring parental or other significant person's presence
4. Maintaining the child's usual routines

RECREATION

Newborn and Infant
- Provide developmentally appropriate mobiles, rattles, and music boxes.
- Hold and talk soothingly to the newborn or infant.
- For the older infant, play "peek-a-boo" and similar games.

Toddler and Preschooler
- Provide developmentally appropriate toys.
- Encourage coloring, singing, use of music, and games.
- Take the toddler or preschooler to the playroom if possible.

School-Age Child
- Encourage participation in peer group activities if possible.
- Provide favorite collection items or encourage a new hobby (collecting stamps or coins, building models, or playing board games for the child who has activity restriction).
- Provide music, video games, or computer access.
- Encourage the child to visit the playroom or recreation room and interact with other hospitalized school-age children.

REST
- Promote a calm, quiet environment to allow for rest periods.
- Establish rituals to help the child prepare for sleep at night—for example, bathing, brushing teeth, reading a story, playing a quiet board game, or watching a favorite TV show (if necessary, record show to play at appropriate time).

RELATIONSHIPS
- Arrange for visits from family members, including siblings.
- Encourage visits from friends.
- If friends are unable to visit, encourage writing, calling, email, or live computer chat to maintain communication.
- Encourage school-age children and adolescents to attend peer support groups.

ROUTINES
- Ask families to inform nursing staff of the child's normal routines.
- Provide transition objects from home, such as a blanket or favorite toy.
- Talk with the older school-age child and adolescent to determine his or her wishes regarding routines (e.g., if the child prefers to perform hygiene in the mornings or evenings).
- Inform the child or adolescent about anticipated changes to provide an opportunity to adapt.

---

should provide sources for oral stimulation, such as pacifiers and age-appropriate teething toys. The infant should be rocked and touched with light stroking to provide tactile stimulation for developmental growth. However, minimize excessive noise and prolonged stimuli to allow the infant periods of rest.

Encourage parents to stay with the hospitalized infant. If family members are unable to remain at the hospital, encourage them to visit their infant as often as possible. Explain and emphasize the importance of parent–infant attachment and bonding to the parents.

Clinical Tip

Children encounter many members of the healthcare team, in addition to other hospital personnel, when hospitalized. Children ages 6 to 18 months perceive these people as strangers and may cry when someone new enters the room. As the child sees a person over and over again, the stranger anxiety for that person subsides. Providing consistent caregivers as much as possible will limit the number of "strangers" that the child encounters while hospitalized.

Toddler

Toddlers are the group most at risk for a stressful experience as a result of illness and hospitalization. This age group is old enough to understand that their routine has been disrupted, but they do not understand why. Separation from parents is the major stressor, and they protest vigorously when their parents depart. When one or both parents cannot be present, they can leave mementos to comfort the child. These might include a piece of cloth scented with the mother's favorite perfume or father's cologne (unless the child has a respiratory condition or another contraindication for this intervention), an object belonging to a parent, or an audio or video recording with messages from the parents.

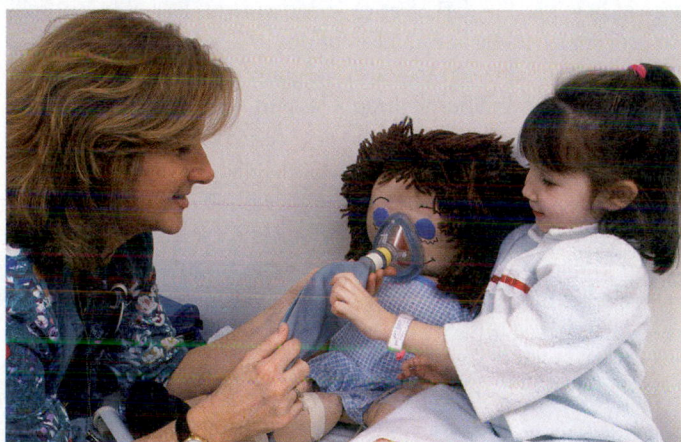

FIGURE 15–1 ■ The pediatric nurse wears a colorful uniform to decrease anxiety associated with white uniforms.

Clinical Tip

Dress code policies that allow or require pediatric nurses to wear colorful uniforms eliminate the anxiety related to "white uniforms" that has existed in the past. Uniforms with familiar characters may serve as a source of comfort and distraction for the child (Figure 15–1 ■ and Box 15–1).

Disruption of routine also causes stress for the toddler. The nurse encourages parents to remain present as much as possible for important rituals such as toileting, carrying out bedtime routines, and singing favorite nursery rhymes. Autonomy is a developmental task of the toddler (see Chapter 5 ⊘). Having their activities limited

BOX 15–1	Research: Uniforms

A study conducted by Roohafza, Pirnia, Sadeghi, et al. (2009) examined anxiety levels of 92 children ages 7 to 15 years who were exposed to nurses in white or colorful uniforms during their hospital stay of 3 to 5 days. Anxiety levels were assessed on admission and at discharge. The children who were exposed to nurses in white uniforms demonstrated higher levels of anxiety at discharge than those exposed to nurses in colorful uniforms.

and being confined especially threaten children in this age group. When possible, maintain the toddler's normal home routines for bathing and other activities. Allow the toddler to have choices when possible, such as choosing the color of Jell-O or which gown or pajamas to wear.

In addition to parental separation and schedule disruption, common stressors for the toddler include fear of pain, fear of invasive procedures, fear of change, and fear of mutilation. The parents' presence plays a large role in diminishing these fears. In addition, therapeutic play with simple explanations can diminish these fears.

Clinical Tip

Toddlers may challenge a nurse by refusing to cooperate with treatments and procedures, including physical assessments. To diffuse such confrontations, encourage cooperation by offering the toddler some sense of control. For example, a nurse might comment, "Once I have listened to your heart, lungs, and stomach you can choose whether you want to ride in the wagon or be pushed in the toy car to the playroom."

Preschooler

The greatest stressors for preschoolers are their fear of being alone, fear of being in the dark, fear of abandonment, fear of loss of self-control related to the body and emotions, and fear of bodily injury or mutilation. Preschoolers may also feel guilty about being sick, or they may view illness and hospitalization as punishment.

Similar to the toddler, preschoolers desire a normal routine. The nurse can partner with the family to maintain routines as much as possible. Developmentally, preschoolers exhibit a sense of initiative (see Chapter 5 🔗) as they explore the world around them. To promote that initiative, the nurse can encourage the preschool child's independence by offering choices such as "Do you want to take the red medicine or the purple medicine first?"

Parents should be encouraged to stay with the child if possible. For those who cannot stay, preschoolers need to know when to expect their parents to return to the hospital. Because most preschoolers lack a concept of time measurements like "2 hours," "half past four," or "3 o'clock," respond with simpler statements of time, such as "after supper" or "before breakfast." Encourage parents to make telephone calls to the preschooler if possible. Some parents are able to make calls from work, and preschoolers get a sense of security from hearing their parent's voice confirming that they will return to the hospital.

Parents often believe it is better to leave the hospital room after their child has fallen asleep so their departure will not stress the child. In fact, the opposite is true. If a child awakens to find the parent gone unexpectedly, he or she may become anxious and develop a lack of trust. Instead, encourage parents to tell their child when they need to leave and why (e.g., has to go to work or go home). By providing honest information to the child, the parents demonstrate that they can be trusted.

School-Age Child

The school-age child relies on parents and others for support and understanding during stressful events and procedures. Although school-age children attempt to maintain their composure during painful or invasive procedures, generally they still require a great deal of support. Major sources of stress for hospitalized school-age children include:

- Loss of control related to body functions
- Privacy issues
- Fear of bodily injury, pain, and concerns related to death
- Separation from family and friends

School-age children understand concepts, so parents who cannot remain at the bedside are encouraged to tell the child when they will return. Parents are encouraged to be available for telephone calls to provide support and comfort to their child. Stressful procedures can lead to regression or other behavioral changes, although this is less likely than with younger patients. Inform the parents that this behavior is normal during stressful situations.

Developmentally, school-age children exhibit a sense of industry (see Chapter 5 🔗), taking pride in their achievements at home, at school, and in sports. To foster that sense of industry, allow these children to participate in their care as much as possible. Encourage them to continue with schoolwork and to engage in creative outlets such as art or crafts.

Adolescent

Major stressors for hospitalized adolescents include loss of independence, control, and privacy; fear of bodily injury or changes in body image; fear of disability, pain, and even death; and separation from peers, home, and school. Preoccupation with appearance and body image are paramount in this age group. By offering education and explanations that focus on these issues, nurses can provide significant reassurance to the adolescent. Adolescents often try to maintain independence and rigid self-control when undergoing painful and invasive procedures. Because hospitalization may increase dependence on their parents, adolescents may respond with frustration and anger. The nurse who respects the adolescent's desire for privacy and independence is often successful in establishing a trusting relationship and assisting the adolescent to cope with the hospitalization and illness. Encourage the adolescent to discuss thoughts and feelings about experiences. Careful listening by the nurse is essential in establishing a positive rapport.

Adolescents are in the process of establishing their identity and becoming independent of their parents' influence (see Chapter 5 🔗), so control over aspects of their care is important. Partner with the family and multidisciplinary team to ensure the adolescent is an active participant in decisions and the plan of care. Privacy and modesty are major concerns, as adolescents' physical characteristics are rapidly changing. To demonstrate respect for their feelings, knock on the door before entering and ask permission before conducting assessments or other procedures. By allowing choices in clothing, hair, and music, the nurse can acknowledge the importance of the adolescent's self-image.

The peer group is a major influence in adolescents' lives. Allowing flexible visiting hours for friends helps teens maintain their social network and provides needed support. When friends are not able to visit, providing teens with Internet access offers a means of accessing their friends for support. Encouraging participation in recreation and teen lounge facilities available during hospitalization provides the adolescent with additional peer group support opportunities.

Family Responses to Hospitalization

The illness and hospitalization of a child disrupt a family's usual routines. Parental roles change when the child is hospitalized and care is being provided by nursing staff. Roles may be altered as one parent remains at the hospital with the child while the other parent or siblings take on additional tasks at home. Family members may experience anxiety and fear, especially when the outcome is unknown or a potentially serious health condition prompted the hospitalization. Parents who perceive their child is in pain find the experience difficult and require support. Family members' ability to cope can be challenged by:

- A serious emergency
- A lengthy illness
- A chronic condition
- A poor prognosis
- Lack of family support
- Lack of financial or community services

The stress on parents can be compounded by the burden of missed work, additional expenses, and concerns about feeding and caring for children at home. (See Chapter 17 🔗 for a description of nursing support for the family of a child with a life-threatening illness or injury.)

Parents have unique needs and stressors; therefore, nurses should individualize care based on these specific needs. Needs frequently identified by both nurses and parents of hospitalized children include the need (Shields, Young, & McCann, 2008):

- For measures to relieve anxiety
- To be able to speak in private to the physician about their child's condition
- For a designated place for parents to sleep
- For information related to discharge and home care
- To be able to spend time with other children

It is essential that nurses assess parental needs and attend to those needs in order to establish a trusting relationship. Parents who have support from nursing staff have less anxiety, have more self-confidence, and are better equipped to make decisions and participate in their child's care.

Nurses also need to be alert to family members' cultural views about health, illness, and the causation of illness, which can influence their response to hospitalization and the family's management of the experience. Cultural influences may also determine which family member is the decision maker regarding healthcare practices, and provide guidelines for acceptable treatments (Spector, 2009).

Siblings' Experience

The siblings of a hospitalized child may receive little attention from the parents who are overwhelmed and anxious about their hospitalized child's health. Factors that affect the sibling's adjustment include (Gursky, 2007; O'Brien, Duffy, & Nicholl, 2009):

- Age
- Gender
- Developmental level
- Perception of the illness
- Severity of the illness
- Prior experience
- Information received about the illness
- Social support
- Parental stress

Younger siblings who do not understand the causes of illness and hospitalization may feel guilty about fighting with or being mean to their brother or sister in the past. Some siblings may fear becoming ill themselves. Some may believe that they played a role in the child's illness or injury and need reassurance that they did not cause it. If siblings did in some way contribute to their brother's or sister's illness or injury, help them to cope with their guilt by providing them with an opportunity to discuss these feelings. Depending on the situation, some may need mental health counseling. Siblings often have nightmares about the illness or injury their brother or sister has sustained and about the ill child dying (see Chapters 17 and 18 🔗).

As hospitalization causes family roles and routines to change, siblings may feel insecure and anxious. Behavioral problems may develop, or school performance may deteriorate. Siblings may feel jealous because the ill brother or sister seems to monopolize the parents' attention. They may demonstrate behaviors ranging from jealousy or envy to resentment, guilt, hostility, anger, insecurity, regression, and fear. The siblings of an ill child can manage well when given support, and parents may need help providing that support.

It is essential that siblings receive information about their brother's or sister's condition and hospitalization using language and concepts appropriate to their ages and developmental levels (Gursky, 2007). Education and support to siblings of hospitalized children promotes coping and adaptation to a sibling's illness.

Preoccupied with their hospitalized child, parents may not consider bringing siblings to visit. Without firsthand knowledge, siblings often assume far worse than what is actually happening at the hospital. The siblings may fantasize about the illness or injury and the appearance of their brother or sister. Siblings who are not adequately informed about the hospitalized child's condition may fear that the child will be disabled or die, even when this is unlikely. To dispel any misconceptions, parents should take any siblings to see the hospitalized child as soon as possible. As appropriate, encourage siblings to visit. Such a visit is especially encouraged if the child could potentially die, as it allows the sibling the opportunity to say good-bye (see Chapter 18 🔗 for further discussion of the dying child). These visits often help to improve the mood of the hospitalized child and assist the sibling to overcome misconceptions or negative emotions. Because children's fantasies are often worse than reality, unfounded fears may be relieved by a visit.

Before the visit, prepare the siblings by explaining what they will likely encounter. Describe the hospital environment, including equipment, sounds, and smells. Describe how the brother or sister will appear. If the hospitalized child acts, moves, talks, or appears differently than before the hospitalization, provide an explanation beforehand. Consider using a doll, drawing pictures, or showing an actual photograph of the child to help prepare the siblings. See Partnering with Families: Strategies for Working with the Sibling of a Hospitalized Child.

During the visit, demonstrate how to talk to and touch the ill child and encourage the siblings to do the same. After the visit, discuss with siblings what they saw and felt, and answer any questions they may have. When siblings cannot visit, contact with the hospitalized child can be maintained by sending pictures, drawings, cards, and messages recorded on iPods, and through email, instant messaging, or webcam. Partner with the family to determine the most appropriate and effective method of communicating if the sibling is unable to visit. If parents are staying at the hospital with the hospitalized child,

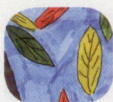

Partnering with Families

Strategies for Working with the Sibling of a Hospitalized Child

The nurse working with siblings of a hospitalized child can implement the following strategies to assist the siblings in understanding:

- Be truthful. Explain why the child is hospitalized, what the treatment involves, and how long the hospitalization is expected to last.
- Assure siblings that they did not cause the illness and that the hospitalized child did nothing wrong. If a sibling had some involvement in or responsibility for the health crisis, referral for mental health counseling may be needed.
- Allow siblings to ask questions and discuss fears and other feelings.

- Encourage siblings to visit if possible. Cover tubes and wires with a sheet. Wash off blood or cover bloody bandages if possible. Prepare them for any equipment, dressing, and procedures they might see, and any sounds they might hear.
- Warn siblings if the hospitalized child is not speaking. Say something like, "John can't talk now. He seems to be sleeping deeply. He may be able to hear, though, so you can touch him and talk to him."
- Encourage siblings to express their feelings related to the disruptive effect of the child's hospitalization on family life.

---

help them establish communication routines for the well siblings. For example, encourage them to call the siblings at home at a regular time each night. Allowing the siblings at home the opportunity to share their day, and to receive an update on the hospitalized child, provides a feeling of connectedness and may minimize feelings of worry and resentment. The phone call offers siblings a consistent link to the parents and the reassurance that they are important and loved.

Clinical Tip

Siblings with fever or other symptoms of infectious disease should not be allowed to visit. Inform the parents and family about any specific policies related to sibling visitation.

Family Assessment

To support the hospitalized child and provide family-centered care, nurses develop an understanding of the family dynamics and individualize the nursing care according to the needs of the child and family. To develop a plan of care that involves all family members, the nurse assesses the impact of the child's illness or hospitalization on the family. Table 15–4 provides a list of questions to guide the nurse in determining the family roles, knowledge of the family, support systems, and effects on siblings (see Chapter 2 for a detailed discussion of family assessment).

Collaborate with the family to determine their resources, such as:

- Coping strategies of family members
- Financial resources
- Access to health care
- Availability of community services

A family with limited financial support may manage quite well because they have effective coping strategies, whereas another family with greater financial resources may have difficulty if their coping strategies are ineffective. Staying with a hospitalized child can be a financial drain for parents if one or both must take a leave of absence from work, miss scheduled workdays, or travel to the hospital. Additional expenses may include hotel rooms, meals, parking fees, and childcare for other children. Assess the family's ability to manage these additional expenses. To evaluate the burden of hospitalization, use a multidisciplinary approach, which may lead to increased access to community resources and support for families.

Assess the family dynamics by evaluating:

- Quality of communication
- Methods of coping with stress

- Risk factors
- Sources of strength

Partner with the family to identify coping mechanisms. Recognize that many children may be hospitalized far from home and the family's usual support systems, creating stress for them and for their family members. Find out where family members are staying, how far they are from home, and what support systems have been disrupted. Parents use a variety of coping mechanisms in these situations, including

---

TABLE 15–4	Family Assessment

Family Roles

- What changes will the child's illness create in the family?
- Will household tasks need to be reallocated?
- What specific burdens will be placed on family members?
- Will one parent stay with the child or spend a great deal of time in the hospital?
- Will one parent or guardian be primarily responsible for communicating with other family members?

Knowledge

- What knowledge does the family have about the child's condition and treatment? Does the family need further information?
- How quickly can discharge planning and teaching begin?

Support Systems

- Does the child or family have health insurance? What percentage of costs will it cover? Will other financial support be needed? Will costs continue for ongoing care after hospitalization? If so, will existing health insurance cover those costs?
- Are close friends or family available to provide care for other children, assist with family tasks, or help in other ways?
- Are there community services such as support groups, camps for children with disabilities, education sessions, or equipment and financial resources to which the nurse can refer the family?

Siblings

- Have siblings been informed of the ill child's condition and the expected outcome?
- Have they been reassured that they did not cause the illness?
- Do they understand the change in roles and family routines?
- Are they able to visit the ill child?
- Have their teachers been informed of the family stress?
- If the hospitalized child's life is threatened, are the siblings involved in a therapy plan to promote coping?

Developing Cultural Competence
Supporting Alternative Health Practices

Many cultural groups use a combination of Western medicine and traditional or folk medicine (Spector, 2009). This information may not be shared with nurses or physicians, both out of respect and in fear that they will be told not to use these methods. Recognizing and supporting use of traditional practices along with Western medicine can promote health and provide comfort for children and families. Ask the families about the use of traditional, complementary, or alternative therapies. Examples include herbal remedies, healers, acupuncture, prayer, and hot and cold foods. Refer to Chapter 3 🕗 for examples specific to certain cultural groups.

reading, relaxation, and exercise. Additional common sources of support include friends, relatives, and pastors as well as hospital chaplains and social workers.

Examine how the family has dealt with the child's health needs if the child has been hospitalized or required home care in the past. (See Developing Cultural Competence: Supporting Alternative Health Practices.) Determine the family members' level of understanding related to the child's hospitalization and anticipated therapy. Collaborate with family members to determine their desired role in the child's care. Assess the family's needs for referral to family service agencies or other community organizations. Evaluate the need for support groups or agencies that provide medical equipment or other assistance.

Teaching the child and family, providing support, and referring them to community resources are key elements in providing family-centered care. Additional resources available for the child and family include social workers, child and family mental health professionals, and advanced practice nurses. Additionally, hospital programs and parent support groups are available to assist families in coping with a child's illness.

NURSE'S ROLE IN THE CHILD'S ADAPTATION TO HOSPITALIZATION

Hospitalization of the child may be planned or unexpected. A child may be hospitalized for any of the following reasons:

- The child develops an acute illness or exacerbation of a chronic illness.
- The child requires diagnostic or treatment procedures or requires elective surgery.
- The child who was previously healthy suffers a serious injury, necessitating unexpected hospitalization.

Planned Hospitalization

When hospitalization is planned, children and their parents have time to prepare for the experience. (See Partnering with Families: Parental Preparation of Children for Hospitalization.) Through preadmission preparation, children and their families are introduced to the acute care setting. Assess the family's knowledge and expectations and provide information about likely experiences. A variety of approaches can be used to provide information and allay fears:

- Tours of the hospital unit or surgical area are helpful. This activity assists the child and family to become familiar with the environment they will encounter. During tours, preschoolers and school-age children can see and handle items with which they will come

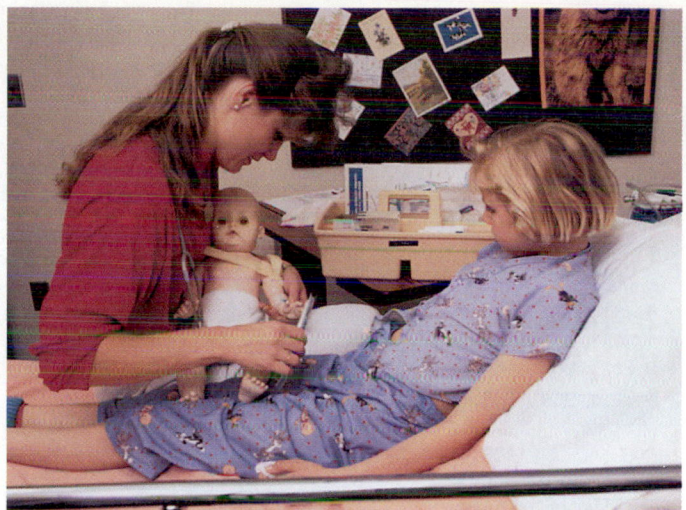

FIGURE 15–2 ■ The child's anxiety and fear often will be reduced if the nurse explains what is going to happen and demonstrates how the procedure will be done by using a doll. Based on your experience, can you list five actions you can take to prepare a school-age child for hospitalization?

in contact. If a tour is not possible, photographs or a DVD can be used to demonstrate the medical setting and procedures.
- The surgical team's attire is less frightening if the child has a chance to try it on and engage in play while wearing the attire.
- Medical equipment is not as frightening when the child learns what it does and observes how it is used, for example, through demonstration on a doll (Figure 15–2 ■).
- Puppets and skits can be used to help explain procedures to children.
- Offer health fairs, as many hospitals do, to explain health procedures to children. During a tour, while hospitalized, or at home, the child can be exposed to books or media that explain in age-appropriate terms what to expect during various procedures (Box 15–2).
- Reinforce teaching through coloring books or other educational materials (Figure 15–3 ■).

Different approaches may be more effective in helping adolescents prepare for hospitalization. In addition to written materials, models, and DVDs, adolescents also learn from talking with peers who have had similar experiences. To demonstrate respect for their sense of independence and privacy, offer adolescents an opportunity to ask questions without their parents present.

BOX 15–2	Examples of Children's Books Regarding Hospitalization

- *The Berenstain Bears Go to the Doctor*, by S. Berenstain & J. Berenstain
- *Clifford Visits the Hospital*, by N. Bridwell
- *Corduroy Goes to the Doctor*, by D. Freeman & L. McCue
- *Curious George Goes to the Hospital*, by M. Rey & H. A. Rey
- *Do I Have to Go to the Hospital? A First Look at Going to the Hospital*, by P. Thomas
- *Franklin Goes to the Hospital*, by P. Bourgeois & B. Clark
- *Going to the Hospital, First Experiences*, by M. Bates
- *Lions Aren't Scared of Shots: A Story for Children About Visiting the Doctor*, by H. J. Bennett & M. S. Weber

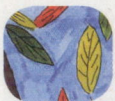

Partnering with Families

Parental Preparation of Children for Hospitalization

The nurse can assist the parents in preparing the child for hospitalization by suggesting the following interventions:

- Read stories to the child about the experience. Numerous books and pamphlets are available.
- Talk about going to the hospital and what it will be like. Talk about coming home.
- Encourage the child to ask questions about the hospital and surgery.
- Encourage the child to draw pictures of what the hospital will be like.

- Visit the hospital unit before hospitalization if possible.
- Let the child touch or see equipment if possible.
- Provide a doctor or nurse kit for the child to play with.
- Provide clothing so the child can dress up like a nurse or doctor if desired.
- Plan for support via parents' presence, telephone calls, and special items of the parents that the child can keep during the stay.
- Be honest.

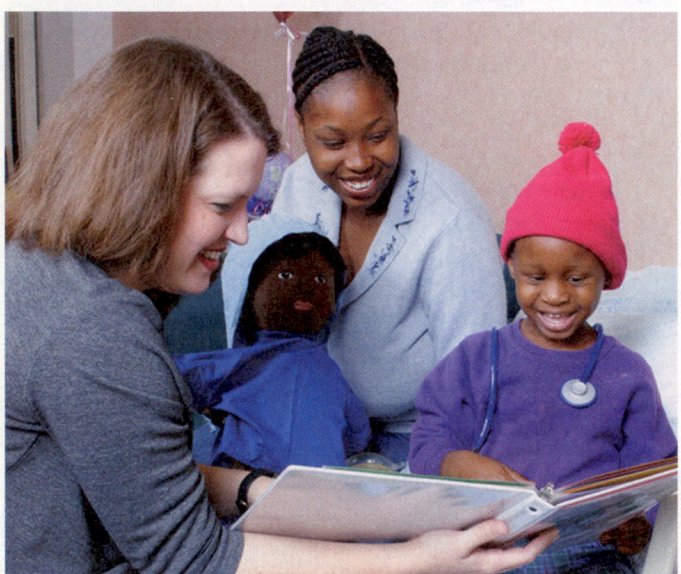

FIGURE 15–3 ■ The nurse reads a story to reinforce teaching about the hospital.

Include the family in preparing the child of any age for hospitalization. Parents can be instrumental in preparing a child for hospitalization by reviewing material presented, being available to answer questions, and being truthful and supportive.

Unexpected Hospitalization

An unanticipated admission places the child at emotional risk for several reasons, including:

- Lack of preparation for the experience
- Uncertainty and unpredictability of events that follow
- Unfamiliarity of the environment
- Heightened anxiety of the child's parents

An admission for exacerbation of a disease, such as cystic fibrosis or leukemia, can provoke feelings of depression or hopelessness.

Assist the child and family who are not prepared for hospital admission to adapt to the experience by orienting them to the environment, providing an opportunity for questions, offering truthful responses, and explaining all procedures and expectations. Discuss the anticipated plan of care for the child, and involve the family in the child's care. Give the family an opportunity to express their fears and concerns. Refer to social services or parent support groups if additional support is needed.

NURSING CARE OF THE HOSPITALIZED CHILD

Family-centered nursing care of the hospitalized child focuses on promoting the child's and family's coping strategies to deal with the stressors of hospitalization, promoting optimal development and safety (see Baccalaureate Essential box), and minimizing disruption of the child's usual routine as much as possible.

Clinical Tip

The hospital environment can pose a variety of safety risks for children, especially toddlers and preschoolers. The nurse should dispose of syringe caps, thermometer covers, gloves, and other equipment that children could chew on or swallow. Latex balloons should not be permitted due to the risk of suffocation. See Box 15–3 for age-specific safety measures.

Special Units and Types of Care

Children admitted to a hospital may be cared for in one or more of the following units:

- General pediatric unit
- Short-stay unit, outpatient unit, or ambulatory surgical unit
- Emergency department
- Neonatal intensive care unit (NICU) or pediatric intensive care unit (PICU)

Baccalaureate Essential II
Basic Organizational and Systems Leadership for Quality Care and Patient Safety

Quality improvement and safety is a priority for healthcare organizations. Nurses at the bedside have a major influence on the quality of care provided and the safety of the patient; however, it is the responsibility of the organization's leadership to provide the staffing and resources so that safe and quality care can be provided (Disch, Dreher, Davidson, et al., 2011). Healthcare providers must advocate for best practices that focus on risks unique to children. Children in the healthcare setting are at risk for harm related to misidentification, adverse effects from high-alert medications, and healthcare-acquired or associated infection (Steering Committee on Quality Improvement and Management & Committee on Hospital Care, 2011). Young children are especially vulnerable to injury because of their developmental immaturity, including the inability to recognize safety risks. It is essential that the hospital environment be free of hazards that pose risks for children.

BOX 15–3	Safety Measures for the Hospitalized Child

NEWBORN AND INFANT

- Use age-appropriate crib and bedding.
- Secure equipment cords under the infant's gown or shirt.
- Do not allow the infant to chew on cords.
- Properly dispose of syringe caps and other small items that may present a choking hazard.
- Establish with parents a list of persons who may visit the child.
- Keep crib rails up when a parent is not at the bedside.

TODDLER AND PRESCHOOLER

- Maintain the bed in low position.
- Keep side rails up when a parent is not at the bedside.
- Do not allow the child to chew on cords.
- Keep the room clutter-free.
- Remove all unnecessary equipment from the child's room.
- Properly dispose of syringe caps and other small items that may present a choking hazard.
- Latex balloons should not be permitted due to the risk of suffocation.
- If toddlers and preschoolers are curious about hospital equipment, provide them the opportunity to explore the equipment safely and with guidance (e.g., syringes without needles, blood pressure cuffs to satisfy curiosity).
- Keep in mind that these children are naturally curious and explorative.
- Instruct family members to inform staff when they are leaving the room to ensure that the toddler or preschooler is being observed.

SCHOOL-AGE CHILD

- Instruct the child to avoid manipulating hospital equipment such as intravenous fluid pumps, patient-controlled analgesia (PCA) pumps, and oxygen gauges.
- Allow the child the opportunity to explore hospital surroundings and equipment with guidance.
- Instruct family members to inform staff when they are leaving the room to ensure that the child is being observed.

ADOLESCENT

- Address issues such as smoking in the room and consuming alcohol, since friends could possibly bring cigarettes or alcohol to the hospitalized adolescent.
- Instruct the adolescent to take only medications given by nurses in the hospital.

BOX 15–4	Nursing Considerations in Preparing Parents and Child for Planned Short-Stay Admission

- Are there special requirements prior to arrival, such as not being permitted food or drink or needing extra fluid intake?
- What time and where must the child appear?
- Are any special forms, insurance numbers, or previous records needed?
- How long will the child stay in the hospital?
- Can the child bring something familiar from home such as a blanket or stuffed animal?
- Are parents expected or encouraged to be with the child or stay in the health facility?
- Is there a chance the child may need to remain longer than expected?
- What will the child's condition be for transfer home?
- Will special equipment or care be needed?
- What symptoms can indicate problems?
- Where can the family go or whom can they call in case of problems or questions?

Nursing care for regular hospital admission includes:

- Orienting the child and family to the unit and procedures
- Adhering to the child's normal routine as much as possible, including child and family in the decision-making process
- Providing direct care to the child
- Promoting a safe environment for the child
- Promoting the child's growth and developmental needs

Short-Stay, Outpatient, and Ambulatory Surgical Units

Hospital stays for children have generally become short. Many procedures are performed in outpatient units, such as minor surgery (in ambulatory surgical centers), diagnostic tests (such as cardiac catheterizations), radiology studies requiring sedation, and treatments (such as chemotherapy). The child may be admitted in the morning and discharged that afternoon. In addition, children who have potentially serious illnesses may be placed on a short-stay or 23-hour observation unit for monitoring or limited treatment, after which medical staff decide either to hospitalize the child for additional treatment or, if improvement occurs, to discharge the child.

These short stays are considered beneficial primarily because they cause minimal disruption of family patterns and are cost-effective for the institution, health insurance company, and family. Nurses assist parents to prepare the child properly for planned admissions, monitor the child during the procedures, encourage family participation in care, and keep families well informed (Box 15–4).

Nursing care of the child in short-stay, outpatient, and ambulatory surgical units is the same as for regular hospital admission. However, time for teaching is compressed, requiring the nurse to implement teaching methods in a minimal amount of time to ensure the family understands discharge instructions. Effective teaching methods on this accelerated schedule include demonstration, videos, pamphlets with verbal review, and informal teaching sessions.

Emergency Care

When a child is brought to an emergency department, the parents are usually frightened and insecure and may even be in a state of shock. The fast pace and critical nature of the unit creates an atmosphere in which parents are hesitant to ask questions and are anxious about

Hospitalized children may require surgical treatment involving preoperative and postoperative care. Children with infectious diseases require isolation precautions. Other children may require rehabilitative care to achieve or restore maximum potential.

General Pediatric Care Unit

Smaller facilities typically incorporate all pediatric care specialties in one unit or area, whereas larger medical centers and children's hospitals have separate medical units for different specialties. Specialized units may include medical and surgical units, orthopedic units, oncology units, mental health units, and units specific to developmental levels (e.g., adolescent unit). Admission to a specialized unit may be the result of an acute condition, such as pneumonia or trauma, or the result of an exacerbation of a chronic condition, such as asthma. Other causes for admissions include surgical procedures requiring longer than 24-hour stays and the need for inpatient treatments and services.

the outcome. Many factors can contribute to the parents' anxiety and stress (see Chapter 17 🔗):

- Unexpected nature of the situation
- Uncertainties in the emergency environment
- Necessity for quick decision making
- Need for numerous procedures, tests, and treatments
- Fear of pain

The nurse keeps both the child and the family informed about what is being done and when more news may be available. The parents and child are encouraged to remain together as much as possible. Parents who wish to remain with a child even during invasive procedures or resuscitation efforts should be allowed to do so, and this option is supported by the Emergency Nurses Association (2009). The nurse collaborates with the family members to determine their desired presence in critical situations and keeps them informed about the health care provided (see Chapter 17).

Intensive Care Unit

Intensive care units provide specialized medical care to neonates, infants, and children requiring advanced technical support and interventions and continuous monitoring (see Chapter 17).

Neonatal intensive care unit The NICU provides specialized care to preterm neonates with complications, those born with congenital defects affecting cardiovascular or respiratory function, and neonates in other life-threatening situations.

Pediatric intensive care unit The PICU provides specialized nursing care to infants and children, including children with life-threatening illnesses and injuries, acute exacerbations of chronic illness (such as severe or life-threatening asthma exacerbation), or any other condition requiring advanced support and continuous monitoring.

Parents of a newborn in the NICU or a child in a PICU are likely to be anxious, particularly since the child's illness may be severe and the prognosis may be guarded. The unfamiliar equipment may create an atmosphere of fear or anxiety. Numerous healthcare professionals work in the intensive care environment, and without effective and open communication, parents may not know whom to question or even what questions to ask. Encourage the family to write down their questions, and direct them to the appropriate source if you are unable to answer the questions.

In summary, nurses in NICU and PICU settings:

- Provide comprehensive direct care to the child
- Provide emotional support to the child and family
- Explain the purpose of treatments and machines
- Help parents to hold or touch their child
- Provide referral to other services if appropriate

Isolation

Children who require isolation to prevent spread of infection may experience lack of stimulation due to limited contact with other children and visitors. Frequent family visits are important and should be encouraged. Family members may be reluctant to wear protective garments either out of fear of using them incorrectly or because they believe they are unnecessary. The nurse ensures that the family understands the reason for isolation and any special procedures. Having contact with and holding the child are encouraged when possible. (Infection control methods are described in Box 22–1 of Chapter 22 🔗.)

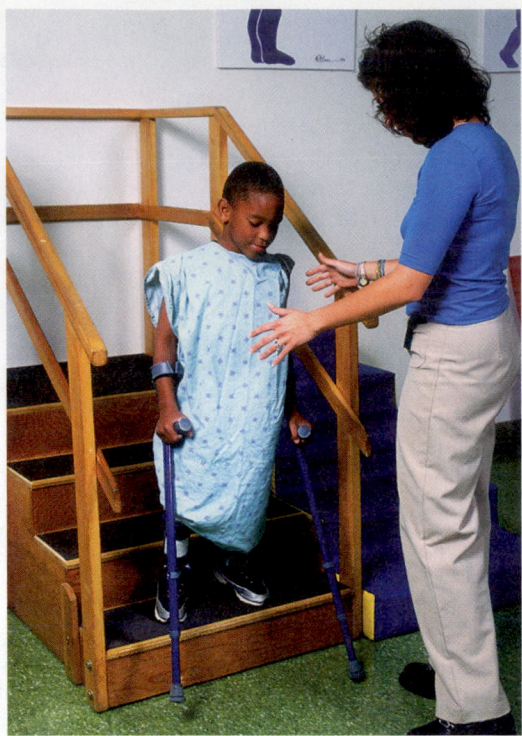

FIGURE 15–4 ■ Rehabilitation units provide an opportunity for the child to relearn such tasks as walking and climbing stairs. They provide an important transition from hospital to home and community.

Rehabilitation

Rehabilitation is the process of assisting a child with physical or mental challenges to reach full potential through therapy and education. Rehabilitation units provide children with ongoing care and support to continue recovery beyond the initial period of illness or injury (Figure 15–4 ■). These may be separate units within a hospital or independent centers. The rehabilitation may be on an inpatient or outpatient basis. Children who experience brain injury, spinal cord injury, near drowning, and burns commonly require extensive rehabilitation. The rehabilitation process can be lengthy; families may need support in adapting to changes in lifestyle, income, finances, and responsibilities.

An important objective of rehabilitation is to assist the child with physical, psychosocial, or educational challenges to reach his or her fullest potential and to promote achievement of developmentally appropriate skills. Collaboration with a multidisciplinary team including parental involvement is essential. Sometimes rehabilitation becomes long term and the child needs care and support for a chronic condition (see Chapter 16 🔗).

Developing Cultural Competence
Support Systems

There are many cultural influences on health beliefs and practices. For example, Mexican Americans view family as a strong support network. Extended family may want to be with a hospitalized child. The father of the child is often the spokesperson, and the mother commonly is influential in decisions regarding child health care. The nurse should incorporate all people the family wishes to have present in the hospital and include them in explanations about health care.

Parental Involvement and Parental Presence

Family members are essential to the child's care during illness. Integrity of the family unit is fostered through parental involvement during the child's hospital stay. Involvement provides parents with control and a feeling that they are active participants in their child's progress, and it also prepares the family for care that will be required when the child goes home. The child benefits greatly from parental presence and participation and experiences reduced emotional distress and anxiety if the parents are present (see Developing Cultural Competence: Support Systems). If parent–child attachment remains uninterrupted, the child experiences a decrease in behavioral maladjustments.

A positive relationship between parents and the healthcare team is an essential component of family-centered care. Parental satisfaction is enhanced when parents' questions about their child's care and condition are answered; when the healthcare team is kind and caring, and takes experiences of parents seriously; and when prompt and consistent care is provided (Fisher & Broome, 2011). Parents need to feel valued. The nurse should partner with the family and multidisciplinary team to determine the extent to which the parents desire to be involved in the child's care (Power & Franck, 2008) and to ensure that accurate and consistent information is given related to hospital care and discharge planning. (See Developing Cultural Competence: Use of Interpreters.) See Chapter 2 ⊘ for more information on family-centered care and family presence. Hospitals have policies on visitation, including the hours of visitation, who can visit, and how many visitors are allowed at a time. Some facilities have adopted policies that do not even use the word "visitor."

Preparation for Procedures

Hospitalized children may experience numerous procedures during hospitalization, from collection of urine or blood specimens to lumbar punctures and surgery. Unfamiliar stressors will be more upsetting for the child than known stressors (Gursky, Kestler, & Lewis, 2010). Maintain a positive attitude when preparing the child, and reassure the child that it is normal to be frightened of unknown experiences. Special techniques can help the child to understand and cope with feelings about these procedures. Techniques used to prepare the child depend on developmental age, coping abilities, and previous experience.

Psychologic Preparation

Preparation may begin a few moments to several days before the procedure, depending on the child's age. In providing sensitive care to the child, nurses assume that a procedure can potentially be traumatic for the child. Even providing urine in a specimen cup or undergoing radiologic examination can be frightening if the child does not understand the reason for the procedure or know what to expect. Administration of medication can also make the child frustrated or anxious. When preparing the child for medication administration using techniques appropriate to the developmental level of the child, the nurse ensures that the medication is safely given (Table 15–5).

Use developmentally appropriate techniques to assess the child's knowledge and feelings about an upcoming procedure. Examples include use of drawings, stories, body outline dolls, anatomically correct dolls, and conversation with the child. When assessing the child's perception about procedures, the nurse should consider the following:

- Does the child know the purpose of the procedure?
- Has the child experienced this procedure before? Was the experience painful, frightening, or reassuring?
- What does the child think will happen? Are the child's beliefs accurate?
- Is the procedure painful?
- What techniques does the child use to gain control in challenging situations?
- Will the parents or other caregiver be present to provide support?

Clinical Tip

An anesthetic cream such as EMLA or ELA-Max is applied before a potentially painful procedure. This can lessen discomfort, thereby alleviating the child's fears (see Chapter 21 ⊘ p. 592).

When explaining a procedure and its purpose, use words that the child understands. (See Chapter 6 ⊘) Older children require explanations geared to their cognitive level and previous experiences. They will want to know what is happening, why, and what they can do to cope during the procedure (Table 15–6).

For adolescents, provide written information, DVDs, and other available media. Schedule time for questions and discussions. Allow adolescents to make choices about their own health care when possible. For example, ask questions such as "Do you want your hand numbed for the IV start?" Maintain a positive attitude when preparing adolescents, and reassure them that it is normal to be frightened of unknown experiences.

Clinical Tip

Procedures should never be performed in a playroom or during a play activity. The nurse acts as the child's advocate by ensuring that treatments by other healthcare professionals (such as blood draws or respiratory treatments) are not performed in the playroom. Assist the child to the treatment room and reassure the child that he or she may return to the playroom after the treatment is completed.

Parental presence can provide comfort and support to the child during procedures. Parents should be allowed to choose whether they want to stay for the procedure. Some parents may feel that they will be too upset to support the child; others will choose to stay. Some adolescents want their parents to be involved in their care, while others prefer to minimize their parents' roles. Ensure that the adolescent's wishes are known regarding parental presence. See Box 15–5.

Physical Preparation

Physical preparation depends on the age of the child and the procedure. Preprocedural sedation may be required. If sedation is required the child will not be able to have anything by mouth (NPO) for a period of time. Young infants might be provided sucrose for procedures (see Chapter 21 ⊘ for pain management). Procedural checklists are often utilized.

Developing Cultural Competence
Use of Interpreters

Nurses in the pediatric acute care environment frequently encounter patients and parents who do not speak English. It is imperative that nurses use appropriate interpreter services to communicate with these families. Use of children and family members to obtain patient history, to provide explanations of illness and treatment, and to obtain informed consent can lead to concerns related to accuracy of the information. In some situations, the family member providing the interpretation might actually withhold information to protect the ill child or the parents (National Center for Cultural Competence, 2010).

A DAY IN THE LIFE
of a Hospital Nurse

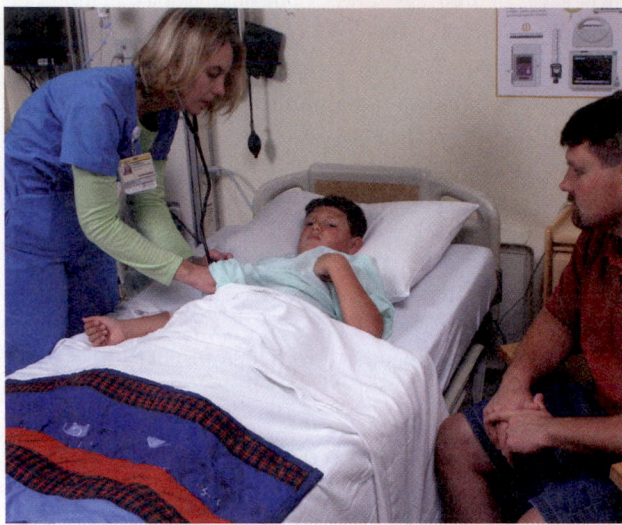

Eight-year-old David was admitted to the inpatient pediatric unit to rule out appendicitis. Rebecca performs her morning assessment on David. The father's presence at the bedside provides comfort to this hospitalized child.

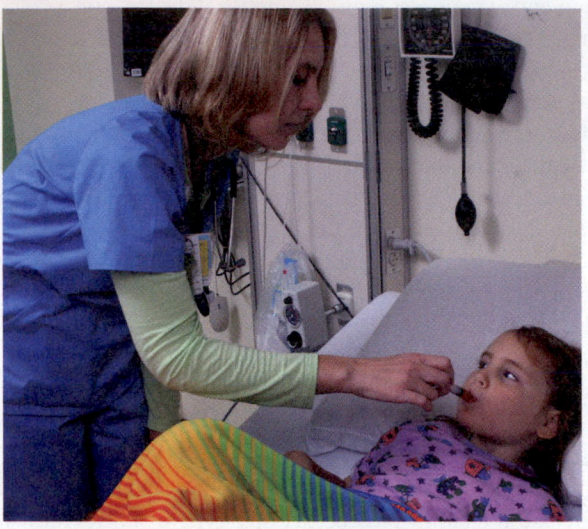

Four-year-old Lana needs medication for an elevated temperature. Notice that the nurse takes into consideration the child's developmental level and uses an oral syringe to administer the medication.

Rebecca Hughes, a pediatric nurse who is employed in a hospital inpatient area, has the opportunity to work in a variety of settings. These settings include general pediatric units, specialty units such as hematology/oncology, adolescent and cardiac units, pediatric intensive care or intermediate care, the emergency department, and pediatric surgical areas. The roles of the pediatric nurse vary depending on the settings in which he or she is employed. Regardless of the setting, all pediatric nurses implement the nursing process to provide developmentally appropriate family-centered care throughout the day while caring for their patients and helping other members of the healthcare team in the care of their patients.

On a general pediatric unit, Rebecca provides care for children of different ages and with a variety of diagnoses. Although she begins the day with a plan, her planned activities are frequently altered because of changes in patient status, emergencies, and new admissions. Flexibility and the ability to prioritize are necessary qualities of the hospital nurse.

The pediatric nurse in the hospital setting:

- Receives a report on each patient at the beginning of the shift
- Assesses each patient at the beginning of the shift and throughout the day

Flexibility and the ability to prioritize are necessary qualities of the hospital nurse.

- Answers questions that the child's parents have about the child's plan of care or condition
- Prepares the child for medical procedures with age-appropriate information
- Administers medications to children using age-appropriate techniques
- Performs required skills such as maintaining nasogastric tubes to suction, changing dressings, starting IVs, and hanging IV fluids
- Teaches parents skills required for home care
- Delegates responsibilities to other members of the healthcare team as needed
- Provides discharge teaching to parents
- Provides a report on each patient at the end of the shift

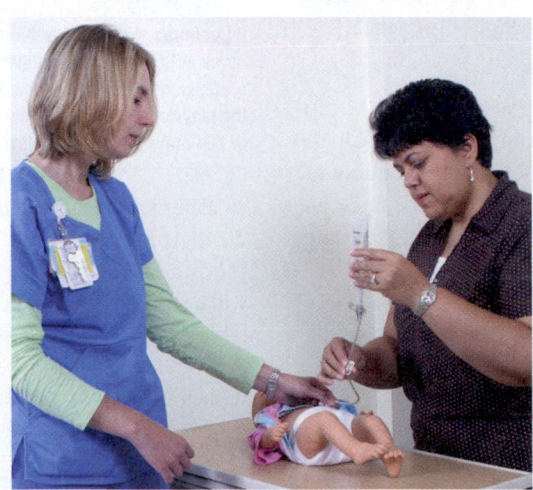

Teaching is an essential aspect of pediatric nursing. The nurse teaches this mother how to administer gastrostomy feedings.

TABLE 15–5	**Variations in Medication Administration to Children**	

ROUTE	DEVELOPMENTAL CONSIDERATIONS	TECHNIQUES
Oral	Children under 5 years cannot generally swallow pills and capsules.	■ Medications are usually given in liquid form (elixir, syrup, or suspension). ■ Avoid putting medications in a bottle of formula since it will be impossible to determine how much medication the child has taken if some of the formula is left in the bottle. ■ Sometimes tablets are crushed or capsules are opened and mixed with a liquid flavoring or small amount of food. Check with the pharmacy to be sure this does not inactivate the drug. Never crush enteric-coated or timed-release medicine. ■ When choosing a vehicle for crushed tablets, use only one spoonful of applesauce, pudding, jelly, or similar food or 1–2 mL of liquid. ■ Use an oral syringe to increase accuracy.
	Children may not want to take medicine.	■ Position young children upright to avoid choking and aspiration. ■ Give liquid medicines slowly by oral syringe (for infants) aimed at the inside of the cheek. ■ A preschooler may prefer to drink the medicine from a medicine cup, but the medication must first be measured using a syringe to ensure accuracy. ■ Have the expectation that the medicine will be taken. Let children choose the type of fluid to drink after, but do not ask if they will take their medicine now.
Rectal	Colon is small.	■ For children under 3 years, the nurse's gloved fifth finger is used for insertion. After this age, the index finger can usually be used. ■ Lubricate the tip of the suppository. The nurse may need to hold the buttocks together for a few minutes to keep the medication from being expelled.
Ophthalmic and otic	Young children may be fearful of medicines placed in the eyes or ears.	■ Adequate immobilization is needed to avoid injury. ■ The nurse's hand can be stabilized by resting the wrist on the child's head. ■ Explanations and therapeutic play can be used with children old enough to understand the process of administration. ■ Have medication at room temperature.
Topical	Skin of infants is thin and fragile.	■ Only prescribed doses and medicines appropriate for young children should be used on the skin. ■ Covering the area or keeping the child's hands occupied may be necessary to ensure adequate contact of medication with the skin.
Intramuscular	Anatomy and physiology of children differ from that of adults.	■ The gluteus maximus muscle (dorsal gluteal site) is not recommended in children due to danger of injury to the sciatic nerve (Tschudy & Arcana, 2011). ■ The vastus lateralis site is preferred for children. ■ Amounts to be administered should be limited to no more than 1–2 mL for the ventrogluteal site, depending on muscle size. Refer to the Clinical Skills Manual ■ for illustrations. ■ The deltoid muscle is rarely used in young children except for the small vaccine doses.
Intravenous	Veins are small and fragile.	■ Careful maintenance of sites is needed. ■ Common infusion sites include hands and feet, although scalp veins are sometimes used in infants. ■ Infusion pumps require frequent monitoring.
	Fluid balance is critical.	■ Syringe pumps are often used when minimal fluid is to be given over an extended period. ■ Central lines are commonly used for long-term intravenous medication therapy.

Source: Bindler, R. C., Ball, J. W., Ladewig, P. W., & London, M. L. (2011). Clinical skills manual for maternal & child nursing care (3rd ed., p. 110). Upper Saddle River, NJ: Pearson.

Performing the Procedure

Procedures on young children are generally performed in a **treatment room** (a room designated for performing treatments such as intravenous starts, blood drawing, and lumbar punctures) to promote the child's sense of security that his or her own room is a "safe" and relatively pain-free site. Older children can be given the option of having a procedure performed in the treatment room or in their own hospital room. Older school-age children and adolescents may prefer to remain in their room for the procedure. See Box 15–6.

Perform the procedure as quickly and efficiently as possible. If the parents wish to participate, ask them to hold the child's hand or stand close by for comfort. Utilize nursing staff instead of parents to immobilize the child as needed. The parents, or another nurse, can be designated to support the child by providing gentle touch, talking, singing, giving reassurance, or illustrating stress reduction techniques.

After the procedure, no matter how the child responded, the child should be praised. A choice of reward often soothes the young child. If the procedure is performed in a treatment room, the child is returned to his or her room for comfort and reassurance. Refer to Chapter 21 for discussion of pain management and sedation for procedures.

TABLE 15–6	Assisting Children Through Procedures	
DEVELOPMENTAL STAGE	**BEFORE PROCEDURE**	**DURING PROCEDURE**
Infant	None for infant. Explain to parents the procedure, the reason for it, and their role. Allow parents the option of being present for procedures. Parents may be able to touch a foot or rub a cheek and talk soothingly to the infant.	■ Nursing staff should immobilize the infant securely and gently. Parents should not be asked to hold the child down. ■ Perform the procedure quickly. Use touch, voice, pacifier, and bottle as distractions. ■ Ask the parent to hold, rock, and sing to the infant after the procedure.
Toddler	Give the explanation just before the procedure, since a toddler's concept of time is limited. Explain that the child did nothing wrong; the procedure is simply necessary.	■ Perform in the treatment room. Nursing staff should immobilize the child securely. ■ Give short explanations and directions in a positive manner. ■ Avoid giving choices when none are available. For example, "We are going to do this now" is better than "Is it okay to do this now?" ■ Allow the child to cry or scream. ■ Comfort the child after the procedure. Give the child a choice of a favorite drink or special sticker.
Preschool child	Give simple explanations of the procedure. Basic drawings may be useful. While providing supervision, allow the child to touch and play with equipment to be used if possible. Since any entry into the body is viewed as a threat, state that the child's body will remain the same, and use adhesive bandages to reassure the child that the body is intact and parts will not "fall out."	■ Perform in the treatment room. Nursing staff should immobilize the child securely. ■ Give short explanations and directions in a positive manner. Encourage control by having the child count to 10 or spell his or her name. ■ Allow the child to cry. Give positive feedback for cooperation and getting through the procedure. ■ Encourage the child to draw afterward to explore the experience.
School-age child	Clear, thorough explanations are helpful. Use drawings, pictures, books, and contact with equipment. Teach stress reduction techniques such as deep breathing and visualization. Offer a choice of reward after the procedure is completed.	■ Be ready to immobilize the child if needed. Allow the child to remain in position by self if he or she is able to be still. Explain throughout the procedure what is happening. Facilitate use of stress control techniques. Praise cooperative efforts.
Adolescent	Give clear explanations orally and in writing. Teach stress reduction techniques. Explore fear of certain procedures, such as staple removal or venipuncture.	■ Assist the adolescent in self-control. Assist with use of stress control techniques. ■ Explain expected outcomes and tell when results of the test will be completed.

BOX 15–5	Research: Psychosocial Preparation for Procedures

Gursky et al. (2010) conducted a quasi-experimental study involving 24 children receiving repair of a laceration in an emergency department setting. Ages ranged from 3 to 13 years with a mean of 7 years. Seven children were in the intervention group and received individualized preparation prior to and distraction during the procedure from a child life specialist. Preparation lasted 15 minutes and included an explanation using a doll and role play of each step of the process using age-appropriate terms. The parent and child were asked about usual coping strategies. The child life specialist provided age-appropriate distraction techniques such as singing, blowing bubbles, and talking that were practiced before the procedure and utilized during the procedure. Children were encouraged to ask questions and verbalize any specific fears. Seventeen children in the comparison group received standard nursing care before and during the procedure. Standard care included wound care, verbal explanations about the procedure, updates, and answering questions. The child's distress was observed during laceration repair. Children who received the intervention showed significantly less distress during the procedure than those in the comparison group, and they had lower distress scores throughout the observation period. Parents of children in the intervention group reported lower levels of distress in their children as compared to levels of distress reported by parents of children in the comparison group.

BOX 15–6	Treatment Room

The treatment room is utilized rather than the child's own hospital room so that the child always has a "safe" environment and comfort zone by knowing that no unpleasant or painful procedures will occur in his or her room.

Pediatric hospitals and large medical centers generally provide treatment rooms on each unit. Smaller hospitals and community hospitals may not provide a specific treatment room designated for pediatrics; however, any room other than the child's own room is an appropriate alternative. If smaller hospitals do not have a treatment room or provide an alternative, nurses acting as a child advocate should be vigilant in encouraging the establishment of such a room to minimize the stressors the hospitalized child experiences.

Preparation for Surgery

A child's surgical experience may be elective, planned in advance, or a result of an emergency or trauma. How a child responds to the experience is related to the psychologic and physical preparation he or she receives. Preoperative preparation decreases anxiety in both the child and the parent (Chahal, Manlhiot, Colapinto, et al., 2009; Frisch, Johnson, Timmons, et al., 2010). The accompanying Nursing Care Plan summarizes key elements of preoperative and postoperative care.

Nursing Care Plan

The Child Undergoing Surgery

INTERVENTION	RATIONALE	EXPECTED OUTCOME

PREOPERATIVE CARE

1. Nursing Diagnosis: Knowledge, Deficient related to preoperative and postoperative events

INTERVENTION	RATIONALE	EXPECTED OUTCOME
NIC Priority Intervention— *Teaching, Preoperative:* Assisting the parent and child to understand and mentally prepare for surgery and postoperative recovery		**NOC Suggested Outcome—** *Knowledge:* Extent of understanding conveyed about treatment regimen

GOAL: *The child and family will acquire knowledge related to the operation.*

INTERVENTION	RATIONALE	EXPECTED OUTCOME
■ Ask questions of the parent and child about surgery.	■ Prior knowledge and understanding can be reinforced and used to guide your presentation.	The child and family are able to verbalize details about expected preoperative and postoperative events. They ask questions that demonstrate understanding.
■ Teach about preoperative and postoperative events using appropriate developmental methods such as dolls, drawings, stories, and tours.	■ Developmental level determines the cognitive approach that works best for teaching.	The child demonstrates skills needed in the postoperative period.
■ Reinforce information the family has received about the purpose of surgery.	■ The physician may have explained the operation.	
■ Have the child demonstrate postoperative events that pertain to his or her case such as deep breathing, putting a bandage on a doll, taping an intravenous line on a doll, and pressing the PCA button.	■ Concrete experience promotes learning.	
■ Allow the parents and child to ask questions.	■ Learners must have the opportunity to ask questions.	

2. Nursing Diagnosis: Anxiety related to planned surgery

INTERVENTION	RATIONALE	EXPECTED OUTCOME
NIC Priority Intervention— *Anxiety Reduction:* Minimizing apprehension, dread, foreboding, or uneasiness related to an unidentified source of anticipated danger		**NOC Suggested Outcome—** *Coping:* Actions to manage stressors that tax an individual's resources

GOAL: *The child and family will show decreased behavior indicating anxiety.*

INTERVENTION	RATIONALE	EXPECTED OUTCOME
■ Question the child about expectations of hospitalization and previous experiences.	■ Previous experiences can influence the present anxiety level.	The child and family demonstrate less anxiety. They verbalize understanding and comfort in hospital routines.
■ Orient the child to the hospital setting, routines, staff, and other patients.	■ Familiarity with the setting and people can decrease anxiety by removing unknown factors.	Parents support the child for traumatic procedures.
■ Institute age-appropriate play and interactions with the child.	■ Play can increase trust level and decrease anxiety.	
■ Explain procedures and prepare for those that might cause trauma. Encourage parents to support the child.	■ The child is more likely to trust caregivers if they are truthful and if parents are present.	
■ Allow the parents and child to ask questions.	■ Questioning provides an opportunity to explain the unknown, which decreases anxiety.	

3. Nursing Diagnosis: Infection and Injury, Risk for related to exposure to infectious agents and use of preoperative medication

INTERVENTION	RATIONALE	EXPECTED OUTCOME
NIC Priority Intervention— *Infection Control and Fall Prevention:* Minimizing the acquisition and transmission of infectious agents, and instituting special precautions with patient at risk of falling		**NOC Suggested Outcome—** *Risk Control:* Actions to eliminate or reduce actual, personal, and modifiable health risks

GOAL: *The child will show no signs of infection.*

INTERVENTION	RATIONALE	EXPECTED OUTCOME
■ Monitor vital signs at least every 4 hours. Inspect skin and respiratory status each shift.	■ Increase in vital sign levels, skin lesions, nasal drainage, or adventitious breath sounds can indicate signs of infection in the child.	The child's vital signs and assessment are within age-appropriate limits.
■ Report any variations from expected vital signs.	■ Symptoms are reported so surgery can be canceled if necessary.	The child is transported safely to the operating room.

(continued)

Nursing Care Plan

The Child Undergoing Surgery, *continued*

INTERVENTION	RATIONALE	EXPECTED OUTCOME
■ Keep side rails up after preoperative medication is given. Maintain NPO status when ordered. Transport the child to the operating room safely secured.	■ Preoperative medication can alter level of consciousness. NPO status prevents aspiration.	

POSTOPERATIVE CARE

4. Nursing Diagnosis: Skin Integrity, Impaired related to disruption of skin surface

NIC Priority Intervention—*Wound Care:* Prevention of wound complications and promotion of wound healing		**NOC Suggested Outcome—***Wound Healing:* The extent to which cells and tissues have regenerated following intentional closure

GOAL: *The child will be free of infection.*

■ Monitor vital signs per hospital routine. Record and report changes from baseline.	■ Changes in vital signs, especially increased temperature and pulse, can indicate infection.	The child shows no signs of infection.
■ Monitor surgical dressing and drains every hour.	■ Excess drainage may indicate infection.	The surgical wound heals without infection.
■ Change or reinforce dressings when wet.	■ Wet dressing can allow organisms to come into contact with the surgical wound.	The intravenous line remains patent without signs of infection.
■ Assess the intravenous site every 2 hours for redness, swelling, pain, or pallor.	■ Intravenous lines may become infiltrated or cause thrombophlebitis.	The child continues to demonstrate no signs of infection at home.
■ Teach parents signs of infection before discharge. Teach parents aseptic technique for dressing change and wound care.	■ Parents report signs of infection and perform home care as needed.	

5. Nursing Diagnosis: Constipation, Risk for related to surgical procedure and anesthetics

NIC Priority Intervention—*Constipation Management:* Establishment and maintenance of regular bowel elimination		**NOC Suggested Outcome—***Bowel Elimination:* Ability of the gastrointestinal tract to form and evacuate stool effectively

GOAL: *The child will achieve and maintain normal bowel functioning by the fourth postoperative day.*

■ Auscultate bowel sounds every 4 hours. Offer liquids only when bowel sounds are present. Assess the abdomen for distention.	■ Restricting fluids avoids distention if peristalsis is not normal.	The child has a bowel movement within 2 to 3 days after surgery with normal pattern by the fourth postoperative day.
■ Document the character and frequency of bowel movements.	■ Knowledge of bowel status ensures early identification of constipation.	
■ Advance the diet as tolerated.	■ Fluids and roughage promote normal bowel functioning.	
■ Increase activity as ordered and tolerated.	■ Physical activity promotes peristalsis.	

6. Nursing Diagnosis: Fluid Volume: Imbalanced, Risk for related to intravenous infusion and NPO status

NIC Priority Intervention—*Fluid Management:* Promotion of fluid balance and prevention of imbalance complications		**NOC Suggested Outcome—***Fluid Balance:* Balance of water in intracellular and extracellular components

GOAL: *The child will achieve and maintain proper circulating volume.*

■ Monitor vital signs per hospital routines.	■ Changes in vital signs, especially pulse or blood pressure, can indicate fluid imbalance.	The child remains in fluid balance with no vomiting in postoperative period.

GOAL: *The child will tolerate oral intake when started, with no nausea, vomiting, or dehydration present.*

■ Record intake and output. Be alert for fluid loss via dressings or watery stools. Evaluate hydration status by skin turgor and mucous membranes.	■ Intake and output are roughly equivalent. Urinary retention sometimes occurs postoperatively as a result of anesthesia. Fluid status can be assessed by skin and mucous membrane hydration.	
■ Monitor laboratory values of hematocrit and hemoglobin.	■ Increased hematocrit and hemoglobin can indicate hemoconcentration and underhydration. Decreased serum values can indicate hemodilution or overhydration.	
■ Begin oral intake after assessment of bowel sounds. Record vomiting. Administer antiemetics if indicated.	■ Vomiting can cause fluid loss.	

Nursing Care Plan | The Child Undergoing Surgery, *continued*

INTERVENTION	RATIONALE	EXPECTED OUTCOME
7. Nursing Diagnosis: Gas Exchange, Impaired related to anesthetics and pain		
NIC Priority Intervention—*Airway Management:* Facilitation of patency of air passages		**NOC Suggested Outcome**—*Respiratory Status:* Ventilation: Movement of air in and out of lungs
GOAL: *The child will maintain adequate ventilation with no respiratory impairment.*		
■ Auscultate lungs every 2 hours. Record rate, rhythm, and quality of respiration. Evaluate respiratory rate after analgesics.	■ Early identification of respiratory difficulty aids early treatment. Analgesics, especially morphine, may slow respiratory rate.	The child moves adequate air in and out of lungs and has an appropriate respiratory rate.
■ Administer oxygen if ordered.	■ Oxygen may facilitate breathing status postoperatively.	
■ Reposition the child every 2 hours.	■ Repositioning ensures expansion of all lung fields.	
■ Encourage deep breathing and coughing every 2 hours. Use incentive spirometer, pinwheels, or other blow toys appropriate for the developmental level of the child.	■ All areas of the lungs must be expanded. Mucus is expectorated.	
■ Ensure proper intake and output.	■ Balanced fluid status ensures liquefication of secretions and prevents excess fluid accumulation.	
8. Nursing Diagnosis: Pain, Acute related to surgical procedure		
NIC Priority Intervention—*Pain Management:* Alleviation of pain or a reduction in pain to a level of comfort that is acceptable to the patient		**NOC Suggested Outcome**—*Pain Control Behavior:* Personal actions to control pain
GOAL: *The child will maintain an adequate comfort level.*		
■ Assess behavioral cues (e.g., crying, movement, guarding).	■ Behavior of preverbal children provides clues to pain experience.	The child's pain is controlled as demonstrated by a low number on the pain assessment tool (behavioral or verbal).
■ Use an appropriate pain assessment tool for verbal and nonverbal children.	■ An age-appropriate pain assessment tool allows verbal children to quantify the amount of pain.	
	■ Pain assessment tools designed for nonverbal children allow the nurse to quantify the amount of pain when the child cannot provide a self-report (see Chapter 21 🔗 for descriptions of a variety of pain assessment tools).	
■ Administer prescribed pain medications around the clock.	■ Narcotics and nonnarcotic analgesics alter pain perception.	
■ Use age-appropriate nonpharmacologic methods of pain control (e.g., distraction, repositioning, massage).	■ Nonpharmacologic interventions interfere with pain perception.	
9. Nursing Diagnosis: Skin Integrity, Risk for Impaired related to limited mobility after surgery		
NIC Priority Intervention—*Skin Surveillance and Pressure Management:* Collection and analysis of patient data to maintain skin integrity and minimize pressure to body parts		**NOC Suggested Outcome**—*Risk Control:* Actions to eliminate or reduce actual personal and modifiable health threats
GOAL: *The child's skin will remain intact.*		
■ Turn and reposition the child every 2 hours.	■ Repositioning takes pressure off the skin and allows increased circulation.	The child develops no pressure areas.
■ Keep linens clean and dry.	■ Clean linen decreases the chance of skin breakdown.	The wound heals without complication.
■ Get the child up and ambulating when ordered.	■ Movement decreases pressure on skin and improves circulation.	
■ Assess the incision for drainage, redness, and intactness of staples or stitches every 4–8 hours.	■ Early identification of infection or problems with wound healing can ensure prompt treatment.	
10. Nursing Diagnosis: Anxiety (Child and Family) related to change in health status and environments		
NIC Priority Intervention—*Anxiety Reduction:* Minimizing apprehension, dread, foreboding, or uneasiness related to an unidentified source of danger		**NOC Suggested Outcome**—*Coping:* Actions to manage stressors that tax an individual's resources

(continued)

Nursing Care Plan   The Child Undergoing Surgery, *continued*

INTERVENTION	RATIONALE	EXPECTED OUTCOME
GOAL: *The child and family will verbalize comfort with postoperative care and outcome.*		
■ Explain monitors, drainage dressings, intravenous lines, and procedures.	■ Knowledge of purpose decreases anxiety.	The child and family demonstrate coping skills to deal with hospitalization.
■ Reassure the child and family that anxiety is a normal response to the stressful event of surgery.	■ Knowledge of what is expected decreases anxiety.	
■ Encourage parental presence and care of the child.	■ The child's anxiety decreases with parental presence.	
■ Use touch and other nonverbal and verbal communication with the child and family.	■ Effective communication reassures the child and family.	

11. Nursing Diagnosis: Knowledge, Deficient related to care at home

NIC Priority Intervention—Teaching: Planning, implementation and evaluation of a teaching program designed to address a patient's particular needs.		**NOC Suggested Outcome**—*Knowledge: Treatment Regimen:* Extent of understanding conveyed about treatment regimen
GOAL: *The child and family will verbalize self-care required at home.*		
■ Provide oral and written home care instructions regarding surgical wound care, medications, activities, and diet.	■ Teaching regarding home care is necessary early in hospitalization.	The child and family demonstrate skills needed for home care following discharge. They verbalize plans for future care.
■ Provide a number to call for questions or concerns. Instruct on follow-up visits.	■ Parents need to know emergency information and that follow-up care is required.	

NANDA-I © 2012

Preoperative Care

Preoperative care of the child includes both psychosocial and physical preparation for surgery. The goal of preoperative teaching is to reduce the fear associated with the unknown and decrease stress and anxiety associated with surgery.

Psychosocial Preparation

Preoperative teaching is geared to the child's developmental level. If child life specialists (discussed later in the chapter) are available, they can also play an important role in preparing the child for surgery. When the child will be transferred to an intensive care unit or recovery room after surgery, a visit to the area before surgery can reduce the fear and anxiety associated with waking up in a strange environment filled with frightening sights, sounds, and smells. The use of DVDs, body outline dolls, anatomically correct puppets and dolls, drawings, and models is encouraged to teach the child about the surgical procedure. For example, a doll was used as a teaching aid in preparing Tiona, the child described in the chapter opening, for surgery. Playing with stethoscopes, gowns, masks, and syringes without needles also helps the child feel more in control (see discussion about therapeutic play later in this chapter). Children are reassured that their parents can accompany them to the operating room floor and will be waiting when they awaken from surgery. Parents should be allowed to carry infants and young toddlers to the pediatric holding area or have them ride in one parent's lap in a wheelchair. Older toddlers and preschoolers should be allowed to ride in a special wagon if possible. Special teddy bears and blankets are generally allowed in the preoperative holding area and provide comfort to the child. The nurse should make sure that the item is labeled with the child's name. Prepare family members for what to

anticipate and what is expected of them. Special equipment such as intravenous setups and monitoring devices are explained. In some hospitals, only one or two immediate family members are allowed to visit the child at one time. Visitors may be required to wear special gowns, shoes, or hats, and they may be restricted to certain areas.

Parental Presence During Anesthesia Induction

Many hospitals now allow parents to be present with their child during anesthesia induction and again in the postanesthesia recovery area. Parents often want to support their child before and immediately after a surgical procedure, and their presence offers reassurance and comfort to the child. The decision to allow parents to be present during induction of anesthesia must be made on an individual basis. Nurses should be open to change in practice and realize that incorporating the option of parental presence during anesthesia induction supports the principles of family-centered care and decreases anxiety in the child (Pruitt, Johnson, Elliott, et al., 2008). The nurse explains expectations, such as surgical gown, cap, shoe covers, and the parent's role during induction. The nurse offers the parents an opportunity to ask questions and voice concerns.

Physical Preparation

Preparation for surgery may occur in designated preoperative areas. Procedures generally conducted in preoperative areas include premedication, intravenous start (if not performed following general anesthesia), and preparation of the surgical site. If urinary catheterization is necessary, it is usually not performed until the child has been anesthetized.

Preoperative procedures and guidelines vary among hospitals and outpatient surgical centers. Preoperative checklists are used in ambulatory and acute care settings to ensure proper physical preparation of patients for surgery. A sample preoperative checklist is provided in Box 15–7. Weigh the preoperative child accurately, measure vital signs, and ask about last fluid intake amount and type. Monitor urinary output. NPO status in an infant and young child is distressing to both the child and the parents. Reinforce teaching regarding necessary NPO status and provide support to the family as needed (see Partnering with Families: Waiting for the Child to Go to Surgery).

Nursing management during the preoperative period includes establishing accurate baseline data, administering prescribed fluids, and performing assessments of fluid status. When an intravenous infusion is prescribed, start the infusion (see the Clinical Skills Manual ⊂▭), ensuring that the type of fluid and flow rate match those that are ordered and that would be expected for the weight of the child.

Of necessity, the young child who undergoes surgery usually is restricted from consuming oral foods and fluids just before, during, and for a period after surgery, thus creating a risk of fluid imbalance. The length of time the child is kept without oral intake prior to surgery varies. Recommendations from the American Society of Anesthesiologists indicate that clear liquids may be given up until 2 hours prior to surgery, breast milk until 4 hours prior to surgery, and infant formula 6 hours prior. Milk and a light meal may be consumed up until 6 hours prior to surgery (Crenshaw & Winslow, 2008). Infants will generally have very specific orders related to what time they should be made NPO for breast milk, formula, and clear liquids. These orders will depend on what time the infant is scheduled for surgery. Because children beyond infancy do not usually eat or drink during the night, orders are usually written for NPO after midnight. If surgery is not scheduled for the morning, however, more specific orders should be written, especially for the toddler and preschool-age child, who will not be as tolerant of an extended NPO status. The ultimate decision on how long the child is NPO lies with the anesthesiologist and may vary depending on personal experiences and beliefs.

Infants are especially unable to conserve fluids; therefore, even a short time of NPO status for a diagnostic test may lead to imbalance. Surgery often causes fluid loss from bleeding, which can further compromise fluid balance. In addition, the child may experience third spacing, a loss or pooling of fluid in a body space such as the abdomen in response to either surgery or the child's condition. Although decisions about the total amount of fluid required are determined by anesthesiologists during the surgery, the nurse needs an understanding of the amount of fluid generally required during the perioperative period. If a child is NPO prior to surgery and no

intravenous line has been started, the child requires additional fluids during and after surgery to compensate for those not taken in during the period of fasting.

Clinical Judgment

Sometimes, due to emergencies, planned surgeries for infants and young children may be postponed for several hours. These children are NPO and generally do not have IV access. What action should the nurse take in this case?

Decisions regarding the types of fluids administered before, during, and after surgery are determined based on the child's condition, length of surgery, and clinical condition. During surgery, nurses continue to administer fluids, measure fluid losses, and assess the child continuously (see Chapter 23 🔗 for fluid requirements for children).

Postoperative Care

Postoperative care of the child includes both physical and psychologic care. In the immediate postoperative period, perform baseline monitoring of vital signs; evaluate evidence of fluid loss via dressings, vomiting, or drainage tubes; and record hourly urinary

BOX 15–7	Preoperative Checklist
_____	Check that consent forms are witnessed and signed and in the patient's chart.
_____	Be sure the child's name band is in place.
_____	Be sure any allergies are prominently noted in the child's chart and on a special name band.
_____	Remove any prosthetic devices, including orthodontic appliances and body piercings.
_____	Check the child's mouth for loose teeth and tongue piercings.
_____	Remove eyeglasses and jewelry.
_____	Bathe and cleanse the operative site if ordered.
_____	Put the child in a hospital gown, allowing the child to wear underwear.
_____	Check that all special tests have been completed and the results are in the child's chart.
_____	Have the child void before surgery.
_____	Keep the child NPO before surgery.
_____	Give the child prescribed medications.
_____	Check vital signs and record on the chart.
_____	Transport the child safely to the operating room.

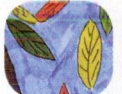

Partnering with Families

Waiting for the Child to Go to Surgery

Waiting for the child to go to surgery can be a very stressful time for both the family and the child. The major stressor for the infant and young child is the need to be NPO. Having a child who is upset because of hunger is very stressful for parents. Other stressors for parents include the risks of the surgery, pain the child will experience after the surgery, and in some cases what diagnosis may be made during or following the operation. Nurses must be sensitive to the concerns of the parents and provide support to these families. If the scheduled time for surgery has passed and no one has come to transport the child to the pediatric holding area, the nurse should call the operating room and see when they might expect that someone will come to get the child for surgery. Although this takes a few minutes, it is an essential aspect of a trusting family-centered environment.

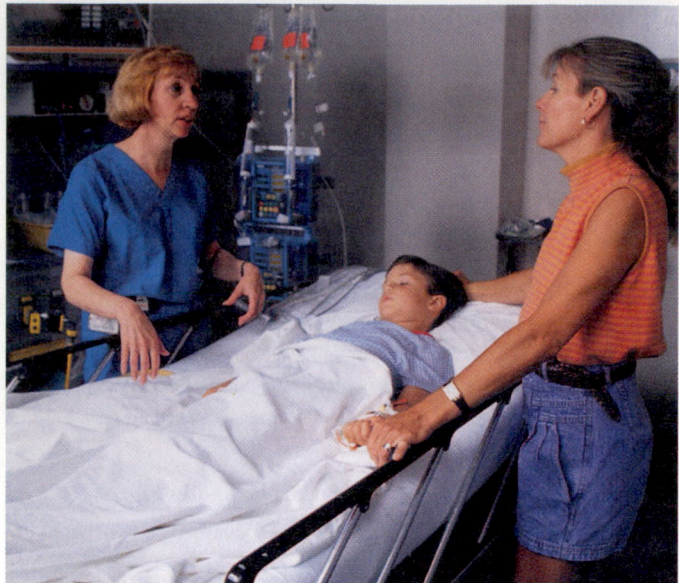

FIGURE 15–5 ■ This child has just undergone surgery and is in the postanesthesia care unit (PACU). Although the child's physical care is immediate and important, remember that both the child and the family have strong psychosocial needs that must also be addressed. It is important to reunite the family as soon as possible after surgery.

output. Maintain effective airway clearance and monitor for evidence of respiratory depression or distress (see Chapter 25 🔗). Examine the postoperative orders and ensure that the child receives the type and amount of intravenous fluid indicated.

The child's level of consciousness is evaluated, and vital signs are assessed frequently according to protocol, generally every 15 minutes for 1 hour, then every 30 minutes for 1 hour, followed by hourly vital signs for 4 hours. The surgical site is observed for drainage, and dressings are monitored for bleeding. The nurse monitors the child's intake and output hourly and provides comfort and pain relief. See Chapter 21 🔗 for details concerning pain management. Resumption of oral intake is dependent on the surgical procedure, the child's condition, and surgeon protocol. Once oral fluids are resumed, monitor for emesis. When the child is consuming adequate fluids, the rate of intravenous fluids is decreased or discontinued according to physician orders.

Parents are encouraged to visit with the child as soon after surgery as possible (Figure 15–5 ■). In some facilities, after surgery, children are brought to the postoperative anesthesia care unit (PACU) or postanesthesia recovery unit (PAR), where the child recovers from anesthesia. Depending on the child's condition, he or she may be discharged home directly from an outpatient surgical procedure or transferred to a general pediatric unit or intensive care unit.

Postoperative Home Care Instructions

Routine postoperative instructions for the family of the child undergoing outpatient or 1-day-stay surgical procedures include monitoring for signs of infection such as drainage, redness, or swelling of the surgical incision; fever; and change in behavior. Instructions for follow-up visits, medications, other treatments, wound care, and signs and symptoms that require medical attention are also provided. Additional instructions are tailored according to the surgical procedure and the child's condition. The nurse ensures the

family understands home care instructions through their return demonstration and statement of understanding.

STRATEGIES TO PROMOTE COPING AND NORMAL DEVELOPMENT OF THE HOSPITALIZED CHILD

During hospitalization, care of the child focuses not only on meeting physiologic needs, but also on meeting psychosocial and developmental needs. Nurses can employ several strategies to help children adapt to the hospital environment, promote effective coping, and provide developmentally appropriate activities: rooming in, child life programs, therapeutic play, and therapeutic recreation.

Rooming In

The practice of **rooming in** involves a parent staying in the child's hospital room during the course of the hospitalization. Some hospitals provide cots, while others have special built-in beds on pediatric units. In some institutions a parent is provided a separate room on the unit. Parents who stay at the bedside usually want to help care for their child (Power & Franck, 2008). Communication between the nurse and family is important so that the parent's desire for involvement is understood and supported.

Rooming in provides the child with the comfort and security of parental presence. Some parents may feel more comfortable staying with their child and participating in care, whereas others may experience more stress if they are missing work and are away from home and their other children. Partner with the parents to establish a rooming-in plan that is beneficial to both the child and family. For example, parents may alternate turns staying with the child. Grandparents, aunts and uncles, and grown siblings may be included in the plan.

Some facilities offer free or reduced-cost meals to the parent rooming in. The parent who does not receive these meals may often skip many meals due to the financial impact on an already overburdened budget related to illness and hospitalization. The nurse should be alert to the parent who never leaves the bedside and should make sure parents are eating. Emphasize the importance of the child's need for a healthy parent. Social services or other departments may be able to assist the family in obtaining meals while rooming in with the hospitalized child.

Parents rooming in with their child for an extended hospitalization can be encouraged to take advantage of facilities such as the Ronald McDonald room, Ronald McDonald house, or other housing available for parents, at some point during the stay as a respite for a few hours. This will provide them with an opportunity for needed rest and privacy.

Child Life Programs

Many hospitals have child life programs that focus on the psychosocial needs of hospitalized children. Professional child life specialists, paraprofessionals, and volunteers staff these departments (Figure 15–6A and B ■). A **child life specialist** plans activities to provide age-appropriate play for children either in the child's room or in a specialized playroom. Some of the planned activities are designed to assist children in working through feelings about illness. Examples include playing with medical equipment, acting out procedures or treatments on dolls, using games to act out feelings, or drawing pictures about hospital treatments (Figure 15–7 ■).

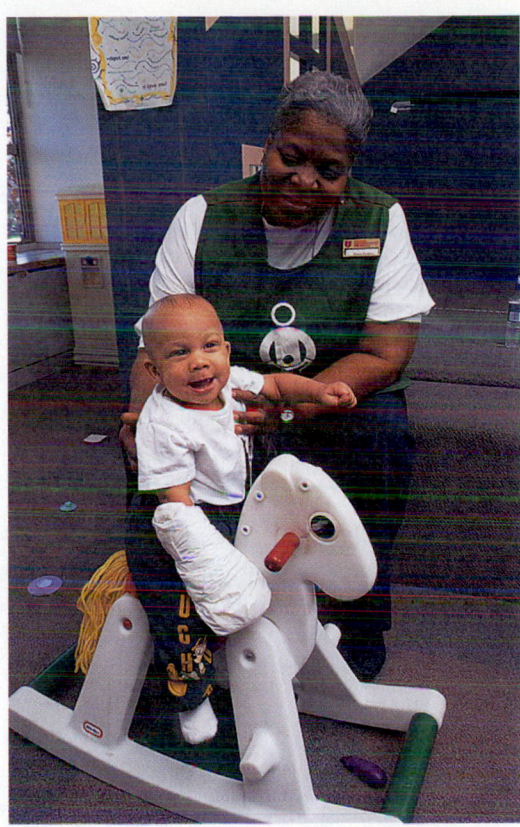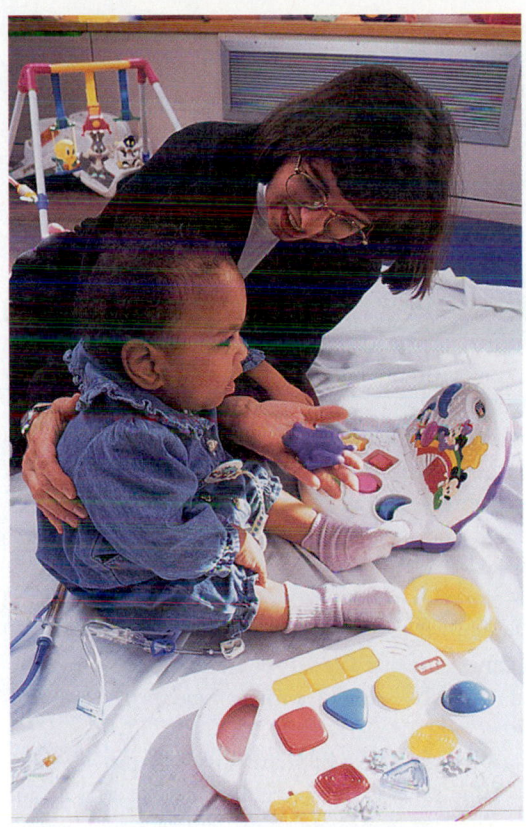

FIGURE 15–6 ■ *A*, Volunteers such as this foster grandmother can provide stimulation and nurturing to help young children adapt to lengthy hospitalizations. *B*, Child life specialists plan activities for young children in the hospital to facilitate play and stress reduction.

Both the child life department and the nursing staff focus on the emotional needs of hospitalized children. Child life specialists and nurses collaborate to formulate a plan to assist children with particular needs. Before engaging in activities, attention is given to the child's level of mobility, fatigue, readiness to participate, and other barriers such as pain. The nurse and child life specialist can work together to determine appropriate methods to promote coping with painful procedures.

Therapeutic Play

Play is a significant component of childhood, and the stress of illness and hospitalization increases the value of play. Hospitals, however, because of the need to contain costs, may minimize their play programs. Therefore, nurses should document the need for and benefits of play. Beyond facilitating normal development, play sessions can provide a means for the child to:

- Learn about health care
- Express anxieties
- Work through feelings
- Achieve a sense of mastery or control over frightening or little-understood situations

Play that presents an opportunity to deal with the fears, concerns, and stressors of health experiences is called **therapeutic play.** Therapeutic play has many benefits for both the child and the health professional. It allows the child an opportunity to relive, understand, and integrate fearful healthcare experiences. The child can achieve a sense of mastery by being in control of the occurrences during play. This helps to lower the child's stress and anxiety about the events. In

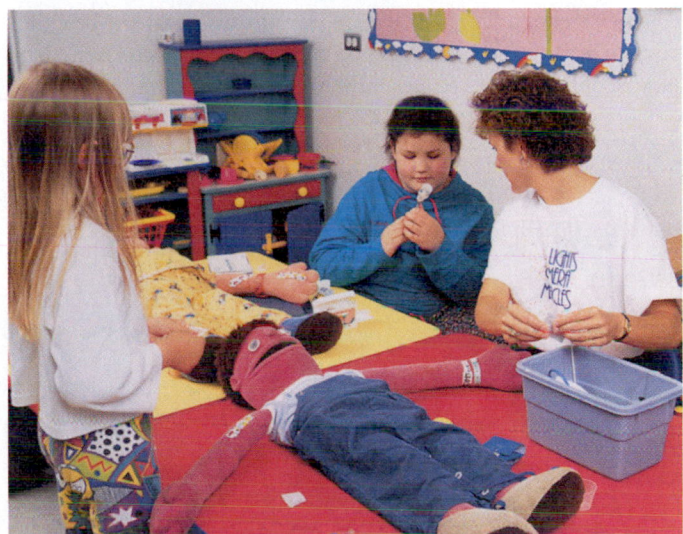

FIGURE 15–7 ■ A child life specialist works with children being treated for cancer. Special dolls are used to familiarize children with the procedures they undergo.

addition, the healthcare professional can observe the child's play to learn more about the type of events that cause anxiety to the child. The child's coping methods can be observed and additional techniques offered to the child. *Play therapy* is a mental health technique used to treat children with mental health problems, rather than normal life events that have caused anxiety. This technique is discussed in Chapter 34 🔗.

Through therapeutic play, the child's knowledge of his or her illness or injury can be assessed. A common technique involves using an outline drawing of the body (Figure 15–8 ■) or having the child draw a picture about the hospitalization. Drawings can be used to determine what the child knows and understands about the hospitalization. In addition to assessment, drawing can be used as a nursing intervention. Demonstrate to the child on a drawing what will occur during surgery or a treatment. The child's drawings of healthcare experiences allow him or her to express fears and gain mastery over the situation.

Dramatic play, in which medical situations encountered are reenacted by the child, often assists the child to cope with painful treatments and intrusive procedures. Safe medical equipment such as bandages and syringes without needles, and scrubs and uniforms for dress up, are effective materials for encouraging dramatic play. Dramatic play offers an outlet for anxiety in children trying to deal with stressful and confusing situations. At the same time, these activities allow the nurses to observe and assess the child's perception of the illness and procedures. The nurse is then able to clarify any of the child's misconceptions.

A variety of techniques may be used to promote therapeutic and dramatic play (Table 15–7), depending on the child's developmental stage. The nurse can ensure that a variety of age-appropriate toys, distraction materials (stress balls, bubbles, music), and "prizes" are available (Box 15–8).

Many hospitals, particularly children's hospitals, provide playrooms on each of the units to allow children a place to play and socialize with same-age peers. These rooms are generally brightly decorated in children's themes and provide numerous opportunities for play, such as board games, video games, supplies for painting or drawing, and age-appropriate toys for each developmental level. For younger children, families may be encouraged to bring the child's favorite age-appropriate toys from home. For older children, there may be options for computer communication with children in other

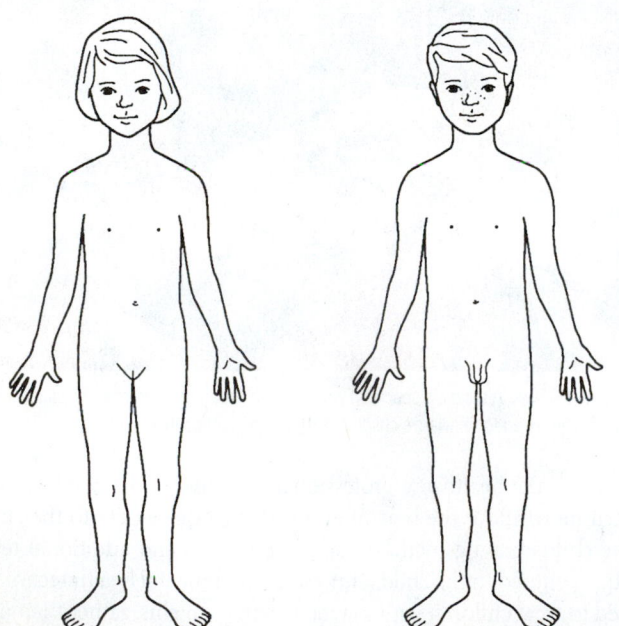

FIGURE 15–8 ■ The nurse can use a simple gender-specific outline drawing of a child's body to encourage children to draw what they think about their medical problem. Such drawings reveal a child's interpretation, which the nurse can work with to provide enhanced teaching.

BOX 15–8 **Prize Basket**

A "prize" basket is an effective method of providing rewards and distraction to the toddler, preschooler, and even school-age child. The basket contains age-appropriate toys, games, and items that the child may choose from as a reward for participating in a procedure. For example, bubbles, stuffed animals, small dolls, coloring books, balls, and books are inexpensive (they may also be donated) items from which the child can choose. Even if the child is uncooperative, once the procedure is completed the child should be praised and offered the opportunity to choose from the prize basket.

---

hospitals. Portable electronic gaming equipment may be available to children in isolation or those unable to come to the playroom or teen lounge. Specific interventions according to developmental level are discussed in the following section.

Newborn and Infant

Newborns and infants require external stimuli for growth. The use of mobiles, music, and mirrors helps to promote stimulation and offer comfort to the newborn or infant. Parents and family members are encouraged to cuddle or rock the infant and sing lullabies. Talking to the infant encourages interaction and play.

Toddler

Through play, toddlers explore the environment and learn to identify with significant people in their lives. Play is also an acceptable way for toddlers to release tensions caused by stress or aggressive impulses.

Approach toddlers slowly and make the initial approach in their parents' presence, if possible, to decrease feelings of stranger anxiety (wariness of strangers). Playing a variation of peek-a-boo or hide-and-seek using the curtain surrounding the toddler's crib or bed helps promote the realization that objects out of sight, such as parents, do return. The use of a familiar blanket or stuffed animal can temporarily substitute for the security of parents. The toddler can be read familiar stories. Repetition of stories promotes a sense of stability in the unfamiliar hospital environment.

A doll can be used to re-create a stressful environment, thereby providing an opportunity for the child to express and work through feelings. Other developmentally appropriate toys for toddlers include familiar objects from home—measuring cups or spoons, wooden puzzles, building blocks, and push-and-pull toys. Playing with safe hospital equipment (bandages, syringes without needles, and stethoscopes) helps toddlers to overcome the anxiety associated with these items. Supervise these play sessions and remove hospital equipment when you leave.

Preschooler

The nurse can intervene to reduce the stress produced by preschoolers' fears through the use of certain kinds of play. A simple outline of the body or a doll can be used to address the child's fantasies and fears of bodily harm. Playing with safe hospital equipment may help preschoolers to work through feelings such as aggression (Figure 15–9 ■).

Preschoolers prefer crayons and coloring books, puppets, felt and magnetic boards, play dough, books, and recorded stories. Preschoolers and older children often enjoy **animal-assisted activity.** Children's hospitals and units can have visits from pets, most commonly dogs, to provide diversion and relaxation (McKenney & Johnson, 2008; Ryan, 2008) (Figure 15–10 ■).

TABLE 15–7	**Therapeutic Play Techniques**	
TECHNIQUE*	**ASSESSMENT**	**INTERVENTIONS**
Stories	Have the child make up a story about a picture. Analyze content and emotional clues in the story. Have the child tell a story about an important experience in a group of other children.	Read or make up stories to explain illness, hospitalization, or other specific aspects of health care. Emotions such as fear can be included.
Drawings	Ask the child to draw a picture about being in the hospital. Consider subject matter, size and placement of items in drawings, colors used, presence or absence of physical barriers, and general emotional feeling.	Use the child's drawings or outlines of the body to explain care, procedures, or conditions. Provide an opportunity for the child to draw pictures of his or her choice, or suggest topics such as a picture of the child's family or healthcare encounter. Ask the child to tell you about the picture. Be alert to the child's emotions. You might say, "This child must be frightened by the big x-ray machine."
Music	Observe types of music chosen and effects of played music on behavior.	Encourage parents and children to bring favorite music to the hospital for stress relief. Have music playing during tests and procedures. Parents can record their voices to play for infants and young children during separations. During longer hospitalizations, children can record messages for siblings or classmates, who are then encouraged to record their responses. Playtime can include the opportunity to play instruments and sing.
Puppets	The puppets can ask questions of young children, who are often more likely to answer the puppet than a person.	Perform short skits to teach children necessary healthcare information. Include emotional content when appropriate.
Dramatic play	Provide dolls and medical equipment, and analyze the roles assigned to dolls by the child, the behavior demonstrated by the dolls in the child's play, and the apparent emotions. Dolls with health problems like those of the child are especially helpful.	Provide dolls and equipment for play sessions. To ensure safety, supervise closely when actual equipment is used. Respond to emotions and behavior shown. Use dolls and equipment such as a cast, nebulizer, intravenous apparatus, and stethoscope to explain care. Use dolls with problems or disabilities similar to those of the child when available. Provide toys that foster expression of emotion, such as a pounding board and indoor darts.
Pets	Provide animal-assisted activity. Watch the interaction between the child and animal.	Respond to emotions the child shows. Facilitate touch and stroking of animals.

*Additional techniques, such as sand or water play, may be appropriate in specific situations.

School-Age Child

Although play begins to lose its importance in the school-age years, the nurse can still use some techniques of therapeutic play to help the hospitalized child cope with stress. Age-appropriate crafts and activities provide diversion and a sense of accomplishment. School-age children often regress developmentally during hospitalization, demonstrating behaviors characteristic of an earlier state, such as separation anxiety and fear of bodily injury. Outlines of the body, anatomically correct dolls, or condition-specific dolls (Figure 15–11 ■) can be used to illustrate the cause and treatment of the child's illness. Terms for body parts that are suitable for older children are used. Drawings provide an outlet for expression of fear and anger.

School-age children enjoy collecting and organizing objects and often ask to keep disposable equipment that has been used in their care. They may use these items later to relive the experience with their friends. Games, books, puzzles, schoolwork, crafts, tape recordings, computers, and video games provide an outlet for stress and increase self-esteem in the school-age child. The type of play used should promote a sense of mastery and achievement.

Adolescent

Many of the special play techniques used with younger children are not suitable for adolescents. However, adolescents do require a planned **therapeutic recreation** program to assist them in meeting developmental needs during hospitalization. Peers are very important to the adolescent, and the isolation of hospitalization can be difficult. Telephone contact with other teenagers and visits from friends should be encouraged. Interactions with other hospitalized teenagers while eating pizza, playing video games, watching a movie,

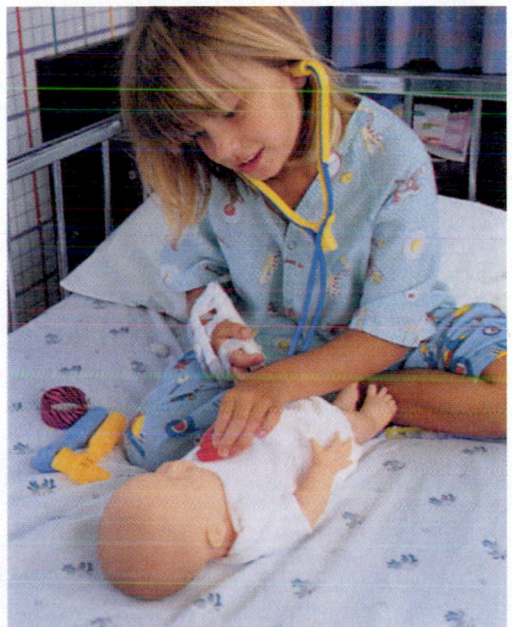

FIGURE 15–9 ■ Age-appropriate play will help the child adjust to hospitalization and care.

or participating in other activities can help adolescents feel a sense of normalcy (Figure 15–12 ■). Physical activities that provide an outlet for stress are recommended. Even adolescents who are on bed rest or who use wheelchairs can play a modified form of basketball. Some hospitals provide a teen room or teen lounge with age-appropriate activities such as a pool table, video games, and computers.

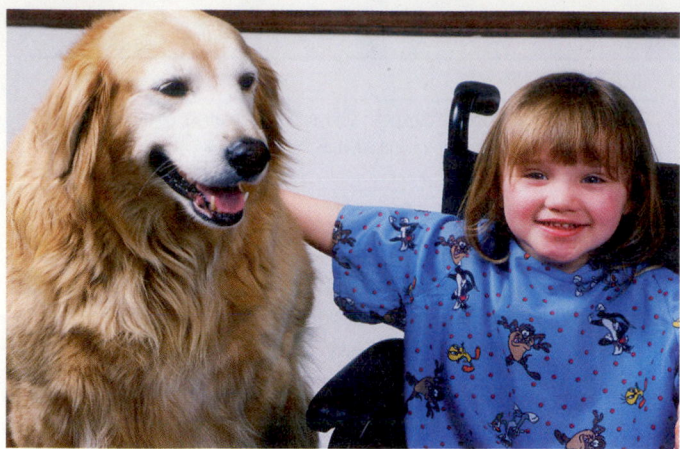

FIGURE 15–10 ■ Hospitals may have animal-assisted activity from specially trained animals to provide comfort and distraction during health care. Both the child and the dog seem to be smiling!

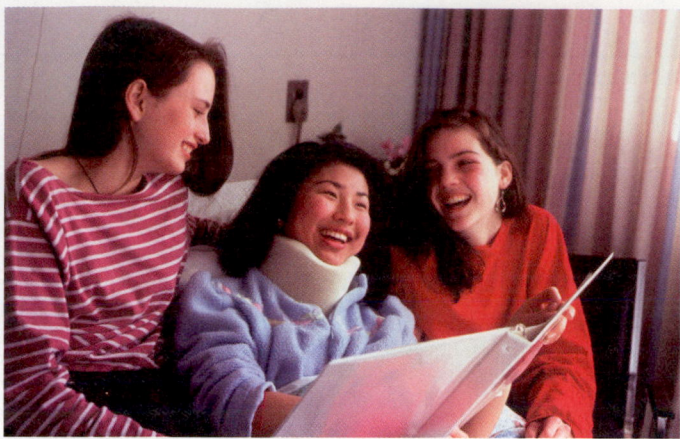

FIGURE 15–12 ■ Having interaction with other hospitalized adolescents and maintaining contact with friends outside the hospital are very important so that the teenager does not feel alone.
Source: *Flirt/Superstock.*

The independence of adolescence is interrupted by illness. Nurses can provide choices for teenagers to assist them in regaining control. Providing adolescents with options and encouraging them to choose an evening recreational activity can promote their feelings of independence.

Strategies to Meet Educational Needs

Some hospitalizations are so short that the absence of the child or adolescent from school and peers is of minimal concern. However, if hospitalization is expected to last longer than a few days or if the child's condition will change, necessitating special school

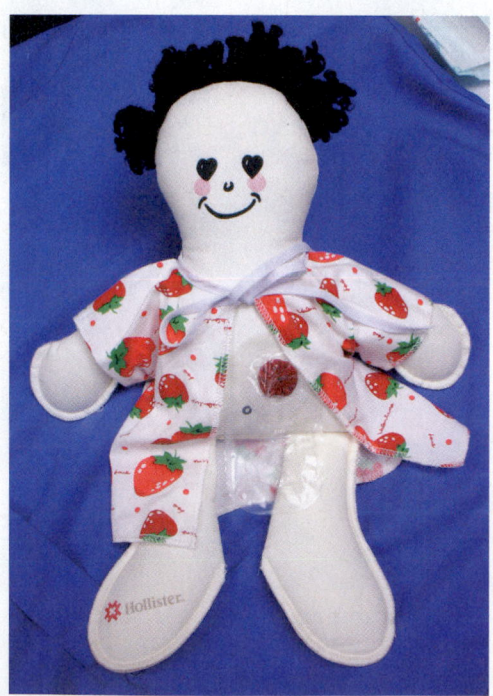

FIGURE 15–11 ■ Having the child play with dolls like this Shadow Buddy that have "conditions" similar to his or her own will help the child adjust. Such play helps the child realize what activities are possible.
Source: *Used with permission from the Shadow Buddies Foundation.*

arrangements, the nurse assesses the effects of hospitalization on the child's education (see Legal and Ethical Considerations: Schooling).

When an elective procedure occurs, partner with families to arrange the extended school absence with teachers. The child can then be provided with schoolwork to complete in the hospital or at home when capable. This minimizes educational deficits and future problems for the child. Pencils, paper, comfortable work areas, computers, and quiet work times are provided to meet the child's educational needs. Telephone calls, Internet connections, and live videoconferencing with teachers can be arranged as needed. Pediatric hospitals generally provide in-house teachers to meet the child's educational needs. The hospital teachers collaborate with the child's school teachers to ensure the child is meeting the educational objectives to avoid deficits upon return to school.

Nurses should also consider the social aspects of school and peers. Peers can be encouraged to visit a hospitalized classmate, send cards and letters, call on the telephone, or communicate via the Internet. Classmates may even want to make a video recording of a class session, allowing everyone the opportunity to send a message to the child. When the child returns to school, the nurse can visit the classroom to provide classmates with information about the child's medical condition or assist the child in creating his or her own presentation about the hospital experience and medical condition.

The hospital nurse may contact the child's school nurse when special arrangements are necessary for situations such as mobility

Legal and Ethical Considerations
Schooling

The Joint Commission on Accreditation of Healthcare Organizations (2009) mandates provision of schooling for the child in a healthcare facility for an extended period.

challenges. For example, the child who is wearing a large cast or who requires medications or other treatments, such as tracheostomy care, may offer challenges in a traditional school setting. Refer to Chapter 14 🔗 for further discussion of caring for the child in the community.

The child with chronic health problems or requiring long-term hospitalization has additional needs with regard to school. Hospitals or rehabilitation units may have classrooms, teachers, and facilities to promote learning. Many school districts provide tutors or computer connections for students who are hospitalized or receiving home care for extended periods. Teachers can visit children at the hospital or at home. Parents are often pivotal in making arrangements to meet the child's educational needs, since they interact with the child, the school, and the healthcare team. Further discussion of meeting the educational needs of the child with a chronic condition is provided in Chapter 16 🔗.

Child and Family Teaching

Teaching is an essential part of the nurse's role in care of hospitalized children and their families. It begins with the initial contact between the family and healthcare providers. Teaching may be informal, as when the nurse integrates an explanation during routine care, or structured, as when the nurse plans and implements a formal teaching program.

Nurses emphasize to the family that most teaching will occur in informal sessions rather than in formalized programs. The family should be aware of the teaching process to encourage active listening and participation. Actively involve the family in the learning process to ensure their understanding. The nurse and family partner together to identify the family's learning needs and appropriate teaching methods to best convey the information. Recall that family members may be at various cognitive and anxiety levels and therefore have needs for different types of teaching. Develop a plan with both the family and other healthcare professionals to facilitate learning among the child and family members.

Teaching directed at children that takes into account their developmental level and is detailed and accurate will be more effective (Gursky et al., 2010). Learning is achieved more successfully when teaching involves more than one sense (such as hearing, vision, and touch).

Teaching about the behaviors observed in hospitalized children and the strategies to deal with these behaviors is helpful for parents. For instance, provide parents of hospitalized toddlers with information on the typical behaviors of hospitalized children and the strategies to assist them. By being informed, the parents should have less anxiety and a greater capacity for involvement and support of their child during hospitalization.

Teaching directed at parents must be geared to their level of understanding. If English is not spoken or is the parents' second language, then an interpreter may be necessary. If interpreters are needed to facilitate understanding, be sure they are arranged and available for teaching sessions (see Chapters 3 and 6 🔗 for further discussion of the use of interpreters).

Depending on the information to be presented, teaching may use the cognitive, psychomotor, or affective domains of learning. Teaching that includes all three domains is more effective. Explanations or reading materials, including pamphlets, booklets, DVDs, and models, are tailored to a level the parent can understand. The choice of tools used varies depending on the child's diagnosis and available materials.

Timing is a critical factor in teaching. Parents and children are less receptive to teaching when they are preoccupied with stress or activities. Collaborating with the parents in scheduling specific times for teaching sessions may be helpful.

Teaching Plans

Teaching plans provide structure for the creation and delivery of patient and family education. By developing a teaching plan, a nurse helps to ensure that all the necessary information is included and taught efficiently. Additionally, this written documentation of teaching allows for continuity of care between nurses and other disciplines. Multidisciplinary teaching plans provide clear communication for all health team members in the teaching process. A teaching plan should include:

- Goals and expected outcomes
- Interventions needed to achieve the specified goals and a method
- Time for evaluation of the expected outcomes
- Teaching methods and types of materials to be used

Nurses individualize teaching plans and sessions according to the child's ability and needs. Adequate assessment of the child's strengths and abilities, along with collaboration with parents and other members of the multidisciplinary team, can assist the nurse to establish an individualized plan of the most effective teaching methods for the child. See Partnering with Families: Standardized Teaching Plan: Preparing the Child for Surgery.

The child's primary caretaker should be an active participant in the development and implementation of the teaching plan. The primary caretaker is most often a parent but may be a close family member (uncle, aunt, or grandparent). Prior to establishing a teaching plan the nurse should assess the child's or parent's knowledge, skills, and feelings by considering the following questions:

- What does the parent/caretaker or child know about the health issue?
- What are the expectations of the child and family?
- What is the cognitive level or ability to learn?
- Is there a desire to learn?
- What previous experiences affect the learning experience, either positively or negatively?
- What previous interventions have been the most useful for the child and family?
- What resources are available to the parents, child, and nurse that enhance understanding of the health condition?
- Are there feelings or beliefs that might interfere with the learning process?
- What complementary care does the family use, and how does this relate to the teaching plan?

The second step involves deciding what knowledge, skill, or change in attitude is desired. Outcome criteria or objectives are established with the parent and child. Possible teaching methods and a range of approaches are explored. A variety of resources,

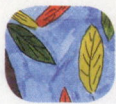

Partnering with Families

Standardized Teaching Plan: Preparing the Child for Surgery

Whether the child is encountered in the clinic, preoperative admissions clinic, emergency department, or pediatric unit, the nurse should prepare the child for surgery as much as possible. While younger children should be told about a planned operation the day before, school-age children and adolescents should be told as soon as the operation is scheduled. Age-specific guidelines should be followed. (See Table 15–6: Assisting Children Through Procedures on page 400, and Nursing Care Plan: The Child Undergoing Surgery.)

GENERAL PRINCIPLES
- Ask the child's parents what they have told their child about the operation.
- Assess the child's perception of the operation using developmentally appropriate activities.
- Teach the child about the operation and what to expect during the pre- and postoperative period, clarifying any misconceptions.
- Reassess the child's perception of the operation.

SAMPLE TEACHING PLAN FOR TIONA, THE 5-YEAR-OLD GIRL SCHEDULED FOR A TONSILLECTOMY AND ADENOIDECTOMY

When: At the preadmissions visit the day prior to surgery
Where: In a quiet room, without distraction
How:
- Ask Tiona's mother what she has told her daughter about the surgery.
- Ask Tiona to draw a picture about going to the hospital.
- Ask Tiona why she needs the operation.
- Using a body outline doll or picture of a body outline, ask Tiona to show you what part is going to be fixed.
- Use pictures, books, dolls, and safe medical equipment to clarify misconceptions and teach Tiona about the operation. Allow Tiona the opportunity to play with safe medical equipment.
- Reassess Tiona's understanding of the operation by allowing her to dress up in scrubs and "operate" on a doll. Include what she will see, hear, taste, smell, and feel in both the preoperative and postoperative period.

---

including written materials (books, pamphlets, handouts, and stories), computer software, audiovisual presentations, and others, are available to encourage interest from the child and family. Refer to Chapter 1 🔗 for information on reading level of patient education materials. In some settings, audiovisual and computer resources may be limited. Small-group teaching sessions (e.g., for children with recently diagnosed diabetes) may be another option and provide the child with an opportunity to interact and learn from peers experiencing the same condition. Gathering two or three parents together on a unit to learn and share experiences may also be helpful.

Clinical Tip
For children who can use multiple senses (hear, touch, see a model or equipment, read, look at pictures, or even smell such items as alcohol swabs), learning is more complete. This is particularly important for the school-age child in the stage of concrete operational thought, who must be able to manipulate materials in order to learn.

For some conditions, standardized teaching plans are available in books and from healthcare agencies. These plans can serve as a guide in developing an individualized teaching plan.

Teaching for Children with Special Healthcare Needs

Children who have disabilities may have special learning needs. If the child has a visual impairment or perceptual difficulty, material is presented in auditory and tactile ways. Children who have hearing deficits require visual and tactile presentations. When psychomotor skill performance is needed to assess a child with neuromuscular conditions, special aids and devices may be necessary to enable the child to hold a syringe, draw up a liquid, or perform other tasks. Children who have learning disabilities may require more frequent reinforcement and shorter teaching sessions. These children are evaluated often for comprehension in order to adjust teaching as necessary.

Children who have chronic conditions or special healthcare needs may have been hospitalized numerous times and have received other health care at home and in the community. They usually have adapted coping mechanisms that help them deal with the chronic illness. Nurses can talk with the child to determine what has helped in the past, provide information about what to expect during the current hospitalization, assign staff members who are familiar when possible, and follow each child's lead in assisting his or her coping.

Do not assume that the child with a history of numerous hospitalizations understands all activities. Each hospitalization is different. Even the most routine activities should be explained. Regularly review the updated plan of care with the parents and child. Provide the child with opportunities to ask questions and to express concerns and fears. Assess the child's individual learning needs. Older children can be asked how they best like to learn. Determine the necessity for special equipment or teaching methods.

PREPARATION FOR HOME CARE

Nurses play an important role in preparing the child and family for discharge home; this preparation starts early during the hospitalization. The nurse works with the social service department, home care agencies, and the family to plan for equipment, procedures, and other home care needs. Home care nurses collaborate with the hospital nurse and assist families to meet the child's healthcare needs.

Assessing the Child and Family in Preparation for Discharge

Preparations for the discharge process are best started upon admission to the hospital. The healthcare team, including the primary healthcare provider, nurse, social worker, and discharge planner, partners with the family to ensure a smooth transition. Assess the family's ability to manage the child's care and if any special adaptation to the home environment is necessary.

When a child who has been hospitalized for an extended time is to be discharged home, the school district is contacted by the hospital teacher (if available) or social worker, and plans for education or reentry into school are made. This involves an assessment of the child by the school district and formulation of an *individualized education plan (IEP)*. The IEP may include home tutors, specialized services from persons such as physical or speech therapists, or arrangements for transport of the child with a disability to the school and provisions for special medical care as needed. An *individualized health plan (IHP)* may also be required. See Chapter 16 ⊘ for definitions and a detailed discussion on IEPs and IHPs.

Some common problems that interfere with successful discharge planning include financial concerns, the family's unavailability for teaching and planning, lack of equipment, and lack of teamwork among involved healthcare disciplines. Nurses who assess for these potential problems from the initial contact with the child and family can intervene and assist the family to resolve them as soon as possible.

Preparing the Child and Family for Discharge

The family may need to learn physical and rehabilitative procedures for the child's care. Short-term care may be necessary until the child regains full function. In other situations, care may be required throughout the child's life. This may involve measuring vital signs or assessing blood glucose levels. Partner with families to teach them about the child's care at home.

Some facilities provide families with the opportunity to provide 24-hour care to the child prior to discharge to help them gain confidence in providing care and allow the nurse to assess for areas requiring further teaching.

For the child requiring complex long-term care, parents may need to learn about intravenous lines, medications, oxygen administration, or ventilators (Figure 15–13 ■). See Chapter 16 ⊘ for discussion of the child with a chronic condition. Parents of children at risk for respiratory or cardiac arrest are encouraged to learn cardiopulmonary resuscitation (CPR) (refer to Appendix F ⊘ and the Clinical Skills Manual ⊂⊃). Individual sessions to teach the family CPR can be arranged. Some families require support and assistance to become providers of end-of-life care (see Chapter 18 ⊘ for discussion of end-of-life care).

Not all children discharged after hospitalization will require additional care. However, these families still need support and education, as they may continue to be anxious or stressed over their child's hospitalization. Standard discharge plans for routine hospital discharge include:

- Follow-up appointment date(s)
- Phone number(s) to call for questions
- Medication instructions
- Signs and symptoms to monitor for that are specific to the condition
- Instructions for care at home

Ensure that the family understands these instructions and has ample time for questions before discharge home.

Preparing the Child and Family for Home Health Care

Children discharged from the hospital may require short- or long-term home health care. Children with multisystem conditions may

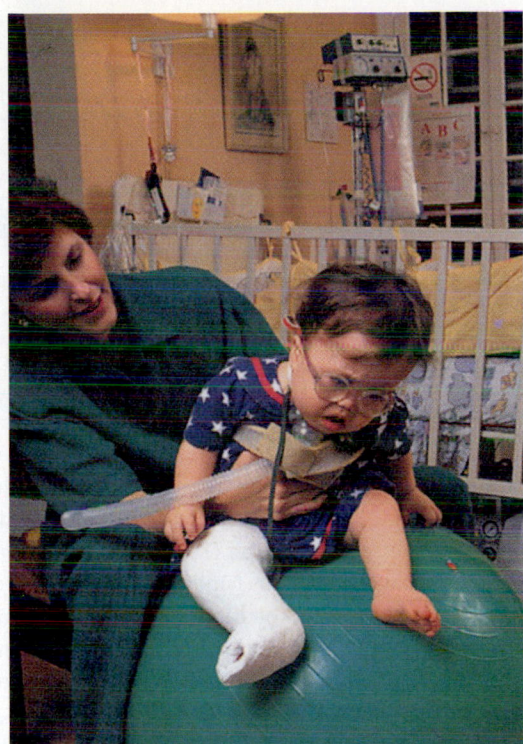

FIGURE 15–13 ■ This child with chronic medical problems is being cared for at home. Are there any legal implications for the hospital and the nurse associated with preparation of the child and family for home care?

require home care involving specialized equipment and personnel. Early planning provides the family time to investigate health insurance benefits, support services in the community, and other needs before discharge. The education provided and the parents' ability to perform care is discussed with a visiting nurse or individual who manages the home care program.

Nurses can support parents during rooming in by making them comfortable and integrating them into discussions and decisions about the child's care; they are collaborators in all of the care involved. Nurses can also view every interaction as a teachable moment and constantly include teaching whenever a parent is present. Explanations related to medications, assessments being performed, and how this will be adapted in the home situation should be included. In addition, resources including phone numbers, parent support groups, reading material, and Internet sources should be provided. The effectiveness of teaching should be evaluated prior to discharge (Weiss et al., 2008) (Box 15–9). Ask parents what care they feel comfortable with and what they need more assistance to perform. Involve them in the decision about referral to a home healthcare nurse or school nurse.

The nurse collaborates with the social service department, home care agencies, and the family to plan for equipment, procedures, and other home care needs. Home care nurses then assume the child's care and assist families to meet the child's healthcare needs. See Chapter 14 ⊘ for further discussion of home health care.

Preparing the Child and Family for Long-Term Care or Rehabilitation

When ill or injured children require long-term care, they are often transferred from an acute care hospital to a rehabilitation center or other long-term care facility. Like discharge planning, the rehabilitation

BOX 15–9   Research: Parental Readiness for Discharge

A study by Weiss, Johnson, Malin, et al. (2008) evaluated readiness for discharge in 135 parents of children who were hospitalized. The parent who was the primary caregiver of the child after discharge from the hospital participated in the study. Results of this study indicated that the nurse's skill in presenting the discharge information was a significant predictor of the parents' readiness for discharge. A higher rating by the parents of the nurse's skill in discharge teaching correlated with a higher level of discharge readiness. The amount of content delivered was not a significant predictor, with 90% of the parents indicating that they actually received more content than needed. Parents who had higher levels of discharge readiness also had less coping difficulty post discharge.

phase of the treatment does not begin at the time of discharge from the acute care hospital but, instead, early in the hospitalization phase. The plan of care is instituted in the hospital, interventions and therapies are begun, and plans are made for continued care. A multidisciplinary team, including the nurse, social worker, and case manager, coordinates the process and collaborates with the family to ensure a transition that causes the least disruption to the child and family. (See Chapter 1 .)

When it becomes apparent that a child will require long-term care, the healthcare team explores with the family the options and resources available to provide the following care:

- Home care with support services such as visiting nurses and physical therapists
- A long-term care facility
- A specialized rehabilitation center that can provide care for an extended period

The nurse supports the family during the decision-making process about which option will be the most beneficial, considering the needs of the child, the financial implications, the roles and supports available to the family unit, and the resources available in the community. Guidelines to assist parents in evaluating rehabilitation centers are available from the Brain Injury Association of America

(2011). Families can also be referred to the Commission on Accreditation of Rehabilitation Facilities.

Families often require assistance in determining the insurance coverage for long-term care or rehabilitation as coverage for these services may be limited. Social services can assist the family in identifying insurance resources. If parents must take a leave of absence from work to provide care for the child, inform them about the coverage provided by the Family Medical Leave Act (U.S. Department of Labor, 2010). Partner with social services to assist the family in completing the applications, if needed.

Nurses in acute care hospitals frequently coordinate services when transfer to another facility occurs. This involves providing information to the new facility about the child's history, plan of care, treatment, and current status. Forms should be available to assist the person responsible for coordinating the transfer. Provide copies of nursing and medical care plans to ensure continuity of care.

Families require support and assistance in dealing with the transfer from the acute care setting to another facility. The family may benefit from a visit to the facility before the child is transferred. Meeting the staff and becoming familiar with the environment can assist the family in preparing the child for a new environment. The family can then provide the child with brochures, pictures, and other materials from the facility and explain what the child can anticipate experiencing upon transfer. If possible, visits from rehabilitation center or long-term care facility nursing staff to the child before transfer can also be beneficial.

Whether the child is discharged home without the need for further care or with the need for home healthcare or rehabilitative care, the nurse maintains a family-centered approach to provide the child and family with information and support during the discharge process. The nurse ensures that the family is prepared for the discharge and that the family understands any treatments and monitoring. Contact information is provided and any support services required are arranged before the child is discharged.

Chapter Highlights

- Hospitalization is a stressful event for all children and their families, especially when the hospitalization is unplanned and sudden.
- Children's understanding about their illnesses and hospitalizations is based on cognitive and psychosocial stage/level, and upon previous healthcare experiences.
- Nurses assess the impact of the child's illness or hospitalization on the family unit and provide individualized family-centered care.
- Families are always disrupted by a child's hospitalization, and various approaches can help them to understand the process and cope more successfully with this challenge.
- When hospitalization is planned, both the child and parents can prepare for the experience. Nurses assist this process by teaching them what to expect.

- A teaching plan includes goals and expected outcomes, interventions needed to achieve the specified goals, and a method and time for evaluation of the expected outcomes. How the teaching plan is implemented depends on the unique characteristics of the child and family to be taught.
- The child is prepared for procedures using a variety of techniques taking into consideration the child's developmental age, coping abilities, and previous experience.
- Strategies such as child life programs, rooming in, therapeutic play, and therapeutic recreation help meet the psychosocial needs of the hospitalized child.
- The nurse assists the family to plan for the child's long-term healthcare needs and home care issues. Culturally competent care is integrated throughout all provisions of care.

Clinical Reasoning in Action

INTRODUCTION

Recall Tiona, the child described in the beginning of the chapter. She is a 5-year-old girl who was admitted to the hospital for a tonsillectomy and adenoidectomy (T&A).

DESCRIPTION

Following Tiona's operation, she refused to drink liquids because it hurt when she swallowed. After receiving intravenous pain medication, Tiona realized that she could swallow without too much pain and began to eat Popsicles and drink liquids. She was then switched to oral pain medication. Later in the day, Tiona was drinking liquids well enough to be discharged home.

DISCUSSION

1. What information should the nurse include in the discharge teaching plan for Tiona's mother?

2. As Tiona and her mother are preparing to leave the hospital, Tiona says, "I am going to be good so I do not have to come to the hospital anymore!" How should the nurse respond?

3. Tiona's mother states that she is worried that her daughter will not drink enough at home. What can the nurse suggest to Tiona's mother to encourage her to drink fluids? What are the symptoms of dehydration that Tiona's mother should watch for over the next few days?

4. Children Tiona's age have many fears and stressors related to hospitalization and surgery. How can her mother assist Tiona to express her feelings about the hospital experience once she is home?

NCLEX-RN® Review

1. The nurse is caring for a female child who is recovering from a motor vehicle accident. The child's parents ask if it is okay to bring the child's siblings to visit. What is the most appropriate response by the nurse?
   1. "No, it would not be good for your child to see her siblings as it may make her worse."
   2. "No, it would be very upsetting for your child's siblings to see her this way."
   3. "Yes, it is okay to bring your child's siblings to see her as long as you bring someone to watch them."
   4. "Yes, it is okay to bring your child's siblings for a visit as long as we educate them on what to expect when they visit.

2. How can the nurse best limit the amount of separation anxiety that the hospitalized toddler will experience?
   1. Reduce the amount of time spent with the child when the parents are not present.
   2. Discourage the amount of time the parents hold their child while hospitalized.
   3. Encourage the parents to leave the child's room when care is being provided.
   4. Encourage parental involvement in the child's care and suggest rooming in if possible.

3. Which behavior by a child's parents is the best indicator that they understand how to administer medication to the child at home following surgery?
   1. The parents sign the written discharge instruction verifying understanding of the instructions.
   2. The parents give the medication to the child using the appropriate technique in the nurse's presence.
   3. The parents state they understand how to administer the medication and deny questions.
   4. The parents state they can give the medication to the child using appropriate technique.

4. The nurse is caring for a 5-year-old male child who will be having a tonsillectomy performed. What teaching method is most appropriate for this child prior to the surgical procedure?
   1. Provide the child's mother with brochure about the procedure.
   2. Sit with the child while he watches a video about the procedure.
   3. Use dolls to teach the child about the procedure.
   4. Allow the child to talk to other children who have had the procedure.

See Appendix I 🔗 for answers.

References

Bindler, R. C., Ball, J. W., Ladewig, P. W., & London, M. L. (2011). *Clinical skills manual for maternal & child nursing care* (3rd ed., p. 110). Upper Saddle River, NJ: Pearson.

Brain Injury Association of America. (2011). *A guide to selecting and monitoring brain injury rehabilitation services.* Retrieved from http://www.biausa.org/Default.aspx?SiteSearchID=1192&ID=/search-results.htm

Chahal, N., Manlhiot, C., Colapinto, K., Alphen, J. V., McCrindle, B. W., & Rush, J. (2009). Association between parental anxiety and compliance with preoperative requirements for pediatric outpatient surgery. *Journal of Pediatric Health Care, 25*(6), 372–377.

Crenshaw, J. T., & Winslow, E. H. (2008). Preoperative fasting and medication instruction: Are we improving? *AORN Journal, 88*(6), 963–976.

Disch, J., Dreher, M., Davidson, P., Sinioris, M., & Wainio, J. A. (2011). The role of the chief nurse officer in ensuring patient safety and quality. *Journal of Nursing Administration, 41*(4), 179–185.

Drahota, A., & Malcarne, V. L. (2008). Concepts of illness in children: A comparison between children with and without intellectual disability. *Intellectual and Developmental Disabilities, 46*(1), 44–53.

Emergency Nurses Association. (2009). *Emergency nursing resource: Family presence during invasive procedures and resuscitation in the emergency department.* Retrieved from http://www.ena.org/IENR/ENR/Documents/FamilyPresenceENR.pdf

Fisher, M. J., & Broome, M. E. (2011). Parent-provider communication during hospitalization. *Journal of Pediatric Nursing, 26*(1), 58–69.

Forsner, M., Jansson, L., & Söderberg, A. (2009). Afraid of medical care: School-aged children's narratives about medical fear. *Journal of Pediatric Nursing, 24*(6), 519–528.

Frisch, A. M., Johnson, A., Timmons, S., & Weatherford, C. (2010). Nurse practitioner role in preparing families for pediatric outpatient surgery. *Pediatric Nursing, 36*(1), 41–47.

Gursky, B. (2007). The effect of educational interventions with siblings of hospitalized children. *Journal of Developmental & Behavioral Pediatrics, 28*(5), 392–398.

Gursky, B., Kestler, L. P., & Lewis, M. (2010). Psychosocial intervention on procedure-related distress in children being treated for laceration repair. *Journal of Developmental and Behavioral Pediatrics, 31*(3), 217–222.

Joint Commission on Accreditation of Healthcare Organizations. (2009). *The Joint Commission: 2010 Accreditation Requirements Chapters: Accreditation Program: Long Term Care*. Retrieved from http://www.jointcommission.org

Jolley, J., & Shields, L. (2009). The evolution of family-centered care. *Journal of Pediatric Nursing, 24*(2), 164–170.

McKenney, C., & Johnson, R. (2008). Unleash the healing power of pet therapy. *American Nurse Today, 3*(5), 29–31.

Myant, K. A., & Williams, J. M. (2005). Children's concepts of health and illness: Understanding of contagious illnesses, non-contagious illnesses and injuries. *Journal of Health Psychology, 10*(6), 805–819.

Myant, K. A., & Williams, J. M. (2008). What do children learn about biology from factual information? A comparison of interventions to improve understanding of contagious illnesses. *British Journal of Educational Psychology, 78*, 223–244.

National Center for Cultural Competence. (2010). *Working with linguistically diverse populations*. Retrieved from http://www11.georgetown.edu/research/gucchd/NCCC/features/language.html

O'Brien, I., Duffy, A., & Nicholl, H. (2009). Impact of childhood chronic illnesses on siblings: A literature review. *British Journal of Nursing, 18*(22), 1358–1365.

Piko, B. F., & Bak, J. (2006). Children's perception of health and illness: Images and lay concepts in preadolescence. *Health Education Research: Theory & Practice, 21*(5), 643–653.

Power, N., & Franck, L. (2008). Parent participation in the care of hospitalized children: A systematic review. *Journal of Advanced Nursing, 62*(2), 622–641.

Pruitt, L. M., Johnson, A., Elliott, J. C., & Polley, K. (2008). Parental presence during pediatric invasive procedures. *Journal of Pediatric Health Care, 22*, 120–127.

Roohafza, H., Pirnia, A., Sadeghi, M., Toghianifar, N., Talaei, M., & Ashrafi, M. (2009). Impact of nurses clothing on anxiety of hospitalised children. *Journal of Clinical Nursing, 18*, 1953–1959.

Ryan, J. (2008). "Pet" projects: Animal-assisted therapy for young patients. *Contemporary Pediatrics, 25*(7), 88.

Salmela, M., Salanterä, S., & Aronen, E. (2009). Child-reported hospital fears in 4 to 6-year-old children. *Pediatric Nursing, 35*(5), 269–276.

Shields, L., Young, J., & McCann, D. (2008). The needs of parents of hospitalized children in Australia. *Journal of Child Health Care, 12*(1), 60–75.

Spector, R. E. (2009). *Cultural diversity in health and illness* (7th ed.). Upper Saddle River, NJ: Pearson.

Steering Committee on Quality Improvement and Management & Committee on Hospital Care. (2011). Policy statement—Principles of pediatric patient safety: Reducing harm due to medical care. *Pediatrics, 127*(6), 1199–1212.

Stubenrauch, J. M. (2010). Hospitalizations of medically complex children rising. *American Journal of Nursing, 110*(12), 15–16.

Tschudy, M. M., & Arcara, K. M. (2011). *The Harriet Lane handbook* (19th ed.). St. Louis: Elsevier Mosby.

U.S. Department of Labor. (2010). *Fact Sheet #28: The Family and Medical Leave Act of 1993*. Retrieved from http://www.dol.gov/whd/regs/compliance/whdfs28.pdf

Weiss, M., Johnson, N. L., Malin, S., Jerofke, T., Lang, C., & Sherburne, E. (2008). Readiness for discharge in parents of hospitalized children. *Journal of Pediatric Nursing, 23*(4), 282–295.

Wilson, M. E., Megel, M. E., Enenbach, L., & Carlson, K. L. (2010). The voices of children: Stories about hospitalization. *Journal of Pediatric Health Care, 24*(2), 95–101.

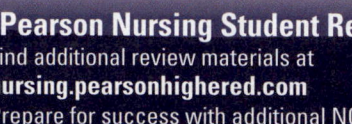

Pearson Nursing Student Resources

Find additional review materials at
nursing.pearsonhighered.com
Prepare for success with additional NCLEX®-style practice questions, interactive assignments and activities, web links, animations and videos, and more!

Nursing Care of the Child with a Chronic Condition

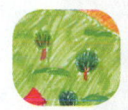 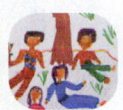 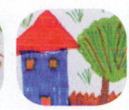

KEY TERMS

Learning Outcomes

After completing this chapter, you will be able to:

1. Explain the causes of chronic conditions in children.

2. Identify the categories of chronic conditions in children.

3. Assess the child with a chronic condition and apply specific nursing interventions for the child at different ages.

4. Assess the family of a child with a chronic condition and analyze the impact of the child's condition on the family.

5. Prepare the family of the child with a chronic condition to effectively care for the child in the home.

6. Summarize nursing management for the child with a chronic condition to support transition to school and adult living.

7. Discuss the family's role in care coordination and case management.

> "I'm excited to finally be going to school, but I'm afraid too. What if the other kids don't like me? Is my mommy going to be okay while I'm gone?"
>
> —*Haley, 8 years old*

Haley Leftwich is an 8-year-old girl with cerebral palsy. She had an intraventricular hemorrhage during her neonatal intensive care unit (NICU) hospitalization for prematurity. Haley lives with her mother and two older siblings, ages 10 and 13. Her parents divorced when Haley was 3 years old. She has frequent contact with her father, who she visits on weekends. Her father is supportive emotionally, physically, and financially in the care of Haley and her siblings.

Haley's mother is the full-time primary care provider. Routine care includes hygiene, supplemental enteral tube feedings to promote adequate nutrition in between oral feedings, range of motion (ROM) exercises, and homeschooling. Haley uses her motorized wheelchair without difficulty, and her mother has decided that she would benefit from social interaction and a structured educational environment at the local public school. Her family asks the clinic nurse and case manager at the cerebral palsy clinic for assistance in helping with planning Haley's entry into school.

How can the clinic nurse and case manager assist Haley and her family in this transition? What special arrangements are needed to permit a child to receive care for a chronic condition while at school? What measures can be taken to ensure an effective transition between home and school?

GENERAL CONCEPTS IN THE CARE OF A CHILD WITH A CHRONIC CONDITION

Although specific chronic conditions are discussed in detail in the chapters addressing body systems, this chapter focuses on general care concepts for the child requiring additional care coordination for a chronic condition. Nurses are essential in providing family-centered care to children with a chronic condition and their families. Nurses may assume many roles in this process, including direct care in the hospital, community setting, home, or school. Nurses often assume the role of care coordinator or case manager to help the family link with appropriate resources, plan care while wisely using health insurance resources, and integrate services needed to promote the best care for the child and family. Nurses apply a broad range of knowledge, assessment, and management skills when caring for these children and families.

Overview of Chronic Conditions

A **chronic condition** is generally thought of as one that is expected to last at least 3 months (Allen, 2010). An estimated 10 million children under the age of 18 in the United States have special healthcare needs related to some type of chronic condition (Betz, 2008). Chronic conditions vary in etiology, manifestations, severity, and their effect on the child's physical, psychosocial, and cognitive development. Chronic conditions develop from multiple causes:

- Genetic or inheritable conditions may be manifested as a chronic condition. Examples include muscular dystrophy, hemophilia, sickle cell disease, and cystic fibrosis.
- Conditions may result from a congenital defect or insult to the infant during fetal development, such as neural tube defect, maternal substance abuse, cleft palate, and cerebral palsy.
- Insult or injury may be associated with birth and care following birth (sepsis, prematurity, intraventricular hemorrhage) that lead to conditions such as bronchopulmonary dysplasia, attention deficit disorder, and vision or hearing impairment.
- Conditions can be acquired through injury or acute medical conditions such as brain injury, cancer, HIV infection, drowning, and mental health problems.

These and additional chronic illnesses are discussed in the systems chapters later in this text. In most cases, these chronic conditions become lifelong disorders, but the impact on the affected child is variable according to the severity of the condition, the stage of growth and development when the condition occurs, and the child's and family's responses to the condition. While some conditions require intense monitoring and technologic support for survival, other conditions cause few limitations and have minimal effect on quality of life.

The wide variety of chronic health conditions experienced by children and the different nature of these conditions affect the child's growth and development and health status in unique ways (Figure 16–1 ■). Chronic conditions have often been defined by diagnostic categories or by functional or social limitations. Examples of categories of chronic conditions include the following (Allen, 2010, p. 7):

- Limitations in function that would typically be expected for the child's age and development
- Disfigurement
- Dependency on medications or a special diet for control of the condition

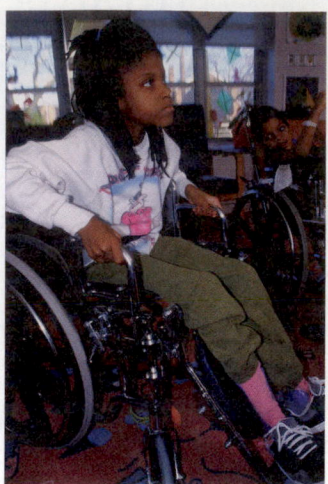
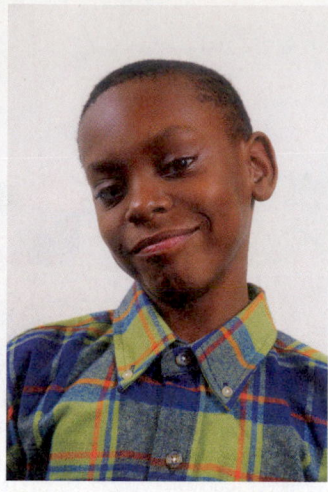

A   **B**

FIGURE 16–1 ■ Children with chronic conditions may have a visible or nonvisible health condition, or a condition that is nonvisible until an acute episode makes it visible. *A,* The child who uses a wheelchair has a visible disability. *B,* The child with a seizure disorder may have no visible signs of the condition unless a seizure is witnessed.

- Dependency on medical technology for functioning
- Need for more medical care and related services than typically used by a healthy child of the same age
- Special ongoing treatments at home or school

See Table 16–1 for examples of chronic conditions that fall into some of these categories. Many children with chronic conditions have special healthcare needs that fall into several of these areas. In the majority of cases, the more severe the chronic condition, the greater the number of categories of special healthcare needs. Many children with a chronic condition and children dependent on technology require specialized health care. The term **children with special healthcare needs (CSHCN)** is applied to "those who have or are at increased risk for a chronic physical, developmental, behavioral, emotional condition and who also require health and related services of a type or amount beyond that required by children generally" (U.S. Department of Health and Human Services, Health Resources and Services Administration, Maternal and Child Health Bureau, 2008). Many of these children have a **disability,** a limitation that interferes with a child's ability to fully participate in society, which can

TABLE 16–1	Examples of Conditions by Special Healthcare Need Category
SPECIAL HEALTHCARE NEED CATEGORY	**CHRONIC HEALTH CONDITION EXAMPLES**
Dependent on medications or special diet	Diabetes mellitus, asthma, seizures, phenylketonuria, organ transplantation, cystic fibrosis
Dependent on medical technology	Renal failure, bronchopulmonary dysplasia
Increased use of healthcare services	Cancer, sickle cell disease, prematurity
Functional limitations	Down syndrome, brain injury, autism, myelodysplasia, cerebral palsy

be related to medical impairment (chronic health condition), functional limitation (mobility, self-care, communication, or learning behavior impairment), or a mental condition that interferes with social interactions.

The prevalence of children in the United States with special healthcare needs increased from 12.8% in 2001 to 13.9% in 2005–2006 (Betz, 2008). Although these children represent a small percentage of the nation's children, they require significantly more healthcare resources than those without special healthcare needs, including more visits to clinics and emergency departments, dental visits, inpatient hospital days, and prescription medications. Efforts to reduce health costs have resulted in fewer hospitalizations and more care in the community for CSHCN. The proposed objectives for *Healthy People 2020* related to healthcare delivery to CSHCN are summarized in Box 16–1.

The child with a life-threatening illness or a chronic condition as the result of a complex illness, prematurity, or a congenital defect may be considered **medically fragile** (Miles, Holditch-Davis, Burchinal, et al., 2011). Some of these children are **technology assisted,** dependent on a medical device that is required to sustain life or to maintain health status (mechanical ventilators, intravenous nutrition or drugs, tracheostomy, suctioning, oxygen, or nutritional support with tube feedings) (Figure 16–2 ■). Other children depend on medical devices that compensate for vital body functions and require nursing care management such as renal dialysis, urinary catheters, and colostomies.

Children assisted by technology can be cared for at home because compact portable equipment is available. Home-based equipment used for the child with a chronic condition may include ventilators, enteral feeding tubes, intravenous catheters, infusion pumps, dialysis equipment, and oxygen. With the support of home health services, parents can learn to manage the child's care. The benefit of home health services to the child is support of physical, emotional, and cognitive growth and development within the home care setting, in a more normal environment.

Clinical Tip

Children who are dependent on technology, such as a feeding pump for nutritional support or a dialysis machine for peritoneal dialysis, might be able to participate in usual childhood activities; however, the equipment or procedure might prohibit them from doing so. If the child is only receiving the medical treatment intermittently, partner with the family to schedule the procedures to allow time for the child to participate in childhood activities, within the limitations of the illness.

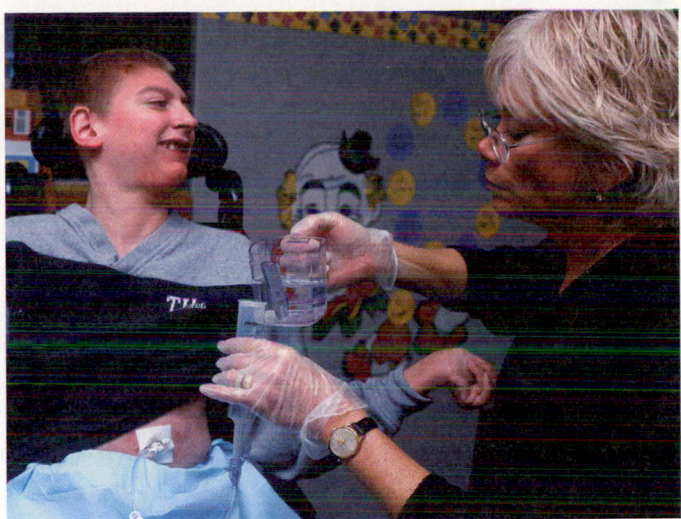

FIGURE 16–2 ■ This child needs a gastrostomy tube to ensure adequate nutrition is obtained to support growth and promote resistance to infection.

All families with children experiencing a chronic condition need to make lifestyle adjustments, ensuring a baseline of care that helps to maintain the child's health status and promotes growth and development. In many cases, the child has a baseline level of home management with episodic exacerbations that require the family to make sudden adjustments in family routines, such as may occur with the child who has seizures or an infection. These exacerbations often cause stress and disrupt family routines. Some chronic conditions, such as cystic fibrosis, diabetes mellitus, bronchopulmonary dysplasia, and significant cognitive impairment, require the family to learn and provide care that is complex and time intensive. These more severe chronic conditions often affect the child's physical and psychologic development. Table 16–2 outlines healthcare needs of these children and families and the nursing implications related to planning health services delivery to children and their families.

THE FAMILY OF A CHILD WITH A CHRONIC CONDITION

Informing the Parents

The way that parents become aware of their child's chronic condition is as variable as the type of chronic condition. Chronic conditions present very differently among infants and children.

- Chronic conditions may be detected prenatally, at birth, or early in infancy. Examples include a neural tube defect, Down syndrome, a condition like phenylketonuria or sickle cell anemia identified by newborn screening, or a complication of care provided in the NICU, such as bronchopulmonary dysplasia.
- Parents may suspect that the infant or child has a problem and seek a diagnosis, such as in cerebral palsy when the infant does not achieve motor developmental milestones or in autism when the child does not achieve appropriate communication skills.

BOX 16–1	*Healthy People 2020* Objectives for Children with Special Healthcare Needs

- Increase the proportion of youth with special healthcare needs whose healthcare provider has discussed transition planning from pediatric to adult health care
- Increase the proportion of children, including those with special health care needs, who have access to a medical home
- Increase the proportion of children with special healthcare needs who receive their care in family-centered, comprehensive, coordinated systems

Source: *U.S. Department of Health and Human Services. (2012).* Healthy People 2020 Objective Topic Areas and Page Numbers. *Retrieved from http://healthypeople.gov/2020/topicsobjectives2020/pdfs/HP2020objectives.pdf*

TABLE 16–2	Healthcare Needs of Children with Chronic Conditions	
HEALTHCARE NEED	**DEFINITION**	**NURSING ACTIONS**
Access to care	Care includes the availability and accessibility of providers with knowledge as well as ancillary services needed by children and their families.	Assist the family in obtaining transportation assistance if required. Assist the family in identifying healthcare providers that provide health promotion and other services to address the child's specific healthcare needs.
Appropriateness of care	Services and care are delivered by individuals with expertise and experience that are developmentally and culturally appropriate for the child and family.	Support the family by outlining educational and health services needed when developing an individualized education plan (IEP) and individualized health plan (IHP).
Comprehensiveness of care	Care includes coverage of the preventive, primary, and tertiary care needs of children, and linkages with other service systems, such as education, social services, and family support systems.	Provide the family with resource contacts such as social services, family support groups, and other systems to help the family manage the child's condition.
Coordination of care	Families are linked to medical care, financial health resources, and educational and community-based services; information is centralized.	Assist the family to identify a care coordinator or to develop the skills to become the care coordinator. See page 434. Provide guidance and resources if the family decides to assume the role of care coordinator. Encourage the family to partner with the healthcare team to ensure continuity of care.
Continuity of care	Care is provided through a medical home or pediatric healthcare home; linkages between primary, specialty, therapeutic, and home care exist throughout childhood.	Facilitate communication between all the child's healthcare providers. Include the family and older child in all decision making.
Degree to which family-centered services are provided	Importance of the family is reflected in the way services are planned and delivered, building on individual and family strengths, and respecting the diversity of each family.	Determine the needs of the child and the family to ensure they are being addressed. Assist the family in identifying local and specialized healthcare providers. Recognize and respect the culture and cultural practices of the child and family.

- Recurrent illnesses may actually be related to a chronic condition such as asthma or cystic fibrosis. A serious injury, such as a traumatic brain injury, can also cause disabilities.
- Some children may start school before their learning or behavior problems are identified.

Clinical Tip

When discussing a child's chronic condition with the family, use the child's name. Avoid labeling the child with a condition, such as "diabetic child"; instead refer to the situation as "the child with diabetes." This places the emphasis on the *child* rather than the *condition*.

See Developing Cultural Competence: Racial Disparities in Family-Centered Care for Children with Special Healthcare Needs.

The following guidelines may be considered when informing parents of the diagnosis of a chronic illness or disability in their child:

1. Inform parents of their child's diagnosis in person, in a private setting, and free from interruptions. Tell both parents together. Offer parents the opportunity to have a relative or friend as a support person during the discussion.
2. Present information in small amounts at a time and at the level of the parents' understanding.
3. Plan and organize the information to be provided. Use simple, direct language without medical jargon. Individualize the pace of the interview and approaches taken to present the explanation, taking into consideration a family's culture and the family's response to the information.
4. Share accurate, up-to-date information about the diagnosis, treatment options, specialty referrals, and community resources.

5. Talk about the strengths and positive attributes of the child, as well as the child's limitations and characteristics due to the illness or disability.
6. Evaluate the discussion to assess whether the family's needs were met and to determine the type of support and additional information that should be provided.
7. Plan a follow-up discussion to repeat and clarify the information provided and to give the parents a chance to get additional questions answered.

Practice Alert

Realize that once parents hear the name of the diagnosis, such as "cancer" or "cystic fibrosis," they may not hear anything else that is said. Observe for cues to this in parents' facial expressions and verbal responses, and alert the healthcare provider or person providing this information of these signals.

Developing Cultural Competence
Racial Disparities in Family-Centered Care for Children with Special Healthcare Needs

Family-centered care (FCC) is an essential component of care of children with special healthcare needs and their families. Findings of a research study by Coker, Rodriquez, and Flores (2010) indicated that Latino and African American children and those from households with a non-English primary language were less likely to receive family-centered care than White children and those from homes with English as a primary language. Components of FCC assessed using a questionnaire included whether the physician listened carefully, spent enough time with the family, was sensitive to family and cultural values, provided adequate information, and helped the family feel like they were a partner in the care of their child. Additionally, parents were asked if an interpreter was available when needed. It is essential that CSHCN receive culturally competent family-centered care regardless of race or ability to speak English.

Informing the Child

Informing the child of a newly acquired chronic condition is individualized and is based on the child's developmental level and age. Questions the child may ask vary but often focus on the cause of the condition, how to make it better, and how it will affect daily life. Provide information tailored to the child's level of understanding and answer questions honestly. (See Chapter 6 🔗.)

Parental Reaction

Parents need time to comprehend the diagnosis and its meaning to their lives after learning about the child's diagnosis. Some parents may feel relieved that a diagnosis is finally identified after all of the concern, diagnostic testing, and uncertainty. They may feel that their concerns have been validated. For many parents, however, the information can be distressing. The parents may question the diagnosis and may even question the accuracy of the test and the competency of the healthcare provider. Reactions to the diagnosis of a chronic illness vary among parents, and may include shock, denial, anger, sadness, sorrow, and depression. Support during this time will facilitate parental coping (Theofanidis, 2007). The nurse should be empathetic and supportive of parental emotional expression.

Clinical Tip

Parents who have just received a diagnosis of a chronic illness may be very angry. Although they are angry at the diagnosis, this anger may be projected to the nursing staff that is providing care to the child. Accept this anger as a normal emotional reaction to receiving bad news and continue to provide support to the family and the child. Refer for counseling and additional assistance as needed.

Parents grieve for the loss of the perfect child and other losses such as the following:

- Loss of family routines and goals
- Loss of the ideal parent–child relationship
- Siblings' loss of some usual childhood routines
- Loss of expectations for the development and life expectancy of the child with the chronic condition
- Child's loss of the parents' expectation of childhood

Parents may blame themselves or their spouse if the condition is genetic. When the child's condition results in a significant disability, the family has a daily reminder of their losses and how they differ from other families. Parents may have difficulty bonding with the affected infant because of guilt or disappointment, because they fear that the infant will not survive, or because the infant looks or behaves differently. Parents report episodes of recurrent sadness, particularly when reminded that their child is different from a healthy child (such as when the child starts school). This sadness has been described as **chronic sorrow** and is believed to be a coping mechanism that allows parents to periodically grieve the child who has a diagnosis that is permanent, progressive, recurring, and cyclic in nature (Gordon, 2009).

Siblings' Reactions

Siblings of children with a chronic condition are affected in a variety of ways, and they demonstrate a variety of emotional responses (Giallo & Gavidia-Payne, 2008; Williams, Piamjariyakul, Graff, et al., 2010). Negative responses predominate and include feelings of jealousy, resentment, anger, depression, worry, and anxiety (Williams et al., 2010). Siblings of chronically ill children are at increased risk for behavioral problems and may demonstrate changes in mood and attention-seeking behaviors. They may also demonstrate lower self-esteem, problems in school, and embarrassment (Williams et al., 2010). Siblings may fear that they themselves will have the same disease or condition as the affected child.

Some siblings have positive responses and demonstrate maturity, empathy, increased family closeness, and sensitivity (Williams, Ridder, Setter, et al., 2009). Siblings who adjust more positively are those who have a more cohesive family, social support, and positive communication with their parents (Williams et al., 2010). See Chapter 15 🔗 for siblings' responses to the child experiencing an illness.

Nurses should help parents to recognize that siblings are at risk for negative outcomes and provide suggestions and resources to parents that decrease this risk (Williams et al., 2010). Provide siblings with information about the illness, and assist parents to recognize the need for parental support and individual time with siblings, which will promote adjustment in the siblings. Maintenance of family routines is helpful in promoting a sense of the normal. Help the family select appropriate ways the sibling can help with the care of the child with a chronic condition, while also recognizing that the sibling needs a childhood with peer interactions, physical exercise, and recreation. Siblings who have difficulty adjusting may benefit from peer support groups, family-based interventions, and counseling (Giallo & Gavidia-Payne, 2008).

STRESSORS ON THE FAMILY

Having a child with a chronic condition places great demands on parents. Parents spend several hours a week providing, arranging, or coordinating care for their child (Gordon, 2009).

Stressors reported by families having a child with a chronic condition include:

- Learning as much as possible about the child's condition and expected progression in severity
- Learning about all the technical aspects of care for the child and how to integrate that care into family routines
- Finding ways each family member can help with the child's care, including extended family members who may live nearby
- Communicating with health professionals and attempting to serve as a full partner in the child's care
- Identifying the most appropriate resources for the child
- Continuing employment while meeting care needs of the child
- Managing a family budget that is drained by expenses for care not covered by health insurance plans and other financial resources
- Attempting to provide siblings as normal a life as possible
- Opening the home to strangers who provide home care to the child
- Coping with episodes when the child's condition worsens and fearing that the child will die
- Working with the child to gradually assume more responsibility for self-care

Certain transitions or events are more stressful for the family, as they disrupt family routines or require adaptation by the family. As mentioned earlier, the time of diagnosis is the initial transition or event that results in changes in a family's expectations. Other times of transition that cause stress or trigger more intense feelings of sorrow include (Gordon, 2009):

- Illness exacerbations
- Hospitalization
- When development milestones do not occur as expected, such as high school graduation

Some families have the strength and resilience to manage the child's healthcare needs and maintain family functioning. Parental relationship stress may be present and further increased by concurrent family illnesses, a death in the family, or the presence of a family conflict. The marriage relationship is at risk for breakdown if the couple is not able to communicate, share in the care for the child and other family members, and have common expectations for the child's condition and abilities to perform self-care.

Caregiver Burden

Caregiver burden is the unrelenting pressure and anxiety related to providing daily care to a child with disabilities while meeting other family obligations. The parents of the child who is medically fragile must perform technical care and complicated procedures, keep records, and be vigilant in monitoring symptoms (Figure 16–3 ■). Parents may feel overwhelmed by the responsibilities of providing this care. Feelings of chronic fatigue, strain, and emotional distress are common in parents, especially mothers (Carnevale, Rehm, Kirk, et al., 2008).

The stressors of parents with a child who is technology dependent vary by the child's functional status, the extent of care needed, the financial burden, the family's strengths and resiliency, and the available resources. Parents have greater personal strain and caregiver distress when the child has poor functional status and when the child's healthcare needs are not met (Aitken, McCarthy, Slomine, et al., 2009) (Box 16–2). See Chapter 15 ⊘ for the discussion of nursing care in the home.

Meeting family obligations can be challenging even when a family support infrastructure exists, as there is a constant struggle to keep the needs of the child and the family in balance. Mothers may be unable or not have the energy to meet their own personal needs for health care. The parent who remains in the home providing care to the child who is chronically ill may experience social isolation. Spousal support is essential to manage all the family and childcare requirements. Employment responsibilities also must be integrated into the schedule, and hours of work often must be negotiated to ensure parental coverage for the child's care.

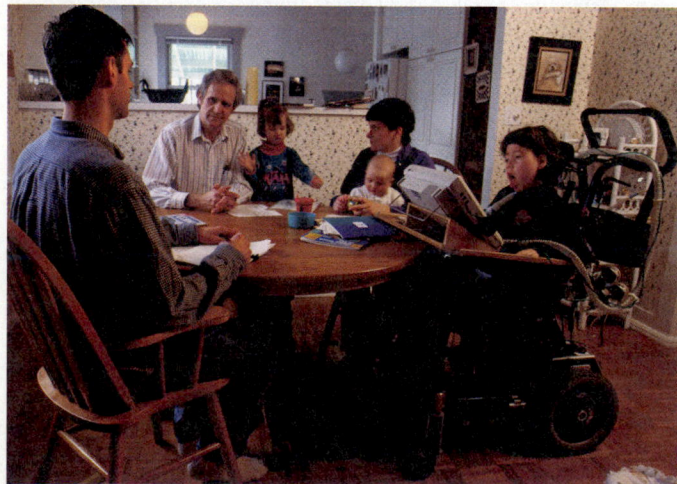

FIGURE 16–3 ■ Daily caregiving demands of the child who is medically fragile continue 24 hours a day, 7 days a week. Parents need to identify ways to share the care of the child and other family care management. When the child lives with a single parent, additional healthcare resources are needed so the parent can sleep.

BOX 16–2 **Research: Coping Methods Used by Fathers of Children with Chronic Illnesses**

A descriptive study of 54 fathers of children with chronic illnesses evaluated coping methods using the Folkman and Lazarus Revised WAYS Questionnaire. This tool was designed to identify thoughts and actions used to cope with stressful events and is composed of eight subscales: confrontive coping, distancing, self-controlling, seeking social support, accepting responsibility, escape-avoidance, planful problem-solving, and positive reappraisal. In addition to the questionnaire, the fathers completed a perceived severity of illness scale. Coping methods used by fathers in relation to parenting a child with a chronic illness were ranked in order of importance. The three highest-ranking subscales were positive reappraisal, planful problem solving, and seeking social support, respectively. Positive reappraisal includes focusing on one's personal growth, and it contains a religious dimension. Planful problem solving involves a deliberate effort to change the situation, and seeking social support involves an effort to seek tangible, emotional, and informational support (Broger & Zeni, 2011).

Knowledge of coping methods used by parents is essential in providing family-centered care to families of children who are chronically ill. The needs of both parents should be identified, and support should be given to both mothers and fathers.

Even when parents develop the capacity and skills to coordinate the child's medical care, the work on behalf of the child remains intensive and must be sustained long term. Administrative work such as scheduling appointments, keeping records, developing and maintaining lists, completing health insurance claim forms, and appealing denied payments may seem never-ending. Advocacy efforts for resources and opportunities are ongoing but should be adapted to changes in the child's condition and developmental stage. See Table 16–3 for nursing actions to assist families with significant stressors.

Maltreatment of the Child with a Chronic Condition

Children with chronic illnesses are at increased risk for child maltreatment, and the risk for abuse increases with the number of chronic conditions in the child (Svensson, Bornehag, & Janson, 2010). Factors that increase the risk of abuse in these children include the following (Hibbard, Desch, & Committee on Child Abuse and Neglect and Council on Children with Disabilities, 2007):

- Higher emotional, physical, economic, and social demands on the family
- Limited social and community support and the inability of parents to cope with the care and supervision responsibilities
- Failure of the child to receive medications, appropriate educational placement, and adequate medical care
- Increased stress related to the child's behavioral characteristics (e.g., communication problems, aggressiveness)
- Lack of adequate breaks or respite from caring for the child

Assess the family for ineffective coping and the potential for abuse of the child with a chronic condition. Make appropriate referrals to support services such as mental health counseling, social services, and respite.

Family Financial Issues

The economic impact of caring for a child with a chronic condition is significant. Even with good insurance coverage, the family still incurs a major financial burden. Approximately 40% of families in the United States who have a child with special healthcare needs experience a financial burden related to their child's illness (Looman, O'Conner-Von, Ferski, et al., 2009). Although health plans claim

Legal and Ethical Considerations
Supplemental Security Income

Children under the age of 18 years who are considered blind or have other disabilities are eligible for Supplemental Security Income (SSI). The child may be eligible at the time of birth or at a later age. When children turn 18 they are evaluated using the criteria for adults with disabilities (U.S. Social Security Administration, 2011).

that home care of these children costs less than care in institutions, families assume responsibility for many out-of-pocket expenses. Examples of additional expenses that families pay out of pocket may include special diets, durable equipment and supplies, transportation to healthcare visits, respite care, and co-payment for health services including prescriptions. Home health nursing care may be needed if both parents continue to work or to cover the night shift so parents can sleep. Home health care may not be covered or may only be partially covered by the family's insurance (Looman et al., 2009).

Another financial concern for the family of a child with a chronic condition in the home is the high incidence of job instability that can occur as a direct result of the child's condition (Looman et al., 2009). Parents may lose their employment due to excessive absences to provide care for the child or may be required to reduce hours worked to make sure the child receives adequate care. Such job instability further threatens the family's access to health insurance for the remainder of the family as well as the child with a chronic condition (see Legal and Ethical Considerations: Supplemental Security Income). See Chapter 1 for information related to the Children's Health Insurance Program (CHIP).

Promoting Healthy Family Coping

Families often engage in a coping strategy called **normalization.** Through normalization, the family views the care of the child with a chronic condition as a "normal" part of life, rather than an inconvenience or something outside of their routine. The family redefines what is normal for them by adopting a "normalcy lens" that enables them to see that their family follows some normal routines like all other families (Knafl & Santacroce, 2010):

- They acknowledge the child's condition and know that it has the potential to threaten the family's lifestyle.
- Their parenting behaviors and family routines are consistent with how they view other families functioning.
- The child's treatment regimen is integrated into the usual routines of the family and child, in a manner that permits the family to seem normal.
- The parents interact with others based on their view of the child and family as normal.

With normalization, the parents may be able to move the child's condition to the subconscious so it does not take a dominant place in the family's life and thoughts. They choose to focus on the normal aspects of the child and the family's life. Through normalization, families are able to develop flexibility in management of the treatment plan, making life easier for the family (Knafl & Santacroce, 2010). Threats to sustaining normalization may include worsening of the child's health status that makes the parents more aware of the child's serious condition, changed management routines, new family additions, or other family situational changes.

Some families are unable to achieve or sustain the sense of normalization, even though it may be seen as a desired goal. In many cases these families are still adjusting to their child's condition, the child's condition may have recently changed, or another family stressor is present. In these families, the child's condition may be a major focus of family life or a source of conflict in the family. The child could be viewed as different from his or her peers, leading parents to modify their parenting style to accommodate their dramatically changed view of their child (Knafl & Santacroce, 2010).

TABLE 16–3	Nursing Interventions for Common Family Stressors
STRESSOR	**NURSING IMPLICATIONS**
Uncertainty	Be honest in responding to the parents' questions. Serve as an advocate to ensure that information from the primary healthcare provider or specialists is being relayed to the family.
Fear of potential loss of the child	If the death of the child is likely or uncertain, support the family and refer to social services or other support to assist the family in anticipatory grieving. Ensure that the family is kept informed about all changes in the child's condition.
High-technology environment of the neonatal or pediatric intensive care unit	Orient the parents to the child's environment. Explain all equipment and procedures. Encourage them to be active participants in the child's care.
Communication with healthcare providers	Serve as the family's advocate to ensure communication is shared between the multidisciplinary team members. Ensure the family understands all communication, and offer clarification if required. Ensure that the parents are fully informed and participate in all decision making regarding the child's care. Provide an interpreter if needed to facilitate communication.
Deciding whom to inform about the chronic condition	Assist the family in identifying all individuals who need to know about the child's condition. Extended family members and friends can offer support and may provide assistance with care. Recommend that childcare or school officials (if school age) be informed since the child is in their care for a majority of the time.
Increased out-of-pocket expenses	Partner with the family to identify cost-effective measures to reduce expenses. Refer the family to social services to determine any available assistance for health care, respite care, meals, or transportation.
Social isolation and role strain	Encourage the family to participate in support groups, including those available online. Parent-to-parent support groups can offer support and guidance. Encourage the family to take respite time from care of the child. Assist the family in determining satisfactory arrangements for respite care (e.g., family member, healthcare or respite provider).
Dividing time between healthy children and child with chronic condition	Encourage parents to take "special time" with healthy siblings. Also encourage the family to include all members in planning family activities and to ensure that each child has an opportunity to plan activities. Identify social supports to help provide transportation and enable participation in recreational or peer group activities.

Complementary Therapy   Hippotherapy

Horses have been used for many years to treat children with conditions such as cerebral palsy, muscular dystrophy, communication disorders, and autism. *Hippotherapy* is a type of physical therapy that uses the movement of a horse to improve the posture, balance, muscle tone, and functional motor skills of the child. Hippotherapy also has psychologic benefits such as empowerment, stress reduction, and increased self-esteem. Social benefits of hippotherapy include learning socially acceptable ways to express feelings and self-control. Educational benefits may include improving the child's capacity to learn and improvement in math skills through the use of games during hippotherapy (Granados & Agís, 2011) (Figure 16–4 ■).

Nurses can be effective in working with families by listening to the issues and offering suggestions (see Complementary Therapy: Hippotherapy). Often the opportunity to talk through the child's management plan will help the family consider different strategies that may be effective. The nurse can also provide links to community resources that may help the family.

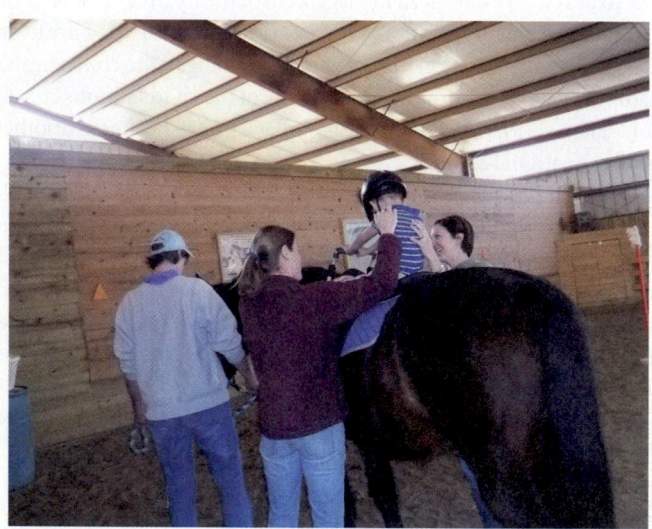

A

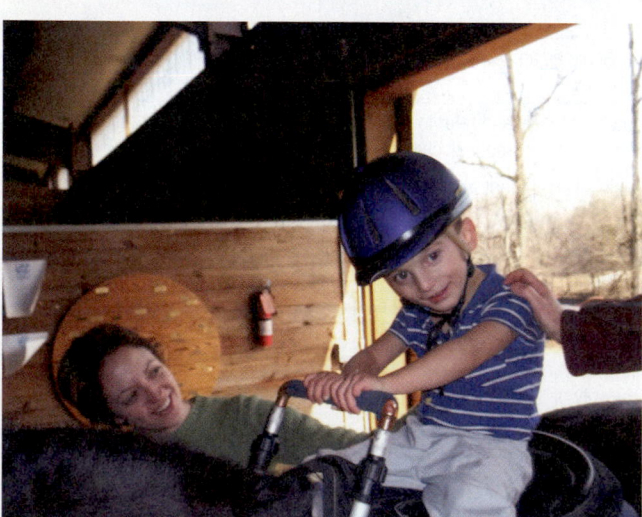

B

FIGURE 16–4 ■ Hippotherapy uses the movement of a horse to improve the posture, balance, muscle tone, and functional motor skills of the child.

Source: *A, B, Photo by Michele Davidson, PhD, CNM.*

THE CHILD WITH A CHRONIC CONDITION
Developmental Considerations

The child with a chronic condition has the same developmental and emotional needs as the healthy child and should be encouraged to achieve the same developmental milestones as a child without a chronic condition. However, the impact of the chronic condition on the child's cognitive, physical, and emotional health may lead to altered developmental achievement expectations. A **developmental delay** results when there is failure to achieve anticipated developmental milestones during specific developmental stages.

Newborn and Infant

Newborns and infants that are medically fragile are at risk for chronic conditions related to brain injury, oxygen deprivation, and respiratory problems. Newborns cared for in the NICU are exposed to an environment of bright lights and high-pitched noises that can negatively affect their development (Figure 16–5 ■) (Kellam & Bhatia, 2008; Lasky & Williams, 2009).

Nurses should promote development and parent–infant bonding by encouraging the parents to spend time with the infant and engage in face-to-face interaction. When the newborn is stable, provide opportunities for parents to touch, soothe, and care for the infant. Provide sensory stimuli such as mobiles, soft music, and different textures for the infant to touch.

Toddler

When the toddler has a chronic condition, parents may need to control and set limits on movement, play, behavior, or social interactions. This interferes with the achievement of autonomy and development of self-control. Some parents are overprotective and may do simple tasks they feel the child is incapable of accomplishing, rather than encouraging the child to try to do things independently. The child can lose independence and lack opportunities to meet developmental tasks (Figure 16–6 ■).

Nurses can promote the development of toddlers with chronic conditions by offering the child choices when possible, such as which color gown to wear or which food to eat first. Help parents recognize the toddler's capabilities, and allow the child to take the time to

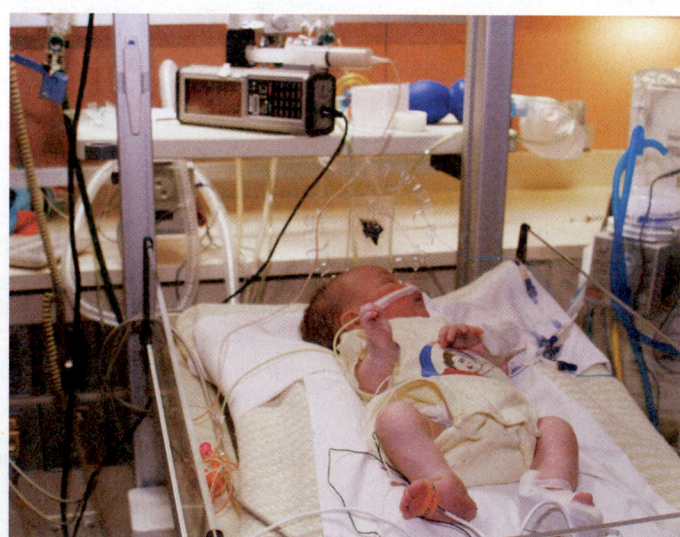

FIGURE 16–5 ■ Development of trust may be disrupted for the infant in the NICU or hospital unit when there are multiple caregivers and experiences of painful stimuli.

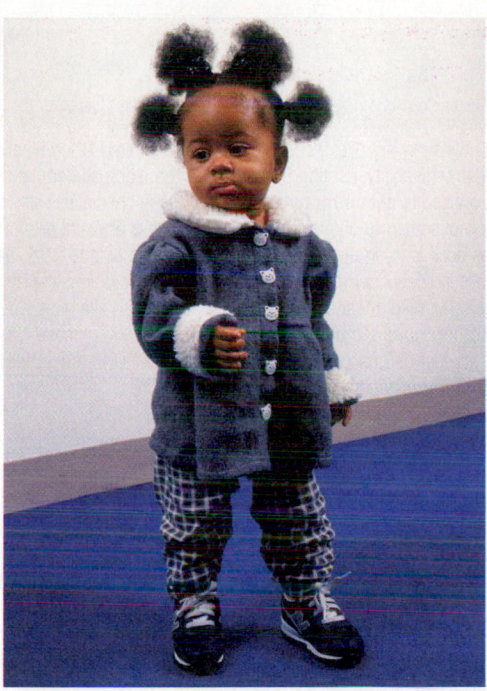

FIGURE 16–6 ■ Toddlers may experience difficulty in adapting to constraints of the condition and treatments related to their disorder. Depending on the condition, toddlers may be unable to achieve developmental milestones such as walking, toilet training, and feeding self. Delays in speech also become apparent during this stage.

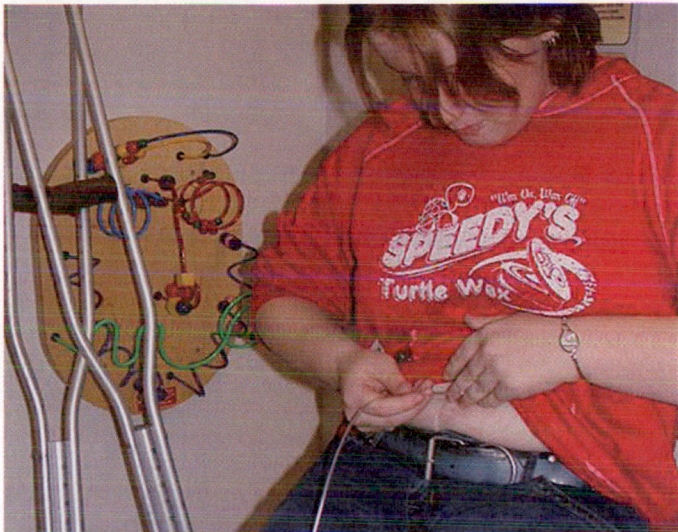

FIGURE 16–7 ■ All adolescents need to learn how to assume responsibility for their personal care and to make good decisions about future life plans. The adolescent with a chronic condition must also learn to independently manage the health condition (such as this girl performing self-catheterization) and to take that condition into consideration when making future life plans. This may be more challenging for adolescents who have a limited life expectancy or when parents are unable to relinquish their control and thus fail to encourage the child to assume more responsibility for self-care.

practice and learn a skill. Identify the next most appropriate developmental tasks for the child to learn, and give the parents some strategies they can use to offer learning opportunities.

Preschooler

Preschool children recognize the association between body parts and problems associated with the chronic condition. The preschooler engages in magical thinking during this stage, and the child may believe that his or her thoughts or behaviors caused the condition. The child may also think the condition is a form of punishment. Decreased energy due to the condition may interfere with the preschooler's ability to learn about the environment, develop social relationships, gain a sense of self-confidence, and learn a sense of purpose (Vessey & Sullivan, 2010).

Nurses can promote development by explaining the purpose of treatments and procedures in terms the preschooler can understand, and by emphasizing that treatments and procedures are not punishment for any wrongdoing. Look for ways to use play so the child can learn an aspect of self-care, perform an activity, and feel a sense of accomplishment. See Chapter 15 ⊘ for ways to use play in the hospital setting. Encourage social interactions with other children when possible. Give positive feedback to the child for appropriate efforts and successes.

School-Age Child

Early school-age children have an increased understanding of their condition and are capable of participating in certain aspects of monitoring and care. Older school-age children begin to understand about managing their condition and the long-term needs associated with their condition. They can assume more responsibility for their care such as serum glucose monitoring, intermittent self-catheterization, or monitoring the condition of skin under braces.

Some children with chronic conditions have learning difficulties and other limitations that interfere with education and social competence. The child needs to gain social skills, interact with peers, master new information, learn to cope with stress, and acquire skills that lead to self-sufficiency in order to develop a sense of industry. Other children may have functional limitations (e.g., communication, mobility, stamina, and self-care) that interfere with participation in school and extracurricular activities and prevent them from developing independence and mastery, and from developing socially (Vessey & Sullivan, 2010). Nurses can promote development of school-age children by encouraging their interaction with children in the same age group. When possible, this should occur with children who have the same type of chronic condition. Link the child to a peer support group to promote social interaction and to help the child recognize that others also have the same condition. When the child has an extended absence from school because of the chronic condition, encourage contact from school peers and friends through cards and computer messages, as well as the completion of school assignments. Begin to identify aspects of the child's care that the child can learn to assume under the parents' supervision. Inform families of the benefit of special camps for children with the chronic condition (when available) to promote recreation, social interaction, and learning skills of self-care.

Adolescent

Adolescence is a stage of profound physical, psychologic, and physiologic changes. The adolescent with a chronic condition has numerous challenges with the rapid changes in growth and sexual maturation; ongoing development of identity, body image, and self-concept; and the need to plan for vocational and healthcare transitions. Cognitive development and abstract thinking skills are achieved during this stage, allowing the adolescent to develop an understanding of the short-term and long-term consequences related to the condition (Figure 16–7 ■).

The adolescent becomes more aware of differences between self and peers. Some adolescents are unable to cope with the recognizable differences between themselves and healthy peers, and they withdraw from social activities and relationships. Others may engage in risky behavior (e.g., alcohol, sexual activity, eating foods that interfere with therapy) that may be harmful to themselves or to management of their condition, just to be accepted by peers.

Nursing actions to promote development of the adolescent include patient education to help the adolescent learn about the chronic condition, care needed to manage or control the condition, and problem solving and specific skills for integrating self-care management into daily life. Parents need to be coached to transition care over to the adolescent and to support the adolescent to make healthy decisions regarding care. Encourage the adolescent to build a safety net of friends who know enough about the chronic condition to assist if a problem occurs, such as a seizure, asthma episode, or insulin reaction. Discuss sexual maturation and the importance of protected sexual activity, and discourage risky behaviors by the adolescent. Provide the adolescent an opportunity to express concerns regarding self-management, vocational planning, and future independent living.

Education and Schooling

All children, including those with chronic conditions and special healthcare needs, are entitled by federal law to a free education that is matched to their developmental and functional capabilities (Individuals with Disabilities Education Act [IDEA] and Section 504 of the Rehabilitation Act of 1973). (See Legal and Ethical Considerations: Federal Laws and Children with Disabilities.) **Early intervention** provides special services for infants and toddlers up to age 3 years who have a developmental delay, have a diagnosed physical or mental condition that has a high probability of resulting in developmental delay, or are at risk for developmental delay. It is a federal program administered by the state (Caley, 2011; Goldstein, Altman, & Zimmerman, 2010). Children are evaluated at age 3 to determine continued eligibility in preschool (Caley, 2011). IDEA has led to support of communities that are developing early childhood education programs and to schools with students who are blind or deaf, have autism, or have traumatic brain injury. Provisions for adolescent transitional planning for adult living, including vocational training and independent living, are also included in the IDEA (U.S. Department of Education, 2010).

Attending school is an important transition for children with chronic conditions and their families. Sending the child to school has several benefits for the child and family, including opportunities for socialization with children and adults outside of the family. School attendance promotes a feeling of normalcy in the family and provides a break for the primary care provider. Haley, the child in the opening vignette, looks forward to attending school but also expresses fears. Her integration into the school system will require the collaboration of her family, school personnel, the nurse, and other members of the healthcare team. (See the Collaborative Care section on page 429.)

Educational System Planning

Careful planning is needed when a child with special needs attends school or receives other education services. Many children have chronic medical conditions that require management during the day in the school environment, such as asthma, diabetes, and attention deficit disorder. Some children simply need medications administered regularly or episodically. Other children require more extensive

Legal and Ethical Considerations
Federal Laws and Children with Disabilities

- The Rehabilitation Act, PL 93-112, of 1973 prohibited discrimination against people with a disability. Section 504 specifies that each student who has a disability is entitled to **accommodations**—services or special assistance provided in the school setting to ensure that a student with a physical or mental impairment has access to an appropriate education and is able to participate as fully as possible in school activities. Examples of accommodations might include additional time to take a test, strategies that decrease an allergic child's exposure to peanuts, or allowing the child to test his or her blood glucose. Students with disabilities must be provided with educational services to meet their needs just as services are provided to those without disabilities. See Chapter 14 for further discussion on the nurse's role in the school setting.

- The Education for All Handicapped Children Act, PL 94-142, of 1975 mandated that all children, including those with disabilities, be provided with free public education and related services. Safeguards were put in place to ensure that the rights of children with disabilities and their parents are protected. Additional purposes of this legislation were to assist states to provide education to children with disabilities and to evaluate the effectiveness of efforts to educate children with disabilities.

- The Education for All Handicapped Children Amendments, PL 99-457, of 1986 expanded the scope of PL 94-142 to include appropriate services for infants and toddlers with disabilities and their families.

- The Individuals with Disabilities Education Act (IDEA), PL 105-17, of 1997 and the Individuals with Disabilities Education Act of 2004, PL 108-446 (reauthorization of the 1997 legislation), ensure that all children with disabilities have available to them a free and appropriate public education that emphasizes special education and related services designed to meet their unique needs and prepare them for employment and independent living. Every child with a disability must have a written individualized education plan (IEP), and parents have the right to question placement decisions and to due process when settling differences. In addition, the 2004 legislation focused more on state and local accountability to educate children with disabilities.

Source: *Data from Fish, W. W. (2008). The IEP meeting: Perceptions of parents of students who receive special education services.* Preventing School Failure, 53(1), 8–14; Selekman, J., & Vessey, J. A. (2010). School and the child with a chronic condition. In P. J. Allen, J. A. Vessey, & N. A. Schapiro, Primary care of the child with a chronic condition (5th ed., pp. 42–59). St. Louis, MO: Mosby; U.S. Department of Education. (2011). Protecting students with disabilities. Retrieved from http://www2.ed.gov/about/offices/list/ocr/504faq.html; U.S. Department of Education. (2010). Thirty-five years of progress in educating children with disabilities through IDEA. Retrieved from http://www2.ed.gov/about/offices/list/osers/idea35/history/index_pg10.html

interventions integrated into the school day, such as blood glucose monitoring or intermittent self-catheterization. The education system is obligated to provide reasonable accommodations to ensure that the child's medical needs are met during the school day. The education system's obligation is negotiated with the family in formalized plans. The school nurse is an active participant on the team that collaborates with the family to develop these formalized plans:

- An **individualized family service plan (IFSP)** is developed for the early intervention process for infants with special healthcare needs and their families. The IFSP contains information about the services required to support a child's development and enhance the family's capacity to facilitate the child's development. The family and education service providers work as a team to plan, implement, and evaluate services specific to the family's unique concerns, priorities, and resources.

- An **individualized education plan (IEP)** is developed for a child with cognitive, motor, social, and communication impairments who needs special education services. The IEP is jointly planned with the school administrator, teacher, parents, and

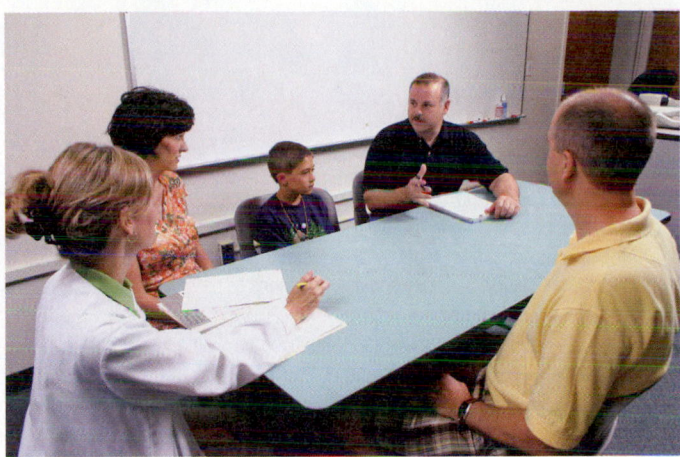

FIGURE 16–8 ■ An annual meeting of the school administrator, teacher, and school nurse, as well as the parents and child, is important in identifying the educational goals for the child and the special education resources to help meet those goals.

other special support professionals as appropriate for the child's condition (Figure 16–8 ■). The child is also included in the process when possible. The plan is developed after an assessment of the child's abilities and specific functional limitations (Box 16–3).

■ An **individualized health plan (IHP)** is developed for the child with medical conditions that need to be managed within the school setting. An IHP may be developed simultaneously with the IEP for the child with a health problem and a co-existing functional impairment. Some children only need an IHP for management of their chronic medical condition at school, such as daily medication administration or glucose monitoring and insulin injection. An order from a licensed healthcare provider is required for medication administration and special

---

BOX 16–3 | Elements of an IEP

- Student's name
- Date of meeting to develop or review the IEP
- Statement of transition service needs of student beginning at age 14 years
- Present level of assessments and education performance, including how the child's disability affects the child's involvement and progress in a general curriculum or participation in appropriate activities
- Measurable annual goals that include benchmarks or short-term objectives in meeting the child's needs that enable the child to be involved in or progress in the general curriculum or participate in appropriate activities
- Special education and related services, supplementary aids and services, and program modifications or supports for school personnel needed to enable the child to make advancements toward attaining annual goals
- Explanation to the extent that the child will or will not participate with children who do not have disabilities
- Any specific modification in the administration of state or district-wide assessments of achievement that are needed for the child to participate in the assessment, or reasons for excluding the child from assessment
- How the child's progress toward annual goals will be measured
- How the child's parents will be regularly informed of the child's progress toward annual goals and the extent to which the child's progress is sufficient to meet goals by the end of the year

Source: *Data from U.S. Department of Education. (2006). Individualized education programs. Retrieved from http://idea.ed.gov/explore/view/p/%2Croot%2Cdynamic%2CTopicalBrief%2C1 0%2C; U.S. Department of Education. (2000). A guide to the individualized education program. Retrieved from http://www2.ed.gov/parents/needs/speced/iepguide/iepguide.pdf*

---

treatments. Learning may be challenged when the child has frequent acute illness episodes that result in missed days of school, and the IHP often integrates methods to prevent the child from being penalized for those absences.

■ An Individualized Section 504 Accommodation Plan may be used rather than an IHP for children with physical or mental impairments. The same process is used for development of the plan.

■ An **individualized transition plan (ITP)** is included in the development of an IEP for each child with a chronic disability who is 14 years or older. The ITP focuses on assisting individuals to receive vocational training and in moving successfully from the home into other community living settings as they grow older.

Parents have an important role in ensuring that their child receives the most appropriate educational services. School systems must provide a full range of educational services for children with special healthcare needs, including services that support cognitive development, self-care skills, mobility, improved communication, and social skills. Because each child's severity and combination of impairments is unique, identifying and matching the specific services for each child requires discussion and negotiation. Parents should make an effort to learn about the different types of educational services that address a child's specific disability in preparation for the IEP meeting. Parents often need a mentor or experienced parent to help with the development of the IEP the first few times. In this way, the parents are better prepared to participate in the educational planning and development of the child's IEP. (See Partnering with Families: Preparing for an IEP Meeting.) School nurses are employees of the school system and may be limited in their advocacy role on behalf of individual students. However, school nurses are in a good position to educate the IEP team about specific interventions needed by children with medical conditions and ways to integrate those interventions into the school day.

Teachers will need to learn to identify specific health problems, such as increased respiratory effort in a child with asthma, or sweating, pallor, and loss of concentration in a child with diabetes. The child's teachers become part of the child's safety net for rapid access to needed healthcare intervention. With support from the school administration and school nurse, teachers can learn about the child's condition and special care that may be needed during the school day, such as a snack for the child with diabetes, management of the child who has a seizure, and ways to reduce the spread of infection within the classroom.

The Child's Response to Entering School

Children with chronic conditions—whether they cause minimal interference in the child's daily life or significant interference, such as dependence on technology—face certain challenges in the school setting. They may for the first time recognize differences between themselves and other children, such as appearance, abilities, social skills, or special treatment needs. Limitations in abilities may cause the child to be shy or embarrassed. Other children may also tease the child because of his or her physical or functional limitations (Marchitto, 2010). Some children, particularly adolescents, may attempt to hide their condition or fail to adhere to necessary recommendations, such as dietary restrictions, to appear like their peers.

Education for Children Who Are Medically Fragile

Children who are medically fragile or technology assisted are also entitled to education and education services in the school setting. The parents and the school system must carefully consider the child's need for skilled supportive nursing care. Parents are often anxious about how

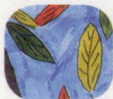

Partnering with Families

Preparing for an IEP Meeting

Parents need to be prepared to meet with the school administrator, teacher, and health professionals when the child's IEP will be developed so they can be effective advocates. Provide parents with the following suggestions:

- Talk with another parent who has experienced the IEP process to help prepare for the meeting. Inquire about what information should be shared about the child and what types of requests for services are appropriate. Parent support groups are a good place to talk with other parents who have gone through the process. Parent information and training programs often have parents who can provide support and mentoring for parents participating in the IEP process for the first time. The National Dissemination Center for Children and Youth with Disabilities website has a state-by-state directory of resources.

- Learn about the range of special education services available. Discussions with parent mentors can provide information about the special education services available for a child with specific disabilities.

- The child must be evaluated prior to the development of the IEP. Provide parental consent for the evaluation and carefully review the results of the evaluation. Ask for assistance in interpreting evaluation results if they are unclear.

- Attend the IEP planning meeting in person, and when appropriate bring the child to the meeting.

- Be prepared to provide a summary of the child's strengths and parental concerns about enhancing the child's education.

- During discussions about potential educational strategies for the child, parents should listen carefully and ask questions to be fully informed about the special education service options.

- Listen to the educational goals and objectives as well as how the child's progress in meeting those goals and objectives will be evaluated. Parents should ask questions or raise issues if they disagree with the IEP goals and objectives.

- Review the written plan to ensure that it matches the discussion during the IEP meeting. If the plan does not seem to match the child's needs, parents have the right to ask for revisions of the IEP. If the parents feel that special education is not being provided as outlined in the child's IEP or a good faith effort is not being made to assist the child to achieve the goals and objectives in the IEP, due process can be initiated.

- Request a new IEP planning meeting if the child appears to have made substantial progress in meeting goals and objectives during the school year. More frequent revisions to the IEP with new goals and objectives may be needed to support the child's progress.

---

well the child will be cared for by others during the school day. Risks for the child in the school setting include safety issues related to ventilators, tracheostomy, and medication therapy, as well as exposure to infectious diseases. The school administration must provide the personnel resources and equipment needed to ensure that care and a care provider are consistently available. Modifications to the school setting for the child, such as wheelchair ramps or an elevator, may be needed. Sometimes the child is placed in a classroom with healthy children, and the teacher is expected to monitor the child with a chronic condition and provide care as needed. Health aides may be assigned to provide care for one or more children with school nurse supervision. Some children are placed in classes composed of children with special healthcare needs where health aides are more available to provide needed care.

Nurses play a key role in assisting the family to understand that a teacher's primary responsibility is to teach, not to provide health care. The teacher is responsible for the health and safety of all children in the classroom. Parents need to have realistic expectations about the level of skilled support services that can be provided to a child who is medically fragile in a classroom. Teachers and education leaders are often challenged to meet the obligations for the child's special education services in balance with the needs of all other children in the classroom.

Homeschooling

The family of a child who is medically fragile or technology dependent may choose the option of homeschooling the child, with resources provided through the school system. Homeschooling may be used for all of the child's education or for periods when the child is experiencing exacerbations or more complications from the condition. The benefits of homeschooling include continuity of education when the child would otherwise be unable to attend

school and reducing the child's stress and fatigue. Potential negative effects of homeschooling include lack of peer and social interaction and decreased opportunity to develop social skills. The family that chooses homeschooling needs to establish a routine for the education process.

Transition to Adulthood

Improved survival rates have led to an increase in the number of adolescents with special healthcare needs transitioning to adulthood, many of whom have difficulty transitioning to adult healthcare services (Lotstein, Ghandour, Cash, et al., 2009). When their chronic condition could affect their future ability to work and live independently, customized **transition** planning is needed in preparation for adulthood and self-determination. A transition plan is developed in collaboration with the family based on the needs that have been identified in relation to the adolescent's goals for health care, employment, and community living. Objectives of a transition plan should include promotion of health and disease prevention, promotion of psychosocial adjustment to adulthood, promotion of independence in daily living as appropriate, maximizing the adolescent's potential, and maintaining continuity of resources (Sanders, Kuo, Levey, et al., 2009). Healthy & Ready to Work services may be particularly helpful to adolescents and families in planning for the transition to adulthood (HRTW National Resource Center, 2009).

Clinical Judgment

Martin is a 17-year-old with sickle cell anemia. As he reaches adulthood, the need to transition from the pediatrician to an adult healthcare provider will arise. What factors should be taken into consideration in deciding when this healthcare transition should occur?

Adolescents need continuous access to health care as young adults to maximize quality of life and lifelong functioning and potential (White & Hackett, 2009). One of the proposed objectives of *Healthy People 2020* focuses on facilitation of healthcare transition for adolescents, including provision of the resources available to make this transition (U.S. Department of Health and Human Services, 2012). Transition planning should focus on identifying and moving the adolescent or young adult from child-centered services to adult-oriented healthcare services. In addition to finding a regular source for health care, transition includes finding adequate insurance, as many young adults experience interruption in coverage once they turn 21 years of age (Lotstein, Inkelas, Hays, et al., 2008). Four domains of transition outcomes for adolescents with special healthcare needs have been identified by Lotstein et al. (2008, p. 24):

- Ongoing access to age- and disease-appropriate healthcare providers
- Access to continuous, affordable health insurance
- Development of disease self-management skills and condition problem-solving skills
- Access to age-appropriate educational and vocational opportunities to allow economic self-sufficiency

These four domains can help guide research and policy development (Park & Irwin, 2008). See the Baccalaureate Essentials box.

Collaborative Care

Care of the child with a chronic condition generally requires a multidisciplinary health professional approach, including physicians, nurse practitioners, nurses, nutritionists, social workers, case workers, physical therapists, occupational therapists, and a case manager.

Hospitalization

Children with chronic disorders are more likely to be hospitalized than children without chronic disorders. Depending on the severity of the condition, long-term hospitalization for months or years may be required for the child with a chronic condition. The family is an integral part of the plan of care for an ill or hospitalized child. Acute hospitalization resulting from exacerbation of the child's disorder places increased demands and stressors on the child and family. The child and parent may fear worsening of the condition or even death. Refer to Chapter 15 🖉 for a discussion of nursing care of the hospitalized child.

Ethical Issues

Ethical issues often arise for children with chronic conditions or disabilities. There is an ongoing debate concerning who ultimately makes the decisions—parents or the primary healthcare providers—about withholding treatments, implementing treatments, and other medical care issues. Issues regarding clinical ethics related to children with chronic conditions or disabilities include the following:

- Withholding and refusal of treatment (see Chapter 1 🖉)
- Advance directives (do-not-resuscitate orders) (see Chapters 1 and 18 🖉 for further discussion)
- Genetic testing and screening programs (see Chapter 4 🖉)
- Sexual and reproductive rights
- Sterilization of adolescents with intellectual disability
- Organ donation and rationing of care
- Research involving individuals with disabilities

Transition Between Hospital and Home

Many families become the primary caregiver for the child with a chronic condition, assuming responsibility for assessment and treatment despite the level of skill and complexity involved in that care. Numerous benefits to home care include the promotion of health, well-being, and development for the child; decreased financial costs to health insurance companies and the healthcare system; and a sense of satisfaction to families when they are able to care for their child at home. However, because of the time required to care for the child at home, parent caregivers are at risk for social isolation, caregiver burden, and caregiver illness (Nicholas & Keilty, 2007). See the previous discussion of caregiver burden on page 422.

The family faces numerous challenges for home care, including modification of the home. Management of the condition involves technologic support, medications, and treatment regimens, all potential necessities to maintain the child in the home. Family members must decide who has responsibility for different aspects of the child's care. Many families must also decide whether both spouses will continue to work or if one parent will stay home to care for the child. Home health nursing care may be needed if both parents continue to work or to cover the night shift so parents can sleep.

Moving the child who is chronically ill, or a technology-assisted child, to the home setting is a life-changing decision for the family and it must be done with collaboration between the family and the healthcare team. Preparation for the child's transition to the home requires that the family receive extensive training and instructions on the child's care.

This transition is often challenging and intimidating for the family who now must assume the role of independent caregiver for

---

Baccalaureate Essential V
Healthcare Policy, Finance, and Regulation

Policy initiatives that promote a positive transition to adulthood are essential for adolescents with special healthcare needs. In addition to being part of *Healthy People 2020*, many professional organizations have developed policy statements related to transition to adulthood for these youth, including the provision that individuals with special healthcare needs have continuous healthcare coverage through adolescence and adulthood (Sanders et al., 2009; Shaw & DeLaet, 2010).

Health insurance helps to ensure that young adults have access to comprehensive healthcare services. Approximately one third of adolescents with disabilities who have been receiving Children's Supplemental Security Income (SSI) will not meet adult criteria for SSI. This jeopardizes their ability to receive Medicaid when they turn 18 years of age. Those who do retain eligibility for Medicaid generally receive a less comprehensive package than they did as children (Park & Irwin, 2008). These potential gaps in coverage and decrease in services make the transition to adulthood difficult. It is essential that a plan for comprehensive healthcare coverage be established before the child reaches adulthood (Sanders et al., 2009).

Recent regulations have been put into place that will decrease the number of adolescents and young adults without health insurance. The Patient Protection and Affordable Care Act of 2010 (PPACA) includes legislation that prevents denial of healthcare benefits based on pre-existing conditions (Laiteerapong & Huang, 2010). This legislation also expands healthcare insurance benefits by allowing young adults to stay on their parents' insurance policies up to age 26 (Collins & Nicholson, 2010).

Nurses who work with adolescents with special healthcare needs should collaborate with the care coordinator, advanced practice nurse, physician, social worker, and other members of the healthcare team to facilitate a successful transition to adulthood without interruption in quality health care and health insurance coverage. Nurses can also work with their professional organizations to develop policies that facilitate a successful transition.

a child who may have been hospitalized for several months. Family members often feel unprepared to handle the complex situation of the chronic condition and technologic supports. The family needs to be highly motivated and possess strength and resiliency factors to overcome the obstacles that will arise. In this way, they will be successful in assuming management responsibility for the child's care.

Barriers to family support services   Parents of children with disabilities often identify barriers that prevent them from receiving adequate family support services. The family of the child with a chronic condition may not initially recognize the barriers that interfere with receiving adequate social support. The nurse assists the family in first recognizing any barriers. Once barriers are identified, appropriate referral (e.g., financial assistance, healthcare providers) and other resources can be recommended. See Table 16–4 for potential barriers and nursing implications.

Health Promotion and Health Maintenance of Children with Chronic Conditions

Most children with chronic conditions are cared for at home with or without home nursing or other healthcare services, and they may rely solely on the family for their support and care. Children with chronic health conditions require regular health promotion, health screening, and health maintenance care, as well as specialized health services to assist the child and family in the condition's management. Parents need education and guidance to reduce risks for further illness and injury and to foster the child's development. The goal is to promote the child's growth and development and permit the child to have as normal a childhood as possible. The child with a chronic condition needs a medical or healthcare home to ensure that all of the child's healthcare needs are met. Ideally this healthcare provider is located in the community where the family resides, making it more convenient for the family to obtain routine health care as well as care for episodic illnesses. Having a regular healthcare provider has many advantages for the family:

- Because the child and family are seen more frequently, a trusting, family-centered relationship can develop. The healthcare provider learns about the family's strengths and coping abilities.
- The healthcare provider sees the child and family when things are going well and during exacerbations. This may enable the healthcare provider to identify strategies that help the family to better coordinate the child's care.
- When the provider is based in the same community as the child, it is likely that information about community resources is known; this will reduce the efforts that families need to make to identify appropriate services for the child.

An optimal healthcare arrangement for the child with a chronic condition exists when the medical or healthcare home provider collaborates with a pediatric team or specialist that specializes in the care of children with a specific chronic condition. Pediatric specialists, advanced practice nurses, and other healthcare providers (e.g., physical therapists, social workers, and nutritionists) often function as a team providing coordinated care to the family and child with a chronic condition, such as spina bifida, cystic fibrosis, or cerebral palsy. These specialty teams are often found in major medical centers, requiring travel to the facility. When communication flows from the team to the child's healthcare provider and back to the team, the child's physician can monitor new treatments, and consultation can be sought if the child's health status changes. See the Collaborative Care section on page 429.

TABLE 16–4   Barriers to Family Support Services

BARRIER	NURSING IMPLICATIONS
Attitudes and beliefs of healthcare providers	Evaluate personal biases and beliefs regarding working with children with special healthcare needs.
Family's awareness of condition and treatment	Assess the family's level of understanding of the child's condition and treatment.
	Offer careful explanation over multiple visits to provide the family opportunities for questions and to develop an understanding.
	Encourage the family to discuss their fears and concerns.
Collaboration and respect between healthcare providers and family members	Be familiar with program policies and standards of practice.
	Encourage a family-centered care team approach between the family and healthcare provider team.
	Demonstrate respect for the family's decisions.
	Demonstrate respect for the family's culture.
	Assist the family in choosing a case manager or in assuming the role of case manager themselves.
Cost of care	Provide the family with information regarding healthcare insurance or health reimbursement options, such as Medicaid or SSI.
Resources	Assist the family to identify appropriate healthcare providers to meet the child's special healthcare needs.
	Refer the family to child and parent advocacy groups.
	Provide families with names, telephone numbers, and addresses of other significant resources.
	Assist the family in identifying local services that are appropriate to meet the child's healthcare needs.
	Refer the family to counseling if appropriate.

Source: Data from FRIENDS National Resource Center for Community-Based Child Abuse Prevention (CBCAP). (2006). Making family support programs accessible to children with disabilities and their families. *Retrieved from* http://www.friendsnrc.org/download/children_disabilities.pdf

Sometimes a pediatric specialist serves as the child's medical or healthcare home. Although this may seem like a good strategy for care, there are some risks that health promotion services will be minimized. It is important to ensure that regular health promotion and health maintenance services, such as immunizations, are not overlooked during the care of acute exacerbations of the chronic condition.

See the Health Promotion & Maintenance Overview on page 431.

Nursing Management

In collaboration with the family and a multidisciplinary healthcare team, the nurse assists the family to manage the child's care at home, provides guidelines to promote the child's health and growth and development, and supports the family by facilitating psychosocial adaptation.

The nurse's role in caring for the child with a chronic condition includes providing health supervision from infancy to transition into adulthood, collaborating with the multidisciplinary healthcare team, partnering with parents or caregivers to manage the child's care at home, referring the family to appropriate community services, assisting with planning for education services, promoting positive

Health Promotion & Maintenance Overview

The Child with a Chronic Condition

The child with a chronic condition requires monitoring and intervention to foster growth and development. The nurse can help promote and maintain health in the following ways.

GROWTH AND DEVELOPMENT SURVEILLANCE

- Monitor the child's growth and developmental patterns.
- Monitor for developmental delays.
- Explain to parents that regression following rehospitalization or exacerbation of the condition in the toddler or older child is normal. Be patient and work with the child to regain developmentally acquired skills.
- Ask the family about financial resources to pay for physical therapy, occupational therapy, speech therapy, and other services that promote the acquisition of developmentally appropriate skills. Financial constraints can impede adherence with recommended therapies; refer the family to resources.

NUTRITION

- Refer the family to a nutritionist and to resources for nutritional supplements or special dietary food, as well as for enteral or parenteral nutrition equipment.
- Assist the mother in learning how to breastfeed the infant or how to continue breastfeeding if desired.

PHYSICAL ACTIVITY/RECREATION

- Encourage the parents to promote physical activities within the child's ability.
- Assist the family in identifying appropriate activities for the child, such as swimming classes for children with disabilities.
- Encourage the child to participate in a camp for children with similar chronic conditions.

ORAL HEALTH

- Encourage regular dental visits for dental caries screening and other oral health issues such as grinding the teeth.
- Teach the parents to provide and promote good dental hygiene.

MENTAL AND SPIRITUAL HEALTH

- Assess the child for self-esteem status related to body image if the condition affects physical appearance. Help the child and family identify strengths that can help enhance self-esteem.
  - Ask the older child about experiences with any teasing associated with the condition or physical appearance. Discuss possible responses when teasing occurs.
- Refer the child for counseling if indicated.

RELATIONSHIPS

- Evaluate the parents for parent–infant bonding.
- Encourage peer interaction.
- Encourage participation in social activities within the child's ability.

DISEASE PREVENTION STRATEGIES

- Teach the family to maintain a record of the child's immunizations, illnesses, and treatments. Ensure that the child obtains additional immunizations appropriate for higher risk status for infection, such as the meningococcal vaccine and palivizumab for respiratory syncytial virus (RSV).
- Ask school personnel to provide information when an increase in acute infectious diseases among classmates is noticed so parents can decide if the child should remain home from school for a few days.
- Encourage good hand hygiene before and after providing care to the child.

INJURY PREVENTION STRATEGIES (SAFETY)

- Assist parents to establish a safe home environment for children with visual or motor difficulties.
- Ensure that parents obtain injury prevention guidance offered to families with healthy children, such as use of car safety seats and seating the child in the back seat of the car.
- Customize injury prevention guidance to the special needs of the child, such as testing bath water temperature for children with reduced sensation in the lower extremities.

---

parenting behaviors and psychosocial adaptation and well-being of the child and family, and promoting growth and development of siblings.

Nursing Assessment and Diagnosis

Physiologic and Developmental Assessment

Conduct a physical assessment of the child, noting general health and also specifically focusing on systems affected by the chronic condition. Perform a developmental assessment to help identify future developmental goals, and offer anticipatory guidance.

Family Assessment

Assess individual family members' level of understanding of the condition, treatment, and anticipated outcome of the condition. Determine the family's stage of acceptance of the child's chronic illness and how well the child's care is integrated into family routines. Evaluate the child's home care environment to determine the potential for abuse, lack of adequate care, or neglect, and opportunities to enhance care provided. Assess the family's strengths, stressors, risk factors, and coping strategies.

Nursing diagnoses that may apply to the family of a child with a chronic condition include:

- Coping: Family, Compromised related to inadequate financial resources for prolonged condition management
- Fatigue related to excessive role demands in caring for the child with a chronic condition and other family members
- Knowledge, Deficient related to a complex condition management plan
- Parenting, Risk for Impaired related to stress with caring for the child with a chronic condition and lack of a social support system
- Caregiver Role Strain related to the child's illness chronicity and 24-hour care responsibility

NANDA-I © 2012

Nursing diagnoses that may apply to the child are provided in the Nursing Care Plan on pages 432–433. Additional nursing diagnoses may be found in the nursing care plans for children with specific chronic conditions in the systems chapters.

Nursing Care Plan   The Child with a Chronic Condition

INTERVENTION	RATIONALE	EXPECTED OUTCOME
1. Nursing Diagnosis: Knowledge, Deficient (Child) related to learning self-care skills		
NIC Priority Intervention—*Individual Teaching:* Planning, implementing, and evaluating a teaching program designed to address a patient's particular need		**NOC Suggested Outcome**—*Knowledge:* Extent of understanding conveyed about treatment regimen
GOAL: *The child will acquire self-care skills for lifetime management.*		
■ Assess the child's developmental level and select an educational approach and self-care activities to match. ■ Review with the child all steps involved in the self-care skill and how to perform the skill. ■ Use demonstration/return demonstration until the child is comfortable with procedures. ■ Help parents develop a planned sequence of self-care skills to teach the child. ■ Discuss a plan for increased responsibility for self-care with the child and parents.	■ Learning goals for the child must match knowledge and skill expectations appropriate for the developmental stage. ■ The child may have watched the routine used by parents many times, and asking the child to list each step helps the nurse identify extra training needed. ■ Evaluation permits positive reinforcement and guidance for modification of techniques. ■ Parents need guidance to identify appropriate self-care skills that the child is developmentally ready to learn. ■ Parents often need encouragement to transition responsibility to the child, becoming a supervisor rather than the person controlling care.	■ The child demonstrates the proper technique in the self-care skill and is able to assume responsibility for that skill with supervision by the parent. Responsibility for self-care increases as new skills are learned.
2. Nursing Diagnosis: Family Processes, Interrupted related to management of a chronic disease		
NIC Priority Intervention—*Normalization Promotion:* Assisting parents and other family members of children with chronic illnesses or disabilities in providing normal life experiences for their children and families		**NOC Suggested Outcome**—*Family Health Status:* Overall health status and social competence of family unit
GOAL: *The child and family will manage the required treatments, monitoring, and medication regimen for the child's condition while maintaining family routines and functioning.*		
■ Assess the child's and family's lifestyle and attempt to fit the child's care needs into those schedules. ■ Discuss the family's routines for special occasions and vacations and any activities important to the child. Identify ways to modify the child's management for these occasions and activities.	■ Fitting the child's care to the child's and family's lifestyle promotes adherence to the regimen and healthier family processes. ■ It is important for the child to participate in special events with the family and peers to promote psychologic development.	■ The child and family maintain important family routines and successfully manage the child's condition.
3. Nursing Diagnosis: Coping, Readiness for Enhanced related to self-care management of a chronic condition		
NIC Priority Intervention—*Resiliency Promotion:* Assisting individuals, families, and communities in development, use, and strengthening of protective factors to be used in coping with environmental and societal stressors		**NOC Suggested Outcome**—*Health-Seeking Behavior:* Personal actions to manage stressors that tax an individual's resources.
GOAL: *The child will develop a support system network.*		
■ Talk with the child about how to tell friends, teachers, and other important persons about the chronic condition. ■ Discuss ways to explain the condition to important persons and how to answer questions. ■ Role-play ways to talk about the condition with friends and teachers. ■ Encourage the child to attend peer support groups or camps specific to the child's condition.	■ These important persons can assist the child in an emergency if they have enough information to assess the problem. ■ Having an opportunity to plan and role-play the conversation will reduce the child's anxiety about condition disclosure. ■ Sharing information about the condition helps others understand changes in lifestyle needed by the child. ■ Learning and support networks developed at camp can promote development of problem-solving skills that increase coping abilities.	■ The child identifies the friends, teachers, and other important persons informed about the chronic condition who can provide support when needed.

Nursing Care Plan   The Child with a Chronic Condition, *continued*

INTERVENTION	RATIONALE	EXPECTED OUTCOME
4. Nursing Diagnosis: Health-Seeking Behaviors (Adolescent) related to learning self-management of a chronic disorder		
GOAL: *The adolescent will develop independent ability to manage his or her condition.*		
■ Allow the adolescent to perform as many self-care procedures as possible at each developmental stage.	■ Gradually learning self-care skills helps make this seem a regular expected behavior.	■ The adolescent performs appropriate daily management of self-care and seeks help to appropriately manage episodic acute problems.
■ Encourage the adolescent to problem solve and make decisions regarding care. Review decisions and provide feedback or appropriate guidance.	■ Problem-solving skills and competence in self-care management develop with positive feedback or corrective guidance.	
■ Encourage parents to stay involved even when the adolescent takes primary responsibility for care.	■ The adolescent is likely to adhere to the treatment plan when the parents continue to show interest and supervise care.	
■ Encourage the adolescent to discuss the condition and care directly with the healthcare provider.	■ The adolescent begins to learn the process for seeking health care and becoming an advocate for own care.	

NANDA-I © 2012

Planning and Implementation

Newborn Care

Promote parent–newborn attachment by demonstrating to parents how to hold (if possible), stroke, touch, rub, and talk to the newborn attached to technologic devices. Explain the purpose of all technology, the sights and sounds, and what they indicate to help reduce anxiety in handling the newborn. Reduce environmental noise and bright lights, but provide developmentally appropriate visual stimulation for the newborn, such as pictures of a face or a patterned design. Ensure adequate pain management for procedures performed (see Chapter 21 🔗). When possible, provide continuity of nursing staff for the newborn to help parents bond with the newborn, to educate the parents about the child's condition, and to begin preparing for home care.

The Child with a Newly Diagnosed Chronic Condition

Just as with the newborn's family, it is equally important to address the fears and concerns of the family of a child with a newly diagnosed chronic condition. Provide the condition-specific education to help prepare the family for care at home and begin discharge planning. Care of the technology-dependent child includes educating the family about equipment use and maintenance, specific tasks associated with treatment, and monitoring of the child. Ongoing assistance may be required to help families deal with financial issues, time management, and other challenges. See the systems chapters later in this textbook for condition-specific family education and discharge planning.

Discharge Planning and Home Care Teaching

As the newborn or child with a newly diagnosed chronic condition transitions to the home, parents often feel overwhelmed with preparations for home care, the anxiety of caring for a newborn with special healthcare needs, grief for the loss of their expectations for a healthy baby, and uncertainty of how to support the child's growth and development needs. Partner with the parents to ensure a smooth transition from hospital to the home environment. Assist the family in the initial discussions with the multidisciplinary team that participates in developing the child's care plan. Ensure that the family understands the role of each care provider. Provide contact numbers for parents to call should any issues arise at home.

Education to provide care of the child at home may be initiated by the hospital nursing staff, and then transitioned to special nurse educators or the home health nurses. Care is taken to ensure that all aspects of management are discussed with the family and that they demonstrate an understanding and ability to perform the care required.

During discharge planning the identification of a parent peer or peer support group may be helpful to provide support to the family. Parent peers who have had similar experiences may be very helpful in identifying strategies for the initial care transition in the home and additional issues that arise over time. If the family has a computer, Internet resources for information and family support should be provided.

Collaborate with the family and healthcare team to ensure that the child has a medical or healthcare home in the local community to provide health promotion and maintenance and to assist with the coordination of local community resources. Promote communication and joint planning of care between the specialty care provider and local healthcare provider. Nurses working in hospital specialty clinics and other community settings can help ensure that children with chronic conditions receive multidisciplinary referrals and have appointments scheduled. Social services may be called to assist the family with identifying financial resources and other community resources for home management.

Coordination of Care

Care coordination is the process of planning and integrating healthcare services among providers in an effort to achieve and promote good health in the child (American Academy of Pediatrics, 2009; Wood, Winterbauer, Sloyer, et al., 2009). Care coordination in a medical home decreases unmet healthcare needs, improves family satisfaction, and decreases hospitalizations (Wood et al., 2009). An additional role of care coordination is the facilitation of transition

Evidence-Based Practice | Care Coordination for Children with Special Healthcare Needs

PROBLEM

Children with special healthcare needs require assistance from a variety of programs and services to maximize their potential. Fragmentation of care may result in the child's needs being unmet.

EVIDENCE

Data were analyzed from the 2005–2006 National Survey of Children with Special Healthcare Needs to determine the association between receiving adequate care coordination, family–provider relations, and outcomes in the child and family. Data indicated that 68.2% of the families reported receiving some type of assistance with care coordination. Of these, 59.2% indicated they received adequate help, and 40.8% indicated the assistance was inadequate. Adequate care coordination was associated with family-centered care, satisfaction with care received, and a partnership with healthcare professionals. Families who reported receiving adequate care coordination were less likely to have problems with specialty referrals, family financial burden, and reduction in work hours. These families also had less out-of-pocket expenses, fewer visits to the emergency department per month, and fewer missed days of school for the CSHCN than families who reported receiving inadequate assistance with care coordination (Turchi, Berhane, Bethell, et al., 2009).

A descriptive study of six pediatric primary care practices was conducted to evaluate the effectiveness of a care coordination measurement tool. Other purposes of the study were to describe care coordination activities that occurred in a pediatric primary care setting, to assess the relationship of care coordination activities in this setting to outcomes related to the use of resources, and to measure personnel costs related to care coordination activities. The study found that care coordination activities were used by patients at all levels of acuity, including children and youth with special healthcare needs; the care coordination tool was used effectively in the pediatric primary care setting; care coordination provided by nurses instead of physicians in this setting decreased costs; and care

coordination by nurses as an integral aspect of each visit decreased the number of visits to the primary care provider and to the emergency department (Antonelli, Stille, & Antonelli, 2008).

A longitudinal study compared the use of pediatric practice-based care coordination to an agency-based model of care coordination. Six pediatric practices participated in the study. Three of the practices continued agency-based care coordination (comparison group) while three practices had a nurse care coordinator placed onsite, who received training and quality improvement (intervention group). Children and youth with special healthcare needs were identified. At baseline, 262 of these families/children were interviewed. At 18 months, 76 families/children in the intervention group and 68 in the comparison group were interviewed. Results of the study indicated that families who received practice-based care coordination reported a higher level of satisfaction with care coordination, were more likely to report that their experience with care coordination had improved, reported fewer barriers to healthcare services, and were treated better by the staff in the office (Wood et al., 2009).

IMPLICATIONS

Practice-based care coordination in which the nurse works with families to facilitate coordination of services is effective and leads to greater satisfaction with care, reduced costs, and fewer barriers to healthcare services. The nurse assists families to identify needed programs and services and is in an excellent position to serve as a liaison between these programs and the family to decrease the risk for fragmentation of care.

CRITICAL THINKING APPLICATION

Why is care coordination a vital aspect of care of CSHCN? What is an example of coordination of services for CSHCN? How do nurses play a vital role in care coordination for CSHCN?

---

from a pediatric healthcare provider to an adult healthcare provider (White & Hackett, 2009). (See Evidence-Based Practice: Care Coordination for Children with Special Healthcare Needs.)

A **case manager,** often a nurse or social worker, may be given responsibility to help the family with care coordination. Case managers are often paid by a healthcare insurer to reduce healthcare costs by coordinating the healthcare team, determining family needs, identifying financial and local support resources, and arranging for needed healthcare services.

Care coordination may also include helping the family modify the home to support required technology, such as mechanical ventilation or wheelchair use. Assistance may be required in purchasing or leasing ventilators, infusion pumps, or other specialized equipment. The coordination plan also includes determining the potential need for home health nursing, physical therapy, or other home health services.

Families become very well educated about their child's condition and the services that would make managing the condition easier. Once management goals are established by the multidisciplinary team, the case manager partners with the family to help in the decision-making process regarding how goals will be met. An important role is helping the family to determine cost-effective strategies to meet healthcare goals and to delay the time when the child reaches the cap on health insurance benefits.

Some families assume the role of care coordinator for their child. It is essential for the family to understand that care coordination is time consuming and requires ongoing assessment and evaluation of the child's status and anticipated outcomes. Support family members

in their decision to lead the care coordination process by helping the parents to become knowledgeable about the child's condition and treatment regimen. Encourage the parents to take an active role in the treatment planning and decision-making process so that they gain confidence in their abilities. Many hospitals have workshops for parents who are managing the complex care of their children. Parent-to-parent support groups can provide advice, support, and suggestions for referrals. Review the care coordination to ensure that the child has access to the most appropriate care and resources. Provide positive feedback to the parents as their advocacy skills increase.

Suggest that the family maintain a log of the healthcare team members, their roles, when the child was seen and any interventions, the results of interventions, and future planned interventions or treatments. The family can use this information when communicating with the healthcare providers, particularly in an emergency, and it may also help eliminate unnecessary duplication of procedures.

Respite Care

Respite care is an important support service to care for the child with a chronic condition while the parents take a short break away from the daily care. Respite allows parents an opportunity for rest so they may sustain their role as caregivers. Care may be provided by extended family, friends, or an agency and may take place in the home or an area outside of the home such as a residential setting or hospice. The length of time may vary from a few hours to several days (Eaton, 2008). An example of respite might be skilled nursing care in a facility or the home so the family can have a weekend away. Assist the family in identifying respite care that meets the individual family's

Weblink | Respite Locator

Legal and Ethical Considerations
Katie Beckett Act

The Tax Equity and Fiscal Responsibility Act of 1982 (PL 97-248), also known as the Katie Beckett Act, provides financial assistance so parents can hire trained care providers for respite care.

needs from the services available in the community. Many states have passed legislation for in-home family support services that include respite care. Because many respite services charge for their assistance, the family may require help in identifying respite waiver subsidies available to them. See Legal and Ethical Considerations: Katie Beckett Act. Reliable childcare and enrollment in school are other mechanisms for families to obtain respite care.

Clinical Tip

The ARCH National Respite Network helps parents locate respite care services in their area.

Support for the Child with a Chronic Condition

Provide the child with opportunities to express concerns about the condition and the effect the condition has on quality of life. The child who has had the chronic condition since birth or early childhood requires assistance in understanding more about the condition as cognitive development and understanding increase. As the child grows, collaborate with the child and family to include the child in self-care management according to cognitive and developmental level, and to participate in the decision-making process. Encourage the child to assume a role in care and management of the condition. This may include maintaining a journal, self-administering medications, or monitoring glucose levels. See Partnering with Families: Developmental Strategies for Promoting the Child's Self-Care for more information.

Support the transition of adolescents to adult health services by introducing the adolescent to members of the healthcare team that will eventually assume a role in providing care. Encourage the adolescent to take a more assertive role in healthcare visits with the pediatric healthcare team in preparation for working with a new healthcare team. Ensure that the adolescent understands the role each new member of the team will assume.

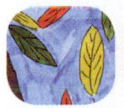

Partnering with Families

Developmental Strategies for Promoting the Child's Self-Care

When the child is cognitively able to learn about the chronic condition and begins to take some responsibility for self-care, knowledge of cognitive and psychomotor development helps in developing strategies to teach the child about self-care. Ideally such learning should begin early in life, but even when the condition develops at a later age, educating the child can still be based on knowledge of the child's development. Education and assumption of self-care responsibility should be appropriately matched to the child's developmental abilities. The ultimate goal is to transition all self-care responsibility to an adolescent who has learned important health skills, has practiced these skills, and has incorporated them into a daily routine, leading to compliant health maintenance behavior (White & Hackett, 2009).

- Toddlers (1 to 3 years) can cooperate with the daily routines of care and assist in simple ways, such as holding an item. The toddler can also learn simple concepts such as foods allowed or not allowed. When a routine is established, the toddler learns what to expect through daily repetition.
- Preschoolers (4 to 5 years) are able to imitate some of the parent's behaviors regarding care, and they can learn simple terms that describe their condition and how they feel when the condition is not well controlled (e.g., weak and dizzy with diabetes, difficulty breathing with asthma).

  Parents can help teach the child simple terms about the condition and have the child practice telling the information to other family members. Help the parent identify a simple task that is part of the management care routine that the child can do to help (e.g., holding the spacer during the asthma treatment, washing the hands, taking supplies out of a bag or box).
- Early school-age children (6 to 9 years) are more aware of physical feelings associated with when the condition is and is not well controlled. The child is also capable of performing some aspects of care (e.g., fingerstick for glucose monitoring, writing the glucose reading in a log, controlling inhalation to use aerosol medication, selecting appropriate foods for a meal or snack), having seen it performed by parents repeatedly or after being taught and coached to do it well.

  The parent can support the child's learning by increasing the information provided about the condition and need for treatment. Give the child an option about which self-care skill to learn first, next, and so on. The parent is then able to select skills appropriate to the child's developmental ability and teach the child to perform them. As the child demonstrates proficiency with a skill, a new skill can be added. The child can take responsibility for learned self-care skills with supervision, and the parent performs other unlearned skills.

- Late school-age children (10 to 12 years) have a greater understanding of how the body works and the impact of the chronic condition. They have the capability of discussing some aspects of care directly with the healthcare provider. By 12 years of age, the child can learn to perform all the psychomotor skills associated with the condition.

  Parents can support the child in assuming more responsibility for self-care by initially providing a list of all steps in the management plan or other tools that will help with decision making (e.g., dose of insulin, adding food to diet on days with soccer practice). Provide corrective feedback as necessary. Continue to answer questions, particularly when problem solving and when decisions need to be made about care. Rather than controlling the discussion, encourage the child to talk independently with the healthcare provider.
- Adolescents can, with the prior steps of preparation, become the primary managers of their daily care. They usually have the cognitive ability to problem solve and make adjustments in the care routine for special occasions or illness and to ask for help when a complex care situation develops. The adolescent should have a network of friends and family who are informed about the condition and able to assist in an emergency.

  Parents should monitor the self-care provided without interfering in the adolescent's care routine unless corrective feedback is needed. Encourage the adolescent to take full responsibility for self-care management, but encourage open communication about the condition and other healthcare concerns. Discuss risky behaviors and the potential impact on general health and the condition specifically. Provide support and assistance during the time the adolescent transitions to adult healthcare providers.

Health Promotion

Review the next stage of expected development with parents and provide suggestions and strategies to help the child with a chronic condition achieve developmental milestones. Partner with the family to ensure that other children in the family are also receiving appropriate care and stimulation to promote their growth and development. Discuss with parents routine health promotion and maintenance needs of all children in the family such as immunizations, dental hygiene, and any screening tests. See Chapters 8 through 13 🔗.

Discuss parenting approaches for the child with a chronic condition. Encourage a structured environment with limitations as developmentally appropriate for the child. Assist the family as needed in providing a nurturing environment and offering praise for achievement of tasks.

Facilitate Education Service Planning

Assist the family with school entry of the child with a chronic condition. Discussions with the family can help them in defining appropriate expectations and goals. The nurse can also communicate with school personnel about any classroom modifications required by the child, and educate teachers and other school personnel about the medical or assistive equipment used by the child. This information is then integrated into the child's IHP, which may be a stand-alone plan or tied to an IEP.

The school nurse can also assist the family with Section 504 planning activities by serving as a liaison between the school and the child's healthcare team. Key health records that are needed to plan the IHP should be assembled after the family provides informed consent. Encourage the family to establish regular communication with the school personnel and school nurse.

Clinical Tip

Special accommodations for the child with disabilities may include extending test-taking times, tutors, note takers, and the use of technologic equipment to assist in the learning environment. Encourage parents to ask questions regarding computer accessibility, arrangements for tutors or note takers, private study areas, and individualized attention. Partner with the child and family to determine the appropriate level of participation in school activities, including after-school activities.

In the case of a do-not-resuscitate (DNR) request for the child at school, encourage collaboration with school personnel, teachers, and other members of the healthcare team as necessary to facilitate an agreement between the school and family. Many school systems do not have a policy that permits honoring a DNR request, and the school nurse is an important liaison in the discussion and development of the policy. Refer to Chapter 18 🔗 for further discussion of DNR requests in school.

Support the Family's Psychosocial Adjustment

A positive relationship between the healthcare team and the family is essential. Provide the child, parents, and siblings an opportunity to discuss how the experience of a chronic illness affects their daily lives. Listening and offering strategies to improve the organization of care, as well as the use of community and family supports, can help enhance the family's coping. Assist the family in identifying support systems, and encourage the family to communicate with those support systems as needed. Help the family see that simple chores performed by friends and extended family such as cooking meals, transporting

siblings to recreational events, or picking up supplies at the supermarket can reduce stress, especially during times when the child is hospitalized. Refer the family to support groups in the community that might offer suggestions and information to the family. Counseling may be helpful to parents experiencing marital stress.

Identify ways to improve accessibility of services to children with chronic conditions and their families. For example, arranging transportation, finding resources closer to home, and arranging for home visits may improve accessibility.

Assist the family to provide information to the siblings about the child's disability at the appropriate developmental level so that the information is tailored specifically to the siblings' level of understanding. Provide instructional materials, videos, books, pamphlets, and other information when available. Inform the parents that siblings of the child with a chronic condition may experience an array of feelings. See the discussion on page 421 regarding sibling reactions.

Clinical Tip

Siblings of children with chronic conditions may feel overwhelmingly guilty about their feelings of jealousy, shame, and anger. Inform the siblings that these feelings are normal and that they are not "bad" for having them.

Emergency Preparedness

Advance planning is needed to ensure that children who are medically fragile and require technology for survival or have the potential for life-threatening episodes have the necessary resources in the event of a disaster. The designated shelter for such children, with health professionals and electric power for the needed equipment, should be identified and known to the family. In the meantime, battery packs for power backup should be available at all times. Additionally, parents need to arrange for durable power of attorney so that consent for emergency medical care can be available as needed. The child and parents may become separated during the disaster, or the parents may become injured and unable to care for the child. Refer to Chapter 14 🔗 for more information related to emergency preparedness.

Evaluation

Expected outcomes for care of the family of a child with a chronic condition may include:

- The child and family establish effective coping mechanisms.
- The child and family experience reduced anxiety.
- The child and family demonstrate understanding and management of the condition.
- Parenting patterns are appropriate and supportive of the child's growth and development.
- Role conflict and caregiver strain are minimized.
- Caregivers achieve adequate rest, sleep, and socialization.
- The child and family adjust to the child's chronic condition.
- The adolescent successfully transitions to adult health services and living arrangements.

NURSE'S REACTIONS TO CARE OF CHILDREN WITH A CHRONIC CONDITION

Nurses and other healthcare professionals generally describe their role in caring for families and children with chronic conditions as very rewarding. However, over time these nurses may experience conflicting feelings, including grief, fatigue, and burnout, particularly if the needs of families and children served are difficult to meet (Aycock & Boyle, 2009; Yoder, 2010). Nurses need to recognize signs of **compassion fatigue,** an emotion that comes from understanding the traumatic events experienced by families and the stress from helping or wanting to help the families. Research by Yoder (2010) identified several trigger situations that could lead to compassion fatigue or burnout in nurses. These situations included caring for patients, system problems (such as workload and decisions by management), and personal issues. The weariness and lack of energy associated with compassion fatigue may become severe and affect the ability to function at work or home if the nurse's coping mechanisms are not effective.

Self-care activities such as exercise, meditation, recreation, maintaining a sense of humor, and social nonwork relationships are beneficial short-term personal coping strategies. Taking vacations to rest and reenergize, changing patient assignments, or transferring to a new work area are other strategies that can help the nurse balance personal mental health with the compassion needed for ongoing work with these families.

Chapter Highlights

- A chronic condition is a long-term, ongoing condition that is expected to last 3 months or more and may involve any of the following alone or in combination: functional limitations, disfigurement, dependence on technology, medications, special diet for management of the condition, and requiring more healthcare services than a healthy child.

- Approximately 10 million children in the United States have special healthcare needs related to some type of chronic condition.

- Chronic conditions can occur as a result of a genetic condition, congenital anomaly, injury during fetal development or at birth, complication of care after birth, serious infection, or significant injury.

- Children who are medically fragile are those dependent on a medical device for survival or prevention of further disability.

- A developmental delay results when there is failure to achieve anticipated milestones during specific developmental stages.

- Parents may experience many of the same responses to the diagnosis of a child's chronic condition as if they had experienced the child's death, including shock, disbelief, anger, denial, and despair. Siblings of the child with a chronic illness may have feelings of jealousy, resentment, anger, depression, and guilt.

- The time of diagnosis is one of the most stressful times for families of children with chronic conditions as the parents wait anxiously for the outcome of diagnostic procedures. Other times associated with significant stressors for the family include developmental milestones, school entry, adolescence, planning for the transition to adult health and vocational services, and planning for long-term guardianship.

- Moving the child who is chronically ill or technology dependent to the home setting is a life-changing decision for the family, and it must be done with collaboration between the family and the healthcare team.

- Caregiver burden, the ongoing pressure of caring for children with special healthcare needs, causes fatigue and makes it difficult for the parents to meet other family obligations.

- The financial burden of caring for a child with special healthcare needs is significant even when the family has health insurance.

- In an effort to cope and feel a sense of control over the family's life, the parents may use normalization, a process of focusing on those aspects of family life and routine that are similar to other families while integrating the needs of the child with a chronic condition.

- Sending the child to school has several benefits for the child and family, including socialization for the child beyond the immediate family, respite for parents, and promotion of a sense of normalization in the family.

- An individualized education plan (IEP) is developed for a child with cognitive, motor, social, or communication impairments who needs special education services in the school setting. An individualized health plan (IHP) is developed for the child with medical conditions that need to be managed within the school setting.

- Children who are medically fragile or dependent on technology are entitled to a free and appropriate education and education services in the school setting. The school administration is obligated to plan for and ensure that the personnel resources and equipment needed to provide care are consistently available.

- An individualized transition plan (ITP) is developed for adolescents with a chronic condition in collaboration with the family to assist in identifying appropriate support programs, living arrangements, and employment for adult life.

- The child with a chronic condition is more likely to be hospitalized than the child without a chronic condition. Sudden hospitalization resulting from exacerbation of the child's disorder places increased demands and stressors on the child and family.

- Children with chronic health conditions require regular health promotion, health screening, and health maintenance care, as well as specialized health services to assist the child and family in the management of the condition.

- The role of the nurse in caring for the child with a chronic condition includes providing health supervision from infancy to transition into adulthood, collaborating with the multidisciplinary healthcare team, and partnering with the family to manage the child's care at home.

- Care coordination involves planning and integrating healthcare services among providers in an effort to achieve and promote good health in the child. Care coordination decreases unmet healthcare needs, improves family satisfaction, and decreases hospitalizations. Care coordination also facilitates transition from a pediatric healthcare provider to an adult healthcare provider.

- Nurses who specialize in caring for children with complex chronic conditions may experience compassion fatigue as they continue their efforts to meet the ongoing needs of these families.

Clinical Reasoning in Action

INTRODUCTION

Recall Haley, the child with cerebral palsy who will be attending school for the first time. Her mother had initially preferred homeschooling for Haley, and now wants to support her social development with other children. Haley's sister is in the local elementary school and, if possible, her mother would like Haley to attend the same school. A case manager is asked to assist with facilitating Haley's entry into school.

DESCRIPTION

The case manager coordinates a multidisciplinary meeting of the clinic nurse, physical therapist, physician, and Haley's family to review her health status and to discuss the transition to school. They also discuss potential accommodations needed for Haley's mobility limitations. A full educational evaluation has not yet been performed, and the family is encouraged to talk with the school system to initiate that process. The multidisciplinary team assists the parents in developing a plan for Haley's transition to school. Once her mother has signed consent, the case worker will ensure that needed medical records are transferred to the school for development of the IEP and IHP.

DISCUSSION

1. What role will the clinic nurse and case manager have in helping develop Haley's IEP and IHP?

2. What role will the school nurse have with the child, caregivers, teacher, and classmates during the facilitation of school entry?

3. Based on Haley's age and developmental stage, what feelings, fears, and concerns might she be expected to experience related to entry into school? What interventions would be beneficial to Haley?

4. What actions will the mother need to take in preparing the school personnel for Haley's health needs?

5. Haley's 10-year-old sister attends the same school. What effects of Haley's entry into school might the sibling experience?

NCLEX-RN® Review

1. Which nursing intervention is directed toward the school-age child's independent management of asthma symptoms?
   1. Encourage the child to use the flow meter and record results every day.
   2. Assess the child and family's level of understanding about asthma.
   3. Discuss with the child how to tell friends about asthma.
   4. Teach the parents proper use of inhalers.

2. A 3-year-old female child with multiple disabilities requires daily tube feedings and tracheostomy suctioning. The nurse has successfully explained available and needed services when the mother makes which statement?
   1. I can call respite caregivers to give me a break from her daily requirements.
   2. I can call my church to get support for my family when we need it.
   3. My daughter needs to have play dates with children her own developmental age.
   4. My family should engage in conversation with a counselor at least twice monthly.

3. The family of a hospitalized child with leukemia believes the child will be cured by prayer alone, and plans to take the child home. Which nursing intervention will address this barrier to care?
   1. Demonstrate respect for the family's wishes.
   2. Evaluate the home for wheelchair accessibility.
   3. Communicate the parents' request to the child's physician.
   4. Assess the family's understanding of leukemia.

4. Which outcome indicates a successful transition from hospital to home for the family of a 2-year-old child with a tracheostomy due to bronchopulmonary dysplasia?
   1. The parents demonstrate proper technique of suctioning the tracheostomy in the hospital.
   2. The child demonstrates self-care skills prior to discharge.
   3. The family provides appropriate home care for the child while maintaining family routines.
   4. The parents demonstrate how to take the child's vital signs at home.

See Appendix I 🫘 for answers.

References

Aitken, M. E., McCarthy, M. L., Slomine, B. S., Ding, R., Durbin, D. R., Jaffe, K. M., . . . CHAT Study Group. (2009). Family burden after traumatic brain injury in children. *Pediatrics, 12*(1), 199–206.

Allen, P. J. (2010). The primary care provider and children with chronic conditions. In P. J. Allen, J. A. Vessey, & N. A. Schapiro, *Primary care of the child with a chronic condition* (5th ed., pp. 3–21). St. Louis, MO: Mosby.

American Academy of Pediatrics. (2009). *Tools for coordinating care.* Retrieved from http://www.medicalhomeinfo.org/tools/coordinating%20care.html

Antonelli, R. C., Stille, C. J., & Antonelli, D. M. (2008). Care coordination for children and youth with special health care needs: A descriptive, multisite study of activities, personnel costs, and outcomes. *Pediatrics, 122*(1), e209–e216.

Aycock, N., & Boyle, D. (2009). Interventions to manage compassion fatigue in oncology nursing. *Clinical Journal of Oncology Nursing, 13*(2), 183–191.

Betz, C. L. (2008). Forthcoming issues to confront as children and youth with special health care needs grow up. *Journal of Pediatric Nursing, 23*(4), 237–240.

Broger, B., & Zeni, M. B. (2011). Fathers' coping mechanisms related to parenting a chronically ill child: Implications for advanced practice nurses. *Journal of Pediatric Health Care, 25*(2), 96–104.

Caley, L. (2011). Risk and protective factors associated with stress in mothers whose children are enrolled in early intervention services. *Journal of Pediatric Health Care.* In Press.

Carnevale, F. A., Rehm, R. S., Kirk, S., & McKeever, P. (2008). What we know (and do not know) about raising children with complex continuing care needs. *Journal of Child Health Care, 12*(1), 4–6.

Coker, T. R., Rodriquez, M. A., & Flores, G. (2010). Family-centered care for US children with special health care needs: Who gets it and why? *Pediatrics, 125*(6), 1159–1167.

Collins, S. R., & Nicholson, J. L. (2010). *Realizing health reform's potential: Young adults and the Affordable Care Act of 2010*. Retrieved from http://www.commonwealthfund.org/~/media/Files/Publications/Issue%20Brief/2010/Oct/1446_Collins_young_adults_and_ACA_ib.pdf

Eaton, N. (2008). "I don't know how we coped before": A study of respite care for children in the home and hospice. *Journal of Clinical Nursing, 17*(23), 3196–3204.

Fish, W. W. (2008). The IEP meeting: Perceptions of parents of students who receive special education services. *Preventing School Failure, 53*(1), 8–14.

FRIENDS National Resource Center for Community-Based Child Abuse Prevention (CBCAP). (2006). *Making family support programs accessible to children with disabilities and their families*. Retrieved from http://www.friendsnrc.org/download/children_disabilities.pdf

Giallo, R., & Gavidia-Payne, S. (2008). Evaluation of a family-based intervention for siblings of children with a disability or chronic illness. *Australian e-Journal for the Advancement of Mental Health, 7*(2), 84–96.

Goldstein, K. P., Altman, S., & Zimmerman, A. (2010). State and federal benefits for children with special healthcare needs. *Pediatric Annals, 39*(4), 240–253.

Gordon, J. (2009). An evidence-based approach for supporting parents experiencing chronic sorrow. *Pediatric Nursing, 35*(2), 115–119.

Granados, A. C., & Agís, I. F. (2011). Why children with special needs feel better with hippotherapy sessions: A conceptual review. *Journal of Alternative and Complementary Medicine, 17*(3), 191–197.

Hibbard, R. A., Desch, L. W., & Committee on Child Abuse and Neglect and Council on Children with Disabilities. (2007). Maltreatment of children with disabilities. *Pediatrics, 119*(5), 1018–1025.

HRTW National Resource Center. (2009). *About HRTW*. Retrieved from http://www.hrtw.org/about_us/index.html

Kellam, B., & Bhatia, J. (2008). Sound spectral analysis in the intensive care nursery: Measuring high-frequency sound. *Journal of Pediatric Nursing, 23*(4), 317–323.

Knafl, K. A., & Santacroce, S. J. (2010). Chronic conditions and the family. In P. J. Allen, J. A. Vessey, & N. A. Schapiro, *Primary care of the child with a chronic condition* (5th ed., pp. 74–89). St. Louis, MO: Mosby.

Laiteerapong, N., & Huang, E. S. (2010). Health care reform and chronic diseases: Anticipating the health consequences. *Journal of the American Medical Association, 304*(8), 899–900.

Lasky, R. E., & Williams, A. L. (2009). Noise and light exposures for extremely low birth weight newborns during their stay in the neonatal intensive care unit. *Pediatrics, 123*(2), 540–546.

Looman, W. S., O'Conner-Von, S. K., Ferski, G. J., & Hildenbrand, D. A. (2009). Financial and employment problems in families of children with special health care needs: Implications for research and practice. *Journal of Pediatric Health Care, 23*(2), 117–125.

Lotstein, D. S., Inkelas, M., Hays, R. D., Halfon, N., & Brook, R. (2008). Access to care for youth with special health care needs in the transition to adulthood. *Journal of Adolescent Health, 43*(1), 23–29.

Lotstein, D. S., Ghandour, R., Cash, A., McGuire, E., Strickland, B., & Newacheck, P. (2009). Planning for health care transitions: Results from the 2005–2006 National Survey of Children with Special Health Care Needs. *Pediatrics, 123*(1), e145–e152.

Marchitto, C. (2010). Transitioning the needs of children with chronic illness: Exploring communication between hospitals and school settings. *Social Work Student Papers*. Paper 61. Retrieved from http://digitalcommons.providence.edu/socialwrk_students/61

Miles, M. S., Holditch-Davis, D., Burchinal, M. R., & Brunssen, S. (2011). Maternal role attainment with medically fragile infants: Part 1. Measurement and correlates during the first year of life. *Research in Nursing and Health, 34*, 20–34.

Moses, M., Gilchrest, C., & Schwab, N. C. (2005). Section 504 of the Rehabilitation Act: Determining eligibility and implications for school districts. *Journal of School Nursing, 21*(1), 48–58.

Nicholas, D. B., & Keilty, K. (2007). An evaluation of dyadic peer support for caregiving parents of children with chronic lung disease requiring technology assistance. *Social Work in Health Care, 44*(3), 245–259.

Park, M. J., & Irwin, C. E. (2008). Youth with special health care needs: Facilitating a healthy transition to adulthood. *Journal of Adolescent Health, 43*(1), 6–7.

Sanders, R. A., Kuo, D. Z., Levey, E., & Cheng, T. L. (2009). Transitioning adolescents to adult care and adulthood: Part 1 of 2. *Contemporary Pediatrics, 26*(11), 46–52.

Selekman, J., & Vessey, J. A. (2010). School and the child with a chronic condition. In P. J. Allen, J. A. Vessey, & N. A. Schapiro, *Primary care of the child with a chronic condition* (5th ed., pp. 42–59). St. Louis, MO: Mosby.

Shaw, T. M., & DeLaet, D. E. (2010). Transition of adolescents to young adulthood for vulnerable populations. *Pediatrics in Review, 31*(12), 497–505.

Svensson, B., Bornehag, C. G., & Janson, S. (2011). Chronic conditions in children increase the risk for physical abuse—But vary with socio-economic circumstances. *Acta Paediatrica, 100*, 407–412.

Theofanidis, D. (2007). Chronic illness in childhood: Psychosocial adaptation and nursing support for the child and family. *Health Science Journal, 1*(2), 1-9.

Turchi, R. M., Berhane, Z., Bethell, C., Pomponio, A., Antonelli, R., & Minkovitz, C. S. (2009). Care coordination for CSHCN: Associations with family–provider relations and family/child outcomes. *Pediatrics, 124*(Suppl. 4), S428–S434.

U.S. Department of Education. (2000). *A guide to the individualized education program*. Retrieved from http://www.ed.gov/parents/needs/speced/iepguide/index.htm

U.S. Department of Education. (2006). *Individualized education programs*. Retrieved from http://idea.ed.gov/explore/view/p/%2Croot%2Cdynamic%2CTopicalBrief%2C10%2C

U.S. Department of Education. (2010). *Thirty-five years of progress in educating children with disabilities through IDEA*. Retrieved from http://www2.ed.gov/about/offices/list/osers/idea35/history/index_pg10.html

U.S. Department of Education. (2011). *Protecting students with disabilities*. Retrieved from http://www2.ed.gov/about/offices/list/ocr/504faq.html

U.S. Department of Health and Human Services, Health Resources and Services Administration, Maternal and Child Health Bureau. (2008). *The National Survey of Children with Special Health Care Needs Chartbook 2005–2006*. Rockville, MD: U.S. Department of Health and Human Services.

U.S. Department of Health and Human Services. (2012). *Healthy People 2020 Objective Topic Areas and Page Numbers*. Retrieved from http://healthypeople.gov/2020/topicsobjectives2020/pdfs/HP2020objectives.pdf

U.S. Social Security Administration. (2011). *Understanding Supplemental Security Income SSI for Children*. Retrieved from http://www.ssa.gov/ssi/text-child-ussi.htm

Vessey, J. A., & Sullivan, B. J. (2010). Chronic conditions and child development. In P. J. Allen, J. A. Vessey, & N. A. Schapiro, *Primary care of the child with a chronic condition* (5th ed., pp. 22–41). St. Louis, MO: Mosby.

White, P. H., & Hackett, P. (2009). On the threshold to the adult medical home: Care coordination in transition. *Pediatric Annals, 38*(9), 513–520.

Williams, P. D., Piamjariyakul, U., Graff, J. C., & Stanton, A. (2010). Developmental disabilities: Effects on well siblings. *Issues in Comprehensive Pediatric Nursing, 33*, 39–55.

Williams, P. D., Ridder, E. L., Setter, R. K., Liebergen, A., Curry, H., Piamjariyakul, U., & Williams, A. R. (2009). Pediatric chronic illness (cancer, cystic fibrosis) effects on well siblings: Parents' voices. *Issues in Comprehensive Pediatric Nursing, 32*(3), 94–113.

Wood, D., Winterbauer, N., Sloyer, P., Jobli, E., Hou, T., McCaskill, Q., & Livingood, W. (2009). A longitudinal study of a pediatric practice-based versus an agency-based model of care coordination for children and youth with special health care needs. *Maternal Child Health Journal, 13*, 667–676.

Yoder, E. A. (2010). Compassion fatigue in nurses. *Applied Nursing Research, 23*, 191–197.

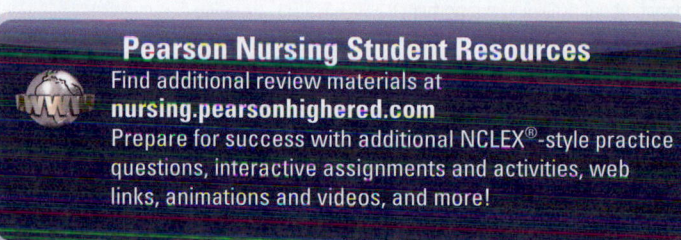

Pearson Nursing Student Resources

Find additional review materials at
nursing.pearsonhighered.com
Prepare for success with additional NCLEX®-style practice questions, interactive assignments and activities, web links, animations and videos, and more!

Learning Outcomes

After completing this chapter, you will be able to:

1. Discuss the variety of settings in which the nurse may encounter a child with a life-threatening condition.

2. Summarize the effects of a life-threatening illness or injury on children.

3. Identify the coping mechanisms utilized by the child and family in response to stress.

4. Examine the family's experience and reactions to having a child with a life-threatening illness.

5. Develop a plan of care for the child with a life-threatening illness and the family.

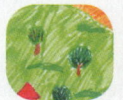 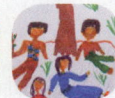 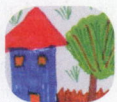
"I was so scared when I saw my sister with all of those tubes in her mouth, arms, and everywhere else. The noise was terrible—every machine in there made weird noises. My mother and daddy are so upset, but they're thankful that I'm okay. I sure hope Alexa wakes up soon."

—*Sharon, age 8*

Alexa Cruz, 6 years old, was a passenger in the back seat of her parents' car when another car struck them broadside, pushing in the back passenger door. Even though Alexa was wearing a lap belt, her head struck the car window. She was unconscious at the scene and had a bruise across her abdomen where the lap belt restrained her. The emergency medical system responded and decided Alexa had injuries serious enough to transport her to the trauma center. A cervical collar was applied in case her cervical spine was also injured. Upon arrival at the trauma center, Alexa's airway, breathing, circulation, and responsiveness were assessed. She was breathing spontaneously, and her heart rate was strong and regular but more rapid than normal. Her blood pressure was appropriate for her age. Because she was not fully responsive, an endotracheal tube was inserted and oxygen was administered. An intravenous line was started and lactated Ringer's solution was administered. Alexa's abdomen was slightly distended, and she flinched and withdrew to touch when her abdomen was palpated in the left upper quadrant. She was admitted to the pediatric intensive care unit (PICU) so she could be monitored carefully for changes to her physiologic status and provided needed treatment. Further evaluation will determine the extent of Alexa's head injury and if she has a spleen laceration or other injury in the abdomen.

What do children like Alexa face after admission to the pediatric intensive care unit? What nursing strategies can help a critically ill or injured child cope with the experience? What stressors will families face during the child's hospitalization? What interventions could help them in this crisis? What strategies should be used to help siblings understand what has happened to their brother or sister? This chapter offers guidance about providing supportive care to critically ill and injured children like Alexa and to their families.

The intense emotional and physical demands placed on the child who is critically ill or injured present a challenge to nurses' attempts to provide developmentally appropriate care. The child's parents and siblings are confronted with a stressful situation. A family-centered care model offers a framework for performing nursing interventions that help to minimize stress and enhance coping by the ill or injured child, parents, and siblings.

LIFE-THREATENING ILLNESS OR INJURY

A **life-threatening condition** is one in which there is a considerable likelihood of death even though treatment may prolong the child's life or the child may have a complete recovery from the illness or injury (Institute of Medicine, 2003; Watters, Sayre, & Silbergleit, 2005). A threat to a child's life may be expected, as in a chronic condition or progressive disabling disease. More often the death is unexpected due to an unintentional injury, the leading cause of death in children, or an acute illness. (See Chapter 1 for the leading causes of death in children in different age groups.) How children, parents, and siblings cope with the threat will depend on the anticipated or unanticipated nature of the event and the conditions surrounding the child's admission to the hospital.

When death results from a chronic condition or terminal illness, the child and family generally have time to adjust to episodes of life-threatening crisis and impending death. Although the child could die unexpectedly during treatment, parents have some knowledge of the condition, the hospital setting, and the healthcare team and have had an opportunity to become involved in the child's therapy as integral members of this team. Emergency admission for an acute illness or unintentional injury, in contrast, brings with it sudden stressors as the child and family are thrust into an unfamiliar environment, confronted with frightening or invasive procedures, and faced with an uncertain outcome.

Nursing care of children and families coping with specific chronic diseases or terminal illnesses such as cancer, cystic fibrosis, or muscular dystrophy, as well as care of the dying child, is discussed in other chapters in this book. The following discussion focuses on the concepts of nursing care for children with acute life-threatening illnesses or injuries.

SETTINGS ENCOUNTERED BY CHILDREN WITH A LIFE-THREATENING CONDITION

Children with a life-threatening condition may experience admission to a variety of healthcare settings. Included are emergency departments, pediatric intensive care units, and neonatal intensive care units. These departments are staffed with nurses who specialize in the care of children with life-threatening conditions.

Emergency Department

Children are taken to the emergency department (ED) for a variety of reasons. Many of these children are treated and sent home (Owens, Zodet, Berdahl, et al., 2008). (See Developing Cultural Competence: Discharge Instructions from the Emergency Department.) According to 2007 data, the leading reasons for visits to the ED for children under the age of 15 were fever, vomiting, and cough. Additionally, there were 121 visits per 10,000 children younger than 5 years of age with a primary diagnosis of asthma (Niska, Bhuiya, & Xu, 2010).

Accidental injury is the leading cause of morbidity and mortality in the pediatric population. Injuries account for a significant percentage of pediatric emergency department visits, with an estimated 9.2 million

---

Developing Cultural Competence
Discharge Instructions from the Emergency Department

Many children seen in the emergency department are sent home after evaluation and treatment. Detailed, clear instructions in the patient's or parents' primary language are essential for positive outcomes. Patel, Kennebeck, Caviness, et al. (2009) evaluated the effectiveness of a bilingual discharge facilitator to verbally reinforce written discharge instructions to English- and Spanish-speaking parents of children ages 3 months to 18 years seen in the emergency department with acute gastroenteritis. While discharge instructions are frequently given to parents hurriedly in a busy emergency department setting, the discharge facilitator spent an average time of 14 minutes with each family reviewing discharge instructions. Both English- and Spanish-speaking parents who were provided verbal reinforcement of discharge instruction by a discharge facilitator demonstrated a higher level of recall than those who received standard discharge instructions. The use of a bilingual discharge facilitator had a greater impact on recall in the Spanish-speaking group, supporting the importance of taking time to review discharge instructions verbally in the parents' primary language.

children visiting the ED annually for unintentional injury. Data from 2000–2006 indicate that in the United States, motor vehicle–related accidents were the leading cause of death in children ages 0 to 19. Falls were the leading cause of nonfatal injury in children ages 0 to 15 (Borse, Gilchrist, Dellinger, et al., 2008). Although most emergency department visits are not due to life-threatening circumstances, the nurse must be prepared to respond to those that are. The American Heart Association offers courses in pediatric advanced life support, in which nurses and other healthcare providers learn the emergency protocols for life-threatening events such as respiratory arrest and hypovolemic shock. The Emergency Nurses Association offers the Emergency Nurse Pediatric Course (ENPC) to provide information about pediatric emergency nursing. See Appendix F and the Skills Manual .

The role of the emergency department nurse includes triaging the child, initiating lifesaving measures (e.g., pediatric advanced life support), collaborating with the multidisciplinary emergency department team, and providing support to the family.

Children and their families may encounter a fast-paced environment in the emergency department, with the child receiving simultaneous care from multiple healthcare providers. The unfamiliar, hectic environment, compounded with the uncertainty of the child's life-threatening condition, can be a frightening experience and a significant source of stress for the family. Each emergency department develops its own set of unique requirements and protocols, which may limit the number of family members who can accompany the child. Family members who are asked to remain in the waiting room while the child receives treatment may experience additional stress and anxiety.

Clinical Tip

In addition to the stressors experienced due to life-threatening injury or illness in their child, parents may also suddenly be faced with the dilemma of arranging for the care of other children. For example, the siblings may be at school and need to be picked up by a certain time. Parents may need assistance to make these arrangements when they are in a state of crisis. They must decide if one of them will leave the hospital to pick up their other children and inform them of their sibling's illness or injury, or whether a family member or friend will do it for them. This may not be an easy decision for the parents and will depend in part on the condition of the hospitalized child. Assist family members in making a decision with which they are comfortable.

The nurse, in addition to other healthcare professionals, should keep the family informed of the care provided and the child's status. Many facilities provide a social worker in the emergency department to coordinate the flow of information and support the families of critically ill children. Other emergency departments have limited personnel, and a nurse may take a leadership role to ensure the family receives adequate support.

Pediatric Intensive Care Unit

The **pediatric intensive care unit (PICU)** is a highly specialized care unit for children with a life-threatening illness or injury. Children undergoing procedures such as thoracic, cardiovascular, airway, craniofacial, and abdominal surgeries, and organ transplants, are often admitted to the PICU postoperatively as well. While the length of stay and the severity of illnesses in children admitted to the PICU have not changed in the past several years, the mortality rate in the PICU has decreased considerably (Namachivayam, Shann, Shekerdemian, et al., 2010).

Not all hospitals are equipped with pediatric intensive care units; therefore, the child and family may experience a transfer from one facility to another that provides specialized care for critically ill children. The child admitted to the PICU experiences multiple sensory stimuli, ranging from constant sounds of monitor alarms and supportive equipment to bright lights, and interventions from multiple healthcare professionals.

The role of the nurse in the PICU includes maintaining life support measures such as ventilatory support and administration of vasoactive medications. The nurse explains the environment and equipment, which may include ventilators, dialysis machines, arterial lines, central venous pressure lines, intracranial pressure lines, and warming/cooling blankets. Families are often overwhelmed by the amount of equipment attached to the child, in addition to the altered appearance of the child requiring these supportive devices. Before the family visits the child for the first time, the nurse prepares the family members for what they will see and hear. It is especially important that the nurse explain any difference in appearance the child may have. For example, the nurse might say, "Alexa will not look like herself because her face is swollen and bruised. She has a tube in her mouth to help her breathe." See Partnering with Families: Terms Commonly Used in Pediatric Intensive Care Units.

Families of children in the intensive care unit may also experience hospital rules regarding visitation. Many children's hospitals support open visitation by parents and siblings and encourage parents to spend as much time as possible with their critically ill child. Other intensive care units may restrict such visitations, limiting the specific hours and length of visits. The number of people who can visit at a time may also be limited. These restrictions are often a source of frustration for families, especially when the child's outcome is uncertain. Nurses can support family-centered care by encouraging their hospitals and specialized units to reduce or remove restrictive visitation policies.

Clinical Tip

Intensive care settings generally have policies on how many people can visit at a time, but there are times when flexibility is essential. For example, a family of four, with one member being the ill or injured child, needs to be together at times. In addition, extended family members visiting from out of town may want to spend time not only with the hospitalized child, but with the parents of the child as well. Extended family members are generally very important to families, and their presence during times of crisis assists the family to cope and adjust to the situation.

Neonatal Intensive Care Unit

Newborns with life-threatening conditions are admitted to the **neonatal intensive care unit (NICU).** Common reasons for NICU admission include premature birth, congenital defects, respiratory

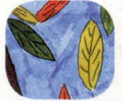

Partnering with Families

Terms Commonly Used in Pediatric Intensive Care Units

Families are often overwhelmed with the terminology used in the PICU. What is everyday language to the healthcare team may be unfamiliar to family members. Understanding the terminology may help to reduce the family's stress. The nurse can provide the family with a list of common terms used in the PICU, clarify their meaning, and encourage family members to ask questions if they do not understand. This list may include the following terms and explanations:

- **Arterial blood gases (ABGs):** A sample of blood from an artery that helps to identify the level of oxygenation and provides a guide for changes necessary in treatment. The blood sample may be obtained through an arterial line.
- **Arterial line:** A catheter inserted into an artery that allows for continuous monitoring of blood pressure and for blood sampling for arterial blood gases.
- **ET tube (endotracheal tube):** The plastic tube that is placed into the child's trachea or airway, either through the nose or through the mouth. The tube is usually connected to a ventilator (breathing machine) to help the child breathe.
- **Isolation:** A method used to prevent the transfer of infections to the child or visitors. Gowns, gloves, mask, and a special isolation room may be included in the isolation guidelines.

- **IV (intravenous) line:** A catheter inserted into a blood vessel. The catheter provides a method to administer fluids, nutrition, and medications. IVs may be inserted into the veins in the hand, arm, or foot, or into the neck, scalp (in infants), chest, or groin area.
- **Monitor:** A screen that shows the child's heart rhythm and rate, blood pressure, and oxygen level.
- **NG tube (nasogastric tube):** A tube that is inserted in the child's nose and into the stomach. The tube can be used to drain stomach fluids and to administer feedings and medications.
- **Oxygen saturation:** A measure of the amount of oxygen in the blood.
- **Pulse ox (pulse oximeter):** A probe that is secured to the child's finger, toe, hand, or foot. Note the red light on the probe. This measures the oxygen saturation in the child's blood.
- **Restraint:** Soft wraps that may be secured around the child's hands to keep them from pulling out tubes.
- **Ventilator:** A machine that is connected to an endotracheal tube (or tracheostomy) that assists the child to breathe.

distress, difficult delivery, and infections (March of Dimes, 2009). In 2008, 523,033 infants were born preterm (prior to 37 weeks' gestation) in the United States. This represents 12.3% of all live births (National Center for Health Statistics, 2011).

The role of the nurse in the NICU is similar to that of the nurse in the PICU, though there are distinct differences. The NICU nurse deals primarily with premature newborns and those with life-threatening congenital defects.

The family of the newborn in neonatal intensive care experiences a unique situation since the newborn is admitted to a critical care unit rather than being sent home with the parents as anticipated. Admission of an infant to the NICU is very stressful for parents. Separation from the infant is difficult, and the potential for impaired parent–newborn attachment exists. Family-centered care promotes active participation in the care of the infant and facilitates parent–newborn attachment. Family-centered care has been implemented in many neonatal intensive care units; however, not all NICUs have embraced this philosophy of care, and its implementation remains inconsistent in many areas (Gooding, Cooper, Blaine, et al., 2011; Wigert, Berg, & Hellström, 2010). Visitation policies may be in place that limit the amount of time parents can spend with their child. Parents may also experience grief over loss of the "perfect child."

CHILD'S EXPERIENCE OF A LIFE-THREATENING ILLNESS OR INJURY

Admission to the hospital, emergency department, or PICU is one of the most frightening experiences a child can have. The critically ill child may appear extremely anxious and fearful, or withdrawn, solemn, and preoccupied with his or her physical condition. The illness or injury often brings pain, decreased energy, and changes in the child's level of consciousness.

Young children admitted to the PICU may be unable to understand what is happening to them (Figure 17–1 ■). The PICU environment appears overwhelming, fast paced, and frightening, secondary to the numerous machines, noises, people, and procedures the child encounters. This type of environment places the child at risk for *sensory overload*, a feeling that results from too much

stimulation. The child's normal sleep patterns can be disrupted due to the lack of day–night patterns in many intensive care units. Being cared for by strangers contributes to the child's anxiety. The child's limited ability to move intensifies feelings of powerlessness and vulnerability. The child might experience a feeling of *sensory deprivation*, resulting from lack of interaction with familiar people and a familiar environment.

Children's developmental levels, past experiences, types of illness, coping mechanisms, and available emotional support influence their responses to stress. Nurses must consider how the child's developmental level and coping skills will influence his or her ability to deal with the emergency department or PICU experience. Successful coping can provide the child with the skills to handle difficult situations in the future.

An unanticipated admission places the child at emotional risk for several reasons, including the lack of preparation for the experience, the uncertainty and unpredictability of events that follow, the unfamiliarity of the environment, and the heightened anxiety of parents. An admission for an acute exacerbation of a disease such as cystic fibrosis or leukemia can provoke feelings of depression or hopelessness. See Chapter 15 for the stressors and responses of children to hospitalization by age group.

The child cared for in the PICU will experience the stressors of a child who is hospitalized. The PICU environment, however, is more intense, placing these children at greater risk for posttraumatic stress disorder (Colville, Kerry, & Pierce, 2008). Children in the PICU are generally sicker and experience numerous invasive procedures. In addition to the stressors associated with their own care, they may hear alarms and other noises associated with the care of other children, increasing the stress they already feel (Ward-Begnoche, 2007). See Box 17–1 for research on posttraumatic stress after the PICU experience.

Coping Mechanisms

Coping refers to the cognitive and behavioral responses that help a person manage specific internal and external demands that exceed personal resources, thus enabling the person to solve problems and to respond appropriately. The child may mirror the parents' behaviors

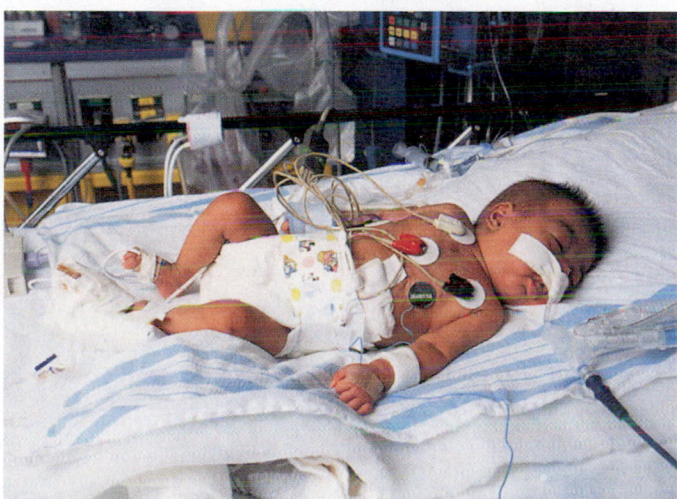

FIGURE 17–1 ■ Jooti feels pain, hears noises, has her sleep disrupted, and has limited mobility because of all the equipment attached to her. What care and comfort can you offer parents who see their child like this?

| BOX 17–1 | **Research: Posttraumatic Stress After the PICU Experience** |

Children and adolescents requiring hospitalization for a serious injury are at risk for posttraumatic stress disorder. In a study by Colville et al. (2008), 102 children between the ages of 7 and 17 years were interviewed about their experience in a pediatric intensive care unit 3 months after their discharge from the unit. Three purposes of the study were to determine if these children experienced delusional or factual memories of their experience, to examine the relationship between these types of memory and medical and demographic variables, and to determine if there was a relationship between the presence of factual or delusional memories and posttraumatic stress. The ICU memory tool and the Impact of Event Scale were utilized. The study found that 63% of the children had at least one factual memory, and 32% had delusional memories (including hallucinations) of the experience. Children who did not have any factual memories were more likely to have had a traumatic brain injury. Children receiving opiates and/or benzodiazepines for 2 or more days were 5 times more likely to have delusional memories, although 10 children who received these medications for less than 2 days reported having delusional memories. Having a factual memory was not significantly related to posttraumatic stress, while children who reported delusional memories had higher posttraumatic stress scores. Refer to Chapter 34 for a detailed discussion on posttraumatic stress disorder (PTSD).

and responses, which may help or hinder the child's response to stress. The child's temperament, previous coping experiences, and availability of support systems all combine to influence his or her ability to cope with the current experience. Coping behavior is influenced by maturation, cognitive development (increased attention span, problem-solving ability, and understanding of cause and effect), and increased impulse control.

The nature and severity of the illness and an emergency admission to the hospital stress a child's coping capabilities. Defense mechanisms displayed by children in these situations include **regression,** or return to an earlier behavior (a common reaction to stress), denial, **repression** (involuntary forgetting), postponement, and bargaining. See Chapter 15 for detailed discussion on coping mechanisms for hospitalized children.

Nursing Management

Nursing care of the child with a life-threatening illness or injury and his or her family includes assessing the child's physical and psychosocial needs, assessing the family's psychosocial needs, providing physical and psychosocial care for the child, and providing support for parental physical and emotional needs.

Nursing Assessment and Diagnosis

Nursing assessment involves, in addition to physiologic parameters, skilled observation of the child's psychosocial and emotional needs.

An understanding of normal psychosocial and cognitive development is necessary to plan developmentally appropriate interventions. Assessment should include the child's response to illness, the environment, coping strategies, and the need for information and support.

The accompanying Nursing Care Plan includes common nursing diagnoses for the child coping with a life-threatening illness or injury. The following nursing diagnoses may also be appropriate:

- Communication: Verbal, Impaired related to the effects of endotracheal intubation and mechanical ventilation
- Spiritual Distress related to the crisis of illness or suffering
- Sleep Pattern, Disturbed related to excessive stimulation, pain, and anxiety caused by the critical care unit environment
- Activity, Deficient Diversional related to forced inactivity

NANDA-I © 2012

Planning and Implementation

Nursing care focuses on promoting a sense of trust, providing education about the illness or injury, preparing the child for procedures, facilitating the use of play, and promoting a sense of control. Physiologic care for the child in the PICU may include the following: frequent physiologic assessment, pain and sedation management, nutritional support, medication administration, management of multiple IV lines and pumps, maintenance of ventilatory and hemodynamic monitoring equipment, and wound care.

Nursing Care Plan | The Child Coping with a Life-Threatening Illness or Injury

INTERVENTION	RATIONALE	EXPECTED OUTCOME
1. Nursing Diagnosis: Anxiety (Child) related to separation from parents, unfamiliar environment, strangers as caretakers, invasive procedures		
NIC Priority Intervention—_Anxiety Reduction:_ Minimizing apprehension, dread, foreboding, or uneasiness related to an unidentified source of anticipated danger		**NOC Suggested Outcome—**_Anxiety Control:_ Ability to eliminate or reduce feelings of apprehension and tension from an unidentified source
GOAL: _The child will exhibit or express an increased sense of security._		
■ Encourage parents to remain at the bedside (open visitation) and to participate in the child's care by touching, talking to, reading to, and singing to the child.	■ Presence of the parents is comforting to the child.	The child appears more relaxed and acknowledges the parents' presence. Behavioral manifestations of anxiety are absent. Restful periods of sleep are noted.
■ Talk with the child. Avoid discussions at bedside that the child should not overhear.	■ The child may overhear and remember, even if unconscious.	
■ Offer to arrange a visit from the chaplain or other spiritual support.	■ Spiritual support often provides comfort and sustenance in a time of crisis.	
■ Provide the child with developmentally appropriate explanations when possible. Encourage the child to ask questions and express concerns.	■ Information reduces anxiety and builds trust.	
■ Make the child's bedside more personal and familiar by encouraging parents to bring in security objects, family photos, and favorite toys from home.	■ Security objects decrease unfamiliarity of the hospital environment. The child derives comfort from the presence of personal items.	
■ Involve the child in play appropriate to developmental age (see Chapter 5 ⟨𝘦⟩).	■ Play provides familiarity, decreases fantasy, and provides motor activity.	
■ Provide care using a primary nursing care model.	■ Consistency in caregivers helps to build the child's trust. Caregivers learn the child's cues.	

Nursing Care Plan | The Child Coping with a Life-Threatening Illness or Injury, *continued*

INTERVENTION	RATIONALE	EXPECTED OUTCOME
2. Nursing Diagnosis: Powerlessness related to inability to communicate, and control relinquished to the healthcare team		
NIC Priority Intervention—*Self-Esteem Facilitation:* Encouraging a patient to assume more responsibility for own behavior		**NOC Suggested Outcome**—*Health Beliefs: Perceived Control:* Personal conviction that one can influence an outcome
GOAL: *The child or adolescent will have an increased sense of control over the situation.*		
■ Provide opportunities for choices when possible. Encourage participation in self-care.	■ Such opportunities provide a sense of control and autonomy through decision making.	The child or adolescent expresses satisfaction over the ability to control some elements of the situation.
■ Prepare the child or adolescent in advance (timing dependent on developmental level) for procedures. Describe the sensations that will be experienced. Allow some choice in timing or method of pain relief.	■ Providing information to the child or adolescent lets them know what to expect. Allowing choices gives them a sense of involvement and lets them know that their input is important.	The child or adolescent participates in self-care and decision making.
■ Provide routines for the child both within a 24-hour period and for scheduled care. When possible, incorporate rituals from home.	■ Self-control is maintained through rituals.	
■ Provide other means of communication to the child who is intubated (e.g., a word board or finger board).	■ Maintaining communication provides autonomy and independence for the child.	
■ Wrap IV lines well and use arm boards to help reduce the need for restraints and im-mobilizers. Provide appropriate explanations, and release at regular intervals if used.	■ Release from restraints or immobilizers helps di-minish the sense of powerlessness that accompanies their use.	
3. Nursing Diagnosis: Pain, Acute related to injuries, invasive procedures, or surgery		
NIC Priority Intervention—*Pain Management:* Alleviation of pain or a reduction in pain to a level of comfort that is acceptable to the patient		**NOC Suggested Outcome**—*Comfort Level:* Feelings of physical and psychologic ease
GOAL: *The child will experience reduced pain and improved comfort.*		
■ Assess the child's pain: location, intensity, what makes it better or worse.	■ Assessment provides baseline information from which a plan of care can be developed.	The child experiences a perceived or actual improvement in comfort level.
■ If appropriate, use a pain assessment scale (see Chapter 21).	■ Use of a scale provides continuity and consistency in monitoring the child's pain.	
■ Provide optimal pain relief with prescribed analgesics. Provide comfort measures—such as position changes and back rubs. Provide diversional activities as appropriate or possible. Incorporate the family in pain relief modality.	■ Physiologic and psychologic methods of pain control can be used in combination to maximally improve outcomes.	

NANDA-I © 2012

Provide Psychosocial Care for the Child

Children admitted to a PICU need support for the stressful experi-ence. Children often feel and hear even when unconscious, so touch and verbal interchanges are important. Nurses play a key role in pro-viding developmentally appropriate support to the child. Nursing interventions are directed at building a trusting relationship, mini-mizing the stressors experienced by the child, and promoting cop-ing skills. Ongoing reassessment of progress in meeting the child's needs is critical. The child life specialist can also assist the child to cope with the PICU environment and procedures through a variety of techniques. See the discussion on pages 406–407 in Chapter 15 🔗. See Complementary Therapy: Music.

Promote a Sense of Security

For children of all ages, feeling secure depends on a sense of physi-cal and psychologic safety. A sense of physical security is difficult to attain within the PICU because of the frequent procedures that are part of the child's treatment plan. Parental presence at the bedside is one of the best ways to decrease anxiety and promote a sense of secu-rity. Including parents as partners in the child's care provides comfort

Complementary Therapy   Music

Nonpharmacologic measures, such as music therapy, may be beneficial in de-creasing stress in children in the pediatric intensive care unit. A literature review by Austin (2010) examined the effects of music therapy in the intensive care environ-ment and found many beneficial effects including distraction, relaxation, promotion of sleep, and reduction of heart and respiratory rate. Music therapy should be used when possible as a method to decrease anxiety in this setting; however, research indicates that music that is familiar to the child should be used (Austin, 2010).

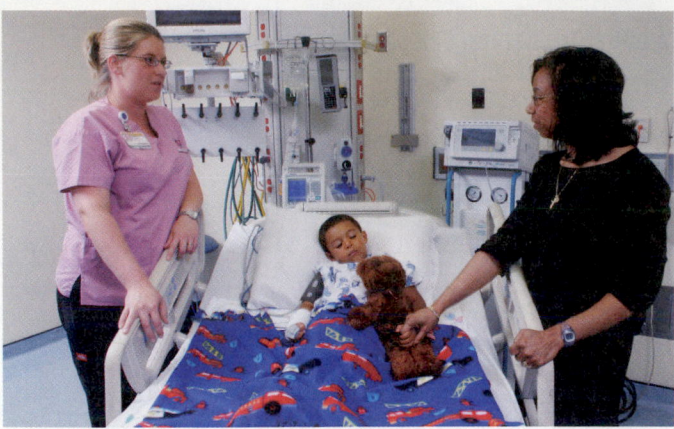

FIGURE 17–2 ■ By their very nature, PICUs are ominous and sterile. To lessen this effect, it helps to personalize the child's space. Being there with the child and parent, answering questions, or just talking can be a comfort to both.

and reassurance to the child. Consistency of staff is invaluable in developing familiarity and a trusting relationship with the child.

Personalizing the child's bedside can also promote comfort and a sense of security. Pictures from home, a favorite blanket or toy, music, or posters can make the environment friendlier and more familiar to the child (Figure 17–2 ■). Religious or spiritual symbols may also provide psychologic support.

Provide Education and Prepare the Child for Procedures

A child's ability to understand the cause of the illness and its treatment depends on cognitive abilities. Help younger children to understand that illness and hospitalization are not a punishment. Preparation for procedures is important at all ages, even for the child who is unconscious or sedated. Toddlers will benefit from being talked to, soothed, and touched during and after the procedure. Provide preschoolers, school-age children, and adolescents with an explanation of the sensations they can expect to experience (temperature, vibrations, sounds, smells, tastes, sight). See Chapter 15 ⊘ for further information about preparation and support of the child during procedures.

Facilitate the Use of Play

Play can be used to alleviate stress and to help children prepare for procedures. The nurse can also use play to assess the child's developmental level. Even within the PICU, therapeutic play provides motor activity and helps the child cope with stressors (see Chapter 15). Children who have limited mobility due to tubes and immobilizers can still feel a sense of accomplishment, for example, by completing a puzzle, even if the nurse points to each piece and the child responds through nods and gestures where it should be placed. Play can help children work through a painful situation, making it more tolerable. Play also provides the child with a sense of normality and confidence in caretakers.

Promote a Sense of Control

Children between toddlerhood and adolescence experience a loss of control during a life-threatening illness. This loss of control may be related to the body, emotions, normal routines, or privacy. Nursing interventions should promote a sense of control over these areas. Chapter 15 discusses nursing interventions to promote a sense of control in hospitalized children in general.

Children hospitalized in an intensive care unit experience a heightened sense of loss of control, secondary to the many machines, noises, and limits on mobility. These children often remove or threaten to remove technologic equipment or devices employed in their care such as an endotracheal tube, peripheral intravenous line or central line, nasogastric tube, or arterial line. The child's actions are often referred to as **treatment interference.** Physical immobilizers are sometimes used in children with altered consciousness to prevent the unintentional removal of technologic devices or equipment (da Silva & de Carvalho, 2010). Although immobilizers are sometimes necessary, they contribute to the child's sense of powerlessness. The Joint Commission requires that hospitals have policies and procedures for the use of restraints or immobilizers and a plan to release them regularly for short periods. Restrain children as little as possible, and explain the rationale for immobilizers, emphasizing that they are not a punishment (see Skills Manual ⫘). Nurses should also position these devices in a way that maintains comfort as much as possible.

Parents and nurses can partner to prevent treatment interference. Intervention strategies by parents include supervision, simple instructions, a calm approach, setting limits, a sense of security, and repositioning. Seek input from the family about the child's preferences and family values regarding music, television, and DVDs that might distract the child (see Chapter 15). Enhance the child's coping skills by teaching the child and family a combination of relaxation, visual imagery, or distraction techniques, and comforting self-talk phrases, such as "This will be over soon," "If I stay calm, it will be all right," and "It will be over faster and then I can do something fun." Help parents become the child's coping coaches.

Evaluation

Expected outcomes of nursing care include:

- A trusting relationship is developed with the child and family.
- The child is given preparation and support for procedures.
- The child's coping is promoted by family presence and therapeutic play.

PARENTS' EXPERIENCE OF A CHILD'S LIFE-THREATENING ILLNESS OR INJURY

The uncertainty and unpredictability of a child's life-threatening illness challenges a family's coping and stability. The sudden loss of the parenting role with the emergency admission of their child causes stress. Families display many different responses and coping mechanisms such as crying, emotional outbursts, fear, and demanding information. Parents are at risk for development of PTSD, depression, and anxiety when the child is hospitalized in an intensive care unit (Colville, Cream, & Kerry, 2010). Parents may find it difficult to support the child if their own needs are not met. They can transmit their anxiety to the child, who then becomes even more anxious. Family-centered care must be provided; if the needs of the family are met, it will help ensure that the needs of the child with a life-threatening condition are met. Clear, concise communication is imperative.

The Family in Crisis

The critical care environment and the implications of a life-threatening illness or injury of a child are far removed from the everyday experiences of most families. The unfamiliarity of the environment and the

Evidence-Based Practice | Parental Anxiety and Stress When the Child Is in the PICU

PROBLEM

Nurses expect parents to experience stress when their child has a life-threatening condition, but what causes the most anxiety and stress for parents of children in the pediatric intensive care unit (PICU)? Does continued presence at the bedside reduce this anxiety and stress?

EVIDENCE

A prospective cohort study by Needle, O'Riordan, and Smith (2009) examined factors that contributed to anxiety in 35 parents or legal guardians of children in the PICU. The effect of anxiety on the parents' ability to comprehend medical information within 24 hours after the child's admission to the PICU was also evaluated. In this study, 34 parents completed the State Trait Anxiety Inventory to measure anxiety, and 28 completed an open-ended questionnaire to assess comprehension of medical information. The ability of the physician to recognize parental anxiety was also evaluated using a multiple-choice questionnaire. Results of the study showed that 60% of the parents demonstrated state anxiety scores higher than a sample of patients with diagnosed anxiety disorder. Having a child on mechanical ventilation was the only significant predictable factor associated with high state anxiety scores. The study also showed that parents with high anxiety do comprehend medical information, with 93% demonstrating fair to excellent retention within 24 hours of their child's admission to the PICU. Physicians did not recognize high anxiety in about one third of parents, but were more likely to do so if the child was mechanically ventilated. The study also found that parents of chronically ill children demonstrated high state anxiety scores.

Experiences of parents admitted to the PICU were evaluated in a qualitative study by Latour, van Goudoever, Schuurman, et al. (2011). In this study, 39 mothers and 25 fathers were interviewed, and six major themes emerged: "attitude of the professionals; coordination of care; emotional intensity; information management; environmental factors; parent participation" (p. 319). The authors noted an association among the themes of professionals' attitude, information management, and emotional intensity. This association suggests that failure to receive adequate information and empathy from staff may result in higher stress in parents.

A comparative descriptive study by Smith, Hefley, and Anand (2007) examined stressors for 86 parents of children in a PICU without bed space for parents, and stressors for 92 parents of children in a new PICU that provided a bed so that one parent could stay at the bedside through the night. Parents in the new unit were also allowed to be present during rounds and report, whereas those in the old unit were required to leave during these times. Parents who were allowed continual presence at the bedside reported lower total stress scores than those who were not allowed to be present at all times. They also reported lower stress scores related to the child's appearance, alteration in their parental role, not being able to see their child, and the overall PICU experience. The most stressful experience for parents in the new unit was witnessing procedures performed on their child.

IMPLICATIONS

Parents with children in the PICU have more stressors than parents of children on a general pediatric unit and are likely to have high anxiety levels. Parents who are not allowed to spend the night in the PICU or to stay in the unit during rounds and report have more stressors than those who are allowed continual presence. After the child is admitted, it is important to provide adequate information regarding the child's care. Identifying ways that the parents can participate in the child's care is important so that a sense of the parental role is maintained. Staff should convey a sense of empathy toward parents and recognize that parents with high levels of anxiety may need additional support.

CRITICAL THINKING APPLICATION

Consider what your response would be if it were your child in the PICU. Would your stressors be different from those reported by these parents because of your nursing education? How would you want the nurse caring for your child to support you? Would you want to stay with your child all the time if it was allowed? After considering your personal responses, does it help you identify nursing care strategies for working with parents of a child with a life-threatening condition?

uncertainty and seriousness of the illness or injury create a **family crisis,** which occurs when the family encounters a problem that seems insurmountable and usual coping skills are not effective. See Evidence-Based Practice: Parental Anxiety and Stress When the Child Is in the PICU.

Since families have little time to prepare for the experience, a sudden admission threatens family integrity by causing enormous stress and separation from loved ones. Interruption of the unique parent–child relationship can be more stressful to parents than the physical PICU environment. Siblings are also affected; see discussion on page 453. In addition, extended family members such as grandparents must be considered. Stresses are further intensified in the case of divorce, separation, and stepparenting. Financial problems, long distance from home to hospital, or another ill or injured family member can compound the crisis. See Chapter 2 🔗 for a discussion on family assessment and family resiliency. In addition, the outcome of the admission may not be positive, and nurses need to be equipped to support families in this situation.

Parental Reactions to Life-Threatening Illness or Injury

When faced with a threat to their child's life, parents typically progress through stages that may include shock and disbelief, anger and guilt, deprivation and loss, anticipatory waiting, and readjustment or mourning. Some families progress through these stages in a linear fashion, while others go back and forth between stages, especially if the child's condition improves and then worsens.

Shock and Disbelief

The universal reaction to a child's life-threatening condition is shock and disbelief. As the familiar is disrupted, parents experience a loss of control and an inability to regain their bearings. The hospital environment, emergency department, or PICU may seem unreal. The emotions parents experience initially are intensified by the physical appearance of their child (particularly after a major injury); the presence of monitors, tubing, and equipment; and the actual injury or illness (Figure 17–3 ■). As Alexa's mother from the opening scenario stated, "I felt distanced, in a daze, in and out of it that first day after the accident."

Shock and disbelief begin in the first few moments after hearing the "news" and can last for days. The shock helps postpone the full impact of the crisis. During this period, parents grope for answers and explanations about the illness or injury. Information must be repeated many times to parents, since in this stage they are often unable to assimilate information easily.

Clinical Tip

When presenting bad news to family members, the nurse and other members of the healthcare team should acknowledge the family's emotions. Be prepared for tears and have tissue nearby (Levetown & Committee on Bioethics, 2008).

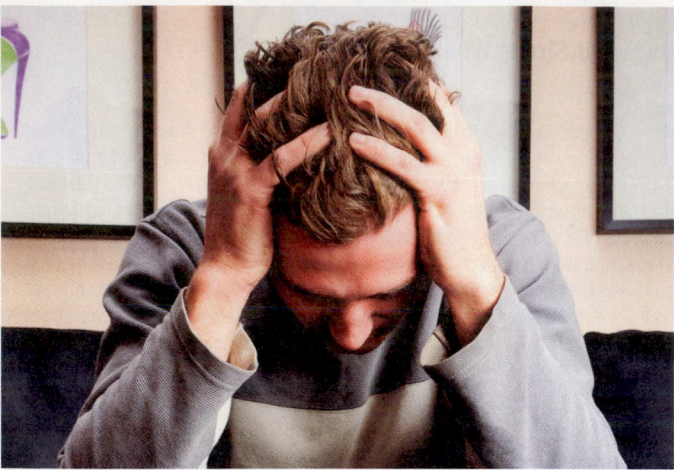

FIGURE 17–3 ■ This father is in a state of shock following his child's injury. He is unable to pay attention to information being provided, so repeat important information until it is understood.

Source: *Shutterstock*

Anger and Guilt

Anger and guilt surface as parents become more aware of their child's illness or injury. Their anger may be directed toward themselves or each other because they could not protect their child. Other individuals may be blamed, such as the driver of a motor vehicle involved in a crash injuring the child. Parents may also be angry with their child. This anger may be a result of injuries the child sustained when breaking known rules such as drinking and driving, playing with matches, or riding a bicycle without a helmet. Lastly, the anger may not be directed at anyone specifically. Injuries caused by natural disasters such as an earthquake, flood, or hurricane provoke as much anger as those that result from the actions of people, and may pose a challenge to the parents' spiritual beliefs.

Parents typically react to their child's illness or injury with some degree of guilt. This reaction may be magnified in the intensive care environment. The fact that the guilt usually has no basis in real events does not lessen the feeling. A question parents frequently ask at this stage is, "Why not me instead of my child?" Parents' feelings of guilt may be related to the following:

1. They may feel responsible for causing the illness or injury. Statements such as, "If only I hadn't sent him to the store on his bike, this wouldn't have happened," or, from the father of a 2-year-old who nearly drowned, "Maybe if I hadn't been working, he would have been in my care and this wouldn't have happened," reflect feelings of guilt for causing or failing to prevent the injury.

2. They may feel guilty about not noticing the onset of an illness or disregarding earlier symptoms of an illness. For example, the mother of a 1-year-old with meningitis repeatedly said, "I shouldn't have waited so long to take her to the doctor!"

Deprivation and Loss

As the shock associated with the child's life-threatening condition slowly recedes, new stressors emerge. Within minutes or hours, parents are deprived of the familiar role of being a parent of a healthy child and find themselves in the unexpected and unfamiliar role of being a parent of a critically ill child.

The difficulty and ambivalence parents feel in releasing a part of their responsibility as the child's primary caretakers to strangers can threaten their self-esteem and self-control. If parents cannot participate in the child's care, they may feel helpless or worthless.

Anticipatory Waiting

Once the child's condition is stabilized and survival seems likely, parents often move into a period of anticipatory waiting. This stage is characterized as "life suspended in time." Parents spend a great deal of time waiting: for test results, for explanations, for their child to become conscious, or for surgery to be over. Parents may fear leaving the area because they may miss an important procedure, physician visit, or decisions or changes in treatment. Lack of mobility decreases the parents' use of typical coping mechanisms, so anxiety and the sense of powerlessness may increase. If the parents have a cell phone, write down that number and assure them that they will be called for any change in the child's condition. This allows parents to feel like they can leave at least for a few minutes. If the parents do not have a cell phone, provide a pager if available.

Parents may have a preoccupation with medical details. During this period, they may ask questions about the long-term effects of the illness or injury on the child, about the potential for brain damage, or about the need for additional surgeries. Parents may place demands on staff and become frustrated when the child's progress is slow.

Readjustment or Mourning

The last stage that parents experience is readjustment or mourning. Readjustment is experienced as the child recovers, improves steadily, and prepares for transfer and discharge. In contrast, parents of the child who dies reenter the cycle of emotions characteristic of grief (see Chapter 18 🔗 for further discussion of end-of-life issues). Parents also mourn when the child remains seriously ill or unresponsive, when the outcome remains uncertain for an extended period, or when long-term care is required.

Table 17–1 lists the most important needs of parents when a child is hospitalized with a life-threatening illness or injury.

Nursing Management

Nursing care of the family includes assessing the family's psychosocial needs and providing support for parental physical and emotional needs.

Nursing Assessment and Diagnosis

Nurses who work with families of children who are critically ill have a unique opportunity to help them adapt and to promote family functioning. Begin by assessing the family's reaction to the illness, their coping skills, stressors, and needs (see Chapter 2 🔗). This initial assessment provides baseline information to develop a care plan and strategies that meet the psychosocial and physiologic needs of the family. Several nursing diagnoses may apply to parents who are dealing with their child's life-threatening illness or injury. Examples include:

- Family Processes, Interrupted related to the impact of a critically ill child on the family system
- Spiritual Distress related to the child's life-threatening illness or injury, suffering, or death
- Fatigue related to extreme stress, sleep deprivation, and crisis
- Hopelessness (parents) related to the child's deteriorating physical condition
- Coping: Family, Compromised related to the severity of the illness or injury in the child

NANDA-I © 2012

TABLE 17–1   Nursing Interventions to Meet Parental Needs When the Child Is Hospitalized with a Life-Threatening Illness or Injury

PARENTAL NEEDS	NURSING INTERVENTIONS
Information	■ Provide information and frequent updates about the child's condition. Repeat the information and provide other materials frequently as parents forget or cannot concentrate on details with all of their stress. ■ Explain the child's condition, equipment being used, and procedures of care. ■ Facilitate a discussion with the physician at least daily. ■ Provide general information about unit policies, team members, and phone numbers.
Proximity to their child	■ Provide permission for the parents to remain at the bedside. ■ Encourage parents to touch and speak with the child, and demonstrate ways if parents are hesitant. ■ Work within the unit to provide open, flexible visiting hours.
Reestablishment of their parental role and control	■ Implement family-centered care so parents feel recognized as important to their child's recovery and as the decision maker for the child's treatment options.
Participation in their child's care	■ Encourage parents to participate in care (e.g., bathing and hair care, diaper changes, feeding, range of motion exercises, massages). ■ Encourage parents to help with diversional activity (e.g., reading, singing, telling stories). ■ Encourage parents to explain equipment and procedures to the child to reduce the child's fears.
Confidence in the treatment plan and caregivers	■ Try to maintain continuity in staffing and healthcare contacts. ■ Demonstrate caring for the child. ■ Provide assurance that the child is receiving appropriate treatment and pain management.
Psychologic support	■ Acknowledge that the situation is difficult. ■ Help parents to focus on the positive or unchanged aspects of the child's appearance. ■ Encourage parents to get rest and nutrition to help them maintain physical resources necessary for coping. ■ Provide space and privacy as needed. ■ Give hope if realistic—an essential component of coping. ■ Offer the choice of other family members to be present. ■ Discuss the possible responses of siblings and the long-term emotional responses of the patient.

Planning and Implementation

Nursing care focuses on providing family-centered care to help meet the needs of families, minimize stress, and enhance family coping. See Chapter 2 ✪, Table 2–1. The challenge to nurses is to blend and balance technology with caring. See page 437 in Chapter 16 for a description of compassion fatigue and Chapter 18 ✪ for a discussion on caring for the dying child.

Provide Information and Build Trust

Orienting parents to the hospital, as well as to the unit routines, helps them to adapt to their surroundings. Parents will gain a sense of control and independence if they know where to get supplies and how to find the lounge, cafeteria, and restrooms.

Provide frequent and accurate information. Deliver information on the child's illness, condition, and plan of care in a manner and language readily understandable to parents. Upon admission, provide parents with an idea of what to expect in the days ahead and be prepared for special procedures or major changes in therapy. Parents also need to be prepared before they see their child for the first time. Explain that tubes and monitors are present and how the child will look and react.

Honesty in discussions with parents is extremely important. If parents feel misled or that information is being withheld, a trusting relationship will be impossible. Informed parents, however, will feel that they are active participants in decision making and care planning for their child. Trust is facilitated when parents believe that the staff truly cares about their child and sees the child as an individual. Trust is especially important when difficult decisions must be made, such as withdrawal of life support. Parents need a sense of hope regarding their child's illness to help them cope. Focus on the positive aspects of the child's condition.

Clinical Judgment

Many different types of equipment are used in the pediatric intensive care setting. Parents may have high levels of anxiety related to the presence of equipment and alarms that may sound. Recall the opening scenario. What can the nurse do to relieve anxiety in Alexa's mother related to equipment and alarms in this setting?

Clinical Tip

Explain to the child and parents in easy-to-understand terms the purpose of equipment being used. Answer alarms quickly. Follow with an explanation of why alarms sound, including the fact that many times monitor alarms will sound when the child moves, if the monitor becomes disconnected, or if the monitor patches are loose.

Facilitate Positive Staff–Parent Relationships and Communication

Given the intensity of the parents' experience when their child is critically ill, it is easy to see that problems can arise between staff and parents. Each healthcare team member must be aware of the child's current status so that parents receive the same information from all staff. A consistent message can instill confidence. Provide explanations geared to the parents' level of understanding, using language the parents can understand. Realize that in stressful times, parents may

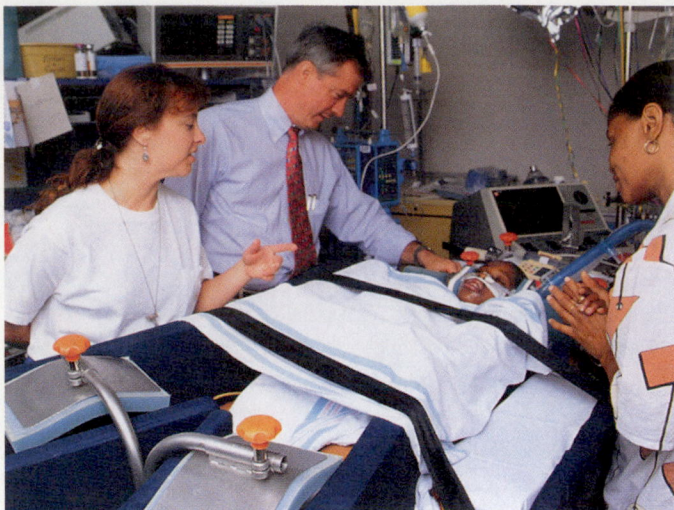

FIGURE 17–4 ■ In times of crisis, everyone likes to know that someone is in charge and who that person is. The parents should meet and talk with the staff physician in charge and the nurses as often as possible. Parents need to know that someone is responsible, even if different people are providing care.

not hear everything that is said. Repetition, written information, and referral to computer sources may be helpful.

Introduce the parents to the nurse and physician with overall responsibility for the child's care. This is especially important in teaching hospitals that have rotating interns and residents. The attending physician with the overall responsibility should meet with parents as often as necessary to talk about changes in the child's condition or treatment plan and to allow time for parents to ask questions (Figure 17–4 ■). Encourage parents to keep a daily log or notebook to record information on the child's care, progress, and needs as well as questions they want to ask the healthcare team. Family care conferences can be helpful when a large number of team members provide care. See Box 17–2.

BOX 17–2   Research: Parental Presence in the NICU

A descriptive study of 67 parents of 42 children in a neonatal intensive care unit that allowed parents to stay as much as they desired examined the time that parents spent in the NICU. Accommodations provided for parents varied and included the maternity ward, a hotel for families, parent rooms at the NICU, and the parents' own home. Parents who stayed in a parent room spent more time at the child's bedside (Wigert et al., 2010).

Specific factors that facilitated parental presence and those that obstructed their presence were identified. Reasons identified by parents for being present in the NICU were the desire to take parental responsibility, the child's condition, wanting to be in control, and wanting to be involved in the child's care. Some of the fathers also identified that they were in the NICU because the mother could not be present due to her postpartum condition. Factors that facilitated family presence included being treated well by the staff, a family-friendly environment, being able to come and go freely, high-quality care, getting information on a regular basis, and being invited by the staff to participate in the care of the child. Factors obstructing family presence included being treated poorly by the staff, ill health of the child's parents, a non-family-friendly environment, care of the home and care of other children at home, lack of information, distance, and a difficult socioeconomic situation (Wigert et al., 2010).

Clinical Tip

Arrange for daily visits by an interpreter if the family does not speak or understand English. Have information about the child's condition and plan of care summarized so the interpreter can communicate this information to the family during the visit. The interpreter should be called to make additional visits to interpret information if the child's condition or plan of care changes.

Promote Parental Involvement

An important role of nurses is to encourage and support parents in their parenting role. The parents' place when possible is at the bedside—their very presence can comfort the child, minimize fears, and reduce the child's experiences with pain during invasive procedures. Being at the child's bedside in the PICU has also been shown to decrease parental stress (Frazier, Frazier, & Warren, 2010). Parents provide continuity and may notice subtle changes that a newly assigned nurse may miss. Throughout the child's hospitalization, parents will continue to need reassurance and encouragement.

Participation in the care of their child is an integral aspect of family-centered care and enhances the family's ability to cope with the child's illness or injury. Open communication with families about their child's treatments and the plan of care facilitates parental involvement in the care of the child (Frazier et al., 2010). See Partnering with Families: Involving Family Members in NICU/PICU Settings. Parents who do not remain at the bedside with their child may feel that they are not important members of the team. When parents are unable to remain at the bedside, it is essential that they be allowed to call the unit at any time to check on their child. See Box 17–3.

Family Presence During Resuscitation or Invasive Procedures

Many hospitals are implementing policies that permit families to be present during resuscitation and invasive procedures. (See Partnering with Families: Presence During Resuscitation.) Healthcare professionals have expressed concern that parents who are allowed to witness resuscitation efforts might lose control and interfere with resuscitation efforts. Another concern is that medical staff, especially those in training, might feel uncomfortable, and that there is an increased risk for litigation (Meeks, 2009). However, reports related to family presence during resuscitation have failed to demonstrate any increase in litigation and have indicated family satisfaction with being allowed at the bedside. In addition, studies have failed to show that family presence interrupts care or interferes with the healthcare

BOX 17–3   Research: Parents' Perceptions of Their Role in the Pediatric Intensive Care Unit

A qualitative interpretive study explored parents' perception of their role in the pediatric intensive care unit. Parents of seven children were interviewed to determine their individual experiences in the PICU. Emotions during the interview process ranged from guilt, fear, and helplessness to relief, hope, and cautious optimism. Ames, Rennick, and Baillargeon (2011) noted a theme among parents of "being present and participating in the child's care" (p. 146), including active caring, providing reassurance and explanations to their child, and just being there to comfort their child. A second theme of "forming a partnership of trust with the PICU healthcare team" (p. 146) included being able to share their expertise as a parent, building a trusting relationship with the team, and being able to take care of themselves. The final theme of "being informed of the child's progress and treatment plan as the person who "knows' the child best" (p. 146) included knowing about their child's status, understanding the care that was being provided to their child, and being aware of what to expect next.

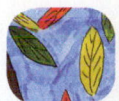

Partnering with Families

Involving Family Members in NICU/PICU Settings

Family participation in the care of the child in the pediatric or neonatal intensive care unit can be extremely beneficial to both the child and family. The child benefits from parental presence and continuity of care, while parents benefit from having some sense of control over their child's situation. Partner with parents of children in the NICU/PICU to become involved in their child's care by incorporating the following strategies:

- Allow unrestricted visitation in the PICU and NICU.
- Provide frequent updates to parents either by phone or in person.
- Provide information that is easy to understand.
- Limit the number of different people providing care to the child as much as possible.

- Allow parents to have an active role in decision making regarding the care of their child.
- Listen to parents' suggestions related to care of the child, such as a favorite position for sleeping.
- Encourage parents to touch, soothe, and hold their infant or child.
- Allow and encourage parents to participate in the physical care of the child as much as possible.
- Invite parents to participate in rounds on their child.
- Provide meal vouchers and a place to sleep for parents.

Source: *Data from Cameron, M. A., Schleien, C. L., & Morris, M. C. (2009). Parental presence on pediatric intensive care unit rounds.* Journal of Pediatrics, 155, *522–528; Frazier, A., Frazier, H., & Warren, N. A. (2010). A discussion of family-centered care within the pediatric intensive care unit.* Critical Care Nursing Quarterly, 33*(1), 82–86; Gooding, J. S., Cooper, L. G., Blaine, A. I., Franck, L. S., Howse, J. L., & Berns, S. D. (2011). Family support and family-centered care in the neonatal intensive care unit: Origins, advances, impact.* Seminars in Perinatology, 35, *20–28; Nyqvist, K. H., & Engvall, G. (2009). Parents as their infant's primary caregivers in a neonatal intensive care unit.* Journal of Pediatric Nursing, 24*(2), 153–163; March of Dimes. (2009). Which babies need care in the NICU? Retrieved from http://www.marchofdimes.com/baby/inthenicu_whichbabies.html; McClement, S. E., Fallis, W. M., & Pereira, A. (2009). Family presence during resuscitation: Canadian critical care nurses' perspectives.* Journal of Nursing Scholarship, 41*(3), 233–240.*

providers' ability to intervene in the care of the child (Emergency Nurses Association [ENA], 2010). Advantages of family presence include the following:

- Facilitates grieving and a sense of closure
- Reassures family that everything possible was done for their child
- Keeps the family together
- Provides an opportunity for education and discussion
- Gives parents a sense of control
- Improves communication with family members
- Improves satisfaction with care

Bowden & Greenberg, 2009; ENA, 2010; Levetown & Committee on Bioethics, 2008; March of Dimes, 2009; McClement, Fallis, & Pereira, 2009

It is essential that a trained support person be with parents who choose to be present during the resuscitation of their child (Bowden & Greenberg, 2009). See Box 17–4.

Clinical Tip

If parents choose not to witness the resuscitation efforts, regular updates (5- to 10-minute intervals) should be provided to the parents as they wait in a private area. The hospital chaplain or other family support team member should be notified so that support can be provided to parents while they wait.

Provide for Parental Physical and Emotional Needs

The experience of having a child with a life-threatening illness or injury drains parents' physical and emotional reserves. Parents often need encouragement to take care of themselves and to periodically take a break. A statement such as, "It is important for you to eat and rest because Alexa is really going to need you when she wakes up," helps parents to realize that becoming exhausted benefits neither them nor the child. Provision of a pager or cell phone may help reduce the parents' anxiety. Record the parents' cell phone numbers on the medical record and at the bedside.

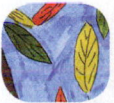

Partnering with Families

Presence During Resuscitation

The Emergency Nurses Association (ENA, 2010) supports the option of family presence during invasive procedures and resuscitation. Parents and other family members (e.g., grandparents) may wish to be present during invasive procedures (such as lumbar puncture) or resuscitation of the child. The nurse partners with the family to determine their needs at the time. To better facilitate the needs of the family, the following is determined:

- Who desires to be present during resuscitation or invasive procedures?
- What role will they play during the procedure (e.g., snuggle child for comfort)?

Healthcare agencies should have established protocols for family presence during invasive procedures or resuscitation (ENA, 2010). The nurse providing family-centered care recognizes that each situation is individualized according to the child's and family's needs. The nurse ensures that a support person from the multidisciplinary team (e.g., another nurse, social worker) is available to stay with the family members during resuscitation (Bowden & Greenberg, 2009).

| BOX 17–4 | **Steps to Follow When Families Are Present During Resuscitation** |

- Prior to entering the room, the parents are informed about what they will see.
- The parents are told that if they feel uncomfortable or if the team is unable to provide necessary care due to their presence, they will be escorted out.
- Once in the room, parents are informed about what is being done for the child and the role of each person present.
- The parents are positioned so they can see the child's face and hold his or her hand. Encourage the parents to tell the child how much he or she is loved.

Source: *Adapted from Levetown, M., & Committee on Bioethics. (2008). Communicating with children and families: From everyday interactions to skill in conveying distressing information. Pediatrics, 121(5), e1441–1460.*

Clinical Tip

Encourage parents to take time for themselves to be alone, alternating times to be away for a short break. Suggest places they can go such as a lounge, meditation room, chapel, or courtyard. There are times when both parents may need to get away together. If parents are hesitant to leave the child alone, ask if another family member or friend might be able to stay with the child for short periods. Hospitals generally have volunteers who can sit with children for a while to allow parents to feel comfortable leaving the child.

Many communities have a residence for families of hospitalized children. This is often an inexpensive but warm and supportive environment for families. The Ronald McDonald Children's Charities supports many of these residences (Figure 17–5 ■). The Ronald McDonald Family Room may be found in some hospitals and is provided as a comfortable setting where families of hospitalized children can get away from the high-tech hospital atmosphere while remaining close to the child. Computer resources in one of these locations or in a family resource center may make it possible for parents to stay in contact with concerned family and friends. When financial burdens are a consideration, family and social service referrals may be needed.

Parents are often at different levels of coping during a crisis. The severity of the child's illness or injury may foster cohesion between the couple and build a stronger relationship. Unfortunately, the

Weblink | Resources for Families

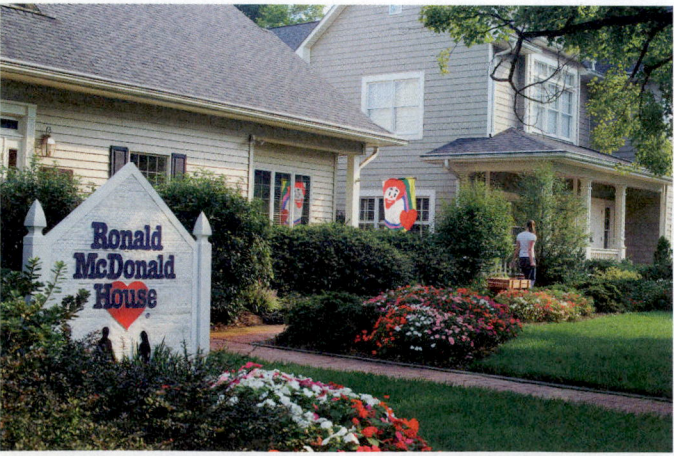

FIGURE 17–5 ■ A Ronald McDonald House provides a place where families of hospitalized children can go to take a break.

Source: *Wake Forest Baptist Health (WFBH) Photography.*

Complementary Therapy **Prayer**

Parents often pray for their child who is ill or injured. Friends and relatives frequently offer support through prayer as well. In the United States, prayer has been reported as the most frequently used form of complementary therapy. Studies show that 45% of Americans pray for health, 43% pray for their own health, and 25% ask other people to pray for them (Nance, Griffin, McNulty, et al., 2010). A study that explored complementary therapy practices of 62 adults, ages 21 to 30, included questions related to four types of prayer: contemplative-meditative (being in God's presence), ritualistic (reciting prayer), petitionary (asking God for something specific), and colloquial (speaking in one's own words to God for guidance). Colloquial prayer was used most often, followed by contemplative-meditative prayer (Nance et al., 2010).

---

reverse may also be true—differences in styles or levels of coping may foster a sense of isolation, placing a strain on the couple's relationship. Nurses should be alert to family dynamics and risk factors, and refer the family for counseling or therapy, if indicated.

Maintain or Strengthen Family Support Systems

Support systems are the extended network of family, friends, and religious and community contacts that provide nurturance, emotional support, and direct assistance to parents, thus enabling them to cope with overwhelming problems and crises. Most parents indicate that having family or friends nearby is crucial as a support system. See Complementary Therapy: Prayer.

Extended family, especially grandparents, and friends frequently offer the family assistance, but parents may need to be reassured that it is all right to ask for help as well. Some parents may be uncomfortable asking for help, instead attempting to handle multiple responsibilities themselves, often to the point of exhaustion. Some parents are so overwhelmed that they are unable to respond to offers of help because it requires too great a mental effort on their part. The nurse should assist the parents in responding to these offers for assistance.

Nurses may need to intervene on parents' behalf when they have inadequate support. People who come unannounced to visit, stay too long, or visit too often may frustrate parents. They may find it difficult to tell well-meaning but insensitive friends and family that they cannot deal with visitors right now. In these situations, it may be helpful for the nurse to offer to serve as a gatekeeper. Partnering with the family to establish suggested "visiting times" for friends and extended family members may help to alleviate some of the parents' frustration and fatigue. An extended family member may be given the responsibility of relaying information to others. See Partnering with Families: Lessening the Burden.

Families of children with a life-threatening illness or injury often have emotional needs beyond the support capabilities of the nurse caring for the child. Referrals to family and professionally led support services or pastoral care may be beneficial in these instances.

Refer to Chapter 18 🕭 for a discussion of nursing care of the family experiencing the death of a child.

If the child recovers and is transferred from an intensive care unit to an intermediate or general acute care setting, parents need to be given specific information related to changes in routines and staffing that will occur. Although transfer from an intensive care setting may be a relief to parents as it is generally a sign that their child is improving, a certain amount of stress, anxiety, and insecurity accompanies

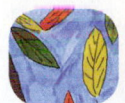

Partnering with Families

Lessening the Burden

Families of critically ill children are often overwhelmed and burdened with well-meaning inquiries from friends, coworkers, and extended family members. Parents are often required to repeat the same information numerous times to those inquiring about the child's condition, and this can be exhausting for the parents. Partner with the family to identify some effective methods of communicating the child's status while reducing the burden on the family. Suggestions can include the following:

- Designate a family member or another person to be responsible for relaying information to others.

- Identify a specific time period for calls and visits to allow for rest (e.g., between 10 a.m. and 12 noon and 6 p.m. and 8 p.m.).
- For prolonged hospitalizations, suggest the family create a website to post updates about the child's condition and treatments. The site can also be used to allow friends and family to provide responses and words of encouragement.
- Develop an email list and send updated messages periodically.

---

this move. These negative feelings are generally related to poor communication and lack of preparation for the transition (Latour et al., 2011). Nursing staff on both the transferring and the receiving unit should take time to inform parents of changes that will occur.

Evaluation

Expected outcomes of nursing care include the following:

- The nurse establishes a trusting relationship and effective communication with the family.
- Parents participate in their child's care as much as desired.
- Parents and extended family members receive emotional support and nurturance needed to sustain them through the child's illness.
- The parents' coping is promoted through education and preparation for procedures.

THE SIBLINGS' EXPERIENCE

As the parents' focus shifts to the critically ill child, they may need support in dealing with the healthy siblings.

Nursing Management

Siblings also need care and may feel left out when everyone's attention is focused on the child who is ill. Siblings of critically ill children may demonstrate behaviors ranging from jealousy or envy to resentment, guilt, hostility, anger, insecurity, regression, and fear. Several nursing diagnoses may apply to siblings of hospitalized children with a life-threatening illness or injury:

- Anxiety (Sibling) related to the unfamiliar environment
- Coping, Ineffective related to sudden change in routines
- Knowledge, Deficient related to the child's illness, injury, and procedures

NANDA-I © 2012

Recognize that siblings may fear becoming ill themselves or may believe that they played a role in the child's illness. Siblings often have nightmares about the illness or injury their brother or sister has sustained and about the ill child dying. Inform siblings about their brother or sister's condition using language and concepts appropriate to their ages and developmental levels. As appropriate, siblings

should be allowed to visit. Visitation provides a sense of comfort for the entire family (Keefe, 2008). Such a visit should be encouraged if the child could potentially die, to allow the sibling to say good-bye. Because children's fantasies are often worse than reality, unfounded fears may be relieved by a visit. These visits often also help to lift the spirits of the ill child.

Preparation for the visit is important (Keefe, 2008). Before the visit, talk with the siblings about what to expect, and describe how their brother or sister will look. If the ill child acts, moves, talks, or looks different than usual, provide an explanation beforehand. Describe the hospital environment, including equipment, sounds, and smells. Using a doll, drawing pictures, or showing an actual picture of the child can help prepare the siblings. (See Chapter 15, Partnering with Families: Strategies for Working with the Sibling of a Hospitalized Child.)

During the visit, the nurse should demonstrate how to talk to and touch the ill child and encourage the siblings to do the same (Figure 17–6 ■). The length of the visit should be relatively short and based on the child's developmental age. After the visit, discuss with siblings what they saw and felt, and answer any questions they may have. When a sibling cannot visit, contact with the ill child can

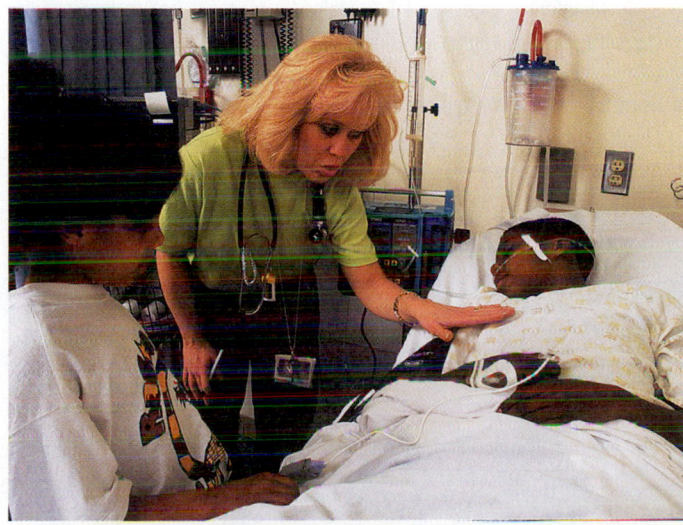

FIGURE 17–6 ■ During the sibling's visit to the ill child, it is important to talk with the sibling and answer any questions asked in an honest manner at a level the child can understand.

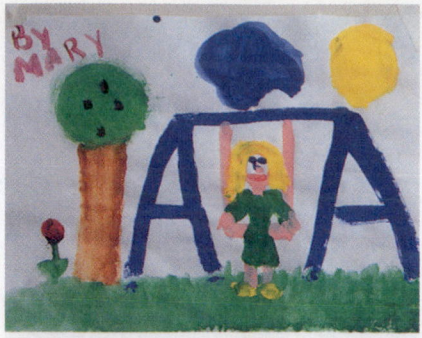

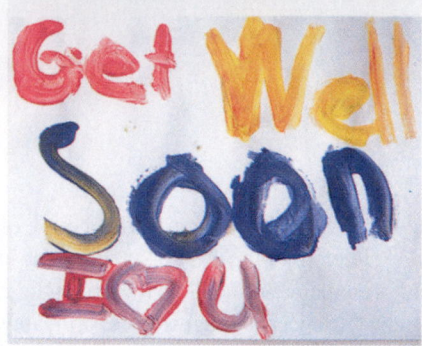

FIGURE 17–7 ■ It is important that parents and siblings feel comfortable communicating with the child who is seriously ill. If siblings cannot visit, they should be encouraged to paint or record messages. They need to be able to express themselves and to feel that they are helping.

be maintained by sending pictures, drawings, cards, and recorded messages, or by using cell phones if allowed (Figure 17–7 ■).

If parents are staying at the hospital with the ill child, encourage them to call the siblings at home daily. Allowing the siblings at home the opportunity to share their day as well as to receive an update on the ill child provides a feeling of connectedness. The phone call offers siblings a consistent link to the parent as well as the reassurance that they are important and loved. Internet contact may also allow for instant messaging and a way to communicate with older siblings. Arrange for access to a computer or the Internet if possible for families that will find this contact supportive.

Evaluation

Expected outcomes of nursing care include:

- The nurse establishes a trusting relationship with siblings.
- Siblings are prepared for visits to the child with a life-threatening illness or injury.
- Siblings receive emotional support and assistance to cope with the unfamiliar environment.

Chapter Highlights

- A life-threatening illness or injury places intense emotional and physical demands on the child and family due to the unfamiliar environment of the emergency department or intensive care unit, frightening or invasive procedures, and an uncertain outcome.
- Defense mechanisms displayed by children in stressful situations such as a life-threatening illness or injury include regression (return to an earlier behavior), denial, repression (involuntary forgetting), postponement, and bargaining.
- Nursing interventions to promote a child's psychologic health include permitting parents to be present, preparing children for procedures, using play to help the child manage anxiety, and allowing the child some choices to gain a sense of control.

- Parents typically progress through the stages of shock and disbelief, anger and guilt, deprivation and loss, anticipatory waiting, and readjustment or mourning when their child has a life-threatening illness or injury.
- A family-centered approach will help meet the needs of families, minimize stress, and enhance family coping. Appropriate nursing care includes providing information and building trust, promoting family involvement (including presence during procedures and resuscitation if desired), encouraging parents to meet physical and emotional needs, facilitating effective communication, and maintaining family support networks.
- The nurse should ensure siblings receive information about their critically ill or injured brother or sister and regular messages from the parents to help them control feelings of jealousy, guilt, fear, and insecurity.

Clinical Reasoning in Action

INTRODUCTION

Recall Alexa in the opening scenario. She is unconscious from hitting her head and has a serious abdominal injury following a motor vehicle crash in which she was a passenger. She is being cared for in the pediatric intensive care unit so that she can be monitored closely for life-threatening complications.

DESCRIPTION

An abdominal (CT) scan has revealed a spleen laceration that is bleeding, so Alexa is being carefully monitored for hypovolemia. She has regained consciousness, but drifts off to sleep frequently. Alexa's mother is at her bedside. Her father, who was driving the car, is being evaluated at another hospital, and Alexa's 8-year-old sister Sharon is staying with a neighbor.

DISCUSSION

1. What are the developmentally appropriate nursing interventions to address Alexa's stressors related to this sudden hospitalization?

2. What physical assessment procedures are used to monitor Alexa's condition?

3. What nursing interventions should be implemented to support Alexa's family?

4. What information should be provided to Sharon to help her understand what has happened to her sister?

NCLEX-RN® Review

1. What is the expected outcome for a hospitalized child experiencing anxiety related to a life-threatening injury and fear of invasive procedures?
   1. The child will appear more relaxed with fewer indications of anxiety.
   2. The child will be able to verbalize the source of the increased anxiety.
   3. The parents will appear more relaxed with fewer indications of anxiety.
   4. The parents will be able to verbalize the source of the increased anxiety.

2. What is the priority intervention for an adolescent admitted to the pediatric intensive care unit following a serious motor vehicle collision?
   1. Frequently touch and talk to the adolescent.
   2. Assign consistent caregivers.
   3. Limit visitors to parents.
   4. Involve the adolescent in planning care goals.

3. The nurse is planning care for a child admitted to the ICU following a penetrating chest injury. Which indicates the priority consideration in planning this care?
   1. Giving pain medications as needed
   2. Empowering the child
   3. Allowing open visitation
   4. Keeping the room quiet

4. A 2-year-old was admitted to the hospital in critical condition after ingesting about 20 children's chewable vitamins with iron 2 days ago. The mother said, "Since they were my child's vitamins, I didn't think they were poison." Which is the most appropriate nursing intervention in this situation?
   1. Explain the open visiting policy for parents and close friends.
   2. Question the mother regarding her knowledge of other child safety risks.
   3. Teach the mother about the dangers of iron poisoning.
   4. Explain the child's condition and what is being done at this time for the child.

See Appendix I 🔗 for answers.

References

Ames, K. E., Rennick, J. E., & Baillargeon, S. (2011). A qualitative interpretive study exploring parents' perception of the parental role in the pediatric intensive care unit. *Intensive and Critical Care Nursing, 27*(3), 143–150.

Austin, D. (2010). The psychophysiological effects of music therapy in intensive care units. *Paediatric Nursing, 22*(3), 14-20.

Borse, N. N., Gilchrist, J., Dellinger, A. M., Rudd, R. A., Ballesteros, M. F., & Sleet, D. A. (2008). *CDC Childhood Injury Report: Patterns of unintentional injuries among 0–19 year olds in the United States, 2000–2006.* Atlanta, GA: Centers for Disease Control and Prevention, National Center for Injury Prevention and Control.

Bowden, V. R., & Greenberg, C. S. (2009). Should family members be present when their child is being resuscitated? *Pediatric Nursing, 35*(4), 254–256.

Cameron, M. A., Schleien, C. L., & Morris, M. C. (2009). Parental presence on pediatric intensive care unit rounds. *Journal of Pediatrics, 155*, 522–528.

Colville, G. A., Cream, P. R., & Kerry, S. M. (2010). Do parents benefit from the offer of a follow-up appointment after their child's admission to intensive care? An exploratory randomised controlled trial. *Intensive and Critical Care Nursing, 26*, 146–153.

Colville, G. A., Kerry, S., & Pierce, C. (2008). Children's factual and delusional memories of intensive care.

American Journal of Respiratory and Critical Care Medicine, 177, 976–982.

da Silva, P. S. L., & de Carvalho, W. B. (2010). Unplanned extubation in pediatric critically ill patients: A systematic review and best practice recommendations. *Pediatric Critical Care Medicine, 11*(2), 287–294.

Emergency Nurses Association (ENA). (2010). *Emergency Nurses Association position statement: Family presence during invasive procedures and resuscitation in the emergency department.* Retrieved from http://www.ena.org/SiteCollectionDocuments/Position%20Statements/FamilyPresence.pdf

Frazier, A., Frazier, H., & Warren, N. A. (2010). A discussion of family-centered care within the pediatric intensive care unit. *Critical Care Nursing Quarterly, 33*(1), 82–86.

Gooding, J. S., Cooper, L. G., Blaine, A. I., Franck, L. S., Howse, J. L., & Berns, S. D. (2011). Family support and family-centered care in the neonatal intensive care unit: Origins, advances, impact. *Seminars in Perinatology, 35*, 20–28.

Institute of Medicine. (2003). Patterns of childhood death in America. In M. J. Field & R. E. Behrman, *When children die: Improving palliative and end-of-life care for children and their families* (pp. 41–71). Washington, DC: National Academy Press.

Keefe, S. (2008). A family affair. *Advance for Nurses, 10*(8), 33–34.

Latour, J. M., van Goudoever, J. B., Schuurman, B. E., Albers, M. J. I. J., van Dam, N. A. M., Dullaart, E., . . . Hazelzet, J. A. (2011). A qualitative study exploring the experiences of parents of children admitted to seven Dutch pediatric intensive care units. *Intensive Care Medicine, 37*(2), 319–325.

Levetown, M., & Committee on Bioethics. (2008). Communicating with children and families: From everyday interactions to skill in conveying distressing information. *Pediatrics, 121*(5), e1441–1460.

March of Dimes. (2009). *Which babies need care in the NICU?* Retrieved from http://www.marchofdimes.com/baby/inthenicu_whichbabies.html

McClement, S. E., Fallis, W. M., & Pereira, A. (2009). Family presence during resuscitation: Canadian critical care nurses' perspectives. *Journal of Nursing Scholarship, 41*(3), 233–240.

Meadors, P., & Lamson, A. (2008). Compassion fatigue and secondary traumatization: Provider self care on intensive care units for children. *Journal of Pediatric Health Care, 22*(1), 24–34.

Meeks, R. (2009). Parental presence in pediatric trauma resuscitation: One hospital's experience. *Pediatric Nursing, 35*(6), 376–380.

Namachivayam, P., Shann, F., Shekerdemian, L., Taylor, A., van Sloten, I., Delzoppo, C., . . . Butt, W. (2010). Three decades of pediatric intensive care: Who was admitted, what happened in intensive care, and what happened afterward. *Pediatric Critical Care Medicine, 11*(5), 549–555.

Nance, J. G., Griffin, M. T. Q., McNulty, S. R., & Fitzpatrick, J. J. (2010, November/December). Prayer practices among young adults.*Holistic Nursing Practice,* 338–344.

National Center for Health Statistics. (2011). *Final natality data.* Retrieved from http://www.marchofdimes.com/peristats/

Needle, J. S., O'Riordan, M., & Smith, P. G. (2009). Parental anxiety and medical comprehension within 24 hours of a child's admission to the pediatric intensive care unit. *Pediatric Critical Care Medicine, 10*(6), 668–674.

Niska, R., Bhuiya, F., & Xu, J. (2010). National Hospital Ambulatory Medical Care Survey: 2007 Emergency Department Summary. *National Health Statistics Reports, 26,* 1–32. Retrieved from http://www.cdc.gov/nchs/data/nhsr/nhsr026.pdf

Nyqvist, K. H., & Engvall, G. (2009). Parents as their infant's primary caregivers in a neonatal intensive care unit. *Journal of Pediatric Nursing, 24*(2), 153–163.

Owens, P. L., Zodet, M. W., Berdahl, T., Dougherty, D., McCormick, M. C., & Simpson, L. A. (2008). Annual report on health care for children and youth in the United States: Focus on injury-related emergency department utilization and expenditures. *Ambulatory Pediatrics, 8*(4), 219–240.

Patel, B., Kennebeck, S. S., Caviness, A. C., & Macias, C. G. (2009). Use of a discharge facilitator improves recall of emergency department discharge instructions for acute gastroenteritis. *Pediatric Emergency Care, 25*(9), 558–564.

Smith, A. B., Hefley, G. C., & Anand, K. J. S. (2007). Parent bed spaces in the PICU: Effect on parental stress. *Pediatric Nursing, 33*(3), 215–221.

Ward-Begnoche, W. (2007). Posttraumatic stress symptoms in the pediatric intensive care unit. *Journal for Specialists in Pediatric Nursing, 12*(2), 84–92.

Watters, D., Sayre, M. R., & Silbergleit, R. (2005). Research conditions that qualify for emergency exception from informed consent. *Academic Emergency Medicine, 12*(11), 1041–1044.

Wigert, H., Berg, M., & Hellström, A-L. (2010). Parental presence when their child is in neonatal intensive care. *Scandinavian Journal of Caring Sciences, 24,* 139–146.

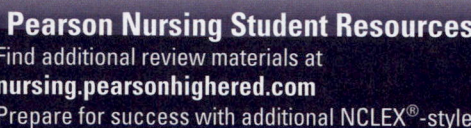

Pearson Nursing Student Resources

Find additional review materials at
nursing.pearsonhighered.com
Prepare for success with additional NCLEX®-style practice questions, interactive assignments and activities, web links, animations and videos, and more!

End-of-Life Care and Bereavement

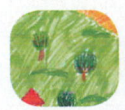 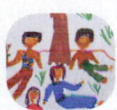 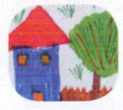

Learning Outcomes

After completing this chapter, you will be able to:

1. Contrast the developing concept of death and loss among infants, toddlers, preschoolers, school-age children, and adolescents.

2. Analyze the cultural and spiritual influences on the child's and family's responses to death, loss, and grief.

3. Demonstrate interventions for the dying child based on developmental responses to his or her impending death.

4. Examine ethical issues associated with the care of a child who is dying.

5. Apply assessment skills to identify the physiologic changes that occur in the child who is dying.

6. Devise a nursing care plan to provide family-centered care for the child who is dying and his or her family.

7. Plan bereavement support for the parents and siblings after the death of a child.

8. Evaluate strategies to support nurses who care for children who die.

> "My daddy told me my baby brother Zach isn't coming home because he is going to die. Mommy stays with Zach in the hospital all of the time. I just wish everyone would come home. Why does Zach have to die anyway?"
>
> —*Marilee, age 7*

Zachary Conway is a 3 1/2-year-old who began experiencing motor difficulties and demonstrating bizarre emotional behavior a few months ago. After a series of diagnostic studies, he was diagnosed with an inoperable, rapidly progressing brain tumor. Zachary underwent radiation and chemotherapy to reduce the size of the tumor, which relieved symptoms for a couple of months. After experiencing a grand mal seizure and becoming dehydrated from poor oral nutritional intake, he was admitted to the oncology unit at the children's hospital.

Zachary's condition has deteriorated and his death is imminent. The nurse is now focused on promoting his comfort and supporting his family during the death vigil. Zachary is awake but appears lethargic. He is receiving enteral feedings, fluids, and pain medication via a nasogastric tube. He interacts very little with anyone other than his mother.

Zachary's mother remains with him at all times, except for short breaks to eat and call family members. His father spends several hours each day at the hospital. Zachary's sister, Marilee, attends school in the second grade. Her grandparents are caring for her after school when her mother and father are with Zachary.

What is the role of the nurse in caring for Zachary and his family? What nursing interventions address the physiologic and psychologic needs of the child who is dying? How can you provide family-centered care?

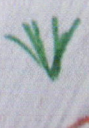

DEATH IN CHILDREN

In the United States, more than 48,033 children and adolescents under 20 years died in 2009, with infants accounting for nearly half of those deaths (Kochanek, Xu, Murphy, et al., 2011). Childhood death may be the result of a low birth weight, congenital malformation, chronic condition, sudden illness, or injury. Approximately 90% of children between 1 and 19 years of age receive hospital-based care during their final weeks of life (Hinds & Kelly, 2010). Refer to Chapter 1 for a thorough discussion of the neonatal, postnatal, and age-specific death rates, and the leading causes of injury deaths in children of all ages.

The death of a child is a devastating, life-altering experience for the parents, siblings, and other family members. The nurse caring for the child and family experiencing death, loss, and **grief** (an individual's intense feelings and behaviors in response to the death of a person or object to whom one is attached) must consider the personal, ethical, legal, spiritual, cultural, and biological influences on these individuals. This enables the nurse to provide supportive and sensitive care to the dying child and family and assist them through the grieving process.

When the family is faced with end-of-life care of a child, this often involves the progressive decline associated with a chronic condition or multiple acute care episodes (Figure 18–1 ■). However, some deaths occur suddenly, such as with a severe acute illness or injury, which limits opportunities for planned end-of-life care. Whether the child's death is the result of a chronic condition or an acute circumstance, the nurse is pivotal in providing valuable care and support to the child and family.

CONCEPTS OF LOSS AND DEATH

Everyone at some point in life experiences loss and death. Children may suffer loss as a result of a changed relationship through death of a parent, separation or divorce of parents, or death of a grandparent.

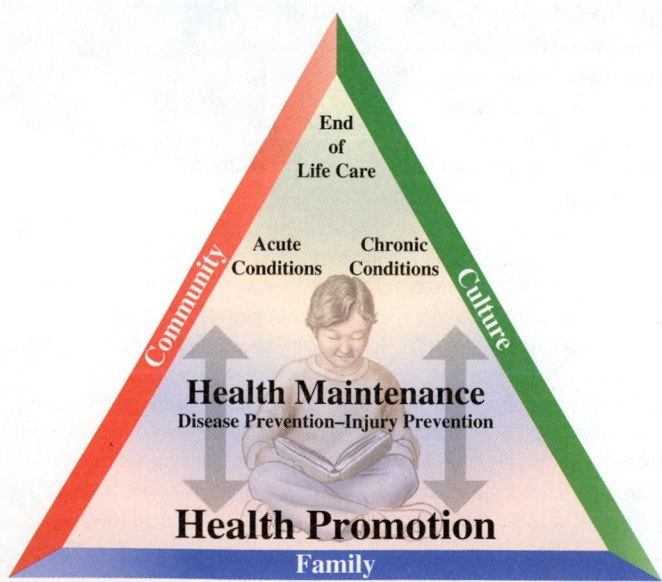

FIGURE 18–1 ■ The Bindler-Ball Child Health Continuum illustrates the paths that may lead to a child's death. In many cases, the child's death is associated with a chronic condition such as cancer or congenital anomalies, but it is important to remember that approximately 27% of deaths of children under age 20 years are sudden and unexpected as a result of injury (Friebert, 2009).

Legal and Ethical Considerations
Determination of Death

The Uniform Determination of Death Act developed the legal definition used for the determination of death in 1980. This act states that a dead individual is one who sustained either irreversible cessation of circulatory and respiratory functions, or irreversible cessation of all functions of the entire brain, including the brainstem (Hills, 2010).

Loss

Loss is an actual or potential change in status of something valued, so that it is no longer available to be experienced. **Anticipatory loss** is experienced before the loss actually transpires. Sources of loss for children may include:

- Loss of a loved one (e.g., parent, sibling, grandparent, friend, childcare provider, pet)
- Loss of an aspect of oneself, such as a body part or function (e.g., amputation, organ failure, hearing or vision loss)
- Loss of an object (e.g., favorite toy)
- Separation from an accustomed environment (e.g., relocation to new neighborhood or new school)

Death

Medicine and society struggle with the definition of death because of the existence of technology and advanced life support systems. Historically, death was defined as the irreversible cessation of circulatory and respiratory functions, and no diagnostic precision was needed to declare death. However, the definition of death needed modification because of technology and ventilators that could sustain respiratory function. The definition of death also needed to become more precise before organs could be harvested for donation. One commonly accepted definition of death in the United States is **brain death,** or the irreversible cessation of all functions of the brain, the master regulating body organ that integrates the person as a whole (Zielinski, 2011). This definition also implies no chance of recovery. See Legal and Ethical Considerations: Determination of Death.

Specific medical protocols for clinical determination of death vary by state and hospital (Hills, 2010). Brain death determination guidelines generally require confirmation by two physicians after evaluating the patient twice. The time interval between evaluations (12 to 48 hours) varies by the age of the child. Before an evaluation is performed, it is essential to make sure that the child is not hypothermic and has no potential conditions that could contribute to brain death findings (e.g., use of paralytic medications, drug overdose, metabolic derangement, and cause of the coma has been diagnosed) (Table 18–1). Additional confirmatory tests may be conducted in some circumstances, such as encephalography and cerebral blood flow scans (Zielinski, 2011).

THE CHILD'S EXPERIENCE WITH DEATH AND LOSS

For children, major losses associated with death include the death of a parent, death of a grandparent, death of a sibling, and death of a friend. The death of a sibling is discussed later in this chapter. Children also experience loss through several circumstances not related to the death of a person, including parental separation or divorce,

TABLE 18–1 Brain Death Criteria

BRAIN FUNCTIONING	CLINICAL SIGNS
Coma	Unconscious, no vocalization
Absent clinical functions of the brain	Flaccid tone and no purposeful movement
	No increase in heart rate with pressure on eyeballs
Absent brainstem function	Pupils midposition or dilated, nonresponsive to light
	No blink response to corneal stimulation
	No spontaneous eye movements with abrupt rotation of head or ice water irrigation in each ear
	No gag reflex with oropharyngeal stimulation
	No cough reflex to tracheal stimulation
	Apnea—no respiratory movements when removed from ventilator

Source: Data from *Lee, K. J. (2011). Brain death. In R. M. Kliegman, B. F. Stanton, J. W. St. Geme, N. F. Schor, & R. E. Behrman, Nelson textbook of pediatrics (19th ed., pp. e63-1–e63-3). Philadelphia: Elsevier; Mathur, M., Petersen, L., Stadtler, M., Rose, C., Ejike, J. C., Petersen, F., . . . Ashwal, S. (2008). Variability in pediatric brain death determination and documentation in Southern California. Pediatrics, 121(5), 988–993; Hills, T. E. (2010). Brain death: A review of evidence-based guidelines. Nursing 2010, 40(12), 34–40.*

loss of a pet, loss of a possession, and relocation. The significance of the loss to the child determines the amount and type of grieving the child experiences. Children differ from adults in their understanding of loss and death, but like adults, they miss the loved one who died. Their understanding and behavioral responses vary according to their developmental level and their previous experience with loss and death. See Table 18–2.

Death of a Parent

The death of a parent is an extremely traumatic event for the child and has a significant impact on the child's self-concept, health, and social and economic circumstances. Children who have lost a parent always have emotional distress, but they may internalize their feelings, leading to insomnia, learning problems, and health issues such as headaches and abdominal pain. The child's reaction to the death of a parent is greatly influenced by the manner in which the surviving parent reacts to the death and supports the child. When the bereaved parent is grieving the loss of a spouse, parenting responsibilities may be overwhelming. Just as with adults, the death of a parent changes the life of the child forever. Children do not quickly bounce back after the death of a parent. Children need continued support, understanding, and counseling over time to prevent negative complications of grief.

Additional losses for the child may occur as the result of a parent's death. The death may bring about relocation or a change in living arrangements. For example, the child may have to live with a noncustodial parent, grandparent, or other extended family member. The family's financial status may change as a result of the loss of a wage earner. Older children may be expected to assume more responsibility for the home or younger siblings, allowing them less time for peers and recreational activities. See Partnering with Families: Leaving Memories for Children.

Death of a Grandparent

The death of a grandparent is often the first experience a child has with death of a significant individual. The child's grandparent may have had a special role in the development of the child's sense of

trust, love, and belonging. With an understanding of a grandparent's death, the child may come to the realization that his or her parents will die also.

Clinical Tip

Communicating with children about death is often a difficult task for parents. The words used to describe death may vary by culture, so learn the terminology used by cultural groups in your community. Parents and other adults should avoid euphemisms such as "she has gone to sleep" since this may confuse children and hinder their understanding of the finality of death. Parents and healthcare providers should not be afraid to use the word *death* or *dead* when explaining these concepts to children. After discussing death with children, provide them with the opportunity to ask questions and express their feelings.

The child's reaction to the loss of a grandparent is dependent on the significance of the grandparent to the child. In many families and cultures, grandparents are important influences in the child's life. Children may be raised by a grandparent, they may be cared for by a grandparent while the parents work, or they may reside in the same household with the grandparent. Grandparents are often a child's link to his or her heritage through storytelling and sharing family history. The influence of the grandparent on the child may therefore have considerable meaning to the child, and the impact of a grandparent's death may be as significant as the death of a parent.

Death of a Friend

Children may experience the death of a friend due to a chronic condition, acute illness, or injury. Since children with chronic and life-threatening conditions are living longer and are able to attend school and engage in social activities, they are likely to have developed close friendships with other children. The childhood friends and schoolmates of children who are chronically ill should be prepared for the potential death according to their developmental level. When a friend dies suddenly, such as through violence or unintentional injury, there is no time for preparation. Whether the death of a friend was anticipated or sudden, the child experiences the same stages of grief as with other losses. The death of a peer may bring about the first realization that the elderly are not the only ones who die. The adolescent's sense of invulnerability may be shaken.

Some schools offer grief support and counseling to provide opportunities for the children's expressions of grief and sadness. The development of a memorial is often helpful for children. Planting a tree, hanging a plaque, or creating a play area at school in memory of the deceased child helps the children to express their grief. (See Table 18–3 for further resources.)

Other Potentially Significant Losses

For many children, the first significant loss is that of a pet. A pet is often viewed by the child as a source of unconditional love and acceptance. The child typically views a pet as a friend, companion, and member of the family. The child may experience a pet's loss through death (anticipated or unexpected), or because the pet ran away or was stolen. How the parents and other adults support the child and handle the loss can affect the manner in which the child learns to cope with loss and death later in life.

Parents should offer honest, simple, and developmentally appropriate explanations to help the child understand what happened. Telling a child that the dog was old and sick, so it had to be "put to

TABLE 18–2	The Child's Developmental Understanding of Death, Potential Behaviors, and Nursing Considerations	
UNDERSTANDING OF DEATH	**POTENTIAL BEHAVIORS**	**NURSING MANAGEMENT**
Infant		
Cognitive Stage: Sensorimotor	Resists cuddling or clings more than usual	Provide a sense of security by holding and hugging the infant.
Death is perceived as separation and abandonment	Protests the disruption in caretaking	Use a soothing voice to tell the infant you will be there to provide care.
Senses disruption in home, emotions of caregivers, and altered routines	May have feeding problems	Help parents to reduce their emotional distress while caring for the infant.
Senses separation	Cries excessively	
	Sleeps more than usual	Try to return to usual routines.
Toddler		
Cognitive Stage: Preoperational	Regresses to younger stage of development	Encourage parents to hold and cuddle the toddler to help reduce the fear of separation.
No understanding of true concept of death	Clingy, does not want to let the parent out of sight	Follow familiar routines.
Aware someone is missing—separation anxiety	May have decreased activity	Be tolerant of regressive behaviors.
Unable to distinguish death from temporary separation or abandonment	Whiny, irritable; may show distress by biting, hitting, or tears	Use distraction (toys, games, videos) when the child is fussy or clingy.
	Problems eating and sleeping	
	Alternates between grieving behavior and playing behavior	
	Fearful	
Preschooler		
Cognitive Stage: Preoperational	Regresses to younger stage of development, such as tantrums, or problems with bowel and bladder control	Be tolerant of regression in developmental tasks.
Believes death is temporary and the dead person will return	Uses play activities to cope with strong feelings	Provide honest and consistent responses to the child's questions.
Confuses death with being away or asleep	Asks when deceased will come back or what the dead "do"	Encourage the return to usual routines and provide reassurance that you will be with the child.
Death may be seen as punishment	May fear going to sleep, has nightmares, afraid of dark	Encourage parents to keep memories alive with pictures and objects that remind the child of the loved one.
Experiences magical thinking (believes his or her thoughts or actions potentially caused the death)	Crying spells, may be mimicking behaviors of adults	Suggest rituals such as going to the cemetery, releasing helium balloons, and planting flowers that might help the child learn to manage the loss.
Has beginning experiences with the death of animals and plants	Seems morbidly fascinated with death	
	Asks a lot of questions	
	Complains of abdominal pain	
School-Age Child		
Cognitive Stage: Concrete Operations	Crying, moody, may become withdrawn and distant; may have angry outbursts or disruptive behaviors	Listen to the child and answer questions honestly.
Understands difference between temporary separation and death	May deny sadness by hiding tears and acting more like adults	Return to usual routines and activities and involvement with the child's social group.
By 6 years, recognizes that death is permanent	Decreased concentration with schoolwork, may refuse to go to school	Make sure the child knows he or she will not be abandoned.
Knows that death occurs in others, but begins to recognize that he or she will also die	May develop a morbid interest in dead things, the symbols of death, and the biologic aspects of death	Encourage parents to keep memories alive through activities such as art, music, creating a memory book, sewing a quilt, and planting a garden.
By 9–10 years, understanding of death is same as adult	May fear another loved person will die	Share Internet resources.
May have guilt or assume blame for the death	May try to comfort parents by taking over tasks	Use coping support groups.
May not realize that death can occur at any age	May have psychosomatic complaints—abdominal pain or headache	Encourage the family to seek faith-based support.
Adolescent		
Cognitive Stage: Formal Operations	May have severe depression, mood swings, withdrawal from friends	Be available and encourage open communication.
Intellectually capable of understanding death	May feel angry or guilty	Encourage the teen to keep memories alive with pictures and other things that remind him or her of the loved one.
Recognizes that all people, including self, must die	Girls may seek comfort from friends	Inform the teen about available counseling and support groups.
Has a better grasp of association between illness and death	Eating and sleeping problems	Share Internet resources.
Sense of invincibility conflicts with fear of death	May attempt to confront or deny death as if it is an adversary, leading to acting-out or risk-taking behaviors	Encourage the child to seek support from his or her faith group.
Able to recognize the effect of death on others	Uses abstract and philosophic reasoning	

Source: *Data from Auman, M. J. (2007). Bereavement support for children. Journal of School Nursing, 23(1), 34–39; Linebarger, J. S., Sahler, O. J. Z., & Egan, K. A. (2009). Coping with death. Pediatrics in Review, 30(9), 350–355; Schum, L. N., & Kane, J. R. (2009). Psychological adaptation of the dying child. In D. Walsh, A. T. Caraceni, R. Fainsinger, K. Foley, P. Glare, C. Goh, . . . L. Radbruch, Palliative medicine (1st ed., pp. 1085–1092). Philadelphia: Saunders Elsevier.*

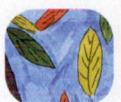

Partnering with Families

Leaving Memories for Children

Dying parents may ask the nurse about leaving memories for their child. Suggestions that the nurse could offer include the following:

- Making video recordings and dating them according to when they wish the child to view them (e.g., special occasions such as birthdays and graduation)
- Journaling or writing to the child about their love for the child and their experience of being a parent
- Writing out birthday cards and providing special gifts for each of the child's birthdays and having family members give them to the child at the appropriate time

- Writing letters and asking family members to mail them to the child at the designated time
- Making a "memory book" of the parent's life with the child from birth
- Sharing special moments (e.g., "I remember the first time you smiled at me," or "I remember the first day you said "mama'") either in writing or on a video recording

sleep" may cause anxiety in the 4-year-old about what will happen when he or she sleeps at night. The 8-year-old who is told "God was lonely, so he took Cocoa to live with him," may become concerned about what other loved ones God may desire.

Suggestions for helping the child cope with the loss of a pet include burying the pet and having a memorial service, talking about good memories of the pet, planting flowers or a tree in memory of the pet, and creating a scrapbook.

FACTORS INFLUENCING FAMILY RESPONSES TO DEATH AND LOSS

Grief is an experience that affects all individuals; however, cultural beliefs, spiritual beliefs, and social support systems are central factors influencing a child's and family's response to death and loss. Other

factors specifically influencing the child's response, including developmental level, are discussed in the following section.

Culture

Recognizing and understanding a family's cultural traditions and practices when they are experiencing the death of a child helps nurses to provide individualized care to the dying child and the family. Each culture has its own way of defining, addressing, and acknowledging death. Customs, ceremonies, religious laws, and beliefs are strongly connected with such events. Culture influences the individual's reaction to loss, and the expression of grief is often determined by the customs of the culture. Some families may believe that grief is a private matter, and they may internalize and repress their feelings. Others may believe that outward demonstration of the expression of

TABLE 18–3	Books for Children Who Experience the Death of a Family Member or Friend	
BOOK	**PUBLISHER**	**AGE GROUP**
A Separate Peace, by John Knowles	New York: MacMillan	12 and up
Blackwater, by Eve Bunting	New York: Harper Collins	12 and up
When a Friend Dies: A Book for Teens About Grieving and Healing, by Marilyn E. Gootman	Minneapolis: Free Spirit Press	12 and up
Bridge to Terabithia, by Katherine Paterson	New York: Harper Collins	10–14
On My Honor, by Marion Dane Bauer	New York: Bantam Doubleday Dell Publishing	8–12
Charlotte's Web, by E. B. White	New York: Harper and Row	5–10
Children Also Grieve: Talking About Death and Healing, by L. Goldman	Philadelphia: Jessica Kingsley	5–10
Gentle Willow: A Story for Children About Dying, by J. C. Mills	Washington: Magination Press	5–10
If Nathan Were Here, by Mary Bahr	Eerdmans Books for Young Readers	5–10
Tell Me Papa: Answers to Questions Children Ask About Death and Dying, by J. Johnson and M. Johnson	Omaha, NE: Centering Corporation	4–10
This Book Is for All Kids, but Especially My Sister Libby. Libby Died, by J. Simon.	Riverside, NJ: Andrews McMeel Publishing	4–8
Missing Hannah: Based on a True Story of Sudden Infant Death Syndrome, by D. Kane	Bloomington, IN: Author House	4–8
Flying Hugs and Kisses (English) or *Besos y abrazos al aire* (Spanish), by J. Sample	Centennial, CO: Lifevest Publishing	4–8
Dancing on the Moon, by Janice Roper	Cheverly, MD: SIDS Educational Services	3–8

Source: From National Sudden and Unexpected Infant/Child Death & Pregnancy Loss Resource Center. (2007). Bereavement resources for children: A selected annotated bibliography. Retrieved from http://www.sidscenter.org/TopicalBib/BereavementForChildren.html; Smith, C. (2010). Death, general: Resource list. Retrieved from http://www.nursingconsult.com/das/patient/view/239299363-2/10072/24810.html/top?sid=1146105885&SEQNO=5

Developing Cultural Competence
Diverse Perspectives on Death

Cultural differences are important to consider when working with families dealing with the death of a loved one. Some examples of differences include the following (Schaffer & Norlander, 2009, pp. 159–168):

- African Americans often place great importance on the presence of their families and the involvement of families in their care. They embrace religion and spirituality. They may be less likely to request medications for pain and other symptoms because of an expectation to suffer. Families may prefer aggressive treatment because of a fear that the predicted prognosis is incorrect.

- Asian families often desire to protect the terminally ill from knowledge of their condition so their final days will be peaceful. Decision making is often based upon what is best for the family, and aggressive treatments may be desired to preserve life. It may be believed that making plans for the child's death could cause the child's premature death.

- Hispanics generally believe the entire family makes important decisions. They see death as a natural part of life, and they do not want to be a burden for their families. Cultural customs related to grief and loss vary. Crying openly is seen as appropriate. Faith is very important in times of death. The anniversary of a loved one's death is observed every year.

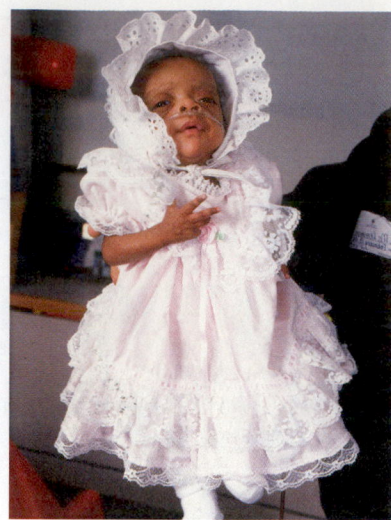

FIGURE 18–2 ■ Religious rituals, such as baptism and blessing of an ill infant, may provide great comfort to the family. When the infant is stable, a traditional baptism may be performed in the home or church with family and friends present. When the infant has a life-threatening illness, baptism may be performed in the hospital by a chaplain or health professional.

grief is acceptable and is even encouraged. However, it is important to note that not all families observe traditional rites and rituals. See Developing Cultural Competence: Diverse Perspectives on Death.

Faith-Based Beliefs and Spirituality

In order for the nurse to provide family-centered care to the dying child and his or her family, the faith or spiritual beliefs of the family should be assessed. An individual's spiritual beliefs and practices considerably influence his or her reactions to loss and subsequent behavior. Faith and spirituality may be a fundamental coping mechanism when a family is dealing with death and dying. Faith-based or spiritual leaders may be helpful to families.

Most death ceremonies and rituals are based on culture and spiritual beliefs. Most faith groups have specific practices related to death, which may be expressed through prayer, meditation, rituals, worship, music, art, and dance. Many cultural groups wish to keep a vigil and prevent the dying person from being alone. Other groups cry loudly and wail, a sign that they care about the dying person. Some families may desire to have the child baptized prior to death (Figure 18–2 ■). See Table 18–4 for an overview of faith-based traditions in mourning and after-death rites.

GRIEF AND BEREAVEMENT

Death or loss causes pain and emotional distress, but one must disengage emotionally from the deceased and adapt to a new life that does not include the deceased. The intense feelings and behaviors of grief are painful, individualized, and exhausting. Many factors influence a person's grief responses, including the perception of the preventability of the illness or injury, the suddenness and other circumstances of the death, previous losses, the nature of the attachment with the person who died, spiritual or faith orientation, and culture. Grief is very individualized. Grief feelings and physical sensations include sadness, anger, fatigue, inability to concentrate, numbness, sleep disturbances, depression, and anxiety. Somatic symptoms may include nausea, anorexia, blurred vision, chest pain, dizziness, dyspnea, palpitations, and syncope.

Anticipatory mourning is the process of emotional preparation for the loss to come, often associated with a diagnosis of terminal illness. Grief, mourning, and sadness all are experienced as the person sees the changes in function of the loved one and recognizes the loss of a certain future. In some cases, families become closer and more cohesive as they cope with these losses and balance conflicting demands. Anticipatory mourning does not necessarily make the actual grief after the death easier or shorter.

Bereavement describes experiencing loss through the death of a loved one, but not the emotional aspect of the loss. **Mourning** is the social ritual and expression of loss, as well as the behavioral and psychologic process of adapting to the loss. Mourning is often influenced by custom, spiritual beliefs, and culture.

Stages of Grieving

Though many theorists have described phases or stages of grieving, one of the more well-known frameworks is Kübler-Ross's (1983) five stages of grieving: denial, anger, bargaining, depression, and acceptance (Buglass, 2010). Rather than stages, these are really emotional states that survivors experience, sometimes repeatedly, as they progress toward acceptance. See pages 447–448 for more explanation about these five stages. Parkes's theory identifies four stages of grieving that have similarities to Kübler-Ross's model: shock or numbness, yearning or pining, disorganization and despair, and recovery (Buglass, 2010). Worden developed his theory of grief with four significant tasks rather than stages:

- Accept the reality of the loss.
- Process the pain of grief.
- Adjust to life without the loved one.
- Find an enduring connection with the deceased in the midst of embarking on a new life.

Worden's theory is a proactive way of managing the loss, grief, and new challenges (Corr & Coolican, 2010). Grief takes time, and the amount of time needed before a person is able to move on to life without the loved one is variable. See Table 18–5 for nursing management associated with the stages or tasks of grieving.

TABLE 18–4   Spiritual Traditions in Mourning and After-Death Rites

FAITH-BASED OR SPIRITUAL GROUP	POSSIBLE BELIEFS AND RITUALS	ORGAN DONATION OR AUTOPSY BELIEFS
American Indians	Beliefs and practices vary widely among tribes	Varies among tribes
	Navajo who touch the body need to have a ceremony to be protected from the deceased's spirit	
	Body must be as whole as possible for afterlife	
Buddhism	Last-rite chanting at bedside	Organ donation is considered act of mercy, autopsy is individual choice
	Cremation is preferred	
Catholicism	Sacrament of the sick	Autopsy, organ donation are acceptable
	Obligated to take ordinary but not extraordinary means to prolong life	
	Burial	
Christian Science	Unlikely to seek medical help to prolong life	Organ donation is not acceptable
	Disposal of body and parts is decided by family	
Hinduism	Death is seen as a passage; rebirth is expected	Autopsy, organ donation are acceptable
	Religious prayers chanted before and after death	
	Thread tied around the neck or wrist signifies a blessing, do not remove	
	Body is bathed and massaged in oils, dressed in new clothes, and then cremated	
	Women may loudly wail, moan, and beat their chests to display grief	
Islam	Attempts to shorten life are prohibited	Organ donation is acceptable
	Deathbed should be turned to face toward Mecca	Autopsy only for medical or legal reasons
	Passages from Quran stressing hope and acceptance are read to dying patient	
	Body is washed only by Muslim of same gender and wrapped in a white shroud	
Jehovah's Witness	Use of extraordinary means to prolong life is individual choice	Autopsy if required by law
	Burial determined by family preference	Organ donation is forbidden
Judaism	Generally desire natural death versus use of technology to prolong life	Autopsy is permitted in certain circumstances
	Dying patient should not be left alone	Organ donation may be acceptable
	Body ritually washed and embalming is prohibited	
	Burial within 24 to 48 hours, all body parts must be buried together	
	Seven-day mourning period (Shiva)	
Mormonism	If death is inevitable, promote a peaceful and dignified death	Autopsy is permitted with permission of next of kin
	Burial in temple clothes	Organ donation is individual choice
Orthodox Christian	Extraordinary means of life support are not required, but euthanasia is not acceptable	Organ donation is permitted
	Cremation is discouraged	
Protestantism	Burial or cremation is individual decision	Organ donation and autopsy are individual decisions
	Preference for prolonging life or natural death is individual choice	
Seventh-Day Adventist	Prefer prolonging life	Autopsy, organ donation are acceptable
	Disposal of body and burial are individual decisions	

Source: Adapted from Spector, R. E. (2009). Cultural diversity in health and illness (7th ed., pp. 136–142). Upper Saddle River, NJ: Pearson Prentice Hall; Purnell, L. D. (2009). Guide to culturally competent health care (2nd ed.). Philadelphia: F. A. Davis Company; Orthodox Church of America. (2011). Death/funerals. Retrieved from http://oca.org/questions/deathfunerals

Complicated grief is an unhealthy grief with symptoms that persist for at least 6 months after the loss. The grief is intensified to the level that it interferes with the individual's ability to function. Characteristics of complicated grief include an intense yearning for the loved one, an inability to accept the death, avoidance of reminders of the loss, feeling emotionally numb or detached from others, having excessive bitterness, feeling that life is meaningless without the loved one and there is no prospect for future fulfillment, and

feeling uneasy about moving on. It occurs in 10% to 20% of the bereaved (Lichtenthal & Kissane, 2009).

Social Support System

Those closest to the grieving child and family can be a great source of physical, emotional, and functional support, which can positively influence the successful resolution of grief. However, some people are uncomfortable or lack experience in dealing with death, and rather

TABLE 18–5	Stages of Grieving and Nursing Management	
STAGE	**BEHAVIORAL RESPONSES**	**NURSING MANAGEMENT**
Denial, shock, numbness	Disbelief, it seems like a bad dream	Be verbally supportive.
	Unable to process information about the death	Do not reinforce denial.
	Questions the reality of the death	Don't argue—allow the child or parents to come to terms in their own time.
	Unable to believe that the child will not come home again	
	May say, "This can't be happening" or "This can't be true."	
Anger, hostile reactions	May direct anger at physicians and nurses who could not save the family member	Recognize that anger is a normal response to feelings of loss and powerlessness.
	May express anger at God or supreme being	Avoid withdrawal or retaliation.
	May be angry about the bad things that have happened to a loved one or the inability to control what happened	Do not take anger personally.
		Remain with the child or parents even though they express anger.
Bargaining, yearning, pining	Yearns for life to return to the way it was	Actively listen, using eye contact and stillness.
	Expresses guilt, focusing on "what if" or "if only" scenarios	Encourage survivors to identify and express their feelings.
	May bargain for life to return to the way it was, or to see the loved one in heaven	Offer spiritual support if appropriate.
		Make follow-up phone calls at regular intervals to the survivors (1 month, 3 months, 6 months, and 1 year).
Depression, disorganization, or despair	Has sadness and lethargy	Assist family and friends to understand the grieving process.
	Daily activities seem pointless	Encourage friends and family to continue making contact.
	May withdraw from social and life activities	
Acceptance, recovery	Comes to terms with the death of the child and learns to live with the loss of the loved one	Encourage the family to create memories.
	Accepts the reality that the loved one is physically gone	Allow the individual to progress through the tasks or stages on his or her own timeline.
	Eventually starts reaching out to others	Encourage participation in activities that have meaning to the family member.

Source: *Data from Kübler-Ross, E., & Kessler, D. (2005). On grief and grieving (pp. 7–28). New York: Scribner; Hardy-Bougere, M. (2008). Cultural manifestations of grief and bereavement: A clinical perspective.* Journal of Cultural Diversity, 15(2), 66–69.

than offering support in the time of need, they may withdraw from the grieving person or family. Others may offer support initially, but as they return to their usual activities, they may cease to provide ongoing support for those still grieving.

Another consideration is that the grieving individual may be unable or unwilling to accept support when it is offered. Social factors that can interfere with grieving include a lack of social recognition of the loss, perceived inability to share the loss, and traumatic circumstances of the loss.

END-OF-LIFE CONSIDERATIONS AND DECISION MAKING

When the family is faced with end-of-life decision making and care because of a child's chronic condition or multiple acute episodes, the family relies on the nurse and other members of the healthcare team to provide honest information about various treatment options and potential outcomes. Depending on cognitive abilities, developmental stage, physical and mental status, and prior experiences in health care, the child should also participate in the decision-making process. As children are informed about their role in healthcare decisions, they gain skills in describing symptoms and home management (Levetown & the Committee on Bioethics, 2008). The family may need to consider issues such as palliative care, hospice care, allow-natural-death requests, and continuation of the child's education.

Baccalaureate Essential I
Liberal Education for Baccalaureate Generalist Nursing Practice

A liberal education fosters the development of a personal values system that enables the nurse to engage in ethical decision making and to act upon those decisions. This may involve applying knowledge of social and cultural factors for the diverse population of children and families served. Nurses who work with children and families with life-limiting conditions develop a personal values system to help families during one of the most difficult times of their lives. They often develop a close relationship, carefully listening and asking sensitive questions to help the child and family identify what is important to them in the time remaining. These nurses work to avoid ethical conflicts when possible by collaborating with the healthcare team to support parents in making end-of-life decisions. Nurses ensure that the family's and child's wishes are respected and provide a source of comfort as difficult decisions are made (Hinds & Kelly, 2010).

Palliative Care

Palliative care is a multidisciplinary care approach to prevent and relieve suffering and to enhance quality of life for patients and their families, regardless of the stage of the disease or the need for other therapies. This approach also aims to optimize the patient's function, help with decision making, and provide opportunities for personal growth. Palliative care may be provided simultaneously with curative care, life-prolonging care, or as the main focus of care (National

| BOX 18–1 | Core Elements of Palliative Care |

- Services are family centered, with the goals and preferences of the patient and family integrated with the support and guidance in decision making by the healthcare team.
- Palliative care ideally begins at the time of diagnosis of a life-threatening or debilitating condition and continues until the child is cured or dies, and into the bereavement period.
- Regular comprehensive assessments are performed to help patients and families understand changes in condition and how those changes affect care goals and future treatment.
- An interdisciplinary care team provides palliative care, and includes physicians, nurses, psychologists, pharmacists, chaplains, social workers, child life therapists, and other needed health professionals. Service coordination is important so that palliative care is provided in all healthcare settings and in the home. Physical symptom management is an important focus, such as relief of pain and suffering (emotional as well as physical symptoms from the condition).
- Effective communication strategies are used to help the child and family develop care goals and make healthcare decisions.
- The healthcare team needs to be skilled in the care of the dying child and bereaved family.
- Palliative care should be provided in all healthcare delivery settings and be accessible to all children in need of services.
- Evaluation of the care processes and outcomes should be performed to promote high-quality care.

Source: *Adapted from National Consensus Project for Quality Palliative Care. (2009). Clinical practice guidelines for quality palliative care (2nd ed., pp. 9–10). Retrieved from http://www.nationalconsensusproject.org*

Consensus Project for Quality Palliative Care, 2009). See Box 18–1 for core elements of palliative care.

The population that could be appropriately targeted for palliative care includes children who die each year due to life-threatening conditions not associated with injury (73% of all pediatric deaths) (Friebert, 2009). Palliative care may occur in the home, hospital, or other facility. Palliative care is appropriate for children receiving curative and life-prolonging care, as well as those transitioning to end-of-life care. Examples of palliative-care cases include cancer, severe congenital heart defects, severe forms of osteogenesis imperfecta, HIV infection, and certain chromosomal disorders. Palliative care is also an option for very preterm neonates and for children with lethal genetic anomalies. Children may require these services for many years.

Barriers to providing effective pediatric palliative care may be attitudinal, educational, institutional, regulatory, or financial factors. In some cases, health professionals feel that palliative care is the same as end-of-life care, rather than a care strategy that should be implemented along with curative care. Many barriers to palliative care exist, and different barriers may be perceived by physicians and nurses, or by healthcare professionals working in different clinical settings. See Evidence-Based Practice: Identifying Barriers to Pediatric End-of-Life Care.

Nurses work in collaboration with the healthcare team to improve palliative care for children. Nursing roles include the following actions (Foster, Lafond, Reggio, et al., 2010):

- Plan nursing care for children with life-threatening medical conditions and their families that matches the child's physical, cognitive, emotional, and spiritual level of development.
- Help families regain control in their lives by actions such as encouraging the child to attend school, having siblings visit the child in the hospital, maintaining discipline for the ill child and siblings, and considering the use of family medical leave from work.
- Provide adequate resources so the family can effectively participate in the decision-making process. Reassure the parents

Evidence-Based Practice   Identifying Barriers to Pediatric End-of-Life Care

PROBLEM
A large majority of children who die due to life-limiting conditions die in the hospital setting, often in the pediatric intensive care unit (PICU). Palliative care is an important feature of care, but many barriers still limit the provision of quality end-of-life care in the hospital setting. The perspectives of nurses are important, so strategies for improving palliative care at the end of life can be identified.

EVIDENCE
Barriers to palliative care for children perceived by 240 physicians and nurses in a large children's hospital was the focus of a survey study. Respondents selected between 26 potential barriers, and the four most common barriers identified were uncertain prognosis, family not ready to acknowledge an incurable condition, language barriers, and time constraints. Physicians were more likely than nurses to select cultural differences and conflict among family and staff members as barriers to palliative care. Nurses were more likely than physicians to note the lack of a palliative care team as a barrier. Providers not based in an intensive care unit (ICU) more frequently identified time constraints, staff shortages, and parental discomfort with withdrawal of nutrition and hydration as barriers compared to ICU providers (Davies, Sehring, Partridge, et al., 2008).

A survey was conducted with a national sample of 985 PICU nurses to identify their perceptions of barriers and supportive behaviors for end-of-life care. The greatest obstacles reported by the 474 respondents were language barriers, parental discomfort with withdrawal of mechanical ventilation, lack of communication between the interdisciplinary team leading to discontinuity in the child's care, and the lack of value perceived by the nurse regarding his or her opinion about the

direction of the patient's care. A supportive behavior prior to the child's death was having the child's code status clearly described in the medical record (Beckstrand, Rawle, Callister, et al., 2010).

A survey of 410 nurses working at a large children's hospital investigated issues regarding palliative care. Higher hours of palliative care education were significantly related to less difficulty in talking about death and dying with children and their families (Freudtner, Santucci, Feinstein, et al., 2007).

IMPLICATIONS
In each of the studies, language or communication challenges were significant barriers to the provision of palliative or end-of-life care. Communication is important between all members of the healthcare team to promote collaboration on the care plan and to ensure that consistent information is communicated to the parents. Making sure that family members hear the same message about the child's prognosis increases trust and reduces any confusion they may have regarding their child's status. Many healthcare providers have difficulty talking with families and children who are dying. Nurses should receive palliative care education to decrease the difficulty associated with talking about death and dying to children and families.

CRITICAL THINKING APPLICATION
Carefully plan an interaction with the family of a child who is dying so that the communication process will be effective. Identify the key points that should be included in the interaction and appropriate behaviors of the participating healthcare professionals.

that whatever decisions they choose to make, they are the right ones for them.

- Provide honest answers to questions asked by the ill child and his or her siblings.
- Encourage families to spend and cherish time with each other. Parents should also spend time alone, with each other, and with their healthy children.
- Consider ways that the healthy siblings could be involved in care of the ill child to reduce the sibling's loneliness or isolation. Make sure the sibling is informed about the child's changes in health status and goals of care.

Advance Care Planning

Advance care planning for a child's death is important as it becomes apparent that there is no realistic chance for cure and that death will occur in the near future. Initiating an advance care process is beneficial for parents and healthcare providers. The advance care planning process supports parents' values and improves their perceptions of good quality care. Parents need clear and accurate information about the child's prognosis to make decisions about treatment options and end-of-life care. For example, parents of children with cancer should be involved in decision making about the following emotional and difficult issues (Baker, Hinds, Spunt, et al., 2008):

- To pursue more chemotherapy versus discontinue disease-directed treatment
- To choose phase I research therapy versus no cancer treatment
- To maintain or withdraw life support
- To adopt a do-not-resuscitate order

Healthcare providers should help the family by describing the expected changes in the child's functional ability and quality of life as the disease progresses. One of the more significant challenges is determining when the child's condition reaches the point at which a decision is needed to shift from aggressive curative therapy to symptom-centered comfort care.

Adolescents should participate in any advance planning discussions (see Legal and Ethical Considerations: The Patient Self-Determination Act). Their experiences with a serious medical condition give them a better understanding of death than their peers (Christenson, Lybrand, Hubbard, et al., 2010). Because of the adolescent's desire for autonomy, information about all choices should be provided. When engaged in advance care planning, the adolescent may express a desire to refuse treatment or request withdrawal of treatment. Open and honest discussion with the adolescent can help parents and the healthcare team to determine if he or she fully understands the implications of terminating curative therapy. If the intent is to avoid more painful procedures, the adolescent should be informed about options for pain relief. However, the adolescent may have reached the acceptance stage in the grieving process and is ready for death to occur. Once parents are satisfied that the adolescent has reached a resolution based on facts, it may be easier for the parents to support and respect the adolescent's wishes.

Hospice Care

Hospice is a philosophy of care for a terminally ill child that is focused exclusively on comfort and ensuring that the remaining time for the child is lived as comfortably and fully as possible. An estimated

Legal and Ethical Considerations
The Patient Self-Determination Act

The Patient Self-Determination Act of 1990 (PSDA) supports the rights of persons 18 years of age or older to make decisions about their medical care. Although many adolescents younger than 18 have the cognitive skills necessary for decision making and are involved in decisions concerning their care, the PSDA limits their legal rights. Creative strategies are needed to develop a model of decision-making rights and responsibilities for adolescents that is built on the PSDA and shared with parents who ultimately will be responsible for decisions on care.

5,000 children in their last 6 months of life could potentially benefit from hospice care on any given day (Friebert, 2009). The child who is terminally ill is maintained as alert as possible without pain, and the family is provided with choices about health care and death with dignity (Clemens, Jaspers, & Klaschik, 2009). Hospice care may be provided in the home, in the hospital, or in a freestanding facility. Families and children receive emotional, spiritual, and medical support from the care team that may include nurses, physicians, religious and faith leaders, social workers, and mental health professionals.

For hospice care to be successful, the child and family, as well as the child's physician, must perceive hospice as a desirable choice. Discussions during advance care planning may ease the way to acceptance of hospice, or aggressive comfort treatment, a term that may be more acceptable to the family. The family may require assistance to view hospice care as an opportunity to focus on the time left with the child. In pediatric hospice, the family learns to focus on the quality of life by keeping communication open between the child and family members. Hospice care or aggressive comfort treatment helps identify the activities that enable the child and family to say their good-byes while choosing how to leave memories. Fears and anxiety about the dying process are addressed. The overall approach is to promote a peaceful death.

For the child who will receive palliative and/or hospice care, the family and healthcare providers collaborate to determine which treatments are appropriate to continue with the child's end-of-life care. These treatments may include total parenteral nutrition (TPN), intravenous fluids, gastric or nasogastric tube feedings, and certain medications. Nurses participate on a multidisciplinary healthcare team to provide comprehensive care to the dying child and the family. Health plan coverage for pediatric palliative/hospice care services or alternative financial assistance is investigated. Hospice also offers assurance that following the death of their child, parents will not have to face their grief alone as counseling and support are provided for 1 year following the death of the child.

Parents may choose hospice home care for their terminal newborn or infant. This provides the infant and family the opportunity to spend time together unencumbered by technical equipment and the presence of strangers. Nurses can encourage the bonding process by allowing the parents to dress the infant, introduce the infant to siblings, and take photographs with the infant as part of the family unit. Special considerations for this family are necessary since they are experiencing the child's entire life cycle in a short duration.

Ethical Issues Surrounding a Child's Death

Because a child's death is so emotionally charged, potential misunderstandings and conflicts can develop between families and healthcare providers. The more common ethical issues that need to be addressed include withdrawal of or withholding treatment, parental treatment refusal, and do-not-resuscitate orders. See Chapter 1 🔗 for ethical decision-making principles and terminology.

Withdrawing or Withholding Treatment

The decision to withdraw or withhold life-sustaining treatments, such as mechanical ventilation or dialysis, from the dying infant or child is extremely difficult and highly emotional for the parents. Some parents misunderstand and believe that withdrawing treatment means that all care is discontinued. Some parents feel that the decision to discontinue aggressive treatment is a form of abandonment, and it may lead them to feel as though they chose the day their child would die (Beckstrand, Rawle, Callister, et al., 2010). Treatments may be withdrawn if the child's outcome is inevitable death and continuation of the treatment causes more suffering than benefit or prolongs the dying process. However, aggressive comfort measures should be provided to the child, including pain medication.

The decision to withhold medically provided nutrition and hydration (through nasogastric or gastrostomy tubes and intravenous catheters) from infants and children is controversial because their provision is associated with nurturing and love. However, they may be withheld in certain cases when food and fluids are of no benefit to the child. An ethics committee should review these cases (Diekema, Botkin, & the Committee on Bioethics, 2009).

Clinical Tip

Care must be used in how parents are asked to withdraw or forgo therapies. An effective communication strategy is to inform parents that an intervention was initiated to give the child the best chance at recovery, but it has not been effective and is not beneficial for the child. When asking to withhold therapy such as cardiopulmonary resuscitation, it is helpful to indicate that the therapy is not effective in reversing overwhelming illness, brain damage, or multiple organ failure (Levetown & the Committee on Bioethics, 2008).

The nurse may feel conflicted when parents and physicians are unable to discontinue aggressive therapies that the nurse feels are extending the child's suffering. Consultation with the hospital ethics committee can help clarify issues involved and reduce the emotions associated with the conflict. During the consultation an unbiased professional collects facts about the child's condition, clarifies the beliefs and values of parents and health professionals, and improves communication while investigating options for compromise.

Conflicts Regarding Parental Refusal of Treatment

Parents and healthcare providers sometimes disagree over what, if any, medical interventions should be provided when the child is dying. Parents may refuse treatments based on religious convictions or because they wish to avoid certain interventions that are unacceptable to them, but they may still want other aggressive care interventions (Duhon & Moazam, 2008; O'Mathúna & Lang, 2008). Initiating highly technical, but possibly futile, interventions may cause emotional and financial stress that can overwhelm young parents.

Consultation with the hospital's ethics committee should also be obtained to help resolve the conflict. The healthcare team requests to have a surrogate legal guardian appointed in certain situations when recommended care is refused. The conflict sometimes makes it difficult for the nurse to have a supportive relationship with the parents, but the nurse should demonstrate proper concern and care of the child in these cases.

Do-Not-Resuscitate Orders

Parents faced with a child's inevitable death as a result of a terminal illness or condition may be asked by a physician to consider a **do-not-resuscitate (DNR) order,** choosing not to have cardiopulmonary resuscitation (CPR) performed or to take other lifesaving interventions for a child who stops breathing. Terms becoming more common are **allow natural death (AND)** and **comfort care,** which involves the continuation of ongoing care, managing pain, and choosing not to initiate CPR if the child stops breathing or the heart stops beating (Box 18–2). For children with end-stage, irreversible life-limiting conditions, the family and healthcare providers must decide if a resuscitation attempt would be in the child's best interest. Factors influencing the decision for a DNR or AND status include allowing the child to die with dignity, and the possibility of causing more harm and suffering if resuscitative measures are implemented. Parents require ongoing support as they may feel they are "giving up" on their child.

When faced with the decision of requesting a DNR or AND for a child, the family requires honest information. It is essential that the family understands that the child will continue to receive palliative care or interventions such as oxygen, suctioning, pain control, and supportive nursing care in the presence of a DNR or AND order. If a child with a DNR order requires anesthesia or surgery, a discussion about maintaining or suspending the DNR order should occur when obtaining informed consent for the procedure.

School considerations The Americans with Disabilities Act of 1990 and the Education for All Handicapped Children Act mandate that all children with disabilities—including those with complex chronic conditions and terminal illnesses—are entitled to the same education as other students. Children with a chronic or terminal illness may be at high risk of dying while at school. School officials have many concerns about accepting a DNR order, including the effect of the student's death on classmates, liability issues, and the potential misinterpretation of the DNR order for an emergency such as choking. Parents may not want their healthy children exposed to death in a classroom or other school setting. The majority of large school districts (80%) and school districts in 31 state capitals do not have policies, regulations, or protocols for dealing with a student's DNR order. However, 46% of schools have health staff that follow DNR orders (Council on School Health & the Committee on Bioethics, 2010).

The best approach for handling DNR requests at school is collaboration between the child, family, nurse and other healthcare providers, school officials, and social workers or other personnel with knowledge or expertise in DNR requests at school. In some cases, the child's individual school health plan may include a DNR statement as well as a list of the care that should be provided if the child develops breathing difficulty.

BOX 18–2	Research: Discussing End of Life

A study investigating the beliefs about the term "allow natural death" among 118 healthcare professionals within a pediatric hospital found that some clarification was needed between the terms "allow natural death" and "withdrawal of care." However, the term "allow natural death" was found to promote ease in approaching family members for an end-of-life discussion (Jones, Parker-Raley, Higgerson, et al., 2008).

Euthanasia

Euthanasia is the action taken with the sole intent of ending a patient's life. The American Nurses Association (ANA) position statement on providing care at the end of life states that euthanasia is illegal and unethical for nurses. However, assistance with dying is an appropriate nursing role, much like palliative care; it involves the relief of physical and emotional suffering during the dying process (American Nurses Association, 2010). The ANA emphasizes the nurse's obligation to provide timely, humane, comprehensive, and compassionate end-of-life care.

END-OF-LIFE NURSING CARE FOR THE CHILD WHO IS DYING

Care of the child who is dying and the family presents one of the greatest challenges to the nurse, requiring the utmost sensitivity and compassion. An understanding of the dying child's experiences during each developmental stage can assist the nurse in delivering individualized care to the child. See Table 18–2. Children as young as 5 years of age can sense when they are seriously ill. A child's awareness of death develops more rapidly when he or she is experiencing the progression of a disease and related medical treatment. Children with life-threatening illnesses often learn about death and their own illness from exposure to other children who are seriously ill and dying during hospitalization or clinic visits.

Awareness of Dying by Developmental Age

Infants and toddlers are not actually aware of death; they are aware of and react to changes in normal routines and parental nonverbal communication. Toddlers may know they "feel bad" but do not understand that their physical symptoms are associated with impending death (Figure 18–3 ■).

Preschool children can see their bodies deteriorate and feel the effects of medications used during disease progression and treatment. Changes in self-concept occur as they perceive these body changes. The preschool child often describes illness in terms of mutilation to the body. The child may realize that he or she is dying because of these physical changes, as well as the reactions of parents and hospital staff.

School-age children also have subtle fears about body integrity and anxieties related to the serious nature of their illness. This greater preoccupation with illness is considered by many professionals as the child's version of **death anxiety,** a feeling of apprehension or fear of death. Children may express death anxiety as a concern with treatments that invade the body or interfere with normal body functions.

Adolescents have a mature understanding of death, but the normal developmental milestones of adolescence add to their challenges in facing a terminal illness. They are struggling to establish their own identity and plans for the future. At a time when body image is extremely important, they may be faced with the possibility of mutilation and disfigurement. Adolescents who are dying are often isolated from their peers during a period when peers are the most essential social group. Adolescents with terminal illnesses may be angry because they recognize their loss at a time when the whole world is opening up to them.

Do not expect adolescents to handle feelings in the same way as adults. They often avoid expressing anger against the family by seeking to control and direct these feelings elsewhere. Adolescents often

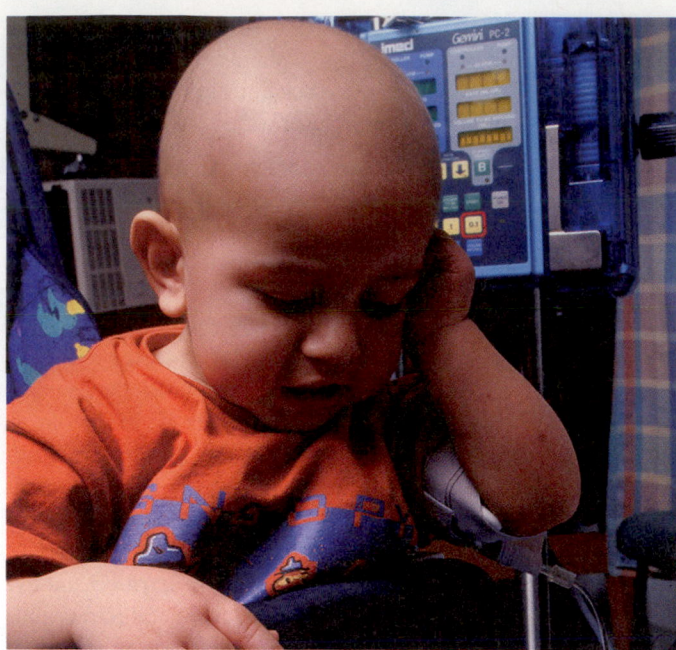

FIGURE 18–3 ■ The toddler with a life-threatening disorder recognizes that he feels bad and that routines are different. His anxiety may increase due to the concern and feelings of sadness exhibited by his parents.

become angry at changes in treatment procedures, lack of explanations, and threats to their independence. As death nears, the adolescent may permit comforting and support and may accept care from warm and loving family members, as long as he or she is not treated condescendingly.

Nursing Management

Nursing care of the dying child and family focuses on providing family-centered support for the physical and psychosocial needs of the child and family members.

Nursing Assessment and Diagnosis

Nursing assessment of the dying child and family includes a physiologic assessment of the child and a psychosocial assessment of all family members, an assessment of cultural and spiritual influences on the child and individual family members, and an assessment of the child and family's social support system.

Physiologic Assessment of the Child Who Is Dying

Assess the child's physiologic status and comfort level. Physiologic changes in the dying child may be directly related to the child's disease process or injury. The signs and symptoms of approaching death are discussed in the Clinical Manifestations table.

Psychosocial Assessment of the Dying Child and Family

Assess the child's awareness of impending death. Examples of questions the child may ask include:

- What will death be like? Will it hurt?
- What will happen to me when I die? What happens after I die?
- Will I be punished for the bad things I have done?
- When will I be with [person(s) closest to child] again?
- Will an angel come to take me away? What does heaven look like?

Clinical Manifestations The Child Who Is Dying

SYSTEM	CLINICAL MANIFESTATIONS
Cardiovascular system (decreased cardiac output and peripheral circulation)	The heart rate may initially increase as hypoxia develops, then the heart rate and blood pressure decrease. A change in pulse pressure and a decrease in the volume of Korotkoff sounds indicate imminent death. Diaphoresis; clammy, cool skin; and changes in skin coloring (mottled to cyanosis) occur. Mottling is a sign of imminent death.
Respiratory system (impaired cardiac function leads to pulmonary congestion)	Tachypnea, diminished breath sounds, and hypoxia occur. Dyspnea may occur; **air hunger,** the most severe form of dyspnea, may cause the child to look panicked, gasp for breath, and sit upright. **Cheyne-Stokes respirations** (periods of shallow breathing alternating with apnea) is a sign of imminent death. As the muscles relax, secretions accumulate in the oropharynx and bronchi, causing noisy breathing as air passes through these secretions. Moaning or grunting with breathing commonly occurs.
Neurologic system (decreased cerebral perfusion, hypoxemia, metabolic acidosis, and accumulation of toxins from renal and liver failure contribute to neurologic dysfunction)	Agitation or restlessness, withdrawal, increasing drowsiness, and confusion may occur. The child may be unconscious during final hours. The child may speak of visions (persons or objects) not visible to others. Hearing and vision acuity may deteriorate, but remember that hearing is considered to be the last of the senses to diminish during death.
Musculoskeletal system	Extreme muscle weakness and fatigue occur. The child may be unable to reposition self and toilet self. Difficulty swallowing occurs. The child may be unable to cough effectively and clear airway secretions.
Renal system (decreased renal function)	Decreased urine production occurs. Parenteral fluids may cause increased edema. Sphincters relax and incontinence can occur.
Gastrointestinal system	Decreased oral fluid intake and anorexia are common. Sphincters relax and bowel incontinence can occur.

BOX 18–3	**Questions to Assess Spiritual Needs and Emotional Resources of the Family**

- Which spiritual rituals and resources have significance to the family?
- Are there any beliefs or cultural practices that bring comfort to the family?
- Should the child's death occur with the immediate family or with an extended family group?
- Where do you (individual family members) get your support?
- What gives you strength and energy?

- Will my parents be all right?
- Can you come with me?
- Will you remember me?

Assess the family for coping skills and the need for social support. Discussions may focus on cultural and spiritual traditions, rituals, and emotional resources related to loss and grieving (Box 18–3). Assess the parents' ability to talk with the child about his or her impending death.

Examples of nursing diagnoses that apply to the dying child and the family include the following:

- Fear (Child) related to unanswered questions and concerns of abandonment
- Anxiety, Death (Child) related to own impending death
- Grieving (Parents) related to imminent death of the child
- Hopelessness (Parental) related to failure of therapies to prolong the child's life

NANDA-I © 2012

Planning and Implementation

Nursing care for the dying child and the family includes providing comfort, assisting the child in a peaceful death, assisting the family and child with coping strategies, and facilitating grief (Figure 18–4 ■). The accompanying Nursing Care Plan provides suggestions for caring for the dying child.

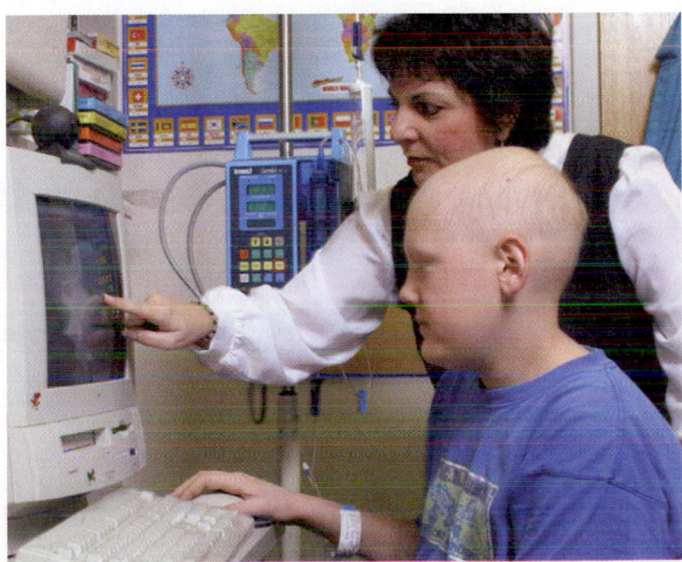

FIGURE 18–4 ■ A child and his mother explore chat rooms for terminally ill children receiving palliative care.

Nursing Care Plan | The Child Who Is Dying

INTERVENTION	RATIONALE	EXPECTED OUTCOME
1. Nursing Diagnosis: Spiritual Distress (Child and Parents) related to the child's impending death		
NIC Priority Intervention— *Spiritual Growth Facilitation:* Facilitation of growth in a patient's capacity to identify, connect with, and call upon the source of meaning, purpose, comfort, strength, and hope in her/his life		**NOC Suggested Outcome**—*Dignified Life Closure:* Personal actions to maintain control and comfort with the approaching end of life
GOAL: *The child and family will interact with a spiritual leader to promote peace and serenity as death approaches.*		
■ Assess the family's cultural, religious, or spiritual beliefs and practices.	■ Assessing beliefs and practices enables the nurse to integrate plans for rituals and support important to the family.	Important ceremonies or rituals associated with death are performed.
■ Ask the family if they would like to have a spiritual leader notified or present.	■ A spiritual leader often provides comfort and enables the family to cope with the death.	Interactions with spiritual leaders promote comfort as evidenced by improved readiness for death.
■ Facilitate the observance of religious, cultural, or spiritual rituals.	■ Some rituals require special permission or need some modification to be safely performed in a hospital setting.	
2. Nursing Diagnosis: Anxiety, Death (Parents) related to the situational crisis of the child's impending death		
NIC Interventions—*Coping Enhancement:* Assisting a patient to adapt to perceived stressors, changes, or threats which interfere with meeting life demands and roles		**NOC Suggested Outcome**—*Acceptance: Health Status:* Reconciliation to significant change in health circumstances
GOAL: *The parents will have reduced anxiety related to remaining with the dying child during the death vigil.*		
■ Provide information to the family about the signs and symptoms of approaching death.	■ Information about expected changes in breathing patterns, consciousness, agitation, ability to swallow, and cool skin reduce anxiety in parents when these changes occur.	Parents will take an active role in caring for the dying child.
■ Encourage parents to invite close family members or friends to share the death vigil.	■ Presence of supportive family and friends reduces parents' feeling of isolation.	Parents seek support of family members or friends during the death vigil.
■ Provide information about the nursing interventions and medications used to keep the child comfortable, and reassure parents that regular assessments of the child's comfort are performed.	■ Parents often fear that the child will have a painful death or that giving the pain medication will cause the child's death.	
■ Provide information about comfort measures parents can provide to the child, such as singing, massage, warm blankets, a cool cloth to the head, praying, or reading.	■ Providing comfort gives the parents an active role in the child's care and a sense of purpose.	
■ Educate the parents about the signs and symptoms of death and what to do if they suspect the child has died.	■ Parents often fear being alone when the child dies and not knowing how to react or what to do.	
3. Nursing Diagnosis: Coping: Family, Disabled related to intense emotional state following the child's death		
NIC Priority Intervention—*Family Support:* Promotion of family values, interests, and goals		**NOC Suggested Outcome**—*Family Coping:* Family actions to manage stressors that tax family resources
GOAL: *The parents will adjust to the death of the child and begin to make funeral or memorial service plans.*		
■ Remove medical supplies, equipment, and tubing from the room. Cover leaking wounds and use a diaper as needed for incontinence.	■ Removing medical supplies helps the family see the child who has died as a loved family member rather than as a patient.	The parents say good-bye to the child and take the next steps in planning a funeral or memorial service.
■ Encourage parents to hold the child, and provide as much time as needed to say good-bye.	■ Providing time will facilitate closure. Time may be needed for other family members to arrive and say good-bye.	

Nursing Care Plan The Child Who Is Dying, continued

INTERVENTION	RATIONALE	EXPECTED OUTCOME
■ Ask the family if they have preferences for the bathing or care of the body or for dressing the child who has died.	■ This honors cultural practices and shows respect for the child and family.	
■ Offer to assist with phone calls to family, friends, and spiritual leaders.	■ Some parents are unable to make needed phone calls immediately and may appreciate assistance.	
■ Assist with decision making for the funeral or memorial service arrangements as needed.	■ Providing options helps promote family choice.	
■ Provide follow-up bereavement support with phone calls and cards. Refer the family to community bereavement resources.	■ Follow-up contact lets the family know that they and the child are not forgotten. An assessment of the need for ongoing bereavement support can be made.	

NANDA-I © 2012

Meeting the Physiologic Needs of the Child

Pain Management

A major goal of care of the dying child is to promote comfort and keep the child pain-free. Opioids may be prescribed and are administered routinely to promote optimal pain relief. For the child who remains alert, delivery of opioids via patient-controlled analgesia (PCA) pump is an option, as this provides the child with some sense of control. Oral, transdermal, or rectal pain medications are also available for families who choose to withhold intravenous fluids. Nurses may also implement complementary therapies for comfort and pain management such as massage, distraction, and guided imagery to children who are able to participate. Parents should be taught to assist with and provide complementary therapies. Refer to Chapter 21 🔗 for detailed discussion of pain management of the child.

Promoting Comfort

If dyspnea or air hunger occurs, place the child in an optimal position for breathing or to maintain the airway. Opening a window or using a circulating fan may help relieve the child's distress. An opioid may be prescribed for air hunger or tachypnea as its action dilates the pulmonary vessels, reduces oxygen consumption, and decreases pulmonary congestion. In some cases, supplemental oxygen or an anxiolytic medication is used. Table 18–6 provides additional information on meeting the physiologic needs of the dying child.

Meeting the Psychologic Needs of the Dying Child and the Family

Promote a trusting nurse–child–family relationship. Be honest in responses to the child and family. Allow opportunities for communication by listening and being present (Box 18–4). The nurse's acceptance of the child's and family's feelings and attitudes helps to promote trust. Demonstrate respect for the child's and family's religion, culture, and values.

Provide the child with opportunities for fantasy play, drawings, and storytelling, without emphasizing or reinforcing death themes. Listen to what children tell you about themselves and their lives. **Death imagery,** references to death or death-related topics (going away, separation, and funerals), or anticipated experiences with treatment may be themes of their stories. These themes are expected and do not reflect repression or other pathology.

Some children who are dying want to leave a legacy so they will be remembered. They can express their good-byes through photography, journals, poetry, writing letters, or music. Some children choose

---

> **BOX 18–4** **Communicating with the Family**
>
> ■ Show compassion and a sense of connection with the child and family members. Be honest and truthful. Encourage and respond to questions.
> ■ Acknowledge the family's emotions and be prepared for tears. Be willing to show your own emotions. Take the time to listen.
> ■ Do not abandon the patient and family. Check with the family periodically to determine if more discussion or support would be helpful.
> ■ Elicit and request the family's values and goals, and provide as much help as possible to achieve them.
> ■ Help patients explore their realistic options. Help them identify persons who will be supportive at this time.
> ■ Be supportive, but avoid offering unrealistic hope.

to make crafts or a memory box for others, or to give away special possessions.

When caring for adolescents, remember that outbursts of anger are common but not personally directed at the nurse. Provide activities to help adolescents channel their feelings. Continue providing support despite their behavior. This approach may encourage adolescents to accept comforting without losing face. Be available to listen when the adolescent wants to talk and express feelings and frustrations. Promote friendships with other adolescents having similar interests or problems. Provide adolescents with as much independence and control over their situation as possible. As described on page 466, include adolescents in the decision-making process and provide them the opportunity to express their feelings, concerns, and wishes.

Wish fulfillment is one way to provide a respite for the family and child from the hospital. Often the entire family, including siblings, participates in the child's wish experience. Children participating in the creation of a wish have the opportunity to make choices and influence decisions. Talking about the experience after the wish is fulfilled may promote opportunities for the family to share their feelings with each other (Ewing, 2009).

Communicating with the Child of His or Her Impending Death

The child who is dying may be aware of impending death even before being told. Many healthcare providers believe it is beneficial to tell the child he or she is dying. When not told he or she is dying, the child may feel isolated and not share his or her thoughts about death. The child may believe that expressing his or her awareness of death

TABLE 18–6	Nursing Care for the Child at the End of Life
PHYSIOLOGIC NEED	**NURSING MANAGEMENT**
Airway clearance	Elevate the head of the bed for the conscious child to promote airway clearance.
	Place the unconscious child in side-lying position to promote airway clearance.
	Suction oral and throat secretions as needed. Scopolamine drops or a patch may be used to help dry up secretions.
	Maintain oxygen as indicated for hypoxia.
Skin and hygiene care	Bathe the perspiring child frequently and change bed linens as needed.
	Provide frequent oral care for dry mouth.
	Apply lotions and creams for dry or itching skin (encourage parents to participate).
	Apply moisture barrier skin preparations for incontinence.
Elimination	Encourage dietary fiber intake as tolerated to avoid constipation.
	Administer stool softeners or laxatives as indicated, especially when opioids are prescribed because constipation is a side effect.
	Provide a call light within reach for assistance onto the bedpan or commode.
	Ensure that the bedpan, urinal, or commode chair is within easy access.
	Place absorbent pads under the child who is incontinent; change linen as often as indicated.
	Perform catheterization if necessary.
	Maintain a clean and odor-free room.
Nutrition	Administer antiemetics for vomiting so that the child may still be able to eat.
	Encourage liquid foods as tolerated.
	Provide the child with preferred foods, including the child's favorite foods from home.
	Encourage family participation at mealtime.
Fatigue/sleep	Prioritize activities of daily living to reduce unnecessary activities.
	Plan rest periods and social interactions to maximize the child's energy for visitors.
	Reduce sleep disruptions.
Physical mobility	Reposition the child on bed rest at frequent intervals (every 2 hours or as indicated) as the child may be too fatigued to move.
	Support the child's position with pillows, blanket rolls, or towels as needed.
	Use pressure-relieving surfaces as indicated.
	If the child is able to sit in a chair, assist the child out of bed periodically.
Sensory	Reduce the frequency of monitoring the child's blood pressure and heart rate.
	Ask the alert child about his or her preference for room lighting.
	Reduce the intrusion of hospital noise and unnecessary personnel in the patient's room.
	Decrease excessive stimulation to reduce restlessness, agitation, or confusion.

and related fears will place an added emotional burden on family members.

Clinical Judgment
What themes might a child have in art or conversations that indicate an awareness that he or she is dying?

Parents may prefer to protect the child from bad news and not talk to the child about his or her serious illness and potential death. Parents may feel incapable of dealing directly with the child's questions about dying. They may feel that talking about the impending death will take away the child's hope. Offer to set up a meeting with the parents and the healthcare team to discuss their fears and concerns about telling their child the truth. Explain that the child needs to trust his or her parents and healthcare providers.

Other parents take on the responsibility to have a discussion with their child. When the family is ready, assist them in role-playing or possible words they can use to talk with their child about his or her death at a developmentally appropriate level (Box 18–5). Emphasize

to the parents that the child may actually need to hear the word *dying* in order to understand. The child needs to know he or she will always be loved and remembered.

Some parents may prefer that the child's questions be answered honestly by a member of the healthcare team. A professional who has special bereavement counseling training can assist children and families with the discussion. Some older children and adolescents may find it easier to talk about death with a friend or a nurse with whom there is a close relationship rather than their parents.

Family Support as the Child Dies
Parents need to be present when possible during the child's actual dying as it is a pivotal event in their parent–child relationship. Some parents choose to be present during resuscitation and other invasive procedures (see Chapter 17 🔗). Parents also prefer to have a familiar nurse provide the care as the child is dying. They wish to contribute positively to their child's death, even if to provide the child a peaceful and comfortable death.

Work closely with the family when the child's death is imminent, because they will remember the experience and words spoken for

BOX 18–5

Strategies for Communicating with the Child Who Is Dying

- Look for opportunities to talk with the child, such as when the child's physical health or behavior is changing (disruptive behavior, withdrawal, anger, hyperalert state, sleeping more than usual). Be receptive when the child initiates a conversation.
- Assess how much the child knows and how much the child wants to know. Identify information that is misunderstood and provide correct information. Be honest with the child when a clear question is asked.
- Recognize that children may not want to share their fears with their parents. A question such as "What are you most worried about?" may start the conversation. Allow the child to express his or her feelings and to be upset. Empathize with the child's feelings.
- Reassure the child that you will be available to listen and give support. Ask the child what is most important to him or her with the time remaining.
- Allow the child to communicate through nonverbal means, such as art, music, and writing.
- Acknowledge that the child's life can be complete, even if it is short. Let dying children know they will always be loved and remembered.
- If the child is old enough to participate in treatment decisions, a conversation about choices provides an opportunity for the child to gain information and empowers him or her in relation to circumstances concerning his or her own death.

Source: Data from Evan, E. E., & Cohen, H. J. (2011). Child relationships. In J. Wolfe, P. S. Hinds, & B. M. Sourkes, Textbook of interdisciplinary pediatric palliative care (pp. 125–134). Philadelphia: Elsevier Saunders; Dunlap, S. (2008). The dying child: Should we tell the truth? Pediatric Nursing, 20 (6), 28–31; Kersun, L. S., & Shemesh, E. (2007). Depression and anxiety in children at the end of life. Pediatric Clinics of North America, 54, 691–708; McSherry, M., Carroll, J. M., & Rourke, M. T. (2007). Psychosocial and spiritual needs of children living with a life limiting illness. Pediatric Clinics of North America, 54, 609–629.

the rest of their lives. Prepare the family for changes in the child's appearance and behavior. Providing parents with a room in which to be alone with the child ensures privacy at this extremely personal time. If the child is in the PICU, using an isolation room may help promote an environment that is calm and serene with lowered lighting and reduced noise (Box 18–6).

Ask the family in a nonjudgmental, supportive manner what is important to them in the last moments or hours of their child's life and what will be important to them in the grief process. Holding the child is a universal request and is always permitted, along with touching, stroking, kissing, and talking soothingly. The family can also be encouraged to lie in the bed and "snuggle" with the dying child. This offers support and comfort to both the child and family. Encourage parents to maintain their parental role by continuing with caregiving activities such as bathing or dressing the child for the last time.

Some parents may feel they need to give the child "permission" to die by telling the child "mommy and daddy are going to be all right," or some other phrase that communicates this message to the child. Many families find that saying good-bye as a group is helpful. Families need the opportunity to cry together and to tell each other how much they will miss each other. Assure them that the death vigil is important, so

the child does not feel isolated or abandoned as death approaches. The dying child should never be left alone when death is imminent.

Clinical Tip
When the child's death is imminent and parents need a short break for a meal or shower, arrange for another family member or close person to remain with the child. If no one is available, a nurse (or other member of the healthcare team with whom the child is familiar) should remain present to ensure that the child does not die alone.

Promote Spiritual and Cultural Needs
The nurse discusses the family's spiritual needs and arranges access to a chaplain, priest, rabbi, or other spiritual leader who can help reduce a child's spiritual fears and promote peace and comfort among family members. The nurse should ask the family about specific cultural and faith beliefs and practices, and facilitate requests, such as baptism of a newborn. Special rites or ceremonies may be requested and should be accommodated when possible. See Developing Cultural Competence: Hmong Rites.

The nurse partners with the family to determine their spiritual and cultural preferences related to rituals following the child's death. It is important for the nurse to determine who will be responsible for carrying out the activities. For example, cultural rituals may include special procedures for washing, dressing, shrouding, and positioning the dead. Some families may choose to have music, while others may use Reiki (a Japanese practice) or chants. Identify which family member will perform the cultural rituals. Refer to Chapter 3 for further discussion of cultural influences on the child and family.

Tissue and Organ Donation
Hospitals that receive reimbursement for care from Medicaid and Medicare are required to refer potential organ donors to their local organ procurement organization (OPO) in a timely manner (Committee on Hospital Care, Section on Surgery, & Section on Critical Care, 2010). Healthcare workers are thus expected to inform the family of potential donors about the option of making an anatomic gift. Nurses can best serve the family of the dying child who could be a potential donor, as well as potential organ recipients, by becoming familiar with national guidelines for organ collection and donation.

Information about organ and tissue donation is discussed in a sensitive manner by identifying the family's needs, beliefs, and desires regarding organ donation. Most facilities have personnel trained in identifying and coordinating the appropriate time to discuss organ and tissue donation, often while brain death testing is occurring or when withdrawal of life support is being discussed with the family. Generally, an OPO coordinator will work in collaboration with the healthcare team to help explain the process of organ donation, but also to assure the family that the organ donation process is separate from the decisions regarding care provided to their child. The OPO

BOX 18–6

Research: Settings for End-of-Life Care
Families need supportive environments during the end-of-life vigils with their child. Environmental needs include privacy, access to the child, adequate space for family members, control of sensory stimuli (lighting, noise, and odors), cleanliness, safety, facilities to care for themselves, and the physical presence of persons who provide professional and personal support (Meert, Briller, Schim, et al., 2008).

Developing Cultural Competence
Hmong Rites
Many culturally influenced rules and customs surround dying. For instance, the Hmong belief system holds that children will live in eternity in the same state in which they existed at the time of death. Therefore, it is important the child's body remain intact at death.

coordinator has an important role in providing family support during the donation process and long-term follow-up of the donor family, along with other members of the healthcare team. The cost of organ donation is paid by the OPO, but recipients pay transplantation costs. Most organ donations are made after declaration of brain death, but in some cases it occurs following cardiac death.

Postmortem Care

Offer ongoing support after the child dies. Questions like the following may help begin the conversation: "I'm sorry for your loss. How can I help?" "What are your traditions when an infant or child dies?" "Is there someone I can call for you?"

Clinical Tip

Although crying with families was once considered unprofessional to some, it is now recognized as an expression of caring and empathy. Nurses should feel free to express their sorrow and grief for the child and family.

The nurse should ask about the family's wishes for postmortem care before performing any care. Ask before removing any jewelry or other item from the child because cultural and spiritual practices may specify that an article remain on the child after death. The nurse should follow the healthcare facility's guidelines for postmortem care. The child should be positioned according to guidelines or cultural/religious practices, the room should be cleaned, and medical equipment should be removed.

Practice Alert

In cases of a sudden violence-related death of a child or adolescent, collection of forensic evidence is required. Removal of medical equipment may not be permitted. Follow facility guidelines for collection of evidence and the chain of possession prior to giving evidence to law enforcement authorities. The family may not be permitted to have as much physical contact with the child's body in these circumstances.

Concerning postmortem care of an infant, wrap the baby in a blanket and offer the mother and other family members the opportunity to hold and rock the baby. If the baby is disfigured, clothe or wrap the baby in a manner that optimizes his or her best physical characteristics. However, many parents may not be as focused on disfigurement and see beauty in their infant. Parents may wish to dress the baby in a special outfit or blanket. Encourage the parents to name their baby. Some mothers may avoid a mother–child relationship and refuse to provide care or hold their dead or dying newborn.

After the child's death, allow the family to spend as much time as they need with the child's body. Never rush family members who are saying good-bye to the child.

Save all of the child's personal items—especially in the case of an infant, whose parents may have few mementos. A lock of hair from the back of the head; a handprint, hand outline, or hand mold; a footprint; the identification band; and the child's weight and height should be collected (Figure 18–5 ■). If grandparents are present, they might also appreciate a set of mementos. Ask for permission before cutting a lock of hair as some cultural and religious groups prohibit it. The last clothes or patient gown worn by the child and blanket used by the infant should be sealed in a plastic bag to retain the child's scent. Use a special remembrance box or container for the child's possessions, as it may be traumatic for the family to receive them. If parents refuse to take the mementos, provide them to another family

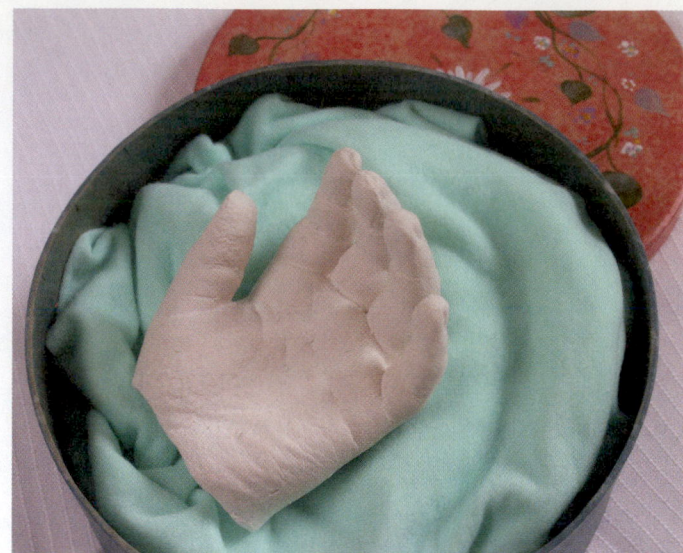

FIGURE 18–5 ■ Nurses can provide families with a memento of the child who dies by creating a plaster cast of the child's hand, or a hand or foot print.

member or retain them. Document the collection of the mementos and who received them in case parents ask for them at a later time.

Autopsy

When the exact cause of death is not clear, an autopsy may be suggested. In the event of an unnatural death, such as suicide or homicide, an autopsy is required by state law. Other situations requiring an autopsy may include the sudden death of an infant or child previously considered healthy, an acute illness resulting in death, and cases of suspected abuse. Because the decision to conduct an autopsy in these situations is not a choice made by parents, the family requires support as they may feel they have relinquished control over their child's body.

Parents may be hesitant to consent to an autopsy because they are uneasy with the prospect of their child's body being further invaded. The family is informed that the autopsy will likely reveal the cause of death, which is especially important if the cause of death is related to a genetic disorder and may affect future childbearing decisions. The findings of the autopsy may help the parents with any guilt by reassuring them of the inevitability of death. Support the family during this decision-making process.

Bereavement Support

A bereavement folder should be provided to parents containing helpful information that includes resources available to help with a memorial service or funeral and potential sibling responses. Include grief counseling resources and encourage the family to use them for the first year after the death. A list of appropriate support groups, books, and articles can be given to parents for later use. Parents can be referred to national organizations, such as the Candlelighters Foundation or Compassionate Friends, and to local support groups for bereaved parents or siblings who may feel isolated and alone. See additional information related to bereavement support on the companion website.

Some healthcare facilities have formal perinatal and pediatric follow-up programs for bereaved parents to encourage a healthy progression through the grieving process. Follow-up occurs at designated time points, such as at 1 month, 3 months, 6 months, the child's birthday, and the anniversary of the child's death. Nurses who were closest to the family often perform the follow-up so that the follow-up is meaningful.

Evaluation

Expected outcomes of caring for the dying child and family may include the following:

- The child is comfortable and pain-free with physiologic needs met.
- The cultural and spiritual needs of the family are met.
- The child and family feel supported during the dying process.
- The nurse gives continued family support after the child's death.

FAMILY CARE AFTER THE DEATH OF A CHILD

Children who die in the hospital have several paths to their deaths, including the following (Hurwitz, Lewandowski, & Hilden, 2009):

- Sudden unexpected death (e.g., sudden infant death syndrome, suicide, septic shock)
- Lethal congenital anomaly (e.g., trisomy 13, anencephaly)
- Potentially curable disease with relapses (e.g., cancer)
- Progressive disease with periodic crises before death (e.g., muscular dystrophy)

Communicating with Parents When a Child Dies Unexpectedly

While 73% of children and adolescents who die each year have a chronic illness or a terminal condition, approximately 27% die suddenly as a result of injury (Friebert, 2009). A sudden or unexpected death, such as one that results from sudden infant death syndrome, injury, illness, suicide, or violence, can place parents at risk for complicated grief (Meert, Donaldson, Newth, et al., 2010). Parents and other family members have not had the opportunity to anticipate the child's death. A child's

suicide produces agonizing anger, guilt, and confusion; the fact that the child ended his or her own life compounds the feelings of guilt because parents may think they missed signs of the child's intentions.

Research indicates that the manner in which parents receive bad news regarding their child's death may influence their ability to cope with the situation, and can have lasting effects. The death of a child should be disclosed in a sensitive manner with compassion and sympathy. A private room in a quiet location is appropriate for discussing the child's death without interruptions or distractions. A physician and nurse who have been directly involved in the child's care and are able to answer the parents' questions are generally the best choice for who should deliver the news. The pagers and cell phones of the physician and nurses participating in the conversation should be placed on vibrate or turned off. Awareness of body language is important for healthcare professionals during the disclosure of the child's death. Eye contact, sitting rather than standing, and providing touch, such as holding a hand or touching an arm, provides the parents with assurance that the focus is on them and their child. Avoid the use of medical jargon; use terms that the family members understand. Frequently evaluate the parents' understanding of what they have been told. Parents should be told everything possible, and uncertainties should be acknowledged. See Partnering with Families: Strategies for Communicating with Parents Whose Child Dies Suddenly.

Family follow-up support is essential to facilitating the family's grief. Especially in the case of an unexpected death, the family may not have understood all of the information provided to them at the time of their child's death. A follow-up visit provides parents the opportunity to ask questions at a later time. If an autopsy has been performed, explaining the results may clarify uncertainties and assist the parents through their grieving process.

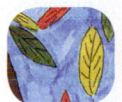

Partnering with Families

Strategies for Communicating with Parents Whose Child Dies Suddenly

The following strategies can assist the nurse in working with parents whose child dies suddenly:

- Identify a family support person or spokesperson for the medical team to keep the family informed during resuscitation efforts.
- Allow as much time as possible for the family to understand the seriousness and worsening of the child's status. Provide several updates during the resuscitation (two or three times over 15 minutes), or allow them to be present during the resuscitation. Prepare them for what is to come.
- Have both parents present if possible for discussions after the death. Have a family support member or friend present for a single parent. Have the discussion in a private place with telephone access.
- The healthcare providers should remove gloves and gowns spattered with blood. All members of the healthcare team should introduce themselves to the family.
- During the discussion, speak plainly and directly about the condition. Use the child's name. Explain any factual details known about what happened at the scene and what was done during the resuscitation. Pause and assess the family's understanding of the information. Allow the family to ask questions.
- Sit close and make eye contact. Notify the family of the child's death, explaining the care provided and that the child's injuries were too severe to survive. Let the family know that everything possible was done to save the child's life. If the child was not in pain or did not suffer, share that information. Share your emotions with the family. Accept whatever emotions the family members express.

- Offer to telephone clergy, family, and friends. Determine how you can help the family at this time.
- After the death, prepare the body for viewing by covering disfiguring wounds and explaining any tubes or lines that must remain because of legal or medical examiner requirements. Escort the family to see the child, and have a healthcare provider stay with the family for some time.
- Provide a time (varies from 15 minutes to 3 hours) and a place for the family to be with the child after death. Sometimes the child and family can be moved to a room with privacy and fewer disruptions. Depending upon cultural preferences, the family may wish to bathe the child or hold and rock the child.
- Convey information to the family about the cause of death, requirements for and value of an autopsy with sudden death, funeral preparations, and the normal grief process. Provide the family with some key information in writing, such as the child's diagnosis, name of the attending physician, and the phone number family may call to ask additional questions.
- Arrange for family follow-up to see how they are responding to the child's loss and to review autopsy findings.

Source: *Data from Levetown, M., & the Committee on Bioethics. (2008). Communicating with children and families: From everyday interactions to skill in conveying distressing information. Pediatrics, 121(5), e1441–e1460; O'Malley, P. J., Brown, K., Krug, S. E., & the Committee on Pediatric Emergency Medicine. (2008). Patient- and family-centered care of children in the emergency department. Pediatrics, 122(2), e511–e521.*

Parents' Reactions to a Child's Death

The death of one's child is likely the most traumatic event a parent will experience. When the loss is sudden and unexpected, the abruptness adds a dimension of shock that may last for 4 to 5 weeks. The shock that accompanies the death of a child may be manifested by shortness of breath, a choking sensation, hollowness in the stomach, hyperventilation, heart palpitations, loss of strength, and crying.

Although parents progress through distinct stages of grief, the timeline and nature of the grief process differ for each individual. The intense pain and shock initially felt by parents gradually give way to feelings of sadness, anger, guilt, depression, and loneliness. Insomnia, fatigue, preoccupation with sleep, and decreased or increased activity level may be experienced during the grieving process. Parents may also experience difficulties in concentration, hallucination experiences, and dreams of the dead child. Parents lose interest in activities that were formerly satisfying. Some parents avoid reminders of the child who has died, and others visit places and cherish objects that remind them of the child (Corr & Coolican, 2010).

Very slowly, and with much support, energy returns and parents again begin to enjoy life experiences. Parents may process grief on different timelines. When spouses experience the stages of grief at different levels or on different timelines, the spouse with more intense grieving may need additional support to prevent a sense of loneliness or isolation.

The Death of a Newborn or Young Infant

In 2009, 26,412 infants died either shortly after birth or during the first year of life (Kochanek, Xu, Murphy, et al., 2011). The death of a newborn forces the parents to experience their child's entire life cycle in a short period, and they are faced with overwhelming grief at a time when they anticipated the experience of joy. The death of a newborn may occur shortly after birth as a result of low birth weight or congenital anomalies, or during the first year of life due to congenital conditions or sudden infant death syndrome (SIDS) (refer to Chapter 25 ✐ for further discussion of SIDS).

In some cases prenatal screening reveals that the fetus has a lethal anomaly, and parents choose to deliver the child rather than terminate the pregnancy. Palliative care is an option for these families so they have the opportunity to be a parent for a short time. Advance care planning regarding initial resuscitation or DNR orders and withholding or withdrawing treatment can be considered (Munson & Leuthner, 2007). The mother experiencing the death of a newborn requires instructions on lactation suppression.

Unique experiences may occur with multiple births, such as the death of one or more of the infants. This can lead to conflicting emotions in the parents. While they grieve about the death of one infant, they must parent and bond with the surviving infant.

Nursing Management

Following the death of a child, parents and families may require ongoing care to assist them in adapting to the loss of the child and dealing with their surviving children. Emphasize to parents that although the period surrounding their child's death is difficult, caring for themselves physically and mentally is important. Parents may experience friction because each may move through the stages of grief at different rates and with different intensity. For example, a father who processes grief by burying himself in work activities may be unable to offer support to a mother experiencing anger or depression. Parents may be unavailable emotionally to their living children, requiring additional family members or close friends to offer support to those children.

Support the family to achieve a positive resolution of the grieving process. Inform parents that certain dates, such as the day of the week the child dies, the child's birthday, or family holidays, will be difficult and may trigger intense sadness. Parents may benefit from keeping a journal of their thoughts and memories, or writing letters or poems to and about their child. It is important to inform grieving parents that although their pain may diminish as time passes, they will revisit the experience repeatedly during their lives. Parents will always have a bond or relationship with the dead child, but some parents may eventually carry forward with a legacy for the child who died, such as a memorial or crusade. See Partnering with Families: Supporting a Healthy Family Grieving Process, and Box 18–7.

Siblings' Reactions to a Child's Death

Siblings who experience the death of a brother or sister require supportive and compassionate care at an appropriate developmental level. Siblings anticipating the addition of a new baby to the family will also feel the loss. In the course of the child's illness, the siblings often have received less attention from parents. Children experiencing the death of a newborn sibling have reported feeling a lack of understanding about the illness, confusion, and anxiety during the dying process, but they also valued opportunities to see or hold the infant (Fanos, Little, & Edwards, 2009). Depending on their stage of development, they may fear that they caused their brother or sister to be injured or become ill, or worry that bad thoughts on their part brought on the illness.

Nurses and other support personnel assist the child in adapting to their parents' grief, distraction, and increased protectiveness of them. Siblings need to hear that their parents' grief in no way diminishes the love they have for them. Recommending a support group for the siblings may also facilitate their bereavement process and let them know they are not alone in experiencing this type of loss. Table 18–2 highlights children's understanding of death at different developmental stages, some of the possible behavioral responses, and nursing considerations for family education.

Nursing Management

When talking with the siblings of a child who is dying, honesty is most important. Children should be provided with information about a newborn sibling's death just as they would for an older sibling's death. Consider the information that Marilee in the opening scenario should be told. Provide explanations in language that is developmentally appropriate. Children have vivid imaginations, so provide information about the child's death in a manner they can understand. Otherwise they may use their imagination to make up their own ideas about what is happening, ideas that may be worse than what actually happened (Hain & Jassal, 2010, p. 239).

Reassure siblings that they did not cause their brother or sister to die (unless they did contribute to the child's death) and that death

---

BOX 18–7	Research: Family Support After Death

A study involving 58 families whose newborn or child died in the prior 12 to 24 months investigated the quality of care provided before, at the time of, and following a child's death. Some priorities for improvement following the child's death included wanting more information about autopsy results, discussions about what happened at the time of death, and a need for follow-up phone calls and information on where to go for counseling. Bereavement support programs may help address these needs (Widger & Picot, 2008).

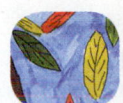

Partnering with Families

Supporting a Healthy Family Grieving Process

Nurses can assist families toward a healthy grieving process after a child's death in the following ways:

- Provide information about the grieving process and explain that grief exerts tremendous stress on even the most loving relationships. Inform families that each person processes grief on his or her own timeline.
- Recommend open lines of communication between parents and bereaved siblings. Encourage parents to show their emotions so young children and adolescents will learn that it is appropriate to share their feelings and to display appropriate grieving behavior.
- Alert parents to the special needs of young children who may feel that they caused the child's death due to their magical thinking.
- Consider having the sibling participate in a bereavement group with other children of a similar age. The sibling may have an opportunity to honestly

talk about his or her feelings and learn more about coping with personal struggles from other children (Davies, Collins, Steele, et al., 2007).

- Advise parents to be watchful for their adolescents' responses to the death and to seek help if any of the following behaviors are noticed: suicidal thoughts or actions, long-standing depression, isolation from friends and family, failing in school or overachieving, major changes in personality or attitude, serious eating problems, use of drugs or alcohol, fighting or criminal behavior, and inappropriate sexual activity (Biddle, Sekula, Zoucha, et al., 2010).
- Explain that many family members and friends may distance themselves because they are uneasy with death and grief.
- Inform families that major holidays, birthdays, and anniversary dates of the child's death may be especially difficult emotional times.

---

was not a punishment for wrongdoing. Allow the siblings to ask questions. Acknowledge the emotions they are feeling and emphasize that it is all right for them to be sad, angry, frightened, or tearful.

The nurse should use the same amount of energy and concern in acknowledging the sibling's grief as in acknowledging the grief of adults. Ask the child how he or she feels about saying good-bye to the dying infant or child, and provide physical and emotional support. Prepare the sibling before seeing the dying brother or sister by briefly explaining what he or she may see, feel, hear, and smell. Answer questions truthfully. The sibling may have to hear the information several times.

Clinical Tip
Young children are likely to ask questions repeatedly, testing to see if the same responses are provided each time. Children need to understand the finality of death—that all body functions have stopped. Simple statements that can be told to children include, "Adam's heart will never beat again," "He will never get cold or hungry," and "He will never come home again."

As appropriate and comfortable for the family, siblings should be permitted to participate in planning the child's memorial or funeral

service. Being able to grieve as a family provides a sense of connection to the parents and provides security at a vulnerable time. If siblings attend the funeral or memorial service, prepare them for what to expect, such as an open casket or the behaviors of mourners. Provide a support person such as a family member or close friend who can monitor the siblings' needs while the parents attend to other matters. Keep the family together as much as possible. Children may ask what happens to their brother's or sister's soul or spirit, and the response to the child is dependent on the family's spiritual and cultural beliefs.

As with their parents, sibling bereavement is a lifelong process. The nurse should encourage parents to make sure other caregivers and teachers know about the sibling's loss. See Partnering with Families: Assisting Children with Grieving.

NURSES' REACTIONS TO CARING FOR THE CHILDREN WHO DIE

Children are highly valued by society because of their potential future contributions. Children are expected to have a normal life span, and the death of a child is often viewed as a tragedy. Caring for children

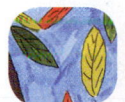

Partnering with Families

Assisting Children with Grieving

Families can help the child express and deal with feelings about the loss of a sibling, parent, or grandparent in a variety of ways. Some examples include the following:

- Children learn to express feelings by watching adults and the way they express feelings. They need to be allowed to grieve with the family. Let children express all feelings, including sadness, guilt, and anger.
- Encourage the child to participate in a support group where stories and feelings can be shared and appreciated by others who have lost a sibling. They learn they are not alone in their thoughts and feelings, and they learn to handle their emotional reactions (Nolbris, Abrahamsson, Hellström, et al., 2010).
- Draw a picture of each family member and show how each person is grieving. An older child could write about how each person is grieving.

- Make a memory garden with favorite flowers and plants.
- Provide a memory object belonging to the deceased or make a keepsake box.
- Create a memory book using art and photos, as well as writing special thoughts and feelings about the family member. A video of the child's life could be developed.
- Allow children to play with toys and act out their feelings.
- Follow suggestions in books that talk about how to help children with grief, such as *It's OK to Cry: A Parent's Guide to Helping Children Through the Losses of Life* by H. Norman Wright, *Helping Children Grieve* by Ruth Arent, or *When Children Grieve* by John James.

who are dying is especially stressful and demanding for healthcare professionals. Nurses caring for the dying child may feel extreme sadness, ambivalence, hopelessness, and pain from watching the overwhelming grief of the parents (Morgan, 2009). They may develop depression and grieve for the loss of the personal relationship with the child (Gerow, Conejo, Alonzo, et al., 2010). Some nurses may cope by distancing themselves socially from the dying child and the family to maintain composure and a professional demeanor and to protect themselves from the pain of repeated loss. These nurses are at risk for compassion fatigue, or *burnout*, which involves feelings of hopelessness, an unwillingness to deal with work, and feeling that one's efforts make no difference.

Caring for the dying child may be especially difficult for nurses with young children of their own. They tend to identify with the child, making it more likely that they will have difficulty dealing with the death in a professional manner. Nurses may not be able to recognize the dying child's anxiety and fears because of their own personal defenses against their sense of helplessness to alter the course of the child's disease.

Nurses who work with children who are terminally ill and their families require special preparation to meet the needs of these individuals and to manage personal stress simultaneously. Mentorship with experienced hospice nurses, as well as additional educational experiences, may help promote professional nursing care. Nurses who work with dying children and their families must learn to cope effectively with grief and to develop empathy, competence, and confidence in their ability to provide more humane and effective nursing care.

Nurses should feel free to express their sorrow and grief for the child and family. Some nurses attend funeral and memorial services when invited by the patient's family or when they personally desire to attend. Attending the services may assist the nurses with their own grieving and promote closure. Additionally, the presence of nurses who provided care to the child may offer the family continued support as this displays a meaningful way of demonstrating their care for the deceased child and the family.

Nurses working in emergency departments caring for children who die suddenly, or in hospice settings and hospital units caring for children who are terminally ill, need support systems to help balance the stresses of working with dying children. The workplace should acknowledge the stress and overwhelming feelings nurses experience when working with children who die. Educational seminars on compassion fatigue may help nurses identify coping strategies for personal care (Meadors & Lamson, 2008). Support systems may include discussions with peers or bereavement debriefing group sessions with mental health professionals that provide an opportunity for nurses and other health professionals to discuss their grief, feelings, and concerns (Figure 18–6 ■). Nurses who participated in one bereavement debriefing program appreciated hearing how other disciplines viewed the child's death from their perspective, and they believed they were better able to manage their grief (Keene, Hutton, Hall, et al., 2010).

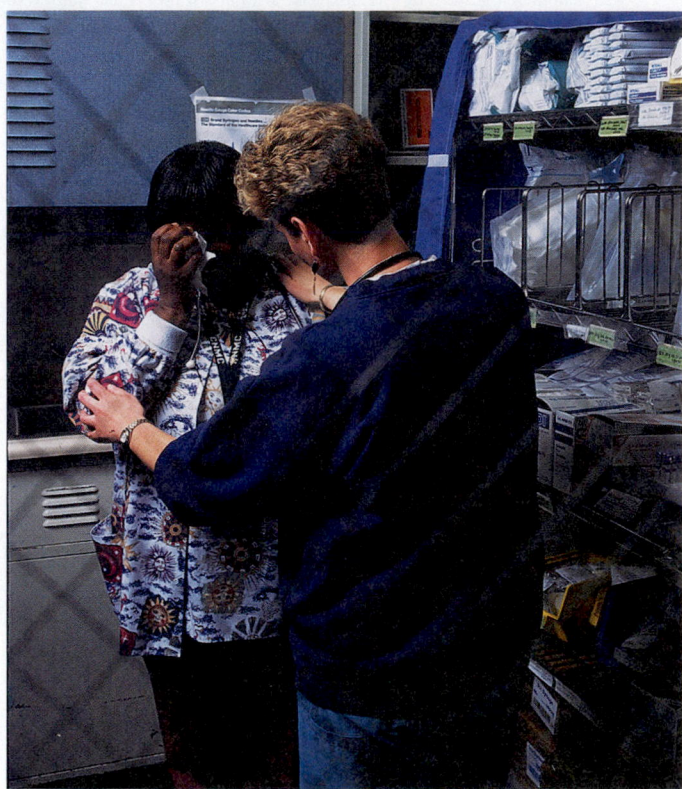

FIGURE 18–6 ■ Nurses need to express their own grief in a supportive environment after a child's death. Sharing the sadness and grief or futility of resuscitation efforts with colleagues can often help nurses continue to provide supportive care to the next families who need compassionate care.

Chapter Highlights

- One commonly accepted definition of death in the United States is brain death, or the irreversible cessation of all functions of the brain, including the cerebral cortex and brainstem.
- Children may experience loss through death of a parent, sibling, grandparent, pet, or friend, and through losses associated with relocation, trauma, and loss of an object.
- The child's developmental level, culture, spirituality, and parental support directly affect the child's response to loss, death, and grief.

- Grief is individualized. Not everyone dealing with a loss will experience all of the stages (denial, anger, bargaining, depression, and acceptance), and individuals who do experience all stages may not experience them in the sequence listed.
- Palliative care is a multidisciplinary care approach to prevent and relieve suffering and to enhance quality of life for patients and their families, regardless of the stage of the disease or the need for other therapies.

- The families of children who are dying face many decision-making issues such as palliative and/or hospice care, advance care planning, the withholding or withdrawal of treatments, and DNR or AND requests.
- Children with life-threatening illnesses often learn about death and their own illness through exposure to other children who are ill and dying. Even if they have not been told they are dying, they will know their condition is worsening with extra treatments, feeling ill, changes to the body, and cues from their parents.
- It is essential to work closely with the family when a child's death is imminent, helping to provide the support and services most important to them in the last moments or hours of their child's life.

- The nurse caring for the child who is dying and the family offers physiologic and psychosocial support during end-of-life care.
- Bereavement support must be provided to the family, making sure that siblings are not overlooked. Allow siblings to participate in planning the memorial service. Encourage parents to allow siblings to express their emotions.
- Caring for a child who is dying is difficult, and nurses need special preparation to meet the needs of the child and family while managing their own personal stress.

Clinical Reasoning in Action

INTRODUCTION

Recall Zachary, the 3-year-old child with an inoperable brain tumor hospitalized and near death. His seizures and dehydration are being treated. He is also receiving morphine for pain. His mother remains at his bedside while his father and other family members visit.

DESCRIPTION

Despite aggressive therapy, Zachary's condition has continued to deteriorate. After consulting with Zachary's healthcare team, the parents agree to discontinue the radiation and aggressive treatment. He will continue to receive antiseizure medications, pain medication, and nutrition. They have requested a DNR order, and the family wishes to have time with Zachary to say good-bye. The parents want guidance to help Zachary's 7-year-old sister Marilee say good-bye.

DISCUSSION

1. What role does the hospital nurse play in facilitating end-of-life care for Zachary?
2. Based on Marilee's developmental level, what is her understanding of Zachary's imminent death? What nursing interventions should be offered to help her say good-bye?
3. What are the physiologic signs indicating that Zachary is approaching death?
4. Develop a family-centered nursing care plan for Zachary's end-of-life care.
5. Develop a family-centered nursing care plan for Zachary's family during end-of-life care.

NCLEX-RN® Review

1. The nurse is planning palliative care for a young child with end-stage liver disease. What should the nurse include in planning care for this child? (Select all that apply.)
   1. Determining whether the family's and child's goals are curative, comfort, or not yet decided.
   2. Helping the family make decisions about medical interventions that are desired.
   3. Identifying the decision makers for the child's health care.
   4. Evaluating the family's understanding of the child's illness and prognosis.
   5. Assisting the family in making funeral arrangements.

2. In developing a plan of family-centered care for a dying child. The nurse should consider which items? (Select all that apply).
   1. Cultural traditions
   2. Financial status
   3. Beliefs related to loss
   4. Coping skills
   5. Spiritual rituals

3. Which is the most appropriate nursing diagnosis for the family of a dying child?
   1. Grieving related to terminal illness
   2. Role Conflict, Parental related to child's hospitalization
   3. Sorrow, Chronic related to child with a terminal illness
   4. Activity Intolerance related to functional changes accompanying the dying process

NANDA-I © 2012

4. A home health nurse needs to make a visit to the home of a child who recently died to close the case. How might the nurse best support this family?
   1. Keep the visit short and businesslike to keep it as painless as possible.
   2. Allow the family to ask questions about the recent events and future expectations.
   3. Ask the family what they have been doing since the child died.
   4. Send another nurse with whom the family is not familiar to keep it impersonal.

See Appendix I ✎ for answers.

References

American Nurses Association. (2010). *Registered nurses' roles and responsibilities in providing expert care and counseling at the end of life.* Retrieved from http://nursingworld.org/MainMenuCategories/EthicsStandards/Ethics-Position-Statements/etpain14426.aspx

Auman, M. J. (2007). Bereavement support for children. *Journal of School Nursing, 23*(1), 34–39.

Baker, J. N., Hinds, P. S., Spunt, S. L., Barfield, R. C., Allen, C., Powel, B. C., . . . Kane, J. R. (2008). Integration of palliative care practices into the ongoing care of children with cancer: Individualized care planning and coordination. *Pediatric Clinics of North America, 55,* 223–250.

Beckstrand, R. L., Rawle, N. L., Callister, L., & Mandleco, B. L. (2010). Pediatric nurses' perceptions of obstacles

and supportive behaviors in end-of-life care. *American Journal of Critical Care, 19*(6), 543–550.

Biddle, V. S., Sekula, L. K., Zoucha, R., & Puskar, K. R. (2010). Identification of suicide risk among rural youth: Implications for the use of HEADSS. *Journal of Pediatric Health Care, 24*(3), 152–167.

Buglass, E. (2010). Grief and bereavement theories. *Nursing Standard, 24*(41), 44–47.

Clemens, K. E., Jaspers, B., & Klaschik, E. (2009). History of hospice. In D. Walsh, A. T. Caraceni, R. Fainsinger, K. Foley, P. Glare, C. Goh, . . . L. Radbruch, *Palliative medicine* (1st ed., pp. 18–22). Philadelphia: Saunders Elsevier.

Christenson, K., Lybrand, S. A., Hubbard, C. R., Hubble, R. A., Ahsens, L., & Black, P. (2010). Including the perspectives of the adolescent in palliative care preferences. *Journal of Pediatric Health Care, 24*(5), 286–291.

Committee on Hospital Care, Section on Surgery, and Section on Critical Care. (2010). Pediatric Organ Donation and Transplantation, *Pediatrics, 125*(4), 822–828.

Corr, C. A., & Coolican, M. B. (2010). Understanding bereavement, grief, and mourning: Implications for donation and transplant professionals. *Progress in Transplantation, 20*(2), 169–177.

Council on School Health & the Committee on Bioethics. (2010). Policy statement—Honoring do-not-attempt-resuscitation requests in schools. *Pediatrics, 125*(5), 1073–1077.

Davies, B., Collins, J., Steele, R., Cook, K., Distler, V., & Brenner, A. (2007). Parents' and children's perspectives of a children's hospice bereavement program. *Journal of Palliative Care, 23*(1), 14–23.

Davies, B., Sehring, S. A., Partridge, J. C., Cooper, B. A., Hughes, A., Philp, J. C., . . . Kramer, R. F. (2008). Barriers to palliative care for children: Perceptions of pediatric health care providers. *Pediatrics, 121*(2), 282–288.

Diekema, D. S., Botkin, J. R., & the Committee on Bioethics. (2009). Clinical report—Forgoing medically provided nutrition and hydration in children. *Pediatrics, 124*(2), 813–822.

Duhon, G., & Moazam, F. (2008). A case study: An uncomfortable refusal. *Hastings Center Report, 38*(5), 15–16.

Dunlap, S. (2008). The dying child: Should we tell the truth? *Pediatric Nursing, 20*(6), 28–31.

Evan, E. E., & Cohen, H. J. (2011). Child relationships. In J. Wolfe, P. S. Hinds, & B. M. Sourkes, *Textbook of interdisciplinary pediatric palliative care* (pp. 125–134). Philadelphia: Elsevier Saunders.

Ewing, B. (2009). Wish fulfillment: Palliative care and end-of-life intervention. *Pediatric Nursing, 35*(2), 81–85.

Fanos, J. H., Little, G. A., & Edwards, W. H. (2009). Candles in the snow: Ritual and memory for siblings of infants who died in the intensive care nursery. *Journal of Pediatrics, 154*(6), 849–853.

Foster, T. L., Lafond, D. A., Reggio, C., & Hinds, P. S. (2010). Pediatric palliative care in childhood cancer nursing: From diagnosis to cure or end of life. *Seminars in Oncology Nursing, 26*(4), 205–221.

Friebert, S. (2009). *NHPCO facts and figures: Pediatric palliative and hospice care in America*. National Hospice and Palliative Care Organization. Retrieved from http://www.nhpco.org/files/public/quality/Pediatric_Facts-Figures.pdf

Freudtner, C., Santucci, C., Feinstein, J. A., Snyder, C. R., Rourke, M. T., & Kang, T. I. (2007). Hopeful thinking and level of comfort regarding providing palliative care: A survey of hospital nurses. *Pediatrics, 119*(1), e186–e192.

Gerow, L., Conejo, P., Alonzo, A., Davis, N., Rodgers, S., & Domian, E. W. (2010). Creating a curtain of protection: Nurses' experiences of grief following patient death. *Journal of Nursing Scholarship, 42*(2), 122–129.

Hain, R. D. W., & Jassal, S. S. (2010). *Pediatric palliative medicine*. New York: Oxford University Press.

Hardy-Bougere, M. (2008). Cultural manifestations of grief and bereavement: A clinical perspective. *Journal of Cultural Diversity, 15*(2), 66–69.

Hills, T. E. (2010). Determining brain death: A review of evidence-based guidelines. *Nursing 2010, 40*(12), 34–40.

Hinds, P. S., & Kelly, K. P. (2010). Helping parents make and survive end of life decisions for their child. *Nursing Clinics of North America, 45*, 465–474.

Hurwitz, C. A., Lewandowski, J. G., & Hilden, J. M. (2009). Neonates, children, and adolescents. In D. Walsh, A. T. Caraceni, R. Fainsinger, K. Foley, P. Glare, C. Goh, . . . L. Radbruch, *Palliative medicine* (1st ed., pp. 1071–1079). Philadelphia: Saunders Elsevier.

Jones, B. L., Parker-Raley, J., Higgerson, R., Christie, L. M., Legett, S., & Greathouse, J. (2008). Finding the right words: Using the terms allow natural death (AND) and do not resuscitate (DNR) in pediatric palliative care. *Journal of Healthcare Quality, 30*(5), 55–63.

Keene, E. A., Hutton, N., Hall, B., & Rushton, C. (2010). Bereavement debriefing sessions: An intervention to support health care professionals in managing their grief after the death of a patient. *Pediatric Nursing, 36*(4), 185–189.

Kersun, L. S., & Shemesh, E. (2007). Depression and anxiety in children at the end of life. *Pediatric Clinics of North America, 54*, 691–708

Kochanek, K. D., Xu, J., Murphy, S. L., Miniño, A. M., & Kung, H. (2011). Deaths: Final Data for 2009, *National Vital Statistics Reports, 60*(3), 1–116.

Kübler-Ross, E. (1983). *On children and death*. New York: Macmillan.

Kübler-Ross, E., & Kessler, D. (2005). *On grief and grieving*. New York: Scribner.

Lee, K. J. (2011). Brain death. In R. M. Kliegman, B. F. Stanton, J. W. St. Geme, N. F. Schor, & R. E. Behrman, *Nelson textbook of pediatrics* (19th ed., pp. e63-1–e63-3). Philadelphia: Elsevier.

Levetown, M., & the Committee on Bioethics. (2008). Communicating with children and families: From everyday interactions to skill in conveying distressing information. *Pediatrics, 121*(5), e1441–e1460.

Lichtenthal, W. G., & Kissane, D. W. (2009). Grief and bereavement. In D. Walsh, A. T. Caraceni, R. Fainsinger, K. Foley, P. Glare, C. Goh, . . . L. Radbruch, *Palliative medicine* (1st ed., pp. 69–74). Philadelphia: Saunders Elsevier.

Linebarger, J. S., Sahler, O. J. Z., & Egan, K. A. (2009). Coping with death. *Pediatrics in Review, 30*(9), 350–355.

Mathur, M., Petersen, L., Stadtler, M., Rose, C., Ejike, J. C., Petersen, F., . . . Ashwal, S. (2008). Variability in pediatric brain death determination and documentation in Southern California. *Pediatrics, 121*(5), 988–993.

McSherry, M., Carroll, J. M., & Rourke, M. T. (2007). Psychosocial and spiritual needs of children living with a life limiting illness. *Pediatric Clinics of North America, 54*, 609–629.

Meadors, P., & Lamson, A. (2008). Compassion fatigue and secondary traumatization: Provider self care on intensive care units for children. *Journal of Pediatric Health Care, 22*(1), 24–34.

Meert, K. L., Briller, S. H., Schim, S. M., & Thurston, C. S. (2008). Exploring parents' environmental needs at the time of a child's death in the pediatric intensive care unit. *Pediatric Critical Care Medicine, 9*(6), 623–628.

Meert, K. L., Donaldson, A. E., Newth, C. J. L., Harrison, R., Berger, J., Zimmerman, J., . . . Shear, K. (2010). Complicated grief, and associated risk factors among parents following a child's death in the pediatric intensive care unit. *Archives of Pediatrics and Adolescent Medicine, 164*(11), 1045–1051.

Michelson, K. N., & Steinhorn, D. M. (2007). Pediatric end-of-life issues and palliative care. *Clinical Pediatric Emergency Medicine, 8*, 212–219.

Morgan, D. (2009). Caring for dying children: Assessing the needs of the pediatric palliative care nurse. *Pediatric Nursing, 35*(2), 86–90.

Munson, D., & Leuthner, S. R. (2007). Palliative care for the family carrying a fetus with a life-limiting diagnosis. *Pediatric Clinics of North America, 54*, 787–798

National Consensus Project for Quality Palliative Care. (2009). *Clinical practice guidelines for quality palliative care* (2nd ed.). Retrieved from http://www.nationalconsensusproject.org/

Nolbris, M., Abrahamsson, J., Hellström, A. L., Olofsson, L., & Enskär, K. (2010). The experience of therapeutic support groups by siblings of children with cancer. *Pediatric Nursing, 36*(6), 298–304.

O'Malley, P. J., Brown, K., Krug, S. E., & the Committee on Pediatric Emergency Medicine. (2008). Patient- and family-centered care of children in the emergency department. *Pediatrics, 122*(2), e511–e521.

O'Mathúna, D. P., & Lang, K. (2008). Medicine vs. prayer: The case of Kara Neumann. *Pediatric Nursing, 34*(5), 413–416.

Orthodox Church of America. (2011). *Death/funerals*. Retrieved from http://oca.org/questions/deathfunerals

Purnell, L. D. (2009). *Guide to culturally competent health care* (2nd ed.). Philadelphia: F. A. Davis Company.

Schaffer, M., & Norlander, L. (2009). *Being present: A nurse's resource for end-of-life communication*. Indianapolis, IN: Sigma Theta Tau International.

Schum, L. N., & Kane, J. R. (2009). Psychological adaptation of the dying child. In D. Walsh, A. T. Caraceni, R. Fainsinger, K. Foley, P. Glare, C. Goh, . . . L. Radbruch, *Palliative medicine* (1st ed., pp. 1085–1092). Philadelphia: Saunders Elsevier.

Smith, C. (2010). *Death, general: Resource list*. Retrieved from http://www.nursingconsult.com/das/patient/view/239299363-2/10072/24810.html/top?sid=1146105885&SEQNO=5

Spector, R. E. (2009). *Cultural diversity in health and illness* (7th ed., pp. 139–142). Upper Saddle River, NJ: Prentice Hall Health.

Widger, K., & Picot, C. (2008). Parents' perceptions of the quality of pediatric and perinatal end-of-life care. *Pediatric Nursing, 34*(1), 53–58.

Zielinski, P. B. (2011). Brain death, the pediatric patient, and the nurse. *Pediatric Nursing, 37*(1), 17–21, 38.

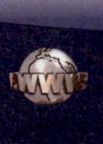

Pearson Nursing Student Resources
Find additional review materials at
nursing.pearsonhighered.com
Prepare for success with additional NCLEX®-style practice questions, interactive assignments and activities, web links, animations and videos, and more!

Nursing Care for Common Health Conditions

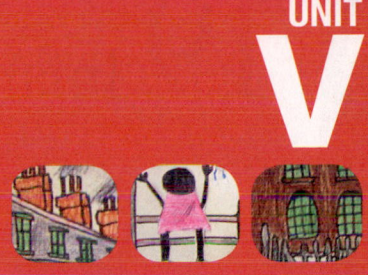

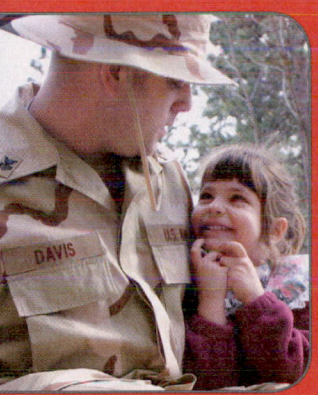 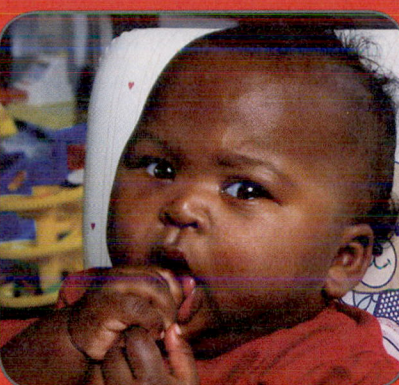 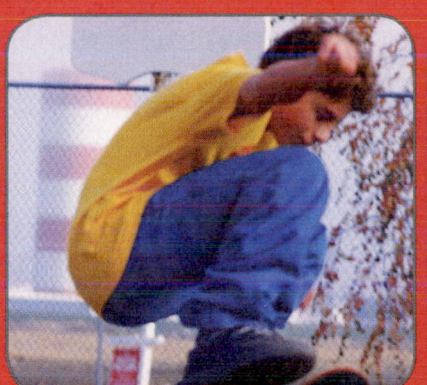 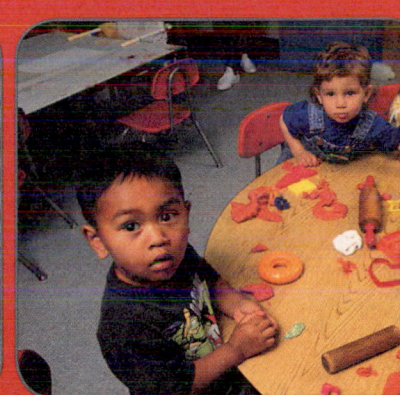

Children experience a wide range of health conditions throughout childhood, whether from nutritional problems, social relationships, influences in the environment, or from communicable diseases. The pediatric nurse partners with the family to identify potential factors that can have an impact on the child's health and to individualize care for the child, promote the child's nutrition, provide a secure and safe environment, and protect the child from communicable diseases. All children are entitled to pain assessment and management to help promote their healing and to reduce stress associated with various health conditions.

19 Infant, Child, and Adolescent Nutrition

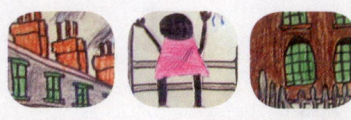

Learning Outcomes

After completing this chapter, you will be able to:

1. Discuss major nutritional concepts pertaining to the growth and development of children.

2. Describe and plan nursing interventions to meet nutritional needs for all age groups from preterm infants through adolescents.

3. Integrate methods of nutritional assessment into care for children and adolescents.

4. Identify and explain common nutritional concerns of children growing up in developed countries.

5. Apply the nursing process to care for children or adolescents with feeding and eating disorders.

6. Prioritize nursing interventions for children with nutritional disorders.

KEY TERMS

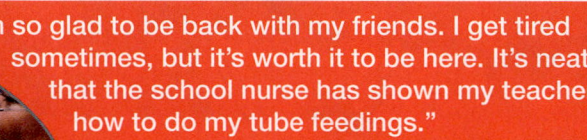

> "I'm so glad to be back with my friends. I get tired sometimes, but it's worth it to be here. It's neat that the school nurse has shown my teacher how to do my tube feedings."
>
> —*Joey, 11 years old*

Joey Jenkins was diagnosed with cerebral palsy early in life. He is now 11 years old and has returned to school after surgery for scoliosis. When evaluated prior to surgery, Joey's nutritional status showed some caloric and nutritional deficits. Joey has limited ability to swallow, related to muscle weakness of cerebral palsy, and was therefore unable to ingest enough calories by mouth to ensure his optimal growth and development. A gastrostomy tube was inserted into his stomach to provide supplementary feedings and maximize his nutritional status prior to surgery. After several weeks of supplemental feedings, Joey was ready for surgery, and he did well in his postoperative recovery.

Joey continues to have supplemental feedings throughout the day. The school nurse has met with his parents and home health nurse to learn about the amount and type of tube feedings he receives, as well as the texture of oral feedings he can manage. The nurse has planned the feeding schedule at school to facilitate adequate nutrition in that setting. In addition, careful ongoing nutritional assessment will be needed to evaluate if Joey is getting the calories and other nutrients he needs for growth and development. How will the school nurse educate the classroom teachers and other school personnel about Joey's unique nutritional requirements? What ongoing communication should take place among school personnel and the family?

dequate nutrition is an essential component of growth and development. The child's nutritional status begins before birth and is related to the mother's nutritional state. After birth and throughout all of childhood, intake influences health. Nurses must assess all children for nutritional status, and then use teaching or other interventions to enhance health. As a nurse, you will provide families with information about normal nutritional needs of infants, children, and adolescents. Common techniques to assess nutrition, such as measuring growth and monitoring hematocrit, provide needed information about whether intake of nutrients is adequate.

All children, their parents, and other care providers can benefit from information about nutritional needs, but some children have additional issues that nurses must consider. A nurse must recognize and respond to the special intake requirements of children with conditions such as food allergies, cystic fibrosis, cerebral palsy, cancer, or diabetes. Nutrition monitoring is provided during health promotion and health maintenance visits throughout childhood so that dietary counseling can be integrated with other teaching to promote development.

When applying concepts of health promotion with families, a nurse may consider common nutritional deficits, as well as the high rate of childhood obesity in North America. But some children have unique nutritional needs due to their social environments. The following contexts—and others—require the nurse to explore specific factors that may affect the child's nutrition:

- If the parents are vegetarian, they may need extra help to ensure their child gets essential nutrients.
- If finances are limited, the family may need resources such as access to food stamps, food banks, or budget planning.
- If the child has been exposed to environmental toxicants, the exposure may have affected nutritional intake.

Whatever the setting in which the nurse is employed, consideration of nutrition should be integrated within nursing care. As we proceed through this chapter, we will address many questions of nursing care and nutrition:

- How can the nurse help parents to monitor food intake in various settings, such as home, childcare settings, schools, and hospitals?
- What interventions will assist families in establishing nutritional habits that foster health promotion?
- How can the nurse help the family prepare to meet nutritional needs of a child who has special nutritional requirements during travel by car or plane?
- How can nurses intervene to help decrease rates of obesity among children?

NUTRITION CONCEPTS
Major Dietary Components

As a nurse, you need to understand and apply basic nutritional concepts with children of widely distributed ages and nutritional needs. Review concepts in this section to provide the background that will form the nursing assessments and interventions in nursing care situations. **Nutrition** refers to taking in food and assimilating it metabolically for use by the body. It is an essential component of life and therefore an important topic to consider in discussions of

TABLE 19–1	Carbohydrates in the Human Diet
SIMPLE CARBOHYDRATES	**EXAMPLES**
Monosaccharides	
Glucose	Corn syrup
Fructose	Honey
	Fruits
Disaccharides	
Sucrose	White sugar
Lactose	Molasses
Maltose	Milk
COMPLEX CARBOHYDRATES	
Polysaccharides	Grains (cereals, breads)
Starch	Pasta
Glycogen	Rice, corn, bulgur
	Legumes
	Potatoes

child growth and development. The body requires a wide array of nutrients. **Macronutrients** are the major building blocks of the body. **Micronutrients** are substances needed in small quantities for healthy body functioning. The need for nutrients is dependent on activity level, state of health, presence of disease or other stress, and age-related needs.

The essential macronutrients are carbohydrates, proteins, and fats. **Carbohydrates** are composed of carbon, hydrogen, and oxygen, arranged in various configurations to form saccharides (sugar molecules). The main function of carbohydrates in the body is production of energy. Indeed, 50% or more of our daily calories come from carbohydrates. See Table 19–1 for common carbohydrates in the human diet. Digestion of carbohydrates occurs in the mouth and small intestine, and monosaccharides are absorbed in the small intestine. Carbohydrates are turned into glucose in the liver and used for energy throughout the body. When there is an excess of glucose, the liver can convert glucose to **glycogen** and store it for use when the body requires energy and food is not being ingested. Remaining carbohydrates are converted to short-chain fatty acids and absorbed in the colon. **Fiber** represents indigestible carbohydrate components that ensure healthy movement of fecal contents through the bowel (Box 19–1). While some carbohydrates are quickly absorbed, causing a rapid rise in blood sugar after ingestion, others are more slowly absorbed, causing a more prolonged blood sugar increase without a high peak (Box 19–2). When insufficient carbohydrates are ingested, the deficiency disease **marasmus** can occur. See the section on dietary deficiencies for further discussion.

Proteins are made of amino acids, compounds that have nitrogen as an essential component, in addition to carbon, hydrogen, and oxygen. Twenty amino acids comprise the proteins in the body. Nine of these are **essential amino acids,** which cannot be manufactured by humans and must be ingested in the diet. Eleven are **nonessential amino acids,** which humans can manufacture when in good health. See Table 19–2 for a list of the amino acids in the body. Proteins are the building blocks of body tissues and are constantly being broken down (**catabolism**) and resynthesized (**anabolism**). When

BOX 19–1	Health Promotion: Dietary Fiber

Dietary fiber has many health benefits. For example, it promotes regular bowel movements, contributes to maintenance of healthy serum lipids and glucose, and decreases rates of duodenal ulcer and colon cancer. Eating whole grains, fruits, vegetables, and legumes is an easy way to increase fiber intake. Most children have a much lower intake of fiber than is recommended, so nurses should recommend increasing fruits, vegetables, and whole grains in the diet. Note below the average intake and recommended intakes for children in the United States (American Academy of Pediatrics Committee on Nutrition, 2009).

AGE	AVERAGE INTAKE (g/DAY)	RECOMMENDED INTAKE (g/DAY)	AVERAGE/RECOMMENDED INTAKE (%)
1–3 years	9.5	19	50%
4–8 years	12.2	25	49%
9–13 years, boys	15.2	31	49%
9–13 years, girls	12.9	26	50%
14–18 years, boys	17.7	38	47%
14–18 years, girls	12.8	26	49%

inadequate carbohydrates and fats are available, the body can break down protein and use components to meet basic energy needs. Since nitrogen is an essential component of amino acids, protein balance is also referred to as **nitrogen balance.** *Positive nitrogen balance* is the term used when more nitrogen is taken into the body than excreted; it occurs during periods of growth during childhood, when additional body tissues are being manufactured, and when the body is replenished after illness or surgery. *Negative nitrogen balance* indicates that the body excretes more nitrogen than it retains; it occurs when dietary intake is limited. **Kwashiorkor** is a deficiency disease that occurs when insufficient protein is ingested. See the section on dietary deficiencies for further discussion.

Fats (or lipids) are the third macronutrient group ingested in the diet. They are complex molecules of several types, consisting of carbon, hydrogen, and oxygen, arranged so that glycerol and fatty acids are the structural subcomponents. The major role of fats is production of body energy, but they are essential in many processes such as cell membrane function, cell signaling, and blood clotting. **Fatty acids** are major components of fats and are referred to as *saturated* (no additional hydrogen atoms could be absorbed by the structure) or *unsaturated* (some additional bonds with hydrogen are possible). Unsaturated fatty acids are further designated as *monounsaturated* (only one potential bond with hydrogen possible) or *polyunsaturated* (two or more potential bonds). *Trans-fatty acids* are formed when food processing is applied to partially hydrogenated unsaturated fatty acids. Unsaturated fatty acids are commonly liquid at room temperature, and hydrogenation hardens them into spreads such as margarine. In recent years it has become evident that these artificially hydrogenated fatty acids (trans-fatty acids) have similar actions to saturated fatty acids in the body; that is, they may raise levels of cholesterol and promote cardiovascular disease. The average intake of trans fat is 5 g daily, but since it has not been separately noted on food labels until recently, the intake for individuals has been difficult to identify or modify. New labeling includes amount of trans fat and assists nurses in instructing individuals about ways to lower this type of dietary fat. Some U.S. cities, and more recently states, have banned or limited use of trans fats in restaurant foods,

BOX 19–2	Health Promotion: Glycemic Index

Glycemic index refers to the blood glucose response to 50 g of carbohydrate from any specific food, as compared to the glucose level after ingestion of white bread or plain glucose. White bread is a "reference food" against which other foods are measured; the glycemic index of white bread is set at 100. A low glycemic index diet (one in which most of the carbohydrates are from low glycemic index foods) has been found to have beneficial effects such as reducing serum lipids, reducing insulin levels, and improving serum glucose control. For this reason, some clinicians recommend a low glycemic diet for persons with or at risk of having diabetes. The American Diabetes Association states that attention to the type of carbohydrate in foods and application of a low glycemic index diet is one method to ensure a healthy diet (American Diabetes Association, 2011).

Beans are an example of a low glycemic index food, whereas white potatoes have a high glycemic index, indicating that the glucose level rises very high soon after ingestion. It is not possible to guess the glycemic index of a food; for example, a baked potato has a glycemic index of 116, whereas a sweet potato has a glycemic index of 70. Charts of glycemic index of common foods have been developed and are available online.

Parents can be taught how to interpret such resources so that glycemic index information about a particular food can be applied to dietary decisions. However, it is difficult to look up every food eaten and rate the entire diet. For most individuals it is wise to simply encourage generous amounts of whole grains, beans and nuts, and fruits and vegetables to provide a diet that has the overall quality of low glycemic index.

TABLE 19–2	Amino Acids

ESSENTIAL AMINO ACIDS	NONESSENTIAL AMINO ACIDS
Isoleucine (Ile)	Alanine (Ala)
Leucine (Leu)	Arginine (Arg)
Lysine (Lys)	Aspartic acid (Asp)
Methionine (Met)	Asparagine (Asn)
Phenylalanine (Phe)	Glutamic acid (Glu)
Threonine (Thr)	Glutamine (Gln)
Tryptophan (Trp)	Glycine (Gly)
Valine (Val)	Proline (Pro)
Histidine (His)	Serine (Ser)
	Cysteine (Cys)
	Tyrosine (Tyr)

TABLE 19–3	Fatty Acids

SATURATED FATTY ACIDS	SOURCES
Butyric	Butterfat, coconut, peanut oil
Caproic	
Caprylic	
Capric	
Lauric	
Myristic	
Palmitic	
Stearic	
Arachidic	
Behenic	

MONOUNSATURATED FATTY ACIDS	
Palmitoleic	Beef, fish, olive oil
Oleic	
Elaidic (trans)	

POLYUNSATURATED FATTY ACIDS	
Linoleic	Safflower, corn, soybean, cottonseed, canola oils, fish
Alpha-linolenic	
Arachidonic	
Eicosapentaenoic	
Docosahexaenoic	

some fast-food restaurants have lowered or eliminated all use of trans fats nationwide, and some popular packaged food items now state on labels that they contain no trans fats. See Table 19–3 for major dietary sources of fatty acids.

Many fats consist of three fatty acids connected to a glycerol base, and are called **triglycerides;** these are the major fats consumed by humans. Cholesterol and lipoproteins are two terms related to fats and are sometimes confused with fats. **Cholesterol** is actually a steroid or sterol compound found only in animal cells and is essential to cell membranes. It may be ingested from foods

and is also manufactured in the body. **Lipoproteins** are combinations of fat and protein that transport fats in the blood. Major lipoproteins include low-density lipoprotein (LDL), high-density lipoprotein (HDL), and very-low-density lipoprotein (VLDL). See Chapter 26 for further description of cholesterol levels in the body. See Table 19–4 for Recommended Dietary Allowances (RDAs) of carbohydrate, protein, fat, and fiber in childhood and adolescence.

In addition to the macronutrients of carbohydrate, protein, and fat, the human body depends on a number of micronutrients, commonly vitamins and minerals. A few vitamins are fat soluble and must have dietary fat for absorption; these include vitamins A, D, E, and K. All other vitamins are water soluble, easily absorbed but readily excreted from the body. They include thiamin, riboflavin, niacin, biotin, and vitamins B_6, B_{12}, and C. See the Clinical Manifestations table for a list of macronutrients, vitamins, minerals, and the clinical manifestations of deficiency or excess in the body. See Appendix C for recommended amounts of micronutrients in the daily diet of children and adolescents.

Nutrition Facts Labels

In 1990, the U.S. federal government first mandated through the Nutritional Labeling and Education Act the information that must be supplied on labels for prepared foods. Since then the law has been updated to provide additional information that is helpful to the consumer, and current debates are occurring about needed revisions to the nutrition facts label. Manufacturers of particular food products provide additional information voluntarily. The label must contain the name of the product; name and address of manufacturer; net contents; ingredients (most common first and then in descending order of amount); serving size; servings per container; amount per serving of calories, fat (including saturated and trans fat), cholesterol, sodium, total carbohydrate (with subcategories for fiber and sugar), protein, vitamin A, vitamin C, calcium, and iron; and percent of daily value for fat, cholesterol, carbohydrate, protein, sodium, potassium, and certain vitamins and minerals based on a 2000 calorie diet. The labels are designed to provide information valuable to children from age 4 years through adulthood. However, it is obvious that some interpretation is needed for the young child not yet consuming a diet

TABLE 19–4	Recommended Dietary Allowances						
	AGE	PROTEIN	CARBOHYDRATE	POLYUNSATURATED FATTY ACIDS n-6	POLYUNSATURATED FATTY ACIDS n-3	TOTAL FAT	FIBER
Infants	0–6 months	1.52 g/kg/d or 9.1 g/d*	60 g/d*	4.4 g/d	0.5 g/d	31 g/d	NE
	7–12 months	1.5 g/kg/d	95 g/d*	4.6 g/d	0.5 g/d	30 g/d	NE
Children	1–3 years	1.1 g/kg/d or 13 g/d	130 g/d	7 g/d (linoleic)	0.7 g/d (α-linolenic)	NE	19 g/d
	4–8 years	0.95 g/kg/d or 19 g/d	130 g/d	10 g/d (linoleic)	0.9 g/d (α-linolenic)	NE	25 g/d
Males	9–13 years	0.95 g/kg/d or 34 g/d	130 g/d	12 g/d (linoleic)	1.2 g/d (α-linolenic)	NE	31 g/d
	14–18 years	0.85 g/kg/d or 52 g/d	130 g/d	16 g/d (linoleic)	1.6 g/d (α-linolenic)	NE	38 g/d
Females	9–13 years	0.95 g/kg/d or 34 g/d	130 g/d	10 g/d (linoleic)	1.0 g/d (α-linolenic)	NE	26 g/d
	14–18 years	0.85 g/kg/d or 46 g/d	130 g/d	11 g/d (linoleic)	1.1 g/d (α-linolenic)	NE	26 g/d

Note: *Values are Adequate Intakes (AIs) rather than Recommended Dietary Allowances (RDAs). All other values on chart are RDAs.

NE = not established

Source: All data from Institute of Medicine. (2006, 2011). Dietary Reference Intakes. Washington, DC: National Academies Press. http://www.nap.edu/iom

Clinical Manifestations Dietary Deficiencies/Excesses

NUTRIENT	DEFICIENCY MANIFESTATION	EXCESS MANIFESTATION
Vitamin A	Night blindness Skin dryness and scaling	Headache Drowsiness Hepatomegaly Vomiting and diarrhea
Vitamin C	Abnormal hair (coiled shape) Skin abnormalities (dermatitis and lesions) Purpura Bleeding gums Joint tenderness Sudden heart failure	Usually none—excess is excreted in urine
Vitamin D	Rib abnormalities Bowed legs	Drowsiness
B vitamins	Weakness Decreased deep tendon reflexes Dermatitis	Usually none—excess is excreted in urine
Protein	Hepatomegaly Edema Scant, depigmented hair	Kidney failure
Carbohydrate	Emaciation Decreased energy Retarded growth and development	Overweight
Iron	Lethargy Slowed growth and developmental progression Pallor	Vomiting, diarrhea, abdominal pain Pallor Cyanosis Drowsiness Shock

Weblink | MyPlate & Alternative Food Guides

of about 2000 calories. See an example of a nutrition facts food label in Figure 19–1 ■.

Recommendations for Dietary Intake

The **Dietary Reference Intakes (DRIs)** are a set of values for macronutrient and micronutrient intake established by the Food and Nutrition Board of the Institute of Medicine and the National Academy of Science that can be used to assess and plan intake for individuals of different ages. They commonly include four different values that can be considered by nurses, nutritionists, and other health personnel (Table 19–5). Although the DRIs are the approach used in the United States, other countries have developed their own approaches to dietary standards. For example, Canada uses *Adequate Intake and Reference Nutrient Intake,* and the United Kingdom uses *Recommended Daily Nutrient Intakes.* The aim of these standards is to provide a method of evaluating individual and population diets, and of planning nutrition programs and education. DRIs are generally specific to males and females in several age categories (Box 19–3).

Although the DRIs provide useful information when evaluating diets, their use can be time consuming. What "quick check" can be performed to provide feedback about the daily diets of children? Become familiar with the U.S. MyPlate food guide. Hang them in schools, clinics, and hospitals. These are fast methods of examining children's intakes for a day to evaluate if they meet most requirements. Instead of calculating amounts of nutrients ingested,

the food guides focus on categories of foods, which readily reflect the actual intake. The numbers of servings from various categories stay constant throughout childhood, but the serving sizes increase as the child gets older. See Figure 19–2 ■ for the U.S. MyPlate food guide, and consult websites for alternative food guides for vegetarians and those from various ethnic groups, such as Hispanic and Native American. (See Developing Cultural Competence: The Mediterranean Diet.)

Developing Cultural Competence
The Mediterranean Diet

Some populations in Greece and southern Italy are renowned for the longevity of their members. Researchers have paid close attention to certain characteristics of the regimen these groups share, known as the Mediterranean diet. This diet encompasses a geographic area called the "Fertile Crescent," which includes sections of Greece, Italy, France, Spain, Portugal, and North Africa. Intake includes many fresh fruits and vegetables, whole grains, and beans; uses nuts, olive oil, and dairy products; has moderate amounts of fish, poultry, and meat; and often includes moderate amounts of wine (Bellisle, 2009). Certain products such as phenols, flavonoids, isoflavonoids, phytosterols, and phytic acid, which have known health effects in the body, are abundant in foods in the Mediterranean diet. In addition, daily physical activity is common. Lower rates of cardiovascular disease, diabetes, and other conditions are associated with the diet. In one study of children with type 1 diabetes, cholesterol profiles improved with training in the Mediterranean diet (Maillot, Issa, Vieux et al., 2011).

Sample label for
Macaroni & Cheese

Nutrition Facts

Serving Size 1 cup (228g)
Servings Per Container 2

Amount Per Serving

Calories 250 | Calories from Fat 110

	% Daily Values*
Total Fat 12g	18%
Saturated Fat 3g	15%
Trans Fat 3g	
Cholesterol 30mg	10%
Sodium 470mg	20%
Total Carbohydrate 31g	10%
Dietary Fiber 0g	0%
Sugars 5g	
Protein 5g	
Vitamin A	4%
Vitamin C	2%
Calcium	20%
Iron	4%

*Percent Daily Values are based on a 2,000 calorie diet. Your Daily Values may be higher or lower depending on your calorie needs.

	Calories:	2,000	2,500
Total Fat	Less than	65g	80g
Sat Fat	Less than	20g	25g
Cholesterol	Less than	300mg	300mg
Sodium	Less than	2,400mg	2,400mg
Total Carbohydrate		300g	375g
Dietary Fiber		25g	30g

FIGURE 19–1 ■ The nutrition facts label of food is based on a typical serving and contains information about fat, cholesterol, sodium, carbohydrate, protein, and selected vitamins. This label is from a box of macaroni and cheese. The daily value information is based on a 2000–2500 calorie diet. What adjustments should be made if the diet has lower calories, such as with young children?

Source: *From U.S. Department of Health and Human Services. (2011). Nutrition facts label. Retrieved from http://www.fda.gov/food/labelingnutrition/consumerinformation/ucm078889.htm*

NUTRITIONAL NEEDS

Nutritional needs evolve during all of infancy and childhood. Nutritional intake:

- Supports growth and development
- Influences the progression of the child along the developmental path

BOX 19–3 **Dietary Reference Intake (DRI) Age Groups**

Pregnancy and Lactation	14–18 years
Birth to 6 months	19–30 years
6–12 months	31–50 years
1–3 years	51–70 years
4–8 years	Over 70 years
9–13 years	

- Helps to maintain the health of the child
- Fosters a state of maximal potential or health promotion

Preterm Infant

Infants who are **preterm** (less than 37 weeks' gestation) and **small for gestational age** (less than 2500 g) have special nutritional needs. They usually need a high calorie/kg intake to provide energy for necessary weight gain. At the same time, immaturity of body systems can make intake and absorption of needed nutrients a challenge. For example, they may lack the neuromuscular ability to adequately swallow and protect the airway. The premature infant has a small stomach size, demonstrates gastrointestinal inability to absorb some nutrients, and lacks the renal maturity needed to handle osmolarity (concentration) of formula and to manage glucose, fluid, and electrolyte excretion dependent on intake. Acute medical problems related to a difficult birth and regulation of body homeostasis offer additional challenges.

Nutrient needs depend both on the specific degree of prematurity and overall health status. The preterm baby who has an illness, such as bronchopulmonary dysplasia (see Chapter 25), sepsis (see Chapter 26), necrotizing enterocolitis (see Chapter 30), or other abnormalities, often has increased metabolic demands. Preterm infants are fed parenterally and/or enterally. The term **parenteral** refers to use of nutrition introduced outside the intestinal tract, usually by the intravenous route, whereas **enteral** refers to nutrition introduced through the intestinal tract, such as in oral or tube feedings.

To provide for energy needs, 50 to 60 kcal/kg per day (parenteral feeding) to 75 kcal/kg per day (enteral feeding) are recommended

TABLE 19–5 **Dietary Reference Intakes (DRIs)**

TERM	DEFINITION	USE	EXAMPLE
Estimated Average Requirement (EAR)	Daily intake needed to meet the requirements of 50% of a certain age and gender group.	Evaluate intake of a group; plan for intake of a group.	Compare the daily intake of vitamin C of a class of children from 24-hour recalls to this number to learn how many do not meet average requirements; plan the daily menu for a childcare center.
Recommended Dietary Allowance (RDA)	Daily intake needed to meet the requirements of most people (97%–98%) of a certain age and gender group.	Set goal for daily intake.	Evaluate the dietary intake of an individual for a nutrient such as vitamin C; make recommendations to an individual for a daily menu.
Adequate Intake (AI)	Used when limited information on the needs for a vitamin is known and EAR is not available, usually because studies on its metabolism in the body are hard to carry out; rather than being based on metabolic studies, it is derived from the average intake of that nutrient by a healthy group of people.	Evaluate intake of a group; plan intake for a group.	See EAR.
Upper Intake (UI)	Upper tolerable intake level; maximum level unlikely to pose a health risk.	Limit fortification levels of foods and provide information to limit dietary supplements.	Consider intake of a fat-soluble vitamin such as vitamin A that is not readily excreted; include both food sources and supplements.

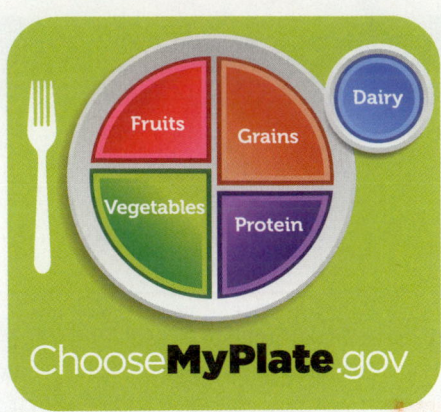

FIGURE 19–2 ■ The U.S. MyPlate food guide is used to provide teaching about amounts of foods recommended for daily intake.

Source: *From U.S. Department of Agriculture and U.S. Department of Health and Human Services. (2011). Retrieved from http://www.choosemyplate.gov*

just to support the infant's resting metabolism; additional amounts are needed for growth, resulting in a requirement of 90 to 120 kcal/kg per day (American Academy of Pediatrics [AAP], 2009). Protein requirements range from 3.4 to 4.4 g/kg daily, and fat intake should be 5 to 7 g/kg daily, or 40% to 55% of total energy ingested by enterally fed infants. The protein/energy ratio is 2.5 to 3.6 g/100 kcal (AAP, 2009). Fluid needs range from 80 to 140 mL/kg/day and are adjusted in response to the infant's condition.

Breast milk is considered the best food whenever the baby can feed adequately to meet requirements. Expressed breast milk can even be placed in a tube feeding for the young infant who receives that form of nutrition. Breast milk provides factors that foster growth of the brain, eyes, and the intestinal tract itself; it enhances cognition and general development. In addition, babies who breastfeed have greater maintenance of temperature and oxygenation, and lower rates of rehospitalization (Ahmed, 2010). While preterm formulas contain essential medium-chain triglycerides and polyunsaturated long-chain triglycerides, additional fatty acids found in breast milk include docosahexaenoic acid (DHA) and arachidonic acid (ARA). DHA is generally 0.1% to 0.3% of total fatty acids in breast milk, and ARA is 0.4% to 0.6% of total fatty acids (AAP, 2009). These fatty acids are major components of neural tissue and retinal photoreceptor membranes, so some companies have started to add these fatty acids

to their formulas. The lipids in human breast milk are well absorbed by the premature baby. Human milk contains the amino acids taurine, glycine, and cystine, which are needed by the premature baby. In addition, breastfeeding provides immunologic protection for the baby against some infections (such as sepsis and necrotizing enterocolitis), promotes positive neurologic development, and fosters positive bonding between mother and newborn (European Society for Pediatric Gastroenterology, Hepatology, and Nutrition [ESPGHAN] Committee on Nutrition, 2009).

When the baby cannot nurse adequately or when the premature infant is less than 1500 grams, human milk fortifiers can be added to breast milk. They can be tailored to meet the baby's particular needs but can include nutrients such as protein, fat, carbohydrate, calcium, phosphorus, and vitamin D. This protein supplementation, accompanied by periodic blood urea nitrogen (BUN) levels, may be helpful to maximize growth of preterm infants (Vlaardingerbroek, van Goudoever, & van den Akker, 2009). In addition, increased mineral content can promote calcium balance and enhanced growth. Fortifiers are intended only for the preterm infant and should not be used in babies beyond 37 weeks' gestation; they are generally discontinued when the infant is 1800 grams or is near discharge from the hospital (AAP, 2009).

Preterm formulas may be needed for some infants and are designed to meet the high-density nutrient needs and to supplement babies with necessary micronutrients. These preparations contain different amounts of some vitamins and minerals than other formulas. They may be used for variable amounts of time, depending on the condition of the baby. Table 19–6 lists common amounts of ingredients in preterm and regular infant formula.

Feeding methods for premature babies may need to be altered until they have acquired necessary neuromuscular and gastrointestinal maturity (Figure 19–3 ■). Some infants need parenteral nutrition for a time, and receive a mixture of carbohydrates, amino acids, fats, electrolytes, vitamins, and minerals via a central line. As the baby gains maturity, enteral feedings begin. Sometimes these are initially through gavage or tube feeding of breast milk or formula, with gradual introduction of oral feedings by breast or bottle. Nurses assist the parents in learning how to successfully achieve enteral feedings for the baby, and perform thorough assessments of the infant's growth and feeding ability. (See Partnering with Families: Feeding the Preterm Infant.) Babies who have been exposed

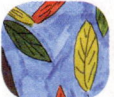 # Partnering with Families

Feeding the Preterm Infant

Parents of preterm infants often need extra support to breastfeed successfully and to feed the infant adequately. The nurse should take careful feeding histories and observe a breastfeeding session. Some suggestions the nurse can provide for the mother include:

■ Begin breast pumping by 6 hours postpartum to ensure adequate milk production.

■ If the infant cannot maintain breastfeeding for 15 minutes, 8 to 10 times daily, the feedings should be followed by use of a breast pump.

■ Babies can be held in skin-to-skin contact with the mother during feedings, even during gavage.

■ Prefeeding and postfeeding weighing of the breastfeeding infant can provide accurate estimates of the infant's ingestion (1 g = 1 mL of milk).

■ The letdown (milk ejection) reflex can be induced before feeding by stimulation of the breast so the infant does not have to suck hard to obtain milk.

■ Assist the baby to place the mouth over the entire areola for feedings, directing the nipple far back to the infant's upper palate.

Source: *Adapted from Ahmed, A. H. (2010). Role of the pediatric nurse practitioner in promoting breastfeeding for late preterm infants in primary care settings. Journal of Pediatric Health Care, 24(2), 116–122.*

TABLE 19–6 **Comparison of Preterm and Infant Formula, Early and Mature Breast Milk (Typical Ingredients per Liter of Liquid)**

NUTRIENT	INFANT FORMULA	PRETERM FORMULA	EARLY MILK (LESS THAN 28 DAYS)	MATURE MILK (28 DAYS AND MORE)
Energy (kcal)	672–680	810–812	varies	650–700
Protein (g)	14.5–16.9	22–24	16	9
Fat (g)	35–36	41–44	varies	39
Polyunsaturated fat (%)	17.7–24	8.4–10.3	13	14–15
Monounsaturated fat (%)	32–38	4.6–4.8	NA	40
Saturated fat (%)	43–45	25–26	43–44	44–45
Carbohydrate (g)	72–76	86–90	42–55	80–82
Calcium (mg)	420–550	1340–1460	250	200–250
Iron (mg)	10.1–12.2	2–13	0.5–1.0	0.3–0.9
Vitamin A	2000–2040 International Units	3330–10,100 USP units	4 mg	0.5–1.2 mg
Vitamin D	400–410 International Units	522–2200 USP units	NA	0.33 mcg
Vitamin E	10–13.6 International Units	27–51 USP units	8–12 mcg	3–8 mcg
Vitamin K (mcg)	54–55	59–97	2–5	2–3
Thiamine (mcg)	405–670	1480–2016	20	200
Riboflavin (mcg)	950–1000	1119–5000	NA	400–600
Pyridoxine (mcg)	410–510	740–2016	NA	90–310
Vitamin B_{12} (mcg)	1.5–2	2–4.4	NA	0.5–1
Niacin (mg)	5–6.8	14.5–40.3	0.5	1.8–6
Folic acid (mcg)	61–108	280–300	NA	80–140
Pantothenic acid (mg)	3–3.4	9.7–15.4	NA	2–2.5
Biotin (mcg)	15–30	32–300	NA	5–9
Vitamin C (mg)	54–81	162–300	NA	80–100
Choline (mg)	81–109	81–97	NA	NA
Inositol (mg)	32–122	45–138	NA	NA

Note: NA = *values not available or highly variable*

Source: *Data summarized from American Academy of Pediatrics, American Academy of Pediatrics (AAP) Committee on Nutrition. (2001). Pediatric nutrition handbook (6th ed.). Elk Grove Village, IL: American Academy of Pediatrics. (2009, pp. 1201–1203, 1245–1246, 1250–1255, 1285–1287)*

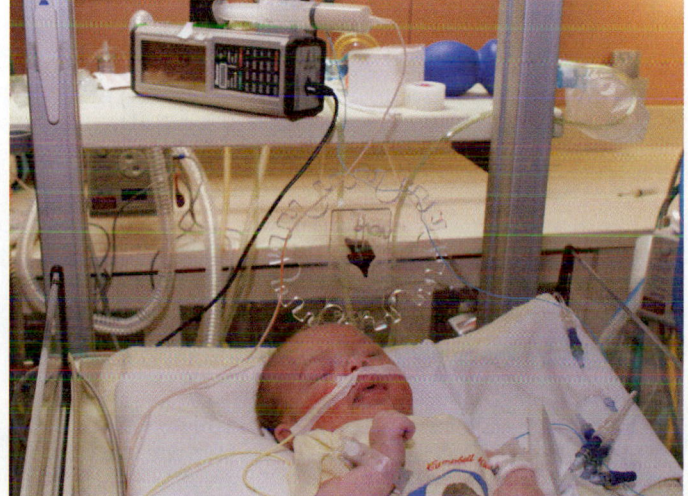

FIGURE 19–3 ■ This premature baby cannot yet coordinate suck and swallow. Gavage feeding is being used until the baby can effectively acquire nutrients.

to illicit drugs prenatally may suck a great deal to meet comforting needs. Careful monitoring of growth and self-consoling ability assists in providing the correct proportions of sucking for nutrition and nonnutritive sucking via pacifier.

Infancy—Birth to 6 Months

From the first feeding of a few ounces of breast milk to a meal of pureed baby foods with the family at 6 months of age, the infant demonstrates an amazing growth in ability to ingest and digest a wide variety of foods. Never again will the individual have such a high metabolic rate or high intake requirements in relation to size. Infants have an extremely fast rate of growth, since birth weight is usually doubled by about 5 months of age. Nevertheless, the small size of the infant's stomach and the immaturity of the digestive system make it a challenge to meet the infant's nutritional needs. (See Chapter 30 for further information about the pediatric differences in the gastrointestinal system.) The great amount of physical activity also necessitates high caloric intake. Nutrient demands for protein and vitamins must be met for the cells of the nervous system and body organs to develop properly. Brain development and normal development also depend on adequate nutritional intake. See Table 19–4 for macronutrient requirements of infants.

Breast and Formula Feeding

The natural first food is breast milk, and its intake should be encouraged for all infants (Figure 19–4 ■). It can be the only food for the first 6 months, and should continue through 12 months of age (Boxes 19–4 and 19–5). The many advantages of breastfeeding for all newborns include excellent nutritional balance, promotion of gastrointestinal function, fostering immune defense, psychologic benefits, and economic advantages. Although breast milk is the best nutritional source for infants, there may be a need for limited supplements. Fluoride and sometimes vitamin D are recommended.

Breastfeeding rates have increased from a low of 20% in the 1970s to nearly 75% at present (Centers for Disease Control and Prevention [CDC], 2011a). However, many mothers do not breastfeed for more than a few weeks, so interventions are needed to increase both rates and length of breastfeeding. Only 43% of infants are still breastfeeding at 6 months, and a mere 13% are exclusively breastfed at 6 months (CDC, 2011a). Nurses are uniquely positioned to encourage and foster breastfeeding. Such information and instruction promotes health of infants by positively influencing the number of women who decide to breastfeed and increasing the number of months they choose to continue breastfeeding. Teaching can emphasize the importance of breastfeeding to the child's well-being. Lower incidences of otitis media, other infections, type 2 diabetes, and, later, cardiovascular diseases and obesity are some of the pediatric benefits that may encourage mothers to breastfeed. Programs for encouraging breastfeeding should involve education and skill/problem-solving information provided by health professionals and trained supportive volunteers. Some hospitals have lactation specialists who assist breastfeeding mothers; in others, staff nurses provide this service. Home visits, phone calls from hospital nursing staff, early visits after the birth to obstetric and pediatric offices, and resources such as La Leche League can provide mothers with needed breastfeeding information and problem-solving suggestions. Provide information so that the mother understands the importance of adequate nutritional intake and sufficient rest. Refer mothers to support programs if they have difficulty breastfeeding, feel unsure how it will fit into family and work life, are very young, or have an infant with problems related to feeding.

The nurse can search out barriers to breastfeeding in the population served and try to address them. For example, ask about family patterns and support of breastfeeding, investigate the mother's work situation, provide ongoing information and assistance for the teen mother, ensure that both hospital and office/clinic healthcare personnel are well trained in breastfeeding support, and evaluate the mother's breastfeeding experience at every healthcare encounter.

The nurse needs to identify barriers among women served and work to decrease them to foster an increased incidence of breastfeeding. Barriers can be related to lifestyle, social and work needs, culture, attitudes, and knowledge. See Chapter 9 🔗 for further guidelines on encouragement of breastfeeding and consult the American Academy of Pediatrics policy on breastfeeding and the use of human milk (AAP, 2009). See Legal and Ethical Considerations: Breastfeeding Laws.

The mother of a hospitalized infant will need special support to continue breastfeeding. The mother should be encouraged to come to the hospital to feed her baby on the same schedule as at home. If the infant cannot breastfeed, the hospital or other agencies may provide an electric pump so the mother can maintain lactation. Many mothers need support at some point during breastfeeding to deal with common challenges (see Partnering with Families: Common Problems

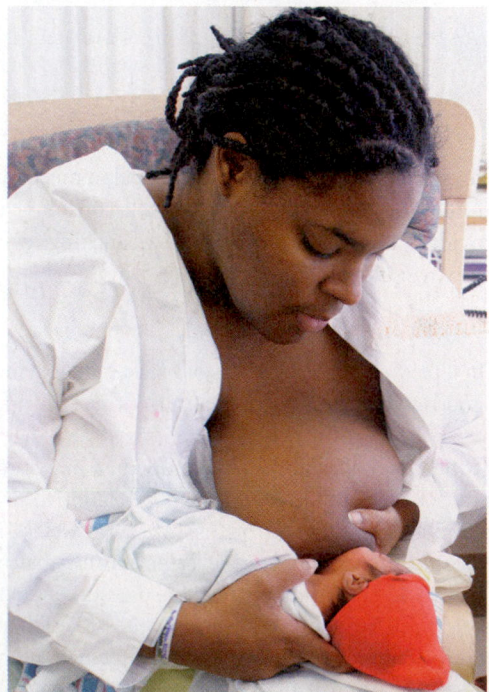

FIGURE 19–4 ■ Breastfeeding offers many physical and emotional benefits for the infant. This new mother is learning to breastfeed her baby. How can nurses encourage mothers to have positive breastfeeding experiences?

BOX 19–4   Breastfeeding Recommendations

The American Academy of Pediatrics states that breastfeeding is the best source of nutrition for babies at least through the first birthday and longer when possible; exclusive breastfeeding for the first 6 months is recommended. Barriers to continued breastfeeding should be identified and minimized (AAP Committee on Nutrition, 2009; American Diabetes Association, 2008). At each healthcare visit with an infant and mother, nurses should inquire about breastfeeding, encourage the mother to continue, or offer resources to assist with successful breastfeeding techniques.

BOX 19–5   Health Promotion: First Foods

Nurses should instruct parents that 4 to 6 months of age is the optimal time to begin supplementary or complementary foods. Many parents begin the first solid foods as early as a few weeks of life. They have often been told by others or read that early food enhances "sleeping through the night" and is more satisfying for the baby. Early introduction of solid food is not needed by the infant, nor does it enhance sleeping for longer periods, health, or any other benefits. Babies are more prone to developing allergies when fed solid food early, and they lack the tongue control and digestive enzymes to take in and metabolize many food products (AAP Committee on Nutrition, 2009).

TABLE 19–7 | Advantages and Disadvantages of Formula Preparations

FORMULA PREPARATION	HOW PACKAGED	ADVANTAGES	DISADVANTAGES
Ready to feed	Bottles or cans	No preparation needed	Most expensive type of formula
Concentrate	Cans of concentrated liquid	Easy to add equal amounts of formula concentrate and water directly into bottle and shake	Can be incorrectly measured, leading to inadequate or unsafe nutrition for infant; requires access to clean water supply such as city tap water or bottled water; well water may have too high a mineral concentration
Powder	Cans	Least expensive type of formula	Can be incorrectly measured, leading to inadequate or unsafe nutrition for infant; requires shaking to mix thoroughly; requires access to clean water supply such as city tap water or bottled water; well water may have too high a mineral concentration

Legal and Ethical Considerations
Breastfeeding Laws

About two thirds of U.S. states now have some laws supporting breastfeeding, such as allowing women to breastfeed in any location (44 states, District of Columbia, and the Virgin Islands), exempting breastfeeding from public indecency laws, or requirements to issue mercury alerts in local fish supplies so breastfeeding women can avoid intake of this toxic mineral. Investigate the laws in your state and community that act as supports or barriers to breastfeeding (National Conference of State Legislatures, 2011).

During Breastfeeding). Some women decide not to breastfeed or are unable to do so. After several months of breastfeeding, some mothers begin to use supplemental bottles of formula when they are away from the infant. Nurses provide these mothers with information about formula preparation and feeding. Three types of formula are available—ready to feed, concentrate, and powder (Table 19–7). All are nutritionally adequate for infants. Iron-fortified infant formula should always be used during the first year of life. Most infants use milk-based formulas, while some who are sensitive to milk are fed soy-based formulas. Many formulas now contain DHA and ARA, two nutrients known to be components of infants' eyes and brains. Some infants, such as those with metabolic disorders, require specialized formulas. For example, casein hydrolysate formula is specially treated (hydrolyzed) to decrease incidence of allergy to casein, the milk protein; amino acid formulas are intended for infants with extreme hypersensitivity to protein; and low phenylalanine formulas are used for infants with phenylketonuria.

Practice Alert

Concentrate or powder formula can be mixed with tap water but must be refrigerated once mixed. Remember to review formula preparation; no water should be added to ready-to-feed formula, while variable amounts are added to concentrate and powder. Be sure that the family is diluting powder and concentrate exactly as recommended to avoid electrolyte and caloric imbalance. Formula that the baby does not drink should be discarded after use and not kept for future feedings. Encourage the parents to prepare only as much formula as the infant is consuming during feedings to minimize waste. This minimizes the chance for bacteria to grow and to cause illness in the baby. When the family lives in older housing, caution them to run tap water for about 2 minutes before using it, and to use only cold water for formula preparation. These practices will minimize the chance that lead is leached from the older pipes in the house (see Chapter 20 🔗 for further discussion of lead poisoning). If the family has a well, the water should be tested for microorganisms before being used for the baby's formula.

Clinical Tip

Cow milk (including evaporated milk) can lead to bleeding and anemia (see Chapter 28 🔗), can interfere with absorption of some nutrients, and has a high solute load (concentration) which immature kidneys can have difficulty excreting. Its use should be avoided during the first year of life.

Breast or formula feeding is discussed at each contact with health professionals to identify potential teaching needs. (See Partnering with Families: Health Promotion—Supplements for Breastfed Babies.) Emphasize to parents the need to hold babies for bottle feeding rather than propping up bottles. This promotes the relationship between parent and child since touch, voice, and eye contact are possible. Caution parents not to let the baby go to sleep with a bottle as this may increase the potential for otitis media (see Chapter 24 🔗) and

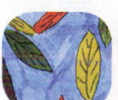

Partnering with Families

Common Problems During Breastfeeding

Most mothers need support during breastfeeding to ask questions and receive suggestions to facilitate the process. Some common issues and solutions include (London, Ladewig, Ball, et al., 2011):

- **Inverted nipples:** Roll nipples between fingers just before feeding. Use breast shields that facilitate nipple protrusion.
- **Breast engorgement:** Have the infant feed until breasts are emptied, or empty using a breast pump. Feed about every 1 1/2 hours. Do not pump between feedings. Use a warm pack before feeding to soften breasts and a cold compress between feedings to slow production if needed.

- **Slow letdown reflex:** Take a warm shower or use a warm compress before feeding. Massage the breast before feeding. Drink fluid before and during feeding. Relax and focus on spending time with the infant.
- **Sore or cracked nipples:** Position the infant correctly with the nipple completely in the infant's mouth. Avoid soaps and other products that can dry nipples. Apply an emollient recommended by a healthcare provider. Ensure diet contains adequate fruits and vegetables.

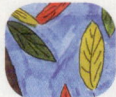

Partnering with Families

Health Promotion—Supplements for Breastfed Babies

- Each baby receives a vitamin K injection after birth to promote adequate blood clotting. After this time no further vitamin K is needed, as the baby manufactures this vitamin in the gut once he or she begins eating.
- Vitamin D, 400 International Units (10 mcg) per day, is recommended for all infants. Those who are breastfed, live in northern climates and urban settings especially in winter, are dark skinned, or are kept well covered when outside are especially at risk for deficiency.

- Iron is not needed unless the infant is not taking in other sources of food with iron by 6 months. The baby may need an iron source earlier if the mother was anemic during pregnancy or while breastfeeding.
- Fluoride 0.25 mg is given after 6 months of age if water is not fluoridated to a level of 0.3 parts per million (ppm), or if the baby is not drinking any water.

promote dental caries. Cereal should not be added to formula unless this has been prescribed for treatment of reflux; the baby needs to learn to eat this more textured food from a spoon.

Infancy—6 to 12 Months

The second 6 months of life are marked by increasing ability to absorb foods and growing nutritional needs. Babies continue breast or formula feeding and gradually add soft and then more textured foods to the diet. Parents who are using formula should continue to select iron-fortified formula for the infant up to 12 months of age. When breastfed babies are not eating foods with iron adequate to meet RDA by 6 months, supplemental iron may need to be added in a dosage of 1 mg/kg/day. Careful dietary assessment and discussion of intake by the nurse at health visits helps the practitioner decide if supplemental iron is needed.

Introduction of Complementary Foods

When should other foods be added to the infant's diet? Although some parents add other foods when the infant is only days or weeks old, it is best to take cues from the infant's developmental milestones. The American Academy of Pediatrics (2009) recommends introducing complementary foods at 4 to 6 months. At this age the extrusion reflex (or tongue thrust) decreases and the infant can sit well with support. The infant is also developing the ability to appreciate texture and to swallow nonliquid foods, and can indicate desire for food or turn away when full. During months 6 through 12, the complementary foods are an addition to the intake of breast milk or formula, rather than replacing that essential intake (Hagan, Shaw, & Duncan, 2008).

The first complementary food added to the infant's diet is usually rice cereal. The advantages of introducing cereal first are that it provides iron at an age when the infant's prenatal iron stores begin to decrease, it seldom causes allergy, and it is easy to digest. One to 2 tablespoons are fed to the infant once or twice daily just before formula or breastfeeding. The infant may appear to spit out food at first because of normal back-and-forth tongue movement. Parents should not interpret this early feeding behavior as indicating dislike for the food. With a little practice, the infant becomes adept at spoon feeding.

Once the infant eats 1/4 cup of cereal twice daily, usually at 6 to 8 months of age, vegetables or fruits can be introduced (Table 19–8). It is wise to introduce only one new food at a time, waiting several days before the next, to clearly identify any food allergies or intolerances.

TABLE 19–8	Health Promotion—Introduction of Solid Foods in Infancy
RECOMMENDATION	**RATIONALE**
Introduce rice cereal at 4–6 months.	Rice cereal is easy to digest, has low allergenic potential, and contains iron.
Introduce fruits or vegetables at 6–8 months. Some healthcare providers recommend vegetable introduction before fruits.	Fruits and vegetables provide needed vitamins. Vegetables are not as sweet as fruits; introducing them first may enhance acceptability to the infant.
Introduce meats at 8–10 months.	Meats are harder to digest, have high protein load, and should not be fed until close to 1 year of age.
Use single-food prepared baby foods rather than combination meals.	Combination meals usually contain more sugar, salt, and fillers.
Introduce one new food at a time, waiting at least 3–4 days to introduce another. Delay feeding eggs, strawberries, wheat, corn, fish, and nut products until close to 2–3 years of age.	If a food allergy or intolerance develops, it will be easy to identify. The foods listed are those most commonly associated with food allergy.
Avoid carrots, beets, and spinach before 6 months of age. Have well water evaluated for nitrates. The recommended level is less than 10 mg/L.	Nitrates in these foods and in water near agricultural runoff can be converted to nitrite by young infants, causing methemoglobinemia.
Infants can be fed mashed portions of table foods such as carrots, rice, and potatoes.	This is a less expensive alternative to jars of commercially prepared baby food; it allows parents of various cultural groups to feed ethnic foods to infants.
Avoid adding sugar, salt, and spices when preparing own baby foods.	Infants need not become accustomed to these flavors; they may get too much sodium from salt or develop gastric distress from some spices.
Avoid honey until at least 1 year of age.	Infants cannot detoxify *Clostridium botulinum* spores sometimes present in honey and can develop botulism.

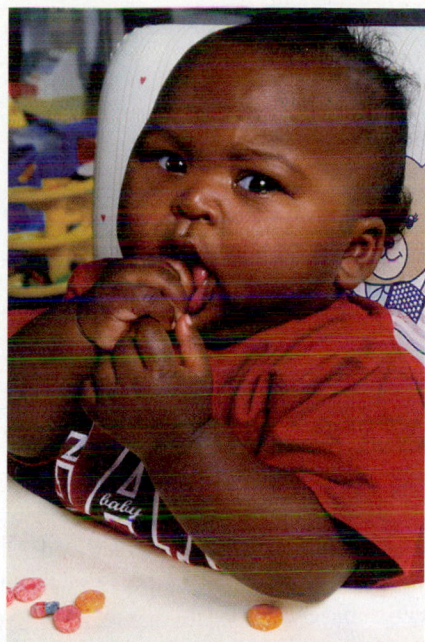

FIGURE 19–5 ■ The baby who has developed the ability to grasp with thumb and forefinger should receive some foods that can be held in the hand.

TABLE 19–9	Infant Nutritional Pattern
Birth to 1 month	■ Eats every 2–3 hours, breast milk or formula ■ Consumes 2–3 oz (60–90 mL) per feeding ■ Has coordinated suck-swallow
2–4 months	■ Has coordinated suck-swallow ■ Eats every 3–4 hours ■ Consumes 3–4 oz (90–120 mL) per feeding
4–6 months	■ Begins baby food, usually rice cereal, 2–3 T, twice daily ■ Consumes breast milk or formula four or more times daily ■ Consumes 4–5 oz (120–150 mL) per feeding
6–8 months	■ Eats baby food such as rice cereal, fruits, and vegetables, 2–5 T, three times daily ■ Consumes breast milk or formula four times daily ■ Consumes 6–8 oz (180–240 mL) per feeding
8–10 months	■ Enjoys soft finger foods three times daily ■ Consumes breast milk or formula four times daily ■ Consumes 6 oz (180 mL) per feeding ■ Uses cup with lid
10–12 months	■ Eats most soft table foods with family three times daily ■ Attempts to feed self with spoon though spills often ■ Consumes breast milk or formula four times daily ■ Consumes 6–8 oz (180–240 mL) per feeding

By 8 to 10 months, most fruits and vegetables have been introduced, and strained meats or other protein (e.g., tofu, cheese, mashed cooked beans) can be added to the infant's diet. Finger foods are introduced during the second half of the first year as the infant's palmar and then finger grasps develop and as teeth begin to erupt (Figure 19–5 ■). Infants enjoy toast, O-shaped cereal, finely sliced meats, cheese and tofu, and small pieces of cooked, softened vegetables. As food and juice intake increase, formula or breastfeedings decrease in amount and frequency (Table 19–9). Certain foods are more commonly associated with development of food allergy, and avoiding them in infancy may decrease allergy incidence. Recommendations for infants at risk due to family history are to delay feeding of cow milk until 1 year, eggs until 2 years, and peanuts, nuts, fish, and shellfish until 3 years (AAP, 2009).

Practice Alert

Advise parents to use caution when providing finger foods to the infant. Hard foods and some soft and malleable foods slip easily into the pharynx and may cause choking. Avoid hot dogs, hard vegetables, candy, whole grapes, and peanut butter. Infants and other young children should always be supervised while eating. Be sure parents are familiar with techniques for airway obstruction removal and have emergency numbers clearly listed on their phones. Refer to the Skills Manual ⬭ for airway obstruction removal information.

Parents who want to make baby foods at home can be encouraged and instructed about how to do so. Some commercially prepared foods have unnecessary additives such as salt, sugar, and food starch, and they may be costly for some families. Parents can easily blend fruits and vegetables the family is eating before adding salt, sugar, or seasoning, as these additives should be avoided in the baby's foods.

Clinical Tip

Caution parents not to use honey in foods for infants, as it can lead to infant botulism. Honey sometimes contains botulinum spores, and the immature gastrointestinal tract of the infant lacks the ability to metabolize and inactivate these spores.

Prepared foods should be used promptly and stored in the refrigerator between feedings. Foods can also be placed into ice cube trays and frozen; a cube or two can be defrosted at mealtime.

Practice Alert

If foods or fluids are microwaved for use with infants or children, there can be "hot spots" that lead to burning. Stirring, shaking, and checking temperature before feeding is needed to protect the child from burns to the mouth. Bottles of formula or breast milk should not be heated in a microwave because of the danger of hot spots, even when the outside of the bottle feels only warm. Placing the bottle in a pan of hot water or under hot tap water for a few minutes is a better alternative.

Weaning has come to be associated with a baby giving up breast-feeding or bottle feeding to drink from a cup, although it can refer to any change in prior patterns. For example, in some cultures and eras, weaning meant to replace the breast with food as the primary nutritional source. Most babies begin to drink from cups sometime in the second half of the first year. By then they can sit upright, like to grasp objects and bring them to their mouths, and are interested in "drinking" in the same manner they see in others. Once most of their liquids are taken from a cup, they are "weaned." There is no perfect time for weaning, but it is good to offer a cup by 8 or 9 months of age. As the baby becomes more adept, the cup can replace or supplement one breast or bottle feeding. The process of weaning is gradual, with both parent and infant making the transition. Some babies prefer to have the comfort of being held for at least one feeding a day well into the second or third year, while others make the transition to cup quickly. Some mothers want to continue breastfeeding for as long as the young child is interested and should be supported in this decision. Others are interested in having the baby weaned by 1 year of age. Ask about the cultural patterns in a family, ask about the parents'

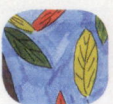

Partnering with Families

Weaning

Weaning is often easy to accomplish, but some parents need assistance in deciding when and how to accomplish this developmental task. Some tips include:

- Once the infant likes to grasp and hold objects, offer water in a cup with a lid.
- If the infant looks around and is preoccupied with other activities during feedings from the breast or bottle, a cup can be offered.

- Start by substituting the cup for one breast or bottle feeding daily and increase to other feedings as the baby seems ready.
- Never provide bottles or cups to carry around or to go to sleep; use them only during feeding times while being held to ensure good dental health.
- Expect the baby to prefer being held for breast or bottle feeding at night, when otherwise tired, or when upset or stressed for a longer period than at other times.

---

desires, and look for clues in the infant. Then provide information to assist the family in the best time and manner in which to wean the baby. See Partnering with Families: Weaning.

Dental Care

Dental care is one of the greatest healthcare needs of children, particularly in the national economic slowdowns when parents often do not have dental insurance through employment or the financial resources to pay for the care. Ask about access to dental care at each child healthcare visit. Refer to low-cost dental programs in the community as appropriate. Keep a list of dental resources to share with families as needed. Some dentists offer care to a certain number of low-income families for reduced rates, and health departments or clinics may offer dental care to children not served by other programs. Review information about early childhood caries (the presence of one or more decayed, lost, or filled tooth surfaces in a primary tooth from birth to 6 years of age), recommendations for cleaning teeth and gums, and food patterns to ensure dental health in Chapters 8, 10, and 11 🖉. See Figure 19–6 ■. Have parents select and establish contact with a dental provider when the child is nearing the end of infancy.

Toddlerhood

Why do parents of toddlers frequently become concerned about the small amount of food their children eat? Why do toddlers seem to survive and even thrive with minimal food intake? The toddler often displays the phenomenon of **physiologic anorexia,** caused when the extremely high metabolic demands of infancy slow to keep pace with the more moderate growth rate of toddlerhood. Although it can appear that the toddler eats nothing at times, intake over days or a week is generally sufficient and balanced enough to meet the body's demands for nutrients and energy.

Parents often need knowledge about types of foods that constitute a healthy diet. During the toddler period, parents play the major role in choosing food intake and socializing the child to eating patterns. Nutritional patterns should be discussed at each healthcare visit. Some easy-to-prepare foods are high in salt and other additives and can lead to exceeding the recommendation of *Healthy People 2020* for sodium intake. Provide alternatives to hot dogs, microwave meals, or fast foods with information about easy preparation of sliced meats, cheese, tofu, fruits, and vegetables. Healthy snacks for young children include yogurt, cheese, milk, slices of bread with peanut butter, thinly sliced fruits, and soft vegetables.

Advise parents to offer a variety of nutritious foods several times daily (three meals and two snacks) and let the toddler make choices from the foods offered. Offer foods only at meal and snack times and have the child eat in a high chair or on a special seat at the table (Figure 19–7 ■). Small portions are most appealing to the toddler. A

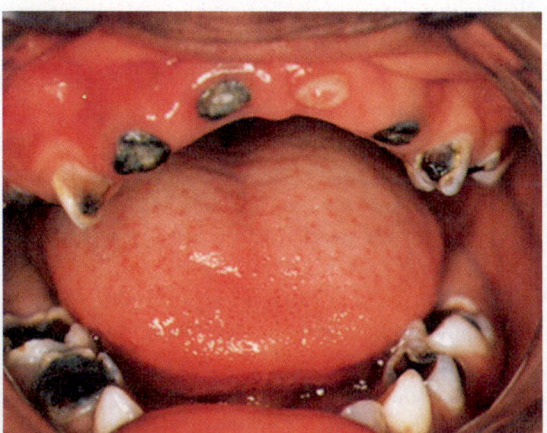

FIGURE 19–6 ■ Early childhood caries. This child has had major tooth decay related to sleeping as an infant and toddler while sucking bottles of juice and milk.

Source: *Courtesy of Dr. Lezley McIlveen, Department of Dentistry, Children's National Medical Center, Washington, DC.*

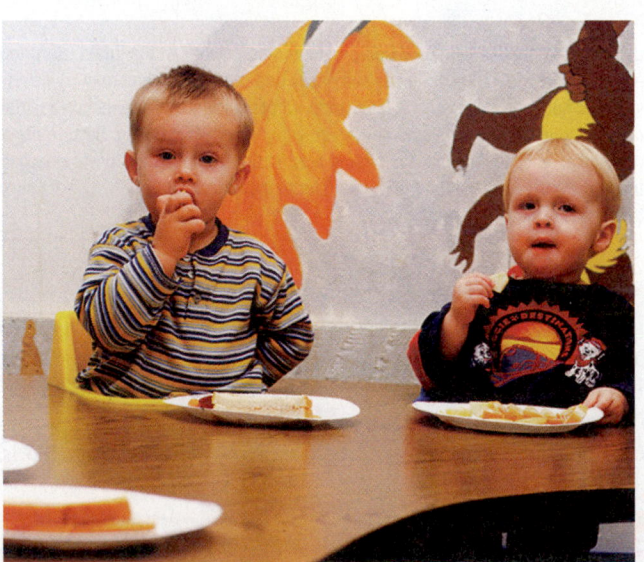

FIGURE 19–7 ■ Toddlers should sit at a table or in a high chair to eat, to minimize the chance of choking and to foster positive eating patterns.

TABLE 19–10	Health Promotion—Typical Daily Intake at Various Ages					
	BREAKFAST	**SNACK**	**LUNCH**	**SNACK**	**DINNER**	**SNACK**
Infant 6 months	2 T rice cereal with 2 oz (60 mL) formula	4 oz (120 mL) formula or breast milk	6 oz (180 mL) formula or breast milk	6 oz (180 mL) formula or breast milk	2 T rice cereal with 2 oz (60 mL) formula, then 6 oz (180 mL) formula or breast milk	4 oz (120 mL) formula or breast milk
12 months	1/4 to 1/2 cup (60–120 mL) apple juice 4 T rice cereal with 4 oz (120 mL) milk	3 crackers 1/2 cup (120 mL) milk	1 thin slice (1/2 oz [14 g]) of turkey 1/2 cup soft cooked carrots 1 cup (240 mL) milk	1/2 slice of cheese 1/2 cup (120 mL) milk or water	1/4 cup plain pasta 1/4 cup thin-sliced apple chunks 1/2 cup (120 mL) milk	1/2 cup yogurt
Toddler	1/4 cup (60 mL) orange juice 1/4 cup cereal with 1/2 cup (120 mL) milk 1/4 banana	5 crackers 1/2 cup (120 mL) milk	2 thin slices (1 oz [28 g]) of turkey with 1/2 slice of bread 1/2 cup soft cooked carrots 1 cup (240 mL) milk	1 slice cheese 1/2 cup (120 mL) juice	1/4 cup plain pasta 1/4–1/2 cup thin-sliced apple chunks 1/2 cup (120 mL) milk	1/2 cup yogurt
Preschooler	1/2 cup (120 mL) orange juice 1/3 cup cereal with 3/4 cup (180 mL) milk 1/2 banana	5 crackers 1/2 orange 1/2 cup (120 mL) milk	3 thin slices (1 1/2 oz [42 g]) of turkey with 1/2 slice bread 1/4 cup cooked carrots 3/4 cup (180 mL) milk	1 slice cheese 1/2 cup (120 mL) juice	1/4–1/2 cup plain pasta with meat sauce 1/2 cup thin-sliced apple chunks 1/2 cup (120 mL) milk	1/2 cup yogurt
School-age child	1/2 cup (120 mL) orange juice 3/4 cup cereal with 1 cup (240 mL) milk 1/2 bagel with jam		4 thin slices (2 oz [56 g]) of turkey with 1 slice bread and condiments Apple 1 cup (240 mL) milk 1 oatmeal cookie	1 1/2 cups popcorn 1 cup (240 mL) lemonade	1/2 cup pasta with meat sauce Dinner salad 1 slice garlic bread 1 cup (240 mL) milk	1 cup pudding or yogurt
Adolescent	1/2 cup (120 mL) orange juice 1 cup cereal 1 cup (240 mL) milk 1 bagel with 1 T peanut butter and jam		3 oz (84 g) meat with 2 slices of bread plus condiments Apple 1 cup (240 mL) milk 1 oatmeal cookie	3 cups popcorn 1 cup (240 mL) lemonade	1 1/2 cup pasta with meat sauce 1 slice garlic bread Salad with dressing 1 cup (240 mL) milk	1 cup pudding Fruit

Note: The young infant should be fed as often as needed rather than on a strict schedule of meals and snacks. The amounts listed for the infant are averages based on a 24-hour recommended intake.

general guideline for food quantity at a meal is 1 tablespoon of each food per year of age (see Table 19–10 for common serving sizes at various ages). The toddler should drink 16 to 24 oz (1/2 to 3/4 L) of milk daily. Caution parents against giving the toddler more than 1 quart (1 L) of milk daily, since this interferes with the desire to eat other foods. Excessive milk consumption leads to dietary deficiencies. Recall that the child should not be placed in bed with a bottle or allowed to carry a bottle of milk or juice around during the day, due to the risk of early childhood caries. Offer water frequently during the day to limit milk intake to recommended amounts.

Parents should be cautioned to use only 100% fruit juice and to limit consumption of this juice to 4 to 6 oz daily for children ages 1 to 6 years to decrease the opportunity for becoming overweight, developing dental caries, and experiencing abdominal discomfort (AAP, 2011). Using water to drink in combination with whole fruits, which provide fiber, is a healthier alternative. Avoid more than one meal weekly from a fast-food restaurant due to the generally high-fat, high-sugar, and low-fiber content of such meals.

Clinical Tip

Toddlers generally eat three meals and two or three snacks daily. Toddlers can drink 2% milk starting at 2 years of age. A maximum of 1 L of milk per day should be consumed. Larger amounts can contribute to obesity and may interfere with the toddler's consumption of a variety of foods, leading to iron deficiency anemia. Cups are recommended for milk and other drinks. Bottle use is generally discontinued by this age although some toddlers continue to breastfeed once or twice daily. The child is learning to use utensils (spoons are best) but may prefer fingers and still needs small serving sizes. Mild flavors are preferred, while spices and bitter tastes are generally disliked.

Practice Alert

Unpasteurized juice should never be fed to young children. It may contain pathogens such as *Escherichia coli*, *Salmonella*, and *Cryptosporidium*, which are particularly harmful to infants, toddlers, and preschoolers (Food Safety Network, 2011).

Learning how to eat with others is an important task of toddlerhood. The toddler displays characteristic autonomy or independence during mealtime. Advise parents to provide opportunities

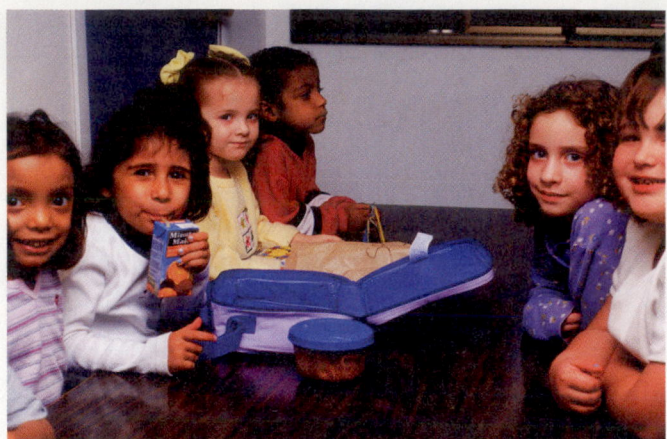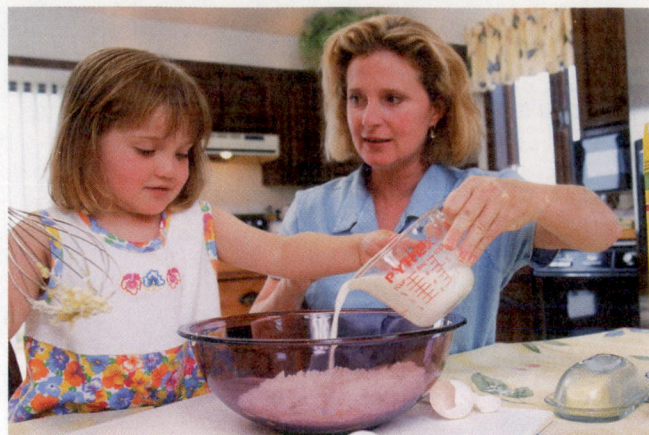

FIGURE 19–8 ■ Preschoolers learn food habits by eating with others. Engaging them in food preparation enhances knowledge of food and promotes intake at meals.

for self-feeding of food with fingers and utensils, and to allow some simple choices, such as type of liquid or cup to use. Young children should eat at a table with others, not be allowed to run and play while eating, and eat at specified meal and snack times. Because social skills are developing, the hospitalized toddler may eat better if allowed to have meals with parents or other hospitalized children. See Chapter 15 ⓔ for further suggestions about management of nutrition in hospitalized children.

Preschool

The diet of the preschooler is similar to that of the toddler, but mealtime is now a more social event, and the child increasingly makes food choices. Preschoolers like the company of others while they eat, and they enjoy helping with food preparation and table setting (Figure 19–8 ■). Involving them in these tasks can provide a forum for teaching about nutritious foods and principles of preparation such as the need for refrigeration, safety around stoves, and cleanliness. Limit visits to fast-food restaurants to about once weekly and use the opportunity to assist the child in making wise choices of nutritionally adequate foods in that setting.

Although the rate of growth is slow and steady during the preschool years, the child has periods of **food jags** (eating only a few foods for several days or weeks) and greater or lesser intake. Advise parents to assess food intake over a 1- or 2-week period rather than at each meal to obtain a more accurate impression of total intake. Food jags can be handled by providing the desired food along with other foods to foster choice. The child who chooses not to eat at snack or mealtime should not be given other foods in between. Hunger will develop and the child will become accustomed to eating when food is provided. Three meals and two or three snacks daily are the norm (see Table 19–10). Limit fruit juice to 8 to 12 oz daily, but begin teaching the "5-a-day" program that supports having five servings of fruits and vegetables each day. Children often spend part of the day in a childcare center or school. Parents need to examine the food provided in these settings and decide how to provide food at home that will supplement the school intake. Times for home meals may need to be altered if the child eats very early or late in the day at school.

The preschool period is a good time to continue encouraging good dental habits. Children can begin to brush their own teeth with parental supervision and help to reach all tooth surfaces. See Chapter 11 ⓔ for recommended doses of fluoride when the water

supply is not fluoridated. If the child has not yet visited a dentist, the first dental visit should be scheduled so the child can become accustomed to the routine of dental care. Nurses in childcare centers can teach toothbrushing techniques and encourage the routine of having all children brush after meals and snacks at the center.

School Age

The school-age years are a period of gradual growth when energy requirements remain at a steady level, although sometime during these years most children experience a preadolescent growth spurt. Girls may begin a growth spurt by 10 or 11 years, and boys a year or so later (Box 19-6). Assessment of pubertal development is important at these ages. Nutritional needs increase dramatically with this spurt, with large numbers of calories and increased amounts of other nutrients required (see Table 19–10 and Appendix C ⓔ for Dietary Reference Intakes).

School-age children are increasingly responsible for preparing snacks, lunches, and other meals. These years are a good time to teach children how to choose nutritious foods and how to plan a well-balanced meal. Because school-age children operate at the concrete level of cognitive thought, nutrition teaching is best presented by using pictures, samples of foods, videos, handouts, and hands-on experience.

School-age children often prefer the types of foods eaten at home and may be resistant to new food items. A hospitalized child may refuse to eat, slowing the recuperative process. Encourage family members to bring favorite foods from home that meet nutritional requirements. This can be especially helpful when the hospital serves food only from the dominant cultural group. A child accustomed to a diet of rice, tofu, and vegetables may not enjoy a hospital meal of

BOX 19–6	**Research: Early Menarche**

Numerous research studies have found a positive relationship between body mass index and early menarche in girls. Additional factors contributing to early menarche may be exposure to environmental endocrine-disrupting chemicals such as phthalates, phytoestrogens, and polychlorinated biphenyls, and the effects of chronic stress (Walvoord, 2010). Early weight monitoring and careful physical assessment are important. The nurse should remain alert for signs of breast development in fourth- or fifth-grade students and early menarche in sixth grade. Such youth may already be overweight and should receive obesity prevention interventions as well as counseling for management of body changes.

hamburger and fries. By school age, food has become strongly associated with social interaction, so it is beneficial to have children eat together or to invite family members to take the child off the unit to eat or to bring in food from home and eat with the child. Many hospitals allow children to plan a pizza night or sponsor other events to encourage eating in a social atmosphere.

Most children consume at least one meal daily in school. Although they may bring lunches to school, many children participate in the school lunch program and perhaps the school breakfast program. Become familiar with the school district's policies in your area for providing foods, snacks, and reduced-price food to students in need. Schools are an excellent setting for educating children about the 5-a-day and other nutritional programs. Classroom teaching and environmental clues in hallways and cafeterias can be used. Establish creative ways to inform and involve parents in nutritional education programs, so that teaching may be reinforced at home. This is also a good age to teach emergency care for choking, since persons of any age can choke and some have been saved by children who learned airway obstruction removal. Nurses working in clinics, offices, and other community settings can partner with school nurses to promote nutritionally adequate services within the school setting.

The loss of the first deciduous teeth and the eruption of permanent teeth usually occur at about 6 years, or at the beginning of the school-age period. Of the 32 permanent teeth, 22 to 26 teeth erupt by age 12, and the remaining molars follow in the teenage years. (See Chapter 7 for the typical sequence of tooth eruption, Chapter 12 for health promotion regarding oral care, and Chapter 24 ⊘ for emergency care for accidental tooth evulsion.) The school-age child should be closely monitored to ensure that brushing and flossing are adequate, that fluoride is taken if the water supply is not fluoridated, that dental care is obtained to provide for examination of teeth and alignment, and that loose teeth are identified before surgery or sports participation. Ask about tooth hygiene, fluoride intake (when pertinent), and loss of teeth at each health maintenance visit.

Adolescence

Most adolescents need well over 2000 calories daily to support the growth spurt, and some adolescent boys require nearly 3000 or more calories daily. When teenagers are active in a variety of sports, these requirements increase further. Because adolescents prepare much of their own food and often eat with friends, they need to learn about good nutrition. Developing a diet that includes a large number of calories, meets vitamin and mineral requirements, and is acceptable to the teen may be a challenge. An adolescent who does not like the hospital lunch and reaches for a soft drink and chips may be receptive to juice and pizza, a more nutritious meal. Small improvements should be viewed positively as they may lead to further changes. The pregnant adolescent has complex nutritional needs; refer to maternity nursing texts for information on working with this population.

Fast food represents a significant intake for many adolescents. Commonly fast food is high in fat, calories, and sodium, and low in essential nutrients such as calcium, folic acid, riboflavin, vitamins A and C, and fiber. Assisting teens to make nutritious selections at fast-food restaurants can be helpful in controlling weight and enhancing intake of nutrients. Some high schools are intervening to improve the health of youth by encouraging students to eat at school rather

BOX 19–7	School Vending Machines

Many school systems in the United States have allowed vending machines for carbonated sweetened beverages and snacks to be installed in public schools. Part of the profits from such machines has enabled revenue-strapped school districts to enhance their incomes. Companies desire exposure to students in order to form their habits to prefer the specific company's products.

However, schools are increasingly challenged about the presence of the machines, especially in light of the growing problem of overweight among youth. Weight status and sweets consumption have been related to vending machines in schools (Minaker, Storey, Raine, et al., 2011; Rovner, Nansel, Wang, et al., 2011). Removing sweetened beverages and sweet/salty snacks from school vending machines has been shown to improve dietary intake both during school hours and at home (Wordell, Daratha, Mandal, et al., 2012).

What is the nursing role in the vending machine issue? Nurses can and do work within schools to inform personnel and students about the problem of obesity, to educate about the sugar content of beverages, and to suggest healthy alternatives. Nurses have been instrumental in working on school nutrition policies that limit hours of vending machine use and types of beverages provided. Parents and nurses can work with school districts to ensure healthy food access for school-age children.

Find evidence to support your decisions about the following questions:

- Should public schools allow vending machines to be placed within schools?
- Is there an age limit for accessibility (should machines be in high schools, middle schools, elementary schools)?
- Should carbonated sweetened beverages and snacks be sold all day, only at certain times such as after lunch periods or after school, or not at all?
- What alternatives exist for fund-raising for districts with insufficient funds for school programs?
- Do schools in your community have vending machines? If so, what beverages and snacks are provided? Does the school, district, or state nutrition policy address sugar-sweetened beverage consumption?

than at nearby fast-food restaurants, decreasing availability of unhealthy foods in school vending machines, and making the school cafeteria a more enticing place to eat (Box 19–7). Although a la carte food items have been integrated into many school lunch programs and are popular with teens, they are often high in fat and calories. Fruit juice should be limited to 8 to 12 oz daily, and adding whole fruits and salads to food programs are healthy alternatives. School nurses play a vital role in helping to tailor a healthy school nutrition program (Figure 19–9 ■). See Evidence-Based Practice: Adolescents and Nutritional Choices.

Remember that peer group influence is important, so group sessions in which adolescents eat lunch together can provide a forum for influencing food habits. Some schools have redecorated lunchrooms to encourage student comfort, socialization, and positive lunch experiences. What other methods can encourage positive nutritional habits among teens?

NUTRITIONAL CHALLENGES

Nutrition is vital for growth and development of all children. Ensuring adequate nutrition, however, is not always as simple as teaching families about dietary needs at various ages. Challenges exist for all families as they strive to obtain and ingest healthy foods. Social, cultural, and political influences all play a part in determining the intake available and acceptable to children and families. Lack of adequate financial resources, widespread availability of fast foods, and mental health problems are discussed throughout this chapter. Nurses can partner with other health professionals to combine knowledge of

Evidence-Based Practice   Adolescents and Nutritional Choices

PROBLEM

Adolescents are largely independent in their food choices. They often eat "on the run" and are influenced by peers and the media. At the same time, rates of obesity are on an escalating upward trajectory. Nurses need to understand and apply evidence-based practices for influencing eating behaviors in adolescents.

EVIDENCE

The HEALTHY study followed nearly 4,000 students in sixth to eighth grades in 42 schools. The intervention schools had a curriculum that focused on healthy drinks, energy balance, exercise, strengthening activities, sedentary behaviors, interpreting media messages, and making choices for life. Researchers found that children in the intervention schools, as compared to control schools not receiving the teaching, had significant positive changes in fruit and water intake (Siega-Riz, El Ghormli, Mobley, et al., 2011).

Another middle-school program with young adolescents, the TEAMS study, began its planning for intervention with a discussion between parents, youth, and school officials on diet and exercise and barriers to healthy food and activity behaviors. The youth understood the importance of healthy diets and exercise but had deficits in knowledge about the characteristics of a healthy diet or exercise program; many misconceptions were found. In addition, the youth often blamed parents and the school for busy schedules, availability of fast foods, and lack of positive role modeling. The TEAMS project used this information to plan for interventions that provided knowledge about food and nutrition and empowered youth to establish their own health goals, thereby influencing the health habits in their families (Power, Bindler, Goetz, et al., 2010).

Communities can engage in healthy weight goals by introducing measures to monitor weight, nutrition, and activity at all health visits. One tool called Passport to Health was developed and implemented successfully by nurse practitioners in a pediatric practice setting. This tool used guidelines from the American Academy of Pediatrics and the National Association of Pediatric Nurse Practitioners to construct a pyramid that helped clinicians classify youth as underweight, healthy weight, overweight, or very unhealthy weight. Goals listed included five fruits and vegetables/day, less than 2 hours of screen time/day, 1 hour of exercise/day, and no sugared beverages. These youth-specific goals were added to the Passport to Health within clinician offices. Nurses audited charts and found that this tool increased the numbers of youth and families who received recorded counseling about weight, healthy eating, and activity (Vaczy, Seaman, Peterson-Sweeney, et al., 2011).

IMPLICATIONS

Nurses and other healthcare providers often assume that youth and families understand recommendations for diet and physical activity. These assumptions are not always true. School programs and healthcare offices/clinics are settings where specific teaching can and should occur. Youth can be encouraged to use the information they receive to identify their own health goals, which can be examined during follow-up healthcare visits and through school programs.

CRITICAL THINKING

- What developmental stages of the adolescent provide challenges to healthy eating and the ability to make wise food choices?
- Construct a list of questions about family food patterns that will help you identify knowledge and knowledge deficits of the child and family.
- Visit a local high school and then travel 1/2 mile in each direction from the school. Record the number of fast-food restaurants, billboards about foods, and any other food-related resources or media.
- Watch 2 hours of television from 3 to 5 p.m., when adolescents frequently arrive home. Record the number of food-related messages, what types of foods are advertised, and other observations.
- How can you assist adolescents to set goals related to healthy diets and physical activity in your potential role as a school nurse at a high school?

---

dietary needs to promote normal growth and development, and the special stresses of particular families to assess and intervene in this important health promotion topic. *Healthy People 2020* recognizes the importance of nutrition and has established several goals related to childhood nutrition. See Table 19–11 for examples of *Healthy People* goals and related health promotion activities of nurses.

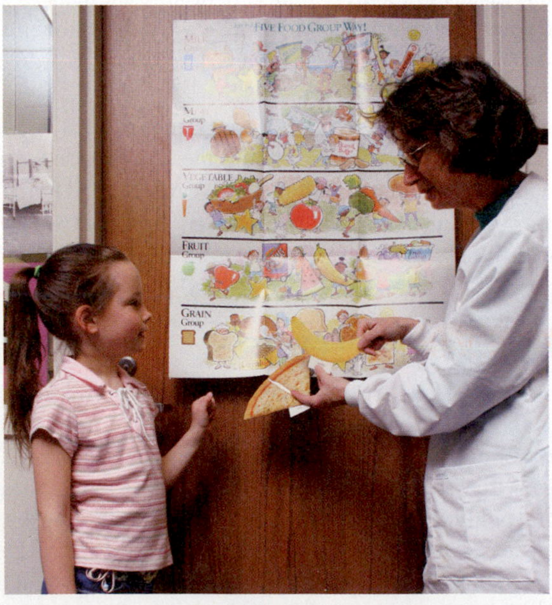

What do you think the likelihood is of reaching the goal regarding the number of children and adolescents with obesity? See the discussion later in this chapter about the increasing incidence of this condition.

NUTRITIONAL ASSESSMENT

What is the best indication that the child's nutrition is adequate? Which data collection methods provide the most accurate information about a child's dietary intake? The nurse plays an important role in assessing the diets of children and in seeking additional evaluation from dietitians and nutritionists in complex situations. Nursing assessments form the basis for establishing health promotion and health maintenance interventions related to nutrition.

Physical and Behavioral Measurement

Growth Measurement

A common method used to evaluate the adequacy of diet is measurement of growth. Preterm infants need a special combination of nutritional assessment techniques (Table 19–12). **Anthropometric measurement** refers to assessment of various parts of the body. Anthropometry of young children commonly includes weight, length, and head circumference. Standing height is substituted for length once the child can stand. Head circumference, also known as occipital-frontal circumference (OFC), is measured until the child is about

FIGURE 19–9 ■ The school nurse provides nutrition posters for the classroom and teaches schoolchildren about healthy food choices.

TABLE 19–11	*Healthy People 2020* Goals Related to Nutrition and Weight Status

GOAL	BASELINE DATA	TARGET	HEALTH PROMOTION NEEDS
Reduce the proportion of children and adolescents who are obese.	2–5 years: 10.7% 6–11 years: 17.4% 12–19 years: 17.9%	2–5 years: 9.6% 6–11 years: 15.7% 12–19 years: 16.1%	■ Dietary intake teaching ■ Encouragement of physical activity ■ Consistent monitoring of growth parameters ■ Provision of information and resources about child intake needs
Increase the contribution of fruits to the diets of the population aged 2 years and older.	0.5 cups/1000 calories	0.9 cups/1000 calories	■ Teaching about benefits and accessibility of fruits ■ Ensuring accessibility to fruits in schools, childcare, and other settings
Increase the variety and contribution of vegetables to the diets of the population aged 2 years and older.	0.8 cups/1000 calories	1.1 cups/1000 calories	■ Teaching about benefits and accessibility of vegetables ■ Ensuring accessibility to vegetables in schools, childcare, and other settings
Increase the contribution of whole grains to the diets of the population aged 2 years and older.	0.3 ounce/1000 calories	0.6 ounce/1000 calories	■ Teaching about benefits and accessibility of grains ■ Ensuring accessibility to whole grains in schools, childcare, and other settings
Reduce consumption of saturated fat in the population aged 2 years and older.	11.3%	9.5%	■ Teaching about sources of saturated fats and alternatives
Reduce consumption of calories from solid fats and added sugars in the population aged 2 years and older.	Solid fats: 18.9% Added sugars: 15.7%	Solid fats: 15.7% Added sugars: 10.8%	■ Teaching about sources of fats and alternatives ■ Teaching about sources of added sugars and alternatives
Reduce consumption of sodium in the population aged 2 years and older.	3641 milligrams/day	2300 milligrams/day	■ Teaching about sources of sodium and alternatives
Increase consumption of calcium in the population aged 2 years and older.	1118 milligrams/day for adolescents	1300 milligrams/day for adolescents	■ Teaching about benefits and sources of calcium
Reduce iron deficiency among young children and females of childbearing age.	1–2 yrs: 15.9% 3–4 yrs: 5.3% Over 12 yrs: 10.4%	1–2 yrs: 14.3% 3–4 yrs: 4.3% Over 12 yrs: 9.4%	■ Teaching about benefits and sources of dietary iron
Increase the number of states with nutrition standards for foods and beverages provided to preschool-aged children in child care. Increase the proportion of schools that offer nutritious foods and beverages outside of school meals.	24 states 9.3%	34 states 21.3%	■ Ensuring nutrition standards for preschools ■ Ensuring school snack machines have healthy alternatives ■ Enabling schools to apply for fruit and vegetable grants to offer these foods to students
Reduce household food insecurity and in so doing reduce hunger.	14.6%	6%	■ Assessing food security in all healthcare settings ■ Teaching about resources for acquisition of foods

Source: Healthy People 2020 *Summary of Objectives (U.S. Department of Health and Human Services, 2011).*

TABLE 19–12	Preterm Newborn Nutrition Assessment Techniques

GROWTH MEASUREMENT	FEEDING PATTERNS	SERUM MEASUREMENTS	OTHER
■ Daily weight ■ Weekly length, crown-heel length, and head circumference ■ Use of special growth charts for preterm infants* ■ Periodic skinfold measurement	■ Abdominal distention/girth ■ Gastric residual ■ Emesis ■ Stool frequency ■ Blood in stool	■ Glucose ■ Electrolytes ■ Alkaline phosphatase, phosphorus, calcium (to detect osteopenia or low bone mass) ■ Hematocrit, hemoglobin, reticulocyte count ■ Proteins and BUN ■ Bilirubin, alanine amino transferase (AST) if on total parenteral nutrition ■ Vitamins or minerals	■ Dual-energy X-ray absorptiometry (DEXA) to evaluate lean-, fat-, and bone-mineral mass

Note: *Special growth charts are described in Olsen, I. E., Groveman, S. A., Lawson, M. L., Clark, R. H., & Zemel, B. S. (2010). New intrauterine growth curves based on United States data. *Pediatrics, 125,* e214–e224.

BOX 19–8	Calculating Body Mass Index

To calculate body mass index (BMI), you must:

1. Be sure that weight is in kilograms. If it is in pounds, divide that number by 2.2 to get kilograms.
2. Change height measurement to meters. Because 1 m = 39.37 in. (or 0.0254 m = 1 in.), you must multiply the child's height in inches by 0.0254 to obtain height in meters.
3. Now square the number of meters.
4. You are ready to calculate BMI. Put kilograms of weight/height in meters squared and divide appropriately.

If a child weighs 26.5 lb, convert to kilograms = 12 kg. The child's height is 34.5 in. = 0.8763 m. Because $m^2 = 0.7679$, BMI = 15.63.

Alternatively, see the Centers for Disease Control and Prevention website for direct calculation of BMI using metric or English units; see the companion website.

5 years of age. Additional measurements that may be included in special circumstances include chest circumference, mid-upper arm circumference, and skinfold measurement at sites such as triceps, abdomen, and subscapular regions. See Chapter 7 and the Skills Manual for detailed descriptions of measurement techniques.

Once the measurements are collected, plot the readings on the appropriate standardized growth curves for weight, length or height, head circumference, and **body mass index (BMI).** BMI is a calculation based on the child's weight and height, or length, and is calculated as kilograms of weight/m^2 of height (Box 19–8). This is a useful calculation for determining if the child's height and weight are in proportion. Identify on the grids where the child falls in percentile for each measurement. Children normally fall between the 10th and 90th percentiles. A measurement below the 5th percentile, especially for BMI, may indicate undernutrition, whereas one over the 85th to 95th percentile may indicate overnutrition (see discussion of overweight later in this chapter). It is important, however, to look at the differences between measurements. A child in the 90th percentile for length and weight is proportional and may be a naturally large child; the BMI will be in about the 50th percentile. On the other hand, a child who is consistently in the 10th percentile for all measurements, but is growing steadily and is at a normal development level, may simply be a small child and will also be at the 50th percentile for body mass index. The BMI numbers change as children grow. Although adults with a BMI of 30 or above are obese, the specific numbers are not descriptive for the child. Only the BMI percentile is used to evaluate growth (Table 19–13).

Much cultural and individual variation exists regarding size. See Appendix A for standardized growth curves by gender and age for infants, children, and adolescents. Visit the companion website to find out more about the growth curves and to access the Centers for Disease Control and Prevention website course in accurate assessment techniques. Plot your measurements on the same growth curve with earlier percentiles for the child (Figure 19–10 ■). When measurements follow the same percentile over time, growth is generally normal for the child and nutrition is likely adequate. However, a sudden or sustained change in percentile may indicate a chronic disorder, emotional difficulty, or a nutritional intake problem. Further assessment of physical status and dietary intake will be needed. See Developing Cultural Competence: Growth Grids.

TABLE 19–13	Body Mass Index Percentiles for Boys and Girls from 5 to 17 Years		
AGE	**BMI PERCENTILE**	**BMI FOR BOYS**	**BMI FOR GIRLS**
5	5th	13.7	13.1
	50th	15.6	15.1
	85th	17.2	16.9
	95th	18.3	18.5
6	5th	13.8	13.4
	50th	15.6	15.2
	85th	17.4	17.2
	95th	19.0	19.3
7	5th	13.9	13.6
	50th	15.8	15.4
	85th	17.8	17.9
	95th	20.0	20.4
8	5th	14.1	13.6
	50th	16.2	15.8
	85th	18.6	18.9
	95th	21.5	21.7
9	5th	14.3	13.7
	50th	16.6	16.4
	85th	19.7	20.1
	95th	23.1	23.0
10	5th	14.6	14.0
	50th	17.2	17.1
	85th	20.9	21.4
	95th	24.6	24.5
11	5th	14.9	14.5
	50th	17.8	17.9
	85th	21.9	22.6
	95th	25.7	26.1
12	5th	15.3	15.1
	50th	18.4	18.8
	85th	22.6	23.6
	95th	26.5	27.5
13	5th	15.9	15.9
	50th	19.1	19.6
	85th	23.2	24.4
	95th	27.1	28.6
14	5th	16.5	16.6
	50th	19.8	20.2
	85th	23.7	24.9
	95th	27.8	29.3
15	5th	17.2	17.1
	50th	20.6	20.6
	85th	24.5	25.2
	95th	28.7	29.6
16	5th	17.9	17.4
	50th	21.3	20.9
	85th	25.4	25.5
	95th	29.8	29.9
17	5th	18.3	17.7
	50th	21.8	21.2
	85th	25.9	25.9
	95th	30.1	31.3

Source: *Reprinted from Rosner, B., Prineas, R., Loggie, J., & Daniels, S. R. Percentiles for body mass index in U.S. children 5 to 17 years of age. Journal of Pediatrics, 132, 211–222. Copyright 1998, with permission from Elsevier.*

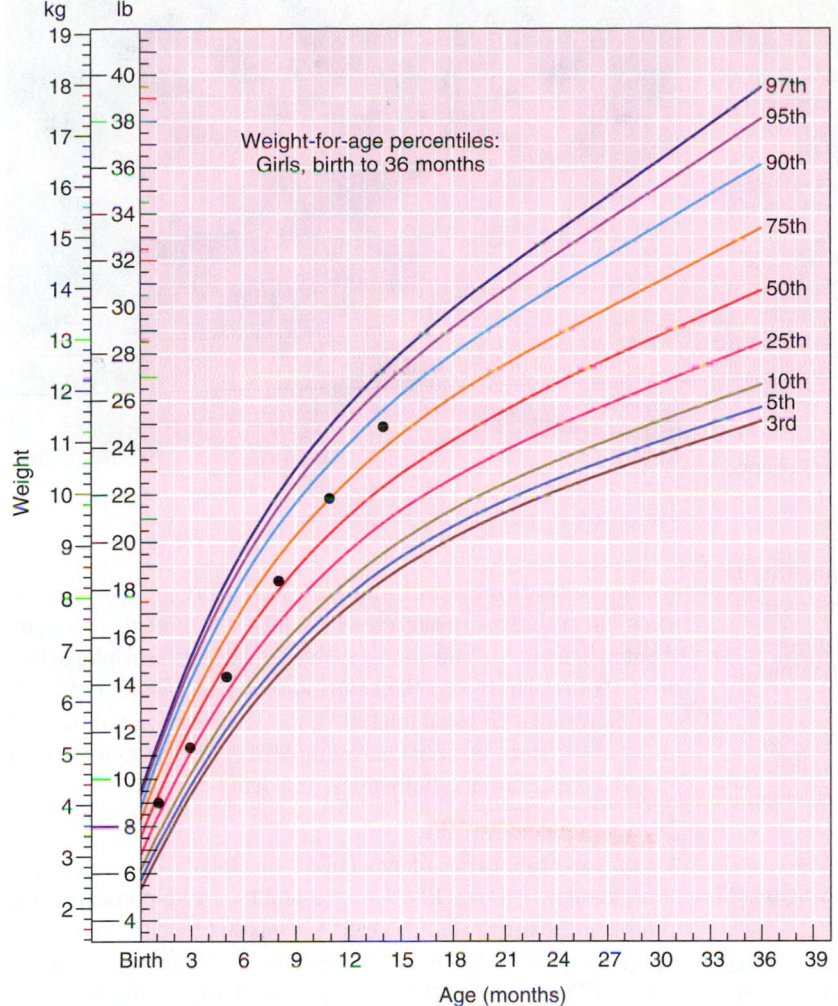

FIGURE 19–10 ■ A growth chart with the first few entries in the same channel and then a change indicated. The growth for the child indicated on this chart remained steady and in the same channel (near the 50th percentile) for some months. Then the weight measurement increased to higher channels. What kind of dietary assessment will you complete with the parents? What could be the possible causes?

Clinical Tip

If you measure a child and find him or her to be in either very low or very high percentiles, try the following:

1. Measure again to check for accuracy.
2. Examine if length or height, weight, and head circumference are in similar percentiles. Is the child proportional?
3. Observe if the parents are very large or very small.
4. Look at the child's chart to see if the patterns have continued over time or if they represent a sudden change.
5. If the percentiles remain either high or low, if there is a lack of body proportion, or if you have other concerns, refer the child to a physician, nurse practitioner, or other healthcare provider. Changes from one channel to another are of concern. For example, if the child has usually been in the 25th percentile for all measurements, and now suddenly is in the 90th percentile for head circumference or weight, additional assessment must be performed to identify the cause.

Additional Physical Measurement

Observations from the physical assessment provide clues to nutritional status. Every body system can be affected by dietary intake, and a combination of certain symptoms may suggest specific nutritional problems. Symptoms of nutritional deficiency may be clear but are often subtle and take years to become manifested (Box 19–9). Common clinical manifestations of deficient and excess nutritional intake are outlined in the Clinical Manifestations table on page 486.

Laboratory measurements can provide useful information when nutritional status is questionable. Some common studies include hematocrit and hemoglobin, serum glucose and fasting insulin, lipids and lipoproteins, and liver and renal function studies. Adding further measurements such as chest circumference and skinfolds (measurement of fat at certain body sites such as triceps, scapular, and abdominal areas) may also be useful (Lee & Nieman, 2010).

Dietary Intake

The mother's dietary intake during pregnancy may provide information about the child's nutritional state, and it can be assessed for pertinent information. Obtain detailed information about the child's dietary intake when there is a potential for nutritional deficiency due to disease, knowledge deficit, or socioeconomic status. After the information is collected, compare the dietary intake with the recommended levels for a child of that age and gender (see Figure 19–2, Table 19–4, and Appendix C ❷ for Recommended Dietary Allowances). The 24-hour recall of intake, food frequency questionnaire, and a dietary screening history provide a good overview of the infant's or child's intake and eating patterns. A food diary provides information about the child's precise food intake.

24-Hour Recall of Food Intake

The 24-hour diet recall is frequently used to assess the adequacy of the diet. People can generally remember their intake in the past day, so results are fairly accurate. It is easy to gather the data and analyze results, and only a few minutes are needed. Ask the parent or child to list all foods eaten during the past 24 hours (Figure 19–11 ■). It is usually helpful to ask for a description of activities in the last day. Then start with the most recent event and move backwards, integrating food intake into the daily schedule. For example, you might begin by saying, "You mentioned you got up early to come to the clinic today. What did Sam eat at home before you left? Did he have a snack as you traveled here or

Developing Cultural Competence
Growth Grids

The growth grids now in use were standardized using a cross section of the U.S. population and are generally reflective of most children. However, children from some other countries or cultures may fall outside these curves. For example, new immigrants or adoptees may be in lower percentiles, and catch up over several months or years. Children of immigrants from developing countries tend to be larger than their parents. Even when small, children should follow normal growth patterns. For example, a child may remain at the 10th or 25th percentile for height, but continue to slowly grow and not fall to a lower percentile.

BOX 19–9	Research: Brain Development

Many studies have confirmed that normal brain development requires good nutrition. Amino acids, carbohydrates, and some vitamins are precursors for neurotransmitters. Essential fatty acids are essential elements in the central nervous system. Trace elements such as zinc are found in the brain and are known to be necessary for memory. Iron is needed for central nervous system **myelinization** (establishment of the myelin or fatty sheath on nerve fibers), which provides for protective and conductive functions of nerve fibers. Iodine is required for normal thyroid function and mental cognition. Cognitive performance, school achievement, and behavioral characteristics are all related to adequate nutritional intake in the early years of life. Reasoning, language, memory, attention, and learning all are affected by nutrition (Laus, Vales, Costa, et al., 2011). Clearly, early nutrition plays a part in child development, and the importance of a good diet cannot be minimized.

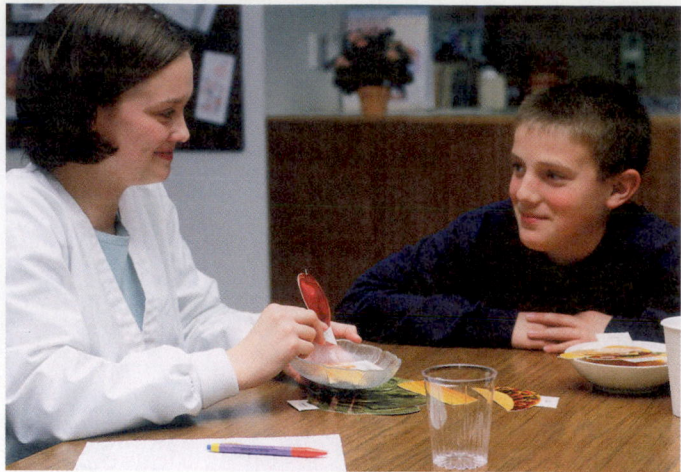

FIGURE 19–11 ■ The nurse is interviewing a child about foods eaten in the last day. Note the models of food and dishes for accurate assessment of serving sizes.

after you arrived?" While asking about the foods eaten, inquire specifically about the following:

- All meals and snacks
- Amounts of each food item consumed (have various sizes of measuring cups, bowls, and plates so accurate amounts can be indicated)
- Types of specific foods used, such as whole milk versus nonfat or 2%, brand names of cereals, specific types of margarine or butter
- Additives used, such as condiments, table salt, spices
- Food preparation methods, including adding fats to cook, removal or retention of fats on meats
- Vitamins and supplements, types, and doses
- Whether the intake is representative of the typical diet (in situations such as illness or vacation, intake may be different than usual)

Prepare questions for the 24-hour recall that will lead to an accurate profile of intake "You said that you ate lunch at school today; what was the school lunch? What type of milk did you have with that?" Include food preparation techniques and condiments used to include added ingredients. When foods are unfamiliar to you, ask where they are obtained so that additional information about nutrient intake can be consulted for later nutritional analysis. Once the 24-hour recall is obtained, conduct an intake analysis:

1. Do a quick check to compare servings of various food types with the MyPlate food guide, as described earlier.
2. Make a detailed analysis to compute calories, carbohydrate, protein, and fat intake and compare them with recommended amounts.

All major vitamins and minerals are also computed and comparisons are made to the DRIs. This computation may be done by hand, using a book of nutrients in common foods, or it may be done on the computer. Several computer programs are available, and the federal government has a website that provides intake levels and comparisons to the RDAs—try computing your own 24-hour recall or that of a child in your clinical setting with the Healthy Eating Index.

Food Frequency Questionnaire

Food frequency questionnaires are available that can be easily administered to parents or children. Usually they ask about how often certain types of foods are eaten in a specified period such as a week or month. Food frequencies provide information about dietary trends for an individual or a group of children. For example, it can answer questions about whether milk or fruit intakes are close to recommended, or whether sugared cereals are commonly ingested. Long

questionnaires can evaluate a total diet, while short ones can focus on specific items such as fruit and vegetable intake. A short questionnaire about milk intake or fruit and vegetable intake may be helpful before the start of a teaching project on nutrition to a class of school-age children. Knowing their usual intake of a food item can provide helpful information for the project. One example of types of questions asked on a food frequency questionnaire is shown in Box 19–10.

Dietary Screening History

Ask the parent about the infant's, child's, or adolescent's eating habits using questions in Boxes 19–11, 19–12, and 19–13. Responses provide information about the family's eating habits and food beliefs beyond that collected on a 24-hour dietary recall or food frequency questionnaire. See Developing Cultural Competence: Dietary Patterns.

Food Diary

Parents are asked to keep a food diary when the child has a nutrition problem or disorder, such as malnutrition, obesity, or diabetes, that requires dietary management. All meals and snacks, with food preparation method and quantities eaten over a 1- to 7-day period, are

---

Developing Cultural Competence
Dietary Patterns

Each culture has eating practices that influence dietary intake. Some groups eat three meals daily and sit with each other for conversation and sharing. Some religious groups may fast at certain parts of the year. Certain foods are more commonly eaten by specific groups. It is important to understand the eating patterns and foods commonly eaten by each cultural group and their contribution to the total nutrition of the child. For example:

- Immigrants from Mexico commonly make their own cheese.
- Native Americans may eat traditional foods such as roots, berries, and wild game or fish.
- Asian groups commonly consume rice as the major carbohydrate source.
- Hindus often do not eat any meat products.
- Muslims may not eat pork and may abstain from alcohol.

Nurses should know common food patterns in cultural groups where they work in order to ask appropriate dietary questions and perform effective teaching. However, it is important to realize that not all members of a particular religious or ethnic group may adhere to the dietary practices common to the group.

| BOX 19–10 | Sample Food Frequency Questions – National Health and Nutrition Examination Survey (NHANES) |

Over the past 12 months, how often did you drink orange juice or grapefruit juice?

- Never
- 1 time per month or less
- 2–3 times per month
- 1–2 times per week
- 3–4 times per week
- 5–6 times per week

How often did you eat pizza?

- Never
- 1–6 times per year
- 7–11 times per year
- 1 time per month
- 2–3 times per month
- 1 time per week
- 2 times per week
- 3–4 times per week
- 5–6 times per week
- 1 time per day
- 2 or more times per day

How often did you eat cold cereal?

- Options as above

How often did you eat potato chips?

- Options as above

How often were the potato chips you ate low-fat or fat-free chips:

- Almost never or never
- About ¼ of the time
- About ½ of the time
- About ¾ of the time
- Almost always or always

Source: *National Cancer Institute (2008).* NHANES Food Questionnaire. *Retrieved from http://riskfactor.cancer.gov/diet/FFQ.English.June0304.pdf*

| BOX 19–11 | Dietary Screening History for Infants |

OVERVIEW QUESTIONS

What was the infant's birth weight?

At what age did the birth weight double and triple?

Was the infant premature?

Does the infant have any feeding problems such as difficulty sucking and swallowing, spitting up, fatigue, or fussiness?

IF INFANT IS BREASTFED

How long does the baby nurse at each breast?

What is the usual schedule for nursing?

Does the baby also take any milk or formula? Amount and frequency? What type?

IF INFANT IS FORMULA FED

What formula is used? Is it iron fortified?

How is it prepared?

Do you hold or prop the bottle for feedings?

How much formula is taken at each feeding?

How many bottles are taken each day?

Does the baby take a bottle to bed for naps or nighttime? What is in the bottle?

IF INFANT IS FED OTHER FOODS

At what age did the baby start eating other foods?

Cereal

Fruit/juices

Vegetables

Finger foods

Meats

Other protein sources

Do you use commercial baby food or make your own?

Does the baby eat any table foods?

How often does the baby take solid foods?

How is the baby's appetite?

Do you have any concerns about the baby's feeding habits?

Does the baby take a vitamin supplement? Fluoride?

Have there been any allergic reactions to foods? Which ones?

Does the baby spit up frequently?

Have there been any rashes?

What types of stools does the baby have? Frequency? Consistency?

| BOX 19–12 | Dietary Screening History for Children |

- What foods or beverages does the child dislike?
- What types of food or beverage does the child especially like?
- What is the child's typical eating schedule? Meals and snacks?
- Does the child eat with the family or at separate times?
- Where does the child eat each meal?
- Who prepares the food for the family?
- What method of cooking is used? Baking? Frying? Broiling? Grilling?
- What ethnic foods are commonly eaten?
- Does the family eat in a restaurant frequently? What type?

- What type of food does the child usually order?
- Is the child on a special diet?
- Does the child need to be fed, feed himself or herself, need assistance eating, or need any adaptive devices for eating?
- What is the child's appetite like?
- Does the child take any vitamin supplements (iron, fluoride)?
- Does the child have any allergies? What types of symptoms?
- What types of regular exercise does the child get?
- Are there any concerns about the child's eating habits?

BOX 19–13   Dietary Screening History for Adolescents

1. Which of these meals or snacks did you eat yesterday?
   _____ Breakfast
   _____ Morning snack
   _____ Lunch
   _____ Afternoon snack
   _____ Dinner/supper
   _____ Evening snack

2. Do you skip breakfast three or more times a week?
   _____ Yes _____ No

3. Do you skip lunch three or more times a week?
   _____ Yes _____ No

4. Do you skip dinner/supper three or more times a week?
   _____ Yes _____ No

5. Do you eat dinner/supper with your family four or more times a week?
   _____ Yes _____ No

6. Do you fix or buy the food for any of your family's meals?
   _____ Yes _____ No

7. Do you eat or take out a meal from a fast-food restaurant two or more times a week?
   _____ Yes _____ No

8. Are you on a special diet for medical reasons?
   _____ Yes _____ No

9. Are you a vegetarian?
   _____ Yes _____ No

10. Do you have any problems with your appetite, like not feeling hungry, or feeling hungry all the time?
    _____ Yes _____ No

11. Which of the following did you drink last week?
    _____ Regular soft drinks
    _____ Diet soft drinks
    _____ Fruit-flavored drinks
    _____ Soy milk
    _____ Whole milk
    _____ Reduced fat (2%) milk
    _____ Low-fat (1%) milk
    _____ Fat-free (skim) milk
    _____ Flavored milk (for example, chocolate, strawberry)
    _____ Coffee/tea
    _____ Tap/bottled water
    _____ Juice
    _____ Sports drinks
    _____ Beer/wine, hard liquor

12. Which of these foods did you eat last week?
    Grains
    _____ Bread   _____ Cereal/grits
    _____ Rolls   _____ Popcorn
    _____ Bagels   _____ Noodles/pasta/rice
    _____ Crackers   _____ Tortillas
    _____ Other:_____
    Vegetables
    _____ Corn   _____ Greens (collard, spinach)
    _____ Peas   _____ Green salad
    _____ Potatoes   _____ Broccoli
    _____ French fries   _____ Green beans
    _____ Tomatoes   _____ Carrots
    _____ Other: _____

Fruits
_____ Apples/juice   _____ Peaches
_____ Oranges   _____ Pears
_____ Grapefruit/juice   _____ Berries
_____ Grapes/juice   _____ Melon
_____ Bananas
_____ Other: _____

Milk and Other Dairy Products
_____ Whole milk   _____ Yogurt
_____ Reduced-fat (2%) milk   _____ Cheese
_____ Low-fat (1%) milk   _____ Ice cream
_____ Fat-free (skim) milk   _____ Flavored milk
_____ Other: _____

Meat and Meat Alternatives
_____ Beef/hamburger   _____ Sausage/bacon
_____ Pork   _____ Peanut butter/nuts
_____ Chicken   _____ Eggs
_____ Turkey   _____ Dried beans
_____ Fish   _____ Tofu
_____ Cold cuts
_____ Other: _____

Fats and Sweets
_____ Cake/cupcake   _____ Chips
_____ Pie   _____ Doughnuts
_____ Cookies   _____ Candy
_____ Other: _____

13. Do you have a working stove, oven, and refrigerator where you live?
    _____ Yes _____ No

14. Were there any days last month when your family didn't have enough food to eat or enough money to buy food?
    _____ Yes _____ No

15. Are you concerned about your weight?
    _____ Yes _____ No

16. Are you on a diet now to lose weight or to maintain your weight?
    _____ Yes _____ No

17. In the past year, have you tried to lose weight or control your weight by vomiting, taking diet pills or laxatives, or not eating?
    _____ Yes _____ No

18. Did you participate in physical activity (for example, walking or riding a bike) in the past week? If yes, on how many days and for how long?
    _____ Yes _____ No

19. Do you spend more than 2 hours per day watching television and videos or playing computer games? If yes, how many hours per day?
    _____ Yes _____ No

20. Do you take vitamin, mineral, herbal, or other dietary supplements (for example, protein powders)?
    _____ Yes _____ No

21. Do you smoke cigarettes or chew tobacco?
    _____ Yes _____ No

22. Do you ever use any of the following?
    _____ Alcohol/beer/wine
    _____ Steroids (without a doctor's prescription)
    _____ Street drugs (marijuana/speed/crack/heroin)

Source: *Adapted from Holt, K., Wooldridge, N., Story, M., & Sofka, D. (Eds.). (2011). Bright futures in practice: Nutrition (3rd ed.). Elk Grove Village, IL: American Academy of Pediatrics.*

recorded. Eating patterns change significantly for holidays or family gatherings, so ask parents to select typical days for the food diary or to record specific events affecting food intake. Food diaries can provide a great deal of helpful information, but take time and motivation to complete accurately (Lee & Nieman, 2010). Be sure instructions are thorough and that the form has a place to record amounts, preparation, events occurring, and where food was eaten. The nurse or parent may need to obtain the school lunch menu and talk with the school lunch personnel to add accurate school intake.

The nurse analyzes data obtained during the assessment. The information is integrated to determine if the child demonstrates risk for nutritional problems. See Box 19–14 for a list of risk alerts. The nurse may consult with or refer the family to a dietitian or nutritionist for additional assessment and teaching.

COMMON NUTRITIONAL CONCERNS

Childhood Hunger

Although most Americans live in a "land of plenty," about 16% of U.S. children live in households that periodically experience **food insecurity,** an inability to acquire or consume adequate quality or quantity of foods in socially acceptable ways, or the uncertainty that one will be able to do so (U.S. Department of Agriculture, 2009). The opposite term, **food security,** is access at all times to enough nourishment for an active, healthy life.

A major cause of hunger in children is poverty. Since one in five children is poor, their families may be unable to provide sustainable

nutrition at all times (Children's Defense Fund, 2010). Many single-income families have a head of household moving into the workforce, so incomes are often not sufficient to provide for family food needs (see Chapter 1 for a description of Temporary Assistance for Needy Families [TANF]). Families may be ineligible for food assistance programs even though they are unable to purchase enough food for all their members. Children with special nutritional needs are at particular risk because it may be more costly to buy and prepare formula or foods for a child with allergies, diabetes, or an immune disorder.

Children who have insufficient dietary intake are at risk for a wide array of health problems. They may become anemic; experience a high rate of infectious disease due to lowered immune response; have slowed developmental maturation, delayed or stunted physical growth, and learning disorders; and be at greater risk of overweight, cardiovascular disease, and diabetes in adulthood (AAP, 2009). Subsequently, the national and individual cost of childhood hunger is great.

Nurses are well positioned to partner with other health professionals such as dietitians and physicians in evaluation of families for food insecurity in a variety of hospital, clinic, school, and home settings. In addition to the assessment of the individual child's nutritional status, further questions can determine families with potential problems. Administer the screening tool to identify risk in families (Box 19–15). Many parents go without food themselves in order to feed their children, so food insecurity may not necessarily directly affect all children. However, anxiety over providing food can be a very stressful event in families, and diet quality deteriorates as insecurity increases. If families have experienced food insecurity or may be likely to at some time, be sure to provide them with access to community agencies and programs that can be of assistance. What resources are available in your community to help families with food insecurity? See Table 19–14.

Overweight and Obesity

After several decades of stable statistics regarding overweight in children, the numbers are now skyrocketing. The current incidence of overweight in the United States is an epidemic and is associated with

BOX 19–14	Risk Alerts for Nutrition

- Consumes
  - Fewer than two servings of fruits daily
  - Fewer than three servings of vegetables daily
  - Fewer than six servings of grains daily
  - Fewer than two to three servings of dairy products daily
  - Fewer than two servings of meat/meat alternative daily
  - Excessive amount of fat
  - Food from fast-food restaurants three or more times weekly
- Has poor appetite
- Skips breakfast, lunch, or dinner three or more times weekly
- Has food jags (eating just a few foods and refusing others for extended periods)
- Has inadequate financial resources to buy food, has insufficient access to food, or lacks access to cooking facilities
- Uses chronic dieting, vomiting, or pills to lose weight
- Is excessively concerned about body size or shape
- Has had significant weight change in past 6 months
- Has BMI less than 5th or greater than 95th percentile
- Is physically inactive (physical activity less than 5 days weekly)
- Participates in excessive physical activity
- Has chronic disease or condition
- Is taking prescription or nonprescription medication
- Uses alcohol, tobacco, or other drugs
- Takes dietary supplements
- Has hyperlipidemia, iron deficiency anemia, or other abnormal serum values
- Has dental caries
- Is pregnant

Source: Adapted from Holt, K., Wooldridge, N., Story, M., & Sofka, D. (Eds.). (2011). Bright futures in practice: Nutrition (3rd ed.). Elk Grove Village, IL: American Academy of Pediatrics.

BOX 19–15	Food Insecurity Screening

1. Does your household ever run out of money to buy food to make a meal?
2. Do you or members of your household ever eat less than you feel you should because there is not enough money for food?
3. Do you or members of your household ever cut the size of meals or skip meals because there is not enough money for food?
4. Do your children ever eat less than you feel they should because there is not enough money for food?
5. Do you ever cut the size of your children's meals or do they skip meals because there is not enough money for food?
6. Do your children ever say they are hungry because there is not enough food in the house?
7. Do you ever rely on a limited number of foods to feed your children because you are running out of money to buy foods for a meal?
8. Do any of your children ever go to bed hungry because there is not enough money to buy food?

Scoring: 5–8 yes = hungry; 1–4 yes = risk of hunger

Source: From the Washington State Department of Health.

TABLE 19–14	Health Promotion—Community Resources for Food
Food Stamp Program	Eligibility based on household size and income; refer students and those with low incomes, especially when they have young children; education services often available
Child Nutrition Programs	School lunch, breakfast, and milk programs; free and lowered cost meals in schools; assist parents to apply
Special Child Programs	Summer programs, Head Start, childcare centers, and homeless children programs may provide nutritional support in some communities
Women, Infants, and Children (WIC)	Supplemental foods and nutrition education to pregnant, breastfeeding, and postpartum women and to their young children; assessment of child growth often included
Nutrition Education and Training Program	Nutrition education for teachers and school food service personnel
Community Services	May include food banks, field gleaning (collecting produce from farmers' fields that will not be sold due to excess or small blemishes), community gardens, and other programs

a wide array of health problems, such as type 2 diabetes, stroke, gallbladder disease, arthritis, cardiovascular disease, sleep disturbances, hypertension, dyslipidemia, respiratory problems, certain cancers, interference with physical activity and activities of daily living, social stigma, discrimination, depression, and lower self-esteem (CDC, 2011b).

A historic high of 17% of children and adolescents are at or above the 95th percentile for BMI (obese), and about the same percentage falls between the 85th and 94th percentiles for BMI (overweight), making about one third of U.S. youth overweight or obese (CDC, 2011b). Even higher rates are seen among specific ethnic groups, with non-Hispanic Blacks, Mexican Americans, and Native Americans showing very high rates. Since overweight in childhood and adolescence frequently tracks into adulthood, the implications for health care are obvious.

Many reasons are cited for the increase in overweight children. The number of calories consumed is not increasing, but children tend to exercise less, particularly on a daily basis. They infrequently walk or ride bikes, either because of the convenience of driving or due to unsafe neighborhoods. Television viewing is very high among youth; movies, the Internet, computer games, social networking, and cell phones are further examples of media commonly used by youth. Children spend over 7 hours daily on such media (Strasburger, Jordan, & Donnerstein, 2010). These are alarming trends because increasing media use is associated with increased rates of obesity. Inactive pursuits do not require high caloric energy, leading to an imbalance in intake and demand for calories. Additionally, sedentary pursuits such as television viewing are often accompanied by ingestion of high-calorie "junk" foods. Many of the sedentary behaviors of youth, such as television viewing and computer use, also subject them to the effects of the media which tends heavily toward food marketing of less healthy foods.

The percentage of calories from fat consumed in the United States is among the highest in the world. Although no more than 25% to 35% of calories should come from total dietary fat, and no more than 10% from saturated fat, over 35% of calories consumed in the United States are supplied by total fat and over 11% by saturated fat (U.S. Department of Health and Human Services, 2011). Most fats should be from polyunsaturated and monounsaturated fatty acids, but current diets contain low amounts of those fats and high amounts of trans-fatty acids (U.S. Department of Health and Human Services, 2011). High levels of dietary fat, particularly trans fat, are associated with higher cholesterol levels and decreased activity. The high rate of dietary fat is related to the large amount of fast food consumed, as fast-food restaurants are convenient and fit well into today's lifestyles. Another contributing factor to overweight is poor snacking habits, which have been on the increase in the last decade. Snacks of choice are often nutrient poor and calorie dense. One study found that single snack items commonly supply 6% to 14% of the day's recommended calories, fat, sugar, and sodium (Lucan, Karpyn, & Sherman, 2010).

What services are available to provide food and nutrition education in your community? *Make a list for use in clinical settings with families.*

Collaborative Care

The goals of collaborative care are identification of children with overweight and partnerships with youth and their families to develop healthy lifestyles. Several diagnostic tests may be indicated when the child is overweight. Height, weight, and body mass index (described earlier in this chapter) are key to accurate diagnosis. Once the child is identified as overweight, a thorough nutrition assessment should be performed. Gather information about physical activity patterns, family history of overweight, cardiovascular disease, hypertension, diabetes, and hypercholesterolemia. Serum cholesterol, triglycerides, glucose, hemoglobin A_{1c}, and insulin may be measured to evaluate risk for cardiovascular disease and type 2 diabetes. Blood pressure must be carefully measured and evaluated with norms to determine the presence of hypertension. See Chapter 26 for cardiovascular measurements and Chapter 32 for a discussion of type 2 diabetes in children.

Although uncommon and controversial in youth, bariatric surgery has been done for morbidly obese individuals in this population. Surgery is considered only after at least 6 months of a supervised weight loss regimen, and only in youth who have skeletal maturity (over 13 years for females or 15 years for males) and have other sequelae of excess weight. Management with low-calorie, low-carbohydrate, and high-protein diets; ongoing psychologic and lifestyle counseling; and family support are needed for the obese teen who has bariatric surgery (Zeller, Guilfoyle, Reiter-Purtill, et al., 2011). (See Legal and Ethical Considerations: Obesity Treatments.)

In the United States, national goals for obesity prevention in children and youth have been established. For all youth, goals include a reduction in incidence of obesity, reduction in average BMI, increase in number of children meeting Dietary Guidelines for Americans,

Weblink   Healthy Eating and Activity Together (HEAT)

Legal and Ethical Considerations
Obesity Treatments

As the rates of obesity increase in youth, new treatments are attempted. Although bariatric surgery has been found to be an effective weight loss strategy in adults, less is known about its effects in children. Bone loss after surgery has been documented (Kaulfers, Bean, Inge, et al., 2011). Some medical centers have developed criteria for performing bariatric surgery on adolescents, but the U.S. Food and Drug Administration does not approve the procedures for use in children (Jen, Rickard, Shew, et al., 2010). Of course, obesity itself and bariatric surgery both include risks for adolescents. What informed consent is needed in these situations? What ethical dilemmas does this treatment present for healthcare providers? Consider how little is yet known about long-term effects of this surgery among youth, and the ongoing nutritional management required after surgery.

and increase in the number meeting physical activity guidelines. For individual children and youth, goals include:

- A healthy weight trajectory
- A diet that is healthful in quantity and quality
- Appropriate amount and type of physical activity
- Achieving physical, psychosocial, and cognitive growth and development milestones

Nursing Management

The goal of nursing management is to prevent new cases of overweight, identify children who are overweight, and support youth and families to establish healthy lifestyles that promote weight loss and maintenance of recommended weights. The nurse should start with a family history of conditions such as hypertension, obesity, and type 2 diabetes to assist in finding children who may be at risk (Benson, Baer, Greco, et al., 2010; Praveen, Kulshreshtha, Khurana, et al., 2010). Assessment includes height, weight, body mass index at each health promotion visit, along with plotting findings on growth charts. Any child who is at or above the 85th percentile for BMI, or who has a change in growth channels, needs further nutritional analysis. Assessment includes (1) measuring and plotting blood pressure; (2) evaluating if parents and siblings are overweight, have elevated blood pressure, exercise infrequently, or are in upper percentiles for weight, BMI, or skinfold, because risks for poor health often cluster in individuals and families; (3) asking about tobacco use in a nonjudgmental manner and inquiring about exposure to environmental tobacco smoke; (4) inquiring about the number of daily hours of television viewing and other screen activities; and (5) asking about sports, how often and for how long the child engages in them, and how vigorously.

Based on the history, the nurse identifies children who are overweight and establishes a profile of the child's associated risks. Both the child's individual health history and family history of obesity and related conditions should be collected. Nursing diagnoses are established based on these data. Several examples are listed in the accompanying Nursing Care Plan. Interventions are directed at all children to promote healthy lifestyles and at children with identified risks to lower the risks for overweight and associated chronic diseases. Nurses can assist parents and children in building good nutritional and exercise habits throughout life, thus decreasing the incidence of overweight and its attendant health risks. Patterns of eating fast foods and meals on the run, and eating while watching television, should be addressed in early health maintenance visits. Caution parents that

television viewing and other screen activities should be limited to a maximum of 2 hours total daily, and that television and video games should not be placed in children's bedrooms. Daily exercise routines starting at 30 minutes and increasing to 60 minutes can be included in most families. This includes walking to school or in the neighborhood, working out with an exercise video, bike riding, taking physical education in school, and performing other similar activities. Also, teach about MyPlate food guide and its integration into a healthy life. Healthy snacks include fruits, vegetables, grains, and nuts. "Super sizing" fast foods and eating out often should be avoided. Recognize that the nurse is often an important role model for healthy eating and physical activity, both for youth and their families.

Nurses can partner with families to encourage weight management. See resources such as "Helping Your Overweight Child" and "Take Charge of Your Health: A Teenager's Guide to Better Health." Review the Healthy Eating and Activity Together (HEAT) guidelines from the National Association of Pediatric Nurse Practitioners.

Some important suggestions include:

- Plan the desired weight goal with your healthcare provider.
- Make changes slowly and only one or two changes at a time.
- Always eat breakfast.
- Include vegetables with each meal.
- Have plenty of fresh fruits, vegetables, and whole grains in the home.
- Limit chips, cookies, carbonated beverages, and other sweetened and fatty snacks.
- Plan meals ahead and eat together as a family.
- Integrate physical activity into daily life.
- Consult with a healthcare provider regularly.

The child who is overweight should be monitored closely to evaluate the success of interventions; implement revisions as needed (Seal & Broome, 2011). Desired outcomes may include weight loss, integration of at least five fruits and vegetables and six servings of whole grains daily, lack of risk factors for cardiovascular disease or type 2 diabetes, and daily exercise of 60 minutes. Consult dietary guidelines for Americans (U.S. Department of Health and Human Services, 2011) for further recommendations. See the Nursing Care Plan for the child who is overweight for additional information on nursing management.

Food Safety

Every year in the United States, about 48 million people (1 in 6) contract foodborne illnesses. Some are quite mild, whereas others can be severe. About 72,000 people are hospitalized and over 1,686 die from these illnesses (CDC, 2011c). Children are at greater risk of severe illness and death from food and water than adults, due to their immature gastrointestinal and immune systems. Children who are immunocompromised are at even greater risk. The most common pathogens are *Campylobacter, Salmonella, Shigella, Cryptosporidium, Listeria, Yersinia,* and *E. coli.* Infants under 1 year are at extremely high risk of *Campylobacter, Rotavirus,* and *Salmonella* illness (CDC, 2011c). A former common cause of food-related illness was hepatitis A. Although still prevalent in some parts of the country, effective management and prevention through immunization has decreased its general incidence (see Chapter 22 🔗).

Nursing Care Plan — The Child Who Is Overweight

INTERVENTION	RATIONALE	EXPECTED OUTCOME
1. Nursing Diagnosis: Nutrition, Imbalanced: More than Body Requirements related to excessive intake in comparison to metabolic needs		
NIC Priority Intervention—*Weight Reduction Assistance:* Facilitating loss of weight and body fat		**NOC Suggested Outcome**—*Weight Control:* Personal actions resulting in achievement and maintenance of optimum body weight for health

GOAL: *The child will demonstrate adequate intake of all nutrients without excessive energy intake.*

INTERVENTION	RATIONALE	EXPECTED OUTCOME
■ Perform thorough nutritional assessment of the child.	■ Assessment assists in identification of dietary risks and strengths as well as health conditions related to nutrition.	The child meets all dietary requirements while achieving weight and body mass index goal.
■ Share results of assessment with the child and family by showing weight, height, and body mass index grids.	■ Many families do not consider their child overweight. Concrete information about the child's size in comparison with recommendations assists in establishing the importance of weight management.	
■ Assess access to sufficient nutritious foods for the family at all times.	■ Food insecurity promotes inadequate intake alternating with excess intake of high-caloric foods.	

■ Identify with the child and family 2–3 target areas to begin weight management. Examples might include:
  ■ Eating fast food only once weekly
  ■ Switching to low-fat dairy products
  ■ Keeping 2 more fresh fruits and vegetables in the house and 2 fewer snack foods
	■ Changing dietary patterns drastically is difficult and may lead to giving up the attempt at weight management. Partnering with the family to set goals enhances chances of success.	

■ Integrate nutrition information into each visit. Examples of topics include:
  ■ Dietary requirements for age group
  ■ Effects of simple sugar and fat intake on weight
  ■ Beneficial effects of fruits, vegetables, whole grains, and nonfat dairy
  ■ Reading food labels
  ■ Healthy choices in fast-food restaurants
  ■ Calculation of fat content of foods
	■ Nutrition information is best learned in an ongoing program.	

■ Use growth grids to help the child and family establish a weight reduction or maintenance goal.	■ Goals motivate families to achieve desired health behaviors. The goal for a young child may be weight maintenance so that as the child grows in height, the correct proportion is reached, whereas weight reduction may be needed for older children or youth who are very obese.	

INTERVENTION	RATIONALE	EXPECTED OUTCOME
2. Nursing Diagnosis: Coping: Family, Readiness for Enhanced related to need to foster health of family member		
NIC Priority Intervention—*Health System Guidance:* Facilitating child's use of appropriate nutrition and health services to foster weight control		**NOC Priority Outcome**—*Health Promoting Behavior:* Actions to promote, sustain, and increase wellness

GOAL: *The family will assist the child to manage stressors and to develop new strategies to support weight control goals.*

INTERVENTION	RATIONALE	EXPECTED OUTCOME
■ Include key family members in some of the counseling sessions with the child who is overweight.	■ Key members of the family are those who purchase foods, provide support for the child, and participate in decisions about health.	The child expresses satisfaction with family understanding and support of weight management goals.
■ Encourage the family to eat together at least once daily if possible or to increase number of meals eaten together weekly.	■ The family is an important support system in weight loss programs. Eating as a family or in a social situation can provide a chance to promote healthy foods; intake is generally lower in fat and calories than when eating alone.	
■ Seek a resource for the child to be monitored about twice monthly; this may be a healthcare provider, nutritionist, school nurse, or other person.	■ This provides an opportunity to monitor the child's progress and to offer support, additional information, and problem-solving techniques.	

Nursing Care Plan | The Child Who Is Overweight, *continued*

INTERVENTION	RATIONALE	EXPECTED OUTCOME
3. Nursing Diagnosis: Activity Intolerance related to sedentary lifestyle		
NIC Priority Intervention—*Exercise Promotion:* Facilitating regular exercise to maintain and increase endurance and energy use		**NOC Priority Outcome—***Endurance:* Extent that energy enables the child to sustain activity

GOAL: *The child will demonstrate activity tolerance by adequate oxygenation, respiratory effort, and ability to speak during brisk walking, biking, or other activity.*

■ Establish daily exercise routine beginning with 15–30 minutes daily of walking.	■ Starting with brief amounts of exercise makes the child feel comfortable and enhances potential for success.	The child demonstrates ability to engage in moderate activity for 60 minutes with minimal respiratory discomfort.
■ Gradually increase activity over 1–2 months until 60 minutes of daily exercise is maintained.	■ A gradual increase as the cardiovascular and respiratory systems adapt is generally comfortable for children; 60 minutes of moderate activity daily is recommended for children.	
■ Use activities enjoyed by the child and suggest options as necessary; refer the family to community resources such as swimming pools, organized sports, and biking groups.	■ Activities the child enjoys will be more likely to remain in usual activity patterns; exercising with others in groups increases motivation.	
■ Have families plan at least 1–2 activities they can do together weekly.	■ This fosters family relationships and provides support and motivation for the child.	
■ Limit screen activities to a maximum of 2 hours daily.	■ Increased use of screen activities is related to poor dietary habits, increased sedentary behaviors, and excess weight.	
■ Have the child keep a log of hours of television, video games, computer, and other similar activities.		
■ Tell the child never to snack while doing screen activities.		
■ Ask about use of tobacco in children in 5th grade or higher.	■ Most adults who smoke began the habit in childhood; middle school years are the most common age for smoking initiation.	
■ Inquire about exposure to environmental tobacco smoke at all ages.	■ Smoking by others in the household can be harmful to children.	
■ Perform teaching to discourage tobacco use or offer cessation programs as needed	■ Smoking decreases respiratory reserves and worsens several cardiovascular disease risks.	

INTERVENTION	RATIONALE	EXPECTED OUTCOME
4. Nursing Diagnosis: Self-Esteem, Chronic Low related to weight		
NIC Priority Intervention—*Self-Esteem Enhancement:* Assisting the child to increase personal judgment of self-worth		**NOC Priority Outcome—***Quality of Life and Self-Esteem:* Expressed satisfaction with life circumstances and positive judgment of self-worth

GOAL: *The child will express positive perception of self-worth and confidence in ability to deal with issues related to weight.*

■ Facilitate development of a positive outlook by exposing the child to others who have been successful with weight loss.	■ A positive outlook increases motivation and feelings of self-efficacy.	The child speaks positively about accomplishments in weight control management.
■ Praise the child for weight loss, weight maintenance, increased physical activity, and other achievements.	■ Praise enhances judgment of self-worth and pride in accomplishments.	
■ Help the child establish rewards for meeting goals, such as purchase of new clothing.		
■ Partner with parents so they understand the value of praise and never label the child by derogatory words such as "fat."	■ Family members are usually the most intimate support system for the child.	

NANDA-I © 2012

Practice Alert

Worldwide, over 3 million people die of illness related to unsafe drinking water each year and most of those deaths are among children. The World Health Organization is focusing on this important health problem. Children are more prone to illnesses such as diarrhea and dehydration when drinking contaminated water. Caution families with children to be sure water supplies are safe during travel or camping and to use bottled or purified water.

Foodborne illness transmission is associated with food preparation and storage practices, lack of adequate training of retail employees regarding foods and hygiene, and increasing amounts and types of foods being imported from other countries. Some examples of contaminated foods in the last few years include undercooked hamburger meat, cross-contamination of salad bars from meats, unpasteurized apple

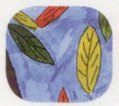

Partnering with Families

Health Promotion Food Safety Guidelines

Four key food preparation safety practices are to:

Clean: Wash hands and surfaces often.
Separate: Avoid cross-contamination.

Cook: Cook to proper temperatures.
Chill: Refrigerate promptly.

Source: *From Partnership for Food Safety Education. (2011). Safe food handling. Retrieved from http://www.fightbac.org*

Weblink   Food Safety

cider, green onions, raw spinach, prepackaged salad and delicatessen meat, berries, and sprouts. Although most infected persons experience acute bloody diarrhea, some can develop serious complications such as hemolytic uremic syndrome (see Chapter 31) or thrombocytic purpura (see Chapter 28). A wide array of other symptoms may include neurologic and respiratory problems, fever, jaundice, or arthritis. Health personnel should integrate teaching regularly so that families can decrease risks of foodborne illness transmitted at home. Recommend that families avoid consumption of unpasteurized milk and fruit juice, raw or undercooked oysters, raw or undercooked eggs, raw or undercooked ground beef, and undercooked poultry (CDC, 2011b). Check the information regarding outbreaks online. See Partnering with Families: Health Promotion Food Safety Guidelines.

Food may carry products other than microorganisms that can be harmful. An example is mercury, which may be concentrated in certain types of fish. This metal can cause harm to the developing nervous system of fetuses, infants, and young children when consumed in large quantities. The U.S. Food and Drug Administration (FDA) and Environmental Protection Agency (EPA) note that fish are an important part of a healthy diet but that certain recommendations should be followed to lower the risk of mercury's detrimental effects. Women who may become pregnant, women who are pregnant or breastfeeding, and young children should take care to do the following (U.S. Food and Drug Administration, 2011):

- Eliminate shark, swordfish, king mackerel, and tilefish from the diet.
- Eat up to 12 oz (two average meals) a week of a variety of low-mercury fish and shellfish such as shrimp, canned light tuna, salmon, pollock, and catfish. Albacore or white tuna has more mercury than light tuna, so limit white tuna to one meal weekly.
- Check for local advisories about the safety of fish caught in your area. In the absence of advice, up to 6 oz (one meal) weekly may be eaten from local waters. Do not eat other fish during that week.

Common Dietary Deficiencies

Although there can be deficits in nearly all nutrients, certain deficiencies are more common in childhood. Either limitations in the food supply or patterns of dietary intake are the cause of most deficiencies. Children with certain disease processes, such as metabolic diseases, may have difficulty absorbing or using nutrients ingested (see Chapter 32 for a discussion of inborn errors of metabolism and Chapter 4 for other genetic conditions that can influence

---

Developing Cultural Competence
Vitamin A

Vitamin A deficiency is common in developing countries. The vitamin is found in liver, dairy products, and fish. Provitamin A sources are yellow and dark green vegetables. The vitamin is fat soluble and stored in the liver. When deficient, children develop night blindness, vision loss, and high rates of infection. Public health efforts have been directed at identifying children with low vitamin A status and providing the vitamin in capsule form or in commonly ingested foods. Nurses should be aware of this health risk when caring for children who have been adopted or otherwise move from developing countries. Adequate nutrition is needed to promote recommended vitamin A intake.

intake or metabolism of food). The nutrient deficiencies present in a population are a result of genetic factors, characteristics of the food supply, and intake patterns of particular groups. See Developing Cultural Competence: Vitamin A.

Iron

Newborns have a store of iron obtained from their mothers in utero, if the maternal nutritional state was satisfactory and the baby is normal gestational age. Breast milk contains little iron, but the iron it does contain has high bioavailability. By 4 to 6 months of age, however, the baby's iron stores begin to decrease and a dietary source of iron must be added. Enriched rice cereal is commonly used to meet these initial iron needs. In babies who do not have adequate iron stores or do not take in enough iron, **anemia** (a reduction in the number of red blood cells) can result (Figure 19–12 ■). Feeding cow milk during infancy can also cause anemia by irritating the gut and leading to small but consistent loss of blood from the gastrointestinal tract. When formulas are used, they should be iron fortified to help avoid iron deficiency anemia (Table 19–15).

Adolescent females comprise the other group most commonly deficient in iron, related to loss of blood in menses, metabolic need of the growth spurt, and poor dietary balance due to sporadic dieting. Further discussion of the symptoms and treatment of iron deficiency anemia can be found in Chapter 28 .

Calcium

Calcium is an essential nutrient for bone development during childhood and adolescence. An increased intake of sweetened carbonated beverages and fruit juices is related to a decrease in calcium intake, especially among adolescents. In addition to displacing milk intake, a high intake of sweetened carbonated beverages

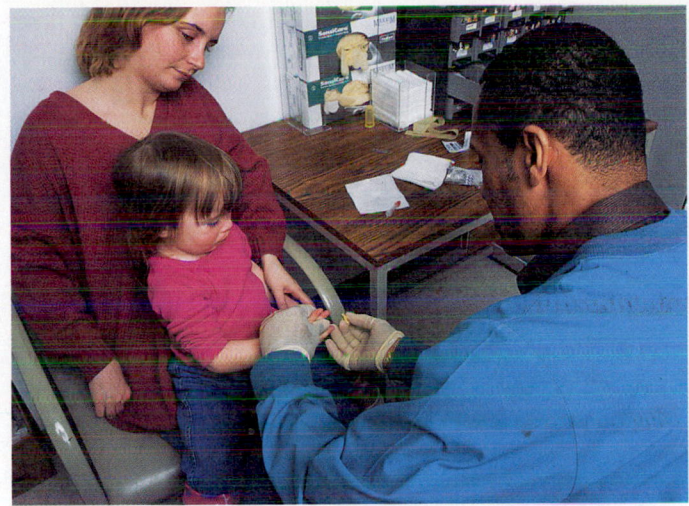

FIGURE 19–12 ■ Most Head Start centers participate in screening programs to identify children at risk for anemia. The child is comfortable sitting on the mother's lap while the nurse does a fingerstick to measure hematocrit.

may decrease calcium absorption because of the high phosphorus content of the beverages. During the adolescent growth spurt, almost 40% of the adult bone mass is accumulated (AAP, 2009). Inadequate intake puts the person at risk for osteoporosis later in life, as there is no ability to make up for earlier deficits. Although genetic variables account for some of the influence on adult bone mass, increasing calcium intake has been shown to promote bone formation. While the recommended daily intake for adolescents is 1300 mg, the average intake for adolescent males is 1145 mg and for females is only 700 to 850 mg—about half of the recommended level (AAP, 2009). See Table 19–15.

Adolescents at highest risk for impaired bone development include female athletes and others who diet to a great degree to maintain slimness. These teens manifest the "female athlete triad" of disordered eating that leads to excessive thinness, poor bone health in spite of excessive exercise, and amenorrhea (Greydanus, Omar, & Pratt, 2010). A high rate of fractures and **osteomalacia** (softening of bones) can result, in addition to an extreme risk of osteoporosis in adulthood (Ackerman & Misra, 2011). Asking about menstrual patterns, as well as exercise and diet, can be combined with physical measurements of height and weight to obtain pertinent information about the teen athlete. See the discussion of the eating disorders anorexia nervosa and bulimia nervosa later in this chapter.

> **BOX 19–16   Growth & Development: Vitamin D**
>
> Vitamin D rickets had virtually disappeared from the United States, but several cases have recently been identified. Suggested reasons for the resurgence include failure to provide vitamin D supplementation when breastfeeding is the sole source of intake for over 6 months, use of nonfortified products such as soy milk, and use of sunscreens or covers when infants are outside. Be alert for infants and toddlers with neurologic conditions such as seizures, low height for age, slowness in learning to walk, delayed tooth eruption and poor tooth enamel, and malformations (bowing) of spine, legs, and arms. Encourage sunscreen use, but be aware that children who are dark skinned or are kept covered due to religious beliefs may be at higher risk. Be certain that breastfed babies receive vitamin D supplements until other vitamin D sources are added to the diet (AAP, 2009; LeFevre, 2010).

Vitamin D

Vitamin D deficiencies were once believed to be rare; however, an increase in cases of vitamin D-deficient rickets has recently been observed, and adequate amounts are needed for bone mineralization. Although the vitamin can be synthesized in the skin upon exposure to sunlight, the amount of sunlight needed for manufacture is variable and determined by the amount of skin exposed, the color of the skin, the latitude, and time of the year. Because of this variability, it is now recommended that all infants from birth to 12 months receive a minimum intake of 400 International Units (10 mcg) daily. All persons older than 12 months should receive 600 International Units (15 mcg) daily (Ross, Taylor, Yaktine, et al., 2011). This vitamin is needed to enhance absorption of calcium, so a lack of vitamin D can contribute to calcium deficiency as well. When rickets is suspected, laboratory studies should include serum calcium, phosphorus, 25-OH vitamin D, alkaline phosphatase, parathyroid hormone, and hematocrit. Radiographs of extremities are performed (LeFevre, 2010). See Box 19–16 for growth and development issues, and see Table 19–15 for dietary sources of vitamin D.

Folic Acid

Epidemiologic evidence has linked increasing folic acid (the most common form of folate in the human body) intake with decreased incidence of neural tube defects such as spina bifida in offspring of mothers. Folate levels are low among adolescents, putting them at particular risk of birth defects when they have babies. The FDA approved fortification of cereals and breads with folate to decrease the population risk of related congenital anomalies. All women from 15 to 45 years should consume 0.4 mg of folic acid daily, and pregnant women should consume 0.6 mg. Teaching for all teens and women

TABLE 19–15	**Food Sources of Selected Nutrients**		
IRON	**CALCIUM**	**VITAMIN D**	**FOLATE**
Meats	Milk and milk products	Milk and formulas fortified with the vitamin	Bread and other products with flour
Iron-fortified formula	Egg yolks	Eggs	Yeast
Iron-fortified baby cereal	Grains	Butter	Spinach, avocado, green leafy vegetables
Iron absorption is enhanced by vitamin C intake if taken together.	Legumes	Margarine	Beans and peas
Iron is present in breast milk in a small amount, but is very well absorbed.	Nuts		Liver
	Soybeans		Fruits

of childbearing age should include common sources and the importance of folate (see Table 19–15).

Protein-Energy Malnutrition

Although micronutrient deficiencies previously described are the most common problems in developed countries, macronutrient deficiencies are the most common nutritional problems worldwide. Whereas kwashiorkor indicates protein deficiency and marasmus indicates a lack of energy-producing calories, both deficiencies often occur together and are referred to as *protein-energy malnutrition (PEM)*. Protein deficiency manifests with edema, leading to the large abdomens and rounded faces seen in severely malnourished children. Other symptoms include scant, depigmented hair; skin changes; and decreased serum proteins. It can occur following severe diarrhea or other infection in susceptible children. Caloric deficiency results in emaciation, decreased energy levels, and retarded development (see the Clinical Manifestations table on page 486). PEM may occur when a child is weaned in order for the mother to provide breast milk to a new baby. Adoptees and immigrants to developed countries sometimes manifest with mild PEM, so careful nutritional assessment is needed to provide adequate nutrition.

Practice Alert

The "female athlete triad" is commonly assumed to occur only in females performing sports that emphasize thinness, but others are also affected. Adolescents with anorexia often exercise excessively in an effort to lose weight. Males may diet because of anorexia or due to participation in a sport with a weight category such as wrestling or horse racing. Good history questions will help you to elicit information about factors influencing extremely thin adolescents.

Celiac Disease

Celiac disease, or gluten-sensitive enteropathy, is a chronic malabsorption syndrome (van Koppen, Schweizer, Cassandra, et al., 2009). About 30% of the population has one of the celiac genetic alterations, and only about 3% develop the disease (Snyder, Young, Green, et al., 2008). It is more common among members of the same family and in children with Down syndrome and Turner syndrome (National Institute of Diabetes and Digestive and Kidney Diseases [NIDDK], 2012).

Etiology and Pathophysiology

Celiac disease is an immunologic disorder (Richey, Howdle, Shaw, et al., 2009) characterized by an intolerance for gluten, a protein found in wheat, barley, rye, and oats. Inability to digest glutenin and gliadin (protein fractions) results in accumulation of the amino acid glutamine, which is toxic to mucosal cells in the intestine. Damage to the villi ultimately impairs the absorptive process in the small intestine.

In the early stages, celiac disease affects fat absorption, resulting in excretion of large quantities of fat in the stools (steatorrhea). Stools are greasy, foul smelling, frothy, and excessive. As changes in the villi continue, the absorption of protein, carbohydrates, calcium, iron, folate, and vitamins A, D, E, K, and B_{12} becomes impaired.

Clinical Manifestations

Symptoms usually occur when solid foods containing gluten are introduced to the child's diet (generally between 6 months to 2 years of age), although celiac disease is sometimes first diagnosed in adulthood. The classic features of celiac disease in infancy include chronic diarrhea, growth impairment, and abdominal distention. The child also demonstrates poor appetite, lack of energy, and muscle wasting with hypotonia.

Atypical features are present in children diagnosed with delayed-onset celiac disease around 5 to 7 years of age. Symptoms include nausea, vomiting, recurrent abdominal pain, bloating, tooth enamel defects, and aphthous ulcers (Rashid, Zarkadas, Anca, et al., 2011). Other symptoms may include delayed growth, iron deficiency, defects in tooth enamel, and abnormal liver function tests. It is common for milder cases to have delayed diagnosis, and therefore the diagnosis can be made at any age (Daitch & Epperson, 2011; Garcia-Manzanares & Lucendo, 2011).

Collaborative Care

Collaborative care focuses on identifying the disorder, nutritional management, and promotion of growth and development.

Diagnostic Tests

Diagnosis is confirmed through measurement of fecal fat content, duodenal biopsy, and improvement with removal of gluten products from the diet. Serum screening tests for IgA antiendomysial antibodies (EMA) and IgA antitissue transglutaminase antibodies (tTGA) are used for diagnosis (NIDDK, 2008). Biopsy of the small intestine may be performed (Garcia-Manzanares & Lucendo, 2011).

Clinical Therapy

Management of the disease is total exclusion of gluten from the diet. This gluten-free diet is a lifetime treatment. Barley, wheat, and rye are completely eliminated; oats are sometimes tolerated. Symptoms generally improve within a few days to weeks. Supplementation with fat-soluble vitamins, vitamin B_{12}, folic acid, calcium, and iron may be needed, depending on results of serum testing (Daitch & Epperson, 2011). Use of probiotics may be helpful (see the discussion of probiotics later in this chapter).

The intestinal villi return to normal in about 6 months. Growth should improve steadily, and height and weight should reach normal range within 1 year. Vitamin and iron supplementation may be needed for a period of time if the child has become malnourished.

Nursing Management

Nursing Assessment and Diagnosis

Assess the child for vomiting, irritability, anemia, hypotonia, and mouth ulcers. Assess growth pattern and developmental achievements. Ask the family about the child's bowel elimination patterns. Observe stool patterns and characteristics.

Nursing diagnoses that apply to the child with celiac disease may include:

- Nutrition, Imbalanced: Less than Body Requirements related to inability to digest gluten and resultant diarrhea
- Growth and Development, Delayed related to altered nutritional status
- Knowledge, Deficient (Parent and Child) related to dietary restrictions

NANDA-I © 2012

Planning and Implementation

Nursing care focuses on supporting the parents in maintaining a gluten-free diet for the child. Partner with the parents and dietitian to establish a nutritional plan for the child.

Thoroughly explain the disease process to the parents. Emphasize the necessity of following a gluten-free diet. Help parents to understand that celiac disease requires lifelong dietary modifications that should not be discontinued when the child is symptom-free. Discontinuation of the diet places the child at risk for growth retardation and the development of gastrointestinal cancers in adulthood. A dietitian should see all children with celiac disease several times during childhood. Nutritional assessment and continued teaching to maintain a gluten-free diet take place at these visits. Substitutions and recipes using potato, rice, soy, quinoa, buckwheat, or bean flours and foods are provided. Dietary management is made difficult by hidden gluten in many prepared foods such as chocolate candy, prepared meats, ice cream, soups, condiments, and food starch.

An infant or toddler's diet is easily monitored at home. When the child enters school, however, ensuring adherence to dietary restrictions becomes more difficult. In addition to easily identified gluten-based foods, such as bread, cake, doughnuts, cookies, and crackers, the child must also avoid processed foods that contain gluten as a filler. School-age children and adolescents are often tempted to eat these foods, especially when among peers. Emphasize the need for compliance while meeting the child's developmental needs.

The child's special dietary needs can place a financial burden on the family. Parents need to purchase prepared rice or corn flour products or make their own bread and bakery products. Advise parents that getting a dietary prescription enables them to deduct the cost of these ingredients and commercially prepared products as a medical expense.

Because the entire family must adapt to the diet, parents and siblings need support and management skills. For information and support, refer parents and children to several organizations, including the American Celiac Society, the Celiac Sprue Association/United States of America, and the Gluten Intolerance Group.

Evaluation

Expected outcomes of nursing care include the following:

- The child receives adequate nutrition to support growth and development needs.
- Growth and developmental milestones appropriate for the child's age are achieved.
- The family demonstrates understanding of dietary restrictions and appropriate meal planning.

Food Reactions

Food reaction encompasses any adverse reaction to foods or substances ingested in foods. The most common food reaction is **food intolerance,** or an abnormal physiologic response to a food that is not immunoglobulin E (IgE) mediated. Examples include indigestion or flatulence upon eating certain foods, a sweating reaction to some spices, rhinitis, and hives with urticaria (Mansoor & Sharma, 2011). Milk and grain products are common causes of food intolerance. Chemical additives, antibiotics, preservatives, and food colorings also can cause food sensitivity reactions. See Developing Cultural Competence: Lactose Intolerance.

The most serious type of food reaction is **food allergy,** an IgE-mediated reaction that is potentially systemic and characteristically rapid in onset. It may be manifested as swelling of the lips, mouth, uvula, or glottis; generalized urticaria; and, in severe reactions, anaphylaxis. Food allergies are the most common cause of anaphylaxis and are most prevalent in children with a

---

Developing Cultural Competence
Lactose Intolerance

Some ethnic groups have a high incidence of lactose intolerance due to low amounts of the enzyme lactase in the gut. Although most members of the group have adequate amounts of lactase in childhood to metabolize milk products, by adulthood 80% to 100% of some groups have become lactose intolerant (AAP, 2009). African Americans, Native Americans, and Asians often have lactase deficiency, which may begin to emerge during childhood. When intolerance to milk products develops, suggest alternative sources of calcium and other nutrients found in milk. Some people who have indigestion with milk are able to eat yogurt without problems.

---

family history of allergic reactions to various substances and foods (**atopy**). The foods that most commonly cause a reaction are fish, shellfish, peanuts, tree nuts, eggs, soy, wheat, corn, strawberries, and cow milk products. About 0.6% of children have an allergy to peanuts, and the incidence has increased in the last two decades (National Institute of Allergy and Infectious Diseases [NIAID], 2011). A majority of the 150 deaths from food allergies that occur annually in the United States are due to peanut allergy. Children who have both food allergy and asthma are most at risk of death from anaphylaxis due to a food allergy. See the Clinical Manifestations table for a list of food allergy symptoms. Individuals with food allergies need to be aware of "hidden" substances in prepared foods. For example, the child who is allergic to peanuts will experience a reaction to a food if peanut extracts were used in preparation of another food in the kitchen at the same time, or if dishes previously containing peanut extract were not adequately washed before preparation of the present food.

Delayed hypersensitivity reactions are attributed to digestive products of food and require a thorough diet history over several days to identify the offending food. These reactions are more difficult to diagnose, because the reaction can occur up to 24 hours after ingestion of the food. There may also be biphasic reactions that occur 1 to 30 hours after an initial anaphylaxis. Such reactions can be severe and life threatening. For these reasons every child with a food allergy who ingests the allergen should be promptly treated with epinephrine and transported to an emergency facility for further management and monitoring.

Note that certain foods can cause either allergy or intolerance so accurate diagnosis is needed. An example is cow milk that can cause an allergy with IgE-mediated systemic reaction, or an intolerance from gastrointestinal response to milk proteins (diarrhea, vomiting, abdominal pain) as a result of lack of the enzyme lactase in the gastrointestinal tract.

Diagnostic tests to identify suspected food allergies include measurement of serum IgE levels, scratch tests, and the **radioallergosorbent test (RAST),** in which radioimmunoassay is used to measure IgE antibodies to specific allergens (see Chapter 27). A diet diary helps to track the date, types of foods eaten, and reactions, if any.

Treatment consists of eliminating the offending foods from the child's diet. Collaborative care involving the child, parents, school, and healthcare providers is needed to ensure that the child with food allergies does not get exposed to the offending allergen and that all children with food reactions can avoid contact with foods to which they are allergic or intolerant. When the child is exposed to the food,

Weblink | Celiac Resources

Clinical Manifestations Food Allergies

SYSTEM	MANIFESTATIONS
Skin and mucous membranes	Urticaria and edema of lips, mouth, throat Hives Reddened cheeks Exacerbated eczema/atopic dermatitis Itching of palms and soles of feet
Circulatory	Hypotension Tachycardia Irregular heartbeat Anaphylaxis
Respiratory	Sneezing Coughing Congestion Difficulty breathing Wheezing Laryngeal edema Recurrent ear infections
Gastrointestinal	Nausea, vomiting, flatulence, diarrhea, abdominal pain
Neurologic	Fatigue Depression, headache Dizziness, syncope Hyperactivity Sleep disturbance Seizures Loss of consciousness, coma, death

Source: *Adapted from Asthma and Allergy Foundation. (2011). Food allergies. Retrieved from* http://www.aafa.org/display.cfm?id=9&cont=286

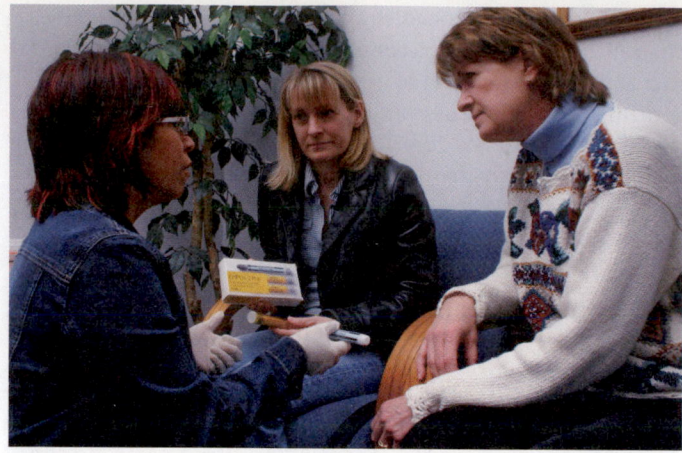

FIGURE 19–13 ■ The school nurse is providing instruction for a mother and teacher about the use of the EpiPen, which may be needed for treatment of a child with food allergy. They have both received prior instruction and practice but need to review techniques before a field trip.

epinephrine should be administered and transport to a treatment center should be immediate. Treatment in the hospital may include additional measures as needed such as bronchodilators, antihistamines, and oxygen therapy (NIAID, 2011). See Chapter 27 🔴 for further information about treatment of anaphylaxis.

Nursing Management

Prevention is the first step. Instruct parents of infants to introduce new foods at a rate of not more than one new food every 3 to 5 days. If a food intolerance is noted, the causative food can be easily identified. Discuss any changes in diet or preparation of formula. Reassure parents that the child's symptoms will disappear when the offending foods are removed from the diet.

Be alert for skin, respiratory, and other characteristic manifestations of food allergy in children. Immediately call 911 for care. Then, all such cases should be referred to an allergist for diagnosis. Assist in testing and instruction. If an allergy is identified, help the family to identify and eliminate the offending foods. Emphasize the importance of reading food labels for hidden foods that can trigger an allergic reaction.

Practice Alert

Every child with a food allergy who ingests the known allergen should be promptly treated with epinephrine and transported to an emergency facility for further management and monitoring. Delayed hypersensitivity and biphasic reactions can lead to life-threatening reaction hours after the ingestion.

Nursing care following diagnosis of a child with food allergy recognizes that the responsibility for preventing ingestion of an allergenic food for a particular child is shared by the child (when old enough to participate), other family members, and the school or other setting. Recognize that food allergies can be life threatening. Plan carefully with the family, childcare facilities, schools, and other community contacts to ensure avoidance of offending foods and to ensure emergency treatment when needed.

Explain to parents all tests, use of a food diary, and care of the child should a reaction occur. The home and school should have an EpiPen or other emergency treatment for the allergic child. It should be available in an accessible place at all times (Figure 19–13 ■). The child with a food allergy should wear medical alert identification. School personnel should know that children should not be given foods at school without parental permission. Some schools have identified peanut-free tables or sections of lunchrooms, or peanut-free classrooms to try to prevent any exposure of susceptible children to peanut products. Be sure that school personnel are informed about the allergy and knowledgeable about the importance of the child's avoidance of the food product. Be certain that the food allergy plan is in place in the school and within each additional setting where the child spends time (see Table 19–16).

Provide resources such as the Food Allergy Network for the family and school personnel. Be alert that food allergies can cause stress for children and families. Particularly if the child has had some life-threatening episodes, the threat of future problems may lead to anxiety in new situations and eating disorders related to fear of eating. The child and parents may therefore need referral to mental health services to manage the stress of a potentially life-threatening disorder.

Feeding and Eating Disorders

Deficiencies in food intake related to available nutrients and safety of the food supply were discussed in the previous section. In addition to these issues of availability, nutrient intake is affected by psychologic issues of individuals as well. Disorders of food intake span the entire developmental spectrum and can affect pregnant women, young children, and adolescents. Some of the most common feeding and eating disorders are discussed here.

TABLE 19–16   Food Allergies—Shared Responsibility

FAMILY RESPONSIBILITY	CHILD RESPONSIBILITY	SCHOOL RESPONSIBILITY
■ Notify and work with the school to develop a Food Allergy Action Plan for the child in all school locations and activities.	■ Do not trade food with other children.	■ Inform all personnel and follow federal, state, and district laws relevant to allergies and sharing medical information.
■ Provide written medical documentation, instructions, and prescribed medications; update, label, and replace as needed (e.g., EpiPen).	■ Do not eat anything known to contain the allergen or when ingredients are unknown.	■ Review health records of all students.
■ Provide a current photo of the child for the Food Allergy Action Plan.	■ Notify an adult immediately if an allergen may have been ingested.	■ Identify a core team to work with the parents and child to establish a Food Allergy Action Plan (may include school nurse, principal, school food service and nutrition manager/director, counselor).
■ Provide emergency contact information.	■ Know the location of emergency medication (e.g., EpiPen).	■ Include the student with a food allergy in school activities.
■ Educate the child to the level possible depending on age and cognition, including safe and unsafe foods, avoiding exposure to unsafe foods, symptoms of allergic reactions, how to tell adults about the problem, and how to read food labels.		■ Implement treatment upon possible ingestion of the allergen; do not wait for a reaction.
■ Institute review of policies/procedure and the Food Allergy Action Plan with the school staff, physician, and child (if old enough) after any reaction.		■ Teach all staff interacting with the child the recognition of food allergy, actions to take in an emergency, and elimination measures of the allergen from meals, snacks, educational tools, and arts and crafts.
		■ Practice the Food Allergy Action Plan and evaluate results.
		■ Work with the school nurse to allow for safe and accessible storage of emergency medicines; arrange instruction for personnel in administration of medication to ensure proper training regardless of time or location.
		■ Students should be allowed to carry their own epinephrine if age appropriate after approval from the physician/clinic, parent, and school nurse, as allowed by state or local regulations.
		■ Include field trips, transportation on school buses, and sports outings in the Food Allergy Action Plan; enforce a no-eating policy on buses.
		■ Ensure emergency communication from all buses, school events, and field trips.
		■ Be alert for, take seriously, and manage threats or harassment against a student with allergy.
		■ Institute a review of the plan after any reaction.

Source: Adapted from Food Allergy and Anaphylaxis Network. (2009). School guidelines for managing students with food allergies. Retrieved from http://www.foodallergy.org/school/guidelines.html

Colic

Colic is a feeding disorder characterized by paroxysmal abdominal pain and severe crying. The crying generally lasts 3 hours or longer and occurs at least 3 days per week. Crying episodes peak around 6 weeks of age and generally resolve by 3 to 4 months of age (Holt, Wooldridge, Story, et al., 2011).

The etiology of colic is unknown. Proposed causes include feeding too rapidly and swallowing large amounts of air.

Characteristically the infant cries loudly and continuously, often for several hours. The infant's face may become flushed. The abdomen is distended and tense. Often the infant draws up the legs and clenches the hands. Episodes occur at the same time each day, usually in the late afternoon or early evening. Crying may stop only when the child is completely exhausted or after passage of flatus or stool.

Symptoms may initially resemble intestinal obstruction or peritoneal infection. These conditions must be ruled out along with sensitivity to formula. Treatment is supportive; no general medical consensus exists on effective treatments or interventions for colic. Some healthcare providers recommend medications such as simethicone (Mylicon) drops. Some recommend formula change to a soy formula or an elemental formula such as Pregestimil.

Nursing care requires a thorough history of the infant's diet and daily schedule and the events surrounding episodes of colicky behavior. Assessment of the infant's feeding patterns and diet includes type, frequency, and amount of feeding (if breastfeeding, maternal diet history), and frequency of burping. Inquire about episodes of colic for onset, duration, and characteristics of cry. Ask the parents what measures are used to relieve crying and their effectiveness.

When possible, observe the feeding method. Parents of infants with colic are often tired and frustrated. They require frequent reassurance that they are not to blame for the infant's condition. Suggest ways of alleviating some of the infant's symptoms and discomfort. (See Partnering with Families: Suggestions for Alleviating Colic.) An important consideration is the significant impact of colic on families. Colic can place extreme stress and fatigue on the family. Active support and counseling for the mother and other family members are essential to reduce the risk of abuse to the infant (Moore, 2009).

Pica

Pica is an eating disorder characterized by ingestion of nonfood items or food items consumed in abnormal quantities or forms. Examples of ingested items include starch, peeling paint, paper, soil components, flour, and coffee grounds. Clinical manifestations include zinc and iron deficiencies as well as symptoms of lead or other heavy metal poisoning (see Chapter 20 ⊘) if these substances are contained in peeling paint or other ingested material. Pica most commonly manifests in pregnancy when women have abnormal cravings for nonfood products, and this can seriously impair the

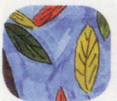

Partnering with Families

Suggestions for Alleviating Colic

- **Provide rhythmic movement:** Front-carrying slings; infant swing (battery-operated swing provides continuous motion); car ride; ride in a stroller.
- **Alternate positions:** Swaddle infant in a soft, stretchy blanket with knees flexed up against abdomen or with legs straight; place infant prone on parent's arm, supporting the body with one hand under the abdomen while cradling the head in the crook of the other arm.
- **Reduce environmental stimuli:** Respond to crying; play quiet, soothing music; prevent sudden loud noises; avoid smoking.

- **Provide various tactile stimuli:** Offer a pacifier; give a warm bath; massage infant's abdomen.
- **Alter intake:** Feed smaller amount and burp frequently; use a bottle with a collapsible bag to prevent sucking air; breastfeeding mothers should eliminate milk products and spicy or gas-producing foods; hold infant upright for 30 minutes after feeding.

---

developing fetus. Some children also manifest ingestion of abnormal amounts of nonfood items and fail to take in adequate nutrients from food. Treatment for children involves removing them from the substances, ensuring an adequate and nutritious diet, and treating any dietary deficiencies noted.

Rumination

Rumination is a rare and serious form of chronic regurgitation of recently ingested food into the mouth, followed by rechewing and reswallowing or expulsion of the material. Chewing movements and mouthing of fingers often precede or accompany regurgitation. Close observation may reveal the infant or child actively initiating gagging with the tongue and fingers.

Rumination is associated with poor maternal–infant bonding and depressive symptoms in children and adolescents (Rood, Roelofs, Bogels, et al., 2009). This behavior is seen in infants deprived of tactile, visual, or auditory stimuli for long periods. The infant substitutes repetitive self-stimulation for the lack of appropriate external stimulation. Rumination can be life threatening because it can lead to weight loss, growth failure, malnutrition, and electrolyte imbalance. During childhood and adolescence, rumination has been associated in some studies with depression.

Diagnostic evaluation focuses on ruling out an organic cause and determining the degree and type of nutritional deficiencies. The child should be observed ruminating to help confirm the diagnosis. Treatment involves correcting the nutritional deficits and developing normal feeding patterns. An interdisciplinary approach with medical and nursing staff and social services is often needed to help parents meet the individual's nutritional and psychologic needs.

Nursing care focuses on establishing a warm, caring relationship with the child and the parents. Making eye contact with the infant, providing food regularly, and stimulating the infant through all the senses are ways to break the pattern of rumination. Children and adolescents should receive depression screening and can be referred for psychologic care (see Chapter 34). Parents need to be included in the infant's or child's care. Discuss proper nutrition and demonstrate feeding techniques and interactions that promote development. Determine the parents' support needs and make a referral to social service agencies as appropriate.

Feeding Disorder of Infancy and Early Childhood (Failure to Thrive)

Feeding disorder of infancy and early childhood, or failure to thrive (FTT), describes a syndrome in which infants or young children fail to eat enough food to be adequately nourished. This disorder accounts for 1% to 5% of pediatric hospitalizations in children under 1 year of age, and many more children are managed in community settings. From 5% to 10% of low-birth-weight infants are affected (Kliegman, Stanton, St. Geme, et al., 2011).

Etiology and pathophysiology The cause of FTT can be organic, as in congenital acquired immunodeficiency syndrome (AIDS) (see Chapter 27), inborn errors of metabolism (see Chapter 32), neurologic disease (see Chapter 33), and esophageal reflux (see Chapter 30). However, most cases of FTT have no organic cause. FTT resulting from nonorganic causes is called feeding disorder of infancy or early childhood.

Infants and children whose parents or caretakers experience poverty, depression, substance abuse, intellectual disability, or psychosis are at risk for this disorder. Parents may be socially and emotionally isolated, or may lack knowledge of infant nutritional and nurturing needs. A reciprocal interaction pattern may exist whereby the parent does not offer enough food or is not responsive to the infant's hunger cues, and the infant is irritable, is not soothed, and does not give clear cues about hunger. The family may lack adequate food resources to provide consistent feedings. Parental neglect is a contributor to the condition. Preterm and small-for-gestational-age babies more commonly have eating disorders (AAP, 2009; Bryant-Waugh, Markham, Kriepe, et al., 2010).

Clinical manifestations The characteristics of this feeding disorder are persistent failure to eat adequately with no weight gain or with weight loss in a child under 6 years of age, which is not associated with other medical conditions or mental disorders and is not caused by lack of or unavailability of food. Weight is generally less than the 5th percentile, and weight for length is less than 80% of ideal weight. Infants with feeding disorders refuse food, may have erratic sleep patterns, are irritable and difficult to soothe, and are often developmentally delayed (Figure 19–14).

Collaborative Care

A thorough history and physical examination are needed to rule out any chronic physical illness. The infant or child may be hospitalized so that healthcare providers can establish a routine for feeding and sleeping. The goals of treatment are to provide adequate caloric and nutritional intake, promote normal growth and development, and assist parents in developing feeding routines and responding to the infant's cues of physical and psychologic hunger.

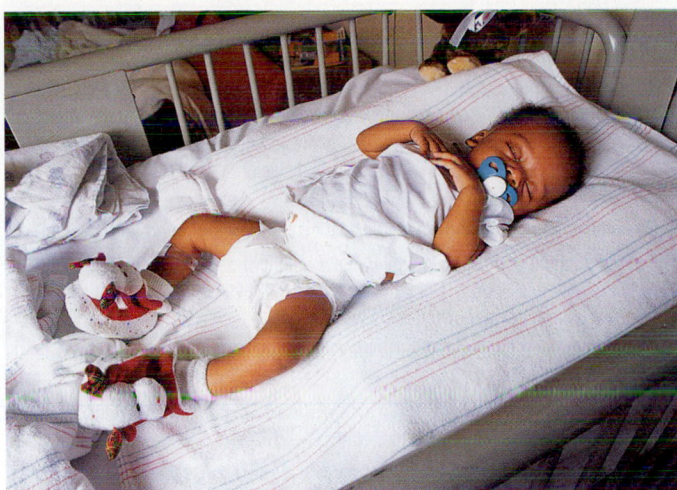

FIGURE 19–14 ■ Infants with failure to thrive may not look severely malnourished, but they fall well below the expected weight and height norms for their age. This infant, who appears to be about 4 months old, is actually 8 months old. He has been hospitalized for feeding disorder of infancy.

Interprofessional teams that include nutrition teaching, home visits, parenting skills information, and other support are most successful (Cole & Lanham, 2011).

Nursing Management

Nursing Assessment and Diagnosis

Assessment of the child by the nurse is essential for establishing the best intervention plan. Accurate measurement of weight and height each time any child is seen for health care provides an important record of growth patterns over time. This helps in identification of the child with an eating disorder. The child's activity level, developmental milestones, and interaction patterns provide important information. When feeding the child, the nurse observes how the child indicates hunger or satiety, the ability of the child to be soothed, and general interaction patterns such as eye contact, touch, and cuddliness. See Developing Cultural Competence: When to Suspect an Eating Disorder.

Parents are questioned about stresses in their lives; these may prevent appropriate interaction with the child. Asking about the pregnancy and delivery can elicit information about early disturbances in the child–parent relationship. Are there other children in the family and have eating problems occurred with them? Are depression, mental illness, or substance abuse present? Observe the child and parent behaviors while they feed the child; cues given by each person and interactional modes such as rocking, singing, talking, and body postures are important.

Following are nursing diagnoses pertinent for the young child with an eating disorder:

- Nutrition, Imbalanced: Less than Body Requirements related to inability to ingest proper amounts of food
- Growth and Development, Delayed related to inadequate food intake
- Parenting, Risk for Impaired related to lack of knowledge about the child's nutritional needs
- Fatigue related to malnutrition

NANDA-I © 2012

Developing Cultural Competence
When to Suspect an Eating Disorder

Each child should maintain a height and weight growth pattern similar to the population standard. Asian American children may normally be below the 5th percentile on growth charts and not have an eating disorder. Suspect an eating disorder when the infant or child falls one standard deviation below his or her own curve and either fails to gain weight or loses weight over several months.

Planning and Implementation

Nursing care centers on performing a thorough history and physical assessment, observing parent–child interactions during feeding times, and providing necessary teaching to enable parents to respond appropriately to their child's needs. The child is often hospitalized initially and evaluated for potential organic causes while staff members feed the child. Accurate weights, nutritional assessments, and developmental evaluation should be done to see if the child grows more normally. Additional diagnostic tests may be carried out at this time to rule out organic causes of the poor growth.

Once a diagnosis of nonorganic failure to thrive is confirmed, parents become involved in feeding the child. Observations of feeding and continued careful physical assessments are needed. The child's intake is accurately recorded at each meal or feeding. Parents are taught how to understand and respond to the child's cues of hunger and satiety. They are taught to hold, rock, and touch the infant during feedings and to establish eye contact with infants and older children.

Upon discharge, referral to an agency that can continue monitoring of the home situation is needed. This provides an opportunity to observe feeding during a home visit and evaluate stresses and behavior patterns among family members. Frequent growth measurement and developmental assessment must be ensured. Parents may need referral to community resources to help them manage stressful situations in their lives and to enhance their parenting skills. Finding a nurturing relationship for the parent may provide the support needed to enhance parenting skills.

Evaluation

Expected outcomes of nursing care include the following:

- Adequate growth and normal development of the infant is achieved.
- An improved parent–child relationship is established.

Anorexia Nervosa

Anorexia nervosa is a potentially life-threatening eating disorder that occurs primarily in teenage girls and young women. An estimated 5% of young women and 1% of young men in the United States are affected by anorexia nervosa or a related eating disorder (AAP, 2009). The typical patient is White and from a middle- to upper-middle-class family. Age at onset varies from 12 years onward but with an average age of 19 years (National Institute of Mental Health, 2010a).

Etiology and pathophysiology Many causes are believed to contribute to the onset of anorexia. Cultural overemphasis on thinness may contribute to the overconcern with dieting, body image, and fear of becoming fat that is experienced by many adolescents. The media in developed countries portray an image of extreme thinness as positive. Chemical changes have been found in the brain and blood of patients with anorexia, leading to theories about a biological cause. Often a significant life stress, loss, or change precedes the onset of anorexia. Stress hormones are commonly elevated in adolescents with anorexia, and immune system function may be disturbed.

Many experts view family issues as contributory to anorexia. Intrafamilial conflicts and dysfunctional family patterns may occur when parents are overcontrolling and perfectionistic. The adolescent's eating behaviors may be an attempt to exercise independence and resolve internal psychologic conflicts.

The adolescent may engage in lengthy and vigorous exercise (up to 4 hours daily) to prevent weight gain. Laxatives or diuretics may be used to induce weight loss. As the disorder progresses, the adolescent perceives the ever thinner body as becoming more beautiful. Youth may share weight loss techniques with friends who are anorectic and search out Internet sites that praise anorexia. The body responds to the abnormal eating behaviors as if starvation were occurring. Leukopenia, electrolyte imbalance, and hypoglycemia develop as a result of protein-energy malnutrition. Once the body mass decreases below a critical level, menstruation ceases.

Clinical manifestations Adolescents with anorexia are characterized by extreme weight loss accompanied by a preoccupation with weight and food, excessive compulsive exercising, peculiar patterns of eating and handling food, and distorted body image. They may prepare elaborate meals for others but eat only low-calorie foods. Characteristically, the fear of becoming fat does not decrease with continued weight loss. Accompanying signs and symptoms of depression, crying spells, feelings of isolation and loneliness, and suicidal thoughts and feelings are common. The disorder is often associated with mental illness such as obsessive-compulsive disorder, anxiety disorders (see Chapter 34), and history of abuse.

Physical findings include cold intolerance, dizziness, constipation, abdominal discomfort, bloating, irregular menses, and malnutrition (see the Photo Story on pages 520–521). Hypothalamic suppression can lead to disturbances of gynecologic function, osteoporosis, decreased bone density, and fractures. Lanugo (fine, downy body hair) may be present. Fluid and electrolyte imbalances, especially potassium imbalances, are common. The child or adolescent is usually energetic despite significant weight loss. Also, extreme weight loss often leads to cardiac arrhythmias (bradycardia).

Collaborative Care

Collaborative care focuses on early diagnosis of the disorder and referral for treatment, with follow-up to ensure continued interventions when needed.

Diagnostic Tests

Diagnosis is based on a comprehensive history, physical examination revealing characteristic clinical manifestations, and the DSM-IV criteria included in Box 19–17. Diagnostic tests commonly include hematocrit and hemoglobin, serum electrolytes, and serum vitamins and vitamin precursors. Bone density examination for females with lengthy amenorrhea is recommended (AAP, 2009).

Clinical Therapy

The goal of treatment is to address the physiologic problems associated with malnutrition, as well as the behavioral and cognitive components of the disorder. A firm focus is placed on reaching a

| BOX 19–17 | **DSM-IV Criteria for Anorexia Nervosa** |

A. Refusal to maintain body weight at or above a minimally normal weight for age and height (e.g., weight loss leading to maintenance of body weight less than 85% of that expected; or failure to make expected weight gain during a period of growth, leading to body weight less than 85% of that expected).

B. Intense fear of gaining weight or becoming fat, even though underweight.

C. Disturbance in the way in which one's weight or shape is experienced, undue influence of body weight or shape on self-evaluation, or denial of the seriousness of the current body weight.

D. In postmenarcheal females, amenorrhea (i.e., the absence of at least three consecutive menstrual cycles).

(A woman is considered to have amenorrhea if her periods occur only following hormone [e.g., estrogen] administration.)

Source: *Reprinted with permission from the* Diagnostic and Statistical Manual of Mental Disorders, *Fourth Edition, Text Revision. Copyright 2000. American Psychiatric Association.*

targeted weight with a gradual weight gain of 0.1 to 0.2 kg/day (0.25 to 0.5 lb/day). Weight gain of 1 to 2 lb/week is a realistic goal (Treasure, Claudino, & Zucker, 2010). Enteral feedings or total parenteral nutrition (TPN) may be necessary to replace lost fluid, protein, and nutrients, although the adolescent often perceives these feedings as a punitive measure.

Individual treatment and family therapy are used to address dysfunctional family patterns and assist the family to accept and deal with the adolescent as an independent and less-than-perfect individual. Family involvement is crucial to effect a lasting change in the adolescent (Brewerton & Costin, 2011; Fisher, Hetrick, & Rushford, 2010; Lock, 2011). Nurses, psychologists, family therapists, and dietitians commonly partner to plan and implement therapy.

Long-term outpatient treatment, in either an individual or a group setting, is frequently necessary. Counseling that engages self-help techniques may be continued for 2 to 3 years to ensure that weight gain and self-image are maintained (Allen & Dalton, 2011). Antidepressant drugs such as imipramine (Tofranil) or desipramine (Norpramin) may be prescribed for co-existing conditions such as depression, anxiety, or obsessive-compulsive disorders. However, they are not generally useful in primary treatment of the disorder (Flament, Bissada, & Spettigue, 2012).

Indications for hospitalization include loss of 25% to 30% of body weight or being at 85% or less of healthy weight, fluid and electrolyte imbalances, hypotension, cardiac arrhythmias, or the need to provide a more intense period of therapy if outpatient treatment fails to produce improvement. Behavior modification techniques are used extensively in combination with counseling and other methods in care of the hospitalized adolescent with anorexia.

Nursing Management

Nursing Assessment and Diagnosis

Obtain a thorough individual and family history. Ask about usual eating patterns, daily caloric intake, exercise patterns, and menstrual history. Ask about medication use; include prescription, nonprescription, and herbal products. Is there a family history of eating disorders? Assess for signs of malnutrition. Obtain height and weight measurements and compare with norms for the general population. Mid-upper arm circumference, skinfold thickness, waist-to-hip ratio, and body composition measurement may all be obtained

(Mattar, Godart, Melchior, et al., 2011). Because the patient with anorexia often wears layers of clothes when being weighed, strive to obtain an accurate measurement.

Nursing diagnoses for the adolescent with anorexia nervosa include the following:

- Nutrition, Imbalanced: Less than Body Requirements related to inadequate intake
- Fluid Volume, Deficient, Risk for related to inadequate fluid intake or fluid volume loss from overuse of laxatives and diuretics
- Thermoregulation, Ineffective related to excessive weight loss and absence of subcutaneous fat
- Constipation related to inadequate food intake and overuse of laxatives
- Body Image, Disturbed related to distorted perception of body size and shape
- Self-Esteem, Chronic Low related to dysfunctional family dynamics
- Coping: Family, Compromised related to parental tendency to be overcontrolling and perfectionistic

NANDA-I © 2012

Planning and Implementation

Nursing care centers on meeting nutritional and fluid needs, preventing complications, administering medications, supporting psychologic interventions, and providing referral to appropriate resources. Specific treatment measures vary depending on physical complications, length and degree of illness, emotional symptoms accompanying the disorder, and family dynamics. Resistance to treatment is common, and nurses who care for adolescents who have anorexia must deal with their own feelings of frustration and anger.

Meet Nutritional and Fluid Needs

Monitor nutritional and fluid intake, encourage consumption of food, and observe eating behaviors at mealtime. Elimination patterns may be altered as a result of increased intake during hospitalization. Monitor for possible problems, including abdominal distention, constipation, or diarrhea. Daily monitoring of serum electrolytes is necessary.

If TPN is administered, watch for complications such as circulatory overload, hyperglycemia, or hypoglycemia. Use strict aseptic technique when changing tubing or dressings.

Administer Medications

Monitor vital signs if the adolescent is receiving antidepressants. Watch for signs of hypertension and tachycardia. Administering medications after meals helps to prevent gastric irritation. Be alert for substance abuse. Patients with anorexia often use products such as excess laxatives or ephedra (also known as ma huang) to induce weight loss. Changes in the central nervous system, vital signs, and other findings may indicate over-the-counter or herbal drug use.

Provide Psychologic Support

Care for the adolescent with anorexia necessarily includes psychologic support as an important component. The nurse will refer the family to a specialist who can counsel and recommend further treatment. Families should be involved in support groups with the youth who has anorexia, and should also receive information about the condition and the youth's plan of care. The adolescent is often treated in individual counseling, and encouragement to participate is needed. Interventions that improve self-concept and lead to a realistic body image are needed. They may include encouragement for

participation in sports, praise for participation in the treatment plan, and immediate referral for relapses as treatment progresses.

Provide Referral to Appropriate Resources

Refer parents and other family members to the American Anorexia and Bulimia Association, National Anorectic Aid Society, and National Association of Anorexia Nervosa & Associated Disorders for further information about the disorder and a list of support groups in their area.

Evaluation

Expected outcomes for nursing care include successful achievement of recommended level for weight gain, maintenance of adequate fluid volume and balanced electrolytes, maintenance of normal blood pressure and heart rhythm, beginning of positive sense of self-esteem, intake of nutritionally balanced diet, and use of psychologic counseling to understand the disorder.

Bulimia Nervosa

Bulimia nervosa is an eating disorder characterized by **binge eating** (a compulsion to consume large quantities of food in a short period of time). Usually the episodes of bingeing are followed by various methods of weight control (purging), such as self-induced vomiting, large doses of laxatives or diuretics, or a combination of methods. Bulimia affects nearly 1% of the general population, with prevalence in young women about three times that in men (National Institute of Mental Health, 2010b). Like anorexia, it affects mainly adolescent girls and young women who are White and in the higher socioeconomic classes (AAP, 2009). The disorder usually begins in middle to late adolescence, at an average age of 20 years.

Etiology and pathophysiology Causes of bulimia nervosa are similar to those of anorexia nervosa: sensitivity to social pressure for thinness, body image difficulties, and long-standing dysfunctional family patterns. Families may be chaotic and distant from the girl, rather than overinvolved as with the girl who has anorexia. Many individuals with bulimia experience depression. It is not clear whether the depression is a cause or a result of the individual's inability to control the bingeing and purging cycles. An adolescent with bulimia often binges after any stressful event.

Bingeing usually occurs in secret for several hours until the individual is stopped by abdominal discomfort, by another person, or by vomiting. At first the episodes of binge eating are pleasurable. Immediately following the binge episode, however, feelings of guilt, shame, anger, depression, and fear of loss of control and weight gain arise. As these feelings intensify, the adolescent becomes increasingly anxious. This usually initiates the purge behaviors.

Purging eliminates the discomfort from bloating and also prevents weight gain. This relieves the feelings of depression and guilt, but only temporarily. Adolescents with bulimia commonly practice the binge–purge cycle many times a day, losing their ability to respond to normal cues of hunger and satiety.

Clinical manifestations Bulimia is often a "silent" disorder since it is easily concealed from healthcare providers; many people engage in bulimia for years before seeking counseling to overcome the disorder. Adolescents with bulimia, like those with anorexia, are preoccupied with body shape, size, and weight. They may appear overweight or thin and usually report a wide range of average body weight over

Weblink

Anorexia and Bulimia Resources

PHOTO STORY...

STACIA: A YOUNG WOMAN'S STRUGGLE WITH ANOREXIA NERVOSA

Consider the effects of this chronic disorder on Stacia and her family and friends. What are the many roles of the nurse in eating disorders?

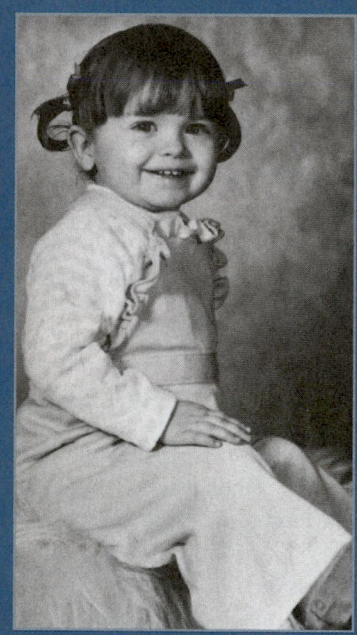

Stacia was a happy child who played an important part in the lives of her parents, brother, and grandparents. She was an outgoing and active young child.

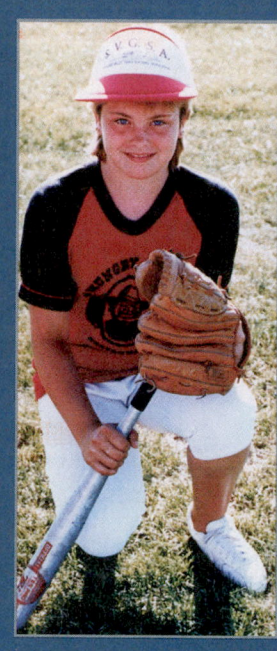

During her school years, Stacia was active in many sports, as demonstrated here in a baseball picture. She had many friends, was popular with classmates, and had an engaging personality.

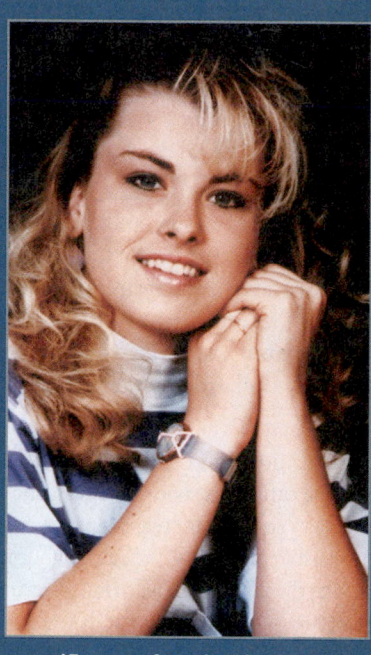

Stacia was 15 years of age in this picture. Her parents had seen no outward signs to cause alarm, but learned at this time that she had been bulimic since she was 12 years of age. Her mother found vomitus concealed in her room and confronted Stacia, who admitted she had engaged in bulimia but that it was "under control."

Although anorexia nervosa is successfully treated among many youth and adults, at times the disease can lead to death. This is the story of a young woman who died of anorexia after what many would call a normal childhood. Stacia lived in a suburban area and had a loving family and many close friends. She was active in sports, engaged in school and extracurricular activities, and had a busy schedule.

Stacia first became ill with bulimia nervosa at age 12 years. She successfully concealed the disease from her parents until she was about 15 years of age. At that point her weight was normal and no outward signs of disturbance were evident. Teens can easily cover up disturbed eating patterns by stating that they are eating with friends during a study time, or that they had a large lunch and will not eat dinner with the family. Such patterns of increasing independence in food choices and schedules are common and expected, although they can easily mask an eating difficulty. Later, her parents discovered that she had undergone several traumatic episodes with neighbors and friends that were not known to them during the early teen years. They believe these traumatic events were held inside and became a major reason for Stacia's eating disorder.

As time progressed, Stacia's bulimia evolved into anorexia nervosa. As her disease became more obvious to her family, she was confronted and agreed to counseling. She continued to tell her family that she could stop being anorexic at any time she wanted and that it was just helpful to be thin in her chosen roles of cheerleader and model. Stacia's concerned family continued to talk with her, and she was finally placed in a residential treatment program. Her parents attended family sessions and attempted to establish a supportive but curative family environment.

Stacia began college and work. She had many friends and a close relationship with a boyfriend. However, as time progressed, she began to show more signs of depression and her anorexia clearly worsened. Her boyfriend broke up with her because it was too painful to see her harming herself. She moved back home and gradually had fewer and fewer friends. She became too weak to work and was obsessed with maintaining control over her food intake. Although she continued to see a therapist, there was no improvement, but rather, a constant deterioration of her condition. Stacia was hospitalized for electrolyte imbalance, dehydration, and other effects of anorexia. She took many medications to treat sleep abnormalities, depression, gastric distress, and other symptoms. Stacia died at age 25 years, weighing 62 pounds.

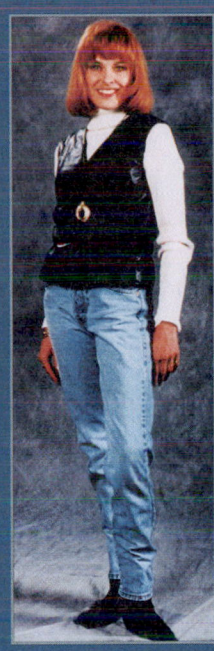

In this photo in her late teen years, Stacia is shown modeling. Most youth who see a photo like this admire the thin appearance of the model and emulate this "look." The praise that thin models receive may positively reinforce anorexic behaviors.

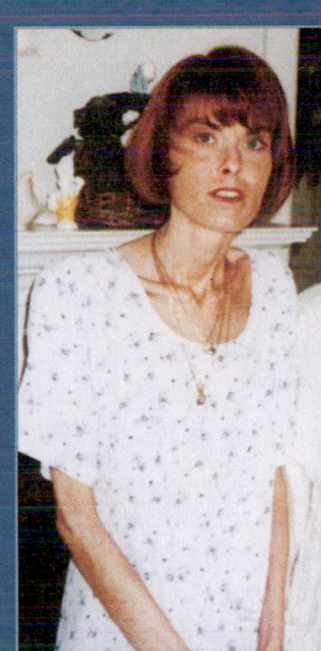

In this photo taken a short time before her death, Stacia demonstrated many symptoms of starvation. She has downy hair on various parts of her body, her skin is pale, her eyes are sunken, and her despair and depression are obvious.

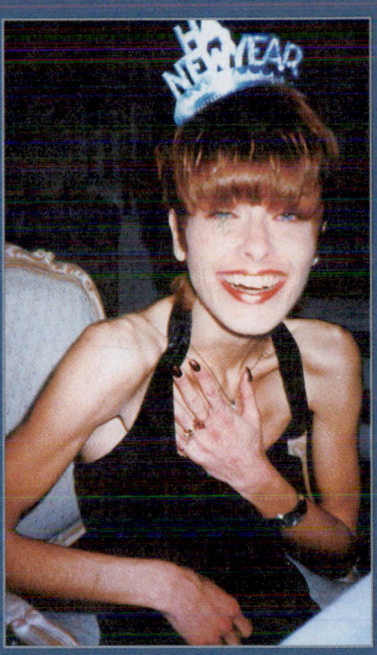

Stacia continued to lose weight slowly over many years. She still looked like an outgoing and fun-loving person, but her cachexia is obvious in this photo.

With gratitude to Stacia's family for sharing photos and her story.

Stacia's mother tells nurses that eating disorders should be confronted and faced early; as the disease progresses, cognition is altered by poor nutrition so treatments are less likely to be successful. She also alerts nurses to websites that encourage and support anorexia; these are very harmful to young people. We are so grateful to Stacia's family for sharing her story.

Consider the effects of this chronic disorder on Stacia and her family and friends. What are the many roles of the nurse in eating disorders, beginning with prevention and early identification, and progressing through treatment phases and the support of family members? How can you help health professionals, school personnel, parents, and youth to understand and deal with eating disorders? What resources are available for you to discuss with a friend who you think may have an eating disorder?

BOX 19–18   **DSM-IV Criteria for Bulimia Nervosa**

A. Recurrent episodes of binge eating. An episode of binge eating is characterized by both of the following:

1. Eating, in a discrete period of time (e.g., within any 2-hour period), an amount of food that is definitely larger than most people would eat during a similar period of time and under similar circumstances

2. A sense of lack of control over eating during the episode (e.g., a feeling that one cannot stop eating or control what or how much one is eating)

B. Recurrent inappropriate compensatory behavior in order to prevent weight gain, such as self-induced vomiting; misuse of laxatives, diuretics, enemas, or other medications; fasting; or excessive exercise.

C. The binge eating and inappropriate compensatory behaviors both occur, on average, at least twice a week for 3 months.

D. Self-evaluation is unduly influenced by body weight and shape.

E. The disturbance does not occur exclusively during episodes of anorexia nervosa.

Source: Reprinted with permission from the Diagnostic and Statistical Manual of Mental Disorders, Fourth Edition, Text Revision. Copyright 2000. American Psychiatric Association.

---

the years. Physical findings depend on the degree of purging, starvation, dehydration, and electrolyte disturbance. Erosion of tooth enamel, increased dental caries, and gum recession, which result from vomiting of gastric acids, are common findings. The back of a hand can have calluses from inducing vomiting. Abdominal distention is often seen. Esophageal tears and esophagitis may also occur.

Collaborative Care

Collaborative care focuses on early diagnosis of the disorder and referral for treatment, with follow-up to ensure continued interventions when needed.

Diagnostic Tests

A comprehensive history is necessary because most adolescents with bulimia appear normal in weight or only slightly underweight. Diagnostic tests include hematocrit, hemoglobin, and serum electrolytes; they may identify signs of altered electrolyte and hematologic status. Lowered potassium levels are related to repetitive vomiting, since gastric contents have a high potassium level. The diagnosis is confirmed by the presence of specific DSM-IV criteria (Box 19–18).

Clinical Therapy

Treatment includes management of physiologic problems, and cognitive-behavior therapy. Medications, such as fluoxetine 60 mg/day for adolescents, may be prescribed (Hay & Claudino, 2012). Management involves a variety of healthcare providers such as physicians, nurses, and therapists. Behavior modification focuses on modifying the dysfunctional eating patterns and restoring normal patterns. Until the episodes of bingeing and purging are under control, feelings of discouragement and hopelessness prevail. Thus, the focus early in treatment is on initiating an immediate behavioral change. Once initial interventions have been successful, group therapy sessions work well for persons with bulimia nervosa. Specific treatment measures may include the following:

- Educating the adolescent about good nutrition (including food choice and caloric content)
- Encouraging the adolescent to keep a log or food journal and assisting the adolescent to make connections between emotional states and stress and the impulse to binge or purge

- Setting up a daily dietary routine of three meals and three snacks a day (using the same foods for each meal and snack every day to change misconceptions about the weight-gaining potential of certain foods and to decrease anxiety about what food must be eaten at the next meal)

Once these initial measures have been taken, the underlying psychosocial issues are explored. The goals of therapy are to provide the bulimic adolescent with adaptive coping skills and to improve self-esteem.

Most adolescents with bulimia do not require hospitalization. Serious abnormalities in fluid and electrolyte levels caused by uncontrollable cycles of bingeing and vomiting, accompanied by depression or suicidal activity, are indications of the need for hospitalization. The prognosis is good with long-term therapy.

Nursing Management

Nursing Assessment and Diagnosis

Obtain a thorough individual and family history, including daily dietary intake and weight fluctuations. Inquire about problems such as abdominal pain or distention, which may indicate an abnormal eating or elimination pattern. Assess the oral mucosa for signs of damage to tooth enamel caused by purging; examine hands for evidence of vomiting-induced calluses.

Following are nursing diagnoses that may be appropriate for the adolescent with bulimia nervosa:

- Nutrition, Imbalanced: Less than or More than Body Requirements related to disordered intake
- Fluid Volume, Deficient, Risk for related to fluid volume loss
- Mucous Membrane: Oral, Impaired related to chemical effects of vomited gastric acids
- Knowledge, Deficient (Adolescent) related to health risks of excessive use of laxatives and diuretics
- Anxiety related to discomfort with weight and eating patterns
- Self-Esteem, Chronic Low related to dysfunctional family dynamics
- Coping, Ineffective related to life stressors

NANDA-I © 2012

Planning and Implementation

Nursing care includes monitoring nutritional intake and elimination patterns, preventing complications, and providing appropriate referrals.

During hospitalization, the patient should keep a food diary. Be alert to the adolescent who hides, gives away, or discards food from the tray or who exits to use the bathroom after meals. The adolescent should be monitored for at least 30 minutes after meals by remaining in a central area in the company of the nurse or other responsible individuals. Withdrawal from laxatives and diuretics is managed with careful observation for alterations in fluid and electrolyte status. Cardiac monitoring may be necessary if potassium levels are seriously altered. Esophageal tearing or esophagitis is treated to promote mucosal healing. Medications such as antidepressants may be administered. Encourage continuation of group and other therapy sessions.

Adolescents with bulimia and their families can be referred to organizations such as those listed in the section on anorexia for assistance and information about the disorder.

Evaluation

Expected outcomes of nursing care for the adolescent with bulimia include manifestation of healthy mucous membranes and skin, adequate intake of fluids and food, balanced food intake, maintenance of normal weight, adequate support and healthy psychologic balance, and absence of bingeing and purging.

Nutritional Support

Providing adequate nutrition for all children can be a challenge for families. Nutritional needs change as children grow and develop, family patterns must be integrated into the child's intake, and many social influences intervene to influence dietary patterns. Some children require even more careful management to ensure that they receive necessary nutrients, either due to increased needs or due to the difficulty in ingesting adequate foods. Several of these particular challenges are discussed here.

Sports Nutrition and Ergogenic Agents

Regular physical activity should be encouraged for all children, with at least 30 to 60 minutes of activity recommended daily. However, during vigorous or prolonged exercise, or during hot weather, there may be special nutritional needs of child and adolescent athletes. A well-balanced diet, reflective of the recommended foods, is needed. A wide variety of fresh fruits and vegetables, grains, and complex carbohydrates usually provides for adequate caloric intake. When the child is hungry, extra calories should come from those food groups, rather than from increased intake of fat. When the child or teen is very active, sports bars or drinks can provide the additional needed calories in a nutritionally balanced manner. Consumption of carbohydrates soon after an athletic event assists in restoring glycogen stores. As always, the height, weight, and BMI percentiles are the best assurance that the individual is growing adequately over time. Adequate energy to perform the sport as well as be attentive and productive at school and for other activities should also be considered (Molinero & Marquez, 2009; Rodriguez, DiMarco, Langley, et al., 2009).

Water should be increased during activity both to minimize the chance of dehydration and to maximize performance. About 1 hour before vigorous exercise, the child should drink one or two glasses (8 to 16 oz) of water and should repeat the same amount of fluid just before the exercise begins. Young children may not feel thirsty and should be encouraged to drink 6 to 12 oz of fluid every 15 to 20 minutes during exercise (AAP Committee on Nutrition, 2009). Water is usually the best replacement, but during extended exercise, sports drinks may be a good alternative for some of the fluid intake. Additional water is needed after activity. Weight loss of 1 lb indicates a loss of about 0.5 quart of fluid. Be sure the child takes in fluid to replace all losses. Some common nutrients that may be deficient in all teens, but even more often in the athlete, are calcium and iron. The increased blood volume common in the well-conditioned person necessitates greater intake. Calcium foods such as milk products and dark green vegetables, and iron foods such as adequate meats and grains, can guard against deficiencies. Many adolescents believe that they need extra protein during athletic seasons; however, most Americans ingest adequate protein to meet even the increased needs of sports, although the vegetarian child or adolescent may need assistance to plan a diet with adequate protein.

Many teens ingest a wide variety of dietary supplements, believing that they act as **ergogenic aids,** or products that enhance performance during sports by influencing energy, alertness, or body composition (Mulcahy, Schiller & Hulstyn, 2010). Most of the claims of these products are unproven, and their safety has not usually been investigated, especially in the young. Effects on youth whose bodies are still developing are particularly unknown and the risks are high for permanent interference with some normal growth patterns. Offer guidance and help the family and teen to investigate claims before choosing to use a product. Be sure that if youth choose to use supplements, they know doses, desired effects, and potential side effects of supplements. Be aware that some sports coaches may encourage small body size and dieting, or encourage use of dietary supplements to increase weight and muscle. Approximately 3.3% of U.S. high school students (4.3% of males and 2.2% of females) report taking illegal anabolic steroids; up to 6.5% in some communities report use (CDC, 2010). These products can have a wide array of side effects. They may stop growth of long bones, lead to endocrine imbalance, and cause increased tendon rupture. They are also illegal in sporting events. Andro and DHEA are steroidal hormones used by some athletes. They can cause masculinization of females, disruption of glucose balance and insulin sensitivity, dyslipidemia, and aggressive behavior (Lumia & McGinnis, 2010).

Some common amino acid nutritional supplements include creatine, carnitine, and glutamine. Although side effects to these substances are minimal, their possible enhancement of performance is temporary and outcomes of long-term use are unknown. Increasing overall nutritional intake to meet needs during high activity is a better alternative. Creatine has been studied more than most supplements; it is made by the body and is present in many protein sources. Supplemental creatine increases the creatine level in muscle and may help to increase performance in short bursts of activity, while not affecting endurance sports. The increase in muscle mass that can occur is actually due to water and will be lost quickly when the supplement is discontinued (Williams, 2006).

Minerals such as chromium, iron, and calcium are used by some youth. Ask about the athlete's social group and whether ergogenic aids are used; this is a strong predictor of use and is reason for additional counseling (Goulet, Valois, Buist, et al., 2010). The nurse can ask careful and sensitive questions, such as "Many athletes take supplements to aid in performance in sports. What supplements do you take or are you considering?" Information can then be provided to enhance the youth's understanding of nutrition and sports performance. Generally, intake of a balanced diet with adequate carbohydrate, protein, and fat will meet the needs of most athletes and lead to maximal sports performance. School nurses can work with physical education teachers and coaches to plan appropriate programs for youth to prevent use of ergogenic aids.

Health-Related Conditions

Many health conditions influence the nutritional state of the child. Conversely, the child's nutritional state can influence the state of health. Figure 19–15 ■ shows some common conditions that influence nutritional needs. These conditions are discussed in various chapters throughout the text. When you read about them, discuss with classmates how you will adjust normal nutritional assessment and teaching due to the presence of a healthcare concern. Which conditions influence absorption of nutrients? Which cause changes in nutritional intake requirements? Some children benefit from special dietary aids, such as eating utensils and cups that are easy to grasp.

Pathophysiology Illustrated
Conditions That Influence Nutritional Needs

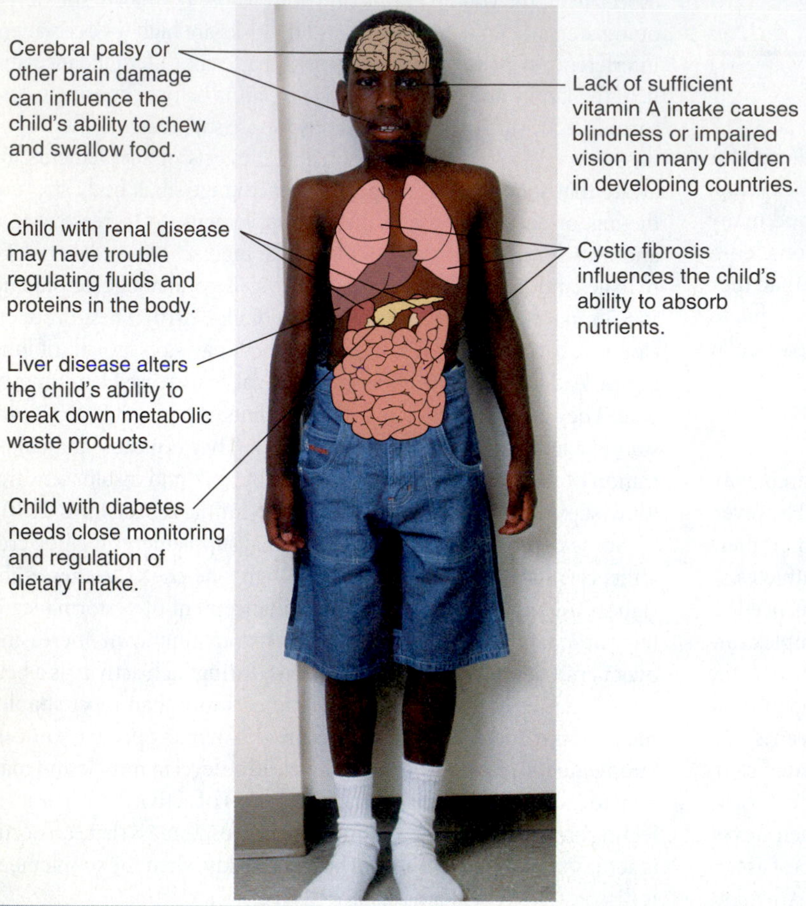

Cerebral palsy or other brain damage can influence the child's ability to chew and swallow food.

Child with renal disease may have trouble regulating fluids and proteins in the body.

Liver disease alters the child's ability to break down metabolic waste products.

Child with diabetes needs close monitoring and regulation of dietary intake.

Lack of sufficient vitamin A intake causes blindness or impaired vision in many children in developing countries.

Cystic fibrosis influences the child's ability to absorb nutrients.

FIGURE 19–15 ■ Although a child's nutritional status influences health, it is also important to consider conditions that may affect the child's nutrition and include this knowledge in your assessment.

Therapists can evaluate and make recommendations about devices that can assist the child at meals. Some genetic conditions affect food intake and metabolism. For example, Prader-Willi syndrome is most commonly caused by a deletion in chromosome 15; among hypotonia, hypogonadism, and other symptoms, it creates a lack of satiety feedback, abnormal ingestion of large amounts of food, and resulting obesity (see Chapter 4 ✏).

Consider the opening scenario and the description of Joey. Often children with cerebral palsy require high caloric intake for health. Constant muscle flexion and the high energy required for movements necessitate higher than normal intake. At the same time, the ability to chew and swallow may be decreased. Youth such as Joey require careful nutritional assessments on an ongoing basis to balance intake with nutritional needs.

Nurses work with families to plan for food access and intake patterns of the child. Some families use herbal products to treat conditions. Nurses inquire about supplements, herbs, and homeopathic remedies and search resources to provide information for families about the effects of these treatments in children. See Complementary Therapy: Herbs and Probiotics.

Vegetarianism

Some families choose to eat vegetarian diets and can be helped and encouraged in their endeavors. Several variations of intake occur. **Vegetarians** eat no poultry, meat, or fish. **Lacto-ovovegetarians** eat eggs and dairy products, and **lactovegetarians** eat dairy products. In contrast, **vegans** are strict vegetarians and eat no animal products. When someone says they are vegetarian, it is best to ask specific questions about what they will and will not eat (Box 19–19).

The vegetarian diet is healthy, is easy to follow, and may even provide extra health benefits (American Dietetic Association, 2009). Some deficiencies may exist; assessment and planning can ensure that they do not develop. Vegans should be sure to include adequate dietary vitamin D and calcium, vitamin B_{12}, minerals such as zinc and iron, fiber, calories, protein, and fat. Completing a 24-hour diet recall for the pregnant or lactating woman, and for vegetarian children, with analysis for RDAs, can be helpful. Provide ideas of various foods to meet nutritional needs and perform other general nutritional teaching. When a vegetarian child is hospitalized, plan with the nutrition department and the child's family to meet intake needs.

Enteral Therapy

Enteral therapy is a form of nutritional support provided when a child cannot take in enough food orally to sustain health. Since it is the closest form of nutritional support to the natural method of eating, it has the least untoward effects and greatest rate of success. Infants, especially preterm or those with medical problems, may need enteral therapy if they cannot ingest adequate nutrients. Some of the children who use enteral therapy are those with cerebral palsy or other neurologic conditions that lead to weakness of the throat and mouth, children with neoplasm or immune dysfunction, those with acute or chronic problems of the gastrointestinal tract, and those in acute states of recovery from accidents or illness. A tube can be inserted into the nasal opening and placed through the esophagus into the stomach; however, a tube that is surgically placed into the stomach through an abdominal opening (gastrostomy), or a jejunal tube, may be chosen for long-term use. As long as the child can absorb and use nutrients, enteral therapy can be successful in providing calories and essential nutrients. Commercially prepared formulas are available, and specially formulated solutions can be adapted for children with specific dietary needs. Nursing care includes care of the gastrostomy tube and entry site to prevent infection and skin breakdown. Ongoing nutritional assessments are needed. The nurse ensures that the tube is correctly placed before each tube feeding. Many families perform enteral feedings at home and school, so teaching and periodic evaluation of techniques are needed. See Chapter 30 ✏ and the Skills Manual ⬭ for further interventions for management of nursing care during tube feedings.

Total Parenteral Nutrition

Parenteral nutrition has made it possible to provide intravenous nutritional support for individuals who cannot eat or are unable to

Complementary Therapy
Herbs and Probiotics

Many families use food products to promote health and treat diseases. These include herbal products that may be acquired from health food stores or the Internet. Herbs are not tested nor regulated by the government, so amounts of ingredients are often not known. Ask families what herbal products they use regularly or to treat disease. Learn about the herbs and any research that has been conducted with children.

Another type of food product is a **probiotic,** a food supplement containing a live microorganism that alters the balance of gut microflora, thereby providing a health benefit. Common probiotics such as *Lactobacillus* and *Bifidobacterium*, which are commonly found in the human gastrointestinal tract, are enhanced by eating yogurt with live cultures and may be helpful in treating diarrhea or atopic dermatitis. Daily intake of pasteurized yogurt with live cultures can safely be encouraged for most children. A **prebiotic** is a nondigestible food ingredient that can stimulate growth or activity of probiotic bacteria (Thomas, Greer, & Committee on Nutrition, 2010). For example, oligosaccharides enhance proliferation of the beneficial *Bifidobacteria*. Probiotics may not be safe in children who are critically ill, have immunodeficiency, or are receiving chemotherapy for cancer.

Inquire about the family's treatment for conditions such as diarrhea. Include questions about food and nutritional supplements in all well-child visits as well as during treatment for children with illnesses.

Weblink — American Dietetic Association

BOX 19–19	Growth & Development: Vegetarian Diet

When a pregnant teen follows a vegetarian diet, additional help will be needed to encourage adequate nutrition. A 24-hour or 2-day diet diary will help identify nutritional needs. Consider additional pregnancy needs for energy, protein, n-3 fatty acids, iron, vitamin D, and calcium; note that vitamin B_{12} is recommended as a supplement. Use the vegetarian planning guides available through the American Dietetic Association.

---

absorb nutrients from the intestinal tract in a normal manner and are at risk of severe malnutrition. Examples of children who benefit from this method of nutrition are those with congenital malformation of the gastrointestinal tract, brain injury, or severe burns. It is also used for support after bone marrow transplant, sepsis, or other critical conditions. A catheter is inserted so that a sterile nutrition solution is infused directly into the bloodstream. A central venous catheter is inserted to promote safe infusion. Fluids usually contain glucose; electrolytes such as sodium, potassium, calcium, magnesium, phosphate, and chloride; vitamins; and proteins. Lipid emulsions are another type of TPN used in some children. Meticulous care is needed, whether in the hospital or at home, to ensure safe TPN infusion and treatment. Possible complications involve infection acquired at the site of infusion or air emboli causing respiratory problems. The nurse performs initial assessment and ongoing evaluation and monitoring of treatment, verifies the solution type and rate of administration, ensures solution storage recommendations are followed, and administers the solutions in hospital or other settings. See the protocols for TPN management in the Skills Manual ⬤▭. See Chapter 23 ✪ for further information about types of intravenous fluids and their use.

Chapter Highlights

- Adequate nutritional intake is necessary for the normal growth and development of children.
- Children with medical or psychosocial conditions require additional nutritional support.
- Dietary intake patterns vary throughout childhood as the child grows, is able to metabolize different types of food, and gains greater gross and fine motor control.
- Nutritional assessment is an essential part of nursing care and may involve approaches such as growth measurement and intake records.
- Common nutritional concerns in childhood include hunger, overweight, foodborne illness, and dietary deficiencies.
- The child with feeding disorder of infancy and childhood requires comprehensive assessment and ongoing management to foster parent–child interaction and adequate nutritional intake.

- The most common eating disorders of adolescents are anorexia nervosa and bulimia nervosa.
- A combination of behavioral management, counseling, and medication is often used in treatment programs for colic, rumination, anorexia, and bulimia.
- Food allergy represents a life-threatening food reaction for children, while food sensitivity/intolerance can lead to uncomfortable but non-life-threatening symptoms.
- Celiac disease requires careful management to eliminate all sources of gluten from the diet.
- Children engaging in sports and those who eat vegetarian diets may need guidance to meet nutritional needs.
- Alternative feeding methods such as enteral and parenteral feedings are required by some children.

Clinical Reasoning in Action

INTRODUCTION

Recall Joey in the opening scenario. He has cerebral palsy, which makes it difficult for him to swallow. This difficulty, in addition to recent surgery for scoliosis, has created nutritional challenges for him. A gastrostomy tube has been inserted so that he can receive supplemental feedings at home and school.

DESCRIPTION

Children with cerebral palsy are often unable to ingest enough nutrients to remain in a healthy nutritional state. The disorder makes it hard to chew and swallow food, and the excess muscular movements of the disorder use extra calories. Surgery has taken an additional toll on Joey. He was unable to eat for several days after the operation for scoliosis, and blood loss of surgery creates negative protein balance. Although he has healed well, nutritional analysis by a nutritionist demonstrated a shortage of calories, calcium, iron, and several other nutrients. Joey can eat soft foods that require little chewing and are easy to swallow. Supplemental feedings by gastrostomy tube have been planned to meet the deficiencies. The feedings will be given every few hours both at home and during school. The family learned how to administer the feedings for Joey in the hospital, and they have partnered with the school nurse so that the teacher can administer them in school. Joey has a hematocrit of 29% and hemoglobin of 10 g/dL.

DISCUSSION

Joey has some nutritional problems, but his care is enhanced by the presence of a supportive family, school nurse, and nutritionist. His teacher has shown competence and understanding in administering feedings in school.

1. Since Joey cannot stand or walk, he is at risk of osteoporosis. What is this disorder and which children are at risk of developing the disorder?
2. What nutrients are especially important to prevent osteoporosis?
3. Formulate nursing interventions that will enhance oral intake of the nutrients that Joey needs. Consider Joey's age and the school setting as you list realistic interventions.
4. How can the school nurse collaborate with the nutritionist and family to plan for Joey's nutritional needs and evaluate outcomes of his care?
5. If Joey's family decides to go on a summer car trip and will need to take feeding solutions and equipment with them, what suggestions can you provide about how to accomplish this?
6. Analyze Joey's hemoglobin and hematocrit. What levels would you expect at his age? How can you foster normal hemoglobin and hematocrit levels? What other nutritional observations can you make that provide clues about Joey's nutritional status?

NCLEX-RN® Review

1. The nurse is teaching a new parent about infant nutrition. The nurse knows that the parent has understood the teaching when the parent states which of the following statements?
   1. "My infant can begin eating with a spoon at 2 weeks of age."
   2. "My infant will only eat from a bottle or breast for 4 to 6 months."
   3. "My baby pushes food out of her mouth with her tongue because she does not like it."
   4. "I can expect my baby to begin eating table food at 3 months of age."

2. The nurse is caring for a child who has been diagnosed with a feeding disorder. Which areas should be included in the nursing assessment? (Select all that apply.)
   1. The child's diet
   2. Food content
   3. Food preferences
   4. Parent feeding practices
   5. Parent's dietary habits

3. The school nurse has established a nursing diagnosis of Imbalanced Nutrition: More than Body Requirements for a student related to excess intake compared to metabolic needs. What is an appropriate outcome for this child?
   1. The child is limited to eating out and fast foods no more than once weekly.
   2. The child loses weight to achieve correct proportion between weight and height on a growth grid.
   3. TV and video gaming are removed from the child's bedroom.
   4. The child demonstrates sufficient intake of all nutrients while achieving or maintaining optimal weight for height.

4. Which statement indicates nutrition counseling has been effective for the mother of a 6-month-old infant?
   1. "I will start my infant on rice cereal since it is iron fortified and has little chance of causing allergy."
   2. "I will start my infant on egg whites since they are high in iron and protein and have little chance of causing allergy."
   3. "I will start feeding fruits and vegetables and progress to whole grain cereals as tolerated."
   4. "I know that I can start feeding my baby strained meats for the iron and protein and progress later to fruits and vegetables."

See Appendix I ⊘ for answers.

References

Ackerman, K. E., & Misra, M. (2011). Bone health and the female athlete triad in adolescent athletes. *Physician and Sportsmedicine, 39*, 131–141.

Ahmed, A. H. (2010). Role of the pediatric nurse practitioner in promoting breastfeeding for late preterm infants in primary care settings. *Journal of Pediatric Health Care, 24*, 116–122.

Allen, S., & Dalton, W. T. (2011). Treatment of eating disorders in primary care: A systematic review. *Journal of Health Psychology.* doi:10.1177/1359105311402244

American Academy of Pediatrics (AAP) Committee on Nutrition. (2009). *Pediatric nutrition handbook* (6th ed.). Elk Grove Village, IL: American Academy of Pediatrics.

American Academy of Pediatrics (AAP). (2011). *Fruit juice and your child's diet.* Retrieved from http://www.healthychildren.org

American Diabetes Association. (2008). Nutrition recommendations and interventions for diabetes. *Diabetes Care, 31*, S61–S78.

American Diabetes Association. (2011). *Glycemic index.* Retrieved from http://www.diabetes.org/food-and-fitness/food/planning-meals/glycemic-index-and-diabetes.html

American Dietetic Association. (2009). Position of the American Dietetic Association: Vegetarian diets. *Journal of the American Dietetic Association, 109*, 1266–1282.

Bellisle, F. (2009). Infrequently asked questions about the Mediterranean diet. *Public Health Nutrition, 12*, 1644–1647.

Benson, L., Baer, H. J., Greco, P. J., & Kaelber, D. C. (2010). When is family history obtained? Lack of timely documentation of family history among overweight and hypertensive paediatric patients. *Journal of Paediatrics and Child Health, 46*, 600–605.

Brewerton, T. D., & Costin, C. (2011). Long-term outcome of residential treatment for anorexia nervosa and bulimia nervosa. *Eating Disorders, 19*, 132–144.

Bryant-Waugh, R., Markham, L., Kriepe, R. E., & Walsh, B. T. (2010). Feeding and eating disorders of childhood. *International Journal of Eating Disorders, 43*, 98–111.

Centers for Disease Control and Prevention (CDC). (2010). Youth risk behavior surveillance—United States, 2009. *Morbidity and Mortality Weekly Report, 59*(SS-5), 1–146.

Centers for Disease Control and Prevention (CDC). (2011a). *Breastfeeding among U.S. children born 1999–2007, CDC National Immunization Survey.* Retrieved from http://www.cdc.gov/breastfeeding/data/NIS_data/

Centers for Disease Control and Prevention (CDC). (2011b). *Overweight and obesity.* Retrieved from http://www.cdc.gov/obesity/childhood/data.html

Centers for Disease Control and Prevention (CDC). (2011c). *2011 estimates of foodborne illness in the United States.* Retrieved from http://www.cdc.gov/Features/dsFoodborneEstimates/

Children's Defense Fund. (2010). *The state of America's children.* Washington, DC: Author.

Cole, S. Z., & Lanham, J. S. (2011). Failure to thrive: An update. *American Family Physician, 83*, 829–834.

Daitch, L., & Epperson, J. N. (2011). Celiac disease. *Clinician Reviews, 21*(4), 49–55.

ESPGHAN Committee on Nutrition. (2009). *Breastfeeding.* Retrieved from http://espghan.med.up.pt/

Fisher, C. A., Hetrick, S. E., & Rushford, N. (2010). Family therapy for anorexia nervosa. *Cochrane Database Systematic Review, 14*(4), CD004780.

Flament, M. F., Bissada, H., & Spettigue, W. (2012). Evidence-based pharmacotherapy of eating disorders. *International Journal of Neuropsychopharmacology, 15*(12), 189–207.

Food Safety Network. (2011). *Safety of unpasteurized fruit juice and cider.* Retrieved from http://www.foodsafetynetwork.ca/aspx

Garcia-Manzanares, A., & Lucendo, A. J. (2011). Nutritional and dietary aspects of celiac disease. *Nutrition in Clinical Practice, 26*, 163–173.

Goulet, C., Valois, P., Buist, A., & Cote, M. (2010). Predictors of the use of performance-enhancing substances by young athletes. *Clinical Journal of Sport Medicine, 20*, 243–248.

Greydanus, D. E., Omar, H., & Pratt, H. D. (2010). The adolescent female athlete: Current concepts and conundrums. *Pediatric Clinics of North America, 57*, 697–718.

Hagan, J. F., Shaw, J. S., & Duncan, P. M. (2008). *Bright futures: Guidelines for health supervision of infants, children, and adolescents* (3rd ed.). Elk Grove Village, IL: American Academy of Pediatrics.

Hay, P. J., & Claudino, A. M. (2012). Clinical psychopharmacology of eating disorders: A research update. *International Journal of Neuropsychopharmacology, 15*(2), 209–222.

Holt, K., Wooldridge, N., Story, M., & Sofka, D. (2011). *Bright futures nutrition* (3rd ed.). Elk Grove Village, IL: American Academy of Pediatrics.

Institute of Medicine. (2006). *Dietary Reference Intakes.* Washington, DC: National Academies Press.

Institute of Medicine. (2011). *Dietary Reference Intakes: Calcium and vitamin D.* Washington, DC: National Academies Press.

Jen, H. C., Rickard, D. G., Shew, S. B., Maggard, M. A., Slusser, W. M., Dutson, E. P., & DeUgarte, D. A. (2010). Trends and outcomes of adolescent bariatric surgery in California, 2005–2007. *Pediatrics, 126*, e746–e753.

Kaulfers, A. M., Bean, J. A., Inge, T. H., Dolan, L. M., & Kalkwarf, H. J. (2011). Bone loss in adolescents after bariatric surgery. *Pediatrics, 127*, e956–e961.

Kliegman, R. M., Stanton, B., St. Geme, J., Schor, N., & Behrman, R. E. (2011). *Nelson textbook of pediatrics* (19th ed.). Philadelphia: Elsevier Saunders.

Laus, M. F., Vales, L. D., Costa, T. M., & Almeida, S. S. (2011). Early postnatal protein-calorie malnutrition and cognition: A review of human and animal studies. *International Journal of Environmental Research and Public Health, 8*, 590–612.

Lee, R. D., & Nieman, D. C. (2010). *Nutrition assessment* (5th ed.). Boston: McGraw-Hill.

LeFevre, M. K. (2010). Rickets: A preventable growth delay. *Journal of Pediatric Health Care, 24*, 408–412.

Lock, J. (2011). Evaluation of family treatment models for eating disorders. *Current Opinion in Psychiatry, 24*, 274–279.

London, M. L., Ladewig, P. W., Ball, J. W., Bindler, R. C., & Cowen, K. J. (2011). *Maternal & child nursing care* (3rd ed.). Upper Saddle River, NJ: Pearson Prentice Hall.

Lucan, S. C., Karpyn, A., & Sherman, S. (2010). Storing empty calories and chronic disease risk: Snack-food products, nutritive content, and manufacturers in Philadelphia corner stores. *Journal of Urban Health, 87*, 394–409.

Lumia, A. R., & McGinnis, M. Y. (2010). Impact of anabolic androgenic steroids on adolescent males. *Physiology & Behavior, 100*, 199–204.

Mansoor, D. K., & Sharma, H. P. (2011). Clinical presentations of food allergy. *Pediatric Clinics of North America, 58*, 315–326.

Maillot, M., Issa, C., Vieux, F., Lairon, D., & Daarmon, N. (2011). The shortest way to reach nutritional goals is to adopt Mediterranean food choices: evidence from computer-generated personalized diets. *American Journal of Clinical Nutrition, 94*, 1127–1137.

Mattar, L., Godart, N., Melchior, J. C., & Pichard, C. (2011). Anorexia nervosa and nutrition assessment: Contribution of body composition measurements. *Nutrition Research Reviews, 24*, 39–45.

Minaker, L. M., Storey, K. E., Raine, K. D., Spence, J. C., Forbes, L. E., Poltnikoff, R. C., & McCargar, L. J. (2011). Association between the perceived presence of vending machines and food and beverage logos in schools and adolescents' diet and weight status. *Public Health Nutrition, 31*, 1–7.

Molinero, O. & Marquez, S. (2009). Use of nutritional supplements in sports: Risks, knowledge, and behavioural-related factors. *Hospital Nutrition, 24*, 128–134.

Moore, D. J. (2009). Inflaming the debate on infant colic. *Journal of Pediatrics, 155*, 772–773.

Mulcahy, M. K., Schiller, J. R., & Hulstyn, M. J. (2010). Anabolic steroid use in adolescents: Identification of those at risk and strategies for prevention. *Physician and Sportsmedicine, 38*, 105–113.

National Association of Nurse Practitioners (NAPNAP). (2010). *History of HEAT mission and objectives.* Retrieved from http://www.napnap.org/ProgramsAndInitiatives/HEAT/HEATmissionAndObjectives.aspx

National Conference of State Legislatures. (2011). *Breastfeeding laws.* Retrieved from http://www.ncsl.org/issues-research/health/breastfeeding-state.laws.aspx

National Institute of Allergy and Infectious Diseases (NIAID). (2011). *Guidelines for diagnosis and management of food allergy in the United States.* Washington DC: U.S. Department of Health and Human Services.

National Institute of Diabetes and Digestive and Kidney Diseases (NIDDK). (2012). Celiac disease. Retrieved from http://digestive.niddk.nih.gov/ddiseases/pubs/celiac/

National Institute of Mental Health. (2010a). *Eating disorders among adults—Anorexia nervosa.* Retrieved from http://www.nimh.nih.gov/statistics/1EAT_ADULT_ANX.shtml

National Institute of Mental Health. (2010b). *Eating disorders among adults—Bulimia nervosa.* Retrieved from http://www.nimh.nih.gov/statistics/1EAT_ADULT_RBUL.shtml

Olsen, I. E., Groveman, S. A., Lawson, M. L., Clark, R. H., & Zemel, B. S. (2010). New intrauterine growth curves based on United States data. *Pediatrics, 125,* e214–e224.

Power, T., Bindler, R., Goetz, S., & Daratha, K. (2010). Obesity prevention in early adolescence: Student, parent, and teacher views. *Journal of School Health, 80,* 13–19.

Praveen, E. P., Kulshreshtha, B., Khurana, M. L., Sahoo, J. P., Gupta, N., Kumar, G., Dwivedi, S. N., & Ammini, A. C. (2010). Obesity and metabolic abnormalities in offspring of subjects with diabetes mellitus. *Diabetes Technologies and Therapeutics, 12,* 723–730.

Rashid, M., Zarkadas, M., Anca, A., & Limeback, H. (2011). Oral manifestations of celiac disease: A clinical guide for dentists. *Journal of the Canadian Dental Association, 77,* b39.

Richey, R., Howdle, P., Shaw, E., & Stokes, T. (2009). Recognition and assessment of coeliac disease in children and adults: Summary of NICE guidelines. *British Medical Journal, 338,* b 1684, doi: 110.1136/bmj.b1684

Rodriguez, N. R., DiMarco, N. M., Langley, S., American Dietetic Association, Dietitians of Canada, & American College of Sports Medicine. *Journal of the American Dietetic Association 109,* 509–527.

Rood, L., Roelofs, J., Bogels, S. M., Nolen-Hoeksema, S., & Schouten, E. (2009). The influence of emotion-focused rumination and distraction on depressive symptoms in non-clinical youth: A meta-analytic review. *Clinical Psychology Review, 29,* 607–616.

Ross, A. C., Taylor, C. L., Yaktine, A. L., & Del Valle, H. B. (Eds.). (2011). *Dietary reference intakes for calcium and vitamin D.* Washington, DC: Institute of Medicine.

Rovner, A. J., Nansel, T. R., Wang, J., & Iannotti, R. J. (2011). Food sold in school vending machines is associated with overall student dietary intake. *Journal of Adolescent Health, 48,* 13–19.

Seal, N., & Broome, M. (2011). Evidence-based interventions for pediatric weight control. *Journal for Nurse Practitioners, 7,* 293–302.

Siega-Riz, A. M., El Ghormli, L., Mobley, C., Gillis, B., Stadler, D., Hartstein, J., . . . HEALTHY Study Group. (2011). The effects of the HEALTHY study intervention on middle school student dietary intakes. *International Journal of Behavioral Nutrition and Physical Activity, 8,* 7.

Snyder, C. L., Young, D. O., Green, P. H. R., & Taylor, A. K. (2008). Celiac disease. In R. A. Pagon, T. C. Bird, C. R. Dolan, & K. Stephens, (eds.). *GeneReviews.* Seattle: University of Washington.

Strasburger, V. C., Jordan, A. B., & Donnerstein, E. (2010). Health effects of media on children and adolescents. *Pediatrics, 125,* 756–767.

Thomas, D. W., Greer, F. R., & Committee on Nutrition. (2010). Probiotics and prebiotics in pediatrics. *Pediatrics, 126,* 1217–1231.

Treasure, J., Claudino, A. M., & Zucker, N. (2010). Eating disorders. *Lancet, 375,* 583–593.

U.S. Department of Agriculture (2009). *Food insecurity in households with children.* Retrieved from http://www.ers.usda.gov/publications/eib56

U.S. Department of Health and Human Services. (2011). *Healthy People 2020.* Washington, DC: U.S. Government Printing Office. Retrieved from http://healthypeople.gov/2020/topicsobjectives2020/pdfs/nutritionandweight.pdf

U.S. Food and Drug Administration. (2011). *What you need to know about mercury in fish and shellfish.* Retrieved from http://www.fda.gov/Food/FoodSafety/

Vaczy, E., Seaman, B., Peterson-Sweeney, K., & Hondorf, C. (2011). Passport to health: An innovative

tool to enhance healthy lifestyle choices. *Journal of Pediatric Health Care, 25,* 31–37.

Van Koppen, E. J., Schweizer, J. J., Csizmadia, C. G., Krom, Y., Hylkema, H. B., van Geel, A. M., . . . Mearin, M. L., (2009). Long-term health and quality-of-life consequences of mass screening for childhood celiac disease: A 10-year follow-up study. *Pediatrics, 123,* e582–e588.

Vlaardingerbroek, H., van Goudoever, J. B., & van den Akker, C. H. (2009). Initial nutritional management of the preterm infant. *Early Human Development, 85,* 691–695.

Walvoord, E. C. (2010). The timing of puberty: Is it changing? Does it matter? *Journal of Adolescent Health, 47,* 433–439.

Williams, M. H. (2006). Sports nutrition. In M. E. Shils, M. Shike, A. C. Ross, B. Caballero, & R. J. Cousins (Eds.), *Modern nutrition in health and disease* (10th ed., pp. 1723–1740). Philadelphia: Lippincott, Williams & Wilkins.

Wordell, D., Daratha, K., Mandal, B., Bindler, R., & Butkus, S. N. (2012). Changes in a middle school food environment affect food behavior and food choices. *Journal of the Academy of Nutrition and Dietetics, 112,* 137–141.

Zeller, M. H., Guilfoyle, S. M., Reiter-Purtill, J., Ratcliff, M. B., Inge, T. H., & Long, J. D. (2011). Adolescent bariatric surgery: Caregiver and family functioning across the first postoperative year. *Surgery in Obesity and Related Diseases, 7,* 145–150.

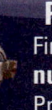

Pearson Nursing Student Resources

Find additional review materials at **nursing.pearsonhighered.com** Prepare for success with additional NCLEX®-style practice questions, interactive assignments and activities, web links, animations and videos, and more!

Social and Environmental Influences on Child and Adolescent Health

 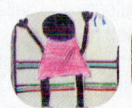 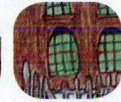

KEY TERMS

Learning Outcomes

After completing this chapter, you will be able to:

1. Identify major social and environmental factors that influence the health of children and adolescents.

2. Apply the ecologic model and resilience theory to assessment of the social and environmental factors in children's lives.

3. Examine the effects of substance use, physical activity, and other lifestyle patterns on health.

4. Evaluate the environment for hazards to children, such as exposure to substances and potential for poisoning.

5. Explore the nursing role in prevention and treatment of child abuse and neglect, and other forms of violence.

6. Plan nursing interventions for children related to social and environmental situations.

> "This school is a lot better than the other one I was in. At least they try to understand you here. It is probably important to get through high school and my parents seem happier that I'm in school. It seems like you can trust the teachers and the nurse more here."
>
> —Amy, 15 years old

Amy Beckman is 15 years old and attends an alternative high school. She recently had an ear piercing that has become painful. She has come to the health room to ask the advice of the school nurse. Upon examination, the area around the piercing is found to be inflamed and mildly edematous. After asking some questions, the nurse learns that Amy's ear was pierced by a friend, using a needle that had been "sterilized" by passing it through a match flame. She has a slight fever but otherwise feels fine.

In Amy's home state, adolescents under 18 years of age must have the signature of a parent for body piercings and tattoos, so she chose to have the procedure done by a friend. She believes this is safe since her friend has done many piercings on others. She admits that her parents are not very pleased with her body art, but that they allow her to do it as long as she agrees to stay in high school. She had previously run away and spent several weeks living on the streets.

What healthcare and social needs does Amy have? How can the nurse support both her and her parents? What signs of resilience does Amy show? This chapter examines the complex social contexts in which children live, learn, and grow, and explores the role of nurses in supporting them to reach their potentials. The challenges of providing comprehensive health care for all children and adolescents, no matter what their lifestyles, are discussed.

Many of the major causes of mortality and morbidity in children are closely linked with social influences in the child's world. The social contexts for young children growing up today are different from those of even a decade ago. Examining the social contexts in which children live and grow can provide insights into the behavior of children and adults, and present opportunities for nursing interventions. All nurses must examine social influences and apply the knowledge gained to plan health care that will benefit youth as they grow into adulthood.

Children and adolescents are also influenced by their environments. The physical setting, exposure to chemical agents, and other environmental factors are increasingly identified as instrumental in determining health. Nurses assess the environment for its risk and protective factors, and then use this information to plan nursing care appropriate to enhance the health status of children and adolescents.

What are the challenges of today's society, some of which children face at a very young age? How can nurses help children to face these challenges and to emerge as healthy and contributing members of society? What roles do nurses play in identifying the protective factors and in minimizing the risk factors of youth? This chapter will help you to examine and apply these concepts in a variety of nursing settings. Social factors are examined first, and then environmental influences. However, realize that the factors overlap and interact with each other. For example, the social condition of poverty may place a child at greater risk of environmental exposure to toxins, and family relationships can be very influential in a child's ability to manage the stress of a natural disaster. Social and environmental factors thus constantly interact and influence each other.

Consider the major causes of death for children from 1 year of age through adolescence that are presented in Chapter 1, Figures 1–11 and 1–12 🔗. Note that most mortality is related to preventable causes linked to present-day lifestyles, including car crashes, fires, drownings, and homicides.

Now examine the major reasons for hospitalization in Table 1–2 🔗. By the time children are 5 years of age, injuries rank as the third cause, and by 10 years, mental disorders and injuries are among the major causes of hospitalization. Respiratory diseases are a leading cause of hospitalization for children from 1 to 9 years. By the teen years, pregnancy and mental disorders are the most common admitting diagnoses to hospitals. All of these conditions leading to hospitalization are related, at least in part, to the social and environmental settings in which we live. These settings and their influences must be examined in order to understand how to best intervene with children. Theories that help us to examine the social and environmental contexts of children and families are discussed earlier in Chapters 2 and 5 🔗 and reviewed below.

THEORETICAL FRAMEWORKS

In this chapter, two main theories will be used to provide a framework in which to examine societal influences on children. These are the ecologic model and the resilience theory, as discussed in Chapter 5. Review them now to assist in evaluating the environmental settings that influence children (see Figure 5–5 and Tables 5–5, 5–8, and 5–9 🔗).

The ecologic theory views the child and the environment as interacting forces, with children influencing systems around them, while they are influenced by these systems (Bronfenbrenner, 2005). Close

| BOX 20–1 | **Research: The Add Health Study** |

The Add Health Study (National Longitudinal Study of Adolescent Health) was conducted during the latter 1990s with over 100,000 adolescents and helped to determine the family, school, and individual characteristics associated with risk factors. Parent–family connectedness, school connectedness, a belief in a higher being, and academic success were predictive of youth having the lowest health risks. Interviews are presently being carried out with the participants who are now young adults; the resulting longitudinal data will show what characteristics and influences persist into adult life (National Institute of Child Health and Human Development, 2010a).

Recall the concept of *attachment* discussed in Chapter 5 🔗. Teens retain attachment and connectedness to family, while testing attachment to peers as support systems (Taylor-Seehafer, Jacobvitz, & Steiker, 2008). Nurses can assist adolescents and their families in establishing a sense of attachment and connectedness to each other. Encourage families to include adolescents in activities, attend their sports and other school events, have meals together regularly, and attend faith-based activities or other community events as a family. Assist the teen to view peers as a safe and supportive resource, but provide support when peer relationships change or do not endure.

systems providing daily contact are microsystems, but other systems encompassing factors such as parental work and political or cultural environments are also important. Understanding these systems, or the forces in which children function, can provide information that guides care providers. For example, if the parents' employers do not provide healthcare insurance, their children may not obtain necessary health care such as immunizations, treatment for diseases, and growth monitoring.

Resilience theory examines risk and protective factors in the child's environment as they influence the child's adaptation to stressful events, and can be modified to lead to more productive and healthy outcomes (Box 20–1). Families may have protective factors that provide strength and assistance in dealing with crises, and risk factors that promote or contribute to healthcare challenges. Risk and protective factors can be identified in children, in their families, and in their communities. The interaction of these factors contributes to health status and determines adaptation to a crisis. For example, if a young child is hospitalized for treatment of an acute infectious illness, protective factors might include the ability of one parent to stay with the child at all times, the ability of a grandmother to care for siblings at home during this time, and the child's ability to adapt to new situations and communicate readily with staff members. On the other hand, risk factors might include lack of comprehensive health insurance to pay for the hospitalization, lack of an identified healthcare "home" (consistent care provider) for the child, and incomplete immunizations.

Theoretical frameworks are useful when examining social and environmental influences on children because they guide us to examine certain factors that can be altered. They suggest assessment data to collect and pertinent nursing interventions. They also help foster partnerships with other care providers who use these and similar theories to plan social, psychologic, and other care for children and their families. Nursing strategies can target risk factors, such as encouraging family behaviors to ensure gun safety by teaching the benefits of gun locks and locked gun cabinets in families with firearms. In addition, protective factors can be emphasized, such as when regular exercise is suggested to help maintain normal weight and cardiovascular function.

SOCIAL INFLUENCES ON CHILD HEALTH

While the genetic characteristics of a child can influence susceptibility to acute or chronic health conditions, the social milieu in which the child grows also has a powerful impact on health. The ecologic model recognizes the inborn characteristics of the child, as well as how these characteristics interact with the child's family, community, and culture. The resilience model suggests methods of evaluating all of the child's characteristics and social characteristics to identify protective factors and risks. Some of the external factors that can directly or indirectly influence child health are discussed in this section.

Poverty

An important risk factor that influences the health of children is poverty. Conversely, basic financial stability is a protective factor that contributes to the general health and well-being of children. However, children are the poorest group in this country, and more children are poor now than at any time in our past. Approximately 19% of children (14.1 million) are poor and live in a family earning less than $21,834 annually for a family of four (Federal Interagency Forum on Child and Family Statistics, 2010).

What is the face of poverty? Some statistics that may prove surprising include:

- The children most likely to be living in poor households are those below 5 years of age.
- About 43% of children living in a single-headed household are poor, while only 9% in married couple households are poor.
- Ethnic variations are startling: One in 10 White children live in poverty, while 1 in 3 Black and Hispanic children live in poverty.
- Poverty rates are higher in suburban and rural areas than in central cities.
- Over 70% of poor children have at least one parent working full time.

Federal Interagency Forum on Child and Family Statistics, 2010

Children who are poor are overrepresented in nearly every health indicator. They are more likely to have unmet health needs, to have difficulty in school, to become teen parents, and to experience multiple health problems, including stunted growth and lead poisoning. Inadequate or unsafe housing, food insecurity, and poor dietary quality are more common.

Nurses should understand the demographics in the areas where they work. What is the poverty rate in the community? What ethnic groups are overrepresented among the poor? Locate resources such as food services, health care for the underserved, and enhanced school programs in order to refer poor families. Recognize that health promotion services may not be high priority when a family lacks adequate housing or food. When a child is seen in any setting, such as in school or in an emergency department or hospital for acute care, refer to health promotion guidelines for the child's age (see Chapters 9 through 13). Measure growth, assess vision and hearing, evaluate dietary intake, and check immunization status. Find out the stresses the family experiences and what resources they need to meet basic necessities. Your nursing care plan should include these health promotion needs and identify nursing diagnoses connected to the acute illness or other health problem.

Homelessness

Poverty leads to homelessness for some children. Children comprise over 25% of the homeless population, and families represent 39%. Families with children are the fastest growing group of homeless people. Each year, from 0.9 to 1.6 million children experience homelessness (National Center on Family Homelessness, 2009). The reasons for homelessness are also common risks for a number of the other challenges to health discussed in this chapter, including poor finances, abuse or other violence, and mental instability. Young children tend to be homeless with their parents. Homeless adolescents are more often alone, having run away, been thrown out of a house, or become street youth.

Children who experience homelessness often have multiple physical and mental health problems, and lack health insurance to provide care for these problems. Some of the common problems faced by homeless children and families include trauma, abuse, substance use, respiratory and skin infections, tuberculosis and HIV, and nutritional disorders. Children may have developmental delays, learning problems, injuries, mental health disruptions, or growth impairment (Coker, Elliott, Kanouse, et al., 2009; Frencher, Benedicto, Kendig, et al., 2010; Kerker, Bainbridge, Kennedy, et al., 2011).

Health problems related to homelessness and other family characteristics continue even after finding a place to live. After families leave homeless shelters, children frequently become separated from their mothers (transition to living with another family member or are sent to foster care) due to parent stress, lack of access to resources, and inability of parents to provide adequate homes for the children. Complex ongoing care is needed. This may begin in a shelter for the homeless, but should continue while the family obtains a place to live, accesses other community services, enrolls the children in school, and attains financial and mental stability. Nurses in all of these settings work with families who are homeless, and they are instrumental in establishing services.

Adolescents who are homeless often have some similarities to younger children but may be dealing with other issues. While some teens may be homeless because parents have lost jobs and homes, others may be homeless because they have had difficulties at home and have chosen to leave or been asked to leave by their families. Recall Amy, who was described in the scenario at the beginning of the chapter. She left home and lived on the streets for several weeks. Teens who have been homeless are more likely to engage in risky behavior, such as unprotected sex with multiple partners and substance use. They are more likely than other teens to need emergency care, to be depressed or have other mental illness, and to become pregnant (National Center on Family Homelessness, 2009). They may be subjected to violence in the areas they choose to live. As with younger children, they may lack adequate food, facilities to maintain hygiene, and health care. Sexually transmitted infections, poor performance or nonattendance at school, and physical or mental illness can all result from patterns of homelessness (National Center on Family Homelessness, 2009).

Nursing management for families with children who are poor or homeless focuses on identification of poverty and homelessness, careful assessment of health risks, and linking the family to resources that can assist with stability and health. Assess eligibility for medical assistance plans and assist in applications as needed. There is often no way to identify poor or homeless children from appearance, and they may hide their status when in school or at healthcare facilities. Addresses given may not be accurate, or the address of a shelter might be used. Children living at shelters or in cars and on the street may not take the school bus, but prefer to walk to avoid stigma. (See Evidence-Based Practice: Developmental and Health Implications of Homelessness.) Be alert for children who have multiple health problems and repeated infectious diseases. They are often hungry and tired, suffer from skin and other infections, and have varying degrees of personal hygiene depending on access to laundry and bathing facilities. See Table 20–1 for examples of nursing care needs for poor and homeless children and families.

Stress

The adverse effect of stress on adults is well documented, and the impact of stress on children has also been recognized. Stress responses are measured by researchers who use salivary cortisol levels (Hunter, Minnis, & Wilson, 2011). Stress can be acute, such as when a child has an argument with a friend, a test in school, or a family crisis. Stress can also become chronic when the family frequently does not have enough food, when fighting or abuse is frequent, or when the child is overscheduled and feels under constant pressure to perform. Children manifest stress in a variety of ways, including regressive behavior, interrupted sleep, hyperactive behavior, gastrointestinal symptoms, crying, and withdrawal from normal events. Common stressful events for children include moving to a new home or school, marital difficulties in the family, abuse, a parent deployment in the military, and being expected to achieve at an extremely high level in school or sports (Figure 20–1 ■). The busy pace of today's lifestyles and the impact of the media in encouraging early development of children may put undue stress upon some children and preteens (Elkind, 2007). Adolescents may be stressed by fulfilling many roles, such as student, part-time worker, and active family member. They may be in school all day, be in sports or music practice for 2 to 3 hours after school, and then have a job for several additional hours. Lack of adequate sleep can add further to stress, in addition to putting the teen at risk for car crashes and poor school performance. For poor families, commonly reported stressors are related to food provision, shelter, transportation, medical care, and personal-time needs.

The child experiencing stress has more frequent respiratory and gastrointestinal illnesses and is more likely to be the victim of an injury. The negative long-term effects of stress on body organs and systems suggest that children under stress are more likely to develop illnesses such as strokes, hypertension, and heart attacks later in life (Balodis, Wynne-Edwards, & Olmstead, 2010).

Nurses help children to manage stress by encouraging good coping strategies and maximizing strengths to foster resilience (Sapienza & Masten, 2011). Healthy lifestyles including good nutrition, exercise, and plenty of sleep can be emphasized with all children. Integrate these topics into each health promotion and health maintenance visit. Consult Chapters 9 through 13 🔗 for detailed interventions with each specific age group.

Partner with military families to assist them when one or both parents are deployed for duty in a remote location. Connect parents with resources for childcare, mental health services, and arrangements that need to be made to prepare for the absence. Due to frequent moves, the family may not be strongly connected to resources in the community. During deployment the remaining parent may return to the home of origin where some family support may be

TABLE 20–1	Common Health Problems and Nursing Management of Children Experiencing Poverty or Homelessness
COMMON HEALTH PROBLEMS	**NURSING MANAGEMENT**
Lack of immunizations	Check immunization records.
	Provide immunizations at schools and in homeless shelters.
Common infectious diseases	Facilitate free clinics in shelters, schools, and community settings.
	Teach hygiene measures.
	Provide resources for disease management.
	Arrange for medications when needed.
	Provide information about resources for bathing and hygiene.
Sleep deficits	Inform parents about respite facilities.
	Arrange for children to have quiet sleep time in school if possible.
Vision and hearing deficits	Perform screening for deficits.
	Provide resources for eyeglasses, hearing aids, and care for ear infections (e.g., service organizations such as Lions Club).
Nutritional deficits	Perform height and weight checks and nutritional assessment.
	Evaluate the family for food security (see Chapter 19 🔗).
	Be sure the child is registered for school breakfast and lunch programs if available.
	Ensure that children are linked to summer food programs at the end of the academic year.
	Refer to the Women, Infants, and Children (WIC) Nutrition Program.
	Inform about resources for meals and field gleaning (harvesting leftover and discarded farm foods) in the community.
Dental care problems	Teach oral hygiene.
	Provide toothbrushes and toothpaste.
	Provide bottled water for use if the child lives in a car or on the street.
	Perform oral assessment.
	Refer to dental programs for people with low incomes.
Injuries	Teach basic safety precautions.
	Visit the living situation if possible to assess for safety hazards.
	Provide helmets, car seats, or other gear needed.
	Teach "street safe" skills (e.g., refusing rides from strangers, avoiding persons with weapons).
	Provide resources for violence prevention and intervention.
Adolescent pregnancy and sexually transmitted infections	Provide sexuality teaching.
	Inform about access to family planning services.
	Assess for child abuse and prostitution.
Mental illness	Assess for depression and other mental illness (see Chapter 34 🔗).
	Evaluate for suicide potential.
	Provide links to mental health services.
	Plan programs to foster self-esteem.
	Arrange for a Big Brother or Big Sister.
	Refer to extracurricular activities in the school and community.
	Arrange for a school bus stop away from a shelter so other students do not stigmatize the homeless child.

Evidence-Based Practice | Developmental and Health Implications of Homelessness

PROBLEM

Children are the age group showing the fastest growth in homelessness. Due to their ages, children are vulnerable to developmental delays, mental health problems, and effects of violence. Families experiencing homelessness may not be able to provide the care children need for healthy growth and development. Most nurses have not been homeless and therefore do not understand the special needs of homeless children.

EVIDENCE

Two nurses reported on the integration of developmental screening tools in a homeless shelter. Language and communication delays were the most common deficits. The researchers concluded that developmental screening is especially critical for homeless children (Chiu & DiMarco, 2010). Other researchers found that long-term consequences of homelessness included poor mental health and poor educational achievement (Shinn, Schteingart, Williams, et al., 2008). In

another nursing study, dental caries were an extremely common health problem among children in homeless shelters, with school-age children having a 34% prevalence of caries (DiMarco, Huff, Kinion, et al., 2009).

IMPLICATIONS

Youth in homeless shelters have multiple healthcare, educational, and social needs. Developmental screening, identification of health issues, and provision of coordinated care are needed.

CRITICAL THINKING APPLICATION

Find at least two agencies that provide health care for persons who are homeless in your community. Are nurses involved in planning health care? What are some of the common health problems treated? What services are provided for families? What links are available to other community resources?

---

present but resources for family members provided on a military base are not available. Help families explain to children why and where the parents are going, and how they will keep in touch during the absence. Children need to know who they will stay with, whether they will attend the same school, and how food and other needs will be met. Parents need family, mental health, and financial support, whether they are being deployed or are remaining at home (Allen, Rhoades, Stanley, et al., 2011; Aranda, Middleton, Flake, et al., 2011).

Parents can be encouraged to provide youth with activities that foster self-esteem and to avoid unrealistic expectations about performance in sports and other activities. Resources to assist with food acquisition, shelter, transportation, and medical care should be

provided for families needing the assistance. Adolescents may benefit from various approaches for stress management such as massage, rest, physical activity, and yoga. See Complementary Therapy: Youth and Yoga.

Families

The families into which children are born influence them profoundly. Children are supported in different ways and acquire different worldviews depending on such factors as whether one or both parents work, how many siblings are present, and whether an extended family is nearby. Note variations in family structure such as adolescent parent, single parent, gay or lesbian parents, extended

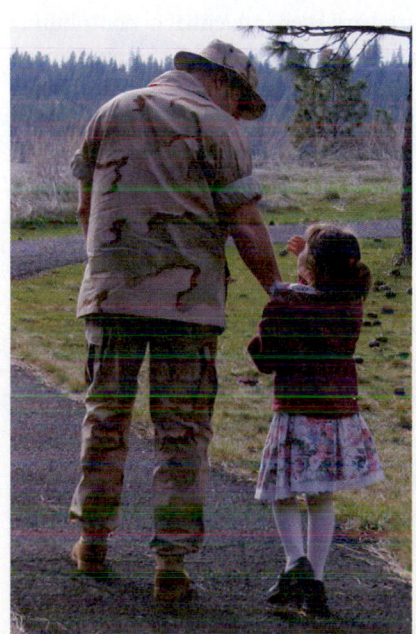

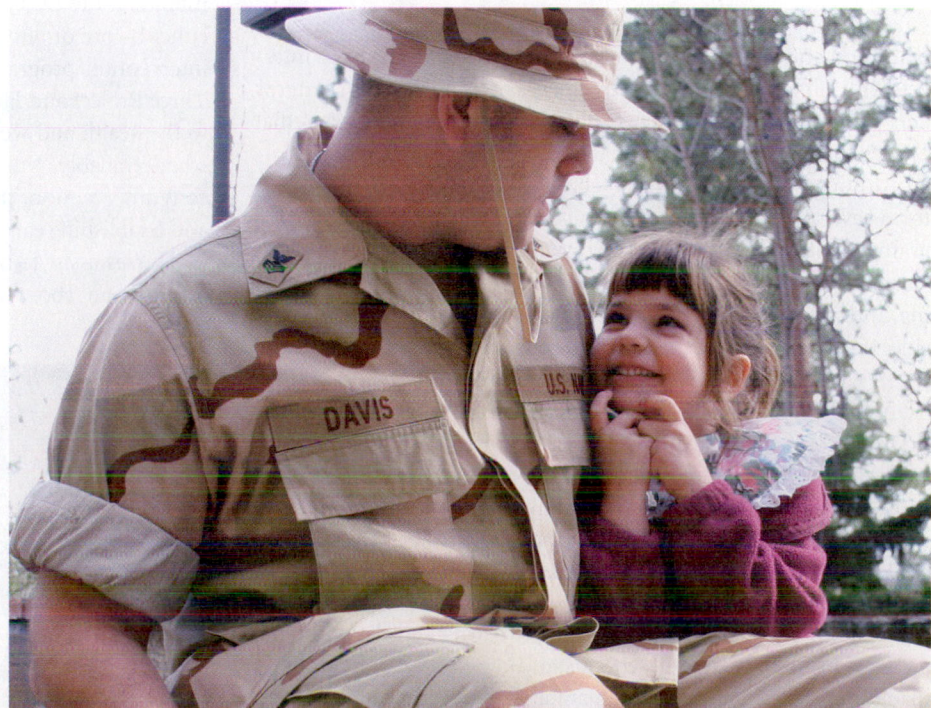

FIGURE 20–1 ■ The special relationship between a father about to be deployed in the military and his young daughter is clear. This father has two other children and is spending time with each of them, as well as with the family together, before leaving. The cycle of leaving and returning home can be stressful for families. Nurses can assist military families in making plans for health care, finances, and communication while gone and providing resources for emotional support for the entire family.

Complementary Therapy **Youth and Yoga**

The health and fitness benefits of yoga have been described previously with adults, and more recently yoga has been introduced to younger populations. Yoga has been used in youth to foster development, promote health, and provide therapy, such as in psychiatric disorders (Kaley-Isley, Peterson, Fischer, et al., 2010). Yoga decreases frequency and intensity of pain in children with functional abdominal pain (Brands, Purperhart, & Deckers-Kocken, 2011). As a physical activity for school-age children, it is calming and may lead to decreased disciplinary problems and improved scholastic performance (White, 2009). Yoga may therefore be a valuable tool for increasing physical activity and enhancing stress reduction among children and adolescents.

family, grandparents caring for grandchildren, and stepparents. Societal changes have affected family life and the needs of children immensely. Working parents often raise children with little time for quality relationships and without the financial resources needed for optimum development. All factors influence the physical and mental health of children and can determine their needs for nursing intervention.

Nurses can complete family diagrams during home visits and in other settings to evaluate the people who are important in a child's life. Both the risk factors of the family (e.g., recent separation, parental stress, and limited healthcare coverage) and the strengths (e.g., loving relationships, influential grandparents or other extended family members, and general good health) should be identified and used in planning care. See Chapter 2 for a thorough discussion of family factors as they relate to family-centered care, and a description of strategies for assessment and intervention with families.

School and Childcare

Once a child is 5 or 6 years of age, several hours daily are spent in a school setting. Physical skills are developed through participation in education and sports. Psychosocial stages are met as the child interacts with children and adults and achieves social interaction patterns and pride in accomplishments. The presentation of concepts that challenge thought processes enhances cognitive development.

Although the primary role of schools is educational, they also perform several health-related functions. School health screening programs identify children with such health problems as hearing loss, visual impairment, and scoliosis. Nurses provide assessment, teaching, and clinical management related to some health problems. Consider the case of Amy in the opening scenario. She went to the school nurse when her body piercing was potentially infected; the nurse examined the site, made suggestions for cleaning, and taught Amy the symptoms that could indicate serious infections. Some schools have clinics that examine and provide even more complete health care for children (Figure 20–2 ■). Many schools teach good nutrition, healthful living, safe sexual practices, and other health-related subjects. A school nurse may be present, at least part time, to plan these classes or to work with teachers. Nurses assist school districts in providing plans for emergency health care when needed. With the increase in mainstreaming, school staff now has the responsibility for administering medications, maintaining urinary catheters, and providing respiratory care and other treatments to ensure the child's proper growth and development. See Chapter 14 for a further discussion of school nurse activities.

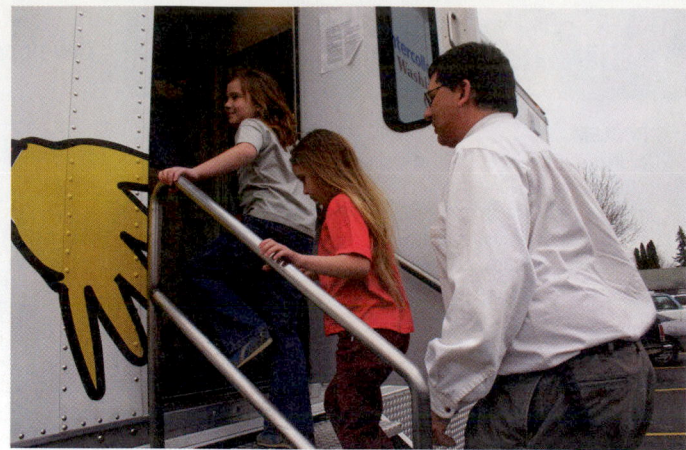

FIGURE 20–2 ■ This father is bringing his two daughters to a mobile van parked near a school to receive health care. Children may receive some of their health care from school-based services including school nurses, clinics, or mobile vans.

Some children spend part or nearly all of their days in childcare settings (Figure 20–3 ■). Over 60% of children under 6 years of age receive some type of childcare regularly. About 19% of children are in childcare up to 9 hours each week, 38% for 10 to 19 hours each week, 36% for 30 to 45 hours each week, and 10% over 45 hours each week. The closeness of the parent–child relationship, the quality of care, and the length of the childcare day are important in determining childcare effects on children. The mother's sensitivity to her child is the best indicator of child behavior regardless of childcare arrangements (ChildStats, 2011; Federal Interagency Forum on Child and Family Statistics, 2010; National Institute of Child Health and Human Development, 2010b).

Nursing management involves helping parents to explore types of childcare options available and to evaluate programs in their communities (Table 20–2). Care options for young school-age children, either before or after school, can also be shared with parents. Early intervention programs with at-risk children, such as the Zero to Three Project and Head Start, have been influential in contributing to the health and welfare of children and should be recommended when available. Nurses frequently manage the health programs in early intervention, providing for screening and health evaluations and establishing early intervention education plans.

Nurses assist families in evaluating childcare centers and share information about accreditation. (See Partnering with Families:

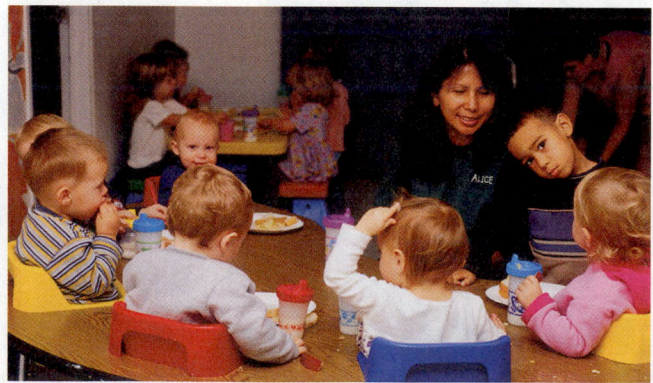

FIGURE 20–3 ■ Most children will spend time in childcare settings. It is important to explore options and find the best fit for the child's needs.

TABLE 20–2	Types of Childcare	
TYPE OF CARE	**DESCRIPTION**	**ADVANTAGE/DISADVANTAGE**
In home	Caretaker comes to home of the child	Child can remain at home Little exposure to infectious diseases No need for alternative care when child is ill Limited contact with other children to encourage development Limited ability to rapidly locate alternative when provider is ill Most costly
Family childcare	Parent brings child to home of a caretaker	Limited number of children Some exposure to other children and encouragement of development Family-type atmosphere Little governmental regulation or examination
Center a. Private, nonprofit (e.g., church, YMCA) b. Public (e.g., Head Start) c. Private proprietary care	Parent brings child to a center where many children receive care	A learning curriculum plan is in place Contact with other children can enhance development Exposure to multiple children increases infectious disease risk

Evaluation of Childcare.) The National Association for the Education of Young Children (2010) has established criteria related to the following:

- Relationships among teachers and families
- Curriculum
- Teaching
- Assessment of child progress
- Health
- Teachers
- Families
- Community relationships
- Physical environment
- Leadership and management

Community

The community in which a child lives may support the child's development or, conversely, expose the child to hazards. Social programs such as Head Start preschools, sports activities, after-school programs, and child abuse treatment centers offer valuable services that improve the experience of growing children. On the other hand, an economically depressed community with scant services and a high homicide rate is unsupportive and hazardous for growing children.

The physical environment is supportive when the child is provided with sidewalks on which to walk to school, open spaces in which to learn and play, and clean air to breathe. Children who must walk to school on unsafe roads, have exposure to contaminated drinking supplies, or live near polluting manufacturing companies or in crowded housing or old structures are at risk for injuries and health problems such as lead poisoning (see the discussion of poisoning and other environmental hazards later in this chapter).

Culture

The child's cultural group may influence the use of traditional and contemporary healthcare practices. If the parents or children are recent immigrants, they may still be learning the English language and finding out about healthcare resources. Even in families that have been in this country for some time, a combination of approaches to health care is common. Children of immigrants may feel stress as they combine their family's traditional culture with the new culture in which the family now lives. They may also have a great deal of responsibility to interpret for the family, since they may speak two languages and understand the practices of the new culture.

Recent immigrants may experience **culture shock,** a state of crisis related to the difference in values and lifestyle between the two cultures they have experienced. This can lead to stress-related symptoms and create a need for healthcare intervention. Children whose parents emigrated from another country may feel different from their peers and develop conflict with their parents, particularly during adolescence.

All cultural groups have rules regarding patterns of social interaction. The number of languages spoken and the amount of speech in the home determine schedules of language acquisition. The particular social roles assumed by men and women in the culture affect school activities and ultimately career choices. Attitudes toward touching and other methods of encouraging developmental skills vary among cultures.

Nurses must become aware of common characteristics of the cultural groups they serve in order to establish culturally competent nursing care. Arrange for interpreters when needed. Be aware that traditional and Western health care may be both accepted and applied; remain nonjudgmental about traditional healing practices. Provide ethnic foods in healthcare facilities. Evaluate youth in immigrant families for conflict between family and societal expectations. See Chapter 3 ⊘ for a thorough discussion of cultural influences on health and the nurse's role in providing culturally competent care.

LIFESTYLE ACTIVITIES AND THEIR INFLUENCES ON CHILD HEALTH

Many of the patterns of daily life play a part in determining the length and quality of one's life. The child's use of tobacco products and controlled substances influences both physical and mental health. Patterns of exercise and use of protective gear help to avoid early disabilities. Media use can influence aggressive behaviors, interfere with need for physical activity, or be a positive force in teaching young

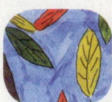

Partnering with Families

Evaluation of Childcare

The nurse can help parents to evaluate childcare options and make decisions about placement for their children. Parents should always be welcome to visit an agency or home childcare—this is essential so they can see the routines in action. Following are suggested questions for them to ask.

ADMINISTRATION

- Is the facility licensed?
- Who are the administrators? What is their training and experience?
- How many staff members are employed? What is their training?
- Is there a parent board? What part does the board play in administering the center?

PHYSICAL ENVIRONMENT, HEALTH, AND SAFETY

- What is the neighborhood like? Is transportation to the center convenient?
- What is the condition of lighting, heat, cooling, and ventilation systems; play spaces (inside and out); and the building's general structure?
- Is playground equipment safe?
- Is there a soft material such as bark, sand, or rubber tiles under climbing equipment?
- Is there always supervision for the children?
- Are there emergency medical forms and signed forms for field trips?
- Who may pick up children? How are they signed in and out?
- What is the immunization policy and how are records examined and maintained?

- Are criminal background checks of staff done for potential child abuse and other problems?
- What is the policy for children with infectious diseases and other illness?
- How are foods prepared? Is staff licensed in food handling?
- What is the state of general cleanliness?
- Who changes diapers? Are recommendations for standard precautions to prevent pathogen transfer followed?
- What arrangements and routines are made for naps and quiet times?

DEVELOPMENTAL APPROACHES

- Is the curriculum appropriate for different age groups?
- Are there materials and plans for gross motor, fine motor, language, and social development?
- How much time do children spend in structured time? Free time?
- How is discipline handled?
- Do the children appear occupied and happy?
- What reading materials are available?
- What type and quantity of field trips are planned?
- What is the educational level and longevity of the childcare workers?
- Is there diversity among the children's backgrounds and experiences?

Source: Adapted from National Association for the Education of Young Children, 2010.

children new concepts. Tattoos that can introduce pathogens are an example of a lifestyle pattern that influences mental and physical health and body image. Excessive sun exposure can lead to skin injury and skin cancer (see Chapter 36 ⊘).

Substance Use

Substance use and abuse occurs in children and adolescents of all socioeconomic levels and is a growing health problem. About 26% of youth currently use tobacco, 42% drank alcohol in the previous month, and 24% engaged in binge drinking during that month (Centers for Disease Control and Prevention [CDC], 2010a). The use of any substance, such as tobacco, alcohol, or illicit drugs, can pose a serious psychologic and physical risk to children and adolescents.

Tobacco Use

Tobacco use is the most preventable cause of adult death in the United States. It leads to 438,000 premature deaths annually and will be responsible for the premature death of 5 million of today's youth as they reach adult years (U.S. Department of Health and Human Services, 2011). Major health problems linked to tobacco use include cardiovascular disease, cancer, chronic lung disease, increased prevalence of car crashes, low birth weight, and other newborn problems. Even passive smoking or environmental tobacco smoke (ETS) is linked to increased heart disease, high blood pressure, respiratory problems, decreased youth academic performance, sudden infant death syndrome, and otitis media (U.S. Environmental Protection Agency, 2010). Cigarette use is most common; however, chewing tobacco, snuff, cigars, and bidis may also be used, and also pose significant health hazards.

Practice Alert

Forms of tobacco other than cigarettes may be popular among certain groups or in specific parts of the country. Smokeless tobacco in forms of chew, snuff, or dip is used regularly by 8.9% of youth. This type of tobacco is even used by students in school without staff being aware of the behavior. Bidis are small, brown, hand-rolled cigarettes that are used by over 2% of youth; they usually have more nicotine than traditional cigarettes and are therefore very addicting (CDC, 2011a). Cigars have been used by 14% of youth (CDC, 2010a). Hookahs, or water pipes, pass smoke through water before it is inhaled. Electronic cigarettes provide electronic mist with flavors and nicotine. Although not regulated at present, the U.S. Food and Drug Administration is concerned about the nicotine they contain with flavors that are enticing to youth, and is considering limiting their sale to young people. Hookahs and electronic cigarettes are used by about 7% of youth (CDC, 2011a). Try to learn the types of tobacco most common in the local community, and plan to integrate history questions during health exams to learn about cigarette and other tobacco use. Never assume that a youth is not using tobacco. Ask every youth questions about it, when parents are not in the room. Consult resources such as the American Academy of Pediatrics and the American Cancer Society to find prevention and cessation materials for youth.

Many nurses view tobacco use as an adult issue, but each day over 3,400 youth try their first cigarette. The major ages for trying tobacco are 9 to 14 years (between sixth and ninth grades). Early initiation of smoking is an extremely risky behavior because nicotine is highly addictive. The majority of adult smokers began smoking before 18 years of age (CDC, 2011a) (Box 20–2).

Although sale of tobacco products to children and advertisements aimed at this age group are forbidden by federal law (except for electronic cigarettes), youth still obtain and use tobacco. The Youth Risk Behavior Surveillance (YRBS) has found that nearly one third of youth use tobacco and one half of all youth have tried tobacco, making this an important health risk (CDC, 2010a).

BOX 20–2   **Research: Youth Risk Behavior Surveillance System**

The Youth Risk Behavior Surveillance System is conducted every other year on large representative numbers of youth by the Centers for Disease Control and Prevention. For example, in 2009, all 50 states and the District of Columbia were included in reported results, including 196 school/local surveys. About 16,410 students were included in that data set, representing a school response rate of 81% and a student response rate of 88% of those questioned (CDC, 2010b). The categories of priority health-risk behaviors investigated in each survey are:

- Behaviors contributing to unintentional and intentional injury
- Tobacco use
- Alcohol and other drug use
- Sexual behaviors that contribute to unintended pregnancy and sexually transmitted infection, including HIV
- Physical activity
- Overweight and weight control

Etiology and pathophysiology Certain characteristics contribute to the likelihood of tobacco use. They include increasing age, male gender, ethnic group, ease of obtaining tobacco products, and smoking among family members (see Developing Cultural Competence: Smoking). Low socioeconomic group membership, access to tobacco products, low price of products, advertising, and lack of parental involvement in the youth's lives are also associated with tobacco use (U.S. Department of Health and Human Services, 2011). Gender differences may exist for youth who are beginning or seeking to quit smoking; maternal smoking contributes to female adolescent initiation of smoking (Sullivan, Bottorff, & Reid, 2011) (Figure 20–4 ■).

Collaborative Care

Many groups work together to both prevent tobacco use and help tobacco users with cessation. Community activists, parents, nurses, school personnel, other health professionals, and even teens themselves partner in youth programs. Successful programs combine several approaches:

- Youth-oriented mass media campaigns about hazards of tobacco use
- Increased tobacco taxes
- Smoke-free policies for schools, restaurants, and other community sites
- Increased regulation of tobacco
- Reduction in youth access to tobacco
- School-based programs in cessation

Developing Cultural Competence
Smoking

Among youth in the United States, White youth are significantly more likely to smoke than either Hispanic or Black peers. About 22.5% of White students reported smoking in the previous month, while 18% of Hispanic and 9.5% of Black students reported this behavior (CDC, 2010a). American Indian and Alaska Natives also have high smoking rates, while Asian Americans have low rates (U.S. Department of Health and Human Services, 2011). There is also regional diversity, with overall smoking rates ranging from 8.5% to 26.1% among various states (CDC, 2010a).

In addition to the Youth Risk Behavior Surveillance that measures smoking and other behaviors among U.S. youth, the Global Youth Tobacco Survey (GYTS) gathers data on 13- to 15-year-old students for the World Health Organization in 132 countries worldwide.

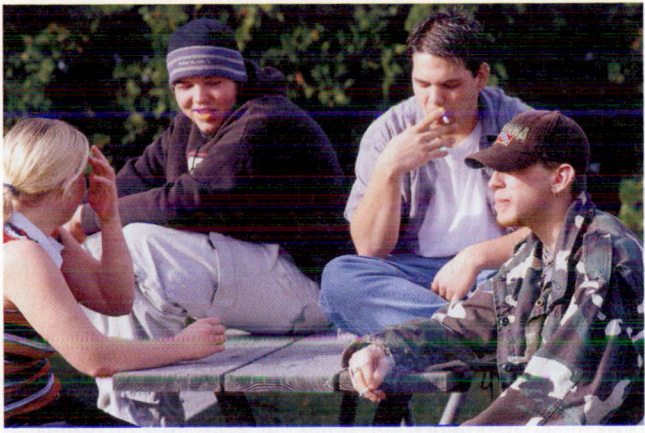

FIGURE 20–4 ■ Approximately 70% of children have tried smoking by their high school years. Early intervention can begin with discussions about smoking starting at 9 or 10 years of age.

Clinical Therapy

Several programs have been developed to encourage youth to avoid tobacco use. In addition, smoking cessation programs are available to assist youth who are already regular smokers. These programs are successful in achieving the goals of cessation or decrease in tobacco use. Use of incentives and counselor-based, individually tailored telephone interventions have been effective (Backinger, Michaels, Jefferson, et al., 2008; CDC, 2009). Once a teen is identified as a smoker, using a biological marker such as urine cotinine (a by-product of tobacco) levels can help to identify the frequency of smoking. This information can be used to make suggestions to the teen about the potential outcomes of the behavior and the cessation program that is most likely to be helpful.

Nursing Management

Nursing management focuses on prevention of tobacco use, early identification of smokers, and referral to treatment and smoking cessation options.

Nursing Assessment and Diagnosis

Nurses are in a unique position to inquire about the incidence of smoking and other tobacco use among youth. Questions should be inserted into all well-child visits, beginning at about 9 to 10 years of age. Inquire about whether family members (especially parents and siblings) smoke or chew, and ask if some of the child's friends have tried smoking. Determine the child's knowledge and beliefs about the benefits and risks of tobacco use. Assess for associated risk behaviors such as alcohol and drug use, sexual behavior, and suicidal thoughts. As the child gets older, more direct and detailed questions are necessary. A nonjudgmental approach will be best to obtain a truthful response. School nurses can make observations about numbers of teens smoking and general attitudes about tobacco use. When children come to hospitals and other health facilities for care, use of tobacco should be part of general admission questions. Remember to include smokeless tobacco use in questioning (chewing tobacco, snuff, dip) and to ask about all forms of smoking.

The following nursing diagnoses may apply to youth who smoke or show potential for this behavior:

- Activity Intolerance related to lowered oxygen supply
- Gas Exchange, Impaired related to ventilation-perfusion imbalance
- Self-Esteem, Chronic Low related to negative self-appraisal

- Knowledge, Deficient Regarding Dangers of Tobacco Use related to developmental focus on the present
- Nutrition, Imbalanced: Less than Body Requirements related to effects of chemical dependence

NANDA-I © 2012

Planning and Implementation

The roles of nurses in preventing and intervening in youth smoking are to inform youth, identify smokers, and implement programs (Table 20–3). Nurses should provide developmentally appropriate information about the hazards of tobacco use in all settings where youth are present. Posters, flyers, and speakers are particularly useful. Include information about short-term problems such as increased rates of upper respiratory infections and worsening of asthma, as well as long-term effects such as addiction, lung cancer, oral cancer, car crashes, emphysema, and other health problems. Addicted teens who share their stories of difficult withdrawal from tobacco, and adults who have had cancer of the lungs or larynx may be effective speakers. Find out where teens obtain tobacco products in the community and where they use the products to target these places. Offer information on available prevention and cessation programs to youth and families in clinics, outpatient surgery centers, community activities, and hospitals. Use opportunities such as care during adolescent pregnancy and illnesses to reinforce the hazardous effects of tobacco on the individual and on those nearby. Adolescent mothers should understand the risks for small-for-gestational-age babies when they smoke in pregnancy, and the increased risk of sudden infant death syndrome (SIDS) when infants are exposed to secondhand smoke (see Chapter 25 ❷ for a detailed discussion of SIDS). Speak to young athletes about the effects of tobacco on athletic performance. Show youth the ways in which this product can interfere with their meeting of life goals. Role-play how to tell other youth "no" when tobacco is offered. Establish programs that increase the sense of self-esteem without tobacco use. Be sure to include parents in the programs so that they see and acknowledge their role in setting an example about tobacco use, and in providing guidelines for the child. The influence of ETS (also known as secondhand smoke) should be discussed.

Adopt a nonjudgmental attitude when asking questions about smoking so that youth who are using tobacco can be identified. Ask questions without parents present and assure youth that the information will not be shared. Ask smokers if they have tried to quit and if they want to "kick the habit." Encourage all youth to cut back and to quit use of tobacco products. Offer direct links to cessation programs to help them in these efforts. Encourage positive behavior changes and coping techniques for youth who are engaged in cessation. Such techniques include keeping busy, avoiding smoking situations, using oral stimulation such as a toothpick or gum, exercising, relaxing,

and using nicotine replacement approaches (Audrain-McGovern, Stevens, Murray, et al., 2011).

Work with the schools and school districts to help establish preventive and cessation programs. There should be clear guidelines about school policies regarding smoking on school grounds. Keeping occasional youth smokers from becoming regular users should be a goal to avoid nicotine addiction. Find out what positive incentives can be offered to youth who are successful in quitting smoking. Contract with them to achieve their goals.

Identify particular youth who are at risk for starting smoking because of parents or other family members who smoke, or peer groups with high smoking rates. Consider the increased risk to youth with chronic disease such as asthma or diabetes who also choose to smoke. Smoking significantly increases the risks of many chronic diseases and complicates treatment (see Chapter 25 ❷ for further information about asthma).

Evaluation

Expected outcomes of nursing interventions regarding tobacco use relate to successful outcomes for communities. They include lowered rates of regular use, delayed initiation of use, and success of cessation programs. Use the following *Healthy People 2020* (U.S. Department of Health and Human Services, 2011) objectives as guidelines:

- Increase smoke-free and tobacco-free environments in schools, including all school facilities, property, vehicles, and school events, to 100%.
- Eliminate tobacco advertising and promotions that influence adolescents and young adults.
- Increase smoking cessation attempts by adolescent smokers to 64%.
- Reduce tobacco use by adolescents to 21%.
- Reduce smokeless tobacco use by adolescents to 6.9%.
- Reduce initiation of tobacco use among adolescents to 5.7%.

Alcohol Use

Alcohol use by the young is common. An estimated 72.5% have tried alcohol, which is the drug of choice and convenience for youth. By 12th grade, 80.3% of females and 79% of males have had alcoholic drinks (CDC, 2010a). Current use is also common, with 42% of high school students admitting to drinking within the last month, and 24% having engaged in binge drinking, or having five or more drinks within a 2-hour period. Even very young adolescents are affected since about 40% of eighth graders have tried alcohol and 11% have had one or more episodes of binge drinking (National Institute on Alcohol Abuse and Alcoholism [NIAAA], n.d.). About 25.6% of high school students report that their first drink was before age 13 years (CDC, 2010a). (See Developing Cultural Competence: Alcohol Use.)

TABLE 20–3	**Nursing Role in Youth Smoking Prevention**	
INFORM	**IDENTIFY**	**IMPLEMENT**
■ Hang posters, provide brochures, and facilitate presentations about smoking risks in all settings where youth are present.	■ Ask questions about smoking and other tobacco use at every health encounter beginning at about 9–10 years of age.	■ Encourage youth tobacco users to quit.
■ Target smokers with special information about the effects of nicotine on their bodies.	■ For users, ask amount and type of tobacco.	■ Facilitate referral to cessation programs.
	■ Learn where youth obtain tobacco and be proactive in stopping sales.	■ Arrange positive rewards for youth who are successful in cessation.

Developing Cultural Competence
Alcohol Use

Among students, Whites have the highest current (within the last 30 days) alcohol use (44.7%), with Hispanics next (42.9%), and Blacks least (33.4%) (CDC, 2010a). Nurses can use this information to target groups most at risk of alcohol ingestion, even at these young ages. Youth will be more likely to listen to members of their own ethnic groups when receiving education on alcohol and drug use.

<table>
<tr><td>BOX 20–3</td><td>Common Inhalant Agents</td></tr>
</table>

AEROSOLS
Cooking spray
Whipped cream
Spray paint
Cosmetic sprays

ADHESIVES
Model glues
Rubber cements

SOLVENTS
Nail polish remover
Paint thinner or cleaner
Lighter fluid
Degreaser

OTHER
Gasoline
Helium

See Clinical Manifestations: Commonly Abused Drugs for symptoms indicating use of inhalant agents.

Numerous health risks are associated with drinking by minors. Perhaps the most common and obvious is that of motor vehicle crashes. About 1,900 young people annually die in alcohol-related injuries from car crashes, 1,600 die in homicides, and 300 die in suicides (NIAAA, n.d.). Others experience assault such as alcohol-related date rape. Alcohol affects the developing brain, decreasing intellectual capacity and increasing the chance for future alcohol use. Additionally, early drinking significantly increases the chance that someone will become an alcoholic later in life. Endocrine problems, liver abnormalities, and decreased bone density can also occur. The neurologic effects of alcohol on the brain are magnified in the young (Alcohol Free Children, 2010). Children are much more likely to try alcohol and to become alcoholic when a family member is alcoholic; this is a significant risk because one in five children grows up in a home with an alcoholic adult (NIAAA, 2009).

Many factors influence the child and adolescent who drink alcohol. Patterns in the family, media advertisements, and social environments in high school and college that honor or expect drinking all contribute to the problem. Access is easy for most youth as older siblings or classmates obtain drinks. It is a "rite of passage" for many at teen birthday parties or college events. Alcohol is the most common and accepted drug in today's society and, as such, youth are exposed to it. They often experiment with alcohol and experience its

effects without understanding or considering the implications of its use. A significant risk factor for initiation of alcohol use is a transition time, such as change from middle to high school, or a major family stress, such as parental separation or divorce.

Drug Use

In addition to alcohol, a variety of other drugs are used by youth. Nearly 37% of students have used marijuana, and 21% have used it in the last month; 6.4% have used cocaine, with nearly 3% having used it in the last month; 6.7% have used ecstasy. Inhalant use of glue, paints, or other substances is more common, with 12% reporting use and 4% having used in the last month. See Box 20–3 for common inhalant agents. Approximately 4% report methamphetamine use, and 2.5% report using heroin (CDC, 2010a). Synthetic drugs such as phencyclidine (PCP), commonly referred to as "designer" drugs, mimic other narcotics, stimulants, and hallucinogens and are also dangerous. Some common contemporary drugs and street names are listed in Table 20–4.

Prescription drugs are increasingly used for nonmedical purposes. For example, methylphenidate (Ritalin) is used for treatment

TABLE 20–4 Common Contemporary Club Drugs, Street Names, and Drug Information

DRUG	ACTION	STREET NAMES	ROUTE	TIME OF ACTION
Methylenedioxymethamphetamine (MDMA)	Stimulant; appetite suppressant; increased pulse, blood pressure (BP), temperature; overhydration, hyponatremia; memory loss	Ecstasy, XTC, X, Adam, Clarity, Hug, Beans, Lover's speed, E	Oral (tablets, capsules)	3–6 hours
Gamma-hydroxybutyrate (GHB) (Xyrem)	Central nervous system (CNS) depressant, euphoria, growth hormone release, hypersalivation, hypotonia	Grievous Bodily Harm, G, Liquid Ecstasy, Soap, Georgia Home Boy, Date-rape drug	Oral (liquid, powder, tablets, capsules)	4 hours
Ketamine	Anesthetic; decreased memory, attention, learning; increased BP; respiratory collapse	Special K, K, Vitamin K, Cat Valiums, Jet	Intravenous, respiratory (injected, snorted, or smoked; liquid or powder)	1–2 hours
Rohypnol (benzodiazepine; flunitrazepam)	Amnesia, sedative; decreased BP, urinary retention; given prior to sexual assault	Roofies, Rophies, Roche, Forget-me Pill	Oral (tablets)	8–12 hours
Methamphetamine	Stimulant; highly addictive; memory loss, violence, psychosis; cardiac and neurologic damage	Speed, Ice, Chalk, Meth, Crystal, Crank, Fire, Glass, Tina, Tweak, Yaba (meth and caffeine)	Oral, respiratory, intravenous (smoked, snorted, injected)	Several hours; long-term permanent effects
Lysergic acid diethylamide (LSD)	Hallucinogen; increased pulse, BP, temperature; psychosis, flashbacks	Acid, Boomers, Blotters, Dots, Yellow Sunshines	Oral (liquid, tablets, capsules), absorbent paper	1–2 hours; trips last 12 hours

Source: *Data from National Institute on Drug Abuse. (2011). NIDA InfoFacts: Club Drugs. Retrieved from http://www.nida/nih.gov/Infofacts/clubdrugs.html and http://www.drugabuse.gov/drugpages .clubdrugs.html*

Complementary Therapy Caffeine Products and Other Stimulants

Youth may be aware of the caffeine content of herbal products and use them in excess. Nearly half of the caffeine overdoses in the United States occur in youth (Seifert, Schaechter, Hershorin, et al., 2011). Guarana is made from cocoa beans and contains caffeine and other drugs such as theophylline. It is available in supplements and is used in some energy drinks. Yerba mate is formulated from a tree and also contains caffeine, theophylline, and other substances. Some noncaffeinated stimulants include panax (Asian ginseng) and ephedra (ma huang). Each family, child, and adolescent should be questioned about intake of caffeine and other stimulants, either in beverages or in herbal forms.

of attention deficit hyperactivity disorder (ADHD) and generally acts as a stimulant. Its unprescribed use among youth has increased dramatically over the past few years. Prescription pain medications are another example of drugs that are abused by youth who find drugs prescribed to family members after surgery or other procedures. Obtainable, over-the-counter (OTC) medications are legal substances that are frequently abused. Easily obtainable at grocery stores and drugstores, these drugs include antihistamines, atropine, bromides, caffeine, ephedrine, pseudoephedrine, phenylpropanolamine, and amphetamine-like substitutes.

Other substances abused are in food sources. Some youth drink multiple servings of coffee, tea, soda pop, and other caffeinated beverages for their psychoactive effects. Certain energy drinks, herbal products, and OTC cold and diet medicines may also be used. Anabolic steroids are the drugs of abuse most commonly used by athletes. See Chapter 19 for further use of enhancing substances. (See Complementary Therapy: Caffeine Products and Other Stimulants.)

Etiology and pathophysiology In most cases, substance abuse represents a maladaptive coping response to the stressors of childhood and adolescence. Individual, peer, family, and community risk factors all contribute to increased incidence of use (American Academy of Child and Adolescent Psychiatry, 2010). A child may begin using drugs or alcohol to deal with stress because family members or peers do so. Children in families with a history of substance abuse are at higher risk of abusing drugs and alcohol. Other risk factors include rebelliousness, aggressiveness, low self-esteem, dysfunctional parental relationships, lack of adequate support systems, academic underachievement, poor judgment, and poor impulse control. Adolescents and young adults use "club drugs" to achieve greater satisfaction during nights dancing, drinking, and attending clubs. Use of these drugs with alcohol can lead to deadly consequences. See Table 20–4 for common club drugs.

Initial experimentation with alcohol or drugs may be unpleasant. With continued use, however, the adolescent learns to "achieve the high," an illusion of power and well-being. The adolescent wants the high more frequently and actively seeks alcohol or drugs. Tolerance to the substance occurs with continued use, and ever-increasing amounts are required to achieve a pleasurable high. Physical and psychologic dependence ensues as the body's tissues require the substance to function properly. Withdrawal symptoms occur when the child or adolescent is deprived of the substance.

Clinical manifestations Substance abuse in children and adolescents is commonly overlooked and underdiagnosed by healthcare providers, due in part to the wide range of clinical presentations. These vary according to type of drug abused, amount, frequency, time of last use, and severity of drug dependence. See Clinical Manifestations: Commonly Abused Drugs for signs and symptoms of substance abuse and potential for dependence.

Common physical manifestations include alterations in vital signs, weight loss, chronic fatigue, chronic cough, respiratory congestion, red eyes, and general apathy and malaise. The mental status examination (refer to Chapter 7) may reveal alterations in level of consciousness, impaired attention and concentration, impaired thought processes, delusions, and hallucinations. Low self-esteem, feelings of guilt or worthlessness, and suicidal or homicidal thoughts are also common.

Poor school performance and changes in mood, sleep habits, appetite, dress, and social relationships are nonspecific characteristics of the child who is abusing substances. These are often the symptoms first noted by family and friends, and should be the subject of questions at each health promotion visit.

Collaborative Care

Multiple psychiatric diagnostic criteria exist for each drug class. Children and adolescents who have other psychosocial disorders commonly use or abuse drugs or alcohol. Therefore, assessment and treatment plans should focus not only on the substance use or abuse, but also on the issues underlying the problem.

Diagnostic Procedures

Diagnosis includes assessment of both the family and the substance-abusing child or adolescent. Physical and psychologic assessments are performed, looking for signs such as change in school performance or friends/family relationships, delinquent behavior, red eyes with dilated or constricted pupils, persistent cough, or alterations in eating or sleeping. Blood and urine levels of substances and metabolites are sometimes measured. The half-life of the substance determines how long after use it can be detected in body fluids, ranging from 1 to 2 days for amphetamines to 2 weeks for barbiturates (American Academy of Child and Adolescent Psychiatry, 2010).

Clinical Therapy

The primary goal of treatment is to teach the child and other family members to develop and sustain positive coping patterns, and to support them during this process. Most treatment programs offer inpatient and outpatient services, as well as aftercare programs. These programs usually consist of peer support focusing on the development of a lifestyle free of drugs or alcohol, healthy family relationships, and positive coping skills. Family involvement is strongly encouraged. Hospitalization is required if the physical dependence is significant and withdrawal places the child at risk for complications such as seizures, depression, or suicidal behavior.

Nursing Management

Nursing management focuses on prevention of substance abuse, early identification of users, and referral to treatment options.

Nursing Assessment and Diagnosis

Mental health assessment of all older children and adolescents requires screening for alcohol and other substances; include screening for over-the-counter and prescription medication use (Gracious, Abe, & Sundberg, 2010; Havens, Young, & Havens, 2011). Maintaining a

Clinical Manifestations Commonly Abused Drugs

DRUG	POTENTIAL FOR DEPENDENCE	CLINICAL MANIFESTATIONS
Depressants Alcohol, barbiturates (amobarbital, pentobarbital, secobarbital)	*Physical and psychologic:* High; varies somewhat among drugs	*Physical:* Decreased muscle tone and coordination, tremors *Psychologic:* Impaired speech, memory, and judgment; confusion; decreased attention span; emotional lability
Stimulants Amphetamines (e.g., Benzedrine), caffeine, cocaine, "bath salts"	*Physical:* Low to moderate *Psychologic:* High; withdrawal from amphetamines and cocaine can lead to severe depression	*Physical:* Dilated pupils, increased pulse and blood pressure, flushing, nausea, loss of appetite, tremors *Psychologic:* Euphoria; increased alertness, agitation, or irritability; hallucinations; insomnia
Opiates Codeine, heroin, meperidine (Demerol), methadone, morphine, opium, oxycodone (Percodan, OxyContin)	*Physical and psychologic:* High; varies somewhat among drugs; withdrawal effects are uncomfortable	*Physical:* Analgesia, depressed respirations and muscle tone, nausea, constricted pupils, overdose may lead to coma or death *Psychologic:* Changes in mood (usually euphoria), drowsiness, impaired attention or memory, sense of tranquility
Hallucinogens Lysergic acid diethylamide (LSD), mescaline, phencyclidine (PCP)	*Physical:* None *Psychologic:* Unknown	*Physical:* Lack of coordination, dilated pupils, hypertension, elevated temperature; severe PCP intoxication can result in seizures, respiratory depression, coma, and death *Psychologic:* Visual illusions and hallucinations, altered perceptions of time and space, emotional lability, psychosis
Volatile Inhalants Glues, typing correction fluid, acrylic paints, spot removers, lighter fluid, gasoline, butane	*Physical and psychologic:* Varies with drug used	*Physical:* Impaired coordination, liver damage (in some cases) *Psychologic:* Impaired judgment, delirium
Marijuana	*Physical:* Low *Psychologic:* Usually low; occasionally moderate to high	*Physical:* Tachycardia, reddened conjunctiva, dry mouth, increased appetite *Psychologic:* Initial anxiety followed by euphoria; giddiness; impaired attention, judgment, and memory

confidential approach will increase the ability to obtain truthful information about use of substances. Assessment tools provide useful information for the healthcare provider. These include the PACES tool and the HEADSS tool. Nurses may encounter the substance-abusing child or adolescent in the emergency department or outpatient clinic, in the school and other community settings, or during hospitalization for an injury or other acute problem. Nursing assessment includes taking a thorough history from the parents and child, observing the child's behavior, and performing a physical examination.

Clinical Tip

PACES provides a framework for areas that should be assessed for each child to identify risk and protective factors related to substance use:

P = Parents, peers
A = Accidents, alcohol/drug use
C = Cigarettes
E = Emotional problems
S = School, sexuality
   Likewise, HEADSS provides a tool for performing youth screening:
H = Home and environment
E = Education, employment
A = Activities
D = Drugs
S = Sexuality
S = Suicide and depression

Source: *Data from Knight, 1997.*

When substance use is known, the history should include the age at which drug use began, pattern of use, length of time the drug has been used, amount of drug used, and psychologic state while on drugs. A history of parental drug use and noninvolvement in parenting puts the child at higher risk for substance abuse, reflecting the combined effects of genetic and environmental influences. Environmental factors such as access to the substance, use with other teens or adults, and resources for treatment are important to consider. Find out what types of addictions are most common in your community so that assessments can be designed to the risks that are highest for youth in those settings (Figure 20–5 ■). See Partnering with Families: Identifying the Youth Who Is Abusing Substances.

Physiologic Assessment

Look for physical signs and symptoms of substance abuse, including bloodshot eyes, dilated or constricted pupils (depending on the substance), slurred speech, and weight loss. The adolescent may appear sleepy or restless, or may show signs of clumsiness or inconsistent behavior. Consider all types of substance abuse, including model glue, gasoline, and other sources. Assess for signs of withdrawal and current intoxication effects.

Practice Alert

Adolescents who have some or all of the following symptoms may be experiencing alcohol withdrawal: anxiety, headache, tremors, nausea and vomiting, malaise or weakness, insomnia, depressed mood or irritability, and hallucinations.

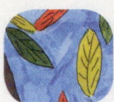

Partnering with Families

Identifying the Youth Who Is Abusing Substances

Families are often confused about the behavior of adolescents and unsure whether it represents normal development or abuse of substances. Some characteristics of normal development that help to differentiate these occurrences are listed here. When concerned about possible substance use, the parent can confront the child or talk with school nurses or counselors.

- Many youth are periodically distant with parents at times, but remain involved with peers in school sports and other activities. Withdrawal from all activities and friends may indicate substance abuse.
- Adolescents often complain about school, but when teachers report the student meets expectations and is consistently performing in the classroom this is normal behavior.

- Teens may be weepy on occasion when having a difficult time with friends or not performing as desired. Continued, consistent weepiness is more likely to indicate depression or substance abuse.
- Teens like to stay up late and are frequently tired in the morning. Abusing teens may "nod off" frequently during the day.
- Many adolescents like to achieve a disheveled look in clothing, but the teen who frequently neglects basic hygiene or does not seem to have the energy to wash and dress may be depressed or abusing substances.
- All teens get some infections, but teens who are abusing substances may have reddened eyes, oral sores, and constant respiratory discomfort from "snorting" substances.

Psychologic Assessment

Changes in social habits may indicate substance abuse. Parents may report a drop in the school-age child's or adolescent's grades or decreased interest in school activities. New friends are not introduced to parents, and the adolescent has less contact with parents, teachers, and other adults who were previously important. Conversely, the youth may appear more energetic, always "on a high," exhibit weight loss, and appear to be high achieving. The child's current drug use, potential for violence, and motivation to make changes are noted. Assess the degree of family support available.

Family Assessment

In families with substance-using adults, children may experience neglect and abuse, as well as exposure to drugs. When family members are substance users, young children may experience periods when adults cannot provide supervision or cannot encourage healthy activities. The children may be exposed to potentially unsafe or violent episodes. When parents are manufacturing products such as methamphetamine, young children are exposed to toxic chemicals and run the risk of suffering burns and other sequelae from home laboratory production and explosions. Be alert for unusual injuries, signs of inconsistent parenting, and delays in or disturbed growth and development. Be prepared to refer parents for care and to follow protocols for child abuse prevention (see section on abuse and neglect later in this chapter).

In addition, when a young person in the family is using drugs, the parents and siblings may be upset, angry, and frustrated. They may feel helpless and worry about the youth who is abusing. Family members may try to protect the youth who is using and shield others from knowing. Such approaches may delay treatment and effective care.

Following are possible nursing diagnoses for children and adolescents who abuse drugs or alcohol:

- Social Interaction, Impaired related to altered thought processes
- Self-Esteem, Chronic Low related to dysfunctional family and social relationships
- Injury, Risk for related to altered perceptions and sensorium
- Violence: Other-Directed or Self-Directed related to physiologic dependence on drugs, alcohol, and other substances

WARNING!

Contaminated
Property

Dangerous Chemicals Have
Been Removed From
These Premises

Entry is Unsafe!

For Information Contact:
Spokane Regional Health District
At: (509) 324-1560

FIGURE 20–5 ■ Methamphetamine is a popular drug because it can be manufactured with items that are available to the lay public such as those shown in the picture. Manufacture of the substance in homes has become a concern of health departments and communities at large. Children can be harmed by the chemicals produced, and may experience neglect and abuse. They may suffer even after the home is found and adults are apprehended as they must be placed in foster homes. Homes must be decontaminated in a lengthy and costly manner before future use after methamphetamine production.

Source: *Photo courtesy of Spokane Regional Health District.*

NANDA-I © 2012

Planning and Implementation

Care of children and adolescents who abuse drugs, alcohol, and other substances is challenging and often frustrating. Long-term mental health counseling may be necessary to resolve underlying issues and foster lifestyle and behavioral changes.

Prevention is the most desirable intervention. The nurse can teach children and their families about substance abuse. Education should begin in primary school and continue with intensification during middle and high school years. Nurses also can play a major role in community education. Various prevention programs have been developed by federal and private organizations.

The youth's protective factors can be identified and used in planning appropriate interventions. For example, a child with goals related to a future career can be helped to see the way in which substance use will interfere with goal attainment. Identifying a strong role model through a program like Big Brothers or Big Sisters can assist children who lack that strength in their families.

The child who has begun to use and abuse drugs needs an intensive intervention program. Referral to a psychiatric health specialist is needed for diagnosis and intervention. Group programs and those that integrate the family are most effective. Find out what resources are present in your community to treat youth who are using alcohol or other drugs. Nurses are active in treatment programs as well as sustaining treatment effects and avoiding relapse during visits to community agencies once the youth returns to family, school, and other surroundings. Referral to support organizations may be beneficial for the child, parents, siblings, and other family members. Self-help groups, which are available in most communities, include Alcoholics Anonymous, Narcotics Anonymous, Al-Anon, Nar-Anon, and Ala-Teen. Parents may receive support from a group such as Parents Anonymous.

The nurse should be aware of the current substance abuse patterns in specific communities. Currently, methamphetamine (meth) use is increasing in many areas and represents a severe threat to youth because it is extremely addictive and resistant to treatment. An increasing awareness of meth's dangers has led to legislation that pseudoephedrine can only be sold as a "behind-the-counter" controlled substance since it is used in home laboratories manufacturing meth. Inappropriate access to prescription medications is another common source of substance abuse. Consult local health departments as well as the National Institute on Drug Abuse and the National Clearinghouse for Alcohol and Drug Information to become aware of current drug abuse patterns and substances so such information can be integrated into screening and intervention methods.

Evaluation

Evaluation about alcohol consumption can be measured by the goals of the Surgeon General's *Call to Action* to prevent and reduce underage drinking. They include:

- Foster changes in American society that facilitate healthy adolescent development and that help prevent and reduce underage drinking.
- Engage parents, schools, communities, all levels of government, all social systems that interface with youth, and youth themselves in a coordinated national effort to prevent and reduce drinking and its consequences.
- Promote an understanding of underage alcohol consumption in the context of human development and maturation that takes into account individual adolescent characteristics as well as environmental, ethnic, cultural, and gender differences.
- Conduct additional research on adolescent alcohol use and its relationship to development.
- Work to improve public health surveillance on underage drinking and on population-based risk factors for this behavior.
- Work to ensure that policies at all levels are consistent with the national goal of preventing and reducing underage alcohol consumption.

Surgeon General, 2007

Expected outcomes of nursing interventions regarding all types of substance abuse include the following:

- The youth abstains from alcohol and street drugs.
- The young person successfully participates in substance abuse treatment programs.
- The child or adolescent displays developmentally appropriate social interactions.
- School performance is at the level of potential.
- The youth is safe from injury.

Physical Inactivity and Sedentary Behavior

In the past few decades, children have become less physically active. This decrease is a reflection of lifestyles in which car travel is valued, computers and televisions are part of daily life, neighborhoods are sometimes unsafe places for play activities, and schools do not routinely require daily physical education (PE) classes (Figure 20–6 ■).

Children and adolescents are subjected to high levels of media exposure, including television, movies, radio, magazines, videos, computers (games and Internet), and a variety of advertising. Media use has dramatically increased in the last few years, and most youth have no restrictions on the amount of use. An astounding 7 hours and 38 minutes is the average amount of time youth use media daily (Kaiser Family Foundation, 2010). This amounts to more than 53 hours per week for most children, and significantly more for some. Frequent use of multitasking allows youth to access TV, computer games, and cell phones all at once. Even at very young ages, children are immersed in various types of media (Box 20–4).

The effects of screen activities include:

- Physical inactivity while viewing
- Lack of active cognition
- Lack of social interaction
- Tendency to eat high-fat snacks and excessive calories while viewing

Physical inactivity leads to many health concerns. A primary outcome is overweight or obesity (see Chapter 19 ⊘). Other outcomes can be an increased rate of type 2 diabetes (see Chapter 32 ⊘), increased exposure to television and computer game violence and sexual activity at early ages (see violence discussion later in this chapter), and early progression of cardiovascular disease (see Chapter 26 ⊘).

Weblink Substance Abuse Resources

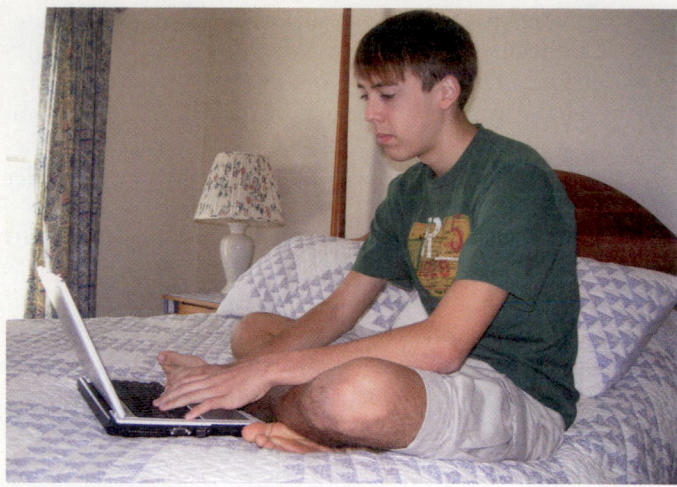
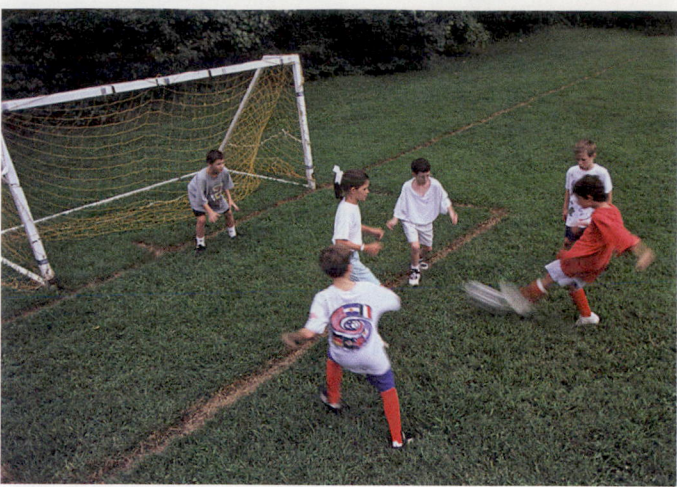

FIGURE 20–6 ■ Physical inactivity is a growing problem among children and can contribute to poor health. It is important to balance sedentary activities, such as playing screen games, with physical and social activities. Sports are an excellent way for children to develop their psychosocial, cognitive, and motor skills.

Source: *B, Wake Forest Baptist Health (WFBH) Photography.*

However, patterns of regular physical activity established in childhood can lead to increased exercise behaviors in adulthood, contributing to lower rates of low back pain, overweight, osteoporosis, heart disease, diabetes, colon cancer, and high blood pressure. Increased exercise behaviors also contribute to a more positive self-image.

Although many children demonstrate low levels of physical activity, a profound decrease in vigorous activity is common in grades 9 through 12. Boys more commonly participate in team sports than girls. Although about 56% of students attend PE classes at least once a week, only 33% have daily PE classes (CDC, 2010a).

Health professionals can integrate assessment of physical activity into all health care and make recommendations to children and families that will help to increase opportunities for physical activity. Nurses assess height, weight, and body mass index to look for signs of overweight (see Chapter 19 ❷). Ask what a typical day is like, and include specific questions about television, computers, and video games. Suggest strategies to lessen the hours spent with media such as increased physical activity and family meals.

Children should be asked about how they like to spend free time. Community and school activities should be encouraged and rewarded. Examples include fun runs, walks that benefit causes, aerobics classes, team sports, roadside cleanups, and fairs and carnivals. Examine the community in which the family lives. Is it possible to walk to the store or ride a bicycle to school? Be sure suggestions are realistic for the particular situation. Help parents and children learn what they can do for physical fitness. Work with school physical education personnel to plan activities both in and out of PE class that promote lifelong exercise routines. Work toward the goal of 60 minutes of daily moderate to vigorous physical activity for all children (American Heart Association, 2008; U.S. Department of Health and Human Services, 2009a). During regular health promotion visits, help children to identify ways to gradually increase physical activity and decrease sedentary time. See Partnering with Families: Physical Activity Guidelines for Youth.

Injury and Protective Equipment

In the discussion of causes of childhood and adolescent morbidities and mortalities in Chapter 1 ❷, unintentional injuries are listed as

---

BOX 20–4   **Research: Young Children and Media Effects**

The use of every component of media, from listening to music to TV to computers and video games, has significantly increased in youth in the last 5 years, while reading books has decreased to less than one half hour daily. Other facts:

- Cell phones are owned by two thirds of youth who operate them as media delivery platforms.
- About 84% of homes have Internet service.
- Nearly one third of youth have a laptop computer.
- Youth who spend more time with media have lower grades and less personal contentment.
- Parents who limit media use have children with lower amounts of usage.
- The largest recent jump in media use is in the 11- to 14-year-old age group.

(Rideout, Foehr, & Roberts, 2010)

These findings are critical for nurses to consider. Physical inactivity or sedentary behavior is linked to obesity, type 2 diabetes, and other chronic disease risks.

Children's ready access to media throughout the day directly interferes with recommended levels of physical activity. In all settings ask parents of young children about their exposure to media. Encourage parents to turn off the television and computer in the house except for select and limited viewing times, avoid media use in the child's bedroom, limit exposure to cell phones, and have the child engaged in physical activity for a greater part of the day than in quiet pursuits. Encourage reading and being read to for young children; parents can schedule reading time to at least equal media viewing. Carefully perform developmental testing on children when exposure to media is high (see Chapter 9 ❷).

CRITICAL THINKING APPLICATION

What other teaching can you identify to address this issue with parents of young children? How can parents integrate media concerns into evaluation of childcare settings? What might the effects be on child growth and development with excessive use of media?

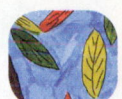

Partnering with Families

Physical Activity Guidelines for Youth

- Engage in 60 minutes or more of physical activity daily.
  - Engage in moderate physical activity (bike riding, walking, baseball, in-line skating) daily.
  - Engage in vigorous physical activity that causes sweating and hard breathing (soccer, running, ice hockey) at least three times weekly.
- Encourage schools to offer physical education to all students, and have students sign up when this is an elective.
- Encourage walking and bike riding to friends' homes and stores when safe.

- Plan physical activities together as a family.
- Get a pet and plan to walk the pet daily.
- Limit television and other similar sedentary activities to no more than 2 hours daily.
- On days home, allow the child to watch television for up to 1 hour, and then insist on 1 hour of reading, 1 hour of physical activity, and 1 hour of socializing with others before returning to more television.

---

a common problem. In fact, a majority of deaths from age 10 years onward result from four causes—motor vehicle crashes, other unintentional injury, homicide, and suicide (National Center for Health Statistics, 2012). (See Developing Cultural Competence: Unintentional Injury Rates.) Homicide is discussed in the violence section later in this chapter; suicide is discussed in Chapter 34 🔗. Chapters 9 through 13 🔗 discuss the frequent injuries seen in children at different developmental ages, and safety precautions to avoid injuries from car crashes, falls, poisonings, and other developmentally related injuries. Many common injuries are preventable with simple use of protective gear and following of safety guidelines (Figure 20–7 ■). These recommendations are explored in the following section.

Clinical Tip

Many sports and activities require safety gear. These include in-line skating, skateboarding, roller hockey, ice hockey, football, soccer, baseball, scooters, all-terrain vehicles, and skiing or snowboarding fast or on jumps. Ask children and adolescents about favorite sports and then explore safety gear used when it is recommended for the activities.

Over 10% of youth rarely or never wear car safety belts in automobiles; 32% of those who ride motorcycles do not wear helmets (CDC, 2010a). The use of safe automobile and motorcycle behaviors must be emphasized again in adolescence, with the recognition that risks increase if driving is combined with use of alcohol and controlled substances, and risk-taking behaviors occur with all wheeled transportation. Adolescents sometimes engage in practices that put them at particular risk, and nurses should be alert for activities in their communities. Examples include car surfing (standing on the trunk, hood, or roof of a moving vehicle), street racing (racing cars down a street at extremely high speed), or "extreme" sports.

About 44 million U.S. children ride bicycles, a beneficial physical activity. However, only about 15% are protected by helmet use, even though bicycles are the most common activity connected with injury (CDC, 2010a). Since almost one half of the U.S. states now have helmet laws, rates of use are highest in states with helmet legislation. Helmets could prevent up to 88% of serious brain injuries from bicycle crashes (National Safe Kids, 2008). Many injuries could be avoided by wearing a helmet, using knee and elbow pads, riding only on smooth surfaces in areas without cars, avoiding riding after

Developing Cultural Competence
Unintentional Injury Rates

Striking ethnic disparities exist in the rates of unintentional injury among children. These differences are due mainly to living in impoverished communities rather than any innate biological variations. Although the unintentional injury rate in children under 14 years declined 39% from 1987 to 2005, the smallest reductions were among American Indian/Alaska Natives (34% decline). Higher reductions were seen in Asian/Pacific Islanders (54% decline), African Americans (48% decline), and White children (44% decline). However, African American and Native American children still have rates of injury 1.5 times those of White children (National Safe Kids, 2008). *What are the major causes of unintentional injury in your community and state?* They may include homicide, motor vehicle crashes, or other causes. *What ethnic and age groups are at greatest risk? How can you integrate teaching in your practice that is specific to the findings in your community?*

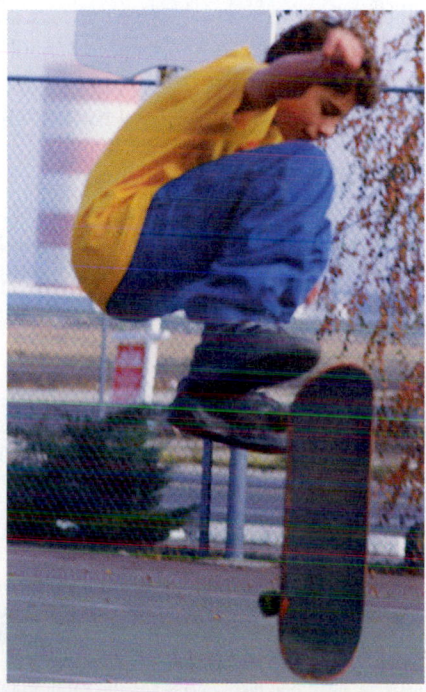

FIGURE 20–7 ■ What protective gear should children use for skateboarding? How would you convince them to use the protection?

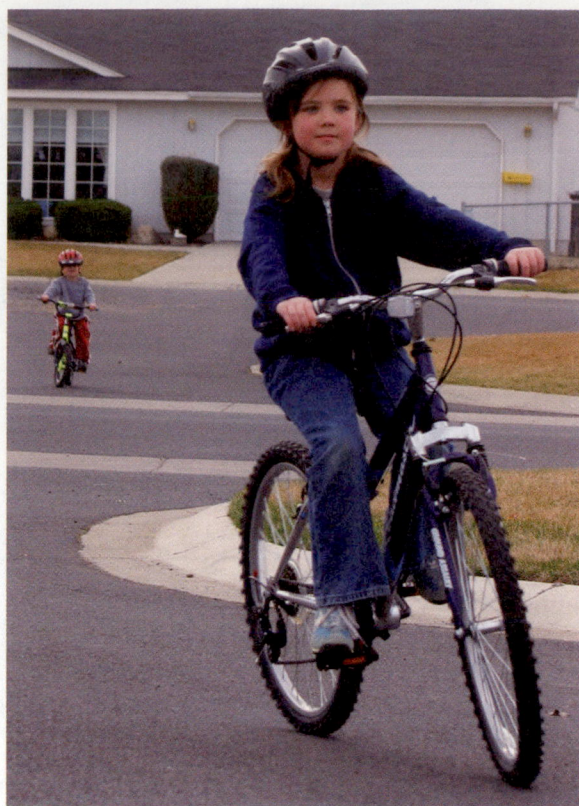

FIGURE 20–8 ■ Having parents insist on helmet use and having friends who also wear bicycle helmets can encourage use by young children.

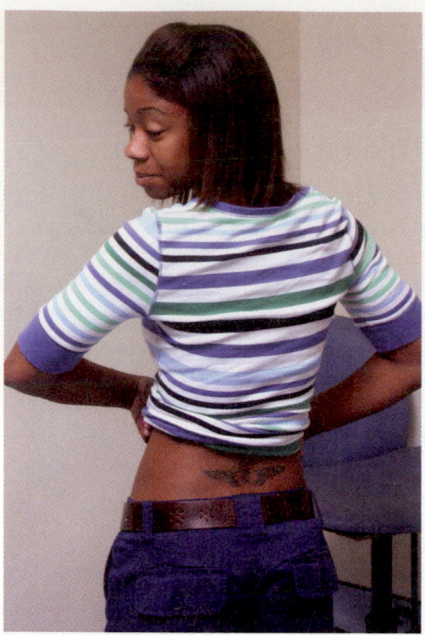

FIGURE 20–9 ■ Youth frequently choose to have tattoos, either in discreet body locations or in visible places such as the arms and neck. Talk openly with adolescents about their health, and teach them to avoid health risks connected with tattoos and piercing.

dark, and using reflective clothing on cloudy days. Strategies to make use of helmets and other protective gear more attractive to children and adolescents are needed (Figure 20–8 ■). Nurses can play a major role in programs to educate and reward children for helmet use, and can assist families to find helmets at a price they can afford. Education should take place in offices and clinics, in school settings, and throughout the community. Nurses can support legislation for helmet use, evaluate proper fits of helmets, and work for incentives and low-cost helmets.

Nurses can be active in identifying behaviors in youth in specific communities and working with schools and other community groups to establish educational programs. Efforts should also include adequate conditioning for sports, proper treatment of injuries, prevention of overuse injuries, and assessment of risky activities.

Practice Alert

A growing number of children engage in "extreme" sports, those that carry a high degree of risk and have not traditionally been common. Some examples are mountain biking, three-wheeling, ski racing, snowboarding through trees and on courses with pikes and other challenges, ice climbing, rock climbing, and wakeboarding. Although the nurse is probably unable to dissuade youth from engaging in these activities, safety measures should be emphasized. Find out what protective gear the youth wears and what is recommended. Keep at hand stories of youth who have been saved by use of such gear. Encourage the youth to engage in sports activities only when responsible adults are present and to have a plan for emergencies, including a working cell phone, leaving information with an adult about plans and expected return, and planning for harsh weather with items such as emergency blankets, gear, and food. Encourage the youth to talk with parents and other adults about the risks and responsibilities of these activities.

Body Art

Humans throughout history have applied body art in the form of painting, tattooing, and piercing. There is a resurgence of interest in this decorative art, especially among teens and young adults (Figure 20–9 ■). Many adolescents have multiple body piercings and tattoos and may even resort to performing these decorations on themselves or friends.

Approximately 25% of adolescents and young adults have tattoos, and even more have at least one body piercing (Armstrong, Roberts, Koch, et al., 2008). In some states, teens must be 18 years of age or have parental permission to obtain body art, but students often report that it is easy to have an adult present who signs and claims to be a parent. Only in some states are tattoo and body piercing businesses required to be licensed and comply with certain regulations. Remember that Amy, who is described in the opening scenario, had her piercing done by a friend. Amy demonstrates some common characteristics of teens who choose to use body art. It may be seen as a way to establish individualism and independence, and helps some teens to feel part of a peer group. Multiple tattoos and piercings are common.

Body art is a common source of infections with skin pathogens, as well as hepatitis B and C (see Chapter 30 ❷ for a discussion of hepatitis). It can be a source of HIV if proper techniques are not followed. Piercings in parts of the body such as the mouth or navel are most prone to bacterial infection and continued redness and irritation. Serious systemic infections such as endocarditis have occurred after some piercings. The pierced site may not appear infected, but transfer of organisms causes serious infection and heart damage. Common infective agents include *Neisseria, Mycobacterium, Streptococcus, Pseudomonas,* and *Staphylococcus* (Bechara, Macheras, Heym, et al., 2010; Kaatz, Elsner, & Bauer, 2008; Kluger, 2010). When noting signs of systemic infection such as fever, weakness, malaise, and arthralgia (see Chapter 26 ❷ for a full discussion of endocarditis), gather history about body piercings and refer for care to the primary healthcare provider. Pierced tongues can lead to chipped teeth or even be

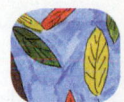

Partnering with Families

Care for Tattoos and Body Piercings

BEFORE THE PROCEDURE

- Visit several studios to make comparisons of technique, quality, and cleanliness.
- Ask to watch a tattoo or piercing done on someone else.
- What are the sterilization and hygiene practices of the artist?
- Is the artist licensed? Trained?
- Look at pictures of completed art and talk with former clients.
- Insist that new, sterile equipment be opened in front of the person to be decorated.
- Consider if this permanent body decoration is desired for a lifetime.
- Consider what the tattoo or piercing will look like in several years.
- Consider the possible side effects such as infection, future dislike for the art, and allergy to dyes or metals.
- Be sure that hepatitis B vaccination is completed before the procedure.
- Be aware that no immunization is available to protect against the health risks of hepatitis C and HIV.

CARE AFTER THE PROCEDURE

- Touch the area only after careful hand washing.
- Keep the area elevated and use ice for the first 2 days to minimize swelling.
- Avoid contact with other persons' body fluids until well healed.
- Turn the piercing jewelry gently several times daily using washed hands.
- Use antibacterial mouthwash, cleaner, or ointment as recommended.
- Avoid pressure and rubbing on the site (such as belts on navel piercings).
- Watch carefully for signs of infection and report them to a healthcare provider:
  - Increased redness
  - Swelling
  - Pain
  - Hot feeling
  - Discharge
- Ask the artist how long healing of a piercing will take. It varies from 2 months in the mouth to 6 to 8 months in the navel.
- Metal is dangerous during some medical procedures such as MRI or during surgery. Be sure to tell doctors and nurses about the piercings when hospitalized or receiving medical care, especially if they are not readily visible.
- If you decide to remove a piece of jewelry soon after placement, then the skin may heal with only a slight scar.

the cause of choking if the jewelry is dislodged from the site. Allergy to dyes, granuloma, and other local skin reactions can also occur (Kaatz et al., 2008).

Another issue that the teen should consider prior to tattooing is the relationship of the tattoo to future lifestyle and identity changes. Advise teens to avoid tattooing the name of a person or musical group since relationships change and tastes in music evolve. Be sure they know the meaning of phrases, foreign words, or symbols. Consider the visibility of the tattoo and its effect on future employment. Tattoos on the face, neck, or other readily visible places may be a detriment during employment interviews. Tattoos should always be considered permanent, since methods for removal may be costly, painful, and unsuccessful. However, requests for tattoo removal are increasing (Armstrong et al., 2008).

Another form of body art that is regarded as disfigurement is **branding** or scarification. Some indigenous cultures use scarification as a form of body art, but the processes have become more prevalent among contemporary youth (Kaatz et al., 2008; Oultram, 2009). In this process, the skin is burned to result in a scar. Usually a desired sign, symbol, or word is inscribed. Results are usually not precise and do not adhere to expected designs. This procedure is done on the self or a friend, using common household metal implements heated in fires or stoves. Others cut themselves in the form of a desired design, a process called **cutting.** This type of self-harm or self-injury is performed with razor blades, knives, scissors, broken glass, needles, or sharp pencils. These practices can result in infection, often do not yield the desired result, and may indicate underlying problems, such as a history of abuse. Healthcare providers should identify cutting or scarring in patterns during examinations, and should be aware that always wearing long sleeves or pants, or seeking to cover body parts during an examination may indicate cutting. Some youth engage in self-injury by cutting that is not intended as art. These youth should

be referred for further assessment and mental health therapy by primary care providers or psychiatric specialists (see Chapter 34 🔗).

Since teens may choose to obtain body art even if parents object and there are state laws to prohibit or make it difficult, nursing care must focus on providing information to the teen, assessing sites, identifying infections, and referring if needed. See Partnering with Families: Care for Tattoos and Body Piercings. Care is almost always provided in community settings such as clinics or schools. Ask teens if they are considering body art, because they often do not seek advice before obtaining the art and may therefore not get adequate teaching. Not all piercings are visible; ask about piercings before all medical procedures since they may need to be removed for surgery, magnetic resonance imaging (MRI), and other tests.

Sexual Orientation

Adolescence is a time of identifying emerging sexuality. Most teens establish relationships with members of the opposite sex and learn how to interact in ways that are guided by their peer group, family, and culture. For some youth, the transition into adult sexuality is more challenging, as they feel emotional and sexual attraction to people of the same sex (**homosexuality**). The term *gay* is often used for homosexual males and *lesbian* for homosexual females. Some youth are *bisexual*, or attracted to both men and women, and some are *transgendered,* an imprecise term for individuals who cross gender lines. The initials **LGBT** are sometimes used to refer to these minority sexuality choices, while the initials **LGBQ** are sometimes used for lesbian, gay, bisexual, or questioning. From 5% to 12% of persons have had a sexual experience with someone of the same sex, and about 3% identify as being LGBT/Q (Chandra, Mosher, Copen, et al., 2011).

Sexual attractions and practices different from the mainstream are not deviant, but may be viewed as part of a continuum of sexual expression. No gene, early life experience, or other event causes homosexuality.

Baccalaureate Essential VIII
Professionalism and Professional Values

Nurses have a long history of altruism, or concern for the welfare of others, belief in autonomy or the right of patients to make their own decisions, and commitment to human dignity or respect for the worth of each individual. Social justice, or fair treatment for all regardless of individual characteristics such as sexual orientation, is a hallmark of nursing care. Nurses therefore bear a responsibility for meeting the needs of youth who are LGBT/Q in a caring and compassionate manner. Integration of knowledge of adolescent development and the special mental health challenges of some LGBT/Q youth are important components of nursing care (Poster & Weber, 2010; Weber, 2009).

Research has demonstrated that the attitudes of nursing and medical students toward LGBT/Q persons often relate to their own background and exposure to individuals who are part of the sexual minority (Chapman, Watkins, Zappia, et al., 2012). Healthcare professionals should examine their own experiences and biases. They should be aware of exclusionary practices in health care that can make LGBT/Q youth uncomfortable or unwelcome (Institute of Medicine, 2011). Then assessment and interventions can successfully be provided so that all youth, regardless of sexual orientation, feel welcome and well cared for in health facilities. Nurses' professional values guide their lifelong learning to ensure value-based behaviors with all patients.

LGBT/Q youth are at risk for a variety of problems related to emotional and physical health. These include rejection by family members and peers, verbal harassment, sexual abuse and physical assault, a high rate of suicide, substance abuse, a high rate of homelessness, and sexual risks of HIV and other sexually transmitted infections. Their health risks need to be identified and appropriate care provided. However, the practice, knowledge, and attitudes of care providers may be barriers to identification of sexual orientation in health practice (see the Baccalaureate Essentials box). Such nondisclosure creates the potential of unmet healthcare needs related to screening, education, counseling, and assessment for health risks (Kitts, 2010).

Nurses can provide health care for LGBT youth in a variety of settings. School nurses and clinics can display a sign that demonstrates they are accepting of persons with minority sexual preferences. These signs include rainbows and triangles, and can be obtained from local gay and lesbian community groups, and other groups such as PFLAG (Parents, Families, and Friends of Lesbians and Gays). Terminology in assessment should be gender-free. Ask the youth, "Do you have one or more sexual partners?" rather than "Do you have a boyfriend?" When youth identify as LGBT, usual care of all kinds should be provided, including preventive care such as immunizations, sports assessments, and injury prevention teaching. Be alert that the youth may have additional health challenges. Ask about peer and parental support; refer to support groups if needed. Significant stress is associated with "coming out," or disclosing sexual preference to family or friends, and sometimes rejection by loved ones occurs. The nurse is often able to provide support both to the youth and to parents during this time. Offer to meet with family or friends if that will assist the teen. Many resources are available to help schools provide safe settings for LGBT/Q youth; nurses can be effective in obtaining such resources for school personnel. Provide resources when the teen is homeless, depressed, or suicidal (see Chapter 34 🔗). Perform testing for sexually transmitted infections if sexual contact is occurring, and teach preventive measures. Foster a positive sense of self-esteem through encouraging activities such as sports, music, and friendships with peers.

EFFECTS OF VIOLENCE

Violence is a threatened or actual use of physical force that leads to potential or actual physical or emotional trauma. In the past several years, adults and children alike have been shocked by violent episodes in schools. Although these incidents have had much media coverage, they are just one type of violence to which children may be exposed. Children can be the recipients of violence during child abuse, bullying, and homicides, and they can perform acts of violence on others. They may be touched by violence when parents, siblings, or other family members are killed in gang conflicts, in terrorist attacks, or in wars. The effects of violence are far reaching and ongoing; they permeate the child's entire lifetime. This section explores certain types of violence affecting children.

Schools and Communities

At a time when firearm deaths are decreasing overall, unintentional deaths and suicides have increased among children. Many of these deaths are committed with firearms found in the home. Over 4,000 youth from 10 to 19 years die from firearm homicides annually, and another approximately 1,500 die from firearm suicide. Firearm homicide is the second leading cause of injury death for youth, and firearm suicide is the fifth leading cause of injury death for youth (CDC, 2011b). Approximately 40% of households with children have guns, and in 25% of those homes the firearms are stored loaded or are not secured under lock. Additionally, parents often report that children do not know firearm locations when the children are actually able to state the locations and have handled the guns (Children's Defense Fund, 2010).

Homicide among children has gained attention in past years due to several shootings at schools and universities. Although homicide is an extreme example, other types of violence exist. Children report being threatened verbally and with guns or knives at home, in schools, and in neighborhoods. They may be beaten up, bullied, or harassed. An estimated 3 to 10 million children are exposed to acts of domestic violence by adults in their homes (U.S. Department of Health and Human Services, 2009b). They may be subjected to dangerous situations in their neighborhoods or during times of homelessness. Date rape or other sexual violence is reported by 9.8% of teens, while 7.4% have been forced to have sexual intercourse (CDC, 2010a).

Practice Alert

When several children are attacked or killed in a school shooting, this tragic occurrence gains media attention. Little do we realize that this tragedy is part of daily life, in separate settings all over the country. A firearm kills about 8 children every day in the United States, or about 56 children per week. An additional 200 to 300 children suffer from nonfatal firearm injuries (Children's Defense Fund, 2010). Nurses must intervene in this national tragedy. Become familiar with firearm injury statistics in your community. Teach families, children, and youth about the dangers of firearms. Urge safe storage. Help schools establish programs to ensure safety for students.

Family risk factors have been identified as more commonly seen in situations when violence has been committed against children (Box 20–5). In addition, children who commit violence more commonly have ready access to firearms, are exposed to violence in the home or community, engage in violent media viewing, and have poor self-esteem or depression.

Realizing the impact of violence on and by children, several federal healthcare initiatives have begun to assist in decreasing violence.

BOX 20–5	**Risk Factors Common in Families with Child Victims of Violence**

- History of mental illness, domestic violence, incarceration, or substance abuse in the home
- Family stresses
- Inadequate childcare or supervision
- Inadequate family social support
- Use of corporal punishment and other inappropriate discipline methods for the child
- Child abuse
- Access to firearms
- Gang membership in family or neighborhood
- High exposure to media violence
- Child hyperactivity and other developmental behavioral disorders

Some programs have been helpful, and incidents of homicides and most other violence have begun to decrease. Programs that are most successful include individual children, parents, schools, and communities. Health and school professionals are instrumental in identifying signs of violence. Provide resources for families and children to decrease violence. Particular types of violence and specific strategies are discussed in the following sections.

War and Terrorism

Internationally, 40 million children experience violence each year, and decreasing violence against children has become a focus of both the World Health Organization and the United Nations (World Health Organization, 2011). Common forms of violence worldwide are war and terrorism. War affects children in several ways: Parents leave home to fight in wars, children may be forced to take on adult roles in families when parents leave, children become orphans when parents are killed, and some children are trained and forced to fight in battles, carry messages, or otherwise engage in combat themselves (UNICEF, 2009). Children who live through wars or have a parent or sibling die in war can be permanently affected by these events. Depression and other mental health problems are common in youth who have experienced war.

Another type of violence is terrorism. The events in the United States of September 11, 2001, and other examples in many countries take a large toll on the mental health of children and adolescents. The response of children to terrorism is not well studied. However, **disasters** such as the World Trade Center attack can lead to sleep and eating problems, fears of entering tall buildings, regression in school performance and other behaviors, and posttraumatic stress disorder (see Chapter 34 for a description of posttraumatic stress and see the discussion in Chapter 14 about disasters). Most children and adolescents who live through terrorism experience profound sadness, cling to adults who provide security, and have a variety of somatic complaints.

Understanding the response of children and adolescents to war and terrorist events can assist healthcare providers in providing interventions to assist children and families. Some key factors include the following:

- Repeated events or more intense experiences, such as being personally involved in a shooting episode, create the greatest

psychologic trauma. Consider that constant exposure by repeated viewing of war and terrorism in the media magnifies the trauma for viewers.
- Children individualize experiences related to their developmental levels. Younger children are very affected by physical separation from parents, whereas older children may worry more about repeat events and their future.
- Some children are resilient in the face of stress, others are affected but recover, and a third group becomes chronically affected. More research will assist understanding of the long-term effects of trauma on various age groups.
- In addition to development, children's prior experiences with stress may contribute to their response to traumatic situations.
- Interventions to assist children can focus on them, their parents, and others in the community, such as teachers. Interventions should be directed at different phases of violence, such as pre-event preparation (emergency preparation and training) and post-event activity (offering special services and resources).

LeBrocque, Hendrikz, & Kenardy, 2010

Several resources have been developed to help families and health professionals help children deal with war and violence. See the resources on the websites of the National Center for Children Exposed to Violence, Society of Pediatric Nurses, and American Academy of Child and Adolescent Psychiatry.

Bullying

One type of violence that frequently occurs in schools is **bullying,** aggressive behavior that is intended to cause harm, exists in a relationship with imbalance of power, and occurs repeatedly. Bullies are aggressive and impulsive, and need to dominate others. Bullying behaviors include verbal abuse (taunting, teasing), name-calling, threats, spreading rumors, social exclusion, and physical abuse (hitting, shoving, kicking, tripping). About 20% of children suffer bullying at school each year, and about 5% did not go to school at least one day in the previous month because of safety concerns due to bullying (CDC, 2010a). Although bullying is most commonly reported in schools, it can occur in neighborhoods as children go to and from school, on school buses, on sports teams, and in other settings.

Bullying can also occur using the Internet and is reported by 20% of young people (Cyberbullying Research Center, 2011). **Cyberbullying** occurs when a child or adolescent is targeted by another via Internet posting or other digital technology, and threatened, tormented, harassed, humiliated, or embarrassed. Personal information may be disclosed or fabricated, persons are excluded, offensive messages are sent, or harmful messages are sent out under the target person's name. Such attacks are socially aggressive and often anonymous.

Bullies are more likely to smoke, drink alcohol, and perform poorly in school; one in four bullies has a criminal record by age 30 (Health Resources and Services Administration, 2009). Bullies are more likely to bring weapons to school, putting other children at risk. Bullying behavior is linked to future delinquent behavior, depression, low self-esteem, loneliness, suicidal ideation, and suicide attempts (Klomek, Marrocco, Kleinman, et al., 2008).

Children who are bullied are more commonly socially isolated and anxious. Health problems such as migraines, stomach pains, suicidal thoughts, and other problems can result. Academic performance commonly deteriorates, and rates of school absenteeism increase. Realizing the serious effects of such behaviors, a number of states have passed legislation that reiterates the rights of all children to attend school in a safe and peaceful manner. Some state education departments mandate school district programs for students about bullying and clear school policies about dealing with the behavior. School antibullying policies are instrumental in decreasing the behaviors (American Academy of Pediatrics, 2011).

A campaign has been developed by the Health Resources and Services Administration Maternal and Child Health Bureau, targeting youth from 9 to 13 years old, to prevent bullying. Access the companion website for information about dealing with this issue in schools in your state.

Incarceration

A growing number of children are entering the judicial system, and many are admitted at young ages. Juveniles are responsible for about 12% of arrests for violent crimes, and their lifestyles and environments place them at a four times greater risk of death than the average teen (Feldman, 2008). Girls represent an increasing number of children in juvenile justice. Children in detention, courts, and other facilities have frequently been victims as well as perpetrators of violence. They often have multiple risks such as substance abuse, early sexual activity, multiple sexual partners, sexual abuse, lack of a healthcare home, and mental health issues such as posttraumatic stress disorder (Feldman, 2008). Nurses may work within the juvenile justice system to provide episodic care for children or to partner with others to establish health-related programs within facilities. Youth who are incarcerated need the following:

- Basic physical care such as immunizations, and vision and hearing screening
- Nutrition assessment and teaching
- Skin assessment and hygiene practice teaching
- Information about sexuality, sexual practices, abstinence, and sexually transmitted infections
- Assessment for substance abuse
- Teaching about hazards of substance use and assistance with quitting
- Mental health services
- Developmental assessment
- Individualized education plans to meet cognitive needs

Abandoned Babies

There are no accurate statistics on numbers of babies that are abandoned in dumpsters, on doorsteps, and in other locations. This tragedy has been addressed by "safe haven" laws in some states that allow women to leave unwanted babies at certain locations such as hospitals and fire stations without legal recrimination. Despite these laws, babies continue to be abandoned, perhaps because mothers do not know about the laws or because they do not believe they will not be found guilty. Young teen mothers may not want others to know they had a baby. In addition, placement of these babies in adoptive homes can be difficult due to paternity suits. Nurses should know their state's safe haven law details. Inform adolescents and young women about the law and post information in community sites frequented by women. Partner with young pregnant women to link them to resources such as adoption agencies when they might not want to keep a baby.

Hazing

Hazing is an activity that is forced upon an individual, causes humiliation, and is required for membership in an organization or group. It is potentially harmful. It is estimated that about 20 to 40 students die annually of events linked to hazing, and even middle and high school athletes engage in hazing activities (Srabstein, 2008). Activities might include removing clothes, drinking large amounts of alcohol, using snuff or other substances, being locked in small places, being beaten, and many other behaviors. In spite of its common practice, many coaches or teachers are unaware of it, and many students do not know what to do about hazing practices. Ask during health visits if the student has ever had to do something to belong to the group or team. Ask about "scary" things others have had them do. Assist schools and colleges in setting up antihazing policies. Encourage students to report hazing. Be aware of the possibility of hazing when seeing children with traumatic injuries.

Domestic Violence

Domestic violence or intimate partner abuse is that which occurs between adult partners in a family. It may involve the parents of a child, or one parent and the significant other. This type of abuse injures the child or adolescent either by witnessing a loved one being abused, or by being the victim. About 3.3 million children annually in the United States are exposed to violence against their mothers or other female care providers. Children who live in homes where intimate partner abuse occurs are significantly more likely to be abused themselves, so the behavior is often a precursor to child abuse. See the additional detailed discussion of child abuse later in this chapter and intimate partner abuse discussions in Chapters 8 through 13 🔗.

Dating Violence

Dating violence is another type of intimate partner abuse that occurs in relationships among youth. Over 9% of adolescent males and females report being victims of dating violence. African American girls more commonly report dating violence than Hispanic or White girls (CDC, 2010a). Girls who report dating violence are also more likely to report other risk behaviors, such as feeling sad, having attempted suicide, or having used substances such as tobacco and drugs. Early sexual activity, having a higher number of sex partners, and being less likely to use birth control are also associated with higher incidence of dating violence. A cluster risk profile may therefore put adolescents more at risk for dating violence.

Date rape is a term used when dating violence takes the form of rape. This can be particularly harmful to females who often do not want to share the event or press charges against the attacker.

Nursing Management

The focus of nursing management is to prevent violence, identify warning signs of violence, intervene with children to decrease effects of violence, and partner with families and other professionals to provide programs and enact legislation that will decrease violence.

Nursing Assessment and Diagnosis

Nurses are in key positions to prevent violence by identifying children who are at risk of being victims of violence. The ecologic framework can be used to assess children. Some questions that can be asked are listed in Table 20–5. It is important to detect both the risks

TABLE 20–5	Assessment Questions to Identify Violence Risk and Protective Factors	
MICROSYSTEM	**MESOSYSTEM**	**EXOSYSTEM**
Have you been hurt by your parents or anyone else at home?	Do your parents attend school meetings? Talk with your teachers?	What stresses do your parents have at work, in your family, or with their health or finances?
When was the last time you were teased or bullied at school? What did you do?	Do you participate in any church, synagogue, or mosque services?	Do you feel like your school helps to keep you safe? Are there plans for handling violent episodes at your school if they were to occur?
Have you ever brought a gun, knife, or other weapon to school?	Do you participate in any community activities? (Examples include clubs, 4H, scouts, volunteering at sporting events, helping at soup kitchens.)	Do you feel safe in your neighborhood?
Do you have access to guns and knives at home? At friends' houses?		Where would you go or who would you call if you felt unsafe or were hurt and no one was at home?
What stresses are there in your family now?		
Tell me about school—what do you like and dislike?		

that lead to vulnerability and the protective factors that can promote resilience and safety. Questions should be adapted to each age group and inserted in every healthcare encounter.

Nurses should screen for violence at each health promotion visit, including gynecologic visits and prenatal care. Ask what is going well and not going well in intimate relationships, and whether the person ever feels unsafe or is forced to do things he or she does not wish to do. Recognize that, although not as common, males may be victims of violence in close relationships. Because alcohol and other drugs are often connected with violence in relationships, ask about their use. Organize peer discussion groups about intimacy in order to help youth develop a sense of self-confidence and self-efficacy that will empower them to refuse activities in relationships in which they do not wish to engage.

Nursing care for violence is discussed in the Nursing Care Plan on the following pages. The following additional nursing diagnoses may be appropriate:

- Violence: Self-Directed Risk for related to history of violence
- Self-Esteem, Chronic Low related to history of abuse
- Family Processes, Interrupted related to situational crises
- Growth and Development, Delayed related to environmental trauma

NANDA-I © 2012

Planning and Implementation

Nurses intervene with individual children and with families in schools, jails, detention centers, and other community settings to increase safety and decrease violence. Children and families are assisted in meeting basic needs and accessing resources to assist with finances, respite care, domestic violence, and other issues. Education is a key element of intervention.

Providing Information

The nurse can teach family members about the dangers of firearms and the necessity for use of gun locks, locked cabinets, storing guns unloaded, and storing guns and ammunition in separate places. Suggest alternative activities to minimize child exposure to violence in the media. Inform parents about rating systems for television and other media and about lockout mechanisms for televisions and computers. Harmful effects of verbal and physical abuse to the child or other family members should be discussed and alternatives explored. See Partnering with Families: Rating Systems for Media on page 554.

Present the school-age child and adolescent with information about bullying and strategies for dealing with the problem. Discuss

school and community resources where the child can go if there are threats of any kind. Date rape and violence are topics for discussion for all teens, as is the importance of reporting the situations when they occur.

Care in the Community

Violence Prevention

Both in schools and in community settings, nurses can plan peer mentoring to provide assistance to children at high risk of experiencing violence. School and community programs for children can be linked and coordinated by nurses to provide for parent involvement and child support. Discuss safety issues, both risks and protective actions, in schools and community groups. Report children who are at risk. Work to establish extended programs for children so they are safe after school. Help children learn behaviors that will help them to be safe in their communities and at home. Teach positive problem solving and conflict management techniques to children and parents.

Special Needs

Youth with special needs are a concern of nurses. Jails and detention centers often have a nurse who visits youth on a regular basis or when health problems occur. Health teaching may be provided in some facilities. Halfway houses and homeless shelters are examples of settings where violence prevention and intervention can occur with youth. Mental health centers and other programs have nurses who work with either child victims of violence (for example, children who have witnessed domestic violence, have witnessed or had a family member murdered, or have been abused at home or school) or perpetrators of violence. See Chapter 34 for a discussion of posttraumatic stress disorder and its effects on the child and adolescent.

War and Terrorism

Partner with families to assist them in dealing with children about war and terrorism. Recognize that youth who have experienced such events are more at risk for mental health disruptions with future events. Answer questions from children honestly, but reassure them that many people are trying to make the situation safe. Other suggestions for parents include:

- Limit television viewing and other media exposure due to constant replaying of the events of terrorism or war. Preschoolers may think the events continue to happen, rather than being a one-time occurrence. Watch television with the child and talk with him or her about what is happening.

Nursing Care Plan   The Child and Violent Behavior

INTERVENTION	RATIONALE	EXPECTED OUTCOME
1. Nursing Diagnosis: Violence: Other-Directed, Risk for related to history of family violence		
NIC Priority Intervention—*Environmental Management: Violence Prevention:* Monitoring and manipulation of the environment to decrease the potential for violent behavior directed toward self, others, or the environment		**NOC Suggested Outcome**—*Impulse Control:* Ability to restrain compulsive or impulsive behavior in child and others
GOAL: *The child demonstrates impulse control.*		
■ Identify violent behaviors in the child.	■ Violence in the child usually develops over time.	■ The child expresses the ability to manage problems in acceptable ways.
■ Provide a safe place for exploration of feelings by referral to school or other counseling, support groups, and other resources.	■ The child needs an opportunity to explore feelings and vulnerability.	
■ Provide strategies for managing anger and alternative ways for coping with problems.	■ Coping strategies can be learned from others and can help in dealing with a stressful home or community.	
■ Refer to and support interventions of mental health specialists.	■ Mental health specialists often manage impulse control and other violence-related behaviors with supportive follow-through by all members of the healthcare team.	
GOAL: *The child is secure in a safe environment.*		
■ Perform thorough assessment of hazards to physical and emotional state in the child's home, neighborhood, and school.	■ Hazards to physical and emotional health promote violence to and from the child.	The child expresses a sense of physical and emotional safety in daily life.
■ Institute actions that will result in removal of the child from unsafe situations.	■ Removal from family, community, or school may be needed to ensure child safety.	
■ Use community resources to provide respite care, teaching for families, and safety instruction for the child.	■ Stress reduction measures may help to decrease violent behaviors.	
2. Nursing Diagnosis: Home Maintenance, Impaired related to insufficient family organization		
NIC Priority Intervention—*Home Maintenance Assistance:* Helping the family to maintain the home as a safe place to live		**NOC Suggested Outcome**—*Role Performance:* Congruence of an individual's role behavior with role expectations
GOAL: *Family members are able to meet role expectations.*		
■ Provide information on the child's developmental needs.	■ Parents need to understand the developmental progression of their children.	Family members meet role expectations, contributing to making the home a safe and secure place for the child.
■ Provide ongoing assessment in the home via home healthcare visits.	■ Assessment is used to identify both risk and protective factors in the home so that strengths can be used in intervention and risks can be mitigated.	
■ Assist the family in identifying hazards in the environment that can impair the child's growth and development.	■ Early identification of hazards can lead to proper interventions to protect the child from harm.	
■ Evaluate the ability of adults to provide a safe, secure, nurturing environment.	■ The family may need respite care, information about the child's needs, financial assistance, or other resources to meet the needs of the child.	
3. Nursing Diagnosis: Hopelessness related to long-term family stress		
NIC Priority Intervention—*Hope Instillation:* Facilitation of the development of a positive outlook in the given situation		**NOC Suggested Outcome**—*Hope:* Presence of internal state of optimism that is personally satisfying and life supporting
GOAL: *The child will have adequate food and sleep, and express satisfaction with life.*		
■ Monitor the child's nutritional state and growth and daily patterns.	■ The child's nutrition, sleep, and other patterns provide clues to the family's ability to perceive hope and provide care for the child.	The child demonstrates normal growth patterns and meets expected developmental outcomes.

Nursing Care Plan | The Child and Violent Behavior, *continued*

INTERVENTION	RATIONALE	EXPECTED OUTCOME
■ Monitor the child's developmental status. ■ Determine adequacy of relationships and support systems.	■ The child needs close personal relationships in order to grow and learn.	

GOAL: *The family will identify resources to achieve life goals.*

INTERVENTION	RATIONALE	EXPECTED OUTCOME
■ Monitor the family's decision-making ability and facilitate goal setting. ■ Provide information on community resources. ■ Refer for psychiatric/mental health and other services if needed.	■ Feeling overwhelmed by daily life events leads to an inability to set goals and make decisions to meet the goals. ■ Resources can assist the family members in setting and achieving realistic goals.	The family establishes realistic goals for growth and development of its members, and takes steps to meet the goals.

4. Nursing Diagnosis: Injury, Risk for related to physical or psychological conditions in the environment

INTERVENTION	RATIONALE	EXPECTED OUTCOME
NIC Priority Intervention—*Safety Behavior:* Family actions to minimize risk of physical or emotional trauma		**NOC Suggested Outcome**—*Parenting: Social Safety:* Parental actions to avoid social relationships that might cause harm or injury; *Risk Control:* Actions to eliminate or reduce actual, personal, and modifiable health risks

GOAL: *Risk for physical and emotional injury to the child is decreased.*

INTERVENTION	RATIONALE	EXPECTED OUTCOME
■ Identify physical and psychologic factors that affect the child's safety. ■ Assist the family to deal with issues such as mental status challenges, fatigue, financial concern, substance abuse, lack of adequate childcare resources, and other factors. ■ Instruct the family on methods of keeping the child safe.	■ Multiple factors in the family can contribute to risk of violence and lack of safety for the child. ■ Families need information about the impact of unsafe settings on the child and methods that can decrease risk of injury.	The child is not injured in physical or emotional ways in the home or other immediate settings.

5. Nursing Diagnosis: Post-Trauma Syndrome related to physical or psychosocial abuse

INTERVENTION	RATIONALE	EXPECTED OUTCOME
NIC Priority Intervention—*Counseling:* Use of an interactive helping process focusing on the needs, problems, and feelings of the child who is a victim of abuse or other violence		**NOC Suggested Outcome**—*Abuse/Violence Recovery:* Healing of psychological and physical wounds of abuse or violence

GOAL: *The child demonstrates recovery from the effects of abuse or violence.*

INTERVENTION	RATIONALE	EXPECTED OUTCOME
■ Refer to a mental health specialist. ■ Assess the child's affect and behaviors. ■ Evaluate social interactions and sense of trust in others. ■ Assist the child in identifying feelings and coping strategies by providing counseling, art therapy, and other strategies.	■ Mental health specialists often manage the care for children with posttrauma syndrome. ■ Disturbed child behaviors can demonstrate a sense of mistrust and insecurity. ■ Evidence of close interactions with others demonstrates reestablishment of a sense of trust. ■ A child who has experienced abuse or other violence needs a therapeutic relationship with a counselor to deal with the trauma and begin to rebuild trust and respect, and to learn coping mechanisms.	The child identifies feelings related to the violent episode(s) and expresses healing of the self.

NANDA-I © 2012

- Continue with structured family events such as meals, recreation, and faith-based activities. Spend time with the child.
- Take cues from the child about how much to discuss. Use words the child or adolescent can understand.
- Partner with the school so teachers know what parents have discussed and parents are aware of how events are discussed at school.
- If youth decide to become active by writing letters or joining campaigns, allow them to participate in this way.

- Be alert for regression in behavior, sleep and eating problems, or other indications of stress. Consider talking with the healthcare provider or a counselor in such situations.
- Expect that even after the child has adjusted, there may be delayed reactions. Anniversaries of events, holidays, and birthdays often bring renewed pain and sadness.
- Realize that adults must care for themselves, obtain stress relief, and talk with others in order to have strength and resources available for children.

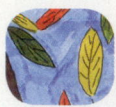

Partnering with Families

Rating Systems for Media

TELEVISION RATING	TELEVISION RATING— MATURE AUDIENCE DETAIL	VIDEO AND COMPUTER	MOVIES	MUSIC
TV-Y: for all TV-Y7: for older children TV-Y7 FV: for older children with fantasy violence content G: general audience TV-PG: parental guidance suggested TV-14: parents strongly cautioned TV-MA: mature audience	FV: fantasy violence L: language V: violence S: sexual situation D: sexual dialogue	EC: for early childhood or those over 3 years E: for everyone over 6 years, mild language E10: for everyone over 10 years, minimal violence T: for teens over 13 years, increased violence and suggestive themes M: for mature viewers over 17 years, intense violence, sexual content, strong language AO: adults only, over 18 years, prolonged violence, sexual scenes, nudity RP: rating pending	G: general PG: parental guidance suggested PG–13: parents strongly cautioned R: restricted to those above 18 years without adult accompaniment NC–17: no one under 18 years admitted, even with adult	Parent Advisory Label: strong language, sex, or substance abuse depicted

Bullying

Nurses can be active in setting up school policies about bullying and integrating assessment and interventions related to bullying into health promotion visits. School programs should:

- Inform all students that bullying is not tolerated.
- Train teachers and other personnel about signs of bullying, such as unexplained injuries, loss of personal belongings, complaints of illness, sleeplessness, and refusal to attend school.
- Assist the school in establishing antibullying protocols, including cyberbullying.
- Ensure adult supervision in hallways, playgrounds, and computer rooms, sites where bullying is most common.
- Teach children to promptly report bullying that is experienced or observed.
- Set up peer support for those who are bullied.
- Arrange therapeutic treatment through school counselors and other resources for those who bully; involve parents in the treatment plan.
- Measure the incidence of bullying, and use data to evaluate the outcomes of policies in schools.

Nurses who are in clinics, offices, and other health promotion settings can also be active in prevention and intervention against bullying:

- Be alert for children with behavior changes (irritability, anxiety, poor self-concept).
- Consider bullying as a potential cause when fear or refusal to attend school is reported by the child or parents.
- Ask questions during visits, such as "Have you ever been afraid to go to school?" or "What are the best and worst things about going to your school?" or "What are the other kids in your neighborhood like?"

- Ask parents what they have done about any situations identified. Partner with the parents to act as a liaison to the school or other agency.
- Refer identified bullies and victims of bullying to mental health specialists.

Exposure to violence takes many forms, and assessment for violence should take place in every healthcare encounter, through both observation and questioning. Activity in the community to decrease violence and to provide information and resources for families is an important nursing role.

Evaluation

Expected outcomes of nursing care for violence prevention include the following:

- A decrease in incidents of homicides, firearm injuries, abuse, date rape, bullying, and other violence is evident among children.
- Programs to decrease violence are established and evaluated.
- Children verbalize what to do if violence occurs and how to solve problems without becoming violent.
- Youth display personal positive judgment of self-worth.
- Youth are able to make positive choices between alternative behaviors.
- The family provides mutual support for each family member.
- Children exhibit healthy adjustment following violent events.

Child Abuse

One of the most common types of violence against children is child abuse. Children from all socioeconomic groups and both males and females are victims of abuse. This type of violence can have implications for both the physical and mental health of children, and can influence

TABLE 20–6 Risk Factors for Child Abuse and Neglect	
FACTORS INCREASING RISK FOR PHYSICAL ABUSE	**FACTORS INCREASING RISK FOR SEXUAL ABUSE**
Poverty	Absence of natural father or having a stepfather
Violence in the family	Being female
Prematurity or low birth weight	Mother's employment outside the home
Unrelated male primary caretaker	Poor relationship with parent
Parents who were abused as children	Parental relationship characterized by conflict
Age less than 3 years	
Child disability or condition that requires a great deal of care (e.g., intellectual disability, attention deficit hyperactivity disorder)	Parental substance abuse or social isolation
Parental substance abuse or social isolation	

their health status long after the abuse has occurred. Physical abuse may come to mind first but is only one part of a larger problem. In addition to physical abuse, the definition of child abuse includes physical neglect, emotional abuse and neglect, verbal abuse, and sexual abuse.

Abuse generally involves an act of commission, that is, actively doing something to a child physically, emotionally, or sexually, such as hitting, belittling, or molesting. Neglect more often involves an act of omission, such as not providing adequate nutrition, emotional contact, or necessary physical care. Because the evidence is often not visible, emotional abuse and neglect are more difficult to identify and prove than physical abuse or neglect. The major types of abuse and neglect are defined below, with a section on medical maltreatment (Munchausen syndrome by proxy) following. Risk factors for abuse and neglect are listed in Table 20–6.

Reported cases of abuse and neglect are likely only a small percentage of the total. There are 3.3 million reports of abuse and neglect annually, with 71% of them due to neglect, 16% from physical abuse, 9% related to sexual abuse, and 7% for emotional abuse (CDC, 2010b). Nearly five children daily (about 1,500 children annually) die from child abuse in the United States (Childhelp, 2011). Infants have the highest rate of abuse (21.7/1,000), with decreasing rates as children get older (12.9/1,000 for 1-year-olds, 11/1,000 for 4- to 7-year-olds, 8.4/1,000 for 12- to 15-year-olds, and 5.5/1,000 for 16- to 17-year-olds) (CDC, 2010b).

Physical Abuse

Physical abuse is the deliberate maltreatment of another individual that inflicts pain or injury and may result in permanent or temporary disfigurement or even death. Common methods of physical abuse in children are listed in Table 20–7.

Physical Neglect

Physical neglect is the deliberate withholding of or failure to provide the necessary and available resources to the child. Behaviors constituting physical neglect include failure to provide for the following basic needs: supervision appropriate for the child's age, adequate nutrition and hydration, hygiene (e.g., clean diapers and clothes, bathing and toileting facilities), shelter (e.g., warmth in winter), and appropriate health care (e.g., immunizations, dental care, medications, eyeglasses). Neglect is the most common type of abuse, especially in infancy when it is responsible for the majority of maltreatment (Brodowski, Nolan, Gaudiosi, et al., 2008).

Emotional Abuse

Emotional abuse usually involves shaming, ridiculing, embarrassing, or insulting the child. It can also include the destruction of a child's personal property, such as tearing up the child's favorite family photographs or letters, or harming, killing, or giving away the child's pet. These actions are frequently used as a means of frightening or controlling the child.

TABLE 20–7 Methods of Physical Abuse in Children	
Hitting, slapping, kicking, or punching	Tying the child to a fence, bed, tree, or other object
Whipping with belts, shoes, or electrical cords **(1)**	Throwing the child against a wall, down stairs, or against a window
Inflicting burns with a lit cigarette or lighter **(2)**	Choking or gagging the child
Immersing child or body part in scalding water (commonly legs, perineal area, hands, or feet: see Figure 36–23 🔗)	Fracturing the legs, arms, ribs, or skull
Shaking the child violently ("shaken child" syndrome)	Deliberately administering excessive doses of prescribed or nonprescribed drugs
	Deliberately withholding prescribed medication

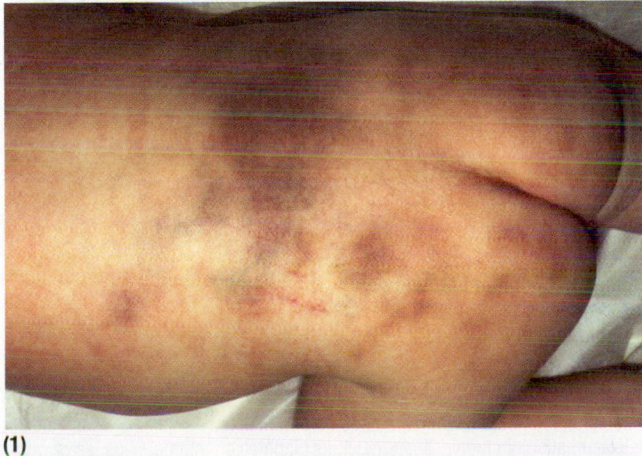

(1)

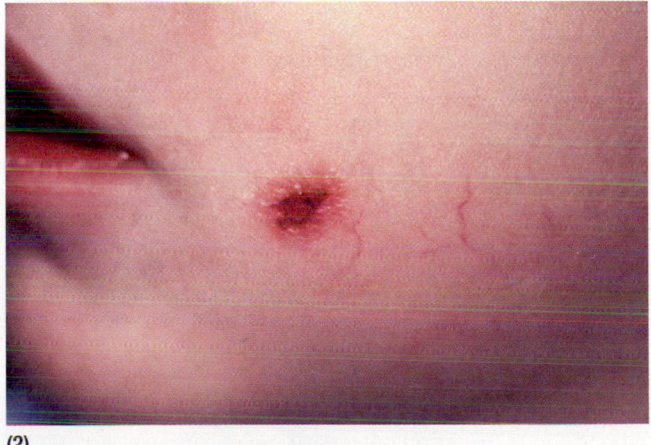

(2)

Source: *(1) BioPhoto Assoc/Photo Researchers; (2) Copyright 2012 NMSB—Custom Medical Stock Photo, All Rights Reserved.*

Verbal abuse is a common method of emotional abuse. Words can be a violent and volatile weapon against a child, eroding the child's fragile sense of self and destroying self-esteem. Common examples of verbal abuse include yelling obscenities at the child, calling the child names, threatening to "put the child away" or to give away or kill the child's pet, telling the child "I wish you were never born" or "You're worthless," and using words to humiliate, shame, or degrade the child.

Emotional Neglect

Emotional neglect is characterized by the caretaker's emotional unavailability to the child. The usual style of interaction is cold and lacking in sensitive personal attention. The child suffers from a lack of nurturance and failure of the parent or caretaker to meet basic dependency needs. Another common example of emotional neglect occurs when the parent is mentally ill, or abusing alcohol or other substances and cannot respond adequately to the child's developmental needs.

Sexual Abuse

Child sexual abuse is the exploitation of a child for the sexual gratification of an adult. About 1.2 per 1,000 children (almost 100,000) in the United States are sexually abused each year. Approximately 10% of schoolchildren report that they have been sexually abused. Many children who are sexually abused are under the age of 5 years, some as young as 3 months. The average age for sexual molestation is 4 years. The perpetrator is sometimes a parent, stepparent, or someone else known to the child such as a friend, neighbor, or baby-sitter. Methods of sexual abuse may be sexual acts, allowing others to commit sexual abuse, threats, exploitation via video or other means, and a variety of other actions (National Center for PTSD, 2011).

The word *child* in sexual abuse and molestation refers to anyone who has not reached the age of consent, even if a teenager. **Incest** is sexual activity between close family members, so that marriage would be legally or culturally prohibited. Abusers often threaten to harm or kill the child or another family member if the child discloses the abuse.

Some abusers are pedophiles, people who have sexual impulses toward preadolescent children. The pedophile is at least 16 years of age and is at least 5 years older than the victim, and the victim is 13 years of age or younger. Another form of sexual abuse is exhibitionism, or obtaining sexual arousal by exposing one's genitals to a stranger. Some children are also victims of prostitution, forced to offer themselves for money or the pleasures of others, either in person or through videos and Internet sources.

Practice Alert

The following are common forms of sexual abuse:

- Oral–genital contact
- Fondling and caressing the genitals
- Anal intercourse
- Vaginal intercourse
- Rape
- Sodomy
- Prostitution
- Forcing viewing of or participation in pornography such as sexually explicit or nude photographs
- Encouraging nude photos or sexual activity via Internet or video

Etiology and pathophysiology Regardless of the type of abuse, the most common abuser is the child's parent or guardian, a male friend

of the child's mother, or another family member or friend. Substance abuse is a major contributor to the problem, with about one half of cases related to parental alcohol or drug abuse (Childhelp, 2011). Risk factors associated with abusive behavior in adults include the following:

- Psychopathology, such as drug addiction or alcoholism, low self-esteem, poor impulse control, and other personality disorders
- Poor parenting experiences, such as abuse in the abuser's own childhood, rejection by the abuser's own parent(s), lack of knowledge of alternative methods of discipline, strong belief in or family tradition of harsh discipline, and lack of parental affection
- Marital stressors and problems with partners, such as hostile-dependent, abusive, or nonsupportive relationships, and one-sided decision making
- Environmental stressors, such as legal, financial, medical, or housing problems
- Social isolation, such as few friends and limited use of sitters, family, or other resources
- Inappropriate expectations for the developmental level of the child

Clinical manifestations Refer to the Clinical Manifestations tables of child abuse and sexual abuse in children and adolescents. Behaviors inconsistent with developmental stage may be apparent. For example, the toddler or preschooler may be indiscriminately friendly with unfamiliar adults, including healthcare providers, rather than demonstrating shyness or anxiety. For the infant or young child with "shaken baby syndrome" or "shaken child syndrome," the symptoms are those of CNS injury from repeated coup and contrecoup injury (see Chapter 33 for further information about shaken baby syndrome 🔗). The high water and gelatinous content of the infant's brain makes it highly vulnerable to injury during shaking. Symptoms include vomiting, irritability, fatigue, poor feeding, bradycardia, apnea, enlarged fontanel, and seizures. Bruises are usually not present,

---

Clinical Manifestations   Child Abuse

- Multiple bruises in various stages of healing
- Scald burns with clear lines of demarcation and in a glove or stocking distribution (see Figure 36–23 🔗)
- Rope, belt, or cord marks, usually seen on the mouth, buttocks, back, legs, and arms (see Figure 1 in Table 20–7)
- Burn scars in various stages of healing, particularly with demarcation suggesting the object used to create the burn
- Multiple fractures in various stages of healing; spiral fractures not explained by accident
- Shortness of breath and distress upon being moved, indicating chest contusions and possible rib fractures
- Cranial injuries
- Abdominal injury
- Change in behavior or school performance
- Fear and avoidance of certain people or situations
- Anger and violent play
- Sedation from overmedication
- Exacerbation of chronic illness (such as diabetes or asthma) because of withholding of medication

Clinical Manifestations Sexual Abuse in Children and Adolescents

- Vaginal discharge
- Blood-stained underpants or diaper
- Genital redness, pain, itching, or bruising
- Difficulty walking or sitting
- Urinary tract infection
- Sexually transmitted infection
- Somatic complaints, such as headaches or stomachaches
- Sleeping problems, such as nightmares or night terrors
- Bed-wetting
- Unwillingness to go to baby-sitter, family member, neighbor, or other person
- Fear of strangers
- New or excessive sexual curiosity or play
- Constant masturbation
- Curling into fetal position
- Phobias about particular places, people, or things
- Abrupt changes in school performance and attendance
- Changes in eating habits
- Abrupt changes in behavior (especially withdrawal)
- Child or adolescent female acts like a wife or mother
- Excessively seductive behavior
- Child or adolescent works as a prostitute

but computed tomography (CT) is often definitive for the diagnosis, with radiographs and MRI used for a thorough diagnostic profile.

Manifestations of physical neglect include undernourishment (evidenced by constantly feeling hungry, hoarding or stealing food, and being underweight), unclean clothes and body, poor dental health (extensive cavities or generally poor condition of teeth), and inappropriate clothing for the season.

Manifestations of emotional abuse, verbal abuse, emotional neglect, and witnessing domestic violence include fear, poor physical growth, and failure to meet appropriate developmental milestones. The child may have difficulty relating to adults, impaired communication skills, and developmental delays. Behavioral manifestations include anxiety, fear, shame, aggression, delinquency, and depression.

Children who have been sexually abused may exhibit a variety of physical and behavioral signs and symptoms. Bruising, bleeding, and laceration of the genital area are obvious signs of trauma (National Center for PTSD, 2011). However, sexual abuse does not always result in apparent injury. Among the many long-term consequences of child sexual abuse are ongoing feelings of shame, guilt, anger, and hostility; decreased self-esteem, which leads to increased self-destructive behavior and risk of suicide; recurrence of victimization experiences; substance abuse; posttraumatic stress disorder (see Chapter 34 ✪); and eating disorders (see Chapter 19 ✪). Children who have been abused are more likely to abuse others in the future. Factors associated with greater psychologic harm to the child include (1) a long period of abuse, (2) use of violent force or threat of violence, (3) abuse involving penetration (intercourse or oral–genital sex), and (4) abuse involving family members, especially the father or stepfather.

Collaborative Care

The diagnosis and management of child abuse is complicated and can involve partnerships among many individuals and groups. Often the child is identified in a healthcare setting with an injury, and physicians, nurses, and others partner to analyze the situation. Sometimes parents suspect abuse by another care provider and seek assistance. At times, suspected abuse is reported to investigating agencies, and social service workers or law enforcement officials investigate. School personnel identify and report suspected abuse. Once verified, treatment may also be complex, involving school counselors, nurses, mental health specialists, physicians, and family members. The child's risk situations and protective situations are identified to build a safety net and manage the mental health issues involved.

Diagnostic Tests

Diagnosis of abuse is made on the basis of a careful history and thorough physical examination. Radiograph, CT, and MRI studies may be ordered to identify signs of recurrent abuse such as healed fractures and other damaged tissues. Laboratory studies may involve urine culture for signs of infection or screening for sexually transmitted infections. Laboratory studies are also used to rule out causes of bleeding such as use of blood studies to test for hemophilia. Genitourinary examination may be performed if sexual abuse is suspected. Some children are admitted directly to the hospital with the diagnosis of suspected abuse or neglect. Less obvious as a victim of abuse is the child admitted with a skull fracture when parents report a simple fall. A mismatch of the degree of injury and the reported incident, or mismatch of the child's developmental level with the injury, indicate a need to report the incident to authorities for further investigation.

Neglect, which is more difficult to define and identify, frequently requires hospitalization with a comprehensive medical, social, and psychiatric evaluation. Five basic categories must be considered when attempting to diagnose neglect: (1) medical care neglect (lack of necessary medical care), (2) gross safety neglect (lack of appropriate supervision), (3) physical neglect (lack of food and shelter), (4) emotional neglect, and (5) educational neglect.

Interviews by mental health specialists may be performed in cases where the child is old enough to communicate verbally or through play techniques. All 50 states have extensive and complex statutes regarding reporting of child abuse and neglect. A specialist must be consulted, especially if the child's testimony will be used in court (see Legal and Ethical Considerations: Child Abuse Laws).

Children do not routinely make false allegations of abuse. If indeed there is reason to believe the allegations are false, a child and adolescent therapist (psychiatrist, psychologist, psychiatric clinical nurse specialist, or social worker) with special expertise should be consulted to determine the truth. Keep in mind that children who

Legal and Ethical Considerations
Child Abuse Laws

Every state has a child abuse law specifying the particular behaviors that define each type of abuse. Any professional who works with children and reasonably suspects that a child has been abused is required to report this suspicion to the local agency for child protective services. Reports made in good faith are not liable to countersuits; however, professionals who suspect abuse and do not report it may be held responsible by the courts. See the U.S. Department of Health and Human Services website for state laws.

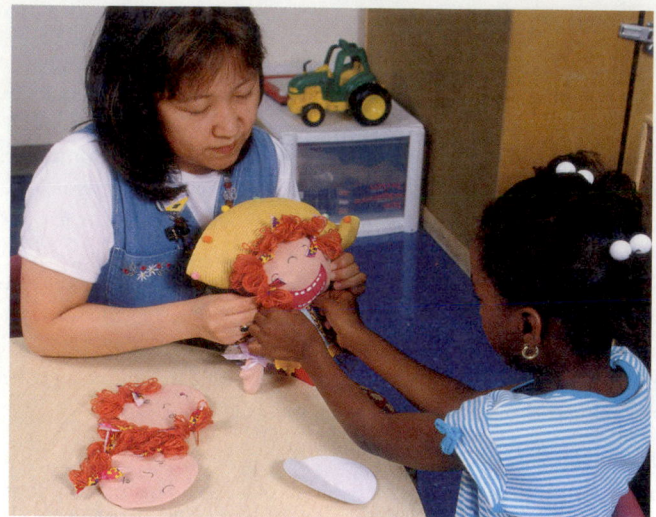

FIGURE 20–10 ■ Therapeutic strategies with young children involve various methods of communication, such as dramatic play and art.

withdraw their accusations have often been threatened or coerced into doing so.

Clinical Therapy

Initial therapy focuses on providing safety. Physical injuries are treated and the child is removed from the abusive situation. Children who have been physically, emotionally, or sexually abused are at risk for major mental health problems, such as depression and posttraumatic stress disorder (see Chapter 34 ⊘). They require skilled care by mental health professionals who are specially trained in this area. Initially the treatment goals include prevention of self-destructive or other dangerous acts. Children must be encouraged to express their fears and feelings in a safe and supportive environment. Equally important is the child's need to build coping skills and self-esteem. The child must be reassured and convinced that he or she is in no way responsible or to blame for what happened.

Individual treatment with art therapy is often used initially because it is the least threatening method in the early stages of treatment, it can easily be tailored to meet the child's individual needs, and it prepares the child for other forms of treatment such as family and group therapy (Figure 20–10 ■). Family or group therapy may be of benefit in exploring the child's concerns and feelings. Anger is common, especially in children who were abused by a trusted adult such as the father or stepfather.

Some children are themselves sexual offenders. An adolescent sexual offender is a minor who commits any sexual act with a person of any age that is against the victim's will, without consent, and/or in an aggressive, exploitive, or threatening manner. Some common characteristics of these youth are prior violence, psychologic/psychiatric problems, history as a victim of abuse, member of a dysfunctional family, and personal characteristics such as loneliness and low self-esteem.

Nursing Management

Nursing Assessment and Diagnosis

Nursing assessment in instances of suspected child abuse or neglect requires a comprehensive history and physical examination, with documentation of findings. Consultation with social service agencies in the community is important if the family is receiving services.

Obtaining the history can be stressful for both the nurse and the parent. Use of therapeutic communication techniques and a quiet, unhurried environment are helpful. Maintaining a nonjudgmental attitude at all times is essential. Obtaining information about abusive and neglectful behaviors requires the nurse to establish a trusting relationship with parents who are often afraid to trust any professional.

Clinical Tip

The nurse should communicate in an open manner. Although this is recommended in all communication interactions, it may be difficult to accomplish in the challenging situation of possible abuse. A clear statement of purpose is needed, for example, "Hello, Mr. S. My name is Joan T. I'm Jonathan's nurse. I will be talking with you and asking you some questions about his overall health."

The health history sequence should include (1) parental concerns, (2) general family history, and (3) specific child history. This sequence begins with nonthreatening topics and allows the nurse to demonstrate concern before asking abuse-related questions. Obtain details about how injuries occurred. The parents' and child's own words should be documented verbatim using quotation marks. Compare reports obtained from each family member for lack of consistency and details that change over time.

It is important to differentiate true child abuse from cultural variations that might inaccurately be assumed to indicate abuse (Figure 20–11A and B ■). For example, traditional treatment practices are sometimes mistaken for signs of physical abuse. The Chinese practice of cupping, which involves heating a bamboo cup and placing it on the skin, is a traditional treatment for headaches or abdominal pain. The Vietnamese practice of cao gio (rubbing out the wind), in which a coin or the fingers are forcefully rubbed on the chest, back, or neck, is used to treat minor ailments. Ask about marks on the skin, how they occurred, and what health practices the family uses.

It is desirable to interview the parent and child both separately and together. Parent–child interaction during an intensive history-taking session provides an opportunity to observe the child's behavior and the parent's method of handling and responding to the child. Interviews may occur in school. The nurse should provide a confidential setting and use a nonjudgmental manner.

Data gathered during history taking are particularly important in light of physical findings. Are there discrepancies between the history and physical assessment data? Do the parents give a history of an uncontrollable, inattentive toddler when the nurse observes a child who is attentive throughout a 15-minute examination? Assess the child's general appearance, including dress and behavior, during the assessment. How do the child's affect, behavior, and development compare with those of other children the same age? Assess the child's interaction and behavior with the parent as well as the parent's behavior and interaction with the child. Be alert for the signs of shaken child syndrome; this may appear as a subtle neurologic condition, or a sudden nonresponsive state. Measure head circumference in children under 3 years, and perform a neurologic examination (see Chapter 7 ⊘).

Be alert for signs of domestic violence. For example, if a mother who brings in a child for care displays signs of abuse, say to the mother, "I see you have a black eye. Can you tell me what happened?" or "You say you are afraid that your boyfriend may hurt Shandra. Has he been hurting you? Do you want to talk about that?" Additionally, use open-ended approaches so that teens who have experienced dating violence know that they can discuss this.

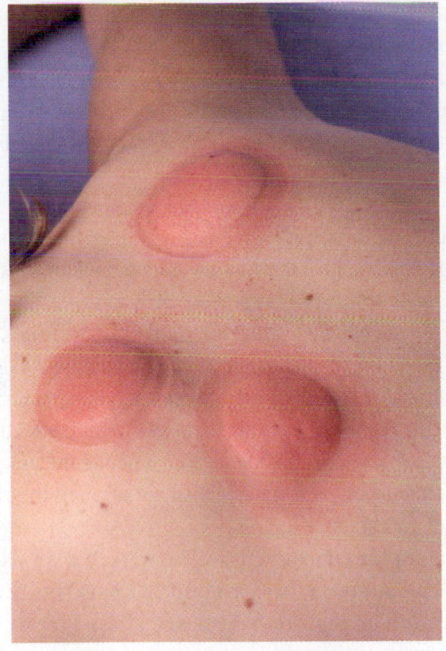

A

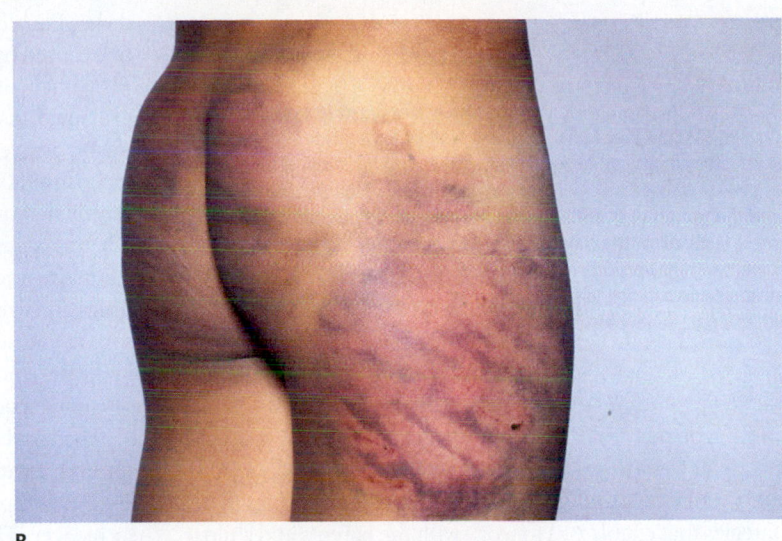

B

FIGURE 20–11 ■ It is important to differentiate cultural practices, such as *A*, cupping, and *B*, coining, from signs of child abuse. Traditional treatment practices are sometimes mistaken for signs of physical abuse. The Chinese practice of cupping, which involves heating a bamboo cup and placing it on the skin, is a traditional treatment for headaches or abdominal pain. The Vietnamese practice of cao gio (rubbing out the wind), in which a coin or the fingers are forcefully rubbed on the chest, back, or neck, is used to treat minor ailments.

Source: *A*, © doc-stock / Alamy; *B*, Biophoto Associates / Photo Researchers, Inc.

Documentation of findings is important in all situations, but it is essential in cases of suspected child abuse and neglect. Record physical findings as observed. Draw diagrams to document skin injuries. Document the location, nature, and extent of injuries with photographs.

Practice Alert

Each person who handles a laboratory specimen or other item (e.g., clothing soiled with semen) in cases of suspected child abuse must be identified in the patient's record, and the specimen must never be left unattended. Special bagging may be required. Forms that document the care of the specimen are sent with it to the police investigating the event. This documented chain of possession is necessary to ensure the admissibility of the evidence in court.

Following are nursing diagnoses that may be appropriate for the physically abused or neglected child:

- Coping, Defensive related to psychological impairment
- Pain, Acute related to inflicted injuries
- Skin Integrity, Impaired related to inflicted injuries
- Growth and Development, Impaired related to lack of supportive parenting and environment
- Nutrition, Imbalanced: Less than Body Requirements related to inadequate caloric intake
- Health Maintenance, Ineffective related to lack of parental provision of child's essential needs
- Fear related to actual physical harm or repeated risk of injury
- Injury, Risk for related to physical abuse
- Violence, Risk for, related to parental inability to manage anger

Additional diagnoses that may apply to the emotionally abused or neglected child include the following:

- Self-Esteem, Chronic Low related to lack of appropriate emotional support from parents

- Coping: Family, Disabled related to dysfunctional family dynamics and pattern of physical abuse

Diagnoses that may apply to the sexually abused child include the following:

- Anxiety related to potential separation from parent
- Rape-Trauma Syndrome related to sexual exploitation
- Role Performance, Ineffective related to domestic violence
- Personal Identity, Disturbed related to interference with usual activities of childhood

NANDA-I © 2012

Planning and Implementation

Nursing care focuses on helping to remove the child from an abusive environment, preventing further injury, providing supportive care, and reinforcing the importance of follow-up care and counseling.

Prevent Further Injury

Work with social services and community agencies to assess the child's home environment, individuals living in the home, and the actions surrounding the abuse. Assist in removing the child from the home to temporary custody of the court or foster care of another relative, if indicated. Counsel family members about abuse and refer for appropriate therapy. Be sure that all people of childbearing age know the law in your state regarding safe places to leave unwanted babies. Teach all dating youth how to deal with violence during dating. Have domestic violence resources in your community readily available at all settings where care is provided for children.

Provide Supportive Care

Protect and treat the child's injuries (e.g., fractures, burns). Include parents in the child's treatment plan and keep them informed about the child's progress. Even if suspected of inflicting injuries to the child, the parent is still the child's primary caretaker. Talk with the parent as you would with any parent. Be supportive of any guilt expressed. Encourage the parent to assist with the child's care. Observe parent–child interactions and document supportive behaviors and the child's response to the parent versus other care providers.

Clinical Tip

When children have been abused, they are often frightened in new situations. Sexually abused children may resist removing clothes for a physical examination or medical test. They may want to wear undergarments to the surgical suite. Members of the gender who abused them may be distrusted. When aware of a history of abuse, ask the parents or guardians how to best facilitate the child's health care. Be sensitive to fears. Allow the child to wear clothing and to have a support person present or whatever may provide a sense of security. Specially trained counselors are available in some settings to provide support. Consistency in nurses assigned to the child may provide for rapport and trust.

Interacting in a nonjudgmental manner with a parent suspected of abusing his or her child can be difficult. Talk with a colleague about anger you feel toward the parents or about the child's injuries or specific actions surrounding the abuse. Use team meetings to develop strategies that enable you to work with the parents and child.

Home Care Teaching

If there is any question about the child returning to a potentially dangerous situation, support the child's removal from the situation, or establishing a safety net in the home. The child may receive supervised care in the home by court order. Childcare, home nursing, and social worker visits may need to be arranged. Parents should be referred to parent effectiveness classes, family therapy, and support groups as necessary. If a neighbor or friend is the abuser, then the family may need support and legal advice when a term of incarceration is finished and the perpetrator returns to the community. Some states and communities have sexual offender laws which require notification when an offender on parole resides within a neighborhood.

Encourage the family to inform other care providers when the child's abuse history may affect a response to care. They should be alert to signs of posttraumatic stress disorder in order to seek assistance if the child has continuing problems (see Chapter 34 🅔).

Evaluation

Expected outcomes of nursing care for the child who has been abused or neglected include maintenance of normal growth and development, establishment of a positive sense of self-esteem, provision of parenting information and stress relief for parents, provision of a nurturing environment for the child, and absence of episodes of abuse.

Munchausen Syndrome by Proxy

Munchausen syndrome by proxy is a potentially deadly form of child abuse that involves the fabrication of signs and symptoms of a health condition in a child. Its prevalence is not well described. In most cases, it is the mother who creates these fictitious signs in her child (the proxy). The victim is usually under 6 years, and commonly under 1 year of age. Frequently the child's symptoms of illness are used to gain entry into the medical system to meet the abuser's own psychologic needs for attention. In some cases the perpetrator induces illness by giving the child medications or other actions such

as adding blood to the child's urine specimen (National Center for Biotechnology Information, 2011).

The issues of abuse are multidimensional. The child is a victim of the feigned illness, repeated hospitalizations, and invasive procedures. Equally disruptive is the deprivation of the child's daily routine caused by the periodic medical crises.

Munchausen syndrome by proxy should be suspected when unexplained, recurrent, or extremely rare conditions occur; illness is unresponsive to treatment; and the history and clinical findings are inconsistent. The most commonly reported signs and symptoms are central nervous system dysfunction, apnea, diarrhea, vomiting, fever, seizures, signs of bleeding (in urine or stool), and rashes. The parent may overdose the child on medications, such as nonprescription drugs and even syrup of ipecac, causing a variety of side effects. Poisoning and suffocation are commonly found. The symptoms occur in the presence of the same caretaker and disappear when the child is separated from that caretaker.

The child often appears uncooperative, extremely anxious, fearful, and negative. The caretaker, who in contrast appears very cooperative, competent, and loving, often expresses a desire for the child to recover. The caretaker may even suggest diagnostic procedures to try to determine "what's wrong." Characteristically the caretaker thrives in the healthcare environment.

The cause of Munchausen syndrome by proxy is often complex and rooted in the caretaker's own abusive or neglectful childhood. The disorder occurs in all socioeconomic classes. Often the perpetrator has some type of healthcare background, such as nursing or another allied health profession. The abuser is often young, married, and of the middle socioeconomic class. A history of insecure attachment is often present (National Institutes of Health, 2009).

A suspicion of Munchausen syndrome by proxy requires a coordinated evaluation by an interdisciplinary team. Members of the team must organize and communicate a strategic plan regarding collection of evidence, confrontation of the abuser, and management of the hospitalized child. The child's safety is the ultimate concern. When medical personnel suspect Munchausen syndrome by proxy, child protection agencies and law enforcement are informed, and a plan is established for management of the case.

Nursing Management

Special care should be taken to maintain a trusting relationship with the caretaker so that he or she does not become suspicious and leave the hospital. Often the best person on the team to function in the role of "trusted other" is a member of the psychiatric consultation team.

Careful documentation of parent–child interactions, presence or absence of symptoms, and other pertinent observations is essential. The child must be closely monitored. If blood is present in the child's urine, stool, or vomitus, careful documentation is needed about whether the nurse was present or whether the parent provided the sample. Covert video surveillance may be ordered by the hospital when the syndrome is highly suspected in a particular situation. Expert consultants may be needed to ensure legal requirements for investigation are met. When enough evidence is collected to prove Munchausen syndrome by proxy, the physician or another member of the psychiatric team confronts the caretaker in planning with law enforcement officials. Once diagnosis is made, the child must be placed in a safe setting. Siblings must be examined and their safety considered by social service and law enforcement groups. Only after legal and psychiatric experts determine that the home setting is safe can children be returned to the parent guilty of medical abuse.

ENVIRONMENTAL INFLUENCES ON CHILD HEALTH
Environmental Contaminants

Chemicals in the environment, both indoor and outdoor, are significant contaminant exposures that children experience every day. Contaminants are **toxins,** harmful or poisonous chemicals produced by metabolism of a biological organism (e.g., ricin), or **toxicants,** environmental hazards from chemical pollutants (Duderstadt, 2009). Many of these chemicals are commonly produced during industrial manufacture. The World Health Organization estimates that more than 3 million children worldwide die each year due to environment-related causes (Magzamen, Van Sickle, Rose, et al., 2011).

Environmental contaminants may be found in the air, water, soil, food, complementary therapies, and various objects, such as jewelry (Galvez, Graber, Sheffield, et al., 2009). Ground and surface water can be contaminated by manufacturing processes, agricultural and urban runoff into streams, sewage treatment, landfills, and particulates in the air.

Chemicals used in manufacturing plastics have recently caused concern for children's health because they have estrogen-mimicking properties. Phthalates are used to make flexible plastic products, such as catheters, intravenous tubing and bags, food packaging, and toys. Bisphenol A (BPA) is used to make hard plastics, such as baby bottles, containers used for microwaving, toys, and linings of food cans. BPA leaches into the food when the items used are heated.

Outdoor air contains many contaminants in solid, liquid, or gas form that can irritate lung tissues. Particulates in these contaminants (smoke, mist, fumes, or smog) often result from motor vehicle exhaust and industrial processes (coal-burning plants, refineries, and chemical plants). Exposure to these contaminants may cause potential acute and chronic health problems in children, such as asthma, bronchitis, infant mortality, and problems in lung development and function (Suwanwaiphatthana, Ruangdej, & Turner-Henson, 2010). See Legal and Ethical Considerations: Clean Air and Toxic Substance Laws.

Contaminant exposure in the child's home, school, or other location is also a significant problem as children are estimated to spend 90% of their time indoors (Suwanwaiphatthana et al., 2010). Examples of potential contaminants in the home include mold, drinking water contaminants, radon, carbon monoxide leaking from a furnace or gas-fueled appliance, and tobacco smoke. Health problems that could result from exposures in the home include allergies, asthma, infection, hypersensitivity disorders, central nervous system problems, and dermatitis (Barnes, Fisher, Postma, et al., 2010).

Some additional potentially harmful environmental exposures across various settings include:

- Pesticides such as organophosphates, organochlorine, carbamates, and pyrethroids. Children may be exposed through home use, parents who work in pesticide manufacturing, garden/farm/agricultural use, and ingestion through food treated with pesticide.
- Fish that contain high amounts of methylmercury (e.g., shark, tile fish, and swordfish).
- Heavy metal exposure, including lead, mercury, arsenic, and chlorine.

It is difficult to measure and draw conclusions about the effects of certain exposures because studies comparing groups of children with exposures to those without exposures cannot be conducted due to ethical reasons. Most knowledge about environmental exposure comes from epidemiologic studies in which large groups of individuals experienced exposure. For example, the National Health and Nutrition Examination Survey (NHANES III) investigated the prevalence of BPA in 2,517 participants. Surprisingly, results revealed that 92.6% of participants age 6 years and older had urinary concentrations of BPA, indicating how pervasive it is in our environment (Erler & Novak, 2010). Human exposure to BPA is of concern with regard to development of the prostate and brain, behavior in infants and children, and early puberty in girls (Erler & Novak, 2010) (Box 20–6).

Children are generally more vulnerable than adults to such environmental exposures because of their developing bodies and metabolism. (See Figure 14–10 in Chapter 14 🔗.) Physiologic reasons for this greater vulnerability include the following:

- Increased exposure to contaminants near to the ground because of smaller size
- Increased ingestion due to common hand-to-mouth behaviors of young children
- Increased absorption of products through thinner skin
- Delayed elimination due to developing enzyme systems that slow the metabolism of some products
- Higher respiratory and cardiovascular rates that increase exposure to carbon monoxide and other air pollutants

Contaminants in the environment can influence children in complex ways. Maternal exposure can affect the developing fetus or the infant being breastfed. Children are exposed to many chemicals on a daily basis through skin contact, inhalation, food, and water.

Legal and Ethical Considerations
Clean Air and Toxic Substance Laws

The Clean Air Act of 1990, Public Law 95–95, requires the U.S. Environmental Protection Agency (EPA) to establish outdoor air quality standards, and set limits for contaminants known to be harmful to the public and the environment. Air quality standards are reviewed every 5 years by the EPA.

The Toxic Substances Control Act of 1976, 15 U.S.C. §2601 et seq, provides the EPA with the authority to require testing and reporting of chemical substances as well as restrictions on mixing toxic substances. The current list includes 83,000 chemical substances, but only 200 have been tested for safety in children and adults, and only 5 have been banned (Duderstadt, 2009).

BOX 20–6   Research: The National Children's Study

The National Children's Study, a federal initiative to study the interactions between genetics and the environment, was authorized by the Children's Health Act of 2000 (PL 106-310). The impact of factors such as air, water, diet, sound, family dynamics, community and cultural influences, and genetics on the growth, development, and health of U.S. children will be studied. Mothers are being recruited during pregnancy, and children born will be followed until age 21 years. This study will help address the limited knowledge about environmental exposures by assessing the physical, chemical, biological, and psychosocial influences on a child's well-being (National Institute of Child Health and Human Development, 2010c).

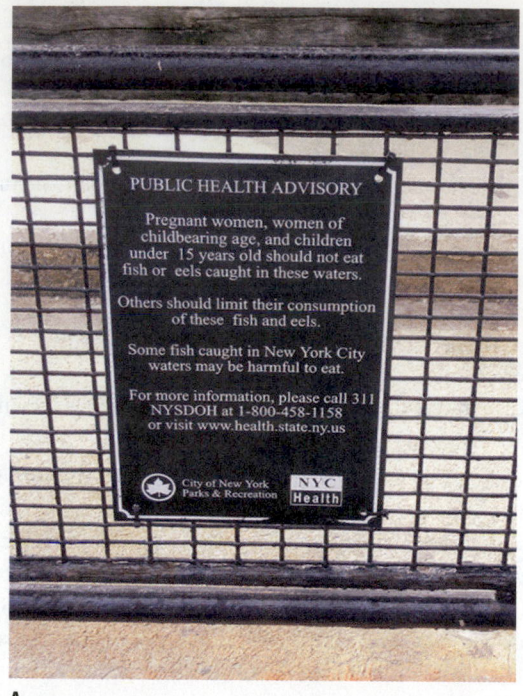

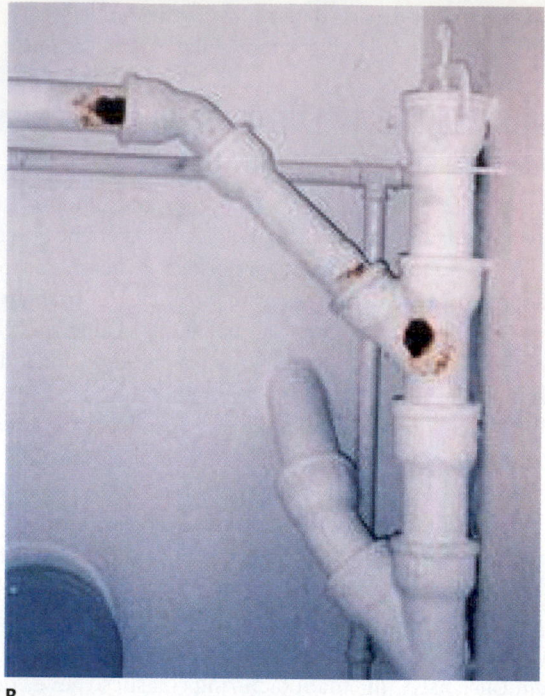

A　　　　　　　　　　　　　　　　　　　　　　　**B**

FIGURE 20–12 ■ Children are most at risk for the effects of environmental toxic agents because of their developing organs and cognition. *A*, Heavy metals such as mercury are harmful, and children may be exposed through manufacturing or by eating fish with high levels of mercury. *B*, Older homes pose risks such as deteriorating pipes that allow lead to enter the water supply. Moist conditions also allow growth of molds that can increase prevalence of asthma symptoms.

Harmful exposures are often difficult to identify (Figure 20–12 ■). Environmental tobacco smoke (ETS) is one known harmful chemical. Prenatal exposure may result in a low-birth-weight infant or sudden infant death syndrome (see Chapter 25 ❷). Exposure after birth is associated with lower respiratory illnesses, middle ear disease, and asthma (Magzamen et al., 2011).

Nursing Management

Nurses are instrumental in identifying exposure to environmental toxic agents. Questions that may help identify exposures to children should focus on the following:

- Occupation of the parents and adults living in the home of the child, and whether it involves harmful substances such as dust and chemicals
- Proximity of the child's home to power plants, industrial plants, or toxic waste areas
- Age of home (homes built before 1978 or renovated in the last 6 months are at risk for contamination with chemicals)
- Safety items used in the home, such as radon, carbon monoxide, and smoke detectors
- Hobbies of the child and family member that require the use of toxic materials, such as lead with stained glass work, glue with model building, or pesticides used with gardening
- Child's consumption of nonfood products

Nurses in all healthcare settings should learn more about the potential for environmental exposures in the child's home and other locations where he or she spends significant time. Consider the possibility of environmental exposure and refer for blood testing and further evaluation whenever delayed development or behavioral problems are evident. Hair, urine, and other testing may also be conducted, depending upon the toxin. Removal of the toxin from the body by drug treatment is possible for some substances (see lead poisoning on page 563).

Community health nurses may become engaged in environmental risk management by evaluating potential hazards in a child's home. Nurses perform an assessment of hazards (e.g., mold, carbon monoxide, and pesticides) and then help the family develop a plan to reduce hazards in the home environment.

Assist parents to reduce their child's exposure to environmental toxins. Children should have their hands washed before all meals and snacks, and they should be discouraged from putting nonfood items in the mouth. If parents work with toxic materials, they should be encouraged to shower and change clothes before leaving work and to wash work clothing separately. Exposure to chemicals used in plastic production can be reduced by choosing glass bottles; using paper plates or glass dishes to microwave foods; using plastics that have numbers 1, 2, 4, and 5 which do not have phthalates or BPA; and not placing acidic foods in plastic containers (Roberts, 2010).

Clinical Tip

Mercury poses a significant environmental hazard. Check to be sure parents have a nonmercury thermometer in the home. If they have a mercury thermometer, inform them to look in the community for a collection or exchange program that accepts mercury devices, such as a waste facility plant.

If a mercury device such as a thermometer breaks, the spill should be cleaned using the following method:

- Remove others (especially children) from the area.
- Open windows and doors to the outside, and then close other internal doors.
- Put on gloves.
- Place broken glass on a paper towel, fold over, and place in a ziplock bag.
- Gather all mercury beads together using a piece of cardboard, stiff index cards, or a squeegee. Get at a low level with a flashlight to locate all beads, and search the entire room as the beads can roll a distance.

- Use an eyedropper to collect the mercury beads, and place them on a damp paper towel. Place the paper towel, mercury, and eyedropper in the ziplock bag.
- Contact the health department, fire department, or waste management agency for disposal directions, and label the bag as directed.
- Dispose of clothing that has had mercury spilled on it. Do not walk around in shoes that might be contaminated with mercury.
- NEVER vacuum or sweep mercury or pour it down a drain.

U.S. Environmental Protection Agency, 2011

Lead Poisoning

Lead poisoning has been successfully prevented in many areas of the United States, with a substantial decline in lead levels from the mid-1970s. The average serum lead level for children is now 1.9 mcg/dL, down from 15 mcg/dL in 1976. The removal of lead from gasoline and paint in the 1970s significantly reduced lead exposure for children. Approximately 450,000 U.S. children (1%) from 1 to 5 years of age have blood lead levels above the recommended upper level of 5 mcg/dL (CDC, 2012). There is no safe level of lead exposure, as even children with blood lead levels lower than 10 mcg/dL have been reported to have a decrease in cognition (Warniment, Tsang, & Galazka, 2010) (Box 20–7).

Etiology and Pathophysiology

Lead in paint is the most common source of lead exposure for preschool children. Children are also exposed to lead when they ingest contaminated food, water, and soil or when they inhale dust contaminated with lead. See Developing Cultural Competence: Sources of Lead Exposure Among Cultural Groups for sources of lead exposure in various products and medications. Other potential sources of lead exposure include:

- Soil from decades of airborne lead deposits
- Drinking water from lead pipes, coolers with lead-soldered or lead-lined tanks, or lead-soldered teapots
- Food stored in lead-soldered cans or leaded crystal, or prepared in improperly fired pottery
- Imported toys, antique toys, cribs, and furniture
- Parental occupations and hobbies that involve exposure to lead (e.g., plumbing, battery manufacturing, highway construction, furniture refinishing, stained glass work, pottery making)
- Airborne lead in areas surrounding smelters and battery manufacturing

Woolf, Goldman, & Bellinger, 2007

Children are at greater risk for elevated blood lead levels because they absorb and retain more lead in proportion to their weight than adults. Many of these children are in families with incomes below the federal poverty rate. Some children live in older homes with lead dust and paint exposure. One recent study found a higher rate of elevated blood lead levels in immigrant children living in New York City (Tehranifar, Leighton, Auchincloss, et al., 2008).

BOX 20–7 Research: Blood Lead Levels

A study conducted in the United Kingdom testing 488 school-age children examined the association of blood lead levels with developmental, behavioral, and standardized education outcomes. No effects were seen in children with blood lead levels less than 5 mcg/dL. Blood lead levels of 5 to 10 mcg/dL were associated with a reduction in scores on reading and writing. Lead levels greater than 10 mcg/dL were also associated with antisocial behavior and hyperactivity (Chandramouli, 2009).

**Developing Cultural Competence
Sources of Lead Exposure Among Cultural Groups**

Potential sources of lead exposure for children from various cultural groups include ayurvedic medicine (traditional medications used by individuals of Indian and South Asian heritage); Chinese and Middle Eastern herbal products for teething, colic, and gastrointestinal distress; and eye cosmetics (kohl, surma) imported from Asia, the Middle East, Africa, and Mexico (Warniment et al., 2010). Amulets or jewelry with lead beads that the child may put in the mouth may be used by some Southeast Asian families to protect the child but increase the child's risk of lead poisoning (CDC, 2011c). Litargirio (lead monoxide), a powder used as an antiperspirant/deodorant by members of the Hispanic community, may be ingested by children who touch the powder residue with their hands (CDC, 2005).

An acute exposure to lead will result in a higher blood lead level that slowly decreases as the lead is stored in the bones. The lead may be in the bones releasing lead to the blood for decades. Lead interferes with normal cell function, primarily of the nervous system, blood cells, and kidneys.

Clinical Manifestations

Clinical manifestations depend on the degree of toxicity. At levels below 10 mcg/dL, the child has no specific signs associated with lead poisoning. However, impaired mental function can occur with blood levels even lower than 10 mcg/dL. Other neurologic effects include decreased IQ scores, cognitive deficits, antisocial behavior, and poor education outcomes (Woolf et al., 2007). Lead ingestion by a woman during pregnancy can result in fetal malformations, reduced birth weight, and premature birth. Severe lead poisoning, although rare, can occur with blood lead levels higher than 70 mcg/dL and can result in encephalopathy, coma, and death.

Collaborative Care

Diagnostic Tests

The Centers for Disease Control and Prevention now recommends screening children enrolled in Medicaid and those at risk for elevated lead levels (based on state or local risk assessment). Screening occurs at 12 and 24 months, as well as for children between 3 and 6 years of age if not previously screened (CDC, 2011c).

A venous blood sample is preferred as it reduces the risk of specimen contamination from lead on the skin. Capillary specimens are used in some cases with careful skin preparation. Any elevation in a capillary specimen must be confirmed by a venous sample. A blood lead (Pb-B) level less than 5 mcg/dL is considered acceptable, although it may still not screen out all children with impaired development due to lead.

Clinical Tip

Blood samples of lead report results in micrograms/deciliter or µg/dL. The symbol of a Greek letter (µ), when written, can be unclear and misinterpreted, so its use is no longer recommended, especially with regard to medication dosages. You may still see µg/dL used in some publications.

Clinical Therapy

Nutritional and environmental education history should be provided to parents of children with Pb-B levels between 5 and 14 mcg/dL. A confirmatory Pb-B level should be obtained in a month with follow-up testing in 3 months. Children with Pb-B levels between

15 and 19 mcg/dL should have a repeat test in a month to confirm the Pb-B level. Educate these children on nutritional and environmental exposure and recommend another Pb-B level test in 2 months. When the Pb-B level is higher than 20 mcg/dL, the child needs a repeat test to confirm the level in 1 week to 1 month. A complete history and physical examination, laboratory testing for iron deficiency anemia, and a radiograph of the abdomen (to see if particles of lead can be seen) are performed. An environmental investigation and removal of sources of lead from the child's environment should be initiated. Chelation therapy is recommended when Pb-B levels are greater than 45 mcg/dL. Children with Pb-B levels greater than 70 mcg/dL are critically ill and require immediate hospitalization and chelation therapy as well as interventions to provide a lead-free environment upon discharge.

Chelation is a reaction in which an organic compound, containing carbonyl (CO) and hydroxyl (OH) groups, interacts with a metal to form a compound that the child can eliminate. Succimer (DMSA) is the preferred agent because it can be given orally, but dimercaprol (BAL in oil) may be used. Calcium disodium ethylenediamine tetraacetate ($CaNa_2$ EDTA) and d-penicillamine may be used in some cases. Chelation therapy has the potential for serious side effects, so consultation with a toxicologist is important before beginning therapy. Children are monitored closely during and after the treatment. BAL can lead to hypertension, tachycardia, headache, fever, or nephrotoxicity. Succimer is associated with gastrointestinal side effects, rash, headache, and neurologic symptoms.

Long-term follow-up of children receiving chelation therapy is essential. The child should never be discharged unless a lead-free home environment has been ensured.

Nursing Management

Nursing care focuses on screening children at risk for lead poisoning, educating parents about good nutrition and actions they can take to reduce environmental lead exposure, and follow-up monitoring of children with elevated blood lead levels.

Nursing Assessment and Diagnosis

Ask parents about the child's development and eating habits. Inquire about and be alert for the child's risk of lead exposure. For example, the dust resulting from renovation of a home built before the 1970s has lead in it. Children should be screened for elevated blood lead levels in the following situations:

- The child is suspected by a parent or a healthcare provider to be at risk for lead exposure.
- The child has a sibling or frequent playmate with an elevated blood lead level.
- The child is a recent immigrant, refugee, or foreign adoptee.
- The child's parent or principal caregiver works professionally or recreationally with lead.
- The child has a household member who uses traditional, folk, or ethnic remedies or cosmetics or who routinely eats food imported informally (e.g., by a family member) from abroad.
- The child's family has been designated at increased risk for lead exposure by the health department because the family has local risk factors for lead exposure (e.g., residence in a designated high-risk zip code or near a known point source).

Wengrovitz & Brown, 2009

Examples of nursing diagnoses for the child at risk of lead poisoning may include the following:

- Contamination related to lead in home environment associated with house renovation
- Development: Delayed, Risk for related to ingestion of lead
- Knowledge, Deficient (Parents) related to essential nutritional requirements for the young child

NANDA-I © 2012

Planning and Implementation

Nurses often work with state and local health officials to plan and implement screening for children at high risk of lead exposure. After children with elevated blood lead levels are identified, educate parents about sources of lead in the environment and techniques to reduce the child's exposure. The following housekeeping interventions should be recommended:

- Damp mop the floors, windowsills, baseboards, and wooden furniture.
- Wash the child's hands and face before meals and naptime.
- Wash toys and pacifiers frequently.
- Remove shoes before entering the house to keep contaminated soil outside.

Teach parents the importance of including foods high in iron in the child's diet, as iron deficiency anemia may make the child more susceptible to injury from lead ingestion (Warniment et al., 2010). Educate the parents about appropriate administration of ferrous sulfate if the child has iron deficiency anemia (see Chapter 28 🔗). The child should eat meals at regular intervals, as lead is absorbed more readily on an empty stomach.

Be sure that parents understand the importance of follow-up blood lead level testing. Referral to a lead prevention program, visiting nurse, or social services may be appropriate.

Nurses who administer chelating drugs are challenged by the complexity of treatment and required care. Chelation should always be managed in consultation with toxicologists. Careful monitoring of liver and kidney function, and cardiac, gastrointestinal, and neurologic systems is important. Administration for some chelating agents is by the intramuscular route and is painful; children will need skilled nursing and child life specialist care.

Evaluation

The *Healthy People 2020* objective can be used to evaluate community efforts at lead poisoning prevention. The national target average blood lead level for children 1 to 5 years of age in 2020 is 1.4 micrograms/dL (U.S. Department of Health and Human Services, 2011).

Expected outcomes of nursing care for the child with lead poisoning include the following:

- The child has normal growth, development, and cognition.
- The child has adequate nutritional intake.
- Lead sources are successfully removed from the child's environment.
- A safe environment is established for the child.

Poisoning

Nearly 2.5 million poisonings occur annually in the United States, with the majority (91%) of these in the person's own residence.

About 39% of poisonings occur in children under 3 years of age and 52% in children under 6 years of age. In 2009, fatalities due to poisonings occurred in 79 children and adolescents up to an age of 20 years (6.8% of all poisoning fatalities in the United States for that year). Two thirds of the 48 reported fatalities for adolescents were suspected suicides (Bronstein, Spyker, Cantilena, et al., 2010).

Etiology and Pathophysiology

Young children are at risk for ingestion of foreign substances because of their characteristic behaviors, which involve exploration of the environment. Infants and toddlers commonly place objects in their mouths. Although most poisons are ingested, other routes of contamination include absorption through the skin, inhalation of dust particles and gases, and contact with the eyes.

The most dangerous toxic substances a small child may ingest include iron, antidepressants, hypoglycemic agents, cardiovascular drugs, salicylates, anticonvulsants, and illicit drugs (McGregor, Parkar, & Rao, 2009). The five most common classifications of poisons ingested by children less than 6 years of age are cosmetics and personal care products, analgesics, household cleaning products, miscellaneous foreign bodies and toys, and topical preparations (Bronstein et al., 2010). Other common causes of poisoning include vitamins, cold and cough preparations, pesticides, and plants (e.g., Boston ivy, poinsettia, philodendron, lily-of-the-valley, daffodil bulbs, azalea, and rhododendron). Some household items are nontoxic and cause little harm; however, items that contain caustic agents or toxic chemicals can cause irreversible damage or death. Substances most often associated with a fatality in children less than age 6 years include analgesics, plants, cold and cough preparations, and hydrocarbons (Bronstein et al., 2010). See Legal and Ethical Considerations: The Poison Prevention Packaging Act.

Practice Alert

Parents who suspect that their child has ingested a poison should immediately call the Poison Control Center (PCC) at 1-800-222-1222. This toll free number can be accessed from anywhere in the United States and Puerto Rico, and the caller is connected to the closest poison control center.

The poison control center will advise parents about treatment to begin at home, and if the child needs treatment in the emergency department. If the child has vomited, the vomitus should be brought to the emergency department. With older children, the possibility of intentional ingestion needs to be considered.

Clinical Manifestations

The manifestations of poisoning depend on the toxin. Some common effects include altered mental status, respiratory or cardiac symptoms, seizures, vital sign changes, and gastrointestinal symptoms. Symptoms may be mild initially. Full effects of the toxin may be delayed as the toxin is absorbed, if the medication has an extended release action or when a toxic metabolite results from breakdown of the ingested substance. See the Clinical Manifestations table for commonly ingested toxic agents.

Legal and Ethical Considerations
The Poison Prevention Packaging Act

The Poison Prevention Packaging Act of 1970 mandates child protective devices for all potentially toxic substances, such as household cleansers and medications. However, many are still ingested by children.

Collaborative Care

Collaborative care focuses on identifying the poison and its source; stabilizing the child's airway, breathing, and circulation; reducing the effects of the exposure or removing the offending agent; and reducing the risk of recurrence.

Diagnostic Tests

A history of medications taken by family members (including over-the-counter medications and complementary therapies) and household toxins that the child could have accessed should be obtained to help guide medical management. Specifically obtain information about the child's potential access to acetaminophen, salicylates, opioids, hydrocarbons, caustic agents, and antidepressants. Retrieve information about where and when the child was found; how long the child was unsupervised; and the child's history of depression or suicide, allergies, and any other medical problems. Various diagnostic tests are used based upon the suspected poison. Blood, urine, and even hair toxicology screens are often performed. Other tests may include serum glucose, an electrocardiogram, serum electrolytes, and arterial blood gases. Testing of vomitus for the presence of medications or poisons may be helpful in determining the amount ingested.

Clinical Therapy

In the emergency department the child's airway, breathing, circulation, and level of consciousness are assessed, as well as the presence of a life-threatening condition (see Appendix F 🔴). Carefully monitor the child for changes in status as some toxins take time to produce symptoms. The goal of treatment is to prevent further absorption of the poison and to reverse or eliminate its effects. The Poison Control Center is consulted to obtain guidance for treatment. An antidote is prescribed if one is available. See Chapter 21 🔴 for treatment of an opioid overdose.

Practice Alert

Antidotes and agonists are available for some ingestions, including the following:

- Acetaminophen—N-acetylcysteine
- Calcium channel blockers—calcium chloride, glucagon
- Digoxin—digoxin immune Fab
- Opioids—naloxone
- Organophosphates—atropine
- Warfarin or rodent killers—vitamin K

McGregor et al., 2009

Gastric lavage and activated charcoal are no longer routine therapy but may be used in some children if within one hour of ingestion. Cathartics or whole bowel irrigation with polyethylene glycol may be used for heavy metals or for long-acting or sustained-release medications (McGregor et al., 2009). Syrup of ipecac is no longer recommended for treating suspected poisoning. Vomiting is rarely induced because too much of the poison may be absorbed before the agent used to cause vomiting is effective.

Children with severe poisoning are admitted to the intensive care unit to carefully monitor the child and provide supportive care for the toxin's effects (e.g., arrhythmias, depressed respirations, seizures, hypotension, hypoglycemia, and electrolyte abnormalities). Potential complications of poisoning, depending on the type of poison, include respiratory and/or cardiac arrest, hypovolemic shock, liver failure, renal failure, seizures, and esophageal or tracheal burns.

Clinical Manifestations   Commonly Ingested Toxic Agents

TYPE	SOURCES	CLINICAL MANIFESTATIONS	CLINICAL THERAPY
Corrosives (strong acids and alkaline products that cause chemical burns of mucosal surfaces)	Batteries Oven cleaners Drain cleaners Clinitest tablets Antirust compounds Toilet bowl cleaners Hair relaxers	Vomiting Drooling, difficulty swallowing Severe burning pain in mouth, throat, or stomach Swelling of mucous membranes; edema of lips, tongue, and pharynx (may cause respiratory obstruction) Agitation	■ Do not induce vomiting! ■ Dilute toxin with water to prevent further damage.
Hydrocarbons (organic compounds that contain carbon and hydrogen; most are distillates of petroleum)	Gasoline Kerosene Furniture polish Lighter fluid Paint thinners	Gagging and coughing Nausea, vomiting Altered mental status Respiratory symptoms associated with aspiration (tachypnea, cyanosis, retractions)	■ Do not induce vomiting! (Aspiration of hydrocarbons places the child at high risk for pneumonia.) ■ Use gastric lavage only for highly toxic hydrocarbons. ■ Provide supportive respiratory care.
Acetaminophen	Many over-the-counter products	Nausea, vomiting, anorexia Sweating Pallor Right upper quadrant abdominal pain and tenderness with liver involvement; coagulation and bilirubin abnormalities	■ Administer the antidote N-acetylcysteine, which binds with the metabolite, preventing absorption and protecting the liver. ■ Activated charcoal may be used.
Salicylates	Products containing aspirin	Nausea, vomiting Dehydration Diaphoresis Tachypnea High temperature Bleeding tendencies Tinnitus Disorientation Agitation, restlessness Confusion, coma	■ Administer activated charcoal. ■ Correct electrolyte imbalances ■ Administer intravenous sodium bicarbonate and fluids (to make the urine alkaline).
Cardiac medications	Calcium channel blockers, beta blockers, digoxin	Bradycardia, arrhythmias, heart block Hypotension, Dizziness, unsteady gait Altered mental status, seizures Nausea, vomiting	■ Administer IV fluids. ■ Administer prescribed medications: ■ Vasopressor therapy ■ Calcium chloride ■ Glucagon, or high-dose regular insulin with supplemental glucose to achieve euglycemia ■ Digoxin immune Fab
Hypoglycemic agent	Sulfonylurea	Hypoglycemia Tachycardia Diaphoresis, clammy skin Mental status changes, coma	■ Administer prescribed medications: ■ Glucagon ■ Octreotide
Iron	Prenatal vitamins Therapeutic iron tablets	Vomiting, diarrhea Abdominal pain Hematemesis and bloody stools with severe ingestions Drowsiness Hypovolemic shock	■ Activated charcoal may be used. ■ Administer intravenous fluids and sodium bicarbonate. ■ Deferoxamine chelation therapy may be used.

Source: Data from O'Donnell, K. A., & Ewald, M. B. (2011). Poisonings, In R. M. Kleigman, B. F. Stanton, J. W. St. Geme, N. F. Schor, & R. E. Behrman, Nelson textbook of pediatrics, (19th ed., pp. 250–270), Philadelphia, PA: Elsevier. McGregor, T., Parkar, M., & Rao, S. (2009). Evaluation and management of common childhood poisonings. American Family Physician, 79(5), 397–403; Smollin, C. G. (2010). Toxicology: Pearls and pitfalls in the use of antidotes. Emergency Medical Clinics of North America, 28, 149–161.

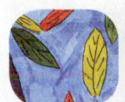

Partnering with Families

Avoiding Childhood Poisoning

Families with children require instructions for avoiding childhood poisoning. Teach family members these interventions to help avoid childhood poisonings:

- Place household cleaners, medications, vitamins, and other potentially poisonous substances out of the reach of children or in locked cabinets.
- Use warning stickers such as Mr. Yuk on all containers.
- Request all prescriptions to have child-resistant caps, and ensure that all over-the-counter medications have child-resistant caps.

- Store products in their original containers. Never place household cleaners or other toxic products in food or beverage containers.
- Remove houseplants from the child's play areas.
- Use caution when visiting other settings that are not childproofed (e.g., grandparents' homes). Remember that visitors may have pills in their purses or pockets that are easily reached by children.

Nursing Management

Nursing care focuses on initial emergent care and stabilization of the child with poisoning and prevention of repeated poisoning.

Nursing Assessment and Diagnosis

Obtain the history from the family or caregiver about the child's suspected ingestion substance, time, amount, and symptoms. Initial assessment focuses on airway, breathing, circulation, and mental status. Perform a complete physical assessment observing for signs of poisoning, such as drooling, diaphoresis, wheezing, increased or depressed respirations, stridor, abnormally large or small pupil size, burns on the lips or mouth, unusual breath odor, and seizures. Assess the vomitus for presence of medication or other ingested substances. Determine the child's height and weight or use a length-based tape to determine medication dosages and equipment sizes.

Clinical Tip

A color-coded tape, called the Broselow tape, can be used to determine a child's length or height quickly in an emergency. The color zones on sections of the tape indicate the dosages of emergency drugs to be used.

Nursing diagnoses for the child with ingestion of a toxic substance may include:

- Airway Clearance, Ineffective related to excessive secretion effect of toxic substance
- Gas Exchange, Impaired related to depressed neurological status
- Aspiration, Risk for related to depressed neurological status and vomiting
- Cardiac Output, Decreased related to arrhythmia effects of toxic substance
- Injury, Risk for related to repeated occurrences of poisoning
- Family Processes, Interrupted related to poisoning of a family member

NANDA-I © 2012

Planning and Implementation

Emergency care focuses on airway and hemodynamic stability, removal of toxic agents, and support of the family. The child is attached to pulse oximetry and a cardiorespiratory monitor. An intravenous line is started for the administration of fluids and an antidote, if available. When activated charcoal is prescribed, it may be in a ready-to-drink solution in an opaque container, or it may need to be mixed with sorbitol or apple juice to encourage the child to drink it. Cover the cup so the child does not see the black liquid, and provide a straw to prevent spillage.

Provide Emotional Support

Provide support to the parents who may have feelings of anger, guilt, or fear regarding the poisoning event. Wait until the child is out of immediate danger before questioning parents in detail about the incident.

Family Education

Discuss with parents the need to supervise infants and young children at all times. Ask parents how medicines and cleaning agents are stored and whether the house contains any plants. Teach parents proper methods of childproofing the home. The poison control number **1-800-222-1222** should be programmed in or placed beside every phone in the house. Suggest measures for preventing recurrence of poisoning. (See Partnering with Families: Avoiding Childhood Poisoning.)

Evaluation

Expected outcomes for nursing care of the child with poisoning include:

- The child maintains an open airway, effective gas exchange, ventilatory function, and stable heart rate and blood pressure.
- The child does not demonstrate wheezing, coughing, pneumonia, or other signs indicating aspiration.
- The child's neurologic status is appropriate for age.
- The family demonstrates effective measures to prevent repeated ingestions and to improve home environment safety.

Ingestion of Foreign Objects

A total of 93,574 cases of ingestion of foreign objects were reported in the United States for children less than 6 years of age in 2009. Coins, parts of toys, button batteries, and glass are common objects ingested by children less than age 6 years. Four pediatric deaths were associated with battery ingestions (Bronstein et al., 2010). Adults often witness infants and young children ingesting foreign bodies, and older children may report swallowing an object. Some small, round, smooth objects do not cause any clinical distress, unless aspirated. See Chapter 25 🔗 for care of children with an aspirated foreign body.

Many foreign body ingestions are asymptomatic, but some cause symptoms. If the foreign body is lodged in the esophagus, children may present with substernal pain, drooling, and dysphagia. Some children may exhibit respiratory symptoms such as wheezing or coughing. Ingestion of a sharp object may result in a perforation. Erosion of the mucosa and strictures may develop at the site of a retained foreign body, such as a button battery. Bowel obstruction may occur in some cases, causing abdominal distention and pain.

Clinical Judgment

If a foreign body is aspirated rather than ingested, what respiratory symptoms would potentially be present?

Many ingested foreign bodies in children are radio-opaque, so radiographs of the neck, chest, and abdomen may be useful in verifying the ingestion and identifying its location in the gastrointestinal tract (Figure 20–13 ■). Most foreign bodies pass through the gastrointestinal tract and are eliminated in the stool. A lodged esophageal foreign body may be removed by endoscopy or advanced into the stomach to reduce complications. Endoscopic examination and retrieval of the ingested foreign body is often urgently performed for sharp objects, magnets, and button batteries.

Nursing Management

Nursing care centers on supporting the child, collaborating in the identification and removal of the foreign body, and teaching the child and family measures to reduce reoccurrence. Assess the child's airway, breathing, and circulatory status. Assess the child for any symptoms of the ingestion, such as drooling, wheezing, substernal pain, dysphagia, and coughing. Obtain a thorough history from the family about the event, what was ingested, and any symptoms that the family witnessed.

Prepare the child for radiologic studies. Explain the procedures and reassure the child and family during the studies. If endoscopic examination or retrieval is necessary, prepare the child and family for the procedure.

When the foreign object is in the stomach and expected to pass through the intestines without complications, teach the family and child how to monitor the stools for the object. Provide and suggest

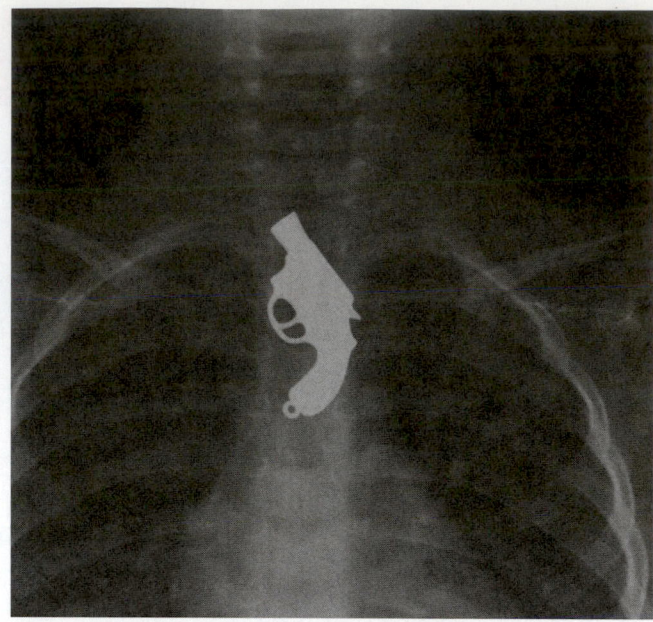

FIGURE 20–13 ■ Radiograph of a toy gun in the esophagus of a child.
Source: *Evelyn Anthony, MD, Department of Radiology, Brenner Children's Hospital, WFUHS.*

the use of tongue blades to examine stools for the foreign body. If the object has not passed in the expected time frame (generally 48 hours), encourage the family to return for a radiologic examination to assess the object's progress through the gastrointestinal tract.

Partner with the family to establish a safe home environment for the child and prevent a future ingestion. Encourage the family to avoid purchasing toys with small and potentially removable parts, to keep all small items out of the child's reach, and to ensure the child is monitored at all times.

Expected outcomes for nursing care of the child with an ingested foreign body include removal of the foreign body, reduced risk for a future ingestion, and family description of preventive measures to promote a safe environment for the child.

Chapter Highlights

- Many of the major morbidities and mortalities of childhood and adolescence are related to social and environmental factors.
- The theory of ecologic development provides a framework to use in assessing the interactions of children with factors in their environments.
- The theory of resilience examines risk and protective factors of children in order to formulate interventions to assist the child dealing with health problems related to social conditions.
- Poverty is a pervasive and important risk factor that influences many health outcomes.
- Some poor families experience homelessness and are at risk for a number of health problems.

- Stressful experiences, family structure, and the community all influence the health of children.
- Tobacco use is high among youth, and the most common time for initiation of tobacco use is the middle school years.
- Tobacco prevention and cessation programs are needed throughout the school years.
- Substance abuse by alcohol and drugs occurs in childhood and adolescence and compounds many health risks.
- A major contributor to overweight and other health problems is the lack of physical activity among children.

- Protective equipment can reduce the number and severity of injuries during risky physical activities.
- Teens need information about body art safety procedures if they choose this method of self-expression.
- Violence can be directed at children, and children can be the perpetrators of violence.
- All families should be regularly assessed for violence, and prevention strategies should be applied when needed.
- Child abuse can take the form of physical abuse or neglect, emotional abuse or neglect, or sexual abuse.
- The nurse plans interventions for an array of abusive situations such as abandoned babies, hazing, domestic violence, and Munchausen syndrome by proxy.

- Environmental contaminants affect the health of children, from the prenatal period through childhood; developmental variations place the child at particular risk.
- Lead in paint is the most common source of lead exposure for preschool children, but other sources include contaminated food, water, and soil or inhaled dust contaminated with lead.
- More than half of all reported poisonings occur in children less than 6 years of age. Numerous medicines, plants, pesticides, and other household products are ingested by children each year.
- Nurses educate parents to avoid accidental ingestion of poisons or foreign objects by children, and to provide emergency and supportive care after ingestions.

Clinical Reasoning in Action

INTRODUCTION

Recall 15-year-old Amy Beckman from the chapter-opening scenario. She has visited the school nurse due to an ear that is painful after a piercing by a friend. The nurse examines all of Amy's piercings on her ears, face, and navel. Amy is talkative and willing to answer the nurse's questions about her body art and her life. She elaborates about her life when she ran away last year and seems to be analyzing her own motives and goals.

DESCRIPTION

The nurse finds that both of Amy's ears have multiple piercings and jewelry. They all appear clean and without inflammation or drainage. The ear that Amy had the nurse check has one new small earring about midway in the ear. Amy admitted that it was hard for her friend to get this piercing in the place desired so her ear was manipulated a great deal during the insertion about 2 days ago. Amy's vital signs are temperature 99.8°F, pulse 76, respirations 18, and blood pressure 118/62.

While gathering data, the nurse inquires about Amy's immunization status. She states that she has no idea what immunizations she has had. The last she remembers were when she was quite small. She had a diagnosis of mild asthma in the past but is not using any inhalers now and has had no exacerbations for about 2 years. She does not really know what asthma is, only that she occasionally had difficulty breathing.

Amy provides information about her weeks spent living on the streets. She left home and school because she felt like no one understood her and she did not like the rules that she had to follow. She spent a few nights with a friend, but left when the friend's mother was going to call Amy's mother to inform her of Amy's whereabouts. She slept under bridges at night and went to a mission for meals and showers. She began smoking and panhandled for money. After a few weeks, while speaking with a nursing student at the shelter, Amy decided that a life on the streets was not for her. She "saw the light," as she describes it. She called her mother and asked to come home. She describes her mother as concerned and caring, and her father as distant and removed. Amy has one older brother who is living and working in another state; she talks with him only on his infrequent visits home. She is sad that she is not closer to her father and older brother. She has a younger brother who is 6 years old, and feels like she needs to be around home for him. At the same time, she discusses her dislike

of rules and states that it is hard to have her mother tell her what time to be home at night.

DISCUSSION

1. Amy seems to have some conflicting feelings. She yearns to be at home with her family members but resists the rules that the family sets. She is troubled that there is not more closeness with her father and brother, but she broke some family ties herself when she ran away. What is Amy's developmental stage, according to Erikson? What tasks does she need to accomplish for healthy development to occur? How is her present setting supportive of accomplishing her developmental tasks? How can the school nurse support Amy's developmental progression?

2. Amy clearly has demonstrated many risk and protective factors for physical and psychosocial health. Recall the theory of resilience described in this chapter and Chapter 5 ⊘. Make a list of Amy's risk factors. What puts her at risk of disease or of developing an unhealthy lifestyle? Then make a list of Amy's protective factors. What strengths does she have? You will use this list to formulate nursing diagnoses and interventions for Amy.

3. Based on your summary of Amy's risk and protective factors, list three nursing diagnoses. Be sure that they encompass both physical and psychosocial health.

4. What immunizations should Amy have at her age? Consult the immunization schedule in Chapter 22 ⊘ for ideas. Think also about the diseases that are common with body art and learn which of these can be prevented by immunization.

5. Amy admitted that she began smoking while living on the street. Phrase some open-ended questions to determine both her present smoking habits and whether she has experimented with drugs.

6. Develop a series of nursing interventions that would enhance Amy's health and prevent disease and mental health problems.

7. Consider the roles played by the school nurse in an alternative school. Discuss the skills needed by that nurse in order to work effectively with teens, families, the school, and the greater community. What partnerships should the nurse develop with each of these groups?

NCLEX-RN® Review

1. A community health nurse has performed an assessment of drug use among teens in a neighborhood. The nurse is going to address some concerns at a meeting with the parents in the neighborhood. Which would be appropriate advice by the nurse?

1. If the teen is using drugs, therapy is not needed if the parents talk to their child.
2. The teen can stay home alone often after the age of 15 years to establish independence.
3. Encourage the parents to set consistent limits and be involved in their children's lives.
4. Methamphetamine use is not a risk for teens, just adults.

2. The nurse is teaching discharge instructions to parents who brought their child in following an accidental overdose of a poisonous substance. Which indicates successful teaching has taken place about prevention?

1. The parents state they will induce vomiting with syrup of ipecac.
2. The parents state the toll-free number for Poison Control.
3. The parents state they will throw all medication away.
4. The parents state they will examine each room of their house to assess the safety risks for their child.

3. While weighing a 12-month-old in the clinic, the nurse notes six nickel-size bruises on the child's buttocks. The bruises range in color from purple to greenish yellow. The nurse also notes a cord mark on the child's thigh. Which would be an appropriate nursing intervention?

1. Report suspected child abuse to the appropriate authority.
2. Inform the parents that abuse is suspected.
3. Document the main findings only.
4. Do nothing, since these findings are normal for a child who is learning to walk.

4. Which intervention will facilitate positive coping in a preschool-age child after a deadly explosion in the neighborhood where the child lives?

1. Postpone planned family events.
2. Accept delayed reactions in the child.
3. Initiate detailed discussion about the event.
4. Let the child watch it on the television often.

See Appendix I 🔴 *for answers.*

References

Add Health Study. (2010). *Add Health. The National Longitudinal Study of Adolescent Health*. Retrieved from http://www.cpc.unc.edu/projects/addhealth

Alcohol Free Children. (2010). *Youth*. Retrieved from http://www.alcoholfreechildren.org/info/youth

Allen, E. S., Rhoades, G. K., Stanley, S. M., & Markman, H. J. (2011). On the home front: Stress for recently deployed army couples. *Family Process, 50,* 235–247.

American Academy of Child and Adolescent Psychiatry. (2010). *Alcohol and drug abuse*. Retrieved from http://www.aacap.org/

American Academy of Pediatrics. (2011). *Bullies beat down self-esteem*. Retrieved from http://www.healthychildren.org

American Heart Association. (2008). *Exercise (physical activity) and children*. Retrieved from http://www.americanheart.org/presenter.jhtml?identifier=4596

Aranda, M. C., Middleton, L. S., Flake, E., & Davis, B. E. (2011). Psychosocial screening in children with wartime-deployed parents. *Military Medicine, 176,* 402–407.

Armstrong, M. L., Roberts, A. E., Koch, J. R., Saunders, J. C., Owen, D. C., & Anderson, R. R. (2008). Motivation for contemporary tattoo removal: A shift in identity. *Archives of Dermatology, 144,* 879–884.

Audrain-McGovern, J., Stevens, S., Murray, P. J., Kinsman, S., Zuckoff, A., Pletcher, J., . . . Wileyto, E. P. (2011). The efficacy of motivational interviewing versus brief advice for adolescent smoking behavior change. *Pediatrics, 128*(1), e101–e111.

Backinger, C. L., Michaels, C. M., Jefferson, A. M., Fagan, P., Hurd, A. L., & Grana, R. (2008). Factors associated with recruitment and retention of youth into smoking cessation intervention studies: A review of the literature. *Health Education Research, 23,* 359–368.

Balodis, I. M., Wynne-Edwards, K. E., & Olmstead, M. C. (2010). The other side of the curve: Examining

the relationship between pre-stressor physiological responses and stress reactivity. *Psychoneuroendocrinology, 35,* 1363–1373.

Barnes, G., Fisher, B., Postma, J., Harnish, K., Butterfield, P., & Hill, W. (2010). Incorporating environmental health into nursing practice: A case study on indoor air quality. *Pediatric Nursing, 36*(1), 33–39, 52.

Bechara, C., Macheras, E., Heym, B., Pages, A., & Auffret, N. (2010). Mycobacterium abscessus skin infection after tattooing: First case report and review of the literature. *Dermatology, 221,* 1–4.

Brands, M. M., Purperhart, H., & Deckers-Kocken, J. M. (2011). A pilot study of yoga treatment in children with functional abdominal pain and irritable bowel syndrome. *Complementary Therapy in Medicine, 19,* 109–114.

Brodowski, M. L., Nolan, C. M., Gaudiosi, J. A., Yuan, Y. Y., Zikratova, L., Oritz, M. J., . . . Hammond, W. R. (2008). Nonfatal maltreatment of infants—United States, October 2005–September 2006. *Morbidity and Mortality Weekly Report, 57,* 336–339.

Bronfenbrenner, U. (2005). *Making human beings human: Bioecologic perspectives*. Thousand Oaks, CA: Sage Publications.

Bronstein, A. C., Spyker, D. A., Cantilena, L. R., Green, J., Rumack, B. H., & Griffen, S. L. (2010). 2009 annual report of the American Association of Poison Control Centers' National Poisoning Data System (NPDS): 27th annual report. *Clinical Toxicology, 48,* 979–1178.

Centers for Disease Control and Prevention (CDC). (2005). Lead poisoning associated with use of litargirio—Rhode Island, 2003. *Morbidity and Mortality Weekly Report, 54*(9), 227–229.

Centers for Disease Control and Prevention (CDC). (2009). *Youth tobacco cessation: A guide for making informed decisions*. Atlanta, GA: Author.

Centers for Disease Control and Prevention (CDC). (2010a). *Youth Risk Behavior Surveillance—United States, 2009*. Retrieved from http://www.cdc.gov/pdf/ss/ss5905.pdf

Centers for Disease Control and Prevention (CDC). (2010b). *Child maltreatment*. Retrieved from http://www.cdc.gov/violenceprevention/pdf/CM-Datasheet-a.pdf

Centers for Disease Control and Prevention (CDC). (2011a). *Youth and tobacco use*. Retrieved from http://www.cdc.gov/tobacco/data_statistics/fact_sheets/youth_data/tobacco_use/index.htm

Centers for Disease Control and Prevention (CDC). (2011b). Violence-related firearm deaths among residents of metropolitan areas and cities—United States, 2006–2007. *Morbidity and Mortality Weekly Report, 60,* 573–578.

Centers for Disease Control and Prevention (CDC). (2011c). Lead poisoning of a child associated with use of a Cambodian amulet—New York City, 2009. *Morbidity and Mortality Weekly Report, 60*(3), 69–71.

Centers for Disease Control and Prevention (CDC). (2012). *Low level lead exposure harms children: A renewed call for primary prevention, a report of the Advisory Committee on Childhood Lead Poisoning Prevention*, Retrieved from http://www.cdc.gov/nceh/lead/ACCLPP/Final_Document_030712.pdf

Chandra, A., Mosher, W. D., Copen, C., & Sionean, C. (2011). Sexual behavior, sexual attraction, and sexual identity in the United States: Data from the 2006–2008 National Survey of Family Growth. *National Health Statistics Report, 36,* 1–36.

Chandramouli, K. (2009). Effects of early childhood lead exposure on academic performance and behavior in school age children. *Archives of Disease in Childhood, 94*(11), 844–884.

Chapman, R., Watkins, R., Zappia, T., Nicol, P. & Sheilds, L. (2012). Nursing and medical students' attitude, knowledge and beliefs regarding lesbian, gay, bisexual and transgender parents seeking health care for their children. *Journal of Clinical Nursing 21*, 938–945.

Childhelp. (2011). *National child abuse statistics*. Retrieved from http://www.childhelp.org/pages/statistics

Children's Defense Fund. (2010). *State of America's Children 2010*. Retrieved from http://www.childrens-defense.org/child-research-data-publications/data/state-of-americas-children-2010-gun-violence.pdf

ChildStats. (2011). *Child care*. Retrieved from http://www.childstats.gov/americaschildren09/famsoc3.asp

Chiu, S. H., & DiMarco, M. A. (2010). A pilot study comparing two developmental screening tools for use with homeless children. *Journal of Pediatric Health Care, 24*, 73–80.

Coker, T. R., Elliott, M. N., Kanouse, D. E., Grunbaum, J. A., Gilliland, M. J., Tortolero, S. R., . . . Schuster, M. A. (2009). Prevalence, characteristics, and associated health and health care of family homelessness among fifth-grade students. *American Journal of Public Health, 99*, 1446–1452.

Cyberbullying Research Center. (2011). *Research*. Retrieved from http://cyberbullying.us/research.php

DiMarco, M. A., Huff, M., Kinion, E., & Kendra, M. A. (2009). The pediatric nurse practitioner's role in reducing oral health disparities in homeless children. *Journal of Pediatric Health Care, 23*, 109–116.

Duderstadt, K. G. (2009). Chemical policy and the impact on child health. *Journal of Pediatric Health Care, 23*(6), 421–424.

Elkind, D. (2007). *The hurried child: 25th anniversary edition*. Cambridge, MA: Da Capo Lifelong Publishing.

Erler, C., & Novak, J. (2010). Bisphenol A exposure: Human risk and health policy. *Journal of Pediatric Nursing, 25*, 400–407.

Federal Interagency Forum on Child and Family Statistics. (2010). *America's children: Key national indicators of well-being 2010*. Washington, DC: U.S. Government Printing Office.

Feldman, J. M. (2008). Caring for incarcerated youth. *Current Opinion in Pediatrics, 20*, 398–402.

Frencher, S. K., Benedicto, C. M., Kendig, T. D., Herman, D., Barlow, B., & Pressley, J. C. (2010). A comparative analysis of serious injury and illness among homeless and housed low-income residents of New York City. *Journal of Trauma, 69*(Suppl. 4), S191–S199.

Galvez, M. P., Graber, N. M., Sheffield, P. E., Forman, J. A., & Balk, S. J. (2009). Hot topics in pediatric environmental health. *Contemporary Pediatrics, 26*(7), 34–47.

Gracious, B., Abe, N., & Sundberg, J. (2010). The importance of taking a history of over-the-counter medication use: A brief review and case illustration of "PRN" antihistamine dependence in a hospitalized adolescent. *Journal of Child and Adolescent Psychopharmacology, 20*, 521–524.

Havens, J. R., Young, A. M., & Havens, C. E. (2011). Nonmedical prescription drug use in a nationally representative sample of adolescents: Evidence of greater use among rural adolescents. *Archives of Pediatrics and Adolescent Medicine, 165*, 250–255.

Health Resources and Services Administration (2009). *The national bullying prevention campaign*. Washington, DC: Author.

Hunter, A. L., Minnis, H., & Wilson, P. (2011). Altered stress responses in children exposed to early adversity: A systematic review of salivary cortisol studies. *Stress, 14*(6), 614–626.

Institute of Medicine. (2011). *The health of lesbian, gay, bisexual and transgender people: Building a foundation for better understanding*. Washington, DC: National Academies Press.

Kaatz, M., Elsner, P., & Bauer, A. (2008). Body-modifying concepts and dermatologic problems: Tattooing and piercing. *Clinics in Dermatology, 26*, 35–44.

Kaiser Family Foundation (2010). *Generation M2: Media in the lives of 8- to 18-year olds*. Retrieved from http://www.kff.org/entmedia/mh012010pkg.cfm

Kaley-Isley, L. C., Peterson, J., Fischer, C., & Peterson, E. (2010). Yoga as a complementary therapy for children and adolescents: A guide for clinicians. *Psychiatry, 7*(8), 20–32.

Kerker, B. D., Bainbridge, J., Kennedy, J., Bennani, Y., Agerton, T., Marder, D., . . . Thorpe, L. E. (2011). A population-based assessment of the health of homeless families in New York City, 2001–2003. *American Journal of Public Health, 101*, 546–553.

Kitts, R. L. (2010). Barriers to optimal care between physicians and lesbian, gay, bisexual, transgender, and questioning adolescent patients. *Journal of Homosexuality, 57*, 730–747.

Klomek, A. B., Marrocco, F., Kleinman, J., Schonfeld, I. S., & Gould, M. S. (2008). Peer victimization, depression and suicidality in adolescents. *Suicide and Life Threatening Behavior, 38*, 166–180.

Kluger, N. (2010) Cutaneous complications related to permanent decorative tattooing. *Expert Reviews in Clinical Immunology, 6*, 363–371.

Knight, J. R. (1997). Adolescent substance use: Screening, assessment, and intervention. *Contemporary Pediatrics, 14*, 45, 51–56, 61–72.

LeBrocque, R. M., Hendrikz, J., & Kenardy, J. A. (2010). The course of posttraumatic stress in children: Examination of recovery trajectories following traumatic injury. *Journal of Pediatric Psychology, 35*, 637–645.

Magzamen, S., Van Sickle, D., Rose, L. D., & Cronk, C. (2011). Environmental pediatrics. *Pediatric Annals, 40*(3), 144–151.

McGregor, T., Parkar, M., & Rao, S. (2009). Evaluation and management of common childhood poisonings. *American Family Physician, 79*(5), 397–403.

National Association for the Education of Young Children. (2010). *Introduction to the NAEYC early childhood program standards and accreditation criteria: Program standards*. Retrieved from http://www.naeyc.org/accreditation

National Center for Biotechnology Information. (2011). *Munchausen syndrome by proxy*. Retrieved from http://www.ncbi.nih.gov/pubmedhealth/PNH0002522/

National Center for Health Statistics & National Vital Statistics System. (2012). *Fatal injury reports, 2008*. Retrieved from http://webapppa.cdc.gov/cgi-bin/broker.exe

National Center for PTSD. (2011). *Child sexual abuse*. Retrieved from http://www.ptsd.va.gov/public/pages/child-sexual-abuse.asp

National Center on Family Homelessness. (2009). *America's youngest outcasts*. Newton, MA: Author.

National Institute of Child Health and Human Development. (2010a). *Add Health Study*. Retrieved from http://www.nichd.nih.gov/health/topics/add_health_study.cfm?renderforprint=1

National Institute of Child Health and Human Development. (2010b). *Study of early child care and youth development*. Retrieved from http://www.nichd.nih.gov/health/topics/seccyd.cfm

National Institute of Child Health and Human Development. (2010c). *What is the national children's study?* Retrieved from http://www.nationalchildrens-study.gov/Pages/default.aspx

National Institute on Alcohol Abuse and Alcoholism (NIAAA). (n.d.). *Snapshot of underage drinking*. Retrieved from http://www.niaaa.nih.gov

National Institute on Alcohol Abuse and Alcoholism (NIAAA). (2009). *Underage drinking research initiative*. Retrieved from http://www.nationalchildrensstudy.gov

National Institute on Drug Abuse. (2011). *NIDA InfoFacts: Club drugs*. Retrieved from http://www.nida/nih.gov/Infofacts/clubdrugs.html and http://www.drugabuse.gov/drugpages/clubdrugs.html

National Institutes of Health. (2009). *Munchausen syndrome by proxy*. Retrieved from http://www.nlm.nih.gov/medlineplus/ency/article/001555.htm

National Safe Kids. (2008). *Report to the nation: Trends in childhood unintentional injury mortality and parental views on child safety*. Retrieved from http://www.usa.safekids.org/assets/docs/ourwork/research/research-report-safe-kids-week-2008.pdf

O'Donnell, K. A., & Ewald, M. B. (2011). Poisonings, In R. M. Kleigman, B. F. Stanton, J. W. St. Geme, N. F. Schor, & R. E. Behrman, *Nelson textbook of pediatrics*, (19th ed., pp. 250–270), Philadelphia, PA: Elsevier.

Oultram, S. (2009). All hail the new flesh: Some thoughts on scarification, children and adults. *Journal of Medical Ethics, 35*, 607–610.

Poster, L., & Weber, S. (2010). Editorial: Special issue on mental health nursing care of LGBT adolescents and young adults. *Journal of Child and Adolescent Psychiatric Nursing, 23*, 1–2.

Rideout, V. J., Foehr, U. G., & Roberts, D. F. (2010). *Generation M²: Media in the lives of 8- to 18-year-olds*. Menlo Park, CA; Kaiser Family Foundation.

Roberts, J. (2010). *Plastics in the environment: How do they affect children?* Retrieved from http://www.medscape.com/viewarticle/725771_print

Sapienza, J. K., & Masten, A. S. (2011). Understanding and promoting resilience in children and youth. *Current Opinion in Psychiatry, 24*, 267–273.

Seifert, S. M., Schaechter, J. L., Hershorin, E. R., & Lipshultz, S. E. (2011). Health effects of energy drinks on children, adolescents and young adults. *Pediatrics, 127*, 511–528.

Shinn, M., Schteingart, J. S., Williams, N. C., Carlin-Mathis, J., Vialo-Karagis, M., Becker-Klein, R., & Weitzman, B. C. (2008). Long-term associations of homelessness with children's well-being. *American Behavioral Scientist, 51*, 789–810.

Srabstein, J. (2008). Deaths linked to bullying and hazing. *International Journal of Adolescent Medicine and Health, 20*, 235–239.

Sullivan, K. M., Bottorff, J., & Reid, C. (2011). Does mother's smoking influence girls' smoking more than boys' smoking? A 20-year review of the literature using a sex- and gender-based analysis. *Substance Use and Misuse, 46*, 656–668.

Surgeon General. (2007). *Surgeon General's call to action to prevent and reduce underage drinking*. Retrieved March 16, 2007, from http://www.surgeongeneral.gov/topics/underagedrinking/about/html

Suwanwaiphatthana, W., Ruangdej, K., & Turner-Henson, A. (2010). Outdoor air pollution and children's health. *Pediatric Nursing, 36*(1), 25–32.

Taylor-Seehafer, M., Jacobvitz, D., & Steiker, L. H. (2008). Patterns of attachment organization, social connectedness, and substance use in a sample of older homeless adolescents: Preliminary findings. *Family and Community Health, 31*(Suppl. 1), S81–S88.

Tehranifar, P., Leighton, J., Auchincloss, A. H., Faciano, A., Alpert, H., ... Wu, S. (2008). Immigration and risk of childhood lead poisoning: findings from a case-control study of New York City children. *American Journal of Public Health, 98,* 92–97.

UNICEF. (2009). *Promoting synergy between child protection and social protection.* Retrieved from http://www.unicef.org/wcaro/wcaro_UNICEF_ODI_5_Child_Protection.pdf

U.S. Department of Health and Human Services. (2009a). *Physical activity guidelines for Americans.* Retrieved from http://www.health.gov.paguidelines/guidelines.default.aspx

U.S. Department of Health and Human Services. (2009b). *Domestic violence and the child welfare system.* Retrieved from http://www.childwelfare.gov/pubs/factsheets/domesticviolence.cfm

U.S. Department of Health and Human Services. (2011). *Healthy People 2020.* Washington, DC: Author.

U.S. Environmental Protection Agency. (2010). *Health effects of exposure to secondhand smoke.* Retrieved from http://www.epa.gov/smokefre.healtheffects.html

U.S. Environmental Protection Agency. (2011). *Mercury releases and spills.* Retrieved from http://publicaccess.supportportal.com/ics/support/default.asp?deptID=23012&task=knowledge&folderID=950

Warniment, C., Tsang, K., & Galazka, S. S. (2010). Lead poisoning in children. *American Family Physician, 81*(6), 751–757.

Weber, S. (2009). Policy aspects and nursing care of families with parents who are sexual minorities. *Journal of Family Nursing 15,* 384–399.

Wengrovitz, A. M., & Brown, M. J. (2009). Recommendations for blood lead screening of Medicaid-eligible children aged 1–5 years: An updated approach to targeting a group at high risk. *Morbidity and Mortality Weekly Report, 58*(RR-9), 1–14.

White, L. S. (2009). Yoga for children. *Pediatric Nursing, 35,* 277–283.

Woolf, A. D., Goldman, R., & Bellinger, D. C. (2007). Update on the clinical management of childhood lead poisoning. *Pediatric Clinics of North America, 54,* 271–294.

World Health Organization. (2011). *Violence and injury prevention and disability: Prevention of child maltreatment.* Retrieved from http://www.who.int/violence_injury_prevention/violence/activities/child_maltreatment/en/

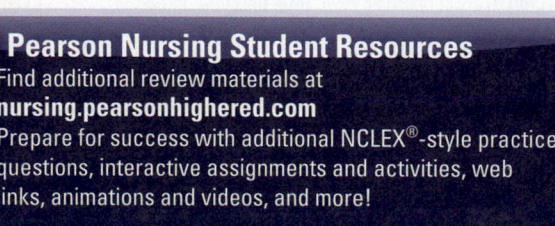

Pearson Nursing Student Resources

Find additional review materials at
nursing.pearsonhighered.com
Prepare for success with additional NCLEX®-style practice questions, interactive assignments and activities, web links, animations and videos, and more!

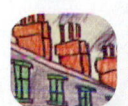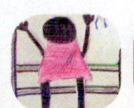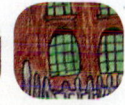

Pain Assessment and Management

KEY TERMS

Learning Outcomes

After completing this chapter, you will be able to:

1. Explain the pathophysiology of pain as well as the physiology that enables nonpainful touch and massage to help reduce pain.

2. Summarize the physiologic and behavioral consequences of pain in infants and children.

3. Analyze the behaviors of an infant or a child to assess for pain.

4. Assess a young child's readiness to use a self-report pain scale.

5. Calculate an opioid dose and describe the methods used to administer opioids to children.

6. Examine the role of nonpharmacologic (complementary) interventions in effective pain management.

7. Plan the nursing care for an infant or child in acute pain that integrates pharmacologic interventions and developmentally appropriate nonpharmacologic (complementary) therapies.

8. Distinguish between the clinical therapies used for acute and chronic pain.

9. Compare the effectiveness of pain management strategies for procedures such as venipuncture and immunizations.

10. Plan the nursing care for the child to be given sedation and analgesia for a medical procedure.

"I don't know how bad the pain will be from this operation. I hardly ever take anything for pain after hurting myself. Is this going to be worse than the time I got a bad cut on my leg?"

—Lucas, age 14

Lucas Aronson, 14 years old, is being prepared to undergo orthopedic surgery to stabilize a slipped capital femoral epiphysis. During his preoperative teaching, the nurse shows Lucas how to use a pain scale, explaining what each of the faces means. The nurse tells Lucas that he will be asked to point to the face that matches how much he hurts several times after his operation. Lucas is asked about the most pain he has ever felt, and what caused that pain. The nurse will use that information to help Lucas identify the amount of pain he has during future pain assessments. Lucas is also encouraged to tell the nurse or his parents when he has pain after the operation so that he can be given medication to relieve the pain.

The nurse also discusses the importance of assessing and treating pain with Lucas's parents, as Lucas will go home after one night in the hospital. The nurse lets them know that controlling Lucas's pain will make it easier for him to move around and it promotes healing.

Why is it important to manage a child's pain? In addition to using a pain scale, what information will the nurse use to assess Lucas's postoperative pain? How is pain treated in children?

very child has his or her own perception of pain. A neurologic response to tissue injury, **pain** is an unpleasant sensory and emotional experience associated with actual or potential tissue damage (Pappagallo & Werner, 2008). Much of the acute pain infants and children feel associated with medical conditions and procedures can be prevented or greatly relieved. Effective pain management is every child's right. Management of pain involves an age-appropriate assessment of pain, selecting and implementing an appropriate method to relieve pain, and evaluating the effectiveness of the intervention (Twycross, 2009). The nurse needs a thorough understanding of pain pathophysiology and pharmacology to select appropriate interventions.

PAIN

Pain may be either acute or chronic. **Acute pain** is sudden pain of short duration; it may be associated with a single event, such as surgery or an injury that can be linked to the pain discomfort. It may also be associated with an acute exacerbation of a condition such as a sickle cell crisis. An immediate pain response occurs right at the time of tissue damage. The inflammatory response following the initial tissue injury helps sustain the pain response. The pain often decreases and ends as healing occurs.

Chronic pain is persistent, lasting longer than 3 months; it is often associated with a prolonged disease process such as juvenile idiopathic arthritis or cancer. Chronic pain may be nociceptive or neuropathic pain. **Nociceptive pain** is the normal processing of pain stimuli caused by tissue injury or damage. **Neuropathic pain** is an abnormal processing of pain stimuli by the peripheral or central nervous system, and may be initiated or caused by a primary lesion or dysfunction of the nervous system. See page 594 for more information on chronic pain.

Pathophysiology of Pain

Nociceptors are free nerve endings at the site of tissue damage that are activated from a chemical, mechanical, or thermal injury. Nociceptors are activated by substances such as bradykinin, prostaglandins, serotonin, histamine, and substance P that make it possible to begin the transmission of pain impulses from the nerve endings to the spinal cord. Two fibers are responsible for the transmission of pain stimuli from the injury site to the dorsal horn of the spinal cord. The large, myelinated A-delta fibers quickly transmit sharp pain that is localized and triggers a protective withdrawal response (Figure 21–1 ■). The small, unmyelinated C fibers slowly transmit pain impulses associated with burning or aching diffuse pain. A-beta fibers transmit touch, movement, and vibration impulses rather than pain impulses between the nerve endings and dorsal horn of the spine (Pasero & McCaffery, 2011, p. 6).

After sensory information reaches the substantia gelatinosa in the dorsal horn of the spinal cord, the pain signal is then transmitted

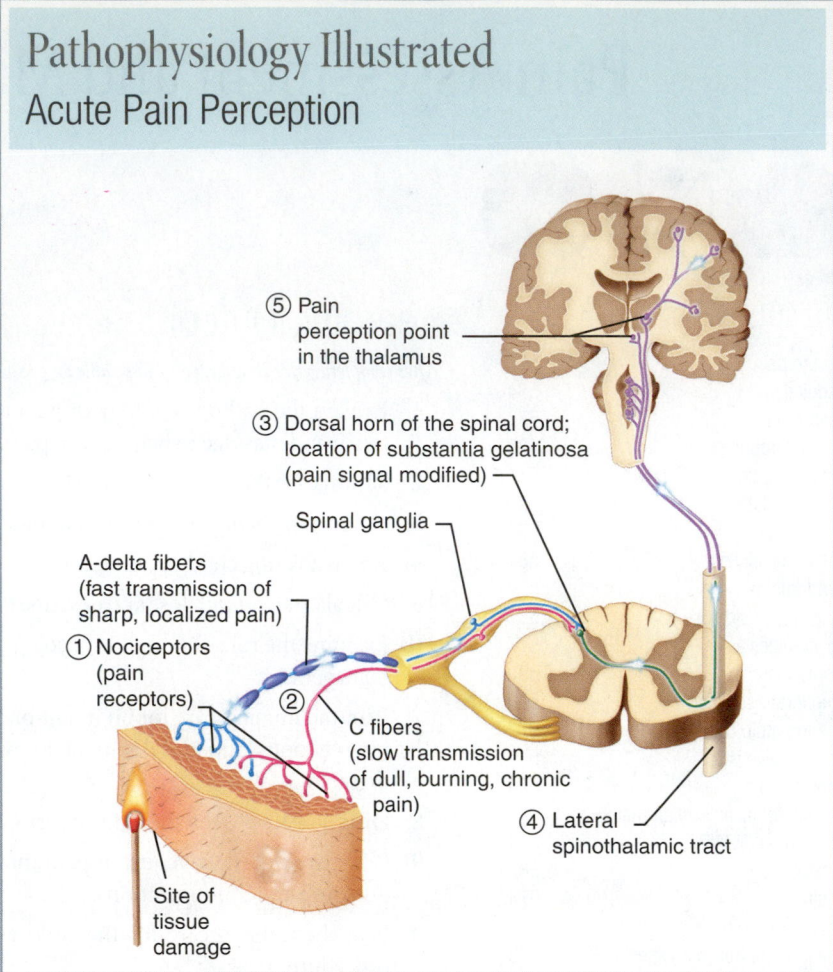

Pathophysiology Illustrated
Acute Pain Perception

⑤ Pain perception point in the thalamus

③ Dorsal horn of the spinal cord; location of substantia gelatinosa (pain signal modified)

Spinal ganglia

A-delta fibers (fast transmission of sharp, localized pain)

① Nociceptors (pain receptors)

②

C fibers (slow transmission of dull, burning, chronic pain)

④ Lateral spinothalamic tract

Site of tissue damage

FIGURE 21–1 ■ 1 Nociceptors (free nerve endings at the site of tissue damage) transmit information via specialized nerve fibers to the spinal cord.
2 Unmyelinated C fibers slowly transmit dull, burning, diffuse pain as well as chronic pain. Large, myelinated A-delta fibers quickly transmit sharp, well-localized pain. Nociceptors are stimulated by mechanical, thermal, and chemical injury. Biochemical mediators (bradykinin, prostaglandin, serotonin, histamine, and substance P) are produced in response to tissue damage. These substances help move the pain impulse from the nerve endings to the spinal cord.
3 After the sensory information reaches the substantia gelatinosa in the dorsal horn of the spinal cord, the pain signal may be modified depending on the presence of other stimuli, from either the brain or the periphery.
4 The pain signal is then transmitted through the lateral spinothalamic tract, to the thalamus of the brain where perception occurs.
5 Once the sensation reaches the brain, interpretation of pain occurs, and emotional responses may increase or decrease the intensity of the pain perceived.

to the thalamus of the brain primarily through the ascending spinal tracts. The thalamus is the main relay station for sensory information. Pain information is then transmitted to the cerebral cortex as well as the reticular and limbic systems for the processing and interpretation of pain, leading to the conscious awareness of pain. The pain signal may be modified depending on the presence of other stimuli, either from the brain or from the periphery.

A two-way control of nociceptive transmission occurs within the brain, spinal tracts, and dorsal horn. Some substances, such as **endorphins** (exogenous opioids), serotonin, and norepinephrine can *modulate* (change or inhibit) the pain perceived. Pain perception can also be modulated when a competing nonpain impulse is sent along the same pathways used for pain transmission.

Neonatal Pathophysiology

Do neonates have the ability to feel pain like other children? Infants at 25 weeks' gestation have activation of the brain cortex in response to pain (Badr, Abdallah, Hawari, et al., 2010). By the middle of the third trimester, the ascending pain-transmitting fibers are fully connected to the brain cortex, and the newborn has functioning pathways for pain sensation (Kennedy, Luhmann, & Zempsky, 2008). However, nociceptive processing by newborns is different due to their neurophysiologic and cognitive immaturity. Since myelination of spinal fibers continues after birth, most pain impulses in newborns are transmitted along the nonmyelinated C fibers rather than the A-delta fibers. The transmitted pain signal is less precise. Even though the pain transmitted is along the slower C fibers, the distance from the site of pain to the brain is shorter than in adults.

Practice Alert

The maturation of the preterm newborn is important with regard to the amount of pain behaviors exhibited by preterm infants. Newborns at less than 28 weeks' gestation may have a dampened pain behavioral response. Frequent painful procedures may also make preterm infants, especially sick newborns, too fatigued to show pain behaviors (Badr et al., 2010).

Misconceptions About Pain in Children

Healthcare professionals once believed that infants and children feel less pain than adults. Underestimation and undertreatment of pain in infants and children was based on this belief. Healthcare professionals now recognize that children of all ages feel pain, just as adults do. Other barriers to effective pain management of infants and children include the difficulty and complexity of pain assessment as well as inadequate research. For a review of past myths and the contrasting reality, see Table 21–1.

Developmental Aspects of Pain Perception, Memory, and Response

Although every infant and child perceives pain, their understanding, response to pain, and memory of painful events change as they develop. A number of factors influence the pain perceived by the child, including maturation of the nervous system, the child's developmental stage, and previous pain experiences. See Table 21–2 to learn more about the child's understanding of pain as well as the behavioral and verbal responses to pain at each age.

Memory of a past painful experience can trigger anticipatory anxiety that elevates a child's pain response (Walco, 2008). The child's memory and response to anticipated pain are also related to developmental stage. As described below, newborns and infants develop a memory of pain. Preschool-age children demonstrate pain memory by making efforts to delay a painful procedure.

Children's responses to acute or chronic pain are influenced by factors such as memory of a past painful experience, their temperament, their ability to control what will happen, their use of a pain coping mechanism, and emotions like fear or anxiety (Walco, 2008). Depending on their developmental stage, children use different

TABLE 21–1	Misconceptions About Pain in Infants and Children
MYTH	**REALITY**
Neonates and infants are incapable of feeling pain. Children do not feel pain with the same intensity as adults because a child's nervous system is immature.	The anatomic and physiologic aspects for pain transmission develop during the third trimester. Preterm and full-term neonates may be more sensitive to pain stimuli. The descending neurotransmitters from the brain to the dorsal horn of the spinal cord are not fully developed at birth, and neonates are less able to modulate pain impulses (Kennedy et al., 2008).
Infants are incapable of expressing pain.	Infants express pain with both behavioral and physiologic cues that can be assessed.
Infants and children have no memory of pain.	It is believed that painful episodes can be encoded into the child's memories, and numerous studies have documented that preterm and full-term neonates have a pain memory. For example, neonates who had numerous heelsticks associated the smell of alcohol with heelsticks and had higher pain responses than neonates without numerous heelsticks (Kennedy et al., 2008).
Parents exaggerate their child's pain.	Parents know their child and are able to identify when the child is in pain.
Children are not in pain if they can be distracted or they are sleeping.	Children use **distraction** (engaging in a pleasant activity to help focus attention on something other than pain) to cope with pain, but they soon become exhausted when coping with pain and fall asleep.
Repeated experiences with pain teach children to be more tolerant of pain and cope with it better. They become accustomed to pain after having it for a while.	Children who have more experience with pain respond more vigorously to pain, rather than tolerating the discomfort. Experience with pain teaches the child how severe the pain can become. For example, children experiencing prior painful cancer treatment procedures reported greater pain during procedures performed later, even when adequate analgesia was used (Kennedy et al., 2008).
Children recover more quickly than adults from painful experiences such as surgery.	Children heal quickly from surgery, but they have the same amount of pain from surgery as an adult.
Children tell you if they are in pain. They do not need medication unless they appear to be in pain.	Children may be too young to express pain or afraid to tell anyone other than a parent about the pain. The child may fear the treatment for pain will be worse than the pain itself.
Children without obvious physical reasons for pain are not likely to have pain.	The cause of pain cannot always be determined. The feeling of pain is subjective and should be accepted by nurses.
Children run the risk of becoming addicted to pain medication when used for pain management.	Addiction is extremely rare when the child is treated for an acute condition (less than 1%) (Twycross, 2009, p. 40).

TABLE 21–2	The Child's Understanding of Pain, Behavioral Responses, and Verbal Descriptions of Pain by Developmental Stage		
AGE GROUP	**UNDERSTANDING OF PAIN**	**BEHAVIORAL RESPONSE**	**VERBAL DESCRIPTION**
Infant			
Under 6 months	No apparent understanding of pain; responsive to parental anxiety	Generalized body movements, chin quivering Facial grimacing Poor feeding	Cries
6–12 months	Has a memory of pain; responsive to parental anxiety	Reflex withdrawal to stimulus Facial grimacing Disturbed sleep, irritability, restlessness	Cries
Toddler			
1–3 years	Lacks understanding of what causes pain and why he or she might be experiencing it	Demonstrates fear of painful situations May resist with entire body or have localized withdrawal Aggressive behavior Disturbed sleep	Cries and wails, cannot describe intensity or type of pain May use common words for pain such as *owie* and *boo-boo* after age 2 years
Preschooler			
3–6 years (preoperational)	Pain is a *hurt* Does not relate pain to illness but may relate pain to an injury Often believes pain is punishment or someone else is responsible for his or her pain Unable to understand why a painful procedure will help him or her feel better	Active physical resistance Directed aggressive behavior, strikes out physically and verbally when hurt Easily frustrated	Has the language skills to express pain on a sensory level Can identify location and intensity of pain May deny pain May believe his or her pain is obvious to others
School-Age Child			
7–9 years (concrete operations)	Understands simple relationships between pain and disease Understands the need for painful procedures to monitor or treat disease May associate pain with feeling bad or angry May recognize psychologic pain related to grief and hurt feelings	Passive resistance Clenches fists, holds body rigidly still Suffers emotional withdrawal Engages in plea bargaining	Can specify location and intensity of pain Can describe pain's physical characteristics in relation to body parts
10–12 years (transitional)	Has a better understanding of the relationship between an event and pain Has a more complex awareness of physical and psychologic pain, such as moral dilemmas and mental pain	May pretend comfort to project bravery May regress with stress and anxiety	Able to describe intensity and location with more characteristics Able to describe psychologic pain
Adolescent			
13–18 years (formal operations)	Has a capacity for sophisticated and complex understanding of the causes of physical and mental pain Recognizes that pain has both qualitative and quantitative characteristics Can relate to the pain experienced by others	Wants to behave in a socially acceptable manner (like adults), shows a controlled behavioral response May immerse self in an activity as a pain distraction May not complain about pain if given cues from nurses and other healthcare providers who believe it should be tolerated	More sophisticated descriptions as experience is gained Uses common meanings of words to describe pain (*pain, hurt, ache*) similar to adults May think nurses are attuned to his or her thoughts, so it is unnecessary to tell the nurse about the pain

coping strategies to deal with their pain (such as escape, postponement or avoidance, diversion, and imagery).

Children may not complain of pain for several reasons:

- Young children are unable to give a detailed description of their pain because of their limited vocabulary and pain experiences.
- Some children believe they need to be brave and do not want to worry their parents.
- Preschoolers and adolescents may assume the nurse knows they have pain.
- Some children are afraid that the pain treatment will hurt more than the pain they are already feeling.

Cultural Influences on Pain

Little evidence exists that there are significant or predictable differences in sensory aspects of pain perception between racial and ethnic groups (Finley, Kristjánsdóttir, & Forgeron, 2009). However, culture and social learning greatly influence a child's expression of pain. Infants and children may express pain, but they are dependent upon parents and caregivers to recognize their pain and respond. Children learn directly and indirectly from their parents and extended family about the normal or right way to respond to pain. They observe family members in pain and try to imitate their responses. By showing approval and disapproval, parents teach their children how to behave

Developing Cultural Competence
Examine Your Own Experience

Think about your childhood pain experiences and how your family encouraged you to be stoic or to express pain. These types of experiences often contribute to a health professional's attitudes about pain management. For example, some healthcare providers (as well as parents) may believe that being in pain for a little while is not so bad, that pain helps build character. However, all nurses need to acknowledge the child's right to pain management, the current standard of care.

when in pain. Children learn how much pain should be tolerated and how much discomfort justifies a complaint. They also learn how to express a complaint of pain and who to approach for pain relief. Depending upon cultural values, some caregivers may not believe that all pain needs treatment while others readily provide pain relief. See Developing Cultural Competence: Examine Your Own Experience.

Many ethnic groups, such as Anglo-Saxon–Germanic, Irish, Amish, and Appalachian, encourage a more stoic response in which expression of pain is diminished. Other ethnic groups, such as people of Italian and Jewish descent, are more likely to use both verbal and nonverbal methods (moans and groans) to express pain freely (Purnell, 2009). Some groups are more comfortable expressing pain to family members than to healthcare providers. However, be careful to avoid stereotyping. Not all members of an ethnic group will demonstrate the same pain response. Children will have individualized responses to pain based on past experiences, and younger children have had less time to acquire culturally learned behaviors.

Physiologic Consequences of Pain

Unrelieved pain is stressful and has many undesirable physiologic consequences on several body systems (Table 21–3). For example, the child with acute postoperative pain takes shallow breaths and suppresses coughing to avoid more pain. These self-protective actions increase the potential for respiratory complications. Unrelieved pain may also delay the return of normal gastric and bowel functions and lead to occult gastrointestinal bleeding. Anorexia associated with pain may delay the healing process. In addition to elevations in vital signs, an increased release of catecholamines, glucagon, and corticosteroids occurs.

Effects on Newborns

Unrelieved pain can result in a catabolic state that can have a serious effect on newborns and young infants with higher metabolic rates and fewer nutritional reserves. Pain in the newborn and infant drains energy resources needed for growth and healing. Stress responses include increases in the vital signs and intracranial pressure. The autonomic nervous system signs include gagging, hiccupping, vomiting, dilated pupils, and forehead and palmar sweating (Zeitzer & Krane, 2011).

Because the newborn's brain is developing so rapidly, repeated painful experiences are thought to alter nerve pathways and lead to hypersensitivity to pain and a greater behavioral response to painful events, such as immunizations (Kennedy et al., 2008). Concerns are increasing that the long-term consequences of repetitive pain in newborns may include an increased pain response, **hyperalgesia** (increased response to a pain stimulus because of peripheral nerves are sensitized) and even **allodynia** (hypersensitivity to light touch) (Walco, 2008).

TABLE 21–3	Physiologic Consequences of Unrelieved Pain in Children	
RESPONSES TO PAIN	**POTENTIAL PHYSIOLOGIC CONSEQUENCES**
Respiratory Changes	
Rapid shallow breathing	Alkalosis
Inadequate lung expansion	Decreased oxygen saturation, atelectasis
Inadequate cough	Retention of secretions
Neurologic Changes	
Increased sympathetic nervous system activity and release of catecholamines	Tachycardia, elevated blood pressure, change in sleep patterns
Metabolic Changes	
Increased metabolic rate with increased perspiration	Increased losses of fluid and electrolytes
	Increased blood glucose and cortisol levels
Immune System Changes	
Depression of immune and anti-inflammatory responses	Increased risk of infection, delayed wound healing
Gastrointestinal Changes	
Decreased gastric acid secretions and intestinal motility	Impaired gastrointestinal functioning, nausea, anorexia, ileus
Altered Pain Response	
Increased pain sensitivity	Hyperalgesia, decreased **pain threshold** (the point at which pain is felt), exaggerated memory of painful experiences

Source: *Data from Greenwald, M. (2010). Analgesia for the pediatric trauma patient: Primum non nocere?* Clinical Pediatric Emergency Medicine, 11*(1), 28–40; Walden, M. (2007). Pain in the newborn and infant. In C. Kenner & J. W. Lott,* Comprehensive neonatal nursing: An interdisciplinary approach *(4th ed., pp. 360–371). Philadelphia: Elsevier Saunders; Huether, S. E. (2010). Pain, temperature regulation, and sensory function. In K. L. McCance & S. E. Huether (Eds.),* Pathophysiology: The biologic basis for disease in adults and children *(6th ed., pp. 481–524). St. Louis, MO: Mosby Elsevier.*

PAIN ASSESSMENT

The goal of pain assessment is to provide accurate information about the location and intensity of pain and its effects on the child's functioning.

Pain History

Parents and caregivers can provide a great deal of information about the child's response to pain and its effects on the child's functioning, such as the following:

- How the child typically expresses pain, both verbally and behaviorally. Children and parents use similar terms to describe pain. Using the same word that the child uses makes communicating with the child easier (Box 21–1).
- The child's previous experiences with painful situations and how the child responded.
- How the child copes with and manages pain. The child with several past pain experiences may not exhibit the same types of stressful behaviors as the child with few pain experiences.
- What works best to reduce the child's pain.
- The parent's and child's preferences for analgesic use and other pain interventions.

Older children may be able to give a history of painful episodes. When attempting to obtain information about the child's pain experiences and present level of pain, keep in mind that many children modify their pain descriptions depending on the type of questions

BOX 21–1	Words Used by Young Children for Pain

Young children are unable to give a detailed description of their pain because of limited vocabulary and pain experiences. Children slowly acquire words for pain over the first 6 years of life. Toddlers and preschoolers use *ouch* and *hurt* to describe pain. Use of the words *pain* and *sore* is not common before 6 years of age (Kuttner, 2010, p. 100). Other pain words include *owie, boo-boo, ache, stinging, cutting, burning, itching, hot,* and *tight*.

asked and what they expect will happen as a result of their response. Some questions to ask the child include:

- "What kinds of things caused hurt in the past? What made the hurt feel better?"
- "What do you tell your mother (or other significant person) when you hurt (or are in pain)? What do you want your mother to do for the hurt?"
- "What would you like the nurse to do when you are hurt? What should the nurse or anyone else do when you are hurt?"
- "Where do you hurt? What does it feel like? What do you think is causing the hurt?"

Pain Assessment Scales

Pain assessment tools for children have been developed and tested primarily to evaluate procedural and postsurgical pain. These tools have been designed to enable developmentally appropriate assessment of pain, and as a result may measure the following:

- Behavioral measures, such as expression, positioning, movement, and crying
- Self-report or how the child quantifies the pain

Physiologic parameters, such as heart rate, respiratory rate and pattern, oxygen saturation, and blood pressure may also be apparent when the child has pain, but no pain assessment tool has yet been developed using these parameters.

Many tools have been tested for **validity** (the extent to which an instrument or scale measures what it is supposed to measure) and **reliability** (the extent to which the same score is obtained when an instrument or scale is used either by different persons or by the same person at different times). Some of the more commonly used pain assessment tools for different age groups with good validity and reliability are presented on the following pages.

Behavioral Pain Scales for Newborns

Assessment tools that combine behavioral and physiologic signs are the most valid for health professionals to use in rating the level of pain in infants and nonverbal children. These scales rely on the nurse's observation of the child. It is important to ensure that all elements of the pain scale can be evaluated; for example, an infant cannot cry if intubated.

Neonatal infant pain scale The Neonatal Infant Pain Scale (NIPS) was developed to evaluate procedural pain in preterm and full-term neonates up to 6 weeks after birth (Table 21–4). The neonate's facial expression, cry quality, breathing patterns, arm and leg position, and state of arousal are observed. The tool has good interrater reliability and validity (Twycross et al., 2009, p. 101).

CRIES scale The CRIES Scale was developed to evaluate postoperative pain in preterm and full-term neonates in the intensive care unit

TABLE 21–4	Neonatal Infant Pain Scale (NIPS)
CHARACTERISTIC	**SCORING CRITERIA**
Facial Expression 0 = Relaxed muscles 1 = Grimace	■ Restful face with neutral expression ■ Tight facial muscles; furrowed brow, chin, and jaw (Note: At low gestational ages, infants may have no facial expression.)
CRY 0 = No cry 1 = Whimper 2 = Vigorous CRY	■ Quiet, not crying ■ Mild moaning, intermittent cry ■ Loud screaming, rising, shrill, and continuous (Note: Silent cry may be scored if infant is intubated, as indicated by obvious facial movements.)
Breathing Patterns 0 = Relaxed 1 = Change in breathing	■ Relaxed, usual breathing pattern maintained ■ Change in breathing, irregular, faster than usual, gagging, or holding breath
Arm Movements 0 = Relaxed/restrained (with soft restraints) 1 = Flexed/extended	■ Relaxed, no muscle rigidity, occasional random movements of arms ■ Tense, straight arms; rigid; or rapid extension and flexion
Leg Movements 0 = Relaxed/restrained (with soft restraints) 1 = Flexed/extended	■ Relaxed, no muscle rigidity, occasional random movements of legs ■ Tense, straight legs; rigid; or rapid extension and flexion
State of Arousal 0 = Sleeping/awake 1 = Fussy	■ Quiet, peaceful, sleeping; or alert and settled ■ Alert and restless or thrashing; fussy

Source: From Lawrence, J., Alcock, D., McGrath, P., et al. (1993). The development of a tool to assess neonatal pain. Neonatal Network, 12(6), 61; Morrow, C. (2010). Reducing neonatal pain during routine heel lance procedures. MCN American Journal of Maternal Child Nursing, 35(6), 346–354.

(ICU). This tool has been demonstrated to have validity and good interrater reliability for procedural and surgical pain (Twycross et al., 2009, p. 101). See the companion website for a copy of this scale.

Behavioral indicators of infant pain The Behavioral Indicators of Infant Pain (BIIP) was developed to evaluate acute pain in preterm infants. Behavioral indicators of pain (sleep/wake state, five facial actions, and two hand actions) that were previously validated for assessing neonatal pain were combined into an assessment tool. The tool has demonstrated validity and interrater reliability for assessing acute pain in preterm infants (Holsti, 2008).

Premature infant pain profile The Premature Infant Pain Profile (PIPP) was developed to evaluate procedural pain in preterm and full-term neonates between 28 and 40 weeks' gestation (Table 21–5). It rates pain behaviors (brow bulge, eye squeeze, and nasolabial furrow), physiologic measures (heart rate and oxygen saturation), and two other parameters (gestational age and behavioral state) with a score from 0 to 3 for each. The tool has been validated for use with procedural pain, and it has good interrater reliability (Stevens, 2010).

TABLE 21–5	Premature Infant Pain Profile			
		Scoring		
INDICATOR	**0**	**1**	**2**	**3**
Gestational age	Greater than or equal to 36 weeks	32 weeks to 35 weeks 6 days	28 weeks to 31 weeks 6 days	Less than 28 weeks
Behavioral state	Active/awake, eyes open, face movements	Quiet/awake, eyes open, no facial movements	Active/sleep, eyes closed, facial movements	Quiet/sleep, eyes closed, no facial movements
Heart rate maximum	0–4 beats per minute increase	5–14 beats per minute increase	15–24 beats per minute increase	Greater than or equal to 25 beats per minute increase
Oxygen saturation minimum	0 to 2.4% decrease	2.5 to 4.9% decrease	5.0 to 7.4% decrease	7.5% decrease or more
Brow bulge	None (less than or equal to 9% of time)	Minimum (10–39% of time)	Moderate (40–69% of time)	Maximum (greater than or equal to 70% of time)
Eye squeeze	None (less than or equal to 9% of time)	Minimum (10–39% of time)	Moderate (40–69% of time)	Maximum (greater than or equal to 70% of time)
Nasolabial furrow	None (less than or equal to 9% of time)	Minimum (10–39% of time)	Moderate (40–69% of time)	Maximum (greater than or equal to 70% of time)

Note: Scoring: Score the gestational age before assessing the infant. Observe the infant for 15 seconds to score the behavioral scale before the potential painful event. Record the baseline heart rate and oxygen saturation. Observe the infant for 30 seconds immediately following the painful event. Score the physiologic and facial changes seen during this time and record immediately. Sum the score for all 7 indicators. The maximum score is 21. The higher the score the greater the pain behavior.

Source: *Stevens, B., Johnston, C., Petryshen, P., & Taddio, A. (1996). Premature infant pain profile: Development and initial validation. Clinical Journal of Pain, 12, 13–22; Stevens, B. (2010). The premature infant pain profile: Evaluation 13 years after development. Clinical Journal of Pain,26(9), 813–830.*

Behavioral Pain Scales for Infants and Young Children

Face, legs, activity, cry, and consolability (FLACC) observational tool The FLACC Observational Pain Assessment Tool is an easily administered tool to assess acute pain in infants and young children following surgery (Table 21–6). This tool is most commonly used in clinical practice with children between 2 months and 7 years, or until the child is able to self-report pain with another pain scale. FLACC is an acronym for the five assessment categories: face, legs, activity, cry, and consolability. To use the FLACC, observe the child during routine care for 1 to 5 minutes, and then select the score that most closely matches the behavior of each category. The scores for the five categories are added together for the total score. The tool has validity and reliability for evaluation of postoperative pain.

Assessing Children with Cognitive Impairment

Assessing the pain of a child with cognitive impairment is equally as challenging as with the nonverbal child. While some children with cognitive impairment may be able to use simple self-report pain tools, others will not. In these cases, pain assessment tools with behavioral and physiologic indicators will be appropriate.

Noncommunicating children's pain checklist The Noncommunicating Children's Pain Checklist (NCCPC) was designed specifically for children with cognitive impairment. The checklist includes numerous items for each of the following categories: vocal sounds, social, facial features, activity, body and limb movements, and physiologic signs. This tool can be used to assess postoperative pain and pain in the home setting (Ghai, Makkar, & Wig, 2008). The child is observed over a 10-minute session to assess how frequently each checklist item is observed. Specific score ranges have been associated with mild and moderate to severe pain (Breau & Burkitt, 2009).

Revised FLACC The FLACC with some modifications can be successfully used by parents to assess postoperative pain in children with cognitive impairment. Before surgery the parent identifies pain behaviors the child displays, such as a specific facial expression, physical body movement, behavioral emotional change, or self-injurious behavior. These behaviors are added to the descriptors for the scores in each of the FLACC categories. This tool has shown good validity and interrater reliability for use in this population (Ghai et al., 2008). Testing has revealed better agreement between parent and nurse scoring using this customized tool than with other pain assessment tools. The Revised FLACC may be more easily adapted for clinical practice than the NCCPC or other pain assessment tools in this population (Voepel-Lewis, Malviya, Tait, et al., 2008).

Self-Report Pain Rating Tools for Children

Self-report assessment tools are considered to be the best method of assessing pain in children and adolescents who can provide such information. Once the child has developed number concepts, a self-report tool to assess pain can be used. Examples of self-report tools developed for children include the Faces Pain Rating Scale, the Oucher Scale, and the Color Analogue Scale.

Assessing readiness to use self-report pain rating tools How will you know if a young child 3 to 5 years old is able to answer to how much pain he or she has? Young children gradually develop the understanding of concepts important in being able to use pain scales. The child must understand the basic concept of a little or a lot of pain well enough to communicate about it. Assess the child's language skills—ability to use words in sequence, follow simple directions, and answer simple questions.

Children 2 to 3 years old are usually able to understand the concept of "more or less." With the development of this concept, the child cannot be given more than three choices on a pain scale (none, some, a lot) to assess the amount of pain. Some children at age 3 to 4 years can understand rank order and magnitude, enabling the child to use a self-report pain rating tool.

TABLE 21–6	FLACC Observational Pain Assessment Tool		
Categories	**Scoring**		
	0	**1**	**2**
Face	No particular expression or smile	Occasional grimace or frown; withdrawn, disinterested	Frequent to constant frown, clenched jaw, quivering chin
Legs	Normal position or relaxed	Uneasy, restless, tense	Kicking or legs drawn up
Activity	Lying quietly, normal position, moves easily	Squirming, shifting back and forth, tense	Arched, rigid, or jerking
Cry	No cry (awake or asleep)	Moans or whimpers, occasional complaint	Crying steadily, screams or sobs; frequent complaints
Consolability	Content, relaxed	Reassured by occasional touching, hugging, or being talked to; distractible	Difficult to console or comfort

Guidelines for Scoring the FLACC

Face

Score 0 if the patient has a relaxed face, makes eye contact, shows interest in surroundings.

Score 1 if the patient has a worried facial expression, with eyebrows lowered, eyes partially closed, cheeks raised, mouth pursed.

Score 2 if the patient has deep furrows in the forehead, closed eyes, an open mouth, deep lines around nose and lips.

Legs

Score 0 if the muscle tone and motion in the limbs are normal.

Score 1 if the patient has increased tone, rigidity, or tension; if there is intermittent flexion or extension of the limbs.

Score 2 if the patient has hypertonicity, the legs are pulled tight, there is exaggerated flexion or extension of the limbs, tremors.

Activity

Score 0 if the patient moves easily and freely, normal activity or restrictions.

Score 1 if the patient shifts positions, appears hesitant to move, demonstrates guarding, a tense torso, pressure on a body part.

Score 2 if the patient is in a fixed position, rocking; demonstrates side-to-side head movement or rubbing of a body part.

Cry

Score 0 if the patient has no cry or moan, awake or asleep.

Score 1 if the patient has occasional moans, cries, whimpers, sighs.

Score 2 if the patient has frequent or continuous moans, cries, grunts.

Consolability

Score 0 if the patient is calm and does not require consoling.

Score 1 if the patient responds to comfort by touching or talking in 30 seconds to 1 minute.

Score 2 if the patient requires constant comforting or is inconsolable.

Interpreting the Behavioral Score

Each category is scored on the 0–2 scale, which results in a total score of 0–10.

0 = Relaxed and comfortable   **4–6** = Moderate pain

1–3 = Mild discomfort   **7–10** = Severe discomfort or pain or both

Source: From Merkel, S. I., Voepel-Lewis, T., Shayevitz, J. R., & Malviya, S. (1997). The FLACC: A behavioral scale for scoring postoperative pain in young children. Pediatric Nursing, 23(3), 293–297; Voepel-Lewis, T., Zanotti, J., & Dammeyer, J. A. (2010). Reliability and validity of the face, legs, activity, cry, consolability behavioral tool in assessing acute pain in critically ill patients. American Journal of Critical Care, 19(1), 55–62. The FLACC scale was developed by Sandra Merkel, MS, RN; Terri Voepel-Lewis, MS, RN; and Shobha Malviya, MD, at C. S. Mott Children's Hospital, University of Michigan Health System, Ann Arbor, MI. Used with permission.

Clinical Tip

The young child's development of number and rank order concepts can be evaluated with either of the following tasks:

- Ask the child which number is larger, 5 or 9? Then ask which number is smaller, 7 or 4?
- Ask the child to place several blocks or pieces of paper of different sizes in a row from biggest to smallest.

If a correct response is given to either task, then the child is ready to use a self-report pain rating tool.

Preschool and school-age children

Faces pain rating scale The Faces Pain Rating Scale has a series of six or seven cartoon-like faces with expressions from smiling (or neutral) to tearful, depending upon the model selected. The Wong-Baker scale is commonly used (Figure 21–2 ■). Children as young as 3 years of age can use this tool if they understand number and rank order concepts. After explanations about the meaning for each face, the child selects the face that is the closest match to the pain felt. The nurse should not use the tool to compare with the child's facial

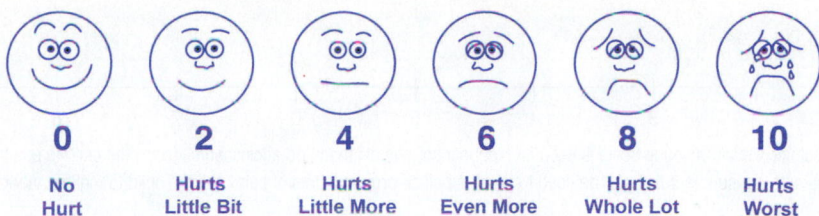

0	**2**	**4**	**6**	**8**	**10**
No Hurt	Hurts Little Bit	Hurts Little More	Hurts Even More	Hurts Whole Lot	Hurts Worst

FIGURE 21–2 ■ The Wong-Baker FACES Pain Rating Scale is valid and reliable in helping children to report their level of pain. After determining that the child has an understanding of number concepts, teach the child how to use the scale. Point to each face and use the words under the picture to describe the amount of pain the child feels. Then ask the child to select the face that comes closest to the amount of pain felt.

Source: Copyright 1983, Wong-Baker FACES® Foundation, www.WongBakerFACES.org. Used with permission. Originally published in Whaley & Wong's Nursing Care of Infants and Children. © Elsevier Inc.

expression to determine pain level. Older children can use the words associated with the tool to provide a pain rating. The Faces Pain Rating Scale has good validity and reliability for measuring pain intensity (Twycross et al., 2009, p. 90).

Oucher scale The Oucher Scale (Figure 21–3 ■) presents a series of six photographs of a child expressing increased intensity of pain in combination with a vertical visual analogue scale with numbers from 0 to 10. The young child selects a face that matches his or her

level of pain. The older child can select a number between 0 and 10. The nurse should not compare the photos with the child's expression to determine a pain level. The tool has been developed and tested in three cultural groups: Caucasian, African American, and Hispanic. It has validity and reliability for children between 3 and 12 years of age (Anthony & Schanberg, 2007).

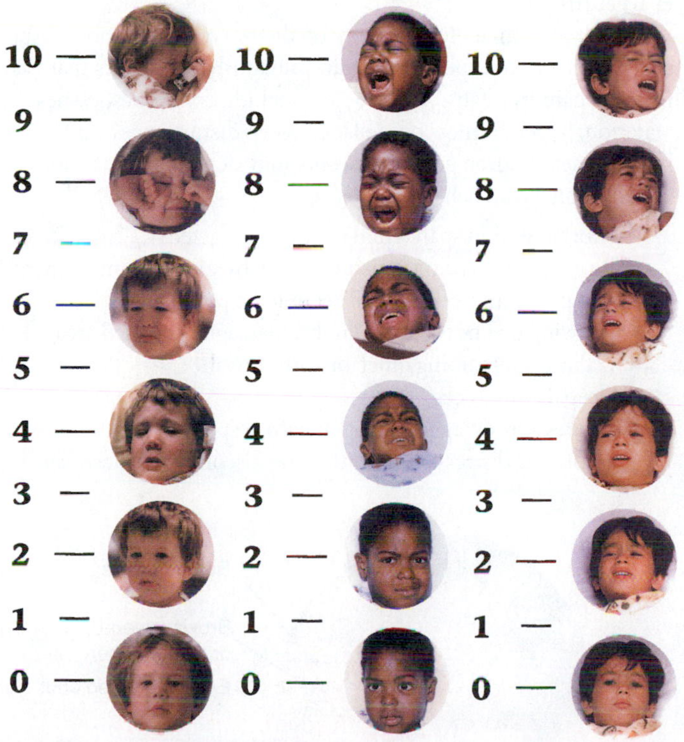

Poker chip scale The Poker Chip Scale uses four checkers or poker chips to quantify acute procedural and hospital-based pains. The child is given four poker chips and is asked to pick the number of chips that match his or her pain. The child is told that one chip is a little pain or hurt and four chips is the most pain he or she could have. Scores tend to correlate with other pain rating tools, and it is especially valuable in children ages 3 and 4 years. It has successfully been used in children from many cultures (Cohen, Lemanek, Blount, et al., 2008).

Older school-age children and adolescents All of the tools listed for infants and children may be used for school-age children. However, older children and adolescents have a better understanding of language and number concepts, so additional tools can be used to assess pain. In each case, the child should be asked about the location of pain and descriptions of the quality or type of pain.

Numeric pain scale The Numeric Pain Scale or Visual Analogue Scale (VAS) is a 10 cm horizontal or vertical line with marks or numbers from 0 to 10 at equal intervals. The line is anchored with "no pain" on the 0 side and "most pain" on the 10 side (Figure 21–4 ■). This tool sometimes has marks at equal intervals to provide a numeric dimension to the tool. A VAS designed as a pain thermometer is appropriate for use in children. The child needs to have good cognitive ability and be 8 years or older to use this pain rating tool (Twycross et al., 2009, p. 94).

Word-graphic rating scale The Word-Graphic Rating Scale uses a horizontal line and has words describing increasing pain intensity across the bottom (Figure 21–5 ■). The child is given instructions to mark the line that is closest to the pain felt. A millimeter ruler can then be used to quantify the pain and record the number as the pain score. This scale can be used to help children understand the concept of increasing pain severity using the five word anchors at specific points along the scale.

Adolescent pediatric pain tool The Adolescent Pediatric Pain Tool includes a human figure drawing, the Word-Graphic Rating Scale (0 to 100 mm), and a list of words to describe the pain. The human figure drawing can be used for the adolescent to indicate the location of all pain sites. The Word-Graphic Rating Scale is used as

FIGURE 21–3 ■ Use the Oucher version that is the best match for the ethnicity of the child. After determining that the child has an understanding of number concepts, teach the child to use the Oucher. Point to each photo and explain that the bottom picture is "no hurt," the second photo is a "little hurt," the third photo is a "little more hurt," the fourth photo is "even more hurt," the fifth photo is "a lot of hurt," and the sixth photo is the "biggest or most hurt you could ever have." The numbers beside the photos can be used to score the amount of pain the child reports.

*In the form presented in this book, the Oucher is for educational purposes only and cannot be used for patient care.

Source: A, The Caucasian version of the Oucher, developed and copyrighted by Judith E. Beyer, RN, Ph.D., 1983. B, The African-American version of the Oucher, developed and copyrighted by Mary J. Denyes, RN, Ph.D., and Antonia M. Villarruel, RN, Ph.D., 1990. Cornelia P. Porter, RN, Ph.D., and Charlotta Marshall, RN, MSN, contributed to the development of the scale. C, The Hispanic version of the Oucher, developed and copyrighted by Antonio M. Villarruel, RN, Ph.D., and Mary J. Denyes, RN, Ph.D., 1990. http://www.oucher.org

Weblink

Human Figure Outline and Pain Word Descriptors

Numeric Pain Scale
9 years–adult

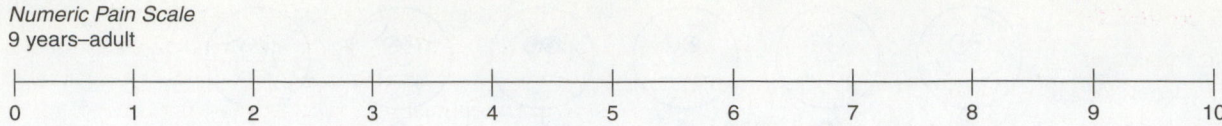

| | | | | | | | | | | |
|0|1|2|3|4|5|6|7|8|9|10|

FIGURE 21–4 ■ The Numeric Pain Scale or Visual Analogue Scale is used for older school-age children and adolescents. Teach the child to use the scale by saying that 0 is no pain and 10 is the most pain ever felt. In between are numbers that can be used to report small or large amounts of pain. Ask the child to make a mark any place along the line that is the best match for the amount of pain felt.

| No Pain | Little Pain | Moderate Pain | Large Pain | Worst Possible Pain |

FIGURE 21–5 ■ The Word-Graphic Rating Scale can be used independently or as part of the Adolescent Pediatric Pain Tool. Words rather than numbers are under the line. Teach the child to use the scale by pointing to the side of the line that is no pain. Then run your finger along the line to the other side and tell the child that this location is the worst possible pain. Ask the child to make a mark along the line that is the best match for the amount of pain felt. Use a millimeter ruler to measure from the "no pain" end of the line to the marked location to identify the pain score. Make sure a line of the same length is used each time pain is assessed for comparison.

Source: Adapted from *Pediatric Nursing*, 1997, Volume 23, Number 1, pp. 31–34. Reprinted with permission of the publisher, Jannetti Publications, Inc., East Holly Avenue, Box 56, Pitman, NJ 08071-0056; (856) 256-2300; FAX (856) 589-7463; Web site: http://www.pediatricnursing.net/ ; For a sample copy of the journal, please contact the publisher.

described above, and the word choices help provide the adolescent with the different ways to characterize the pain felt. It was originally developed for postoperative pain, but it is also used for assessment of acute and chronic pain related to disease. It has good validity and reliability, and can be used in children as young as 5 years (Twycross et al., 2009, p. 95).

Pain Location

Young children (3 years and older) can localize pain if given a body outline facing front and back (see Figure 15–8 in Chapter 15). The child can be asked to mark all places where the pain is located or to color the area of pain with crayons. Ask the child to use one color for the place where it hurts the most, and then to choose a different color for areas with less pain. Children often use red, black, or purple to indicate severe pain; however, it is important to ask the child about the colors selected and used to indicate different pain intensities.

ACUTE PAIN

Children experience acute pain related to a variety of illnesses and injuries, surgery, and invasive procedures. Just as with adults, children must have their pain assessed and managed.

Clinical Manifestations

Physiologic Indicators

Acute pain stimulates the adrenergic nervous system and results in physiologic changes, including tachycardia, tachypnea, hypertension, flushing or pallor, pupil dilation, peripheral vasoconstriction, pallor, increased perspiration, and decreased oxygen saturation (Huether, 2010). Changes in these physiologic signs demonstrate a complex stress response. These signs are not specific to pain, so they cannot be used for monitoring acute pain. However, some of these signs can be used to assess pain when combined with behavioral changes and self-reporting.

Clinical Tip

When the body adapts physiologically to acute pain, vital signs return to near normal and perspiration decreases after several minutes. Thus changes in vital signs are not a reliable indicator of pain in children because they last such a short time and they may also be an indication of anxiety or fear. Chronic pain of long duration that is persistent or continuous permits physiologic adaptation so normal heart rate, respiratory rate, and blood pressure levels are often seen (Huether, 2010).

Behavioral Indicators

Newborns and infants demonstrate a large number of behaviors when in acute pain. These behaviors include knitted brows, squinted eyes with cheeks raised, eyes closed, crying, jerky or flailing movements, and stiff posture (Figure 21–6 ■). A less mature or sick newborn may have a weaker cry or a less expressive face, or not have the energy to make as many body movements as the well infant (Badr et al., 2010).

Children with acute pain may be distressed and anxious, especially if they have experienced pain previously. Behaviors that may indicate pain in infants and toddlers include crying, restlessness or agitation, hyperalertness or vigilance, sleep disturbances, and irritability. Older children and adolescents may demonstrate the following additional pain behaviors:

- Short attention span (child is easily distracted)
- Posturing (guarding a painful joint by avoiding movement), remaining immobile, or protecting the painful area
- Drawing up knees, flexing limbs, massaging affected area
- Lethargy, remaining quiet, or withdrawal
- Sleep disturbances
- Depression or aggressive behavior, especially for those with emotional distress and fear that the discomfort will worsen

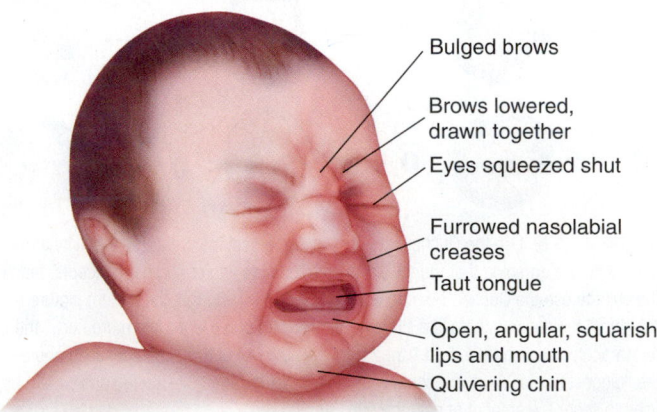

Bulged brows
Brows lowered, drawn together
Eyes squeezed shut
Furrowed nasolabial creases
Taut tongue
Open, angular, squarish lips and mouth
Quivering chin

FIGURE 21–6 ■ Neonatal characteristic facial responses to pain include bulged brow; eyes squeezed shut; furrowed nasolabial creases; open, angular, squarish lips and mouth; taut tongue; and a quivering chin.

Source: Redrawn from Carlson, K. L., Clement, B. A., & Nash, P. (1996). Neonatal pain: From concept to research questions and the role of the advanced practice nurse. *Journal of Perinatal Neonatal Nursing, 10(1)*, 64–71.

Collaborative Care

Diagnostic Procedures

Behavioral pain scales and self-report pain rating tools are used to evaluate pain in children (see pages 578–582). Even though acute pain is associated with tachycardia, tachypnea, and elevated blood pressure, existing conditions such as infection, trauma, and anemia or stress may also be responsible for these vital sign changes. No laboratory tests are used routinely to assess pain. However, prolonged, severe pain produces a physiologic stress response that includes the chemical release of catecholamines, cortisol, aldosterone, and other corticosteroids. Elevated blood glucose levels also occur (Huether, 2010).

Clinical Therapy

Pain management includes both pharmacologic and nonpharmacologic (complementary) therapies. Although children need adequate pharmacologic pain medication, nonpharmacologic therapies can enhance the pain management and ultimately reduce the amount of pain medication needed. See page 587 for complementary therapies.

Opioids **Opioids** are analgesics commonly given for severe pain, such as after surgery or a significant injury. Opioids such as morphine and codeine may be administered by oral, subcutaneous, intramuscular (IM), and intravenous (IV) routes. In some cases opioids can be administered topically, such as a fentanyl patch. Oral and intravenous routes are preferred for use in children because the intramuscular and subcutaneous routes cause pain and stress at the time of administration. Administration of opioids by an oral route is as effective as by intramuscular and intravenous routes when the drug is given in an **equianalgesic dose** (the amount of drug, whether given by oral or parenteral routes, needed to produce the same analgesic effect). See the Medications table for opioids commonly used for children. The optimal analgesic dose varies widely among patients in all age groups (American Pain Society, 2008). Meperidine is rarely used in children because its metabolite has the potential to cause seizures (American Pain Society, 2008).

Practice Alert

The morphine per dose maximum varies by age group to reduce the risk for respiratory depression (Taketomo, Hodding, & Kraus, 2010):

- Newborns = 0.1 mg/kg/dose
- Infants older than 3 months = 2 mg/dose
- Children 1 to 6 years = 4 mg/dose
- Children 7 to 12 years = 8 mg/dose
- Adolescents = 15 mg/dose

Opioid side effects Common side effects include sedation, nausea, vomiting, constipation, urinary retention, and itching. These should be treated by rotating the opioids used or with specific therapies as follows:

- **Sedation**—supplement lower opioid dose with nonsedating analgesia (Pasero & McCaffery, 2011, p. 512)
- **Nausea and vomiting**—antiemetic, alternate opioid
- **Constipation**—stool softener, stimulant laxative, increased fluids and dietary fiber
- **Urinary retention**—bethanechol, catheterization

Medications Opioid Analgesics and Recommended Doses for Children and Adolescents*

DRUG	APPROXIMATE EQUIANALGESIC ORAL DOSE	APPROXIMATE EQUIANALGESIC PARENTERAL DOSE	RECOMMENDED STARTING DOSE (ADULTS GREATER THAN 50 KG)		RECOMMENDED STARTING DOSE (CHILDREN[a] & ADULTS LESS THAN 50 KG)	
			ORAL	PARENTERAL	ORAL	PARENTERAL
Morphine	30 mg	10 mg	15–30 mg every 3–4 hours	10 mg every 3–4 hours	0.3 mg/kg every 3–4 hours	0.05–0.1 mg/kg every 3–4 hours
Codeine	120 mg	75 mg IV or subcutaneous	30–60 mg every 3–4 hours	60 mg every 2 hours	0.5–1 mg/kg every 3–4 hours[a]	NR
Hydromorphone (Dilaudid)	7.5 mg	1.5 mg	5–10 mg every 3–4 hours	1.5 mg every 3–4 hours	0.03–0.08 mg/kg every 4 hours	0.01–0.015 mg/kg every 3–4 hours
Levorphanol (Levo-Dromoran)	4 mg (acute) 1 mg (chronic)	2 mg (acute) 1 mg (chronic)	2–4 mg every 6–8 hours	2 mg every 6–8 hours	0.04 mg/kg every 6–8 hours	0.02 mg/kg every 6–8 hours
Methadone (Dolophine, others)	10 mg (acute) 2–4 mg (chronic)	5 mg (acute) 2–4 mg (chronic)	5–10 mg every 8 hours	10 mg every 8 hours	0.1–0.2 mg/kg every 12–36 hours	0.1–0.2 mg/kg every 12–36 hours
Oxycodone (Roxicodone)	20 mg	NA	5 mg every 3–4 hours	NA	0.1–0.2 mg/kg every 3–4 hours[a]	NA
Fentanyl	NA	0.1 mg	5 mcg/kg Lozenge	50–100 mcg every 1–2 hours	5–15 mcg/kg Oralet[b]	0.5–1 mcg/kg every 1–2 hours

NR = Not recommended, NA = Not available

*For all parenteral opioids, start with the low dose and titrate to effective pain control.

[a] Caution: Doses of aspirin and acetaminophen in combination with opioid/NSAID preparation must also be adjusted to the patient's body weight.

[b] Oralet is not widely used because of nausea and vomiting side effects.

Source: *Data from American Pain Society. (2008).* Principles of analgesic use in the treatment of acute pain and cancer pain *(6th ed., pp. 14–17). Glenview, IL: Author; Kraemer, F. W., & Rose, J. B. (2009). Pharmacologic management of acute pediatric pain.* Anesthesia Clinics, 27*(2), 241–268; Taketomo, C. K., Hodding, J. H., & Kraus, D. M. (2010).* Pediatric dosage handbook *(17th ed., p. 949). Hudson, OH: American Pharmacists Association.*

- **Pruritus**—antihistamine, alternate opioids, or naloxone 0.1–0.2 mcg/kg/hr continuous IV infusion (given simultaneously with opioid) (Pasero & McCaffery, 2011, p. 500)

A more serious opioid adverse effect is respiratory depression. When the child's condition is unstable, as with trauma or a critical illness, the dosage of opioids must be carefully calculated to match the child's cardiorespiratory status. Frequent assessments and cardiorespiratory monitoring or pulse oximetry are important safety guidelines when the infant or child has a condition that puts him or her at increased risk for respiratory depression. See the Practice Alert box for more information on respiratory depression. See Developing Cultural Competence: Codeine Use. **Addiction,** a patient's loss of control over the use of a substance with a compulsive use of the substance despite harm, is a rare complication in children treated for painful conditions (American Pain Society, 2008).

Practice Alert

Respiratory depression (unresponsiveness and progressively decreasing respiratory rate) may progress to respiratory arrest and is the major life-threatening complication of opioid administration. Clinical signs that predict the development of respiratory depression include sleepiness, small pupils, and shallow breathing. Children at higher risk for opioid-induced respiratory depression are those with an altered level of consciousness, an unstable circulatory status, a history of apnea, or a known airway problem such as obstructive sleep apnea. Respiratory depression is most likely to occur when the child is sleeping, a state that augments the depressant effect on the respiratory center and potential airway obstruction by the tongue (American Pain Society, 2008, p. 31).

Identify the time interval before drug-specific peak respiratory depression occurs, and then carefully monitor the child's vital signs during that period. Remember that pulse oximetry does not measure ventilation, so monitoring the respiratory rate is essential. Naloxone is the drug used for reversal of opioids' adverse effects. In children weighing less than 40 kg, use a 10 mcg/kg solution of naloxone diluted in saline, administered at a rate of 0.5 mcg/kg every 2 minutes to gradually reduce the opioid effects without causing withdrawal symptoms (American Pain Society, 2008, p. 31).

When opioids are given over an extended period (a week or two), children develop **physical dependence,** the physiologic adaptation to an analgesic or sedative drug at the peripheral and central neurons. Physical dependence is not addiction. These children may experience **withdrawal,** the physical signs and symptoms that occur when a sedative or analgesic medication is stopped suddenly. **Tolerance** is an adaptation to an opioid dosage that results in a shorter duration of drug effectiveness over time, and an increasing dosage is needed to produce the same level of pain relief. For example, a child might develop physical dependence or tolerance after being in an intensive care setting long term with pain management for life-threatening injuries, multiple surgeries, and invasive procedures. See the Clinical Manifestations table for signs and symptoms of withdrawal.

Acetaminophen and nonsteroidal anti-inflammatory drugs Nonsteroidal anti-inflammatory drugs (NSAIDs) such as ibuprofen, primarily given orally, are medications with analgesic properties effective for the relief of mild to moderate pain and chronic pain. Acetaminophen is a nonnarcotic analgesic that is used like an NSAID. It works by raising the pain threshold and is equal to aspirin in analgesic properties. The Medications table on page 585 presents recommended dosages of these drugs. They are most commonly used for bone, inflammatory, and connective tissue conditions. An NSAID may be prescribed in combination with an opioid to increase the effectiveness of the opioid and to reduce the amount of opioids needed for pain relief.

Acetaminophen is a nonnarcotic analgesic and antipyretic that is used like NSAIDs; however, it does not have systemic anti-inflammatory action. It produces analgesia by inhibiting the synthesis of prostaglandins in the central nervous system and peripherally blocks pain. Ibuprofen may be more effective than acetaminophen for painful conditions associated with inflammation because of its anti-inflammatory properties. See Box 21–2.

Drug administration Pain from surgery, major trauma, acute episodes such as vaso-occlusive crisis, or cancer will be present for predictable periods because of the effects of tissue damage (Box 21–3). Pain relief should be provided around the clock. Every effort should be made to

---

Developing Cultural Competence
Codeine Use

Codeine gets its analgesic properties with its conversion to morphine by the liver; however, about 10% of Caucasians and varying percentages of other ethnic groups are unable to convert codeine to morphine because they lack the CYP2D6 enzyme (Pasero & McCaffery, 2011, p. 330). Children with these genetic differences may have limited or no analgesic response to codeine. This demonstrates why response to pain medications must be carefully monitored.

Clinical Manifestations Opioid Withdrawal

SYSTEM	SIGNS AND SYMPTOMS	NURSING MANAGEMENT
Central nervous system	Irritability, increased wakefulness, tremulousness, hyperactive deep tendon reflexes, clonus, inability to concentrate, frequent yawning, sneezing, delirium, hypertonicity, visual or auditory hallucinations	■ Slowly wean the child off opioids over 2 to 4 weeks to prevent withdrawal symptoms. One plan is to switch the child to oral opioids and reduce the daily dose by 10% over several days. The longer the child has been taking opioids, the longer the tapering should take. ■ Clonidine may reduce some symptoms of opioid withdrawal.
Gastrointestinal system	Nausea, feeding intolerance with vomiting, abdominal cramps, diarrhea, salivation, uncoordinated suck and swallow	
Sympathetic nervous system	Tachycardia, tachypnea, increased blood pressure, nasal stuffiness, lacrimation, chills alternating with hot flashes, sweating, fever	

Source: *Data from American Pain Society. (2008).* Principles of analgesic use in the treatment of acute pain and cancer pain *(6th ed.). Glenview, IL: Author; Pasero, C., & McCaffery, M. (2011).* Pain assessment and pharmacologic management. *St. Louis: Mosby Elsevier.*

Medications Recommended Doses of Acetaminophen and NSAIDs for Children and Adolescents

ORAL MEDICATIONS PEAK ACTION TIME	USUAL ADULT DOSE	USUAL PEDIATRIC DOSE	NURSING MANAGEMENT
Nonopioid analgesic			
Acetaminophen 0.5–2 hours oral	500–1000 mg every 4–6 hours	10–15 mg/kg every 4–6 hours	Lacks the peripheral anti-inflammatory activity of other NSAIDs; rectal suppository available. Do not exceed five doses a day.
NSAIDs			
Aspirin 1–2 hours oral	500–1000 mg every 4–6 hours	10–15 mg/kg every 4 hours Maximum daily dose = 4 g	Do not use in children under 19 years with possible chicken pox or flu viral illness due to link with Reye syndrome (see Chapter 33 🔗); may cause gastric upset and bleeding; rectal suppository available
Choline magnesium trisalicylate (Trilisate) 2 hours oral	1000–1500 mg every 12 hours	25 mg/kg every 12 hours	Does not increase bleeding time like other NSAIDs; also available as oral liquid. Give with food to avoid gastrointestinal upset.
Ibuprofen (Motrin, Advil) 1–2 hours oral	200–400 mg every 4–6 hours	5–10 mg/kg every 6 hours	Available as oral suspension; do not use in children with bleeding disorders; give with food to decrease gastrointestinal upset.
Naproxen (Naprosyn, Aleve) 2–4 hours oral	500 mg initially, then 275 mg every 6–8 hours	5–10 mg/kg every 12 hours	Available as oral liquid; give with food to decrease gastrointestinal upset; use no longer than 3 days unless prescribed by healthcare provider.
Ketorolac (Toradol) 1–3 minutes IV 45 minutes IM	30–60 mg IV loading dose, then 15–30 mg every 6 hours	1 mg/kg IV loading dose up to 60 mg, then 0.5 mg/kg up to 30 mg IV every 6 hours	Use no longer than 5 days; should not be used for children with bleeding disorder or at risk for bleeding complications.

Source: *Data from American Pain Society. (2008).* Principles of analgesic use in the treatment of acute pain and cancer pain *(6th ed., pp. 6–10). Glenview, IL: Author; Taketomo, C. K., Hodding, J. H., & Kraus, D. M. (2010).* Pediatric dosage handbook *(17th ed., p. 949). Hudson, OH: American Pharmacists Association.*

give the child analgesics without causing more pain. The preferred routes of administration are intravenous, local nerve block, and oral.

Continuous-infusion analgesia is recommended to maintain pain control for children with continuous or persistent pain as it keeps drug blood levels constant. Analgesics may also be given intravenously on a scheduled basis (e.g., every 3 to 4 hours). Delays in giving analgesics on a scheduled basis increase the chances of **breakthrough pain** (pain that emerges as the pain medication wears off, resulting in the loss of pain control) and the subsequent anticipation of pain. Giving analgesics on an as-needed (PRN) basis for acute pain also results in the loss of pain control. More medications are often needed to restore pain control than would have been required for continuous-infusion analgesia.

Patient-controlled analgesia Patient-controlled analgesia (PCA) is a method of administering an intravenous analgesic, such as morphine, using a computerized pump that is programmed by the healthcare professional and controlled by the child. After initial pain

control has been achieved with a continuous IV infusion of morphine (basal dose) by the nurse, the child presses a button to receive a smaller analgesic dose (bolus dose) for episodic pain relief (Figure 21–7 ■). This method of pain management is especially useful for pain control in the first 48 hours after surgery or until oral pain management is possible. Safety features to prevent overdoses include the ability to set the maximum number of bolus infusions per hour and the maximum amount of drug received in a specific time period. Additional pain medication may be ordered as needed to supplement the continuous and patient-administered infusion when pain control is not maintained. The IV may be maintained for weaning bolus infusions during the transition to oral medications to ensure that the child has adequate analgesia (see the Skills Manual 🔗).

Children selected for PCA should be able to push the injection button and have the cognitive ability to understand that pushing the button will give them medication that will relieve pain after a slight delay. Children and adolescents benefit from PCA by receiving continuous pain control and having the ability to control their comfort level with no trauma from injections. Once children can take oral analgesics, PCA is discontinued.

BOX 21–2   Research: Pain Management for a Fracture

In a study of 336 children ages 4 to 18 years with uncomplicated arm fractures, each child was given either ibuprofen or acetaminophen with codeine for pain during the first 72 hours after injury. Parents assessed the child's pain using a faces pain scale before giving medication and an hour later. Pain scores and the time of medication administration were recorded in a pain diary. A rescue pain medication was available to the child if the pain medication was inadequate. Ibuprofen had similar effectiveness in pain management to acetaminophen with codeine; however, the child using ibuprofen had fewer adverse effects (Drendel, Gorelick, Weisman, et al., 2009).

BOX 21–3   Easing Abdominal Pain

Analgesics were often withheld from children with acute abdominal pain for fear that physical examination findings would be changed and delay the diagnosis of potential need for surgery. Studies involving children with acute appendicitis revealed that giving morphine did not delay the diagnosis or cause complications associated with opioid use (Greenwald, 2010). Be an advocate for pain management in these children.

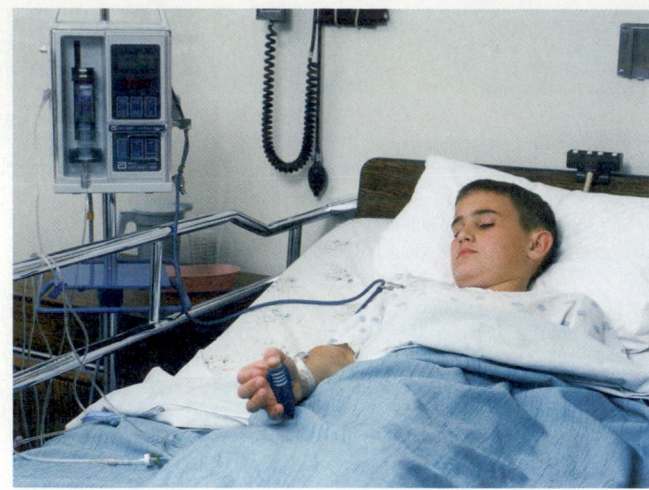

FIGURE 21–7 ■ By using patient-controlled analgesia, the older child is able to regulate the intake of an intravenous analgesic such as morphine.

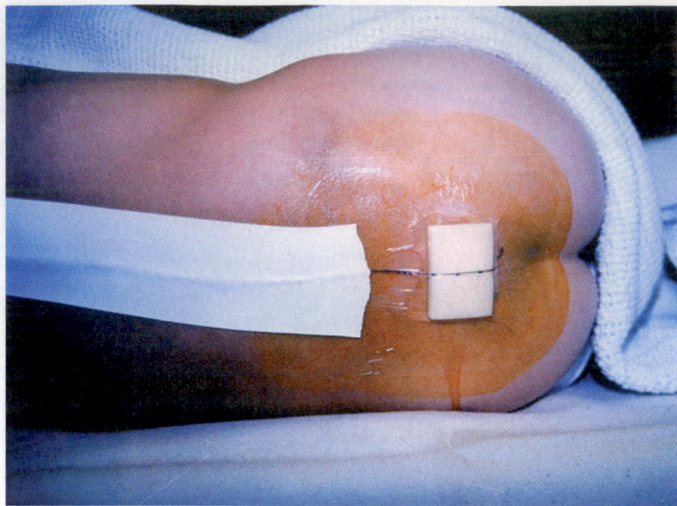

FIGURE 21–8 ■ An epidural pain block is one example of a regional analgesia used for postoperative pain management. Once the epidural catheter is placed, it is taped and wrapped securely; small doses of pain medication are then continuously infused by a pump.

PCA is prescribed mostly for children ages 7 years and older but may be offered to children as young as 5 years. The child is less likely to administer an overdose as the effect of the medication causes sedation. In rare cases, PCA by proxy, with a parent or nurse given the responsibility for pushing the injection button, may be used for a child with disabilities or a child too young to take responsibility for PCA. To reduce the potential for an adverse event, the parent or nurse must follow special guidelines for making pain assessments when responsible for pushing the PCA button (Howard, Lloyd-Thomas, Thomas, et al., 2010; Kraemer & Rose, 2009). Some studies have reported a higher risk for adverse events (bradypnea, oxygen desaturation, and oversedation) in children using PCA by proxy (Franson, 2010). See Partnering with Families: Teaching About Patient-Controlled Analgesia (PCA).

Regional pain management Epidural pain control provides selective analgesia and has become more common for postoperative pain management. An epidural catheter is inserted during general anesthesia into either the lumbar or the caudal space, and advanced up to the space close to the dermatomes to be blocked (Kraemer & Rose, 2009) (Figure 21–8 ■). Analgesia may be administered by intermittent bolus, continuous infusion by a small pump, or PCA to maintain pain control for the first 24 to 48 hours after surgery. Opioids

alone or in combination with a local anesthetic may be used. Stable plasma opioid levels can be maintained. Only minute doses of drugs are needed because of the high concentration achieved at the opioid receptors in the spinal cord's dorsal horn (Pasero & McCaffery, 2011, p. 415). Potential adverse effects of epidural opioids include nausea, vomiting, pruritus, sedation, and respiratory depression, just as with other routes of administration (Box 21–4).

Local nerve blocks, such as a femoral or popliteal block for anesthesia and analgesia of a leg or interscalene (in a muscle of the

BOX 21–4	Research: Epidural versus Intravenous Opioid Use

A meta-analysis of four prospective, randomized controlled trial design studies was conducted to investigate the efficacy of postoperative continuous epidural analgesia for adolescents having scoliosis surgery. The comparison patients received intravenous opioids by PCA. The visual analogue scale (VAS) was used to assess pain at 24, 48, and 72 hours. VAS scores were significantly lower in the epidural analgesia group on all 3 postoperative days. Side effects of nausea and pruritus were also lower in the epidural analgesia group, and patient satisfaction scores were higher in the epidural analgesia group (Taenzer & Clark, 2010).

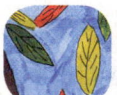

Partnering with Families

Teaching About Patient-Controlled Analgesia (PCA)

- What is PCA? Analgesia means pain relief: You get to control the amount of medicine you receive by using the machine.
- The machine gives the medicine by passing it through the tube that is connected to your intravenous line. When you push the button, the machine pumps pain medicine into the intravenous line to make you feel better.
- The machine limits the amount of medicine you can get, up to the amount ordered by the physician. You can get any amount up to the maximum by pushing the button repeatedly. The push button will not let you make a mistake if you drop it or roll on it. Do not let another family member push the button.

- Whenever you feel pain, hurt, or discomfort, push the button to get more medicine. You should be the only one to push the button.
- No needles for pain shots are needed as long as the intravenous line is in place.
- The PCA may not relieve all of your pain, but it should make you feel comfortable. Let the nurse know if you think your PCA is not working.
- The PCA will be used until you can take pills or drink liquid pain medicine.

cervical vertebrae) for the upper extremity, are used more frequently for pain control after surgery. The regional block is most often performed when the child is anesthetized. A subcutaneous catheter is inserted into the local area for infusion of the analgesia. A single dose or a continuous infusion of the analgesia with a pump may be used (Kraemer & Rose, 2009). Pain control is achieved without systemic side effects from the anesthesia. Tingling felt in the fingers or toes of the affected limb is the first sign that the nerve block is receding.

Nonpharmacologic Methods of Pain Management

Complementary therapies are nonpharmacologic methods used for pain management that can enhance the effect of analgesics and potentially reduce the dose of analgesia required. One or more of these therapies may provide adequate pain relief when the child has low levels of pain. See Complementary Therapy: Pain Control.

Complementary therapies may involve cognitive or behavioral methods; however, techniques such as touch, heat or cold applications, and a sugar-coated pacifier should not be overlooked for enhancing pain management. Partner with other providers who can assist with the use of complementary therapies, such as child life personnel who can perform therapeutic play, and physical therapists.

Cognitive behavioral therapies Various techniques are used to reduce fear, pain, and anxiety while increasing the child's sense of control. Such therapies involve the use of a specific technique before, during, and after a procedure. In some cases dolls, role-playing, role modeling, and practicing desirable behavior may be combined with relaxation, hypnosis, and guided imagery to promote coping with multiple invasive procedures in children with cancer and chronic illness. See page 409 in Chapter 15 🔵 for more information.

Distraction Distraction involves engaging a child in a wide variety of pleasant activities that help focus attention on something other than pain and anxiety associated with a medical procedure. Examples of distraction activities are listening to music, singing a song, playing a game, blowing bubbles, watching television or a video, and playing a computer game. Guided imagery and breathing techniques may be forms of distraction for school-age children and adolescents. Parents can serve as effective distraction coaches when given guidance about how to interact with their children. Developmentally appropriate activities for the child should be selected for distraction. Children in severe pain cannot be distracted; but do not assume the pain is gone if a child can be distracted.

Guided imagery Imagery is a mind-body therapy, or a cognitive behavioral process that encourages the child to relax (often with progressive muscle relaxation techniques) and focus concentration on vivid mental images as if they were real, and to ignore things such as a painful procedure. Exploring a favorite place, remembering a funny story, or being a superhero are all images that can be used. This method is most effective in children over 6 years of age. Ask the child to think about all the sights, sounds, smells, tastes, and feelings that will help him or her to create an image and to experience the favorite place, activity, or story. Imagery has been used successfully by children and adolescents to reduce pain and anxiety associated with surgery (Huth, Daraisch, Henson, et al., 2009).

Relaxation techniques Relaxation techniques are used to reduce muscle tension because pain is often aggravated when muscles are tensed. Progressive muscle relaxation is one relaxation technique. The child is asked to tense a muscle group for 10 seconds and notice how it feels. Then the child is asked to relax the muscle group for 10 seconds and compare it to how it felt when tensed. Teach the child to tense and relax different muscle groups, starting with the hands or feet, and then moving to more central muscles in the arms or legs. The exercise is best done in a quiet location with the child focusing on something pleasant. With practice, the child should be able to detect the difference between tense and relaxed muscles and then to reduce the tension.

Breathing techniques Breathing techniques can be used for either distraction or muscle relaxation during a painful procedure or to reduce stress and anxiety. Ask the child to take slow regular deep breaths with the diaphragm. Have the child place the hands on the abdomen while he or she looks at and feels the abdomen rise and fall slowly with each deep breath. Alternatively, the child or adolescent can take a deep breath, hold it for 5 seconds, and blow out through the mouth to push the tension out or the needle away. The young child can be encouraged to take shallow breaths in through the nose and out through the mouth while thinking of a particular image. The image could be a train, and short breaths could be the "toot, toot" of the train engine.

Hypnosis Hypnosis is an altered state of awareness facilitating heightened concentration, decreased awareness of external stimuli, increased relaxation, and increased suggestibility. The hypnotic suggestion often uses muscle relaxation and guided imagery, and post-hypnotic suggestions are given for the relief of anxiety, tension, and pain. Language such as "you are the boss of your body and can help make this headache not bother you any more" helps the child gain mastery over physical symptoms. Children more easily respond to hypnosis than adults because of their imaginative powers for fun and fantasy, and to cope with fears and challenges. Hypnosis has been successful in assisting children and adolescents to manage the stress and pain associated with invasive medical procedures and chronic pain such as daily headaches (Accardi & Milling, 2009; Kohen, 2011).

Cutaneous stimulation Gently rub the painful area, massage the skin gently, and hold or rock the child. Touching provides a stimulus to compete with the pain stimuli that are transmitted from the peripheral nerves to the spinal cord and brain. These actions may reduce the pain felt by the child. Swaddling, kangaroo care, and skin-to-skin contact between mother and preterm neonate are methods to reduce the pain responses of neonates.

Sucrose solution Concentrated sucrose solutions (2 mL of 24% solution) have been proven effective for pain relief during painful procedures in preterm and term newborns up to 1 month of age, and for immunizations given to infants up to 12 months of age (Harrison,

---

Complementary Therapy Pain Control

A simple explanation of the gate control theory of pain helps explain how the pain impulses to the brain may be inhibited at the level of the dorsal horn of the spine. Stimulation of the larger A-beta fibers by ice or nonpainful touch and pressure such as massage causes the substantia gelatinosa in the dorsal horn of the spinal cord to "close the gate" and decrease the transmission of pain impulses to the brain (Huether, 2010). Cognitive-behavioral therapies, such as distraction and hypnosis, inhibit transmission of pain perception between the brain and dorsal horn of the spine (Kuttner, 2010, p. 50).

Bueno, Yamada, et al., 2010). Sucrose is thought to activate the endogenous opioid system through taste (Taddio, Shah, Hancock, et al., 2008). The solution should be given 2 minutes before the procedure, and the analgesic effect of sucrose lasts approximately 3 to 5 minutes. Allow the infant to continue sucking on a pacifier or to breastfeed during the procedure to further reduce distress.

Application of heat and cold Heat application promotes dilation of blood vessels, and the increased blood circulation enables pain neurotransmitters and metabolites to be removed from the site (Lane & Latham, 2009). Heat also promotes muscle relaxation, breaking the pain-spasm-pain cycle. To reduce edema, do not apply heat in the first 24 hours after an injury.

The application of cold is believed to slow the ability of pain fibers to transmit pain impulses, reducing the number of pain signals that reach the brain. Cold also controls pain during its acute stage by decreasing bleeding, edema, inflammation, and muscle spasm (Lane & Latham, 2009). Cover cold packs with a towel to reduce the risk for a cold injury. Apply for 20 to 30 minutes and then remove for about 10 minutes before continuing therapy. Assess the skin for redness or signs of irritation. Discontinue cold applications immediately if the skin alternately blanches and reddens afterward or if blisters or redness do not subside between applications.

Electroanalgesia Also known as transcutaneous electrical nerve stimulation (TENS), **electroanalgesia** delivers small amounts of electrical stimulation to the skin by electrodes. This electronic stimulation is stronger than the pain impulses and, because of the gate control theory, is thought to interfere with the transmission of pain impulses from the peripheral nerves to the spinal cord and brain. TENS may be used for both acute and chronic pain management, as well as prior to physical therapy. The only known side effect is skin irritation at the electrode site.

Acupuncture A traditional Chinese treatment for pain relief, acupuncture has been gaining greater acceptance in Western medicine. Acupuncture is based on the theory that energy, or chi, flows along channels through the body (meridians) that are connected by acupuncture points. Pain occurs with obstruction of the energy flow, and inserting needles at the appropriate acupuncture points restores the energy flow (Kundu & Berman, 2007). Placement of acupuncture needles at specific pain points releases endogenous opioid peptides (Wu, Sapru, Stewart, et al., 2009). Limited research has been conducted about the effectiveness of acupuncture use in children.

Nursing Management

Nurses have an ethical obligation to relieve a child's suffering. Unrelieved pain has consequences, and appropriate pain management may have benefits such as earlier mobilization, shortened hospital stays, and reduced costs. To provide effective nursing care of children in pain, anticipate the presence of pain and acknowledge the child's rights to pain management.

Nursing Assessment and Diagnosis

The perception of pain and the response to it make pain a unique experience for each infant, child, and adolescent. When assessing pain in children, keep the following questions in mind:

- What is happening in tissues that might cause pain? Assume that children who have had surgery, an injury, a vaso-occlusive

episode, or illness are experiencing pain since these events also cause pain in adults. Are there multiple injury sites?
- What external factors could be causing pain? For example, is the cast too tight or is the child poorly positioned in bed?
- Are there any indicators of pain, either physiologic or behavioral?
- How is the child responding emotionally?
- How does the child or parent rate the pain?

Physiologic symptoms such as nausea, fatigue, dyspnea, bladder and bowel distention, and fever may also influence the intensity of pain felt by a child. The child's behavior or responses to pain stimuli may also be affected by fear, anxiety, separation from parents, anger, culture, age, or a previous pain experience.

When working with an infant or child, determine which pain assessment tool is most appropriate for the circumstance and developmental stage of the infant or child. When using a self-report pain scale, use the same tool each time you assess for pain and for evaluation of pain management, so reported pain levels may be compared.

Clinical Tip

When assessing pain using a behavioral pain scale, first consider if the child is expected to have pain because of surgery, injury, or other health condition. Then, if the score on the behavioral scale is low, consider if the tool being used is appropriate to assess the child's pain (for example, can all elements of the behavioral pain scale be assessed?). If the answer is no, one strategy is to have the parent identify behaviors indicating that the child is in pain. If pain is suspected, provide analgesia and evaluate the child's response by observing changes in behavior.

School-age children and adolescents may not exhibit distress in direct proportion to their pain intensity. Thus, behavioral measures may not match the child's self-report of pain intensity. Children may have coping skills that help them stay calm and expressionless. They may limit movement after surgery to reduce pain. However, their self-assessment may reveal moderate to severe levels of pain. Because children in these age groups can accurately report pain intensity, use the self-report as the valid pain assessment.

Surgery and trauma can result in multiple sites of pain (e.g., incision or laceration, cut or bruised muscles, interrupted blood supply, nasogastric tube placement, insertion sites of intravenous lines). When using pain scales in the assessment of a verbal child, attempt to identify all sites of pain, and then identify the intensity of pain at each site.

Examples of nursing diagnoses for children in pain may include the following:

- Pain, Acute, related to injury and femur fracture
- Anxiety related to anticipation of pain from an invasive procedure
- Mobility: Physical, Impaired related to pain
- Nausea related to opioids used for pain management

NANDA-I © 2012

See the Nursing Care Plan for the child with postoperative pain for more nursing diagnoses.

Planning and Implementation

Nursing management involves several actions to increase and maintain patient comfort once the assessment is completed and nursing diagnoses are developed. Pain management involves the use of analgesic and anesthetic medications, as well as nonpharmacologic or complementary therapies. The nurse must also monitor, evaluate, and document the effectiveness of pain control measures to provide optimal comfort. See Evidence-Based Practice: Challenges to

Nursing Care Plan

The Child with Postoperative Pain

INTERVENTION	RATIONALE	EXPECTED OUTCOME
1. Nursing Diagnosis: Pain, Acute, related to surgery and injury		
NIC Priority Intervention—*Pain Management:* Alleviation of pain or a reduction in pain to a level of comfort that is acceptable to the patient		**NOC Suggested Outcome**—*Comfort Level:* Feelings of physical and psychologic ease
GOAL: *The child will report pain relief.*		
■ Have the child select a pain scale and rate the amount of pain perceived before and 30–60 minutes after analgesia is given to ensure pain relief.	■ The child's pain rating is the best indicator of pain relief. Maintenance of pain control requires less analgesia than treating each acute pain episode.	The child reports pain relief after administration of analgesia, indicated by a lower level on a pain assessment scale.
■ Assess pain control each hour to ensure that the child's pain is relieved.	■ Frequent monitoring identifies inadequate pain control before it becomes significant.	
■ Reposition the child every 2 hours to maintain good body alignment.	■ New positions decrease muscle cramping and skin pressure.	
■ Provide therapeutic touch or massage. Encourage the parents to read a story or play favorite music.	■ Complementary therapy reduces stress and enhances the analgesic action.	
2. Nursing Diagnosis: Sleep Pattern, Disturbed, related to inadequate pain control and physical discomfort		
NIC Priority Intervention—*Sleep Enhancement:* Facilitation of regular sleep-awake cycles		**NOC Suggested Outcome**—*Sleep:* Extent and pattern of sleep for mental and physical rejuvenation
GOAL: *The child will experience fewer disruptions of sleep caused by pain.*		
■ Give analgesia by continuous infusion or every 3–4 hr around the clock.	■ Pain breakthrough occurs even during sleep and disturbs its healing effects.	The child sleeps for the age-appropriate number of hours per day, undisturbed by pain.
3. Nursing Diagnosis: Therapeutic Regimen Management: Family, Ineffective, related to self-management of pain control and use of nonpharmacologic pain control measures		
NIC Priority Intervention—*Self-Modification Assistance:* Reinforcement of self-directed change initiated by the patient to achieve personally important goals		**NOC Suggested Outcome**—*Treatment Behavior Pain Control:* Personal actions to palliate or eliminate pain
GOAL: *The child and family will effectively use patient-controlled analgesia (PCA) and complementary therapies.*		
■ Teach the child how the PCA works and when to push the button.	■ The child must know that pain can be relieved by pushing the PCA button and how the button works.	The child's pain rating stays low.
■ Teach the family and the child how to use age-appropriate imagery, distraction, relaxation techniques, and other complementary therapy pain relief measures.	■ Complementary therapies enhance the effect of analgesia, reduce the amount of pain medication needed, and help the child cope with anxiety from the pain episode.	The child and family independently use complementary therapies for pain control.
GOAL: *The child and family will use appropriate analgesia after discharge.*		
■ Discuss appropriate pain control to use at home after discharge.	■ The family and child need information about assessing pain and pain management to use at home.	The family demonstrates pain assessment and states appropriate dosage and frequency of analgesic to use at home.
4. Nursing Diagnosis: Breathing Pattern, Ineffective, related to opioid overdose		
NIC Priority Intervention—*Respiratory Monitoring:* Collection and analysis of patient data to ensure airway patency and adequate gas exchange		**NOC Suggested Outcome**—*Vital Signs Status:* Temperature, pulse, respirations, and blood pressure within expected range for the individual
GOAL: *The child will maintain adequate ventilations.*		
■ Verify that the correct dose of opioid analgesia is given for the child's weight.	■ Respiratory depression is a significant complication of opioid analgesia when too much analgesia is given.	The child has no episode of respiratory depression associated with analgesia.

(continued)

Nursing Care Plan   The Child with Postoperative Pain, *continued*

INTERVENTION	RATIONALE	EXPECTED OUTCOME
■ Monitor vital signs and depth of inspirations before the opioid is administered and at the time of peak drug action. Withhold opioid if vital signs fall within parameters established by the physician or policy.	■ A respiratory depression episode must be identified before progression to respiratory arrest occurs. All opioids act on the brainstem center that decreases responsiveness to CO_2 tension.	
■ Calculate the agonist dose ordered by the physician to be sure it will reverse respiratory depression, but not counteract the effect of analgesia.	■ Valuable time will be saved if the agonist is needed for an episode of respiratory depression. complete reversal of analgesia will cause the child to have significant pain.	

5. Nursing Diagnosis: Constipation, Risk for, related to opioid administration and decreased motility of gastrointestinal tract

NIC Priority Intervention—*Constipation Management:* Prevention and alleviation of constipation		**NOC Suggested Outcome**—*Bowel Elimination:* Ability of gastrointestinal tract to form and evacuate stool effectively

GOAL: *The child will have minimal constipation.*

■ Assess bowel sounds and abdominal distention, and then palpate the abdomen.	■ Signs of constipation must be anticipated and identified.	The child has bowel movements at least every 2 days while on opioid pain control.
■ Request a physician order for a stimulating laxative and stool softener.	■ Opioids increase the transit time of feces and interfere with bile enzymes needed for evacuation.	
■ Provide fluids of choice to increase fluid intake when IV fluids are decreased.	■ Extra fluids will counteract the opioid action of increasing the absorption of water from the large intestine.	
■ Inform the family and child that constipation is a side effect of pain medication.	■ Parents can become partners in encouraging fluid intake and monitoring bowel movements.	

NANDA-I © 2012

Adequate Pain Management. Also see Legal and Ethical Considerations: Standards for Pain.

Pharmacologic Intervention

Healthcare facility guidelines for pharmacologic intervention of pain often suggest that the child have a specific pain rating or higher before administering analgesia. Give analgesics as prescribed by the physician, ensuring that the dose is appropriate for the child's weight and medical situation. When administering an opioid by intravenous infusion, PCA, or PCA by proxy, monitor the flow rate and the site for infiltration. Follow institutional guidelines for monitoring the child's vital signs, and use a pulse oximeter or cardiorespiratory monitor with an audible alarm set for children at risk for respiratory depression. An end tidal CO_2 monitor may be used when the child is intubated. Vital signs (heart rate and blood pressure) may not change in response to effective analgesia when infection, trauma, and other stressors keep them elevated. Make sure analgesic antagonists such as naloxone are available should adverse effects develop. The dose should be precalculated and the medication immediately available when an opioid is used.

Clinical Tip

Naloxone may be used to treat respiratory depression caused by an opioid drug at a dose and slow infusion rate that does not reverse the opioid's pain control effects. A continuous infusion or repeated doses may be needed for severe adverse effects. Dosages are available for all ages, including neonates.

Check for the presence of other side effects of analgesics, such as sedation, nausea, vomiting, itching, urinary retention, and constipation. If side effects occur, either prescribe an alternative opioid or manage the side effects with other medications when analgesia is needed long term.

Oral NSAIDs are generally ordered for less severe pain or chronic pain. These medications may mask fever. Be alert to the potential complication of gastrointestinal hemorrhage in children with critical illnesses or injuries, as they may have increased gastric acids as a physiologic response to stress.

Evaluating Pain Management

Use the following questions to evaluate the child's pain management:

- What is the child's pain behavioral score or self-report score 15 to 30 minutes following intravenous pain medication, and 1 hour after oral pain medication is administered? Has adequate pain control been achieved?
- Is the child being assessed at appropriate intervals for pain intensity and pain management response? Is the child's comfort level maintained?
- Is the timing of the medication administration appropriate to prevent breakthrough pain?
- Does the child have any side effects to the analgesic? Is the nurse prepared to manage any adverse effects that might occur?

Use a flow sheet to document pain assessments, medication administration, complementary therapies, and results of pain control measures to guide ongoing nursing actions.

Dramatic reductions in pain should occur, but not all pain may be eliminated. Many children sleep after receiving an analgesic. This sleep is not a side effect of the drug or a sign of an overdose, but the result of pain relief. Pain interrupts sleep, and once pain is relieved, the child can sleep comfortably. However, sleep does not always indicate

Evidence-Based Practice

Challenges to Adequate Pain Management

PROBLEM

A one-day survey of pain prevalence in a Canadian children's hospital revealed that 77% of 248 interviewed children had pain during admission. Moderate to severe pain was reported by 27% of the children at the time of the survey, and another 64% reported moderate to severe pain in the prior 24 hours. While analgesics were administered to 58% of the children, only 25% of children got doses of analgesia throughout the day (Taylor, Boyer, & Campbell, 2008). Why does inadequate management of children with acute pain continue to occur?

EVIDENCE

Findings of a national study in which three vignettes were used to assess the responses of 334 pediatric nurses to children's pain did not reveal any personal or professional characteristics of nurses (years of clinical experience, continuing education about pain, education level, and age) related to pain management (Griffin, Polit, & Byrne, 2008). A recent study used a conceptual content cognitive mapping method to explore what pediatric nurses (n = 87) think about pain assessment and management. Two vignettes were used with 10-year-old boys self-reporting a pain score of 8 after a surgical procedure. One boy was grimacing and the other boy was smiling. The expected outcome was for the nurse to accept the child's self-report of pain and to select the appropriate dose of morphine to administer IV from the prescribed range. While the majority of nurses believed the child's self report (88.5% for the grimacing child and 72.4% for the smiling child), a larger proportion selected to administer the correct dose of morphine (versus undermedicating) to the grimacing child (73.6%) than to the smiling child

(41.4%). The study had two significant predictors of administration of the correct dose of analgesia: agreement with the patient's self-reported pain rating and fewer years of experience in pediatric nursing (Van Hulle Vincent, Wilkie, & Szalacha, 2010).

IMPLICATIONS

Pain management is a complex process that requires the nurse to assess the child and make clinical judgments about treatment. Research findings regarding nurse characteristics associated with better pain management are inconsistent. The Van Hulle Vincent, Wilkie, and Szalacha study reveals much about the characteristics of nurses, such as a higher focus on pain behaviors than self-report to assess pain. Additionally, even when nurses agreed with the child's self-report of pain, many did not select to administer the correct analgesia dose. It is uncertain what additional support may be needed to ensure that children are adequately treated for pain. Potentially more infrastructure support is needed within hospitals to provide guidance for the pain management of children, but nurses still need to make the correct decisions regarding adequate pain management.

CRITICAL THINKING APPLICATION

In the clinical setting, identify the infrastructure supports to promote pain management of children, such as pain assessment tools, pain flow sheets, pain management policies and guidelines, education, and resources for complementary therapies. What additional supports would help you as an inexperienced nurse to gain competence in pediatric pain management?

Legal and Ethical Considerations
Standards for Pain

In 2001, the Joint Commission introduced standards for the assessment and management of pain in patients. All patients have the right to assessment and management of pain, pain screening must occur during their initial assessment and as appropriate during follow-up visits in all health care settings, and patient education should include managing pain (Joint Commission, 2011).

---

pain control. A child in pain may fall asleep in exhaustion. Look for other symptoms of pain, such as excess movement or moaning.

Become an advocate for children when the dose or type of analgesic ordered is inadequate. A decrease in an opioid's effect over time or the need for increasing amounts of the opioid to produce or maintain the same level of pain relief or sedation effect occur when children with severe pain have been taking opioids or sedatives for several days. The duration of effective analgesia is shorter than expected, and breakthrough pain occurs. An increase in dosage may be needed to achieve the previous level of pain relief. Analyze all of the information about the child's pain management before asking the physician to change the analgesia dosage. Review the child's record for documentation that the prescribed drug has been given at the appropriate dose and frequency and that the child's pain relief is ineffective despite the drug administration. After verifying the record, provide the physician with information about the characteristics of the child's pain and ask that the medication be changed.

Regional Nerve Block

When an epidural or regional nerve block is used following surgery, the analgesic effect does not recede for several hours after the catheter is removed, but the time of effectiveness varies by type of analgesia used. In some cases when an epidural catheter is maintained for a

day or more, such as following scoliosis surgery, continuous infusion or patient-controlled epidural anesthesia may be used. A transparent sterile dressing is placed over the catheter site as a barrier against infection, and this dressing is not usually removed or changed. Inspect the site daily for inflammation around the catheter site.

Assess the extremity for color, temperature, and capillary refill. Assess motor function by asking children if they can move their legs, wiggle their toes, and lift their buttocks off the bed. Ensure proper positioning of the extremity to prevent nerve damage. Be careful when ambulating the child with a regional nerve block in the extremity. Protect the extremity from injury because the child has reduced feeling in the limb. The affected limb may be placed in a splint or sling while the nerve block is working to protect it. Monitor the child at least every 2 hours for tingling of fingers or toes, an indication that the analgesic effect is receding. Regular assessment for pain is still important as breakthrough pain can occur with a nerve block. Effective oral analgesia should be initiated to maintain pain control before the nerve block recedes.

Clinical Tip

Pain is one of the presenting symptoms of many common health problems (e.g., otitis media, pharyngitis, and urinary tract infection). Often the only medication prescribed is an antibiotic to clear the infection. This may leave the child in pain for 48 to 72 hours until the antibiotic brings the infection under control. Give parents recommendations for pain control and comfort measures during this period.

- Make sure parents have acetaminophen or ibuprofen in an appropriate formulation (drops, elixir, or tablets) for the child's age, and that the medication's expiration date has not passed.
- Inform the parents about the correct amount of pain medication to use and how frequently it can be given. Ensure that parents have the appropriate medication measuring device.
- Suggest complementary therapies appropriate for the child's age to help manage the child's pain.

Nonpharmacologic Intervention

Complementary therapies are nonpharmacologic methods of pain management that can be used with or without analgesia. One or more of these methods may provide adequate relief of low levels of pain. When used with analgesics, nonpharmacologic methods often increase the effectiveness of the analgesic or reduce the dosage required (see page 587).

Parents are one of the most powerful nonpharmacologic methods of pain relief available to children (Figure 21–9 ■). The parent helps reduce the child's anxiety, and children often feel more secure telling parents about their pain and anxiety. When parents are actively participating in the child's care during hospitalization, make sure they know the appropriate interventions for pain relief. Parents can rate their child's pain using a quantitative scale, so involve them in their child's pain management. Teach them about how complementary therapies can be used to enhance the child's pain management, and help the parent select the age-appropriate complementary therapies for the child. Encourage children and parents to use the techniques that work best for them. See Partnering with Families: Helping a Child Cope with Pain.

Increase Comfort during Painful Procedures

Help the child cope with a painful procedure by explaining what sensations to expect and what will happen during the procedure. This reduces stress more effectively than just providing information about the procedure. Chapter 15 ⏳ gives methods for preparing children of different developmental ages for procedures.

Make every effort to increase the child's comfort during painful procedures, including the use of complementary therapies. Topical anesthetics can be used to reduce the pain associated with an immunization, other injection, intravenous insertion, venipuncture, heel lance, or the first needlestick of another procedure. Consider the amount of time for the topical anesthetic to become effective when a procedure is scheduled. Some mechanisms for administration of topical anesthetics include the following:

- Vapocoolant sprays can be used for injections. They are generally effective almost immediately. The product may also be applied to intact skin using a cotton ball saturated with the spray. The action is short, usually less than a minute. The spray contains chemicals that are eye irritants, so avoid spraying near the eyes.
- EMLA (eutectic mixture of local anesthetics) cream, a mixture of 2.5% lidocaine and 2.5% prilocaine in an emulsion, is

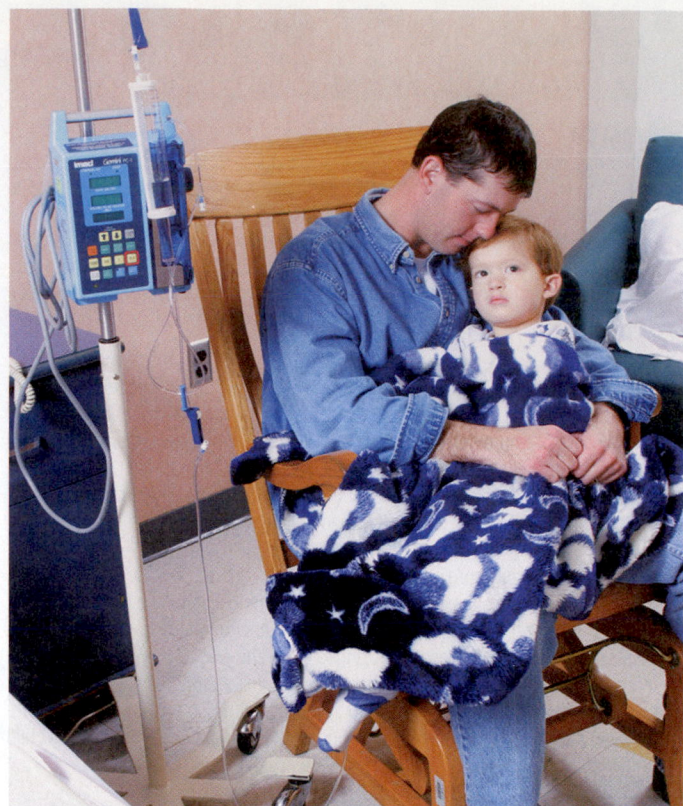

FIGURE 21–9 ■ The presence of the parent is important for pain management and is a significant complementary therapy. Parents help their children cope just by being present. Children are more likely to relax and enable other pain modalities to be more effective. Children often feel more secure telling parents about their pain and anxiety.

effective if applied 1 to 2 hours before a needlestick procedure on intact skin, or 5 to 10 minutes on genital mucosa for neonatal circumcision (Bell, 2009). See Figure 21–10 ■ . Blanching of the skin may be seen due to the vasoconstrictive action on capillaries in the skin. Methemoglobinemia may occur when used in young infants (Zempsky, 2008).

- L-M-X4, 4% liposomal lidocaine (formerly called ELA-MAX), is effective if applied 30 minutes before needlestick. It can be used with or without an occlusive dressing. L-M-X4 is available without a prescription.

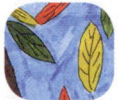

Partnering with Families

Helping a Child Cope with Pain

Parents provide security and help reduce the child's anxiety associated with pain and hospitalization. Children often feel more secure telling their parents about their pain and anxiety. When parents are actively participating in the child's care during hospitalization, teach them how complementary therapies can be used to enhance the child's pain management. Help the parents select the age-appropriate complementary therapy for the child:

- **Infants**—holding, cuddling, sucking a pacifier, massage
- **Toddlers**—massage, stories, bubbles, touch, holding and rocking, music (Figure 21–9)

- **Preschoolers**—engaging in play, stories, music, imagining being a superhero, watching television or a video
- **School-age children**—rhythmic breathing, muscle relaxation, guided imagery, talking about pleasant experiences, playing games, listening to radio, watching television or a video
- **Adolescents**—rhythmic breathing, muscle relaxation, guided imagery, having visitors, playing games, watching television, listening to CD player or iPod

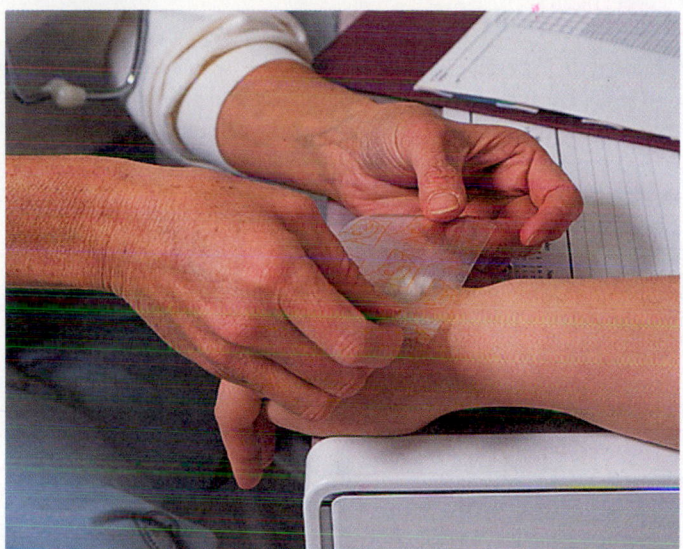

FIGURE 21–10 ■ When painful procedures are planned, use EMLA cream to anesthetize the skin where the painful stick will be made. Apply a thick layer of cream over intact skin (one half of a 5-g tube). Cover the cream with a transparent adhesive dressing, sealing all the sides. The cream anesthetizes the dermal surface in 45 to 60 minutes.

- **Iontophoresis** involves a patch containing 10% lidocaine hydrochloride and 0.1% epinephrine that is placed over the planned needlestick site. A small machine generates low-voltage electric current to transport anesthetic into the skin in about 10 minutes to a depth of 6.4 mm (Zempsky, 2008). The child may have transient skin blanching under the patch. Pain or burn sensations have been experienced on rare occasions by children.
- The Synera anesthetic patch, which contains 70 mg of lidocaine and 70 mg of tetracaine, has an integrated heating component that causes warming (up to 40°C), and adhesive to stick to the skin. The heating component is activated when the patch is exposed to oxygen. It should not be used on mucous membranes or broken skin. The patch is applied for 20 to 30 minutes prior to the procedure but may be applied up to 60 minutes for deeper anesthesia (Zempsky, 2008).
- A needle-free powder lidocaine delivery system produces rapid analgesia for IV starts and venipuncture within 1 to 3 minutes. The system has a sterile, single use, prefilled, and disposable cartridge that is pressed against the skin. Pressurized helium gas ruptures the cartridge and forces lidocaine particles to penetrate the skin. Minor erythema and petechiae may be seen where the delivery system was used (Zempsky, Bean-Lijewski, Kauffman, et al., 2008).

Clinical Tip

Teach parents about the use of L-M-X4 when the child is scheduled for an immunization or venipuncture. L-M-X4 cream can be applied to the skin before departing for the healthcare visit. Provide directions regarding the correct placement of the cream on the arm or leg. Have the parents follow the directions from the package regarding the amount to use and how to cover the site with plastic wrap during the trip to the health center.

A local anesthetic may be injected (e.g., lidocaine buffered by sodium bicarbonate or bupivacaine) or applied topically (e.g., lidocaine, epinephrine, and tetracaine [LET]) to provide analgesia for emergent invasive procedures, such as a laceration repair or lumbar puncture.

Complementary Therapy   A Pain Management Kit

Assemble a pain management kit to promote distraction, imagery, and relaxation in children. Items that might be included are "magic" wands, pinwheels, bubble liquid, a slinky spring toy, a foam ball, party noisemakers, and pop-up books. It may also be helpful to include items for therapeutic play such as syringes with needles removed, adhesive bandages, alcohol swabs, and other supplies from a medical kit. The pain management kit may be especially helpful for children who are being prepared for surgery or for painful procedures and need to be distracted. Parents can also help the child to cope with mild or moderate pain during a procedure by using items in this kit that match the child's developmental stage and individual interests.

Lidocaine can also be injected subcutaneously in a small area to reduce the pain of deeper needle insertion. Use of a topical anesthetic reduces the pain of the injected anesthetic. Some settings do not yet use topical anesthetic agents for an unexpected intravenous insertion, injection, or venipuncture. Support practice change to provide pain management for simple procedures. Such change often requires provider training, policy change, readily available anesthetic agents, and sometimes charging a fee for the anesthetic agent applied.

Complementary therapies, especially imagery, relaxation techniques, and distraction, may reduce the anxiety associated with the anticipation of the procedure, even when topical anesthetics are used. Teach parents and children to use these therapies before procedures. Help children to control their anxiety through therapeutic play. See Complementary Therapy: A Pain Management Kit.

Clinical Judgment

What complementary therapies might work best in a preschool-age child having an intravenous start? What about a school-age child?

Newborn Pain Management

Pain assessment and management of newborns in an intensive care nursery has different challenges, but valid and reliable pain assessment tools exist (see page 578). Select the tool that is best for the neonate's gestational age, such as the PIPP. Pain management is important because newborns in the neonatal ICU experience many painful procedures on a daily basis, such as heel lancing to obtain blood specimens, as well as surgical procedures. When possible, minimize the number of painful procedures or cluster them to reduce neonatal distress. The administration of intravenous opioids requires special training to understand their actions and potential adverse effects in neonates that require monitoring. Advocate for the development of guidelines for neonatal pain management when they do not exist. Use topical anesthetics for procedure pain when possible. EMLA is approved for use in neonates with a gestational age of 37 weeks and later (Walden & Carrier, 2009). Complementary therapies, such as sucrose solution, breastfeeding, and skin-to-skin contact, should also be used to help the neonate cope with painful procedures. Evaluate all pain management interventions for effectiveness.

Discharge Planning and Home Care Teaching

Children are frequently discharged from the hospital, emergency department, or healthcare center with oral analgesics following surgery, injury, or treatment of acute medical conditions. Teach parents and children about the dosage and frequency of administration and the side effects of the analgesic ordered (Box 21–5).

| BOX 21–5 | Research: Analgesia Use by Parents |

A study involving 132 parents of children who had elective outpatient surgery investigated the parents' pain assessment and management practices. Parents indicated that their child experienced significant pain, but on average they provided only 1 dose of analgesia in the first 48 hours after surgery. Reasons that parents gave for not giving more doses of analgesia included the following: concern that analgesics were addictive, worry about side effects, and belief that the analgesia would work better if fewer doses were given. Parent teaching should address these concerns (Rony, Fortier, Chorney, et al., 2010).

Practice Alert

Acetaminophen has a new liquid concentration for infants. It was previously manufactured with higher concentrated drops for infants (80 mg/1 mL or 80 mg/0.8 mL) while the pediatric concentration is 160 mg/5 mL. In 2011, the U.S. Food and Drug Administration guidance directed manufacturers to label the concentration of liquid acetaminophen (160 mg/5 mL) for infants to reduce the risk for accidental overdose (U.S. Food and Drug Administration, 2011). Manufacturers voluntarily agreed to stop producing the more concentrated formulation. Ask parents to carefully check the label of liquid acetaminophen for the concentration before giving a recommended dose of acetaminophen because parents may still have some of the higher concentration acetaminophen in homes. Emphasize the need to use the syringe provided in the packaging to ensure that a correct dose is given to infants and children. Ask about other medications taken by the child to identify any that have acetaminophen as an ingredient, such as a cold product, to prevent an overdose. Make sure parents know to follow dosage guidelines to avoid exceeding the maximum dose which can cause liver toxicity.

Parents have the responsibility to provide adequate pain control for their child after day surgery. As the child leaves the surgical center pain-free, the parents may not anticipate pain. Because of cultural values, certain parents may feel the child should learn to tolerate some amount of pain. Provide guidance to help parents assess their child's pain and directions for giving pain medications. (See Partnering with Families: Pain Management for the Child at Home.)

Evaluation

Expected outcomes of nursing care include the following:

- Children at risk for pain are assessed and undergo implementation of pain management.
- The child with pain experiences improved and maintained comfort.
- The nurse successfully advocates for additional pain medication dosage when needed.
- The child experiences enhanced comfort with the use of age-appropriate complementary methods of pain management.
- Parents maintain pain management after discharge.

CHRONIC PAIN

Children do experience medical conditions that cause chronic pain and recurrent acute pain with possible variation in severity and quality. Chronic pain can occur in one or more body systems. Medical conditions such as juvenile idiopathic arthritis, sickle cell anemia, cancer, headaches, recurrent abdominal pain, and HIV infection all cause chronic and recurrent pain. Girls are more likely than boys to experience chronic pain with greater pain intensity and in multiple locations (Lynch, Kashikar-Zuck, Goldschneider, et al., 2007). Approximately 15% to 20% of children and adolescents have chronic pain (American Pain Society, 2011). Children and adolescents with chronic and recurrent pain have functional limitations related to school, social activities and relationships, physical activity, and family responsibilities (Palermo, 2009).

Etiology and Pathophysiology

Chronic pain may be nociceptive or neuropathic, which is caused by abnormal functioning of the central nervous system. The sympathetic nervous system is not aroused in the same way as with acute pain. Ongoing stimulation of nociceptors can sensitize the peripheral and central nervous systems, resulting in altered or enhanced transmission of pain sensory information. Specific nerve fibers become irritated and more sensitive, leading to hyperalgesia in which a pain sensation is felt as more painful. Allodynia, a normally nonpainful sensation felt as pain, may also occur. Headache, abdominal pain, and musculoskeletal pain account for the majority of recurring pain. In some cases in which chronic pain is associated with vague and nonspecific symptoms, there is no easily identifiable cause.

Clinical Manifestations

Physical signs and symptoms should be viewed together. Behavioral indicators of chronic pain may include inactivity, posturing, depression, and difficulty concentrating and sleeping. Chronic pain of long duration that is persistent or continuous permits physiologic adaptation so normal heart rate, respiratory rate, and blood pressure levels are often seen (Huether, 2010). Many of these children have anxiety, depression, and low self-esteem (Meldrum, Tsao, & Zeltzer, 2009). Varying levels of disability may also exist.

Selected Chronic Pain Conditions

Information about selected chronic pain conditions and pain management strategies is provided below.

Sickle Cell Disease

Sickle cell disease is an inherited blood disorder that causes red blood cells to change from round to sickle shaped. Vaso-occlusive episodes

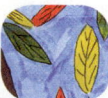

Partnering with Families

Pain Management for the Child at Home

- Review the child's pain behaviors and the fact that the child may still have pain even though watching television, playing, or sleeping.
- Discuss why pain management is important and how uncontrolled pain can slow recovery.
- Discuss the need for scheduled pain medication rather than waiting for the onset of pain to begin treatment.

- Review the child's pain management plan.
- Inform parents that a sudden increase in pain intensity could mean a complication has developed that needs medical attention. Provide healthcare provider contact information to report the increasing pain.
- Review the complementary therapies and the role they play in pain management.

occur as the sickle-shaped blood cells obstruct small blood vessels and deprive the tissues of oxygen and cause inflammation. These episodes are associated with significant recurrent pain that may last for hours to weeks. Painful vaso-occlusive episodes are often unpredictable. Some children develop severe pain that requires an emergency department visit or hospitalization when all usual home interventions have been used. No standard pain management exists for sickle cell disease. Intravenous opioids are commonly used for acute sickle cell crisis. For home management of pain, children are often prescribed NSAIDs and oral opioids that are equianalgesic to parenteral dosages, such as codeine, hydromorphone, and oxycodone. Additional strategies to manage pain at home to prevent hospitalization include fluids and complementary therapies such as distraction, relaxation techniques, guided imagery, deep breathing, and self-hypnosis. Parents and children make efforts to prevent painful episodes with several strategies as described on page 915 🔗.

Cancer Pain

Children with cancer may have acute, chronic, and intermittent pain. Children with cancer undergo numerous invasive procedures and treatments that cause pain and distress, such as bone marrow aspiration, lumbar puncture, chemotherapy, and radiation. The effect of these cumulative procedures may have a significant impact on the child's suffering, as multiple sites of pain may be present simultaneously. As cancer progresses, pain may become persistent, and eventually require 24-hour pain control. Breakthrough pain may also occur. The amount of pain and suffering that a child with cancer experiences may be underestimated, especially toward the end of life when aggressive life-prolonging therapies are used. See page 962 🔗.

A pain management program is important for children with cancer. Children and families should participate in pain assessments and in developing goals for pain management. Acetaminophen and NSAIDs may be the first pain medications prescribed with the addition of opioids. Medications are given as needed when pain episodes are intermittent. When pain is persistent throughout the day, 24-hour pain control is initiated and dosing should be determined by the amount of medication needed to relieve pain without causing intolerable adverse reactions (American Pain Society, 2008, p. 23). Breakthrough pain medication may also be prescribed. Side effects such as sedation, nausea, constipation, pruritus, and respiratory depression must be managed.

Complex Regional Pain Syndrome

Complex regional pain syndrome is a neuropathic pain syndrome in which excessive pain is out of proportion to the injury or event that preceded the pain. The pain syndrome is often located in an extremity and includes sensory disturbances such as allodynia/hyperalgesia, autonomic dysfunction, and motor dysfunction. The actual pathophysiologic mechanism is not known. Girls between 8 and 16 years of age are most commonly affected (Stanton-Hicks, 2010). A history of minor trauma or repeated stress injury, such as that which could occur in competitive sports, is sometimes reported. The child has burning pain; exaggerated sensitivity to cold; paresthesia; loss of feeling secondary to a thermal, tactile, or vibratory sensation; or allodynia. Signs of autonomic dysfunction in the affected body region include edema, skin color and temperature changes, or abnormal sweating.

Treatment is focused on improving function with aggressive physical and occupational therapy and cognitive behavioral therapy to teach the child coping skills for controlling responses to pain while attempting to relieve pain. Some children need additional therapies coordinated by a pediatric pain specialist, such as long-term epidural analgesia. Tricyclic antidepressants and antiseizure medications may be prescribed to promote sleep and to help assist with pain management (Stanton-Hicks, 2010).

Collaborative Care

Diagnostic Testing

No tools have been developed to assess chronic pain for any child age group. It may be valuable to use multiple tools to assess pain, including a body outline where all pain scales can be marked, a self-report pain rating tool, and a list of words that describe pain characteristics. Having the child keep a pain diary, including pain characteristics, may also be helpful for assessment of recurrent pain. Assess the child for muscle spasms, trigger points, and areas of somatic sensitivity (sensitive to light touch).

Clinical Therapy

Children with chronic pain need an individualized pain treatment plan with a primary focus on improved function and improved comfort. In some cases a multidisciplinary pain management team works with the child and family to identify optimal pain therapies for the child. Analgesic medications are prescribed, including NSAIDs, acetaminophen, and opioids, often in combination. Transdermal fentanyl patches may be used for some children with more severe chronic pain needing long-term pain management. Complete pain relief may not be possible, and the child may need additional pain medication for acute flares of the condition. Tricyclic antidepressants may be prescribed for their analgesic properties and because depression may be a co-existing condition. Gabapentin, an antiseizure medication, has efficacy in treating neuropathic pain (Hollan, 2007). Exercise and physical therapy are important to help promote improved function in the child with chronic pain. Cognitive behavioral therapies are used to help the child cope with pain and enhance pain management.

Nursing Management

Nursing Assessment and Diagnoses

When assessing chronic pain in the child, approach pain as if it is the primary problem for attention. Assessment and evaluation of chronic pain in children should include the following aspects (American Pain Society, 2011):

- Approach pain as the primary present problem. The physical, behavioral, and psychologic signs and symptoms should be viewed together.
- Obtain the history of pain onset, its development over time, intensity, duration, location, what makes it worse or relieves it, and its impact on daily life (sleeping, appetite, school, and social interactions). Identify any stressful events, family discord, moves, deaths, or other changes, such as a new school.
- Identify the amount of distress the child and family experience with pain, including anxiety, depression, and hopelessness.
- Determine what the family and child believe causes the pain and their response to it.
- Identify past pain problems in the family and the current methods of treatment.
- Observe the child's appearance, posture, gait, and emotional and cognitive state.
- Assess muscle spasms, trigger points, and areas sensitive to light touch, and perform a complete neurologic examination.

Date	Time	Pain Intensity	Pain Medication Taken	How Much	Other Pain Relief Methods	Amount of Pain 1 Hour Later

FIGURE 21–11 ■ A pain diary is an important tool to help record the painful episodes experienced with chronic conditions such as rheumatoid arthritis or episodic conditions such as sickle cell disease. Have the child choose a pain scale to record pain intensity 1 hour after intervention.

Older children with recurrent episodes of pain can be encouraged to keep a written or online diary or log to describe the characteristics, timing, activities, and potential triggers of their pain, as well as their response to pain treatment measures. Encourage them to use a pain assessment tool to rate the pain intensity before and after medications and other pain control measures are used. See Figure 21–11 ■. This record can help improve pain management.

Examples of nursing diagnoses for children with chronic pain include:

- Pain, Chronic (Hand), Pain related to arthritic joint inflammation and degeneration
- Sleep Pattern, Disturbed related to ineffective management of chronic pain
- Mobility: Physical, Impaired, related to ineffective management of chronic pain
- Constipation, Risk for, related to opioid medication and limited activity

NANDA-I © 2012

Planning and Implementation

Children with chronic conditions such as arthritis, sickle cell disease, cancer, and recurrent headaches often need long-term pain management, and in some cases care by a pain management team. Planning the pain management care for the child and family should be individualized to the child's condition and pain experience. It should also integrate the family's beliefs and values, as well as cultural preferences for care. Because pain can affect the child's psychologic health, assessment and care for depression should be implemented. (See Chapter 34 🔗.) Psychologic support may also be helpful to promote coping skills.

Additional strategies for chronic pain management include the following:

- Explain and validate pain and its causes.
- Discuss treatment goals with the child and family, and jointly develop a care plan that integrates pharmacologic and non-pharmacologic (complementary) methods.
- Develop a care plan for painful episodes associated with acute flares of their condition.
- Provide effective preventive pain management for procedural pain, as many of these children have numerous medical procedures. If the child's chronic pain is managed with opioids, special consideration is needed to manage the child's procedural pain.

Work with the family to proactively manage constipation when the child takes opioids for pain. Constipation is a side effect that does not improve over time. Fluids and fiber should be added to the diet, and the child should also take a stimulating laxative and potentially a stool softener.

Monitor pain intensity at each office visit and frequently during hospitalizations. It is important to identify when the child needs additional pain management interventions proactively to improve the quality of life.

Assist the child and family to identify age-appropriate and acceptable complementary therapies to help cope with discomfort such as massage, distraction, biofeedback, relaxation, and self-hypnosis. Additionally, exercise should be integrated into the child's daily routine to promote function. Physical therapy may be necessary to enable the child to maintain or regain function. The parents may want to consider whether an individual health plan for pain management at school should be initiated.

Evaluation

Expected outcomes of nursing care include the following:

- The child uses selected complementary therapies to help manage chronic pain.
- The nurse, family, and child recognize the need for additional pain management interventions with frequent assessments.
- The child's side effects of pain management, such as constipation, are managed.

SEDATION AND PAIN MANAGEMENT FOR MEDICAL PROCEDURES

Children undergo a wide variety of painful diagnostic and treatment procedures in the hospital and in outpatient settings. Procedures such as chest tube insertion, arterial puncture, lumbar puncture, bone marrow aspiration, insertion of a central or peripheral intravenous line, fracture reduction, laceration repair, and burn debridement cause significant pain in children. The anticipation of these procedures causes anxiety and emotional distress that can lead to greater intensity of pain. For example, children who have experienced prior pain associated with painful cancer-treatment procedures may have greater pain during later procedures, even when provided with adequate analgesia (Kennedy et al., 2008).

Sedation is a medically controlled state of depressed consciousness (light to deep) used for painful diagnostic and therapeutic procedures and analgesia. The state of sedation ranges from light to deep. Children often need light sedation for minimally painful procedures. Children undergoing painful procedures such as burn debridement, laceration repair, bone marrow aspiration, and fracture

Medications Used for Sedation

MEDICATION	ACTION	NURSING MANAGEMENT
Benzodiazepines Midazolam (Versed) Lorazepam (Ativan) Diazepam (Valium) May be reversed by flumazenil	Midazolam is preferred for its rapid and short action time (within 2 to 3 minutes of IV administration). It produces skeletal muscle relaxation, amnesia, and moderate sedation. Pain is still perceived. Routes of administration: oral, intranasal, IV, IM, and rectal	▪ Analgesia should be co-administered to manage pain associated with the procedure. ▪ Simultaneous administration of potent opiates such as fentanyl or morphine may increase the depth of sedation and increase the risk of hypotension and respiratory depression. ▪ May cause paradoxical reaction in some children (hysteria, restlessness, inconsolability, and agitation).
Hypnotics (barbiturates) Thiopental Methohexital Pentobarbital	Thiopental and methohexital are ultra-short-acting and produce hypnosis and sedation useful for painless diagnostic procedures. Pentobarbital is a short-acting barbiturate that produces deep sedation. Routes of administration: rectal and IV	▪ May cause hypotension, hypoventilation, and apnea in children, so the child may need positioning, supplemental oxygen, and assisted ventilation. ▪ May increase pain sensation.
Analgesics Fentanyl Alfentanil May be reversed by naloxone or nalmefene	Fentanyl is an opioid preferred for its short action for procedural analgesia in combination with midazolam. Route of administration: IV	▪ Rapid administration may lead to rigidity of the chest wall, bradycardia, and hypotension. ▪ Other side effects include pruritus, nausea, and vomiting. ▪ Children appear to be asleep, but may be able to maintain awareness.
Ketamine	Acts by dissociating the central nervous system from external stimuli (e.g., pain, sight, and sound). Has analgesic, sedative, and amnesic properties while maintaining cardiovascular stability. Child appears awake with eyes open but does not respond behaviorally. Routes of administration: IV, oral, IM	▪ Airway reflexes and respirations are unimpaired. Upper airway secretions are increased. May have random movements. Encourage an older child to plan a pleasant dream as this may decrease unpleasant recovery reactions. ▪ The child may need positioning to maintain the airway during sedation. ▪ May have vomiting, agitation, muscular hypertonicity, transient apnea or respiratory depression, or transient laryngospasm with emergence from sedation. IV ondansetron may reduce incidence of vomiting.
Propofol (Diprivan)	Sedative, hypnotic, and muscle relaxant with very rapid onset (30 seconds) and quick recovery (6 minutes). Mild antiemetic. Route of administration: IV	▪ May be combined with fentanyl to add analgesia, but this combination may increase the risk of respiratory depression. ▪ Take care to avoid contamination as the lipid emulsion promotes bacterial growth. ▪ Causes pain when administered IV push unless co-administered with lidocaine. Contraindicated in children with hypersensitivity to eggs and soy products.
Dexmedetomidine	Alpha-2 agonist with sedative and analgesic effects. Routes of administration: IV, oral, and transmucous (buccal and intranasal)	▪ May be associated with initial hypertension with reflex bradycardia that usually stabilizes to a level below baseline. ▪ May be effective in sedating patients with autism.
Etomidate	Ultra-short-acting hypnotic sedative and amnesic medication without analgesic properties that has a short recovery time. Route of administration: IV	▪ May cause episodes of nausea, vomiting, agitation, myoclonus, and respiratory depression. ▪ Has less effect on the heart rate and blood pressure than other medications.
Chloral Hydrate	Sedative, hypnotic with analgesic properties that is used for painless diagnostic procedures. Routes of Administration: oral and rectal	▪ Time to peak sedation is 30 minutes with a recovery time of an additional 1 to 2 hours. The child may have a residual motor imbalance and agitation. ▪ Should not be used in children with neurodevelopmental disorders. ▪ Drug is most reliable in children under 4 years of age.

Source: *Data from Green, S. M., Roback, M. G., Kennedy, R. M., & Krauss, B. (2011). Clinical practice guideline for emergency department ketamine dissociative sedation: 2011 update. Annals of Emergency Medicine, 57(5), 444–461; Miner, J. R., & Burton, J. H. (2007). Clinical practice advisory: Emergency department procedural sedation with propofol. Annals of Emergency Medicine, 50(2), 182–187; Kost, S., & Roy, A. (2010). Procedural sedation and analgesia in the pediatric emergency department: A review of sedative pharmacology. Clinical Pediatric Emergency Medicine, 11(4), 233–243; McCarty, E. C., & Mencio, G. A. (2008). Anesthesia and analgesia for the ambulatory management of children's fractures. In N. E. Green & M. F. Swiontkowski, Skeletal trauma in children (4th ed., pp. 609–620). Philadelphia, PA: Saunders Elsevier.*

reduction should be premedicated with analgesia and sedation. Benzodiazepines such as diazepam (Valium), midazolam (Versed), and pentobarbital are commonly used for sedation. Ketamine, propofol (Diprivan), and etomidate may also be used for sedation. Inhaled nitrous oxide may be used in association with local anesthesia for procedural sedation. Chloral hydrate may be used for children under age 4 years for painless procedures (Mace, Brown, Francis, et al., 2008). Analgesia should be used in combination with sedation when procedures are painful. See the Medications table for sedation medications.

Clinical Manifestations Light, Moderate, and Deep Sedation

ASSESSMENT FACTORS	LIGHT SEDATION	MODERATE SEDATION	DEEP SEDATION
Airway	Maintains airway independently and continuously	Maintains airway independently and continuously	Impaired ability to maintain airway, may need assisted ventilation
Cough and gag reflexes	Reflexes intact	Reflexes intact	Partial or complete loss of reflexes
Level of consciousness	Responds normally to verbal stimuli	Purposeful response to verbal or gentle tactile stimulation	Purposeful response after repeated or painful stimuli

Source: *Data from Mandt, M. J., & Roback, M. G. (2007). Assessment and monitoring of pediatric procedure sedation. Clinical Pediatric Emergency Medicine, 8, 223–231; Diaz, L. K., & Jones, L. (2009). Sedating the child with congenital heart disease. Anesthesiology Clinics, 27, 301–319; Tschudy, M. M., & Arcara, K. M. (2012). Harriet Lane Handbook (19th ed., p. 143). Philadelphia, PA: Elsevier.*

When sedatives are given in lower doses, **moderate sedation** (formerly called conscious sedation) occurs in which the child maintains protective reflexes, retains the ability to independently and continuously maintain a patent airway, and retains the ability to respond to tactile and verbal stimuli. **Deep sedation** is a controlled state of depressed consciousness or unconsciousness in which protective airway reflexes are lost. See the Clinical Manifestations table for the characteristics of different levels of sedation.

The goals of procedural sedation and analgesia are to prevent or relieve pain and anxiety, make it easier to do the medical procedures, and prevent complications such as respiratory distress, an obstructed airway, aspiration, or an adverse reaction to the medications used. The level of sedation is actually a continuum, and the child may progress from one level to a deeper level, which is why the child must be carefully monitored during sedation. Every healthcare facility where pediatric sedation is performed should have guidelines to ensure safe healthcare practices. These guidelines often require health professionals monitoring the child to have specific qualifications, such as training in pediatric advanced life support. The child must be carefully monitored for respiratory depression and signs of deep sedation because the child may lose protective reflexes and need assisted ventilation. Antagonist agents are available for opioids (naloxone) and benzodiazepines (flumazenil) when the effects of sedation and respiratory depression need to be reversed.

Nursing Management

The nurse has an important role in advocating for safe and effective sedation and pain management for the child undergoing an invasive diagnostic or therapeutic procedure. Educate parents about the time a child with scheduled sedation should fast prior to the procedure, following agency procedure guidelines for the age of the child. Use complementary therapies such as distraction and imagery to help reduce the child's anxiety while waiting for the sedation to take effect. Prevent anticipated procedure-related pain with an analgesic, and give time for the medication to become effective. When possible, administer drugs by a nonpainful route (oral, transmucosal, or intravenous). When procedures must be repeated (e.g., bone marrow aspirations for children with leukemia), give optimal sedation and analgesia for the first procedure to reduce anxiety about future procedures. To prevent increased anxiety, avoid delays in performing procedures. Make sure the results of pain management are documented.

When the child receives sedation, monitoring the child's status for respiratory depression or airway obstruction is important during the procedure and until the medication wears off. Nursing assessments include *visual* confirmation of respiratory effort, color, and vital signs. Pulse oximetry and capnography (to monitor ventilation) may also be used for monitoring, but this equipment must not replace visual assessment. Vital signs must be checked every 15 minutes until the child regains full consciousness and level of functioning. If light sedation progresses to deep sedation, airway management is essential, and vital signs should be checked every 5 minutes. Resuscitation equipment must be available and drug antagonists must be precalculated and ready to administer; see the Skills Manual 🔗.

Practice Alert

When moderate sedation is administered, be sure to have the resources available to monitor the child's vital signs and to provide advanced life support if the child should progress to deep sedation. All healthcare facilities have special protocols for management of children receiving sedation.

If complications occur, the following equipment should be immediately available: suction apparatus, a bag-valve mask for assisted ventilation with capability of 90% to 100% oxygen delivery, an oxygen supply, a defibrillator, drugs for advanced life support, and drug antagonists (Mandt & Roback, 2007).

Criteria for discharge after sedation include the following:

- The child has satisfactory and stable cardiovascular function and airway patency.
- The child arouses easily and has intact protective reflexes.
- The child is adequately hydrated.
- The infant is able to hold the head up and sit up unassisted if old enough to do so, or the child can stand and walk without assistance.
- The discharge status is the same as admission status.

Parents should be informed to anticipate the possibility that the child may have mild adverse effects from sedation, such as crying, lethargy, and vomiting. When ketamine is used the child may have sleep disturbances, crying, and headaches (Steurer & Luhmann, 2007).

Chapter Highlights

- Pain is an unpleasant sensation that is either acute or chronic, perceived in response to tissue damage. Neuropathic pain is one form of chronic pain.
- Unrelieved pain is stressful for newborns, infants, and children, causing many undesirable physiologic consequences on body systems.
- A child's responses to and understanding of pain depend on age, stage of development, culture, and prior painful experiences.
- Children learn how and when to seek help for pain and how to cope with pain by observing other family members.
- Pain assessment should include physical, behavioral, and emotional factors to obtain the most accurate information about the location and intensity of the child's pain and how the child responds to it.
- Pain assessment should include the use of a valid and reliable pain assessment tool that is appropriate for the child's age and condition.
- Every infant, child, and adolescent has the right to adequate pain control.
- Pharmacologic interventions for pain control include opioids, nonsteroidal anti-inflammatory drugs (NSAIDs), and acetaminophen.
- Opioids are equally effective when administered by oral, intramuscular, and intravenous routes when an equianalgesic dose is used.
- Analgesia for continuous or severe pain should be given around the clock to maintain pain control. Patient-controlled analgesia is one method of administering an opioid medication around the clock and allowing the child to infuse small doses when pain is felt.
- Complementary therapies for pain management include the following: parental presence, distraction, cutaneous stimulation, sucrose solution, electroanalgesia, guided imagery, breathing techniques, progressive muscle relaxation techniques, hypnosis, application of heat and cold, biofeedback, and acupuncture.
- Epidural and regional nerve blocks are used more frequently for postsurgical pain management because they have fewer side effects than systemic medications.
- Many diagnostic and therapeutic procedures cause pain and anxiety in children. Provide optimal prophylactic pain management to reduce the anxiety associated with future procedures.
- Parents need education and preparation to provide pain control for children who are discharged home following surgery and injuries.
- Children with recurrent and chronic painful conditions need to have an individualized pain management plan that includes analgesics and complementary therapies.
- Sedation is used to reduce the child's anxiety associated with nonpainful or painful procedures. Analgesia is given with sedation when the procedure will cause pain or discomfort to the child.

Clinical Reasoning in Action

INTRODUCTION

Recall Lucas, the 14-year-old at the beginning of the chapter, who is to have orthopedic surgery for a slipped capital femoral epiphysis (see Chapter 35 🔗). He will go home the same day of surgery.

DESCRIPTION

Lucas received a dose of IV morphine in the postanesthesia unit at 10 a.m. He has an order for a repeat dose at 2 p.m. prior to discharge. He will be sent home with acetaminophen with codeine for pain every 3 to 4 hours.

DISCUSSION

1. What are the most appropriate pain assessment tools for Lucas to use to report his level of pain to the nurse?

2. What complementary pain therapies are of value for Lucas's condition and age?

3. Lucas weighs 52 kg. What is the appropriate dose of morphine for Lucas and the calculated volume (concentration of 2 mg per mL) to be administered?

4. Describe the important nursing assessments for Lucas following morphine administration.

5. Develop a teaching plan for Lucas's home pain management and expected medication side effects. When should Lucas receive his first dose of acetaminophen with codeine?

NCLEX-RN® Review

1. The nurse takes the vital signs of an infant who has just returned from surgery. What indicates that the infant may have acute pain requiring nursing intervention?
   1. The infant eagerly takes the bottle.
   2. The infant watches the crib mobile.
   3. The infant has a heart rate of 180.
   4. The infant responds to the parents.

2. The nurse is caring for a 12-year-old child who injured his leg in a backyard football game. He is currently complaining of mild pain at the site and has received oral pain medication. What is the most appropriate complementary therapy for pain management for this child?
   1. Wrap the child in a blanket.
   2. Offer the child a sugary drink.
   3. Offer bubbles to the child.
   4. Teach progressive muscle relaxation.

3. During rounds, the nurse is performing an initial assessment on a 12-year-old child with sickle cell disease. The nurse notes that he child has hypoactive bowel sounds and is grimacing in pain. How can the nurse best assist this patient?

1. Ensure the child has pain medication for uncontrolled pain.
2. Ask the child when the last bowel movement occurred.
3. Make sure the child ambulates every 2 hours.
4. There is no need to provide any intervention at this time.

4. A 3-year-old is scheduled to return to the clinic in one week to have blood drawn by venipuncture to reassess electrolyte values. The child's parents ask if there is anything they can do to decrease the child's discomfort from the procedure. Which would be the most appropriate action by the nurse?

1. Suggest distraction techniques the parents can use for the child during the procedure.
2. Suggest the parents reassure the child the procedure will not hurt as long as he or she holds completely still.
3. Suggest that the parents obtain L-M-X4 from a pharmacy, and instruct them how to use it.
4. Suggest therapeutic play prior to the procedure to ensure the child understands what will occur.

See Appendix I 🔗 for answers.

References

Accardi, M. C., & Milling, L. S. (2009). The effectiveness of hypnosis for reducing procedure-related pain in children and adolescents: A comprehensive methodological review. *Journal of Behavioral Medicine, 32*, 328–339.

American Pain Society. (2008). *Principles of analgesic use in the treatment of acute pain and cancer pain* (6th ed.). Glenview, IL: Author.

American Pain Society. (2011). *Pediatric chronic pain.* Retrieved from http://www.ampainsoc.org/advocacy/pediatric.htm

Anthony, K. K., & Schanberg, L. E. (2007). Assessment and management of pain syndromes and arthritis pain in children and adolescents. *Rheumatic Disease Clinics of North America, 33*, 625–660.

Badr, L. K., Abdallah, B., Hawari, M., Sidani, S., Kassar, M., Nakad, P., & Breidi, J. (2010). Determinants of premature infant pain responses to heel sticks. *Pediatric Nursing, 36*(3), 129–136.

Bell, E. A. (2009). Update on topical anesthetics. *Infectious Diseases in Children, 22*(7), 12.

Breau, L. M., & Burkitt, C. (2009). Assessing pain in children with intellectual disabilities. *Pain Research and Management, 14*(2), 116–120.

Cohen, L. L., Lemanek, K., Blount, R. L., Dahlquist, L. M., Lim, C. S., Palermo, T. M., . . . Weiss, K. E. (2008). Evidence-based assessment of pediatric pain. *Journal of Pediatric Psychology, 33*(9), 939–955.

Diaz, L. K., & Jones, L. (2009). Sedating the child with congenital heart disease. *Anesthesiology Clinics, 27*, 301–319.

Drendel, A. L., Gorelick, M. H., Weisman, S. J., Lyon, R., Brousseau, D. C., & Kim, M. K. (2009). A randomized clinical trial of ibuprofen versus acetaminophen with codeine for acute pediatric arm fracture pain. *Annals of Emergency Medicine, 54*(4), 553–560.

Finley, G. A., Kristjánsdóttir, Ó., & Forgeron, P. A. (2009). Cultural influences on the assessment of children's pain. *Pain Research & Management, 14*(1), 33–37.

Forshee, B. A., Clayton, M. F., & McCance, K. L. (2010). Stress and disease. In K. L. McCance & S. E. Huether (Eds.), *Pathophysiology: The biologic basis for disease in adults and children* (6th ed., pp. 336–359). St. Louis, MO: Elsevier Mosby.

Franson, H. E. (2010). Postoperative patient-controlled analgesia in the pediatric population: A literature review. *AANA Journal, 78*(5), 374–378.

Ghai, B., Makkar, J. K., & Wig, J. (2008). Postoperative pain assessment in preverbal children and children with cognitive impairment. *Pediatric Anesthesia, 18*, 462–477.

Green, S. M., Roback, M. G., Kennedy, R. M., & Krauss, B. (2011). Clinical practice guideline for emergency department ketamine dissociative sedation: 2011 update. *Annals of Emergency Medicine, 57*(5), 449–461.

Greenwald, M. (2010). Analgesia for the pediatric trauma patient: Primum non nocere? *Clinical Pediatric Emergency Medicine, 11*(1), 28–40.

Griffin, R. A., Polit, D. F., & Byrne, M. W. (2008). Nurse characteristics and inferences about children's pain. *Pediatric Nursing, 34*(4), 297–305.

Harrison, D., Bueno, M., Yamada, J., Adams-Webber, T., & Stevens, B. (2010). Analgesic effects of sweet-tasting solutions for infants: Current state of equipoise. *Pediatrics, 126*(5), 894–902.

Hollan, M. (2007). A practical way to manage chronic pain. *Clinical Advisor, 10*(1), 51–59.

Holsti, L. (2008). Is it painful or not? Discriminant validity of the Behavioral Indicators of Infant Pain (BIIP) scale. *Clinical Journal of Pain, 24*(1), 83–88.

Howard, R. F., Lloyd-Thomas, A., Thomas, M., Williams, D. G., Saul, R., . . . Peters, J. (2010). Nurse-controlled analgesia (NGA) following major surgery in 10,000 patients in a children's hospital. *Pediatric Anesthesia, 20*, 126–134.

Huether, S. E. (2010). Pain, temperature regulation, sleep, and sensory function. In K. L. McCance, S. E. Huether, V. L. Brasher, & N. S. Rote (Eds.), *Pathophysiology: The biologic basis for disease in adults and children* (6th ed., pp. 481–524). St. Louis, MO: Elsevier Mosby.

Huth, M. M., Daraisch, N. M., Henson, M. A., & McLeod, S. M. (2009). Evaluation of the Magic Island: Relaxation for kids compact disc. *Pediatric Nursing, 35*(5), 290–295.

Joint Commission. (2011). *Facts about pain management.* Retrieved from http://www.jointcommission.org/pain_management/

Kennedy, R. M., Luhmann, J., & Zempsky, W. T. (2008). Clinical implications of unmanaged needle-insertion pain and distress in children. *Pediatrics, 122* (Suppl. 3), S130–S133.

Kohen, D. P. (2011). Chronic daily headache: Helping adolescents help themselves with self-hypnosis. *American Journal of Clinical Hypnosis, 54*, 32–46.

Kost, S., & Roy, A. (2010). Procedural sedation and analgesia in the pediatric emergency department: A review of sedative pharmacology. *Clinical Pediatric Emergency Medicine, 11*(4), 233–243.

Kraemer, F. W., & Rose, J. B. (2009). Pharmacologic management of acute pediatric pain. *Anesthesiology Clinics, 27*, 241–268.

Kundu, A., & Berman, B. (2007). Acupuncture for pediatric pain and symptom management. *Pediatric Clinics of North America, 53*, 885–899.

Kuttner, L. (2010). *A child in pain: What health professionals can do to help.* Bethel, CT: Crown House Publishing Limited.

Lane, F., & Latham, T. (2009). Managing pain using heat and cold therapy. *Pediatric Nursing, 21*(6), 14–18.

Lawrence, J., Alcock, D., McGrath, P., Kay, J., MacMurray, S. B., & Dulberg, C. (1993). The development of a tool to assess neonatal pain. *Neonatal Network, 12*(6), 61.

Lynch, A. M., Kashikar-Zuck, S., Goldschneider, K. R., & Jones, B. A. (2007). Sex and age differences in coping styles among children with chronic pain. *Journal of Pain and Symptom Management, 33*(2), 208–216.

Mace, S. E., Brown, L. A., Francis, L., Godwin, S. A., Hahn, S. A., Howard, P. K., . . . Clark, R. M. (2008). Clinical policy: Critical issues in the sedation of pediatric patients in the emergency department. *Annals of Emergency Medicine, 51*(4), 378–399.

Mandt, M. J., & Roback, M. G. (2007). Assessment and monitoring of pediatric procedure sedation. *Clinical Pediatric Emergency Medicine, 8*, 223–231.

McCarty, E. C., & Mencio, G. A. (2008). Anesthesia and analgesia for the ambulatory management of children's fractures. In N. E. Green & M. F. Swiontkowski, *Skeletal trauma in children* (4th ed., pp. 609–620). Philadelphia, PA: Saunders Elsevier.

Meldrum, M. L., Tsao, J. C. I., & Zeltzer, L. K. (2009). "I can't be what I want to be": Children's narratives of chronic pain experiences and treatment outcomes. *Pain Medicine, 10*(6), 1018–1034.

Merkel, S., Voepel-Lewis, T., Shayevitz, J. R., & Malviya, S. (1997). The FLACC: A behavioral scale for scoring postoperative pain in young children. *Pediatric Nursing, 23*(3), 293–297.

Miner, J. R., & Burton, J. H. (2007). Clinical practice advisory: Emergency department procedural sedation with propofol. *Annals of Emergency Medicine, 50*(2), 182–187.

Morrow, C. (2010). Reducing neonatal pain during routine heel lance procedures. *MCN American Journal of Maternal Child Nursing, 35*(6), 346–354.

Palermo, T. M. (2009). Assessment of chronic pain in children: Current status and emerging topics. *Pain Research & Management, 14*(1), 21–26.

Pappagallo, M., & Werner, M. (2008). *Chronic pain: A primer for physicians*. Chicago: Remedica.

Pasero, C., & McCaffery, M. (2011). *Pain assessment and pharmacologic management*. St. Louis, MO: Elsevier Mosby.

Purnell, L. D. (2009). *Guide to culturally competent care* (2nd ed.). Philadelphia, PA: F. A. Davis.

Rony, R. Y. Z., Fortier, M. A., Chorney, J. M., Perret, D., & Kain, Z. N. (2010). Parental postoperative pain management: Attitudes, assessment, and management. *Pediatrics, 125*(6), e1372–1378.

Stanton-Hicks, M. (2010). Plasticity of complex regional pain syndrome (CRPS) in children. *Pain Medicine, 11,* 1216–1223.

Stevens, B. (2010). The premature infant pain profile: Evaluation 13 years after development. *Clinical Journal of Pain, 26*(9), 813–830.

Stevens, B., Johnston, C., Petryshen, P., & Taddio, A. (1996). Premature infant pain profile: Development and initial validation. *Clinical Journal of Pain, 12*(1), 13–22.

Steurer, L. M., & Luhmann, J. (2007). Adverse effects of pediatric emergency sedation after discharge. *Pediatric Nursing, 33*(5), 403–407.

Taddio, A., Shah, V., Hancock, R., Smith, R. W., Stephens, D., Atenafu, E., . . . Katz, J. (2008). Assessing postoperative pain in neonates: A multicenter observational study. *Pediatrics, 118*(4), e992–e1000.

Taenzer, A. H., & Clark, C. (2010). Efficacy of postoperative epidural analgesia in adolescent scoliosis surgery: A meta-analysis. *Pediatric Anesthesia, 20,* 135–143.

Taketomo, C. K., Hodding, J. H., & Kraus, D. M. (2010). *Pediatric dosage handbook* (17th ed., p. 949). Hudson, OH: American Pharmacists Association.

Taylor, E. M., Boyer, K., & Campbell, F. A. (2008). Pain in hospitalized children: A prospective cross-sectional survey of pain prevalence, intensity, assessment, and management in a Canadian pediatric teaching hospital. *Pain Research & Management, 13*(1), 25–32.

Tschudy, M. M., & Arcara, K. M. (2012). *Harriet Lane Handbook* (19th ed., p. 143). Philadelphia, PA: Elsevier.

Twycross, A. (2009). Why managing pain in children matters. In A. Twycross, S. J. Dowden, & E. Bruce (Eds.), *Managing pain in children*. United Kingdom: Wiley-Blackwell.

U.S. Food and Drug Administration. (2011). *FDA Drug Safety Communication: Addition of another concentration of liquid acetaminophen marketed for infants*. Retrieved from http://www.fda.gov/Drugs/DrugSafety/ucm284741.htm#sa

Van Hulle Vincent, C., Wilkie, D. J., & Szalacha, L. (2010). Pediatric nurses' cognitive representations of children's pain. *Journal of Pain, 11*(9), 854–863.

Voepel-Lewis, T., Malviya, S., Tait, A. R., Merkel, S., Foster, R., & Krane, E. J. (2008). A comparison of the clinical utility of pain assessment tools for children with cognitive impairment. *Pediatric Anesthesia, 106*(1), 72–78.

Voepel-Lewis, T., Zanotti, J., & Dammeyer, J. A. (2010). Reliability and validity of the face, legs, activity, cry, consolability behavioral tool in assessing acute pain in critically ill patients. *American Journal of Critical Care, 19*(1), 55–62.

Walco, G. A. (2008). Needle pain in children: Contextual factors. *Pediatrics, 122*(Suppl. 3), S125–S129.

Walden, M. (2007). Pain in the newborn and infant. In C. Kenner & J. W. Lott, *Comprehensive neonatal nursing: An interdisciplinary approach* (4th ed., pp. 360–371). Philadelphia, PA: Elsevier Saunders.

Walden, M., & Carrier, C. (2009). The ten commandments of pain assessment and management in preterm neonates. *Critical Care Nursing Clinics of North America, 21,* 235–252.

Wu, S., Sapru, A., Stewart, M. A., Milet, M., Hudes, M., Livermore, L., & Flori, H. (2009). Using acupuncture for acute pain in hospitalized children. *Pediatric Critical Care Medicine, 10*(3), 291–296.

Zeitzer, L. K., & Krane, E. J. (2011). Pediatric pain management. In R. M. Kleigman, B. F. Stanton, J. W. St. Geme, N. F. Schor, & R. E. Behrman, *Nelson textbook of pediatrics* (19th ed., pp. 360–375). Philadelphia, PA: Elsevier Saunders.

Zempsky, W. T. (2008). Pharmacologic approaches for reducing venous access pain in children. *Pediatrics, 122* (Suppl. 3), S140–S153.

Zempsky, W. T., Bean-Lijewski, J., Kauffman, R. E., Koh, J. L., Malviya, S. V., Rose, J. B., . . . Gennevois, D. J. (2008). Needle-free powder lidocaine delivery system provides rapid effective analgesia for venipuncture or cannulation pain in children: Randomized, double-blind comparison of venipuncture and venous cannulation pain after fast-onset needle-free powder lidocaine or placebo treatment trial. *Pediatrics, 121*(5), 979–987.

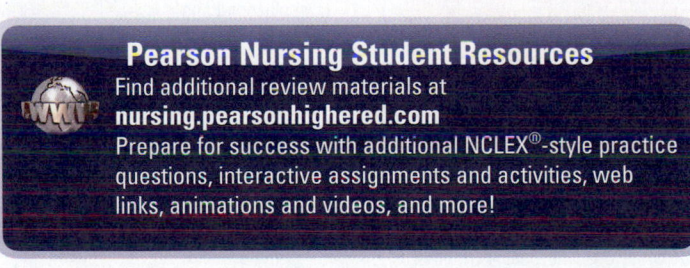

Pearson Nursing Student Resources

Find additional review materials at
nursing.pearsonhighered.com
Prepare for success with additional NCLEX®-style practice questions, interactive assignments and activities, web links, animations and videos, and more!

22 Immunizations and Communicable Diseases

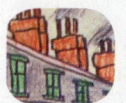 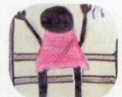 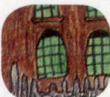

Learning Outcomes

After completing this chapter, you will be able to:

1. Compare the vulnerability of children and adults to communicable diseases.

2. Propose strategies to control the spread of infection in healthcare and community settings.

3. Examine the role that vaccines play in reduction and elimination of communicable diseases.

4. Plan the nursing care for children of all ages needing immunizations.

5. Design a plan to maintain the potency of vaccines.

6. Differentiate between common communicable diseases and vector-borne diseases.

7. Describe the medical and nursing management of common communicable diseases.

8. Create a parent education session that includes important considerations in administering acetaminophen and ibuprofen to infants and children with a fever.

9. Analyze the pathophysiology of sepsis to guide the nursing assessment of infants and children with this disorder.

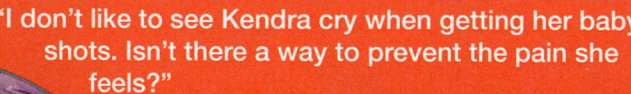

> "I don't like to see Kendra cry when getting her baby shots. Isn't there a way to prevent the pain she feels?"
>
> —*LaNaya King, mother*

Kendra King, 4 months old, has been brought by her parents to the community health center for her well-baby checkup and next immunizations. Kendra was born at full term, and she is healthy and growing at an appropriate rate. She has not yet had any illnesses. Her parents have enjoyed watching her grow and she has gained new developmental skills over the past 4 months. During Kendra's health visit, the pediatric nurse practitioner talks with her parents about her food intake and describes how well she is growing.

Kendra's mother reveals that she has heard information on the radio that concerns her about the safety of vaccines and asks for more information. She also wants to know why so many shots are given at a time. The nurse practitioner discusses vaccine safety with Kendra's parents and talks about the importance of each of the vaccines Kendra is to receive. She then obtains consent to administer each of the vaccines.

What factors determine the timing of vaccines for administration to infants and children? Why are infants and children at higher risk for infectious diseases? What methods should parents use to reduce the number of infectious diseases in their children? What are signs of a serious infection in an infant and in a child?

COMMUNICABLE DISEASE AS A HEALTH PROBLEM

A **communicable disease** is an illness that is passed via **direct transmission** (from one person or animal to another by contact with body fluids), via **indirect transmission** (to a person by contact with contaminated objects), or by *vectors* (ticks, mosquitoes, other insects). An **infectious disease** is any communicable disease caused by microorganisms that are commonly transmitted from one person to another or from an animal to a person. Communicable diseases are a major cause of morbidity in infants and children in the United States. Children can develop complications or secondary infections that require healthcare intervention, and in some cases these infections result in death.

For a communicable disease to occur, an *infectious agent* (pathogen) must be present and by direct or indirect transmission pass to a susceptible host (Figure 22–1 ■). Nurses have an important health promotion role in reducing the transmission of infectious diseases by immunization and in educating families to interrupt the transmission of infection in other ways, such as quarantine or hand hygiene.

Special Vulnerability of Newborns and Infants to Infection

Infants in particular are susceptible to infection for several reasons:

- **Their immune systems are not fully developed at birth.** The lymphatic organs of full-term neonates produce a large number of T and B lymphocytes, but very few of these cells have been exposed to **antigens** (foreign substances that trigger an immune system response) that would enable production of

antibodies (proteins capable of responding to specific infectious agents) for an immune response. See Chapter 27 for more information on the development of the immune system.

- **Passively acquired maternal antibodies provide limited protection.** Immunoglobulin G (IgG) is transferred through the placenta beginning at 20 weeks' gestation (Wynn & Levy, 2010). Preterm infants are at greater risk of communicable disease because they receive fewer maternal antibodies prior to birth and their immune system is even less mature (Hall, Noble, & Smith, 2009). Other immunoglobulins involved in immunity (IgA and IgM) do not cross the placenta. Placental transfer of antibodies (**passive immunity**) provides the newborn with protection from viruses and organisms to which the mother has been exposed. Breastfeeding provides some continuing passive protection, but many infants are not breastfed. Passive immunity decreases in the newborn in the months after birth.
- **Disease protection through immunization is incomplete.** The timing of immunizations is tied to the responsiveness of the infant to specific vaccines and the waning protection from maternal antibodies.

Newborns are at risk for infection before, during, and immediately after birth. In the prenatal period, the newborn may be exposed to a maternal infection that is transmitted through the placenta, such as rubella, varicella, or parvovirus. Pathogens may also be introduced to the fetus through the cervix during preterm labor. In the perinatal period, pathogens may be introduced to the neonate through an internal fetal monitor, premature rupture of the membranes, or vaginal examinations of the mother. Assisted delivery with forceps or vacuum extractor may cause skin lacerations. Maternal infection, such as streptococcus B, herpes simplex, or HIV, can also be transmitted as the fetus moves through the birth canal. After birth, the newborn may be exposed to pathogens through skin breakdown, invasive equipment, and exposure to infected healthcare personnel.

Vulnerabilities of Children to Infection

The poor hygiene behaviors of young children promote the transmission of communicable diseases in environments where children are in close contact (Figure 22–2 ■). The fecal-oral and respiratory routes are the most common sources of transmission in children. Young children may not wash their hands after toileting unless closely supervised. They then put their fingers in the mouth or rub their nose and eyes. Diapers may leak stool, exposing children to fecal organisms. In some cases, the child may be contagious before disease symptoms occur (e.g., varicella and parvovirus B-19) and before the child can be isolated. See the table beginning on page 626 for more information about these and other communicable diseases.

Infants and children develop **active immunity,** antibody development for specific infections through immunization or exposure to the natural disease. Subsequent exposure to the same type of organism often results in resistance or in a less severe infection. (Refer to "Anatomy and Physiology" and "Pediatric Differences" in Chapter 27.) See Developing Cultural Competence: Beliefs about Disease Causation.

Pathophysiology Illustrated
The Chain of Infection

FIGURE 22–1 ■ An effective chain of transmission for infection requires a suitable habitat, or reservoir, for the pathogen. A reservoir may be living or nonliving. Transmission may be direct or indirect. Direct transmission involves physical contact between the source of the infection and the new host. Indirect transmission occurs when pathogens survive outside humans before causing infection and disease. To prevent or control the spread of infection (achieve infection control), one of the links in the chain must be broken, for example, by eliminating one or more of the habitats or reservoirs (e.g., insecticide spraying to kill mosquitoes that carry malaria). Isolating an infected individual interferes with disease transmission, and killing the pathogen eliminates the causal agent.

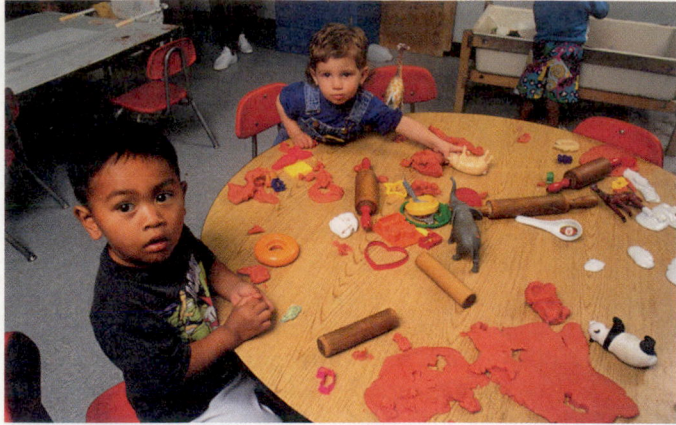

FIGURE 22–2 ■ Communicable diseases are easily transmitted in settings such as childcare centers where children handle common objects after coughing, sneezing, or drooling on them. The organisms survive to be picked up by another child handling the same object. The second child then may rub his or her eyes, nose, or mouth and introduce the infection. Young children depend upon caregivers to help break the chain of infection.

Public Health and Communicable Diseases

Common preventable communicable diseases are a significant public health problem. Major public health efforts that have decreased the occurrence of communicable diseases include safer drinking water, better sanitation, improved standards of living, and increased immunization.

Reducing the number of preventable childhood illnesses is a major national goal of *Healthy People 2020,* and nurses are important partners in this effort. Specific objectives are targeted at the reduction or elimination of the following infectious diseases (U.S. Department of Health and Human Services, 2010):

- Reduce, eliminate, or maintain elimination of congenital rubella syndrome, *Haemophilus influenzae* type b invasive disease, measles, mumps, pertussis, rubella, and varicella.
- Reduce new invasive cases of pneumococcal infections in children under 5 years.

Developing Cultural Competence
Beliefs About Disease Causation

In some cultures, infectious diseases are seen as punishment or the result of curses or evil spirits. For example, Native Americans traditionally view illnesses as the result of disharmony or displeasing the spirits. They may not believe in the germ theory of disease causation.

These national objectives reflect the significance of these preventable diseases as a public health problem. When infectious diseases are not prevented, the impact on the family and the healthcare system is significant. Health insurers must cover the cost of conditions that might have been prevented, and families may accrue costs for medications and treatments. Parents miss work while caring for the child and may miss more time from work if they become ill themselves. Children are directly affected when they miss time from school and interrupt their learning.

Public health authorities conduct **disease surveillance,** monitoring patterns of disease occurrence from the reported cases of communicable diseases in the United States. National disease surveillance efforts have increased in response to concerns of bioterrorism and potential **pandemics,** the emergence and worldwide spread of an infection (e.g., H1N1 influenza) that causes significantly increased morbidity and mortality (see page 626).

Infection Control

Preventing the spread of communicable diseases is a process that involves several strategies that must be well coordinated. Proper hand hygiene is one of the most important strategies for everyone. Nurses have a significant role in this process and are responsible for implementing several infection control strategies, such as standard precautions and transmission-based precautions (Box 22–1). Other strategies for infection control include the following:

- Promote and provide immunizations. See the immunization schedule on pages 611–613.

BOX 22–1	Infection Control Methods

STANDARD PRECAUTIONS

- Wash hands with soap and water when visibly dirty or contaminated by blood or other body fluids, and after using the toilet (World Health Organization, 2009). See Figure 22–3 ■ .
- Use alcohol-based hand rubs to decontaminate the hands when not visibly soiled, or after cleansing with soap and water in all other clinical situations (World Health Organization, 2009).
- Wear gloves when contact with blood, body fluids, secretions, excretions, nonintact skin, or mucous membranes might occur. Change gloves each time they are contaminated with these substances, washing hands before regloving.
- Wear additional protective equipment such as gown, mask, and goggles if body fluid splashes can occur.
- Wear the protective equipment to clean up body fluid spills. Discard waste in appropriate body substance waste containers. Clean the area with bleach or another acceptable cleaner. Bag contaminated laundry in secured and labeled bags.
- Discard needles, scalpels, and lancets in labeled sharps containers without recapping.
- Separate or isolate ill children from well children. Frequently assess children in waiting rooms of clinics and physician's offices to identify children who should be isolated. Separate hospitalized children with infections from children with a high risk for infection, such as those with compromised immune systems.

TRANSMISSION-BASED PRECAUTIONS

- Use airborne precautions for diseases transported by the airborne route, such as measles, chicken pox, or tuberculosis. Care providers use high-efficiency particulate air filter respirators (or other respirators that filter inspired air) for protection. In addition, a negative airflow ventilation system room is needed for tuberculosis. The patient in airborne precautions must wear a surgical mask when leaving the room to filter expired air. Keep the patient's room door closed.
- Use droplet precautions for diseases transmitted by the droplet route, such as *Haemophilus influenzae* type b, pneumonia, rubella, and pertussis. A surgical mask is needed when coming within 3 feet of the patient. The patient wears a mask when leaving the room. The room door can remain open, and special respirators are not required.
- Use contact precautions for diseases, such as hepatitis A, *E. coli*, and gonorrhea, that spread by direct contact with the skin or by indirect contact with a contaminated object in the patient's environment. Apply gloves for all care. Use antimicrobial soap for hand washing after removing gloves, and do not touch potentially contaminated surfaces or items in the patient's room. Gowns are worn if the healthcare professional's clothing may come in contact with contaminated surfaces or the patient. Patients should be placed in a private room or with other patients with the same pathogen.

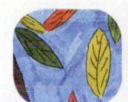

Partnering with Families

Reducing the Transmission of Infection

Teach families to reduce transmission of infection among family members with the following practices:

- Use disposable tissues and discard immediately after use.
- Wash hands thoroughly with soap and water or cleansing gels after all contact with the child's diaper, used tissues, runny nose, and mucous membranes.
- Teach children to cough or sneeze into their upper arm or elbow rather than into their hands.
- Teach children to wash their hands with soap and water after toileting and before eating.
- Do not allow children to share dishes and utensils.
- Wipe kitchen counters and surfaces where food is prepared and eaten with a disinfectant such as Lysol or a bleach solution.

- Wash hands well before preparing food, and wash hands several times during the food preparation process. Follow guidelines for safe food preparation and storage.
- Wash dishes and cutting boards in warm soapy water or use the sanitizing cycle on the dishwasher.
- Wipe counters and surfaces that are used for diaper changes or that the child touches with a disinfectant such as a bleach solution, Lysol, or isopropyl alcohol. Make sure the diaper-changing area is well away from food preparation areas.
- Dispose of diapers in closed containers.

- Eliminate the habitat or reservoir of the host (e.g., eliminate standing water where mosquitoes breed).
- Kill the pathogen (e.g., sanitize toys and surfaces exposed to organisms).
- Educate parents and caregivers of children about the need for hand hygiene and standard precautions, safe food preparation and storage, taking action to avoid exposure to certain organisms (e.g., ticks that cause Lyme disease), and the importance of immunizations. See Partnering with Families: Reducing the Transmission of Infection.

IMMUNIZATION

The development and widespread availability of vaccines has been one of the great breakthroughs of modern medicine. The average infant born in 2012 receives immunizations for 14 childhood diseases by the age of 6 years. The 14 childhood diseases for which vaccines are routinely recommended include the following: measles, mumps, rubella, polio, pertussis (whooping cough), diphtheria, tetanus, *Haemophilus influenzae* type b, hepatitis A, hepatitis B, influenza, pneumococcus, rotavirus, and varicella (chicken pox). In addition, vaccines have been developed recently for older children, adolescents, and adults to protect against pertussis, meningococcus, and the human papillomavirus. Administering these vaccines greatly improves the health of children and reduces the parental burden of caring for ill children. For example, the rate of pneumonia hospitalizations in children less than age 2 years decreased by 35% after the introduction of the pneumococcal conjugate vaccine in 2000 (Grijalva, Griffin, Nuorti, et al., 2009).

Before the 1950s, when infant and childhood immunization programs were initiated, the annual impact of communicable diseases in the United States was staggering. Thousands of children died or had permanent disabilities as a result of being infected from diseases such as polio, rubella, measles, diphtheria, pertussis, and *Haemophilus influenzae* type b (Children's Hospital of Philadelphia, 2010). See Legal and Ethical Considerations: Vaccine Assistance Acts.

Etiology and Pathophysiology

Immunization introduces an antigen into the body in the form of a vaccine. The person then naturally produces antibodies and develops active immunity without becoming sick with the disease. Some children need antibodies faster than the body can develop them with a vaccine, such as an unimmunized toddler receiving chemotherapy for cancer who becomes exposed to chicken pox. Passive immunity is needed to prevent the disease from occurring or to reduce its severity. In the case

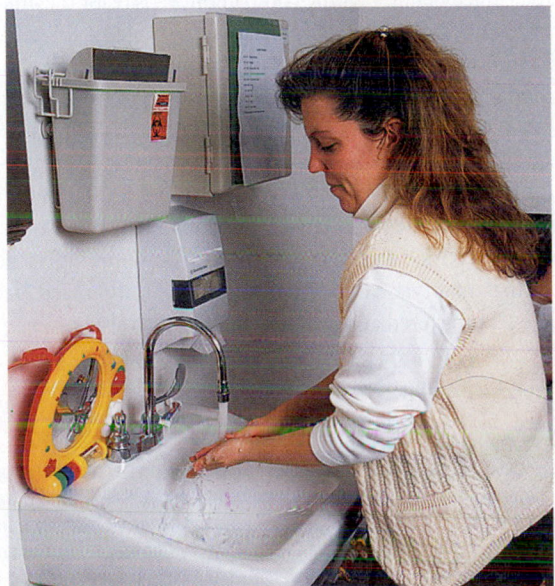

FIGURE 22–3 ■ Proper hand washing with soap and water for 1 to 2 minutes is one of the most effective measures in preventing transmission of microorganisms. Alcohol-based hand sanitizers, which take less than 30 seconds to use, are a good alternative to hand washing. Selecting a hand sanitizer with an emollient may reduce dryness and cracking of the skin. Placing dispensers in convenient locations generally increases the number of times the hands are cleaned.

Legal and Ethical Considerations
Vaccine Assistance Acts

The Polio Vaccination Assistance Act of 1955 established the first national program to support states and communities to acquire and provide polio vaccines. The Vaccine Assistance Act of 1962 authorized the Centers for Disease Control and Prevention to support immunization campaigns (Immunization Action Coalition, 2010).

of the toddler exposed to chicken pox, varicella immune globulin is given by injection to reduce the child's risk for developing the disease, which could be fatal in this child. Passive immunity does not confer lasting immunity, so varicella vaccine is administered at a later time to start the process of antibody development (active immunity).

Since the first vaccines were developed in the late 1800s, many diseases have decreased dramatically in incidence. For example, the introduction of the pneumococcal conjugate vaccine in 2000 was found to be 97.4% efficacious in protecting fully vaccinated infants against invasive pneumococcal disease caused by the specific serotypes included in the vaccine (Nuorri & Whitney, 2010). Two doses of varicella are 98.3% effective in preventing chicken pox (Shapiro, Vazquez, Esposito, et al., 2011).

Types of vaccines against childhood illnesses used in the United States include the following:

- **Killed virus vaccine**—a vaccine that contains a microorganism that has been killed but is still capable of inducing the human body to produce antibodies (e.g., inactivated poliovirus vaccine).
- **Toxoid**—a toxin that has been treated (by heat or chemical, such as formaldehyde) to weaken its toxic effects but retain its antigenicity (e.g., tetanus toxoid).
- **Live virus vaccine**—a vaccine that contains a microorganism in live but attenuated, or weakened, form (e.g., measles and varicella vaccines).
- **Recombinant vaccine**—a vaccine in which an organism has been genetically altered for use in vaccines (e.g., hepatitis B and **acellular pertussis vaccine** [proteins from pertussis rather than the whole bacterial cell are used to stimulate the process of active immunity]).
- **Conjugate vaccine**—a vaccine in which an altered organism is joined with another substance to increase the immune response (e.g., pneumococcal conjugate vaccine). For example, the *Haemophilus influenzae* type b (Hib) vaccine is conjugated with a protein carrier such as tetanus toxoid, but these vaccines confer no immunity to tetanus.

Improvements in vaccine technology continue to increase the safety and efficacy of immunization against an increasing number of diseases. Today's vaccines are often produced synthetically by means of recombinant DNA technology or genetic engineering. This technology offers the benefit of decreased side effects while providing immunity for diseases. Many other vaccines are in development, including group A streptococcal vaccine, respiratory syncytial virus vaccine, *Chlamydia trachomatis* vaccine, and a salmonella vaccine.

Clinical Manifestations

Children receiving vaccines can have a variety of reactions as the body responds to the injected antigen, which stimulates the immune response. Children receiving vaccines commonly have a local reaction that includes erythema, swelling, pain, and induration at the site of the injection. This reaction shows that the child is responding to the antigen and developing protection to the disease. Systemic reactions that often occur include fever, fussiness or irritability, malaise, and anorexia. A rash or arthralgia may occur with some vaccines. Adolescents may experience syncope or vasovagal reaction within 15 minutes of immunization, leading to fall-related secondary injuries such as brain injury (Kroger, Sumaya, Pickering, et al., 2011).

Local allergic reactions, such as wheal, urticaria, or transient petechiae, can occur in minutes to hours after the injection. Anaphylaxis is a life-threatening allergic reaction that occurs rarely, in about 0.26 to 0.65 cases per million doses of vaccine (Purssell, 2009). It is manifested by hypotension, generalized urticaria, angioedema, and laryngeal edema. The reactions to specific vaccines can be found on the Medications table listing common pediatric immunizations on pages 607–610. See Chapter 27 🔗 for more information about anaphylaxis.

Collaborative Care

Vaccines should be administered at specific ages and intervals. The timing for the first vaccines is determined by the age at which **transplacental immunity** (passive immunity transferred from mother to infant) decreases or disappears, and when the immune system of the infant or child is developed enough to produce antibodies in response to the vaccine. Scientists continue to study the duration of protection from vaccines. Most vaccines do not confer lifelong immunity. For example, a second dose of the MMR and varicella vaccine is required.

Immunization Schedule

Before a vaccine is added to the approved vaccine schedule for children, the U.S. Food and Drug Administration (FDA) must license the vaccine, and the Centers for Disease Control and Prevention's Advisory Committee on Immunization Practices (ACIP) must recommend the vaccine for use. In addition, the U.S. government must decide to include the vaccine in the Vaccines for Children program.

The recommended schedule for childhood immunizations is reviewed and updated at least annually to reflect new vaccines and the need for repeat immunization. Experts from the ACIP, the American Academy of Pediatrics (AAP), and the American Academy of Family Practitioners (AAFP) collaborate to create a uniform vaccination schedule. See Figure 22–4 and Figure 22–5 ■ on pages 611–612 for the recommended schedules for the 2012 immunization of children in the United States. Because the vaccine schedule changes at least annually in the United States, visit the companion website for the link to the most current recommended immunization schedule for U.S. children.

The immunization recommendations and schedule vary for children who begin immunizations later in childhood or need catch-up doses. See Figure 22–6 ■ on page 613. Supplemental immunizations for meningococcal (MCV4) and pneumococcal (PPSV23) infections are recommended for certain children at high risk for invasive disease.

Pediatric healthcare providers—physicians, nurses, advanced practice nurses, and physician associates—use the immunization schedules to ensure that infants and children become fully immunized. Vaccines should be administered at specific ages and intervals; however, when a child receives immune globulins or blood products to treat various conditions, the timing of vaccine administration is altered.

Practice Alert

Immune globulin and blood products inhibit the child's response to live virus vaccines such as measles, mumps, rubella, and varicella. Ask about recent administration of immune globulin and blood products. Refer to the most current guidelines from the Centers for Disease Control and Prevention's Advisory Committee on Immunization Practices (ACIP) to identify the correct interval (3 to 11 months) between the administration of the blood product or immune globulin, or completion of immunosuppression therapy and administration of a live virus vaccine (Kroger et al., 2011).

Similarly, if immune globulin must be given within 14 days after administration of a live virus vaccine, the vaccine should be readministered after the period specified, unless serologic testing determines that the child developed adequate serum antibodies (AAP, 2012, p. 37).

Medications Recommended Pediatric Immunizations

IMMUNIZATION TYPE	SIDE EFFECTS	CONTRAINDICATIONS	NURSING MANAGEMENT
Diphtheria and Pertussis Vaccines and Tetanus Toxoid (DTaP, Tdap) *Type:* Inactivated. *Route:* Intramuscular. *Dosage:* 0.5 mL. *Age(s) Given:* 2, 4, 6, 15–18 months; 4–6 years (five doses); 11–12 years (Tdap). Do not restart the series, no matter when prior dose(s) were given. For a prior serious reaction to the pertussis component of DTaP vaccine, use DT (children less than 7 years) and Td (children 7 years and older) vaccines. May give at same time as all other vaccines, in a separate site. *Storage:* Refrigerate, irreversible loss of potency if frozen. Daptacel stopper contains latex. Pediarix[a] stopper vial is latex-free.	*Common:* Redness, pain, swelling, nodule at injection site; fever to 38.3°C (101°F); drowsiness, irritability, fussiness; anorexia within 2 days of injection. Increase in frequency and magnitude of local reactions with doses 4 and 5, e.g., entire limb swelling. *Serious:* Allergic reaction, anaphylaxis; shock or collapse (an episode with sudden loss of muscle tone, pallor, fever, and unresponsiveness), fever above 40.5°C (104.8°F); febrile seizure; persistent inconsolable crying.	Immediate anaphylactic reaction. Encephalopathy not associated with another cause within 7 days of vaccine dosage. Gelatin allergy (do not use Tripedia). *Precautions* for DTaP and Tdap administration and if the child has the following reactions within the listed time frame after the previous dose: ■ Fever of 40.5°C (105°F) or higher within 48 hours ■ Inconsolable crying lasting 3 hours or longer within 48 hours ■ Collapse or shock-like state within 48 hours ■ Guillain-Barré syndrome less than 6 weeks after previous dose ■ Progressive neurologic disorder ■ Seizure within 3 days of dose Delay administration until moderate to severe febrile illnesses have resolved. Postpone Tdap to adolescents with a progressive neurologic disorder, encephalopathy, or uncontrolled epilepsy until the condition is stabilized.	Use same brand for all doses when possible. Ask about previous reactions to immunization. Shake vaccine before withdrawing. Solution will be cloudy. Do not use if any clumps are present. DTaP may coincide with or hasten the recognition of a seizure disorder. In children with a history of seizures with or without fever, give acetaminophen at the time of vaccine and then every 4 hours for 24 hours. Inform parents of the chance of an increased reaction to the fourth and fifth doses. Since different product preparations (e.g., single and combination vaccines) may be used for all, one, or some doses, read package inserts carefully. A tetanus booster may be given in the case of a contaminated wound or burn, if 5 or more years have elapsed since the last dose.
Haemophilus Influenzae Type b Vaccine (Hib) *Type:* Inactivated. *Route:* Intramuscular. *Dosage:* 0.5 mL. *Age(s) given:* 2, 4, 6, 12–15 months for PRP-T (ActHIB[a]) *or* 2, 4, 12–15 months (three doses for PRP-OMP (PedvaxHIB[a]). Do not restart the series, no matter when the prior dose(s) were given. May give at same time as all other vaccines in a separate site. *Storage:* Refrigerate, irreversible loss of potency if frozen.	*Common:* Pain, redness, or swelling at site. *Serious:* Anaphylaxis (extremely rare); fever.	Prior anaphylactic reaction to this vaccine or vaccine component. *Precautions:* Moderate or severe acute illness with or without fever	Solution is clear and colorless. Since different product preparations (e.g., single and combination vaccines) affect the immunization schedule, read package inserts carefully. Use the same vaccine preparation for all doses of the primary series when possible. Follow directions for reconstituting, refrigerating, and discarding unused reconstituted vaccine.
Hepatitis A Vaccine (HepA) *Type:* Inactivated. *Route:* Intramuscular. *Dosage:* 0.5 mL (1.0 mL over 18 years). *Age(s) given:* 12–23 months or 2–18 years, first dose followed by second dose 6–12 months later. Do not restart the series, no matter when the prior dose was given. May give at same time as all other vaccines in a separate site. *Storage:* Refrigerate, irreversible loss of potency if frozen.	*Common:* Pain, tenderness, induration at injection site.	Known hypersensitivity to any component. Prior hypersensitivity or anaphylactic reaction to prior vaccine dose. *Precautions:* Pregnancy. Moderate or severe acute illness with or without fever.	Shake well, slightly opaque white suspension. Can be given for postexposure prophylaxis against hepatitis in persons not previously immunized. Immune globulin and vaccine can be given at the same time in different sites. Vaccine brands can be interchanged. Vaqta vials have a latex stopper.

(continued)

Medications Recommended Pediatric Immunizations (*continued*)

IMMUNIZATION TYPE	SIDE EFFECTS	CONTRAINDICATIONS	NURSING MANAGEMENT
Hepatitis B Vaccine (Hep B) *Type*: Inactivated. *Route*: Intramuscular. *Dosage*: 0.5 mL (1 mL at 20 years). *Age(s) given*: Birth, 1–2 months, 6–18 months (three doses). A three-dose series can be started at any age. Do not restart the series, no matter when the prior dose(s) were given. May give at same time as all other vaccines in a separate site. *Storage*: Refrigerate, irreversible loss of potency if frozen. Engerix-B[a] and Recombivax HB[a] are single-vaccine preparations. Only a monovalent (single vaccine) preparation should be used in infants from birth to 6 weeks of age.	*Common*: Pain, redness at injection site, fever. *Serious*: Anaphylaxis is uncommon.	Prior anaphylaxis reaction. Serious hypersensitivity reaction to past dose, perhaps due to yeast hypersensitivity. *Precautions:* Infant weight less than 2000 g. Moderate or severe acute illness with or without fever.	If mother has HBsAg+ or unknown status, give vaccine to infant within 12 hours of birth along with hepatitis B immune globulin in another site. Shake vaccine before withdrawing. Solution will appear cloudy. Various formulations (pediatric, adult, dialysis) and combination vaccines are available. Read package insert carefully and follow directions for the product used. Infants of HBsAg+ mothers should have anti-HBs levels checked at the visit after completion of the HepB series. Infants who are HBsAg− and anti-HB levels less than 10 mIU/mL should be reimmunized with three doses at 2-month intervals and then retested (AAP, 2012, p. 388). Vaccine brands can be interchanged for three-dose series.
Human Papillomavirus Vaccine (HPV4) (Quadrivalent) *Type*: Recombinant. *Route*: Intramuscular. *Dosage*: 0.5 mL. *Age(s) given*: 11–12 years, second dose 2 months later, third dose 6 months after the first dose. Minimum age for the vaccine administration is 9 years. May be administered with hepatitis B vaccine in separate site. *Storage*: Refrigerate, irreversible loss of potency if frozen.	*Common*: Pain, swelling, erythema at the injection site, headache, nausea, pruritus, and fever. *Less Common:* Syncope (vasovagal reaction). *Potential Serious Reactions:* Guillain-Barré syndrome, blood clot, bronchospasm, asthma, arthritis.	Hypersensitivity to any vaccine components (e.g., yeast). Pregnancy. *Precautions:* Moderate to severe acute illness with or without fever.	Solution is a white cloudy liquid. Shake well before use. Protect vaccine from light to protect its potency. Adolescent should be seated or lying down for vaccine administration, and then observed for 15 minutes when seated because of risk of fainting and syncope. Vaccine series should be completed before onset of sexual activity. Educate parents and adolescents about this vaccine's potential to prevent cervical cancer and human papillomavirus infections. Some families may refuse the vaccine for young adolescents due to concerns that it might encourage sexual behavior (Thomas, 2008).
Influenza Vaccine *Type:* Inactivated (TIV), live attenuated for intranasal use (LAIV). *Route:* TIV—intramuscular (all ages), LAIV—intranasal (2 years and older). *Dosage:* 0.25 mL in infants 6–35 months, 0.5 mL beginning at 3 years. *Age(s) given:* Annually beginning at 6 months of age. May give at same time as all other vaccines in a separate site. *Storage:* Both TIV and LAIV should be refrigerated, do not freeze.	*Common after TIV:* May have soreness or swelling at injection site. *Mild systemic symptoms:* Fever, muscle aches, nausea, lethargy, headache, and chills. Febrile seizures may occur in children ages 6 to 23 months (U.S. Food and Drug Administration, 2011). Life-threatening allergic reactions are rare. *Common after intranasal vaccine:* Runny nose or nasal congestion, fever, headache or muscle aches, abdominal pain and occasional vomiting.	*TIV and LAIV:* Severe allergic reaction (anaphylaxis) to prior dose or to egg or chicken protein, Guillain-Barré syndrome within 6 weeks of prior dose. LAIV is also contraindicated in children with immunosuppression or certain chronic conditions. *Precaution:* Postpone vaccine when child has acute febrile illness until asymptomatic, but may be given with minor illness, with or without fever.	Thawed intranasal vaccine is pale yellow, clear to slightly cloudy. Administered annually in autumn at the time recommended by the Centers for Disease Control and Prevention (CDC). Intranasal dose is split (0.25 mL) with a dose divider clip. Administer in each nostril while child is sitting in an upright position. Insert the tip of the sprayer inside the nose and depress the plunger to spray. Children between 6 months and 9 years who are receiving the influenza vaccine for the first time should get two doses separated by at least 4 weeks (injectable) and 6 weeks (intranasal). TIV should be used for any child living in a household with a severely immunocompromised person.

Medications Recommended Pediatric Immunizations (*continued*)

IMMUNIZATION TYPE	SIDE EFFECTS	CONTRAINDICATIONS	NURSING MANAGEMENT
Measles, Mumps, Rubella Vaccines (MMR) *Type:* Live attenuated. *Route:* Subcutaneous. *Dosage:* 0.5 mL. *Age(s) given:* 12–15 months; 4–6 years (two doses). May give at same time as all other vaccines in a separate site. *Storage:* Refrigerate, do not freeze. When reconstituted, keep refrigerated and away from light; discard if unused within 8 hours. Diluent can be refrigerated or stored at room temperature. MMR may be combined with the varicella vaccine (MMRV).	*Common:* Elevated temperature 1–2 weeks after immunization, redness or pain at injection site, noncontagious rash, joint pain. *Serious:* Allergic reaction or anaphylaxis, febrile seizure, meningitis (usually mild), encephalopathy, thrombocytopenic purpura, and rare cases of coma and permanent brain damage. Children, ages 12–23 months, receiving the MMRV vaccine have an increased risk of febrile seizures 7–10 days after administration, compared to children receiving MMR and varicella vaccines separately (Klein, Fireman, Yih, et al., 2010).	Severe allergic reaction (e.g., anaphylaxis) after a prior vaccine dose or to vaccine component (e.g., neomycin, or gelatin). Pregnancy. Severe immunodeficiency due to malignancy, congenital immunodeficiency disease, long-term immunosuppressive therapy, or child with HIV infection who is severely immunocompromised. *Precautions:* Receipt of immune globulin or blood product in last 3–11 months, but specific interval depends on product received (Kroger et al., 2011, p. 40). History of thrombocytopenia or thrombocytopenic purpura. Moderate or severe acute illness with or without fever.	Reconstituted vaccine is a clear, yellow solution. Give entire contents of reconstituted vial even if more than 0.5 mL. May be given to child with an egg allergy (Kroger et al., 2011, p. 42). Inquire about immunosuppression. Children with HIV infection should receive the vaccine. Instruct adolescent girls of childbearing age to avoid pregnancy for 3 months after immunization. If giving a tuberculin (TB) test, administer at same time as MMR or 4–6 weeks later. If MMR and Varivax are not given on the same day, space them more than 28 days apart. Ensure that adolescents going to college receive a second MMR dose.
Meningococcal Vaccine (MCV4) *Type:* Inactivated. *Route:* MCV4—intramuscular, MPSV4—subcutaneous. *Dosage:* 0.5 mL. *Age(s) given:* 11–12 years, and second dose 5 years later. May be given at same time as other vaccines. *Storage:* Refrigerate, do not freeze. Refrigerate MPSV4 diluent. MCV4 is the preferred vaccine in children and adolescents.	*Common:* Pain at injection site, irritability, headache, and fatigue. *Severe:* Guillain-Barré syndrome occurring within 6 weeks after vaccine.	Severe allergic reaction (e.g., anaphylaxis) after prior dose or to a vaccine component (e.g., diphtheria toxoid). *Precautions:* Moderate or severe acute illness with or without fever.	Protect vaccine from light. Vial stopper contains latex. May be given to children ages 2 years and older when immunosuppressed by disease, asplenia, or medication. Give two doses at least 8 weeks apart with booster dose every 5 years thereafter. Alternate approved vaccine is meningococcal conjugate vaccine MenACWY.
Pneumococcal Conjugate Vaccine (PCV13) *Type:* Conjugate. *Route:* Intramuscular. *Dosage:* 0.5 mL. *Age(s) given:* 2, 4, 6, 12–15 months. Do not restart the series, no matter when the prior dose(s) were given. *Storage:* Refrigerate, irreversible loss of potency if frozen.	*Common:* Pain, redness, swelling, induration at injection site; fever; irritability, decreased appetite, increased or decreased sleep. *Severe:* Allergic reaction or anaphylaxis.	Severe allergic reaction (e.g., anaphylaxis) after a prior dose of PCV7, PCV13, or vaccine containing diphtheria toxoid, or a component of one of the listed vaccines. *Precaution:* Moderate or severe acute illness with or without fever.	Clear, colorless, or slightly opalescent liquid. PCV13 includes 13 serotypes accounting for 60% of the causes of invasive pneumococcal disease (Hayden, 2010). If the series was started with the older PCV7 vaccine with 7 serotypes, complete it with PCV13. If the child completed the PCV series, give one supplemental dose of PCV13. Give one supplemental dose of PCV13 to any child up to age 6 years with a chronic health condition who received PPSV23. Give a single dose of PCV13 to children 6 to 18 years at risk for invasive pneumococcal disease because of chronic disease or immunocompromising conditions (Hayden, 2010).

(*continued*)

IMMUNIZATION TYPE	SIDE EFFECTS	CONTRAINDICATIONS	NURSING MANAGEMENT
Pneumococcal Polysaccharide Vaccine (PPSV23) *Type:* Inactivated. *Dose:* 0.5 mL. *Route:* Intramuscular or subcutaneous. *Age(s) given:* May be given as young as age 2 years, second dose 5 years after first dose. May be given at the same time as other vaccines. *Storage:* Refrigerate.	*Common:* Soreness, erythema, warmth, swelling and induration, fever. *Less common:* Malaise, nausea, vomiting, headache, muscle aches, rash, urticaria. *Serious:* Hypersensitivity reactions (anaphylaxis), Guillain-Barré syndrome.	Hypersensitivity to any vaccine component. *Precautions:* Delay administration if acute febrile illness is present. Pregnancy.	Clear, colorless solution. Used for children ages 2 years and older at high risk for invasive pneumococcal disease (sickle cell disease, asplenia, cochlear implants, HIV infection, congenital immune deficiency). Give 2 weeks prior to elective splenectomy, cochlear implant, or other immunocompromising therapy. Child should also receive full series of PCV7 or PCV13. Duration of vaccine protection is unknown.
Poliovirus Vaccine (IPV) *Type:* Inactivated. *Route:* Subcutaneous or intramuscular; follow manufacturer's guidance for vaccine used. *Dosage:* 0.5 mL. *Age(s) given:* 2, 4, 12–18 months; 4–6 years (four doses). Do not restart the series, no matter when prior dose(s) were given. May give at same time as all other vaccines in a separate site. *Storage:* Refrigerate; do not freeze.	*Common:* Swelling and tenderness, irritability, tiredness. *Serious:* Allergic reaction or anaphylaxis.	Severe allergic reaction (e.g., anaphylaxis) after prior dose or to vaccine components (neomycin, streptomycin, or polymyxin B). *Precautions:* Pregnancy. Moderate or severe acute illness with or without fever. Oral polio vaccine is no longer licensed for use in the U.S. or Canada, but may still be used in developing countries. Prior doses of oral polio vaccine are not a contraindication for IPV.	Prior to immunization, ask if the child has an allergy to the antibiotic contained in the specific IPV product available. Clear, colorless suspension. Do not use if it contains particulate matter, becomes cloudy, or changes color. All doses must be separated by at least 4 weeks. IPV can be given to an infant or child when a family member is immunocompromised.
Rotavirus Vaccine (PRV, RV5) *Type:* Live. *Route:* Oral. *Dosage:* 1 mL or 2 mL. *Age(s) given:* 2, 4, and 6 months (three doses). Do not start the series if the infant is 15 weeks of age or older. May give at same time as all other vaccines. *Storage:* Refrigerate; do not freeze. Use the same manufacturer for all vaccine doses.	*Common:* Vomiting, diarrhea, irritability. *Potential serious adverse reactions:* Seizures, bronchiolitis, gastroenteritis, pneumonia, fever, urinary tract infection. Surveillance since approval of PRV and RV5 has identified a potential low increased risk of intussusception and monitoring continues (CDC, 2010c).	Severe allergic reaction (anaphylaxis) after a previous dose or to a vaccine component. Severe combined immunodeficiency disorder (SCID). Prior history of intussusception. *Precautions:* Altered immunocompetence other than SCID. Chronic gastrointestinal disease. Spina bifida or bladder exstrophy. Moderate or severe acute illness with or without fever. Preexisting gastrointestinal disease.	Pale yellow clear liquid in single-dose tube for direct oral administration. Protect vaccine from light. Squeeze the liquid into the infant's mouth toward the inner cheek until the dosing tube is empty. If the infant spits out or regurgitates a small amount, do not repeat the dose. No restrictions on the infant's intake of formula, breast milk, or food before or after vaccine. Discard the empty tube and cap into an approved biological waste container. Complete all three doses of vaccine by 32 months of age.
Varicella Virus Vaccine (Var) *Type:* Live attenuated. *Route:* Subcutaneous. *Dosage:* 0.5 mL. *Age(s) given:* 12–15 months; and 4–6 years (two doses). 13 years and older (two doses 4–8 weeks apart) if not previously vaccinated. *Storage:* Keep frozen. Diluent can be stored in refrigerator or at room temperature.	*Common:* Pain or redness at injection site, fever. Less commonly a vaccine-related rash (mild exanthem of two to five lesions that last for 2–3 days) may appear during the first month after the injection. *Severe:* Allergic reaction or anaphylaxis; thrombocytopenia; febrile seizure; central nervous system manifestations.	Severe allergic reaction (e.g., anaphylaxis) after a prior dose or to a vaccine component (e.g., neomycin or gelatin). Known severe immunodeficiency due to malignancy, chemotherapy, congenital immunodeficiency disorder, long-term immunosuppressive therapy, or patients with HIV infection who are severely immunocompromised. Pregnancy. *Precautions:* Receipt of antibody-containing blood products or immune globulin within past 3–11 months (interval depends upon the product used). Moderate or severe acute illness with or without fever.	Prior to immunization, ask if child is immunodeficient or on immunosuppression treatment or had an allergy to a vaccine component. Clear, colorless to pale yellow liquid when reconstituted. If MMR and varicella vaccines are not given the same day, space the vaccines by at least 28 days. Instruct adolescent girls of childbearing age to avoid pregnancy for 3 months after immunization. Antiviral agents should not be used 1 day before or for 21 days after vaccine. Give vaccine to unimmunized child exposed to varicella within 3 days to help build immunity quickly.

[a]Trade names.

Source: *Data from American Academy of Pediatrics. (2012). Red Book: Report of the Committee on Infectious Disease (29th ed.). Elk Grove Village, IL: Author; Kroger, A. T., Sumaya, C. V., Pickering, L. K., & Atkinson, W. L. (2011). General recommendations on immunization: Recommendations of the Advisory Committee on Immunization Practices (ACIP). Morbidity and Mortality Weekly Report, 60(2), 1–62; Centers for Disease Control and Prevention (CDC). (2011a). Immunization schedules. Retrieved from http://www.cdc.gov/vaccines/recs/schedules/default.htm; Merck & Co. (2011). Pneumovax 23: Pneumococcal vaccine polyvalent. Retrieved from http://www.fda.gov/downloads/BiologicsBloodVaccines/Vaccines/ApprovedProducts/UCM131661.pdf; Centers for Disease Control and Prevention (CDC). (2011d). Vaccine storage and handling guide. Retrieved from http://www.cdc.gov/vaccines/recs/storage/guide/vaccine-storage-handling.pdf*

FIGURE 1: Recommended immunization schedule for persons aged 0 through 6 years—United States, 2012 (for those who fall behind or start late, see the catch-up schedule [Figure 3])

Vaccine ▼ Age ▶	Birth	1 month	2 months	4 months	6 months	9 months	12 months	15 months	18 months	19–23 months	2–3 years	4–6 years	
Hepatitis B[1]	Hep B	HepB			HepB								Range of recommended ages for all children
Rotavirus[2]			RV	RV	RV[2]								
Diphtheria, tetanus, pertussis[3]			DTaP	DTaP	DTaP		see footnote[3]	DTaP				DTaP	
Haemophilus influenzae type b[4]			Hib	Hib	Hib[4]		Hib						Range of recommended ages for certain high-risk groups
Pneumococcal[5]			PCV	PCV	PCV		PCV				PPSV		
Inactivated poliovirus[6]			IPV	IPV		IPV						IPV	
Influenza[7]						Influenza (Yearly)							
Measles, mumps, rubella[8]							MMR		see footnote[8]			MMR	Range of recommended ages for all children and certain high-risk groups
Varicella[9]							Varicella		see footnote[9]			Varicella	
Hepatitis A[10]							Dose 1[10]				HepA Series		
Meningococcal[11]							MCV4 — see footnote[11]						

This schedule includes recommendations in effect as of December 23, 2011. Any dose not administered at the recommended age should be administered at a subsequent visit, when indicated and feasible. The use of a combination vaccine generally is preferred over separate injections of its equivalent component vaccines. Vaccination providers should consult the relevant Advisory Committee on Immunization Practices (ACIP) statement for detailed recommendations, available online at http://www.cdc.gov/vaccines/pubs/acip-list.htm. Clinically significant adverse events that follow vaccination should be reported to the Vaccine Adverse Event Reporting System (VAERS) online (http://www.vaers.hhs.gov) or by telephone (800-822-7967).

1. **Hepatitis B (HepB) vaccine.** (Minimum age: birth)
   At birth:
   - Administer monovalent HepB vaccine to all newborns before hospital discharge.
   - For infants born to hepatitis B surface antigen (HBsAg)–positive mothers, administer HepB vaccine and 0.5 mL of hepatitis B immune globulin (HBIG) within 12 hours of birth. These infants should be tested for HBsAg and antibody to HBsAg (anti-HBs) 1 to 2 months after completion of at least 3 doses of the HepB series, at age 9 through 18 months (generally at the next well-child visit).
   - If mother's HBsAg status is unknown, within 12 hours of birth administer HepB vaccine for infants weighing ≥2,000 grams, and HepB vaccine plus HBIG for infants weighing <2,000 grams. Determine mother's HBsAg status as soon as possible and, if she is HBsAg-positive, administer HBIG for infants weighing ≥2,000 grams (no later than age 1 week).
   Doses after the birth dose:
   - The second dose should be administered at age 1 to 2 months. Monovalent HepB vaccine should be used for doses administered before age 6 weeks.
   - Administration of a total of 4 doses of HepB vaccine is permissible when a combination vaccine containing HepB is administered after the birth dose.
   - Infants who did not receive a birth dose should receive 3 doses of a HepB-containing vaccine starting as soon as feasible (Figure 3).
   - The minimum interval between dose 1 and dose 2 is 4 weeks, and between dose 2 and 3 is 8 weeks. The final (third or fourth) dose in the HepB vaccine series should be administered no earlier than age 24 weeks and at least 16 weeks after the first dose.

2. **Rotavirus (RV) vaccines.** (Minimum age: 6 weeks for both RV-1 [Rotarix] and RV-5 [Rota Teq])
   - The maximum age for the first dose in the series is 14 weeks, 6 days; and 8 months, 0 days for the final dose in the series. Vaccination should not be initiated for infants aged 15 weeks, 0 days or older.
   - If RV-1 (Rotarix) is administered at ages 2 and 4 months, a dose at 6 months is not indicated.

3. **Diphtheria and tetanus toxoids and acellular pertussis (DTaP) vaccine.** (Minimum age: 6 weeks)
   - The fourth dose may be administered as early as age 12 months, provided at least 6 months have elapsed since the third dose.

4. **Haemophilus influenzae type b (Hib) conjugate vaccine.** (Minimum age: 6 weeks)
   - If PRP-OMP (PedvaxHIB or Comvax [HepB-Hib]) is administered at ages 2 and 4 months, a dose at age 6 months is not indicated.
   - Hiberix should only be used for the booster (final) dose in children aged 12 months through 4 years.

5. **Pneumococcal vaccines.** (Minimum age: 6 weeks for pneumococcal conjugate vaccine [PCV]; 2 years for pneumococcal polysaccharide vaccine [PPSV])
   - Administer 1 dose of PCV to all healthy children aged 24 through 59 months who are not completely vaccinated for their age.
   - For children who have received an age-appropriate series of 7-valent PCV (PCV7), a single supplemental dose of 13-valent PCV (PCV13) is recommended for:
     — All children aged 14 through 59 months
     — Children aged 60 through 71 months with underlying medical conditions.
   - Administer PPSV at least 8 weeks after last dose of PCV to children aged 2 years or older with certain underlying medical conditions, including a cochlear implant. See MMWR 2010:59(No. RR-11), available at http://www.cdc.gov/mmwr/rr/rr5911.pdf.

6. **Inactivated poliovirus vaccine (IPV).** (Minimum age: 6 weeks)
   - If 4 or more doses are administered before age 4 years, an additional dose should be administered at age 4 through 6 years.
   - The final dose in the series should be administered on or after the fourth birthday and at least 6 months after the previous dose.

7. **Influenza vaccines.** (Minimum age: 6 months for trivalent inactivated influenza vaccine [TIV]; 2 years for live, attenuated influenza vaccine [LAIV])
   - For most healthy children aged 2 years and older, either LAIV or TIV may be used. However, LAIV should not be administered to some children, including 1) children with asthma, 2) children 2 through 4 years who had wheezing in the past 12 months, or 3) children who have any other underlying medical conditions that predispose them to influenza complications. For all other contraindications to use of LAIV, see MMWR 2010:59(No. RR-8), available at http://www.cdc.gov/mmwr/pdf/rr/rr5908.pdf.
   - For children aged 6 months through 8 years:
     — For the 2011–12 season, administer 2 doses (separated by at least 4 weeks) to those who did not receive at least 1 dose of the 2010–11 vaccine. Those who received at least 1 dose of the 2010–11 vaccine require 1 dose for the 2011–12 season.
     — For the 2012–13 season, follow dosing guidelines in the 2012 ACIP influenza vaccine recommendations.

8. **Measles, mumps, and rubella (MMR) vaccine.** (Minimum age: 12 months)
   - The second dose may be administered before age 4 years, provided at least 4 weeks have elapsed since the first dose.
   - Administer MMR vaccine to infants aged 6 through 11 months who are traveling internationally. These children should be revaccinated with 2 doses of MMR vaccine, the first at ages 12 through 15 months and at least 4 weeks after the previous dose, and the second at ages 4 through 6 years.

9. **Varicella (VAR) vaccine.** (Minimum age: 12 months)
   - The second dose may be administered before age 4 years, provided at least 3 months have elapsed since the first dose.
   - For children aged 12 months through 12 years, the recommended minimum interval between doses is 3 months. However, if the second dose was administered at least 4 weeks after the first dose, it can be accepted as valid.

10. **Hepatitis A (HepA) vaccine.** (Minimum age: 12 months)
    - Administer the second (final) dose 6 to18 months after the first.
    - Unvaccinated children 24 months and older at high risk should be vaccinated. See MMWR 2006:55(No. RR-7), available at http://www.cdc.gov/mmwr/pdf/rr/rr5507.pdf.
    - A 2-dose HepA vaccine series is recommended for anyone aged 24 months and older, previously unvaccinated, for whom immunity against hepatitis A virus infection is desired.

11. **Meningococcal conjugate vaccines, quadrivalent (MCV4).** (Minimum age: 9 months for Menactra [MCV4-D], 2 years for Menveo [MCV4-CRM])
    - For children aged 9 through 23 months 1) with persistent complement component deficiency; 2) who are residents of or travelers to countries with hyperendemic or epidemic disease; or 3) who are present during outbreaks caused by a vaccine serogroup, administer 2 primary doses of MCV4-D, ideally at ages 9 months and 12 months or at least 8 weeks apart.
    - For children aged 24 months and older with 1) persistent complement component deficiency who have not been previously vaccinated; or 2) anatomic/functional asplenia, administer 2 primary doses of either MCV4 at least 8 weeks apart.
    - For children with anatomic/functional asplenia, if MCV4-D (Menactra) is used, administer at a minimum age of 2 years and at least 4 weeks after completion of all PCV doses.
    - See MMWR 2011:60:72–6, available at http://www.cdc.gov/mmwr/pdf/wk/mm6003. pdf, and Vaccines for Children Program resolution No. 6/11-1, available at http://www. cdc.gov/vaccines/programs/vfc/downloads/resolutions/06-11mening-mcv.pdf, and MMWR 2011:60:1391–2, available at http://www.cdc.gov/mmwr/pdf/wk/mm6040. pdf, for further guidance, including revaccination guidelines.

This schedule is approved by the Advisory Committee on Immunization Practices (http://www.cdc.gov/vaccines/recs/acip), the American Academy of Pediatrics (http://www.aap.org), and the American Academy of Family Physicians (http://www.aafp.org).
Department of Health and Human Services • Centers for Disease Control and Prevention

FIGURE 22–4 ■ Recommended immunization schedule for children 0 to 6 years, United States, 2012.

Source: From http://www.cdc.gov/vaccines/recs/schedules/child-schedule.htm#printable

FIGURE 2: Recommended immunization schedule for persons aged 7 through 18 years—United States, 2012 (for those who fall behind or start late, see the schedule below and the catch-up schedule [Figure 3])

Vaccine ▼ Age ▶	7–10 years	11–12 years	13–18 years	
Tetanus, diphtheria, pertussis[1]	1 dose (if indicated)	1 dose	1 dose (if indicated)	Range of recommended ages for all children
Human papillomavirus[2]	see footnote[2]	3 doses	Complete 3-dose series	
Meningococcal[3]	See footnote[3]	Dose 1	Booster at 16 years old	
Influenza[4]	Influenza (yearly)			Range of recommended ages for catch-up immunization
Pneumococcal[5]	See footnote[5]			
Hepatitis A[6]	Complete 2-dose series			
Hepatitis B[7]	Complete 3-dose series			
Inactivated poliovirus[8]	Complete 3-dose series			Range of recommended ages for certain high-risk groups
Measles, mumps, rubella[9]	Complete 2-dose series			
Varicella[10]	Complete 2-dose series			

This schedule includes recommendations in effect as of December 23, 2011. Any dose not administered at the recommended age should be administered at a subsequent visit, when indicated and feasible. The use of a combination vaccine generally is preferred over separate injections of its equivalent component vaccines. Vaccination providers should consult the relevant Advisory Committee on Immunization Practices (ACIP) statement for detailed recommendations, available online at http://www.cdc.gov/vaccines/pubs/acip-list.htm. Clinically significant adverse events that follow vaccination should be reported to the Vaccine Adverse Event Reporting System (VAERS) online (http://www.vaers.hhs.gov) or by telephone (800-822-7967).

1. **Tetanus and diphtheria toxoids and acellular pertussis (Tdap) vaccine.** (Minimum age: 10 years for Boostrix and 11 years for Adacel)
   - Persons aged 11 through 18 years who have not received Tdap vaccine should receive a dose followed by tetanus and diphtheria toxoids (Td) booster doses every 10 years thereafter.
   - Tdap vaccine should be substituted for a single dose of Td in the catch-up series for children aged 7 through 10 years. Refer to the catch-up schedule if additional doses of tetanus and diphtheria toxoid–containing vaccine are needed.
   - Tdap vaccine can be administered regardless of the interval since the last tetanus and diphtheria toxoid–containing vaccine.
2. **Human papillomavirus (HPV) vaccines (HPV4 [Gardasil] and HPV2 [Cervarix]).** (Minimum age: 9 years)
   - Either HPV4 or HPV2 is recommended in a 3-dose series for females aged 11 or 12 years. HPV4 is recommended in a 3-dose series for males aged 11 or 12 years.
   - The vaccine series can be started beginning at age 9 years.
   - Administer the second dose 1 to 2 months after the first dose and the third dose 6 months after the first dose (at least 24 weeks after the first dose).
   - See *MMWR* 2010;59:626–32, available at http://www.cdc.gov/mmwr/pdf/wk/mm5920.pdf.
3. **Meningococcal conjugate vaccines, quadrivalent (MCV4).**
   - Administer MCV4 at age 11 through 12 years with a booster dose at age 16 years.
   - Administer MCV4 at age 13 through 18 years if patient is not previously vaccinated.
   - If the first dose is administered at age 13 through 15 years, a booster dose should be administered at age 16 through 18 years with a minimum interval of at least 8 weeks after the preceding dose.
   - If the first dose is administered at age 16 years or older, a booster dose is not needed.
   - Administer 2 primary doses at least 8 weeks apart to previously unvaccinated persons with persistent complement component deficiency or anatomic/functional asplenia, and 1 dose every 5 years thereafter.
   - Adolescents aged 11 through 18 years with human immunodeficiency virus (HIV) infection should receive a 2-dose primary series of MCV4, at least 8 weeks apart.
   - See *MMWR* 2011;60:72–76, available at http://www.cdc.gov/mmwr/pdf/wk/mm6003.pdf, and Vaccines for Children Program resolution No. 6/11-1, available at http://www.cdc.gov/vaccines/programs/vfc/downloads/resolutions/06-11mening-mcv.pdf, for further guidelines.
4. **Influenza vaccines (trivalent inactivated influenza vaccine [TIV] and live, attenuated influenza vaccine [LAIV]).**
   - For most healthy, nonpregnant persons, either LAIV or TIV may be used, except LAIV should not be used for some persons, including those with asthma or any other underlying medical conditions that predispose them to influenza complications. For all other contraindications to use of LAIV, see *MMWR* 2010;59(No.RR-8), available at http://www.cdc.gov/mmwr/pdf/rr/rr5908.pdf.
   - Administer 1 dose to persons aged 9 years and older.

   - For children aged 6 months through 8 years:
     — For the 2011–12 season, administer 2 doses (separated by at least 4 weeks) to those who did not receive at least 1 dose of the 2010–11 vaccine. Those who received at least 1 dose of the 2010–11 vaccine require 1 dose for the 2011–12 season.
     — For the 2012–13 season, follow dosing guidelines in the 2012 ACIP influenza vaccine recommendations.
5. **Pneumococcal vaccines (pneumococcal conjugate vaccine [PCV] and pneumococcal polysaccharide vaccine [PPSV]).**
   - A single dose of PCV may be administered to children aged 6 through 18 years who have anatomic/functional asplenia, HIV infection or other immunocompromising condition, cochlear implant, or cerebral spinal fluid leak. See *MMWR* 2010:59(No. RR-11), available at http://www.cdc.gov/mmwr/pdf/rr/rr5911.pdf.
   - Administer PPSV at least 8 weeks after the last dose of PCV to children aged 2 years or older with certain underlying medical conditions, including a cochlear implant. A single revaccination should be administered after 5 years to children with anatomic/functional asplenia or an immunocompromising condition.
6. **Hepatitis A (HepA) vaccine.**
   - HepA vaccine is recommended for children older than 23 months who live in areas where vaccination programs target older children, who are at increased risk for infection, or for whom immunity against hepatitis A virus infection is desired. See *MMWR* 2006;55(No. RR-7), available at http://www.cdc.gov/mmwr/pdf/rr/rr5507.pdf.
   - Administer 2 doses at least 6 months apart to unvaccinated persons.
7. **Hepatitis B (HepB) vaccine.**
   - Administer the 3-dose series to those not previously vaccinated.
   - For those with incomplete vaccination, follow the catch-up recommendations (Figure 3).
   - A 2-dose series (doses separated by at least 4 months) of adult formulation Recombivax HB is licensed for use in children aged 11 through 15 years.
8. **Inactivated poliovirus vaccine (IPV).**
   - The final dose in the series should be administered at least 6 months after the previous dose.
   - If both OPV and IPV were administered as part of a series, a total of 4 doses should be administered, regardless of the child's current age.
   - IPV is not routinely recommended for U.S. residents aged 18 years or older.
9. **Measles, mumps, and rubella (MMR) vaccine.**
   - The minimum interval between the 2 doses of MMR vaccine is 4 weeks.
10. **Varicella (VAR) vaccine.**
   - For persons without evidence of immunity (see *MMWR* 2007;56[No. RR-4], available at http://www.cdc.gov/mmwr/pdf/rr/rr5604.pdf), administer 2 doses if not previously vaccinated or the second dose if only 1 dose has been administered.
   - For persons aged 7 through 12 years, the recommended minimum interval between doses is 3 months. However, if the second dose was administered at least 4 weeks after the first dose, it can be accepted as valid.
   - For persons aged 13 years and older, the minimum interval between doses is 4 weeks.

This schedule is approved by the Advisory Committee on Immunization Practices (http://www.cdc.gov/vaccines/recs/acip), the American Academy of Pediatrics (http://www.aap.org), and the American Academy of Family Physicians (http://www.aafp.org).
Department of Health and Human Services • Centers for Disease Control and Prevention

FIGURE 22–5 ■ Recommended immunizations schedule for children and adolescents 7 to 18 years, United States, 2012.

Source: From http://www.cdc.gov/vaccines/recs/schedules/child-schedule.htm#printable

FIGURE 3. Catch-up immunization schedule for persons aged 4 months through 18 years who start late or who are more than 1 month behind—United States • 2012

The figure below provides catch-up schedules and minimum intervals between doses for children whose vaccinations have been delayed. A vaccine series does not need to be restarted, regardless of the time that has elapsed between doses. Use the section appropriate for the child's age. **Always use this table in conjunction with the accompanying childhood and adolescent immunization schedules (Figures 1 and 2) and their respective footnotes.**

Persons aged 4 months through 6 years					
Vaccine	Minimum Age for Dose 1	Minimum Interval Between Doses			
		Dose 1 to dose 2	Dose 2 to dose 3	Dose 3 to dose 4	Dose 4 to dose 5
Hepatitis B	Birth	4 weeks	8 weeks and at least 16 weeks after first dose; minimum age for the final dose is 24 weeks		
Rotavirus[1]	6 weeks	4 weeks	4 weeks[1]		
Diphtheria, tetanus, pertussis[2]	6 weeks	4 weeks	4 weeks	6 months	6 months[2]
Haemophilus influenzae type b[3]	6 weeks	4 weeks if first dose administered at younger than age 12 months / 8 weeks (as final dose) if first dose administered at age 12–14 months / No further doses needed if first dose administered at age 15 months or older	4 weeks[3] if current age is younger than 12 months / 8 weeks (as final dose)[3] if current age is 12 months or older and first dose administered at younger than age 12 months and second dose administered at younger than 15 months / No further doses needed if previous dose administered at age 15 months or older	8 weeks (as final dose) This dose only necessary for children aged 12 months through 59 months who received 3 doses before age 12 months	
Pneumococcal[4]	6 weeks	4 weeks if first dose administered at younger than age 12 months / 8 weeks (as final dose for healthy children) if first dose administered at age 12 months or older or current age 24 through 59 months / No further doses needed for healthy children if first dose administered at age 24 months or older	4 weeks if current age is younger than 12 months / 8 weeks (as final dose for healthy children) if current age is 12 months or older / No further doses needed for healthy children if previous dose administered at age 24 months or older	8 weeks (as final dose) This dose only necessary for children aged 12 months through 59 months who received 3 doses before age 12 months or for children at high risk who received 3 doses at any age	
Inactivated poliovirus[5]	6 weeks	4 weeks	4 weeks	6 months[5] minimum age 4 years for final dose	
Meningococcal[6]	9 months	8 weeks[6]			
Measles, mumps, rubella[7]	12 months	4 weeks			
Varicella[8]	12 months	3 months			
Hepatitis A	12 months	6 months			
Persons aged 7 through 18 years					
Tetanus, diphtheria/ tetanus, diphtheria, pertussis[9]	7 years[9]	4 weeks	4 weeks if first dose administered at younger than age 12 months / 6 months if first dose administered at 12 months or older	6 months if first dose administered at younger than age 12 months	
Human papillomavirus[10]	9 years	Routine dosing intervals are recommended[10]			
Hepatitis A	12 months	6 months			
Hepatitis B	Birth	4 weeks	8 weeks (and at least 16 weeks after first dose)		
Inactivated poliovirus[5]	6 weeks	4 weeks	4 weeks[5]	6 months[5]	
Meningococcal[6]	9 months	8 weeks[6]			
Measles, mumps, rubella[7]	12 months	4 weeks			
Varicella[8]	12 months	3 months if person is younger than age 13 years / 4 weeks if person is aged 13 years or older			

1. **Rotavirus (RV) vaccines (RV-1 [Rotarix] and RV-5 [Rota Teq]).**
   • The maximum age for the first dose in the series is 14 weeks, 6 days; and 8 months, 0 days for the final dose in the series. Vaccination should not be initiated for infants aged 15 weeks, 0 days or older.
   • If RV-1 was administered for the first and second doses, a third dose is not indicated.
2. **Diphtheria and tetanus toxoids and acellular pertussis (DTaP) vaccine.**
   • The fifth dose is not necessary if the fourth dose was administered at age 4 years or older.
3. **Haemophilus influenzae type b (Hib) conjugate vaccine.**
   • Hib vaccine should be considered for unvaccinated persons aged 5 years or older who have sickle cell disease, leukemia, human immunodeficiency virus (HIV) infection, or anatomic/functional asplenia.
   • If the first 2 doses were PRP-OMP (PedvaxHIB or Comvax) and were administered at age 11 months or younger, the third (and final) dose should be administered at age 12 through 15 months and at least 8 weeks after the second dose.
   • If the first dose was administered at age 7 through 11 months, administer the second dose at least 4 weeks later and a final dose at age 12 through 15 months.
4. **Pneumococcal vaccines.** (Minimum age: 6 weeks for pneumococcal conjugate vaccine [PCV]; 2 years for pneumococcal polysaccharide vaccine [PPSV])
   • For children aged 24 through 71 months with underlying medical conditions, administer 1 dose of PCV if 3 doses of PCV were received previously, or administer 2 doses of PCV at least 8 weeks apart if fewer than 3 doses of PCV were received previously.
   • A single dose of PCV may be administered to certain children aged 6 through 18 years with underlying medical conditions. See age-specific schedules for details.
   • Administer PPSV to children aged 2 years or older with certain underlying medical conditions. See MMWR 2010:59(No. RR-11), available at http://www.cdc.gov/mmwr/pdf/rr/rr5911.pdf.

5. **Inactivated poliovirus vaccine (IPV).**
   • A fourth dose is not necessary if the third dose was administered at age 4 years or older and at least 6 months after the previous dose.
   • In the first 6 months of life, minimum age and minimum intervals are only recommended if the person is at risk for imminent exposure to circulating poliovirus (i.e., travel to a polio-endemic region or during an outbreak).
   • IPV is not routinely recommended for U.S. residents aged 18 years or older.
6. **Meningococcal conjugate vaccines, quadrivalent (MCV4).** (Minimum age: 9 months for Menactra [MCV4-D]; 2 years for Menveo [MCV4-CRM])
   • See Figure 1 ("Recommended immunization schedule for persons aged 0 through 6 years") and Figure 2 ("Recommended immunization schedule for persons aged 7 through 18 years") for further guidance.
7. **Measles, mumps, and rubella (MMR) vaccine.**
   • Administer the second dose routinely at age 4 through 6 years.
8. **Varicella (VAR) vaccine.**
   • Administer the second dose routinely at age 4 through 6 years. If the second dose was administered at least 4 weeks after the first dose, it can be accepted as valid.
9. **Tetanus and diphtheria toxoids (Td) and tetanus and diphtheria toxoids and acellular pertussis (Tdap) vaccines.**
   • For children aged 7 through 10 years who are not fully immunized with the childhood DTaP vaccine series, Tdap vaccine should be substituted for a single dose of Td vaccine in the catch-up series; if additional doses are needed, use Td vaccine. For these children, an adolescent Tdap vaccine dose should not be given.
   • An inadvertent dose of DTaP vaccine administered to children aged 7 through 10 years can count as part of the catch-up series. This dose can count as the adolescent Tdap dose, or the child can later receive a Tdap booster dose at age 11–12 years.
10. **Human papillomavirus (HPV) vaccines (HPV4 [Gardasil] and HPV2 [Cervarix]).**
   • Administer the vaccine series to females (either HPV2 or HPV4) and males (HPV4) at age 13 through 18 years if patient is not previously vaccinated.
   • Use recommended routine dosing intervals for vaccine series catch-up; see Figure 2 ("Recommended immunization schedule for persons aged 7 through 18 years").

Clinically significant adverse events that follow vaccination should be reported to the Vaccine Adverse Event Reporting System (VAERS) online (http://www.vaers.hhs.gov) or by telephone (800-822-7967). Suspected cases of vaccine-preventable diseases should be reported to the state or local health department. Additional information, including precautions and contraindications for vaccination, is available from CDC online (http://www.cdc.gov/vaccines) or by telephone (800-CDC-INFO [800-232-4636]).

FIGURE 22–6 ■ Recommended immunization schedule for children and adolescents (4 months to 18 years) who start late or who are more than 1 month behind, United States, 2012.

Source: From http://www.cdc.gov/vaccines/recs/schedules/child-schedule.htm#printable

Immunization of immune compromised children A small number of children have primary immunodeficiency diseases, such as DiGeorge syndrome. Other children can become immune compromised for many reasons, such as malignancy, hematopoietic stem cell transplantation (HSCT), solid organ transplantation, and HIV infection treated with antiretroviral therapy. Administration of live virus vaccines may be less safe for a child receiving 2 mg/kg per day of prednisone or equivalent for more than 14 days (Tamma, 2010). Each child's immunization plan must be individualized to the condition present. Some general guidelines for immunization practices include the following (Nield, Troischt, & Kamat, 2009; Tamma, 2010):

- Children with altered immunocompetence should generally receive the influenza vaccine; the age-appropriate polysaccharide-based vaccines of pneumococcal, meningococcal, and *Haemophilus influenzae* type b; and all other inactivated vaccines (Kroger et al., 2011).

- Severely immunocompromised children should not receive live viral or bacterial vaccines (Tamma, 2010). Passive immunization may be the only option for children with severe immunosuppression or children unable to mount an antibody immune response.

- Vaccines should be postponed until 3 months after immunosuppression drugs have been stopped.

- Healthy survivors of HSCT can be immunized with inactivated vaccines after 1 year and live virus vaccines after 2 years. Some providers repeat all immunizations after HSCT.

- Children receiving solid organ transplantation should receive age-recommended immunizations prior to surgery. Live virus vaccines should be administered at least 4 weeks prior to surgery.

- Children with HIV on stable highly active antiretroviral therapy (HAART) can be immunized with inactive vaccines. Measles and varicella vaccines may be given when children have mild clinical disease.

- Children living with or having other close contacts with persons having altered immunocompetence should receive all age-appropriate vaccines. Other live virus vaccines (measles, mumps, rubella, varicella, and rotavirus vaccines) should be administered (Kroger et al., 2011).

Immunization of internationally adopted children
Approximately 18,500 children are adopted each year from other countries (Spicer & Powell, 2010). The recommended immunization schedule in some countries varies because of the higher risk of vaccine-preventable diseases, sometimes giving vaccines in shorter intervals which could interfere with a child's immune response. Children less than 10 years of age who are internationally adopted may not have written proof of immunizations prior to entry into the United States. In such cases, adoptive parents are required to indicate their intent to have the child become fully immunized when proof is not available (AAP, 2012, p. 191). Often vaccines are administered according to the catch-up schedule when no immunization record exists or if there is doubt about the potency of the vaccines given.

Improving immunization rates
The effort to increase the numbers of children protected from vaccine-preventable diseases and to monitor immunization status is a national public health initiative. *Healthy People 2020* states important goals for reduction

---

Legal and Ethical Considerations
Vaccination Laws

No federal vaccination laws exist, but all 50 states require certain vaccinations for children entering public schools. Depending on the state, children must be vaccinated against some or all of the following diseases: mumps, measles, rubella, diphtheria, pertussis, tetanus, and polio (CDC, 2010a).

---

of vaccine-preventable diseases (U.S. Department of Health and Human Services, 2010):

- Achieve and maintain effective vaccination coverage levels for universally recommended vaccines among young children.
- Increase the proportion of children ages 19 to 35 months who receive the recommended doses of all recommended vaccines.
- Maintain vaccination coverage levels for children in kindergarten.
- Increase routine vaccination coverage levels for adolescents.
- Increase the percentage of children and adults who are vaccinated annually against seasonal influenza.

Many missed opportunities to immunize children have been identified. Children (and siblings present) should have their immunization status assessed during all healthcare visits, during hospitalizations, and in schools (see Legal & Ethical Considerations: Vaccination Laws). Efforts to increase immunization levels among children are also supported by healthcare payers that require contracted healthcare providers to comply with the pediatric immunization standards. Patient records are audited to ensure compliance.

The reported level of full immunization (four doses of DTP/DT/DTaP, three doses of poliovirus vaccine, one measles-mumps-rubella vaccine, three doses of Hib vaccine, three doses of hepatitis B vaccine, one dose of varicella vaccine, and four doses of PCV7) for children between 19 and 35 months of age in 2009 was 70.5%. This is a significant improvement over the reported level of full immunization with the same vaccines in 2005 of 47.3%. The reported percentage of children who had no immunizations was 0.6%. Variations were found by racial and ethnic groups, with PCV coverage being lower for Black and Asian children (Wooten, Kolasa, Singleton, et al., 2010).

Adolescents, a group recently targeted for additional immunizations, present many challenges for full immunization. Adolescents more commonly seek health care for acute illnesses and injuries rather than health promotion. In 2009, adolescents 13 to 17 years of age were found to have the following vaccination coverage: one dose Tdap since 10 years (76.2%), one to two doses of meningococcal vaccine (53.6%), two doses of MMR (89.1%), three or more doses of HepB (80.9%), two doses of varicella or disease (75.7%), and three or more doses of HPV (26.7%) (Dorrell, Stokley, Yankey, et al., 2010). The lower rate for meningococcal vaccine may be associated with limited availability of the vaccine during the year. The lower rate for HPV vaccine may be reflective of its recent addition to the vaccine schedule and parental concerns about it. See Evidence-Based Practice: Adolescent Immunization Challenges.

Challenges in achieving optimal immunization rates Lower immunization rates of children are often associated with economic factors, limited access to health care, lack of healthcare services at hours convenient for working parents, inadequate education regarding the importance of immunization, and cultural or religious prohibitions.

Evidence-Based Practice Adolescent Immunization Challenges

PROBLEM

Adolescents are often not receiving all the needed immunizations, including the human papillomavirus (HPV) vaccine, despite the fact that this vaccine can help prevent cervical cancer, genital warts, and HPV. It is important to identify the strategies that improve the rate of immunization for this age group.

EVIDENCE

A questionnaire was sent to 6,000 parents of middle school children exploring their willingness to permit their child to receive specific vaccines in the school setting. A total of 615 (10%) questionnaires were returned, predominantly from Hispanic families. Specific vaccines listed on the questionnaire included Tdap, varicella, measles-mumps-rubella, influenza, human papillomavirus, hepatitis B, and meningococcus. Parents were most willing to have their child receive the influenza vaccine at school and least willing to permit the child to receive the HPV vaccine (Middleman & Tung, 2010).

Another study reviewed the immunization records of 17,349 children ages 12 to 18 years who received health care in either a community health center (n = 9,132) or a school-based health clinic (SBHC) (n = 8,217). This population was predominantly Latino and had either no insurance or coverage through Medicaid or SCHIP. Adolescents seen in the SBHCs were more likely to be up to date for the following vaccines: Tdap, varicella, MMR, and HPV for adolescents 16 to 18 years of age. No difference was seen in immunization rates for the hepatitis A or meningococcal vaccines. The adolescents in the SBHCs were also more likely to have received multiple doses to complete a vaccine series, especially the HPV vaccine in 16- to 18-year-olds (Federico, Abrams, Everhart, et al., 2010).

A third study explored factors associated with the decision making to get the HPV vaccine among 156 adolescent females in grades 9 through 12 attending a college preparatory high school and a public co-educational high school. Students completed a questionnaire with a focus on immunization status and decision making, health visits, sources of information about the HPV vaccine, sociodemographic information, and vaccine-related knowledge. Findings revealed that 48.4% of the adolescent respondents participated in the decision to get the vaccine. Of the 156 adolescents surveyed, 39.2% opted to receive the vaccine and 9.2% opted not to receive the vaccine. Adolescents who chose not to receive the vaccine were more likely to consider the vaccine to be unsafe. Adolescents who participated in decision making stated the most important sources of information were their parents, doctors or nurses, and their own reading (Mathur, Mathur, & Reichling, 2010).

IMPLICATIONS

The increased number of vaccines recommended for adolescents has resulted in efforts to identify strategies that will increase immunization rates for this population. Adolescents do not have as many health promotion visits as younger children. The increased use of SBHCs or immunization programs in the school setting may be an effective strategy. For example, SBHCs often provide immunizations without a fee, target medically underserved youth, and do not require parents to miss work. In this setting, adolescents are more likely to be provided with age-appropriate education about health issues and sexual behavior, and they may be encouraged to take a larger role in decision making about getting vaccines.

CRITICAL THINKING APPLICATION

Use the vaccine information in the Medications table and information about human papillomavirus in Chapter 31 🔗 to design a brochure targeted to both adolescent males and females about the HPV vaccine, its safety, and its importance for long-term health.

The federal Vaccines for Children program provides free vaccines for qualified children and adolescents less than 19 years of age and has resolved some of the economic factors associated with vaccine coverage. See Legal and Ethical Considerations: Vaccines for Children Program. However, the cost of vaccines is a barrier for children with private health insurance. Physicians are not always reimbursed by health insurers for the full cost, and their reimbursement is often delayed. As a result, physicians may have difficulty keeping vaccines in stock while waiting for reimbursement to order the next batch of vaccines.

Vaccine shortages Vaccine shortages interfere with the goal of achieving high immunization levels. Some vaccines are produced by only one manufacturer who may not meet the demand, or may have a problem with vaccine production. The CDC's Advisory Committee on Immunization Practices and the American Academy of Pediatrics develop guidelines for immunizing children when vaccine shortages occur, to ensure coverage for all children.

Legal and Ethical Considerations
Vaccines for Children Program

The estimated cost of fully immunizing a child through the adolescent years in 2011 is estimated to be $2,026.68 for all approved vaccines in the private healthcare setting (CDC, 2011b). The Vaccines for Children (VFC) program was created by the Omnibus Budget Reconciliation Act of 1993 as an entitlement program required in each state's Medicaid plan. This program makes immunizations available at no cost to children who are uninsured and Medicaid recipients. The CDC buys the vaccines at a discount and distributes them by way of public health agencies to private physicians and public health clinics registered as VFC providers (CDC, 2011c).

Vaccine refusals An increasing number of parents are choosing not to immunize their children for philosophic reasons. Some of these reasons include the following (Amer, 2009):

- Belief that the diseases vaccines prevent may not be dangerous, and they occur rarely today
- Concerns about the safety of vaccines and fear that the child could be harmed
- Concerns that giving so many vaccines at one time may overwhelm the immune system of an infant
- Concerns about adverse effects of vaccines, which are widely publicized, but not hearing about the millions of children who have no adverse effects
- Lack of trust in the doctors and government recommending vaccines, believing that pharmaceutical companies and the government mainly promote vaccines for profit
- Religious reasons related to the fact that some vaccines are grown in human embryo fibroblasts (from tissue cultures, not human embryos) needed for mass replication

See Table 22–1 for common misconceptions some parents have about vaccines and the correct information.

Vaccine Safety

Serious reactions to vaccines may occur in rare instances, for which the National Vaccine Injury Compensation Program was established. See Legal and Ethical Considerations: Vaccine Safety for more information. The range of serious reactions and disabilities that may occur include the following: anaphylaxis, encephalopathy, bacterial neuritis, chronic arthritis, thrombocytopenic purpura, and death. The significant reactions eligible for compensation specific to each vaccine are listed in Table 22–2.

TABLE 22–1	Vaccine Safety Information
MISINFORMATION	**CORRECT INFORMATION**
Vaccine-preventable diseases have been eliminated.	Even though the incidence of vaccine-preventable diseases is low in the United States, most diseases are never completely eliminated. These diseases still occur in developing countries. With airline travel, a traveler can reintroduce a disease from a country or another community where the disease still exists. Recent outbreaks of diseases such as measles and pertussis have been linked to groups of children not immunized because of religious and personal beliefs (Smith & Marshall, 2010). If numerous parents in one community decide not to immunize their children, the **herd immunity** (protection provided by persons with immunity to an infection to others who are susceptible or not protected) level drops and children in that community are at higher risk of infection (Nield, et al., 2009). If the infected person comes into contact with only immunized individuals, the susceptible person is indirectly protected. Herd immunity is especially important for higher risk children being treated for conditions (e.g., leukemia) that affect their immune status.
Immunization weakens the immune system. Multiple vaccines overload the immune system and cause harmful effects.	Vaccination uses the body's immune system to prevent a future infection. Vaccines contain many fewer antigens to protect against infections than in the past. The young infant is capable of generating protective immune responses to multiple vaccines simultaneously. These vaccine immune challenges are less than the number of environmental exposures children face every day (Amer, 2009).
Thimerosal use in vaccines may cause mercury poisoning.	Thimerosal, a bacteriostatic agent that contains ethyl mercury, was previously used to sterilize vaccines in multidose vials. Because ethyl mercury could possibly cause nerve and brain damage in the developing child, vaccine manufacturers eliminated thimerosal from most vaccines in 2001. Only the multidose influenza vaccine continues to have trace amounts of thimerosal (Amer, 2009). Fears about thimerosal should no longer be a reason for parents to refuse immunizations for their children.
It would be better to let the child get the disease than get immunized.	Many parents have never seen some of the vaccine-preventable diseases, and they do not understand the potential dangers of these diseases. Many diseases can cause suffering, permanent disability, and even death. Children who are not immunized are at a much greater risk of becoming infected if a disease outbreak occurs, and also at higher risk for secondary infections like pneumonia. Additionally, these children may transmit the infection to pregnant women and high-risk infants and children.
Vaccines do not work. Children still get the disease.	No vaccine is 100% effective, and immunity does wane over time, leading to the need for subsequent immunizations.
Vaccines may cause serious conditions, such as autism.	Numerous studies have confirmed the lack of association between the measles vaccine and autism, as well as thimerosal in vaccines and autism (Amer, 2009; Hensley & Briars, 2010).

The Vaccine Safety Datalink project, linking the Centers for Disease Control and Prevention with eight managed care organizations, allows monitoring regarding the adverse effects of vaccines. This data system contains data from 9 million people who did and did not get a vaccine, and did or did not experience adverse events. This system makes it possible to identify rare adverse events to vaccines (Smith & Marshall, 2010). The Vaccine Safety Datalink project supplements the Vaccine Adverse Event Reporting System, which enables notification of serious vaccine adverse events from all providers. Both systems are important for monitoring vaccine safety.

Nursing Management

Nursing management focuses on the health promotion activities of immunization by teaching parents about vaccines and their possible side effects, addressing their fears about possible reactions, obtaining consent, administering vaccines, and reporting adverse reactions.

Nursing Assessment and Diagnosis

Nurses are responsible for reviewing a child's immunization record to determine whether the child needs immunization. Inquire about the child's preventive care as well as health problems. Review the child's history carefully, identifying any previous reactions to immunizations, allergies, and immune diseases.

Screening for Vaccine Administration

When talking with a parent to identify if an infant or child who needs an immunization has any contraindications to receiving a vaccine, the following questions can help:

- Is the child sick today?
- Does the child have allergies to medications, food, a vaccine component (e.g., eggs, neomycin, gelatin, or yeast), or latex?
- Has the child had a serious reaction to a vaccine in the past?
- Has the child had a health problem with lung, heart, kidney, or metabolic disease (e.g., diabetes); asthma; or a blood disorder? Is he or she on long-term aspirin therapy?
- If the child to be vaccinated is between the ages of 2 and 4 years, has a healthcare provider told you that the child had wheezing or asthma in the past 12 months?
- Has the child, a sibling, or a parent had a seizure? Has the child had brain or other nervous system problems?
- Does the child have cancer, leukemia, HIV infection, or any other immune system problem?
- Has the child taken cortisone, prednisone, other steroids, or anticancer drugs or had radiation treatments in the past 3 months?
- Has the child received a transfusion of blood or blood products, or been given immune (gamma) globulin or an antiviral drug in the past year?
- Is the child/adolescent pregnant, or is there a chance she could become pregnant in the next month?
- Has the child received any vaccinations in the past 4 weeks?

Legal and Ethical Considerations
Vaccine Safety

Vaccines must be thoroughly tested for safety prior to licensure by the FDA. The National Childhood Vaccine Injury Act of 1986 provides compensation for a family if a link between a child's immunization and a serious adverse effect is found. The Vaccine Adverse Event Reporting System (VAERS) was established in 1988 to track serious vaccine reactions. Follow-up of the patient's condition occurs at 60 days and 1 year after the adverse event.

TABLE 22–2 | *National Vaccine Injury Act—Vaccine Injury Table*

VACCINE	ADVERSE EVENT COVERED	TIME INTERVAL FOR FIRST SYMPTOM OR MANIFESTATION OF ONSET—FOR COMPENSATION
Tetanus toxoid–containing vaccines (e.g., DTaP, Tdap, DTP-Hib, DT, Td, or TT)	Anaphylaxis or anaphylactic shock	4 hours
	Bacterial neuritis	2–28 days
	Any acute complication or sequela (including death) of above events occurring in the specified time period	Not applicable
Pertussis antigen–containing vaccines (e.g., DTaP, Tdap, DTP, P, DTP-Hib)	Anaphylaxis or anaphylactic shock	4 hours
	Encephalopathy (or encephalitis)	72 hours
	Any acute complication or sequela (including death) of above events occurring within the specified time period	Not applicable
Measles, mumps, rubella virus–containing vaccines in any combination (e.g., MMR, MR, M, R)	Anaphylaxis or anaphylactic shock	4 hours
	Encephalopathy (or encephalitis)	5–15 days
	Any acute complication or sequela (including death) of above events occurring within the specified time period	Not applicable
Rubella virus–containing vaccines (e.g., MMR, MR, R)	Chronic arthritis	7–42 days
	Any acute complication or sequela (including death) of above events occurring within the specified time period	Not applicable
Measles virus–containing vaccines (e.g., MMR, MR, M)	Thrombocytopenic purpura	7–30 days
	Vaccine strain measles viral infection in an immunodeficient recipient	6 months
	Any acute complication or sequela (including death) of above events occurring within the specified time period	Not applicable
Polio live virus-containing vaccines (OPV)	Paralytic polio:	
	■ In a non-immunodeficient recipient	30 days
	■ In an immunodeficient recipient	6 months
	■ In a vaccine-associated community case	Not applicable
	Vaccine-strain polio viral infection:	
	■ In a non-immunodeficient recipient	30 days
	■ In an immunodeficient recipient	6 months
	■ In a vaccine-associated community case	Not applicable
	Any acute complication or sequela (including death) of above events	Not applicable
Polio inactivated virus–containing vaccines (e.g., IPV)	Anaphylaxis or anaphylactic shock	4 hours
	Any acute complication or sequela (including death) of above events occurring within the specified time period	Not applicable
Hepatitis B vaccines	Anaphylaxis or anaphylactic shock	4 hours
	Any acute complication or sequela (including death) of above events occurring within the specified time period	No limit
Haemophilus influenzae type b polysaccharide conjugate vaccines	No condition specified	Not applicable
Hepatitis A vaccines	No condition specified	Not applicable
Varicella vaccine	No condition specified	Not applicable
Rotavirus vaccine	No condition specified	Not applicable
Pneumococcal conjugate vaccine	No condition specified	Not applicable
Meningococcal vaccines	No condition specified	Not applicable
Trivalent influenza vaccines	No condition specified	Not applicable
Human papillomavirus (HPV) vaccines	No condition specified	Not applicable
Any new vaccine recommended by the CDC for routine administration to children after publication by the Secretary of the Department of Health and Human Services of notice of coverage	No condition specified	Not applicable

Effective date: July 22, 2011. For guidance in further interpretation of this table, visit the website below.
Source: *From Health Resources and Services Administration. (2011).* National Vaccine Injury Compensation Program. *Retrieved from http://www.hrsa.gov/vaccinecompensation/vaccineinjurytable.pdf*

Contraindications include a moderate to severe acute illness with or without fever, hypersensitivity reaction to specific vaccine components (e.g., eggs, neomycin, gelatin), anaphylactic reaction to a vaccine, immune globulin therapy in the last 3 to 11 months, cancer treatment, and pregnancy. See the Medications table on pages 607–610 for specific vaccine contraindications.

Identifying Vaccines Needed

Nurses are responsible for reviewing a child's immunization record and determining if the child needs any vaccines. Make sure the most current immunization guidelines are used to review the child's record. New vaccines or different vaccine requirements may have been approved leading to modification of the immunization schedule. If the child has not received all appropriate immunizations for age, determine the best combination of vaccines to give at this visit to better protect the child. If catching up on immunizations, make sure that an adequate interval has passed between doses of a vaccine by using the catch-up guidelines (see Figure 22–6). Identify opportunities to give needed immunizations to siblings accompanying the family on the visit. A minor illness should not deter the nurse from giving an immunization to the child seeking care or to a sibling.

Clinical Tip

Make every effort to stay current on immunization guidelines and information about vaccines, safe administration, adverse effects, and so on. Major resources provide more extensive information about immunization schedules and specific vaccines, as well as infectious and communicable diseases. The American Academy of Pediatrics *Red Book: Report of the Committee of Infectious Diseases* is updated about every 3 years. See the companion website for the *Pink Book*, published by the Public Health Foundation which has comprehensive information on communicable diseases and vaccines. The revised immunization schedule is published each January in several pediatric medical and nursing journals. The CDC maintains a regularly updated website with detailed information about immunizations, the most recent vaccine schedule, and infectious and communicable diseases.

Clinical Tip

Preterm and low-birth-weight infants are vulnerable to infection. The latest research regarding the ability of preterm and low-birth-weight infants to develop protection from vaccines has revealed that although their immune response may be somewhat decreased, they do respond adequately and develop full immunity by the end of the vaccination series. Therefore, preterm and low-birth-weight infants who are medically stable should receive all routinely recommended vaccines at the same chronologic age and in the same dosage as full-term infants.

The only difference in immunization recommendations is for a delay in initiation of hepatitis B vaccine for infants weighing less than 2000 g whose mother is hepatitis B negative. The hepatitis B vaccine should be given at 30 days of age to a medically stable infant when the infant has ability to respond to the vaccine. If the mother is hepatitis B positive, the newborn should receive the hepatitis B vaccine and immune globulin, but the dose of vaccine should not be counted toward completion of the hepatitis B vaccine. An infant hospitalized through 6 weeks of age should have rotavirus vaccine administered at the time of discharge (Kroger et al., 2011).

The accompanying Nursing Care Plan explores four potential nursing diagnoses that may apply to the child needing immunizations. Additional nursing diagnoses may include the following:

- Anxiety related to fear of needles
- Skin Integrity, Risk for Impaired related to vaccine response
- Health Maintenance, Ineffective related to cultural beliefs regarding routine immunization

NANDA-I © 2012

Planning and Implementation

Nurses should be strong advocates for immunization. Being well informed about immunizations, their potential side effects, and recommended schedules assists immunization efforts.

Improving Immunization Rates

To avoid missed opportunities in administering immunizations, be sure to evaluate the child's immunization record (as well as the record of siblings present) in all healthcare settings: on acute care units in the hospital, in the emergency department, in health clinics, and in school. If a child is underimmunized at 3 months of age, it is a strong predictor of being underimmunized at 2 years of age (Stevenson, 2009). A designated nurse vaccine manager is one way to promote an effective immunization program. This nurse can take responsibility for educating staff and developing protocols for immunization, tracking inventory, and ensuring safe storage of vaccines. To reduce the number of missed opportunities for full immunization of children, use the following guidelines (Kroger et al., 2011):

- Reminders should be placed in the child's health record to remind healthcare providers about the child's need for immunizations. All healthcare agencies (schools, urgent care centers, hospitals, and community clinics) should fully evaluate immunization status and provide immunizations when they are needed.
- A call-back system should be established or reminders sent to parents about the child's need for immunizations when due or overdue.
- Immunizations can be given when the child has a minor illness with or without a low-grade fever, and with antibiotic treatment. Recent exposure to an infectious disease is not a reason to defer a vaccine.
- Several vaccines can be given at the same visit at different anatomic sites. Two injections can be given in different sites on the same extremity, one inch apart.
- Combination vaccines can reduce the overall number of injections needed in the first 2 years from 20 to 13. See Table 22–3 on page 620.
- Immunizations can be given when there was a local reaction to a prior vaccine or a family member had an adverse response.

Protect Vaccine Potency

Take special care to ensure vaccine potency. An improperly stored vaccine may have reduced potency or be rendered ineffective, resulting in the child having an inadequate immune response, or even no response. When accepting new shipments of vaccine, check for damage to the packaging and identify if any delay in the shipment could have resulted in exposure to temperatures that could damage the vaccine potency.

Some vaccines are frozen; others are refrigerated. Read the package inserts of vaccines to determine proper storage conditions. Vaccines should be stored in a refrigerator that has separate doors for the refrigerator and freezer units. The refrigerator should maintain a consistent temperature in the range of 35°F to 46°F (2°C to 8°C). The freezer should maintain a consistent temperature of 5°F (15°C) or lower. Keep jugs of water in the refrigerator and trays of ice in the freezer to help keep the temperature of the units consistent. Store the vaccines in the middle of the refrigerator and freezer where the temperature is maintained in the desired range. Check the expiration date of the vaccines, and place older vaccines in front to be used first.

Nursing Care Plan | The Child Needing Immunizations

INTERVENTION	RATIONALE	EXPECTED OUTCOME
1. Nursing Diagnosis: Infection, Risk for related to incomplete immunization series		
NIC Priority Interventions—*Immunization Vaccination Management: Administration:* Monitoring immunization status, facilitating access to immunizations, and provision of immunizations to prevent communicable disease		**NOC Suggested Outcome—*Immune Status:*** Adequacy of natural and acquired appropriately targeted resistance to internal and external antigens
GOAL: *The child will be adequately protected from disease-preventable illnesses.*		
■ Review the child's immunization record for needed vaccines at each healthcare visit. ■ Identify all due vaccines that can be provided simultaneously. ■ Identify potential contraindications to needed vaccines. Review past reactions to vaccines.	■ Children who have missed needed vaccines can be identified. ■ Giving multiple vaccines at the same visit more adequately protects the child. ■ Identifying contraindications and reviewing past reactions reduces the risk for adverse vaccine reactions.	The child is adequately protected from vaccine-preventable illnesses.
2. Nursing Diagnosis: Immunization Status, Readiness for Enhanced related to family seeking vaccines for the child		
NIC Priority Intervention—*Decision-Making Support:* Providing information and support for a patient who is making a decision regarding health care.		**NOC Suggested Outcome—*Knowledge Treatment: Regimen:*** Extent of understanding conveyed about a specific treatment regimen.
GOAL: *Parents will sign consent for vaccines to be given.*		
■ Educate the parents and adolescents about the need for specific vaccines and the risk if not received. Obtain signed consent before giving vaccines.	■ Informed consent is required for all treatments.	The parent(s) complete(s) the consent form, which is placed in the child's file.
GOAL: *Parents and adolescents will state the side effects of vaccines given.*		
■ Review past reactions to vaccines and describe common potential reactions and why they occur. ■ Describe serious side effects that should be reported to the healthcare provider.	■ Parents should expect common reactions and know they indicate the child's body is building protection to the illness. ■ Parents need to be prepared for potential serious side effects so they can obtain care if needed.	Parents report all serious side effects to the healthcare provider.
GOAL: *Parents will manage common side effects of vaccines.*		
■ Teach parents general comfort measures for common side effects, for example: ■ Cool pack to immunization site(s) ■ Acetaminophen or ibuprofen for fever and discomfort ■ Rocking and holding the infant ■ Gentle movement of affected extremity	■ Parents will know how to make the child more comfortable during the 24–48 hours after the vaccine is given.	The child is given comfort measures after vaccine administration.
3. Nursing Diagnosis: Pain, Acute related to injection and associated anxiety		
NIC Priority Intervention— *Pain Management:* Alleviation of pain or a reduction in pain to a level of comfort that is acceptable to the patient		**NOC Suggested Outcome—*Pain Control:*** Personal actions to control pain
GOAL: *The child's anxiety and pain associated with immunizations are reduced.*		
■ Prepare all immunization injections and supplies enabling injections to be given quickly. ■ Provide guidelines for parents to hold the child and provide distraction and reassurance during and immediately following injections. ■ Right before giving injections, tell the child what to expect, that it is okay to cry, and how to cooperate.	■ Shortening exposure to syringes and needles reduces the child's anxiety. ■ Distraction and security of being held by a parent provides comfort and reduces anxiety. ■ Information about what will happen and how to cooperate helps the child manage anxiety.	The time the child cries during and after injections is brief. The child is easily comforted.

(continued)

Nursing Care Plan   The Child Needing Immunizations, *continued*

INTERVENTION	RATIONALE	EXPECTED OUTCOME
■ Apply firm pressure over the injection site, or use vapocoolant spray on injection sites before the injection.	■ Pressure or spray will reduce needlestick pain.	
■ Inform the child when all injections have been completed and offer praise and comfort.	■ Information and comfort lets the child know when to relax.	

4. Nursing Diagnosis: Injury, Risk for related to vaccine reaction

NIC Priority Intervention—*Risk Identification:* Analysis of potential risk factors, determination of health risks, and prioritization of risk reduction strategies for an individual or group		**NOC Suggested Outcome**—*Risk Control:* Personal actions to prevent, eliminate, or reduce actual modifiable health threats

GOAL: *The child's potential vaccine reactions will be safely managed.*

■ Prepare for life-threatening reactions by having resuscitation drugs and equipment immediately available.	■ Anaphylactic reactions must be managed quickly and effectively.	The child has no reaction or has a severe reaction to a vaccine that is managed effectively.
■ Monitor the child for 15 minutes after the vaccine administration before letting the child go home.	■ A life-threatening response will usually become apparent within this time frame.	
■ Assess the child for extreme anxiety and injection fearfulness.	■ These are potential signs the child may have a vasovagal response to the injection.	
■ Have the fearful child sit or lie down until symptoms of vasovagal response have disappeared.	■ The child who faints and falls may sustain a brain injury.	
■ Report all serious vaccine-related reactions to the appropriate agency using the standard form.	■ This is a legal requirement for all healthcare providers.	

NANDA-I © 2012

Check the temperature of the refrigerator and freezer units twice daily, and record the temperatures on a log to determine that the required temperature is constantly maintained. Review the temperature log weekly, and keep the logs on file for 3 years (Kroger et al., 2011). Automatic temperature measurement systems are available that check and record temperatures at established times. Make sure the facility has an emergency plan for safe storage of vaccines in case of a power outage or natural disaster. If an outlet tied to an emergency power system is available, keep the refrigerator and freezer plugged into that outlet. Manufacturers of the vaccine and the CDC can be consulted for advice about how to handle vaccine that has been subjected to a power outage.

Family Education and Informed Consent

Federal legislation requires written consent to be obtained before administering a vaccine. In most healthcare settings, the nurse has the responsibility to inform the parents or the child's legal guardian, and supply the most current Vaccine Information Statement (VIS) for each vaccine to be administered. See Legal and Ethical Considerations: Vaccine Information Statements.

TABLE 22–3	Combination Vaccines	
VACCINE NAME	**VACCINE COMPONENTS**	**AGES USED**
Comvax	Hib and HepB	2, 4, and 12–15 months of age; three doses
TriHIBit	DTaP and Hib	15–18 months, fourth dose of Hib and DTaP series
Twinrix	HepA and HepB	18 years and older
Pediarix	DTaP, HepB, and IPV	2, 4, and 6 months of age; three doses
ProQuad	MMR and Varicella	12–15 months of age and 4–6 years of age
Kinrix	DTaP and IPV	4–6 years, fifth dose of DTaP and fourth dose of IPV
Pentacel	DTaP, IPV, and Hib	2, 4, 6, and 15–18 months of age; four doses

Source: *Adapted from Kroger, A. T., Sumaya, C. V., Pickering, L. K., & Atkinson, W. L. (2011). General recommendations on immunization: Recommendations of the Advisory Committee on Immunization Practices (ACIP). Morbidity and Mortality Weekly Report, 60(2), 37.*

Legal and Ethical Considerations
Vaccine Information Statements

A Vaccine Information Statement (VIS) must be given to parents for each vaccine the child will receive as directed by the National Vaccine Injury Act of 1986 and 1993. The VIS provides concise information about the vaccine, risks and benefits of the vaccine, its recommended schedule, what to do if adverse effects occur, where to find more information, and a description of the National Vaccine Injury Compensation Program. The VIS for each vaccine is updated by the Centers for Disease Control National Immunization Program, and they are available through the program's website.

Developing Cultural Competence
Vaccine Information Statements

Consider literacy and reading level when giving a VIS to a parent. Although written at a sixth-grade level, parents may have difficulty reading the VIS or they may not be able to read. It is acceptable to read the VIS to parents and make sure that parents understand the information. The VIS has been translated into 30 languages, but make sure the parent can read the preferred spoken language before assuming the parent will understand the translated VIS. Answer questions when necessary, and supplement the VIS with other teaching materials such as videos or DVDs.

It is the nurse's responsibility to make sure that the most current VIS is provided to the parents about each vaccine to be administered. When teaching about immunizations, make sure that the parents understand the information in the VIS, and answer any questions they might have. Identify vaccines due to be given at this visit and on the next visit so that the parents know their child's immunization status. It may save time to give parents the VIS for the next vaccines to take home and review prior to the next visit. See Developing Cultural Competence: Vaccine Information Statements.

Additional education should focus on the fact that immunization is one of the most important ways the parents can protect their child. Vaccines prevent diseases that previously killed children, or caused serious illnesses such as pneumonia. If children were no longer immunized, the diseases would come back. If a child is not immunized, he or she could get very sick or die from a disease; the child could also infect other children, especially those with chronic conditions such as leukemia who are at higher risk of serious infection. Provide parents with recommendations for trustworthy information about immunizations on the Internet. For example, the CDC and the Children's Hospital of Philadelphia have trustworthy vaccine information for parents and patients. See Partnering with Families: Preparing the Child for Immunizations.

Discuss the risks and benefits of each vaccine with parents, as well as common local reactions. There are risks with every vaccine, but most risks are mild. The child might have a fever, redness, or pain in the leg. Each vaccine can cause an allergic reaction or seizure, but these are rare events. It is the nurse's responsibility to know the potential adverse consequences of vaccines and to be informed about the latest research regarding potential vaccine-related conditions.

In order for parents to provide informed consent, the nurse needs to answer questions to their satisfaction. Parents may have heard sensational stories about the consequences of vaccines, and correct information is needed to help them make informed decisions. With more information, the parents who have philosophic reasons for not immunizing their children may see the value of getting some or all of the recommended vaccines.

For each vaccine administered, the nurse is required to record the (1) month, day, and year of administration, (2) vaccine given, (3) manufacturer, (4) lot number and expiration date of the immunization given, (5) site and route of administration, and (6) name, title, and address of the person who administers the vaccine. Obtain written consent from the parent or guardian to give the needed vaccines on the healthcare facility's standardized form. Provide parents with a record of the child's immunizations, and enter the information on vaccines administered into the healthcare agency's official records.

Parents have the right to refuse vaccines for their children, but if there is a disease outbreak, the nonimmunized child must be kept out of school or childcare. Local, city, or state courts decide how to settle any conflicts. If the parent chooses not to have the child receive a particular vaccine, document the informed refusal. This is one method to communicate the seriousness of not allowing the child to be protected from a vaccine-preventable disease. A form that can be used for documentation of informed refusal is available from the American Academy of Pediatrics.

Clinical Judgment
What information would be included in an informed refusal documentation?

Provide guidelines for managing expected mild reactions at home. (See Partnering with Families: Care of the Child After Immunizations.) See recommended acetaminophen and ibuprofen doses for children of various ages in the Clinical Tip on page 641. Make sure that parents have the correct dosage information for the acetaminophen or ibuprofen formulation that is in the home (Box 22–2). Schedule the child's next appointment for a health supervision visit and inform parents of the need for the next immunizations.

Preparing Vaccines for Administration
Check the expiration date of the vaccines to be used. When reconstituting vaccines, it is important to use the solution provided or follow the manufacturer's directions. Write the date and time on the

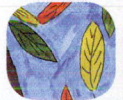

Partnering with Families

Preparing the Child for Immunizations

Parents can help make the immunization experience less stressful for the child with some planning. Encourage the parents to be honest about the purpose of the healthcare visit and the need for the immunization. Parents can take these extra steps to reduce the child's anxiety (Luthy, Sperhac, Faux, et al., 2010):

- Take a favorite toy or blanket along on the visit that can help comfort the child during the immunization.

- Stay with the child during the injections, either holding or sitting beside the child. Remain calm and distract the child with activities such as counting, singing, reading, playing with a toy, or making funny faces.
- Let the child know that crying is acceptable behavior but that kicking and screaming are not acceptable.
- Provide comfort after the injection(s).
- Plan a reward for the child, such as a sticker or a visit to a favorite place.

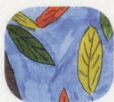

Partnering with Families

Care of the Child After Immunizations

After your child receives an immunization, observe for any reactions that might occur.

- Check the injection sites. Local pain, redness, and swelling are common. Ice can be put on the sites to help reduce swelling and pain.
- The child may have a fever, joint pain, muscle aches, or fatigue within hours to days after the vaccine is given. Acetaminophen or ibuprofen may be given to reduce a fever and pain. The symptoms should disappear in a day or two. Call your healthcare provider if you are concerned about the symptoms. See Chapter 33 🖉 for information about aspirin and Reye syndrome.

- If your child has a mild allergic reaction to the vaccine, you might notice a few hives around the injection site. A severe allergic reaction is indicated by a flushed face; swelling of the face, mouth, or throat; wheezing or other difficulty breathing; shock (confusion, lack of movement or response, or unconsciousness); and abdominal cramping. If these symptoms occur, call 911 or your emergency number so your child can be taken to the emergency department for treatment. While waiting for the ambulance to arrive, lay the child on his or her back and raise the legs to promote blood return to the vital organs.

BOX 22–2	Research: Acetaminophen and Vaccine Response

A recent study explored the effect of giving prophylactic rectal acetaminophen (paracetamol) with immunization on infant febrile reaction and vaccine responses. Half of the 459 infants were randomly assigned to receive prophylactic rectal acetaminophen every 6 to 8 hours in the first 24 hours after immunization. The other infants received no prophylactic acetaminophen. Therapeutic acetaminophen was used in the control group if the parent desired or physician recommended. Fever greater than 39.5°C was uncommon in either group of children. The prophylactic acetaminophen group had lower antibody responses to the vaccines. It is possible that acetaminophen given at the time of immunization can exert a direct effect on cell-mediated responses. Additional studies are needed to verify these findings. However, it might be appropriate to give acetaminophen only when the child has a febrile response (Prymula, Siegrist, Chlibek, et al., 2009).

bottle if it is a multidose vial. Reconstituted vaccines may have a short shelf life, so to ensure potency reconstitute the vaccine just prior to administration. If the reconstituted single-dose vaccine is not used within the time specified by the manufacturer, it should be discarded (Kroger et al., 2011). See vaccine-specific information in the table on pages 607–610.

Use of longer needles (25 mm rather than 16 mm) reduces the rate of local reactions and tenderness in infant immunizations (Table 22–4). A recent study concluded that 25 mm needles reduced local reactions to the fifth DTaP vaccine, whether the deltoid or vastus lateralis muscle was used (Jackson, Starkovich, Dunstan, et al., 2008). If the child has extra adipose tissue, stretch the skin to decrease the amount of subcutaneous tissue the needle must go through. This may ensure that the intramuscular vaccine is given deeper into the muscle mass. Some vaccines are given subcutaneously at a 45° angle with a 5/8-inch 23 to 25 gauge needle. Subcutaneous injections should be made into the upper thigh of infants less than 12 months of age, and into the upper outer triceps region for all other ages (Kroger et al., 2011).

Practice Alert

When giving the diphtheria, tetanus, and pertussis vaccines, ensure that you are using the correct preparation. DTaP has a higher dose of diphtheria and is to be used for children under age 7 years, especially for the initial three doses to stimulate an effective antibody response. If DTaP is given to adolescents rather than Tdap, the vaccine is effective, but adverse effects are more likely (Bell, 2010).

Reducing Pain and Anxiety

Prepare the parents to help reduce the anxiety and pain of the immunizations. Let them know it is okay to be anxious, but to try to stay calm for the child. Give the appropriate immunizations to the child as efficiently as possible, while providing support to the child (Figure 22–7 ■).

Be alert for adolescents who are anxious and may develop syncope. Be prepared to catch them to prevent injury. Nurses should make efforts to reduce the pain associated with vaccine injections,

TABLE 22–4	Recommended Length of 22 to 25 Gauge Needles for Intramuscular Immunization and Preferred Injection Site

AGE AND INJECTION LOCATION	INTRAMUSCULAR NEEDLE SIZE
Newborns and preterm infants—anterolateral thigh[¶]	5/8 inch (16 mm)
Infants 1 to 12 months—anterolateral thigh[§]	1 inch (25 mm)
Toddlers 1 to 2 years—anterolateral thigh[§]	1 to 1 1/4 inch (25–32 mm)
deltoid muscle of arm	5/8 to 1 inch (16–25 mm)
Children and adolescents 3 to 18 years—deltoid muscle[§]	5/8 to 1 inch (16–25 mm)
anterolateral thigh	1 to 1 1/4 inch (25–32 mm)
Adolescents 19 years and older—deltoid muscle	
Weight less than 60 kg (130 lb)	5/8 inch (16 mm)
Weight of 60 to 70 kg (130 to 152 lb)	1 inch (25 mm)
Females weighing 70 to 90 kg (152 to 200 lb)	1 to 1 1/2 inch (25–38 mm)
Males weighing 60 to 118 kg (152 to 260 lb)	1 to 1 1/2 inch (25–38 mm)
Females weighing more than 90 kg (200 lb) and males weighing more than 118 kg (260 lb)	1 1/2 inch (38 mm)

[¶]If skin is stretched tight to avoid bunching subcutaneous tissue

[§]Preferred injection site

Source: *From Kroger, A. T., Sumaya, C. V., Pickering, L. K., & Atkinson, W. L. (2011). General recommendations on immunization: Recommendations of the Advisory Committee on Immunization Practices (ACIP).* Morbidity and Mortality Weekly Report, 60(2), 15–16.

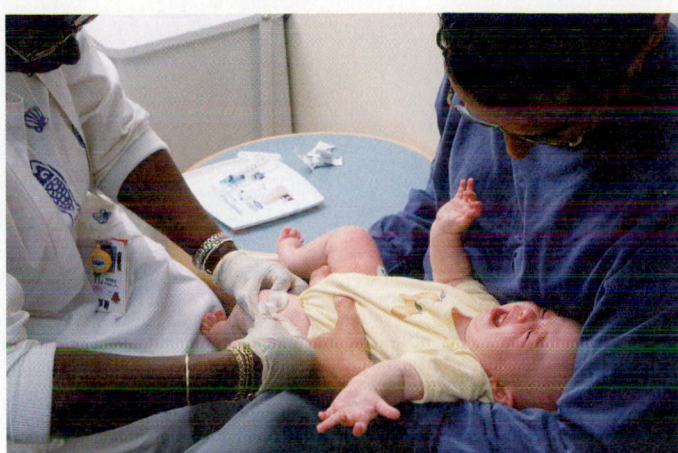

FIGURE 22–7 ■ Give immunizations quickly and efficiently. Do not prolong the wait and let fear grow. The child will be anxious, especially when more than one injection is to be given.

especially since infants and children must return for more injections in the future. Reducing pain will also lessen the anxiety associated with future visits for health care. Suggestions for pain management include the following techniques:

- Give infants up to 4 months of age 24% sucrose water to suck (use a prepared solution, e.g., Sweet-Ease, or mix 1 packet of table sugar with 10 mL of tap water) immediately before the injection. Sucrose water has been demonstrated to reduce pain in newborns and young infants. See Chapter 21 🕑. Then allow the infant to suck on a pacifier or breastfeed during the injections.
- Apply pressure at the site for 10 seconds before the injection.
- Provide information about obtaining L-M-X4 (a topical anesthetic available without a prescription) prior to the next visit. Instruct parents how to apply L-M-X4 cream to one or more sites prior to the child's appointment. See Chapter 21 for information regarding use of L-M-X4.
- Use vapocoolant spray immediately before the injection. Spray on the planned injection site for 3 to 7 seconds from a distance of 3 to 9 inches. Alternatively, spray it on a cotton ball and hold it against the skin for a couple of minutes.
- Have two providers each give an injection simultaneously in different extremities to reduce the time children have to be anxious about multiple injections.
- Use age-appropriate distraction techniques (see Chapter 21).
- Do not prolong the process of giving immunizations, and give the child honest answers that the needles will cause some pain.
- Let the child select the arm or leg for the injection and type of distraction to promote coping. After the injections are completed, let the parent comfort the child.

Practice Alert

Adolescents are at a greater risk of syncope or vasovagal response after a vaccine injection. Fainting increases the risk for traumatic brain injury. Provide the injection when the adolescent is sitting or lying down. Observe the adolescent while sitting or lying down for 15 minutes to help protect the adolescent from secondary injury in case of syncope.

Preparation for Emergencies

Anaphylaxis following immunization is a rare event. However, the office or clinic setting should have standing orders for nurses to perform initial management of vaccine reactions, including anaphylaxis. Keep epinephrine 1:1000 and resuscitation equipment immediately available. The dose for epinephrine (aqueous 1:1000) is 0.01 mL/kg per dose up to 0.5 mL intramuscularly. The dose can be repeated every 10 to 20 minutes for up to a total of three doses until symptoms subside or other emergency care interventions are initiated (AAP, 2012, p. 68). Regularly check the shelf-life date of available epinephrine to be assured of its potency. Ensure that specific serious reactions following immunization are reported to the U.S. Department of Health and Human Services, as required by law.

Evaluation

Expected nursing outcomes include the following:

- The parent provides fully informed consent for immunizations.
- The child receives all age-appropriate immunizations at each health visit, including catch-up immunizations if needed.
- The parents are educated to manage mild reactions to immunizations at home.
- The parents know how to identify and report serious reactions to immunizations.

COMMUNICABLE DISEASES IN INFANTS AND CHILDREN

Communicable diseases cause acute illnesses. These diseases are caused by bacterial, viral, protozoan, or fungal organisms. As noted earlier, infants and children develop communicable diseases more frequently than adults do. Active immunity to microorganisms does not occur until there is natural exposure or immunization that leads to the development of antibodies. Therefore, infants and children are more susceptible to the large number of infectious organisms to which they have no resistance.

Etiology and Pathophysiology

Microorganisms (bacterial, viral, fungal, and protozoan) use the human body to reproduce. In some cases they have a mutually beneficial relationship, such as occurs with the bacteria in the gastrointestinal tract that help with digestion. Other microorganisms are pathogens that cause communicable diseases. They enter the body through direct contact with mucous membranes and injured skin, inhalation, and ingestion. **Vectors,** biting insects or animals, can transmit infectious organisms into the skin and blood. The microorganisms spread through the lymph and blood to other tissues and organs where they multiply.

When a microorganism succeeds in invading the body through its defenses (such as the skin and mucous membranes), the inflammatory response is initiated (Figure 22–8 ■). Neutrophils are the predominant phagocytic cell in the early inflammatory response (ingesting bacteria, dead cells, and cellular debris). Monocytes and macrophages also serve a role in phagocytosis in later stages. Cytokines, such as interleukins and interferons, enhance the inflammatory response by increasing the microbicidal activity of the macrophages. Natural killer cells specifically work to kill cells infected with viruses. Interferons help prevent viruses from infecting healthy cells by attaching to neighboring cells of the virus-invaded cell, stimulating the healthy cells to produce an antiviral protein. Antimicrobials also prevent the growth of or destroy microorganisms that have not developed antibiotic resistance. See Chapter 27 🕑 for more information about the inflammatory and immune response.

Pathophysiology Illustrated
Inflammatory Response

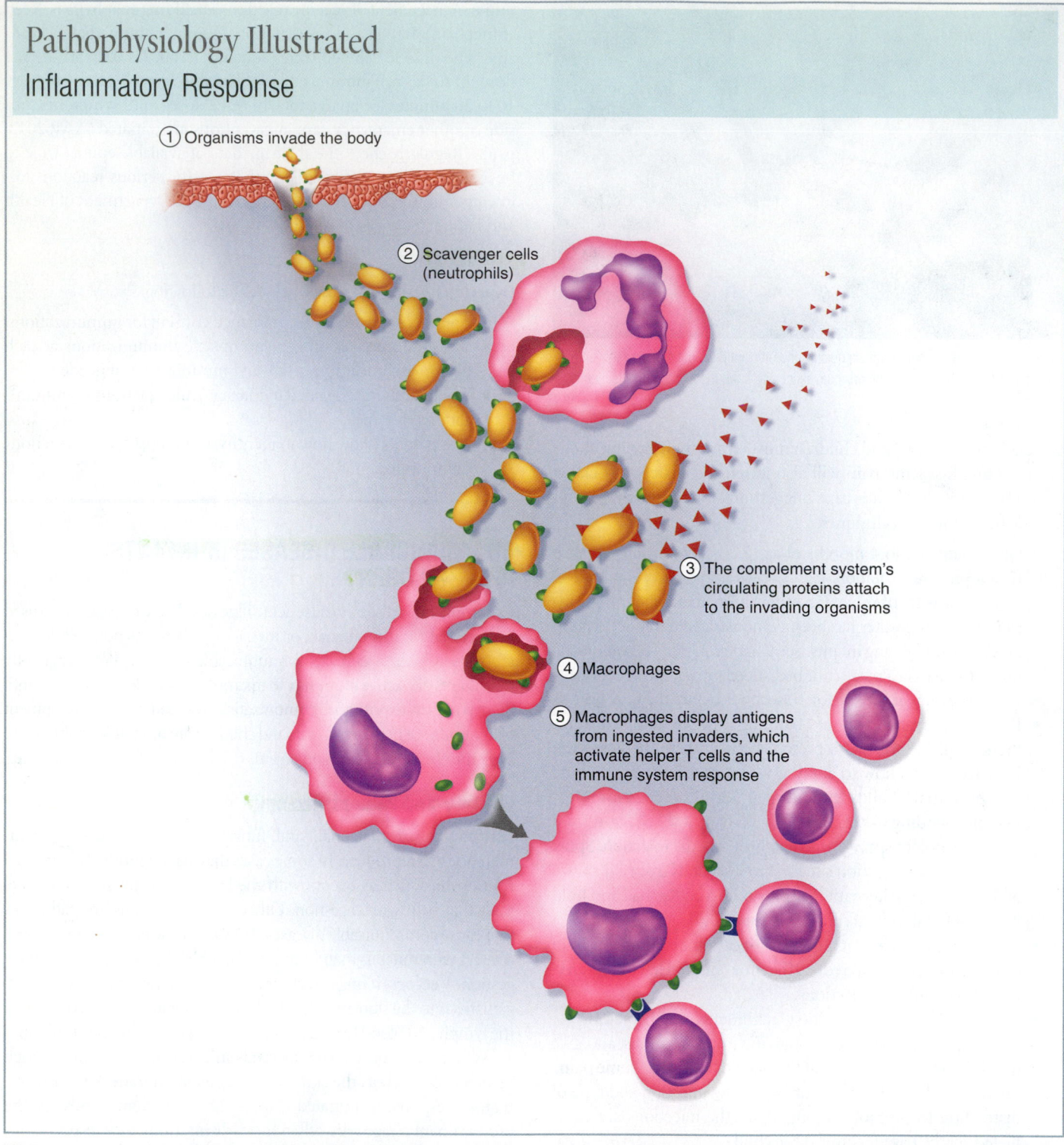

① Organisms invade the body

② Scavenger cells (neutrophils)

③ The complement system's circulating proteins attach to the invading organisms

④ Macrophages

⑤ Macrophages display antigens from ingested invaders, which activate helper T cells and the immune system response

FIGURE 22–8 ■ After the body is invaded by microorganisms, neutrophils, the complement system proteins, and macrophages rush to the site. Neutrophils act as scavenger cells and engulf microorganisms. Macrophages also engulf microorganisms and trigger the immune system to respond. The complement system's proteins attach to the microorganisms, leading to their death.

When antibodies have developed to a specific microorganism to which the child is exposed, they protect the child by:

- Activating the inflammatory response
- Neutralizing bacterial toxins by serving as an antitoxin, preventing the toxin from binding with the tissues
- Preventing the initial attachment and entrance of viruses into the cells

- Producing a substance (opsonin) that makes the bacterial outer capsule susceptible to **phagocytosis** (the engulfment and destruction of microorganisms, dead cells, and foreign particles)

Bacteria

The initial response of the body to invasion by bacteria is inflammation. Endotoxins increase capillary permeability and trigger fever.

Most bacteria have found ways to prevent destruction by the inflammatory and immune systems and cause disease in the following ways:

- By producing toxins that kill phagocytes and injure cells or tissues, as occurs with staphylococcus
- By producing a thick capsule of carbohydrate or protein that prevents efficient phagocytosis, as occurs with the polysaccharide covering of the pneumococcus

Viruses

Viruses are the most common cause of infections in humans. They are parasitic organisms that invade the cells and take them over for their own survival and reproduction. The cell's protein synthesis is halted. Viruses usually hide in the cells and avoid the typical inflammatory and immune responses. They penetrate the cell and release the viral genetic material into the cytoplasm. The cell's lysosomal membrane is disrupted, releasing enzymes that can kill the cell. As they reproduce cell to cell, eventually the body's immune response to the virus overwhelms it and the infection is cured. In some cases the virus reproduces at such a slow rate that the infected person is asymptomatic and becomes a carrier of the virus. Secondary bacterial infection can occur in virus-damaged cells. See Chapter 27 for more information about the immune response and viral infections such as HIV.

Fever

Fever is an increased body temperature of 38°C (100.4°F) or higher taken by rectal or tympanic route, and 37.8°C (100°F) or higher by the oral route. In cases of infection, the body temperature is regulated at a higher level, resulting in fever. The hypothalamus is the control center for the regulation of body temperature and is frequently compared to a thermostat due to its regulatory function (Figure 22–9). As blood circulates through the hypothalamus, this brain structure regulates body temperature by directing body systems to conserve or dissipate heat, depending on the temperature of the blood.

Pyrogens (substances that stimulate fever) may include toxins, products of viral or bacterial metabolism, antigen–antibody complexes, and complement components. The pyrogens stimulate monocytes, macrophages, and other inflammatory cells to release pyrogenic cytokines (interleukins, interferons, and tumor necrosis factor) into circulation. This activity results in an increased production of prostaglandin which raises the body's thermoregulatory set point, thus causing the fever to occur (Avner, 2009).

A rise in the hypothalamus's set point leads to a process of heat generation and heat conservation. Involuntary shivering generates body heat. Vasoconstriction of the blood vessels close to the skin surface and seeking a warmer environment (e.g., extra clothing, assuming a fetal position) are methods of heat conservation. When the temperature is elevated, the heart rate, respiratory rate, and metabolic rate increase. Vasodilation occurs and the skin flushes, becoming warm to the touch.

Communicable diseases differ in their epidemiology, transmission, and incubation period. Many infections are communicable

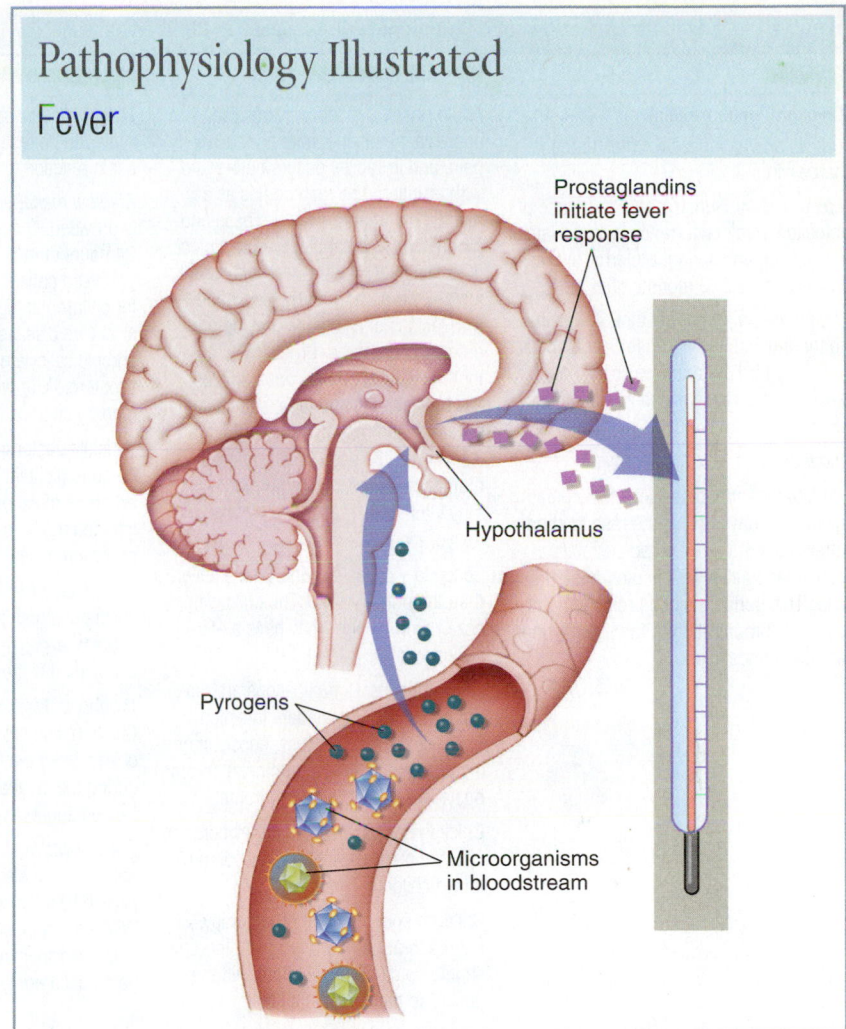

Pathophysiology Illustrated
Fever

FIGURE 22–9 ■ The hypothalamus functions as the body's thermostat, directing the body to conserve or dissipate heat. When microorganisms invade the body, endogenous pyrogens are released into the bloodstream. These substances travel to the hypothalamus, where they trigger the production and release of prostaglandins, which initiate the fever response. Blood is diverted from the extremities to more central vessels. This helps increase the core body temperature by decreasing heat loss. Shivering, the rapid contraction and relaxation of the skeletal muscles, burns energy and produces heat until the blood is the temperature of the altered temperature set point in the hypothalamus. The body then maintains the temperature at the new set point until antipyretics are given or the organisms causing the fever are eliminated.

between humans, but many are vaccine preventable. The epidemiology, clinical manifestations, treatment, prevention, and nursing care of selected communicable diseases of childhood are detailed in Table 22–5 starting on page 626. Some communicable diseases are transmitted by insects or animals (**zoonosis**) and are not transmitted from person to person. See Table 22–6 on page 638. See Chapter 24 for information about conjunctivitis; Chapter 25 for information on tuberculosis; Chapter 27 for information on HIV infection; Chapter 30 for information on hepatitis A, B, and C, and parasites; Chapter 31 for information on sexually transmitted infections; and Chapter 36 for information about impetigo, methicillin-resistant *Staphylococcus aureus*, scabies, and lice.

Clinical Manifestations

The child with a communicable disease has several symptoms. Fever is the most common sign. Other common signs and symptoms

TABLE 22-5	Selected Infectious and Communicable Diseases in Children		
DISEASE	**CLINICAL MANIFESTATIONS**	**CLINICAL THERAPY**	**NURSING MANAGEMENT**
Chicken Pox (Varicella)*[+] *Causal agent:* Varicella-zoster, human herpesvirus 3. *Epidemiology:* Humans are the source of infection. Peak occurrence is in the late fall, winter, and spring. Maternal antibodies disappear 2–3 months after birth. *Transmission:* Direct contact of the virus to the mucous membranes or conjunctiva primarily through airborne spread of secretions and occasionally with lesion contact. *Incubation period:* 14–21 days. *Period of communicability:* Most contagious 1–2 days before the rash to shortly after onset of rash. Contagious state continues until all lesions are crusted over. This period may be prolonged after passive immunization or in children who are immunodeficient.	Acute onset of mild fever, malaise, anorexia, headache, mild abdominal pain, and irritability occurs before and with eruption. The rash begins as a macule on an erythematous base and progresses to a papule, then to a clear, fluid-filled vesicle. The rash may erupt for 1–5 days and is itchy. Up to 250 to 500 lesions of all stages may be present at any one time. Crusts may remain for 1–3 weeks. The lesions begin on the trunk, scalp, and face, and then spread to the rest of the body. Ulcerative lesions may be seen in the mucous membranes. Lesions in the mouth may lead to decreased fluid intake and dehydration. Secondary cases are often more severe than the primary case. The child with eczema or sunburn may have a more severe rash. *Complications:* Complications are rare but can include secondary infection (cellulitis, local abscesses, sepsis, meningitis, encephalitis, pneumonia), thrombocytopenia, and Reye syndrome. Chicken pox can be fatal in newborns of infected mothers and immunocompromised children. Children undergoing chemotherapy, steroid treatment, or transplant therapy should be carefully monitored after exposure to the disease.	*Diagnostic testing:* Fluid from vesicle or scab can be tested using polymerase chain reaction for diagnosis. *Medical management:* Supportive care is provided. IV acyclovir is used within 24 hours of rash onset for immunocompromised patients. Oral acyclovir is used for children at high risk of moderate or severe disease (e.g., treated with chronic salicylate therapy, aerosol corticosteroids, or with chronic skin or pulmonary condition) (AAP, 2012, p. 778). Varicella-zoster immune globulin or immune globulin IV is given within 96 hours of exposure to newborns of infected mothers and to exposed immunocompromised, unimmunized children. The vaccine may be given to healthy children without immunity within 72 hours of exposure to prevent or significantly modify the disease. *Prognosis:* Most children recover fully. Children who are immunocompromised or who were treated with corticosteroids during the incubation period must be treated aggressively. *Prevention:* Varicella is vaccine preventable. See the Medications table on page 610 for vaccine information. Wild virus (varicella strain not covered in the vaccine) cases occur in vaccinated children.	▪ Use airborne and contact precautions while children are contagious. ▪ Upon admission to the hospital, inquire about varicella immunization or recent exposure. Place all exposed children in isolation to protect newborns and immunocompromised patients. ▪ Nurses should have documented immunity. ▪ When treated at home, isolate the child from all susceptible individuals, especially medically fragile and immunocompromised children or adults, and women early in pregnancy. Notify the school or childcare facility of the child's illness. ▪ Give acetaminophen or ibuprofen to control fever. ▪ Give oral antihistamines for relief of itching. Oatmeal and Aveeno baths are soothing. Caladryl lotion applied to lesions may also provide relief. ▪ Keep the child's fingernails short and clean. Young children may need to wear soft cotton mittens when itching cannot be controlled. ▪ Change bed linens frequently. Wash linen in mild soap and rinse well. ▪ Reassure the child that the lesions are temporary and will go away, but some scars may develop. ▪ Observe the child closely for symptoms of complications such as drowsiness, meningeal signs, respiratory distress, and dehydration. Disorientation and restlessness may indicate viral encephalitis. ▪ Monitor for acyclovir side effects: nausea, vomiting, diarrhea, abdominal pain, as well as allergic skin reactions or headache. Monitor renal function if the child has renal insufficiency.

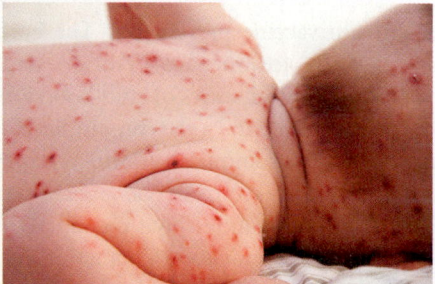

Skin lesions of chicken pox, in all stages of development.

Source: *Phanie Agency/Photo Researchers.*

*Indicates that a vaccine or antitoxin is available for use in high-risk or as-needed situations.
[+]Indicates that the disease has a safe and effective vaccine.

TABLE 22–5 | **Selected Infectious and Communicable Diseases in Children** *(continued)*

DISEASE	CLINICAL MANIFESTATIONS	CLINICAL THERAPY	NURSING MANAGEMENT
Diphtheria* *Causal agent: Corynebacterium diphtheriae.* *Epidemiology:* Occurs mostly in colder months in unimmunized or inadequately immunized persons. Cases of cutaneous and wound diphtheria occur sporadically in the tropics. The disease is endemic in parts of Africa, Latin America, Asia, the Middle East, and states of the former Soviet Union. *Transmission:* Contact with respiratory droplets, nasal or eye discharge, or skin lesion; or less commonly by indirect contact with contaminated items or unpasteurized milk. *Incubation period:* 2–7 days or longer. *Period of communicability:* Usually 2–4 weeks or until 4 days after antibiotics are started.	The characteristic lesion is an adherent grayish pharyngeal membrane that in severe cases may extend into the trachea or cause airway obstruction. Attempts to remove the membrane result in bleeding. Symptoms can be mild or severe with a gradual onset over 1–2 days. A sore throat and enlarged tender cervical lymph nodes are present. The child may have a swollen neck. *Complications:* The organism produces an endotoxin that causes myocarditis and peripheral neuropathy (diplopia, slurred speech, difficulty swallowing, or paralysis of the palate) or ascending paralysis that may be confused with Guillain-Barré syndrome.	*Diagnostic testing:* A culture may be obtained from the nose or throat, or from a cutaneous lesion. *Medical management:* Administration of IV equine antitoxin (for respiratory diphtheria) occurs after the child is tested for sensitivity. The dose is based upon the duration of symptoms. Antibiotic therapy is provided for 14 days with IV or IM penicillin G, changing to oral erythromycin when the child can swallow. *Prognosis:* Mortality of 5–10% with respiratory diphtheria, even with treatment (Heymann, 2008). *Prevention:* Diphtheria is a vaccine-preventable disease. See the Medications table on page 607. Booster doses are needed every 10 years after the primary series. This is a reportable disease. The disease does not confer immunity.	■ Isolate the child and use transmission-based precautions. ■ Monitor closely for signs of increasing respiratory distress, as well as cardiac and neurologic complications. ■ Have emergency airway equipment available. Provide humidified oxygen as necessary. ■ Administer antitoxin and antibiotics as prescribed. ■ Use oral suction gently as necessary. ■ Allow children to use mouthwash if desired. Gargling is not permitted because it can irritate the pharyngeal surfaces. ■ Encourage liquids as tolerated. Intravenous fluids may be necessary. ■ Provide emotional support to the family. ■ Initiate the search for patient contacts to give antibiotics and immunization boosters.
Enteroviruses *Causal agent:* Group A and B Coxsackieviruses, human enteroviruses. *Epidemiology:* Occurs worldwide, most commonly in summer and early fall. More common in settings with poor hygiene and overcrowding. Immunity to specific virus probably occurs after infection, but duration is unknown. *Transmission:* Fecal-oral and respiratory routes. *Incubation period:* 3–6 days. *Period of communicability:* Viral shedding may occur for weeks or months after infection onset.	Each of the viruses causes different manifestations. Herpangina—sudden fever onset, sore throat, and small, discrete grayish papulovesicular ulcerative pharyngeal lesions that gradually increase in size. Hand, foot, and mouth disease—diffuse lesions may occur on the mouth buccal surfaces and tongue; papulovesicular lesions on the hands and feet; last for 7–10 days. Irritability, fever, anorexia, dysphagia, malaise, and a sore throat. *Complications:* Children with immune deficiencies may have more severe manifestations.	*Diagnostic testing:* A polymerase chain reaction or culture of stool, throat, or other primary site may be obtained. *Medical management:* Care is supportive. Immune globulin IV is used in children with severe immunodeficiency disorders (AAP, 2012, p. 317). *Prognosis:* Recovery is generally good with supportive care. *Prevention:* Avoid contact with infected persons early in the disease.	■ Use standard precautions if the child is hospitalized. ■ Use good hand hygiene. ■ Apply topical lotions and give systemic medications as ordered to lessen the pain and relieve the irritation. ■ Offer cool drinks and soft, bland foods (no citrus, salty, or spicy foods). Swallowing may be painful. ■ Offer warm saline mouth rinses. ■ Observe for dehydration. ■ Give nonaspirin antipyretics for fever. ■ Keep the child out of school or child-care while the child is febrile.
Erythema Infectiosum (Fifth Disease) *Causal agent:* Human parvovirus B19. *Epidemiology:* Occurs worldwide, most often in winter and spring. The disease also occurs in epidemics, every 3–7 years (Heymann, 2008). The incidence is highest in children between the ages of 5 and 14 years. *Transmission:* Respiratory secretions and blood. *Incubation period:* 4–21 days. *Period of communicability:* Most infectious before the rash appears.	Stage 1 begins as a mild illness (fever, headache, malaise, and body ache) lasting 2–3 days. A symptom-free period of 1–7 days follows. Stage 2 occurs with a fiery-red rash on the cheeks giving a "slapped face" appearance. Circumoral pallor is seen. A lacelike symmetric, erythematous, maculopapular rash appears on the trunk and spreads to the extremities, sparing the palms and soles. The rash may be mildly pruritic. Stage 3 lasts 1–3 weeks as the rash fades but can reappear if the skin is irritated or exposed to sunlight. *Complications:* Children with hemolytic conditions may have transient aplastic crisis. Polyarthropathy is rare in children.	*Diagnostic testing:* Diagnosis is made by physical signs, or a positive serum immunoglobulin (Ig) M parvovirus B19-specific antibody (important when exposure to a pregnant woman is likely). *Medical management:* Medical care is supportive and recovery is usually spontaneous. Children with hemolytic conditions may need blood transfusions if an aplastic crisis occurs. Immunodeficient patients may develop a chronic infection and may be treated with IV immune globulin therapy (AAP, 2012, p. 541).	■ Use standard and droplet precautions if hospitalized. Isolation is needed only for children with aplastic crisis or when immunosuppressed. ■ Nonaspirin antipyretics may be given to control fever. ■ Use soothing oatmeal or Aveeno baths if the rash is pruritic. Antipruritics may also help to relieve itching. ■ Encourage rest and offer frequent fluids. ■ Keep children out of direct sunlight if possible. Use protective, light, loose clothing if exposure to sunlight cannot be avoided.

(continued)

TABLE 22–5	Selected Infectious and Communicable Diseases in Children *(continued)*		
DISEASE	**CLINICAL MANIFESTATIONS**	**CLINICAL THERAPY**	**NURSING MANAGEMENT**

Erythema Infectiosum (Fifth Disease) (continued)

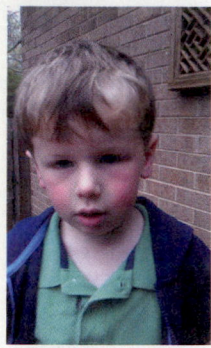

Bright red rash on the cheeks, as if the child's face has been slapped.

Source: *Courtesy of Maura Connor, Nursing EIC/Pearson Education.*

CLINICAL THERAPY

Prognosis: Fetal infection may result in fetal hydrops, anemia, or spontaneous abortion.

Prevention: Avoid contact with infected persons.

NURSING MANAGEMENT

- The immune-competent child can return to school or child care once the rash has appeared (AAP, 2012, p. 541).
- Explain the three stages of rash development to parents.
- Exposed pregnant women should promptly seek medical attention.

Haemophilus Influenzae, Type B⁺

Causal agent: Coccobacilli *H. influenzae* bacteria, which has several serotypes and can be encapsulated or nonencapsulated.

Epidemiology: Occurs most often in the spring and summer. Unimmunized and inadequately immunized infants and young children are most commonly affected. Neonates may acquire the organism by aspirating amniotic fluid or contact with vaginal secretions.

Transmission: Direct contact with respiratory secretions or droplet inhalation. The organism frequently colonizes in the respiratory tract.

Incubation period: Unknown.

Period of communicability: 3 days from onset of symptoms.

CLINICAL MANIFESTATIONS

The illness begins with a viral upper respiratory infection. The organism passes through the mucosal barrier to directly invade the bloodstream. It can cause several severe invasive illnesses, including meningitis, epiglottitis, pneumonia, septic arthritis, and cellulitis. It may cause sepsis in infants. Other illnesses caused by the organism include sinusitis, otitis media, bronchitis, and pericarditis. Each disease has very specific clinical manifestations.

Invasive disease has decreased 99% since introduction of the vaccine (AAP, 2012, p. 346).

Complications: Illness caused by *H. influenzae* type b responds to antibiotic therapy. Left untreated, the disease causes severe sequelae and death, especially in young infants from conditions such as meningitis, epiglottitis, sinusitis, pneumonitis, and cellulitis.

CLINICAL THERAPY

Diagnostic testing: Cultures of the blood, cerebrospinal fluid, or middle ear aspirate may be obtained.

Medical management: Treatment for invasive disease is IV antibiotics for 10 days. Dexamethasone may be given to reduce the neurologic sequelae of meningitis. Infections such as otitis media can be managed with oral antibiotics.

Rifampin may be given to unprotected household contacts if another child 4 years or younger has not completed immunizations.

Prognosis: With rapid diagnosis and treatment, recovery occurs. When treatment is delayed, disability may occur.

Prevention: H. influenzae type b is a vaccine-preventable infection. See the Medications table on page 607 for vaccine information.

NURSING MANAGEMENT

- Use droplet precautions until 24 hours after the initiation of antibiotics.
- Identify potential contacts and review their immunization status. Determine the need for vaccine dose or rifampin. Instruct parents to seek health care rapidly if the exposed child becomes ill.
- Administer antipyretics to help the child feel more comfortable.
- Closely monitor IV sites for patency and infiltration.
- Perform nursing care measures specific to the illness.
- Inform family members that rifampin turns urine and other body fluids orange, and it will cause stains.

Herpes Simplex Virus

Causal agent: Herpes simplex, type 1 (HSV-1).

Epidemiology: Worldwide distribution with an infection rate higher in lower socioeconomic populations (70–80%) than in higher (40–60%) among adults in the United States, with the prevalence increasing with age (Chayavichitsilp, Buckwalter, Krakowski, et al., 2009). The virus remains latent in the trigeminal ganglion.

Transmission: The virus is transmitted through exposure of the mucous membranes or skin to an active lesion or mucosal secretions of an infected individual. It can also be transmitted by respiratory droplets or by exposure to the secretions of an asymptomatic person shedding the virus.

CLINICAL MANIFESTATIONS

Mild cases may be asymptomatic. Prodromal symptoms include burning or paresthesia at the site, lymphadenopathy, fever, malaise, myalgia, loss of appetite, and headaches.

Herpes labialis (fever blisters or cold sores) is manifested as small vesicles on an erythematous base along the outer vermillion border of the lips. The vesicles rupture, leaving painful erosions with or without crusting.

Herpetic gingivostomatitis involves multiple round ulcers or superficial erosions on the palate, tongue, and gingival surface. The child may have diffuse erythema and swelling of the gingivae, drooling, foul smelling breath, and anorexia. Dehydration may result from poor fluid intake.

CLINICAL THERAPY

Diagnostic testing: Cell cultures can be grown in special transport media. Direct fluorescent antibody (DFA) stain and enzyme immunoassay of cells may confirm the diagnosis.

Medical management: Treatment is supportive, including pain management (viscous lidocaine), to encourage fluid intake and rehydration.

Oral acyclovir reduces viral shedding and shortens the healing time. Acyclovir also shortens the duration of lesions during a recurrence.

Prognosis: Treatment does not result in a cure. Disseminated neonatal herpes causes a high rate of disability and mortality. In children this is a self-limiting primary infection with reactivation of the latent virus.

NURSING MANAGEMENT

- Use standard precautions and contact precautions if mucosal lesions are present.
- Teach parents how to reduce the risk of infecting other family members.
- Demonstrate how to apply viscous lidocaine to oral lesions before encouraging the child to drink fluids.
- Encourage the intake of cold soft foods and cool liquids with low acidity to reduce pain, such as gelatin, applesauce, pudding, popsicles, and white grape or apple juice. Help parents set goals for fluid intake so that dehydration is avoided.
- Encourage the child to rinse the mouth frequently to soothe the mucous membranes.

---

*Indicates that a vaccine or antitoxin is available for use in high-risk or as-needed situations.
⁺Indicates that the disease has a safe and effective vaccine.

TABLE 22–5	Selected Infectious and Communicable Diseases in Children *(continued)*		
DISEASE	**CLINICAL MANIFESTATIONS**	**CLINICAL THERAPY**	**NURSING MANAGEMENT**
Herpes Simplex Virus *(continued)* *Incubation period:* 2–12 days. *Period of communicability:* The virus is usually shed for a week or longer.	Herpetic whitlow, an inflamed finger with a single or multiple vesicles, can occur if the infected child sucks a thumb or finger and spreads the infection to a location where the skin is broken. Neonatal herpes is manifested in the first 4 weeks of life with signs that occur in the skin, eye, and mouth; central nervous system; or disseminated to other body organs (liver, adrenal glands, lungs). *Complications:* Immunocompromised children are at increased risk for secondary infection.	*Prevention:* Avoid direct contact with individuals with lesions. No vaccine exists.	■ Monitor the child for dehydration (see Chapter 23 🔗) and contact the health professional if concerned. ■ Children with herpes labialis should not be excluded from school or child-care. Children with gingivostomatitis should be excluded until drooling stops (AAP, 2012, p. 408). ■ Teach children and adolescents with active skin lesions to avoid contact with others during contact sports.
Influenza ✓ *Causal agent:* Orthomyxoviruses, types A, B, and C. Type A can be subtyped based on surface proteins: hemagglutinin (H) and neuraminidase (N). *Epidemiology:* Prevalent in the United States from October to March, but the virus is active in other parts of the world year-round. The influenza A virus genetically alters each season. The number of infections peak in about 3 weeks from the initial case and continue for about 3 months. Incidence of infection is often greater in young children who have fewer prior influenza infections and antibodies. *Transmission:* Spreads by aerosolized particles and direct contact with respiratory secretions or contaminated surfaces. *Incubation period:* 1–4 days, average of 2 days. *Period of communicability:* Greatest in first 3 to 5 days of illness. Virus shedding occurs for up to 7 days in children.	Abrupt onset of fever (38–40°C), chills, dry cough, runny nose, sore throat, malaise, aches, headache, and anorexia. Children may have nausea and vomiting, diarrhea, and abdominal pain. Recovery usually occurs in 3–5 days. *Complications:* Pneumonia, otitis media, asthma exacerbation, tracheitis, myocarditis, myositis, febrile seizures, sinusitis, and neurologic conditions such as encephalitis or encephalopathy. Children with chronic pulmonary, hematologic, metabolic, and cardiovascular conditions are at greater risk of severe infection. The estimate of H1N1 infection among children ages 0 to 17 years in 2009 was about 18 million cases, 78,000 hospitalizations, and 1,180 deaths (Woo, 2010).	*Diagnostic testing:* Rapid antigen testing from throat swabs, nasopharyngeal washings, and sputum are widely available and detect antigens of influenza A and B. Viral cultures may also be performed, along with direct fluorescent antibody or indirect immunofluorescent antibody staining. *Medical management:* Treatment is supportive. Antiviral therapy for children includes (AAP, 2012, pp. 443-444): 1 year and older—oseltamivir (Tamiflu) and amantadine; 7 years and older—zanamivir (Relenza); 13 years and older—rimantadine. Recommendations for antiviral therapy may change each season. Antiviral therapy has a greater benefit if started within 48 hours, reducing the duration of symptoms. *Prognosis:* Most children recover from the infection. *Prevention:* An annual influenza immunization is recommended for children beginning at age 6 months. The vaccine becomes effective within 10 to 14 days of administration. See the Medications table on page 608 for information about the influenza vaccine.	■ Use droplet and contact precautions for hospitalized infants and children. ■ For home care, encourage the parents to frequently wash their hands and to isolate the child from other family members. ■ Provide fluids to keep nasal secretions moist and to prevent dehydration. ■ Provide acetaminophen or ibuprofen for fever management and mild pain. ■ If antiviral medications are given, be alert for nausea and vomiting. Zanamivir can exacerbate asthma. ■ Provide rest and quiet diversional activities. ■ Children should be kept home until 24 hours after fever is gone. ■ Teach parents to be alert to signs of influenza complications. ■ Become familiar with community pandemic infection plans. See the companion website.
Measles (Rubeola)*+ ✓ *Causal agent:* Morbillivirus, a member of the paramyxovirus group. *Epidemiology:* No longer endemic in the United States. Cases primarily occur due to importation of the virus from other countries and transmission to susceptible individuals (CDC, 2012). In 2008, 91% of cases occurred in unimmunized persons or those of unknown status (CDC, 2008a). Passive maternal immunity lasts until the infant is age 6–9 months (Heymann, 2008). Measles is an endemic disease in developing countries. Global measles control is a World Health Organization goal.	The prodrome stage usually consists of nonspecific anorexia and malaise. Stage 2 includes the development of Koplik spots (1–3 mm gray or blue-gray spots on an erythematous base that appear on the oral mucosa, usually opposite the second molars on the buccal mucosa). They slough before or during the onset of the rash. This stage lasts 1–3 days. Stage 3 has the sudden onset of a high spiking fever, conjunctivitis, coryza, cough, and rash, reaching their peak 2–4 days after onset. A characteristic dark red to purple, blotchy, maculopapular rash becomes confluent. The rash begins on the face and spreads to the trunk and extremities. It is mildly pruritic.	*Diagnostic testing:* Diagnosis can be made by a serologic test for immunoglobulin (Ig) M measles antibody. *Medical management:* Treatment is supportive. Vitamin A may be given to malnourished children to reduce mortality. No antiviral therapy is available. Antibiotics are used for secondary bacterial infections. Immune globulin, administered up to 6 days after exposure, may be helpful in preventing or reducing disease severity for infants less than 12 months of age, immunocompromised children, and pregnant women.	■ Maintain airborne precautions when the child is hospitalized. ■ Use a cool-mist vaporizer to help clear respiratory passages. ■ Suction the nose and oral cavity very gently as necessary. ■ Give nonaspirin antipyretics for fever and antipruritics for itching. ■ Antitussives may be ordered to control coughing. ■ Teach parents to observe for complications and to seek care as needed.

(continued)

TABLE 22–5	Selected Infectious and Communicable Diseases in Children *(continued)*		
DISEASE	**CLINICAL MANIFESTATIONS**	**CLINICAL THERAPY**	**NURSING MANAGEMENT**

Measles (Rubeola)* *(continued)*

Transmission: Direct contact with respiratory droplets and airborne spread.

Incubation period: About 7–14 days.

Period of communicability: Begins 2–4 days before the rash and continues until the fever is gone.

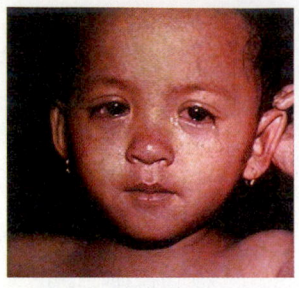

Confluent maculopapular rash with measles.

Source: *Courtesy of Centers for Disease Control and Prevention/Barbara Rice. http://phil.cdc.gov/phil/details.asp?pid5989*

CLINICAL MANIFESTATIONS:

Other symptoms include fatigue, photophobia, and generalized lymphadenopathy.

Complications: Diarrhea, otitis media, pneumonia, bronchitis, laryngotracheobronchitis, encephalitis, and death. Complications and death more commonly occur in children who are severely malnourished or immunocompromised. The younger the child, the greater the risk for complications.

CLINICAL THERAPY:

Prognosis: Increased risk of death in children under age 5 years and immunocom promised persons (AAP, 2012, p. 489).

Prevention: Measles is a vaccine-preventable disease. See the Medications table on page 609 for vaccine information. Prevent exposure to susceptible persons. This is a reportable disease.

NURSING MANAGEMENT:

- Maintain bed rest and provide diversional activities. Elevate the head of the bed. Keep the room cool with good air circulation. Use light, nonirritating blankets.
- Keep skin clean and dry. Avoid the use of soaps.
- Offer small amounts of cool liquids frequently. Blended, pureed, and mashed foods are most easily tolerated.

Meningococcus⁺

Causal agent: Neisseria meningitidis, a gram-negative diplococcus.

Epidemiology: Occurs most often in the winter or early spring. Serogroups B, C, Y, or W-135 cause most infections in the United States. Highest rates occur in children under 2 years of age and among adolescents 15–18 years. Persons living in poverty or crowded conditions are at higher risk. Outbreaks have occurred in childcare centers, college dormitories, and military recruit camps.

Transmission: Spread by inhalation or respiratory droplets from human carriers.

Incubation period: 2–10 days.

Period of communicability: Until 24 hours of treatment with an antibiotic to which the organism is sensitive.

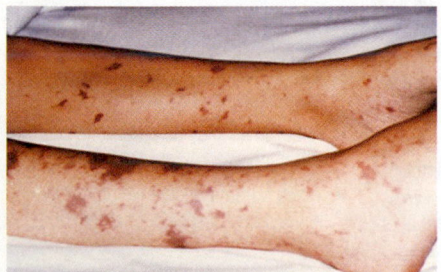

Purpura with meningococcemia.

Source: *Courtesy of Meningitis Trust.*

CLINICAL MANIFESTATIONS:

Children may develop meningitis or meningococcemia, or the two conditions may occur together.

Begins with an abrupt onset of fever, chills, malaise, muscle aches, vomiting, and **prostration** (extreme exhaustion).

Meningitis neurologic signs include decreased mental status, seizures, or coma.

In meningococcemia, a maculopapular rash becomes petechial and may progress to purpura and sepsis. The condition may further deteriorate to septic shock with leg pain, cold extremities, and pallor (Mola, Nield, & Weisse, 2009).

Complications: The condition can progress to septic shock, disseminated intravascular coagulation, and loss of digits or limbs due to gangrenous necrosis. Other complications include hearing loss, neurologic disabilities (increased intracranial pressure, cranial nerve palsies, obstructive hydrocephalus), and scarring.

CLINICAL THERAPY:

Diagnostic testing: Cultures of the blood and cerebrospinal fluid are obtained. A Gram stain of petechial skin scrapings may also be performed.

Medical management: IV antibiotics include penicillin G (or alternatively cefotaxime, ceftriaxone, and ampicillin). Chloramphenicol is used for children allergic to penicillin.

The child is managed aggressively in the intensive care unit to maintain the airway, assist ventilation, and manage shock with IV fluids and vasopressors. Plasma, blood, or platelets are used to treat the disseminated intravascular coagulation.

Prognosis: About 10% of all patients with invasive disease die (AAP, 2012, p. 500).

Prevention: See the Medications table on page 609 for vaccine information. Close contacts are given rifampin, ceftriaxone, ciprofloxacin, or azithromycin.

The vaccine may also be used to prevent secondary cases if the primary case is caused by a serotype covered in the vaccine (AAP, 2012, p. 505). This is a reportable disease.

NURSING MANAGEMENT:

- Use standard and droplet precautions until the effective antibiotic has been administered for 24 hours.
- Be alert for the development of shock and respiratory compromise as the disease progresses rapidly. Have emergency equipment available.
- Avoid overloading the child with fluids when giving IV fluids and blood products. Monitor for signs of increased intracranial pressure.
- Help the family mobilize its support system, and keep the family informed of the child's status and treatment as the disease progresses.
- Help identify close contacts that should receive prophylactic antibiotics. Educate them about the expected side effects (i.e., orange urine and tears with rifampin).
- Teach close contacts to be observant for signs of illness and to seek health care promptly if they occur.
- Help coordinate rehabilitation for the child.

*Indicates that a vaccine or antitoxin is available for use in high-risk or as-needed situations.

⁺Indicates that the disease has a safe and effective vaccine.

TABLE 22–5 | **Selected Infectious and Communicable Diseases in Children** *(continued)*

DISEASE	CLINICAL MANIFESTATIONS	CLINICAL THERAPY	NURSING MANAGEMENT
Mononucleosis ✓ *Causal agent:* Epstein-Barr virus (EBV), human herpesvirus type 4. *Epidemiology:* The virus infects the oral mucosa and salivary glands. EBV infection occurs worldwide in no seasonal pattern. Infection commonly occurs early in life, and spread among family members is common. Infection during adolescence and young adulthood is common in the United States (King, 2009). *Transmission:* Direct contact with saliva or through blood transfusion. EBV can survive in saliva for several hours outside the body. *Incubation period:* Estimated to be 4–6 weeks. *Period of communicability:* The virus may be shed from the oral mucosa and saliva for 6–18 months (King, 2009).	In very young children mononucleosis may be mild and have no distinguishing clinical signs. In other children, the disease is characterized by fever, malaise, headache, anorexia, abdominal pain, a painful sore throat (exudative pharyngotonsillitis), and cervical lymphadenopathy. Hepatosplenomegaly and elevated liver function tests may occur. The syndrome typically lasts 2–3 weeks, but fatigue may continue in some children for weeks longer. *Complications:* Rare side effects include central nervous system symptoms such as encephalitis, aseptic meningitis, cranial nerve palsies, and Guillain-Barré syndrome. Hematologic complications such as splenic rupture, thrombocytopenia, or hemolytic anemia can also occur. Lymphomas and death can occur. EBV causes complex syndromes in immunocompromised children, such as those with transplants.	*Diagnostic testing:* The serologic Monospot test or a heterophil antibody response test is used to confirm the diagnosis. However, signs may be present for up to 4 weeks before the Monospot test is positive (King, 2009). A complete blood count with leukocytosis with greater than 10% atypical lymphocytes may be seen. *Medical management:* Treatment is supportive. Corticosteroids may be used to control tonsillar swelling and pain from an impending airway obstruction, hemolytic anemia, and severe thrombocytopenia. Ampicillin and amoxicillin should be avoided as a nonallergic rash often develops (AAP, 2012, p. 321). *Prognosis:* Rarely fatal. After recovery, the virus remains latent in the lymphoid system and can be reactivated during periods of immunosuppression. *Prevention:* No known prevention.	■ Use standard precautions if the child is hospitalized. ■ Give antipyretics and analgesics for fever and sore throat. Offer warm salt water for gargling. Offer soft foods and encourage fluids. ■ Maintain bed rest during the acute phase. ■ Reassure adolescents who may be worried about keeping up with schoolwork that they can return to school when the fever is gone and swallowing is normal. Fatigue may persist for a few weeks. ■ Educate the teen to avoid intimate contact and not to share food and beverages until recovered. ■ Contact sports and strenuous activity (e.g., weight lifting) should be avoided until the liver and spleen are normal-sized, usually in about 4 weeks. ■ If splenomegaly is present, alcohol should be avoided for 3 months after liver function test results return to normal.
Mumps (Parotitis)+ ✓ *Causal agent:* Rubulavirus in the Paramyxoviridae family. *Epidemiology:* Occurs worldwide in unvaccinated children, most often in winter and spring. Infection and vaccination induce lifelong immunity. Maternal antibodies begin to disappear in infants at the age of 12–15 months. *Transmission:* Contact with respiratory tract secretions. *Incubation period:* 12–25 days. *Period of communicability:* 1–2 days before parotid swelling until 9 days after swelling subsides.	Acute onset of malaise, fever, and swelling of one or more salivary glands (parotid, sublingual, or submaxillary) are the classic signs. Other signs include earache, headache, pain with chewing, and decreased appetite and activity. Mumps may also be asymptomatic in some children. *Complications:* Aseptic meningitis, sensorineural hearing loss, and orchitis (inflammation of the epididymis, pain on testicular palpation, and scrotal swelling—most often unilateral) may occur in 20–30% of postpubertal males, but sterility is relatively rare (Heymann, 2008).	*Diagnostic testing:* A viral culture may be taken from the throat, urine, or cerebrospinal fluid. A serologic test for mumps-specific IgM antibodies may be performed. *Medical management:* Therapy is supportive, focused on symptom relief. *Prognosis:* Mumps is usually self-limiting. *Prevention:* Mumps is a vaccine-preventable disease. See the Medications table on page 609 for vaccine information. This is a reportable disease. A 2009 outbreak in a summer camp in New York occurred after the index case became infected in the United Kingdom, resulting in 1,521 cases as of January 2010 (CDC, 2010b).	■ Use standard and droplet precautions for hospitalized children while contagious. ■ Children cared for at home are generally uncomfortable but are rarely very ill. ■ Avoid exposure to immunocompromised or susceptible individuals. ■ Give nonaspirin analgesics and antipyretics to control fever and pain. ■ Encourage fluid intake. Offer soft foods as swallowing and chewing may be painful. Avoid foods and beverages that increase salivary flow and cause pain (e.g., citrus, spices, and candies). ■ Talking may be painful. Provide a bell or other attention-getting device. ■ Educate parents about when to seek health care for signs of complications. ■ Keep children out of school or child-care until 5 days after onset of parotid swelling (CDC, 2008b).

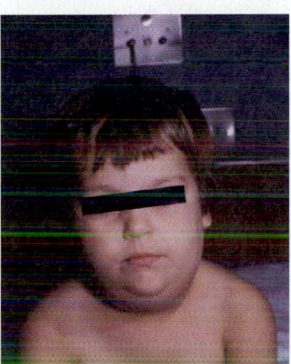

Parotid gland swelling with mumps.

Source: *Courtesy of Centers for Disease Control and Prevention.*

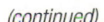

(continued)

TABLE 22–5	Selected Infectious and Communicable Diseases in Children *(continued)*		
DISEASE	**CLINICAL MANIFESTATIONS**	**CLINICAL THERAPY**	**NURSING MANAGEMENT**
Pertussis (Whooping Cough)[+] *Causal agent:* Bordetella pertussis, a gram-negative coccobacillus. *Epidemiology:* Occurs worldwide. Since the 1980s, the number of reported cases has steadily increased in infants and adolescents. More than 13,000 cases of pertussis were reported in 2008 (Spratling & Carmon, 2010). Pertussis may occur in adolescents and adults who have waning immunity, and they then can spread the disease to unimmunized infants. *Transmission:* Inhalation or direct contact with respiratory droplets. *Incubation period:* 7–10 days. *Period of communicability:* Begins about 1 week after exposure. The disease is most contagious before the paroxysmal cough stage. Communicable for 5 days after antibiotic therapy is initiated.	The onset is insidious. *Catarrhal stage:* The disease begins with nasal congestion, a runny nose, low-grade fever, and a mild nonproductive cough, lasting 1–2 weeks. *Paroxysmal stage:* The cough is more severe at night with coughing spasms. A forceful inspiration through a narrowed glottis causes stridor or "whooping." Infants less than 6 months of age may have gagging, gasping, or apnea rather than whooping. Sucking on a bottle may trigger the coughing spell. Coughing may be accompanied by flushing; cyanosis; vomiting; and profuse drainage from the nose, eyes, and mouth. Paroxysmal coughing may last 1–6 weeks or more. Dehydration may result from decreased oral intake. Adolescents often have upper respiratory symptoms with persistent coughing spasms lasting 3–9 weeks (Edwards & Johnson, 2007). *Convalescent stage:* The cough gradually improves over 2–3 weeks. *Complications:* Pneumonia, atelectasis, encephalopathy, seizures, and death.	*Diagnostic testing:* A culture from the nasopharynx, polymerase chain reaction (PCR), direct fluorescent antibody (DFA), and serology are used for diagnosis. *Medical management:* Macrolide antibiotics (erythromycin, azithromycin, and trimethoprim-sulfamethoxazole) are recommended by the CDC. Symptoms are reduced if initiated in the catarrhal state. If started later they may only reduce communicability (Spratling & Carmon, 2010). *Prognosis:* The disease is most severe in infants under 6 months of age, and most deaths occur in this age group. *Prevention:* Pertussis is a vaccine-preventable disease. An acellular vaccine is approved for adolescents and adults. See the Medications table on page 607 for vaccine information. Immunity wanes 5–10 years after vaccination and 7–20 years after natural infection. This is a reportable disease. Close contacts should be treated with macrolide antibiotics for prophylaxis	■ When hospitalized, use droplet precautions until 5 days after starting antibiotics. ■ Continually assess respirations and oxygen saturation with a cardiac monitor and pulse oximetry. The smaller the child, the greater the risk for respiratory distress and apnea. ■ Meet infant needs promptly to reduce crying which can precipitate coughing. Remain with the child during coughing spells, when hypoxic and apneic episodes are most likely. Give oxygen if ordered. Have emergency equipment available. ■ Provide humidification. Gentle suctioning may be necessary. ■ Give nonaspirin antipyretics as needed for fever. ■ Encourage frequent rest periods. ■ Provide small frequent feedings of desired foods. ■ Encourage the child to take fluids. The child may need IV hydration if oral intake is not tolerated. ■ Provide emotional support to parents. ■ Teach parents to watch for signs of respiratory failure and dehydration if the child is managed at home.
Pneumococcal infection[+] *Causative agent:* Streptococcus pneumoniae, a gram-positive diplococcus, many serotypes. *Epidemiology:* The organism is found in the nasopharynx of healthy people. Outbreaks occur in the winter and spring. In temperate climates, 8 of 90 serotypes account for most of the invasive pediatric diseases. Children less than age 2 years have the highest rates of invasive pneumococcal disease (Bolton & Barson, 2010). Exposure to a respiratory viral infection or secondhand smoke exposure may predispose the respiratory epithelium to invasion (Bolton & Barson, 2010). *Transmission:* Person-to-person spread of respiratory droplets. *Incubation period:* Unknown, may be 1–3 days. *Period of communicability:* Unknown. Probably less than 24 hours after beginning effective antibiotic therapy.	The signs and symptoms are related to the focal area of infection. The organism causes otitis media, sinusitis, pharyngitis, laryngotracheobronchitis, pneumonia, meningitis, and bacteremia. See Chapter 24 🕮 for signs of otitis media, sinusitis, and pharyngitis. See Chapter 25 🕮 for signs of laryngotracheobronchitis and pneumonia. See Chapter 33 🕮 for signs of meningitis. In bacteremia, high fever without an obvious source and an elevated white blood cell count occur. Individuals with immunodeficiency (e.g., asplenia, malignancy, sickle cell disease, HIV infection, and nephrotic syndrome) and children with cochlear implants are at higher risk of invasive disease. *Complications:* Meningitis, mastoiditis, bacteremia, pneumonia, empyema, septic arthritis, osteomyelitis, infective endocarditis, and brain abscess.	*Diagnostic testing:* Bacterial cultures are performed from site of infection. *Medical management:* Symptomatic care specific to the focus of infection is provided. Antibiotic selection is based upon culture sensitivity. Many pneumococcal strains are resistant to penicillin, cefotaxime, and ceftriaxone. Vancomycin may be required. Dexamethasone may be an adjunctive therapy for meningitis. *Prognosis:* Pneumococcal meningitis is associated with neurologic sequelae (e.g., hearing loss, motor deficits). Pneumonia is the leading cause of death worldwide. *Prevention:* Many serotypes are preventable with immunization. See the Medications table on page 609 for vaccine information. It is hoped that the new vaccine PCV13 will result in a significant reduction in invasive disease, just as the prior vaccine PCV7 did.	■ If the child is hospitalized, maintain standard precautions. ■ Provide nonaspirin antipyretics for control of fever and comfort. ■ Encourage fluids, and monitor intake and output. ■ Monitor vital signs and level of consciousness to identify signs of worsening condition. ■ Educate parents about the need for the vaccine, as the unimmunized child could become infected repeatedly with different serotypes. ■ Many children with mild disease will be treated at home. Educate parents about signs indicating a need to seek urgent medical attention, appropriate medication administration, and comfort measures for the child.

*Indicates that a vaccine or antitoxin is available for use in high-risk or as-needed situations.
[+]Indicates that the disease has a safe and effective vaccine.

TABLE 22–5	Selected Infectious and Communicable Diseases in Children *(continued)*		
DISEASE	**CLINICAL MANIFESTATIONS**	**CLINICAL THERAPY**	**NURSING MANAGEMENT**
Poliomyelitis[+] ✓ *Causal agent:* Poliovirus is an enterovirus with three serotypes. *Epidemiology:* Global eradication efforts have eliminated polio in all but four countries (Afghanistan, India, Nigeria, and Pakistan), and nearly all cases occur in children less than 5 years of age (Heymann, 2008). Imported polio is a threat to inadequately immunized children. *Transmission:* Primarily by the fecal-oral route, but also the respiratory route. *Incubation period:* Usually 7–10 days. *Period of communicability:* Highest before and right after clinical symptoms develop. The virus is excreted in the feces for 3–6 weeks.	More than 90% of infections are asymptomatic. The child may have a nonspecific minor illness with a low-grade fever and sore throat. This minor illness may be followed by aseptic meningitis and paresthesias. Asymmetric flaccid paralysis may occur acutely in up to 2% of cases. The site of paralysis depends on the location of injury to the brainstem or spinal cord. Residual paralysis may occur in more than half of those affected (AAP, 2012, p. 588). *Complications:* Permanent motor paralysis, respiratory arrest, myocardial failure, aseptic meningitis, and postpolio syndrome.	*Diagnostic testing:* Cell cultures from stool or throat swabs are performed. *Medical management:* Treatment is supportive. No chemotherapeutic agents are available that directly kill the poliovirus. *Prognosis:* If paralysis of the respiratory or swallowing muscles occurs, it is life threatening. Motor paralysis may result in long-term disability. *Prevention:* Poliomyelitis is a vaccine-preventable disease. See the Medications table on page 610 for vaccine information. The vaccine confers lifelong immunity. This is a reportable disease.	■ Use standard and contact precautions for hospitalized children. ■ Observe the child closely for respiratory paralysis (ineffective cough, talking with frequent pauses, shallow and rapid respiratory rate). Keep emergency equipment at bedside. Assist ventilations as needed until mechanical ventilation is set up. ■ Use moist hot packs, which may relieve discomfort. ■ Encourage fluids. ■ Keep the child on bed rest, and position the child to promote body alignment. ■ Perform range-of-motion exercises to prevent contractures after the acute phase. Help coordinate rehabilitation. ■ Provide emotional support to the child and family. Keep the child and family informed about the illness and what is happening to the child.
Roseola (Exanthem Subitum, Sixth Disease) ✓ *Causal agent:* Human herpesvirus type 6 (HHV-6) or type 7 (HHV-7). *Epidemiology:* Occurs worldwide, primarily in children 6–24 months of age (after maternal antibodies decline). No seasonal pattern. *Transmission:* Contact with saliva or respiratory secretions. *Incubation period:* 9–10 days. *Period of communicability:* Healthy persons shed the virus (AAP, 2012, p. 415).	Sudden, high fever up to 39.5°C (103°F) for 3–7 days, during which the child does not appear toxic (normal appetite and behavior) and has no rash or disease-specific signs. An erythematous maculopapular rash appears after the fever resolves, and lasts hours to days. The child's appetite is normal. *Complications:* Febrile seizures are common. Encephalopathy or encephalitis may occur.	*Diagnostic testing:* Polymerase chain reaction (PCR) testing for HHV-6 in the blood or cerebrospinal fluid may be performed. *Medical management:* Roseola is self-limiting, and treatment is supportive. *Prognosis:* Roseola is benign in most cases. Nearly all children over 3 years of age have a positive antibody titer to HHV-6 (AAP, 2012, p. 415).	■ Children are rarely hospitalized, but use standard precautions if they are. ■ Give nonaspirin antipyretics to control fever. ■ Observe the child closely for any seizure activity, especially during the acute febrile periods. ■ Encourage fluids to maintain hydration. ■ Reassure parents that the rash will disappear in a few days.
Rotavirus[+] ✓ *Causal agent:* RNA viruses of the Reoviridae family. Groups A, B, and C infect humans. *Epidemiology:* Occurs more often in cool periods of the year. Most common cause of severe diarrhea in children less than age 5 years. *Transmission:* Fecal-oral route, and possibly the respiratory route. *Incubation:* 1–3 days. *Period of communicability:* Virus is found in stool for up to 30 days in immunocompromised children (Heymann, 2008).	Acute onset of fever and vomiting followed by watery diarrhea 1–2 days later. Up to 10–20 diarrheal stools a day. Symptoms last 3–8 days. *Complications:* Dehydration and electrolyte disturbances. Immunocompromised children may develop persistent infection and diarrhea (AAP, 2012, p. 626). Death occurs in rare circumstances.	*Diagnostic testing:* Enzyme immunoassay or latex agglutination assay is used to detect group A rotavirus antigen in a stool specimen. *Medical management:* Treatment involves adequate fluid and electrolyte replacement with oral rehydration solution. Antimotility drugs should not be used as they slow bowel transit and increase exposure to infectious toxins (Heymann, 2008). If severely dehydrated, IV fluid resuscitation is performed. No antiviral therapy is available. *Prevention:* The disease is vaccine preventable. See the Medications table on page 610 for vaccine information. Naturally acquired infection protects against reinfection that causes severe diseases.	■ Use standard and contact precautions if the child is hospitalized. ■ Encourage parents to use good hand hygiene with soap and water or gel hand sanitizers. ■ Clean and disinfect contaminated surfaces. ■ Assess hydration status frequently. ■ Breastfeeding is continued during oral rehydration therapy, but wait up to 24 hours before giving formula. ■ Older children can be fed complex carbohydrates and lean meats, yogurt, fruits, and vegetables after 24 hours of oral rehydration therapy.

(continued)

TABLE 22–5	Selected Infectious and Communicable Diseases in Children *(continued)*		
DISEASE	**CLINICAL MANIFESTATIONS**	**CLINICAL THERAPY**	**NURSING MANAGEMENT**
Rubella (German Measles)[+] *Causal agent:* An RNA virus, member of the family Togaviridae, genus *Rubivirus.* *Epidemiology:* Occurs worldwide and is most prevalent in the winter and spring. No longer endemic in the United States (AAP, 2012, p. 630). Most U.S. cases occur among foreign-born children and adults from countries that have poor rubella vaccination coverage. Congenital rubella syndrome is thought to occur due to lack of immunization. *Transmission:* Droplet spread, direct contact with infected persons, or contact with articles soiled by nasal secretions. *Incubation period:* 14–21 days (most commonly 16–18 days). *Period of communicability:* Several days before the rash onset up until 2 weeks after rash onset. Infants with congenital rubella may continue to shed the virus for up to a year after birth.	May be asymptomatic. Rubella is generally a mild disease. Prodromal symptoms include a low-grade fever along with lymphadenopathy (postauricular, cervical, and suboccipital). Forschheimer spots (discrete, erythematous pinpoint or larger lesions on the soft palate) are seen during the prodromal phase. Then the characteristic pink, nonconfluent, maculopapular rash first appears on the face and neck 1–5 days later, and then progresses to the rest of the body within 24 hours. The rash generally fades in the same sequence or all at once. *Complications:* Polyarthritis and polyarthralgia may occur in postpubertal females. Pregnant females infected during the first trimester may have a fetus that develops congenital rubella syndrome. Neonatal signs of congenital rubella syndrome include growth retardation, radiolucent bone disease, hepatosplenomegaly, thrombocytopenia, and purpuric skin lesions (giving a "blueberry muffin" appearance).	*Diagnostic testing:* Enzyme immunoassays, a latex agglutination test, a cell culture from a nasal swab, and detection of rubella-specific IgM or IgG antibodies may be performed. *Medical management:* Treatment is supportive. Rubella is generally self-limiting in children. *Prognosis:* Disease is usually mild and benign. The major risk is to the fetus of a mother infected in the first trimester. Congenital rubella syndrome may result in fetal death or congenital anomalies (ophthalmologic, cardiac, auditory, and neurologic). *Prevention:* Rubella is a vaccine-preventable disease. See the Medications table on page 609 for vaccine information. Females of childbearing age need to be immunized to reduce the risk for congenital rubella syndrome. 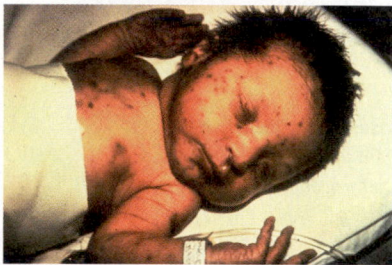 "Blueberry muffin" appearance in infant with congenital rubella syndrome. **Source:** *Courtesy of Centers for Disease Control and Prevention.*	■ Maintain standard and droplet precautions for contagious children. ■ Maintain contact precautions for infants with congenital rubella syndrome until 1 year of age unless nasopharyngeal and urine cultures are repeatedly negative after 3 months of age (AAP, 2012, p. 631). ■ Children are usually treated at home and should be isolated from pregnant women. ■ Give nonaspirin analgesics and antipyretics for any pain and fever. ■ Encourage the child to drink preferred fluids and food. ■ Provide quiet activities. ■ Exclude children from childcare or school for 7 days after onset of rash. School and childcare facilities should be notified of the child's illness.
Streptococcus A *Causal agent:* Group A streptococci (GAS) numerous serotypes. *Epidemiology:* Pharyngeal infections tend to occur more in late fall, winter, and spring when closer person-to-person contact occurs. Pyodermal infections tend to occur in warmer seasons because of the association with minor skin trauma and insect bites. Different strains are associated with pharyngeal and pyodermal infections, and with rheumatic fever and acute glomerulonephritis (AAP, 2012, p. 669). *Transmission:* Contact with respiratory secretions for pharyngitis or direct contact with skin lesions. *Incubation period:* Pharyngeal: usually 2–5 days; pyodermal: usually 7–10 days. *Period of communicability:* Highest during acute infection. Noncontagious within 24 hours of starting antibiotics.	*Pharyngeal:* Abrupt onset with a sore throat, dysphagia, tender cervical nodes, malaise, high fever, headache, abdominal pain, anorexia, and vomiting. The pharynx is beefy red with exudates, and palatal petechiae may be seen. Absence of cough or rhinitis in most cases. *GAS respiratory tract infection:* Children under 3 years may develop serous rhinitis, moderate fever, irritability, and anorexia rather than pharyngitis. *Scarlet fever:* A characteristic erythematous, confluent, pinpoint, sandpaper rash most often occurs with pharyngitis. The rash blanches with pressure, concentrates in flexor skin creases, and spares the circumoral area. In 3–4 days, the rash begins to fade and the tips of the toes and fingers begin to peel. The classic strawberry tongue is seen on day 4–5. *Pyodermal:* Lesions (impetigo) are honey-colored crusts at the site of open lesions. *Complications:* If untreated, acute otitis media, sinusitis, peritonsillar or retropharyngeal abscess, cervical lymphadenitis, acute rheumatic fever, and acute glomerulonephritis. Invasive disease with toxic shock syndrome, bacteremia, and necrotizing fasciitis or myositis can be fatal.	*Diagnostic testing:* A rapid strep antigen test or culture of secretions from the pharynx and tonsils is performed. Cultures of skin lesions are not indicated (AAP, 2012, p. 673). *Medical management:* Prompt antibiotic treatment. Oral penicillin V is the drug of choice for pharyngitis. Oral cephalosporin or a macrolide or azalide antibiotic is used if the child is allergic to penicillin. Uncomplicated nonbullous impetigo is treated with mupirocin or retapamulin ointment. Invasive strains causing necrotizing fasciitis or myositis need IV antibiotics and surgical intervention (exploration and debridement of dead tissue). *Prognosis:* Recovery is usually good with antibiotic therapy. Some healthy children become chronic carriers of streptococcus A in the pharynx. *Prevention:* None. 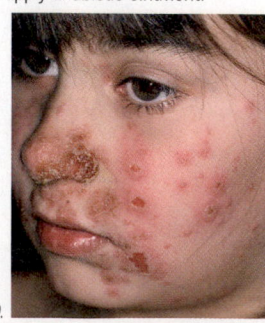 Impetigo. **Source:** *Courtesy of Jason L. Smith, M.D.*	■ Use standard and droplet precautions for pharyngeal infections and contact precautions for skin infections if the child is hospitalized. ■ Promote bed rest during the febrile stage. ■ Give nonaspirin antipyretics to control fever. Teach parents important signs of a worsening condition. ■ For pharyngeal infections, offer warm salt water for gargling. Encourage cool, clear, nonacidic fluids and a soft diet. Swallowing may be difficult. ■ Emphasize to parents the importance of giving the child the full course of antibiotics. ■ Encourage family members with sore throats to have throat cultures taken. ■ For impetigo, teach the parents to wash the skin, remove crusts, and apply antibiotic ointment.

*Indicates that a vaccine or antitoxin is available for use in high-risk or as-needed situations.
[+]Indicates that the disease has a safe and effective vaccine.

TABLE 22–5 | Selected Infectious and Communicable Diseases in Children *(continued)*

DISEASE	CLINICAL MANIFESTATIONS	CLINICAL THERAPY	NURSING MANAGEMENT
Streptococcus B ✓ *Causal agent:* Group B streptococci (GBS), a gram-positive, aerobic diplococcus. *Epidemiology:* The gastrointestinal tract is the reservoir for GBS and the source of vaginal colonization, but it may also be colonized in the pharynx. Rates of colonization during pregnancy are between 15% and 35% (AAP, 2012, p. 681). Risk of neonatal infection is increased for preterm infants (less than 37 weeks of gestation), in cases of prolonged rupture of membranes, and in mothers with intrapartum fever, chorioamnionitis, or GBS bacteriuria during the pregnancy. The incidence of early-onset GBS infection in term neonates is 0.3 per 1,000 live births (Koenig & Keenan, 2009). *Transmission:* Not sexually transmitted. Intrauterine infection of fetus can occur. Neonatal infection may occur before or during birth. *Incubation period:* For early onset neonatal disease, fewer than 7 days; for late onset neonatal disease, unknown. *Period of communicability:* Unknown.	The mother is usually asymptomatic. *Early-onset neonatal disease:* The newborn becomes acutely ill, often within 24 hours of birth with a range of 0–6 days. The infant often has signs of systemic infection that include respiratory distress, apnea, shock, pneumonia, and sometime meningitis. *Late-onset neonatal disease:* Newborn between 3 and 4 weeks of age (range 7–89 days) may develop signs of bacteremia, meningitis, or signs of other focal infection such as osteomyelitis, septic arthritis, pneumonia, adenitis, or cellulitis (AAP, 2012 p. 680). *Complications:* Death, developmental delay, blindness, deafness, and other neurologic impairments (Koenig & Keenan, 2009).	*Diagnostic tests:* Complete blood count, chest radiograph, cultures of body fluids, including blood, urine, cerebrospinal fluid, and breaks in the skin or open lesions. *Medical management:* Ampicillin plus an aminoglycoside are used in newborns when GBS infection is suspected and before culture results are known. Penicillin G may be used if the organism is sensitive. Duration of treatment is dependent upon focus of infection. *Prognosis:* GBS early-onset disease remains a significant cause of death in the preterm population (19.9%), with the highest mortality observed in very-low-birth-weight neonates (35%) (Koenig & Keenan, 2009). *Prevention:* Current guidelines recommend screening all pregnant women to identify GBS carriers who should then receive IV intrapartum antibiotics followed by careful monitoring of the newborns for signs of infection. No strategies prevent late-onset GBS in neonates.	■ Use standard precautions for infected newborns. Wash hands after each contact with the infant. Adhere to all infection control guidelines to reduce the risk of transmitting the infection to other newborns. ■ Ensure that the appropriate IV antibiotic dosage is administered at the correct rate and on time to maintain optimal blood levels. ■ Monitor the newborn for side effects and toxicity associated with the antibiotic. ■ Maintain a neutral thermoregulatory environment. ■ Monitor vital signs, and observe for signs indicating progression or resolution of the infection. Monitor for development of complications. ■ Provide adequate fluid and caloric intake. Monitor weight, urine output, and urine specific gravity. ■ Provide honest information and support the parents. Permit parents to touch the baby and participate in care as much as the newborn's condition permits.
Tetanus*+ ✓ *Causal agent: Clostridium tetani,* an anaerobic gram-positive bacillus. *Epidemiology:* The bacillus is common and exists as a spore in soil, dust, and animal excretions. The organism produces an endotoxin that affects the central nervous system. *Transmission:* The organism is transmitted to humans through puncture wounds or broken skin. Newborns in developing countries can acquire tetanus when the mother is unimmunized and an unsterile tool is used to cut the umbilical cord, or if the ritual dressing placed on the cord is unknowingly contaminated with tetanus spores (Heymann, 2008). *Incubation period:* 3 days–3 weeks (average 10 days). *Period of communicability:* Not direct person-to-person contact.	Acute onset of stiffness of the neck and jaw, with painful facial and neck muscle spasms, difficulty chewing and swallowing over a few days, and headache. Noise or sudden movement may stimulate spasms. Spasms of facial muscles may produce a grinning expression (risus sardonicus). Localized prolonged and painful muscle contraction may occur at the site of the wound. Eventual rigidity of the abdomen and trunk produces **opisthotonos** (rigid hyperextension of the entire body). Respiratory muscles can be affected and cause airway obstruction and suffocation. Newborns have difficulty with sucking, progressing to an inability to suck, irritability, and nuchal rigidity. *Complications:* Laryngospasm, respiratory distress, death.	*Diagnostic testing:* The disease is diagnosed clinically rather than by laboratory tests. *Medical management:* Tetanus immune globulin is given intramuscularly to unimmunized persons as soon as possible. Tetanus toxoid is given at the same time in a separate site. The wound is cleaned and debrided. Intensive care is provided with cardiorespiratory monitoring, assisted ventilation, nutrition, and supportive care. Medications used to treat tetanus include IV metronidazole and penicillin G. Complete recovery may take weeks. *Prognosis:* Neonatal mortality is high, especially when intensive care is unavailable. *Prevention:* Tetanus is a vaccine-preventable disease. See the Medications table on page 607 for vaccine information. After the primary series, tetanus boosters should be updated every 10 years, or in 5 years if experiencing a potentially contaminated wound. Proper surgical debridement of wounds decreases the chance of infection.	■ Use standard precautions when the child is hospitalized. ■ Assist with wound debridement. ■ Monitor the child's condition. Handle as little as possible. Reduce stimulation by placing the child in a quiet, darkened room. ■ Offer skin and respiratory care. The child may need an endotracheal tube, suctioning, and supplemental oxygen for airway support. ■ Provide feedings via total parenteral nutrition or feeding tube. ■ Maintain hydration with IV fluids and electrolytes. ■ Try to reduce the child's anxiety, as mental status may be unaffected. ■ Prepare the family for a possible poor prognosis.

TABLE 22–6	Selected Communicable Diseases Transmitted by Insect or Animal Hosts (Zoonosis)		
DISEASE	**CLINICAL MANIFESTATIONS**	**CLINICAL THERAPY**	**NURSING MANAGEMENT**
Lyme Disease* *Causal agent:* Borrelia burgdorferi, a spirochete. *Epidemiology:* Occurs in 47 states and the District of Columbia. Most cases occur in the Northeastern, Mid-Atlantic, and North Central states. Exposure occurs in any outdoor setting where ticks are endemic. Lyme disease occurs year-round, with the highest incidence between April and October and in U.S. children between 5 and 9 years of age (AAP, 2012, p. 475). *Transmission:* The tick transmits the infected spirochete after feeding for 36 hours. Lyme disease is the most common vector-borne illness in North America. *Incubation period:* 1–55 days after an infected tick bite. A rash in 48 hours is an allergic reaction or infection, not Lyme disease. *Period of communicability:* The infection is not contagious from person to person.	*Early localized disease (ELD):* Erythema migrans, a painless expanding single annular red rash, starts as a red macule or papule and expands over days or weeks to 5–15 cm in diameter. It sometimes has a partial central clearing (bull's eye). The rash may look like a bruise in patients with dark skin. It occurs in about 50% of cases and may appear at the site of the tick bite or elsewhere on the body (Savely, 2010). The patient may have fever, body aches, headache, and malaise. *Early disseminated disease (EDD):* In 3–10 weeks after the tick bite, multiple smaller erythema migrans lesions may be seen. The following signs may develop: fever, headache, neck pain, malaise, conjunctivitis, enlarged lymph nodes, and cranial nerve palsies. Carditis and meningitis may occur. *Late disseminated disease (LDD):* In 2–12 months, Lyme arthritis develops, commonly in the knee with pain, swelling, and effusion. The child may develop encephalitis, polyneuritis, and memory problems. *Complications:* Left untreated, Lyme disease progresses to late disseminated disease with carditis, encephalitis, or meningitis (Kest & Pineda, 2008).	*Diagnostic testing:* Diagnosis of ELD is by presence of erythema migrans. An enzyme-linked immunosorbent assay (ELISA) plus the Western blot test may be used in EDD or LDD. *Medical management:* Treatment involves the use of oral amoxicillin, cefuroxime, or doxycycline for 14–21 days for ELD, 21–28 days for EDD, and 28 days for LDD. Intravenous antibiotics may be administered for up to 28 days for persistent arthritis, carditis, meningitis, or encephalitis. *Prognosis:* Lyme disease may result in significant morbidity. There is no acquired immunity, so reinfection may occur. *Prevention:* Avoid areas that are heavily tick infested, and wear protective clothing. Check for ticks (especially hidden in hair) after every outing. Remove ticks as soon as possible. Check pets as they may carry home ticks that could be transferred to the child. No vaccine is currently available.	■ Use standard precautions if the child is hospitalized. ■ Educate parents about the importance of giving the complete course of antibiotics. ■ Tell parents to have the child avoid sun exposure when taking doxycycline. ■ Nonaspirin analgesics and antipyretics may provide relief of mild fevers, headaches, and muscle and joint aches. ■ Children with Lyme disease may tire easily. Promote rest and avoid vigorous activities that may be difficult. ■ Educate parents and children about the disease and early recognition of the symptoms. ■ Teach parents to safely remove ticks. Grasp the tick gently but firmly with fine-point tweezers where the mouthparts are attached. Pull gently until the tick releases. Clean the area with soap and water. ■ Use tick prevention on pets, and check pets for ticks.

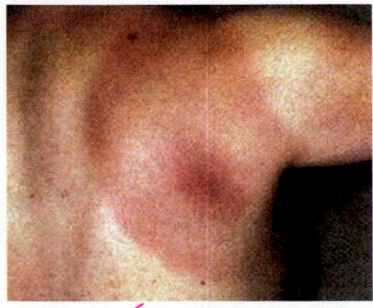

Erythema migrans with Lyme disease.
Source: *Reproduced with permission.* © *Pfizer Inc..*

Malaria *Causal agent:* Plasmodium, four species (P. falciparum, P. vivax, P. ovale, P. malariae). *Epidemiology:* Occurs in tropics and subtropics in Africa, Americas, Asia, and Oceania. Children have the highest mortality. The disease is acquired during travel to an endemic area. P. falciparum causes the most serious disease. In 2008, 18.9% of cases in the United States occurred in children 18 years and younger (Mali, Steele, Slutsker, et al., 2010).	Malaria begins with nonspecific signs such as high fever alternating with chills, profuse diaphoresis, and fatigue. Periods of symptomatic improvement may be seen between cycles lasting 48 or 72 hours depending upon type of infection. Children may also have anorexia, vomiting, splenomegaly, and anemia. Additional symptoms include nausea, vomiting, diarrhea, cough, tachypnea, arthralgia, and body aches. Attacks may recur over the course of the year after infection, but the parasites die out gradually if reinfection does not occur.	*Diagnostic testing:* Blood smears for parasites, or a polymerase chain reaction assay. A rapid malaria test is available. Laboratory tests often reveal anemia and thrombocytopenia. *Medical management:* The child is hospitalized for fluid replacement, anemia management, and antipyretics. The blood is regularly monitored for parasite density.	■ Use standard precautions for the hospitalized patient. ■ Maintain fluid intake. Monitor intake and output. ■ Monitor the hematocrit and hemoglobin, as well as the blood glucose level. ■ Observe for signs of increasing illness severity such as confusion, seizures, and shock. Be prepared to provide emergency support with an airway and supplemental oxygen until the child can be transferred to the ICU.

*Indicates that a vaccine or antitoxin is available for use in high-risk or as-needed situations.
+Indicates that the disease has a safe and effective vaccine.

TABLE 22–6	Selected Communicable Diseases Transmitted by Insect or Animal Hosts (Zoonosis) *(continued)*		
DISEASE	**CLINICAL MANIFESTATIONS**	**CLINICAL THERAPY**	**NURSING MANAGEMENT**
Malaria *(continued)* *Transmission:* The bite of an infected female *Anopheles* mosquito introduces the parasite to the person. The parasite infects the hepatic cells and reproduces. When the hepatic cell ruptures, parasites are released and infect the red blood cells. Transmission can occur by blood transfusion or transplacentally. *Incubation period:* Varies by type, generally 8–25 days after a mosquito bite, but may be up to 1 year. *Period of communicability:* Communicable by blood or blood product transfusion, or the transplantation of organs from an infected person.	Children who live in endemic areas and survive the first 5 years of life develop immunity to the severe effects of the disease as long as they have frequent reexposure to the infection. *Complications:* Severe anemia in young children. Cerebral malaria occurs in children 3–6 years of age. Older children and adolescents more commonly have pulmonary edema, respiratory failure, renal failure, spontaneous bleeding, and shock. Children with asplenia are at high risk for death. In 2008, 863,000 deaths occurred, primarily among children under 5 years of age living in sub-Saharan Africa (Mali et al., 2010).	Antimalarial medication is selected based on drug resistance by malaria species and includes: chloroquine, quinine sulfate and tetracycline, clindamycin, doxycycline, mefloquine, and atovaquone-proguanil. Medications may be given orally or by IV. Hypoglycemia may result from quinine treatment or because parasites consume large quantities of glucose. Intensive care is needed in severe disease. Children may need blood transfusions for severe anemia. *Prognosis:* Certain species have dormant liver-stage parasites, which can reactivate and cause malaria several months or years after the infecting mosquito bite. *Prevention:* While traveling in endemic areas use DEET insect repellent, screened rooms, DEET-treated mosquito netting, and cover the body with light-colored clothing. Antimalarial chemoprophylaxis may be prescribed prior to travel in an endemic region. No vaccine is available. Malaria is a reportable disease.	■ Administer antipyretics to control the fever and promote comfort. ■ Provide information and emotional support to parents. ■ Educate families traveling to endemic areas about the importance of antimalarial chemoprophylaxis. Explain the need to take the medication correctly despite the common side effects of nausea and vomiting. ■ Discuss the need to protect children during nocturnal feeding times of mosquitoes with protective clothing, mosquito repellent, and mosquito netting around the bed.
Rabies (Hydrophobia)* *Causal agent:* Lyssavirus in the Rhabdoviridae family, two types (urban, in dogs; wild, in wildlife). *Epidemiology:* Occurs worldwide. Urban rabies is generally controlled by vaccination of dogs and cats. The most common carriers of rabies are raccoons, bats, skunks, and foxes (Snow, 2011). Four cases were reported in the United States and Puerto Rico in 2009 (Snow, 2011). *Transmission:* Infected saliva from bite of rabid animal introduces the virus into the wound. The virus travels along the nerves to the brain where it multiplies and migrates along the efferent nerves to the salivary glands. Human-to-human transmission is rare, e.g., by organ transplant. *Incubation period:* Highly variable, but usually 3–8 weeks. *Period of communicability:* 3–7 days before the onset of symptoms and throughout the disease course.	Children may be free of symptoms during the long incubation period. The prodromal period lasts 2–10 days with the following signs and symptoms: fever, headache, malaise, apprehension, and paresthesia at the site of the bite. Classic signs of acute neurologic involvement include excitability, hydrophobia (spasms of muscles used for swallowing), delirium, and seizures. Paralysis of the extremities and respiratory muscles occurs in some cases. The patient progresses to coma and respiratory failure. *Complications:* Usually results in death.	*Diagnostic testing:* Confirmed by fluorescent antibody staining of the dead animal's brain tissue or detection of the virus in the patient's saliva or cerebrospinal fluid. *Medical management:* Immediately wash animal bites thoroughly with soap and water and irrigate well with a virucidal agent such as povidone-iodine. Avoid suturing the wound (Heymann, 2008). Postexposure prophylaxis with human rabies immune globulin (HRIG) and human diploid cell rabies vaccine (HDCV) should be given as soon as possible to all persons bitten by animals that may be rabid. Half of the HRIG is infiltrated around the wound, and the remainder is given IM. HDCV is repeated on days 3, 7, and 14, after the bite (four doses). If the person has altered immune competence, five doses of the HDCV should be given with the fifth dose given on day 28 after the bite (Rupprecht, Briggs, Brown, et al., 2010). The HDCV series may be stopped if the animal is found free of rabies. The vaccine is of no value once rabies symptoms are present. *Prognosis:* If symptoms develop, usually results in death. No drug improves the prognosis. *Prevention:* Immunize all domestic animals against rabies.	■ Alert local animal control to find and quarantine any animal suspected of having rabies, if possible. ■ Provide emotional support to the family while reinforcing the urgency for the vaccine and the need for a series of injections. ■ Ensure that the vaccine is injected into the muscle to prevent vaccine failure. ■ Educate parents and the child about the side effects of the vaccine—irritation at the injection site, itching, headache, muscle aches, nausea, and dizziness. ■ If the child acquires rabies, he or she will be hospitalized. Institute contact and droplet precautions. ■ Make the child as comfortable as possible. ■ Keep liquids out of sight of the child with hydrophobia. ■ Provide emotional support to the family of the dying child. ■ Participate in local education about rabies and safe interactions with dogs. See Chapter 36 ⊘. ■ Teach children to avoid contact with all unknown animals, dead or alive.

(continued)

| TABLE 22–6 | Selected Communicable Diseases Transmitted by Insect or Animal Hosts (Zoonosis) *(continued)* |

DISEASE	CLINICAL MANIFESTATIONS	CLINICAL THERAPY	NURSING MANAGEMENT
Rocky Mountain Spotted Fever (Tickborne Typhus Fever, Sao Paulo Typhus) *Causal agent: Rickettsia rickettsii,* a gram-negative coccobacillus. *Epidemiology:* Occurs throughout the United States, southern Canada, and Central and South America. Most infections generally occur between April and September. *Transmission:* Transmitted by a dog or wood tick bite after the tick has been attached for 4–6 hours. The organism localizes and multiplies in the endothelial cells of blood vessels and causes vasculitis. *Incubation period:* 2–14 days (most commonly 7 days) after bite of an infected tick. *Period of communicability:* No person-to-person transmission.	Onset may be gradual or rapid with vague signs that mimic other diseases. Early symptoms are nonspecific fever, malaise, headache, muscle aches, anorexia, nausea, vomiting, and diarrhea. The characteristic erythematous maculopapular rash that blanches usually appears between the third and fifth day of the illness, but it may be absent in 10% of cases (Chen & Sexton, 2008). It usually appears first on the wrist and ankles and spreads to the palms and soles before becoming widely disseminated. The rash may be difficult to see on children with dark skin. Confusion, seizures, photophobia, transient deafness, meningoencephalitis, and other focal neurologic problems may occur (Chen & Sexton, 2008). *Complications:* Disseminated intravascular coagulation (DIC) and acute respiratory distress syndrome. Partial paralysis of lower extremities may occur. Gangrene may require amputation of digits or extremities.	*Diagnostic testing:* Thrombocytopenia may be present and is an important diagnostic clue. Immunofluorescent antibody testing is commonly performed. Direct immunofluorescence or immunoperoxidase tests may be performed on skin biopsies. *Medical management:* Treatment of choice is doxycycline regardless of patient age for 5–7 days or until the child has been afebrile for 3 days (Chen & Sexton, 2008). Hospitalization is necessary in a patient with severe disease or needing IV antibiotics. *Prognosis:* Delay in treatment can cause a more severe disease. A mortality rate of 5% is associated with delayed treatment (Chen & Sexton, 2008). Infection induces immunity. *Prevention:* Avoid areas that are heavily tick infested, and wear protective clothing. Check children for ticks and if found remove promptly.	■ Use standard precautions when the child is hospitalized. ■ When the child is hospitalized, have hemodynamic monitoring equipment and emergency supplies readily available. ■ Administer antibiotics as prescribed. ■ Observe for purpura development or any abnormal bleeding. ■ Make the child as comfortable as possible. ■ Provide quiet diversion activities. ■ Provide emotional support, and keep parents informed about the child's condition. ■ Educate parents about prevention and the appropriate technique for tick removal.

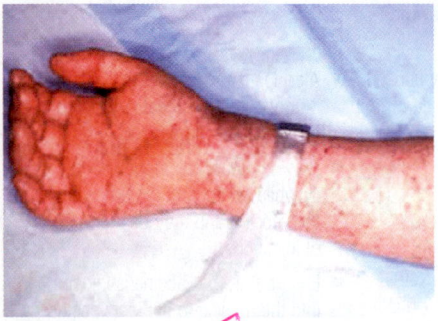

Petechia and purpura with Rocky Mountain spotted fever.

Source: *Reproduced with permission.*
© *Pfizer Inc. Courtesy of Pfizer Central Research.*
(1989). Lyme disease. Groton, CT: Author.

DISEASE	CLINICAL MANIFESTATIONS	CLINICAL THERAPY	NURSING MANAGEMENT
West Nile Virus *Causative agent:* An RNA *Flavivirus.* *Epidemiology:* Infected wild birds (crow family) and the mosquitoes that feed on them carry the illness. The infection has been reported in all states except Alaska and Hawaii, several Canadian provinces, Mexico, Central America, and the Caribbean. The majority of the cases occur during summer months. The elderly and those with weak immune systems are at greatest risk. *Transmission:* Through bite of infected mosquito. May also occur by blood transfusion or organ transplant from an infected donor. *Incubation period:* 2–15 days, but may range to 21 days in immunocompromised patients. *Period of communicability:* Not transmitted from person to person.	Only 20% of infected individuals develop West Nile Virus symptoms (AAP, 2012, p. 792). Signs include an abrupt onset of fever, headache, body aches, and weakness. Abdominal pain, nausea, vomiting, and diarrhea often occur. Some patients have a transient maculopapular rash. While most symptoms last several days, the fatigue, malaise, and weakness may last weeks. Approximately 1% of infected people develop neurologic infections and disease such as aseptic meningitis, encephalitis, or flaccid paralysis (Rossi, Ross, & Evans, 2010). *Complications:* Encephalitis, meningitis, or acute flaccid paralysis. Death may occur in less than 1% of infected persons (AAP, 2012, p. 792).	*Diagnostic testing:* Serum or cerebrospinal fluid is tested for West Nile Virus specific IgM antibodies. Viral culture can be performed. *Medical management:* Treatment is supportive. For severe cases the patient will be in intensive care and supported with IV fluids, airway management, respiratory support, management of cerebral edema, and management of secondary infections. *Prognosis:* Most who develop West Nile virus recover completely, but those with encephalitis or flaccid paralysis may have permanent neurologic deficits. *Prevention:* There is no vaccine. Donor blood is screened. Reduce potential mosquito breeding locations by changing standing water in birdbaths, pet water bowls, and wading pools at least weekly. Use DEET and wear protective clothing, especially in the dawn and twilight hours when mosquitoes bite. This is a reportable disease.	■ Use standard precautions if the child is hospitalized. ■ Provide supportive care for those with encephalitis and meningitis. ■ Be prepared to provide emergency airway and respiratory support. ■ Teach families to control mosquito breeding and to protect children and adults from mosquito bites.

*Indicates that a vaccine or antitoxin is available for use in high-risk or as-needed situations.
⁺Indicates that the disease has a safe and effective vaccine.

Clinical Manifestations   Infection in Infants and Children by Age Group

SYSTEM	INFANTS		CHILDREN	
Central nervous system	Irritable Decreased responsiveness Lethargy Bulging anterior fontanel High-pitched cry	Muscle weakness *Additional Signs in Newborns:* Seizures Subtle changes in muscle tone or hypotonia	Irritable or combative Stiff neck Back pain Decreased responsiveness	Photophobia Brudzinski sign Kernig sign Malaise
Cardiovascular	Tachycardia Decreased perfusion Weak peripheral pulses Pallor or mottled skin Flushed, dry skin	Delayed capillary refill time *Additional Signs in Newborns:* Cyanosis Hypotension Bradycardia	Tachycardia Decreased perfusion Weak peripheral pulses Pallor or flushed, dry skin Delayed capillary refill time	
Respiratory	Tachypnea Increased work of breathing with retractions and nasal flaring Crackles Cough Stridor Decreased oxygen saturation	Irregular breathing *Additional Signs in Newborns:* Apnea (new onset or increased episodes) Increased or new-onset oxygen requirement Grunting	Tachypnea Dyspnea Retractions Nasal flaring Crackles	Cough Stridor Decreased oxygen saturation
Gastrointestinal	Vomiting Diarrhea Abdominal distention Poor feeding	*Additional Signs in Newborns:* Abdominal wall discoloration Paralytic ileus Bloody stool Jaundice or hepatosplenomegaly	Nausea and vomiting Diarrhea Abdominal discomfort Abdominal distention Poor appetite	
Renal	White blood cells (WBCs) and bacteria in urine *Additional Signs in Newborns:* Decreased urine output Hematuria, proteinuria		WBCs and bacteria in urine	
Hematopoietic (See Appendix D 🔗 for expected laboratory values by age.)	Neutropenia Increased immature WBCs (bands) in bacterial infections Lymphocytosis in viral infections *Additional Signs in Newborns:* Fraction of band cells greater than 0.2 Thrombocytopenia		Leukocytosis Increased immature WBCs (bands) in bacterial infections Lymphocytosis in viral infections	
Metabolic	Hyperthermia or hypothermia Hypoglycemia or hyperglycemia		Hyperthermia Chills Hypothermic in septic shock	
Other	Rash Dry mucous membranes Poor skin turgor Sunken anterior fontanel Petechiae or purpura		Rash Petechiae and/or purpura Dry mucous membranes Poor skin turgor	

include fatigue, malaise, weakness, body aches, poor appetite, nausea and vomiting, diarrhea, headache, and reduced responsiveness or ability to concentrate. See the Clinical Manifestations table above for signs and symptoms of infection in infants and children by the system involved.

Collaborative Care

For many infectious and communicable diseases, management is supportive. In addition to diagnostic tests, collaborative care includes fever management, promoting the child's comfort, antibiotic administration for bacterial infections, and in some cases antiviral agents for specific viral illnesses.

Diagnostic Procedures

Diagnostic tests include bacterial, viral, or fungal cultures from sites where the infection may potentially be located, such as the blood, skin, pharynx, urine, feces, and cerebrospinal fluid. See the Skills Manual 🔗 for guidelines related to collection of specimens. Blood may be obtained to perform tests for condition-specific immunoglobulin antibodies. In some cases, radiographs or special imaging may be used to identify localized infection in an organ such as the lungs.

Clinical Therapy

A fever can be a beneficial physiologic response, helping to slow the growth of organisms that thrive at lower body temperatures. A fever decreases the serum levels of zinc, iron, and copper needed by bacteria for reproduction. It helps to mobilize the immune response by increasing neutrophil production and enhancing phagocytosis (Huether, 2010). Fever is not inherently harmful until it reaches 41°C (105.9°F). For this reason, medical management may include postponing treatment of low-grade fevers under 38.9°C (102°F) in otherwise healthy children to promote the body's natural defenses against an infection.

Fevers are often treated, especially in children with pulmonary or cardiac disorders who may be unable to tolerate the higher metabolic rate and oxygen need. Fevers may also be treated if associated with discomfort. Acetaminophen and ibuprofen are the preferred antipyretics for children. Aspirin is no longer recommended for children because of its association with Reye syndrome. Antipyretics reduce fever by inhibiting prostaglandin synthesis, which results in lowering of the body's temperature set point. See Complementary Therapy: Fever Treatment.

Antibiotic use Administration of antibiotics is often another component of clinical therapy for communicable diseases. Before the introduction of antibiotics, children used natural defenses to fight infection, and often died as the result of overwhelming sepsis. Antibiotics have been responsible for significant decreases in morbidity and mortality from infections among children. However, strains of bacteria have developed resistance to many antibiotics due to the overuse of antibiotics. Examples include community-acquired methicillin-resistant *Staphylococcus aureus* and community-acquired pneumonia caused by pneumococcus. Antibiotic resistance is associated with treatment failure, increased costs associated with using a second and more expensive antibiotic, and in some cases, lack of an effective antibiotic for the pathogen. In addition, fewer new antibiotics are in development than in prior years. Children with chronic illnesses such as cystic fibrosis, sickle cell disease, and acquired immunodeficiency syndrome (AIDS) are particularly susceptible to infection by antibiotic-resistant pathogens. Many specialty organizations and medical centers have developed guidelines for best practices associated with the use of antibiotics for the treatment of common infections, such as acute otitis media. See Chapter 24 🔗.

Antiviral medications, such as acyclovir, may be ordered for certain types of viral infections, such as varicella (chicken pox), herpes simplex virus type 1 and 2, influenza, and others. In cases when the child is immunocompromised, the antiviral medication needs to be provided very early in the infectious period to minimize the potentially life-threatening consequences of the infection.

Some cases of communicable disease must be reported to the state health department for disease surveillance and to determine the effectiveness of certain preventive measures, such as vaccines. For example, data about immunization rates in a community or state can be matched with reported cases of disease to evaluate public health and health promotion interventions. Cases can be reported on state-designated websites.

Nursing Management

The goal of nursing management is to assess the child for initial symptoms and potential progression in severity of the infection. Nursing care is focused on managing the child's symptoms, promoting the child's hydration, and preventing the spread of infection.

Nursing Assessment and Diagnosis

Assess the child's hydration status and fluid intake, vital signs, comfort level, and appetite, and observe for seizures and for a **toxic appearance** (lethargy, poor perfusion, hypoventilation or hyperventilation, and cyanosis). The child with a fever may be irritable and restless, sleep fitfully, and have nonspecific muscular pain. Identify those children who may be at higher risk for a serious illness in association with a fever, in particular:

- Infants and children having a toxic appearance
- Neonates less than 28 days of age with a temperature over 38°C (100.4°F)
- Children less than 4 years of age with a temperature over 41°C (105.8°F)
- Children with conditions such as a ventriculoperitoneal shunt, congenital heart disease, asplenia, and sickle cell disease

Observe the child for other signs of infection, such as a rash, nausea and vomiting, or diarrhea, as well as generalized symptoms of a poor appetite, body aches, and malaise.

Examples of nursing diagnoses that may be appropriate for children with infectious and communicable diseases are as follows:

- Hyperthermia related to infectious disease process
- Skin Integrity, Impaired related to hyperthermia and scratching of skin lesions
- Mucous Membrane: Oral, Impaired related to infectious disease process
- Fluid Volume, Deficient related to repeated episodes of vomiting and diarrhea
- Therapeutic Regimen Management: Family, Ineffective related to complexity of care required by the child

NANDA-I © 2012

Planning and Implementation

Most children with communicable diseases are cared for at home; however, children may be evaluated in various healthcare settings. The nurse's role includes assisting with the collection of cultures, treating the infection, administering antibiotics or antiviral agents on schedule, promoting the child's comfort, and educating parents. The nurse also monitors the child's response to therapy, staying alert for signs that the infection is worsening. Be sure that infants and children have pain management for painful diagnostic procedures such as lumbar punctures. Encourage parents to assist with their child's care.

Prevent Disease Transmission

Nursing care of children with communicable diseases in healthcare settings focuses on preventing the spread of infection. Children with suspicious rashes and respiratory infections should be isolated from other children. Draining wounds should be covered and dressings should be

---

Complementary Therapy

Fever Treatment

Many cultures subscribe to the hot and cold theory of disease causation. "Hot" and "cold" do not refer to temperature but to categories. Fever, a hot condition, is treated by giving the patient cold substances (foods or medicines). Cold foods include dairy products, fresh vegetables, fruits, chicken, goat meat, and fish. Cold medicines include orange flower water, linden, and sage. Ask parents how they think the illness should be treated. Encourage them to use that treatment as long as it is not known to cause harm. Check current literature for guidance when needed. Teach parents about additional Western medicine treatments they can use. (See Chapter 3 🔗.)

disposed of appropriately. All items with which the infected child comes into contact are considered contaminated (e.g., linens, toys, medical equipment). The fecal-oral and respiratory routes are the most common sources of infection. Use standard precautions and good hand hygiene. Wipe down hard surfaces in the examining room with an antiseptic solution before another child uses the room. If possible, wipe down toys in the waiting room daily with a nontoxic antiseptic solution. Dispose of linens in appropriately marked linen bags. Ensure that all healthcare professionals are fully immunized or that unimmunized or pregnant healthcare professionals are not exposed to children with certain infections (e.g., pertussis, rubella, or varicella). See page 605 for information to teach families about reducing the transmission of infection.

Children are often admitted to the hospital for treatment of severe infections. In addition, countless numbers of **nosocomial infections** (hospital-acquired infections) occur each year. Follow the facility's standard precautions and transmission-based precautions to reduce the spread of infectious diseases to staff and other patients. Bring any questions and concerns to the hospital's infection control nurse. (Refer to the Skills Manual for more detailed information.)

Fever Management

Nursing care for treatment of fever includes administering antipyretics, removing unnecessary clothing, and careful continued monitoring of the child's temperature. Identify clear fluids the child prefers to drink, and encourage the intake of extra fluids.

Practice Alert

While alternating acetaminophen with ibuprofen in the care of children with fever has been the subject of studies, this practice increases the risk of harm to the child. The potentially synergistic effects of the two medications on the kidneys can cause renal tubular toxicity when used repeatedly for an illness (Miller, 2007). An important patient safety initiative to reduce the risk for overdosing is to encourage parents to use only one antipyretic with the correct dose and administration interval for fever management.

Care in the Community

Teach parents to care for their child at home, including how and when to give antipyretics, over-the-counter medications, and antibiotics if ordered; what foods and beverages are appropriate; and how to care for rashes and other topical symptoms. Provide guidelines about the types of fluids to encourage. Identify the antipyretic available in the home and provide the parents with guidelines for the correct dosage.

Clinical Tip

Acetaminophen and ibuprofen preparations commonly available in the home are infant drops, liquid syrup, chewable tablets, and adult strength tablets or capsules. Concentration in liquids and dosage in tablets vary by the type of preparation. The dose of acetaminophen to treat fever is 10 to 15 mg/kg/dose every 4 to 6 hours, not to exceed five doses in 24 hours. For children 12 years and older the maximum daily dose is 4 g. The dose of ibuprofen is 4 to 10 mg/kg/dose every 6 to 8 hours with a maximum daily dose of 40 mg/kg.

Acetaminophen	Ibuprofen
Infant's liquid—160 mg/5 mL using package dispenser	Infant drops—50 mg/1.25 mL, using package dropper
Children's liquid—160 mg/5 mL	Children's liquid—100 mg/5 mL
Chewable tablets—80 mg and 160 mg	Chewable and junior tablets—50 mg and 100 mg
Adult tablets or caplets—325 mg and 650 mg	Adult tablets or caplets—200 mg

Parents often fear a fever, believing it is a disease rather than a symptom of an illness. Provide information and reassurance. Help them to recognize signs of the child's worsening condition in association with the child's specific disease. See Partnering with Families: Guidelines for Evaluating and Treating Fever in Children.

Teach parents the importance of proper use of antibiotics when ordered to help reduce the development of antibiotic-resistant bacteria:

- Give all the antibiotic dosages as prescribed for the full number of days ordered. Help parents select the best times to give each prescribed dose to keep blood levels constant. This will help ensure that the bacteria causing the infection are eradicated, rather than having some bacteria left alive to mutate and resist the antibiotic in the future.
- Make sure parents know whether to give the antibiotic with food or without food to promote optimal absorption.
- Discard any remaining antibiotic when all prescribed doses have been given. Antibiotics have an expiration date and lose potency after that date.
- Do not share the antibiotic with any other family member. If that family member is ill, there will not be enough antibiotic to fully treat the infection, even if the same bacteria is causing the infection.

Educate parents about methods to reduce disease transmission in the home, such as good hygiene. Encourage parents to limit the exposure of elderly family members, infants, and visitors to the ill child. Make sure that the ill child's dishes and utensils are washed in hot soapy water or sanitized in a dishwasher. Place dressings with drainage in a plastic bag for disposal to prevent contact by other family members.

Encourage children to rest. Provide quiet diversional activities such as board games, DVDs, and music. Promote fluid intake and provide foods that the child prefers and do not cause discomfort. Reduce itching of rashes with lukewarm baths with Aveeno or oatmeal and topical lotions. Keep the child's hands clean and nails trimmed. Cover the hands with clean socks or mittens if scratching cannot be controlled.

Correct any misconceptions parents and childcare workers may have about the occurrence or cause of the infectious disease in their child. The parents and other providers may believe that they have exposed the child to certain germs or bacteria. Teach them that infection control will reduce exposure of other children and family members to the infectious disease.

Evaluation

Expected outcomes of nursing care include the following:

- Opportunities for the spread of infection between patients and family members are minimized.
- The fever is managed effectively with antipyretics.
- The full antibiotic treatment course is completed, if ordered.

SEPSIS

Sepsis or septicemia is a systemic inflammatory response syndrome (SIRS) in the presence of infection, such as bacteria invading the bloodstream. Infants in the perinatal period and during the first year of life are at a high risk for developing sepsis, especially those with low birth weight and those who have several invasive procedures performed. Older infants and children who develop sepsis often have a chronic condition, burns, invasive catheters, or compromised

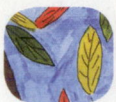

Partnering with Families

Guidelines for Evaluating and Treating Fever in Children

ABOUT FEVERS

- A fever is not a disease; it is the body's physiologic response to an infection. A fever means the child's body is using natural defenses to fight an infection and kill viruses and bacteria.
- If the child has a fever and does not look sick, it may be better to let the child use the natural defenses to fight off the virus or bacteria causing the fever, but follow guidelines about when to contact the child's healthcare provider.

CARE FOR A FEVER

- Use a thermometer to check the child's temperature every 4 to 6 hours, or more often if the fever returns. See the Skills Manual ⬭ .
- Use either acetaminophen or ibuprofen (do not use aspirin) to lower the temperature. Use the correct dose and preparation for the child's weight, and keep track of the times when the medication is given. Do not alternate the medications. Alternating the medications increases the risk that the infant or child will get an overdose that could cause harm. If the child is taking a cold medication with acetaminophen, call the healthcare provider for advice about acetaminophen dosage.
- Remove all but a light layer of the child's clothing to help lower the temperature.
- Monitor the child's behavior and response to the fever medication. The medication will reduce the child's temperature. The temperature may rise again in 4 to 6 hours after the medication has worn off. Check the temperature and give another dose of medication. Do not give more than the number of doses a day recommended on the medicine bottle. The temperature will not return to normal until the child is recovering from the illness.
- Sponging is not routinely recommended. The lukewarm water may increase shivering and discomfort. Do not sponge the child using alcohol.

- Provide generous amounts of fluids for the child to drink and allow the child to rest.

CALL YOUR HEALTHCARE PROVIDER IMMEDIATELY IF:

- The infant is under 2 months old and has a fever higher than 38.0°C (100.4°F).
- The child has a fever over 40.1°C (104.2°F), and the following symptoms are present:
  - The child is crying inconsolably or whimpering. The child cries when moved or otherwise touched by the parent or other family members.
  - The child is difficult to awaken.
  - The child's neck is stiff.
  - There are purple spots present on the skin.
  - Breathing is difficult and no better after the nose is cleared.
  - The child is drooling saliva and is unable to swallow anything.
  - The child has a convulsion or seizure.
  - The child acts or looks very sick.

CALL YOUR HEALTHCARE PROVIDER WITHIN 24 HOURS IF:

- The child is 2 to 4 months old (unless fever occurs within 48 hours of a DTaP shot and the infant has no other serious symptoms).
- The fever is higher than 40.1°C (104.2°F) (especially if the child is under 3 years old).
- The child complains of burning or pain with urination.
- The fever has been present more than 24 hours without an obvious cause or location of infection.
- The fever went away for more than 24 hours and then returned.
- The fever has been present for more than 72 hours.

---

immune system, or are taking antibiotics long term (Hazinski, Mondozzi, & Baker, 2010). Severe sepsis that progresses to septic shock is a significant health problem with an estimated in-hospital mortality rate of up to 10% (Czaja, Zimmerman, & Nathans, 2009).

Etiology and Pathophysiology

Common microorganisms associated with sepsis include group B streptococcus, *E. coli, Haemophilus influenzae,* and staphylococcus. Newborns can acquire infections during the prenatal and perinatal periods, as well as during the first weeks of life because they have inadequately developed inflammatory and immune system responses, enabling microorganisms to rapidly invade, spread, and multiply (see Chapter 27 ⊘). Low-birth-weight infants often have invasive procedures performed that increase their risk for infections.

Mediators along with procoagulation factors initiate inflammation and coagulation, inhibit fibrinolysis, and lead to disseminated intravascular coagulation (see Chapter 28 ⊘). White blood cells multiply throughout the body and macrophages produce cytokines, which dilate the blood vessels and increase permeability. Fibrin deposits impede blood flow. Blood flow congestion occurs in some tissue beds, reducing the delivery of oxygen and nutrients to the tissues, and bacteria may be trapped and multiply unchecked. Dysfunction of the microvascular system may result in leaking capillaries, peripheral edema, and fluid accumulation in the lungs (Rubarth, 2010).

The sepsis inflammatory cascade also triggers vasodilation and constriction that can cause cellular hypoxia and organ dysfunction (e.g., myocardial, respiratory, renal, hepatic, or neurologic dysfunction).

Clinical Manifestations

Symptoms of sepsis in newborns are often nonspecific, such as feeding problems (decreased intake, poor sucking, or lack of interest in feeding); subtle changes in color, tone, and activity; abdominal distention; and vomiting and diarrhea. Rather than a fever, newborns often have hypothermia. Nonspecific respiratory distress or apnea may be noted, especially if group B streptococcus is the causative organism. See the Clinical Manifestations table on page 639 for signs of infection in newborns by body system. Early signs of sepsis in children include fever or hypothermia, tachycardia, and tachypnea.

As septic shock begins, the child may initially have a fever, tachycardia, tachypnea, warm extremities, bounding pulses, brisk capillary refill, and normal urine output. Responsiveness may be altered. As septic shock progresses, hypotension, prolonged capillary refill time, mottled cool extremities, weak pulses, progressive mental status changes, and decreasing urine output are seen, along with fever or hypothermia. Shock may progress to cardiac arrest if interventions are unsuccessful.

Collaborative Care

Care focuses on diagnosis of sepsis and aggressive therapy to promote the infant's survival and to reduce the potential consequences such as neurologic damage.

Diagnostic Procedures

Diagnosis is often suspected from clinical signs and symptoms. The diagnostic clinical signs of an initial systemic response in a newborn less than 1 month of age are as follows: a low temperature or fever, tachycardia, respiratory rate greater than or equal to 60 beats/min and increasing respiratory distress, and elevated white blood cells with an increase in immature neutrophils (Rubarth, 2010).

Because a focal site of infection is usually not apparent, culture specimens are obtained from the blood, urine, cerebrospinal fluid, and skin lesions. Radiographs of the lungs and other potential sites may reveal signs of infection. Blood is obtained for a complete blood count and white blood cell differential. A high white cell count with low neutrophil and high band (immature white blood cell) counts indicate the presence of an infection. A C-reactive protein level may be elevated.

Clinical Therapy

Clinical therapy focuses on preserving vital organ function with oxygen, aggressive intravenous fluid resuscitation, and vasopressor medications to manage vasodilation and improve renal perfusion. Acid-base, glucose, and electrolyte levels are monitored, and imbalances are managed. Packed red blood cells may be given to maintain the child's hemoglobin level. Antibiotics are initiated immediately and changed if necessary to target the specific microorganism causing the infection, once the culture and sensitivity results are known. Cardiorespiratory monitoring and temperature regulation of the environment are performed. Enteral or parenteral nutritional support may be initiated early.

Nursing Management

Nursing care of the infant or child with sepsis occurs in the neonatal or pediatric intensive care unit (NICU or PICU). Nursing care is focused on identifying the infant with signs of infection, monitoring the newborn's status during clinical therapy, and preventing the development of sepsis in low-birth-weight newborns. Nursing care of children with sepsis involves careful assessment of the child's response to clinical therapy and support to the family of the child with a life-threatening infection.

Nursing Assessment and Diagnoses

Maintain a high level of suspicion for the development of sepsis in high-risk newborns. Monitor the newborn's condition for signs and symptoms of infection and sepsis, especially high-risk newborns that have invasive procedures performed or are assisted with various types of technology (e.g., ventilator or central line).

Assess and monitor the vital signs and temperature of infants and children with sepsis. Monitor perfusion, intake and output, and weight. Check for perfusion using capillary refill time and temperature of the extremities. Ensure that the cardiorespiratory monitor leads are attached so that episodes of apnea in the neonate or bradycardia in the older infant and child are detected. Note any petechiae or purpura that could be associated with disseminated intravascular coagulation. Monitor laboratory tests (glucose, electrolytes, acid-base

balance) to identify any significant changes needed in clinical therapy. Observe for signs that the condition is worsening or resolving.

Examples of nursing diagnoses may include the following:

- Thermoregulation, Ineffective related to inflammatory illness
- Breastfeeding, Interrupted related to infant illness
- Protection, Ineffective related to inadequately developed inflammatory and immune system response
- Fluid Volume, Deficient related to fever and poor intake
- Gas Exchange, Impaired related to respiratory distress syndrome
- Family Processes, Interrupted related to situational crisis with child's life-threatening illness

NANDA-I® 2012

Planning and Implementation

Ensure that antibiotics and other medications are administered as prescribed. Monitor for side effects of antibiotics, especially when they may cause renal or other organ system damage. Make sure that the newborn's environmental temperature is maintained. Carefully manage the IV fluid administered to ensure that the infant or child receives the volume needed to maintain perfusion. Ensure that the child's airway is maintained and oxygen and ventilatory support are provided as prescribed.

Assist in the care of infants and children during diagnostic procedures. Ensure the provision of pain management (see Chapter 21). Soothe the infant afterward with positioning, a pacifier, low lighting, and swaddling. Soothe the child with gentle touch, holding, and music.

Provide support to parents who are stressed, because the newborn has the potential for development of disabilities or progression of the condition to severe sepsis or septic shock. Provide information about the newborn's illness and treatment plan. Encourage the parents to participate in the newborn's care as much as possible.

Prevention of nosocomial infection is a significant role of the nurse and includes good hand hygiene by all persons touching the newborn, use of aseptic technique for all procedures, and limiting exposure to individuals with infections. Other measures to reduce the risk of infection in neonates include skin care with barriers that maintain skin integrity.

Discharge planning includes educating parents about the need to administer antibiotics until the full course is completed. Teach parents to identify signs and symptoms that the infection is not resolving as expected. Encourage the parents to keep healthcare appointments so that the infant can be monitored for signs of neurologic impairment.

Evaluation

Expected outcomes of nursing care include:

- Early signs of sepsis are recognized.
- Treatment is initiated rapidly to minimize potential sequelae.
- The newborn's temperature-regulation mechanism is stabilized.
- The parents are educated to complete the child's antibiotic medications and to return for healthcare visits to monitor the child for sequelae.

EMERGING INFECTION CONTROL THREATS

Public health officials regularly perform disease surveillance, continuous monitoring and tracking of the incidence and patterns of infections, to identify emerging infections. Pandemic influenza, a worldwide influenza epidemic, has been the most recent focus of

Bioterrorism and Emerging Infections Resources

Weblink

attention, but other rare infectious diseases such as avian influenza have been past concerns. See Table 22–5 for influenza information. Special disease surveillance attention is also directed at infectious agents that could be weapons of terrorists (anthrax, smallpox, plague, botulism, hemorrhagic fever, or tularemia). See the Clinical Manifestations table for potential biological terrorism agents.

Collaborative Care

Along with the United States, many countries have a response plan in case any of these infectious diseases are identified. Once an infectious disease outbreak is identified, health professionals are notified through the national Health Alert Network (HAN) to be alert for patients with signs and symptoms, to isolate the infected, and to refer those most seriously ill to designated hospitals or centers of care. The Centers for Disease Control and Prevention and state health departments have developed guidelines for infection control management and are partnering with hospitals and local health providers to prepare them to manage hundreds of ill patients in an epidemic. See Chapter 14 🔗.

Nursing Management

Nurses have a responsibility for maintaining a high level of suspicion when numerous individuals with similar signs and symptoms are present in school or seek care in any healthcare facility. Initiating infection control measures such as airborne and contact precautions may help reduce the transmission of infection. Instituting isolation is appropriate before a definitive diagnosis when the level of suspicion is high. Assess children and provide supportive nursing care for the identified infection.

Nurses should regularly review guidelines posted by the Centers for Disease Control and Prevention about the management of specific health threats and plans for pandemic flu. They should also participate in planning for the healthcare facility's preparedness to respond to potential epidemics as a partner in the state and local emergency preparedness planning.

Clinical Manifestations | Potential Biological Terrorism Agents

ORGANISMS	CLINICAL MANIFESTATIONS	CLINICAL THERAPY
Anthrax *Causal agent:* *Bacillus anthracis* *Cutaneous anthrax.*	■ Cutaneous—papule that progresses to a vesicle and then to a skin ulcer with a depressed black scab area in the center. Not painful. Child may have fever, malaise, headache, and regional lymphadenopathy. ■ Gastrointestinal—nausea, loss of appetite, bloody diarrhea, hematemesis, fever, stomach pain, severe abdominal pain followed by fever and septicemia. ■ Inhalation—brief prodrome with respiratory symptoms like a sore throat, mild fever, malaise, and muscle aches followed by development of dyspnea, chest pain, shortness of breath, and systemic symptoms. Shock, pleural effusion, sepsis, or meningitis may develop, and death may occur without treatment.	■ IV ciprofloxacin or doxycycline for patients over 12 years. For children under 12 years, IV ciprofloxacin plus clindamycin and penicillin G. ■ Corticosteroids are recommended in all patients who have pulmonary edema, respiratory failure, and meningitis (Kman & Nelson, 2008). ■ Postexposure prophylaxis is 60 days of ciprofloxacin or doxycycline. ■ Vaccine approved only for persons over 18 years (three doses at 0, 2, and 4 weeks) (Moran, Talan, & Abrahamian, 2008).
Botulism *Causal agent:* *Clostridium botulinum*	■ Begins with cranial nerve palsies, often beginning with ptosis, diplopia, blurred vision, and sluggishly reactive pupils. ■ Progressive descending paralysis with speech and swallowing problems, loss of gag reflex, and then symmetric descending flaccid paralysis. ■ Confusion may be present. ■ May be preceded by abdominal cramps, nausea, vomiting, or diarrhea.	■ Slow IV infusion of equine antitoxin diluted in normal saline may halt progression of symptoms, but paralysis will not be reversed. ■ Epinephrine and diphenhydramine for serum sickness or urticaria.
Hemorrhagic Fever *Causal agent:* Ebola or Marburg virus	■ Abrupt onset of fever, myalgia, headache, nausea, vomiting, abdominal pain, photophobia, diarrhea, chest pain, cough, and pharyngitis. ■ Maculopapular rash prominent on trunk soon after fever; petechiae, ecchymosis, subconjunctival hemorrhages; shock and circulatory collapse in short period. ■ Ghostlike appearance, looks critically ill.	■ Fluid resuscitation to manage hypotension and shock; then maintain fluid and electrolyte balance. ■ Blood, platelets, and plasma administration for severe hemorrhage. ■ Ribavirin, but the U.S. Food and Drug Administration has not approved its use for this purpose.
Pneumonic Plague *Causal agent:* *Yersinia pestis*	■ Severe respiratory illness with high fever, chills, headache, cough, and breathing difficulty. ■ Rapidly developing pneumonia with bloody or watery sputum. May lead to respiratory failure and shock. ■ May have gastrointestinal symptoms, such as nausea, vomiting, diarrhea, and abdominal pain.	■ Gentamicin IV or streptomycin IM. Alternative antibiotics include IV doxycycline, ciprofloxacin, or chloramphenicol. ■ May require aggressive fluid resuscitation, vasopressors, and monitoring in the ICU. ■ Prophylaxis with oral doxycycline or quinolone for 6 days.

Clinical Manifestations Potential Biological Terrorism Agents (*continued*)

ORGANISMS	CLINICAL MANIFESTATIONS	CLINICAL THERAPY
Smallpox *Causal agent:* Variola major virus 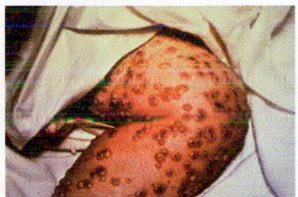 *Smallpox, lesions all in same stage of development.*	■ Prodrome 2–4 days before rash: abrupt onset with fever (38.3°C [101°F] or higher), malaise, headache, muscle pain, nausea and vomiting, and backache. ■ Rash begins with red spots in the mouth and on the tongue that develop sores and break open. Then a few macules, known as herald spots, appear on the forehead, face, and extremities, spreading to become a generalized rash. Macules progress to papules, to tense vesicles, to tense deep pustules with an umbilicated appearance. Lesions are firm, all in same stage of development. See comparison to chicken pox on page 626. The temperature usually falls and the patient feels better. ■ The pustules form scabs by the end of the second week, and the scabs fall off after 3–4 weeks.	■ Supportive care. ■ Antibiotics for secondary infection. ■ The vaccine can be effective if given within the first few days after exposure.
Tularemia *Causal agent:* *Francisella tularensis*	■ Fever, fatigue, chills, headache, malaise, and body aches. ■ Cough, substernal pain, dyspnea, and chest pain. ■ May develop hemorrhagic inflammation of airways that progresses to bronchopneumonia, pleuritis, and hilar lymphadenopathy. ■ May also have pharyngitis, bronchiolitis, and pneumonia with systemic symptoms.	■ Supportive care. ■ Gentamicin IV or streptomycin IM, alternative antibiotics include IV doxycycline, ciprofloxacin, or chloramphenicol. ■ Prophylaxis with doxycycline or ciprofloxacin.

Source: *Kman, N. E., & Nelson, R. N. (2008). Infectious agents of bioterrorism: A review for emergency physicians.* Emergency Medicine Clinics of North America, 26, *517–547; Moran, G. J., Talan, D. A., & Abrahamian, F. M. (2008). Biologic terrorism.* Infectious Disease Clinics of North America, 22, *145–187; Senior, K. (2008). Yersinia pestis: A force to be reckoned with.* Lancet Infectious Diseases, 8(12), *746. Photos courtesy of the Centers for Disease Control and Prevention.*

Chapter Highlights

- Reducing the number of preventable childhood illnesses is a major national public health goal.
- A communicable disease is an illness caused by microorganisms that are commonly transmitted from one host (animal or human) to another.
- Newborns and infants are especially vulnerable to infectious diseases because their immune systems are immature, their passively acquired maternal antibodies provide limited protection, and disease protection through immunization is not yet complete.
- For a child to acquire a communicable disease, the following need to be present: an infectious agent or pathogen, an effective means of transmission, and a susceptible host.
- Infection control measures that caregivers can take include the following: performing good hand hygiene with soap and water or alcohol-based gels, disinfecting hard surfaces touched by the child or the child's body fluids, disinfecting toys the child has mouthed before letting other children play with them, and making sure all children are fully immunized.
- Major public health efforts that have decreased the occurrence of infectious and communicable diseases include safer drinking water, better sanitation, improved standards of living, and increased immunization.
- The average infant born in 2012 will receive immunizations for 14 childhood diseases by 6 years of age. In the United States, immunizations protect children from diphtheria, tetanus, pertussis, polio, hepatitis B, *Haemophilus*

influenzae type b, influenza, measles, mumps, rubella, varicella, rotavirus, and pneumococcus.
- Vaccines must be given at specific ages and intervals. Immunization timing is related to decreasing maternal antibody protection, to the child's developing ability to make antibodies in response to a vaccine, and to whether the vaccine provides lifelong immunity or requires a booster for prolonged immunity.
- The Vaccines for Children program provides free immunizations for low-income children to ensure that finances are not a barrier to full immunization for those children.
- When parents resist immunizations for religious or philosophic reasons, the nurse should provide them with accurate information and help them understand that their child may be at significant risk for an infection with potential serious consequences if not immunized.
- The potency of vaccines must be protected with storage in the refrigerator or freezer at the appropriate temperature.
- The National Vaccine Injury Acts of 1986 and 1993 provide compensation if a link between immunization and a serious adverse effect is found. The Vaccine Adverse Event Reporting System has been established to track serious vaccine reactions.
- Immunization information is updated frequently. It is the nurse's responsibility to regularly obtain current information about vaccines, the immunization schedule, and important information to share with parents and adolescents.

- Infectious and communicable diseases are caused by bacterial, viral, protozoan, or fungal organisms.
- Fever is often a sign of infectious disease in children. When pathogens invade the body, the hypothalamus functions as the body's thermostat, directing the body to conserve or dissipate heat. Pyrogens released into the bloodstream lead to an increased production of prostaglandin which raises the body's thermoregulatory set point, thus causing the fever to occur.
- The child with a toxic or septic appearance has the following signs: lethargy, poor perfusion, tachypnea or bradypnea, and pallor or cyanosis.

- The appropriate use and administration of antibiotics to help reduce the development of antibiotic-resistant bacteria includes the following: Give antibiotic dosages as prescribed for the full number of days ordered, do not share with other family members who might be ill, and discard when all doses have been given.
- Sepsis is a systemic response to infection that has a high mortality rate.
- The public health system is conducting disease surveillance to detect the emergence of rare infections, an epidemic, or the presence of infectious disease potentially caused by terrorists.

Clinical Reasoning in Action

INTRODUCTION

Recall the scenario at the beginning of the chapter involving 4-month-old Kendra and her parents who came to the health center for Kendra's immunizations and health assessment. Kendra's growth and development is occurring as appropriate for her age.

DESCRIPTION

Kendra has previously received the following vaccines: two doses of HepB, and one dose each of DTaP, IPV, Hib, RV, and PCV13. Kendra's parents need information to help console and comfort her during and after the immunizations.

DISCUSSION

1. List the vaccines that Kendra should receive today. When should she return for the next needed vaccines?

2. What are the nurse's responsibilities before giving Kendra her needed vaccines? How will the nurse ensure that the vaccines given have full potency?

3. What are some potential methods to reduce the pain associated with the vaccine injections?

4. What preparation should the health center have in case Kendra has a serious allergic reaction to one of the vaccines?

5. Develop a teaching plan for Kendra's care at home following the immunizations.

NCLEX-RN® Review

1. Regardless of age, which is the priority nursing diagnosis for children in need of immunizations?
   1. Injury, Risk for related to immunization reaction
   2. Immunization Status, Readiness for Enhanced related to planned health promotion visit
   3. Infection, Risk for related to inadequate acquired immunity
   4. Anxiety related to receiving scheduled immunizations

NANDA-I © 2012

2. The nurse is planning the equipment needs for a new pediatric clinic where immunizations will be given, among other services. Which indicates the priority consideration?
   1. A new office is not allowed to have vaccines for at least one year.
   2. Educating staff on vaccine administration.
   3. Cabinet space should be allocated specifically for vaccines.
   4. A medication refrigerator is necessary for vaccine storage.

3. A child presents in the emergency department experiencing a high fever alternating with chills, profuse diaphoresis, and fatigue that has been occurring over the last 48 hours. The child has recently returned from a trip to South America. What infectious disease does the nurse suspect based upon the symptoms and history of the child?
   1. Lyme disease
   2. Malaria
   3. Tetanus
   4. Rubella

4. The nurse assesses a 4-year-old who was adopted from Russia and had no immunizations. The child does not appear ill, but has a fine, pink, maculopapular rash that progressed from the face to the neck, chest, and back, then to the extremities within 3 days. Which communicable disease would the nurse suspect?
   1. Scarlet fever
   2. Rubella (German measles)
   3. Meningococcus
   4. Varicella

See Appendix I ⊘ for answers.

References

Amer, A. (2009). Point-counterpoint: Responding to common reasons for vaccine refusal. *Consultant for Pediatricians, 8*(Suppl. 10), S15–S18.

American Academy of Pediatrics (AAP), Committee on Infectious Disease. (2012). *Red book: Report of the Committee on Infectious Disease* (29th ed.). Elk Grove Village, IL: Author.

Avner, J. R. (2009). Acute fever. *Pediatrics in Review, 30*(1), 5–13.

Bell, E. A. (2010). DTaP or Tdap: Vaccine and drug name confusion. *Infectious Diseases in Children, 23*(10), 12.

Bolton, M., & Barson, W. (2010). Invasive pneumococcal disease and the need for the new 13-valent pneumococcal vaccine. *Pediatric Annals, 39*(8), 497–503.

Centers for Disease Control and Prevention (CDC). (2008a). Update: Measles—United States, January–July 2008. *Morbidity and Mortality Weekly Report, 57*(33), 893–896.

Centers for Disease Control and Prevention (CDC). (2008b). Updated recommendations for isolation of persons with mumps. *Morbidity and Mortality Weekly Report, 57*(40), 1103–1105.

Centers for Disease Control and Prevention (CDC). (2010a). *State vaccination requirements.* Retrieved from http://www.cdc.gov/vaccines/vac-gen/laws/state-reqs.htm#other

Centers for Disease Control and Prevention (CDC). (2010b). Update: Mumps outbreak—New York and New Jersey, June 2009–January 2010. *Morbidity and Mortality Weekly Report, 59*(5), 125–129.

Centers for Disease Control and Prevention (CDC). (2010c). *Vaccines and preventable diseases: Statement regarding Rotarix and RotaTeq rotavirus vaccines and intussusception.* Retrieved from http://www.cdc.gov/vaccines/vpd-vac/rotavirus/intussusception-studies-acip.htm

Centers for Disease Control and Prevention (CDC). (2011a). *Immunization schedules.* Retrieved from http://www.cdc.gov/vaccines/recs/schedules/default.htm

Centers for Disease Control and Prevention (CDC). (2011b). *CDC price list.* Retrieved from http://www.cdc.gov/vaccines/programs/vfc/cdc-vac-price-list.htm#pediatric

Centers for Disease Control and Prevention (CDC). (2011c). *Vaccines for Children program.* Retrieved from http://www.cdc.gov/vaccines/programs/vfc/

Centers for Disease Control and Prevention (CDC). (2012). Measles, 2011. *Morbidity and Mortality Weekly Report, 61*(15), 253–257.

Chayavichitsilp, P., Buckwalter, J., Krakowski, A. C., & Friedlander, S. F. (2009). Herpes simplex. *Pediatrics in Review, 30*(4), 119–129.

Chen, L. F., & Sexton, D. J. (2008). What's new in Rocky Mountain spotted fever? *Infectious Disease Clinics of North America, 22,* 415–432

Children's Hospital of Philadelphia. (2010). *Vaccine education center.* Retrieved from http://www.chop.edu/service/vaccine-education-center/home.html

Czaja, A. S., Zimmerman, J. J., & Nathans, A. B. (2009). Readmission and late mortality after pediatric severe sepsis. *Pediatrics, 123*(3), 849–857.

Dorrell, C., Stokley, S., Yankey, D., & Cohn, A. (2010). National, state, local area vaccination coverage among adolescents aged 13–17 years—United States, 2009. *Morbidity and Mortality Weekly Report, 59*(32), 1018–1023.

Edwards, K. M., & Johnson, D. R. (2007). Rising to the challenge of pertussis persistence. *Clinical Advisor, 10*(6), 58–77.

Federico, S. G., Abrams, L., Everhart, R. M., Melinkovich, P., & Hambidge, S. J. (2010). Addressing adolescent immunization disparities: A retrospective analysis of school-based health center immunization delivery. *American Journal of Public Health, 100*(9), 1630–1634.

Grijalva, C. G., Griffin, M. R., Nuorti, J. P., & Walter, N. D. (2009). Pneumonia hospitalizations among young children before and after introduction of pneumococcal conjugate vaccine—United States, 1997–2006. *Morbidity and Mortality Weekly Report, 58*(01), 1–4.

Hall, M., Noble, A., & Smith, S. (2009). *A foundation for neonatal care: A multi-disciplinary guide.* New York: Radcliff Publishing.

Hayden, G. F. (2010). The newly licensed pneumococcal conjugate vaccine: Questions and answers. *Consultant for Pediatricians, 9*(6), 203–206.

Hazinski, M. F., Mondozzi, M. A., & Baker, R. A. U. (2010). Shock, multiple organ dysfunction syndrome and burns in children. In K. L. McCance, S. E. Huether, V. L. Brashers, & N. S. Rote, *Pathophysiology: The biologic basis for disease in adults and children* (6th ed., pp. 1727–1754). St. Louis, MO: Elsevier Mosby.

Health Resources and Services Administration. (2011). *National Vaccine Injury Compensation Program.* Retrieved from http://www.hrsa.gov/vaccinecompensation/vaccineinjurytable.pdf

Hensley, E., & Briars, L. (2010). Closer look at autism and the measles-mumps-rubella vaccine. *Journal of the American Pharmacists Association, 50*(6), 736–741.

Heymann, D. L. (2008). *Control of communicable diseases manual* (19th ed.). Washington, DC: American Public Health Association.

Huether, S. E. (2010). Pain, temperature regulation, sleep, and sensory function. In K. L. McCance, S. E. Huether, V. L. Brashers, & N. S. Rote, *Pathophysiology: The biologic basis for disease in adults and children* (6th ed., pp. 481–524). St. Louis, MO: Mosby Elsevier.

Immunization Action Coalition. (2010). *Historic dates and events related to vaccines and immunization.* Retrieved from http://www.immunize.org/timeline/

Jackson, L. A., Starkovich, P., Dunstan, M., Yu, O., Nelson, J., Dunn, J., . . . Decker, M. (2008). Prospective assessment of the effect of needle length and injection site on the risk of local reactions to the fifth diphtheria-tetanus-acellular pertussis vaccination. *Pediatrics, 121*(3), e646–e652.

Kest, H. E., & Pineda, C. (2008). Lyme disease: Prevention, diagnosis, and management. *Contemporary Pediatrics, 25*(6), 56–64.

King, J. (2009). Infectious mononucleosis: Update and considerations. *Nurse Practitioner, 34*(11), 42–45.

Klein, N. P., Fireman, B., Yih, W. K., Lewis, E., Kulldorff, M., Ray, P., . . . Weintraub, E. (2010). Measles-mumps-rubella-varicella combination vaccine and the risk of febrile seizures. *Pediatrics, 126*(1), e1–e8.

Kman, N. E., & Nelson, R. N. (2008). Infectious agents of bioterrorism: A review for emergency physicians. *Emergency Medicine Clinics of North America, 26,* 517–547.

Koenig, J. M., & Keenan, W. J. (2009). Group B Streptococcus and early-onset sepsis in the era of maternal prophylaxis. *Pediatric Clinics of North America, 56,* 689–708.

Kroger, A. T., Sumaya, C. V., Pickering, L. K., & Atkinson, W. L. (2011). General recommendations on immunization: Recommendations of the Advisory Committee on Immunization Practices (ACIP). *Morbidity and Mortality Weekly Report, 60*(2), 1–62.

Luthy, K. E., Sperhac, A. M., Faux, S. A., & Miner, J. K. (2010). Improving immunization rates in the clinic and community. *Contemporary Pediatrics, 27*(9), 54–60.

Mali, S., Steele, S., Slutsker, L., & Arguin, P. M. (2010). Malaria surveillance—United States, 2008. *Morbidity and Mortality Weekly Report, 59*(SS-7), 1–3.

Mathur, M. B., Mathur, V. S., & Reichling, D. B. (2010). Participation in the decision to become vaccinated against human papillomavirus by California high school girls and the predictors of vaccine status. *Journal of Pediatric Health Care, 24*(1), 14–24.

Merck & Co. (2011). *Pneumovax 23: Pneumococcal vaccine polyvalent.* Retrieved from http://www.fda.gov/downloads/BiologicsBloodVaccines/Vaccines/ApprovedProducts/UCM131661.pdf

Middleman, A. B., & Tung, J. S. (2010). Urban middle school parent perspectives: The vaccines they are willing to have their children receive using school-based immunization programs. *Journal of Adolescent Health, 47*(3), 249–253.

Miller, A. A. (2007). Alternating acetaminophen with ibuprofen for fever: Is this a problem? *Pediatric Annals, 36*(7), 384–388.

Mola, S. J., Nield, L. S., & Weisse, M. E. (2009). Meningococcal disease: Suspect it, treat it, prevent it. *Consultant for Pediatricians, 8*(4), 116–120.

Moran, G. J., Talan, D. A., & Abrahamian, F. M. (2008). Biologic terrorism. *Infectious Disease Clinics of North America, 22,* 145–187.

Nield, L. S., Troischt, M. J., & Kamat, D. (2009). Vaccinating the immunocompromised child. *Consultant for Pediatricians, 8*(Suppl. 10), S7–S14.

Nuorti, J. P., & Whitney, C. G. (2010). Prevention of pneumococcal disease among infants and children—Use of 13-valent pneumococcal conjugate vaccine and 23-valent pneumococcal polysaccharide vaccine. *Morbidity and Mortality Weekly Report, 59*(RR-11), 1–20.

Prymula, R., Siegrist, C., Chlibek, R., Zemlickova, H., Vackova, M., Smetana, J., . . . Schuerman, L. (2009). Effect of prophylactic paracetamol administration at time of vaccination on febrile reactions and antibody responses in children: Two open-label, randomized controlled trials. *Lancet, 374*(9698), 1339–1350.

Purssell, E. (2009). Uncertainties and anxieties about vaccination, answering parent's concerns. *Journal of Pediatric Nursing, 24*(5), 433–440.

Rossi, S. L., Ross, T. M., & Evans, J. D. (2010). West Nile virus. *Clinical Laboratory Medicine, 30,* 47–65.

Rubarth, L. B. (2010). Sepsis, pneumonia, and meningitis: What is the difference? *Newborn and Infant Reviews, 10*(4), 177–181.

Rupprecht, C. E., Briggs, D., Brown, C. M., Franka, R., Katz, S. I., Kerr, H. D., . . . Centers for Disease Control and Prevention (CDC). (2010). Use of a reduced (4 dose) vaccine schedule for postexposure prophylaxis to prevent human rabies. *Morbidity and Mortality Weekly Report, 59*(RR-2), 1–10.

Savely, V. (2010). Lyme disease: A diagnostic dilemma. *Nurse Practitioner, 35*(7), 44–50.

Senior, K. (2008). *Yersinia pestis*: A force to be reckoned with. *Lancet Infectious Diseases, 8*(12), 746.

Shapiro, E. D., Vazquez, M., Esposito, D., Holabird, N., Steinberg, S. P., Dziura, J., . . . Gershon, A. A. (2011). Effectiveness of 2 doses of varicella vaccine in children. *Journal of Infectious Disease, 203*(3), 312–315.

Smith, M. J., & Marshall, G. S. (2010). Navigating parental vaccine hesitancy. *Pediatric Annals, 39*(8), 476–482.

Snow, M. (2011). Human rabies: Treatment and prevention. *Nursing 2011, 41*(4), 65–66.

Spicer, K. B., & Powell, D. A. (2010). Immunizations for internationally adopted children. *Pediatric Annals, 39*(8), 517–524.

Spratling, R., & Carmon, M. (2010). Pertussis: An overview of the disease, immunization, and trends for nurses. *Pediatric Nursing, 36*(5), 239–243.

Stevenson, A. M. (2009, November). Factors influencing immunization rates. *Clinical Advisor*, 19–26.

Tamma, P. (2010). Vaccines in immunocompromised patients. *Pediatrics in Review, 31*(1), 38–40.

Thomas, T. L. (2008). The new human papillomavirus (HPV) vaccine: Pros and cons for pediatric and adolescent health. *Pediatric Nursing, 34*(5), 429–431.

U.S. Department of Health and Human Services. (2010). *Healthy People 2020*. Retrieved from http://www.healthypeople.gov/2020/topicsobjectives2020/overview.aspx?topicid=23

U.S. Food and Drug Administration. (2011). *Fluzone vaccine safety*. Retrieved from http://www.fda.gov/BiologicsBloodVaccines/SafetyAvailability/VaccineSafety/ucm240037.htm

Woo, T. M. (2010). 2009 H1N1 influenza pandemic. *Journal of Pediatric Health Care, 24*(4), 258–266.

Wooten, K. G., Kolasa, M., Singleton, J. A., & Shefer, A. (2010). National, state, and local area vaccination coverage among children aged 19–35 months—United States, 2009. *Morbidity and Mortality Weekly Report, 59*(36), 1171–1177.

World Health Organization. (2009). *World Health Organization guidelines on hand hygiene in health care* (p. 151). Geneva, Switzerland: Author. Retrieved from http://whqlibdoc.who.int/publications/2009/9789241597906_eng.pdf

Wynn, J. L., & Levy, O. (2010). Role of innate host defenses in susceptibility to early-onset neonatal sepsis. *Clinics in Perinatology, 37*, 307–337.

Pearson Nursing Student Resources
Find additional review materials at
nursing.pearsonhighered.com
Prepare for success with additional NCLEX®-style practice questions, interactive assignments and activities, web links, animations and videos, and more!

Nursing Care of Specific Health Conditions

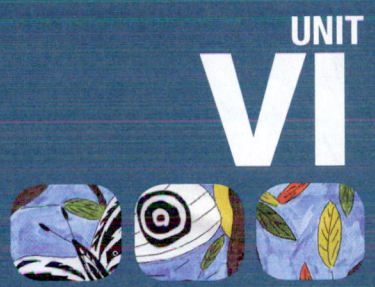

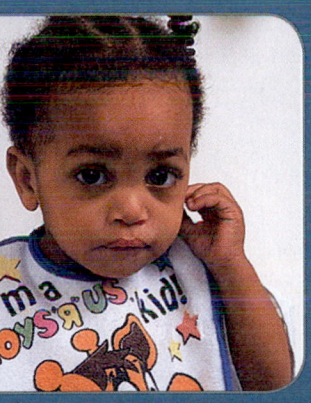 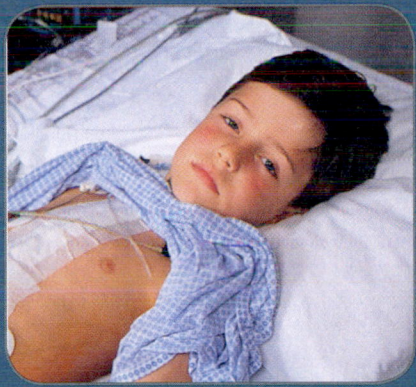 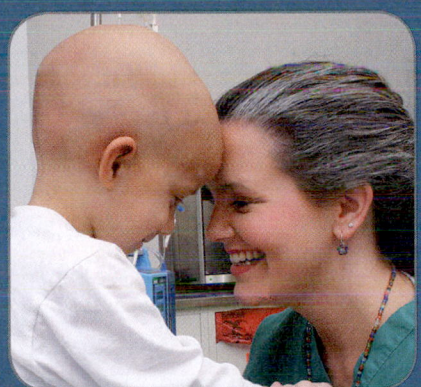 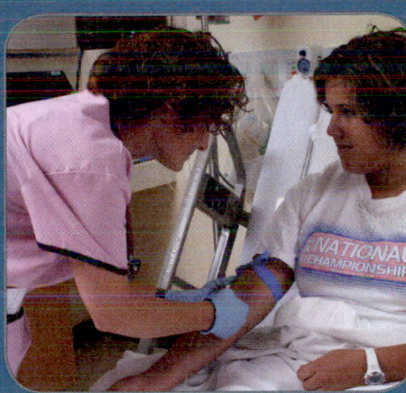

A child's healthcare needs are determined by the developmental level and specific health condition. The child may experience a health alteration related to any one body system, or may experience health alterations to several body systems simultaneously. The nurse applies knowledge of growth and development, anatomy, and pathophysiology in assessing the child with an altered health status. Psychosocial care is integrated into assessments and interventions. The nurse partners with the family in establishing a plan of care that will promote optimal achievement of growth and development, which may be affected by specific health conditions. The nurse also collaborates with other health professionals to provide individualized health care to the child and family.

CHAPTER 23

Alterations in Fluid, Electrolyte, and Acid–Base Balance

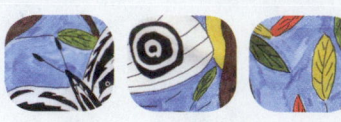

Learning Outcomes

After completing this chapter, you will be able to:

1. Describe normal fluid and electrolyte status for children at various ages.

2. Identify regulatory mechanisms for fluid and electrolyte balance.

3. Interpret threats to fluid and electrolyte balance in children.

4. Analyze assessment findings to recognize fluid-electrolyte problems and acid–base imbalance in children.

5. Integrate assessment information to plan appropriate interventions for children experiencing fluid-electrolyte problems and acid–base imbalance.

> "Vernon didn't want to play. Grandma says Mommy took him to the clinic so they can make him better."
>
> —*Shawna, age 4*

Vernon Smith is 18 months old. Several days ago he developed vomiting and diarrhea. His parents tried to get him to eat, but he had little appetite. He drank a few sips of water and juice, but the next morning he was listless and would not drink anything. The diarrhea continued.

Vernon's mother brought him to the urgent care center. Vernon is irritable on arrival, and his mother reports that he has been alternately irritable and lethargic. His mucous membranes and tongue appear dry, and skin turgor over the abdomen is slightly decreased. His mother notes that Vernon has had only two wet diapers today and says the urine in his diapers was dark in color. She also reports that he weighed 26 lb (12 kg) at the clinic last week. However, when the nurse weighs him, the scale reads only 24.5 lb (11 kg). Vernon is moderately dehydrated and needs rapid replacement of the proper type of fluids. He is started on oral replacement therapy at the urgent care center and is expected to stay several hours for monitoring. His mother makes arrangements for someone to care for her 4-year-old daughter, Shawna, at home for the day.

What happens inside the body when dehydration occurs? How can a nurse recognize dehydration? What laboratory studies provide clues to the degree of Vernon's dehydration? What types of fluid does Vernon need? What nursing management is important for his recovery? Why are young children at greater risk for dehydration than adults? What do parents need to be taught to prevent and manage dehydration? This chapter presents information that will enable you to answer these questions.

urses need to thoroughly understand fluid, electrolyte, and acid–base homeostasis and imbalances when providing care to pediatric patients like Vernon, in the preceding scenario. In this chapter, we present information about the processes that maintain fluid and electrolyte balance, and describe the common imbalances that may occur in children. We also describe how the body regulates acid–base status and explain the management of acid–base imbalances.

Many health conditions cause changes in body fluids and electrolytes, or alter acid–base balance, including gastroenteritis, burns, respiratory problems, and kidney disorders. Sometimes management of fluid status in the home or in a short-term ambulatory facility can prevent more serious illness or hospitalization. Children who cannot take in normal fluids by mouth due to surgery need short-term management of fluid by intravenous (IV) route. In specialized areas such as newborn and pediatric intensive care units, emergency rooms, and operative suites, nurses provide intensive and careful management of fluids. When children with a chronic condition cannot ingest adequate fluids due to neuromuscular conditions, gastrostomy feeding tubes and other measures can ensure balanced intake. In all of these cases, nursing care is essential to evaluate intake, assess the child, and plan and implement appropriate interventions.

Although disruptions in fluid balance usually occur during an illness, at other more predictable times the child may require management to prevent fluid imbalance. For example, athletes and those exercising in hot weather need management of intake to promote fluid and electrolyte balance. The nurse is well positioned to work with families to promote health by maintenance of fluid balance and can use a preventive approach to ensure fluid balance. Nurses also partner with childcare centers and schools to plan for offering appropriate fluid for children. In all clinical settings, nurses partner with parents so they are aware of fluid needs for children of various ages in differing environments and who have different degrees of activity.

ANATOMY AND PHYSIOLOGY

Physiology of Fluid and Electrolyte Balance

Fluid in the body is in a dynamic state, necessary to achieve proper balance of fluids and electrolytes. In persons of all ages, fluid continuously leaves the body through the skin, in feces and urine, and during respiration. Much of the human body is composed of water. **Body fluid** is body water that has solutes dissolved in it. Some of the solutes are **electrolytes,** or charged particles (ions). Electrolytes such as sodium (Na^+), potassium (K^+), calcium (Ca^{++}), magnesium (Mg^{++}), chloride (Cl^-), and inorganic phosphorus (Pi) ions must be present in the proper concentrations for cells to function effectively.

In persons of all ages, body fluid is located in several compartments. The two major fluid compartments contain the **intracellular fluid** (fluid inside the cells) and the **extracellular fluid** (fluid outside the cells). The extracellular fluid is made up of **intravascular fluid** (the fluid within the blood vessels) and **interstitial fluid** (the fluid between the cells and outside the blood and lymphatic vessels). Extracellular fluid accounts for about one third of total body water, and intracellular fluid accounts for about two thirds. The concentrations of electrolytes in the fluid differ depending on the fluid compartment. For example, extracellular fluid is rich in sodium ions; intracellular fluid, by contrast, is low in sodium ions but rich in potassium ions (Table 23–1).

TABLE 23–1	Electrolyte Concentrations in Body Fluid Compartments		
	EXTRACELLULAR FLUID (ECF)		**INTRACELLULAR FLUID (ICF)**
COMPONENTS	**VASCULAR**	**INTERSTITIAL**	
Na^+	High	High	Low
K^+	Low	Low	High
Ca^{++}	Low	Low	Low (higher than ECF)
Mg^{++}	Low	Low	High
Pi	Low	Low	High
Cl^-	High	High	Low
Proteins	High	Low	High

Fluid moves between the intravascular and interstitial compartments by a process called **filtration.** Water moves into and out of the cells by the process of **osmosis.** These processes are discussed later in the chapter. Electrolytes move over cell membranes both by **diffusion** of particles from a location of greater to less concentration, and by **active transport.** Active transport requires metabolic energy cost but is effective even against the concentration gradient; it therefore enables electrolytes to move from lower to higher areas of concentration.

Physiology of Acid–Base Balance

Normal acid–base balance is necessary for proper function of the cells and the body. The number of hydrogen ions (H^+) present in a fluid determines its acidity. Increasing the hydrogen ion concentration makes a solution more acidic. Because the hydrogen ion concentration in body fluids is very low, acidity is expressed as **pH** (the negative logarithm of the hydrogen ion concentration) rather than as the hydrogen ion concentration itself. The range of possible pH values is 1 to 14, with a pH of 7 being neutral. The lower the pH, the more acidic the solution. The higher the pH, the more basic the solution. Body fluids are normally slightly basic.

The pH of body fluids is regulated carefully to provide a suitable environment for cell function. The pH of the blood influences the pH inside the cells. **Acidemia** refers to a blood pH below normal levels, whereas **alkalemia** is an increased blood pH. For the enzymes outside the cells to function optimally, the pH must be in the normal range. If the pH inside the cells becomes too high or too low, then the speed of chemical reactions becomes inappropriate for proper cell function. Cell protein function relies on the correct level of hydrogen ions. Thus acid–base imbalances result in clinical signs and symptoms, and, in severe cases, they may cause death.

In the course of their normal function, all cells in the body produce two kinds of acids: carbonic acid (H_2CO_3) and metabolic (noncarbonic) acids. Carbonic acid is eliminated by the lungs in the form of carbon dioxide and water. Common metabolic acids include pyruvic acid, sulfuric acid, acetoacetic acid, lactic acid, hydrochloride acid, and beta-hydroxybutyric acid. These acids are released into the extracellular fluid and must be neutralized or excreted from the body to prevent dangerous accumulation. They can be neutralized to some degree by the buffers in body fluids and are excreted by the kidneys.

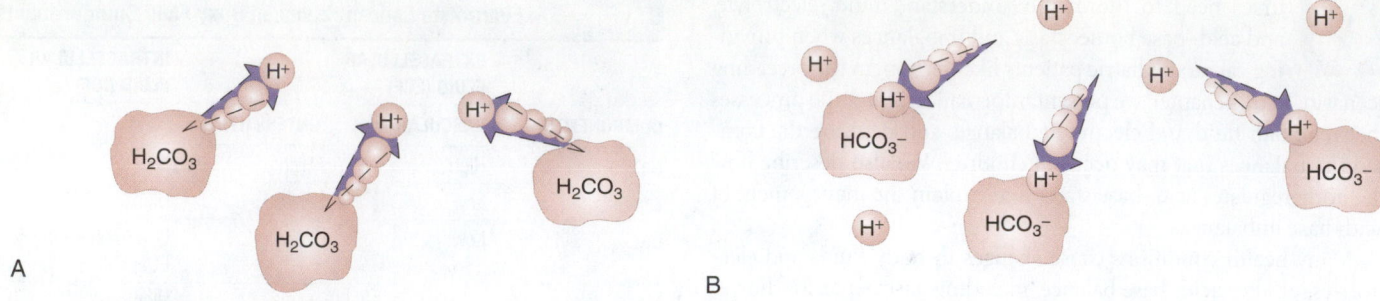

FIGURE 23–1 ■ *A,* How buffers respond to an excess of base. If the blood has too much base, the acid portion of a buffer pair (e.g., H_2CO_3 of the bicarbonate buffer system) releases hydrogen ions (H^+) to help return the pH to normal. *B,* How buffers respond to an excess of acid. If the blood has too much acid, the base portion of a buffer pair (e.g., HCO_3^- of the bicarbonate buffer system) takes up hydrogen ions (H^+) to help return the pH to normal.

Buffers

The maintenance of hydrogen ions within normal range relies heavily on buffers. A **buffer** is a compound that binds hydrogen ions when their concentration rises and releases them when the concentration falls (Figure 23–1 ■). Several kinds of buffers are present in the body (Table 23–2). Various body fluids have buffers to meet their special needs. The bicarbonate buffer system neutralizes metabolic acids (Figure 23–2 ■).

All buffer systems have limits. For example, if there are too many metabolic acids, the bicarbonate buffers become depleted. The acids then accumulate in the body until the kidneys excrete them. Clinically, this is seen as a decreased serum bicarbonate concentration and decreased blood pH.

Role of the Lungs

The lungs are responsible for excreting excess carbonic acid from the body. A child breathes out carbon dioxide and water, the components of carbonic acid, with each breath. With faster and deeper breaths, more carbonic acid is excreted. Since carbonic acid is converted in the body to carbon dioxide and water by the enzyme carbonic anhydrase, an indirect laboratory measurement of carbonic acid is $\mathbf{Pco_2}$, the partial pressure of carbon dioxide in arterial blood.

Although a child can voluntarily increase or decrease the rate and depth of respirations, they are usually involuntarily controlled. The $\mathbf{Po_2}$ (partial pressure of oxygen in arterial blood), Pco_2, and pH of the blood are monitored by chemoreceptors in the hypothalamus of the brain and in the aorta and carotid arteries. The input from the chemoreceptors is combined with other neural input to change breathing according to needs. Rate and depth increase or decrease according to the amount of carbonic acid that needs to be excreted.

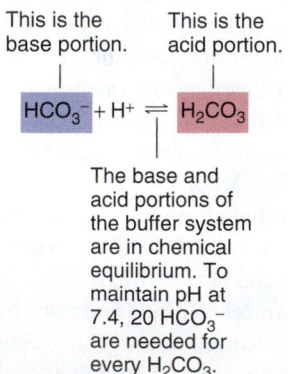

This is the base portion. This is the acid portion.

$$HCO_3^- + H^+ \rightleftharpoons H_2CO_3$$

The base and acid portions of the buffer system are in chemical equilibrium. To maintain pH at 7.4, 20 HCO_3^- are needed for every H_2CO_3.

FIGURE 23–2 ■ The bicarbonate buffer system.

If a child has a condition that decreases the excretion of carbonic acid or causes breathing to be too slow or shallow (such as overmedication following surgery), carbonic acid accumulates in the blood. Clinically, this manifests as an increased blood Pco_2 and is a form of respiratory acidosis. The reverse will also be true in the child breathing excessively or deeply, which leads to decreased Pco_2 and respiratory alkalosis.

Role of the Kidneys

The kidneys regulate metabolic acids from the body in two ways. They reabsorb filtered bicarbonate to prevent its loss in the urine, and they regenerate bicarbonate when needed to restore balance. Bicarbonate is formed when acids and ammonium combine with extra ions. Blood bicarbonate concentration is an indicator of the amount of metabolic acids present, because bicarbonate is used in buffering the acids. When the concentration is normal, metabolic acids are present in usual amounts (Figure 23–3 ■).

Fluid homeostasis is maintained by several body systems that influence the kidneys. Excess elimination of body fluid is prevented by *antidiuretic hormone* (ADH), which is secreted by the hypothalamus in response to osmolality of extracellular fluids and fluid volume in intravascular spaces. The *renin-angiotensin system* regulates fluid status by a complex hormone balance system. The kidneys release *renin* when intravascular fluid volume is low; renin acts on a substance released by the liver to produce *angiotensin*; angiotensin constricts blood vessels and promotes secretion of *aldosterone* from the adrenal cortex; aldosterone then causes the kidneys to increase reabsorption of sodium and water. See Chapter 31 🖉 for further information regarding kidney regulation.

In a healthy child, the result of these renal processes is excretion of metabolic acids and maintenance of blood bicarbonate concentration within normal limits. When acidosis occurs, these processes may take several hours to days to be effective in restoring balance. In the child whose kidneys are not producing enough urine, metabolic acids may not be effectively excreted. Accumulation of these acids uses

TABLE 23–2	Important Buffers
BUFFER	**MAJOR LOCATIONS IN THE BODY**
Bicarbonate	Plasma; interstitial fluid
Protein	Plasma; inside cells
Hemoglobin	Inside red blood cells
Phosphate	Inside cells; urine

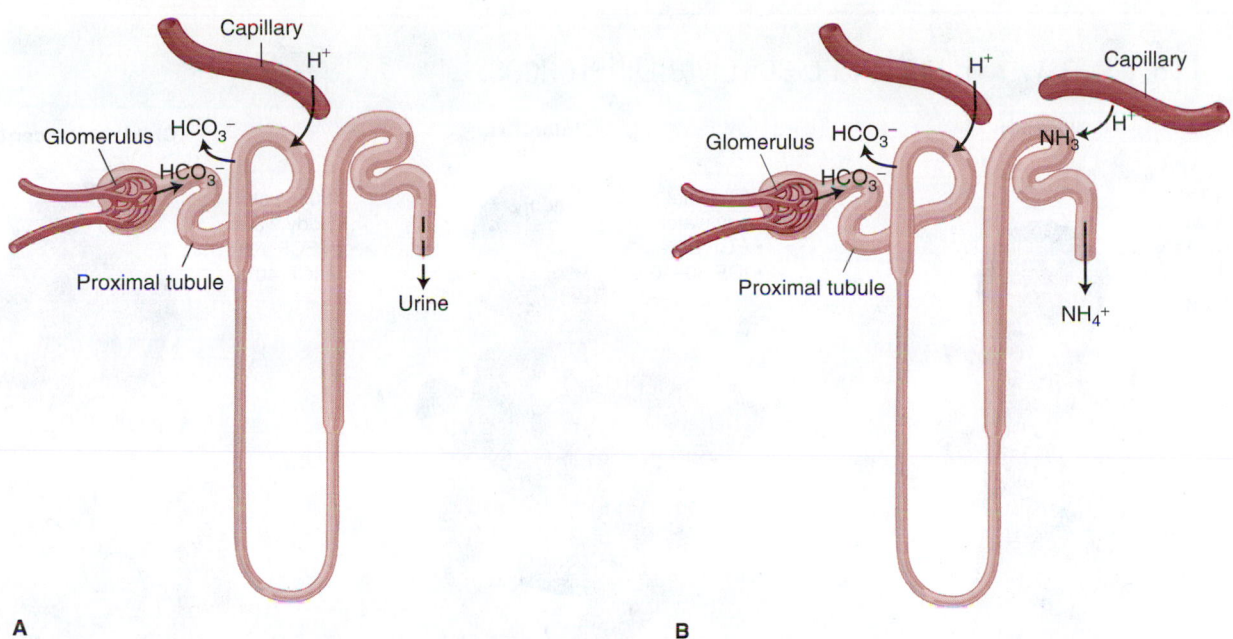

A
B

FIGURE 23–3 ■ The kidneys and metabolic acids. *A*, Recycling of bicarbonate by the kidneys. Bicarbonate ions that are in the blood are filtered into the renal tubules at the glomerulus. In the proximal tubules, bicarbonate ions are reabsorbed into the blood at the same time that hydrogen ions are transported from the blood into the renal tubular fluid. *B*, Secretion and buffering of hydrogen ions in the kidneys. If the urine is too acidic, the cells that line the urinary tract could be damaged. To prevent this problem, hydrogen ions secreted into the distal tubules are neutralized by phosphate buffers or bound to ammonia and excreted in the form of ammonium ions.

up many of the available bicarbonate buffers, resulting in a decreased serum bicarbonate concentration and metabolic acidosis.

Role of the Liver

The liver plays a role in maintaining acid–base balance by metabolizing protein, which produces hydrogen ions. It also synthesizes proteins needed to maintain osmotic pressures in the fluid compartments.

PEDIATRIC DIFFERENCES

The physiology of infants and young children makes them more vulnerable than adults to fluid, electrolyte, and acid–base imbalances. The percentage of body weight that is composed of water varies with age (Figure 23–4 ■). The percentage is highest at birth (and higher in premature than in full-term infants) and decreases with age (see Figure 23–5 ■ As They Grow: Fluid and Electrolyte Differences). Neonates and young infants have a proportionately larger extracellular fluid volume than older children and adults because their brain and skin (both rich in interstitial fluid) occupy a greater proportion of their body weight. Much of our extracellular fluid is exchanged each day. During infancy, there is a high daily fluid requirement with little fluid volume reserve; this makes the infant vulnerable to dehydration. As an infant grows, the proportion of water inside the cells increases, the extracellular amount decreases in comparison, and the risk of fluid imbalance begins to decrease.

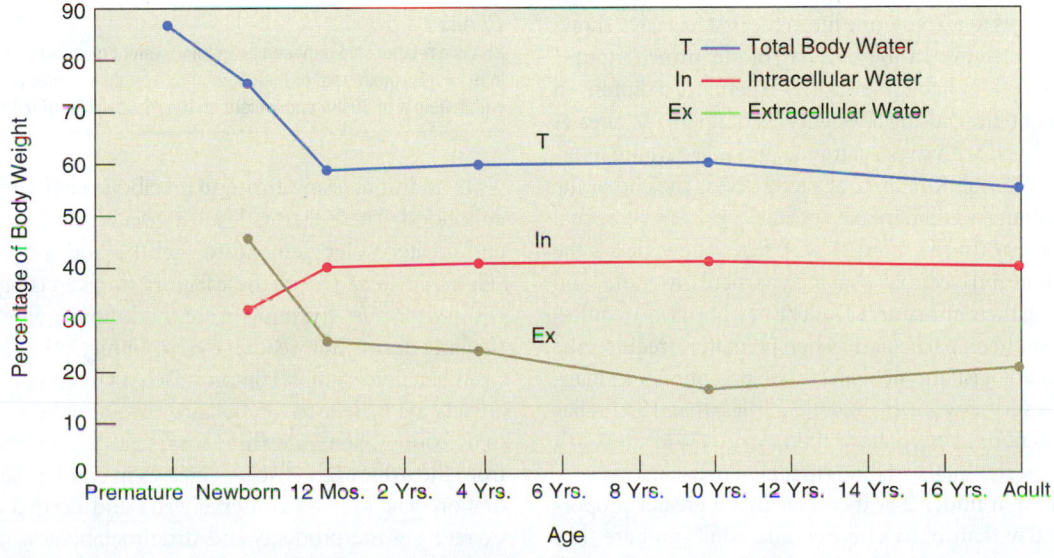

FIGURE 23–4 ■ The major body fluid compartments at various ages. *Extracellular* fluid is composed mainly of intravascular fluid (fluid in blood vessels) and interstitial fluid (fluid between the cells and outside the blood and lymphatic vessels). *Intracellular* fluid is that within cells.

Source: *From Bindler, R., & Howry, L. (2005). Pediatric drug guide. Upper Saddle River, NJ: Prentice Hall.*

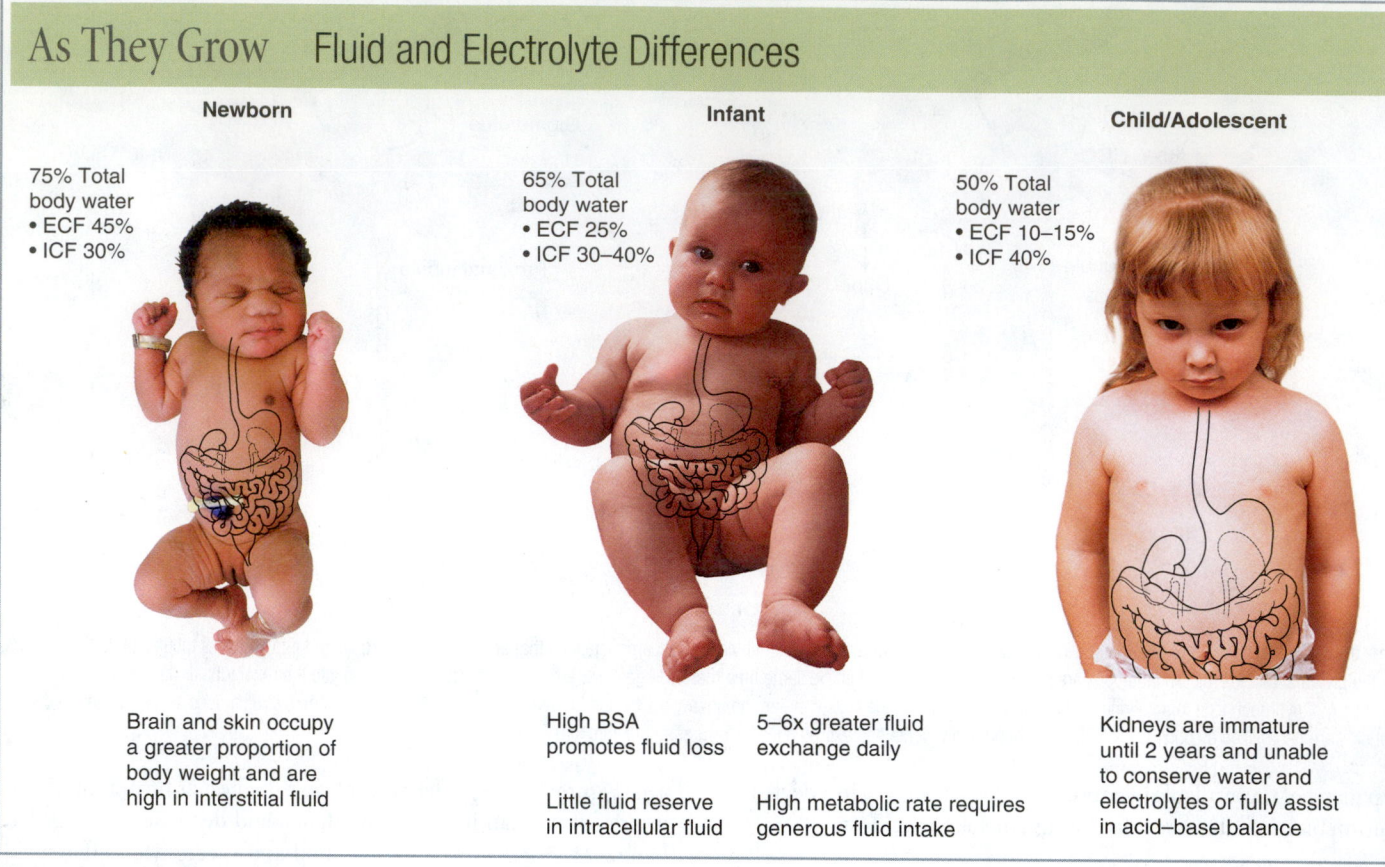

As They Grow   Fluid and Electrolyte Differences

Newborn

75% Total
body water
• ECF 45%
• ICF 30%

Brain and skin occupy
a greater proportion of
body weight and are
high in interstitial fluid

Infant

65% Total
body water
• ECF 25%
• ICF 30–40%

High BSA
promotes fluid loss

Little fluid reserve
in intracellular fluid

5–6x greater fluid
exchange daily

High metabolic rate requires
generous fluid intake

Child/Adolescent

50% Total
body water
• ECF 10–15%
• ICF 40%

Kidneys are immature
until 2 years and unable
to conserve water and
electrolytes or fully assist
in acid–base balance

FIGURE 23–5 ■ The newborn and infant have a high percentage of body weight composed of water, especially extracellular fluid, which is lost from the body easily. Note the small stomach size which limits ability to rehydrate quickly.

The newborn has the most striking differences in fluid status from older infants. These include:

- Basal metabolic rate twice that of children
- Approximately 4 to 5 times greater water intake needs/kg of body weight
- Only 10% of the ability to excrete sodium (Gardner, Carter, Enzman-Hines, et al., 2010)

The newborn adapts to extrauterine life in the first few days, showing variations in fluid status. In the first day of life, urine output is limited and body weight is stable. Newborns experience a diuresis in the first 3 to 5 days of life, causing a weight loss of up to 7%. Greater weight loss is associated with hypernatremia and may require intervention (Kusuma, Agrawal, Kumar, et al., 2009). Near the end of the first week, urine output and fluid intake become approximately equal in amount. Prematurity (born before 37 weeks' gestation) delays the ability to manage fluid and electrolyte balance, particularly due to fluid and heat loss through their immature skin. The newborn who requires surgery or other treatment, particularly when premature, requires the expertise of a neonatologist and neonatal nurse practitioner to manage fluid needs. The very-low-birth-weight baby (less than 1500 g) has an even greater than normal loss of body fluid in the period after birth and often requires greater intake of fluids to maintain balance.

Infants and children under 2 years of age lose a greater proportion of fluid each day than older children and adults and are thus more dependent on adequate intake. They have a greater amount of skin surface or **body surface area (BSA)** (relationship between height and weight measured in squared meters) and thus have greater

insensible fluid loss through the skin. Because of this large BSA, they are also at greater risk when burned. See the Skills Manual 🔗 and Appendix G 🔗 for further description of BSA, which is often considered when determining fluid needs of infants and children over 10 kg in weight, and can be used to calculate medication dosages for children.

Clinical Tip

BSA is a relationship between height and weight measured in squared meters. BSA in m^2 = the square root of [height in cm × weight in kg]/3600. For example, a child with a height of 80 cm and weight of 10 kg has a BSA of 0.48 m^2.

In addition, respiratory and metabolic rates are high during early childhood. These factors lead to greater water loss from the lungs and greater water demand to fuel the body's metabolic processes (Figure 23–6 ■). Due to these factors, the exercising child dehydrates easily and must consume more fluid during physical activity, particularly during hot weather (Mayo Clinic, 2011).

When fluid status is compromised, a number of body mechanisms are activated to help restore balance. Several of these mechanisms occur in the kidney. **Sensible fluid loss,** that which is measurable, such as from the urine and bowels, decreases in compensation during dehydration. The kidneys conserve water and needed electrolytes while excreting waste products and drug metabolites. In children under 2 years of age, however, the glomeruli, tubules, and nephrons of the kidneys are immature. They are thus unable to conserve or excrete water and solutes effectively (see Chapter 31 🔗). Because more water is

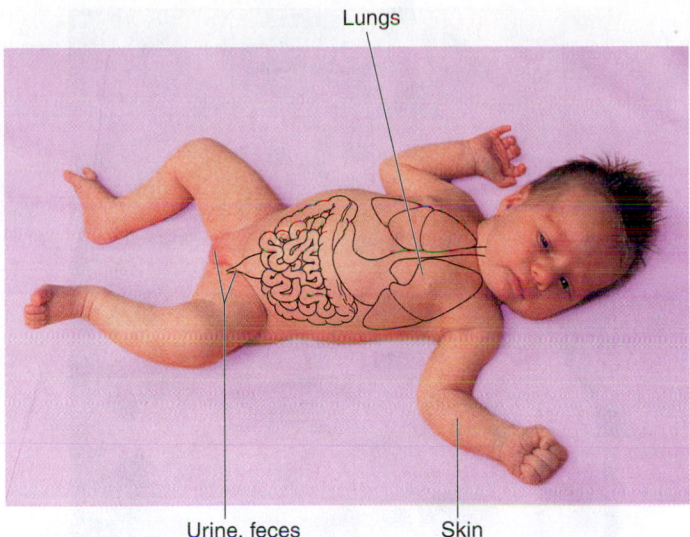

Lungs

Urine, feces   Skin

FIGURE 23–6 ■ Normal routes of fluid excretion from infants and children.

generally excreted, the infant and young child can become dehydrated quickly or develop electrolyte imbalances. In addition, infants have a weaker transport system for ions and bicarbonate, placing them at greater risk for acidosis and acid–base imbalances. Children under 2 years of age also have difficulty regulating electrolytes such as sodium and calcium. Renal response to high solute loads is slower and less developed, with function improving gradually during the first year of life.

Finally, in addition to the immaturity of physiologic processes, many health conditions make young children more vulnerable to fluid deficit (Box 23–1). See Table 23–3 for assessment categories for these body functions. See Table 23–4 for common laboratory tests used to assess fluid, electrolyte, and acid–base balance.

FLUID VOLUME IMBALANCES

When fluid excretion and losses are matched by the proper volume and type of fluid intake, fluid balance will be maintained. If, however, fluid output and intake are not matched, fluid imbalance may occur rapidly. The major types of fluid imbalances are extracellular fluid volume deficit (**dehydration**), extracellular fluid volume excess, and interstitial fluid volume excess (**edema**).

Extracellular Fluid Volume Imbalances

Extracellular Fluid Volume Deficit (Dehydration)
Extracellular fluid volume deficit occurs when there is not enough fluid in the extracellular compartment (intravascular and interstitial).

BOX 23–1	Health Conditions Contributing to Fluid Imbalance

- Radiant heat (phototherapy) used to treat hyperbilirubinemia increases insensible fluid loss through the skin.
- The increased respiratory rate in some illnesses leads to excessive water loss from the lungs.
- Fever increases the metabolic rate and, therefore, the water demands due to increased metabolism.
- Vomiting and diarrhea increase fluid and electrolyte losses from the gastrointestinal system.
- Fistulas, blood loss, and drainage tubes contribute to fluid deficits.
- Renal disease can influence rates of fluid excretion and urine concentration.

TABLE 23–3	Assessment Guidelines for the Child with a Fluid, Electrolyte, or Acid–Base Alteration*
ASSESSMENT FOCUS	**ASSESSMENT GUIDELINES**
Body weight	■ Has weight decreased since the last measurement or weight reported by the family?
	■ If so, how much? What percent of body weight is the weight loss?
Skin and mucous membranes	■ What are the temperature, turgor, and moistness of the skin?
	■ Examine skin turgor where most descriptive for children (chest, abdomen, upper thighs).
	■ Describe moistness of oral mucous membranes.
	■ Describe moistness of the eyes and presence of tears.
	■ Is edema present in any body parts?
Cardiovascular and respiratory systems	■ What are the pulse and blood pressure?
	■ Test capillary refill time. Capillary refill is tested on the forehead, chest, abdomen, or palm of the hand.
	■ What is the respiratory rate? Is the rate regular?
Gastrointestinal system	■ Does the child have nausea, vomiting, or diarrhea? If so, how often and for how long has it continued?
	■ Is the child eating and drinking? How much and what types of foods and fluids?
Urinary system	■ What is the child's urinary output?
	■ What is the urine specific gravity?
Musculoskeletal system	■ Describe muscle tone and symmetry.
Neurologic system	■ Describe the child's state of alertness and any changes observed.
	■ What is the level of consciousness?
	■ Is the anterior fontanel at the skin surface or does it appear sunken?

Note: *Refer to Chapter 7 🖉 for the actual techniques of assessment mentioned in this table.

TABLE 23–4	Diagnostic Procedures and Laboratory Tests for Fluid, Electrolytes, and Acid–Base Balance*
LABORATORY TEST	**PURPOSE**
Serum electrolyte panel (e.g., sodium, potassium, chloride, bicarbonate)	The variety of electrolytes measured in the serum can reflect imbalances in water and electrolyte values. They provide the basis for further assessment and diagnosis of the condition and for the types of fluids needed during management to reestablish balance.
Arterial blood gases	Arterial blood can be analyzed for pH, partial pressure of carbon dioxide (Pco_2), partial pressure of oxygen (Po_2), and serum bicarbonate (HCO_3^-). Levels are analyzed for information about acid–base balance.
Urinary specific gravity	This measure of urine's density is used to assess its concentration. An increasing number indicates higher concentration of molecules, signifying lower levels of hydration.

Note: *See Appendix D and E 🖉 for information about these diagnostic procedures and for expected laboratory tests values.

Depending on the cause of dehydration, sodium may be at a normal, low, or elevated level. (Hyponatremia and hypernatremia are described later in the chapter, on pages 670–673.) The state of body water deficit is called dehydration. There are three major types of dehydration:

- **Isotonic dehydration (isonatremic dehydration)** occurs when fluid loss is not balanced by intake, and the loss of water and loss of sodium are in proportion. The serum sodium is therefore within normal limits even though the circulating blood volume is lowered. Most of the fluid lost is from the extracellular component. This type of dehydration is commonly manifested in the illnesses of young children such as vomiting and diarrhea.

- **Hypotonic dehydration (hyponatremic dehydration)** occurs when fluid loss is characterized by a proportionately greater loss of sodium than water. Serum sodium is below normal levels. Compensatory fluid shifts occur from the extracellular to intracellular components in an attempt to establish normal proportions, thus leading to even greater extracellular dehydration. Severe and prolonged vomiting and diarrhea, burns, and renal disease can lead to this condition, as well as administration of intravenous fluid without electrolytes in treatment of dehydration.

- **Hypertonic dehydration (hypernatremic dehydration)** occurs when sodium loss is proportionately less than water loss. Serum sodium is above normal levels. Compensatory fluid shifts occur from the intracellular to extracellular components in an attempt to establish normal proportions. The extracellular component therefore remains fairly normal, delaying the onset of signs and symptoms of dehydration until the condition is quite serious. Neurologic symptoms such as altered level of consciousness, confusion, lethargy, and dizziness, reflecting intracellular imbalance, may occur simultaneously with more common symptoms of dehydration. The condition may be caused by an uncommon health problem such as diabetes insipidus (see Chapter 32 🔗) or administration of intravenous fluid or tube feedings with high electrolyte levels.

The body continuously attempts to compensate for fluid and electrolyte imbalance by shifting fluid and electrolytes from one component to another. Therefore, it is rare for only one type of dehydration to occur. The child's fluid and electrolyte status and symptoms are constantly changing, so ongoing assessment and management will be needed when an imbalance is discovered.

Etiology and pathophysiology Extracellular fluid volume deficit is usually caused by the loss of sodium-containing fluid from the body. The situations that most often cause loss of fluid containing sodium are vomiting, diarrhea, nasogastric suction, hemorrhage, and burns. Vomiting and diarrhea are common manifestations of disease in children throughout the world, and each year up to 5 million children die from dehydration related to diarrhea. About 300 to 500 die annually in the United States from this problem, about 220,000 are hospitalized (accounting for 9% of pediatric hospitalizations), and about 1.5 million receive care on an outpatient basis (Canavan & Arant, 2009; Diggins, 2008). See Chapter 30 🔗 for a detailed description of gastroenteritis (vomiting and diarrhea) in children.

Young children who enter a parked car and are unable to get out, or are left in a closed car by parents, are at risk of dehydration and

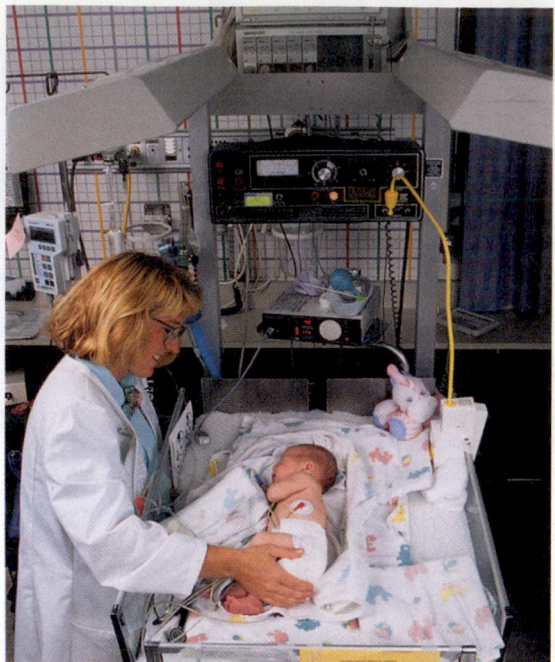

FIGURE 23–7 ■ Use of an overhead warmer or phototherapy increases insensible fluid excretion through the skin, thus increasing the fluid intake needed.

even death. Another cause of extracellular fluid volume deficit in infants is increased water loss in low-birth-weight infants who are kept under radiant warmers to maintain heat (Figure 23–7 ■). Their high BSA puts them at risk of dehydration due to insensible fluid loss through the skin. Less frequently, adrenal insufficiency, accumulation of extracellular fluid in a third space such as the peritoneal cavity (**third-spacing**), or overuse of diuretics may be the cause. The latter etiology is most often seen in adolescents who are bulimic for weight control (see Chapter 19 🔗).

Among young children, excessive activity during very hot weather without sufficient fluid replacement can lead to fluid and electrolyte imbalance. Children are more prone than adults to imbalance from exercise because of several of the physiologic differences described earlier in the chapter. Because children have a greater BSA than adults, they can gain more heat from the environment when it is hot, and lose more when it is cold. In addition, the high metabolic rate of children is further increased during exercise so that fluid lost in metabolism is significant. Young children do not sweat effectively and may be unable to eliminate heat by this method. Children may not feel thirsty and so fail to drink even when dehydrated (Centers for Disease Control and Prevention, 2009). Additional risk factors include obesity; vigorous outdoor activity in heat; and a combination of high temperature, high humidity, wind, and exposure to radiant heat (Centers for Disease Control and Prevention, 2010).

Burns involve complex health problems that are described in Chapter 36 🔗. Burns of the skin usually involve huge loss of body fluids, including water and electrolytes, particularly sodium. Hypotonic dehydration is the type most commonly seen in the initial period after a burn. Serum proteins are also lost so body fluid is more likely to leak into interstitial spaces, causing edema and further contributing to the fluid deficit. The kidneys decrease urine production because of their decreased blood flow leading to decreased urinary output. While the fluid imbalance of burns is therefore complicated, the first imbalance encountered is often that of dehydration with accompanying hyponatremia.

For burns, gastroenteritis, and other illness, initial dehydration in the first 3 days reflects a high loss of extracellular fluid. About 80% of the fluid loss is extracellular; about 20% is intracellular. With time, however, the relationship begins to change so that in illnesses over 3 days, about 60% of fluid loss is extracellular while 40% is intracellular (Tschudy & Arcara, 2011). Since the electrolyte composition of extracellular and intracellular fluids differs (see Table 23–1), electrolyte management will need to change for long-term conditions.

Clinical Tip
Many conditions that cause dehydration are accompanied by fever, which produces additional demands for fluid. For each degree of Celsius increase above 37°, 0.42 mL/kg/hr of additional fluid is needed.

Clinical manifestations The signs of dehydration relate to the severity or degree of the body water deficit (Table 23–5). They are a result of both the decreased fluid (e.g., diminished turgor and mucous membrane moisture) and the body's response to the fluid deficit (e.g., pulse and blood pressure changes). See page 658 for clinical manifestations of extracellular fluid volume deficit and page 658 for clinical manifestations of exertional heat illness.

Mild dehydration is hard to detect, because children appear alert and have moist mucous membranes. Infants may be irritable, and older children are thirsty. In moderate dehydration, the child is often lethargic and sleepy, but may have periods of restlessness and irritability, especially if an infant. Skin turgor is diminished, mucous membranes appear dry, and urine is dark in color and diminished in amount. Pulse rate is usually increased and blood pressure can be normal or low. Vernon, described at the beginning of this chapter, was displaying symptoms of moderate dehydration. His urine output

was decreased, and he had lost about 8% of his body weight. What other signs and symptoms of moderate dehydration can you identify in the opening scenario? What additional assessments would you want to perform on Vernon?

Clinical Tip
Normal urinary output is 0.5 to 1 mL/kg/hr for children and 2 mL/kg/hr for infants. Based on the child's weight in kg, calculate an expected urinary output. When output is less than that, be alert for other signs of dehydration and for reasons that dehydration may be occurring. In addition, consider the timing and frequency of voiding. Generally, lack of voiding for 4 hours, with no urge to void, indicates decreased urinary output and dehydration.

Severe dehydration is manifested by increasing lethargy, altered consciousness or nonresponsiveness, low to markedly decreased blood pressure, rapid thready pulse, poor skin turgor, dry mucous membranes, and markedly decreased (oliguria) or absent (anuria) urinary output.

Recall that in hypertonic dehydration, the more common symptoms of mild and moderate dehydration may be delayed since fluid is being moved from the intracellular to the extracellular component. Some of the first manifestations of dehydration may therefore indicate severe dehydration as compensatory mechanisms fail. Level of consciousness alterations, seizures, or profoundly decreased urinary output may manifest quickly.

Collaborative Care

Nurses work with other healthcare providers to provide care for the child with dehydration. Physicians, nurse practitioners, and physician assistants often provide primary care in hospitals, urgent care centers, and clinics to the child with extracellular fluid volume deficit. You will provide ongoing assessments, administer intravenous and oral fluids,

TABLE 23–5	Severity of Clinical Dehydration		
CLINICAL ASSESSMENT	**MILD**	**MODERATE**	**SEVERE**
Percent of body weight lost	Up to 5% (40–50 mL/kg)	6–9% (60–90 mL/kg)	10% or more (greater than 90 mL/kg)
Level of consciousness	Alert, restless, thirsty	Irritable or lethargic (infants and very young children); alert, thirsty, restless (older children and adolescents)	Lethargic to comatose (infants and young children); often conscious, apprehensive (older children and adolescents)
Blood pressure	Recommended level for age	Recommended or low; postural hypotension (older children and adolescents)	Low to undetectable
Pulse	Regular and strong	Rapid	Rapid, weak to nonpalpable
Skin turgor	Immediate; less than 2 seconds return after pinching skin	Poor; 2–3 seconds return after pinching skin	Very poor; 3–4 seconds return after pinching skin
Mucous membranes	Moist	Dry	Parched
Urine	Usual output	Decreased output (less than 1 mL/kg/hr), dark color; increased specific gravity	Very decreased or absent output
Thirst	Slightly increased	Moderately increased	Greatly increased unless lethargic
Fontanel	Usual for age	Sunken	Sunken
Extremities	Warm; rapid capillary refill of less than 2 seconds	Delayed capillary refill (greater than 2 seconds)	Cool, discolored; delayed capillary refill (greater than 3–4 seconds)
Respirations	Regular; usual rate	Usual or rapid rate	Changing rate and regularity
Eyes	Moist; usual appearance	Slightly sunken, decreased tears	Deeply sunken, absent tears

Source: *Data from Chameides, L., Samson, R. A., Schexnayder, S. M., & Hazinski, M. F. (2011).* PALS: Pediatric advanced life support provider manual. *Dallas, TX: American Heart Association; and Kliegman, R. M., Stanton, B. F., St. Geme, J., & Behrman, R. E. (2011).* Nelson textbook of pediatrics *(19th ed.). Philadelphia, PA: Saunders.*

Clinical Manifestations Exertional Heat Illness

CONDITION	ETIOLOGY	SIGNS AND SYMPTOMS
Exercise-associated muscle cramps (heat cramps)	Dehydration from profuse sweating Electrolyte imbalance with sodium losses replaced by hypotonic fluid Neuromuscular fatigue	Acute, painful skeletal muscle cramps often in lower legs Thirst Fatigue
Heat syncope	Loss of sodium and water Peripheral vasodilation Reduced cardiac output Cerebral ischemia	Tunnel vision Pale, sweaty skin Decreased pulse Dizziness, faintness
Heat exhaustion	Elevated core body temperature (but below 105°F) Sodium loss	Sweating, pallor (eventually decreased sweating) Dehydration Muscle cramps Nausea, anorexia, diarrhea Decreased urinary output Weakness, fainting, dizziness
Heatstroke	Elevated core temperature (greater than 105°F) Temperature regulation overwhelmed by heat production or absence of adequate heat loss Organ system failure from overheating (medical emergency)	Altered mental status, seizures, coma Tachycardia Hypotension Sweating Hyperventilation Vomiting, diarrhea Death can occur from severe acidosis, hyperkalemia, renal failure, and disseminated intravascular coagulation
Exertional hyponatremia	Serum sodium less than 130 mmol/L Exercise over 4 hours with water or other low-solute fluids for replenishment	Disorientation, headache, lethargy Swollen extremities Vomiting Pulmonary or cerebral edema Death can occur from sodium imbalance

Source: *Data from American Academy of Pediatrics. (2010). Exertional heat-related illness. Retrieved from http://www.healthychildren.org; Council on Sports Medicine and Fitness and Council on School Health. (2011). Policy statement—Climatic heat stress and exercising children and adolescents. Pediatrics, 128, e741–e747; Pagnotta, K. D., Mazerolle, S. M., & Casa, D. J. (2010). Exertional heat strokes and emergency issues in high school sport. Journal of Strength and Conditioning Research, 24(7), 1707–1709.*

and collect necessary laboratory specimens. Nurses also instruct parents about prevention, recognition, and treatment of dehydration.

Diagnostic Tests

The diagnosis of dehydration is best accomplished by clinical observations, as described in Table 23–5. A major indicator to the degree of dehydration is percent of weight loss. The serum electrolyte panel may be helpful in severe and continuing dehydration that is complicated by electrolyte imbalance or acidosis. The tests include serum electrolytes, creatinine, and glucose. Elevated blood urea nitrogen (greater than 17 mg/dL) and low serum bicarbonate (less than 16 to 17 mEq/L or 16 to 17 mmol/L) are useful to identify moderate and

Clinical Manifestations Extracellular Fluid Volume Deficit

ETIOLOGY	CLINICAL MANIFESTATIONS
Decreased fluid volume	Weight loss
	Sunken fontanel (infant)
Inadequate circulating blood volume to offset the force of gravity when in upright position	Postural blood pressure drop (older children) Dizziness
Decreased intravascular volume	Delayed capillary refill time Flat neck veins when supine (older children)
Inadequate circulation to the brain	Dizziness, syncope
Inadequate circulation to the kidneys	Oliguria
Cardiac reflex response to decreased intravascular volume	Thready, rapid pulse
Decreased interstitial fluid volume	Decreased skin turgor

Evidence-Based Practice

Oral Rehydration Therapy

PROBLEM

In spite of recommendations that children with mild or moderate dehydration be treated with oral rehydration therapy for gastroenteritis, many healthcare facilities and providers administer intravenous fluids to these children.

EVIDENCE

A nursing review of current literature reviewed recommendations from the American Academy of Pediatrics (AAP) and the World Health Organization (WHO) for treatment of childhood dehydration (Diggins, 2008). In the United States alone, gastroenteritis leads to 3 million healthcare visits annually. However, most children can effectively be treated with a solution of glucose, electrolyte, and water. Such treatment is less invasive and less painful for young children and is safe, effective, and easy to administer. A clinical pathway for nursing care in an emergency department that included assessment and oral rehydration initiation for dehydrated children decreased the length of visits (Doan, Chan, Leung, et al., 2010). Such treatment is less costly in addition to being easier to administer and more comfortable for the child (Pershad, 2010).

IMPLICATIONS

Nurses can partner with other healthcare professionals to establish clinical pathways for dehydration treatment that follow recommendations. Implementing oral rehydration therapy immediately after assessment of the child assists in effective treatment. Appropriate oral rehydration solutions should be available in pediatric units, emergency departments, and all homes with children.

CRITICAL THINKING APPLICATION

What questions can you ask a parent and what assessments will you perform to accurately evaluate if the child has mild or moderate dehydration? What oral rehydration solutions can the parent have available in the home setting? How will you inform colleagues of the current recommendations for treatment of children with dehydration?

---

severe diarrhea (Madati & Bachur, 2008). The results can be used to target the fluid type and amount to best meet the imbalances identified. Urine specific gravity may be elevated.

Clinical Judgment

Urine specific gravity, which reflects the concentration of urine, usually increases in older children who are dehydrated. However, due to the inability of the child under 2 years of age to concentrate urine effectively, do you think a rising specific gravity is commonly seen in the child under 2 years who is dehydrated? Why or why not?

Clinical Therapy

Prevention is best and allows for early identification of gastroenteritis and climatic heat stress (Council on Sports Medicine and Fitness & Council on School Health, 2011). Medical management depends on accurate identification of the degree of dehydration. The treatment for extracellular fluid volume deficit is administration of fluid containing sodium. This may be accomplished by oral rehydration therapy or by intravenous fluids.

Oral rehydration therapy has been used for many years in developing countries without an accessible supply of intravenous fluids. The benefits of using this therapy early to prevent severe dehydration and to treat mild and moderate dehydration in children in developed countries have now been recognized. The therapy is successful in treating the dehydration caused by many gastrointestinal illnesses and prevents hospitalization for many infants and young children. It is the treatment of choice for children with diarrhea who have mild to moderate dehydration (Colletti, Brown, Sharieff, et al., 2010; Tschudy & Arcara, 2011). Solutions are available commercially that contain water, carbohydrate (sugar), sodium, potassium, chloride, and lactate. Some clinicians allow lactose-free milk, breast milk, or half-strength milk to be given in addition to oral rehydration therapy solution. The WHO/UNICEF solution was developed for use with cholera and is not generally used for diarrhea treatment in the United States, as its sodium and chloride loads are higher than those of other commercial solutions. See Evidence-Based Practice: Oral Rehydration Therapy.

When the child is severely dehydrated, intravenous fluid is administered, often accompanied with oral rehydration. The intravenous fluid is often Ringer's lactate or 0.9% normal saline, followed by or accompanied with dilute saline, such as one-half or one-quarter normal saline. The fluid combination replenishes the extracellular fluid volume and adds solutes to return the body fluid to normal. See Table 23–6 for a description of the most common types of intravenous fluids, and see the Clinical Skills Manual for intravenous fluid initiation and management. The child may be hospitalized or treated with intravenous fluids in a short-stay unit until the dehydration is controlled. Once hydration is completed, the child may resume an age-appropriate diet. Children with profuse vomiting may be treated with one or more doses of a medication such as ondansetron (Zofran) to decrease vomiting and enhance the control of dehydration.

In developing countries with a high rate of diarrheal diseases in childhood, supplementation with zinc has been associated with less persistent and severe disease, and zinc supplementation in healthy children is associated with fewer episodes of diarrhea and respiratory disease (Passariello, Terrin, DeMarco, et al., 2011; Patel, Mamtani, Badhoniya, et al., 2011; Yakoob, Theodoratou, Jabeen, et al., 2011). The mineral is commonly found in meats, liver, eggs, and seafood. In addition, certain functional foods that contain normal intestinal bacterial flora (probiotics), or substances that promote normal flora, are under investigation for preventing diarrhea in children at risk of fluid and electrolyte imbalance from gastrointestinal disease.

Nursing Management

Nurses assess children of all ages for signs of fluid imbalance. Partnering with parents to prevent fluid imbalance is important. Nurses provide information on normal needs of infants and children and special needs during exercise or illness, and help parents to recognize imbalances. Nurses collaborate with other healthcare providers to perform and analyze laboratory tests for diagnosis, administer intravenous and oral fluids as needed, and provide comfort measures for the child experiencing imbalance.

Nursing Assessment and Diagnosis

Prevention of dehydration is the major aim. Teach parents of all newborns and infants how to identify the problem. This age group is most at risk for dehydration, and the signs are hardest to detect. When the

TABLE 23–6	Common Intravenous Solutions, Uses, and Components

IV SOLUTION	USES	COMPONENTS							
		CHO (G/100 ML)	PROTEIN (G/100 ML)	CAL/L	NA⁺ (MEQ/L)	K⁺ (MEQ/L)	CL⁻ (MEQ/L)	HCO₃ (MEQ/L)	CA⁺⁺ (MEQ/L)
D_5W	Restores water loss and plasma volume, has minimal calories, lowers sodium levels	5	—	170	—	—	—	—	—
Normal saline (0.9% NaCl)	Restores water and sodium loss, maintains sodium and chloride at present levels	—	—	—	154	—	154	—	—
Ringer's solution	Expands intracellular fluid, replaces extracellular losses	0–10	—	0–340	147	4	155.5	—	4
Lactated Ringer's solution	Replaces fluid loss from burns, bleeding, and severe diarrhea	0–10	—	0–340	130	4	109	28	3
Albumin 25% (salt poor albumin)	Restores major plasma protein in blood loss that has been treated with NS (plasma expander)	—	25	1000	100–160	—	Less than 120	—	—

Note: *Variations and combinations are available to tailor intake to needs of the child. For example, $\frac{1}{2}$ NS (0.45% NaCl) or $\frac{1}{4}$ NS (0.225% NaCl) are often used in young children; the lower sodium content helps to avoid inadvertent hypernatremia. $D_5\frac{1}{2}$ NS and $D_5\frac{1}{4}$ NS are combinations of D_5W and NS; they provide both carbohydrate and sodium. Amino acid 8.5% is an additional plasma expander to restore loss of plasma proteins.*

Source: *Information adapted from Tschudy, M. M., & Arcara, K. M. (2011). The Harriet Lane handbook (19th ed.). Baltimore: Johns Hopkins University Press; and LeMone, P., & Burke, K. M. (2011). Medical surgical nursing (5th ed.). Upper Saddle River, NJ: Prentice Hall Health.*

child is admitted to a facility, weigh the child without clothing and with the same scale as used for previous weights. If hospitalized, continue with daily weights at the same time each day.

Clinical Tip
One liter of fluid weighs about 1 kg. The approximate amount of fluid deficit can be calculated using this formula. In the opening scenario, Vernon has lost 1 kg of weight, so he has lost approximately 1 L of fluid from his body.

Compare to past weights and calculate weight loss. Carefully measure intake and output, urine specific gravity, level of consciousness, pulse rate and quality, skin turgor, mucous membrane moisture, quality and rate of respirations, and blood pressure (Figure 23–8 ■). Recognize that the child with renal disease may not show increased urine specific gravity due to the kidney's inability to concentrate urine.

Clinical Tip
A way to estimate urinary output is to weigh a dry diaper before placing it on an infant, and then after the infant has voided. Each gram of increased weight is approximately equivalent to 1 mL of urine. Be sure to weigh the diaper on the same scale, and change it quickly after urination before the fluid has evaporated. When precise measures are needed, a urine bag may be placed on the infant to measure urinary output (see the Skills Manual ⊂⊃).

To obtain urine from an infant for testing specific gravity, place two cotton balls in the diaper. When they are wet, put on gloves, push them into a 10-mL syringe, and squeeze out the urine with the plunger.

Compare the blood pressure when the child is supine with the pressure when the child is sitting with legs hanging down or standing. If the child is dehydrated, the sitting or standing blood pressure will be lower than the supine blood pressure, because blood accumulates in the dependent legs.

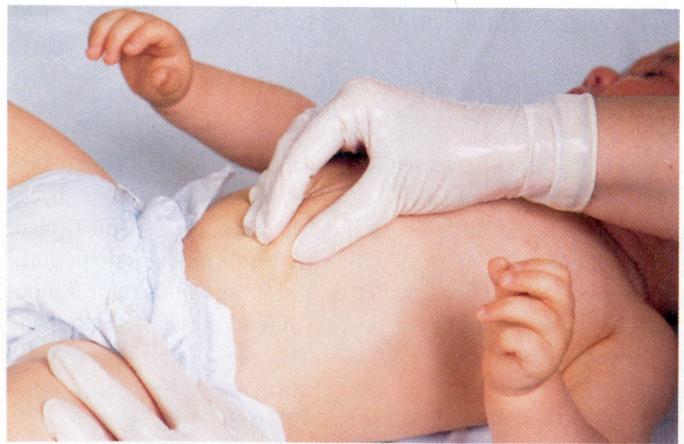 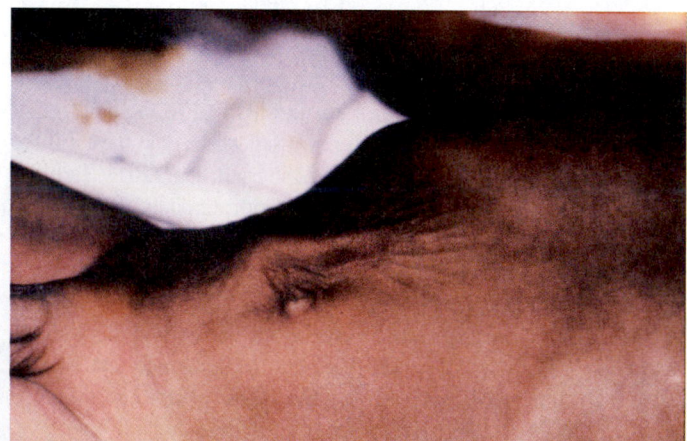

FIGURE 23–8 ■ Assessing skin turgor takes skill and practice. *A,* In moderate dehydration the skin may have a doughy texture and appearance. *B,* Later, in severe dehydration, the more typical "tenting" of skin is observed. Diminished turgor is most easily assessed in infants or children with little subcutaneous fat; it is more difficult to assess in those with larger amounts of fat. The chest, abdomen, and upper thighs are locations to measure turgor.

Evaluate the alertness of the child and any signs of lethargy or weakness. The nurse will obtain samples of urine and blood as needed for laboratory tests.

The nursing diagnosis Deficient Fluid Volume applies to all children who have an extracellular fluid volume deficit. Other diagnoses depend on the severity of the condition and the age of the child. Several nursing diagnoses that might be appropriate for the child who is mildly to severely dehydrated are included in the accompanying Nursing Care Plans. Additional care of the child with dehydration from gastroenteritis can be found in Chapter 30 🥚. Specific examples of nursing diagnoses include the following:

- Fluid Volume, Deficient related to active fluid volume loss or failure of regulatory mechanisms
- Tissue Perfusion: Peripheral, Risk for Ineffective related to hypovolemia
- Injury, Risk for related to postural hypotension

NANDA-I © 2012

Planning and Implementation

Nursing care of the dehydrated child focuses on preventing dehydration when possible, providing oral rehydration fluids, teaching parents oral rehydration methods, and, if necessary, administering intravenous fluids and medications to decrease vomiting and restore fluid balance. The accompanying Nursing Care Plan summarizes care of the child with mild to severe dehydration. Daily weights at the same time each day, frequent vital signs, neurologic assessments, and intake and output measures are important components of care that provide data needed for care management. The nurse should document findings and report changes in condition. Take measures to ensure the child's safety such as keeping side rails up and providing assistance when out of bed. Administer fluids and electrolyte solutions by intravenous and oral routes as prescribed.

Prevent Dehydration

Nursing care can often prevent dehydration. Carefully monitor temperature probes in radiant warmers and incubators for newborns to prevent overheating and resulting dehydration. Teach parents proper clothing for infants to prevent overheating. Teach parents to keep automobiles locked when not in use and to never leave a child in a closed car for any length of time. Such measures would prevent heat-related deaths of young children confined in cars.

Nursing Care Plan   The Child with Mild or Moderate Dehydration

INTERVENTION	RATIONALE	EXPECTED OUTCOME
1. Nursing Diagnosis: Therapeutic Regimen Management: Family, Ineffective related to family knowledge deficit about diarrhea and vomiting		
NIC Priority Intervention—*Family Involvement:* Facilitate family participation in care of the child		**NOC Suggested Outcome**—*Participation: Healthcare Decisions:* Personal involvement in selecting healthcare options
GOAL: *Parents will describe appropriate home management of fluid replacement for diarrhea and vomiting.*		
■ Explain how to replace body fluid with an oral rehydration solution. Encourage parents to keep the solution at home and begin use with the first sign of diarrhea.	■ Use of an oral rehydration solution can enable successful treatment of vomiting and diarrhea at home.	Parents are successfully able to treat the child's diarrhea and vomiting at home. The child is adequately hydrated.
■ Teach parents to continue the child's normal diet in addition to providing replacement fluids for diarrhea.	■ Diet plus fluid supplementation leads to faster recovery.	
■ Provide verbal and written instructions to parents at each well-child visit.	■ Parents are provided with a reference for later use.	
2. Nursing Diagnosis: Knowledge, Deficient (Parent) related to causes of dehydration		
NIC Priority Intervention—*Teaching:* Teach causes of dehydration		**NOC Suggested Outcome**—*Knowledge:* Extent of understanding conveyed about treatment regimen
GOAL: *Parents will state common causes of childhood dehydration.*		
■ Teach parents childhood conditions that commonly lead to dehydration.	■ If parents recognize situations that can lead to dehydration, they will be more alert to its appearance.	Parents recognize conditions of risk for dehydration in children.
3. Nursing Diagnosis: Fluid Volume: Deficient, Risk for related to worsening of child's condition		
NIC Priority Intervention—*Fluid Management:* Promote fluid balance		**NOC Suggested Outcome**—*Fluid Balance:* Balance of water in extra- and intracellular compartments of body
GOAL: *Parents will seek health care for the child's worsening condition.*		
■ Teach parents to seek care when the child's vomiting or diarrhea worsens, or the child's mental alertness changes.	■ Severe dehydration may occur if milder forms are not successfully treated.	Parents seek prompt attention for the child's worsening condition, preventing the development of severe dehydration.
■ Teach parents to recognize symptoms of dehydration.		

Nursing Care Plan   The Child with Severe Dehydration

Intervention	Rationale	Expected Outcome
4. Nursing Diagnosis: Fluid Volume: Deficient related to excess losses and inadequate intake		
NIC Priority Intervention—*Fluid Management:* Promote fluid balance		**NOC Suggested Outcome**—*Fluid Balance:* Balance of water in extra- and intracellular components of the body
GOAL: *The child will return to normal hydration status and will not develop hypovolemic shock.*		
▪ Monitor weight daily, using the same scale, and with no clothes on the child. Assess intake and output every shift. Assess heart rate, postural blood pressure, skin turgor, capillary refill time, fontanel (infant), and urine specific gravity every 4 hours or more frequently as indicated.	▪ Frequent assessment of hydration status facilitates rapid intervention and evaluation of the effectiveness of fluid replacement.	The child has signs of normal hydration.
▪ Administer intravenous fluids as ordered. Monitor for crackles in dependent portions of the lungs.	▪ Replace fluid lost from the body. Excessive replacement of sodium-containing fluids could cause extracellular fluid volume excess.	
5. Nursing Diagnosis: Injury, Risk for related to decreased level of consciousness		
NIC Priority Intervention—*Fall Prevention:* Institute special precautions		**NOC Suggested Outcome**—*Fall Prevention:* Minimize risk factors that precipitate falls
GOAL: *The child will not experience injury.*		
▪ Raise the side rails of the bed. Ensure that a small child does not become tangled in bed covers.	▪ Safety measures protect the child.	The child does not fall or suffer other injury.
▪ Monitor level of consciousness every 2–4 hours or more often as indicated.	▪ Frequent assessment provides evidence of the need for safety interventions and of the effectiveness of therapy.	
▪ Monitor serum sodium concentration daily or more often.	▪ Elevated serum sodium concentration causes brain cell shrinkage and decreased level of consciousness.	
▪ Have the child sit before rising from bed and assist to stand slowly.	▪ Slow adjustment to upright posture reduces light-headedness (dizziness) from decreased blood volume.	
6. Nursing Diagnosis: Activity Intolerance related to bed rest/immobility		
NIC Priority Intervention—*Activity Therapy:* Plan activities to meet child's developmental needs		**NOC Suggested Outcome**—*Energy Conservation:* Manage energy to sustain activity
GOAL: *The child will engage in normal activity for age.*		
▪ Plan activities appropriate for the age of the child that can be done in bed.	▪ Activities will provide distraction and promote recovery.	The child engages in normal developmental activities and receives adequate rest.
▪ Group nursing interventions to provide time for the child to rest.	▪ The child will require more rest than usual.	
▪ Provide assistance during meals and other activities as needed.	▪ Prevention of overexertion will conserve body fluid and promote healing.	

NANDA-I © 2012

Nurses play an important role in educating parents, youth, school personnel, and coaches about the dangers of heat-related illness. Prevention is essential, so that children can exercise safely. Prior to a new exercise regimen, perform an assessment for risk factors, including medical conditions that put the child at high risk, such as cystic fibrosis, diabetes, obesity, or intellectual disability. Prior history of heat-related illness or a recent change from a cooler to hotter environment increases risk. Long exercise periods increase the stress upon the body. Adolescents who drink alcohol or have an alcoholic binge are in danger of dehydration from alcohol effects; since they usually hide such behavior from coaches and parents, they may be at particular risk when participating in sports during hot weather. Major nursing interventions involve partnering with families and athletic coaches to prevent problems by identifying those at risk and teaching youth the dangers of alcoholic dehydration. Nurses also teach those working with youth to recognize and treat dehydration promptly. See Partnering with Families: Preventing Heat-Related Illness. Recognize that heat syndromes can result in death, so prevention, prompt recognition, and treatment are essential.

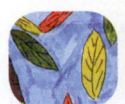

Partnering with Families

Preventing Heat-Related Illness

Teach parents, coaches, and youth the following preventive techniques:

- Precede exercise programs with a physical examination designed to identify risks.
- Reduce intensity of activity when temperature or humidity is high.
- Allow a 10- to 14-day period of acclimatization to higher temperatures with gradual increase in duration and intensity of exercise before reaching the usual exercise level.
- Ensure hydration before activity begins.
- During activity, stop for fluids every 15 to 20 minutes. Children up to 90 lb should drink 150 mL (5 oz), and those over 90 lb should drink 250 mL (9 oz). A combination of water and sports drink is best.
- Recognize low urine volume or dark color as a sign of dehydration.
- Wear light-colored, light clothing. Never use rubber clothing designed to promote weight loss through sweating.
- Maintain adequate sleep and nutritional status; avoid alcohol use.

Additional tips for coaches:

- Weigh all children before and after a vigorous event to evaluate if weight and therefore fluids are maintained; use the findings to instruct children in proper intake.
- Be familiar with signs of heat-related illness.
- Have cell phones or other mechanisms available to call for emergency assistance.

- At least two adults should always be present at exercise sessions.
- Keep adequate fluids and sports drinks readily available.
- During all-day practices, allow 2 to 3 hours of rest during the middle of the day with fluids and food provided.
- Practice in shade or use fans if possible.
- Obtain and use a wet-bulb globe temperature (WBGT) risk measurement that considers humidity (70% of heat stress), radiation (20% of heat stress), and temperature (10% of heat stress). For WBGT less than 50°F, normal activities are generally safe; for 50°F to 65°F, activities are generally safe but exertional heatstroke (EHS) can occur; by 65°F to 72°F, risk of EHS increases; from 72°F to 78°F, EHS risk is increased for all; from 78°F to 82°F, the risk is high for those not acclimatized; and by 82°F, activities should be cancelled. As the WBGT reading increases, enforce longer rest periods in the shade every 15 minutes, limit activities for all children, and eliminate activity for those not acclimatized.
- Understand symptoms for recognition of all heat-related problems.
- Obtain prompt first aid treatment for any heat-related problems.

Source: *Data from Armstrong, Casa, Millard-Stafford, et al., 2007. Exertional heat illness during training and competition. Medicine & Science in Sports & Exercise, 39, 556–572; and Landry, G. L. (2011). Heat injuries. In R. M. Kliegman, B. F. Stanton, J. W. St. Geme, N. F. Schor, & R. E. Behrman, Nelson textbook of pediatrics (19th ed., pp. 2420–2421). Philadelphia, PA: Saunders Elsevier.*

Provide Oral Rehydration Fluids

In mild or moderate dehydration, oral rehydration fluid should be the first intervention (Box 23–2) (Canavan & Arant, 2009). It is given in frequent small amounts; for example, 1 to 3 teaspoons of fluid every 10 to 15 minutes is a useful guideline for starting oral rehydration. For the first 2 to 4 hours of treatment, 50 mL of fluid for each kilogram of the child's weight should be the target intake. Instruct parents to continue to administer 1 teaspoon every 2 to 3 minutes even if the child vomits, as small amounts of the fluid may still be absorbed.

Children are often treated in special sections of emergency departments or outpatient clinics for several hours to begin hydration. Oral or nasogastric tube feedings may be used to regulate the intake of oral rehydration fluid. Once the child is adequately hydrated and able to take oral fluids, the child can be discharged with instructions for parents to continue therapy at home, thus avoiding hospitalization.

Practice Alert

Sugar facilitates the absorption of sodium in oral rehydration fluids. Tell parents not to give diet beverages for oral rehydration, because they contain no sugar and will not be effectively absorbed. On the other hand, if an oral rehydration solution is too concentrated, it can worsen diarrhea. Juice and cola are highly concentrated and should be diluted to half strength when given to a child with diarrhea. Encourage parents to keep an oral rehydration solution in liquid or powder form on hand at all times and to use these solutions rather than juice or soda when the child first develops diarrhea. In settings where this is not possible, such as developing countries, oral rehydration solution is made by thoroughly mixing 8 teaspoons of sugar, 1 teaspoon of salt, and 1 liter of clean or boiled water (Rehydration Project, 2008).

Teach Parents Oral Rehydration Methods

Instruct parents about the types of fluids and amounts to be given. See Partnering with Families: Oral Rehydration Therapy Guidelines on page 670. Begin teaching with parents of all newborns and reinforce teaching at each well-child visit. Advise parents to continue the child's normal diet in addition to providing the rehydration solution. Cereals, starches, soups, fruits, and vegetables are allowed. Tell parents to avoid simple sugars, which can worsen diarrhea because of osmotic effects, including soft drinks (if used, soft drinks should be diluted with equal parts of water), undiluted juice, Jell-O, and sweetened cereal.

Repeated vomiting of large volumes of fluid or a worsening of the child's condition can indicate the need for intravenous therapy. Teach parents when to seek further medical care. If the child's condition worsens or does not improve after 4 hours of oral rehydration therapy, parents should contact a healthcare professional. (See Complementary Therapy: Probiotics.)

BOX 23–2	Oral Rehydration and Maintenance Fluids for Mild and Moderate Dehydration

- Ceralyte
- Equalyte
- Hydralyte
- Infalyte
- KaoLectrolyte
- Lytren
- Naturalyte
- Pedialyte

- Pediatric Oral Maintenance Solution
- Rehydralyte
- Resol
- ReVital
- Ricelyte
- WHO/UNICEF oral rehydration solution

Complementary Therapy Probiotics

Probiotics are live organisms that when ingested provide some health benefit. Probiotics have been explored for their possible beneficial effects in treating diarrheal diseases, and many have been tried among youth. Some of the common probiotics used for gastrointestinal illness include forms of *Lactobacillus* and *Bifidobacterium*, gram-positive bacteria that are part of the normal intestinal flora. There is some evidence that probiotics are effective in treating diarrhea from viral gastroenteritis or diarrhea caused by oral antibiotics, but ongoing research on safety in various conditions is needed (Thomas, Greer, & Committee on Nutrition, 2010). Ask parents if they have used any of these probiotics for treatment of themselves or their children, since some families are routinely adding them to formula. See Chapter 19 🅔 for further information on probiotics.

Monitor Intravenous Fluid Administration

Ill neonates usually receive all fluids intravenously, and many babies and children in intensive care units receive most fluids intravenously. See the Clinical Skills Manual ⬭ for information on the initiation and management of intravenous fluids. The child hospitalized for dehydration usually requires administration of intravenous fluids. Be sure that the amount of fluid administered to all infants and children corresponds with the diagnosed dehydration state and maintenance fluid needs of the child (Box 23–3). Verify that the type of fluid administered is that which is prescribed. Usually, about half of the 24-hour total maintenance and replacement needs will be given to a dehydrated child in the first 6 to 8 hours, with a slower rate infused for the remainder of the 24 hours. During the first 1 to 3 hours, the infusion rate may be highest to rapidly expand the vascular space. Rapid infusion of a 20 mL/kg isotonic crystalloid solution (normal saline or lactated Ringer's) bolus over 20 minutes is sometimes used in outpatient settings, followed by a further bolus or oral fluids (Chameides et al., 2011; Kliegman, Stanton, St. Geme, et al., 2011). When oral fluids are tolerated, the decision for discharge can be made and hospitalization avoided.

Maintain the intravenous line carefully so fluid infusion can be kept on schedule (refer to the Skills Manual ⬭). Use a pump to prevent inadvertent, rapid infusion, which can lead to fluid overload and electrolyte imbalance (Figure 23–9 ▪). The site is wrapped to avoid inadvertent dislodgment, but the dressing must be removed to observe and adequately assess the intravenous site. Play with the toddler and preschool child frequently and use diversionary methods, as necessary, to distract the child from the intravenous line. Monitor the child carefully and implement safety precautions as necessary. Once the child begins to tolerate some oral fluids, oral rehydration therapy is substituted for intravenous fluid administration, and frequent administration of appropriate fluids is needed.

Maintain Safety Precautions

The child who is dehydrated is often light-headed and lethargic. Keep side rails up and supervise and assist the child when getting up. Have parents stay at the bedside while the child is being treated in ambulatory units and instruct them to maintain safety precautions as they take the child home.

Discharge Planning and Home Care Teaching

Prevention of dehydration is the best approach when possible. Encourage breastfeeding because it is associated with a decreased incidence of gastroenteritis. During health promotion and health

---

BOX 23–3 Calculation of Intravenous Fluid Needs

1. First, calculate the maintenance fluid needs of the child, according to the following guideline.

USUAL WEIGHT	MAINTENANCE AMOUNT
Up to 10 kg	100 mL/kg/24 hr
11–20 kg	1000 mL + (50 mL/kg for weight above 10 kg)/24 hr
Greater than 20 kg	1500 mL + (20 mL/kg for weight above 20 kg)/24 hr

Example: *Vernon's weight is 12 kg. He needs 1000 mL + (50 × 2), or 1100 mL/24 hr for maintenance fluid.*

2. Next, calculate replacement fluid for that loss.

Example: *Vernon has lost 1 kg (8%) of his body weight. Multiplying the percentage of body weight × 10 yields the mL/kg/24 hr required:*

$$8 \times 10 = 80 \text{ mL/kg/24 hr}$$

$$80 \text{ mL/kg} \times 12 \text{ kg} = 960 \text{ mL}$$

Thus, Vernon's replacement fluid needs are 960 mL/24 hr or 40 mL/hr. It is also helpful to know that 1 liter of fluid weighs about 1 kilogram. In Vernon's case, since he has lost 1 kg of weight, his replacement fluid need is roughly equivalent to 1 L (1000 mL). This is very close to the 960 mL calculated in the previous formula.

3. Finally, calculate continued losses and add to the total maintenance and replacement needs.

Note: *These fluid needs are for most children who have a problem causing dehydration. In special circumstances, such as very-low-birth-weight infants, or children with problems such as renal disease, the maintenance amounts need to be adjusted. Consult with specialists treating the child and specialized references to learn about fluid needs in these situations.*

---

maintenance visits, encourage all parents to keep oral rehydration fluids at home in case they are needed at some time; they are available in most grocery stores and pharmacies. Address the need for increasing fluids in hot weather and when the child is exercising. Reinforce safety teaching to decrease the incidence of burns, an important

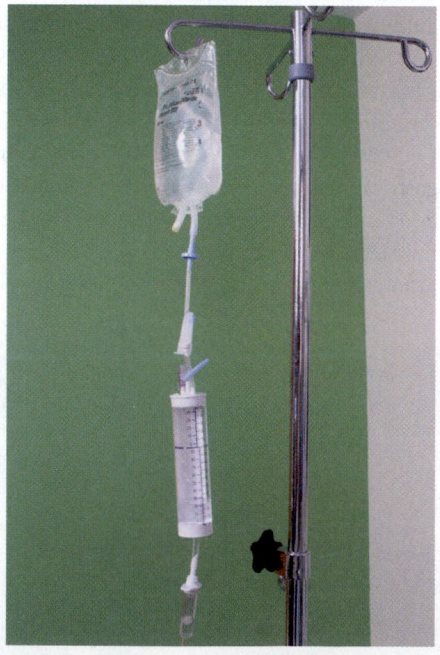

FIGURE 23–9 ▪ The use of a volume control device with an intravenous saline infusion is important to prevent a sudden extracellular fluid volume overload.

cause of dehydration. Teach the signs and symptoms of vomiting and diarrhea so parents recognize these problems accurately.

Prior to discharge from the hospital or outpatient facility after dehydration treatment, parents need instructions about types of fluids and amounts to encourage. Teach the signs of dehydration that parents can recognize such as increasing lethargy, dry mucous membranes, decreased urine output, and either increased thirst or anorexia. Parents should seek help immediately when these symptoms occur. Emphasize that the newborn and infant are at highest risk and that prompt care is needed if dehydration persists. After treatment, instruct parents to begin the child's normal diet once hydration is complete, determined by adequate urinary output and normal behaviors. Review methods of minimizing the child's chance of acquiring gastrointestinal infections (e.g., avoiding contact with other children who are infected; using careful hand washing and dishwashing procedures when a child in the home is affected). See Chapter 30 🔗 for further discussion of gastrointestinal illness and Chapter 22 🔗 for infectious and communicable diseases. Nurses should be alert for children in the community who have other health conditions that predispose them to fluid and electrolyte imbalance, such as those with cancer, diabetes, AIDS, cystic fibrosis, anorexia or bulimia, and renal disease. When these children are seen for health promotion and health maintenance visits, or because of a health complication, they should be evaluated for fluid and electrolyte imbalance.

Evaluation

Expected outcomes of nursing care for the child with dehydration include the following:

- Water and electrolytes are balanced in intracellular and extracellular compartments.
- Urinary output is within normal limits.
- Adequate fluid intake meets maintenance needs.
- Vital signs are within normal limits.

Extracellular Fluid Volume Excess

Extracellular fluid volume excess occurs when there is too much fluid in the extracellular compartment (intravascular and interstitial). This imbalance may also be called saline excess or extracellular volume overload. If this disorder occurs by itself (without saline disturbance), the serum sodium concentration is normal. There is simply too much extracellular fluid, even though it has a normal concentration.

Infants and children who develop an extracellular fluid volume excess have a condition that causes them to retain **saline** (sodium and water), or they have been given an overload of sodium-containing isotonic intravenous fluid (Figure 23–10 ■).

Clinical Tip

A normal saline solution is a salt solution that has the same percentage of salt as the human body. This is a 0.9% solution of sodium chloride. The term *normal* indicates that there is the same weight, in grams, of sodium and chloride in the solution. There are 154 mEq/L of sodium and 154 mEq/L of chloride in normal saline. Normal (isotonic) saline or Ringer's lactate (Ringer's lactate contains carbohydrate and additional electrolytes) is often used for early rehydration to avoid the risk of hyponatremia (Kannan, Lodha, Vivekanandhan, et al., 2011; Moritz & Ayus, 2011; Yung & Keeley, 2009). More dilute sodium solutions are the choice of treatment once rehydration has begun; solutions such as $^1/_2$ normal saline or $^1/_4$ normal saline are used then. If the child is not taking in oral fluids or food, dilute saline solutions with glucose may be prescribed (for example, $D_5{}^1/_2$ NS which is 5% dextrose in $^1/_2$ strength normal saline).

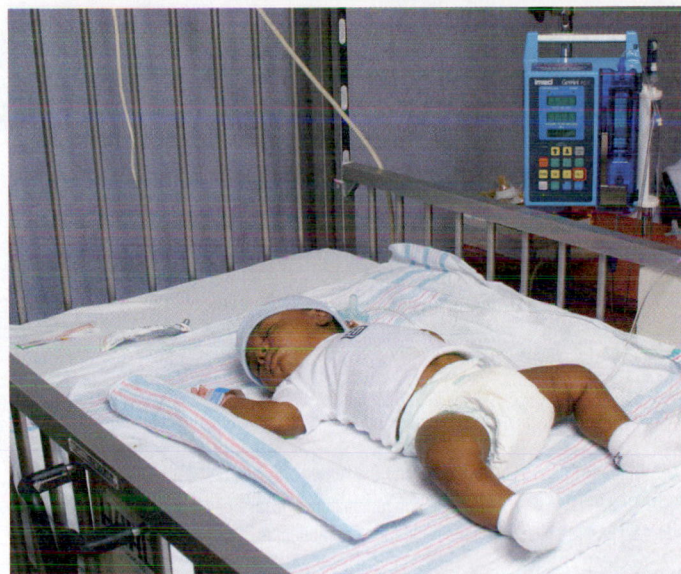

FIGURE 23–10 ■ If isotonic fluid containing sodium is given too rapidly or in too great an amount, an extracellular fluid volume excess will develop. Carefully monitor fluid intake, excretion, and retention in infants and children.

What conditions cause retention of saline? The hormone aldosterone is secreted by the adrenal cortex. One of its normal functions is to cause the kidneys to retain saline in the body (Figure 23–11 ■). Saline excess can be caused by any condition that results in excessive aldosterone secretion, such as adrenal tumors that secrete aldosterone, congestive heart failure, liver cirrhosis, and chronic renal failure (Figure 23–12 ■). Most glucocorticoid medications, such as prednisone, have a mild saline-retaining effect when taken long term. Intravenous fluid volume regulation is important, especially in young children. Either inaccurate calculation of needed fluid or inadvertent infusion of excess fluids can cause overload.

Because fluid has weight, extracellular fluid volume excess is characterized by weight gain.

Clinical Tip

You can tell if a child's weight gain is due to normal growth or to the development of extracellular fluid volume excess by looking at the speed with which the increase develops. Sudden weight gain (e.g., 0.5 kg [approximately 1 lb] in 1 day) is due to the accumulation of fluid. Gain of 0.5 kg overnight is due to retention of about 500 mL of saline.

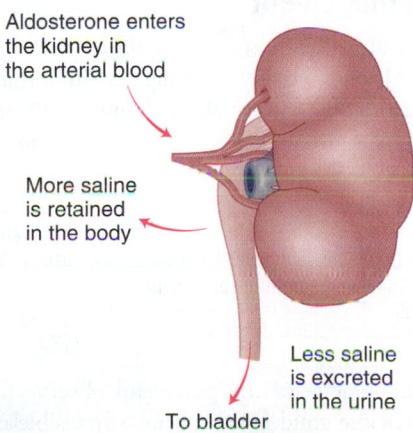

Aldosterone enters the kidney in the arterial blood

More saline is retained in the body

Less saline is excreted in the urine

To bladder

FIGURE 23–11 ■ Aldosterone has a saline-retaining effect. Increased aldosterone secretion can be caused by adrenal tumors or congestive heart failure.

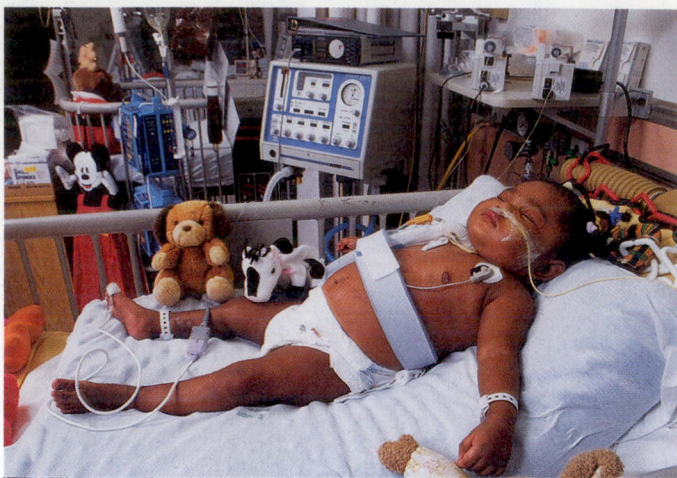

FIGURE 23–12 ■ This infant with congenital heart disease has signs of generalized edema. Note the fluid retention in the face and abdomen.

An overload of fluid in the blood vessels and interstitial spaces can cause clinical manifestations such as bounding pulse, distended neck veins in children (not usually evident in infants), hepatomegaly, dyspnea, orthopnea, and lung crackles. Edema is the sign of overload of the interstitial fluid compartment (see description later in the chapter). In an infant, edema is often generalized or distributed throughout the body. Edema in children with extracellular fluid volume excess occurs in the dependent parts of the body, that is, in the parts closest to the ground. Thus, edema is evident in sacral areas in a child supine in bed. Edema that develops from other causes is described in the next section of this chapter.

Diagnosis of extracellular fluid volume excess is determined by clinical evaluation of weight gain and other manifestations. Serum electrolyte panels aid in diagnosis, and studies of liver or renal function may provide information about the cause of the condition.

Clinical therapy for extracellular fluid volume excess focuses on treating the underlying cause of the disorder. For example, a child who has congestive heart failure is given medications to strengthen the heart's ability to contract (see Chapter 26 🔗 for further discussion of management of fluid volume excess in congenital heart disease). In addition, diuretics may be given to remove fluid from the body, thus reducing the extracellular fluid volume directly.

Nursing Management

Rapid weight gain is the most sensitive index of extracellular fluid volume excess. Therefore, daily weighing is an important nursing assessment. Measure the child's intake and output. When treatment is successful, output is greater than intake.

Clinical Tip
The infant's urine output is important to monitor both dehydration and edema. Weigh the diaper before and after use. A 1-g weight increase in the diaper equals 1 mL of urine volume. Change the diaper frequently to minimize urine loss from evaporation.

Assess the character of the pulse and observe for neck vein distention when the child is sitting (usually visible only in older children). Monitor for signs of pulmonary edema (an indication of severe imbalance) by listening to lung sounds in the dependent lung fields (crackles) and assessing for respiratory distress (rapid respiratory rate, use of accessory muscles of respiration). Observe for edema.

The potential for a child to develop a fluid overload is present whenever an isotonic intravenous solution containing sodium is being administered. Examples include normal saline (0.9% NaCl), Ringer's solution, and lactated Ringer's solution. In such cases, monitor the infusion rate frequently and carefully, and use a pump when possible to aid in accurate administration.

Practice Alert
Occasionally intravenous fluid is infused too rapidly, causing extracellular fluid volume excess and endangering the fluid and electrolyte status of a young child. The nurse can take the following measures to minimize this risk:

- Use small bags of fluid, so if the fluid were to infuse quickly, the amount infused would be limited.
- Always use infusion pumps when available so that the rate is programmed and monitored.
- Check and double-check the machine after setting to be sure it was properly programmed.
- Have another nurse check your calculation of rates and total fluid to be infused until you are certain of your skill in this area.
- Finally, remember that even mechanical pumps can have faulty performance so check the intravenous line, bag, and rate frequently.
- If an infusion pump is not available, use a volume control chamber or burette.

If an excess of fluid has already developed, administer the medical therapy as prescribed and monitor for any complications of the therapy. For example, many diuretics increase potassium excretion in the urine, an increase that may lead to an abnormally low plasma potassium concentration unless potassium intake is increased. (Refer to the discussion of hypokalemia on pages 676–677.) It is also important to monitor for the development of extracellular fluid volume deficit as a result of diuretic therapy.

If edema is present, provide careful skin care and protection for edematous areas. Teach parents how to provide skin care and perform position changes at home. See the following section for additional interventions related to edema.

If a child has a long-term condition such as chronic renal failure that predisposes to extracellular fluid volume excess, fluid restriction and a dietary sodium restriction may be prescribed (see Chapter 31 🔗 for further detail). Teach parents how to manage sodium restriction. See Developing Cultural Competence: Low-Sodium Diets. Plan low-sodium meals that fit the family's cultural practices. If the child is old enough to participate, incorporate games into the teaching. If a scale is available, teach parents to take and record an accurate daily weight.

Expected outcomes include electrolyte balance, maintenance of intact skin, and dietary intake as prescribed.

Interstitial Fluid Volume Excess (Edema)
Edema is an abnormal increase in the volume of interstitial fluid. It may be caused by an extracellular fluid volume excess or it may be due to other causes.

The causes of edema are best understood in the context of normal capillary dynamics. Fluid moves between the vascular and interstitial compartments by the process of filtration. Filtration is the net result of forces that tend to move fluid in opposing directions. The strongest forces will determine the direction of fluid movement.

Developing Cultural Competence
Low-Sodium Diets

To adapt teaching about low-sodium diets to the cultural practices of a family, ask patients what types of food they usually eat. Help them to choose low-sodium foods from their diets and to avoid high-sodium foods. This approach is more effective than giving the same list of restricted foods to each family.

For example, some Asians may use monosodium glutamate to flavor foods and can be encouraged to add this at the table for family members who can have extra sodium rather than during cooking. Many Hispanic groups use large amounts of cheese that can provide significant sodium. Encourage them to look for low-sodium cheese and substitute cottage cheese for other types since it is lower in sodium. Canned foods tend to have high sodium, so teach all families to use fresh or frozen produce rather than canned when possible. Low-sodium milk is available and a good option for young children. Teach families how to read and interpret food labels to learn about sodium content. Realize that many people do not know that "sodium" on a label indicates content of "salt."

At the capillary level, two forces (blood hydrostatic pressure and interstitial osmotic pressure) tend to move fluid from the capillaries into the interstitial fluid, while two other forces (blood colloid osmotic pressure and interstitial fluid hydrostatic pressure) tend to move fluid in the opposite direction (from the interstitial fluid into the capillaries). The net result of these forces usually moves fluid from the capillaries into the interstitial compartment at the arterial end of the capillaries, and fluid from the interstitial compartment back into the capillaries at the venous end of the capillaries. This process brings oxygen and nutrients to the cells and removes carbon dioxide and other waste products.

Edema occurs if the balance of these four forces is altered so that excess fluid either enters or leaves the interstitial compartment in an imbalanced manner (Figure 23–13 ■ Pathophysiology Illustrated: Capillary Dynamics and Edema). This may occur through any of the following:

1. Increased blood hydrostatic pressure
2. Decreased blood colloid osmotic pressure
3. Increased interstitial fluid osmotic pressure
4. Blocked lymphatic drainage

Various clinical conditions are associated with these altered forces (Table 23–7):

1. **Increased blood hydrostatic pressure.** When extracellular fluid volume excess occurs, the increased fluid volume in

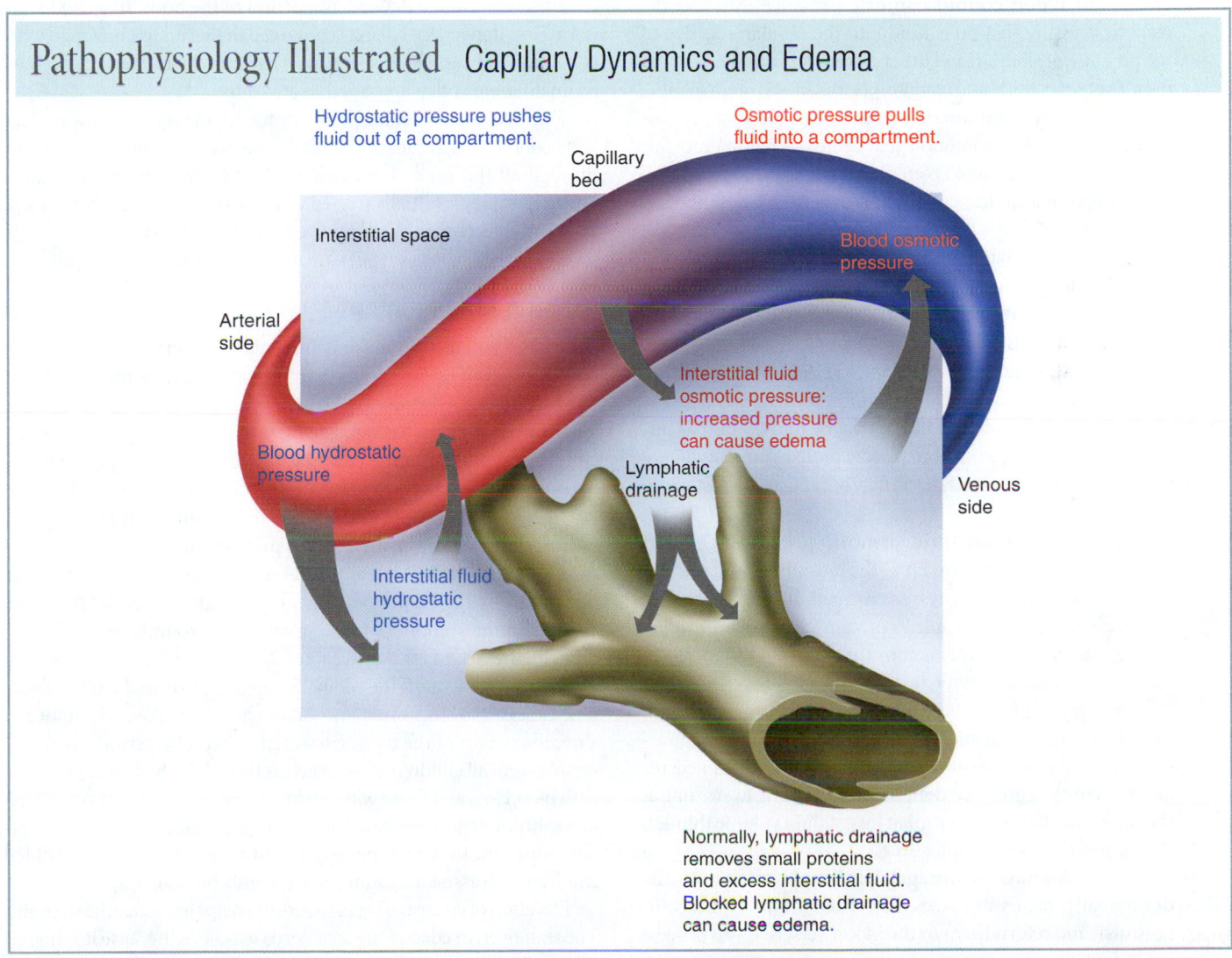

Pathophysiology Illustrated   Capillary Dynamics and Edema

Hydrostatic pressure pushes fluid out of a compartment.

Osmotic pressure pulls fluid into a compartment.

Capillary bed

Interstitial space

Blood osmotic pressure

Arterial side

Interstitial fluid osmotic pressure: increased pressure can cause edema

Blood hydrostatic pressure

Lymphatic drainage

Venous side

Interstitial fluid hydrostatic pressure

Normally, lymphatic drainage removes small proteins and excess interstitial fluid. Blocked lymphatic drainage can cause edema.

FIGURE 23–13 ■ With normal capillary dynamics, fluid moves out of the compartment by the force of hydrostatic pressure in the blood vessel and is pulled out by interstitial osmotic pressure. Fluid is forced into the compartment by interstitial hydrostatic pressure and pulled in by compartment osmotic pressure. Abnormal capillary dynamics can cause edema.

TABLE 23–7   Clinical Conditions That Cause Edema

EDEMA DUE TO INCREASED BLOOD HYDROSTATIC PRESSURE	EDEMA DUE TO DECREASED BLOOD OSMOTIC PRESSURE	EDEMA DUE TO INCREASED INTERSTITIAL FLUID OSMOTIC PRESSURE	EDEMA DUE TO BLOCKED LYMPHATIC DRAINAGE
■ Increased capillary blood flow	■ Increased albumin excretion	■ Increased capillary permeability	■ Tumors
■ Inflammation	■ Nephrotic syndrome (albumin leaks into urine)	■ Inflammation	■ Goiter
■ Local infection	■ Protein-losing enteropathies (excess albumin in feces)	■ Toxins	■ Parasites that obstruct lymph nodes
■ Venous congestion	■ Decreased albumin synthesis	■ Hypersensitivity reactions	■ Surgery that removes lymph nodes
■ Extracellular fluid volume excess	■ Kwashiorkor (low-protein, high-carbohydrate starvation diet provides too few amino acids for liver to make albumin)	■ Burns	
■ Right-sided heart failure	■ Liver cirrhosis (diseased liver unable to make enough albumin)		
■ Venous thrombosis			
■ External pressure on vein			
■ Muscle paralysis			

the vascular compartment congests the veins. The pressure against the sides of the capillary is increased, and more fluid then enters the interstitial compartment.

2. **Decreased blood colloid osmotic pressure.** Much of the osmotic pressure that pulls fluid into the capillaries is due to the presence of albumin and other plasma proteins made by the liver. The part of the blood osmotic pressure that is due to plasma proteins is often called **oncotic pressure** or blood colloid osmotic pressure. Any condition that decreases plasma proteins will decrease blood colloid osmotic pressure and cause edema. For example, if a clinical condition causes large amounts of albumin to leak into the urine, the liver will not be able to make albumin fast enough to replace it. As a result, the plasma protein level will fall, decreasing the blood osmotic pressure. Without this pulling force to return fluid to the capillaries, edema will occur. This is the cause of the edema that occurs in children who have nephrotic syndrome (see Chapter 31 🔗). Another cause in children is prolonged surgical procedures with significant blood loss. Intravenous fluids and blood may be infused during surgery to replace those losses, but plasma proteins are lost and not fully restored by infusion. Edema may be seen in the postoperative period.

3. **Increased interstitial fluid osmotic pressure.** Ordinarily, only a few small proteins enter the interstitial fluid, and the interstitial fluid osmotic pressure is small. If the capillary becomes abnormally permeable to proteins, however, the influx of large amounts of proteins into the interstitial fluid causes a dramatic increase in interstitial fluid osmotic pressure. This increased pulling force keeps an abnormal amount of fluid in the interstitial compartment. This mechanism plays an important part in the edema caused by a bee sting or a sprained ankle. It occurs to a greater extent in burns, leading to swelling at the same time that there is a great loss of fluid volume through the burned skin (see Chapter 36 🔗).

4. **Blocked lymphatic drainage.** The lymph vessels normally drain small proteins and excess fluid from the interstitial compartment and return them to the blood vessels. If this process is blocked, fluid accumulates in the interstitial compartment. This may occur when a tumor blocks lymphatic drainage.

Edema causes swelling, which may be localized or generalized. The swelling of tissue may cause pain and restrict motion. Edema that is due to extracellular fluid volume excess or right-sided heart failure usually occurs in the dependent portion of the body. In a child who is walking, dependent edema is observed in the ankles; in a child who is bedfast and supine, it is seen in the sacral area. The skin over an edematous area often appears thin and shiny.

The main focus of clinical therapy for edema is to treat the underlying condition that caused the edema. Such conditions are discussed throughout this book. For example, the edema from inflammation due to an injury is initially treated with cold to reduce capillary blood flow and thus reduce blood hydrostatic pressure (see Chapter 35 🔗 for a description of this type of treatment in musculoskeletal injury).

Nursing Management

A child or parent may make comments that alert the nurse to the development of edema. Shoes may become tight by the end of the day (dependent edema); the waistband of pants or a skirt may be "outgrown" suddenly (generalized edema or ascites, which is accumulation of fluid in the peritoneal cavity); the eyes may be puffy (periorbital edema); a ring may be too tight; fingers may "feel like sausages." In many cases visual inspection is sufficient to recognize edema. Observe for the presence of **pitting edema,** a "pit" or concave indentation that remains after an edematous area is pressed downward by the examiner's fingers for about 5 seconds. To detect changes in the amount of swelling, measure around the edematous part (Figure 23–14 ■). See Chapter 7 🔗 for further description of assessment of edema. If the edema is caused by extracellular fluid volume excess, daily measurements of weight and intake and output are a necessary part of the daily assessment. Carefully perform such assessments in all children at risk, such as those who had recent surgery with blood loss and those with health conditions such as heart failure or nephrotic syndrome. Nursing assessment should also focus on the integrity of the skin, presence of pain, and restricted motion. In older children, also assess alterations in the child's body image.

Elevation of an area of localized edema helps to reduce the swelling. The skin over an edematous area needs extra care because it is fragile (Figure 23–15 ■). Carefully position an infant or child who is on bed rest and turn frequently to prevent pressure sores. Use sheepskin and

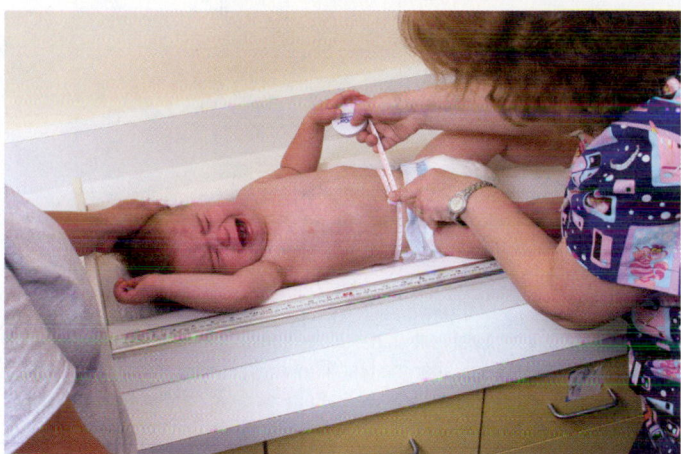

FIGURE 23–14 ■ Finding the same location each day for measuring circumference to assess edema can be accomplished by use of a reference point. An indelible marker may be used to mark the measurement location on the skin, if this is acceptable to the child and parents.

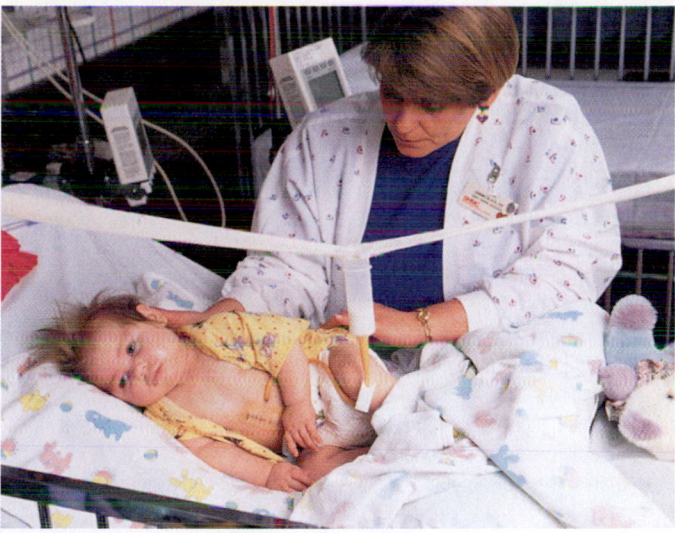

FIGURE 23–15 ■ Edematous tissue is easily damaged. It must be kept clean and dry and free of pressure.

special mattresses to decrease pressure on the skin. Turning must be performed carefully to avoid skin abrasion by rubbing against the sheets. Pat the skin dry after cleansing rather than rubbing it. Trim the child's fingernails smooth to prevent scratching. Teach parents skin care for the child at home and recommend checking for redness or skin breakdown several times daily. Teach older children to inspect their skin carefully to identify areas needing special care. Prevention and care of pressure ulcers is described in Chapter 36 ⊘.

If restricted mobility is a problem, specific plans to help the child manage activities are needed. For example, if an edematous finger restricts hand movement, food can be cut into bite-size portions before the meal is served, so that the child can still eat independently.

Discomfort from edema may require creative interventions by the nurse. Distraction with toys or activities appropriate to the child's developmental level can be useful. Interventions to treat the underlying problem can also reduce the edema and its accompanying discomfort. Interventions for edema should be added to the nursing management of the underlying condition that causes the edema. Administration of the prescribed medical therapy and observation for the complications of therapy are nursing responsibilities.

It is important to help the child comply with prescribed fluid restrictions and teach the parents how to do this at home. See Partnering with Families: Interventions for a Child Who Has a Fluid Restriction. Allow the child to choose favorite fluids to drink.

Discuss with school-age children and adolescents feelings of embarrassment about the edematous appearance. They need to understand the reason for edema and be able to explain it to peers. Arrange for the child to meet other children with similar concerns.

Desired outcomes of care include maintenance of intact skin, normal respiratory sounds and effort, normal weight patterns, and maintenance of fluid and electrolyte balance.

ELECTROLYTE IMBALANCES

All body fluids contain electrolytes, although the concentration of those electrolytes varies, depending on the type and location of the fluid. When a serum electrolyte value is reported from the laboratory, it provides information about the concentration of that electrolyte in the blood. It may not necessarily reflect the concentration of the electrolyte in other body compartments. Each laboratory has standard values based on the machines and assay techniques used. Refer to local laboratory norms and realize that levels in references are general or average levels that may differ slightly from a specific laboratory standard. Refer to Table 23–1 to see which electrolytes are highest and lowest in concentration in the blood and other fluid compartments. Recognize that values of normal have ranges. A child can have a value slightly out of the range and not be in a health crisis. Clinical manifestations and the entire profile of the child are considered. Notice that levels listed in this chapter for conditions such as hyperkalemia,

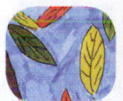

Partnering with Families

Interventions for a Child Who Has a Fluid Restriction

- Give cold rather than lukewarm fluids.
- Use an insulated glass that looks bigger than it is. This works well with preschoolers and school-age children.
- Be sure that extra fluids are removed from meal trays before the child sees them.

- Have the child swish fluids around in the mouth before swallowing to relieve thirst. School-age children and adolescents can often use this intervention.
- Provide frequent oral care.
- Suggest eating meals without fluids, saving them to drink between meals.
- Provide a chart so an older child can keep intake records.

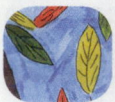

Partnering with Families

Oral Rehydration Therapy Guidelines

Calculate the specific amounts required for individual children based on the following guidelines, and instruct parents in terminology they understand. Provide measuring devices with proper amounts marked.

- Children with diarrhea and no dehydration should be continued on age-appropriate diets.
- For minimal dehydration, if the child weighs less than 10 kg, give 60 to 120 mL oral rehydration solution (ORS) for each diarrheal stool or vomiting episode. If over 10 kg in weight, give 120 to 240 mL ORS for each diarrheal stool or vomiting episode. Meanwhile, continue breastfeeding, or resume the age-appropriate diet after initial hydration.
- Start with small amounts, administering 3 to 5 mL in a small cup or spoon every few minutes. Increase amounts gradually if no vomiting occurs.
- Recommend or provide samples of oral rehydration therapy (ORT) solutions. Suggest ready-to-feed or powdered forms for choice by parents.

- For moderate dehydration, give 50 to 100 mL/kg ORS in the first 3 to 4 hours and replace fluids in each stool or vomiting episode.
- For severe dehydration, the child is hospitalized and treated with intravenous fluids. When hydrated adequately or concurrently with intravenous rehydration, begin oral rehydration therapy with 100 mL/kg of fluid in 4 hours and stool replacement as described above.
- Recalculate fluid needs after the first 4 hours and adjust as needed. If the child is not taking increased fluids and otherwise improving by this time, contact the healthcare provider.
- When rehydration is complete, resume a normal diet.

Source: *Data from Canavan, A., & Arant, B. S. (2009). Diagnosis and management of dehydration in children.* American Family Physician, *80(7), 692–696; Children's Mercy Hospital. (2011). Guidelines for oral rehydration. Retrieved from http://www.childrensmercy.org/Content/view.aspx?id=8130*

hypokalemia, hypernatremia, hyponatremia, and others are a bit above or below the normal ranges for the electrolytes to which they refer. These levels are critical values, indicating values significantly out of the normal range and usually requiring immediate healthcare intervention.

Electrolytes are normally gained and lost in relatively equal amounts so the body remains in balance. However, when a child has an abnormal route of loss, such as vomiting, wound drainage, or nasogastric suction, electrolyte balance can be disturbed. In addition, supplementation with electrolytes via IV fluids in proportion different than body fluids can also cause electrolyte imbalance. Children with disease states that interfere with normal mechanisms of electrolyte regulation, such as renal disease, also have disturbance in

electrolyte levels. Monitoring for signs of imbalance becomes important in all of these cases.

Sodium Imbalances

The serum sodium concentration reflects the **osmolality** of body fluids, that is, their degree of concentration or dilution. It refers to the number of moles of the substance per kilogram of water in the solution. Serum sodium concentration reflects the proportion of water and sodium in the extracellular compartment. When the osmolality of body fluids becomes abnormal, the cells swell or shrink. These cell size changes are due to osmosis, the movement of water across a semipermeable membrane into an area of higher particle concentration (Figure 23–16 ■). Sodium levels are maintained at high

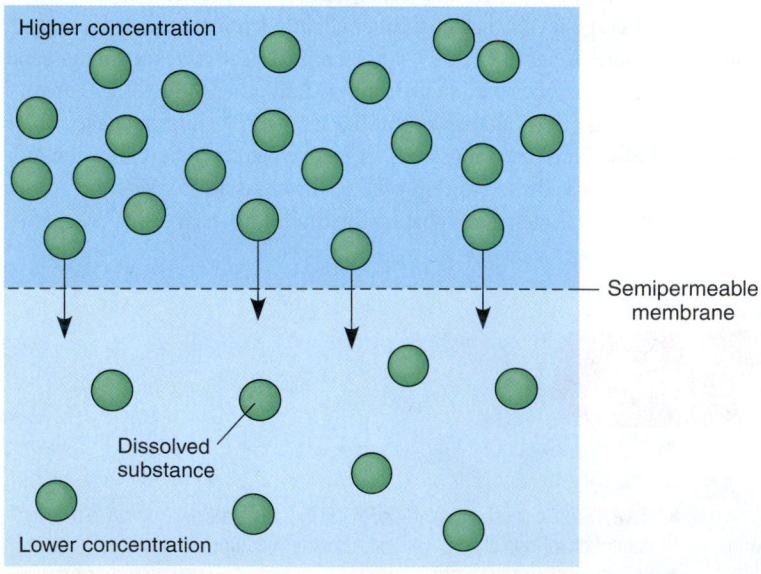

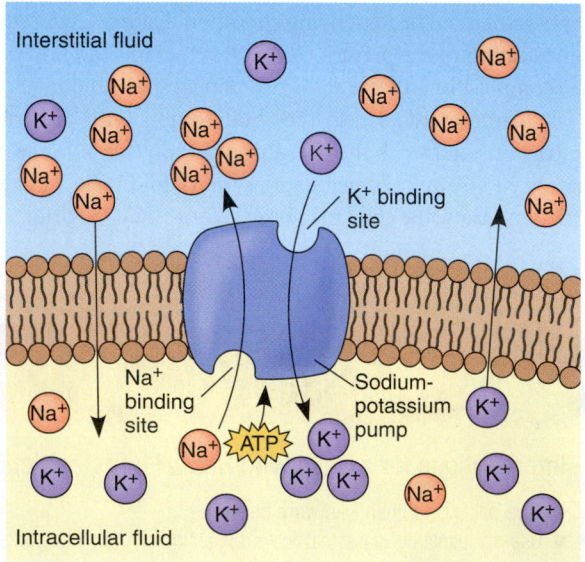

FIGURE 23–16 ■ *A,* Water balance is maintained by the simple passage of molecules from greater to lesser concentration across cell membranes. *B,* Sodium levels are maintained by an active transport system, the sodium-potassium pump, which moves these electrolytes across cell membranes in spite of their concentrations.

extracellular and low intracellular levels by the sodium-potassium pump, which moves these electrolytes against their expected concentration gradients.

Sodium plays several important roles in the body and is an important **cation** (positively charged particle). It is important in blood pressure regulation and maintenance of fluid volume. Most oral ingestion of sodium is in the form of sodium chloride where the cation is joined with the **anion** (negatively charged particle) of chloride (Cl^-), in the form NaCl.

Hypernatremia

Hypernatremia is a condition of increased osmolality of the blood. The body fluids are too concentrated, containing excess sodium relative to water. Sodium level generally falls between 134 and 143 mmol/L. A serum sodium level above 145 mmol/L in children is diagnostic of hypernatremia (Greenbaum, 2011; Tschudy & Arcara, 2011).

Etiology and pathophysiology Hypernatremia results from conditions that cause the body to lose relatively more water than sodium or to gain relatively more sodium than water (Table 23–8). Examples include children who do not have access to adequate water or are developmentally delayed and do not perceive thirst. Special circumstances in which a high solute intake may occur without adequate water include an infant formula that is too concentrated or one that is prepared with salt instead of sugar. A breastfed baby not receiving adequate breast milk who has normal water loss may develop hypernatremic dehydration. This is a particular risk at 2 to 3 days of age, when babies generally have diuresis, if the baby does not feed well or the mother does not yet produce an adequate amount of breast milk (Box 23–4). Newborns in the neonatal intensive care unit usually do not require sodium in intravenous infusions until about day 3 of life, when newborn diuresis occurs; earlier administration of sodium may lead to hypernatremia. Preterm infants under 27 weeks' gestation are more likely to develop hypernatremia than older infants (Kusuma et al., 2009; Unal, Arhan, Kara, et al., 2008).

Clinical manifestations An infant or child who has hypernatremia is generally thirsty. The urine output is low unless the hypernatremia is caused by diabetes insipidus. A decreased level of consciousness manifested by confusion, lethargy, or coma results from shrinking of the brain cells. Seizures can occur when hypernatremia occurs rapidly or is severe. Symptoms in the neonate include decreased activity

TABLE 23–8	Causes of Hypernatremia
LOSS OF RELATIVELY MORE WATER THAN SODIUM	**GAIN OF RELATIVELY MORE SODIUM THAN WATER**
Inadequate intake from breastfeeding with normal output	Inability to communicate thirst
Diabetes insipidus (not enough antidiuretic hormone)	Limited or no access to water
Diarrhea or vomiting without fluid replacement	High solute intake without adequate water (e.g., tube feedings)
Excessive sweating without fluid replacement	Improper formula preparation leading to excessive concentration
High solute intake without adequate water (causes kidneys to excrete water)	Intravenous hypertonic saline
Increased aldosterone	

BOX 23–4   **Research: Causes of Hypernatremia**

In recent years, the major causes of hypernatremia in infants have changed. Formerly, untreated diarrhea was a common cause. Recently, there has been an increase in the number of breastfed babies diagnosed with hypernatremia in the newborn period. When babies have the normal diuresis at 2 to 3 days of age but are not able to feed well or the mother does not have adequate breast milk, hypernatremia can occur. Decrease in activity and alertness, seizures, and excessive weight loss (10% or more of birth weight) in the first few days are symptoms in the neonate (Kusuma et al., 2009). Nurses teach mothers of newborns how to evaluate the feeding behaviors of their babies, how to weigh babies especially when early discharge after delivery occurs, and how to perform careful physical assessments to find infants with decreased neurologic response.

Another potential cause of hypernatremia is inadequate provision or offering of water to children who are hospitalized or who have chronic disease that interferes with their ability to express thirst. Nurses should ensure that children, especially those with developmental delays or who are unable to care for themselves, are offered adequate amounts of fluid. Assess intake and output and be alert for signs of neurologic change.

and alertness, loss of 10% or more of birth weight, and seizures. Severe hypernatremia can be fatal.

Collaborative Care

The major laboratory test that is diagnostic of sodium imbalance is serum sodium. The normal level for newborns is 131 to 144 mmol/L, and for children it is 134 to 143 mmol/L. See Table 23–9 for normally acceptable laboratory values for electrolytes. Specific gravity of urine is concentrated in hypernatremia and dilute in hyponatremia. The normal levels are 1.001 to 1.018 in infants to 2 years of age, and 1.010 to 1.030 for children over 2 years. Antidiuretic hormone (ADH) levels and 24-hour urinary output are helpful in diagnosing diabetes insipidus as the cause (see Chapter 31 🔗).

Clinical Tip

Specific gravity compares the density of urine with the density of water (water density is 1.000). The infant's kidney is less able to concentrate urine, so the urine is more dilute. The child under 2 years is less able to concentrate urine even when dehydrated, so specific gravity may not indicate the true severity of the infant's fluid and electrolyte imbalance.

Hypernatremia is treated by intravenous administration of **hypotonic fluid,** or fluid that is more dilute than normal body fluid. This therapy dilutes the body fluids back to normal concentration. If a child is dehydrated, **isotonic fluids** (those with the osmolality of body fluids) may be ordered first to replenish the volume, followed by hypotonic fluid to correct the osmolality. The underlying cause of the disorder is also treated.

Nursing Management

Teaching can prevent many cases of hypernatremia. Be sure the breastfeeding mother has instruction and resources about lactation before discharge after delivery. If discharged soon after birth, be sure the infant has an appointment to have weight checked within the first few days, and alert the parents to expected output of four to six wet diapers daily. By about 10 days, infants should have regained the birth weight. Assess the infant's alertness and general neurologic status (see Chapter 7 🔗).

When an infant is sick or developing slowly, parents sometimes want to feed the infant more concentrated formula to build the child's

TABLE 23–9	Normal Serum Values for Electrolytes in Infants and Youth	
	NEWBORN	**INFANT AND CHILD**
Sodium	131–144 mmol/L (131–144 mEq/L)	134–143 mmol/L (134–143 mEq/L)
Potassium	Premature 4.5–7.2 mmol/L (4.5–7.2 mEq/L)	3.7–5.0 mmol/L (3.7–5.0 mEq/L)
	Term 3.2–5.7 mmol/L (3.2–5.7 mEq/L)	
Calcium (total)	Premature 1.7–2.3 mmol/L (6.8–9.2 mg/dL or 3.4–4.6 mEq/L)	2.18–2.68 mmol/L (8.7–10.7 mg/dL or 4.36–5.36 mEq/L)
	Term 1.98–2.68 mmol/L (7.9–10.7 mg/dL or 3.96–5.36 mEq/L)	
Magnesium	0.65–1.02 mmol/L (1.6–2.5 mg/dL or 1.30–2.04 mEq/L)	0.66–0.99 mmol/L (1.6–2.4 mg/dL or 1.32–1.98 mEq/L)
Phosphorus	Newborn 1.55–2.65 mmol/L (4.8–8.2 mg/dL)	1–3 years 1.23–2.10 mmol/L (3.8–6.5 mg/dL)
		4–11 years 1.20–1.81 mmol/L (3.7–5.6 mg/dL)
		12–15 years 0.94–1.74 mmol/L (2.9–5.4 mg/dL)
		16–19 years 0.87–1.52 mmol/L (2.7–4.7 mg/dL)

Laboratories may have slightly different levels of normal depending on assays performed. Always consult the normal values for your particular laboratory.

Source: *From Greenbaum, L. A. (2011). Electrolyte and acid–base disorder. In R. M. Kliegman, B. F. Stanton, J. W. St. Geme, N. F. Schor, & R. E. Behrman, Nelson textbook of pediatrics (19th ed., pp. 212–242). Philadelphia, PA: Saunders Elsevier; Soldin, S. J., Wong, E. C., Brugnara, C., & Soldin, O. P. (2011). Pediatric reference ranges (7th ed.). Washington, DC: AACC Press.*

strength. Parents and caregivers of bottle-fed babies should be taught never to give undiluted formula concentrate or evaporated milk due to the high sodium content.

Clinical Tip
Careful teaching about how to mix powdered formula so it is not too concentrated can help prevent hypernatremia. Pictures are an important teaching tool if the parents are not able to read labels or instructions. Ask for return demonstration to evaluate ability to mix formula accurately.

Children with delayed development are at risk for hypernatremia since they may not be able to recognize thirst or obtain fluids when dehydrated. Teach parents about the child's fluid requirements (use Box 23–3 to calculate), and offer adequate fluids when the child is hospitalized.

Parents should be cautioned to keep salt out of reach, because eating handfuls of salt has caused hypernatremia. Teach parents to offer extra fluids during hot weather. See Partnering with Families: Preventing Heat-Related Illness on page 663. Teach oral rehydration therapy for use at home during mild vomiting and diarrhea (see page 670).

When a child is hospitalized for hypernatremia, monitor serum sodium level and measure intake and output and urine specific gravity. Specific gravity changes toward normal levels as therapy progresses. Frequently assess responsiveness to monitor the effect of hypernatremia on brain cells. As the concentration of body fluids returns to normal, the child will become more alert and responsive. Watch for rebound hyponatremia while monitoring the fluid replacement. Implement safety interventions such as raised bed rails for protection. Ensure adequate rest and introduce developmentally appropriate activities when the child is alert.

Water deprivation is a form of child neglect or abuse. In neglect, the parents simply do not provide adequate water for the child. A form of child abuse that sometimes includes water deprivation is Munchausen syndrome by proxy (see Chapter 20 🔗). A small child who is hospitalized with hypernatremia that does not have a detectable cause may be subject to water deprivation. Assess the child's general condition, developmental tasks, the family dynamics, and the parent's understanding of formula preparation and the child's fluid intake needs.

Nurses can prevent hypernatremia in hospitalized infants and children by administering water between tube feedings, keeping water available, and offering it frequently. Offering frequent small amounts and using frozen juice pops and other creative interventions can increase children's intake.

Desired outcomes of treatment for hypernatremia include balance of electrolytes and fluid in the intracellular and extracellular compartments, and alert level of consciousness.

Hyponatremia

In hyponatremia, the osmolality of the blood is decreased. The body fluids are too dilute, containing excess water relative to sodium. Hyponatremia is the most common sodium imbalance in children (Kliegman et al., 2011). A serum sodium level below 134 to 135 mmol/L in children (131 mmol/L in newborns) is diagnostic of hyponatremia (Greenbaum, 2011).

Etiology and pathophysiology Hyponatremia results from conditions that cause gain of relatively more water than sodium or loss of relatively more sodium than water (Table 23–10). Intake of excessive water without sodium is called **water intoxication.** As an example, oral intake of water causes hyponatremia in unusual conditions such

TABLE 23–10	Causes of Hyponatremia	
GAIN OF RELATIVELY MORE WATER THAN SODIUM	**LOSS OF RELATIVELY MORE SODIUM THAN WATER**
Excessive intravenous D₅W (5% dextrose in water)	Diarrhea or vomiting with replacement by tap water only instead of fluid containing sodium
Excessive tap water enemas	Excessive sweating such as in cystic fibrosis
Irrigation of body cavities with distilled water	Diuretics, especially thiazides
Excessive antidiuretic hormone	
Forced excessive oral intake of tap water	
Congestive heart failure	

as forced fluid intake. More commonly, parents feed an infant only water or dilute formula to save money instead of regular-strength formula or breast milk. Excessive swallowing of swimming pool water by an infant can have the same effect. Infants are vulnerable to the type of hyponatremia caused by water intoxication, because they have a poorly developed thirst mechanism and may continue to drink, and then are unable to excrete excess water quickly due to immature kidney function. Exercise-associated hyponatremia can occur when persons in prolonged physical activity such as marathon running consume hypotonic fluids in the form of water or very dilute sports drinks above the levels lost in respiratory, gastrointestinal, skin, and urinary routes (Hew-Butler, Ayus, Kipps, et al., 2008).

Clinical manifestations The child with hyponatremia has a decreased level of consciousness, which results from swelling of brain cells. This can be manifested as anorexia, nausea, vomiting, headache, muscle weakness, decreased deep tendon reflexes, agitation, lethargy, or confusion. The condition can progress to respiratory arrest, dilated pupils, decorticate posturing, and coma. If hyponatremia arises rapidly or is extreme, seizures may occur. Hyponatremia is a frequent cause of seizures in infants under 6 months of age. Severe hyponatremia can be fatal.

Collaborative Care

Nurses partner with other healthcare providers to gather laboratory specimens helpful in assessing for sodium imbalance. Careful correction of fluid and electrolyte balance is managed by the nurse, physician, neonatal nurse practitioner, pediatric nurse practitioner, and other care providers.

Diagnostic Tests

Serum sodium is the major diagnostic test. ADH levels and 24-hour urinary output are helpful in diagnosing diabetes insipidus as the cause of hyponatremia.

Clinical Therapy

Hyponatremia should be prevented in hospitalized children receiving intravenous solutions (particularly postoperatively) by administering isotonic rather than hypotonic solutions. In cases of improper formula preparation or fluid intake, hyponatremia is treated by feeding proper formula or restricting the intake of water. This therapy allows the kidneys to correct the imbalance by excreting excess water from the body. If a child is having seizures from hyponatremia, intravenous **hypertonic fluid** (more concentrated than body fluid) may be administered. Use of this concentrated saline is a way to rapidly increase body fluid concentration, but it must be monitored carefully because it can easily cause rebound hypernatremia. For exercise-associated hyponatremia, intravenous access is established at the first aid site, hypertonic saline is administered, and oxygen is delivered (American Academy of Pediatrics, 2010; Council on Sports Medicine and Fitness, 2011; Pagnotta, 2010).). In cases of diabetes insipidus, treatment for the condition is needed (see Chapter 31 @). Careful administration and monitoring are needed to avoid rebound hypernatremia.

Nursing Management

Nurses carefully assess all infants and children who are at risk for hyponatremia and promptly report symptoms to the primary care provider. Appropriate fluids with electrolytes are administered and monitored closely.

Nursing Assessment and Diagnosis

Monitor serum sodium level and measure intake and output. If an infant with hyponatremia has normal ADH levels, and other causes have been ruled out, careful questioning about proper preparation of formula and feeding practices is needed. A toddler or school-age child may be subjected to forced fluid intake as a form of child abuse. Sensitive interviewing and a caring manner on the part of the nurse can help identify such problems in a family.

Because hyponatremia is characterized by decreased level of consciousness, frequent assessment of responsiveness will be necessary to monitor the response to therapy. The child will become more alert and responsive as the concentration of body fluids returns to normal.

The highest priority nursing diagnosis for hyponatremia addresses the Risk for Injury related to the child's decreased level of consciousness. The following diagnoses might also apply:

- Self-care Deficit related to weakness and tiredness
- Health Maintenance, Ineffective related to parental information misinterpretation about infant formula
- Breastfeeding, Ineffective related to inadequate sucking by infant or inadequate milk production

NANDA-I © 2012

Planning and Implementation

Nurses can prevent hyponatremia in hospitalized children by using normal saline instead of distilled water for irrigations and by avoiding tap water enemas. Verify intravenous types and amounts and question use of hypotonic fluids in a child with no intake of sodium (Crawford & Harris, 2011). Teach parents to replace body fluids lost through diarrhea or vomiting with oral electrolyte solutions (see discussion of oral rehydration therapy earlier in this chapter). The child with a disease such as cystic fibrosis or who takes thiazide diuretics needs fluid and sodium intake above that recommended for other children. The child who is being treated for hyponatremia needs careful monitoring to avoid hypernatremia. Verify infusion rates and types of solutions. Take vital signs and evaluate level of consciousness every 15 to 30 minutes during infusion of sodium-containing solutions. Record and report results. As the child's condition returns to normal and sodium balance is returned, be certain that the infusion type and rate is also adjusted by the prescriber.

Evaluation

Expected outcomes of nursing care for hyponatremia include the following:

- The child remains safe from injury.
- Balance of fluid and electrolytes is maintained.
- Proper intake of formula, breast milk, and other fluids is established.

Potassium Imbalances

Potassium is an essential cation that performs many necessary functions in the body. It is present in high levels in intracellular fluids and is active in enzyme performance in cells. It is needed for contractility of heart and skeletal muscle. Potassium intake in healthy children comes from potassium-rich foods such as fruits and vegetables. Potassium is absorbed easily from the intestine. A potassium imbalance arises when the serum potassium concentration rises or falls outside the normal range. Potassium imbalances are caused by alterations in potassium intake, distribution, or excretion; or by loss of potassium

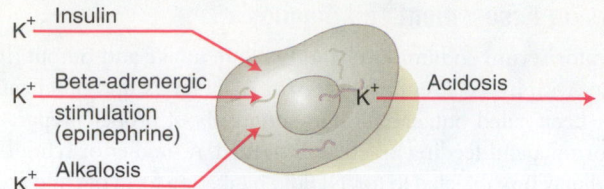

FIGURE 23–17 ■ Factors that shift potassium ions into or out of cells.

through an abnormal route such as burns, emesis, nasogastric suction, or renal failure.

Most of the potassium ions in the body are found inside the cells. The sodium-potassium pump in cell membranes moves potassium ions into cells to maintain the high intracellular potassium concentration (see Figure 23–16). Potassium ions can be shifted into or out of cells by various physiologic factors (Figure 23–17 ■). Potassium is excreted from the body through urine, feces, and sweat. The hormone aldosterone increases potassium excretion in the urine.

Hyperkalemia

Hyperkalemia is an excess of potassium in the blood. Potassium levels generally fall between 3.2 and 5.7 mmol/L for newborns, and 3.7 to 5.0 mmol/L for infants and children. Hyperkalemia is reflected by a level above 5.7 mmol/L in newborns or 5.5 mmol/L or above in children.

Etiology and pathophysiology Hyperkalemia is caused by conditions that involve increased potassium intake, shift of potassium from cells into the extracellular fluid, and decreased potassium excretion. Indeed, renal insufficiency is a primary cause of hyperkalemia. Premature infants commonly have low systemic blood flow and resultant poor renal function, leading to hyperkalemia. Increased potassium intake is usually due to intravenous potassium overload. Excessive or too rapid intravenous administration of potassium-containing solutions can occur if the potassium requirement is overestimated or if the intravenous infusion infuses too quickly.

Blood transfusion is another source of potassium intake that may cause hyperkalemia. Potassium ions leak out of red blood cells that are stored in a blood bank. The longer the blood is stored, the more potassium leaks out of cells and accumulates in the fluid portion of the transfusion. Hyperkalemia from administration of stored blood arises when multiple units are transfused, as when infants receive exchange transfusions or children receive multiple blood transfusions after a serious injury or in surgery.

Shift of potassium from cells into the extracellular fluid occurs when there is massive cell death, as with a crush injury, in sickle cell anemia (hemolytic crisis), in severe acidosis causing respiratory failure and organ failure, or when chemotherapy for a malignancy is rapidly effective. In these situations, the dead cells release their high-potassium contents into the extracellular fluid. Potassium ions also shift out of cells in metabolic acidosis caused by diarrhea and in diabetes mellitus when insulin levels are low.

Decreased potassium excretion occurs with acute or chronic oliguria during renal failure, prematurity, severe hypovolemia, and conditions that decrease the secretion of aldosterone by the adrenal cortex (lead poisoning, Addison disease, hypoaldosteronism). Several medications can lead to hyperkalemia.

Practice Alert

The following medications can cause hyperkalemia:

- Potassium-containing preparations
- Cytotoxic agents
- Potassium-sparing diuretics
- Angiotensin-converting enzyme (ACE) inhibitors
- Nonsteroidal anti-inflammatory analgesics
- Beta-blockers
- Heparin
- Trimethoprim-sulfamethoxazole antibiotic

Clinical manifestations All clinical manifestations of hyperkalemia are related to muscle dysfunction because potassium plays a vital role in muscle activity. Hyperactivity of gastrointestinal smooth muscle causes intestinal cramping and diarrhea in some children. The skeletal muscles become weak, beginning typically with leg weakness and ascending. Weakness can progress to flaccid paralysis. The child is often lethargic. Dysfunction of cardiac muscle causes cardiac arrhythmias such as tachycardia and may result in heart failure and cardiac arrest. Abnormalities in the electrocardiogram include a prolonged QRS complex, a peak in T waves, atrioventricular (AV) block, and ventricular tachycardia.

Collaborative Care

Nurses collaborate with other healthcare providers to perform accurate diagnosis of hyperkalemia, to treat the underlying conditions that cause the imbalance, and to restore electrolyte balance.

Diagnostic Tests

The major diagnostic test is serum potassium. In addition, observations of symptoms and abnormal electrocardiograph are indicative of hyperkalemia.

Clinical Tip

If an infant's hyperkalemia was diagnosed using blood obtained from a heelstick, intracellular fluid may have contaminated the sample. Intracellular fluid has a higher level of potassium which may leak into the extracellular fluid if cells are hemolyzed during the draw. A venous sample should be obtained to verify the potassium level. Additionally, it is possible for a blood sample to be damaged and show increased potassium when tested. If there is an absence of symptoms in the child, obtain a repeat sample for analysis to verify results.

Clinical Therapy

Hyperkalemia is treated by management of the underlying condition that caused the imbalance. If the serum potassium concentration is very high or is causing dangerous cardiac arrhythmias, treatment to decrease the serum potassium level may be ordered. These treatments may remove potassium from the body or drive it from the extracellular fluid into the cells. Potassium is removed from the body by peritoneal dialysis or hemodialysis, by potassium-wasting diuretics, or with a cation exchange resin (Kayexalate) that is administered orally or rectally. Medical treatments that drive potassium ions into cells are intravenous sodium bicarbonate, intravenous insulin, glucose, and calcium gluconate.

Nursing Management

Nursing management for the child with hyperkalemia is focused on restoring electrolyte balance and maintaining safety and health until normal potassium levels return.

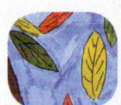

Partnering with Families

Potassium-Rich Foods

When the child is hyperkalemic, teach the parents about some common foods that contain high amounts of potassium so they can be avoided.

- Apricots
- Bananas
- Cantaloupe
- Cherries
- Coconut water
- Dates
- Figs
- Molasses
- Orange juice
- Peaches
- Potatoes
- Prunes
- Raisins
- Strawberries
- Tomato juice

Nursing Assessment and Diagnosis

Monitor serum potassium levels. Ongoing assessment of muscle strength is important, because the muscle weakness may progress to flaccid paralysis. (This paralysis is reversible on correction of the potassium imbalance.) Diarrhea can occur in infants and children. An older child may complain of intestinal cramping. Monitor the pulse rate carefully. Monitor urinary output in those with renal disease and in all infants, especially premature babies.

Nursing diagnoses for a child who has hyperkalemia depend on the severity of the clinical manifestations. The cause of the imbalance may also lead to useful diagnoses that guide teaching for the child and the parents regarding safety measures and accurate medication administration. The following nursing diagnoses may apply:

- Activity Intolerance related to decreased cardiac output secondary to cardiac arrhythmias
- Injury, Risk for related to muscle weakness
- Self-Care Deficit: Bathing and Dressing related to neuromuscular impairment
- Anxiety related to change in health status
- Health Maintenance, Ineffective related to parental lack of knowledge of dietary sources of potassium intake for a child with chronic renal failure
- Therapeutic Regimen Management: Family, Ineffective related to complexity of therapy

NANDA-I © 2012

Planning and Implementation

Nursing care includes measures to prevent hyperkalemia from developing in hospitalized children. If hyperkalemia does develop, care shifts to administering intravenous solutions, continuous monitoring of cardiopulmonary status, ensuring safety, promoting adequate nutrition, and preparing the child and family for discharge. Provide for easy bathroom access for older children and frequently check diapers for younger children. For the child in the community, potassium levels are monitored when the child is taking a drug that causes hyperkalemia, such as those used for cancer treatment.

Prevent Hyperkalemia

Any child who is receiving an intravenous infusion that contains potassium is at risk for hyperkalemia. Check that urine output is normal before administering intravenous potassium solutions. Observe the child closely and perform cardiorespiratory monitoring.

Be sure blood or packed red blood cells are fresh, especially for the child receiving multiple transfusions, and for all neonates. Use a cardiac monitor during infusion of these products to watch for arrhythmias. Be alert for hyperkalemia in any child receiving a medication that may cause the condition.

Administer Intravenous Solutions

Once a child is diagnosed as hyperkalemic, ensure that any infusions with added potassium are stopped. Several infusions may need to be managed, including glucose, sodium bicarbonate, and calcium gluconate. Maintain the infusion at the ordered rate and monitor the child's condition frequently.

Monitor Cardiopulmonary Status

Upon diagnosis of hyperkalemia, an electrocardiogram is performed and a cardiac monitor applied. Monitor for any changes in cardiac status and for cardiac arrhythmias. Report to the managing healthcare provider abnormal rate and character of pulse as well as shortness of breath.

Ensure Safety

Since the child is weak, side rails should be raised. Position the child carefully. Assist the child with activities requiring leg muscle strength, such as climbing into bed or pushing up in bed. Encourage quiet activities with frequent rest periods, considering both the child's developmental level and the degree of muscle involvement. Document and report any change in muscle weakness.

Promote Adequate Nutritional Intake

Adequate caloric intake is necessary to prevent tissue breakdown and the resultant potassium release from cells. Offer the child nourishing snacks if his or her appetite is decreased. Restrict potassium-rich foods. See Partnering with Families: Potassium-Rich Foods.

Discharge Planning and Home Care Teaching

If the child has chronic renal failure or another condition that decreases aldosterone secretion, parents and the child need to be taught to restrict foods that are high in potassium. Most oral rehydration solutions, including Pedialyte, contain potassium and should not be used to provide fluid for the child. Likewise, cola drinks contain potassium and should be avoided. Instruct the family not to use salt substitutes, which commonly contain potassium. Parents should check with the care provider and pharmacist before giving even over-the-counter products to the child, as some of these medications contain potassium.

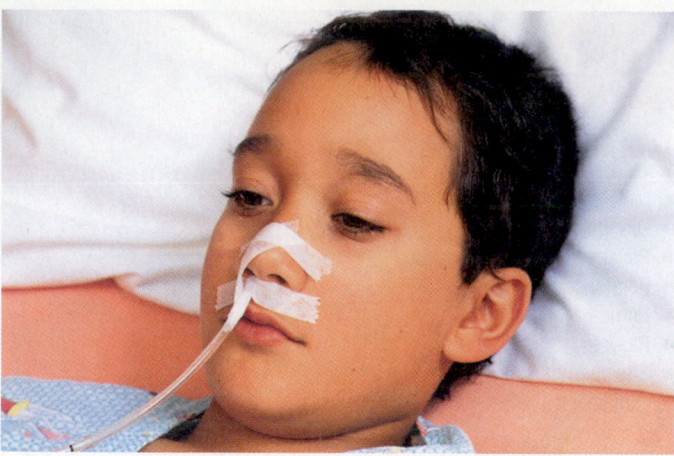

FIGURE 23–18 ■ Because this child has a nasogastric tube in place that requires suctioning, it is important to monitor his potassium levels.

Management of renal failure at home with frequent visits for dialysis and other treatments can be challenging. Refer to Chapter 31 ⊘ for further suggestions to help parents handle this condition.

Evaluation

Expected outcomes of nursing care for hyperkalemia include the following:

- The child returns to a state of fluid and electrolyte balance.
- Environmental safety is maintained.
- Adequate nutritional intake is maintained to provide essential potassium.
- Normal cardiac rate and rhythm are assessed.

Hypokalemia

Hypokalemia occurs when the serum potassium concentration is too low. Total body potassium may be decreased, normal, or even increased when the serum level is low, depending on the cause of the imbalance. Serum potassium levels below 3.7 mmol/L in children (3.2 mmol/L for newborns) are diagnostic of hypokalemia.

Etiology and pathophysiology Hypokalemia is caused by conditions that involve increased potassium excretion, decreased potassium intake, shift of potassium from the extracellular fluid into cells, and loss of potassium by an abnormal route.

Increased potassium excretion through the gastrointestinal tract is the major cause of hypokalemia in children. Loss of potassium occurs through vomiting and diarrhea (gastroenteritis). This is a major cause of the electrolyte imbalance and child mortality in developing countries. In the chapter-opening vignette, what caused Vernon's increased potassium excretion? Causes can include diarrhea, self-induced vomiting, and excessive stooling in bulimia. Nasogastric suctioning (Figure 23–18 ■) and intestinal decompression can cause potassium loss.

Causes of increased urinary potassium excretion are osmotic diuresis (glucose present in urine), hypomagnesemia, increased aldosterone (hyperaldosteronism, congestive heart failure, nephrotic syndrome, cirrhosis), and increased cortisol (Cushing disease and syndrome). Eating large amounts of black licorice made from the root of *Glycyrrhiza glabra* increases renal retention of sodium and excretion of potassium. A number of medications are also associated with hypokalemia (Sarafidis, Georgianos, & Lasaridis, 2010).

Practice Alert

Drugs that may cause hypokalemia include:

- Beta-adrenergic agonists
- Insulin
- Potassium-wasting diuretics
- Parenteral penicillins
- Glucocorticoids
- Aminoglycoside antimicrobials
- Systemic antifungals
- Antineoplastics
- Laxatives, especially when abused
- Osmotic diuretics (mannitol)

Decreased potassium intake will lead to hypokalemia slowly, or more rapidly if combined with increased excretion or loss of potassium. Hospitalized children may be placed on NPO status and receive prolonged intravenous therapy without potassium. Adolescents concerned about weight loss or those with anorexia nervosa may embark on diets low in potassium and may take medications that induce diuresis or diarrhea.

Shift of potassium from the extracellular fluid into cells occurs in alkalosis and hypothermia (unintentional or induced in surgery). Hyperalimentation often causes hypersecretion of insulin, which also shifts potassium into cells.

Clinical manifestations Since the ratio of intracellular to extracellular potassium determines the responsiveness of muscle cells to neural stimuli, it is not surprising that the clinical manifestations of hypokalemia involve muscle dysfunction. Gastrointestinal smooth muscle activity is slowed, leading to abdominal distention, constipation, or paralytic ileus. Skeletal muscles are weak and unresponsive to stimuli, and weakness may progress to flaccid paralysis. The respiratory muscles may be impaired. Cardiac arrhythmias can occur. Polyuria results from changes in the kidney caused by hypokalemia. Symptoms may include mild fatigue, particularly a prolonged QT interval, depressed ST segment, and flat or inverted T waves. Polyuria, polydipsia, and decreased urine specific gravity result from changes in the kidney caused by hypokalemia.

Collaborative Care

Nurses and other healthcare professionals collaborate to perform accurate laboratory tests to identify hypokalemia and to treat the causes in order to restore normal balance.

Diagnostic Tests

Serum measurement of potassium is the major diagnostic tool. See normal values in the previous section on hyperkalemia and in Table 23–9. In addition, observations of symptoms and an abnormal electrocardiograph are indicative of hypokalemia.

Clinical Therapy

Medical management of hypokalemia focuses on replacement of potassium while treating the cause of the imbalance. Potassium replacement may be given intravenously or orally.

Nursing Management

Nurses collect serum specimens for analysis, monitor for signs and symptoms of the imbalance, and intervene to ensure the child's safety and restore potassium balance.

Nursing Assessment and Diagnosis

Monitor serum potassium levels. Observe for muscle weakness, which is frequently detected first in the legs. Parents may report that muscle weakness restricts the child's activities and impairs interactions with peers. Skeletal muscle strength can be difficult to assess if the child is lethargic, as shown with Vernon at the beginning of the chapter.

Muscle weakness may affect the respiratory muscles. Assess the child frequently to determine the need for assisted ventilation. Cardiac monitoring is important for continued assessment of hypokalemia-associated arrhythmias.

Assess for diminished bowel sounds. Ask the parents if the child has recently been awakening to use the toilet at night or has begun bed-wetting after previously being dry at night. These may be symptoms of polyuria associated with underlying disease, which has led to hypokalemia.

The most important nursing diagnoses in the child with severe hypokalemia relate to cardiac arrhythmias and respiratory muscle weakness. The following nursing diagnoses may apply:

- Activity Intolerance, Risk for related to decreased cardiac output secondary to cardiac arrhythmia
- Breathing Pattern, Ineffective related to respiratory musculoskeletal impairment
- Injury, Risk for related to muscle weakness
- Self-care Deficit: Bathing and Dressing related to neuromuscular impairment
- Constipation related to decreased motility
- Anxiety related to change in health status
- Health Maintenance, Ineffective related to management of potassium supplements or high-potassium diet
- Therapeutic Regimen Management: Family, Ineffective related to complexity of potassium therapy
- Nutrition, Imbalanced: Less than Body Requirements related to lack of basic nutritional knowledge regarding safe weight-loss diet

NANDA-I © 2012

Planning and Implementation

Nursing care of the child with hypokalemia focuses on ensuring adequate potassium intake, monitoring cardiopulmonary status, promoting normal bowel function, ensuring safety, providing dietary counseling, and preparing the child and family for discharge.

Ensure Adequate Potassium Intake

Since potassium is excreted from the body every day, daily potassium intake is necessary to prevent hypokalemia. A child with hypokalemia who is able to eat should be given a high-potassium diet. Teach parents (and the child if old enough) which foods are high in potassium and how to incorporate them into the daily diet (see Partnering with Families on page 675).

Children who have no oral intake for a period of time should receive intravenous fluids that contain potassium. Calculate the dosage to ensure accuracy, and be sure that the infusion pump runs as scheduled. Sometimes the child will complain of burning along the vein when potassium is infused. The infusion may need to be slowed temporarily to alleviate pain and maintain the intravenous line. Remain vigilant to maintain patency of the vein to avoid infiltration which can cause tissue damage. A central line is a better choice than a peripheral line in order to decrease side effects of administration. Consult the hospital formulary for dilution and administration

---

| BOX 23–5 | Growth & Development: Bradycardia |

Bradycardia occurs at different levels for children of various ages. For infants, a pulse rate below 100 beats per minute (beats/min) is considered bradycardia. For young children, 80 beats/min may be the identified number, whereas for adolescents, a pulse below 60 beats/min is bradycardia. Look at the child's age and normal pulse range to find changes that indicate bradycardia.

---

guidelines; slow administration is needed to avoid arrhythmias and cardiac arrest. Ensure adequate fluid output for the child's age to avoid hyperkalemia from potassium infusion.

Check serum potassium for high or low potassium levels. Monitor urine output. A child who is oliguric can develop hyperkalemia when receiving supplements.

Monitor Cardiopulmonary Status

Hypokalemia potentiates digitalis toxicity. A child with hypokalemia who is receiving digitalis needs careful surveillance for digitalis toxicity, which is manifested as anorexia, nausea, vomiting, and bradycardia (Box 23–5). Observe for these effects. Take the pulse rate and rhythm regularly. Monitor respirations and ease of breathing to watch for decreased respiratory muscle activity.

Promote Normal Bowel Function

Ensure adequate fluids and fiber in the diet. Monitor and record the number of stools and report inadequate stools.

Ensure Safety

Keep side rails up. Assist the child as needed to move into and out of bed. Reposition the child frequently to preserve skin integrity of limbs that are not moved regularly. Perform passive range of motion if the child is not moving. Use supportive pillows to position the child properly.

Provide Dietary Counseling

The adolescent who is trying to lose weight and not consuming a nutritious diet needs dietary teaching. More intensive treatment will be needed for teens who are anorexic or bulimic (see Chapter 19 🔴 for interventions in these cases).

Discharge Planning and Home Care Teaching

Teach parents how to give potassium supplements, if prescribed. Liquid or powdered potassium supplements can be mixed with juice or sherbet to improve the bitter taste. The parent should call the mixture "medicine" so that the child does not learn to dislike all juices. Teach the parents signs of both hypokalemia and hyperkalemia and whom to call to report these symptoms. The signs must be reported promptly so medications can be adjusted.

Evaluation

Expected outcomes of nursing care during hypokalemia include the following:

- The child has normal rate and rhythm of heart and respiratory system.
- Regular bowel movements occur.
- Safety is maintained.
- Knowledge of child and family regarding food sources of potassium is adequate.

Pathophysiology Illustrated   Calcium Imbalance

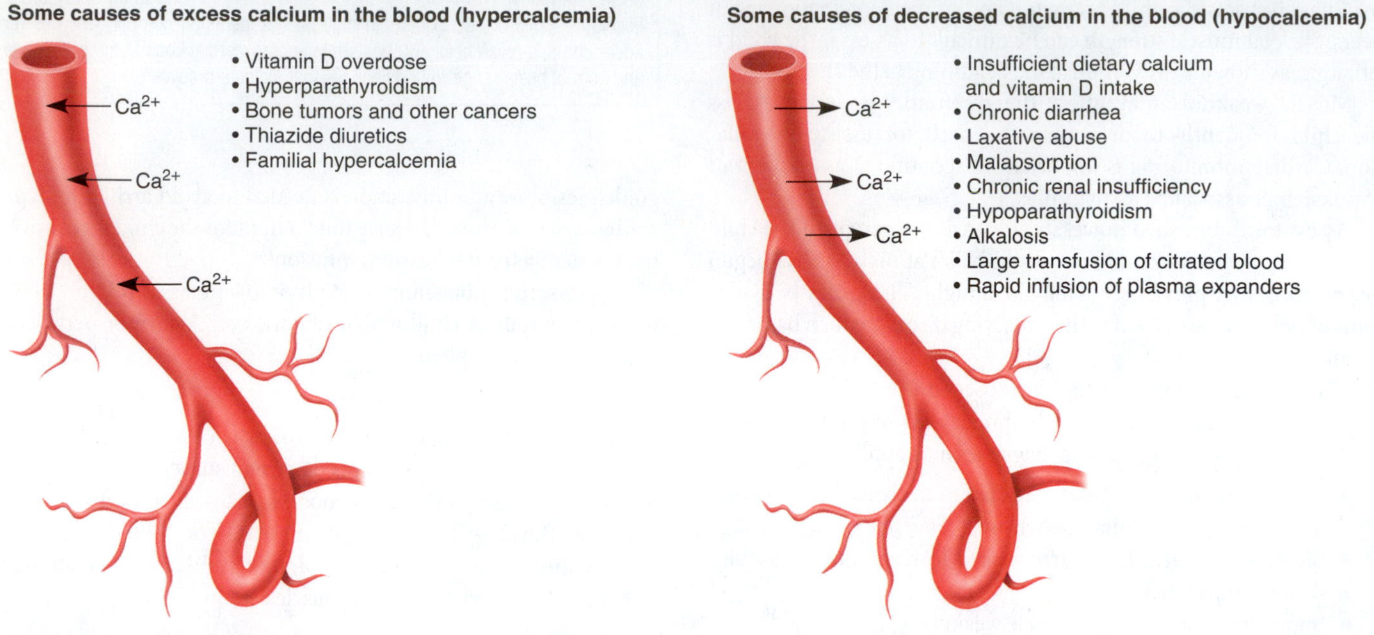

Some causes of excess calcium in the blood (hypercalcemia)

- Vitamin D overdose
- Hyperparathyroidism
- Bone tumors and other cancers
- Thiazide diuretics
- Familial hypercalcemia

Ca^{2+}

Ca^{2+}

Ca^{2+}

Some causes of decreased calcium in the blood (hypocalcemia)

- Insufficient dietary calcium and vitamin D intake
- Chronic diarrhea
- Laxative abuse
- Malabsorption
- Chronic renal insufficiency
- Hypoparathyroidism
- Alkalosis
- Large transfusion of citrated blood
- Rapid infusion of plasma expanders

Ca^{2+}

Ca^{2+}

Ca^{2+}

FIGURE 23–19 ■ A variety of conditions can lead to hypercalcemia and hypocalcemia.

Calcium Imbalances

A normal serum calcium concentration is important for many physiologic functions, including muscle and nerve function, secretion of hormones, bone formation and strength, and clotting of the blood. Calcium is the most abundant mineral in the body, with about 99% of it being present in bones (American Academy of Pediatrics, 2009). There are three forms of calcium in plasma—calcium bound to protein, calcium bound to small organic ions (e.g., citrate), and free ionized calcium (Ca^{++}), the only physiologically active form. A discussion of dietary calcium intake and its importance in bone formation can be found in Chapter 19 🔗. Also see Developing Cultural Competence: Calcium Intake and Osteoporosis.

Calcium imbalances are caused by alterations in calcium intake, absorption, distribution, or excretion. Calcium absorption requires vitamin D for maximum efficiency and is greatest in the duodenum. Calcium distribution involves calcium entry into and exit from bones

and the distribution of different forms of calcium in the plasma. Excretion of calcium occurs in urine, feces, and sweat (Figure 23–19 ■). Parathyroid hormone is the major regulator of the plasma calcium concentration. It increases this concentration by increasing calcium absorption, increasing calcium withdrawal from bones, and decreasing calcium excretion in the urine. The plasma calcium concentration has an important influence on cell membrane permeability and influences the threshold potential of excitable cells. For this reason, calcium imbalances alter neuromuscular irritability.

Hypercalcemia

Hypercalcemia refers to a plasma excess of total calcium (above 5.3 mEq/L [2.7 mmol/L]). Because so much calcium is stored in the bones, however, the serum levels of calcium may not reflect body stores.

Etiology and pathophysiology Hypercalcemia is caused by conditions that involve increased calcium intake or absorption, shift of calcium from bones into the extracellular fluid, and decreased calcium excretion. Hypercalcemia due to increased calcium intake or absorption may occur if an infant is fed large amounts of chicken liver (source of vitamin A) or is given megadoses of vitamin D or vitamin A, or if a child or adolescent consumes large amounts of calcium-rich foods concurrently with antacids (milk-alkali syndrome). Infants with very low birth weight can develop hypercalcemia if they have inadequate phosphorus intake, as bone phosphorus and calcium will be resorbed. Hypercalcemia may also occur when children receiving total parenteral nutrition are given doses of calcium that are too high.

Most cases of hypercalcemia in children are due to a shift of calcium from bones into the extracellular fluid. The excessive amounts of parathyroid hormone produced in hyperparathyroidism cause calcium withdrawal from bones. Prolonged immobilization also

Developing Cultural Competence
Calcium Intake and Osteoporosis

Ingestion and absorption of calcium is important in the growing child to ensure formation of strong bones. Adolescents who ingest more calcium have less risk of osteoporosis later in life. It has been noted that Black women have less bone loss and fewer fractures than White women. Studies with Black and White individuals have demonstrated that Blacks absorb more calcium from the diet, and lose less in their urine, leading to increased bone density. However, this has led to an underidentification of osteoporosis in Black women who have relative risks of lactose intolerance and low dairy intake. Assess calcium intake for all and suggest appropriate interventions for your population group and individuals (NIH Osteoporosis and Related Bone Diseases National Resource Center, 2011).

causes withdrawal of calcium from bones. Often, the excess calcium ions are excreted in the urine. However, if calcium is withdrawn from bones faster than the kidneys can excrete it, hypercalcemia results. Hypercalcemia also occurs with many types of malignancies such as leukemias. The malignant cells produce substances that circulate in the blood to the bones and cause bone resorption. The calcium from the bones then enters the extracellular fluid, causing hypercalcemia. Bone tumors and chemotherapy destroy bone directly, leading to the release of calcium. In spite of high calcium in the blood, the levels in bone are low and the child is prone to fractures. Familial hypercalcemia and infantile hypercalcemia are rare congenital disorders.

Thiazide diuretics (e.g., thiazide and hydrochlorothiazide) decrease calcium excretion in the urine and may contribute to development of hypercalcemia. Other drugs that can cause hypercalcemia include lithium and theophylline (Ruppe, 2011).

Clinical manifestations Hypercalcemia may have nonspecific symptoms, making diagnosis difficult. Many of the signs and symptoms of hypercalcemia are manifestations of decreased neuromuscular excitability. Constipation, anorexia, nausea, and vomiting can occur. Fatigue and skeletal muscle weakness predominate. Confusion, lethargy, and decreased attention span are common, and polyuria develops. Renal calculi may form due to the high calcium levels. Severe hypercalcemia may cause cardiac arrhythmias and arrest. Neonates with hypercalcemia have flaccid muscles and exhibit failure to thrive. Hypercalcemia increases sodium and potassium excretion by the kidneys and can lead to polyuria and polydipsia.

Collaborative Care

Nurses collaborate with other healthcare providers to assess for hypercalcemia. Treatments focus on medications and care during dialysis when this treatment is needed.

Diagnostic Tests

Serum calcium is tested although the blood levels may not reflect bone stores. Additional diagnostic laboratory analyses to assist in diagnosis of the cause include albumin, phosphate, magnesium, alkaline phosphate, electrolytes, blood urea nitrogen, creatinine, and parathyroid hormone.

Hypercalcemia is treated by increasing fluids and administering the diuretic furosemide (Lasix) to increase excretion of calcium in the urine. Treatment to decrease intestinal absorption of calcium involves effective use of glucocorticoids. Bone resorption can be decreased by administration of glucocorticoids and calcitonin. Phosphate is sometimes given to treat hypercalcemia, but it may cause dangerous precipitation of calcium phosphate salts in body tissues. Dialysis may be used, if necessary. Treatment of the underlying cause for the disorder is needed as well.

Nursing Management

The nurse assesses calcium status and plans nursing care to help in establishing normal calcium balance.

Nursing Assessment and Diagnosis

Nursing assessment of a child with hypercalcemia includes monitoring serum calcium levels, level of consciousness, gastrointestinal function, urine volume, specific gravity, cardiac rhythm, and pH. Recall that there are several types of calcium, and notice that laboratory results may provide total calcium or ionized calcium; refer to the laboratory normal ranges for proper interpretation. With chronic hypercalcemia, assessment of activity tolerance and developmental level becomes important.

Many nursing diagnoses are appropriate for children who have hypercalcemia. Diagnoses that address cardiac and neuromuscular manifestation are especially important. The following nursing diagnoses may apply:

- Activity Intolerance, Risk for related to decreased cardiac output secondary to cardiac arrhythmia
- Injury, Risk for related to decreased level of response
- Injury, Risk for related to neuromuscular impairment
- Injury, Risk for related to possibility of spontaneous fractures
- Self-Care Deficit: Bathing and Dressing related to neuromuscular impairment
- Anxiety related to change in health status
- Constipation related to decreased motility
- Nutrition, Imbalanced: Less than Body Requirements related to anorexia and nausea
- Urinary Elimination, Impaired related to renal calculi

NANDA-I © 2012

Planning and Intervention

Carefully calculate calcium in total parenteral nutrition and other solutions, administer these solutions with caution, and use cardiac monitoring to prevent hypercalcemia in hospitalized children.

Interventions to increase fluid intake are important for children with hypercalcemia or those who are immobilized. A generous fluid intake, appropriate to the child's age, is necessary to keep the urine dilute and to help reduce constipation (a common symptom of hypercalcemia). An acidic urine helps to keep calcium from forming stones. Because urinary tract infections may cause the urine to be alkaline, nursing interventions to prevent urinary tract infection are necessary. Thiazide diuretics, which decrease calcium excretion, should not be given to the child with hypercalcemia. Provide a high-fiber diet to help reduce constipation.

Increasing mobility through assisted weight bearing helps to decrease the withdrawal of calcium from bones that is caused by immobility. If the hypercalcemia is caused by withdrawal of calcium from bones, the child is at risk for fractures with minor trauma and must be handled with special care. See Chapter 35 🔗 for further discussion of care following fractures and prolonged casting. A further description of metabolic emergency with hypercalcemia during cancer treatment can be found in Chapter 29 🔗.

Teach parents to avoid giving calcium-rich foods and calcium antacids (e.g., Tums) to children with hypercalcemia. Suggest juices and frozen fruit desserts as an alternative to milk and ice cream. Vitamin D supplements should be avoided as they increase calcium absorption from the gastrointestinal tract.

Evaluation

Expected outcomes of nursing care include the following:

- Cardiac pump effectiveness is demonstrated by absence of arrhythmias.
- Safety is ensured to prevent fractures.
- Normal bowel excretion is assessed.
- Adequate nutritional status is maintained.

Hypocalcemia

Hypocalcemia is a serum deficit of calcium (below 4.3 mEq/L [2.1 mmol/L] in children, 4 mEq/L [2 mmol/L] in newborns, or 3.4 mEq/L [1.7 mmol/L] in premature infants). Recall that serum calcium levels may not reflect body stores of this mineral, as most of the body's calcium is stored in bone.

Etiology and pathophysiology Hypocalcemia is caused by conditions that involve decreased calcium intake or absorption, shift of calcium to a physiologically unavailable form, increased calcium excretion, and loss of calcium by an abnormal route.

Decreased calcium intake or absorption causes hypocalcemia in children with chronic generalized malnutrition, or with a diet that is low in vitamin D and calcium. Female adolescents trying to lose or maintain a low weight often decrease foods that contain calcium and may develop chronic hypocalcemia. In these cases, premature bone loss and inadequate bone formation occur. (See Chapter 19 🔗 for further discussion of calcium intake during adolescence.) This deficit cannot be made up later in life, thus increasing the risk of osteoporosis.

Even with a normal calcium intake, hypocalcemia occurs if the mineral is not absorbed. If a child does not have enough vitamin D, calcium is not absorbed efficiently from the duodenum. Sunlight speeds formation of vitamin D in the skin. Children who are institutionalized without access to sunlight (e.g., children with severe developmental delays), those with very dark skin, or children kept well covered when outside may become hypocalcemic due to lack of vitamin D (see Chapter 19). Uremic syndrome is another cause of vitamin D deficiency. It interferes with the kidney's ability to activate vitamin D. High phosphate intake can cause hypocalcemia. Chronic diarrhea and steatorrhea (fatty stools) also reduce calcium absorption from the gastrointestinal tract.

About 40% of calcium is bound to proteins and is not available for interactions, 10% is bound to small organic ions such as citrate, and about 50% is ionized and physiologically active. The shift of calcium into a physiologically unavailable form occurs when calcium shifts into bone, or free ionized calcium in plasma binds to proteins or small organic ions in the plasma. Conditions leading to hypocalcemia include the following:

- Too much calcium shifts into bones in various types of hypoparathyroidism, including DiGeorge syndrome (congenital absence of the parathyroid glands; see Chapter 32 🔗 for further description of this syndrome).
- Alkalosis causes more calcium to bind to plasma proteins and become physiologically inactive. For example, citrate, found in transfused blood, can bind to body calcium.
- Ionized hypocalcemia, which is due to an increased binding of plasma ionized calcium during alkalosis, occurs rapidly. The ionized hypocalcemia persists until the alkalosis resolves or the citrate is metabolized by the liver.
- Hypomagnesemia impairs parathyroid hormone function and may cause hypocalcemia. Some types of neonatal hypocalcemia are associated with delayed parathyroid hormone function or hypomagnesemia.
- A genetic abnormality can result in calcium-sensing receptor defect.
- Infants of mothers with diabetes may have hypocalcemia in response to glycosuria that leads to hypomagnesemia.

- Very-low-birth-weight babies and newborns with respiratory impairment are prone to develop hypocalcemia.
- Calcium shifts rapidly into bone when rickets is treated.
- A high plasma phosphate concentration causes plasma calcium to decrease.
- Children who receive liver transplants are hypocalcemic for several days due to impaired citrate metabolism.

Increased calcium excretion occurs in steatorrhea, when calcium secreted into the gastrointestinal fluid binds to the fecal fat in addition to the dietary calcium bound in the feces. A similar situation occurs in acute pancreatitis.

Loss of calcium by an abnormal route may contribute to hypocalcemia as calcium is lost from the body through burn or wound drainage or sequestered in acute pancreatitis. Many different medications can cause hypocalcemia.

Practice Alert

Drugs that may cause hypocalcemia include:

- Antacids (if overused)
- Laxatives (if overused)
- Oil-based bowel lubricants
- Anticonvulsants
- Phosphate-containing preparations
- Protein-type plasma expanders during rapid infusion
- Antineoplastics

Clinical manifestations. The signs and symptoms of hypocalcemia are manifestations of increased muscular excitability (tetany). In children they include twitching and cramping, tingling around the mouth or in the fingers, carpal spasm, and pedal spasm. Infants may demonstrate tremors, muscle twitches, and brief tonic-clonic seizures. Laryngospasm, seizures, and cardiac arrhythmias are more severe manifestations of hypocalcemia and may be fatal. Hypocalcemia may cause congestive heart failure, especially in neonates.

Although these symptoms are diagnostic of acute calcium deficiency, a more common state in children and adolescents is chronic low intake of calcium. This may be manifested by spontaneous fractures in infants and in adolescents who exercise excessively. See Chapter 19 for further information about osteoporosis and osteopenia in youth.

Collaborative Care

Laboratory measurements of serum calcium are the most useful diagnostic tool. Cardiac monitoring may be performed to observe for cardiac arrhythmias.

Hypocalcemia is treated by oral or intravenous administration of calcium. See the Medication table. The original cause of the imbalance is also treated. If the hypocalcemia is due to hypomagnesemia, the magnesium must be replenished before the calcium replacement can be successful. When the cause is chronic low dietary intake, counseling is needed about high-calcium foods, and perhaps the necessity for vitamin D intake or supplements.

Nursing Management

Nurses assess diets and partner with families to ensure adequate calcium intake by children and adolescents. When medical conditions put the child at risk of hypocalcemia, careful ongoing assessments of the

Medication Used to Treat Acute Hypocalcemia

MEDICATION	ACTION	NURSING MANAGEMENT
10% calcium gluconate IV	Calcium is a normal body electrolyte and may need to be infused in infants or young children with health problems leading to low calcium. It is also used during exchange transfusion in neonates since citrate in the blood transfusion can bind body calcium. In the form of CaCl, calcium may be used during resuscitation. Calcium regulates excitability of muscles and nerves, and therefore affects cardiac function (inotropic effect); is necessary for blood clotting; plays a role in storage and release of neurotransmitters, in renal function, and in maintaining cell membranes; and is an antidote to excessive magnesium infusion.	Verify dose and preparation carefully with the prescriber and another nurse. Monitor heart rate and rhythm—hypotension and bradycardia can occur. Use extreme caution if given in cardiac or renal disease. Maintain IV carefully to avoid extravasation; do *not* administer by peripheral infusion, scalp vein, IM, or SC. Precipitates when given in infusion with bicarbonate.

child are needed. Acute hypocalcemia is treated, associated problems monitored, and medications administered to restore calcium balance.

Nursing Assessment and Diagnosis

Carefully assess growth in infants and children as a marker of adequate calcium intake, and nutritional status in general. When an adolescent female is dieting or very thin, be sure to ask about excessive sports and other activities, and about regularity of menstrual periods. If periods are irregular or not occurring, collect additional dietary information to help determine whether the girl is lacking in intake of calcium, calories, and other nutrients. These assessments are needed even if serum calcium values are normal. Look for signs of inadequate nutrition such as fat and muscle wasting, dry hair, and cold hands and feet.

In those who may have acute hypocalcemia, assess for muscle cramps, stiffness, and clumsiness; grimacing caused by spasms of facial muscles; twitching of arm muscles; and laryngospasm. Increased neuromuscular excitability may be detected by testing for Trousseau sign or Chvostek sign. Many healthy newborns have a positive Chvostek sign; however, this assessment should be reserved for children over several months of age. Monitor serum calcium levels and perform continuous cardiac monitoring to observe for cardiac arrhythmias.

The effects of increased neuromuscular excitability in the child with hypocalcemia are the basis for the following nursing diagnoses:

- Injury, Risk for related to potential for fractures
- Risk for Breathing Pattern, Ineffective related to laryngospasm

- Activity Intolerance related to decreased cardiac output secondary to cardiac arrhythmias
- Environmental Interpretation Syndrome, Impaired related to electrolyte imbalance
- Nutrition, Imbalanced: Less than Body Requirements related to lack of basic nutritional knowledge of sources and recommended amounts of calcium intake

NANDA-I © 2012

Planning and Implementation

To correct calcium deficiency in the hospitalized child, give oral or intravenous calcium as ordered. Monitor for complications of calcium supplementation. A 10% IV calcium gluconate solution should be readily available for emergency use in severe hypocalcemia. Calcium is never given intramuscularly because it causes tissue necrosis.

Take measures to ensure safety for the child who is hospitalized with hypocalcemia. Seizure precautions may be necessary. Explain the cause of muscle cramps to parents and older children.

Counsel the family about dairy products and nondairy foods rich in calcium (see Partnering with Families: High-Calcium Foods). For the adolescent female whose weight is low and menstrual patterns show irregularities, total calories and calcium intake should be increased. Teaching may also be needed about proper calcium intake and its importance both to athletic performance and to prevention of osteoporosis. Encourage three glasses of nonfat milk per day. Teach ways to use milk in the diet. For example, sprinkle nonfat dry milk on cereal and other

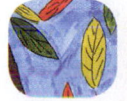

Partnering with Families

High-Calcium Foods

When a child needs to increase sources of calcium, parents may be unfamiliar with the variety of foods that contain calcium. Although they are aware that dairy products have high calcium, there are many other foods that add a significant amount of calcium to the diet. Some may be more acceptable to families in certain cultures. Possible sources of calcium include the following:

- Milk
- Cheese
- Yogurt
- Pudding
- Egg yolks

- Legumes
- Nuts
- Figs
- Chicken
- Salmon (canned with bones)
- Grains (Cream of Wheat, farina, bran muffins)
- Sardines (canned)
- Tofu
- Fruit drinks with added calcium

foods. If the child is lactose intolerant, emphasize nondairy sources of calcium and advise parents to purchase special milk treated with lactase. This milk is more costly, and inadequate family finances may be an impediment to its use. If a child has a health condition leading to chronic diarrhea, encourage increased intake of calcium-rich foods. Calcium supplements in the form of calcium carbonate tablets may be used.

Clinical Tip

To test for Trousseau sign, a blood pressure cuff may be inflated for about 3 minutes. If a carpal spasm occurs, the Trousseau sign is positive. To test for Chvostek sign, the skin is tapped lightly just in front of the ear (over the facial nerve). If the corner of the mouth draws up because of muscle contraction, the Chvostek sign is positive. These findings may be indicative of hypocalcemia or hypomagnesemia.

Practice Alert
Oral Calcium

Calcium tablets and powders are available for relief of acid indigestion and to increase calcium intake when it is deficient. Popular products contain calcium carbonate (e.g., Tums), calcium acetate, calcium citrate, tricalcium phosphate, calcium lactate, calcium gluconate, and calcium polycarbophil. Since so many forms exist, be sure that chewable tablets are chewed, sustained-release tablets are swallowed whole, and powders are mixed and administered as recommended. The most common side effect is constipation; other side effects are hypercalcemia and renal calculi.

Intravenous Calcium

Intravenous calcium is administered to treat severe hypocalcemia such as in tetany due to parathyroid disease, in cardiac resuscitation, during exchange transfusions in newborns, and to relieve muscle cramps caused by insect bites. Intravenous calcium has several serious potential side effects, so nursing care centers on maintaining an intact intravenous line, continuous cardiorespiratory monitoring, and monitoring calcium and phosphate levels.

Evaluation

Expected outcomes of nursing care for hypocalcemia include the following:

- Ingestion of recommended dietary allowances for calcium occurs.
- Discomfort from muscle spasms related to calcium imbalance does not occur.
- The child is free from injury due to fractures.

Magnesium Imbalances

Magnesium is necessary for enzyme function in cells, acetylcholine release, glycolysis, stimulation of adenosine triphosphate enzymes (ATPases), and bone formation. Magnesium is a component of chlorophyll; thus, magnesium intake is aided by eating dark green leafy vegetables. Nuts and grains are also good sources of this mineral. Magnesium is absorbed primarily from the terminal ileum. It is distributed among the extracellular fluid (small amounts), the cells (larger amounts), and the bones (largest amounts). Magnesium excretion occurs in urine, feces, and sweat.

Magnesium imbalances are caused by alterations in magnesium intake, distribution, or excretion; by loss through an abnormal route; or by a combination of these factors. The plasma magnesium concentration influences the release of acetylcholine at neuromuscular junctions. Thus, magnesium imbalances are characterized by alterations in neuromuscular irritability.

Hypermagnesemia

Hypermagnesemia occurs when the plasma magnesium concentration is too high (above 2.4 mg/dL [0.99 mmol/L]). Keep in mind that the serum levels measured in the laboratory may not reflect body magnesium stores, because most of the magnesium in the body is located in the bones and inside the cells.

Hypermagnesemia is caused by conditions that involve increased magnesium intake and decreased magnesium excretion. Impaired renal function leading to decreased magnesium excretion is the most common cause of hypermagnesemia in children. In both oliguric renal failure and adrenal insufficiency, magnesium ions that cannot be excreted in the urine accumulate in the extracellular fluid.

Less frequently, increased magnesium intake may cause hypermagnesemia. Magnesium sulfate ($MgSO_4$) given to treat eclampsia in the mother before delivery causes hypermagnesemia in the newborn. Abnormally high amounts may also be taken in magnesium-containing enemas, laxatives, antacids, and intravenous fluids. Epsom salt is a readily available product and is a nearly pure magnesium sulfate preparation; its use as an enema has caused death in children. It has been used as a cathartic in the treatment of poisoning in the past but due to its potential for overdose, sorbitol is now preferred. Aspiration of seawater, as in drowning, is an uncommon but potentially serious source of excessive magnesium intake. Children with Addison disease can have abnormally high magnesium levels.

Clinical manifestations of hypermagnesemia include decreased muscle irritability, hypotension, bradycardia, drowsiness, lethargy, and weak or absent deep tendon reflexes. In severe hypermagnesemia, flaccid muscle paralysis, fatal respiratory depression, cardiac arrhythmias, and cardiac arrest occur (Musso, 2009).

Hypermagnesemia is managed primarily by increasing the urinary excretion of magnesium. This is usually accomplished by increasing fluid intake (except in oliguric renal failure) and by the administration of diuretics. Dialysis may sometimes be necessary.

Nursing Management

The goal of nursing management is to provide assessment of magnesium status in infants and children at risk of imbalance, and to intervene to restore balance when necessary. Monitor serum magnesium levels. Take the child's blood pressure (to monitor for hypotension), heart rate and rhythm (to monitor for bradycardia and cardiac arrhythmias), respiratory rate and depth (to observe for respiratory depression), and deep tendon reflexes (to assess muscle tone and paralysis or movement). Keep the side rails of the bed raised. Children with hypermagnesemia or oliguria should not be given magnesium-containing medications or sea salt.

Teach parents of children with chronic renal failure that these children should never be given milk of magnesia, antacids that contain magnesium, or other sources of magnesium. Parents should learn to read labels carefully to look for products that contain magnesium. When hypermagnesemia is treated with diuretics, monitor potassium levels to watch for hypokalemia.

Expected outcomes of nursing care include maintenance of electrolyte balance, normal neuromuscular tone, safety, and regular heart rate and rhythm.

Hypomagnesemia

Hypomagnesemia refers to a plasma magnesium concentration that is too low (below 1.6 mg/dL [0.66 mmol/L]). Remember that the serum levels of magnesium may not reflect body stores, as most of the magnesium in the body is found in cells and bones.

Partnering with Families

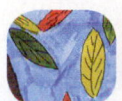

Magnesium-Rich Foods

Magnesium is a mineral with which most families are not familiar. When a child needs to increase magnesium intake, families can be encouraged to add two to three of the following foods to the child's daily diet:

- Whole grain cereal
- Dark green vegetables
- Soy
- Almonds
- Peanut butter
- Bananas
- Egg yolk

Hypomagnesemia is caused by conditions that involve decreased magnesium intake or absorption, shift of magnesium to a physiologically unavailable form, increased magnesium excretion, and loss of magnesium by an abnormal route. Hypocalcemia often accompanies and contributes to hypomagnesemia.

Neonates whose mothers are diabetic sometimes develop hypomagnesemia in the newborn period. Decreased magnesium intake or absorption can occur if a child who is not eating has prolonged intravenous therapy without magnesium. Chronic malnutrition is another cause of decreased magnesium intake. Magnesium absorption is decreased in chronic diarrhea, short bowel syndrome, malabsorption syndromes, and steatorrhea.

A shift of magnesium to a physiologically unavailable form may occur after transfusion of many units of citrated blood products, because magnesium bound to the citrate is not physiologically active. Such transfusions cause prolonged hypomagnesemia in liver transplant patients who have impaired citrate metabolism. Magnesium shifts rapidly into bones that have been deprived of adequate stores.

Increased magnesium excretion in the urine occurs with diuretic therapy, the diuretic phase of acute renal failure, diabetic ketoacidosis, and hyperaldosteronism. Chronic alcoholism, occasionally seen in adolescents, increases urinary magnesium excretion. Magnesium contained in gastrointestinal secretions is bound to fat and excreted in the stool.

Loss of magnesium by an abnormal route occurs with prolonged nasogastric suction and through sequestration of magnesium in acute pancreatitis. Several medications may cause hypomagnesemia, such as magnesium-wasting diuretics, some antineoplastic agents, systemic antifungals, aminoglycoside antibiotics, and laxatives.

Hypomagnesemia is characterized by increased neuromuscular excitability (tetany). The clinical manifestations are hyperactive reflexes, skeletal muscle cramps, twitching, tremors, and cardiac arrhythmias. Seizures can occur with severe hypomagnesemia. Hypomagnesemia is associated with high mortality for children in the pediatric intensive care unit.

Magnesium serum levels are measured, along with serum calcium and potassium, since these electrolyte disturbances often occur together. See the normal level for serum magnesium in the previous section. Hypomagnesemia is managed by administering magnesium and treating the underlying cause of the imbalance.

Nursing Management

In addition to monitoring serum magnesium levels, nursing assessment of hypomagnesemia includes monitoring deep tendon reflexes, testing for Trousseau and Chvostek signs, monitoring cardiac function, and observing for muscle twitching. Children who are able to talk will report muscle cramping. Because magnesium levels are not routinely measured in many settings, request the test for any child who has risk factors and early manifestations of hypomagnesemia. When intramuscular or intravenous magnesium is ordered, administer carefully as directed and monitor vital signs. Electrocardiogram and renal studies may precede drug administration. Have resuscitative drugs and equipment readily available during drug administration.

Teach parents of a child with hypomagnesemia or continuing risk factors such as chronic diarrhea to include magnesium-rich foods in the diet (see Partnering with Families: Magnesium-Rich Foods). Before administering magnesium supplements, verify that the child's urine output is adequate. Monitor deep tendon reflexes if intravenous magnesium is given, and observe for complications of magnesium supplementation.

Practice Alert
Oral Magnesium

Magnesium tablets, capsules, solution, and suspension are available for relief of acid indigestion and to stimulate peristalsis. Popular products contain magnesium citrate, magnesium hydroxide, magnesium oxide, and magnesium salicylate. When used as a cathartic, administer the recommended amount of water to ensure bowel evacuation. The most common side effect is abdominal cramping accompanied by diarrhea; other side effects are dehydration, respiratory depression, and electrolyte imbalance.

Intravenous Magnesium

Intravenous magnesium is administered in the form of magnesium sulfate to treat severe hypomagnesemia, refractory hypocalcemia, and intractable seizures. Intravenous magnesium has side effects of hypermagnesemia, respiratory depression, hypotension, and central nervous system (CNS) depression. This form of therapy requires close monitoring of body systems and electrolyte status.

Expected outcomes for nursing care include restoration and maintenance of electrolyte balance.

Phosphorus Imbalances

Phosphorus plays an important role in cellular metabolism and is an important component of bone. Phosphorus circulates as the phosphate ion in blood, and the inorganic form (Pi) is measured in laboratory samples. Normal levels are highest in infants and decrease with age (Johnson, 2010).

Hyperphosphatemia is manifested by a Pi level above 1.8 mmol/L (5.6 mg/dL). It is associated with hypoparathyroidism, inadvertent excess administration of phosphate such as intravenously or via enemas, and tumor lysis syndrome (see Chapter 29 for further description of this syndrome in cancer chemotherapy). Symptoms are similar to those for hypocalcemia (see previous discussion). The condition is treated with phosphate binders; dialysis can be used when the condition is severe (Greenbaum, 2011).

Hypophosphatemia is manifested by a Pi level below 0.91 mmol/L (2.8 mg/dL). It is associated with starvation states, corticosteroid drugs, and vitamin D deficient rickets (see Chapter 19 🔗), and is seen in very premature infants. Neurologic symptoms are most common. Oral or intravenous potassium phosphate is used for treatment.

Clinical Evaluation of Fluid and Electrolyte Imbalance

How can you evaluate children appropriately for fluid and electrolyte imbalance without thinking through the clinical manifestations of every possible disorder one after the other? First, perform a rapid risk factor assessment on each child to see which factors are present (Tables 23–11 and 23–12). Remember that most imbalances influence other factors so it is common to find more than one type of fluid and electrolyte problem. Examining several body systems such as cardiovascular, respiratory, and neurologic will be necessary to get a comprehensive picture of the child.

A risk factor assessment may be performed mentally during routine tasks. Look for factors that alter the intake, retention, and loss of isotonic fluid and water. This information is used to evaluate which fluid imbalance is most likely to occur in a particular child. Next, look for factors that alter electrolyte intake and absorption, distribution between plasma and other electrolyte pools, excretion, and abnormal routes of electrolyte loss. This information is used to evaluate which electrolyte imbalances are most likely to occur in the child. A review of pathophysiology is important to understand the role of the other electrolytes and substances, such as phosphorus, in the body. Apply growth and development principles to identify what types of problems might be most common in various age groups. For example, the newborn is more likely to be dehydrated due to lack of adequate intake, while the toddler more commonly suffers fluid loss from nausea and vomiting.

After evaluating possible imbalances for the child, perform a clinical assessment. Assessment of fluid imbalances is performed by assessing weight changes, vascular volume, interstitial volume, and cerebral function (Table 23–13). Assessment of electrolyte imbalances is performed by assessing serum electrolyte levels, skeletal muscle strength, neuromuscular excitability, gastrointestinal tract function, and cardiac rhythm (Table 23–14). Next, check for other manifestations that are specific to a particular high-risk imbalance (e.g., polyuria in hypokalemia). Evaluate any serum laboratory values available. This method of risk factor assessment followed by clinical assessment provides a rapid yet thorough approach to assessment for fluid and electrolyte imbalances.

ACID–BASE IMBALANCES

There are four acid–base imbalances. Two are the result of processes that cause too much acid in the body and are referred to as **acidosis.** The other two imbalances are the result of processes that cause too little acid in the body and are called **alkalosis.** An acid–base disorder caused by too much or too little carbonic acid is called a respiratory acid–base imbalance. A disorder caused by too much or too little metabolic acid is called a metabolic acid–base imbalance (Box 23–6). Mixed imbalances—acidosis concurrent with alkalosis—are possible as well.

Arterial blood gas measurements (ABGs) provide a laboratory evaluation of a child's current acid–base status. In addition, oxygenation saturation, or the percentage of hemoglobin saturated with arterial blood, is normally 95% to 100%. See Table 23–15 for normal values for each measurement and Box 23–7 for a method that can help to interpret the pH, P_{CO_2}, and bicarbonate concentrations, which are the most important acid–base measures. Capillary blood gases are commonly used with neonates and infants to decrease the amount of blood used for samples. End-tidal CO_2 can provide a continuous noninvasive measurement. Remember that P_{CO_2} reflects carbonic acid status, and bicarbonate concentration reflects the metabolic acid status (Dzierba & Abraham, 2011).

Respiratory Acidosis

Respiratory acidosis is caused by the accumulation of carbon dioxide in the blood. Since carbon dioxide and water can be combined into carbonic acid, respiratory acidosis is sometimes called carbonic acid excess. The condition can be acute or chronic. It is controlled by the lungs.

TABLE 23–11	Risk Factor Assessment for Fluid Imbalances
ISOTONIC FLUID (EXTRACELLULAR FLUID VOLUME IMBALANCES)	**WATER**
Is there a source of increased intake?	Is there a source of increased intake?
Is aldosterone secretion increased or decreased?	Is antidiuretic hormone secretion increased or decreased?
Is there a source of loss from the body?	Is there a source of unusual loss from the body?

TABLE 23–12	Risk Factor Assessment for Electrolyte Imbalances		
ELECTROLYTE INTAKE AND ABSORPTION	**ELECTROLYTE SHIFTS**	**ELECTROLYTE EXCRETION**	**ELECTROLYTE LOSS BY ABNORMAL ROUTE**
Is it increased? Is it decreased?	Has it shifted from the electrolyte pool to plasma? Has it shifted from plasma to the electrolyte pool?	Is excretion increased? Is excretion decreased?	Do any of the following exist: ▪ Vomiting? ▪ Diarrhea? ▪ Nasogastric suction? ▪ Wound? ▪ Burn? ▪ Excessive sweating?

TABLE 23–13 | Summary of Clinical Assessment of Fluid Imbalances

ASSESSMENT CATEGORY	SPECIFIC ASSESSMENTS	CHANGES WITH FLUID IMBALANCES
Rapid changes in weight	Daily weights at same time each day	Weight gain—extracellular volume excess
		Weight loss—extracellular volume deficit; clinical dehydration
Vascular volume	Capillary refill time	Increased—extracellular volume deficit; clinical dehydration
	Character of pulse	Bounding—extracellular volume excess
		Thready—extracellular volume deficit; clinical dehydration
	Postural blood pressure measurements	Postural drop—extracellular volume deficit; clinical dehydration
	Lung sounds in dependent portions	Crackles—extracellular volume excess
	Central venous pressure	Increased—extracellular volume excess
		Decreased—extracellular volume deficit; clinical dehydration
	Tenseness of fontanel (infants)	Bulging—extracellular volume excess
		Sunken—extracellular volume deficit; clinical dehydration
	Neck vein filling (older children)	Full when upright—extracellular volume excess
		Flat when supine—extracellular volume deficit; clinical dehydration
Interstitial volume	Skin turgor	Skin tents—extracellular volume deficit; clinical dehydration
	Presence or absence of edema	Edema—extracellular volume excess
Cerebral function	Level of consciousness	Decreased—clinical dehydration
	Neurologic function	Impaired—cerebral edema

TABLE 23–14 | Summary of Clinical Assessment of Electrolyte Imbalances

ASSESSMENT CATEGORY	SPECIFIC ASSESSMENTS	CHANGES WITH ELECTROLYTE IMBALANCES
Skeletal muscle function	Muscle strength	Weakness, flaccid paralysis—hyperkalemia; hypokalemia
Neuromuscular excitability	Deep tendon reflexes	Depressed—hypercalcemia; hypermagnesemia
		Hyperactive—hypocalcemia; hypomagnesemia
	Chvostek sign (except in infants)	Positive—hypocalcemia; hypomagnesemia
	Trousseau sign	Positive—hypocalcemia; hypomagnesemia
	Paresthesias	Digital or perioral—hypocalcemia
	Muscle cramping or twitching	Present—hypocalcemia; hypomagnesemia
Gastrointestinal tract function	Bowel sounds	Decreased or absent—hypokalemia
	Elimination pattern	Constipation—hypokalemia; hypercalcemia
		Diarrhea—hyperkalemia
Cardiac rhythm	Arrhythmia	Irregular—hyperkalemia; hypokalemia; hypercalcemia; hypocalcemia; hypermagnesemia; hypomagnesemia
	Electrocardiogram	Abnormal—hyperkalemia; hypokalemia; hypercalcemia; hypocalcemia; hypermagnesemia; hypomagnesemia
Cerebral function	Level of consciousness	Decreased—hyponatremia; hypernatremia

BOX 23–6 | Acid–Base Imbalances

Acidosis: Relatively too much acid in the body

Respiratory acidosis: Relatively too much carbonic acid

Metabolic acidosis: Relatively too much metabolic acid

Alkalosis: Relatively too little acid; excess base and bicarbonate in the body

Respiratory alkalosis: Relatively too little carbonic acid

Metabolic alkalosis: Relatively too little metabolic acid; excess base

Etiology and Pathophysiology

Any factor that interferes with the ability of the lungs to excrete carbon dioxide can cause respiratory acidosis. These factors may interfere with the gaseous exchange within the lungs, may impair the neuromuscular pump (respiratory muscles and their innervation that moves air in and out of the lungs), or may depress the respiratory rate (Table 23–16; Figure 23–20 ■).

As the P_{CO_2} begins to increase, the pH of the blood begins to decrease. Compensatory mechanisms begin to act in the form of nonbicarbonate buffers, additional hydrogen ion excretion by the kidneys, and formation and decreased bicarbonate excretion by the kidneys.

BOX 23–7	**Critical Thinking: How to Interpret Arterial Blood Gas Measurements**

Ask the following questions to analyze blood gas results:

1. What is the pH? If the pH is normal, the child has no imbalance or has compensated for an imbalance. If the pH is below normal, the child has acidosis. If the pH is above normal, the child has alkalosis.

2. What is the Pco_2? If the Pco_2 is normal, the child does not have a respiratory acid–base imbalance. If the Pco_2 is above normal, the child has respiratory acidosis. This may be the primary disorder or may be a compensatory response to metabolic alkalosis. Looking at the bicarbonate concentration helps you decide. If the Pco_2 is below normal, the child has respiratory alkalosis. Again, this can be the primary disorder or may be a compensatory response to metabolic acidosis.

3. What is the bicarbonate concentration? If the bicarbonate concentration is within normal range, the child does not have a metabolic acid–base imbalance. If the bicarbonate is above normal, the child has metabolic alkalosis. This can be a primary disorder or can be compensatory in respiratory acidosis. When bicarbonate is below normal, the child has metabolic acidosis, either as a direct disorder or as a compensatory response to respiratory alkalosis.

4. What do the results together tell you? If the pH is abnormal and either the Pco_2 or bicarbonate concentration is normal, there is an uncompensated acid–base disorder. If all three values are abnormal, the child has a partially compensated disorder and the pH will provide the definitive answer. If Pco_2, pH, and bicarbonate are all decreased, then partially compensated metabolic acidosis is most likely. If pH is normal and Pco_2 and bicarbonate are abnormal, there is a fully compensated acid–base disorder.

5. What are the child's history and clinical signs? Does your interpretation fit with what you know about the child's medical condition and with assessments you are making? This last step helps you to integrate laboratory data with the clinical picture to strengthen your nursing care of the child with an acid–base imbalance.

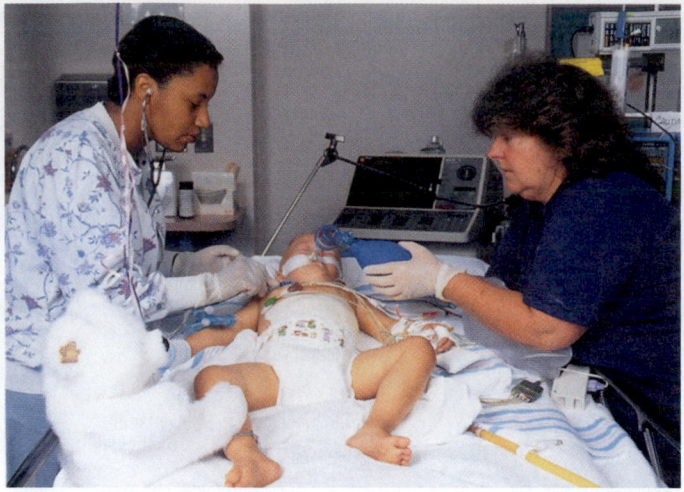

FIGURE 23–20 ■ This child may develop respiratory acidosis or respiratory alkalosis. If the tidal volume is set too low during mechanical ventilation, carbon dioxide (carbonic acid) will accumulate in the body (respiratory acidosis) because it is not being excreted by the lungs. If the tidal volume is set too high, carbon dioxide will be depleted in the body (respiratory alkalosis) because it is being excreted in great quantities.

These compensatory mechanisms may take several days to become clinically evident in most situations, depending on the underlying cause and the amount of compensation occurring.

Clinical Manifestations

Acidosis in the brain cells causes CNS depression, manifested by confusion, lethargy, headache, increased intracranial pressure, and even coma. Acute respiratory acidosis can lead to tachycardia and

TABLE 23–15	Normal Blood pH and Gases		
	INFANTS	**CHILDREN**	**ADOLESCENTS**
Arterial blood pH	7.18–7.5	7.27–7.49	7.35–7.41
Arterial blood Po_2	60–70 mmHg (8–9.3 pKa)	80–108 mmHg (10.7–14.4 pKa)	80–100 mmHg (10.7–13.3 pKa)
Arterial blood Pco_2	27–41 mmHg (3.6–5.5 pKa)	32–48 mmHg (4.3–6.4 pKa)	32–48 mmHg (4.3–6.4 pKa)
Arterial blood Hco_3^- (bicarbonate)	19–24 mmol/L	18–25 mmol/L	20–29 mmol/L

TABLE 23–16	Causes of Respiratory Acidosis		
FACTORS AFFECTING THE LUNGS	**FACTORS AFFECTING THE NEUROMUSCULAR PUMP**	**FACTORS AFFECTING CENTRAL CONTROL OF RESPIRATION**
Aspiration	Botulism	Brain tumor
Atelectasis	Congenital diaphragmatic hernia	Central sleep apnea
Bronchopulmonary dysplasia	Flail chest	General anesthesia
Croup	Guillain-Barré syndrome	Head injury
Cystic fibrosis	High cervical spinal cord injury	Sedative overdose
Epiglottitis	Hypokalemic muscle weakness	
Laryngeal edema	Kyphoscoliosis	
Pulmonary edema	Mechanical underventilation	
Pulmonary embolism	Muscular dystrophy	
Severe pneumonia	Pneumothorax or hemothorax	
Spasm of the airways	Poliomyelitis	
	Tetanus	

TABLE 23–17	Laboratory Values in Acid–Base Imbalance		
IMBALANCE	**PCO$_2$**	**PH**	**HCO$_3^-$**
Respiratory Acidosis			
Uncompensated	Increased	Decreased	Normal
Partially compensated	Increased	Decreased but moving toward normal	Increasing
Fully compensated	Increased	Normal	Increased
Respiratory Alkalosis			
Uncompensated	Decreased	Increased	Normal
Partially compensated	Decreased	Increased but moving toward normal	Decreasing
Fully compensated	Decreased	Normal	Decreased
Metabolic Acidosis			
Uncompensated	Normal	Decreased	Decreased
Partially compensated	Decreasing	Decreased but moving toward normal	Decreased
Fully compensated	Decreased	Normal	Decreased
Metabolic Alkalosis			
Acute condition; uncompensated	Normal	Increased	Increased
Partially compensated	Increasing	Increased but moving toward normal	Increased
Fully compensated	Full compensation limited by the need for oxygen	Full compensation limited by the need for oxygen	Full compensation limited by the need for oxygen

cardiac arrhythmias. The child's arterial blood gases always show an increased Pco$_2$, the laboratory sign of increased carbonic acid. Serum pH can be decreased or normal.

Collaborative Care

Laboratory tests involve arterial blood gases as described in Table 23–15. Treatment of respiratory acidosis requires correction of the underlying cause. For example, treatment may include bronchodilators for bronchospasm, mechanical ventilation for neuromuscular defects, decreasing sedative use, or surgery for kyphoscoliosis (Table 23–17).

Nursing Management

The nurse assumes an important role in assessment of the child with an acid–base problem. Early identification of increasing imbalance is key to early therapeutic interventions. Nursing interventions focus on keeping the child safe, monitoring effects of treatment, and ensuring management of respiratory, cardiovascular, renal, and other body systems.

Nursing Assessment and Diagnosis

Nursing assessment plays a pivotal role in decisions about interventions for respiratory acidosis, especially in chronic conditions such as cystic fibrosis and kyphoscoliosis. Assess respiratory rate, rhythm, and depth carefully. Take the apical pulse and be alert for tachycardia or arrhythmia. A cardiac monitor may be used. Obtain serial arterial blood gas measurements in acute conditions to evaluate changing status. Assess the level of consciousness and energy. Observe for chronic fatigue, headache, or decreased level of consciousness.

Several nursing diagnoses may apply to the child with respiratory acidosis. The most important of these addresses the child's risk for injury. Other nursing diagnoses depend on the specific clinical manifestation and the particular cause of the acidosis. Examples include:

- Injury, Risk for related to decreased level of consciousness
- Activity Intolerance related to decreased cardiac output secondary to cardiac dysrhythmias

- Breathing Pattern, Ineffective (hypoventilation) related to neuromuscular impairment
- Pain, Acute (headache) related to cerebral vasodilation
- Therapeutic Regiment Management: Family, Ineffective related to complexity of bronchodilator therapy

NANDA-I © 2012

Planning and Intervention

Prevention is a major focus of nursing care for the child at risk of respiratory acidosis. When the condition has developed, the nurse engages in measures to correct the acidosis and maintain safety for the child.

Care in the Community

Teach children at risk for respiratory acidosis and their parents preventive measures to use at home. For the child with a chronic condition such as cystic fibrosis, muscular dystrophy, or kyphoscoliosis, demonstrate deep breathing and encourage its use several times each day. Teach the family signs of infection—including fever, increased respiratory secretions, and discomfort with breathing—so the problems can be treated promptly to prevent further respiratory involvement. Position the child to facilitate chest expansion (Figure 23–21 ■). Teach parents about proper administration of any necessary medications. For example, the child with cystic fibrosis may receive antibiotics to prevent respiratory infections. Teach parents and older children about home respirator use (Figure 23–22 ■).

Hospital-Based Care

For the hospitalized child, the focus is on ensuring safety. Keep side rails raised, and turn and position the child frequently. Evaluate mental status and document and report any changes in alertness. When laboratory values of blood pH and Pco$_2$ are available, evaluate them promptly and report any changes or abnormalities. Administer medications as ordered. Carefully watch the doses of sedatives to avoid further respiratory depression. Provide suctioning as needed and encourage deep breathing. It is usually difficult to get a young child to do deep breathing or to use the "blow bottle" that is often given to older

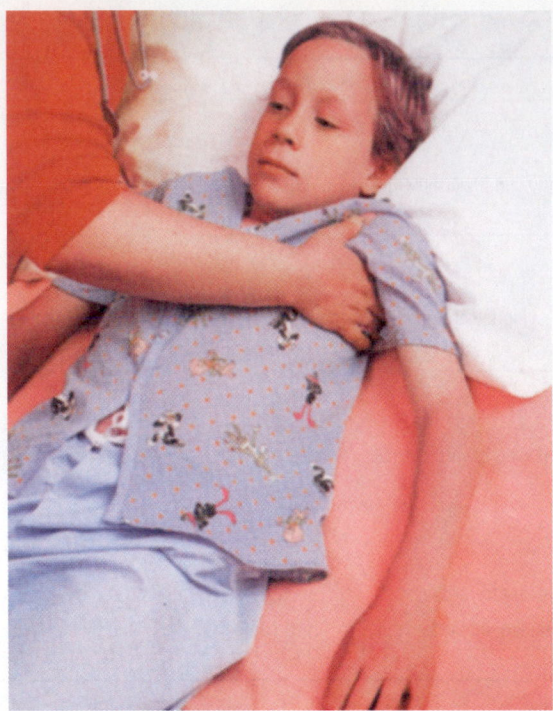

FIGURE 23–21 ■ Positioning to facilitate chest expansion. If the child is positioned to avoid chest compression or slumping to the side, this will help correct respiratory acidosis.

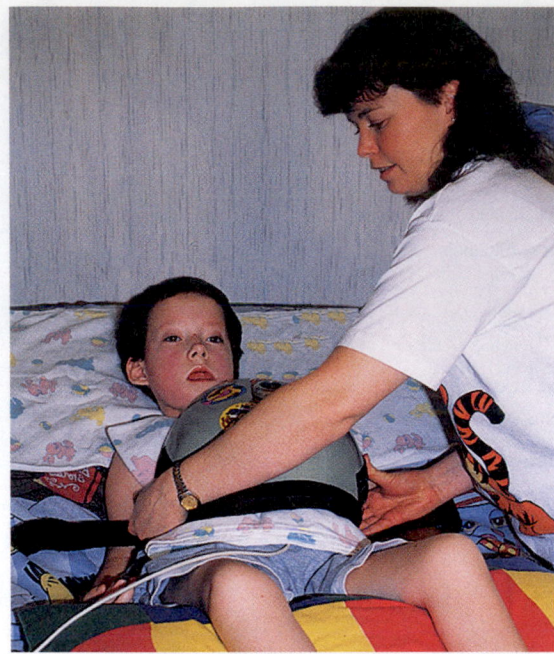

FIGURE 23–22 ■ This child, who has muscular dystrophy, uses a "turtle" respirator at home to assist with breathing. His parents required instructions from the nurse on use of the respirator. The family has a generator to provide electricity for the respirator during power outages.

children and adults. To make deep breathing fun, use a pinwheel and have the child turn it during play. Alternatively, give a child a straw and have him or her blow bubbles in a glass of water, or have the child use the straw to blow scraps of paper across the bedside table.

Evaluation

Expected outcomes of nursing care for the child with respiratory acidosis include the following:

- Safety is maintained in the environment.
- The rate and rhythm of respirations is adequate.
- Causative disorders of respiratory acidosis are adequately managed.

Respiratory Alkalosis

Respiratory alkalosis occurs when the blood contains too little carbon dioxide. It is sometimes called carbonic acid deficit. Some of the most common causes in young children are hypoxia such as that from severe asthma, salicylate poisoning, and sepsis.

Excess carbon dioxide loss is caused by hyperventilation, in which more air than normal is moved into and out of the lungs. Common causes of hyperventilation include:

- Hypoxemia
- Anxiety
- Pain
- Fever
- Salicylate poisoning
- Meningitis
- Encephalitis
- Septicemia caused by gram-negative bacteria
- Mechanical overventilation

In many cases, respiratory alkalosis lasts for several hours only. Renal compensation does not occur, as these compensatory mechanisms take several days to begin action. An example is the hyperventilation that occurs with acute anxiety. If the condition persists, however, the kidneys will begin to retain more acid and excrete more bicarbonate. Hydrogen ions will be released from body buffers to decrease plasma bicarbonate. While the imbalance continues, cellular function is thus protected by returning pH to normal levels.

Arterial blood gas measurements show a decreased Pco_2 in respiratory alkalosis. Blood pH is generally elevated. The lack of carbon dioxide causes neuromuscular irritability and paresthesias in the extremities and around the mouth. Muscle cramping and carpal or pedal spasms can occur. The child may be dizzy or confused.

Clinical therapy focuses on correcting the condition that caused the hyperventilation, sepsis, hypoxia, or other condition so that the body's compensatory mechanisms can return carbon dioxide levels to normal. Oxygen therapy may be helpful in some cases of hypoxia. Salicylates are removed from the body (see Chapter 20 🔵 for treatment during poisoning), drugs that have interfered with breathing are stopped, and sepsis is treated with effective medications. Anxiolytic medications may also be prescribed to treat anxiety.

Nursing Management

Nursing Assessment and Diagnosis

Assess the child's level of consciousness and ask if the child feels lightheaded or has tingling sensations or numbness in the fingers, in the toes, or around the mouth. Assess the rate and depth of respirations. Monitor the hospitalized child's Po_2 with serial arterial blood gas measurements to evaluate changes in status. A careful assessment is needed regarding the cause of hyperventilation. Did an occurrence cause anxiety for the child? Is pain present (see Chapter 21)? Has

TABLE 23–18 Techniques for Reducing Anxiety in Children with Paresthesias

INFANT	TODDLER OR PRESCHOOLER	YOUNG SCHOOL-AGE CHILD	OLDER SCHOOL-AGE CHILD OR ADOLESCENT
Calming touch	Stuffed toy to hug	Talking quietly about a happy event	Explaining the reason for the tingling and that it will go away
Quiet voice	Singing familiar quiet nursery songs	Telling a familiar story	Use of guided imagery
Swaddling	Acknowledging the child's feelings	Reading a familiar book together	Familiar music on iPod or radio
Holding quietly	Holding calmly	Explaining that the tingling will go away	Asking what the child does when anxious or scared
		Use of simple guided imagery and supportive listening	Talking about coping strategies

the child received salicylates in any form? Is the child mechanically ventilated? Is there a CNS infection such as meningitis?

Planning and Implementation

Nursing care for the child with respiratory alkalosis centers on teaching stress management techniques, maintaining pain control, promoting respiratory function, ensuring safety, maintaining fluid status, and providing health supervision and home care.

Practice Alert

The Po₂ must be checked before any therapy for respiratory alkalosis is started, because it is dangerous to stop hyperventilation if oxygenation is poor. When Po₂ is low, the child's hyperventilation may be a protective mechanism to increase blood oxygenation. Other measures such as oxygen therapy or mechanical ventilation may need to start first, followed by treatment for the cause of respiratory alkalosis.

Teach Stress Management Techniques

When anxiety is the cause of respiratory alkalosis, instruct the child to breathe slowly, in rhythm with your own breathing. Teach stress control techniques such as relaxation or imagery, and use other developmentally appropriate interventions for situations that cause anxiety in children and adolescents (Table 23–18).

Maintain Pain Control

Use medications, imagery, distraction, positioning, massage, and other techniques to decrease pain and maintain pain management. Chapter 21 describes these and other measures to assist with pain control.

Promote Respiratory Function

Have the child cough, or suction as needed. Be certain that mechanical ventilation systems are working properly. See Chapter 25 for detailed information about management of respiratory function.

Ensure Safety

Provide a safe environment for the child who has a decreased level of consciousness. Be sure the child is supervised when sitting or standing up. Keep bed rails raised.

Regulate Fluid Status

Renal compensation to manage ongoing respiratory alkalosis requires adequate urinary output. Regulate fluid intake to ensure urine output unless fluids are restricted due to medical condition.

Care in the Community

Teach parents to keep aspirin and other salicylate products out of reach of children, preferably in a locked medicine box. Instruct parents to call the poison control center immediately in case of poison ingestion.

Evaluation

Expected outcomes of nursing care for the child with respiratory alkalosis include the following:

- Normal respiratory rate and rhythm are maintained.
- Environmental safety is maintained.
- Fluid status is adequately managed.

Metabolic Acidosis

Metabolic acidosis is a condition in which there is an excess of any acid other than carbonic acid. For this reason, it is sometimes called noncarbonic acid excess.

Etiology and Pathophysiology

Metabolic acidosis is caused by an imbalance in production and excretion of acid or by excess loss of bicarbonate (Table 23–19). Excess accumulation occurs by one of two mechanisms. First, a child can eat or drink acids or substances that are converted to acid in the body. Examples include aspirin, boric acid, and antifreeze. Second, cells can make abnormally high amounts of acid that cannot be excreted. This is the case in ketoacidosis of untreated diabetes mellitus, in untreated growth hormone deficiency, in children with bladder construction that uses part of the bowel, or in the starvation that can occur in anorexia or bulimia. A disorder of excretion occurs in conditions such as oliguric renal failure (Figure 23–23).

Bicarbonate can be lost from the body through the urine or through excessive loss of intestinal fluid. Diarrhea, fistulas, and ileal drainage are all possible sources. Carbonic anhydrase inhibitors also can cause loss of excess bicarbonate in the urine.

When the pH of the blood decreases below normal, the chemoreceptors in the brain and arteries are stimulated and respiratory

TABLE 23–19 Causes of Metabolic Acidosis

GAIN OF METABOLIC ACID	LOSS OF BICARBONATE
Diabetic ketoacidosis	Diarrhea
Distal renal tubular acidosis	Intestinal or pancreatic fistula
Hyperalimentation	Proximal renal tubular acidosis
Ingestion of acid precursors (e.g., antifreeze)	
Ingestion of acids (e.g., aspirin)	
Oliguria (e.g., renal failure)	
Some inborn errors of metabolism (e.g., maple syrup urine disease)	
Starvation ketoacidosis	
Tissue hypoxia (lactic acidosis)	

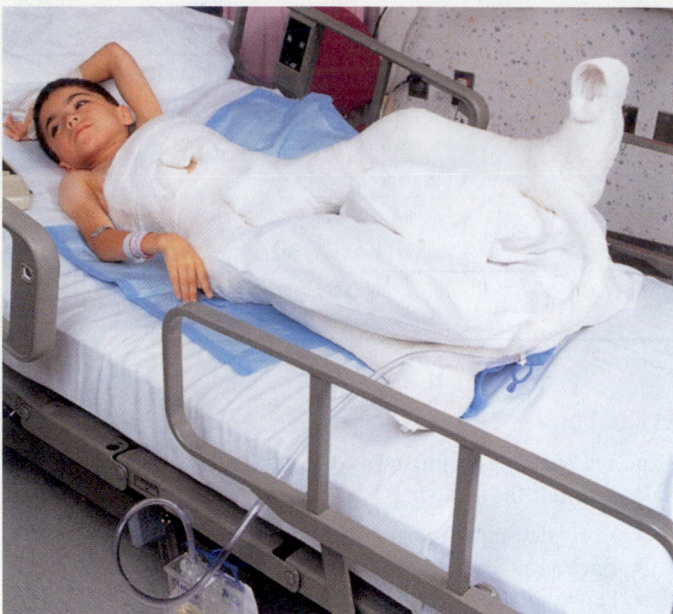

FIGURE 23–23 ■ With any child who is postoperative or immobilized, it is important to monitor urine output to detect oliguria. If the kidneys do not produce very much urine, the metabolic acids accumulate in the body and cause metabolic acidosis. Inadequate fluid intake in the postoperative or immobilized child can lead to oliguria and, potentially, metabolic acidosis. Note this child's urine collection device.

compensation begins. The child's rate and depth of breathing increase, and carbonic acid is removed from the body. The blood pH shifts to a more normal range even though the cause is not corrected. The underlying condition and the degree of compensation will alter the clinical laboratory values observed.

Clinical Manifestations

Laboratory values show decreased blood pH and decreased HCO_3 and Pco_2. An attempt at respiratory compensation causes one of the most important signs of metabolic acidosis, increased rate and depth of respirations (hyperventilation) or **Kussmaul respirations.** Severe acidosis can cause decreased peripheral vascular resistance and resultant cardiac arrhythmias, hypotension, pulmonary edema, and tissue hypoxia. Confusion or drowsiness may result, as well as headache or abdominal pain.

Collaborative Care

Laboratory tests include blood pH and blood gases, as described in the preceding clinical manifestations section. (Review Table 23–15 on page 686.) Treatment of metabolic acidosis depends on identification and treatment of the underlying cause. For example, renal failure would be treated with medications or dialysis, an intestinal fistula would be repaired, and hyperalimentation formula would be regulated to decrease acidosis. In severe metabolic acidosis, intravenous sodium bicarbonate may be used to increase the pH and to prevent cardiac arrhythmias. This treatment is difficult to manage, because renal excretion can cause excess retention of bicarbonate; therefore, intravenous sodium bicarbonate is used only in severe situations, such as prolonged cardiac arrest.

Nursing Management

Nurses seek to prevent metabolic acidosis by partnering with families to avoid accidental ingestion of harmful substances by young children and to avoid complications of diabetes when possible. Nursing interventions seek to restore balance, and include monitoring of arterial blood gases and body systems.

Nursing Assessment and Diagnosis

When families bring a young child in for a health promotion visit, assess the risk of poisoning in the home and the family's knowledge of prevention techniques. For the child being treated for acidosis, assess the rate and depth of respirations. Evaluate the child's level of consciousness frequently. Be alert for signs or complaints of headache and abdominal pain. Serial arterial blood gas measurements will usually be obtained to evaluate changes in status.

The following nursing diagnoses can apply to the child with metabolic acidosis:

- Injury, Risk for related to confusion/drowsiness or decreased responsiveness
- Cardiac Output, Decreased related to cardiac dysrhythmias
- Tissue Perfusion: Cerebral, Risk for Ineffective related to tissue hypoxia
- Therapeutic Regimen Management: Family, Ineffective related to complexity of management of diabetes mellitus

NANDA-I © 2012

Planning and Implementation

Ensure safety, taking into account the child's level of consciousness and alertness. Turn the child and change his or her position to prevent pressure on the skin. Limit the child's activities to decrease cardiac workload.

Position the child to facilitate chest expansion. Provide oral care during rapid respirations because the mouth may become dry. Monitor intravenous solutions and laboratory values indicating acid–base balance. Report changes promptly.

Once the child is stabilized, provide teaching to compensate for knowledge deficits. Teach parents of young children to keep medications and acids locked in a secure place and out of reach to prevent poisoning (Figure 23–24 ■). This includes medicines with aspirin as well as substances commonly kept in the garage for car maintenance. Teach about home management of diabetes and about early identification and treatment to avoid diabetic ketoacidosis. Expected outcomes of nursing care relate to prevention of acidosis and restoration of normal body balance during disease processes.

Metabolic Alkalosis

Metabolic alkalosis occurs when there are too few metabolic acids, a condition sometimes called noncarbonic acid deficit.

A gain in bicarbonate or a loss of metabolic acid can cause metabolic alkalosis (Table 23–20). Bicarbonate is gained through excessive intake of bicarbonate antacids or baking soda or through metabolism of bicarbonate precursors such as the citrate contained in blood transfusions. Increased renal absorption of bicarbonate can occur with diuretic use, in profound hypokalemia, in primary hyperaldosteronism, or with extreme deficit in extracellular fluid volume. A more current cause is the use of enhanced water to constitute powdered formula (Eby, 2009). Acid can be lost through severe vomiting, such as that seen in infants with pyloric stenosis and in continued removal of gastric contents through suction.

When the chemoreceptors in the brain and arteries detect the rising pH of metabolic alkalosis and respirations decrease, carbonic acid is retained in the body. This carbonic acid can neutralize the bicarbonate and return pH toward normal.

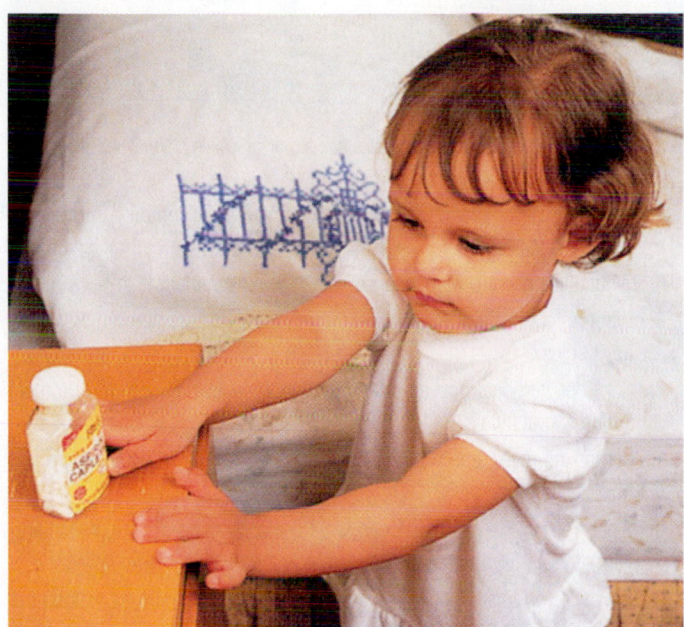

FIGURE 23–24 ■ Teaching parents to use safety latches on cabinets to keep aspirin away from small children can prevent one cause of metabolic acidosis.

TABLE 23–20	Causes of Metabolic Alkalosis	
GAIN OF BICARBONATE	**LOSS OF METABOLIC ACID**
Ingestion of baking soda	Prolonged vomiting (e.g., pyloric stenosis)
Ingestion of large quantities of bicarbonate antacids	Nasogastric suction
Exchange transfusion or massive transfusion (citrate is metabolized to bicarbonate)	Cystic fibrosis
	Hypokalemia
Increased renal absorption of bicarbonate	Diuretic therapy
	Hyperaldosteronism
	Adrenogenital syndrome
	Cushing syndrome

Blood pH, bicarbonate, and Pco_2 are usually elevated in metabolic alkalosis. Hypokalemia often occurs simultaneously (refer to page 676 to review signs of hypokalemia). Respiratory rate and depth usually decrease. Increased neuromuscular irritability, cramping, paresthesia, tetany, seizures, and excitation can occur. Finally, this state can progress to weakness, confusion, lethargy, and coma.

See Table 23–15 for laboratory findings. Clinical therapy is directed at treating the underlying cause of the condition. Increasing the extracellular fluid volume with intravenous normal saline is used to facilitate renal excretion of bicarbonate. Medications such as acetazolamide increase renal excretion of bicarbonate as well.

Nursing Management

Assess the child's level of consciousness frequently. Alertness may decrease after an initial period of excitement, so regular assessments are needed. Monitor neuromuscular irritability. Observe for nausea and vomiting. Assess the rate and depth of respirations carefully. Obtain serial arterial blood gas measurements as ordered.

Facilitate ease of respirations. Ensure safety by keeping bed rails elevated and by turning the child frequently. Position the child on the side to avoid aspiration of vomitus.

If antacids or improper formula constitution were the cause of the alkalosis, teach the child and parents about correct use of these medications.

Mixed Acid–Base Imbalances

It is possible for two acid–base imbalances to occur simultaneously. For example, a child with cystic fibrosis can, at the same time, develop respiratory acidosis from lung problems with metabolic alkalosis from vomiting during an illness. Treatment with diuretics may cause concurrent metabolic alkalosis resulting from extracellular volume depletion and hypokalemia in a child with congestive heart failure and chronic respiratory acidosis. In these cases, all underlying causes must be identified and treated. Care of children with mixed acid–base imbalances is often complicated, requiring hospitalization and careful management. Upon discharge, the nurse can teach parents about signs of imbalance that need to be reported and treated to prevent further complications. Evaluation of care is based on outcomes of adequate respiratory ventilation and metabolic balance.

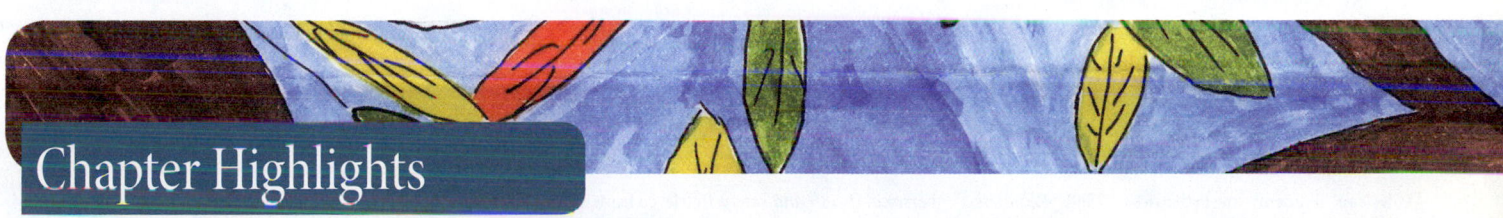

Chapter Highlights

- Young children are at risk for fluid and electrolyte imbalance due to differences in body fluid compartments and regulation systems.
- Nurses institute health promotion and health maintenance measures to maintain normal body fluids for children who exercise in hot weather and those undergoing surgery.
- Extracellular fluid volume deficit manifests as dehydration.
- Extracellular fluid volume excess is due to an excess of saline in the body.
- Interstitial fluid volume excess manifests as edema and weight gain.

- Nurses carefully manage fluid status of young children and teach parents prevention and treatment of fluid imbalances caused by gastroenteritis and other disease states.
- The most common electrolyte imbalances are hypernatremia and hypokalemia, and thus involve sodium and potassium.
- Normal acid–base balance is necessary for proper function of cells in the body.
- The lungs, kidneys, and liver play a role in maintaining acid–base balance.
- Acid–base imbalance can involve alkalosis or acidosis; either can have a respiratory or metabolic origin.

Clinical Reasoning in Action

INTRODUCTION

Consider the scenario involving 18-month-old Vernon at the chapter beginning. He has had vomiting and diarrhea for several days. Assessment of body weight loss, skin turgor, and level of activity suggests moderate dehydration. His mother has arranged childcare for today for her 4-year-old daughter.

DESCRIPTION

Vernon refuses attempts at feeding him orally. His pulse becomes rapid and his blood pressure decreases. After several hours in the monitoring unit, he has not voided and has a capillary refill of about 4 seconds.

DISCUSSION

1. What type of dehydration is Vernon likely experiencing now?
2. Has he lost both water and sodium in proportion (isotonic dehydration), or relatively more water (hypotonic dehydration) or sodium (hypertonic dehydration)?

3. Does Vernon have any signs of alkalosis or acidosis? Which might be expected to occur in his condition?
4. What type of intravenous fluid might be ordered for Vernon if intravenous therapy is started?
5. What is his needed maintenance fluid? His replacement fluid?
6. What amount of oral rehydration therapy (ORT) is recommended as therapy begins?
7. Consider Vernon's age and developmental stage. How will you promote intake of oral fluid?
8. Vernon improves and is to be sent home tonight. Instruct his mother about how to continue the ORT.
9. Since Vernon has gastroenteritis, what precautions do you suggest to prevent other family members from becoming affected?
10. How will you assist Vernon's mother to plan care for him as well as her 4-year-old daughter?

NCLEX-RN® Review

1. A nurse obtains a history from a breastfeeding mother with a small 3-month-old infant who has been vomiting. Which would give the nurse an indication that this infant has severe dehydration?
   1. The infant is having a seizure.
   2. The pulse rate is slightly elevated.
   3. Skin turgor is normal.
   4. Mucous membranes are dry.

2. The nurse is caring for a child who has been diagnosed with extracellular fluid volume excess related to congestive heart failure. The child's parents ask the nurse what can be done to treat the condition. What is a correct response from the nurse? (Select all that apply.)
   1. "Your child may be placed on medication to strengthen the heart."
   2. "Your child may be given a diuretic."
   3. "Your child will be started on an IV drip of lactated Ringer's."
   4. "Your child will be given an oral rehydration solution."
   5. "Your child will be given a bronchodilator."

3. An 11-month-old child presents with a sodium level of 150 mmol/L. The nurse would expect which finding?
   1. Adequate fluid intake
   2. Child neglect or abuse
   3. Developmental delay
   4. Poor fluid intake

4. The nurse is assessing an 11-year-old child admitted for status asthmaticus. The child's respiratory rate is 56 and the pulse is 112. Which can the nurse expect to find in the child's lab results?
   1. A CBC with white blood cell count of 19.8.
   2. A potassium of 4.2 on the chemistry.
   3. An ABG with a pH of 7.2, an HCO3 of 35, and a CO2 of 50.
   4. A blood urea nitrogen of 15 mg/dL.

See Appendix I 🔗 *for answers*.

References

American Academy of Pediatrics. (2009). *Pediatric nutrition handbook* (6th ed.). Elk Grove Village, IL: Author.

American Academy of Pediatrics. (2010). *Exertional heat-related illness*. Retrieved from http://www.healthychildren.org

Bindler, R., & Howry, L. (2005). *Pediatric drug guide*. Upper Saddle River, NJ: Prentice Hall.

Canavan, A., & Arant, B. S. (2009). Diagnosis and management of dehydration in children. *American Family Physician, 80,* 692–696.

Centers for Disease Control and Prevention. (2009). *Extreme heat: A prevention guide to promote your personal health and safety*. Retrieved from http://www.bt.cdc.gov/disasters/extreme heat_guide.asp

Centers for Disease Control and Prevention. (2010). Heat illness among high school athletes—United States, 2005–2009. *Morbidity and Mortality Weekly Report, 59,* 1009–1013.

Chameides, L., Samson, R. A., Schexnayder, S. M., & Hazinski, M. F. (2011). *PALS: Pediatric advanced life support provider manual*. Dallas, TX: American Heart Association.

Children's Mercy Hospital. (2011). *Guidelines for oral rehydration*. Retrieved from http://www.childrensmercy.org/Content/view.aspx?id=8130

Colletti, J. E., Brown, K. M., Sharieff, G. Q., Barata, I. A., Ishimine, P., & ACEP Pediatric Emergency Medicine Committee. (2010). The management of children with gastroenteritis and dehydration in the emergency department. *Journal of Emergency Medicine, 38,* 686–698.

Council on Sports Medicine and Fitness & Council on School Health. (2011). Policy statement—Climatic heat stress and exercising children and adolescents. *Pediatrics, 128,* e741–e747.

Custer, J. W., & Rau, R. E. (2009). *The Harriet Lane handbook* (18th ed.). Philadelphia, PA: Elsevier.

Crawford, A., & Harris, H. (2011). I.V. fluids: What nurses need to know. *Nursing, 41*(5), 31–38.

Diggins, K. C. (2008). Treatment of mild to moderate dehydration in children and oral rehydration therapy. *Journal of the American Academy of Nurse Practitioners, 20*, 402–406.

Doan, Q., Chan, M., Leung, V., Lee, E., & Kissoon, N. (2010). The impact of an oral rehydration clinical pathway in a paediatric emergency department. *Pediatric and Child Health, 15*, 503–507.

Dzierba, A. L., & Abraham, P. (2011). A practical approach to understanding acid–base abnormalities in critical illness. *Journal of Pharmacy Practice, 24*, 17–26.

Eby, A. K. (2009). Metabolic alkalosis after using enhanced water to dilute powdered formula. *MCN, 34*, 290–294.

Gardner, S., Carter, B., Enzman-Hines, M., & Hernandez, J. (2010). *Merenstein and Gardner's handbook of neonatal intensive care.* St. Louis, MO: Elsevier Mosby.

Greenbaum, L. A. (2011). *Electrolyte and acid–base disorder.* In R. M. Kliegman, B. F. Stanton, J. W. St. Geme, N. F. Schor, & R. E. Behrman, *Nelson textbook of pediatrics* (19th ed., pp. 212–242). Philadelphia, PA: Saunders Elsevier.

Hew-Butler, T., Ayus, J. C., Kipps, C., Maughan, R. J., Mettler, S., Meeuwisse, W. H., . . . Exercise Associated Hyponatremia Panel. (2008). Statement of the second international exercise-associated hyponatremia consensus development conference, New Zealand, 2007. *Clinical Journal of Sports Medicine, 18*, 111–121.

Johnson, V. L. (2010). Disorders of phosphorus homeostasis. In L. G. Feld & F. J. Kaskel, *Fluid and electrolytes in pediatrics* (pp. 173–210). New York, NY: Human Press.

Kannan, L., Lodha, R., Vivekanandhan, S., Bagga, A., Kabra, S. K., & Kabra, M. (2011). Intravenous fluid regimen and hyponatraemia among children: A randomized controlled trial. *Pediatric Nephrology, 25*, 2303–2309.

Kliegman, R. M., Stanton, B. F., St. Geme, J., & Behrman, R. E. (2011). *Nelson textbook of pediatrics* (19th ed.). Philadelphia, PA: Saunders.

Kusuma, S., Agrawal, S. K., Kumar, P., Narang, A., & Prasad, R. (2009). Hydration status of exclusively and partially breastfed near-term newborns in the first week of life. *Journal of Human Lactation, 25*, 280–286.

Landry, G. L. (2011). *Heat injuries.* In R. M. Kliegman, B. F. Stanton, J. W. St. Geme, N. F. Schor, & R. E. Behrman, *Nelson textbook of pediatrics* (19th ed., pp. 2420–2421). Philadelphia, PA: Saunders Elsevier.

Madati, P. J., & Bachur, R. (2008). Development of an emergency department triage tool to predict acidosis among children with gastroenteritis. *Pediatric Emergency Care, 24*, 822–830.

Mayo Clinic. (2011). *Dehydration and youth sports.* Retrieved from http://www.mayoclinic.com

Moritz, M. L., & Ayus, J. C. (2011). Intravenous fluid management for the acutely ill child. *Current Opinion in Pediatrics, 23*, 186–193.

Musso, C. G. (2009). Magnesium metabolism in health and disease. *International Urology and Nephrology, 41*, 357–362.

NIH Osteoporosis and Related Bone Diseases National Resource Center. (2011). *Osteoporosis and African American women.* Retrieved from http://www.niams.nih.gov/Health_Info/Bone/Osteoporosis/Background/default.asp

Pagnotta, K. D., Mazerolle, S. M., & Casa, D. J. (2010). Exertional heat stroke and emergency issues in high school sport. *Journal of Strength and Conditioning Research, 24*(7), 1707–1709.

Passariello, A., Terrin, G., DeMarco, G., Cecere, G., Ruotolo, S., Marino, A., . . . Berni Canani, R. (2011). Efficacy of a new hypotonic oral rehydration solution containing zinc and prebiotics in the treatment of childhood acute diarrhea: A randomized controlled trial. *Journal of Pediatrics, 158*, 288–292.

Patel, A. B., Mamtani, M., Badhoniya, N., & Kulkami, H. (2011). What zinc supplementation does and does not achieve in diarrhea prevention: A systematic review and meta-analysis. *BMC Infectious Diseases, 11*, 122.

Pershad, J. (2010). A systematic data review of the cost of rehydration therapy. *Applied Health and Economic Policy, 8*, 203–214.

Rehydration Project. (2008). *Oral rehydration solutions.* Retrieved from http://www.rehydrate.org

Ruppe, M. D. (2011). Medications that affect calcium. *Endocrine Practice, 17*(Suppl. 1), 26–30.

Sarafidis, P. A., Georgianos, P. I., & Lasaridis, A. N. (2010). Diuretics in clinical practice. Part II: Electrolyte and acid–base disorders complicating diuretic therapy. *Expert Opinion in Drug Safety, 9*, 259–273.

Thomas, D. W., Greer, F. R., & Committee on Nutrition. (2010). Clinical report—Probiotics and prebiotics in pediatrics. *Pediatrics, 126*, 1217–1231.

Tschudy, M. M., & Arcara, K. M. (2011). *The Harriet Lane Handbook* (19th ed.). Baltimore: Johns Hopkins University Press.

Unal, S., Arhan, E., Kara, N., Uncu, N., & Allefendioglu, D. (2008). Breast-feeding-associated hypernatremia: Retrospective analysis of 169 term newborns. *Pediatrics International, 50*, 29–34.

Yakoob, M. Y., Theodoratou, E., Jabeen, A., Imdad, A., Eisele, T. P., Ferguson, J., . . . Bhutta, Z. A. (2011). Preventive zinc supplementation in developing countries: Impact on mortality and morbidity due to diarrhea, pneumonia, and malaria. *BMC Public Health, 13*(Suppl. 3), S23.

Yung, M., & Keeley, S. (2009). Randomised controlled trial of intravenous maintenance fluids. *Journal of Paediatrics and Child Health, 45*, 9–14.

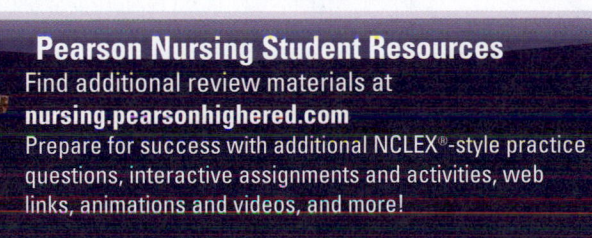

Pearson Nursing Student Resources

Find additional review materials at
nursing.pearsonhighered.com

Prepare for success with additional NCLEX®-style practice questions, interactive assignments and activities, web links, animations and videos, and more!

CHAPTER 24

Alterations in Eye, Ear, Nose, and Throat Function

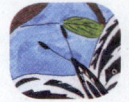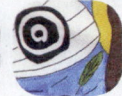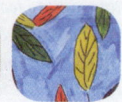

Learning Outcomes

After completing this chapter, you will be able to:

1. Identify anatomy and physiology, as well as pediatric differences in the eyes, ears, nose, and throat of children and adolescents.

2. Describe abnormalities of the eyes, ears, nose, throat, and mouth in children.

3. Plan for screening programs and identification of children with vision and hearing abnormalities.

4. Integrate evidence-based research to plan comprehensive nursing care for children with vision or hearing impairments.

5. Apply current recommendations when implementing care and teaching for children with abnormalities of the eyes, ears, nose, throat, and mouth.

6. Prioritize preventive and treatment principles when implementing care for children related to the eyes, ears, nose, and throat.

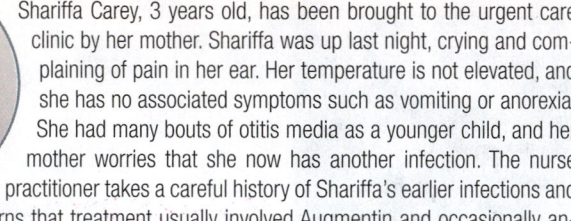

"What is that thing? Don't put it in my ear."
—Shariffa, age 3

Shariffa Carey, 3 years old, has been brought to the urgent care clinic by her mother. Shariffa was up last night, crying and complaining of pain in her ear. Her temperature is not elevated, and she has no associated symptoms such as vomiting or anorexia. She had many bouts of otitis media as a younger child, and her mother worries that she now has another infection. The nurse practitioner takes a careful history of Shariffa's earlier infections and learns that treatment usually involved Augmentin and occasionally another antibiotic. Mrs. Carey has worried about whether Shariffa's hearing was affected by the earlier infections. She recently enrolled her daughter in a Head Start program and is eager to see how they evaluate Shariffa's hearing and language.

The nurse practitioner demonstrates the otoscope to Shariffa to promote her comfort with the examination. A diagnosis of acute otitis media is made. The nurse informs Mrs. Carey that most children get better in 2 to 3 days, and instructs her in administration of the correct dose of acetaminophen. She asks her to call the clinic in 2 days to report on Shariffa's condition. Since Mrs. Carey was familiar with former treatment with antibiotics upon diagnosis, the nurse practitioner carefully explains why practitioners now wait for 2 to 3 days before beginning antibiotics. She also offers to make another appointment to review Shariffa's admission findings from Head Start and to further evaluate Shariffa's hearing and language development.

The eye, ear, nose, throat, and mouth are connected; therefore, a malformation, infection, or other condition in one of these structures may affect another of these body parts. Intact sensory structures are necessary for attainment of developmental milestones; thus alterations, especially to the eye and ear, may delay a child's development. In the preceding scenario, Shariffa's frequent otitis media when she was younger may have had an influence on her language development as a preschooler. Fortunately, her early childhood program offers screening and interventions to help her develop normally. As demonstrated by the scenario, most children with eye, ear, nose, and throat disorders are treated at home or in the community rather than in the hospital. Most screening for disorders occurs in newborn nurseries, clinics, and schools.

Infections of the eye, ear, and upper respiratory system are common abnormalities, and most pediatric nurses will need to be experts in assessment and interventions for these conditions. Health promotion and health maintenance settings provide an opportunity for screening to identify alterations, for teaching to prevent injuries, and for applying interventions that capitalize on sensory capabilities to enhance development.

How are conditions of the eye, ear, nose, and throat or mouth related? Which conditions have the potential to affect a child's growth, development, and behavior? What important testing during the newborn period can lead to early identification and intervention with children who may have an abnormality in this system? In what settings do children with eye, ear, nose, throat, and mouth conditions receive care? This chapter will explore the answers to these questions. It will present the screening guidelines for hearing, vision, and speech; the treatment for common disorders of the eye, ear, nose, throat, and mouth (including upper respiratory infections); nursing interventions that can prevent problems; and methods of partnering with parents and other health professionals to foster development of children with alterations in this body system.

ANATOMY AND PHYSIOLOGY

Sight, hearing, taste, and smell depend on proper functioning of receptor organs and interpretation by the brain. Thus, certain cranial nerves are also an integral part of the anatomy and physiology of the eye, ear, nose, throat, and mouth. Children are prone to both congenital and acquired sensory alterations, as well as a wide array of infections and injuries that can affect the eye, ear, nose, throat, mouth, and upper respiratory system.

Eye

The eye is a complex structure composed of the eyeball and its supporting structures. The *sclera,* or white part of the eye, is the outermost layer. It is transparent in the anterior eye to form the *cornea,* which allows light to enter. The *iris,* or colored part of the eye, is muscular, allowing it to change the size of the *pupil* and regulate the light that enters the eye. The *lens* is located behind the pupil and focuses light onto the retina. The *anterior chamber,* or the space between the cornea and iris, is filled with a fluid called *aqueous humor.* The *posterior chamber* is located behind the lens and is filled with *vitreous humor.* The innermost, posterior section of the eye is the *retina,* which has an inner layer that receives light impulses and an outer neural layer that transports visual images to the brain by the optic nerve (cranial nerve II). The *rods* in the retina perceive vision

in dim light and allow for peripheral vision; the *cones* perceive vision in bright light and are responsible for color discernment. See Figure 24–1 ■ for normal structures of the child's eye.

The eye has several supporting structures that assist in the sensation of vision. *Eyebrows, eyelids,* and *eyelashes* protect the eye and add touch sensation. The *conjunctiva* lines the cornea and the inside of the eyelids, lubricating the eye and keeping it viable. The lacrimal apparatus and ducts bathe the eye and produce tears. A series of six muscles allow the eye to move to all planes and maintain the shape of the eyeball. They are innervated by the oculomotor, trochlear, and abducens nerves (cranial nerves III, IV, and VI).

Ear

The ear is responsible for the sensory ability of hearing, and it establishes the sense of equilibrium. The *external ear* contains the *auricle,* which is visible outside the body; the *external canal;* and the *tympanic membrane.* These structures collect sound waves and direct them to the middle and inner ear. The *middle ear* lies behind the tympanic membrane and contains three bones necessary for sound vibrations: the *incus, malleus,* and *stapes.* Another part of the middle ear, the *eustachian tube,* connects to the nasopharynx and equalizes middle ear pressure. The *inner ear* contains the bony labyrinth, which in turn houses the *vestibule, semicircular canals,* and the *cochlea.* The vestibule and semicircular canals are responsible for the sense of equilibrium. The cochlea contains the *organ of Corti,* which contains sensory hair cells that are innervated by the vestibulocochlear (acoustic) nerve (cranial nerve VIII).

Nose, Throat, and Mouth

The structures of the nose, throat, and mouth are important to all humans. Mucous membranes bathe these body parts and have a high rate of growth. They help to maintain hygiene and protect the body from infectious agents. Salivary apparatus and taste buds are essential parts of the mouth and tongue. The nasal passages contain external nostrils, the sinuses, and the pharynx (or throat). The olfactory, facial, glossopharyngeal, and vagus nerves (cranial nerves I, VII, IX, and X) are responsible for the sense of smell, taste, coordinated swallowing, and the gag reflex, respectively.

PEDIATRIC DIFFERENCES
Eye

How are the eyes of children different from those of adults? Chapter 7 ⊘ provides a detailed discussion of the assessment of the eyes. **Visual acuity** is the ability to discriminate letters or other objects. The eyes of neonates differ from the eyes of adults in several ways. Visual acuity in neonates ranges between 20/100 and 20/400. The lens is more spherical and cannot accommodate to both near and far objects, which means that the neonate sees best at a distance of about 20 cm (8 in.). Because the optic nerve is not yet completely myelinated, the ability to distinguish color and other details is decreased. If the infant is preterm, especially less than 32 weeks' gestation, retinal vascularization, particularly in the periphery of the retina, may be incomplete. Retinal surface area doubles from week 24 of gestation until term, and most retinal development occurs from 24 to 40 weeks' gestation (Graven & Browne, 2008). Pupillary reflex reaction is detected by about 28 to 30 weeks' gestation and so may be sluggish in preterm infants. The rectus muscles that control

As They Grow The Eye

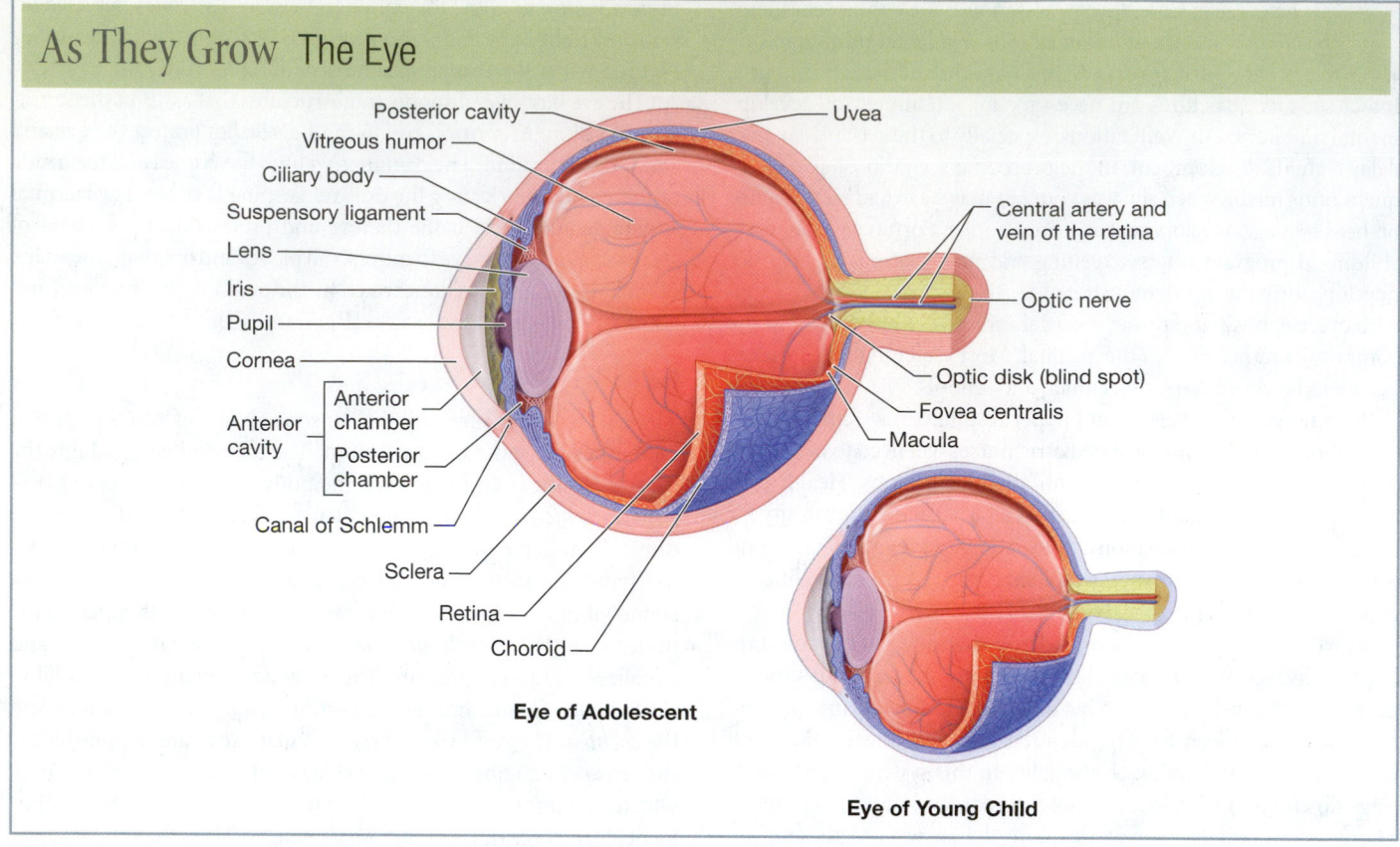

Eye of Adolescent

Eye of Young Child

FIGURE 24–1 ■ The eye is well developed at birth, but there are some variations in the visual acuity of the infant and young child. What influence would the young child's visual acuity have on the types of toys and books that should be made available?

binocular vision may be somewhat uncoordinated at birth. The eyes should be aligned and movement coordinated by the age of 3 months. Transient **nystagmus** (involuntary rapid eye movement) and **esotropia** (momentary turning inward of eyes) are common in neonates but decrease in incidence during the first few months of life. Conjunctival and retinal hemorrhages may be observed in the newborn as a result of the trauma of birth; they usually improve gradually and have no lasting effects. The red reflex is examined in children because it is a key method for identifying the presence of retinoblastoma (see Chapter 7 🔗 for the method to evaluate the red reflex and Chapter 29 🔗 for a description of retinoblastoma). Since premature infants must continue eye development after birth, in an environment with many medical risks, conditions such as strabismus, retinopathy of prematurity, refractive errors, and color identification deficits are more common among children who were born prematurely (Graven & Browne, 2008).

The cornea of the infant and young child occupies a larger portion of the orbit than in the adult; the eyeball is about three fourths of its adult size. Because the eye is relatively unprotected laterally, it is more easily injured. The sclera of the neonate is thin and translucent with a bluish tinge, and the iris is blue or gray. Eye color changes during the first 6 months of life. Infants produce tears to nourish and oxygenate the outer layers of the cornea. However, parents do not see tears when a young infant cries because the infant's lacrimal system drains them efficiently into the nasal cavity.

As infants grow, their eyes mature and their vision improves. By the age of 2 or 3 years, most children have a visual acuity of 20/50, and by the age of 6 or 7 years, it is 20/20. See Figure 24–1 for a summary

of pediatric differences of the eye. Visual acuity is measured using standardized letter or picture charts (see Chapter 7 🔗 and the Skills Manual 🔗). **Vision** refers to the complex process of acquiring meaning from what is seen, involving the eye, brain, and related neurologic and physiologic structures. Cognitive development interacts with a child's maturing physiologic system to bring increasing meaning to objects in sight (Table 24–1). The first few years of life are considered critical for the formation of normal vision. As acuity improves, the brain learns to interpret messages received from the eyes. Disturbances in vision, even in one eye, can affect the retinal nerve function, muscle function in the eye, or the brain's ability to interpret visual input.

Ear

Why do infants and young children have more ear problems than adults? The eustachian tube, which connects the nasopharynx to the middle ear, is proportionately shorter, wider, and more horizontal in infants than in older children or adults (Figure 24–2 ■). During sucking, yawning, and other movements, the tube opens for milliseconds, allowing free passage of air between the nasopharynx and the middle ear. These factors predispose young children to development of otitis media or middle ear infection.

The fetus can hear at about 20 weeks' gestation, and the auditory nerve function is mature at about 5 months of age in the infant. Before 34 weeks' gestation, the external ear is soft with little cartilage apparent. The external ear canal is small at birth, although the internal ear and middle ear are relatively large. As a result, the tympanic membrane is close to the surface and can be easily injured.

TABLE 24–1	Visually Related Developmental Milestones
AGE	**MILESTONE**
Term neonate	Demonstrates alertness to light and visual stimulus presented 8–12 in. (20–30 cm) from eyes
1 month	Follows an object 60 degrees horizontally and 30 degrees vertically, blinks at an approaching object
2 months	Follows a person or moving object for 180 degrees from 6 ft (2 m) away, smiles in response to a face, raises head 30 degrees from prone
3 months	Tracks an object through 180 degrees, regards own hand, begins visual-motor coordination
4–5 months	Social smile, reaches for a cube 12 in. (30 cm) away, notices a raisin 12 in. (30 cm) away, stares at own hand
7–8 months	Reaches and grasps an object, picks up a raisin by raking, transfers objects from hand to hand
8–9 months	Pokes at holes in a peg board, well-developed pincer grasp, crawls, uncovers toy after seeing it hidden
12–14 months	Stacks blocks, places a peg in a round hole, stands and walks

Source: Data from Rudolph, C., Rudolph, A., Lister, G., First, L., & Gershon, A. (2011). Rudolph's pediatrics (22nd ed.). New York, NY: McGraw-Hill; Kliegman, R. M., Stanton, B., St. Geme, J., Schor, N., & Behrman, R. E. (2010). Nelson textbook of pediatrics (19th ed.). Philadelphia, PA: Saunders.

Nose, Throat, and Mouth

Up to the age of 6 months, infants are primarily nasal breathers. Edema and nasal discharge may interfere with adequate air intake and feeding. Mucosal swelling and exudate may block the small nasal passages of young children. The immature immune system of young children (see Chapter 27 🌐 for further description) and the frequent exposure to other children with illnesses cause a high rate of upper respiratory infections in this population.

The palatine tonsils, which are visible on oral examination, are located on each side of the oropharynx. (The method for examining a child's throat is discussed in Chapter 7 🌐.) Although tonsils vary in size considerably during childhood, they are normally large, especially in school-age children. The nasopharyngeal tonsils (adenoids) lie in the posterior wall of the nasopharynx, just above the oropharynx. In children, the adenoids may become enlarged, harboring bacteria and interfering with breathing.

The mouth is an important organ for the infant as strong muscles are needed for sucking and thereby receiving nutrients. Sucking is an important developmental skill that promotes the muscles needed for later speech development. Taste sensation is present before birth, as evidenced by increased swallowing of amniotic fluid that has been sweetened. Taste sensations increase during childhood. By about 6 months of age the first tooth emerges, and by about 2 years the full set of 20 primary teeth is present. Tooth loss of the primary set begins about 5 to 6 years, and gradually the secondary teeth (32 total) erupt during childhood. See Chapter 7 for a further description of teeth eruption.

Assessment guidelines for the child with an alteration of the eye, ear, nose, or throat are provided in Table 24–2. See Chapter 7 for assessment techniques appropriate for each age group. For example, safe restraint practices and creative approaches to promote child understanding and cooperation are needed. See Table 24–3 for common diagnostic tests used; the tests and nursing implications are thoroughly described in Appendix E 🌐.

DISORDERS OF THE EYE
Infectious Conjunctivitis

Conjunctivitis is an inflammation of the conjunctiva, the clear membrane that lines the inside of the lid and sclera. There are several types of conjunctivitis, depending on the cause of inflammation. Bacteria, viruses, allergies, trauma, or irritants cause the conjunctiva to become swollen and red with a clear, yellow, or white discharge (Figure 24–3 ■). Parents commonly refer to all conjunctivitis as "pink eye."

Ophthalmia Neonatorum

Conjunctivitis in an infant under 30 days of age is called ophthalmia neonatorum. These infections are usually acquired from the mother during vaginal delivery as a result of contact with infected vaginal discharge containing organisms such as *Chlamydia trachomatis* and *Neisseria gonorrhoeae*. Such infections can cause serious damage to the eye and lead to permanent corneal damage. Antibiotics are instilled into the eyes of newborns soon after birth as a prophylactic measure against ophthalmia neonatorum (see Legal & Ethical Considerations: Prophylactic Eye Treatment).

Additional Neonate Eye Conditions

Chemical conjunctivitis occasionally occurs in newborns as a reaction to prophylactic medication. It is considered as a possible

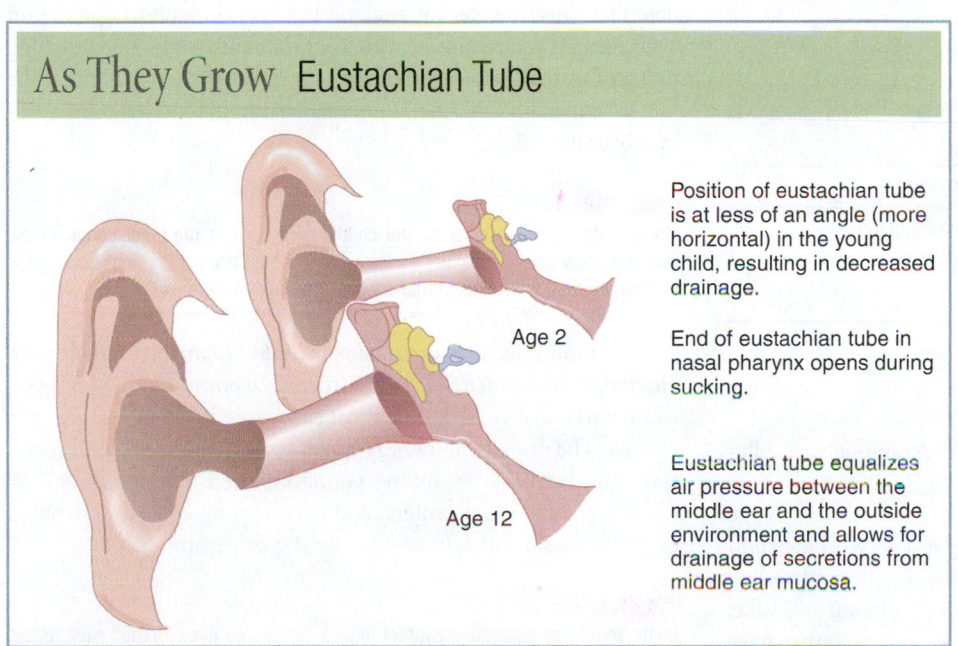

As They Grow Eustachian Tube

Age 2

Age 12

Position of eustachian tube is at less of an angle (more horizontal) in the young child, resulting in decreased drainage.

End of eustachian tube in nasal pharynx opens during sucking.

Eustachian tube equalizes air pressure between the middle ear and the outside environment and allows for drainage of secretions from middle ear mucosa.

FIGURE 24–2 ■ Of the three anatomic differences in the eustachian tube between adults and small children (shorter, wider, more horizontal), which do you think could cause more problems for the child and why? Answer: More horizontal. Small children who are bottle-fed in a supine position have a greater probability of developing otitis media because the eustachian tube opens when the child sucks and the horizontal angle provides easy access to the middle ear. In older children the greater angle helps keep foreign substances and germs away from the middle ear.

TABLE 24–2	Assessment Guidelines for the Child with an Alteration of the Eye, Ear , Nose, or Throat*	
ASSESSMENT FOCUS	**ASSESSMENT GUIDELINES**	
Eyes	■ Describe eye structures and symmetry.	
	■ Describe visual acuity using a screening test appropriate for age.	
	■ Measure extraocular movements to all quadrants. Evaluate corneal light reflex, cover–uncover test, and visual fields.	
	■ Using the ophthalmoscope, elicit and evaluate the red reflex bilaterally.	
	■ Observe for and report abnormalities such as eye drainage, cloudiness of lens, or abnormal eye movement.	
Ears	■ Describe placement and symmetry of the external ear.	
	■ Describe auditory acuity using a screening test appropriate for age.	
	■ Using the otoscope, evaluate the ear canal and tympanic membrane.	
	■ Ask about ear pain, drainage, and discomfort.	
Nose	■ Describe the symmetry and placement of the nose. Are the nares bilaterally patent? Are there lesions or drainage?	
	■ Are several smells identified?	
	■ Are signs of sinus infection present, such as facial edema or pain, headache, and tenderness upon palpation over sinus areas?	
Mouth and throat	■ Are oral mucous membranes intact?	
	■ How many primary/secondary/loose teeth are present? Are there visible caries? Are there broken or chipped teeth?	
	■ Evaluate the soft and hard palate for intactness.	
	■ Describe the throat and size/appearance of tonsils.	
	■ Palpate cervical lymph nodes, noting size and tenderness.	

*Refer to Chapter 7 🔴 for the actual techniques of assessment mentioned in this table.

TABLE 24–3	Diagnostic Procedures and Laboratory Tests for the Eye, Ear, Nose, and Throat*
DIAGNOSTIC PROCEDURES	**LABORATORY TESTS**
Audiologic screening	Complete blood count (CBC)
Newborn hearing screening	Culture and sensitivity
Tympanogram	

*See Appendixes D and E 🔴 for information about these diagnostic procedures and for expected laboratory tests values.

cause when conjunctivitis develops within 24 to 48 hours after instillation of the medication.

Infants who have frequent tearing and mattering (eyelid discharge that has formed a crust) on awakening may have a *plugged lacrimal duct*, a condition that can mimic conjunctivitis. Treatment involves massaging the tear duct every 4 hours when the infant is awake. Lacrimal ducts that remain plugged after the age of 1 year may have to be opened surgically.

Bacterial Conjunctivitis

Bacterial conjunctivitis can occur in children of any age. It is characterized by edema of the eyelid, red conjunctiva, and enlarged

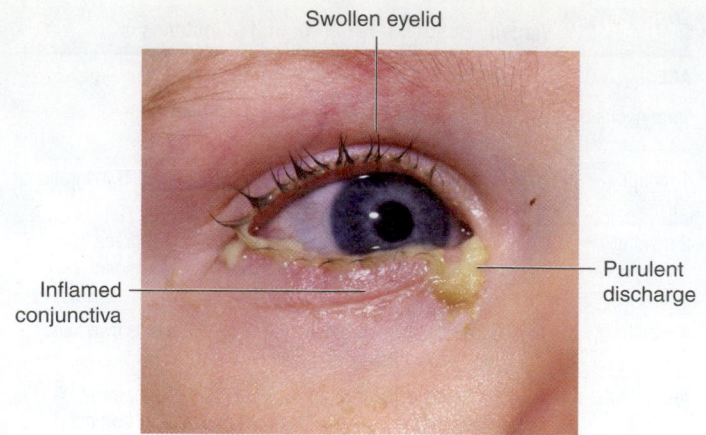

FIGURE 24–3 ■ Acute conjunctivitis. The major difference between bacterial and viral conjunctivitis is that bacterial conjunctivitis has a purulent discharge that may result in crusting whereas the discharge from viral conjunctivitis is serous (watery). Allergic conjunctivitis produces watery to thick drainage and is characterized by itching. Which type of conjunctivitis is seen in this picture?

Source: Dr. P. Marazzi / Science Source.

Legal and Ethical Considerations
Prophylactic Eye Treatment

By federal law, all infants born in the United States are given prophylactic eye treatment soon after delivery to help prevent ophthalmia neonatorum. The nurse is responsible for administering this eye ointment. Penicillin, tetracycline, erythromycin, or povidone-iodine ointments are most commonly used.

preauricular lymph glands. There is usually mucopurulent exudate that causes mattering, making the eyes difficult to open upon awakening. Older children with conjunctivitis complain of itching or burning, mild photophobia, and a feeling of scratching under the lids. Although bacterial conjunctivitis can be bilateral, it is more commonly unilateral.

Clinical Tip

Place a gloved index finger on the child's nose next to the inner corner of the eye and apply gentle pressure for several seconds. If mucopurulent drainage is discharged from the eye, bacterial conjunctivitis may be present.

Common infectious organisms include *Staphylococcus aureus*, *Haemophilus influenzae*, *Streptococcus pneumoniae*, and *Moraxella catarrhalis* (Gold, 2011). Most cases are caused by hand-to-eye contact. The disease can rapidly spread when groups of youth spend time together, such as among young children and adolescents in schools and childcare centers, and even among college students in dormitories, sororities, fraternities, and sports teams.

Practice Alert

Some youth use decorative contact lenses, and some even "trade" such lenses with other youth. Contact lenses should only be prescribed and fitted by a qualified eye professional. There have been reports of bacterial conjunctivitis, corneal damage, and allergic reactions to these cosmetic lenses. The U.S. Food and Drug Administration (FDA) has informed practitioners to be alert for dangers that occur due to improperly obtained lenses.

Viral Conjunctivitis

Other infections, most commonly in older children, can be caused by viruses. Viral conjunctivitis is commonly bilateral. Adenovirus is a common cause and spreads from respiratory adenovirus infection in a hand-to-eye manner. Signs and symptoms are similar to those of bacterial conjunctivitis, although sometimes milder in severity and slower in onset.

Herpes simplex virus (HSV) can also cause infection, either by transfer from a herpes-infected mother to a neonate during birth or by contact with an infected person in infants or children of any age. Ophthalmic herpes infection is often unilateral, painful, and accompanied by characteristic vesicular lesions on the eyelids and skin of the face (Wagner, 2011). A culture of the lesions is performed for diagnosis, and any accompanying conjunctivitis is assumed to be caused by herpes virus. For the infection caused by HSV, prompt and vigorous treatment is needed to prevent eye injury or blindness, which can occur in children with recurrent herpes virus infections as a result of antibody reaction to the viral antigen. Herpes virus infections commonly recur, so periodic treatment and sometimes prophylaxis may be needed.

Allergic Conjunctivitis

Allergic conjunctivitis is a common cause of eye discomfort (Bielory, 2010). When conjunctivitis is caused by an allergy, the child complains of intense itching. Examination reveals red eyes with watery discharge, and the conjunctivae have a "cobblestone" appearance. The eyes may also appear edematous.

Collaborative Care

The goal of collaborative care is prompt diagnosis and treatment of any conjunctivitis to prevent both continued discomfort for the baby or child and any long-term damage to the eye. Medications are given in the form of otic drops or ointment for direct delivery to the eye and minimization of systemic effects.

In most cases, a diagnosis of the cause of conjunctivitis is made based on the history and symptoms. Cultures can be taken, especially in infants or in cases suspected of being unusual bacterial illness or herpes viruses. A Gram stain of discharge and conjunctival scraping for potential *Chlamydia* or herpes is performed. Infants and children must be promptly referred to primary care providers or eye specialists for treatment of possible eye infections. When diagnosed in the neonatal intensive care unit, the infant is isolated to prevent spread to other infants.

Antibiotic eye medication is prescribed in droplet or ointment form if a bacterial infection is suspected. Treatment may be started after a laboratory sample is obtained but before the results are known. Fluoroquinolones are frequently used to treat bacterial conjunctivitis; drops or ointment can be used (Tepedino, 2010). Other drugs used to treat bacterial infections include sulfonamides, aminoglycosides, polymyxin B/trimethoprim, and azithromycin (Granet, 2011; Pichichero, 2010). When gonococcal conjunctivitis occurs in newborns, ceftriaxone is recommended; the disease is resistant to penicillin (Tigchelaar, Kannikeswaran, & Kamat, 2008). Chlamydial infections are treated with oral erythromycin or tetracycline. Careful total evaluation of the newborn with any conjunctivitis is also performed to watch for other signs of infection. Instructions for instilling eye medications are given in the Skills Manual ⊂▭⊃.

Viral conjunctivitis may be treated with comfort measures such as cleaning drainage away with a warm clean cloth, avoiding bright lights, and avoiding reading. Ophthalmic antibiotics are sometimes given to prevent bacterial invasion due to frequent rubbing of the eyes. Herpes simplex virus infections of the eye are treated promptly by an ophthalmologist, neonatologist, or other professional trained in this serious disease. Topical drugs are used, and often are combined with a systemic antiviral agent such as acyclovir. Neonatal herpes simplex virus is treated vigorously with parenteral acyclovir for 21 days (or longer if central nervous system involvement is found upon lumbar puncture) and with topical ophthalmic medication (trifluridine, iododeoxyuridine, or vidarabine). Recurrent lesions may necessitate suppressive or prophylactic treatment with oral acyclovir (Corey & Wald, 2009).

If an allergen is diagnosed as the cause of conjunctivitis, systemic or topical antihistamines may be prescribed. Topical steroids and vasoconstrictors may also be used. Decongestants can be combined with systemic antihistamines for short-term therapy. More current treatment involves use of mast-cell stabilizers to decrease the activation of mast cells that accompanies allergic reactions. Most mast-cell stabilizers have been tested and found to be safe in children 3 years of age and older. See the Medications table on page 700.

Practice Alert

Topical steroids can be used to treat allergic conjunctivitis. However, these drugs could mask the symptoms of an infection with herpes virus, leading to serious eye damage. Any red eye should be diagnosed by an ophthalmologist or well-trained pediatric care provider so that viral infections are ruled out before use of steroids. *How do steroids work? Why could masking a herpes infection have important implications?*

Nursing Management

Nurses routinely instill prophylactic antibiotics into the eyes of newborns after birth. A careful examination should occur so that any cases of ophthalmia neonatorum are referred promptly to an ophthalmologist. Women infected with gonococcus or chlamydia should be identified so their babies can receive attention and medication at birth to prevent infection. Infants born at home should have ocular examinations soon after birth.

Nurses also perform assessments of the eyes of infants and children in many settings and refer for care those with identified redness, edema, and discharge. Because bacterial conjunctivitis is contagious, advise parents that children should not return to childcare or school until symptoms abate. For all types of conjunctivitis, teach parents the importance of careful hand hygiene and the avoidance of shared towels. Inform parents that children should not rub their eyes; soft cotton mittens may help prevent infants from doing so. Toddlers may be distracted by activities that keep their hands busy.

Teach parents the proper techniques for instilling eye medications. Answer questions about types of infections; some parents do not understand that most viral infections are not treated with antibiotics. For children with allergies, alert parents to signs of infection such as increased redness and thickness of discharge, so if the child gets an eye infection, prompt treatment will be obtained. For the child at the appropriate developmental level, the itching of allergic conjunctivitis may be relieved by laying clean washcloths with very cold water over the eyes for several minutes two to three times daily. It is best not to use contact lenses during periods of allergic conjunctivitis since they can further exacerbate the condition. See Partnering with Families: Instilling Eye Medications.

Medications Used to Treat Conjunctivitis

MEDICATION	ACTION/INDICATION	NURSING MANAGEMENT
Fluoroquinolones (e.g., besifloxacin, norfloxacin, ciprofloxacin, ofloxacin, levofloxacin, moxifloxacin, sparfloxacin) Other antibiotics (erythromycin, tobramycin, polymyxin B)	Antibiotics effective against a broad spectrum of gram-positive and gram-negative organisms; generally interfere with enzymes needed for DNA replication in bacteria causing eye infections.	If a culture and sensitivity test is ordered, perform the test before beginning the antibiotic. Teach parents correct administration of drops or ointment. Be alert for signs of reactivity to medication which might be manifested as local burning, crusting, itching, and edema.
Acyclovir	Antiviral drug effective against herpes simplex virus (HSV).	Most viral conjunctivitis infections are not treated with medication; good hygiene practices are followed and the infection clears without treatment by medication. However, HSV infections must be treated because they can harm vision. Acyclovir is administered intravenously to neonates and some children with HSV; ongoing suppressive oral therapy is used for recurrent infections. Teach the family to recognize characteristic herpes skin lesions and report them and all eye redness immediately. Ensure that family and other care providers understand the possible chronic nature of HSV and engage in careful hygiene to prevent spread when infections are active. Prepare and administer IV form as ordered, over at least 1 hour. Shake oral suspension when that form is used for children.
Mast-cell stabilizers (e.g., cromolyn, nedocromil, olopatadine)	Inhibit release of histamine from mast cells, thereby decreasing allergic response. Used to treat itching and other symptoms of allergic conjunctivitis.	Teach the family the correct instillation of medication. Encourage other methods to decrease itching such as cool compresses several times daily to the eyes. Avoid rubbing eyes, which can introduce bacteria or virus to the already inflamed eyes. If medication does not provide relief or additional eye symptoms appear, consult again with the healthcare provider.

Periorbital Cellulitis

Periorbital cellulitis is an infection of the eyelid and surrounding tissues that is usually caused by bacteria. It is an uncommon complication of sinusitis in some children. The average age for occurrence is 5 to 7.5 years (Cohen, 2011; Hauser & Fogarasi, 2010; Yang, Quah, Seah, et al., 2009). Children present with edematous, tender, red or purple eyelids; restricted, painful movement of the area around the eye; and fever. A CT scan may be performed to rule out other abscesses . Periorbital cellulitis should be treated promptly to prevent the spread of the infection to the posterior orbit; ampicillin/sulbactam or cefuroxime is commonly prescribed. Orbital cellulitis is a serious outcome that can lead to bacterial meningitis and all of its possible sequelae (see Chapter 33). Clinical therapy includes hospitalization for intravenous administration of antibiotics and the application of hot packs. Children usually respond favorably within 48 to 72 hours.

Nursing management of periorbital cellulitis begins with identification of potential cases and prompt referral for treatment. When the child is hospitalized, the nurse administers antibiotics, provides supportive care, monitors vital signs, and teaches the family about the infection. Desired outcomes are rapid resolution of the infection and return to normal daily activity with no impairment in eye function. See Chapter 36 for additional information about cellulitis in other body parts.

Visual Disorders

Vision, the complex process of acquiring meaning from what is seen, depends on many factors. The eyes must move quickly and in a coordinated manner (see Chapter 7 for discussion of eye movement assessment). They must function together for clear, single vision to occur. If this ability, called **binocularity,** is not present (perhaps due to strabismus or amblyopia), the child may have double vision and the

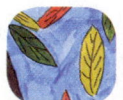

Partnering with Families

Instilling Eye Medications

It can be challenging to safely instill medication into the eyes of young children. Give parents the following suggestions:

- Wash hands well.
- Be sure the medicine is warmed at least to room temperature.
- Remove any drainage from the eye with a clean or sterile moist, warm cloth or gauze.
- Wash hands again.
- Have the child lie on the back with eyes closed.

- Gently pull the lower lid down to form a small pocket.
- Apply a thin string (for ointment) or drops (for liquid) of the medicine.
- Allow the eyelid to return to normal position.
- Have the child keep the eye closed (but not squeezed shut) for several seconds.
- Help prevent spread of the infection by keeping the child's hands clean.
- Enhance comfort by keeping the head elevated to decrease swelling and by avoiding exposure to bright light.

brain cannot make sense of the images it receives. Normally, the perceptions of objects seen are integrated with other senses through eye–hand coordination, and with the brain through visual imagery and discrimination of objects. Although visual acuity is essential, the child's movements, mental processes, and other senses all interact to give meaning to objects that are viewed. About 5% to 10% of young children have some type of vision impairment. If uncorrected, early visual impairment interferes with learning, developmental progression, and school performance; it may even lead to further deterioration of vision, total blindness, and adult visual problems (Davidson & Quinn, 2011).

Etiology and Pathophysiology

Several of the common visual disorders involve errors of refraction (Figure 24–4 ■). As light enters the eye, it is bent or refracted to fall on the retina. Variations in shape of the eyeball are often genetic in nature and can cause light rays to fall in another area of the eye, where they cannot be interpreted. Common refractive errors include:

- **Hyperopia (farsightedness).** Light rays focus posterior to the retina, resulting in an inability to focus on nearby objects. All children have some degree of hyperopia until 9 to 10 years of age. However, their eyes can accommodate sufficiently to enable them to see near objects clearly. Blurring of vision occurs only in children with excessive hyperopia, or a difference in accommodation between the two eyes. Amblyopia, or weakened vision of the poorer eye, can occur in these children if treatment is not obtained.
- **Myopia (nearsightedness).** Light rays focus anterior to the retina, resulting in an inability to see far-off objects. Although children of any age can manifest myopia, it most commonly develops at about 8 years of age. The child may complain of headaches and often squints to improve distance vision.
- **Astigmatism.** Light rays are refracted differently depending on their place of entry to the eye. The curvature of the cornea or lens is not uniformly spherical, causing blurred images. The child with astigmatism often holds pages very close to the face to obtain the best visual image.

Other common visual disorders in children are characterized by abnormal musculature that causes asymmetric eye movement and by other anatomic abnormalities. They include:

- **Strabismus**—abnormal turning of the eye, usually inward or outward, due to a weak eye muscle. The eyes are misaligned so that binocularity of vision does not occur. The condition is usually present at birth and up to approximately 6 months of age, but can develop as a result of amblyopia, described next. When strabismus is the primary disorder, it may also lead to amblyopia since the eye with abnormal musculature may lose its ability to see normally.
- **Amblyopia**—reduced vision of the eye. Generally one eye has much poorer vision than the other, resulting in loss of binocularity. As noted, the child's muscle in the poorer eye may fail to function normally over time, resulting in strabismus. Amblyopia is usually genetic and appears at birth. At times it is the result of another eye abnormality such as glaucoma, cataract, or even eye injury.
- **Cataracts**—lens opacity. Some cataracts are present at birth, whereas others are acquired during childhood. Some of the causes of acquired cataracts include retinopathy of prematurity (described later in this chapter), metabolic diseases such

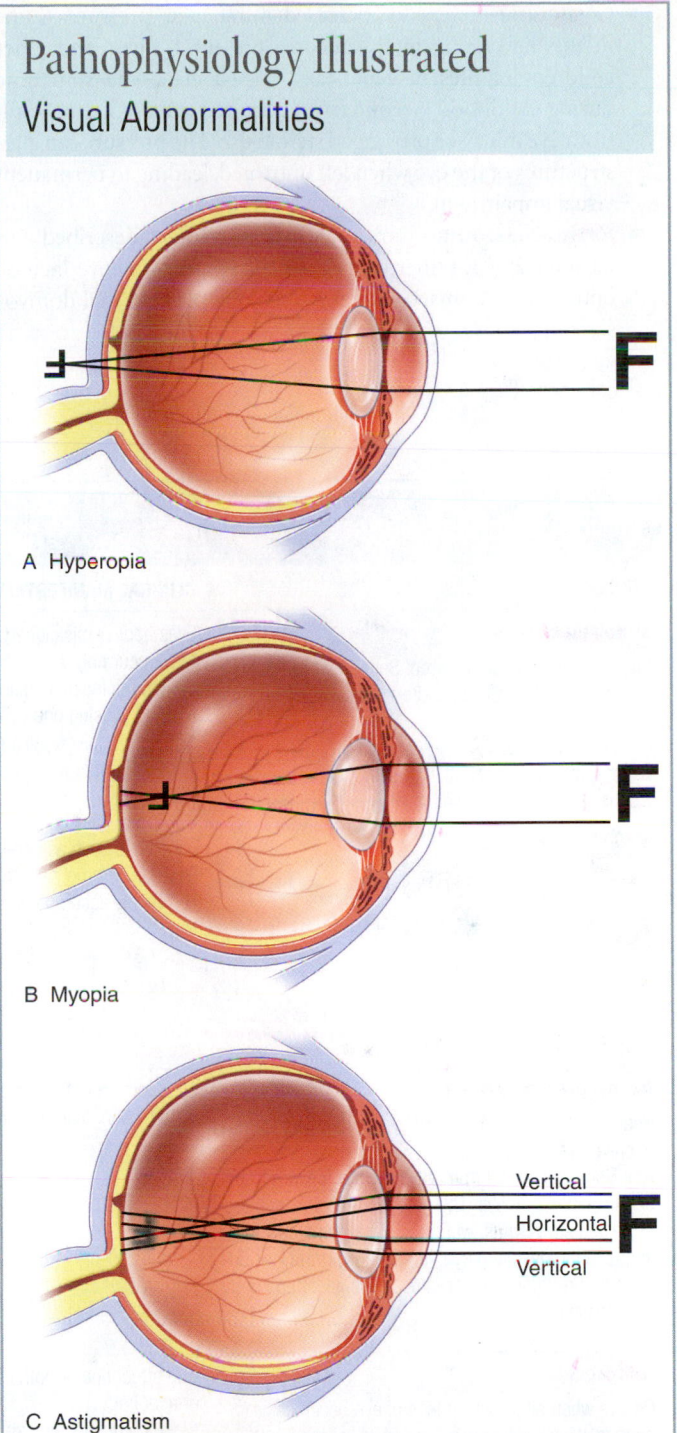

Pathophysiology Illustrated
Visual Abnormalities

A Hyperopia

B Myopia

C Astigmatism

FIGURE 24–4 ■ In hyperopia, light rays focus behind the retina, making it difficult to focus on objects at close range. In myopia, light rays focus in front of the retina, making it difficult to focus on objects that are far away. In astigmatism, light rays do not uniformly focus on the eye due to abnormal curvature of the cornea or lens.

as galactosemia, diabetes mellitus, and long-term use of corticosteroids. A major cause of congenital cataracts in the past was congenital rubella syndrome, the mother's infection with rubella during gestation. Since children and women now receive rubella vaccine, there are very few cases of rubella in pregnant women and consequently few cases of cataracts from the syndrome. Genetic abnormalities have now become the most common cause (Trumler, 2011).

- **Glaucoma**—refers to increased intraocular pressure. Some infants have congenital glaucoma present at birth, and other children manifest a genetically caused glaucoma sometime during childhood. Secondary or acquired glaucoma can result from eye injury or prolonged steroid use. The pressure can alter structures of the eye when left untreated, leading to permanent visual impairment.

- **Retinoblastoma**—tumor of the retina, described in Chapter 29 🔗. Other cancers that may affect the eye include optic nerve glioma, optic nerve meningioma, and rhabdomyosarcoma.

Clinical Manifestations

Children with eye abnormalities may show a variety of behaviors. An infant who notices objects only on one side or consistently holds the head more to one side may have a decrease in vision in the other eye. Cataracts may be visualized as the lens appears cloudy. Muscular problems may be evident when the eyes do not move symmetrically or one eye deviates inward or outward. Some children squint, cover one eye, hold toys or books close to the face, or have watering eyes. For further detail on clinical manifestations of specific eye conditions, see the Clinical Manifestations table.

Clinical Manifestations Visual Disorders

ETIOLOGY	CLINICAL MANIFESTATIONS	CLINICAL THERAPY
Strabismus Can be congenital or acquired. Seen in up to 4% of all children; 30–50% of children with strabismus develop amblyopia. Most common types: **Esotropia:** inward deviation of eyes ("crossed eyes") **Exotropia:** outward deviation of eyes ("wall-eyes") 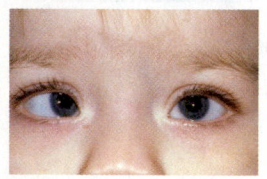 Strabismus **Source:** Biophoto Associates / Photo Researchers, Inc.	Eyes appear misaligned to observer. May occur only when child is tired. Symptoms include squinting and frowning when reading; closing one eye to see; having trouble picking up objects; dizziness and headache. Corneal light reflex and cover–uncover tests confirm diagnosis. Child may have no other abnormalities, but certain conditions such as cerebral palsy, hydrocephalus, Down syndrome, and seizure disorder are more commonly accompanied by strabismus.	Occlusion therapy (patching the fixating or good eye for 1–2 hours daily to force use of the weak eye). Compensatory lenses. Surgery of the rectus muscles to correct muscle imbalance. Eyedrops to cause blurring of the good eye. Prisms. Vision therapy (eye exercises). If treatment is begun before 24 months of age, amblyopia (reduced vision in one or both eyes) may be prevented.
Amblyopia ("lazy eye") Reduced vision in one or both eyes; affects up to 4% of children. Amblyopia can result from anything that causes visual deprivation to one eye. The most common causes are untreated strabismus, with the child "tuning out" the image in the deviating eye, congenital cataract, or uncorrected refractive errors causing visual differences between eyes.	Symptoms are the same as for strabismus. Vision testing can be used to diagnose condition.	Compensatory lenses. Occlusion therapy for 2–6 hours daily through patching the eye or eye glass. Occasionally vision therapy (eye exercises) is used in an attempt to improve the weaker eye. Atropine 1% 1 drop/day in unaffected eye. Treatment is discontinued when visual acuity no longer improves; 20/20 acuity rarely attained. Treatment is most successful if received by 5–6 years of age.
Cataracts Occurs when all or part of lens of eye becomes opaque, which prevents refraction of light rays onto retina. Seen in 2/10,000 newborns. 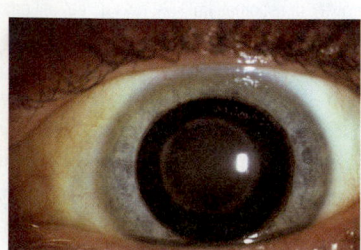 Congenital cataract **Source:** Sue Ford / Science Source / Photo Researchers, Inc.	Can affect one or both eyes and may be congenital or acquired. Clouding of lens indicates presence of cataract; however, cataracts are not always visible to naked eye. Symptoms included distorted red reflex, symptoms of vision loss (see strabismus), white pupil (leukocoria). May be present alone but sometimes associated with other conditions such as fetal alcohol syndrome, Down syndrome, and Turner syndrome.	Must be diagnosed at a young age for successful treatment; many cases are missed. Specific treatment depends on age at diagnosis, whether one or both eyes are affected, extent of clouding, and presence of other ocular abnormalities. Surgical removal of lens and corrective lenses; contact lenses frequently used; results of surgery are good; surgery before the age of 2 months is associated with the best results; visual acuity in 55% of children is 20/40 or better. Lens implant may be used. Eye protectors and restraints are used postoperatively to prevent injury; antibiotic or steroid drops may be used for several weeks; treatment for amblyopia may be necessary.

Clinical Manifestations Visual Disorders (*Continued*)

ETIOLOGY	CLINICAL MANIFESTATIONS	CLINICAL THERAPY
Glaucoma Increased intraocular pressure damages eye and impairs visual function; ciliary body of eye produces aqueous fluid that flows between iris and lens into anterior chamber; if enough fluid accumulates, blindness results; affects 1/100,000 newborns. May be congenital (occurring in first 3 years of life) or juvenile (occurring from 3–30 years) and affect one or both eyes. Primary glaucoma (50% of cases) is an isolated anomaly of drainage; secondary glaucoma (50% of cases) is associated with other ocular or systemic abnormalities.	Symptoms of congenital glaucoma include tearing, blinking, corneal clouding, eyelid spasms, and progressive enlargement of eye; photophobia (extreme sensitivity to light). Symptoms of juvenile glaucoma include constant bumping into objects in child's periphery (painless visual field loss); seeing halos around objects. Diagnosis is made using tonometer, which measures intraocular pressure.	Surgery to reduce intraocular pressure is treatment of choice, since medications used to combat glaucoma in adults are not as effective in children. Compensatory lenses are used following surgery. Treatment is not always successful, especially if the child has congenital glaucoma, so parents' feelings regarding care of a child with visual impairment should be explored.

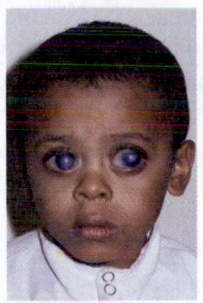

Congenital glaucoma

Source: *Copyright 2012—Custom Medical Stock Photo, All Rights Reserved.*

Source: *Data from Nield, L. S., Mangano, L. M., & Kamat, D. (2008, January). Strabismus: A close-up look. Consultant for Pediatricians, 17–25; Granet, D. B., & Khayali, S. (2011). Amblyopia and strabismus. Pediatric Annals, 40(2), 89–94; Mickler, C., Boden, J., Trivedi, R. H., & Wilson, M. E. (2011). Pediatric cataract. Pediatric Annals, 40(2), 83–87; Kliegman, R. M., Stanton, B., St. Geme, J., Schor, N., & Behrman, R. E. (2010). Nelson textbook of pediatrics (19th ed., pp. 2152–2181). Philadelphia, PA: Saunders.*

Collaborative Care

The goal of collaborative care for visual disorders is early detection of abnormalities and prompt treatment. Since vision is developing in early childhood, a problem with one eye can affect permanent visual acuity if not detected and treated.

Diagnostic Tests

Visual disturbances must be diagnosed and treated promptly to prevent impairment or loss of vision. Most children undergo a simple test for visual acuity during healthcare visits as soon as they can cooperate with the examiner. Once in school, children's visual acuity is screened every 2 to 3 years during the elementary years. Table 24–4 provides a series of questions that can be asked to identify visual disturbances in children. A child who does not pass vision screening is referred to an ophthalmologist or optometrist for more detailed examination of near and far vision, eye structure and movement, and color discrimination. During health promotion visits, infants and young children should be examined by using the cover–uncover test, and the red reflex should be examined with an ophthalmoscope. See Chapter 7 🔗 for thorough descriptions of both of these tests.

TABLE 24–4	Assessment Questions for Identifying Visual Disturbances in Children	
INFANT	**YOUNG CHILD**	**SCHOOL-AGE CHILD**
Ask the parents:	Ask the parents:	Ask the parents:
Does your baby follow an object from one side to the other?	Does your child follow you with his or her eyes as you come into a room?	Does your child like to look at pictures and read?
What is your baby's reaction when you are directly in front and close?	Are other objects followed with ease?	Does your child hold toys or books close, or sit very close to the television?
Does the baby seem to notice an object to the right and left sides?	Do both eyes work together or does one seem to wander off?	Does your child squint or rub the eyes?
Do your baby's eyes ever appear to move asymmetrically?	At what age did your baby sit, stand, walk?	Is he or she performing at grade level in all subjects?
What is your baby learning to do right now?	Does your child have any difficulty picking up objects?	Has your child demonstrated any learning difficulties?
	Do the child's eyes appear crossed in photos?	Does he or she use a computer, watch television, or play computer games?
		Does your child play sports and games at the same level of ability as peers?

Clinical Therapy

Compensatory lenses are prescribed for many visual disorders, particularly refractive disorders. A significant difference in visual acuity between the eyes is often a result of amblyopia or strabismus, and further treatment by patching or surgery may be needed. The visual acuity of a child with compensatory lenses should be reevaluated every 1 to 2 years. More frequent visits to an eye specialist are needed when a child is being treated for amblyopia or strabismus.

Cataracts are generally treated surgically with removal of the lens, placement of lens transplant, or use of corrective contact lenses. Glaucoma frequently requires surgery in children to provide outflow for fluid and resultant decrease in intraocular pressure. The variety of cancers are treated with surgery and chemotherapy.

Nursing Management

The nurse focuses activities on identification of children with eye problems, and on partnering with parents and other professionals to provide care for the child with a visual disorder.

Nursing Assessment and Diagnosis

The nurse plays an important role in identifying eye disorders in children. Ask questions that will help to identify the child with a decrease in visual acuity (see Table 24–4). You will perform careful eye examinations of newborns and children. Observe for symmetry of placement and movement, ability to follow objects with each eye, and any abnormalities in appearance. The light reflex test, cover–uncover test, and visual acuity testing are essential for every child. See Chapter 7 🔗 for a description of eye examination and the Skills Manual 🔗 for visual acuity tests. Vision screening should be conducted at birth and at all well-child visits.

Nurses in schools plan and carry out visual acuity screening on children. Generally certain grades (such as kindergarten, 2, 5, and 8) are screened annually along with any children new to a district. The nurse performs and records the screening results, and informs the school and families of any children with abnormal results who are referred to an eye specialist for care. An important part of the screening process is following up on referrals to be certain that children receive the diagnostic care they need. See Chapter 14 🔗 for the nurse's role in referral in community agencies.

Potential nursing diagnoses related to visual problems are as follows:

- Injury, Risk for Disturbed Sensory Perception related to error of refraction
- Growth and Development, Delayed related to effects of visual impairment
- Self-Esteem, Situational Low related to poor school performance resulting from visual impairment

NANDA-I © 2012

Planning and Implementation

When abnormalities are found on screening, nurses refer families to the care of an eye specialist. When prescriptive lenses are used, the nurse instructs the parent and child on correct wear practices and care. See the Skills Manual 🔗 for information about contact lens care. Sometimes nurses partner with community resources to provide financial assistance for care. The Lions Club and other groups may be able to provide glasses for children if the family cannot afford them.

Provide explanations for parents who are confused about the diagnosis or treatment. Instruct parents in patching for the recommended period of time daily (usually 2 to 6 hours) for the child with amblyopia.

If surgery is required, surgical and postoperative follow-up are needed. This will include pain control, observing for signs of infection (ophthalmic or systemic), and administering needed eye medications. Sterile technique is used postoperatively to provide eye care. Promptly report deviations from normal such as increased pain, redness, discharge, or edema of the eye; increased temperature or pulse, which may indicate infection; increased sensitivity to light; or other abnormalities. Children are usually discharged home with instructions to minimize vigorous activities for a certain period of time. Perform postoperative and discharge teaching and emphasize the importance of follow-up visits.

Evaluation

The nurse evaluates the effectiveness of vision screening and treatment for individuals and groups of children. Use the *Healthy People 2020* (U.S. Department of Health and Human Services, 2010) objectives related to vision as a guide to evaluation of programs (Table 24–5). See the section on visual impairment later in the chapter for information on the child with a diagnosed decrease in vision.

Color Blindness

Color blindness is an X-linked recessive disorder found in 10% of males and very rarely in females; it is more common in White than Black males. The most common form affects the ability to distinguish between the colors red and green. Blue-yellow discrimination and other colors can also be involved. Preschool boys are tested for color blindness in some clinics to identify those with the disorder. The Ishihara color blindness test is often used and consists of numbers embedded in a background that are difficult for persons with color blindness to see (Choi & Hwang, 2009). Color blindness is not treatable, and management focuses on issues of safety (e.g., problems in distinguishing red and green traffic signals) and techniques to improve discrimination of colors in the affected color groups.

Retinopathy of Prematurity

Retinopathy of prematurity (ROP) occurs when immature blood vessels in the retina constrict and become necrotic. This condition, which may occur in infants of low birth weight or of short gestation, can heal completely or lead to mild myopia or retinal detachment and blindness.

Etiology and Pathophysiology

Retinopathy of prematurity results from injury to the developing capillaries of the retina. Oxygen therapy is associated with the development of ROP (Figure 24–5 ■), but other factors such as respiratory distress, assisted ventilation, apnea, bradycardia, heart disease, multiple blood transfusions, infection, hypoxia, hypercarbia, acidosis, shock, and sepsis have been linked with the disorder. Cerebral palsy is sometimes an associated factor, and more cases are seen in multiple births. It is most common in male infants born before 28 weeks' gestation and weighing under 1600 g (3 lb, 8 oz) at birth. A genetic link may be present as White infants are more commonly affected than those of African heritage, and Alaska Natives have a high rate of the disorder. In developed countries, ROP is the second most common cause of blindness, occurring in 12.5% of infants born from 23 to 26 weeks' gestation. In infants weighing less than 1250 g, ROP's incidence is 66%, and in infants less than 1000 g, the incidence is 82% (Askin & Diehl-Jones, 2009).

TABLE 24–5	*Healthy People 2020* Objectives Related to Vision in Children
OBJECTIVE	**NURSING IMPLEMENTATION**
Increase the proportion of preschool children aged 5 years and under who receive vision screening.	■ Establish programs to screen preschoolers in childcare centers for visual acuity, symmetry of eye movement, and ability to focus. ■ Sponsor programs at schools, clinics, vans, religious organizations, and other settings to screen vision of young children.
Reduce visual impairment due to uncorrected refractive errors.	■ Establish a referral and follow-up plan for children who do not pass screening. ■ Post resources on bulletin boards, websites, and other places where parents look for health information.
Reduce visual impairment.	■ Ensure that pregnant women obtain recommended prenatal care in order to reduce prematurity which is a risk factor for visual impairment. ■ Perform screening for visual impairment during each health encounter. ■ Refer children to eye specialists when parents are concerned about a child's vision or any abnormalities are noted.
Increase the use of personal protective eyewear in recreational activities and hazardous situations around the home.	■ Assist families to understand that most eye injuries are preventable. ■ Partner with families to plan for protection during sports such as hockey and racquetball, as well as yard work. ■ Include teaching about emergency care for eye injuries to teachers, coaches, and parents.
Increase the use of vision rehabilitation services and assistive/adaptive devices by persons with visual impairments.	■ Screen children with glasses or contact lenses in place. ■ Check for fit of glasses; check strap to keep glasses on toddler. ■ Encourage annual visits to an eye specialist for children with visual impairment. ■ Assist families and school personnel to provide safe and stimulating environments for children with visual impairment.

Source: Adapted from U.S. Department of Health and Human Services. (2010). Healthy People 2020. Washington, DC: U.S. Government Printing Office. Retrieved from http://www.healthypeople.gov/2020/

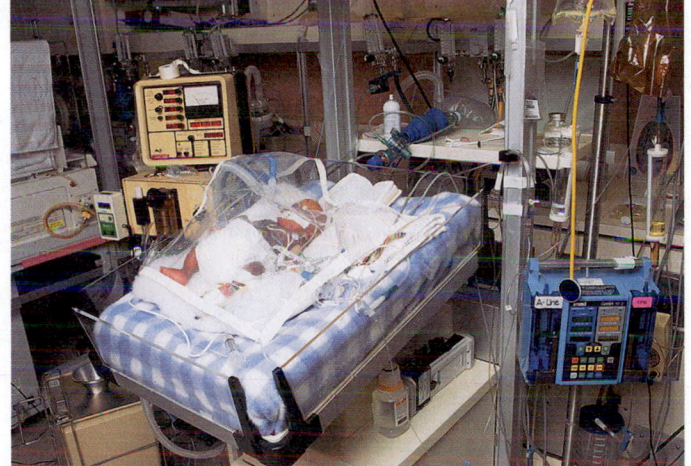

FIGURE 24–5 ■ This premature infant in the neonatal intensive care unit is receiving artificial ventilation—a risk factor for retinopathy of prematurity. The infant will need careful management of oxygen therapy, determined by oxygen saturation readings, as well as periodic eye examinations.

The retina is normally vascularized by about 8 months' gestation. For the premature infant, however, this process must continue after birth and the environmental and other conditions listed in the preceding paragraph appear to affect its course. Arteriole constriction, followed by vascular proliferation of abnormal vessels, occurs. In most cases, the abnormal vessels gradually regress and normal vascularization occurs. Sometimes, however, the abnormal vascularization continues into the vitreous cavity, causing abnormalities of the retina, optic disc, and macula. It is not known why the disease progresses in some cases, but progression is directly linked to lower birth weight, greater prematurity, and duration (not necessarily concentration) of oxygen therapy.

Although the developing capillaries are lost, in up to 90% of cases some degree of revascularization occurs late. The degree of visual loss, varying from slight to total, is determined by the degree of revascularization that occurs.

Clinical Manifestations

ROP is characterized by progressive changes in the retinal blood vessels, and in severe disease, by retinal detachment. Premature and low-birth-weight infants at risk for the disease are given frequent ocular examinations to ensure early detection of these changes. For infants who do not receive ophthalmologic examinations, resulting visual impairment may be detected only later in infancy when the child progresses slowly in meeting developmental milestones, fails to reach for objects, and does not follow objects or faces with the eyes. When visual impairment is present, the child usually manifests myopia. Total loss of vision can occur in the child who suffers a retinal detachment.

Collaborative Care

The goals of collaborative care are to provide ongoing evaluation of infants at risk for ROP, to provide care for the disorder to minimize effects, and to support the child who has visual impairment due to the disorder.

Diagnostic Tests

Diagnosis is made by ophthalmologic examination. A classification system that includes zone, stage, and plus disease is used to describe the location, extent, and severity of the disease (Table 24–6).

In general, the more posterior the disease, and the larger the amount of retinal tissue involved, the more severe the disease and the greater risk of vision loss (Salvin, Lehman, Jin, et al., 2010).

All infants at risk—those under 1500 g (3 lb, 7 oz) or born before 32 weeks' gestation, and those at risk with birth weight from 1500 to 2000 g (3 lb, 7 oz to 4 lb, 3 oz) born after 32 weeks' gestation—are assessed frequently using binocular indirect ophthalmoscopy, by an ophthalmologist who is experienced with the condition. The disease is not manifested before 4 to 6 weeks after birth, so it is important that the infant receive regular eye examinations until the risk is discounted. Eye examinations continue every 1 to 3 weeks, with the frequency determined by the location of disease, the progress of disease, and the infant's degree of immature vascularization.

TABLE 24–6	Diagnosis of Retinopathy of Prematurity		
ZONE (AREA OF RETINA INVOLVED WITH ABNORMAL VASCULATURE)	**STAGE (SEVERITY OF ROP WHEREVER IT IS PRESENT)**	**PLUS DISEASE (VASCULAR DILATION AND TORTUOSITY NOTED IN POSTERIOR POLE IN AREA NEAR OPTIC NERVE)**	**THRESHOLD (MEASURE OF SEVERITY OF DISEASE; USED TO JUDGE WHEN TREATMENT IS NEEDED)**
Zone I (most posterior and near optic nerve head)	Stage 1 (line divides vascular and avascular retina)	Present	Threshold I (Stage 3 ROP in Zone I or II and five continuous or eight cumulative "clock hour" areas with plus disease; treatment is required)
Zone II (outside or area anterior to Zone I)	Stage 2 (line of demarcation is elevated)	Absent	
Zone III (only present on temporal side of eye; nasal quadrants are adequately vascularized)	Stage 3 (new vascularization is present in the demarcation area)		

Source: Data from Alme, A. M., Mulhern, J. L., Hejkal, T. W., Meza, J. L., Qui, F., Ingvoldstad, D. D., & Margalit, E. (2008). Outcomes of retinopathy of prematurity patients following adoption of revised indications for treatment. *BMC Ophthalmology, 13*(8), 23.

Involvement of blood vessels in the periphery of the retina rarely leads to visual impairment. With involvement in other areas of the retina, risk of visual problems is more common.

Clinical Therapy

Treatment of infants with severe ROP often involves laser therapy to stop progression of the disease process. Other surgical procedures such as a scleral buckle procedure and vitrectomy have been used in retinal detachments. A threshold or measure of severity of disease is based on zone, stage, and plus disease levels (see Table 24–6), and used to determine the timing and type of treatment.

Associated problems such as strabismus, amblyopia, and myopia should be managed to promote maximal development.

Nursing Management

Nursing management focuses on referring the infant at risk for ROP for ophthalmoscopic evaluation and assisting the family in coping with visual impairment when that is a result of the disorder.

Nursing Assessment and Diagnosis

Assessment of the infant at risk for ROP begins at birth by identifying infants who may require oxygen therapy or assisted ventilation. Look for risk factors such as prematurity and low birth weight. Assess the infant's breathing efforts and report any changes. Be certain the ventilation equipment is properly set to deliver the correct ventilatory pressure and amount of oxygen, evaluated by pulse oximetry saturation. Oxygen is increased in small increments to manage desaturations below target level. Ventilatory equipment is meticulously monitored. The nurse weans the infant from oxygen as indicated by the oxygen saturation reading in concordance with standing orders in the neonatal intensive care unit. Note the cumulative risks in a particular case (greater prematurity and longer exposure to higher levels of oxygen increase risk) and suggest the need for a referral to an ophthalmologist. See Tables 24–6 and 24–7 for referral criteria for assessment and classification of cases.

The accompanying Nursing Care Plan outlines several nursing diagnoses for a child with a visual impairment secondary to ROP. Following are other nursing diagnoses that may be appropriate for an infant with the potential to develop ROP or a child with resulting visual impairment:

- Social Interaction, Impaired related to altered transmission of visual impulses
- Gas Exchange, Impaired related to ventilation-perfusion imbalance
- Growth and Development, Delayed related to effects of visual impairment
- Family Processes, Interrupted related to a child with a visual impairment

NANDA-I © 2012

TABLE 24–7	Assessment and Treatment for Retinopathy of Prematurity	
INITIAL ASSESSMENT	**FOLLOW-UP ASSESSMENT**	**TREATMENT**
Who? All infants less than 1500 g or less than 32 weeks' gestation; babies from 1500–2000 g who have other risk factors	Every 2–3 weeks if vasculature is immature and extends to Zone II but no retinopathy is present; Stage 1 or 2 ROP, Zone III; or regressing ROP in Zone III*	Ablative therapy with laser therapy is most common. Treatment within 72 hours of identification of treatable disease is needed to minimize risk of retinal detachment.
When? From 4–9 weeks postnatal age, or 31–36 weeks of postmenstrual age, depending on the gestational age of the infant at birth	Every 2 weeks if ROP is Stage 1, Zone II, or regressing ROP in Zone II*	Earlier ablation with cryotherapy was used, and is still available in some developing countries that do not have access to laser therapy.
What? Pupil dilation using binocular indirect ophthalmoscopy by an ophthalmologist experienced in ROP; one examination is satisfactory only if full retinal vascularization is seen bilaterally	Every 1–2 weeks if no ROP but having incomplete vasculature in Zone I; Stage 2 ROP, Zone II; regressing ROP, Zone I* Every week for infants with ROP in Stage 1 or 2; Zone I, Stage 3 ROP, Zone II*	Surgery is needed in some cases.

*See Table 24–6 for a description of stages and zones for ROP.

Source: Data from American Academy of Pediatrics Section on Ophthalmology. (2006). Screening examination of premature infants for retinopathy of prematurity. Pediatrics, 117, 572–576.

Nursing Care Plan

The Child with a Visual Impairment Secondary to Retinopathy of Prematurity

INTERVENTION	RATIONALE	EXPECTED OUTCOME
1. Nursing Diagnosis: Environmental Interpretation Syndrome, Impaired related to altered reception, transmission, and integration of visual images		
**NIC Priority Intervention—*Visual Deficit Enhancement:* ** Assistance in accepting and learning alternate methods for living with diminished vision		**NOC Suggested Outcome—*Developmental Progression:* ** Compensate for sensory deficits by maximizing use of impaired senses
GOAL: *The child will receive adequate sensory input.*		
■ Provide kinesthetic, tactile, and auditory stimulation during play and in daily care (e.g., talking and playing). Provide music while bathing an infant, using bells and other noises on each side of the infant. Verbally describe to a child all actions being carried out by the adult.	■ Because visual sensory input is not present, the child needs input from all other senses to compensate and provide adequate sensory stimulation.	The child demonstrates minimal signs of sensory deprivation.
2. Nursing Diagnosis: Injury, Risk for related to impaired vision		
**NIC Priority Intervention—*Fall Prevention:* ** Instituting special precautions with patients at risk for injury		**NOC Suggested Outcome—*Risk Control:* ** Actions to eliminate or reduce modifiable health threats
GOAL: *The child will be protected from safety hazards that can lead to injury.*		
■ Evaluate the environment for potential safety hazards based on age of child and degree of impairment. Be particularly alert to objects that give visual cues to their dangers (e.g., stairs, stoves, fireplaces, candles). Eliminate safety hazards and protect the child from exposure. Take the child on a tour of new rooms (e.g., schools, hotel room, hospital room).	■ The child may be at risk for injury related both to developmental stage and inability to visualize hazards.	The child will experience no injuries.
3. Nursing Diagnosis: Growth and Development, Delayed related to impaired vision		
**NIC Priority Intervention—*Developmental Enhancement:* ** Facilitating or teaching parents and caregivers to facilitate optimal growth and development of children		**NOC Suggested Outcome—*Child Growth and Development:* ** Milestones of developmental progression
GOAL: *The child has experiences necessary to foster normal growth and development.*		
■ Help parents plan early, regular social activities with other children. ■ Provide opportunities and encourage self-feeding activities. ■ Provide an environment rich in tactile and auditory sensory input. ■ Assess growth and development during regular examinations to identify the child's strengths and needs.	■ The child with a visual impairment benefits developmentally from contact with other children. ■ To obtain adequate nutrients, the child needs to feel comfortable feeding self. ■ Sensory input is needed for normal development to occur. ■ Regular examinations aid in early identification of growth problems or developmental delays, so that appropriate interventions can be planned.	The child demonstrates normal growth and development milestones.
4. Nursing Diagnosis: Family Processes, Interrupted Coping related to child's prolonged disability from sensory impairment		
**NIC Priority Intervention—*Family Mobilization:* ** Utilization of family strengths to influence child's health positively		**NOC Suggested Outcome—*Positive Coping:* ** Extent to which family can mobilize resources to deal with the child's needs
GOAL: *The family identifies methods for coping with their child who has a visual impairment.*		
■ Provide explanation of visual impairment as appropriate. ■ Refer parents to organizations, early intervention programs, and other parents of children with visual impairment. ■ Assist parents to plan for meeting developmental, educational, and safety needs of their visually impaired child. Offer resources for enhancing the home environment to assist the child with a visual impairment.	■ The parents may feel guilt about the child's visual impairment, which can be allayed by knowledge of the cause. ■ The parents will receive needed information and support from others. ■ The child may require an enhanced environment to foster developmental progress.	The family successfully copes with the experience of having a child with a visual impairment.

NANDA-I © 2012

Planning and Implementation

The nurse plays an important role in preventing ROP. Encourage early and regular prenatal care to prevent unnecessary premature births. Administer oxygen only to newborns who need it, and in the amount specified by the physician to maintain prescribed oxygen saturation. Ensure that the proper ventilatory settings are used. Be alert for infants with multiple risk factors and refer them, when appropriate, for ophthalmologic examination. Parents of infants at risk for ROP require information about the disorder, as well as support, as the long-term effects on the child's vision are often identified only after subsequent examinations as the child grows. Families may be frustrated that a prognosis cannot be made at the time of the first eye examination. Explanations and consistent updates on the infant's condition can be reassuring.

The accompanying Nursing Care Plan summarizes care for the child with a visual impairment resulting from ROP. The nurse is instrumental in case management for such children. Reinforce to parents the importance of follow-up eye examinations. Teach methods of stimulating development for the child with visual impairment (refer to the next section in this chapter).

Evaluation

Expected outcomes of nursing care for the child with retinopathy of prematurity are:

- Visual impairment is identified early in life.
- The child achieves normal developmental milestones.
- The family effectively manages the child's visual condition.

Visual Impairment

Visual impairment related to refractive errors, amblyopia, strabismus, and astigmatism occurs in 5% to 10% of young children (Granet & Khayali, 2011). About 500,000 children in the United States have visual impairment and about 60,000 are legally blind (vision 20/200 or worse) (American Foundation for the Blind, 2011).

Many conditions discussed earlier in this chapter lead to temporary or permanent visual impairment. Infants who are premature; whose mothers were infected prenatally with rubella, toxoplasmosis, or other viruses; and who have certain congenital and hereditary conditions have a high risk of visual problems (Table 24–8). Fetal alcohol syndrome (FAS) is a major cause of visual disturbance; 90%

TABLE 24–8 Common Causes of Visual Impairment in Children	
CONGENITAL OR HEREDITARY	**ACQUIRED**
Cataracts	Injury to eye or head
Glaucoma	Infections
Tay-Sachs disease	Rubella
Marfan syndrome	Measles
Down syndrome	Chicken pox
Fetal alcohol syndrome	Brain tumor
Prenatal infections (maternal infection)	Retinopathy of prematurity
Rubella	Cerebral palsy
Toxoplasmosis	
Herpes simplex	
Retinoblastoma	

TABLE 24–9 Signs of Visual Impairment	
INFANTS	**TODDLERS AND OLDER CHILDREN**
May be unable to follow lights or objects	May rub, shut, or cover eyes
Do not make eye contact	Tilt or thrust head forward
Have a dull, vacant stare	Blink frequently
Do not imitate facial expressions	Hold objects close
	Bump into objects
	Squint

of children with FAS have eye abnormalities (see Chapter 34 🔗 for further description of FAS).

The signs of visual impairment depend on the cause and degree of the problem and the age of the child (Table 24–9). The child's eyes may appear crossed or watery, and the lids may be crusty. Verbal children may complain of itching; dizziness; headache; or blurred, double, or poor vision.

Collaborative Care

Diagnostic tests include vision screening, followed by referral to an eye specialist for full examination. Tests that are commonly performed include responses to visual stimuli, symmetry of eye movements, location of corneal light reflex, cover–uncover testing, visual field testing, and funduscopic examination of the retina. The U.S. Preventive Services Task Force (2011) recommends screening to detect amblyopia, strabismus, and defects in visual acuity in children at least once between 3 and 5 years of age. The American Academy of Pediatrics recommends age-appropriate eye evaluations at health visits from birth to 3 years and age-appropriate visual acuity testing and ophthalmoscopy in children 3 years and older (Hagan, Shaw, & Duncan, 2008).

Clinical therapy depends on the child's condition and may include surgery, medication, and supportive aids. In the case of a disorder that results in permanent visual impairment, an interdisciplinary team of specialists works with the child and family. Nurses have an important role in this team, collaborating not only with families but with other healthcare professionals to plan appropriate interventions.

Nursing Management

The nurse plays a key role in identifying children with visual impairment and in partnering with families to provide an environment for the child with visual impairment that fosters normal growth and development.

Nursing Assessment and Diagnosis

Prevention of low vision, early identification of the condition, and interventions to enhance development of children with low vision provide the focus for nursing care (see Evidence-Based Practice: Nursing Role in Vision Screening and Follow-Up). Vision screening facilitates early detection and treatment of conditions that can lead to vision loss. Visual testing can be done at any age, including immediately after birth. Developmental milestones that require vision, such as following bright lights, reaching for objects, or looking at pictures in a book, can be used to assess vision. For children over the age of 3 years, visual acuity is most frequently measured by means of an age-appropriate acuity test (see Chapter 7 🔗 and the Skills Manual 🔗). The photo

Evidence-Based Practice   Nursing Role in Vision Screening and Follow-Up

PROBLEM

Screening for visual ability is important to identify children with impairments. The American Academy of Pediatrics recommends that children be screened at every well-child visit, beginning in the newborn period, to include vision history, vision assessment, external inspection of the eyes and lids, eye movement assessment, pupil examination, and elicitation of the red reflex. Once the child can cooperate, usually by about 3 years, a vision test such as HOTV or tumbling E, along with ophthalmoscopic examination, should be added to the examination (Chou, Dana, & Bougatsos, 2011; U.S. Preventive Services Task Force, 2008). Nurses are often the health professionals that conduct vision examinations, evaluate results, and provide follow-up care. They participate in well-child health visits and often perform assessments of vision in schools. More than 20% of school-age children have some kind of vision problem, and youth from lower income families and minority groups are more likely to have undiagnosed vision problems (Basch, 2011).

EVIDENCE

A study of school screening found that when two nurses performed vision screening using the E chart, agreement on findings for 6- to 7-year-olds was just 78%, while agreement was 86% for 13- to 14-year-olds (Ore, Tamir, Stein, et al., 2009). In response to findings such as these, there is a proposal that school nurses should all take a course in vision screening to become experts in performing this important task (Proctor, 2009). A study of the outcomes of school vision screening of 2,726 children found that 3 children in 100 were identified with a vision problem, such as myopia, hyperopia, and astigmatism (Kemper, Helfrich, Talbot, et al., 2012). This study also found that no follow-up on the outcome of referral for a full eye examination was obtained for 35% of the children with problems.

IMPLICATIONS

Nurses play a vital role in ensuring that children receive early, periodic, and regular visual and eye screening. Evidence suggests there may be a lack of reliable testing, particularly for young schoolchildren and those from minority groups or low-income families. While identification of problems is important, the nursing roles of referring for care, identifying barriers to care, and ensuring that follow-up care has been received are also integral to vision care.

CRITICAL THINKING APPLICATION

What vision screening methods are available in the offices, clinics, and schools in your community? Does your state provide guidelines to assist school nurses in managing school vision programs? How could you perform vision screening in the hospital setting if a child did not demonstrate expected visual ability for age? Design a follow-up program for a school that screens all kindergartners and first graders for visual acuity. What questions will you ask parents during a well-child visit for a 2-year-old to determine if vision is normal? How will you combine your knowledge of developmental milestones with screening for vision?

---

screener is a device that can take a photo of the child's eyes and is useful for infants, toddlers, and preschoolers. The photo can be used to diagnose refraction errors, eye opacities, and misalignment. Visual fields and the ability to discriminate colors are tested at school age, when children can cooperate with the testing.

Children who are visually impaired may lag in development of cognitive and other skills. Children who are sighted learn the word *cup* using four senses—sight, touch, hearing, and taste—to obtain the information necessary to connect the word with the object it represents. In contrast, children with visual impairments rely on only three senses—touch, hearing, and taste. They learn concepts through differences in sounds, textures, and shapes (Box 24–1).

In addition, many visual disorders are linked with other conditions that influence development. Thus, a child with cerebral palsy or fetal alcohol syndrome should be assessed frequently to identify a visual disorder, as well as to evaluate normal developmental milestones.

Nursing diagnoses for the child with impaired vision may include the following:

- Health Maintenance, Ineffective related to altered sensory perception
- Injury, Risk for related to poor vision
- Growth and Development, Delayed related to visual impairment
- Family Processes, Interrupted Coping related to demands of a child with a sensory impairment

NANDA-I © 2012

BOX 24–1	Growth & Development: Visual Impairment

Infants with visual impairment use kinesthesia, touch, and language to socialize. They will appreciate and use touch more than other children and will respond to verbal explanations when others use nonverbal communication. Vision affects both fine and gross motor skills, so skills such as hand-to-mouth coordination and walking may be delayed in children who are visually impaired.

Planning and Implementation

The first intervention used by nurses in all settings is prevention of visual impairment when possible, both in children with normal sight and those with some visual impairment in order to prevent further damage. Prevent visual deficits by teaching safety in activities that can injure the eye. Encourage protective eyewear in sports such as hockey, handball, and football. Work with school personnel to establish guidelines for protective eyewear for chemistry or other science or industrial education courses that may present a risk to eyes. Keep laser pointers away from children since they can cause retinal damage, especially when stared at for 10 seconds. Young children do not blink as often as adults or older children and so are at greater risk of retinal damage from lasers.

Several strategies can be used by nurses who work with children who are visually impaired. Nursing care focuses on encouraging the child's use of all senses, promoting socialization, helping parents to meet the child's developmental and educational needs, and providing emotional support to parents. Refer the parents to an early intervention program upon diagnosis. Be sure that a regular series of developmental screening is performed either in the early intervention program or during healthcare visits. Developmental screening should be done about every 2 months during infancy, and every 6 months from 1 to 5 years. As the child grows, assess for physical activity, since children with visual impairments are less likely than sighted children to achieve physical activity milestones. Suggest exercise that is safe and continues to challenge physical development. Dancing, balance and coordination activities, and running can all be encouraged. Nearly all care will occur in community and home settings.

Encourage Use of All Senses

Children who are partially sighted or blind use other senses to a great extent. Encouraging the use of the eyes as much as possible is important even if a child has poor vision (Figure 24–6 ■). See Partnering with Families: Enhancing Development of the Child Who Is Visually Impaired.

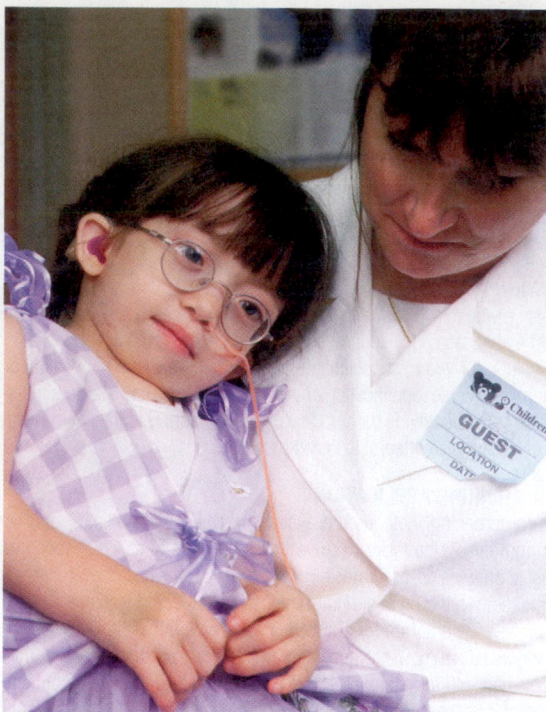

FIGURE 24–6 ■ This child with a visual impairment needs ongoing developmental assessments and a comprehensive individual education plan. Note that she is receiving tube feedings and therefore has other healthcare needs.

Promote Socialization

The child's interactions and socializations should be as normal as possible (i.e., similar to those of sighted children of the same age and development).

- Stroke, rock, and hug infants and children who are visually impaired. Sing and talk to them. Infants with visual impairment appreciate and use touch and verbal interactions more, both in interactions with others and when exploring new objects. The infant does not make eye contact and has facial lack of expression. Encourage parents to plan for interactions between the child and a variety of other children.

- Teach parents to read body language and vocalization as expressions of emotion. Facial expressions give a great deal of information, but infants and children with low vision do not have the ability to learn by visual imitation. Show parents how to use tactile means to teach appropriate facial expressions. For example, a touch on the arm can be soft and stroking to indicate a smile, but firmer to indicate dismay or a frown.

- Explain to parents that discipline and rewards for children with poor vision should be the same as those for other children in the family. The child should be given age-appropriate tasks.

- Encourage contact with peers as the child grows older. Teach the child to look directly at persons who are talking to him or her. Play, sports, and other activities can be modified to give the child the same social experiences as a sighted child.

- Foster physical activity for children with visual impairments by encouraging involvement in early intervention programs; recommending programs that increase cardiovascular strength, endurance, upper body strength, and flexibility; and facilitating participation in and reward for sports and athletics.

Clinical Tip

The following strategies can be used by nurses working with the child who is visually impaired:

- Call the child's name and speak before touching the child.
- Tell the child when you are leaving the room.
- Describe what each procedure will feel like (e.g., blood pressure cuff, otoscope).
- Let the child touch the equipment to establish familiarity.
- Describe what foods are present and their locations on the food tray.

Care in the Community

Public laws require that each state provide educational and related services for children with disabilities (see Chapter 1 🔗). Parents and professionals should develop an individualized education plan (as discussed in Chapter 14 🔗) that maximizes the child's learning ability. If possible, the child with a vision problem should attend childcare and preschool with children who have normal visual acuity. Although some developmental skills such as feeding and dressing may be slower

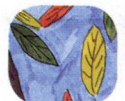

Partnering with Families

Enhancing Development of the Child Who Is Visually Impaired

- Encourage a toddler or preschooler who is visually impaired to look at pictures in well-lit settings. Have a school-age child read large-print books. Computers designed for the visually impaired are also available. The Optacon (a device that raises print so it can be felt by the child) and View Scan (which magnifies print) are instruments that improve the ability to read.
- Expose the infant and child to everyday sounds.
- Encourage the infant to use the sense of touch to explore people and objects. Have the parents purchase toys with sound and texture in mind. Directional concepts can be taught using games. Responding to the infant's and child's vocalizations encourages the use of speech.
- Teach specific techniques for toileting, dressing, bathing, eating, and safety.
- When the child becomes mobile, furniture and other objects in the environment should be kept in the same positions so the child can safely move

around independently. Extra care must be taken to prevent injuries when a child does not see.
- Emphasize the child's abilities. Adolescents can use seeing-eye dogs or a white cane to function independently.
- Encourage the child to function independently within normal developmental parameters.
- If in the hospital or another unfamiliar environment, orient the child to the placement of objects and do not rearrange them.
- Teach those around the child to:
  - Announce their presence to the child when approaching.
  - When walking with a child who is blind, walk slightly ahead of the child so he or she can sense the person's movements.
  - Let the child hold the seeing person's arm rather than the reverse.
  - Identify the contents of meals and encourage the child to feed self.

to develop than in sighted children, plans for encouraging development tailored to the child's needs can assist in learning skills.

Provide parents with information about educational options before their child reaches school age. Education should take place in a setting that allows the child to have contact with other children and to participate in social activities. Familiarize the child with the new environment and allow time for adjustment. The child may be mainstreamed with a tutor, be partially mainstreamed in a resource room, attend special classes, or be tutored at home. If the child is to attend public school, suggest to parents that they contact the school well before enrollment to ensure that school personnel understand the child's disability.

Make sure that items such as large-print books, Braille materials, audio equipment, or an Optacon (described earlier) are available. Ensure that frequent eye examinations are performed, and assist with proper use and care of prescribed glasses or contact lenses, as necessary.

As the child enters middle and high school, it may be challenging to move to new schools or communities unfamiliar to the child. Help the parents to plan activities that will enable the youth to meet new friends.

Provide Emotional Support

Family members often need help to understand the child's abilities and disabilities. Having a child with visual impairment can be a challenge for parents, causing anxiety about the child's future, worry about ability to meet the child's needs, financial concerns, and insufficient time for the marital partner and other family members. Support them as they learn about the child's visual problems, tell friends and family, and then adjust to providing a nurturing environment for the child. Assist them in explaining the child's visual impairment to school personnel or other children in a classroom. Some specific interventions include the following:

- Encourage habilitation as soon as realistically possible. Make the adjustment easier by providing information about the child's specific type of visual impairment, available community services, and groups or associations for children with similar vision conditions. Suggest resources to families of children with visual disorders.
- Listen to the family's concerns regarding the child's visual deficit, and offer information about resources that can assist the family.
- Ensure that parents meet their own physical and emotional needs so they are better able to care for and provide support to their child. Support groups, respite care, and financial resources in the community may all lower stress for parents.

Evaluation

Expected outcomes of nursing care for the child with a visual impairment include the following:

- The child is prevented from injury.
- Growth and development occurs to the child's maximum potential.
- An individualized education plan is developed for the child.
- The family uses effective stress management techniques.

Injuries of the Eye

In the United States, eye injuries are common in children of all ages, especially from 11 to 14 years, and particularly in males. Sports, darts,

BOX 24–2	Community Care

Inform parents, children, coaches, teachers, and others that many sports require eye protection, such as:

- Badminton
- Baseball
- Basketball
- Bicycling
- Fencing (face cage)
- Football
- Hockey (field, ice, roller, street)
- Handball
- Lacrosse
- Racquetball
- Soccer
- Squash
- Swimming (swim goggles)
- Tennis

fireworks, air-powered BB guns, blunt and sharp objects, chemical and thermal burns, physical irritants, and abuse are causes of eye trauma. Sports injuries are most common, with 100,000 occurring annually; they are a common cause of blindness in children (National Eye Institute, n.d.).

Prevention is an important part of health promotion. Protective eyewear should be used by participants in all sports with a risk of eye injury (Box 24–2). The most common injuries occur in basketball and baseball, with less risk from fishing, swimming, bicycling, soccer, and football (Pieper, 2010).

Practice Alert

Be sure to check the immunization status of the child with an eye injury. If the child has not had a tetanus booster within 5 years, this immunization should be given. A tetanus-diphtheria (Td) or tetanus-diphtheria-pertussis (Tdap) booster should be administered in most cases. See Chapter 22 for a full description of immunizations.

When athletes have the best-corrected visual acuity of worse than 20/40 in the lowest vision eye, they should wear eye protection during all sports. Some injuries can be treated at home, but many necessitate a trip to the emergency department or require hospitalization. Personnel take careful history of the injury, perform assessment of the eye, and measure visual acuity. See the Clinical Manifestations table for a summary of clinical manifestations and emergency treatment of common eye injuries.

Nursing Management

The nurse's role in eye injuries has two main components. First, perform teaching at each health promotion examination about ways to prevent eye injuries in children. Second, be well informed about emergency treatment of eye injuries and provide necessary information to school personnel and families. This information is important for all children but is especially vital for those with impaired vision or with only one functional eye. When the extent of injury is not clear, always recommend that the child be evaluated in an emergency care facility.

Visual impairment caused by trauma is largely preventable. Scissors, knives, and other sharp objects should be out of the reach of young children. They should be supervised when using scissors, pencils, and other sharp objects. Parents should be aware of sharp and exploding parts of toys and purchase only those intended for the age of the child. Keep household products with harmful chemicals and solutions out of reach of young children. All children should be encouraged to wear protective eyewear during sports that most commonly lead to eye injury. School nurses can ensure that students use

Clinical Manifestations Eye Injuries and Emergency Treatment

CONDITION AND ETIOLOGY	CLINICAL MANIFESTATIONS	CLINICAL THERAPY
Subconjunctival hemorrhage (caused by coughing, mild trauma, or increased physical activity)	Reddened area in conjunctiva	Usually heals spontaneously; child should see ophthalmologist if most of sclera is covered or if condition does not clear up in 1–2 weeks.
Periorbital ecchymosis	"Black eye" or bruising of the skin around the eye	Apply ice to eye area (both eyes) for 5–15 minutes every hour for the first 1–2 days after injury (even if only one eye is affected, both eyes may discolor); then apply warm compresses beginning the second day after injury.
Foreign body on conjunctiva	Intense pain or feeling of something in the eye	Do not let child rub eye; remove material on surface of eye by closing upper lid over lower lid, irrigating or everting upper lid, visualizing material, and removing it with a slightly damp handkerchief; patch eye and transport child to emergency department if foreign body cannot be removed.
Corneal abrasion	Intense pain and redness	Superficial corneal abrasions are diagnosed by touching a sterile fluorescein strip to lower conjunctiva; dye remains where corneal epithelial cells are disrupted; most corneal abrasions heal spontaneously although antibiotic ointment may be prescribed and eyes patched in some children.
Burns (alkaline burns readily penetrate cornea and are more serious than acid burns)	Pain and/or complaints of "blindness" or vision loss	For child with chemical burn, irrigate eye for 15–30 minutes; transport child to emergency department, where irrigation should continue (see Skills Manual ⬭); pupils are dilated to reduce pain and prevent adhesions; after irrigation is complete, eyes are patched and antibiotics are prescribed.
Penetrating and perforating injuries	Pain	Obtain medical assistance immediately; never try to remove an object that has penetrated the child's eye; such objects should be removed by an ophthalmologist; prevent the child from rubbing injured eye; cover both eyes with shield before transportation to emergency department.
Eye injuries caused by severe blows to head and eye (blunt trauma can seriously injure all eye structures, including orbit, which can be fractured)	Pain and redness	Transport immediately to ophthalmologist's office or emergency department for evaluation and treatment. Personnel should be aware that retinal hemorrhage is a common presentation of the type of child abuse called "shaken child syndrome." (See Chapter 20 🔴 for further discussion of child abuse.)

protective eye gear in chemistry classes and that emergency treatment for injury is posted in classrooms. When eye injury does occur, the nurse may care for the child at home and in the community. The permanent loss of vision from an injury can cause feelings of guilt and anger in the child and family, and the nurse may need to provide emotional support.

DISORDERS OF THE EAR

Otitis Media

Otitis media, or inflammation of the middle ear, is sometimes accompanied by infection. This condition is one of the most common childhood illnesses. About 84% of infants have at least one case of acute otitis media by 3 years of age (Shaikh & Hoberman, 2010). Otitis media occurs more frequently among boys and in children who attend childcare centers, in those with allergies, in children exposed to tobacco smoke, and in those who use pacifiers several hours daily. It is most common during the winter months. Children with conditions such as cleft lip and palate or Down syndrome more often experience otitis media. Breastfeeding appears to be protective against otitis media. In the past decade, an increased number of cases have been observed, and recent changes have been made in recommendations for treatment.

Etiology and Pathophysiology

The specific cause of otitis media is unknown, but it appears to be related to eustachian tube dysfunction. Often an upper respiratory infection precedes the development of otitis media. This infection causes the mucous membranes of the eustachian tube to become edematous. As a result, air that normally flows to the middle ear is blocked, and the air in the middle ear is reabsorbed into the bloodstream. Fluid is pulled from the mucosal lining into the former air space, providing a medium for the rapid growth of pathogens. The tympanic membrane and fluid behind it become infected. The most common causative organisms are *Streptococcus pneumoniae,* *Haemophilus influenzae,* and *Moraxella catarrhalis* (Pichichero, Casey, Hoberman, et al., 2008).

Conditions such as enlarged adenoids or edema from allergic rhinitis can also obstruct the eustachian tube and lead to otitis media. Pacifier use raises the soft palate and thus alters dynamics in the eustachian tube, providing for entry of microorganisms from the nasopharynx. Recurrent otitis media has an increased frequency in children of parents who smoke. Children with multiple siblings and those who attend childcare centers have increased rates of recurrent acute otitis media (Daly, Hoffman, Kvaerner, et al., 2009). Ethnicity appears to play a role in the incidence of otitis media. See Developing Cultural Competence: Otitis Media.

Clinical Manifestations

Otitis media is the general term for inflammation of the middle ear. *Acute otitis media* (AOM) is diagnosed when the child has acute onset of ear pain, marked redness of the tympanic membrane upon otoscopy, and middle ear effusion (Figure 24–7 ■). Recurrent acute otitis media indicates repeated bouts of AOM, such as three in 6 months, or four in 12 months. *Otitis media with effusion* (OME) is evidence of fluid in the middle ear without inflammation (Figure 24–8 ■). OME sometimes becomes chronic in nature (continuing more than

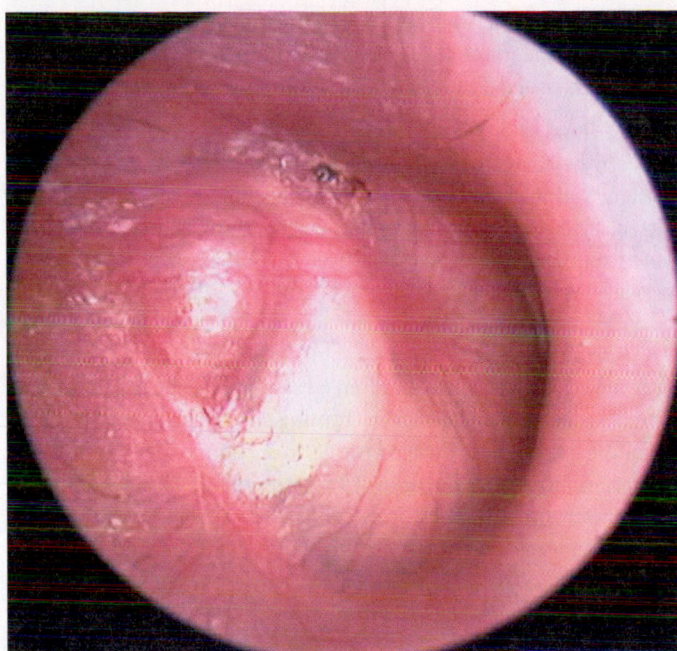

FIGURE 24–7 ■ Acute otitis media is characterized by abrupt onset, pain, middle ear effusion, and inflammation. Note the injected vessels and altered shape of cone of light. See Chapter 7 🔗 for a normal tympanic membrane.

Source: *Courtesy of Kevin Kavanagh, MD, FACS.*

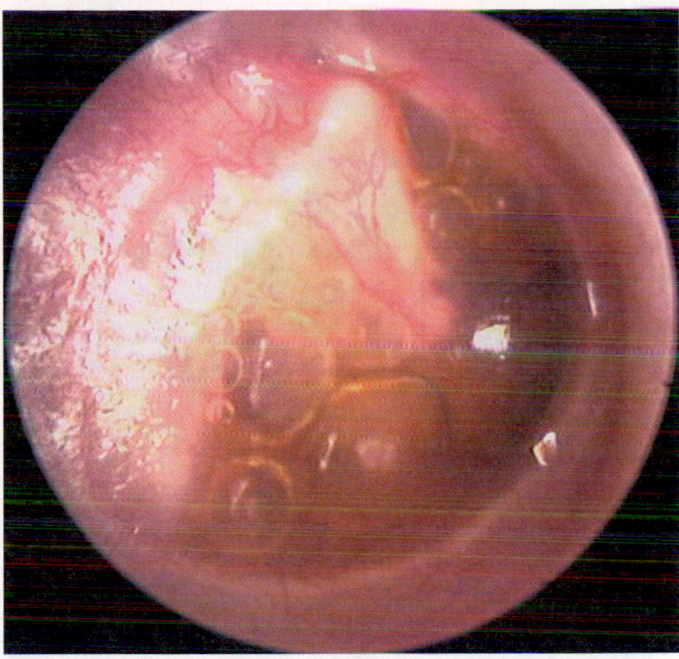

FIGURE 24–8 ■ Otitis media with effusion is noted on otoscopy by fluid line or air bubbles. Pneumatic otoscopy or tympanometry shows a nonmobile tympanic membrane. Note that the light reflex is not in the expected position due to a change in tympanic membrane shape from air bubbles. Where would you expect to see the light reflex? (See Chapter 7 🔗 for a description of normal findings.)

Source: *Courtesy of Kevin Kavanagh, MD, FACS.*

Developing Cultural Competence
Otitis Media

American Indian and Alaska Native children have a very high rate of otitis media, perhaps due to culturally related bony structure of the ear, nose, and mouth. Black children have a higher incidence of the condition than White children. However, White children are more likely to have tympanostomy tube insertion for treatment of otitis media. The major risk factor for frequent otitis media is low socioeconomic status, regardless of ethnicity (Smith & Boss, 2010). Be alert for risk factors, plan prevention programs, and ensure prompt care and teaching about treatments for families of children affected. *What prevention measures would you emphasize for families?* See the nursing management section on otitis media for suggestions of preventive approaches.

3 months) and is more commonly associated with hearing loss. See the Clinical Manifestations table below.

Infants and young children have characteristic behaviors that indicate otitis media may be present. Pulling at the ear is a sign of ear pain (Figure 24–9 ■). Diarrhea, vomiting, and fever are typical of otitis media. Irritability and "acting out" may be signs of a related hearing impairment. The child with otitis media often has night awakenings with crying due to increased pressure when prone or supine. See the Clinical Manifestations table for further detail.

Clinical Manifestations Acute Otitis Media and Otitis Media with Effusion

ETIOLOGY	CLINICAL MANIFESTATIONS	CLINICAL THERAPY
Acute otitis media—bacterial infection in the middle ear from pathogens transferred from the nasopharynx; most common infectious agents are *S. pneumoniae, H. influenzae, M. catarrhalis.*	*Behavioral*—ear pain, pulling at ear, rapid onset, irritability, malaise, poor feeding. *Examination*—bulging tympanic membrane, air or fluid bubbles present behind tympanic membrane; immobile or poorly mobile tympanic membrane, red (or other color change such as white, gray, or yellow as long as bulging is present) tympanic membrane, reduced visibility of tympanic membrane landmarks with displaced light reflex.	Treat ear pain with anesthetic eardrops, herbal pain products instilled into the auditory canal, or systemic acetaminophen or ibuprofen. Verify that the tympanic membrane is intact before inserting eardrops. Observe the child's condition for 48–72 hours and if not improved, treat with course of antibiotics.
Otitis media with effusion—collection of fluid in the middle ear behind the tympanic membrane which is not infected with bacteria.	*Behavioral*—difficulty hearing or responding as expected to sounds. *Examination*—signs of acute inflammation are NOT present; tympanic membrane is retracted or neutral; immobile or partly mobile tympanic membrane; yellow or gray tympanic membrane; opaque or thickened tympanic membrane with visibility of landmarks reduced.	Provide symptomatic treatment of pain. Carefully assess hearing acuity over several months. Assess speech if loss of hearing acuity occurs. Assess development.

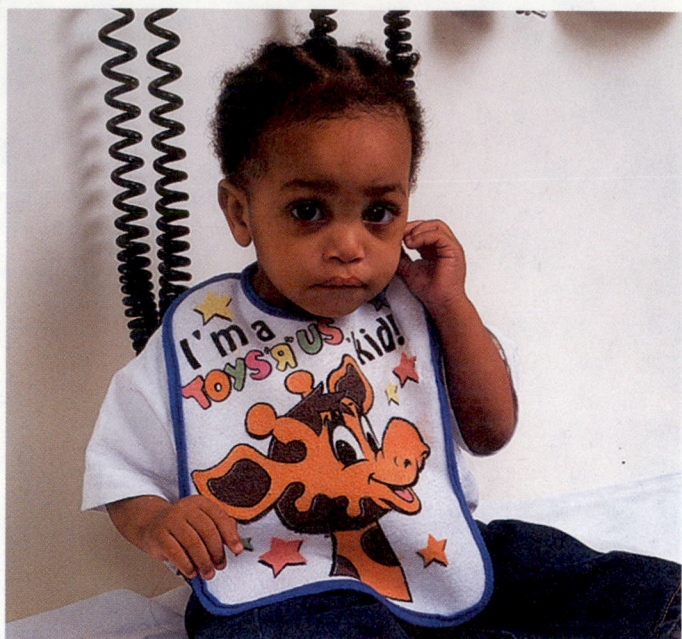

FIGURE 24–9 ■ This young child is pulling at the ear and acting fussy, two important signs of otitis media. Ask the parents about the presence of fever and night awakenings, additional signs that are often observed in children with this condition.

Collaborative Care

Health professionals collaborate in care for children to accurately diagnose children with otitis media and to implement current guidelines for treatment.

Diagnostic Tests

Diagnosis of otitis media is based on otoscopic examination. Acute otitis media is diagnosed with certainty when there is a history of acute onset, presence of middle ear effusion (bulging or decreased mobility of the tympanic membrane, fluid behind the membrane, or otorrhea or discharge), and signs and symptoms of inflammation (erythema of the tympanic membrane or discomfort that makes sleep and other activities difficult for the child) (Shaikh & Hoberman, 2010). Otoscopic examination includes visualization and pneumatic otoscopy. The trained clinician can perform pneumatic otoscopy in which positive and negative air pressure in the external canal reveals contour and movement of the tympanic membrane (see Chapter 7 🔗 for a further description of this technique).

Special gradient acoustic reflectometry (SGAR) measures the condition of the middle ear by introducing a sound and measuring the tympanic membrane response. A flat tympanogram, indicating absence of normal movement for the tympanic membrane, is also suggestive of otitis media. (The tympanogram is described in the section on hearing impairment later in this chapter.)

Occasionally, the middle ear fluid is cultured so that the causative organism can be identified. If the tympanic membrane is not intact, the culture is easy to obtain from drainage in the auditory canal; in cases with repeated antibiotic treatment failure, a tympanocentesis may be done to aspirate some fluid from the middle ear through the tympanic membrane.

Since otitis media with effusion may only involve fluid in the middle ear without inflammation, it is best diagnosed by pneumatic otoscopy and tympanometry. Since this type of otitis media is most commonly associated with hearing loss, audiologic testing should be performed in the pediatric healthcare home (medical home) if the effusion persists for 3 months or longer. A referral to an audiologist should be made for children who fail testing in the office or are less than 4 years of age (Otitis Media with Effusion, 2004).

Clinical Therapy

Concern has developed about the increasing appearance of drug-resistant antimicrobials as causative agents in otitis media. Based on current knowledge, the American Academy of Pediatrics and the American Academy of Family Physicians established joint recommendations in 2004 (American Academy of Pediatrics, Subcommittee on Management of Acute Otitis Media, 2004). Acute otitis media is now treated with antibiotic therapy for 10 days in children under 6 years, and 5 to 7 days for children 6 years and over. Consistent with current guidelines, analgesics are administered but acute otitis media antibiotic treatment is delayed for 48 to 72 hours after diagnosis in children 6 months to 2 years with nonsevere illness at presentation AND uncertain diagnosis, or in children 2 years and older without severe symptoms OR with uncertain diagnosis (Hoberman, Paradise, Rockette, et al., 2011).

Clinical Judgment

Consider the case of Shariffa in the opening scenario. What assessments did the nurse practitioner consider to decide upon treatment? Was delayed treatment the best option? Why did the nurse practitioner instruct the mother to call back with information about Shariffa's course of illness?

When antibiotic therapy is not prescribed initially, the child can be given ibuprofen, acetaminophen, or topical aural analgesic drops for pain relief; the child should return for further treatment if symptoms continue (Spektor, 2010). (See Complementary Therapy: Naturopathic Extract for Ear Pain in Otitis Media.)

When prescribed, the choice of antibiotic depends on the probable organism, ease of administration, cost, previous effectiveness, and any history of allergies. First-line therapy is amoxicillin at a dose

---

Complementary Therapy   Naturopathic Extract for Ear Pain in Otitis Media

Since many children with otitis media experience ear pain that can disrupt their sleep and that of family members, anesthetic eardrops have been used for their analgesic effect on the tympanic membrane. Since some families might prefer use of natural remedies for ear pain, a study comparing Herbal Extract Ear Drops (a naturopathic herbal extract of *Allium sativum, Verbascum thapsus, Calendula flores, Hypericum perforatum,* lavender, and vitamin E) with a local anesthetic of amethocaine and phenazone was conducted. About half of the total 171 children received each of the pain treatments, and parents rated the children after training with a pain tool. Both treatments were effective in decreasing ear pain over the 3 days of the study. There was no significant difference in success rates of local anesthetic and naturopathic agent; in fact, the naturopathic agent was as effective or more effective than anesthetic at each measurement period. It was concluded that herbal pain control may be beneficial for treatment of ear pain and can help to decrease the need for antibiotic treatment for every case of otitis media (Sarrell, Cohen, & Kahan, 2003). However, in a collective analysis of several studies (called a meta-analysis), it was concluded that there is as yet insufficient evidence to confirm whether naturopathic treatment is effective for treatment of ear pain in children. Unfortunately, further studies have not been done to confirm or deny effectiveness of either prescription or over-the-counter medications for ear pain. Nurses can provide information for parents about study results, monitor closely the treatments used for individual children and their effectiveness, and review literature frequently for reports of future studies on the efficacy of naturopathic treatment of pain in otitis media.

Medications Used to Treat Acute Otitis Media

MEDICATION	ACTION/INDICATION	NURSING MANAGEMENT
Amoxicillin	Broad-spectrum antibiotic that inhibits mucoprotein synthesis in cell wall of bacteria; used to treat some gram-positive and gram-negative infections.	Assess for previous allergy to drug, penicillins, or cephalosporins. Take as instructed for entire period prescribed. If oral suspension is given, refrigerate and shake well before administration. Teach parents how to administer drug to the child. Have family report side effects such as rash and diarrhea.
Amoxicillin and clavulanate potassium	Action and use are similar to amoxicillin. However, clavulanate is a β-lactamase inhibitor that enhances the effect of amoxicillin.	See amoxicillin.
Cefuroxime	A second-generation cephalosporin that binds to one or more of the penicillin-binding proteins in cell walls of bacteria; useful in treatment of most gram-negative and some gram-positive infections.	See amoxicillin.
Allergen eardrops	The topical solution (antipyrine and benzocaine) reduces pain, congestion, and edema to relieve otitis media pain.	Fill the external ear canal with 2–4 drops every 1–2 hours as needed. Insert a cotton pledget in the ear canal after administering. Do not use if the tympanic membrane is perforated or if tympanostomy pressure equalizing (PE) tubes are in place.

of 80 to 100 mg/kg/day. Amoxicillin with clavulanate or cefuroxime are second-line drugs. If an intramuscular drug is preferred, cefdinir at 14 mg/kg/day, cefpodoxime at 10 mg/kg/day, or cefuroxime at 30 mg/kg/day can be prescribed (Custer & Rau, 2009; Dagan, 2010). See the Medications Used to Treat Acute Otitis Media table for more details about common medications used.

OME is not treated with antibiotics but is evaluated periodically to be sure there is not an additional AOM that needs treatment. Children with OME generally improve within 3 months. Since this type of otitis is more commonly associated with hearing loss and cochlear damage, follow-up with audiology is essential. If hearing is abnormal, speech testing should be performed. Smoking should not take place near the child (Farboud, Skinner, & Pratap, 2011; Otitis Media with Effusion, 2004; Williamson, 2011).

Neither decongestants nor antihistamines have been shown to be effective in the treatment of otitis media with or without effusion. Steroids also do not appear to have any long-term beneficial effect. If infection recurs despite antibiotic treatment for acute otitis media or if OME continues 4 months or more with persistent hearing loss present, **myringotomy** (surgical incision of the tympanic membrane) may be performed and **tympanostomy tubes** (pressure-equalizing tubes) may be inserted to drain fluid from the middle ear.

Nursing Management

Nursing management in the child with otitis media focuses on prevention of infection when possible, prompt identification of treatment, and teaching for the family so that the child is successfully treated.

Nursing Assessment and Diagnosis

The tympanic membrane is assessed at each health promotion visit and during examinations for illness. Examine the color, transparency, mobility, presence of landmarks, and light reflex. Ask the parents if the child has had a fever, been fussy, or been pulling at the ears. Assess for signs of impaired hearing, observing for the child's ability to hear whispered or soft sounds.

Inquire about what the family has done at home to treat the ear infection and its associated pain. Some home remedies, such as rocking and singing to the child in pain, are safe. Some other practices may be harmful.

Several nursing diagnoses that may apply to the child with otitis media are included in the accompanying Nursing Care Plan on page 716. Additional nursing diagnoses may include the following:

- Body Temperature: Imbalanced, Risk for Hyperthermia related to infectious process
- Fatigue (Child and Parent) related to sleep deprivation
- Communication: Verbal, Impaired related to chronic ear infections and altered sensory reception

NANDA-I © 2012

Practice Alert

Some parents engage in a home treatment called "ear wicking" in which a specially designed candle with a narrow end is placed in the ear canal. The larger end remains outside the ear and is lit. As the candle burns slowly it is thought to "melt" ear wax so that it is easily removed. Dangers include burning of hair or skin, especially in young children who move during the procedure, and melting of candle wax into the ear which blocks the canal and must be surgically removed. Ear wicking should be discouraged for all, but especially in children.

Planning and Implementation

Preventive measures should be emphasized. Exposure to environmental tobacco smoke (secondhand smoke) in the home increases the incidence of otitis media in children; therefore, parents who smoke should be encouraged to avoid smoking near the child or in the home. Provide resources for smoking cessation since even the clothing and hair of a smoker creates exposure for the child. Wood-burning stoves should also be avoided when possible. If young children are in childcare with fewer than 10 children, incidence of otitis media decreases; some parents will choose childcare based on this information. Breastfeeding provides some protection from the condition, and this information can be used to encourage this practice during all of infancy. Placing babies to sleep with a pacifier may

Nursing Care Plan | The Child with Otitis Media

INTERVENTION	RATIONALE	EXPECTED OUTCOME
1. Nursing Diagnosis: Pain, Acute related to inflammation and pressure on tympanic membrane		
NIC Priority Intervention—*Pain Management:* Alleviation or reduction in pain to a level of comfort acceptable to patient and family		**NOC Suggested Outcome—*Pain Level:*** Amount of reported or demonstrated pain
GOAL: *The child or parent will indicate absence of pain.*		
■ Give analgesic such as acetaminophen. Use analgesic eardrops. ■ Have the child sit up, raise head on pillows, or lie on unaffected ear. ■ Apply heating pad or warm hot water bottle. ■ Have the child chew gum or blow on balloon to relieve pressure in ear.	■ Analgesics alter perception or response to pain. ■ Elevation decreases pressure from fluid. ■ Heat increases blood supply and reduces discomfort. ■ Attempts to open the eustachian tube may help aerate the middle ear.	The verbal child states that pain is relieved. The nonverbal child has improved disposition and comfort.
2. Nursing Diagnosis: Infection related to presence of pathogens		
NIC Priority Intervention—*Infection Control:* Minimizing the acquisition and transmission of infectious agents		**NOC Suggested Outcome—*Risk Control:*** Actions to eliminate or reduce health threats
GOAL: *The child will be free of infection.*		
■ Encourage breastfeeding of infants. ■ Instruct the parents to administer antibiotics exactly as directed and to complete the prescribed course of medication. ■ Telephone the parents 2–3 days after initial examination. ■ Examine the ear 3–4 days after completion of antibiotic treatment and provide symptomatic treatment.	■ Breastfeeding affords natural immunity to infectious agents. ■ Taking antibiotics as prescribed minimizes the chance for overgrowth of pathogens. ■ If symptoms have not improved in 36 hours, treatment should be evaluated. ■ A checkup determines if treatment is effective.	The child's temperature is normal, symptoms have disappeared, and the tympanic membrane shows no signs of infection.
3. Nursing Diagnosis: Caregiver Role Strain, Risk for related to chronic disease		
NIC Priority Intervention—*Caregiver Support:* Provision of necessary support, information, and advocacy to facilitate care by parents		**NOC Suggested Outcome—*Caregiver Performance:*** Provision by family care provider of health care for child
GOAL: *The parents will manage the child's condition with minimal stress.*		
■ Determine the parents' ability to manage the condition. Provide frequent information and feedback. ■ Encourage parental input in managing care. ■ Listen carefully to parental expressions of frustration and fatigue and try to understand parents' feelings.	■ Many parents can treat children at home. Knowledge of the condition allows parents to make informed decisions and to manage the condition effectively. ■ Active participation increases confidence and the ability to manage the condition. ■ Reacting empathetically encourages parents to communicate.	The parents express confidence about treating the child and state that stress is reduced.
4. Nursing Diagnosis: Growth and Development, Delayed related to hearing loss		
NIC Priority Intervention—*Developmental Enhancement:* Facilitating optimal growth and development of the child		**NOC Suggested Outcome—*Growth and Development:*** Milestones of developmental progression
GOAL: *The child will have normal hearing and normal motor and language development.*		
■ Assess hearing ability frequently. ■ Assess motor and language development at each healthcare visit.	■ Monitoring detects hearing loss early. ■ Early detection of developmental delays can lead to appropriate intervention.	The child's general health and hearing improve, and incidence of the condition decreases. The child has language and motor development within norms for age group.

NANDA-I © 2012

increase incidence and should be avoided, particularly in the infant with prior infections. Encourage immunizations as recommended for young children. The Hib vaccine is effective in preventing otitis media and other diseases caused by *Haemophilus influenzae* type b, and the pneumococcal vaccine (Prevnar) is effective against some strains of *Pneumococcal pneumoniae*. See Chapter 22 for further detail about these immunizations.

Most children with otitis media are not hospitalized; therefore, nursing management centers on care of the child in the home. Parents may not understand why the child with a possible infection is not given antibiotics. Explain the problem of developing resistant strains of bacteria, and that new research indicates most children improve after 48 to 72 hours even without antibiotics. Encourage them to bring the child back for care if the condition worsens or has not improved in the recommended time. Teach them proper use of analgesic eardrops, ibuprofen, or acetaminophen, as recommended by the prescriber.

When antibiotics are prescribed, review administration techniques with parents and emphasize that the entire course of medication should be given to the child as prescribed. Discuss the side effects of the medication, and have parents contact the healthcare provider to report side effects or other concerns. Schedule an appointment to have the ears examined again after the medication is complete (Box 24–3).

Likewise, parents of children with OME need explanations about why there is a waiting period of about 3 months with no medications or other medical care. Explain that antibiotics, steroids, and antihistamines/decongestants have not been effective treatment and that most children improve in 3 months. Assure them that if the effusion continues beyond that time, the child will be tested for hearing acuity, and if indicated, for speech development.

The chronic nature of otitis media in some children can create problems for the family. The child's waking at night with ear pain results in lack of sleep and parental fatigue. Parents often become frustrated and disillusioned because of the inability of the healthcare system to cure the child and may fear a permanent hearing impairment. Reassure parents that as the child grows older, the recurrent infections eventually cease. Teach pain relief techniques such as correct administration of eardrops, oral administration of acetaminophen, and positioning the baby with the head slightly elevated, which often decreases pressure and pain. Provide hearing and language examinations at regular intervals, inform parents of results, and refer

---

BOX 24–3	**Research: Emerging Strains of Bacteria**

Drug resistance to antibiotics has developed as some organisms evolve to interfere with the actions of medications. Some organisms inactivate antibiotics by producing beta-lactamase, an enzyme that breaks through the beta-lactam ring of penicillin and related drugs. For example, a common infectious agent in otitis media, *Streptococcus pneumoniae*, has been effective in inactivating common antibiotics; it has also been able to reduce permeability of cells to some antibiotics and increase production of penicillin-binding proteins that decrease drug action. Study of drug resistance has led to current recommendations for treatment of otitis media.

Knowledge of antibiotic use and emerging strains of bacteria causing otitis media continues to develop. Widespread use of antibiotics for otitis media has contributed to drug resistance so that some bacteria have developed resistance to commonly used antibiotics. These antibiotics then become ineffective in treating infections in persons with conditions such as immune suppression or frequent infections (Centers for Disease Control and Prevention, 2011). Healthcare providers sometimes use drugs not approved for pediatric use to treat otitis media that is resistant to treatment. Fluoroquinolone antibiotics are examples of drugs that have been used in such cases, and these drugs are not adequately tested for use in children.

Nurses play a major role in ensuring that parents understand why an antibiotic might not always be ordered, and in instructing about proper measurement and administration of antibiotics that are prescribed. Review the literature regularly to learn about resistant strains of bacteria identified, treatments recommended, and actions versus side effects of medications used.

---

to an audiology specialist if hearing problems are identified. For the child with some hearing loss due to otitis media with effusion, a home environment that fosters cognitive skills can overcome the effects of lowered hearing during the time of infection. Nurses should focus interventions on helping parents to read and talk frequently with children who have otitis media with effusion.

The child who is having tympanostomy tubes inserted is generally treated in a day surgery setting. (See Partnering with Families: Care of the Child with Tympanostomy Tubes.) Occasionally, children admitted to the hospital for other problems have a concurrent ear infection. The accompanying Nursing Care Plan summarizes nursing care for the child with otitis media.

Evaluation

Expected outcomes of nursing care for the child with otitis media include:

- The child returns to normal sleep and feeding patterns.
- The young child demonstrates normal hearing and speech development.

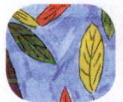

Partnering with Families

Care of the Child with Tympanostomy Tubes

AFTER SURGERY
- Encourage the child to drink generous amounts of fluids.
- Reestablish a regular diet as tolerated.
- Give pain medication (acetaminophen) as ordered for discomfort and at bedtime.
- Place drops in the child's ears if prescribed.
- Restrict the child to quiet activities.

FOLLOWING POSTOPERATIVE PERIOD
- Follow the physician's instructions regarding swimming and water (some caution against swimming and other activities that might get water in ears; others do not).
- Earplugs can be used to prevent water from getting into ears.
- Be alert for tubes becoming dislodged and falling out, and alert the physician (they usually fall out within 1 year).
- Report purulent discharge from the ear, which may indicate a new ear infection. Contact the care provider.

- Effective pain management and temperature management are manifested.
- Parents demonstrate an understanding of the treatment regimen.

Otitis Externa

Otitis externa is an inflammation of the skin and surrounding soft tissue of the ear canal. It is sometimes called "swimmer's ear" because it is common in children who swim frequently, especially during hot and humid weather. The ear canal can also be injured by use of cotton-tipped applicators, foreign objects, or sprays used near the face. If the tympanic membrane is not intact because of tympanostomy tubes or breakage of the membrane, there may be drainage visible in the canal; this drainage may irritate the canal and lead to otitis externa. Any irritation of the canal can become infected with bacteria, virus, or fungi; sometimes it represents an allergic reaction. The child usually complains of pain and itching, and may have intense pain when the examiner presses on the tragus, or skin tab in front of the ear. Sometimes the ear appears swollen, and redness or drainage of the canal may be seen upon otoscopic examination.

Treatment of otitis externa requires removing the dried and flaking epithelium and cerumen. Burrows solutions or normal saline are used to irrigate and clean the canal if the tympanic membrane is intact. Steroid eardrops are used to decrease inflammation, and antibiotic drops are used if a bacterial infection is suspected. If the child has tympanostomy tubes or a perforated tympanic membrane, non-ototoxic ear antibiotics such as quinolone antibiotic eardrops are used. Ibuprofen or acetaminophen is commonly used for pain control. The child should be seen by the healthcare provider if the condition has not improved by 48 to 72 hours. The child should not return to swimming for about 5 days. The ear canal should then be kept dry by using earplugs or a swim cap for swimming and gently blow-drying the canal after bathing. Cotton-tipped applicators or other objects should not be placed in the ear canal so that the skin in the canal can heal. If hair sprays or other solutions are irritating, they should not be used by the child or adolescent.

Nurses should be aware of the signs of otitis externa such as a painful ear, drainage, and irritated canal. Verify that the tympanic membrane is intact during otoscopic examination. Teach families to avoid the irritants identified such as cotton-tipped applicators, sprays, and frequent swimming. Demonstrate proper instillation of drops (see the Skills Manual ⬭⬭⬭) and give instructions for use of acetaminophen for pain relief in the acute period.

Hearing Impairment

Approximately 1 million children in the United States have some form of hearing impairment. Hearing loss is present in 3 out of every 1,000 births (Gaffney, Eichwald, Grosse, et al., 2010). These hearing impairments are expressed in terms of **decibels (dB),** which are units of loudness, and rated according to severity (Table 24–10). Children who have only a mild hearing loss (35 to 40 dB) may miss 50% of everyday conversation and are considered at high risk for school failure. Children with a hearing loss of more than 90 dB are considered legally deaf.

Etiology and Pathophysiology

About 50% of hearing loss is genetically caused, generally in a recessive inheritance pattern with GJB2 gene abnormalities (American

TABLE 24–10	Severity of Hearing Loss	
TYPE OF LOSS	**DECIBEL LEVEL (DB)**	**HEARING ABILITY**
Slight/mild	20–40	Some speech sounds are difficult to perceive, particularly unvoiced consonant sounds.
Moderate	41–60	Most normal conversational speech sounds are missed.
Severe	61–80	Speech sounds cannot be heard at a normal conversational level.
Profound	81–90	No speech sounds can be heard.
Deaf	91 and above	No sound at all can be heard.

Source: *Data from American Speech-Language-Hearing Association. (2008).* Type, degree, and configuration of hearing loss. *Retrieved from http://www.asha.org/public/hearing/disorders/types.htm*

Speech-Language-Hearing Association, 2011). Another 25% is due to causes around the time of birth or after birth such as prematurity, toxemia, intrauterine infection, and anoxia. Acquired causes are due to injury or disease later in life such as frequent ear infections, infectious diseases, ototoxic drugs, head injury, and noise exposure (American Speech-Language-Hearing Association, 2011). This type of loss is increasing; hearing loss among 12- to 19-year-olds has increased from 14.9% in 1988–1994 data to 19.5% today (Shargorodsky, Curhan, Curhan, et al., 2010).

Known risk factors for infant hearing loss include:

- A family history of permanent childhood hearing loss*
- Positive titer for TORCH infections (toxoplasmosis, rubella, cytomegalovirus, syphilis, herpes)*
- Craniofacial abnormalities (pinna, ear canal, ear tags, ear pits, temporal bone anomalies)
- Very low birth weight (less than 1500 g)*
- Neonatal intensive care unit for over 5 days, or need for extracorporeal membrane oxygenation (ECMO), assisted ventilation, administration of ototoxic medications (gentamicin, tobramycin) or loop diuretics (furosemide), or hyperbilirubinemia that requires exchange transfusion*
- Chemotherapy, particularly aminoglycoside medication administration for over 5 days*
- Low Apgar score at 1 or 5 minutes*
- Bacterial or viral meningitis*
- Mechanical ventilation for more than 5 days
- Presence of syndromes associated with hearing loss (Down syndrome, Pierre Robin syndrome, Arnold-Chiari malformation, neurofibromatosis, osteopetrosis, Hunter syndrome, and others)*
- Physical findings associated with conditions known to be associated with hearing loss (e.g., white forelock)
- Head trauma, especially basal skull/temporal bone fractures requiring hospitalization*
- Caregiver concerns regarding speech, language, hearing, developmental delay*

*Associated with delayed-onset hearing loss (Joint Committee on Infant Hearing, 2007, 2008).

Hearing disorders can be classified according to the location of the deficit. **Conductive hearing loss** occurs when conditions in the external auditory canal or tympanic membrane prevent sound from reaching the middle ear. **Sensorineural hearing loss** occurs when the hair cells in the cochlea or along the vestibulocochlear (acoustic) nerve (cranial nerve VIII) are damaged. This leads to permanent hearing loss. A **mixed hearing loss** indicates a hearing loss having a combination of conductive and sensorineural causes.

Common causes of conductive hearing loss include impacted cerumen, the most frequent reason for conductive loss; outer ear infection ("swimmer's ear"); trauma; or a foreign body. Conductive loss also occurs if the tympanic membrane does not fully vibrate, as in otitis media. In these cases hearing loss may be restored after the infection clears. Chronic and untreated ear infections may lead to ear structural changes and permanent hearing impairment. The loss of acuity may be gradual or rapid and results in diminished hearing in all ranges.

Conditions leading to sensorineural hearing loss may be congenital (maternal rubella), genetic (Tay-Sachs disease), or acquired (such as from ototoxic drugs, bacterial meningitis, or loud noise). In sensorineural hearing loss, high-frequency sounds are most affected. Such hearing loss may be preceded by **tinnitus** or ringing in the ears. Teenagers who use earphones at high volumes or attend many rock concerts are at risk for hearing loss (Figure 24–10 ■). Other noise hazards include firecrackers, guns, and power and farm equipment (Box 24–4).

Clinical Manifestations

Hearing is both an innate and a learned behavior. Infants and children who are hearing impaired exhibit a range of behaviors, depending on

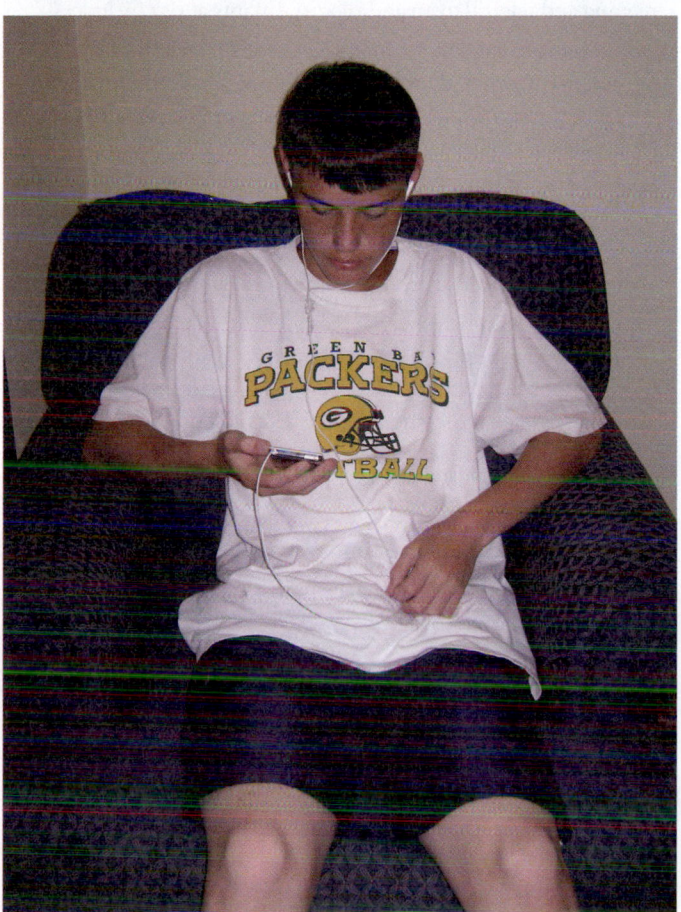

FIGURE 24–10 ■ Listening to loud music with headphones or at rock concerts is a frequent cause of hearing loss among teenagers and young adults. This adolescent needs to be informed about the possible outcomes of this activity, and methods to minimize risk for loss of hearing.

BOX 24–4	Research: Noise-Induced Hearing Loss

Children and adolescents may have hearing impairments due to noise exposure from loud music, often in ranges not screened during school auditory testing (Zhao, Manchaian, French, et al., 2010). A study of respondents to an MTV survey showed one half had experienced symptoms such as tinnitus or hearing loss after loud music exposure, but most did not recall hearing about prevention of hearing loss (Quintanilla-Dieck, Artunduaga, & Eavey, 2009). Music-induced hearing loss (MIHL) is a preventable public health condition. Consider music and other health risks; nurses should identify and find sources of noise in the child's environment. They may include stereos, rock concerts, airplanes, firearms, power tools, machinery, and toys. Encourage the use of ear protection during hazardous activities (Quintanilla-Dieck et al., 2009). Be aware of the potential harm from listening to iPods or other music using headphones since the sound is in very close contact with the ear, usually loud and directed into the ear canal with no dissipation into surrounding air. Additionally, the current practice of using headphones for extended parts of the day increases the risk of injury. How will you plan to identify and teach about risks of loud noise with all preadolescents and adolescents?

the child's age and the severity of the deficit. Infants who hear normally respond to sound in both obvious and subtle ways that do not occur in those who are hearing impaired (Table 24–11). As children with hearing impairments mature, language skills are affected. Hearing loss is often manifested as a cognitive deficit, a behavioral problem, or both.

Collaborative Care

Care focuses on preventing hearing impairment when possible and providing an environment that supports development for the child with a hearing impairment.

TABLE 24–11	Behaviors Suggestive of Hearing Impairment
AGE	**BEHAVIOR**
Infant	Has a diminished or absent startle reflex to loud sound
	Does not awaken when environment is very noisy
	Awakens only to touch
	Does not turn head to sound at 3–4 months
	Does not localize sound at 6–10 months
	Babbles little or not at all
Toddler and preschooler	Speaks unintelligibly, in a monotone, or not at all
	Communicates needs through gestures
	Appears developmentally delayed
	Appears emotionally immature, yells inappropriately
	Does not respond to doorbell or telephone
	Appears more interested in objects than people and prefers to play alone
	Focuses on facial expressions rather than verbal communications
School-age child and adolescent	Asks to have statements repeated
	Answers questions inappropriately, except when able to view speaker's face
	Daydreams and is inattentive
	Performs poorly at school or is truant
	Has speech abnormalities or speaks in a monotone
	Sits close to or turns television or radio up loudly
	Prefers to play alone

Diagnostic Tests

Early identification of hearing loss is a key element in successful treatment (Box 24–5). Normal hearing is indicated when infants and young children respond automatically with a blink or the startle reflex to unexpected or loud noises. As they mature, they localize the sound source and look in its direction, then understand speech sounds, and finally, by about 1 year of age, begin to communicate verbally. Detection of hearing loss in infants is important to ensure optimal development. Universal newborn hearing screening is recommended before 1 month of age, with diagnostic audiologic evaluation before 3 months in those not passing screening, and beginning of early intervention programs by 6 months of age for those with hearing impairment (U.S. Preventive Services Task Force, 2008). Children identified in these universal screening programs have earlier referral, diagnosis, and treatment, and better language skill development (Nelson, Bougatsos, & Nygren, 2008). Some infants with hearing abnormalities are missed on the first screening, and cases of late-onset hearing loss also occur. Therefore, all children should be evaluated for communication development beginning at 2 months of age during all well-child visits (Harlor, Bower, & the Committee on Practice and Ambulatory Medicine, 2009).

Observations of response to noise in all newborns should be accompanied by more sophisticated testing such as auditory brainstem response or transient evoked otoacoustic emissions. One or two screenings are administered before hospital discharge. Additionally, some centers rescreen all infants within one month of discharge (Figure 24–11 ■). See Table 24–12 for a description of the common tests used for newborn hearing.

TABLE 24–12	Screening Tests for Newborn Hearing
TEST	**MECHANISM OF ACTION**
Otoacoustic emission (OAE) (either transient-evoked [TEOAE] or distortion-product [DPOAE])	A measure of low-intensity sounds from the cochlear hair cells in response to clicks from a probe placed in the ear canal
	Sensitive in frequency range above 1500 Hz
	May show false negative for loss below 1000–1500 Hz
	Detects inner ear hearing loss by evaluating cochlear and hair cell function
	Does not detect neural damage to cranial nerve VIII
	Can be sensitive to outer ear canal obstruction or middle ear effusion, leading to false-positive result
Auditory brainstem response (ABR)	Electrical response to auditory stimuli from three surface scalp electrodes
	Reflects activity of cochlea, cranial nerve VIII, and auditory brainstem pathways
	Detects hearing loss from 1000–8000 Hz
	May show false-negative results for losses in the 500–2000 Hz levels
	Will give a positive result (indicating hearing loss) if there is damage to cranial nerve VIII or brainstem pathways even if cochlear loss is not present

Infants and children at risk of hearing loss must have ongoing screening and referral to an audiologist. Infants at risk include:

- Infants admitted to the intensive care unit (ICU)
- Infants readmitted to the hospital in the first month with a risk factor for hearing loss, for example, hyperbilirubinemia
- Infants or children with cytomegalovirus infection, meningitis, and syndromes associated with hearing loss, trauma, chemotherapy, or ECMO treatment

Joint Committee on Infant Hearing, 2007, 2008

These at-risk infants need the following evaluations:

- Child and family history of risks
- Frequency-specific auditory brainstem response (ABR) via air and bone conduction
- Click-evoked ABR when there is risk of neural hearing loss
- Otoacoustic emission (OAE)—distortion product or transient evoked
- Tympanometry
- Clinical observation of sound response

Further, at-risk children need the following during healthcare visits from 6 to 36 months of age:

- Child and family history of risks
- Parental report of auditory, visual, and communication ability
- Behavioral audiometry
- OAE testing
- Tympanometry and acoustic reflex thresholds
- ABR testing if not previously performed

Joint Committee on Infant Hearing, 2007, 2008

An otoscopic examination and a tympanogram can be performed to determine conductive hearing loss. The **tympanogram** is a test performed with a machine called a tympanometer that provides a graph of the ability of the middle ear to transmit sound. An airtight probe is inserted into the external ear canal and a tone is emitted. The

BOX 24–5	Growth & Development: Hearing Loss

Children with hearing loss can easily fall behind their peers in language milestones since they cannot hear and speak in the same manner as other children. Without interventions to enable them to learn language, they can also fail to develop reading and literacy skills, related cognitive processes, and social-emotional skills (Joint Committee on Infant Hearing, 2007). Carefully evaluate hearing and all developmental milestones during each regularly scheduled healthcare visit. Refer infants and children with abnormalities for further evaluation. When hearing loss is identified as a cause of delayed development, interventions guided by healthcare professionals with expertise in hearing loss are needed.

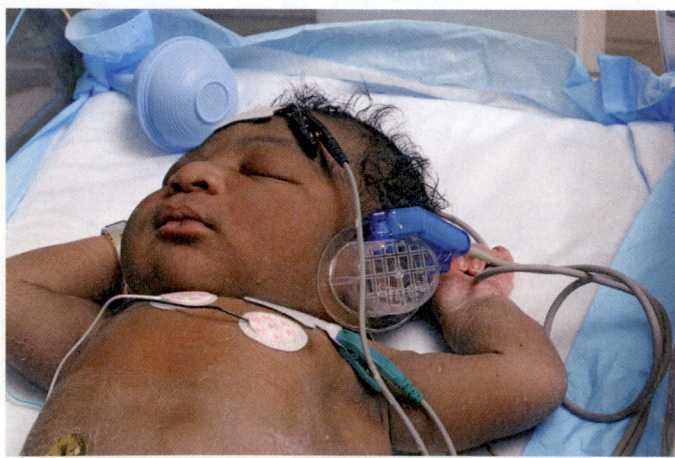

FIGURE 24–11 ■ Newborn hearing screening is an effective tool in diagnosing some cases of hearing impairment very early in life.

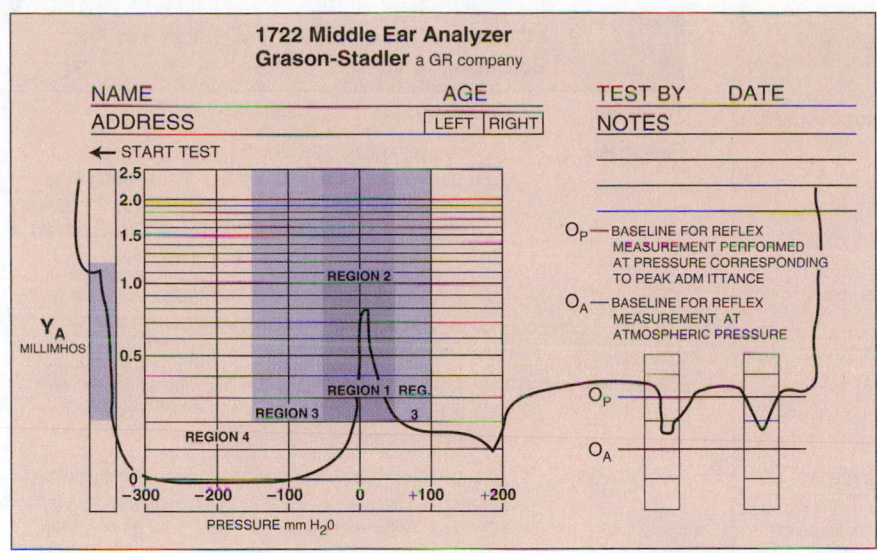

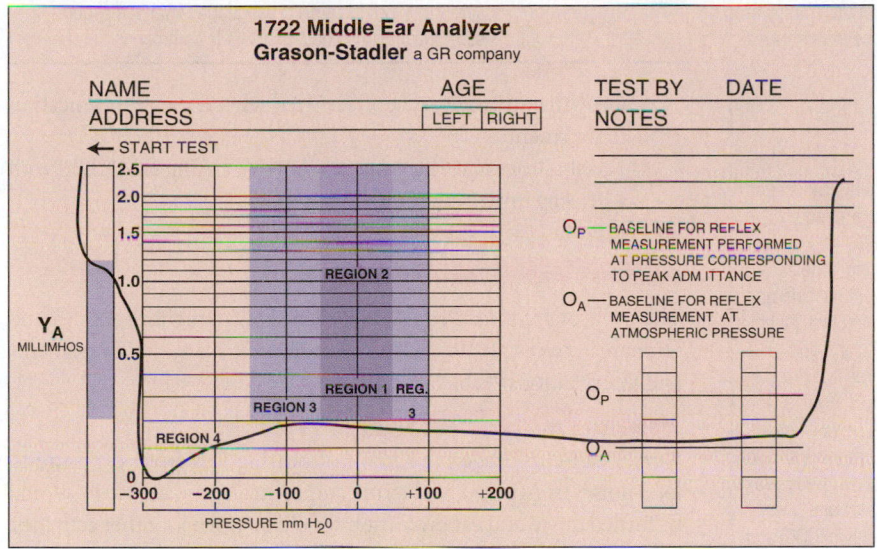

FIGURE 24–12 ■ *A,* This tympanogram demonstrates normal hearing as evidenced by the curve showing the tympanic membrane's movement when a sound wave is emitted into the ear canal. Mobility is between 0.2 mL and 1 mL, the normal range. *B,* In contrast, note the flat pattern in the second tympanogram, which shows very restricted mobility of the tympanic membrane in response to sound.

pressure is measured by the probe and plotted on a graph. A flat tympanogram suggests that the tympanic membrane cannot move normally due to fluid behind it and is therefore indicative of conductive hearing loss (Figure 24–12 ■).

Audiography can be used with cooperative children over 3 years of age. Sounds of various frequencies and intensities are presented to the child through earphones with a machine called an audiometer, and the child is instructed to raise a hand upon hearing the sound. (See the Skills Manual ⊂⊃ .) Audiography cannot detect hearing loss caused by middle ear effusion but can indicate sensorineural loss. The hearing of preschool and school-age children is tested by asking them to repeat whispered words. Hearing of school-age children and adolescents also is assessed with the Weber and Rinne tests (see Chapter 7 ❂).

Clinical Therapy

If a hearing loss is uncorrectable, a multidisciplinary team of pediatrician, audiologist, otolaryngologist, speech-language pathologist, nurse, teacher, and social worker should assist the child and family

with adaptation to the disability. If the deficit is due to recurrent otitis media with effusion, tympanostomy tube insertion may improve hearing. Extra verbal stimulation by parents and care providers may help the child with otitis media with effusion to have improved cognitive and verbal performance.

A hearing aid may be prescribed for a conductive loss. It collects and magnifies the sound that is presented to the auditory nerve. A sensorineural loss is more difficult to treat, but cochlear implants and bone conduction hearing aids have been used in some children. Cochlear implants are increasingly being used in children and have restored hearing in some who are profoundly deaf. (See Box 24–6 for more information on cochlear implants; see Legal & Ethical Considerations: Deafness and Cochlear Implants.)

For children with uncorrectable hearing loss, several approaches are used to enhance communication (Table 24–13). Children with hearing impairment may receive speech therapy and instructions in lipreading, sign language, cuing, and fingerspelling.

Nursing Management

Nursing roles include partnering with families to prevent hearing loss when possible, administering diagnostic tests and assessing development to identify hearing loss, and supporting the family of a child with hearing impairment to maximize communication skills and developmental progression.

Nursing Assessment and Diagnosis

Nurses conduct newborn hearing tests soon after birth and make observations of the infant's responses to sound. As the child grows, hearing should be assessed at every well-child visit. The best judges of hearing are parents; ask them if they have concerns about their child's hearing. Be alert for parents who believe their children do not have normal hearing, since they are often the first to diagnose a hearing impairment. An infant's reaction to rattles, bells, or handclapping 30 cm (12 in.) from the ear is an important observation. Language milestones should be evaluated when the older infant and child are examined. Language development is a major area of focus in children who are deaf. Infants who are deaf begin to babble at about 5 to 6 months of age, the same age as hearing infants. However, this babbling decreases and then ceases several months later in the child with a hearing impairment.

School nurses use audiometers to evaluate hearing during screening programs in schools and refer children who do not pass the screening test. See the Skills Manual ⊂⊃ for techniques in performing hearing screening. Nurses in offices often use tympanometers to evaluate ear function.

Following are common nursing diagnoses for the child with impaired hearing:

- Communication: Verbal, Impaired related to hearing loss
- Injury, Risk for related to abnormal sound receptivity

| BOX 24–6 | Cochlear Implants |

WHAT IS A COCHLEAR IMPLANT?

A cochlear implant is a small electronic device that helps to provide sound for those who are deaf or profoundly hard of hearing. It consists of the following:

1. A microphone to pick up sound that is located outside the body, worn as a headpiece behind the ear
2. A speech processor which organizes sound from the microphone; worn behind the ear or on a belt
3. A transmitter that transfers the sound into electrical impulses; part of the headpiece behind the ear
4. Electrodes which send the signals to the brain; receiver implanted in the skin behind the ear with a wire leading to the cochlear fluid in the middle ear

WHEN CAN CHILDREN GET COCHLEAR IMPLANTS?

The minimum age to receive an implant in the United States is 12 months, upon recommendation of the National Institutes of Health (NIH, 2011), although most children who receive an implant are 2 to 6 years old. The reason for allowing the surgery at this young age is the recognition that most speech foundations are laid by 2 years of age, and younger children have more success in language acquisition following the implant. About 28,400 cochlear implants have been performed on children in the United States (NIH, 2011).

WHAT FOLLOW-UP IS NEEDED FOR CHILDREN AFTER COCHLEAR IMPLANT?

Children with implants receive carefully planned speech therapy, and families are taught how to promote speech development. Regular assessments by speech specialists with adjustment of the early intervention program are needed. The major complication following surgery is an infection of the insertion site or associated meningitis. There is an elevated risk of bacterial meningitis following implant, so all children with implants must receive pneumococcal vaccine and *Haemophilus influenzae* type b vaccine prior to surgery for the implant (Rubin, Papsin, & Committee on Infectious Diseases and Section on Otolaryngology—Head and Neck Surgery, 2010). Children under 2 years should receive Prevnar, the pneumococcal conjugate vaccine, before surgery. Children over 2 years who have already received Prevnar vaccine should get one dose of the polysaccharide pneumococcal vaccine (Pneumovax 23). Children from 24 to 50 months should receive two doses of Prevnar, 2 or more months apart, followed by Pneumovax 23 at least 2 months later. Children 5 years and older should receive one dose of Pneumovax 23. Consult the Centers for Disease Control and Prevention (CDC) and the Canadian Health Network for updates on immunization recommendations.

Legal and Ethical Considerations
Deafness and Cochlear Implants

Many people who are deaf consider deafness a culture, similar to an ethnic group or a group with other common traits and experiences. They believe they are fully functional, communicate and socialize with others satisfactorily, and do not view deafness as a defect. They believe it is an affront to their culture to consider that someone should try to change from being deaf to hearing. Others note that only a select few can obtain cochlear implants due to their cost and the fact that health insurance may not cover the surgery or instrumentation or speech therapy. Other people are opposed to use of cochlear implants for children because of the surgical risk involved and the fact that children are not old enough to make their own decision about choosing the surgery. However, the earlier the child has the surgery and hears sounds, the more likely speech is to develop. Read about the controversy; imagine the difficulty parents have as they try to make the choice about treatment for the child who is hearing impaired (Pray & Jordan, 2010). Consider the ethical implications of the information parents need to receive about potential benefits and risks, the course of treatment, and the lack of information about long-term effects. How can nurses support the family as they consider alternatives and make decisions, and then once the treatment decision is made?

TABLE 24–13	Communication Techniques for Children Who Are Hearing Impaired
TECHNIQUE	**DESCRIPTION**
Cued speech	Supplement to lipreading; eight hand shapes represent groups of consonant sounds, and four positions about the face represent groups of vowel sounds; based on the sounds the letters make, not the letters themselves; child can "see-hear" every spoken syllable a hearing person hears.
Oral approach	Uses only spoken language for face-to-face communication; avoids use of formal signs; uses hearing aids and residual hearing.
Total communication	Uses speech and sign, fingerspelling, lipreading, and residual hearing simultaneously; child selects communication technique depending on the situation.
Sign language	A separate language that allows the user to communicate quickly and accurately with others who understand signs. The signs or hand movements represent words or concepts. When a sign is not available, the word can be spelled out using signs. American Sign Language (ASL) is most often used; British Sign Language (BSL) is common in Europe.

- Growth and Development, Delayed related to communication impairment
- Family Processes, Interrupted related to caring for a child with a hearing impairment

NANDA-I © 2012

Planning and Implementation

The goals of *Healthy People 2020* (U.S. Department of Health and Human Services, 2010) can guide nurses in planning assessments and interventions (Table 24–14).

Prevention and Early Identification

Nurses can encourage prevention of hearing loss from exposure to loud noises from power and farm equipment and music. Music should be turned down and ear protection should be worn for other activities. School nurses should be active in hearing conservation education programs in school. The nurse should develop and deliver hearing conservation curricula to children at elementary, middle, and high school levels; inform teachers and other professionals about noise-induced hearing loss; and train volunteers to assist with school programs.

Early identification of hearing loss in infants and children is facilitated by newborn screening, developmental assessment, and childhood screening programs. Infants should be tested for hearing loss by 1 month of age. In cases of loss, intervention should begin before 6 months of age (Joint Committee on Infant Hearing, 2007, 2008). Some newborns pass the universal hearing screening examination but are later found to have hearing loss, so ongoing evaluation at all healthcare visits is essential (Young, Reilly, & Burke, 2011). Be alert for expected language milestones during early childhood as this can be a clue to hearing impairment (see Table 24–11).

Care in the Community

Most of the care for children with hearing impairment takes place in the community. The nurse integrates special care into the health promotion and health maintenance visits of children with hearing impairments. Nursing care of the child with a hearing impairment focuses on facilitating the child's ability to receive spoken language and to send information, on helping parents to meet the child's schooling needs, and on providing emotional support to parents. Refer the parents to

TABLE 24–14 *Healthy People 2020* Objectives Related to Hearing in Children

OBJECTIVE	NURSING IMPLEMENTATION
Increase the proportion of newborns who are screened for hearing loss by no later than age 1 month, have audiologic evaluation by age 3 months, and are enrolled in appropriate intervention services by age 6 months.	Perform screening of newborns in nurseries. Evaluate results of hearing tests during health promotion visits and home visits to families with infants. Refer newborns with abnormal results for further screening. Refer infants with diagnosed hearing impairment to early intervention programs before they are 6 months of age.
Decrease otitis media in children and adolescents.	Partner with families to provide treatment as prescribed for otitis media. Provide teaching on correct administration of medications, need for immunizations that prevent against types of otitis media, and comfort measures for children with ear pain.
Increase the proportion of persons with hearing impairments who use hearing aids or assistive listening devices or who have cochlear implants.	Refer families to audiologic counseling to receive an overview of services helpful to the child. Explain and interpret services available. Assist the family in identifying useful services and the financial resources to assist in their use. Partner with families to liaison with schools to explain the adaptive devices used by the child and to form an individualized education plan.
Increase the proportion of persons who have had a hearing examination on schedule.	Perform screening in newborn nurseries and at each health promotion or home visit for infants. Organize school screening programs to screen children at least at each age prescribed by state laws (often kindergarten and grades 2, 5, and 8 for new children to the district).
Increase the use of hearing protection practices.	Teach all children about ear protection. Be alert for signs of hearing loss such as tinnitus. For those at risk of hearing loss, ensure regular audiometric testing.
Reduce the proportion of adolescents who have elevated hearing thresholds, or audiometric notches, in high frequencies (3, 4, or 6 kHz) in both ears, signifying noise-induced hearing loss.	Integrate hearing conservation instruction into each health maintenance visit. Ask about use of earphones, participation in rock bands, and attendance at rock concerts. Inquire about use of a cell phone directly on one ear. Assist schools to establish regular curricula related to hearing conservation.

Source: Adapted from U.S. Department of Health and Human Services. (2010). Healthy People 2020. *Washington, DC: U.S. Government Printing Office. Retrieved from http://www.healthypeople.gov/2020/*

an early intervention program as soon as the diagnosis of hearing impairment is made, in order to foster the child's development.

If a cochlear implant is planned, the child needs surgical care and follow-up to monitor results and integrate sound gradually into the child's life. See the Photo Story on page 724. Parents often need help to decide on the best method for hearing and language enhancement for the child. The nurse may need to interpret information, refer to the Internet and other resources, and help parents partner with other parents who have chosen various approaches for their own children. Children with cochlear implants need regular speech therapy after surgery. Refer parents to appropriate resources. Keep the child up to date for immunizations. Pneumococcal and meningococcal meningitis are more common among those who are not adequately immunized (Melton & Backous, 2011). Teach parents signs and symptoms of meningitis so they can seek prompt care if needed. See the Health Promotion & Maintenance Overview on page 725.

Nurses may be active in the community to encourage access for those with hearing impairment. This may include attending and requesting classes in American Sign Language at local community colleges and schools, or arranging for sign language interpretation at public events.

Facilitate Ability to Receive Spoken Language

Be aware of how the child compensates for hearing loss, and use the following strategies in communication:

- If hearing loss is mild or temporary or if the child reads lips, first obtain the child's visual attention by lightly touching the child or saying the child's name.
- Position your face 1 to 2 m (3 to 6 ft) from the child's face and make sure that the child's eyes are focused on your face and lips.

Make sure the room is well lit, with no backlighting. Speak at a normal rate and tone, and use facial expressions that show caring or concern. If the child does not understand, rephrase the information in shorter, simpler sentences. Use specific, concrete explanations, and give the child time to comprehend. Watch for subtle signs of misinterpretations, and give consistent and immediate feedback because only 30% of the English language is visible on the lips (Figure 24–13 ■).

- Be familiar with the different types of hearing aids. Hearing aids, which are microphones that amplify all sounds, can be worn in or behind the ear, in the frame of glasses, or on the body with a wire attached to the ear. When talking to a child with a hearing aid, speak slowly and be positioned 15 to 45 cm (6 to 18 in.) from the microphone using a normal conversational tone. Talk to the child even if the child is not looking at you. Make sure the batteries are fresh for the best reception. All sound is amplified, so reduce background noise as much as possible. (See Partnering with Families: Care of the Hearing Aid on page 726.)
- Acoustic feedback, an audible whistling sound that cannot always be heard by the child, is a common problem with hearing aids. To eliminate this sound, readjust the hearing aid to ensure that it is inserted properly and that no hair or earwax is caught between the ear mold and canal. Turning down the volume may also help.
- A remote microphone system is another type of device designed to improve hearing. This is often used in the classroom situation because it eliminates background noise. The speaker wears a transmitter that picks up the voice and transmits it to a receiver worn by the child.

PHOTO STORY...

COMMUNICATING WITH A COCHLEAR IMPLANT

Kate is 5 years old and has had decreased hearing ability from birth. She was born at term and had no risk factors for hearing loss. When she was several months old, Kate's parents suspected that she was hard of hearing. Her father designed an experiment: He crashed pans together behind her and found no response. The family was devastated but sought care and explored options to assist Kate with communication. They decided on a cochlear implant in her inner ear when Kate was 2 years of age. The implant connects to a microphone that is placed outside her head. She wears a sound processor on her belt that codes signals so that she can receive them in the implant. Kate communicates verbally now and visits a speech therapist each week who helps her learn how to listen for sounds, solve problems, and respond verbally. As an example, the therapist, Kate, and her

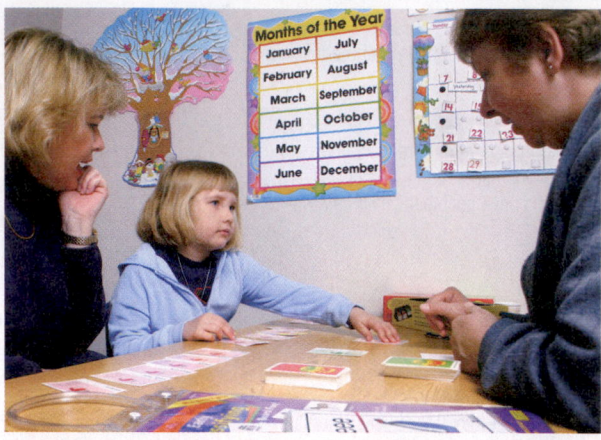

Kate is playing a card game with the speech therapist while her mother sits next to her. Notice her visual attention to the therapist which enhances her interpretation of speech.

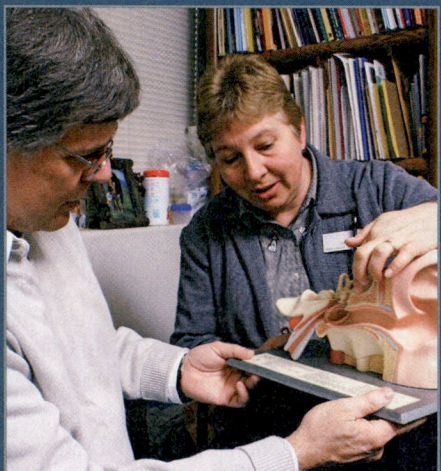

The speech therapist reinforces prior teaching about cochlear implants with Kate's father.

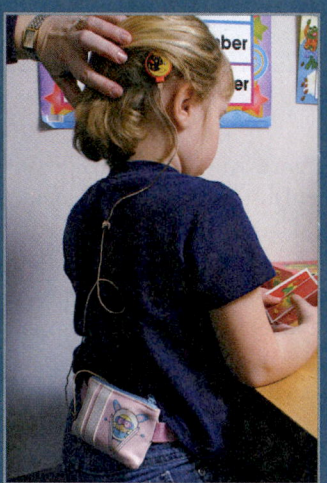

Notice the belt pack that Kate is wearing. Her microphone connects to the sound processor which enables her to hear and make sense of sounds.

mother work on a card game that combines problem solving, visual recognition, and verbal skills. Kate's father attends most of the speech therapy visits also and appreciates the therapist's willingness to periodically review with him the anatomy of the ear so that he can better understand his daughter's impairment and surgery. Recall that teaching needs to be repeated and expanded upon as the family is able to understand the condition more fully. Kate will attend kindergarten next year and continue to receive speech therapy to enhance her ability to listen, comprehend, and verbalize.

The experience of Kate's family is quite typical. Although there are risk factors for development of hearing impairment such as an infant who is premature or has a family history of impairment, the majority of children with a hearing impairment do not have any known risk factors. Because of this, healthcare providers are often not proficient at identifying the impairment

during infancy, when institution of sign language and other methods of communication is most effective. Nurses are instrumental in performing hearing testing on all newborns, carefully monitoring developmental progression, and testing response to sounds during all healthcare visits. Parents are usually the first to notice the child's inability to hear normally, as demonstrated by the case of Kate's father. Ask them about their perceptions of the child's hearing ability.

What other healthcare needs can you identify for Kate now that she is 5 years old? Recall that she is at risk for infection, so immunizations such as pneumococcal vaccine and *Haemophilus influenzae* type b need to be up to date. As Kate begins kindergarten, what do her teachers and classmates need to know? How can the family and school nurse establish an individualized education plan to enhance Kate's learning?

Health Promotion & Maintenance Overview

The Child with a Hearing Impairment

GROWTH AND DEVELOPMENTAL SURVEILLANCE

- Ensure that the child receives all immunizations at scheduled times. All children with cochlear implants should have pneumococcal vaccine (PCV7 for under 5 years or PPV23 for over 5 years); meningococcal vaccine should be considered. *Haemophilus influenzae* type b vaccine should be administered on recommended schedule. The immunizations should be completed 2 weeks before surgery for cochlear implant. Children should be up to date on all immunizations, but rubella, mumps, and measles are especially important since infections with the diseases could cause further hearing loss.
- Complete a developmental assessment, including receptive and expressive verbal skills, at each visit.
- Teach about safety precautions for those with hearing impairment, such as inability to hear announcements at school, fire alarms at home, or sirens when in travel. Assist the family to install visual stimuli for fire alarms and other safety needs.

COMMUNICATION

- Review the type of communication used by the child, and the family's satisfaction with it.
- Ask about relationships with other children, both hearing impaired and those with normal hearing.
- Review discipline techniques used by the parents and consistency of limit setting.

NUTRITION AND PHYSICAL ACTIVITY

- Complete a 24-hour diet recall and be sure the child receives adequate nutrition appropriate in energy for activities.

- Review the child's exercise patterns since some children with hearing impairment may avoid interactions with other children in sports.
- Refer the family to community activity programs as needed.

MENTAL HEALTH

- Find out stressors for the child, parents, and other family members.
- Locate community resources for early intervention and ongoing programs.
- Assist the youth and family to plan for moves to new schools and communities, and for plans related to transition to young adulthood, including college, trade schools, or work in the community.

DISEASE PREVENTION STRATEGIES

- Be sure signs of ear infection such as fever, irritability, disturbed sleep, rubbing an ear, or ear drainage are promptly evaluated in the pediatric healthcare home.
- Teach parents to administer antibiotics for ear infections exactly as prescribed.
- Encourage breastfeeding of infants and avoiding smoking to minimize incidence of ear infections.
- Be sure the child has all recommended immunizations.

INJURY PREVENTION STRATEGIES

- Encourage the family to preserve any hearing the child may have by avoiding exposure to loud sounds; when children are old enough to understand be sure they safeguard against exposure to loud music, guns, and other risks.
- Teach the child and family to plan for safety when crossing streets, driving cars, escaping house fires, and other situations that normally rely on hearing.

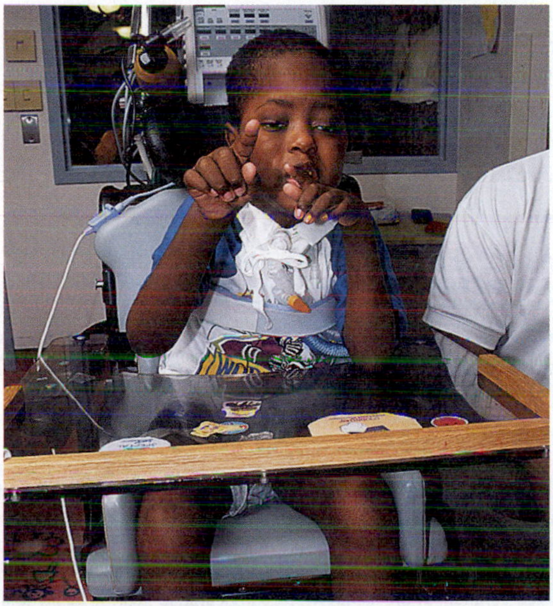

FIGURE 24–13 ■ This child with a hearing impairment and tracheostomy is communicating by means of American Sign Language.

Facilitate Ability to Send Information

Maintain the child's hearing aid in proper condition (Figure 24–14 ■). Many children with impaired hearing communicate using speech, which is enhanced through speech therapy. In addition, they are taught to sign, fingerspell, or use cued speech. Articulation may be difficult, and understanding what the child is trying to say may be frustrating for both the nurse and the child. Taking time to listen carefully is important.

Measures to promote speech and communication development as well as safety are implemented. Ask the parents to explain the child's communication techniques and to help interpret words. Have younger children point to pictures. Use assisted technologies such as a computer or picture board, as well as drawings or gestures if necessary. This technique is especially helpful for communicating feelings of pain and hunger during hospitalization. If the child signs or fingerspells, be sure you understand the signs for important functions. Give older children paper and pencil to write requests. People other than parents should be able to understand what the child is trying to communicate. Have an interpreter available if the child uses American Sign Language. Learn some common signs yourself to communicate simple words or phrases. Orient the child carefully to new settings such as the hospital room or a new school.

Help Parents to Meet Child's Educational Needs

Public laws apply to the education of children who are hearing impaired (see Chapter 1). After diagnosis, the parents and professionals together agree on an individualized education plan (see discussion in Chapter 14). Childcare and preschool are recommended for children with hearing problems to foster socialization skills and increase time for communicating with others. Some parents may choose to send the child to a separate program or school for the deaf and may need assistance to find such resources.

- Provide parents with information about adjustments that may have to be made for the child with a hearing impairment who

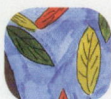

Partnering with Families

Care of the Hearing Aid

Families need to know how to maintain the child's hearing aid in proper condition to ensure its function. They can be taught when the child receives the first hearing aid, with at least annual updates to check on knowledge and questions. Items to include in teaching are as follows:

- The three types of hearing aid are those that fit totally in the ear canal, those that fit in the external ear canal, and those that fit behind the ear.

- The hearing aid should be cleaned each day with a damp cloth. Change the batteries as needed, usually about once a week. Disconnect the battery when not in use.
- Place the hearing aid in the ear with the volume off, then slowly turn up to half volume. Adjust as needed.
- Be sure the hearing aid fit is checked yearly, as the child's growth may necessitate a new fitting.

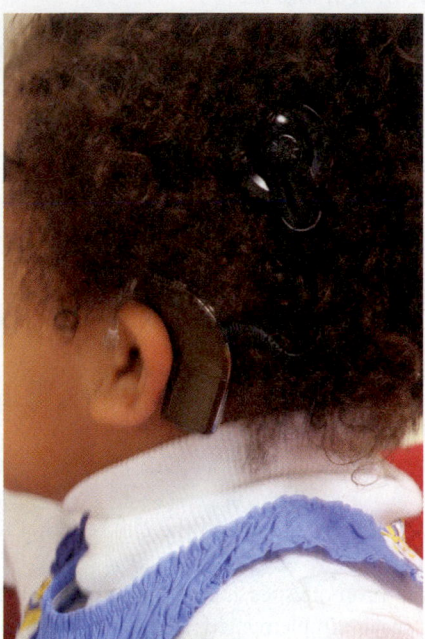

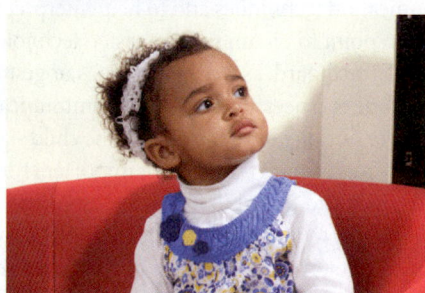

FIGURE 24–14 ■ *A,* Claretia has had a cochlear implant and is acquiring more speech rapidly since her surgery. Her device is shown in place. *B,* Note that her mother uses a headband to prevent this active toddler from dislodging her external device.

attends public school. By sitting at the front of the classroom, the child can hear and see more clearly. The teacher should always face the child when speaking, and background noise should be reduced.

- Tell parents that children who are hearing impaired have the same intelligence quotient (IQ) distribution as children without hearing impairment. However, communication and learning can be difficult, and extra support is needed.
- Children with hearing impairment should reach their intellectual potential, although development in certain areas may take place more slowly than it does in children with no hearing impairment.

Provide Emotional Support

By recognizing the effects of the diagnosis on the family, the nurse can help family members deal with their reactions to the child's hearing loss. Supporting healthy coping is an important intervention to help the parents carry on with their lives.

- Help the parents understand the child's hearing ability and its effect on speech and language development. Provide accurate information about their concerns. Work jointly with other healthcare professionals and social service workers if necessary.
- Tell the family about the community services available for medical, nursing, psychologic, and financial assistance. Link the family with the deaf or hearing-impaired community and resources.

Evaluation

Expected outcomes of nursing care for a child with hearing impairment include the following:

- The child successfully establishes a chosen communication method.
- The child manifests growth and development to maximum potential.
- An individualized education plan is established for the child.
- The family accesses resources and deals positively with stress.

Injuries of the Ear

Ear injuries of many types commonly occur in children. Lacerations, infections, and hematomas may occur in the external ear structures, especially the pinna. Children may place foreign objects in the ear, and insects may enter the ear canal.

Practice Alert

Parents and children should be instructed never to put any object in the child's ear. Some parents believe that the ear canal should be cleaned with a cotton-tipped swab. However, if the cleaning is too vigorous or the child moves unexpectedly, a ruptured tympanic membrane could result. This method of cleaning can also lead to impacted cerumen in the canal, which can decrease hearing ability and lead to discomfort.

If an alkaline button battery (like those found in many toys or watches) is inserted in a child's ear, it can rapidly destroy tissue, causing perforation of the tympanic membrane, destruction of the ossicles, and local tissue ulceration. Removal should be performed with the child under sedation or general anesthesia.

Rupture of the tympanic membrane may result from head injuries, blows to the ear, or insertion of objects into the ear canal. Serous drainage from the ear can indicate a basilar skull fracture. Be alert for ruptured tympanic membranes in combination with conjunctival

TABLE 24–15	Emergency Treatment of Ear Injuries
INJURY	**TREATMENT**
Pinna	
Minor cuts or abrasions	Wash thoroughly with soap and water and rinse well; leave exposed to air if possible or apply adhesive bandage, monitor for infection.
Hematomas	Needle aspiration should be performed and pressure dressing applied; undrained hematomas may become fibrotic; "cauliflower ear" deformity may develop.
Cellulitis or abscesses	Apply moist heat intermittently; make sure that prescribed antibiotic is taken; minor surgery may be performed for an abscess.
Deep lacerations	Apply pressure to stop bleeding; transport to physician's office or emergency department for suturing.
Ear Canal	
Foreign bodies	Have child lie on back and turn head over edge of bed, with affected side down; wiggle earlobe and have child shake head; foreign object may fall out as result of gravity; if object remains in ear, call physician; do not try to remove foreign body with tweezers since this may push the object further into the ear.
Insects	Shine flashlight into ear to try to attract insect; instilling a few drops of mineral oil, olive oil, or alcohol kills insect, and irrigating ear canal gently may remove dead insect (see Skills Manual 🔗).
Tympanic Membrane	
Ruptures	Call physician if child has persistent ear pain after blow, blast injury, or insertion of foreign object; cover external ear loosely with piece of sterile cotton or gauze; if the tympanic membrane has been ruptured, systemic or topical antibiotics are prescribed.

hemorrhage and other signs of shaken child syndrome (see Chapters 20 and 33 🔗 for further discussion of this type of child abuse).

See Table 24–15 for information on the emergency treatment of ear injuries. Any injury resulting in earache, decreased hearing, imbalance problems, persistent bleeding, or other discharge should be seen by a physician.

DISORDERS OF THE NOSE AND THROAT

A variety of disorders affect the nose and throat of children. They commonly relate to infection or trauma. The areas are anatomically connected, and with the trachea and upper bronchi they comprise the upper respiratory system. Several of the disorders of the upper respiratory system are discussed in the following section.

Epistaxis

Epistaxis, or nosebleed, is common in school-age children, especially boys. Kiesselbach's plexus, an area of plentiful veins located in the anterior nares, is a usual source of bleeding, commonly caused by irritation from nose picking, foreign bodies, or low humidity. Other causes include forceful coughing, allergies, or infections resulting in congestion of the nasal mucosa. Posterior nosebleeds have a variety of causes, some of which may indicate systemic disease (i.e., bleeding disorder) or injury. Bleeding from the posterior septum is more serious and may be life threatening. Hospitalization may be necessary.

Children with nosebleeds are sometimes brought to the emergency department by a parent who has been unable to stop the flow of blood within a few minutes. Both parent and child may be frightened. Ask the parent briefly about any history of nosebleeds and other contributing factors, including medications. Take the child's pulse and blood pressure to monitor for hypovolemia when there is excessive blood loss. Carefully examine the nasal mucosa by asking the child to blow any clots out gently, if possible. Suctioning may be necessary.

Observing the flow may help determine if the blood is coming from an anterior or a posterior location. A nosebleed confined to one side of the nose is almost always anterior, but posterior bleeding can flow on one or both sides. If blood cannot be seen, the child may be swallowing it and may become nauseated. Suspect posterior bleeding in children who have sustained blunt trauma to the head.

The child with anterior bleeding should sit upright quietly. The head should be tilted forward to prevent blood from trickling down the throat, which can lead to vomiting. The nares should be squeezed just below the nasal bone and held for 10 to 15 minutes while the child breathes through the mouth. An ice bag can be applied to the nose or back of the neck. If the bleeding does not stop, a cotton ball or swab soaked with Neo-Synephrine, epinephrine, thrombin, or lidocaine may be inserted into the affected nostril to promote topical vasoconstriction or anesthesia. Once the bleeding has stopped, the nostril may have to be cauterized with silver nitrate or electrocautery. If the bleeding cannot be stopped, absorbable packing may be used.

Posterior bleeding must also be stopped by packing, and the child must be monitored carefully. Arterial ligation is occasionally needed. Repeated or severe nosebleeds need further evaluation (Montague, Whymark, Howatson, et al., 2011).

Nursing Management

Assess the child's hematocrit or hemoglobin if significant bleeding has occurred. Report abnormal results to the primary care provider. Children with frequent epistaxis should have a complete history taken and physical examination performed to rule out systemic disease.

After the nosebleed has stopped, the child is more vulnerable to recurrent bleeding and should avoid bending over, stooping, strenuous exercise, hot drinks, and hot baths or showers for the next 3 to 4 days. Sleeping with the head elevated on two or three pillows and humidifying the air with a vaporizer may also prevent a recurrence. Provide parents with suggestions for prevention and home management of epistaxis. See Partnering with Families: Prevention and Home Management of Epistaxis.

Nasopharyngitis

Nasopharyngitis, also known as upper respiratory infection (URI) or the common cold, causes inflammation and infection of the nose and throat and is probably the most common illness of infancy and childhood. More than 200 viruses and numerous bacteria can cause this condition. The most common viruses include rhinovirus and coronavirus, and the most frequently occurring bacterium is group A streptococcus. See Chapter 25 🔗 for a discussion of respiratory

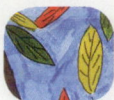

Partnering with Families

Prevention and Home Management of Epistaxis

PREVENTION

- Humidify the child's room, especially during the winter.
- Discourage the child from picking or rubbing the nose or inserting foreign objects in the nose.
- Instruct the child to blow the nose gently and release sneezes through the mouth.

HOME MANAGEMENT

- Keep the child calm.
- Sit the child upright with head tilted slightly forward so blood does not run down the nasopharynx.

- Press a roll of cotton under the upper lip to compress the labial artery.
- Apply steady pressure to both nostrils just below the nasal bone with the thumb and forefinger for 15 to 20 minutes. Time by the clock.
- Apply an ice pack or cold compress to the bridge of the nose or the back of the neck.
- Call the healthcare provider if the bleeding does not stop.
- Avoid vigorous exercise and aspirin or other anticoagulant drugs during the first few days after an episode of epistaxis.

Source: *Adapted from Melia, L., & McGarry, G. W. (2011). Epistaxis: Update on management.* Current Opinion in Otolaryngology & Head and Neck Surgery, 19, *30–35.*

---

syncytial virus (RSV), a common cause of both upper and lower respiratory illness. The organisms causing nasopharyngitis incubate in 1 to 3 days, and the infection is communicable several hours before symptoms develop and for 1 to 2 days after they begin. Symptoms may last 4 to 10 days or longer. The pathogens are believed to spread when the infected person touches the hand of an uninfected person, who then touches his or her mouth or nose, resulting in self-inoculation with infected droplets.

A red nasal mucosa with clear nasal discharge and an infected throat with enlarged tonsils may be apparent in children with nasopharyngitis. Vesicles may be present on the soft palate and in the pharynx. Accompanying symptoms may vary, depending on the child's age (Table 24–16).

Between episodes of nasopharyngitis, the child should be asymptomatic. If a child continues to have upper respiratory infections or a chronic cough, the presence of an underlying condition such as allergy, asthma, or polyps should be ruled out.

Nursing Management

For infants who cannot breathe through the mouth, normal saline nosedrops can be administered every 3 to 4 hours, especially before feeding. (Refer to the Skills Manual 🔗 for instructions on how to administer nosedrops.) For infants over 9 months of age, nasal stuffiness can be treated with normal saline nosedrops. The nosedrops followed by suction with a bulb syringe may be needed before feedings.

TABLE 24–16 | Symptoms of Nasopharyngitis

INFANTS YOUNGER THAN 3 MONTHS OF AGE	INFANTS 3 MONTHS OF AGE OR OLDER	OLDER CHILDREN
Lethargy	Fever	Dry, irritated nose and throat
Irritability	Vomiting	Chills, fever
Feeding poorly	Diarrhea	Generalized muscle aches
Fever (may be absent)	Sneezing	Headache
	Anorexia	Malaise
	Irritability	Anorexia
	Restlessness	Postnasal drip
		Thin nasal discharge, which may later become thick and purulent
		Sneezing

Complementary Therapy
Nasopharyngitis Treatments

Many families use home and herbal remedies for treatment of nasopharyngitis ("colds"). *American ginseng root extract* has been helpful in adults with respiratory tract infections. It has also been demonstrated to be safe in children from 3 to 12 years (Vohra, Johnston, Laycock, et al., 2008). *Echinacea* is a product derived from a plant that has been used as an immune stimulant; it is available in capsules, juice, tea, and other preparations. Some studies of *Echinacea* have not identified effectiveness in treating upper respiratory tract infections with the product (Barrett, Brown, Rakel, et al., 2010). Other studies have found that the product was effective in reducing symptoms or duration of respiratory infection (Hart & Dey, 2009). Vitamin C may decrease the duration but not the severity of nasopharyngitis (Heimer, Hart, Martin, et al., 2009). Future studies with children may help to further define the efficacy of vitamin C.

Some products taken for nasopharyngitis may actually be harmful. Herbal products that contain aristolochic acid, a substance that can cause cancer and kidney disease, can be found on numerous Internet sites, and several are marketed as cold remedies (U.S. Department of Health and Human Services, 2011).

Some Hispanic and Asian cultural groups believe in the "hot and cold" theory of disease, in which health problems are viewed as the result of imbalance. For example, some Mexican Americans traditionally treat a "cold disease" such as an earache or common cold with "hot" substances. Ask families if they prefer to eat certain foods during an illness. Incorporating such preferences can promote the child's health and increase the family's confidence in healthcare providers. (Refer to Chapter 3 🔗 for further information.)

Home treatments known to promote comfort during nasopharyngitis include antipyretics, humidified air, and increased fluid intake.

Nurses should assess home or herbal remedies used to treat a child's upper respiratory infection and check to be sure these products are safe for use in children. Integrate preferences whenever possible. What questions can you ask to obtain the necessary information? Where will you go to obtain information about the safety of complementary treatments? Refer to Chapter 3 for further information on helping families evaluate safety of products used.

Children over 6 years of age can use nasal sprays. See Complementary Therapy: Nasopharyngitis Treatments.

Decongestant nosedrops and sprays should not be used for more than 4 or 5 days or more often than recommended. Antihistamines may be helpful for children with allergic rhinitis or profuse nasal drainage. Long-acting nasal sprays and medications with several ingredients are not recommended. See Partnering with Families: Teaching About Over-the-Counter Cough and Cold Medications.

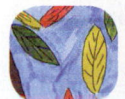
Partnering with Families

Teaching About Over-the-Counter Cough and Cold Medications

Parents may try to treat children who have upper respiratory infections with the same medications they are accustomed to taking for a cold. Prepare them during a health promotion visit and help them plan for how to handle medications for the child. Guidelines are as follows:

- Do NOT use cough and cold products in children under 2 years unless given specific directions to do so by a healthcare provider.
- Read the label to be sure the medication is recommended for the child's age and condition. Give only the dose recommended for the age and weight of the child. Do NOT use products packaged for adults.
- Be sure you know how to measure the medication. Tablespoon and teaspoon are *not* the same, and using household spoons may lead to incorrect dosing. Use the measuring device that is provided with liquid medications for greatest accuracy. If one is not provided, purchase one at the pharmacy that is precisely labeled. Use only a measuring device with the precise marking to match the dose you need to give.
- Consult the pharmacist, nurse, or doctor if you have questions, if the child is taking other medicines, if the medication is not recommended for the

age of your child, if the child's condition does not improve, or if other symptoms appear.

- Use the child-resistant cap after each opening of the bottle. Store the medication out of reach of all children, preferably in a locked location.
- Inspect containers and do not buy those that may have tears, imperfections, or tampering.
- Review all of the information in the "Drug Facts" box on the package label.
- If you use home remedies or other herbal products to treat colds, be sure to check on their safety with your healthcare provider first.
- If the child becomes more ill or does not improve, stop the medicine and contact the healthcare provider. If you do not understand instructions on the package, contact a healthcare provider before using it.

Source: *Adapted from Goldman, R. D. (2009). Cough and cold medications are risky for children. Journal of Pediatrics, 155(3), 451–452; and U.S. Food and Drug Administration. (2011). Public Health Advisory—FDA recommends that over-the-counter (OTC) cough and cold products not be used for infants and children under 2 years of age. Retrieved from http://www.fda.gov/drugs/drugsafety*

Room humidification may help prevent drying of nasal secretions. Antipyretics such as acetaminophen or ibuprofen reduce fever and make the child more comfortable. Aspirin is not recommended because of its association with Reye syndrome (refer to Chapter 33).

Children should avoid strenuous physical activity and engage in quiet play such as reading, listening to music or stories, or watching television or DVDs. Children should not be forced to eat, but the intake of favorite fluids to liquefy secretions should be encouraged. Parents should be told that no medicine or vaccine can prevent the common cold, but eliminating contact with infected persons can reduce the spread of infection. Proper hand washing and disposal of tissues help to decrease the spread of infection. Cleaning counters, toys, door knobs, and other surfaces on a daily basis can also decrease the spread of infections. Discourage sharing of food, dishes, and utensils at meals.

Sinusitis

Sinusitis is an inflammation of one or more of the paranasal sinuses. These sinuses, which have respiratory epithelium and are continuous with the respiratory tract, are air-filled hollow sterile cavities and include the maxillary, ethmoid, frontal, and sphenoid sinuses (Box 24–7). The sinuses commonly become infected following a viral upper respiratory infection, and therefore sinusitis is a common occurrence in children (DeMuri & Wald, 2010). It is important to differentiate viral from bacterial sinusitis. In both cases, the child's history reveals an upper respiratory infection for several days, followed by improvement in symptoms and a decrease in nasal drainage. In bacterial infection, the upper respiratory infection improves but an increase in purulent nasal drainage may be observed, with an elevated temperature about 102°F (39°C). The symptoms persist over 10 days with accompanying facial pain, headache, and fever. The most common infectious agents are the same as those for otitis media, namely *Streptococcus pneumoniae, Haemophilus influenzae,* and *Moraxella catarrhalis* (Edmondson & Parikh, 2008). Chronic sinusitis may occur in children with uncontrolled allergies and asthma.

BOX 24–7	Growth & Development: Sinuses

The ethmoid and maxillary sinuses form during gestation by about month 3 to 4, and are present at birth. Ethmoid sinuses continue to develop after birth and are fully formed by the midteen years. Frontal sinuses form from 5 to 8 years of age but are not complete until adolescence. Sphenoid sinuses begin development at age 6 and are mature in young adulthood. Children over 1 year of age can experience sinusitis following upper respiratory infections, but the sinuses involved are dependent on development of the paranasal sinuses (Edmondson & Parikh, 2008).

Signs and symptoms of sinusitis in children are sometimes nonspecific. A history of recent upper respiratory infection is common, persistent cough from postnasal drip can occur, and nasal discharge or swelling may be apparent. Malodorous breath, fever, mouth breathing, headache, hyponasal speech, and cervical lymphadenopathy may be present (DeMuri & Wald, 2010). Young children may be anorexic or have difficulty feeding, and older children may complain of headache or fatigue.

A diagnosis of sinusitis is usually based on history and physical examination findings. Percussion and illumination of sinuses are not generally useful in children. Computed tomography (CT), magnetic resonance imaging (MRI), and radiographs may be done, but they can be costly, they require sedation of young children, and results may not be conclusive. For the child with repeated sinusitis or who appears toxic, aspiration of sinus exudate may be performed for culture by an otolaryngologist.

Although most primary care providers treat suspected sinusitis with antibiotics, many cases will clear spontaneously without treatment. Amoxicillin is the first choice for therapy; amoxicillin/clavulanate, cefuroxime, cefdinir, azithromycin, and clarithromycin are also sometimes used (DeMuri & Wald, 2010). Children with recurrent and chronic (lasting 12 weeks or longer) sinusitis should be referred for further care by an otolaryngologist and allergy specialist, as inflammatory disease can be present and medication treatment can be challenging (Brook, 2010).

Parents whose child has persistent and purulent nasal drainage should be told to see a healthcare provider, particularly if the drainage is accompanied by facial pain, headache, and fever. Teach parents to correctly administer antibiotics (e.g., to take medications for the full course) if prescribed, and to use saline nosedrops if needed for comfort. Infants may need the nose cleared with nosedrops and a bulb syringe prior to feedings. (Refer to the Skills Manual ⬭ for correct use of a bulb syringe.) Antipyretics can be given for fever and to relieve pain.

Pharyngitis

Acute pharyngitis is an infection that primarily affects the pharynx, including the tonsils. It is seen most frequently in children 4 to 7 years and is rare in children less than 1 year. Viruses cause approximately 80% of these infections; the rest are caused by bacteria. Bacterial pharyngitis is commonly known as strep throat, because about 20% to 40% of bacterial pharyngitis is caused by group A beta-hemolytic streptococcus (GABHS) (Bonsignori, Chiappini, & DeMartino, 2010; Martin, 2010).

The major complaint is a sore throat. Children with minimal throat redness and pain, exudate, mild lymphadenopathy, and a low-grade fever, and who have been exposed to someone who has strep pharyngitis, should have a throat culture. The classic signs of purulent drainage and white patches are not present in all cases of strep throat.

A child who finds swallowing difficult or extremely painful, who drools, or who exhibits signs of dehydration or respiratory distress should be seen by a physician immediately. These signs could be indicators of serious conditions such as epiglottitis (see Chapter 25 ⬭) or diphtheria (see Chapter 22 ⬭). Peritonsillar abscess (a tonsil infection that spreads into surrounding tissues and causes cellulitis) and retropharyngeal abscess (an infection of the lymph nodes that drain the adenoids, nasopharynx, and paranasal sinuses) are other serious conditions. These conditions may have additional symptoms such as decreased neck movement, neck edema or pain, and respiratory distress (Galioto, 2008; Page, Bauer, & Lieu, 2008). CT scan or MRI may be helpful in diagnosis of abscess. See the Clinical Manifestations table for manifestations of viral pharyngitis, strep throat, peritonsillar abscess, and retropharyngeal abscess.

Collaborative Care

The diagnosis of strep throat is made by throat culture, using the rapid or traditional strep tests. Results of the rapid strep test may be available within minutes; those for the traditional test are available in 24 to 48 hours (Gunder, Lee, & Maner, 2010). A negative rapid test is followed by a traditional test to verify the rapid results.

Clinical Tip

Throat cultures must be properly performed for accurate diagnosis. A sterile cotton-tip applicator is swabbed across the tonsils, posterior edge of the soft palate, and uvula. Cooperative children can be asked to put their hands under their buttocks, open their mouth, and laugh or pant like a dog. The throat is quickly swabbed. Uncooperative and young children are placed on their back with their hands next to their head and held by a parent or an assistant. The tongue is gently depressed with a tongue blade and the throat is swabbed. Be sure to swab both tonsils.

Pharyngitis caused by group A beta-hemolytic streptococcus should be treated with oral penicillin for 10 days or by long-acting penicillin given in one injection. If the child is allergic to penicillin, erythromycin is given. Azithromycin and clarithromycin are additional examples of antibiotics used for treatment. Acute symptoms should resolve within 24 hours of therapy, at which time the child is no longer contagious. For pharyngitis that is caused by a virus, symptomatic treatment alone is used.

Peritonsillar abscess is treated by draining the abscess, providing antibiotics effective in treating the fluid cultured from the abscess, and hydration. Commonly administered antibiotics include ampicillin/sulbactam, penicillin G, and clindamycin. Once treatment has been achieved, the child is evaluated for possible tonsillectomy (Galioto, 2008). Retropharyngeal abscess is also frequently treated by drainage of the abscess, although intravenous antibiotics alone are effective in some cases. Ampicillin/sulbactam, clindamycin, cephalosporin, and penicillin are common antibiotics. Respiratory management may be needed (Page et al., 2008).

Clinical Manifestations Viral Pharyngitis, Strep Throat (Group A Beta-Hemolytic Streptococcus [GABHS]),[a] Peritonsillar Abscess, and Retropharyngeal Abscess

VIRAL PHARYNGITIS	STREP THROAT	PERITONSILLAR ABSCESS	RETROPHARYNGEAL ABSCESS
Nasal congestion	Abrupt onset	Fever	Fever
Mild sore throat	Tonsillar exudate[b]	Malaise	Sore throat
Conjunctivitis	Painful cervical lymphadenopathy[b]	Sore throat, more severe on one side	Inability to eat
Cough	Anorexia, nausea, vomiting, abdominal pain	Marked erythema and edema, especially of one side of throat and soft palate	Neck pain and edema
Hoarseness	Severe sore throat	Mouth odor	Pharyngitis
Mild pharyngeal redness	Headache, malaise	Difficulty speaking	Respiratory distress and stridor
Minimal tonsillar exudate	Fever above 38.3°C (101°F)	Difficulty opening mouth wide	
Mildly tender anterior cervical lymphadenopathy	Petechial mottling of soft palate	Cervical lymphadenitis	
Fever below 38.3°C (101°F)		Ear pain	

[a]Children 6 months to 3 years of age may have streptococcus with symptoms that resemble those of viral pharyngitis. Children with scarlet fever have the symptoms of strep throat plus a sandpaper-textured erythematous generalized rash and pallor around the lips.

[b]Classic signs of strep throat.

Source: *Data from Galioto, N. J. (2008). Peritonsillar abscess. American Family Physician, 77, 199–202, 209; Page, N. C., Bauer, E. M., & Lieu, J. E. C. (2008). Clinical features and treatment of retropharyngeal abscess in children. Otolaryngology—Head and Neck Surgery, 138, 300–306.*

Nursing Management

Nursing care focuses on symptomatic relief. Acetaminophen reduces throat pain and generalized fever. Cool, nonacidic fluids and soft foods, ice chips, or frozen juice pops given frequently in small amounts facilitate swallowing and prevent dehydration. Humidification, chewing gum, and gargling with warm salt water (5 g to 250 mL water; 1/4 teaspoon to 8 oz water) soothe an irritated throat.

Clinical Tip

Children may be more willing to gargle with salt water if the mixture is placed in a spray bottle and sprayed gently toward the throat. Do you know why? The salt water bypasses the salt sensation on the outer part of the tongue and is not as distasteful. The gentle spray does not stimulate a gag reflex; it delivers the salt solution directly to the throat area where it can be gargled and then spit out.

Commercial throat sprays or throat lozenges are not generally more effective than these home remedies. Encourage the child to rest and conserve energy to promote recovery.

Teach parents the importance of completing the entire course of antibiotics if prescribed for bacterial pharyngitis. After about 2 days on the medication, have the parents replace the child's toothbrush with a new one to avoid reinfection by bacteria that can survive on the moist brush. Reinforce to parents the importance of treating streptococcal infections, as untreated infections may lead to rheumatic fever, cervical adenitis, sinusitis, glomerulonephritis, or meningitis.

Tonsillitis and Adenoiditis

Tonsillitis is an infection or inflammation (hypertrophy) of the palatine tonsils. Although most children with pharyngitis have infected tonsils, they do not necessarily have inflammation that indicates tonsillitis. The adenoids are lymphatic tissue located on the posterior pharyngeal wall and are sometimes called the pharyngeal tonsils; they can manifest with acute or chronic infection.

Etiology and Pathophysiology

Like pharyngitis, tonsillitis and adenoiditis may be caused by a virus or bacterium. The primary site of infection is the tonsils. The condition tends to recur several times in certain children.

Clinical Manifestations

Symptoms suggestive of tonsillitis include frequent throat infections with breathing and swallowing difficulties, persistent redness of the anterior pillars, and enlargement of the cervical lymph nodes. If children breathe through their mouths continuously, the mucous membranes may become dry and irritated. Adenoiditis is characterized by nasal stuffiness, discharge, and postnasal drip, which results in coughing or excessive clearing of the throat.

Collaborative Care

The goal of treatment is relief from discomfort for the child. Symptomatic treatment, antibiotics, and occasionally surgery are used.

Diagnostic Tests

Diagnosis is made on the basis of visual inspection and clinical manifestations. Tonsils appear large and inflamed. Enlarged adenoids are diagnosed by radiologic studies (Box 24–8). A diagnosis of tonsillitis requires enlarged tonsils with pain and inflammation.

Clinical Therapy

Symptomatic treatment for tonsillitis is the same as for pharyngitis. Tonsillectomy is the third most common surgery in children, with 530,000 surgeries annually. Recent guidelines provide clear

---

BOX 24–8	Growth & Development: Tonsils

During normal development, children often have a growth of tonsillar tissue that makes the tonsils appear large. However, a diagnosis of tonsillitis requires enlarged tonsils accompanied by pain and inflammation. Observe the tonsils of many school-age children to learn the variation in size of tonsils that is commonly seen.

recommendations for surgery involving repeated infections and sleep-disordered breathing. Watchful waiting is recommended in most cases. Tonsillectomy can be considered when there are at least seven episodes of tonsillitis in the previous year, at least five episodes per year for 2 years, or at least three episodes annually for 3 years. In these cases, tonsillitis diagnosis requires a sore throat and at least one of the following symptoms: temperature above 38.3°C (101°F), cervical adenopathy, tonsillar exudate, and positive group A beta-hemolytic streptococcus infection (Baugh et al., 2010). Sleep-disordered breathing that exists with tonsillar hypertrophy and a condition such as growth abnormality, poor school performance, enuresis, or behavioral problem is also appropriate reason for surgical tonsillectomy (Mitka, 2011). One intraoperative dose of intravenous dexamethasone is recommended, but routine operative antibiotics are not needed.

Nursing Management

The goal of nursing care in tonsillitis and adenoiditis is promotion of comfort for the child and successful treatment of infection. If surgical removal is indicated, the nurse prepares the family and child for the surgery, provides postoperative care, and teaches information needed for postsurgical home care.

Nursing Assessment and Diagnosis

Assess the throat carefully during each physical examination. Observe for tonsils that are simply large (a common finding in childhood) and those that are inflamed as well as larger than expected for age (refer to Figure 7–28 in Chapter 7 🔗). Look for the degree of redness and presence of exudate. Ask if the child has pain or difficulty swallowing. Ask about the history of past tonsillar infections and the length of time of the present discomfort. Collect information about snoring, restlessness, or repeated night wakenings.

If surgery is indicated, take a complete history of the child preoperatively. Remember to evaluate for loose teeth and report them to the surgeon since they are common in children of this age. Monitor vital signs and observe for respiratory distress, hemorrhage, and dehydration postoperatively. Ask about medication usage.

The following nursing diagnoses may apply to the child with tonsillitis:

- Pain, Acute related to inflammation of the pharynx
- Fluid Volume: Deficient, Risk for related to inadequate intake
- Breathing Pattern, Ineffective related to obstruction by enlarged tonsils
- Swallowing, Impaired related to inflammation and pain
- Knowledge, Deficient (Parents) related to home care following discharge

NANDA-I © 2012

Planning and Implementation

The nurse provides general supportive care and, if medication is prescribed, encourages completion of the full course of treatment. The nursing management of children with tonsillitis is similar to that of children with pharyngitis (see earlier discussion).

If surgery is indicated, the nurse helps parents prepare their child for a short-term surgical procedure with a possible overnight stay in the hospital (see Chapter 15 ✏). Children should be free of sore throat, fever, or upper respiratory infection for at least 1 week before surgery. They should not be given aspirin or other medications that alter bleeding time for 10 days to 2 weeks prior to surgery, as these medications can increase postoperative bleeding (American Academy of Otolaryngology—Head and Neck Surgery, 2012). Check if any herbal medications are taken and report them to the physician and anesthesiologist, because some may interfere with anesthetic drugs used in surgery or interfere with normal blood clotting.

Discharge Planning and Home Care Teaching

Discharge planning includes teaching parents about pain management, fluid and nutrition intake, activity restrictions, and possible complications in the postoperative period. Most children will have a sore throat for 7 to 10 days after tonsillectomy. Advise parents how to relieve the child's throat pain.

Children may experience ear pain, especially when swallowing, between 4 and 8 days after tonsillectomy. Advise parents that this pain is the result of referred pain from the tonsillar area and does not indicate an ear infection.

Emphasize to parents the importance of adequate fluid intake. Children should be given any liquid they prefer for the first week, except citrus juices, which may produce a burning sensation in the throat. Soft foods such as gelatin, applesauce, frozen juice pops, and mashed potatoes can be added as tolerated.

Children do not need to be confined to bed, but vigorous exercise should be avoided for the first week after surgery. Advise parents that the child may return to school approximately 10 days after tonsillectomy.

Any surgery carries with it the risk of postoperative complications. Teach parents the normal signs of healing in the postoperative period, as well as signs of complications. (See Partnering with Families: Care After Tonsillectomy, and Complications of Tonsillectomy and Adenoidectomy.)

Evaluation

Expected outcomes of nursing care for the child with tonsillitis include:

- The child is able to consume adequate food and fluids.
- Pain and fever are managed to a level of comfort for the child.
- The child does not experience postoperative complications such as bleeding, hemorrhage, and dehydration.
- The child heals without complication.

DISORDERS OF THE MOUTH

The mouth is an important structure that is directly linked to both the gastrointestinal and respiratory systems. Structural problems can occur in the mouth, often in conjunction with other defects. See Chapter 30 ✏ for a description of tracheoesophageal fistula and cleft lip and palate. Both of these defects are commonly connected with structural defects of the mouth, most notably a cleft or opening in

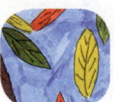

Partnering with Families

Care After Tonsillectomy

After a child's tonsillectomy, the parent can institute measures to increase the child's comfort.
- Have the child drink adequate cool fluids or chew gum, as this reduces spasms in the muscles surrounding the throat.
- Give acetaminophen elixir or other analgesic as prescribed.

- Apply an ice collar around the child's neck.
- Have the child gargle with a solution of 2.5 g (0.5 teaspoon) each of baking soda and salt in 8 oz of water.
- Have the child rinse the mouth well with viscous lidocaine, if prescribed by the surgeon, and then swallow the solution.

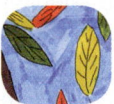

Partnering with Families

Complications of Tonsillectomy and Adenoidectomy

BLEEDING
- To prevent bleeding, aspirin or other drugs that alter bleeding should not be given for pain for the first postoperative week. Use acetaminophen or ibuprofen as directed instead.
- Bleeding is most likely to occur within the first 24 hours or 7 to 10 days after the tonsillectomy, when the scar is forming. Report any trickle of bright red blood as well as increased swallowing to the physician immediately.

INFECTION
- The back of the throat will look white and have an odor for the first 7 to 8 days after the surgery. The child may also have a low-grade fever. These are not signs of infection.

- For temperatures over 38.3°C (101°F), acetaminophen may be used.
- Call the physician if the child develops a fever above 38.8°C (102°F).

PAIN
- Administer acetaminophen or other analgesic as prescribed.
- Offer frequent small amounts of cool liquids. Avoid citrus juice.
- Provide for rest and quiet activities for several days.

the palate. See Chapter 7 🔗 for a description of examination of the mouth and tongue in neonates and older children to identify structural problems. Dental caries and oral health are thoroughly discussed in the Health Promotion chapters.

A second type of mouth disorder in children is ulceration. Children sometimes have changes in the mucous membranes of the mouth, associated with illnesses or infections, or as a side effect of drug treatments. These disorders are discussed later in the chapter.

Trauma is a third cause for mouth disorders in children. Accidents can cause fractures of the jaw or other trauma. Fractures are discussed in Chapter 35 🔗. Trauma that leads to dental emergencies is discussed later in this chapter.

Mouth Ulcers

A variety of conditions can cause mouth ulcers in children. They commonly occur in conjunction with certain medications or diseases (Figure 24–15 ■). Oral mucosa has a fast rate of growth, so conditions that impair cell synthesis will cause breakdown in the mucosa with lack of new tissue growth. The growth of mucosal tissue requires adequate moisture, so dehydration is a risk factor for development of oral ulcers.

Trauma is another cause of oral ulcers. See the Clinical Manifestations table for the etiology, clinical manifestations, and clinical therapy for conditions leading to oral ulcers in children.

Collaborative Care

The goals of collaborative care are relief from pain and promotion of ulcer healing.

Diagnostic Tests

Most mouth ulcers and other oral lesions are diagnosed by history and appearance. Culture of exudate may be helpful in identifying an

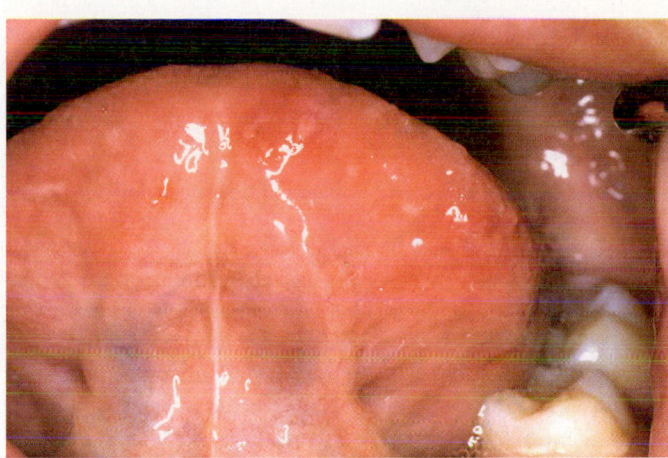

FIGURE 24–15 ■ The child with aphthous ulcers in the mouth has discomfort and pain that interfere with ingestion of food and fluids. These ulcers can be caused by infectious organisms and are most common in children with immune suppression. Frequent oral assessment and meticulous oral care are needed by all children at risk of oral ulcers.
Source: *Copyright 2012 Edward H. Gill—Custom Medical Stock Photo, All Rights Reserved.*

infective cause. Biopsy may be performed if the cause is not clear or a mouth cancer is possible. Occasionally laboratory blood analysis is done and may show leukocytosis in infectious cases and Stevens-Johnson syndrome.

Clinical Therapy

Most mouth ulcers are treated symptomatically. Since the oral mucosa is fast growing, the cells can rapidly heal. Keeping the mouth clean and administering systemic or topical analgesics can assist with comfort. Foods should be mild and nonirritating. Acyclovir may be administered for treatment of herpes infections. Antibiotics are needed for bacterial infection of oral lesions. Stevens-Johnson

Clinical Manifestations   Mouth Ulcers in Children

DISORDER	ETIOLOGY	CLINICAL MANIFESTATIONS
Chemotherapy-related oral mucositis	Many chemotherapy drugs used to treat cancer attack all rapidly growing cells in the body. Lack of intake of sufficient fluids to provide adequate hydration exacerbates the development of mucositis.	The oral mucosa may have painful ulcers that bleed, become infected, or interfere with food intake.
AIDS-related oral mucositis	Some of the drugs used to treat HIV infections and the poor nutritional state of children with AIDS can promote the development of oral ulcers.	Painful oral ulcers further interfere with adequate food intake.
Stevens-Johnson syndrome (see Chapter 36 🔗)	Erythema multiforme is a rare mucocutaneous disease, and erythema multiforme major is also known as Stevens-Johnson syndrome. After a prodromal period with fever, malaise, fatigue, and sore throat, the characteristic lesions of the disease erupt. Stevens-Johnson syndrome may occur with recurrent herpes virus infection, *Mycoplasma pneumoniae,* or as a reaction to drugs such as nonsteroidal anti-inflammatories, anticonvulsants, and sulfonamides.	Endothelial cells, epithelial cells, and mucosal cells are affected, causing blisters and erosion of conjunctiva, oral cavity, and genital mucosa. A bullous erythematous rash also is common and pneumonia can result.
Aphthous ulcers	These lesions are commonly called "canker sores." An allergic or autoimmune cause is suspected, but herpes gingivitis should be ruled out.	They often recur in the same child over time. Ulcers are on the inside of the lips or throughout the mouth; about 1–3 ulcers occur at a time.
Herpes simplex gingivostomatitis (see Chapter 22 🔗)	Herpes virus is the causative organism. Herpes simplex infections of the face and nose are referred to as "cold sores."	Multiple ulcers and vesicles of the gingiva, palate, buccal mucosa, lips, and tongue appear. They may be accompanied by skin vesicular lesions characteristic of herpes on the face.
Traumatic ulcers	Trauma to the oral mucosa can lead to ulcers. Children may bite the side of the mouth, may poke a pencil or other object into the mucosa, or can have burns from hot liquids or acidic substances.	One or more ulcerations are visible and may become infected due to source of trauma.

syndrome necessitates removing the drug that causes the reaction, and treating the child with oral antihistamines and supportive therapy.

Nursing Management

Nurses assess oral mucosa and implement treatments for oral ulcers.

Nursing Assessment and Diagnosis

Nurses assess the oral cavity of all children beginning in the neonatal period. Structural abnormalities are promptly referred for further diagnostic work. Mouth ulcers are examined for size, location, drainage, and pain. For those at risk, such as children on chemotherapy, regular careful examination of the oral mucosa is an important part of care. Some of the appropriate nursing diagnoses for children with oral ulcers include:

- Pain, Acute related to injury of oral cavity
- Mucous Membrane: Oral, Impaired related to chemotherapy or infection
- Nutrition, Imbalanced: Less than Body Requirements related to inability to ingest adequate foods

NANDA-I © 2012

Planning and Implementation

Nurses play an important role in treatment of oral ulcers. Most ulcers are treated symptomatically and will heal rapidly. Ensure that children have good oral care, including brushing teeth with a soft bristle brush or by use of mouth sponges. Rinse the mouth after all meals and snacks. Teach the family correct administration of oral medications and topical preparations designed to treat infection or provide comfort. When oral mucosa ulcers are predicted, such as with chemotherapy or in AIDS, begin oral protocols before lesions occur to decrease their appearance and severity. Encourage a diet that has only mild foods, avoiding spices and very sweet, sour, and acidic items. Cold foods may be better accepted. Monitor hydration status to ensure adequate fluid intake. Teach parents correct administration of acetaminophen or other analgesic treatment. Use standard precautions to protect the child from infections and prevent their flora from being transferred to other children or family members. Encourage parents to keep children with herpes gingivostomatitis out of contact with other children if active lesions or drooling are present.

Evaluation

Desired outcomes of nursing care for children with oral problems include:

- There are decreased reports of oral pain or disruptive effects on dietary intake.
- Structural intactness and normal function of oral mucosal membranes is observed.
- The child ingests adequate fluids and nutrients.

Mouth and Dental Emergencies

Children may have trauma to the mouth and teeth during sporting activities and during other injuries. Some cases occur in the toddler years as children become more mobile, while avulsions are most common from 7 to 14 years (Trope, 2011). Nurses inform parents of proper treatment for injuries and may provide emergency treatment in schools and other community settings. Injury prevention is encouraged through use of protective gear during sports. See Chapter 20 🔗 for a discussion of protective sporting gear and of body piercing which may include the oral cavity. Mouth guards can be helpful to prevent dental damage. The best guards are custom made by dentists because they fit the mouth well and are more likely worn because of their comfort.

Because the mouth has a profuse blood supply, bleeding may be extensive for even minor injuries. It is best to use clean cloths to absorb the blood and prevent choking on it, and get the child to an emergency facility to have the lesion carefully examined.

Dental injuries may involve fracture of a tooth, luxation (partial extrusion), or avulsion (complete removal). The periodontal ligament holds the tooth in the socket, but its attachment is torn during a tooth avulsion. The child should be transported immediately to an emergency facility. If otherwise stable, an emergency dental visit is the best choice. When avulsion has occurred, fast care improves the chance that a permanent tooth can be reimplanted and kept alive. When reimplanted within 30 minutes, the chances of survival of the tooth are best (American Association of Endodontists, 2010). Nurses can perform care or teach parents what to do in case of dental emergency. Referral to dental resources may be needed. See Chapters 8 to 13 🔗 for specific dental care needs for health promotion and health maintenance at each age during childhood and adolescence. See Partnering with Families: Care of a Tooth Avulsion.

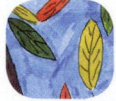

Partnering with Families

Care of a Tooth Avulsion

When a tooth is removed during an injury, prompt treatment may influence the chance that it can be reimplanted. If the child's condition is stable, try to reimplant the tooth and then transfer the child to an emergency dental facility.

- Handle the tooth only by the crown (its top) rather than the root to avoid further damage.
- Gently rinse the tooth with a stream of sterile saline. Do not place it under running water.
- Insert the tooth into the socket.
- Have the child provide gentle pressure by biting a piece of gauze or a moistened tea bag.

- If the child is unstable or has other injuries, enlist emergency medical transportation (call 911). In this case, the tooth is transported with the child and kept moist.
- If a dental aid kit is available, it may contain a transport liquid such as Viaspan or Hank's Balanced Salt Solution. If these are not available, alternatives include cold milk, saline, saliva, or water with a pinch of salt. Place the tooth in one of these transfer liquids to keep it moist and send it with the child to the healthcare facility.

Source: *Adapted from American Association of Endodontists. (2010). Emergency steps for saving a knocked-out tooth. Retrieved from http://www.aae.org/patients/patientinfo/references/avulsed.htm*

Chapter Highlights

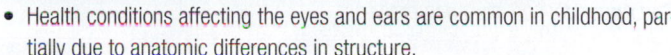

- Health conditions affecting the eyes and ears are common in childhood, partially due to anatomic differences in structure.
- Disorders of the eye and ear can lead to developmental and communication delays.
- Conjunctivitis can occur throughout childhood, and can be caused by bacteria, viruses, and allergy.
- Conjunctivitis in the newborn, ophthalmia neonatorum, can be acquired during birth from the mother and can pose a serious health threat.
- Children manifest a wide array of visual disorders such as hyperopia, myopia, and astigmatism.
- Conditions that can seriously affect vision are strabismus, amblyopia, cataracts, and glaucoma.
- An iatrogenically caused visual disorder is retinopathy of prematurity.
- Nurses commonly screen vision of children in schools and health facilities to identify those with visual impairment.
- Interventions for the child with visual impairment center on providing input through other senses to maximize child development.

- Otitis media is the most common childhood health condition, and has increased in incidence in the past decade.
- Overgrowth of resistant organisms has made treatment of otitis media difficult.
- Treatment of otitis media may begin with up to 3 days of monitoring, followed by antibiotic therapy if the child's condition worsens.
- Newborns should be screened for response to sounds; those at high risk of hearing impairment should be carefully monitored in early childhood.
- Hearing loss may be conductive, sensorineural, or mixed.
- Nursing plan interventions maximize development and communication in the child with a hearing impairment.
- Common disorders of the nose and throat in children include epistaxis, nasopharyngitis, pharyngitis, and tonsillitis.
- Common disorders of the mouth in children are structural abnormalities and oral ulcers.
- Nurses are influential in providing care in dental emergencies and referring families for adequate dental care.

Clinical Reasoning in Action

INTRODUCTION

Consider the opening scenario with Shariffa, who presented with pain in her ear and was diagnosed with acute otitis media.

DESCRIPTION

Shariffa is about to begin preschool after having been cared for by her mother and an aunt for the first 3 years of her life. Shariffa has one older brother who is 6 years old, and they spend every other weekend across town with their father. Shariffa's mother has been concerned about her daughter's communication abilities. She knows some words, but her vocabulary is limited. Her mother is not certain that she always responds to sounds.

DISCUSSION

The nurse practitioner must explain why an antibiotic is not immediately prescribed for Shariffa. It is also important to know if Shariffa has relief from the ear pain within the next 2 to 3 days. As Shariffa begins attendance at a preschool,

what new challenges will her family face? How can you help them to learn about and become oriented to this new facility? What help might Shariffa's mother need as she makes a transition to her planned part-time job?

Use Bronfenbrenner's ecological theory (Chapter 5 🔗) to develop questions about Shariffa's microsystem, mesosystem, exosystem, and macrosystem that will influence her health care and support.

1. What observations will you make in the clinic to provide clues to Shariffa's communication abilities? How will you assess Shariffa's hearing acuity? What developmental test can you administer? (See Chapter 8 🔗 for further information about developmental tests.)
2. Plan the information you can provide to the mother to explain current treatment for otitis media. When should Shariffa's condition be reevaluated?
3. Plan a program for Shariffa's family that includes reading, encouraging language, and fostering communication abilities. Describe the expected receptive and expressive speech at her age.

NCLEX-RN® Review

1. The nurse is caring for a child with vision impairment. Which is a priority nursing intervention for this child?
   1. Encourage the child to use all five senses.
   2. Teach the parents to read body language.
   3. Teach the parents special safety measures.
   4. Perform screening at every checkup.

2. After a discussion with the nurse about common ear and hearing disorders in children, which statement by the parent indicates that correct learning has taken place?
   1. "Prevention is the key."
   2. "Antibiotics are needed immediately for otitis media."
   3. "Herbal eardrops should not be given to children."
   4. "Loud music cannot cause hearing loss."

3. The nurse is caring for a child with a hearing impairment. Which action is the focus of care for this child?

1. Facilitating communication
2. Preparing for cochlear implant
3. Referring the parents to community services
4. Preparing the individualized education plan (IEP)

4. The parents of a child who had a tonsillectomy 3 days ago call about concerns with symptoms they are seeing. Which symptom would alert the nurse that the child may be having a postoperative problem?

1. The child has white crusts on the back of the throat.
2. The child is having increased swallowing.
3. The child will only eat Popsicles.
4. The child complains of throat pain.

See Appendix I ⬤ for answers.

References

Alme, A. M., Mulhern, M. L., Hejkal, T. W., Meza, J. L., Qui, F., Ingvoldstad, D. D., & Margalei, E. (2008). Outcome of retinopathy of prematurity following adoption of revised indications for therapy. *BMC Ophthalmology, 8*, 23.

American Academy of Otolaryngology—Head and Neck Surgery. (2012). *Tonsillectomy pain management.* Retrieved from http://www.entnet.org/AboutUs/Q-A-TAPainManagement.cfm

American Academy of Pediatrics, Section on Ophthalmology. (2006). Screening examination of premature infants for retinopathy of prematurity. *Pediatrics, 117*, 572–576.

American Academy of Pediatrics, Subcommittee on Management of Acute Otitis Media. (2004). Diagnosis and management of acute otitis media. *Pediatrics, 113*, 1451–1465.

American Association of Endodontists. (2010). *Emergency steps for saving a knocked-out tooth.* Retrieved from http://www.aae.org/patients/patientinfo/references/avulsed.htm

American Foundation for the Blind. (2011). *Children and youth with vision loss.* Retrieved from http://www.afb.org/Section/asp?SectionID=15&TopicID=411&DocumentID=4896

American Speech-Language-Hearing Association. (2008). *Type, degree, and configuration of hearing loss.* Retrieved from http://www.asha.org/public/hearing/disorders/types.htm

American Speech-Language-Hearing Association. (2011). *Causes of hearing loss in children.* Retrieved from http://www.asha.org/public/hearing/disorders/causes.htm

Askin, D. F., & Diehl-Jones, W. (2009). Retinopathy of prematurity. *Critical Care Nursing Clinics of North America, 21*, 213–233.

Barrett, B., Brown, R., Rakel, D., Mundt, M., Bone, K., Barlow, S., & Ewers, T. (2010). Echinacea for treating the common cold: A randomized trial. *Annals of Internal Medicine, 153*, 769–777.

Basch, C. E. (2011). Vision and the achievement gap among urban minority youth. *Journal of School Health, 81*, 599–605.

Baugh, R. F., Archer, S., Mitchell, R. B., Rosenfeld, R. M., Amin, R., Burns, J. J., . . . Bielory, L. (2010). Allergic conjunctivitis and the impact of allergic rhinitis. *Current Allergy and Asthma Reports, 10*, 122–134.

Bielory, L. (2010). Allergic conjunctivitis and the impact of allergic rhinitis. *Current Allergy and Asthma Reports, 10*(2), 122–134.

Bonsignori, F., Chiappini, E., & DeMartino, J. (2010). The infections of the upper respiratory tract in children. *International Journal of Immunopathology and Pharmacology, 23*(Suppl. 1), 16–19.

Brook, I. (2010). Chronic sinusitis in children. *Pediatric Annals, 39*(1), 41–47.

Centers for Disease Control and Prevention. (2010). Identifying infants with hearing loss—United States, 1999–2007. *Morbidity and Mortality Weekly Report, 59*, 220–223.

Centers for Disease Control and Prevention. (2011). *Facts about antibiotic resistance.* Retrieved from http://www.cdc.gov/getsmart/antibiotic-use/fast-facts.html

Choi, S. Y., & Hwang, J. M. (2009). Ishihara test in 3- to 6-year-old children. *Japan Journal of Ophthalmology, 53*, 455–457.

Chou, R., Dana, T., & Bougatsos, C. (2011). *Screening for visual impairment in children ages 1–5 years: Systematic review to update the 2004 U.S. Preventive Services Task Force recommendation.* Agency for Healthcare Research and Quality. Report No. 11-05151-EF-1.

Cohen, S. M. (2011). Orbital cellulitis as a complication of sinusitis. *Journal for Nurse Practitioners, 7*, 38–44.

Corey, L., & Wald, A. (2009). Maternal and neonatal herpes simplex virus infections. *New England Journal of Medicine, 361*, 1376–1385.

Custer, J. W., & Rau, R. E. (2009). *The Harriet Lane handbook* (18th ed.). St. Louis, MO: Elsevier Mosby.

Dagan, R. (2010). Appropriate treatment of acute otitis media in the era of antibiotic resistance. *Paediatric Drugs, 12*(Suppl. 1), 3–9. doi:10.2165/11538720-S0-000000000-00002

Daly, K. A., Hoffman, H. J., Kvaerner, K. J., Kvestad, E., Casselbrant, M. L., Homol, P., & Rovers, M. M. (2009). Epidemiology, natural history and risk factors: Panel report from the 9th international research conference on otitis media. *International Journal of Pediatric Otolaryngology, 74*, 231–240.

Davidson, S., & Quinn, G. E. (2011). The impact of pediatric vision disorders in adulthood. *Pediatrics, 127*, 334–339.

DeMuri, G., & Wald, E. R. (2010). Acute sinusitis: Clinical manifestations and treatment approaches. *Pediatric Annals, 39*(1), 34–40.

Edmondson, N. E., & Parikh, S. R. (2008). Complications of acute bacterial sinusitis in children. *Pediatric Annals, 37*(10), 680–685.

Farboud, A., Skinner, R., & Pratap, R. (2011). Otitis media with effusion ("glue ear"). *British Medical Journal, 343*. doi:10.1136/bmj.d3770

Gaffney, M., Eichwald, J., Grosse, S.D., & Mason, C.A. (2010). Identifying infants with hearing loss—United States 1999–2007. *Morbidity and Mortality Weekly Report 59*, 220–223.

Galioto, N. J. (2008). Peritonsillar abscess. *American Family Physician, 77*, 199–202, 209.

Giordano, T., Litman, R. S., Li, K. K., Mannix, M. E., Schwartz, R. H., Setzen, G., . . . Patel, M. M. (2011). Clinical practice guideline: Tonsillectomy in children. *Otolaryngology—Head and Neck Surgery, 144*. doi:10.1177/0194599810389949

Gold, R. S. (2011). Treatment of bacterial conjunctivitis in children. *Pediatric Annals, 40*, 95–105.

Goldman, R. D. (2009). Cough and cold medications are risky for children. *Journal of Pediatrics, 155*(3), 451–452.

Granet, D. B. (2011, May). Treating bacterial conjunctivitis. *Infectious Diseases in Children,* 10–15.

Granet, D. B., & Khayali, S. (2011, February). Amblyopia and strabismus. *Pediatric Annals,* 89–94.

Graven, S. N., & Browne, J. V. (2008). Visual development in the human fetus, infant, and young child. *Newborn & Infant Nursing Reviews, 8*, 194–201.

Gunder, L., Lee, L., & Maner, D. (2010, Summer). Rapid strep testing in ambulatory care. *Clinician Reviews,* 12–14.

Hagan, J. F., Shaw, J. S., & Duncan, P. M. (2008). *Bright futures* (3rd ed.). Elk Grove Village, IL: American Academy of Pediatrics.

Harlor, A. D., Bower, C., & the Committee on Practice and Ambulatory Medicine. (2009). Clinical report—Hearing assessment in infants and children: Recommendations beyond neonatal screening. *Pediatrics, 124*, 1252–1263.

Hart, A., & Dey, P. (2009). Echinacea for prevention of the common cold: An illustrative overview of how information from different systematic reviews is summarized on the internet. *Preventive Medicine, 49*(2–3), 78–82.

Hauser, A., & Fogarasi, S. (2010). Periorbital and orbital cellulitis. *Pediatric Review, 31*, 242–249.

Heimer, K. A., Hart, A. M., Martin, L. G., & Rubio-Wallace, S. (2009). Examining the evidence for the use of vitamin C in the prophylaxis and treatment of the common cold. *Journal of the American Academy of Nurse Practitioners, 21*, 295–300.

Hoberman, A., Paradise, J. L., Rockette, H. E., Shaikh, N., Wald, E. R., Kearney, D. H., . . . Barbadora, K. A. (2011). Treatment of acute otitis media in children under 2 years of age. *New England Journal of Medicine, 364*, 105–115.

Joint Committee on Infant Hearing. (2007). Year 2007 position statement: Principles and guidelines for early hearing detection and intervention programs. *Pediatrics, 120*, 898–921.

Joint Committee on Infant Hearing. (2008). *Clarification for Year 2007 JCIH position statement.* Retrieved from http://www.jcih.org/clarification%20year%20207%20statement.pdf

Kamat, D. M. (2010, October). Orbital cellulitis. *Consultant for Pediatricians*, 374–375.

Kemper, A. R., Helfrich, A., Talbot, J., & Patel, N. (2012). Outcomes of an elementary school-based vision screening program in North Carolina. *Journal of School Nursing, 28*, 24–30.

Kliegman, R. M., Stanton, B., St. Geme, J., Schor, N., & Behrman, R. E. (2010). *Nelson textbook of pediatrics* (19th ed.). Philadelphia, PA: Saunders.

Martin, J. M. (2010). Pharyngitis and streptococcal throat infections. *Pediatric Annals, 39*, 22–27.

Melia, L., & McGarry, G. W. (2011). Epistaxis: Update on management. *Current Opinion in Otolaryngology & Head and Neck Surgery, 19*, 30–35.

Melton, M. F., & Backous, D. D. (2011). Preventing complications in pediatric cochlear implantation. *Current Opinion in Otolaryngology & Head and Neck Surgery, 19*(5), 358–362.

Mickler, C., Boden, J., Trivedi, R. H., & Wilson, M. S. (2011, February). Pediatric cataract. *Pediatric Annals*, 83–87.

Mitka, M. (2011). Guideline cites appropriateness criteria for performing tonsillectomy in children. *Journal of the American Medical Association, 305*, 661–662.

Montague, M. L., Whymark, A., Howatson, A., & Kubba, H. (2011). The pathology of visible blood vessels on the nasal septum in children with epistaxis. *International Journal of Otorhinolaryngology, 75*, 1032–1034.

National Eye Institute. (n.d.). *Sports-related eye injuries*. Retrieved from http://www.nei.nih.gov/sports/pdf

National Institutes of Health (NIH). (2011). *Cochlear implants*. Retrieved from http://www.nidcd.nih.gov/health/hearing/coch.asp

Nelson, H. D., Bougatsos, C., & Nygren, P. (2008). Universal newborn hearing screening: Systematic review to update the 2001 U.S. Preventive Services Task Force recommendation. *Pediatrics, 122*, e266–276.

Nield, L. S., Mangano, L. M., & Kamat, D. (2008, January). Strabismus: A close-up look. *Consultant for Pediatricians*, 17–25.

Ore, L., Tamir, A., Stein, N., & Cohen-Dar, M. (2009). Reliability of vision screening tests for school children. *Journal of Nursing Scholarship, 41*, 250–259.

Otitis Media with Effusion. (2004). Clinical practice guideline. *Pediatrics, 113*, 1412–1429.

Page, N. C., Bauer, E. M., & Lieu, J. E. C. (2008). Clinical features and treatment of retropharyngeal abscess in children. *Otolaryngology—Head and Neck Surgery, 138*, 300–306.

Pichichero, M. E. (2010, June). AOMT: Changing incidence, changing pathogens. *Infectious Diseases in Children*, 10–12.

Pichichero, M. E. (2011). Bacterial conjunctivitis in children: Antibacterial treatment options in an era of increasing drug resistance. *Clinical Pediatrics, 50*(1), 7–13.

Pichichero, M. E., Casey, J. R., Hoberman, A., & Schwartz, G. (2008). Pathogens causing recurrent and difficult-to-treat acute otitis media, 2003–2006. *Clinical Pediatrics, 47*, 901–906.

Pieper, P. (2010). Epidemiology and prevention of sports-related eye injuries. *Injury Prevention, 36*, 359–361.

Pray, J. L., & Jordan, I. K. (2010). The deaf community and culture at a crossroads: Issues and challenges. *Journal of Social Work in Disability and Rehabilitation, 9*, 168–193.

Proctor, S. E. (2009). A course in vision screening for school nurses. *NASN School Nurse, 24*, 254–261.

Quintanilla-Dieck, M. L., Artunduaga, M. A., & Eavey, R. D. (2009). Intentional exposure to loud music: The second MTV.com survey reveals an opportunity to educate. *Journal of Pediatrics, 155*, 550–555.

Rubin, L. G., Papsin, B., & Committee on Infectious Diseases and Section on Otolaryngology—Head and Neck Surgery. (2010). Cochlear implants in children: Surgical site infections and prevention and treatment of acute otitis media and meningitis. *Pediatrics, 126*, 381–391.

Rudolph, C., Rudolph, A., Lister, G., First, L., & Gershon, A. (2011). *Rudolph's pediatrics* (22nd ed.). New York, NY: McGraw-Hill.

Salvin, J. H., Lehman, S. S., Jin, J., & Hendricks, D. H. (2010). Update on retinopathy of prematurity: Treatment options and outcomes. *Current Opinion in Ophthalmology, 21*, 329–334.

Sarrell, E. M., Cohen, H. A., & Kahan, E. (2003). Naturopathic treatment for ear pain in children. *Pediatrics, 111*, e574–579.

Shaikh, N., & Hoberman, A. (2010, January). Update: Acute otitis media. *Pediatric Annals*, 28–33.

Shargorodsky, J., Curhan, S. G., Curhan, G. C., & Eavey, R. (2010). Change in prevalence of hearing loss in U.S. adolescents. *Journal of the American Medical Association, 304*, 772–778.

Smith, D. F., & Boss, E. F. (2010). Racial/ethnic and socioeconomic disparities in the prevalence and treatment of otitis media in children in the United States. *Laryngoscope, 120*, 2306–2312.

Spektor, Z. (2010, June). AOE: Predisposing factors and pathogens. *Infectious Diseases in Children*, 3–6.

Subcommittee on Management of Acute Otitis Media, American Academy of Pediatrics. (2004). Diagnosis and management of acute otitis media. *Pediatrics, 113*, 1451–1465.

Tepedino, M. E. (2010). Consider new fluoroquinolone for the treatment of bacterial conjunctivitis. *Infectious Diseases in Children, 23*(9), 56–61.

Tigchelaar, H., Kannikeswaran, H., & Kamat, D. M. (2008, June). Gonococcal conjunctivitis. *Consultant for Pediatricians*, 241–243.

Trope, M. (2011). Avulsion of permanent teeth: Theory to practice. *Dental Traumatology, 27*, 281–294.

Trumler, A. A. (2011). Evaluation of pediatric cataracts and systemic disorders. *Current Opinion in Ophthalmology, 22*, 365–379.

University of the State of New York. (2011). *School vision screening guidelines*. Albany, NY: Author.

U.S. Department of Health and Human Services. (2010). *Healthy People 2020*. Retrieved from http://www.healthypeople.gov

U.S. Department of Health and Human Services (2011). *Report on carcinogens* (12th ed.). Retrieved from http://ntp.niehs.nih.gov/ntp/roc/twelfth/roc12.pdf

U.S. Food and Drug Administration. (2011). *Public Health Advisory—FDA recommends that over-the-counter (OTC) cough and cold products not be used for infants and children under 2 years of age*. Retrieved from http://www.fda.gov/drugs/drugsafety

U.S. Preventive Services Task Force. (2008). Universal screening for hearing loss in newborns: U.S. Preventive Services Task Force recommendation statement. *Pediatrics, 122*, 143–148.

U.S. Preventive Services Task Force. (2011). *Vision screening*. Retrieved from http://www.ahrq.gov/news/visioneng.htm

Vohra, S., Johnston, B. C., Laycock, K. L., Midodzi, W. K., Dhunnoo, I., Harris, E., & Baydala, L. (2008). Safety and tolerability of North American ginseng extract in the treatment of pediatric upper respiratory tract infection: A phase II randomized, controlled trial of 2 dosing schedules. *Pediatrics, 122*, e402–410.

Wagner, R. S. (2011, May). Differentiating bacterial conjunctivitis from allergic and viral conjunctivitis. *Infectious Diseases in Children*, 4–9.

Williamson, I. (2011, January 12). Otitis media with effusion in children. *Clinical Evidence*, pii:0502 .

Yang, M., Quah, B. L., Seah, L. L., & Looi, A. (2009). Orbital cellulitis in children—Medical treatment versus surgical management. *Orbit, 28*(2–3), 124–136.

Young, N.M., Reilly, B.K., & Burke, L. (2011). Limitations of universal newborn screening in early identification of pediatric cochlear implant candidates. *Archives of Otolaryngology, Head and Neck Surgery 137*, 230–234.

Zhao, F., Manchaian, V. K., French, D., & Price, S. M. (2010). Music exposure and hearing disorders: An overview. *International Journal of Audiology, 49*, 54–64.

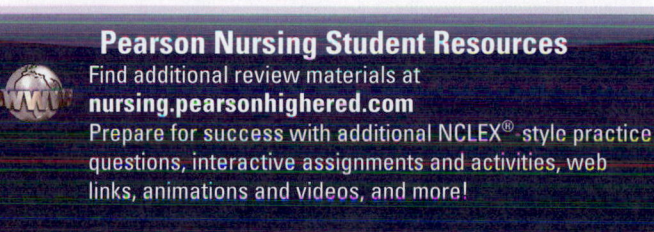

Pearson Nursing Student Resources

Find additional review materials at
nursing.pearsonhighered.com
Prepare for success with additional NCLEX® style practice questions, interactive assignments and activities, web links, animations and videos, and more!

CHAPTER 25
Alterations in Respiratory Function

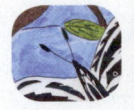 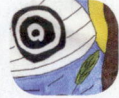 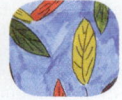

Learning Outcomes

After completing this chapter, you will be able to:

1. Describe unique characteristics of the pediatric respiratory system's anatomy and physiology and apply that information to the care of children with respiratory conditions.

2. Contrast respiratory conditions and injuries that can cause respiratory distress in infants and children.

3. Distinguish between mild, moderate, and severe respiratory distress, and plan the appropriate nursing care for each level of respiratory distress severity.

4. Assess the child's respiratory status and analyze the need for oxygen supplementation.

5. Differentiate between the signs and symptoms of a child with an upper airway and lower airway respiratory condition.

6. Create a nursing care plan for a child with a common acute respiratory condition.

7. Plan the nursing care for a child with a chronic respiratory condition.

8. Demonstrate the nursing assessment for a child with an acute lung injury.

> **"It scares me when Hannah has trouble breathing. Usually she gets better pretty fast when she uses her inhaler. Mom and Dad were really scared when she was in the hospital."**
>
> —*Simon, age 6*

Hannah McGregor, a 9-year-old with asthma, lives at home with her parents and two brothers who are 6 and 4 years old. Hannah developed asthma at about 5 years of age and has had wheezing episodes that were generally controlled by rescue medications. Two weeks ago Hannah had a severe asthma episode that started at school and was possibly associated with the paint or glue used on a project. She did not have any quick-relief medications at school, and she delayed going to the school nurse to finish her project. By the time her mother arrived to pick her up, she was in respiratory distress. After receiving treatment in the emergency department, Hannah was admitted to the pediatric intensive care unit (PICU).

Two weeks later, Hannah and her mother are in the health center to meet with the nurse practitioner to learn more about asthma management. At today's visit her lungs are clear to auscultation, and her peak expiratory flow reading is in the green zone. Mrs. McGregor reports that she has given all prescribed medications since the hospitalization. Both Hannah and her mother are motivated to prevent a future hospital admission if possible. The nurse practitioner uses a model to show Hannah how asthma narrows her airway and makes it difficult to breathe. She then works with Mrs. McGregor and Hannah to develop a plan for asthma control with daily medications.

What are the current recommendations for managing Hannah's asthma and to help prevent asthma episodes? How should Hannah handle future episodes that start at school? What arrangements are needed for Hannah to have access to her medications at school?

This chapter explores several special factors in the child's respiratory system that create ongoing threats to respiratory function and overall health. Most respiratory problems in children produce mild symptoms, last a short time, and can be managed at home. Other respiratory conditions are chronic and have a significant impact on the child's growth and development. Pediatric respiratory conditions may occur as a primary problem or as a complication of nonrespiratory conditions. They may be life threatening or have long-term implications. Respiratory conditions are the most common cause of hospitalization in children between birth and 9 years of age and a leading cause in youth between 10 and 17 years of age (Yu, Wier, & Elixhauser, 2011).

Respiratory conditions may be a result of structural problems, functional problems, or a combination of both. Structural problems involve alterations in the size and shape of parts of the respiratory tract. Functional problems involve alterations in gas exchange and threats to this normal process from irritants (such as large particles and chemicals) or invaders (such as viruses or bacteria). Alterations in other organ systems, especially the immune and neurologic systems, may also threaten respiratory function. Nurses must learn to assess the child's current respiratory status quickly, monitor progress, and anticipate potential complications. When reading this chapter, keep in mind the distinction between structural and functional problems to help you understand what is normal and what is abnormal about the child's maturing respiratory system. Refer to Chapter 24 🔴 for information on upper respiratory conditions such as colds, otitis media, sinusitis, and pharyngitis.

ANATOMY AND PHYSIOLOGY

The respiratory system is composed of both the upper and lower airways. The upper airway, containing the nasopharynx and oropharynx, serves as the pathway for gases exchanged during **ventilation,** the movement of oxygen into the lungs and carbon dioxide out of the lungs. The airway has a mucosal lining covered with cilia (tiny hairs) that assists in the humidification of inspired air. Mucosal secretions and cilia movements promote the removal of foreign particles from the air as it travels to the lungs. The larynx divides the upper and lower airways. The lower airways (trachea, bronchi, and bronchioles) serve as the pathway of gases to the alveoli of the lungs. The left lung is divided into two lobes, and the right lung is divided into three lobes. Alveolar sacs surrounded by capillaries are located at the end of the airways and are the site of gas exchange, where oxygen diffuses across the alveolocapillary membrane. Surfactant secreted by alveolar cells coats the inner surface of the alveolus to allow expansion during inspiration. The lung tissue surrounding the airways keeps them from collapsing as the oxygen moves in and carbon dioxide moves out during ventilation. The lungs are positioned in the thoracic cavity, where the ribs and muscles protect the lungs from injury.

The intercostal muscles work with the diaphragm to perform the work of breathing. The diaphragm is a muscle that separates the abdominal and thoracic cavity contents. When the diaphragm contracts, it creates negative pressure that increases the thoracic cavity's volume and pulls air into the lungs. The lungs and chest wall have the ability to expand during inspiration (**compliance**) and then to recoil or return to the resting state with expiration. The work of breathing is tied to the muscular effort required for ventilation, which can be increased in cases of disorders that increase stiffness of the lungs or obstruct the airways.

The respiratory center in the brain controls respiration, sending impulses to the respiratory muscles to contract and relax. Breathing is usually involuntary as the nervous system automatically adjusts the ventilatory rate and volume to maintain normal gas exchange (Brashers, 2010b). Chemoreceptors monitor the pH, $PaCO_2$, and PaO_2 in the arterial blood and send signals to the respiratory center to increase ventilation in cases of arterial hypoxemia. Effective gas exchange requires a near even distribution of ventilation and **perfusion** (oxygenated blood flow to all portions of the lungs). As oxygen diffuses across the alveolocapillary membrane, it dissolves in the plasma and the resulting pressure (PaO_2) helps bind the oxygen to the hemoglobin molecules where it is then transported to the cells for metabolism. Carbon dioxide produced by cellular metabolism is dissolved in the plasma (PCO_2) and/or as bicarbonate and travels back to the lungs where it diffuses across the alveolocapillary membrane (Brashers, 2010b).

PEDIATRIC DIFFERENCES

The child's respiratory tract constantly grows and changes until about 12 years of age. The young child's neck is shorter than an adult's, resulting in airway structures that are closer together.

Upper Airway Differences

The child's tracheal airway is shorter and narrower than an adult's airway. These differences create a greater potential for obstruction (Figure 25–1 ■). The infant's airway is approximately 4 mm in diameter, about the width of a drinking straw, in contrast to the adult's airway diameter of 20 mm. The child's little finger is a good estimate for the child's tracheal diameter and can be used for a quick assessment of airway size. The trachea primarily increases in length rather than diameter during the first 5 years of life. The tracheal division of the right and left bronchi is higher in a child's airway and at a different angle than the adult's (Figure 25–2 ■). The cartilage that supports the trachea is more flexible, and the airway may become compressed if the head and neck are not appropriately positioned.

The child's narrower airway causes a greater increase in **airway resistance,** the effort or force needed to move oxygen through the trachea to the lungs. As air moves from the child's nares down the trachea to the distal airways (alveoli), it must flow through a relatively small area. Friction and increasing resistance are generated as air passes through the airway. When edema and swelling of the trachea occur in response to a virus, bacterium, or other irritant, the airway is further narrowed, and air is inspired more quickly to maintain oxygenation status (Figure 25–3 ■). The resulting negative pressure in the airway draws tissues closer together, further narrowing the airway and increasing airway resistance.

Newborns are obligatory nose breathers. The only time a newborn breathes through the mouth is when he or she is crying. The coordination of mouth breathing is controlled by maturing neurologic pathways; thus, infants up to 2 to 3 months of age do not automatically open the mouth to breathe when the nose is obstructed. It is essential to keep the newborn's nose patent for such activities as breathing and eating. Infants, children, and adults can breathe through either the nose or the mouth.

As They Grow Comparison of Airway Structures

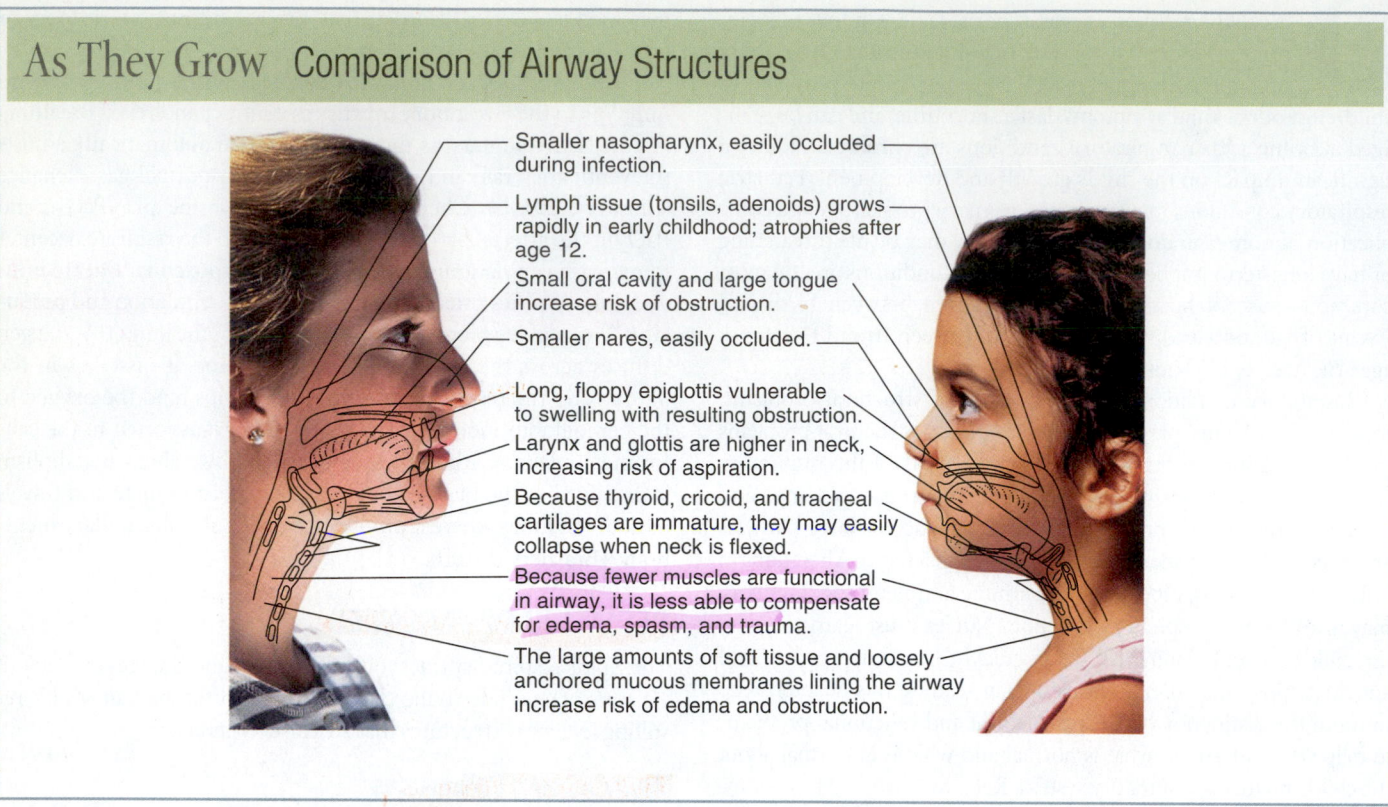

Smaller nasopharynx, easily occluded during infection.

Lymph tissue (tonsils, adenoids) grows rapidly in early childhood; atrophies after age 12.

Small oral cavity and large tongue increase risk of obstruction.

Smaller nares, easily occluded.

Long, floppy epiglottis vulnerable to swelling with resulting obstruction.

Larynx and glottis are higher in neck, increasing risk of aspiration.

Because thyroid, cricoid, and tracheal cartilages are immature, they may easily collapse when neck is flexed.

Because fewer muscles are functional in airway, it is less able to compensate for edema, spasm, and trauma.

The large amounts of soft tissue and loosely anchored mucous membranes lining the airway increase risk of edema and obstruction.

FIGURE 25–1 ■ It is easy to see that a child's airway is smaller and less developed than an adult's airway, but why is this important? The infant and child are more vulnerable to the consequences of an upper respiratory tract infection, enlarged tonsils and adenoids, an allergic reaction, positioning of the head and neck during sleep, and small objects that can be aspirated. All can cause an airway obstruction that results in respiratory distress.

As They Grow Trachea Position

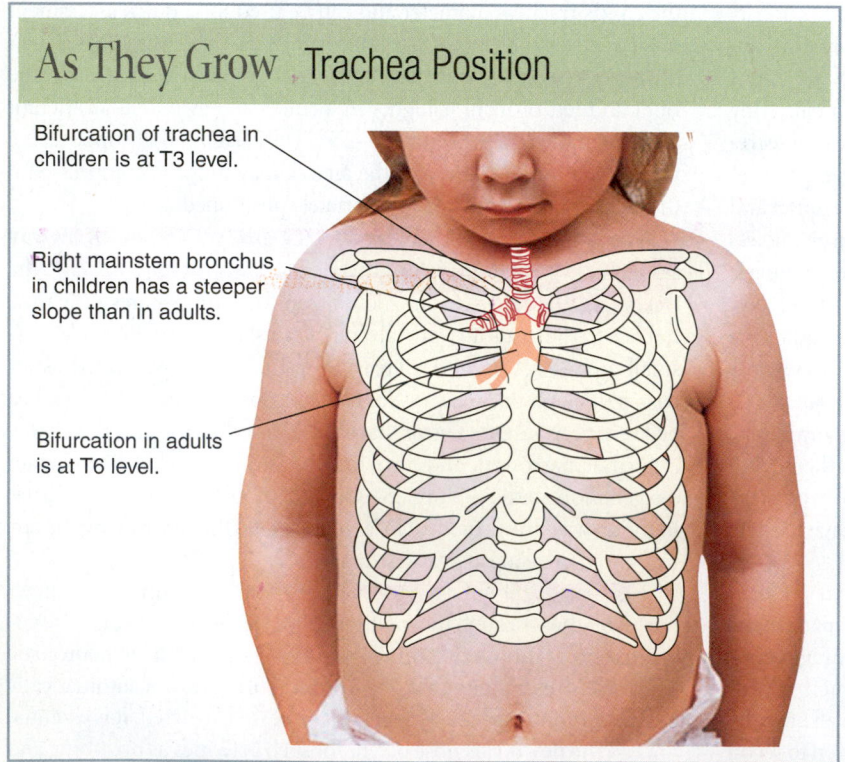

Bifurcation of trachea in children is at T3 level.

Right mainstem bronchus in children has a steeper slope than in adults.

Bifurcation in adults is at T6 level.

FIGURE 25–2 ■ In children, the trachea is shorter and the angle of the right bronchus at bifurcation is more acute than in the adult. Where is an aspirated foreign body likely to land? When you are resuscitating or suctioning, you must allow for the differences in the length of the trachea because it is easier to slip into the right bronchus with an endotracheal tube or suction catheter.

Lower Airway Differences

While the tracheobronchial tree is complete in a full-term newborn, the child's lower airway is also constantly growing. Gas exchange cannot occur in preterm infants before 24 weeks' gestation because lung sacs have not yet developed. By 32 weeks' gestation, developed lung sacs begin differentiating into alveoli (Smith, McKay, van Asperen, et al., 2010). Full-term newborns have only 25 million alveoli. These alveoli are not fully developed, and the distal bronchioles that extend to the alveoli are narrow and fewer in number than in an adult. After 8 years of age the alveoli begin increasing in size and complexity. The number of alveoli increases to 300 million by adulthood (Brashers, 2010b).

The bronchi and bronchioles are lined with smooth muscle, but these are undeveloped in newborns. By 5 months of age an infant has sufficient muscles to react to irritants by bronchospasm and muscle contraction.

Children under 6 years use the diaphragm to breathe because the intercostal muscles are immature. By 6 years of age the child uses the intercostal muscles more effectively. The ribs are primarily cartilage and very flexible. In cases of respiratory distress, the negative pressure caused by the diaphragm movement causes the chest wall

Pathophysiology Illustrated Airway Diameter

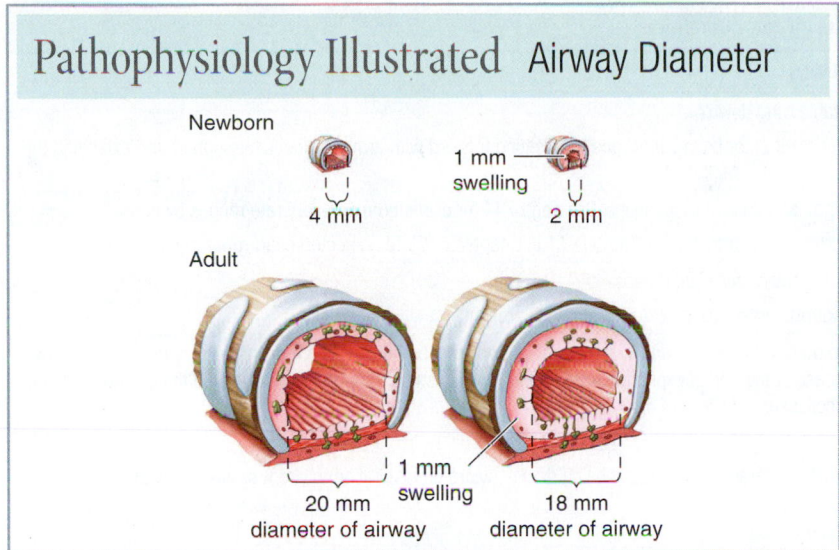

FIGURE 25–3 ■ The diameter of an infant's airway is approximately 4 mm, in contrast to an adult's airway diameter of 20 mm. An inflammatory process in the airway causes swelling that narrows the airway, and airway resistance increases. Note that swelling of 1 mm reduces the infant's airway diameter to 2 mm, but the adult's airway diameter is only narrowed to 18 mm. Air must move more quickly in the infant's narrowed airway to get the same amount of air to the lungs. The friction of the quickly moving air against the side of the airway increases airway resistance. The infant must use more effort to breathe and breathe faster to get adequate oxygen.

Pathophysiology Illustrated Retraction Sites

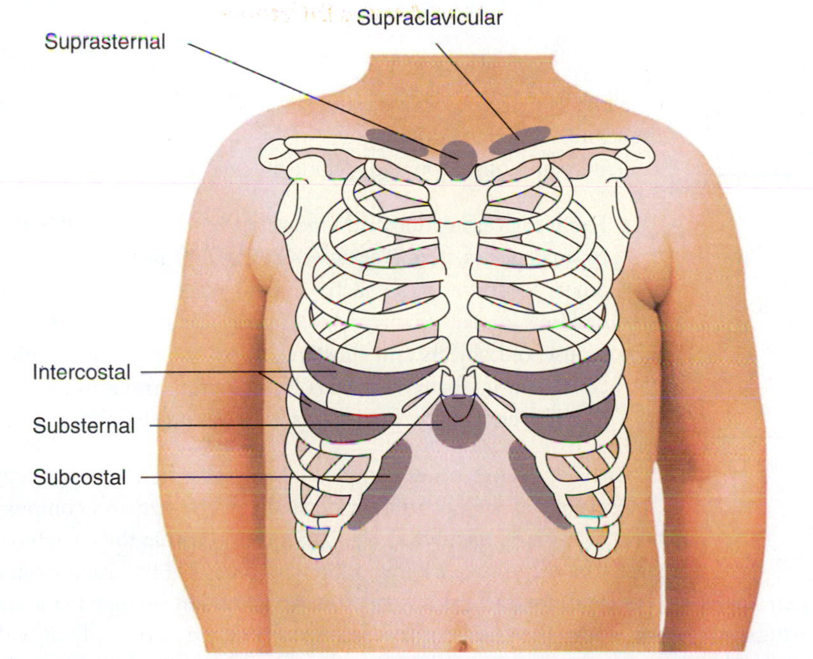

Suprasternal

Supraclavicular

Intercostal

Substernal

Subcostal

FIGURE 25–4 ■ The chest wall is flexible in infants and young children because the chest muscles are immature and the ribs are cartilaginous. With respiratory distress, the negative pressure created by the downward movement of the diaphragm to draw in air is increased, and the chest wall is pulled inward causing retractions. Intercostal retractions are seen in mild respiratory distress. As the severity of respiratory distress increases, retractions can be seen in the substernal and subcostal areas. In cases of severe distress, accessory muscles (sternocleidomastoid and trapezius muscles) are used, and retractions are seen in the supraclavicular and suprasternal areas.

to be drawn inward causing **retractions,** seen as sunken areas between the ribs during inspiration. See Figure 25–4 ■ for sites of retractions associated with respiratory distress.

Oxygen consumption is higher in children than adults because of their greater metabolic rate. This rate of oxygen consumption increases when the child is in respiratory distress. The child also has fewer muscle glycogen reserves, leading to more rapid muscle fatigue when accessory muscles must be used for breathing (Gott & Froh, 2010).

Respiratory Assessment

Performing a nursing assessment of the child with a potential or actual respiratory condition involves a careful review of the signs and symptoms in many body systems and analysis of their relationship to respiratory functioning. Use the guidelines in Table 25–1 to perform a comprehensive assessment of a child with a respiratory condition. Numerous diagnostic procedures and laboratory tests are used for the diagnosis of respiratory conditions (Table 25–2). Additional information about these diagnostic procedures and laboratory tests can be found in Appendixes D and E ⓔ.

RESPIRATORY DISTRESS AND RESPIRATORY FAILURE

Many conditions associated with the respiratory system progress from difficulty breathing to respiratory distress. If the condition is not managed effectively, it can progress further to respiratory failure. Recognition of the child's respiratory signs and symptoms is a critical nursing role so that appropriate care is provided to prevent the progression to respiratory failure. Foreign body aspiration is a common cause of airway obstruction and respiratory distress.

Foreign Body Aspiration

Airway obstruction exists when the air passage in the respiratory tract and lungs is slowed or blocked. Foreign body aspiration is the inhalation of any object (solid or liquid, food or nonfood) into the respiratory tract. In young children, aspiration occurs most often during feeding and reaching activities, while crawling, or during playtime. It is a major health threat for infants and young toddlers because of their increasing mobility and tendency to place small objects in the mouth. However, aspiration may occur in children of any age.

Foreign body aspirations are a common cause of unintentional injury in the home among children. In 2007 in the United States, 162 children less than 20 years of age died from foreign body aspiration, and 37% of these deaths were related to food aspiration. Nearly 75% of these children were younger than age 3 years (Levin & Smith, 2010).

TABLE 25–1	Assessment Guidelines for the Child with a Respiratory Condition*
ASSESSMENT FOCUS	**ASSESSMENT GUIDELINES**
Position of comfort	■ Is the child comfortable lying down? ■ Does the child prefer to sit up or be in **tripod position** (sitting forward with arms on knees for support and extending the neck)?
Vital signs	■ Assess the rate, depth, and ease of respirations. See page 744 for expected respiratory rate ranges by age. ■ Assess the pulse for rate and strength. See Table 7–11 in Chapter 7 🖉 for expected heart rate ranges by age.
Lung auscultation	■ Are breath sounds bilateral, diminished, or absent? ■ Are **adventitious sounds** (wheezes, crackles, or rhonchi) present?
Respiratory effort (work of breathing)	■ Is **stridor** (audible crow-like inspiratory and expiratory breath sounds) present? Is there **grunting** (a sound produced by the rapid breath release at the end of expiration after the newborn has used the vocal cords to hold the expiratory breath to prevent alveolar collapse)? ■ Is breathing labored? ■ Are retractions (visible appearance of the chest being drawn inward on inspiration) present or are accessory muscles used to breathe? ■ Is nasal flaring present? ■ Is **tachypnea** (abnormally rapid respiratory rate) present? ■ Can the child say a full sentence, or is a breath needed every few words? Is the cry strong or weak? ■ Do the chest and abdomen rise simultaneously with inspiration, or is **paradoxical breathing** present in which the chest and abdomen do not rise simultaneously?
Color	■ What is the color of the mucous membranes, skin, and nail beds? Pink, pale, cyanotic, or **mottled** (patches of pink, pale, and cyanotic skin)? ■ Does crying improve or worsen the color?
Cough	■ Is the cough dry (nonproductive), wet (productive, mucousy), brassy (noisy, musical), or croupy (barking, seal-like)? ■ Is the coughing effort forceful or weak?
Behavior change	■ Is irritability, restlessness, or change in level of responsiveness present?
Family history	■ Is there a family history of asthma or cystic fibrosis?

Note: *Refer to Chapter 7 🖉 for the actual techniques of assessment mentioned in this table.

TABLE 25–2	Diagnostic Procedures and Laboratory Tests for the Respiratory System*
DIAGNOSTIC PROCEDURES	**LABORATORY TESTS**
Bronchoscopy	Arterial blood gas analysis
Chest radiograph	Cultures
Polysomnography (sleep study)	Neonatal screening for cystic fibrosis
Pulse oximetry	Protein-purified derivative (PPD), the Mantoux test
Spirometry (pulmonary function tests)	
Sweat chloride test	

Note: *See Appendixes D and E 🖉 for information about these diagnostic procedures and for expected laboratory tests values.

Etiology and Pathophysiology

In infants and young children, aspiration may be caused when small objects are placed in the child's mouth. Coordinated chewing and swallowing does not fully develop until 4 years of age (Levin & Smith, 2010). Foreign body aspiration may also occur more commonly in children with neuromuscular disorders, developmental delay, or any condition that may impair chewing and swallowing. Many aspirations occur when young children, who have something in their mouths, take a deep and rapid inspiration after bumping their heads

or falling. Children also have a cough that is less effective at removing the aspirated foreign body.

Items commonly aspirated include the following:

- Foods such as hot dogs, nuts, popcorn, hard candy, meat bones, or small pieces of raw vegetables and fresh fruit
- Small, loose toy parts such as small wheels, bells, and latex balloons
- Household objects and substances such as beads, safety pins, coins, buttons, batteries, and colorful liquids (mouthwash, perfume) in enticing packages (small screw bottle tops)

Partial and sometimes complete airway obstruction may occur. The severity of the obstruction depends on the size and composition of the object or substance and its location within the respiratory tract. The majority of aspirated foreign bodies (AFBs) usually cause bronchial, not tracheal, obstruction. An object lodged high in the airway above the vocal cords is frequently coughed out easily or with some assistance (such as use of chest thrusts and back blows or the abdominal thrust). The right lung is the more common site of lower airway aspiration because of the sloped angle of its bronchus (see Figure 25–2). Objects may migrate from higher to lower airway locations. An object may also move back up to the trachea, creating extreme respiratory difficulty. When an object is lodged in the trachea

Clinical Manifestations   Airway Obstructions in Different Locations

LOCATION OF AIRWAY OBSTRUCTION	CLINICAL MANIFESTATION
Nasopharyngeal obstruction, enlarged tonsils or adenoids	Sonorous snoring
Partially obstructed upper airway (in or above the larynx, and upper trachea)	Inspiratory stridor
Obstruction of the mid to lower trachea and central bronchus	Expiratory stridor or wheeze, croupy or low-pitched cough
Fixed obstruction at site of larynx or subglottic space	Inspiratory and expiratory stridor
Obstructed vocal cords	Hoarseness, weak cry

Source: Data from Gott, K., & Froh, D. K. (2010). Alterations in pulmonary function in children. In K. L. McCance, S. E. Huether, V. L. Brashers, & N. S. Rote, Pathophysiology: The biologic basis for disease in adults and children (6th ed., p. 1311). St. Louis, MO: Mosby.

it is a life-threatening situation. If the obstruction causes severe hypoxia, brain damage may occur.

Clinical Manifestations

The child may initially have a sudden onset of choking, spasmodic coughing, or shortness of breath without fever or other symptoms of illness. After the AFB moves into the airway, compression of the trachea may lead to signs of increased respiratory effort such as **dyspnea** (difficulty breathing), tachypnea (increased respiratory rate), nasal flaring, and retractions. The child may also have neck or throat pain. As respiratory distress progresses, the child may have a concentrated focus on breathing or an anxious expression, signs of air hunger. The child may also sit in a forward position with the neck extended, as if to straighten out the airway. Retractions may not be present if air movement is diminished. As the child becomes increasingly hypoxic, behavior changes such as irritability and decreased responsiveness will be seen.

The older child who aspirates and has an airway obstruction may clutch the neck, the universal sign for choking. Coughing, choking, gagging, **dysphonia** (muffled, hoarse, or absent voice sounds), and wheezing may be brief or may persist for several hours if the object drops below the trachea into one of the mainstem bronchi. The child may also have unilateral decreased breath sounds if the object lodges in the right mainstem bronchus.

In some cases the child becomes asymptomatic after coughing for 15 to 30 minutes as the child's airway adapts to the foreign body. See the Clinical Manifestations table above for signs associated with obstructions in various locations of the airway. If the foreign body drops into the lower airway and is not removed, the child may present weeks later with complications of the aspiration, such as a chronic cough, persistent or recurrent pneumonia, or a lung abscess.

Collaborative Care

Initial management is focused on maintaining a patent airway and relieving the airway obstruction.

Diagnostic Tests

Children are usually brought to the hospital after a sudden episode of coughing. A careful history is taken to determine whether aspiration actually occurred. Coughing, gagging, or choking in a child associated with feeding or crawling on the floor is usually a confirming event for an aspiration. The physical examination may reveal

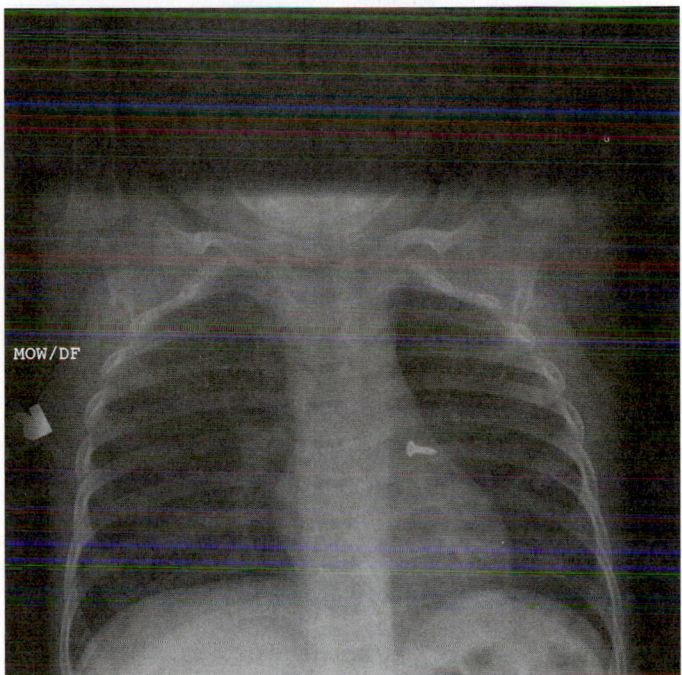

FIGURE 25–5 ■ An aspirated screw is clearly visible in the child's left mainstem bronchus on this chest radiograph.

Source: Courtesy of Evelyn Anthony, MD, Department of Radiology, Brenner Children's Hospital, Wake Forest University Health Sciences.

decreased breath sounds, stridor, and respiratory distress in the child without a witnessed aspiration.

A chest radiograph is performed. When the object aspirated is radiopaque, it can be seen on the radiograph (Figure 25–5 ■). Because most objects aspirated are organic, only 15% of the objects are radiopaque (Srivastava, 2010). A forced expiratory radiograph may be ordered to detect local hyperinflation (air trapping) and a mediastinal shift away from the affected side, abnormalities that can be caused by the AFB. Air trapping occurs when the AFB acts as a valve, allowing more air to be inspired than expired.

Clinical Therapy

When a life-threatening total airway obstruction occurs, efforts to clear the obstruction include back blows and chest thrusts in an infant, or abdominal thrusts in older children. In the emergency department, oxygen is administered. When the foreign body is positioned above the larynx, efforts are made to visualize it with a laryngoscope and remove it with Magill forceps. Whenever possible, the child is taken to the operating room so that optimal conditions exist to protect and maintain the child's airway during removal of the foreign body. When a partial airway obstruction exists, fluoroscopy and fiber-optic bronchoscopy may be used to identify, locate, and extract the foreign body.

Following removal of the foreign body, the child is stabilized and observed for a few hours in a short-stay unit. Depending on the type of object, location of the object, and degree of obstruction, surgical removal and hospitalization may be required.

In some cases children are initially treated for pneumonia or asthma without recognizing that a foreign body is the cause of respiratory distress. This occurs more often when the AFB is not visualized on a radiograph. When the child is nonresponsive to medications, further diagnostic testing may reveal the foreign body (Srivastava, 2010). See the section on pneumonia, page 765, for clinical therapy for the child having complications from aspiration.

Nursing Management

Nursing management is focused on assessing and monitoring the child until the obstruction can be removed, supporting the child and family during the crisis, and preventing future airway obstructions.

Nursing Assessment and Diagnosis

Physiologic Assessment

The child with an acute AFB will be in respiratory distress. Perform the respiratory assessment following guidelines in Table 25–1. See Table 25–3 for expected respiratory rates by age. If the object remains lodged in the airway, observe the child for signs of increasing respiratory distress, especially vital signs, altered mental status, and audible wheezing on auscultation. Identify the types of retractions present to help determine the severity of respiratory distress. If the obstruction occurs above the trachea, inspiration is more affected. If the obstruction occurs below the trachea, expiration is more affected. Changes in breath sounds, from noisy to decreasing to absent, on the affected side may be noted. This can indicate that the object is moving and blocking a mainstem bronchus.

Practice Alert

If the child cannot say "P" in words like *Pluto* or *Peter Pan*, the expiratory effort is noticeably diminished as a result of the foreign body.

The depth and location of retractions is associated with the severity of respiratory distress. Isolated intercostal retractions indicate mild distress. Subcostal, suprasternal, and supraclavicular retractions indicate moderate distress. These retractions accompanied by use of accessory muscles in the neck indicate severe distress.

Attach the child to a cardiorespiratory monitor and **pulse oximeter** (a transcutaneous assessment method to detect the amount of hemoglobin saturated with oxygen [SpO_2]) to assess the child for subtle signs of increasing hypoxia associated with the airway obstruction (Figure 25–6 ▪). See Box 25–1 for guidelines to increase the accuracy of pulse oximeter readings. Constant assessment is performed as the child may develop a complete obstruction. Refer to the Skills Manual ⊂⊃.

TABLE 25–3	Normal Respiratory Rate Ranges by Age
AGE	**RESPIRATORY RATE PER MINUTE**
Newborn	30–60
1 year	20–40
3 years	20–30
6 years	16–22
10 years	16–20
17 years	12–20

BOX 25–1 **Guidelines for Increasing the Accuracy of Pulse Oximetry Readings**

- Place the sensor over clean and dry skin, such as a finger, toe, or earlobe. Avoid sites with blue, black, or green nail polish that can interfere with the sensor.
- Check the SpO_2 when the child is not moving or shivering to avoid false readings.
- Avoid exposing the sensor probe to bright light or sunshine as this may falsely increase the reading.
- Check the child's hemoglobin level. If the child has anemia, a normal pulse oximetry reading may not reflect good oxygen transport to the tissues.
- Make sure the heart rate detected by the pulse oximeter matches the child's heart rate by direct assessment for accuracy.
- Keep the child warm. The sensor may be unable to accurately detect pulsatile blood flow if the child has decreased perfusion, such as from shock or cold extremities.
- If checking the SpO_2 intermittently, be sure to place the sensor on the extremity opposite the one used to measure the blood pressure to avoid inaccurate readings.

Source: Data from Clark, A. P., Giuliano, K., & Chen, H. M. (2006). Pulse oximetry revisited: "But his O_2 was normal!" Clinical Nurse Specialist, 20(6), 268–272; Mininni, N. C., Herzer, T. D., Marino, M. L., & Kohler, W. (2009). Why continuous pulse oximetry is a must in critical care. American Nurse Today, 4(9), 34–36.

Practice Alert

These signs and symptoms signal the body's response to increased metabolic demands for oxygenation as a result of stress or impending illness:

- Increasing restlessness, irritability, unexplained sudden confusion
- Rapid heart rate accompanied by a rapid respiratory rate

Psychosocial Assessment

The unexpected and acute nature of the event creates anxiety for parents and child. The child will be anxious and fearful because of the difficulty breathing. Parents may experience a variety of other emotions—fear, anger, or guilt. Assess the family's level of distress and coping ability.

Developmental Assessment

As the child's condition stabilizes, observe how well the child's developmental abilities match the parents' understanding of age-appropriate behaviors. See Chapters 10 and 11 ⊘.

Common nursing diagnoses for a child with an AFB include the following:

- Airway Clearance, Ineffective related to obstruction by a foreign body
- Ventilation: Spontaneous, Impaired related to respiratory muscle fatigue

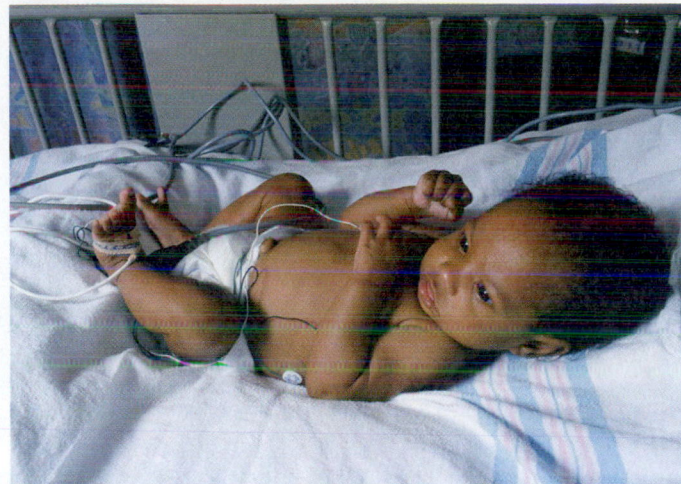

FIGURE 25–6 ■ Attach the pulse oximetry sensor over an area of the body that is clean and dry, and where blood vessels are relatively close to the skin, such as the foot of this infant. Alternative sites include a fingernail or toenail that has dark nail polish removed, or an earlobe.

- Anxiety (Child) related to difficulty breathing, unfamiliar surroundings, and procedures
- Injury, Risk for related to small objects in the environment

NANDA-I © 2012

Planning and Implementation

When the airway is totally obstructed, administer chest thrusts and back slaps to an infant, or abdominal thrusts to a child in an effort to remove the AFB. See Appendix F 🔗.

If the child has a partially obstructed airway, the period immediately after aspiration and until the foreign body can be removed is critical. The nurse should promptly report and document subtle changes in the child's respiratory and mental status during this period. A nurse must remain with the child who has significant airway obstruction, and emergency resuscitation equipment must be immediately accessible.

Allow the child to select the position of comfort. In many cases this will be sitting upright or a semi-Fowler position. Avoid performing any procedures that will increase the child's anxiety or stress. Sudden movements or increased respiratory effort may cause the obstruction to move and completely obstruct the airway. Keep the child and family informed about planned procedures and provide them with emotional support. Provide a quiet environment and encourage the presence of the parents to help reduce the child's fear and anxiety.

After the AFB is removed, the child is observed for a few hours in a short-stay unit to ensure that inflammation of the airway from the procedure and removed foreign body does not lead to a respiratory complication.

Discharge Planning and Home Care Teaching

Prevention of future foreign body aspirations is a major focus for nursing care. Provide education or reinforce information about developmental characteristics of the child and potential safety hazards in the environment. Encourage the parents to learn cardiopulmonary resuscitation (CPR), choking prevention techniques, and back blows, chest thrusts, or abdominal thrusts.

Evaluation

Expected outcomes of nursing care include the following:

- The child spontaneously ventilates after removal of the foreign body.
- Parents and children learn how to prevent future aspiration incidents.

Respiratory Failure and Acute Respiratory Distress Syndrome

Respiratory failure occurs when the body can no longer maintain effective gas exchange. It often results from a serious acute or chronic respiratory or neuromuscular condition.

Etiology and Pathophysiology

The physiologic process that ends in respiratory failure begins with hypoventilation of the alveoli. Hypoventilation occurs when the body's need for oxygen exceeds actual oxygen intake, such as when the airway is partially occluded, lung injury has occurred, or the exchange of oxygen and carbon dioxide in the alveoli is disrupted. This disruption may occur for any of the following reasons:

- A malfunction of the respiratory center stimulation occurs (the alveoli do not receive the message to diffuse, such as may occur with opioid overdose).
- The muscles of ventilation are fatigued and do not work effectively (e.g., a severe asthma episode or muscular dystrophy).
- The relationship between ventilation and perfusion (blood flow to the alveoli) is impaired (Figure 25–7 ■).

Poor ventilation of the alveoli results in **hypoxemia** (lower than normal blood oxygen level) and **hypercapnia** (an excess of carbon dioxide in the blood). See Appendix D 🔗 for expected laboratory values by age. When the blood levels of oxygen and carbon dioxide reach abnormal levels, **hypoxia** (lower than normal oxygen level in the tissues) occurs and respiratory failure begins.

Children may develop acute respiratory distress syndrome (ARDS), an acute respiratory failure (severe hypoxemia) caused by lung injury that does not respond to supplemental oxygen. The lung injury causes an inflammatory-immune response and alveolar-capillary membrane damage. Examples of conditions that injure the lungs include sepsis, pneumonia, meconium aspiration, aspiration of stomach contents, smoke inhalation, and near drowning. Information on most of these conditions is provided later in the chapter. See Chapter 33 🔗 for information on near drowning.

The increased permeability of the damaged alveolar-capillary membrane allows fluid and protein to accumulate in the alveoli, resulting in pulmonary edema. This in turn results in decreased lung compliance and functional residual capacity, reducing airflow and causing a ventilation-perfusion mismatch and hypoxemia (Gott & Froh, 2010). Other body systems may also contribute directly or indirectly to an increased workload, causing the respiratory system to fail.

Clinical Manifestations

Signs of respiratory distress worsen with impending respiratory failure and include irritability, lethargy, mottled color or cyanosis, diaphoresis, and increased respiratory effort such as dyspnea (difficulty breathing), tachypnea (increased respiratory rate), nasal flaring, and retractions. Grunting in infants is a sign of severe distress and the

Pathophysiology Illustrated Ventilation-Perfusion Ratio

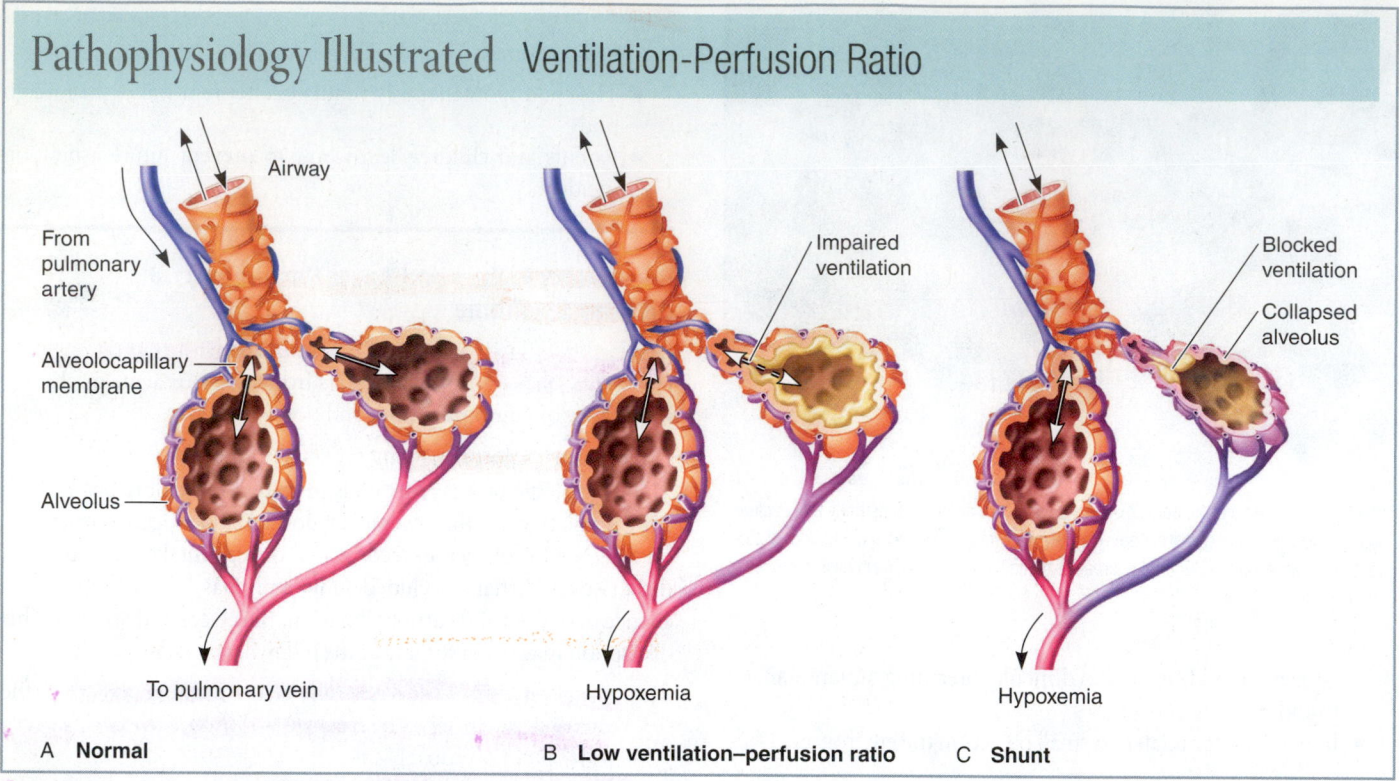

FIGURE 25–7 ■ A ventilation-perfusion mismatch can occur when an infant or child has an abnormal distribution of ventilation or perfusion. *A*, Children with normal lung function and circulation have a ventilation-perfusion ratio of 0.8 to 0.9 because perfusion is greater than ventilation (air exchange) in the lung bases. *B*, When ventilation is inadequate to well-perfused areas of the lungs, the ventilation-perfusion ratio is low or mismatched, resulting in shunting. Blood passing through the pulmonary capillaries gets less oxygen exchange than normal, and hypoxemia occurs. This is the case in asthma due to bronchoconstriction and in pneumonia because alveoli are filled with fluid. *C*, In the case of neonatal acute respiratory distress syndrome, ventilation does not occur because the alveoli are collapsed, so blood passes through the alveolar capillaries and no oxygenation occurs. The ventilation-perfusion ratio is very low with significant shunting that does not respond to oxygen therapy because the capillary bed never gets exposed to the supplemental oxygen (Brashers, 2010a).

Clinical Manifestations Respiratory Failure and Imminent Respiratory Arrest

PHYSIOLOGIC CAUSE	CLINICAL MANIFESTATIONS
Initial Respiratory Failure The child is attempting to compensate for an oxygen deficit and airway blockage. The oxygen supply is inadequate; behavior and vital signs reflect compensation and beginning hypoxia.	Restlessness Tachypnea Tachycardia Diaphoresis
Early Decompensation The child uses accessory muscles to assist oxygen intake; hypoxia persists and efforts now waste more oxygen than is obtained.	Nasal flaring Retractions Grunting Wheezing Anxiety and irritability Mood changes Headache Hypertension Confusion
Severe Hypoxia and Imminent Respiratory Arrest These signs occur because the oxygen deficit is overwhelming and beyond spontaneous recovery. Cerebral oxygenation is dramatically affected; central nervous system changes are ominous.	Dyspnea Bradycardia Cyanosis Stupor and coma

potential need for mechanical ventilation (Prodhan, Sharoor-Karni, Lin, et al., 2011). See the clinical manifestations table for signs of respiratory failure and imminent respiratory arrest.

Practice Alert

When the child in respiratory distress has had increased respiratory effort over a prolonged period, a decreasing respiratory rate is a critical sign of impending respiratory arrest. The ventilatory muscles are so fatigued that the child will soon stop breathing.

Collaborative Care

Physicians, nurses, and respiratory therapists collaborate on treating the respiratory failure and its cause in an effort to prevent its progression to death.

Diagnostic Tests

The child's history, vital signs, and respiratory signs provide important clues about the progression from respiratory distress to respiratory failure. Arterial blood gases help to identify hypoxemia and hypercapnia. Pulse oximetry provides a transcutaneous estimate of the hemoglobin saturated by oxygen (SpO_2), and it is expressed as the percentage of hemoglobin capable of transporting oxygen. Pulse oximetry helps to assess oxygenation, but not ventilation, and it helps determine when an arterial blood gas is needed. See Figure 25–8 ■ for guidelines to interpret pulse oximetry readings. See Appendix D 🔗 for normal ranges of arterial blood gases. Refer to Chapter 23 🔗 for

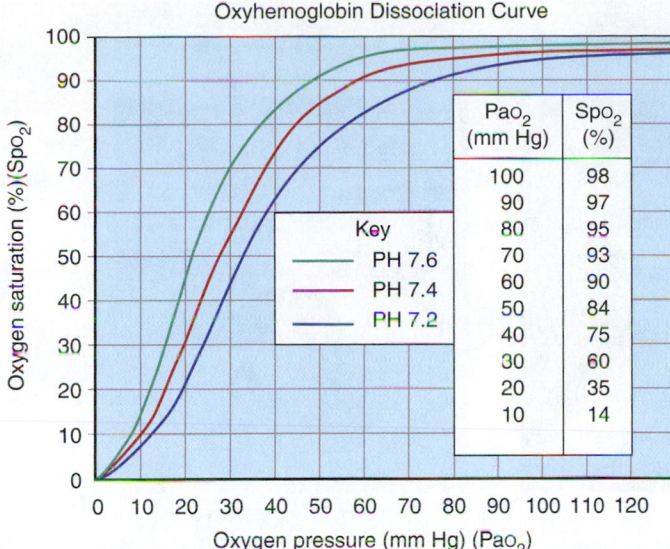

FIGURE 25–8 ■ The relationship between the partial pressure of oxygen in arterial blood (PaO₂) and pulse oximetry reading (SpO₂) is not linear. When hypoxia exists, the hemoglobin releases oxygen in the body tissues. When hypoxia does not exist, oxygen remains bound to the hemoglobin. A fall in pulse oximetry reading is associated with a more dramatic reduction in PaO₂. The oxyhemoglobin dissociation curve demonstrates the relationship between the SpO₂ and PaO₂ and is important in correctly interpreting the pulse oximetry reading. For example,

- When cardiac output is normal, the hemoglobin concentration is adequate, and the pH is normal (7.4), an SpO₂ above 93% to 95% is associated with a PaO₂ of 90 mmHg or adequate oxygen delivery.
- An SpO₂ of 90% or less indicates hypoxemia with a PaO₂ of 60 mmHg or less.
- An SpO₂ of 60% or less indicates severe hypoxemia with a PaO₂ of less than 30 mmHg.
- If anemia or low cardiac output is present, an SpO₂ greater than 95% can indicate inadequate oxygen delivery.
- If the child has a higher pH, the hemoglobin does not as easily release the oxygen to the tissues. In this case the oxyhemoglobin dissociation curve shifts to the left, and the SpO₂ of 90% is associated with a PaO₂ of 50 mmHg.
- If the child has a lower pH, the hemoglobin more readily releases oxygen to the tissues. In this case the oxyhemoglobin dissociation curve shifts to the right, and the SpO₂ of 90% is associated with a PaO₂ of greater than 70 mmHg.

interpretation of acidosis and alkalosis that must be considered simultaneously with assessment of oxygenation status. Hypercarbia in the presence of acidosis is a sign of respiratory failure. Hypoxemia unresponsive to supplemental oxygen is also a sign of respiratory failure.

Clinical Therapy

Medical management is focused on treating the cause of respiratory failure and reversing the severe hypoxemia with oxygen, mechanical ventilation, and positive end-expiratory pressure (PEEP) to increase functional residual capacity. These children are admitted to the pediatric intensive care unit (PICU).

As the child becomes more hypoxic, the level of responsiveness deteriorates and the child's ability to keep the airway patent decreases. As the level of responsiveness decreases, insertion of an endotracheal tube is needed to stabilize the airway. The tube must be protected and stabilized to prevent its displacement. End-tidal CO₂ monitoring is used to measure carbon dioxide expiration to ensure that the endotracheal tube is appropriately positioned in the trachea. See the Clinical Skills Manual ⬭. A **tracheostomy,** the creation of a surgical opening into the trachea through the anterior neck at the

cricoid cartilage, is often performed if long-term airway management is needed.

Assisted ventilation must be provided until the child breathes spontaneously or until mechanical ventilation is initiated. Children are often sedated to optimize ventilation. Continuous positive airway pressure (CPAP) is one form of PEEP used to improve oxygenation and lung compliance. When respiratory failure cannot be managed, it results in cardiopulmonary arrest.

When acute respiratory failure becomes life threatening, extracorporeal membrane oxygenation (ECMO) may be initiated (Ayad, Dietrich, & Mihalov, 2008). ECMO is a cardiopulmonary bypass system with external oxygenation and a pump mechanism that provides respiratory and hemodynamic support. It allows the lungs to rest and heal. However, several significant complications may result from its use, such as bleeding, stroke, renal insufficiency, hypertension, seizures, electrolyte abnormalities, pneumothorax, cardiac dysfunction, and infection (Ayad et al., 2008). This is a complex and expensive treatment available in special centers, so the child may have to be transferred to another hospital to receive this therapy.

Nursing Management

Nursing care is focused on the recognition of progression from respiratory distress to respiratory failure and supportive care to the child and family.

Nursing Assessment and Diagnosis

Monitor the child for changes in vital signs, respiratory status, and level of responsiveness. Perform the respiratory assessment using guidelines in Table 25–1. Signs and symptoms of respiratory compromise may progress rapidly. Detection of earlier subtle signs is important so interventions can be initiated to prevent progression to respiratory failure. Attach a cardiorespiratory monitor and pulse oximeter. Serial blood gases may be needed to monitor the child.

Practice Alert

When the child has a chronic respiratory or neuromuscular condition, development of respiratory failure may be gradual as muscles associated with breathing may be weakened. Signs will be subtle. Be particularly alert to behavior changes in addition to respiratory signs. Pulse oximetry and serial blood gases may be needed to monitor the child.

If the child has an endotracheal tube or tracheostomy tube, assess for secretions that may further obstruct the airway.

Examples of nursing diagnoses associated with respiratory failure include:

- Breathing Pattern, Ineffective associated with prolonged tachypnea and muscle fatigue
- Airway Clearance, Ineffective related to sedation and loss of protective cough reflex
- Communication: Verbal, Impaired related to artificial airway
- Family Processes, Interrupted related to child's life-threatening illness

NANDA-I © 2012

Planning and Implementation

Position the child with respiratory distress in an upright position (by elevating the head of the bed) with the head in midline to help maintain the airway. Administer oxygen as ordered (Figure 25–9 ■).

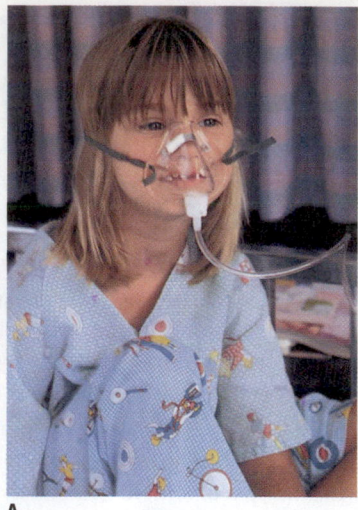
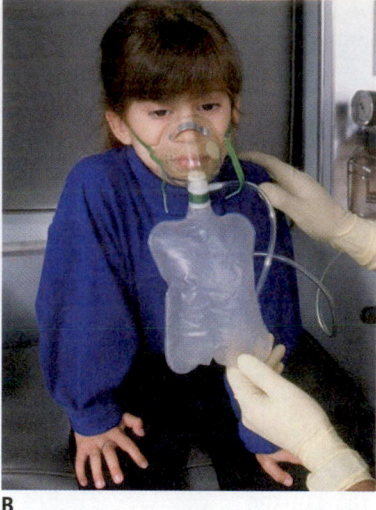
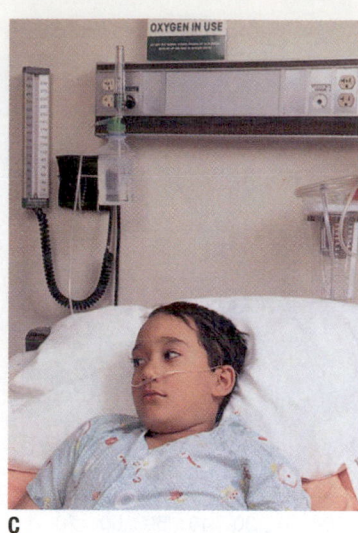

A **B** **C**

FIGURE 25–9 ■ Various oxygen delivery devices are used to provide supplemental oxygen to children. *A*, Simple face mask; *B*, Nonrebreather mask; *C*, Nasal cannula. Oxygen delivery devices are selected to match the concentration of oxygen needed by the child. In respiratory failure, a higher concentration of oxygen is needed to reverse the hypoxemia. Which oxygen delivery devices should be used? Are there any contraindications to oxygen use in a child who is hypoxic?

See the Skills Manual ⊂⊃ for a review of oxygen delivery systems and amount of oxygen delivered by each. Keep a bag-valve mask and emergency equipment readily available at the bedside to assist ventilations if respiratory status deteriorates.

Clinical Tip
Excessive crying and anxiety deplete metabolic reserves and increase oxygen demand. Comfort the child and avoid invasive procedures that will increase distress. Assisted ventilation and vigorous crying may both cause the stomach to become distended and impede diaphragmatic function. A nasogastric tube may be inserted to prevent stomach distention.

Because endotracheal and tracheostomy tubes prevent vocal cord vibration, children who are intubated cannot cry or talk. Once infants and young children who are intubated recover from the sedation or anesthesia, they often express initial frustration and fear when they cannot communicate verbally. Explain the reasons for the inability to cry and talk to the child and parents. When the child is alert, give suggestions for ways to make noise and gain attention when needed, such as striking the mattress. For older children obtain and demonstrate the use of a communication board. Keep the call light within easy reach.

Suction airway secretions as needed, and provide tracheostomy care if present. See the Skills Manual ⊂⊃ for tracheostomy care procedures. Provide good skin care around the endotracheal tube or tracheostomy to prevent breakdown over pressure points. Chest physiotherapy may also be prescribed.

Provide support to parents and children. The parents are stressed because of the life-threatening nature of the disorder. See Chapter 17 ❷. If the child's condition progresses, provide end-of-life care. See Chapter 18 ❷. Help the family identify resources and support to care for other children so parents may spend more time with the child who is critically ill. Provide age-appropriate information to the child once sedation wears off to reduce fear, and permit the parents to be with the child as much as possible.

Once the child begins responding to clinical therapy, the child is weaned from the ventilator and the endotracheal tube is removed. The child will be moved to the pediatric nursing unit for the remainder of treatment for the condition causing respiratory failure.

Discharge Planning and Home Care Teaching
Many children are discharged from the hospital and cared for at home for an extended period with a tracheostomy tube in place. It is essential to teach parents how to maintain and suction the airway, clean the tracheostomy site, and change the tube. They must demonstrate competence in all aspects of tracheostomy care, as well as emergency resuscitation skills adapted to the tracheostomy. Make a referral to a home health agency and supply company. Referral to social work for planning the financial needs related to home care is often needed. A home healthcare nurse can provide follow-up care and support for the child and family. See the Skills Manual ⊂⊃ for management of the tracheostomy tube.

Evaluation
Expected outcomes of nursing care include the following:

- The child's airway is supported and ventilated until the respiratory failure is reversed.
- A communication method for an alert child unable to talk is provided.
- Skin integrity around the artificial airway and pressure surfaces on the body is maintained.
- Family education and support for provision of home tracheostomy care is provided.

APNEA
Newborns normally have **periodic breathing,** an irregular rhythm with occasional pauses of up to 20 seconds between breaths. This breathing pattern is not apnea. **Apnea** is the cessation of respiration lasting longer than 20 seconds, or any pause in respiration associated with cyanosis, marked pallor, hypotonia, or bradycardia. Apnea can be characterized in the following ways:

- *Central apnea*—complete cessation of breathing effort
- *Obstructive apnea*—absence of nasal airflow when respiratory efforts are present (Remember that newborns are nasal breathers, and they do not open their mouths to breathe.)
- *Mixed apnea*—central respiratory pause that either precedes or follows airway obstruction

Apnea may be the first major sign of respiratory dysfunction in the neonate. Two types of apnea occur during infancy, but they are different conditions: apnea of prematurity and apparent life-threatening event.

Apnea of Prematurity

Apnea of prematurity (AOP) is defined as apnea in an infant born before 37 weeks' gestation, and it is often associated with immature respiratory control. Although the cause is unknown, it may occur when the infant's baseline CO_2 level (the physiologic stimulus for breathing) decreases below the apnea threshold (Al-Saif, Alvard, Manfreda, et al., 2008). Apneic episodes often occur during periods of active sleep.

Diagnostic procedures performed include a pneumogram and other tests to identify potential underlying conditions contributing to the AOP such as gastroesophageal reflux, sepsis, metabolic errors or electrolyte abnormalities, poor thermoregulation, seizures, and anatomic abnormalities.

Infants are treated with methylxanthines (usually caffeine). See Box 25–2 for research on caffeine therapy in low-birth-weight infants. Ventilator support may be used when apnea episodes are severe, and CPAP may be used when obstructive apnea is suspected. Episodes often disappear when the newborn's respiratory system matures, usually by 37 weeks' gestational age (Silvestri, 2009).

Nursing Management

Nurses play an important role in evaluating signs and symptoms associated with potential underlying conditions as well as monitoring the infant for apneic episodes.

Supportive care for AOP includes placing the neonate with the head at midline and the neck in the neutral position or slightly extended to minimize upper airway obstruction. Tactile stimulation, such as rubbing the infant's back or feet, often is enough to halt an apneic episode.

The medication dosage administered is small and must be carefully titrated. Monitor vital signs and clinical response. These drugs increase oxygen consumption and can diminish weight gain. Observe the infant for signs of caffeine toxicity, such as tachycardia, tachypnea, jitteriness, tremors, and unexplained seizures and vomiting.

BOX 25–2	Research: Caffeine Therapy in Low-Birth-Weight Infants

The Caffeine for Apnea of Prematurity randomized placebo-controlled trial involving 2,006 preterm infants (birth weights of 500 to 1250 g) was conducted to identify potential effects of prolonged administration of caffeine on the development of the brain and other organs. Caffeine significantly improved the infant's survival. Evaluation of infants at a corrected age of 18 to 21 months indicated that caffeine use did not place the infants at higher risk for neurodevelopmental disability. Caffeine also shortened the duration of supplemental oxygen therapy and assisted ventilation as well as reduced the incidence of bronchopulmonary dysplasia (Davis, Schmidt, Roberts, et al., 2010). When the same infants were evaluated at 5 years of age, caffeine did not result in significant differences in mortality and disability outcomes when compared to infants assigned to the placebo group (Schmidt, Anderson, Doyle, et al., 2012). The use of caffeine has also been found to be more cost-effective than the placebo treatment (Dukhovny, Lorch, Schmidt, et al., 2011).

Apparent Life-Threatening Event

An apparent life-threatening event (ALTE) is defined as a frightening episode of apnea accompanied by a skin color change (e.g., cyanosis or pallor), limp muscle tone, choking, or gagging. Infants at a median age of 2 months, but less than 12 months, are more commonly affected (Silvestri, 2008). The reported incidence for ALTE is about 0.6 to 9.4 per 1,000 live births (Bonkowsky & Tieder, 2009).

Etiology and Pathophysiology

Of ALTE episodes found to have a diagnosis, the most commonly associated conditions include gastroesophageal reflux, seizures, and lower respiratory tract infections. Less common associated conditions include trauma, metabolic disease, cardiac arrhythmias, sepsis, pertussis, and medication dosage error. Child abuse should also be considered as a potential cause of ALTE. ALTE and sudden infant death syndrome (SIDS) have different clinical and epidemiologic factors (Bonkowsky & Tieder, 2009).

Clinical Manifestations

The most common signs and symptoms include apnea, cyanosis, hypotonia, unresponsiveness, labored breathing, and lethargy. The infant may have pallor, or occasionally erythema rather than cyanosis. The parents are frightened by the episode and may fear the infant is dying. These episodes may occur during sleep, wakefulness, or feeding. The infant usually has no signs at the time of examination following the episode.

Collaborative Care

Once the stability of the child's cardiorespiratory system has been ensured, a detailed history is taken in an effort to detect potential conditions or causes of the ALTE.

Diagnostic Tests

The history should attempt to determine if the episode was associated with central apnea (the part of the brain that controls breathing during sleep does not function properly); central cyanosis (seen in the core of the body, tongue, and lips); or seizure activity versus obstructive apnea after choking, perioral cyanosis, or pallor. No minimum set of diagnostic tests has been identified for evaluation of the infant experiencing ALTE; however, initial tests may include an electrocardiogram, complete blood count with differential, serum electrolytes, cultures, serum ammonia levels, and a chest radiograph. **Polysomnography,** a sleep study, may be requested. Child abuse screening may include an ophthalmologic examination and computed tomography of the head. No cause is found for about 50% of ALTE cases (Bonkowsky & Tieder, 2009).

Clinical Therapy

Physical stimulation or emergency resuscitation may be required to revive the infant. A cardiorespiratory monitor and pulse oximeter are attached. The infant who appears to be well is rarely admitted to the hospital, but admission may be appropriate for young infants with prematurity, cases of suspected child abuse, infections, recurrent ALTEs, or a family history of genetic or metabolic conditions. Treatment is targeted toward the underlying condition, such as seizures, infection, or a metabolic condition. Some children with positive polysomnography testing may be sent home with cardiorespiratory monitors and event recorders to detect future events. Although home apnea monitoring is considered unnecessary for the child with no identifiable cause of ALTE, some children will be sent home with an apnea monitor for 4 to 6 weeks (Silvestri, 2009).

Nursing Management

Nursing care includes collecting a detailed history of the event, observing and monitoring cardiorespiratory status, providing supportive care to the infant and family, facilitating the diagnostic process, and anticipating the need for emergency resuscitation and for the diagnostic process.

Nursing Assessment and Diagnosis

Establish rapport with the parents to create a sense of trust. Do not give parents the impression that their parenting skills are being judged or questioned. Important historical information to collect is listed in Box 25–3. Additional information about birth history or perinatal insults, and medical conditions should also be collected. Consider if the story told about the event has any inconsistencies that raise the suspicion of potential child abuse.

Assess the infant's responsiveness and behavior, identifying irritability, decreased responsiveness, or unexplained sleepiness. Monitor vital signs, and assess the child's growth. The focus of the physical examination is to detect signs of injury, infection, neurologic abnormalities, or features suggestive of a genetic or metabolic syndrome. Attach a cardiorespiratory monitor and pulse oximeter to continuously assess the heart rate, respiratory rate, and oxygenation status while the infant is awake and asleep.

Examples of nursing diagnoses associated with ALTE include:

- Breathing Pattern, Ineffective related to airway obstruction or metabolic disorder
- Coping: Family, Compromised related to infant's potential life-threatening episode
- Breastfeeding, Interrupted related to infant's hospitalization and change in established routines
- Anxiety (Parents) related to concerns that another ALTE episode will occur

NANDA-I © 2012

BOX 25–3	Topics to Address in a Focused History for Infants with ALTE

- Before the event, what was the child doing (sleeping or awake, eating, coughing, crying, or vomiting)?
- What was observed during the event (apnea, choking, change in muscle tone, rhythmic shaking, eye deviation, change in mental status, change in skin color)?
- Who observed the event? How long did the event last? Was gentle stimulation or active resuscitation needed to end the event?
- Has the child had a prior ALTE episode and evaluation?
- Was the infant premature or have any conditions needing treatment after birth?
- Is there a family history of seizures, cardiac conditions, neurologic, genetic, or metabolic disorders?
- What medications does the child take? Could any medications have been given to the infant (e.g., cold medications)?
- What is the infant's interest in feeding and the feeding pattern? Is there any gagging or coughing with feeding?

Source: Data from Silvestri, J. M. (2008). Apparent life-threatening events in the young infant and neonate. Clinical Pediatric Emergency Medicine, 9, 184-190; Bonkowsky, J. L., & Tieder, J. S. (2009). A pragmatic approach to ALTEs. Contemporary Pediatrics, 26(11), 60; Marc, D., Berg, M. D., Nadkarni, V. M., Gausche-Hill, M., Kaji, A. H., & Berg, R. A. (2010). Apparent life threatening events. In J. A. Marx, R. S. Hockberger, R. M. Walls, J. G. Adams, W. G. Barsen, . . . E. J. Newton, Rosen's emergency medicine (7th ed., pp. 73–76). Philadelphia, PA: Elsevier Mosby.

Planning and Implementation

Provide Emotional Support

Establishing rapport and open communication with the family is essential for creating a sense of trust. Parents are naturally fearful and anxious if they witnessed the infant's episode and are concerned about a serious medical condition. Explanations of tests and treatment help to decrease parental anxiety and increase their understanding of the situation.

If the infant is hospitalized, encourage parents to hold and cuddle the infant to provide a sense of security and well-being. Encouraging parents' participation in the infant's care helps to meet these needs and promotes family bonding. Often parents are hesitant to touch the infant because they are afraid of disconnecting the monitoring cable. Wrapping the cable inside the infant's blanket helps secure the wires, increasing parents' feelings of confidence when handling the infant.

Assist the mother to continue breastfeeding and maintaining the supply of breast milk by pumping if necessary. Support the mother's desire to continue breastfeeding by ensuring that she gets adequate fluids and nutrition. Provide privacy for breast pumping, and store breast milk for future feedings.

Anticipate Emergency Resuscitation

Because the infant who has had an ALTE continues to be at risk for cardiopulmonary arrest, emergency resuscitation equipment and drugs should be readily accessible at all times.

Discharge Planning and Home Care Teaching

Address home care needs early in anticipation of the infant's discharge. Some infants will be sent home with an apnea monitor, and parents need to learn how to operate it. Review guidelines for safe sleep positioning. See Partnering with Families: Home Care Instructions for the Infant Requiring a Cardiorespiratory Monitor. Parents also need to learn what to do if the infant has another apneic episode as well as techniques for choking intervention. Teach parents to perform cardiopulmonary resuscitation and first aid for choking prior to discharge. Talk with parents about how to manage this new family stressor and still meet the needs of other family members. Refer to the Skills Manual ⌕.

Evaluation

Expected outcomes of nursing care include:

- The apneic episode is promptly managed and respirations are restored.
- Parents know how to identify and manage future apneic episodes.
- Breastfeeding is maintained, if the mother prefers.
- The infant's sense of security and development is promoted.

Obstructive Sleep Apnea

Obstructive sleep apnea syndrome (OSAS) is a disorder of breathing during sleep that is characterized by recurrent episodes of partial and complete obstruction of the upper airway that disrupts sleep and interferes with adequate respiration (Perez & Ward, 2008). This results in breathing difficulty and snoring when the child sleeps. OSAS occurs more commonly between 3 and 6 years of age when the tonsils and adenoids are at their largest in contrast to the airway's size. It is equally common in boys and girls. OSAS is believed to affect 1% to 3% of school-age children (Loghmanee & Sheldon, 2010).

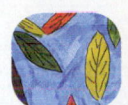

Partnering with Families

Home Care Instructions for the Infant Requiring a Cardiorespiratory Monitor

EMERGENCY PREPARATION

- Have an emergency plan and complete an emergency information form about the infant's health problem. Notify the telephone company, electric company, local rescue squad, and local emergency department (establishes priority status).
- Post or enter important phone numbers by or in all phones (e.g., rescue squad, physician, equipment company, power company, neighbor, parent work numbers).
- Learn CPR, back blows, and chest thrusts for airway obstruction
- Keep the monitor battery fully charged.

SAFETY PRECAUTIONS

- Place the monitor on a firm surface away from water; keep away from other appliances (television, microwave oven).
- Ensure that alarms are audible from all locations.
- Ensure that the monitor and event recorder are turned on.
- Thread cable and wires through the lower end of the infant's clothes.

ROUTINE CARE

- Understand reasons for the monitor and frequency of use. Review the manual for troubleshooting. The monitor should be used all the time, but if removed periodically, it should always be used while the infant is sleeping.

- Learn how to attach and detach the infant chest leads and belt. Care for the skin by moving patches correctly, and do not use oils or lotions on the chest. Evaluate the skin for irritation or sores under the electrodes, and move the electrode if the skin is irritated.

RESPONDING TO AN ALARM

- First observe the infant's respiratory movement to determine if the alarm is a real event or a loose lead.
- Stimulate the infant if respiration is absent or the infant is lethargic. Start by calling the infant's name and gently touching; proceed to vigorous touch if needed.
- If no response, proceed with CPR.

LOOSE LEAD

- Check electrode patches. Is one loose? Dirty? Is the belt loose?
- Check wires from the electrode or monitor cable.
- Check the power supply. Is the battery low? Power failure? Monitor malfunctioning?

Etiology and Pathophysiology

The upper airway contains about 30 muscles that permit the pharynx to collapse, enabling the child to talk and swallow, but also maintain airway patency. When the child is awake, muscle tone is maintained and the airway remains patent even when obstructions such as enlarged adenoids and tonsils, craniofacial anomalies, or obesity are present. During sleep, the airway muscles relax, the pharynx becomes obstructed, and airway resistance is increased, leading to snoring. Breathing during sleep is also less deep as the ventilatory drive decreases. During non–eye movement sleep the **tidal volume** (the amount of air inhaled and exhaled during a normal breath) and respiratory rate are lower, resulting in a lower volume breathed each minute (minute ventilation). During rapid eye movement sleep, the skeletal muscles relax and the respiratory rate is irregular. The combination of decreased intercostal muscle activity, a variable respiratory rate, and tidal volume predisposes the child to hypoxemia.

The severity of OSAS may range from a continuous partial airway obstruction to episodes of total obstruction with no air movement despite breathing effort. Some children arouse from sleep repeatedly to increase airway muscle tone so that they can breathe. Other children snore without arousals and thus sleep with a partial airway obstruction resulting in prolonged hypoventilation over several hours. In both cases, the child experiences hypoxemia, hypercapnia, acidemia, and hemodynamic alterations, such as elevated blood pressure and increased pulmonary arterial pressure in association with apneic episodes. Cerebral blood flow is also decreased during sleep.

Hypertrophy of the adenoids and tonsils is the most common cause of OSAS. Other children at risk for OSAS include those with macroglossia (e.g., Down syndrome, Beckwith-Wiedemann

syndrome), craniofacial anomalies (e.g., Apert syndrome, Pierre Robin sequence, Treacher Collins syndrome, Crouzon syndrome), obesity, neuromuscular disorders (e.g., cerebral palsy, muscular dystrophy), Prader-Willi syndrome, and mucopolysaccharidosis.

Clinical Manifestations

Children with OSAS snore and have signs of labored breathing during sleep such as retractions and paradoxical breathing. After pauses in snoring or lack of airflow, the child may be noted to snort, gasp, choke, move, or arouse to take a breath. Sleep is restless and the child may sleep in unusual positions to hyperextend the neck and airway. The child may mouth breathe when awake. Daytime sleepiness and other symptoms of sleep deprivation (poor attention, increased activity, aggression, acting-out behavior, and poor school performance) may be noted. The child may also have enuresis and report a morning headache resulting from carbon dioxide retention.

The child may be obese, have normal weight, or even have failure to thrive. Growth impairment may occur, potentially due to increased energy needed for the work of breathing. Without treatment, complications develop that can include pulmonary hypertension, **cor pulmonale** (obstruction of pulmonary blood flow that leads to right ventricular hypertrophy and heart failure), pulmonary edema, systemic hypertension, and cognitive impairment.

Collaborative Care

Clinical management is focused on diagnosing children with OSAS and selecting the appropriate therapy for the child.

Diagnostic Tests

Health professionals need to be proactive in inquiring about snoring and its characteristics during examinations. See Box 25–4 for

BOX 25–4	History Questions for Assessment for Obstructive Sleep Apnea Syndrome

- Does the child snore? If so, how often, and how loudly?
- Have you observed the child struggling to breathe during sleep? Gasp? Snort? Choke? Or stop breathing at night or during naps?
- Does the child become restless during sleep, sleepwalk, have night terrors, or act confused during arousals?
- Does the child assume unusual sleep positions? Upright? On multiple pillows?
- Does the child wet the bed after a period of being dry at night?
- Does the child exhibit signs of being excessively sleepy or tired during the day? At school?
- Does the child complain of morning headaches and dry mouth upon awakening?
- Is the child having difficulty with schoolwork or relationships? Are there any signs of behavior problems such as hyperactivity or aggressiveness?
- Does the child fall asleep in less than 30 minutes in a motor vehicle?

Source: Data from Peeke, K., Hershberger, M., & Marriner, J. (2006). Obstructive sleep apnea syndrome in children. Pediatric Nursing, 32(5), 489–494; Rosen, D. (2010). Obstructive sleep apnea in children: Accurate diagnosis, effective treatment. Consultant for Pediatricians, 9(4), 128–133.

screening questions to use for OSAS and associated problems. Physical examination findings may be normal, but mouth breathing and enlarged tonsils and adenoids may be seen. Diagnosis is made by polysomnography, a sleep study that simultaneously records the sleep state, gas exchange, breathing efforts, cardiac rhythm, and muscle activity and movement. The number of hypopnea and apnea episodes, and associated oxygen desaturation and sleep disturbances are measured.

Clinical Therapy

Adenotonsillectomy is the most common treatment for OSAS, and resolution of the condition occurs in up to 71% of children (Loghmanee & Sheldon, 2010). Some children are at higher risk for respiratory complications in the immediate postoperative period, such as those younger than 3 years of age and those with severe OSAS, cardiac complications due to OSAS, failure to thrive, obesity, prematurity, craniofacial abnormalities, and neuromuscular disorders. These children need extubation and CPAP or hospital admission until postoperative swelling has receded and the upper airway is stable. Polysomnography is usually repeated about 6 to 8 weeks after surgery to determine if any residual OSAS remains.

Weight loss strategies are implemented for children who are obese. CPAP, bi-level positive airway pressure (BiPAP), or a high-flow open nasal cannula system is used for children with surgical contraindications or those with persistent OSAS after adenotonsillectomy. Pressure levels are adjusted until apneic episodes, sleep arousals, and hypoxemia are eliminated, and they may need to be changed as the child grows. Craniofacial surgery or even tracheostomy may be treatment options in rare cases. Dental appliances, intranasal corticosteroids, and leukotriene modifiers are being investigated for their role in reducing the inflammatory aspects of OSAS (Loghmanee & Sheldon, 2010).

Recurrence of sleep-disordered breathing in children 1 year after adenotonsillectomy is greater in children who are obese, necessitating long-term follow-up of these children (Loghmanee & Sheldon, 2010).

Nursing Management

The goal of nursing care is to identify children at risk for OSAS and to support the family during surgery or initiation of other therapies.

Nursing Assessment and Diagnosis

In the community setting, all children should be screened for snoring as part of their routine health care. Assess the child for signs of nasal obstruction, mouth breathing, and enlarged tonsils. Determine if the child has symptoms of sleep deprivation or if a condition is present that places the child at high risk for OSAS. When snoring is present, encourage the family to keep a sleep diary. Coordinate referral to a sleep center for polysomnography evaluation.

Prior to surgery, review the child's history and symptoms to identify higher risks for complications following surgery. Following adenotonsillectomy, the child is placed on a cardiorespiratory monitor and continuous pulse oximetry to detect oxygen desaturation.

The following nursing diagnoses might be appropriate for the child with OSAS:

- Gas Exchange, Impaired related to airway obstruction associated with enlarged tonsils and adenoids
- Tissue Perfusion: Cerebral, Risk for Ineffective related to hypoventilation
- Therapeutic Regimen Management: Family, Ineffective related to nonadherence in use of continuous positive airway pressure

NANDA-I © 2012

Planning and Implementation

Nursing care in the community is initially focused on educating the parents about the potential serious complications associated with OSAS and the interventions that can resolve or control the condition. Explain the purpose of polysomnography evaluation and how to prepare the child for the strange setting and the wires that will be attached during the sleep study. Most pediatric centers will allow the parent to stay with the child during the study. Encourage the family to return for a follow-up sleep study after adenotonsillectomy to determine if the condition is resolved or if additional intervention is needed.

An initial intervention may be weight loss to help reduce airway obstruction. See Chapter 19 🕑 for nutritional guidelines for weight loss appropriate for the child's age. Ongoing growth and development is monitored to observe for improved growth patterns and behavior after intervention begins.

Following adenotonsillectomy, the hospital nurse monitors the child for bleeding, edema, respiratory compromise, respiratory distress, and episodes of oxygen desaturation. Pain is often managed by nonopioid analgesics (acetaminophen) and complementary therapies to avoid additional respiratory depression. See Chapter 24 🕑 for care of the child undergoing adenotonsillectomy. The child should be carefully monitored postoperatively at home, particularly 2 to 3 days after surgery when obstructive apnea may occur.

Sleep center nurses provide education and support to families of children who need to use CPAP, BiPAP, or the high-flow open nasal cannula system to treat the OSAS. The nurse helps identify the best fitting mask or nasal prong system for positive-airway-pressure delivery. Parents may need guidance about helping children to use the device until they are accustomed to it. See Box 25–5.

BOX 25–5 | **Research: OSAS and Use of Continuous Positive Airway Pressure**

A small study of 12 children, 5 to 15 years of age, investigated the use of warm humidified air delivered through an open nasal cannula in children with OSAS and without adenotonsillectomy. This therapy reduced the amount of inspiratory flow limitation, improved oxygen stores, and decreased arousals. It is believed to be an alternative to CPAP therapy, but more studies are needed before it is widely implemented (McGinley, Halbower, Schwartz, et al., 2009).

Evaluation

Expected outcomes of nursing care include the following:

- No significant complications are experienced by the child following adenotonsillectomy.
- The child has minimal snoring and undisturbed sleep due to apnea episodes.
- Catch-up growth occurs in cases of failure to thrive.
- The child's behavior and school performance improves.

Sudden Infant Death Syndrome

Sudden infant death syndrome (SIDS) is defined as the sudden death during sleep of an infant under 1 year of age that remains unexplained after a thorough investigation, including an autopsy, a review of the circumstances of death, and the clinical history. In 2009, SIDS was the third leading cause of death in infants less than 12 months of age (Kochanek, Xu, Murphy, et al., 2011). Most SIDS deaths occur in infants between 2 and 4 months of age. It is currently unpredictable and in some cases unpreventable.

Etiology and Pathophysiology

The interaction of multiple factors may lead to SIDS or infant asphyxia (Kinney & Thach, 2009; Trachtenberg, Haas, Kinney, et al., 2012):

- An underlying vulnerability of the infant (e.g., a genetic cardiac dysrhythmia such as long QT syndrome, or a defect in neural networks that control respirations, sleep, and arousal)
- A critical developmental period (such as before cardiorespiratory system maturation)
- An additional stressor (e.g., rebreathing exhaled air, bed sharing, being overheated, or a respiratory infection)
- A more recent theory is that many cases result from abnormalities associated with the neurotransmitter serotonin in the medulla oblongata which may interfere with the brainstem-mediated protective responses (e.g., arousal) during sleep in a critical development period (Duncan, Paterson, Hoffman, et al., 2010).
- Recent research has revealed that cerebral oxygenation is depressed in healthy term infants when they sleep in the prone position, making them more difficult to arouse (Wong, Witcombe, Yiallourou, et al., 2011).

See Box 25–6 for infant and maternal factors that place infants at risk for SIDS. Protective factors may be completed immunizations for age and use of a pacifier when the infant is put down to sleep (Adams, Good, & Defranco, 2009).

BOX 25–6 | **Risk Factors for Sudden Infant Death Syndrome**

INFANT RISK FACTORS

- Preterm and low birth weight
- Native Americans and Black infants at a higher risk (may be a genetic factor); Whites and Asians at a lower risk
- Males at a higher risk (may be a genetic factor)
- Maternal smoking, alcohol intake, or substance abuse
- Socioeconomic disadvantages (e.g., single parenthood, younger mother, fewer years of education, unemployment)

ENVIRONMENTAL RISK FACTORS

- Sleeping in a prone or side-lying position
- Secondhand smoke exposure
- Bed sharing
- Soft bedding or the use of pillows, quilts, or soft toys with bedding

Source: Data from Kinney, H. C., & Thach, B. T. (2009). The sudden infant death syndrome. New England Journal of Medicine, 361(8), 795–805; Behm, I., Kabir, Z., Connolly, G. N., & Alpert, H. R. (2012). Increasing prevalence of smoke-free homes and decreasing rates of sudden infant death syndrome in the United States: An ecological association study. Tobacco Control, 21, 6–11; Trachtenberg, F. L., Haas, E. A., Kinney, H. C., Stanley, C., Krous, H. F. (2012). Risk Factor Changes for Sudden Infant Death Syndrome After initiation of the back to sleep campaign, Pediatrics, 129(4), 630–638.

Clinical Manifestations

The first symptom is cardiopulmonary arrest. Clinical findings include evidence of a struggle or change in position and the presence of frothy, blood-tinged secretions from the mouth and nares. Typically parents find the infant dead in the crib in the morning or after a nap, and they report having heard no cries or disturbances during the sleep interval.

Collaborative Care

The Back to Sleep Campaign, encouraging the placement of infants in supine position for sleeping, was initiated in 1992 to reduce the incidence of SIDS. The American Academy of Pediatrics and the Centers for Disease Control and Prevention recommend that infants be placed on their back to sleep. The dramatic decrease in SIDS deaths, 50% since 1992, has been attributed to the success of educational campaigns about placing infants to sleep on their backs (Carrier, 2009).

Nursing Management

The sudden, unexpected nature of the infant's death is often addressed in the emergency department. The nurse's role is to be empathetic and provide support to the family during one of its greatest crises. Special support is needed during communication of bad news and the family's response to the shock of their infant's death. See the companion website and Chapter 18 🔗 for guidelines to support the bereaved family.

Clinical Tip

Guidelines for support of families experiencing SIDS should include baptism services, religious support, grief counseling, assistance with funeral arrangements, and counseling on cessation of breastfeeding, if appropriate. Giving parents information about the potential reactions of siblings can help them respond to their needs.

Reassure the parents that they are not responsible for the infant's death, and assist them in contacting other family members and

Weblink | *SIDS Resources*

Evidence-Based Practice   Infant Sleep Positioning

PROBLEM

In 2008, 15% of all infants were estimated to sleep in the prone position; however, the rate of prone or side-lying sleep is much higher among African American infants (38%) (Carrier, 2009). What will help encourage African American parents to place their infant to sleep on its back?

EVIDENCE

Interviews were conducted with 708 mothers with infants under 8 months of age enrolled in the WIC supplemental nutrition program in four major cities to investigate infant sleep location. While room sharing with the infant in a separate bed was reported by 48.6% of all mothers, 37.2% of African American mothers reported bed sharing, higher than all other races. Bed sharing was also reported by a higher percentage of teenage mothers (Fu, Colson, Corwin, et al., 2008).

A qualitative study, using focus groups and individual interviews, investigated the beliefs and perceptions of 73 African American mothers with infants under 6 months of age from all socioeconomic levels regarding sudden infant death syndrome. Three major themes emerged. Mothers did not see a plausible connection between SIDS and sleep position, especially since the cause of SIDS cannot be explained. Mothers also believed SIDS occurred randomly and could be "God's will." They also believed their own vigilance was the best protection for their baby. Some mothers reported placing the infant in bed with them to more closely monitor the infant (Moon, Oden, Joyner, et al., 2010).

A study used focus groups and interviews with 83 African American mothers from both upper and lower socioeconomic groups to learn about surfaces and soft bedding used for their infants. Findings revealed that parents had different interpretations of firm bedding, and they believed that soft bedding (pillows, blankets, and crib bumper pads) would increase the infant's comfort and in some cases safety. For example, parents believed that the surface was firm if a pillow or blanket was placed between the mattress and the sheet and the sheet was tucked tautly around the pillow or blanket. Misconceptions about firm and soft bedding increase the risk for suffocation and SIDS as the infant sleeps (Ajao, Oden, Joyner, et al., 2011).

IMPLICATIONS

The Back to Sleep campaign has been very successful in increasing awareness of the importance of placing infants to sleep in a supine position. African American mothers reported being aware of this recommendation, but do not necessarily believe it (Oden, Joyner, Ajao, et al., 2010). Nurses need to consistently work with parents to encourage a safe sleep position and location. One project evaluated an effort to improve nurse modeling of safe sleep practices in seven hospitals in an urban area with a large population of African American parents. This project worked with hospitals to implement policies regarding supine sleep position for newborns and other infants, educated nurses about sleep position recommendations, and conducted crib audits to assess changes in infant sleep positioning. The policy change and education resulted in nurses changing their behavior, positioning infants on their back to sleep, and increasing the effort to educate parents about safe sleep positioning (Shaefer, Herman, Frank, et al., 2010).

CRITICAL THINKING APPLICATION

Identify if policies exist for infant sleep position in the maternity and pediatric sections of your hospital. Conduct an audit of cribs and bassinets to determine what proportion of infants are sleeping in supine position.

---

mobilizing support. Older children may need reassurance that SIDS will not happen to them. They may also believe that bad thoughts or wishes about their baby brother or sister caused the death. Support groups can help parents, siblings, and other family members express these fears and work through their feelings about the infant's death. The First Candle organization can help families locate a support group in their geographic area. Parents may need extra support at a later time with the birth of a subsequent newborn.

Prevention of SIDS

Nurses can play an important role in educating the public about the link between SIDS and infant sleep positioning. Hospitalized infants should be placed to sleep in the supine position rather than side-lying or prone. Parents often model the sleep position used by nurses. Encourage parents who smoke tobacco products to stop smoking or to avoid smoking in areas where the infant sleeps and spends time. Visit the companion website for infant sleep position resources. See Evidence-Based Practice: Infant Sleep Positioning.

Educate all parents of neonates and infants about the recommended sleep position for their infants at home, and ask them to make sure this sleep position is used when the infant is cared for by another family member, baby-sitter, or childcare center. In addition to sleep position, parents and care providers should place the infant on a firm mattress and avoid the use of loose bedding, toys, and pillows. Bed sharing with the parent should be discouraged. Use a sleeper rather than a blanket to keep the infant warm while sleeping, but avoid overheating the infant with too many covers or clothes. The American Academy of Pediatrics recommends the use of a pacifier for bedtime and naptime. Pregnant women and mothers who smoke should be educated that fetal and infant tobacco exposure increases the infant's risk for SIDS. See Box 25–7.

BOX 25–7   Research: SIDS Prevention

A recent population-based case-control study in 11 California counties explored how the use of a fan or open window affected the risk for SIDS. It was thought that fan use could reduce the infant's risk of rebreathing exhaled carbon dioxide trapped by the bedding near the airway. Fan use during last sleep was associated with a 72% reduction in the rate of SIDS among the studied population. The effect was greater when the infant was in a warmer environment, shared a bed, and was not using a pillow (Coleman-Phox, Odouli, & De-Jun, 2008).

Parents should also be encouraged to give the infant supervised tummy time when awake to promote motor development and to reduce infant skull flattening. See Chapter 33 for information related to positional plagiocephaly (infant skull flattening).

CROUP SYNDROMES

Croup is a term applied to a broad classification of upper airway illnesses that result from inflammation and swelling of the epiglottis and larynx. The swelling usually extends into the trachea and bronchi. See Figure 25–3. Viral croup syndromes include spasmodic laryngitis (spasmodic croup) and laryngotracheobronchitis. Bacterial croup syndromes include bacterial tracheitis and epiglottitis (Figure 25–10 ■).

Laryngotracheobronchitis (LTB) and bacterial tracheitis affect a large number of children across all age groups in both sexes. Epiglottitis, previously a common serious respiratory illness, is rare in the United States because of immunization for *Haemophilus influenzae* type b. LTB is the most common disorder, but epiglottitis and bacterial tracheitis are more serious. The subglottic area is the only region of the airway that has a complete cartilaginous ring, preventing

Pathophysiology Illustrated
Airway Changes with Croup

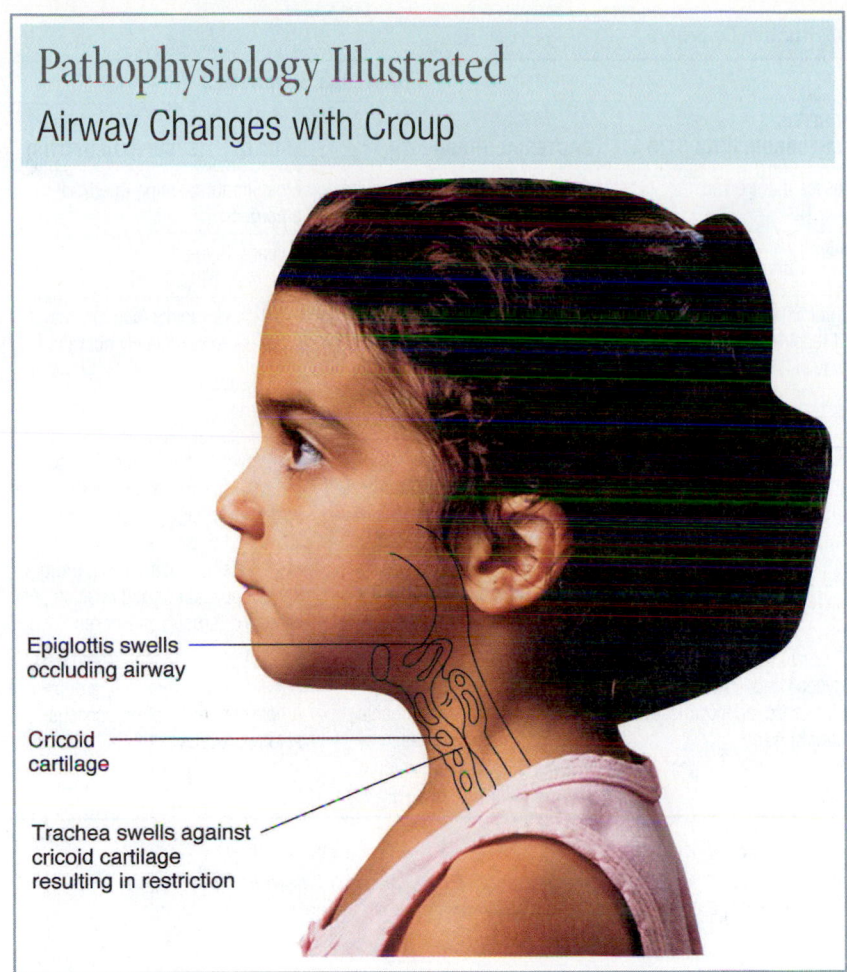

Epiglottis swells
occluding airway

Cricoid
cartilage

Trachea swells against
cricoid cartilage
resulting in restriction

FIGURE 25–10 ■ Two important changes in the upper airway occur with croup: the epiglottis swells, thereby occluding the airway, and the trachea swells against the cricoid cartilage, causing constriction.

outward expansion of an edematous airway. Thus, 1 mm of swelling can reduce the normal airway size by more than 50%, leading to major symptoms (Sobol & Zapata, 2008). The initial symptoms of all three conditions include inspiratory stridor, a "seal-like" barking cough, and hoarseness. See Table 25–4 and the following sections for comparisons between the different croup syndromes.

Laryngotracheobronchitis

The term *croup* is most often used to refer to laryngotracheobronchitis, a viral invasion of the upper airway that extends throughout the larynx, trachea, and bronchi. Table 25–4 compares LTB and other croup syndromes. However, spasmodic laryngitis is often difficult to clinically differentiate from LTB.

Etiology and Pathophysiology

Acute viral LTB is most common in children under 6 years of age, with a peak incidence from 7 to 36 months of age (Wald, 2010). Boys are affected more often than girls. LTB is of greatest concern in infants and children under the age of 6 years, because of potential airway obstruction. The causative organism is usually parainfluenza virus type I, II, or III, which appears during late fall and winter months in clustered outbreaks. Other viruses causing this disorder include influenza, respiratory syncytial virus, adenoviruses, *Mycoplasma pneumoniae*, herpes simplex I, human metapneumovirus, and human coronavirus (Wald, 2010).

The tracheal and laryngeal airway tissues respond to the invading virus with inflammation and edema. Copious, tenacious secretions further increase the child's respiratory distress. The laryngeal inflammation causes the airway diameter to narrow in the subglottic area, the site of the smallest upper airway diameter. Even small amounts of mucus or edema can quickly obstruct the airway. During inspiration, the walls of the inner airway are pulled together, further irritating the inflammation and respiratory distress.

Clinical Manifestations

Most children brought to the emergency department with LTB have been ill for a couple of days with upper respiratory symptoms. These symptoms progress to a cough and hoarseness. Low-grade fever and an inflamed pharynx may or may not be present. Symptoms may be worse at night. Common presenting signs are runny nose, tachypnea, inspiratory stridor, and a seal-like barking cough. The presence of expiratory stridor, severe tachypnea, retractions, and oxygen desaturation are associated with a more severe airway inflammation and swelling. Changes in mental status indicate the development of hypoxemia and potential respiratory failure. Table 25–5 can be used to assess the severity of croup.

Collaborative Care

Diagnostic Procedures

Diagnosis is often made by history and clinical signs. Pulse oximetry is used to detect hypoxemia. If the diagnosis of LTB is in question and the airway is not threatened, anteroposterior (AP) and lateral radiographs of the upper airway may be taken; these may show a tapered symmetric subglottic narrowing called a "steeple sign" in some children. Another reason to do the radiograph is to rule out the presence of a foreign body that could be causing symptoms.

Practice Alert

Throat cultures and visual inspection of the inner mouth and throat are contraindicated in children with LTB and epiglottitis. These procedures can cause **laryngospasms** (spasmodic vibrations that close the larynx) to occur as a result of the child's anxiety or of probing this reactive and already compromised area. A complete airway obstruction may result from the laryngospasm.

Clinical Therapy

Management consists of maintaining and improving respiratory effort with medications and airway supplemental oxygen when the SpO$_2$ level is less than 92%. See Medications Used for Symptomatic Treatment of Laryngotracheobronchitis.

Children who respond well to medications are often sent home from the emergency department after an observation period. Children with persistence of moderate to severe symptoms after nebulizer medications are admitted for further observation and treatment. Airway obstruction is a potential complication of severe LTB. The child may require intubation and transfer to the PICU to maintain airway patency if total obstruction is imminent. Most children, however, respond positively to the medications and oxygen therapy and are discharged within 48 to 72 hours.

TABLE 25–4 Summary of Acute Infectious Upper Airway Obstructive Disorders

| | VIRAL SYNDROMES | | BACTERIAL SYNDROMES | |
	ACUTE SPASMODIC LARYNGITIS (SPASMODIC CROUP)	LARYNGOTRACHEITIS/ LARYNGOTRACHEOBRONCHITIS (LTB)	BACTERIAL TRACHEITIS	EPIGLOTTITIS (SUPRAGLOTTITIS)
Severity	Least serious	Serious; progresses if untreated	Can be life threatening; requires close observation	Most life threatening (medical emergency)[a]
Age group	3 months–3 years	3 months–8 years	1 month–13 years[a], mean age of 5–7 years	2 years–8 years
Onset	Abrupt nighttime onset; usually a well child, but may be associated with upper respiratory infection (URI); resolves over 24–48 hours; recurs[a]	Gradual onset; starts as URI, progresses to symptoms of respiratory distress and obstructed airway in 24–48 hours	Progressive from URI over 2–5 days; may present like LTB	Progresses rapidly (hours)[a]; may progress to completely obstructed airway
Clinical manifestations	Afebrile; hoarseness, mild respiratory distress; barking-seal cough; noisy inspiration; anxiety	*Early:* mild fever (less than 40.0°C [104°F]); cough has barking-seal, brassy, or croupy character; hoarseness; rhinorrhea; sore throat; stridor (inspiratory); apprehension; restless/irritable May progress to retractions, increasing stridor; cyanosis	High fever (greater than 39.0°C [102.2°F]); toxic appearance, URI appears as viral croupy cough; croup initially; stridor (tracheal); thick, copious, purulent secretions; patient often prefers to lie flat, no drooling or dysphagia	High fever (greater than 39.0°C [102.2°F]); URI; intense sore throat; dysphagia[a], drooling[a]; increased pulse and respiratory rate; patient appears toxic; prefers upright position (tripod position with chin thrust)[a], cherry red epiglottis
Etiology	Unknown; suspect viral with allergic/emotional influences	Parainfluenza, types I and II, respiratory syncytial virus, influenza, adenoviruses, or *Mycoplasma pneumoniae*	Staphylococcus, *Moraxella catarrhalis*, and non-typeable *Haemophilus influenzae*; may follow viral LTB as a bacterial superinfection	*Haemophilus influenzae*, group A beta-hemolytic streptococcus, staphylococcus

[a]Classic parameter or key point (distinguishes condition).

Source: *Data from Roosevelt, G. E. (2007). Acute inflammatory upper airway obstruction (croup, epiglottitis, laryngitis, and bacterial tracheitis). In R. M. Kliegman, R. E. Behrman, H. B. Jenson, & B. F. Stanton, Nelson textbook of pediatrics (18th ed., pp. 1762–1767). Philadelphia, PA: Elsevier Saunders; and Wald, E. L. (2010). Croup: Common syndromes and therapy. Pediatric Annals, 39(1), 15–21.*

Nursing Management

Nursing Assessment and Diagnosis

The initial and ongoing physical assessment of the child with LTB focuses on adequacy of respiratory functioning. Table 25–1 provides guidelines for the assessment of respiratory distress. Attach a cardiorespiratory monitor and pulse oximeter, and monitor frequently.

The child should be in an area where continuous visual monitoring is possible to identify changes in airway patency. Particular attention should be paid to the child's respiratory effort, breath sounds, preferred position, and responsiveness. Note any change in behavior

such as agitation or irritability. Physical exhaustion can diminish the intensity of retractions and stridor. As the child uses the remaining energy reserve to maintain ventilation, breath sounds may actually diminish. Responsiveness will decrease as hypoxemia increases. Noisy breathing (audible airway congestion, coarse breath sounds) in this situation verifies adequate energy stores.

The following nursing diagnoses might be appropriate for the child with acute LTB:

- Breathing Pattern, Ineffective related to airway narrowing, decreased energy, and fatigue
- Fluid Volume: Deficient, Risk for related to inadequate fluid intake prior to admission
- Fear (Child) related to dyspnea, unfamiliar surroundings, procedures, and separation from support system
- Knowledge, Readiness for Enhanced (Home Management of Croup) related to care for any future episodes

NANDA-I © 2012

Planning and Implementation

Skillful nursing care can greatly assist children with LTB and their families to cope with the symptoms of the illness. Nursing care focuses on maintaining airway patency, promoting fluid balance, reducing stress, and teaching the family how to care for the child at home.

Maintain Airway Patency

Supplemental oxygen with humidity may be needed for hypoxemia, but cool mist and humidified air have not been proven to be of benefit (Wald, 2010). Allow the child to assume a position of comfort,

TABLE 25–5 Assessment of Croup Severity

LEVEL OF SEVERITY	CHARACTERISTICS
Mild	Occasional barking cough, no audible stridor at rest, no retractions
Moderate	Frequent barking cough, audible stridor at rest, mild retractions at rest, no agitation
Severe	Frequent barking cough, prominent stridor, tachypnea, marked retractions, agitation, and/or distress
Impending respiratory failure	Frequent barking cough, stridor at rest, retractions, lethargy or decreased level of consciousness, cyanosis. Cough, stridor, and retractions may not be present due to respiratory fatigue and airway compromise.

Source: *Data from Wald, E. L. (2010). Croup: Common syndromes and therapy. Pediatric Annals, 39(1), 18. Printed with permission from SLACK Incorporated.*

Medications Used for Symptomatic Treatment of Laryngotracheobronchitis

MEDICATION	ACTION/INDICATION	NURSING MANAGEMENT
Beta-agonists and beta-adrenergics (albuterol, racemic epinephrine). Aerosolized through face mask	Rapid-acting bronchodilator, decreases bronchial and tracheal secretions and mucosal edema. Used to decrease symptoms of moderate to severe respiratory distress, and constriction of subglottic mucosa and submucosal capillaries. Reduces need for artificial airway.	■ Signs and symptoms improve in about 30 minutes, but relief is only temporary; lasts about 2 hours providing time for the corticosteroid to work. ■ Monitor the child for tachycardia (160–200 beats/min), hypertension, dizziness, headache, and nausea; may necessitate stopping medication.
Corticosteroids (e.g., dexamethasone). IM, PO, nebulized budesonide	Anti-inflammatory used to decrease edema; has a long half-life of 36–54 hours. The child less frequently needs an emergency airway, and stridor resolves faster.	■ Monitor for cardiovascular symptoms (hypertension), observing closely for individual response.

which will most likely be sitting upright or lying with the head elevated. Be immediately available to attend to the child's respiratory needs, and keep resuscitation equipment at the bedside. Administer medications.

Communication

An important developmental consideration is the child's ability to communicate reliably. The nurse must be immediately available to attend to the child's respiratory needs during emergency department or outpatient care. If hospitalization is needed, place the child in a room near the nurses' station. Parents are helpful in providing support to the child and alerting the nurse when the respiratory symptoms worsen. A means of communication (sign language or simple word cues) may help the older child to alert nursing staff about respiratory difficulty.

Meet Fluid and Nutritional Needs

The illness preceding the emergency department visit may have interfered with the child's ability and desire to drink fluids, compromising the fluid status. Recognizing the potential fluid deficit and monitoring the child's hydration and nutritional status are essential. Fluids help thin secretions and provide calories for energy and metabolism.

Children with LTB usually prefer cool, noncarbonated, nonacidic drinks such as oral rehydration fluids or fruit-flavored drinks. Remember that gelatin, ice, and fruit-flavored ice pops are also fluids. Parents can be encouraged to gain the child's cooperation in taking oral fluids. An intravenous infusion may be necessary to rehydrate the child, maintain fluid balance, or provide emergency medication access. The child should be observed closely for difficulty in swallowing or drooling, which may be an early sign of epiglottitis or bacterial tracheitis.

Discharge Planning and Home Care Teaching

During the child's observation period, the nurse should take every opportunity to assess the parents' knowledge of symptoms of LTB and discuss actions to take if symptoms recur. For example, instruct parents to call the child's healthcare provider if the following occurs:

- Mild symptoms do not improve after 1 hour of exposure to cool night air or air conditioning.
- The child's breathing is rapid and labored.
- The child does not drink adequate liquids, and urine output is reduced.

Evaluation

Expected outcomes of nursing care include the following:

- The child experiences decreased respiratory distress.
- The child's fear and anxiety reduce after family support and explanations about care.

Epiglottitis (Supraglottitis)

Epiglottitis (also known as supraglottitis) is an inflammation of the tissues surrounding the epiglottis, the long narrow structure that closes off the glottis during swallowing. Because edema in this area can rapidly (within minutes or hours) obstruct the airway by occluding the trachea, epiglottitis is considered a potentially life-threatening condition. (Table 25–4 compares epiglottitis with other acute upper airway infectious disorders.)

Etiology and Pathophysiology

Epiglottitis is caused by bacterial invasion of the soft tissue of the supraglottic area by streptococcus, staphylococcus, or *Haemophilus influenzae* type b (Hib) in unimmunized children or those with vaccine failure. The resulting inflammation causes swelling in the tissues surrounding the epiglottis, leading to airway obstruction. Since use of the Hib vaccine has become widespread, there has been a 10-fold decrease in the incidence of epiglottitis (D'Agustino, 2010).

Clinical Manifestations

Characteristically, a previously healthy child suddenly becomes very ill. The child initially develops a high fever (greater than 39°C [102.2°F]), with a severe sore throat. The four classic signs of epiglottitis in order of their appearance are:

- Dysphonia, muffled, hoarse, or absent voice sounds; talking is painful
- **Dysphagia,** difficulty in swallowing
- Drooling, the child refuses fluids or resists swallowing due to intense throat pain
- Distressed respiratory effort with inspiratory stridor

To fully open the airway and improve air intake, the child sits up and leans forward with the jaw thrust forward in the classic "sniffing" or tripod posture and refuses to lie down (Figure 25–11 ■). As airway

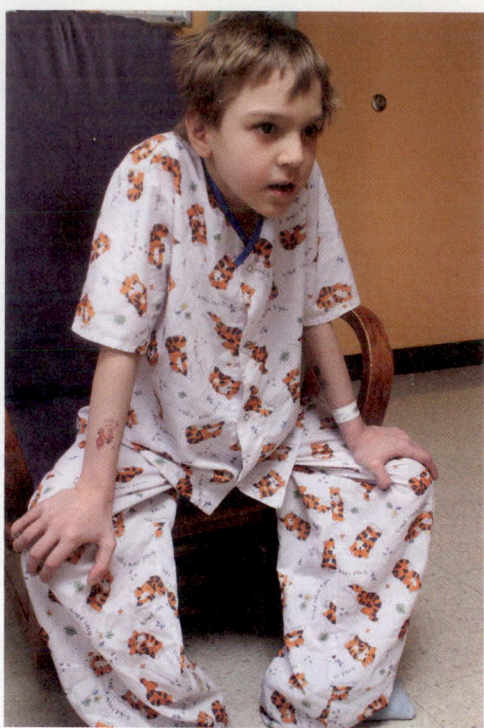

FIGURE 25–11 ■ Children with severe respiratory distress and a narrowed airway often sit in a tripod position, leaning forward with arms on the legs. The head and neck are extended with the jaw thrust forward to help keep the airway open. This position may also be seen in a child with an acute asthma flare.

obstruction progresses, the child becomes anxious and develops cyanosis and mental status changes associated with hypoxia.

Collaborative Care

Care of the child with suspected epiglottitis is focused on rapid diagnosis and ensuring an emergency airway.

Diagnostic Procedures

Diagnosis is often based on physical signs and a lateral neck radiograph with hyperextension of the head and neck.

Practice Alert

Visual inspection of the mouth and throat is contraindicated in children with suspected epiglottitis because of the risk for laryngospasm and airway obstruction. No anxiety-provoking examinations or procedures are performed until the airway is secured.

Clinical Therapy

Immediate clinical therapy usually involves insertion of an endotracheal tube to maintain the airway, usually in the operating room or intensive care unit. At the same time, the airway is inspected and a direct culture of the supraglottic tissue is taken. Antibiotics effective for gram-positive organisms and *H. influenzae* (ceftriaxone, cefotaxime, or ampicillin plus sulbactam) are given until blood culture sensitivities are available, at which time the antibiotic may be changed to one more specific for the organism. Racemic epinephrine and corticosteroids are not effective. If *H. influenzae* is the causative organism, rifampin prophylaxis should be given to any child under 48 months who is not completely immunized against *H. influenzae* or who is immunocompromised (American Academy of Pediatrics [AAP], 2012, p. 347).

Nursing Management

Nursing management consists of airway management, drug therapy, hydration, and emotional and psychosocial support of the child and parents.

Nursing Assessment and Diagnosis

Until the child is intubated, allow the child to assume a position of comfort, often sitting. The child's respiratory and airway status should be observed closely and continuously. The child often breathes slowly and with great concentration as the airway obstruction increases. Note any change in the child's level of consciousness—from anxiety to lethargy to stupor as hypoxia increases—and notify the physician immediately.

Practice Alert

Observe the child continuously for inability to swallow, absence of voice sounds, increasing respiratory distress, and acute onset of drooling (an ominous sign of supraglottic obstruction). If any of these signs occur, get medical assistance immediately. The quieter the child, the greater the cause for concern.

Examples of nursing diagnoses include the following:

- Airway Clearance, Ineffective related to increased swelling of the epiglottis and drooling
- Anxiety (Child) related to increasing difficulty breathing
- Coping: Family, Compromised related to sudden onset of life-threatening illness

NANDA-I © 2012

Planning and Implementation

Until intubated, the child is never left unattended or transported away from equipment or personnel who can perform emergency airway interventions. Allow the child to sit upright or assume a position of comfort to maintain the airway patency and breathe more easily. Provide a quiet environment with as little stress as possible to decrease anxiety and crying. Anxiety-provoking procedures, such as a throat culture or venipuncture, are postponed until the airway is secure. Crying stimulates the airway, increases oxygen consumption, and can precipitate laryngospasm. Supplemental humidified oxygen may be used initially to reverse hypoxemia.

Provide support to parents as they cope with the sudden onset of a life-threatening illness. Dyspnea and loss of voice, or even the inability to create sounds, can be frightening to a child. The unfamiliar hospital environment and strange equipment can create stress for child and parent alike. It is important to reassure the parents that the child's voice loss is temporary and to explain the need for the various pieces of equipment. Identify ways to help parents notify family members and ensure that other children are cared for during the crisis. Keep parents informed about the child's status, and permit them to stay with the child to help keep the child calm.

The child is cared for in an intensive care unit after the airway has been stabilized. Administer prescribed antibiotics to treat the infection and IV fluids to provide hydration. Because the child was febrile with a sore throat before admission, fluid intake may have been compromised. Most children show rapid improvement once oxygen, antibiotics, and fluid therapy are started. The endotracheal tube will be removed in 1 to 2 days, and home care may involve completing the course of antibiotics. Refer to the Skills Manual ⬭. Parents need instructions on proper administration and potential side effects of drug therapy.

Evaluation

Expected outcomes of nursing care include the following:

- The acute infection resolves and the endotracheal tube is removed.
- Support is provided to the child and parents.

Bacterial Tracheitis

Bacterial tracheitis occurs as a secondary infection of the upper trachea following an initial viral LTB. The secondary infection may be caused by *Staphylococcus aureus*, group A streptococcus, *Moraxella catarrhalis*, or *Haemophilus influenzae* (usually in unvaccinated children).

Characteristic signs of the disorder include signs of viral croup for several days before a productive cough, high fever, and a toxic appearance. Dysphagia and drooling are rarely present, and the child can lie flat. Table 25–4 compares bacterial tracheitis and other croup syndromes.

Diagnosis is often made by blood cultures after the child is not responsive to usual LTB management. Endoscopic examination may be performed on children with minimal airway symptoms. The subglottis is edematous with ulceration, and thick mucopurulent exudate may obstruct the trachea and main bronchi. The majority of children are intubated, and then culture and sensitivities are obtained.

Because of the similarity of symptoms, bacterial tracheitis may be misdiagnosed initially as LTB. Instead of improving with nebulized epinephrine, the child's condition worsens. Antibiotics are given for 10 to 14 days. Supplemental oxygen may be ordered. Frequent suctioning, humidification, and monitoring for patency of the endotracheal tube are required.

Nursing Management

The child with bacterial tracheitis is cared for in the intensive care unit until the endotracheal tube is removed. The child must have airway patency assessed frequently because of the thick tracheal secretions that pool high in the upper airway. The endotracheal tube and airway should be suctioned as needed, and humidified air or oxygen should be provided. (See the Clinical Skills Manual ⬭ .) Children generally prefer lying flat to sitting up. This seems to be a position of comfort that allows the child to conserve energy. Antibiotics are administered as ordered.

The earlier section on epiglottitis discusses other nursing care interventions that may also be appropriate for the child with bacterial tracheitis.

LOWER AIRWAY DISORDERS

The lower airway, or bronchial tree, lies below the trachea and includes the bronchi, bronchioles, and alveoli. Lower airway disorders occur because a structural or functional problem interferes with the lungs' ability to complete the respiratory cycle. Lower airway disorders include neonatal respiratory distress syndrome, meconium aspiration, bronchopulmonary dysplasia, bronchitis, bronchiolitis, pneumonia, and tuberculosis.

Neonatal Respiratory Distress Syndrome

Neonatal respiratory distress syndrome (RDS), also known as hyaline membrane disease, is the most common cause of respiratory distress in preterm infants in the United States. The incidence is highest in infants of lower gestational age at birth; RDS affects 60% of preterm infants less than 28 weeks' gestation, 30% of preterm infants between 28 and 34 weeks' gestation, and less than 5% of infants greater than 34 weeks' gestation (Maitra, 2010). RDS may also occur in infants born to mothers with diabetes, born by cesarean section, and in cases of maternal hemorrhage or perinatal asphyxia. The incidence is increased in males and in White infants (Gott & Froh, 2010).

Etiology and Pathophysiology

RDS develops as a result of immature lung development with inadequate alveolar surface areas for gas exchange, and deficiency of **surfactant** (a lipid-protein secreted in the lungs that lowers the alveolar surface tension, making it difficult to inflate the alveoli). In utero, the fetal lungs are filled with fluid that is expelled during vaginal birth. When the infant takes the first breath after birth, this fluid is expelled from the alveoli. Most of the fetal lung fluid is moved to the interstitial spaces and absorbed. Less fluid is expelled by preterm newborns because their small size results in fewer mechanical forces during passage through the vagina. With the onset of breathing, inspiration and negative thoracic pressures fill the alveoli with air.

Without sufficient surfactant, fluid droplets remaining in the alveoli cause the surface tension to increase, and the sides of the alveoli collapse or stick together on expiration. Significant negative pressure is needed for the newborn to breathe and reopen the alveoli. Preterm infants also have a compliant chest wall and stiff lungs, and the repeated breaths with negative pressure lead to **atelectasis** (collapse of a portion of the lung). As a consequence the newborn uses more energy to breathe, becomes exhausted, and is unable to sustain the work of breathing. Decreased air movement and hypoxia occur, resulting in vasoconstriction of the pulmonary vascular beds, increased pulmonary vascular resistance, respiratory acidosis, and partial return to fetal circulation. See information on fetal circulation in Chapter 26 🔗. Metabolic acidosis develops following a prolonged lack of oxygen at the cellular level. Several factors are associated with the development of chronic lung disease following RDS such as long-term ventilatory support, oxygen administration, and infections.

Clinical Manifestations

Signs and symptoms become apparent within minutes of birth. They include tachypnea (at rates greater than 60 breaths/min), nasal flaring, intercostal and subcostal retractions, grunting, crackles, cyanosis, slow capillary refill, paradoxical breathing, decreased breath sounds, and labored breathing. Apnea and irregular breathing are seen as the newborn tires.

Collaborative Care

Care focuses on identifying and treating the fetus at risk for RDS and providing surfactant and ventilatory support to neonates with the disorder.

Diagnostic Procedures

Diagnosis is often made within minutes of birth when resuscitation is needed for severe respiratory distress in a preterm infant. Tracheal aspirates of amniotic fluid may be evaluated for the lecithin-sphingomyelin (L/S) ratio. Blood gases are monitored for signs of hypoxemia. A chest radiograph may show diffuse fine granular densities with portions of an air-filled tracheobronchial tree as early as 6 hours after birth. An echocardiogram may be used to assess for a vascular shunt (patent ductus arteriosus) that enables blood to bypass the lungs.

Clinical Therapy

Management for a fetus less than 34 weeks' gestation involves glucocorticoid administration to the mother while efforts are made to stop preterm labor. This therapy accelerates the fetus lung development. After birth, management includes resuscitation airway management, temperature control, and assisted ventilation with nasal CPAP to expand the alveoli and preserve respiratory function. Surfactant is administered by nebulization or CPAP every 12 hours for several days. Supplemental oxygen may be administered based on clinical need.

Ventilatory support is provided with CPAP and PEEP or with mechanical ventilation. Arterial blood gases and pH are measured frequently. Careful monitoring is needed, especially when supplemental oxygen is used, to reduce the risk of adverse effects of hyperoxia, such as bronchopulmonary dysplasia and retinopathy of prematurity. Inhaled nitric oxide therapy for preterm infants undergoing mechanical ventilation has been associated with decreased oxygen use, fewer days of ventilation, a lower incidence of bronchopulmonary dysplasia, and reduced risk of brain injury in infants with birth weight of 1250 g or less (Gott & Froh, 2010). Intravenous fluid therapy, nutrition, prophylactic antibiotics, maintenance of blood pressure, and management of the patent ductus arteriosus are other therapies used to support function of the respiratory and other body systems. See Chapter 26 🔗 for patent ductus arteriosus therapy. Most infants survive with treatment, but chronic lung disease is a significant complication in very-low-birth-weight infants. See page 783 for information on chronic lung disease.

Nursing Management

The newborn is cared for in a neonatal intensive care nursery. The oxygenation status and acid–base balance of the infant with RDS is closely monitored using pulse oximetry and blood gases. Nursing assessment focuses on identifying changes in respiratory status, such as quality of respirations and pulse, breath sounds, grunting respirations, nasal flaring, increasing retractions, apnea, overall color, signs of dehydration, and changes in the infant's behavior.

Care of the infant is organized to eliminate any unnecessary physical stimulation, as this additional stress contributes to respiratory compromise. The CPAP is lost when the infant cries, so crying should be minimized. The infant is usually placed in a warmer to stabilize the temperature and to reduce metabolic demands. Fluid management is critical as excess fluids can lead to pulmonary edema. Airway suctioning should be performed within the endotracheal tube only to prevent injury to the trachea. Provide fluids and nutrition to help meet energy needs. Position the infant to facilitate breathing. Parents need clear explanations about the infant's health status and planned interventions. By remaining available to parents and answering their questions, the nurse establishes a positive relationship and facilitates essential communication.

Discharge planning involves helping parents gain confidence in their care of the infant. Because of the potential for respiratory distress and chronic lung disease after discharge, parents should be taught CPR, administration of needed medications, and oxygen administration if ordered. See page 786. Home care nursing may be needed to provide follow-up support. Parents may benefit from a referral to a support group.

Meconium Aspiration Syndrome

Meconium is the greenish black, sticky material present in the bowels of the fetus. It is composed of amniotic fluid, mucus, lanugo, bile, exfoliated cells, glycoproteins, various enzymes, minerals, and lipids. In cases of fetal distress, the meconium may be released into the amniotic fluid and then aspirated while in utero, during labor, or during delivery. An estimated 13% of infants are born with meconium-stained amniotic fluid, and 0.61 per 1,000 live births require mechanical ventilation for meconium aspiration syndrome (MAS). A higher risk for meconium aspiration syndrome (MAS) is associated with advanced gestational age, greater than 40 weeks (Singh, Clark, Powers, et al., 2009).

Etiology and Pathophysiology

Aspiration of thick meconium can lead to partial or complete airway obstruction, atelectasis, air trapping with increased functional residual capacity, and air leaks. Meconium may cause small airway obstruction, surfactant dysfunction, and a chemical inflammation of the airway leading to pulmonary edema. Some areas of the lungs may be hyperinflated while others collapse, leading to a ventilation-perfusion mismatch and hypoxemia. See page 746. All of these pathophysiologic changes lead to hypoxia, hypercapnia, and respiratory and metabolic acidosis. Severe MAS is associated with a high risk for air leaks and pulmonary hypertension.

Clinical Manifestations

Newborns may range from mild respiratory distress to more severe respiratory distress with tachypnea, grunting, gasping respirations, flaring, retractions, and cyanosis. Yellowish staining of the skin, nails, and umbilical cord is usually present if meconium was present in the amniotic fluid in utero for more than 3 hours. The infant may have a barrel chest due to hyperinflated lungs. Rales and rhonchi may be heard on auscultation. Signs of neurologic depression are also apparent.

Collaborative Care

Diagnostic Procedures

Typical findings on chest radiograph are patchy infiltrates, areas of consolidation, and hyperinflation. The chest radiograph may also reveal a pneumothorax or air leak when present. An umbilical arterial line is inserted to monitor the arterial blood pressures, blood pH, and blood gases as needed.

Clinical Therapy

Intubation is performed if the infant has decreased or absent respirations, bradycardia, and hypotonia. Suctioning of the nasopharynx, the oropharynx, and the trachea through the endotracheal tube is no longer recommended at the time of birth (Wiswell, 2008). IV fluids, blood, and medications may be infused through an umbilical arterial line. Surfactant replacement therapy may be used. Various modes of mechanical ventilation are used. If the newborn progresses to respiratory failure and is not responding to other therapies, transfer to a neonatal intensive care unit for nitric oxide or ECMO therapy may be necessary.

Nursing Management

The newborn with MAS is cared for in a neonatal intensive care nursery. Nursing management follows guidelines previously described for RDS with careful attention to changes in respiratory signs. Actions involve carefully assessing and monitoring the newborn for hypoglycemia, signs of complications, and response to treatment. Place the neonate in a quiet area to reduce environmental stimuli. Organize care to the infant to eliminate any unnecessary physical stimulation. Regulation of the environmental temperature and maintenance of adequate oxygenation and ventilation are essential. Meeting caloric requirements and administering IV fluids and medications are nursing care priorities.

Provide support to families who must cope with suddenly changed expectations about having a healthy baby. Help them understand the infant's health problems and rationale for the treatment provided.

Transient Tachypnea of the Newborn

Transient tachypnea of the newborn is a progressive respiratory distress disorder that may resemble respiratory distress syndrome. It may develop in infants large for gestational age and term, as well as those born by cesarean section without spontaneous labor. Fetal lung fluid is typically absorbed before and during delivery. Vaginal birth newborns less commonly develop the disorder because their thorax is compressed during delivery, forcing out some of the lung fluids. This condition occurs in 11 per 1,000 live births (Nash & Smith, 2008).

While the cause of transient tachypnea of the newborn is unknown, the fetal lung fluid that remains leads to transient pulmonary edema, or a wet lung syndrome. The lung fluid is believed to decrease pulmonary compliance (lung stiffness increases) and tidal volume (dead space increases). A few infants progress to develop respiratory failure and pulmonary hypertension. It is sometimes difficult to distinguish this condition from RDS.

The newborn has no initial breathing difficulties at birth. Tachypnea with rates greater than 60 breaths, and up to 100 breaths, per minute develops within 6 hours of birth. Respiratory distress may develop with signs including expiratory grunting, nasal flaring, retractions, and mild cyanosis when on room air. Air trapping may increase the anterior-posterior diameter of the chest. No crackles or rhonchi are heard on auscultation. These infants often do not appear to be severely ill. Condition improvement begins within 12 to 24 hours of age, with recovery by 72 hours of age.

Diagnosis is based upon absence of adventitious breath sounds and a chest radiograph which may show small pleural fluid collections. Blood gas and electrolyte levels may be obtained. The chest radiograph findings clear within 48 to 72 hours. Clinical therapy sometimes involves supplemental oxygen (30% to 50% concentration) with an oxyhood, fluids, and electrolytes.

Nursing Management

Nursing assessment and management for transient tachypnea of the newborn is the same as for RDS during the acute care phase. Monitor and identify changes in the newborn's respiratory status, as well as fluid and electrolyte levels. Attach a cardiorespiratory monitor and pulse oximeter. Monitor oxygen delivery and the infant's response to supplemental oxygen.

Organize care to the infant to eliminate any unnecessary physical stimulation. The infant is usually placed in a warmer to stabilize the temperature and to reduce metabolic demands. Feedings may be postponed because of the rapid respiratory rate and risk for aspiration. Support the mother's effort to breastfeed as soon as the infant's condition allows it. Parents need clear explanations about the infant's health status and planned interventions. Help parents to identify changes in the infant's condition indicating recovery.

Bronchitis

Acute bronchitis, inflammation of the trachea and bronchi, rarely occurs in childhood as an isolated problem. The bronchi can be affected simultaneously with adjacent respiratory structures during a respiratory illness. Bronchitis occurs most commonly in winter months.

The classic symptom of bronchitis is a dry, hacking cough, which increases in severity at night. The cough may or may not be productive. The child may swallow sputum and vomit as a result. The chest and ribs may be painful because of the deep and frequent coughing. Over several days breath sounds may become coarse with fine crackles, and some scattered high-pitched wheezing may be heard. Treatment is palliative unless the child develops a fever and a secondary bacterial infection which requires antibiotic therapy.

Nursing Management

Nursing management includes supporting respiratory function through rest, humidification, hydration, and symptomatic treatment. Refer to the sections on asthma and pneumonia for detailed information on treatment measures.

Home care should emphasize the self-limiting nature of the disorder. Parents who smoke should be advised that quitting or refraining from smoking in the child's presence may benefit the child.

Bronchiolitis and Respiratory Syncytial Virus

Bronchiolitis is a lower respiratory tract illness that occurs when an infecting agent (virus or bacterium) causes inflammation and obstruction of the small airways, the bronchioles. At least 1 in 7 infants develop bronchiolitis during the first year of life, and approximately 100 infants die each year from this condition (Alverson & Ralston, 2011). Children with bronchiolitis have an increased risk for wheezing and asthma later in childhood (Sorce, 2009).

Etiology and Pathophysiology

Bronchiolitis is associated with the respiratory syncytial virus (RSV) in 70% of cases and the metapneumovirus in 5% to 15% of cases (Zorc & Phelan, 2008). Other viruses known to cause bronchiolitis include the adenovirus, parainfluenza virus, coronavirus, rhinovirus, and influenza virus. Some infants are infected with more than one virus, especially those who are more ill.

RSV occurs in annual epidemics from October to March. It is transmitted through direct contact with respiratory secretions or contaminated surfaces. The virus is shed by the infected child for 3 to 8 days, and the incubation period is 2 to 8 days. Nearly all children have been infected with RSV by 2 years of age, and reinfection is common as infection does not confer immunity (AAP, 2012, pp. 609). Infants at high risk for severe infection with RSV include those who are immunosuppressed or have lung disease, severe neuromuscular disease, or complicated congenital heart defects, or were very low birth weight (Miller, 2010).

Viruses, acting as parasites, invade the mucosal cells that line the small bronchi and bronchioles. The invaded cells die when the virus bursts from inside the cell to invade adjacent cells. The membranes of the infected cells fuse with adjacent cells, creating large masses of cells or "syncytia." The resulting cell debris clogs and obstructs the bronchioles and irritates the airway. In response, the airway lining swells and produces excessive mucus. Despite this protective response by the bronchioles, the actual effect is partial airway obstruction during expiration and bronchospasms.

The cycle is repeated throughout both lungs as the airway cells are invaded by the virus. The partially obstructed airways allow air in, but the mucus and airway swelling block expulsion of the air. This creates the wheezing and crackles in the airways. Air trapped below the obstruction also interferes with normal gas exchange, leading to a ventilation-perfusion mismatch and hypoxemia. See page 746. The child with RSV is therefore at risk for apnea and respiratory failure as hypoxemia and hypercarbia develop.

Clinical Manifestations

Some children have mild symptoms such as rhinitis, cough, low-grade fever, wheezing, tachypnea, poor feeding, vomiting, and diarrhea. Dehydration may be present if the child has been sick for several days. Parents report that the infant or child is acting more ill—appearing sicker, less playful, and less interested in eating. Infants, especially, may refuse to feed or may spit up what they eat along with thick, clear mucus.

The infant or child with a more severe infection has tachypnea greater than 70 breaths per minute, grunting, increased wheezing, retractions, nasal flaring, irritability, lethargy, poor fluid intake, and a distended abdomen from overexpanded lungs. As hypoxia develops, the infant becomes cyanotic and has decreasing mental status. As the airflow continues to decrease, breath sounds diminish. Thus the noisier the lungs, the better, as this indicates that the child is still able to move air in and out of the lungs. Airway hyperresponsiveness may persist for weeks after the virus has resolved.

Collaborative Care

Care is focused on providing oxygen, fluids, and medications to support the infant and young child until the infection resolves.

Diagnostic Procedures

The history and physical examination provide the data needed to diagnose bronchiolitis. Chest radiographs show hyperinflation, patchy atelectasis, and other signs of inflammation. Enzyme-linked immunosorbent assay (ELISA) or immunofluorescent assay performed on the posterior nasopharyngeal specimen are the laboratory tests used to identify the virus causing bronchiolitis (see the Clinical Skills Manual ⟨▭▭⟩).

Clinical Therapy

Treatment is supportive as no effective therapy for RSV bronchiolitis exists. Hospitalized children who test positive for RSV are isolated or roomed together to minimize the spread of the virus to other hospitalized children. Humidified oxygen is recommended if the SpO_2 reading falls below 90% in previously healthy infants (Selden & Scarfone, 2009). The delivery method chosen is based upon the desired concentration of oxygen, the degree of humidity, and the child's response. Other supportive care includes hydration with oral or intravenous fluids and nasal suctioning to facilitate breathing. Continuous positive airway pressure may be used in the child with moderate to severe bronchiolitis. Chest physiotherapy is not used because research has revealed that it does not decrease oxygen requirements, reduce severity, or shorten length of hospital stay (Selden & Scarfone, 2009).

Few medications are prescribed for RSV and bronchiolitis. Emergency department treatment with nebulized epinephrine and systemic corticosteroids have been found to have no effect on reducing hospitalizations when used individually, but when used in combination, there was some reduction in hospitalizations (Selden & Scarfone, 2009). Bronchodilators can be offered to see if a clinical response occurs. Nebulized hypertonic saline (3%) is currently being investigated for effectiveness after several studies had conflicting outcomes (Selden & Scarfone, 2009). Antipyretics may be used. Antibiotics are not used routinely unless the child also has a bacterial infection. Ribavirin, an aerosol antiviral drug specifically available for RSV treatment, is reserved for select cases of severe disease; however, it does not reduce the length of hospitalization or need for mechanical ventilation. Ribavirin is also toxic to exposed health professionals (Todd, Roberg, & Welliver, 2010).

Although RSV bronchiolitis resolves in 5 to 7 days, recurrent wheezing episodes or problems with pulmonary function can be complications. These complications may be associated with the child's predisposition to asthma rather than a direct association with RSV infection (AAP, 2012, p. 609).

Prevention of RSV

Prevention of RSV is a focus for children at high risk for severe bronchiolitis, including the following (AAP Committee on Infectious Disease, 2009):

- Children under 24 months of age with chronic lung disease of prematurity who have needed medical therapy within 6 months of the start of RSV season
- Children under 24 months of age with significant congenital heart disease requiring medical therapy
- Infants born at 28 weeks' gestation or less during their first 12 months of life
- Infants born at 29 to 32 weeks' gestation up to 6 months of age
- Infants born at 32 to 35 weeks' gestation with either of the following risk factors: childcare attendance or a sibling less than 5 years of age

Intramuscular palivizumab (Synagis) is used for prophylaxis for children in the high-risk category. A dose of 15 mg/kg is given every 30 days for 5 months beginning in October or November at the onset of the RSV season. Prophylactic treatment is expensive, but it costs less than hospitalization for an infant with RSV. Palivizumab does not interfere with administration of normal recommended childhood vaccines (AAP, 2012, p. 616).

Nursing Management

Nurses have a role in prevention of RSV by educating parents and caregivers about methods to reduce exposure and transmission of the disease by frequent hand hygiene and by eliminating exposure to crowds, other children, and cigarette smoke.

Nursing Assessment and Diagnosis

Physiologic Assessment

Assess airway and respiratory function carefully. Astute observation skills are important to ensure timely interventions for worsening respiratory symptoms and prevention of respiratory failure (see Table 25–1 and Clinical Manifestations: Respiratory Failure and Imminent Respiratory Arrest on page 746). Attach a cardiorespiratory monitor and pulse oximeter. A decreased oxygen saturation level below 90% is the best indicator of severe disease. Assess the child's skin and mucous membranes for hydration status. Weigh the child daily, and monitor the intake and output.

Practice Alert

Practice Alert

RSV bronchiolitis often increases in severity before beginning to resolve. Stay alert for signs of increased respiratory distress and a greater need for oxygen. Signs of life-threatening illness in the infant with bronchiolitis include central cyanosis, respiratory rate greater than 70 breaths per minute, listlessness, and apneic episodes. The chest is hyperinflated, and air exchange is so poor that breath sounds are very diminished on auscultation.

Psychosocial Assessment

Children and their parents should be observed for signs of fear and anxiety. The unfamiliar hospital environment and procedures can increase stress. Parents' questions, as well as their nonverbal cues, help direct nursing interventions during admission and throughout hospitalization.

The accompanying Nursing Care Plan lists common nursing diagnoses for the child with bronchiolitis. The following diagnoses might also be appropriate:

- Airway Clearance, Ineffective related to increased airway secretions in bronchioles
- Activity Intolerance related to imbalance between oxygen supply and demand
- Family Processes, Interrupted related to sudden acute illness of the infant

NANDA-I © 2012

Clinical Judgment

What assessment should be initiated if you notice that an infant who has had tachypnea for several hours begins breathing slower than the expected rate for age?

Planning and Implementation

Nursing management of the hospitalized child focuses on maintaining respiratory function, supporting overall physiologic function and hydration, reducing the child's and family's anxiety, and preparing the family for home care. Prevent the transmission of RSV and other organisms by using airborne and standard precautions. See Chapter 22 🔗, Box 22–1.

Maintain Respiratory Function

Close monitoring of the child's respiratory status is essential to evaluate the child's improvement or to spot early signs of deterioration. Supplemental oxygen with humidity may be provided via nasal cannula, mask, hood, or tent. When the child resists or is frightened by the oxygen apparatus on the face, engage the parent to soothe the child and promote acceptance of the therapy. Patent nares are important to promote oxygen intake. A bulb syringe and saline nosedrops can be used to quickly and easily clear the nasal passages. The head of the bed should be elevated to ease the work of breathing and drain mucus from the upper airways.

Support Physiologic Function

The grouping of nursing tasks promotes the child's physiologic function by decreasing stress and promoting rest. Rest is a key component in improving the child's breathing and overall health. Medications may be administered to control fever and promote comfort as needed.

Infants may have feeding difficulties and are at risk for aspiration. Suction the nasal passages before giving oral feedings. Smaller volumes and more frequent feedings will help conserve energy for infants with bronchiolitis who are formula-fed and breastfed. When tachypnea is present, oral feedings are withheld. Nasogastric tube feedings may be used to provide nutrition. An intravenous infusion may be ordered to rehydrate and maintain fluid balance until the child is capable of taking sufficient oral fluids.

Reduce Anxiety

The need for hospitalization and assistive therapies creates anxiety and fear in the child and parents. The parents may be frightened by the child's continued respiratory difficulty and the presence of assistive equipment at bedside. Infants may respond to their parents' anxiety and be more irritable. An important part of nursing care is anticipating, recognizing, and acting to decrease the child's and parents' anxiety. Provide parents with regular updates and explanations, and answer questions they may have about planned care.

Partner with parents to care for the child in the hospital. Their presence and ability to calm the infant or child can be helpful in the child's recovery. They should be reassured that holding or touching the child will not dislodge wires or tubing. If the child has been ill for a few days before admission, the parents are likely to be tired. Acknowledging parents' physical and emotional needs facilitates a spirit of caring and enhances communication between staff and family. Encourage the parents to take turns at the child's bedside and to take breaks for meals and rest.

Discharge Planning and Home Care Teaching

Children are discharged once they show sufficient stability in maintaining adequate oxygenation saturation without supplemental oxygen (as evidenced by easing of respiratory effort and decreased mucous production). In most children, symptoms decrease within 24 to 72 hours; however, resolution of all symptoms may take weeks. Coughing may continue for a few weeks postdischarge. Teach the parents that all who interact with the infant should wash their hands frequently to reduce exposure to other organisms. Educate parents about proper administration of medications. Acetaminophen may be prescribed for persistent low-grade fevers and general discomfort. Advise parents that RSV infection can recur; therefore, they need to know how to recognize signs and symptoms of respiratory distress and when to call the physician. See Partnering with Families: Discharge Teaching for Bronchiolitis.

Prevention

Another important nursing role is to educate parents of infants at high risk for RSV to obtain monthly injections of palivizumab and to promptly seek care if respiratory symptoms develop. Nurses in health centers administer palivizumab and should be aware that the injections are painful. Efforts to reduce the pain of the injection should be made. See Box 25–8. See Chapter 21 🔗.

Evaluation

In addition to the expected outcomes of nursing care provided on the accompanying Nursing Care Plan, the infant at high risk receives all doses of palivizumab.

BOX 25–8	Research: Reducing Pain of Palivizumab Injections

A recent study involving 55 infants and toddlers evaluated the use of EMLA cream and nitrous oxide for pain management of palivizumab injections. Each child randomly received one of three analgesic choices at each of the first 3 monthly injections: EMLA cream and air inhalation, nitrous oxide/oxygen plus an application of placebo cream, and nitrous oxide/oxygen plus EMLA. Nitrous oxide/oxygen inhalation was effective in decreasing pain associated with the injection, but the combined use of nitrous oxide/oxygen and EMLA cream was more effective than either treatment used alone (Carbajal, Biran, Lenclen, et al., 2008).

Nursing Care Plan The Child with Bronchiolitis

INTERVENTION	RATIONALE	EXPECTED OUTCOME
1. Nursing Diagnosis: Breathing Pattern, Ineffective related to increased work of breathing		
NIC Priority Intervention—*Respiratory Monitoring:* Collection and analysis of patient data to ensure airway patency and adequate gas exchange		**NOC Suggested Outcome—***Vital Signs Status:* Temperature, pulse, respiration, and blood pressure within expected range for the child's age
GOAL: *The child will return to respiratory baseline and will not experience respiratory failure.*		
■ Assess respiratory status (Table 25–1) when the child is calm and not crying at least every 2–4 hours, or more often as indicated for an increasing or decreasing respiratory rate and episodes of apnea. ■ Attach a cardiorespiratory monitor and pulse oximeter with alarms set. Record and report changes promptly to the physician.	■ Changes in breathing pattern occur quickly when the child's energy reserves are depleted. Baseline and subsequent assessments help detect changes in the respiratory rate and quality of respiratory effort. ■ The alarm can alert the nurse to any sudden respiratory changes and lead to more rapid interventions.	The child returns to respiratory baseline within 48–72 hours.
GOAL: *The child's oxygenation status will return to baseline.*		
■ Administer humidified oxygen via mask, nasal cannula, hood, or tent. ■ Assess and compare the child's SpO_2 level when on room air and on supplemental oxygen. ■ Note the child's response to ordered medications. ■ Position the head of the bed up, or place the child in a position of comfort on the parent's lap, if crying or struggling in the crib or bed. ■ Assess tolerance to feeding and activities.	■ Humidified oxygen loosens secretions, helps maintain oxygenation status, and eases respiratory distress. ■ Comparison of SpO_2 levels provides information to assess condition improvement. ■ Medications act systemically to improve oxygenation and decrease inflammation. ■ Position facilitates improved aeration and promotes decreased anxiety (especially in toddlers) and energy expenditure. ■ This provides an assessment of condition improvement.	The child's respiratory effort eases. The SpO_2 level remains at 95% or higher during treatment. The child tolerates therapeutic measures with no adverse effects. The child rests quietly in a position of comfort.
2. Nursing Diagnosis: Fluid Volume: Deficient, Risk for related to inability to meet body requirements and increased metabolic demand		
NIC Priority Intervention—*Fluid Management:* Promotion of fluid balance and prevention of complications resulting from abnormal or undesired fluid levels		**NOC Suggested Outcome—***Hydration:* Amount of water in intracellular and extracellular compartments of body
GOAL: *The child's immediate fluid deficit is corrected.*		
■ Evaluate need for intravenous fluids. Maintain IV, if ordered.	■ Previous fluid loss may require immediate replacement.	The child's hydration status improves during the acute phase of illness as demonstrated by appropriate urine output and moist mucous membranes.
GOAL: *The child will be adequately hydrated, be able to tolerate oral fluids, and progress to a normal diet.*		
■ Calculate maintenance fluid requirements and give oral fluids, IV fluids, or both. ■ Offer clear fluids and incorporate parents in care. Offer fluid choice when tolerated. ■ Maintain strict intake and output monitoring and evaluate specific gravity at least every 8 hours. ■ Perform daily weight measurement on the same scale at the same time of day. ■ Assess mucous membranes and presence of tears. Evaluate skin turgor.	■ Assessment of fluid requirements enables the nurse to maintain hydration while transitioning the child to oral fluids. ■ A choice of fluid offered by the parent gains the child's cooperation. ■ Monitoring provides objective evidence of fluid loss and ongoing hydration status. ■ Weight measurement provides further evidence of improvement of hydration status. ■ Moist mucous membranes and tears are signs of adequate hydration.	The child takes adequate oral fluids to maintain hydration. The child accepts the beverage of choice from the parent or nursing staff. The child's weight stabilizes after 24–48 hours; skin turgor is supple. The child shows evidence of improved hydration.

Nursing Care Plan | The Child with Bronchiolitis, *continued*

INTERVENTION	RATIONALE	EXPECTED OUTCOME
3. Nursing Diagnosis: Anxiety (Child and Parent) related to acute illness, hospitalization, uncertain course of illness and treatment, and home care needs		
NIC Priority Intervention—*Anxiety Reduction:* Minimizing apprehension, dread, foreboding, or uneasiness related to an unidentified source of anticipated danger		**NOC Suggested Outcome—***Anxiety Control:* Ability to eliminate or reduce feelings of apprehension and tension from an unidentifiable source
GOAL: *The child and parents will demonstrate behaviors that indicate less anxiety.*		
■ Encourage parents to express fears and ask questions; provide direct answers and discuss care, procedures, and condition changes.	■ Parents have the opportunity to vent feelings and receive timely, relevant information. This reduces parents' anxiety and increases trust in nursing staff.	Parents and child show less anxiety as symptoms improve and as the child and parents feel more secure in the hospital environment. The parent freely asks questions and participates in the child's care. The child cries less and allows staff to hold or touch him or her.
■ Incorporate parents in the child's care. Encourage parents to bring familiar objects from home. Ask about and incorporate in the care plan the home routines for feeding and sleeping.	■ Familiar people, routines, and objects decrease the child's anxiety and increase parents' sense of control over an unexpected, uncertain situation.	
GOAL: *Parents will verbalize knowledge of bronchiolitis symptoms and use of home care methods before the child's discharge from the hospital.*		
■ Explain symptoms, treatment, and home care of bronchiolitis.	■ Anticipating the potential for recurrence assists the family to be prepared for a potential recurrence of respiratory symptoms after discharge.	Parents accurately describe respiratory symptoms and initial home care actions.
■ Provide written instructions for follow-up care arrangements, as needed.	■ Written and verbal instructions reinforce knowledge. Parents may not "hear" and remember details if only given verbally.	
■ Make sure parents can read the instructions, provided in the family's primary language.	■ Many families have reading difficulty and may read a language other than English.	

NANDA-I © 2012

Pneumonia

Pneumonia is an inflammation or infection of the bronchioles and alveolar spaces of the lungs. It occurs most often in infants and young children. The incidence of pneumonia in the United States is 35 to 40 cases for every 1,000 children younger than 5 years of age, and 7 cases for every 1,000 adolescents 12 to 15 years of age (Durbin & Stille, 2008). Pneumonia can be community-acquired or hospital-acquired (e.g., associated with mechanical ventilation). Children at higher risk for community-acquired pneumonia are those exposed to cigarette or woodstove smoke and those with chronic conditions, such as sickle cell disease, asthma, bronchopulmonary dysplasia, cystic fibrosis, congenital heart disease, and immunodeficiency.

Etiology and Pathophysiology

Pneumonia may be viral, mycoplasmal, or bacterial in origin. In children under 5 years of age, pneumonia is most often caused by viruses such as RSV, influenza A and B, parainfluenza virus, adenovirus, and human metapneumovirus. Bacterial pneumonia is more common in children older than 5 years of age, but it can occur in all age groups. Common bacterial organisms include *Streptococcus pneumoniae*, *Chlamydophila pneumoniae*, and *Staphylococcus aureus*. Group B *streptococcus*, enteric gram-negative bacilli, and *Chlamydia trachomatis* are found in infants younger than age 3 months.

The infection often follows an upper respiratory tract infection with inhalation of organisms colonized in the nasopharynx or bacteremia that spreads the organisms to the lung tissue. The lower airway

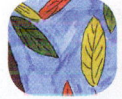

Partnering with Families

Discharge Teaching for Bronchiolitis

General care instructions:
■ Use a bulb syringe to clear the nares of an infant under 1 year of age.
■ Give fluids to help keep secretions thin and provide small frequent feedings.
■ Encourage active toddlers to rest and take naps during recovery; however, toddlers usually recognize their own activity limits and rest.
■ Make sure the infant gets adequate rest and nutrition. Limit the time upright in infant seats and swings (Coffman, 2009).

Advise parents to call the healthcare provider if:
■ Breathing is rapid or difficult.
■ Respiratory symptoms interfere with sleep or eating.
■ Symptoms persist in a child who is less than 1 year old, has heart or lung disease, or was premature and had lung disease after birth.
■ The child acts sicker—appears tired, less playful, and less interested in food (parents just "feel" the child is not improving).

has physiologic defense mechanisms (mucociliary clearance, coughing, and secretion of IgA) that promote its ability to retain a sterile environment, in addition to immune mechanisms. Some noninfectious causes of pneumonia include aspiration of food, emesis, gastric reflux, and hydrocarbon ingestions. These substances cause **pneumonitis,** a chemical injury, and an inflammatory response sets the stage for bacterial invasion.

Bacterial pathophysiology. When bacterial invaders circulate through the bloodstream to the lungs, they attach to the respiratory epithelium and cause cell destruction. An inflammatory response and edema usually result. Cellular debris and mucus cause airway obstruction. This leads to the proliferation of organisms that spread within the bronchial tree. Bacteria may be distributed evenly throughout one or more lobes of a single lung, a pattern termed *unilateral lobar pneumonia*. Potential complications of bacterial pneumonia include pleural effusion, empyema, pericarditis, and bacteremia.

Viral pathophysiology. Viruses frequently enter from the upper respiratory tract, infiltrating the alveoli nearest the bronchi of one or both lungs. The virus invades alveolar cells, replicating and bursting out forcefully, killing the cells and sending out cell debris. Airway obstruction occurs due to swelling, abnormal secretions, and cellular debris. The viral cells rapidly invade adjacent areas, distributing themselves in a scattered, patchy pattern, often referred to as bronchopneumonia. The small airway in infants increases the risk for progression to atelectasis, edema, a ventilation-perfusion mismatch, and hypoxemia. The resulting lung injury makes the child susceptible to secondary bacterial pneumonia.

Clinical Manifestations

Pneumonia is often preceded by an upper respiratory tract infection including rhinitis and a cough. Regardless of the causative agent, symptoms include fever (usually a lower temperature is associated with viral pneumonia), cough, and tachypnea. Other signs and symptoms include crackles, wheezes, dyspnea, restlessness, and decreased breath sounds if consolidation exists. Newborns and infants may have grunting, nasal flaring, irritability, lethargy, and a diminished appetite. Diminished breath sounds may be noted. Children with bacterial pneumonia may have chest pain and try to splint the chest when coughing. As the condition increases in severity, the infant or child will have increased work of breathing, cyanosis, retractions, and use of accessory muscles. See the Clinical Manifestations table below. A child's age, severity of symptoms, and presence of an underlying lung, cardiac, or immunodeficiency disease may result in variations from classical clinical findings.

Collaborative Care

Diagnostic Procedures

Diagnosis is made based upon history, physical signs, and symptoms. Chest radiography helps distinguish the type of pneumonia present. See the Clinical Manifestations table below for characteristic radiographic findings. A blood culture may be obtained when the child has a high fever. Children over 8 years of age may be able to produce enough sputum for culture. Younger children may have a nasopharyngeal aspirate tested with polymerase chain reaction or immunofluorescence tests to identify respiratory viruses. A white blood cell count greater than 20,000 may be a sign of bacterial cause. A tuberculin test should be performed in any child with known exposure or risk factors for tuberculosis (see page 767). Children with recurrent pneumonia (two or more episodes in a year or a lifetime total of three or more episodes) need to be evaluated for immunodeficiency syndromes, foreign body aspiration, obstruction or compression of the airway, anatomic abnormality, cystic fibrosis, and asthma (Durbin & Stille, 2008).

Clinical Therapy

Clinical management for all types of pneumonia includes symptomatic therapy (pain and fever control) and supportive care through airway management, fluids, fever management, and rest. Community-acquired pneumonia is initially treated with oral amoxicillin, clindamycin, or cefixime. If hospitalization is required, IV ampicillin, clindamycin, or cefotaxime is used. Vancomycin is reserved for complicated pneumonia in hospitalized children (Kronman & Shah, 2009). The child hospitalized with community-acquired pneumonia receives supplemental oxygen and IV fluids to maintain hydration. When complications such as an **empyema** (a collection of pus in the pleural space) or pleural effusion develop, a thoracostomy tube may be inserted for drainage. Refer to the Skills Manual ⊂▭⊃.

Clinical Manifestations Pneumonia by Causative Organism		
ETIOLOGY	**CLINICAL MANIFESTATIONS**	**CHEST RADIOGRAPH FINDINGS**
Mycoplasma pneumoniae	Insidious onset, malaise, muscle aches, headache, fever, sore throat, rhinorrhea, dry hacking cough that becomes productive, fine crackles, anorexia	Bilateral patchy infiltrates and mild pleural effusions
Viral pneumonia	Sudden or insidious onset, rhinorrhea, slight cough that may become productive, low-grade fever and chills, crackles, and wheezes	Bilateral interstitial infiltrates and hyperinflation
Streptococcus pneumoniae	Sudden onset, high fever, productive cough, chest pain, tachypnea, nasal flaring, retractions, fine crackles, decreased breath sounds in affected area and dullness on percussion, fremitus; may have emesis and abdominal pain	Lobar consolidation, may have pleural effusions
Staphylococcus aureus	Upper respiratory infection and abrupt change in condition, high fever, cough, toxic appearance, lethargy, chest pain, nasal flaring, retractions, fine crackles, dullness on percussion, fremitus	Limited patchy infiltrate, multilobar consolidation
Chlamydia pneumoniae	Insidious onset, minimal or absent fever, tachypnea, malaise, persistent cough, pharyngitis	Pleural effusions and lobar infiltrates

Nursing Management

Most children with pneumonia are cared for at home. For those infants and children who are hospitalized, the goal of nursing care is to monitor the child's condition for increasing respiratory distress and to restore optimal respiratory function. Nursing measures for the child with bronchiolitis are generally applicable to the child with pneumonia.

Nursing Assessment and Diagnosis

Assess the infant's or child's condition, paying particular attention to respiratory rate, heart rate, and temperature, and observe color for pallor or cyanosis. Attach a pulse oximeter to monitor the SpO_2 level. Assess hydration status. Assess for the presence of pain with coughing.

Examples of nursing diagnoses include the following:

- Fatigue related to respiratory distress, coughing, and sleep deprivation
- Airway Clearance, Ineffective related to exudate in the alveoli
- Fluid Volume: Imbalanced, Risk for related to increased metabolic rate, fever, and respiratory distress

NANDA-I © 2012

Planning and Implementation

The goal of nursing care is to restore optimal respiratory function. Assist the child to take deep breaths to fully aerate the lungs and to promote coughing to clear secretions and cellular debris. The child may need relief of pain when coughing and deep breathing. Teach the child and parent how to splint the chest, by hugging a small pillow, teddy bear, or doll, to make coughing less painful. Pain medication (acetaminophen or ibuprofen) can provide the added benefits of temperature control and may aid in sleep.

Maintain hydration by offering preferred clear fluids. Administer IV fluids when the infant or child is unable to maintain an adequate fluid intake. Encourage small amounts of soft foods when tolerated. Give antibiotics as prescribed.

Discharge Planning and Home Care Teaching

Discharge planning should be addressed early in the hospital stay. Medications, especially antibiotics, must be taken at prescribed intervals and for the full course. Make sure parents learn the proper administration of drugs and any side effects. Inform parents of signs indicating the infant's or child's condition may be worsening such as increased difficulty breathing and refusal to take fluids. Provide contact information in case parents have questions or are concerned about the child's condition. A chest radiograph may be obtained during a follow-up visit to see if the lungs are clear. Symptoms of pneumonia usually disappear long before the lungs are completely healed. Some children continue to have worsening reactive airway problems or abnormal results on pulmonary function tests. Most children, however, recover uneventfully.

Preventive measures against pneumonia are limited; however, the *Haemophilus influenzae* type b vaccine has dramatically reduced the incidence of pneumonia due to that organism. The new pneumococcal conjugate vaccine (PCV13), now regularly administered to infants, is expected to further reduce the incidence of pneumonia due to strains of *Streptococcus pneumoniae* beyond that of the previous vaccine (PCV7). The 23-valent pneumococcal vaccine is recommended for children over 2 years of age who are immunosuppressed or have chronic diseases (sickle cell disease, other types of functional or anatomic asplenia, HIV infection, or primary immunodeficiency) and for children who are receiving immunosuppressive therapy. See Chapter 22 for information about immunization schedules and a discussion on pertussis.

Tuberculosis

Tuberculosis (TB), caused by the organism *Mycobacterium tuberculosis*, is a major world public health problem. In 2000, the estimated number of new cases of TB in the world was 8.3 million, and 884,019 (11%) were in children under 15 years of age (Marais & Schaaf, 2010). The epidemic of HIV infection has had a significant effect on the rates of children with TB in developing countries. In 2007, 820 children under 15 years of age in the United States acquired TB (Cruz & Starke, 2010). In 2010, the TB rate was 11 times greater among foreign-born persons in the United States than among U.S.-born persons. Rates were also higher among Hispanics, non-Hispanic Blacks, and Asians than among non-Hispanic Whites (Centers for Disease Control and Prevention [CDC], 2011a). For both U.S.-born and foreign-born children and adolescents, children under 5 years of age had the highest rate of TB, but foreign-born adolescents had a rate 20 times higher than U.S.-born adolescents (Menzies, Winston, Holtz, et al., 2010).

Etiology and Pathophysiology

Children usually acquire a TB infection from infected adults who cough, sneeze, speak, or sing, and send out tiny droplets containing the bacillus. When the child inhales these droplets, the bacillus is small enough to travel directly to the alveoli and cause infection; however, many bacilli are trapped in the upper airway, preventing infection. When the bacillus reaches the alveoli, an immune response is initiated. Macrophages surround the bacillus and wall it off where it multiplies within a small hard capsule, called a tubercle. The tubercle bacilli grow slowly, dividing every 25 to 32 hours. The bacilli grow for 2 to 12 weeks until they number 1,000 to 10,000, at which point the cellular immune response to TB can be elicited by a response to the TB skin test.

In persons with intact cell-mediated immunity, activated T cells and macrophages form granulomas that limit multiplication and spread of the organism. Proliferation of TB is arrested once cell-mediated immunity develops, but small numbers of viable bacilli may remain in the granuloma. These individuals have latent tuberculosis infection (LTBI) with a positive tuberculin skin test and no clinical or radiographic signs of disease. They are not infectious and cannot transmit the disease.

Active TB can develop as the bacilli grow, divide within the macrophage, and break free of the macrophage. Infants and adolescents have the greatest risk of transitioning from LTBI to active TB. Factors increasing that risk include immunosuppressive therapy, HIV co-infection, malnutrition, vitamin D deficiency, chronic medical conditions, and TB infection in the past 2 years (AAP, 2012, p. 738; Newton, Brent, Anderson, et al., 2008). The greatest risk for LTBI transition to active TB (including meningitis and disseminated TB) occurs within 2 to 12 months after initial infection (Ranganathan & Sonnappa, 2009). Children younger than 10 years of age with active TB are rarely contagious because they have small pulmonary lesions and an unproductive cough from which few or no bacilli are expelled (AAP, 2012, pp. 738–739).

Extrapulmonary TB occurs in 10% to 20% of children (Peredo-Pinto & Jacobs, 2008). Tuberculosis meningitis can occur 3 to 6 months after primary infection and is one of the most severe forms of childhood TB (Newton et al., 2008). If a tubercle extends into a blood vessel, TB can also spread to the liver, spleen, kidneys, or bone marrow.

Clinical Manifestations

Infants, children, and adolescents with LTBI are asymptomatic. Infants with pulmonary TB may have a persistent cough, decreased appetite, weight loss or failure to gain weight, low-grade fever, and fatigue. Wheezing and decreased breath sounds may be present, but respiratory distress is uncommon. Children with active TB may have fatigue, cough, anorexia, weight loss or growth delay, night sweats, chills, a low-grade fever, and enlarged lymph nodes. Hemoptysis is a late sign of advanced pulmonary TB.

When TB has spread outside the pulmonary system, signs are specific to the system invaded:

- **Superficial lymphadenitis:** firm, nontender, or minimally tender lymph nodes measuring 2 to 4 cm; matting of nodes; may have overlying violet-colored skin discoloration
- **Pleural effusion:** fever, fatigue, respiratory distress, chest pain, diminished breath sounds, and dullness to percussion; more common on right side; occurs more often in older children and adolescents
- **Central nervous system and miliary:** occurs most commonly in children under age 2 years; high fever, vomiting, lethargy, headache, seizures, nuchal rigidity, cranial nerve palsies, and irritability; also hepatosplenomegaly and generalized lymphadenopathy
- **Osteoarticular:** inflammation, pain, swelling, fever, and limited range of motion of the affected bone or joint

Collaborative Care

Diagnostic Procedures

Screening to identify an infant's or child's risk for LTBI should occur during the first health visit, then every 6 months until 2 years of age, and then annually. Administer an intradermal tuberculin skin test (TST) with 5 tuberculin units of purified protein derivative (PPD, the Mantoux test) if one or more of these risk factors are present (AAP, 2012, p. 740):

- The child was born in any country or region with endemic infection, e.g., Asia, Middle East, Africa, Latin America, and countries of the former Soviet Union.

- The child traveled outside the United States and had contact with the resident population for more than a week in any country or region listed above.
- The child has a family member or contact with confirmed or suspected contagious TB.

A positive test (induration of 15 mm or greater) indicates that the child has been exposed to and infected with TB, and antibodies have been produced against the bacillus (AAP, 2012, p. 742).

An interferon-gamma release assay, QuantiFERON-TB Gold (QFT-G), may be beneficial to support TST findings. It is most useful when a child vaccinated with bacille Calmette-Guérin (BCG) has a borderline positive response to the PPD, when a repeat PPD may cause a boost response, or when the child cannot return in 48 to 72 hours for a PPD reading (Ranganathan & Sonnappa, 2009). Like the PPD, the QFT-G cannot distinguish between latent or active TB. See Table 25–6 for other diagnostic procedures that may be used to confirm the diagnosis. Acid-fast stains of blood, gastric aspirate, and sputum cultures reveal the bacillus. Chest radiographic findings vary depending upon the child's condition, and may include a granuloma, calcification, intrathoracic lymphadenopathy, atelectasis or infiltrate of a segment or lobe, pleural effusion, cavitary lesions, or miliary (disseminated) disease. For infants, children, and adolescents with active TB, a chest radiograph should be obtained after 2 to 3 months of therapy to evaluate response.

Clinical Therapy

Management focuses on diagnosis and treatment of active and latent TB with antitubercular drugs, including isoniazid, rifampin, pyrazinamide, and ethambutol. See Medications Used to Treat Latent and Active TB in Children on page 769. Drug resistance to these medications has occurred because infected individuals did not complete courses of medications, permitting the TB bacillus to develop resistance. Therapy for active TB usually involves a 6-month regimen consisting of isoniazid, rifampin, pyrazinamide, and ethambutol for the first 2 months, and isoniazid and rifampin for the remaining 4 months.

TABLE 25–6	Diagnostic Procedures for Tuberculosis
DIAGNOSTIC TEST	**INDICATION AND RATIONALE**
Intradermal injection of purified protein derivative (PPD)	Confirms infection (latent or active) with the TB organism (3–12 weeks after exposure); however, the child must return in 48–72 hours for the test to be read and interpreted. The response is boosted if positive and used a second time.
QuantiFERON-TB Gold (QFT-G)	Confirms infection (latent or active) with the TB organism through blood analysis within 24 hours. Does not boost patient's response if used a second time.
Chest radiograph (anteroposterior and lateral views)	Confirms presence of pulmonary TB (small, seed-like opacities may be visible); however, radiologic changes may look like other chronic lung conditions.
Blood cultures for *Mycobacterium tuberculosis*	Proves diagnosis; defines specific drug sensitivity.
Gastric washings (nasogastric tube aspirates), performed in early morning before ambulation or feeding on 3 separate days	Confirms active pulmonary TB. Used in children under 12 years who cannot produce sputum.
Sputum cultures (expectorated, from bronchoscopic examination, or induced sputum using aerosolized hypertonic saline)	Confirms active pulmonary TB.
Biopsy of pleura, lymph nodes, liver, other tissues for culture and tissue examination	Taken when lymphadenopathy, pleural effusion, or other extrapulmonary signs are present.
Lumbar puncture	Tests cerebrospinal fluid to confirm meningeal TB.

Source: *Data from the American Academy of Pediatrics. (2012). Red Book: 2012 Report of the Committee on Infectious Diseases (29th ed., pp. 739–740). Elk Grove Village, IL: Author; Marais, B. J., & Schaaf, H. S. (2010). Childhood tuberculosis: An emerging and previously neglected problem. Infectious Disease Clinics of North America, 24, 727–749.*

Medications Used to Treat Latent and Active TB in Children

MEDICATION AND CLASSIFICATION	NURSING MANAGEMENT
Isoniazid (bactericidal)	■ Obtain baseline bilirubin and liver function studies as hepatotoxicity can occur. ■ Obtain a baseline weight. ■ Assess ophthalmologic and hematopoietic status studies. ■ Give 1 hour before or 2 hours after meals unless gastrointestinal irritation occurs, then give with food. Tablets can be crushed. ■ Interferes with hepatic metabolism of phenytoin, may cause toxicity. ■ Monitor for symptoms of hypersensitivity, signs of hepatotoxicity (anorexia, fever, malaise, nausea, vomiting, diarrhea, weight loss), dark urine, and jaundice. ■ Adolescent should avoid alcohol. ■ Pyridoxine supplementation (vitamin B_6) is recommended for children and adolescents with meat- and milk-deficient diets, children with nutritional deficiencies, infants being exclusively breastfed, and adolescents who are pregnant or HIV infected to prevent peripheral neuritis and seizures.
Rifampin (bactericidal)	■ Obtain baseline bilirubin and liver function studies as this drug can alter the pharmacokinetics and serum concentrations of other drugs. ■ Assess medications taken for interaction with rifampin (i.e., diazepam, beta-adrenergics, barbiturates, analgesics, corticosteroids, digitalis, and others). ■ Assess renal and hematopoietic status studies. ■ Give 1 hour before or 2 hours after meals unless gastrointestinal irritation occurs, then give with food. Capsule contents can be sprinkled on applesauce or suspended in flavored syrup. ■ Monitor for symptoms of jaundice and other side effects. ■ Inform parents and child about orange-colored body fluids. ■ Contact lens will become permanently discolored if used. ■ Adolescent females who are sexually active should not use oral contraceptives as rifampin makes them ineffective.
Pyrazinamide (bacteriostatic)	■ Obtain baseline liver function studies, and renal and hematopoietic status studies. Monitor for symptoms of hepatotoxicity. ■ Monitor blood glucose level in children with diabetes as glycemic control may be affected. ■ When used in combination with isoniazid and rifampin, a 6-month course of therapy is possible.
Ethambutol (bacteriostatic or bactericidal, depending upon dosage used)	■ Obtain baseline liver function studies, and renal and hematopoietic status studies. ■ Perform a baseline and monthly ophthalmologic test of visual acuity, visual fields, and color discrimination as the drug may cause reversible or irreversible optic neuritis, particularly in children with impaired renal function. ■ Give with meals if gastrointestinal irritation occurs. ■ Inform parents and child to report any vision changes.

LTBI is treated with a single daily dose of isoniazid for 9 months (or rifampin for 6 months if TB is drug resistant to isoniazid). Therapeutic agents are modified if a drug-resistant strain of TB is causing the infection. Other drugs are used less commonly for treatment of drug-resistant TB, including amikacin, capreomycin, cycloserine, ethionamide, kanamycin, levofloxacin, moxifloxacin, para-aminosalicylic acid, and streptomycin (AAP, 2012, p. 748–749).

TB is a major public health problem, especially with the number of drug-resistant strains developing worldwide. By law, cases of active TB must be reported immediately to the public health department so that disease contacts can be traced to help prevent further spread. If a child is diagnosed with TB, it is considered a sentinel case, and an adult contact with active TB must be identified.

Nursing Management

Nurses have an important role in identifying children with one or more risk factors for TB, such as foreign-born children and children with potential exposure, so infected children can get prompt treatment.

Nursing Assessment and Diagnosis

Assessment focuses on retaining a level of suspicion that certain children are at higher risk for exposure to TB and for developing the infection, and considering appropriate screening guidelines using the information on page 768. In addition, consider the child's immunosuppression status and exposure to individuals with HIV infection. Children at risk should have a PPD applied and read within 48 to 72 hours.

Carefully evaluate infants and young children who have a tuberculin skin test conversion as they are at greater risk to develop active TB over the next few months. When the ill child presents for health care, perform a complete physical assessment, but carefully assess for weight loss, fever, fatigue, coughing, and respiratory status. If TB is suspected, implement airborne isolation precautions until the infection status is known.

When the child is hospitalized with active TB, assess the child's respiratory status, energy level, nutritional intake, and weight. The child with no cough and negative sputum acid-fast bacillus smears does not need to be isolated (AAP, 2012, p. 756). If the patient is contagious, airborne isolation is needed. The nurse assists with the collection of blood, sputum, and gastric aspirate cultures so that drug sensitivity can be identified.

Examples of nursing diagnoses that might be appropriate include the following:

- Infection, Risk for (Active TB) related to positive tuberculin skin test
- Nutrition, Imbalanced: Less than Body Requirements related to anorexia and active infection
- Therapeutic Regimen Management: Family, Ineffective related to poor adherence to medication administration regimen

NANDA-I © 2012

Planning and Implementation

Nursing care centers on administering medications and providing supportive care. Teach parents and children about the disease process, medications, possible side effects, and the importance of long-term therapy for the prescribed 6 to 12 months. Offer suggestions for medication administration to resistant infants and toddlers. Emphasize the importance of taking medications as prescribed on an empty stomach.

Clinical Tip

Children with active TB should receive "directly observed drug therapy" administered by a nurse or other healthcare provider to ensure that the drug is being taken. Direct observation should occur 2 or 3 times a week for the duration of treatment (Ranganathan & Sonnappa, 2009). Even children with LTBI should receive directly observed drug therapy twice a week.

The nurse works with the families of children and adolescents with LTBI to encourage completion of therapy. Help the family to develop a strategy that enables them to remember to give the medication on alternating days with directly observed drug therapy. In the case of an adolescent, the nurse encourages increased responsibility for health care. While parents need to be involved, the adolescent can make choices about the time of day to take the medication and can set up a reminder system to take it. Parents can support the adolescent by establishing a contract with incentives when the adolescent takes all medications in the established time period.

Unless the child is seriously ill, hospitalization is not needed. In most cases when the child is hospitalized, standard precautions are maintained as the child is not infectious. If the child or adolescent has extensive pulmonary infection, positive sputum cultures, or suspected congenital tuberculosis, airborne precautions are used, including an airborne infection isolation room and a "fitted" and "sealed" particulate respirator for all healthcare providers. Airborne precautions are used until culture smears indicate a diminishing number of organisms and the older child's or adolescent's cough is improving (AAP, 2012, p. 756). Limit visitors to people who have been medically evaluated for TB to reduce the risk of infection to other children and hospital staff. Family members should use masks (reverse airborne precautions) when visiting the child in the hospital until it is determined that they are not infectious. Facilitate tuberculin skin testing of family members and close contacts followed by chest radiographs as necessary.

Encourage proper nutrition and rest to promote normal growth and development. The child can return to school or childcare when effective therapy has been instituted, adherence to therapy has been documented, and clinical symptoms have diminished substantially (AAP, 2012, p. 758). Most children who have been successfully treated for TB are able to lead essentially normal lives. The sections

on pneumonia on page 767 and on meningitis in Chapter 33 🔗 discuss other nursing measures appropriate for the child with TB.

Evaluation

Expected outcomes of nursing care may include:

- The child completes the full course of TB medications.
- The child regains energy and appetite, and catch-up growth occurs.
- TB testing of all family members and close contacts occurs, followed by treatment as appropriate.

CHRONIC LUNG DISEASES

Asthma

Asthma is a chronic disorder of the airways that is complex and characterized by variable and recurring symptoms, airflow obstruction, bronchial hyperresponsiveness, and an underlying inflammation (National Asthma Education and Prevention Program, 2007, p. 12). Asthma is one of the most common chronic disorders affecting children, and the **prevalence** (the percentage of the population that has a condition at a specific point in time) of asthma remains at historic high levels since the late 1990s. In the United States, the rate of asthma prevalence for children ages 0 to 17 years continues to rise, from 8.7% in 2001 to 9.6% (7.1 million) in 2009; however, this rate is higher among children in lower socioeconomic families. Boys more commonly have asthma than girls, but during adolescence the prevalence of asthma in girls is similar to that of boys. Of these children, 57.2% reported an asthma episode in the past 12 months (Akinbami, Moorman, & Liu, 2011; CDC, 2011b).

Asthma has a significant impact on children and their families. In 2009, 59.1% of children with a reported asthma episode missed at least one day of school due to asthma, and the average number of school days missed was 3.8. An asthma episode resulted in an emergency department visit by 32.5% of children, and 8% were hospitalized (CDC, 2011b). In the United States, a total of 6.7 million visits for asthma episodes were made by children to private physician offices, and 0.8 million visits were made by children to hospital outpatient departments. An average number of 174 deaths per year are due to asthma in the United States (Akinbami et al., 2011). See Developing Cultural Competence: Asthma Prevalence.

Developing Cultural Competence
Asthma Prevalence

The prevalence of asthma among children in the United States varies by racial and ethnic group. Non-Hispanic White children have a prevalence of 8.2%. In contrast, non-Hispanic Black children have a prevalence rate of 11.1%. When all subgroups of Hispanic children are considered together, their prevalence rate is 6.3%; however, Puerto Rican children have the highest prevalence (16.6%). Mexican children have the lowest prevalence rates (4.9%) of all Hispanic groups. Asian children have an asthma prevalence of 5.3%, and American Indians and Native Alaskans have a prevalence rate of 8.8% (Akinbami et al., 2011). The higher rate in non-Hispanic Black children may be associated with a higher percentage of these children living in urban and low socioeconomic areas as well as being exposed to emotional stress, such as living in a community with a high level of violence (Hines, 2011). One potential explanation for the higher prevalence rate of Puerto Rican children is an ethnic-specific genetic predisposition associated with the inflammatory cascade along with physical and socioeconomic exposures (e.g., molds, traffic-related emissions, and maternal smoking) (Watts & Schechter, 2010).

Pathophysiology Illustrated Asthmatic Episode

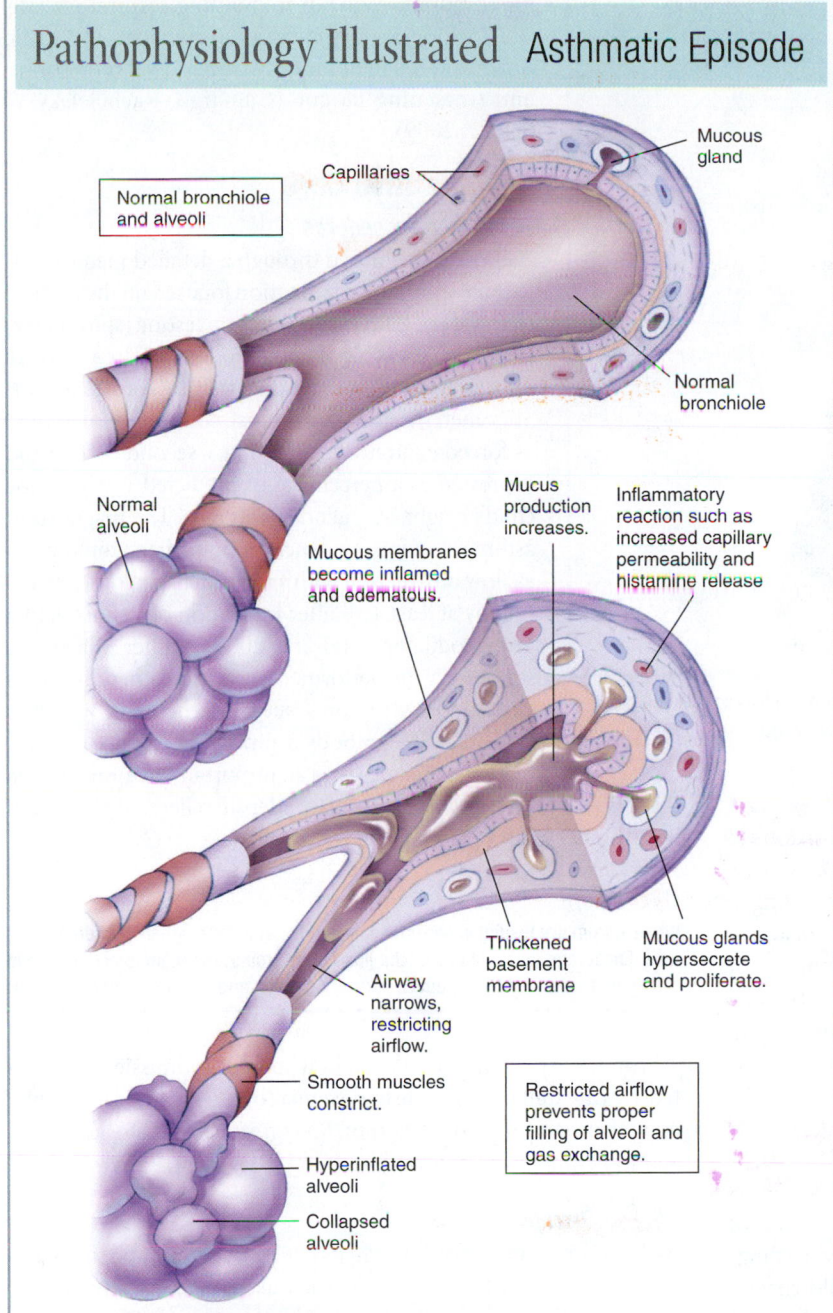

FIGURE 25–12 ■ What can cause an asthmatic episode? Some asthma triggers are exercise, infection, and allergies. This illustration shows how asthma obstructs airflow through bronchoconstriction and inflammatory changes, narrowing the airway and thus increasing production of mucus.

According to the hygiene hypothesis, these protective factors increase exposure to infections in early life that enable the child's immune system to develop along a nonallergic pathway (National Asthma Education and Prevention Program, 2007, p. 23).

Inflammation causes the normal protective mechanisms of the lungs (mucous formation, mucosal swelling, and airway muscle contraction) to overreact in response to a stimulus and cause an acute asthma episode (sudden onset of breathing difficulty with cough, wheeze, or breathlessness) and airway obstruction. The **trigger,** a stimulus initiating an acute asthma episode, can be inflammatory or noninflammatory. Triggers increase the frequency and severity of smooth muscle contraction (bronchospasm), and airway responsiveness is enhanced through inflammatory mechanisms. Asthma triggers include exercise, viral or bacterial agents, allergens (mold, dust, pollen, furry pets, birds), fragrances, food additives, pollutants, weather changes (humidity and temperature), and emotions or stress. The asthma triggers may vary for individual children.

With exposure to a trigger, IgE and sensitized mast cells may be activated, leading to the release of many inflammatory mediators (e.g., histamines, prostaglandins, and leukotrienes). The inflammatory mediators release pro-inflammatory cytokines, causing chronic airway inflammation that may be associated with **airway remodeling** (permanent airway damage that involves thickening of the subbasement membrane, subepithelial fibrosis, airway smooth muscle hypertrophy and hyperplasia, blood vessel proliferation and dilation, and mucous gland hyperplasia and hypersecretion) (Brashers, 2010a). This results in decreased airway elasticity and decreased lung function. These permanent alterations are not prevented by or fully responsive to currently available treatments (Brashers, 2010a; National Asthma Education and Prevention Program, 2007, pp. 16–19). The reactive airway responses to stimuli are present before the trigger initiates the physiologic sequence that results in an asthma episode.

Airway narrowing results from bronchial constriction, airway swelling, and production of copious amounts of mucus. Mucus clogs small airways, trapping air below the plugs (Figure 25–12 ■). Decreased perfusion of the alveolar capillaries results from hypoxic vasoconstriction and increased pressure due to hyperinflation of the alveoli. Hypoxemia leads to an increased respiratory rate with a reduced minute volume (air breathed per minute) because of airway resistance.

Etiology and Pathophysiology

Asthma is a chronic inflammatory disease of the lungs in children who are genetically susceptible. More than 100 genes are associated with the susceptibility and pathogenesis of asthma (Brashers, 2010a). Some of these genes regulate the inflammatory process. It is caused by the interplay of multiple factors, including indoor air contaminants (e.g., tobacco smoke, pet dander, and cockroach feces), outdoor air pollutants, recurrent respiratory viral infections, and allergic disease (e.g., atopic eczema, hay fever, and food allergies). Protective factors that reduce the risk for asthma include a large family size, later birth order, childcare attendance, dog in the family, and living on a farm.

Clinical Manifestations

The sudden appearance of breathing difficulty (cough, wheeze, or breathlessness) is often referred to as an acute asthma episode, asthma flare, or asthma attack. The infant or child who has had frequent episodes of coughing or frequent respiratory infections should also be evaluated for asthma. Frequent coughing, especially at night, is the warning signal that the child's airway is very sensitive to stimuli; it may be the only sign in "silent" asthma.

Pathophysiology Illustrated Barrel Chest

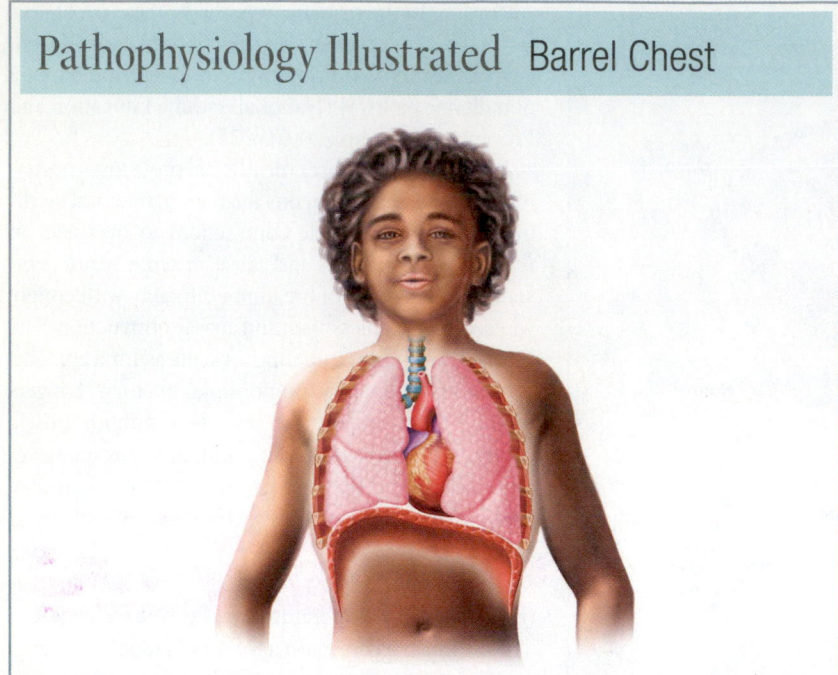

FIGURE 25–13 ■ A barrel chest may result from chronic respiratory conditions such as asthma or bronchopulmonary dysplasia, in which chronic air trapping or hyperinflation of the alveoli occur.

During an acute episode, respirations are rapid and labored and the child often appears tired because of the ongoing effort required to breathe. Nasal flaring and intercostal retractions may be visible. The child exhibits a productive cough and expiratory wheezing, a prolonged expiratory phase, decreased air movement, use of accessory muscles, and respiratory fatigue. The child may complain of chest tightness. Moderate anxiety occurs as the asthma episode begins, and increases as the episode intensifies. Severe anxiety, in turn, intensifies physical responses and symptoms, and a vicious cycle is established.

In cases of severe obstruction, wheezing may not be heard because of the lack of airflow. Head bobbing may be seen in young children with the use of accessory muscles (sternocleidomastoids) to breathe. The resulting hypoxia, as well as the cumulative effect of previously administered medications, contributes to behaviors ranging from wide-eyed agitation to lethargic irritability. In children who have repeated acute asthma episodes, a barrel chest (hyperinflation of the thorax) and the use of accessory muscles of respiration are common findings (Figure 25–13 ■). **Pulsus paradoxus,** when the arterial blood pressure decreases during inspiration by 10 mmHg, may be present in severe asthma episodes.

The symptoms of exercise-induced bronchospasm are cough, wheeze, chest pain or tightness, shortness of breath, and fatigue. Symptoms peak 5 to 10 minutes after completing the exercise session, and subside within 30 to 60 minutes (Cuff & Loud, 2008).

Life-Threatening Asthma Exacerbation

In some cases, unrelenting, severe respiratory distress and bronchospasm persists despite pharmacologic and supportive interventions. These children are in acute respiratory distress. Clinical manifestations include the use of accessory muscles, restlessness and anxiety, altered mental status, inability to say more than a word or two without gasping for breath, diaphoresis, and cyanosis. Signs of impending respiratory failure include an inability to speak, inability to lie down, altered mental status, intercostal retractions, and worsening fatigue (Camargo, Rachelefsky, & Schatz, 2009).

Collaborative Care

Diagnostic Procedures

Asthma is diagnosed through a detailed medical history and physical examination focused on the respiratory system. Pulmonary function testing (spirometry) is used to assess airway function in children who are old enough to cooperate, generally by age 5 to 6 years. Spirometry readings are most commonly measured as forced expiratory volume in 1 second (FEV_1) and expressed as a percentage of predicted FEV_1 for the child's height, age, gender, and race. The diagnosis of asthma requires evidence of episodic symptoms of airflow obstruction with a reversal of airflow obstruction by at least 12% after inhalation of a short-acting bronchodilator (Stewart, 2008). Other diagnostic studies may be performed to exclude other diagnoses with similar symptoms, such as a chest radiograph to rule out a foreign body aspiration. Evidence of atopy (eczema or allergies) is an important factor in asthma diagnosis. Skin testing may be used to identify allergens that could be asthma triggers.

Clinical Tip

When spirometry testing is performed, coach the child to give the best effort each time. Encourage the child to seal the lips tightly around the mouthpiece. The child is then instructed to breathe out as hard as possible, and then to breathe in deeply.

Laboratory findings for the child who needs admission to an intensive care unit may include hypoxemia (may be masked by supplemental oxygen), a $Paco_2$ of 42 mmHg or greater, respiratory acidosis, and sometimes metabolic acidosis (Gott & Froh, 2010).

Clinical Therapy

Asthma is a disorder that varies in its course over time and the symptoms experienced by individuals, such as remission or increasing severity. Asthma severity is classified by the amount of respiratory impairment present and risk (e.g., the number of episodes needing oral systemic corticosteroid therapy). See Tables 25–7 and 25–8 for the classification of asthma severity in children of different ages. The asthma severity classification guides the recommended therapy protocol. Although current asthma treatment, including inhaled corticosteroids, is effective in controlling symptoms, reducing airflow limitations, and preventing exacerbations, it does not appear to prevent the underlying severity of asthma (National Asthma Education and Prevention Program, 2007, p. 28).

Clinical therapy includes medications, hydration, education, and support of parents and child. Pharmacologic therapies are matched to the severity of asthma for long-term control and for management of acute episodes. See Medications Used to Treat Asthma on pages 778–779. The goal is to maintain asthma control long term using the least amount of medication, thus reducing the risk for adverse effects.

TABLE 25–7 | **Classification of Asthma Severity for Children Between Birth and 4 Years of Age**

		CLASSIFICATION OF ASTHMA SEVERITY (0–4 YEARS OF AGE)			
			PERSISTENT		
	COMPONENTS OF SEVERITY	INTERMITTENT	MILD	MODERATE	SEVERE
Impairment	Symptoms	2 or fewer days a week	Greater than 2 days a week, but not daily	Daily	Throughout the day
	Nighttime awakenings	0	1–2 times a month	3–4 times a month	Greater than 1 time a week
	Short-acting beta$_2$-agonist (SABA) use for symptom control (not for prevention of exercise-induced bronchospasm)	2 or fewer days a week	Greater than 2 times a week, but not daily	Daily	Several times a day
	Interference with normal activity	None	Minor limitation	Some limitation	Extremely limited
Risk	Exacerbations requiring oral systemic corticosteroids	0–1 time a year	← 2 or more times a year →		
		← Consider severity and interval since last exacerbation →			
		Frequency and severity may fluctuate over time for patients in any severity category.			
Recommended step for initiating therapy (see Figure 25–14A ■)		Step 1	Step 2	Step 3 and consider short course of oral systemic corticosteroids	
		In 2–6 weeks, depending on severity, evaluate level of asthma control that is achieved. If no clear benefit is observed in 4–6 weeks, consider adjusting therapy or alternative diagnoses.			

Source: *From National Asthma Education and Prevention Program. (2007). Expert panel report 3: Guidelines for the diagnosis and management of asthma (p. 307). Bethesda, MD: National Heart Lung and Blood Institute, National Institutes of Health. Retrieved from http://www.nhlbi.nih.gov/guidelines/asthma/index.htm*

A stepwise approach to medication therapy is recommended that matches the child's asthma severity, adding or changing specific medications if the severity progresses. In some cases reducing or stepping down medications is considered if the child's asthma has been well controlled for at least 3 months (Williams, 2009). The child's response to therapy after 2 to 6 weeks guides the need to further step up medications in an effort to control symptoms. See Figure 25–14A, B, and C ■ on pages 775–777 for the nationally recommended stepwise approach to managing asthma in children by age group 0 to 4 years, 5 to 11 years, and 12 years to adulthood. Children with persistent asthma are recommended to use daily inhaled corticosteroids, and additional long-term control medications are added as severity increases. Children with intermittent asthma may only need short-acting beta$_2$-agonists. If the child's asthma control is difficult to achieve, referral to an asthma specialist should be considered.

Clinical Tip

Signs of well-controlled asthma in all pediatric age groups include symptoms 2 or fewer days a week; nighttime awakenings no more than once a month (twice a month in 12 years and older); no interference with normal activity, school, or exercise; use of a short-acting beta$_2$-agonist for symptom control 2 or fewer days a week; greater than 80% of predicted peak flow (in children 5 years and older); and no more than one acute asthma episode a year requiring oral system corticosteroids (Vanhoose & Wood, 2009).

The proper use of a peak expiratory flow meter (PEFM) can help monitor the child's airway changes to identify signs of worsening lung function and the beginning of an acute asthma episode, especially in children who may not recognize the onset of an asthma episode (Callahan, Panter, Hall, et al., 2010). A PEFM reading of less than 30% to 50% of the predicted level indicates severe airway obstruction.

Response to home treatment during an acute asthma episode is also possible. This device provides a simple quantitative and reproducible measurement of the maximum flow of air that the cooperative child can push forcefully out of the lungs. See page 781 for the technique and interpretation of PEFM readings.

Children should have a detailed written asthma action plan for use at school and at home that includes indicators of worsening asthma, a list of specific symptoms, and recommendations for treatment. The plan indicates when the child should use rescue medications (short-acting beta$_2$-agonists), initiate oral systemic corticosteroids, and contact the healthcare provider or go to the emergency department. The patient's measured personal best peak flow reading is a good value to use for medication administration guidelines in the patient's asthma action plan, and the effectiveness of treatment is confirmed by improved PEFM readings. Children should be involved in development of their asthma action plans as much as possible.

Exercise-induced asthma. Children should be encouraged to participate in physical activities and exercise. Children with **exercise-induced asthma** have a history of coughing, breathlessness, chest pain, or wheezing that occurs during and after exercise. A spirometry or PEFM reading of a 15% decrease in peak flow with exertion is usually noted. Pretreatment with short-acting beta$_2$-agonists immediately before exercise often prevents exercise-induced asthma and provides relief for up to 3 hours (Robinson & Van Asperen, 2009).

Acute asthma episodes. Most children with acute exacerbations respond to aggressive management in the emergency department, including continuous albuterol by nebulizer, oral systemic corticosteroids, and inhaled ipratropium. Chest physiotherapy is not beneficial and it causes unnecessary stress to the child. Children who do not

TABLE 25–8	Classification of Asthma Severity in Children 5 to 11 Years of Age and 12 Years to Adulthood

	COMPONENTS OF SEVERITY	CLASSIFICATION OF ASTHMA SEVERITY (5–11 YEARS OF AGE AND 12 YEARS–ADULTHOOD)			
		INTERMITTENT	PERSISTENT		
			MILD	MODERATE	SEVERE
Impairment	Symptoms	2 or fewer days a week	Greater than 2 days a week, but not daily	Daily	Throughout the day
	Nighttime awakenings	2 times or less per month	3–4 times a month	Greater than 1 time a week, but not nightly	Often 7 times a week
	Short-acting beta$_2$-agonist (SABA) use for symptom control (not for prevention of exercise-induced bronchospasm)	2 or fewer days a week	Greater than 2 times a week, but not daily	Daily	Several times a day
	Interference with normal activity	None	Minor limitation	Some limitation	Extremely limited
	Lung function (**5–11 years**)	■ Normal FEV$_1$ between exacerbations ■ FEV$_1$ greater than 80% predicted ■ FEV$_1$/FVC greater than 85%	■ FEV$_1$ equals greater than 80% predicted ■ FEV$_1$/FVC greater than 80%	■ FEV$_1$ equals 60–80% predicted ■ FEV$_1$/FVC equals 70–80%	■ FEV$_1$ less than 60% predicted ■ FEV$_1$/FVC less than 75%
Normal FEV$_1$/FVC: 8–19 years 85%	Lung function (**12 years to adulthood**)	■ Normal FEV$_1$ between exacerbations ■ FEV$_1$ greater than 80% predicted ■ FEV$_1$/FVC normal	■ FEV$_1$ equals greater than 80% predicted ■ FEV$_1$/FVC normal	■ FEV$_1$ equals 60–80% predicted ■ FEV$_1$/FVC reduced 5%	■ FEV$_1$ less than 60% predicted ■ FEV$_1$/FVC reduced more than 5%
Risk	Exacerbations requiring oral systemic corticosteroids	0–1 time a year?	← 2 or more times a year →		
		← Consider severity and interval since last exacerbation →			
		Frequency and severity may fluctuate over time for patients in any severity category.			
Recommended step for initiating therapy (5–11 years) (see Figure 25–14B ■)		Step 1	Step 2	Step 3, medium dose inhaled corticosteroid option Consider short course of oral system corticosteroids.	Step 3, medium dose inhaled corticosteroid option, or step 4
Recommended step for initiating therapy (12 years–adulthood) (see Figure 25–14C ■)		Step 1	Step 2	Step 3 Consider short course of oral system corticosteroids.	Step 4 or 5
For both age groups, evaluate level of asthma control achieved in 2–6 weeks and adjust therapy accordingly.					

*FEV$_1$ = forced expiratory volume in 1 second; FVC = forced vital capacity

Source: *Adapted from National Asthma Education and Prevention Program. (2007). Expert panel report 3: Guidelines for the diagnosis and management of asthma (pp. 308, 344). Bethesda, MD: National Heart Lung and Blood Institute, National Institutes of Health. Retrieved August 30, 2007, from http://www.nhlbi.nih.gov/guidelines/asthma/index.htm*

respond or who are already being managed at home on corticosteroids have a greater chance of hospital admission.

Severe asthma exacerbations. Some children with severe (potentially life-threatening) asthma exacerbations need aggressive and immediate intervention in the intensive care unit, such as those who had an emergency department or private physician visit in the prior 24 hours. These children may progress to respiratory failure and die. The child is placed on a cardiorespiratory monitor and pulse oximeter. Intravenous magnesium sulfate may be used in addition to other medications used for the acute exacerbation. Heliox (70% helium, 30% oxygen) may be used to drive the nebulizer (Robinson & Van Asperen, 2009). Some children will need mechanical ventilation or CPAP.

Nursing Management

The goal of nursing management is to perform assessments and interventions to support the child during acute asthma episodes and to assist the child and family to control asthma symptoms.

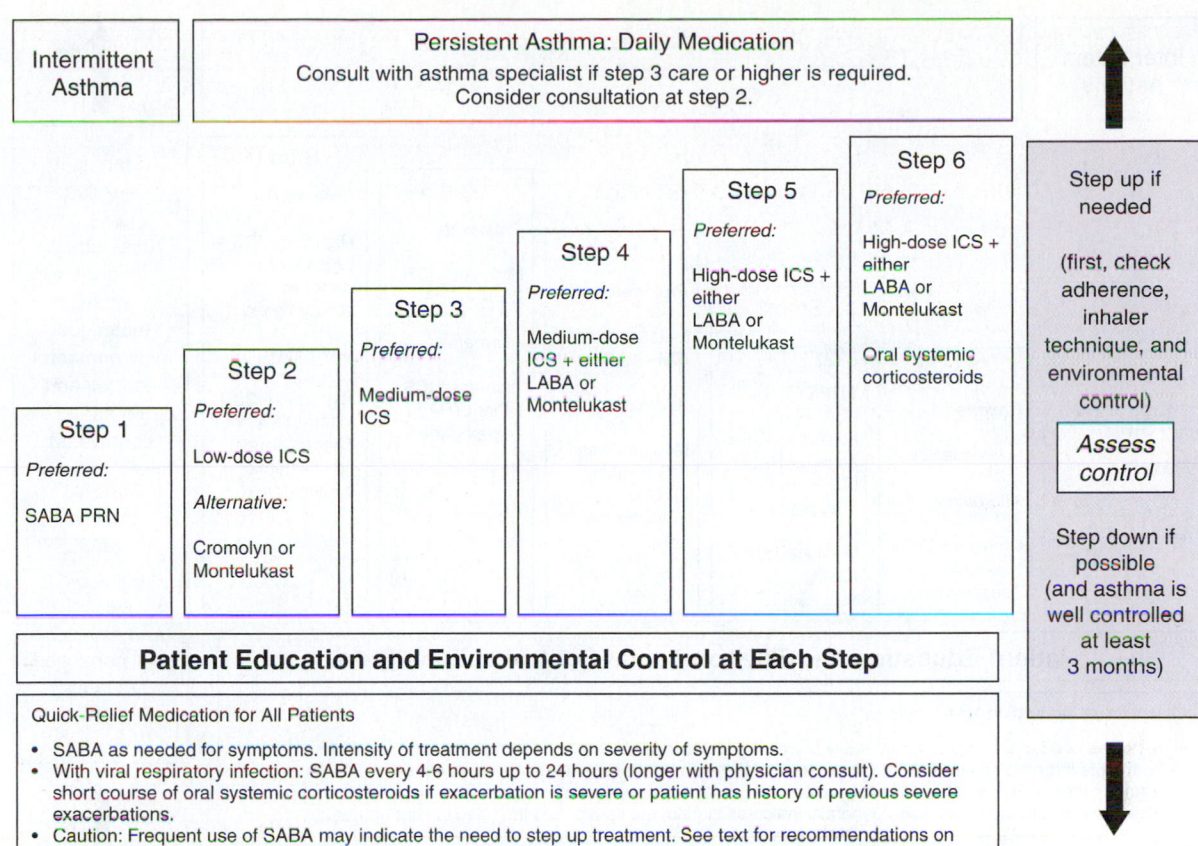

FIGURE 25–14A ■ Stepwise approach for managing asthma in children 0 to 4 years of age.

Source: *From National Asthma Education and Prevention Program. (2007). Expert panel report 3: Guidelines for the diagnosis and management of asthma (p. 305). Bethesda, MD: National Institutes of Health, National Heart Lung and Blood Institute. Retrieved August 30, 2007, from http://www.nhlbi.nih.gov/guidelines/asthma/index.htm*

Nursing Assessment and Diagnosis

Hospital-Based Care

The nurse usually encounters the child and family in the emergency department, nursing unit, or health center. Acute care has become necessary because the child's level of respiratory compromise cannot be managed at home.

Physiologic Assessment

Identify the child's current respiratory status first by assessing the ABCs—airway, breathing, and circulation—to make sure that the child's condition is not life threatening. If the child is moving air or talking, assess the quality of breathing and respiratory effort. Assess the respiratory rate and auscultate the lungs for the quality of breath sounds and for the presence or absence of wheezing. Inspect the chest for retractions to assess the severity of respiratory distress. Note whether a cough or stridor is present. Is the child in a tripod position or comfortable reclining with head elevated? Observe the child's color and assess the heart rate. Only after no life-threatening respiratory distress is found should the assessment move on to other systems.

Attach a pulse oximeter to monitor oxygen saturation. An SpO_2 reading less than 92% indicates hypoxemia. Assess skin turgor, intake and output, and urine specific gravity. The child may be in too much respiratory distress to use the PEFM. Because asthma can be a symptom of another illness, a head-to-toe assessment should be performed to identify other associated problems. See Table 25–1 for assessment guidelines.

Assess Asthma Management

Key questions to consider asking parents and older children or adolescents include the following (National Asthma Education and Prevention Program, 2007, p. 332):

— Which medicines is the child currently taking? How often?
— How is the medication administered?
— How many times a week is a medication dose missed?
— What issues have you had related to giving the medicine (cost, time, lack of perceived need)?
— What concerns do you have about the prescribed asthma medication?
— What other treatments for asthma are you using (e.g., complementary therapies)?

Psychosocial Assessment

Assess the child's anxiety or fear related to the asthma flare or hospitalization. How are the parents responding to the latest episode? Are they anxious, concerned, or frustrated? Do they have concerns about finances, missing work, or other family members at home? Assess whether the child thinks this flare could have been avoided if

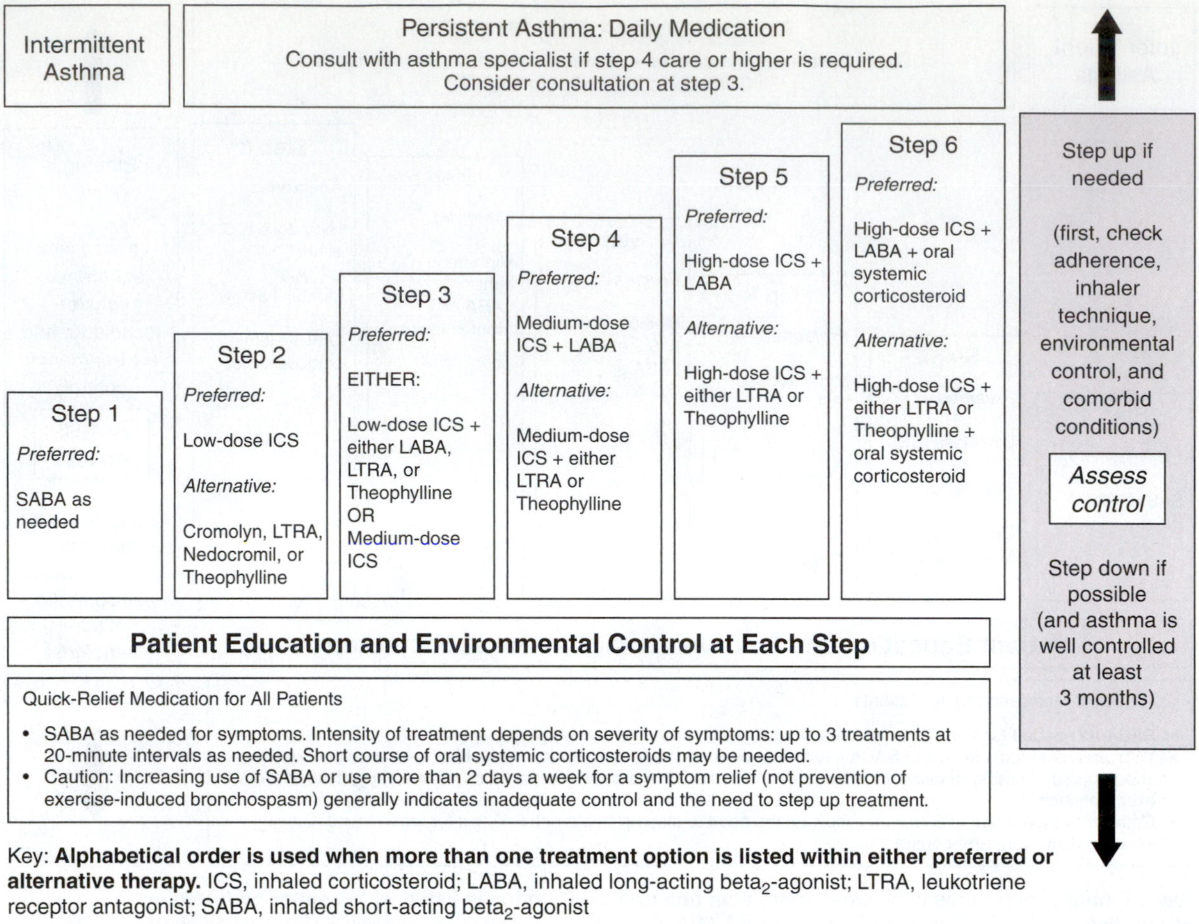

Intermittent Asthma	Persistent Asthma: Daily Medication Consult with asthma specialist if step 4 care or higher is required. Consider consultation at step 3.

Step 1

Preferred:

SABA as needed

Step 2

Preferred:

Low-dose ICS

Alternative:

Cromolyn, LTRA, Nedocromil, or Theophylline

Step 3

Preferred:

EITHER:

Low-dose ICS + either LABA, LTRA, or Theophylline OR Medium-dose ICS

Step 4

Preferred:

Medium-dose ICS + LABA

Alternative:

Medium-dose ICS + either LTRA or Theophylline

Step 5

Preferred:

High-dose ICS + LABA

Alternative:

High-dose ICS + either LTRA or Theophylline

Step 6

Preferred:

High-dose ICS + LABA + oral systemic corticosteroid

Alternative:

High-dose ICS + either LTRA or Theophylline + oral systemic corticosteroid

Step up if needed

(first, check adherence, inhaler technique, environmental control, and comorbid conditions)

Assess control

Step down if possible (and asthma is well controlled at least 3 months)

Patient Education and Environmental Control at Each Step

Quick-Relief Medication for All Patients

- SABA as needed for symptoms. Intensity of treatment depends on severity of symptoms: up to 3 treatments at 20-minute intervals as needed. Short course of oral systemic corticosteroids may be needed.
- Caution: Increasing use of SABA or use more than 2 days a week for a symptom relief (not prevention of exercise-induced bronchospasm) generally indicates inadequate control and the need to step up treatment.

Key: **Alphabetical order is used when more than one treatment option is listed within either preferred or alternative therapy.** ICS, inhaled corticosteroid; LABA, inhaled long-acting beta$_2$-agonist; LTRA, leukotriene receptor antagonist; SABA, inhaled short-acting beta$_2$-agonist

FIGURE 25–14B ■ Stepwise approach for managing asthma in children 5 to 11 years of age.

Source: *From National Asthma Education and Prevention Program. (2007). Expert panel report 3: Guidelines for the diagnosis and management of asthma (p. 306). Bethesda, MD: National Institutes of Health, National Heart Lung and Blood Institute. Retrieved August 30, 2007, from http://www.nhlbi.nih.gov/guidelines/asthma/index.htm*

medications had been taken. The nurse should look for clues to hidden stress and self-blaming.

Common nursing diagnoses for the child experiencing an acute asthma flare include the following:

- Airway Clearance, Ineffective related to airway compromise, copious mucous secretions, and coughing
- Gas Exchange, Impaired related to airway obstruction
- Fluid Volume: Deficient, Risk for related to difficulty in taking adequate fluids with respiratory distress
- Anxiety (Child and Parents) related to difficulty breathing and change in health status
- Therapeutic Regimen Management: Family, Ineffective related to lack of understanding about and need for daily management of a chronic disease

NANDA-I © 2012

Planning and Implementation

Pharmacologic and supportive therapies are used to reverse the airway obstruction and promote respiratory function. Nursing interventions focus on maintaining airway patency, meeting fluid needs, promoting rest and stress reduction for the child and parents, supporting the family's participation in care, and providing the child and family with information to enable them to manage the child's disease and ongoing developmental needs.

Maintain Airway Patency

If the child is exhibiting breathing difficulty, give supplemental oxygen by nasal cannula or face mask. Humidified oxygen should be used to prevent drying and thickening of mucous secretions. The child should be placed in a sitting (semi-Fowler) or upright position to promote and ease respiratory effort. The effectiveness of positioning, response to medications, and oxygen administration is evaluated by pulse oximeter and by observing for improved respiratory status.

Clinical Judgment

If the mental status of a child with an asthma episode changes to less responsive, what could be the cause and what nursing actions should be initiated?

The respiratory distress and need for supplemental oxygen can be stressful for parents and child alike (Figure 25–15 ■). Encouraging the parents' presence can be reassuring for the child. The parents should be kept informed of procedures and results, and their input should be obtained in developing the treatment plan.

Most medications are given by inhalation route (Figure 25–16 ■). This route of administration enables the pulmonary blood vessels to rapidly absorb the medication while minimizing the systemic effects. (See the Clinical Skills Manual ⬭ .) The inhaled droplets provide the added benefit of moisture. Continuous inhalation treatments by nebulizer may be used for some children with severe exacerbations.

Intermittent Asthma	Persistent Asthma: Daily Medication Consult with asthma specialist if step 4 care or higher is required. Consider consultation at step 3.

Step 1

Preferred:

SABA as needed

Step 2

Preferred:

Low-dose ICS

Alternative:

Cromolyn, LTRA, Nedocromil, or Theophylline

Step 3

Preferred:

Low-dose ICS + LABA OR Medium-dose ICS

Alternative:

Low-dose ICS + either LTRA, Theophylline, or Zileuton

Step 4

Preferred:

Medium-dose ICS + LABA

Alternative:

Medium-dose ICS + either LTRA, Theophylline, or Zileuton

Step 5

Preferred:

High-dose ICS + LABA

AND

Consider Omalizumab for patients who have allergies

Step 6

Preferred:

High-dose ICS + LABA + oral corticosteroid

AND

Consider Omalizumab for patients who have allergies

Step up if needed

(first, check adherence, environmental control, and comorbid conditions)

Assess control

Step down if possible (and asthma is well controlled at least 3 months)

Each step: Patient education, environmental control, and management of comorbidities.

Step 2–4: Consider subcutaneous allergen immunotherapy for patients who have allergic asthma (see notes).

Quick-Relief Medication for All Patients

- SABA as needed for symptoms. Intensity of treatment depends on severity of symptoms: up to 3 treatments at 20-minute intervals as needed. Short course of oral systemic corticosteroids may be needed.
- Use of SABA more than 2 days a week for symptom relief (not prevention of EIB) generally indicates inadequate control and the need to step up treatment.

Key: **Alphabetical order is used when more than one treatment option is listed within either preferred or alternative therapy.** EIB, exercise-induced bronchospasm; ICS, inhaled corticosteroid; LABA, inhaled long-acting beta$_2$-agonist; LTRA, leukotriene receptor antagonist; SABA, inhaled short-acting beta$_2$-agonist

FIGURE 25–14C ■ Stepwise approach for managing asthma in children 12 years of age and older.

Source: *From National Asthma Education and Prevention Program. (2007). Expert panel report 3: Guidelines for the diagnosis and management of asthma (p. 343). Bethesda, MD: National Institutes of Health, National Heart Lung and Blood Institute. Retrieved August 30, 2007, from http://www.nhlbi.nih.gov/guidelines/asthma/index.htm*

See Box 25–9 on page 780 for growth and development considerations in administering medications with inhalation devices. Monitor the child for medication side effects. The frequency of vital sign assessment is determined by the severity of symptoms.

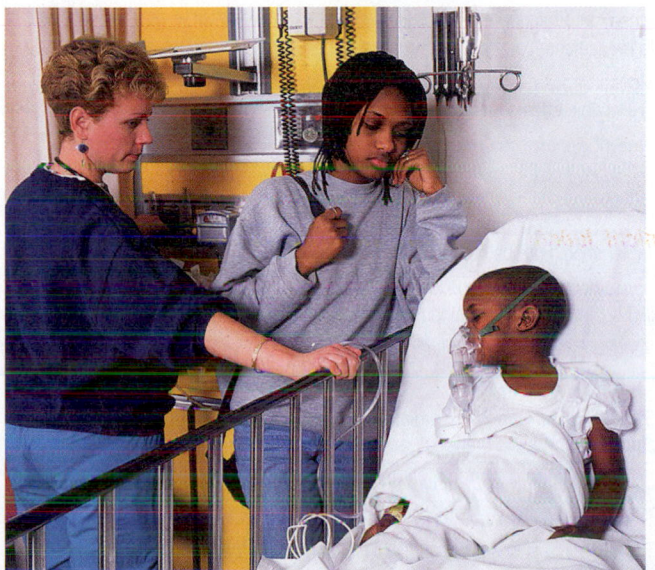

FIGURE 25–15 ■ Acute exacerbations of asthma may require management in the emergency department. The child is placed in a semisitting position to facilitate respiratory effort. Providing support to both the child and parent is an important part of nursing care during these acute episodes. The mother is exhausted after a sleepless night of caring for her son.

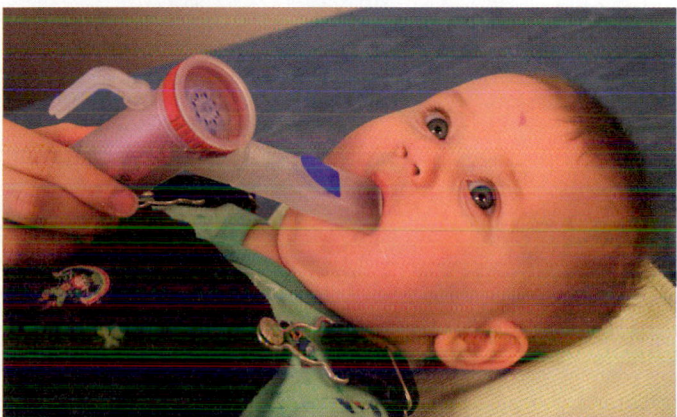

FIGURE 25–16 ■ Medications given by aerosol therapy allow infants and children to get optimal therapy without injections and their associated pain and stress. Parents can hold the nebulizer and reduce the infant's fear. Alternatively a face mask could be attached to the nebulizer.

Medications Used to Treat Asthma

QUICK-RELIEF MEDICATION	ACTION/INDICATION	NURSING MANAGEMENT
Short-Acting Beta$_2$-Agonists (SABA) Albuterol Levalbuterol Pirbuterol: *Metered dose inhaler (MDI) or nebulizer*	Relaxes smooth muscle in airway leading to rapid bronchodilation (within 5–10 minutes) and mucus clearing Drug of choice for acute therapy and for prevention of exercise-induced bronchospasm	■ Use this rescue medication before inhaled steroid, wait 1–2 minutes between puffs, wait 15 minutes to give inhaled steroid. Child should hold breath 10 seconds after inspiring. Then rinse mouth and avoid swallowing medication. Use a spacer. ■ Differences in potency exist, but all products are comparable on a per puff basis. ■ Some dose-related side effects include tachycardia, nervousness, nausea and vomiting, and headaches. ■ Regular use more than 2 days a week for symptom control indicates a loss of control and need for additional therapy.
Corticosteroids Methylprednisolone Prednisone Prednisolone: *Oral*	Diminishes airway inflammation, secretions, and obstruction, enhances bronchodilating effect of beta$_2$-agonists Used for acute asthma episodes that are not completely responsive to beta$_2$-agonists; helps reduce rate of hospitalization	■ Short-term therapy should continue until child achieves 80% peak expiratory flow rate personal best or symptoms resolve. ■ Give with food to reduce gastric irritation. ■ Give oral dose in early morning to mimic normal peak corticosteroid blood level. ■ Assess for potential adverse effects of long-term therapy: decreased growth, unstable blood sugar, and immunosuppression.
Anticholinergic Ipratropium: *Metered dose inhaler (MDI) or nebulizer*	Inhibits bronchoconstriction and decreases mucus production with an onset of action in 30–90 minutes	■ Do not use for primary emergency treatment because of delayed onset. ■ Rinse mouth afterward to get rid of bitter taste. ■ Side effects include increased wheezing, cough, nervousness, dry mouth, tachycardia, dizziness, headache, and palpitations. ■ Prevent medication contact with eyes.

DAILY CONTROL MEDICATIONS	ACTION/INDICATION	NURSING MANAGEMENT
Long-Acting Beta$_2$-Agonists (LABA) Salmeterol Formoterol: *Dry powder inhaler (DPI)*	Relaxes smooth muscles in airway, used for nocturnal symptoms and prevention of exercise-induced bronchospasm. These medications should not be used as single therapy for asthma in children, but prescribed in combination with corticosteroids (U.S. Food and Drug Administration, 2010).	■ Do not use for acute asthma episode. ■ Take pre-exercise dose 30–60 minutes before activity. Do not use additional dose before exercise if already using twice-daily doses which should be 12 hours apart. ■ Caution against overdosage as side effects such as tachycardia, tremor, irritability, and insomnia will last 8–12 hours. ■ Report failure to respond to usual dose as this may indicate a need for stepped-up therapy.
Inhaled Corticosteroids (ICS) Beclomethasone Budesonide Flunisolide Fluticasone Mometasone Triamcinolone: *Metered dose inhaler (MDI) or nebulizer*	Anti-inflammatory, controls seasonal, allergic, and exercise-induced asthma Effectively reduces mucosal edema in airways	■ Administer with spacer or holding chamber. ■ Separate parts and clean inhaler daily. ■ Rinse mouth and gargle following treatment to remove drug from oropharynx to reduce chance of cough, thrush, and dysphonia. ■ Monitor growth; however, recommended doses do not have long-term or irreversible effects on vertical growth (Fong & Levin, 2007). ■ Prevent eye exposure through proper MDI, nebulizer, or DPI administration. ■ Monitor for headache, gastrointestinal upset, dizziness, and infection. ■ Use exactly as prescribed.
Methylxanthines Theophylline: *Oral*	Relaxes muscle bundles that constrict airways; dilates airway; provides continuous airway relaxation; sustained release for prevention of nocturnal symptoms	■ Tablet should not be crushed or chewed. ■ Use for long-term control. Works best when a therapeutic serum level (10–20 mcg/L) is maintained; give same time each day. ■ Requires serum level monitoring and dose adjustment. ■ Limit caffeine intake. ■ Side effects include tachycardia, dysrhythmias, restlessness, tremors, seizures, insomnia, hypotension, severe headaches, vomiting, and diarrhea.
Mast-Cell Inhibitors Cromolyn sodium Nedocromil: *Metered dose inhaler (MDI) or nebulizer*	Anti-inflammatory, inhibits early and late phase asthma response to allergens and exercise-induced bronchospasm; may be used for unavoidable allergen exposure. May be used as a substitute for inhaled corticosteroids in mild persistent asthma, but evidence of their effectiveness for pediatric asthma is weak (Robinson & Van Asperen, 2009).	■ Do not use at time of symptom development or acute exacerbation. ■ The patient must use up to 4 times a day to be effective. ■ Therapeutic response is seen in 2 weeks; maximum benefit may not be seen for 4–6 weeks. ■ Adverse reactions include wheezing, bronchospasm, throat irritation, nasal congestion, and anaphylaxis. Immediately report these symptoms to physician.

Medications Used to Treat Asthma (*Continued*)

DAILY CONTROL MEDICATIONS	ACTION/INDICATION	NURSING MANAGEMENT
Leukotriene Receptor Antagonist (LTRA) Montelukast Zafirlukast: *Oral*	Reduces inflammation cascade responsible for airway inflammation Improves lung function and diminishes symptoms and need for rescue medications Adjunct to inhaled corticosteroids in moderate to severe persistent asthma or substitute for inhaled corticosteroids in mild persistent asthma	■ Granules for infants and chewable tablets for young children are available. ■ Administer montelukast in the evening; may be given with food or without. ■ Make sure child chews montelukast chewable tablet rather than swallowing whole; granules may be mixed in applesauce or ice cream; do not mix medication in a liquid. ■ Administer zafirlukast 1 hour before or 2 hours after a meal. ■ Family needs to report fever, acute asthma episodes, flulike symptoms, severe headaches, or lethargy. ■ Take as prescribed; do not withdraw abruptly.
Immunotherapy Omalizumab: *Subcutaneous*	A therapeutic anti-immunoglobulin E monoclonal antibody that targets IgE, blocking it from causing allergic reactions leading to asthma symptoms; when added to recommended therapy for inner-city children with moderate or severe asthma, it further improved asthma control (Busse, Morgan, Gergen, et al., 2011).	■ It is approved for children 12 years and older with moderate or severe persistent asthma. ■ Injections are required every 2–4 weeks based on serum IgE levels. ■ Be alert for anaphylaxis; it should be administered in a site prepared to treat anaphylaxis.
Hyposensitization (allergy shots) *Subcutaneous*	Series of injections that can reduce sensitivity to unavoidable allergens (e.g., mold, pollen); gradual dose increase over time increases the child's tolerance to allergic substances	■ They may be of value for a child with persistent asthma having allergies that can be addressed by immune therapy.

Source: *Data from Wilson, B. A., Shannon, M. T., & Shields, K. M. (2011). Nurse's drug guide 2011. Upper Saddle River, NJ: Pearson; Banasiak, N. C. (2007). Childhood asthma: Part two: Management update. Journal of Pediatric Health Care, 21(3), 184–191; Robinson, P. D., & Van Asperen, P. (2009). Asthma in childhood. Pediatric Clinics of North America, 56, 191–226; Fong, E. W., & Lewin, R. H. (2007). Inhaled corticosteroids for asthma. Pediatrics in Review, 28(6), e30–e35; Stewart, L. J. (2008). Pediatric asthma. Primary Care: Clinics in Office Practice, 35, 25–40.*

Meet Fluid Needs

Fluid therapy is often necessary to restore and maintain adequate fluid balance. Adequate hydration is essential to thin and break up trapped mucous plugs in the narrowed airways. If an adequate oral intake is not possible because of the child's compromised respiratory status, an intravenous infusion may be needed. Additional medications and glucose may also be provided through the IV. Monitor the child's intake and output to avoid overhydration and to prevent pulmonary edema in severe asthma episodes.

As respiratory difficulty diminishes, oral fluids can be offered slowly. Involving the parents can help gain the child's cooperation in taking oral fluids. The child's fluid preferences should be determined and choices provided where possible.

Clinical Tip

Iced beverages precipitate bronchospasms in some children with asthma. It is safest to offer the child room-temperature or slightly cooled fluids without ice.

Promote Rest and Stress Reduction

The child who has had an acute asthma episode is usually very tired when admitted to the nursing unit. Labored breathing and low oxygenation often leave the child exhausted. Place the child in a quiet, private room, if possible, to promote relaxation and rest. By grouping tasks, nurses can avoid repeatedly disturbing the child.

Support Family Participation

The parents may stay with the child, but they may be exhausted after spending hours with their child in respiratory distress. Give parents the option of assisting with the child's treatments, rather than expecting them to do the care in addition to comforting the child. Provide frequent updates about the child's condition and encourage the parents to take breaks as needed.

Length of hospitalization depends on the child's response to therapy. Any underlying or accompanying health problem, such as preexisting lung disease or pneumonia, can complicate and extend the child's hospital stay. Communicate with the family of the hospitalized child frequently about the child's condition.

Discharge Planning and Home Care Teaching

Parents need a thorough understanding of asthma—how to prevent acute episodes and how to follow the asthma action plan to manage the child's acute asthma episodes earlier to avoid unnecessary hospitalization. When possible, educate parents when they are rested, but refer the parents and child to a healthcare provider who can provide more comprehensive education, as occurred with Hannah in the chapter-opening scenario. Make sure the child receives an appointment with an allergist or asthma specialist if moderate to severe persistent asthma exists. Support of the parents and child should focus on helping them to understand and cope with the diagnosis and the need for daily management to promote near-normal respiratory function while the child continues to grow and develop normally. See Developing Cultural Competence: Asthma Control.

Care in the Community

Nurses provide care to children with asthma in pediatricians' offices, specialty asthma clinics, schools, and summer camps. Nurses have a major role in increasing the family's knowledge about the disease, medication therapy, and the need for follow-up care according to guidelines of the National Asthma Education and Prevention Program. The goal is to help reduce the number of asthma episodes the

BOX 25–9	Growth & Development: Medication Administration

Metered dose inhalers (MDIs), nebulizers, and dry powder inhalers (DPIs) are the devices used for inhalation therapy. Even with proper technique, much of the medication delivered by inhalation is deposited in the oropharynx and swallowed. These devices cause special challenges for administration to infants and young children. Many devices require cooperation, coordination, and appropriate technique that is taught and reinforced frequently.

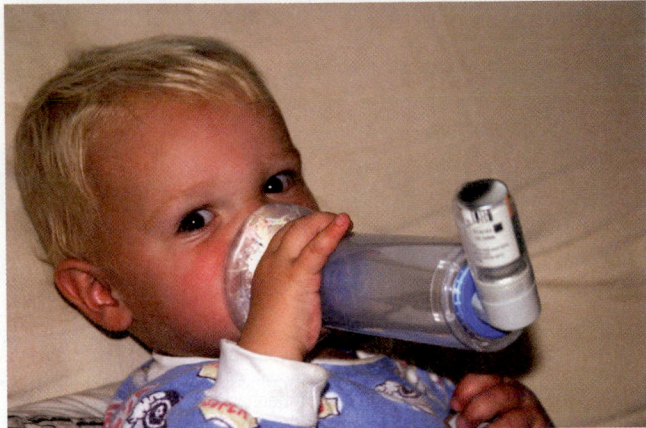

Source: © David Wall / Alamy.

- Children over 5 years usually have the ability to use an MDI, coordinating medication release and inspiration; however, they may prefer to use a holding chamber or spacer with a valve. Spacers enhance the amount of drug delivered to the lungs and reduce the amount of drug deposited in the mouth and throat (Zagaria, 2010). Valves prevent the escape of medication during use. Spacers have a mouthpiece or mask attachment. When selecting a spacer for infants and young children, choose one with a mask because they tend to be nasal breathers. Choose a mask that fits the child's face and has a flexible seal to prevent an air leak around the facial features. When the young child is uncooperative, it may be difficult to maintain a seal. Work with young children to improve cooperation for medication delivery with play and distraction. Crying leads to prolonged exhalation and short inspiratory efforts which reduces lung deposition. The plastic spacer should be washed with household detergent and permitted to air-dry to reduce any electrostatic charge that could attract medication particles.

- Steps in using an MDI include the following: shake the canister, breathe out, and close the mouth around the mouthpiece between the lips and teeth. The child should begin to inhale slowly as a puff of the MDI is released. The breath should be deep over 3 to 5 seconds, and the breath should then be held for 10 seconds. When teaching the child to use an MDI without a spacer, let the child learn to breathe slowly through a straw. When a spacer is used, release a puff of medication, and immediately put the mask on the face or the mouthpiece in the mouth, and have the child take 4 to 6 breaths. Remove the spacer

mask from the child's face or mouthpiece from the child's mouth, and have the child hold his or her breath for 10 seconds (Asthma Initiative of Michigan for Healthy Lungs, 2011). When a spacer with a face mask is used, the child's face should be washed after inhalation.

- Some inhaler and spacer brands have a whistle on inhalation indicating that a breath is too fast or too shallow, but in others it indicates an adequate breath has been taken. When teaching the child and family about inhaler use, make sure you know what the whistle indicates.

- A nebulizer is a device that changes liquid medication into aerosol particles. No coordination of breathing is required, making nebulizers easier for young children to use. An added benefit is the humidification provided during the treatment. While nebulizers are not more efficient than MDIs with a spacer, they may lead to better outcomes because the child only needs to breathe normally. The nebulizer mouthpiece should be in the child's mouth, and mouth breathing is important for drug delivery. If the child cannot coordinate mouth breathing, a tightly fitting face mask can be used. If the mouthpiece is away from the mouth, lung deposition of the medication is reduced and the eyes may be exposed to the medication. Nebulizers are expensive, need a power source, and take 8 to 10 minutes for the treatment. Infants and young children may have difficulty cooperating for the duration of the nebulizer treatment. Crying may decrease delivery of the medication to the lungs.

- DPIs are activated when the patient takes a breath, so puffs do not need to be coordinated with inhalation. No spacer is required and no propellant is used. The child must be able to take rapid, deep, and sustained breaths to effectively use the device (Fong & Levin, 2007). They can generally be used by children 5 years and older. Drug delivery to the lower airway varies between 15% and 30% dependent upon the type of inhaler. Children less than 6 years of age who are wheezing may not be able to inspire at a rate fast enough to obtain the optimal amount of medication. Essential steps for using a DPI include the following: remove the lid, load the dose (puncturing the blister or capsule), fully breathe out away from the device, put the mouthpiece between the lips and teeth, and breathe in deeply and forcefully. Hold the breath for 10 seconds and remove the mouth from the device (Asthma Initiative of Michigan for Healthy Lungs, 2011). One way to teach the child to inhale forcefully is to have the child place a paper tissue over the open mouth and inhale deeply for a count of 5 seconds. The tissue should be attached to the mouth without being held for the duration of the breath. The child who cannot do this maneuver is unable to correctly use a DPI device (Amirav, 2010).

Source: *Data from Zagaria, M. A. E. (2010). Inhalant agents for asthma, bronchospasm, and COPD: Focus on delivery devices and inhalation technique. American Journal for Nurse Practitioners, 14 (3), 21–25; Everard, M. L. (2006). Aerosol delivery to children. Pediatric Annals, 35(9), 630–636; Virchow, J. C. (2005), What plays a role in the choice of inhaler device for asthma therapy, Current Medical Research and Opinion, 21(Suppl. 4), S19–S25. Sleath, B., Ayala, G. X., Gillette, C., Williams, D., Davis, S., Tudor, G., . . . Washington, D. (2011). Provider demonstration and assessment of child device technique during pediatric asthma visits. Pediatrics, 127(4), 642–648; Asthma Initiative of Michigan for Healthy Lungs. (2011). How to use a metered-dose inhaler the right way. Retrieved from http://www.getasthmahelp.org/inhalers_main.asp*

Developing Cultural Competence
Asthma Control

Black and Latino children are less likely to use asthma daily control medication than White children. A telephone and mail interview study conducted in English and Spanish with 668 parents of children with persistent asthma revealed some interesting differences. Parents of Black and Latino children had lower expectations for their child's functioning with asthma (e.g., a greater number of symptomatic days was expected) than White parents. Black and Latino parents were also more concerned than White parents about medication effects of prescribed daily control medications, which may lead to less regular use. This study suggests that different health beliefs may be a factor in asthma management (Wu, Smith, Bokhour, et al., 2008).

child experiences. The required lifestyle changes may be difficult for the child and parents.

Discuss the quick-relief medications used to manage acute asthma episodes, as well as control medications for daily management. Regularly review the child's technique for using an inhaler to ensure that proper technique is used. Assess how often the child uses the quick-relief inhaler by how frequently a new inhaler is purchased. There are 200 puffs per inhaler, and if one inhaler per month (or 6 to 7 puffs per day) is used, further investigation is needed. This could reflect poor asthma control or poor technique in using the inhaler so that full benefit of the medication is not gained. Encourage school-age children to assume more responsibility for care, including avoidance

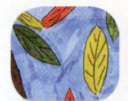

Partnering with Families

Using a Peak Expiratory Flow Meter

Use of a peak expiratory flow meter (PEFM) can help assess the severity of asthma. This device measures the child's ability to push air forcefully out of the lungs. Changes in PEFM readings signal worsening lung function and the beginning of an asthma episode. To use a PEFM:

- Set the device at zero or the base level.
- Stand up and take as deep a breath as possible.
- Put the mouthpiece of the meter in the mouth and firmly close the lips around it. Do not cough or let your tongue block the mouthpiece.
- Blow out as hard and fast as possible over 1 to 2 seconds.

- Write down the reading.
- Repeat the process two times and record the highest of three numbers on the chart.
- Measure and record the best PEFM reading twice a day for 2 to 3 weeks to determine the child's personal best reading. (The child should be using all prescribed asthma medications during the day so the best reading is obtained.) The child's personal best will change as the child grows taller, so this process will need to be repeated at least every year.
- The physician will use the child's personal best average readings to individualize the color zones to guide treatment in the child's action plan.

ZONE	PEFM RATE (BEST AND PREDICTED FOR AGE)	ACTION NEEDED
Green	80–100%	Good asthma control. Relatively free of asthma symptoms. Follow the asthma management plan and take usual medications.
Yellow	50–80%	"Caution," as your asthma is worsening. Contact your allergist to fine-tune your therapy.
Red	Less than 50%	"Danger," your asthma management and treatment program isn't controlling your symptoms. Use your inhaled bronchodilator. If peak flow readings do not return to at least the yellow zone, contact your allergist.

Source: *Adapted from American Academy of Allergy, Asthma, and Immunology (AAAAI). (2013). Peak flow meter. Retrieved from http://www.aaaai.org*

of known triggers, early symptom recognition, relaxation breathing, and the proper use of inhaled medications. The family should be reassured that most children with asthma can lead a normal life with some modifications.

Parents of children (4 to 11 years old) who have been diagnosed with asthma or have had quick-relief or daily control medications should be encouraged to complete the Childhood Asthma Control test. The 5 questions ask about how much symptoms interfere with daily activities, how frequently shortness of breath and nighttime symptoms occur, frequency the quick relief medication is used, and how the parent rates the child's asthma control. The nurse can download a copy of this test and assist the parent to complete the test. This recently validated tool can help the healthcare provider obtain basic information about the child's asthma control (Chipps, Zeiger, Murphy, et al., 2011).

Review the family's daily plan for monitoring the child's respiratory status. Encourage the school-age child or parent of younger children to use a symptom diary to note the daytime and nighttime symptoms, including peak flow measurements for 2 weeks prior to a health visit. Evaluate the child's technique with the PEFM and the parent's ability to identify the timing and type of stepped-up care needed to manage worsening symptoms. The goal is to bring acute asthma episodes under control with stepped-up care before emergency care is needed. This can be achieved only with daily monitoring. See Partnering with Families: Using a Peak Expiratory Flow Meter. This provides guidelines for appropriate technique that should be used to teach and reinforce technique at each visit. To help toddlers learn how

to use a peak flow meter, have them practice by blowing into party favors (e.g., noisemakers).

Health Maintenance

Ensure that the child gets regular health promotion and maintenance care, including routine immunizations; however, live virus vaccines may need to be postponed if the child has used oral corticosteroids recently. Monitor the child's growth if the child is treated with an inhaled corticosteroid (ICS) and courses of oral corticosteroid because the disease and these medications may affect overall growth. Low- and medium-dose inhaled corticosteroids are usually associated with only a small reduction in growth velocity, about 1 cm the first year, and this growth reduction is not usually progressive over time. Higher doses of ICS administered for prolonged times may be associated with a greater decrease in height, especially if combined with frequent courses of oral corticosteroids (National Asthma Education and Prevention Program, 2007, p. 289).

Physical activity and exercise is important for all children for physical fitness and to maintain appropriate body weight. Assess the amount of activity and exercise children with asthma are getting and any symptoms they experience such as chest tightening, wheezing, or shortness of breath. Exercise-induced asthma typically occurs 5 to 10 minutes after stopping the activity and resolves in another 20 to 30 minutes. Children who have symptoms with usual play activities should get a step up in treatment or be moved to the next level of medication management (National Asthma Education and Prevention Program, 2007, p. 297). First determine that the child gets some

Weblink | Childhood Asthma Control Test

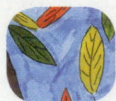

Partnering with Families

Home Care for the Child with Asthma

IDENTIFY CURRENT KNOWLEDGE ABOUT THE CONDITION AND ITS IMPACT ON THE CHILD

a. Review the parents' and older child's understanding of asthma pathophysiology and its effect on the child. Ask:

- What causes asthma? What happens in the lungs during an acute asthma episode?
- What are the early warning signs of an acute asthma episode in your child?
- What are your child's symptoms and how does he or she respond to them? Does your child wake up at night? Does your child cough a lot? When?
- Is your child involved in any exercise activity? If no, why not? Do asthma symptoms occur?
- Does asthma interfere with social activities or activities with friends?

b. What are the child's personal asthma triggers? (Suggest that the parents and child keep a written log of symptoms that occur during the day and night, as well as when and where symptoms occur to help identify triggers, e.g., home, school, outdoors, with exercise.)

SET UP A SCHEDULE FOR PARENTS TO LEARN ASTHMA MANAGEMENT

- Make sure the parents understand that asthma is a chronic condition that needs daily management and environmental control to reduce or prevent acute asthma episodes.
- Work with the physician to develop an asthma action plan for daily management, quick relief, and when to call the physician or seek emergency care.
- Assess the child's technique when using a peak expiratory flow meter (PEFM), and correct technique as needed. Discuss when to use the PEFM

and how to interpret and use the results for asthma control. Keep a record of PEFM readings for 2 weeks prior to each health visit.

REVIEW PARENTS' UNDERSTANDING OF MEDICATION THERAPY

- Provide information about medications: name, type of drug, dose, method of administration, expected effect, and possible side effects. Make sure families understand that daily control medication helps prevent acute asthma episodes, so the child will not feel them working as he or she does with quick-relief medications. Address the parents' fears about maintaining their child on "steroid" medication, and make sure they understand this is different from the anabolic steroids used and abused by athletes.
- Assess the child's technique for the use of an MDI or DPI and correct as needed.
- When parents use a nebulizer treatment for an infant or young child, suggest diversions that might help the child cooperate during the 8- to 10-minute treatment.

ADDRESS ASSOCIATED ISSUES

- What are the financial considerations of medication cost and lifestyle changes?
- Has the childcare provider or school and teacher been notified? What arrangements have been made for the child's use of medications at childcare or school?
- Does the child with persistent asthma have a medical identification bracelet or tag?
- Would a self-help group or camp experience be helpful for the child?

---

exercise, and then identify how frequently the child has symptoms of asthma and compare that to the classification of asthma severity in Tables 25–7 and 25–8. For example, exercise-induced asthma symptoms that occur daily would put the child in the *moderate persistent* category. Make sure the daily control and quick-relief medication asthma action plan is used by the child. See Complementary Therapy: Exercise and Asthma.

Child and Family Education

Once the stress of the acute asthma episode has passed, take advantage of opportunities to provide more extensive education at each health visit. See Partnering with Families: Home Care for the Child with Asthma for a guide to topics that should be discussed in asthma education.

Engage the child in learning about how the lungs work and what happens when an asthma episode occurs. Teach the child about asthma and how to begin steps toward self-management as appropriate. Teaching relaxation breathing may be helpful during an asthma flare to help manage symptoms until the rescue medication is effective. An activity book or coloring book may be a good teaching tool. Encourage the child to ask questions about his or her asthma. Make sure the parents and the child understand that asthma is a chronic and progressive condition rather than an episodic illness. Teach the child and family about the importance of the daily control

> ### Complementary Therapy   Exercise and Asthma
>
> Although exercise is a frequent trigger of asthma symptoms in the majority of patients, the benefits of routine exercise, such as running and swimming, on asthma symptoms are improved fitness and decreased severity of asthma symptoms (Rance & O'Laughlen, 2011). A study with 45 children evaluated the safety of a 9-week program of vigorous swimming and moderate-intensity golf. Benefits found were reduced childhood asthma symptoms and physician office visits (Weisgerber, 2008).

medication program, and develop a written plan to help the family manage asthma. Discuss strategies that may help the family remember to give the child the daily asthma medications. See Box 25–10. The plan should include the daily control medications, quick-relief medications to take once symptoms of an asthma episode are identified, and when to call the health professional. Determine if the family uses any complementary and alternative therapies for asthma management. Special summer camps are available that help children with asthma learn to manage their disease.

Provide printed educational materials and referral to a local support group to help parents gain additional knowledge and confidence that will enable them to help their child lead a normal life. Many hospitals have family resource centers that can assist the parents to find helpful information on the Internet.

| BOX 25–10 | Research: Asthma Management Routines |

A study involving 226 children and their families focused on the effect of asthma management routines in adherence to medications used to treat asthma. Routines include factors such as house cleaning, medication administration, medical visits, and filling prescriptions. Medication routines involved regularity, predictability, and planning medication use. Results revealed that the greater the number of routines related to medication management, the better the adherence to asthma medication use (Peterson-Sweeney, Halterman, Conn, et al., 2010). Nurses should try to identify routines to help with medication administration and adherence, such as keeping medications where they will be seen at mealtime.

Legal and Ethical Considerations
Self-Administration of Asthma Medications in Schools

All 50 states have passed legislation that entitles a child with asthma to carry and self-administer asthma medications at school (Allergy and Asthma Network, 2010). Families of children old enough to recognize worsening asthma symptoms and to self-administer rescue medications should make sure the school knows about the state law. See the companion website for links to specific state laws.

Preventing Acute Asthma Episodes

Environmental control is an important part of asthma management. When possible, pets and plants should not be kept in the home (and never in the child's bedroom). Active dust mite control should be attempted, but is very challenging as mites live in the carpets, mattresses, upholstered furniture, bedcovers, soft toys, and clothes. Particular attention should be directed at controlling dust mites in the child's bed and bedroom. The child's mattress and pillow should be encased in plastic covers. Pets in the home should be bathed frequently to reduce pet dander. Cockroach eradication should be initiated. Smoke from cigarettes, woodstoves, and fireplaces should be eliminated. See Partnering with Families: Removing Common Allergens from the Home on page 895 in Chapter 27.

Childcare and School Management

Help parents to communicate with the childcare provider or school personnel regarding the child's condition. The child should have an individualized health plan (that includes an asthma action plan) developed so that medications are given as needed, including in preparation for exercise. An actual physician order is needed to treat the child's asthma symptoms at school (see Legal & Ethical Considerations: Self-Administration of Asthma Medications in Schools). Make sure the child has a supply of medications at school or childcare as well as at home. For example, the older child or adolescent may use a cell-phone case to carry the inhaler. Many schools are attempting to become "asthma-friendly" through efforts to reduce asthma triggers by improving the environment, provide asthma education and awareness programs for students and staff, and coordinate with families to better manage asthma and reduce absenteeism due to asthma (CDC, 2008). Help the young child learn the early signs of an asthma episode (coughing, breathlessness) so that treatment can be obtained before signs become more serious. Make sure teachers of young children can recognize signs of an asthma episode and reduce a child's anxiety about going to the nurse for quick-relief medications.

Assess family support systems and family response to the chronic illness. Work to establish a partnership with the child and family that supports their ability to perform and maintain daily control medication regimens. In one study, adolescents who perceived greater family support (e.g., by facilitating communication with the healthcare provider and by providing strategies to encourage the adolescent to use the medication) were associated with greater asthma control and quality of life (Rhee, Belyea, & Brasch, 2010).

Refer to the Nursing Care Plan for the child with asthma in the community setting.

Evaluation

Expected outcomes of nursing care include the following:

- The child or parents recognize early asthma symptoms and promptly use rescue medications, hydration, and relaxation breathing to prevent severe respiratory distress.
- Asthma triggers are identified and efforts are made to avoid asthma triggers.
- The family implements the prescribed asthma daily treatment plan, and an asthma action plan is used to treat acute episodes.
- The child has improved asthma control with fewer asthma episodes.
- The child with a severe acute asthma episode responds to oxygen, fluids, and medication therapy and avoids hospital admission.

Bronchopulmonary Dysplasia (Chronic Lung Disease)

Bronchopulmonary dysplasia (BPD), also called chronic lung disease, is defined as the need for supplemental oxygen for at least 28 days after premature birth. Its severity is determined by the respiratory support interventions required at birth. BPD is one of the most serious chronic lung diseases in infants. The typical infant who develops BPD has a birth weight of 1000 g or less and a gestational age at birth of less than 28 weeks (Fakhoury, Sellers, Smith, et al., 2010). BPD is estimated to occur in a third of newborns with a birth weight less than 1500 g, despite improvements in neonatal care; however, its incidence decreased by 4.3% annually between 1993 and 2006 (Stroustrup & Trasande, 2010). BPD is a major cause of mortality and long-term morbidity in infants.

Etiology and Pathophysiology

BPD usually develops in premature neonates with a gestational age of less than 28 weeks who receive mechanical ventilation, often on the day of birth. In this group of neonates, abnormal pulmonary development or arrested lung development is also believed to be a factor in development of BPD. The infant has fewer and larger alveoli with less functional surface area and abnormal development of capillaries in the alveolar region (Gott & Froh, 2010). Potential contributing factors are intrauterine infection or a patent ductus arteriosus that leads to increased pulmonary blood volume, both factors resulting in an influx of inflammatory cells. Other potential causes of BPD include pneumonia, sepsis, meconium aspiration syndrome, and diaphragmatic hernia (Baraldi & Filippone, 2007). Ventilation-perfusion mismatch occurs, and the infant requires oxygen supplementation and respiratory intervention to support the work of breathing. Antenatal corticosteroids, surfactant replacement therapy, and gentle ventilation techniques have reduced the incidence of BPD in more mature preterm infants (Geary, Caskey, Fonseca, et al., 2008).

Nursing Care Plan   The Child with Asthma in the Community Setting

Intervention	Rationale	Expected Outcome

1. Nursing Diagnosis: Family Processes, Readiness for Enhanced related to increased control of asthma with daily medication

Intervention	Rationale	Expected Outcome
NIC Priority Intervention—*Normalization Promotion:* Assisting parents and other family members of children with chronic illnesses or disabilities in providing normal life experiences for their children and families		**NOC Suggested Outcome**—*Family Normalization:* Ability of family to maintain routines and management strategies that contribute to optimal functioning when a family member has a chronic illness or disability

GOAL: *The child and parents will work in partnership with the nurse to improve the child's asthma management.*

Intervention	Rationale	Expected Outcome
■ Listen to the family's concerns about asthma management and respond with information to correct any misconceptions.	■ The parents' concerns may not be the same as the nurse's. If the parents' concerns are not addressed, the parents may not adhere to recommended care.	The parents express greater confidence in averting and managing their child's asthma episodes.
■ Teach the family skills (assessment, use of equipment, and giving medications) for managing the child's asthma.	■ Proper use of equipment and appropriate medication dosage will help alleviate asthma symptoms.	
■ Provide telephone consultation to the parents during management of the first few asthma episodes.	■ Support and reinforcement of learning during an asthma episode will increase the parents' confidence in managing future episodes.	
■ Educate the parents about when to call for future medical advice or to seek emergency treatment.	■ Parents need guidelines for judging the severity of asthma episodes.	Parents appropriately call to ask questions about initiating home management or going to the emergency department for an asthma flare.

2. Nursing Diagnosis: Knowledge, Readiness for Enhanced (Asthma Management) related to concerns over recent asthma hospitalization

Intervention	Rationale	Expected Outcome
NIC Priority Intervention—*Health Education:* Developing and providing instruction and learning experiences to facilitate voluntary adaptation of behavior conducive to health in individuals, families, groups, or communities		**NOC Suggested Outcome**—*Knowledge: Health Promotion:* Extent of understanding conveyed about information needed to obtain and maintain optimal health

GOAL: *The child and parents will recognize early signs of an asthma episode and begin appropriate treatment following the child's asthma action plan.*

Intervention	Rationale	Expected Outcome
■ Teach the child and parents to use a peak expiratory flow meter.	■ The peak expiratory flow meter helps quantify changes in respiratory status before symptoms are detected.	The number of asthma episodes requiring medical intervention is reduced.
■ Help the child recognize his or her personal best peak expiratory flow reading and the range indicating asthma symptoms.	■ Identifying a personal best peak expiratory flow reading helps establish the ranges to be used for future symptom identification.	
■ Teach the family and child to give medications when the peak expiratory flow reading falls to the yellow range.	■ Giving medications before an asthma episode becomes established may help avert the actual episode.	
■ Teach the child and family to monitor the child's response to medications with the peak expiratory flow meter.	■ Monitoring the response gives the family information to determine when home care is inadequate and medical intervention is needed.	

3. Nursing Diagnosis: Health Maintenance, Ineffective related to lack of school asthma action plan

Intervention	Rationale	Expected Outcome
NIC Priority Intervention—*Health System Guidance:* Facilitating a patient's location and use of appropriate health services		**NOC Suggested Outcome**—*Health Promoting Behavior:* Actions to sustain or promote optimal wellness, recovery, and rehabilitation

GOAL: *An individualized health plan (IHP) with an asthma action plan will be developed to help control and manage the child's asthma symptoms.*

Intervention	Rationale	Expected Outcome
■ Provide the family with educational materials to give to the school nurse and school administrators.	■ School personnel need the latest information about effective asthma management in school settings.	Implementation of the IHP reduces the number of school absences for asthma episodes that occur during school hours and increases participation in school activities.
■ Advocate for all children with asthma to have an asthma action plan developed.	■ Establishing a school policy will help all children with asthma receive appropriate care.	
■ Support the family to have an IHP that includes the healthcare provider's written orders customized for the child.	■ The child with asthma needs an asthma action plan to treat asthma episodes at school.	
■ Include in the IHP participation in regular school/class activities such as field trips and physical education, and what to do if asthma symptoms occur at school.	■ Participation, even with modification or premedication prior to activities, promotes self-esteem and peer relationships.	

Nursing Care Plan — The Child with Asthma in the Community Setting, *continued*

Intervention	Rationale	Expected Outcome
■ Help the family to obtain extra equipment and medications that can be provided to the school.	■ Schools will provide care, but the families must provide all supplies, equipment, and medications.	
■ Work with the parents and school nurse to teach the specific asthma interventions to a designated person in the school nurse's absence.	■ School nurses often travel between several schools. The school administrator or secretary often serves as the backup care provider.	

4. Nursing Diagnosis: Self-Esteem, Situational Low, Risk for (Child) related to need to seek special care during school hours

NIC Priority Intervention—*Self-Esteem Enhancement:* Assisting a patient to increase his or her personal judgment of self-worth		**NOC Suggested Outcome**—*Self-Esteem:* Personal judgment of self-worth

GOAL: *The child's improved control over asthma will increase his or her self-esteem and peer relationships.*

■ Assess the child's peer relationships and opportunities for age-appropriate interactions, including sports.	■ Assessment is important to identify the best strategies to support the child and family.	The child establishes friendships and engages in activities with peers.
■ Motivate the child and family to gain increased control of asthma so the child can participate in normal childhood activities and sports.	■ Motivation may increase compliance with recommended daily asthma control interventions.	

NANDA-I © 2012

Severity of BPD in infants with a gestational age less than 32 weeks is categorized by the need for supplemental oxygen for at least 28 days plus these characteristics (Askin & Diehl-Jones, 2009):

- **Mild**—breathing room air at 36 weeks' postmenstrual age or at discharge
- **Moderate**—needs less than 30% supplemental oxygen at 36 weeks' postmenstrual age or at discharge
- **Severe**—needs greater than or equal to 30% supplemental oxygen and/or positive pressure ventilation or nasal CPAP at 36 weeks' postmenstrual age or at discharge

Clinical Manifestations

The infant with BPD has persistent signs of increased respiratory effort, including tachypnea, nasal flaring, grunting, retractions, and irritability. The infant may have wheezing, crackles, and pulmonary edema. Feeding can create increased oxygen demands the infant cannot meet, fatigue, and poor intake leading to failure to thrive. The infant has intermittent bronchospasms, mucous plugging, and air trapping that may lead to episodes of sudden respiratory deterioration. The air trapping persists and in time causes the chest to assume a barrel shape. Cyanosis may be seen in severe cases.

Collaborative Care

Care is focused on supporting the infant's lung function and providing care for episodes of respiratory compromise until lung healing and development occur.

Diagnostic Procedures

The diagnosis of lung injury is evident by the dependence on supplemental oxygen, respiratory support, and other clinical manifestations. A chest radiograph is often obtained.

Clinical Therapy

Initial medical management of the very-low-birth-weight infant involves surfactant instillation by the endotracheal tube, continuous positive airway pressure with nasal prongs, supplemental oxygen flow to maintain the oxygen saturation between 90% and 95%, IV fluids, early amino acid supplementation, and parenteral nutrition followed in a few days by enteral feeds. Low-dose indomethacin may be provided to reduce the risk for intraventricular hemorrhage and to close the patent ductus arteriosus (Geary et al., 2008).

Once BPD has developed, affected children may have frequent respiratory illnesses, feeding difficulties, growth failure, and rehospitalizations. Medical management involves the treatment of symptoms that supports respiratory function and good nutrition, which helps accelerate lung maturity. Supplemental oxygen with humidity is used. A tracheostomy may be needed for long-term airway management to prevent narrowing of the trachea. Infants with severe BPD are carefully weaned off assisted ventilation.

Increased calories are provided to support growth, but fluids are restricted to prevent pulmonary edema. Some children require gastrostomy or nasogastric feeding to get adequate calories. Chest physiotherapy and medications (diuretics, bronchodilators, anti-inflammatories, and methylxanthines) are also used. See the Medications table on page 786. Antibiotics are used to aggressively treat infections. With improvement and adequate weight gain, the child is weaned off oxygen, diuretics, and bronchodilators.

Infants with BPD may die due to respiratory failure and infection. Recurrent infections and their complications may occur. Efforts should be made to reduce environmental exposure to viral illnesses. Pulmonary function may remain abnormal for several years, with gradual improvement potentially beginning at school age. BPD is a significant risk factor for poor functional outcomes such as difficulties with motor and cognitive skills (Kelly, 2010).

Nursing Management

The goals of nursing management are to assess and manage the infant's acute episodes, ensure adequate nutritional support, and promote the infant's growth and development.

Medications   Used to Treat Bronchopulmonary Dysplasia

MEDICATION	ACTION/INDICATION	NURSING MANAGEMENT
Bronchodilators (beta₂-adrenergic agonists, anticholinergics, theophylline, albuterol nebulizer)	Decreases airway resistance, increases expiratory flow in small airways, stimulates mucous clearance; different drugs work together for best response	■ Monitor vital signs and potential signs of toxicity. ■ Medications should be given at the same time each day. ■ Encourage fluid intake.
Anti-inflammatory agents (cromolyn sodium)	Decreases inhibition of inflammatory mediators from mast cells	■ Ensure parents use proper technique for inhaler and spacer. ■ Clean inhaler daily, rinsing and drying parts.
Diuretics (furosemide, chlorothiazide, spironolactone)	Helps remove excess fluid from lungs; decreases pulmonary resistance and increases pulmonary compliance; may cause electrolyte imbalances	■ Follow guidelines for allowable fluid intake. ■ Monitor serum potassium and sodium levels. ■ Teach families about sodium and potassium-rich foods to eat or avoid, depending upon diuretic prescribed.
Potassium chloride	Prevents electrolyte imbalances associated with diuretics	■ Monitor serum potassium level. ■ Teach families about potassium-rich foods to avoid or use in moderation.
Methylxanthines (caffeine, theophylline)	Increases respiratory drive, decreases apnea, and relaxes muscle bundles that constrict airways	■ Monitor vital signs and respiratory status. ■ Monitor for adverse effects such as irritability, tremor, tachycardia, nausea, and vomiting.
Palivizumab (Synagis)	Protects infant from respiratory syncytial virus	■ Teach family the importance of monthly injection beginning in the fall.

Nursing Assessment and Diagnosis

The infant with chronic BPD may become acutely ill at any time. At each healthcare visit, assess the child's respiratory status, any signs of infection, as well as growth and development. Many of these infants have poor weight gain because the work of breathing requires extra calories. Assess how well the family is managing care for the child in the home and any stressors that might exist. Evaluate development regularly as the infant may develop motor, language, and cognitive delays. Coordinate a periodic assessment of hearing and vision.

Infants with BPD may become acutely ill at any time and require hospitalization. Assess airway and respiratory function, vital signs, color, and behavior changes to identify signs of worsening respiratory symptoms even when oxygen is provided. During hospitalization for an acute episode, a cardiorespiratory monitor and pulse oximeter are used. Observe for airway obstruction when the infant has a tracheostomy, and suction as needed.

Nursing diagnoses that may be appropriate include:

- Gas Exchange, Impaired related to ventilation-perfusion imbalance
- Caregiver Role Strain related to 24-hour responsibility for infant with BPD
- Nutrition, Imbalanced: Less than Body Requirements related to high metabolic needs and fatigue associated with feeding
- Development: Delayed, Risk for related to chronic condition and limited opportunities to practice motor skills

NANDA-I © 2012

Planning and Implementation

Care of the hospitalized infant is organized to eliminate any unnecessary physical stimulation, as this additional stress contributes to respiratory compromise. Position the infant to facilitate breathing and administer humidified oxygen if ordered. Provide daily tracheostomy care, observe for airway obstruction, and suction as needed. See the Skills Manual ⬤.

Administer medications as ordered. Management of fever will help minimize energy needs. Provide fluids and nutrition to help meet energy needs. Careful management of administered fluid volumes is critical as excess fluids can lead to pulmonary edema. Support the mother who desires to breastfeed. Some children receive nasogastric or enteral feedings.

Provide toys and mobiles that are age appropriate, but do not encourage excessive activity so that growth and development is promoted. Support the parents with clear explanations about the infant's health status and planned interventions to reduce anxiety.

Discharge Planning and Home Care

Plans for care at home must be carefully coordinated early in the child's hospitalization. Once home, many infants need ventilation therapy, oxygen, tracheostomy care, multiple medications, fluid restrictions, and high-calorie feedings (Figure 25–17 ■). Including parents in the infant's care early prepares them for home care responsibilities. Make referrals for needed oxygen, respiratory supplies, medications, and follow-up care. Some families require home health nursing assistance, especially during the initial transition period. Teach parents to provide the complex care needed by the infant. Inform families of the need for RSV prophylaxis, and provide the first injection prior to discharge if during RSV season.

Care in the Community

It is important to provide for the infant's normal development through rest, nutrition, stimulation, and family support. Help families identify additional family members who might be willing to learn how to care for the infant so that the parents can have a few hours of respite during the week. Families may need assistance in planning a schedule that ensures the infant receives needed care and leaves some time free for other children and family activities. Refer the family to an early intervention program (e.g., Child Find) as infants with severe BPD are at risk for delayed development.

Frequent rehospitalization may occur. While the lungs may function adequately, they remain vulnerable throughout childhood to common respiratory illnesses. Infants with BPD do not have the same respiratory reserve as healthy infants and can become very ill rapidly. Teach parents to identify signs of respiratory compromise indicating a need for rapid intervention. Help the parents to develop an emergency care plan for use in those cases when the infant becomes suddenly ill and emergency care is needed. A model emergency information form for emergency care providers is available from the American Academy of Pediatrics.

Nutritional requirements to support growth must be balanced with fluid restrictions to prevent the development of pulmonary edema. A high-caloric formula (24 to 30 calories/oz) or a formula supplemented with carbohydrates and medium-chain triglycerides may be given to promote weight gain. Some children need nasogastric or enteral feedings to get adequate nutrition when cyanosis is noted with feeding. Oral tactile hypersensitivity that interferes with feeding may be a problem in these children because of the long-term use of nasogastric, orogastric, and endotracheal tubes. See Chapter 9 . Electrolytes may be monitored monthly. All infants with BPD need more frequent health promotion visits and all immunizations. See the Health Promotion and Maintenance Overview: Bronchopulmonary Dysplasia.

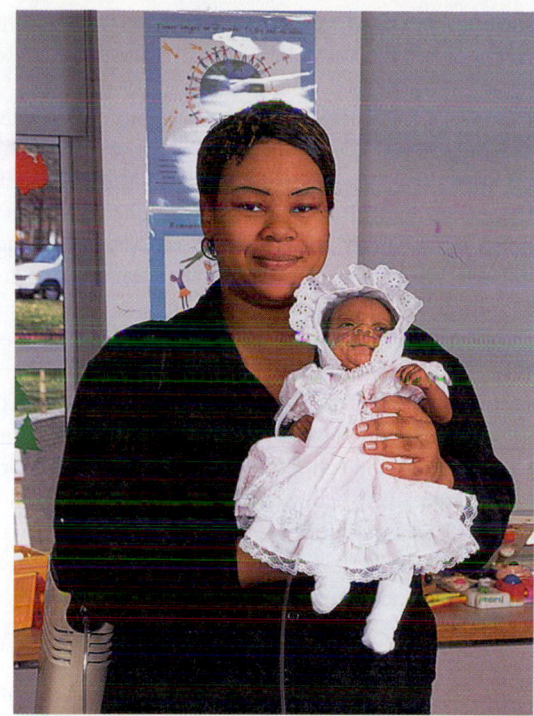

FIGURE 25–17 ■ Many children with BPD are cared for at home, with the support of a home care program to monitor the family's ability to provide airway management, oxygen, and support. This premature infant girl, who is now 4 months old but weighs only about 5 pounds, requires respiratory support with oxygen.

Health Promotion & Maintenance Overview

Bronchopulmonary Dysplasia

HEALTH SUPERVISION
- Assess blood pressure to detect abnormal findings associated with pulmonary hypertension.
- Perform hematocrit frequently during the first year of life to assess for anemia.
- Perform routine hearing assessment at each visit.
- Coordinate vision screening by an ophthalmologist every 2 to 3 months during the first year of life. Myopia and strabismus are common in premature infants.
- Coordinate pulmonary function tests annually or as needed for clinical condition.
- Perform other screening tests as recommended for age.

GROWTH AND DEVELOPMENTAL SURVEILLANCE
- Assess growth and plot measurements on a growth chart corrected for gestational age. Even if length and weight are lower than normal, monitor for continued growth following the growth curves.
- Perform the Denver II and record the developmental assessment corrected for gestational age.

NUTRITION
- Review caloric intake and ensure that intake is optimal for growth. Assess difficulties with feeding related to oral motor function. Refer to a nutritionist as necessary.

PHYSICAL ACTIVITY
- Organize care so that the child has time to rest during the day.
  - Suggest strategies for parents to promote the infant's normal motor development.

FAMILY INTERACTIONS
- Identify ways to coordinate care during the night to reduce the number of times the child and family have sleep disturbed.
- Provide discipline appropriate for developmental age.
- Encourage development. Provide developmentally appropriate toys and activities.

DISEASE PREVENTION STRATEGIES
- Reduce exposure to infections. If out-of-home childcare is used, select a provider caring for a small number of children. If possible, avoid the use of childcare centers during RSV season.
- Immunize the child with the routine schedule based on chronologic age.
- Give the 23-valent pneumococcal vaccine at 2 years of age.
- Provide monthly injections of palivizumab throughout the RSV season to protect the child from respiratory syncytial virus.

CONDITION-SPECIFIC GUIDANCE
- Develop an emergency care plan for times when the infant's condition rapidly worsens.

Evaluation

Expected outcomes of nursing care may include:

- Adequate calories are provided to sustain growth in length and weight following introduction of oral foods.
- The family rapidly identifies acute illness episodes.
- Emergency care is provided to prevent or manage the infant's respiratory decompensation.
- The infant's development is promoted.

Cystic Fibrosis

Cystic fibrosis (CF) is a common inherited autosomal recessive disorder of the exocrine glands that results in physiologic alterations in the respiratory, gastrointestinal, and reproductive systems. The incidence of cystic fibrosis varies by race—1 in 3,200 Caucasians, 1 in 8,000 Hispanics, 1 in 15,000 African Americans, and 1 in 31,000 Asian Americans (Gott & Froh, 2010; Hazle, 2010). Gender is not a factor in incidence. Approximately 30,000 children and adults have cystic fibrosis in the United States, and approximately 45% are older than age 18 years. More than 70% of children with cystic fibrosis are diagnosed by 2 years of age. In 2009, the median life span for individuals with cystic fibrosis in the United States was mid-30s, compared to elementary school age in the 1950s (Cystic Fibrosis Foundation, 2011a).

Etiology and Pathophysiology

A gene isolated on the long arm of chromosome 7 directs the function of the transmembrane conductance regulator (CFTR) protein. This protein controls the movement of chloride and sodium in and out of the cells that line the organs. Mutations of this gene alter the structure, function, and production of the protein that is essential for normal functioning of the respiratory, digestive, and reproductive systems. More than 1,700 mutations of the CFTR gene on chromosome 7 have been recorded that can cause cystic fibrosis (Lomas & Fowler, 2010). The most common cystic fibrosis gene mutation for the North American population is ΔF508 (delta F508), but this mutation can vary in how severely it affects someone with cystic fibrosis (O'Sullivan & Freedman, 2009). Some less common mutations of the CF gene may cause milder symptoms (Cystic Fibrosis Foundation, 2011b). An estimated 1 in 31 persons in the United States is a carrier of a defective CFTR gene, and carriers are healthy (Gott & Froh, 2010).

With a defective CFTR protein, chloride-ion transport across the exocrine and epithelial cell membranes is impaired, and increased sodium absorption reduces water movement across cell membranes. Body secretions become thickened in the sweat ducts, airway, pancreatic duct, intestine, biliary tree, and vas deferens. The lungs become clogged with mucus, leading to infections. Obstructions in the pancreas stop the flow of natural enzymes that enable the body to digest and absorb food. While the exact mechanism of how the gene alteration causes disease symptoms is unknown, one theory maintains that excessive reabsorption of salt and water away from the airway dehydrates and thickens the airway mucus. The lubricating layer between the epithelium and mucus inhibits normal ciliary action and cough clearance. This thickened mucus can then harbor bacteria (O'Sullivan & Freedman, 2009).

Obstructions in the airways lead to air trapping, hyperinflation, and atelectasis. Secondary respiratory infections occur. Even with antibiotics and a good response, over time the airways develop chronic bacterial and fungal colonization, bronchiectasis, and respiratory failure. Pneumothorax and hemothorax may occur in older children. The rate of progression is variable among affected children. Respiratory failure is the leading cause of mortality.

The majority of children with CF have a genotype that affects the pancreas. Pancreatic ducts become damaged, resulting in failure to secrete the natural enzymes necessary to digest fats, fat-soluble vitamins, and proteins. Nutritional deficits may result in failure to thrive. As some children get older, the pancreas may stop producing sufficient insulin, and glucose intolerance results, leading to the development of cystic fibrosis–related diabetes mellitus.

The intestinal tract is also affected by failure to secrete enough chloride and fluid into the intestines. This causes meconium ileus (an intestinal obstruction) in 15% of newborns with cystic fibrosis (O'Sullivan & Freedman, 2009). Older children may have intermittent and recurrent episodes of partial small bowel obstruction that can progress to total obstruction, abdominal distention, and vomiting. Chronic inflammation may occur in the intestines, as it does in the lungs, and lead to the development of Crohn's disease. About 5% of children with cystic fibrosis develop liver disease (O'Sullivan & Freedman, 2009).

Metabolic function is altered as a result of the imbalances created by excessive electrolyte loss through perspiration, saliva, and mucous secretion. These children are at risk for hyponatremic dehydration secondary to electrolyte imbalance.

Clinical Manifestations

One of the first signs of cystic fibrosis noticed by parents is a salty taste to the skin. A meconium ileus may be found in the newborn. Other primary symptoms are associated with the production of thick, sticky mucus. See the Clinical Manifestations table on the next page.

Most children with cystic fibrosis have a voracious appetite but have difficulty maintaining and gaining weight because of malabsorption of food and an increased metabolic rate associated with frequent infections. Infants and children may have a delayed bone age, short stature, and delayed onset of puberty.

Some adolescents and young adults in later stages of cystic fibrosis report chronic pain. Chest pain is most commonly reported and may be musculoskeletal in origin, related to regular use of accessory muscles for breathing. Unilateral chest pain of sudden onset associated with shortness of breath is an indication of pneumothorax. Bleeding, bruising, and hemoptysis may result from impairment of coagulation factors with liver cirrhosis (Wiehe & Arndt, 2010).

Collaborative Care

Diagnostic Procedures

Cystic fibrosis is usually diagnosed in infancy or early childhood with one of four major presentations: newborn meconium ileus, malabsorption or failure to thrive, chronic respiratory infections, or fecal impaction and intussusception ("telescoping" of the bowel) (see Chapter 30).

Newborn screening is performed on dried blood samples (the same ones used for other neonatal screening tests) to detect immunoreactive trypsinogen (IRT) concentrations (enzyme produced by the pancreas), which are high in infants with cystic fibrosis. If the reading is high, a second IRT test may be performed at 2 to 3 weeks of age to see if the IRT concentration is still high. Some states perform both an IRT and a DNA analysis on the same blood sample if the IRT concentration is high. The DNA analysis identifies the potential existence of

Clinical Manifestations Cystic Fibrosis

BODY SYSTEM	PATHOPHYSIOLOGY	CLINICAL MANIFESTATIONS
Upper respiratory	Thickened mucus clogs sinuses	Nasal polyps Chronic sinusitis, frontal headaches, purulent nasal discharge, post-nasal discharge
Lower respiratory	Thickened mucus reduces ciliary clearance; obstructs the airways; leads to air trapping and hyperinflation; permits bacteria to colonize Chronic fibrotic changes in lungs	Chronic moist, productive cough, wheezing, coarse crackles Frequent infections Shortness of breath, decreased exercise tolerance Barrel chest Clubbing of fingers and toes (Figure 25–18 ■)
Pancreas	Thickened mucus damages pancreatic ducts and obstructs enzymes necessary to digest fats, fat-soluble vitamins, and proteins Enzymes produced damage the pancreas, and fibrosis leads to failure to produce adequate insulin	Food is poorly digested Large quantity of greasy, bulky stools (steatorrhea) that are frothy, foul smelling, and floating Deficiency of vitamins A, D, E, and K Poor weight gain or failure to thrive; delayed onset of puberty Cystic fibrosis–related diabetes
Gastrointestinal	Thickened intestinal secretions and decreased motility of the gut Obstruction of bile ducts	Meconium ileus at birth Abdominal distention Constipation or intestinal obstruction Rectal prolapsed Liver cirrhosis
Reproductive	Males—absence of vas deferens in males, low levels of sperm in semen Females—thick vaginal discharge and decreased cervical secretions	Males—infertility Females—may have difficulty conceiving
Sweat glands	Excess electrolyte loss in the sweat, especially chloride and sodium	Salty sweat Salt depletion, hyponatremia

Source: Data from O'Sullivan, B. P., & Freedman, S. D. (2009, May 30). Cystic fibrosis. Lancet, 373, 1891–1904; Kelly, M. M. (2010). Prematurity. In P. J. Allen, J. A. Vessey, & N. A. Shapiro, Primary care of the child with a chronic condition (5th ed., pp. 756–771). St. Louis, MO: Mosby Elsevier; Wiehe, M., & Arndt, K. (2010). Cystic fibrosis: A systems review. AANA Journal, 78(3), 246–251.

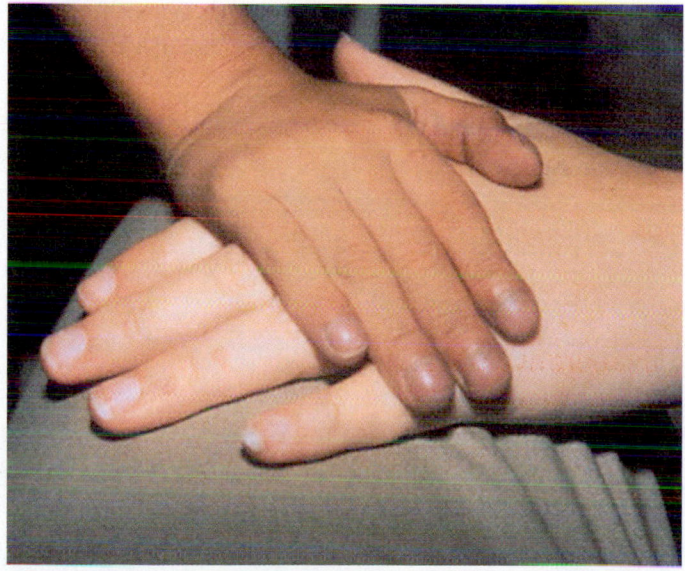

FIGURE 25–18 ■ Digital clubbing.

a chromosome mutation that causes cystic fibrosis (Rock & Sharp, 2010). The IRT and chromosome mutation analysis is considered a screening test for cystic fibrosis. Newborn screening for CF is performed in all 50 states and the District of Columbia (Cystic Fibrosis Foundation, 2011c). Genetic testing is also available for adults with a positive family history, partners of individuals with cystic fibrosis, and couples seeking prenatal testing to identify carriers of cystic fibrosis gene mutations.

A sweat chloride test by pilocarpine iontophoresis is considered the gold standard for diagnosis of cystic fibrosis, even when newborn screening tests are positive (see Appendix E 🔗). A chloride level greater than 60 mEq/L is diagnostic with other signs (meconium ileus, high IRT level, or positive family history), and a level of 50 to 60 mEq/L is suspicious. The test is often repeated to confirm the diagnosis (Figure 25–19 ■).

A spirometer is used on children older than 6 years to monitor pulmonary function. Forced vital capacity (FVC) and forced expiratory volume in one second (FEV_1) readings are taken. Sputum cultures are obtained to identify organisms and sensitivities for antibiotic treatment.

Clinical Therapy

Clinical therapy focuses on maintaining respiratory function, managing infection, promoting optimal nutrition and exercise, and preventing intestinal obstruction. See Table 25–9. Newly diagnosed children who begin treatment before the onset of symptomatic lung disease are aggressively treated to slow the development of chronic respiratory infections and reduction in pulmonary function, and to improve nutrition and support growth.

Treatment is focused on controlling infection and inflammation, and on reducing mucus accumulation. Various forms of bronchial hygiene therapy, such as manual chest physiotherapy, are used

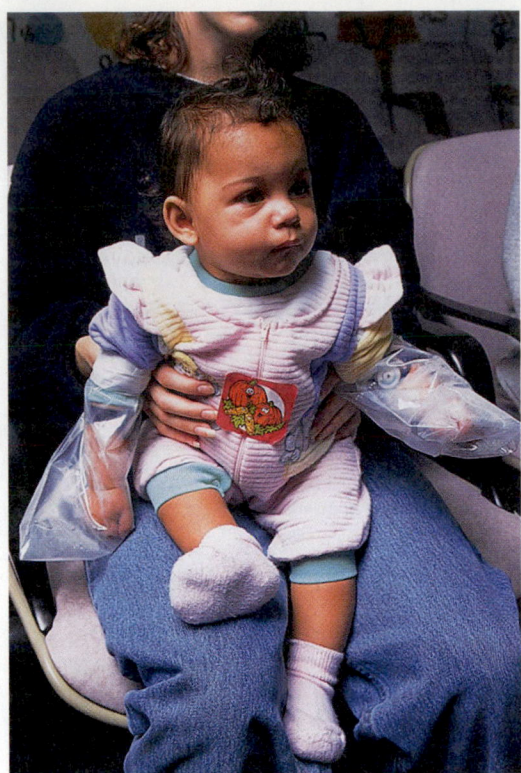

FIGURE 25–19 ■ The parent may hold and reassure the infant or small child being evaluated for cystic fibrosis with a sweat chloride test. To collect the sweat, pilocarpine is applied to a small area on the arm or leg. An electrode with weak electrical current is placed on the area to stimulate the child to sweat. The area is cleaned and a piece of filter paper is placed over the area and covered in plastic. The filter paper is removed after 30 minutes and the sweat content is analyzed.

regularly to reduce the accumulation of mucus in the lungs. See Box 25–11 for the various types of chest physiotherapy used by children with cystic fibrosis.

Frequent prolonged courses of antibiotics for infections may be prescribed to improve pulmonary function, exercise tolerance, and quality of life. Inhaled tobramycin, colistimethate (Coly-Mycin M), or Cayston is given to children with chronic *Pseudomonas aeruginosa* infection to suppress bacterial growth; it is given in alternating months (Montgomery & Howenstine, 2009). Children who have evidence of *Pseudomonas aeruginosa* or *Burkholderia cepacia* infections have a poorer outcome. Medications are used to reduce sputum viscosity and to dilate the airways before administration of inhaled antibiotics and before airway clearance techniques are performed. Anti-inflammatory treatment is sometimes prescribed. Vitamins and pancreatic enzymes are also provided to improve the child's nutritional status. See Medications Used to Treat Cystic Fibrosis on the next page.

Collaborative care with physicians, nurses, respiratory therapists, and nutritionists has led to improvements in medical management and optimal nutrition that have prolonged the lives of children and adults with cystic fibrosis. However, complications such as cystic fibrosis–related diabetes mellitus (often with insulin insufficiency and insulin resistance) must be carefully managed along with the progression of the disease (see Chapter 32 ⊘). Cystic fibrosis–related diabetes occurs in 20% of adolescents with cystic fibrosis, but is rare earlier in childhood (Moran, Becker, Casella, et al., 2010). This disorder is challenging to manage because the child needs a large caloric intake that must be balanced by insulin dosage. End-stage lung disease is the cause of death in 80% of patients with cystic fibrosis (O'Sullivan & Freedman, 2009).

Lung transplantation may be performed, and approximately 60% of cases survive for the first 5 years (Hazle, 2010). Approximately 120 to 150 lung transplants are performed in individuals with cystic fibrosis each year in the United States (Wiehe & Arndt, 2010). Immunosuppressive medications can cause significant problems in individuals infected with *Pseudomonas* or *Burkholderia cepacia,* making them ineligible for lung transplant at many centers. The major complication of lung transplantation is chronic rejection, also known as **bronchiolitis obliterans,** involving irreversible changes to the small airways that are unresponsive to immunologic medication management.

TABLE 25–9	Clinical Therapy for Cystic Fibrosis
CLINICAL THERAPY	**RATIONALE**
Respiratory Therapy	
Exercise and physical fitness	■ Promotes maintenance of lung function
Airway clearance techniques—chest physiotherapy twice a day for all lung segments (percussion or vibration with child positioned to promote sputum drainage), oscillating chest vests, or other expiratory techniques (see page 791)	■ In association with coughing and breathing techniques, airway clearance techniques help secretions move to the bronchi from smaller airways
Immunizations	■ Prevention of viral and some bacterial infections
Chest tube drainage of air leaks	■ Resolves pneumothorax
Thoracostomy to sew over ruptured alveoli	■ Repairs area of recurrent pneumothorax and prevents future flare in same location
Lung transplantation	■ Reversal of respiratory failure
Gastrointestinal Tract Therapy	
Acid suppression preparation	■ Gastroesophageal reflux worsens lung function; enteric coating of enzyme supplements is affected by high acid levels in duodenum
Hyperosmolar enemas, isotonic fluid lavage of the intestines (oral or by nasogastric tube)	■ Enema relieves meconium ileus in most infants; fluid lavage reduces distal intestinal obstruction
Nutrition	
Well-balanced diet with 110–200% of Recommended Dietary Allowance (RDA) for calories (Stallings, Stark, Robinson, et al., 2008)	■ Promotes essential nutrient balance for health, growth, and weight maintenance, as well as increased lung capacity and survival

BOX 25–11	Bronchial Hygiene Therapy

Various methods of airway clearance can be used to clear mucus and secretions from the lungs to improve lung function and gas exchange and to prevent infection. The most recent research reports that there is no significant difference between airway clearance techniques for short-term and long-term management of increasing mucus transport out of the lungs (Pryor, Tannenbaum, Scott, et al., 2010). For the child with cystic fibrosis, it is important to find an airway clearance technique that the family and child will be most likely to fit into the daily routine for disease management.

- **Chest physiotherapy.** A parent or therapist percusses or applies vibration over each lung segment for 3 to 5 minutes while the child is maintained in different positions. Gravity promotes drainage of the secretions loosened by percussion or vibration. This method is preferred for infants and toddlers, but it is very time consuming. See the Skills Manual ⊂⊃ for correct techniques and positions.

- **Forced expiratory technique.** This technique (huffing) is performed by making two to three forced exhalations without closure of the glottis, like exhaling to steam up a mirror, followed by relaxed breathing. The lower airway compression associated with huffing is a good alternative when coughing causes small airways to collapse due to intrathoracic pressure.

- **Oscillating positive expiratory pressure (PEP).** The child breathes in and out about 15 times through a mouthpiece or mask attached to a device with a special expiratory valve. For example, a flutter or acapella valve provides intermittent positive pressure in the airways during exhalation that vibrates the airway walls to loosen secretions. It is believed to improve mucus clearance by increasing pressure behind secretions or by preventing airway collapse during expiration. Deep breathing and breath holding or huffing can then be performed to help move mucus to the larger airways for coughing up.

- **High-frequency chest wall oscillation.** The patient puts on an inflatable vest that creates an oscillating motion against the chest wall by an air pulse generator that rapidly inflates and deflates the vest. This method helps remove secretions by generating differences between expiratory and inspiratory flow and velocity. The child should stop the machine every 5 minutes to perform deep breathing and coughing to help remove the mucus. Children older than 4 years can use this method.

- **Active cycle of breathing technique (ACBT).** The child adopts a set of breathing techniques that helps get air behind the mucus, lowers airway spasm, and clears the mucus. Breathing control, normal gentle breathing with the lower chest while relaxing the upper chest and shoulders, is performed first and intermittently between other breathing techniques. The child then takes in deep breaths, holding each for 3 seconds to get more air behind the mucus. Chest percussion or vibration may be performed during this stage, followed by breathing control. Forced expiratory techniques such as huffing can then be performed, followed by breathing control (Cystic Fibrosis Foundation, 2011d).

- **Autogenic discharge.** Varied airflows are used to move mucus from different lung areas. For example, the child does a series of huffing and coughs to move mucus from the small airways to the larger airways for clearance (O'Sullivan & Freedman, 2009). This technique works best in children over age 8 years.

Medications Used to Treat Cystic Fibrosis

MEDICATIONS	ACTIONS	NURSING MANAGEMENT
Bronchodilators (beta-adrenergic agonists, anticholinergics) *Aerosol*	Opens large and small airways; few studies exist to demonstrate their effectiveness.	■ Use before airway clearance techniques. Have the child hold the breath 10 seconds after inhalation. ■ Avoid swallowing the medicine, and rinse the mouth afterward.
Dornase alfa (DNase or Pulmozyme) *Aerosol*	Loosens, liquefies, and thins pulmonary secretions	■ Keep refrigerated until placed in the nebulizer. ■ Monitor for improvement in dyspnea and mucus clearance.
Hypertonic saline (7%) *Aerosol*	Hydrates the airway mucus and stimulates coughing (Montgomery & Howenstine, 2009)	■ Use following the bronchodilator.
Ibuprofen *Oral*	Slows the rate of pulmonary function decline (Flume, O'Sullivan, Robinson, et al., 2007)	■ Educate the child and parents to monitor for signs of gastrointestinal bleeding. ■ Ensure that the child does not take aspirin or other NSAIDs unless approved by the physician.
Antibiotics *Oral, IV, inhalation*	Used to treat and suppress infections; selected based upon culture and sensitivities	■ Higher doses than normal and prolonged courses may be needed because of rapid clearance. ■ Teach the child and family to develop a schedule to give the correct dose at appropriate intervals.
Pancreatic enzyme supplements (Cotazym-S, Pancrease, Viokase) *Oral*	Assists in digestion of nutrients decreasing fat and bulk; given prior to food ingestion	■ Give prior to food ingestion. ■ Ensure that enzymes are taken with meals and snacks.
Vitamins A, D, E, and K *Oral*	Cystic fibrosis interferes with vitamin production; supplements are required in water-soluble form for better absorption (vitamins A, D, E, and K are naturally fat soluble); iron deficiency results from malabsorption syndrome.	■ Ensure that vitamins are prescribed in non-fat-soluble form to promote absorption. ■ Give twice a day.
Recombinant human growth hormone *Subcutaneous*	May improve height and weight, and pulmonary function in prepubertal children; its value in treating cystic fibrosis is still not clear (Phung, Coleman, Baker, et al., 2010).	■ Rotate injection sites in the abdomen and thighs. ■ Monitor height growth regularly. ■ Monitor blood glucose level in children with a family history of diabetes.

Nursing Management

The goal of nursing management is to partner with the family to manage the chronic disease by promoting optimal nutrition and reducing the incidence of infection. Care of the child with previously diagnosed cystic fibrosis is the focus of the following discussion.

Nursing Assessment and Diagnosis

Physiologic Assessment

Physical assessment of the child focuses on the adequacy of respiratory function. Inquire about the frequency and character of the child's cough and sputum characteristics. Compare this information with the child's baseline. Changes in the cough may be more important than its presence or absence related to the development of a new infection. Auscultate the chest for breath sounds, crackles, and wheezes. Note any cyanosis or clubbing of the extremities. Obtain oxygen saturation and spirometry readings if changes in respiratory status are suspected.

Evaluate the child's growth, plotting the weight and height on a growth curve. Determine whether the child is maintaining an appropriate growth pattern. Children with significantly lower percentiles for height and weight on the growth curve should be considered malnourished. Inquire about the child's appetite and dietary intake. Ask about nutritional supplements, pancreatic enzymes, and vitamins used. Observe the adolescent for the appearance of secondary sexual characteristics, which are often delayed due to the nutritional status.

Assess the child's stooling pattern. Identify whether the child has problems with abdominal pain or bloating, and whether these problems can be related to eating, stooling, or other activities. Palpate the abdomen for liver size, fecal masses, and evidence of pain.

Psychosocial Assessment

Inquire about the family's and child's emotional and psychosocial responses to managing the illness. The emotional stress of this chronic disease may not be readily apparent on hospital admission or in the clinic settings, particularly if the child's symptoms are mild and not imminently life threatening. Ongoing observation of the child's and parents' behavior helps direct nursing interventions. Parents may feel guilt as carriers of the disease. Siblings may also show signs of difficulty in dealing with the illness, particularly if not affected by the disease. Siblings with cystic fibrosis may be affected if the child is showing signs of significant deterioration, being forced to acknowledge their own future course with the disease. In some cases, one parent may also have cystic fibrosis and need additional support with personal disease management as well as their child's (Lomas & Fowler, 2010).

The nurse should ask parents about how the child's illness has affected day-to-day functioning, potential conflicts with family activities, and how they have adapted to the child's plan of care. Investigate the need and options for respite. Identify what parents of young children have told the child and siblings about the disease. What kind of questions have the child and siblings asked about cystic fibrosis, and how have parents answered them? Has the child ever asked about his or her life expectancy? If not, what would parents say if asked?

Common nursing diagnoses for the child with cystic fibrosis include the following:

- Airway Clearance, Ineffective related to thick mucus in lungs
- Infection, Risk for related to the presence of mucous secretions conducive to bacterial growth
- Nutrition, Imbalanced: Less than Body Requirements related to the need for increased calories to meet growth and metabolic needs
- Role Conflict, Parental related to interruptions in family life due to the home care regimen and child's frequent exacerbations

NANDA-I © 2012

Planning and Implementation

Nursing management involves supporting the child and family initially, when the diagnosis is made, during subsequent hospitalizations, and during visits to specialty and primary healthcare providers. The nurse's role begins with implementing specific medical therapies and providing nursing care to meet the child's physiologic and psychosocial needs. Airway clearance techniques, medications, and nutrition must be coordinated to promote optimal body function. Psychosocial support and reinforcement of the child's daily care needs are important in preparation for home care.

Children with cystic fibrosis require periodic hospitalization when a severe infection occurs or for a pulmonary and nutritional assessment. The child is usually placed in a private room to reduce the spread of infectious organisms with standard precautions. Children with cystic fibrosis are not co-roomed to reduce the risk for transmission of *Pseudomonas aeruginosa* and *Burkholderia cepacia*.

Respect the parents' experiences as the child's primary care providers and include them in the child's routine care as much as possible. However, parents may view the hospital stay as a break from the rigorous daily pulmonary care routine at home and need support to take advantage of the respite. While the family is often proficient at providing physical care to the child, the nurse should take the opportunity provided during rehospitalization to review basic and new information about airway clearance techniques, medications, and nutrition. This is especially important as the child matures and begins to assume some self-care responsibilities. Keeping lines of communication open and validating parents' understanding of their child's disease and care needs are important steps in preparing the family to cope with this chronic health challenge.

Provide Respiratory Therapy

Chest physiotherapy or an airway clearance technique is usually performed one to three times per day before meals to facilitate the removal of secretions from the lungs, as coughing may stimulate vomiting (Figure 25–20 ■). Aerosol treatments with a bronchodilator, as well as DNase and hypertonic saline to help thin respiratory secretions, precede chest physiotherapy. Respiratory therapists and nurses often collaborate in teaching parents and other family members the skills for these necessary treatments. Older children use an oscillating vest or other airway clearance technique while hospitalized rather than chest physiotherapy. Refer to the Skills Manual ⌘ .

Administer Medications

Antibiotics for an acute exacerbation are provided by oral, inhalation, and intravenous routes. Because children with cystic fibrosis have an increased clearance of most antibiotics, they need higher doses and long treatment courses, often for at least 14 days until the child achieves the best possible lung function. Because of the higher antibiotic dosages, renal function needs to be monitored. Serum drug levels of antibiotics may be ordered to ensure therapeutic dosing. In some cases, a portacath or peripherally inserted central catheter (PICC line) is placed so that IV antibiotics may be given at home to enable an earlier discharge.

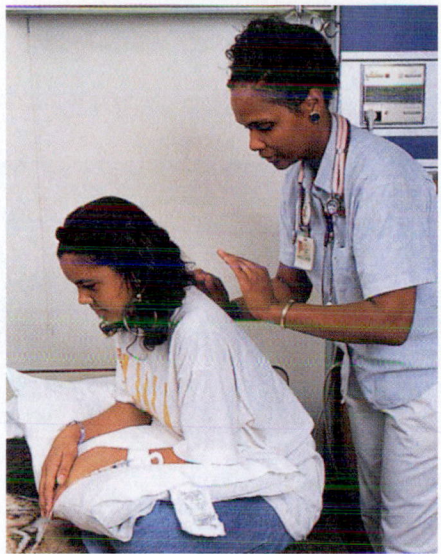

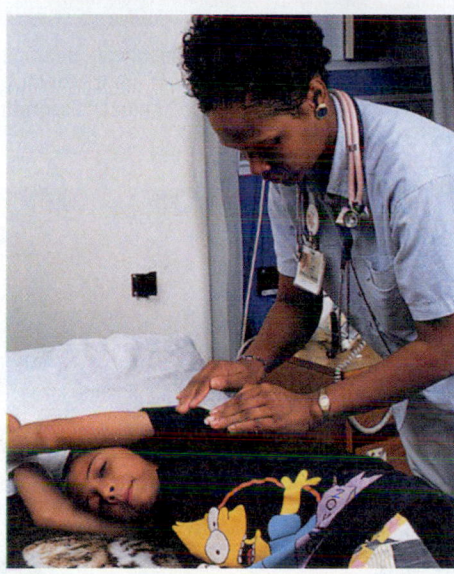

FIGURE 25-20 ■ Postural drainage can be achieved by clapping with a cupped hand on the chest wall over the segment to be drained. This action creates vibrations that are transmitted to the bronchi so that secretions are loosened and drain by gravity to the bronchi. *A,* If the obstruction is in the posterior apical segment of the lung, the nurse can do this with the child sitting up. *B,* If the obstruction is in the left posterior segment, the child should be lying on the right side. Several other positions can be used depending on the location of the obstruction. See the Skills Manual.

Meet Nutritional Needs

Digestive problems can be eased with pancreatic enzymes and dietary modification. Pancreatic enzyme supplements come in powder sprinkles and capsule form and are taken orally with all meals and large snacks. The amount needed is individualized based on the child's nutritional needs and digestive response to these supplements.

Parents need to learn what foods if any should be avoided or eliminated because of the child's gastrointestinal problems. The goal is to achieve near-normal, well-formed stools and adequate weight gain. Referral should be made to a nutritionist before the time of discharge. Fat-soluble vitamins (A, D, E, and K) are not completely absorbed from food; therefore, they must be taken in water-soluble form. Multivitamins taken twice daily usually are sufficient to prevent vitamin deficiency.

> **BOX 25-12** | **Research: Cystic Fibrosis and Self-Care Indicators**
>
> A study with 123 adolescents with cystic fibrosis investigated predictors of universal health self-care (e.g., eating a nutritious diet) and of CF-related self-care (e.g., airway clearance techniques and taking medications). Satisfaction with family was a predictor of universal self-care and CF-related self-care. A greater sense of life being meaningful and manageable, plus ego strength, attention to health, health knowledge, and decision-making capabilities were predictive of universal self-care. Adolescents who engaged in higher levels of universal self-care were more likely to engage in CF-related self-care (Baker & Denyes, 2008).

Respiratory complications necessitate additional energy expenditure. Some children require nutritional supplements or supplemental nasogastric or gastrostomy feedings to gain and maintain weight. The diet should be well balanced, with an emphasis on high caloric value. Children with CF may require 1.5 times the daily caloric requirements. Fats and salt are both necessary in the diet. Balanced with pancreatic enzyme supplements, moderate fat intake adds an important source of calories.

Psychosocial Support

The nurse should assist the parents and child to learn ways to promote health after discharge. Emotional support is essential because the diagnosis of this disorder creates anxiety and fear in both the parents and the child. The child and parents need assistance with emotional and psychosocial issues relating to discipline, body image (stooling and odor, clubbing, barrel chest), frequent rehospitalization, the potential fatal nature of the illness, the child's feeling of being different from friends, and overall financial, social, and family concerns. Because the disorder is inherited, families may have more than one child with cystic fibrosis. Parents may have unspoken feelings of anger and guilt, blaming themselves for their children's condition. Refer families to genetic counseling and to support groups. See Box 25–12.

Discharge Planning and Home Care Teaching

The financial burden of medications, supplies, and medical follow-up may not be recognized immediately by a family overwhelmed by the diagnosis. Initially, parents need assistance in obtaining necessary equipment. If the family requires financial assistance, they should be referred to the appropriate social services and to the Cystic Fibrosis Foundation. Home care of the child with cystic fibrosis is expensive and can be draining on the family's finances.

Community Care

Nurses may encounter the child in specialty clinics, health centers, and schools. Assess the child as described on page 792. Observe the child's physical appearance, noting overall body proportions and any changes characteristic of cystic fibrosis. Respiratory function tests are usually performed every 6 months during cystic fibrosis center visits. Assess hearing acuity on a regular basis, especially if the antibiotic tobramycin is used because this medication has been associated with hearing loss.

A psychosocial assessment is especially important when the child is going through major developmental stages. School-age children and adolescents often are embarrassed at being viewed as different from peers. Ask how the child or adolescent feels about the need for a special diet and to eat so much more than his or her peers, medications, and the daily routine of respiratory management.

Review the child's use of bronchodilators and airway clearance techniques. If additional short-term therapies are prescribed to help

PHOTO STORY...
MANAGING CYSTIC FIBROSIS

Management of cystic fibrosis takes a lot of time each day, whether at home or in the hospital.

Shaun, a 13-year-old with cystic fibrosis, has a challenging time managing all the aspects of his disease. Shaun has an older sister who does not have cystic fibrosis. He lives with his mother and sister in a town about 50 miles from the cystic fibrosis center at the university medical center. Shaun is in the seventh grade at a local middle school, where he manages to keep his grades at a C level despite occasional school absences because of infection flare-ups. He plays on a Little League baseball team and enjoys riding his bicycle, but he usually spends a few days in the hospital each year for intensive therapy sessions to clear his lungs.

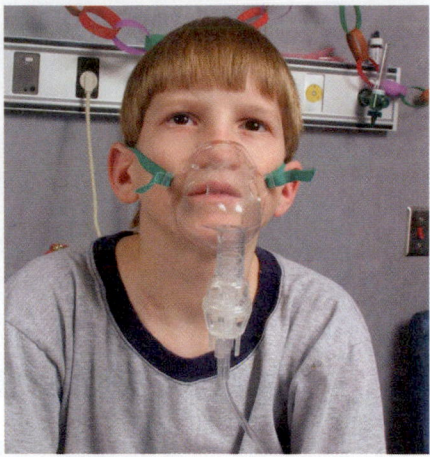

Shaun takes his nebulizer treatment with DNase prior to chest physiotherapy to increase the moisture of mucous secretions and ease expectoration.

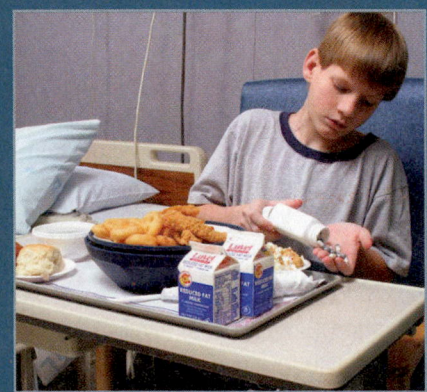

Shaun needs lots of calories and takes his pancreatic enzymes prior to eating lunch which is composed of double portions and high-calorie foods.

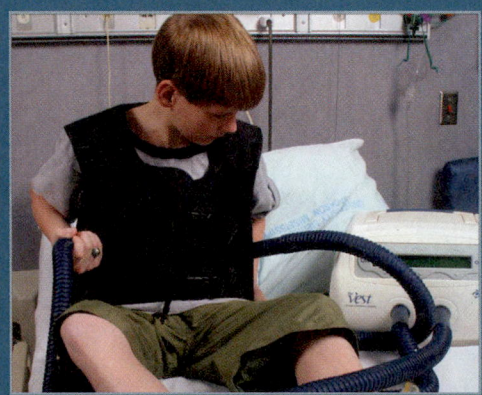

Shaun performs chest physiotherapy two times a day when at home. He uses a vest that he can independently set up and control.

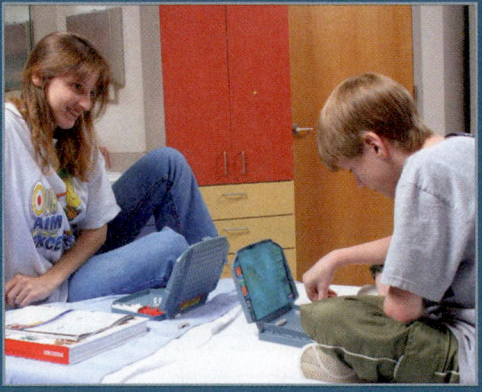

Shaun and his mother take time for recreation with a game to break the monotony of his time in the hospital.

Management of cystic fibrosis takes a lot of time each day, whether at home or in the hospital. All of his care must be scheduled around school and recreation. In most cases, the treatments cut in to his recreational time. Shaun has learned to manage many aspects of his care, relieving his mother of some responsibility. For example, Shaun can set up his nebulizer treatment and even measure the amount of DNase to use. After the nebulizer treatment, he uses an oscillating vest for chest physiotherapy for about 30 minutes per treatment. Coughing up sputum during and after the treatment is very tiring.

Shaun needs many extra calories to grow as well as meet metabolic demands. His mother works hard to prepare and provide the extra calories he needs throughout the day. He must take pancreatic enzymes to help him digest the foods. Because Shaun sometimes has difficulty getting enough calories, he has a gastrostomy tube for nighttime feedings. This has made it possible to get enough calories to help support his adolescent growth spurt.

improve pulmonary status, partner with the child and family to identify the best time to fit the additional treatment into the daily schedule and review the techniques to use. The airway clearance technique selected for use three or four times a day has a significant impact on family time. An alternative to chest physiotherapy such as an oscillating vibration vest may be more easily accepted by the family, especially since the parent does not have to physically perform the percussion and vibration. A regular vigorous exercise regimen is also beneficial in improving lung function, respiratory muscle strength, endurance, and airway clearance. Aerobic fitness is a significant factor in longer survival and quality of life for patients with cystic fibrosis.

Managing the child's nutritional needs is important and takes time and energy. Parents often have a difficult time encouraging the child with cystic fibrosis to eat the extra calories needed for optimal nutrition, setting the stage for a potential mealtime battleground. To be successful, parents need guidance about managing negative mealtime behaviors, in addition to guidelines for preparing nutritional calorie-dense foods and snacks. Increase calorie intake by offering high-calorie snacks between meals and before bed.

Clinical Tip

Use of cream or half and half added to soups, casseroles, and puddings; cream cheese spread on breads, muffins, and crackers; sour cream added to casseroles; and powdered milk added to regular milk, meatloaf, and custards are all ways to increase the calories in food eaten. Ensure Plus, Boost, or Carnation Instant Breakfast can be added to ice cream and fruit to make a milk shake (Pitts, Flack, & Goodfellow, 2008).

The child's diet is often customized by a nutritionist to plan high-calorie meals and snacks that will meet the child's calorie needs. Extra intervention, such as a gastrostomy tube for nighttime feedings, may be needed when the child's weight is 85% to 90% of ideal weight for height. Children with adequate nutrition have a longer life expectancy.

Children with cystic fibrosis lose more than normal amounts of salt in their sweat. This loss can become intensified during hot weather, strenuous exercise, and fever. During periods of exercise and increased sweating, the child should be encouraged to drink more fluids and increase salt intake. Parents should allow the child to add extra salt to food and should permit some salty snacks (pretzels with salt, pickles, carbonated soda). Teach parents to recognize early symptoms of salt depletion, including fatigue, weakness, abdominal pain, and vomiting, and to contact the child's healthcare provider if these symptoms occur.

Adolescents have special developmental issues and needs that must be addressed since the median survival rate has increased to more than 35 years of age. Gradual assumption of responsibility for daily disease management is necessary and may be challenging when there is rebellion and defiance to treatment. Individualized planning to achieve their daily care regimen may be helpful to these adolescents and still enable them to interact with peers at school.

Adolescents with cystic fibrosis know they are different from their peers and must learn how to cope with that difference. They also need to develop normal relationships and establish intimacy with a partner. Information about potential infertility must be provided along with the guidelines for safe sexual practices to reduce the risk for sexually transmitted diseases. Females may potentially be able to conceive and should be given contraception.

Adolescents must deal with the fact that they have a terminal condition, and they often need help to establish appropriate educational and occupational goals for their future. Transitioning to adult healthcare services and planning for independent life with a chronic disease requires support and planning. Palliative care planning should be initiated in adolescents and young adults as the disease progresses to respiratory failure. See Chapter 18 🔗. Discussions about options such as a lung transplant may be initiated with those considered to be candidates for the surgery. The patients who receive a transplant are not cured, but trade the problems of end-stage cystic fibrosis for lifelong immunosuppression and all the resulting complications.

Cystic fibrosis affects all family members and disrupts activities of daily living for everyone. It is important to refer families to counseling and group therapy with families of other children with cystic fibrosis if indicated. The Cystic Fibrosis Foundation is a source for information on current advances in the disorder. Local chapter activities also provide emotional support for parents and children.

Evaluation

Expected outcomes of nursing care include the following:

- The child and family become proficient in providing the daily pulmonary care, reducing the incidence of respiratory infections.
- A schedule and routine for daily pulmonary care is developed that fits into family and school activities.
- The child consumes adequate calories and pancreatic enzymes to support growth and to stay within desirable weight ranges.
- The child and family cope effectively with the child's disease.

INJURIES OF THE RESPIRATORY SYSTEM

Airway compromise after an unintentional injury can cause death if not managed quickly and effectively. Children are vulnerable to changes in respiratory function after injury because the small size of their airway makes it vulnerable to obstruction. The airway may be obstructed by the tongue or small amounts of blood, mucus, or foreign debris or swelling in the respiratory tract or adjacent neck tissue, leading to hypoxia and respiratory failure. If the child's neck is flexed or hyperextended, the soft laryngeal cartilage may compress and obstruct the airway. See Appendix F 🔗 for emergency airway management.

Practice Alert

Never allow the neck of an injured child to hyperextend (bend completely backward) or hyperflex (bend completely forward). Hyperextension flattens the trachea because there is no firm cartilage to provide structural support. Hyperflexion can kink and compress the trachea. Both maneuvers obstruct rather than open the airway.

Smoke Inhalation Injury

Exposure of the child's face and airway to fire or thermal conditions leads to dramatic responses in the child's respiratory tract. Inhalation injury from smoke and heat increases the child's risk for airway obstruction, carbon monoxide poisoning, acute respiratory distress syndrome, and late complications such as pneumonia and pulmonary embolism (Antoon & Donovan, 2007). Children are more vulnerable to smoke inhalation injury because their smaller airway diameter can be obstructed by edema, and a higher respiratory rate increases their exposure to noxious chemicals.

Weblink

Cystic Fibrosis Foundation

Etiology and Pathophysiology

The severity of a smoke inhalation injury is influenced by the type of material burned and whether the child was exposed in an open or closed space. The composition of materials determines how easily it ignites, how fast it burns, and how much heat is released. These factors influence the production of smoke and toxic gases. Smoke, a product of the burning process that is composed of gases and particles, is generated in varying volumes and density, and it consumes oxygen from the air. The type and concentration of invisible toxic gases affect the severity of pulmonary damage. The duration of exposure to the smoke produced and any toxic gases contribute significantly to the child's prognosis.

Exposure to extreme heat, common in house fires, leads to surface injury and upper airway damage. The upper airway normally removes heat from inhaled gases, sparing the lower airway from thermal damage when the patient is conscious. However, this action results in marked edema, placing the young child at particular risk for airway obstruction. Edema develops rapidly over a few hours and may lead to acute respiratory distress syndrome.

Carbon monoxide (CO) is a clear, colorless, odorless gas that is present in all fire conditions as the fire consumes oxygen. This is a significant concern when the child is trapped in a closed space fire. The CO molecule binds more firmly to hemoglobin than does oxygen. As a result, it replaces oxygen in circulation and rapidly produces tissue hypoxia in the child. The longer the exposure to CO, the greater the hypoxia. The brain receives inadequate oxygen, resulting in confusion. This accounts for the inability of fire victims to escape as confusion progresses to loss of consciousness. The process can be rapidly reversed, however, if 100% supplemental oxygen or hyperbaric oxygen treatment is provided before hypoxia becomes too severe (Baum, 2008).

Damage to the lower airway most often results from chemicals or toxic gas inhalation. Soot is carried deep into the lungs and often contains corrosive chemicals formed by combustion of various substances. The soot combines with surface water in the lungs to deposit acid-producing chemicals on the lung tissue. These acids burn the tissue, causing loss of cilia, loss of surfactant, and edema. Tissue destruction, pulmonary edema, and disruption of gas exchange produce the initial insult to the lungs and potential airway obstruction. Days later, the damaged tissue sloughs off, obstructing the airways. Because the cilia that normally help in removing debris have been destroyed, the lungs become a breeding ground for microorganisms. Pneumonia becomes a major health concern. The damaged alveoli heal by scar tissue formation. This can greatly reduce the future functioning of the lungs.

Clinical Manifestations

Burns of the face and neck, singed nasal hairs, soot around the mouth or nose, and hoarseness with stridor or voice change all indicate inhalation injury, even when the child initially has no respiratory distress. Edema develops rapidly over a few hours and may lead to airway obstruction with signs such as tachypnea, stridor, coughing, wheezing, and drooling. Respiratory distress develops and can lead to respiratory failure. If carbon monoxide poisoning is present the child will be confused or unconscious, and have cardiac arrhythmias.

Collaborative Care

Diagnosis is based upon history of the child being exposed to smoke in a closed area, as well as signs of soot around the nose and mouth. If the child has minimal signs and symptoms when seen in the emergency department, admission for close observation and monitoring for progression of respiratory distress is often indicated. Initial treatment is 100% humidified oxygen administered through a nonrebreather mask. Arterial blood gases and a carboxyhemoglobin level are obtained. With the development of respiratory distress, aggressive airway management with endotracheal tube insertion, mechanical ventilation, and monitoring are provided in the pediatric intensive care unit. Chest physiotherapy and suctioning may be provided in collaboration with respiratory therapists in an effort to keep the airway clear. All other injuries sustained in the fire are treated.

Nursing Management

Nursing assessment for respiratory distress is a key initial role. Check vital signs frequently. Attach a pulse oximeter to monitor the oxygen saturation. Auscultate the lungs for crackles, wheezes, and decreased breath sounds. Assess for level of consciousness and behavior changes that could indicate increasing hypoxia.

Provide oxygen as ordered. Position the child to promote respiratory function. If the child's condition deteriorates, assist with procedures to secure the child's airway and prepare the child for transfer to the intensive care unit. Assess the family's response to the life-threatening crisis and offer support with information about the child's condition. See Chapter 17 🔗.

Blunt Chest Trauma

Blunt chest trauma in children often occurs with other system injuries. Infants and toddlers most often receive blunt chest trauma due to motor vehicle crashes and abuse. School-age children are more commonly injured in incidents related to bicycles, scooters, skateboards, and skates. Adolescents are most often injured in high-energy motor vehicle crashes. Chest injuries may not be obvious and can be extremely difficult to evaluate.

Most children who die after sustaining severe blunt trauma were hypoxic because of poor airway and ventilatory control. A child's elastic, pliable chest wall and thin abdominal muscles provide minimal protection to underlying organs. This elasticity of the ribs often prevents fractures; however, the presence of a rib fracture in a child under age 12 years indicates trauma of significant force. The energy from blunt trauma is transferred directly to the internal organs, often causing a pulmonary contusion or pneumothorax. Children also have a more mobile mediastinum permitting structures in the chest to shift, such as occurs with a tension pneumothorax. See page 797.

Pulmonary Contusion

A pulmonary contusion is the most common reported injury associated with blunt chest trauma. It is defined as bruising damage to the tissues of the lung that often occurs without bony injury to the thorax. The lung tissue bruising causes bleeding from the capillaries into the alveoli, which may lead to capillary rupture in the air sacs. Pulmonary edema develops in the lower airways as blood and fluid from damaged tissues accumulate over a couple of days. Acute respiratory distress syndrome and long-term respiratory dysfunction may result (see page 745).

Initially the child may appear asymptomatic. Respiratory distress, along with fever, wheezing, **hemoptysis** (coughing up blood from the respiratory tract), and crackles, may develop over several hours. Careful observation is required during the first 12 hours after the injury to detect decreased perfusion related to ventilatory impairment.

Pathophysiology Illustrated   Pneumothorax

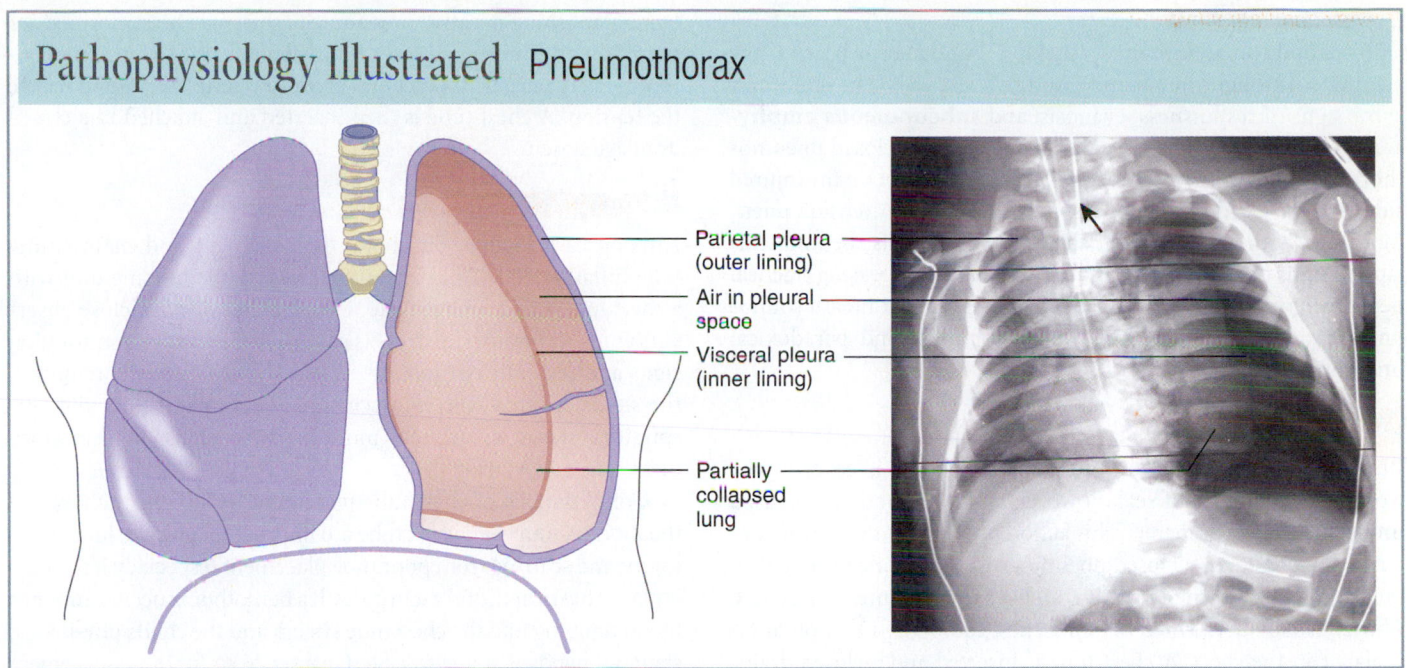

FIGURE 25–21 ■ *A,* A pneumothorax is air in the pleural space that causes a lung to collapse. Whether the air results from an open injury or from bursting of alveoli due to a blunt injury or hyperinflation, it is important to focus on airway management and maintain lung inflation. *B,* Pneumothorax, note the collapsed lung on the patient's left side and mediastinal shift of the trachea and heart toward the right side.

Source: *Courtesy of Dorothy Bulas, M.D., Children's National Medical Center, Washington, DC.*

Chest radiographs or computed tomography are used to diagnose a pulmonary contusion, but it may take several hours for evidence to appear on radiographic images. Therapy includes fluid restriction, supplemental oxygen, pain control, incentive spirometry, and avoiding prolonged immobilization. Children with severe injury to the lungs will require mechanical ventilation with low airway pressures. Pneumonia is a potential complication.

Nursing Management

Nursing centers on providing the necessary physiologic support, such as supplemental oxygen, positioning, incentive spirometry, fluid management, and comfort measures.

Observe for hemoptysis, dyspnea, decreased breath sounds, wheezes, crackles, and transient temperature elevation. The child's level of consciousness is an excellent indicator of respiratory function. Agitation and lethargy can signal increasing hypoxia. The thorax should be inspected for symmetric chest wall movement and equal presence of breath sounds in both lungs. The child may initially appear stable but requires careful and thorough monitoring to detect signs of deterioration. When monitoring the status of a child who has a pulmonary contusion, do not rely on the child's color as an indicator of adequate oxygenation. Cyanosis in children is often a late indicator of respiratory distress.

Children with significant injuries are cared for in the intensive care unit. Some children require ventilator support as the pulmonary tissues heal. Fluids are carefully managed to avoid increasing pulmonary edema. Diuretics may be given to decrease edema in the interstitial pulmonary tissue. Incentive spirometry should be performed while assisting the child to reduce discomfort associated with coughing.

Support the parents who are anxious about the potential life-threatening nature of the child's injury. See Chapter 17 🔗 for suggested support for families and siblings.

Pneumothorax

A **pneumothorax** occurs when air enters the pleural space because of tears in the tracheobronchial tree, the esophagus, or the chest wall. If blood collects in the pleural space, it is called a *hemothorax*. If blood and air collect, it is called a *pneumohemothorax*.

Etiology and Pathophysiology

Pneumothorax may develop as a complication of mechanical ventilation or high peak inspiratory or end-expiratory pressure used to achieve adequate oxygenation and ventilation. It may also occur in chronic lung conditions such as neonatal respiratory distress syndrome, status asthmaticus, and cystic fibrosis in which there is gas trapping and alveolar hyperinflation. A pneumothorax is one of the more common thoracic injuries in pediatric trauma patients.

The three types of pneumothorax are open, closed, and tension.

- An open pneumothorax, sometimes referred to as a sucking chest wound, results from any penetrating injury that exposes the pleural space to atmospheric pressure.
- A closed pneumothorax is sometimes caused by blunt chest trauma with no evidence of rib fracture. The chest may be compressed against a closed glottis (such as may occur with breath holding), causing a sudden increase in pressure within the thoracic cavity. The pressure increase is transferred to the alveoli, causing them to burst. A single burst alveolus may be able to seal itself off, but with the destruction of many alveoli the lung collapses.
- A tension pneumothorax is a life-threatening emergency that results when air leaks into the chest during inspiration but cannot escape during expiration. Internal pressure continues to build, compressing the chest contents and collapsing the lung. Venous blood return to the heart is impaired as the trachea, heart, vena cava, and esophagus are compressed toward the unaffected lung when the mediastinum shifts, leading to decreased cardiac output (Figure 25–21 ■).

Clinical Manifestations

With an open pneumothorax, a sucking sound may be heard as the air moves through the opening on the chest wall. The child may show signs of restlessness, cyanosis, and **subcutaneous emphysema** (air leakage in the tissue). The child with a closed pneumothorax may have breath sounds decreased or absent on the injured side, and the child may be in respiratory distress. A tension pneumothorax with a mediastinal shift may be seen as the lung collapses. Signs of tension pneumothorax include increasing tracheal deviation, respiratory distress, decreased or absent breath sounds on one side, decreased chest wall movement, and paradoxical breathing.

Collaborative Care

Immediate treatment for an open pneumothorax is covering the wound with an airtight seal; however, a gloved hand can be used until a bandage is prepared. This action prevents more air from entering the chest. For a closed pneumothorax, a needle or tube thoracostomy is performed rapidly to relieve the pressure in the chest. This is usually performed before a chest radiograph that often reveals air in the chest. A chest tube is inserted and a closed drainage system is attached to help remove the air and reinflate the lung by reestablishing negative pressure. Surgery may be performed for persistent or recurrent air leaks. Immediate care for a tension pneumothorax is a needle thoracentesis to allow air to escape and relieve the tension. A chest tube is then inserted and attached to a closed drainage system.

Nursing Management

Nursing care focuses on airway management and maintaining lung inflation. The child usually arrives on the nursing unit with a chest tube and drainage system in place. Continued close observation for respiratory distress is essential. Carefully monitor vital signs and respiratory function. When the chest tube is removed, the site is covered with an occlusive dressing and the child's respiratory status is carefully monitored for signs of respiratory distress.

Complications of chest tube placement include hemothorax (if the thoracostomy and chest tube are improperly placed), lung tissue injury, and scarring from poor tube placement (especially if the tube is placed too near the breast in girls). If a hemothorax occurs, monitor blood draining into the chest tube system and the child's physiologic status for hypovolemic shock. See Chapter 26 for the management of a child in hypovolemic shock.

Chapter Highlights

- Respiratory conditions are the most common cause of hospitalization in children between 1 and 9 years of age and a leading cause in children between 10 and 19 years of age.
- The child's airway is shorter and narrower than an adult's. These differences create a greater potential for obstruction. The lungs have no muscles of their own, so respiration is powered by the diaphragm and intercostal muscles.
- Foreign body aspiration is most often caused by small objects that make their way into the child's mouth, such as foods, small toy parts, or household objects like beads, safety pins, coins, or buttons. The increasing mobility and tendency to put small objects in the mouth makes this a major health problem for infants and toddlers.
- Signs of impending respiratory failure in infants and children include worsening respiratory distress, irritability, lethargy, mottled color or cyanosis, diaphoresis, and increased respiratory effort such as dyspnea (difficulty breathing), tachypnea (increased respiratory rate), nasal flaring, grunting, and retractions.
- Apnea is cessation of respiration lasting longer than 20 seconds, or any pause in respiration associated with cyanosis, marked pallor, hypotonia, or bradycardia.
- Three types of apnea are noted in neonates: central apnea, in which there is complete cessation of breathing; obstructive apnea, in which there is an absence of nasal airflow when respiratory efforts are present; and mixed apnea, in which a central respiratory pause either precedes or follows airway obstruction.
- Obstructive sleep apnea syndrome is a disorder of breathing during sleep that in children is commonly caused by enlarged tonsils and adenoids. Children have symptoms of sleep deprivation such as daytime sleepiness, poor attention, increased activity, aggression or acting-out behavior, and poor school performance.

- Sudden infant death syndrome (SIDS) is a leading cause of death in infants. Onset of the fatal episode occurs during sleep and remains unexplained after a thorough investigation, including an autopsy, a review of the circumstances of death, and the clinical history.
- Laryngotracheobronchitis (LTB) is a viral croup syndrome with signs of an upper respiratory illness, hoarseness, tachypnea, inspiratory stridor, and a seal-like barking cough. Fever may or may not be present.
- Epiglottitis is caused by bacterial invasion of the soft tissue of the larynx, causing inflammation and edema of the epiglottis and surrounding tissues that can result in life-threatening airway obstruction. Classic signs of epiglottitis include dysphonia, dysphagia, drooling, and distressed respiratory effort.
- Neonatal respiratory distress syndrome is the most common cause of respiratory distress in preterm infants, and the incidence increases to 60% of all preterm infants with a gestational age of less than 28 weeks.
- A higher risk for meconium aspiration syndrome occurs in neonates of advanced gestational age, greater than 40 weeks. The meconium causes a chemical inflammation of the airway that can lead to pulmonary edema, small airway obstruction, and persistent pulmonary hypertension.
- Respiratory syncytial virus (RSV) is the most common cause of bronchiolitis, a lower respiratory tract illness that occurs when an infecting agent (virus or bacterium) causes inflammation and obstruction of the bronchioles.
- Symptoms of pneumonia in infants and children include elevated temperature, crackles, wheezes, cough, dyspnea, tachypnea, restlessness, and decreased breath sounds if consolidation occurs.

- Children under 2 years have an increased risk of developing tuberculosis, and if untreated have a greater chance of progressing to active TB and spreading beyond the lungs (e.g., meningitis and disseminated TB).
- Asthma is one of the most common chronic respiratory disorders in childhood. The respiratory difficulties of an acute asthma episode result from inflammation that causes the normal protective mechanisms of the lungs (mucous formation, mucosal swelling, and airway muscle contraction) to overreact in response to a stimulus and cause airway obstruction.
- Bronchopulmonary dysplasia (BPD) usually develops in neonates with a birth weight of 1000 g or less and a gestational age at birth of less than 28 weeks who are treated with oxygen and positive-pressure ventilation for respiratory failure or respiratory distress syndrome. Treatment leads to inflammation and damage to the bronchioles, resulting in fibrosis, edema of the bronchioles, and smooth muscle hypertrophy.

- In cystic fibrosis, defective chloride-ion transport across the exocrine and epithelial cell walls results in an abnormal accumulation of viscous, dehydrated mucus that affects the respiratory, gastrointestinal, and reproductive systems.
- Signs of smoke inhalation injury in children include burns of the face and neck, singed nasal hairs, soot around the mouth or nose, and hoarseness with stridor or voice change.
- Pulmonary contusion occurs in association with blunt chest trauma. The energy from the injury often bruises the lung tissue in the absence of rib fractures. Although the child may appear initially asymptomatic, respiratory distress often develops within a few hours.
- A pneumothorax may become life threatening if internal pressure from a closed pneumothorax is not vented. Air leaking into the chest cavity during inspiration cannot escape during expiration, increasing compression. Venous blood return to the heart is impaired as the mediastinum shifts toward the unaffected lung.

Clinical Reasoning in Action

INTRODUCTION

Return to the scenario at the beginning of the chapter. Hannah and her mother are learning more about asthma management during a health center visit with the nurse practitioner. She has no asthma symptoms during today's visit, and has taken all medications prescribed since her recent hospitalization.

DESCRIPTION

Prior to the acute asthma episode that occurred at school, Hannah had used only short-acting beta$_2$-agonists for symptoms, about once a week. During her hospitalization she needed systemic corticosteroids and was sent home with oral corticosteroids that were tapered and discontinued 3 days ago. Because of the severity of her asthma episode, Hannah's daily treatment will be changed from step 1 for intermittent asthma to step 2 for mild persistent asthma.

DISCUSSION

1. Describe the signs and symptoms that would indicate that Hannah's asthma is progressing in severity. Develop an asthma action plan that provides guidance for daily management as well as managing asthma symptoms to avoid an emergency department visit.

2. Identify information about the family's lifestyle and home environment that could be potential triggers for Hannah's asthma.

3. Develop an asthma education plan that corresponds to Hannah's stage of development, and identify appropriate self-care responsibilities to begin teaching her.

4. Describe the essential elements of an individualized health plan for Hannah and the actions that must be taken to have one developed in collaboration with the school nurse.

NCLEX-RN® Review

1. The nurse is caring for an infant who was admitted to the hospital for the treatment of RSV bronchiolitis. What assessment item would the nurse report immediately to the healthcare provider?
   1. Increased temperature
   2. Increased heart rate
   3. Decreased pulse oximeter saturations
   4. Decreased bowel sounds

2. The neonatal nurse is giving discharge instructions to parents of an infant diagnosed with bronchopulmonary dysplasia (BPD). Teaching was ineffective if which statement is made by one of the parents?
   1. "I can expect my baby to require diuretic therapy."
   2. "I can expect my baby to be on oxygen therapy for the rest of his life."
   3. "I can expect my baby to receive respiratory treatments at least once daily."
   4. "I can expect to come to the office monthly during winter months for at least 1 year."

3. An 8-year-old child is diagnosed with viral pneumonia and sent home from the clinic without an antibiotic prescription. The symptoms worsen, and the child returns to the clinic a week later with signs of a higher fever, listlessness, and a harsh, productive cough. The child's mother states, "I knew a prescription for antibiotics was needed." Which indicates the nurse's most appropriate response?
   1. "It is better to wait to make sure so we don't use antibiotics unnecessarily. This approach also saves healthcare dollars."
   2. "Sometimes we just do not know. I'm glad you came back in."
   3. "You do not want to expose your child to medication unnecessarily. Now it is necessary, because it is bacterial pneumonia."
   4. "Antibiotics are not effective for viral pneumonia. Bacteria can grow later in the duration of the illness, making antibiotics necessary later."

4. The nurse is caring for a pediatric patient who may be experiencing obstructive sleep apnea syndrome. What questions are appropriate to include in the history assessment for this child? (Select all that apply)
   1. "Does your child sleep on his/her back?"
   2. "Does your child complain of evening headaches?"
   3. "Does your child have any signs of hyperactivity?"
   4. "Does your child have difficulty with schoolwork?"
   5. "Does your child wet the bed?"

See Appendix I 🖉 for answers.

References

Adams, S. M., Good, M. W., & Defranco, G. M. (2009). Sudden infant death syndrome. *American Family Physician, 79*(10), 870–874.

Ajao, T. I., Oden, R. P., Joyner, B. L., & Moon, R. Y. (2011). Decisions of black parents about infant bedding and sleep surfaces: A qualitative study. *Pediatrics, 128*(3), 494–502.

Akinbami, L. J., Moorman, J. E., & Liu, X. (2011, January 12). Asthma prevalence, health care use, and mortality: United States, 2005–2009. *National Health Statistics Reports, 32*, 1–16.

Allergy and Asthma Network. (2010). *Medications at school.* Retrieved from http://aanma.org/advocacy/meds-at-school/

Al-Saif, S., Alvard, R., Manfreda, J., Kwatkowsky, K., Cates, D., Qurashi, M., & Rigato, H. (2008). A randomized controlled trial of theophylline versus CO_2 inhalation for treating apnea of prematurity. *Journal of Pediatrics, 153*(4), 513–518.

Alverson, B., & Ralston, S. L. (2011). Management of bronchiolitis: Focus on hypertonic saline. *Contemporary Pediatrics, 28*(2), 30–38.

American Academy of Allergy, Asthma, and Immunology (AAAAI). (2013). *What is a peak flow meter?* Retrieved from http://www.aaaai.org/

American Academy of Pediatrics (AAP). (2012). *Red book: 2012 Report of the Committee on Infectious Diseases* (29th ed.). Elk Grove Village, IL: Author.

American Academy of Pediatrics (AAP) Committee on Infectious Disease. (2009). Policy statement—Modified recommendations for use of palivizumab for prevention of respiratory syncytial virus infections.

Amirav, I. (2010). To inhale or not to inhale: Is that the question? A simple method of DPI instruction. *Journal of Pediatrics, 156*(2), 339–339e1.

Antoon, A. Y., & Donovan, M. K. (2007). Burn injuries. In R. M. Kliegman, R. E. Behrman, H. B. Jenson, & B. F. Stanton, *Nelson textbook of pediatrics* (18th ed., pp. 450–458). Philadelphia, PA: Elsevier Saunders.

Askin, D. F., & Diehl-Jones, W. (2009). Pathogenesis and prevention of chronic lung disease in the neonate. *Critical Care Nursing Clinics of North America, 21*, 11–25.

Asthma Initiative of Michigan for Healthy Lungs. (2011). *How to use a metered-dose inhaler the right way.* Retrieved from http://www.getasthmahelp.org/inhalers_main.asp

Ayad, O., Dietrich, A., & Mihalov, L. (2008). Extracorporeal membrane oxygenation. *Emergency Medical Clinics of North America, 26*, 953–959.

Baker, L. K., & Denyes, M. J. (2008). Predictors of self-care in adolescents with cystic fibrosis: A test of Orem's theories of self-care and self-care deficit. *Journal of Pediatric Nursing, 23*(1), 37–48.

Banasiak, N. C. (2007). Childhood asthma: Part two: Management update. *Journal of Pediatric Health Care, 21*(3), 184–191.

Baraldi, E., & Filippone, M. (2007). Chronic lung disease after premature birth. *New England Journal of Medicine, 357*(19), 1946–1955.

Baum, C. R. (2008). What's new in pediatric carbon monoxide poisoning? *Clinical Pediatric Emergency Medicine, 9*, 43–46.

Behm, I., Kabir, Z., Connolly, G. N., & Alpert, H. R. (2012). Increasing prevalence of smoke-free homes and decreasing rates of sudden infant death syndrome in the United States: An ecological association study. *Tobacco Control, 21*, 6–11.

Bonkowsky, J. L., & Tieder, J. S. (2009). A pragmatic approach to ALTEs. *Contemporary Pediatrics, 26*(11), 54–63.

Brashers, V. L. (2010a). Alterations in pulmonary function. In K. L. McCance, S. E. Huether, V. L. Brashers, & N. S. Rote, *Pathophysiology: The biologic basis for disease in adults and children* (6th ed., pp. 1266–1309). St. Louis, MO: Mosby Elsevier.

Brashers, V. L. (2010b). Structure and function of the pulmonary system. In K. L. McCance, S. E. Huether, V. L. Brashers, & N. R. Rote, *Pathophysiology: The biologic basis for disease in adults and children* (6th ed., pp. 1242–1265). St. Louis, MO: Mosby Elsevier.

Busse, W. W., Morgan, W. J., Gergen, P. J., Mitchell, H. E., Gern, J. E., Liu, A. H., . . . Sorkness, C. A. (2011). Randomized trial of omalizumab (Anti-IgE) for asthma in inner-city children. *New England Journal of Medicine, 364*(11), 1005–1015.

Callahan, K. A., Panter, T. M., Hall, T. M., & Slemmons, M. (2010). Peak flow monitoring in pediatric asthma management: A clinical practice column submission. *Journal of Pediatric Nursing, 25*, 12–17.

Camargo, C. A., Rachelefsky, G., & Schatz, M. (2009). Managing asthma exacerbations in the emergency department: Summary of the National Asthma Education and Prevention Program Expert Panel Report 3: Guidelines for the management of asthma exacerbations. *Journal of Allergy and Clinical Immunology, 124*, S5–S14.

Carbajal, R., Biran, V., Lenclen, R., Epaud, R., Cimerman, P., Thibault, P., . . . Fauroux, B. (2008). EMLA cream and nitrous oxide to alleviate pain induced by palivizumab (Synagis) intramuscular injections in infants and young children. *Pediatrics, 121*(6), e1591–e1598.

Carrier, C. T. (2009). Back to sleep: A culture change to improve practice. *Newborn & Infant Nursing Reviews, 9*(3), 163–168.

Centers for Disease Control and Prevention (CDC). (2008). *Initiating change: Creating an asthma-friendly school.* Retrieved from http://www.cdc.gov/HealthyYouth/asthma/creatingafs/index.htm

Centers for Disease Control and Prevention (CDC). (2011a). Trends in tuberculosis—United States, 2010. *Morbidity and Mortality Weekly Report, 60*(11), 333–337.

Centers for Disease Control and Prevention (CDC). (2011b). Vital signs: Asthma prevalence, disease characteristics, and self-management education—United States, 2001–2009. *Morbidity and Mortality Weekly Report, 60*(17), 547–552.

Chipps, B., Zeiger, R. S., Murphy, K., Mellon, M., Schatz, M., Kosinski, M., . . . Ramachandran, S. (2011). Longitudinal validation of the Test for Respiratory Asthma Control in Kids in pediatric practices. *Pediatrics, 127*(3), e737–e747.

Clark, A. P., Giuliano, K., & Chen, H. (2006). Pulse oximetry revisited: "But his O_2 was normal!" *Clinical Nurse Specialist, 20*(6), 268–272.

Coffman, S. (2009). Late preterm infants and risk for RSV. *Maternal and Child Nursing, 34*(6), 378–384.

Coleman-Phox, K., Odouli, R., & De-Jun, L. (2008). Use of a fan during sleep and risk of sudden infant death syndrome. *Archives of Pediatrics and Adolescent Medicine, 162*(10), 963–968.

Cruz, A. T., & Starke, J. R. (2010). Pediatric tuberculosis. *Pediatrics in Review, 31*(1), 13–25.

Cuff, S., & Loud, K. (2008). Exercise-induced bronchospasm. *Contemporary Pediatrics, 25*(9), 88–95.

Cystic Fibrosis Foundation. (2011a). *About cystic fibrosis: What you need to know.* Retrieved from http://www.cff.org/AboutCF/

Cystic Fibrosis Foundation. (2011b). *About cystic fibrosis: Frequently asked questions.* Retrieved from http://www.cff.org/AboutCF/Faqs/

Cystic Fibrosis Foundation. (2011c). *Screening for cystic fibrosis.* Retrieved from http://www.cff.org/AboutCF/Testing/NewbornScreening/ScreeningforCF/

Cystic Fibrosis Foundation. (2011d). *Airway clearance techniques.* Retrieved from http://www.cff.org/treatments/Therapies/Respiratory/AirwayClearance/

D'Agustino, J. (2010). Pediatric airway nightmares. *Emergency Medical Clinics of North America, 28*, 119–126.

Davis, P. G., Schmidt, B., Roberts, R. S., Doyle, L. W., Asztalos, E., Haslam, R., . . . Tin, W. (2010). Caffeine for apnea of prematurity trial: Benefits may vary in subgroups. *Journal of Pediatrics, 156*(3), 382–387.

Dukhovny, D., Lorch, S. A., Schmidt, B., Doyle, L. W., Kok, J. H., Roberts, R. S., . . . Zupancic, J. A. F. (2011). Economic evaluation of caffeine for apnea of prematurity. *Pediatrics, 127*(1), e146–e155.

Duncan, J. R., Paterson, D. S., Hoffman, J. M., Mokler, D. J., Borenstein, N. S., Belliveau, R. A., . . . Kinney, H. C. (2010). Brainstem serotonergic deficiency in sudden infant death syndrome. *Journal of the American Medical Association, 303*(5), 430–437.

Durbin, W. J., & Stille, C. (2008). Pneumonia. *Pediatrics in Review, 29*(5), 147–158.

Everard, M. L. (2006). Aerosol delivery to children. *Pediatric Annals, 35*(9), 630–636.

Fakhoury, K. F., Sellers, C., Smith, E. O., Rama, J. A., & Fan, L. L. (2010). Serial measurements of lung function in a cohort of young children with bronchopulmonary dysplasia. *Pediatrics, 125*(6), e1441–e1447.

Flume, P. A., O'Sullivan, B. P., Robinson, K. A., Goss, C. H., Mogayzel, P. J., Willey-Courand, D. B., . . . Cystic Fibrosis Foundation, Pulmonary Therapies Committee (2007). Cystic fibrosis pulmonary guidelines: Chronic medications for maintenance of lung health. *American Journal of Respiratory and Critical Care Medicine, 176*, 957–969.

Fong, E. W., & Levin, R. H. (2007). Inhaled corticosteroids for asthma. *Pediatrics in Review, 28*(6), e30–e35.

Fu, L. Y., Colson, E. R., Corwin, M. J., & Moon, R. Y. (2008). Infant sleep location: Associated maternal and infant characteristics with sudden infant death syndrome prevention recommendations. *Journal of Pediatrics, 153*(4), 503–508.

Geary, C., Caskey, M., Fonseca, R., & Malloy, M. (2008). Decreased incidence of bronchopulmonary dysplasia after early management changes, including surfactant and nasal continuous positive airway pressure treatment at delivery, lowered oxygen saturation goals, and early amino acid administration: A historical cohort study. *Pediatrics, 121*(1), 89–96.

Gott, K., & Froh, D. L. (2010). Alterations in pulmonary function in children. In K. L. McCance, S. E. Huether, V. L. Brashers, & N. R. Rote (Eds.), *Pathophysiology: The biologic basis for disease in adults and children* (6th ed., pp. 1310–1343). St. Louis, MO: Mosby Elsevier.

Hazle, L. A. (2010). Cystic fibrosis. In P. J. Allen, J. A. Vessey, & N. A. Shapiro, *Primary care of the child with a chronic condition* (5th ed., pp. 405–426). St. Louis, MO: Mosby Elsevier.

Hines, A. B. (2011). Asthma: A health disparity among African American children: The impact and implications for pediatric nurses. *Journal of Pediatric Nursing, 26*(1), 25–33.

Kelly, M. M. (2010). Prematurity. In P. J. Allen, J. A. Vessey, & N. A. Shapiro, *Primary care of the child with a chronic condition* (5th ed., pp. 756–771). St. Louis, MO: Mosby Elsevier.

Kinney, H. C., & Thach, B. T. (2009). The sudden infant death syndrome. *New England Journal of Medicine, 361*(8), 795–805.

Kochanek, K. D., Xu, J., Murphy, S. L., & Kung, H. (2011). Deaths: Final data for 2009, *National Vital Statistics Reports, 60*(3), 1–116.

Kronman, M. P., & Shah, S. S. (2009). Pediatric community-acquired pneumonia. *Contemporary Pediatrics, 26*(9), 40–43.

Levin, R. A., & Smith, G. A. (2010). Choking prevention among young children. *Pediatric Annals, 39*(11), 721–724.

Loghmanee, D. A., & Sheldon, S. H. (2010). Pediatric obstructive sleep apnea: An update. *Pediatric Annals, 39*(12), 784–789.

Lomas, P. H., & Fowler, S. B. (2010). Parents and children with cystic fibrosis: A family affair. *American Journal of Nursing, 110*(8), 30–37.

Maitra, A. (2010). Diseases of infancy and childhood. In V. Kumar, A. K. Abbas, N. Fausto, & J. C. Aster, *Pathologic basis of disease* (8th ed., pp. 456–481). Philadelphia, PA: Saunders Elsevier.

Marais, B. J., & Schaaf, H. S. (2010). Childhood tuberculosis: An emerging and previously neglected problem. *Infectious Disease Clinics of North America, 24*, 727–749.

Marc, D., Berg, M. D., Nadkarni, V. M., Gausche-Hill, M., Kaji, A. H., & Berg, R. A. (2010). Apparent life threatening events. In J. A. Marx, R. S. Hockberger, R. M. Walls, J. G. Adams, W. G. Barsen, . . . E. J. Newton, *Rosen's emergency medicine* (7th ed., pp. 73–76). Philadelphia: Elsevier Mosby.

McGinley, B., Halbower, A., Schwartz, A. R., Smith, P. L., Patil, S. P., & Schneider, H. (2009). Effect of a high-flow open nasal cannula system on obstructive sleep apnea in children. *Pediatrics, 124*(1), 179–188.

Menzies, H. J., Winston, C. A., Holtz, T. H., Cain, K. P., & MacKenzie, W. R. (2010). Epidemiology of tuberculosis among US- and foreign-born children and adolescents in the United States, 1994–2007. *American Journal of Public Health, 100*(9), 1724–1729.

Miller, S. (2010). A community health concern: Respiratory syncytial virus and children. *Journal of Pediatric Nursing, 25*, 551–554.

Mininni, N. C., Herzer, T. D., Marino, M. L., & Kohler, W. (2009). Why continuous pulse oximetry is a must in critical care. *American Nurse Today, 4*(9), 34–36.

Montgomery, G. S., & Howenstine, M. (2009). Cystic fibrosis. *Pediatrics in Review, 30*(8), 302–309.

Moon, R. Y., Oden, R. P., Joyner, B. L., & Ajao, T. (2010). Qualitative analysis of beliefs and perceptions about sudden infant death syndrome in African-American mothers: Implications for safe sleep practices. *Journal of Pediatrics, 157*(1), 92–97.

Moran, A., Becker, D., Casella, S. J., Gottlieb, P. A., Kirkman, M. S., Marshall, B. C., . . . CFRD Consensus Conference Committee. (2010). Epidemiology, pathophysiology, and prognostic implications of cystic fibrosis-related diabetes. *Diabetes Care, 33*(12), 2677–2683.

Nash, P., & Smith, J. R. (2008). Common neonatal complications. In K. R. Simpson & P. A. Creehan, *AWHONN's perinatal nursing* (3rd ed., pp 612–646). Philadelphia, PA: Lippincott, Williams & Wilkins.

National Asthma Education and Prevention Program. (2007). *Expert panel report 3: Guidelines for the diagnosis and management of asthma*. Bethesda, MD: National Institutes of Health, National Heart Lung and Blood Institute. Retrieved from http://www.nhlbi.nih.gov/guidelines/asthma/index.htm

Newton, S. M., Brent, A. J., Anderson, S., Whittaker, E., & Kampmann, B. (2008). Pediatric tuberculosis. *Lancet Infectious Diseases, 8*(8), 498–510.

Oden, R. P., Joyner, B. L., Ajao, T. I., & Moon, R. Y. (2010). Factors influencing African American mothers' decisions about sleep position: A qualitative study. *Journal of the National Medical Association, 102*(10), 870–880.

O'Sullivan, B. P., & Freedman, S. D. (2009, May 30). Cystic fibrosis. *Lancet, 373*, 1891–1904.

Peeke, K., Hershberger, M., & Marriner, J. (2006). Obstructive sleep apnea syndrome in children. *Pediatric Nursing, 32*(5), 489–494.

Peredo-Pinto, H., & Jacobs, N. M. (2008). A 17-month infant with a calf lesion and generalized hypotonia. *Pediatric Annals, 37*(2), 96–98.

Perez, I. A., & Ward, S. L. D. (2008). The snoring child. *Pediatric Annals, 37*(7), 465–470.

Peterson-Sweeney, K., Halterman, J. S., Conn, K., & Yoos, H. L. (2010). The effect of family routines on care for inner city children with asthma. *Journal of Pediatric Nursing, 25*, 344–351.

Phung, O. J., Coleman, C. I., Baker, E. L., Scholle, J. M., Girotto, J. E., Makanji, S. S., . . . White, C. M. (2010). Recombinant human growth hormone in the treatment of patients with cystic fibrosis. *Pediatrics, 126*(5), e1211–e1226.

Pitts, J., Flack, J., & Goodfellow, J. (2008). Improving nutrition in the cystic fibrosis patient. *Journal of Pediatric Health Care, 22*(2), 137–140.

Prodhan, P., Sharoor-Karni, S., Lin, J., & Noviski, N. (2011). Predictors of respiratory failure among previously healthy children with respiratory syncytial virus infection. *American Journal of Emergency Medicine, 29*, 168–173.

Pryor, J. A., Tannenbaum, E., Scott, S. F., Burgess, J., Cramer, D., Gyi, K., & Hodson, M. E. (2010). Beyond postural drainage and percussion: Airway clearance in people with cystic fibrosis. *Journal of Cystic Fibrosis, 9*, 187–192.

Rance, K., & O'Laughlen, M. (2011). Obesity and asthma: A dangerous link in children. *Journal for Nurse Practitioners, 7*(4), 287–292.

Ranganathan, S. C., & Sonnappa, S. (2009). Pneumonia and other respiratory infections. *Pediatric Clinics of North America, 56*, 135–156.

Rhee, H., Belyea, M. J., & Brasch, J. (2010). Family support and asthma outcomes in adolescents: Barriers to adherence as a mediator. *Journal of Adolescent Health, 47*, 472–478.

Robinson, P. D., & Van Asperen, P. (2009). Asthma in childhood. *Pediatric Clinics of North America, 56*, 191–226.

Rock, M. J., & Sharp, J. K. (2010). Cystic fibrosis and CRMS screening: What the primary care pediatrician should know. *Pediatric Annals, 39*(12), 759–768.

Roosevelt, G. E. (2007). Acute inflammatory upper airway obstruction (croup, epiglottitis, laryngitis, and bacterial tracheitis). In R. M. Kliegman, R. E. Behrman, H. B. Jenson, & B. F. Stanton, *Nelson textbook of pediatrics* (18th ed., pp. 1762–1767). Philadelphia, PA: Elsevier Saunders.

Rosen, D. (2010). Obstructive sleep apnea in children: Accurate diagnosis, effective treatment. *Consultant for Pediatricians, 9*(4), 128–133.

Schmidt, B., Anderson, P. J., Doyle, L. W., Dewey, D., Gruneau, R. E., Asztalos, E. V., . . . Caffeine for Apnea of Prematurity (CAP) Trial Investigators. (2012). Survival without disability to age 5 years after neonatal caffeine therapy for apnea of prematurity. *Journal of the American Medical Association, 307*(3), 275–282.

Selden, J. A., & Scarfone, R. J. (2009). Bronchiolitis: An evidence-based approach to management. *Clinical Pediatric Emergency Medicine, 10*, 75–81.

Shaefer, S. J. M., Herman, S. E., Frank, S. J., Adkins, M., & Terhaar, M. (2010). Translating infant safe sleep evidence into nursing practice. *Journal of Obstetric, Gynecologic, and Neonatal Nursing, 39*(6), 618–626.

Silvestri, J. M. (2008). Apparent life-threatening events in the young infant and neonate. *Clinical Pediatric Emergency Medicine, 9*, 184–190.

Silvestri, J. M. (2009). Indications for home apnea monitoring (or not). *Clinical Perinatology, 26*, 87–99.

Singh, B. S., Clark, R. H., Powers, R. J., & Spitzer, A. R. (2009). Meconium aspiration syndrome remains a significant problem in the NICU: Outcomes and treatment patterns in term neonates admitted for intensive care during a 10 year period. *Journal of Perinatology, 29*, 497–503.

Sleath, B., Ayala, G. X., Gillette, C., Williams, D., Davis, S., Tudor, G., . . . Washington, D. (2011). Provider demonstration and assessment of child device technique during pediatric asthma visits. *Pediatrics, 127*(4), 642–648.

Smith, L. J., McKay, K. O., van Asperen, P. P., Selvadurai, H., & Fitzgerald, D. A. (2010). Normal development of the lung and premature birth. *Paediatric Respiratory Reviews, 11*(3), 135–142.

Sobol, S. E., & Zapata, S. (2008). Epiglottitis and croup. *Otolaryngology Clinics of North America, 41*, 551–566.

Sorce, L. R. (2009). Respiratory syncytial virus: From primary care to critical care. *Journal of Pediatric Healthcare, 23*(2), 101–108.

Srivastava, G. (2010). Airway foreign bodies in children. *Clinical Pediatric Emergency Medicine, 11*(2), 67–72.

Stallings, V. A., Stark, L. J., Robinson, K. A., Feranchack, A. P., Quinton, H., & Clinical Practice Guidelines for Growth and Nutrition Subcommittee: Ad Hoc Working Group. (2008). Evidence-based practice recommendations for nutrition-related management of children and adults with cystic fibrosis and pancreatic insufficiency: Report of a systematic review. *Journal of the American Dietetic Association, 108*(5), 832–839.

Stewart, L. J. (2008). Pediatric asthma. *Primary Care: Clinics in Office Practice, 35*, 25–40.

Stroustrup, A., & Trasande, L. (2010). Epidemiologic characteristics and resource use in neonates with bronchopulmonary dysplasia: 1993–2006. *Pediatrics, 126*(2), e291–e287.

Todd, F. E., Roberg, K. A., & Welliver, R. C. (2010, November). Preventing RSV infection in at-risk infants: Current and emerging strategies. *Journal of Pediatric Nursing, 25*(Suppl. 5), 1–16.

Trachtengerg, F. L., Haas, E. A., Kinney, H. C., Stanley, C., Krous, H. F. (2012). Risk factor changes for sudden infant death syndrome after initiation of the back to sleep campaign, *Pediatrics, 129*(4), 630-638.

U.S. Food and Drug Administration. (2010). *FDA Drug Safety Communication: New safety requirements for long-acting inhaled asthma medications called long-acting beta-agonists (LABAs)*. Retrieved from http://www.fda.gov/Drugs/DrugSafety/PostmarketDrugSafetyInformationforPatientsandProviders/ucm200776.htm

Vanhoose, K. J., & Wood, A. F. (2009). Current insight into childhood asthma: Implications for practice. *American Journal for Nurse Practitioners, 13*(9), 10–18, 42.

Virchow, J. C. (2005), What plays a role in the choice of inhaler device for asthma therapy, *Current Medical Research and Opinion,* 21(Suppl. 4), S19–S25.

Wald, E. L. (2010). Croup: Common syndromes and therapy. *Pediatric Annals, 39*(1), 15–21.

Watts, K. D., & Schechter, M. S. (2010). Origins of outcome disparities in pediatric respiratory disease. *Pediatric Annals, 39*(12), 793–798.

Weisgerber, M. (2008). Moderate and vigorous exercise programs in children with asthma: Safety, parental satisfaction, and asthma outcomes. *Pediatric Pulmonology, 43*(12), 1175–1182.

Wiehe, M., & Arndt, K. (2010). Cystic fibrosis: A systems review. *AANA Journal, 78*(3), 246–251.

Williams, D. M. (2009). Management of pediatric asthma: Focus on the Expert Panel Report 3. *Journal of Pediatric Health Care, 23*(6), 357–368.

Wilson, B. A., Shannon, M. T., & Shields, K. M. (2011). *Nurse's drug guide 2011.* Upper Saddle River, NJ: Pearson.

Wiswell, T. E. (2008). Delivery room management of the meconium-stained newborn. *Journal of Perinatology, 28,* S19–S26.

Wong, F. Y., Witcombe, N. B., Yiallourou, S. R., Yorkston, S., Dymowski, A. R., Krishnan, L., . . . Horne, R. S. C. (2011). Cerebral oxygenation is depressed during sleep in healthy term infants when they sleep prone. *Pediatrics, 127*(3), e558–e565.

Wu, A. C., Smith, L., Bokhour, B., Hohman, K. H., & Lieu, T. A. (2008). Racial/ethnic variation in parent perceptions of asthma. *Ambulatory Pediatrics, 8*(2), 89–97.

Yu, H., Wier, L. M., & Elixhauser, A. (2011). *Hospital stays for children, 2009.* HCUP Statistical Brief #118. Rockville, MD: Agency for Healthcare Research and Quality. Retrieved from http://www.hcup-us.ahrq.gov/reports/statbriefs/sb118.pdf

Zagaria, M. A. E. (2010). Inhalant agents for asthma, bronchospasm, and COPD: Focus on delivery devices and inhalation technique. *American Journal for Nurse Practitioners, 14*(3), 21–25.

Zorc, J. J., & Phelan, K. J. (2008). An update on the AAP's bronchiolitis guidelines and the latest evidence on assessment and treatment. *Contemporary Pediatrics, 25*(2), 55–62.

Pearson Nursing Student Resources
Find additional review materials at
nursing.pearsonhighered.com
Prepare for success with additional NCLEX®-style practice questions, interactive assignments and activities, web links, animations and videos, and more!

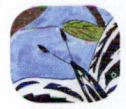 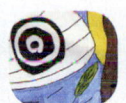 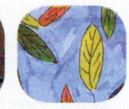

Alterations in Cardiovascular Function

KEY TERMS

Learning Outcomes

After completing this chapter, you will be able to:

1. Explain the transition from fetal to pulmonary circulation.

2. Describe the anatomy and physiology of the cardiovascular system, focusing on the flow of blood and action of the heart valves.

3. Contrast the pathophysiology associated with congenital heart defects having increased pulmonary circulation, decreased pulmonary circulation, and obstructed systemic blood flow.

4. Create a nursing care plan for the child with a congenital heart defect cared for at home prior to corrective surgery.

5. Plan the nursing care for the child undergoing open heart surgery.

6. Recognize the signs and symptoms of congestive heart failure in an infant and child.

7. Differentiate between heart diseases that are acquired during childhood and congenital heart defects.

8. Distinguish between the pathophysiology of hypovolemic shock, distributive shock, and cardiogenic shock.

> "I've already given up so much because of my heart condition, like swimming and biking with my friends. Depending on a pacemaker to make my heart work better is hard to get used to. I wonder what will happen next."
>
> —*Tim, age 16*

Tim Howard, who is 16 years old, was diagnosed with tetralogy of Fallot at birth. He had a surgical repair for this defect as an infant. His parents were anxious when he was born and throughout his early childhood because of their concern about his heart defect and the possible disabilities that he might have. Other than the usual childhood illnesses, Tim grew and developed as expected during childhood. His parents were careful to make sure he had regular health promotion care. Until the revised American Heart Association guidelines were released, he always received antibiotic prophylaxis for infective endocarditis before dental care. His parents tried to follow the pediatrician's advice to treat him as a normal child.

One year ago, Tim felt dizzy and tired more quickly with exercise and activity, indicating the potential development of a rhythm disturbance. After a comprehensive cardiac evaluation, Tim was found to have an episodic slow ventricular heart rate. A pacemaker was determined to be his best treatment option. Tim's exercise limitations are no strenuous activities, competitive sports, or biking, which had been a favorite activity. He is now seen every 6 months in the pediatric cardiac clinic to monitor for further changes in his condition.

Tim, a junior in high school, is trying to figure out these new limitations on his life and how they will affect his relationships with friends. He has average grades in school, and he has no idea if his heart condition will be a problem as he begins to think about future jobs. He has lots of friends, but wonders if he will keep them with his new activity limitations. His parents have always made the decisions about his visits and treatment. What other information does Tim need as he prepares for his future? What types of school activities could Tim be involved in with his friends? What kinds of jobs should Tim consider?

Alterations in cardiovascular function may be the result of a congenital defect, acquired infection, or injury. Congenital heart disease occurs in approximately 1% of all live births, but it is the leading cause of death related to a birth defect during the first year of life; 70% of these deaths occur in the first 28 days of life (Petrini, Broussard, Gilboa, et al., 2010). It is estimated that about one third of children born with congenital heart disease die as a result of their cardiac disease, and about a third of those deaths occur in the first year of life (McDaniel, 2010). Nearly 1 million adults with congenital heart defects are living today in the United States (Sable, Foster, Uzark, et al., 2011). Improved survival is attributed to diagnostic advances, surgical technique refinement, and intensive care. Because children are having surgery at younger ages, nursing care required to identify and manage responses of infants and children with heart disease has become more challenging.

ANATOMY AND PHYSIOLOGY

The heart is divided into four chambers: two atria and two ventricles. Atrioventricular valves (tricuspid and mitral) separate the atria from the ventricles. They open and close to control the flow of blood to the ventricles. The semilunar valves (pulmonary and aortic) open when the ventricles pump blood and close to prevent the backflow of blood to the ventricles. The great arteries (aorta and pulmonary artery) carry blood away from the heart to either the body or the lungs. Pulmonary veins and the superior and inferior vena cavae return blood to the heart. See Figure 26–1 ■ for the anatomy of the heart.

The heart is the pump that circulates the blood through the systemic and pulmonary systems. Blood flows to the lungs for oxygen and carbon dioxide exchange. The oxygen-saturated blood then returns to the heart to be pumped out to the systemic circulation to oxygenate the tissues. Figure 26–1 illustrates the oxygen saturation of blood in each heart chamber and pressures generated by each chamber. See Table 26–1 for **hemodynamics** (passage of blood through the heart and pulmonary system and pressures generated by blood against the chamber walls) of the normal heart. The heart's electrical conduction system controls the rhythmic pumping (Figure 26–2 ■).

TABLE 26–1	Hemodynamics of the Normal Heart	
ACTION	**RIGHT SIDE OF HEART**	**LEFT SIDE OF HEART**
Blood return to heart	Systemic circulation by way of the superior and inferior vena cavae.	Lungs by way of the left and right pulmonary veins.
Diastolic phase	Pulmonary valve closes and tricuspid valve opens.	Aortic valve closes and mitral valve opens.
	Blood flows from the vena cavae through the right atrium and tricuspid valve into the right ventricle.	Blood flows from the pulmonary veins through the left atrium and mitral valve into the left ventricle.
Systolic phase	Tricuspid valve closes and pulmonary valve opens.	Mitral valve closes and aortic valve opens.
	Blood is pumped from the right ventricle into the pulmonary artery and passes into the right and left pulmonary arteries and lungs.	Blood is pumped from the left ventricle into the aorta where it enters the systemic circulation.

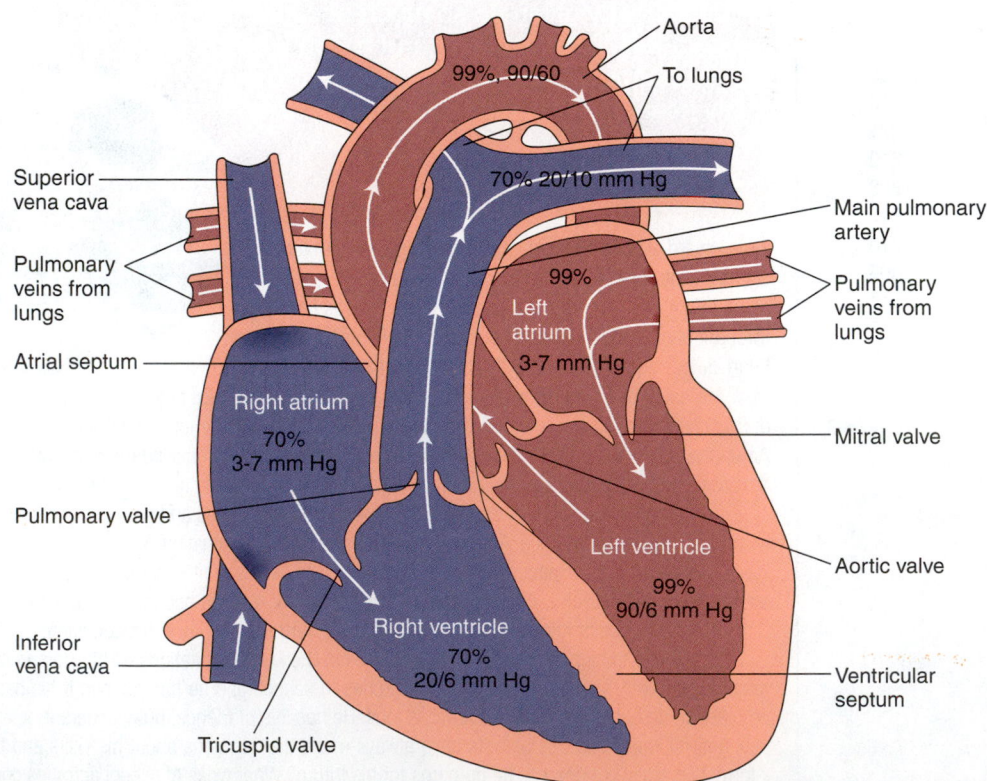

FIGURE 26–1 ■ Anatomy of the heart, direction of blood flow, and normal pressure gradients and oxygen saturation levels in the heart chambers and great arteries. The right ventricle has a lower pressure during systole than the left ventricle because less pressure is needed to pump blood to the lungs through the rest of the body.

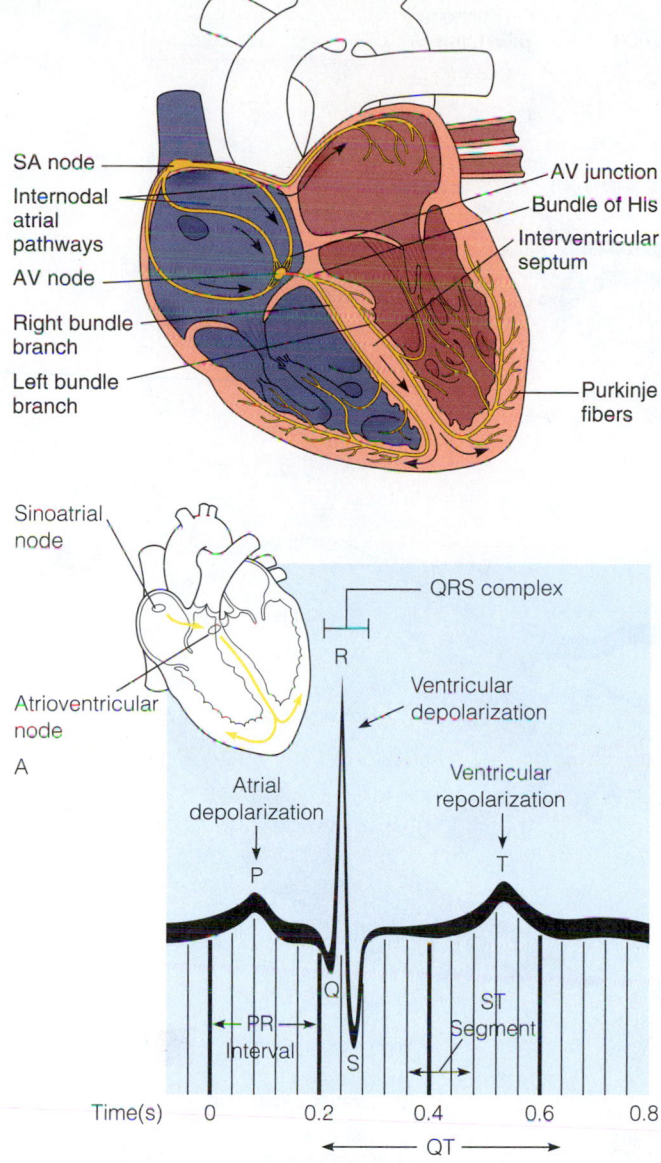

FIGURE 26–2 ■ *A*, Electrical conduction system of the heart. Depolarization normally follows a sequence that begins in the sinoatrial (SA) node and travels through the atrial muscle to the atrioventricular (AV) junction, and then through the AV node to the ventricular muscles. The pathway in the ventricles begins in the bundle of His and divides into the right and left bundle branches. The pathway terminates in the Purkinje system so that the impulse spreads across the myocardium. *B*, Normal electrocardiogram pattern.

P wave—atrial depolarization

P-R interval—time from the beginning of atrial depolarization to the beginning of ventricular depolarization

QRS complex—ventricular depolarization

T wave—ventricular repolarization

ST segment—period between ventricular depolarization and repolarization

PEDIATRIC DIFFERENCES

Fetal Circulation

Blood flows from the placenta to the fetus through the umbilical vein. Blood flow through the **ductus venosus** (the fetal vascular channel between the umbilical vein and the inferior vena cava) permits the blood to enter the right atrium of the heart. The **foramen ovale,**

an opening between the atria in the fetal heart, allows blood to flow from the right to the left atrium, and then into the left ventricle. Blood is then pumped into the aorta and the systemic circulation. Some blood returns from the head and upper extremities to the superior vena cava and right atrium. It flows to the right ventricle where it is pumped to the pulmonary artery. The majority of the blood passes through the **ductus arteriosus,** the fetal vascular channel between the pulmonary artery and the descending aorta, to enter the systemic circulation. A small amount of the blood from the pulmonary artery goes to the fetal lungs. Blood eventually returns to the placenta by way of the umbilical arteries. See Figure 26–3 ■ .

During fetal circulation, the blood with the highest oxygen content goes to the heart and the brain. The constricted pulmonary vessels limit blood flow to the lungs (high pulmonary vascular resistance). Blood, however, flows easily to the extremities because systemic vascular resistance is low. After the umbilical cord has been cut, the newborn must quickly adapt to receiving oxygen from the lungs.

Transition from Fetal to Pulmonary Circulation

The transition from fetal to pulmonary circulation occurs within just a few hours after birth. The first breath expands the lungs, and blood that previously passed through the ductus arteriosus begins flowing to the lungs. Increased pulmonary blood flow and decreased pulmonary vascular resistance results. Pressure in the left atrium increases as increased blood flow is returned from the lungs through the pulmonary veins.

Systemic vascular resistance (the force or resistance of the blood in the body's blood vessels that helps return blood to the heart) increases and right atrial pressure falls after the umbilical cord is cut. Increased pressure in the left atrium stimulates closure of the foramen ovale. The flaps of the foramen ovale close and fibrin deposits permanently seal the opening unless there is excess pressure on the right side of the heart. Table 26–2 provides a comparison of fetal and neonatal circulation, and Figure 26–4 ■ illustrates the differences. The ductus arteriosus, responding to higher oxygen saturation, normally constricts and closes within 10 to 15 hours after birth. Permanent closure usually occurs by 10 to 21 days after birth. If the infant's oxygen saturation remains low, the ductus arteriosus closure may be delayed or prevented. Fetal tissues are accustomed to low oxygen saturation. This may explain why newborns with cyanotic heart disease appear relatively comfortable when their arterial partial pressure of oxygen (PaO$_2$) is very low.

Heart Hemodynamics

Once the transition to extrauterine life is complete, the blood travels through the heart and lungs with each side of the heart working in parallel. Review the normal heart hemodynamics to understand the pathophysiology of various heart conditions. See Figure 26–1.

Cardiovascular Changes as the Child Grows

The infant's cardiovascular system is proportionately larger in relation to body size than an adult's. The right ventricle is larger than the left at birth because the high pulmonary resistance during fetal life forced the right ventricle to be as muscular and strong as the left ventricle. As the pulmonary resistance drops, the right ventricle muscle reduces in size to equal that of the left ventricle by 1 month of age (McDaniel, 2010). The higher systemic vascular pressures force the left ventricle to develop quickly.

The decreasing pulmonary vascular resistance at birth leads to thinning of the small pulmonary arteriole lining, and increases the

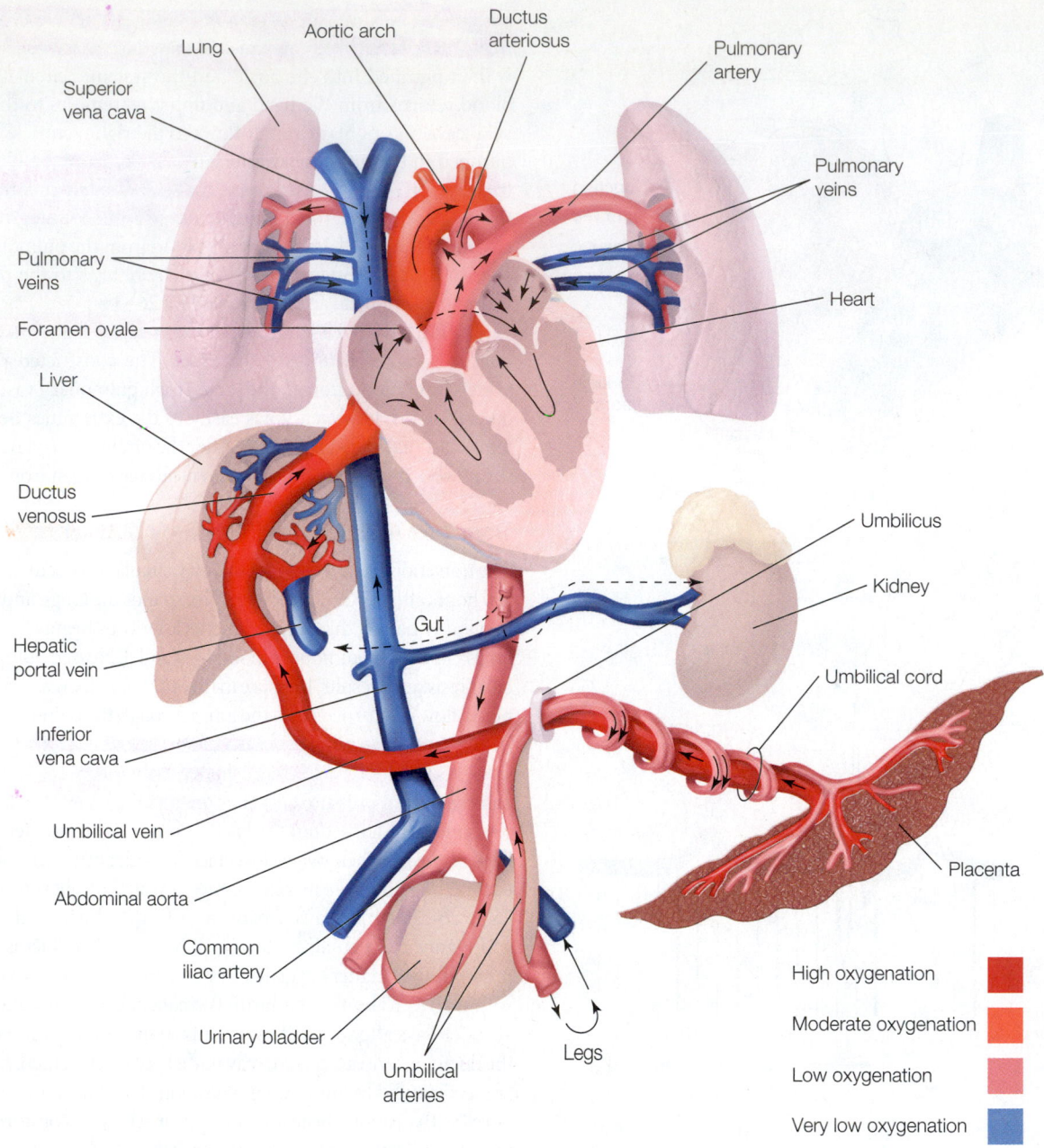

FIGURE 26–3 ■ Fetal circulation. Blood leaves the placenta and enters the fetus through the umbilical vein. The ductus venosus, the foramen ovale, and the ductus arteriosus allow the blood to bypass the fetal liver and lungs. After circulating through the fetus, the blood returns to the placenta through the umbilical arteries.

Source: *From Davidson, M. R., London, M. L., & Ladewig, P. A. W. (2012). Maternal-newborn nursing and women's health (9th ed.). Upper Saddle River, NJ: Pearson.*

TABLE 26–2	Comparison of Fetal and Neonatal Circulation	
BLOOD VESSELS AND CHANNELS	**FETAL**	**NEONATAL**
Pulmonary blood vessels	Constricted, with very little blood flow; lungs not expanded.	Vasodilation and increased blood flow; lungs expanded; increased oxygen stimulates vasodilation.
Systemic blood vessels	Dilated, with low resistance; blood mostly in placenta.	Arterial pressure rises due to loss of placenta; increased systemic blood volume and resistance.
Ductus arteriosus	Large, with no tone; blood flow from pulmonary artery to aorta.	Reversal of blood flow; now from aorta to pulmonary artery because of increased left atrial pressure. Ductus arteriosus is sensitive to increased oxygen and body chemicals and begins to constrict.
Foramen ovale	Patent, with increased blood flow from right atrium to left atrium.	Increased pressure in left atrium attempts to reverse blood flow, closing flaps on the one-way valve.
Ductus venosus	Patent, blood flow from placenta to liver and inferior vena cava.	Blood flow stops when umbilical cord is cut; ductus venosus begins to constrict.

Source: *From London, M. L., Ladewig, P. W., Ball, J. W., Bindler, R. C., & Cowen, K. J. (2011). Maternal & child nursing care (3rd ed., p. 539). Upper Saddle River, NJ: Pearson Education, Inc.*

As They Grow   Transition of Fetal Circulation to Postnatal Pulmonary Circulation

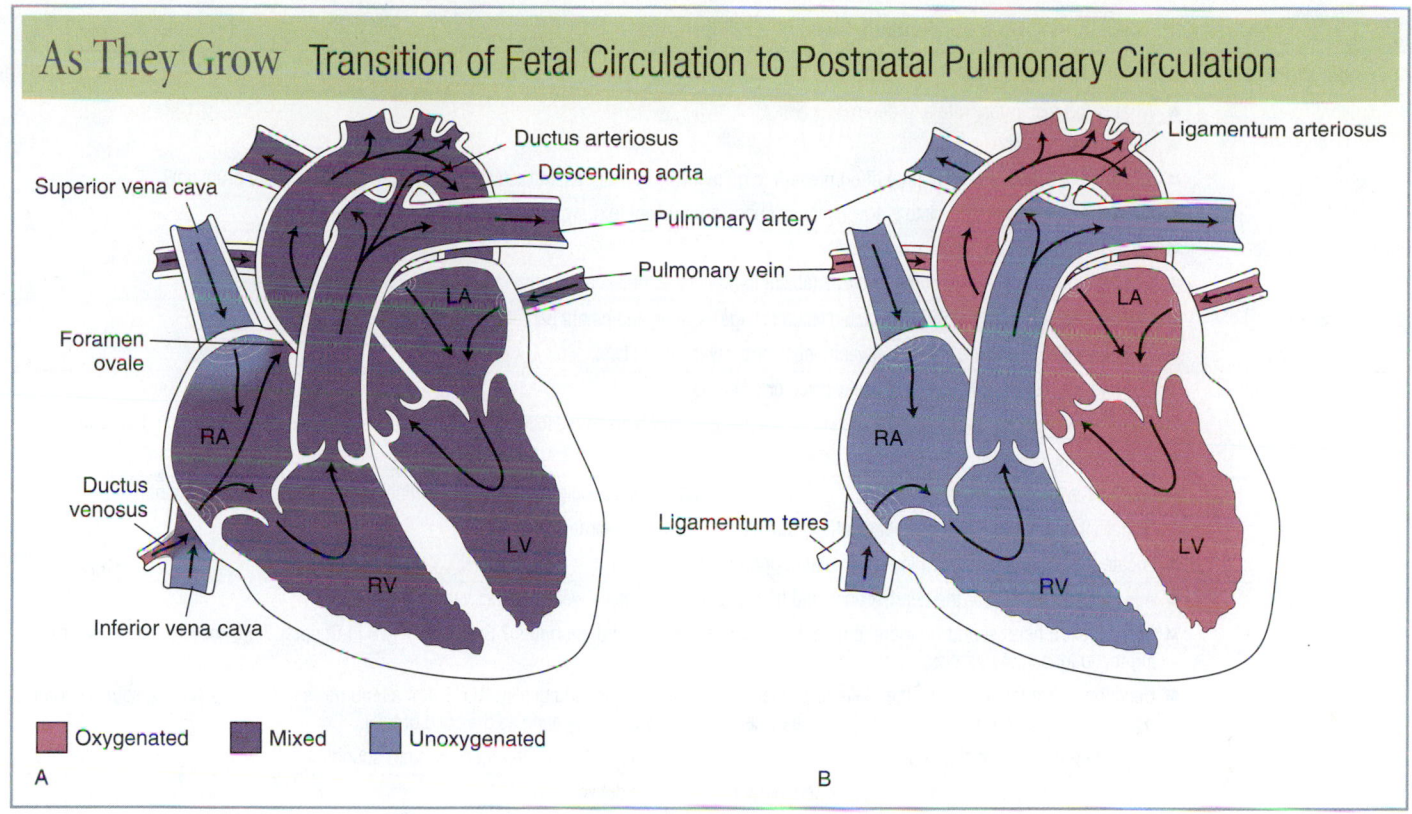

FIGURE 26–4 ■ The arrows indicate the flow of blood through the heart while the color indicates the level of oxygen saturation in the blood. *A,* Fetal (prenatal) circulation. *B,* Pulmonary (postnatal) circulation. *LA,* left atrium; *LV,* left ventricle; *RA,* right atrium; *RV,* right ventricle.

diameter in these blood vessels. The pulmonary bed also develops in response to lung growth. Both changes result in development of pulmonary resistance of adult levels by 2 months of age. However, the neonate who experiences conditions such as alveolar hypoxia, acidosis, and hypothermia may develop prolonged pulmonary vasoconstriction that results in pulmonary hypertension (McDaniel, 2010).

The decreased left ventricular strength is one reason for the neonate's low systolic blood pressure (approximately 39 to 59 mmHg). The heart muscle fibers develop during early childhood and by 9 years of age, the weight of the heart has increased by six times (McDaniel, 2010). As the child's heart grows and develops, the systolic blood pressure rises, reaching adult levels by puberty.

Oxygenation

Oxygen bound to hemoglobin is transported to the tissues by the systemic circulation. Hematocrit and hemoglobin concentrations appropriate for the child's age are necessary for adequate oxygen transport (see Chapter 28 🔗). The arterial **oxygen saturation** is the amount of oxygen that can potentially be delivered to the tissues. **Desaturated blood** results when oxygenated and unoxygenated blood mix due to a congenital heart defect. Cyanosis, which indicates **hypoxemia** (lower than normal amounts of oxygen in the blood), results from an increased concentration of arterial deoxygenated hemoglobin. Cyanosis can be seen only after the deoxygenated hemoglobin in the veins is reduced by 5 g/100 mL. However, the arterial oxygen saturation level at which cyanosis is seen depends upon whether the child has anemia, normal blood levels, or polycythemia. Cyanosis is seen at higher arterial oxygen saturations when the child has more polycythemia and at much lower levels when the child has anemia (Park, 2008, pp. 140–141).

Clinical Tip

A pulse oximeter provides a noninvasive measurement of the percutaneous arterial oxygen saturation level (SpO_2) and may provide an early sign of hypoxia before cyanosis is visualized. A reading of 95% to 98% is normal in children. Refer to Box 25–1 and Figure 25–6 🔗 for a review of pulse oximetry use and interpretation.

The child's bone marrow responds to chronic hypoxemia by producing an excess number of red blood cells, known as **polycythemia,** to increase the amount of hemoglobin available to carry oxygen to the tissues. A hematocrit value of 50% or higher is common in children who have heart defects causing cyanosis because their bodies attempt to increase available oxygen to the tissues by increasing red blood cell production. Extreme polycythemia is determined by a hemoglobin concentration greater than 20 g/dL. Polycythemia is also associated with a platelet dysfunction that increases the risk for thromboembolism, especially if the child becomes dehydrated.

Practice Alert

Children respond to severe hypoxemia with bradycardia. Cardiac arrest in children often results from prolonged hypoxemia related to respiratory failure or shock rather than from a primary cardiac arrhythmia as in adults (Zideman & Hazinski, 2008). Bradycardia is therefore a significant warning sign that cardiac arrest is imminent. Appropriate management of hypoxemia often reverses bradycardia and prevents cardiac arrest.

Cardiac Functioning

The infant's metabolic rate and oxygen requirements double at birth, so a higher heart rate is required to maintain a high **cardiac output** (volume of blood ejected from the left ventricle each minute) and

TABLE 26–3   Assessment Guidelines for the Child with a Cardiac Condition*

ASSESSMENT FOCUS	ASSESSMENT GUIDELINES
Respirations	■ What is the respiratory rate and depth? ■ Is a cough present? ■ Are signs of increased respiratory effort present (e.g., tachypnea, dyspnea, retractions, nasal flaring, or expiratory grunting)? ■ Auscultate breath sounds: Note if adventitious sounds are present (e.g., wheezes, crackles).
Pulse characteristics	■ Assess the pulse rate, rhythm, and quality. ■ Compare pulse sites for strength and rate (apical to brachial or radial, and femoral).
Blood pressure	■ Compare the blood pressure to expected value for age, gender, and height percentile. (See Appendix B 🔗.) ■ Compare blood pressure values between upper and lower extremities.
Color	■ Observe overall color: Note pallor, dusky color, or cyanosis. ■ Compare the color in peripheral and central locations (e.g., nail beds to mucous membranes). Does crying improve or worsen the color? ■ Assess pulse oximetry.
Chest	■ Inspect the anterior and posterior chest for any skeletal abnormalities, bulging, or *heaving* (lifting of the chest wall during contraction). ■ Palpate the chest wall over the heart for any pulsations, heaves, or vibrations. ■ Locate the point of maximum intensity using topographic landmarks.
Heart auscultation	■ Auscultate the heart for the heart sounds and their quality (loud versus weak, distinct versus muffled). ■ Are any extra heart sounds present (e.g., a third or fourth heart sound, murmurs)? See Table 7–13 in Chapter 7 🔗 for information on grading the loudness of murmurs. ■ Describe murmurs present by their intensity, location, radiation, timing, and quality. NOTE: Not all murmurs indicate pathology; some children have a functional murmur (not related to a heart defect, and often disappearing as the child grows). ■ Auscultate the heart with the child in sitting and reclining positions to detect differences in heart sounds.
Fluid status	■ Observe for signs of periorbital, facial, or peripheral edema, or for dehydration. ■ Observe for abdominal distention. ■ Palpate the liver to detect hepatomegaly. ■ Assess capillary refill.
Activity and behavior	■ Determine if exercise intolerance is present or if the child tires with feeding. ■ Note presence of diaphoresis and when it occurs. ■ Identify changes in activity level.
General	■ Assess pattern of growth.

*Refer to Chapter 7 🔗 for the actual assessment techniques mentioned in this table.

adequate oxygen transport. Cardiac output is controlled by four interrelated actions:

- Heart rate
- **Preload,** the volume of blood in the ventricle at the end of diastole that stretches the heart muscle before contraction
- **Contractility,** the ability of the heart muscle fibers to contract forcefully
- **Afterload,** the systemic resistance to the ventricular ejection of blood

Cardiac output in newborns and young children depends primarily on heart rate until the heart muscle is fully developed at 5 years of age. Infants have less **compliance** (amount of distention or expansion the ventricles can achieve to increase stroke volume) of the heart muscle, meaning that **stroke volume** (the amount of blood ejected with each contraction) cannot increase substantially. During stress, exercise, fever, or respiratory distress, infants and children become tachycardic, which increases their cardiac output. The infant has little cardiac reserve capacity until oxygen requirements begin to decrease at about 2 months of age (McDaniel, 2010). Infants have a greater risk of heart failure than older children because the immature heart is more sensitive to volume or pressure overload.

Cardiac Assessment

Performing a nursing assessment of the child with a potential or actual cardiac condition involves a careful review of the signs and symptoms in many body systems and analysis of their relationship to cardiac functioning. Use the guidelines in Table 26–3 to perform a comprehensive assessment of a child with a cardiac condition. Numerous diagnostic procedures and laboratory tests are used for the diagnosis of cardiovascular conditions. See Table 26–4. Additional information about these diagnostic procedures and laboratory tests can be found in Appendixes D and E 🔗.

CONGENITAL HEART DISEASE

Congenital heart disease refers to a defect in the heart or great vessels, or persistence of a fetal structure after birth. Congenital heart defects are one of the most common birth defects, with an incidence of approximately 6 to 8 per 1,000 live births; however, 96% of newborns with congenital heart defects who survive the first year of life will still be alive at 16 years of age (Sadowski, 2009). Infants (48.1%) and children ages 1 to 17 (12.4%) account for the majority of all mortality due to congenital heart disease. Deaths due to congenital heart disease in infants, children, and adults declined approximately

TABLE 26–4	Diagnostic Procedures and Laboratory Tests for the Cardiovascular System*	
DIAGNOSTIC PROCEDURES	**LABORATORY TESTS**	
Cardiac catheterization	Complete blood count	
Chest radiograph	Arterial blood gases	
Echocardiogram (transthoracic and transesophageal)	Antistreptolysin-O antibody titer	
Exercise testing	Erythrocyte sedimentation rate	
Ambulatory electrocardiography (Holter monitor)	C-reactive protein	
	Serum lipid panel	
Hyperoxitest	Serum drug tests (e.g., digoxin)	
Computed tomography		
Magnetic resonance imaging		

Note: *See Appendixes D and E 🔗 for information about these diagnostic procedures and tests.

3% per year between 1999 and 2006 (Gilboa, Salemi, Nembhard, et al., 2010). More than 35 types of congenital heart defects have been documented.

Etiology and Pathophysiology

The fetal heart begins forming on day 18 of pregnancy as the heart tube develops. The septum between the atria and ventricles forms during the fourth and fifth week of fetal life, and the blood vessels begin forming (McDaniel, 2010; Sadowski, 2009). Most cardiac congenital defects develop during the first 8 weeks of gestation, the time when the fetus is most susceptible to teratogens. Many congenital heart defects result from a combined or interactive effect of genetic and environmental factors, such as the following (McDaniel, 2010):

- Fetal exposure to drugs such as phenytoin, lithium, warfarin, and valproic acid
- Fetal exposure to alcohol—tetralogy of Fallot, atrial septal defect, ventriculoseptal defect
- Fetal exposure to secondary tobacco smoke—septal and right-sided defects (Malik, Cleves, Honein, et al., 2008)
- Maternal systemic viral infections such as rubella (patent ductus arteriosus, pulmonic stenosis, coarctation of aorta) or coxsackie B5 (endocardial fibroelastosis)

- Increased maternal age—ventriculoseptal defect, tetralogy of Fallot
- Maternal metabolic disorders such as phenylketonuria (coarctation of aorta and patent ductus arteriosus), diabetes mellitus (ventricular septal defects, cardiomegaly, transposition of great arteries), and hypercalcemia (aortic stenosis, pulmonic stenosis, aortic hyperplasia)
- High altitude—patent ductus arteriosus, atrial septal defect
- Maternal complications of pregnancy such as increased age and antepartal bleeding
- Genetic factors—family recurrence patterns
- Prematurity—patent ductus arteriosus, ventricular septal defect

Congenital heart defects can occur as an isolated defect or as a malformation associated with a genetic syndrome (Table 26–5). Chromosomal abnormalities are associated with at least 25% of children with congenital heart defects. Common examples include trisomy syndromes (13, 18, and 21), Turner syndrome, Noonan syndrome, DiGeorge syndrome, and cri du chat syndrome. While some conditions develop due to mutations of genes, others are transmitted in an autosomal dominant or autosomal recessive pattern. See Chapter 4 🔗 for more information on genetic transmission. Because of this genetic component, the incidence of congenital heart defects may slowly rise as persons with some of these defects survive and have children of their own. An increased incidence of congenital heart defects occurs in families. If one child has a congenital defect, the risk for a congenital defect in subsequent children having the same parents is increased (McDaniel, 2010).

Congenital heart defects are generally categorized by the pathophysiology and hemodynamics, rather than by whether a defect causes cyanosis. The categories of defects include the following:

- Increased pulmonary blood flow (see page 813)
- Decreased pulmonary blood flow (see page 820)
- Obstructed systemic blood flow (see page 828)

Mixed defects are those that fall into one of the three previous classifications, but the infant's survival is dependent upon mixing of systemic and pulmonary blood (see page 820). Because children with mixed defects and decreased pulmonary blood flow have similar clinical therapy and nursing management, these two categories of defects will be discussed together.

TABLE 26–5	Congenital Heart Defects Commonly Associated with Genetic Disorders
GENETIC DISORDER	**ASSOCIATED CONGENITAL HEART DEFECTS***
Trisomy 13	VSD, ASD, PDA, dextrocardia, double outlet right ventricle
Trisomy 18	VSD, ASD, PDA, PS, TOF
Down syndrome (trisomy 21)	AV canal, VSD, ASD, TOF, PDA
Cri du chat	PDA, VSD, ASD
Turner syndrome (monosomy 23)	AS, COA, bicuspid aortic valve, mitral valve prolapse, HLHS, aortic root dilation/dissection
Noonan syndrome (chromosome 12q24 region mutation)	Valvular pulmonic stenosis, AS, ASD, VSD
DiGeorge syndrome, velocardiofacial syndrome (chromosome 22q11 microdeletion)	Interrupted aortic arch, aortic arch abnormalities, VSD, TOF, truncus arteriosus

*AS—aortic stenosis, ASD—atrial septal defect, AV canal—atrioventricular canal (endocardial cushion defect), COA—coarctation of aorta, HLHS—hypoplastic left heart syndrome, PDA—patent ductus arteriosus, PS—pulmonic stenosis, TGA—transposition of the great arteries, TOF—tetralogy of Fallot, VSD—ventriculoseptal defect

Source: *Data from: D'Alessandro, L.C.A., Peyvandi, S., Schachtner, S, & Goldmuntz, E. (2012). The genetics of abnormal cardiac development, In M. M. Gleason, J. Rychik, & R. Shaddy, Pediatric Practice Cardiology, (pp. 79-81). New York, NY: McGraw Hill Medical; Park, M. K. (2008). Pediatric Cardiology for Practitioners, (5th ed., pp. 10-13), Philadelphia, PA: Mosby Elsevier; and Zeigler, V. L. (2008). Congenital heart disease and genetics. Critical Care Clinics of North America, 20, 159–169.*

Clinical Manifestations Heart Defects by Pathophysiology

ETIOLOGY	TYPES OF DEFECTS	CLINICAL MANIFESTATIONS
Increased pulmonary blood flow	Patent ductus arteriosus, atrial septal defect, ventricular septal defect, atrioventricular canal defect (endocardial cushion defect)	Tachypnea, tachycardia, murmur, congestive heart failure, poor weight gain, diaphoresis, periorbital edema, frequent respiratory infections
Decreased pulmonary blood flow	Pulmonic stenosis, tetralogy of Fallot, pulmonary atresia, tricuspid atresia	Cyanosis, hypercyanotic episodes, poor weight gain, polycythemia
Obstruction to systemic blood flow	Coarctation of aorta, aortic stenosis, hypoplastic left heart syndrome, mitral stenosis, interrupted aortic arch	Diminished pulses, poor color, delayed capillary refill time, decreased urine output, congestive heart failure with pulmonary edema
Mixed defects—all are within one of the above categories, but the difference is that postnatal survival is dependent upon mixing of systemic and pulmonary blood	Transposition of great arteries, total anomalous pulmonary venous connection, truncus arteriosus, double outlet right ventricle	Cyanosis, poor weight gain, pulmonary congestion, congestive heart failure may occur with increased shunting

Clinical Manifestations

The presence of a heart murmur is often the first indication of a congenital heart defect. A loud murmur indicates blood is flowing with higher pressure than normal to get through a narrowed valve or vessel, or through a **shunt** (movement of blood between the systemic and pulmonary circulation through an abnormal anatomic opening, such as between the ventricles). Other clinical manifestations and the timing of their appearance vary by the pathophysiology and severity of the defect (see the Clinical Manifestations table for heart defects by pathophysiology). Newborns may be initially asymptomatic but develop symptoms in the first few days of life. Other newborns are symptomatic as soon as the umbilical cord is cut. Some infants and children may be asymptomatic except for a heart murmur, such as with a small atrial septal defect. See Chapter 7 🔗 for assessment of murmurs. Signs and symptoms of congenital heart disease in older children include exercise intolerance, chest pain, arrhythmias, **syncope** (transient loss of consciousness and muscle tone after exercise or activity), and sudden death.

Practice Alert

Exercise-induced dizziness or syncope in older children and adolescents with congenital heart disease is a serious sign indicating a need for medical evaluation. This may be a symptom of a serious condition that could lead to death if not identified and treated; however, sudden death may also occur.

Collaborative Care

Diagnostic Procedures

The history and physical examination may lead to a suspicion of congenital heart disease. Multiple tests and procedures are used to diagnose heart defects, including a chest radiograph, electrocardiogram (ECG), two-dimensional echocardiogram, transthoracic echocardiogram, cardiac catheterization, exercise testing, computed tomography (CT), magnetic resonance imaging (MRI), and a hyperoxia test. Information about the purpose and nursing considerations associated with these diagnostic procedures is in Appendix E 🔗. Blood tests include hematocrit and hemoglobin. Arterial blood gases may be obtained for some children, especially when cyanosis or a complex heart defect is suspected.

Cardiac catheterization as a diagnostic procedure enables precise measurement of oxygen saturation within the heart's chambers and great arteries, and pressure gradients in each of these structures. Contrast material is used to identify the anatomy and blood flow patterns through angiography. In some cases, a biopsy of the heart muscle may also be obtained to evaluate muscle function problems, inflammation, or heart transplant rejection.

Genetic testing should be provided to patients and their families so they have accurate information and receive counseling about the cause and risks for recurrence in subsequent pregnancies.

Clinical Therapy

One third of infants born with congenital heart defects develop life-threatening symptoms in the first few days of life. Treatment for congenital heart defects depends on the severity of symptoms and whether the condition is imminently life threatening.

Interventional cardiac catheterization Interventional cardiac catheterization is performed to correct some congenital heart defects. A balloon may be used to create a larger opening in the atrial septum (atrial septostomy), to perform a **valvuloplasty** dilating a **stenotic** (narrowed or small) pulmonic or aortic valve, or expanding a coarctation of the aorta. See Figure 26–5 ■ and Table 26–6. Another

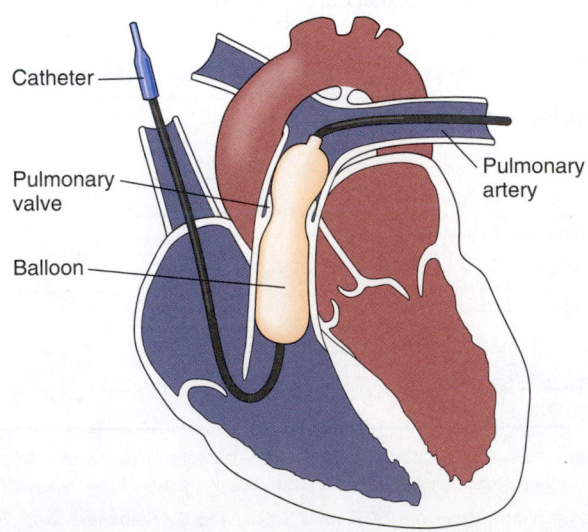

Catheter

Pulmonary valve

Balloon

Pulmonary artery

FIGURE 26–5 ■ One form of interventional cardiac catheterization: balloon valvuloplasty to open the pulmonary valve in cases of pulmonic stenosis.

TABLE 26–6	Clinical Interventions for Congenital Heart Defects*
CARDIAC CATHETERIZATION PROCEDURES AND THERAPEUTIC USE	**DESCRIPTION**
Balloon Atrial Septostomy—Rashkind, or with transatrial needle puncture and balloon dilation Palliative for TGA	Creation of larger defect (at the foramen ovale) between atria to increase mixing of oxygenated and deoxygenated blood, performed during cardiac catheterization.
Balloon Dilation Procedure Corrective for PS and MS; palliative for AS, COA	A deflated balloon is inserted and inflated in the opening of a narrowed valve or blood vessel to stretch it open. A stent may be inserted to keep the vessel open.
Device Closure Corrective for PDA, ASD, VSD	Closure of ductus arteriosus by an umbrella or coil device, and closure of a septal defect by a septal occluder.
SURGICAL PROCEDURES AND THERAPEUTIC USE	**DESCRIPTION**
Aorta End-to-End Anastomosis Corrective for COA	Resection of the narrowed section of the aorta and connecting the proximal and distal sections.
Blalock-Taussig Shunt, Modified Palliative for TOF, single ventricle lesions with pulmonary outflow obstruction	Creation of aortopulmonary conduit (from the brachiocephalic artery to pulmonary artery) to increase pulmonary blood flow.
Brock Corrective for PS	Blind incision of pulmonary valve.
Damus-Kaye-Stansel (pulmonary artery-to-aortic anastomosis) Corrective for TGA, complex single ventricle defects	Pulmonary artery is cut in two with the proximal section attached to the ascending aorta; the distal section is sewn over, and a shunt is created between the systemic circulation and the pulmonary artery to send blood to the lungs.
Fontan Palliative for HLHS, single ventricle defects	Creation of a conduit between the inferior vena cava and pulmonary artery to increase pulmonary blood flow—total right heart bypass. This permits the single ventricle to assume the responsibility for the systemic circulation and eject blood into the aorta.
Glenn, Bidirectional Glenn Palliative for HLHS, single ventricle defects	Superior vena cava connected to the right pulmonary artery along with closure of the aortopulmonary shunt. Systemic venous blood from the head is sent to the lungs directly without ventricular pumping.
Jatene (arterial switch) Corrective for TGA	Aorta and pulmonary arteries are transected and reattached to the opposite stumps; coronary arteries are moved to new aorta area.
Norwood Palliative for aortic hypoplasia, single ventricle defects, e.g., HLHS	Atrial septectomy, anastomosis of the main pulmonary artery to the aorta, and an arterial-pulmonary shunt, e.g., the modified Blalock-Taussig shunt.
Norwood with Sano modification Palliative for HLHS	Creation of a right ventricle to pulmonary artery conduit so that both the direct pulmonary and aorta blood flow originates in the right ventricle.
Patch Aortoplasty Corrective for COA	Insertion of a Dacron patch or opened left subclavian vein to expand the lumen of the aorta.
Pulmonary Artery Banding Palliative for VSD, AV canal, single ventricle defects	Placement of constricting band around pulmonary artery to reduce pulmonary blood flow and pressure.
Rastelli Corrective for TGA with pulmonic stenosis, TOF, tricuspid atresia, truncus arteriosus, and some cases of double outlet right ventricle	Creation of a conduit between the right ventricle to pulmonary artery with closure of the ventricular septal defect. In the case of truncus arteriosus, the pulmonary arteries are removed from the truncus.
Ross Corrective for AS	The diseased aortic valve is replaced with the patient's pulmonic valve (pulmonary autograft), and a homograft (valve from a human donor) replaces the pulmonic valve.
Subclavian Flap Aortoplasty Corrective for COA	Division of the distal subclavian artery and insertion of a flap into the aorta through the coarcted segment.
Transplant Corrective for HLHS, complex defects, cardiomyopathies	Replacement of diseased heart with donor heart.

*AS—aortic stenosis, ASD—atrial septal defect, AV—atrioventricular, COA—coarctation of aorta, HLHS—hypoplastic left heart syndrome, MS—mitral stenosis, PDA—patent ductus arteriosus, PS—pulmonic stenosis, TOF—tetralogy of Fallot, TGA—transposition of great arteries, VSD—ventricular septal defect

intervention involves inserting a stent into a patent ductus arteriosus to maintain patency as an alternative to long-term prostaglandin E_1 (PGE_1) infusion. Insertion of an expandable stent may also be used to treat a stenotic **hypoplastic** (underdeveloped structure) pulmonary artery or coarctation of the aorta.

A coil can be used to occlude a patent ductus arteriosus and other vessels, and a septal closing device can be used for some atrial septal and ventriculoseptal defects (Figure 26–6 ■). Rare complications of patent ductus arteriosus (PDA) occlusion include embolism or malposition of the device and hemolysis due to persistent shunting of blood across a partially occluded PDA. Complications are rare following the septal closure of an atrial septal defect, and they include device displacement, arrhythmias, and stroke due to thrombus formation. Anticoagulant therapy may be ordered during the procedure

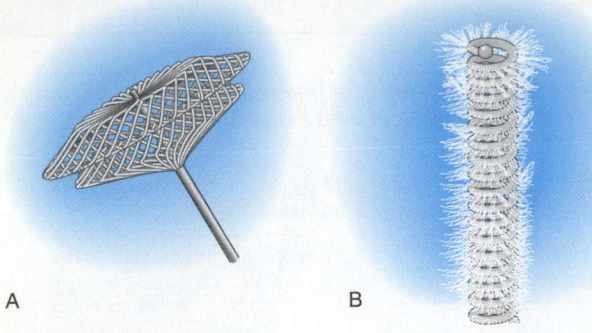

A   B

FIGURE 26–6 ■ *A,* Example of a septal occluder used to close an atrial septal defect (ASD) and less commonly to close a ventricular septal defect (VSD). *B,* Example of a coil used to close a patent ductus arteriosus (PDA). The coil of wire covered with tiny fibers occludes the ductus arteriosus when a thrombus forms in the mass of fabric and wire.

and for several months following the placement of the occlusion device.

Surgical interventions Many heart defects can be surgically repaired with restoration of normal hemodynamics and physiology. A **palliative procedure** (a surgical or interventional catheterization procedure that does not create normal anatomic or hemodynamic results) may be performed in children with a potentially fatal or lethal condition. The palliative procedure may also be performed as an initial procedure, allowing an infant to grow before definitive corrective surgery. Table 26–6 lists the types of surgical and interventional cardiac catheterization interventions performed on children with congenital heart defects.

Nursing Management of the Child Undergoing a Cardiac Catheterization

Cardiac catheterization is often performed on an outpatient basis; however, some children will be admitted for observation to monitor for complications or for scheduled surgery. Various diagnostic tests may be performed before the procedure, such as a chest radiograph, ECG, echocardiogram, complete blood count, and electrolytes. The child is given nothing by mouth (NPO) for several hours, except for medications, and arrives at the catheterization laboratory 1 to 2 hours before the procedure. In preparation for the procedure, the child is asked to void and is given an oral sedative. Infants and young children usually need deeper sedation to keep them still during the procedure.

Nursing Assessment and Diagnosis

Physiologic Assessment

Before the procedure, assess the child using the assessment guidelines in Table 26–3. Pay particular attention to the child's vital signs, hematocrit and hemoglobin concentrations, and capillary refill time. In addition, collect baseline data on skin temperature and color, and strength of the pedal and popliteal pulses for comparison with post-catheterization assessments.

For several hours after the procedure, monitor the child for potential complications such as arrhythmia, bleeding, hematoma development, thrombus formation, and infection. No bleeding should occur at the catheterization site. Assess vital signs and perfusion of the lower extremities (pedal and popliteal pulses, skin temperature, color, capillary refill, and sensation), and compare to precatheterization status. The child's temperature and vital signs should remain stable. Monitor intake and output because the contrast medium may cause diuresis.

Clinical Tip

A pressure dressing is a thick layer of gauze pads covered by a tight adhesive placed over a site where bleeding must be controlled. The dressing should be monitored frequently (every 5 minutes for 15 minutes, then every 15 minutes for an hour, and then hourly, or as directed by physician orders). Observe for signs of blood or wetness of the dressing, but do not remove the dressing to view the site until the time has elapsed for the pressure dressing order. Check under the buttocks to make sure blood does not ooze out and run under the child.

Practice Alert

Ileofemoral artery injury associated with cardiac catheterization is more common in newborns and young infants. Reduced limb warmth and decreased pedal perfusion in the extremity following transfemoral cardiac catheterization is an indication of potential arterial occlusion and limb ischemia. Immediate medical intervention is needed to prevent permanent neurovascular damage to the extremity.

Psychosocial Assessment

Assess the parents' need for emotional support. This may be the first invasive procedure performed on a newborn with a congenital heart defect. The parents have had little time to understand and cope with the infant's condition. It is also possible that this may be a procedure performed on an asymptomatic child, such as a child with an atrial septal defect when transcatheter closure is planned. The child may have anxiety about separation from parents and fears about all the equipment and people performing an invasive procedure while awake. The child may also have fears due to past hospital experiences.

The following nursing diagnoses may apply to the child who undergoes cardiac catheterization:

- Fear related to separation from support system in a stressful situation
- Anxiety (Family) related to potential for serious diagnosis
- Fluid Volume: Imbalanced, Risk for related to preprocedure NPO status and diuretic effect of contrast medium
- Tissue Perfusion: Peripheral, Risk for Ineffective related to mechanical reduction of arterial and venous blood flow to lower extremity

NANDA-I © 2012

Planning and Implementation

Prepare the parents for the procedure and what to expect with regard to their child. Engage the parents in preparing the child for the procedure. Use age-appropriate information to prepare the child for cardiac catheterization, and plan the timing of education to the child's developmental age. A tour of the catheterization laboratory for a school-age child may reduce the child's fears about the large equipment. Because the child will be sedated but arousable for the procedure, explain the sensations that he or she will experience (e.g., restraints on arms, equipment noises, cold liquid cleanser for catheter site, and warm feeling of contrast injection). Older children and adolescents can be taught coping strategies to manage their anxiety during the procedure.

Nursing care during a cardiac catheterization focuses on monitoring the child's vital signs, reassuring the child, and providing emergency care if necessary. Talking with the child or playing music during the procedure may provide distraction. After the catheters and guide wires are removed at the end of the procedure, direct pressure must be applied for 15 minutes. A pressure dressing is then placed over the site for several hours. Regular assessment of the site of catheterization and distal extremity is performed for several hours after the

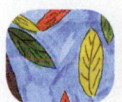

Partnering with Families

Home Care After Cardiac Catheterization

Check for signs of complications several times in the first 24 hours after catheterization and notify the physician if any of these signs are noted:

- Fever
- Bleeding or a bruise increasing in size at the catheterization site
- Foot on side of catheterization site is cooler than other foot
- Loss of feeling in foot on side of catheterization

If the child is treated with diuretics, observe for signs of dehydration:

- Dry mucous membranes
- Absence of tears
- Strong urine

Encourage fluids to help flush the dye out of the body and to prevent dehydration. Allow no rough or active play for the first 24 hours. Permit quiet play such as crayons or markers, board games, puzzles, books, music, and videos.

---

procedure. Contact the physician if bleeding occurs or circulation is impaired in the distal extremity.

The child is kept on bed rest for 4 to 6 hours with an effort to keep the leg straight for several hours. Avoid elevating the head of the bed as flexion of the hips is not permitted during this period. Activity is then limited for 24 hours, and in some cases the child is hospitalized overnight. Provide quiet activities to keep the child occupied.

Encourage the intake of small amounts of clear liquids initially, and then progress to other fluids and food as the child tolerates them. Maintaining hydration is important because the contrast medium used during the procedure has a diuretic effect. The child's intake and output should be balanced. Infants and children treated with diuretics have a greater potential for dehydration, and identification of excessive urinary excretion is important so that additional fluids can be provided.

Discharge Planning and Home Care Teaching

Children are usually discharged several hours after the cardiac catheterization. Teach the parents to watch the child for signs of complications, and make sure they know when to notify the physician. See Partnering with Families: Home Care After Cardiac Catheterization.

Evaluation

Expected outcomes of nursing care include the following:

- Any potential complications (thrombosis or hemorrhage) are rapidly identified and managed following cardiac catheterization.
- The child's fluid balance is maintained.

CONGENITAL HEART DEFECTS THAT INCREASE PULMONARY BLOOD FLOW

The most common congenital heart defects result from a connection between the left and right side of the heart (septal defect) or between the great arteries (patent ductus arteriosus) that allows blood to flow between the left and right side of the heart.

Etiology and Pathophysiology

The pressures on the left side of the heart are higher than on the right side. When a connection occurs between the left and right side of the heart, blood will shunt from the left side to the right side and increase the amount of blood that is pumped to the lungs. The size of the connection and how much blood passes through it determine if or how quickly the child will develop signs associated with congestive heart failure (see page 829). The increased pulmonary blood flow

causes increased pulmonary vascular resistance (constriction of the pulmonary vascular bed) in an effort to reduce the blood flow, and pulmonary artery hypertension (see page 840). Right ventricular hypertrophy develops to counteract the increasing pulmonary vascular resistance and deliver the increased volume of blood to the lungs.

Clinical Manifestations

The infant's heart rate, respiratory rate, and metabolic rate are increased due to the high pulmonary blood flow. Sucking breast milk or formula takes energy, and diaphoresis may be noted with feeding. Often the infant is unable to obtain enough calories to support the metabolic rate and growth, so poor weight gain may be noted. Congestive heart failure may develop if the pulmonary system is overloaded with blood, leading to dyspnea, tachypnea, intercostal retractions, and periorbital edema. Frequent respiratory infections occur because the wet environment in the lungs supports bacterial growth. The symptoms of congestive heart failure appear earlier when the heart defect is more severe and complex. See Table 26–7 for the pathophysiology, clinical manifestations, and clinical therapy for the congenital heart defects that increase pulmonary blood flow.

Collaborative Care

Diagnostic Procedures

See Table 26–7 for tests used to diagnose the different congenital defects in this category. Coagulation studies, platelet counts, and serum electrolytes are commonly obtained for children in preparation for open heart surgery, in addition to a chest radiograph, complete blood count, and urinalysis.

Clinical Therapy

Surgery to correct or manage defects that cause significant increased pulmonary blood flow is performed early in infancy to prevent irreversible pulmonary artery hypertension, the major complication of these defects. Unless complications develop before surgery, the child should make a complete recovery without limitations. Table 26–7 provides the clinical therapy for the individual with congenital heart defects that increase pulmonary blood flow.

Conservative treatment, such as waiting until the child is symptomatic or older, may be selected initially for some children with these defects. For example, a small ventricular septal defect may close spontaneously, or atrial septal defect closure is postponed until preschool or early school-age years. Ibuprofen or indomethacin may be given to preterm infants with a patent ductus arteriosus when immediate

TABLE 26–7	Pathophysiology, Clinical Manifestations, and Clinical Therapy for Heart Defects That Increase Pulmonary Blood Flow

DEFECT PATHOPHYSIOLOGY

Patent Ductus Arteriosus (PDA)

Common congenital defect caused by persistent fetal circulation that occurs in 5–10% of all infants with congenital heart disease (Khalid & Busse, 2011). When pulmonary circulation is established and systemic vascular resistance increases at birth, pressures in the aorta become greater than in the pulmonary arteries. Blood is then shunted from the aorta to the pulmonary arteries, increasing circulation to the pulmonary system. In normal newborns, the ductus closes by day 2 or 3 of life. PDA is a common problem of preterm infants with an incidence of 8 per 1,000 live births due to physiologic effects of prematurity, such as respiratory distress syndrome and hypoxia, that work to keep the ductus arteriosus open (Khalid & Busse, 2011).

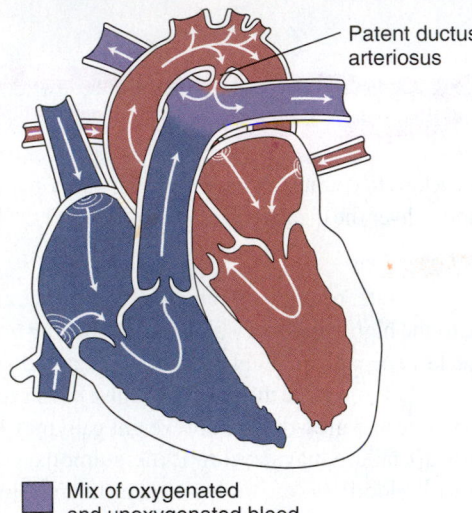

Patent ductus arteriosus

■ Mix of oxygenated and unoxygenated blood

CLINICAL MANIFESTATIONS AND CLINICAL THERAPY

Clinical Manifestations

Dyspnea; tachypnea; tachycardia; full, bounding pulses; widened pulse pressure; hypotension may be noted when cardiac output is low. May be asymptomatic.

Congestive heart failure (CHF), intercostal retractions, hepatomegaly, and poor growth may be seen when a large PDA exists.

A continuous "machinery" murmur is auscultated during both systole and diastole, and a thrill may be palpated in the pulmonic area.

The infant is at risk for frequent respiratory infections and pneumonia.

Diagnostic Procedures

The chest radiograph and ECG show left ventricular hypertrophy.

The PDA can be visualized, and left to right shunt can be measured on echocardiogram.

Clinical Therapy

Ligation of PDA by open thoracostomy or video-assisted thoracoscopic surgery is the standard treatment, but an obstructive device inserted during catheterization is used in some children.

Intravenous ibuprofen or indomethacin often stimulates closure of the ductus arteriosus in premature infants, but cannot be used in all cases, such as when CHF is present.

Prognosis: No long-term sequelae occur if treated before pulmonary vascular disease develops. If PDA is not treated, the child's life span is shortened because pulmonary hypertension and pulmonary vascular obstructive disease develop.

Atrial Septal Defect (ASD)

The opening in the atrial septum permits left to right shunting of blood. Three types of ASDs occur: secundum (in the central portion of the atrial septum), primum (an endocardial cushion defect with anomalies of the tricuspid and/or mitral valves), and sinus venosus (near the inferior or superior vena cava junction). The opening may be small, as when the foramen ovale fails to close, or large, as when the septum is completely absent. Of children with congenital heart disease, 33–50% have an ASD in combination with other defects, but it may occur as an isolated defect in 6% of children (Abdulla & Hanrahan, 2011).

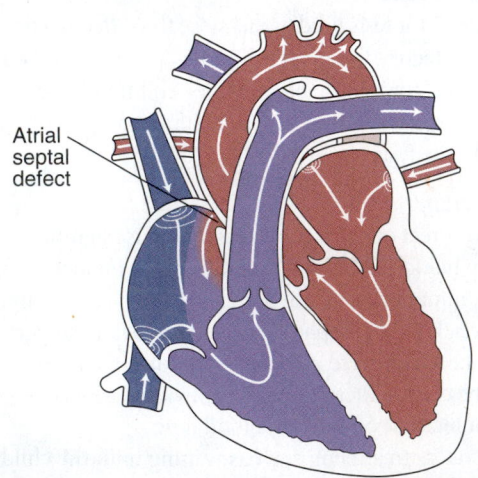

Atrial septal defect

Clinical Manifestations

Infants and young children usually have no symptoms. Small and midsize ASDs may not be diagnosed until preschool years or later.

Large ASDs may cause CHF, easy tiring, and poor growth.

A soft systolic ejection murmur occurs in the pulmonic area with fixed wide splitting of S_2 through all phases of respiration.

Diagnostic Procedures

An echocardiogram identifies a dilated right ventricle due to blood overload and the shunt size.

The chest radiograph and ECG reveal little information unless the ASD is large, or excessive shunting and right ventricular hypertrophy is present.

Clinical Therapy

Spontaneous closure of some types of ASDs occurs within the first 4 years of life. No activity limitations are needed. ASDs larger than 8 mm rarely close spontaneously.

Surgery to close or patch the ASD is performed when significant increased pulmonary blood flow causes CHF, or when spontaneous ASD closure has not occurred by 2 years of age.

Secundum ASDs may be closed by a device (septal occluder) during cardiac catheterization.

Prognosis: Many persons with uncorrected small and midsize ASDs have lived to middle age without symptoms; however, a risk for stroke exists. Small clots that commonly develop in the right atrium are usually filtered out by the lungs, but instead pass directly into the left atrium through the ASD. CHF and pulmonary hypertension may also develop in untreated adults. Atrial arrhythmias may occur in untreated adults.

| TABLE 26–7 | Pathophysiology, Clinical Manifestations, and Clinical Therapy for Heart Defects That Increase Pulmonary Blood Flow (*continued*) |

DEFECT PATHOPHYSIOLOGY

Ventricular Septal Defect (VSD)

An opening in the ventricular septum results in increased pulmonary blood flow. Blood is shunted from the left ventricle directly across the open septum into the pulmonary artery. This most common congenital heart defect occurs in approximately 15–20% of cases either in isolation or in combination with other defects (Khalid & Abdulla, 2011). It can occur in any area of the ventricular septum.

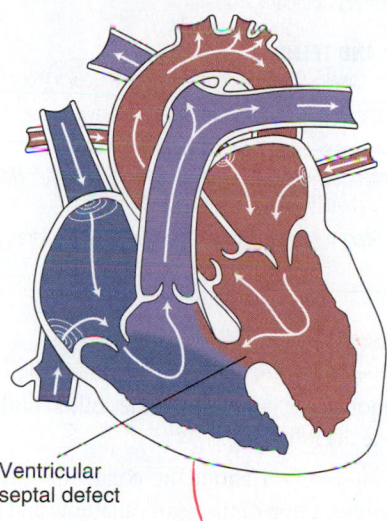

Ventricular
septal defect

Atrioventricular Canal (Endocardial Cushion Defect)

Endocardial cushions are fetal growth centers for mitral and tricuspid valves and atrioventricular (AV) septum. AV canal refers to a combination of defects in the atrial and ventricular septa and portions of the tricuspid and mitral valves. The most complex AV canal malformation results in one AV valve and large septal defects between both atria and ventricles. Approximately 4% of children with congenital heart disease have an AV canal, and 70% of these children have trisomy 21 (Khalid & Mehrota, 2011).

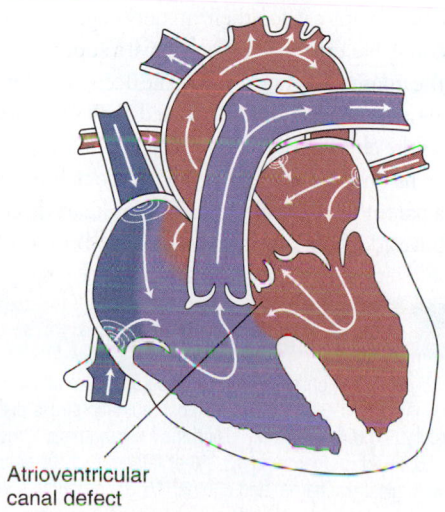

Atrioventricular
canal defect

CLINICAL MANIFESTATIONS AND CLINICAL THERAPY

Clinical Manifestations

Moderate and large VSDs may be associated with CHF (with symptoms such as tachypnea, dyspnea, and poor growth), an increased number of pulmonary infections, and pulmonary hypertension.

A systolic murmur is auscultated at the third or fourth left intercostal space at the sternal border.

Diagnostic Procedures

A chest radiograph and ECG reveal few abnormal findings when VSDs are small. An enlarged heart and pulmonary vascular markings on chest radiograph may be seen when a large VSD causes shunting. Right and left ventricular hypertrophy may be seen on ECG.

Echocardiogram establishes the diagnosis if shunting is present.

Cardiac catheterization is rarely used for diagnosis but may be used to assess pulmonary vascular resistance.

Clinical Therapy

Most small VSDs close spontaneously within the first 6 months of life. Treatment is conservative when no signs of CHF or pulmonary hypertension are present.

The child who develops CHF will be treated with furosemide, digoxin, and angiotensin-converting enzyme (ACE) inhibitors. Palliative pulmonary artery banding may be used to reduce blood flow to the lungs and CHF until surgery. Patching of the VSD occurs at 3–12 months of age.

Device closure of VSD during cardiac catheterization is attempted for some defects.

Prognosis: Highest risk associated with surgical repair is in the first few months of life. Children respond well to surgery and experience substantial catch-up growth. Tachyarrhythmias, right bundle branch block, and complete heart block are possible complications.

Clinical Manifestations

The severity of symptoms depends on the amount of left to right shunting of blood across the septum.

Infants may develop CHF, tachypnea, tachycardia, poor growth, recurrent respiratory infections, and repeated respiratory failure.

A **holosystolic** murmur (heard during the entire phase of systole) is loudest at the left lower sternal border, and the intensity reflects the amount of mitral regurgitation. S_1 is accentuated and S_2 is split.

Diagnostic Procedures

On chest radiograph, **cardiomegaly** (enlargement of the heart by hypertrophy of its walls) and pulmonary vascular markings are present.

On ECG, atrial enlargement, right ventricular hypertrophy, and an incomplete right bundle branch block are noted.

Echocardiogram reveals dilation of the ventricles, septal defects, and details of the valve malformation.

Cardiac catheterization reveals increased oxygen in the right atrium and increased right ventricle and/or pulmonary artery pressure.

Clinical Therapy

Surgery is usually performed by 3 months of age to prevent pulmonary vascular disease. Patches are placed over septal defects, and valve tissue is used to form functioning tricuspid and mitral valves.

Palliative pulmonary artery banding may be used to reduce blood flow to the lungs and CHF, enabling the infant to grow before surgery.

In some cases, a Glenn shunt is performed at 4–8 months of age followed by a Fontan procedure at 12–24 months of age.

The child with CHF will be treated with furosemide, digoxin, and ACE inhibitors until surgery.

Infective endocarditis prophylaxis is required until 6 months after corrective surgery.

Prognosis: Arrhythmias and mitral valve regurgitation, a residual septal defect, and subaortic stenosis may occur postoperatively. Short-term survival rates between infants with and without Down syndrome are similar.

closure of the ductus is needed. Interventional catheterization may be performed for these defects (see Table 26–6).

Postpericardiotomy syndrome is a potential complication in 25% to 30% of children when surgery involves an incision through the pericardium, leading to pericardial and pleural inflammation (Park, 2008, p. 377). It is believed to result from an autoimmune response to damaged myocardium or pericardium, or blood in the pericardial sac. The syndrome generally develops within a few weeks to a few months after surgery, more often in children over age 2 years. It is characterized by a high fever up to 40°C (104°F), fatigue, decreased appetite, nausea, vomiting, and sometimes severe chest pain that worsens with deep inspiration and in supine position. The median duration of the condition is 2 to 3 weeks. Mild cases are treated with bed rest and nonsteroidal anti-inflammatory drugs (NSAIDs) or indomethacin. Severe cases may need corticosteroids or emergency pericardiocentesis (Bernstein, 2011).

Nursing Management Prior to Surgery

Nursing Assessment and Diagnosis

Physiologic Assessment

Prior to surgery the infant or child is seen regularly to assess growth and to detect signs of congestive heart failure (CHF). Many infants with a small atrial septal defect or ventricular septal defect will have no growth problems. Failure to gain weight is an indication of an increased metabolic rate and inability to consume adequate calories for both metabolic function and growth. Be concerned if the infant or child has increased respiratory effort, poor feeding, diaphoresis, fatigue, recurrent pulmonary infections, and signs of CHF. Assessment of length and head circumference growth is also important to determine the full impact of the condition on growth.

Psychosocial Assessment

Assess the ability of the parents to cope with the diagnosis of their infant's congenital heart defect. Initially parents may be in shock and feel guilty or anxious. The newborn may initially look healthy and have few symptoms. Parents need an opportunity to express their feelings and to begin learning to cope with their child's illness. The initial period of diagnosis, hospitalization or frequent cardiac clinic visits, and early care of the infant at home is very stressful. Parents need special support if their infant has a life-threatening heart defect.

Following are examples of nursing diagnoses associated with heart defects having increased pulmonary blood flow and their complications:

- Fluid Volume: Excess related to heart failure and pulmonary vasculature overload
- Infant Feeding Pattern, Ineffective related to shortness of breath and fatigue
- Infection, Risk for related to pulmonary vascular congestion and chronic illness
- Family Processes, Interrupted related to crisis of child's serious illness

NANDA-I © 2012

Planning and Implementation

Nursing management of the child with a large defect prior to surgery may be similar to the care provided for CHF. See page 834 for specific nursing interventions.

BOX 26–1	Resources for Parents and Children with Congenital Heart Defects

FOR PARENTS

It's My Heart by the Children's Heart Foundation, 2004

A Parent's Guide to Children's Congenital Heart Defects by Gerri Freid Kramer and Shari Maurer, Three Rivers Press, 2001

The Heart of a Child: What Families Need to Know About Heart Disorders in Children by C. A. Neill, E. A. Clark, and C. Clark, Johns Hopkins Press, 2001

Heart Defects in Children: What Every Parent Should Know by C. J. Wild, Chronimed Publishing Company, 1999

FOR CHILDREN AND TEENS

Pump the Bear by Gisella Olivo Whittington, Brown Books (Young Children)

Blue Lewis and Sasha the Great by Carol Donsky Newell, Cally Press (Young Children)

Overcoming Challenges! Congenital Heart Defects: Life After Heart Surgery by Melissa Curnel, Gorham Printing (Children and Teens)

A Night Without Stars by James Howe, Camelot (Older Children, Teens, and Adults)

Family Education

Participate with members of the cardiology team to provide information and education to the family about the child's condition. Information may include the following:

- General information about the congenital heart disease, including a description of the heart's anatomy and physiology and the defect (Box 26–1)
- Information about genetic and environmental influences associated with the child's specific defect
- Sample case histories with good and poor prognoses
- Overview of the child's prognosis and timing of medical and surgical interventions
- Interventions for CHF, if it develops (see page 832 for care guidelines.)

Psychosocial Support

Parents may need support for their anxiety regarding an uncertain surgical outcome. Determine if parents have a support system as they learn about the infant's diagnosis and make decisions about the child's surgery. Some parents may be concerned that signing consent for surgery places the child in even more danger of illness or even death. Identify some resources for support, such as social services, pastoral services, or a parent whose child has a similar heart defect, if the parents do not have adequate support systems. See Box 26–2.

BOX 26–2	Research: Posttraumatic Stress Disorder in Parents

A study of 128 parents of children with cardiac surgery requiring cardiopulmonary bypass was conducted to assess for posttraumatic stress disorder (PTSD) following surgery and 6 months later. Using the Posttraumatic Stress Diagnostic Scale (PDS), 16.4% of mothers and 13.3% of fathers met full criteria for PTSD at the time of surgical discharge, and another 15.7% of mothers and 13.3% of fathers met partial criteria. At 6 months after surgery, the number of parents who met PTSD criteria declined to 14.9% of mothers and 9.5% of fathers. These rates are similar to other studies performed with parents of children with life-threatening illness. Unfortunately, no assessment of parents was performed prior to surgery to determine if some pre-existing psychologic issues were present (Helfricht, Latal, Fischer, et al., 2008).

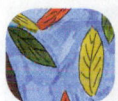

Partnering with Families

Home Care of Children with Congenital Heart Defects Before Surgery

ROUTINE HEALTH CARE

- Wash hands frequently or use alcohol or cleansing gels to prevent transmission of infections to the infant.
- Provide well-child care and all immunizations, including influenza vaccine and monthly injections of palivizumab for respiratory syncytial virus during the fall and winter. Live virus vaccines may need to be postponed for 3 months if surgery is scheduled and blood products will be used.
- Brush the teeth twice a day and provide fluoride treatment if the water is not fluoridated. Have the child visit the dentist beginning at 2 to 3 years of age for preventive dental care.

ADMINISTRATION OF MEDICATIONS

- Give medications safely with a dosage schedule that fits the family's routine.

- Keep digoxin locked up to prevent ingestion by the patient or other children in the family.

SIGNS OF ILLNESS

- Notify the physician if the child has fever, vomiting, or diarrhea. It is important to maintain adequate hydration.
- Notify the physician if the infant or child begins feeding poorly. This may be the initial sign of congestive heart failure.

ACTIVITY

- Allow the child to set his or her own activity level. Children with congenital heart defects usually do not overexert themselves.

Parents should be offered genetic counseling if planning a future pregnancy. Parents may need support and care during pregnancy as fetal echocardiography can identify structural heart defects as early as 18 to 20 weeks' gestation.

Home Care

Children are often managed at home until surgery. The initial important focus is on growth. The parents should encourage feeding but allow the infant to breastfeed or take formula for no longer than 30 minutes, or for the length of time directed by the health provider for infants with complex congenital heart defects or CHF. Breastfeeding is encouraged because of its beneficial effects for the infant, and it is less stressful than bottle-feeding (Cook & Higgins, 2010). Infants should be held at a 45-degree angle to reduce tachypnea. If the infant has difficulty gaining weight, pumping the breasts and supplementing breast milk with calorie fortification may be encouraged. Feedings through a transpyloric, nasogastric, or gastrostomy tube may also be given at night or 24 hours a day to ensure that adequate calories are ingested. Even when tube feedings are used, encourage the infant to take some formula orally to provide positive oral stimulation. See feeding suggestions for the infant with CHF on page 836.

Efforts should be made to reduce the infant's exposure to infectious diseases because illness can further increase the stress on the child's cardiac system. Encourage frequent hand hygiene with soap and water or alcohol gels.

Practice Alert

When children with complex congenital heart defects develop an infection, they may experience problems that cause extra concern such as the following (Cook & Higgins, 2010):

- Severe respiratory infections make hypoxemia worse in children with cyanosis.
- Fever increases the metabolic rate and oxygen demands, which increase the work of the heart.
- Vomiting and diarrhea can lead to dehydration, especially in the infant or child on diuretics.
- If the child has polycythemia, dehydration can lead to thrombus formation.

Regular health promotion visits are important, and all immunizations are provided according to the recommended schedule. Monthly prophylaxis for respiratory syncytial virus with palivizumab should be provided during the peak season for infants less than 24 months of age with congenital heart defects being treated for congestive heart failure or with complex congenital heart defects (American Academy of Pediatrics, 2009). See Chapter 25 🕮. See Partnering with Families: Home Care of Children with Congenital Heart Defects Before Surgery.

Preparation for Surgery

When preschool age or older, prepare the child for the settings, equipment, and experiences to expect during anesthesia induction and in the postoperative period. Pictures or a visit to the intensive care unit (ICU) will be helpful. Follow guidelines for preoperative treatment described in Chapter 15 🕮. If an infant or toddler is having surgery, provide parents with information about how the child will look, equipment that will be used, and what care will be provided in the immediate postoperative period.

Evaluation

Expected outcomes of nursing care include the following:

- The child receives adequate nutritional intake by oral feedings and supplemental tube feeding as necessary.
- The child's growth pattern follows the established growth curve percentile.
- The child receives all age-appropriate immunizations and respiratory syncytial virus (RSV) prophylaxis.
- The parents effectively cope with the stress of the child's condition.

Nursing Management at the Time of Surgery

Children with these heart defects are hospitalized either because of complications, such as congestive heart failure, or for surgery. The goal of nursing management is to perform assessments, provide supportive care to the family, and meet the child's nursing care needs before and after surgery.

Nursing Assessment and Diagnosis

At the time of surgery, the child needs a careful history and physical examination to detect the presence or potential development of any acute illnesses. Assess the child's behavioral patterns, cardiac function, respiratory function, weight, and fluid status. Refer to Table 26–3 on page 808 for additional assessment guidelines for the child with a congenital heart defect of increased pulmonary blood flow.

Critical Care

In the immediate postoperative period the child will be cared for in the ICU. The child's condition is carefully monitored with invasive hemodynamic techniques, laboratory tests (e.g., arterial blood gases, hematocrit, electrolytes, acid–base balance), and physical examination (e.g., vital signs, temperature, SpO$_2$, level of consciousness, peripheral perfusion, and respiratory effort). The heart is auscultated for clarity of heart sounds, and lungs are auscultated to assess breath sounds. Assess for arrhythmias (e.g., tachyarrhythmias, ventricular arrhythmias, and complete heart block) that are common after cardiac surgery involving coronary bypass, or with hemodynamic dysfunction or electrolyte disturbances (Payne, Ziegler, & Gillette, 2011). Monitoring cardiac output is especially important because the child's history of increased pulmonary blood flow can result in increased pulmonary vascular reactivity associated with pulmonary artery hypertension. Monitor fluid intake and output. Monitor the chest or mediastinal tube drainage to ensure the tubes are patent and that bleeding is not occurring. Regularly assess the child's level of pain. See Chapter 21 🔗.

General Nursing Unit

After the child's transfer to the general nursing unit, assessment focuses on signs of surgical complications such as infection, arrhythmias, and impaired tissue perfusion (Figure 26–7 📷). The child may have a cardiac monitor attached or pacer wires in place. Monitor the child's temperature and inspect the surgical incision site if exposed. Fever, excessive incisional pain, spreading erythema around the incision, and wound drainage beginning 3 to 4 days postoperatively may be early signs of infection. Assess the chest and lungs for breath sounds, respiratory effort, and signs of distress that may indicate pneumonia or fluid in the pleural space. Monitor the vital signs, including blood pressure, as well as the SpO$_2$.

Monitor the child's heart rate by auscultating the apical pulse to detect an irregular heart rate or bradycardia. Either condition is an indication of reduced cardiac output that requires immediate intervention. To assess for impaired tissue perfusion, check pulse oximetry (SpO$_2$), capillary refill, extremity warmth, pedal pulses, level of consciousness, and urine output. Reduced urine output is a sign of decreased cardiac output. Continue to assess the child's pain.

Examples of nursing diagnoses following cardiac surgery include the following:

- Breathing Pattern, Ineffective related to respiratory muscle fatigue
- Pain, Acute related to surgical incision and expansion of chest with coughing and deep breathing exercises
- Fluid Volume: Imbalanced, Risk for related to impact of surgery on heart's pumping action
- Infection, Risk for related to surgery and chronic disease status

NANDA-I © 2012

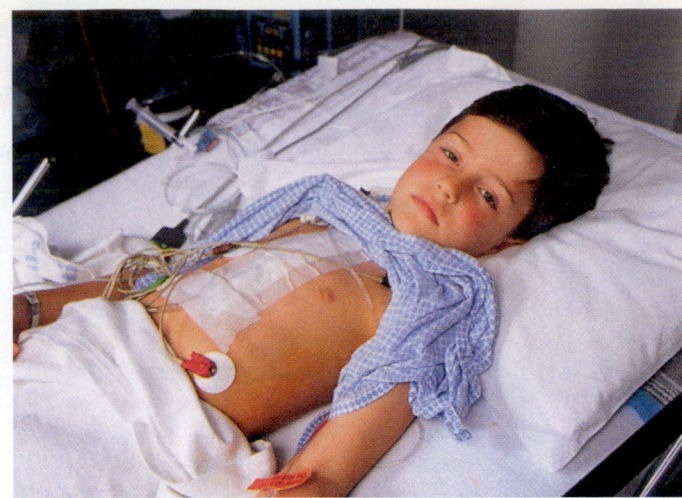

FIGURE 26–7 ■ A child with atrial septal defect repair. Surgery is performed with this type of defect to prevent pulmonary vascular obstructive disease as an adult.

Planning and Implementation

Critical Care Unit

Nursing care following surgery focuses on promoting the child's recuperation. Following surgical correction of the heart defect, the child is usually cared for in an ICU until stable. Depending upon the complexity of surgery and potential complications, the ICU stay may be 1 or more days. The child will be initially intubated and on a ventilator. When the child is stable and able to breathe independently, the ventilator will be turned off. The endotracheal tube will be removed when the child is able to maintain the airway. Suctioning is performed as needed until the child can handle secretions. Several intravenous lines will be placed after the child is under anesthesia to monitor arterial and venous pressures, and to infuse fluids. Nontraumatic blood samples may be obtained from the arterial line. Chest or mediastinal tubes will be placed to drain air, fluids, and blood from around the heart and lungs. Radiant heat warmers may be used to help maintain a child's temperature when unstable or to gradually rewarm a child when hypothermia has been used during surgery. Measures to reduce an elevated body temperature are taken to prevent additional increases in the metabolic rate and oxygen consumption. Electrolyte imbalances are corrected. Enteral nutrition may be initiated to provide essential nutrients and to improve the immune response. Prophylactic antibiotics are usually given postoperatively. Arrhythmias are managed with antiarrhythmia medications.

Pain Management

Pain management with 24-hour intravenous opioids should be provided for 1 to 2 days postoperatively, or until the child is taking fluids. Once the child is taking oral fluids and foods, transition to oral analgesics occurs, and these should also be administered around the clock. Follow the guidelines for pain management provided in Chapter 21 🔗. Teach parents and caregivers to lift and move the child without lifting under the arms to reduce stress on the incision and potential pain.

Promote Respiratory Function

Encourage the child to take deep breaths and cough or to perform spirometry exercises regularly to promote full lung expansion. Bubbles or pinwheels may help young children to take deep breaths. Provide tips for splinting the chest (a pillow or stuffed animal) to

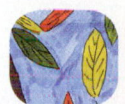

Partnering with Families

Home Care of the Child After Cardiac Surgery

- Place infants in car safety seats for travel home from the hospital. Place a small blanket over the incision to prevent the straps from rubbing the incision area.
- Sponge bathe the infant or use a tub bath with low water level to bathe the child. Avoid soaking the incision until the sutures are out, the Steri-Strips fall off, or the Dermabond has flaked off and the incision is healed. Clean the incision daily with gentle baby or pH-balanced soap as directed by the healthcare provider. Do not use oils, creams, lotions, or ointments on the incision. Cover the incision with a clean shirt or bib to keep it clean and dry. In infants, make a special effort to keep the area under the chin clean and dry to reduce the risk of infection.
- Pick up infants and young children by placing one hand under the head and the other hand under the hips. Avoid picking the child up with hands placed under the arms because this puts stress on the incision and causes pain.
- Allow the child to increase activity gradually as tolerated, starting with quiet play for the first week at home. Report increased fatigue or decreased activity tolerance to the physician. Postpone rough play, bike riding, and strenuous activities for 6 weeks until the sternum incision has healed completely. The child may be allowed to return to school in about 3 weeks; no backpack should be used for several additional weeks.
- Acetaminophen or ibuprofen can be given for pain control. Use the dose appropriate for the weight of the infant or child or as directed by the healthcare provider.

- Encourage a nutritious diet and snacks so the infant or child has an opportunity to catch up for previous growth deficits.
- Call the healthcare provider about any concerns regarding the child's health and recovery.
  - Report any signs of wound infection (redness, swelling, tenderness, or drainage around the incision), fever over 40.3°C (101°F), flulike symptoms, a change in appetite or activity level, irritability, or an increased respiratory rate.
  - High fever, chest pain, and increased respiratory and heart rates occurring within a few weeks of surgery may indicate postpericardiotomy syndrome. The child needs to be evaluated for severity of the condition.
- Antibiotic prophylaxis for infective endocarditis should be given for dental and invasive respiratory procedures as directed for 6 months after corrective surgery when a prosthetic heart valve or prosthetic material is used. See the Medications table on page 843. Report any unexplained fever or illness during the first 2 months following surgery to the child's healthcare provider.
- Live virus vaccines should be postponed after cardiac surgery when blood products have been administered (5 months for packed red cells, 6 months for whole blood) (American Academy of Pediatrics, 2012 p. 38).

reduce the pain associated with coughing and deep breathing. Chest physiotherapy may be performed in children under 3 years of age. See the Skills Manual ⌐⊐.

Manage Fluids and Nutrition

Encourage the infant or child to begin oral fluids and nutrition when permitted. Although oral fluids are rarely limited, intake and output should be assessed carefully. Ask parents to bring in favorite foods to encourage the child to eat when such foods can be tolerated. Promote bowel elimination following surgery, especially when opioids are used for pain management.

Administer antibiotics as ordered. If intravenous antibiotics are continued after the child's oral intake is established, the intravenous line can be converted to a heparin or saline lock; see the Skills Manual ⌐⊐.

Encourage the child to increase activity gradually with longer periods out of bed every day. However, ensure adequate rest periods to promote healing. Provide diversional activities and opportunities for therapeutic play so the child can better manage the stresses associated with pain and frightening procedures.

Discharge Planning and Home Care Teaching

Infants and children may be discharged from the hospital within a few days of surgery. Parents need information to prepare for continuing care of the child at home such as the following:

- Information about the specific cardiac defect, the surgery, and prognosis
- Medications prescribed and their administration
- Care of the incision and identification of worrisome symptoms of infection

- Nutrition and feeding strategies
- Health promotion (activity guidelines, need for hearing screening, ways to promote development)
- Bacterial endocarditis prophylaxis if prescribed

Spreading the education over several days rather than at one session enables the parents to hear information more than once and to identify questions and concerns. See Partnering with Families: Home Care of the Child After Cardiac Surgery.

Prepare parents for potential behavior problems of young children that may result from the stressful experience of the hospitalization. It is not unusual for children to experience nightmares, separation anxiety, and overdependence on parents. Encourage parents to reassure children about their security and to promote play and other means to deal with their feelings. When the child's symptoms continue for several weeks, referral for psychologic assessment and support may be needed for posttraumatic stress disorder. See Chapter 34 ⊚.

Reassure parents of children with complete correction of their cardiac defect that they should have no further cardiovascular problems. Encourage parents to allow the child to live a normal and active life after recovery from surgery. The normalization of the child's life should be reinforced at the surgical follow-up visits.

Evaluation

Examples of expected outcomes of nursing care include the following:

- The child's pain is effectively managed.
- Full lung expansion is regained with spirometry exercises or chest physiotherapy.
- The child's incision heals without infection.

- The child's growth catches up to expected height and weight over the next few months to years.
- The child recovers from the psychologic effects of surgery.

DEFECTS CAUSING DECREASED PULMONARY BLOOD FLOW AND MIXED DEFECTS

Information about these two defect categories is combined in this section because the clinical therapy and nursing interventions are similar. Distinguishing features of each defect are described by etiology, pathophysiology, and clinical manifestations.

Etiology and Pathophysiology

Defects Causing Decreased Pulmonary Blood Flow

Defects or an embryologic failure that obstructs the flow of blood from the right side of the heart to the lungs decreases pulmonary blood flow. This results in little or no blood reaching the lungs to get oxygenated. If an atrial or ventricular septal opening exists between the left and right side of the heart, right-sided pressures exceed those on the left, resulting in right to left shunting. Evidence of cyanosis that does not respond as expected to oxygen is a classic sign of decreased pulmonary blood flow related to congenital heart disease.

Clinical Judgment

Why would the child with decreased pulmonary blood flow not respond to supplemental oxygen with decreased cyanosis?

The kidneys produce the erythropoietin hormone that stimulates the bone marrow to produce more red blood cells, resulting in polycythemia, an excessive increase in the production of red blood cells to increase the amount of hemoglobin available to carry oxygen to the tissues. Chronic polycythemia can result in sluggish blood flow through the small vessels, placing infants and children at increased risk for thromboembolism in the cerebral and pulmonary vessels. Over time the survival time of platelets is reduced, and the synthesis of vitamin K–dependent clotting factors is impaired. These factors increase the infant's risk of bleeding with surgery.

Brain abscesses are more common in children with polycythemia and septal defects associated with decreased pulmonary blood flow. Bacteria in the unoxygenated blood may cross into the systemic circulation through the septal defect, since that portion of the blood does not get filtered by the lung capillaries which serve that function (Park, 2008, p. 145).

When infants and children with cyanosis rise in the morning, they may experience an abrupt decrease in systemic vascular resistance and pulmonary blood flow. This physiologic change can trigger a **hypercyanotic** (hypoxic or "tet") **episode** when combined with a sudden increase in cardiac output and venous return that occur with activities such as crying, feeding, exercise, a warm bath, and straining with defecation. The partial pressure of oxygen (PO_2) is lowered, and the partial pressure of carbon dioxide (PCO_2) rises. In this severe decompensation the hypoxemia becomes progressively worse as the respiratory center in the brain overreacts, increasing the respiratory effort. The additional respiratory effort further increases the cardiac

output and contributes to a life-threatening decline unless rapid intervention is successful.

Mixed Defects

Many complex congenital heart defects involve a combination of defects that fall into one of the previous two categories (defects that increase or decrease pulmonary blood flow). What is unique about them is that the newborn is dependent upon mixing of the pulmonary and systemic circulations for survival during the postnatal period. This mixing of oxygen-saturated and desaturated blood results in a general desaturated systemic blood flow and cyanosis. Pulmonary congestion occurs because of increased pulmonary blood flow and obstruction of systemic flow.

Clinical Manifestations

Defects Causing Decreased Pulmonary Blood Flow

Clinical manifestations in infants initially include cyanosis shortly after birth, dyspnea, and a loud murmur. Cyanosis often occurs when the ductus arteriosus closes, causing hypoxemia. The skin may initially be ruddy or mottled before cyanosis is observed. Cyanosis that does not respond to supplemental oxygen is a classic sign. Signs and symptoms of chronic hypoxemia include fatigue, clubbing of the fingers and toes, exertional dyspnea, and delayed developmental milestones. See Figure 25–18 on page 789 🔗. Infants may need to stop sucking periodically during feedings to breathe, and diaphoresis may be seen with the increased work of eating. These infants have a higher metabolic rate, and inadequate calories may be consumed resulting in poor weight gain. See Table 26–8 for the pathophysiology, clinical manifestations, and clinical therapy for the congenital heart defects that decrease pulmonary blood flow.

Clinical Tip

Cyanosis is typically observed when the amount of reduced hemoglobin in the veins reaches a level of about 5 g/100 mL in a child with a normal hemoglobin level. The ratio of oxygenated and deoxygenated blood is related to the amount of pulmonary blood flow. When there is less pulmonary blood flow, cyanosis is more significant. Cyanosis may also be greater when the tissues demand more oxygen (e.g., crying, feeding, or a higher metabolic rate with fever).

When the infant or child has severe obstruction to pulmonary blood flow, hypercyanotic episodes can occur suddenly. Toddlers with uncorrected cyanotic heart disease often squat to relieve dyspnea (Figure 26–8 ■). The knee–chest or squatting position reduces the cardiac output by decreasing the venous return from the lower extremities and by increasing the systemic vascular resistance. Hypercyanotic episodes usually appear between 2 months and 2 years of age. Signs include:

- Increased rate and depth of respirations
- Increased cyanosis, pallor, and poor tissue perfusion
- Increased heart rate
- Diaphoresis
- Irritability and crying
- Seizures and loss of consciousness

Older children with decreased pulmonary blood flow defects that are not totally corrected may have additional symptoms. Exercise-induced dizziness and syncope are serious signs indicating a need for medical evaluation.

TABLE 26–8 Pathophysiology, Clinical Manifestations, and Clinical Therapy for Heart Defects with Decreased Pulmonary Blood Flow

DEFECT PATHOPHYSIOLOGY

CLINICAL MANIFESTATIONS AND CLINICAL THERAPY

Pulmonic Stenosis

Stenosis is narrowing of a valve, valve area, or great artery above the valve. Stenosis obstructs blood flow into the pulmonary artery, which increases preload (the volume of the blood in the ventricle at the end of diastole) and results in right ventricular hypertrophy. Pulmonic stenosis is the second most common congenital heart defect, accounting for 8% of all cases, and it occurs in combination with 30–50% of other congenital heart defects (Hoffman, Mehrota, & Buckvold, 2011). Stenosis may progress as the heart muscle grows and develops in the subvalvular area.

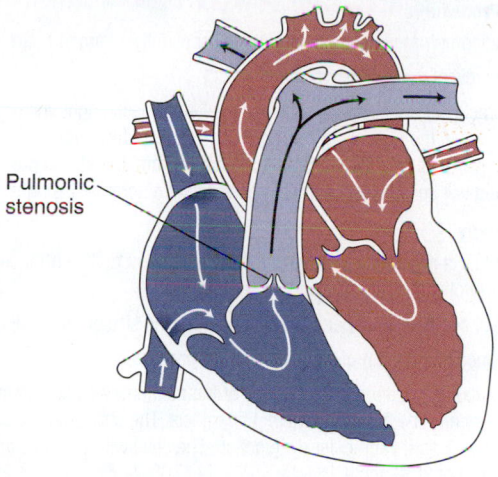

Pulmonic stenosis

■ Decreased unoxygenated blood flow

Clinical Manifestations

Children with mild stenosis may have no symptoms and grow normally.

In moderate stenosis, dyspnea and fatigue occur on exertion. Signs of CHF and hepatosplenomegaly are rare but may result from chronic pressure overload. Heart failure and chest pain on exertion may occur in severe cases.

A loud systolic ejection murmur with a widely split S_2 and thrill may be found in the pulmonic listening area.

Diagnostic Procedures

The chest radiograph may show an enlarged pulmonary artery with normal heart size and normal pulmonary vascularity.

The ECG may demonstrate right atrial enlargement and right ventricular hypertrophy.

The echocardiogram provides information about the pressure gradient across the valve and size of valve ring.

Cardiac catheterization findings include increased right ventricular pressure and a normal or slightly lowered pulmonary artery pressure.

Clinical Therapy

Dilation by balloon valvuloplasty, performed during cardiac catheterization, treats simple pulmonic stenosis.

Surgical valvotomy may still be used, especially when other defects such as VSD are present.

Surgical resection may be needed for narrowing above the valve area. Pulmonary regurgitation may result but is not a significant problem.

Prognosis: Pulmonic stenosis does not typically increase in severity. Lifelong infective endocarditis prophylaxis is needed.

Tetralogy of Fallot

Four defects—pulmonic stenosis, right ventricular hypertrophy, ventricular septal defect (VSD), and overriding of aorta—make up the condition. This results from underdevelopment or hypoplasia of the outflow portion of the right ventricle. Some children have a fifth defect: open foramen ovale or atrial septal defect. It is one of the most common congenital heart defects causing cyanosis and accounts for about 6% of all cases of congenital heart disease (Luxenberg & Torchen, 2011). Elevated pressures in the right side of the heart cause a right to left shunt. The overriding aorta and VSD allow unoxygenated blood to pass into the systemic circulation.

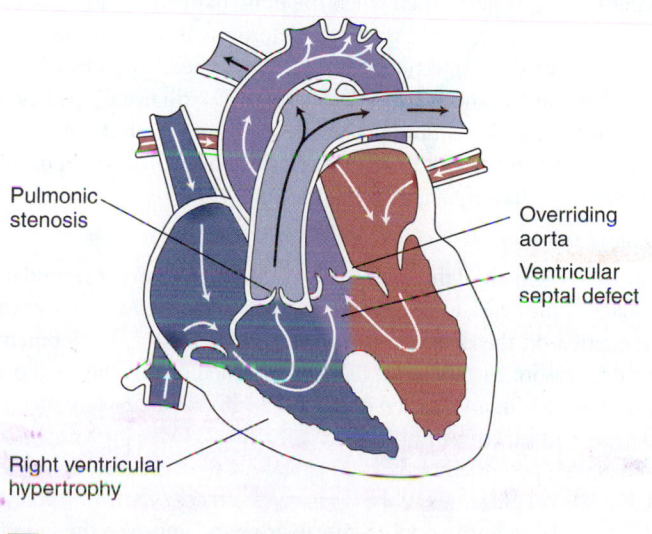

Pulmonic stenosis

Overriding aorta

Ventricular septal defect

Right ventricular hypertrophy

■ Decreased unoxygenated blood flow

■ Mixed oxygenated and unoxygenated blood

Clinical Manifestations

As ductus arteriosus closes, the infant becomes hypoxic and cyanotic. The degree of pulmonary stenosis determines severity of symptoms.

A systolic murmur is heard in the pulmonic area, and a single S_2 is heard. A thrill may also be palpated in the pulmonic area.

Polycythemia, hypoxic episodes, metabolic acidosis, poor growth, clubbing, and exercise intolerance may develop.

Toddlers with uncorrected defects instinctively squat (assume a knee–chest position) to decrease the return of systemic venous blood to the heart. See Figure 26–8.

Diagnostic Procedures

A chest radiograph shows the boot-shaped heart due to the large right ventricle, decreased pulmonary vascular markings, and a prominent aorta.

The ECG shows right ventricular hypertrophy.

The echocardiogram shows the VSD, obstruction of pulmonary outflow, an overriding aorta, and the size of the pulmonary arteries. The condition may be detected by fetal echocardiography.

Cardiac catheterization is usually not performed prior to surgery.

Blood tests reveal an increased hematocrit and hemoglobin levels and an increased clotting time.

Clinical Therapy

Management of hypercyanotic episodes is provided on page 825. Monitoring the child for metabolic acidosis or prolonged unconsciousness is critical.

Many infants have total corrective surgery at about 4–6 months of age, unless a hypercyanotic episode occurs at a younger age. A few children with severe defects may have palliative surgery (modified Blalock-Taussig shunt) performed first to allow the infant to grow prior to surgery.

If prosthetic material is used for the corrective surgery, infective endocarditis prophylaxis is required until 6 months after corrective surgery.

Prognosis: Not all children are cured by surgery, but most have improved quality of life and improved longevity. Right bundle branch rhythm pattern may result from surgery. Ventricular arrhythmias may occur many years after surgery and may cause sudden death (Park, 2008, p. 243).

(continued)

TABLE 26-8	Pathophysiology, Clinical Manifestations, and Clinical Therapy for Heart Defects with Decreased Pulmonary Blood Flow *(continued)*

DEFECT PATHOPHYSIOLOGY

Tricuspid or Pulmonary Atresia

In tricuspid atresia, the tricuspid valve is absent, resulting in no communication between the right atrium and the right ventricle. The right ventricle is hypoplastic (small and nonfunctional). Blood flows to the left side of the heart through a patent foramen ovale. The ductus arteriosus provides the only flow of blood to the pulmonary arteries. Tricuspid atresia accounts for 2.5–3% of congenital heart defects (McDaniel, 2010).

Pulmonary atresia, the absence of communication between the right ventricle and the pulmonary artery, either at the site of the pulmonary valve or in the main pulmonary artery, is a severe form of pulmonary stenosis (McDaniel, 2010).

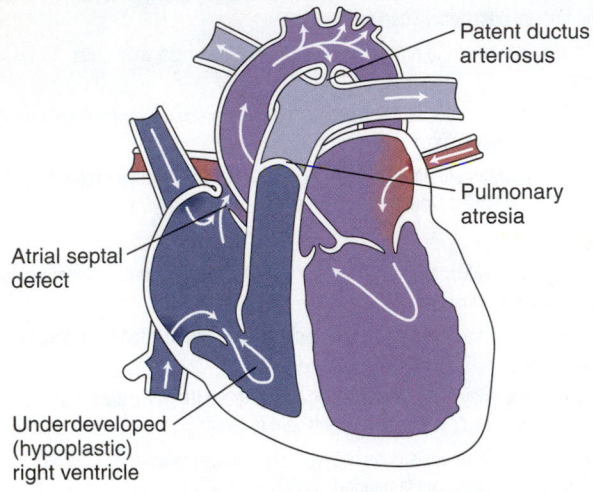

Patent ductus arteriosus

Pulmonary atresia

Atrial septal defect

Underdeveloped (hypoplastic) right ventricle

■ Decreased unoxygenated blood flow

■ Mixed oxygenated and unoxygenated blood

CLINICAL MANIFESTATIONS AND CLINICAL THERAPY

Clinical Manifestations

Cyanosis is present at birth.

Tachypnea, CHF, pulmonary edema, hepatomegaly, acidosis, hypoxic episodes, clubbing, polycythemia, and growth delays occur.

A continuous murmur from the PDA is heard in the pulmonic area. A single S_2 is heard in the aortic area. A harsh systolic murmur may be heard in the tricuspid area in pulmonary atresia.

Diagnostic Procedures

The chest radiograph may reveal a normal-size or slightly enlarged heart.

The ECG may reveal right atrial hypertrophy.

The transthoracic echocardiogram shows a small hypoplastic right ventricular cavity and tricuspid valve, the absence of the right ventricular outflow tract, a dilated right atrium, and right to left shunting across the atrial septum. If a VSD is present, right to left shunting will be detected with the possibility of a normal-size right ventricle.

Clinical Therapy

Prostaglandin E_1 is given immediately to maintain a patent ductus arteriosus. Digoxin and diuretics may be given.

A balloon atrial septostomy is performed to increase the size of the atrial opening.

A Rastelli or modified Fontan procedure results in improved survival.

Prognosis: Outcome depends upon the size of the pulmonary outflow tract developed by surgery and the fibrosis in the right ventricle. The child is at increased risk for arrhythmia and right ventricular dysfunction. The child with tricuspid atresia has a 5-year survival of 80% and a 10-year survival of 70% (Park, 2008, p. 262).

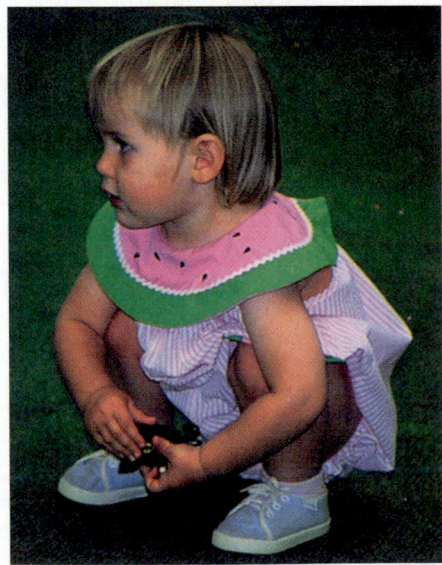

FIGURE 26–8 ■ A child with an unrepaired defect of decreased pulmonary blood flow squats (assumes a knee–chest position) to relieve hypercyanotic episodes.

Mixed Defects

Infants with these complex congenital heart defects have varying degrees of cyanosis and CHF. See Table 26–9 for the pathophysiology, clinical manifestations, and clinical therapy for these complex mixed defects.

Collaborative Care

Diagnostic Procedures

Specific diagnostic procedures are listed in Tables 26–8 and 26–9. A hyperoxia test is performed when the pulse oximetry reading is less than 93% or cyanosis is apparent to determine if the cyanosis is related to the cardiac condition or another cause. See Appendix E ✿. If the infant has a cyanotic heart defect, the PaO_2 will usually be below 150 mmHg and the saturations will be less than 85%, but test results will be higher if the condition is respiratory or neurologic in origin (Hartas, Tsounias, & Gupta-Malhotra, 2009).

Clinical Therapy

Early management of these defects is important to prevent secondary damage to the heart, lungs, and brain, including the adverse effects of hypoxemia on the child's cognitive and psychomotor development. For this reason, corrective surgery is performed during the newborn period or early infancy, when possible. A palliative procedure such as an atrial balloon septostomy may be performed first to preserve life in infants with potentially lethal congenital heart defects and those defects with complications so that corrective surgery can be postponed. This gives the infant an opportunity to grow and improves the success of corrective surgery. See Figure 26–9 ■ for various palliative shunts (surgically created channels for blood flow) that may be performed. Congestive heart failure is treated aggressively (see page 832). See Tables 26–8 and 26–9 for clinical therapy for specific congenital heart defects.

TABLE 26-9	Pathophysiology, Clinical Manifestations, and Clinical Therapy for Mixed Defects

DEFECT PATHOPHYSIOLOGY

CLINICAL MANIFESTATIONS AND CLINICAL THERAPY

Transposition of the Great Arteries (TGA)

In this disorder the pulmonary artery is the outflow tract for the left ventricle, and the aorta is the outflow tract for the right ventricle, creating parallel circulations. This condition is life threatening at birth, and survival initially depends on an open ductus arteriosus and foramen ovale. This condition is one of the most common congenital heart defects causing cyanosis and accounts for up to 10% of all defects (McDaniel, 2010). An ASD or VSD may also be present with TGA.

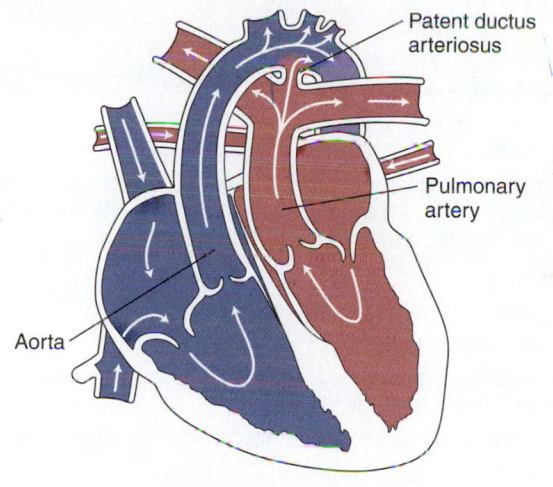

Clinical Manifestations

Cyanosis, apparent soon after birth; progresses to hypoxia and acidosis. Cyanosis does not improve with supplemental oxygen; however, cyanosis may be less apparent when a large VSD is also present.

CHF may develop immediately or over days or weeks.

Tachypnea (60 breaths/min) is often present without retractions or other signs of dyspnea.

A systolic murmur is heard if a VSD is present; otherwise no murmur is generally heard. S$_2$ is loud.

Infants take a long time to feed and need frequent rest periods because of a rapid respiratory rate and fatigue.

Growth failure may be evident as early as 2 weeks of age if corrective surgery is not performed.

Diagnostic Procedures

A chest radiograph may reveal a classic egg-shaped heart on a string (narrow superior mediastinum) with enlarged ventricles and increased pulmonary vascular markings.

The ECG reveals right ventricular hypertrophy.

The echocardiogram reveals the abnormal positioning of the great arteries when the position of arteries arising from ventricles is visible.

Cardiac catheterization shows increased right ventricular pressure, and the catheter can enter the aorta through the right ventricle.

Blood laboratory tests reveal increased hematocrit and hemoglobin levels or polycythemia.

Clinical Therapy

Prostaglandin E$_1$ is initially ordered to maintain a patent ductus arteriosus until a palliative procedure can be performed. Oxygen is administered for severe hypoxia.

Balloon atrial septostomy may be performed during cardiac catheterization in newborns as a first stage to permit oxygenated and unoxygenated blood to mix until surgery is performed. The septostomy is later corrected surgically.

Corrective surgery (arterial switch) is usually performed between 1 and 3 weeks of age.

Prognosis: Survival without surgery is impossible. Few complications occur with the arterial switch procedure. Arrhythmias (sick sinus syndrome, atrial flutter, and atrial fibrillation), decreased right ventricular function, pulmonary vascular disease, and sudden death may be long-term complications associated with previously used surgical procedures (e.g., Mustard and Senning) (Park, 2008).

Truncus Arteriosus

A single large vessel empties both ventricles and provides circulation for the pulmonary, systemic, and coronary circulations. A VSD is usually present. This occurs in approximately 2% of congenital heart defects (McDaniel, 2010).

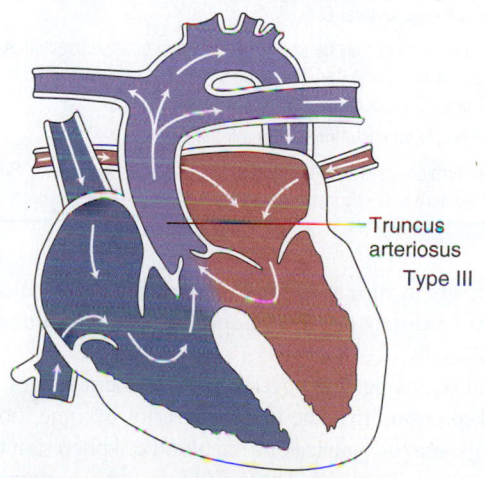

■ Mixed oxygenated and unoxygenated blood

Clinical Manifestations

Cyanosis develops soon after birth; however, this is also a condition of increased pulmonary blood flow. Severe CHF, tachypnea, dyspnea, retractions, fatigue, poor feeding, poor growth, polycythemia, clubbing, increased pulse pressure, bounding peripheral pulses, a widened pulse pressure, frequent respiratory infections, and cardiomegaly also occur.

The VSD produces a harsh systolic murmur in the lower sternal border. A systolic click may be auscultated in the apex and pulmonic area.

Diagnostic Procedures

The chest radiograph shows cardiomegaly, a large aorta, and increased pulmonary vascular markings.

The ECG reveals right and left ventricular hypertrophy.

The echocardiogram shows a VSD, a large single great artery, and one semilunar valve.

Clinical Therapy

Rastelli procedure is performed to close the VSD, enabling the left ventricle to empty into the single large great artery and creating a passage to the pulmonary arteries. Repeated surgery is necessary to enlarge the pulmonary artery conduit as the child grows.

Digoxin and diuretics are given.

Prognosis: Survival from surgery ranges from 10–30% (Park, 2008, p. 281). The long-term prognosis is unknown. Ventricular arrhythmias may develop. The child should not participate in competitive or strenuous sports.

(continued)

TABLE 26–9 Pathophysiology, Clinical Manifestations, and Clinical Therapy for Mixed Defects (*continued*)

DEFECT PATHOPHYSIOLOGY	CLINICAL MANIFESTATIONS AND CLINICAL THERAPY

Total Anomalous Pulmonary Venous Return

The pulmonary veins empty into the right atrium or systemic circulation leading to the right atrium rather than into the left atrium. The foramen ovale must remain patent for mixed blood from the right atrium to pass to the systemic circulation. Any obstruction of the pulmonary veins increases severity of the condition. This occurs in about 1% of all congenital heart defects (McDaniel, 2010).

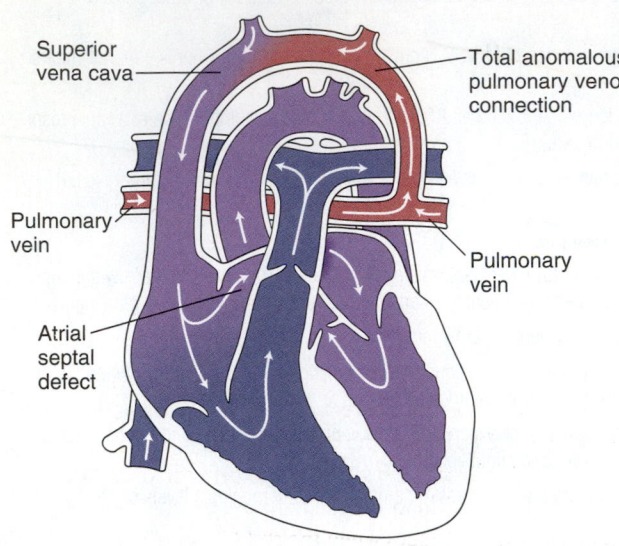

Superior vena cava

Total anomalous pulmonary venous connection

Pulmonary vein

Pulmonary vein

Atrial septal defect

Clinical Manifestations

The infant may have mild cyanosis and tachypnea. Increased cyanosis may occur with feedings as the filled esophagus compresses the common pulmonary vein. When the pulmonary veins are compressed, increased pulmonary blood flow results in tachycardia, dyspnea, pulmonary edema, retractions, crackles, hepatomegaly, poor feedings, irritability, and failure to thrive.

A precordial bulge may be palpated.

The S_2 has a wide, fixed split when there is no pulmonary vein obstruction.

A gallop rhythm is present, and an ejection murmur may or may not be auscultated.

Diagnostic Procedures

The chest radiograph may show cardiac enlargement, and the lung fields may reveal pulmonary edema.

The ECG reveals hypertrophy of the right atrium and ventricle.

The echocardiogram shows a dilated right atrium and ventricle, smaller left-sided chambers, dilated pulmonary arteries, and a patent foramen ovale. It can determine the type of pulmonary drainage and if the pulmonary venous return is obstructed.

Clinical Therapy

Prostaglandin E_1 is given to maintain a patent ductus arteriosus.

Digoxin and diuretics are given to treat CHF.

Balloon atrial septostomy may be performed to increase blood flow to the left side, so surgery can be delayed until the infant is stabilized.

Surgery to reconnect or baffle the pulmonary veins to the left atrium is performed.

Prognosis: Survival without surgery is not possible. Children may develop pulmonary vein obstruction or atrial arrhythmias.

Double Outlet Right Ventricle

The aorta and pulmonary artery both arise from the right ventricle, and the only outlet for the left ventricle is a large VSD. Increased pulmonary blood flow and reduced systemic blood flow occur unless pulmonic stenosis is present. This occurs in less than 1% of all congenital heart defects (Park, 2008, p. 287).

Clinical Manifestations

Cyanosis, tachypnea, and signs of CHF occur in the neonatal period. Failure to thrive occurs.

A loud S_2 and a systolic murmur are heard at the upper left sternal border, with or without a systolic thrill.

Diagnostic Procedures

Chest radiography may show a normal heart size or cardiomegaly. Pulmonary vascular markings may be decreased or increased, and a prominent pulmonary artery segment may be seen.

The ECG shows right axis deviation, right atrial hypertrophy, right ventricular hypertrophy, and right bundle branch block. First-degree AV block may be present.

An echocardiogram shows the origin of both great arteries from the anterior right ventricle, the absence of the left ventricle outflow, and the ventricular septal defect.

Clinical Therapy

Digoxin and diuretics are used to treat CHF.

A modified Blalock-Taussig shunt may be performed when cyanosis is severe. A balloon atrial septostomy is performed when the VSD is too small. Surgery performed is the arterial switch or Rastelli procedure, depending upon co-existing defect.

Infective endocarditis prophylaxis is often required for life.

Prognosis: Ventricular arrhythmia should be treated to prevent sudden death. Some patients need future surgery to revise the surgical correction.

If closure of the ductus arteriosus causes life-threatening shock in newborns, such as those with tricuspid atresia, pulmonary atresia, transposition of great arteries, and truncus arteriosus, prostaglandin E_1 (PGE$_1$) is prescribed to reopen the ductus arteriosus. These infants depend on a patent ductus arteriosus for survival or improvement in pulmonary or systemic blood flow. Treatment with PGE$_1$ provides time for the newborn to be transferred to a cardiac center for diagnostic evaluation and surgical intervention. Response time to PGE$_1$ varies depending on the type of defect.

Adverse effects include respiratory depression and apnea, so the infant must be closely monitored and sometimes ventilation must be assisted.

The child's hemoglobin level and hematocrit values must be monitored to ensure that the blood does not become too viscous. Polycythemia may be managed by red blood cell pheresis if the blood viscosity becomes too high. These children are also monitored for anemia, as they do not tolerate the lower hemoglobin and oxygen-carrying capacity.

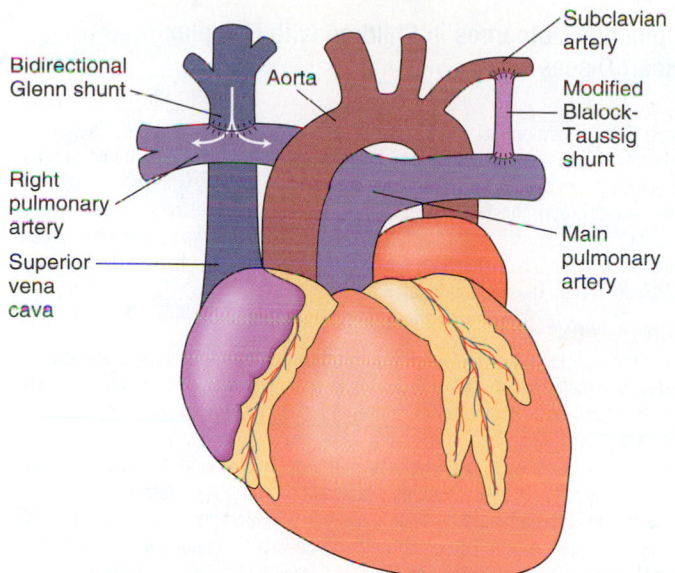

FIGURE 26–9 ■ Anatomic location of the modified Blalock-Taussig and Glenn shunts for palliative procedures.

Labels on figure: Bidirectional Glenn shunt, Aorta, Subclavian artery, Modified Blalock-Taussig shunt, Right pulmonary artery, Main pulmonary artery, Superior vena cava

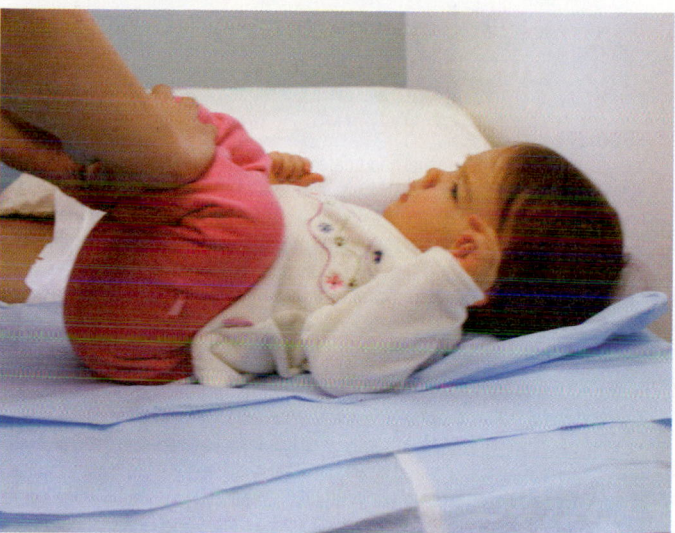

FIGURE 26–10 ■ Place the infant who has a hypercyanotic episode in the knee–chest position. This position increases systemic vascular resistance in the lower extremities.

Infective endocarditis Prophylactic antibiotics for infective endocarditis are required for most children with complex cardiac defects prior to surgery and for 6 months after surgery. See Box 26–3 for the children who need lifelong prophylaxis. See Medications Used for Infective Endocarditis Prophylaxis for Dental and Invasive Respiratory Procedures on page 843.

Hypercyanotic episodes Oral propranolol may be prescribed to prevent hypercyanotic episodes (Park, 2008, p. 239). Hypercyanotic episodes are treated aggressively. To increase the systemic vascular resistance, the child is placed in the knee–chest position (Figure 26–10 ■). Reduce any irritating or painful stimuli, and make efforts to calm the child. Supplemental oxygen is provided. If the hypercyanotic episode is not relieved with these measures, more aggressive treatment is initiated. Start an intravenous line to provide sedation, morphine to decrease agitation, and a fluid bolus to increase central venous pressure.

BOX 26–3	**Cardiac Conditions Needing Infective Endocarditis Antibiotic Prophylaxis**

- Previous infective endocarditis
- Unrepaired cyanotic congenital heart defect
- For 6 months following complete repair of a congenital cardiac defect using prosthetic material during surgery or cardiac intervention.
- Use of a prosthetic cardiac valve or prosthetic material for valve repair
- Use of prosthetic materials for repair of complex congenital heart defects, including palliative shunts and conduits (e.g. for single ventricle defects), or a residual effect remains near or at the site of the prosthetic material that inhibits endothelialization
- Heart transplantation after which the recipient develops cardiac valve dysfunction

Source: *From Wilson, W., Taubert, K. A., Gewitz, M., Lockhart, P. B., Baddour, L. M., et al. (2007). Prevention of infective endocarditis: Guidelines from the American Heart Association Rheumatic Fever, Endocarditis, and Kawasaki Disease Committee, Council on Cardiovascular Disease in the Young, and the Council on Clinical Cardiology, Council on Cardiovascular Surgery and Anesthesia, and the Quality of Care and Outcomes Research Interdisciplinary Working Group. Circulation, 116, 1736–1754; Duval, X., & Lepert, C. (2008). Prophylaxis of infective endocarditis: current tendencies, continuing controversies. Lancet, 8, 225–232; and McDonald, J. R. (2009). Acute infective endocarditis, Infectious Disease Clinics of North America, 23(3), 643–664.*

A beta-blocker may be given to reduce the heart rate and reduce any heart muscle spasms. Dopamine or phenylephrine may be used to increase systemic vascular resistance. Metabolic acidosis is treated if present. Packed red blood cells may be administered to improve oxygen delivery to the tissues when the child is anemic. Postpone all unpleasant procedures. Once a hypercyanotic episode has occurred, immediate palliative or corrective surgery is often scheduled.

Long-term clinical therapy Children with complex congenital heart defects require lifelong assessment and medical care following palliative or corrective heart surgery. Some need multiple stages of surgery, revisions of previous surgeries, valve replacements, or interventional cardiac catheterization to reopen valves or vessels that have become stenotic. An implanted pacemaker may be needed for arrhythmias associated with anomalies of the conduction system or unavoidable surgical incisions in the areas of the sinoatrial node or sinoventricular node. The Mustard, Senning, and Fontan procedures, as well as TOF repairs, are associated with increased risk of arrhythmias. A pacemaker may be used in older children with potentially life-threatening AV block or ventricular arrhythmias, as described for Tim in the opening scenario (Park, 2008, pp. 451–455). Why would these children be at greater risk for arrhythmias?

Outcomes and prognosis Most children with congenital heart disease have normal IQ scores, and children with corrected simple defects can lead normal lives; however, neurologic insults can occur for many reasons. Conditions such as congestive heart failure and cyanosis can affect gross motor development. Infants with complex congenital heart defects are at risk for preoperative neurologic insult. Inadequate nutrition during the first year of life, when rapid brain development occurs, places the infant at greater risk. Some infants are at risk for neurodevelopmental problems because of structural brain abnormalities, abnormal cerebral blood flow, chromosomal abnormalities, and cerebral ischemia. Infants with cyanosis who also have iron deficiency anemia may develop a cerebrovascular accident. Another potential cause of a stroke is thrombus formation during cardiac catheterization or surgery that may become an embolus (Cook & Higgins, 2010). Cardiopulmonary bypass and deep hypothermic circulatory arrest used in most surgery for congenital heart disease may

Evidence-Based Practice

Neurodevelopmental Outcomes in Children with Complex Congenital Heart Disease

PROBLEM

Infants with serious congenital heart defects are exposed to pathophysiology (prolonged hypoxemia, profound acidosis, and low cardiac output) because of the timing of surgical interventions. In addition, nutrition may have been less than adequate for their metabolic rate and brain growth. With the rising potential for children with complex congenital heart defects to have developmental and cognitive problems, parents and school officials need information to evaluate and plan for educational supports as necessary.

EVIDENCE

A longitudinal study of 131 infants with complex congenital heart defects explored neurologic and developmental outcomes. It specifically excluded infants that were expected to have neurologic problems prior to surgical intervention (e.g., prematurity, chromosomal abnormalities, and radiographic evidence of brain malformation). Infants were assessed prior to surgery, and 56% had abnormalities on the neurologic examination; similar findings were found on the postoperative examination. Upon follow-up of 94 children at school entry, 28.4% had neurologic abnormalities and 5% had severe impairments. Mean intelligence quotient (IQ) scores were found to be in the low-normal range (in the 90s). Approximately 20% of the children had cognitive difficulties. Behavior problems (e.g., withdrawal, anxiety, sadness, somatic symptoms) were common in this population. A majority of parents (75%) expressed concerns about their child's development. Education supports were provided to 22% of the children and 23% were receiving rehabilitation services. This study revealed that a large percentage of children with complex congenital heart defects have neurodevelopmental abnormalities prior to surgery (Majnemer, Limperopoulos, Shevell, et al., 2008; Majnemer, Limperopoulos, Shevell, et al., 2009).

Another study evaluated the neurocognitive functioning of 45 European children between ages 6 and 16 years scheduled for elective open heart surgery compared with 41 healthy peers. Children diagnosed with genetic syndromes, cognitive impairment (IQ < 70), and severe learning disabilities were excluded. Results revealed that the children with scheduled cardiac surgery demonstrated neurocognitive deficits in motor planning and visual memory when compared with the control group. This finding was true in patients scheduled for their first surgery as well as those scheduled for follow-up surgery. It was speculated that these deficits may be associated with the cardiac disease rather than cardiac surgery (Van der Rijken, Hulstijn-Dirkmaat, Kraaimaat, et al., 2009).

IMPLICATIONS

The pathophysiologic effects of congenital heart defects and surgery are associated with motor and cognitive problems in some children. Affected children may have difficulties with executive functioning skills such as problem solving and memory, as well as visual-spatial and visual-motor skills. Children with heart defects that are related to poor systemic perfusion beginning in the fetal period are more likely to have lower IQ scores (Majnemer et al., 2008). These cognitive deficits may lead to learning disabilities in children who have congenital heart defects. Regular developmental screening of these children is important to identify the specific neurodevelopmental problems that could be present. Evaluations should be conducted over time to identify behavior problems and learning disabilities. Children may need to have an individualized education plan (IEP) developed when disabilities affect learning.

CRITICAL THINKING APPLICATION

Develop an outline of important information for a parent of a child with a complex congenital heart defect to discuss with the child's teacher and school officials when the child enters school. Using information about developing an IEP in Chapter 16 🔗, identify important steps for a parent to take when it is anticipated that a child could have a learning disability resulting from the congenital heart defect and surgery.

---

contribute to the development of neurodevelopmental problems (Cook & Higgins, 2010). See Evidence-Based Practice: Neurodevelopmental Outcomes in Children with Complex Congenital Heart Disease.

Nursing Management

Nursing management of the hospitalized child focuses on monitoring PGE₁ therapy (for newborns only; used until palliative surgery is performed), treating hypercyanotic episodes, and providing postsurgical care. Nursing management also involves supporting parents to care for the child at home until initial or subsequent surgery is to be performed by reducing parental anxiety, providing guidelines for adequate nutrition, helping parents recognize signs of illness or progression of the child's condition, and formulating a plan for emergency treatment.

Nursing Assessment and Diagnosis

Physiologic Assessment Prior to Surgery

The cardiovascular status of infants receiving PGE₁ therapy needs to be closely monitored in the neonatal intensive care unit. Assess vital signs, heart rhythm, skin color, peripheral pulses, and capillary refill time. Observe for signs of improvement in vital signs and color as the oxygen saturation increases and acidosis decreases following the initial treatment, as well as adverse effects. In some cases these infants need endotracheal intubation and assisted ventilation. Because these infants are at risk for CHF, additionally monitor for tachycardia, tachypnea, crackles, frothy secretions, low urine output, and pulmonary edema.

Practice Alert

Common side effects of PGE₁ therapy include cutaneous vasodilation, bradycardia, tachycardia, hypotension, seizure activity, fever, and apnea.

Prior to or between stages of surgery, the infant or child is seen regularly to assess growth and to assess for signs of progressive deterioration in cardiac status. Monitor physiologic status using the assessment guidelines in Table 26–3. These children are at risk for growth problems that affect height, weight, and head circumference. The child's weight, length, and head circumference measurements are plotted on a growth curve to monitor the significance of the growth problems.

The child who has not had corrective surgery needs careful observation for signs of increased cyanosis in the morning or at other high-risk times. Observe for neurologic signs of thromboembolitic complications from polycythemia such as headache, dizziness, excessive irritability, and paralysis. Older children with cyanotic defects may have clubbing of the fingers and toes (see Figure 25–18 on page 789 🔗).

Assessment Following Surgery

Children are admitted to the intensive care unit following surgery. Children undergoing video-assisted thoracostomy surgery may go to the postanesthesia unit and a short-stay unit for discharge the same day. Refer to the section on nursing assessment of the child with increased pulmonary blood flow on page 816 for nursing care guidelines. Once the child is transferred to the general nursing unit, monitor the child's heart functioning. Assess vital signs, pulse oximetry, skin color, perfusion of the skin by capillary refill, and distal pulses. Monitoring fluid intake and output following surgery is critical. A sudden sustained increase in pulse and respirations and a decrease in peripheral perfusion may be early signs of hemorrhage. Note any signs of respiratory distress that may indicate the development of a pneumothorax or CHF.

Psychosocial Assessment

Assess the parents' need for information and emotional support. In some cases, the infant's condition is first identified at birth; however, congenital heart defects are also being identified by fetal sonogram or echocardiogram. The parents will be grieving the loss of a perfect newborn and will be extremely anxious about the infant's condition and prognosis.

Examples of nursing diagnoses that may apply to a child with decreased pulmonary blood flow include:

- Cardiac Output, Decreased related to ventricular restriction and an obstructed outflow tract
- Infection, Risk for related to unfiltered bacteria in the blood and sites of blood shunting that promote bacterial growth
- Pain, Acute related to palliative or corrective surgery
- Caregiver Role Strain related to care of a child with chronic illness
- Activity Intolerance related to cyanosis and dyspnea on exertion
- Growth and Development, Delayed related to profound hypoxemia
- Therapeutic Regimen Management: Family, Ineffective related to complexity of therapeutic regimen: assessment and management of unpredictable hypercyanotic episodes

NANDA-I © 2012

Planning and Implementation

Home Care of the Child Before Surgery

Infants with tetralogy of Fallot and other defects are often managed at home initially as they grow and potentially improve surgical outcome. Parents are usually anxious because of the need to wait before surgery can be performed. They often fear that the infant will not survive until surgery or that they will be unable to manage any problems the infant may have. Provide parents with information and teach them how to care for the child at home. Some infants have such special home care needs that home health nursing and other community services are required. Many of these children require supplemental nutrition and oxygen for emergencies. These children maintain a low oxygen saturation rate because unoxygenated blood mixes with oxygenated blood, and oxygen has no effect on improving the oxygen saturation level.

Promoting Development

Cyanosis with or without CHF often results in delayed gross motor skills. Parents become concerned that the level of cyanosis will damage the brain. Make referrals to community-based early intervention programs so that developmental specialists can help parents set realistic developmental goals for the child.

Encourage parents to treat the infant as normally as possible. Children with mild cyanotic lesions do not need to adjust activity. The child with moderate to severe disease should be able to tolerate crying for a few minutes without difficulty.

Clinical Tip

Crying may improve cyanosis caused by lung disease or disorders of the central nervous system. In children with heart defects that cause cyanosis, crying usually makes cyanosis worse. Prolonged crying should not be permitted because it causes fatigue and further hypoxia.

Caring for a Hypercyanotic Episode

Hypercyanotic episodes become life threatening if not treated immediately. The child becomes progressively more hypoxic and limp, loses consciousness, is likely to have a seizure or cerebrovascular accident, and may die. These episodes commonly develop between 4 and 6 months of age. Teach parents to observe for signs of worsening cyanosis, particularly in the morning, that could signal the beginning of a hypercyanotic episode. Some families may be provided with a pulse oximeter to assess oxygen saturation daily. Knowledge of the child's typical SpO_2 is important to help parents identify a change that may indicate an emergency.

Provide guidelines for the initial management of the hypercyanotic episode. The parents should call for an ambulance and try to calm and reassure the infant. The infant should be placed in knee–chest position; parents should hold the infant facing the parent's chest, place one arm under the infant's knees, fold the infant's legs up toward the infant's chest, and use the other arm to support the infant's back. Alternatively, the infant can be placed supine with the knees bent up toward the chest (see Figure 26–10). If oxygen is available, provide it in a manner that does not further upset the infant. If none is available in the home, the emergency medical technicians will administer oxygen during transport to the emergency department.

Clinical Tip

Develop an emergency care plan for the infant in anticipation of acute problems such as a hypercyanotic episode or respiratory distress. Parents should learn cardiopulmonary resuscitation. Provide parents with a card or brief history form with information about the child's condition, medications, necessary emergency care, and the physician's name, so emergency care providers have vital information for the initial treatment of the child. The American Academy of Pediatrics has a model emergency information form in English and Spanish. See the companion website.

Managing Illnesses

Teach parents to promptly report signs of illness to the physician. Fever increases the metabolic rate and causes further stress on the heart. Vomiting and diarrhea may lead to dehydration, a particular risk in children with polycythemia that can make the blood become even more viscous and potentially cause a thrombus. Additionally, dehydration leads to decreased systemic vascular resistance, resulting in a further decreased blood flow to the pulmonary system and increased cyanosis. Aggressive management with antipyretic medication and fluid volume replacement is necessary.

Teach parents to observe the child for signs of infective endocarditis, including low-grade fever, fatigue, and malaise. They need to notify the physician if these symptoms occur within 2 months of surgery or a high-risk procedure. Educate parents about the need to request antibiotic prophylaxis for the child.

Although parents may travel with children who are cyanotic, they should not take them to areas of high altitude without first consulting with the physician. Supplemental oxygen when traveling on an airplane may be necessary.

Hospital-Based Care of Infant and Child

Care of the Newborn

Monitor and carefully maintain the central, umbilical, or peripheral intravenous lines in the newborn receiving continuous infusion of PGE_1. Observe the infant for side effects of prostaglandin treatment. Have intubation equipment and a resuscitation bag and mask at bedside in case of apnea. Have intravenous fluids available to control hypotension.

Infants and Toddlers Prior to Surgery

Avoid any unpleasant or anxiety-provoking procedures in an effort to prevent a hypercyanotic episode. If a hypercyanotic episode occurs, follow guidelines for treatment on page 825. Immediately notify the physician for further orders if these procedures are ineffective and the episode continues.

Following Surgery

The child is initially cared for in the intensive care unit as described on page 818. Postoperative bleeding is a potential risk in children with polycythemia, because bleeding times are prolonged and platelet counts are low. Chest tube output is monitored carefully for bright red blood or excessive volume. Bright red blood in the chest tube is a significant sign of hemorrhage. Fluids and diuretics are used to maintain preload in the right ventricle whereas **inotropic medications** (agents that improve the velocity of heart contractility) are used to support cardiac output. Children are transferred to the general nursing unit once heart function has stabilized.

Once the child returns to the general nursing unit, nursing care is the same as described for the child having surgery for increased pulmonary blood flow. See page 818.

Community-Based Care After Surgery

Adolescents need to be supported as they transition to assuming responsibility for their own care. Practice guidelines now recommend coordination of care of adults with complex congenital heart disease between the primary care provider and a cardiologist based in a regional center with expertise in the care of adults with congenital heart disease (Sable et al., 2011). See the Health Promotion & Maintenance Overview on page 829.

Evaluation

Examples of expected nursing care outcomes include the following:

- Appropriate emergency treatment is provided to the child with a hypercyanotic episode.
- The parents effectively manage medical illnesses and fever at home to prevent dehydration and thromboembolism.
- The family copes with stress of the child's condition and other family demands.
- The child demonstrates developmental progress in gross motor, fine motor, and language skills following surgery.

DEFECTS OBSTRUCTING SYSTEMIC BLOOD FLOW

Etiology and Pathophysiology

An anatomic stenosis (narrowing of a valve, the area around the valve, or in the great artery above the valve) causes obstruction to blood flow and results in a pressure load on the left ventricle and decreased cardiac output. The greater the narrowing, the more obstructed the blood flow is to the systemic circulation. Neonates with severe left outflow obstruction or left ventricular dysfunction often develop decreased cardiac output and shock.

Clinical Manifestations

Clinical manifestations of these congenital heart defects are those associated with a low cardiac output: diminished pulses, poor color, delayed capillary refill time, and decreased urinary output. The blood cannot move past the obstruction, so it backs up into the left atrium and then into the lungs, causing congestive heart failure and pulmonary edema. With mild obstructions, the child may have leg cramps, cooler feet than hands, and stronger pulses and higher blood pressure in the upper extremities than the lower extremities. Decreased blood supply to the gastrointestinal tract may result in necrotizing enterocolitis. See Chapter 30 ⬤. See Table 26–10 for the pathophysiology, clinical manifestations, and clinical therapy for the congenital heart defects that obstruct systemic blood flow.

Clinical Tip

The blood pressure, which is usually 10 to 15 mmHg higher in the legs than the arms, may be lower in the legs than the arms when the child has coarctation of the aorta, a defect that obstructs systemic blood flow.

Collaborative Care

Neonates with critical left outflow obstruction or left ventricular dysfunction may develop decreased cardiac output and shock. PGE_1 and inotropes may be required to support the systemic circulation until the obstruction is relieved or ventricular function improves.

Nursing Management

Children with aortic stenosis and coarctation of the aorta should have nursing care as described in the nursing management sections in Congenital Heart Defects That Increase Pulmonary Blood Flow on page 813. Infants with hypoplastic left heart syndrome should have nursing care as described in the nursing management sections in Defects Causing Decreased Pulmonary Blood Flow and Mixed Defects on page 820. (See Complementary Therapy: Medication Interactions on page 831.)

Parents of children with life-threatening defects such as hypoplastic left heart syndrome are under intense pressure to make a decision about the best treatment for their child. For this condition there is no cure, and a decision must be made that is best for their individual situation (the Norwood or Sano surgical procedure, a heart transplant, or palliative care). Many newborns must be transferred to a regional cardiac surgery center. Parents are faced with the potential death of the newborn before having an opportunity to grieve the loss of a healthy infant or cope with their emotions. Parents attempting to understand the newborn's condition may have difficulty fully understanding informed consent for palliative procedures. Unless the congenital heart defect was diagnosed through fetal echocardiogram, the parents do not have much time to carefully weigh the information about the various treatment options. Nurses have an important role in supporting parents through this difficult decision-making period. Share the following information with parents so they are fully informed for decision making: treatment options and their associated mortality, the intense care that the surviving child will need, the potential for neurocognitive and neurodevelopmental disabilities, and unknown long-term survival. Seek the support of other family members, clergy, or social workers to assist the parents through this period. Infant hearts for transplant are often not available. Many parents feel the need to give the newborn the best chance of survival with surgery. See Box 26–4 on page 831. If parents choose comfort or palliative care, interventions such as PGE_1 are discontinued, and the infant is given appropriate pain medication and comfort. The newborn may be cared for at home with hospice support services. (See Chapter 18 ⬤.) Reassure parents that they are good parents, no matter what decision they make.

Health Promotion & Maintenance Overview

The Adolescent with Congenital Heart Disease

DISEASE PREVENTION STRATEGIES

- Ensure that the adolescent completes all immunizations, including the influenza vaccine annually.
- Encourage visits to the dentist twice a year for cleaning and restoration of decayed teeth as needed. Make sure the adolescent knows this is one way to reduce endocarditis risk.
- Ensure that the adolescent has a healthcare home for general health and illness care. Provide appropriate health screening according to recommended schedules (see Chapter 13 📎).
- Discuss the future treatment needed for the condition and frequency of cardiac evaluations.
- Encourage female adolescents to initiate gynecologic care to ensure that appropriate care is provided for sexual health and contraception. For example, estrogen-based contraception is contraindicated for many females with complex congenital heart defects because of the risk of thromboembolism (Sable et al., 2011). Ensure that the adolescent understands that special care during pregnancy may be needed to reduce risks to the mother and fetus.
- Provide counseling about health risks associated with tobacco use, alcohol and drug use, and unprotected sex.

NUTRITION

- Encourage the adolescent to eat nutritious meals and snacks, and to avoid excess weight gain that could stress the heart function.
- Adolescents with polycythemia should drink adequate water to maintain hydration.

PHYSICAL ACTIVITY

- Inquire about the adolescent's preferred exercise and activity level. An individualized assessment with graded exercise testing on a treadmill or bicycle should be performed in all adolescents with congenital heart disease, and an exercise prescription with heart rate goals should be provided. Repeat exercise testing if new symptoms or changes in clinical status develop (Sable et al., 2011).
- Discuss any activity or other limitations, such as strenuous work or sports participation.

ENDOCARDITIS RISK AND PROPHYLAXIS

- For adolescents at increased risk for infectious endocarditis, discuss situations that could contribute to the development of endocarditis such as body piercing, tattooing, acupuncture, electrolysis, dental care, intrauterine device for contraception, and various diagnostic and surgical procedures. Teach adolescents about the signs and symptoms of endocarditis so they can seek medical care promptly.
- Provide education about antibiotic prophylaxis and the need to inform all healthcare providers about the heart condition if prophylaxis is needed. Provide the adolescent with the guidelines for medications used for endocarditis prophylaxis published by the American Heart Association. See page 843.

MENTAL AND SPIRITUAL HEALTH

- Discuss the adolescent's concerns for the future, as there may be significant uncertainty about the disease course and outcome.
  - Identify and refer adolescents as needed for counseling or to a support group of adolescents of similar age with congenital heart disease.
  - Begin the process of transitioning the adolescent to adult health care in which full responsibility for ongoing health care will become the role of the individual rather than the parents.

PATIENT EDUCATION

- Provide education directed to the adolescent about the specific nature of the congenital heart defect, surgeries that have been performed, and the types of symptoms resulting. Provide information about specific signs that require a physician to be notified. Remember that previous education has been targeted to the parents. Correct any misperceptions that prior surgery has resulted in a normal heart if that is not the case.
- Provide a written summary of the key points regarding medical management of the adolescent's condition that can be used when visiting other health professionals (e.g., surgeons, dentists, other medical specialists). This summary should include diagnosis, surgeries or other interventions, current cardiac status, medications, baseline functional status, recommended restrictions, and expectations regarding disease progression (Sable et al., 2011).
- Discuss the medications needed and why, and develop plans for the adolescent to assume responsibility for self-administration. Educate the adolescent to seek guidance before using over-the-counter medications and herbal medications because of the potential for medication interaction.
- Discuss the genetic aspects of the condition and provide resources for genetic counseling if desired.
- Discuss the danger signs of the condition (such as arrhythmias, or the potential of dehydration in an adolescent with cyanosis) and how to seek urgent or emergency care. Role-play may help the adolescent gain confidence in seeking advice from health professionals.

VOCATIONAL EDUCATION

- Reassure the adolescents who have had complete repairs of the congenital heart defect and have no disabilities that they have no limitations in their career or vocational selection.
- Provide career and vocational counseling to adolescents with cardiac disabilities that match their interests, academic abilities, and clinical limitations, and encourage preparation for employment that can be maintained throughout the working career. If a job application asks about disabilities, the adolescent does not need to disclose the heart problem if it will not interfere with the job being sought.
- Inform adolescents with congenital heart disease–related disabilities about their rights under the Americans with Disabilities Act of 1990.
- Families and patients should be informed to research health insurance options before the adolescent is no longer eligible for coverage on the parents' plan. Adolescents should be informed that healthcare coverage is an important benefit to investigate when considering any future job change.

CONGESTIVE HEART FAILURE

Congestive heart failure (CHF) is a disorder of circulation in which cardiac output is inadequate to support the body's circulatory and metabolic needs. It may result from a congenital heart defect that causes either increased pulmonary blood flow or obstruction to the systemic outflow tract, from problems with heart contractility and arrhythmias, or from pathologic conditions that require high cardiac output, such as severe anemia, acidosis, or respiratory disease. CHF

TABLE 26–10 Pathophysiology, Clinical Manifestations, and Clinical Therapy for Heart Defects That Obstruct the Systemic Blood Flow

DEFECT PATHOPHYSIOLOGY	CLINICAL MANIFESTATIONS AND CLINICAL THERAPY

Aortic Stenosis

Narrowing of the aortic valve obstructs blood flow to systemic circulation. The narrowing may be subvalvular, at the valve, or supravalvular. Aortic stenosis accounts for 10% of all cases of congenital heart defects (Park, 2008). This defect is often associated with a bicuspid (two valve leaflets) rather than normal tricuspid valve. The pressure gradient across the valve usually increases during periods of rapid growth with the associated increase in cardiac output because the valve does not grow at a comparable rate. The left ventricle hypertrophies to force the blood past the narrowed valve opening, and it may progress to left ventricular failure (Holmes & McCarville, 2011).

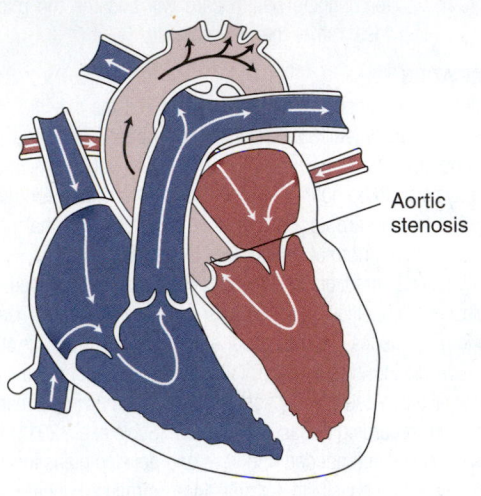

Aortic stenosis

☐ Decreased oxygenated blood flow

Clinical Manifestations

A majority of infants and young children are asymptomatic and grow and develop normally. Some newborns have life-threatening aortic stenosis noted at birth. CHF develops in infants with significant stenosis.

The blood pressure is normal, but a narrow pulse pressure may be noted. Peripheral pulses may be weak.

Occasionally the child complains of chest pain and dyspnea after exercise, but exercise intolerance is uncommon. Fainting and dizziness are serious signs that require intervention.

A systolic heart murmur and thrill occur in the aortic or pulmonic listening areas with transmission to the neck. An ejection click may be heard. Splitting of the S_2 may be noted with severe aortic stenosis. Aortic insufficiency may result from interventions, causing a high-pitched diastolic decrescendo murmur along the left sternal border near the mitral area.

Diagnostic Procedures

The chest radiograph is usually normal but may reveal a slight prominence of the left ventricle and aorta with increased severity.

The ECG is usually normal in mild cases but may show mild left ventricular hypertrophy and inverted T waves with increased severity.

An echocardiogram reveals the number of the valve cusps, pressure gradient across the aortic valve, and size of the aorta.

Exercise testing may be used in asymptomatic children to determine amount of obstruction present and allowable exercise for the child.

Clinical Therapy

Newborns with life-threatening aortic stenosis need PGE_1 to maintain a patent ductus arteriosus until the aortic valve can be dilated.

The aortic valve may be successfully dilated by balloon valvuloplasty or by surgical valvotomy. Surgical treatment is palliative rather than curative. Aortic valve replacement (Ross procedure) is performed when stenosis is severe or if significant regurgitation results from other interventions.

Prognosis: Chest pain, syncope, and sudden death can occur in symptomatic children, particularly during vigorous exercise. Increasing left-side obstruction or aortic insufficiency may develop as the child ages. Stenosis may reoccur following intervention and may worsen as the valve calcifies. Valve replacement may be necessary once adulthood is reached, often requiring lifelong anticoagulant therapy. Lifelong infective endocarditis prophylaxis is required.

Coarctation of the Aorta

Narrowing or constriction of the descending aorta, often near the ductus arteriosus or left subclavian artery, obstructs systemic blood outflow. This defect is relatively common, occurring in 5–8% of all children with congenital heart disease. The defect occurs in 30% of children with Turner syndrome (Awad & McCarville, 2011).

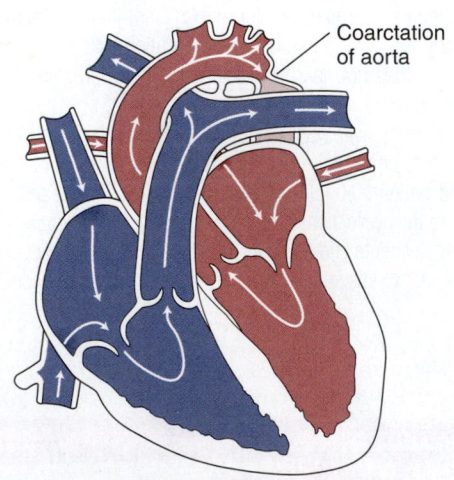

Coarctation of aorta

Clinical Manifestations

Many children are asymptomatic and grow normally, but infants with severe constriction may show signs of cyanosis in the lower extremities, heart failure, and shock as the ductus arteriosus closes. Renal failure and necrotizing enterocolitis may develop. Infants with moderate constriction may have poor feeding, failure to thrive, increased respiratory effort, and CHF.

Reduction in blood flow through the descending aorta causes lower blood pressure in legs and higher blood pressure in arms, neck, and head. Brachial and radial pulses are typically bounding, but femoral pulses are weak or absent.

Older children may complain of weakness and pain in the legs after exercise.

S_2 is loud and single on auscultation. A systolic ejection murmur may be heard at the upper right and middle or lower left sternal border. A thrill may be palpated in the suprasternal notch.

Diagnostic Procedures

The chest radiograph may reveal cardiomegaly, pulmonary venous congestion, and indentation of descending aorta. Rib notching (change in the smooth contour of the rib apparent on radiograph) from collateral vessels is rarely seen before 10 years of age.

ECG shows left ventricular hypertrophy, and right ventricular hypertrophy may be seen in severe cases.

Echocardiogram permits measurement of the size of the aorta and the actual coarctation, and it assesses the functioning of the aortic valve and left ventricle.

CT scan and MRI show the site of the coarctation as well as better imaging of the aortic arch and collateral circulation.

TABLE 26–10	Pathophysiology, Clinical Manifestations, and Clinical Therapy for Heart Defects That Obstruct the Systemic Blood Flow (*continued*)
DEFECT PATHOPHYSIOLOGY	**CLINICAL MANIFESTATIONS AND CLINICAL THERAPY**

Coarctation of the Aorta, continued

Clinical Therapy

In symptomatic newborns, PGE_1 is given to reopen the ductus arteriosus and promote blood flow to the lower extremities. Treatment to prevent congestive heart failure may be initiated with inotropic medications, diuretics, and oxygen (Park, 2008). Surgical resection is often preferred initially rather than balloon dilation to reduce the risk for coarctation. Balloon dilation may be performed for re-coarctation (Park, 2008). Some older children are treated with balloon angioplasty with stent placement in the coarctation segment (Awad & McCarville, 2011).

Prognosis: Balloon dilation and surgical resection are palliative, as coarctation may recur with either procedure. Lifelong follow-up is necessary. Persistent hypertension occurs in some children.

Hypoplastic Left Heart Syndrome

Absence or stenosis of mitral and aortic valves is associated with an abnormally small left ventricle and a small aortic arch. It accounts for about 1.5% of congenital heart defects (Awad & Busse, 2011). As one of the most severe congenital heart defects, an estimated 45% of children with this defect die prior to 5 years of age (Park, 2008, p. 273).

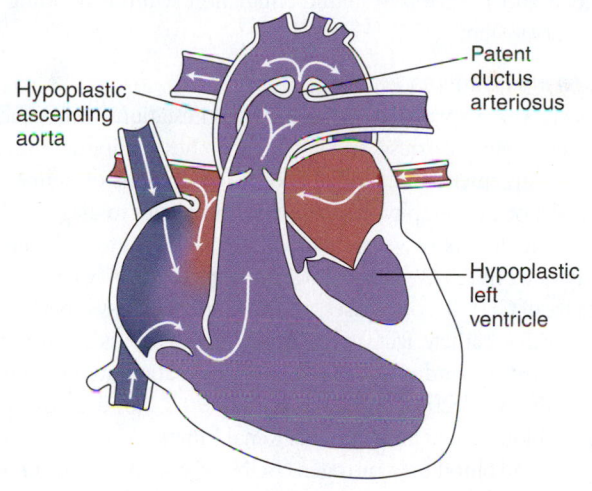

Hypoplastic ascending aorta

Patent ductus arteriosus

Hypoplastic left ventricle

■ Mixed oxygenated and unoxygenated blood

Clinical Manifestations

With closure of ductus arteriosus, the newborn develops progressive cyanosis, tachycardia, tachypnea, dyspnea, retractions, and decreased peripheral pulses.

Poor peripheral perfusion, respiratory distress, pulmonary edema, and CHF eventually lead to shock, metabolic acidosis, and death.

A single loud heart sound is present, and often no murmur is present.

Diagnostic Procedures

The chest radiograph shows cardiomegaly and increased pulmonary venous congestion.

The echocardiogram shows the small left ventricle. Fetal echocardiography can diagnose this condition.

Clinical Therapy

Prostaglandin E_1 is given immediately to maintain a patent ductus arteriosus.

Supplemental oxygen is avoided.

Three treatment options are currently available for these infants: the Norwood and Sano procedures, a heart transplant (see page 840), and comfort or palliative care.

Surgery is performed in three stages. The Norwood stage 1 procedure is performed in the first week of life (reconstruction of the aorta, committing the right ventricle to pumping blood through the pulmonary valve to the aorta, and creating a Sano shunt to get adequate blood to the lungs). The Norwood stage 2, connecting the superior vena cava directly to the pulmonary artery (Glenn shunt), is performed at about 3–6 months of age. The stage 3 Fontan procedure, performed at 2–3 years of age, connects the inferior vena cava to the pulmonary circulation, ending the mixing of oxygenated and deoxygenated blood.

Few infant hearts are available for transplantation, but this procedure adds complications of immune suppression, graft rejection, and coronary artery disease (Awad & Busse, 2011).

Prognosis: Survival is not possible without intervention, and survival after the 3-stage surgery is low. The child having successful surgery will have some limitations in physical activity because of a single ventricle. Many of these children have significant cognitive and neurologic impairment (see page 826).

---

also results from acquired heart disease, such as cardiomyopathy or Kawasaki disease. The incidence is unknown, but an estimated 15% to 25% of children with congenital heart defects develop CHF (Madriago & Silberbach, 2010).

Complementary Therapy **Medication Interactions**

Caution parents of children with congenital heart defects treated with anticoagulants, digoxin, or diuretics to avoid using complementary therapies such as herbal products because of their potential interaction with prescribed medications. Ginkgo and ginseng increase the effect of anticoagulants. St. John's wort interacts with warfarin (Coumadin) to decrease the drug's effect. Ginseng may interact with furosemide and cause drug resistance. St. John's wort interacts with digoxin and decreases the drug level (Holcomb, 2009).

BOX 26–4 **Research: Perceptions of Cost for Families**

A study involving interviews with parents of 20 children (ages 1 day to 5 years) hospitalized after surgery for congenital heart disease investigated out-of-pocket and nonmedical costs associated with the child's condition and its effect on family functioning. Financial impact on the family included dramatic reductions in income when a job was changed or lost because childcare was not available. Unpredictable out-of-pocket expenses included food and lodging for travel to the cardiac center, prescriptions, prescribed formula, parking fees and other costs during hospitalization, and medical charges not covered by health insurance. The social and emotional costs to the family were high, including taking siblings out of social and school activities to decrease the ill child's exposure to infection. The family's emotional and financial burden increased with greater disease complexity. Family uncertainty was a major theme as parents felt the need to be prepared for anything that could happen (Connor, Kline, Mott, et al., 2010).

Etiology and Pathophysiology

Blood volume overloads associated with congenital heart defects are the most common cause of CHF in infants. Many infants with this pathophysiology develop CHF within the first 6 months of life (McDaniel, 2010). Some defects shunt blood from the left side of the heart to the right when the left ventricle contracts so that extra blood must be pumped to the pulmonary system rather than through the aorta. This overloads the pulmonary system, and if prolonged can lead to pulmonary artery hypertension, an often irreversible condition leading to life-threatening pulmonary vascular resistance (see page 840). Obstructive congenital defects (e.g., pulmonary or aortic stenosis) restrict the flow of blood, so the ventricles hypertrophy and work harder to force blood through these structures. Eventually the heart muscle cannot keep up with the demand. Several congenital heart defects can cause congestive heart failure during the first months of life, such as hypoplastic left heart syndrome, aortic atresia, transposition of the great arteries, coarctation of aorta, a large ventricular septal defect, atrioventricular canal, and tricuspid atresia (McDaniel, 2010).

When cardiac output remains insufficient, the body's organs and tissues do not receive adequate oxygen. The renin-aldosterone-angiotensin system, the sympathetic nervous system, and cytokine-induced inflammation are activated. The decreased cardiac output leads to production of metabolites in various organ systems, which in turn stimulate vasodilation and decreased blood pressure. The falling blood pressure stimulates angiotensin and kidney mechanisms to retain fluid, as well as stimulating an increase in systemic vascular resistance. Tachycardia, enhanced myocardial contractility, and hypertrophy of the myocardium result from activation of the sympathetic nervous system and increased release of catecholamines. These actions initially improve the cardiac output and maintain blood pressure, a form of compensated shock. Yet, this continuing increased work for the heart worsens symptoms (Madriago & Silberbach, 2010). Ultimately, the heart muscle cannot stretch the fibers any further to accommodate increased volume in the ventricles, and the force of contractions is decreased. This leads to progressive systemic edema and pulmonary congestion. Initially the right or left side of the heart may fail, but eventually failure is bilateral.

Clinical Manifestations

Initial signs of CHF may be subtle and not immediately recognized. The infant tires easily, especially during feeding. Weight loss or lack of normal weight gain, diaphoresis, irritability, and frequent respiratory infections may be evident. Older children may have exercise intolerance, dyspnea, abdominal pain or distention, and peripheral edema. Skin color changes such as mottling or pallor are seen.

As the disease progresses, symptoms such as tachypnea, tachycardia, pallor or cyanosis, nasal flaring, grunting, retractions, cough, or crackles may occur. An S_3 **gallop** (a third heart sound that produces a rhythm like the gait of a horse) may be auscultated. Generalized fluid volume overload is seen more commonly in toddlers and older children. Periorbital and facial edema and hepatomegaly are signs of fluid volume excess. Exercise intolerance, anorexia, cough, wheezing, crackles, and jugular venous distention are seen in older children. See the Clinical Manifestations table on congestive heart failure for more detail.

Cardiomegaly, enlargement of the heart by hypertrophy of its muscles, is a compensatory mechanism as the heart attempts to maintain cardiac output. Cyanosis, weak peripheral pulses, cool extremities, hypotension, and heart murmur are precursors of cardiogenic shock, which can occur if CHF is not adequately treated. (Cardiogenic shock is discussed beginning on page 859.)

Collaborative Care

The goals of medical management are to make the heart work more efficiently and to remove excess fluid. This decreases the cardiac workload and improves systemic circulation without flooding the pulmonary system.

Diagnostic Procedures

Diagnosis is based primarily on clinical manifestations such as tachycardia, respiratory distress, and crackles. A chest radiograph reveals cardiac enlargement and venous congestion or signs of pulmonary edema. Echocardiography confirms CHF and helps to diagnose specific cardiac defects or ventricular dysfunction and to estimate the severity of CHF. An electrocardiogram helps to identify an arrhythmic cause of CHF. In some cases, an endocardial biopsy is performed during cardiac catheterization to diagnose myocarditis or cardiomyopathies. See Appendix E ❷ for more information about diagnostic procedures. Electrolytes, lactic acid, arterial blood gases, and a complete blood count are obtained. Renal function is evaluated with creatinine and blood urea nitrogen (BUN) levels. Liver function tests may be elevated. See Appendix D ❷ for expected laboratory values.

Clinical Therapy

The first goal of medical management is to treat the cause of CHF, such as stopping an arrhythmia. The next goal is to maximize cardiac output and tissue perfusion while enabling the heart to work more efficiently and to remove excess fluid. This decreases the heart's work and improves systemic circulation without flooding the pulmonary system. Diuretics, such as furosemide, bumetanide, chlorothiazide, and spironolactone, are given to promote fluid excretion and

Clinical Manifestations Congestive Heart Failure	
ETIOLOGY	**CLINICAL MANIFESTATIONS**
Pulmonary venous congestion	Mild resting tachypnea, wheezing, crackles, retractions, cough, grunting, nasal flaring, cyanosis, recent onset of poor feeding, increased tachypnea and diaphoresis during feeding
Systemic venous congestion	Tender and enlarged liver, ascites, periorbital edema, peripheral edema, and weight gain associated with retained fluids; jugular vein distention and dependent edema in older children
Impaired cardiac output	Tachycardia, weak pulses, hypotension, capillary refill time greater than 2 seconds, pallor, cool extremities, oliguria, tiring with play, restlessness, irritability
High metabolic rate	Failure to thrive or slow weight gain, diaphoresis

Medications Used to Treat Congestive Heart Failure

DRUG	ACTION	NURSING MANAGEMENT
Digoxin (Lanoxin)	Increases myocardial contractility, improving systemic circulation	Assess the heart rate for 1 minute prior to giving a dose to detect bradycardia or changes in heart rhythm or quality. Have the dose verified by a second nurse. Monitor the child for digoxin toxicity. See page 834 for more nursing management.
Furosemide (Lasix)	Rapid diuresis; blocks reabsorption of sodium and water in renal tubules	Monitor patients during rapid diuresis for vital signs, intake and output, and fluid and electrolyte imbalances. Monitor for hypokalemia. Assess for digoxin toxicity if hypokalemia is present.
Thiazides (Diuril): Chlorothiazide (suspension) Hydrochlorothiazide (tablets)	Maintenance diuresis, decreases absorption of sodium, water, potassium, chloride, and bicarbonate in renal tubules	Monitor blood pressure and intake and output rates and patterns. Monitor lab values for hypokalemia. Assess for digoxin toxicity if hypokalemia is present.
Spironolactone (Aldactone)	Maintenance diuresis (potassium sparing)	Assess for signs of fluid and electrolyte imbalance, and digitoxicity.
ACE (angiotensin-converting enzyme) inhibitor (Captopril, Enalapril)	Promotes vascular relaxation and reduced peripheral vascular resistance, reduces afterload	Monitor for hypotension with initiation of therapy and dosage changes. Assess for common side effects such as cough, hyperkalemia, and worsening renal function.
Propranolol (Inderal)	Increases contractility	Monitor vital signs and peripheral perfusion. Monitor intake and output ratio and daily weight. Dietary sodium is usually restricted.
Carvedilol (Coreg)	Improves left ventricular function, promotes vasodilation of systemic circulation for chronic heart failure and dilated cardiomyopathy	Give with food. Assess the heart rate for bradycardia when the dose is increased. Monitor for hypotension in the first hour after administration. Assess cardiac output by monitoring tissue perfusion, peripheral pulses, blood pressure, and urine output. Plasma digoxin concentration may be increased with this drug. Monitor for digoxin toxicity. Monitor liver function periodically.

Source: Data from Wilson, B. A., Shannon, M. T., & Shields, K. M. (2011). Pearson nurses' drug guide 2011. New York, NY: Pearson; and Torres, M., & Nieves, J. A. (2009). Progress in congenital cardiac care for newborns and infants: The emerging role of "off-label" medications. Newborn and Infant Nursing Reviews, 9(1), 18–30.

decrease preload. Because most diuretics (except for spironolactone) cause potassium loss, serum potassium levels are monitored and potassium supplements may be ordered.

Inotropic medicines and afterload-reducing agents (such as ACE inhibitors) are sometimes used to lessen the workload of the heart and help it to work more efficiently. Digoxin is the drug most commonly used to slow the heart rate, increase cardiac filling time, and therefore increase cardiac output. Occasionally a higher than normal dose is given initially, followed by a lower maintenance dose. This process, called **digitalization,** speeds the child's response to the drug to achieve therapeutic blood levels more quickly. The safety and effectiveness of beta-blockers, such as propranolol and carvedilol, were tested in a randomized controlled trial in children, but these drugs failed to make significant improvements in the clinical severity of cases versus controls managed by placebo (Madriago & Silberbach, 2010).

Surgery or interventional catheterization to correct a congenital heart defect may become the treatment of choice when congestive heart failure is difficult to manage. Cardiac transplantation may be performed for children with end-stage cardiomyopathy or complex congenital heart defects such as hypoplastic left heart syndrome (see page 831).

Other medical therapy is supportive. Airway management, ventilatory support, rest, and fluid and dietary management are also part of the treatment plan. Oxygen may be ordered (Figure 26–11 ■). Most children improve rapidly after medication is administered. See Medications Used to Treat Congestive Heart Failure.

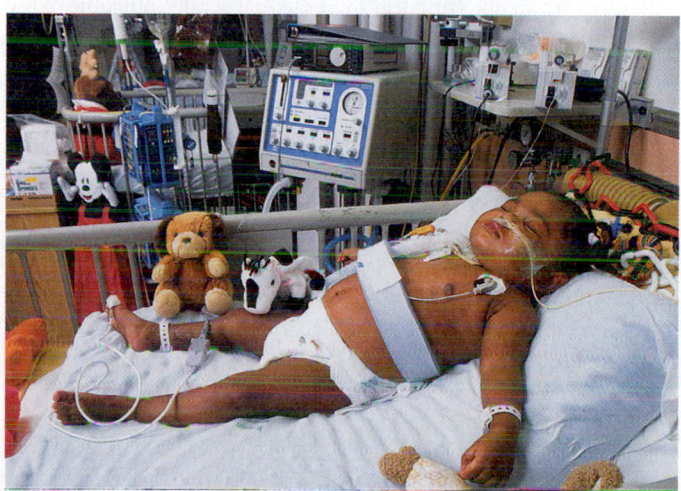

FIGURE 26–11 ■ This infant is receiving intravenous fluids and being ventilated with supplemental oxygen. Note the generalized edema. Her condition is being continuously monitored for congestive heart failure following open heart surgery.

Nursing Management

The focus of nursing care is careful assessment of the child and family, promoting oxygenation and cardiovascular functioning, safely administering medications, fostering growth and development, and helping the family plan to care for the child at home.

Nursing Assessment and Diagnosis

Physiologic Assessment

As diagnosis of CHF depends primarily on physical symptoms, nursing observations are important. Assess the child's behavioral patterns, cardiac function, respiratory function, and fluid status using the guidelines on page 808. Use the age-specific heart and respiratory rates in Chapter 7 to identify tachycardia and tachypnea. Obtain a detailed history of the onset of symptoms from the parents, as CHF often develops slowly. Be suspicious of developing CHF if feedings take 30 minutes or longer.

Clinical Judgment

What changes in vital signs, behavior, and fluid status would indicate that an infant's or child's CHF is progressing in severity?

Measure intake and output carefully. Weigh the infant's diapers before use and after changing. The difference in weight provides information about output (1 g = 1 mL urine). Weigh the child at the same time each day because fluid volume varies throughout the day. Assessment of weight and weight gain is important to determine the child's response to treatment and need for surgical intervention. Some children have difficulty gaining weight as inadequate calories are consumed for the energy expended feeding. In other children weight gain may be noticed, and it is important to determine if it is fluid or growth accounting for the weight gain.

Observe for changes in peripheral edema and circulation. If ascites is present, take serial abdominal measurements to monitor changes (see the Skills Manual ⬭ for guidelines). Turn the child frequently to assess the skin for redness and breakdown.

Family Assessment

Take a history of the child's previous hospitalizations and assess the family's knowledge about the child's condition. Families of children with CHF are anxious and fear the potential serious outcome of the problem and the need to provide ongoing care. Assess the family's anxiety level and coping strategies. Evaluate the family's economic status. Medication is crucial to treatment, and a family's inability to afford or obtain the necessary medications jeopardizes the child's ability to survive.

Assess the parents' understanding of the child's condition and ability to provide the necessary care at home. Correct medication dosage is critical. Extensive time is needed to feed the infant so that adequate nutrition is obtained. Identify the parent's or caregiver's ability to make the observations of change in the child's condition as well as to provide needed care. Find out if another family member is available who could support young parents to ensure that the child's needs are met or to provide respite care.

Developmental Assessment

Because fatigue limits the activities of the child with CHF, he or she does not have the opportunity to practice the skills needed to attain normal developmental milestones. Perform developmental assessment with a tool such as the Denver II (see Chapter 8 ⬭). In addition, parents can provide information about the attainment of expected developmental milestones such as sitting, manipulating objects, standing, or walking. When CHF is well controlled, the child's energy level increases and developmental skills often improve. In infants and toddlers, assessments every 2 to 3 months are useful to observe development and evaluate disease management.

Parents may limit the child's contact with other children because of frequent infections and exercise intolerance. Ask parents about contact and play with other children and a typical day's activity schedule.

Several nursing diagnoses that may apply to the child with congestive heart failure are given in the accompanying Nursing Care Plans. The primary nursing diagnosis is Cardiac Output, Decreased related to cardiac anomaly.

Planning and Implementation

Nursing care for the child with CHF focuses on administering and monitoring effects of medications, maintaining adequate oxygenation and myocardial function, promoting rest, fostering development, providing adequate nutrition, and providing emotional support to the child and family.

Administer and Monitor Prescribed Medications

Children with CHF usually receive digoxin and diuretics. These medications are potent and must be administered correctly. Before giving the digitizing dose of digoxin, establish baseline vital signs, assess the quality of the peripheral pulses and clinical symptoms, and also obtain an electrocardiogram. Check serum electrolytes, and monitor serum potassium (if diuretics are given as a low potassium level increases the risk for digoxin overdose) and hepatic and renal function. Assess hydration status, and hydrate if hypovolemic.

Before giving any dose of digoxin, take the apical pulse for 1 minute. Call for a physician's advice *before* administering the digoxin in the following conditions:

- The heart rate is less than 60 to 100 beats/min, depending upon age (e.g., less than 100 in infants), or is higher or lower than the guideline noted in the physician's order.
- Changes in heart rhythm or quality are noted.

Practice Alert

Observe the child carefully for signs of digoxin toxicity. Early signs include cardiac arrhythmias in children. Early indicators in adults (nausea, vomiting, anorexia, diarrhea, visual disturbance) are rarely the initial signs of toxicity in children. Obtain a serum digoxin level at least 6 hours after the daily dose. Monitor the serum digoxin levels closely during antibiotic therapy as altered intestinal flora may precipitate digoxin toxicity.

Maintain Oxygenation and Myocardial Function

Oxygen therapy may be ordered. Ensure that tubing is patent, the oxygen flow rate is correct, the oxygen delivery device is working properly, and humidification is provided. Keep the child calm and quiet. Place the child in a semi-Fowler or 45-degree angle position to promote maximum oxygenation.

Promote Rest

Group assessments and interventions together to ensure that the child has some uninterrupted rest each hour. Rocking is restful and comforting for infants. Encourage older children to engage in quiet activities such as playing board or computer games or watching videos and reading.

Nursing Care Plan | The Child Hospitalized with Congestive Heart Failure

INTERVENTION	RATIONALE	EXPECTED OUTCOME
1. Nursing Diagnosis: Cardiac Output, Decreased related to cardiac anomaly (VSD)		
NIC Priority Intervention—*Hemodynamic Regulation:* Optimization of heart rate, preload, afterload, and contractility		**NOC Suggested Outcome**—*Cardiac Pump Effectiveness:* Extent to which blood is ejected from the left ventricle per minute to support systemic perfusion pressure
GOAL: *The child's cardiac output will be sufficient to meet the body's metabolic demands.*		
■ Administer digoxin as ordered.	■ Digoxin increases contractility of the heart and force of contraction.	The child's cardiac output is sufficient as indicated by increased energy, adequate feeding intake, and decreased edema.
	■ Digoxin may cause bradycardia. Pulse and heart sounds provide information about heart functioning.	
■ Use a cardiac monitor if prescribed.	■ The monitor notes bradycardia and arrhythmias.	
■ Monitor the serum potassium level and for digitoxicity.	■ Hypokalemia increases the risk of digitoxicity.	The child maintains normal serum potassium levels and therapeutic levels of digoxin.
■ Provide for rest periods each hour.	■ Rest decreases the need for high cardiac output.	The child rests hourly and has adequate energy to eat and play.
GOAL: *The child will manifest adequate oxygenation.*		
■ Evaluate respiratory rate and lung sounds. Use pulse oximetry to determine oxygen saturation readings.	■ Respiratory rate, lung sounds, and pulse oximetry provide information about oxygenation and ease of respiration.	The child maintains a normal SpO_2 level and respiratory rate for age without evidence of adventitious sounds or diaphoresis.
■ Provide oxygen and humidification if prescribed. Observe for diaphoresis, a sign of increased respiratory effort.	■ Supplemental oxygen decreases tachypnea, and humidification moistens secretions to keep the airway clear.	
■ Place the child in a semi-Fowler position.	■ This position facilitates lung expansion.	
2. Nursing Diagnosis: Fluid Volume: Excess related to heart failure		
NIC Priority Intervention—*Fluid Management:* Promotion of fluid balance and prevention of complications resulting from abnormal or undesired fluid levels		**NOC Suggested Outcome**—*Fluid Balance:* Balance of water in the intracellular and extracellular compartments of the body
GOAL: *Intake and output will be balanced once excess fluid is excreted.*		
■ Administer diuretics as ordered.	■ Diuretics mobilize fluids and facilitate excretion.	The child's intake and output are proportional, and electrolyte levels remain within normal ranges.
■ Measure intake and output carefully. Weigh diapers to assess output of infants. Weigh daily. Measure abdominal girth daily. Observe for peripheral edema.	■ Adequate output is a good indicator of renal perfusion. Assessments demonstrate effectiveness of treatment.	
■ Monitor electrolytes.	■ Electrolyte imbalance is common when diuretics are given.	
■ Maintain fluid restrictions if prescribed.	■ Fluid restriction is sometimes used to decrease cardiac load.	
3. Nursing Diagnosis: Skin Integrity, Risk for Impaired Related to Altered Fluid Status		
NIC Priority Intervention—*Pressure Management:* Minimizing pressure to body parts		**NOC Suggested Outcomes**—*Tissue Integrity: Skin and Mucous Membranes:* Structural intactness and normal physiologic function of skin and mucous membranes
GOAL: *The child's peripheral and central edema will decrease.*		
■ Provide frequent skin care for edematous body parts and elevate extremities.	■ Edematous skin injures easily. Elevation promotes return of fluid from extremities.	The child has no skin breakdown after edema resolves.
■ Change the child's position frequently.	■ Position change promotes circulation to skin over pressure points.	
■ Inspect skin frequently for redness and skin breakdown over pressure points.	■ Inspection identifies earliest stages of skin breakdown.	

(continued)

Nursing Care Plan   The Child Hospitalized with Congestive Heart Failure, *continued*

INTERVENTION	RATIONALE	EXPECTED OUTCOME
4. Nursing Diagnosis: Nutrition, Imbalanced: Less than Body Requirements related to high metabolic needs and rapid tiring while feeding		
NIC Priority Intervention—*Nutrition Management:* Assistance with or provision of a balanced dietary intake of food and fluids		**NOC Suggested Outcome**—*Nutrition Status:* Extent to which nutrients are available to meet metabolic needs
■ Hold the infant at a 45-degree angle for feeding.	■ Position facilitates breathing while eating.	The infant or child gains recommended weight according to growth grids. All dietary requirements are met, and mealtimes are pleasant.
■ Record intake carefully.	■ Evaluation of intake indicates whether caloric and other nutritional needs are met.	
■ Weigh the child daily.	■ Weight indicates growth (in absence of fluid retention).	
■ Give frequent small meals with rest periods in between.	■ Digesting small meals requires less energy.	
■ Use high-calorie formula or give high-calorie snacks.	■ High-calorie formulas and snacks provide calories efficiently.	
■ Use soothing approaches such as holding infants for feeding and having parents eat with the older child.	■ A restful approach facilitates intake with minimum cardiac work.	
■ Transition to supplemental tube feedings if the infant is not able to gain weight.	■ Tube feedings provide added calories without taxing the infant's energy.	
5. Nursing Diagnosis: Coping: Family, Compromised related to unknown nature of child's disease		
NIC Priority Intervention—*Caregiver Support:* Provision of necessary information, advocacy, and support to facilitate primary patient care by someone other than healthcare professional		**NOC Suggested Outcome**—*Family Coping:* Family actions to manage stressors that tax an individual's resources
GOAL: *Parents will express lessened anxiety as hospitalization proceeds.*		
■ Encourage parents to room in or stay with their child. Explain procedures and treatment. Involve parents in care as much as possible. Have parents plan the child's play periods.	■ Involvement in the child's care lessens parental anxiety and fear of the unknown.	Parents participate in developing and implementing the treatment plan and providing care to the child.
■ At discharge, provide clear instructions and information about what to do in an emergency, and whom and where to call with questions.	■ Having resources available provides feelings of security.	
■ Allow parents to verbalize questions, concerns, and feelings. Refer parents to support groups or other resources as needed.	■ Emotional support is needed to lessen anxiety.	

NANDA-I © 2012

Foster Development

Encourage parents to play with the child, using toys to stimulate eye–hand coordination and fine motor movements. Such toys include rattles, blocks, and stuffed animals for infants, and books, paper and pencil, and dolls for older children. Encourage sitting, standing, or walking for short periods with adequate rest afterward to promote the development of large muscles. Singing, talking, and playing music encourage the development of cognitive and language skills.

Provide Adequate Nutrition

Teach parents about feeding techniques. The mother who chooses to breastfeed the infant should not be discouraged. The antibodies contained in breast milk reduce infections, and the milk is naturally low in sodium. However, the sucking involved in feeding may cause dyspnea and force the infant to rest frequently during feeding. Frequent small feedings may be the best approach. Infants should be burped frequently to permit rest and prevent vomiting. Make sure parents understand that changes in feeding habits (decreased intake, vomiting, sleeping through feedings, increased perspiration with feedings) may indicate deteriorating cardiac status.

Clinical Tip

Ways to decrease the work of feeding, either with breast or bottle, include the following (Cook & Higgins, 2010):

■ Hold the infant at a 45-degree angle. If the parent gets fatigued due to the long feeding time, the infant can be shifted to an infant seat at a 45-degree angle. This position helps to decrease venous return to the heart and reduce metabolic demand.

■ Limit feeding time to 30 to 40 minutes so the infant does not get overtired. Some children may need the feeding time limited to 20 minutes.

■ Permit the infant to set the rhythm for feeding and resting.

■ Follow the infant's cues for hunger, satiety, and tiring.

Attempting to have the infant eat adequate calories to satisfy hunger and to support growth puts a lot of pressure on the parents. Encourage parents to use the feeding time for nurturing and bonding with the infant, as they learn the infant's cues for hunger and satiety.

Adequate nutrition is needed to support the infant's growth. These infants often require up to 150 kcal/kg or more per day for their increased metabolic rate and to sustain weight gain. Some infants need a higher caloric formula (24 to 30 cal/oz) to obtain adequate nutrition or to meet fluid restrictions. If the amount of fluid cannot be increased, powdered formula, low-osmolarity glucose polymers, or medium-chain triglyceride (MCT) oil may be added to standard formula; however, because the renal solute load must be considered, follow guidelines provided by a nutritionist or cardiologist (Cook & Higgins, 2010).

It is not unusual for infants with heart problems to develop failure to thrive as the result of feeding difficulties (see Chapter 19). When infants have significant dyspnea with feeding, special feeding techniques are needed. Other infants require nutritional supplementation by transpyloric, nasogastric, or gastrostomy tube (Figure 26–12 ■). Parents are often advised to give the infant a chance to feed normally for a specific period, such as 20 to 30 minutes, depending on how much dyspnea the infant has with feeding. The remainder of the formula is then given by tube feeding.

Provide Emotional Support

When a child is hospitalized with CHF, the family is often anxious about his or her condition. Give parents an opportunity to express concerns. Explain the child's treatment regimen, and make sure family members understand the child's need for nutrition and rest. Answering questions about the child's prognosis and the ultimate outcome can be reassuring to some families. Provide family members with information, and relay questions to the physician. Refer parents to appropriate support groups, as talking to other parents of children with cardiac conditions may be a source of emotional support.

Discharge Planning and Home Care Teaching

Home care needs should be identified and addressed as early as possible before discharge. While the child is hospitalized, teach the family about the administration of medications and signs of a worsening condition. Arrange for home care nursing visits to reinforce the education provided for home care management and to monitor the child's condition. Ensure that the family has a phone contact for emergency assistance if they live a distance from the healthcare provider.

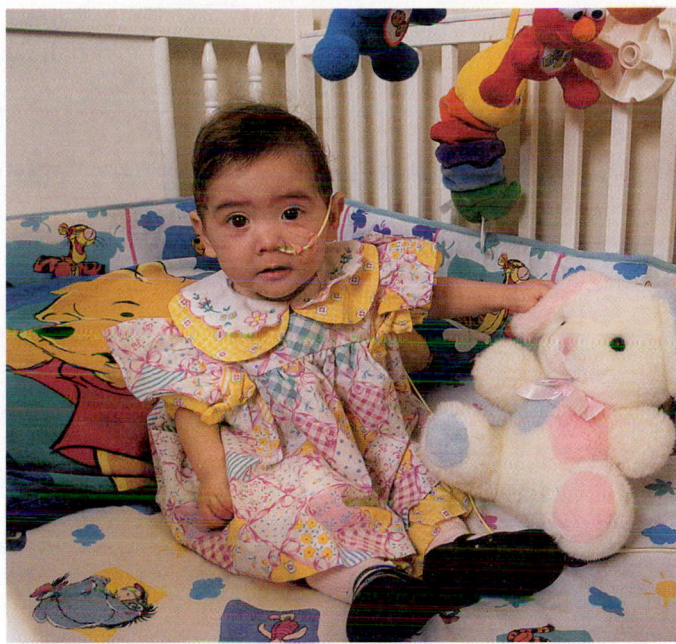

FIGURE 26–12 ■ Infants with cardiac conditions often require supplemental feedings to provide sufficient calories for growth and development. The parents of this infant girl have been taught how to give her tube feedings at home.

Medication Administration

Demonstrate administration of drugs, and then supervise while the parents measure and administer medications. Make sure parents have oral syringes or other appropriate measuring devices to ensure that the infant receives the correct dose. Teach parents about the toxic effects of digoxin and other drugs and provide an information sheet for home reference. See Partnering with Families: Administering Digoxin.

Assessment for Worsening Condition

Show parents how to feed the child to maximize nutritional intake. Tell them to watch for symptoms such as increased feeding difficulty, irritability, lethargy, breathing difficulty, and puffiness around the eyes or extremities, which indicate that CHF is worsening. Parents are frequently taught to take the child's pulse and to report any significant change to the physician. An increase in pulse rate can signal CHF, and a decrease in pulse rate can indicate digoxin toxicity. Teach parents to

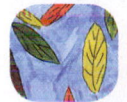

Partnering with Families

Administering Digoxin

- Take the child's pulse prior to giving digoxin. Report to the physician when the pulse rate falls below or rises above guidelines provided.
- Administer the medication exactly as prescribed at the same time each day. The parents can decide to give the medication with food or without food, but they must be consistent in giving it the same way each day.
- Do not repeat the digoxin dose if the child vomits unless directed to do so by the physician.
- Do not give the child over-the-counter medications for colds, coughs, allergies, gastrointestinal upset, or obesity without approval.

- Do not give the child herbal preparations such as ginseng, ma-huang, or ephedra. They interact with digoxin and may cause digoxin toxicity or arrhythmias.
- Keep the medication locked and out of reach of children. In case of accidental ingestion, immediate medical care is needed. Be sure to record the poison control center number on all phones.
- Remind the child's healthcare providers about the potential interaction between digoxin and certain antibiotics (e.g., tetracycline, erythromycin, rifampin, neomycin) so that safe antibiotics can be prescribed when needed (Park, 2008, p. 471).

Nursing Care Plan

The Child with Congestive Heart Failure Being Cared for at Home

INTERVENTION	RATIONALE	EXPECTED OUTCOME
1. Nursing Diagnosis: Growth and Development, Delayed related to effects of physical disability		
NIC Priority Intervention—*Developmental Enhancement:* Teaching parents to facilitate optimal gross motor, fine motor, language, cognitive, social, and emotional growth of preschool children		**NOC Suggested Outcome—***Child Development* (2 years): Milestones of physical, cognitive, and psychosocial progression by 2 years of age
GOAL: *The child will meet developmental milestones for age group.*		
■ Perform baseline developmental assessment.	■ Assessment provides comparison for later assessments and a basis for planning specific games, toys, and activities.	The child displays normal language, fine motor skills, and gross motor activity.
■ Plan for short play periods after rest.	■ Short play periods maintain energy and facilitate play.	
■ Introduce age-appropriate toys and activities such as rattles and blocks for infants and art projects for older children.	■ Play activities facilitate learning and mastery of developmental tasks.	
■ Plan for interactions with healthy children.	■ Social skills are learned through contact with others.	
2. Nursing Diagnosis: Therapeutic Regimen Management: Family, Ineffective related to complexity of therapeutic regimen		
NIC Priority Intervention—*Mutual Goal Setting:* Collaborating with the family to identify and prioritize care goals, and then developing a plan for achieving those goals		**NOC Suggested Outcome—***Compliance Behavior:* Actions taken on the basis of professional advice to promote wellness, recovery, and rehabilitation
GOAL: *Parents will demonstrate correct administration of medications.*		
■ Have parents prepare the medication dosages and administer the digoxin, diuretics, and other medications to the child under the supervision of the home health nurse.	■ Demonstrating techniques used to pour and administer medications enables the nurse to identify dosage errors and to suggest methods to help ensure the child gets all needed medications.	The child receives the appropriate dosage of all medications.
GOAL: *Parents will state side effects of medications and symptoms of congestive heart failure.*		
■ Describe side effects of medications. Give parents handouts with a telephone number to call to ask questions or report side effects.	■ If side effects are understood, serious complications can be avoided.	Parents report that the child continues to demonstrate improvement and adequate cardiac output without signs of congestive heart failure.
■ Describe subtle onset of CHF and its symptoms (increasing weakness, exhaustion, irritability, difficulty feeding, cough or difficult respirations, edema).	■ Parents can evaluate the child regularly and note subtle changes requiring medical management.	
3. Nursing Diagnosis: Nutrition, Imbalanced: Less than Body Requirements related to chronic illness and tiring while feeding		
NIC Priority Intervention—*Weight Gain Assistance:* Facilitation of body weight gain		**NOC Suggested Outcome—***Nutritional Status: Food and Fluid Intake:* Amount of food and fluid taken into the body over a 24-hour period
GOAL: *The infant or child will demonstrate normal weight gain for age.*		
■ Teach parents methods to promote food intake related to positioning, size of feedings, and food choices.	■ Positioning, frequency of feedings, size of feedings, and use of high-caloric foods can enhance nutritional intake.	The infant or child shows normal weight gain.
■ Observe feeding during a home visit.	■ Feedback can assist parents in integrating positive feeding techniques.	Parents report and demonstrate successful feedings of the child.
4. Nursing Diagnosis: Activity Intolerance (Child) related to poor cardiac output		
NIC Priority Intervention—*Energy Management:* Regulating energy use to treat or prevent fatigue and optimize function		**NOC Suggested Outcome—***Energy conservation:* Extent of active management of energy to initiate or sustain activity
GOAL: *The child will perform all necessary activities of daily living without undue tiring.*		
■ Suggest activities that parents can alternate with rest throughout the child's day.	■ Activities to promote development must be alternated with rest due to decreased cardiac output.	The child performs necessary activities and rests frequently each day.

Nursing Care Plan · The Child with Congestive Heart Failure Being Cared for at Home, *continued*

INTERVENTION	RATIONALE	EXPECTED OUTCOME
■ Have parents limit the child's exposure to persons with contagious disease.	■ When the child is ill and tired, the immune system can be compromised.	
■ Help the family plan quiet surroundings to promote the child's rest.	■ The home setting may need to be altered to promote rest.	

5. Nursing Diagnosis: Caregiver Role Strain (Parent) related to 24-hour responsibility for child's care

NIC Priority Intervention—*Caregiver Support:* Provision of the necessary information, advocacy, and support to facilitate primary patient care by someone other than a healthcare professional		**NOC Suggested Outcome**—*Caregiver Endurance Potential:* Factors that promote family care provider continuance over an extended period of time

GOAL: *Parents will express the ability to meet their own needs.*

■ Assess family and community supports. Provide information related to respite care.	■ Family members or community agencies may provide respite care.	Parents report some time away from the child and report renewal in caring for the child.
■ Encourage parents to seek activities to meet personal needs.	■ Parents need time to meet their own personal needs in order to successfully care for their child.	

NANDA-I © 2012

identify signs of dehydration when the child is managed on diuretics. An acute illness could lead to dehydration more quickly when the child takes these medications.

Care in the Community

The second of the two accompanying Nursing Care Plans outlines home care of the child with CHF. Parents play a critical role in the care of the child with heart disease by facilitating normal development and limiting the development or consequences of CHF.

Home care nurses often collaborate with cardiac specialists and advanced practice nurses in the hospital outpatient setting to support the family and child so that the child's condition is appropriately managed in the home. These children are evaluated frequently for progression in signs and symptoms, appropriate weight gain, and developmental progress. Families are evaluated for their ongoing ability to manage the child's condition and coping with the stress of caring for a sick child. Additional needs for psychosocial support or for financial resources are monitored. Daily care of these children is taxing and usually requires that a parent or caregiver be present 24 hours a day. Identify how the family is managing the needs of other children.

Evaluate family resources so that adequate child or respite care can be arranged if needed. Periodically review how the family assesses the child's energy level, physical condition for progressively worsening signs, and feeding problems. Observe medication administration and correct any errors. Watch the child feeding and provide suggestions as necessary. Reinforce any education or guidance that will help the family in the daily plan of care for the child.

Evaluation

Expected outcomes of nursing care can be found in the Nursing Care Plans.

CARDIOMYOPATHY

Cardiomyopathy is a serious disorder of the heart's muscle that affects chamber size, wall thickness, or contraction and leads to problems with ventricular systolic or diastolic function.

Dilated Cardiomyopathy

Dilated cardiomyopathy is the most common form of cardiomyopathy in infants and children. In children, the incidence is estimated to be 0.57 per 100,000 per year, but it occurs more often in boys than girls, in Blacks than Whites, and in infants under age 1 year (Jeffries & Towbin, 2010). The cause may be genetic, acquired, or secondary to myocardial disorders resulting from systemic or multi-organ disorders. An autosomal dominant inheritance accounts for about 30% to 48% of cases; however, X-linked inheritance patterns also exist, such as with muscular dystrophy (Jeffries & Towbin, 2010). In this form of cardiomyopathy, the ventricles stretch or dilate to accommodate increased blood volume. Over time, the heart muscle becomes weaker and does not pump blood effectively. The atrium may also dilate. Blood pools in the heart and clots may form, placing the child at risk for emboli to the lungs and the brain. Ventricular arrhythmias, atrial fibrillation, and mitral regurgitation may develop.

The child usually presents in CHF with tachypnea, wheezing, and poor cardiac output. Arrhythmias may develop that can cause cardiac arrest. The goals of treatment are to improve the heart's functional status, treat CHF, and prevent disease progression. Treatment involves digoxin, an ACE inhibitor, diuretics, antiarrhythmics, anticoagulants, and carvedilol or metoprolol. Ultimately a heart transplant may be considered. An implantable cardioverter/defibrillator is used in some children.

Hypertrophic Cardiomyopathy

Hypertrophic cardiomyopathy is a relatively common form of cardiomyopathy with about 50% of cases genetically transmitted as an autosomal dominant trait (Park, 2008). This form is associated with the enlargement or hypertrophy of the left ventricle and the ventricular septum, making the ventricular walls rigid. Enlargement may cause obstruction of the blood outflow tract, diastolic dysfunction of the left ventricle, myocardial ischemia, and/or mitral regurgitation. Sudden death may occur in athletes with this condition, resulting from a malignant ventricular arrhythmia that is triggered by intense exercise (Berger, Dhala, & Dearani, 2009).

Clinical manifestations vary depending upon the pathophysiology of the cardiomyopathy, such as how much obstruction to the outflow tract exists. Some children are asymptomatic, but others have symptoms of cardiac failure (exertional dyspnea, shortness of breath when supine, chest pain, and general fatigue), atrial fibrillation, or sudden death.

Treatment involves beta-blockers, which slow the heart rate and improve ventricular filling time; however, they do not change the prognosis. Vasodilators are used with extreme caution as they lower the systemic vascular resistance and worsen the obstruction in the outflow tract. An implantable cardioverter/defibrillator has proven effective for some children at risk for sudden death. Surgical septal myectomy is performed in some children with severe obstruction of the outflow tract when medical treatment is unsuccessful (Berger et al., 2009). A heart transplant may ultimately be needed for some children.

Nursing Management

Nursing management for dilated cardiomyopathy is the same as for children with congestive heart failure unless or until a heart transplant is performed. Nursing management for hypertrophic cardiomyopathy involves frequent visits to assess the child's condition and to review progress with beta-blocker medication.

HEART TRANSPLANTATION

Heart transplantation is now considered an acceptable treatment option for children with end-stage cardiac failure, complex congenital heart defects with failed surgical correction, or congenital heart defects for which surgery is not an option because of the risks of surgery or survival outcomes are worse than transplantation. Approximately 450 heart transplants are performed on children each year in the United States. In infants the reason for heart transplantation is higher for congenital heart disease (63%) than for cardiomyopathy (31%). Cardiomyopathy is more often the reason for heart transplantation in children ages 1 to 10 years (55%) and adolescents (64%) (Conway & Dipchand, 2010). Unfortunately for infants and children, waiting for donor hearts has the highest rate of waiting-list mortality of all solid organ recipients. Survival rates following heart transplantation are improving, but the greatest risk of death is within the first 6 months following surgery. The overall 20-year survival rate for children receiving heart transplants is 40%, with a 1-year survival rate of 80%, a 5-year survival rate of 68%, and a 10-year survival rate of 58% (Conway & Dipchand, 2010).

Children may have improved linear growth following transplantation, but these children may not reach population norms for growth. Developmental assessment has revealed that these children have deficits in the area of expressive language, short-term memory, visual-motor integration, and fine motor skills. Cognitive testing has revealed a 10- to 15-point reduction in IQ scores compared to children in a control group (Conway & Dipchand, 2010). Children often have a good quality of life until significant morbidity develops. Children need to be monitored for behavioral, social, and psychologic problems as some children and families need support to promote optimal psychologic functioning.

Acute rejection is a leading cause of mortality, especially within the early years after transplantation. The immunosuppression regimen usually includes calcineurin inhibitors (cyclosporin or tacrolimus), azathioprine or mycophenolate mofetil, and corticosteroids. Signs of acute organ rejection in infants and children are often nonspecific. Tachycardia and irregular rhythm are associated with acute rejection. Endomyocardial biopsy is performed during cardiac catheterization frequently during the first year after transplant to detect rejection, and then annually if no rejection occurs.

Practice Alert

Signs of acute rejection of a transplanted heart include the following: low-grade fever, increasing resting heart rate, fatigue, abdominal pain, nausea, vomiting, and decreasing exercise tolerance. Chronic rejection involves rapidly progressive coronary artery narrowing.

Hyperlipidemia and blood vessel thickening in the transplanted heart has become the leading cause of death for long-term survivors. Statin medications are prescribed to control hyperlipidemia, and hypertension is treated with calcium channel blockers. Because the transplanted heart does not have the usual nerve connections, the child or adolescent does not usually experience chest pain (Sudan, Bacha, John, et al., 2007).

Infection is another cause of mortality and morbidity. Bacterial, fungal, and viral (e.g., cytomegalovirus) infections cause the most problems, but some common childhood illnesses (e.g., acute otitis and upper respiratory infections) may be well tolerated. Care should be taken to ensure that any new medications prescribed do not interfere with immunosuppression treatment, such as antibiotics in the macrolide category.

Nursing Management

Depending upon the age at time of transplant, the child may not have had all immunizations (see Chapter 22 🔗). Live virus vaccines are contraindicated in children with heart transplants. Help parents arrange for school and childcare center administrators to immediately alert the family if any cases of measles, mumps, rubella, and chicken pox occur. Preventive treatment for the child can be provided as necessary. Good hand hygiene to reduce the spread of infection should be encouraged at home and at school.

After recovery from surgery, the child may have near-normal exercise capabilities and normal heart function, enabling the child to return to school and other activities. Immunosuppressive medications will be continued long term and can cause a variety of side effects such as hair growth, gum hyperplasia, weight gain, moon face, acne, rashes, and osteoporosis. Children and adolescents may need support to develop positive self-esteem.

Organ rejection is a major concern of families. Educate the parents and child about the need to adhere to the immunosuppression protocol and to keep appointments for procedures to assess rejection status. Adolescents need special attention to promote adherence to the immunosuppression protocol.

PULMONARY ARTERY HYPERTENSION

Pulmonary artery hypertension (PAH) causes a sustained increase in pulmonary artery pressure. Conditions that may lead to PAH include congenital cardiac defects (e.g., endocardial cushion defect, truncus arteriosus, or a large ventricular septal defect), pulmonary diseases (e.g., meconium aspiration syndrome or acute respiratory distress in a newborn), and congenital diaphragmatic hernias.

Etiology and Pathophysiology

The response to excessive pulmonary blood flow is pulmonary vascular vasoconstriction to decrease the blood flow to the lungs. The smooth muscle in the small pulmonary arteries hypertrophies to sustain vasoconstriction if the excess pulmonary blood flow is not controlled, such as by banding the pulmonary artery. Hypoxemia resulting from pulmonary hypertension helps maintain the vasoconstriction.

In response, the child develops right ventricular hypertrophy to increase the pulmonary artery pressure and to push blood across the constricted pulmonary vascular bed. Inflammation, hypertrophy of small pulmonary arteries, and fibrosis develop. The increased pressure leads to a right to left shunt, and right heart function is impaired. Right-sided heart failure can occur. PAH may become irreversible and progressive (Rothstein, Paris, & Quizon, 2009). Without treatment, the median estimated survival time after diagnosis is less than 1 year in children (van Loon, Roofthooft, Delhaas, et al., 2010).

Clinical Manifestations

The infant displays tachypnea, cyanosis, retractions, and fatigue. Tiring with feeding and failure to thrive is seen. Fluid and electrolyte imbalance is likely. As right-sided heart failure occurs, signs of CHF develop. Older children may have dyspnea, chest pain, and syncope on exertion.

Jugular distention, hepatomegaly, or peripheral edema may be seen if the child has CHF caused by severe PAH.

Collaborative Care

Diagnostic procedures include ECG, radiographic imaging with MRI to identify precise pulmonary vascular anatomy associated with the condition, pulmonary function tests, and a number of laboratory tests. A sleep study may be ordered when the child has a history of snoring or sleep apnea. Cardiac catheterization is the diagnostic procedure used to determine the severity of PAH, assess the prognosis, and select appropriate treatment. Clinical therapy involves surgery to correct an obstructive lesion or close a defect. If surgery is performed before the pulmonary vascular changes become fixed with hypertrophy and fibrosis of the small pulmonary arteries, PAH may be reversed. Medications used to treat PAH include diuretics, ACE inhibitors, calcium channel blockers, and anticoagulants. Therapy for pulmonary hypertension related to pulmonary conditions involves supplemental oxygen and correcting the pulmonary condition causing pulmonary hypertension. Newborns may be treated with supplemental oxygen, inhaled nitrous oxide, or extracorporeal membranous oxygenation. Pulmonary vasodilator drugs without U.S. Food and Drug Administration (FDA) approval for children (sildenafil and bosentan) are included in formal studies of effectiveness for children (van Loon et al., 2010). No cure is available, but life can be prolonged with these measures.

Nursing Management

Nursing care focuses on promoting rest for oxygen conservation, monitoring fluid intake and output carefully, and administering medications and oxygen. Airplane travel may be possible with supplemental oxygen. Exercise should be tailored to avoid dyspnea. Give parents needed support and information about their child.

ACQUIRED HEART DISEASES

Infective Endocarditis

Infective endocarditis is a potentially life-threatening but uncommon infection in an individual with endocardial cell damage. Infectious endocarditis may be associated with a congenital heart defect, rheumatic heart disease, a central venous catheter, heart surgery, or

Pathophysiology Illustrated
Infective Endocarditis

— Vegetation

— Bicuspid aortic valve

FIGURE 26–13 ■ The endocardium is injured by high velocity through a stenotic valve, by turbulent blood flow across a septal defect, or by the positioning of a central venous catheter. Fibrin and platelets migrate to the site of the endothelial damage, becoming the foundation for nonbacterial thrombotic emboli where the infective organisms settle. In some cases, a vegetation forms near the site of the injury, in this case around the aortic valve.

intravenous drug abuse. It is believed that the rate of endocarditis in children has increased, potentially because of improved surgical management, greater survival of children with congenital heart disease, and an increased incidence of hospital-acquired endocarditis (Saiman, 2009).

Etiology and Pathophysiology

In children with congenital heart disease, a high velocity or turbulent blood flow can injure the endocardium and result in deposition of platelets and fibrin on the surface of the endothelium or valve. See Figure 26–13 ■. Bacteria in the bloodstream, introduced by various dental or medical procedures or by injury, may then adhere to **endocardium** (the tissue lining the heart chambers) and colonize. The most common bacteria associated with infectious endocarditis include *Streptococcus viridans, enterococci, Staphylococcus aureus, Staphylococcus epidermidis, Haemophilus influenzae,* and gram-negative bacteria (Lennox, 2012). These bacteria multiply and trigger further deposition of platelets and fibrin, causing a vegetation. An increasing number of children with infective endocarditis have had corrective or palliative surgery with or without implanted vascular grafts, patches, or prosthetic valves that can serve as a locus of infection. Indwelling central venous catheters positioned in the right side of the heart also damage the endocardium or valve endothelium. In some cases, the organism causes a vegetation on the valve leaflets, causing regurgitation and heart failure. The vegetation can break off and become an embolus that travels to the vital organs.

Clinical Manifestations

Symptoms can be mild and develop slowly, or they can be severe and develop rapidly. The most common presenting sign in children is a recurrent fever. Other symptoms are fatigue, weakness, weight loss, headache, joint and muscle aches, and diaphoresis. Other signs may include a new heart murmur, hepatosplenomegaly, and congestive heart failure. Petechiae, splinter hemorrhages under nails, Roth spots (exudative lesions of the retina), Osler nodes (red, painful nonhemorrhagic nodules on the pads of the fingers and toes), and Janeway lesions (nontender, blanching macular lesions on the palms and soles) may be seen in adolescents (Lennox, 2012). Children with indwelling catheters may initially have pulmonary symptoms or signs related to septic pulmonary embolism.

Collaborative Care

Diagnostic Procedures

The Duke Criteria are used for the diagnosis of infective endocarditis (Box 26–5). Infective endocarditis is diagnosed primarily by blood culture. An elevated erythrocyte sedimentation rate, anemia, elevated C-reactive protein level, and increased white blood cell count may also be present, Transesophageal and transthoracic echocardiography detect the presence of vegetation or infective lesions in the heart, the extent of valve damage, and cardiac function.

Clinical Therapy

Clinical therapy consists of administering high doses of bactericidal antibiotics such as penicillin G, ceftriaxone, vancomycin, nafcillin, oxacillin, gentamicin, ciprofloxacin, and cefazolin. Intravenous administration is preferred, with therapy continuing for 4 to 8 weeks until the infective organism is eradicated. Serum levels of antibiotics are monitored to maintain a therapeutic range. Surgery is often necessary to replace a heart valve or because of the risk of embolism. If CHF occurs because of damage to a heart valve, bed rest and medications such as digoxin and furosemide are prescribed initially until it is determined whether medical therapy is adequate or if surgery will be required. Most children are cured with appropriate medical and surgical treatment (Saiman, 2009).

Prevention of infective endocarditis is preferred, and antibiotic prophylaxis is recommended for dental procedures (involving manipulation of gingival tissue or periapical region of teeth, or the perforation of the oral mucosa) and invasive respiratory procedures (involving incision or biopsy) for selected individuals at highest risk for adverse outcomes

from infective endocarditis. Antibiotic prophylaxis is no longer routinely recommended for gastrointestinal or genitourinary procedures. See Box 26–3 on page 825 for children who should receive antibiotic prophylaxis for dental and invasive respiratory procedures. Maintenance of good oral hygiene and regular dental care are major methods recommended to reduce the risk for infective endocarditis (Wilson, Taubert, Gewitz, et al., 2007). See Medications Used for Infective Endocarditis Prophylaxis for Dental and Invasive Respiratory Procedures.

Nursing Management

When the child has infective endocarditis, nursing care focuses on assessing the child's condition, monitoring for complications, administering medications, and teaching the parents about the child's care.

Nursing Assessment and Diagnoses

Assessment focuses on the child's respiratory and cardiovascular status. Pay careful attention to the vital signs, oxygen saturation, and level of consciousness because CHF and embolism may occur. The child will be on a cardiac monitor and pulse oximeter. Monitor the child's temperature, intake and output, and level of comfort. Monitor for the development of complications such an embolus. The parents will be very anxious about the child's condition, especially if this occurs following surgery for a congenital heart defect or in a critically ill child or newborn. Monitor the parents' coping skills and need for information.

Nursing diagnoses that may be associated with infective endocarditis include the following:

- Self-Care, Readiness for Enhanced related to requesting infectious endocarditis antibiotic prophylaxis
- Infection, Risk for related to central venous catheter
- Caregiver Role Strain related to child's increasing care needs
- Spiritual Distress, Risk for (Parents) related to child's deteriorating health status and challenge to their belief and values system

NANDA-I © 2012

Planning and Intervention

Nursing care focuses on preventing infective endocarditis for those cases when it is preventable. Parents of children and adolescents need to tell every healthcare provider about the risk for infective

---

BOX 26–5   Duke Criteria for Diagnosis of Infective Endocarditis

MAJOR CRITERIA

1. Positive blood culture from two or more separate blood cultures or single positive blood culture for *Coxiella burnetii*, or antiphase 1 IgG antibody titer greater than 1:800

2. Evidence of endocardial involvement noted on echocardiogram of an intracardiac mass on a valve or supporting structure, abscess, or new partial dehiscence of a prosthetic valve; alternatively new valvular regurgitation is discovered

MINOR CRITERIA

1. Predisposing heart condition or injectable drug abuse
2. Temperature of 38.0°C (100.4°F) or higher
3. Vascular phenomena such as major arterial emboli, septic pulmonary infarcts, mycotic aneurysm, intracranial hemorrhage, conjunctival hemorrhages, and Janeway lesions
4. Immunologic phenomena such as glomerulonephritis, Osler nodes, Roth spots, and rheumatoid factor

5. Microbiological evidence of positive blood culture but does not meet major criteria or serologic evidence of active infection with organism consistent with infectious endocarditis

Diagnosis is confirmed using the Duke Criteria when pathologic evidence of a vegetation or intracardiac abscess exists plus one of the following clinical criteria:

- Two major criteria
- One major criterion and three minor criteria
- Five minor criteria

Infectious endocarditis should be considered when one major criterion and one minor criterion or three minor criteria are present.

Source: *Saiman, L. (2009). Endocarditis and intravascular infections. In S. S. Long, L. K. Pickering, & C. G. Prober, Principles and practice of pediatric infectious diseases (3rd ed., pp. 269–277). New York, NY: Elsevier Churchill Livingstone; McDonald, J. R. (2009). Acute infectious endocarditis. Infectious Disease Clinics of North America, 23, 643–664; American Heart Association, Baddour, L. M., Wilson, W. R., Bayer, A. S., Fowler, V. G., Bolger, A. F., et al. (2005). Infective endocarditis: Diagnosis, antimicrobial therapy, and management of complications. Circulation,111, e394–e433.*

Medications Used for Infective Endocarditis Prophylaxis for Dental and Invasive Respiratory Procedures

SITUATION	ANTIBIOTIC RECOMMENDATIONS	NURSING MANAGEMENT
Oral	Amoxicillin	■ One large dose is given 30–60 minutes before the procedure. If the preprocedure dose is not taken, the dose may be taken up to 2 hours postprocedure. ■ Teach parents and the child to keep at least one dose in the home to take before dental visits or for dental emergencies. ■ Have parents inform each healthcare provider of the child's heart defect and need for prophylaxis. ■ Dentists and physicians can write the prescription.
Unable to take oral medication—use IV or IM preparations	Ampicillin OR Cefazolin or ceftriaxone	
Allergic to penicillin or ampicillin	Cephalexin OR Clindamycin OR Azithromycin or clarithromycin	
Allergic to penicillin or ampicillin and unable to take oral medication—use IV or IM preparations	Cefazolin or ceftriaxone OR Clindamycin	

Source: *Modified from Wilson, W., Taubert, K. A., Gewitz, M., Lockhart, P. B., Baddour, L. M., et al. (2007). Prevention of infective endocarditis: Guidelines from the American Heart Association Rheumatic Fever, Endocarditis, and Kawasaki Disease Committee, Council on Cardiovascular Disease in the Young, and the Council on Clinical Cardiology, Council on Cardiovascular Surgery and Anesthesia, and the Quality of Care and Outcomes Research Interdisciplinary Working Group. Circulation, 116, 1736–1754.*

endocarditis. They need to become advocates and ask for prophylaxis, specifically prior to procedures such as professional teeth cleaning, other dental procedures, tonsillectomy or adenoidectomy, bronchoscopy, and surgery on the respiratory system. Make sure the family has copies of the wallet card produced by the American Heart Association that can be shared with healthcare providers.

Administer medications as ordered and monitor serum antibiotic levels. Monitor for side effects of antibiotics and for infiltration or extravasation at the infusion site. Keep invasive procedures to a minimum. Use careful aseptic technique when managing central lines and venous access devices.

The child is often lethargic and on bed rest. Encourage parents to assist with the child's care and plan quiet age-appropriate activities. Make sure the parents are fully informed about the child's care and potential for complications. Permit time for them to express their feelings and frustrations over the development of this infection. Identify ways that parents can contribute to the care of the child.

Discharge Planning and Home Care Teaching

Begin discharge planning and education for the care of the child at home as soon as possible. Home infusion antibiotic therapy may be ordered so that care can be provided on an outpatient basis. At discharge, arrange home health nursing and instruct parents about care needed for the child's recuperation. Homeschooling will be needed during the recovery period. Help parents to maintain contact with the child's friends and encourage social interactions. Reinforce the need for follow-up visits. Explain the importance of informing physicians and dentists about the child's history of endocarditis so that care is taken to prevent infection before invasive procedures.

Evaluation

Expected outcomes of nursing care include the following:

■ Infective endocarditis is prevented in the child with a complex congenital heart disease.
■ Complications associated with infective endocarditis are rapidly detected.

Rheumatic Fever

Rheumatic fever is an inflammatory connective tissue disorder that results from an autoimmune response to an infection with M serotypes of group A beta-hemolytic streptococci. While this is a significant health problem in developing countries, the incidence is very low in the United States, most likely due to hygiene and access to medical care (Gerber, Baltimore, Eaton, et al., 2009; Steer & Carapetis, 2009).

Epidemiology

Only a small number of individuals infected with the strain of group A streptococcus develop acute rheumatic fever. It is believed that individuals who develop rheumatic fever have a genetic susceptibility to the disease. An estimated 60% of patients with acute rheumatic fever develop rheumatic heart disease (Steer & Carapetis, 2009).

Clinical Manifestations

One to 3 weeks after an untreated streptococcal infection, the hallmark signs of rheumatic fever may occur. Major manifestations include the following:

■ Carditis may be detected by the development of a new murmur which indicates involvement of the mitral or aortic valve. Chest pain may be caused by pericardial inflammation.
■ Polyarteritis, in which two or more large joints become inflamed with pain, swelling, tenderness, erythema, and heat, occurs. The signs may shift from joint to joint (migratory polyarthritis). Subcutaneous nodules may develop and be palpated over bony prominences and along extensor tendons.
■ Erythema marginatum, a nonpruritic skin rash with pink macules and blanching in the middle of the lesions, appears on the trunk but never on the face and hands. Heat darkens the rash.
■ Sydenham chorea (St. Vitus dance), characterized by aimless movements of the extremities plus facial grimacing, occurs when the central nervous system is affected.

Collaborative Care

Diagnostic Procedures

Diagnosis is based on clinical signs (Jones criteria; Table 26–11) and evidence of preceding group A streptococcal infection by either (1) a positive throat culture or rapid streptococcal antigen test or (2) an elevated or rising streptococcal (antistreptolysin-O) antibody titer. An elevated antistreptolysin-O titer of 333 Todd units in children indicates a recent streptococcal infection (Brashers, 2010).

TABLE 26–11	Jones Criteria: Guidelines for Diagnosis of Initial Attack of Rheumatic Fever	
MAJOR MANIFESTATIONS	**MINOR MANIFESTATIONS**	
Carditis	*Clinical findings*	
Polyarthritis	Arthralgia	
Chorea	Fever	
Erythema marginatum	*Laboratory findings*	
Subcutaneous nodules	Elevated acute-phase reactants	
	Elevated erythrocyte sedimentation rate	
	Elevated C-reactive protein	
	Prolonged PR interval on ECG	

Interpretation: If supported by evidence of preceding group A streptococcal infection by culture or rising antistreptolysin-O titer, the presence of two major manifestations or one major and two minor manifestations indicates a high probability of acute rheumatic fever.

Source: *Data from Park, M. K. (2008). Pediatric cardiology for practitioners (5th ed., pp. 382). St. Louis, MO: Elsevier Mosby; Ferrieri, P. (2002). Proceedings of the Jones Criteria workshop. Circulation, 106, 2521–2523; and Brashers, V. L. (2010). Alterations in cardiovascular function. In K. L. McCance, S. E. Huether, V. L. Brashers, & N. R. Rote, Pathophysiology: The biologic basis for disease in adults and children (6th ed., pp. 1142–1208). St. Louis, MO: Mosby Elsevier.*

Clinical Therapy

Clinical therapy includes antibiotics (penicillin, sulfadiazine, or erythromycin) to eradicate the streptococcal infection. Aspirin is used for fever, arthritis, and arthralgias. Corticosteroids may be used for severe carditis causing CHF (Park, 2008). Carditis occurs more often in children than in adolescents or adults (Steer & Carapetis, 2009). Most children in the United States receiving early treatment recover fully, but they are at risk for subsequent episodes of rheumatic fever. Children should be monitored carefully by echocardiogram for potential cardiac complications. Long-term antibiotic prophylaxis (intramuscular benzathine penicillin, oral penicillin V, or oral sulfadiazine in persons allergic to penicillin)to reduce the risk for recurrent episodes is given well into adulthood. Children with heart valve damage need antibiotic prophylaxis for infective endocarditis.

Nursing Management

The most important role of the nurse is prevention of rheumatic fever. Nurses in clinics, offices, and schools need to ensure that all children with possible streptococcal infections have a throat culture. Even if the sore throat is mild, a culture is needed if family members or other contacts have had a streptococcal infection. Emphasize to the family the importance of giving the entire 10-day course of antibiotics when a culture is positive.

In a case of severe rheumatic fever, the child will be hospitalized for a period of time. Nursing care focuses on assessing the child's condition, promoting recovery, and ensuring adherence to the treatment regimen.

During the acute inflammatory phase, take the child's temperature at least every 4 hours and monitor vital signs. The child is on bed rest while monitoring for the onset of carditis, and for 4 weeks if carditis develops. Auscultate the child's heart and note any unusual sounds. Observe the child for changes in skin, joints, or behavior. Family members should have throat cultures done to identify possible asymptomatic streptococcal carriers.

Administer the antibiotic, aspirin, and corticosteroid as ordered. The child is usually lethargic and often has joint pain. Aspirin often relieves pain dramatically after a few doses. Place the child's joints in neutral position and handle them carefully. Provide quiet activities,

and encourage visits or telephone calls from family members and friends. For the child with chorea, provide emotional support because the purposeless involuntary movements that can last for 5 to 15 weeks can be disturbing. Encourage the family to participate in the child's hospital care.

During the recovery phase, the child will generally be cared for at home. Activities may be limited, especially if heart damage is suspected. Help parents plan quiet activities, such as playing board games, working with computers, or reading, and arrange rest periods after the child returns to school. Reassure the child and parents that the effects of chorea will eventually subside.

On discharge, a daily oral low-dose antibiotic is prescribed or a monthly long-acting antibiotic injection is given. Make sure the child and parents understand the importance of taking prescribed medication well into adulthood to prevent future infection and possible heart damage from recurrent rheumatic fever. Stress the importance of telling future healthcare providers, including dentists and surgeons, about the child's rheumatic fever history so prophylactic antibiotics can be given when needed to prevent infective endocarditis.

Make sure the parents understand that the child's future sore throats may be streptococcal and that a throat culture should be taken even when the child is taking daily antibiotics. The child may need additional antibiotics for the infection. Emphasize the importance of follow-up care to prevent new infections and to monitor heart function.

Kawasaki Disease

Kawasaki disease is an acute febrile, systemic vascular inflammatory disorder that affects small and midsize arteries, including the coronary arteries. It is the leading cause of acquired heart disease in children in the United States (McLellan & Baker, 2011). The disorder occurs more commonly in males than females. Children under 5 years of age account for 80% of cases, and 50% of cases occur in children under 2 years (American Academy of Pediatrics, 2012, p. 457). This disorder is most commonly found in Asian and Pacific Islander children in the United States, but it can occur in children of all races (McLellan & Baker, 2011).

Etiology and Pathophysiology

The etiology of Kawasaki disease is unknown. It is believed that a genetically susceptible child has a self-limiting inflammatory response to an infectious trigger. The specific infectious agent has not been identified. A seasonal distribution of cases occurs with the greatest incidence in the winter and spring. The disorder occurs in three phases. The acute phase, from onset to resolution of the fever, is associated with widespread inflammation of the blood vessels. This multisystem inflammatory disease involving the small and midsize arteries sometimes causes aneurysms in the coronary arteries as well as other arteries. Without treatment, approximately 1 in 5 affected children will develop coronary artery aneurysms (Baker, Lu, Minich, et al., 2009). Other complications may include myocarditis, impaired left ventricular function, valve regurgitation, arrhythmia, and pericardial effusion (McLellan & Baker, 2011).

Clinical Manifestations

The three stages of the disease are acute, subacute, and convalescent.

- The acute stage of Kawasaki disease, lasting 1 to 2 weeks, is characterized by irritability, high fever that persists for more than 5 days, conjunctival hyperemia, red throat, swollen hands

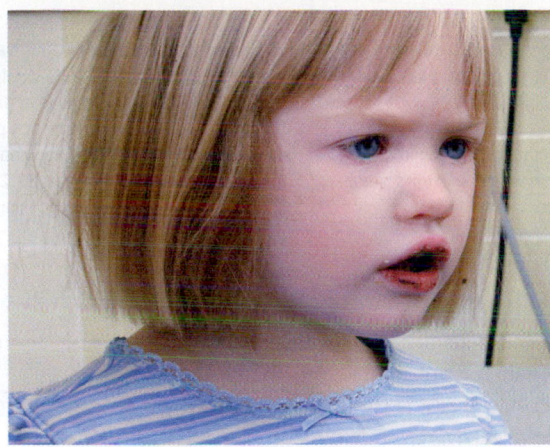

FIGURE 26–14 ■ This child has returned for one of her frequent follow-up visits to assess her cardiac status after treatment for Kawasaki syndrome. Notice the lips that show the inflammation and cracking.

TABLE 26–12	Diagnostic Criteria for Kawasaki Disease When Fever Is Present 5 Days or Longer and Includes Four of Five Principle Features
BODY PART AFFECTED	**PRINCIPAL FEATURES**
Eyes	Bilateral bulbar conjunctivitis without exudate
Oropharyngeal	Intense erythema of the buccal and pharyngeal surfaces with dry, swollen, cracked, and fissuring lips and a strawberry tongue
Skin	Erythema of the palms and soles, edema of the hands and feet, and then desquamation after 2 or more weeks of symptoms
	Polymorphic rash—dermatitis of the trunk with an erythematous maculopapular rash
Lymph nodes	Cervical lymphadenopathy, frequently unilateral, with a lymph node over 1.5 cm in diameter found early in the disease

Source: *Data from McLellan, M. C., & Baker, A. L. (2011). At the heart of the fever: Kawasaki disease.* American Journal of Nursing, 111*(6), 57–63; American Heart Association. (2010). Kawasaki disease. Retrieved from http://www.heart.org/HEARTORG/Conditions/More/CardiovascularConditionsofChildhood/Kawasaki-Disease_UCM_308777_Article.jsp; and Vetter, V. L. (2006). Kawasaki disease. In V. L. Vetter,* Pediatric cardiology: The requisites in pediatrics *(p. 132). St. Louis, MO: Elsevier Mosby.*

and feet, maculopapular or erythema multiforme-like rash on the trunk and perineal area, unilateral enlargement of the cervical lymph nodes, diarrhea, and hepatic dysfunction.

- The subacute stage, lasting 2 to 4 weeks, is characterized by cracking lips and fissures, desquamation of the skin on the tips of the fingers and toes, joint pain, cardiac disease, and thrombocytosis (Figure 26–14 ■).
- In the convalescent stage, 6 to 8 weeks after disease onset, the child appears normal but lingering signs of inflammation may be present.

Some cases have an atypical or incomplete presentation. Other clinical manifestations may include arthralgias, abdominal pain, diarrhea, and vomiting, as well as signs of hepatic dysfunction, gallbladder hydrops, aseptic meningitis, and rarely sensorineural hearing loss.

Collaborative Care

Diagnostic Procedures

No specific laboratory test is diagnostic for Kawasaki disease. The disorder is diagnosed when a high spiking fever over 39°C (102.2°F) for 5 days or longer is present along with four of five principal features not explained by another disease process (Table 26–12). When fewer than four criteria are present, but echocardiography or angiography reveals coronary artery abnormalities, Kawasaki disease is also diagnosed.

Initial blood studies show signs of systemic inflammation (an elevated white cell count with a predominance of granulocytes, an erythrocyte sedimentation rate greater than 40 mm/hr, and C-reactive protein greater than 3 mg/dL). Platelet counts, the bilirubin level, and the alanine aminotransferase level may also be elevated. White blood cells may be found in the urine, but this is often associated with sterile pyuria (McLellan & Baker, 2011). Echocardiography is used to identify specific vascular changes in the heart and coronary arteries. Repeat echocardiograms are performed frequently to monitor the development of coronary lesions during the acute phases of the disease, and then periodically during recovery and long-term follow-up to observe for resolution of coronary artery lesions.

Clinical Therapy

Kawasaki disease is treated with intravenous immune globulin (IVIG), ideally within 7 to 10 days of onset to reduce the risk for coronary artery aneurysm. The 2 g/kg single infusion is given over

an 8- to 12-hour period. To reduce the risk of allergic response to this product, some children are administered IV diphenhydramine before the IVIG dose is started. High doses of aspirin (80 to 100 mg/kg/day in four divided doses) are given while the fever is high to promote comfort. The dose is decreased to 2 to 5 mg/kg once daily once the child has been afebrile for 2 to 3 days. This lower dose of aspirin may be prescribed until the platelet count is normal or continued on a long-term basis if cardiac abnormalities occur. High doses of immune globulin and aspirin given before the 10th day of fever have been shown to reduce the incidence of coronary artery lesions and aneurysms, and the duration of fever (McLellan & Baker, 2011). When the fever persists or returns within 36 hours after the first administration of immune globulin, a second infusion of IVIG at 2 g/kg may be given. When the second dose of immune globulin is ineffective, no therapy is considered optimal. Infliximab, a monoclonal antibody, has recently been evaluated in a small number of children having IVIG-resistant Kawasaki disease after a first dose of IVIG. The study's children were found to have a shorter duration of fever and hospitalization and similar sequelae to those treated with a second dose of IVIG (Son, Gauvreau, Burns, et al., 2011).

Children are usually hospitalized for 3 or more days, depending on the presence of cardiac lesions and persistence of the fever. Most children recover fully. Careful monitoring for cardiac disease continues for several weeks or months. Coronary aneurysms may develop in 5% of children treated with IVIG, but about 50% to 67% of coronary artery aneurysms resolve within 2 years (McLellan & Baker, 2011). Some children with large coronary artery aneurysms are less likely to have resolution of aneurysms, and stenosis of these coronary arteries may occur over time.

Nursing Management

Nursing care focuses on promoting comfort, monitoring for early signs of complications or disease progression, and supporting the family.

Nursing Assessment and Diagnoses

Assessment is important in identifying signs of Kawasaki disease, as the acute phase of this disorder is commonly confused with other diseases. The nurse in the community must be alert to early signs and symptoms.

When the child is hospitalized, take the temperature every 4 hours and before each dose of aspirin. Carefully assess the extremities for edema, redness, and desquamation every 8 hours. Examine the eyes for conjunctivitis and the mucous membranes for inflammation. Monitor the child's dietary and fluid intake and weigh the child daily. Carefully assess heart sounds and rhythm.

Nursing diagnoses that may be appropriate for the child with Kawasaki disease include:

- Mucous Membrane: Oral, Impaired related to inflammation and decreased fluid intake
- Skin Integrity, Impaired related to edema, diaphoresis, and skin desquamation
- Body Temperature: Imbalanced, Risk for related to inflammatory process
- Family Processes, Interrupted due to the child's acute and potentially life-threatening illness

NANDA-I © 2012

Planning and Implementation

Administer aspirin and immune globulin as prescribed. Monitor for side effects of aspirin such as bleeding and gastrointestinal upset. Administer IVIG as a blood product, carefully regulating the infusion rate to run slowly according to the physician's orders, and monitoring for any reactions to the infusion. The infusion rate may initially be slow at 0.5 mL/kg/hr for 30 minutes and then gradually increased to 2 mL/kg/hr. If symptoms of reaction are noted, stop the infusion immediately (see Chapter 27 🔗).

Promote the child's comfort. Assess pain and provide analgesics and complementary therapies to manage pain. Keep the child's skin clean and dry, and lubricate the lips. Use cool compresses to make the feverish child more comfortable. Change the child's clothes and bed linens frequently. Give frequent small feedings of soft foods and liquids that are neither too hot nor too cold.

Use passive range of motion exercises to facilitate joint movement. Because the child with Kawasaki disease is frequently lethargic and irritable, plan rest periods and quiet, age-appropriate activities. Encourage the parents to participate in their child's care to promote comfort and reassurance for the child. Provide the parents with information about the disease and the child's treatment.

Discharge Planning and Home Care Teaching

Before the child is discharged, teach the parents to administer aspirin as ordered and to watch for side effects. Have them measure the child's temperature daily for the first 2 weeks and record it on a log. Any fever above 38.3°C (101°F) should be reported to the physician. Advise the parents that after recuperation, the child may need to avoid contact sports or other activities that could cause bleeding, especially if aspirin is continued long term or warfarin is prescribed. Emphasize the need for follow-up care to monitor for cardiac complications. These children should also be monitored for risk factors of hypertension and hyperlipidemia. If the child recovers without cardiovascular complications, encourage the child to live an active lifestyle without exercise limitations. Limitation of strenuous activity is recommended for all children with coronary aneurysms or coronary artery stenosis.

Practice Alert

Postpone the immunization of a child with Kawasaki disease with live vaccines (e.g., measles or varicella) for 11 months after IVIG administration as it interferes with the child's immune response to the live virus vaccine. If the child is at high risk of exposure to measles or varicella, immunize the child before this time has passed, then reimmunize the child 11 months after IVIG treatment. Do not postpone immunization with inactivated vaccines (American Academy of Pediatrics, 2012 p. 38).

Evaluation

Examples of expected nursing care outcomes include the following:

- Comfort in the child with acute symptoms, rash, fever, and irritability is promoted.
- Periods of rest and quiet activity are balanced to promote the child's recovery.

CARDIAC ARRHYTHMIAS

Cardiac **arrhythmias** (abnormal heart rhythms or dysrhythmias) occur frequently in children, but less commonly than in adults. Based on the child's pulse rate, pediatric arrhythmias have three categories (Inaba & Horeczko, 2009):

- Fast—tachyarrhythmias (sinus tachycardia)
- Slow—bradyarrhythmias (sinus bradycardia)
- No pulse (ventricular tachycardia, ventricular fibrillation, pulseless electrical activity, or asystole)

Less common arrhythmias are often associated with postoperative complications of congenital heart disease, Kawasaki disease with coronary artery involvement, rheumatic heart disease, cardiomyopathy, and electrolyte abnormalities (Inaba & Horeczko, 2009).

Arrhythmias must be recognized because they can cause decreased cardiac output and congestive heart failure or further progress to an even more serious arrhythmia that could result in sudden death. Review Figure 26–2 for the normal electrical conduction system to determine where specific stimulation or interruption occurs in association with various arrhythmias.

Etiology and Pathophysiology

Tachyarrhythmias (e.g., sinus tachycardia) often occur with acute conditions, such as hypoxia, anemia, hypovolemia, shock, hyper- or hypokalemia, hyperthyroidism, catecholamine medications, and stimulant or illicit drug use.

The most common cause of bradyarrhythmias (e.g., sinus bradycardia) is hypoxemia. Other potential causes include hypothermia, increased intracranial pressure, heart block, hypothyroidism, sick sinus syndrome, and various medications and toxins (e.g., digoxin, beta-blockers, calcium channel blockers, and cholinergic agents) (Inaba & Horeczko, 2009). These types of arrhythmias generally resolve once the underlying condition is treated.

Some arrhythmias result from genetic conditions, such as forms of supraventricular tachycardia and long QT syndrome. Neonates and young children may be predisposed to supraventricular tachycardia (SVT) because of an accessory atrioventricular pathway for the heart's electrical system or Wolff-Parkinson-White syndrome. Healthy infants and children usually tolerate short periods of SVT. Prolonged episodes of SVT (e.g., 24 to 48 hours) may progress to CHF or cardiogenic shock if untreated (see page 859) (Schlechte, Boramanand, & Funk, 2008).

Cardiac output is affected because blood returning during diastole cannot keep pace with such a rapid heart rate.

Long QT syndrome is a rhythm disturbance of autosomal dominant and autosomal recessive inheritance (caused by several distinct gene defects) that puts children at risk for ventricular fibrillation and sudden death. Some of these gene defects are mutations that have an effect on the potassium, sodium, and calcium channels (Shimizu, 2008). In long QT syndrome, the ventricular tachycardia with a prolonged QT interval impairs cardiac output, leading to syncope or seizures. It is thought to be associated with some cases of sudden infant death syndrome (Samson & Atkins, 2008).

Clinical Manifestations

Bradycardias

Bradycardia is a heart rate less than the lower limit of normal for the child's age, usually a rate less than 80 beats/min in infants and less than 60 beats/min in children and adolescents, that is associated with poor systemic perfusion (Inaba & Horeczko, 2009). Some athletes may normally have a heart rate of 60. Refer to Chapter 7 🔗 for normal heart rate ranges by age. General symptoms of bradycardia include fatigue, exercise intolerance, dizziness, and syncope.

Tachycardias

Supraventricular tachycardia (SVT), the most common pathologic tachycardia in infants and children, is the abrupt onset of a rapid, regular heart rate. The presenting heart rate in infants with SVT will be greater than 220 beats/min. In older children, heart rates will be greater than 180 to 240 beats/min. Early signs of SVT in infants include poor feeding, irritability, and pallor. Older children may have palpitations, chest pain, dizziness, shortness of breath, decreased exercise tolerance, and syncope. Chest pain associated with arrhythmias generally results from decreased cardiac output leading to myocardial ischemia. Adolescents report many of the same signs as older children, but may also have pallor, a feeling of palpitations in the neck, and diaphoresis. Recurrent attacks are common.

Long QT Syndrome

The arrhythmia may be triggered by demanding physical exercise, a strong emotional reaction, or an abrupt loud noise (e.g., doorbell or alarm clock). In some genetic forms, the arrhythmia is not triggered by exercise but more often occurs during rest or sleep. Hypokalemia may trigger long QT arrhythmia in one genetic form of the disorder. Arrhythmia may occur without warning and result in sudden death. Presenting signs include episodic dizziness, palpitations, syncope, seizure, or cardiac arrest.

Signs and symptoms of different classifications of arrhythmias can be found in the Clinical Manifestations table.

Collaborative Care

Diagnostic Procedures

An electrocardiogram is initially used to diagnose an arrhythmia. If symptoms are episodic, a 24-hour Holter monitor or an event monitor may be used to capture the arrhythmia. With an event monitor, the patient can push a button on the monitor to activate the mark of the ECG tracing at the time of the symptoms. The event monitor retains the ECG tracing immediately before and during the episode. The ECG record can then be transmitted by telephone for immediate interpretation. Stress testing may also be performed when exercise either triggers or is associated with the symptoms.

Invasive procedures may be needed to diagnose some arrhythmias.

- Electrophysiologic cardiac catheterization allows electrode catheters to be placed in the right side of the heart. Areas of the heart can be selectively stimulated to trigger the arrhythmia. Medications can then be given intravenously to identify which medication can be used to effectively treat the arrhythmia.
- Transesophageal recording involves passing an electrode catheter into the lower esophagus to stimulate and record the arrhythmia.

Long QT syndrome If the child is resuscitated or evaluated because of early signs, the arrhythmia is commonly detected by electrocardiogram that reveals a ventricular tachycardia and **torsades de pointes** (a distinct form of ventricular tachycardia in patients with marked QT prolongation on the ECG, appearing as a "twisting of the points"). A cardiology evaluation carefully reviews the family history for any unexplained death and fainting triggered by exercise or loud noise. An epinephrine QT test is performed in which the child is given epinephrine during an ECG to detect an abnormal QT interval. Long QT genetic testing is also performed to detect genes with mutations for potassium channels, sodium channels, or calcium channels.

Clinical Therapy

Treatment for arrhythmias depends upon the type and severity.

Bradycardias For sinus bradycardia due to an acute condition, oxygen, ventilation, and medications such as epinephrine or atropine are used until the condition resolves. Other chronic bradycardias due to heart block often require a pacemaker.

Tachycardias Supraventricular tachycardia episodes are initially treated with vagal maneuvers to slow the heart rate when the infant or child is stable. In infants, the application of ice or iced saline solution to the face or rectal stimulation with a thermometer may reduce the heart rate. An older child can perform a **Valsalva maneuver,** a forced expiratory effort against a closed airway (e.g., holding the breath and bearing down as if to have a bowel movement or blowing forcefully on the thumb), which increases intrathoracic and venous pressures and thus slows the heart rate. Adenosine may be given intravenously when the vagal maneuvers are unsuccessful. Amiodarone and procainamide may be used in some children. See Medications Commonly Used to Treat Arrhythmias on page 849. When the child does not return to sinus rhythm after vagal maneuvers and medications, the child is sedated and invasive maneuvers are used.

- In **synchronized cardioversion,** the timed administration of a calibrated electrical charge by a defibrillator to coincide with the peak of the QRS complex is used in unstable patients to convert the tachyarrhythmia to a sinus rhythm.
- With esophageal overdrive pacing, an electrode is inserted into the esophagus and positioned behind the left atrium. The heart is stimulated at a very rapid rate to interrupt the tachycardia.

Recurrent episodes of SVT are common, and long-term digoxin, verapamil, propranolol, procainamide, or amiodarone may be given to reduce the frequency of episodes (Anderson & Vetter, 2010). Radiofrequency ablation may be performed in the cardiac catheterization laboratory with specialized electrophysiology equipment. A catheter is guided to the site of the accessory conduction system pathway triggering the tachycardia. Radiofrequency energy is transmitted to the muscle cells through which the accessory conduction system passes. The muscle cells in that small area die and block the

Clinical Manifestations Arrhythmias

ETIOLOGY	CLINICAL MANIFESTATIONS	CLINICAL THERAPY
Sinus node dysfunction—surgical injury to the sinoatrial node or its arterial supply, right atrial dilatation, myocarditis, antiarrhythmic medications	Bradycardia, fatigue, exercise intolerance, dizziness, syncope	Adequate ventilation, oxygenation Medications: epinephrine, atropine, isoproterenol, glucagon Temporary or permanent pacemaker
Incomplete conduction of impulses through the atrioventricular node, surgery for transposition of great arteries, tetralogy of Fallot, endocardial cushion defect, ventricular septal defect, subaortic resection, aortic valve replacement, inflammation due to myocarditis, Lyme disease, rheumatic fever	Heart block (first, second, or third degree), slow ventricular heart rates, atrial rate may be faster than the ventricular rate Congestive heart failure, fatigue, exercise intolerance, dizziness, syncope 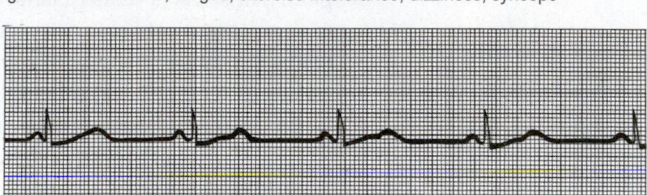	Temporary or permanent pacemaker
Reentrant circuit with or without an accessory conduction pathway, or an ectopic focus; Wolff-Parkinson-White syndrome	Sustained tachyarrhythmia of 130–300 beats/min depending on age and etiology, supraventricular tachycardia, atrial flutter in some cases Infants: irritability, lethargy, poor feeding, tachypnea, signs of congestive heart failure Older children: palpitations, chest discomfort, abdominal pain, dizziness, syncope, cardiac arrest 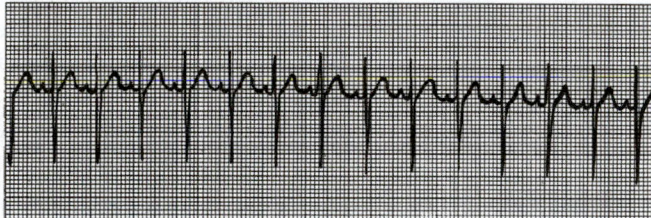	Vagal maneuvers Medications: adenosine, amiodarone, digoxin, beta-blockers Synchronized cardioversion **Radiofrequency ablation,** the use of radio energy (heat) to destroy a very small section of the myocardium through which an accessory conduction pathway passes Implantation of an antitachycardia pacemaker or cardioverter-defibrillator
Severe electrolyte or metabolic abnormalities, hypoxia, hypothermia, drug toxicity, cardiomyopathy, ventriculotomy for congenital heart defect, long QT syndrome	Ventricular tachycardia with abrupt onset, torsades de pointes, heart rate greater than 220 beats/min, cardiac arrest Infants: lethargy, tachypnea, poor feeding, pallor or cyanosis, diaphoresis Older children: palpitations, chest discomfort, dizziness, nausea, syncope, sudden cardiac death 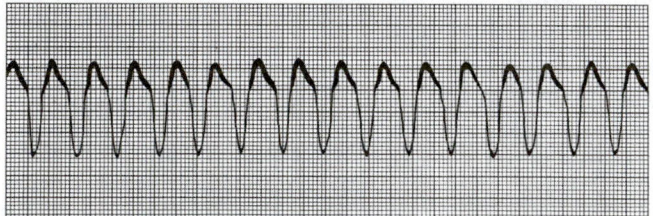	Medications: amiodarone, procainamide, or lidocaine Synchronized cardioversion, implantable pacemaker, or cardioverter-defibrillator Radiofrequency ablation in a few cases Surgical intervention (revision of previous heart surgery, cryoablation, transplant)
Hypovolemia, febrile illness, drugs or stimulant medications	Sinus tachycardia, gradual onset, heart rate less than 200 beats/min	Fluids or blood replacement Antipyretic
Inheritance of one or more genes associated with long QT syndrome	A prolongation of the QT interval on ECG, torsades de pointes, syncope with exertion or emotional upset or loud noises, palpitations, seizure, cardiac arrest	Medications: beta-blocker (propranolol, atenolol), sodium channel blockers Exercise restrictions Avoid triggers and drugs that cause QT interval to be prolonged Pacemaker or cardioverter-defibrillator

Source: *Data from Inaba, A. S., & Horeczko, T. (2009). Cardiac disorders. In J. A. Marx, R. S. Hockberger, R. M. Walls, J. G. Adams, W. G. Barsan, M. H. Biros, . . . E. J. Newton,* Rosen's emergency medicine *(7th ed., pp. 2152–2158). St. Louis, MO: Elsevier Mosby; Shimizu, W. (2008). Genetics of congenital long QT syndrome and Brugada syndrome. Future of Medicine, 4(4), 379–389; Doniger, S. J., & Sharieff, G. Q. (2006). Pediatric dysrhythmias. Pediatric Clinics of North America, 53, 85–105.*

Medications Commonly Used to Treat Arrhythmias

MEDICATION	USE AND ACTION	NURSING MANAGEMENT
Epinephrine Alpha- and beta-adrenergic agonist	Used for bradycardia and low cardiac output Strengthens myocardial contraction, restores cardiac rhythm	Place the child on a cardiac monitor to assess heart rate and potential arrhythmias. Monitor the blood pressure.
Atropine Anticholinergic	Used for sinus bradycardia, asystole during cardiac resuscitation Blocks vagal impulse to the heart; decreases AV conduction time, shortens PR interval, increases heart rate	Monitor for paradoxical bradycardia that may occur within the first 1–2 minutes of IV administration. It may be used prior to intubation in young children to prevent bradycardia due to vagal stimulation.
Adenosine Class IA antiarrhythmic	Used to restore sinus rhythm for cases of supraventricular tachycardia, atrial flutter Slows conduction through the atrioventricular and sinoatrial nodes, interrupts reentry pathways through the AV node	Medication is administered rapidly by IV push and followed by a saline flush. Monitor heart rate, blood pressure, and cardiac rhythm continuously as the drug is administered. Run an ECG strip as the medication is administered to monitor conversion from arrhythmia to sinus rhythm.
Amiodarone Class III antiarrhythmic (potassium channel blocker) with Class I and Class II properties	Used for life-threatening ventricular tachycardia, supraventricular tachycardia, atrial flutter, and ventricular fibrillation Slows conduction time through the atrioventricular node, prolongs the refractory period, and increases coronary blood flow	Rate of administration varies with each of two loading doses and maintenance doses. Monitor the ECG for expected slowing of rate and ECG changes. Monitor for adverse effects of hypotension, nausea and vomiting, and bradycardia.
Propranolol Class II antiarrhythmic	Used for supraventricular tachycardia, and tachyarrhythmias Reduces myocardial irritability, depresses automaticity of sinus node, decreases atrioventricular and intraventricular conduction velocity	Monitor blood glucose levels in neonates and infants. Monitor for other side effects such as hypotension, bradycardia, and nausea. Neonates are susceptible to respiratory depression.
Digoxin Inotropic, antiarrhythmic	Used for atrial fibrillation, atrial flutter, and some cases of SVT Decreases conduction velocity through the atrioventricular node; increases force and velocity of myocardial systolic contraction	Monitor for digoxin toxicity and side effects such as bradycardia, tachyarrhythmia, nausea, anorexia, sleepiness, and vision changes. Monitor calcium level which influences sensitivity to digoxin.
Verapamil Class IV antiarrhythmic	Used for refractory supraventricular tachycardia and ventricular tachycardia Not used in infants under 1 year of age and for chronic therapy in patients with Wolff-Parkinson-White syndrome Decreases and slows sinoatrial and atrioventricular node conduction	An ECG is needed to monitor for bradycardia. Monitor the blood pressure for hypotension. Monitor for other adverse effects such as headache, dizziness, and constipation. Keep the child in bed for an hour after IV administration to prevent effects of hypotension.
Procainamide Class IA antiarrhythmic (sodium channel blocker)	Used for supraventricular tachycardia, ventricular tachycardias, and atrial tachycardias Decreases myocardial excitability and conduction velocity, increases duration of refractory period	Administer IV drug slowly with an infusion pump. Discontinue drug temporarily when arrhythmia is interrupted. Monitor for hypotension and ventricular arrhythmias if given intravenously. Do not use with amiodarone which will also cause QT prolongation.
Lidocaine Class IB antiarrhythmic	Used for ventricular arrhythmias Suppresses automaticity of His-Purkinje conduction system, increases electrical stimulation threshold of the ventricles during diastole	The drug is given by intravenous or intraosseous routes in a bolus dose. Stop infusion immediately if cardiac depression occurs (prolonged PR or QRS interval, worsening of arrhythmia). Monitor respiratory and neurologic status, blood pressure, and ECG for signs of potential overdose and toxicity. Cimetidine and beta-blockers may increase effect of lidocaine.

Source: *Data from Samson, R. A., & Atkins, D. L. (2008). Tachyarrhythmias and defibrillation. Pediatric Clinics of North America, 55, 887–907; Wilson, B. A., Shannon, M. T., & Stang, C. L. (2011). Pearson nurse's drug guide 2011. Upper Saddle River, NJ: Pearson; Gahart, B. L., & Nazareno, A. R. (2012). 2012 intravenous medications (28th ed.). St. Louis, MO: Elsevier Mosby.*

transmission of the extra impulses triggering the tachycardia. This procedure is frequently successful, and medications to control the tachycardia can be discontinued. In some cases, however, a cardioverter-defibrillator may need to be implanted.

Long QT syndrome Initial treatment may include cardiopulmonary resuscitation, intravenous magnesium, a lidocaine infusion,

correcting electrolyte imbalances, cardiac pacing, and withdrawing medications that prolong the QT interval. Beta-blockers (e.g., propranolol) are often effective in treating the condition. Medications that prolong the QT interval should not be prescribed. Children with the condition should not engage in competitive sports, and swimming should be supervised. In some cases, the child is given a pacemaker or cardioverter-defibrillator.

Nursing Management

The focus of nursing care is assessment of the child, preparing the child and family for diagnostic procedures, and educating the parents about medications and other interventions for the specific rhythm problem.

Nursing Assessment and Diagnoses

The child suspected of having an arrhythmia should have the level of consciousness, heart rate, and other vital signs monitored. A cardio-respiratory monitor and pulse oximetry should be used to identify deterioration of the child's condition. Changes in color, weakness, irritability, and changes in feeding pattern may indicate the development of hypoxia.

Practice Alert

When the heart rate reaches 180 beats/min in a child (220 beats/min in an infant) and is sustained for a long period, cardiac output falls. The time needed for blood to fill the ventricles during diastole is too short. Oxygen delivery to the myocardium is decreased because perfusion of the coronary arteries is compromised during the short diastolic phase, leading to syncope. Without treatment, cardiac output is decreased and congestive heart failure may develop (Anderson & Vetter, 2010).

Any child in the community found to have an abnormal ECG finding, unusual heart rhythm, syncope (especially with exercise), or dizziness with palpitations should be referred to a pediatric cardiologist for evaluation.

Nursing diagnoses that may be considered for the child with arrhythmias include:

- Cardiac Output, Decreased related to dysfunctional electrical system conduction
- Coping: Family, Compromised related to recurrent life-threatening arrhythmia in infant
- Development: Delayed, Risk for related to repeated illness episodes
- Social Interaction, Impaired related to ban from team sports

NANDA-I © 2012

Planning and Implementation

The child will be treated in the emergency department or intensive care unit, depending upon the type of arrhythmia and how stable the child is while being treated. Attach the cardiorespiratory monitor or external pacing leads and equipment as ordered. Assist the child with Valsalva maneuvers if ordered for SVT, and monitor for recurrence of the arrhythmia. Administer medications as ordered and observe for response. Provide for rest and adequate nutrition. Have emergency medications and resuscitation equipment readily available at the bedside.

Practice Alert

When applying ice or iced saline to the face of an infant, take care to avoid pressure on the eyes as retinal damage could occur. Also ensure that the child's airway is unobstructed by the ice packs.

Prepare the child and family for procedures. When sedation is ordered for invasive procedures such as synchronized cardioversion, follow the institution's guidelines for frequent assessment and intervention.

Discharge Planning and Home Care Teaching

Episodes of arrhythmia are frightening for both the child and parents, as is the unpredictability of recurrent episodes and risk for sudden cardiac death with some arrhythmias. Provide support and encourage the parents to promote the child's normal development between episodes. Emphasize that medications help prevent or reduce episode frequency.

Carefully explain the treatment plan and home care. Teach parents to take the child's apical pulse. Describe and provide written instructions about the danger signs indicating a recurrence of the acute condition and how to seek emergency care. Make sure parents are trained in CPR and, if appropriate, in how to perform Valsalva maneuvers. Provide telephone numbers of emergency medical facilities and help parents plan how to seek emergency care.

Make sure the parents and child with SVT understand the need to avoid using cardiac stimulant drugs such as decongestants as these drugs might trigger another episode. Provide preparation for the child and family for procedures such as radiofrequency ablation, or pacemaker or cardioverter-defibrillator implantation.

Make sure the parents and child with long QT syndrome know to avoid triggers that cause arrhythmia episodes such as competitive athletics, loud noises, and extreme emotional stress. Teach the parents and adolescents to remind the primary care provider about prescription medications that should be avoided (e.g., antihistamines and macrolide antibiotics). An updated list of these medications can be found online.

Clinical Tip

Kara Mia, by Maryann Anglim and Walter Allan, MD, tells the story of an adolescent who experiences a cardiac arrest and anoxic injury as a result of long QT syndrome and provides information about the disorder.

Evaluation

Expected outcomes of nursing care include the following:

- Arrhythmia episodes decrease in frequency because of adherence to prescribed medications.
- Parents respond appropriately when an arrhythmia episode occurs.

DYSLIPIDEMIA

Dyslipidemia is an abnormal concentration of one or more lipids (total cholesterol, low-density lipoproteins, triglycerides, or high-density lipoproteins) in the blood. Although children do not usually die of atherosclerotic heart disease, it is important to identify children who have a genetic history or lifestyle that makes them more susceptible to future coronary heart disease and to implement preventive health measures to reduce their risk of disease and premature death as adults. Autopsy studies have revealed that fatty streaks are present in the aorta by 10 years of age and in the coronary arteries by 20 years of age (Zappalla & Gidding, 2009).

Epidemiology and Pathophysiology

Significant risk factors for dyslipidemia include increased level of low-density lipoproteins, decreased level of high-density lipoproteins, elevated blood pressure, type 1 or 2 diabetes mellitus, cigarette smoking, and obesity (Daniels, Greer, & the Committee on Nutrition, 2008). Certain conditions are associated with accelerated atherosclerosis in children and adolescents: familial hypercholesterolemia, type 1 and 2 diabetes mellitus, Kawasaki disease, and heart transplantation (Zappalla & Gidding, 2009). Improving lipid and lipoprotein concentrations during childhood and adolescence may help lower the child's risk of adult cardiovascular disease.

Dietary fat is absorbed from the small intestine and transported to the liver. Triglycerides may be stored in adipose tissue or used by muscles as an energy source. The liver produces the lipoproteins (cholesterol, triglycerides, low-density and high-density lipoproteins). The low-density lipoprotein (LDL) particles collect beneath the endothelial layer of the arteries where oxidation occurs and an inflammatory and immune response is initiated. Excess LDL particles are engulfed by macrophages, and the macrophages with lipids combine with T cells to form the fatty streak, the first stage of atherosclerosis.

LDLs are associated with increased cardiovascular risk if high levels are present in the blood. High-density lipoproteins (HDLs), associated with reduced cardiovascular risk, attract free cholesterol and support the transfer of cholesterol from the lower density lipoproteins and peripheral tissues to the liver. Abnormalities in the lipid levels may be the result of excessive production, lack of clearance of the lipoprotein particles, a genetic defect in lipid metabolism, or other defects such as enzyme deficiencies.

Some children have primary dyslipidemia due to familial hypercholesterolemia. Obesity is the leading secondary cause of dyslipidemia. Examples of secondary causes include hypothyroidism, diabetes, nephritic syndrome, and certain drugs such as corticosteroids, beta-blockers, and isotretinoin (Brashers, 2010). Most commonly, children have milder lipid abnormalities that arise from a combination of heredity and lifestyle factors.

Clinical Manifestations

Children and adolescents rarely have signs or symptoms of dyslipidemia, and the condition is usually only discovered during blood screening tests.

Collaborative Care

Diagnostic Tests

Dyslipidemia is identified by a blood test. Total cholesterol, high-density lipoprotein cholesterol (HDL-C), and triglycerides are measured. The LDL-C level is calculated using an equation based on the triglyceride, HDL-C, and total cholesterol levels. See Table 26–13 for recommended levels and levels of higher risk. A C-reactive protein level may also be obtained in some adolescents as this marker of inflammation is associated with cardiovascular disease risk (Wijnstok, Twisk, Young, et al., 2010).

Lipid screening recommendations for children and adolescents vary among organizations, such as the American Academy of Pediatrics (AAP); the National Heart, Blood, and Lung Institute; and the U.S. Preventive Services Task Force. The AAP recommends that all children between 2 and 10 years of age be screened for dyslipidemia with a fasting lipid profile when the following risk factors are present (Daniels et al., 2008):

- A family history of premature cardiovascular disease before age 55 years in parents or grandparents
- A parent with high blood concentrations of cholesterol
- An unknown family history
- Other risk factors for cardiovascular disease in children such as hypertension, obesity (body mass index greater than 85th percentile), or diabetes mellitus

TABLE 26–13	Laboratory Values for Assessment of Dyslipidemia in Children Between 2 and 19 Years Old	
TEST	**RECOMMENDED LEVEL**	**LEVELS OF HIGHER RISK**
Total cholesterol	Under 170 mg/dL	Borderline: 170–199 mg/dL
		Abnormal: 200 mg/dL or higher
LDL-C	Under 110 mg/dL	Borderline: 110–129 mg/dL
		Abnormal: 130 mg/dL or higher
Triglyceride		
0 to 9 years	Under 75 mg/dL	Borderline: 75–99 mg/dL
		Abnormal: 100 mg/dL or higher
10 to 19 years	Under 90 mg/dL	Borderline: 90–129 mg/dL
		Abnormal: 130 mg/dL or higher
HDL-C	45 mg/dL or higher	Borderline: 40–45 mg/dL
		Abnormal: Under 40 mg/dL

Source: *Adapted from National Heart Lung and Blood Institute (NHLBI). (2011).* Expert Panel on Integrated Guidelines for Cardiovascular Health and Risk Reduction in Children and Adolescents. *Retrieved from http://www.nhlbi.nih.gov/guidelines/cvd_ped/index.htm*

Clinical Therapy

Primary prevention of atherosclerosis should begin during childhood. The primary management of dyslipidemia in most children includes dietary modifications, exercise, and other changes in lifestyle. The child's diet is carefully analyzed and changes are made to satisfy the dietary guidelines so that saturated fats are less than 7% of total caloric intake, and cholesterol intake is less than 200 mg per day for treatment of elevated LDL-C levels. If the child is obese, weight loss of about 10% of the body mass index is encouraged (Zappalla & Gidding, 2009). Regular exercise is also prescribed.

If the child continues to have high serum lipid levels, a lipid specialist should be consulted. Lipid-lowering medications (cholestyramine or colestipol, niacin, and statins) may be considered for children over 8 years of age at the highest risk for early-onset cardiovascular disease. Several statins (e.g., lovastatin, simvastatin, atorvastatin, and pravastatin) have been approved by the FDA for children over 10 years who have familial hypercholesterolemia. The initial goal is to lower the LDL-C concentration to less than 160 mg/dL. However, the target LDL concentration may be as low as 130 mg/dL, or even 110 mg/dL when a strong family history of cardiovascular disease and other risk factors exist (Daniels et al., 2008). Children and adolescents taking statins should have a baseline lipid panel, creatine kinase, and liver transaminases and then have them reevaluated in 4 weeks, and then on a periodic basis.

Nursing Management

Nursing care focuses on identifying children at risk for dyslipidemia, providing education about diet and exercise, and monitoring eating patterns. Identification and management of dyslipidemia takes place in a variety of community agencies. Office and clinic nurses identify children at risk who need to have serum lipids measured. Nurses in schools provide education on ways to reduce risk factors. The child's history of exercise patterns, weight and body mass index percentiles, and dietary intake provides important information. See Box 26–6. Obtain data on familial heart disease, hypertension, diabetes, and smoking to determine risk factors. Total cholesterol level screening does not require fasting, but the child will need to fast for 12 hours before blood is drawn for a complete lipid evaluation.

BOX 26–6	Research: Cardiovascular Risk Factors

A study of 474 children, adolescents, and young adults between 11 and 23 years of age without diabetes mellitus was conducted to determine if those with carotid artery thickness and stiffness could be predicted by the presence of cardiovascular risk factors. Carotid artery thickness and stiffness was assessed by ultrasound. The presence of the following cardiovascular risk factors was assessed in all study subjects: body mass index greater than 95th percentile; blood pressure greater than 95th percentile based on age, gender, and height; fasting glucose of 100 mg/dL or more or fasting insulin at the 95th percentile; and the presence of dyslipidemia at levels similar to those in the high-risk category in Table 26–13. Subjects with two to four risk factors were considered high risk, and those with one or none were considered low risk. The high-risk group with more risk factors had significantly greater artery thickness and stiffness than the low-risk group. However, one risk factor, BMI greater than 95th percentile, was also associated with thicker and stiffer arteries (Shah, Dolan, Gao, et al., 2011).

Work with nutritionists to provide dietary teaching and monitor family eating patterns. The food plan for the child and entire family should consist primarily of fruit, vegetables, whole grains, low-fat and nonfat dairy products, lean meat and fish, legumes, and nuts. Processed foods and those with simple carbohydrates (sugar and white flour) should be limited because they worsen triglyceride and HDL-C levels (Zappalla & Gidding, 2009). Help parents recognize that modeling food choices will help children learn to eat better foods and reduce lipid levels. For children with familial hypercholesterolemia, lifelong dietary control is essential.

Encourage parents to promote physical activity, limit sedentary time for their children, and serve as role models. Help the child select an enjoyable moderate to intense activity for daily participation in addition to 30 minutes of vigorous, aerobic activities (e.g., jogging, swimming, bicycling, in-line skating, or soccer) at least three to four times a week to promote cardiovascular fitness. When 30 minutes is not possible, encourage two 15-minute exercise periods. The exercise will help control the child's weight and blood pressure, reduce the risk of diabetes, and help raise the HDL cholesterol level. Discourage smoking by the child or the parents as it increases the risk for cardiovascular disease.

Children and adolescents taking statin medications should be educated to inform their healthcare provider promptly if any of these adverse effects are noted: myalgia, muscle soreness, weakness, tenderness, or dark-colored urine. Signs of hepatic dysfunction should also be reported (nausea, anorexia, fatigue, vomiting, pain in right upper abdomen, and jaundice). Adolescent females should be cautioned that statins are not to be used if pregnant.

Since many affected children have family members with dyslipidemia, it is important to include the entire family in the treatment plan. Lifestyle changes such as diet and exercise are difficult for a single family member to implement. The family of a child with dyslipidemia requires continual teaching and reinforcement. Nutrition assessments and evaluation of family diet should be performed periodically.

HYPERTENSION

Hypertension in children and adolescents is defined as a systolic or diastolic blood pressure reading that is equal to or greater than the 95th percentile for age, gender, and height (see Appendix B 🔴 for blood pressure tables). Normal blood pressure is defined as a systolic or diastolic reading that falls below the 90th percentile for age, gender, and height. Hypertension is now estimated to occur in 5% of the pediatric population, possibly related to the number of children who are obese (Brady, Siberry, & Solomon, 2008). The increasing rate of hypertension in childhood is a significant concern because it is a major risk factor for heart disease and stroke during adulthood.

Etiology and Pathophysiology

Primary hypertension is less common in children than in adults. The most common causes of secondary hypertension in children include coarctation of the aorta, renal disorders, neoplasms, endocrine disorders, and obstructive sleep disorder (Brady et al., 2008). Primary or essential hypertension may be associated with a genetic or familial predisposition and obesity.

Renal disorders associated with hypertension include glomerulonephritis, renal insufficiency, hypoplastic kidney, polycystic kidney disease, and reflux nephropathy. Other less common causes of secondary hypertension include endocrinopathies (hyperthyroidism, adrenal hyperplasia, Cushing syndrome, and pheochromocytoma), increased intracranial pressure, and certain medications. See Table 26–14 for medications and other agents that can cause an elevated blood pressure. See Developing Cultural Competence: Blood Pressure.

TABLE 26–14	Medications and Other Agents That May Elevate the Blood Pressure
CLASSIFICATION OF AGENT	**SPECIFIC MEDICATIONS AND AGENTS**
Over-the-counter medications	Caffeine
	Ephedrine
	Pseudoephedrine
	Nonsteroidal anti-inflammatory drugs (ibuprofen, meloxicam, naproxen)
Prescription medications	Cyclosporin, tacrolimus
	Dexedrine
	Erythropoietin
	Glucocorticoids
	Methylphenidate
	Oral contraceptives
	Phenylephrine
	Antidepressants (venlafaxine, bupropion, desipramine, phenelzine)
Herbal Supplements	Ephedra (ma-huang)
	Ginseng
	Guarana
	Licorice
	St. John's wort
Illicit Drugs	Cocaine
	Methamphetamines
	Ecstasy (MDMA)
	Anabolic steroids
	Phencyclidine

Source: *Adapted from the MayoClinic.com article,* Medications and supplements that can raise your blood pressure. *Retrieved from http://www.mayoclinic.com/health/blood-pressure/MY00256*

Developing Cultural Competence
Blood Pressure

A recent study investigated risk factors for 184 children of diverse racial background who had been diagnosed with primary hypertension. Among the group of children less than age 13 years, no differences were found between Black children and non-Black children. For the group of children 13 years of age and older, Black adolescents had greater blood pressure elevations than non-Black adolescents by both episodic and 24-hour ambulatory blood pressure monitoring. In this case, age and potentially pubertal status had a significant association with cardiovascular risk status in Black adolescents (Brady, Fivush, Parekh, et al., 2010).

Clinical Manifestations

Children rarely have symptoms of hypertension, and the condition is usually detected during a health examination. Children with hypertension may have sleep-disordered breathing with obstructive apnea (see Chapter 25). Symptoms of severe hypertension may include headaches, nausea, vomiting, dizziness, epistaxis, visual changes, and diplopia.

Collaborative Care

Diagnostic Procedures

The diagnosis of hypertension is based on three or more separate readings a week apart in which the systolic or diastolic reading is greater than or equal to the 95th percentile for gender, age, and height (Council on Sports Medicine and Fitness, 2010). The child with an elevated blood pressure should initially have a urinalysis, serum creatinine, and serum electrolyte levels performed. If one of these is abnormal, a urine culture and renal ultrasound should be performed. A lipid panel should be obtained to detect secondary causes of hypertension. See Chapter 31 for more information about assessment of kidney functioning. Fasting glucose and serum insulin may be evaluated in children who are overweight. Thyroid and adrenal hormone levels may be obtained to rule out hyperthyroidism. An echocardiogram can be performed to assess for coarctation of the aorta or left ventricular hypertrophy. Polysomnography may be performed to identify a sleep disorder. A drug screen may be appropriate to identify substances that could cause hypertension (Brady et al., 2008).

Clinical Therapy

Nonpharmacologic measures for reduction of blood pressure focus on lifestyle changes that include weight reduction and 30 to 60 minutes of physical activity each day. Dietary modification to reduce sodium is recommended, along with provision of three to five fruit servings daily and adequate intake of calcium and dietary fiber. Less than 10% of calories should come from saturated fats. The Dietary Approaches to Stop Hypertension (DASH) diet that is low in sodium and enriched in calcium and potassium is effective for adolescents with elevated blood pressure (Couch, Saelens, Levin, et al., 2008). Smoking, alcohol, and illicit drugs should be strongly discouraged.

Medications are used for children with persistent, severe hypertension that is not resolved with nonpharmacologic therapies. End-organ damage (left ventricular hypertrophy, retinopathy, or microalbuminuria) is another indication for pharmacologic therapy. While all classifications of antihypertensive agents work in children, ACE inhibitors and calcium channel blockers are most commonly prescribed for children because of their low side effects (Brady et al., 2008).

Nursing Management

Nursing care focuses on detecting the child with hypertension and helping the child and family make lifestyle changes that help prevent hypertension or control the blood pressure when hypertension occurs.

Nursing Assessment and Diagnosis

Take a complete history for the child with borderline hypertension and other associated diseases. Are parents or siblings hypertensive? Is the child obese? How many servings of fruit does the child eat daily? What is the number of servings of dairy products? What is the child's daily salt intake? What are the child's daily exercise routines? Does the child have any sleep problems (e.g., nighttime wakening, snoring, daytime sleepiness)? Review any medications or other potential agents used by the child or adolescent.

When assessing the child for hypertension, consistently use the right arm (this is the standard arm used for the blood pressure tables) and make sure to use the appropriate cuff size (see the Clinical Skills Manual). Have the child sit quietly for 5 minutes before taking the blood pressure. Make sure at least one blood pressure reading is made using the leg, to assess for coarctation of the aorta. The systolic reading in the leg is normally 5 to 10 mmHg higher than the arm reading (Park, 2008, p. 22). Measure the child's height and identify the height percentile from the growth curve (see Appendix A). Compare the child's systolic and diastolic readings to the blood pressure table for gender, age, and height percentile to determine if the blood pressure is elevated (see Appendix B). See Box 26–7.

Monitor the blood pressure of the child with borderline hypertension every 3 to 6 months. Take at least two readings during the visit and average them if they differ.

Examples of nursing diagnoses for the child with hypertension include the following:

- Health Behavior, Risk Prone related to failure to modify lifestyle factors that contribute to hypertension
- Nutrition, Imbalanced: More than Body Requirements related to excess calorie and salt intake
- Health Maintenance, Ineffective related to lack of daily physical activity

NANDA-I © 2012

Planning and Implementation

Teach the child and parents the importance of weight reduction and dietary modifications (see Chapter 19). Provide suggestions about substitute seasonings for salt and lists of salty foods to avoid. Encouraging these children to follow a low-salt diet is important. Increasing intake of low-fat dairy products and fruits can contribute to blood pressure control.

BOX 26–7 | **Research: Unrecognized Elevated Blood Pressure**

A recent study examined the records of 726 children with a blood pressure reading of 120/80 mmHg or higher or at the 90th percentile or higher and no prior diagnosis of hypertension to identify how many were recognized as having an elevated blood pressure. Healthcare providers recognized only 17% of cases of elevated blood pressure. Factors associated with failure to recognize an elevated blood pressure included absence of obesity, family history of cardiovascular disease, and an obviously elevated blood pressure (Brady, Solomon, Neu, et al., 2010).

PHOTO STORY...

REDUCING BLOOD PRESSURE

Marielle is 4 1/2 years old and is in the health center today for a more complete evaluation of her elevated blood pressure. Over the past 2 months, Marielle has been in the health center three times to have her blood pressure measured, and each time it has been elevated. Her blood pressure readings have been 108/70, 110/68, and 108/68 on each of the prior visits. Today her blood pressure reading is 106/70. In each case either the systolic or the diastolic reading is at the 95th percentile for age, gender, and height. The blood pressure reading in her leg was higher than the reading in her arm, as is expected, and this finding did help rule out coarctation of the aorta as a cause of her elevated blood pressure. Her urinalysis and urine culture are negative, but additional urine tests are being ordered today to identify any potential renal problem.

Marielle weighs 25 kg (50 lb) and is 104 cm (41 in.) tall. She is at the 97th percentile for weight and the 50th percentile for height. Her body mass index (BMI) is 20.9, or greater than the 99th percentile for her age, sex, and height percentile. Mrs. Hudson, Marielle's mother, reports that her husband has high blood pressure that is controlled with medication. When reviewing Marielle's diet, her mother reports that she is a good eater. She eats few fruits, but likes milk and juices; she has four to five glasses of each daily. She also loves salty foods such as pretzels and chips. Mrs. Hudson prepares most of the meals for the family, and uses rice or potatoes, some vegetables, and meats to prepare various dishes. She uses salt in all foods she prepares.

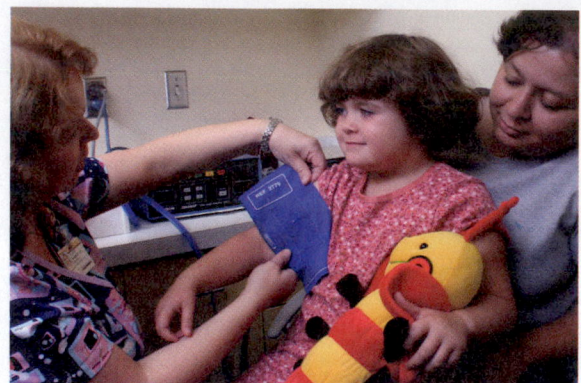

Because obtaining an accurate reading of Marielle's blood pressure is important, the nurse is identifying the correctly sized blood pressure cuff to use. In this case, an oscillometric reading will be taken.

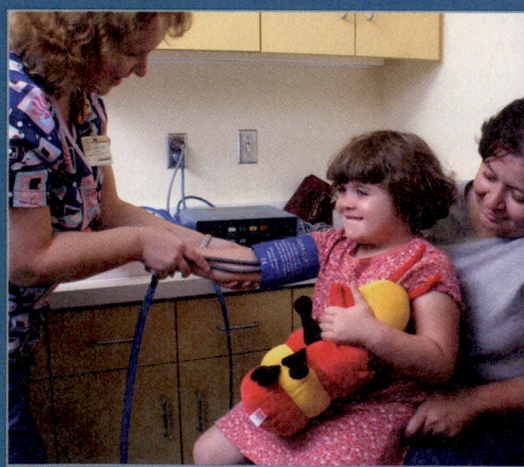

The nurse is holding Marielle's right arm level with her heart to obtain the blood pressure reading. This is the standardized position and arm used for development of the blood pressure tables. Notice that Marielle looks relaxed for the blood pressure reading, which should help avoid an elevated reading due to stress or fear.

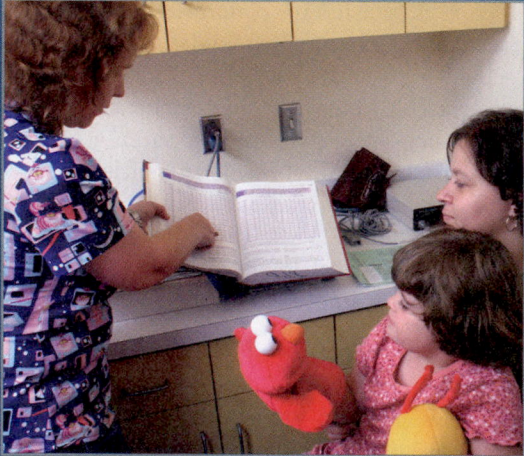

After obtaining Marielle's blood pressure, the nurse looks at the blood pressure table for gender, age, and height percentile to interpret the reading. She shows Mrs. Hudson Marielle's reading.

Marielle does not go to preschool. She stays with her grandmother during the day while her parents work. She has cousins that she plays with during the day, but her activities are limited to the small backyard.

The focus is now on helping Marielle reduce her blood pressure through dietary changes to allow her height to move into proportion with her weight, thus lowering her BMI. The amount of milk and juice she drinks every day must be reduced to recommended levels, and all dairy products should be low fat or nonfat. She needs to have access to fresh fruit for snacks rather than chips and pretzels. Mrs. Hudson is also encouraged to reduce the amount of salt she adds to food while it is being prepared as this may help control both her husband's and Marielle's blood pressure. Mrs. Hudson is also encouraged to explore ways to increase Marielle's activity, such as a family walk in the neighborhood each evening, gradually working up to 30 to 60 minutes of moderate activity daily.

Complementary Therapy   Breathing Awareness Meditation for Blood Pressure Control

Chronic stress has been associated with essential hypertension as well as hyperactivity of the systemic nervous system and an associated increase in sodium appetite. A study involving 166 African American high school students with elevated blood pressures investigated the use of breathing awareness meditation on blood pressure and urinary excretion of sodium. One comparison group received health education training about cardiovascular risk factor modification, and a second control group received lifestyle training that focused on problem solving, conflict resolution, and anger management. Interventions occurred over a 3-month period. Ambulatory blood pressure measurement, heart rate, and urine sodium levels were measured before and after interventions. The students participating in breathing awareness meditation had significantly greater decreases in school blood pressure and in 24-hour systolic blood pressure readings than students in the other groups. They also had significantly greater decreases in the 24-hour diastolic blood pressure and heart rate than the life skills training group. While urine sodium excretion was decreased more in the study group than either control group, it was not at a significant level (Gregoski, Barnes, Tingen, et al., 2011).

Discuss ways to increase activity and reduce time watching television or playing computer games. Provide suggestions for the management of stress and stressful situations (see Complementary Therapy: Breathing Awareness Meditation for Blood Pressure Control). Emphasize the importance of avoiding smoking, alcohol, and drugs. Teaching that involves the entire family is usually the most effective. Instruct the family on correct administration of prescribed medications when used.

Evaluation

Expected outcomes of nursing care include the following:

- The child maintains an appropriate weight for age and height and consumes a low-fat diet.
- The child and family recognize foods high in sodium by the child and family.
- The child and family adhere to scheduled follow-up visits for hypertension evaluation and treatment.

INJURIES OF THE CARDIOVASCULAR SYSTEM

Shock is an acute, complex state of progressive circulatory dysfunction resulting in failure to deliver sufficient oxygen and other nutrients to meet cell and tissue demands. It can be caused by a variety of conditions such as hemorrhage, dehydration, sepsis, obstruction of blood flow, and cardiac pump failure.

Hypovolemic Shock

Hypovolemic shock is a clinical state of inadequate tissue and organ perfusion resulting from the movement of blood or plasma out of the intravascular compartment, leading to an inadequate intravascular volume (Figure 26–15 ■). The blood or plasma in the vascular space may be decreased because of hemorrhage or fluid movement into the interstitial spaces.

Etiology and Pathophysiology

Major causes of decreased intravascular blood volume include the following:

- Hemorrhage from a significant injury (e.g., splenic or hepatic rupture, major vessel injury) or surgery

- Plasma loss from burns, nephrotic syndrome, and sepsis
- Fluid and electrolyte loss associated with dehydration, diabetic ketoacidosis, and diabetes insipidus

Shock results in inadequate delivery of oxygen (hypoxia and ischemia) and nutrients to cells and the accumulation of toxic wastes in the capillaries. This reduction in intravascular volume leads to decreased systemic blood return to the heart and ventricular filling. Lower stroke volume results, leading to a decrease in cardiac output and mean arterial pressure. The child has both intravascular and interstitial fluid loss. Cellular hypoxia and acidosis develop simultaneously. The accumulation of toxins and inadequate tissue oxygenation cause cellular damage.

When the brain perceives inadequate oxygen delivery, the child's body attempts to compensate with adrenergic and renal mechanisms in the following ways:

- Catecholamine and cortisol levels dramatically rise, which increase the heart rate, blood pressure, and myocardial contractility.
- The renin-angiotensin-aldosterone system is stimulated to retain sodium and intravascular fluid when kidney perfusion is reduced.
- The antidiuretic hormone is secreted when the atria have reduced blood volume, and this leads to oliguria.
- Glucagon is released to increase the blood sugar level for energy to support life-preserving functions.
- The respiratory rate increases to improve oxygenation and decrease waste accumulation in the cells.
- The hydrostatic pressure falls, permitting fluid to shift into the vascular space and increase the circulating blood volume.
- The peripheral vasculature constricts to maintain the systemic vascular resistance, which increases left ventricular afterload and provides perfusion of the brain, heart, and lungs as long as possible.

The compensatory efforts increase the myocardium's consumption of oxygen. Tachycardia may impair coronary blood flow, potentially causing myocardial ischemia if rapid intervention does not occur. The child is able to compensate until 20% to 25% of volume loss occurs, and then hypotension results, a sign of severe decompensated shock (Hazinski, Mondozzi, & Baker, 2010). Life-threatening end-organ failure may result if therapy is not immediately initiated.

Clinical Manifestations

Signs of early hypovolemic shock in children are nonspecific, but they need to be recognized before hypotension occurs. Signs indicating that the child is compensating for a decreased blood volume are persistent tachycardia, usually sustained at a rate greater than 130 beats/min, increased respiratory effort, prolonged capillary refill time (greater than 2 sec), weak peripheral pulses, pallor or mottled color, and cold extremities (signs of decreased perfusion). The blood pressure is often within normal values for age until compensatory mechanisms are exhausted. The infant and child may be irritable and anxious and then become progressively less responsive as hypovolemia increases. Urine output decreases due to the reduced renal blood flow. Low urine output is less than 2 mL/kg/hr in infants, less than 1 mL/kg/hr in children, and less than 0.5 mL/kg/hr in adolescents (Hazinski et al., 2010). In cases of dehydration, dry mucous membranes and poor skin turgor are also present.

Pathophysiology Illustrated
Hypovolemic Shock

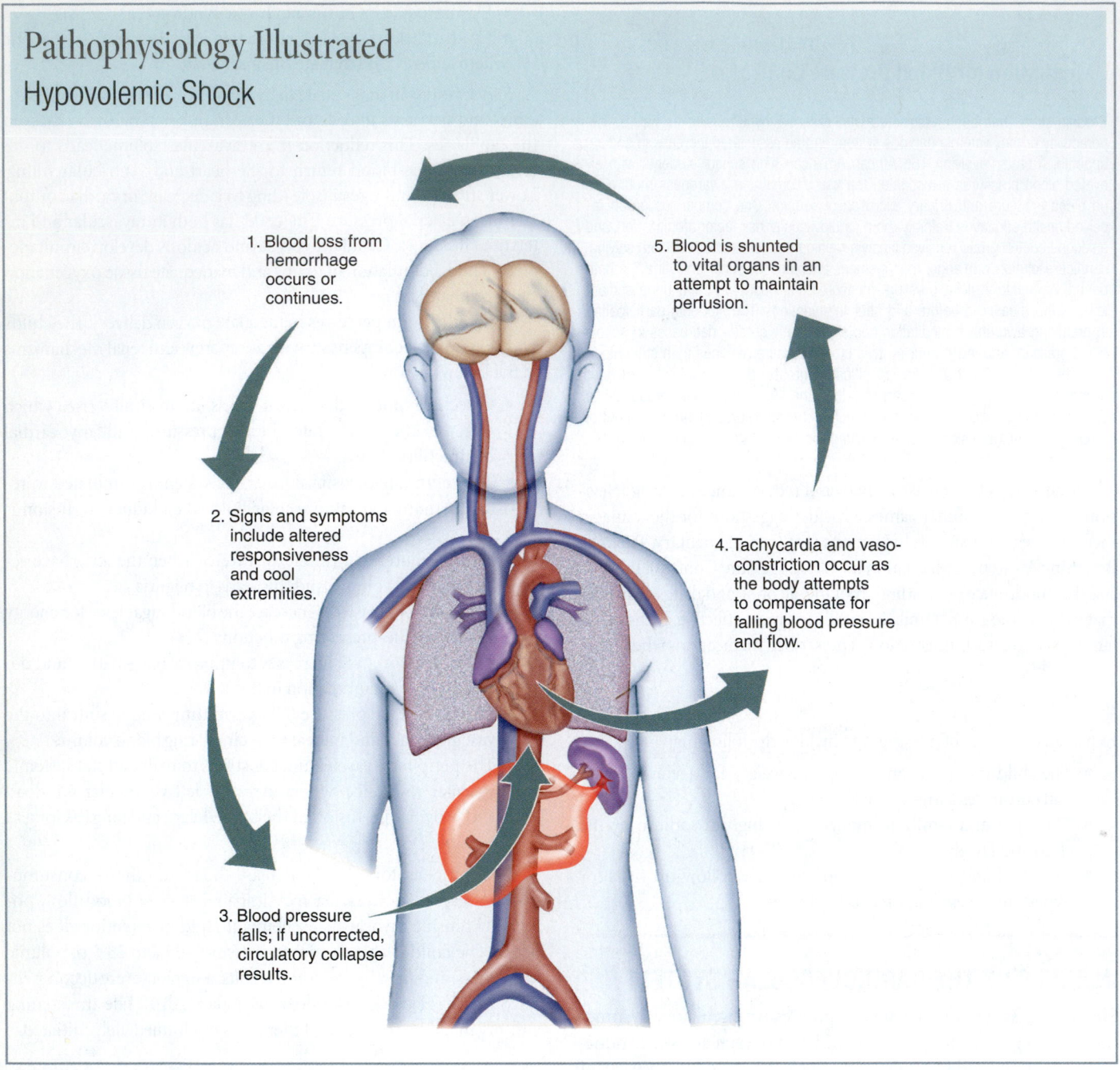

1. Blood loss from hemorrhage occurs or continues.

2. Signs and symptoms include altered responsiveness and cool extremities.

3. Blood pressure falls; if uncorrected, circulatory collapse results.

4. Tachycardia and vasoconstriction occur as the body attempts to compensate for falling blood pressure and flow.

5. Blood is shunted to vital organs in an attempt to maintain perfusion.

FIGURE 26–15 ■ If hemorrhage reduces the circulating blood volume sufficiently then the compensatory mechanisms support blood circulation by increasing the heart rate and constricting the peripheral blood vessels. This response shifts the remaining blood to larger blood vessels so that the vital organs continue to be perfused. When the blood loss exceeds 20% to 25%, the child's body can no longer compensate; blood pressure falls and circulatory collapse is imminent.

If treatment is not initiated, the condition progresses until the child can no longer compensate. At that time, the systolic blood pressure drops and the pulse pressure decreases. The reduced cerebral blood flow causes diminished level of consciousness. The condition can progress to cardiopulmonary failure. The Clinical Manifestations table compares the signs associated with early, uncompensated, and profound shock.

Collaborative Care

Diagnostic Procedures
No laboratory values can be used to evaluate the volume deficit rapidly enough to diagnose hypovolemic shock. The child is examined for characteristic signs to confirm the diagnosis. Laboratory tests commonly performed after hypovolemic shock is diagnosed and treatment is initiated include hematocrit and hemoglobin, arterial blood gases, serum electrolytes, glucose, osmolality, BUN, and urinalysis. The BUN and specific gravity are usually elevated when dehydration is the cause of hypovolemia. The type and severity of dehydration present influence the serum sodium and osmolality levels (see Chapter 23 for more information about dehydration and electrolyte levels).

Clinical Therapy
Emergency care focuses on improving tissue perfusion by correcting the intravascular volume deficit and providing supplemental oxygen.

Clinical Manifestations Hypovolemic Shock

SYSTEM	EARLY COMPENSATED SHOCK	MODERATE UNCOMPENSATED SHOCK	SEVERE UNCOMPENSATED SHOCK
Cardiac	Mild tachycardia, weak distal pulses, strong central pulses, normal blood pressure	Moderate tachycardia, thready distal pulses, weak central pulses, decreasing systolic blood pressure	Extreme tachycardia, absent distal pulses, thready central pulses, hypotension
Respiratory	Mild tachypnea	Moderate tachypnea	Severe tachypnea
Neurologic	Normal, anxious, irritable	Confusion, agitation, combative behavior, lethargy, decreased pain response	Comatose state
Skin	Mottled appearance; capillary refill time greater than 2 sec; cool, clammy extremities	Pallor, capillary refill time greater than 3 sec; cold, dry extremities, sunken eyes	Pale, cold skin, cyanosis, capillary refill greater than 5 sec
Renal	Decreased urine output, increased specific gravity in older infants and children	Oliguria, increased specific gravity	No urine output

Source: *Data from Ralston, M., Hazinski, M. F., Zaritsky, A. L., Schexnayder, S. M., & Kleinman, M. E. (2006). Pediatric advanced life support: Provider manual (p. 100). Dallas, TX: American Heart Association; Hazinski, M. F., Mondozzi, M. A., & Baker, R. A. U. (2010). Shock, multiple organ dysfunction syndrome, and burns in children. In K. L. McCance, S. E. Huether, V. L. Brashers, & N. R. Rote, Pathophysiology: The biologic basis for disease in adults and children (6th ed., pp. 1727–1754). St. Louis, MO: Mosby Elsevier; and Steffen, K. M. (2011). Trauma, burns, and common critical care emergencies. In M. M. Tschudy, & K. M. Arcara, The Harriet Lane handbook (19th ed., p. 109). Philadelphia, PA: Elsevier Mosby.*

An open airway is established, oxygen is administered, and ventilation is assisted if necessary. Bleeding is controlled, and an intravenous or intraosseous line is started to provide large volumes of crystalloid fluids (Ringer's lactate or normal saline). A fluid volume of 20 mL/kg is administered rapidly over 5 minutes. The same amount of fluid is given in 5 minutes if the child's physiologic condition does not improve after fluid is first administered. If no improvement is seen after the second or third fluid bolus, packed red blood cells are usually ordered. Some children need inotropic medications provided in intravenous drips to sustain cardiac output and increase renal perfusion while the cause of hypovolemic shock is identified and treated. Once the child's physiologic condition is stabilized, the cause of the hypovolemic shock becomes the focus of examination and treatment.

Clinical Tip

Initial signs that a child with hypovolemic shock is responding to fluid resuscitation include slowing of the heart rate, improved color, improved responsiveness, increased warmth of the extremities, and a faster capillary refill time. The systolic blood pressure should increase.

Nursing Management

Nursing care is focused on early detection of hypovolemic shock so that intervention is initiated before the blood pressure falls.

Nursing Assessment and Diagnosis

Ask the parent (or child, if appropriate) about possible injuries or the duration and severity of acute illnesses. If no external bleeding is evident, determine whether an injury may be causing internal bleeding. For example, the liver and spleen are highly vascular organs that have little protection from direct blunt forces. Significant bleeding from injury to one of these organs can cause hypovolemic shock without direct evidence of bleeding. An acute illness such as gastroenteritis with prolonged vomiting and diarrhea can also result in dehydration and hypovolemic shock. If external bleeding is apparent, determine the amount of blood lost. Although children lose the same amount of blood from a laceration as adults, the total volume of blood lost is proportional to their weight.

Clinical Tip

The child has approximately 80 mL of blood for every kilogram of body weight. When estimating blood loss, consider the following blood volumes in children:

- Newborn—3 kg × 80 mL = 240 mL (1 cup)
- 5-year-old—25 kg × 80 mL = 2000 mL (2 quarts)
- 13-year-old—50 kg × 80 mL = 4000 mL (1 gallon)

Frequently assess the child's heart rate, respiratory rate, blood pressure, capillary refill time, level of consciousness with the Glasgow Coma Scale (see Chapter 33 🔗), color, and skin temperature to identify any changes that indicate improvement or deterioration in the child's condition. Monitor urine output and specific gravity hourly. Signs of the child's improved status include the following:

- A decrease in heart rate, respiratory rate, and capillary refill time
- An increase in systolic blood pressure and urine output
- Improved color, level of consciousness, and skin temperature
- Regaining of lost weight

Practice Alert

When an injured child is admitted to the hospital for a problem such as a liver or spleen laceration, assess the child's circulatory status frequently. Current medical treatment for these injuries is conservative. Surgeons give the liver or spleen a chance to heal spontaneously rather than perform immediate surgery to control bleeding and repair the laceration. Even if the child's circulatory condition was stabilized during emergency care, shock can develop again if bleeding continues.

Assess the parents' response and coping mechanisms to the potentially life-threatening injury of their child. Families are unprepared for the abrupt change in the child's condition because of the unpredictability of the injury. See Chapter 17 🔗.

The following nursing diagnoses may apply to the child with hypovolemic shock:

- Cardiac Output, Decreased related to hypovolemia
- Fluid Volume: Deficient related to active fluid volume loss due to vomiting and diarrhea

- Tissue Perfusion: Cerebral, Risk for Ineffective related to impaired transport of oxygen across the alveolar and capillary membrane
- Airway Clearance, Ineffective related to altered level of consciousness
- Coping: Family, Compromised related to life-threatening condition of the child

NANDA-I © 2012

Planning and Implementation

Nurses in the emergency department and intensive care unit participate in the resuscitation of the child in hypovolemic shock, often having guidelines or protocols for nursing actions. Assist with the child's assessment and the establishment of intravenous access. Calculate and prepare the amount of warmed intravenous fluid needed for administration according to the child's weight (20 mL/kg). Ensure rapid fluid administration by intravenous push or pressure bag. Monitor the child's physiologic response to the fluid bolus within 5 minutes. Prepare a second and third fluid bolus. Warmed intravenous fluids are used for resuscitation because hypothermia may interfere with the child's response to treatment. Keep the child covered or use heat lamps to reduce body heat loss.

When packed red blood cells are administered, verify that the correct blood has been obtained for the child. Change the intravenous fluid to normal saline solution to prevent clotting during blood administration. Assess the child carefully for a transfusion reaction (see Chapter 28 ❷). Monitor the child's physiologic circulatory responses for improvement or deterioration in status. Notify the physician of any deterioration.

Provide support to the child and family during the acute phase of treatment. Parents and children with hypovolemic shock resulting from injury or severe dehydration are usually apprehensive. The child may be fearful because of the sudden hospitalization or may be agitated because of an altered level of consciousness. Determine the causes of the child's anxiety. The parents often fear for the child's life in cases of severe injury. In cases when the parent is present during the resuscitation, ensure that a healthcare provider is assigned to give information and support during the emergency care provided. Update the parents about the child's condition frequently if the parent is in the waiting area. Explain the care being provided and how it helps the child. Listen to their concerns and correct any misconceptions.

Evaluation

Examples of expected nursing care outcomes include the following:

- Progression to uncompensated shock is prevented by fluid resuscitation.
- The family copes with the stress of the child's injury.

Distributive Shock

Distributive shock is an abnormal distribution of blood volume usually resulting from a decrease in systemic vascular resistance and a

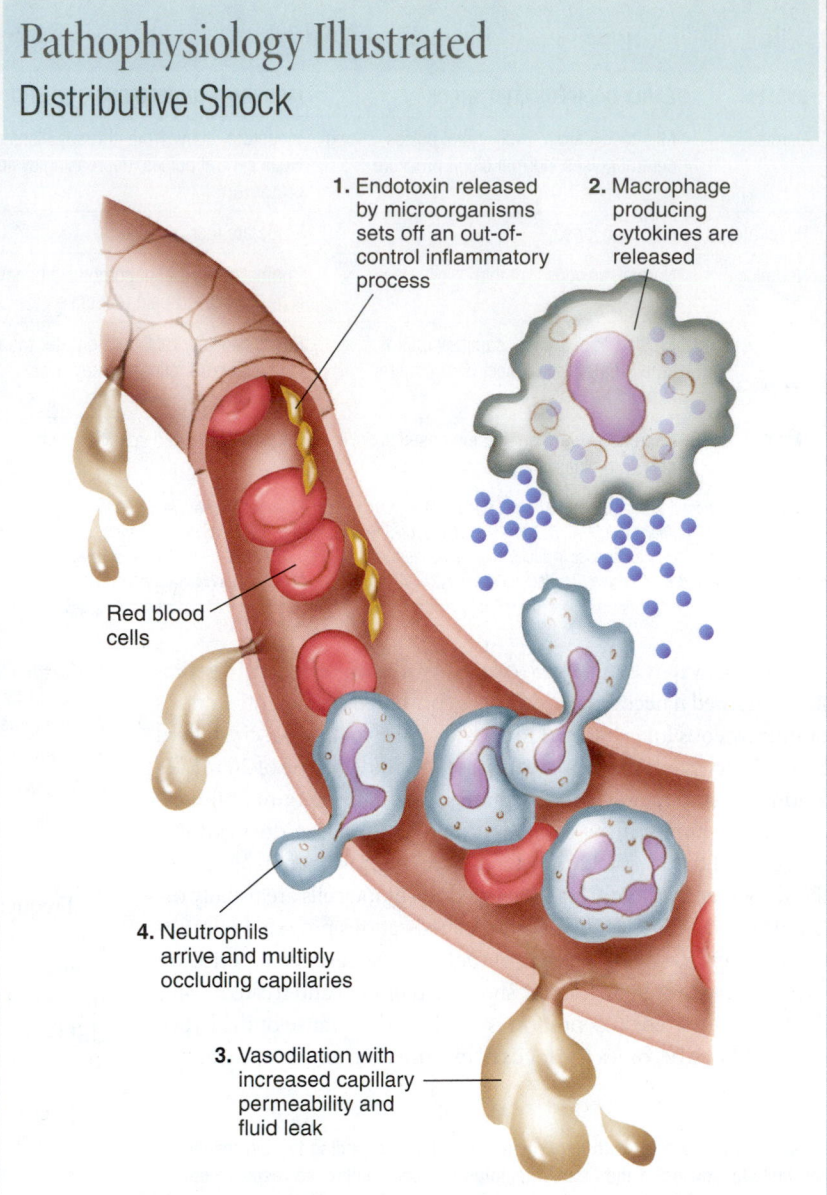

Pathophysiology Illustrated
Distributive Shock

1. Endotoxin released by microorganisms sets off an out-of-control inflammatory process

2. Macrophage producing cytokines are released

Red blood cells

4. Neutrophils arrive and multiply occluding capillaries

3. Vasodilation with increased capillary permeability and fluid leak

FIGURE 26–16 ■ In neurogenic shock, blood pools in the extremities because the vascular tone is lost with spinal cord injury. Blood flow becomes sluggish because inadequate blood is returned to the heart to maintain the needed cardiac output. The tissues receive inadequate amounts of oxygen for cell metabolism.

maldistribution of blood flow to the extremities because of vasodilation and capillary permeability. Less blood is returned to the heart, so preload drops and cardiac output falls. Blood flow is inadequate to all tissue beds. The child attempts to compensate for low systemic vascular resistance by increasing cardiac output to maintain the blood pressure.

Causes of distributive shock include the following:

- Neurogenic in which vasodilation occurs with loss of vasomotor tone, such as occurs with a spinal cord injury or various medications (morphine, beta-blockers, barbiturates, antihypertensives, anesthetic agents) (Figure 26–16 ■).
- Anaphylaxis with vasodilation due to loss of vasomotor tone and capillary leak resulting from the release of mediators from the tissue mast cells in an immediate hypersensitivity reaction. See Chapter 27 ❷.
- Sepsis that may result from these organisms: beta-hemolytic streptococcus, *Haemophilus influenzae* type b, *Neisseria*

Pathophysiology Illustrated
Obstructive Shock

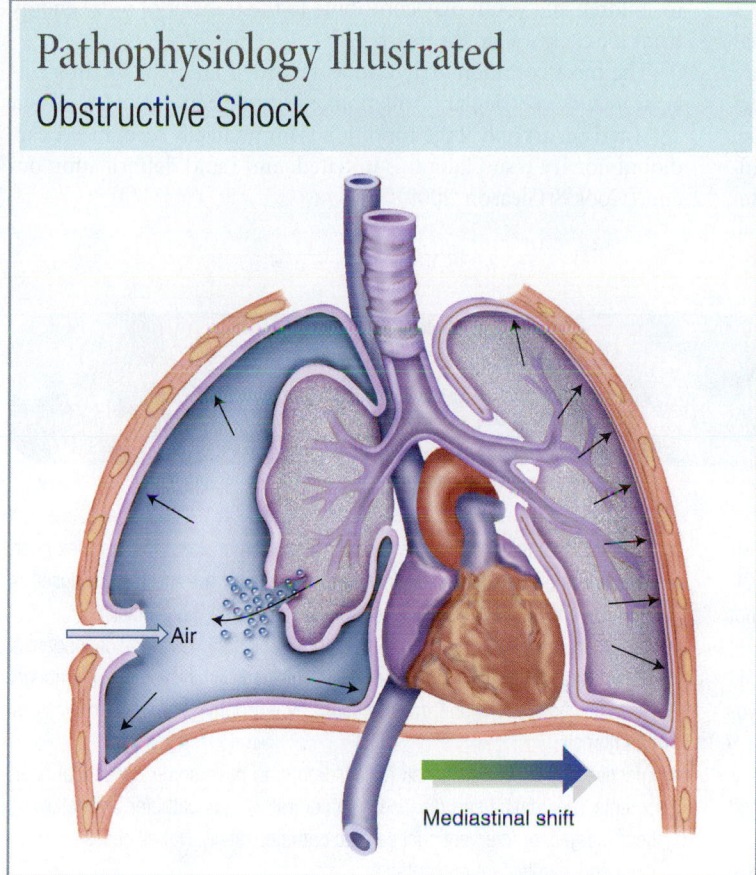

Air

Mediastinal shift

FIGURE 26–17 ■ Compression of the vena cavae or great arteries can occur when a tension pneumothorax causes a mediastinal shift. The shifting heart and lungs obstruct blood flow to and from the heart, leading to obstructive shock.

meningitidis, Streptococcus pneumoniae, Staphylococcus aureus, Staphylococcus epidermidis, Pseudomonas, and *Candida.* Low systemic vascular resistance results from the child's response to the invading organisms.

Nursing Management

The child with distributive shock is cared for in the intensive care unit. Nursing care focuses on detecting and managing subtle changes in the child's physiologic status to improve the child's condition. Parents are supported as described in Chapter 17 🐙. Please see Chapter 22 🐙 for nursing care of sepsis and septic shock.

Obstructive Shock

Obstructive shock occurs from a mechanical blockage of blood flow into and through the heart and great vessels (Figure 26–17 ■). Causes in children include compression of the vena cava, pericardial tamponade, pulmonary embolism, tension pneumothorax, pleural effusion, and congenital heart defects with outflow obstruction (e.g., severe aortic stenosis). Management is focused on treatment of the underlying condition.

Nursing Management

The child is usually cared for in the intensive care unit with nursing care focused on supporting the child's respiratory and cardiovascular functioning. See Chapter 25 🐙 for care of the child with a tension pneumothorax.

Cardiogenic Shock

Cardiogenic shock is an impairment of myocardial function that interferes with the heart's ability to maintain adequate cardiac output and tissue perfusion. Causes of cardiogenic shock in children may include severe obstructive congenital heart disease such as hypoplastic left heart syndrome, cardiomyopathy, myocarditis, severe electrolyte or acid–base imbalance, a complication of shock, and early septic shock (Hazinski et al., 2010).

Clinically, cardiogenic shock resembles hypovolemic shock with low cardiac output. Tachycardia, tachypnea, increased respiratory effort, decreased oxygen saturation, normal or low blood pressure, weak or absent peripheral pulses, prolonged capillary refill time, cool and pale extremities, and oliguria are common signs. Disorientation and restlessness occur as the compensatory mechanisms fail. Compensatory responses divert blood to the heart and brain; however, reduced blood flow to the kidneys, liver, and intestines can lead to ischemia and end-organ failure. Increased systemic vascular resistance puts more stress on the failing heart. Each contraction causes more blood to accumulate in the heart and pulmonary vessels, eventually leading to CHF, reduced perfusion of the coronary arteries and myocardial ischemia, metabolic acidosis, and circulatory collapse. Multisystem organ failure can occur from persistent ischemia.

An enlarged heart and pulmonary congestion may be seen on a chest radiograph. The goal of medical treatment is to improve myocardial function and cardiac output. Diuretics and vasodilators are given along with adequate ventilatory support, sedatives, analgesics, and antipyretics. Inotropic agents may be used in some cases.

Nursing Management

The child is cared for in the intensive care unit. Nursing care focuses on monitoring and supporting the child's respiratory and cardiovascular status, fluid management, and medication administration. See Chapter 17 🐙 for care of the child with a life-threatening condition.

Myocardial Contusion

Myocardial contusion, a rare injury in children, results from a strong, blunt force against the chest wall that injures the heart muscle, usually the right ventricle. Blood flow to areas of the heart muscle is disrupted, or myocardial cells are directly destroyed. This potentially life-threatening condition is often associated with a motor vehicle–related injury, a crush injury, or a fall.

A myocardial contusion should be suspected in cases of injury to the anterior chest. The child has chest wall tenderness and chest pain because of fractured ribs or chest wall contusion. An electrocardiogram reveals arrhythmias or signs of myocardial infarct. A two-dimensional echocardiogram may show an abnormality in heart wall movement. Cardiac enzymes (troponin I) are often elevated. Because of the risk of sudden arrhythmias, the child is admitted to the intensive care unit for cardiac monitoring.

Commotio Cordis

Commotio cordis, also known as a cardiac concussion, is a blunt, nonpenetrating blow to the precordium that causes ventricular fibrillation and sudden death. Most injuries occur in male children and adolescents (Cook & Gleason, 2009). The majority of victims are healthy children and youth without an underlying cardiovascular disease participating in sports such as baseball, softball, ice hockey, and lacrosse. In some cases the event is triggered by physical contact with another person, such as a fist, elbow, knee, or head. The timing of the impact on the precordium is believed to coincide with the vulnerable period of cardiac repolarization. The narrower anteroposterior diameter of the chest and increased compliance of the chest wall in children and youth may contribute to the transfer of more energy from the chest wall to the heart.

The most common arrhythmias recorded after the victim's collapse include ventricular fibrillation or asystole. Survival is low, about 13%, and occurs only if the condition is immediately recognized, cardiopulmonary resuscitation is initiated, and rapid defibrillation occurs (Cook & Gleason, 2009).

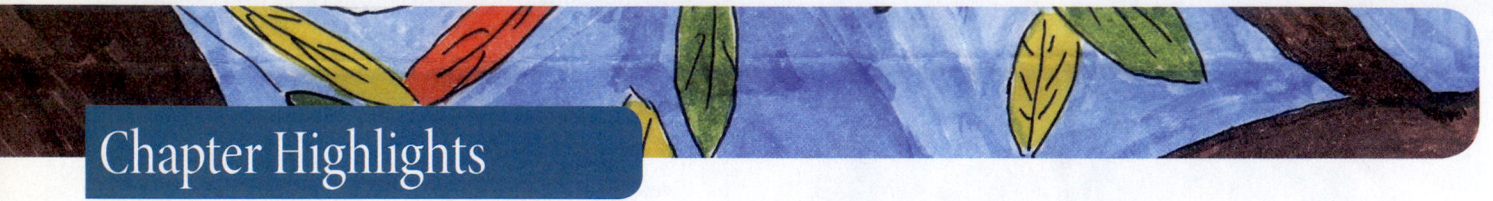

Chapter Highlights

- Infants are at risk of heart failure because their immature heart is more sensitive to volume or pressure overload. The heart muscle fibers are less developed and the ventricles have less compliance so that stroke volume cannot increase substantially.
- Increasing cardiac output is primarily heart rate dependent in infants and children under 5 years of age. After that age, the muscle fibers in the myocardium are developed enough to stretch and increase ventricular volume.
- Most congenital heart defects develop during the first 8 weeks of pregnancy, and they are often the result of a combined or interactive effect of genetic and environmental factors.
- Congenital heart defects are categorized by pathophysiology and hemodynamics:
  - Defects that increase pulmonary blood flow include patent ductus arteriosus, atrial septal defect, ventricular septal defect, and atrioventricular canal.
  - Defects that decrease pulmonary blood flow include pulmonic stenosis, tetralogy of Fallot, pulmonary atresia, and tricuspid atresia.
  - Defects that decrease systemic blood flow include aortic stenosis, coarctation of the aorta, and hypoplastic left heart syndrome.
  - Transposition of the great arteries and truncus arteriosus are examples of mixed defects that require mixing of the pulmonary and systemic circulations for neonates to survive.
- Cardiac catheterization provides a means for the evaluation of the anatomy, as well as the hemodynamics and pressure gradients within the heart. Some heart defects can be corrected through interventional cardiac catheterization.
- Some children have complex congenital heart defects that require multiple stages of surgery to improve the quality of life.
- Infants with congenital heart defects that increase pulmonary blood flow are at high risk for development of congestive heart failure. Pulmonary artery hypertension can develop if the defect is not corrected at an early age.
- The child with a congenital heart defect that decreases pulmonary blood flow may have life-threatening hypercyanotic episodes requiring emergency treatment.
- Congenital heart defects that obstruct systemic blood flow cause signs and symptoms associated with low cardiac output: diminished pulses, poor color, prolonged capillary refill time, and decreased urinary output.
- Blood volume overloads associated with congenital heart defects are the most common causes of congestive heart failure in infants.
- Signs of congestive heart failure may include tachypnea, tachycardia, pallor or cyanosis, nasal flaring, grunting, retractions, cough, crackles, periorbital and facial edema, jugular vein distention, and hepatomegaly.
- Cardiomyopathy during childhood occurs most often in infancy and adolescence.

- Heart transplantation is performed in infants and children for complex heart defects or cardiomyopathy. Rejection and infection are the major causes of mortality and morbidity during the first year following the transplant.
- Pulmonary artery hypertension is a life-threatening complication of congenital heart disease with excessive pulmonary blood flow. Irreversible pulmonary vascular changes include inflammation, hypertrophy of pulmonary vessels, and fibrosis.
- Infective endocarditis is a risk for children who have some congenital heart defects, rheumatic heart disease, or a central venous catheter, and following heart surgery or interventional cardiac catheterization. Not all cases of infectious endocarditis are preventable.
- Rheumatic fever is an inflammatory connective tissue disease following a streptococcal infection that may affect the heart, joints, skin, or central nervous system. Long-term antibiotic therapy is prescribed after the acute phase of the illness to prevent repeated infections.
- Kawasaki disease is an acute febrile, systemic inflammatory illness with an unknown etiology and potential complication of coronary artery aneurysm. It is the most common acquired cardiovascular disease in childhood in the United States.
- Two potentially life-threatening cardiac arrhythmias are supraventricular tachycardia and long QT syndrome.
- Some children have familial or lifestyle-related dyslipidemia that causes undesirable levels of cholesterol or triglycerides. These children need dietary intervention and exercise regimens to reduce the risk of coronary artery disease as an adult.
- Hypertension in children and adolescents is defined as a systolic or diastolic blood pressure reading that is equal to or greater than the 95th percentile for age, gender, and height.
- Shock is an acute, complex state of circulatory dysfunction resulting in failure to deliver sufficient oxygen and other nutrients to meet cell and tissue demands.
- Signs that a child is in compensated hypovolemic shock include tachycardia, increased respiratory effort, prolonged capillary refill time, weak peripheral pulses, pallor, and cold extremities.
- Distributive shock is an abnormal distribution of the blood volume that results from a decrease in vascular resistance. It may be caused by anaphylaxis, sepsis, or spinal cord injury.
- Obstructive shock occurs from a mechanical blockage of blood flow into and through the heart and great vessels.
- Myocardial contusion results from a strong, blunt force against the chest wall that injures the heart muscle. Blood flow to areas of the heart muscle may be disrupted, or myocardial cells may be directly destroyed.

Clinical Reasoning in Action

INTRODUCTION

Recall Tim, 16 years old, in the opening scenario who was born with the tetralogy of Fallot congenital heart defect. Despite successful corrective surgery as an infant, he recently had a pacemaker placed to help manage the episodic slow ventricular heart rate.

DESCRIPTION

Tim is the oldest of two children in his family; his brother is 10 years old. Tim had been able to participate in all usual school and childhood activities except sports until the past year. He has many friends, both boys and girls. Tim is becoming more aware of how different he is from his peers due to his heart defect and recent pacemaker implantation. Tim's parents had previously made all of his healthcare decisions, but at the time the pacemaker was needed, Tim became more involved in the patient education and decision-making process. Now Tim is realizing that he must become much more involved in his health care, but he does not know how to assume that responsibility.

DISCUSSION

1. What is the potential explanation for the development of an arrhythmia so many years after the original heart surgery?
2. What physical limitations and ongoing care needs does Tim have?
3. What emotional and behavioral responses should be expected from Tim when learning more about his physical limitations and future healthcare needs?
4. Develop a teaching plan to educate Tim about his congenital heart condition and self-management to maintain his health status.
5. Develop a transition plan for Tim to begin taking primary responsibility for all aspects of his health care.

NCLEX-RN® Review

1. The nurse is caring for an infant taking digoxin (Lanoxin). Which would alert the nurse to hold the digoxin and notify the healthcare provider?
   1. A heart rate of 90
   2. A digoxin level 1.25 ng/mL
   3. Palpable peripheral pulses
   4. A potassium level of 4.0 mEq/L

2. The nurse is caring for a 4-month-old infant with congestive heart failure. Knowing that the infant will tire easily, what nursing intervention is priority?
   1. Encourage visitors to provide support to the infant.
   2. Provide toys from home.
   3. Feed the infant prior to other interventions.
   4. Bathe the infant before feeding.

3. Prior to heart surgery, an older infant with Tetrology of Fallot is fed formula through a nasogastric tube 24 hours a day in the home to ensure adequate calories. What teaching by the home health nurse will aid in this infant's appropriate growth and development?
   1. Try to wean the child from the bottle to the cup.
   2. Start an infant playgroup.
   3. Delay the administration of the respiratory syncytial virus (RSV) vaccine.
   4. Encourage the infant to take a small amount of formula by mouth each day.

4. The nurse is assessing a child with vascular disruption for hypovolemia. What assessment parameter is most appropriate?
   1. Cardiopulmonary monitoring
   2. Capillary refill
   3. Pulse
   4. History of the injury

See Appendix I ⊘ for answers.

References

Abdulla, R., & Hanrahan, A. (2011). Atrial septal defect. In R. Abdulla (Ed.), *Heart disease in children* (pp. 91–102). New York, NY: Springer.

American Academy of Pediatrics, Committee on Infectious Diseases (AAP). (2009). Policy statement—Modified recommendations for use of palivizumab for prevention of respiratory syncytial virus infections. *Pediatrics, 124*(6), 1694–1701.

American Academy of Pediatrics, Committee on Infectious Diseases (AAP). (2012). *Red book: Report of the Committee on Infectious Disease* (29th ed.). Elk Grove Village, IL: Author.

American Heart Association. (2010). *Kawasaki disease*. Retrieved from http://www.heart.org/HEARTORG/Conditions/More/CardiovascularConditionsofChildhood/Kawasaki-Disease_UCM_308777_Article.jsp

Anderson, B. R., & Vetter, V. L. (2010). Arrhythmogenic causes of chest pain in children. *Pediatric Clinics of North America, 57*, 1305–1329.

Awad, S. M. M., & Busse, J. (2011). Hypoplastic left heart syndrome. In R. Abdulla (Ed.), *Heart disease in children* (pp. 273–282). New York, NY: Springer.

Awad, S. M. M., & McCarville, M. A. (2011). Coarctation of the aorta. In R. Abdulla (Ed.), *Heart disease in children* (pp. 159–166). New York, NY: Springer.

Baddour, L. M., Wilson, W. R., Bayer, A. S., Fowler, V. G., Bolger, A. F., et al. (2005). Infective endocarditis: Diagnosis, antimicrobial therapy, and management of complications. *Circulation, 111*, e394–e433.

Baker, A. L., Lu, M., Minich, L. L., Atz, A. M., Klein, G. L., Korsin, R., . . . Pediatric Heart Network Investigators. (2009). Associated symptoms in the ten days before diagnosis of Kawasaki disease. *Journal of Pediatrics, 154*, 592–595.

Berger, S., Dhala, A., & Dearani, J. A. (2009). State-of-the-art management of hypertrophic cardiomyopathy in children. *Cardiology in the Young, 19*(Suppl. 2), 66–73.

Bernstein, D. (2011). General principles of treatment of congenital heart disease. In R. M. Kliegman, B. F. Stanton, N. F. Schor, J. W. St. Geme, & R. E. Behrman, *Nelson textbook of pediatrics* (19th ed., pp. 1602–1605). Philadelphia, PA: Elsevier Saunders.

Brady, T. M., Solomon, B. S., Neu, A. M., Siberry, G. K., & Tarekh, R. S. (2010). Patient-, provider-, and clinic-level predictors of unrecognized elevated blood pressure in children. *Pediatrics, 125*(6), e1286-e1293.

Brady, T., Siberry, G. K., & Solomon, B. (2008). Pediatric hypertension. *Contemporary Pediatrics, 25*(11), 46–56.

Brady, T. M., Fivush, B., Parekh, R. S., & Flynn, J. T. (2010). Racial differences among children with primary hypertension. *Pediatrics, 126*(5), 931–937.

Brashers, V. L. (2010). Alterations in cardiovascular function. In K. L. McCance, S. E. Huether, V. L. Brashers, & N. R. Rote, *Pathophysiology: The biologic basis for disease in adults and children* (6th ed., pp. 1142–1208). St. Louis, MO: Mosby Elsevier.

Connor, J. A., Kline, N. E., Mott, S., Harris, S. K., & Jenkins, K. J. (2010). The meaning of cost for families of children with congenital heart disease. *Journal of Pediatric Health Care, 24*(5), 318–325.

Conway, J., & Dipchand, A. I. (2010). Heart transplantation in children. *Pediatric Clinics of North America, 57*, 353–373.

Cook, C. C., & Gleason, T. G. (2009). Great vessel and cardiac trauma. *Surgical Clinics of North America, 89*, 797–820.

Cook, E. H., & Higgins, S. S. (2010). Congenital heart disease. In P. J. Allen, J. A. Vessey, & N. A. Shapiro, *Primary care of the child with a chronic condition* (5th ed., pp. 385–404). St. Louis, MO: Elsevier Mosby.

Couch, S. C., Saelens, B. E., Levin, L., Dart, K., Faloglia, G., & Daniels, S. R. (2008). The efficacy of a clinic-based behavioral nutrition intervention emphasizing a DASH-type diet for adolescents with elevated blood pressure. *Journal of Pediatrics, 152*, 494–501.

Council on Sports Medicine and Fitness. (2010). Policy statement—Athletic participation by children and adolescents who have systemic hypertension. *Pediatrics, 125*(6), 1287–1293.

D'Alessandro, L.C.A., Peyvandi, S., Schachtner, S, & Goldmuntz, E. (2012). The genetics of abnormal cardiac development, In M. M. Gleason, J. Rychik, & R. Shaddy, *Pediatric Practice Cardiology*, (pp.79-81). New York, NY: McGraw Hill Medical.

Daniels, S. R., Greer, F. R., & the Committee on Nutrition. (2008). Lipid screening and cardiovascular health in childhood. *Pediatrics, 122*(1), 198–208.

Doniger, S. J., & Sharieff, G. Q. (2006). Pediatric dysrhythmias. *Pediatric Clinics of North America, 53*, 85–105.

Duval, X., & Lepert, C. (2008). Prophylaxis of infective endocarditis: current tendencies, continuing controversies. *Lancet, 8*, 225–232.

Gahart, B. L., & Nazareno, A. R. (2012). *2012 Intravenous Medications* (28th ed.). St. Louis, MO: Elsevier Mosby.

Gerber, M. A., Baltimore, R. S., Eaton, C. B., Gewitz, M., Rowley, A. H., Shulman, S., & Taubert, K. A. (2009). Prevention of rheumatic fever and diagnosis and treatment of acute streptococcal pharyngitis. *Circulation, 119*, 1541–1551.

Gilboa, S. M., Salemi, J. L., Nembhard, W. N., Fixler, D. E., & Correa, A. (2010). Mortality resulting from congenital heart disease among children and adults in the United States, 1999–2006. *Circulation, 122*, 2254–2263.

Gregoski, M. J., Barnes, V. A., Tingen, M. S., Harshfield, G. A., & Treiber, F. A. (2011). Breathing awareness meditation and Lifeskills training programs influence upon ambulatory blood pressure and sodium excretion among African American adolescents. *Journal of Adolescent Health, 48*, 59–64.

Hartas, G., Tsounias, E., & Gupta-Malhotra, M. (2009). Approach to diagnosing congenital cardiac disorders. *Critical Care Nursing Clinics of North America, 21*, 27–36.

Hazinski, M. F., Mondozzi, M. A., & Baker, R. A. U. (2010). Shock, multiple organ dysfunction syndrome, and burns in children. In K. L. McCance, S. E. Huether,

V. L. Brashers, & N. R. Rote, *Pathophysiology: The biologic basis for disease in adults and children* (6th ed., pp. 1727–1754). St. Louis, MO: Mosby Elsevier.

Helfricht, S., Latal, B., Fischer, J. E., Tomaske, M., & Landolt, M. (2008). Surgery-related posttraumatic stress disorder in parents of children undergoing cardiopulmonary bypass surgery: A prospective cohort study. *Pediatric Critical Care Medicine, 9*(2), 217–223.

Hoffman, J. F., Mehrota, S. M., & Buckvold, S. M. (2011). Pulmonary stenosis. In R. Abdulla (Ed.), *Heart disease in children* (pp. 133–147). New York, NY: Springer.

Holcomb, S. S. (2009). Common herb drug interactions: What you should know. *Nurse Practitioner, 34*(5), 21–29.

Holmes, K. W., & McCarville, M. A. (2011). Aortic stenosis. In R. Abdulla (Ed.), *Heart disease in children* (pp. 149–158). New York, NY: Springer.

Inaba, A. S., & Horeczko, T. (2009). Cardiac disorders. In J. A. Marx, R. S. Hockberger, R. M. Walls, J. G. Adams, W. G. Barsan, M. H. Biros,…E. J. Newton, *Rosen's emergency medicine* (7th ed., pp. 2152–2158). St. Louis, MO: Elsevier Mosby.

Jeffries, J. L., & Towbin, J. A. (2010). Dilated cardiomyopathy. *Lancet, 375*, 752–762.

Khalid, O. M., & Abdulla, R. (2011). Ventricular septal defect. In R. Abdulla (Ed.), *Heart disease in children* (pp. 103–111). New York, NY: Springer.

Khalid, O. M., & Busse, J. (2011). Patent ductus arteriosus. In R. Abdulla (Ed.), *Heart disease in children* (pp. 113–121). New York, NY: Springer.

Khalid, O. M., & Mehrota, S. M. (2011). Atrioventricular canal. In R. Abdulla (Ed.), *Heart disease in children* (pp. 123–132). New York, NY: Springer.

Lennox, E. G. (2012). Cardiology. In M. M. Tschudy & K. M. Arcara, *The Harriet Lane handbook* (19th ed., p. 191). Philadelphia, PA: Elsevier Mosby.

London, M. L., Ladewig, P. W., Ball, J. W., & Bindler, R. C. (2011). *Maternal & child nursing care* (3rd ed.). Upper Saddle River, NJ: Pearson.

Luxenberg, D. M., & Torchen, L. (2011). Tetralogy of Fallot. In R. Abdulla (Ed.), *Heart disease in children* (pp. 167–176). New York, NY: Springer.

Madriago, E., & Silberbach, M. (2010). Heart failure in infants and children. *Pediatrics in Review, 31*(1), 4–11.

Majnemer, A., Limperopoulos, C., Shevell, M. I., Rohlicek, C., Rosenblatt, B., & Tchervenkov, C. (2008). Developmental and functional outcomes at school entry in children with congenital heart disease. *Journal of Pediatrics, 153*, 55–60.

Majnemer, A., Limperopoulos, C., Shevell, M. I., Rohlicek, C., Rosenblatt, B., & Tchervenkov, C. (2009). A new look at outcomes of infants with congenital heart disease. *Pediatric Neurology, 40*(3), 197–204.

Malik, S., Cleves, M. A., Honein, M. A., Romitti, P. A., Botto, L. D., Yang, S.,… National Birth Defects Prevention Study. (2008). Maternal smoking and congenital heart defects. *Pediatrics, 121*(4), e810–e816.

McDaniel, N. L. (2010). Alterations in cardiovascular function in children. In K. L. McCance, S. E. Huether, V. L. Brashers, & N. R. Rote, *Pathophysiology: The biologic basis for disease in adults and children* (6th ed., pp. 1209–1241). St. Louis, MO: Mosby.

McDonald, J. R. (2009). Acute infective endocarditis. *Infectious Disease Clinics of North America, 23*(3), 643–664.

McLellan, M. C., & Baker, A. L. (2011). At the heart of the fever: Kawasaki disease. *American Journal of Nursing, 111*(6), 57–63.

National Heart Lung and Blood Institute (NHLBI). (2011). Expert Panel on Integrated Guidelines for Cardiovascular Health and Risk Reduction in Children and Adolescents. *Retrieved from http://www.nhlbi.nih.gov/guidelines/cvd_ped/index.htm*

Park, M. K. (2008). *Pediatric cardiology for practitioners* (5th ed.). St. Louis, MO: Elsevier Mosby.

Payne, L., Ziegler, V. L., & Gillette, P. C. (2011). Acute cardiac arrhythmias following surgery for congenital heart disease: Mechanisms, diagnostic tools, and management. *Critical Care Clinics of North America, 23*, 255–272.

Petrini, J. R., Broussard, C. S., Gilboa, S. M., Lee, K. A., Oster, M., & Honein, M. A. (2010). Racial differences by gestational age in neonatal deaths attributable to congenital heart defects—United States, 2003–2006. *Morbidity and Mortality Weekly Report, 59*(37), 1208–1211.

Ralston, M., Hazinski, M. F., Zaritsky, A. L., Schexnayder, S., & Kleinman, M. E. (2006). *Pediatric advanced life support: Provider manual*. Dallas, TX: American Heart Association.

Rothstein, R., Paris, Y., & Quizon, A. (2009). Pulmonary hypertension. *Pediatrics in Review, 30*(2), 39–45.

Sable, C., Foster, E., Uzark, K., Bjornsen, K., Canobbio, M. M., Connolly, H. M.,… Williams, R. G. (2011). Best practices in managing transition to adulthood for adolescents with congenital heart disease: The transition process and medical and psychosocial issues. *Circulation, 123*, 1454–1485.

Sadowski, S. L. (2009). Congenital cardiac disease in the newborn infant: Past, present, and future. *Critical Care Clinics of North America, 21*, 37–48.

Saiman, L. (2009). Endocarditis and intravascular infections. In S. S. Long, L. K. Pickering, & C. G. Prober, *Principles and practice of pediatric infectious diseases* (3rd ed., pp. 269–277). New York, NY: Elsevier Churchill Livingstone.

Samson, R. A., & Atkins, D. L. (2008). Tachyarrhythmias and defibrillation. *Pediatric Clinics of North America, 55*, 887–907.

Schlechte, E. A., Boramanand, N., & Funk, M. (2008). Supraventricular tachycardia in the pediatric primary care setting: Age-related presentation, diagnosis, and management. *Journal of Pediatric Health Care, 22*(5), 289–299.

Shah, A. S., Dolan, L. M., Gao, Z., Kimball, T. R., & Urbina, E. M. (2011). Clustering of risk factors: A simple method of detecting cardiovascular disease in youth. *Pediatrics, 127*(2), e312–e318.

Shimizu, W. (2008). Genetics of congenital long QT syndrome and Brugada syndrome. *Future of Medicine, 4*(4), 379–389.

Son, M. B., Gauvreau, K., Burns, J. C., Corinaldesi, E., Tremoulet, A. H., Watson, V. E.,… Newburger, J. W. (2011). Infliximab for intravenous immunoglobulin resistance in Kawasaki disease: A retrospective study. *Journal of Pediatrics, 158*(4), 644–649.

Steer, A. C., & Carapetis, J. R. (2009). Acute rheumatic fever and rheumatic heart disease in indigenous populations. *Pediatric Clinics of North America, 56*, 1401–1419.

Steffen, K. M. (2011). Trauma, burns, and common critical care emergencies. In M. M. Tschudy & K. M. Arcara, *The Harriet Lane handbook* (19th ed., p. 109). Philadelphia, PA: Elsevier Mosby.

Sudan, D., Bacha, E. A., John, E., & Bartholomew, A. (2007). Childhood organ transplantation. *Pediatrics in Review, 28*(12), 439–453.

Torres, M., & Nieves, J. A. (2009). Progress in congenital cardiac care for newborns and infants: The emerging role of "off-label" medications. *Newborn and Infant Nursing Reviews, 9*(1), 18–30.

Towbin, J. A., Lowe, A. M., Colan, S. D., Sleeper, L. A., Orav, E. J., Clunie, S., . . . Lipshultz, S. E. (2006). Incidence, causes, and outcomes of dilated cardiomyopathy in children. *Journal of the American Medical Association, 296*(15), 1867–1876.

Van der Rijken, R., Hulstijn-Dirkmaat, G., Kraaimaat, F., Nabuurs-Kohrman, L., Daniëls, O., & Maassen, B. (2009). Evidence of impaired neurocognitive functioning in school-age children awaiting cardiac surgery. *Developmental Medicine and Child Neurology, 52*(6), 552–558.

van Loon, R. L. E., Roofthooft, M. T. R., Delhaas, T., van Osch-Gevers, M., ten Harkel, A. D., Strengers, J. L., . . . Berger, R. M. F. (2010). Outcome of pediatric patients with pulmonary arterial hypertension in the era of new medical therapies. *American Journal of Cardiology, 106,* 117–124.

Vetter, V. L. (2006). Kawasaki disease. In V. L. Vetter, *Pediatric cardiology: The requisites in pediatrics* (pp. 131–144). St. Louis, MO: Elsevier Mosby.

Wijnstok, N. J., Twisk, J. W. R., Young, I. S., Woodside, J. V., McFarlane, C., McEneny, J., . . . Boreham, C. A. G. (2010). Inflammation markers are associated with cardiovascular diseases risk in adolescents: The Young Hearts Project 2000. *Journal of Adolescent Health, 47,* 346–351.

Wilson, B. A., Shannon, M. T., & Shields, K. M. (2011). *Pearson nurse's drug guide 2011.* New York, NY: Pearson.

Wilson, W., Taubert, K. A., Gewitz, M., Lockhart, P. B., Baddour, L. M., Levison, M., . . . The Council on Scientific Affairs of the American Dental Association. (2007). Prevention of infective endocarditis: Guidelines from the American Heart Association Rheumatic Fever, Endocarditis, and Kawasaki Disease Committee, Council on Cardiovascular Disease in the Young, and the Council on Clinical Cardiology, Council on Cardiovascular Surgery and Anesthesia, and the Quality of Care and Outcomes Research Interdisciplinary Working Group. *Circulation, 116,* 1736–1754.

Zappalla, F. R., & Gidding, S. S. (2009). Lipid management in children. *Endocrinology Clinics of North America, 38,* 272–283.

Zeigler, V. L. (2008). Congenital heart disease and genetics. *Critical Care Clinics of North America, 20,* 159–169.

Zideman, D. A., & Hazinski, M. F. (2008). Background and epidemiology of pediatric cardiac arrest. *Pediatric Clinics of North America, 55,* 847–859.

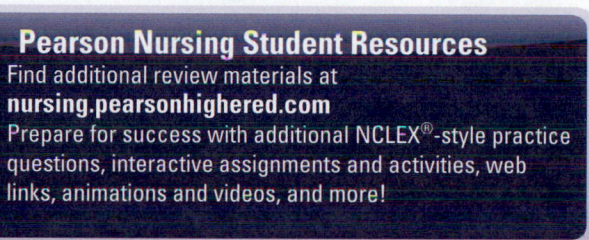

Pearson Nursing Student Resources

Find additional review materials at
nursing.pearsonhighered.com
Prepare for success with additional NCLEX®-style practice questions, interactive assignments and activities, web links, animations and videos, and more!

CHAPTER
27 Alterations in Immune Function

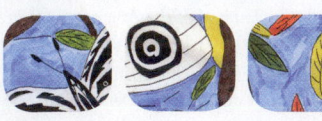

Learning Outcomes

After completing this chapter, you will be able to:

1. Describe the structure and function of the immune system.

2. Apply knowledge of the immune system to the care of children with immunologic disorders.

3. Explain the differences between primary and secondary immune deficiency.

4. Summarize infection control measures needed for children with an immunodeficiency.

5. Develop a nursing care plan in partnership with the family for a child with human immunodeficiency virus (HIV) infection.

6. Contrast immune deficiency diseases and autoimmune diseases.

7. Plan nursing care for the child with an autoimmune condition such as systemic lupus erythematosus or juvenile arthritis.

8. Describe exposure prevention measures for the child with latex allergy.

9. Apply nursing interventions and prevention measures for the child experiencing hypersensitivity reactions.

KEY TERMS

> ### "My knees are very stiff in the morning and they hurt a lot too!"
> —*Rachel, age 8*

Eight-year-old Rachel Dustin has a 6-week history of pain in both knees. She has been exercising some at school but stopped 2 weeks ago because of the pain. Her parents attributed the knee pain to this activity but are now concerned because her pain is getting worse. Rachel does not have a history of recent injury, but she complains of her legs being stiff in the morning. In addition, her mother recently noticed that Rachel's knees are slightly swollen. The pediatrician ordered radiographs that ruled out injury and a complete blood count (CBC) that ruled out an acute infection. Rachel is referred to a pediatric rheumatologist who orders further lab work including tests for antinuclear antibody (ANA), human leukocyte antigen (HLA), and rheumatoid factor. The erythrocyte sedimentation rate (ESR) and C-reactive protein (CRP) are also evaluated. Based on Rachel's history, physical examination, and lab results, she is diagnosed with juvenile idiopathic arthritis, which the rheumatologist further classifies as oligoarthritis. What should medical management include? What are the goals of management? What complications might occur? What should the nurse include in teaching for Rachel and her family?

Signs and symptoms of immunologic disorders in children are often nonspecific. The immune system is one of the few body systems that regulate, either directly or indirectly, all other body functions. Thus, a problem with the immune system can result in multisystem consequences and may be life threatening. The child with recurring infections may have an undiagnosed immunologic disorder. Congenital abnormalities sometimes signal a defect in cellular immunity. In this chapter, we will examine the more common disorders of immune function and discuss nursing care of families and children who have these diseases.

ANATOMY AND PHYSIOLOGY

The function of the immune system is to recognize any foreign substances within the body—in simple terms, to distinguish "nonself" from "self"—and to eliminate foreign substances as efficiently as possible. When the body recognizes the presence of a substance that it cannot identify as part of itself, the body protects itself through the immune response. Normally, the immune system responds to an invasion of foreign substances, or antigens, in numerous ways (Table 27–1). It produces **antibodies,** or proteins that work against **antigens,** the foreign substances that trigger the immune response. There are many types of antibodies, which are described later in this section. The immune system also produces other types of cells, such as T lymphocytes and natural killer (NK) cells.

Immunity is either natural or acquired. **Natural immunity** is composed of the defenses present at birth, such as intact skin, body pH, natural antibodies from the mother, and inflammatory and phagocytic properties. **Acquired immunity** consists of humoral (antibody-mediated) and cell-mediated immunity and is not fully developed until a child is about 6 years of age.

Humoral immunity is responsible for destroying bacterial antigens. B lymphocytes, produced in the bone marrow, gut, and other lymphoid tissue, are the central factor in humoral immunity and develop into plasma cells that produce antibodies. Antibodies are a type of protein called **immunoglobulins,** of which there are five types: IgM, IgG, IgA, IgD, and IgE (Table 27–2). IgM, IgG, and IgA act to control a number of body infections, whereas IgE is useful in combating parasitic infections and is part of the allergic response. The role of IgD is unknown (Diamond & Grimaldi, 2009).

Antibodies are found in serum, body fluids, and certain tissues. When a child is first exposed to an antigen, the B-lymphocyte system begins to produce antibodies that react specifically to that antigen (Figure 27–1 ■). It takes approximately 3 days for this process, known as the **primary immune response,** to occur. Subsequent encounters with the antigen trigger memory cells, resulting in a **secondary immune response** within 24 hours.

Cellular immunity or *cell-mediated immunity* uses T lymphocytes, produced mainly in the thymus, to provide cellular immunity and protect against most viruses, fungi, slowly developing bacterial infections such as tuberculosis, and tumors. In addition, they control the timing of the response in delayed hypersensitivity reactions, such as the purified protein derivative (PPD) test, and are responsible for the rejection of foreign grafts, such as transplants. Specialized types of

TABLE 27–1	Cells and Tissues of the Immune System	
COMPONENT	**LOCATION**	**FUNCTION**
Leukocytes		
Granulocytes		
Neutrophils	Circulation	Phagocytosis and chemotaxis
Eosinophils	Circulation, respiratory tract, and gastrointestinal tract	Phagocytosis
		Protection against parasites
		Involved in allergic response
Basophils	Circulation	Release of chemotactic substances
Monocytes and macrophages	Circulation (monocytes) and body tissue, such as skin (histiocytes), liver (Kupffer cells), alveoli, spleen, tonsils, lymph nodes, bone marrow, brain	Trapping and phagocytizing of foreign substances and cellular debris
		Secretion of interleukin-1 to stimulate lymphocyte growth
Lymphocytes		
T cells (mature in thymus gland)	Circulation, lymph system, tissues	Activation of T and B cells
		Control of viral infections and destruction of cancer cells
		Involved in hypersensitivity reactions and graft tissue rejection
B cells (mature in bone marrow)	Circulation, spleen	Production of antibodies (immunoglobulins) to specific antigens
NK (natural killer) cells	Circulation	Cytotoxic; killing of tumor cells, fungi, viral-infected cells, and foreign tissue
Lymphoid Tissues		
Primary or central lymphoid structures	Bone marrow and thymus gland	Production of immune cells; sites for cell maturation
Secondary or peripheral lymphoid structures	Lymph nodes, spleen, tonsils, intestinal lymphoid tissue, lymphoid tissue in other organs	Sites for activation of immune cells by antigens

Source: From LeMone, P., Burke, K., & Bauldoff, G. (2011). Nursing care of patients with infection. In Medical-surgical nursing: Critical thinking in patient care (4th ed., pp. 269–305). Upper Saddle River, NJ: Pearson.

TABLE 27–2	Classes of Immunoglobulins	
IMMUNOGLOBULIN	LOCATION	ACTION
IgM	Present in intravascular spaces (blood and lymph)	Mediates cytotoxic response and activates complement
		First antibody produced with primary immune response
IgG	Present in all body fluids	Active against bacteria, bacterial toxins, and viruses
		Activates complement
		Only immunoglobulin to cross the placenta
IgA	Present in secretions of gastrointestinal, respiratory, and genitourinary tracts	Prevents binding of viruses to cells of the respiratory and gastrointestinal tracts
IgD	Present in blood, lymph, and surfaces of B cells	Function not fully understood
IgE	Present in internal and external body fluids	Releases chemical mediators responsible for immediate hypersensitivity response

T lymphocytes include killer T cells, suppressor T cells, and helper T cells. Suppressor T cells inhibit B lymphocytes from differentiating into plasma cells. Helper T cells aid in the proliferation and immunologic function of other cells. T lymphocytes have proteins on their surfaces that attract and trap receptors; they can be used to measure the immune activity of these cells. NK cells (also known as non-B/non-T lymphocytes) originate in the bone marrow and thymus and migrate to the blood and spleen. They play a role in control of viral infection, tumors, and autoimmune disease.

Complement is a component of blood serum consisting of 11 protein compounds. It is an inactive enzyme that activates in response to antigen–antibody functions, resulting in a generalized

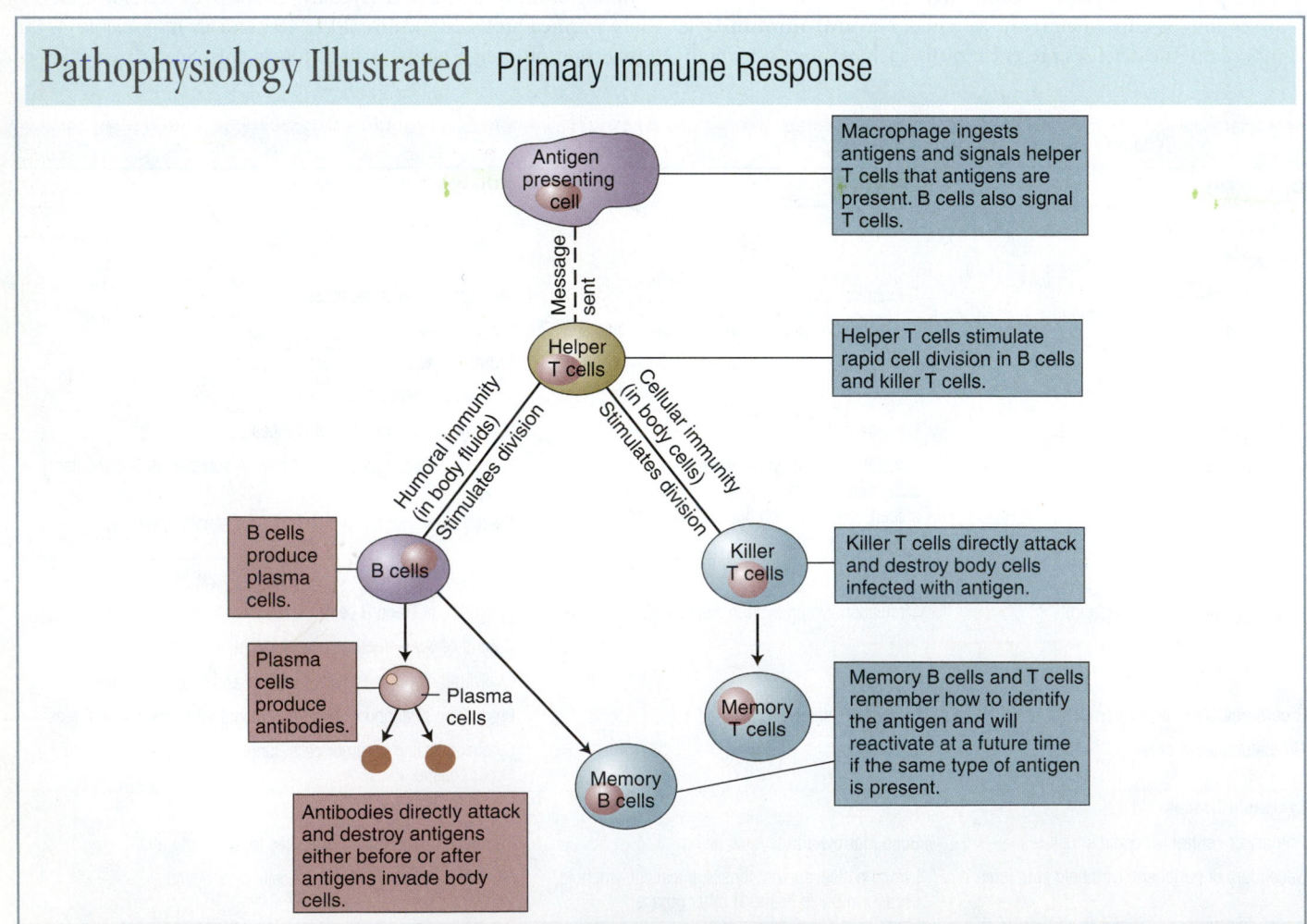

Pathophysiology Illustrated Primary Immune Response

Antigen presenting cell

Macrophage ingests antigens and signals helper T cells that antigens are present. B cells also signal T cells.

Message sent

Helper T cells

Helper T cells stimulate rapid cell division in B cells and killer T cells.

Humoral immunity (in body fluids)
Stimulates division

Cellular immunity (in body cells)
Stimulates division

B cells produce plasma cells.

B cells

Killer T cells

Killer T cells directly attack and destroy body cells infected with antigen.

Plasma cells produce antibodies.

Plasma cells

Memory T cells

Memory B cells and T cells remember how to identify the antigen and will reactivate at a future time if the same type of antigen is present.

Memory B cells

Antibodies directly attack and destroy antigens either before or after antigens invade body cells.

FIGURE 27–1 ■ The primary response encompasses a cascade of events that involve humoral and cellular immunity. What part of the response enables the body to react quickly the next time a specific antigen is sensed in the body?

inflammatory reaction that kills foreign cells. It also plays a role in causing some autoimmune diseases.

Immune cells also secrete proteins called **cytokines** that carry messages for immune system function. Lymphocytes, monocytes, and macrophages all secrete cytokines that have a variety of effects on the target cells. Effects may include stimulation of growth through proliferation of cells, differentiation of cellular actions, production of inflammation, sensitization to pain, and other actions. Interleukins, a type of cytokine, were first identified in white blood cells but now are known to be present in many cells. Many types of interleukins have been identified and some are known to influence the function of the immune system.

PEDIATRIC DIFFERENCES

Infants and children have differing amounts of some immunoglobulins. IgG is the only immunoglobulin that crosses the placenta; as a result, a newborn's levels are similar to those of the mother's (Buckley, 2011). This maternal IgG disappears by 6 to 8 months of age. The infant's IgG then increases gradually until mature levels are reached at 7 to 8 years. IgM levels are low at birth, rise markedly at 1 week of age, and continue to increase until adult levels are reached at about 1 year. IgA and IgE are not present at birth. Manufacture of these immunoglobulins begins by 2 weeks of age; however, normal values are not achieved until 6 to 7 years. It is thus easy to see why children under 6 years of age become ill so often—they do not have a full complement of immunoglobulins.

In contrast, cell-mediated immunity achieves full function early in life. The thymus begins producing T cells in the fetus, and by birth many of these cells are present. The thymus is large at birth, grows during childhood, reaches peak size just before puberty, and then decreases in size (Buckley, 2011). Other lymphoid tissue such as the spleen and tonsils are also comparatively large in young children. Because of the well-developed cellular immunity, any blood infused into newborns is generally irradiated to prevent **graft-versus-host disease** (a series of immunologic reactions in response to transplanted cells) from transfused lymphocytes (Figure 27–2 ■).

Newborns have somewhat lower numbers of NK cells than older children and adults, decreasing their ability to respond to certain antigens. See Figure 27–3 ■ for the differentiation between B and T lymphocytes and NK cells. The levels of some complement proteins are lower in newborns than in older children and adults, thus delaying and hampering response to certain infections. Newborns are most prone to development of infection, particularly when born premature, since they have lower levels of their own immunity. Breast milk provides increased immunity to the infant and provides more immunity to the infant than commercial formula (Verhasselt, 2010).

Nurses play an important role in preventing infections in newborns and promptly identifying infections in children of all ages. See Table 27–3 for assessment guidelines that provide information about the immune system. See Table 27–4 for laboratory tests providing information about the immune system. See Appendix D 🖱 for more specific information related to CBC, complement, and immunoglobulin values.

IMMUNODEFICIENCY DISORDERS

Immunodeficiency, a state of decreased responsiveness of the immune system, can occur to varying degrees in response to any number of events. Children with congenital immune deficiency, or **primary immune deficiency,** are born with a failure of humoral antibody formation (B-cell disorder), a deficient cellular immune

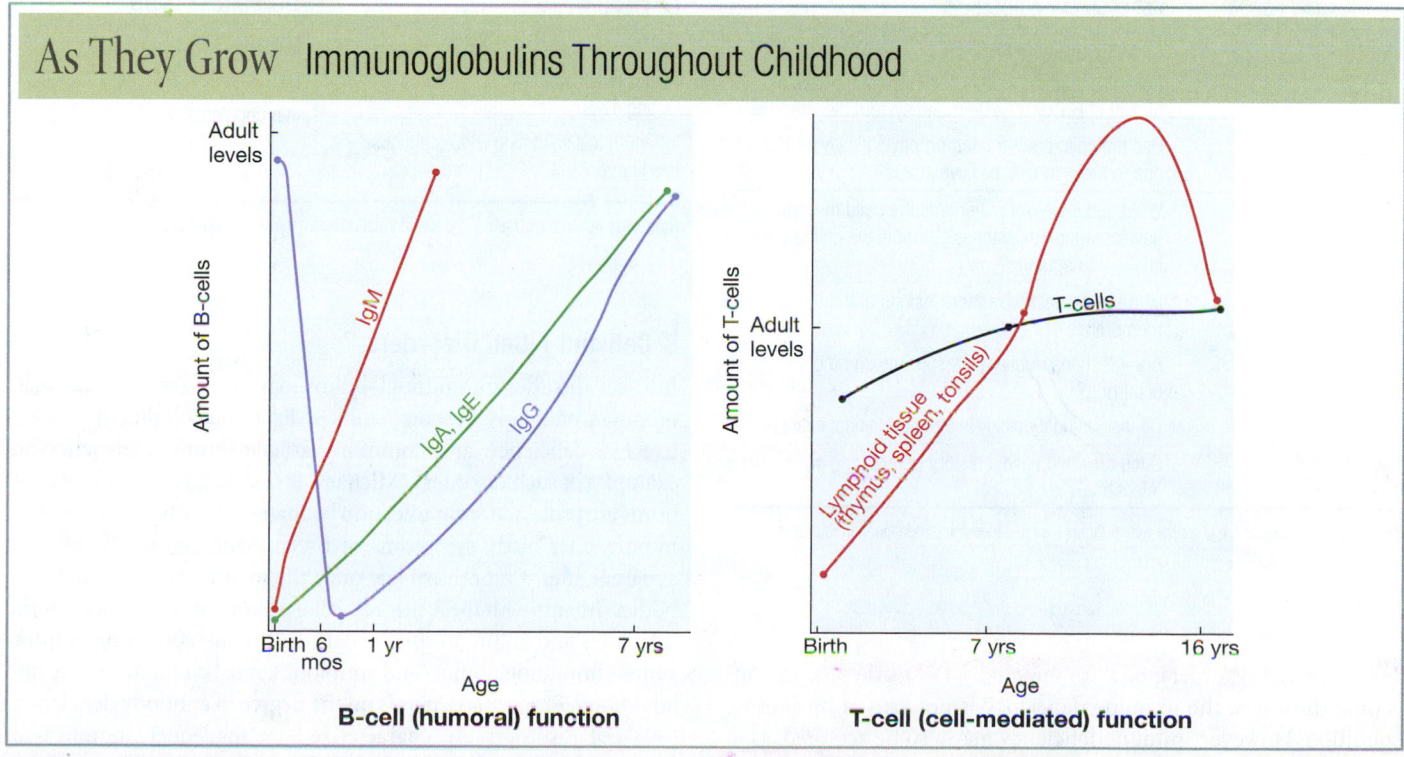

As They Grow Immunoglobulins Throughout Childhood

B-cell (humoral) function

T-cell (cell-mediated) function

FIGURE 27–2 ■ Different types of immunoglobulins mature at variable times throughout childhood. Children have high levels of some types of immunoglobulins, while others may be low at certain periods during development.

FIGURE 27–3 ■ Development and differentiation of lymphocytes from the lymphoid stem cell (lymphoblasts). The cells circulate, mature in lymph tissue, and are activated to their specific functions when exposed to antigens.

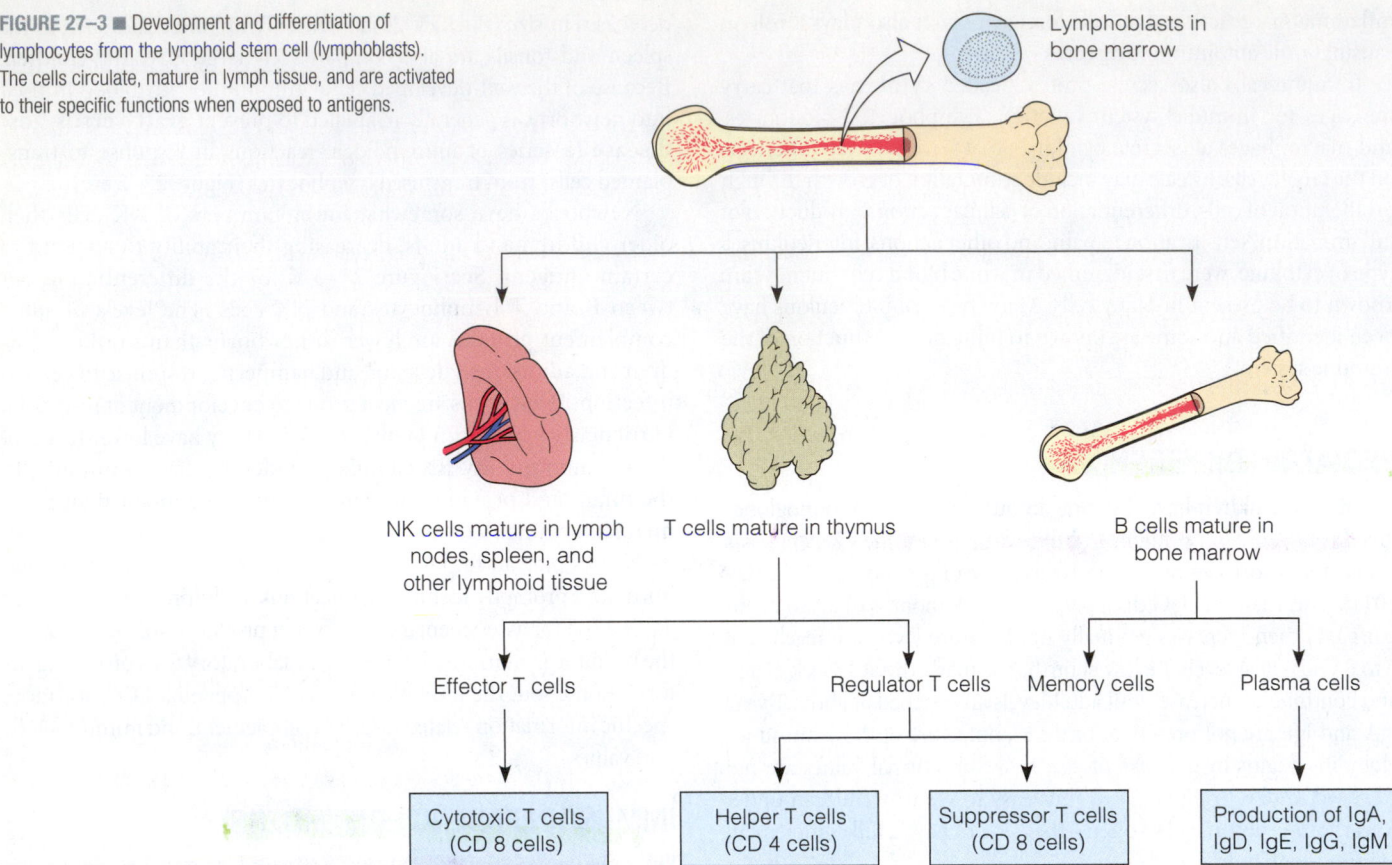

TABLE 27–3	Assessment Guidelines for the Child with an Immune System Condition*
ASSESSMENT FOCUS	**ASSESSMENT GUIDELINES**
Family history	Does a family member have a history of allergy?
	Does the mother or other family member have a history of HIV or other immune system disorder?
	Has the child been treated prophylactically for HIV due to the mother's positive status?
Growth and development	What is the growth pattern? Is the child meeting developmental milestones? What is the child's food intake and appetite?
Skin and mucous membranes	Is the skin intact? Are there lesions of the mucous membranes?
	Are infections or allergic responses commonly occurring?
	Do lesions heal quickly without additional infection?
Evidence of diseases	Does the child have a history of recurring or unusual infections?

Note: *Refer to Chapter 7 ⟳ for the actual techniques of assessment mentioned in this table.

TABLE 27–4	Diagnostic Procedures and Laboratory Tests for the Immune System*
DIAGNOSTIC PROCEDURES	**LABORATORY TESTS**
HIV tests—see Table 27–8	Complete blood count
Radioallergosorbent testing (RAST)—see page 893	Circulating IgE antibodies
Intradermal skin testing (skin reactions)—see Figure 27–10	Immunoglobulins

Note: *See Appendixes D and E ⟳ for information about these diagnostic procedures and tests.

B-Cell and T-Cell Disorders

In B-cell disorders, immunoglobulins may be present in inadequate numbers or nearly absent. X-linked agammaglobulinemia, selective IgA deficiency, and common variable immunodeficiency are examples of such disorders (Michaels & Green, 2011). Because newborns are protected from infection by maternal antibodies in the first months after birth, symptoms of B-cell disorders usually become apparent after 3 months of age once the infant loses maternal antibodies. Infants with these disorders have frequent recurrent bacterial infections and failure to thrive. With treatment, consisting of intravenous immunoglobulins and antibiotics, most children survive into adulthood. Prognosis depends on the degree of antibody deficiency.

T-cell disorders are characterized by inadequate numbers of T lymphocytes or absence of T-cell functions. Isolated T-cell disorders are rare, are usually accompanied by a B-cell disorder, and may

system (T-cell disorder), or a combination of both defects. In congenital disorders, the immune deficiency is not caused by another condition. However, immunodeficiency may also be acquired, as in HIV infection. Acquired immune deficiency is also called **secondary immune deficiency.**

be associated with congenital abnormalities (as in DiGeorge syndrome) or of unknown cause. Table 27–6 reviews laboratory studies for immune conditions.

DiGeorge Syndrome

DiGeorge syndrome, a T-cell disorder caused by chromosome deletion at 22q11.2, is usually diagnosed soon after birth. The estimated incidence is 1 per 3,000 to 6,000 births (McDonald-McGinn & Sullivan, 2011). The syndrome is characterized by absence (complete DiGeorge) or hypoplasia (partial DiGeorge) of parathyroid or thymus glands, hypocalcemia with tetany within 24 to 48 hours after birth, cardiac defects, low-set ears, hypertelorism (widely set eyes), and viral and bacterial infections in the neonatal period (Buckley, 2011, 2008). There is generally a mild to moderate decrease in T-cell counts (McDonald-McGinn & Sullivan, 2011). Prophylactic antibiotics are used to prevent bacterial infections. Children with partial DiGeorge are treated with calcium and vitamin D supplements. Those with complete DiGeorge need thymus transplantation to survive (Buckley, 2008).

Immunodeficiency with Hyper-IgM

Immunodeficiency with hyper-IgM is a T-cell disorder that affects mainly males and causes decreased T-cell function, variable abnormal levels of immunoglobulins, and high titers of some antibodies. It is usually X linked but may be autosomal in some cases. Recurrent bacterial infections including pneumonia, upper respiratory tract infections, and otitis media occur in children with this disorder (Lewis, Nadeau, & Cohen, 2009). Intravenous immune globulin (IVIG) therapy is helpful in decreasing the frequency of lower respiratory tract infections and severe infections but does not affect the frequency of upper respiratory infections or other infections (Park, 2010). Hematopoietic cell transplantation decreases the morbidity and mortality associated with this disorder (Lewis et al., 2009).

TABLE 27–5	Laboratory Findings for Selected Congenital Immunodeficiency Disorders
DISORDERS	**LABORATORY FINDINGS**
B Cell	
X-linked hypogammaglobulinemia	Reduced IgA, IgM, IgE, IgG (less than 100 mg/dL), absence of B cells in peripheral blood, normal T cells
Selective IgA deficiency	IgA less than 10 mg/dL
Common variable immunodeficiency	Reduced IgG, IgA, and IgM
T Cell	
DiGeorge syndrome	Lymphopenia; absent T-cell functions, decreased T cells, normal B cells
Immunodeficiency with hyper-IgM	Reduced IgG, IgA; elevated IgM; mutations in T-cell surface proteins
Combined	
Severe combined immunodeficiency syndrome (SCID)	Complete absence of T- and B-cell and NK immunity
Wiskott-Aldrich syndrome	Thrombocytopenia, low platelet volume, nonfunctional B cells, normal IgG, decreased IgM, increased IgA, increased IgE; inability to respond to polysaccharide antigens

Severe Combined Immunodeficiency Disease

Severe combined immunodeficiency disease (SCID), the most severe form of primary immune deficiency, is a congenital condition characterized by absence of both humoral and cellular immunity that is manifested by lack of appropriately functioning T cells and B cells (Joshi & Davies, 2009; Yee, DeRavin, Elliott, et al., 2008). SCID occurs in X-linked recessive and autosomal recessive forms. In some cases, SCID may be the result of chromosomal abnormalities. The disorder is much more common in males than females and is estimated to occur in 1 per 50,000 live births. Without appropriate treatment, children born with SCID usually do not survive more than 1 year (Buckley, 2011; Joshi & Davies, 2009).

Etiology and Pathophysiology

SCID is caused by genetic mutations that lead to impaired lymphoid development in children with low T and NK cells. The B lymphocytes present may appear normal in number, but their function is compromised due to the severe T-cell deficiency (Ochs & Notarangelo, 2010).

Clinical Manifestations

Symptoms of SCID develop early in life. The infant often demonstrates a susceptibility to infection, presenting during the first few months of life with persistent respiratory infections and diarrhea (Buckley, 2011). Recurrent oral candidiasis, failure to thrive, and skin infections are also frequently seen in these children. Additionally, failure to completely recover from infection, frequent reinfection, and infection with viruses such as cytomegalovirus and the bacterium *Pneumocystis carinii* (*jiroveci*) are common in the child with SCID (Buckley, 2011). Children are also highly susceptible to serious infections such as meningitis, skin or organ infection, osteomyelitis, or sepsis.

Collaborative Care

The goal of clinical therapy is to restore immune function. In addition to diagnostic studies, collaborative care includes preventing and treating systemic infection, promoting skin integrity, managing medication therapy, and providing parental support. The family of the child undergoing hematopoietic stem cell transplantation will require additional education and support.

Diagnostic Tests

A marked reduction in lymphocyte counts is indicative of SCID. Patients with SCID generally have very few T cells and NK cells (Joshi & Davies, 2009). The B-lymphocyte count may be decreased, elevated, or normal, although these cells do not function normally. Immunoglobulin levels are significantly reduced (Joshi & Davies, 2009). Diagnosis is usually made only after extensive laboratory testing. In addition to a complete blood count, erythrocyte sedimentation rate, and B- and T-cell lymphocyte counts, other studies may be performed, including IgA, IgG, and IgM antibody titers to immunizations received and neutrophil count. A chest radiograph is conducted to assess thymus size.

Clinical Therapy

The standard therapy for SCID is the administration of intravenous immune globulin, which is administered to provide protection until humoral immunity is established. Hematopoietic stem cell transplantation (see Chapter 28 🔗) offers the best hope for children with SCID. T-cell function is restored with the transplantation, and

TABLE 27–6	Cells Evaluated in Laboratory Studies for Immune Conditions	
TEST AND TYPE OF CELL EVALUATED/NORMAL VALUES	**ACTION**	**IMPLICATION OF INCREASED OR DECREASED LEVELS**
White Blood Cell (WBC) Count		
Neutrophil (polys) (54–62%)	Phagocytic cell that defends against bacteria	Increased in bacterial infection, inflammatory processes, and some malignancies
Eosinophil (1–3%)	Associated with antigen–antibody reaction	Increased in allergic reaction; decreased in children receiving corticosteroids
Lymphocytes (T, B, non-B/non-T [NK]) (25–33%)	Major components of immune system	Increased in many infections; decreased in children with immune deficiency
Immunoglobulins		
IgM, IgG, IgA, IgD, IgE (See Appendix D for age-specific values)	Many roles in a number of immunologic reactions	Increased in presence of infection or allergic response; decreased in children with immune deficiency

new cells appear 3 to 4 months after infusion of the donor stem cells. Prognosis for the child is poor without aggressive therapy and transplant.

With the identification of the genetic defect for SCID in recent years, gene therapy has been successfully attempted to treat a small number of children. Although serious side effects occur in some children, gene therapy offers hope for the future and could become the treatment of choice for children with SCID (Buckley, 2011).

Prevention and prompt treatment of infection are essential. Antibiotic therapy is targeted at infectious agents. Antibiotic prophylaxis and special immunization recommendations are needed. Children with T-cell deficiencies should receive lymphocyte-depleted and irradiated blood products due to the risk of infection and graft-versus-host disease from lymphocytes in the donor blood (Schwartz & Sinha, 2011).

Nursing Management

Nursing care is focused on preventing the spread of infection, promoting proper nutrition and skin care, supporting the family, and promoting growth and development.

Nursing Assessment and Diagnosis

Obtain a thorough history of infections, including age of onset, type of causal organism, frequency, and severity. Assess family history and determine if the child has had any unusual reactions to vaccines, medications, or foods. Measure the child's height and weight and plot on a growth chart to identify failure to thrive. Assess the child's nutritional intake and fluid and electrolyte balance. Assess for evidence of infections involving the skin, subcutaneous tissues, respiratory system, and mucous membranes. Palpate the abdomen for hepatomegaly and the lymph nodes for lymphadenopathy. Perform a developmental assessment and assess for delays in achievement of developmental milestones. Assess family support systems and coping mechanisms when a child is diagnosed with the disorder.

The primary nursing diagnosis for a child with SCID is Risk for Infection related to immunodeficiency. Other nursing diagnoses may include the following:

- Nutrition, Imbalanced Less than Body Requirements related to illness
- Skin Integrity, Risk for Impaired related to immunologic deficit

- Caregiver Role Strain, Risk for related to a child with a chronic, life-threatening illness
- Development: Delayed, Risk for related to physical disability and chronic illness

NANDA-I © 2012

Planning and Implementation

Nursing care of the child who is immunodeficient focuses on preventing infection. However, even with the use of environmental controls, such as maintaining children inside special units (positive-pressure rooms) to maintain a sterile environment, these children are prone to **opportunistic infections** (those caused by normally nonpathogenic organisms in persons who lack normal immunity).

Prevent Systemic Infection

Frequent and thorough hand hygiene is essential. Standard precautions are always used and transmission-based precautions are established when indicated; see the Skills Manual 🔗. Implement sterile aseptic technique when caring for all sites where needles, catheters, central lines, endotracheal tubes, pressure-monitoring lines, peripheral intravenous lines, or other invasive equipment enters the child's body. Food and other items entering the hospital room may require special treatment. The child should be placed in a positive-pressure isolation room, and contact with infectious individuals should be avoided. Inform parents that because of the risk of infection to the child, live vaccines are avoided for the child as well as siblings, parents, and other household members. Refer to the current recommendations for immunizations for the immunocompromised child.

Promote Skin Integrity

The skin is the only intact defense that many immunodeficient children have. Provide thorough and frequent skin care, and observe all possible pressure areas closely for signs of breakdown or infection. Implement measures to avoid skin trauma. Reposition the child frequently and encourage range of motion exercises.

Promote Nutritional Balance

Encourage adequate fluid and nutritional intake. Provide foods that the child prefers and those with high nutritional value. Offer small frequent feedings of high-calorie, protein-rich foods. Protein intake can be increased by adding dried milk powder to foods. Adding small amounts of fats and special nutritional formulas to the diet can increase energy intake. Only pasteurized milk products should be used to avoid potential infection. Refer to a dietitian as needed to plan with parents for the best, individualized diet for the child.

Manage Medication Therapy

Many of the medications used in the long-term treatment of children with SCID have numerous side effects. Monitor closely for side effects of antibiotics, such as overgrowth of resistant organisms (e.g., thrush infections in the mouth, *Clostridium difficile* infections of the gastrointestinal tract), and administer IVIG safely (Table 27–7).

Provide Emotional Support and Referrals

SCID is a life-threatening and devastating disease. Even with aggressive therapy, the prognosis is poor for children who do not receive hematopoietic stem cell transplant. Evaluate the family's knowledge about the disease and provide education on infection control measures and signs of infection. Encourage the parents to assist in and manage care for their child. (See Partnering with Families: Reducing Risk of Infection.) The parents may experience guilt because of the genetic nature of the disease and the difficulties of treatment. Partner with the family and provide them the opportunity to discuss their feelings and concerns. Listen closely to their concerns and encourage them to discuss their fears. Offer referrals to an appropriate support group or counselor if needed. Genetic counseling should be encouraged (see Chapter 4).

Evaluate the family's ability to care for the child at home. Provide opportunities for the child to have contact with other children when it is safe to do so. Suggest activities that will foster development. Offer financial resource information and other referrals as needed. See Chapter 17 for information about assisting the family in care of the child with a life-threatening illness.

The family of a child who undergoes hematopoietic stem cell transplantation requires additional information, support, and referrals. The transplantation procedure involves surgery for both the ill child and the donor, which is often another child in the family. After the transplant, the ill child will be hospitalized for several months until T-lymphocyte levels are sufficient to provide resistance to infection. During this period, parents may need to rely on social services to help manage the family situation, particularly if the child is hospitalized at a medical center far from the family's home. Assess the family's situation and make appropriate referrals to social services and to support groups. Introduce parents to other families undergoing hematopoietic stem cell transplantation. (See Chapter 28 for discussion of hematopoietic stem cell transplantation.)

Evaluation

Expected outcomes of nursing care include the following:

- The child is free of infection.
- The child demonstrates adequate nutritional status as determined by normal growth patterns.
- Intact skin is maintained.
- The family demonstrates adaptive coping to the demands of a chronic illness.
- The child demonstrates developmental progress consistent with expectations.

Wiskott-Aldrich Syndrome

A combined congenital immunodeficiency syndrome, Wiskott-Aldrich syndrome (WAS) is an X-linked recessive disorder that occurs in males and causes mutation in the WAS gene and changes in the WAS protein. The gene resides on Xp11.22–11.23 (Buckley, 2011). The incidence is 4 in 1 million live male births (Dibbern & Routes, 2010). The IgM levels are low, IgG levels are normal or slightly low, and IgA and IgE levels are elevated (Buckley, 2011). The diagnosis is made in the early neonatal period on the basis of thrombocytopenia, which leads to bleeding as evidenced by petechiae, hematuria, bloody diarrhea, and hematemesis. In addition to thrombocytopenia and related symptoms, Wiskott-Aldrich syndrome is characterized by eczema and recurrent infections in infancy and childhood. Infections including otitis media, bacterial pneumonia, and skin infections are common (Albert, Notarangelo, & Ochs, 2011; Schwartz & Siperstein, 2011).

Treatment is supportive and includes antibiotic prophylaxis, platelet transfusions, and intravenous immune globulin (IVIG). Splenectomy may reduce the risk of bleeding. However, this is done sparingly due to the risk of life-threatening infection following the procedure.

TABLE 27–7	Nursing Considerations in the Administration of Intravenous Immune Globulin (IVIG)	
USE	**SIDE EFFECTS**	**NURSING MANAGEMENT**
Intravenous immune globulin is prepared from pools of multiple samples of human plasma and contains globulin (primarily IgG). It is used in immune thrombocytopenic purpura, Kawasaki disease, primary immunodeficiency disorders, hemolytic anemia, AIDS, and other disorders. Some types of immune globulin are given IM and are effective against specific diseases. For example, hepatitis B immune globulin (HBIG) is effective in preventing infection after exposure to hepatitis B. Palivizumab (Synagis) is effective in providing passive immunity against RSV in high-risk infants.	Local inflammatory reaction with erythema, urticaria, malaise, headache, fever, nausea, vomiting, arthralgia; hypersensitivity reaction with fever, chills, anaphylaxis; infusion reaction with nausea, flushing, chills, headache, wheezing, difficulty breathing, pain in back or abdomen, anaphylaxis.	■ Have emergency drugs and equipment readily available to treat a hypersensitivity reaction or infusion reaction. ■ Treat with an antipyretic or antihistamine before the infusion as prescribed. ■ Follow the manufacturer's directions for reconstitution, dilution, and intravenous infusion rates. ■ Do not mix with other medications for infusion. ■ Monitor vital signs throughout the infusion. Stop the infusion immediately and notify the physician if there are any signs of hypersensitivity. ■ Activate the emergency system as needed. ■ Have the family instruct healthcare providers about IVIG therapy because immunization recommendations will be altered.

Source: *Data from Wilson, B. A., Shannon, M. T., & Shields, K. M. (2011).* Nurse's drug guide 2011. *Upper Saddle River, NJ: Pearson; Wilson, B. A., Shannon, M. T., & Shields, K. M. (2011).* Intravenous drug guide 2011–2012. *Upper Saddle River, NJ: Pearson.*

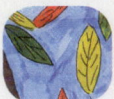

Partnering with Families

Reducing Risk of Infection

Teach family members the following practices to reduce the risk of transmission of infection:

- Wash all bottles, nipples, and pacifiers with hot water and soap, or in the dishwasher.
- Do not allow the child to share utensils, cups, bottles, or pacifiers.
- Use safe food preparation practices such as peeling fruit and vegetables and using different surfaces and utensils for preparing meats vs. other foods.

- Change diapers frequently. Cleanse the skin with mild soap and dry thoroughly.
- Perform hand hygiene before handling the child, after changing diapers, and before feeding the child.
- Maintain clean pets and keep the pet's environment clean.
- Avoid exposing the child to illnesses of other family members and friends, such as colds.

The treatment of choice and the only cure for Wiskott-Aldrich syndrome is hematopoietic stem cell transplantation (HSCT). Following HSCT, the child is at risk for both rejection and graft-versus-host disease (see page 897) (Albert et al., 2011; Schwartz & Siperstein, 2011).

Nursing Management

Nursing care is similar to that for the child with SCID. Assess for splenomegaly, cervical lymphadenopathy, and hepatomegaly. Observe for excessive bleeding from any wounds or bleeding from the gastrointestinal tract.

Refer the parents for genetic counseling to help them understand the disease transmission and the probability of having another child with the same disorder (see Chapter 4 🔴). Arrange for psychologic support for those parents who may be overwhelmed with guilt from learning that the illness is inherited.

Partner with the family and assist them with establishing coping skills to deal with the knowledge that the child has a chronic and potentially fatal illness. Referral to family counseling may be appropriate. Provide support during the process of HSCT transplantation. Expected outcomes are the child's return to normal immunologic function, absence of hemorrhage, and successful coping with a life-threatening illness.

Human Immunodeficiency Virus and Acquired Immune Deficiency Syndrome

Acquired immune deficiency syndrome (AIDS) is caused by the human immunodeficiency virus (HIV-1 primarily, HIV-2 less commonly) (American Academy of Pediatrics [AAP], 2009). As HIV destroys the body's ability to fight infection, opportunistic infections that would normally not affect healthy people destroy the immune system. AIDS, the advanced stages of HIV infection, may result if treatment is not initiated.

Most cases of HIV in children are the result of perinatal transmission. The Centers for Disease Control and Prevention (CDC) estimates that 131 infants were born with HIV infection in the United States in 2009 (CDC, 2011a) as compared to the peak incidence of 1,650 in 1991 (CDC, 2007). This improvement is primarily due to more effective identification and treatment of mothers who are infected with HIV and infants exposed to HIV.

The leading cause of newly acquired HIV infection in teens is unprotected sexual intercourse, while use of injectable drugs is responsible for most other cases. In many cases, both of these factors are involved.

Figure 27–4A and B ■ shows that the number of cases of HIV infection in adolescents ages 15 to 19 has increased since 2006 as has the number of people living with HIV infection in this age group (CDC, 2011b) (see Developing Cultural Competence: HIV/AIDS in Africa).

Etiology and Pathophysiology

Children can acquire HIV in a form of **vertical transmission** from their mothers transplacentally or during delivery. Transmission can occur during birth from blood, amniotic fluid, and exposure to genital tract secretions, and after birth through breast milk from mothers

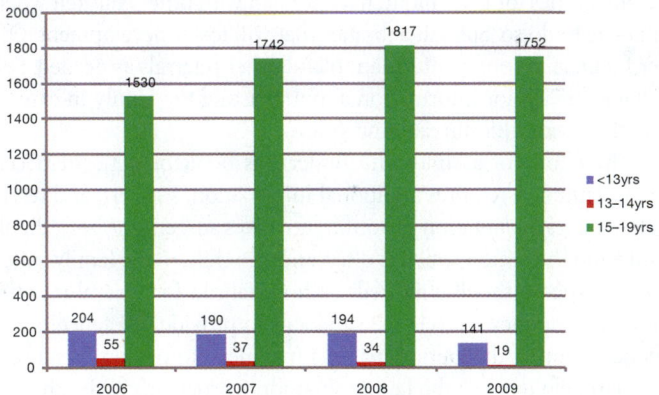

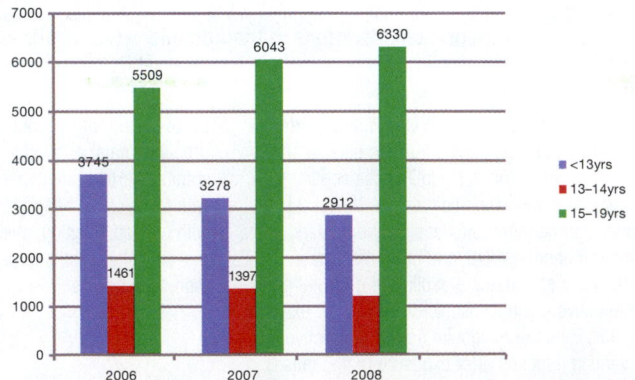

FIGURE 27–4 ■ *A,* Estimated number of cases of HIV in children and adolescents by year of diagnosis based on data from 40 states with confidential name-based HIV reporting. *B,* Estimated number of children and adolescents living with HIV/AIDS during 2006–2008 based on data from 40 states with confidential name-based HIV reporting.

Source: *Data from Centers for Disease Control and Prevention (CDC). (2011b). Diagnosis of HIV infection and AIDS in the United States and dependent areas, 2009. Retrieved from http://www.cdc.gov/hiv/surveillance/resources/reports/2009report/index.htm#1*

Developing Cultural Competence
HIV/AIDS in Africa

While major inroads have been made in the United States and other developed countries to stem the numbers of cases of HIV/AIDS in children, less developed countries still have large numbers of affected children. HIV/AIDS is especially a problem in sub-Saharan Africa. In 2007, approximately 88% of the 2.5 million children less than 15 years of age who have HIV/AIDS lived in Africa. In 2007, an estimated 370,000 African children were infected with HIV. Health professionals who treat children with HIV/AIDS are in short supply in Africa. The Pediatric AIDS Corps is a program that focuses on the placement of pediatricians and other physicians in African countries for at least a year to provide pediatric and family HIV/AIDS treatment and care (Kline, Ferris, Jones, et al., 2009).

who are infected with HIV. However, risk for perinatal transmission has been significantly reduced since mothers identified as infected receive antiretroviral therapy (ART) during pregnancy, undergo a cesarean section, and are advised not to breastfeed. If the mother is not treated, there is a 25% chance that the newborn will be infected (National Institute of Allergy and Infectious Diseases, 2008) compared to a 2% or less chance when the mother begins treatment early in the pregnancy (CDC, 2011c). Prenatal testing is essential to further reduce the incidence of HIV infection in children (Box 27–1).

The virus affects multiple systems and eventually destroys the ability of the child's immune system to respond to infection. An understanding of the natural history of HIV disease is still evolving, and there are several important differences in the disease progression and clinical manifestations of pediatric and adult HIV infection.

HIV selectively targets and destroys T cells, thereby decreasing and eventually eliminating cellular immunity and affecting humoral immunity as well (Figure 27–5 ■). HIV destroys the CD4 T cells (helper cells) which are crucial to normal function of the immune system. The child is left unprotected against a myriad of bacterial, viral, fungal, and opportunistic infections, which are ultimately fatal. Every organ system can be affected.

BOX 27–1 HIV Screening Recommendations

In 2006, the CDC issued revised recommendations for HIV screening, advising routine screening for all patients between 13 and 64 years of age. Patients must still be informed that testing is a routine part of screening and be given information related to the testing that includes an explanation about the disease, the meaning of positive and negative results, and an opportunity to decline. Separate written consent is not required, as general consent for medical care is sufficient (Hahn, 2009). The CDC also recommends that HIV testing be a part of prenatal screening of all pregnant women (CDC, 2011c).

Clinical Manifestations

The neonate is asymptomatic at birth. The time period for the development of opportunistic infections varies; however, the interval from HIV infection to the onset of overt AIDS is shorter in children than in adults. See Clinical Manifestations: Human Immunodeficiency Virus in Children.

Most children with HIV infection have nonspecific findings, including lymphadenopathy, hepatosplenomegaly, oral candidiasis, failure to thrive and weight loss, delayed development, swelling of the parotid gland, and chronic diarrhea (AAP, 2009; Smith, 2011). Recurrent bacterial infections, lymphoid interstitial pneumonitis (LIP), and progressive neurologic deterioration are more common in children than adults. *Pneumocystis jiroveci* pneumonia (formerly known as *Pneumocystis carinii*) is also common and may present early in infancy (Smith, 2011).

Collaborative Care

There is no cure for HIV or AIDS. Care focuses on prevention of HIV transmission, detection of the presence of HIV, aggressive therapy to reduce progression to AIDS, and promotion of the infant or child's growth and development and survival.

Diagnostic Tests

Most children with HIV infection are diagnosed early in life. Virologic tests for detection of the virus are monitored in infants born to mothers infected with HIV. These tests are performed at 14 to 21 days. Infants who are at high risk for infection should have virologic

Clinical Manifestations Human Immunodeficiency Virus in Children

ETIOLOGY	CLINICAL MANIFESTATIONS	NURSING MANAGEMENT
Frequent, chronic, or unusual infections due to poor immune response	Chronic bilateral otitis media Oral candidiasis *Pneumocystis jiroveci* pneumonia (PCP) Skin disorders Fever Parotitis	Teach families the importance of antimicrobial therapy for treatment of infections and the need for recommended immunizations. Limit exposure to groups of people or to individuals with known infections of any kind.
Poor nutritional intake due to lack of appetite caused by disease and medications	Failure to thrive (eating disorder of childhood) Weight and body mass index below 10th percentile Chronic diarrhea Skin irritation	Monitor growth. Provide supplemental intake such as enteral feedings at night, and total parenteral nutrition (TPN) if needed. Provide meticulous skin care to prevent breakdown.
Immune system overgrowth to compensate for lack of proper immune response	Hepatosplenomegaly and lymphadenopathy	Assess abdomen frequently. Teach about safe transport to avoid injury to the liver and spleen.

Note: *Be alert for the possibility of HIV infection in infants with combinations of listed clinical manifestations, especially in infants known to be at risk.*

Source: *Data from American Academy of Pediatrics (AAP). (2009). Red book: Report of the Committee on Infectious Diseases (28th ed.). Elk Grove Village, IL: Author; Smith, S. (2011). Infectious diseases. In K. J. Marcdante, R. M. Kliegman, H. B. Jenson, & R. E. Behrman, Nelson essentials of pediatrics (6th ed., pp. 355–462). Philadelphia, PA: Elsevier Saunders.*

Pathophysiology Illustrated Human Immunodeficiency Virus

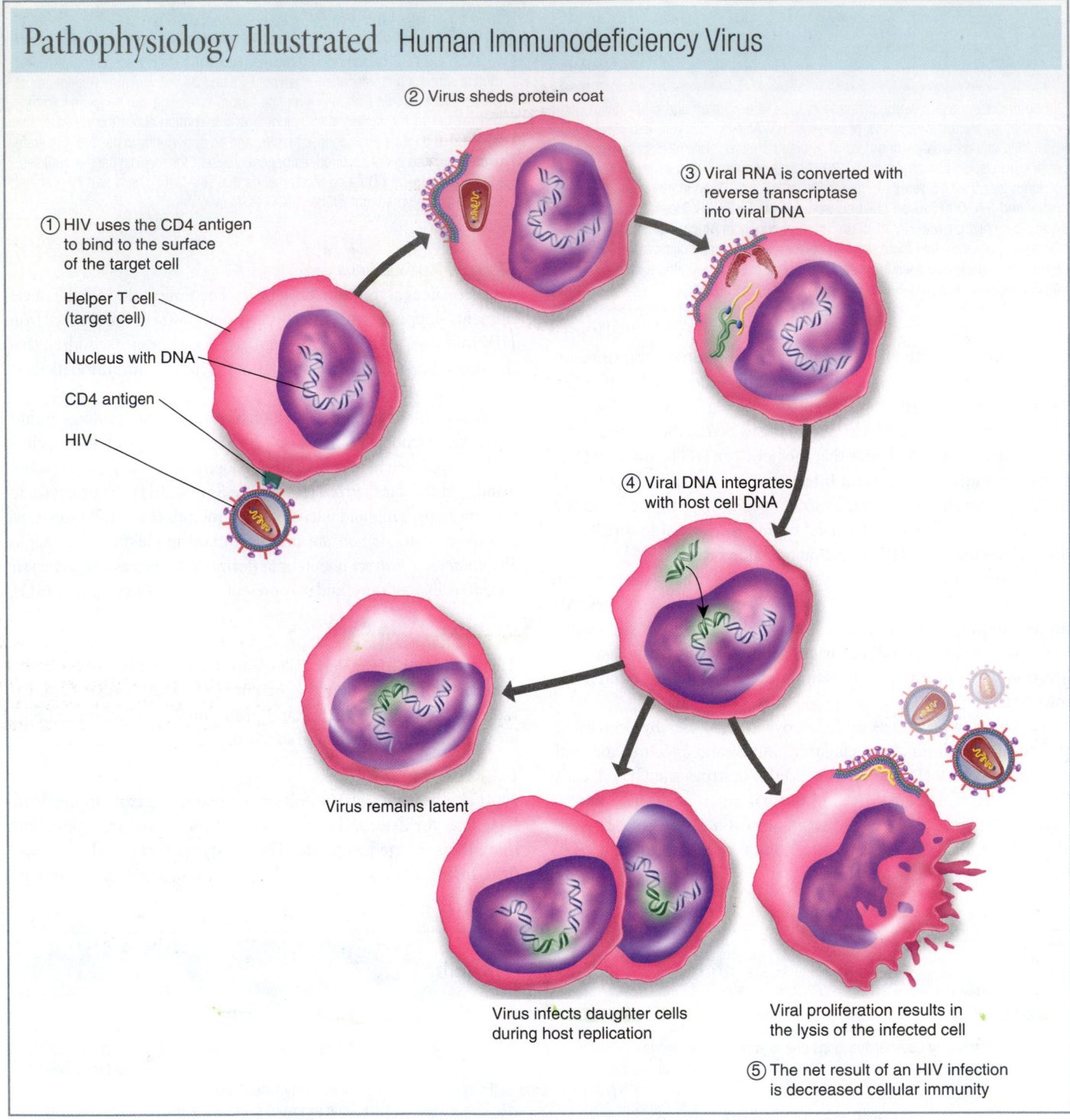

② Virus sheds protein coat

③ Viral RNA is converted with reverse transcriptase into viral DNA

① HIV uses the CD4 antigen to bind to the surface of the target cell

Helper T cell (target cell)

Nucleus with DNA

CD4 antigen

HIV

④ Viral DNA integrates with host cell DNA

Virus remains latent

Virus infects daughter cells during host replication

Viral proliferation results in the lysis of the infected cell

⑤ The net result of an HIV infection is decreased cellular immunity

FIGURE 27–5 ■ The human immunodeficiency virus gains entry into helper T cells, uses the cell DNA to replicate, interferes with normal function of the T cells, and destroys the normal cells.

testing at birth. Infants with initially negative tests should be retested at 1 to 2 months. Infants who are negative at 14 to 21 days and at 1 to 2 months should be tested again at 4 to 6 months. See Table 27–8. The preferred tests are the HIV DNA polymerase chain reaction (PCR) or the HIV RNA assay (viral load). Any positive result is confirmed by retesting. In addition, CD4+ percentage or counts should be performed at least every 3 to 4 months to evaluate the child's immune status (U.S. Department of Health and Human Services, 2010).

In infants who have had repeated negative virologic tests for detection of the virus, an antibody test to see if the maternal HIV antibodies

have disappeared should be performed at 12 months of age. If the antibody test is still positive, it should be repeated at 15 to 18 months of age. Antibody tests that are used include enzyme-linked immunosorbent assay (ELISA) or enzyme immunoassay (EIA). These tests are confirmed with the Western blot test or the indirect immunofluorescence assay (IFA) (U.S. Department of Health and Human Services, 2010). The CDC considers children less than 13 years of age to be infected if their symptoms meet the CDC criteria for HIV infection. The CDC criteria address two issues: the diagnosis of HIV and the clinical classification of children infected with HIV (AAP, 2009) (Table 27–9).

TABLE 27–8	**Commonly Used HIV Tests**
TEST	**DESCRIPTION**
CD4+ cell counts and percentages	Used to assess immune status at diagnosis and ongoing.
HIV DNA polymerase chain reaction (PCR)	A test that makes copies of a DNA sequence which can then be analyzed; useful to detect HIV or other conditions with only small amounts of blood. Preferred for detection of HIV infection in infants.
HIV RNA assay (viral load)	A test that makes copies of an RNA sequence which can then be analyzed to evaluate the severity of the infection at diagnosis and the response to treatment. May be used to confirm HIV infection in infants.
Western blot test	The definitive and confirmatory test for HIV. Allows visualization of particular antibodies to each viral protein.
Rapid HIV tests	Rapid HIV tests may use blood or saliva and produce results in 3–20 minutes. Useful for quick screening but results must be confirmed with serum tests as false positives can occur. See Box 27–2.
Enzyme immunoassay (EIA) and enzyme-linked immunosorbent assay (ELISA)	A test that is used to identify HIV; detects antibodies to the virus. Positive results are verified by the Western blot test.

Source: *Data from Hahn, E. K. (2009). Incorporating the CDC recommendations for adolescent HIV screening into practice. Journal for Nurse Practitioners, 5(4), 265–273; U.S. Department of Health and Human Services. (2010). Guidelines for the use of antiretroviral agents in pediatric HIV infection. Retrieved from http://aidsinfo.nih.gov/contentfiles/PediatricGuidelines.pdf*

TABLE 27–9	**Clinical Categories for Children Younger than 13 Years of Age with Human Immunodeficiency Virus (HIV) Infection**

Diagnosis of HIV Infection in Children

- HIV infected (two or more positive tests for HIV or clinical signs and symptoms of HIV infection or an AIDS-defining illness)
- Perinatally exposed (born to a mother known to be infected with HIV)
- Seroconverter (born to a mother known to be infected with HIV but has had two negative HIV tests)

Classification of Children with HIV

- **Category N**—not symptomatic, with no signs or symptoms of HIV infection or only one of the conditions in Category A
- **Category A**—mildly symptomatic with two or more of the following but none of those listed in Category B or C:
  - Lymphadenopathy
  - Hepatomegaly
  - Splenomegaly
  - Dermatitis
  - Parotitis
  - Recurrent or persistent upper respiratory infection, sinusitis, or otitis media
- **Category B**—moderately symptomatic with conditions other than those listed in Category A and C that are attributed to HIV infection:
  - Anemia
  - Bacterial meningitis, pneumonia, sepsis
  - Candidiasis, oropharyngeal (thrush)
  - Cardiomyopathy
  - Cytomegalovirus infection
  - Diarrhea, recurrent or chronic
  - Hepatitis
  - Herpes simplex virus (HSV) stomatitis
  - HSV bronchitis, pneumonitis, or esophagitis
  - Herpes zoster
  - Leiomyosarcoma (neoplasm of smooth muscle)
  - Lymphoid interstitial pneumonia (LIP) or pulmonary lymphoid hyperplasia complex
  - Nephropathy
  - Nocardiosis
  - Persistent fever
  - Toxoplasmosis
  - Varicella, disseminated
- **Category C**—severely symptomatic, manifested by:
  - Multiple, recurrent serious bacterial infections
  - Candidiasis, esophageal or pulmonary
  - Coccidioidomycosis, disseminated (fungal infection caused by *Coccidioides immitis*)
  - Cryptococcosis, extrapulmonary (fungal infection caused by *Cryptococcus neoformans*)
  - Cryptosporidiosis or isosporiasis (parasitic disease caused by *Cryptosporidium*)
  - Cytomegalovirus
  - Encephalopathy
  - HSV infection, persistent
  - Histoplasmosis
  - Kaposi sarcoma
  - Lymphoma
  - *Mycobacterium* tuberculosis, disseminated
  - *Mycobacterium*, other species or unidentified species infection
  - *Pneumocystis jiroveci* pneumonia (PCP)
  - Progressive multifocal leukoencephalopathy
  - *Salmonella* septicemia, recurrent
  - Toxoplasmosis of the brain
  - Wasting syndrome

Source: *Used with permission of the American Academy of Pediatrics. Red book: 2009 report of the Committee on Infectious Diseases (28th ed., pp. 382–390). Elk Grove Village, IL: Author. Copyright American Academy of Pediatrics, 2009.*

| BOX 27–2 | **Rapid HIV Tests** |

Many people who are at risk of HIV infection may not have HIV testing readily available. To reduce barriers to early detection of the virus, rapid HIV tests have been made available. Specimens are obtained from saliva or from a blood sample. Oral fluids are obtained by gently swabbing both the upper and lower outer gums of the mouth. Results are available in 3 to 20 minutes. Some FDA-approved options include OraQuick Advance Rapid HIV-1/2 Antibody Test, Reveal G3 HIV-1 Antibody Test, Uni-Gold Recombigen HIV Test, and Multispot HIV-1/HIV-2. Health professionals must be prepared to offer counseling during the same visit as when the test is administered. Traditional laboratory tests are used to confirm positive rapid HIV tests (Hahn, 2009).

Clinical Therapy

Medical management begins with prevention of the spread of HIV from mother to newborn. Due to the rapidity of disease progression in perinatally transmitted HIV infection, early identification of infected infants is important to ensure the most effective treatment. Mothers infected with HIV should be identified during pregnancy, and their infants should undergo periodic laboratory testing, as described earlier. All infected mothers should receive combination antiretroviral therapy after the 14th week of pregnancy (AAP, 2009).

Early identification of mothers infected with HIV and implementation of antiretroviral therapy will lead to a decrease in the number of infants and children with HIV infection.

Medication Therapy

All infants of infected mothers with indeterminate HIV infection status should start prophylaxis against *Pneumocystis jiroveci* pneumonia by the age of 4 to 6 weeks and continue to 1 year of age unless the diagnosis of HIV infection is excluded. Prompt therapy with anti-infectives is used for bacterial and viral opportunistic infections. The need for prophylaxis after 1 year of age is dependent on the child's degree of immunosuppression (AAP, 2009).

Treatment for the child diagnosed with HIV involves highly active antiretroviral therapy (HAART). Initial medication therapy should include a combination of several antiretroviral (AVR) drugs. At least three drugs from a minimum of two different categories should be used. See Medications Used to Treat Human Immunodeficiency Virus in Children for information related to antiretroviral drugs that may be used in children. Families should be advised that these drugs neither cure HIV nor prevent transfer from the person infected to others.

Children on antiretroviral therapy should be monitored closely for side effects and toxicity related to the medications. In addition to

Medications Used to Treat Human Immunodeficiency Virus in Children

MEDICATION	ACTION	NURSING MANAGEMENT
Nucleoside/Nucleotide Reverse Transcriptase Inhibitors (NRTIs)		
Abacavir Didanosine Emtricitabine Lamivudine Stavudine Zidovudine (AZT)	Inhibits action of viral reverse transcriptase, an enzyme in the conversion of RNA to DNA	■ Baseline data include physical assessment and laboratory studies (especially measurement of white and red blood cell counts). Monitor at least monthly for changes. ■ Common side effects include fever, headache, insomnia, myalgia, nausea, vomiting, diarrhea, anorexia, bone marrow suppression with resulting granulocytopenia and anemia, dyspnea, cough, and skin rash. ■ Teach signs and symptoms of infection.
Protease Inhibitors		
Atazanavir Darunavir Fosamprenavir Lopinavir/Ritonavir Nelfinavir Ritonavir Tipranavir	Blocks the function of the enzyme protease needed for viral formation and growth	■ Baseline data include physical assessment and laboratory studies such as serum electrolytes, CBC, liver function studies, blood glucose, hemoglobin A$_{1c}$, serum amylase, and creatine phosphokinase (CPK). Monitor at least monthly for changes. ■ Monitor for specific side effects of the particular drug administered. ■ Side effects include central nervous system changes, cardiovascular changes, life-threatening hematologic changes, respiratory distress, and allergy. Oral forms are taken within 2 hours of a full meal.
Nonnucleoside Reverse Transcriptase Inhibitors (NNRTIs)		
Efavirenz Nevirapine	Binds to viral reverse transcriptase and disrupts the conversion of RNA to DNA	■ Baseline data include physical assessment and laboratory studies (such as liver and kidney function tests, CBC and differential). Monitor at least monthly for changes. ■ Side effects include fever, headache, nausea, diarrhea, hepatitis, altered liver function, anemia, neutropenia, drowsiness and fatigue, altered mental status, rash, and Stevens-Johnson syndrome. ■ Teach the family to notify the healthcare provider immediately if rash appears.
Fusion Inhibitors		
Enfuvirtide	Prevents viral entry	■ This medication requires subcutaneous injection twice a day. ■ There is a high incidence of local reaction at the injection site, limiting the use of this medication in children.

Source: *Data from U.S. Department of Health and Human Services. (2010). Guidelines for the use of antiretroviral agents in pediatric HIV infection. Retrieved from http://aidsinfo.nih.gov/contentfiles/ PediatricGuidelines.pdf;* Marón, G., Gaur, A. H., & Flynn, P. M. (2010). Antiretroviral therapy in HIV-infected infants and children. Pediatric Infectious Disease Journal, 29(4), 360–363.

information obtained from a history and physical, a complete blood count and blood chemistry should be evaluated prior to beginning treatment, 4 to 8 weeks later, and then every 3 to 4 months. In addition, CD4+ cell counts and HIV RNA levels are recommended at the same time intervals to evaluate compliance with the medication regimen and effectiveness of the treatment. A lipid panel is also recommended every 6 to 12 months to monitor for signs of elevated cholesterol and triglyceride levels (U.S. Department of Health and Human Services, 2010).

The earlier the child develops AIDS, the poorer the prognosis. An estimated 20% of children with HIV infection develop AIDS in the first year of life, and most of them die by 4 years of age. The other 80%, however, may not develop serious disease until adolescence. With rapid advances in the treatment of HIV infection, the life span of children and adolescents cannot be predicted as these treatments are significantly extending their lives (Plowfield, 2007).

Nursing Management

Nurses are involved in administering HIV tests, counseling pregnant women, teaching youth about measures to decrease risk of the disease, and providing care for the children affected by the disease. The initial goal of nursing management is to implement health promotion measures to reduce the risk of transmission of HIV to newborns, infants, children, and adolescents. Once a child with HIV infection is identified, nursing care is focused on managing the child's symptoms, promoting growth and development, reducing the child's exposure to infectious organisms, and preventing further transmission of HIV. End-of-life care is administered when needed, and nurses provide solace and assistance for families managing the complex disease of HIV infection.

Nursing Assessment and Diagnosis

For infants at risk of HIV infection, obtain the HIV test results of the mother if available. When the mother's results are positive, the infant should be screened for HIV infection according to the CDC guidelines as described in the previous section. Facilitate the screening and explain the necessity to the family.

Physiologic Assessment

Assessment centers on observation and evaluation of potential sites of infection. Assess breath sounds, respiratory status, level of consciousness, and mental status and report any abnormal findings. Assess the child's height and weight frequently. Observe for signs of failure to thrive and assess for anemia. Assess for *Candida* infections in the mouth and the diaper area. Note any developmental delays in motor skills or intellectual functioning, which could result from encephalopathy and poor nutrition, and can signal an increasing severity in symptom level. These findings should be reported immediately so that further medical evaluation can be implemented.

Psychosocial Assessment

Assess family support systems and coping mechanisms. The stressors of caring for a child with HIV infection may overwhelm the parents. Assess the family's ability to care for the child. Inquire about the extended family's ability to provide daily care as well as emotional support. Support the family when they decide to inform a school-age child or adolescent of the diagnosis. When assessing an adolescent with HIV infection, evaluate the teen's understanding of how HIV is transmitted and the response to the diagnosis. See Partnering with Families: Informing the Child of HIV Status.

The accompanying Nursing Care Plan includes common nursing diagnoses that may apply to a child hospitalized with HIV infection. Other nursing diagnoses may include the following:

- Diarrhea related to gastrointestinal infection, malignancy, or drug reactions
- Gas Exchange, Impaired related to pulmonary disease
- Growth and Development, Delayed related to chronic infection and poor nutrition
- Coping: Family, Compromised related to child's life-threatening illness

NANDA-I © 2012

Planning and Implementation

Nursing care centers on preventing infection and providing emotional support and developmentally appropriate health promotion and health maintenance. The first step in managing HIV infection is prevention. Nurses must be active in evaluating test results and instituting measures to prevent perinatal transmission of HIV to the infants of infected mothers. Adequate testing, prophylaxis to protect HIV-exposed infants from opportunistic infections, and follow-up visits for evaluation of general health and development for all infants at risk of the disease are advised.

Education related to HIV infection, transmission of the disease, and testing should be a routine part of anticipatory guidance provided to adolescents. Adolescents who are sexually active should be offered HIV testing. Some states have provisions that allow teens to be tested for HIV without parental knowledge (Hahn, 2009). Peer education has been found to be effective in teaching adolescents about

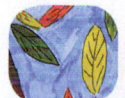

Partnering with Families

Informing the Child of HIV Status

Older school-age children and adolescents with HIV should be informed of their diagnosis and counseled appropriately regarding sexual transmission (AAP, 2009). Telling the child is difficult for parents and they often avoid doing so. Because parents usually want to be the ones to tell the child, they need help to plan how to discuss the issue and ongoing support in the process of communication. Nurses can assist in the following ways:

- Help parents understand the need to discuss the diagnosis with the child.

- Provide information about how to tell the child. Role-play with the parents how to tell the child. Use information at the child's level of developmental understanding, and assist parents to be honest.
- Provide sources of hope—the success of treatment, children living with HIV, and maintaining an active life.
- Assist the family to join support groups or web-based groups.
- Provide emotional support for this difficult task and allow for ongoing opportunities to express concerns, fears, and anxieties.

Nursing Care Plan   The Child with Acquired Immune Deficiency Syndrome

INTERVENTION	RATIONALE	EXPECTED OUTCOME
1. Nursing Diagnosis: Infection, Risk for related to immunosuppression		
NIC Priority Intervention—*Infection Control:* Minimizing the acquisition and transmission of infectious agents		**NOC Suggested Outcome**—*Risk Control:* Answers to eliminate or reduce actual, personal, and modifiable health threats
GOAL: *Risk factors for infection will be reduced as evidenced by absence of signs of infection.*		
■ Assess the child every 2–4 hours for fever; lesions in the mouth; and redness, inflammation, soreness, and lesions on the skin or around intravenous lines.	■ Fever is one of the few signs of infection in the immunosuppressed child who does not have a sufficient number of white blood cells.	The child has no fever and shows no other signs of infection.
■ Auscultate for changes in breath sounds every 2 hours. Perform pulmonary toilet (coughing, deep breathing, incentive spirometry) every 2–4 hours.	■ Pneumonia is a likely infection in the child with HIV infection.	
■ Enforce good hand hygiene. Allow no fresh flowers, fruits, or vegetables in the child's room. Screen visitors for colds or recent exposure to varicella. Use blood and body fluid precautions (refer to the Clinical Skills Manual ⊂⊃). Practice strict asepsis for dressing changes and suctioning.	■ Control of environmental factors helps prevent infection.	
■ Coordinate patient care assignments to avoid exposing the child to individuals with recent infections or immunizations.	■ Planning minimizes chances for infection.	
■ Organize patient care activities to allow for adequate periods of rest.	■ Rest periods allow the child to regain energy.	
■ Follow recommendations of the CDC and AAP for immunizing children who are immunosuppressed. Avoid the varicella vaccine. Perform annual TB testing.	■ Special recommendations consider the child's decreased immune response and the danger of acquiring disease from certain live virus vaccines.	
2. Nursing Diagnosis: Nutrition, Imbalanced Less than Body Requirements related to loss of appetite and decreased absorption of nutrients		
NIC Priority Intervention—*Nutrition Management:* Assistance with or provision of a balanced dietary intake of food and fluids		**NOC Suggested Outcome**—*Nutritional Status:* Extent to which nutrients are available to meet metabolic needs
GOAL: *The child will demonstrate adequate nutritional status to meet metabolic needs as evidenced by adequate weight gain for age.*		
■ Encourage frequent small meals to promote nutritional and fluid intake.	■ Additional nutrition is required to rebuild the immune system.	The child eats frequent meals of adequate nutritional content.
■ Maintain nasogastric tube feeding, if ordered. Total parenteral nutrition may be necessary to ensure adequate nutrition.	■ Supplementation may be needed to ensure adequate calories.	Periodic weight evaluation reveals no weight loss.
■ Eliminate unpleasant stimuli and odors from the environment during meals.	■ Unpleasant stimuli decrease the desire for food.	
■ Monitor skin turgor every shift.	■ Skin turgor reflects hydration status.	
■ Weigh daily. Involve a nutritionist in planning a diet for the child that includes favorite foods.	■ Including favorite foods encourages intake.	
3. Nursing Diagnosis: Skin Integrity, Risk for Impaired related to skin infection, immobility, or diarrhea		
NIC Priority Intervention—*Skin Surveillance:* Collection and analysis of patient data to maintain skin integrity		**NOC Suggested Outcome**—*Tissue Integrity:* Skin and mucous membranes: Structural intactness and normal physiological function of skin and mucous membranes
GOAL: *The child will have intact skin.*		
■ Observe all pressure areas closely for signs of infection or breakdown.	■ Skin care is important in the immunocompromised child. The skin may be the only intact defense the child has.	The child is free of preventable skin breakdown.
■ Keep skin clean and dry. Provide perineal care to minimize irritation from diarrhea.	■ Skin care prevents breaking or cracking of skin.	

Nursing Care Plan

The Child with Acquired Immune Deficiency Syndrome, *continued*

INTERVENTION	RATIONALE	EXPECTED OUTCOME
4. Nursing Diagnosis: Knowledge, Deficient related to home care of the child with AIDS		
NIC Priority Intervention—*Teaching, Treatment*: Preparing a patient and family to understand and mentally prepare for a treatment		**NOC Suggested Outcome—*Knowledge, Treatment Regimen*:** Extent of understanding conveyed about treatment of HIV infection
GOAL: *The parent(s) will demonstrate knowledge about home care including medication regimen, measures to prevent infection, and signs and symptoms to report to healthcare providers.*		
■ Explain the importance of optimizing the child's health status and reducing the risk of complications through diet, rest, and meticulous personal hygiene. Be sure that parents and other family members understand how HIV infection is spread and take appropriate precautions.	■ Knowledge about the disorder and preventive measures is necessary to provide safe and effective home care for the child.	The parent describes appropriate home care and preventive measures for a child with AIDS.
■ Inform the family about signs and symptoms of infection that should be reported promptly to the physician or nurse (fever, chills, cough, mild erythema).	■ Knowledge of signs and symptoms increases compliance and ensures prompt treatment.	
5. Nursing Diagnosis: Caregiver Role Strain related to anxiety about the child's condition and demands of providing care		
NIC Priority Intervention—*Caregiver Support*: Provision of the necessary information, advocacy, and support to facilitate primary patient care by someone other than a health professional		**NOC Suggested Outcome—*Caregiver Emotional Health*:** Feelings, attitudes, and emotions of a family care provider while caring for the child over an extended period of time
GOAL: *The parent(s) will demonstrate emotional health as evidenced by decreased anxiety related to the child's condition and care.*		
■ Encourage family members to express fears and concerns regarding the child's prognosis.		The parent states decreased anxiety.

NANDA-I © 2012

HIV prevention (Mahat, Scoloveno, DeLeon, et al., 2008). Nurses can be instrumental in developing educational programs related to HIV prevention in school settings.

If the child is diagnosed with HIV, close health supervision is needed to ensure medications are given and examinations are carried out. When HIV progresses to clinical AIDS, nursing care is similar to that of a child with any serious chronic, life-threatening disease. Nursing care centers on preventing infection, managing pain, promoting respiratory and other organ function, promoting adequate nutritional intake, and providing emotional support to the parents and child, while promoting the child's growth and development.

Prevent Infection

Children who are immunosuppressed become infected with bacteria as well as other organisms that are common in the environment. Protect the neonate from HIV-infected maternal secretions. Bathe the newborn as soon as possible after delivery and wash the eyes and face before administration of prophylactic eyedrops or ointment. Avoid invasive procedures in the newborn and encourage the mother to formula-feed the baby rather than breastfeed. See Developing Cultural Competence: Breastfeeding and HIV/AIDS.

Properly dispose of needles and contaminated materials to reduce the transmission of HIV (Figure 27–6 ■). Standard precautions (see Chapter 22 ⊘) are implemented in all healthcare encounters to prevent exposure to HIV. See the Skills Manual ⊂⊃ .

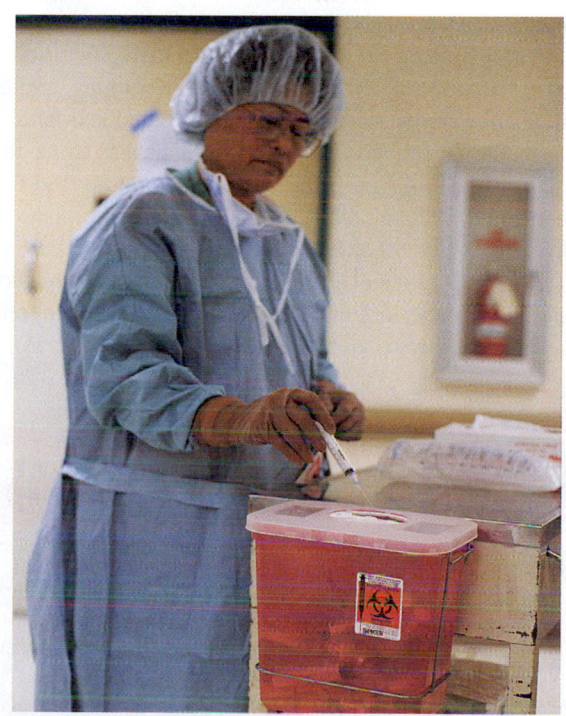

FIGURE 27–6 ■ This nurse is disposing of a needle and syringe in a biohazard container, a necessary practice to avoid the transmission of HIV through needlesticks with contaminated needles.

Developing Cultural Competence
Breastfeeding and HIV/AIDS

In countries such as the United States, where infant formula and clean water are readily available, it is recommended that the HIV-infected mother formula-feed instead of breastfeed her infant. In developing countries where infant formula is not available or in areas where hygiene and sanitation conditions are poor and access to clean water to wash bottles and to reconstitute formula is not available, the benefits of breastfeeding outweigh the risk of transmission of HIV from the mother to the infant (National Institute of Allergy and Infectious Diseases, 2008; Shalo, 2008).

Developing Cultural Competence
HIV/AIDS and Blacks

According to data at the end of 2007, Blacks accounted for 46% of people living with a diagnosis of HIV infection in the 37 states and five U.S. dependent areas with long-term HIV reporting. In addition, Blacks comprised 45% of new infections in the United States in 2006. During 2005–2008, the HIV diagnosis rate among Blacks increased from 68/100,000 to 74/100,000, more than any other race or ethnicity. The CDC has established several activities to address this concern, including the Act Against AIDS campaign (CDC, 2010). Nurses need to be aware of the incidence of HIV infection and AIDS in the Black population and focus on opportunities for education and prevention.

Frequent hand hygiene and limiting exposure of the child to individuals with upper respiratory or other infections are the best interventions to protect the child with HIV from acquiring other infections. See Partnering with Families: Childcare Center Safety Precautions.

Because the risk of serious outcomes for measles disease is great, a live measles-mumps-rubella vaccine is administered at 12 to 15 months unless the child is severely immunosuppressed. Vaccination with the live varicella vaccine is considered safe and effective in children with no or mild symptoms of HIV infection. The benefits and risks of the vaccine are weighed, and the child should receive the immunization if appropriate. Tuberculosis is more common in children with AIDS; therefore, annual skin tests that are performed and read by health professionals are recommended (AAP, 2009). See Chapter 22 🔵 for immunization recommendations for the child who is immunocompromised. Educate sexually active adolescents on the importance of practicing safe sex and the ramifications of high-risk sexual behaviors and intravenous drug abuse (see Chapter 20 🔵). See Developing Cultural Competence: HIV/AIDS and Blacks.

Promote Medication Regimen Adherence

A treatment regimen including antiretroviral therapies for the child with HIV infection may be complex, time consuming, and costly, presenting an overwhelming challenge to the child and family. Adherence to the prescribed antiretroviral regimen is imperative as nonadherence will likely result in increased morbidity and mortality (Khan, Song, Williams, et al., 2009). Some common reasons for nonadherence include frequent dosing, restrictions on daily schedules, caregiver nonadherence, the child's displeasure with medication (e.g., pill size, number of pills or amount of liquid, bad taste), side effects, and dietary restrictions (Khan et al., 2009; Malee, Williams,

Montepiedra, et al., 2011; Purdy, Freeman, Martin, et al., 2008). Strategies for achieving optimal management of the treatment regimen include educating the parent or care provider, and child when developmentally appropriate, about the purpose of the medication, the benefits of adhering to the regimen, and the potential consequences of failure to adhere to the regimen. Behavior modification techniques, using positive reinforcement, can be very effective in promoting the child's adherence. Provide support to the family, and tailor the medication regimen to the family's routine when possible. Praise should be offered to the child and parent for adhering to the regimen. If problems exist in management of the treatment regimen, carefully listen to the family to help determine the cause. Collaborate with the family in establishing goals to help meet the prescribed treatment regimen. If further intervention is required, options include direct observational therapy or home visits. See Box 27–3 and Evidence-Based Practice: Adolescents with HIV Infection and Medication Regimen Adherence.

BOX 27–3	Research: Adherence to Antiretroviral Therapy

A study of 46 children between the ages of 6 and 18 years who had acquired HIV infection perinatally and had been receiving antiretroviral therapy (ART) for at least 1 year evaluated three adherence measures. Pharmacy refill, caregiver report, and appointment maintenance data were evaluated as they relate to viral-load suppression. Although individual measures were not predictive of viral response, when all three measures were in agreement, viral suppression could be predicted (Burack, Gaur, Marone, et al., 2010). Since adherence is essential for positive outcomes in these patients, nurses must continue to evaluate methods of promoting medication regimen adherence in children and adolescents with HIV infection.

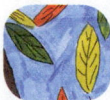

Partnering with Families

Childcare Center Safety Precautions

Because children with HIV or other bloodborne infections may be enrolled in childcare centers, staff in these centers should use standard precautions in handling blood and body fluids. Partner with the family and childcare centers to provide instructions to childcare center personnel in use of these precautions. Assist childcare centers in establishing procedures to notify all parents when a child with an infectious disease has been at the center.

Encourage parents of immunocompromised children to take any necessary precautions to minimize the chances of their children becoming ill. Parents of children who are infected with HIV must be very cautious to limit the exposure of their children to infectious diseases. Parents should consider using smaller family childcare centers to reduce the number of children the child is exposed to.

Evidence-Based Practice

Adolescents with HIV Infection and Medication Regimen Adherence

PROBLEM

HIV infection is a significant health problem among adolescents in the United States (Mahat et al., 2008). Adherence to highly active antiretroviral therapy (HAART) has been shown to decrease morbidity and mortality; however, adolescents have poorer adherence to medication regimens compared to younger children (Khan et al., 2009). What factors are most frequently associated with medication nonadherence in adolescents with HIV infection?

EVIDENCE

A cross-sectional observational study by Rudy, Murphy, Harris, et al. (2009) examined factors that contribute to nonadherence to antiretroviral therapy in 396 adolescents and young adults ages 12 to 24 who were infected with HIV after age 9. Among the subjects in this study, 62.6% were adherent to HAART and 37.4% were nonadherent. Personal barriers to adherence examined in this study were mental health barriers, the presence of structural barriers, and self-efficacy and outcome expectancy. Results of this study showed that having a mental health disorder was not associated with adherence. Structural barriers significantly associated with adherence were problems with medical insurance, problems with transportation to pick up medications and to get to clinic appointments, problems getting prescriptions filled, problems related to jobs or school, and problems with family or taking care of children. Not having a place to sleep at night was not significantly associated with adherence. The number of structural barriers was also associated with adherence. Among subjects with no structural barriers, 72.7% were adherent, while 62.1% of subjects with one barrier were adherent and 40.2% of subjects with two or more barriers were adherent. This study also examined the subjects' self-efficacy (confidence in one's ability to adhere to the medication regimen) and outcome expectancy (impression of the effect of taking antiretroviral medications). Adherence was significantly higher in subjects with higher self-efficacy and outcome expectancy related to treatment. The study further examined nonadherent subjects and found that of those who had low self-efficacy and low outcome expectancy and had at least one structural barrier and a mental health disorder, 68.8% were nonadherent with HAART.

Another study by Rudy et al. (2010) examined how these same factors contributed to HAART nonadherence in 368 adolescents and young adults, ages 12 to 24, who were infected perinatally. Among the subjects in this study, 74.5% were adherent to their medication regimen and 25.5% were nonadherent. As with the previous study, having a mental health disorder was not associated with adherence. Additionally, adherence was significantly higher in subjects with higher self-efficacy and outcome expectancy. The only structural barriers associated with nonadherence in this study were problems with medical insurance, problems related to school, and problems with family or taking care of children. The number of barriers was associated with adherence with 80.4% of subjects with no barriers being adherent, 65.8% with one barrier being adherent, and 59.2% with two or more barriers being adherent. Higher nonadherence rates were found in over half of the subjects who had low self-efficacy and outcome expectancy, a mental health disorder, and a structural barrier.

Murphy, Lam, Narr-King, et al. (2010) examined health literacy and adherence to antiretroviral therapy in 186 adolescents infected with HIV. Adequate functional health literacy was demonstrated in 85% of the subjects, 2.7% had marginal literacy, and 11.8% had inadequate literacy. Of the subjects who demonstrated adequate functional health literacy, 35.7% were adherent to the medication regimen, 23.8% were less than adherent, and 40.5% were totally nonadherent. Of those subjects who had demonstrated either marginal or inadequate functional health literacy, 23.5% were adherent, 41.2% were less than adherent, and 35.3% were totally nonadherent. Health literacy was not associated with adherence to the antiretroviral medication regimen. Health literacy, however, was associated with medical care that was received. Subjects with higher health literacy received medical care more frequently.

IMPLICATIONS

Adherence to the HAART regimen is problematic in the adolescent population. Research indicates that adherence to the HAART regimen significantly improves outcomes. Barriers to adherence must be identified, and interventions should be developed to decrease these barriers (Rudy et al., 2010). It is essential that adolescents have adequate medical care and receive comprehensive education related to the importance of adherence to their medication regimen and the positive effects of adhering to antiretroviral therapy. Access to a pharmacy to fill prescriptions at each medical appointment is essential. Measures that increase the adolescent's confidence in the ability to comply with the treatment plan should be implemented. Discuss strategies with adolescents that will assist them in remembering to take their medication.

CRITICAL THINKING APPLICATION

What barriers does your health center address in its care of children with HIV (e.g., literacy, pharmacy on site, enrollment in the State Children's Health Insurance Program [SCHIP], support for transportation) that may lead to medication nonadherence in the adolescent who is HIV infected? What support does the adolescent need to improve medication adherence? What measures can the nurse take to improve medication adherence in the adolescent?

Clinical Tip

Work with the family of the child with HIV infection to establish a plan for medication administration. Assist them to establish a time schedule that limits the administration of several large amounts of medication at the same time. Stress the importance of disguising the taste of bitter medications to increase the child's willingness to take the medication.

Promote Respiratory Function

Because many children with HIV infection develop pneumonia, encourage the child to cough and deep breathe every 2 to 4 hours. In the community, regular physical activity encourages lung aeration. When in the hospital, blowing cotton balls with a straw, blowing bubbles, or other games may engage the interest of a younger child. Reposition infants frequently so all areas of the lungs can fully expand. Rest periods to conserve energy and lower the body's demand for oxygen should be included in the plan of care.

Promote Adequate Nutritional Intake

Because many children with HIV infection have failure to thrive, nutrition is an important part of their care. (See Chapter 19 🔵 for information to include in a detailed nutritional assessment.) A nutritionist should be involved in planning an appropriate diet for the child that provides necessary calories, protein, and other nutrients. Vitamins may be especially lacking in the diets of children with HIV infection. Antioxidants (vitamin A, vitamin E, zinc, and selenium) are known to enhance general immune system function and should be consumed at recommended levels. It is important, however, to verify that there are no interactions between specific vitamins and the child's prescribed antiretroviral medications. Periodic dietary analysis and teaching are needed. Hyperalimentation, nasogastric feeding, or gavage feeding sometimes provides adequate nutrition.

Diarrhea resulting from gastrointestinal infection and lactose intolerance is a common finding in children with HIV infection and complicates other nutritional disturbances. Alternative infant formulas may be recommended. Although antidiarrheal medications are not generally used in infants, they may be prescribed for older children. Carefully monitor hydration status, skin turgor, and urine output. Provide careful perineal skin care to prevent infection.

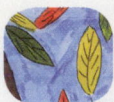

Partnering with Families

Food Safety and HIV

The child with HIV infection is more prone to foodborne disease. Instruct parents to practice the following:

- Use a separate cutting board exclusively for meats, and wash it with hot soapy water after use.
- Wash all utensils with hot soapy water between any uses.
- Wash and peel fresh fruits and vegetables. Consider use of canned varieties to limit exposure to microorganisms.

- Use a disposable cloth or a cloth that is washed after each meal to clean dishes. A sponge can harbor organisms and should not be used.
- Have well water checked for contaminants regularly if that is the source of drinking water.
- Do not allow the child to eat raw or undercooked meats, fish, eggs, or cookie dough. Avoid natural honey.
- Bleach solution (2 tablespoons liquid chlorine bleach added to 1 quart cold water) is a good low-cost sanitizer for cleaning surfaces in the kitchen.

The frequency of *Candida* infections leads to blisters, cracking, and discharge involving the oral mucous membranes. Mouth care with a nonalcohol-based solution such as normal saline to keep the child's lips and mouth moist should be performed every 2 to 4 hours. The child may need a prescription mouthwash. Precautions to guard against foodborne illness are particularly important for the child who is HIV infected. See Partnering with Families: Food Safety and HIV.

Provide Emotional Support

The family of the child with HIV infection is under emotional stress; this is compounded if others in the family are infected. The infected teen may see progression of disease in the parent and lose hope. Integrate social services and support groups into the care of the child as soon as the diagnosis is made. Provide the family an opportunity to discuss their fears and feelings. In many parts of the United States, HIV infection still carries a tremendous stigma, and the family may not be able to discuss their feelings outside the healthcare environment. Safeguard the wishes of the family regarding privacy of the diagnosis. See Legal & Ethical Considerations: Confidentiality.

Clarify any misconceptions the older child with HIV infection may have about transmission of the disease. Routes of transmission and the need for safe sexual practices must be clearly discussed with adolescents. Providing support for adolescents is particularly important, as the dependence that this chronic and terminal disease brings can make it difficult to meet the developmental task of independence. Adolescents may benefit from contact with other infected peers. See Partnering with Families: Supporting the Family of a Child with HIV Infection.

Discharge Planning

The diagnosis of HIV infection is surrounded by strong emotions and fears. Be honest and direct. Education is essential and begins at

Legal and Ethical Considerations
Confidentiality

Disclosure of patient information is a breach of confidentiality that may subject a nurse to legal action. Disclosure of confidential information occurs when a patient's condition—for example, a diagnosis of HIV infection—is discussed inappropriately with any third party. In addition, privacy must be provided when calling individuals in for office visits and in all provisions of care.

the time of admission or diagnosis. Explain that there is no evidence that casual contact among family members can spread the infection. For the child who has been hospitalized, home care needs should be identified in advance of discharge.

Discuss the family's finances as well as health insurance coverage for the child's care. Assess the family's ability to provide nutritious food, pay for required medications, and ensure a supportive environment. Refer to services as needed to ensure provision of quality care for the child after discharge.

Support groups, home healthcare nursing services, financial assistance, and psychologic counseling are usually needed at some point during the child's illness, and the family should be aware of the availability of such services. Assist the family with coping mechanisms to deal with feelings of guilt about the child's condition.

Care in the Community

Much of the care of the child with HIV infection takes place in the community. With the continued success of aggressive therapy, the majority of children infected with HIV can be expected to attend childcare and school. Additionally, a substantial number of these

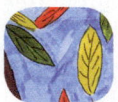

Partnering with Families

Supporting the Family of a Child with HIV Infection

The majority of children infected with HIV acquired the infection as a result of perinatal transmission. This presents a challenge for the family because both the child and the mother are infected. The mother may be burdened with strong emotional and physical barriers that could interfere with the ability to provide the appropriate care to the child. Partner with the family to determine

support systems, available assistance, needs of the child, and needs of the mother. Referrals to social services as well as other services may assist the family in obtaining the needed support for providing care to both the mother and the child. The child may require foster care if the mother is too ill or has died as a result of the HIV infection.

children will reach adolescence, and some will reach adulthood. Assess the family and community support systems and provide resources and referrals as needed to help parents provide adequate care for their child and to assist adolescents as they transition to adulthood (see Chapter 16 🔗). Many children with HIV infection are placed in foster homes, and these families require careful instruction to manage this multifaceted illness.

School attendance guidelines recommend unrestricted school attendance and childcare center attendance for children with HIV infection. In addition, children should be allowed to participate in all activities to the extent that their health and other recommendations for management of infectious diseases permit (AAP, 2009). Contraindications to school attendance include lack of control over body secretions, biting, and open wounds that cannot be covered. CDC guidelines for standard precautions should always be followed in the school, childcare, and home settings. The nurse or assigned school personnel may be responsible for providing medicines or other care at school for the child infected with HIV (Plowfield, 2007). It is recommended that children with HIV take part in school sports. While injuries are possible, it is unlikely that large quantities of blood are present in sports injuries. Additionally, coaches and others should be instructed in and follow universal precautions for all injuries in any individual in sports events.

Even though the child's HIV status is confidential, in certain instances the HIV status of a child attending childcare or school is known. Parents of other children, schoolteachers, other school personnel, classmates, and others in the community may express concerns regarding the school attendance of a child infected with HIV. The child infected with HIV may face social stigma and fear associated with the disease. An important role for the nurse is to educate individuals about the disease and its transmission. Factual information presented in a professional manner and the opportunity to ask questions may reduce the potential for ostracizing the child in this situation.

Assist the family in altering the home environment to provide standard precautions during care. Ensure that the child and family understand that HIV is transmitted through blood, urine, stool, and other body fluids. Educate family members about the importance of hygiene measures. Encourage careful hand hygiene and instruct parents to use recommended precautions when handling body fluids. Explain that they should wear gloves when changing diapers; disposing of urine, stool, and emesis; or treating the child's cuts and scrapes. Wash hands immediately after contact with blood or other body fluids. Instruct parents to use a bleach solution for disinfection of objects when necessary and to avoid contact with persons with infectious illnesses.

Parents will also require instruction on correct administration and side effects of any medications the child is taking. Giving a child a complicated combination of drugs can be challenging for all families; therefore, teaching is tailored to the particular family and is followed by repeated evaluation of the family's success with medication administration.

Emphasize the importance of promoting the child's development. Periodic screening should be performed to assess for delays in growth and development. Provide the parents with information on how to support the child in achieving developmental milestones. Encourage contact with other children and adults, provide for appropriate toys, teach parents how to encourage the child's communication, and

praise the family for what the child has already accomplished. Children who manifest decreasing achievement of developmental milestones or other neurologic symptoms should be referred immediately to the primary healthcare provider to be assessed for signs of HIV-related encephalopathy. The nurse's record of the child's development will be of great importance in this situation. The child must receive regular health maintenance care, such as child health supervision visits, immunizations, and care for any other health conditions. See the Health Promotion & Maintenance Overview on page 884.

Practice Alert

When a child has been diagnosed with HIV, even common childhood infections are a cause for concern. Conditions such as respiratory infection, fever, chicken pox, or gastrointestinal illness can progress rapidly to a life-threatening stage. Teach families to seek prompt treatment with the development of fever or any other sign of illness. The parent's close observation and feeling that something is not right should be cause for concern and medical evaluation.

Evaluation

There are many desired outcomes of care for the child with HIV infection or AIDS. Expected outcomes of nursing care include the following:

- The numbers of cases of pediatric HIV due to vertical transmission from known infected mothers decrease.
- Infectious diseases are prevented in children with HIV infection.
- The child has adequate respiratory function and perfusion.
- Nutritional intake of affected children supports normal growth patterns and prevents malnutrition.
- The family who has a child with HIV adequately copes with the stress of chronic disease.
- The child attends school and receives other supports in the educational process.

AUTOIMMUNE DISORDERS

In an immune system damaged by pathologic changes, an immune response may occur to some of the body's own proteins, resulting in the production of autoantibodies. These pathologic conditions in which the body directs the immune response against itself—identifying "self" as "nonself"—are called **autoimmune disorders.**

The primary feature of autoimmune disorders is tissue injury caused by a probable immunologic reaction of the host with its own tissues. Structural or functional changes occur as immune cells attack other cells in the body. Autoimmune disorders are grouped into systemic and organ-specific diseases. Systemic diseases, which generally involve more than one organ, include systemic lupus erythematosus and juvenile arthritis, which are discussed in this chapter. Organ-specific diseases, which primarily affect a single organ, include type 1 diabetes (discussed in Chapter 32 🔗) and thyroiditis. Immune thrombocytic purpura is an immune disease affecting blood platelets and clotting, as discussed in Chapter 28 🔗. Psoriasis is a T-cell mediated autoimmune disease of the skin and is discussed in Chapter 36 🔗.

Systemic Lupus Erythematosus

Systemic lupus erythematosus (SLE) is a chronic inflammatory, autoimmune disease of unknown origin that involves many organ

Health Promotion & Maintenance Overview

The Child with HIV or AIDS

GROWTH AND DEVELOPMENT SURVEILLANCE
- Monitor and record growth, including head circumference, monthly until 2 to 3 years of age. Monitor the body mass index and note decreasing growth as expected for age.
- Assess for developmental delay using the Denver Developmental Screening Test.
- Teach the family techniques to encourage development.
- Refer the family to a local early intervention program if delayed development is present.
- Refer the family to special services if required (e.g., speech or physical therapy).
- Assist the family in establishing a home care and childcare plan for the infant, toddler, and preschooler, and an individualized education plan for the school-age child.
- Emphasize the need for routine vision and hearing examinations.
- Refer the adolescent to appropriate sources to assist with transition into adulthood.

NUTRITION
- Monitor for failure to thrive with careful measurements of height and weight.
- Encourage the use of dietary supplements if needed.
- Teach the family proper care of enteral or tube feedings.
- Monitor the child for diarrhea, vomiting, and weight loss.
- Develop strategies to foster a well-balanced diet.

PHYSICAL ACTIVITY
- Encourage the child to engage in physical activity appropriate for age. Ensure precautionary measures if the child is thrombocytopenic.

ORAL HEALTH
- Teach the family that dental caries are a source of infection and that the child should be screened beginning at age 2 to 3 years, and every 6 months thereafter.

- Teach the family how to provide proper oral care to the child.

MENTAL AND SPIRITUAL HEALTH
- Ask the child or adolescent to describe feelings related to having a chronic disease.
- Refer the child to counseling if appropriate.
- Encourage the child to participate in peer support groups.
- Ask the child and family to identify sources of spiritual strength.

RELATIONSHIPS
- Discuss the transmission of HIV through sexual contact.
- Ask the adolescent who is sexually active to identify his or her methods of safe sex.
- Refer the adolescent to counseling if required since adolescence is the period of sexual identity and a time for sexual experimentation.

DISEASE PREVENTION STRATEGIES
- Refer to the current CDC recommendations for immunizations in children with HIV infection.
- Teach the family about standard blood and body fluid precautions.
- Instruct the family to avoid exposing the child to persons with infections.

INJURY PREVENTION STRATEGIES
- Teach the family how to properly and safely store medications.
- Encourage frequent hand hygiene by all family members. Suggest placing small bottles of antibacterial hand sanitizer throughout the house.
- Monitor the child's platelet count.
- Encourage the use of car safety seats, seat belts, bicycle helmets, and other protective equipment as indicated.

---

systems (Silverman & Eddy, 2011). Although it is primarily diagnosed in adulthood, approximately 20% of cases are diagnosed prior to age 16 (Brunner, Higgins, Wiers, et al., 2009). SLE affects 1.5 million people in the United States. It is more common among Blacks, Native Americans, Hispanics, and Asians than Whites. More severe disease and higher mortality and morbidity are seen in Black patients (Mattingly, 2011). SLE is 7 times more common in females than males (Brunner et al., 2009).

Etiology and Pathophysiology

The exact etiology of SLE is unknown. A genetic component is suspected because the disease is often more common in certain families. It is believed that in those genetically predisposed an outside environmental agent causes the body to initiate an abnormal immune system response to its own tissues (Lupus Foundation of America, 2011; Silverman & Eddy, 2011). The body produces autoantibodies and combines with antigens to form immune complexes. These antigen–antibody complexes are deposited in the connective tissue, triggering an inflammatory response. The chronic inflammation then destroys connective tissue. The tissue damage varies according to the organ involvement, though the tissues most likely to be affected

are the small blood vessels, glomeruli, joints, spleen, and heart valves. Because many systems can be affected simultaneously, organ damage with subsequent multisystem failure may occur.

Clinical Manifestations

Manifestations may be acute, with onset of nephritis, arthritis, or vasculitis, or may be noted as a gradual onset with nonspecific symptoms. Symptoms depend on the organ involved and the amount of tissue damage that has occurred and include fever, fatigue, malaise, and weight loss. Other clinical manifestations include a rash, arthritis, and nephritis (Defendi, 2011; Mattingly, 2011). A butterfly rash on the face, consisting of a pink or red rash over the bridge of the nose extending to the cheeks, is a characteristic finding (Figure 27–7 ■). Children with SLE may have anemia, leukopenia, and thrombocytopenia (Mattingly, 2011). Renal disease, the leading cause of morbidity and mortality in these children, is evident at diagnosis in 50% of children with SLE and in 80% to 90% within the first year of diagnosis. Central nervous system disorders may occur in children with SLE and include headaches, mood disorders, seizure disorders, and cerebrovascular disease (Silverman & Eddy, 2011). See the Clinical Manifestations table on page 885 for a comprehensive list of possible manifestations.

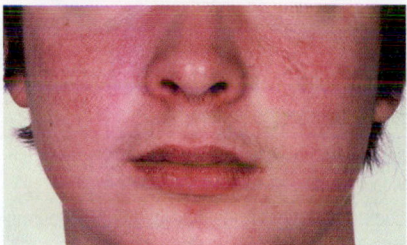

FIGURE 27–7 ■ This child displays a "butterfly" rash across the cheeks and bridge of the nose. It is often seen in the child with SLE.

Source: *Copyright 2012 Wellcome Trust Library—Custom Medical Stock Photo, All Rights Reserved.*

SLE is characterized by periods of remission and exacerbation (flares). Flares are triggered by a variety of causes including sun exposure, an upper respiratory infection or other infection, and stress. The child or family may be able to identify other triggers to flares, such as particular events, activities, or situations.

Collaborative Care

The goals of clinical therapy are to create a remission of symptoms, to prevent exacerbations of the disease, and to prevent complications.

Diagnostic Tests

Blood tests reveal anemia, elevated blood urea nitrogen (BUN), abnormal plasma proteins, abnormal erythrocyte sedimentation rate (ESR), presence of antinuclear antibodies, and a positive lupus erythematosus (LE) cell reaction, which indicates nonspecific inflammation. The Coombs test is positive. Radiologic examinations include chest radiographs and computed tomography (CT) scans, as well as magnetic resonance imaging (MRI) of affected joints. A 24-hour urine collection and imaging studies, as well as renal biopsies, may be performed to evaluate lupus nephritis. Urinalysis may reveal proteinuria. Diagnosis is established based on the presence of at least four of the following criteria (Mattingly, 2011; Silverman & Eddy, 2011):

- Butterfly (malar) rash
- Red raised patches (discoid rash)
- Photosensitivity
- Mouth or nasal ulcers
- Arthritis
- Serositis
- Renal disorders
- Neurologic disorders
- Blood disorders
- Immunologic disorders
- Positive antinuclear antibody

Clinical Therapy

See the Medications table on page 886 for pharmacologic therapy for systemic lupus erythematosus. Diet may be restricted if the child has excessive weight gain or fluid retention from steroids and renal damage. See Partnering with Families: Side Effects of Corticosteroids.

The prognosis depends on the severity of the internal organ involvement. Whereas SLE was once considered a fatal disease, 5-year survival rates for SLE are as high as 100%, and 10-year survival rates of 85% have been cited (Defendi, 2011). Survival rates decrease to 80% at 15 years after diagnosis (Mattingly, 2011). Kidney failure is managed by hemodialysis or peritoneal dialysis. Renal transplantation

Clinical Manifestations	Childhood-Onset Systemic Lupus Erythematosus
SYSTEM	**CLINICAL MANIFESTATIONS**
Integumentary	A butterfly rash on the face, consisting of a pink or red rash over the bridge of the nose extending to the cheeks (a characteristic finding) Photosensitivity Alopecia Mouth or nose ulcers
Hematologic	Fatigue Fever Easy bruising Bloody stools Nosebleeds Anemia
Musculoskeletal	Joint pain Swollen inflamed joints Myalgias Muscle weakness
Neurologic	Headache Peripheral neuropathy Psychosis Seizures Mood disorder Cognitive disorder Stroke
Pulmonary	Chest pain Dyspnea Pulmonary hypertension Pulmonary embolism
Cardiac	Arrhythmias Chest pain Friction rub Raynaud phenomenon (fingers turning white and/or blue in the cold)
Renal	Hematuria Hypertension Proteinuria Edema
Gastrointestinal	Abdominal pain (may rotate to the shoulder)

Source: *Adapted from Mattingly, E. (2011). Lupus in adolescents. Advance for NPs & PAs, 2(4), 27–32; Klein-Gitelman, M. S. (2010). Systemic lupus erythematosus. Retrieved from http:// emedicine.medscape.com/article/1008066-overview; Silverman, E., & Eddy, A. (2011). Systemic lupus erythematosus. In J. T. Cassidy, R. E. Petty, R. M. Laxer, & C. B. Lindsley, Textbook of pediatric rheumatology (6th ed., pp. 315–343). Philadelphia, PA: Elsevier Saunders.*

has been very successful for treatment of renal failure secondary to lupus nephritis. See Chapter 31 🔗 for a discussion of renal failure.

Nursing Management

Nursing management focuses on identifying triggers, reducing exacerbations (flares), minimizing complications associated with the disease process, and promoting optimal growth and development.

Nursing Assessment and Diagnosis

Since systemic lupus erythematosus generally consists of multiorgan involvement, careful assessment of each of the systems is essential to detect any complications as early as possible. A thorough physiologic assessment as well as a thorough psychosocial assessment is essential.

Medications Used to Treat Systemic Lupus Erythematosus

MEDICATION	ACTION/INDICATION	NURSING MANAGEMENT
Corticosteroids Prednisone Methylprednisolone	To control inflammation	▪ Monitor for side effects including weight gain, mood changes, insomnia, and elevated serum glucose. ▪ Caution: Corticosteroids may interfere with normal growth and increase susceptibility to infection. ▪ Do not give live vaccines in the child on high-dose steroids. ▪ Ensure that the family is notified if a case of chicken pox, measles, or mumps occurs in the school or childcare setting so the child can be given appropriate care.

Antimalarial preparations:
Hydroxychloroquine (Plaquenil)
	To treat symptoms associated with skin lesions and renal and arthritic pain (Although the exact action of these drugs on SLE is not known, they often permit continued remission with a lowered dose of steroids.)	▪ Administer with milk or meals to reduce gastric irritation.
		▪ Teach the family to report the following serious side effects:
		  ▪ Weakness
		  ▪ Visual symptoms
		  ▪ Hearing loss
		  ▪ Bruising
		  ▪ Unusual bleeding
		  ▪ Skin eruptions

Nonsteroidal anti-inflammatories (NSAIDs) Naproxen Ibuprofen	To relieve muscle and joint pain	▪ Monitor for side effects including abdominal pain, bleeding, and gastrointestinal complications. ▪ Teach the family to monitor for side effects and to avoid administration of additional NSAIDs. ▪ NSAIDS should be taken with food.
Immunosuppressants Cyclophosphamide Azathioprine Methotrexate Cyclosporine Mycophenolate mofetil	To help control SLE during acute exacerbations	▪ Monitor for infection. ▪ Implement measures to reduce risk of infection. ▪ Monitor for thrombocytopenia. ▪ Monitor for GI symptoms including nausea, vomiting, diarrhea, and epigastric pain. ▪ Teach the family to protect the child from exposure to sunlight and wear sunscreen and sunglasses. ▪ Avoid live vaccines.

Source: *Data from Ilowite, N., & Laxer, R. M. (2011). Pharmacology and drug therapy. In J. T. Cassidy, R. E. Petty, R. M. Laxer, & C. B. Lindsley,* Textbook of pediatric rheumatology *(6th ed., pp. 71–126). Philadelphia, PA: Elsevier Saunders; Klein-Gitelman, M. S. (2010). Systemic lupus erythematosus. Retrieved from http://emedicine.medscape.com/article/1008066-overview; Mattingly, E. (2011). Lupus in adolescents. Advance for NPs & PAs, 2(4), 27–32; Silverman, E., & Eddy, A. (2011). Systemic lupus erythematosus. In J. T. Cassidy, R. E. Petty, R. M. Laxer, & C. B. Lindsley,* Textbook of pediatric rheumatology *(6th ed., pp. 315–343). Philadelphia, PA: Elsevier Saunders.*

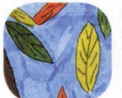

Partnering with Families

Side Effects of Corticosteroids

The side effects of the corticosteroids, immunosuppressants, and antimalarial drugs used in the treatment of children with SLE include hair loss, susceptibility to infection, "moon face," retinal damage, and bone loss. These are significant side effects for the adolescent who is commonly concerned about appearance. Special teaching, guidance, and support may be needed for teens with SLE. The adolescent may benefit from peer interaction with others who have the same experiences. Encourage the adolescent to find methods to explain the side effects and appearance. For example, a science teacher or health teacher may allow the adolescent the opportunity to present information about the disease and treatment.

Physiologic Assessment

Assess the child's nutritional status including comparison of prior and current weight for evidence of recent weight loss or weight gain. The skin is assessed for rashes, ulcers, photosensitivity, ecchymosis, petechiae, cyanosis, and hair loss. Respiratory assessment includes breath sounds and respiratory rate and assessing for extra sounds associated with pleural effusion or pleuritis. Cardiovascular assessment includes vital signs and assessing heart tones and for signs of pericarditis or friction rub. Musculoskeletal assessment includes joint pain, joint swelling, joint deformity, pain, weakness, and ability to perform activities of daily living. Assess the neurologic system for changes in affect or cognitive abilities and seizure activity.

Psychosocial Assessment

Because SLE is a chronic disease that primarily affects adolescents, psychosocial assessment is indicated. Assess family interactions, exploring stressful situations such as divorce or trauma. Treatment-related restrictions associated with medications, and changes in appearance such as weight gain, cushingoid appearance, and skin rashes can lead to withdrawal, depression, and risk for suicide. Perform psychologic assessments periodically as the child grows and adapts to the disorder or faces new developmental challenges with a chronic disease. Evaluate school performance. Additional suggestions include:

- Prepare the teen for side effects and changes in appearance.
- Have teens role-play about ways to explain the effect of medications to peers.
- Identify ways to adapt attire to address some appearance issues (e.g., scarves for head, loose clothing).
- Talk about ways to reduce bone loss.

The following nursing diagnoses may apply to the child with systemic lupus erythematosus:

- *Skin Integrity, Risk for Impaired* related to photosensitivity
- *Activity Intolerance* related to joint pain and fatigue
- *Body Image, Disturbed* related to side effects of medications and skin alterations
- *Infection, Risk for* related to immunosuppressive medications
- *Pain, Acute* related to joint inflammation and injury

NANDA-I © 2012

Planning and Implementation

The goals of nursing care are to assist the child to manage and cope with a chronic disease, prevent infection, promote adequate nutrition, facilitate a remission, and recognize and avoid triggers for flares.

Prevent Infection

Infections are a leading cause of death for patients with systemic lupus erythematosus. Prophylactic antibiotics may be required for dental work and surgical procedures. Instruct the patient and family to inform all healthcare providers of the disease in order to plan for prophylactic measures. Emphasize the importance of receiving recommended immunizations, including pneumococcal, meningococcal, and influenza. Instruct the family on hand hygiene and infection control measures in the home. Warn adolescents about the dangers of tattooing and body piercing because of the risk of infection.

Maintain Fluid Balance

Because most children with SLE have renal involvement, nursing care includes maintaining accurate intake and output measurements and frequent evaluation of the child's fluid and electrolyte status and weight.

Promote Adequate Nutrition

Currently, there are no specific dietary plans for the child with SLE; however, the diet may be restricted depending on renal involvement, weight gain, weight loss, or other complications. The child is at risk for weight gain associated with treatment with steroids and a decreased activity level during exacerbations of this disease. A well-balanced, nutritious diet with calcium and vitamin D supplements to support bone density as well as appropriate fluid intake for age should be encouraged.

Promote Skin Integrity

The presence of ulcers on mucous membranes can cause weakening of the tissues, placing the child at increased risk for infection. Provide instructions on oral care to maintain intact oral mucosa. Encourage the use of good hygienic measures and a mild soap for the skin. Recommend that adolescents limit their use of cosmetics, especially oil based. Reinforce the importance of avoiding sunlight as much as possible and the use of sun protection factor (SPF) of 30 or higher at all times when in the sun. Encourage the child to wear protective clothing to limit exposure to sunlight (see Chapter 36 🔗 for discussion of sun exposure). Additionally, avoidance of unprotected fluorescent lighting should be included since exacerbations of SLE have been reported following this exposure. Educate adolescents that the use of tanning beds will cause the same reaction as sun exposure. Provide instructions on oral care to maintain intact oral mucosa. Provide instructions on the care of the head if alopecia occurs.

Promote Rest and Comfort

The child with SLE experiences fatigue and joint pain, leaving little energy reserve during acute episodes of the disease. Encourage frequent rest periods and a nutritious diet to maximize energy stores. A physical therapist can plan a therapeutic exercise program to encourage mobility and increase muscle strength. Implement measures such as application of heat to painful areas. See Complementary Therapy: SLE and Stress.

Manage Side Effects of Medications

Observe for side effects of medications used for treatment, and teach the child and family about these effects. For example, immunosuppressant drugs can reduce the body's resistance to infection, and nonsteroidal anti-inflammatory drugs commonly cause gastric distress and bleeding of the gastrointestinal tract. The antimalarial drug hydroxychloroquine increases the risk of retinopathy and blindness; therefore, eye examinations should be performed every 6 months (Ilowite & Laxer, 2011). Corticosteroid side effects include cushingoid effects, weight gain, and hypertension. Sulfa drugs should be avoided because they increase photosensitivity.

Provide Emotional Support

Adolescents may have an altered body image as a result of rash, alopecia, arthritic changes in the joints, and chronic disease. Referral to a lupus support group, social services, or counseling may be helpful. The Lupus Foundation of America can provide information to help parents and children adjust to the disease. Internet support groups are also available for those with SLE.

Weblink | Lupus Foundation of America

Complementary Therapy **SLE and Stress**

Systemic lupus erythematosus exacerbations have been linked to stress. Stress-reducing techniques such as guided imagery, reading, yoga, and quiet games can benefit the child or adolescent and reduce exacerbations of SLE. The nurse can review the child's activities and partner with the child and family to evaluate the need for stress reduction. It may be necessary to discontinue a sport, music lesson, or other activity temporarily to provide a chance for the child to relax each day. *What stressors are common to children, and how can they be reduced in the child with SLE?*

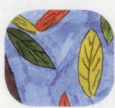

Partnering with Families

SLE and Pregnancy

The female adolescent with systemic lupus erythematosus may express concern about her future ability to have children. Explain that there is no reason that a female with lupus should not get pregnant, unless she has moderate to severe organ involvement (e.g., central nervous system, kidney, or heart and lungs) which would place her (the mother) at risk. However, because of the increased risk of disease activity during or immediately after (3 to 4 weeks) pregnancy, those who have SLE should plan pregnancy with prepregnancy care, and those who are pregnant and have SLE should be carefully monitored by their healthcare provider.

Avoidance of Triggers for Disease Flares

Many children and their parents can recognize the signs of an impending flare and the triggers that precede them. Some of the triggers that might cause a flare include sunlight, stress, illness, and medications. Partner with the parents and child to implement measures to avoid these triggers. See Care in the Community, which follows. Female adolescents who are sexually active should avoid birth control pills that contain the hormone estrogen, because the extra estrogen may exacerbate symptoms. In addition, alternative birth control methods should be discussed with the adolescent. See Partnering with Families: SLE and Pregnancy.

Care in the Community

Care of the child with systemic lupus erythematosus occurs primarily in the community since the child is generally hospitalized only for acute exacerbations or a co-existing health condition. The parents and child should be taught the avoidance of triggers and stressors and the signs and symptoms of impending flares. Teach parents the importance of infection control measures in the home and environment. Partner with the parents to promote the child's growth and development and to establish an individualized education plan if needed. Encourage the parents to allow the child to participate in activities as long as the child is physically capable and measures to prevent sun exposure are implemented (e.g., wide-brim hats, long sleeves, sunscreen). Instruct the parent to notify the primary healthcare provider of any of the following symptoms: bloody stools, easy bruising (with or without nosebleeds), seizures, new or high fever, and chest or abdominal pain. Refer the adolescent and family to appropriate sources for vocational counseling. Refer the family to the Lupus Foundation of America and other resources.

Evaluation

Successful outcomes of nursing care involve management of this chronic disease. Expected outcomes of nursing care include the following:

- No signs of infection are evident.
- Adequate intake and output levels are maintained, with demonstrated fluid and electrolyte balance and renal function.
- Intact skin is maintained.
- A balance of rest and activity is maintained to promote development.
- The child or adolescent develops a positive body image.

Juvenile Idiopathic Arthritis

Arthritis in children has long been referred to as juvenile rheumatoid arthritis or JRA in the United States. In recent years, the International League of Associations for Rheumatology has adopted the term juvenile idiopathic arthritis (JIA) to describe arthritis with an unknown cause in children (Nistala, Woo, & Wedderburn, 2009).

Juvenile idiopathic arthritis refers to inflammation involving one or more joints, lasting more than 6 weeks, diagnosed prior to 16 years of age, and without any other known cause (Coren, Ciervo, & Mason, 2008; Nistala et al., 2009). This disease results in decreased mobility, swelling, and pain. The peak age of onset for JIA is between 1 and 3 years of age, with the illness occurring twice as often in females as in males (Nistala et al., 2009). Approximately 1 out of every 1,000 children in the United States has JIA (Stanley & Ward-Smith, 2011). It is estimated that 40% to 60% of children with JIA will continue with symptoms into adulthood (Sarma, Misra, & Aggarwal, 2008).

Juvenile arthritis affects joints and surrounding tissues in addition to potential effects on other organs such as the heart, lungs, liver, and eyes. During the disease's course, the child may experience pain, impaired mobility, and interference with normal growth and development. Children may enter remission or manifest continued symptoms of a chronic disease. Remission may last for months, years, or a lifetime. Rarely, the disease is unresponsive to treatment or the child may suffer lasting impairment such as bone and joint changes. Children with early onset have a better prognosis for complete recovery.

Etiology and Pathophysiology

The cause of JIA is unknown, but it is thought to have an autoimmune basis. Inflammation begins in the joint and leads to pain and swelling (Figure 27–8 ■). Scar tissue eventually develops, resulting in limited range of motion. Altered growth related to early closure of epiphyseal plates, small joint contractures, and synovitis may occur. Although terminology varies among the different classifications, the three major types of juvenile arthritis under the most current classification of JIA are oligoarthritis, polyarthritis, and systemic arthritis (Nistala et al., 2009).

- *Oligoarthritis* involves four or fewer joints. Approximately 60% of children with JIA have oligoarthritis (Sanzo, 2008). **Uveitis** (inflammation of the middle layer of the eye) occurs in approximately 30% of children with oligoarthritis (Nistala et al., 2009). Recall Rachel in the chapter opener who had involvement of two joints and was diagnosed with oligoarthritis.
- *Polyarthritis* involves five or more joints. This type of arthritis affects approximately 30% of the children with JIA. This

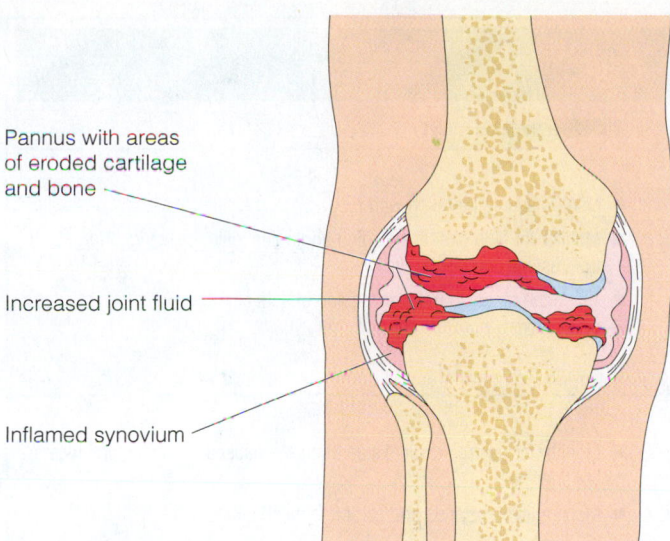

FIGURE 27–8 ■ Joint inflammation and destruction in juvenile arthritis.

Pannus with areas of eroded cartilage and bone

Increased joint fluid

Inflamed synovium

classification is further identified as rheumatoid factor positive or negative. Uveitis occurs in approximately 10% of children with polyarthritis (Nistala et al., 2009).

- *Systemic arthritis* is characterized by high fever; swollen, painful joints; and rash. Systemic arthritis affects internal organs and joints. Approximately 10% of children with JIA have systemic arthritis (De Benedetti & Schneider, 2011; Sanzo, 2008).

Clinical Manifestations

JIA may be restricted to a few joints or be systemic with involvement of multiple joints. Symptoms can include fever, rash, lymphadenopathy, splenomegaly, and hepatomegaly. The child may develop a limp or obviously favor one extremity over the other. A slow rate of growth or uneven growth of extremities may also be noted. Pain, stiffness, loss of motion, and swelling occur in the large joints such as the knees. Older children may develop symmetric involvement of the small joints of the hand. The disease is frequently chronic, extending over several years after an initial manifestation with pain and other symptoms. Remissions and exacerbations are characteristic.

Collaborative Care

Diagnosis is made primarily on the basis of the history and assessment findings.

Diagnostic Tests

No specific laboratory tests to confirm the presence of juvenile arthritis exist; however, some tests help to support the diagnosis. The child may present with anemia and leukocytosis. Erythrocyte sedimentation rate (ESR) and C-reactive protein (CRP) tests may be helpful in determining the amount of inflammation. Rheumatoid factor and antinuclear antibody (ANA) tests may be positive (Petty & Cassidy, 2011). Radiographs are generally performed to exclude other causes, such as fractures, rather than as a definitive diagnosis, though the radiographs are useful in monitoring for joint damage and bone development.

Clinical Therapy

The goals of treatment are to relieve pain, control inflammation, preserve joint function, prevent deformities, achieve remission of the disease, minimize side effects of the disease and treatment, and

promote normal growth and development (Petty & Cassidy, 2011). Pharmacologic management of juvenile arthritis is provided in the Medications table on page 890.

Physical and occupational therapy are performed to increase strength and mobility of joints while protecting them from injury. The physical therapist or occupational therapist tailors an exercise regimen specifically to the child. Range of motion exercises are essential to maintain joint mobility. The therapist may recommend the use of splints or other special equipment to protect joints from injury associated with excessive use or to maintain function. Exercise such as swimming is encouraged because it involves a majority of the muscles and joints with minimal impact and stress on joints. Surgery is occasionally performed to relieve pain and maintain or improve joint function in children with joint contractures.

Complications such as chronic uveitis, which results from chronic inflammation, may occur in children with juvenile arthritis. Children with oligoarthritis and polyarthritis will need eye exams either every 3 to 4 months or 4 to 6 months depending on their age and the presence or absence of ANA. Because uveitis is rare in children with systemic arthritis, the recommended frequency for eye exams is every 12 months (Petty & Rosenbaum, 2011).

Growth interference for the child with juvenile arthritis is a potential complication. The specific disorder may result in bone growth disturbance such as contractures or effusions, and the administration of corticosteroids long term can also inhibit growth.

Nursing Management

Nursing care focuses on pain relief, maintaining joint mobility, preventing deformities, promoting self-care, and promoting growth and development.

Nursing Assessment and Diagnosis

A careful history is important because it is sometimes the primary mode of diagnosis. Assess for joint swelling and deformities, pain, decreased mobility, morning stiffness, fever, nodules under the skin, growth delays, and enlarged lymph nodes.

The following nursing diagnoses may apply to the child with juvenile arthritis:

- Activity Intolerance related to chronic pain
- Mobility: Physical, Impaired related to joint stiffness and inflammation
- Anxiety related to stress of chronic illness
- Pain, Chronic related to joint inflammation
- Body Image, Disturbed related to condition and physical appearance

NANDA-I © 2012

Planning and Implementation

Nursing care focuses on promoting mobility, encouraging adequate nutrition, and teaching the parents and child about the disease and its management. Most care will occur in the community, including physical therapy, with only occasional hospitalizations at the time of an exacerbation of the disease or in the presence of a co-existing condition.

Promote Improved Mobility

The goals of physical therapy are to maintain joint function, strengthen muscles, increase tone, maintain body alignment, and prevent permanent deformities such as contractures. Range of

Medications Used to Treat Juvenile Arthritis

MEDICATION	ACTION/INDICATION	NURSING MANAGEMENT
Nonsteroidal Anti-Inflammatory Drugs (NSAIDs)		
Ibuprofen Naproxen Indomethacin Diclofenac Piroxicam Meloxicam	To reduce inflammation and pain	■ NSAIDs should be taken with food. ■ Monitor for side effects including abdominal pain, bleeding, and gastrointestinal complications. ■ Teach the family to monitor for side effects and to avoid administration of additional NSAIDs.
Disease-Modifying Antirheumatic Drugs (DMARDs)		
Methotrexate (MTX) (the most commonly used DMARD in children) Sulfasalazine	May be prescribed in combination with NSAIDs or used alone when NSAIDs are ineffective in relieving symptoms of joint pain and swelling	■ Monitor for gastrointestinal side effects—nausea, vomiting, oral ulcers, and diarrhea. ■ Monitor liver enzymes and complete blood count. ■ Live virus vaccines should not be administered to the child receiving methotrexate. Consult the CDC for immunization recommendations.
Corticosteroids		
Prednisone (oral) Methylprednisolone (intravenous) Triamcinolone hexacetonide (intra-articular)	Generally prescribed to children with the more severe forms of juvenile arthritis to control symptoms until a DMARD takes effect	■ Side effects include weight gain, mood changes, insomnia, and elevated serum glucose. ■ Caution must be taken with corticosteroids if used long term as they may interfere with normal growth and increase susceptibility to infection.
Biologic Response Modifiers		
Etanercept (Enbrel) Infliximab (Remicade) Adalimumab (Humira)	Tumor necrosis factor (TNF) inhibitor	■ Monitor for side effects of itching, redness, or swelling at injection site. ■ Do not administer live vaccines. ■ Do not administer medication during active infection.

Source: *Data from Nistala, K., Woo, P., & Wedderburn, L. R. (2009). Juvenile idiopathic arthritis. In G. S. Firestein, R. C. Budd, E. D. Harris, I. B. McInnes, S. Ruddy, & J. S. Sergent,* Kelley's textbook of rheumatology *(8th ed., pp. 1657–1675). Philadelphia, PA: Elsevier Saunders; Petty, R. E., & Cassidy, J. T. (2011). Chronic arthritis in childhood. In J. T. Cassidy, R. E. Petty, R. M. Laxer, & C. B. Lindsley,* Textbook of pediatric rheumatology *(6th ed., pp. 211–235). Philadelphia, PA: Elsevier Saunders; Sanzo, M. (2008). The child with arthritis in the school setting.* Journal of School Nursing, 24*(4), 190–196; Stanley, L. C., & Ward-Smith, P. (2011). The diagnosis and management of juvenile idiopathic arthritis.* Journal of Pediatric Health Care, 25,*191–194.*

motion exercises, stretching, hydrotherapy, and swimming help to prevent deformities (Figure 27–9 ■). Encourage the child to perform activities of daily living. Exercise may be painful or even difficult for the child; however, it strengthens and stretches the muscles and prevents potential contractures. Emphasize the importance of establishing a regular exercise and activity routine. Encourage periods of rest during exacerbations, as the child fatigues more easily. Medications may be given to reduce joint swelling and inflammation. In addition, warm compresses to the involved joints are soothing. See Complementary Therapy: Juvenile Arthritis.

During exacerbations, the activities will be modified and individualized according to the child's ability and comfort level. Teach the child methods to reduce stress on joints, such as using wrist splints when lifting. If the child requires splints, a schedule for removal should be established. See Partnering with Families: Reducing Joint Stiffness.

Encourage Adequate Nutrition
Promote general health by encouraging a well-balanced diet. Children with decreased mobility may have reduced metabolic needs,

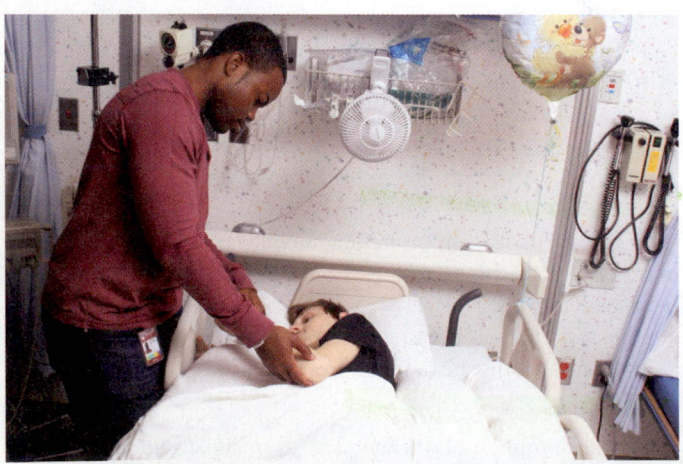

FIGURE 27–9 ■ Passive range of motion exercises are an important aspect of physical therapy for a child or adolescent with juvenile idiopathic arthritis.

Complementary Therapy Juvenile Arthritis

Complementary therapy may be used to help relax muscles in the child with arthritis. Relaxation techniques including imaging, massage, yoga, and controlled breathing may be used for temporary relief of pain associated with arthritis (Stanley & Ward-Smith, 2011).

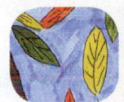

Partnering with Families

Reducing Joint Stiffness

The child with juvenile arthritis experiences joint stiffness which is generally more severe in the mornings upon awakening. Teach the child and family the following steps to help reduce joint stiffness:

- Maintain proper body alignment while in bed to promote pain relief and prevention of contractures.
- Medications may be given to reduce joint swelling and inflammation.

- Warm compresses to the involved joints and warm baths or showers each morning are soothing since heat promotes relief of pain and joint stiffness.
- Moist heat may also include the use of whirlpools, hot tubs, or heated paraffin baths.
- Some children may prefer cold packs applied to joints rather than heat packs.

---

and excess weight causes additional muscle strain. Pain may also reduce the child's appetite. The child's emotional status may affect nutritional intake. Encourage adequate hydration and fiber to reduce the risk of constipation associated with immobility. Dietary consultation will help ensure that the child receives adequate calories and a well-balanced diet. Monitor the child's food and liquid intake. Periodically perform diet recalls and nutritional assessments. Plot growth carefully and watch for changes in growth percentiles (see Chapter 8 for additional information regarding nutrition assessment).

Manage Side Effects of Medication

Aspirin and corticosteroids may lead to gastric irritation. To decrease the risk of stomach irritation or pain, the medications should be administered with food, milk, or a prescribed antacid. Since high doses of aspirin are given, monitor for signs and symptoms of aspirin toxicity, including tinnitus, decreased hearing, nausea, vomiting, drowsiness, irritability, and rapid, deep breathing. The family is cautioned against simultaneous use of other NSAIDs.

Clinical Judgment

Children with JIA may receive methotrexate as part of their treatment regimen, placing them at increased risk for infection. Which vaccines should be avoided when the child is on this medication?

Care in the Community

The child with JIA may never, or rarely, be hospitalized. Most care takes place during visits to healthcare offices, clinics, and physical therapy. Educate parents on the child's condition and prognosis, and answer their questions about the child's treatment. The child may need support to adjust to the diagnosis of a chronic illness (see Chapter 16). Allow the child to express anger and frustration about the diagnosis of arthritis. Allow the opportunity for the child and parents to express feelings regarding the crippling effects of the disease. Social services, a child life specialist, or a psychologist is consulted as needed.

Encourage the child to maintain contact with peers and to attend school when possible. Partner with the child and family to assist in identifying activities of interest for the child to engage in and provide them with opportunities for social contacts. Arts and science clubs, swim club, choir, scouts, and other similar organizations can provide the child social activities. Encourage parents to allow the child to participate in desired activities as long as the child is following the recommendations of the primary healthcare provider and physical or occupational therapist. Explain to the child and parents that overexertion may lead to exacerbation of the disease. Inform parents about

possible complications of JIA, such as altered growth related to early closure of epiphyseal plates, small joint contractures, and synovitis.

Partner with the family and school officials to meet the child's needs (Table 27–10). Accommodations at school may include providing a set of books for the home so that the child is not required to carry the books home daily. Additional time may be required for the child to move from class to class. Adaptive computers and tutors during exacerbations may be helpful. School nurses work with the child, family, and school personnel to establish the child's individualized education plan (IEP) (Sanzo, 2008).

Parents and children can be referred to the Arthritis Foundation and the American Juvenile Arthritis Organization for further information and support. Refer the adolescent for vocational counseling and offer support for transition into adult services.

Evaluation

Expected outcomes of nursing care for the child with juvenile arthritis include the following:

- The child participates in desired activities without difficulties.
- The child maintains joint mobility with no joint deformity.
- The child is free from infection.
- The child does not experience pain.
- The child develops a positive body image.
- Parents express adequate understanding, support, and management of the therapeutic regimen.

ALLERGIC REACTIONS

For unclear reasons, an increasing number of children are being diagnosed with some type of allergy, such as allergic rhinitis and asthma. Why are some children allergic to cats, for instance, although no one else in the family has allergies? To answer this question, the nurse requires a basic understanding of the mechanisms of allergy. This section provides an overview of allergic reactions, anaphylaxis, and latex allergies. Other allergic reactions, including atopic dermatitis, contact dermatitis, erythema multiforme, and Stevens-Johnson syndrome, are discussed in Chapter 36 . Food allergies are discussed in Chapter 19 . Asthma is discussed in Chapter 25 .

Allergy is an abnormal or altered reaction to an antigen. Antigens responsible for clinical manifestations of allergy are called **allergens** (see Box 27–4 for a list of common childhood allergens). Allergens can be ingested in food or drugs, injected, absorbed through contact with unbroken skin, and inhaled. Having a family member with an

TABLE 27–10	Mobility Issues for the Child and Adolescent with Juvenile Arthritis
NURSING DIAGNOSIS	**NURSING MANAGEMENT**
Mobility: Physical, Impaired related to inability to walk hallways, climb stairs, open locker, obtain lunch, carry books	■ Work with the school to identify methods of transport such as wheelchair access, use of elevators, and placement/opening of locker. ■ Identify methods of carrying items such as lunch and books. ■ Consider having two sets of books and other items—one at home and one at school, to eliminate the need to carry these items—or use a wheeled book bag. ■ Explore with the child access to supportive shoes to facilitate adequate support when walking. ■ If arthritic symptoms worsen upon inactivity, arrange for the child to rise, walk, or exercise on a schedule that facilitates mobility.
Communication, Impaired related to inability to raise hand or write	■ Partner with school personnel to establish an IEP for the child that includes methods of communication appropriate to the condition such as an alternative signaling method. ■ Evaluate the child for use of a computer or recording device at home and school, and ensure access to these resources if needed. ■ Refer to an occupational therapy specialist if special pens or pencils could enhance writing ability. ■ Consider the use of a cell phone or other device that the child can manipulate and use to call identified persons for help if needed.
Self-Care Deficit: Toileting and Self-Care Deficit: Dressing related to weakness and inability to manipulate clothing	■ Partner with occupational therapy to plan clothing and fasteners that the child can manipulate. ■ Locate a toilet in the school that provides room, adequate space, and privacy for the child who needs extra time for toileting activities. ■ Identify a member of the school staff who the child can turn to for assistance in completing dressing or other activities.
Pain, Chronic related to stiffness of joints and inactivity secondary to prolonged sitting	■ Encourage the child to stretch arms and legs every 30 minutes. ■ Plan activities that require the child to get up and move. ■ Partner with the teacher to identify opportunities for the child to move (e.g., going to the restroom, passing out papers, writing on the board) and to seat the child in a location that will allow for standing and walking without disturbing the class.
Development: Delayed, Risk for related to effects of physical condition	■ Plan methods to help the child maintain independence and meet developmental milestones. ■ Enlist help of peers to assist the child with mobility in school and transferring items as needed. ■ Refer children to others who have had arthritis as a source of support. ■ Refer to summer camps and other special programs for children with arthritis.

NANDA-I © 2012

Source: *Data from Jones, K. B., & Higgins, G. C. (2010). Juvenile rheumatoid arthritis. In P. J. Allen, J. A. Vessey, & N. A. Schapiro,* Primary care ofthe child with a chronic condition *(5th ed., pp. 587–606).* St. Louis, MO: Mosby/Elsevier; Sanzo, M. (2008). The child with arthritis in the school setting. *Journal of School Nursing, 24(4), 190–196.*

allergy increases the chance that a child will be affected, even to different allergens or by showing different bodily manifestations. An allergic reaction is an antigen–antibody reaction and can manifest itself as anaphylaxis, atopic disease, serum sickness, or contact dermatitis. Therefore, the symptoms can be mild to severe or life threatening and they can be localized or systemic. Characteristic findings in children with allergies are summarized in the Clinical Manifestations table on page 893.

The **hypersensitivity response,** an overreaction of the immune system, is responsible for allergic reactions. Hypersensitivity reactions have been classified into four types (Table 27–11). Type I hypersensitivity reactions, the most common allergic reactions, occur within seconds or minutes of exposure to the antigen and may progress to anaphylaxis. The release of chemical substances such as histamine is responsible for the signs and symptoms exhibited. The first time a child is exposed to the allergen, there is no reaction. With every exposure thereafter, however, the child who is allergic may have a reaction to the allergen.

Type II sensitivity reactions occur within 15 to 30 minutes after exposure to the antigen. Type III hypersensitivity (immune complex) reactions may be difficult to distinguish from type II reactions. Hypersensitivity reactions generally peak within 6 hours. Type IV reactions are delayed responses that do not appear until several hours after exposure and require 24 to 72 hours to develop fully. A type IV reaction, which is not confined to any specific tissue, is elicited by relatively complex antigens such as those of bacteria and viruses and by simple antigens such as drugs and metals. (See Chapter 36 ℮ for a description of contact dermatitis.)

BOX 27–4	Common Childhood Allergens

Common childhood allergens include:

- Animal dander
- Cockroaches
- Cow milk
- Dust
- Egg whites
- Medications (e.g., penicillin)
- Mites
- Mold
- Plant pollens
- Peanuts
- Seafood
- Shellfish
- Soy
- Tree nuts
- Wheat

Clinical Manifestations Allergic Reactions in Children

SYSTEM	CLINICAL MANIFESTATIONS
Respiratory system	Wheezing Rhinitis (seasonal and perennial) Cough Adventitious breath sounds Inspiratory stridor Edema of glottis Nasal congestion or discharge
Gastrointestinal system	Abdominal pain and colic Mouth sores Diarrhea Bloody stools Geographic tongue Vomiting
Skin	Angioedema Urticaria Eczema and atopic dermatitis Erythema multiforme Purpura Drug and food rashes Contact dermatitis
Nervous system	Headache Tension Fatigue Seizures Tremors Irritability Sleep disorders Decreased concentration
Eyes	Conjunctivitis Ciliary spasm Iritis Itching of eyes Tearing
Hematologic	Thrombocytopenic purpura Hemolytic anemia Leukopenia Agranulocytosis
Musculoskeletal system	Arthralgia Myalgia Torticollis
Genitourinary system	Dysuria Vulvovaginitis Enuresis
Miscellaneous	Anaphylactic shock Serum sickness

Collaborative Care

Assessment of the child with allergy includes a complete physical examination; laboratory, radiograph, and pulmonary function studies; tests of nasal function; and skin testing. See Box 27–5. Treatment generally involves avoidance of the allergen, such as substitution of a different drug when the child has a drug allergy. Desensitization may sometimes be used with increasing doses of the allergen administered subcutaneously in an office where resuscitation is readily available. This treatment is useful for allergy to bees or some pollen.

BOX 27–5   **Allergy Testing**

Direct skin testing and RAST testing are available for some antigens. While the radioimmunoassay test is no longer used, the blood test to detect IgE antibodies is still referred to as RAST. This test measures circulating IgE antibodies to many allergens and generally correlates well with skin test results. Although RAST results take longer than skin tests, RAST is safer with no likelihood of anaphylaxis, and results are not affected by medications. In addition to quicker results, advantages of skin testing include the ability to test for many allergens (Huang, 2010).

For skin allergies, the allergen is avoided, skin is kept well lubricated, and topical steroids may be used. Oral antihistamines are sometimes used to treat allergy. Emergency medical care may be required to treat anaphylaxis. See Legal & Ethical Considerations: Anaphylaxis Medications at School.

Nursing Management

The child with allergies requires a thorough assessment, including a complete past medical history, family history, personal and social history, and review of symptoms. The history focuses on the following areas:

- What symptoms does the child experience? Encourage the child to describe the difficulty in his or her own words.
- Are the symptoms continuous or intermittent? What are the frequency and duration of episodes?
- When did the child first begin to experience symptoms? Did the child have eczema/atopic dermatitis or a feeding problem in infancy or childhood? Did the infant have frequent bouts of colic or skin problems when new foods were introduced? Was there a change in symptoms at puberty? Are the symptoms becoming worse or spontaneously improving?
- What known agents in the environment are known to cause difficulties?
- Are there seasonal variations in symptoms? At what time of the day or night do symptoms usually occur?

The nurse may be responsible for performing intradermal skin tests for allergies (Figure 27–10 ■). Nursing care focuses on treating the symptoms, alleviating the anxiety of the child and parents, and identifying the allergens. Educating the child and family on methods to minimize or avoid exposure to allergens is important. Parents of children who have had severe reactions to bee or wasp stings should be taught how to take precautions (avoid bright colored clothing and avoid perfumed soaps and lotions) and how to provide emergency treatment if the child is stung. See Chapter 36 ⏚. An EpiPen may be prescribed, and the parents and child will require instructions on its proper use. (See Partnering with Families: Using an EpiPen.)

Partner with the family to determine effective measures to allergy-proof the home. Pets, dust, carpets, fabrics, feather pillows

Legal and Ethical Considerations
Anaphylaxis Medications at School

Forty-eight states have passed legislation that allows students to carry their medications for anaphylaxis including an epinephrine auto-injector (Allergy & Asthma Network, 2009). This legislation eliminates a delay in receiving medication for anaphylaxis and is potentially lifesaving for the child.

TABLE 27–11	Types of Hypersensitivity Reactions		
TYPE	**MECHANISM OF ACTION**	**CLINICAL MANIFESTATIONS**	**EXAMPLES**
Type I Localized or systemic reactions	Antibodies bind to certain cells, causing release of chemical substances that produce an inflammatory reaction.	Hypotension, wheezing, spasm of smooth muscle, stridor, wheal, urticaria, edema, vomiting, diarrhea	Anaphylaxis Extrinsic asthma
Type II Tissue-specific reactions	Antibodies cause activation of complement system, which leads to tissue damage.	Variable; may include dyspnea or fever	Transfusion reaction ABO incompatibility Hemolytic anemia
Type III Immune-complex reactions	Immune complexes are deposited in tissues, where they activate complement, which results in a generalized inflammatory reaction.	Urticaria, fever, joint pain	Acute glomerulonephritis Serum sickness
Type IV Delayed reactions	Antigens stimulate T cells that release lymphokines, which cause inflammation and tissue damage.	Variable; may include fever, erythema, pruritus, contact dermatitis, blistering	Contact dermatitis Tuberculin skin test Stevens-Johnson syndrome Graft-versus-host disease Allograft rejection

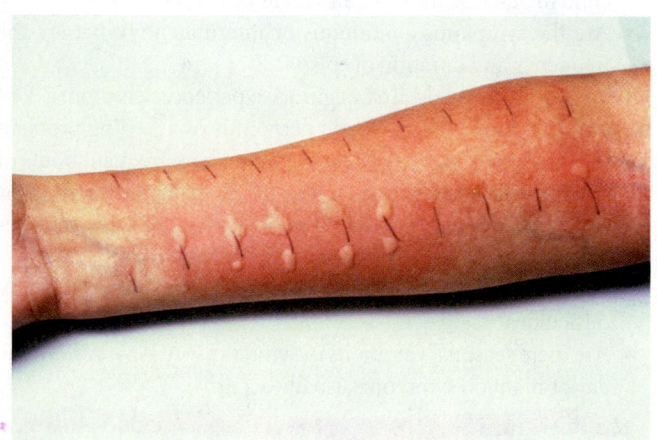

FIGURE 27–10 ■ Results of intradermal skin testing on the forearm. Injections are given on each side of the markings. Note the positive results marked by induration and erythema in response to certain antigens.

Source: *Images and Text Copyright © 2012 Photo Researchers, Inc. All Rights Reserved. Southern Illinois University/Science Source.*

and bedding, and cigarette smoke can all cause allergic reactions. If families are reluctant to give up pets, frequent baths can reduce dander, which is the usual allergen. (See Partnering with Families: Removing Common Allergens from the Home.) When the child has type I reactions to an environmental substance, avoidance of the allergen is most critical. In addition, care providers, families, and school personnel must be able to treat anaphylaxis if exposure to the allergen occurs. School nurses keep records regarding children's allergies and inform school personnel about the allergies and cautions that should be followed. Be sure to label the child's chart and bed, and apply a red armband to alert others to allergies when the child is hospitalized. Nurses must be aware of the resuscitation procedures and equipment in all facilities such as hospital units, offices, childcare centers, and schools. See Chapter 25 🔗 for airway maintenance. Refer to the Skills Manual 🔗 for resuscitation procedures.

Anaphylaxis

Anaphylaxis is a potentially life-threatening systemic reaction to an allergen. Symptoms can occur within minutes or up to 2 hours after exposure to an allergy-causing substance. The disorder is rare in

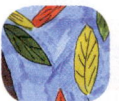

Partnering with Families

Using an EpiPen

If the child has had a severe or systemic reaction in the past, ensure that the parents know how to handle an anaphylactic reaction if the child experiences another reaction.

- Kits with syringes of premeasured epinephrine are available by prescription.
- Ensure that family members understand how to use the kit.
- Instruct the family on proper storage of the kit and to avoid exposing the kit to the sun or high temperatures.
- Instruct the family to frequently check the expiration date of the epinephrine.

- Encourage the child to wear a medical alert bracelet.
- Emphasize to the family that a kit should be readily available at school, camp, childcare, or other settings, with someone instructed in its use. If the kit is available at school, an individualized health plan (IHP) should be on file that includes administration of medications.
- Inform the family to call 911 if the EpiPen is used because the effect is good for only 20 minutes. Emergency medical services (EMS) will have a second dose and can get the child to care quickly.

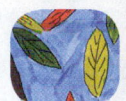

Partnering with Families

Removing Common Allergens from the Home

Reducing exposure to the known allergens in the home setting is important. Instruct the family to take the following measures to minimize contact with allergens:

- Keep pets out of the child's bedroom.
- Clean frequently with moist cloths, dusters, and mops to remove dust.
- Use plastic covers on mattresses and pillows.
- Avoid carpeting when possible.

- Avoid toys that collect dust (plastic and wood toys are better alternatives than stuffed fabric toys, unless they can be washed).
- Use high-efficiency air filters.
- Repair homes to prevent entry of water and subsequent mold development.
- Consider dehumidification in moist climates, especially in the child's bedroom.

---

children. The annual incidence of anaphylactic reactions is approximately 50 per 100,000 individuals (including adults) (Sampson & Leung, 2011). Those with asthma, eczema, or hay fever are at greater relative risk of experiencing anaphylaxis (Food Allergy and Anaphylaxis Network, 2011).

Etiology and Pathophysiology

In the hospital setting, anaphylaxis in children is generally caused by medications and latex. In the community, however, the most common cause of anaphylaxis is allergy to foods, primarily peanuts (Sampson & Leung, 2011). See the discussion of food allergy in Chapter 19 🔗.

The child does not experience anaphylaxis with the first exposure to an allergen, but rather produces immunoglobulin E (IgE) antibodies against the antigen. Following a subsequent exposure, the antigen reacts with the IgE antibodies, causing a disruption in cellular integrity. Histamine is released in large quantities, causing increased capillary permeability and massive vasodilation, resulting in hypotension and eventual vascular collapse. Respiratory distress occurs as histamine causes constriction of the bronchioles. As serotonin is released, the capillary permeability in the lungs is increased, leading to plasma leakage into the alveoli, resulting in pulmonary edema. Death can occur within minutes if severe anaphylaxis is not treated immediately.

Clinical Manifestations

Anaphylaxis is an exaggerated hypersensitivity reaction that is characterized by sudden onset of airway, breathing, or circulation problems, or a combination of these problems. Changes in the skin and mucosa may also occur (Younker & Soar, 2010). Specific symptoms include urticaria, pruritus, angioedema, wheezing, stridor, dyspnea, cyanosis, soft-tissue swelling, cough, pallor, sweating, and tachycardia. Severe reactions may lead to respiratory or cardiac arrest and death (Linton & Watson, 2010; Younker & Soar, 2010). See page 896 for clinical manifestations of anaphylaxis.

Collaborative Care

The immediate recognition and treatment of anaphylactic reaction is essential to preservation of life. Procurement of a stable airway and intravenous access are established. Epinephrine is the medication of choice for treating an anaphylactic reaction (Sampson & Leung, 2011). Epinephrine may be administered subcutaneously, intramuscularly, or via endotracheal tube. Epinephrine reverses the symptoms of an anaphylactic reaction by causing vasoconstriction and reversing airway constriction.

Antihistamines, such as diphenhydramine (Benadryl), and steroids are often administered to the child experiencing an anaphylactic reaction. Though antihistamines and steroids may be administered with epinephrine, they are never prescribed as a substitute for epinephrine since they take longer to act and cannot reverse many of the symptoms of anaphylaxis (Food Allergy and Anaphylaxis Network, 2011).

Intravenous access is obtained for fluid resuscitation, because large volumes of fluid may be required to treat hypotension caused by increased vascular permeability and vasodilation. Oxygen is administered. The child may require endotracheal intubation and mechanical ventilation (see Chapter 25 🔗).

Prevention of reexposure to the allergen is essential. Determining the cause of anaphylaxis, if uncertain, may require numerous diagnostic studies and allergy testing under controlled circumstances. Previous tolerance of a substance does not rule it out as the trigger.

Nursing Management

The goal of nursing care is to recognize and immediately treat anaphylaxis and educate the child and family to avoid exposure to allergens. The child may need care in the pediatric intensive care unit (PICU).

Nursing Assessment and Diagnosis

Assess the child for respiratory distress, hypotension, tachycardia, and edema. Assess breath sounds for wheezing, and monitor oxygen saturation. Assess all vital signs including peripheral pulses. Monitor urine output hourly. Assess skin temperature, color, and moisture.

Nursing diagnoses that apply to the child with anaphylaxis include:

- Cardiac Output, Decreased related to profound hypotension and shock
- Tissue, Perfusion: Cardiac, Risk for Decreased related to decreased blood flow, hypotension, and shock
- Fluid Volume: Imbalanced, Risk for related to vasodilation and capillary permeability
- Anxiety (Parental and Child) related to life-threatening emergent condition

NANDA-I © 2012

Planning and Implementation

Nursing roles involve preventing anaphylactic reactions by partnering with families to minimize exposure to allergens and by alerting all healthcare personnel in hospitals and clinics to the child's allergy.

Clinical Manifestations Anaphylaxis

SYSTEM	CLINICAL MANIFESTATIONS	NURSING MANAGEMENT
Respiratory	Wheezing Stridor Dyspnea Laryngospasm Bronchospasm Pulmonary edema Cyanosis	Monitor respiratory status. Monitor breath sounds. Monitor arterial blood gases. Administer medications as prescribed; administer oxygen and fluids. Provide ventilatory support as needed.
Cardiovascular	Profound hypotension Tachycardia Dysrhythmias	Monitor heart rate, blood pressure, and cardiac rhythm. Monitor peripheral pulses. Manage fluid intake and output.
Neurologic	Anxiety Restlessness Lethargy Progression to coma	Conduct neurologic assessment at regular intervals. Assess for changes in level of consciousness. Assess for changes in anxiety level.
Gastrointestinal	Vomiting Diarrhea Abdominal pain	Assess for vomiting or diarrhea. Assess for abdominal pain. Assess bowel sounds and limit intake when not present.
Integumentary	Edematous face, lips, tongue, hands, feet Warm skin	Assess for edema and rashes. Assess skin temperature. Ensure comfort measures.
Renal	Oliguria progressing to anuria	Monitor intake hourly. Adjust intake and medications to maintain normal urinary output. Monitor serum BUN and creatinine.

In addition, knowledge of emergency procedures and frequent evaluation of emergency equipment and response is important in all facilities such as schools, homes, and hospitals.

Emergency management of anaphylaxis consists of administration of epinephrine, oxygen, and intravenous fluids. Maintain the child on bed rest immediately following anaphylaxis until the observation period has concluded, which may be several hours or longer. Provide the child and family the opportunity to express anxiety and concerns.

For home care, partner with the family to ensure that the child and family members can properly administer epinephrine. Emphasize to the family that the child should always wear a medical identification tag and have an EpiPen available for emergencies. Ensure that the childcare providers or school officials can recognize the signs and symptoms of anaphylaxis and can appropriately administer epinephrine. Instruct the child and family to activate the emergency medical system (911) as soon as epinephrine is administered.

Evaluation

Expected outcomes of nursing care of the child with anaphylaxis include:

- Cardiac output is stabilized and vital signs are within baseline limits.
- Tissue perfusion to all organs is stabilized.
- Fluid balance is restored.
- The child and family express anxiety and utilize effective coping mechanisms.

Latex Allergy

Latex is a sap from the rubber tree. It is prevalent in the environment and is a component of many commercial products, including medical products (Gavin & Patti, 2009). Latex allergy is caused by an IgE-mediated response that develops after repeated exposure to latex. A reaction to latex products can be manifested as an irritant reaction of the skin; as a type IV delayed hypersensitivity with eczema or contact dermatitis 48 to 96 hours after exposure; or as a type I hypersensitivity, which is immediate and often has systemic manifestations (itchy eyes, urticaria, bronchospasm, or anaphylaxis) (De Queiroz, Combet, Berard, et al., 2009; Deval, Ramesh, Prasad, et al., 2008; Pollart, Warniment, & Mori, 2009).

Latex allergy is present in approximately 1% to 2% of the general population (Pollart et al., 2009). It is more common among certain occupations, including healthcare workers, and in specific types of patients. An estimated 5% to 15% of healthcare workers and approximately 60% of children with spina bifida are allergic to latex (Asthma and Allergy Foundation of America, 2010). In addition, children who have frequent medical procedures or multiple surgeries involving latex are at increased risk of developing allergy to latex (Asthma and Allergy Foundation of America, 2010; De Queiroz et al., 2009).

Practice Alert

In 1998, the U.S. Food and Drug Administration ordered that warning labels be placed on any medical products that contain latex, advising that use of the product might cause an allergic reaction (United States Food and Drug Administration 2012). Check product labels in your healthcare facility for this warning. What products should have a label?

| BOX 27–6 | Measures to Protect Against Latex Allergy |

Healthcare personnel are at high risk of developing latex allergy because of intense exposure to products containing latex. Nurses can protect themselves by using the following measures:

- Decrease exposure by choosing alternative products when available (use synthetic rubbers, polyethylene, nitrile, neoprene, vinyl gloves).
- Use powder-free gloves if using latex gloves (the powder has high amounts of latex, which can be inhaled).
- Avoid use of oil-based hand creams and lotions before putting on latex gloves, as these preparations break down the latex.
- When symptoms of sensitivity to latex occur on exposure (rash, hives, nasal congestion, conjunctivitis, cough, or wheeze), contact the employee health department of your facility.
- If diagnosed as latex allergic, avoid all contact and wear a medical alert bracelet.

Collaborative Care

Children and adolescents at high risk should receive allergy testing for latex. When a positive skin test has occurred or when a person has had a reaction to latex, all latex products must be removed from the individual's environment. Alternative products, such as nonlatex gloves and catheters, must be used when providing health care. See Box 27–6.

Nursing Management

Assess the child for risk factors for latex allergy. Alternative products, such as nonlatex gloves and catheters, must be used when providing health care. Emphasize to the family that the child with latex allergy should wear a medical alert identification bracelet at all times and should have an epinephrine kit readily available at home and school.

Be alert for any signs of hypersensitivity when the child is receiving health care, and be prepared with drugs and equipment to treat anaphylaxis. This is especially important in operative settings when acute anaphylaxis is often life threatening. Emphasize to parents and children that many everyday products contain latex, including latex balloons and condoms (Table 27–12).

GRAFT-VERSUS-HOST DISEASE

Graft-versus-host disease can occur when organs are transplanted or when bone marrow or stem cells are transfused into a recipient, typically as treatment for leukemia or severe combined immunodeficiency disease.

Etiology and Pathophysiology

In a child with severe immunodeficiency disease, lymphocyte production does not occur or is impaired. For a child with leukemia, the child's lymphocyte production is blocked by irradiation or chemotherapy that purposefully destroys bone marrow function. The child then receives donor bone marrow or stem cells by intravenous infusion. After a period of time in isolation to prevent infection, the new cells attach to the child's bone marrow and begin production. The child's lymphocyte production increases and immune response develops. (See further description of this treatment's use for cancer in Chapter 29 .) However, despite blood and tissue typing, sometimes the donor cells are incompatible with the recipient cells and the new cells begin to mount an immunologic response in the child

who has received the transplant. The incidence of the disease is less in matched siblings than in matched nonsibling transplants.

In graft-versus-host disease, the host is immunocompromised whereas the donor tissue is immunologically competent. The host, or recipient, cannot raise a defense to the infused and incompatible cells; however, the donor cells release cytokines and become enlarged or inflamed, leading to tissue damage in many body organs such as the gastrointestinal system and the skin. The process is further worsened by the recipient's general tissue condition. The preparatory irradiation or chemotherapy has already caused tissue damage and release of the child's own inflammatory cytokines in these tissues (Velardi & Locatelli, 2011).

Clinical Manifestations

Graft-versus-host disease may be either acute or chronic. Acute disease has generally been thought of as occurring during the first 100 days after transplant, while chronic disease has been labeled as occurring 100 days posttransplant. This classification however is not all inclusive, since acute disease can occur after 100 days posttransplant, chronic disease can occur before 100 days, and the two can overlap. Current classifications focus on presentation of symptoms (Liu & Hockenberry, 2011).

In acute disease, the skin, liver, and upper and lower gastrointestinal tract are affected. The disease is classified according to severity of symptoms. Symptoms of the skin range from an erythematous maculopapular rash to bulla formation and desquamation. Gastrointestinal symptoms include anorexia, nausea, vomiting, and diarrhea. The diarrhea may be voluminous and in severe situations life threatening. Liver enzymes and bilirubin are also elevated (Carpenter & MacMillan, 2010).

Chronic graft-versus-host disease is similar to an autoimmune reaction in the recipient's body and affects multiple systems, including skin, oral cavity, eyes, gastrointestinal tract, liver, lungs, and joints (Baird, Cooke, & Schultz, 2010; Liu & Hockenberry, 2011). Recurrent infections, skin reactions, and thrombocytopenia are frequent occurrences. Specific symptoms may include but are not limited to an erythematous rash, mucositis, diarrhea, anorexia, nausea, jaundice, pulmonary infiltrates, pruritus, muscle weakness and pain, and photophobia (Baird et al, 2010).

Collaborative Care

The aim of collaborative care is to prevent graft-versus-host disease when possible—to identify it early and to intervene to decrease the immune response in the recipient.

Diagnostic Tests

Careful physical examination and laboratory tests assist in determining presence of the disease and stage of reaction. Clinical staging ranges from stage I for mild disease to stage IV for severe disease. Mild skin involvement includes presence of rash on less than 25% of skin surface. Severe involvement is indicated when much of the body is affected with blisters and desquamation. Mild liver involvement is evident with a bilirubin of 2 to 3 mg/dL, while severe disease is indicated with a bilirubin of more than 15 mg/dL (see Appendix C for additional expected liver function test results in children). Mild diarrhea indicates some gastrointestinal involvement, whereas severe diarrhea and abdominal pain indicate advanced disease (Carpenter & MacMillan, 2010; Velardi & Locatelli, 2011).

TABLE 27–12	Sources of Possible Latex Contact in the Home and Community
FREQUENTLY CONTAIN LATEX	**EXAMPLES OF LATEX-SAFE ALTERNATIVES/BARRIERS**
School/Office/Art supplies: paints, glue, erasers, fabric paints	Elmers (School Glue, Glue-All, GluColors, Carpenters Wood Glue, Sno-Drift paste); FaberCastel erasers; Crayola (except stamps, erasers); Liquitex paints; DickBlick tempera; acrylic paints and soap erasers; Play-Doh; Pro-Craft; Clic Eraser; Pentel erasers, pens, and pencils; 3M Post-it Notes; Scotch Magic Tape
Balloons	Mylar balloons, self-sealing Myloons, Mister Balloon
Balls: Koosh balls, tennis balls, bowling balls, ball pits	PVC (Headstrom Sports Ball), Nerf Foam Ball, Gertie Balls, Googlie Imperial Toys
Carpet backing, gym floor, gym mats	Broadloom carpets contain no NRL. For other products, provide barrier cloth or mat
Chewing gum	Bubblicious, Trident (Warner-Lambert), Wrigley gums (check new products), Bazooka gum, Bubble Yum, Ice Breakers gum
Clothes: liquid appliqués on tee-shirts, elastic on socks, underwear, sneakers, sandals	Cloth-covered elastic, neoprene (Decent Exposures, NOLATEX Industries), Buster Brown elastic-free socks (Vermont Country Store)
Condoms, contraceptive sponges, diaphragm	Polyurethane (Avanti), female condom (Reality), Wideseal Silicone Diaphragms (Milex), Trojan Supra Condom, FemCaps
Costumes: masks, face paint, nail polish	Check all products
CPR manikins and medical training aids	Most Laerdal products
Crutches: tips, axillary pads, hand grips	Cover with cloth, tape
Dental dams, cups, bands, root canal material, orthodontic rubber bands	PURO/M27 intraoral elastics (Midwest Orthodontic), wire springs, sealant (Delton), dams (Meer Dental, Hygenic Corp), John O Butler, Earloop masks (Richmond)
Diapers, incontinence pads, rubber pants	Huggies, First Quality, Gold Seal, Tranquility, Always, *some* Attends, Drypers Diapers (not training pants), Confidence (Paper-Pak), Pampers, Luvs
Feeding nipples	Silicone, vinyl (*selected* Gerber, Evenflo, MAM, Ross, Mead Johnson)
Food handled with latex gloves	Synthetic gloves for food handling
Handles on racquets, tools, bicycles	Vinyl, leather handles, or cover with cloth or tape
Kitchen cleaning gloves	PVC MYPLEX (Magla), cotton liners (Allerderm)
Mattress, pressure relief	Check each one for latex content
Miscellaneous items	Some medical stickers by MediBadge, UAL, Cushie Tushie Potty Seat, Bumbo Seat
Newsprint, ads, coupons, lottery scratch tickets	None
Pacifiers	Soothies (Children's Med Ventures), *selected* Binky, Gerber, Infa, Kip, MAM
Paints, sealants, stains, etc.	There is no natural rubber in latex paint, though it may be present in some waterproof paints and sealants.
Play pits, playground surfaces	Natural rubber latex may be a component of surfaces, Boundless Playgrounds
Rubber bands, bungee cords	Plasti bands
Toothbrushes, infant massager	Soft bristle brush or cloth, Gerber/NUK, all Oral B products
Toys—Stretch Armstrong, old Barbies	Jurassic Park figures (Kenner), 1993 Barbie, Disney dolls (Mattel), many toys by Fisher Price, Little Tikes, Playschool, Discovery, Trolls (Norfin), Silly-putty
Water toys and equipment: beach thongs, masks, bathing suits, caps, scuba gear, goggles	PVC, plastic, nylon, Suits Me Swimwear
Wheelchair cushions	Jay, ROHO cushions, Sof Care bed/chair cushions (Gaymar)
Wheelchair tires	Recommend using leather gloves
Zippered plastic storage bags	Waxed paper, plain plastic bags, Ziploc bags, Glad Press N' Seal

Note: *Associated allergies: Foods include banana, avocado, chestnut, kiwi, and pear. Plants include poinsettia and milk weed pods.*

Source: *From Spina Bifida Association. (2009). Latex in the hospital environment and latex in the home and community. Retrieved from http://www.spinabifidaassociation.org/atf/cf/%7BEED435C8-F1A0-4A16-B4D8-A713BBCD9CE4%7D/LatexList09.pdf*

Clinical Therapy

The first therapy is prevention of the disease by tissue typing. Studies are being conducted to identify further differentiation of tissue types that may be helpful in preventing disease. Early identification is key to beginning therapy and stopping progression of the disease. Several drugs are used in treatment, commonly cyclosporine, tacrolimus, and prednisone or methylprednisolone (Carpenter & MacMillan, 2010).

Nursing Management

Nursing management focuses on careful physical assessment to assist in early identification of the disease process, and partnering with other health professionals and families to ensure treatment for the child. All body systems can be involved, especially in chronic disease, so frequent and thorough assessments are needed. Place particular emphasis on skin examination and reporting rashes that occur. Monitor gastrointestinal functioning by asking about nausea, vomiting, diarrhea, abdominal pain, bloody stools, and dietary intake. Weigh and measure the child and compare to earlier findings. Auscultate the lungs and be alert for signs of infection. Inquire about pain in joints or other body parts. Perform regular eye examinations and ask about burning or itching of eyes.

Nursing care for the child who has had a bone marrow or stem cell transplant is complex. Emphasize the need for regular examinations to identify any signs of disease. Provide resources if the family needs transportation or financial assistance to obtain these examinations. Teach the family the importance of obtaining immunizations as recommended; children with immunosuppression may require special additional immunizations and may require prophylaxis to infections such as pneumonia. Instruct the family on administration of medications if the child receives immunosuppressants. Have the family report fever, change in behavior or neurologic functioning, dietary intake changes, gastrointestinal symptoms, or other concerns. Have the child avoid contact with infectious individuals and settings such as shopping malls. Help the family arrange for a home tutor and an individualized education plan if the child must remain out of school for a period of time.

Medications used to treat graft-versus-host disease have many side effects. Assist families to administer medications properly and become familiar with side effects. Educate them about the importance of regular monitoring such as blood tests (which may include drug levels), height and weight, developmental assessments, and other necessary evaluations.

The desired outcomes for care of the child with a hematopoietic stem cell transplant include adequate blood cell production and healthy immune response, prevention and early treatment of graft-versus-host disease, and normal growth and development without sequelae of disease.

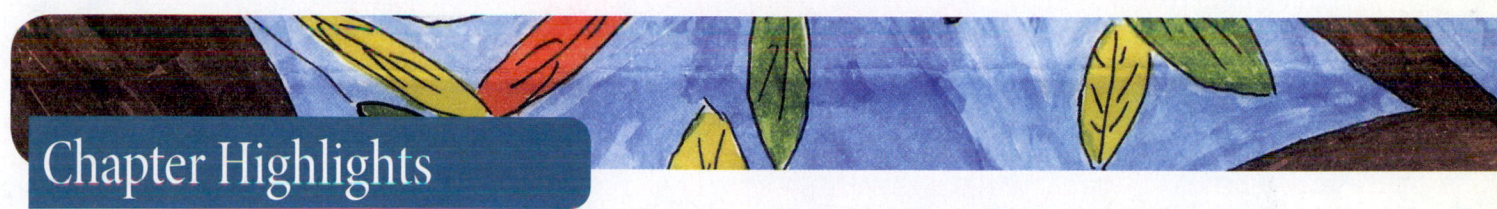

Chapter Highlights

- The infant is born with natural immunity from the mother, and develops acquired immunity gradually in the first 6 years of life.
- Acquired immunity is humoral (antibody mediated) and cell mediated.
- B cells, T cells, natural killer (NK) cells, and complement proteins are the major components of a healthy immune system.
- Disorders of the immune system can be due to genetic causes (primary immune deficiency) or can be acquired (secondary immune deficiency).
- Severe combined immunodeficiency disease (SCID) is life threatening and requires careful medical and nursing management.
- Human immunodeficiency virus (HIV) can lead to acquired immune deficiency syndrome (AIDS); care focuses on prevention of this major viral infection.
- When the child is infected with HIV, support for nutrition, infection control, and developmental stimulation is needed.
- Nurses provide support for families of children with severe immune deficiency with a focus on finances, provision of complex medical care, and emotional support.
- Autoimmune disorders such as juvenile idiopathic arthritis and systemic lupus erythematosus occur when the body perceives its own tissue as foreign and mounts a defense against it.

- Systemic lupus erythematosus (SLE), a generalized disorder mainly occurring in females, is a chronic inflammatory, autoimmune disease of unknown origin that involves many organ systems.
- Juvenile idiopathic arthritis is a chronic autoimmune inflammatory disease characterized by joint inflammation resulting in decreased mobility, swelling, and pain that occurs slightly more often in girls than in boys.
- Although progress is slow, the body may return to normal after manifestation of an autoimmune disorder.
- There continues to be a rise in the number of children diagnosed with some types of allergy. A thorough assessment and careful teaching can help the child with allergies to successfully manage reactions.
- Allergy to latex products is commonly seen in children, healthcare workers, and the general population. Children most at risk for latex allergy include those with myelodysplasia and congenital urinary tract anomalies.
- Graft-versus-host disease can occur when organs are transplanted or when bone marrow or stem cells are transfused into a recipient.

Clinical Reasoning in Action

INTRODUCTION

Recall Rachel, the 8-year-old introduced at the beginning of this chapter, who was diagnosed with juvenile idiopathic arthritis after a 6-week history of knee pain. Based on the fact that only two joints were involved, Rachel's arthritis was further classified as oligoarthritis.

DESCRIPTION

To decrease the inflammation and pain, naproxen was prescribed for Rachel. She will also be referred to a physical therapist. The physician recommends that Rachel participate in regular physical activity such as swimming. In addition, an appointment with an ophthalmologist is scheduled.

DISCUSSION

1. What should be included in patient teaching related to the medication prescribed for Rachel? What other medications might be prescribed if the naproxen is not effective?
2. Why does Rachel need to see an ophthalmologist?
3. How will swimming and physical therapy benefit Rachel?
4. What adaptations might the school nurse need to arrange for Rachel?

NCLEX-RN® Review

1. The nurse is caring for child who is experiencing respiratory difficulty following the administration of a medication. What drug should the nurse initially plan to administer to this child if indicated?
1. Give epinephrine through an EpiPen.
2. Give prednisone immediately.
3. Give oxygen.
4. Give diphenhydramine (Benadryl).

2. When discussing care requirements for a child with human immunodeficiency virus (HIV infection), the nurse discusses infection control precautions. Which statement indicates the need for further instruction?
1. "I should make sure to wash my hands frequently."
2. "The temperature should be taken rectally every day."
3. "When I perform diaper changes, I will wear gloves."
4. "I will not allow anyone with colds to visit."

3. The nurse is teaching a family about ways to minimize contact with allergens. What items should the nurse include in the teaching?
1. Keeping pets outside
2. Using cloth covers on mattresses and pillows
3. Avoiding hardwood floors in the home
4. Cleaning frequently with moist cloths

4. When providing dietary guidance to a child with spina bifida with a known allergy to latex, the nurse should make the suggestion that which foods be avoided?
1. Oranges
2. Broccoli
3. Kiwi fruit, bananas, and avocados
4. Carrots

See Appendix I ⊘ for answers.

References

Albert, M. H., Notarangelo, L. D., & Ochs, H. D. (2011). Clinical spectrum, pathophysiology and treatment of the Wiskott–Aldrich syndrome. *Current Opinion in Hematology, 18,* 42–48.

Allergy & Asthma Network. (2009). *Medications at school.* Retrieved from http://www.aanma.org/advocacy/meds-at-school/

American Academy of Pediatrics (AAP). (2009). *Red book: Report of the Committee on Infectious Diseases* (28th ed.). Elk Grove Village, IL: Author.

Asthma and Allergy Foundation of America. (2010). *Latex allergy.* Retrieved from http://www.aafa.org/display.cfm?id=9&sub=21&cont=383

Baird, K., Cooke, K., & Schultz, K. R. (2010). Chronic graft-versus-host disease (GVHD) in children. *Pediatric Clinics of North America, 57*(1), 297–322.

Brunner, H. I., Higgins, G. C., Wiers, K., Lapidus, S. K., Olson, J. C., Onel, K., . . . Seid, M. (2009). Health-related quality of life and its relationship to patient disease course in childhood-onset systemic lupus erythematosus. *Journal of Rheumatology, 36*(7), 1536–1545.

Buckley, R. H. (2008). DiGeorge. In *Merck Manual Online.* Whitehouse Station, NJ: Merck Research Laboratories. Retrieved from http://www.merckmanuals.com/professional/sec14/ch175/ch175h.html?qt=DiGeorge&alt=sh

Buckley, R. H. (2011). The T-, B-, and NK-cell systems. In R. M. Kliegman, B. F. Stanton, J. W. St. Geme III, N. F. Schor, & R. E. Behrman, *Nelson textbook of pediatrics* (19th ed., pp. 722–738). Philadelphia, PA: Elsevier Saunders.

Burack, G., Gaur, S., Marone, R., & Petrova, A. (2010). Adherence to antiretroviral therapy in pediatric patients with human immunodeficiency virus (HIV-1). *Journal of Pediatric Nursing, 25*(6), 500–504.

Carpenter, P. A., & MacMillan, M. L. (2010). Management of acute graft-versus-host disease in children. *Pediatric Clinics of North America, 57,* 273–295.

Centers for Disease Control and Prevention (CDC). (2007). *Mother to child (perinatal) HIV transmission and prevention.* Retrieved from http://www.cdc.gov/hiv/topics/perinatal/resources/factsheets/pdf/perinatal.pdf

Centers for Disease Control and Prevention (CDC). (2010). *HIV among African Americans.* Retrieved from http://www.cdc.gov/hiv/topics/aa/resources/factsheets/pdf/aa.pdf

Centers for Disease Control and Prevention (CDC). (2011a). *HIV/AIDS statistics and surveillance.* Retrieved from http://www.cdc.gov/hiv/topics/surveillance/resources/reports/

Centers for Disease Control and Prevention (CDC). (2011b). *Diagnoses of HIV infection and AIDS in the United States and dependent areas, 2009.* Retrieved from http://www.cdc.gov/hiv/surveillance/resources/reports/2009report/index.htm#1

Centers for Disease Control and Prevention (CDC). (2011c). *One test, two lives. HIV screening for prenatal care.* Retrieved from http://www.cdc.gov/Features/1Test2Lives/

Coren, J. S., Ciervo, C. A., & Mason, D. (2008, June). Ten-month-old with joint swelling in left hand and left knee. *Consultant for Pediatricians, 7*(6), 245–247.

De Benedetti, F., & Schneider, R. (2011). Systemic juvenile idiopathic arthritis. In J. T. Cassidy, R. E. Petty, R. M. Laxer, & C. B. Lindsley, *Textbook of pediatric rheumatology* (6th ed., pp. 237–248). Philadelphia, PA: Elsevier Saunders.

De Queiroz, M., Combet, S., Berard, J., Pouyau, A., Genest, H., & Mouriqua, P. (2009). Latex allergy in children: Modalities and prevention. *Pediatric Anesthesia, 19,* 313–319.

Defendi, G. L. (2011). Systemic lupus erythematosus. *Consultant for Pediatricians, 10*(1), 26– 27.

Deval, R., Ramesh, V., Prasad, G. B. K. S., Jain, A. K. (2008). Natural rubber latex allergy. *Indian Journal of Dermatology, Venereology & Leprology, 74*(4), 304–310.

Diamond, B., & Grimaldi, C. (2009). B cells. In G. S. Firestein, R. C. Budd, E. D. Harris, I. B. McInnes, S. Ruddy, & J. S. Sergent, *Kelley's textbook of rheumatology* (8th ed., pp. 177–199). Philadelphia, PA: Elsevier Saunders.

Dibbern, D. A., & Routes, J. M. (2010). *Wiskott-Aldrich syndrome.* Retrieved from http://www.emedicine.com/med/topic1162.htm

Food Allergy and Anaphylaxis Network. (2011). *Anaphylaxis.* Retrieved from http://www.foodallergy.org/section/a

Gavin, M., & Patti, P. J. (2009). Issues in latex allergy in children and adults receiving home healthcare. *Home Healthcare Nurse, 27*(4), 231–239.

Hahn, E. K. (2009). Incorporating the CDC recommendations for adolescent HIV screening into practice. *Journal for Nurse Practitioners, 5*(4), 265–273.

Huang, S. W. (2010, March). Allergy testing in children: Which test when? *Consultant for Pediatricians, 9*(3), 93–100.

Ilowite, N., & Laxer, R. M. (2011). Pharmacology and drug therapy. In J. T. Cassidy, R. E. Petty, R. M. Laxer, & C. B. Lindsley, *Textbook of pediatric rheumatology* (6th ed., pp. 71–126). Philadelphia, PA: Elsevier Saunders.

Jones, K. B., & Higgins, G. C. (2010). Juvenile rheumatoid arthritis. In P. J. Allen, J. A. Vessey, & N. A. Schapiro, *Primary care of the child with a chronic condition* (5th ed., pp. 587–606). St. Louis, MO: Mosby/Elsevier.

Joshi, S. A., & Davies, S. M. (2009). Hematopoietic stem cell transplantation for immunodeficiencies and genetic diseases. In R. Hoffman, E. J. Benz, S. J. Shattil, B. Furie, L. E. Silberstein, P. McGlave, & H. Heslop, *Hematology: Basic principles and practice* (5th ed., pp. 1577–1586). Philadelphia, PA: Churchill Livingstone-Elsevier.

Khan, M., Song, X., Williams, K., Bright, K., Sill, A., & Rakhmanina, N. (2009). Evaluating adherence to medication in children and adolescents with HIV. *Archives of Disease in Childhood, 94,* 970–973.

Kline, M. W., Ferris, M. G., Jones, D. C., Calles, N. R., Mizwa, M. B., Schwarzwaldk, H. L., . . . Schutze, G. E. (2009). The Pediatric AIDS Corps: Responding to the African HIV/AIDS health professional resource crisis. *Pediatrics, 123*(1), 134–136.

Klein-Gitelman, M. S. (2010). *Systemic lupus erythematosus*. Retrieved from http://emedicine.medscape.com/article/1008066-overview

Lewis, D. B., Nadeau, K. C., & Cohen, A. C. (2009). Disorders of lymphocyte function. In R. Hoffman, E. J. Benz, S. J. Shattil, B. Furie, L. E. Silberstein, P. McGlave, & H. Heslop (Eds.), *Hematology: Basic principles and practice* (5th ed., pp. 721–745). Philadelphia, PA: Churchill Livingstone-Elsevier.

Linton, E., & Watson, D. (2010). Recognition, assessment and management of anaphylaxis. *Nursing Standard, 24*(46), 35–39.

Liu, Y.-M., & Hockenberry, M. (2011). Review of chronic graft-versus-host disease in children after allogeneic stem cell transplantation: Nursing perspective. *Journal of Pediatric Oncology Nursing, 28*(1), 6–15.

Lupus Foundation of America. (2011). *About lupus.* Retrieved from http://www.lupus.org/webmodules/webarticlesnet/templates/new_learnunderstanding.aspx?articleid=2232&zoneid=523

Mahat, G., Scoloveno, M. A., DeLeon, T., & Frenkel, J. (2008). Preliminary evidence of an adolescent HIV/AIDS peer education program. *Journal of Pediatric Nursing, 23*(5), 358–363.

Malee, K., Williams, P., Montepiedra, G., McCabe, M., Nichols, S., Sirois, P. A., . . . Kammerer, B. (2011). Medication adherence in children and adolescents with HIV infection: Associations with behavioral impairment. *AIDS Patient Care and STDs, 25*(3), 191–200.

Marón, G., Gaur, A. H., & Flynn, P. M. (2010). Antiretroviral therapy in HIV-infected infants and children. *Pediatric Infectious Disease Journal, 29*(4), 360–363.

Mattingly, E. (2011). Lupus in adolescents. *Advance for NPs & PAs, 2*(4), 27–32.

McDonald-McGinn, D. M., & Sullivan K. E. (2011). Chromosome 22q11.2 deletion syndrome (DiGeorge syndrome/velocardiofacial syndrome). *Medicine, 90*(1), 1–18.

Michaels, M. G., & Green, M. (2011). Infections in immunocompromised persons. In R. M. Kliegman, B. F. Stanton, J. W. St. Geme III, N. F. Schor, & R. E. Behrman, *Nelson textbook of pediatrics* (19th ed., pp. 902–903). Philadelphia, PA: Elsevier Saunders.

Murphy, D. A., Lam, P., Narr-King, S., Harris, D. R., Parsons, J. T., & Muenz, L. (2010). Health literacy and antiretroviral adherence among HIV-infected adolescents. *Patient Education and Counseling, 79*, 25–29.

National Institute of Allergy and Infectious Diseases. (2008). *HIV infection in infants and children.* Retrieved from http://www.niaid.nih.gov/topics/HIVAIDS/Understanding/Population%20Specific%20Information/Pages/children.aspx

Nistala, K., Woo, P., & Wedderburn, L. R. (2009). Juvenile idiopathic arthritis. In G. S. Firestein, R. C. Budd, E. D. Harris, I. B. McInnes, S. Ruddy, & J. S. Sergent, *Kelley's textbook of rheumatology* (8th ed., pp. 1657–1675). Philadelphia, PA: Elsevier Saunders.

Ochs, H. D., & Notarangelo, L. D. (2010). Immunodeficiency diseases. In K. Kaushansky, M. A. Lichtman, E. Beutler, T. J. Kipps, U. Seligsohn, & J. T. Prchal,

Williams hematology (8th ed., pp. 1153–1173). New York, NY: McGraw-Hill.

Park, C. L. (2010). *X-linked immunodeficiency with hyper IgM.* Retrieved from http://emedicine.medscape.com/article/889104-overview

Petri, M., & Magder, L. (2004). Classification criteria for systemic lupus erythematosus: A review. *Lupus, 13*, 829–837.

Petty, R. E., & Cassidy, J. T. (2011). Chronic arthritis in childhood. In J. T. Cassidy, R. E. Petty, R. M. Laxer, & C. B. Lindsley, *Textbook of pediatric rheumatology* (6th ed., pp. 211–235). Philadelphia, PA: Elsevier Saunders.

Petty, R. E., & Rosenbaum, J. T. (2011). Uveitis in juvenile idiopathic arthritis. In J. T. Cassidy, R. E. Petty, R. M. Laxer, & C. B. Lindsley, *Textbook of pediatric rheumatology* (6th ed., pp. 305–314). Philadelphia, PA: Elsevier Saunders.

Plowfield, L. A. (2007). HIV disease in children 25 years later. *Pediatric Nursing, 33*(3), 273–278.

Pollart, S. M., Warniment, C., & Mori, T. (2009). Latex allergy. *American Family Physician, 80*(12), 1413–1418.

Purdy, J. B., Freeman, A. F., Martin, S. C., Ryder, C., Elliott-DeSorbo, D. K., Zeichner, S., & Hazra, R. (2008). Virologic response using directly observed therapy in adolescents with HIV: An adherence tool. *Journal of the Association of Nurses in AIDS Care, 19*(2), 158–165.

Rudy, B. J., Murphy, D. A., Harris, D. R., Muenz, L., & Ellen, J. (2009). Patient-related risks for nonadherence to antiretroviral therapy among HIV-infected youth in the United States: A study of prevalence and interactions. *AIDS Patient Care and STDs, 23*(3), 185–194.

Rudy, B. J., Murphy, D. A., Harris, D. R., Muenz, L., & Ellen, J. (2010). Prevalence and interactions of patient-related risks for nonadherence to antiretroviral therapy among perinatally infected youth in the United States. *AIDS Patient Care and STDs, 24*(2), 97–104.

Sampson, H. A., & Leung, D. Y. M. (2011). Anaphylaxis. In R. M. Kliegman, B. F. Stanton, J. W. St. Geme III, N. F. Schor, & R. E. Behrman, *Nelson textbook of pediatrics* (19th ed., pp. 816–818). Philadelphia, PA: Elsevier Saunders.

Sanzo, M. (2008). The child with arthritis in the school setting. *Journal of School Nursing, 24*(4), 190–196.

Sarma, P. K., Misra, R., & Aggarwal, A. (2008). Physical disability, articular, and extra-articular damage in patients with juvenile idiopathic arthritis. *Clinical Rheumatology, 27*, 1261–1265.

Schwartz, R. A., & Sinha, S. (2011). *Pediatric severe combined immunodeficiency.* Retrieved from http://emedicine.medscape.com/article/888072-overview

Schwartz, R. A., & Siperstein, R. (2011). *Pediatric Wiskott-Aldrich syndrome.* Retrieved from http://emedicine.medscape.com/article/888939-overview

Shalo, S. (2008). For HIV-positive mothers: To breastfeed or not to breastfeed? *American Journal of Nursing, 108*(11), 20.

Silverman, E., & Eddy, A. (2011). Systemic lupus erythematosus. In J. T. Cassidy, R. E. Petty, R. M. Laxer, & C. B. Lindsley, *Textbook of pediatric rheumatology* (6th ed., pp. 315–343). Philadelphia, PA: Elsevier Saunders.

Smith, S. (2011). Infectious diseases. In K. J. Marcdante, R. M. Kliegman, H. B. Jenson, & R. E. Behrman, *Nelson essentials of pediatrics* (6th ed., pp. 355–462). Philadelphia, PA: Elsevier Saunders.

Spina Bifida Association. (2009). *Latex (natural rubber) in the hospital environment and latex (natural rubber) in the home and community.* Retrieved from http://www.spinabifidaassociation.org/atf/cf/%7BEED435C8-F1A0-4A16-B4D8-A713BBCD9CE4%7D/LatexList09.pdf

Stanley, L. C., & Ward-Smith, P. (2011). The diagnosis and management of juvenile idiopathic arthritis. *Journal of Pediatric Health Care, 25*, 191–194.

U.S. Department of Health and Human Services. (2010). *Guidelines for the use of antiretroviral agents in pediatric HIV infection.* Retrieved from http://aidsinfo.nih.gov/contentfiles/PediatricGuidelines.pdf

Velardi, A., & Locatelli, F. (2011). Graft versus host disease (GVHD) and rejection. In R. M. Kliegman, B. F. Stanton, J. W. St. Geme III, N. F. Schor, & R. E. Behrman, *Nelson textbook of pediatrics* (19th ed., pp. 760–762). Philadelphia, PA: Elsevier Saunders.

Verhasselt, V. (2010). Neonatal tolerance under breastfeeding influence: The presence of allergen and transforming growth factor-b in breast milk protects the progeny from allergic asthma. *Journal of Pediatrics, 156*, S16–20.

United States Food and Drug Administration (2012). New type of latex glove cleared. Retrieved from http://www.fda.gov/ForConsumers/ConsumerUpdates/ucm048052.htm

Wilson, B. A., Shannon, M. T., & Shields, K. M. (2011). *Nurse's drug guide 2011.* Upper Saddle River, NJ: Pearson.

Wilson, B. A., Shannon, M. T., & Shields, K. M. (2011). *Intravenous drug guide 2011–2012.* Upper Saddle River, NJ: Pearson.

Yee, A., DeRavin, S. S., Elliott, E., Ziegler, J. B., & Contributors to the Australian Pediatric Surveillance Unit. (2008). Severe combined immunodeficiency: A national surveillance study. *Pediatric Allergy and Immunology, 19*, 298–302.

Younker, J., & Soar, J. (2010). Recognition and treatment of anaphylaxis. *Nursing in Critical Care, 15*(2), 94–98.

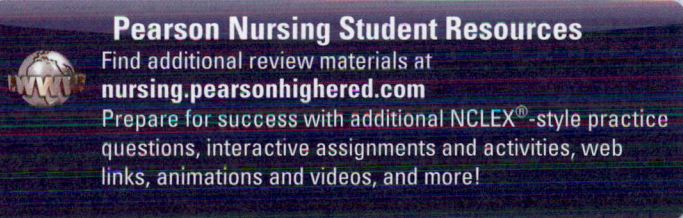

Pearson Nursing Student Resources
Find additional review materials at
nursing.pearsonhighered.com
Prepare for success with additional NCLEX®-style practice questions, interactive assignments and activities, web links, animations and videos, and more!

28 Alterations in Hematologic Function

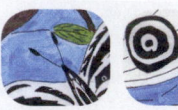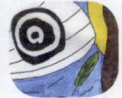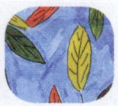

Learning Outcomes

After completing this chapter, you will be able to:

1. Describe the function of red blood cells, white blood cells, and platelets.

2. Discuss the pathophysiology and clinical manifestations of the major disorders of red blood cells affecting the pediatric population.

3. Discuss the pathophysiology and clinical manifestations of the major disorders of white blood cells affecting the pediatric population.

4. Discuss the pathophysiology and clinical manifestations of the major bleeding disorders affecting the pediatric population.

5. Compare and contrast the major bleeding disorders, disorders of red blood cells, and disorders of white blood cells affecting the pediatric population.

6. Develop a family-centered nursing care plan for the management of a child with a hematologic disorder.

7. Prioritize nursing interventions for a child receiving hematopoietic stem cell transplantation (HSCT).

> **"I am fine most of the time, I feel just like a normal kid until I get sick. Then the pain reminds me that I am not a normal kid. I have a disease and it hurts—a lot."**
>
> —*Michael, age 12*

Michael Draper is a 12-year-old boy who is admitted to the hospital with severe abdominal pain. He was diagnosed with sickle cell anemia as an infant. Although Michael is in relatively good health, he was hospitalized on two previous occasions related to complications of the disease. Recently, Michael has had several viral illnesses, leading his primary care provider to suspect that his spleen has become fibrotic (a complication associated with sickle cell anemia), leading to impairment of his immune function.

Michael is small for his age and has several bruises on his lower legs. His respirations are rapid and he appears anxious. Michael's parents are knowledgeable about sickle cell anemia. They understand that Michael is experiencing an episode of sickle cell crisis.

An intravenous infusion is started and Michael is medicated for pain. The nurse performs multiple tests and procedures together to allow Michael time to rest in between. Michael is receiving oxygen by nasal cannula to increase his oxygen saturation to normal levels.

What immediate and long-term care does Michael require? What do Michael and his parents need to know about his crisis? How will you help them manage the challenges of this condition? This chapter will assist you in planning care for children like Michael who have disorders of the hematologic system.

The hematologic system is one of a few body systems that regulate, directly or indirectly, all other body functions. Because blood is involved in the function of all tissues and organs, changes in the blood may result in altered functioning of many body organs and structures. This chapter discusses the most common disorders of the blood and blood-forming organs in children. See Chapter 29 🔗 for a discussion of leukemia.

ANATOMY AND PHYSIOLOGY

Blood has two components: a fluid portion called plasma and a cellular portion known as the formed elements of the blood. Plasma contains proteins, electrolytes, clotting factors, antibodies, and anticoagulants. The cellular elements are red blood cells (**erythrocytes**), white blood cells (**leukocytes**), and platelets (**thrombocytes**) (Figure 28–1 ■). A summary of normal values for these and other blood components in children is provided in Table 28–1 and Appendix D 🔗.

Red Blood Cells

Red blood cells (RBCs), or erythrocytes, are the most abundant of the cellular elements of blood. They are formed through a process called **erythropoiesis.** The primary function of red blood cells is to transport oxygen from the lungs to the tissues. These cells also help to carry carbon dioxide from the tissues back to the lungs. Hemoglobin, a red pigment composed of protein and iron, which is contained in the RBC, is essential to its function. The normal life span of the RBC is 120 days. Upon destruction of the RBC by the spleen, most of the iron from the cell is stored for later use in development of new red blood cells. **Erythropoietin** is a hormone produced by the kidney that stimulates RBC production (Figure 28–2 ■).

Polycythemia is an above-average increase in the number of red cells in the blood. (See Chapter 26 🔗 for discussion of polycythemia.) Any condition that causes the quantity of oxygen transported to the tissues to decrease ordinarily increases the rate of red blood cell production. When a child becomes anemic secondary to hemorrhage,

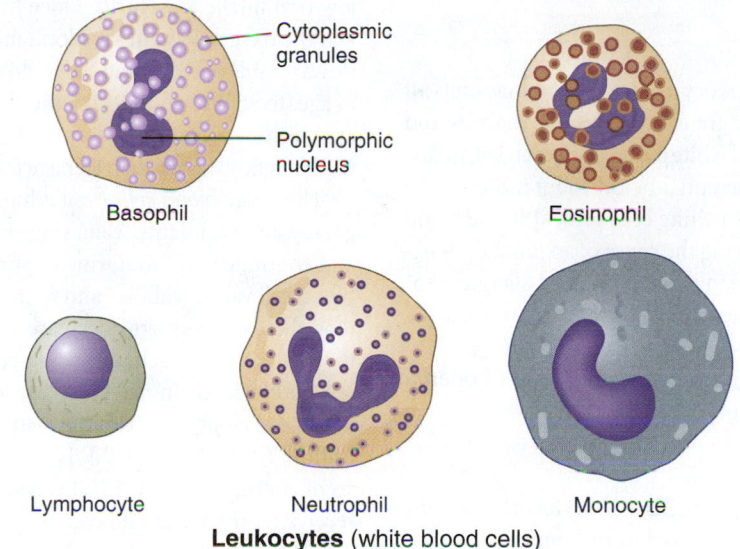

Basophil — Cytoplasmic granules, Polymorphic nucleus

Eosinophil

Lymphocyte   Neutrophil   Monocyte

Leukocytes (white blood cells)

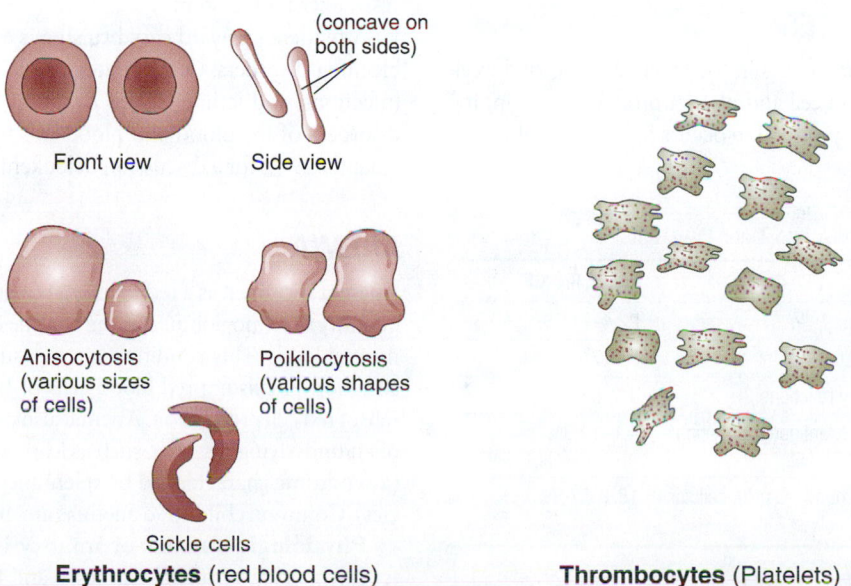

Front view   Side view (concave on both sides)

Anisocytosis (various sizes of cells)   Poikilocytosis (various shapes of cells)

Sickle cells

Erythrocytes (red blood cells)

Thrombocytes (Platelets)

FIGURE 28–1 ■ Types of blood cells.

TABLE 28–1	Mean Values for Common Hematology Tests in Children
TEST	**MEAN VALUE**
Red blood cell (RBC)	$3.8–5.03 \times 10^{12}$/L
Hemoglobin (Hb)	10.2–13.4 g/dL
Hematocrit (HCT)	31.7–39.8%
White blood cell (WBC)	$4.86–11.4 \times 10^{9}$/L
Platelets	$203–367 \times 10^{9}$/L

Source: *Adapted from Soldin, S. J., Wong, E. C., Brugnara, C., & Soldin, O. P. (2011). Pediatric reference ranges (7th ed.). Washington, DC: AACC Press; data from Kliegman, R. M., Stanton, B. F., St. Geme, J. W., Schor, N. F., & Behrman, R. E. (2011). Nelson textbook of pediatrics (19th ed., Table 708.6). Philadelphia, PA: Elsevier Saunders.*

for instance, the bone marrow immediately begins to produce large quantities of red blood cells. **Anemia** is a reduction in the number of red blood cells. The various types of anemia will be discussed in this chapter.

White Blood Cells

White blood cells (WBCs), or leukocytes, are the mobile units of the body's protective system. They are formed in bone marrow and lymph tissue. There are five types of white blood cells, each with a distinct function (Table 28–2). A differential blood count indicates the percentages of the different types of white cells present in the blood and is sometimes useful in identifying the cause of an illness. For example, infections cause an increase in neutrophils, and allergies produce an increase in eosinophils. The role of lymphocytes is discussed with acquired immunodeficiency syndrome in Chapter 27 🔗.

A decrease in the number of white blood cells is called **leukopenia** and can be caused by immune or bone marrow disorders.

Platelets

Platelets, or thrombocytes, are cell fragments that can form hemostatic plugs to stop bleeding. They are synthesized from components in the red bone marrow and are stored in the spleen. A deficiency of platelets can lead to a bleeding disorder and is termed **thrombocytopenia.**

PEDIATRIC DIFFERENCES

Production of *red blood cells* occurs in the fetus by the second week of gestation, with white blood cell and platelet production beginning at 8 weeks. Most of this early production occurs first in the embryonic

TABLE 28–2	White Blood Cells and Their Functions	
CELL TYPE	**FUNCTION**	**VALUE RANGE**
Neutrophils	Phagocytosis	22.4–74.7%
Eosinophils	Allergic reactions	0–4.7%
Basophils	Inflammatory reactions	0.1–0.6%
Monocytes (macrophages)	Phagocytosis, antigen processing	4.1–12.3%
Lymphocytes	Humoral immunity (B cell), cellular immunity (T cell)	18.1–57.8%

Source: *Adapted from Soldin, S. J., Wong, E. C., Brugnara, C., & Soldin, O. P. (2011). Pediatric reference ranges (7th ed.). Washington, DC: AACC Press.*

yolk sac and then in the liver; however, by 20 to 24 weeks' gestation, liver production decreases as bone marrow production begins to predominate (Christensen & Ohls, 2011). At birth, **hematopoiesis,** or blood cell production, occurs in the marrow of almost every bone. The flat bones, such as the sternum, ribs, pelvic and shoulder girdles, vertebrae, and hips, retain most of their hematopoietic activity throughout life.

Fetal RBCs contain fetal hemoglobin which has a high level of affinity for oxygen. The fetus must extract oxygen from the maternal circulation, which has lower oxygen saturation than the atmosphere, so the developing fetus needs this enhanced ability. Fetal hemoglobin is present in decreasing amounts after birth, with normal hemoglobin levels gradually increasing.

Blood volume of the newborn infant is 85 mL/kg of body weight (London, Ladewig, Ball, et al., 2011). At birth, the newborn has a naturally occurring elevation in RBCs and hemoglobin due to a high level of erythropoietin, which stimulates red cell production. Additional contributors to these higher levels are the transfusion of blood from the placenta at birth and low extracellular fluid volume from low oral intake after birth. Once the newborn begins breathing air and the oxygen level in the blood increases, hemoglobin production slows. Levels of RBCs and hemoglobin fall until about 2 to 3 months of age (to about 9 to 11 g/dL) and then begin increasing. Adult levels are reached during adolescence. Teenage males have red blood cell levels slightly higher than teenage females.

The *white blood cell* count is highest at birth, although levels vary greatly among infants. Values begin to decline after 12 hours of life and continue to do so during the first week. By 1 week of age, white blood cell values stabilize and remain stable until 1 year of age. After that, there is a very slow decrease in the white blood cell count until the adult value is reached in adolescence (Newberger & Boxer, 2011).

Platelet levels in newborns are lower than in older children and adults. Levels of many clotting factors are also lower in infants (Scott, Raffini, & Montgomery, 2011). Vitamin K is required for the synthesis of clotting factor II, VII, IX, and X. For this reason, all newborns receive a prophylactic injection of vitamin K at birth (Greenbaum, 2011). Examples of diagnostic and laboratory tests used to evaluate the hematologic system are provided in Appendixes D and E 🔗. (See Box 28–1.) Use the guidelines in Table 28–3 to perform a nursing assessment of this system.

A tendency toward easy bruising is a characteristic sign of many bleeding disorders. Other signs include nosebleeds, pallor, frequent infections, and lethargy. This chapter discusses the most common disorders of the blood and blood-forming organs in children. (See Chapter 29 🔗 for a discussion of leukemia.)

ANEMIA

Anemia is defined as a reduction in the number of red blood cells, the quantity of hemoglobin, and the volume of packed red cells to below-normal levels. This condition can be caused by increased loss or destruction of existing red blood cells or by an impaired or decreased rate of red cell production. Anemia also can be a clinical manifestation of an underlying disorder, such as lead poisoning or **hypersplenism** (a syndrome characterized by splenomegaly and blood cell deficiencies). Common childhood anemias are discussed in this section.

Physiologic anemia of infancy is a normal occurrence. After birth, erythropoietin synthesis, and therefore production of red blood cells, abruptly decreases in response to the higher oxygenation

Pathophysiology Illustrated Erythropoietin Feedback Mechanism

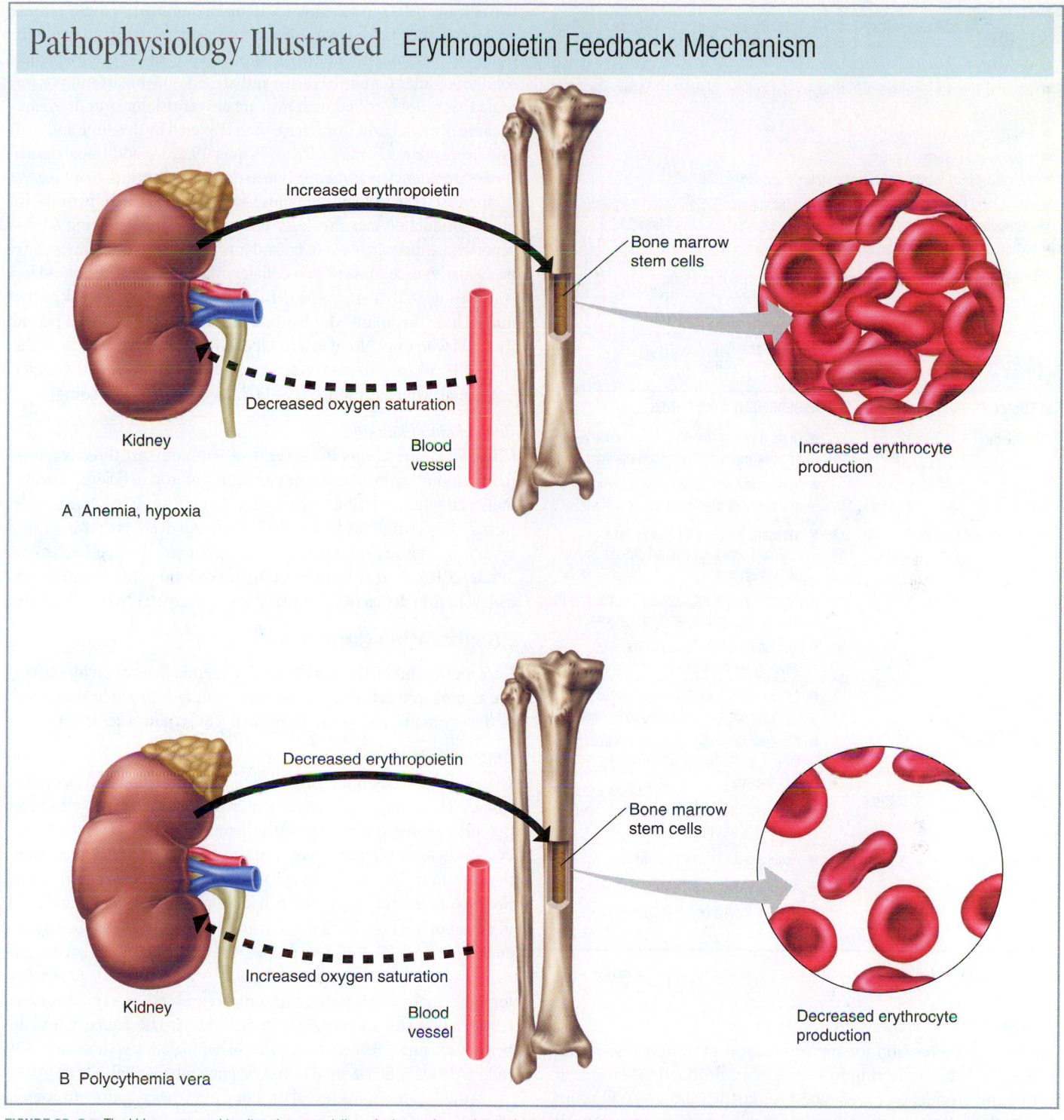

Increased erythropoietin

Bone marrow
stem cells

Kidney

Blood
vessel

Increased erythrocyte
production

A Anemia, hypoxia

Decreased oxygen saturation

Decreased erythropoietin

Bone marrow
stem cells

Kidney

Blood
vessel

Decreased erythrocyte
production

B Polycythemia vera

Increased oxygen saturation

FIGURE 28–2 ■ The kidneys respond to altered oxygen delivery by increasing or decreasing erythropoietin, which stimulates red blood cell production. *A,* As a compensatory mechanism, alterations such as anemia and hypoxia prompt the kidneys to increase erythropoietin, which in turn stimulates the bone marrow to increase red blood cell production. *B,* For conditions in which there is an excess production of red blood cells, such as in polycythemia vera, the kidneys decrease erythropoietin release, which in turn stimulates the bone marrow to decrease red blood cell production.

of tissues. In the following 8 to 12 weeks, the hemoglobin reaches its lowest level, approximately 11 g/dL. The erythropoietin production is again naturally stimulated, red blood cell production increases, and iron stores are adequate until approximately 20 weeks of age regardless of iron intake (Learner, 2011).

Iron Deficiency Anemia

Iron deficiency anemia is the most common type of anemia and the most common nutritional deficiency in children. It occurs most in children ages 6 months to 3 years and in adolescence (Becherer & White, 2010).

BOX 28–1	Laboratory Tests for the Hematologic System*

- Complete blood count
- Clotting indices—prothrombin time, thrombin time, platelets, reticulocyte count
- Fetal hemoglobin level
- Hemoglobin electrophoresis
- Iron indices—ferritin, iron, iron-binding capacity
- Red blood cell indices—mean corpuscular volume (MCV), mean corpuscular hemoglobin (MCH), mean corpuscular hemoglobin concentration (MCHC)
- White blood cell count and differential

*See Appendixes D and E 🖉 for information about these laboratory tests.

TABLE 28–3	Assessment Guidelines for the Child with a Hematologic Condition*
ASSESSMENT FOCUS	**ASSESSMENT GUIDELINES**
Family history	■ Does a family member have sickle cell anemia/trait or other blood disorder? ■ Does a family member have hemophilia or other inherited clotting alteration?
Growth and development	■ Measure height and weight on a regular basis and plot on standardized growth charts. ■ Perform nutritional assessment to see if the child is getting enough calories. ■ Assess the child for attainment of developmental milestones.
Skin	■ Assess for pallor, flushing, rashes, ecchymosis, purpura, and petechiae. ■ Observe for prolonged bleeding/clotting time, easy bruising, and frequent nosebleeds.
Joints	■ Observe for edema, pain, inflammation, and range of motion.
Additional assessments	■ Assess pain in various body parts. ■ Identify frequency of infections. ■ Assess for history of fatigue and lethargy.

Note: *Refer to Chapter 7 🖉 for the actual techniques of assessment mentioned in this table.

Etiology and Pathophysiology

The body requires iron for the production of hemoglobin. Insufficient quantities of iron limit hemoglobin production, in turn affecting the production of red blood cells. RBCs are needed to carry oxygen throughout the body, so anemia results in less oxygen reaching the cells and tissues (Becherer & White, 2010).

Iron deficiency anemia can occur secondary to blood loss, malabsorption, or poor nutritional intake. The full-term newborn receives iron stores from the mother during pregnancy; this generally provides sufficient iron for the infant for about 4 to 6 months after birth (Baker, Greer, & the Committee on Nutrition, 2010). Premature infants do not have as much time in utero; therefore, they have smaller iron stores that become depleted earlier in postnatal life. Increased iron deficit correlates with decreased gestational age (Baker et al., 2010). This is sometimes called **anemia of prematurity.** In addition, when mothers have inadequate nutritional status during pregnancy, give birth to

two or more babies in a pregnancy, or have several pregnancies in close succession, their babies may not have sufficient iron stores that last the usual 4 to 6 months after birth. Infants who do not consume adequate solid foods after 6 months of age and are fed only breast milk or formula that is not fortified with iron are also at risk for iron deficiency because neonatal iron stores have been depleted by this time and their iron needs are not being met. See Chapter 19 🖉 for additional discussion of iron deficiency anemia due to deficits in nutritional intake.

Increased physiologic demands (such as rapid growth periods) for blood production can also lead to anemia. Rapidly growing adolescents whose diets are high in fat and low in vitamins and minerals are particularly susceptible to iron deficiency anemia. Chronic blood loss is also a potential cause of iron deficiency anemia. Those at risk of anemia include the infant who has had bleeding in the neonatal period; the child who loses blood as a result of conditions such as Crohn's disease, celiac disease, or parasitic gastrointestinal illness; and the adolescent female who has **menorrhagia** (heavy menstrual bleeding).

Clinical Manifestations

Clinical manifestations and severity of symptoms are directly related to the amount of iron deficiency or degree of iron deficiency anemia. Pallor, fatigue, and irritability are characteristic findings. Nail bed deformities, growth retardation, developmental delay, tachycardia, and systolic heart murmur can occur with prolonged anemia (Becherer & White, 2010). *Pica*, or consumption of nonfood items, is also associated with iron deficiency anemia (Borgna-Pignatti & Marsella, 2008).

Collaborative Care

Care for the child with iron deficiency anemia focuses on identifying the anemia, correcting the cause, and treating with medications and/or dietary management until a normal RBC count is achieved.

Diagnostic Tests

Diagnosis is made on the basis of clinical presentation and laboratory studies. The hemoglobin, hematocrit, red blood cell count, mean corpuscular volume, mean corpuscular hemoglobin (MCH) and reticulocyte count are evaluated to confirm the diagnosis and help determine the cause of anemia (see Developing Cultural Competence: Chi). Serum iron, serum ferritin, and transferrin levels reflect iron storage and assist in a diagnosis of iron deficiency anemia (Baker et al., 2010). Microscopic analysis (Figure 28–3 ■) reveals that RBCs are microcytic (small) and hypochromic (pale) (Borgna-Pignatti & Marsella, 2008). A diet history and analysis can provide information related to food intake; see Chapter 19 🖉 for guidelines about diet history. The degree of iron deficiency anemia is related to the value of hemoglobin, with a value of 10 to 11 g/dL identified as mild iron deficiency anemia (Baker et al., 2010).

Reticulocyte counts reveal the bone marrow's response to anemia (Box 28–2). For children consuming cow milk, the stool is tested for occult blood. Iron deficiency anemia increases lead absorption (Baker et al., 2010). Serum lead levels may be tested to rule out lead poisoning in a child with anemia (Janus & Moerschel, 2010) (see Chapter 20 🖉 for a full description of lead poisoning).

Anemia is a common symptom associated with a variety of diseases, disorders, and dietary deficiencies. A review of hemoglobin and hematocrit levels, red blood cell indices, and serum ferritin levels may not be sufficient to determine the severity of the underlying problem. Additional blood tests such as total iron binding capacity (TIBC) and transferrin saturation levels are needed to confirm the diagnosis (Appendix D 🖉). If lead poisoning has occurred, removal

Developing Cultural Competence
Chi

According to traditional Chinese beliefs, a person who does not feel well is lacking in chi (inner energy) and blood. Those who follow traditional practices may be hesitant to have blood drawn for laboratory studies for fear of causing bodily weakness.

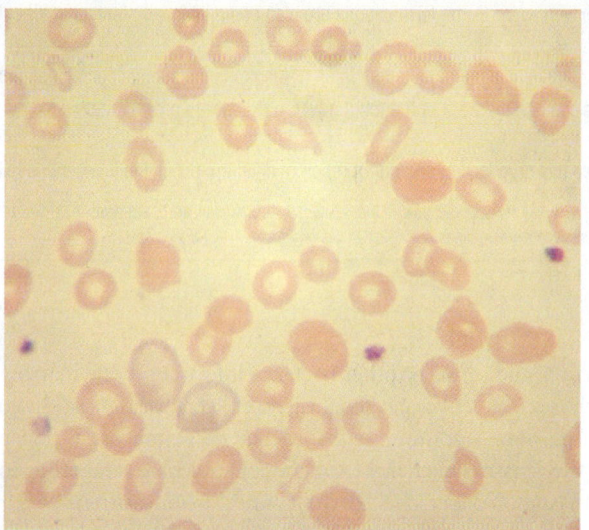

FIGURE 28–3 ■ In iron deficiency anemia, red blood cells appear hypochromic as a result of decreased hemoglobin synthesis.

Source: *Courtesy of Dr. Ed Wong, Laboratory Medicine, Children's National Medical Center, Washington, DC.*

from the source is needed. In severe cases, chelation therapy is considered (see Chapter 20 ⊘).

Clinical Therapy

Treatment involves correction of iron deficiency anemia with oral elemental iron preparations for about 4 months. Ferrous sulfate at a dose of 3 to 6 mg/kg/day for about 4 weeks is a common treatment, followed by evaluation for its effectiveness (Borgna-Pignatti & Marsella, 2008). Oral iron preparations cause several side effects, such as constipation and gastrointestinal discomfort; therefore, the child may receive iron medications (to restore blood levels of iron) while the iron content of the diet is increased above the Recommended Dietary Allowances (RDAs). Oral iron medications can then be tapered off once the child's food intake can supply the needed iron; the child is evaluated in about 6 months for recurring anemia. See Medications Used to Treat Iron Deficiency Anemia.

Nursing Management

Nursing care focuses on screening for the disorder and educating the parents and children about the causes of iron deficiency anemia, dietary management, and the importance of complying with the medication regimen.

Nursing Assessment and Diagnosis

Screening for anemia is recommended at 9 to 12 months of age and at 15 to 18 months of age for young children. During adolescence, males should be screened at routine physical examinations during peak growth spurts. Females should be screened at all routine physical examinations during adolescence (American Academy of Pediatrics,

---

BOX 28–2 Reticulocyte Counts

Reticulocytes are immature or newly released red blood cells. Elevated reticulocyte counts indicate the bone marrow is responding to anemia by releasing new RBCs into the circulation. A low reticulocyte count in the presence of anemia indicates that the bone marrow is not responding appropriately to anemia. Further testing is needed to find the cause of decreased red blood cell production.

Committee on Nutrition, 2009). A hematocrit or hemoglobin is obtained for screening. More detailed tests, such as those identified in the preceding Diagnostic Tests section, are performed if the blood test is abnormal. Children at high risk for nutritional deficiencies, such as those in low-income groups and in Women, Infants, and Children (WIC) programs, may require tests earlier. Nurses screen most children in Head Start annually. In addition, children showing signs of anemia such as low energy and pallor should be screened. Height and weight measurements are obtained at each healthcare visit, plotted on growth charts, and compared with percentiles obtained at previous visits. Slow downward trends in percentiles are of concern and require further nutritional analysis. A diet history and analysis provide information related to food intake (see Chapter 19 ⊘ for guidelines about diet analysis). Developmental screening tests should be performed to assess for developmental delays (see Chapter 8 ⊘).

Nursing diagnoses that may apply to the child with iron deficiency anemia include:

- *Nutrition, Imbalanced: Less than Body Requirements* related to dietary intake
- *Activity Intolerance* related to decreased blood oxygen-carrying capacity
- *Growth and Development, Delayed* related to decreased tissue perfusion
- *Knowledge, Readiness for Enhanced* related to management of iron deficiency anemia

NANDA-I © 2012

Planning and Implementation

The goal of nursing care is centered on educating the family on dietary management, medication therapy, and prevention.

Dietary Management

Dietary management is the preferred long-term treatment for iron deficiency anemia. Teach the child and family to plan for foods that are rich in iron. Include teaching about foods with vitamin C since this vitamin enhances absorption of iron (Borgna-Pignatti & Marsella, 2008) (Table 28–4). The infant over 6 months of age should have a diet that includes breast milk or iron-fortified formula and baby cereals with iron fortification. Avoid cow milk in the first year of life since it can cause bleeding from the gastrointestinal tract, contributing to anemia. If the older infant or toddler consumes large quantities of milk and refuses to eat solid food, restrictions on milk intake may be required. Older infants and toddlers are provided with finger foods such as thinly sliced meats. Adolescents can be encouraged to eat foods with high iron content and vitamin C, such as hamburgers with a slice of tomato. Protein is needed for blood cells, and folic acid helps to convert iron from ferritin to hemoglobin; encourage adequate amounts of these nutrients in the diet.

Medication Therapy

Oral iron preparations, usually ferrous sulfate, are given to correct anemia. Instruct the family about side effects such as black, green, or

Medications Used to Treat Iron Deficiency Anemia

MEDICATION	ACTION/INDICATION	NURSING MANAGEMENT
Ferrous sulfate	Corrects anemia caused by iron deficiency Available in a variety of doses and preparations, such as tablets, capsules, syrup, elixir, and drops	Give on an empty stomach if possible; if gastric distress occurs, give with or immediately after meals. Do not crush tablets. Do not empty capsule contents. Mix liquid preparations with water. Some formulations are also compatible with fruit juice. Check directions on the label. Do not administer with milk. Give through a straw placed on the back of the tongue with a dropper to prevent teeth staining and mask the taste. Instruct families to keep this drug locked and out of reach of children; poisoning is a serious risk.

Source: *Data from Taketomo, C. K., Hodding, J. H., & Kraus, D. M. (2011). Pediatric & neonatal dosage handbook (18th ed.). Hudson, OH; Lexi-Comp; Wilson, B. A., Shannon, M. T., & Shields, K. M. (2011). Nurse's drug guide 2011. Upper Saddle River, NJ: Pearson; Wilson, B. A., Shannon, M. T., & Shields, K. M. (2011). Intravenous drug guide 2011–2012. Upper Saddle River, NJ: Pearson.*

TABLE 28–4   Food Sources of Iron and Vitamin C

IRON-RICH FOODS	VITAMIN C–RICH FOODS
Meats, fish, poultry	Orange juice
Vegetables	Citrus fruits
Dried fruits	Strawberries
Legumes	Tomatoes
Enriched grain products	Broccoli
Whole grain cereals	Green leafy vegetables
Iron-fortified dry cereals	Potatoes
	Some dry cereals

"tarry" stools; constipation; and a foul aftertaste. Emphasize the importance of drinking fluids and eating foods high in dietary fiber to minimize constipation.

Iron overdose can occur if the treated child or others in the family ingest excessive amounts of the drug. Abdominal pain, vomiting, bloody diarrhea, shortness of breath, and shock can occur. Teach safe storage of the medication to avoid poisoning.

Evaluation

Expected outcomes of nursing care for the child with iron deficiency anemia include:

- The child's laboratory results demonstrate a normal red blood cell level.
- The family verbalizes understanding of the treatment regimen.
- The child consumes the recommended dietary intake of iron and vitamin C.
- The child is free of side effects of oral iron therapy.

Normocytic Anemia

In normocytic anemia, there is an increase in the destruction of red blood cells or decreased production of red blood cells. This type of anemia may be related to infections such as parvovirus B19, HIV infection, and sepsis or other bacterial infections; bone marrow disorders such as leukemia; renal disease, liver disease, and hypothyroidism; some autoimmune disorders; G6PD (glucose-6-phosphate dehydrogenase) deficiency (Appendix D 🔗); or several other conditions (Janus & Moerschel, 2010). Clinical manifestations of normocytic anemia are similar to those seen in iron deficiency anemia, with the possible occurrence of hepatomegaly and splenomegaly.

Collaborative Care

Microscopic examination of red blood cells confirms diagnosis. The reticulocyte count will provide information related to bone marrow function and aids in differential diagnosis (Janus & Moerschel, 2010). Treatment of normocytic anemia depends on the underlying cause. When the anemia is associated with inflammation or infection, the underlying condition is treated. When hemorrhage is the underlying cause, the source of the bleeding is identified and treated. In acute emergencies, blood products are infused to make up for some of the losses.

Nursing Management

Nursing management of normocytic anemia depends on the cause of the decreased red blood cells. Children with inflammatory or infectious diseases require careful assessment and management of medication and other treatment regimens. Administer blood products and other intravenous fluids as ordered to restore blood volume. Follow-up and home visits are conducted to assess hematocrit, hemoglobin, and dietary intake.

Sickle Cell Disease

Sickle cell disease is a hereditary **hemoglobinopathy** characterized by the partial or complete replacement of normal hemoglobin with abnormal hemoglobin S (Hb S) in red blood cells. This causes occlusion of small blood vessels, ischemia, and damage to affected organs. Sickle cell trait (carrying one gene for the disease) affects approximately 2 million Americans or 1 in 12 African Americans and 1 in 16 Hispanic Americans (American Sickle Cell Anemia Association, 2010). Individuals with sickle cell trait have one sickle cell hemoglobin gene and one normal hemoglobin gene. They are carriers of the

TABLE 28–5	Types of Sickle Cell Disease (SCD)
DISORDER	**CHARACTERISTICS**
Sickle Cell Anemia (Hb SS)	Most common type of sickle cell disease (65% of SCD cases).
	RBCs are crescent shaped.
	Homozygous condition (child has two sickle hemoglobin genes).
	Child is subject to sickle cell crises.
	Average life span is 45 years of age.
Sickle C Disease (Hb SC)	Child inherits one HbS gene and one HbC gene (25% of SCD cases).
	RBCs are C shaped.
	Anemia is generally milder than in Hb SS disease.
	Painful crises occur about 50% as often as in Hb SS disease.
	Average life span is 65 years of age.
Sickle Beta + Thalassemia Disease (Hb+Sβ) and Sickle Beta 0 Thalassemia Disease (Hb0 Sβ)	Combination of sickle cell trait and thalassemia trait. In sickle cell beta+ there is a reduced amount of hemoglobin A, and life span is near normal. In sickle cell beta 0 there is no hemoglobin A and the life span is mid-50s.

Source: *Data from Debaun, M. R., Frei-Jones, M., & Vichinsky, E. (2011). Hemoglobinopathies. In R. M. Kliegman, B. F. Stanton, J. W. St. Geme III, N. F. Schor, & R. E. Behrman, Nelson textbook of pediatrics (19th ed., pp. 1662–1677). Philadelphia, PA: Saunders Elsevier; Rees, D. C., Williams, T. N., & Gladwin, M. T. (2010). Sickle-cell disease. Lancet, 376, 2018–2031; Saunthararajah, Y., & Vichinsky, E. P. (2009). Sickle cell disease: Clinical features and management. In R. Hoffman, E. J. Benz, S. J. Shattil, B. Furie, L. E. Silberstein, P. McGlave, & H. Heslop (Eds.), Hematology: Basic principles and practice (5th ed., pp. 577–601). Philadelphia, PA: Churchill Livingstone-Elsevier.*

disease and generally do not have symptoms, although symptoms have been known to occur when the body is in extreme conditions (Natarajan, Townes, & Kutlar, 2010).

An estimated 1,000 children are born with sickle cell disease each year in the United States (Sickle Cell Disease Association of America, 2011). Characteristics of the different types of sickle cell disease are summarized in Table 28–5. Sickle cell anemia (Hb SS disease) is the most common type and will be the focus of this discussion. It affects an estimated 70,000 to 100,000 people in the United States. Sickle cell anemia occurs in about 1 of 500 African American infants and in more than 1 of every 36,000 Hispanic children born in the United States (U.S. Department of Health and Human Services, 2011).

Prognosis depends on the severity of the child's disease; children with more frequent exacerbations and hospitalizations have a poorer prognosis. Neonatal screening, early intervention, prophylactic antibiotics, and parent education have extended life spans in individuals with sickle cell disease with an average life span of 45 years for those with Hb SS disease and 65 for those with Hb SC (Gill, Lavin, & Sim, 2010). The life span of individuals with sickle cell trait is normal (Natarajan et al., 2010).

Etiology and Pathophysiology

Sickle cell anemia is an autosomal recessive disorder. If both parents have the trait, with each pregnancy the risk of having a child with the disease is 25%. (Refer to Chapter 4 🔗 for a discussion of recessive gene transmission.)

In sickle cell anemia, the hemoglobin in the red blood cell acquires an elongated crescent or sickle shape (Figure 28–4 ■). Any condition that increases the body's need for oxygen or alters the transport of

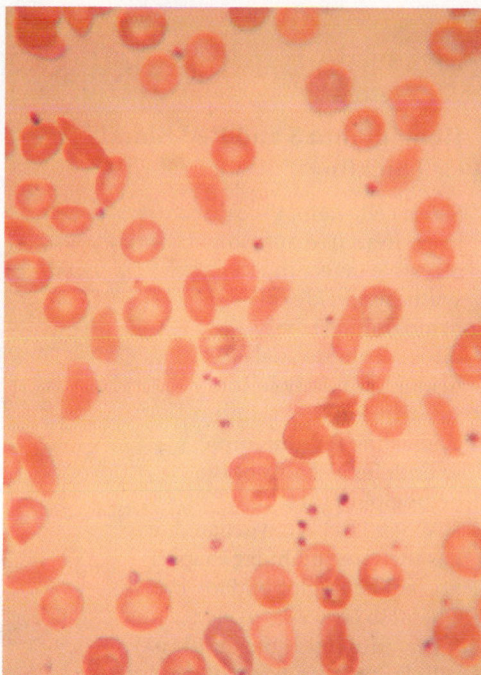

FIGURE 28–4 ■ Many of these red blood cells show an elongated crescent shape characteristic of sickle cell anemia.

Source: *Courtesy of Dr. Ed Wong, Laboratory Medicine, Children's National Medical Center, Washington, DC.*

oxygen may result in sickle cell crisis. The sickled cells are rigid and obstruct capillary blood flow. Microscopic obstructions lead to engorgement and tissue ischemia. This local tissue hypoxia causes further sickling and ultimately large infarctions. See Box 28–3 for factors that may contribute to sickling.

Sickled cells can resume a normal shape when rehydrated and reoxygenated. The membrane of these cells becomes more fragile, however, and cell life is shortened to about 10 to 20 days rather than the usual 120 days (Addis, 2010; Arnold, Alson, Asrat, et al., 2011). In response, bone marrow spaces enlarge to produce more red blood cells. Continuous formation and destruction of the child's red blood cells contributes to the severe hemolytic anemia that is characteristic of sickle cell anemia (Arnold et al., 2011). See Figure 28–5 ■ for further information.

BOX 28–3	Factors Contributing to Sickling

- Fever
- Dehydration
- Altitude
- Extremes in temperature
- Vomiting
- Emotional distress
- Fatigue
- Alcohol consumption
- Pregnancy
- Elevated hemoglobin levels
- Elevated reticulocyte counts
- Excessive exercise or physical activity
- Acidosis

Animation

Sickle Cell Disease

Pathophysiology Illustrated Sickle Cell Anemia

Hemoglobin S and Red Blood Cell Sickling

Sickle cell anemia is caused by an inherited autosomal recessive defect in Hb synthesis. Sickle cell hemoglobin (HbS) differs from normal hemoglobin only in the substitution of the amino acid valine for glutamine in both beta chains of the hemoglobin molecule.

When HbS is oxygenated, it has the same globular shape as normal hemoglobin. However, when HbS loses its oxygen, it becomes insoluble in intra-cellular fluid and crystallizes into rodlike structures. Clusters of rods form polymers (long chains) that bend the erythrocyte into the characteristic crescent shape of the sickle cell.

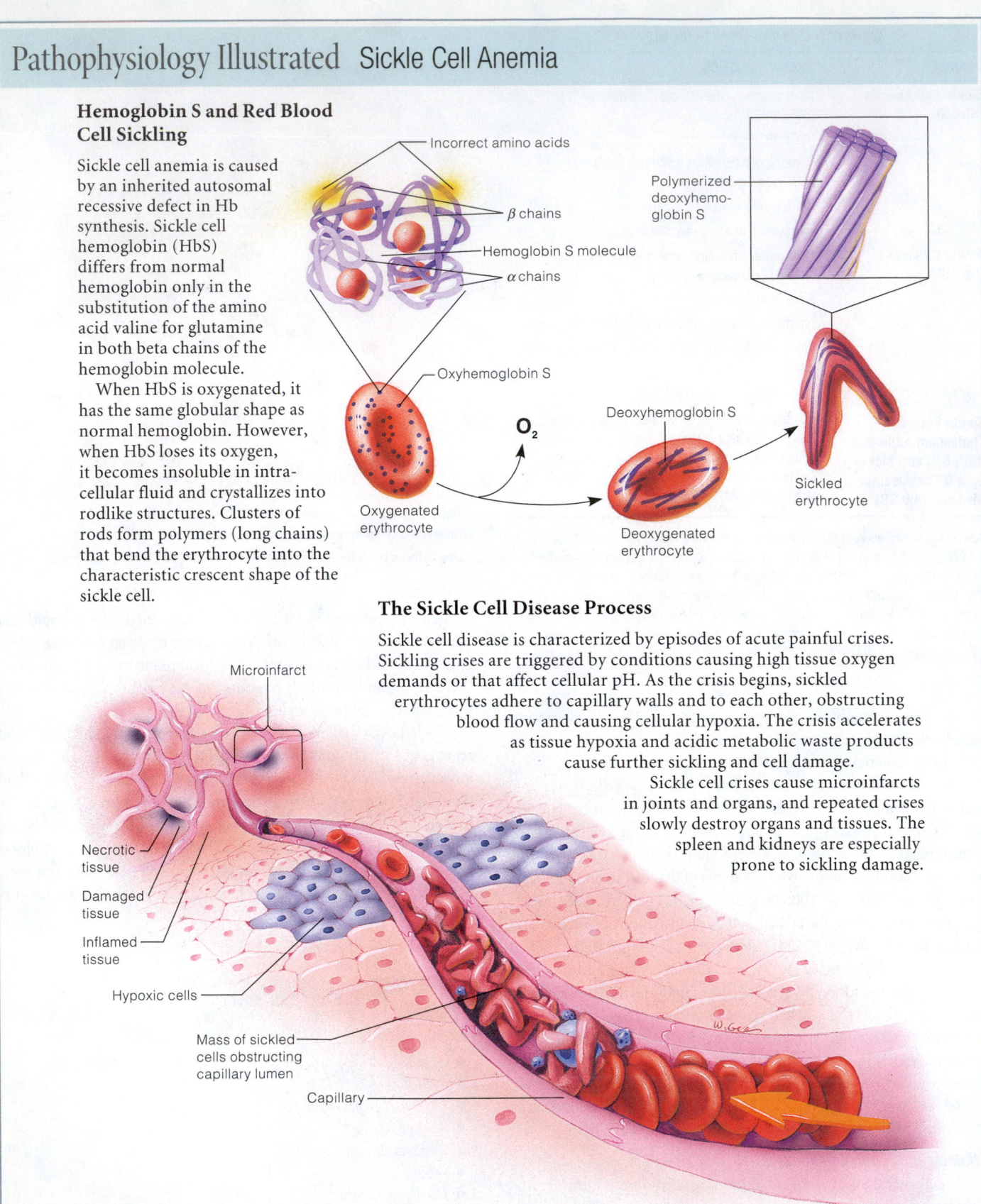

Incorrect amino acids

β chains

Hemoglobin S molecule

α chains

Polymerized deoxyhemo-globin S

Oxyhemoglobin S

O₂

Deoxyhemoglobin S

Oxygenated erythrocyte

Deoxygenated erythrocyte

Sickled erythrocyte

The Sickle Cell Disease Process

Sickle cell disease is characterized by episodes of acute painful crises. Sickling crises are triggered by conditions causing high tissue oxygen demands or that affect cellular pH. As the crisis begins, sickled erythrocytes adhere to capillary walls and to each other, obstructing blood flow and causing cellular hypoxia. The crisis accelerates as tissue hypoxia and acidic metabolic waste products cause further sickling and cell damage.

Sickle cell crises cause microinfarcts in joints and organs, and repeated crises slowly destroy organs and tissues. The spleen and kidneys are especially prone to sickling damage.

Microinfarct

Necrotic tissue

Damaged tissue

Inflamed tissue

Hypoxic cells

Mass of sickled cells obstructing capillary lumen

Capillary

FIGURE 28–5 ■ The etiology, pathophysiology, and disease process of sickle cell anemia.

Organ tissues become damaged by infarctions leading to scarring and impaired function. The spleen is the first organ affected by sickling. Most children with Hb SS disease will have functional asplenia by 5 years of age (DeBaun, Frei-Jones, & Vichinsky, 2011). Children with sickle cell anemia may suffer from splenic sequestration when blood is trapped in the spleen, a life-threatening complication. Many children must undergo splenectomy in early childhood, leading to severely compromised immunity. Infection rate is subsequently high due to impaired immunity. Bacterial infections are the leading cause of death in young children with sickle cell disease.

A cerebrovascular event or stroke occurs in some children with sickle cell disease. Approximately 11% of children experience this complication by 20 years of age (Rees, Williams, & Gladwin, 2010). Stroke can lead to neurocognitive impairment including deficits in memory and speech (Natarajan et al., 2010). Other complications of sickle cell disease may include acute chest syndrome with pulmonary infiltrate and infection, aplastic crisis or temporary cessation of bone marrow blood cell production, **priapism** or sustained and painful penile erection, and gallstone formation (Gill et al., 2010; Inati, Koussa, Taher, et al., 2008). See Table 28–6.

Clinical Manifestations

The manifestations of sickle cell disease range over nearly all of the organ systems. Pathologic changes occur in most body systems and result in multiple signs and symptoms (Figure 28–6 ■). Affected

TABLE 28–6	Complications Associated with Sickle Cell Anemia	
COMPLICATION	**CLINICAL MANIFESTATIONS**	**CLINICAL THERAPY**
Infection, sepsis, and meningitis	■ Bacterial infections are a major cause of morbidity and mortality for the child with sickle cell disease. ■ *Streptococcus pneumoniae* septicemia/meningitis is the most common cause of death during early childhood. ■ Fever in a child younger than 5 years of age with Hb SS disease often indicates a life-threatening bacterial infection.	■ Routine immunization schedule. ■ Pneumococcal vaccine. ■ Prophylactic penicillin. ■ Aggressive treatment of infection.
Limp	■ Gait abnormality. ■ Often the presenting symptom in a child, especially the preverbal child. ■ Consider septic arthritis or other bone or joint infections. ■ Consider bone infarct or osteomyelitis.	■ Depends on underlying cause. ■ Refer to orthopedic or neurologic consults.
Osteomyelitis	■ Increased incidence of infections of the bones and joints in Hb SS disease. ■ Tenderness, swelling, warmth, erythema, or other signs of infection may indicate osteomyelitis. ■ Systemic symptoms include fever, weight loss, and recurrent pain. ■ Leukocytosis and elevated erythrocyte sedimentation rate (ESR).	■ Bone biopsy or aspiration to identify organism. ■ Aggressive intravenous antibiotic therapy lasting approximately 6–8 weeks.
Acute anemia	■ Usually triggered by suppression of the bone marrow from viral or other infections, pooling of blood in the spleen or liver, or increased intravascular hemolysis. ■ Usually presents with acute onset of weakness, lethargy, pallor, breathlessness, palpitations, abdominal pain, and occasionally increased jaundice. ■ Other manifestations include tachycardia, tachypnea, pallor, jaundice, suddenly enlarged spleen/liver, S_3 gallop, and/or congestive heart failure.	■ Compare hemoglobin, hematocrit, reticulocyte count, and bilirubin with baseline values. ■ Treatment is individualized according to degree of anemia and clinical status.
Chest pain and acute chest syndrome	■ Acute chest syndrome describes new pulmonary findings on radiograph; a leading cause of death and morbidity and mortality. ■ Common causes are infarction of bones of the thoracic cage and/or acute pulmonary disease. ■ Common symptoms include pain, cough, fever, and occasional abdominal pain. ■ Signs include tachypnea and shallow respirations. ■ Lungs may be clear to auscultation, or rales may be present. ■ Palpate chest to identify swelling, warmth, and erythema, which may indicate rib and/or vertebral infarction.	■ Hematology referral. ■ Analgesics. ■ Hydration. ■ Incentive spirometry. ■ Pulse oximetry. ■ Oxygen. ■ Antibiotics. ■ Transfusion for severe anemia or hypoxemia.
Cerebrovascular accident (CVA)	■ Ischemic strokes are more common in children with Hb SS disease. ■ Transient ischemic attacks (TIAs) may occur. ■ Mortality is unusual from a first ischemic stroke; however, morbidity may be substantial with severe motor and neuropsychologic deficits. ■ Intracranial hemorrhage in sickle cell patients has a 25% mortality rate. ■ Approximately 15% of children with Hb SS disease have "silent infarcts" in which magnetic resonance imaging (MRI) is suggestive of infarction but there are no overt neurologic deficits. ■ Ischemic stroke most commonly presents with sudden onset of numbness or weakness of an arm and/or leg on one side of the body. ■ Children are most susceptible to stroke between the ages of 2 and 10 years.	■ Computed tomography (CT) scan or MRI should be performed immediately upon suspicion of CVA. ■ Rule out meningitis. ■ Neurosurgical consultation. ■ Chronic transfusions are generally prescribed.

(continued)

TABLE 28–6	Complications Associated with Sickle Cell Anemia (*continued*)	
COMPLICATION	**CLINICAL MANIFESTATIONS**	**CLINICAL THERAPY**
Transfusion therapy	■ Alloimmunization. ■ Transmission of infectious diseases such as hepatitis and HIV.	■ Phenotyping. ■ Monitor transfusion history. ■ Use sickle cell negative blood for transfusion.
Surgery and anesthesia	■ Increased risk of perioperative complications. ■ Surgical procedures that have an increased probability of ischemia or hypoxia deserve special attention (cardiothoracic surgery, techniques associated with hypotension, hypothermia, hyperventilation, and vascular surgery). ■ Laparoscopic surgery appears to lower the postoperative complications of Hb SS disease and should be used when available.	■ Evaluation by anesthesiologist. ■ Maintenance fluids at least 12 hours before surgery. ■ Transfusion if necessary. ■ Monitor pulmonary function tests and measure oxygen saturation by pulse oximetry. ■ Echocardiogram. ■ Renal and liver function. ■ Incentive spirometry preoperatively and postoperatively.
Heart disease	■ Caused by chronic anemia, pulmonary arterial occlusion leading to cor pulmonale, and myocardial damage resulting from small infarcts and iron deposition. ■ Cardiomegaly is seen in most children with Hb SS disease by the age of 5. ■ Signs and symptoms include exercise intolerance, cardiomegaly, pulmonary hypertension, and cor pulmonale after recurrent acute chest syndrome.	■ Baseline cardiac screening. ■ Treat hypertension, valvular disease, mitral valve prolapse, and cor pulmonale. ■ Limits on activity are generally set by the child.
Ocular involvement	■ Red blood sickling can occur in the microvasculature of the eye. ■ Signs may be demonstrated in the conjunctiva, uvea, retina, and optic nerve. ■ Proliferative sickle cell retinopathy may cause vitreous hemorrhage and retinal detachment with loss of vision.	■ Regular ophthalmologic evaluations starting at age 10 years. ■ Small lesions can be treated to avoid large lesions. ■ Laser therapy to obliterate aberrant vessels to prevent retinal hemorrhage and to treat detached retina.
Priapism	■ Persistent painful erection of the penis. ■ Common in Hb SS disease. ■ Can occur at any age. ■ May persist for hours, days, or even weeks. ■ Episodes often begin during sleep. ■ May be associated with dehydration, hypoventilation, and/or a full bladder. ■ Major episodes can last several days and are associated with a high risk of erectile dysfunction.	■ Males should seek medical attention if episodes exceed 3 hours in length or are recurrent. ■ Priapism should be managed by a urologist and hematologist familiar with sickle cell disease. ■ Management of prolonged episode includes hospitalization, hydration, analgesia, and often transfusions.
Avascular necrosis (AVN)	■ Avascular necrosis of the humeral and femoral heads is accompanied by varying degrees of pain and disability. ■ AVN of the humeral head is usually less disabling than femoral head AVN as the shoulder is a non-weight-bearing joint. ■ May also be seen in other bones such as the knees and spine. ■ Symptoms include acute pain in the hips, buttocks, or shoulders with motion limitation because of pain. ■ Pain is intermittent or persistent.	■ Analgesics (nonsteroidal anti-inflammatory drug or narcotic), local heat, and restriction of weight bearing. ■ Healing has been reported in children and teenagers. ■ Hip fusion or reconstruction may be required.
Liver/hyperbilirubinemia	■ Chronic hemolysis leads to icteric sclera, production of gallstones. ■ Acute attacks with pain in right upper quadrant or diffuse abdominal pain, nausea, vomiting, icteric sclera, fever, and leukocytosis. ■ Acute hepatomegaly may occur during a painful crisis. ■ Note: Hepatomegaly is present in 40–80% of patients with Hb SS disease.	■ Management is indicated by symptomology and will include intravenous fluids/NPO, analgesics, intravenous antibiotics, and transfusions. ■ Elective cholecystectomy within 6 weeks after attacks subside.
Kidney/urinary tract	■ Renal intravascular sickling is common in Hb SS disease. ■ Occurs early in life and continues throughout the patient's life. ■ Chronic renal failure may occur. ■ Renal disease is frequently asymptomatic.	■ Regular urinalysis monitoring for proteinuria and/or microscopic hematuria. ■ Urine cultures. ■ Treat urinary tract infections with vigorous antibiotic therapy.

Source: *Adapted from the Sickle Cell Advisory Committee of the Genetic Network of New York, Puerto Rico and the Virgin Islands. (2002, March). Guidelines for the treatment of people with sickle cell disease. Used with permission of the New York State Department of Health.*

Pathophysiology Illustrated Clinical Manifestations of Sickle Cell Anemia

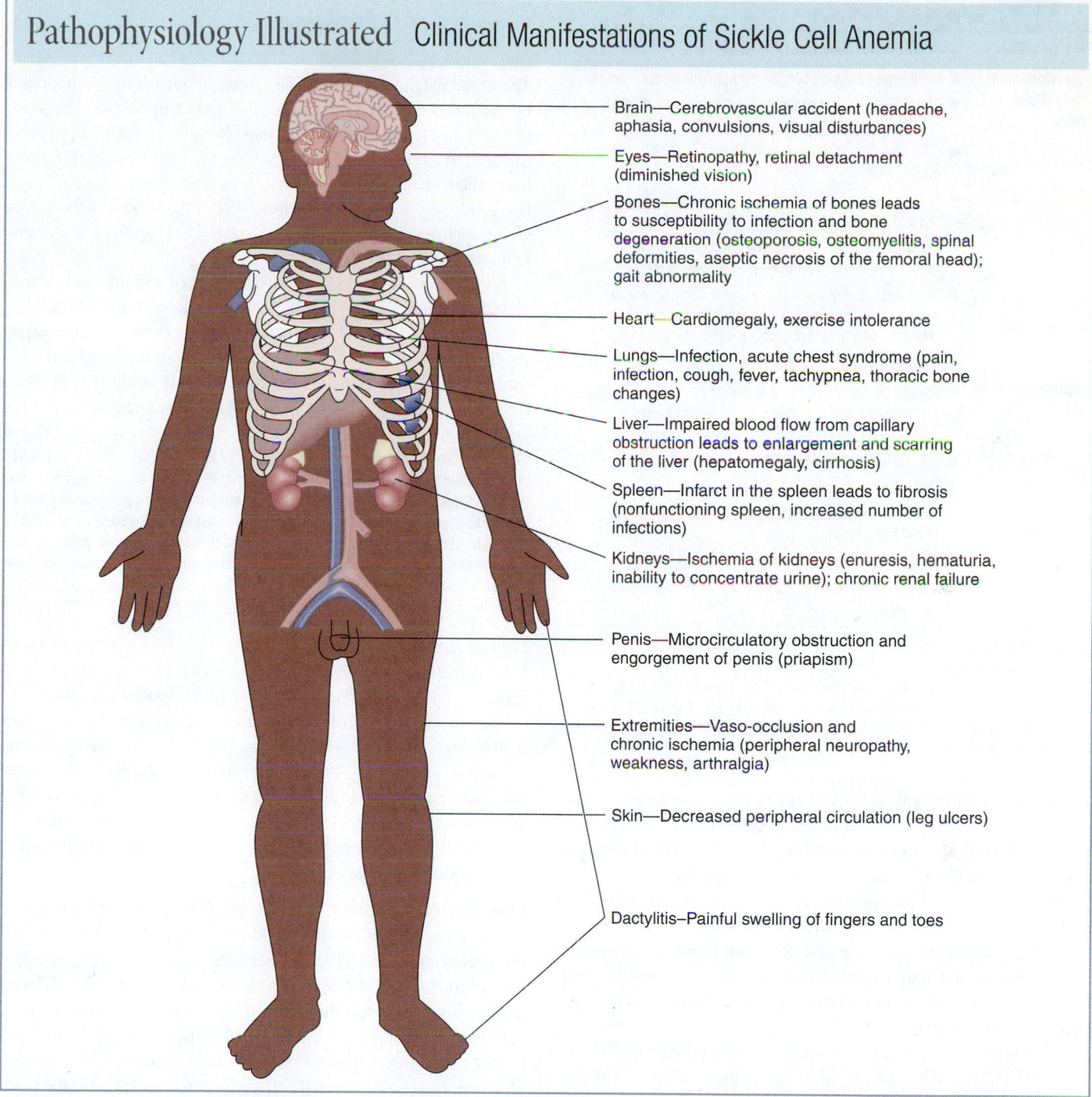

Brain—Cerebrovascular accident (headache, aphasia, convulsions, visual disturbances)

Eyes—Retinopathy, retinal detachment (diminished vision)

Bones—Chronic ischemia of bones leads to susceptibility to infection and bone degeneration (osteoporosis, osteomyelitis, spinal deformities, aseptic necrosis of the femoral head); gait abnormality

Heart—Cardiomegaly, exercise intolerance

Lungs—Infection, acute chest syndrome (pain, infection, cough, fever, tachypnea, thoracic bone changes)

Liver—Impaired blood flow from capillary obstruction leads to enlargement and scarring of the liver (hepatomegaly, cirrhosis)

Spleen—Infarct in the spleen leads to fibrosis (nonfunctioning spleen, increased number of infections)

Kidneys—Ischemia of kidneys (enuresis, hematuria, inability to concentrate urine); chronic renal failure

Penis—Microcirculatory obstruction and engorgement of penis (priapism)

Extremities—Vaso-occlusion and chronic ischemia (peripheral neuropathy, weakness, arthralgia)

Skin—Decreased peripheral circulation (leg ulcers)

Dactylitis–Painful swelling of fingers and toes

FIGURE 28–6 ■ The clinical manifestations of sickle cell anemia result from pathologic changes to structures and systems throughout the body.

children are usually asymptomatic until 4 to 6 months of age because sickling is inhibited by high levels of fetal hemoglobin. Clinical manifestations are directly related to the shortened life span of blood cells (hemolytic anemia) and tissue destruction resulting from **vaso-occlusion** (blockage of a blood vessel). Illness results from recurrent vaso-occlusive events that involve painful crises and chronic organ damage. Sickle cell crises are acute exacerbations of the disease that vary markedly in severity and frequency. Table 28–7 outlines the most common types of crises affecting children with sickle cell disease. Notice that infections, impaired respirations, neurologic

symptoms, pain, and skin changes are common manifestations of the disease. Crises in these systems may occur individually or in combination. Michael, the boy described at the beginning of this chapter, is in sickle cell crisis. Both his lungs and spleen are affected by the present crisis.

The most common reason for hospitalization of the child with sickle cell anemia is acute painful episodes (Inati et al., 2008). The sickled RBCs cause vaso-occlusion, microinfarction, and tissue ischemia. Pain results from avascular necrosis of the bone marrow and tissue ischemia. Pain is typically experienced in the back, abdomen, chest,

TABLE 28–7	Types of Sickle Cell Crises
TYPE OF CRISIS	**CHARACTERISTICS AND CLINICAL MANIFESTATIONS**
Vaso-Occlusive Crisis (Pain Crisis)	■ Most common type of crisis; may last for days or weeks. ■ Precipitated by dehydration, exposure to cold, acidosis, or localized hypoxemia. ■ Caused by stasis of blood with clumping of cells in the microcirculation, ischemia, and infarction. ■ Thrombosis and infarction of local tissue may occur if the crisis is not reversed. ■ Cerebral occlusion can result in stroke, manifested by paralysis and/or other central nervous system complications. ■ Extremely painful; symptoms include fever, tissue engorgement, painful swelling of joints in hands and feet, priapism, and severe abdominal pain.
Splenic Sequestration	■ Life-threatening crisis; death can occur within hours. ■ Caused by pooling of blood in the spleen; since the spleen can hold much of the body's blood supply, cardiovascular collapse can result. ■ Clinical manifestations include profound anemia, hypovolemia, and shock.
Aplastic Crisis	■ Diminished erythropoiesis and increased destruction of red blood cells. ■ Triggered by viral infection or depletion of folic acid. ■ Clinical manifestations include profound anemia, pallor, and fatigue.

Source: *Data from De, D. (2008). Acute nursing care and management of patients with sickle cell. British Journal of Nursing, 17(13), 818–823; Geller, A. K., & O'Connor, M. K. (2008). The sickle cell crisis: A dilemma in pain relief. Mayo Clinic Proceedings, 83(3), 320–323; Gill, V., Lavin, J., & Sim, M. (2010). Managing sickle cell disease. Nursing Made Incredibly Easy, 8(6), 24–33; Inati, A., Koussa, S., Taher, A., & Perrine, S. (2008). Sickle cell disease: New insights into pathophysiology and treatment. Pediatric Annals, 37(5), 311–321.*

and joints. Children with sickle cell anemia can also develop acute chest syndrome (ACS), a life-threatening complication of sickle cell disease. ACS is the second most common reason for hospitalization in children with sickle cell disease (Gladwin & Vinchinsky, 2008).

Pain intensity and duration varies depending on the individual and the location. Pain may be transient in a localized area, such as the wrist, or it may be severe, generalized pain that lasts for several days or weeks and may require hospitalization. The pain is often severe enough to require opioid analgesics and the use of a patient-controlled analgesic (PCA) pump.

Children with sickle cell trait rarely have sickle cell crises. However, they are at risk for splenic infarction at high altitudes. There is also an increased risk for urinary tract infections and venous thrombosis (Saunthararajah & Vichinsky, 2009).

Clinical Judgment

During the initial assessment of a 10-year-old with sickle cell anemia, the nurse notes that the child's breathing is shallow and his respiratory rate is 32 breaths per minute. The child rates the pain in his chest a 4 on a scale of 1 to 10, and he has a temperature of 100.5°F. What complication of sickle cell anemia is the nurse most concerned about based on these symptoms? What actions should the nurse initiate?

Collaborative Care

Management of sickle cell anemia is primarily supportive care aimed at the prevention and treatment of sickling episodes and management of pain. Preventing exposure to infections, preventing exposure

to cold, preventing acidosis, and maintaining normal hydration are important steps in avoiding crises.

Diagnostic Tests

The initial diagnosis of sickle cell disease in newborns is often made by testing cord blood using hemoglobin electrophoresis. The sickle turbidity test (Sickledex) may be used for quick screening purposes in children over 6 months of age, once the fetal hemoglobin levels have fallen. Hemoglobin electrophoresis is performed to verify positive Sickledex test results. Newborn screening of infants for hemoglobinopathies now occurs in most states. (See Developing Cultural Competence: Sickle Cell Disease.)

Serum blood analysis reveals the degree of anemia, with hemoglobin between 5 and 11 g/dL characteristic of sickle cell anemia (Natarajan et al., 2010). Reticulocyte values are elevated, demonstrating the marrow activity that attempts to replace destroyed and nonfunctional red cells. These values are monitored regularly to measure the response of the bone marrow and state of the anemia.

Clinical Tip

When a child with sickle cell anemia is admitted with a reticulocyte count that is lower than the child's normal level, this signifies that the marrow may not be responding appropriately. Parvovirus may be suspected (DeBaun et al., 2011). The child should be placed on isolation precautions per hospital policy to prevent spread of the disease. If parvovirus is ruled out, isolation precautions can be discontinued.

Clinical Therapy

Management focuses on pain control, hydration, oxygenation, prevention of infection, and prevention of associated complications. Treatment of crises involves aggressive hydration, oxygen, pain management, and bed rest to reduce energy expenditure. Neonatal screening, early intervention, prophylactic antibiotics, and parent education have allowed children with sickle cell disease to live into adulthood. The prognosis depends on the severity of the child's disease; children with more frequent exacerbations and hospitalization have a poorer prognosis.

Pain control, hydration, and oxygenation Parenteral analgesics, such as morphine and hydromorphone (Dilaudid), are generally administered around the clock or via patient-controlled analgesia. Pain medications should not be ordered solely on a PRN (as needed) basis, as this allows pain breakthrough and leads to an increased amount of pain medication to regain pain control (Chapter 21 🔗). In addition to parenteral opioids the child may also receive intravenous ketorolac (Toradol) or oral ibuprofen (Motrin) every 6 hours around the clock

Developing Cultural Competence
Sickle Cell Disease

Historically, sickle cell disease has been thought of as only occurring in the African American population. In recent years, the disease has been diagnosed in those of Mediterranean, South American, Arabian, and East Indian descent. All newborns should be screened for sickle cell disease as part of the newborn screening panel (March of Dimes, 2008). While African American families may be familiar with the need for screening, parents of children from other cultures may question this practice. Explain the importance of early diagnosis of sickle cell disease and reinforce the fact that heritage cannot be predicted from appearance or name alone.

Complementary Therapy   **Massage in Children with Sickle Cell Disease**

Management of pain for children with sickle cell disease is a major challenge, both for healthcare providers and families. In addition to pain medications, families might use other comfort measures to alleviate pain in these children. Massage improves circulation and joint movement, provides pain relief, and promotes relaxation (Lemanek, Ranalli, & Lukens, 2009). A study by Lemanek et al. (2009) examined the short-term effectiveness of massage in youth with sickle cell disease. Caregivers provided massage to the child in the home setting. Results of the study showed that massage over a 30-day period decreased depression, anxiety, and pain in youth with sickle cell disease. Nurses can ask families what nonpharmacologic methods they use to decrease pain in their children. Suggest massage as something parents can add to the list of interventions the family can try, and then partner with them to evaluate results. Continue to emphasize medical care while integrating the other comfort measures the family and child find helpful into nursing care plans.

Legal and Ethical Considerations
Blood Transfusions and Religious Beliefs

Jehovah's Witnesses are opposed to transfusion of blood products. Ethical issues arise when blood transfusion is the treatment of choice for childhood disease, since parents may choose not to consent to treatment. Parents have the legal power to refuse treatment for their child; however, when there is a conflict between the parents' wishes and what the healthcare team feels is best for the child, the matter should be referred to the courts to intervene in the best interests of the child. Parents should be kept informed of the intent to obtain a court order (Effa-Heap, 2009). The courts generally accept that the child's life is of the greatest importance and temporarily make the child a ward of the court to allow medical personnel to administer the needed blood product. Recent advances in transfusion alternatives have decreased the incidence of disagreement between religious and medical interventions.

BOX 28–4   Chronic Blood Transfusion

Regularly scheduled transfusions are given to children with SCD who have had a stroke as prophylaxis against recurrent stroke. Chronic blood transfusions are also indicated as a means of stroke prevention in children with SCD who have abnormal cranial Doppler ultrasound, chronic pulmonary hypertension, and refractory congestive heart failure. Simple blood transfusions every 2 to 4 weeks may be adequate to supply red blood cells to the child but at some point may result in iron overload. Other transfusion techniques are as follows:

- Rapid partial exchange transfusion removes whole blood from one arm while donor cells are transfused into the other.
- Exchange transfusion/red cell pheresis (erythrocytapheresis) is an automated RBC procedure that removes sickled cells and replaces them with normal cells (Inati et al., 2011).

as adjunctive therapy. Oral and intravenous fluid replacement also promotes pain relief since dehydration is often a cause of crisis. Fluids reduce the viscosity of the blood, so adequate hydration is essential. Oxygen is usually administered to provide comfort and decrease the incidence of pulmonary complications. See Complementary Therapy: Massage in Children with Sickle Cell Disease.

Prevention and treatment of infection To prevent life-threatening infection it is essential that the child with sickle cell disease receive recommended immunizations including the pneumococcal conjugate vaccine, Hib vaccine, and influenza vaccine (see Chapter 22 🔵). In addition, children with SCD 2 years of age and older should have the 23-valent pneumococcal vaccine (Yanni, Grosse, Yang, et al., 2009). Children 2 years of age and older with anatomic or functional asplenia should also receive the meningococcal vaccine (Centers for Disease Control and Prevention, 2011).

Penicillin prophylaxis is recommended for children from 2 months to 5 years of age to prevent a potentially life-threatening infection with the *Streptococcus pneumoniae* bacteria. The medication may be continued past 5 years of age if the child has had a splenectomy, if the child has a history of severe pneumococcal sepsis, or if the healthcare provider feels the child is still at high risk for infection caused by *S. pneumoniae* (Saunthararajah & Vichinsky, 2009).

Infection in a child with sickle cell anemia is a serious condition requiring immediate attention. When an infection is suspected, cultures (blood, urine, and throat) are obtained to identify the source of infection and the offending organism. Aggressive antibiotic therapy is implemented immediately.

Transfusion of red blood cells Some indications for red blood cell transfusion in the child with sickle cell anemia include splenic sequestration, stroke, acute chest syndrome, severe anemia, and surgery. Blood transfusions improve tissue oxygenation, reduce sickling, and temporarily reduce the percentage of Hb S (Inati, Khoriaty, & Musallam, 2011; Rees et al., 2010). Chronic transfusions may be indicated in the child with sickle cell anemia who has had a stroke (Mirre, Brousse, Berteloot, et al., 2010). See Legal and Ethical Considerations: Blood Transfusions and Religious Beliefs. See Box 28–4 for more information on chronic blood transfusions.

A complication associated with frequent transfusions is iron overload. The iron is stored in tissues and organs (**hemosiderosis**),

because the body has no way of excreting it. For this reason, an iron-chelating drug such as deferoxamine (Desferal), which binds excess iron so it can be excreted by the kidneys, is administered. An oral chelator, deferasirox (Exjade), has been used in some patients since approval by the U.S. Food and Drug Administration (FDA) in 2005 and has demonstrated similar efficacy to deferoxamine infusion (Alvarez, Rodriguez-Cortes, Robinson, et al., 2009). Deferasirox could potentially simplify treatment and improve compliance by use of once-daily oral administration for patients requiring chelation therapy. Side effects of deferasirox can be treated and generally resolve spontaneously. Examples of side effects include diarrhea, abdominal pain, nausea, vomiting, skin rash, elevated serum creatinine levels, neutropenia, and thrombocytopenia (Ault & Jones, 2009). See Box 28–5 for research on compliance with deferasirox therapy.

Another complication of multiple transfusions is the development of red blood cell alloimmunization, which occurs when the child's immune system reacts against antigens on the donated tissues (e.g., blood and stem cells) (see Chapter 27 🔵). The risk for alloimmunization in patients with sickle cell disease is related to differences between ethnic origins of the patient and the donor. To reduce the incidence of alloimmunization, many institutions perform an extended cross-match for ABO, full Rhesus, and Kell blood groups (Rees et al., 2010).

Other therapies Treatment with hydroxyurea has been helpful in adults, and is now being used more frequently in children. This cytotoxic medication improves fetal hemoglobin levels (Brawley, Cornelius, Edwards, et al., 2008). The presence of fetal hemoglobin reduces sickling and subsequently the frequency of painful crises secondary

BOX 28–5	Research: Compliance with Deferasirox Therapy

The use of once-a-day oral deferasirox (DFX) has the potential to simplify treatment of iron overload caused by chronic transfusions. Twenty-one patients ages 7 to 21 years with sickle cell anemia were enrolled in a prospective study to evaluate adherence to the DFX regimen. Intake of greater than or equal to 80% of the prescribed dose was defined as good adherence. Adherence was evaluated by pill counts, calendars, and questionnaires at regular intervals over a 12-month period. Pill counts indicated continued good adherence in only 43% of the patients because of poor bottle return at follow-up visits. Questionnaire responses indicated 71% compliance over the study period. Overreporting may have occurred through the self-report method; thus, true adherence was difficult to evaluate. Reasons for noncompliance included forgetting to take the medication and undesirable side effects associated with the medication. Adherence was better when parents were involved with medication administration and in patients 16 years of age or younger (Alvarez et al., 2009).

to vaso-occlusion. Although studies have demonstrated the effectiveness of hydroxyurea in children, the U.S. Food and Drug Administration (FDA) labeling related to indications for the use of this drug refers only to adults, necessitating off-label usage in the pediatric population (Ware & Aygun, 2009). Side effects of hydroxyurea include leukopenia, thrombocytopenia, anemia, nausea, and skin rash. It is essential that the child on hydroxyurea have frequent monitoring of lab values (Brawley et al., 2008).

Hematopoietic stem cell transplantation Hematopoietic stem cell transplantation (HSCT) is the only known cure for sickle cell anemia and has been used in children with severe complications related to the disease. Only a few hundred people with sickle cell disease have received stem cell transplant worldwide as a cure for sickle cell disease because its use is limited to those children who have a human leukocyte antigen (HLA)-compatible sibling. The survival rate for children with sickle cell disease who have been able to receive a stem cell transplant is 92% to 94% (Rees et al., 2010). (See the discussion regarding HSCT later in this chapter.)

Nursing Management

Nursing care is focused on identifying children at risk for sickle cell disease, recognizing and managing sickle cell crisis, teaching how to prevent crisis, promoting growth and development, preventing complications associated with the disease, and supporting the child and family.

Nursing Assessment and Diagnosis

The nurse with a specialty in genetics may be involved in sickle cell gene testing and counseling to identify and inform carriers and children who have the disease. Once a child is diagnosed with the disease, a comprehensive physical assessment is essential because sickle cell anemia can affect any body system.

Physiologic Assessment

In children who are known to have sickle cell anemia, obtain a detailed history from the parents or child about past crises, precipitating events, medical treatment, and home management. Measure the child's height and weight accurately and compare with past measurements, since failure to thrive is common. Ask about chronic or acute pain that the child is experiencing. Pain may occur in nearly any body part, but most commonly manifests as headache, extremity pain, or abdominal discomfort. Use a pain scale appropriate to the child's age,

and identify pain perception in each body part where pain exists (see Chapter 21 🔗). Assess the pain management protocols the family has used and what has been most successful.

The ill child with sickle cell disease should receive a careful multisystem assessment. Fever, neurologic changes such as decreased alertness or behavioral changes, and respiratory symptoms are emergency conditions that necessitate prompt treatment. When the child is in crisis, assess pain and note the presence of any signs of inflammation or infection. Carefully monitor the child for signs of shock (refer to Chapter 26 🔗).

Practice Alert

For the child who is unable to ambulate during a pain crisis, it is important to encourage the use of an incentive spirometer to prevent pulmonary complications or worsening of pulmonary disease. For the young child who may be unable to use incentive spirometry, having the child blow bubbles or a pinwheel is an effective alternative.

Psychosocial Assessment

The child with sickle cell disease experiences a chronic illness that interferes with activities of daily living. Disturbed self-concept and body image, guilt about disturbing the family routines, depression, and isolation can occur. Carry out an assessment of the child's developmental status with a concentration on friends, family support, and self-concept.

The family of a child with sickle cell disease requires a thorough psychosocial assessment. Ask if other family members have the diagnosis. If the child is newly diagnosed with the disorder, the family will need assistance to deal with feelings related to the serious, life-threatening nature of the disease. Assess parents' understanding of the disease transmission and ask whether genetic counseling has been obtained. Determine whether the family has adequate health-care coverage to pay for the child's medical expenses. Ask older children about their knowledge of the disease, and explore feelings related to the management of a chronic condition. When siblings or other family members are carriers, counseling is needed periodically during the life span so that implications for marriage and having children are understood.

Several nursing diagnoses that may apply to the child with sickle cell anemia are presented in the accompanying Nursing Care Plan. Other nursing diagnoses may include the following:

- Tissue Perfusion: Cerebral, Risk for Ineffective related to interrupted blood flow
- Growth and Development, Delayed related to effects of physical disability
- Caregiver Role Strain related to child's chronic illness
- Mobility: Physical, Impaired related to pain

NANDA-I © 2012

Planning and Implementation

The accompanying Nursing Care Plan summarizes nursing care for the child with sickle cell anemia. Nursing management for the child in crisis focuses on promoting increased tissue perfusion, promoting hydration, controlling pain, preventing infection, ensuring adequate nutrition, preventing complications related to the disease, and providing emotional support to the child and family. Refer back to Michael in the opening scenario to determine how many of the following interventions apply in his situation.

Nursing Care Plan   The Child with Sickle Cell Anemia

INTERVENTION	RATIONALE	EXPECTED OUTCOME
1. Nursing Diagnosis: Tissue Perfusion, Ineffective related to altered affinity of hemoglobin for oxygen		
NIC Priority Intervention—*Circulatory Care:* Promotion of arterial and venous circulation		**NOC Outcome**—*Tissue Perfusion:* Extent to which blood flows through the vessels of the body vasculature and maintains tissue function

GOAL: *The child will show few signs and symptoms of tissue hypoxia.*

■ Instruct the child to avoid physical exertion, emotional stress, low-oxygen environments (e.g., airplanes, high altitudes), and known sources of infection.	■ Decreased activity and exposure reduce the body's need for oxygen.	The child has no shortness of breath and shows no signs of hypoxia.
■ Administer blood transfusions as ordered.	■ Packed cells increase the number of red blood cells available to carry oxygen to tissue cells. Transfusions promote circulation.	
■ Perform several caregiving activities together when possible.	■ Grouping activities allows for optimum rest.	
■ Give oxygen as ordered.	■ A high concentration of oxygen in the alveoli increases diffusion of gas across membranes.	

GOAL: *Repeated strokes will be avoided.*

■ Administer prophylactic transfusions for the child who has had a stroke.	■ Prophylactic transfusions lower the potential for a future stroke.	The child does not suffer a stroke.

2. Nursing Diagnosis: Fluid Volume: Deficient related to inadequate fluid intake and dehydration		
NIC Priority Intervention—*Fluid Management:* Promotion of electrolyte balance and prevention of complications resulting from abnormal or undesired fluid levels		**NOC Suggested Outcome**—*Hydration:* Amount of water in the intracellular and extracellular compartments of the body

GOAL: *The child will maintain or be restored to adequate hydration.*

■ Calculate the child's daily fluid require-ments. Monitor the child's usual fluid consumption and make necessary adjust-ments. Encourage the child to take fluids, providing fluids of choice. Observe for signs of dehydration.	■ Optimizing fluid intake helps prevent dehydration which exacerbates crises.	The child shows signs of adequate hydration.
■ Record intake and output.	■ Recording enables you to monitor daily fluid intake and spacing throughout the day.	
■ Instruct the family to report fever, vomiting, diarrhea, or other signs of fluid imbalance immediately.	■ Early intervention can be effective in minimizing complications from dehydration. The child may need oral or intravenous rehydration therapy.	

3. Nursing Diagnosis: Pain, Chronic related to physical disability and clustering of sickled cells		
NIC Priority Intervention—*Pain Management:* Alleviation of pain or a reduction in pain to a level of comfort acceptable to the patient		**NOC Suggested Outcome**—*Comfort Level:* Feelings of physical and psychological ease

GOAL: *The child will verbalize that pain is controlled.*

■ Administer analgesics, such as morphine or hydromorphone (Dilaudid), as ordered. Continuous intravenous infusion is used for the duration of a painful crisis.	■ The pain of sickle cell crises is excruciating.	The child is pain-free, or pain control is significantly improved.
■ Position carefully.	■ Joints and extremities can be extremely painful.	
■ Ask the family what pain relief measures are helpful and integrate them into care for the child.	■ Complementary therapy such as holding the child, massage, warmth, distraction, and other measures may be instrumental in managing the child's pain.	

(continued)

Nursing Care Plan   The Child with Sickle Cell Anemia, *continued*

INTERVENTION	RATIONALE	EXPECTED OUTCOME
4. Nursing Diagnosis: Infection, Risk for related to chronic disease and splenic malfunction		
NIC Intervention—*Infection Control:* Minimizing the acquisition and transmission of infectious agents		**NOC Suggested Outcome**—*Risk Control:* Actions to eliminate or reduce actual, personal, and modifiable health threats
GOAL: *The child will not develop infection.*		
■ Ensure adequate nutrition by providing a high-calorie, high-protein diet. Ensure that the child's immunizations are up to date and that children less than age 5 years are receiving prophylactic antibiotics. Report any signs of infection to a physician immediately.	■ Children with a chronic illness are at greater risk of infection.	The child is free of infection.
■ Isolate the child from possible sources of infection. Instruct parents about signs of infection and encourage them to seek prompt health care.	■ Restriction of persons with infection decreases the child's contact with infectious agents. Prompt care for infection reduces the chance of sickle cell crisis.	
5. Nursing Diagnosis: Knowledge, Deficient (Child and Parent) related to lack of exposure about cause and treatment of sickle cell anemia		
NIC Intervention—*Teaching Disease Process:* Assisting the patient to understand information related to a specific disease process		**NOC Suggested Outcome**—*Knowledge:* Extent of understanding conveyed about sickle cell disease
GOAL: *The child and family will verbalize understanding of risk factors for sickle cell crises and how to minimize them.*		
■ Review the basics of sickle cell disease. Teach the child and family about signs and symptoms of crises.	■ Knowledge of the disease helps ensure adherence with treatment regimen and adherence to preventive measures.	The child and parent can verbalize precipitating events of crises.
■ Arrange for genetic counseling and testing for sickle cell trait for family members if desired.	■ Questions and concerns regarding future pregnancies can be allayed through knowledge of disease and transmission.	

NANDA-I © 2012

Promote Increased Tissue Perfusion

Administer blood transfusions and oxygen as ordered. To prevent hemolysis, the intravenous fluid used before and after a blood transfusion must be saline rather than D_5W. It is important for all health facilities to have current guidelines for transfusion protocols. Become familiar with the policies and procedures where you work. For example, two nurses should check the child's blood type and patient identification before starting the infusion (Figure 28–7 ■).

Practice Alert

Nurses should consider the following principles when administering blood and blood products:

■ Become familiar with the transfusion policies and procedures at your workplace.

■ Verify the blood type, patient number, donor number, and Rh factor with another registered nurse.

■ Check the blood for sediment, or any nonuniform or unusual characteristics.

■ Use a blood-warming coil to bring blood to room temperature as infusion of cold blood may increase sickling.

■ Assess the child's history for previous transfusion reactions.

■ Blood reactions can occur as soon as the blood transfusion begins. Administer the first 20 mL of blood slowly and observe the child carefully for a reaction.

■ Repeatedly assess the child, including vital signs, according to hospital policy.

■ Remain with the child during the first 20 minutes of the transfusion to monitor for undesirable reactions.

■ If a transfusion reaction occurs, immediately discontinue the transfusion, change the IV to normal saline, and notify the primary healthcare provider.

Refer to the Skills Manual ⊂▭⊃ for further information related to administering blood or blood products.

In small children, blood is usually infused without saline because they cannot manage the extra volume. Monitor for transfusion reactions; see the Clinical Manifestations table. Work with the child and family to avoid emotional stress. Plan with the family for trips to the healthcare facility. Any activities that increase cellular metabolism also result in tissue hypoxia. Schedule caregiving activities and play periods to allow the child the opportunity to obtain optimal rest.

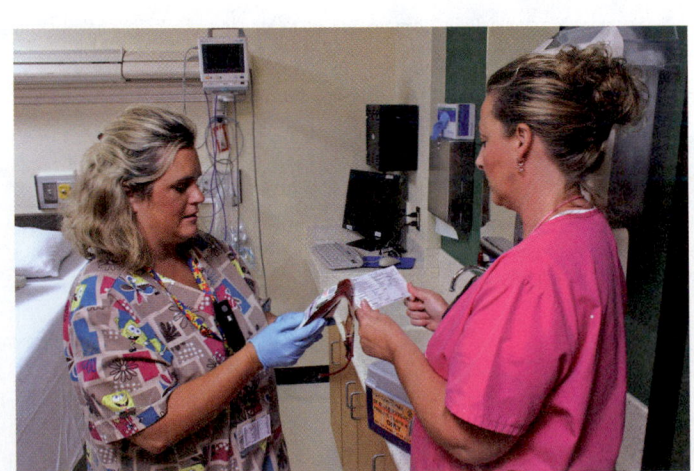

FIGURE 28–7 ■ Blood must be checked by two nurses prior to administration to verify that the child is receiving the correct blood product.

Clinical Manifestations Blood Transfusion Reactions

TYPE OF REACTION AND ETIOLOGY	CLINICAL MANIFESTATIONS	NURSING MANAGEMENT
Allergic reaction related to immune response to protein in the blood	Urticaria, itching, respiratory distress	Stop the transfusion; call the physician; administer antihistamines as ordered. Monitor vital signs; keep intravenous line open with normal saline; check urine for hematuria.
Hemolytic reaction related to mismatched blood, history of multiple transfusions, or infusion with a solution containing dextrose or other additives	Fever, chills, hematuria, headache, chest pain; can progress to shock	
Febrile or septic related to contamination of blood; may also be caused by idiopathic conditions	Chills, fever, headache, decreased blood pressure, nausea and/or vomiting, leg and back pain	Call the physician. Administer medications as ordered.
Circulatory overload related to infusion of excessive amounts of fluid or too rapid administration	Labored breathing, chest or lower back pain, productive cough with rales heard on auscultation, distended neck veins; central venous pressure may increase	Call the physician. Administer diuretics if ordered.

Promote Hydration

The child with sickle cell anemia is adversely affected by dehydration. Calculate the child's fluid maintenance requirements (minimum daily fluid intake) (see Chapter 23 🔘) and monitor the child's oral fluid intake. Administer intravenous fluids as ordered. Adjust oral intake as necessary to keep the child well hydrated.

Pain Management

Administer prescribed analgesics around the clock during crises. If patient-controlled analgesia is used, be sure that basal infusions run as ordered and that the parent or child understands the use of the button for dosing when needed (refer to Chapter 21 🔘 for additional information on chronic pain management). Help the child to assume a comfortable position. Avoid putting stress on painful joints. See Evidence-Based Practice: Sickle Cell Anemia and Pain Management.

Practice Alert

Neither hot nor cold compresses should be used for pain management in the child who has sickle cell anemia. Ischemic tissue is fragile and has reduced sensation, increasing the risk of burn injury. Cold compresses promote sickling.

Prevent Infection

Infection makes the child more susceptible to a crisis, and the crisis, in turn, increases susceptibility to infection. Teach the parents how to administer antibiotics for prophylaxis or for treatment of infection. Partner with the parents to ensure that they have the necessary resources to obtain and give daily antibiotics. Because infections can be particularly virulent and can cause death in these children, parents should be instructed to obtain immediate care when the child is ill. Emphasize the importance of immunizations. See the earlier discussion on page 915 and Chapter 22 🔘 for further information about recommended and supplemental immunizations.

Ensure Adequate Nutrition

Emphasize the importance of adequate nutrition to promote growth. Encourage the child to eat a high-protein, high-calorie diet. Stress the importance of folic acid and vitamin C supplements as prescribed. Perform regular growth measurements. If slow growth is apparent, perform 24-hour recalls and other nutritional assessments.

Prevent Complications of Crises

Observe the child for signs of increasing anemia and shock (mental status change, pallor, vital sign changes). Maintain ongoing monitoring of the child's neurologic status for evidence of altered cerebral function. Assess for an enlarged spleen by gentle palpation. Administer blood transfusions and observe the child for any adverse reaction. Assess growth and developmental milestones.

Provide Emotional Support

Sickle cell anemia is a chronic disease that is accompanied by life-threatening episodic crises. Family members often need help to deal with their feelings about the diagnosis and its implications. For example, consider the effects of sickle cell anemia on Michael (the child in the opening scenario) and his family. Referrals to support groups and contact with others with the disease can be helpful.

Collaborate care with family members and provide them with ongoing support to deal with the stress of having a child with a chronic condition. (See Partnering with Families: Home Care Considerations for the Child with Sickle Cell Anemia.) Provide resources, respite care for parents, and information as needed for siblings. Sickle cell disease and some other hematologic disorders of childhood require that parents provide ongoing monitoring and care for their children with chronic conditions. Refer to Chapter 16 🔘 for a discussion regarding transition of a child with a chronic disorder into adulthood. Refer parents to support groups such as the Sickle Cell Disease Association of America for further information.

Discharge Planning and Home Care Teaching

Partner with the family to identify and address home care needs well in advance of discharge. Provide parents with information about sickle cell disease and the child's treatment. Even parents of a child previously diagnosed with the disorder may benefit from information about the disease process and its management. Explain the basic effect of tissue hypoxia and the effects of RBC sickling on circulation. Partner with the family to explore resources in the home and community and determine if parents will be able to administer medications and fluids and to provide adequate nutrition. Assess their knowledge of signs of infection and of sickle cell crisis and when to seek medical care for the child. Refer the parents for genetic counseling, particularly if they plan to have more children. Encourage adolescents and

Weblink Sickle Cell Disease Association of America

Evidence-Based Practice | Sickle Cell Anemia and Pain Management

PROBLEM

Severe episodes of sickle cell pain crises require hospitalization for pain management. Relief of pain is the primary goal for healthcare providers and is most significant to the child experiencing pain. Research has found that children and adolescents do not always receive adequate pain relief (Jacob & Mueller, 2008). What strategies will ensure that pain levels in children with sickle cell anemia are appropriately assessed and that these children receive adequate pain relief?

EVIDENCE

Zempsky, Loiselle, McKay, et al. (2010) performed a retrospective chart review of 77 patients with sickle cell disease (SCD) who had 152 visits to the emergency department (ED) for pain and compared them to 219 patients who had 221 visits to the ED for a long bone fracture. Ages of patients ranged from 3 to 21 years. Results of the study showed that patients with SCD spent less time in the waiting room than those with fractures. Patients with SCD also had higher pain scores in the ED and were given higher doses of opiates initially than those with fractures. The time from triage in the ED to initial administration of pain medication was not statistically significant between the two groups, with patients in both groups waiting an average of over 60 minutes for administration of opiate analgesics.

Retrospective chart review of the same population identified above evaluated the relationship between pain scores and time to administration of pain medication. Triage pain scores using the visual analog scale (VAS) in the ED for patients with sickle cell disease averaged 7.7 while those for patients with long bone fractures averaged 6.7. For every point increase on the VAS for patients with fractures, the time to administration of pain medication decreased by 5.6 minutes. There was no relationship between the pain score for patients with SCD and time to administration of pain medication (Zempsky, Corsi, & McKay, 2011).

Jacob and Mueller (2008) evaluated pain experiences of 10 children with SCD who were hospitalized with a painful episode. Data from 29 hospital admissions among these 10 subjects were available for review. The sample consisted of 5 males and 5 females with an average age of 14.7 years. Sixteen of the episodes reviewed were for hospital stays of 10 days or less, while 13 were longer than 10 days. Pain intensity and pain management were examined for patients with a hospital stay less than or equal to 10 days and for those with hospital stays greater than 10 days. Pain intensity ratings and patterns of analgesic use including PCA regimens were also examined. Results of the study showed that the mean highest pain intensity score in

the ED was 9.4 while patients had pain for an average of 4.1 days at home prior to coming to the ED. High pain intensity ratings continued throughout the hospital stay. Pain intensity ratings were not significantly different between those with shorter versus longer hospital stays. Morphine delivered through a PCA pump and long-acting morphine were the most frequently used pain medications. Some patients received intermittent doses of morphine. Patients also received other medications such as ketorolac and ibuprofen. Loading doses and basal rates for morphine PCA were on the lower range of recommended doses. Intermittent push doses and lock-out parameters were within recommendations, but the study found that patients were only self-administering approximately 33% of the amount of morphine they could have.

IMPLICATIONS

Children and adolescents with sickle cell disease who present to the emergency department with a painful episode have high levels of pain. These patients may have been in pain for several days prior to coming to the hospital. They may wait for a period of time before receiving opioid pain medication. Pain regimens may not be adequate for these children. Children and adolescents who self-administer pain medication via PCA may undermedicate themselves and therefore fail to achieve adequate pain relief.

Protocols should be established to ensure that children and adolescents who present to the ED with a painful episode receive pain medication in a timely manner. Once the child is hospitalized, pain intensity should be evaluated on a regular basis and the pain regimen adjusted as needed. If the child using a PCA is not pushing the button as often as needed and the pain is not relieved, consider whether a higher dosage in the basal infusion would help pain control. For patients receiving intravenous and oral analgesics administered on an as-needed basis by the nurse, collaborate with the healthcare provider to determine if administering these medications on a scheduled basis increases pain control.

CRITICAL THINKING APPLICATION

How will you determine if the child in sickle cell crisis is obtaining adequate pain relief? (Consult Chapter 21 🔗 for ideas.) What personal beliefs of healthcare providers may influence effective pain management? How can these beliefs be addressed? If the primary healthcare provider has prescribed a subtherapeutic dosage of pain medication for a child in sickle cell crisis, what action should you take?

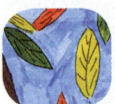

Partnering with Families

Home Care Considerations for the Child with Sickle Cell Anemia

- Follow recommended schedules for health promotion visits.
- Keep scheduled appointments with the child's hematologist.
- Be sure the child is up to date with immunizations, including hepatitis B, annual influenza, pneumococcal and meningococcal vaccines, and *Haemophilus influenzae* type b (Hib).
- Special testing, such as heart and eye examinations, may be needed periodically to check for any sequelae of the disease.
- Follow instructions for antibiotic administration.
- Assess the child's pain and give pain medication as prescribed for acute and chronic pain

- Ensure that the child gets extra fluids in hot weather, when ill, during physical activity, and during travel. Dehydration can lead to crisis.
- As the child develops, provide information about the disease and encourage self-care.
- Be sure the school personnel understand the child's diagnosis and any care required during school hours.
- Contact your healthcare provider if the child has a fever, a common illness that lasts more than a day, seizures, change in behavior, severe pain, abnormal skin color or breathing pattern, or any other symptoms of concern.
- Inform all care providers of the child's condition and need for special planning prior to surgery.

young adults in the family to receive genetic counseling and testing as well.

Partner with the family to be sure they understand the importance of monitoring for signs of dehydration, such as dry mucous

membranes, weight loss, and dark and strong-smelling urine. Provide specific instructions regarding how many ounces of liquid the child needs to drink each day. Emphasize that increased fluid intake is needed to replace the fluids lost from overheating or exposure to hot weather. Make sure both the child and family understand the triggers and precipitating factors for sickle cell crises. Encourage the avoidance of situations that cause crises. Instruct the child and parents about signs and symptoms of crises and that these signs should be reported to their healthcare provider.

When regular blood transfusions are required, the resulting iron overload is damaging to body organs. Provide the family with instructions about the treatment for iron overload. Tell parents that it is important to inform all treating physicians and dentists of the child's medical condition. Special precautions are necessary when the child undergoes surgery of any kind, as hypoxia resulting from anesthesia is a major surgical risk. The child should also wear a medical identification bracelet.

Play and social interactions that promote learning and development are important. Promote peer contact through support groups or website interactions.

Encourage older children with sickle cell anemia to participate in activities with other children between crises, but to avoid strenuous physical exertion and contact sports. Play and social interactions that promote learning and development are important. Situations such as flying at high altitudes may result in sickling. The child and family should be aware of this risk. Recommend discussing flights and travel to higher altitudes with the primary healthcare provider before any plans are made.

Care in the Community

The child may receive home care nursing for transfusion therapy or may need to travel frequently for infusions at a medical center. The nurse partners with the child and family to establish a plan of care. An individualized school health plan will need to be established. The nurse can assist the family and school with establishing this plan.

After the development of an individualized health plan, the nurse can partner with key staff members in the school to ensure that all staff members understand needed management actions. School personnel should be educated about sickle cell disease and signs of complications so that the child can receive medical attention promptly (Knight-Madden, Lewis, Tyson, et al., 2010). Contact numbers for parents should be readily available. Assist the family and school to plan an appropriate schedule of activities without overprotecting the child.

Children who have episodes of sickle cell crisis miss school for prolonged and repeated periods. In addition, if they have experienced strokes as a disease complication, they often have difficulty with speech and language and cognitive deficits (Knight-Madden et al., 2010). Teachers may have difficulty understanding why children with a blood disease are frequently absent and why they may have trouble with concepts in the classroom that they previously understood. School and other community-based nurses can provide information to teachers about sickle cell disease so that they understand the challenges faced by children with the disease.

Clinical Tip

Although an individualized education plan has been developed for the child with sickle cell disease, additional support is needed from teachers, administration, and parents to maximize educational outcomes in these children (Knight-Madden et al., 2010). The school nurse can work with teachers to teach them about the disease, its complications, and how sickle cell disease might affect school attendance and cognitive ability.

Clinical Tip

Care of the child with sickle cell disease requires a multidisciplinary team approach to maximize benefits to the child and the family. Essential team members include the hematologist, nurse (to include clinical nurse specialist/nurse practitioner, hospital nurse, clinic nurse, school nurse, and/or home health nurse), social worker, and counselor. A nurse who serves as a case manager may be in the best position to facilitate coordination of the healthcare team. Consider your role in the care of the patient and family with sickle cell anemia.

Evaluation

Expected outcomes of nursing care for the child with sickle cell anemia include the following:

- The child reports effective pain management.
- The child demonstrates adequate hydration to prevent cell sickling.
- The child displays no side effects of disease in the respiratory system, central nervous system, and body organs.
- The child has normal immune status and freedom from infection.
- The family and healthcare personnel promptly recognize and treat complications of the disease.
- The child meets normal growth and developmental milestones.
- The family demonstrates adequate knowledge of the disease and treatment regimens.

Thalassemias

The thalassemias are a group of inherited blood disorders of hemoglobin synthesis characterized by anemia that can be mild to severe. They affect one of the two pairs of polypeptide chains (alpha and beta polypeptides) in the hemoglobin chain. There are three types of beta-thalassemias (β-thalassemias). β-thalassemia major, also known as Cooley anemia, is the most common type. Alpha-thalassemias (α-thalassemias) vary from the trait to the fatal disorder α-thalassemia major, in which all four alpha-forming genes are defective.

The thalassemias occur most often in people who live in the Mediterranean basin and those who live in tropical and subtropical regions of Asia and Africa, with the prevalence in these areas ranging from 2.5% to 15% of the population (Giardina & Forget, 2009). β-thalassemia is an autosomal recessive disorder, so if both parents carry the abnormal gene, with each pregnancy there is a 25% chance of passing the disorder on to the child.

Etiology and Pathophysiology

Beta-thalassemia In β-thalassemia, defective hemoglobin is synthesized as a result of impaired production of the beta chain of hemoglobin A (Hb A). To compensate for decreased Hb A, production of Hb F (fetal hemoglobin) increases. The RBCs are fragile and are easily destroyed, shortening their life span (Figure 28–8 ■). As hemolysis increases, **hemosiderin** (iron-containing pigment accumulated from hemoglobin as the red blood cells are destroyed) is deposited in the skin, causing a bronze appearance. Chronic anemia leads to hyperplasia of the bone marrow cavity and thinning of the bone marrow cortex as the bone marrow attempts to compensate for the anemia. Pathologic fractures and skeletal deformities may occur as a result of these bone marrow changes. Splenomegaly results from hyperactivity in removing damaged RBCs and from pooling of cells.

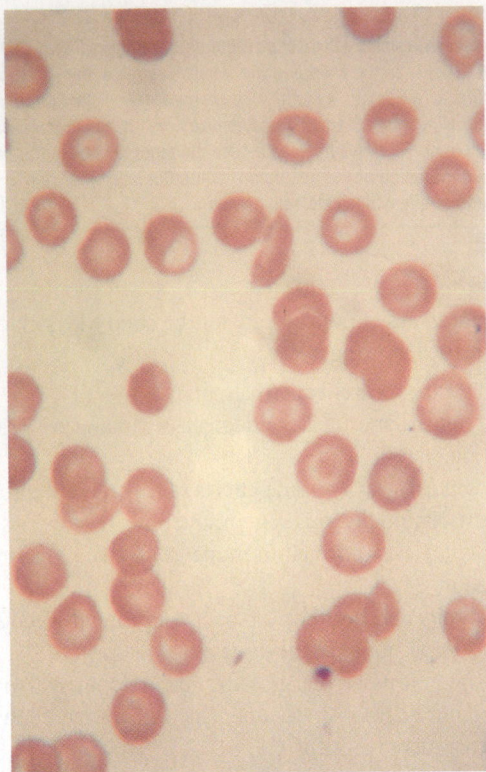

FIGURE 28–8 ■ Red blood cell appearance in β-thalassemia. What characteristic abnormalities can be seen on this microscopic view?

Source: *Courtesy of Dr. Ed Wong, Laboratory Medicine, Children's National Medical Center, Washington, DC.*

The three types of β-thalassemia are (Cunningham, 2008; Muncie & Campbell, 2009; Pinto & Pravikoff, 2011):

- β-thalassemia minor, or thalassemia trait (produces mild anemia or may be asymptomatic)

- β-thalassemia intermedia (produces moderate anemia, may require transfusions)
- β-thalassemia major (produces severe anemia, requires blood transfusions)

Long-term complications related to hemosiderosis include liver failure, endocrine complications, and heart failure. Cardiac complications are the leading cause of death in patients with thalassemia (Cunningham, 2008; Muncie & Campbell, 2009). Other causes of death include liver disease and infection. With improved treatment including adequate transfusion and chelation, individuals with severe forms of thalassemia are surviving longer. However, individuals who are not compliant with therapy or do not have access to chelation have a poor prognosis for survival past the second decade of life (Weatherall, 2010).

Alpha-thalassemia In α-thalassemia, the defect occurs on the alpha chain of adult hemoglobin. As with β-thalassemia, the severity of the disorder is dependent on the number of genes that are defective.

The four types of α-thalassemia are (DeBaun et al., 2011):

- α-thalassemia silent trait—defect in a single alpha chain–forming gene
- α-thalassemia trait—defect in two genes
- Hemoglobin H disease—defect in three genes
- α-thalassemia major—defect in all four alpha-forming genes

Clinical Manifestations

Beta-thalassemia Clinical manifestations of β-thalassemia are caused by the defective synthesis of hemoglobin, structurally impaired red blood cells, and the shortened life span of the RBCs. The infant with β-thalassemia major manifests pallor, failure to thrive, hepatosplenomegaly, and severe anemia that leads to chronic hypoxemia (Richardson, 2007). See Clinical Manifestations of β-thalassemia.

Clinical Manifestations β-Thalassemia

BODY ORGANS	CLINICAL MANIFESTATIONS	NURSING MANAGEMENT
Red Blood Cells (anemia)	Pallor Fatigue Folic Acid Deficiency	Administer blood transfusions as prescribed. Administer folic acid and increase dietary consumption of folic acid and vitamin C.
Skeletal changes	Delayed growth Frontal bossing Maxilla hyperplasia Flat nasal bridge Pathologic bone fractures	Assess growth and plot on a chart—monitor for delays in growth. Teach safety precautions to avoid fractures.
Heart	Shortness of breath Congestive heart failure Murmurs	Assess heart sounds for regularity and presence of murmur. Evaluate the child for signs of congestive heart failure (see Chapter 26 🖉).
Liver/gallbladder	Hepatomegaly Jaundice	Assess skin and sclera for presence of jaundice.
Spleen	Splenomegaly	Monitor for signs of infection.
Endocrine system	Delayed sexual maturation Symptoms of diabetes (see Chapter 32 🖉)	Assess sexual maturation using the Tanner staging.
Skin	Darkening of skin	Assess for skin changes.

Source: *Data from DeBaun, M. R., Frei-Jones, M., & Vichinsky, E. (2011). Hemoglobinopathies. In R. M. Kliegman, B. F. Stanton, J. W. St. Geme III, N. F. Schor, & R. E. Behrman,* Nelson textbook of pediatrics *(19th ed., pp. 1662–1677). Philadelphia, PA: Saunders Elsevier; Muncie, H. L., & Campbell, J. S. (2009). Alpha and beta thalassemia.* American Family Physician, 80*(4), 339–344; Pinto, S., & Pravikoff, D. (2011). Thalassemia, beta. Cinahl Information Systems.*

The liver enlarges as a result of hemosiderosis, and the spleen enlarges as a result of extramedullary hematopoiesis and increased hemolysis of red blood cells.

Alpha-thalassemia The child with a one-gene defect (alpha-thalassemia silent carrier) is generally symptom-free. The child with a two-gene defect (alpha-thalassemia trait) may have mild anemia. Manifestations of hemoglobin H disease include anemia and splenomegaly. Alpha-thalassemia major results in hydrops fetalis, intrauterine congestive heart failure, cardiomegaly, hepatomegaly, and death. Hematopoietic stem cell transplant is the only cure (DeBaun et al., 2011).

Collaborative Care

The goal of collaborative care is to maintain normal hemoglobin levels and to prevent long-term complications associated with the disorder.

Diagnostic Tests

Diagnosis is made by hemoglobin electrophoresis, which reveals a decreased production of one of the globin chains in hemoglobin and an elevated F and A hemoglobin. A complete blood count (CBC) reveals a decreased hemoglobin, hematocrit, and reticulocyte count (DeBaun et al., 2011). Thalassemia can be detected early in infancy. Characteristic erythrocyte cell changes are often recognized in infants by 6 weeks of age. Prenatal testing using chorionic villus sampling (CVS) or amniocentesis can detect or rule out thalassemia in the fetus. Additional diagnostic testing to evaluate the effects of thalassemia on organs of the body include chest radiographs to evaluate heart size; electrocardiogram and echocardiogram to assess heart function; and MRI or CT scans to evaluate the liver, gallbladder, and spleen. A liver biopsy may also be performed to evaluate liver function.

Clinical Therapy

Treatment for thalassemia is supportive. A hypertransfusion program, in which blood transfusions are administered every 2 to 4 weeks, is the conventional therapy used to treat children with severe disease. Since iron overload is a side effect of this treatment, children may be required to receive an iron-chelating drug such as deferoxamine (Desferal) or Exjade. (See previous discussion beginning on page 915.) A splenectomy may be required for the child with splenomegaly. Hematopoietic stem cell transplantation (HSCT) may be offered as an alternative therapy for children newly diagnosed with the disorder. See Box 28–6.

Nursing Management

Nursing care focuses on observing for complications of transfusion therapy, supporting the child and family in dealing with a chronic life-threatening illness, and referring the family for genetic counseling.

BOX 28–6 β-Thalassemia and Transplantation

The only cure for β-thalassemia major is allogeneic hematopoietic stem cell transplantation (HSCT) (Muncie & Campbell, 2009). (See page 932 for a description of different types of HSCT.) The number of people who can receive transplantation is limited to the availability of an HLA-matched donor. An estimated 1 out of 4 siblings is HLA identical; however, the use of cord blood stem cells and donors who are not related has increased the number of people with thalassemia who can receive a transplant (Cunningham, 2008). Overall survival rates range from 62% to 95% depending on the risk classification at the time of transplant (Giardina & Forget, 2009).

Nursing Assessment and Diagnoses

Assess for the classic manifestations, which are pallor, failure to thrive, severe anemia, skin discoloration, and hepatosplenomegaly. Assess for signs of infection including frequent evaluation of temperature. Assess for signs of congestive heart failure, including respiratory distress, fatigue, and edema (see Chapter 26).

Nursing diagnoses for the child with thalassemia may include:

- Infection, Risk for related to splenectomy or functional asplenia
- Knowledge, Deficient related to disease process and management
- Activity Intolerance related to anemia
- Body Image, Disturbed related to discoloration of skin
- Ineffective Tissue Perfusion (All Systems) related to anemia

NANDA-I © 2012

Planning and Implementation

Care for the child receiving blood transfusions as previously discussed. Teach the parents techniques for administration of deferoxamine or the regimen for oral deferasirox to prevent iron overload. See the discussion on pages 915–916.

Chronic toxicity may result from usually high doses of deferoxamine, and resulting complications include hearing loss and renal calcium loss. Blurred vision, decreased visual acuity, and night blindness may occur. Blurred vision should be immediately reported. Periodic ophthalmologic examinations are recommended. Inform the parents and child that deferoxamine discolors urine to a reddish color.

Diet is normal for age and should include folic acid and ascorbic acid (vitamin C). Iron should not be administered and foods rich in iron should be avoided.

If the child has undergone a splenectomy, the risk for infection is increased. Teach the parents and child infection control measures, including proper hand washing and aseptic technique for infusion. Long-term prophylactic antibiotics are generally prescribed.

Provide parents information about thalassemia and its treatment, and encourage them to obtain genetic counseling. The nurse provides emotional support to the child and parents and assists them in coping with a chronic life-threatening illness (see Chapters 16 and 17).

Encourage parents to take an active role in the child's treatment regimen. Partner with the parents and child to provide opportunities for physical activities, such as swimming, that do not increase the risk of fractures. Collaborate with the family and school to establish individualized health and education plans. Discuss potential body image changes with the child and provide an opportunity for the child to express concerns. The child may require referral for counseling in helping to cope with the body image changes.

Compliance with transfusion therapy often becomes an issue as children reach adolescence. Offering the adolescent a choice regarding treatment options, such as when to undergo transfusion, can help to improve compliance. Adolescents with β-thalassemia and parents of newly diagnosed children can be referred to the Thalassemia Action Group of the Cooley's Anemia Foundation.

Evaluation

Expected outcomes of nursing care for the child with thalassemia include:

- The child is free of infection.
- The family verbalizes understanding of the treatment regimen and signs of potential complications.

- The child participates in age-appropriate, safe activities.
- The child develops a positive body image.
- The child demonstrates signs of effective tissue perfusion throughout the body.

Hereditary Spherocytosis

Hereditary spherocytosis (HS) is an autosomal dominant hemolytic disorder occurring in 1 in 5,000 births in North America and Northern Europe (Tracy & Rice, 2008). The red blood cell membrane is fragile due to a defect in the protein spectrin. The red blood cell assumes a spherical doughnut shape. The blood cells are sequestered and hemolyzed in the spleen, leading to anemia in the child (Gallagher, 2010; Linker, 2008).

Clinical manifestations appear in the neonatal period or during early infancy. Severity of the anemia varies, but mild jaundice is usually evident. Aplastic crisis (discussed in the sickle cell section) is the most serious complication the child experiences. Gallstones are a complication associated with hereditary spherocytosis. Complete blood count reveals anemia, and microscopic examination reveals the abnormally shaped cells (Iolascon, Piscopo, & Boschetto, 2008).

Treatment of children with hereditary spherocytosis includes daily folic acid and red blood cell transfusions when indicated. Children with mild, uncomplicated disease may be managed without surgery (Gonzalez & Eichner, 2012). Splenectomy is indicated in children with severe disease with significant signs of anemia, growth failure, and skeletal changes (Abdullah, Zhang, Camp, et al., 2009; Gallagher, 2010; Gonzalez & Eichner, 2012). Removal of the spleen increases the risk of infection and sepsis. Infants and young children are especially at risk. Delaying the surgery until 5 to 9 years of age or at least until age 3 is recommended if possible (Gallagher, 2010). Nursing care for the child with hereditary spherocytosis is the same as care for the child with anemia.

Aplastic Anemia

Aplastic anemia is a deficiency in the number of blood cells resulting from failure of the bone marrow to produce adequate numbers of circulating blood cells. The condition may be congenital or acquired. While aplastic anemia can be related to a congenital marrow disorder, or chemical exposure, most cases are idiopathic (Audino, Blatt, Carcamo, et al., 2010).

Etiology and Pathophysiology

Congenital aplastic anemia (Fanconi anemia) is a rare autosomal recessive syndrome consisting of multiple congenital anomalies. Children with congenital aplastic anemia are at risk for developing malignancies such as acute leukemia (Freedman, 2011).

Acquired aplastic anemia in children can develop after treatment with radiation or chemotherapy or after ingestion of drugs such as chloramphenicol or antiepileptics. This type of anemia can also be a result of an infectious process such as viral hepatitis, mononucleosis, or cytomegalovirus (Hord, 2011).

Clinical Manifestations

Regardless of the etiology, manifestations vary depending on the degree of thrombocytopenia, anemia, and **neutropenia** (decreased neutrophils). The most common symptom is bleeding secondary to thrombocytopenia such as **petechiae** (small pinpoint red or purple spots on the mucous membranes or skin), **purpura** (irregular bluish purple areas of bleeding into the tissues), bloody stools, epistaxis, or retinal bleeding. Other symptoms include weakness and tachycardia. Symptoms associated with anemia include pallor, fatigue, tachycardia, and congestive heart failure. Symptoms related to neutropenia include fever and bacterial infections. Death can result from complications associated with hemorrhage, sepsis, and malignancy.

Collaborative Care

Management includes identifying the child with aplastic anemia; removing any causal agents and treating the underlying disorder or infection; preventing complications associated with neutropenia, thrombocytopenia, and anemia; and supporting the family and child with a life-threatening illness.

Diagnostic Tests

Diagnosis is made by complete blood count studies, which reveal anemia, leukopenia with marked neutropenia, thrombocytopenia, and pancytopenia. Serum iron is elevated. Bone marrow aspiration reveals yellow, fatty bone marrow instead of red bone marrow.

Clinical Therapy

For acquired aplastic anemia, determine risk factors such as exposure to a toxin or chemical, current medications, or previous viral infection, and prevent further exposure to the causal agent. Supportive treatment may include transfusions of packed cells and/or platelets.

Immunosuppressive drug therapy is effective for many children because it is believed the child's immune system is attacking the bone marrow. See Chapter 27 ⊘. Immunosuppressive agents generally include antithymocyte globulin (ATG) and cyclosporine. Tacrolimus and high-dose cyclophosphamide have also been shown to be effective immunosuppressive agents for these patients (Alsultan, Goldenberg, Kaiser, et al., 2009; Audino et al., 2010). Antibiotics are administered if infection is confirmed. The treatment of choice is HSCT from a compatible sibling or family member donor.

Nursing Management

Nursing care is similar to care provided for the child with leukemia (see Chapter 29 ⊘). Nursing actions focus on preventing bleeding, administering and monitoring blood transfusions, preventing infection, encouraging mobility as tolerated, educating the parents and child about the disorder, and providing emotional support.

The nurse partners with the child and family to assist the child with activities of daily living. Cluster patient care to conserve energy since fatigue, poor tissue oxygenation, and weakness may be experienced. Observe for complications associated with administration of blood products, including transfusion reaction and fluid overload. For the child receiving hematopoietic stem cell transplantation, refer to the section discussing HSCT later in this chapter.

Families require support in dealing with a child who has a life-threatening disease. A collaborative approach including social services, spiritual care, and other support services offers comfort and education to families with these special needs. Expected outcomes of nursing care include absence of infection, no bleeding, and parental education related to the disease and treatment.

BLEEDING DISORDERS

The body depends on a complex mechanism to ensure proper clotting of blood and to prevent prolonged bleeding. Platelets and several clotting factors are required. Platelets can be decreased (the condition known as thrombocytopenia) for several reasons:

- Injury of the bone marrow or inability to produce platelets (see the aplastic anemia discussion on page 924)
- Loss or excessive dilution of blood
- Pooling of blood in the spleen (see the description of sickle cell disease beginning on page 908)
- A variety of medical conditions such as disseminated intravascular coagulation (see page 928), hemolytic uremic syndrome (see Chapter 31 🔗), or infection
- Immune response (immune thrombocytopenic purpura; see discussion beginning on page 930)

Clotting factors are most often deficient due to genetic causes; see the discussions of hemophilia and von Willebrand disease that follow.

Hemophilia

Hemophilia refers to a group of hereditary bleeding disorders that result from a deficiency in specific clotting factors. Hemophilia A, or classic hemophilia, is caused by a deficiency of clotting factor VIII in the blood and occurs in 1 in 5,000 live male births. Hemophilia B, also known as Christmas disease, is caused by a deficiency of factor IX and occurs in 1 in 30,000 live male births (Nguyen & Takenaka, 2009). Hemophilia A accounts for 85% of persons with hemophilia, and 10% to 15% have hemophilia B (Scott & Montgomery, 2011). The severity of the disease may range from mild to severe bleeding tendencies. Hemophilia C, a deficiency in factor XI, is an autosomal recessive disease, occurring equally in males and females. The bleeding in factor XI deficiency is generally less severe than in factors VIII and IX deficiencies (Siegel, 2009). The following discussion is focused on hemophilia A and B.

Etiology and Pathophysiology

Genes for clotting factors VIII and IX are located near the terminal long arm of the X chromosome (Scott & Montgomery, 2011). Hemophilia A and B are X-linked recessive disorders, which manifest almost exclusively as affected males and carrier females. A daughter who inherits the gene from her father has a 50% chance at each pregnancy of transmitting the disorder to her sons (refer to Chapter 4 🔗 for a description of genetic transmission). However, as many as one third of the children affected by hemophilia do not have a family member with a history of a clotting disorder. In these cases, the disorder is caused by a new mutation (Scott & Montgomery, 2011).

The degree of bleeding is related to the amount of clotting factor, which is dependent upon the phase of coagulation affected and the severity of the injury (Table 28–8). Potential complications of hemophilia include internal hemorrhaging, transfusion reactions, hypovolemic shock, and death.

Clinical Manifestations

Hemophilia is manifested in different children by bleeding tendencies that range from mild to moderate or severe. Children with hemophilia often do not demonstrate symptoms until after 6 months of age as they become more mobile and incur injuries and bleeding from falls or from tooth eruption. Spontaneous bleeding, **hemarthrosis**

TABLE 28–8	Classification of Hemophilia	
SEVERITY	**FACTOR LEVEL**	**FREQUENCY OF BLEEDING EPISODES**
Mild	5–40%	Occurs with surgery or trauma
Moderate	1–5%	After trauma
Severe	Less than 1%	Spontaneous

Source: *Data from Nguyen, D. D., & Takenaka, K. (2009). Evaluation and management of hereditary hemophilia in the emergency department.* Journal of Emergency Nursing, 35(5), 437–441.

(bleeding into a joint space), and deep tissue hemorrhage occur. Affected children frequently experience bleeding into the joint spaces of the knees, ankles, and elbows (Nguyen & Takenaka, 2009). Bleeding into joint spaces or bursae causes the child to have limited motion because of pain, tenderness, and swelling. Bone changes, contractures, and disabling deformities can result from immobility and from the effects of blood in the joint structures.

Male children may have bleeding after circumcision. Other signs or symptoms include easy bruising (**ecchymosis**), nosebleeds, hematuria, spontaneous bleeding, and bleeding after tooth extraction, minor trauma, or minor surgical procedures. Subcutaneous, intramuscular hemorrhages and gastrointestinal bleeding can occur. Intracranial bleeding may also occur and has an 18% to 30% mortality rate (Nguyen & Takenaka, 2009). Females who carry the trait for hemophilia do not usually manifest symptoms of the disease. However, they may have prolonged bleeding during dental work, surgery, or trauma.

Collaborative Care

The goal of medical management is to control bleeding by replacing the missing clotting factor and to prevent complications associated with bleeding.

Diagnostic Tests

Diagnosis of affected children and carriers can be done before birth through chorionic villus sampling or amniocentesis. Genetic testing of family members is increasingly being used to identify carriers. Diagnosis can also be made on the basis of the history, physical examination, and laboratory data. Laboratory tests will show low levels of factor VIII or IX, and prolonged activated partial thromboplastin time (aPTT). Prothrombin time (PT), thrombin time (TT), fibrinogen, and platelet count are normal. See Table 28–9.

TABLE 28–9	Diagnostic Tests for Clotting Disorders
TEST*	**NORMAL VALUE**
Fibrinogen	175–400 mg/dL
Partial thromboplastin time, activated (aPTT)	22–34 seconds
Platelet count	202–367 × 10⁹/L
Prothrombin time (PT)	11–15 seconds
Thrombin time	14–16 seconds

Note: *See Appendixes D and E 🔗 for information about these diagnostic procedures and tests.

Source: *Data from Kliegman, R. M., Stanton, B. F., St. Geme, J. W., Schor, N. F., & Behrman, R. E. (2011). Nelson textbook of pediatrics (19th ed., Table 708.6). Philadelphia, PA: Elsevier Saunders; Corbett, J. V. (2008). Laboratory tests and diagnostic procedures with nursing diagnoses (7th ed.). Upper Saddle River, NJ: Pearson Prentice Hall.*

Developing Cultural Competence
Treatment of Hemophilia in Developing Countries

Many children with hemophilia in poor countries do not survive into adulthood. Some are not diagnosed and many are undertreated. While children with severe hemophilia in the United States and Europe generally receive coagulation factor three times a week to prevent bleeding into joints, children in developing countries may only receive factor replacement at the time of joint bleeding. The World Federation of Hemophilia (WFH) is working toward improving care of people with hemophilia in developing countries. This includes patient education and support and programs designed to educate healthcare professionals. The Global Alliance for Progress in hemophilia was launched by the WFH in 2003 to increase the number of individuals diagnosed and provided treatment in developing countries over a period of 10 years (Gruppo, 2010).

TABLE 28–10   **Types of Blood and Blood Products for Administration to Children with Hematologic Disorders**

TYPE OF BLOOD OR BLOOD PRODUCT	INDICATION FOR USE
Whole blood	To replace blood volume
	Generally given in hypovolemic shock
Packed red blood cells	To increase oxygen-carrying capacity in anemia and some leukemias, also given in cases of hypovolemic shock
Fresh frozen plasma	To expand blood volume
Albumin	To expand blood volume in shock and trauma
Factor VIII concentrate	To treat factor VIII deficiency (hemophilia A) and von Willebrand disease
Factor IX concentrate	To treat factor IX deficiency (hemophilia B)

Clinical Therapy

The goal of medical management is to control bleeding by replacing the missing clotting factor. Desmopressin (DDAVP), an analog of vasopressin, stimulates the release of factor VIII stored in the blood vessels, thereby increasing the percentage of available factor by approximately threefold. DDAVP is effective in some patients with mild and moderate hemophilia A (Manno & Larson, 2009).

The child with severe hemophilia may be on a prophylactic regimen of factor replacement therapy, whereas the child with mild to moderate hemophilia may only receive episodic therapy. Even with prophylaxis, the child with severe hemophilia may have a bleeding episode and need episodic treatment as well (Manco-Johnson, Abshire, Shapiro, et al., 2007). In addition to decreasing bleeding episodes, prophylaxis decreases joint damage that may result from repeated episodes of hemarthrosis (Rodriguez & Hoots, 2008). See Developing Cultural Competence: Treatment of Hemophilia in Developing Countries.

The outlook for children with hemophilia has been greatly improved by the availability of transfusion therapy. In the past, many children with factor VIII deficiency died in the first 5 years of life. Today, children with moderate or mild hemophilia can lead normal lives. See Table 28–10 for types of blood products available for infusion in hemophilia and other disorders. Additional products have recently been approved for treatment of hemophilia (see Boxes 28–7 and 28–8).

BOX 28–7   **New Products for Treatment of Hemophilia A**

Xyntha, a recombinant antihemophilic factor, is used to prevent and control bleeding episodes in hemophilia A and is produced without the use of additives such as albumin, decreasing the risk for infection after use of this product (Thompson, 2008). Kogenate FS is a version of factor VIII that was first approved in 1993 to control bleeding or prevent bleeding episodes during surgery. Recently it has been approved for use in children with severe hemophilia A to decrease the frequency of bleeding episodes and to reduce joint damage. Clinical trials demonstrated that boys who received daily doses of Kogenate FS had 6 times less joint damage and 8 times less bleeding than boys who only received the product at the time of a bleeding episode (Foster, 2008).

BOX 28–8   **Research: Gene Therapy**

Gene therapy is being explored for treatment of hemophilia. Efforts in animal models are in process. Techniques are improving that reduce the side effects without compromising effectiveness. Gene therapy offers hope for an eventual cure of hemophilia. These research approaches offer the promise of new treatment options in the future (Mátrai, Chuah, & VandenDriessche, 2010).

Nursing Management

Nursing care focuses on identifying the child with hemophilia, implementing measures to prevent or control bleeding, and collaborating with the child and family to reduce the risk of complications associated with the disorder.

Nursing Assessment and Diagnosis

Nursing assessment centers on signs and symptoms that indicate bleeding, achievement of expected growth and development stages, and the child's and family's coping strategies.

Physiologic Assessment

Obtain a complete medical history from the parents or child. In particular, inquire about previous episodes of bleeding and the occurrence of hemophilia or any other bleeding disorders in family members. The history of bleeding will vary depending on the severity of the disease. Observe for prolonged bleeding or oozing of blood. At times, children with mild disorders are diagnosed after incidents such as prolonged nosebleeds or seeping after a venipuncture.

Assess the child for any joint pain, swelling, or permanent deformity, particularly around the knees, elbows, ankles, and shoulders. Assess for pain in any body part. Note the presence of hematuria and mild flank pain. Assess skin for evidence of ecchymoses or petechiae. A neurologic assessment is conducted, as the risk for intracranial hemorrhage and bleeding can lead to peripheral neuropathies.

Psychosocial Assessment

It is difficult for families to manage care of the child with hemophilia, especially if the disease is severe. Assess the family's coping mechanisms and support systems. Determine the family's ability to manage procedures and treatments; the factor concentrates and infusion equipment are costly. Determine if the parents have respite care that enables them to take time for themselves while knowing that the child is cared for safely. Assess older children's understanding of the disease, limitations, and their adaptation to the disease.

Developmental Assessment

Because the child with hemophilia may have physical activity restrictions, physical skills may be delayed. Perform frequent

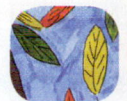

Partnering with Families

Activities and Safety

Parents of children with hemophilia may be hesitant to allow their child to participate in activities for fear of a bleeding episode. Assist the family in identifying safe activities in which the child and adolescent can participate. Encourage children with hemophilia to participate in leisure activities such as computer games, reading clubs, crafts, and social clubs such as Boy Scouts. Swimming, bicycle riding, hiking, and other noncontact sports are excellent options for the child. Knee pads, elbow pads, and helmets should always be used when participating in any physical sports. Activities important to development can be encouraged when coaches, teachers, and others know how to treat bleeding episodes.

Help the family and school to plan an appropriate schedule of activities without overprotecting the child. Children with hemophilia should not engage in contact sports such as football and hockey, which may result in injury and trauma.

---

developmental assessments, being particularly attentive to fine and gross motor skills.

The most important nursing diagnosis for the child with hemophilia is Risk for Injury related to bleeding disorder. Following are other nursing diagnoses that may apply:

- Pain, Acute or Chronic related to bleeding into the joints
- Injury, Risk for related to excessive bleeding
- Mobility, Physical, Impaired related to joint stiffness or contractures
- Knowledge, Deficient related to disease and management
- Family Processes, Interrupted related to family role shift required to care for a child with a chronic illness
- Growth and Development, Delayed related to effects of physical disability

NANDA-I © 2012

Planning and Implementation

The goals of nursing care include preventing and controlling bleeding episodes, limiting joint involvement and managing pain, and providing emotional support to the child and family. Both short-term interventions and long-term management are necessary.

Prevent and Control Bleeding Episodes

Bleeding problems are rare in infants with hemophilia. As children learn to walk and develop other motor skills, however, they often fall and suffer cuts and bruises. Emphasizing to parents the need for close supervision and a safe environment can reduce the risk of injury. Parents should encourage children to play with toys that are safe and age-appropriate. The home environment should be adapted to promote safety, such as by removing rugs that cause tripping and padding furniture with sharp edges. See Partnering with Families: Activities and Safety.

If dental surgery or tooth extraction is necessary, it is performed in a controlled environment by experienced staff. Use of a dental irrigation device is often recommended if the child has excess bleeding from gums. Advise adolescents to shave with an electric razor.

Control any superficial bleeding by applying pressure to the area for at least 15 minutes. Immobilize and elevate the affected area, and apply ice packs to promote vasoconstriction. Follow prescriptions for administration of factor replacement. Carefully monitor the child's condition for any side effects when factor replacement therapy is administered. If the child sustains a head, abdominal, or other major injury, immediate medical attention is required.

When the child is hospitalized, use nursing approaches to minimize the chance of bleeding. Ensure that the hospital environment is safe by orienting the child to the room and keeping the floor and room clear of hazards as much as possible.

Practice Alert

Take the following precautions when caring for children with bleeding disorders:

- Avoid taking temperatures rectally or giving suppositories.
- Avoid intramuscular injections unless absolutely necessary and only after factor replacement has been given. Children should receive recommended immunizations subcutaneously with firm pressure to the injection site for 5 minutes following the injection.
- Apply firm, continuous pressure to venipuncture sites 5 minutes after any venipuncture procedure.
- Do not give aspirin or aspirin-containing products.

Limit Joint Involvement and Manage Pain

During bleeding episodes, hemarthrosis is managed by the administration of factor replacement as quickly as possible, elevating and immobilizing the joint, applying ice packs, and administering analgesics for pain. Once bleeding has been controlled, range of motion exercises are performed to strengthen muscles and joints and to prevent flexion contractures. Physical therapy may be required. Because excessive weight can place an added stress on joints, encourage the child to maintain an appropriate weight. Oral (or in some situations, intravenous) opioids may be required for pain relief. Refer to nursing management of sickle cell anemia pain (earlier in this chapter) for more information.

Clinical Tip

Use the acronym RICE (Rest, Ice, Compression, Elevation) to help you remember important measures to control a bleeding episode.

Provide Emotional Support

The needs of families with children who have hemophilia are best met through a comprehensive partnership approach. Refer the parents for genetic counseling as soon as possible after diagnosis. It is important to identify family members who carry the trait, as they may have excessive bleeding during surgery.

Encourage parents to verbalize their feelings. Be understanding and sensitive to their needs. Mothers may feel guilty about having transmitted the disease to the child and may benefit from assistance in dealing with these feelings. Refer to counseling as appropriate. Partner with the family to explain the disorder and how it affects both the child and other family members. Refer the parents and child to organizations such as the National Hemophilia Foundation for further information.

Discharge Planning and Home Care Teaching

The child may be hospitalized briefly during the first manifestation of bleeding for diagnosis and management. Most care will subsequently take place in the home. Home care needs are identified and addressed well in advance of discharge. Advise parents to have the child wear a medical identification bracelet. Dentists and all other healthcare providers should be aware of the diagnosis.

Explain the cause of bleeding so both the child and parents understand the disease process. Teach the child and family how to identify internal bleeding. Signs and symptoms such as joint pain, abdominal pain, and obvious bleeding are indicators for immediate factor infusion. Make sure the child and parents know what situations could cause bleeding to occur. Teach parents to give acetaminophen for pain instead of aspirin or aspirin-containing products.

Instruct the parents and the child, when appropriate, in the preparation and administration of factor concentrate. If infusion of the missing factor is scheduled on a regular basis, bleeding episodes can be controlled or reduced. Have the parents demonstrate the procedure and make sure they can administer the product properly. As the child advances in age, he or she can assume some of the management responsibilities of care. Ensure that parents know where they can get the factor concentrate.

The child will need an individualized school health plan (see Chapter 15 ⊘). Members of the school staff should be instructed in management of emergencies. The nurse can identify key staff members in the school and teach them the actions that need to be taken.

Help the family and school to plan an appropriate schedule of activities for the child. Refer back to Partnering with Families: Activities and Safety on page 927. Explain how parents can coordinate their child's care with a number of health professionals. Provide ongoing case management, assisting the family to take on this task, if able.

Hemophilia is a debilitating disorder for the child, and it can also be financially draining for the family. Frequent outpatient visits, emergency department visits, hospital admissions, and the cost of factor concentrate can exhaust a family's resources. If indicated, referral should be made to appropriate social services (e.g., the state's maternal and child health program for children with special health-care needs) and organizations such as the National Hemophilia Foundation. Sharing experiences with other families of children with hemophilia can provide support. Investigate the availability of summer camps for children and teens with hemophilia, and provide this information to families.

Evaluation

Expected outcomes of nursing care may include the following:

- The child is free from injury that could cause bleeding.
- Normal joint mobility is maintained.
- Pain is successfully managed to a level of comfort for the child.
- Safe and timely infusions are provided as needed to treat the disease and prevent complications.
- The child demonstrates normal growth and developmental progression.
- The child demonstrates adequate knowledge of disease management, including recognition of bleeding and prompt initiation of infusions.

- Family members verbalize that they have adequate support to provide care to the child with hemophilia and to deal with the genetic implications of the disease.

Von Willebrand Disease

Von Willebrand disease is the most common hereditary bleeding disorder (Hyatt, Wang, Kerlin, et al., 2009; Robertson, Lillicrap, & James, 2008). A variety of subtypes of this disorder are classified based on the amount and functionality of the von Willebrand factor (vWF), a plasma protein and the carrier for clotting factor VIII. The most common form of the disorder is transmitted as an autosomal dominant trait, and can occur in both males and females. The gene for the disease is located on chromosome 12 (Geil, 2009).

Normally, vWF concentration increases in the area of an injury and binds to platelets to facilitate their binding to the damaged vessel wall. With von Willebrand disease, the vWF is not sufficient in quantity or is dysfunctional. Therefore, clot forming and bleeding control is impaired.

The characteristic manifestations are prolonged and excessive mucocutaneous bleeding. In children, this is generally exhibited through gingival bleeding, epistaxis, bruising, and minor wounds or lacerations. Increased bleeding also occurs during surgery and dental extractions. The disease may not be diagnosed until a surgical or dental procedure leads to excessive bleeding. Affected teenage girls may have menorrhagia (increased menstrual bleeding) (Robertson et al., 2008). Gastrointestinal bleeding may also occur. Hemarthrosis is uncommon.

Collaborative Care

Management focuses on identifying the child with von Willebrand disease, restoring clotting function, and preventing complications associated with bleeding.

Diagnosis of von Willebrand disease is made after laboratory studies reveal decreased von Willebrand factor levels, von Willebrand factor antigen levels, and factor VIII activity; reduced platelet agglutination; and prolonged or normal activated partial thromboplastin time (APTT).

Treatment is similar to that for the child with hemophilia and involves infusion of von Willebrand protein concentrate. Desmopressin (DDAVP) is administered to promote release of stored vWF and to prevent bleeding associated with dental or surgical procedures (Thiagarajan, 2011).

Nursing Management

Nursing care is the same as for a child with hemophilia (refer to previous discussion). Teach parents about the disorder and instruct them not to give the child aspirin or other drugs that can cause bleeding or inhibit platelet function. Teach management of bleeding episodes and intravenous infusion techniques, which are the same as for hemophilia. The prognosis is good, and children with von Willebrand disease usually have a normal life expectancy. Expected outcomes of nursing care include prompt management of bleeding and prevention of disease complications.

Disseminated Intravascular Coagulation

Disseminated intravascular coagulation (DIC) is a life-threatening disease which occurs as a complication of other serious illnesses in infants and children.

Weblink National Hemophilia Foundation

Etiology and Pathophysiology

DIC is an acquired pathologic process in which the clotting system is abnormally activated, resulting in widespread clot formation in the small vessels throughout the body. The most common cause of DIC is sepsis. Infections caused by gram-negative and gram-positive bacteria, fungi, viruses, and protozoa may lead to DIC (LeMone, Burke, & Bauldoff, 2011).

The disorder results from increased protease activity which is caused by unregulated release of thrombin. Excess thrombin is generated, followed by deposition of fibrin strands in body tissues (Kumar & Gupta, 2008). Excess thrombin interferes with natural anticoagulants and leads to unrestricted clotting. The circulating fibrin fragments later begin to interfere with platelet aggregation and other aspects of the clotting mechanism, resulting in bleeding or hemorrhage (LeMone et al., 2011). The disease process commonly interferes with function in the pulmonary, renal, hepatic, and central nervous systems (Kumar & Gupta, 2008).

Clinical Manifestations

The clinical manifestations of DIC result from bleeding and clotting disorders. The manifestations range from minor oozing to hemorrhage (see the Clinical Manifestations table).

Collaborative Care

Treatment of DIC focuses on controlling bleeding, identifying and correcting the primary cause of the disorder, and preventing further activation of clotting mechanisms.

Diagnostic Tests

The prothrombin time, thrombin time, and activated partial thromboplastin time are prolonged; fibrin and/or fibrinogen degradation products are high; and platelet count and fibrinogen levels are decreased (Buckley & Pravikoff, 2010; Kumar & Gupta, 2008).

Clinical Therapy

Management is supportive and includes identification and treatment of the underlying disorder; replacement of depleted coagulation factors, fibrinogen, and platelets; and anticoagulant therapy (heparin).

Nursing Management

DIC is a complex disorder that is managed by a critical care team. Nursing care focuses on assessing for bleeding, preventing further injury, and administering prescribed therapies while treating the underlying disorder.

Clinical Manifestations   Disseminated Intravascular Coagulation

ETIOLOGY	CLINICAL MANIFESTATIONS	NURSING MANAGEMENT
Cardiovascular System		
Decreased perfusion, shock	Tachycardia Weakness, malaise Hypotension Circulatory collapse Major vessel thrombosis	Administer fluids as ordered; monitor intake and output. Monitor vital signs. Cluster care to allow for rest periods. Maintain bed rest.
Respiratory System		
Impaired gas exchange due to microclots in the pulmonary vasculature	Tachypnea Decreased breath sounds	Monitor respiratory status. Maintain ventilatory support if required.
Central Nervous System		
Impaired cerebral perfusion	Confusion Coma Seizures	Conduct neurologic assessment every 2 hours during critical period, then every 4 hours until stabilized.
Urinary System		
Impaired renal perfusion Impaired clotting mechanisms, leading to bleeding	Oliguria Anuria Renal failure Hematuria	Monitor urine output hourly. Maintain patent urinary catheter. Monitor urine for blood.
Gastrointestinal System		
Impaired clotting mechanisms, leading to bleeding	Gastrointestinal bleeding Occult blood in stool or emesis Abdominal distention Bleeding from mucous membranes	Monitor for occult blood in stools and emesis. Monitor for overt signs of bleeding from gums. Provide oral care. Measure abdominal girth every 4 hours.
Integumentary System		
Impaired clotting mechanism, leading to bleeding Impaired tissue perfusion	Petechiae Purpura Ecchymosis Bleeding or oozing from wounds, intravenous access site, or body orifices Pallor Cool extremities Cyanosis of extremities Gangrene	Monitor skin for evidence of bleeding. Protect from injury. Monitor distal pulses, temperature, and capillary refill.

Nursing Assessment and Diagnosis

Because all body systems can be involved, careful assessment of all systems is needed on a continual basis. Assess extremities for capillary refill, warmth, and pulses. Frequently assess vital signs and level of consciousness. Observe for petechiae, ecchymoses, and all body orifices and skin breaks for oozing blood every 1 to 2 hours. Careful monitoring of dependent areas is essential, as blood will pool in these locations. Intravenous sites are particularly prone to oozing and should be assessed every 15 minutes. Examine stool for the presence of blood, and measure blood loss as accurately as possible. Assess intake and output. Monitor urine for the presence of blood. Blood urea nitrogen (BUN) and creatinine are monitored to assess renal function.

Nursing diagnoses for the child with disseminated intravascular coagulation may include:

- Tissue Perfusion: Ineffective related to decreased circulating blood volume
- Gas Exchange, Impaired related to decreased perfusion of the lungs
- Skin Integrity, Impaired related to bleeding
- Fear (Parental) related to critically ill child

NANDA-I © 2012

Planning and Implementation

The child with DIC requires critical care nursing. Institute bleeding control precautions and administer replacement therapy of blood products as prescribed. Monitor vital signs frequently and report any signs of complications. Monitor for signs of hypovolemic shock.

Monitor oxygen saturation and arterial blood gases. The child may require mechanical ventilation. Maintain patency of the airway and implement safety measures to preserve endotracheal tube position.

Implement measures to maintain skin integrity, such as gentle and frequent repositioning. Identify the family's coping strategies and support systems to facilitate their ability to manage this life-threatening crisis.

Evaluation

Expected outcomes of nursing care for the child with DIC may include:

- The child regains adequate perfusion of all body systems.
- The child regains adequate gas exchange.
- The child maintains intact skin integrity.
- Family members verbalize that they have adequate support to effectively cope with the child's life-threatening illness.

Immune Thrombocytopenic Purpura

Immune thrombocytopenic purpura (ITP), also known as idiopathic thrombocytopenic purpura, is a bleeding disorder characterized by increased destruction of platelets in the spleen, even though platelet production in the bone marrow is normal. Platelets are destroyed as a result of the binding of autoantibodies to platelet antigens (Hunt, 2010). When the rate of platelet destruction exceeds the rate of platelet production, the number of circulating platelets decreases and blood clotting slows. ITP occurs annually in 4 to 5 per 100,000 children (Vranou, Platokouki, Pergantou, et al., 2008).

The cause of ITP is unknown, but it usually follows an infectious illness. It is seen as an uncommon complication in 1 in 25,000 children after the measles-mumps-rubella vaccination (Blanchette & Bolton-Maggs, 2008).

Symptoms include multiple ecchymoses and petechiae. Mucosal bleeding such as in the mouth or nose is a common presentation. The child has typically been well, has a history of recent viral illness, and then develops onset of bruising and bleeding that concerns parents (Blanchette & Bolton-Maggs, 2008).

Collaborative Care

Management of idiopathic thrombocytopenic purpura focuses on identifying the disorder, preventing bleeding and associated complications, and restoring platelet count.

Diagnosis is made by history and through physical and laboratory findings, which reveal a decreased platelet count (generally less than 20,000 mm³/dL) (Diz-Kucukkaya, Chen, Geddis, et al., 2010). The child has normal hemoglobin and white blood cell counts. A bone marrow aspiration may be performed to rule out other diagnoses (Barrows & Kraj, 2010).

Patients with a platelet count greater than 10,000 and little bleeding may be carefully observed without the need for additional treatment (Segel & Feig, 2009). Families need instructions to identify bleeding, especially intracranial, and to seek care immediately. Children must avoid contact sports until platelet counts return to normal. Intracranial hemorrhage in children with ITP is rare, occurring in only 0.1% to 1% of affected children (Diz-Kucukkaya, Chen, Geddis, et al., 2010). This complication, however, is very serious and accounts for most deaths related to ITP (Choudhary, Naithani, Mahapatra, et al., 2009).

The modalities of treatment for ITP vary among healthcare providers, but may include corticosteroids, intravenous immune globulin (IVIG), and intravenous anti-D immunoglobulin (Blanchette & Bolton-Maggs, 2008; Son, Jeon, Yang, et al., 2008). Platelet administration is not usually indicated unless bleeding is life threatening (Segel & Feig, 2009). With ITP, platelet administration will control bleeding temporarily, since the administered platelets will be destroyed.

It is estimated that 20% to 25% of patients with ITP will develop chronic disease (Blanchette & Bolton-Maggs, 2008). Children who fail to respond to treatment for acute ITP and persist with thrombocytopenia for longer than 8 to 12 months are considered to have chronic ITP (Segel & Feig, 2009). Splenectomy may be an option for children with persistent or chronic disease, significant bleeding, lack of response to drug therapy, or altered quality of life (Neunert, 2011).

Nursing Management

Nursing care focuses on controlling and reducing the number of bleeding episodes. Assess vital signs and level of consciousness. Assess for evidence of bleeding, including petechiae and ecchymosis. The abdomen is assessed for hepatosplenomegaly. Monitor for nosebleeds, oozing at intravenous sites, gastrointestinal bleeding, and indications of intracranial bleeding. Signs of intracranial bleeding include changes in the level of consciousness, vomiting, and seizures; refer to page 1153 for clinical manifestations.

Measures to prevent bleeding are similar to those for the child with hemophilia. Teach parents to use acetaminophen to manage pain and fever, rather than aspirin or other drugs that influence bleeding times. The child should avoid contact sports and other activities that may increase risk of injury. Ensure that the family and child are aware of the signs and symptoms indicating bleeding, including signs of intracranial bleeding. Expected outcomes of nursing care are prevention of bleeding and restoration of normal coagulation patterns with no serious sequelae.

Henoch-Schönlein Purpura

Henoch-Schönlein purpura (HSP) is described as a **vasculitis** (inflammation of the blood vessels) of the small vessels. It is the most common vasculitis in children, affecting approximately 14 children per 100,000 each year (Lee, Bearie, & Lee, 2009). The disease predominates in childhood with a peak incidence of 5 to 6 years of age (Barillas-Arias, Adams, & Lehman, 2008; Reamy, Williams, & Lindsay, 2009). Most of the children affected are under 10 years of age. HSP is twice as common in males as it is in females (Lee et al., 2009).

The cause of HSP is unknown; however, IgA is known to play a role in the development of the illness which generally follows an upper respiratory infection. Other precipitating factors include immunizations, insect bites, foods, and some medications (Barillas-Arias et al., 2008).

The child with HSP typically presents with slightly raised purpuric lesions (palpable purpura, Figure 28–9 ■), arthralgias (joint pain), and colicky abdominal pain. The purpuric lesions commonly appear first on the buttocks, elbows, and legs and do not disappear when pressure is applied (Penny, Fleming, Kazmierczak, et al., 2010). Other symptoms may include bloody stools, hematuria, proteinuria, fever, malaise, vomiting, and headache (Barillas-Arias et al., 2008; Lee et al., 2009; Penny et al., 2010; Treadwell, 2008). HSP is generally a self-limiting disease. Recurrence is seen in approximately 35% of patients. The severity of the renal involvement is the primary prognostic factor and is seen in 20% to 30% of patients (Barillas-Arias et al., 2008). HSP leads to end-stage renal disease in 1% to 5% of children affected (Lee et al., 2009).

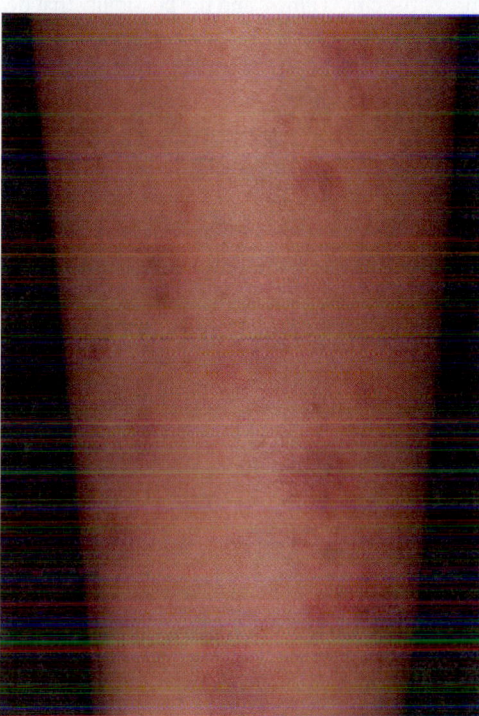

FIGURE 28–9 ■ There are elevated areas of purpura (palpable purpura) on the legs of this patient with Henoch-Schönlein purpura (HSP).

Source: *Courtesy of Daniel P. Krowchuk, MD, Professor of Pediatrics and Dermatology, Department of Pediatrics, Wake Forest School of Medicine, Winston-Salem, NC.*

Collaborative Care

There is no specific laboratory test to confirm the diagnosis. The triad of symptoms described above leads to suspicion of HSP. Tests should be performed to rule out other causes of the child's presenting symptoms and include evaluation of the platelet count, coagulation studies, metabolic panel, complete blood count, erythrocyte sedimentation rate, and C-reactive protein (Barillas-Arias et al., 2008; Dixson, 2010). Imaging studies and surgical consultation may be needed to rule out other causes of the abdominal pain (Barillas-Arias et al., 2010).

Management of HSP is primarily supportive and focuses on controlling gastrointestinal symptoms, joint pain, and renal involvement. Specific management includes hydration, bed rest, and analgesia. The child is also monitored for gastrointestinal and renal complications (Penny et al., 2010). Corticosteroids have been used successfully in controlling both gastrointestinal and joint pain. They are helpful in managing the severity of the nephritis, but not in preventing its development (Barillas-Arias et al., 2008).

Nursing Management

Nursing care for the child with HSP is centered on management of the presenting symptoms. The nurse assesses the child's skin for changes in the purpuric lesions. Careful abdominal assessment is necessary to detect increased abdominal pain and distention that might be associated with gastrointestinal hemorrhage or nephritis. Assess the joints for swelling. Management of joint pain is an essential aspect of care and promotes comfort and tolerance of symptoms. Stools should be evaluated for occult blood. Evaluation of urinary output is essential in monitoring the child's renal function. Test urine for the presence of blood and protein. The child should have daily weights and careful assessment for the development of edema associated with renal involvement. Monitor the child's blood pressure for hypertension (Penny et al., 2010). A full multisystem assessment aids in detection of complications related to hemorrhage in body systems. Any abnormalities should be reported to the physician.

Teaching related to corticosteroid therapy is essential. If the child is being discharged on steroids or is being managed at home (in mild cases), the family must understand the dosage schedule and the side effects of this medication (see Chapter 31 ⊘). HSP generally is self-limiting, but the nurse should be diligent not only in monitoring the child for progression of the disease but in supporting the family during the illness (Penny et al., 2010).

Meningococcemia

Meningococcemia is a virulent disease process that develops in some individuals infected with *Neisseria meningitidis* (see Chapter 22 ⊘ for further discussion on meningococcal disease). Meningococcemia occurs primarily in young children and has a mortality rate of approximately 8% to 10%, with another 11% to 19% suffering sequelae such as limb amputation and hearing loss (Charnock & Sutter, 2008).

Etiology and Pathophysiology

N. meningitidis is a gram-negative bacteria that is transmitted primarily via the respiratory route (Granoff & Gilsdorf, 2011). In meningococcemia, the bacteria are located primarily in the systemic circulation. This gram-negative sepsis leads to clinical shock. The bacteria multiply and release an endotoxin (lipopolysaccharide). This endotoxin triggers other events such as altered immune response, DIC, and circulatory collapse. Endotoxins from the bacteria are thought to impair protein C, which causes thrombosis formation. The virulence of meningococcal disease is 50 to 100 times that of other gram-negative infections (Milonovich, 2007).

Clinical Manifestations

Onset of manifestations is sudden. Often, a respiratory infection is followed by fever, myalgias, weakness, headache, diarrhea, and vomiting. The petechial rash characteristic of this disease may develop before other serious symptoms and progresses rapidly (Granoff & Gilsdorf, 2011; Milonovich, 2007). The child's condition may deteriorate rapidly within a few hours. The clotting cascade is initiated, resulting in bleeding and thrombosis in the tissues (Milonovich, 2007). The child is critically ill and demonstrates multisystem disease. Frequently the skin is pink and then black as the tissues are damaged from reduced oxygen delivery.

Collaborative Care

Care is focused on identifying the disease without delay in order to improve outcome. The mortality rate for meningococcemia is high, particularly when there is a delay in treatment.

Diagnostic Tests

Blood cultures reveal *N. meningitidis*, a gram-negative organism. The organism may also be found in cerebrospinal fluid and synovial fluid (Granoff & Gilsdorf, 2011).

Clinical Therapy

Isolation is implemented per hospital protocol to prevent spread of infection. Treatment consists of antibiotics such as penicillin G, ceftriaxone, or cefotaxime; removal from sources of infection; and multisystem shock management (McGrath, Petropolis, & West, 2010; Milonovich, 2007). (See Chapter 26 ✏ for a description of distributive shock.) Prompt administration of antibiotics to the child who manifests fever with purpura can decrease the severity of outcome. Fluid volume replacement is essential to support blood pressure and correct hypovolemic shock. For the child in septic shock (see Chapter 22 ✏), an arterial catheter is inserted for constant monitoring of blood pressure, and a pulmonary artery catheter may be considered to monitor fluid volume status. Inotropic agents are administered for hypotension and to decrease vascular resistance in vital organs (Milonovich, 2007).

Depending on the child's condition, total parenteral nutrition, sedation and pain relief, dialysis, or amputation may be required. See the previous discussion for management of DIC. Close contacts of the child should receive prophylaxis with rifampin every 12 hours for 2 days. Individuals over 17 may receive a single dose of ceftriaxone or ciprofloxacin (Milonovich, 2007). Antibiotics should be started as soon as possible. The individual should be monitored closely for fever or other signs and symptoms of developing infection.

Nursing Management

Nursing care of the child with meningococcemia is complex. Treatment must begin quickly, and the child generally has a lengthy hospitalization in a pediatric intensive care unit followed by years of care that may involve plastic surgery or prosthetic adaptation.

Nursing Assessment and Diagnosis

Thorough assessments of all body systems are performed. Ongoing assessment of vital signs is essential. Continually assess for changes in level of consciousness. Urinary output is measured to evaluate renal function. Assess for alterations in tissue perfusion by noting cold extremities and circumoral cyanosis. Assess oxygen saturation levels and arterial blood gas values as performed. Assess for indications of seizure activity.

Appropriate diagnoses for the child with meningococcemia may include:

- Tissue Perfusion, Ineffective (All Systems) related to shock
- Fluid Volume, Deficient related to hypovolemia
- Anxiety, Parental related to critically ill child
- Injury, Risk for related to seizures
- Body Image, Disturbed related to effect of disease on body parts

NANDA-I © 2012

Planning and Implementation

Meningococcal vaccine can prevent some cases of the disease. See Chapter 22 ✏ for recommendations related to this vaccine. Nursing care centers on managing fluids, maintaining respiratory support, administering medications, and monitoring for complications associated with meningococcemia. Intravenous infusions must be administered when ordered to ensure correct and timely administration of fluids, antibiotics, and other therapies such as vasopressive agents. Meticulous skin care is necessary to preserve the integrity of tissues. Care is taken to prevent further infections. Nutritional support in the form of total parenteral nutrition is common. Maintain ventilatory support and arterial lines if they are present. Implement safety precautions for seizures (refer to nursing care of seizures in Chapter 33 ✏). Include padding on the crib or side rails and suction equipment at bedside. Assist with wound care debridement as required. Maintain sterile technique.

The nurse offers the family support to deal with the changing critical nature of the child's illness and the possibility that death or permanent, severe deformities will result. When the child improves, continuing comprehensive care in the hospital and then in the community is needed to manage complex issues related to growth, development, nutrition, amputations, and prosthetics. Refer to Chapter 33 ✏ for nursing care of the child with meningitis.

Evaluation

Expected outcomes of nursing care for the child with meningococcemia include:

- The child demonstrates adequate tissue perfusion to all systems.
- Fluid balance is restored.
- The child is free from injury.
- The child demonstrates a positive body image.
- The child's family verbalizes fear and anxiety and receives appropriate support.

HEMATOPOIETIC STEM CELL TRANSPLANTATION (HSCT)

Hematopoietic stem cell transplantation is a treatment used for diseases such as severe combined immunodeficiency disease, severe and unresponsive aplastic anemia, and leukemia (refer to Chapters 27 and 29 ✏). Hematopoietic stem cells exist primarily in the bone marrow but also circulate in the peripheral blood. These cells can grow into new body cells, and have become useful in treatment of immune and hematologic diseases when restoration of normal cells is needed. Stem cells can be obtained from bone marrow, cord blood, or peripheral blood (Peters, Cornish, Parikh, et al, 2010).

Collaborative Care

Hematopoietic stem cell transplants are either autologous or allogeneic. In **autologous transplantation,** the child's own marrow is taken, treated, stored, and reinfused after the child has received chemotherapy. **Allogeneic transplantation** may be **syngeneic** (from an identical twin), related, or unrelated. In allogeneic transplantation, the donor, often a sibling (related), has a compatible human leukocyte antigen (HLA). Human leukocyte antigens are proteins found on the surface of nearly all nucleated cells within the body, and they are responsible for regulating the immune response. When no relative is found to match the child, a histocompatible donor (unrelated) may be sought from the National Marrow Donor Program or a cord blood bank (Brunstein & Wagner, 2008; Petersdorf & Anasetti, 2008). With the development of this registry, bone marrow transplantation from HLA-matched unrelated donors has become possible for some children.

Clinical Therapy

Pretransplant phase After a thorough evaluation of the child, including HLA typing, evaluation of organ functions, and laboratory studies, the child receives high doses of chemotherapy and, sometimes, total body irradiation directed at destroying circulating blood cells and the diseased bone marrow in the ill child. Common chemotherapeutic agents used include cyclophosphamide, busulfan, etoposide, melphalan, cytarabine, and thiotepa. The chemotherapy program for destruction of bone marrow ranges from 7 to 10 days (Moore & Ikeda, 2010). During this time, the child is cared for in strict isolation in a special unit that provides a positive-pressure environment (Figure 28–10 ■).

Transplant phase Following the immunosuppression procedure, the child receives an intravenous transfusion with the donor stem cells. This procedure is similar to administration of a blood product. The healthy stem cells migrate to the bone marrow. Healthy bone marrow, capable of making blood cells, is the anticipated result. If the transplantation is successful, the cells implant in the child's marrow and begin to produce blood cells within approximately 2 to 4 weeks.

Posttransplant phase **Pancytopenia** (marked decrease in RBCs, WBCs, and platelets) lasts for several weeks following the transplantation. The major risks during this period are infection, anemia, bleeding, and severe mouth sores. Transfusion of red blood cells and platelets may be required. The child's illness and the side effects related to the chemotherapy may alter nutritional status. Total parenteral nutrition (TPN) may be implemented to meet the child's nutritional needs during this period.

Except for children receiving syngeneic transplants, immunosuppressive agents are administered to prevent graft-versus-host disease. Once the bone marrow begins to produce new cells, graft-versus-host disease (rejection) is the major threat. Refer to Chapter 27 🔗 for a discussion of this disease.

Nursing Management

Supportive care after the transplantation procedure focuses on preventing infection, controlling bleeding, maintaining adequate

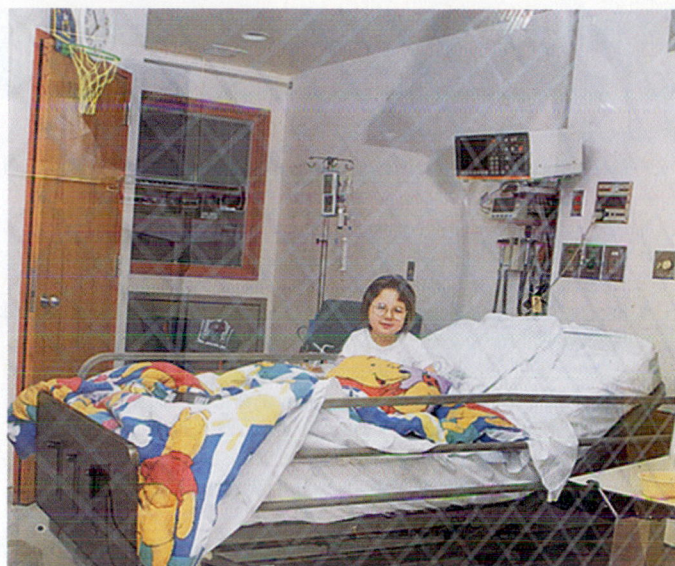

FIGURE 28–10 ■ The child undergoing bone marrow transplantation is hospitalized in a special sterile unit while receiving chemotherapy before the transfusion. The child remains in the unit for several weeks afterward until the new marrow produces enough cells to maintain health.

nutrition and hydration, monitoring for signs of rejection, and providing psychosocial support. This care is provided in a specialized unit in the hospital.

Nursing Assessment and Diagnosis

Monitor the child undergoing HSCT by assessing the skin, mucous membranes, gastrointestinal function, respiratory function, cardiac function, and hydration status. Multisystem assessment is needed. Because graft-versus-host disease may occur at any time, even after the child returns home, frequent thorough assessments are necessary after discharge. Refer to Chapter 27 🔗 for a discussion of graft-versus-host disease.

Nursing diagnoses that apply to the child undergoing HSCT include:

- Infection, Risk for related to immunocompromised state
- Anxiety (Parent and Child) related to life-threatening condition and procedures
- Growth and Development, Delayed related to social isolation with lengthy hospitalization and illness
- Social Isolation related to isolation procedures

NANDA-I © 2012

Planning and Implementation

The treatment is lengthy, the child is often critically ill, and parents may have traveled to a medical center many miles from home for the procedure. Ask parents about other family members and how they are managing. Provide information about inexpensive housing available near the medical center, such as a Ronald McDonald house. Encourage parents to discuss their feelings with other parents of children receiving bone marrow transplantation. Organizations such as the Bone Marrow Transplant Family Support Network can serve as resources for families.

Because hospitalizations of children undergoing bone marrow transplantation are usually lengthy, the child experiences interruptions in developmental achievements. Evaluate the child's age and

Weblink Bone Marrow Transplant Family Support Network

Health Promotion & Maintenance Overview

The Child with Hematopoietic Stem Cell Transplantation

GROWTH AND DEVELOPMENT

- Measure and plot height and weight at each visit using standard growth curve charts.
- Measure onset and progression of puberty using Tanner staging.
- An individualized education plan (IEP) should be performed yearly to identify learning problems.
- Routine hearing screening is advised since hearing loss may occur as a result of ototoxic drug therapy.
- Vision should be screened at each primary care visit since corticosteroid use can cause cataracts. Graft-versus-host disease can result in keratoconjunctivitis, and cytomegalovirus (CMV) can cause retinitis.
- Blood pressure should be monitored at each visit since children are commonly placed on medication for hypertension after HSCT because of nephrotoxic medications.
- Instruct parents to measure and record blood pressure at home if necessary.

NUTRITION

- Teach the family to avoid foods with potential vectors for infection, such as unpasteurized products and undercooked meats.
- A low-sodium diet may be required if the child has hypertension.
- Calcium supplements may be administered to reduce the risk of osteopenia.

PHYSICAL ACTIVITY

- If the child has thrombocytopenia, physical activity may be restricted.
- The child may experience fatigue. Identify the activities tolerated, and encourage those that may promote development.

ORAL HEALTH

- Dental screening and any required restorative care should be done before transplant to reduce potential sources of infection.
- Routine dental care is resumed once the child's immune system is restored. Ask the family about the child's routine dental care.

MENTAL AND SPIRITUAL HEALTH

- Apply developmental approaches to assess the child's feelings after HSCT.
- Ask the child about coping with being in the hospital and at home rather than attending school.

- Many physical changes occur with treatment that may interfere with body image. Assess the child's or adolescent's body image in a manner appropriate to age.

RELATIONSHIPS

- In-hospital or in-home schooling is required after HSCT for 6 to 12 months until immune function has been obtained to reduce the risk of infection. Prevent exposure to family members and peers with any infections.
- Encourage peer contact, telephone calls, email, and letters to reduce the child's feelings of isolation.
- On returning to school, the child is encouraged to participate fully in school activities.
- For the adolescent, sex education is important, especially to avoid sexually transmitted infections.

DISEASE PREVENTION STRATEGIES

- Teach the family that hand hygiene is essential to prevent the spread of infection.
- Dishes should be washed in a dishwasher. Teach safe food preparation techniques.
- In-home childcare is recommended because of the risk of infection in other childcare settings.
- Teach the family that the child should have minimal direct contact with animals to avoid infections.
- Determine the child's need for an altered immunization schedule after HSCT.
- Instruct parents to monitor the child for infection and to report any temperature elevation to the physician.
- Encourage the family to obtain an influenza vaccine annually for the child and all household or close contacts.
- Teach signs and symptoms of infection, and stress the importance of prompt reporting.

INJURY PREVENTION STRATEGIES

- Review safe medication storage with the family.
- Help the family develop a plan for the safe disposal of used needles and syringes.

---

developmental stage and establish developmental goals to be met during the hospitalization. Implement nursing plans to meet the child's developmental needs and encourage further growth. When the child is ready for discharge, be sure the family is prepared to administer medications, recognize signs of graft-versus-host disease, provide adequate nutrition for the child, and perform other necessary care. Arrange for follow-up visits and provide the names of local healthcare contacts who can offer support and provide information. The child may need tutors or other educational assistance to promote integration back into the school setting. See Health Promotion &

Maintenance Overview: The Child with Hematopoietic Stem Cell Transplantation.

Evaluation

Expected outcomes of nursing care include:

- The child is free of signs of infection.
- The family verbalizes that they have adequate support.
- The child achieves appropriate developmental milestones.
- The child has appropriate interaction and contact with family and peers.

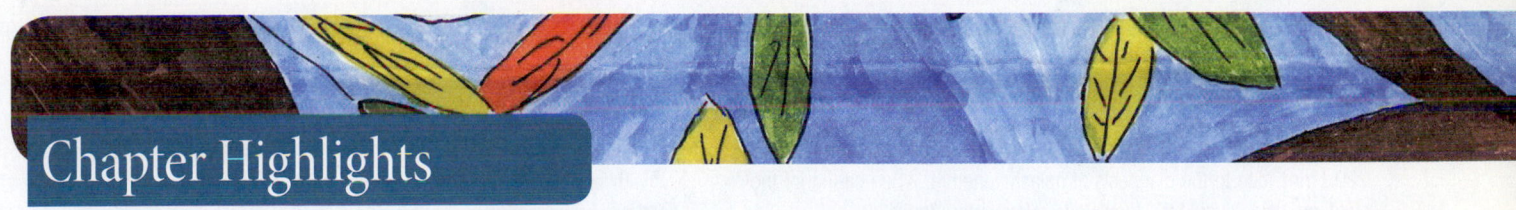

Chapter Highlights

- Erythrocytes (red cells) are a major component of the blood and transport oxygen from the lungs to body tissues.
- Polycythemia is an increase in the number of red blood cells. Anemia is characterized by a decrease in red blood cell number. Leukocytes (white cells) are important in the cell's defenses against disease.
- Thrombocytes (platelets) are necessary for normal clotting of blood.
- The major anemias of childhood include iron deficiency anemia, thalassemia, aplastic anemia, normocytic anemia, and sickle cell anemia.
- Sickle cell anemia is a genetic disease in which an abnormal shape, or sickling, of red blood cells prevents the normal flow of blood.
- Major complications of sickle cell anemia include pain, strokes, retinopathy, enlarged liver and spleen, urinary complications, poor peripheral blood flow, and osteoporosis.
- Nurses assist families in dealing with chronic diseases such as sickle cell anemia by providing information about the disorder and resources that can provide assistance, monitoring child growth and development, instituting preventive care, and managing exacerbations of the disease.
- Hereditary spherocytosis is an autosomal dominant disorder caused by an abnormality of proteins by an unknown cause. The cells have an unusual characteristic cell structure and become sequestered and hemolyzed in the spleen.
- The thalassemias are a group of genetic diseases of red blood cells, which cause defective synthesis of hemoglobin.
- Aplastic anemia is a deficiency of all blood cells related to poor bone marrow function; it can be congenital or acquired after exposure to certain drugs or harmful environmental toxins.
- Hemophilia is a bleeding disorder transmitted by genes; hemophilia A is most common and results in a decrease in clotting factor VIII.
- The goal of treatment for hemophilia is to control bleeding by preventive care and replacement of the missing factor.

- Major nursing concerns for the child with hemophilia include managing bleeding episodes, controlling pain during bleeds, minimizing physical immobility, supporting the family in learning management of this chronic disease, and explaining genetic implications of the disease.
- Von Willebrand disease is a hereditary bleeding disorder characterized by a deficiency of von Willebrand factor, a plasma protein that is a carrier for clotting factor VIII.
- Disseminated intravascular coagulation is a serious condition in which clotting mechanisms are disturbed, leading to extensive clotting and tissue damage.
- Immune thrombocytopenic purpura causes destruction of platelets and most frequently follows a childhood viral disease.
- Management of immune thrombocytopenic purpura includes corticosteroids and immunoglobulins since the disease is considered to be autoimmune in nature.
- Henoch-Schönlein purpura is a small vessel vasculitis that occurs primarily in the pediatric population.
- Occasionally, infection with organisms such as *Neisseria meningitidis* is followed by a severe systemic disease known as meningococcemia.
- Meningococcemia is manifested by sudden high fever, rash, skin and mucosal hemorrhage, and shock; prompt treatment with antibiotics is needed.
- Hematopoietic stem cell transplant (HSCT) is a useful treatment in some diseases of the hematologic system and some cancers; it involves infusion of bone marrow, peripheral stem cells, or neonatal stem cells from a donor into the blood of the recipient where it circulates, implants into the bone marrow, and begins making new blood cells.
- Nursing care before and after HSCT includes infection prevention, careful physical assessment, administration of medications, and support for the family.

Clinical Reasoning in Action

INTRODUCTION

Recall Michael, the child in the opening scenario who is admitted with sickle cell crisis. Michael is receiving intravenous and oral fluids, oxygen, and opioids via a continuous infusion with a PCA pump for bolus infusions. His hemoglobin on admission was 7.7 g/dL, hematocrit was 22%, and WBC count was elevated at 22,000. Michael's father has returned to work and he visits in the evenings. Michael's mother remains at the hospital with her son.

DESCRIPTION

Two days after Michael's admission, he is converted to oral opioids at a lower equianalgesic dosage. He acknowledges achieving adequate pain relief, though he still "aches" all over. His respirations, heart rate, and blood pressure are all within Michael's normal baseline. Michael's WBC count is dropping after receiving intravenous antibiotics.

DISCUSSION

1. Considering Michael's age and developmental stage, what communication techniques will the nurse implement when teaching Michael about his disease and treatment?
2. Refer to Chapter 21 🔗 and plan the pain assessment and management techniques that can be used with Michael for acute and chronic pain management.
3. What are the expected levels of hemoglobin and hematocrit at Michael's age? Why are his levels abnormal? Describe how sickle cell disease influences blood values.
4. What are the most immediate care needs while Michael is hospitalized? What additional care will he require at home?

NCLEX-RN® Review

1. A 3-year-old child has neutropenia as noted by a white blood cell count of 2200 mm³ due to the diagnosis of aplastic anemia. When caring for the child, on which should the family and nursing care focus?
   1. Preventing bruising
   2. Preventing infection
   3. Preventing fatigue
   4. Developmental issues

2. The nurse is caring for a child who has a decreased level of oxygen-carrying blood cells. Which blood cell is deficient?
   1. Erythrocytes
   2. Leukocytes
   3. Thrombocytes
   4. Granulocytes

3. The nurse and the family take special precautions when caring for a child with any bleeding disorder. Which statement indicates teaching about these precautions was not effective?
   1. "My child will have a saline lock if frequent blood draws are anticipated."
   2. "I should provide gentle mouth care at least every 3 hours."
   3. "There is a paper tape that will be easier on my child's skin."
   4. "I will make sure my child has a rectal temperature every 4 hours."

4. The parent of a child diagnosed with sickle cell anemia asks the nurse about air travel with the child. Which is the best response?
   1. "Flying presents a higher risk for infection for a child with sickle cell anemia."
   2. "Flying at high altitudes causes decreased oxygen, causing increased sickling."
   3. "Flying does not pose any particular risks for the child with sickle cell anemia."
   4. "Air travel is not recommended because there are fewer available fluids on flights."

See Appendix I 🔗 for answers.

References

Abdullah, F., Zhang, Y., Camp, M., Rossberg, M. I., Bathurst, M. A., Colombani, P. M., . . . Chang, D. C. (2009). Splenectomy in hereditary spherocytosis: Review of 1657 patients and application of the pediatric quality indicators. *Pediatric Blood & Cancer, 52*(7), 834–837.

Addis, G. (2010). Sickle cell disease, part 1: Understanding the condition. *British Journal of Nursing, 5*(5), 231–234.

Alsultan, A., Goldenberg, N. A., Kaiser, N., Graham, K. K., & Hays, T. (2009). Tacrolimus as an alternative to cyclosporine in the maintenance phase of immunosuppressive therapy for severe aplastic anemia in children. *Pediatric Blood and Cancer, 52*, 626–630.

Alvarez, O., Rodriguez-Cortes, H., Robinson, N., Lewis, N., Sang, C. D. P., Lopez-Mitnik, G., & Paley, C. (2009). Adherence to deferasirox in children and adolescents with sickle cell disease during 1 year of therapy. *Journal of Pediatric Hematology/Oncology, 31*(10), 739–744.

American Academy of Pediatrics, Committee on Nutrition. (2009). Iron. In *Pediatric nutrition handbook* (6th ed., pp. 403–422). Elk Grove Village, IL: American Academy of Pediatrics.

American Sickle Cell Anemia Association. (2010). *How common is sickle cell anemia?* Retrieved from http://www.ascaa.org/How_Common_Is_Sickle_Cell_Anemia.asp

Arnold, J. L., Alson, R., Asrat, W., Bertolone, S., Chew, F. S., Choi, M. H. J., . . . Young, G. M. (2011). *Sickle cell anemia.* Retrieved from http://emedicine.medscape.com/article/205926-overview

Audino, A. N., Blatt, J., Carcamo, B., Castaneda, V., Dinndorf, P., Wang, W. C., . . . Hord, J. D. (2010). High-dose cyclophosphamide treatment for refractory severe aplastic anemia in children. *Pediatric Blood and Cancer, 54*, 269–272.

Ault, P., & Jones, K. (2009). Understanding iron overload: Screening, monitoring, and caring for patients with transfusion-dependent anemias. *Clinical Journal of Oncology Nursing, 13*(5), 511–517.

Baker, R. D., Greer, F. R., & the Committee on Nutrition. (2010). Diagnosis and prevention of iron deficiency and iron-deficiency anemia in infants and young children (0–3 years of age). *Pediatrics, 126*(5), 1040–1050.

Barillas-Arias, L., Adams, A., & Lehman, T. (2008). Pediatric vasculitic syndromes: Henoch-Schonlein purpura. *Consultant for Pediatricians, 7*(9), 361–367.

Barrows, E., & Kraj, B. (2010). Idiopathic autoimmune thrombocytopenic purpura in a 12-year-old boy. *Clinical Laboratory Science, 23*(4), 201–204.

Becherer, S. A., & White, A. (2010). Iron deficiency anemia in the pediatric emergency department. *Journal of Emergency Nursing, 36*(2), 130–133.

Blanchette, V., & Bolton-Maggs, P. (2008). Childhood immune thrombocytopenic purpura: Diagnosis and management. *Pediatric Clinics of North America, 55*, 393–420.

Borgna-Pignatti, C., & Marsella, M. (2008). Iron deficiency in infancy and childhood. *Pediatric Annals, 37*(5), 329–337.

Brawley, O. W., Cornelius, L. J., Edwards, L. R., Northington, G. V., Green, B. L., Inturrisi, C., . . . Schori, M. (2008). National Institutes of Health Consensus Development Conference Statement: Hydroxyurea treatment for sickle cell disease. *Annals of Internal Medicine, 148*, 932–938.

Brunstein, C. G., & Wagner, J. E. (2008). Umbilical cord blood transplantation. In R. Hoffman, E. J. Benz, S. J. Shattil, B. Furie, L. E. Silberstein, P. McGlave, & H. Heslop (Eds.), *Hematology: Basic principles and practice* (5th ed., pp. 1643–1664). Philadelphia, PA: Churchill Livingstone-Elsevier.

Buckley, L. L., & Pravikoff, D. (2010). Disseminated intravascular coagulation (DIC). *Cinahl Information Systems.*

Centers for Disease Control and Prevention. (2011). *Summary of recommendations for child/teen immunization.* Retrieved from http://www.immunize.org/catg.d/p2010.pdf

Charnock, K., & Sutter, D. E. (2008, February). 5-year-old boy with abdominal pain and fever. *Infectious Diseases in Children.* Retrieved from http://www.pediatricsupersite.com/view.aspx?rid=35711

Choudhary, D. R., Naithani, R., Mahapatra, M., Kumar, R., Mishra, P., & Saxena, R. (2009). Intracranial hemorrhage in childhood immune thrombocytopenic purpura. *Pediatric Blood and Cancer, 52*, 529–531.

Christensen, R. D., & Ohls, R. K. (2011). Development of the hematopoietic system. In R. M. Kliegman, B. F. Stanton, J. W. St. Geme III, N. F. Schor, & R. E. Behrman, *Nelson textbook of pediatrics* (19th ed., pp. 1648). Philadelphia, PA: Saunders Elsevier.

Corbett, J. V. (2008). *Laboratory tests and diagnostic procedures with nursing diagnoses* (7th ed.). Upper Saddle River, NJ: Pearson Prentice Hall.

Cunningham, M.J. (2008). Update on Thalassemia: Clinical Care and Complications. *Pediatric Clinics of North America, 55*, 447–460.

De, D. (2008). Acute nursing care and management of patients with sickle cell. *British Journal of Nursing, 17*(13), 818–823.

DeBaun, M. R., Frei-Jones, M., & Vichinsky, E. (2011). Hemoglobinopathies. In R. M. Kliegman, B. F. Stanton, J. W. St. Geme III, N. F. Schor, & R. E. Behrman, *Nelson textbook of pediatrics* (19th ed., pp. 1662–1677). Philadelphia, PA: Saunders Elsevier.

Diz-Kucukkaya, R., Chen, J., Geddis, A., & Lopez, J. A. (2010). Thrombocytopenia. In M. A. Lichtman, T. J. Kipps, U. Seligsohn, K. Kaushansky, & J. T. Prchal, *Williams hematology* (8th ed., pp. 1891–1928). New York, NY: McGraw Hill Medical.

Dixson, M. (2010). Pediatric rash and joint pain: A case review. *Journal of Emergency Nursing, 36*(6), 591–593.

Effa-Heap, G. (2009). Blood transfusion: Implications of treating a Jehovah's Witness patient. *British Journal of Nursing, 18*(3), 174–177.

Foster, M. (2008). FDA approves use of blood product for patients with hemophilia. *Infectious Diseases in Children, 21*(11), 15.

Freedman, M. H. (2011). The inherited pancytopenias. In R. M. Kliegman, B. F. Stanton, J. W. St. Geme III, N. F. Schor, & R. E. Behrman, *Nelson textbook of pediatrics* (19th ed., pp. 1684–1690). Philadelphia, PA: Saunders Elsevier.

Gallagher, P. G. (2010). The red blood cell membrane and its disorders: Hereditary spherocytosis, elliptocytosis, and related disorders. In M. A. Lichtman, T. J. Kipps, U. Seligsohn, K. Kaushansky, & J. T. Prchal, *Williams hematology* (8th ed., pp. 617–646). New York, NY: McGraw Hill Medical.

Geil, J. D. (2009). *Von Willebrand disease.* Retrieved from http://emedicine.medscape.com/article/959825-overview

Geller, A. K., & O'Connor, M. K. (2008). The sickle cell crisis: A dilemma in pain relief. *Mayo Clinic Proceedings, 83*(3), 320–323.

Giardina, P. J., & Forget, B. G. (2009). Thalassemia syndromes. In R. Hoffman, E. J. Benz, S. J. Shattil, B. Furie, L. E. Silberstein, P. McGlave, & H. Heslop (Eds.), *Hematology: Basic principles and practice* (5th ed., pp. 535–563). Philadelphia, PA: Churchill Livingstone-Elsevier.

Gill, V., Lavin, J., & Sim, M. (2010). Managing sickle cell disease. *Nursing Made Incredibly Easy, 8*(6), 24–33.

Gladwin, M. T., & Vinchinsky, E. (2008). Pulmonary complications of sickle cell disease. *New England Journal of Medicine, 359*(21), 2254–2265.

Gonzalez, G., & Eichner, E. R. (2012). *Hereditary spherocytosis.* Retrieved from http://emedicine.medscape.com/article/206107-overview

Granoff, D. M., & Gilsdorf, J. R. (2011). Neisseria meningitidis. In R. M. Kliegman, B. F. Stanton, J. W. St. Geme III, N. F. Schor, & R. E. Behrman, *Nelson textbook of pediatrics* (19th ed., pp. 929–935). Philadelphia, PA: Saunders Elsevier.

Greenbaum, L. A. (2011). Vitamin K deficiency. In R. M. Kliegman, B. F. Stanton, J. W. St. Geme III, N. F. Schor, & R. E. Behrman, *Nelson textbook of pediatrics* (19th ed., pp. 209–211). Philadelphia, PA: Saunders Elsevier.

Gruppo, R. A. (2010). Treatment of hemophilia in developing countries—A journey of a thousand miles. *Pediatric Blood and Cancer, 54*(3), 348–349.

Hord, J. D. (2011). The acquired pancytopenias. In R. M. Kliegman, B. F. Stanton, J. W. St. Geme III, N. F. Schor, & R. E. Behrman, *Nelson textbook of pediatrics* (19th ed., pp. 1691–1692). Philadelphia, PA: Saunders Elsevier.

Hunt, C. W. (2010). Immune thrombocytopenia purpura. *MEDSURG Nursing, 19*(4), 237–239.

Hyatt, S. A., Wang, W., Kerlin, B. A., & O'Brien, S. H. (2009). Applying diagnostic criteria for type 1 von Willebrand disease to a pediatric population. *Pediatric Blood and Cancer, 52*, 102–107.

Inati, A., Koussa, S., Taher, A., & Perrine, S. (2008). Sickle cell disease: New insights into pathophysiology and treatment. *Pediatric Annals, 37*(5), 311–321.

Inati, A., Khoriaty, E., & Musallam, K. M. (2011). Iron in sickle-cell disease: What have we learned over the years? *Pediatric Blood and Cancer, 56*, 182–190.

Iolascon, A., Piscopo, C., & Boschetto, L. (2008). Red cell membrane disorders in pediatrics. *Pediatric Annals, 37*(5), 295–301.

Jacob, E., & Mueller, B. U. (2008). Pain experience of children with sickle cell disease who had prolonged hospitalizations for acute painful episodes. *Pain Medicine, 9*(1), 13–21.

Janus, J., & Moerschel, S. K. (2010). Evaluation of anemia in children. *American Family Physician, 81*(12), 1462–1471.

Kliegman, R. M., Stanton, B. F., St. Geme, J. W., Schor, N. F., & Behrman, R. E. (2011). *Nelson textbook of pediatrics* (19th ed., Table 708.6). Philadelphia, PA: Elsevier Saunders.

Knight-Madden, J. M., Lewis, N., Tyson, E., Reid, M. E., & MooSang, M. (2010). The possible impact of teachers and school nurses on the lives of children living with sickle cell disease. *Journal of School Health, 81*(5), 219–222.

Kumar, R. & Gupta, V. (2008). Disseminated intravascular coagulation. *Indian Journal of Pediatrics 75* (7), 733–738.

Learner, N. B. (2011). Physiologic anemia of infancy. In R. M. Kliegman, B. F. Stanton, J. W. St. Geme III, N. F. Schor, & R. E. Behrman, *Nelson textbook of pediatrics* (19th ed., pp. 1654–1655). Philadelphia, PA: Saunders Elsevier.

Lemanek, K. L., Ranalli, M., & Lukens, C. (2009). A randomized controlled trial of massage therapy in children with sickle cell disease. *Journal of Pediatric Psychology, 34*(10), 1091–1096.

Lee, L. H., Bearie, B., & Lee, C. (2009). Henoch-Schönlein purpura. *Consultant for Pediatricians, 8*(10), 377.

LeMone, P., Burke, K. M., & Bauldoff, G. (2011). Nursing care of patients with hematologic disorders. In P. LeMone, K. Burke, & G. Bauldoff, *Medical surgical nursing: Critical thinking in patient care* (4th ed., pp. 1068–1115). Upper Saddle River, NJ: Pearson.

Linker, C. A. (2008). Hematology. In S. J. McPhee, M. A. Papadakis, & L. M. Tierney, Jr., *Current medical diagnosis and treatment 2008*. McGraw-Hill's Access Medicine.

London, M. L., Ladewig, P. W., Ball, J. W., Bindler, R. C., & Cowen, K. J. (2011). *Maternal & child nursing care* (3rd ed.). Upper Saddle River, NJ: Prentice Hall Health.

Manco-Johnson, M. J., Abshire, T. C., Shapiro, A. D., Riske, B., Hacker, M. R., Kilcoyne, R., ... Evatt, B.L. (2007). Prophylaxis versus episodic treatment to prevent joint disease in boys with severe hemophilia. *New England Journal of Medicine, 357*(6), 535–544.

Manno, C. S., & Larson, P. J. (2009). Transfusion therapy for coagulation factor deficiencies. In R. Hoffman, E. J. Benz, S. J. Shattil, B. Furie, L. E. Silberstein, P. McGlave, & H. Heslop (Eds.), *Hematology: Basic principles and practice* (5th ed., pp. 2247–2256). Philadelphia, PA: Churchill Livingstone-Elsevier.

March of Dimes. (2008). *Sickle cell disease*. Retrieved from http://www.marchofdimes.com/professionals/14332_1221.asp

Mátrai, J., Chuah, M. K. L., & VandenDriessche, T. (2010). Preclinical and clinical progress in hemophilia gene therapy. *Current Opinion in Hematology, 17*, 387–392.

McGrath, B. M., Petropolis, C., & West, P. (2010). Answer: Can you identify this condition? Meningococcemia. *Canadian Family Physician, 56*(9), 895.

Milonovich, L. M. (2007). Meningococcemia: Epidemiology, pathophysiology, and management. *Journal of Pediatric Health Care, 21*(2), 75–80.

Mirre, E., Brousse, V., Berteloot, L., Lambot-Juhan, K., Verlhac, S., Boulat, C., . . . De Montalembert,M. (2010). Feasibility and efficacy of chronic transfusion for stroke prevention in children with sickle cell disease. *European Journal of Haematology, 84*(3), 259–265.

Moore, T., & Ikeda, A. K. (2010). *Bone marrow transplantation*. Retrieved from http://emedicine.medscape.com/article/1014514-overview

Muncie, H. L., & Campbell, J. S. (2009). Alpha and beta thalassemia. *American Family Physician, 80*(4), 339–344.

Natarajan, K., Townes, T. M., & Kutlar, A. (2010). Disorders of hemoglobin structure: Sickle cell anemia and related abnormalities. In M. A. Lichtman, T. J. Kipps, U. Seligsohn, K. Kaushansky, & J. T. Prchal, *Williams hematology* (8th ed., pp. 617–646). New York, NY: McGraw Hill Medical.

Neunert, C. (2011). Idiopathic thrombocytopenic purpura: Advances in management. *Clinical Advances in Hematology & Oncology, 9*(5), 404–406.

Newberger, P. E., & Boxer, L. A. (2011). Leukopenia. In R. M. Kliegman, B. F. Stanton, J. W. St. Geme III, N. F. Schor, & R. E. Behrman, *Nelson textbook of pediatrics* (19th ed., pp. 746–752). Philadelphia, PA: Saunders Elsevier.

Nguyen, D. D., & Takenaka, K. (2009). Evaluation and management of hereditary hemophilia in the emergency department. *Journal of Emergency Nursing, 35*(5), 437–441.

Penny, K., Fleming, M., Kazmierczak, D., & Thomas, A. (2010). An epidemiological study of Henoch-Schönlein purpura. *Pediatric Nursing, 22*(10), 30–35.

Peters, C., Cornish, J. M., Parikh, S. H., & Kurtzberg, J. (2010). Stem cell source and outcome after hematopoietic stem cell transplantation (HSCT) in children and adolescents with acute leukemia. *Pediatric Clinics of North America, 57*, 27–46.

Petersdorf, E. W., & Anasetti, C. (2008). Unrelated donor hematopoietic cell transplantation. In R. Hoffman, E. J. Benz, S. J. Shattil, B. Furie, L. E. Silberstein, P. McGlave, & H. Heslop (Eds.), *Hematology: Basic principles and practice* (5th ed., pp. 1619–1631). Philadelphia, PA: Churchill Livingstone-Elsevier.

Pinto, S., & Pravikoff, D. (2011). Thalassemia, beta. *Cinahl Information Systems*.

Reamy, B. V., Williams, P. M., & Lindsay, T. J. (2009). Henoch-Schönlein purpura. *American Family Physician, 80*(7), 697–703.

Rees, D. C., Williams, T. N., & Gladwin, M. T. (2010). Sickle-cell disease. *Lancet, 376*, 2018–2031.

Richardson, M. (2007). Microcytic anemia. *Pediatrics in Review, 28*(1), 5–14.

Robertson, J., Lillicrap, D., & James, P. D. (2008). Von Willebrand disease. *Pediatric Clinics of North America, 55*, 377–392.

Rodriguez, N. I., & Hoots, W. K. (2008). Advances in hemophilia: Experimental aspects and therapy. *Pediatric Clinics of North America, 55*, 357–376.

Saunthararajah, Y., & Vichinsky, E. P. (2009). Sickle cell disease: Clinical features and management. In R. Hoffman, E. J. Benz, S. J. Shattil, B. Furie, L. E. Silberstein, P. McGlave, & H. Heslop (Eds.), *Hematology: Basic principles and practice* (5th ed., pp. 577–601). Philadelphia, PA: Churchill Livingstone-Elsevier.

Scott, J. P., Raffini, L. J., & Montgomery, R. R. (2011). Hemostasis. In R. M. Kliegman, B. F. Stanton, J. W. St. Geme III, N. F. Schor, & R. E. Behrman, *Nelson textbook of pediatrics* (19th ed., pp. 1693–1699). Philadelphia, PA: Saunders Elsevier.

Scott, J. P., & Montgomery, R. R. (2011). Factor VIII or factor IX deficiency (hemophilia A or B). In R. M. Kliegman, B. F. Stanton, J. W. St. Geme III, N. F. Schor, & R. E. Behrman, *Nelson textbook of pediatrics* (19th ed., pp. 1699–1702). Philadelphia, PA: Saunders Elsevier.

Segel, G. B., & Feig, S. A. (2009). Controversies in the diagnosis and management of childhood acute immune thrombocytopenic purpura. *Pediatric Blood and Cancer, 53*, 318–324.

Sickle Cell Advisory Committee of the Genetic Network of New York, Puerto Rico, and the Virgin Islands. (2002, March). *Guidelines for the treatment of people with sickle cell disease.*

Sickle Cell Disease Association of America. (2011). *Sickle cell disease global*. Retrieved from http://www .sicklecelldisease.org/index.cfm?page=scd-global

Siegel, J. E. (2009). *Factor XI deficiency*. Retrieved from http://emedicine.medscape.com/article/209984-overview

Soldin, S. J., Wong, E. C., Brugnara, C., & Soldin, O. P. (2011). *Pediatric reference ranges* (7th ed.). Washington, DC: AACC Press.

Son, D. W., Jeon, I., Yang, S. W., & Cho, S. H. (2008). A single dose of anti-D immunoglobulin raises platelet count as efficiently as intravenous immunoglobulin in newly diagnosed immune thrombocytopenic purpura in Korean children. *Journal of Pediatric Hematology/ Oncology, 30*(8), 598–601.

Thiagarajan, P. (2011). *Platelet disorders*. Retrieved from http://emedicine.medscape.com/article/201722-overview#aw2aab6c21

Thompson, C. A. (2008). Additional antihemophilic factor to be available. *American Journal of Health-System Pharmacy, 65,* 592.

Tracy, E. T., & Rice, H. E. (2008). Partial splenectomy for hereditary spherocytosis. *Pediatric Clinics of North America, 55*(2), 503–519.

Treadwell, P. A. (2008). Spot the rash. *Infectious Diseases in Children, 21*(3), 20, 52.

U.S. Department of Health and Human Services. (2011). *Who is at risk for sickle cell anemia?* Retrieved from http://www.nhlbi.nih.gov/health/dci/Diseases/Sca/ SCA_WhoIsAtRisk.html

Vranou, M., Platokouki, H., Pergantou, H., & Aronis, S. (2008). Recurrent idiopathic thrombocytopenic purpura in childhood. *Pediatric Blood and Cancer, 51,* 261–264.

Ware, R. E., & Aygun, B. (2009). Advances in the use of hydroxyurea. *Hematology/ the Education Program of the* American Society of Hematology, 62–69.

Weatherall, D. J. (2010). The thalassemias: Disorders of globin synthesis. In M. A. Lichtman, T. J. Kipps, U. Seligsohn, K. Kaushansky, & J. T. Prchal, *Williams hematology* (8th ed., pp. 675–707). New York, NY: McGraw Hill Medical.

Yanni, E., Grosse, S. D., Yang, Q., & Olney, R. S. (2009). Trends in pediatric sickle cell disease-related mortality in the United States, 1983–2002. *Journal of Pediatrics, 154*(4), 541–545.

Zempsky, W. T., Loiselle, K. A., McKay, K., Lee, B. H., Hagstrom, J. N., & Schechter, N. L. (2010). Do children with sickle cell disease receive disparate care for pain in the emergency department? *Journal of Emergency Medicine, 39*(5), 691–695.

Zempsky, W. T., Corsi, J. M., & McKay, K. (2011). Pain scores: Are they used in sickle cell pain? *Pediatric Emergency Care, 27*(1), 27–28.

Pearson Nursing Student Resources
Find additional review materials at
nursing.pearsonhighered.com
Prepare for success with additional NCLEX®-style practice questions, interactive assignments and activities, web links, animations and videos, and more!

The Child with Cancer

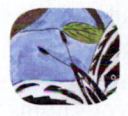 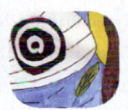 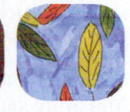

Learning Outcomes

After completing this chapter, you will be able to:

1. Describe the incidence, known etiologies, and common clinical manifestations of cancer.

2. Synthesize information about diagnostic tests and clinical therapy for cancer to plan comprehensive care for children undergoing these procedures.

3. Integrate information about oncologic emergencies into plans for monitoring all children with cancer.

4. Recognize the most common solid tumors in children, describe their treatment, and plan comprehensive nursing care.

5. Plan care for children and adolescents of all ages who have a diagnosis of leukemia.

6. Recognize the most common soft tissue tumors in children, describe their treatment, and plan comprehensive care.

7. Analyze the impact of cancer survival on children and use this information to plan for ongoing physiologic and psychosocial care.

8. Recommend methods for an oncology team including nurses, social workers, psychologists, and child life specialists to partner with school personnel, children and adolescents, families, and others to meet the needs of children with cancer.

> "We don't like it when Sam is sick and our mom has to be away with him so much. It's sort of scary—I wonder if I could get sick like that too."
>
> —*Carolee, Sam's sister, age 8*

Sam Chastain, 4 years old, had bruises on his legs that puzzled his parents since he had not been engaged in any activities that would have caused them. He also appeared to be lethargic and developed a respiratory infection. Suspecting an influenza infection, Sam's parents brought him to the pediatric office. The physician's assessment found hepatosplenomegaly, so a complete blood count was obtained. Low amounts of red blood cells and platelets were seen with high levels of white blood cells. The physician suspected acute lymphoblastic leukemia and referred Sam to the oncology center that afternoon. Sam's mother was devastated; she had never suspected this diagnosis.

The next few days were a blur of making phone calls, arranging care for two older children, and then staying with Sam during his lumbar puncture, bone marrow aspiration, body scans, and placement of a central line. Sam remained in the hospital for initiation of therapy and then was discharged home. He is now returning for his series of consolidation therapy treatments at the oncology clinic. The nurse who planned care in the immediate diagnostic period and during induction therapy prepared him well for every procedure and now sees Sam at clinic visits to provide information and answer questions. The two older siblings were able to attend a recent clinic visit, which allowed them to understand Sam's condition. The nurse identified the family's greatest need as knowledge, since they have many questions at each encounter.

ancer is a daunting diagnosis at any age, but in children it seems even more profound. The diagnosis and treatment are met with shock and disbelief. They require a change in the roles of everyone in the family, and challenge all children and families involved in many ways. Treatments for cancer have improved the prognosis in many cases, but in some, the prognosis still requires that the family deal with a life-threatening illness (see Chapter 17). Nurses who work in pediatric oncology have unique opportunities to assist children and families in mobilizing resources and learning about maximizing physical, emotional, and developmental health while dealing with the challenges of the illness and treatment. Collaboration often involves oncology physicians, clinical nurse specialists and other advanced practice nurses, and a variety of other health professionals.

ANATOMY AND PHYSIOLOGY

Abnormal cellular growth can occur in any area of the body. Why are some growths called cancer and others not? Changes in cellular growth within the body are called **neoplasms** (meaning new growth). A neoplasm is further classified as benign or malignant. **Benign** means that a growth does not endanger life or health; it tends to not recur after treatment. **Malignant** means that if not treated, a growth will recur, continue to grow, and spread to other sites in the body (**metastasis**), ending in death. The common term for this type of cellular growth is *cancer*.

PEDIATRIC DIFFERENCES

Cancers in children often have different etiology than those in adults. Most adult cancers are epithelial in origin, whereas in children, non-epithelial or embryonal cell types predominate. While many adult cancers are slow-growing and result from exposure to carcinogens over time, most childhood cancers are fast-growing. A child who appears healthy may suddenly appear ill over a period of days or weeks. Cancer in adults is often the result of dietary practices or habits such as smoking. Some adult-onset cancers are the result of oncogenic responses to stimuli—that is, responses that stimulate cancerous changes in cells. Other cancers that occur in adults result from prolonged exposure to toxins such as coal dust and asbestos. Some cancers are known to be related to genetic causes. In adults, prevention through general lifestyle changes is a major focus of interventions. In children, however, cancer is usually embryonic (occurring during development of the fetus) or oncogenic in origin (see description of oncogenes on pages 942–943). Thus, lifestyle changes that begin in childhood have little effect on the incidence of childhood cancer, although they may have a positive influence on the incidence of later cancer or other diseases. Occasionally, an environmental exposure is linked to the incidence of cancer in children. Different types of cancers predominate at various ages in childhood, demonstrating the multiple causes and their relationship to age and development (Figure 29–1).

Although not common, some neonates and young infants have cancer that is diagnosed soon after birth. The types of cancers most common in this age group include central nervous system (CNS) tumors, neuroblastoma, leukemia, retinoblastoma, renal or hepatic tumors, sarcomas, and teratomas (arising from primary germ layers). The close proximity of these events to embryogenesis suggests that inherited or acquired genetic susceptibility plays a part. Parental exposure to teratogens is one possible acquired cause. Management of cancer in infancy is demanding, the physiologic needs of the young

infant are complex, and when combined with multifaceted treatment plans, healthcare professionals require special skills.

A major physiologic difference between adults and children that affects cellular growth involves the immune system and how well it functions in the body's defense. The rate of cell growth in children also can play a role in the rapidity with which some childhood cancers progress. The continuing presence of fetal cells in small children is related to some cancers.

The immune system defends the body against foreign organisms and substances through two responses: nonspecific and specific. In a nonspecific response, the components of the immune system attack a variety of targets. Nonspecific components include phagocytic (cell destroying) cells such as mononuclear leukocytes, polymorphonuclear (PMN) leukocytes, natural killer (NK) cells, and complements (noncellular proteins) that work together to destroy invading cells and substances. During the first month of a child's life, the nonspecific response is immature, so phagocytic cells have little ability to move toward cancer cells and fulfill their function. The nonspecific response is also impaired in premature and small-for-gestational-age (SGA) infants.

In a specific response, T lymphocytes and immunoglobulin (Ig) attack only one type of invader. The specific response capability is also immature in infants. B-cell production of various proteins called immunoglobulins (IgM, IgG, and IgA) is below adult levels, so the infant is vulnerable to bacterial and viral infections. (For a detailed discussion of immune function, see Chapter 27 .)

In children, many cells are growing quickly; this fast growth can lead to the proliferation of both cancerous and normal cells. Cell division that is out of control may normally trigger a mechanism called **apoptosis,** whereby the cell "realizes" something is wrong and destroys itself. The process of apoptosis or physiologic cell death limits the growth of cancerous cells. However, this recognition of abnormality and subsequent destruction of cells may not be well developed in young children.

Use the assessment guidelines in Table 29–1 to identify and monitor alterations in cellular growth. Examples of diagnostic and laboratory tests used for cancer are listed in Table 29–2.

CHILDHOOD CANCER

The care of children who have cancer is a challenging specialty in pediatric nursing. For several years, the child undergoes aggressive treatments that may be life threatening and cause serious illness. Often the prognosis is quite hopeful; at other times, a terminal prognosis is expected. For some types of cancer, the child is cared for at home with outpatient visits for treatment and occasional hospitalization when needed for conditions such as fever and neutropenia. The periods of hospitalization are times of intense physical vulnerability for the child and intense emotional vulnerability for both the child and the family. For some cancers, multiple hospitalizations are needed to carry out therapy. To monitor the child closely, nurses need a sound knowledge of physiologic and psychologic responses, medical interventions, and nursing care. Effective communication skills are necessary to partner with the child and family and promote realistic hope.

In the United States, cancer is diagnosed in approximately 11,000 children under 15 years of age, and about 1,500 die from cancer annually (American Cancer Society, 2011; National Cancer Institute, 2008). In children under 15 years of age, cancer is the leading cause of

As They Grow Types of Cancer by Age Group

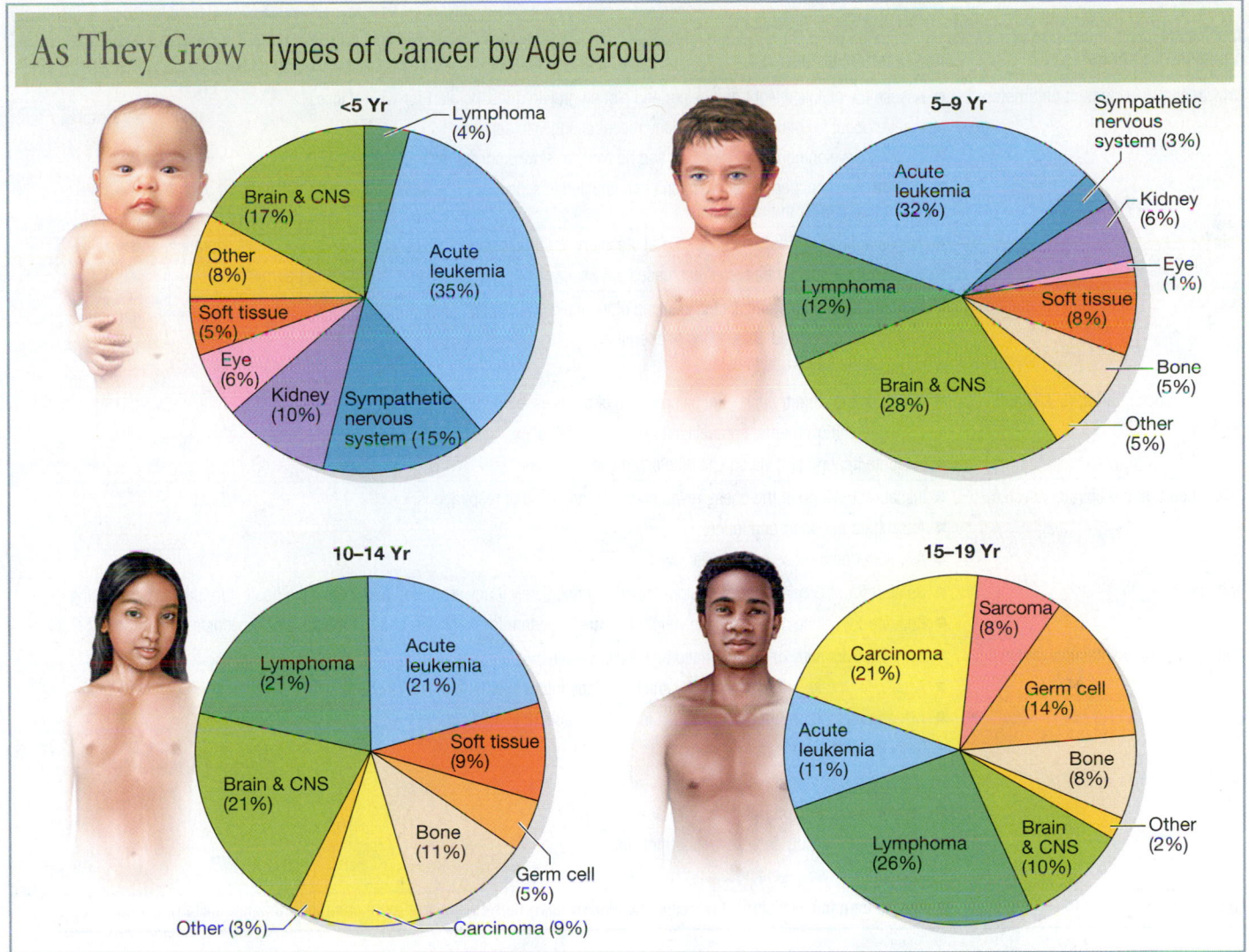

FIGURE 29–1 ■ Percentage of primary tumors by site of origin for different age groups. Notice that in the early years of life, in addition to leukemia, cancers that derive from embryonic cells such as sympathetic nervous system (neuroblastoma) and eye (retinoblastoma) are diagnosed. As the child grows, lymphoma becomes more common in the school years, and germ cell cancers of ovary and testes emerge as more common causes in teens.

Source: Data from Asselin, B. (2011). Epidemiology of childhood and adolescent cancer. In R. M. Kliegman, B. F. Stanton, J. W. St. Geme, N. F. Schor, & R. E. Behrman, Nelson textbook of pediatrics (19th ed., pp. 1725–1727). Philadelphia, PA: Elsevier Saunders.

disease-related death and the second leading cause of overall death, following unintentional injury (American Cancer Society, 2011) (see Chapter 1 🔗). Mortality rates have declined by about 47% since 1975, and the rates for many cancers continue to improve. Children treated in the 1980s, 1990s, and 2000s had significantly lower mortality rates than those treated in the 1960s and 1970s due to multimodal therapies including multiagent chemotherapy, surgery, radiation therapy, and immune system treatments. The overall survival rate is 80% for childhood cancer. Survival rates vary for different types of cancer, ranging from 66% overall for neuroblastoma to 95% overall for Hodgkin disease. The stage at diagnosis and cell histology of cancer also greatly influence survival outcomes. Survival rates are generally lower for males than females, for those diagnosed before 5 years of age, and for children with a central nervous system tumor or certain types of leukemia. Ethnic disparity also exists with Hispanics having lower survival rates than non-Hispanics, and Whites and

Blacks having lower survival rates than Asians/Pacific Islanders and American Indians/Alaska Natives (American Cancer Society, 2011). Both genetics and environment likely play a role in the disparity.

Etiology and Pathophysiology

Alterations in cellular growth occur in response to external and internal stimuli. Neoplasms are caused by one or a combination of three factors: (1) external stimuli that cause genetic mutations, (2) innate immune system and gene abnormalities, and (3) chromosomal abnormalities.

External Stimuli

External stimuli may affect the child's general health and cause mutations in body cells. **Carcinogens** are chemicals or industrial processes that, when combined with genetic traits and in interaction with one another, result in cancer. Several carcinogens cause cancers

TABLE 29–1   Assessment Guidelines for the Child with Cancer*

ASSESSMENT FOCUS	ASSESSMENT GUIDELINES
Growth and development parameters	■ Assess the child's weight and height and plot on growth grids; be alert for weight loss.
	■ Inquire about nutritional intake and any recent changes in appetite.
	■ Perform developmental assessment and be alert for slow progress or regression.
	■ Ask about school performance for children enrolled in school; include this data in every assessment of children who were treated for cancer in the past.
Pain	■ Pain is abnormal if there is no known acute injury or chronic condition; assess any pain for length, duration, and type.
	■ Be alert for limping, headache, decreased activity level, or other symptoms indicative of pain.
Skin	■ Evaluate skin for bruising, petechiae, and other signs of bleeding.
	■ Be alert for pallor and other signs of anemia.
	■ Describe skin lesions.
Eyes, ears, nose, throat (EENT) and sensory	■ Inspect the symmetry and general condition of the eyes, ears, mouth, throat, head, and neck.
	■ Inspect eye movements, corneal light reflex, and red reflex.
	■ Evaluate hearing and vision and note any recent changes.
Chest, heart, and respiratory system	■ Inspect the shape of the chest, respiratory rate, and ease of respirations.
	■ Auscultate the heart and lungs.
	■ Ask about endurance and activity levels.
Abdomen	■ Be alert for abdominal masses. Stop palpation immediately if any are noted and inform the healthcare provider managing care.
	■ Repeated vomiting, anorexia, and weight loss are important for diagnosis and to monitor for side effects of treatment.
Urinary and gastrointestinal systems	■ Evaluate frequency of urination and bowel elimination.
	■ Assess for intake and evidence of vomiting or food intolerance.
	■ Ask about blood or other discoloration in urine or stool.
	■ Be alert for urinary tract infections.
Musculoskeletal system	■ Observe for expected developmental tasks.
	■ Be alert for asymmetry of bone or muscle.
	■ Observe for limping and other abnormalities.
	■ Assess for muscle weakness, tingling, or numbness.
Family history	■ Assess for a family history of any cancer and particularly those that occur more commonly in families (Table 29–3).

Note: *Refer to Chapter 7 🔗 for the actual techniques of assessment mentioned in this table.

TABLE 29–2   Diagnostic Procedures and Laboratory Tests for Alterations in Cellular Growth*

DIAGNOSTIC PROCEDURES	LABORATORY TESTS
Biopsy	Complete blood count (CBC)
Bone marrow aspiration	Red blood cell indices
Computed tomography (CT) or computed axial tomography (CAT)	Serum chemistry panel
Lumbar puncture	Tumor markers in blood or urine—for example, urine for vanillylmandelic acid (VMA)
Magnetic resonance imaging (MRI)	Urinalysis
Positron emission tomography (PET) scan and single-photon emission computed tomography (SPECT)	
Radiograph (x-ray)	
Nuclear medicine scans	
Ultrasound	

Note: *See Appendixes D and E 🔗 for information about these diagnostic procedures and for expected laboratory test values.

that are diagnosed during childhood. Others cause cancers that begin in childhood but are not identified until adulthood. Some chemicals suspected of causing childhood cancer include diethylstilbestrol or DES (maternal use of therapeutic estrogen hormones), anabolic androgenic steroids, alkylating chemotherapy agents, and immunosuppressants used for organ transplantation. Radiation exposure has been known to cause cancers such as leukemia and thyroid tumors in children exposed to nuclear fallout from atomic bombs, other nuclear accidents, and other excessive radiation sources.

External stimuli may also lead to secondary cancers in children, or those occurring after treatment for a primary cancer and of a different cellular type than the primary cancer. Secondary cancers can result when the child is treated for a primary cancer with high doses of radiation. Excessive exposure to ultraviolet radiation from the sun predisposes children to development of skin cancer in adolescence and adulthood. See Chapter 36 🔗 for a discussion of sunburn and the risk of melanoma.

Immune System and Gene Abnormalities

One critical function of a normal immune system is immune surveillance, in which phagocytic cells circulate throughout the body, detecting and destroying abnormal and cancerous cells. Children with congenital immune deficiencies, such as Wiskott-Aldrich syndrome, in which

cellular growth and development (called **proto-oncogenes**) to related genes that allow unregulated cell division and cancerous growth (called **oncogenes**). Among the cancers thought to be linked to virus action and the change of proto-oncogenes to oncogenes are certain leukemias, rhabdomyosarcoma, Burkitt lymphoma, and some forms of Hodgkin disease.

Genetic changes can include autosomal dominant, autosomal recessive, and X-linked transfer. In these cases, the resulting cancers often occur relatively early in life. Cancers of these types are typically aggressive since the child has inherited the abnormal gene so it is within each cell, rather than a single mutation of one gene in a specific cell. Due to progress made in the Human Genome Project (see Chapter 4 🔗), there is increasing ability to perform genetic testing for certain familial cancers. Examples of cancers that are sometimes caused by genetic abnormalities within families include retinoblastoma (described later in this chapter), Wilms tumor (described in this chapter), multiple endocrine neoplasia type 2 (thyroid cancer), and familial adenomatous polyposis (invasive colon cancer). For example, as noted in Table 29–3, children who are missing a band of genetic material on chromosome 13 more frequently have retinoblastoma. Similarly, a Wilms tumor often develops in children missing part of the genetic material from chromosome 11. See Table 29–3 for several examples of cancers that are sometimes genetically linked within families.

Tumor suppressor genes counteract the effect of oncogenes, keeping cellular growth within normal limits. When tumor suppressor genes are missing, unregulated cellular growth can occur. These genes are commonly missing in children with retinoblastoma and Wilms tumor.

Chromosomal Abnormalities

Normal chromosomes undergo change as a part of the genetic process. Most of the changes are not harmful, although some result in chromosomal abnormalities such as hyperploidy (more than the normal number of chromosomes), deletion, translocation, and breakage.

Some other chromosomal abnormalities have been linked to an increased incidence of cancer. Children with the chromosomal disorder of Down syndrome have a relative risk 20 to 30 times higher for developing leukemia than nonaffected children; acute myeloid and lymphoblastic leukemia are the most common types (Zwaan, Reinhardt, Hitzler, et al., 2010). Children who are missing a band

Pathophysiology Illustrated
Proto-Oncogene Alteration

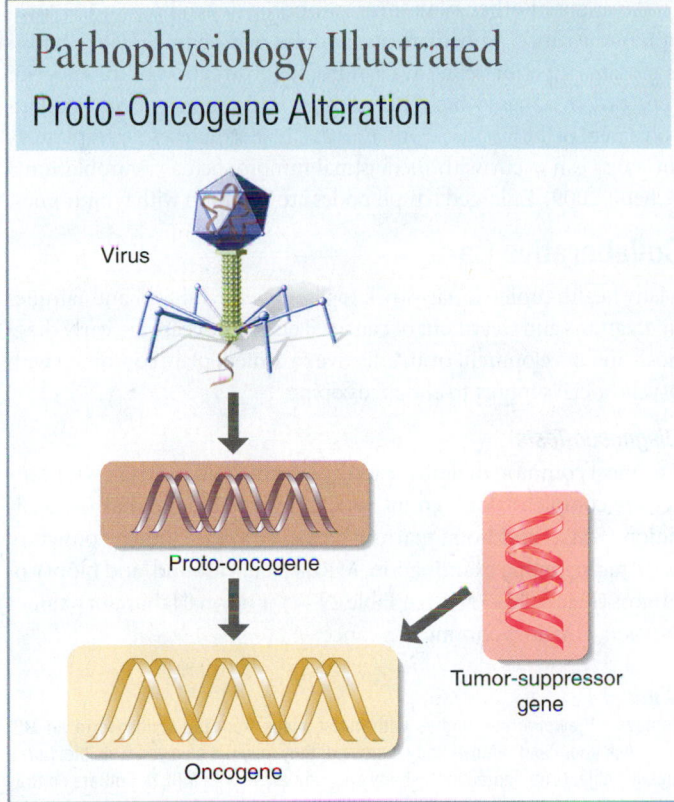

Virus

Proto-oncogene

Tumor-suppressor gene

Oncogene

FIGURE 29–2 ■ A proto-oncogene normally regulates cellular growth and development. When altered by a virus or other external cause, it can change to an oncogene, which allows unregulated genetic activity and tumor growth. Tumor-suppressor genes regulate the effects of oncogenes to decrease wildly proliferating cellular growth.

immune surveillance may fail, are at high risk for cancer. A form of non-Hodgkin lymphoma develops in some children treated with drugs that suppress the immune system. Children with acquired immunodeficiency syndrome (AIDS) may be at higher risk of certain types of cancer, such as Hodgkin disease, non-Hodgkin lymphoma, leiomyosarcoma, and Kaposi sarcoma (Sigel, Dubrow, Silverberg, et al., 2011).

Viruses and other substances may act in the body to alter the immune system, thereby allowing cancer to occur (Figure 29–2 ■). Their action is based on changing certain genes that normally regulate

TABLE 29–3	Types of Familial Cancers	
TYPE OF CANCER	**GENETIC LOCATION**	**DESCRIPTION**
Retinoblastoma	Chromosome 13q14, RB1 gene	Tumor of the eye retina
Wilms tumor	Chromosomal band 11p13, WT1 gene	Tumor of the kidney
Beckwith-Wiedemann syndrome	Chromosome 11p15, genes CDKN1C, KCNQ10T1, LIT1, H19, IGF2	Multiple abnormalities including tumors of kidney, liver, and adrenals; omphalocele, macroglossia
Multiple endocrine neoplasia, type 2	Chromosome 11q13, proto-oncogene RET mutation	Medullary thyroid cancer
Familial adenomatous polyposis	APC tumor suppressor gene mutation on chromosome 5q21	Invasive widespread colon polyps
Li-Fraumeni syndrome	Chromosome 17p13.1, 22q12.1, gene TP53 and CHEK2	Early-onset breast and other soft tissue cancers
Von Hippel–Lindau disease	VHL gene on chromosome 3p26-p35	Hemangioblastoma of retina, cerebellum, or spinal cord; renal cell carcinoma; pheochromocytoma

Source: *Data from Rao, A., Rothman, J., & Nichols, K. E. (2008). Genetic testing and tumor surveillance for children with cancer predisposition syndromes.* Current Opinion in Pediatrics, 20, *1–7.*

of genetic material on chromosome 13 often have retinoblastoma. Similarly, a Wilms tumor often develops in children missing a part of the genetic material from chromosome 11. While only about 10% of cancers are familial, careful history taking to identify cases of cancer in the family can lead to increased surveillance.

Regardless of the location and cause of abnormal cellular growth, the pathophysiologic process of cancer is similar. The altered cell begins to multiply as directed by the altered genetic structure of its DNA and the absence or inactivation of tumor suppressor genes. Each new cell transmits the altered pattern to the next generation. As the abnormal cells replicate, they form a growing neoplastic mass. Normal cells usually die as the increased metabolic rate of the neoplastic cells depletes available nutrition. The altered DNA in the tumor cells may also cause the abnormal cells to invade adjoining tissue. Through continued growth, the mass invades, disrupting a major vessel or a vital organ.

Clinical Manifestations

Each type of childhood cancer signals its presence differently. Because many of the presenting signs and symptoms of cancer are typical of common childhood illnesses, a delay in diagnosis can occur. In some cases, no symptoms are noted until the cancer is advanced. Children more commonly present with metastases (spread of the cancer to a site other than its origin) at time of diagnosis than do adults due to this difficulty in recognition of the disease. Common presenting symptoms of cancer are as follows:

- *Pain* may be the result of a neoplasm either directly or indirectly affecting nerve receptors through obstruction, inflammation, tissue damage, stretching of visceral tissue, or invasion of susceptible tissue. The pain may be in any body part, such as abdominal pain, bone and joint discomfort, or headache.
- **Cachexia** is a syndrome characterized by anorexia, weight loss, anemia, asthenia (weakness), and early satiety (feeling of being full).
- *Anemia* may be experienced during times of chronic blood loss or iron deficiency. In chronic illness the body uses iron poorly. Anemia is also present in cancers of the bone marrow when the number of red blood cells is reduced, in part because of the presence of large numbers of other bone marrow products. Treatment of cancer often promotes further anemia due to bone marrow suppression.
- *Infection* is usually a result of an altered or immature immune system. In addition, infection occurs when bone marrow cancers inhibit maturation of normal immune system cells. Infection may also occur in children who are treated with corticosteroids. Because their immune response is altered, the normal signs of infection may not appear.
- *Bruising* (*ecchymosis*) can occur if the bone marrow cannot produce enough platelets. Petechiae may be present. Prolonged bleeding can occur after minor trauma.
- *Neurologic symptoms* may result from impingement on the brain or nervous system. Signs of increased intracranial pressure, decreased or altered consciousness, eye abnormalities, or other neurologic or behavior changes may be evident.
- *A palpable mass* may be present for certain cancers. This is most commonly abdominal but may be in the neck, along lymph nodes, or in other sites.

A variety of other symptoms can occur depending on the location of the cancer. Subcutaneous nodules may appear if leukocytosis is present. Superior vena cava syndrome (obstruction of the superior vena cava by a mass which leads to increased venous pressure and involvement of the lungs and other mediastinal structures) or respiratory difficulty can occur with mediastinal tumors such as neuroblastoma (Cheng, 2009). Enlarged lymph nodes are common with lymphomas.

Collaborative Care

Many health professionals work together with children and families in diagnosis and treatment of cancer. The goals of care are early diagnosis and development of an effective treatment plan, combined with psychosocial support to enhance coping.

Diagnostic Tests

The most common diagnostic tests performed on children with cancer are complete blood count with differential, bone marrow aspiration (BMA) and bone marrow biopsy (BMBX), lumbar puncture (LP), radiographic examination, MRI, CT, ultrasound, and biopsy of tumors (Figure 29–3 ■). See Table 29–4 for normal laboratory values and abnormalities common in cancer.

Clinical Tip

Remove all jewelry and clothes with metal snaps from the child before an MRI scan. Ask about and remove body piercings; they may not always be visible. Some metallic objects implanted in the body are compatible with MRI, but others contraindicate the use of MRI. Metallic objects include orthodontic braces, metal dental bridgework, cochlear implants, surgical clips or plates, and orthopedic rods. When there are metal objects in the body, be certain to report them to the managing healthcare provider and radiology technician so they can determine if MRI is safe.

Additional tests of serum may be helpful in diagnosis. Studies useful for certain cancers include ultrasound, nuclear medicine

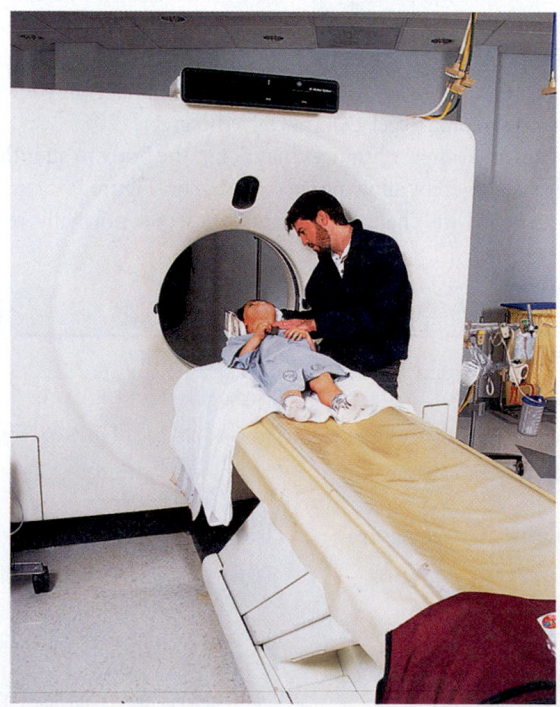

FIGURE 29–3 ■ Computed tomography (CT) can be a frightening procedure for children. This 2-year-old boy is comforted by his father before the procedure.

TABLE 29–4	Selected Diagnostic Tests for Childhood Cancer		
TEST *	**PURPOSE**	**NORMAL LABORATORY VALUES**	**DIAGNOSTIC VALUES**
Bone marrow aspiration	Examines bone marrow	Less than 5% blast cells (immature)	Greater than 25% blast cells in acute lymphoblastic leukemia, most with hypercellular marrow
Lumbar puncture	Examines cerebrospinal fluid	Cell count (in microliters) Polymorphonuclear leukocytes 0 Monocytes 0–5 RBCs 0–5	Presence of malignant cells indicates central nervous system involvement
Complete blood count and differential	Examines cellular components of blood	WBC less than 10,000/microliter Platelets 150,000–400,000/microliter Hemoglobin 12–16 g/dL	WBC less than 10,000/microliter Platelets 20,000–100,000/microliter Hemoglobin 7–10 g/dL
Absolute neutrophil count (ANC)	Blood component ratio: % of segmental neutrophils plus % of bands (immature neutrophils) times WBC count	ANC greater than 1,000	ANC less than 500 indicates risk of infection

Note: *See Appendixes D and E 🔗 for information about these diagnostic procedures and tests.

scans with radioactive isotopes such as gallium or iodine, bone scan with technetium 99m, or positron emission tomography (PET) and single-photon emission computed tomography (SPECT) that combine nuclear medicine with CT (Roach, Alberini, Pecking, et al., 2010). Specific tests such as pulmonary function tests and echocardiograms may be used at baseline to ensure normal organ function before initiating therapy.

The blood work is detailed and includes the following:

- Red blood cell (RBC) count, white blood cell (WBC) count, platelets (CBC with differential)
- Hemoglobin and hematocrit
- RBC indices such as mean corpuscular volume (MCV), mean corpuscular hemoglobin concentration (MCHC), and mean corpuscular hemoglobin (MCH)
- WBC indices (manual differential), which include the percent of all five types (basophils, eosinophils, monocytes, lymphocytes, and neutrophils; neutrophils are further divided into segmented and banded)
- Absolute neutrophil count (ANC) using both the segmented (mature) and band (immature) neutrophils as a measure of the body's infection-fighting capability
- Serum chemistry, which includes electrolytes, including sodium, potassium, chloride, calcium, magnesium, phosphorus, and carbon dioxide
- Additional studies that provide important diagnostic clues in some cases (for example, renal function studies such as blood urea nitrogen [BUN] and creatinine; liver studies such as total bilirubin, alanine aminotransferase [ALT], aspirate aminotransferase [AST], lactic dehydrogenase [LDH], and BUN; alkaline phosphatase may be elevated; uric acid is commonly elevated in leukemia)
- Certain substances, or markers, that are elevated with some specific tumors (for example, α-fetoprotein may be elevated in liver tumors, vanillylmandelic acid [VMA] and homovanillic acid [HVA] may be elevated in adrenal tumors, and elevated catecholamines are found in neuroblastoma)

Urinalysis is performed. It may show abnormal cells such as RBCs (hematuria) that may assist in diagnosis of kidney tumors. Histologic or laboratory analysis of tumor cells is often critical in diagnosis. A needle biopsy or endoscopic procedures of some tumors can be performed to obtain tumor cells. If the tumor is removed during surgery, the entire tumor is available for study. The borders are examined to be certain it has been totally removed, and lymph nodes may also be removed to analyze possible spread via lymph system.

The tests are aimed at identifying the source of the cancer and any metastases to additional sites. This enables the oncology specialist to stage the cancer. **Staging** refers to the process of labeling the type of cancer cells, severity, and spread, to determine the recommended treatment. Stage 1 indicates less severe cancer without spread to other parts of the body, and higher stages 2 through 4 indicate greater severity and spread to other sites.

Clinical Therapy

Clinical therapy for cancer is extremely complex and is managed by a specialist in pediatric oncology. The cancer itself is treated, its effects on the body are addressed, and side effects of treatment require management. Examples of the effects of cancer on the body include altered nutritional status from anorexia due to the cancer diverting nutrients to itself, decreased immune response from impaired manufacture of white blood cells and other immune components, and a variety of symptoms as a tumor presses on vital organs. In addition, cancer treatment itself has many potential side effects that require constant monitoring and adjustments in treatment.

Cancer is treated with one or a combination of several therapies including surgery, chemotherapy, radiation, biotherapy, and hematopoietic stem cell transplantation. Many families also choose some type of complementary therapy, in addition to traditional medical approaches. The treatment plan is determined by the type of cancer, site of primary tumor, and sites of metastasis (spread to other sites in the body).

The goal of treatment may be curative, supportive, and/or provision of end-of-life care. Curative treatment rids the child's body of the cancer. Supportive treatment includes transfusions, pain management, antibiotics, and other interventions to assist the body's defenses and increase the child's comfort. End-of-life treatment is designed to make the child as comfortable as possible when no curative treatment is possible (see Chapter 18 🔗 for a detailed discussion of end-of-life

Pathophysiology Illustrated Chemotherapy Drug Action

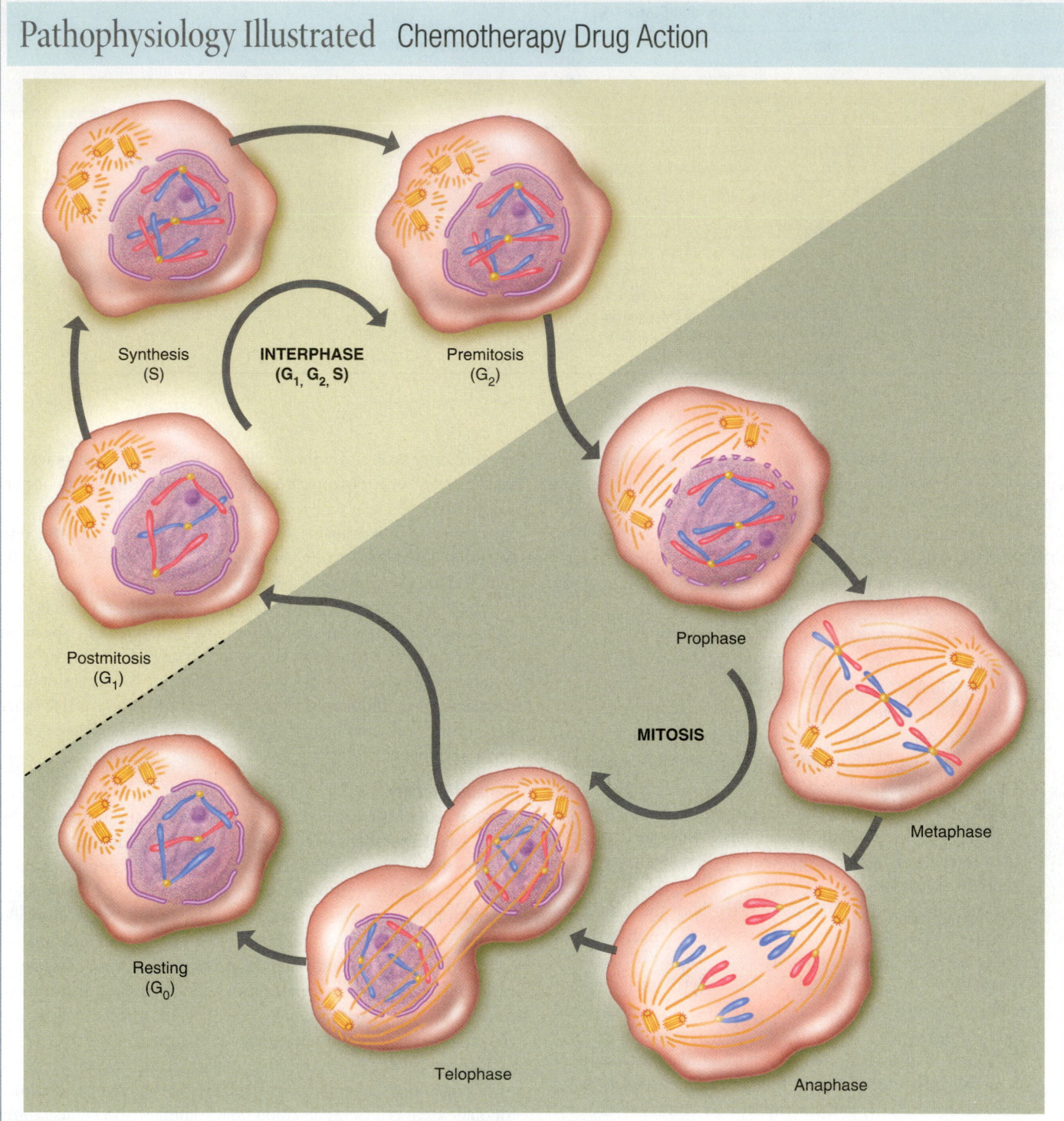

Synthesis
(S)

**INTERPHASE
(G₁, G₂, S)**

Premitosis
(G₂)

Postmitosis
(G₁)

Prophase

MITOSIS

Metaphase

Resting
(G₀)

Telophase

Anaphase

FIGURE 29–4 ■ Chemotherapy drugs either act at specific parts of the cell cycle or are nonspecific for action (act throughout all cell phases).

care for children). Whatever combination of treatment is used, families will have questions and need resources for information.

Surgery Surgery is used to remove or **debulk** (reduce the size of) a solid tumor. An example of a cancer that is commonly treated with surgery is a Wilms tumor. Surgery is also used to determine the stage and type of cancer since the tumor cells can be examined microscopically once removed, and various body organs can be inspected for signs of cancer during the surgery.

Chemotherapy **Chemotherapy** is the administration of specific drugs that kill both normal and cancerous cells. The administration of various chemotherapeutic drugs is timed to achieve the greatest cellular destruction. The schedule is determined by the cell's cycle of replication (Figure 29–4 ■). Several chemotherapeutic drugs are administered simultaneously to maximize their lethal impact on cells at all stages of activity. See the Medications table on pages 947–948.

Whereas DNA in a normal cell can repair itself after chemotherapy, the DNA in a neoplastic cell cannot. The particular chemotherapy

Medications Used for Cancer Chemotherapy

MEDICATION	ACTION/INDICATION	NURSING MANAGEMENT
Cell Cycle Specific Agents		
Antimetabolites ■ 5-Azacytidine ■ 5-Fluorouracil ■ 6-Mercaptopurine ■ 6-Thioguanine ■ Cytosine arabinoside (cytarabine) ■ Hydroxyurea ■ Methotrexate	The antimetabolites work at the synthesis phase of cell division, interfere with function of nucleic acid, and inhibit DNA or RNA synthesis.	Most common side effects are nausea and vomiting, myelosuppression, and mucositis. Specific agents such as methotrexate and cytarabine can cause neurologic toxicity with high doses. Consult drug books and package inserts for a detailed list of side effects. Obtain baseline CBC, liver function, and renal function. Monitor intake and output (I&O) and body weight. Ensure hydration and output levels ordered by the oncologist. Monitor vital signs (VS) and cardiovascular and respiratory function. Watch for ecchymosis or petechiae and signs of infection. Monitor carefully during administration for signs of anaphylaxis.
Vinca alkaloids ■ Etoposide ■ Teniposide ■ Irinotecan ■ Paclitaxel ■ Vinblastine ■ Vincristine	Act during mitosis; bind with cell proteins to inhibit nucleic acid and protein synthesis.	Common side effects include nausea and vomiting, abdominal cramping and diarrhea, constipation, paralytic ileus, hair loss, hypotension or hypertension, peripheral neuropathy, and neurologic toxicity (latter especially with vinblastine and vincristine). Obtain a baseline laboratory analysis of blood. Consult specific drug information for the period of maximum myelosuppressive effect. Be alert for bruising, petechiae, infection, and other signs of myelosuppression. Monitor carefully during administration for signs of anaphylaxis, particularly with etoposide and paclitaxel.
Miscellaneous—G_1 phase activity ■ L-asparaginase	Causes depletion of asparagine, needed by cancer cells; makes cell in G_1 phase vulnerable to other agents; interferes with prosynthesis. Used in combination with other agents in leukemia and other cancers.	Administer intravenously or intramuscularly. Major side effects are severe nausea and vomiting, renal failure, myelosuppression, and acid–base imbalance. Because of the risk of life-threatening hypersensitivity reactions, emergency medications and care must be immediately available. CBC, serum amylase, glucose, coagulation factors, bone marrow function, and liver function tests are performed before therapy and twice weekly. Monitor I&O, neurologic status, gastrointestinal symptoms, and abdominal pain.
Miscellaneous—G_2 phase activity ■ Etoposide	Works at G_2 phase; binds cellular proteins to cause metaphase arrest; also acts on S phase of DNA synthesis. Used with other agents, particularly in recurrent disease.	Administer orally and intravenously. Common side effects are nausea and vomiting, myelosuppression, hair loss, and diarrhea. Can cause anaphylaxis, hypotension, and IV site pain with rapid infusion. Perform baseline CBC, and liver and renal function tests. Check the IV site frequently since extravasation can cause necrosis. Monitor VS during infusion and stop drug if hypotension occurs. Keep emergency drugs and equipment readily available.
Cell Cycle Nonspecific Agents		
Alkylating agents ■ Cyclophosphamide ■ Carboplatin ■ Cisplatin ■ Busulfan ■ Chlorambucil ■ Ifosfamide ■ Thiotepa ■ Mechlorethamine ■ Melphalan ■ Procarbazine ■ Dacarbazine	Substitute an alkyl group for a hydrogen atom, leading to blockage of DNA replication. Used for treatment of many cancers, either alone or in conjunction with other agents.	Most are administered orally and/or intravenously. An array of side effects depends on the specific drug. Some common side effects are nausea and vomiting, diarrhea, myelosuppression, hair loss, neuropathies, pulmonary toxicity, hemorrhagic cystitis, and renal damage; secondary tumors later in life are associated with some agents. Obtain CBC and full blood analysis before and during treatment. Monitor for side effects of the specific agents administered. Ensure generous hydration, monitor for blood in urine, and evaluate I&O. Mesna may be administered with some alkylating agents to lower the risk of hemorrhagic cystitis. Teach the family the importance of long-term monitoring for secondary tumors.

(continued)

Medications Used for Cancer Chemotherapy (*continued*)

MEDICATION	ACTION/INDICATION	NURSING MANAGEMENT
Antibiotics ■ Doxorubicin ■ Mitomycin-C ■ Dactinomycin ■ Bleomycin ■ Daunorubicin ■ Idarubicin ■ Mitoxantrone	Interfere with nucleic acid, inhibiting DNA or RNA synthesis. Used in combination with other agents to treat leukemia and other childhood cancers.	Most are administered intravenously. Common side effects include nausea and vomiting, myelosuppression, mucositis, and skin and pulmonary toxicity. Several have cumulative dose toxicity, such as cardiac abnormalities (doxorubicin) and skin/pulmonary abnormalities (bleomycin); the total dose the child has received must be monitored. Obtain baseline CBC and other blood studies and monitor throughout therapy. Monitor VS, lung function, cardiac function, and neurologic status throughout and following therapy. Be alert for signs of myelosuppression and mucositis.
Nitrosoureas ■ Carmustine ■ Lomustine	Cross breakage in DNA strands so that DNA and RNA replication cannot occur. Used in lymphomas and other childhood cancers. Can cross blood-brain barrier.	Administer orally (lomustine) or intravenously (carmustine). The major side effect is myelosuppression. Others include pulmonary fibrosis, eye infarction, skin changes, hair loss, nausea, and vomiting. Obtain baseline and periodic CBC and other studies. Monitor pulmonary function, skin, and signs of infection or bleeding such as ecchymosis or petechiae.
Hormones ■ Prednisone ■ Prednisolone ■ Dexamethasone	Analog of hydrocortisone; anti-inflammatory; delayed and depressed immune response. Used in conjunction with other agents for many types of childhood cancer.	Often administered orally. Numerous side effects include edema, moon face, mood lability, increased appetite, disturbed sleep, immunosuppression, disturbed glucose control, and osteoporosis. Teach the child and family the effects of the drug. Minimize exposure to persons with infection. Monitor for infections in all systems. Monitor weight regularly. Take VS. Teach to take as directed. Drug must be tapered slowly at the end of therapy.
Topoisomerase I inhibitor ■ Irinotecan ■ Mitoxantrone ■ Topotecan	Inhibit the enzyme topoisomerase I in the cell nucleus, relaxing DNA and preventing its duplication. Used in conjunction with other agents to treat acute lymphocytic leukemia and other childhood cancers.	Administer intravenously; topotecan can be given intrathecally. Common side effects include nausea and vomiting, diarrhea, fever, dehydration, and myelosuppression. Can alter liver function and cause skin changes. Obtain baseline and periodic CBC and other studies, including liver function. Monitor for signs of myelosuppression, gastrointestinal distress, and change in liver function.

treatment protocol used is based on research into different types of cancer cells. A **protocol** is a plan of action for chemotherapy that is based on the results of staging: type of cancer, its stage and location, and the particular cell type (Figure 29–5 ■).

Other drugs used in the treatment of children with cancer include colony-stimulating factors, antiemetics, and nutritional supplements. Colony-stimulating factors are hormone-like glycoproteins that enhance blood cell production and counteract the myelosuppressive effects of chemotherapy drugs. (See the Medications table on page 949.) For example, erythropoietin is produced in the kidney, and a recombinant form (epoetin) can be used to treat anemia of cancer, thereby decreasing the number of transfusions needed. Filgrastim (Neupogen) increases production of neutrophils by the bone marrow. Antiemetics, such as ondansetron (Zofran), can be used to treat the nausea and vomiting that are common side effects of therapy. Nutritional supplements can be given to maintain nutritional status. Some children may need periodic treatment with antibiotics or antiviral drugs to treat infections that occur as a result of decreased immune response.

Cancer chemotherapy is complex and requires care by specialists in oncology. Many drugs have severe side effects during the administration period. These side effects may require administration of other drugs for their treatment. Some medications may have late side effects that occur after therapy is completed, while others are associated with different cancers in the future. The chemotherapeutic regimen often becomes even more complicated with very young children due to their inability to metabolize and excrete certain drugs. Administration of chemotherapy drugs requires specialized knowledge by the nurse. Follow the guidelines for handling of substances posing occupational hazard from the Occupational Safety and Health Administration (OSHA) and guidelines from the Association of Pediatric Hematology/Oncology Nurses.

Radiation Radiation therapy involves the use of unstable isotopes that release varying levels of energy to cause breaks in the DNA molecule and thereby destroy cells. Radiation has been used as a treatment method since the early 1900s, shortly after its discovery. It is often used for the local and regional control of cancer, and in combination with surgery and chemotherapy. It may be either curative or palliative. Examples of cancers treated with radiation include Hodgkin disease, Wilms tumor, retinoblastoma, rhabdomyosarcoma, and CNS

Protocol = Map or plan of action

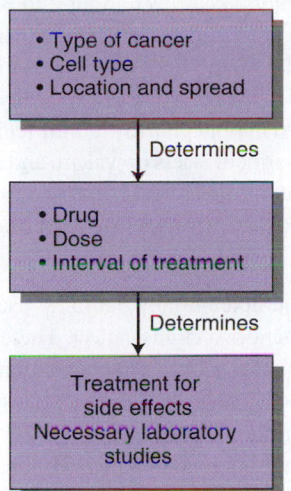

FIGURE 29–5 ■ Chemotherapy protocol. A protocol is a map or plan of action that directs therapy by identifying the drug and its accompanying treatment.

disease in leukemia. Tumors that have a low sensitivity to radiation, such as osteosarcoma and soft tissue sarcomas, require higher doses of radiation or may be treated by other therapies.

The area to be irradiated (treatment field) includes the tumor site and sometimes other involved areas, such as lymph glands. The goal is to irradiate the tumor but not healthy adjacent tissue. The total dose of radiation is divided (or fractionated) and given over several weeks. A common course of radiation treatment might be once daily 4 or 5 days per week for a period of 2 to 7 weeks.

Clinical Tip
Nurses who care for a child receiving implant radiation or who work in a radiation department wear a dosimeter film badge at all times to measure their exposure to radiation. The cumulative radiation exposure is thus measured. The nurse must avoid radiation exposure for a period of time if recommended levels are exceeded.

Biotherapy **Biotherapy** is the use of biological retooling and molecular intervention to produce targeted cancer therapy. Biological retooling uses parts of the human body that are programmed to destroy cells, and applies them to the cancer cells. An example of this technique includes development of antibodies that are tumor specific to certain cancers and produced by the body in response to antigens of cancer cells (Hantel, Lewrick, Schneider, et al., 2010). These antibodies promote apoptosis or death of the cancerous cells. Another example is the group of drugs that stimulate the body's own immune response (Fry & Lankester, 2008). The actions of many biotherapy agents are not completely understood, and some agents have more than one effect. For example, interferon has both antiviral and antiproliferative effects on some malignant cells. Interferon and tumor necrosis factor (TNF) are undergoing clinical trials to study their effectiveness and to develop protocols for their safe use against selected

Medications Used During Cancer Treatment: Colony-Stimulating Factors

MEDICATION	ACTION/INDICATION	NURSING MANAGEMENT
Epoetin alfa (human recombinant erythropoietin)	This glycoprotein stimulates the bone marrow in RBC formation; useful when numbers of RBCs are low due to chemotherapy effects.	Give subcutaneously or intravenously. Do not shake and do not use if discolored or particles are present. Vials are used for a single dose only so any unused medication should be discarded. Obtain CBC before therapy and periodically after; improvement in hematocrit should be seen in 7–14 days. Monitor blood pressure before and during therapy as hypertension can result. Monitor for changes in neurologic response and headache; both seizures and strokes are possible side effects.
Filgrastim (Neupogen) and pegfilgrastim (Neulasta)	This human granulocyte colony-stimulating factor (G-CSF) increases production of neutrophils by the bone marrow.	Administer subcutaneously or intravenously; prepare as directed for IV infusion to prevent its absorption by IV tubing. Single-dose vials only, so discard any solution that is not used. Incompatible with many medications; check package insert; do not give within 24 hours before or after chemotherapy drugs or their effect may be decreased. Obtain baseline and twice-weekly CBC. Monitor for side effects such as bone pain and heart arrhythmias; report fevers and be alert for other signs of infection when neutrophil count is low.
Oprelvekin (Neumega)	A hematopoietic growth factor, interleukin-11, that increases platelet count; useful in low platelet count due to chemotherapy effects on bone marrow.	Administer subcutaneously. Single-dose vials only, so discard any solution that is not used. Obtain baseline CBC and platelet count; monitor platelets throughout treatment. Monitor for side effects such as edema, fever, CNS changes, tachycardia, respiratory problems, and skin rash. Take daily weights and monitor for fluid retention.

The National Center for Complementary and Alternative Medicine Website

Weblink

cancers. Cancer vaccines are under development that may work to help the body fight cancers; a first in this group is human papillomavirus vaccine (see Chapter 22 for further detail).

Molecular targeting involves interference with metabolic pathways (for example, through enzyme disruption) in the tumor cells. It may therefore disturb the cell's growth and development and thereby depress proliferation. For example, the signaling system in cancer cells that leads to proliferation is triggered by kinases, a specific type of enzyme that leads to transfer of phosphates among molecules. Drug therapy can interfere with the action of kinases, leading to cancer cell proliferation arrest (Hu, Lee, Qiu, et al., 2009).

An additional type of biological therapy is gene therapy, or attempting to replace a faulty gene with one that is normal. Genetic technology is rapidly growing and shows promise for future treatment of cancer and other childhood diseases. This complex field includes research to identify genes that lead to disease, recombinant techniques to enable genetic engineering, and studies of enzymes active in DNA and RNA formation. Nurses need to have enhanced knowledge of this important work as technologies are increasingly applied in cancer treatment (National Human Genome Research Institute, 2009).

Bone marrow and hematopoietic stem cell transplantation

Bone marrow and hematopoietic stem cell transplantation (HSCT) are used to treat leukemia, neuroblastoma, and some noncancerous conditions such as aplastic anemia (National Cancer Institute, 2008). The goal of therapy is to administer a lethal dose of chemotherapy and radiation that will kill the cancer, and then to resupply the body with stem cells either from the child's own bone marrow that was previously removed (autologous transplant) and stored or from a compatible donor (allogeneic transplant). Umbilical cord blood is another source of stem cells used for transplant. Peripheral blood stem cells are increasingly being used for transplant. The donor, whether autologous or allogeneic, can be given growth factors prior to donation to stimulate production of stem cells. An advantage of peripheral stem cells is that they can be collected somewhat less painfully and invasively than by the procedure of a bone marrow aspiration; however, a catheter is required to collect the blood stem cells.

Transplantation has become the treatment of choice for some cancers when a relapse occurs while the child is receiving another form of cancer therapy and for primary treatment of certain cancers. First, a histocompatible donor must be located. The child then receives intensive chemotherapy, often followed by total body irradiation. Beginning 7 to 10 days before the transplant, the treatment kills all circulating blood cells and bone marrow contents. Supportive care is needed to treat the effects of nausea, diarrhea, and pain. Following this treatment, the child is intravenously transfused with the transplant stem cells. New blood cells usually form within 2 to 8 weeks. (See Chapter 27 for a description of care for the child undergoing transplantation.)

Stem cells that become established in the host child's bone marrow can also be obtained from newborn umbilical cord blood. For some children this has become a better option than waiting for a matching bone marrow donor. Cord blood can be easily collected at birth from a sibling of the ill child, as histocompatible matches often occur in siblings, or cord blood banks may offer a match. The umbilical cord blood is then infused into the child undergoing treatment and

the same mechanism occurs as in transplantation of bone marrow—implantation of the stem cells into the child's bone marrow and production of normal blood cells over about 2 to 6 weeks. Advantages of umbilical cord blood are that, unlike bone marrow collection, it is not painful for the donor and does not require anesthesia; there is an opportunity to easily collect samples from many ethnic groups that are underrepresented in bone marrow donor registries; graft-versus-host disease after treatment is less prevalent; and storage of umbilical cord blood for use later in life is possible. A variety of federally funded and private blood banks are available to store and provide umbilical blood.

Complementary therapies

Many families use **complementary therapies** in treatment of a child's cancer. These approaches to care are also referred to as alternative or unconventional, and may involve nutritional supplements, oral herbal supplements, touch therapy, and mind–body interventions. Little research has been done on complementary therapies, although up to 80% of children have used at least one such therapeutic approach (Decker, 2008; Paisley, Kang, Insogna, et al., 2011).

Mind–body therapies and touch, such as meditation, prayer, and yoga, are the most frequently used approaches. Some people use nutrition and herbal therapies with foods such as vitamins, carrots, garlic, green tea, cabbage, citrus fruits, ginger root, and willow bark (Decker, 2008; Tomlinson, Hesser, Ethier, et al., 2011). Healthcare providers should be aware of these practices, inquire in a nonjudgmental manner about what therapies are used, and attempt to learn about specific therapies and practices. Although some herbal and nutritional products such as St. John's wort may decrease serum concentration of chemotherapeutic agents, or some may act as hormones in the body, most are not known to negatively affect contemporary medical treatment (see Complementary Therapy: Cancer Prevention). Intake of fruits and vegetables is associated with lower cancer incidence in adults, and some foods such as garlic and oranges may slow cancer growth or enhance medical chemotherapy. Some individuals use herbal supplements to treat cancer; these include cat's claw (bark of a tree root), mistletoe, and shark cartilage. The U.S. Food and Drug Administration (FDA) has allowed testing of the efficacy of some herbal treatments for cancer. Some herbs are useful in treatment of nausea and vomiting, and others can boost the immune system's function. Several cancer drugs such as vincristine and paclitaxel are obtained from plant products.

End-of-life care

Despite modern medical practices and complementary therapies, some children do not survive childhood cancer. In these cases, the focus of health care is to provide comfort and emotional support for the child and family. Too often, healthcare providers feel uncomfortable when a child is expected to die and may withdraw from close contact with the child or family, fail to provide adequate comfort measures, and leave the family without access to needed resources. When delay in the recognition of prognosis occurs, children can experience greater suffering and potentially less integration of end-of-life (or palliative) care. Some of the symptoms for which children are commonly undertreated include pain, dyspnea, nutrition, elimination, and fatigue. Additionally, care may be required from a wide array of specialists, which can lead to fragmentation of care and lack of integrated palliative approaches (Baker, Hinds, Spunt, et al., 2008).

Complementary Therapy Cancer Prevention

Many parents ask what they can do to decrease the incidence of cancer in children as they grow into adulthood. The major teaching areas address complementary health practices. They are:

1. Have children increase intake of fruits and vegetables. Most children do not eat recommended amounts of these foods, and increased intake is associated with lower rates of many cancers. Aim for a minimum of five servings daily.

2. Protect skin with sunscreen. Early excessive exposure to sun, and having had one or repeated severe sunburns during childhood, increases chances of skin cancers developing in adulthood. Tanning bed exposure is a prime risk factor for skin cancer; all children and adolescents, and particularly those with cancer, should strictly avoid tanning beds (Greinert & Boniol, 2011).

3. Discourage smoking among children and be sure children are not exposed to environmental tobacco smoke. This will decrease the future chance of developing lung cancer.

4. Have homes tested for radon. Be alert for exposure to any potential hazardous substances in the home or on parents' clothes if they work in industries with chemicals or other harmful substances.

5. When there is a history of cancer in the family, particularly if it is a type associated with familial incidence such as some breast or ovarian cancers, encourage the family to learn more about the cancer and teach children to receive regular surveillance as they enter young adulthood.

6. Inform youth in all families about screening such as the Papanicolaou test, breast self-examination, and testicular examination that can lead to early detection.

The presence of an end-of-life care team and an integrated plan of care; collaboration between families, the primary care provider, and other practitioners; and focus on the child's developmental level and the needs of the family can enhance the care provided for the child who is dying. An advance directive that outlines the care plans for the child is helpful in preserving the child's quality of life and increasing the child's and family's comfort. See Chapter 18 ⊘ for a detailed description of end-of-life care for children with terminal disease.

Special Issues in Childhood Cancer

Oncologic emergencies Oncologic emergencies result from the cancer itself or as a side effect of treatment. They can be organized into three groups: metabolic, hematologic, and those involving space-occupying lesions. Overall, the most common oncologic emergencies are tumor lysis syndrome, septic shock, brain herniation, spinal cord compression, and superior vena cava compression from a superior mediastinal mass.

Metabolic emergencies Metabolic emergencies result from the lysis (dissolving or decomposing) of tumor cells, a process called *tumor lysis syndrome*. This cell destruction releases high levels of uric acid, potassium, calcium, and phosphates into the blood, resulting in hyperuricemia, hyperphosphatemia, hypocalcemia (due to precipitation with available phosphates to create calcium phosphate), and hyperkalemia. Low levels of sodium result, potentially leading to metabolic acidosis, cardiac arrhythmias, and renal failure. Tumor lysis syndrome is seen most commonly in children with non-Hodgkin lymphoma (especially the subtype Burkitt lymphoma) and acute lymphocytic leukemia (Zonfrillo, 2009). See the Clinical Manifestations table below for laboratory findings and management of tumor lysis syndrome.

A second type of metabolic emergency is septic shock. During periods of immune suppression the child is vulnerable to overwhelming infection, resulting in circulatory failure, hypothermia or hyperthermia, tachypnea, mental changes, inadequate tissue perfusion, and hypotension. Septic shock can be fatal (see Chapter 26 ⊘ for a full description of septic shock), so early and aggressive therapy is needed (Da Silva, Koch Nogueira, Russo Zamataro, et al., 2008). Factors contributing to massive infection include inadequate neutrophil production, abnormal granulocytes (not able to be actively phagocytic), erosions through normal barriers such as blood vessels and mucous membranes, and altered bone marrow production caused by chemotherapy and some forms of radiation. Such infections must be vigorously treated with antimicrobial therapy and hydration management.

A third type of metabolic emergency occurs when large amounts of bone are destroyed by treatment, resulting in hypercalcemia (elevated calcium in the serum). Hypercalcemia is most common in older children with acute lymphoblastic leukemia. Treatment includes hydration and adequate intake of phosphate by oral supplement (Trehan, Cheetham, & Bailey, 2009).

Clinical Manifestations and Management of Tumor Lysis Syndrome

ETIOLOGY	CLINICAL MANIFESTATIONS	CLINICAL THERAPY	NURSING MANAGEMENT
Breakdown of malignant cells releases intracellular components into blood.	Hyperuricemia Hyperkalemia Hyperphosphatemia Hypocalcemia	■ Vigorous hydration with 2–4 times maintenance fluid ■ Correction of electrolyte imbalances ■ Administration of allopurinol or urate oxidase (rasburicase) to reduce conversion of metabolic by-products to uric acid ■ Administration of calcium to treat hypocalcemia and resultant tetany	■ Administer fluids, beginning before therapy. ■ Carefully measure intake and output. ■ Check weight daily. ■ Urine specific gravity should remain less than 1.010. ■ Monitor for desired and side effects of drug therapy.
Electrolyte imbalance causes metabolic acidosis and serious abnormalities.	Cardiac arrhythmias Impaired renal function Tetany, neurologic and mental status changes	■ ECG monitoring ■ Medications such as furosemide to facilitate potassium excretion ■ Dialysis may be needed	■ Administer electrolytes and medications. ■ Urine pH should remain 7.0 to 7.5. ■ Perform Trousseau and Chvostek signs for tetany monitoring and assess neurologic function (see Chapter 33 ⊘). ■ Perform mental status examination. ■ Obtain laboratory specimens as needed.

Some children develop syndrome of inappropriate antidiuretic hormone (SIADH) and have excessive release of ADH. The resulting decreased urinary output leads to water intoxication. See Chapter 32 🔗 for a detailed description of SIADH.

Hematologic emergencies Hematologic emergencies result from bone marrow suppression or infiltration of brain and respiratory tissue with high numbers of leukemic blast cells (hyperleukocytosis). Bone marrow suppression results in anemia and **thrombocytopenia** (decreased platelets) with resultant coagulation disturbance and hemorrhage. Disseminated intravascular coagulation (DIC) occurs in some children and is a life-threatening complication. (See Chapter 28 🔗 for a thorough description of this condition.) Gastrointestinal and central nervous system bleeding (strokes) can occur. Hyperviscosity of the blood can result from increased blood cellular components. For example, disruption of normal WBCs may result in hyperleukocytosis or leukostasis.

Treatment involves infusion of packed red blood cells for anemia and platelet transfusion, vitamin K, and fresh frozen plasma for thrombocytopenia and hemorrhage. Hyperviscosity is treated by plasmapheresis, hydroxyurea, and close management of chemotherapy. Respiratory and other vital support is needed (Granger & Kontoyiannis, 2009; Lewis, Hendrickson, & Moynihan, 2011).

Space-occupying lesions Extensive tumor growth may result in spinal cord compression, increased intracranial pressure, brain herniation, seizures, massive hepatomegaly, gastrointestinal obstruction, cardiac and respiratory complications, and superior vena cava syndrome (obstruction of the superior vena cava by tumor). These emergencies are often caused by neuroblastoma, medulloblastoma, astrocytoma, Hodgkin disease, or lymphoma. After biopsy of the mass, treatment involves radiation therapy, chemotherapy, and corticosteroids.

Psychosocial needs

The diagnosis of cancer is devastating for families. They cannot believe that their vibrant, young child or adolescent has a potentially life-threatening disease. Families are in a state of crisis when the diagnosis is made, with the first response one of shock. At the same time that they are in a state of shock about the diagnosis, parents must gather resources to support the child, make treatment decisions, and adjust family life to integrate the needs of the child with cancer. Some families need to travel a great distance for the child's treatments, and others may have financial constraints that make healthcare costs a major concern. For nearly everyone, parental work schedules and arrangements for other children must be adjusted. Both father and mother should be included in plans of care; extended families may also be important. Most cancer treatment will last for a minimum of several months up to several years, necessitating nearly constant adaptation.

The child reacts to the diagnosis based on age:

- Infants and toddlers are unaware of the severity of the disease and deal with issues such as pain and separation from parents.
- Preschoolers are beginning to understand illness. However, they may think they caused their illness, and they may be confused about why the parent cannot make the illness go away.
- School-age children can understand a diagnosis of cancer and benefit from opportunities to talk about the experience.
- Adolescents find contact with others who have gone through their experience reassuring and supportive.

Nearly all children are hospitalized after diagnosis, and care should include close proximity to parents, involvement in self-care appropriate for age, positive relationships with staff, and emotional care. Programs such as group therapy sessions, computer programs about cancer and treatment, and school reintegration can assist youth who are adjusting to cancer.

There has been some controversy about whether children with cancer have higher depression rates than other children. It is not clear whether the rates differ. Measurements of depression in children who are getting treatments that influence physical comfort are often not reliable. Anxiety about the disease or treatment may be interpreted as depression, and medications for cancer treatment may influence mood or affect (Kurtz & Abrams, 2010; National Cancer Institute, 2011a). Careful assessment of all children with cancer and communication with families to compare the child's present mood to that prior to treatment is important.

Cancer survival

Children with cancer have a variety of common psychologic and physiologic problems, regardless of their specific type of cancer. They and their families are dealing with a complex illness that influences their lives for years. The impact of this experience extends into all areas of function. Over the past 20 to 30 years, treatment for childhood cancers has been increasingly successful, and 80% of children with cancer are now expected to have long-term survival (Oeffinger, Nathan, & Kremer, 2008). The success of new modalities and treatment combinations has, however, created special healthcare needs for many survivors.

Surgery can have many results. Body organs may be removed and manipulated, leading to adhesions, intestinal obstruction, visual impairment, neurologic disruption, and sterility. Removal of the spleen can lead to serious infections. Amputation necessitates the need for prosthetic devices and physical rehabilitation.

Radiation has several long-term effects. It can impair the growth of bones and teeth, leading to conditions such as scoliosis, leg length discrepancy, osteoporosis, or poor dental health. Chronic pain can result from skeletal toxicity (Kaste, 2008). Hypothyroidism can be observed in those who have had head and neck radiation. Cardiotoxicity and pulmonary toxicity can result from mediastinal radiation, while delayed puberty and sterility can result from radiation effects to the cranium and spinal regions. Impaired neurocognitive performance, such as learning difficulties and behavioral change, may occur as long-term effects of treatment, especially with higher doses of radiation (American Cancer Society, 2009).

Secondary cancers, most commonly solid tumors, occur in some survivors. Secondary cancers are also called second malignant neoplasm (SMN). They occur subsequent to the primary cancer and treatment but are of a different histologic type. Although radiation is responsible for most secondary tumors, some chemotherapy drugs have also been implicated. Cancers of the CNS, skin, breast, bone, and thyroid are examples of secondary neoplasms (Reulen, Frobisher, Winter, et al., 2011). Most of these cancers can be effectively treated, emphasizing the need for thorough and frequent monitoring of the treated cancer patient. Other chronic conditions, such as heart failure, congestive heart failure, and cognitive dysfunction, are more common in cancer survivors who are adults than in the general population, while cardiovascular risk and insulin resistance may even be more prevalent in child cancer survivors (Steinberger, Sinaiko, Kelly, et al., 2012). Reproductive health can pose problems as the survivor reaches young adulthood and wishes to have children.

Chemotherapy can cause a wide variety of effects, both during its administration and for years afterward. See the Clinical Manifestations table on page 961. Cardiomyopathy can occur with some drugs, especially the anthracyclines. Temporary or permanent pulmonary toxicity and renal complications can develop. Neurologic effects of some drugs can lead to hearing loss (e.g., cisplatin and ifosfamide), cataracts, and paraplegia (e.g., intrathecal methotrexate for leukemia). Learning disabilities and change in intelligence quotient (IQ) occur in some children. Infertility may result. The effects of cancer and its treatment can manifest in childhood and may continue to adulthood, influencing employment and health (Kirchhoff, Krull, Ness, et al., 2011).

The diagnosis and stress of treatment, along with the risk of recurrence, are significant stressors for the child with cancer. Families may find it difficult to obtain full insurance coverage for the child who has had a prior cancer. Employment can be a potential problem for cancer survivors if employers have concerns about the earlier cancer diagnosis. Most people with cancer report fear of recurrence of the disease, which is a stressor. Some children report decreased quality of life (QOL) and emotional distress (Kurtz & Abrams, 2010; Winick, 2011; Zeltzer, Recklitis, Buchbinder, et al., 2009).

Conversely, hopefulness and the sense of having an added purpose in life can be positive outcomes for many cancer survivors. Some survivors meet with others who have a recent diagnosis, and both children and their families sometimes participate in fund-raising events that financially support cancer research. Survivorship services and care plans promote positive health outcomes (Eshelman-Kent, Kinahan, Hobbie, et al., 2011).

Barriers to optimal care for cancer survivors include inadequate time and programs to deal with survivor assessments, lack of knowledge about survivorship by healthcare professionals, and limited information and research on survivorship issues. Therefore, additional education of healthcare professionals, survivors, and the public, as well as research into survivor issues, is recommended (Eshelman-Kent et al., 2011; Soliman & Agresta, 2008).

Nursing Management

The complex nature of cancer is reflected in multifaceted nursing care. Oncology nursing is a specialty chosen by some nurses who manage the nursing care of children during the diagnostic and treatment phases. Other nurses such as those in schools, home health care, offices/clinics, and hospice care partner with oncology nurses to plan and provide for the child and family undergoing cancer treatment. Advanced practice nurses such as nurse practitioners often play key roles in both hospital and community management. Nursing interventions focus on preventive teaching for all families about risk factors for cancer, health promotion and health maintenance of the child undergoing cancer treatment, carrying out the treatment interventions, managing health problems related to both cancer and the side effects of treatment, and partnering with families to manage the challenging psychosocial needs that emerge when cancer is diagnosed.

Nursing Assessment and Diagnosis
History

During health promotion visits of all children, nurses are aware of the importance of a history of cancer in the family. Particularly when more than one person has had cancer, and when young children in the extended family have been affected, complete a pedigree to isolate cases in the family. (See Chapter 4 🔗.) A history of exposure to known carcinogens is also important. Does a parent work in an industry with chemicals or asbestos that might remain on clothing worn home? Was the child treated with radiation or chemotherapy for a previous cancer? Does the child have an identified condition such as Down syndrome? Does the child have any recognized congenital anomalies? A number of conditions are more commonly associated with certain types of cancer (see Table 29–3).

Physiologic Assessment

When performing any physiologic assessment on children, the nurse considers the possible signs and symptoms of cancer. These include anemia, frequent infections, bleeding disorders, loss of weight, fatigue, pain, and changes in mental health and neurologic status. Assessment of children with the most significant types of childhood cancers is presented in separate sections throughout this chapter.

Once cancer has been diagnosed, a thorough physical assessment of all systems is needed to help in identifying the presence and extent of cancer (see Chapter 7 🔗). Systems needing particularly thorough assessments are neurologic, respiratory, cardiac, and gastrointestinal. Assess hydration status and the tumor site if it is visible. These assessments will be completed regularly at each treatment and monitoring visit. Height and weight should be carefully measured and compared with prior findings for the child. Nutritional intake histories may be pertinent. Assess immunization status, developmental milestones, gait and coordination, and any changes in mental status. Evaluate pain, fatigue, infections, bruising, petechiae, shortness of breath, and elimination problems. Periodic laboratory studies will be performed.

Psychosocial Assessment

Assessment of stress and coping abilities, knowledge of the condition and cognitive level, support systems, developmental level, and body image provides data that help determine the appropriate nursing interventions for the child with cancer and the family.

Stress and Coping

The diagnosis of cancer is a major stressor for both the child and the family. Although each child's prognosis and each family's coping mechanisms are unique, most families deal with the diagnosis in a manner similar to that of other families who have a child with a life-threatening illness (see Chapter 17 🔗). Consider that some families are competent and adapt to stresses with supportive surroundings. They demonstrate resilience and the ability to assist the child and all of their members. Other families, however, may be experiencing multiple stresses, making adaptation to the new diagnosis particularly difficult. Individualization of assessment and intervention approaches will be needed to facilitate psychosocial care.

Assess the family (and child if old enough) for understanding and acceptance of the diagnosis. Evaluate if the family has told the child about the diagnosis and whether the family needs assistance in deciding how to do this. Ask what they have told siblings, and if they need suggestions, help, and support to decide how and when to share information with the child's siblings.

Assess the level of anxiety during healthcare visits and scheduled treatments (Figure 29–6 ■). Evaluate the family's resilience and methods of coping, such as the ability to integrate relaxing and meaningful activities into family life, the use of support systems in the extended family and community, and the ability to alter expectations to take into account the child's health status. Concurrent stressors increase

Weblink | The Association of Pediatric Hematology and Oncology Nurses Website

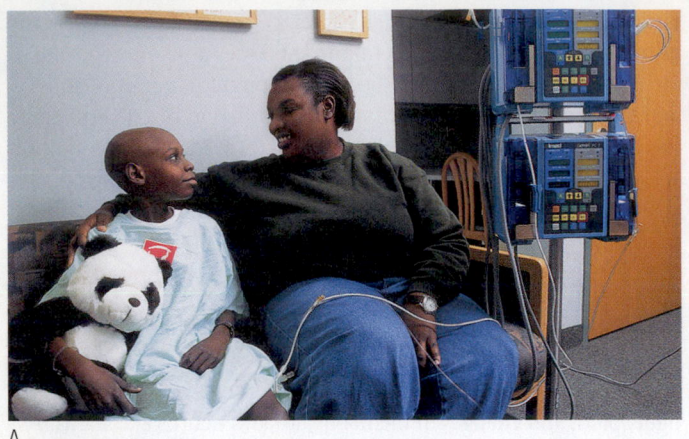

A

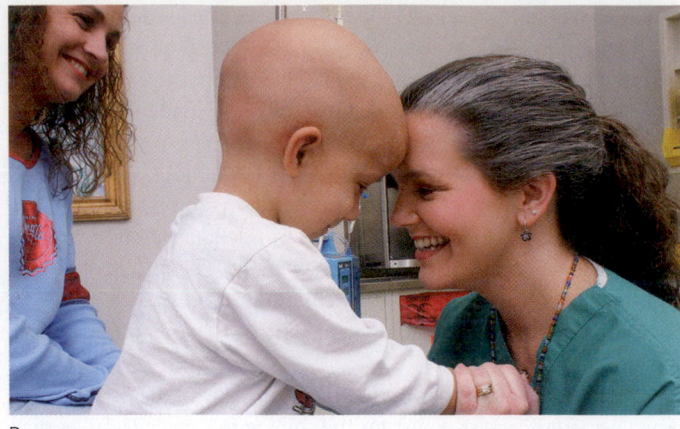

B

FIGURE 29–6 ■ *A*, The child with cancer depends on parents and family members to provide support. *B*, A special relationship often develops between the nurse and the child receiving treatment.

the family's difficulty in coping with childhood cancer. Evaluate the family for stressors such as illness or death of another family member, occupational changes, financial problems, relocation, and change in vacation plans. Evaluate the family's knowledge of the U.S. Family and Medical Leave Act, which enables parents to use sick time, vacation, and leave without pay to care for an ill family member while safeguarding employment.

Knowledge

People who are anxious tend to narrow their scope of attention and may read unintended messages into the behaviors of healthcare personnel. Anxiety also limits a person's ability to retain information.

The child's knowledge of cancer and its treatment should be assessed throughout the treatment period. As the child matures cognitively, new evaluations of knowledge are needed. Cancer and its treatment are complex topics, and parents are exposed to information in various forms, including written material, news reports, discussions with others, and Internet websites and resources. Evaluate their knowledge and information sources, providing them with opportunities to ask questions. Evaluate the learning style of the child and family in order to adapt approaches to meet their needs.

Support Systems

Cancer treatment generally occurs over a long period of time. The extended family is crucial in providing necessary support to the child, parents, and siblings. Identify key persons in the family. They may be the parents, grandparents, or aunts and uncles. Thoroughly assess the coping strategies used by the family to meet the various challenges posed by the child's illness. This information helps to predict the success of interventions, such as home care with intravenous medications, and to decide when referrals for other supportive therapies are needed.

Assess family resources to identify support systems available to help the family during crises and if a child is expected to die. Extended supports include friends, jobs, insurance coverage, religious affiliations, cultural support systems, and the school system (Figure 29–7 ■). Inquire if the insurance carrier provides for a case manager in complex health needs such as cancer. Parents commonly lose contact with close friends following the diagnosis of cancer in a child. This is an additional stressor for the family. Jobs are often a source of support because coworkers may have gone through the same experience. It may

also be comforting for parents to return to a job where they can feel a sense of security in tangible accomplishments. However, jobs can also be a source of stress if employers are unsympathetic to the demands of the child's hospitalization and clinic or office visits.

Faith-based affiliations can be an important source of support. Evaluate whether such affiliations are meaningful for the family and, if so, plan for visits from the appropriate clergy. In some cultures, spiritual leaders are an important part of the family's support. Enable a healer to visit the child and conduct a healing ceremony if that will be supportive to the family and child.

The return to school may pose difficulties for the child with cancer, or it may be a source of support to be connected again to peers. The child is encouraged to go to school, even if only for half a day per

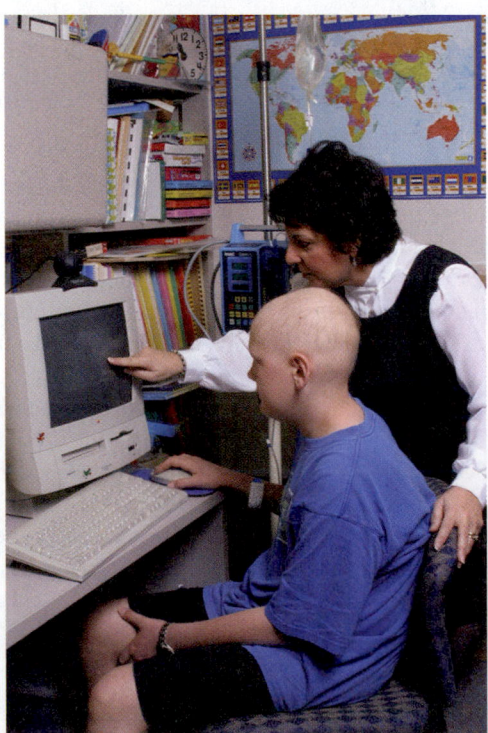

FIGURE 29–7 ■ This teacher comes to the pediatric oncology center to work with students while their chemotherapy is administered. What are the benefits of having her work in this setting?

week, to stay connected to peers. Evaluate the ability of the school to accept a child who is medically vulnerable into the classroom. Nurses who work in the oncology department of the hospital or clinic can ask if the family would give consent to visit the school, meet with the school nurse, and plan together to meet the child's educational needs. Assess whether the other children and teachers have been prepared for the appearance and needs of the child with cancer; suggest that the oncology nurse visit the class to meet with the children and explain the expectations. Arrangements can be made for tutors to help the child keep up with schoolwork if he or she cannot attend school. An individualized education plan is needed (see a description of the IEP in Chapter 14 🔗). Parents need information about the legal right to this plan since the child is newly ill and they will likely not have been exposed to this in the past.

Body Image

Body image is dependent on the child's age and prior experiences (Box 29–1). Body image disturbances occur when a child cannot integrate changes and continues to cling to old images despite their inconsistency with reality. Common means for assessing body image are drawings, colored pictures cut out by the child to form a collage, discussion, and observation. Drawing is an especially powerful tool that assists children in handling the stress of the disease and enhances communication with healthcare providers. See Chapter 15 🔗 for further discussion of these and other assessment techniques that can be used with children.

Hair loss, surgical scars, and cushingoid changes are three common treatment-induced threats to body image. Most children being treated for cancer experience hair loss (Figure 29–8 ■). Children who have cranial surgery lose hair as part of the surgical preparation. Chemotherapy frequently results in some degree of hair loss. The speed of hair loss is unique to the child and can be as rapid as overnight or slower, evidenced by hair left on the pillow and in the hairbrush. Radiation may cause permanent hair loss or thinning. Assess for hair loss and assist the child in the coping method he or she chooses.

A second challenge to the child's body image is surgery. The scars of cranial and neck surgery are obvious, as are amputation and limb salvaging. Abdominal surgery for lymphoma is more easily concealed but is still a threat to the child's body image. A central line that is inserted for medications after surgery involves integration of this line to body image for a time.

A third source of altered body image is the cushingoid features such as round and flushed face, prominent cheeks, double chin, and generalized obesity that result from the use of corticosteroids. As the child's weight increases, stretch marks similar to those of pregnancy may occur. These stretch marks often remain after the corticosteroids are decreased.

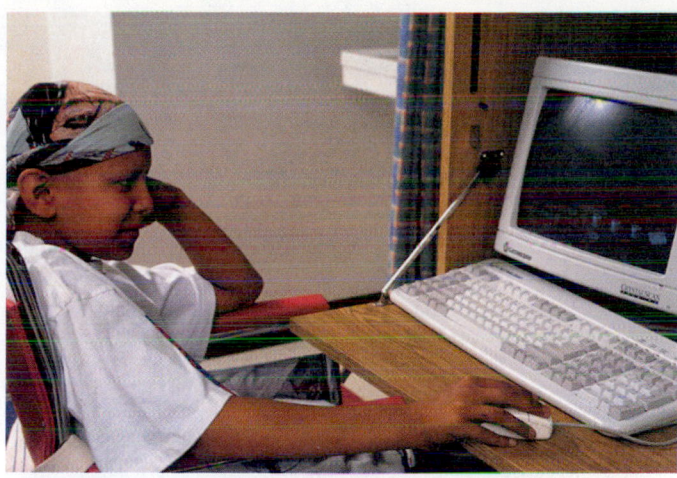

A

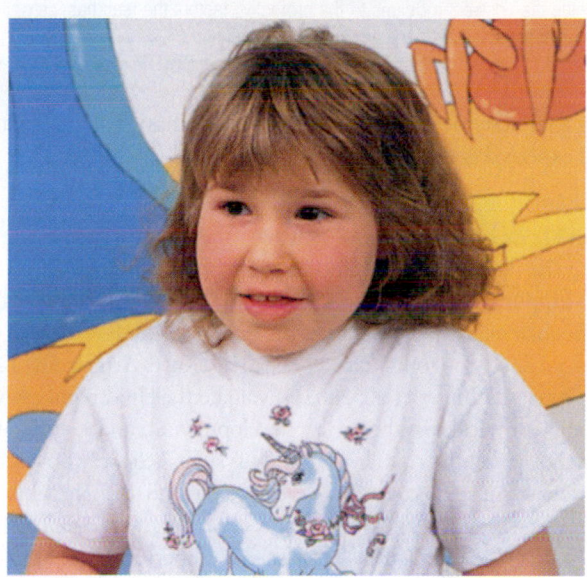

B

FIGURE 29–8 ■ *A,* One of the most common threats to a child's body image at any age is hair loss induced by chemotherapy. Use of hats can improve self-concept. *B,* The child with cushingoid features has a rounded face and prominent cheeks. This change in body image can be a challenge for some children.

Developmental Assessment

Developmental assessment of children should be performed regularly during treatment for cancer, at times when the child feels well so that results are accurate. Children under 6 years of age who have cancer should receive regular developmental assessment with a standardized tool such as the Denver II Developmental Screening Test (see Chapter 8 🔗). Testing can be performed by a home healthcare nurse or by a nurse in the pediatric healthcare home (medical home) who sees the child for a general health supervision visit. Appropriate assessment techniques are used for older children (Box 29–2). Assessment of the child's physical and neurologic development helps in determining the progress made during treatment and provides a baseline for evaluating the long-term effects of treatment. Recommend referral to a neuropsychologist for testing early in treatment and if changes in developmental performance are noted. Observe developmental milestones at each contact with the child and refer for further assessment if regression has occurred. Performance in school

BOX 29–1	**Growth & Development: Cancer and Age Considerations for Body Image**

Children of different ages experience differing threats to body image as a result of cancer treatment. A preschool girl may be most upset at hair loss, since she will look like a boy. A school-age child has the most difficult time with changes that interfere with the developmental task of industry. An amputation, which decreases the child's ability to participate in activities such as sports, dancing, and schoolwork, can be a major challenge during the school-age years. Teenagers are often most worried about such changes as hair loss and cushingoid features, which cause them to look different from peers.

BOX 29–2	Growth & Development: Adolescents Diagnosed with Cancer

During much of childhood, parents are told first about the child's diagnosis and then assisted in determining what the child can understand and planning how the information is best relayed. However, the adolescent is more independent in decision making and establishing support systems. Therefore, joint discussions between the healthcare providers, parents, and teen are generally helpful, followed by individual sessions when the adolescent can meet individually with the healthcare team and have questions answered. The teen needs information about the diagnosis and treatment regimens, as well as an atmosphere where feelings can be discussed and assistance offered in locating other teens with cancer for further discussion and support. Adolescence is a distinct developmental stage that overlaps both childhood and adulthood. Asking for adolescents' perspectives may be the best way of understanding the experience of cancer and offering the support they need. Two questions are suggested: "During treatment there are good days and there are bad days. What makes a good day for you?" and "How has being sick been for you?" The nurse can ask these questions and examine the answers for clues to the protective factors the teen has, as well as areas that require assistance and further intervention.

and social activities with friends provides important information about expected developmental milestones in older children.

Assessment for Impact of Cancer Survival

Nurses are involved with families when a diagnosis of cancer is made, during the therapy process, and in the years that follow. The family needs support as treatment concludes and the child is integrated back into his or her usual home and community roles. For a child who survives cancer, ongoing care is essential (Kurt, Armstrong, Cash, et al., 2008; Oeffinger et al., 2008). Evaluate the child regularly with thorough physical, psychosocial, developmental, and cognitive assessments. Carefully monitor all body systems (e.g., cardiovascular; respiratory; musculoskeletal; eye, ear, nose, and throat; genitourinary). Record height and weight and general growth patterns. Ask about the child's interactions with peers and performance at school. Children who have received cranial radiation and intrathecal chemotherapy need regular scholastic evaluations. Be alert for signs and symptoms that could indicate a secondary tumor.

Assess the need for physical rehabilitation, support related to visual impairment, or treatment for cardiac or musculoskeletal abnormalities. Facilitate periodic evaluation in a healthcare agency so that serious outcomes of treatment can be identified early. Ask the parents about insurance coverage and other financial difficulties during ongoing care.

The accompanying Nursing Care Plan includes several diagnoses that may be appropriate for the child with cancer. Among the many other diagnoses that may be appropriate for a child with cancer are the following:

- Diarrhea related to radiation therapy and toxins
- Urinary Elimination, Impaired related to chemotherapy
- Pain, Acute related to impaired mucous membranes from chemotherapy and radiation therapy
- Skin Integrity, Impaired related to altered nutritional state, effects of medication, radiation, and immobilization
- Coping, Ineffective related to situational crises of chronic and acute illness
- Sleep Pattern, Disturbed related to biochemical agents, anxiety, and unfamiliar surroundings
- Body Image, Disturbed related to chronic illness and treatments

- Knowledge, Deficient (Child or Parents) related to lack of exposure to disease or treatments
- Grieving related to actual or potential loss of significant other

NANDA-I © 2012

Planning and Implementation

The nursing care of children newly diagnosed with cancer and their families includes immediate physiologic and psychologic support, along with anticipatory guidance about imminent and future medical interventions. The family should be assisted and supported in making decisions about types of treatment that are appropriate for the child.

Nursing care of the hospitalized child with cancer and the child receiving ongoing therapy at home is summarized in the accompanying Nursing Care Plan. This care plan is designed for the child who has progressed beyond the cancer diagnosis phase and is receiving chemotherapy.

Physiologic care of the hospitalized child focuses on providing support during treatment. This includes ensuring optimal nutritional intake, administering medications, managing the multiple side effects of chemotherapy and radiation, ensuring adequate hydration, preventing infection, and managing pain.

Ensure Optimal Nutritional Intake

The high metabolic rate of cancer growth depletes the child's nutritional stores so that many children are cachectic at the time of diagnosis. In addition, the catabolic effect of chemotherapy and radiation on normal cells necessitates additional cellular replacement. The child needs increased nutritional intake at a time when nausea and vomiting are occurring as drug side effects, and when decreased activity and general health status result in diminished appetite. This often leads to extreme concern on the part of parents, and they may focus excessive attention on the child's intake. See Partnering with Families: Nutrition and the Child with Cancer.

Care is complicated by the fact that in early treatment the child is often hospitalized and may find hospital food unpalatable or different from usual intake. As time progresses, the child with cancer is more at risk for obesity, diabetes, and osteoporosis, due to both disturbed eating patterns and side effects of treatment (Cohen, Wakefield, Fleming, et al., 2011; Houlston, Buttery, & Powell, 2009). The goals of nutrition therapy during treatment for cancer are to prevent or reverse any nutritional deficiencies, preserve the child's lean body mass, minimize any side effects that influence nutritional state, allow for the child's growth needs, establish or maintain healthy nutritional habits, and improve overall quality of life.

Administer antiemetic drugs to lessen nausea from chemotherapy. Offer frequent, small meals. It may be helpful to offer the child's favorite foods at times when nausea and vomiting are decreased. Ask the family what treatments they use to decrease the child's nausea and vomiting, and inform them of techniques that may enhance intake. Perform 24-hour dietary recalls to assess the child's intake, and evaluate height and weight regularly. Special nutritional products may be given orally, nasogastric or nasoduodenal tube feedings may be given, or total parenteral nutrition may be necessary. When the child's nutritional status is deteriorating or parenteral nutrition is used, perform weekly studies of serum electrolytes, liver chemistry, glucose, and triglycerides. Partner with both the oncologist and the dietitian to plan interventions appropriate for meeting the needs of individual children.

Nursing Care Plan

Hospital Care of the Child with Cancer

INTERVENTION	RATIONALE	EXPECTED OUTCOME
1. Nursing Diagnosis: Pain related to tissue injury		
NIC Priority Intervention—_Pain Management:_ Alleviation or reduction in pain to a level of comfort acceptable to patient		**NOC Suggested Outcome—**_Comfort Level:_ Feelings of physical and psychological ease
GOAL: _The child will report reduced pain that is manageable._		
■ Give analgesics as ordered.	■ Adequate medications can reduce pain.	The child experiences pain reduced to the level that allows the child to interact appropriately and gain rest.
■ Teach relaxation techniques, deep breathing, and distraction.	■ Nonpharmacologic methods work with the medication to reduce pain.	
2. Nursing Diagnosis: Nutrition, Imbalanced: Less than Body Requirements related to inability to ingest or digest food or absorb nutrients		
NIC Priority Intervention—_Nutrition Management:_ Assistance with and provision of a balanced dietary intake		**NOC Suggested Outcome—**_Nutritional Status:_ Extent to which nutrients are available to meet metabolic needs
GOAL: _The child will maintain adequate nutritional intake._		
■ Record all intake and output.	■ Intake and output recordings can assist with early detection of problems.	The child maintains admission weight.
■ Offer small feedings. Encourage favorite foods. Refer to a dietitian for special meals. Weigh daily.	■ These measures can increase caloric intake. Taste changes and mouth sores alter desire for food.	
GOAL: _The child will experience reduced effects of chemotherapy (i.e., nausea and vomiting)._		
■ Teach the child distraction and relaxation techniques. Give antiemetics according to orders.	■ Pharmacologic and nonpharmacologic methods are effective in helping to reduce nausea.	The child has minimal side effects of nausea and vomiting.
3. Nursing Diagnosis: Constipation, Risk for related to change in usual foods and eating patterns		
NIC Priority Intervention—_Constipation Management:_ Prevention and alleviation of constipation		**NOC Suggested Outcome—**_Bowel Elimination:_ The ability of the gastrointestinal tract to form and evacuate stool effectively
GOAL: _The child will reestablish a normal bowel pattern._		
■ Record all output by size and description. Administer stool softeners. Test stool for guaiac. Report changes in stool to the managing healthcare provider. Encourage adequate fluid intake.	■ Chemotherapy or tumor may create constipation, diarrhea, or blood in stool.	The child has a normal bowel pattern.
4. Nursing Diagnosis: Fluid Volume: Excess or Deficient related to medications		
NIC Priority Intervention—_Fluid Management:_ Promotion of fluid balance and prevention of complications resulting from abnormal fluid levels		**NOC Suggested Outcome—**_Fluid Balance:_ Balance of water in the intracellular and extracellular compartments of the body
GOAL: _The child will be adequately hydrated._		
■ Record all intake and output. Monitor intravenous rate and solution as appropriate.	■ Some drugs (e.g., cyclophosphamide) necessitate a high level of fluid intake to prevent complications.	The child demonstrates adequate hydration. Mucous membranes are hydrated.
■ Test specific gravity of urine daily.	■ Renal function may be affected by chemotherapy.	Specific gravity remains within the normal range.
5. Nursing Diagnosis: Infection, Risk for related to immunosuppression, invasive procedures, malnutrition, or pharmaceutical agents		
NIC Priority Intervention—_Infection Protection:_ Prevention and early detection of infection in patient at risk		**NOC Suggested Outcome—**_Risk Control:_ Actions to eliminate or reduce health threats
GOAL: _The child will remain free of infection._		
■ Wash and sanitize hands often. Maintain in isolation if needed.	■ Hand hygiene is effective to reduce organisms. Transmission-based precautions may be needed to safeguard the child.	The child remains infection-free.

(continued)

Nursing Care Plan   Hospital Care of the Child with Cancer, *continued*

INTERVENTION	RATIONALE	EXPECTED OUTCOME
■ Monitor temperature. Report elevations over 38°C (101°F). Use a cooling mattress and other methods as needed.	■ Elevated temperature is a sign of infection.	
■ Administer intravenous antibiotics as ordered.	■ Multiple antibiotics are needed to deal with bacterial and lung infections during neutropenia. Blood cultures may be taken to identify the organism.	The child with an infection is effectively treated.

6. Nursing Diagnosis: Coping, Ineffective related to situational crisis

NIC Priority Intervention—*Coping Enhancement:* Assisting a patient to adapt to stressors which interfere with meeting life demands and roles		**NOC Suggested Outcome**—*Coping:* Actions to manage stressors that tax an individual's resources

GOAL: *The child will demonstrate normal adaptive coping methods.*

■ Encourage drawings and other therapeutic play for expression of feelings. Allow for expression of angry feelings, such as hitting dolls and throwing sponge balls. Discuss how to behave during treatments.	■ Play is a normal way for the child to express self and ideas. Expression of feelings helps identify avoidance coping for further intervention. Misinterpretations can be corrected. Knowledge of appropriate and helpful behaviors supports self-esteem.	The child continues to use usual coping strategies expected for developmental stage.

NANDA-I © 2012

End-of-life care is administered when a child is not expected to live. Nutritional support becomes especially important during this time to improve quality of life, enhance comfort, and support the immune system. Children should be offered foods that they like and are easy to eat. Soft, nonspicy foods such as puddings, eggs, and purees provide high-energy density, ease in consumption, and digestibility. Ensure adequate fluids, and supplement fluids with powdered milk or energy supplements.

Administer Medications

One important intervention of the oncology nurse is administering medications safely, and often several chemotherapeutic drugs are used in combinations. Most chemotherapeutic drugs are prescribed and calculated as dose per meter squared (dose/m^2), with m^2 calculated from the child's height and weight. (Refer to the section on administering medications in the Skills Manual ⬤▭.)

Practice Alert

A treatment known as *leucovorin rescue* is used in conjunction with high-dose methotrexate chemotherapy. Leucovorin (citrovorum factor) is a form of folic acid that helps to protect normal cells from the destructive action of methotrexate. It is started 24 hours after methotrexate administration and is given along with hydration therapy (Warnick & Auger, 2009).

Chemotherapy drugs are prepared with special techniques under laminar flow devices to minimize potential toxic effects on healthcare

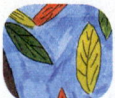

Partnering with Families

Nutrition and the Child with Cancer

Because of the effects of cancer and chemotherapy or other treatment, the child often has a poor appetite. Mucosal sores lead to difficulty chewing and swallowing. Parents can enhance the child's nutritional intake in the following ways:

- Provide frequent small feedings rather than three meals daily.
- Integrate the child's favorite foods into daily menus.
- Have nutritious snacks available for times when the child feels like eating.
- Sprinkle dried milk on top of cereals and other foods to increase calcium and caloric intake.
- Serve smooth, soft foods. Milkshakes with added peanut butter, puddings, and soft casseroles may be well tolerated and preferred. Try a variety of liquid protein-calorie supplements to find those the child likes.
- Avoid making food an area for disagreement. Do not force foods, but make them readily available.
- If the child is vomiting due to therapy, do not encourage food at that time. Food aversions may develop to foods that are vomited.

- Administer antiemetics as ordered during therapy because they can prevent nausea and vomiting. Pharmacologic mouthwashes may promote comfort for oral membranes.
- Report weight loss and increased fatigue.
- Bring the child in for scheduled health visits so growth, development, and effects of therapy can be monitored.
- Request a temporary feeding tube to ensure adequate nutrition. Feedings at night can often increase intake and promote health. Occasionally a central line is inserted to provide total parenteral nutrition.
- Recognize that supplements and tube feedings will usually be covered by insurance if the provider writes an order for them.
- Offer healthy foods, and as the child improves, encourage a nutritious diet that meets requirements for growth.

PHOTO STORY...

SURVIVORS OF CHILDHOOD CANCER

Note that Alysha wears her own clothes for the day; this allows her a feeling of independence and self-expression . . .

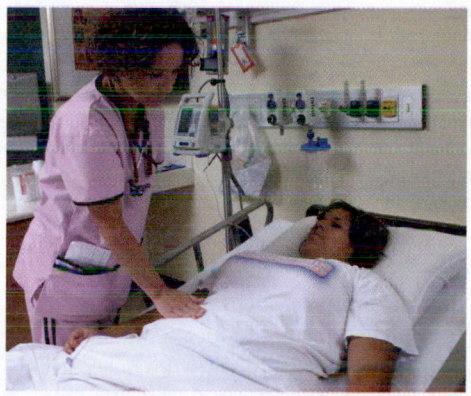

Most children survive the diagnosis and treatment of cancer. Each child and family has a unique way of coping with the challenges they face. The role of the nurse is to identify and draw upon the strengths of the family and provide resources to help increase coping skills. Alysha, 15 years old, has osteogenic sarcoma and had a limb salvage procedure. She is now receiving chemotherapy as the follow-up to treat any remaining cancer in her body. Alysha comes to the oncology clinic for her treatment and is familiar with all of the nurses who administer her care. Note that Alysha wears her own clothes for the day; this allows her a feeling of independence and self-expression that would be

The nurse performs a thorough physical and mental health assessment on Alysha. She completes a head-to-toe assessment and is shown here palpating Alysha's abdomen, noting any tenderness, masses, or other abnormalities.

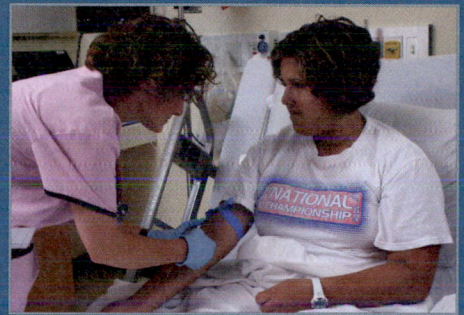

After the assessment is complete, the nurse starts an intravenous infusion for hydration. After the fluid is running, Alysha's medication will be started through a central line.

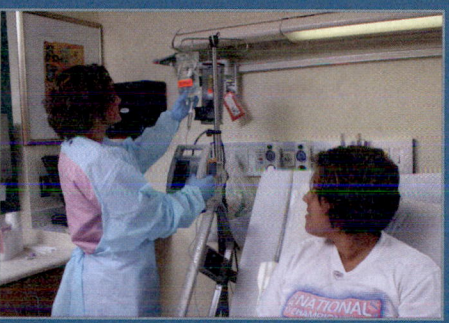

When starting Alysha's infusion, the nurse carefully checks the bag and label to verify that the correct infusion is being used.

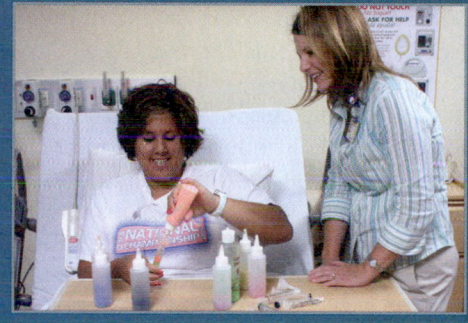

While Alysha is receiving her infusion, the child life specialist brings colored sand and has Alysha engage in sand play. She has told the specialist that she enjoys art and trying different media, and she clearly enjoys this new type of art. Notice that the specialist has integrated syringes into this therapeutic activity, allowing Alysha the opportunity to work with the equipment that is being used for her care, thus understanding and feeling a sense of mastery over this equipment.

lost if she had to wear a hospital gown. While completing the assessment the nurse talks with Alysha, evaluating her psychologic status. She asks her about school, her adjustment to activities with friends, and her family interactions. The nurse carefully explains all procedures so that Alysha understands what is being done. Notice that Alysha is very interested in her care and watches all

steps in the process. Alysha is doing well with her therapy and a complete recovery is expected. Managing the treatment in a positive way is a major goal of the present care. She will also need to be monitored during ongoing visits for any signs of recurrence of cancer, and for any of the possible long-term outcomes of cancer therapy.

providers. Gloves and other hazardous drug protocols are used. Care must be taken to avoid **extravasation** of intravenous drugs (leakage into the soft tissue around the infusion site), as permanent tissue damage can result.

Clinical Tip

Many precautions are needed when administering chemotherapy drugs. The child has a central line or implantable port so that extravasation risk is decreased with these medications, which are potentially harmful if they inadvertently leak into peripheral tissues. The central line must be maintained carefully (see the Skills Manual ⬤━). Healthcare providers must avoid inadvertent contact with chemotherapy drugs. OSHA publishes an instruction manual entitled *Controlling Occupational Exposure to Hazardous Drugs* that outlines general guidelines, protective equipment, and procedures.

In addition to chemotherapy drugs, the nurse administers other medications, such as antiemetics to control nausea, vitamin supplements, and antibiotics. Antiemetics such as ondansetron are given prophylactically when a cancer agent is administered that has known emetic effects. Parents are asked about complementary therapy and medications they are obtaining from other sources and using at home.

All medications must be safely administered and the child should be monitored for side effects. Techniques such as generous hydration accompanying medications help to decrease side effects. **Polypharmacy** (the use of several drugs at one time to treat multiple health conditions) can lead to multiple side effects and can challenge the body's ability to metabolize and excrete drugs. (See Clinical Manifestations: Common Side Effects of Chemotherapy.)

Some children receive fluids and medications at home via central lines, or intramuscular or subcutaneous injection. Consider referral to home healthcare infusion agencies for monitoring of these treatments and provision of supplies for home use.

Parents and children must become well informed about the drugs to be administered and the side effects that may occur. Telephone numbers, websites, and other resources are needed for information

BOX 29–3 Research: Phases of Drug Trials

The nurse who cares for children receiving treatment for cancer must have a good understanding of the phases of drug trials and be able to interpret this information for families deciding on participation.

Phase 1—This is the first clinical trial to involve people; it seeks to answer the question: "Is the treatment safe, and what are its pharmacokinetics?" It is the phase with the greatest risk since the drug has not previously been tested in people.

Phase 2—Once a drug has been found to be reasonably safe, phase 2 trials seek to establish its degree of effectiveness for specific conditions. Side effects and risks are closely monitored.

Phase 3—If a drug is found to be generally safe and effective, in phase 3 it is compared to other standard treatments. It seeks to establish safety, efficacy, and dosage in a variety of patients and settings. After this phase, the FDA deliberates and decides if the drug should be approved.

Phase 4—The approved drug is still tested in phase 4 to determine if there are better ways to prescribe it, regarding dosage, length of treatment, and other factors.

Source: *American Cancer Society, 2010.*

Legal and Ethical Considerations
Clinical Trials

When unapproved investigational drugs are given in a clinical trial, consent by parents is mandatory. They should know the potential benefits and harm to the child. Children who are cognitively able should also give assent verbally or in writing. This assent can usually be obtained from children by the age of 7 to 9 years, depending on the child's level of understanding. Conferences are held with the families, including children, to discuss the disease and potential treatment, identify risks and benefits of treatment, and ensure that the choices are voluntarily made. Participants can decide to withdraw from the research at any time. Even when the family has given consent for a clinical trial, they may have additional questions. Nurses can clarify information and refer the family to the research investigator for further explanations (American Cancer Society, 2009; Unguru, Coppes, & Kamani, 2008).

when questions arise. Inform the family about the phases of drug trials if the child is asked to participate. (See Box 29–3 and Legal and Ethical Considerations: Clinical Trials.)

Manage Treatment Side Effects

All cancer treatments affect some normal body cells as well as cancer cells, causing a wide variety of side effects. Effects of cancer and treatments on the blood include anemia, neutropenia, and thrombocytopenia. Know all side effects of specific drugs administered and monitor for them. Realize that some side effects are late and may be seen after therapy is completed. Emphasize the importance of all follow-up visits scheduled in the future for monitoring of late effects. Refer to the Clinical Manifestations table on common side effects of chemotherapy.

A frequent occurrence is **myelosuppression** or suppression of blood cell production in the bone marrow. Be alert for signs of a decreased white blood cell count, such as infections. **Neutropenia** is present when the absolute neutrophil count (ANC) is less than 500 cells/mm^3 or if between 500 and 1,000 cells/mm^3 when chemotherapy is being given and falling levels are anticipated. At these levels, children will be given a broad-spectrum antibiotic; G-CSF may be given (see the Medications table on page 949). Take the child's temperature, isolate the child from others with infections, and perform serum laboratory studies and cultures as prescribed. All cultures should be completed before antibiotic therapy is begun.

Protect the child from bruises and be alert for hemorrhage or signs of bleeding such as petechiae, nosebleeds, dark colored or bloody stools, and presence of blood in vomit and urine; these are all effects of thrombocytopenia or decreased platelets. The child may need to receive infusions of platelets if thrombocytopenia is severe. When thrombocytopenia occurs, minimize needlesticks and other intrusive procedures. Be ready to deal with nosebleeds and watch for bleeding gums. Report any bleeding, ecchymosis, or petechiae to the oncology specialist. Be sure parents know that the child should avoid contact sports or other rough activities and that any healthcare provider, such as a dentist, should be informed of the child's treatment and condition. Infusions to increase platelets are sometimes administered.

Inadequate red blood cell production can result in anemia. Encourage the child to eat iron-rich foods, and administer nutritional

Clinical Manifestations Common Side Effects of Chemotherapy

SIDE EFFECT	CLINICAL MANIFESTATIONS	CLINICAL THERAPY
Bone marrow suppression	Evidence of suppression usually appears 7–10 days after administration of chemotherapy; recovery is usually complete within 3–4 weeks.	Transfusions of RBCs or platelets are administered based on laboratory findings of CBC and platelets as well as the clinical condition of the child. Some institutions use a low-microbial diet to decrease the possibility that infectious organisms will colonize the intestine during neutropenia. Trimethoprim/sulfamethoxazole (e.g., Septra or Bactrim) is used for *Pneumocystis carinii* pneumonia prophylaxis; nystatin is used for antifungal and antibacterial prophylaxis during neutropenia. Instruct the family and child about the importance of protecting the body from activities that could lead to bruising during periods of mild to moderate thrombocytopenia (platelet count less than 5,000/mm^3). Careful hand hygiene is essential to prevent infection during periods of neutropenia. Encourage use of masks if the family or staff have nasopharyngeal infections, in order to prevent infections during neutropenia. Monitor vital signs to detect infection.
Nausea and vomiting	Symptoms may occur immediately, a few hours later, or any time during treatment.	Antiemetics, such as Zofran, Kytril, Reglan, and Benadryl, are used to treat this side effect. Teach relaxation techniques, hypnosis, and systematic desensitization (a hypnotic process that progressively reduces reactions to objects that cause strong emotional or physical responses) to help decrease the child's symptoms. Encourage mild exercise and change of diet (eating only easily digestible foods) 12 hours before chemotherapy. Be alert for assessment findings that indicate the child has an illness such as influenza which is causing the symptoms.
Anorexia and weight loss	These may occur at any time.	Hyperalimentation is necessary if dietary changes are unsuccessful in halting the child's weight loss. Pay careful attention to changes in taste that affect food preferences. Referral to a dietitian may be helpful to achieve successful modification of the child's diet.
Mucositis	Oral mucositis resulting from chemotherapy usually occurs within 3–4 days and is often a contributing factor in anorexia.	Antifungal agents, such as nystatin or clotrimazole, lessen the possibility of candidal infection. Promote good oral hygiene. Use a soft foam wand or water irrigation to clean teeth. Commercial mouthwashes are not recommended because they contain alcohol and increase drying of the oral cavity; a specially formulated pharmacologic mouthwash may promote comfort.
Constipation	Constipation can occur at any time in treatment but becomes more common as therapy progresses and dietary intake and physical activity decrease.	Stool softeners and laxatives are used to treat this side effect (e.g., MiraLax). Advise parents to increase fluids and fibrous foods in the child's diet.
Pain	Pain can occur at any time and is best understood by subjective explanations of the child.	Acetaminophen, morphine, steroids, nonsteroidal anti-inflammatory drugs, and antidepressants may be used to manage pain. Careful pain assessment is important. The location of the pain may provide a clue to its cause, for example, metastasis to the skull, infiltration of joints, or damage to soft tissue. Pain associated with chemotherapy may also be related to oral mucositis, myalgia, or tumor embolization; painful polyneuropathy can follow treatment with vincristine or cisplatin. Acetaminophen for pain can mask the presence of fever, which signals infection; careful and complete physical assessment is needed to identify infection. Pharmacologic, nonhypnotic (deep breathing, self-control), and hypnotic methods of pain control may be used; the nonpharmacologic methods often prove helpful to children with pain from multiple etiologies.

supplements as needed. RBC transfusions are sometimes needed to treat severe anemia.

Chemotherapy affects all rapidly growing cells in the body, but especially those of the mucous membranes. Provide good oral hygiene with a soft toothbrush, foam wand, or water irrigation device. Report oral breakdown promptly. Partner with the oncologist, dentist, and nutritionist to plan treatment strategies to protect the oral health and erupting teeth of children. See Partnering with Families: Oral Care for common techniques to manage oral hygiene.

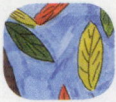

Partnering with Families

Oral Care

Since cancer treatment and poor nutritional status can adversely affect the oral status of children, families need help to plan and carry out prophylactic and treatment measures. Children continue to lose teeth, have new teeth erupt, and require nutrients to help in building teeth not yet erupted, even during cancer treatment. Some suggestions are:

- Provide a visit to the dentist early in treatment for assessment, for treatment of dental disease, and to establish a prevention plan.
- Floss and brush teeth twice daily with a soft bristle brush and rinse with water.

- When granulocyte counts fall below 500/mm^3 or platelets fall below 40,000/mm^3, Toothettes or gauze can be used to clean the teeth. Avoiding brushes will help to prevent bleeding and infection.
- Toothpaste can be used unless it causes discomfort.
- Medications may be used to prevent infection. They may include antibacterial mouthwash, nystatin, or fluconazole. Continue oral fluoride if it is not present in the drinking water.
- If bleeding, infection, or other oral care needs emerge, consult with the dentist and pediatric oncologist to develop a treatment plan.

Evaluate the effects of hair loss or other body image changes on the child. Evaluate sleep, mental status, and developmental progression since all can be affected by chemotherapy.

Radiation can cause burns to the skin. Examine the skin daily during hospitalization or weekly when making home visits. Leave the marks on the skin that outline the radiation target area. Avoid use of lotions, powders, and soaps on the target skin area. Some children may need to be anesthetized to ensure correct positioning for radiation; postanesthesia care will then be needed. Other side effects of radiation include hair loss to the irradiated area, profound fatigue, nausea and vomiting, and additional effects on organs in the irradiated area. Perform comprehensive and ongoing assessments for side effects so they can be managed as needed.

Ensure Adequate Hydration

Hydration management can be a challenge as the child may not be thirsty but is excreting large numbers of cell fragments and other substances as a result of treatment. Offer frequent, small amounts of fluid. Include frozen ice pops or other fluid-containing foods such as Jell-O. Measure intake and output. To ensure adequate excretion, a number of chemotherapy drugs are given with intravenous fluids. It is important to administer fluids as ordered and ensure that the recommended urinary output excretion rate is maintained after drug administration.

Prevent and Treat Infection

Children with cancer have an altered immune system, both from the disease and from the effects of immunosuppressant drugs, and must be kept away from persons with known infections. Teach parents to avoid taking the child to places that attract large gatherings of people, such as department stores, once the child returns home. Emphasize the need to report any exposure to contagious disease, especially chicken pox. Some drugs may mask signs of infection, so be alert for any signs of mild infections. Fever, malaise, and mild respiratory infection must be reported promptly.

Follow recommendations for the immunization of children with cancer as published by the Centers for Disease Control and Prevention (CDC) and the American Academy of Pediatrics (AAP). Usually no immunizations are given to the child until 6 months after completing chemotherapy. Immunity may be lost from some prior immunizations, requiring titer levels and repeat immunization later.

Teach administration of any drugs being used to prevent infection such as pentamidine or sulfa preparations for pneumocystis pneumonia prophylaxis. Management of infections is critical. Children are often hospitalized and central lines are used for antibiotic administration. Blood cultures and cultures of infected body parts help to establish the causative organisms (refer to the Skills Manual ⬭). Due to lowered immune status, unusual agents are sometimes identified. Administer medication treatment on time and as ordered. Ensure that standard precautions and transmission-based precautions are followed. Assess temperature, vital signs, and all body systems at admission and at least every 4 hours.

Manage Pain

The child with cancer may experience pain from the disease itself and from the medical interventions, such as lumbar puncture, bone marrow aspiration, and frequent intravenous infusions and blood draws. Use all possible pain management techniques to keep the child comfortable, as this will assist with comfort and encourage cooperation throughout the long treatment period. (See Chapter 21 ⓔ for suggestions on methods of pain management.) Nurses must examine research on effective pain management for children and integrate findings into practice (Shepherd, Woodgate, & Sawatzky, 2010). See Figure 29–9 ■.

Sedation may be used for some procedures. Administer sedation as prescribed for young children who are undergoing lumbar

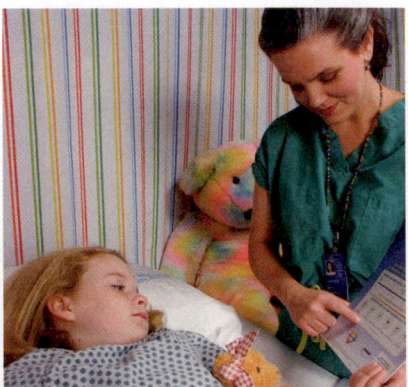

FIGURE 29–9 ■ The nurse is having the child rate her pain by pointing to the face that most closely matches the way she feels. Note her stuffed animals that provide comfort.

punctures, radiation, and other procedures, and monitor them after the procedure. Coordinate painful or intrusive tests so they can be done while the child is sedated. Topical anesthetics such as EMLA cream may be used to numb the skin before a blood draw or an intravenous start.

Clinical Tip

EMLA cream, or eutectic mixture of local anesthetics, is a combination of lidocaine 2.5% and prilocaine 2.5% in an emulsion. Apply a thick layer of the cream to intact skin and cover with an occlusive dressing. Leave in place 1 hour for minor procedures and 2 hours for major procedures. Do not use EMLA on infants who are a gestational age of less than 37 weeks, under 20 kg, or under 12 months and receiving treatment with methemoglobin-inducing agents. Be certain that parents who administer the drug at home prior to the child's scheduled appointment for a procedure realize the importance of limiting the area and duration as ordered and keeping the cream in a safe place to avoid ingestion by any children. (See Chapter 21 for further information about pain control and other local anesthetics.)

Other pain prevention measures include fast-acting sprays, intradermal injection of anesthesia with lidocaine, iontophoresis (local anesthetic and electrical current), and sedation (see the Skills Manual for sedation monitoring).

When possible, include the parents in comforting the child during and after painful procedures. Ask what techniques work at home to relieve pain, and integrate them into care of the child in the health facility. See Complementary Therapy: Pain Management.

Provide Psychosocial Support

A diagnosis of cancer brings with it many emotions for the family. Initially parents experience shock and anger. They need basic information about the disease and the purpose of the tests that will be performed. Instructions often need to be repeated as parents may not process information the first time it is presented due to their increased stress levels. Assist the parents to plan how and when to tell the child the diagnosis. What the child needs to know is based on his or her developmental level and understanding.

After progressing from the initial state of shock about the diagnosis, the family needs to learn more about the disease, including the pathophysiology, treatment, and expected outcome or the prognosis.

Complementary Therapy
Pain Management

Children have many painful and invasive procedures during cancer treatment. In addition to use of medication they will be helped by a variety of other pain management techniques. These include the following:

- The parent's presence during procedures as a support person can be very helpful to manage pain.
- Either a parent or healthcare provider can work with the child to integrate distraction and relaxation techniques such as singing, counting, telling stories, and blowing bubbles. Children and teens can be taught to visualize positive scenes, use rhythmic breathing, or listen to music.
- Hypnosis has been used successfully to manage both pain and nausea/vomiting during cancer treatment with children from 5 to 18 years.

Clarify the family's understanding of these areas and be ready to answer questions. Provide both verbal explanations and written material. Parents may talk with friends, purchase books, or search the Internet for information. Find out where they are getting information and provide additional resources when appropriate. Correct misconceptions and misinformation.

The family needs many strategies to deal with the challenge of long-term treatment for cancer. As the child experiences remissions and exacerbations or complications, the family feels alternately hopeful and discouraged. Help the family to identify support systems, and intervene as needed to enhance these systems. Facilitate contact with extended family members who might be of help, faith-based or spiritual connections, social service agencies, and other resources such as Internet and parent support groups. Assist parents who are concerned about job obligations and finances. Consider the impact on siblings when a child is being treated for cancer. They may alternately resent and feel guilty for the sibling's illness. They may not understand the treatments or disease. School progress may be slowed and teachers may not be aware of the sibling's stress. See Evidence-Based Practice: Cancer, Sleep, and Fatigue.

Evidence-Based Practice   Cancer, Sleep, and Fatigue

PROBLEM

Inadequate amounts and quality of sleep are common problems among youth. Busy schedules and use of screen technologies contribute to poor sleep habits. Daytime sleepiness and other outcomes can result (Sadeh, Dahl, Shahar, et al., 2009). The child or adolescent with cancer is even more likely to have disturbed sleep, due to cancer itself, the treatment protocols, and associated symptoms. What assessments and interventions should the nurse implement to understand sleep needs in the child with cancer?

EVIDENCE

A systematic review by nurses examined the measurement of sleep in adolescents with cancer by measures such as questionnaires, sleep diaries, and actigraphy (a watch-like device that measures movement and accurately displays sleep time). Primary reasons for disturbed sleep in cancer treatment included pain, frequent awakenings or fragmented sleep, and symptoms such as nausea (Erickson, Beck, Christian, et al., 2011). Another study by nurses found that adolescent fatigue related to cancer treatment negatively affected both activity level and mood (Erickson, Beck, Christian, et al., 2011).

Sleep disturbance may even continue after cancer treatment is completed due to brain changes that resulted from a tumor, or from treatment such as radiation or chemotherapy (Rosen, Shor, & Geller, 2008). In over 1,400 survivors of childhood cancer, fatigue and poor sleep quality were identified (Clanton, Klosky, Jain, et al., 2011).

IMPLICATIONS

Cancer interfaces with normal developmental progression in several ways, one of which is sleep. Question sleep patterns at each oncology visit, provide suggestions for sleep hygiene, and refer the teen for sleep intervention as needed. Inquire about daytime sleepiness and fatigue. Have the youth remove televisions and cell phones from the bedroom, rest for periods each day, and maintain routines that enable sleep. (See Chapter 8 for further information about sleep hygiene.)

CRITICAL THINKING APPLICATION

Plan a series of questions to ask an adolescent about the amount of sleep obtained on weekdays and weekends, patterns of sleep, use of screen media during the night, and any changes in sleep since the cancer was diagnosed. What sleep hygiene measures can assist in acquiring needed sleep time and quality?

Weblink Make-a-Wish Foundation

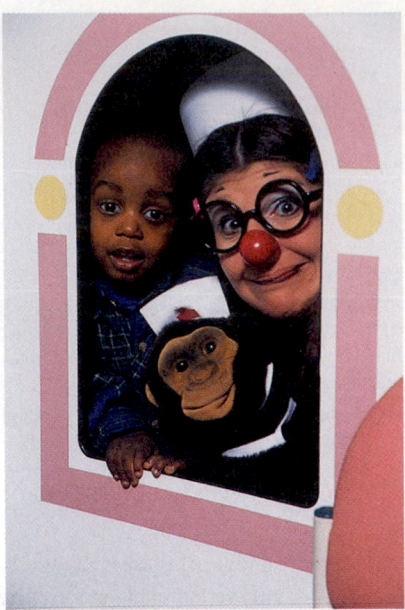

FIGURE 29–10 ■ Clowns from the Big Apple Clown Care Unit can help to ease the stress of hospitalization for seriously ill children and their families. Here, a clown doctor and her puppet distract a toddler who is waiting for his clinic appointment.

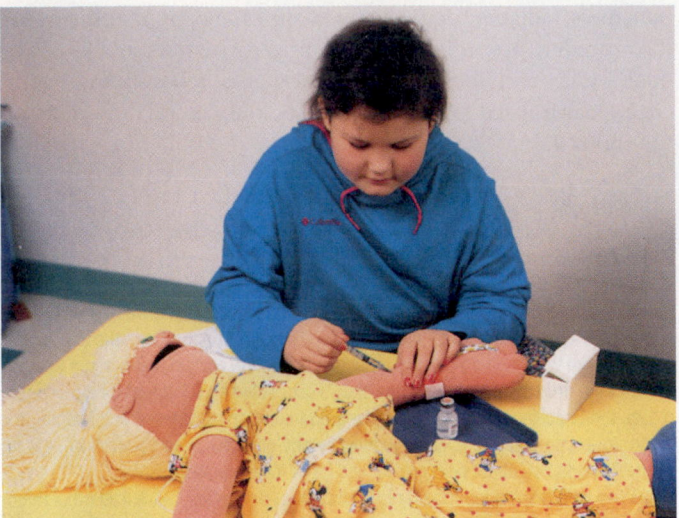

FIGURE 29–11 ■ A child in a pediatric oncology clinic gives injections to a doll. This type of play therapy helps the child deal with fear, thus lowering her stress level.

The child undergoing treatment for cancer needs support appropriate to his or her developmental stage and cognitive level (Figure 29–10 ■). (See Chapters 5 and 15 🔗 for developmental levels and effective support strategies for children of different ages.) Younger children primarily need support during painful procedures and separation from parents. Older children need intervention strategies to assist in working through feelings related to treatments (Figure 29–11 ■). A major developmental task of adolescence is to attain independence and control, but cancer often interferes with adolescents' ability to achieve this task. Therefore, plan nursing strategies that empower adolescents as much as possible. This might include asking them whether they prefer morning or afternoon appointments, placing them on a teen unit where they can receive treatments with other teens, and encouraging parents to allow them choices about issues at home.

For many parents, especially those with daughters, the loss of the child's hair during treatment can be devastating. Ask the parents and the child what this issue is like for them. Prepare them for the fact that it can be rapid or slow. Find out how they plan to cope. Some children want the hair cut very short so its loss will not be as traumatic. Offer resources for wigs, hats, or other ideas. Put them in touch with children who have lost hair and with those who have now regrown it.

Clinical Judgment

Children with hair loss need to protect the bare head from sun exposure and need to be comfortable with their appearance. How will you plan with children at different ages to meet these needs?

Talk with the child's teachers before the return to school after treatment to explain the child's condition and assist with plans to prepare the other children. Role-play with the child how to tell friends about any changes in appearance. A nurse or child life specialist could attend the class of a young child to explain what the child is experiencing. Arrange for tutors if necessary to assist the child with schoolwork

during hospitalization and home care. Explore the option of summer camp for children with cancer. The Make-a-Wish Foundation strives to make dreams come true for children who are ill by sponsoring them for a desired activity or outing. Refer the child to this foundation if appropriate.

The siblings of a child who has cancer may be stressed by the changes in the family. They may grieve over the ill brother or sister and may feel sad and depressed. They also can experience anger, guilt, or resentment and may have a lack of knowledge about the disease and treatment. Inquire about siblings and ask what they know about the child's condition. Find out who is caring for siblings and whether their teachers have been informed about the family situation. Include siblings in care when possible. Invite them to visit and to participate both during hospitalization and at home care visits. They can be involved in play therapy sessions and recreational activities with the ill child. Ask the parents if the siblings are demonstrating symptoms such as depression, behavioral changes, or decrease in school performance and suggest interventions as appropriate. They may benefit from speaking with a school counselor or can be referred to a support group for siblings of children with cancer. Some cancer summer camps welcome siblings as well as children with cancer.

The family of a child with cancer is faced with a life-threatening illness. Refer to Chapter 17 🔗 for strategies to assist the family in coping with this stressor. For many types of cancer, the child may experience a remission with treatment but then a recurrence of disease later as cancer cells grow again. The family may become angry or depressed about the relapse. Repeated treatments challenge the family's support systems. Waiting for the outcome of diagnostic tests can be an especially challenging time. Provide information as soon as possible. If the child's illness progresses, refer the family to hospice to assist them in caring for the child who is terminally ill and in working through the grieving process. Explore support groups and information related to cancer in order to share this information with families.

Care in the Community

Nurses care for children with cancer in community settings and prepare the family for care at home. The Association of Pediatric Hematology/Oncology Nurses (APHON) has established guidelines for

Weblink

The Association of Pediatric Hematology/Oncology Nurses (APHON)

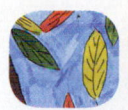

Partnering with Families

Cancer Therapy

Most parents are not aware of the effects of cancer treatment and how they can help children through this experience. Depending on the stage and type of treatment, the following suggestions are for parents:

- Children in radiation and chemotherapy are fatigued. Provide extra rest periods with shorter activity periods between them.
- Have an overnight bag ready in case the child develops a complication and needs to be taken to stay in the hospital for a few days. Several hospital stays of a few days are normal during treatment.
- When concerned about a symptom in the child, ask the care provider. Parents are often key in identifying problems early.

- Parents are usually concerned about central line care but feel more comfortable after a few days of caring for the line.
- Children have poor appetites at times so nutritional intake is needed when they are hungry.
- Remember that children are still at the normal developmental age. Treat them as a reflection of their ages, not as if they are older or younger.
- Try to maintain contact with the child's peer group and family members.
- Seek information from other parents and resources on cancer care.
- Remind parents to get time away and relax so that parental energy remains high and they are better able to deal with the child's therapy.

---

patient safety and quality of care in the ambulatory setting that address staffing resources, chemotherapy and biotherapy administration, telephone triage, and patient education (APHON, n.d.).

Preparation for home care centers on creating a normal environment while supporting the child's physiologic and psychosocial responses to the cancer and treatments. Education is a primary focus of discharge planning and ambulatory interventions. (See Partnering with Families: Cancer Therapy.) Teach the parents how to ensure adequate nutritional intake, to be alert for signs of infection, to protect the child from exposure to communicable disease during times of neutropenia, to administer medications at home, and to handle vomiting and pain. Assist the parents and child to deal with any obstacles to normal development and functioning. Teach the parents and family about symptoms that need to be treated immediately. (See Partnering with Families: Reportable Events for Children Receiving Chemotherapy.)

Home management of a vascular access device or central line, such as a Broviac catheter (refer to the Skills Manual ⊂⊃), is an initial challenge for parents (Figure 29–12 ■). Alternatively, an implanted port may be used and allows the child freedom to swim and engage in other activities. Parents need information about whatever device the child has received. Details about cleaning the site, instilling heparin in the line or reservoir, and other needed care should be demonstrated and reviewed prior to discharge to home. After teaching the parents, observe them performing the procedure before the child is discharged from the hospital or during ambulatory visits.

Clinical Judgment

The child with cancer usually has several episodes of neutropenia during treatment when the WBC count is low. What specific teaching is needed for the child and family during these periods to avoid infection? What signs and symptoms of infection are important for the family to understand?

Emphasize the need for the child and family to have fun and engage in as many normal activities as possible. Play distracts the child and is essential in reducing fears. Children, parents, and siblings often benefit from participation in cancer support groups and cancer summer camps. These activities create additional support systems, build the child's self-esteem, and enhance coping skills through role modeling.

Make home visits to evaluate the family's strengths and needs in the home setting. The presence of a palliative care team; an integrated plan of care; collaboration between families, the primary care provider, and other practitioners; and focus on the child's developmental level and the needs of the family can enhance the care provided when cure is no longer expected. Be sure that the family has adequate support from a hospice and other end-of-life services when the child's condition is terminal. See Chapter 18 ⊘.

Health Promotion and Maintenance

Treatment for cancer is generally a long process. Most children are treated for 2 to 3 years. Since normal developmental stages progress during this time, health promotion and health maintenance visits should still occur. Some usual care may have to be altered, but many

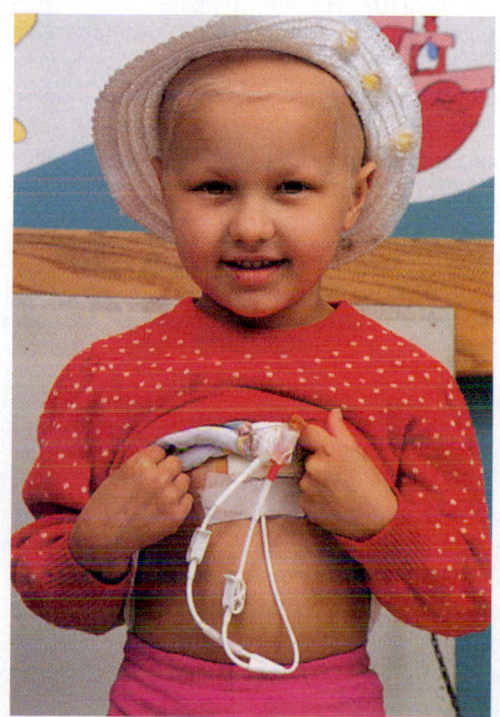

FIGURE 29–12 ■ A vascular access device allows chemotherapeutic agents to be administered without the need for repeated "sticks" to the child.

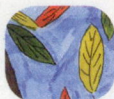

Partnering with Families

Reportable Events for Children Receiving Chemotherapy

Parents require verbal and written instructions about signs and symptoms to report to the child's oncologist while the child is receiving chemotherapy.

Have parents report the following events to the child's oncologist if they occur while the child is receiving chemotherapy:

- Temperature above 38°C (101°F)
- Any bleeding, such as nosebleeds, blood in stool or urine, petechiae, or ecchymosis
- Pain or discomfort with urination or defecation
- Sores in the mouth
- Vomiting or diarrhea

- Persistent pain anywhere, including headache
- Signs of infection, such as cough, fever, runny nose, and tugging at ears
- Signs of infection in central lines, such as redness, drainage, or tenderness
- Exposure to communicable diseases, especially varicella (chicken pox)

Inform dentists and other healthcare providers that the child is receiving chemotherapy prior to procedures. Prophylactic antibiotics should be given before and after dental care.

Source: *Adapted from Bindler, R. M., & Howry, L. B. (2005).* Pediatric drug guide. *Upper Saddle River, NJ: Prentice Hall Health.*

---

of the same developmental concerns of all children should be addressed. Help parents to view the child as a "normal" child who is ill for a period of time but still needs to have limits set on behavior, to develop healthy lifestyles, and to have environmental stimulation to learn to talk, read, or perform motor and cognitive tasks. See the Health Promotion & Maintenance Overview on page 967 for a summary of health promotion and health maintenance needs during cancer treatment.

After the treatment is complete, the child should be closely monitored for any sequelae of cancer survivorship (see the section earlier in the chapter about issues of survivorship). The child should be on a regular schedule for survivorship health visits. Continued surveillance promotes ongoing optimal health and development (Quillen, Crawford, Plummer, et al., 2011). The possibility of treatment-related physical and psychologic side effects necessitates clear instruction for the family, with increasing information provided to the child as cognitive development proceeds. Periodic laboratory and diagnostic tests may be needed, in addition to thorough physical and psychologic examinations. Guidelines for healthcare professionals and survivors have been developed by the Children's Oncology Group, and vary according to the type of cancer and the therapies received (Armstrong, 2010; Leigh, 2008; Oeffinger et al., 2008; Quillen et al., 2011). When the child transitions to a healthcare professional that serves adults, provide a clear and complete summary of the cancer and treatment so that appropriate follow-up can be maintained.

Evaluation

The following expected outcomes of nursing care for the child with cancer relate to the specific disease, treatments, and responses:

- The child has adequate intake to promote normal growth.
- Hydration is sufficient to support body processes and ensure drug and cancer cell product elimination.
- The nurse adapts prompt identification and treatment to minimize treatment side effects.
- Management of pain achieves a level of comfort satisfactory to the child and family.
- The family uses resources to provide necessary support during hospitalizations and treatments.

- The family demonstrates knowledge of management of treatment regimens.
- All family members have adequate support to accept the prognosis of the child's condition.

SOLID TUMORS

Brain Tumors

Central nervous system or brain tumors are the most commonly occurring solid tumors in children and the second most common malignancy, after leukemia. Brain tumors can also be benign; in these cases treatment is required and the prognosis is positive. Each year about 1,300 children under 5 years and 2,200 youth up to 20 years (or 3 to 6 in 100,000) are diagnosed with tumors of the brain and central nervous system, accounting for one in five childhood cancers. The overall survival rate is 70%; although this rate has increased in the last decades, it still is a lower survival rate than for most cancers of childhood (JNCI, 2011; Kuttesch, Rush, & Ater, 2011; McLendon, Adekunle, Rajaram, et al., 2011).

Etiology and Pathophysiology

The cause of most brain tumors is unknown. About 5% to 10% of brain tumors are genetic in origin, and epigenetic techniques are increasingly identifying mechanisms of brain cancers. Exposure to radiation is a known risk factor, such as CNS radiation used for treatment of some other cancers. There is a higher incidence in children with certain other cancers or diseases such as retinoblastoma, renal tumors, neurofibromatosis, tuberous sclerosis, or endocrine syndromes (Faria, Rutka, Smith, et al., 2011; Pollack & Jakacki, 2011).

Brain tumors in children usually occur below the roof of the cerebellum and involve the cerebellum, midbrain, and brainstem (Figure 29–13 ■). In contrast, brain tumors in adults are usually located above the areas between the cerebrum and cerebellum.

The most common brain tumors in children are medulloblastoma; gliomas of the cerebrum or brainstem; cerebral, cerebellar, and supratentorial astrocytoma; ependymoma (from ependymal cells lining the brain ventricles and spinal cord canal); and craniopharyngioma (McLendon et al., 2011).

Health Promotion & Maintenance Overview

The Child Receiving Cancer Treatment

Cancer treatment often extends for several years, so the child needs to continue health promotion and health maintenance visits.

GROWTH AND DEVELOPMENT SURVEILLANCE

- The child is assessed for height, weight, and body mass index. This provides information about growth patterns which may be altered by cancer treatment. If indicated, 24-hour diet recalls and other nutritional assessments are performed.
- Teaching is provided about age-appropriate foods. Since appetite may be impaired during periods of treatment, the child may be lacking fruits, vegetables, or other foods, as well as the nutrients they include. Encourage parents to be sure the child has a well-balanced diet during periods of remission.
- Perform developmental screening of young children. Provide suggestions for parents about the stimulation that is appropriate for the child's age. Include quiet activities that can be used when the child is fatigued or receiving therapy. These might include reading books, listening to music, and working on a computer. Have the parent plan for these activities on days that the child goes for chemotherapy or other treatment.
- Ask about the school-age child's progress in school. Performance may be altered due to neurologic effects of treatment as well as missing school. Plan for the family to partner with the school personnel for provision of tutors, computer programs, or other needed assistance.
- Encourage continued social contact with peers when blood counts are adequate to prevent infection.

PHYSICAL ASSESSMENT AND SCREENING

- Careful physical assessments are performed to identify any abnormalities that may result from cancer or its treatment. Be alert for signs of anemia, neutropenia, and thrombocytopenia; refer for treatment and suggest preventive measures such as infection control for neutropenia. Cardiopulmonary and neuromuscular assessments are particularly important. Vision and hearing should be assessed prior to treatment and periodically throughout. Include measurements of fine and gross motor activity.

ELIMINATION

- Toddlers may have an interruption in toilet training during periods when they do not feel well. Help parents to understand this regression, and encourage them to start again when the child is feeling better.
- Some medications cause diarrhea or constipation, so evaluate bowel patterns and provide guidance as needed. Skin care instruction may be needed if the child has diarrhea and is relatively immobile. Increasing fluids and fiber foods may be needed for constipation.
- Evaluate urinary output since many medications have effects on kidney function. Encourage adequate fluids for age to ensure elimination of medications.

SLEEP AND FATIGUE

- Children undergoing treatment often have disturbed sleep patterns. Parents of young children may become exhausted working all day, getting the child to treatments, and having disturbed sleep at night. Assess both the child's sleep patterns and the family's experiences. Encourage plans for respite care to enable rest periods. Provide cots, rocking chairs, and other comfortable settings for the child and family members during treatments.
- Both the child and parents may not expect or understand the profound fatigue that occurs during cancer treatment. They can be helped to plan for providing quiet times, eliminating electronic media at sleep time, and replenishing energy through naps, massage, relaxing baths, and spending time with family.

PHYSICAL ACTIVITY

- Since the child has periods of fatigue, patterns of physical activity may decrease. Emphasize the importance of integrating physical activity when the child feels well, since it is needed for learning gross motor skills, facilitating blood flow, improving mental status, and setting patterns for the future.

DISEASE AND INJURY PREVENTION STRATEGIES

- The child with cancer has the same safety hazards as other children of the same age, and such topics as car safety seats, fire prevention, water safety, and violence prevention should be addressed.
- An important hazard for children with cancer is infection due to decreased immune response and neutropenic episodes. Keep records of immunization status. Follow the recommendations of the CDC and AAP for other immunizations. Teach the hazards of exposure to large groups and those with infections when the child's immune system is compromised and neutropenia is present. Teach care of central lines and other potential sources of infection. Have families report signs of infection and exposure to known illnesses promptly.

MENTAL AND SPIRITUAL HEALTH

- Evaluate the child and family for signs of anxiety and depression. Ask how they are managing the cancer treatment and what poses the greatest challenges. Refer to other families with similar circumstances for support.
- Ensure that the child has contact with friends through childcare or school, or via phone, letters, and computer.
- Find out the impact of the child's cancer on the parents' jobs. Ask how the siblings have been coping, what changes there are in school performance, and whether teachers and others are aware of the stress the sibling may be experiencing.

TRANSITIONAL CARE

- As the child's treatment ends, instruct them about needed periodic follow-up with the oncologist. Continue to perform neurologic examinations and ascertain school performance. Be alert for signs of secondary tumors.
- Ask about worries regarding the future. As teens grow older, have them take over more responsibility for informing care providers of their cancer history and assist them to transition to adult healthcare providers.

Pathophysiology Illustrated Sites of Brain Tumors in Children

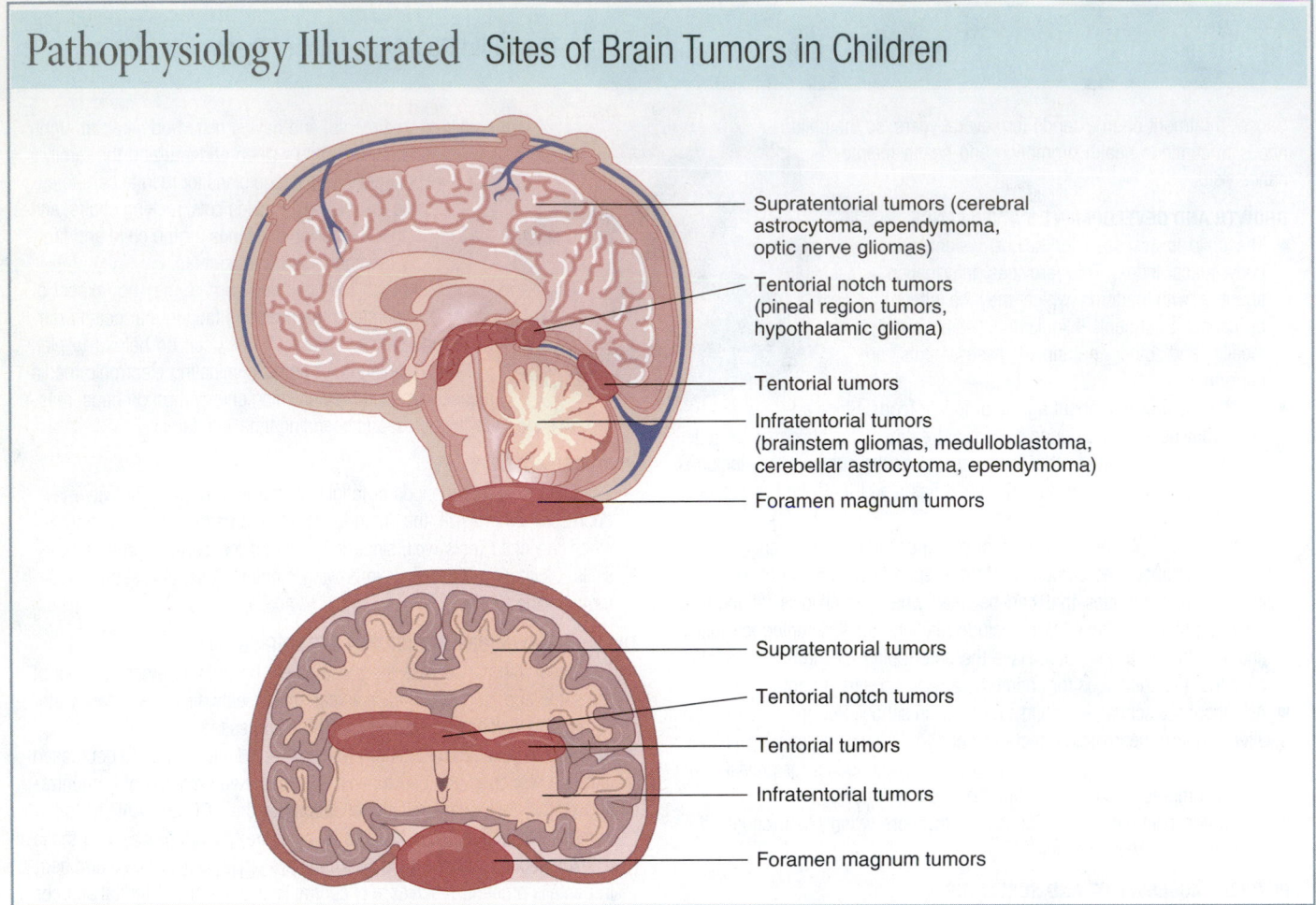

Supratentorial tumors (cerebral astrocytoma, ependymoma, optic nerve gliomas)

Tentorial notch tumors (pineal region tumors, hypothalamic glioma)

Tentorial tumors

Infratentorial tumors (brainstem gliomas, medulloblastoma, cerebellar astrocytoma, ependymoma)

Foramen magnum tumors

Supratentorial tumors

Tentorial notch tumors

Tentorial tumors

Infratentorial tumors

Foramen magnum tumors

FIGURE 29–13 ■ Approximately 1,700 children under the age of 14 years are diagnosed annually as having tumors of the brain and central nervous system. The four most common brain tumors in children are medulloblastoma, cerebral astrocytoma, ependymoma, and brainstem glioma.

Clinical Manifestations

Children with brain tumors can manifest behavioral and neurologic changes; these are frequently a result of increased intracranial pressure and may occur rapidly or slowly and subtly. Some common symptoms include headache (most common manifestation), nausea, vomiting, abnormalities of gait and coordination, dizziness, change in vision or hearing, irritability, fatigue, and mental status changes, such as educational or behavioral problems.

Clinical Tip

Some children with brain tumors have nonspecific signs. They may have a subtle behavior change, fatigue easily, have mild headaches, perform poorly at school, or show some incoordination. For infants, the nonspecificity of symptoms may be even more pronounced. Subtle changes such as increased irritability, anorexia, and developmental delays may occur. Meningitis or other causes may be suspected initially. If the fontanels are open, symptoms may develop more slowly since the skull allows for expansion of the brain. Be alert to subtle signs and to the parents' statement that they notice a change in the child. Report such findings so appropriate assessments can be made.

Brainstem tumors can present with weight deficits and may be mistakenly diagnosed as an eating disorder of infancy and childhood (failure to thrive). This may delay proper treatment. See the Clinical Manifestations table on page 969 for common manifestations of certain types of tumors.

Medulloblastomas are brain tumors in the external layer of the cerebellum. They account for 35% to 40% of childhood brain tumors, and commonly occur in children age 5 to 6 years. They are fast-growing and therefore often present with fast onset of symptoms such as increased intracranial pressure, manifested by increased head circumference in infants, vomiting, headache, ataxia, and vision changes. *Astrocytomas* arise from glial cells and can be either above or below the area between the cerebrum and cerebellum. They comprise 35% to 40% of childhood brain tumors, and vary from low-grade cerebellar to low-grade cerebral to high-grade tumors. The presenting symptoms vary depending on the location of the tumor. Endocrine (including precocious puberty), vision, and behavioral changes are all possible, as well as hemiparesis, increased intracranial pressure, and seizures. *Ependymomas* commonly occur in the fourth ventricle of the posterior fossa and comprise 10% to 15% of childhood brain tumors. Impaired growth, hydrocephalus, seizures, and cranial nerve impairments are the most common manifestations. *Brainstem gliomas* are located in the pons and typically spread into the surrounding tissue. They account for 10% to 15% of childhood brain tumors. Cranial nerve impairments, mental status changes, and motor symptoms occur (Kuttesch et al., 2011).

Collaborative Care

Collaborative care is needed to identify children with brain tumors and provide for them the comprehensive treatment required.

Clinical Manifestations Brain Tumors

TUMOR	ETIOLOGY	CLINICAL MANIFESTATIONS	CLINICAL THERAPY
Medulloblastoma	External layer of cerebellum	Headache, vomiting, ataxia	Surgery; chemotherapy with lomustine, vincristine, cisplatin; radiation
Astrocytomas	Glial cells, supratentorial or infratentorial	Seizures, visual disturbances, increased intracranial pressure, vomiting	Surgery; chemotherapy with vincristine, dactinomycin; radiation
Ependymoma	Fourth ventricle, posterior fossa	Hydrocephalus	Surgery, radiation
Brainstem gliomas	Pons	Cranial nerve (VI and VII) tract signs, nystagmus, ataxia, motor symptoms	Surgery, radiation

Diagnostic Tests

The first step in diagnosing brain tumors is a detailed health history and physical examination. Onset of symptoms, severity, and presentation of neurologic symptoms is recorded. Brain tumors are then definitively diagnosed by means of CT (Figure 29–14A ■), MRI (Figure 29–14B ■), positron emission tomography (PET), single-photon emission computed tomography (SPECT), myelography, and angiography. These tests are used to assess sensory pathway integrity and disease- or drug-related sensory dysfunction. New technologies combine imaging with angiography to more specifically image the lesion. Examples include magnetic resonance angiography (MRA), magnetic resonance spectroscopy (MRS), perfusion and diffusion imaging, digital subtraction angiograph (DSA), and CT angiography (CTA) (Paldino, Faerber, & Poussaint, 2011). Neurophysiologic tests (electroencephalography and brainstem evoked potentials) are used to assess sensory pathway integrity and disease- or drug-related sensory dysfunction. Other tests that may be performed are examination for serum tumor markers such as α-fetoprotein and human chorionic gonadotropin. Analysis of DNA is useful in some types of cancer when a genetic basis is related to cancer type. Such analysis raises ethical and legal issues, particularly with children (see Legal and Ethical Considerations: Genetic Testing and Children). Lumbar puncture is used to identify abnormal cells in the cerebrospinal fluid. Bone marrow aspiration and bone scans identify any extracranial primary neoplastic growth, as cancers in other sites can metastasize to or from the brain.

Clinical Therapy

Treatment depends on the type of brain tumor. Surgery is a common treatment and may be performed to obtain a biopsy specimen, to debulk (reduce the tumor size by partial removal) or excise the tumor, or to treat any hydrocephalus that may be present. During surgery, radiology images allow the neurosurgeon to see computed images of the brain while stimulating nerves to determine their functioning. These techniques provide rapid feedback to the neurosurgeon. Laser surgery, which has delicate, precise control and accuracy, is used when tumors are close to sensitive neural or vascular structures.

Radiation is commonly used in treatment of brain tumors, but its use is delayed when possible for children under 5 years of age to

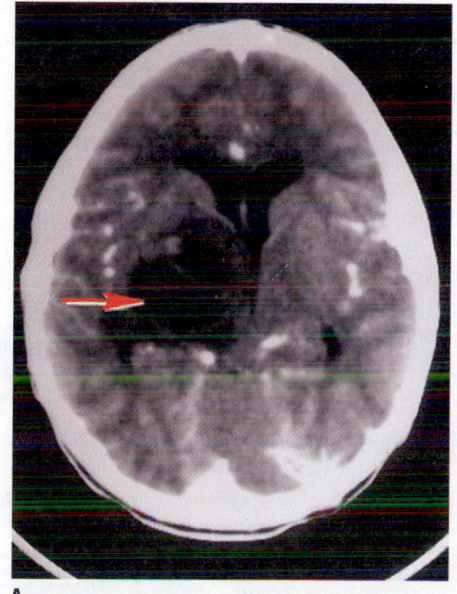

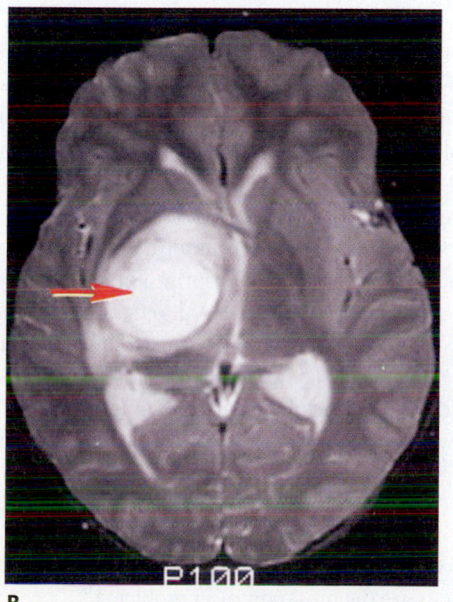

A   **B**

FIGURE 29–14 ■ Radiologic imaging of a child with a brain tumor. *A*, CT scan. *B*, MRI.

Source: *Courtesy of Carlos Sivit, M.D., Children's National Medical Center, Washington, DC.*

Legal and Ethical Considerations
Genetic Testing and Children

The explosion of knowledge related to genomics has been astounding in the area of cancer (see Chapter 4 🔗). Treatments more specifically target the cause of a cancer. Testing of those with familial cancers can provide information that assists in early detection and treatment. When children are tested for a genetic disease, the decision is made by parents, taking away the child's inherent rights to decide whether to have the test. Embryos can even be tested for cancer predispositions. The American Medical Association finds that parents can generally make the decisions about their children and that prenatal genetic testing is acceptable when there is an elevated risk of fetal genetic disorders. Clear communication of the results and their complex meaning is needed. However, the implications of such testing are complex (Patrick-Miller, Bradbury, & Terry, 2010). Will an individual be discriminated against in school, the family, or employment if there is a genetic mutation? Will every individual with a positive genetic test manifest the disease? How and when do parents or health professionals relay test results to children as they get older? Informed consent is an essential part of genetic testing and involves disclosure of procedures, risks, and benefits; understanding by the consumer; voluntary decision making; and clear consent by the parent of a minor child. Nurses must help parents to better understand their decisions and implications, and support them as they decide whether to consent for genetic testing for their children.

minimize long-term undesired effects. A combination of radiation and chemotherapy following surgery has improved the survival of children with medulloblastoma and ependymoma. Intrathecal administration of chemotherapy is useful in some cases. However, the blood-brain barrier is a factor in the effectiveness of chemotherapy for children with brain tumors. For example, when methotrexate is administered intrathecally (in the spinal canal), only a small amount crosses normal brain capillaries. Common chemotherapeutic drugs include vincristine, etoposide, cisplatin, carboplatin, cyclophosphamide, nitrosoureas, methotrexate, and temozolomide. Bone marrow and stem cell transplantation is an increasingly used treatment option.

Numerous new approaches are being investigated and will be used increasingly in the years ahead. New combinations of chemotherapeutic agents, precision-guided delivery of medications and radiotherapy, gene therapy, cytokine-producing therapy to activate the immune system, molecular analysis and epigenetic markers to guide treatment, and blood-brain barrier disruption are examples of emerging treatments (Faria et al., 2011; Pollack, 2011).

Complications of treatment for children with brain tumors are significant. They include severe infections (commonly associated with high-dose chemotherapy), seizure activity, sensorimotor defects, hydrocephalus, and growth problems. Care is taken to treat infections early and aggressively. If a cerebrospinal shunt is used, infection or blockage can occur (see Chapter 33 🔗 for further discussion of cerebrospinal shunts in children). Anticonvulsants are commonly given prophylactically following surgery. Endocrine problems, such as growth hormone changes, hypothyroidism, and panhypopituitarism, may occur when the tumor is in the hypothalamic-pituitary area. Treatment may also lead to impaired cognitive function and emotional or behavioral problems in some children. Memory deficits and selective attention deficits are the most common problems.

Diabetes insipidus is a special consideration in children with midline brain tumors, such as those that compress the hypothalamus, pituitary stalk, or posterior pituitary gland. Manifestations of diabetes insipidus include voiding of large amounts of dilute urine with a specific gravity of less than 1.005 to 1.010 (see Chapter 32 🔗).

Nursing Management

The goals of nursing management are to administer treatment, monitor for side effects, and support the child and family when a brain tumor occurs.

Nursing Assessment and Diagnosis

The focus of physiologic assessment of the child with a brain tumor is determined by its presentation (Table 29–5). Presenting signs can be categorized as follows:

- Nonspecific signs related to increasing intracranial pressure
- Secondary signs related to displacement of intracranial structures
- Focal signs suggesting direct involvement of the brain and cranial nerves

Thorough neurologic examination before surgery is essential to provide a record of baseline functioning and allow the evaluation of the child's changing physiologic status before surgery. Ask if the child has manifested slow changes over time or has had quickly developing symptoms. Measurement of head circumference and assessment of the anterior fontanel are necessary in children under the age of 18 months.

Perform developmental screening on young children using the Denver II or other developmental tests (see Chapter 8 🔗). Ask about the child's social interactions, school performance, and any behavior changes that have occurred.

The following nursing diagnoses may be identified for the child with a brain tumor, depending on the type and location of the tumor:

- Nutrition, Imbalanced: Less than Body Requirements related to loss of appetite
- Mobility: Physical, Impaired related to tumor pressure on coordination centers
- Growth and Development, Delayed related to effects of disability
- Memory, Impaired related to neurological disturbance
- Pain, Acute related to compression of brain tissue

NANDA-I © 2012

Planning and Implementation

The child with a brain tumor requires multidisciplinary care with partnerships among a neurologist, neurosurgeon, pediatrician, dietitian, social worker, other specialists, and the family. The nurse can act

TABLE 29–5	Physiologic Assessment of Brain Tumors
CLINICAL MANIFESTATIONS	**ASSESSMENT**
Nonspecific signs: headache, morning vomiting, somnolence, irritability	Level of consciousness, pupil response, pupil shape and size
Secondary signs: disturbances of cranial nerves; other signs depend on site of tumor	All cranial nerves
Focal signs: truncal ataxia (midline brain tumors), general nystagmus, head tilting	Motor ability, head positions when watching television or looking at people, double vision, sixth cranial nerve involvement

as a case manager to coordinate the complex care needed by the child and help the family to understand the treatment.

For the nursing care of children immediately following surgery, refer to Chapter 15 🔗. In addition, close monitoring of neurologic status is needed postoperatively (see Chapter 33 🔗). Subtle alterations such as visual differences, behavior or alertness variations, and gait changes can herald serious problems from the tumor or pressure in the brain. Many children return from surgery with a ventricular-peritoneal shunt. Be especially alert for signs of increased intracranial pressure and infection. Observe for seizure activity. Administer drugs such as antibiotics, steroids, and anticonvulsants as ordered.

Signs and symptoms of diabetes insipidus may occur following brain surgery (see Chapter 32 🔗 for a description of diabetes insipidus). Nursing care includes hourly measurement of intake and output, measurement of serum sodium levels every 4 to 6 hours, accurate fluid replacement, and frequent assessment of neurologic status. An indwelling urinary catheter is useful for accurate measurement of urinary output.

Having a child with a diagnosis of brain tumor can be devastating to family members. While some tumors have a good prognosis, others do not. Whatever the prognosis, the surgery and other treatment protocols will be frightening to parents. Explain procedures, the purpose of lines, and the use of sedation to keep the child restful, and answer any questions. Ask parents about resources such as other family members, available sick leave from work, and places to stay if they live far from the hospital. Suggest periods of napping and rest, use of facilities to stay near the hospital, and other resources.

Discharge Planning and Care in the Community

Teach the parents to watch for an increase in voiding of dilute urine. Be sure they can recognize the signs of infection and changes in the child's neurologic status. Once the child is ready for discharge, chemotherapy or radiation may begin; inform parents of the reason and potential side effects of these treatments. Assist the family in obtaining any special equipment they may need to care for the child at home, such as a wheelchair, bed rails, or dressings. The American Cancer Society is a potential resource for assistance with these needs.

Children with brain tumors, especially those who have received radiation, often have some permanent sequelae. They may have slowed development, loss of coordination, learning disabilities, or other effects. These sequelae are most common in children who are 3 years of age or younger at the time of radiation therapy. Perform accurate height and weight measures at each healthcare visit. Assess developmental milestones. Ask about progress in school and any special services that might be needed. Perform thorough neurologic assessments. Support the family as they learn to deal with unknown or changed expectations for the child's performance.

Evaluation

Expected outcomes of nursing care for the child with a brain tumor depend on the site of the tumor, clinical therapy, and medical outcome. Possible outcomes include the following:

- Nutritional intake is adequate to support growth and prevent malnutrition.
- A safe environment is maintained for the child.
- Physical mobility is maintained to the limits of developmental level and alterations of disease.

- An environment that supports normal developmental milestones within capability of the child is maintained.
- Pain is managed to a comfort level.
- Parents understand the diagnosis and treatment plan.

Neuroblastoma

Neuroblastoma is the solid tumor most commonly occurring outside the cranium of children. It is responsible for 8% to 10% of childhood cancers and 15% of cancer deaths in children. The average age at diagnosis is 17 to 22 months; it is the most common tumor in infants during the first year of life. Nearly all cases (90%) are diagnosed before 5 years of age (Park, Eggert, & Caron, 2008; Zage & Ater, 2011). Prognosis varies, depending on the staging of the tumor (Table 29–6) and the age of the child, with more favorable outcomes in infants under 1 year of age, and in presenting sites in the pelvis or thorax. Less favorable outcomes are associated with presence of N-myc oncogene amplification. Survival rates are over 90% for stages 1 and 2, but drop to 25% to 35% for stage 4 (Zage & Ater, 2011). As compared to Whites, Hispanics, and Asians, more Black and Native American children have advanced disease upon diagnosis and therefore lower survival rates (Henderson, Bhatia, Pinto, et al., 2011). It is unknown if genetic differences or lack of consistent primary care contributes to this disparity.

Neuroblastoma is commonly a smooth, hard, nontender mass that can occur anywhere along the sympathetic nervous system chain. A frequent location is the abdomen, although other sites are the adrenal, thoracic, and cervical areas.

Etiology and Pathophysiology

Neuroblastoma originates in primitive neurocrest cells of the autonomic nervous system that form the adrenal medulla, paraganglia, and sympathetic nervous system of the cervical sympathetic chain and the thoracic chain. Approximately 50% of neuroblastomas

TABLE 29–6	International Neuroblastoma Staging System
STAGE	**DESCRIPTION**
1	Localized tumor confined to the area of origin; complete gross excision, with or without microscopic residual disease; identifiable ipsilateral and contralateral lymph nodes negative microscopically
2A	Unilateral tumor with incomplete gross excision; identifiable ipsilateral and contralateral lymph nodes negative microscopically
2B	Unilateral tumor with complete or incomplete gross excision; with positive ipsilateral regional lymph nodes; identifiable contralateral lymph nodes negative microscopically
3	Tumor infiltrating across the midline with or without regional lymph node involvement; or unilateral tumor with contralateral regional lymph node involvement; or midline tumor with bilateral regional lymph node involvement
4	Dissemination of tumor to distant lymph nodes, bone, bone marrow, liver, and/or other organs (except as defined in stage 4S)
4S	Localized primary tumor as defined for stage 1 or 2 with dissemination limited to liver, skin, and/or bone marrow in child under 1 year; bone marrow involvement should be minimal (less than 10% of cells)—if greater this would be stage 4 disease

Source: *Data from National Cancer Institute. (2011b). Stages of neuroblastoma. Retrieved from* http://www.cancer.gov/cancertopics/pdq/treatment/neuroblastoma/HealthProfessional/page3

Weblink — American Cancer Society

develop in the adrenal medulla; 30% develop in the cervical, thoracic, or pelvic ganglia; and the remaining are elsewhere along the sympathetic chain (Zage & Ater, 2011). Lymph node metastasis is common.

The cause of neuroblastoma is unknown. A genetic defect found in many cases of neuroblastoma is a deletion of the short arm of chromosome 1 (1p del); other chromosomal abnormalities may include 11q, 14q, and 17q. Amplification of the proto-oncogene N-myc or mutation of Phox2B and ALK genes may be seen (Shuangshoti, Shuangshoti, Nuchprayoon, et al., 2011; Zage & Ater, 2011).

Clinical Manifestations

The location of the mass determines the symptoms. Altered bowel and bladder function occur when the mass is retroperitoneal; characteristic signs are weight loss, abdominal distention, enlarged liver, irritability, fatigue, and fever. Dyspnea or infection may occur when the tumor is mediastinal. Neck and facial edema may result from vena cava syndrome if the tumor is mediastinal and large. Intracranial lesions may be present with periorbital ecchymosis. Malaise, fever, and a limp can occur if there has been metastasis to the bone. Bone marrow disease can manifest as **pancytopenia** (abnormal depression of all cellular blood components) with neutropenia (causing infections) and anemia (causing fatigue). Metastatic spread can result in an array of symptoms affecting multiple organs.

Collaborative Care

The goal of care in neuroblastoma is early identification of disease so that it can be treated in its beginning stages. Support for the family during treatment is a focus of the entire care management team.

Diagnostic Tests

Diagnosis of neuroblastoma begins with a careful history and physical examination to identify changes in behaviors of the young child. The International Neuroblastoma Staging System (INSS) recommends different diagnostic and laboratory evaluations for diagnosis of the primary disease and of metastases (Table 29–7). Routine blood cell counts are needed, including CBC with differential. The test may reveal anemia and thrombocytopenia. There is no classic WBC response, although thrombocytopenia may occur in association with disseminated intravascular coagulation. **Leukocytosis** (higher than normal leukocyte count) and **leukopenia** (lower than normal leukocyte count) have been observed with bone marrow involvement. Serum electrolytes, liver function studies, LDH, coagulation studies, and urinalysis are performed. Baseline cardiac function is evaluated if doxorubicin will be used in treatment.

Tumor markers include vanillylmandelic acid (VMA), homovanillic acid (HVA), dopamine, ferritin, NSE (an enzyme in neural tissue), LDH, and a ganglioside GD2. VMA and HVA are by-products of adrenal hormones, and their levels are usually elevated in the urine and blood (see Appendix D 🔗 for normal values). A variety of laboratory findings are used initially to diagnose the disease and later to follow its progress. A biopsy or surgical removal of the tumor will be followed by analysis of its type and genetic abnormalities. Areas of necrosis and calcification in major organs are readily identifiable with radiologic tests and MRIs. These tests also help in staging of disease by identifying metastases.

Clinical Therapy

The stage of the tumor (see Table 29–6) determines the treatment protocol. Surgical excision of the mass is performed and may be the only treatment in low-risk stages. With higher risk, surgery is followed by chemotherapy with a combination of drugs. Several courses of chemotherapy may be needed prior to surgery when the mass is large or wrapped around major blood vessels. Chemotherapy may include:

- Cyclophosphamide
- Ifosfamide
- Doxorubicin
- Cisplatin
- Carboplatin
- Teniposide
- Etoposide

Radiation is often used, especially in disseminated disease or when tumors are not receptive to chemotherapy. Autologous stem cell transplantation may be performed for advanced disease, sometimes followed by the biological modifier *cis*-retinoic acid and fenretinide (to promote apoptosis). The age of the child, tumor stage, and molecular characteristics of the tumor all guide treatment protocols (Zage & Ater, 2011).

Nursing Management

Nursing management focuses on careful assessment of symptoms in this potentially multisystem disease. Physiologic and psychologic support during treatment are complex for the young child and family.

Nursing Assessment and Diagnosis

The presenting site of the tumor, such as the neck or abdomen, is assessed by observation and inspection. Palpation is contraindicated. Carefully document related functioning, such as bowel and bladder function. Take vital signs to watch for elevated temperature and vital sign changes caused by a thoracic mass. Observe gait and coordination. Take weight and height (or length for infant) and compare with earlier percentiles for the child. Specific assessments during treatment will depend on the treatment methods used (refer to the earlier discussions of chemotherapy and radiation treatment). Psychosocial assessment and emotional assessment of the family are needed.

The following nursing diagnoses may be appropriate for the child with neuroblastoma, depending on the location and extent of the presenting disease:

- Gas Exchange, Impaired related to ventilation-perfusion imbalance
- Mobility: Physical, Impaired related to neuromuscular impairment
- Nutrition, Imbalanced: Less than Body Requirements related to loss of appetite and high metabolic demands of tumor

TABLE 29–7 Diagnostic Tests for Neuroblastoma	
TESTS FOR INITIAL DIAGNOSIS	**TESTS FOR METASTASES**
Tumor tissue diagnosis by light microscopy, *or*	Bone marrow aspirate and biopsy
Biopsy of tumor cells plus laboratory evaluation showing increased urine or serum catecholamines (two separate measures each more than 3 standard deviations above the norm for age) (See Appendix D 🔗 for usual laboratory values)	Radiolabeled scanning with metaiodobenzylguanidine (MIBG)
	Bone scan
	Skeletal radiograph CT or MRI of abdomen, liver, brain, eye orbits
	MRI of spine
	Chest radiograph, with added CT or MRI if radiograph shows lesions

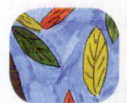

Partnering with Families

The Child with Neuroblastoma

SURGERY PHASE

- Teach the parents to observe for signs of infection at the wound site and to take the child's temperature, if necessary.
- Assist the family to provide pain management including medication administration and various comfort measures.
- Teach the parents the importance of keeping accurate records of urine output and bowel movements and to notify the healthcare provider if the child does not have a bowel movement at least every 3 days.
- Continue with progression to a regular diet.

CHEMOTHERAPY PHASE

- The child frequently has a central line placed early in the chemotherapy phase. The central line greatly reduces the emotional trauma associated with chemotherapy and blood tests. When it is present:
    - Teach the child how to help the parents with cleaning of the central line.

- Teach the child how to protect the central line.
- Teach the parents how to clean and dress the site of the central line.
- Have the parents practice central line care with a model and then on the child before discharge to increase the parents' confidence.
- Give the parents written and illustrated information about care of a central line.
- Arrange for home care dressing supplies before discharge.
- Give the parents detailed chemotherapy information.
- Teach administration of any medications that the parent will perform via central line or other routes.
- Refer the family to the American Cancer Society for coloring books and other resources for children receiving chemotherapy.

- Pain related to tumor pressure and injury
- Grieving (Family) related to potential loss of significant person

NANDA-I © 2012

Planning and Implementation

The nursing management of the child with neuroblastoma can encompass the three phases of medical treatment: chemotherapy, surgery, and radiation. Specific postsurgical care depends on the size and site of the tumor. Normal postoperative care includes providing fluid support and respiratory care and preventing infection.

Nursing care during the chemotherapy phase includes minimizing side effects, preventing infection, teaching parents about the medications their child is receiving, and monitoring physical and emotional growth and development of the young child. When radiation is part of the treatment, use common nursing measures described earlier in the chapter. Topics for parent and family teaching and discharge planning are presented in Partnering with Families: The Child with Neuroblastoma.

Ongoing support and connection to resources to assist in management of the child's treatment at home will be needed. Long-term sequelae following surgery and other treatments require ongoing care. When the prognosis is poor, parents may appreciate referrals to hospice, to other parents who have experienced similar child illnesses, and to other community resources. See Chapter 18 🔗 for additional nursing care for the end of life.

Evaluation

Expected outcomes of nursing care for the child with neuroblastoma include the following:

- Ventilatory exchange is adequate to support daily activities.
- Physical mobility is maintained to the level possible considering developmental age.
- Sensory/perceptual alterations are managed to provide for safety and sensory input.
- Pain is managed to a level of comfort.
- Family members accept and integrate the diagnosis.

Wilms Tumor (Nephroblastoma)

Nephroblastoma, an intrarenal tumor of which the most common type is called Wilms tumor, is a common abdominal tumor of childhood and accounts for 6% of all childhood tumors. The incidence of nephroblastoma is approximately 7.6 cases per 1 million children annually. Wilms tumor occurs most frequently between 2 and 3 years of age, with young ages more commonly seen in bilateral disease (Buckley, 2011).

Etiology and Pathophysiology

Wilms tumor is associated with several congenital anomalies: aniridia (absence of the iris), hemihypertrophy (abnormal growth of half of the body or a body structure), genitourinary anomalies, nevi, and hamartomas (benign, nodulelike growths). This connection suggests a genetic link; chromosome deletions at 11p13 and 11p15 (locations for WT1 and WT2 genes) have been associated with Wilms tumor. TP53, a tumor suppressor gene; CTNB1, an oncogene; and other genetic conditions have been related to Wilms tumor (Buckley, 2011; Huff, 2011). It has a high incidence in Beckwith-Wiedemann syndrome, which is characterized by macroglossia, hemihypertrophy, visceromegaly, and hypoglycemia. However, most children with Wilms tumor have no other abnormalities. Wilms tumor grows very quickly, doubling its size in 11 to 13 days. Such fast growth generally contributes to a large tumor by the time of diagnosis. However, chemotherapy drugs have significantly increased survival rates for children with Wilms tumor, with 90% survival rates (Anderson, Dhamne, & Huff, 2011).

Clinical Manifestations

Wilms tumor is usually an asymptomatic, firm, lobulated mass located to one side of the midline in the abdomen. Often a parent discovers the mass when bathing or handling the child, or may notice that the child's clothing is tight around the abdomen. Hypertension caused by increased renin activity related to renal damage is reported in 25% of cases. Hematuria or abdominal pain is sometimes present.

Collaborative Care

Care by many professionals is needed for prompt diagnosis and treatment of Wilms tumor.

Diagnostic Tests

The diagnosis of Wilms tumor is based on an ultrasound study of the abdomen and an intravenous pyelogram. CT scanning or MRI of the lungs, liver, spleen, and brain may be performed to identify any metastases (Geller & Kochan, 2011). This information is used in staging the tumor (Table 29–8). A complete blood count is obtained, as well as BUN and creatinine levels. Liver function tests are performed. Histologic examination is performed for tissue typing once the tumor is removed.

Clinical Therapy

Treatment is multifaceted and increasingly successful. About 90% of early stages and 70% of metastatic cases have long-term survival (Anderson et al., 2011). Surgery is performed to remove the affected kidney, to examine the opposite kidney, to remove lymph nodes for examination, and to look for other sites of metastases. The total tumor is removed, taking care not to rupture the tumor capsule. Generally the entire kidney is removed, but when the disease is bilateral, a kidney-sparing procedure is needed. Such procedures are being examined for their success in treating unilateral disease as well. Chemotherapy or radiation therapy, alone or in combination, is sometimes used before surgery to reduce the size of the tumor. Children with stage III and IV disease often receive vincristine, dactinomycin, and doxorubicin; cyclophosphamide is sometimes added. Radiation may also follow surgery, especially in disseminated disease. Children whose tumors are almost completely excised and who have a favorable prognosis do not require irradiation of the tumor bed and may receive limited chemotherapy.

Long-term complications of treatment include liver damage, portal hypertension, and mild cirrhosis, which may occur in children treated for right-sided Wilms tumor. Radiation damage (such as thinning or weakening) of the skeleton, pelvis, and thorax has been reported. Kyphosis and scoliosis may occur from irradiation of vertebral bodies and the pelvis. Glomerular damage to the remaining kidney may also occur. Second malignancies in the original radiation field have occurred with orthovoltage radiation, but recent changes in radiation therapy have reduced this risk.

Nursing Management

Nursing management focuses on referring the child with abdominal mass or other symptoms for prompt evaluation, supporting the child and family during therapy, and being alert for any further signs of cancer.

Nursing Assessment and Diagnosis

Perform a thorough baseline assessment of the child. Do not palpate the abdomen because of the potential for spreading the cancerous cells. Monitor the child's blood pressure carefully as hypertension is a common finding that may require treatment.

Practice Alert

If a mass is felt during palpation of a child's abdomen, stop palpating immediately and report the finding to the physician or advanced practice nurse overseeing the child's care. Never palpate the liver or abdomen of a child with Wilms tumor as this could cause a piece of the tumor to dislodge. Place a sign on the child's bed and in the chart alerting health providers not to palpate the child's abdomen.

Nursing diagnoses for a child with Wilms tumor will differ depending on the phase of treatment. Common nursing diagnoses may include the following:

- Infection, Risk for related to inadequate defenses
- Urinary Elimination, Impaired related to anatomic obstruction
- Tissue Perfusion: Cardiac, Ineffective related to hypertension caused by mechanical reduction of blood flow
- Caregiver Role Strain, Risk for related to child's illness severity
- Home Maintenance, Impaired related to demands of child's disease

NANDA-I © 2012

Planning and Implementation

Nursing management can be divided into two phases: the postrenal surgery phase and the chemotherapy phase. (See Chapter 15 🔗 for general care of the child after surgery.) Drawings and special teaching dolls with removable kidneys can be used to teach young children about the surgery. Although chemotherapy may occur at two different times, before and after surgery, nursing management considerations remain the same.

Nursing care during the postrenal surgery phase focuses on pain management and close monitoring of fluid levels. A large incision is necessary to remove the kidney, and the resultant postoperative shift

TABLE 29–8	National Wilms Tumor Study Staging System
STAGE	**DESCRIPTION**
I	The tumor is limited to the kidney and completely excised.
	The surface of the renal capsule is intact. The tumor is not ruptured before or during removal. No residual tumor is apparent beyond the margins of the excision.
II	The tumor extends beyond the kidney but is completely excised. Regional extension of the tumor is present, i.e., penetration through the outer surface of the renal capsule into the perirenal soft tissues. Vessels outside the kidney substance are infiltrated or contain tumor thrombus. Biopsy may have been performed on the tumor, or local spillage of tumor confined to the flank has occurred. No residual tumor is apparent at or beyond the margin of excision.
III	Residual nonhematogenous tumor is confined to the abdomen. Any of the following may occur: ■ Lymph nodes on biopsy are found to be involved in the hilus, the periaortic chains, or beyond. ■ Diffuse peritoneal contamination by the tumor has occurred, such as by spillage of tumor beyond the flank before or during surgery, or by tumor growth that has penetrated through the peritoneal surface. ■ Implants are found on peritoneal surfaces. ■ The tumor extends beyond the surgical margins either microscopically or grossly. ■ The tumor is not completely resectable because of local infiltration into vital structures.
IV	Hematogenous metastasis: deposits are present beyond stage III (e.g., lung, liver, bone, and/or brain).
V	Bilateral renal involvement is present at diagnosis. An attempt should be made to stage each side according to the above criteria on the basis of extent of disease before biopsy.

Source: Data from National Cancer Institute. (2011c). Wilms tumor. Retrieved from http://www.cancer.gov/cancertopics/pdq/treatment/wilms/HealthProfessional/page3

of organs and fluid in the abdominal cavity may create discomfort for the child. Frequently reposition the child and use noninvasive and pharmacologic pain interventions to improve the child's comfort. Gentle handling is important. Monitor fluids closely following surgery to prevent hypovolemia and to assess the shift of fluids out of the third space and out of the body. Assess daily weight, intake and output, and urine specific gravity. Monitor the function of the remaining kidney. Take blood pressure measurements frequently to watch for signs of shock and to assess the functioning of the remaining kidney.

During the chemotherapy phase, monitor the child for side effects of drugs, the potential for infection from the central line site, and the function of the remaining kidney. Advise parents about home care needs, administration of medications, monitoring for drug side effects, and ongoing needs for health monitoring. Be sure care is well coordinated among all healthcare providers.

Evaluation

Desired outcomes for nursing care of the child with nephroblastoma include balanced intake and output, normal vital signs, recovery from surgery, and successful family management of postsurgical care and ongoing treatments.

Bone Tumors

Osteosarcoma (or Osteogenic Sarcoma)

Osteosarcoma is the most common tumor affecting the skeleton of children, with an incidence of 7 cases per 1 million children. Its peak incidence is during the rapid growth years, at 13 years for girls, and 14 years for boys (Arndt, 2011). The tumor is usually located at the metaphysis of the distal femur, proximal tibia, or proximal humerus.

Etiology and pathophysiology Bone tissue produced by osteosarcoma never matures into normal compact bone. Although the cause of osteosarcoma is unknown, radiation exposure (either environmental or treatment related) is associated with its development. Survivors of retinoblastoma have a greatly increased incidence of osteosarcoma. An abnormality of gene p53 has been noted in some cases of this cancer, leading to oncogene malformations and possibly to an absence of tumor suppressor genes (Heare, Hensley, & Dell'Orfano, 2009).

Clinical manifestations The common initial symptoms of osteosarcoma are pain, swelling, and a limp. The pain can be referred to the hip or back, which can delay diagnosis. Deep bone pain causing night awakenings should be investigated (Arndt, 2011). Pulmonary metastasis occurs in up to 20% of cases. Other metastatic sites include kidney, adrenals, brain, and pericardium. When lung metastasis is the only site, lung resection may be successful for treatment. Disseminated metastases and bone lesions have poorer prognoses.

Collaborative Care

Partnerships among professionals will enable the child with a bone tumor to obtain accurate diagnosis, treatment, and necessary rehabilitation.

Diagnostic Tests

Diagnosis of osteosarcoma is made through radiographic studies of the affected area and bone scan. CT or MRI scans of involved bone and other potential sites are performed. Radionucleotide bone scans

are performed. A complete blood count, liver studies, and renal studies are performed for clues to potential metastases. A blood test is included for serum alkaline phosphatase or lactic dehydrogenase (levels may be elevated), and tumor biopsy is performed to confirm the diagnosis. Arteriography may be performed if limb-sparing surgery is contemplated. MRI and other studies are carried out to identify the tumor's relationship to blood vessels, nerves, joints, and soft tissue. Cardiac assessments are performed to establish baseline function prior to treatment with doxorubicin, and CT is carried out to identify possible metastases (Arndt, 2011).

Clinical Therapy

Treatment involves both surgery and chemotherapy. The surgery is either a limb salvage procedure or limb amputation. A limb salvage procedure is possible if a neurobundle (area where several nerves converge) is not involved in the tumor. The tumor is removed, and a bone graft or internal prosthesis may be used. Bone grafts may be autograft (coming from the child and usually obtained from the pelvis) or allograft (coming from another individual). The major risks with a limb salvage procedure are infection and nonunion of the grafted bone with the bone cells in the extremity (Manfrini, Tiwari, Ham, et al., 2011). When limb salvage is not possible, an amputation is performed. Physical rehabilitation will be needed after either amputation or a limb-sparing procedure. Both require careful monitoring as the child grows. For example, in limb salvage with an internal prosthetic, growth of the surrounding bone can impair function; expanding prostheses are now used in some cases. The child with an amputation needs new prostheses and fittings to accommodate growth. Aggressive chemotherapy following surgery has improved the survival rate. At the time of diagnosis, most children have metastases (even though they may not be identifiable), so chemotherapy is needed. Chemotherapy is started before surgery to shrink the tumor, especially in cases where limb salvage (also called limb sparing) surgery is performed. It is also given postoperatively to treat and prevent metastasis. Drugs commonly used for osteosarcoma include:

- Doxorubicin
- Cisplatin
- Ifosfamide with mesna
- Methotrexate with leucovorin rescue

Radiation is generally not effective in treating osteosarcoma although it may be used with chemotherapy for recurrence at other sites.

Ewing Sarcoma

Ewing sarcoma is a malignant, small, round cell tumor usually involving the diaphyseal (shaft) portion of the long bones. The most common sites are the femur, pelvis, tibia, fibula, ribs, humerus, scapula, and clavicle, but any bone may be involved. Ewing sarcoma occurs in two children per 1 million, is most common in Whites and Hispanics, and is less common in Black and Asian children. The incidence is highest in children between the ages of 5 and 20 years, with a median of 14 years. Translocations on chromosomes 11 and 22 have been identified in children with Ewing sarcoma; these are t(11;22)(q24;q12). In addition, these tumors express a proto-oncogene, c-myc (Heare et al., 2009).

The symptoms are similar to those of osteosarcoma and may include pain, swelling, fever, an elevated WBC count, elevated erythrocyte sedimentation rate, and elevated C-reactive protein. Some children present with a fracture of the affected bone. A tumor biopsy is necessary for diagnosis. Diagnostic tests are the same as those for osteosarcoma.

Initial treatment for Ewing sarcoma is chemotherapy to reduce the tumor, followed by surgical removal of the entire bone or intensive high-dose irradiation of the entire bone. Limb-sparing procedures are now commonly performed rather than amputation. Surgery is preferred because of the possibility of a secondary cancer from radiation. Chemotherapy is always used following initial treatment, as undetectable metastases are commonly present. Medications used to treat Ewing sarcoma include:

- Vincristine
- Doxorubicin
- Cyclophosphamide
- Dactinomycin
- Etoposide
- Ifosfamide

Nursing Management

The goals of nursing management for bone tumors are to provide support during treatment and help the child adjust to any changes in body function.

Nursing Assessment and Diagnosis

Carefully evaluate any child or adolescent who has a limp or complains of pain in an extremity. Confirm the onset and whether the symptoms were associated with injury. Refer for further evaluation if the discomfort persists or is not associated with injury. Physiologic assessment of the child with a bone tumor includes assessment of the site before surgery. Assess the child's pain or discomfort, mobility, and gait. Take careful vital signs, especially noting temperature and respirations. Psychologic assessment of the child and family is needed, especially if amputation is planned. Body image disturbances occur when a limb is lost, particularly with school-age children and adolescents. Assess the child's understanding of the treatment and of care after surgery. Inquire about support systems that are available for assistance.

Observe the wound postoperatively for infection and hemorrhage. Assess circulation above and below the operative site. If edema is found, elevate the limb. If a limb salvage procedure is performed, the child's extremity will be intact but it will not function as before, because muscle insertion sites and mass have been removed with the tumor during surgery. Detailed charting of the condition of the surgical site and limb function is important.

If the limb has been amputated, assess the child for the following signs indicating a disturbed body image:

- Refusal to look at or touch the altered or missing body part
- Preoccupation with loss or change
- Feelings of shame or embarrassment, either verbalized or demonstrated
- Distorted perception of normal body (easily seen in the child's drawings of the body)
- Fears of rejection or unwanted attention from others
- Overexposure or hiding of the affected body part
- Actual or perceived change in the structure and function of the body or body parts

Psychosocial assessment of the child and family is discussed in more detail earlier in the general section on childhood cancer (see pages 953–955).

Appropriate nursing diagnoses for the child with a bone tumor are based on the treatment and needs of each child.

- Infection, Risk for related to amputation or limb salvage procedure
- Skin Integrity, Impaired related to mechanical forces of prosthesis
- Mobility: Physical, Impaired related to musculoskeletal impairment
- Body Image, Disturbed related to treatment and injury
- Pain related to physical injury of tissues

NANDA-I © 2012

Planning and Implementation

Care of the child after surgery involves general postoperative care (see Chapter 15 🔗). The child who has had an amputation or limb salvage has special needs regarding skin care and rehabilitation. Inspect the dressing for intactness and bleeding. When the dressing is changed (usually several days after surgery), inspect tissue at the surgical site, using sterile technique. Turn the child at least every 2 hours. The site needs to heal completely before chemotherapy can begin and a prosthesis can be made. Pain management is a major nursing care need. When amputation has occurred, the adolescent will often experience **phantom pain.** This is pain that feels as if it is in the amputated extremity and is caused by trauma to the nerves in the area of the amputation. Acknowledge the pain as real since the nerve endings are intact and the patient perceives real discomfort. Medicate adequately and use additional pain control measures such as repositioning the limb using gentle movement, supporting the limb, and using distraction or deep breathing.

Discuss insurance and other financial arrangements with the parents, as prosthetics can be expensive. Physical therapy will be needed as well. Referral to a Shriners Hospital is an option for some families.

Implement plans to help the child deal with body image disturbance. Plan for a visit from another child who is well adjusted to a prosthesis. Help the child to gradually learn how to care for the stump. Slow progress may be made as the child first looks briefly, then for longer periods, and finally is willing to touch the stump. Show the child how it is possible to continue with sports such as baseball, skiing, or biking with a prosthesis. A discussion group with others can be very useful for adolescents. Plan with the child how to tell friends about the surgery and what issues he or she may face upon return to school. Make plans for elevator access if needed and emergency evacuation procedures. Some children or adolescents may need referral for counseling to assist in dealing with body image disturbance.

The child will receive physical rehabilitation while hospitalized and after discharge. When the child is discharged, explain to the family the importance of bringing the child for outpatient chemotherapy and physical rehabilitation visits. Special arrangements may be needed at the child's school to facilitate a wheelchair, crutches, or ambulation with a new prosthesis. Coordinate with the school nurse about the evaluation of the presence of buttons to open doors, wide doorways to facilitate passage, and any limitations of the building. Contact the school nurse or other school personnel to plan the child's return. The child will need careful management of a schedule that permits both healing of the surgical site with rehabilitation and then the demands of chemotherapy.

Follow-up care is needed to monitor for progress and to be alert for signs of metastases. Fracture may be a sign of recurrent tumor. All body systems such as lungs, heart, kidneys, and liver are monitored for signs of recurrence.

Evaluation

The following expected outcomes of nursing care for the child with a bone tumor focus on the treatments required and adaptation to changes in lifestyle:

- The surgical site heals with no signs of infection.
- The child adapts to changes in mobility status.
- The child successfully adjusts to changes required in school settings.
- Positive body image is achieved.
- Pain is managed to a comfort level.

LEUKEMIA

Leukemia is the most commonly diagnosed pediatric malignancy in children under 14 years of age. A cancer of the blood-forming organs, leukemia is characterized by a proliferation of abnormal white blood cells in the body. Several types of leukemia are differentiated, depending on the blood cells affected. The main types are acute lymphoblastic leukemia (ALL), acute myelogenous leukemia (AML), and the rare chronic leukemias of childhood.

The most common type of childhood leukemia is ALL, which accounts for 25% of all childhood cancer and 78% of leukemias in children. Sam, described in the opening scenario, has ALL. The peak age at onset is 2 to 3 years. ALL is more common in Whites and in boys (Figure 29–15 ■) (Tubergen, Bleyer, & Ritchey, 2011). Subtypes of ALL are based on the French-American-British (FAB) system of classification. The three types of ALL in the FAB system are L1, L2, and L3.

AML refers to all leukemias from myeloid cells. About 17% of childhood leukemias are AML. AML is most common in children younger than 2 years of age and in adolescents. It is more common in males than females, and in Asians/Pacific Islanders, Hispanics, and Whites than in Blacks. Following are subtypes of AML in the FAB classification:

- M0 = acute nonlymphocytic leukemia without maturation
- M1 = acute nonlymphocytic leukemia with poor maturation

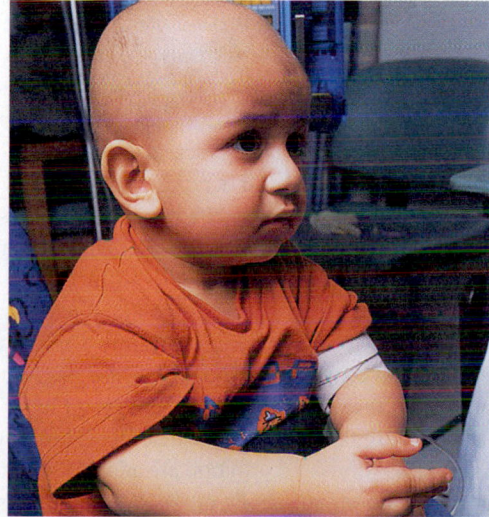

FIGURE 29–15 ■ Acute lymphoblastic leukemia is the most common type of leukemia in children and the most common cancer affecting children under 5 years of age.

- M2 = acute nonlymphocytic leukemia with maturation
- M3 = acute promyelocytic leukemia
- M4 = acute myelomonocytic leukemia
- M5 = acute monocytic leukemia
- M6 = erythroleukemia
- M7 = acute megakaryocytic leukemia

Because chronic leukemias such as chronic myelocytic, chronic myelomonocytic, and chronic lymphocytic leukemia are rare in children, the following discussion will focus on ALL and AML.

Etiology and Pathophysiology

The causes of leukemia are not well understood. Some investigators theorize that exposure to infectious agents can predispose children to leukemia. Genetic factors are believed to play a role in some types of the disease. For instance, children with chromosomal defects such as Down syndrome, neurofibromatosis type I, Bloom syndrome, and Shwachman syndrome have an increased incidence of ALL, and chromosomal abnormalities such as hyperploidy, hypodiploidy, tranlocations, and deletions are present in most children with ALL (Pieters & Carroll, 2008). Children with immune deficiency states, such as ataxia-telangiectasia, congenital hypogammaglobulinemia, and Wiskott-Aldrich syndrome, have an increased risk of ALL. Certain ethnic groups have poorer outcomes from leukemia. (See Developing Cultural Competence: Outcomes of Leukemia.)

Ionizing radiation exposure when in utero, and chemical agents from treatment of an earlier cancer with chemotherapy (alkylating agents and topoisomerase II inhibitors), are thought to play a role in the development of AML. There are several chromosomal and genetic abnormalities associated with AML.

Leukemia occurs when the stem cells in the bone marrow produce immature WBCs that cannot function normally. These cells proliferate rapidly by cloning instead of normal mitosis, causing the bone marrow to fill with abnormal WBCs. The abnormal cells then spill out into the circulatory system where they steadily replace the normally functioning WBCs. As this occurs, the protective lymphocytic functions such as cellular and humeral immunity are reduced, leaving the body vulnerable to infections. The malignant WBCs rapidly fill the bone marrow, replacing stem cells that produce erythrocytes (red blood cells) and other blood products such as platelets, thereby decreasing the amount of these products in circulation. The stem cells are replaced by leukemic clones, eventually resulting in anemia. Children with leukemia commonly experience abnormal bleeding, ecchymosis, or petechiae because of the reduced platelet amounts.

Developing Cultural Competence
Outcomes of Leukemia

Black, Hispanic, and Native American children have statistically poorer outcomes from leukemia treatment than do White and Asian children. Analysis of 5-year survival rates demonstrated poorer outcomes for Black children than White children with AML (Bhatia, 2011). It is unclear whether racial and ethnic groups with poorer outcomes have particular genetic characteristics placing them at risk, do not obtain treatment as soon, have more complications from the disease, enroll less often in clinical trials, or have less access to care at oncology centers. Clearly more research is needed to describe and then eliminate the racial and ethnic disparity in leukemia treatment outcomes.

Clinical Manifestations

Children with ALL and AML usually have fever, pallor, ecchymosis, petechiae, bleeding, lethargy, malaise, anorexia, and large joint or bone pain. Enlargement of the liver and spleen (hepatosplenomegaly) and changes in the lymph nodes (lymphadenopathy) are common. If the leukemia has infiltrated the central nervous system (entered it by means of the circulatory or lymphoid system), the child may exhibit signs such as headache, vomiting, papilledema, and sixth cranial nerve palsy (inability to move the eye laterally). These findings are caused by the leukemic cells massing and putting pressure on nerves. The testicles, spinal cord, and bone marrow are common sites for infiltration. The leukemic cells in the testicle become a mass that causes the testicle to enlarge, often painlessly.

Collaborative Care

Many care providers join together as leukemia is diagnosed and treated. Periodic exacerbations or side effects from treatment require intensification in care. Partnerships with families are needed to provide the lengthy care required.

Diagnostic Tests

Diagnosis is based initially on blood counts and bone marrow aspiration. Blood counts reveal anemia, thrombocytopenia, and neutropenia. Bone marrow aspiration is the definitive test and reveals immature and abnormal lymphoblasts and hypercellular marrow. The percentage of blast cells in marrow is measured. Neutropenia, thrombocytopenia, and anemia are commonly noted (Box 29–4). Other abnormal laboratory findings include elevated serum uric acid and elevated calcium, potassium, and phosphorus levels. New laboratory studies such as rapid flow cytometric assay are making the measurement of even very small numbers of leukemic cells possible, so that treatment can be used to improve prognosis in children with minimal residual disease. Leukemic cells are examined and classified by FAB type, and DNA analysis may provide clues about genetic changes; all of these considerations are used to establish the protocol for treatment. Blood cells of children with ALL are B cell or T cell; these classifications are also used to establish treatment protocols (Box 29–4).

Clinical Therapy

Both ALL and AML are now approached by analysis of molecular targeting for the origin and type of disease identified (Loh, 2010; Masetti, Kleinschmidt, Biagi, et al., 2011; Pui, Carroll, Meshinchi, et al., 2011). Treatment of ALL involves radiation and chemotherapy combinations, using information from these targeted molecular approaches (Rabin & Poplack, 2011). Radiation is used for central nervous system disease, in T-cell leukemia, and for testicular

involvement. Chemotherapy is organized into four phases; some commonly administered drugs are used in each phase:

1. Induction
   - Prednisone
   - Vincristine
   - L-asparaginase
   - Daunorubicin
2. Consolidation
   - L-asparaginase
   - Doxorubicin
3. Delayed intensification
   - Vincristine
   - Ara-C
   - Cyclophosphamide
4. Maintenance of remission
   - 6-mercaptopurine
   - 6-thioguanine
   - Methotrexate

An additional drug used for treatment of central nervous system disease or prophylaxis is intrathecal methotrexate.

Maintenance therapy may continue for 2 to 3 years, causing decreased resistance to infection for this prolonged period of time.

Treatment of AML commonly involves use of the following drugs during the induction and consolidation phases:

1. Induction phase
   - Daunorubicin
   - Doxorubicin
   - Mitoxantrone
   - Cytarabine
2. Consolidation phase
   - Etoposide
   - Teniposide

Maximum cell death occurs during the *induction phase*. The cells that remain after this period are more resistant to treatment. After 3 to 4 weeks, when a remission has occurred, central nervous system prophylaxis begins. Drugs are used in combination with cranial irradiation. During the *consolidation phase*, chemotherapy with L-asparaginase and doxorubicin is administered. *Delayed intensification* uses additional drugs to target the leukemic cells that have survived. Treatment during the *maintenance phase* is aimed at destroying the remaining leukemic cells. Combinations of active drugs are used to prevent resistance. Many complications can occur with such high doses and combinations of drugs, so much of the clinical therapy is aimed at managing these effects. In addition, long-term complications such as central nervous system toxicity; damage to pituitary, liver, kidneys, gastrointestinal tract, heart, lungs, gonads, blood, and immune system; and secondary malignancies can occur.

The prognosis for children with leukemia is much improved with current therapy. An important factor is the initial leukocyte count; the higher the leukocyte count (over 50,000/mm^3) at diagnosis, the worse the prognosis. For children in the low-risk group, the probability of prolonged survival is as high as 90%; even higher risk ALL has a 75% to 80% cure rate with current treatments (Tubergen et al., 2011). Treatment methods and duration are adjusted for each child, depending on that child's metabolic analysis and other risk factors (Rabin & Poplack, 2011). More aggressive treatment is undertaken for those in the higher risk groups.

BOX 29–4	Laboratory Values in Leukemia	
	NORMAL	**COMMON VALUES IN LEUKEMIA**
Leukocytes	Less than 10,000/microliter	Greater than 10,000/microliter
Platelets	150,000–400,000/microliter	20,000–100,000/microliter
Hemoglobin	12–16 g/dL	7–11 g/dL

Approximately 15% to 20% of children have a relapse within a year after completing treatment (Tubergen et al., 2011). Treatment for relapse consists of additional chemotherapy drugs. The prognosis is best if the relapse occurs late after the initial diagnosis and after the initial treatment is completed. Hematopoietic stem cell transplant (HSCT) is a treatment option for the child who has a relapse with ALL who then achieves a second remission; the transplant is given when the child is in remission. Transplant is also used for children with AML; they do not need to be in remission for the transplant to be performed. Overall, 80% of children with leukemia are cured.

Chemotherapy itself can create numerous complications, affecting all body organs. Secondary malignancies sometimes occur later in life. See the section on cancer survival earlier in this chapter.

Nursing Management

Nursing management for the child with leukemia is complex due to the multisystem effects of the disease and the long period required for therapy. Normal growth and development and prevention of sequelae from treatment are major goals.

Nursing Assessment and Diagnosis

A thorough physical assessment is important to ensure prompt identification of problems without injuring the child who has deficient coagulation and immune function. Perform assessments every 8 hours or more often depending on the chemotherapy regimen. Observe carefully for bruising, petechiae, and other signs of bleeding, and fever or other signs of infection. Once chemotherapy has begun, closely monitor renal functioning through specific gravity, intake and output, and daily weight measurement. Monitor dietary intake, nausea, vomiting, and constipation. Observe for mucosal sores in the mouth. A central line is usually in place for intravenous infusion of medications, so careful assessment of the line for proper functioning and for signs of infection is needed. Ask the parents about any behavioral changes. Central nervous system infiltration can affect the child's level of consciousness, causing irritability, vomiting, and lethargy. However, these nonspecific signs can also be induced by chemotherapeutic drugs and antiemetics. Frequent treatments, bone marrow aspirations, and lumbar punctures require pain assessment and an evaluation of the level of knowledge and coping skills of the child and family.

Leukemia causes many changes in the body, and confirmation of the disease is difficult for families to face. Among the many nursing diagnoses that might be appropriate for the child with leukemia are the following:

- Nutrition, Imbalanced: Less than Body Requirements related to inability to ingest food
- Infection, Risk for related to altered immune system functioning
- Injury, Risk for related to bleeding
- Activity Intolerance related to generalized weakness
- Pain related to chemotherapy and disease process
- Sleep Pattern, Disturbed related to chemotherapy drugs and disease process
- Anxiety (Child and Parent) related to change in health status

NANDA-I © 2012

Planning and Implementation

Bone marrow suppression may necessitate transmission-based precautions due to neutropenia (refer to the Skills Manual ⬡). Instruct parents in the prevention of infection and use nursing care measures to prevent infection also. Perform careful hand hygiene; take temperature and other vital signs frequently; give mouth care with antibacterial mouthwashes; and inspect skin, mouth, rectal area, and central line site for any signs of infection. The child should not have subcutaneous or intramuscular injections or rectal suppositories. Fresh fruits and vegetables, particularly with skin, are avoided, and fresh plants or flowers are not allowed near the child. The Nursing Care Plan, earlier in this chapter, presents care for mucositis and other side effects of chemotherapy.

Special attention to renal function is needed when the child receives cyclophosphamide. Gross hematuria is a side effect of this drug. Hydration with intravenous fluids to attain a specific gravity of less than 1.010 prevents or reduces the severity of hematuria. It also prepares the kidneys to manage products of tumor cell breakdown. To achieve the desired specific gravity, the child receives intravenous fluids at 1.5 times maintenance volume for at least 6 to 8 hours before and at least 1.5 hours after administration of the drug. Other chemotherapy drugs have different infusion times while some do not require hydration prior to infusion. Check drug references carefully for recommendations with each drug. Evaluate the infusion site before and frequently during infusion. Although extravasation is not as common with central lines used in cancer treatment as in peripheral lines, it still can occur. Many chemotherapy agents are extremely toxic to tissues. In addition, lysis of the cancer cells can produce toxic side effects (see oncologic emergencies described earlier in the chapter). Careful monitoring of intake and output is required to record the intravenous fluids, assess kidney functioning, and monitor excretion of by-products from destroyed tumor cells. Monitor specific gravity every 8 hours, as well as before and during administration of the drug, and when the intravenous fluids are reduced to maintenance volume levels. Daily weight measurements are important to assist in planning adequate hydration during chemotherapy, as well as to measure nutritional status.

Drug side effects may necessitate infusion of platelets or packed red blood cells. See the Skills Manual ⬡ for techniques and cautions to be used in these situations.

Many children are treated in an oncology clinic, staying in the hospital only on the day of intravenous drug administration and receiving oral medications at home. The time at the hospital is used to assess how the family is managing issues such as nutrition, sleep, medication administration, and obtaining psychosocial support. Careful teaching for the family is needed to ensure safe drug administration and identification of issues requiring further care (Box 29–5).

Nurses play a key role in the long-term multidisciplinary treatment of children with leukemia. The impact of a diagnosis of leukemia and the long-term nature of treatment can severely stress the

BOX 29–5	Research: Education for Families of Children with Cancer

Hospitalizations are brief, so parents take on complex management of the disease soon after diagnosis. Few studies have examined the experience of these families. One nursing study reviewed literature on nursing staff education patterns for families who had newly diagnosed children with leukemia. The study found that early emphasis on educational discharge needs, with consideration of the educational level of the family, age of the child, disease, and treatment, was effective in helping families manage the challenges of cancer (Aburn & Gott, 2011).

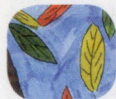

Partnering with Families

Chemotherapy for Leukemia

PHYSICAL CARE

- Schedule rest periods each day.
- Avoid areas of exposure to people with illnesses.
- Drink generous amounts of water.
- Eat a healthy diet, using frequent, small, and nutritious meals to obtain enough nutrients.
- Take medicines prescribed to decrease nausea.
- Maintain good oral hygiene with a soft toothbrush and water irrigation device.
- Avoid sun exposure and check skin each day for any signs of bruises, pressure areas, cuts, or scratches.

- Promote bowel elimination through regular dietary and toileting practices.
- Report any signs of infection, changes in condition, or other concerns.

EMOTIONAL CARE

- Prepare for loss of hair with plans for hats, wigs, or other alternatives.
- Continue contact with friends via phone or Internet, and in person when possible.
- Try relaxation techniques to aid in sleep and management of treatments.
- Talk with clergy, teachers, parents, counselors, friends, or other supportive people about the experience of having leukemia.
- Keep a journal to record feelings and experiences.

coping abilities of both the child and the family. Ongoing psychosocial assessment and emotional support are essential (see the general discussion of psychosocial assessment in the Childhood Cancer section on pages 953–955). Referral to support groups and social services may be beneficial. Assist the family in exploration of alternative therapies such as relaxation, imagery, and nutritional support that may aid the child. Be alert for any interactions that could occur between alternative therapies and the medical regimen. Partner with other health professionals so that a survivorship care plan is established to monitor for late effects of the disease or treatment (Fulbright, Raman, McClellan, et al., 2011). (See Partnering with Families: Chemotherapy for Leukemia, and Complementary Therapy: Nursing Role in CAM Studies.)

Evaluation

Following are expected outcomes for nursing care of the child with leukemia:

- Infection and other secondary complications of chemotherapy are prevented.
- Adequate hydration is maintained.
- Normal urinary output is manifested.
- Blood values are within normal limits.

Complementary Therapy
Nursing Role in CAM Studies

Complementary medicine practices are commonly used by families to increase children's comfort during therapeutic treatment. About one half of families queried used some type of complementary and alternative medical (CAM) treatments for their children with cancer (Bishop, Prescott, Chan, et al., 2010; Post-White, Fitzgerald, Hageness, et al., 2009). Approaches include spiritual and mental practices and herbal or vitamin remedies. Nurses play a major role in identifying families and children who may wish to participate in studies of CAM, informing the families fully about the study, answering questions, and possibly conducting the data gathering to provide the definitive results. Additionally, nurses inquire about treatments that the family is using or those about which they need further information. Inquire about massage, vitamins, herbs, prayer, music, and other techniques. How can you phrase your questions in an open and nonthreatening manner to elicit the information from families?

- The family adapts successfully to parenting a child with chronic illness.
- Parents demonstrate adequate knowledge related to the disease process.

SOFT TISSUE TUMORS

About 12% of pediatric cancers are lymphoma. Of these, 40% to 45% are Hodgkin and 55% to 60% are non-Hodgkin. Other soft tissue tumors discussed in this section are retinoblastoma and rhabdomyosarcoma. Adolescents can develop tumors of the cervix or ovaries (females) or testes (males); the student is referred to adult oncology texts for management of these soft tissue cancers.

Hodgkin Disease

Hodgkin disease, a disorder of the lymphoid system, usually arises in a single lymph node or an anatomic group of lymph nodes (Figure 29–16 ■). Hodgkin disease is rare before 10 years of age. It accounts for just 5% of cancers in children under 14 years, but 15% of cancer in youth from 15 to 19 years. The disease has a bimodal peak with higher incidence in the early 20s and after 50 years (Waxman, Hochberg, & Cairo, 2011). Three forms of the disease exist: that in young persons under 14 years, the young adult form in persons from 15 to 34 years, and the older adult form in those over 50 years. There is a slightly increased incidence in males, which is more pronounced in the disease manifested in younger children (Carbone, Spina, Gloghini, et al., 2011).

Etiology and Pathophysiology

Hodgkin disease occurs in clusters and has been reported in families. This suggests a possible genetic link as well as an infectious agent (virus infections, such as herpes or Epstein-Barr virus, have been linked as precursors) or environmental hazard (Waxman et al., 2011).

Clinical Manifestations

The main symptom of Hodgkin disease is nontender, firm lymphadenopathy, usually in the supraclavicular and cervical nodes but occasionally in the mediastinal area. A mediastinal growth can cause respiratory difficulty because of pressure on the trachea or

Pathophysiology Illustrated
Hodgkin Disease

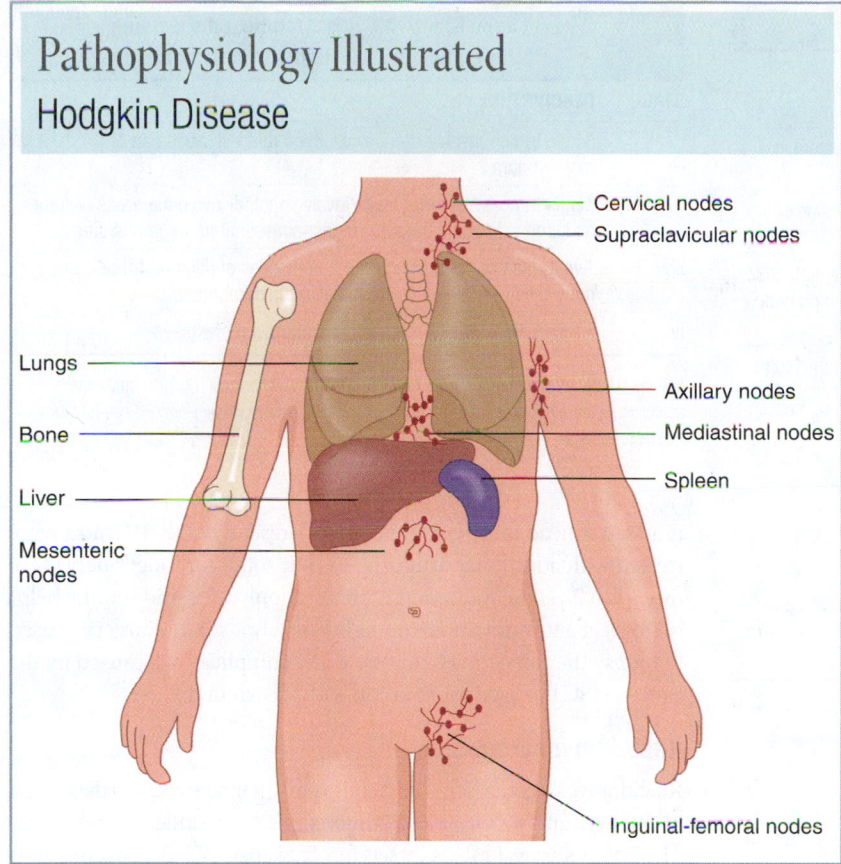

- Cervical nodes
- Supraclavicular nodes
- Lungs
- Bone
- Liver
- Mesenteric nodes
- Axillary nodes
- Mediastinal nodes
- Spleen
- Inguinal-femoral nodes

FIGURE 29–16 ■ Lymph nodes and organs affected in Hodgkin disease in children.

bronchi. A characteristic large cell with multiple nuclei, called the Reed-Sternberg cell, is characteristic of Hodgkin, though the cell is found also in infectious mononucleosis and some other lymphomas. Fever, night sweats, and weight loss occur in one third of children with Hodgkin disease and are associated with a more aggressive form of the disease. The leukocyte count and erythrocyte sedimentation rate (ESR) may be elevated.

Collaborative Care

Primary care providers, diagnostic services, and oncologists work together when lymphoma occurs. Nurses provide ongoing care and monitoring for the child.

Diagnostic Tests

Diagnosis is based on lymph node biopsy; Reed-Sternberg cells are present. A staging classification is used to determine disease severity (Table 29–9). The basis for staging is data obtained from the history, physical examination, radiographic study (for metastasis), chest CT scan, CT or MRI scans of the retroperitoneal nodes, lymphangiogram if there is retroperitoneal involvement, laboratory studies (CBC, ESR, C-reactive protein, alkaline phosphatase, serum copper level, liver and renal function tests), PET, bone scans, and a radionuclide scan with gallium. Bone marrow biopsy, bone scan, or a staging laparotomy may be performed in certain situations when advanced disease is suspected (Waxman et al., 2011). Minimally invasive surgery can be used to biopsy or remove the spleen for diagnosis, avoiding the complications of major surgery.

Clinical Therapy

Treatment is commonly performed in outpatient settings unless complications develop that require hospitalization. Chemotherapy using a four-drug combination has been found to be the most effective drug treatment.

Drugs commonly used in combinations include:

- Doxorubicin
- Bleomycin
- Vinblastine
- Dacarbazine
- Etoposide
- Prednisone
- Cyclophosphamide
- Procarbazine
- Methotrexate
- Mechlorethamine

Radiation is commonly added, with low doses for children who are still growing, and larger doses for those who are physically mature or those whose disease is more advanced at diagnosis. The 5-year survival rate is approximately 85% to 90%, depending on the stage of the disease at diagnosis. Autologous stem cell or allogeneic stem cell transplant is a treatment option in children with advanced disease or relapse. Long-term survivor complications can occur as a result of chemotherapy or radiation.

Non-Hodgkin Lymphoma

The four types of pediatric non-Hodgkin lymphoma (NHL) are (1) lymphoblastic lymphoma, (2) small noncleaved cell (Burkitt) lymphoma, (3) diffuse large B-cell lymphoma, and (4) anaplastic large cell lymphoma (Waxman et al., 2011). Lymphomas of all types are the third most common group of malignancies in children, following leukemia and brain tumors (see Figure 29–1). Non-Hodgkin lymphomas are malignant tumors of lymphoreticular (internal framework of the lymph system) origin. The peak incidence for lymphomas occurs between the ages of 7 and 11 years. It is three times more common in boys than in girls. The cure rate is 85% to 90% (Waxman et al., 2011).

Etiology and Pathophysiology

Lymphoblastic non-Hodgkin lymphomas are caused by T-cell abnormalities. These abnormal T cells are diffuse, highly malignant, and aggressive, and they do not mature. T-cell lymphomas produced by these cells often occur in children with congenital or acquired immunodeficiency states, chronic immune stimulation, or autoimmune disease. Some lymphomas have B-cell abnormalities, most specifically Burkitt lymphoma; 8q24 chromosomal translocation may be found in these cases (Gore & Trippett, 2010; Waxman et al., 2011).

The incidence of lymphomas shows geographic variability. For example, a high incidence of Burkitt lymphoma is found in equatorial Africa, where it causes 50% of childhood cancer. Incidence in Hispanic children is higher than in Whites, and Blacks have the lowest incidence. Males are affected more than females, and children with immune system compromise are most commonly affected. Epstein-Barr virus has been associated with Burkitt lymphoma, but in most cases of NHL there are no known genetic or environmental contributors.

TABLE 29–9   Staging System for Hodgkin Disease

STAGE	DESCRIPTION
I	Disease within a single lymph node region
IE	Disease within a single organ or site outside the lymphatic system (extralymphatic organ)
II	Disease within two or more lymph node regions on the same side of the diaphragm
IIE	Disease within an extralymphatic organ, and of one or more lymph node regions on the same side of the diaphragm; the number of lymph node regions involved may be indicated by subscript
III	Disease of lymph node regions on both sides of the diaphragm; stage III(1) indicates involvement of the upper abdomen above the renal vein while stage III(2) indicates involvement of pelvic or other lower abdomen nodes
IIIE	Disease of lymph node regions on both sides of the diaphragm with involvement of an extralymphatic organ
IIIS	As in III, plus disease within the spleen
IIIS+E	As in III, plus disease in extralymphatic organs and the spleen
IV	Disseminated disease within one or more lymphatic organs with or without lymph node involvement

Source: Data from National Cancer Institute. (2011d). Staging and diagnostic evaluation. Retrieved from http://www.cancer.gov/cancertopics/pdq/treatment/childhodgkins/HealthProfessional/page4/

Clinical Manifestations

Children with non-Hodgkin lymphoma frequently present with fever and weight loss. The lymph glands are usually enlarged or nodular, with the most frequent sites being the cervical, axillary, inguinal, and femoral nodes. However, the disease may be diffuse, without nodular glands. The anterior mediastinum is the primary site for T-cell lymphomas. Tumors that occur in this area may compress the airway (causing breathing difficulty) or superior vena cava (leading to swelling of the face, neck, or arms), and can cause pain. Jaw involvement is common in Burkitt lymphoma. An abdominal mass may cause pain, nausea, and vomiting.

Collaborative Care

Comprehensive, collaborative care aims to treat the illness and prevent complications.

Diagnostic Tests

The symptoms of lymphoma are often nonspecific. Treatments may already have been tried with antibiotics, if a mass is thought to be an infection, or other medication. A careful history will help determine the progression and possible location of disease. CBC is performed; additional blood tests include renal and liver function, electrolytes, uric acid, and LDH. Bone marrow aspiration and lumbar puncture are performed. Chest radiograph, bone scan, gallium scan, CT, and MRI can help to isolate affected body organs. Diagnosis is confirmed by tissue biopsy.

Clinical Therapy

A staging system is used to describe the tumor mass and extension to other body areas (Table 29–10). Treatment is tailored to the type of cancer and its stage. Stages I and II may be treated with drugs such as cyclophosphamide, vincristine, prednisone, and doxorubicin (COPAD) or cyclophosphamide, vincristine, methotrexate, 6-mercaptopurine, and prednisone (COMP). Intrathecal medication

TABLE 29–10   St. Jude Children's Research Hospital Staging Classification for Non-Hodgkin Lymphoma

STAGE	DESCRIPTION
I	Single tumor or node area involved; no tumor in abdomen or mediastinum
II	Single tumor with lymph node involvement; or two node areas or tumor on same side of diaphragm; or gastrointestinal tumor in one site
III	Two tumors or node areas on different sides of diaphragm; or a primary mediastinal, intra-abdominal, or epidural tumor
IV	Any involvement with CNS or bone marrow metastases

Source: Adapted from National Cancer Institute. (2011e). Childhood non-Hodgkin lymphoma treatment. Retrieved from http://www.cancer.gov/cancertopics/pdq/treatment/child-non-hodgkins/HealthProfessional/

is added if head and neck cancers are present. Stages III and IV are treated with additional drugs (up to nine total) for longer periods of time (1 to 2 years). Radiation is uncommonly used and may be helpful to treat a tumor that is impinging on a body part. Surgery is used to biopsy the tumor mass and treat any complications caused by the cancer. HSCT is used for children with recurrent disease.

Rhabdomyosarcoma

Rhabdomyosarcoma is the most common soft tissue sarcoma diagnosed in children, and is especially common in children under 5 years of age. The 5-year survival rate is 70% (Huh & Skapek, 2010). It occurs most often in the muscles around the eyes (extraorbital), in the neck, and less commonly in the abdomen, the genitourinary tract, and the extremities. Genitourinary, bladder, and prostate cancers are more common in children under 5 years, while paratesticular and extremity cancer is more common among adolescents. Rhabdomyosarcoma occurs more often in Whites than in Blacks or Asians. It is uncommon in newborns; if it presents in this age group, abdominal or pelvic sites are most common.

Etiology and Pathophysiology

The cause of rhabdomyosarcoma is unknown. It is more common in children with neurofibromatosis and Li-Fraumeni syndrome, and those whose mothers have breast cancer. Mutations in a tumor suppressor gene p53 are sometimes seen. The abnormal cells arise from mesenchyme which normally grows into muscle, fat, and bone.

Clinical Manifestations

Tumors occurring close to the eye produce swelling, ptosis, visual disturbances, and eye movement abnormalities (Figure 29–17 ■). When the tumor occurs in the genitourinary tract, the result can be urinary obstruction, hematuria, dysuria, vaginal discharge, and a protruding vaginal mass. Rhabdomyosarcoma occurring in the abdomen may be asymptomatic. There is rapid metastasis to the lungs, bones, bone marrow, and distant lymph nodes.

Collaborative Care

Soft tissue tumors that occur in young children require astute observations for early diagnosis. Providers then partner with parents to ensure both treatment and fostering of the young child's development.

Diagnostic Tests

Diagnosis is confirmed by CT, MRI, PET, bone marrow aspiration, and biopsy. CBC, renal and liver studies, and urinalysis are

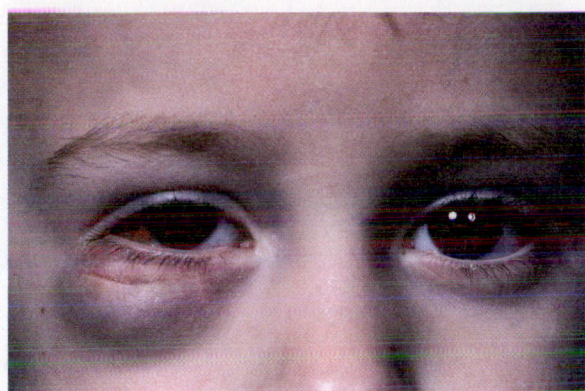

FIGURE 29–17 ■ Rhabdomyosarcoma is characterized by ptosis and swelling.

Source: *Copyright 2012 Wellcome Trust Library—Custom Medical Stock Photo, All Rights Reserved.*

TABLE 29–11	Classification of Rhabdomyosarcoma
GROUP	**DESCRIPTION**
I	Localized tumor, completely resected disease
II	Total gross resection with regional microscopic spread
III	Locally extensive tumor with residual microscopic spread
IV	Any size primary tumor with distant metastatic disease present

Source: *Data from National Cancer Institute. (2011f). Childhood rhabdomyosarcoma treatment. Retrieved from http://www.cancer.gov/cancertopics/pdq/treatment/childrhabdomyosarcoma/ HealthProfessional/*

performed. Lumbar puncture may be used in head and neck tumors. A useful biologic marker, desmin, allows differentiation of rhabdomyosarcoma from other round cell tumors. A significant number of children have metastatic disease at the time of diagnosis, so chest and lung CT scans are performed; regional lymph node biopsies also help to establish the extent of disease (Arndt, 2011).

Clinical Therapy

Treatment includes surgical removal of the tumor when possible. However, if the tumor involves other structures removal may not be possible. Many children have metastasis at time of diagnosis, so the primary tumor is removed. Surgery is followed by wide-field radiation and chemotherapy with a combination of drugs. Common drugs include:

- Vincristine
- Actinomycin
- Cyclophosphamide (VAC therapy)

Prognosis depends on the site, staging (Table 29–11), and histologic findings.

Retinoblastoma

Retinoblastoma is an intraocular malignancy of the retina. It may be bilateral (20% to 30%) or unilateral. In 40% of children, the disease is inherited by an autosomal dominant gene. Family history is collected and retinal examinations are performed, although many cases occur with no family history of the cancer (Zage & Herzog, 2011).

Etiology and Pathophysiology

The tumor arises from embryonic retinal cells. It may be a new mutation of the RB1 gene or may be passed on to offspring of affected individuals in an autosomal dominant manner (Lohmann, 2010; Shields & Shields, 2010). The retinoblastoma gene, RB1, is on chromosome 13q14 and encodes retinoblastoma protein, a tumor suppressor.

Clinical Manifestations

The first sign of retinoblastoma is a white pupil, termed leukokoria or cat's-eye reflex (Figure 29–18 ■). The red reflex is absent, asymmetric, or of a differing color in the affected eye. Other symptoms may include a fixed strabismus (a constant deviation of one eye from the other), orbital inflammation, glaucoma, and heterochromia (irises of different colors).

Retinoblastoma is usually diagnosed when the child is between 1 and 2 years of age. A family history should alert healthcare providers so that regular ophthalmologic examinations can be performed frequently on infants and young children in the family. The appearance of a unilateral tumor demands regular examinations of the healthy eye since bilateral disease can develop. In some children a pineal gland tumor can also develop, causing central nervous system symptoms. The overall tumor-free survival rate is 95% (Zage & Herzog, 2011).

Collaborative Care

Families work with healthcare professionals to identify and treat the disease, as well as support the child after treatment.

Diagnostic Tests

Children at risk for retinoblastoma due to family history can be tested for the RB1 gene. Diagnostic tests for the cancer include full ocular examination and CT, MRI, or ultrasound scans of the eye orbit. All children with a history of retinoblastoma in the family should be examined by an ophthalmologist after birth, at 6 weeks, every 2 to 3 months until 2 years, then every 4 months until 3 years, and then annually to aid in early diagnosis. Tumors are classified according to a staging system, from a very small, localized tumor (group I) to tumors involving more than half the retina and with seeding into the vitreous (group V).

Clinical Therapy

Treatment for retinoblastoma may include removal of the eye (enucleation) when there is permanent retinal damage or failure to respond to other treatment. Other surgical treatments involve cryotherapy or photocoagulation (argon laser therapy). Radiation is nearly always used, either as the sole treatment or before surgery to shrink the tumor. Chemotherapy is sometimes used but is often ineffective as the drugs often fail to penetrate sufficiently into the eye. Chemotherapy

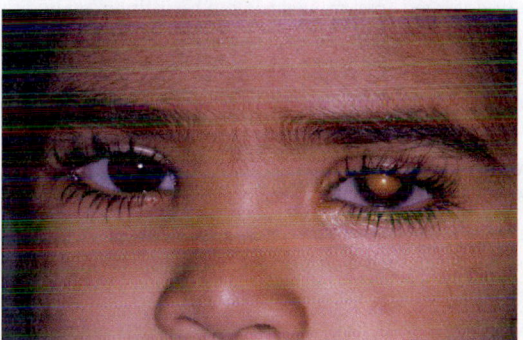

FIGURE 29–18 ■ Retinoblastoma is characterized by leukokoria, a white reflection in the pupil.

Source: *Copyright 2012—Custom Medical Stock Photo, All Rights Reserved.*

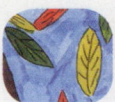

Partnering with Families

Care of the Child with a Soft Tissue Tumor

- Teach the family about the chemotherapy drugs and their side effects.
- Teach about the care of surgically placed venous access devices.
- Provide written and illustrated information about the chemotherapy protocol(s).

- Provide the family with radiation and surgery education specific to the tumor treatment.
- Refer the family to nutrition resources such as dietitians for ways to promote the child's adequate intake of food and fluid.

drugs include carboplatin, etoposide, vincristine, and cyclosporine. Multiple therapies are more commonly used in children with bilateral retinoblastoma. Children with retinoblastoma are at increased risk of developing a secondary tumor, including another retinoblastoma or a sarcoma, most commonly osteogenic sarcoma. However, most young children who have been treated for the disease have good health and normal mental abilities several years after treatment. The most common sequela of retinoblastoma is decrease in visual acuity.

Nursing Management

Nursing management of the child with a soft tissue tumor involves supporting the child and family through the treatment for disease, and monitoring the child over time for recurrence of the primary tumor or for a secondary tumor. (See Partnering with Families: Care of the Child with a Soft Tissue Tumor.)

Nursing Assessment and Diagnosis

Physiologic Assessment

Careful family histories can sometimes identify children at risk who need frequent physical examinations. For example, if a family history of retinoblastoma is present, the child should receive frequent eye examinations. Physiologic assessment of the child with a soft tissue tumor, such as Hodgkin disease, non-Hodgkin lymphoma, rhabdomyosarcoma, and retinoblastoma, focuses on the child's general condition. Accurate height and weight measurements are essential to provide a baseline against which to measure the child's growth during treatment, as well as for calculation of chemotherapeutic drug dosages.

Observe the area of the tumor, such as the face, neck, and abdomen, and describe any changes. Monitor respiratory status if the tumor is on the face or neck. Report any changes in respiratory pattern to the healthcare provider managing care. Avoid palpation of any tumor site or enlarged area; metastasis can be influenced by injudicious palpation and manipulation of a tumor site. Notify the healthcare provider of a change of symmetry in any lymph node or other area of the body.

Gastrointestinal and genitourinary function can be altered by the presence of a tumor and by treatment such as chemotherapy and radiation. Careful monitoring of the child's intake and output is essential. Abdominal and pelvic tumors may affect defecation, so charting of all bowel movements is important. Explain to the family and child why keeping accurate records is necessary.

Observe wounds closely for lack of healing as a result of chemotherapy or radiation. Examine the mouth and extremities for wounds or mucositis. Nutritional changes caused by treatment will affect the body's ability to support healthy cells and heal wounds.

A thorough eye examination is warranted for any child who has a family history of retinoblastoma or has undergone treatment for a prior tumor. Assess color and position of the iris, eye movements, cover–uncover test, and other eye tests as described in Chapter 7 ⊘. Be sure that the child has recommended evaluations by an ophthalmologist.

Psychosocial Assessment

Assessment of the family's psychosocial status and coping mechanisms is an essential component of nursing care. Refer to the general discussion of psychosocial assessment earlier in this chapter. Assessment of body image is needed when the child has a soft tissue tumor affecting appearance of the head and neck. Even after treatment is successfully completed, lasting mental health or cognitive changes such as stress and learning difficulties can be apparent. Screen for symptoms of depression such as loneliness, lack of interest, anxiety, and suicidal thoughts (see Chapter 34 ⊘).

The location and type of soft tissue tumor determine the specific nursing diagnoses for a particular child. Common nursing diagnoses may include the following:

- Tissue Perfusion: Peripheral, Risk for Ineffective related to interruption of blood flow
- Breathing Pattern, Ineffective related to effect of tumor deformity on neck or chest wall
- Swallowing, Impaired related to tumor
- Growth and Development, Delayed related to effects of treatment
- Body Image, Disturbed related to illness and treatment

NANDA-I © 2012

Planning and Implementation

Nursing management of children with soft tissue tumors varies depending on the specific tumor. Children with lymphoma affecting the mediastinum may need respiratory support. Position the child so that the head is elevated. Administer chemotherapy drugs as ordered, maintaining adequate fluids to facilitate excretion of the resultant breakdown products. Monitor the central line used for chemotherapy administration, and teach parents care of the central line when the child is at home.

For the child with a rhabdomyosarcoma involving the bladder, monitor urinary output carefully. Report hematuria and painful urination. Monitor the changes that occur during therapy. For example, in children with eye tumors, observe for a decrease in ptosis, which may indicate successful treatment. Administer pain medications as needed and use distraction and other techniques to decrease the child's discomfort. Emphasize to parents the need for follow-up CT and MRI scans after completion of treatment.

When the child with retinoblastoma undergoes removal of the eye, the parents and child will need detailed instructions on postsurgical care. Demonstrate to the parents care of the socket and use of a conformer to maintain the eye socket shape. When healing is complete and the child receives a prosthetic eye, instruct parents about its insertion and care. The child can gradually be taught to take over this care when old enough. Encourage periodic healthcare visits to monitor for signs of a tumor in the other eye. It may be necessary to adapt developmental interventions to accommodate for sensory alterations. Attention is directed at the body changes of the cancer and its treatment. Children and adolescents may need suggestions to deal with hair loss, disfigurement, and living with serious illness. Referral to other children and teens with similar concerns may be helpful. Parents of all children with cancer need help to encourage normal development in the child.

The child with a soft tissue tumor often receives chemotherapy or radiation, or sometimes both modalities. Nursing management during chemotherapy and radiation is discussed earlier in this chapter in the general sections on these treatment measures (see pages 958–960) and in the Nursing Care Plan for Hospital Care of the Child with Cancer. Generally, the family will need help to adjust to the diagnosis of a life-threatening disease and to the care of the ill child. Refer to Chapter 15 🖉 for a description of postsurgical care. Consult Chapter 24 🖉 for strategies to assist the child and family if the child has a visual impairment resulting from a retinoblastoma. Topics for parent and family teaching and discharge planning are similar to those previously presented. Referral resources to support the families of children with these types of cancer can be found on the companion website.

Care in the Community

Reinforce with families the importance of long-term follow-up after treatment for a soft tissue tumor. Increased risk for secondary cancers for 20 to 30 years is possible, and early identification can help with prompt diagnosis. Partner with other healthcare providers to provide instructions to families as the child transitions from oncology treatment back to the pediatrician so they understand the importance of telling all care providers about the cancer and treatment. Establish care plans for survivors. As children grow into teen and young adult years, help them to take over this important task in their care. Recommended annual examinations include:

- CBC
- Physical examination with special attention to skin, abdomen, and thyroid
- Monitoring for signs of hypo- and hyperthyroidism
- Neurologic and developmental examinations; monitoring of school performance
- First mammogram at 25 years in those with chest radiation
- Pap and pelvic exams for teen girls and young adult women
- Mental status assessment

Evaluation

The following expected outcomes of nursing care for the child with a soft tissue tumor are examples that illustrate the varied tumor presentations:

- Side effects of treatment are effectively managed.
- The surgical site heals with no signs of infection.
- The child adapts successfully to sensory loss if that results from cancer or treatment.
- The child adapts to an altered self-image.
- The child achieves growth and development to maximum potential.
- In cases of terminal disease, parents receive adequate support for the process of anticipatory grieving.

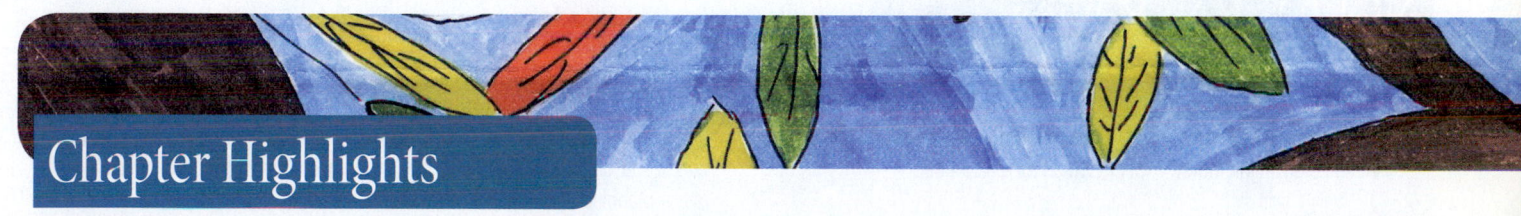

Chapter Highlights

- Cancer is a leading cause of illness and death among children.
- Cancer may be influenced by chromosomal or genetic messages, environmental carcinogens, or infectious processes. Often a combination of factors seems to be present.
- Cancer treatments include surgery, chemotherapy, radiation, biotherapy, and alternative therapies. Palliative care is needed when disease has relapsed and cure is no longer possible.
- Oncologic emergencies are life-threatening conditions caused by cancer or its treatment.
- The main types of oncologic emergencies are metabolic, hematologic, or space occupying.
- Key signs of childhood cancer are pain, cachexia, anemia, infection, bruising, petechiae, and neurologic symptoms.
- A protocol is a plan of action for chemotherapy that is based on the type of cancer, its stage, and the particular cell type.

- Nursing assessment for children with cancer involves detailed physical data, as well as psychologic factors and developmental achievements.
- Common physical nursing interventions for children with cancer involve nutrition, medication administration, hydration, infection prevention, pain management, and measures to decrease side effects of treatment. Families require ongoing psychosocial support, information, and referral to diverse resources when caring for a child with cancer.
- While the number of children who are long-term survivors continues to grow, some of these children experience lasting effects such as cognitive or behavioral problems, recurrent or secondary cancers, or discrimination.
- Nursing care after cancer treatment is completed includes monitoring for any long-term physiologic or psychosocial sequelae.
- Common brain tumors in children include medulloblastoma, astrocytoma, ependymoma, and gliomas.

- Headache, vomiting, ataxia, seizures, increased intracranial pressure, hydrocephalus, and sensory disturbances are the major clinical manifestations of brain tumors.
- Neuroblastoma is a tumor that is located along the sympathetic nervous system chain.
- Nephroblastoma (Wilms tumor) is an intrarenal tumor; when suspected, the abdomen should not be palpated.
- Common bone tumors in childhood are osteosarcoma and Ewing sarcoma; both are most common among adolescents.

- Leukemia is a common childhood malignancy, with the major types being acute lymphoblastic leukemia (ALL) and acute myelogenous leukemia (AML).
- A variety of soft tissue tumors are seen in children and adolescents; they include Hodgkin disease, non-Hodgkin lymphoma, rhabdomyosarcoma, and retinoblastoma.
- Nurses are in a key position to assist families during a diagnosis for cancer, while therapy is carried out, in adjustment to school and other life tasks, and in providing palliative care for children who do not survive.

Clinical Reasoning in Action

INTRODUCTION

Recall 4-year-old Sam, who was described in the opening scenario. He was recently diagnosed with acute lymphocytic leukemia (ALL) and has begun treatment. Both his mother and father are strong supports and his older siblings, Jeffrey (6 years) and Carolee (8 years), are worried about and protective of their younger brother.

DESCRIPTION

On a recent clinic visit, Sam's hemoglobin was found to be 6 g/dL. Sam's parents are eager for information and they want to know what the hemoglobin number means and what normal values are for Sam's age. They have begun to explore the Internet and have questions about complementary care they read about on websites.

DISCUSSION

1. Sam has had several procedures already that are painful and have required sedation. Plan to prepare him for a lumbar puncture for which he will be sedated. Consider his age as you plan how far ahead to tell him, how to explain the room he will be in, and how you will include his parents in the procedure.

2. Lack of all blood cellular components is a side effect of leukemia treatment. Explain why Sam's hemoglobin is low. What is the expected level? What colony-stimulating factor might be used in his treatment to increase RBCs? How will you explain all of this to his parents? What dietary teaching can you do to enhance hemoglobin levels?

3. Infection is a common complication of treatment for leukemia. During Sam's clinic visit, what assessments will you make to monitor for infection? What would you expect his WBC count to be?

4. Jeffrey and Carolee are attending one of Sam's clinic visits when he receives chemotherapy. What questions and activities will you plan for them during the visit? Relate these plans to their developmental levels. What can you do to increase their knowledge and help them feel like they are part of Sam's care? Could their concern for Sam influence their own school performance? What should their teachers know about the fact that they have a sibling who has leukemia?

NCLEX-RN® Review

1. A child is being treated with dexamethasone in conjunction with other chemotherapy for treatment of leukemia. On a follow-up visit, the pediatric oncology clinic nurse expects which as a side effect?
   1. Weight gain
   2. Decreased blood pressure
   3. Anorexia
   4. Improved mood

2. When developing a plan of care for a child who is receiving chemotherapy for acute lymphocytic leukemia, which indicates the priority intervention?
   1. Weigh weekly.
   2. Call physician if urine specific gravity > 1.020.
   3. Provide antiemetics only every 8 hours.
   4. Administer intravenous fluids.

3. A child with leukemia has a white blood cell count of 10,000/microliter, a red blood cell count of 5 ($\times 10^{12}$/L), and platelets of 20,000/microliter. The child is also fairly active, visiting the playroom twice a day. When planning this child's care, which risk should the nurse consider most significant?
   1. Infection
   2. Anemia
   3. Hemorrhage
   4. Pain

4. A 7-year-old female returns to school after yearlong radiation treatments due to a brain tumor. She seems to have difficulty grasping the concepts in most of her classes. Which plan should the school nurse institute?
   1. Create an individualized health plan (IHP) and organize a meeting with the child's teachers.
   2. Advise the parents to keep the child at home and ask social work to arrange tutoring.
   3. Inform the child she must make up all of her schoolwork within 1 month.
   4. Offer homeschooling for 1 to 2 weeks to allow slow integration back to school.

See Appendix I 🔗 *for answers.*

References

Aburn, G., & Gott, M. (2011). Education given to parents of children newly diagnosed with acute lymphoblastic leukemia: A narrative review. *Journal of Pediatric Oncology Nursing, 28,* 300–305.

American Cancer Society. (2009). *Childhood cancer: Late effects of cancer treatment.* Retrieved from http://www.cancer.org/docrot/cri/content/

American Cancer Society. (2010). *Clinical trials: What you need to know.* Retrieved from http://www.cancer.org/acs/groups/cid/documents/webcontent/003006-pdf.pdf

American Cancer Society. (2011). *Cancer in children.* Retrieved from http://www.cancer.org

Anderson, P. M., Dhamne, C. A., & Huff, V. (2011). Wilms tumor. In R. M. Kliegman, B. F. Stanton, J. W. St. Geme, N. F. Schor, & R. E. Behrman, *Nelson textbook of pediatrics* (19th ed., pp. 1760–1762). Philadelphia, PA: Elsevier Saunders.

Armstrong, G. T. (2010). Long-term survivors of childhood central nervous system malignancies: The experience of the Childhood Cancer Survivor Study. *European Journal of Pediatric Neurology, 14,* 298–303.

Arndt, C. A. S. (2011). Neuroblastoma. In R. M. Kliegman, B. F. Stanton, J. W. St. Geme, N. F. Schor, & R. E. Behrman, *Nelson textbook of pediatrics* (19th ed., pp. 1763–1768). Philadelphia, PA: Elsevier Saunders.

Arndt, C. A. S. (2011). Soft tissue sarcomas. In R. M. Kliegman, B. F. Stanton, J. W. St. Geme, N. F. Schor, & R. E. Behrman, *Nelson textbook of pediatrics* (19th ed., pp. 1760–1762). Philadelphia, PA: Elsevier Saunders.

Asselin, B. (2011). Epidemiology of childhood and adolescent cancer. In R. M. Kliegman, B. F. Stanton, J. W. St. Geme, N. F. Schor, & R. E. Behrman, *Nelson textbook of pediatrics* (19th ed., pp. 1725–1727). Philadelphia, PA: Elsevier Saunders.

Association of Pediatric Hematology/Oncology Nurses (APHON). (n.d.). *APHON position paper on ambulatory pediatric hematology/oncology nursing practice.* Glenview, IL: Author.

Baker, J. N., Hinds, P. S., Spunt, S. L., Barfield, R. C., Allen, C., Powell, B. C., . . . Kane, J. R. (2008). Integration of palliative care practices into the ongoing care of children with cancer: Individualized care planning and coordination. *Pediatric Clinics of North America, 55,* 223–250.

Bhatia, S. (2011). Disparities in cancer outcomes: Lessons learned from children with cancer. *Pediatric Blood & Cancer, 56,* 994–1002.

Bindler, R. M., & Howry, L. B. (2005). *Pediatric drug guide.* Upper Saddle River, NJ: Prentice Hall.

Bishop, F. L., Prescott, P., Chan, Y. K., Saville, J., von Elm, E., & Lewith, G. T. (2010). Prevalence of complementary medicine use in pediatric cancer: A systematic review. *Pediatrics, 125,* 768–776.

Buckley, K. S. (2011). Pediatric genitourinary tumors. *Current Opinion in Oncology, 23,* 297–302.

Carbone, A., Spina, M., Gloghini, A., & Tirelli, U. (2011). Classical Hodgkin's lymphoma arising in different host's conditions: Pathobiology parameters, therapeutic options, and outcome. *America Journal of Hematology, 86,* 170–179.

Cheng, S. (2009). Superior vena cava syndrome: A contemporary review of a historic disease. *Cardiology Review, 17,* 16–23.

Clanton, N. R., Klosky, J. L., Jain, N., Srivastava, D. K., Mulrooney, D., Zeltzer, L., . . . Krull, K. R. (2011). Fatigue, vitality, sleep, and neurocognitive functioning in adult survivors of childhood cancer: A report from the childhood cancer survivor study. *Cancer.* doi:10.1002/cncr.25797

Cohen, J., Wakefield, C. E., Fleming, C. A., Gawthorne, R., Tapsell, L. C., & Cohn, R. J. (2011). Dietary intake after treatment in child cancer survivors. *Pediatric Blood & Cancer.* doi:10.1002/pbc.23280

Da Silva, E. D., Koch Nogueira, P. C., Russo Zamataro, T. M., de Carvalho, W. B., & Petrilli, A. S. (2008). Risk factors for death in children and adolescents with cancer and sepsis/septic shock. *Journal of Pediatric Hematology and Oncology, 30,* 513–518.

Decker, G. M. (2008). The marriage of conventional cancer treatments and alternative cancer therapies. *Nursing Clinics of North America, 43,* 221–242.

Erickson, J. M., Beck, S. L., Christian, B., Dudley, W. N., Hollen, P. J., Albritton, K., . . . Godder, K. (2011). Fatigue, sleep-wake disturbances, and quality of life in adolescents receiving chemotherapy. *Journal of Pediatric Hematology and Oncology 33,* e17–e25.

Eshelman-Kent, D., Kinahan, K. E., Hobbie, W., Landier, W., Teal, S., Friedman, D., . . . Freyer, D. R. (2011). Cancer survivorship practices, services, and delivery: A report from the Children's Oncology Group (COG) nursing discipline, adolescent/young adult, and late effects committees. *Journal of Cancer Survivorship, 5*(4), 345–357.

Faria, C. M., Rutka, J. T., Smith, C., & Kongkham, P. (2011). Epigenetic mechanisms regulating neural development and pediatric brain tumor formation. *Journal of Neurosurgery: Pediatrics, 8,* 119–132.

Fry, T. J., & Lankester, A. C. (2008). Cancer immunotherapy: Will expanding knowledge lead to success in pediatric oncology? *Pediatric Clinics of North America, 55,* 147–168.

Fulbright, J. M., Raman, S., McClellan, W. S., & August, K. J. (2011). Late effects of childhood leukemia therapy. *Current Hematologic Malignancy Reports, 6,* 195–205.

Geller, E., & Kochan, P. S. (2011). Renal neoplasms of childhood. *Radiology Clinics of North America, 49,* 689–709.

Gore, L., & Trippett, T. M. (2010). Emerging non-transplant-based strategies in treating pediatric non-Hodgkin's lymphoma. *Current Hematologic Malignancy Reports, 5,* 177–184.

Granger, J. M., & Kontoyiannis, D. P. (2009). Etiology and outcome of extreme leukocytosis in 758 nonhematologic cancer patients: A retrospective, single-institution study. *Cancer, 115,* 3919–3923.

Greinert, R., & Boniol, M. (2011). Skin cancer—Primary and secondary prevention (information campaigns and screening)—With a focus on children and sunbeds. *Progress in Biophysics and Molecular Biology, 107*(3), 473–476.

Hantel, C., Lewrick, F., Schneider, S., Zwermann, O., Perren, A., Reiricek, M., . . . Beuschlein, F. (2010). Anti insulin-like growth factor 1 receptor immunoliposomes: A single formulation combining two anticancer treatments with enhanced therapeutic efficiency. *Journal of Clinical Endocrinology and Metabolism, 95,* 943–952.

Heare, T., Hensley, M. A., & Dell'Orfano, S. (2009). Bone tumors: Osteosarcoma and Ewing's sarcoma. *Current Opinion in Pediatrics, 21,* 365–372.

Henderson, T. O., Bhatia, S., Pinto, N., London, W. B., McGrady, P., Grotty, C., . . . Cohn, S. L. (2011). Racial and ethnic disparities in risk and survival in children with neuroblastoma: A Children's Oncology Group study. *Journal of Clinical Oncology, 29,* 76–82.

Houlston, A., Buttery, E., & Powell, B. (2009). Cook to order: Meeting the nutritional needs of children with cancer in hospital. *Pediatric Nursing, 21*(4), 25–27.

Hu, K., Lee, C., Qiu, D., Fotovati, A., Davies, A., Abut-Ali, S., . . . Dunn, S. E. (2009). Small interfering RNA library screen of human kinases and phosphatases identifies polo-like kinase 1 as a promising new target for the treatment of pediatric rhabdomyosarcoma. *Molecular Cancer Therapeutics, 8,* 3024–3035.

Huff, V. (2011). Wilms tumours: About tumour suppressor genes, an oncogene and a chameleon gene. *Nature Reviews Cancer, 11,* 111–121.

Huh, W. W., & Skapek, S. X. (2010). Childhood rhabdomyosarcoma: New insight on biology and treatment. *Current Oncology Reports, 12,* 402–410.

JNCI. (2011). Brain tumor incidence in the U.S. *Journal of the National Cancer Institute, 103*(9), 707.

Kaste, S. C. (2008). Skeletal toxicities of treatment in children with cancer. *Pediatric Blood & Cancer, 50*(Suppl. 2), 469–473, 486.

Kirchhoff, A. C., Krull, K. R., Ness, K. K., Armstrong, G. T., Park, E. R., Stovall, M., . . . Leisenring, W. (2011). Physical, mental, and neurocognitive status and employment outcomes in the childhood cancer survivor study cohort. *Cancer Epidemiology and Biomarkers Prevention, 20,* 1838–1849.

Kurt, B. A., Armstrong, G. T., Cash, D. K., Krasin, M. J., Morris, E. B., Spunt, S. L., . . . Hudson, M. M. (2008). Primary care management of the childhood cancer survivor. *Journal of Pediatrics, 152,* 458–466.

Kurtz, B. P., & Abrams, A. N. (2010). Psychiatric aspects of pediatric cancer. *Child and Adolescent Psychiatric Clinics of North America, 19,* 401–421.

Kuttesch J. F., Rush, S. Z., & Ater, J. L. (2011). Brain tumors in children. In R. M. Kliegman, B. F. Stanton, J. W. St. Geme, N. F. Schor, & R. E. Behrman, *Nelson textbook of pediatrics* (19th ed., pp. 1746–1753). Philadelphia, PA: Elsevier Saunders.

Leigh, S. A. (2008). The changing legacy of cancer: Issues of long-term survivorship. *Nursing Clinics of North America, 43,* 243–258.Ω

Lewis, M. A., Hendrickson, A. W., & Moynihan, T. J. (2011). Oncologic emergencies: Pathophysiology, presentations, diagnosis, and treatment. *CA: A Cancer Journal for Clinicians, 61,* 287–314.

Loh, M. L. (2010). Childhood myelodysplastic syndrome: Focus on the approach to diagnosis and treatment of juvenile myelomonocytic leukemia. *Hematology, 2010,* 357–362.

Lohmann, D. (2010). Retinoblastoma. *Advances in Experimental Medicine and Biology, 685,* 220–227.

Manfrini, M., Tiwari, A., Ham, J., Colangeli, M., & Mercuri, M. (2011). Evolution of surgical treatment for sarcomas of proximal humerus in children: Retrospective review of a single institute over 30 years. *Journal of Pediatric Orthopedics, 31,* 56–64.

Masetti, R., Kleinschmidt, K., Biagi, C., & Pession, A. (2011). Emerging targeted therapies for pediatric myeloid leukemia. *Recent Patents on Anticancer Drug Discovery, 6,* 354–366.

McLendon, R. E., Adekunle, A., Rajaram, V., Kocak, M., & Blaney, S. M. (2011). Embryonal central nervous system neoplasms arising in infants and young children. *Archives of Pathology and Laboratory Medicine, 135,* 984–993.

National Cancer Institute. (2008). *Bone marrow transplantation and peripheral blood stem cell transplantation.* Retrieved from http://www.cancer.gov/cancertopics/factsheet/Therapy/bone-marrow-transplant

National Cancer Institute. (2011a). *Pediatric considerations for depression.* Retrieved from http://www.cancer.gov.cancertopics

National Cancer Institute. (2011b). *Stages of neuroblastoma.* Retrieved from http://www.cancer.gov.cancertopics/pdq/treatment/neuroblastoma/Patient/page2

National Cancer Institute. (2011c). *Wilms tumor and other childhood kidney tumors treatment: Stage information.* Retrieved from http://www.cancer.gov.cancertopics/pdq/treatment/wilms/HealthProfessional/page3

National Cancer Institute. (2011d). *Childhood Hodgkin lymphoma treatment: Staging and diagnostic evaluation.* Retrieved from http://www.cancer.gov.cancertopics/pdq/treatment/childhodgkins/HealthProfessional/page4

National Cancer Institute. (2011e). *Childhood non-Hodgkin lymphoma treatment: Stage information.* Retrieved from http://www.cancer.gov.cancertopics/pdq/treatment/child-non-hodgkins/HealthProfessional/

National Cancer Institute. (2011f). *Childhood rhabdomyosarcoma treatment: Stage information.* Retrieved from http://www.cancer.gov.cancertopics/pdq/treatment/childrhabdomyosarcoma/HealthProfessional

National Human Genome Research Institute. (2009). *Essential nursing competencies and curricula guidelines for genetics and genomics.* Retrieved from http://www.genome.gov/17517037

Ness, K. K., Armenian, S. H., Kadan-Lottick, N., & Gurney, J. G. (2011). Adverse effects of treatment in childhood acute lymphoblastic leukemia: General overview and implications for long-term health. *Expert Review in Hematology, 4,* 185–197.

Oeffinger, K. C., Nathan, P. C., & Kremer, L. C. M. (2008). Challenges after curative treatment for childhood cancer and long-term follow up of survivors. *Pediatric Clinics of North America, 55,* 251–274.

Paisley, M. A., Kang, T. I., Insogna, I. G., & Rheingold, S. R. (2011). Complementary and alternative therapy use in pediatric oncology patients with failure of frontline chemotherapy. *Pediatrics & Blood Cancer, 56,* 1088–1091.

Paldino, M. J., Faerber, E. N., & Poussaint, T. Y. (2011). Imaging tumors of the pediatric central nervous system. *Radiology Clinics of North America, 49,* 589–616.

Park, J. R., Eggert, A., & Caron, H. (2008). Neuroblastoma: Biology, prognosis, and treatment. *Pediatric Clinics of North America, 55,* 97–120.

Patrick-Miller, L., Bradbury, A. R., & Terry, M. B. (2010). Controversies in communication of genetic screening results for cancer. *Cancer Epidemiology Biomarkers & Prevention, 19,* 624–627.

Pieters, R., & Carroll, W. L. (2008). Biology and treatment of acute lymphoblastic leukemia. *Pediatric Clinics of North America, 55,* 1–20.

Pollack, I. F. (2011). Multidisciplinary management of childhood brain tumors: A review of outcomes, recent advances, and challenges. *Journal of Neurosurgery: Pediatrics, 8,* 133–148.

Pollack, I. F., & Jakacki, R. I. (2011). Childhood brain tumors: Epidemiology, current management and future directions. *Nature Reviews Neurology, 7,* 495–506.

Post-White, J., Fitzgerald, M., Hageness, S., & Sencer, S. F. (2009). Complementary and alternative medicine use in children with cancer and general and specialty pediatrics. *Journal of Pediatric Oncology Nursing, 26,* 7–15.

Pui, C. H., Carroll, W. L., Meshinchi, S., & Arceci, R. J. (2011). Biology, risk stratification, and therapy of pediatric acute leukemias: An update. *Journal of Clinical Oncology, 29,* 551–565.

Quillen, J., Crawford, E., Plummer, B., Bradley, H., & Glidden, R. (2011). Parental follow-through of neuropsychological recommendations for childhood-cancer survivors. *Journal of Pediatric Oncology Nursing, 28,* 306–310.

Rabin, K. R., & Poplack, D. G. (2011). Management strategies in acute lymphoblastic leukemia. *Oncology, 25,* 328–335.

Rao, A., Rothman, J., & Nichols, K. E. (2008). Genetic testing and tumor surveillance for children with cancer predisposition syndromes. *Current Opinion in Pediatrics, 20,* 1–7.

Reulen, R. C., Frobisher, C., Winter, D. L., Kelly, J., Lancashire, E. R., Stiller, C. A., ... Hawkins, M. M. (2011). Long-term risks of subsequent primary neoplasms among survivors of childhood cancer. *Journal of the American Medical Association, 305,* 2311–2319.

Roach, M., Alberini, J. L., Pecking, A. P., Testori, A., Verrecchia, F., Soteldo, J., ... Gottlieb, R. (2010). Diagnostic and therapeutic imaging for cancer: Therapeutic considerations and future directions. *Journal of Surgical Oncology, 103,* 587–601.

Rosen, G. M., Shor, A. C., & Geller, T. J. (2008). Sleep in children with cancer. *Current Opinion in Pediatrics, 20,* 676–681.

Sadeh, A., Dahl, R.E., Shahar, G. & Rosenblat-Stein, S. (2009). Sleep and the transition to adolescence: A longitudinal study. Sleep 32, 1602-1609.

Shepherd, E., Woodgate, R. L., & Sawatzky, J. A. (2010). Pain in children with central nervous system cancer: A review of the literature. *Oncology Nursing Forum, 37,* E318–E330.

Shields, C. L., & Shields, J. A. (2010). Retinoblastoma management: Advances in enucleation, intravenous chemoreduction, and intra-arterial chemotherapy. *Current Opinion in Ophthalmology, 21,* 203–212.

Shuangshoti, S., Shuangshoti, S., Nuchprayoon, I., Kanjanapongkul, S., Marrano, P., Irwin, M. S., & Thorner, P. S. (2011). Natural course of low risk neuroblastoma. *Pediatrics & Blood Cancer.* doi:10.1002/pbc.23325

Sigel, K., Dubrow, R., Silverberg, M., Crothers, K., Braithwaite, S., & Justice, A. (2011). Cancer screening in patients with HIV. *Current HIV/AIDS Report, 8,* 142–152.

Soliman, H., & Agresta, S. V. (2008). Current issues in adolescent and young adult cancer survivorship. *Cancer Control, 15,* 55–62.

Steinberger, J., Sinaiko, A. R., Kelly, A. S., Leisenring, W. M., Steffen, L. M., Goodman, P., ... Baker, K. S. (2012). Cardiovascular risk and insulin resistance in childhood cancer survivors. *Journal of Pediatrics, 160*(3), 494–499.

Tomlinson, D., Hesser, T., Ethier, M. C., & Sung, L. (2011). Complementary and alternative medicine use in pediatric cancer reported during palliative phase of disease. *Support Care Cancer, 19*(11), 1857–1863.

Trehan, A., Cheetham, R., & Bailey, S. (2009). Hypercalcemia in acute lymphoblastic leukemia: A review. *Journal of Pediatric Hematology and Oncology, 31,* 424–427.

Tubergen, D. G., Bleyer, A., & Ritchey, A. K. (2011). The leukemias. In R. M. Kliegman, B. F. Stanton, J. W. St. Geme, N. F. Schor, & R. E. Behrman, *Nelson textbook of pediatrics* (19th ed., pp. 1732–1739). Philadelphia, PA: Elsevier Saunders.

Unguru, Y., Coppes, M. J., & Kamani, N. (2008). Rethinking pediatric assent: From requirement to ideal. *Pediatric Clinics of North America, 55,* 211–222.

Warnick, E. & Auger, D. (2009). Management of patients with primary central nervous system lymphoma treated with high-dose methotrexate. *Clinical Journal of Oncology Nursing 13,* 177–180.

Waxman, I. M., Hochberg, J., & Cairo, M. S. (2011). Lymphoma. In R. M. Kliegman, B. F. Stanton, J. W. St. Geme, N. F. Schor, & R. E. Behrman, *Nelson textbook of pediatrics* (19th ed., pp. 1739–1753). Philadelphia, PA: Elsevier Saunders.

Winick, N. (2011). Neurocognitive outcome in survivors of pediatric cancer. *Current Opinion in Pediatrics, 23,* 27–33.

Zage, P. E., & Ater, J. L. (2011). Neuroblastoma. In R. M. Kliegman, B. F. Stanton, J. W. St. Geme, N. F. Schor, & R. E. Behrman, *Nelson textbook of pediatrics* (19th ed., pp. 1753–1757). Philadelphia, PA: Elsevier Saunders.

Zage, P. E. & Herzog, C. E. (2011). Retinoblastoma. In R. M. Kliegman, B. F. Stanton, J. W. St. Geme, N. F. Schor, & R. E. Behrman, *Nelson textbook of pediatrics* (19th ed., pp. 1768–1769). Philadelphia, PA: Elsevier Saunders.

Zeltzer, L. K., Recklitis, C., Buchbinder, D., Zebrack, B., Casillas, J., Tsao, J. C. I., ... Krull, K. (2009). Psychological status in childhood cancer survivors: A report from the Childhood Cancer Survivor Study. *Journal of Clinical Oncology, 27,* 2396–2402.

Zonfrillo, M. R. (2009). Management of pediatric tumor lysis syndrome in the emergency department. *Emergency Medical Clinics of North America, 27,* 497–504.

Zwaan, M. C., Reinhardt, D., Hitzler, J., & Vyas, P. (2010). Acute leukemias in children with Down syndrome. *Pediatric Clinics of North America, 55,* 53–70.

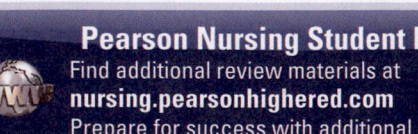

Pearson Nursing Student Resources

Find additional review materials at
nursing.pearsonhighered.com
Prepare for success with additional NCLEX®-style practice questions, interactive assignments and activities, web links, animations and videos, and more!

Alterations in Gastrointestinal Function

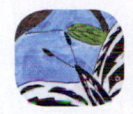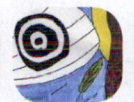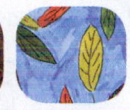

KEY TERMS

Learning Outcomes

After completing this chapter, you will be able to:

1. Describe the anatomic and physiologic characteristics of the developing gastrointestinal system.

2. Discuss the pathophysiologic processes associated with specific gastrointestinal disorders in the pediatric population.

3. Identify signs and symptoms that may indicate a disorder of the gastrointestinal system.

4. Summarize preoperative and postoperative family-centered care for the child born with cleft lip/palate.

5. Contrast nursing management and plan care for disorders of the gastrointestinal system for the child needing abdominal surgery versus the child needing nonoperative management.

6. Analyze developmentally appropriate approaches for nursing management of gastrointestinal disorders in the pediatric population.

7. Summarize etiology, pathophysiology, symptoms, and management for the child with a parasitic or viral infection of the gastrointestinal system.

8. Plan nursing care for the child with an injury to the gastrointestinal system.

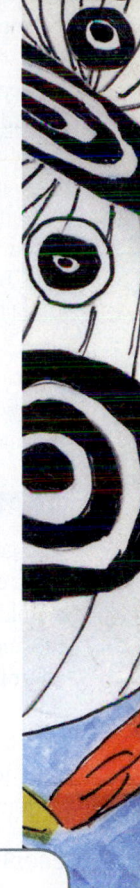

> **"My tummy hurts so bad. I wanted Mommy to make it better."**
>
> *—Jenna, age 4*

Jenna Baker is a 4-year-old who has just been admitted to the pediatric unit following surgery for a ruptured appendix. She complained of her stomach hurting last night, but this morning her condition was worse and she had a temperature of 102°F. Worried that this was not just a virus, Jenna's mother took her to the pediatrician. On the way to the doctor's office, Jenna told her mother that her pain "just went away." While at the pediatrician's office she complained of feeling bad all over. On examination her abdomen was rigid and no bowel sounds were heard. A complete blood count revealed a white blood cell (WBC) count of 22,000 mm³. The pediatrician diagnosed Jenna with appendicitis and most likely a ruptured appendix. He referred Jenna to the emergency department for assessment and surgical consultation. A computed tomography (CT) scan confirmed a diagnosis of appendicitis. During surgery the appendix was found to have ruptured.

Jenna had an open appendectomy with wound closure. A dry dressing is in place. Jenna now has a peripherally inserted central catheter (PICC) line for intravenous fluids, pain medication, and intravenous antibiotics. She also has a nasogastric tube to suction and a Foley catheter.

Jenna's parents feel guilty that the appendix was ruptured and wonder if they could have done something to prevent it. This is Jenna's first hospitalization. Jenna's parents are worried that she will have a lot of pain and wonder how she will cope with the hospitalization. Extended family members, including Jenna's great grandmother, have offered to stay with Jenna part of the time, so her parents can get some rest. What is the priority of nursing care for Jenna in the immediate postoperative period? What should the nurse include when teaching Jenna's parents about the postoperative course?

Through the gastrointestinal (GI) tract, a child ingests and absorbs the foods and fluids necessary to sustain life and promote growth. Most gastrointestinal disturbances produce symptoms that are short term and interfere with nutrition and fluid balance for only a brief period such as the case of Jenna in the opening scenario. Some disorders or severe defects lead to complications that prevent optimal nutrition and adequate growth. (See Chapter 23 🖉 for a discussion of specific fluid imbalances that may accompany gastrointestinal infections.)

Gastrointestinal disorders can result from a congenital defect, acquired disease, infection, or injury. Structural problems may occur when development is altered or ceases in the first trimester of gestation. Because various parts of the gastrointestinal system are developing at this point in gestation, it is not unusual for infants to have more than one structural defect of the gastrointestinal system. Infections can cause an increase or decrease in motility and prevent proper absorption of nutrients. This chapter will describe common gastrointestinal disorders and appropriate management of these disorders.

ANATOMY AND PHYSIOLOGY

The gastrointestinal tract includes the mouth, esophagus, stomach, pancreas, small intestine, and large intestine. Through the GI tract, a child ingests and absorbs the foods and fluids necessary to sustain life and promote growth. Elimination of waste products is another role of the GI tract. The organs of the GI tract are located in the abdomen. Other organs located in the abdominal region include the gallbladder, liver, and spleen. The abdomen is generally divided into four quadrants for purposes of assessment. See Figure 30–1 ■ for the abdominal organs and structures in each quadrant.

Esophagus and Stomach

The esophagus is a continuous tube that allows food to pass to the stomach. Food enters the esophagus through the mouth, where it is chewed. Initial enzyme secretion then begins food digestion. (See Chapter 24 🖉 for more information related to the mouth and pharynx.) The stomach is located in the left upper quadrant (LUQ) of the abdomen. The role of the stomach is to store food and to secrete enzymes and digestive juices that aid in digestion of the food (Table 30–1). Hydrochloric acid stimulates the stomach's pepsinogens to become pepsins which break down proteins and are active in acidic levels (pH of 3 or less). The stomach propels food that is partially digested into the duodenum (a part of the small intestine).

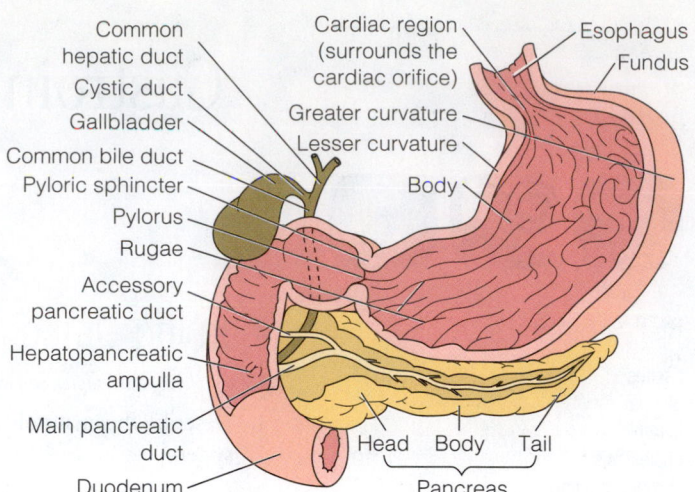

FIGURE 30–1 ■ The internal anatomic structures of the stomach, including the pancreatic, cystic, and hepatic ducts; the pancreas; and the gallbladder.

Pancreas

The pancreas is located behind the stomach and has several functions. The pancreas secretes enzymes, electrolytes, and bicarbonates that aid in the digestion and absorption of fats, proteins, and carbohydrates (Werlin, 2011).

Liver and Gallbladder

The liver, the largest organ in the abdomen, is located in the right upper quadrant (RUQ). Its primary functions include production of blood clotting factors, fibrinogen, and prothrombin; secretion of bile and **bilirubin** (yellow pigment produced from the breakdown of red blood cells); metabolism of fat, protein, and carbohydrates; detoxification of hormones, drugs, and other substances; and storage of vitamins A, D, E, and K and glycogen. The gallbladder is a small organ located behind the liver. The gallbladder stores and concentrates the bile that is produced in the liver. It then releases stored bile as needed into the duodenum. Bile includes a variety of substances such as water, salts, bilirubin, and cholesterol. A major role of bile is to emulsify fats so that fatty acids can be absorbed (Miethke & Balistreri, 2011).

Spleen

The spleen is located high in the LUQ of the abdomen and is a very vascular organ. The spleen may contain more than 500 mL

TABLE 30–1	Enzymes Used in Digestion	
ENZYME	**SOURCE**	**FUNCTION**
Amylase	Secreted by salivary glands	Converts starches to disaccharides
Hydrochloric acid	Secreted by stomach	Stops action of amylase; converts pepsinogen to pepsin that is instrumental in converting proteins to polypeptides
Amylase	Secreted by pancreas	Converts starches to disaccharides
Enterokinase	In small intestine	Converts chymotrypsinogen and trypsinogen to trypsin
Chymotrypsin and trypsin	In small intestine	Converts polypeptides to di- and tripeptides and then to amino acids
Bile salts	From bile and secreted to small intestine	Emulsifies fats
Lipase	From pancreas	Converts fats to fatty acids and glycerol

Source: *Data from Chamley, C. A., Carson, P., Randall, D., & Sandwell, M. (2005). Developmental anatomy and physiology of children. St. Louis, MO: Elsevier; Thibodeau, G. A., & Patton, K. T. (2010). The human body in health & disease (5th ed.). St. Louis, MO: Mosby.*

of blood. Defense against infection is another key role of the spleen. Through phagocytosis, infectious organisms are filtered from the blood (Thibodeau & Patton, 2010).

Small and Large Intestine

The small intestine consists of the duodenum, the jejunum, and the ileum. Each part of the small intestine plays a vital role in the digestion and absorption of carbohydrates, amino acids, and fats (Thibodeau & Patton, 2010). The intestinal wall is covered with small villi, the brush border, through which absorption occurs. Absorption occurs both through diffusion (commonly monosaccharides, amino acids, fatty acids, and glycerol) and through active transport (commonly disaccharides, dipeptides, and tripeptides). A complex system of innervation and secretions maintains a basic pH that facilitates metabolism and absorption. The large intestine includes the cecum, the appendix, the colon (consisting of ascending, transverse, descending, and sigmoid portions), and the rectum which passes to the exterior through the anus. The primary function of the large intestine is reabsorption of fluid and electrolytes from the GI tract and excretion of wastes (Liacouras, 2011). Bacteria in the large intestine synthesize vitamin K and facilitate some vitamin B absorption.

PEDIATRIC DIFFERENCES

Although the fetus makes sucking and swallowing movements in utero and ingests amniotic fluid, the GI system is immature at birth. The processes of absorption and excretion do not begin until after birth because the placenta provides nutrients and removes waste. Sucking is a primitive reflex that occurs whenever the lips or cheeks are stroked. The infant does not have voluntary control over swallowing until about 6 weeks of age.

The stomach capacity of the newborn is quite small, and intestinal motility (**peristalsis**) is greater than in older children (Figure 30–2 ■). These characteristics explain the newborn's need for small, frequent feedings and the increased frequency and liquid consistency of bowel movements. Because of the relaxed cardiac sphincter, infants frequently regurgitate small amounts of feedings.

Digestion takes place in the duodenum. Infants have a deficiency of several enzymes: amylase (which digests carbohydrates), lipase (which enhances fat absorption), and trypsin (which catabolizes protein into polypeptides and some amino acids). Enzymes are usually not present in sufficient quantities to aid digestion until 4 to 6 months of age. Thus, abdominal distention from gas is common.

As They Grow Stomach Capacity Increases Throughout Childhood

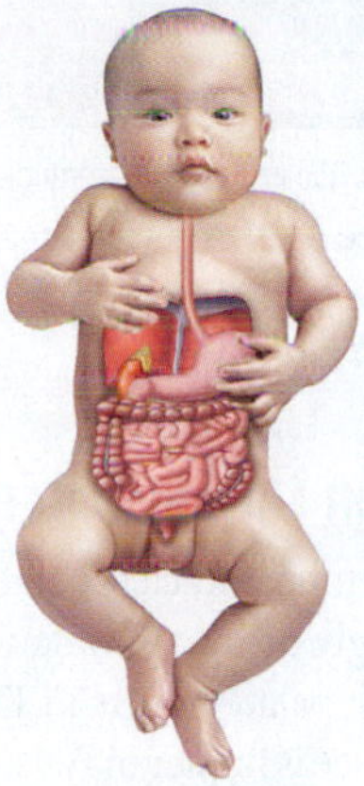

Stomach capacity throughout early childhood

Age	Capacity (mL)
Newborn	10 to 20
1 week	30 to 90
2 to 3 weeks	75 to 100
1 month	90 to 150
3 months	150 to 200
1 year	210 to 360
2 years	500

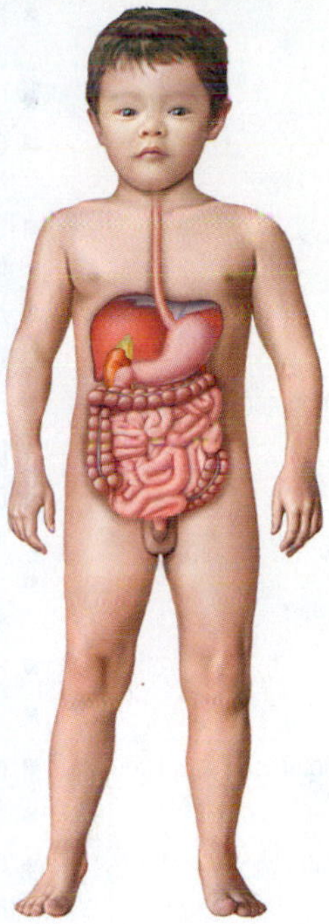

FIGURE 30–2 ■ The young infant has a small stomach capacity as compared to the older child or adolescent. A 30-day term infant has a stomach capacity of only 90 mL (Collopy & Friese, 2010). As the infant grows their stomach capacity increases, decreasing the frequency with which they need to be fed (AAP, 2011). Stomach capacity increases to 360 mL around 1 year of age (Collopy & Friese, 2010), to 500 mL by 2 years of age and to 1500 mL by 16 years of age (Moules & Ramsay, 2008). An adult stomach holds 2–3 liters (Collopy & Friese, 2010; Moules & Ramsay, 2008).

Liver function is also immature. After the first few weeks of life the liver is able to conjugate bilirubin and excrete bile. The processes of **gluconeogenesis** (formation of glycogen from noncarbohydrates), plasma protein and ketone formation, vitamin storage, and **deamination** (removal of amino group from amino compound) remain immature during the first year of life.

By the second year of life, digestive processes are fairly complete. Stomach capacity increases to accommodate a three-meals-per-day feeding schedule. Around 18 months of age, the child becomes aware of a full rectum and is physically able to have some control over excretory functions (Goldson & Reynolds, 2011). See Table 30–2 for guidelines for assessment of the gastrointestinal system. Table 30–3 lists diagnostic tests and laboratory procedures for the gastrointestinal system.

STRUCTURAL DEFECTS

Structural defects can involve one or more areas of the gastrointestinal tract. These defects occur when growth and development of fetal structures are interrupted during the first trimester. This can leave the structure incomplete, resulting in **atresia** (absence or closure of a normal body orifice), malposition, nonclosure, or other abnormalities. The structural defects discussed in this section are cleft lip and cleft palate, esophageal atresia and tracheoesophageal fistula, pyloric stenosis,

TABLE 30–2	Assessment Guidelines for the Child with a Gastrointestinal Condition*
ASSESSMENT FOCUS	**ASSESSMENT GUIDELINES**
Abdomen—inspection	■ Observe the shape of the abdomen.
	■ Note any abdominal distention. Measure abdominal girth.
	■ Observe the umbilicus for protrusion.
	■ Observe for peristaltic waves (visible rhythmic contractions of the intestinal wall smooth muscle).
	■ Observe for jaundice, bruising, and increased bleeding.
Abdomen—auscultation	■ Auscultate for bowel sounds in all four quadrants prior to palpation.
Abdomen—palpation	■ Palpate the abdomen and note if it is soft or firm.
	■ Palpate the size of the umbilical ring.
	■ Does the child complain of pain or tenderness during palpation? Does the infant cry?
	■ Describe any masses palpated by location, shape, size, and consistency.
	■ Palpate the liver for size and tenderness.
	■ Palpate the spleen for size and tenderness.
Mouth and esophagus	■ Note the presence of increased oral secretions.
	■ Note the presence of cleft lip or palate.
Nutrition	■ Note tolerance of feedings, spitting up, emesis, and recurrent respiratory infections.
	■ Observe amount, color, and frequency of emesis.
	■ Note if emesis is associated with feeding and whether it is projectile.
	■ Note amount of intake, frequency of feedings, and growth.
Stool	■ Observe color, consistency, and size of stool. Note any changes in stool patterns.
Family history	■ Ask about history of gastrointestinal illness with genetic influences such as celiac disease and inflammatory bowel disease.

Note: *See Chapter 7 🔗 for actual techniques and order of abdominal assessment.

TABLE 30–3	Diagnostic Procedures and Laboratory Tests for the Gastrointestinal System*
DIAGNOSTIC PROCEDURES	**LABORATORY TESTS**
Abdominal ultrasound	Complete blood count
Barium or contrast enema	Bilirubin
CT of the abdomen	Electrolytes
Endoscopy	Liver enzymes
GI series	Stool for occult blood
Intraesophageal pH probe monitoring	Stool for ova and parasites
Abdominal Radiographs	

Note: *See Appendixes D and E 🔗 for information about these diagnostic procedures and tests.

gastroesophageal reflux and gastroesophageal reflux disease, abdominal wall defects, intussusception, volvulus, Hirschsprung disease, and anorectal malformations. Ostomies, a common surgical intervention during correction of structural defects, are discussed on page 1014.

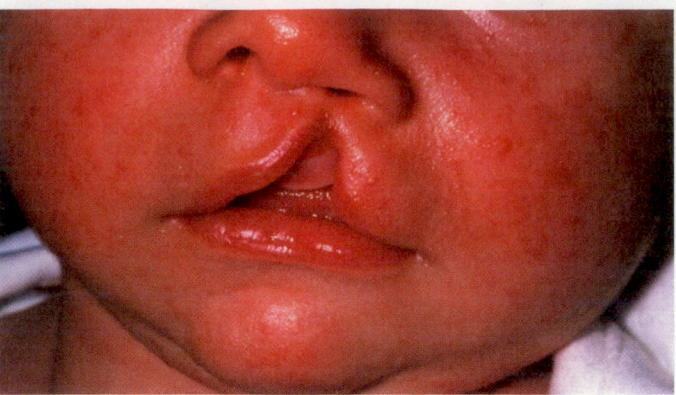

FIGURE 30–3 ■ Unilateral cleft lip.
Source: *Dr. P. Marazzi / Science Source / Photo Researchers, Inc.*

Cleft Lip and Cleft Palate

Cleft lip and cleft palate are two distinct facial defects that can occur singly or in combination (Figure 30–3 ■). Cleft lip with or without cleft palate occurs in 1 out of every 750 to 1,000 live births. The incidence is higher in Asians (1 in 500) than in Caucasians (1 in 750). The defect is less common in African Americans, with an incidence of 1 out of every 2,000 live births. Cleft lip and palate occur together in approximately 45% of cases, while cleft palate occurs alone approximately 35% of the time, and cleft lip occurs alone approximately 20% of the time (Patel, Ramaswamy, Grasseschi, et al., 2009).

Etiology and Pathophysiology

Cleft lip with or without cleft palate results from a failure of the maxillary processes to fuse with the elevations on the frontal prominence during the sixth week of gestation. Normally union of the upper lip is complete by the seventh week. Fusion of the secondary palate occurs between 5 and 12 weeks of gestation. Failure of the tongue to move downward at the correct time will prevent the palatine processes from fusing. The intrauterine development of the hard and soft palates is completed in the first trimester. It is during this time that other major organ systems develop. Although cleft lip or palate occurs as a feature in many different syndromes, a majority of children with these orofacial defects do not have an associated syndrome or other birth defect (Wehby & Cassell, 2010).

There is an increased incidence in families with a prior history of cleft lip or palate. The cause is believed to be multifactorial, involving a combination of environmental and genetic influences. Etiologic factors include smoking during pregnancy and maternal use of alcohol, anticonvulsants such as phenytoin, steroids, or illegal drugs such as cocaine during pregnancy (Slator, Russell, Cole, et al., 2009; Wiet, Sie, Biavati, et al., 2010). Additionally studies have suggested that folate intake during pregnancy may reduce the incidence of cleft lip and palate (Blanton, Henry, Yuan, et al., 2011).

Clinical Manifestations

A cleft that involves the lip is readily apparent at birth. The defect may be a simple dimple in the vermilion border of the lip or a complete separation extending to the floor of the nose. The defect may be unilateral or bilateral and may occur alone or in combination with a cleft palate defect. Incomplete cleft lip has a bridge of tissue connecting the central and lateral lip. Varying degrees of nasal deformity may also be present.

TABLE 30–4	Complications Associated with Cleft Lip or Cleft Palate	
COMPLICATION	**ETIOLOGY**	**NURSING MANAGEMENT**
Feeding problems	The child is unable to suck successfully. Excess air intake results in gastrointestinal distress.	Refer to a nurse specialist for assessment of feeding and evaluation of the need for special nipples. Support mothers who want to breastfeed. Encourage the mother to express her breast milk if the child is unable to nurse. Teach parents to encourage slow feeding with the baby in an upright position, and to burp frequently. Measure frequently to evaluate adequacy of growth.
Otologic	There is a high risk for otitis media due to decreased pharyngeal heights and horizontal positioning of the eustachian tubes. The cleft allows bacteria to enter the eustachian tube. Hearing loss may occur as a result of repeated otitis media.	Monitor for ear infections. Teach the family measures to prevent infections. Use antibiotics to treat ear infections. The child may need tympanostomy tubes placed to promote drainage. Audiology screening is conducted on a regular basis.
Dental and orthodontic	The child may have a delay in eruption of primary teeth. Teeth may erupt in an abnormal pattern and may be small, pointed, or missing. The child is at higher risk for tooth decay. Teeth may be crooked and difficult to clean. Scar tissue may also make toothbrushing difficult.	Promote good oral hygiene and regular visits to a dentist experienced in caring for children with cleft lip/cleft palate. Encourage brushing of teeth from the time teeth begin to erupt. Provide fluoride supplements if needed. Encourage a healthy diet, low in sugar.
Speech development	Abnormalities with the palate, faulty dentition, and hearing problems secondary to frequent ear infections may lead to speech problems.	Evaluate speech and language development on a regular basis.

Source: *Data from Cole, A., Tomlinson, J., Slator, R., & Reading, J. (2009). Understanding cleft lip and palate. 3: Feeding the baby. Journal of Family Health Care, 19(5), 157–158; Owens, J. (2008). Parents' experiences of feeding a baby with cleft lip and palate. British Journal of Midwifery, 16(12), 778–784; Slator, R., Russell, J., Bridges, M., Tomlinson, J., Cole, A., & Morton, J. (2009b). Understanding cleft lip and palate. 2: The first five years. Journal of Family Health Care, 19(4), 122–125; Wiet, G. J., Sie, K., Biavati, M. J., & Rocha-Worley, G. (2010). Reconstructive surgery for cleft palate. Retrieved from http:// emedicine.medscape.com/article/878062-overview#a0102*

Cleft palate defects are less obvious when they occur without a cleft lip and may not be detected at birth. Clefts of the hard palate form a continuous opening between the mouth and nasal cavity and may be unilateral or bilateral, involving just the soft palate or both the soft and hard palates.

Collaborative Care

A multidisciplinary team is involved in cleft lip and palate management since these children have an increased risk for impairment in speech, hearing, and tooth development (Cassell, Daniels, & Meyer, 2009). Coordinated care by specialists in plastic and oral surgery, audiology, speech, otolaryngology, and orthodontics is necessary (Table 30–4).

Diagnostic Tests

Cleft lip and cleft palate are generally diagnosed prenatally, at birth, or during the newborn assessment. Successful imaging of the face via ultrasound can be performed as early as 13 weeks' gestation. Use of three-dimensional ultrasound allows for the most accurate diagnosis of the anomaly (Maarse, Bergé, Pistorius, et al., 2010). After the child is born, cleft lip and cleft palate are diagnosed by characteristic physical findings. The inner and outer surfaces of the lip should be examined. The examiner may use a finger to feel for a cleft palate. Visual examination of the mouth using a light and a tongue depressor is also an effective method for detecting a cleft palate (Slator, Russell, Cole, et al., 2009).

Because clefts may be involved in many life-threatening malformations, immediate diagnostic studies to detect ear deformities, skeletal deformities, heart defects, and genitourinary defects are conducted.

Clinical Therapy

The cleft lip is usually repaired during the first 6 months of life (Cassell et al., 2009) (Figure 30–4 ■). The technique used to repair the lip

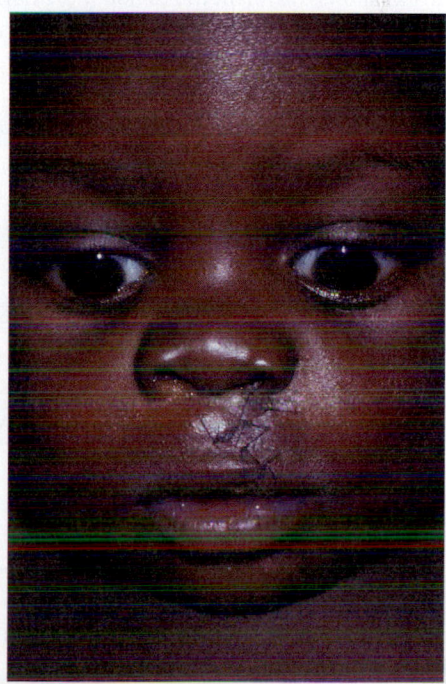

FIGURE 30–4 ■ Repaired unilateral cleft lip.

Source: *Ansary / Custom Medical Stock Photo.*

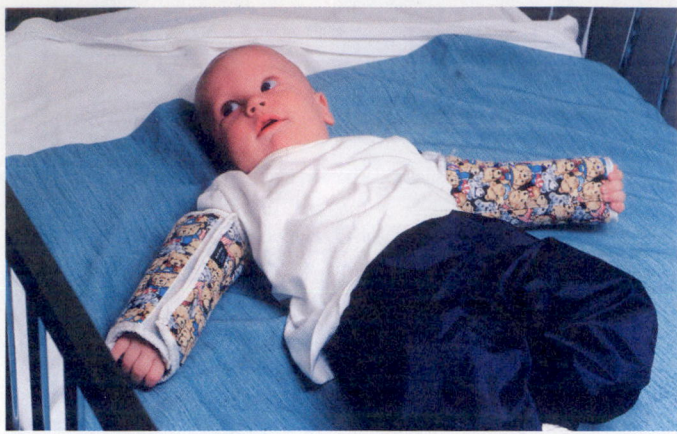

FIGURE 30–5 ■ Elbow immobilizers prevent flexion of the arm and are used to protect the surgical incision postoperatively for cleft lip or palate repair.

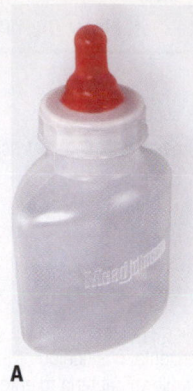
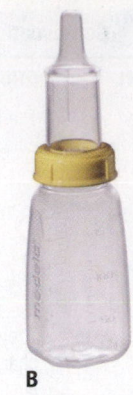

A   **B**

FIGURE 30–6 ■ Special bottles and nipples for the child with cleft lip and/or cleft palate. The cleft palate nurser (*A*) and the SpecialNeeds Feeder (*B*) both have longer, softer nipples and make it easier for the child to feed from a bottle.

Source: *A, photo courtesy of Mead Johnson Nutritional; B, courtesy of Medela AG.*

varies depending on the severity of the defect (Tibesar, Black, & Sidman, 2009). If the defect is severe, the child may need more than one operation to achieve total repair. After surgery, soft elbow immobilizers are used for 2 weeks to prevent the child from thumb sucking or putting fingers in the mouth, which could disrupt the suture line (Kasten, Schmidt, Zickler, et al., 2008) (Figure 30–5 ■) (refer to the Skills Manual ⬭). The child should receive distraction and pain medication as needed to prevent crying, as prolonged crying may disrupt the suture line.

Early closure of the lip enables the infant to form a better seal around the nipple for feeding. The sucking motion strengthens the muscles necessary for speech. Special feeding devices such as longer nipples with enlarged holes are available to help meet the infant's nutritional needs before surgical correction.

Timing of the cleft palate repair varies among surgeons and depends on the size and severity of the cleft. The palate should be closed by 18 months of age (Cassell et al., 2009). This protects the formation of tooth buds and allows the infant to develop more normal speech patterns. Repair of cleft palate may require additional staged reconstructions if the cleft was severe.

Both surgical procedures require the use of general anesthesia, and the hospital stay is dependent upon the child's postoperative progress. Postoperative feeding protocols vary from the use of special nipples or syringes to breastfeeding. Infants with cleft lip and cleft palate are prone to recurrent otitis media, which can lead to tympanic membrane scarring and hearing loss.

Nursing Management

Nursing care involves facilitating feeding, providing emotional support, performing preoperative and postoperative care, assisting parents to coordinate care and maintain a healthy home environment, and making appropriate referrals.

Nursing Assessment and Diagnosis

Physiologic Assessment

A cleft lip defect is observable at birth. A cleft palate defect is usually noted during the newborn assessment by palpation of the palate with the finger (Slator, Russell, Cole, et al., 2009). A description of the location and extent of the defect helps the nurse determine the correct method of feeding. Thorough and complete physical assessment is required since additional defects are sometimes present.

Psychosocial Assessment

Assessment of the family's reactions is an integral part of the overall nursing assessment. Physical deformities, especially of the face, can be devastating to parents. A poorly corrected defect can lead to the development of low self-esteem in the older child. Assess the child's developmental level and social interactions with peers.

The accompanying Nursing Care Plan lists common nursing diagnoses for the infant with a cleft lip and/or palate. Other diagnoses that may be appropriate include:

- Anxiety (parent) related to situational crisis and threat to self-concept
- Attachment, Risk for Impaired Parent/Infant related to newborn's structural defect
- Pain, Acute related to surgical repair of defect
- Growth and Development, Delayed related to structural defect and altered nutritional intake

NANDA-I © 2012

Planning and Implementation

Nursing care involves providing emotional support, performing postoperative care, helping parents coordinate care and maintain a healthy home environment, and making appropriate referrals. See Nursing Care Plan: The Infant with a Cleft Lip and/or Palate for a summary of nursing care.

Facilitate Feeding

Feeding problems for the infant with cleft lip or cleft palate depend on the severity of the anatomic defect. Infants with cleft lip, cleft palate, or both are generally able to breastfeed or bottle-feed with assistance and education related to positioning and feeding techniques (Cole, Tomlinson, Slator, et al., 2009; Owens, 2008). If breastfeeding is not possible, the mother can be assisted to pump her breasts in order for the milk to be fed by a special nurser.

For infants requiring assistance to feed, several wide-based nipples, squeezable bottles, and other special bottles are available (Figure 30–6 ■). Some infants may require a device placed in the mouth to enable them to establish suction. Several companies provide special nursers that may be helpful for children with cleft lip or palate. See Partnering with Families: Feeding the Infant with Cleft Lip or Cleft Palate.

Nursing Care Plan — The Infant with a Cleft Lip and/or Palate

INTERVENTION	RATIONALE	EXPECTED OUTCOME
PREOPERATIVE CARE		
1. Nursing Diagnosis: Aspiration, Risk for related to anatomic defect		
NIC Priority Intervention—*Aspiration Precautions:* Prevention or minimization of risk factors in the patient at risk of aspiration		**NOC Suggested Outcome**—*Respiratory Status: Ventilation:* Movement of air in and out of the lungs
GOAL: *The infant will have no episodes of gagging or aspiration.*		
■ Assess respiratory status and monitor vital signs at least every 2 hours.	■ Frequent assessment allows for early identification of problems.	The infant exhibits no signs of respiratory distress.
■ Keep suction equipment and a bulb syringe at the bedside.	■ Suctioning may be necessary to remove milk or mucus.	
■ Position upright for feedings.	■ Upright positioning minimizes passage of feedings through the cleft.	
■ Feed slowly and use adaptive equipment as needed.	■ This approach facilitates intake while minimizing the risk of aspiration.	
■ Hold upright for 30 minutes after feeding.	■ Holding the infant upright prevents aspiration of feedings.	
■ Burp frequently (after every 15–30 mL of fluid).	■ Frequent burping helps to prevent regurgitation and aspiration.	
2. Nursing Diagnosis: Coping: Family, Compromised related to birth of a child with a defect		
NIC Priority Intervention—*Caregiver Support:* Provision of the necessary information, advocacy, and support to facilitate primary patient care by someone other than a healthcare professional		**NOC Suggested Outcome**—*Family Coping:* Family actions to manage stressors that tax family resources
GOAL: *Parents will begin the bonding process with the infant.*		
■ Help parents to hold the infant and facilitate the feeding process.	■ Contact is essential for bonding.	Parents hold, comfort, and show concern for the infant.
■ Point out positive attributes of the infant (e.g., hair, eyes, alertness).	■ Emphasizing positive attributes helps parents see the child as a whole, rather than concentrating on the defect.	
■ Explain the surgical procedure and expected outcome. Show pictures of other children's cleft lip repair.	■ Eliminating unknown factors helps to decrease anxiety.	
GOAL: *The family's coping ability will be maximized. Parents will verbalize the nature and sequelae of the defect.*		
■ Assess parents' knowledge of the defect, their degree of anxiety and level of discomfort, and the interpersonal relationships among family members.	■ Assessing the parents' knowledge helps to determine the appropriate timing and amount of information to be given regarding the child's defect.	The family demonstrates the ability to cope with and manage the newborn's care.
■ Provide information about the etiology of cleft lip and palate defects and the special needs of these infants. Encourage questions.	■ Concrete information allows parents time to understand the defect and reduces guilt.	
■ Explore the reactions of extended family members.	■ Extended family is an important source of support for most parents of a newborn. Family members can often help promote acceptance and compliance with the treatment plan.	
■ Support rooming in.	■ Rooming in allows parents to continue the bonding process.	
■ Encourage parents to participate in caretaking activities (holding, diapering, feeding).	■ Participation in infant care decreases anxiety and provides parents with a sense of purpose.	
■ Refer to parent support groups.	■ Support groups allow parents to express their feelings and concerns, to find people with concerns similar to their own, and to seek additional information.	

(continued)

Nursing Care Plan

The Infant with a Cleft Lip and/or Palate, *continued*

INTERVENTION	RATIONALE	EXPECTED OUTCOME
3. Nursing Diagnosis: Nutrition: Imbalanced: Less than Body Requirements related to the infant's inability to ingest nutrients		
NIC Priority Intervention—*Nutrition Management:* Assistance with or provision of a balanced dietary intake of foods and fluids		**NOC Suggested Outcome**—*Nutrition Status:* Amount of food and fluid taken into the body over a 24-hour period
GOAL: *The infant will gain weight steadily.*		
■ Assess fluid and calorie intake daily. Assess weight daily (same scale, same time, with infant completely undressed). Teach parents signs of adequate fluid intake such as frequency of wet diapers.	■ Daily assessment provides an objective measurement of whether the infant is receiving sufficient caloric intake to promote growth. Using the same scale and procedure when weighing the infant provides for comparability between daily weights.	The infant maintains adequate nutritional intake and gains weight appropriately.
■ Observe for any respiratory impairment.	■ Any symptoms of respiratory compromise will interfere with the infant's ability to suck. Feedings should be initiated only if there are no signs of respiratory distress.	
■ Provide weight-appropriate calories and fluid amounts. If the infant needs an increased number of calories to grow, referral to a nutritionist should be made. Higher calorie concentration formulas are available.	■ The infant needs optimal calories and fluids for growth and hydration.	
■ Facilitate breastfeeding.	■ Breast milk is recommended as the best food for an infant. The process of breastfeeding helps to promote bonding between mother and infant.	Successful breastfeeding is achieved if desired.
■ Hold the infant in an upright position.	■ An upright position facilitates swallowing and minimizes the amount of fluid return from the nose and into the eustachian tubes.	Feeding is a positive experience for parents and infant.
■ Give the mother information on breastfeeding the infant with a cleft lip and/or palate such as plugging the cleft lip and eliciting a letdown reflex before nursing.	■ Information and specific suggestions may encourage the mother to persist with breastfeeding.	
■ Contact the La Leche League for the name of a support person.	■ The La Leche League promotes breastfeeding for all infants. It can provide support people with experience who will aid the mother.	
■ If the mother is unable to breastfeed (or prefers not to), initiate bottle feeding.		
■ Place the nipple against the inside cheek toward the back of the tongue. If needed, use a premature nipple (slightly longer and softer than a regular nipple with a larger opening) or special cleft feeder.	■ Use of longer, softer nipples makes it easier for the infant to suck. Special cleft feeders decrease the amount of pressure in the bottle and make the formula flow more easily.	
■ Initiate nasogastric feedings if the infant is unable to ingest sufficient calories by mouth.	■ Adequate nutrition must be maintained. Use of a feeding tube allows the infant who has difficulty with oral feeding to receive adequate nutrition for growth.	
4. Nursing Diagnosis: Knowledge, Deficient (Parent) related to lack of exposure and unfamiliarity with resources		
NIC Priority Intervention—*Teaching, Disease Process:* Assisting the patient to understand information related to cleft lip/palate		**NOC Suggested Outcome**—*Knowledge:* Extent of understanding conveyed about cleft lip/palate treatment
GOAL: *Before discharge, parents will verbalize home care methods for care of the infant with cleft lip and palate defect.*		
■ Explain care and treatment (both short term and long term). Discuss potential complications.	■ This information assists the family to deal with the physical and psychosocial aspects of a child with a congenital defect.	Parents demonstrate appropriate care of the child including feeding technique, verbalization of complications that may occur, and verbalization of a plan for follow-up.
■ Demonstrate feeding techniques and alternatives. Allow parents to demonstrate before discharge.	■ Demonstration provides visual instructions. Redemonstration confirms learning.	
■ Provide written instructions for follow-up care arrangements.	■ Written instructions reinforce verbal instructions and provide a reference after discharge.	

Nursing Care Plan

The Infant with a Cleft Lip and/or Palate, *continued*

INTERVENTION	RATIONALE	EXPECTED OUTCOME
■ Introduce the parents (if possible) to a primary care provider in the setting where the infant will receive follow-up care after discharge.	■ Continuity of care is important. Since the infant will require long-term follow-up, a contact with the new provider is helpful.	

POSTOPERATIVE CARE

5. Nursing Diagnosis: Breathing Pattern, Ineffective related to surgical correction of defect

NIC Priority Intervention—*Airway Management:* Facilitation of patency of air passages		**NOC Suggested Outcome**—*Vital Signs Status:* Temperature, pulse, respiration, and blood pressure within expected range for the infant/child

GOAL: *The infant will maintain an effective breathing pattern.*

■ Assess respiratory status and monitor vital signs at least every 4 hours.	■ Frequent assessment allows for early identification of problems.	The infant shows no signs of respiratory infection or compromise.
■ Apply a cardiorespiratory monitor.	■ The monitor enables early detection of abnormal respirations, facilitating prompt intervention.	
■ Keep suction equipment and a bulb syringe at the bedside. Gently suction the oropharynx and nasopharynx as needed; avoid suture areas.	■ Gentle suctioning will keep the airway clear. Suctioning that is too vigorous can irritate the mucosa.	
■ Provide cool mist for the first 24 hours postoperatively if ordered.	■ A mist moisturizes secretions to reduce pooling in the lungs. It also moisturizes the oral cavity.	
■ Reposition every 2 hours.	■ Repositioning ensures expansion of all lung fields.	

6. Nursing Diagnosis: Nutrition, Imbalanced: Less than Body Requirements related to inability to ingest nutrients

NIC Priority Intervention—*Nutrition Management:* Assistance with or provision of a balanced dietary intake of food and fluids		**NOC Suggested Outcome**—*Nutritional Status:* Extent to which nutrients are available to meet metabolic needs

GOAL: *The infant will receive adequate nutritional intake.*

■ Maintain intravenous infusion as ordered.	■ The IV provides fluid when the child is NPO (nothing by mouth).	The infant receives adequate nutritional intake. The infant resumes usual feeding patterns and gains weight appropriately.
■ Begin with clear liquids, then give half-strength breast milk or formula as ordered.	■ It is important to ensure adequate fluids and nutrients.	
■ Use an Asepto syringe or dropper in the side of the mouth.	■ Use of a syringe or dropper avoids the suture line and resultant accumulation of milk or formula in that area.	
■ Give high-calorie soft foods after cleft palate repair.	■ Rough foods, utensils, and straws could disrupt the surgical site.	

7. Nursing Diagnosis: Infection, Risk for related to location of surgical procedure

NIC Priority Intervention—*Infection Control:* Minimizing the acquisition and transmission of infectious agents		**NOC Suggested Outcome**—*Wound Healing: Primary Intention:* The extent to which cells and tissues have regenerated following intentional closure

GOAL: *The infant's mucosal tissue will heal without infection.*

■ Assess vital signs every 4 hours.	■ Elevated temperature may indicate infection.	The infant remains free of infection in the oral cavity. Tissues remain intact and pink.
■ Assess the oral cavity every 2 hours or as needed for tenderness, reddened areas, lesions, or presence of secretions.	■ Frequent assessment aids in identifying infection.	
■ Cleanse the suture line with normal saline or sterile water if ordered.	■ Cleansing helps decrease the presence of bacteria.	The healing process progresses without adverse events in the postoperative period.
■ Cleanse the cleft areas by giving 5–15 mL of water after each feeding.	■ Cleansing prevents accumulation of carbohydrates, which encourage bacterial growth.	
■ If a crust has formed, use a cotton swab to apply a half-strength peroxide solution.	■ The solution helps loosen the crust, aiding in removal.	
■ Apply antibiotic cream to the suture line as ordered.	■ Antibiotic cream counteracts the growth of bacteria.	
■ Use careful hand hygiene and sterile technique when working with the suture line.		

(continued)

Nursing Care Plan | The Infant with a Cleft Lip and/or Palate, *continued*

INTERVENTION	RATIONALE	EXPECTED OUTCOME
8. Nursing Diagnosis: Tissue Integrity, Impaired related to mechanical factors		
NIC Priority Intervention—*Wound Care:* Prevention of wound complications and promotion of wound healing		**NOC Suggested Outcome**—*Wound Healing:* The extent to which cells and tissues have regenerated following intentional closure
GOAL: The lip and/or palate will heal with minimal scarring or disruption.		
■ Position the infant with cleft lip repair on the side or back only.	■ Prone positioning allows the infant to rub the suture line.	The lip/palate heals without complications.
■ Use soft elbow immobilizers. Remove every 2 hours and replace. Do not leave the infant unattended when immobilizers are removed.	■ Immobilizers prevent the infant's hands from rubbing the surgical site. Regular removal allows for skin and neurovascular checks.	
■ Maintain the suture line or Steri-Strips placed over cleft lip repair.	■ Maintaining the suture line will minimize scarring.	
■ Avoid metal utensils or straws after cleft palate repair.	■ These devices may disrupt the suture line.	
■ Do not allow pacifiers.	■ Sucking can disrupt the suture line.	
■ Keep the infant well medicated for pain in the initial postoperative period. Have parents hold and comfort the infant.	■ Good pain management minimizes crying, which can cause stress on the suture line; increases bonding; and soothes the child to decrease crying.	
■ Provide developmentally appropriate activities (e.g., mobiles, music).	■ Appropriate activities soothe and keep the infant calm.	

NANDA-I © 2012

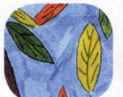

Partnering with Families

Feeding the Infant with Cleft Lip or Cleft Palate

The nurse assists the family to maintain feeding methods to promote the infant's growth and development. Inform parents of the following:

■ The infant with a cleft may require additional time to feed, which may produce fatigue. Allow the child additional time to eat, and provide opportunities for rest after feeding.

■ Feed the infant with the head and chest elevated since gravity helps to prevent milk from coming through the baby's nose or going up the eustachian tubes.

■ Breastfeeding is encouraged if possible; special techniques can help to achieve success.

■ Burp the baby frequently because infants with cleft palate tend to swallow air during feedings.

■ A feeding specialist is available to assist, and can suggest specially designed bottles and other feeding techniques to facilitate feeding the baby.

■ Maintain follow-up appointments so that the infant is weighed and evaluated for growth and development.

■ Inform the primary care provider if the infant has difficulty feeding or develops a problem such as vomiting or respiratory difficulty.

Provide Emotional Support

When a child is born with a cleft lip/cleft palate, parents may grieve for the loss of the ideal child that they expected. Parents may need assistance to view their infant as a whole person, rather than focusing solely on the physical defect. Promote parent–infant bonding by explaining the nature of the structural defect and the procedure for correction. Interact with and speak to the infant in the parents' presence and point out positive attributes such as alertness, soft skin, or active movements. Self-blame is common among parents. Parents can also be referred to the Cleft Palate Foundation for information about the disorder. Pictures of children who have had repair are available at this website. Seeing pictures of children who have had a successful repair offers reassurance to parents.

Parental anxiety is a typical response when children undergo surgery, and it is heightened when the surgery involves an infant. To minimize anxiety, give clear, concise explanations to parents. Allow sufficient time for parents to ask questions. Encourage parents to hold and cuddle the infant before surgery (see Chapter 15 🔗).

Provide Postoperative Care

Provide general postoperative care for the infant. (See Nursing Care Plan: The Infant with a Cleft Lip and/or Palate in this chapter and Nursing Care Plan: The Child Undergoing Surgery in Chapter 15 🔗.) Assess vital signs frequently and maintain the infant's airway. Measure intake and output. When oral fluids with clear liquids are started, they may be given through a dropper, syringe, or special feeder.

Weblink | Cleft Palate Foundation

Developing Cultural Competence
Cleft Lip and Cleft Palate

In many developing countries, infants do not have access to surgery for correction of cleft lip and palate. They may grow into childhood and adulthood with these abnormalities. Medical teams from the United States, Canada, and other countries sometimes travel to developing nations for short medical missions, performing surgery on the children and teaching local doctors surgical techniques. *Are there medical mission teams from your area that perform these surgeries? What is the planning required for such trips to perform surgery safely and care for the children? What is the impact on the communities served?*

Position the infant in a sitting position for the feedings to avoid aspiration. Frequently burp the infant during feedings. The infant then progresses to half-strength breast milk or formula. After each feeding, cleanse the suture line with water or normal saline to avoid accumulation of feedings.

It is important to maintain the suture line to ensure healing. Prevent the infant from rubbing the suture line on the bedding by positioning the infant in a supine position. Keep elbows in soft immobilizers. Maintain the suture line or Steri-Strips placed over the incision. Place antibiotic ointment on the incision site as ordered. Medicate the infant as prescribed to control pain and to minimize crying and stress on the suture line. After cleft palate surgery, avoid the use of metal utensils or straws, which may disrupt the surgical site.

Clinical Tip
An infant who has had a cleft lip repair needs stimulation to provide distraction. This approach will minimize crying, which can damage the suture line. Soft, colorful toys, mobiles, and other visual objects are helpful. Music also can be used to soothe the infant. Parental presence is comforting and reassuring.

Discharge Planning and Home Care Teaching
Identify and address home care needs well in advance of discharge. Discuss all aspects of the infant's care with the parents throughout hospitalization and after surgery. Involve parents in the infant's care to increase their comfort level before discharge and to promote bonding. Teach feeding techniques, how to recognize signs of infection, how to position the infant, and how to care for the suture line.

Discuss with the parents the financial implications of long-term care. Private insurance does not always cover all the costs of care necessary for the child. Refer parents to social services familiar with programs and financial aid for which the parents and child may be eligible. Relief of financial worries enables parents to concentrate on caring for the child. See Developing Cultural Competence: Cleft Lip and Cleft Palate.

Teach parents how to care for the child after discharge. If the child has siblings, emphasize that they will need preparation to accept the child. Sibling rivalry can be heightened when one child receives more attention in the home. Remind parents of the importance of setting limits and of spending time with each child. Determine whether additional family supports are necessary. Provide parents with information on support groups, physicians, social workers, Internet resources, and local services that can help maintain family continuity.

Discuss ways to prevent the infant from touching the suture line. Teach parents how to bundle an infant in a blanket with arms tucked inside the blanket. A front-sling baby carrier may also be used to immobilize the arms. Front-sling carriers provide the additional benefits of comforting the infant through contact with the parent and of holding the infant upright, which aids in optimal positioning after feedings.

After surgical repair, parents need to be taught how to feed the infant and identify signs of complications (fever, vomiting, respiratory distress). Referral to a home healthcare agency for support may be helpful. Encourage follow-up visits with healthcare professionals. The child may need further evaluation of speech development, assessment for presence of ear infections, or a recommendation for plastic surgery. See Health Promotion & Maintenance Overview for the child with cleft lip or palate on page 1000.

Care in the Community
Children need regular monitoring through early childhood to promote good cosmetic outcomes, good dentition, and speech development. In addition to hospital, clinic, and home health nurses, members of the healthcare team often include specialists such as the plastic surgeon, orthodontist, dentist, social worker, audiologist, speech pathologist, and pediatrician (Kasten et al., 2008). The parents are the best coordinators of the child's care. Encourage them to keep a diary listing the professionals with whom they talk and the content of the discussions.

Clinical Judgment
Nurses can provide compassionate care to the family of the child born with cleft lip or cleft palate by pointing out the infant's positive aspects rather than focusing on the cleft. What are examples of appropriate statements the nurse could make to the family?

Evaluation
Expected outcomes of nursing care are provided on the accompanying Nursing Care Plan.

Esophageal Atresia and Tracheoesophageal Fistula

Esophageal atresia is a malformation that results from failure of the esophagus to develop as a continuous tube during the fourth and fifth weeks of gestation. Esophageal atresia occurs in approximately 1 in 4,000 neonates with 90% of those affected also having a tracheoesophageal fistula (Khan & Orenstein, 2011).

Etiology and Pathophysiology
In esophageal atresia, the foregut fails to lengthen, separate, and fuse into two parallel tubes (the esophagus and trachea) during fetal development. Instead the esophagus may end in a blind pouch or develop as a pouch connected to the trachea by a fistula (tracheoesophageal fistula) (Figure 30–7 ■).

Esophageal atresia is often associated with a maternal history of polyhydramnios. Associated anomalies may occur, including congenital heart defects, gastrointestinal or urinary tract anomalies, and musculoskeletal abnormalities (De Jong, de Haan, Gischler, et al., 2010; Khan & Orenstein, 2011).

Clinical Manifestations
Symptoms in the newborn include excessive salivation and drooling, often accompanied by three signs classic for this defect: cyanosis, choking, and coughing. Sneezing may also be manifested. During feeding, the infant returns fluid through the nose and mouth. Aspiration places

Health Promotion & Maintenance Overview

The Child with Cleft Lip or Cleft Palate

The child with cleft lip or cleft palate requires close monitoring and intervention to foster growth and development. The nurse partners with the child and family to achieve healthy outcomes.

GROWTH AND DEVELOPMENT SURVEILLANCE

- Monitor the child's growth and developmental patterns.
- Monitor for developmental delays.
- Explain to parents that behavior regression following surgery in the toddler or older child is normal.

NUTRITION

- Refer the family to sources for nipples, nursers, and other special feeding devices.
- Assist the mother with learning how to express breast milk and facilitate breastfeeding.
- Teach parents to avoid foods that can pose a choking hazard to the child.
- Teach parents to feed the infant in an upright position and to burp the child frequently during feedings.

PHYSICAL ACTIVITY

- Activity for the child having surgical procedures to correct cleft palate is generally restricted for approximately 2 to 3 weeks to allow for healing.
- After healing has occurred, encourage the parents to promote the child's activities as they would any child without cleft lip or cleft palate.

ORAL HEALTH

- The child should be routinely screened for dental caries. Ask the family about dental visits.
- Teach the parents to provide good dental hygiene to the child.
- Routine dental/orthodontic evaluation is necessary for the child with cleft palate.

MENTAL AND SPIRITUAL HEALTH

- Monitor the child's awareness of differences between self and other children and signs of poor self-esteem.
  - Be alert for the child who has had experiences with teasing associated with articulation or physical appearance. Encourage adherence to speech therapy and practice at home.
  - Refer parents to websites such as Project Smile and other resources.
- Refer the child for counseling if indicated.

RELATIONSHIPS

- Evaluate the parents for parent–infant bonding.
- Promote bonding by encouraging the parents to participate in the infant's care, to hold the infant, and to recognize the infant's positive attributes.

DISEASE PREVENTION STRATEGIES

- Teach the family to recognize signs and symptoms of ear or other infections and to seek immediate evaluation. Treatment of acute otitis media is necessary to prevent long-term effects of repeated infections.
- Emphasize to the parents the importance of audiology screening for children with cleft lip and palate to evaluate conductive hearing loss.

INJURY PREVENTION STRATEGIES (SAFETY)

- Assist parents to properly apply elbow immobilizers to protect the suture line in the postoperative period.
- Teach parents to avoid straws, metal spoons, and other sharp utensils that may damage the palate.
- Ask the parents about eating utensils the child uses.

---

the infant at risk for pneumonia. Depending on the type of defect, the infant's abdomen may be distended due to air trapping.

Collaborative Care

Collaborative care includes immediate identification of the defect, prevention of complications such as aspiration, respiratory and nutritional support as needed, and surgical intervention to correct the defect.

Diagnostic Tests

Diagnosis is usually confirmed by attempting to pass a nasogastric or orogastric tube into the stomach. In most cases, the tube meets resistance and can be advanced only minimally. Specific defects and associated anomalies are determined by radiologic examination. Careful examination of the lungs is needed. A delay in diagnosis can be fatal since ingested fluid or secretions may enter the lungs and lead to pneumonia (Khan & Orenstein, 2011).

Clinical Therapy

After diagnosis, a nasogastric tube is inserted to suction the upper pouch. Intravenous antibiotics and fluids are begun. Surgery is performed as soon as possible. Surgical correction may be accomplished in several stages. The first stage usually involves ligation of the fistula and insertion of a gastrostomy tube. In the second stage, the two ends of the esophagus

are reconnected, if possible. When surgical closure (anastomosis) is not possible, a gastrostomy tube must remain in place for use in feeding. Potential postoperative complications include gastroesophageal reflux, aspiration, and stricture formation. The prognosis is usually good with surgery; however, some conditions are complicated, requiring repeated surgeries and long-term management. If the two ends of the esophagus cannot be reconnected, colonic, jejunal, or gastric segments may be used to lengthen the esophagus (Khan & Orenstein, 2011).

Nursing Management

Nursing care consists of collaborative identification of the defect in the immediate newborn period, preventing complications such as aspiration, providing preoperative and postoperative care, teaching the family about the disorder and its treatment, and providing emotional support to the family. Ongoing care is also required to facilitate feeding and promote development.

Nursing Assessment and Diagnosis

The nurse may recognize the signs and symptoms in the immediate newborn period. Assess for difficulty feeding and excessive drooling. Assess for the classic signs of choking, coughing, and cyanosis. Assess for respiratory distress and assess the lung sounds carefully.

Pathophysiology Illustrated
Esophageal Atresia and Tracheoesophageal Fistula

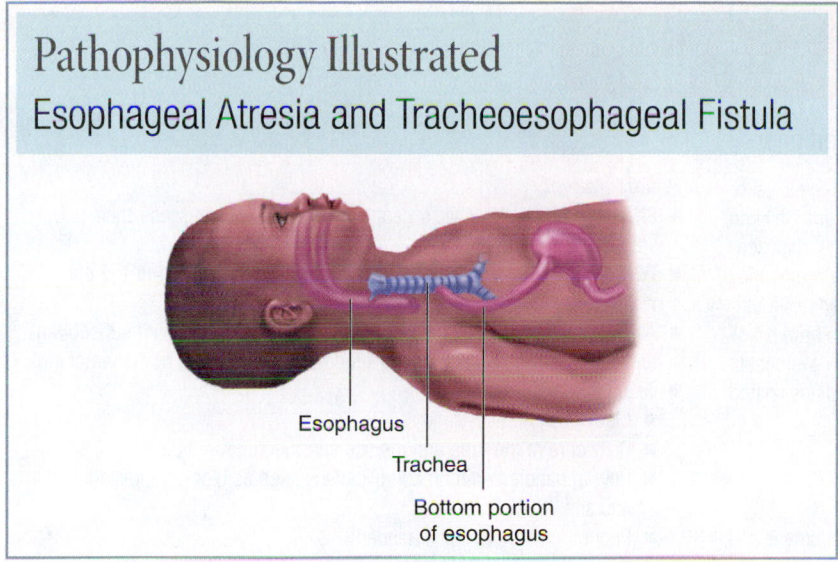

Esophagus

Trachea

Bottom portion
of esophagus

FIGURE 30–7 ■ In the most common type of esophageal atresia and tracheoesophageal fistula, the upper segment of the esophagus ends in a blind pouch connected to the trachea; the fistula connects the lower segment to the trachea.

Esophageal atresia is a surgical emergency. Preoperatively the infant requires close observation and intervention to maintain a patent airway.

Nursing diagnoses that may be appropriate for the infant with esophageal atresia or tracheoesophageal fistula include:

- Aspiration, Risk for related to regurgitation
- Fluid Volume: Deficient related to NPO status
- Nutrition, Imbalanced: Less than Body Requirements related to NPO status
- Infection, Risk for related to aspiration
- Attachment, Risk for Impaired Parent/Infant related to the neonate's emergency surgery

NANDA-I © 2012

Planning and Implementation

Surgical intervention for a newborn is a stressful situation for the parents and family. The parents require emotional support throughout the infant's hospitalization. All procedures should be clearly explained. Assist parents to bond with the infant by stroking and talking to the child. Eliciting questions and allowing parents to participate in the infant's care, especially feeding (when permitted), can facilitate bonding and help to prepare parents for care of the infant after discharge.

Preoperative Nursing Care

Suction should be readily available to remove any secretions that accumulate in the nasopharyngeal airway. Place the infant with the head of the bed slightly elevated to minimize aspiration of secretions into the trachea. Use continuous or low intermittent suction to remove secretions from the blind pouch. Withhold oral fluids and provide maintenance intravenous fluids. Constant monitoring of vital signs and the infant's condition is needed.

Postoperative Nursing Care

After surgery, measure gastrostomy drainage and administer intravenous fluids and antibiotics. Total parenteral nutrition may be required until gastrostomy or oral feedings are tolerated. Monitoring and assessment of feeding tolerance is ongoing. Feedings are introduced slowly and in small amounts. Assess for respiratory difficulty during reintroduction of feedings. Monitor weight and growth and developmental achievements.

Some infants may have one surgery and progress without further complications, whereas others may require several surgical procedures and long-term intervention to ensure adequate nutrition, growth, and development.

Discharge Planning and Home Care Teaching

Once enteral feedings have been established, the infant may be discharged from the hospital with a gastrostomy tube in place (Figure 30–8 ■). (Refer to the Skills Manual ⊂⊃ for care of the child with a gastrostomy tube.) Collaborate with the parents regarding home care needs and teach them about gastrostomy tube care and feeding, signs of infection, and how to prevent postoperative complications. The family of an infant requiring multiple surgical procedures requires ongoing support. The infant is evaluated frequently for adequate nutrition, and growth and development patterns. See Partnering with Families: Teaching the Family About Gastrostomy Tube Feedings.

Evaluation

Outcomes of nursing care depend on the extent of the defect and correction. Examples include:

- The child does not experience respiratory distress and maintains normal respirations.
- The child achieves and maintains a normal weight.
- Positive parent–infant bonding is established.
- The parent has knowledge of the defect, its corrections, and the child's needs.

Pyloric Stenosis

Pyloric stenosis is a hypertrophic obstruction of the circular muscle of the pyloric canal. Pyloric stenosis occurs in approximately 1.8 of

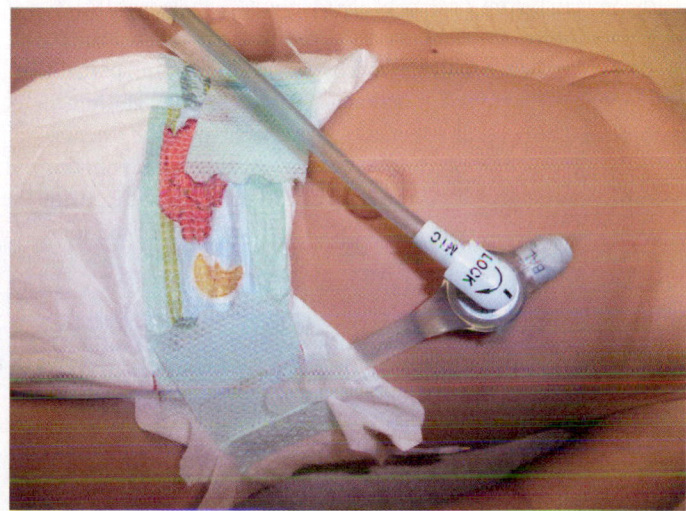

FIGURE 30–8 ■ A gastrostomy tube is used to feed the child with a gastrointestinal disorder such as esophageal atresia.

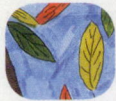

Partnering with Families

Teaching the Family About Gastrostomy Tube Feedings

The infant or child who has difficulty swallowing, consuming oral feedings, or gaining weight may be a candidate for gastrostomy tube placement. Children with chronic conditions such as failure to thrive, cystic fibrosis, neuromuscular disorders, severe gastroesophageal reflux, and genetic syndromes may need to have a gastrostomy tube placed for long-term enteral feedings (Goldberg, Barton, Xanthopoulos, et al., 2010). Parents of children who have or will receive a gastrostomy tube need clear instructions to maximize the benefit of the device to the child. See Chapter 15 🔗 for general guidelines related to teaching plans.

GENERAL PRINCIPLES

Preoperatively

- Assess what the family knows about gastrostomy tube placement and what methods will be most effective in teaching care of the gastrostomy tube and enteral feedings.
- Show the family pictures or dolls with gastrostomy tubes and explain what the child's abdomen will look like in the immediate postoperative period.
- Provide the family with a booklet about gastrostomy tubes and enteral feedings.

Postoperatively

- Show the family the child's gastrostomy tube and reassess their understanding of the tube.
- When feedings are ordered, demonstrate the first feeding to the parents while explaining each step.
- Actively involve a family member in the second feeding. With subsequent feedings, have a family member feed the child with the nurse watching.
- Teach the family about:
  - Medication administration
  - Daily care of the tube and the site surrounding the tube
  - How to handle common complications such as blockage, dislodgment, and site irritation
  - Phone numbers to call if needed
  - When to seek medical care related to the gastrostomy tube
- All family members who are involved in care of the child should practice feeding the child and administering medications to the child prior to discharge. This allows the nurse to assess for understanding of the procedure and gives the family confidence in their ability to care for the child. Some children will need bolus feedings, others may have continuous feedings via a feeding pump, and others may have bolus feedings during the day and continuous feedings at night.

Source: *Data from Goldberg, E., Barton, S., Xanthopoulos, M. S., Stettler, N., & Liacouras, C. A. (2010). A descriptive study of complications of gastrostomy tubes in children.* Journal of Pediatric Nursing, *25(2), 72–80; Saavedra, H., Losek, J. D., Shanley, L., & Titus, M. O. (2009). Gastrostomy tube related complaints in the pediatric emergency department identifying opportunities for improvement.* Pediatric Emergency Care, *25(11), 728–732.*

every 1,000 births. Males are affected more often than females by a 4:1 ratio (Mooney & Hogan, 2011). There is an increased incidence in firstborn White males (Hunter & Liacouras, 2011).

Etiology and Pathophysiology

The exact cause of pyloric stenosis is unknown, although frequently there is a family history of the disorder. **Hypergastrinemia** (too much gastrin in the blood) is thought to play a role in the development of pyloric stenosis. Studies have indicated a higher incidence of the disorder in infants who received oral erythromycin before 2 weeks of age (Mooney & Hogan, 2011).

Hypertrophy of the circular pylorus muscle results in stenosis of the passage between the stomach and the duodenum, partially obstructing the lumen of the stomach (Figure 30–9 ■). The lumen becomes inflamed and edematous, which narrows the opening until the obstruction becomes complete. At this time, vomiting becomes more forceful. As the obstruction progresses, the infant becomes dehydrated and electrolytes are depleted, resulting in metabolic imbalances.

Clinical Manifestations

Symptoms usually become evident 2 to 8 weeks after birth, although onset may vary (Askew, 2010; Mooney & Hogan, 2011). Initially the infant appears well or regurgitates slightly after feedings. The parents may describe the infant as a "good eater" who vomits occasionally. Formula intolerance or allergy may be assumed, leading to multiple changes in formula. Gastroesophageal reflux may also be diagnosed or suspected, especially in the early stages of pyloric stenosis. As the obstruction progresses,

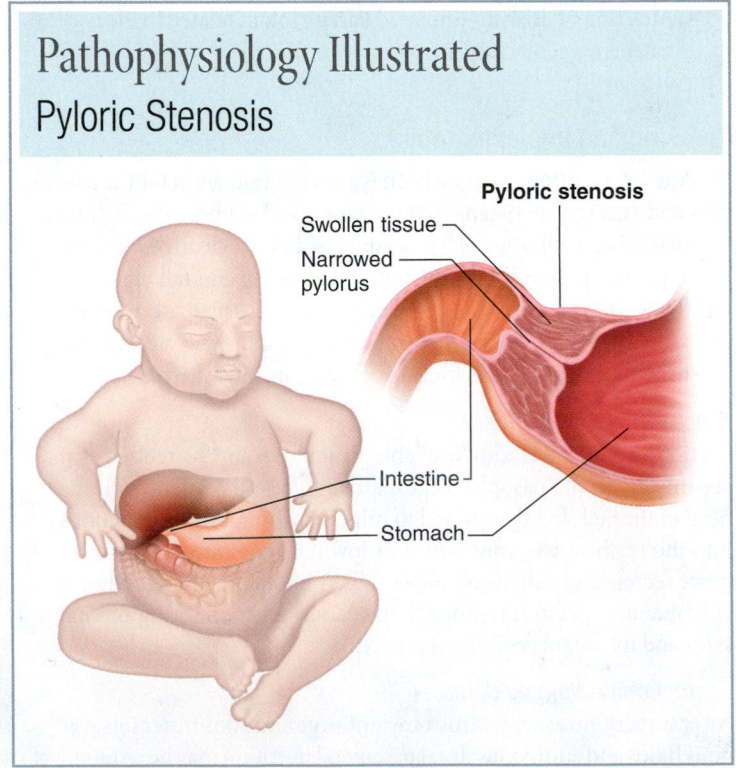

Pathophysiology Illustrated
Pyloric Stenosis

Pyloric stenosis

Swollen tissue

Narrowed pylorus

Intestine

Stomach

FIGURE 30–9 ■ In pyloric stenosis, the hypertrophied pyloric muscle causes symptoms of projectile vomiting and visible peristalsis.

the vomiting becomes projectile. In **projectile vomiting,** the contents of the stomach may be ejected up to 3 feet from the infant. The vomitus is nonbilious and may become blood tinged secondary to repeated irritation of the esophagus.

The infant generally appears hungry, especially after emesis, is irritable, fails to gain weight, and has fewer and smaller stools. Loss of gastric secretions results in dehydration and potentially metabolic alkalosis. On physical examination, peristaltic waves may be observed across the abdomen and an olive-sized mass in the right upper quadrant may be evident (Mooney & Hogan, 2011).

Collaborative Care

Collaborative care includes restoring fluid and electrolyte balance, correcting the defect, and preventing complications associated with the disorder.

Diagnostic Tests

An abdominal ultrasound, to determine the diameter and length of the pyloric muscle, is usually performed to confirm the diagnosis. A pyloric muscle with a thickness of 4 mm, a length of 14 mm, and a diameter of 12 mm or greater is diagnostic for pyloric stenosis. An upper gastrointestinal (UGI) study using contrast medium may be performed. The UGI reveals a lengthened pylorus and a narrow pyloric channel (Mooney & Hogan, 2011).

Blood tests determine the degree of dehydration, electrolyte imbalance, and anemia (see Chapter 23). Common findings are hypochloremia, hypokalemia, and metabolic alkalosis (Askew, 2010; Mooney & Hogan, 2011). Early diagnosis will decrease the frequency with which infants present with an alteration in electrolytes.

Clinical Therapy

Surgical correction (pyloromyotomy) is the treatment of choice. Preoperatively the infant's condition is stabilized with intravenous fluids and electrolytes. A nasogastric tube may be inserted for gastric decompression if emesis is excessive (Askew, 2010).

The surgery is performed as soon as possible after the infant's fluid and electrolyte balance is restored. Open pyloromyotomy is performed through a periumbilical incision or a small, transverse upper abdominal incision. Laparoscopic pyloromyotomy is currently used in many cases and has been shown to be equally as successful as open pyloromyotomy (Hunter & Liacouras, 2011). With both procedures, the pyloric muscle is split to allow the passage of food and fluid.

The prognosis is good. The infant is usually taking fluids within a few hours following surgery and discharged on full-strength formula within 24 hours after surgery.

Nursing Management

Nursing care focuses on collaborative identification of the infant with pyloric stenosis, preventing complications such as dehydration, and preoperative and postoperative management.

Nursing Assessment and Diagnosis

Observe the infant's abdomen for the presence of peristaltic waves. Bowel sounds are hyperactive on auscultation. Auscultate before palpating the abdomen since palpation can cause a change in bowel patterns. Palpation reveals an olive-shaped mass in the right upper quadrant of the abdomen.

Assess the infant's history of vomiting, vital signs, weight, and nutritional status. Assess skin turgor, fontanels, urinary output (weigh diapers), urine specific gravity, capillary refill, and mucous membranes to determine whether hydration is adequate. Describe vomiting episodes and estimated emesis amount. Be alert for signs of an electrolyte imbalance; particularly low levels of serum chloride, sodium, and potassium; and an elevated pH. Because gastric fluid is high in potassium, hypokalemia can result. The infant is also at risk for metabolic alkalosis secondary to loss of hydrochloric acid. (See Chapter 23 for a discussion of these electrolyte imbalances.) Assess parental anxiety related to the child's condition. The child is usually hungry and tries to feed. Crying and general discomfort are frequently observed.

Nursing diagnoses that may be appropriate for the child with pyloric stenosis include:

- Fluid Volume: Deficient related to vomiting
- Nutrition, Imbalanced: Less than Body Requirements related to vomiting and inability to ingest nutrients
- Sleep Pattern, Disturbed related to discomfort and hunger
- Anxiety, Parental related to surgery
- Pain, Acute related to surgical incision

NANDA-I © 2012

Planning and Implementation

Nursing care centers on meeting the infant's fluid and electrolyte needs, minimizing weight loss, promoting rest and comfort, preventing infection, and providing supportive care for parents.

Meet Fluid and Electrolyte Needs

Withhold oral feedings preoperatively because projectile vomiting will continue until the obstruction is relieved. Emphasize to the parents the importance of maintaining an NPO status preoperatively. Intravenous fluid therapy is administered to correct fluid and electrolyte imbalances and to maintain adequate hydration. Maintain patency of the nasogastric tube and measure aspirated contents. Inform parents that all diapers will be weighed to measure the infant's output of urine and stool.

Minimize Weight Loss

The infant loses weight because of frequent vomiting. Monitor weight daily preoperatively and postoperatively. Begin feedings postoperatively according to the healthcare provider's orders. Some surgeons prefer an NPO period following pyloromyotomy, with slow, incremental increases in volume and strength of feedings once feeding has resumed. Others will implement an earlier postoperative feeding approach.

Promote Rest and Comfort

During the preoperative period the infant is hungry and cries often. The infant is swaddled to maintain warmth and provide comfort. Encourage the parents to hold and cuddle the infant. Provide a pacifier to meet the infant's need to suck.

Postoperatively the infant is uncomfortable due to the surgical incision. Analgesics can be administered to relieve discomfort as ordered. (See Chapter 21 for a discussion of pain management.) Instruct parents to avoid pressure on the incision. When diapering the infant, slide the diaper gently under the buttocks rather than lifting the legs. Swaddling, rocking, and use of a pacifier provide comfort to the infant.

Prevent Infection

Postoperatively the incision is covered with collodion or Steri-Strips and should be kept clean and dry. Inspect the incision site for redness, swelling, or discharge. Monitor the infant's temperature every 4 hours. Auscultate lungs to assess for any adventitious breath sounds.

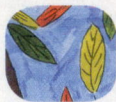

Partnering with Families

Home Care Instructions Following Pyloromyotomy

The infant is generally discharged home the day after surgery with the following home feeding and care instructions:

- The infant may bottle-feed or breastfeed.
- An infant will sometimes vomit after feedings following surgery—this does not mean the surgery was unsuccessful.
- If the infant vomits, offer breast or bottle as soon as interest in feeding occurs.
- The infant should be burped after every 1 to 2 ounces during feeding. If breastfeeding, burp the infant every 5 to 10 minutes.
- After feeding, place the baby in an upright position, holding for approximately 30 minutes, or position the infant on the right side with the head and upper body slightly elevated.
- The infant should not play or be rocked for 30 minutes following feedings.

- Administer analgesics as prescribed. Inform the healthcare provider if the infant is not obtaining adequate pain relief.
- Keep the surgical wound area clean and dry. The bandage or strips may fall off, which is normal. If not, they will be removed at the follow-up visit.
- The infant should be sponge bathed only. Tub baths are avoided until the wound has healed or as instructed by the healthcare provider.
- Notify the healthcare provider if the infant demonstrates any of the following:
  - Redness, drainage, bleeding, or swelling at the surgical site
  - Temperature higher than 100°F
  - Decreased number of wet diapers
  - Inconsolable behavior
  - Vomiting the majority of two consecutive feedings

Provide Supportive Care

The need for hospitalization and surgery creates anxiety for parents. Encourage them to participate in the infant's care and to discuss their fears and concerns. Provide simple and clear explanations about the infant's condition and care. Advise parents that occasional vomiting after surgery may occur.

Discharge Planning and Home Care Teaching

Instruct parents to observe the incision for redness, swelling, or discharge and to notify the healthcare provider immediately if these occur or if the infant develops a fever. To reduce the possibility of infection, advise parents to fold the infant's diaper so that it does not touch the incision. Continued vomiting and signs of dehydration should be reported promptly. See Partnering with Families: Home Care Instructions Following Pyloromyotomy.

Evaluation

Expected outcomes of nursing care of the infant with pyloric stenosis include:

- The child achieves and maintains fluid and electrolyte balance.
- The child has adequate intake of formula or breast milk without vomiting.
- The child's pain is effectively managed.
- The incision heals without infection.

Gastroesophageal Reflux and Gastroesophageal Reflux Disease

Gastroesophageal reflux (GER), the return of gastric contents into the esophagus, is the result of relaxation of the lower esophageal sphincter (Anderson, 2010). GER is one of the most common gastrointestinal disorders in children, affecting approximately 50% of infants ages 0 to 3 months (International Pediatric Endosurgery Group [IPEG], 2008a). There is a higher incidence in premature infants, and males are affected three times more often than females. Children with neurologic impairments, such as cerebral palsy, more commonly experience GER. Some "spitting up" after feedings is considered normal in newborn infants, because of the weak cardiac sphincter of the stomach. However, regurgitation that continues and increases in frequency may be caused by GER and requires further investigation.

Gastroesophageal reflux disease (GERD) is a more serious manifestation of GER. Infants and younger children present with a history of poor weight gain, recurrent vomiting, generalized irritability, and refusal to feed. Infants may also have a history of arching, and respiratory symptoms such as wheezing and apnea (IPEG, 2008a; van der Pol, Smits, van Wijk, et al., 2011; Weill, 2008). Additional symptoms seen in older children and adolescents include heartburn, abdominal/epigastric pain, nausea, and regurgitation (Linton, 2011; Malaty, O'Malley, Abudayyeh, et al., 2008).

Etiology and Pathophysiology

The lower esophageal sphincter of the gastrointestinal tract contains a band of smooth muscle that relaxes during feeding but remains contracted between meals to prevent reflux of stomach contents into the esophagus. If the esophageal sphincter relaxes inappropriately, GER results. Transient lower esophageal sphincter relaxations (TLESRs) occur after eating and during normal digestion; however, children who have GERD may have an increased incidence of reflux secondary to this relaxation (Anderson, 2010). The smaller stomach, shorter esophagus, and immaturity of the lower esophageal sphincter muscle in infants account for the frequency of GER in this population (Weill, 2008).

Clinical Manifestations

Regurgitation or vomiting is the most common sign of gastroesophageal reflux in infants (IPEG, 2008a). Children with gastroesophageal reflux are frequently hungry and irritable. They eat often but still lose weight. Infants with reflux are at risk for aspiration and apnea. Refer to the Clinical Manifestations table on page 1005.

Collaborative Care

Collaborative care includes identifying gastroesophageal reflux, preventing complications associated with the disorder, and treatment through dietary and pharmacologic management or surgical intervention.

Clinical Manifestations Gastroesophageal Reflux and Gastroesophageal Reflux Disease in Infants

CLINICAL MANIFESTATIONS	CLINICAL THERAPY	NURSING MANAGEMENT
Gastroesophageal Reflux Regurgitation or "spitting up" with normal weight gain No signs and symptoms of esophagitis, respiratory infection, or excessive crying	Modify feeding schedule. Thicken feedings with rice cereal or use commercially prepared thickened formula (Enfamil AR). Consider change to hypoallergenic formula if condition persists.	Teach parents of infants to: ■ Give smaller, more frequent feedings. ■ Thicken feedings as directed or use commercially prepared formula. ■ Burp infant every 1 to 2 ounces of formula or after breastfeeding on each side. ■ Hold infant upright for 30 minutes after feeding. Avoid use of infant seat or car seat after feeding. Use car seat only for traveling. The semisitting position complicates GER. Monitor weight gain. Monitor growth and development. Assess for feeding difficulties.
Gastroesophageal Reflux Disease Regurgitation with poor weight gain or failure to thrive Persistent irritability and excessive crying Arching of the neck while feeding Respiratory symptoms such as apnea, cyanosis, wheezing, pneumonia, cough	All methods listed above. Laboratory studies and diagnostic testing. Treatment with histamine H_2 receptor antagonists (H2RAs) or proton pump inhibitors (PPIs) (see Medications table on page 1006). Nissen fundoplication if inadequate response to medications and other interventions.	All nursing interventions as listed above. Teach parents about all medications. Include information specific to amount, frequency, dosage, side effects, and toxic effects. Provide preoperative teaching (see Chapter 15). Provide postoperative care as described previously for the child having abdominal surgery. Teach parents gastrostomy tube care if appropriate.

Source: *Data from Srivastava, R., Jackson, W. D., & Barnhart, D. C. (2010). Dysphagia and gastroesophageal reflux disease: Dilemmas in diagnosis and management in children with neurological impairment. Pediatric Annals, 39(4), 225–231; Weill, V. (2008). Gastroesophageal reflux in infancy. Advance for Nurse Practitioners, 16(1), 47–50; Riffe, I., Sayre, J., Waller, T., Brinker, T., & Roberts, P. (2007). Gastroesophageal reflux disease in infants. Family Practice Recertification, 29(9), 28–33; Tipnis, N. A., & Tipnis, S. M. (2009). Controversies in the treatment of gastroesophageal disease in preterm infants. Clinical Perinatology, 36, 153–164.*

Diagnostic Tests

Diagnosis is confirmed by a thorough history of the child's feeding patterns and by diagnostic evaluation. Although a barium swallow is useful in evaluating the cause of vomiting, it lacks specificity in the diagnosis of GER. Esophageal pH monitoring is the preferred test in the diagnosis of GER and the frequency of reflux episodes. Gastric emptying studies are also useful in the diagnosis of GER (IPEG, 2008a).

Clinical Therapy

Treatment depends on the severity of the condition. Generally, feeding modification, thickened feeding, and positioning are effective management for milder cases. A smaller feeding volume may prove beneficial to avoid overdistention of the abdomen and subsequent reflux. The infant should be burped after every 1 to 2 ounces (Weill, 2008). Rice cereal is sometimes placed in the infant's bottle to thicken feedings to a consistency similar to nectar. Note that breast milk will not readily thicken with addition of cereal. Prethickened formulas are commercially available. For example, Enfamil AR contains added rice and is nutritionally balanced (Weill, 2008). These formulas can be administered without enlarging the nipple hole. Formula change to semi-elemental formula, such as Pregestimil, Nutramigen, or Alimentum, may be recommended (Orenstein & McGowan, 2008). Fatty foods and citrus juices are avoided.

See the Medications table on page 1006. Use of medications to treat GERD in children varies among healthcare providers.

Treatment for severe cases of GERD such as those with recurrent life-threatening aspiration, failure to thrive, and esophagitis may include surgery to create a valve mechanism by wrapping the greater curvature of the stomach (fundus) around the distal esophagus (Nissen fundoplication) (IPEG, 2008a). A gastrostomy tube is frequently inserted during surgery to serve as an access for gastric venting, to prevent postoperative bloating, and as a means for nutritional support if needed (Srivastava, Jackson, & Barnhart, 2010). The gastrostomy tube may be removed after a few weeks or may be left in long term if needed for feedings.

Nursing Management

Nursing management of the infant or child with gastroesophageal reflux or gastroesophageal reflux disease focuses on supporting the infant's or child's nutritional intake, promoting interventions to reduce associated complications, and supporting the family.

Nursing Assessment and Diagnosis

Obtain a thorough history of the child's feeding patterns. Observe vomiting episodes and document amount, color, and consistency of emesis.

Monitor the infant's weight and plot progress on a growth chart. Observe for any signs of respiratory distress and keep the infant's nose and mouth clear of emesis.

Nursing diagnoses that may apply to the infant with gastroesophageal reflux include:

- Aspiration, Risk for related to reflux
- Fluid Volume: Deficient related to reflux
- Nutrition, Imbalanced: Less than Body Requirements related to reflux and NPO status
- Infection, Risk for related to reflux
- Knowledge, Deficient (Parent) related to feeding techniques

NANDA-I © 2012

Planning and Implementation

Adequate nutrition must be maintained for the child to achieve normal growth and development. Infants receiving oral feedings are administered smaller feedings. Elevate the head of the bed to prevent

Medications Used to Treat Gastroesophageal Reflux Disease

MEDICATION	ACTION/INDICATION	NURSING MANAGEMENT
Histamine H₂ Receptor Antagonists		
Zantac (ranitidine) Pepcid (famotidine)	Inhibition of the histamine H₂ receptor on the gastric parietal cell, thus blocking gastric acid secretion	Administer with or without food. If antacids are prescribed, administer 2 hours before or after H₂ antagonists. Teach parents to avoid OTC medications without checking with a healthcare provider. Monitor for side effects: Bradycardia, Fatigue, Rash; Constipation, Headache, Confusion; Diarrhea, Irritability, Thrombocytopenia; Nausea, Dizziness
Proton Pump Inhibitors		
Prevacid (lansoprazole) Prilosec (omeprazole)	These powerful inhibitors of gastric acid secretion alleviate symptoms and help to heal esophagitis. Blocks the final common pathway of acid production by inhibiting activated proton pumps in the gastric parietal cells	Administer in the morning on an empty stomach. Antacids may be administered with omeprazole. Monitor for side effects: Abdominal pain, Fatigue, Nausea; Diarrhea, Headache, Proteinuria; Dizziness, Hematuria, Rash; Constipation, Anorexia. Teach the family to inform the primary healthcare provider if severe diarrhea occurs. Teach the family to inform the primary healthcare provider if changes in urinary elimination, such as pain or discomfort associated with urination, occur.

Source: *Data from Riffe, I., Sayre, J., Waller, T., Brinker, T., & Roberts, P. (2007). Gastroesophageal reflux disease in infants. Family Practice Recertification, 29(9), 28–33; Weill, V. (2008). Gastroesophageal reflux in infancy. Advance for Nurse Practitioners, 16(1), 47–50; Wilson, B. A., Shannon, M. T., & Shields, K. M. (2011). Pearson nurse's drug guide 2011. New York, NY: Pearson.*

aspiration if vomiting should occur. If the child has a gastrostomy tube, maintain skin integrity around the stoma site.

Practice Alert

Prone positioning decreases reflux; however, because of the risk of sudden infant death syndrome with this position, parents are advised to place their infants supine. Parents are encouraged to hold their infant in an upright position for 30 minutes following feedings. Minimize seated positioning such as in an infant seat because this increases intra-abdominal pressure and promotes reflux (Weill, 2008). Front infant pack carriers may be used for younger infants, and backpack carriers may be used for older infants.

Discharge planning focuses on instructing parents how to feed and position the infant, as well as providing comfort and emotional support. Encourage parents to hold and cuddle the infant during all feedings. Providing the infant with a pacifier helps to meet nonnutritive sucking needs. Teach parents how to suction the nose and mouth if vomiting occurs.

Practice Alert

In older children, a pattern of chronic vomiting (low-grade nearly daily emesis) or cyclic vomiting (repeated severe vomiting of an episodic nature) can occur. These patterns differ from vomiting seen in colic or gastroesophageal reflux. Chronic vomiting is often associated with upper gastrointestinal tract diseases such as gastritis and esophagitis, whereas cyclic vomiting (also called cyclic vomiting syndrome) is a functional disorder characterized by recurrent episodes of severe nausea and vomiting. The child has symptom-free periods between episodes (Forbes & Fairbrother, 2008). Continuous vomiting of any nature should be evaluated.

Evaluation

Expected outcomes of nursing care of the child with gastroesophageal reflux and GERD include:

- The child does not exhibit signs or symptoms of respiratory distress or aspiration.
- Fluid and electrolyte balance is maintained.
- The child has adequate intake of nutrition to meet growth and developmental needs.
- No signs and symptoms of infection are evident.
- The parents demonstrate proper feeding techniques.

Abdominal Wall Defects

In early fetal life, the intestines are extra-abdominal. They move intra-abdominally by about 11 weeks of gestation. The two most common congenital defects of the anterior abdominal wall are omphalocele and gastroschisis, which are discussed in this section.

Omphalocele

Omphalocele is a congenital malformation in which intra-abdominal contents herniate through the umbilical cord (Figure 30–10 ■). An omphalocele results when the intestines fail to return to the abdomen when the abdominal wall begins to close by the tenth week of gestation. The size of the sac varies depending on the extent of the protrusion. Large defects may contain the intestines, stomach, liver, and spleen (Hood & Zimmerman, 2013). Omphalocele occurs at the base of the

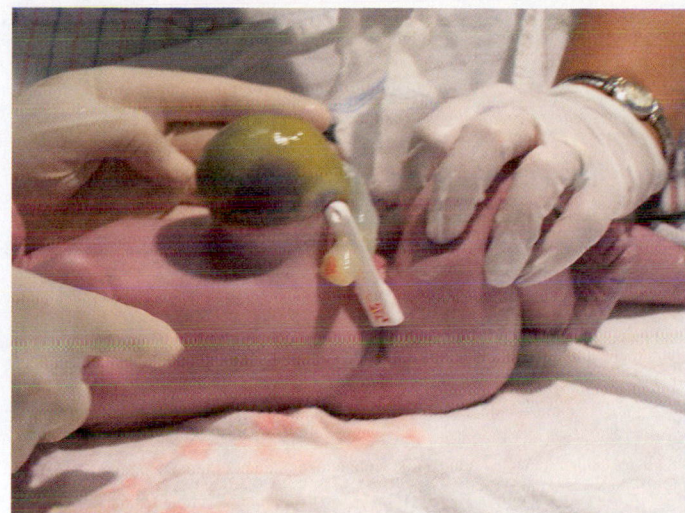

FIGURE 30–10 ■ In omphalocele, the size of the sac depends on the extent of the protrusion of abdominal contents through the umbilical cord.
Source: *Courtesy of Carol Harrigan, RNC, MSN, NNP.*

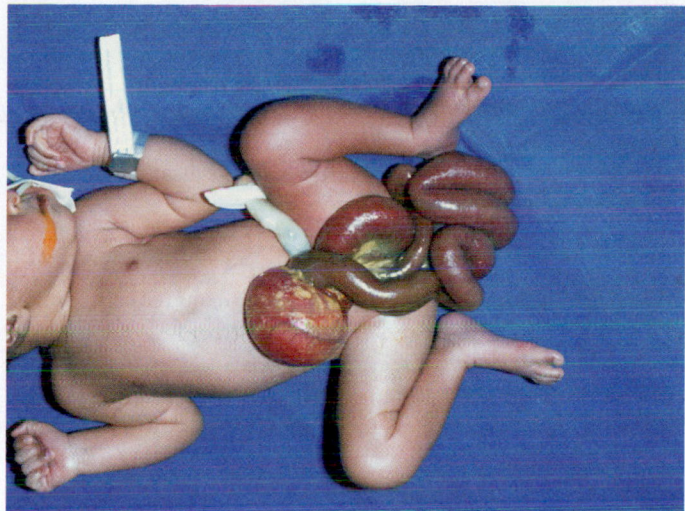

FIGURE 30–11 ■ The newborn with gastroschisis has abdominal contents located outside the abdominal wall.
Source: *Copyright 2012—Custom Medical Stock Photo, All Rights Reserved.*

umbilical cord. The abdominal contents are covered with peritoneum and amniotic membrane (Khan, 2011). Rupture of the sac results in evisceration of the abdominal contents. Omphalocele with herniation of intestines into the umbilical cord occurs in 1 in 5,000 births, while omphalocele with herniation of liver and intestines occurs in 1 in 10,000 births (Carlo, 2011). Between 50% and 70% of infants with omphalocele will have an associated anomaly such as bladder exstrophy, cardiac defects, and Meckel diverticulum (Razmus, 2011).

Gastroschisis

Gastroschisis is a congenital defect of the ventral abdominal wall, characterized by protrusion of bowel through a defect in the abdominal wall to the side (most often to the right) of the umbilicus (Ruano, Picone, Bernardes, et al., 2011). The most common abdominal organs involved are the small intestine and ascending colon. Unlike the omphalocele, no membrane covers the organs (Fillingham & Rankin, 2008) (Figure 30–11 ■). Gastroschisis occurs in approximately 1 in 4,000 live births (Christison-Lagay, Kelleher, & Langer 2011). Approximately 20% of infants with gastroschisis have an associated anomaly, most often atresia or intestinal stenosis (Razmus, 2011).

Collaborative Care

Care of the child with gastroschisis or omphalocele centers on protecting the protruding abdominal organs, correcting the defect, and preventing complications such as hypothermia, infection, and injury to involved organs.

Diagnostic Tests

Elevated maternal serum alpha-fetoprotein (MSAFP) levels are seen in both gastroschisis and omphalocele. Routine prenatal determination of MSAFP and ultrasonography lead to early diagnosis and education to the family, and coordination of the team of specialists needed to manage these congenital anomalies (Razmus, 2011).

Clinical Therapy

The immediate action upon birth is to protect the sac (in omphalocele) or exposed abdominal contents (in gastroschisis) from injury by placing the infant feet first into a bowel bag (large sterile clear bag)

that extends to the nipple line and is secured with ties. The bag is filled with warm saline to decrease heat loss and to keep organs moist, and it allows for visualization of the defect (Razmus, 2011). The child will often be transferred to a neonatal intensive care unit (NICU) with surgical capability for this defect.

Temperature regulation is needed for the newborn due to heat loss through exposed viscera. Fluids are required to replace those lost through viscera. Blood cultures are performed before administering antibiotics. An orogastric or nasogastric tube may be inserted to prevent distention. A thorough examination is performed to rule out cardiac and other abnormalities.

Surgical repair of omphalocele and gastroschisis may occur in one or two stages depending on the severity of the defect. One surgery may be all that is needed to repair a small defect. For larger defects, the first stage of repair may involve nonoperative placement of the abdominal contents or sac into a Silastic silo. Once the abdominal cavity can accommodate the intestinal contents the child will have surgery to close the abdominal wall (Razmus, 2011).

Nursing Management

Nursing care of the newborn with omphalocele or gastroschisis centers on protecting the sac or protruding organs, preventing hypothermia, preventing and identifying infection, providing preoperative and postoperative care, and supporting the family.

Nursing Assessment and Diagnosis

Be alert for signs of associated congenital anomalies. (Refer to the discussions of tracheoesophageal fistula earlier in this chapter, to genitourinary anomalies in Chapter 31, and to congenital heart defects in Chapter 26 ✪.) Assess the integrity of the sac in omphalocele. Assess vital signs at least every hour, paying particular attention to temperature. Urine output is measured to assess fluid needs.

Nursing diagnoses that apply to the newborn with omphalocele or gastroschisis include:

- Fluid Volume, Deficient related to fluid loss through exposed abdominal organs
- Infection, Risk for related to exposed abdominal organs

- Hypothermia related to heat loss through exposed abdominal organs
- Pain, Acute related to surgical incision
- Attachment, Risk for Impaired Parent/Infant related to congenital defect, emergent surgery, and potential loss of neonate
- Anxiety (Parent) related to threat to infant's health status

NANDA-I © 2012

Planning and Implementation

During hospitalization of their child, parents require clear, accurate explanations about the infant's condition. Partner with the family to help the parents deal with the crisis of an acutely ill newborn, provide emotional support, and encourage parents to express their feelings. When the child has multiple anomalies, parents require ongoing support for the lengthy treatment, numerous hospitalizations, and management of nutritional intake. Referral to a counselor or social services may be helpful to the family. In addition, the nurse provides intensive care to the infant before and after correction of the defect. Important nursing actions include monitoring health status and providing comfort measures and nutritional support.

Preoperative Nursing Care

Immediately after birth, follow physician protocol for maintaining the omphalocele sac or for the exposed abdominal contents in gastroschisis as discussed previously. Monitor vital signs at least hourly, paying close attention to temperature, as the infant can lose heat through the sac. The child should be in a warmer or isolette for maintenance of temperature control. Inspect the area for signs of infection. Because the infant is NPO preoperatively, maintain fluid and electrolyte balance with intravenous fluids.

Postoperative Nursing Care

Postoperative care includes measures to control pain, prevent infection, maintain fluid and electrolyte balance, and ensure adequate nutritional intake. Attainment of bowel motility and function varies and is often delayed for weeks after surgery. Total parenteral nutrition for the infant is used until full bowel function has returned (Hood & Zimmerman, 2013).

Evaluation

Expected outcomes of nursing care depend on the severity of the defect and its correction, but may include:

- Fluid volume balance is maintained.
- The incision heals without signs of infection.
- Stable thermoregulatory function is maintained.
- Effective pain management is achieved.
- Parent/infant bonding and attachment is demonstrated.

Intussusception

Intussusception occurs when one portion of the intestine prolapses and then invaginates or telescopes into another. It is one of the most frequent causes of intestinal obstruction during infancy and occurs at a rate of 1 in 2000 infants and children. Intussusception is more common in males. An estimated sixty-five percent of cases occur in children prior to 1 year of age (Deloach & Farber, 2013).

Etiology and Pathophysiology

Ninety percent of cases of intussusception in children are idiopathic, as a direct cause is not generally identified. While the exact cause is

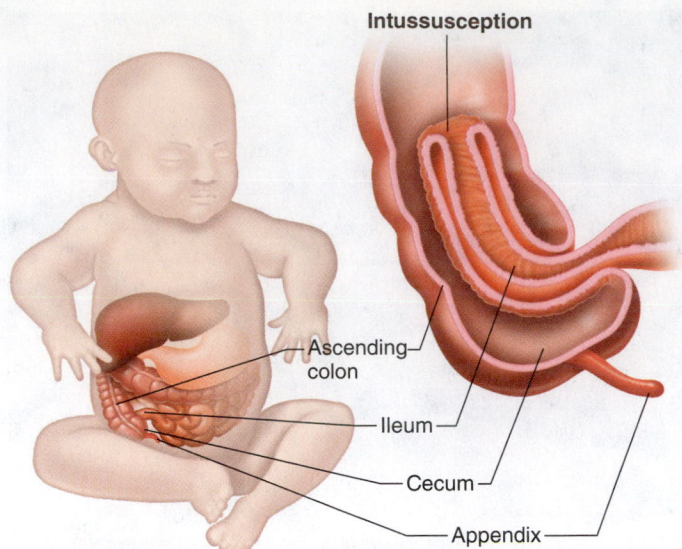

FIGURE 30–12 ■ In infants, intussusception is commonly associated with viral illnesses and gastroenteritis.

unknown, there is frequently a current or recent enteritis or upper respiratory infection (Pepper, Stanfill & Pearl, 2012).

The most common site of intussusception is the ileocecal valve (Cochran, Higgins, & Strout, 2011). Telescoping of the intestine obstructs the passage of stool. The walls of the intestine rub together, causing inflammation, edema, and decreased blood flow. This can lead to bowel ischemia, perforation, peritonitis, and possibly death if not treated promptly (Kairam, Kaiafis, & Shih, 2009) (Figure 30–12 ■).

Clinical Manifestations

The onset of intussusception is usually abrupt. A previously healthy infant or child suddenly experiences acute abdominal pain with vomiting and passage of brown stool. The infant may experience periods of comfort between acute episodes of pain. As the condition worsens, painful episodes increase. The child may have bilious emesis and a palpable abdominal mass. The stools become red and resemble currant jelly because of the mixture of blood and mucus (Cochran et al., 2011; Deloach & Farber, 2013; Saverino, Lava, Lowe, et al., 2010).

Collaborative Care

Collaborative care focuses on reducing the intussusception and restoring fluid and electrolyte balance.

Diagnostic Tests

Diagnosis is made on the basis of the history and confirmed by radiographs and ultrasound of the abdomen. A contrast enema using air or barium can be both diagnostic and therapeutic. An air (or pneumatic) enema reduces the intussusception in approximately 90% of cases and is considered safer than a barium enema because of the decreased risk of perforation (Pepper, et al., 2012).

Clinical Therapy

A nasogastric tube is inserted for gastric decompression. If reduction of the intussusception does not occur during the air or barium enema surgical intervention to reduce the invaginated bowel and remove any necrotic tissue is necessary. Surgery is generally successful in correcting the problem; however, intussusception can recur after hydrostatic reduction or surgical correction.

Nursing Management

Nursing management focuses on maintaining or restoring fluid and electrolyte balance. Intravenous fluids are initiated immediately. Serum electrolyte monitoring is essential to manage imbalances.

Nursing Assessment and Diagnosis

Preoperative assessment includes vital signs, monitoring for abdominal distention, and auscultating for bowel sounds every 4 hours. Monitor intravenous intake. Monitor urine output and measure any vomitus. Assess for number and characteristics of stools. Assess the infant or child for guarding of the abdomen. Monitor serum electrolytes.

Practice Alert

The passage of a normal brown stool may indicate that an intussusception has been reduced. Report this finding to the primary care provider immediately, as the course of treatment may be altered, especially in the case of a planned surgical reduction.

Postoperative assessment includes vital signs, bowel sounds, and intake and output. Assess the surgical incision site. Assess for evidence of pain.

Nursing diagnoses that may apply to the child with intussusception include:

- Pain, Acute related to bowel compression
- Perfusion: Gastrointestinal, Risk for Infective related to bowel compression
- Fluid Volume, Deficient related to vomiting and inability to consume foods/fluids with painful episodes
- Anxiety (Parent and Child) related to child's emergency condition

NANDA-I © 2012

Planning and Implementation

Preoperative care focuses on relieving the child's pain, maintaining patency of the nasogastric tube, and preparing the child and family for the surgical procedure. Postoperative care focuses on monitoring for early signs of infection, managing the child's pain, and maintaining nasogastric tube patency. Feeding protocols vary among practitioners. Generally, after normal bowel function returns, clear liquid feeding or breastfeeding is begun. Feedings are then advanced to half-strength milk and other foods as the infant or child tolerates them.

Discharge occurs shortly after the infant or child begins taking full feedings. Partner with the family to ensure parents understand how to monitor the child for signs of infection, such as fever, wound drainage, and fussiness, and the importance of notifying the primary healthcare provider if symptoms recur or appetite decreases.

Evaluation

Expected outcomes for nursing care of the child with intussusception include the following:

- Effective pain management is achieved.
- Adequate bowel function is demonstrated.
- Fluid and electrolyte balance is maintained.

Volvulus

During the 7th to 12th week of gestation the small intestine undergoes rapid growth. In normal development the intestine rotates counterclockwise as it settles into its permanent position inside the abdominal cavity. Malrotation of the intestine occurs in approximately 3.9 out of every 10,000 live births (Applegate, 2009). When malrotation of the intestine occurs, the child is at risk for **volvulus,** a twisting of the intestine. Volvulus disrupts blood flow in the intestines and can lead to necrosis of the bowel, short bowel syndrome, and death. Volvulus is considered a surgical emergency. Early diagnosis and treatment is necessary to preserve the bowel and to save the child's life (Markowitz & Dancel, 2008).

Symptoms of volvulus in the infant include bilious vomiting, firm abdomen with distention, irritability secondary to pain, and passage of bloody stools. Confirmation of malrotation of the intestine, through upper GI series or contrast studies, supports a diagnosis of volvulus. Emergency exploratory surgery to untwist the bowel is essential (Zerpa & Shapiro, 2013). If a portion of the bowel is necrotic, that portion of the bowel is removed. An ostomy may need to be created, depending on the amount of bowel removed. See the section on ostomies on page 1014. The child is at risk for developing short bowel syndrome if a significant amount of bowel is removed (see page 1032).

Nursing Management

The infant or child who presents to the emergency department with bilious vomiting and a firm and distended abdomen should be assessed quickly to determine the cause of the symptoms. Once volvulus has been diagnosed, nursing management focuses on keeping the child NPO, administering intravenous fluids, assessing vital signs, and reporting symptoms of a worsening condition. The child who has had surgery to correct uncomplicated volvulus will need care similar to that described for the child with intussusception. If the child had necrotic bowel removed, he or she may have an ostomy for a period of time.

Hirschsprung Disease

Hirschsprung disease, also known as congenital aganglionic megacolon, is a congenital anomaly in which inadequate motility causes mechanical obstruction of the intestine. The disease occurs in approximately 1 in 5,000 live births and is more common in males than females. Hirschsprung disease can occur as a single anomaly or in combination with other anomalies such as congenital heart defects and Down syndrome (Kenny, Tam, & Garcia-Barcelo, 2010).

Etiology and Pathophysiology

Hirschsprung disease is the congenital absence of ganglion cells in the wall of a variable segment of rectum and colon. The absence of autonomic parasympathetic ganglion cells in the colon prevents peristalsis at that portion of the intestine, resulting in the accumulation of intestinal contents and abdominal distention. In most cases, the area lacking ganglion cells is limited to the rectosigmoid region of the colon (Fiorino & Liacouras, 2011; Kenny et al., 2010).

Clinical Manifestations

Clinical manifestations of Hirschsprung disease vary depending on the child's age at onset. In newborns, symptoms include failure to pass meconium in the first 48 hours after birth, abdominal distention, and bilious vomiting (Holder & Jackson, 2013; Nelville, 2010). **Enterocolitis** (inflammation of the intestines) is a complication of

Hirschsprung disease that can be fatal if not recognized and treated early. Symptoms of enterocolitis include fever, foul-smelling and/or bloody **diarrhea** (frequent, watery stools), pain, and vomiting (Nelville, 2010).

The older infant or child may have a history of failure to gain weight, malnutrition, chronic progressive **constipation** (difficult and infrequent defecation with passage of hard, dry stool), and recurrent fecal impaction (Nelville, 2010).

Collaborative Care

Collaborative care focuses on identification of Hirschsprung disease, surgical removal of the aganglionic section, promotion of nutrition for growth and development, and achievement of normal bowel elimination patterns.

Diagnostic Tests

Diagnosis is made on the basis of the history, bowel patterns, *anorectal manometry* (reaction of the anal sphincter to distention of the rectum), radiographic contrast studies, and rectal biopsy for presence or absence of ganglion cells. Anorectal manometry demonstrates absence of relaxation of the internal sphincter, an expected response to rectal distention. Normally, distention of the rectum produces relaxation of the internal sphincter. Abdominal radiograph and contrast studies reveal a distended small bowel and proximal colon with an empty rectum. Rectal biopsy, revealing the absence of ganglionic cells and the presence of hypertrophic nerve bundles, has proven to be the most reliable test for confirmation of the diagnosis (Fiorino & Liacouras, 2011).

Clinical Therapy

Primary repair of Hirschsprung disease to remove the aganglionic portion of the bowel using a transanal endorectal pull-through or a transanal pull-through procedure is appropriate in most infants and children. Depending on the amount of bowel affected, a primary repair may not be possible. In that case, a temporary colostomy is created and will be closed when the definitive surgery takes place (Georgeson, 2010).

The return of normal bowel function depends on the amount of bowel involved. Some fecal incontinence and constipation may persist following surgery. Enterocolitis is a serious complication that can occur before or after surgery, resulting in ischemia and ulceration of the bowel wall. Treatment for enterocolitis associated with Hirschsprung disease includes rectal irrigations and antibiotics (Holder & Jackson, 2013).

Nursing Management

Nursing care focuses on collaborative identification of Hirschsprung disease; preoperative and postoperative nursing care, including nutritional support; and supporting the family.

Nursing Assessment and Diagnosis

Nursing assessment in the newborn period includes careful observation for the passage of meconium. Because newborns are often discharged within 24 hours of birth, tell parents to notify the physician if no stool is passed within 48 hours of birth or if the abdomen becomes distended.

When the disease is diagnosed later in infancy or in childhood, obtain a thorough history of weight gain, nutritional intake, and bowel elimination habits. Assess the child's growth and developmental achievements. Assess the child for abdominal distention and severe constipation alternating with diarrhea and vomiting. Assess the stool appearance.

Nursing diagnoses that may apply to the child with Hirschsprung disease include:

- Fluid Volume: Deficient, Risk for related to ineffective bowel function, NPO status, and surgical intervention
- Nutrition, Imbalanced: Less than Body Requirements related to ineffective bowel function, NPO status, and surgical intervention
- Pain, Acute related to surgical incision
- Anxiety (Parent) related to child's illness and required surgical intervention

NANDA-1 @ 2012

Planning and Implementation

Nursing management consists of carefully monitoring fluid and electrolyte balance, maintaining nutrition, providing preoperative and postoperative care, providing pain relief, and promoting bowel elimination.

Preoperative Nursing Care

When Hirschsprung disease is diagnosed, nursing care includes monitoring for infection, managing pain, maintaining hydration, measuring abdominal circumference to detect any distention, and providing support to the child and family. Preoperative oral intake varies depending on the surgeon; however, intake is generally restricted to clear fluids the day before surgery. Rectal irrigations may be performed to evacuate the bowel prior to surgery.

Postoperative Nursing Care

Initial postoperative nursing care is the same as for any other infant or child having abdominal surgery. Maintain intravenous fluids and nasogastric tube, and monitor intake and output. Administer pain medications as prescribed and assess at least every hour for evidence of pain utilizing a pain scale and documenting assessment. If a colostomy was performed, the stoma should be assessed frequently as well as the return of bowel function. See the section on ostomies on page 1014.

Clinical Tip

Following colostomy closure in the child who has had a colostomy for several months, the perineal area is not accustomed to contact with stool. Without meticulous skin care, breakdown is very likely. Teach parents to change diapers frequently, cleanse the perineal area carefully, and apply a protective barrier ointment or cream at each diaper change.

Children occasionally develop constipation, and parents may need guidance to adapt the diet and fluid intake to manage this complication. Because some children develop malabsorption, be alert for signs of poor growth or malnutrition. See Chapter 19 🔗.

Evaluation

Expected outcomes of nursing care of the child with Hirschsprung disease may include the following:

- Fluid and electrolyte balance is maintained.
- Adequate nutritional intake to promote growth and development is evident.

- Adequate bowel function is demonstrated.
- The child's pain is managed effectively.
- The parents demonstrate effective coping with the stress of the child's condition.

Anorectal Malformations

Anorectal malformations refer to anomalies of the rectum and distal anus, the urinary tract, and the genital tract. They have an incidence of approximately 1 in 3,500 to 5,000 live births (Upadhyaya, Gangopadhyay, Srivastava, et al., 2008). Anorectal malformations are frequently associated with anomalies of the musculoskeletal system. Chromosomal abnormalities such as trisomy 13, 18, or 21 may co-exist, and some babies have VACTERL conditions. VACTERL refers to the presence of three or more of the following anomalies: vertebral anomalies, anal atresia, congenital heart disease, tracheoesophageal fistula, renal anomalies, and limb defects (Stafford & Klein, 2011).

The term *imperforate anus* (absence of the anal opening) is frequently used to refer to anorectal malformations and is classified according to the specific defect. Males with imperforate anus frequently have a rectourethral fistula, and girls generally have a rectovestibular fistula (Wilson, Etheridge, Soundappan, et al., 2010). Additional minor defects that may occur include anal stenosis (narrowing of the anus) and anal membrane (skin covering the anal opening) (Pakarinen & Rintala, 2010).

Imperforate anus affects males and females equally. Perineal inspection at birth reveals the absent anal opening. Failure to pass meconium within the first 24 hours of birth may be indicative of imperforate anus. Stool in the urine usually indicates the presence of a fistula between the colon and urinary tract. Cloacal malformations in females, in which the urinary tract, vagina, and rectum fuse together, forming a common channel, may occur. The child with a cloacal malformation has one opening in the perineum (Bischoff, Levitt, Lim, et al., 2010).

Collaborative Care

Collaborative care focuses on preservation of bowel, urinary, and sexual function, as well as treatment of any associated abnormalities.

Diagnostic Tests

Diagnosis of anorectal malformation is usually made at birth or during the newborn assessment of anorectal structures and rectal patency. Ultrasound and lower gastrointestinal radiographic studies confirm the diagnosis and demonstrate the extent of the anomaly. Anorectal manometry may be performed. Careful physical examination of all body systems is performed to identify any associated abnormalities.

Clinical Therapy

Management depends on the extent of the malformation and presence of associated conditions. Anal stenosis may be treated with dilation alone. An imperforate anal membrane is excised surgically, followed by daily manual dilations. A single operation anoplasty may be used to repair rectoperineal defects (previously known as low defects). Higher defects require a three-stage procedure. A temporary colostomy in the newborn period provides for bowel decompression and for protection of the surgical site when the anomaly is repaired. Reconstructive surgery is accomplished via a posterior sagittal anorectoplasty (PSARP) (Levitt & Peña, 2010). Timing of the repair varies. Some surgeons prefer to perform the surgery at 1–3 months (Levitt & Peña, 2010) while others recommend waiting until 3–6 months (Orr, 2011). When the operative site has healed, approximately 2 weeks after surgery, anal dilatations are begun. When the desired size of the anal opening has been achieved, approximately 6 to 8 weeks after surgery, the colostomy is closed (Orr, 2011). Colostomy closure involves anastomosis of the bowel. The child will require irrigations of the colostomy and be on clear liquids by mouth beginning the day prior to surgery. Prophylactic antibiotics will be administered during anesthesia induction and for 48 hours following surgery. The child who has had a colostomy takedown will require pain management and intravenous fluids. The child may have a nasogastric tube in place and will remain NPO until bowel function returns (Guardino & Pieper, 2013).

Nursing Management

Nursing care focuses on newborn assessment of anal patency, preoperative and postoperative care, and family support.

Nursing Assessment and Diagnosis

During the initial newborn assessment, the perineal area is inspected for a poorly developed anal dimple or sacral anomalies. Observe and record passage of meconium. Carefully assess all body systems and promptly report abnormal findings. Be particularly alert for cardiac, respiratory, and urinary output problems. Postoperatively observe the operative area for signs of infection.

Practice Alert

For the child who has had posterior sagittal anorectoplasty, it is very important that nothing be placed in the rectum, including thermometers and suppositories. A sign should be placed on the patient's bed to alert all staff caring for the infant.

Accurate intake and output is essential. Assess vital signs at least every 4 hours. Assess the child for evidence of pain.

Nursing diagnoses that may apply to the infant with anorectal malformation include:

- Pain, Acute related to surgical incision
- Anxiety (Parent) related to infant's health status
- Infection, Risk for related to impaired skin integrity (surgical incision)
- Fluid Volume: Deficient, Risk for related to NPO status
- Knowledge, Deficient (Parent) related to care of stoma

NANDA-I © 2012

Planning and Implementation

Once the diagnosis of anorectal malformation has been made, intravenous fluids are initiated and a nasogastric tube is inserted to decompress the stomach. Monitor the child's intake and output and cardiorespiratory functioning. Provide emotional support to the parents and information about the planned treatments and surgery.

Postoperative care specific to the child who has had the PSARP procedure centers on protection of the surgical site. A Foley catheter will be in place for 5 days to protect the new anal opening from urine. The colostomy that is still in place protects the surgical site from stool. Provide adequate pain management for the child. Intravenous fluids will be given until the child is able to take liquids by mouth.

Nursing care for the child who has had colostomy closure is more complex due to the fact that the bowel has been manipulated during surgery. Maintenance of the nasogastric tube to low wall suction until bowel function returns is essential. Intravenous fluids or total parenteral nutrition through peripheral or central venous access will be provided until the child is able to take fluids by mouth. Intake and output is monitored. The child will frequently have a Foley catheter in place for accurate measurement of urine output.

Clinical Judgment

Following creation of a new anal opening through the PSARP procedure, the child should have nothing placed in the rectum. What specific procedures should be avoided? What measure will remind others of this contraindication? How can the nurse position the child to avoid pressure on the surgical site?

Care of the operative site may include dressing changes in addition to assessment for signs of infection. As the child begins to pass stool through the anal opening for the first time, skin breakdown is likely. The perineal area should be protected with a barrier cream or paste.

Intravenous pain medication should be provided on a regular basis. The nurse is also responsible for administering prescribed antibiotics that protect the child from infection.

The child with associated abnormalities may need several surgeries and interventions to treat all of the conditions present. Partnering with families and the group of healthcare providers will assist in case management that facilitates the child's health and development. Health promotion and health maintenance should include supporting family members, ensuring immunizations, and monitoring developmental status.

Discharge Planning and Home Care Teaching

Infants are increasingly discharged shortly after birth, so parents need clear instructions about normal newborn stools and what abnormalities to report so that anorectal defects not obvious at birth are identified early.

If a colostomy is performed in the newborn period, teach parents how to care for the ostomy site (see the discussion of ostomies on page 1014). Reassure parents that the colostomy will be closed in the future, and help them plan for that hospitalization. Refer them to ostomy support groups in the community or online. Discuss follow-up care and long-term management. Arrange follow-up visits and home care visits to evaluate the child's ostomy site and monitor growth.

After surgery to create the anal opening, teach parents how to take the infant's temperature using the axillary route. Once anal dilatations have begun, the family will be taught how to perform them at home. After the final surgical procedure, discuss feeding regimens and bowel habits necessary to maintain adequate nutrition for growth and development. Advise parents that children with anorectal malformations may have difficulty achieving bowel control. Patience in toilet training is important. When the child reaches an age appropriate for toilet training, encourage the family to speak with a healthcare provider to discuss the child's progress. (See Evidence-Based Practice: Imperforate Anus.)

Evidence-Based Practice   Imperforate Anus

PROBLEM

Despite successful surgery for imperforate anus, the child may have long-term problems with constipation and fecal soiling. Parents may also experience stressors related to their child's condition (Nisell, Öjmyr-Joelsson, Frenckner, et al., 2009). How does a history of imperforate anus affect children and their parents psychosocially?

EVIDENCE

A cross-sectional retrospective study by Nisell, Öjmyr-Joelsson, Frenckner, et al. (2009) examined the psychosocial experiences and potential positive experiences of families who had children born with high or intermediate imperforate anus (IA). Twenty-five mothers and 20 fathers of children with IA participated in the study. Parents of children with juvenile chronic arthritis (JCA) served as the comparison group. Significant findings from the study revealed that mothers of children with IA felt that their social relationships were affected more than mothers of children with JCA. They also reported less respect for their child's will. There were no significant differences in the responses of fathers of children with IA as compared to those of children with JCA. Positive experiences were identified by 48% of mothers and 35% of fathers of children with IA, with no statistical differences when compared to parents of children with JCA. Although 28% of mothers and 25% of fathers had received psychologic care in relation to their child's congenital anomaly, this did not correlate with a higher percentage of positive experiences. Positive experiences focused on the development of the child, personal development of the parent, and strengthening of family unity.

Further research by Nisell, Igl, Öjmyr-Joelsson, et al. (2009) examined the psychosocial experiences of children with a history of high or intermediate imperforate anus. Questionnaires were completed by the same parents utilized in the previous study. While parents of children with IA were more positive in the description of their child's academic adjustment as compared to parents of children with JCA or those with no chronic condition, these parents indicated that their children were not as socially integrated as children in the other groups. Teachers of these children also completed a questionnaire. Children with IA received lower scores

from teachers on questions related to academic performance and adaptive functioning than children with JCA or children with no chronic condition.

Nisell, Öjmyr-Joelsson, Frenckner, et al. (2008) also compared how the child with high or intermediate imperforate anus and his or her mother viewed the child's psychosocial functioning. The same families served as participants in this study as in the previous two studies examined. Responses of 25 children with IA and their mothers were compared with responses of 30 children with chronic arthritis and their mothers and 32 children admitted to the day surgery unit for a minor surgical procedure and their mothers. Results of the study showed disagreement between children in all groups and their mothers, especially in questions related to psychologic issues such as feelings of sadness, anger, and thoughts of inconvenience. Mothers thought their children had more sadness and anger than the children did, and children thought less about their inconvenience than their mothers thought they did. Only mothers of children with IA thought more of their child's health problem than their children perceived. In addition, only mothers of children with IA thought their children had more self-confidence than the children reported that they had. Social variables that were statistically significant between mothers and their children in all groups included being teased and being bullied, with mothers reporting that they thought this happened more often than the children reported its occurrence.

IMPLICATIONS

Nurses who care for children with a history of high or intermediate imperforate anus should assess whether the child continues to have difficulty with constipation and soiling. For those children with continued problems related to IA, assess the impact this condition has on the psychosocial functioning of the child and the family and provide support as appropriate.

CRITICAL THINKING APPLICATION

What age group would be most affected psychosocially by continued problems with fecal soiling related to IA? How can the nurse facilitate coping in the parent and the child?

Evaluation

Expected outcomes of nursing care include:

- The child's pain is effectively managed.
- The parents demonstrate effective coping with the stress of the child's condition.
- Incisions heal without signs of infection.
- Fluid and electrolyte balance is maintained.
- Adequate bowel function is demonstrated.
- The parents demonstrate an understanding of ostomy care and other treatment protocols.

HERNIAS

A **hernia** is the protrusion or projection of an organ or a part of an organ through the muscle wall of the cavity that normally contains it. This protrusion may result from the failure of normal openings to close during fetal development or from weakness in the supporting musculature. When intra-abdominal pressure increases (as when the infant cries or strains to pass stool), the weakened area separates, causing a protrusion of underlying organs. Inguinal hernias are the most common type of hernia occurring in children (see Chapter 31 🕗). Other hernias occurring frequently in children are congenital diaphragmatic hernias and umbilical hernias, which are discussed in this section.

Congenital Diaphragmatic Hernia

In a diaphragmatic hernia, abdominal contents protrude into the thoracic cavity through an opening in the diaphragm. Sites of herniation include the substernal space, the posterolateral region, and the esophageal hiatus.

Etiology and Pathophysiology

The cause of diaphragmatic hernia is a delay or failure in closure of the pleuroperitoneal musculature which forms the diaphragm. Intestines and other abdominal structures enter the thoracic cavity through the opening in the diaphragm. The overall incidence of diaphragmatic hernia is 1 in 2,200 births (Rollins, 2012). Associated anomalies are present in up to 30% of children with diaphragmatic hernia (Maheshwari & Carlo, 2011).

Clinical Manifestations

A diaphragmatic hernia is a life-threatening condition with an overall mortality rate of 20-35% in infants born alive with this condition (Rollins, 2012). Severe respiratory distress secondary to pulmonary hypoplasia occurs shortly after birth. As the infant cries, abdominal organs extend into the thorax, decreasing the size of the thoracic cavity. The infant becomes dyspneic and cyanotic. Characteristic findings include a barrel-shaped chest and sunken abdomen. Diminished or absent breath sounds are noted on the affected side. Bowel sounds may be auscultated over the chest. Heart tones may be auscultated on the right side of the chest. Pneumothorax may be an associated complication.

Collaborative Care

Collaborative care centers on immediate preservation of life, establishing ventilatory support, supporting fluid balance, and surgical correction of the defect.

Diagnostic Tests

Congenital diaphragmatic hernia is diagnosed in utero by ultrasound in approximately 2/3 of patients (Rollins, 2012). If it is not identified prenatally, the condition is first identified postnatally by physical signs and symptoms; confirmation is made by chest radiologic examination (Tsao & Lally, 2010).

Clinical Therapy

The infant is transferred to a NICU as soon as possible. Ventilator support is necessary to manage respiratory compromise. Conventional mechanical ventilation, high-frequency oxygen ventilation, nitric oxide, and extracorporeal membrane oxygenation (ECMO) are the main methods used to treat respiratory failure in these children (Rollins, 2012; Sluiter, van de Ven, Wijnen, et al., 2011).

The infant is positioned with the head and thorax higher than the abdomen to facilitate downward movement of abdominal organs. A nasogastric tube is inserted to decompress the stomach. Intravenous fluids are administered through an umbilical artery catheter.

Once the infant's condition is stabilized, the defect is corrected surgically. The chance for a successful repair and survival is affected by the size of the defect. Children who survive will generally continue to have health concerns and should have continued evaluation of pulmonary, gastrointestinal, nutritional, and neurodevelopmental related problems (Rollins, 2012).

Nursing Management

Nursing care centers on maintaining ventilatory support of the infant, preoperative preparation, postoperative care, and supporting the family during this life-threatening event.

Nursing Assessment and Diagnosis

Assess the infant's vital signs and respiratory status by continuous monitoring. Assess for worsening of respiratory compromise. Assess cardiac rhythm by physical assessment and the cardiorespiratory monitor. Assess breath sounds—note presence of bowel sounds in the thoracic cavity, and note presence of heart tones on the right side of the chest. Assess for cyanosis and altered mental status.

Nursing diagnoses that may apply to the infant with diaphragmatic hernia include the following:

- Breathing Pattern, Ineffective related to compression of lungs by intra-abdominal organs
- Fluid Volume, Deficient, Risk for related to NPO status
- Anxiety (Parent) related to life-threatening condition of neonate
- Attachment, Risk for Impaired Parent/Infant related to infant's life-threatening condition, surgery

NANDA-I © 2012

Planning and Implementation

The infant with a diaphragmatic hernia is admitted to the NICU and requires continuous monitoring. The critical need for emergency surgical intervention and the poor survival rate place great stress on parents and other family members. Offer support and refer the family to appropriate resources for stress management and support.

Preoperative Care

Preoperative management centers on providing supportive care to the infant and parents. Maintain intravenous fluid administration. Place the child on a cardiorespiratory monitor and note the infant's vital signs and pulse oximetry every 30 minutes. Observe for worsening of respiratory compromise. Promote decreased stimulation to keep the infant calm and thus maintain low abdominal pressure. Keep parents informed about the infant's condition, and provide emotional support both before and after surgery.

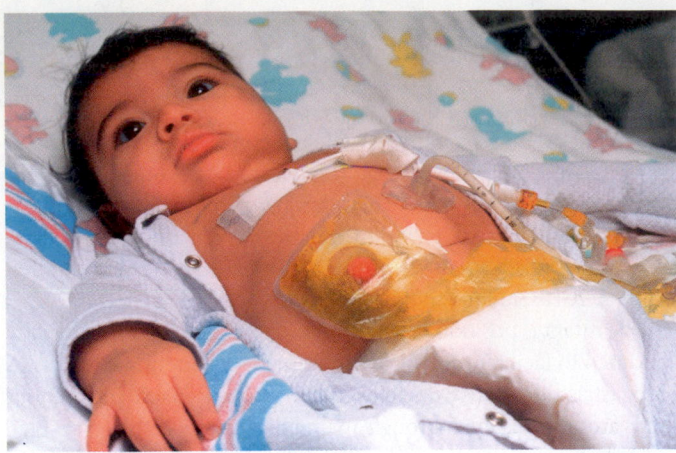

FIGURE 30–13 ■ This infant has several gastrointestinal problems and requires ostomies both for gastric feedings and for drainage of fecal material. Note the appearance of a healthy stoma.

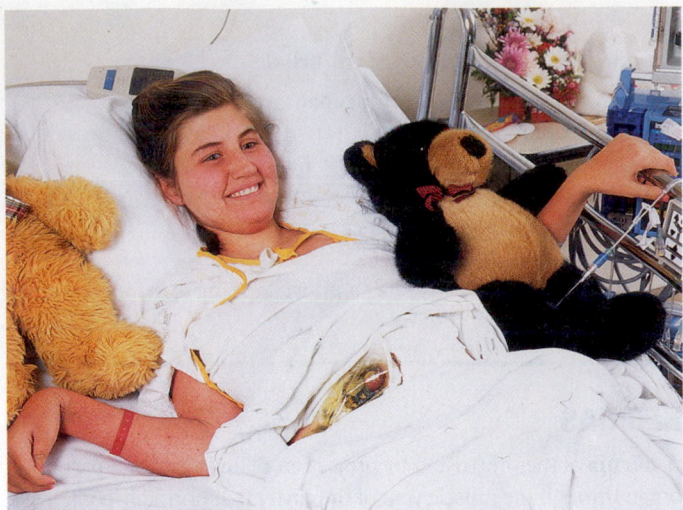

FIGURE 30–14 ■ Nursing strategies to address altered perception of body image and increased feelings of dependence are important when working with adolescents who have ostomies. Support groups or a visit from another teenager who has had an ostomy can facilitate positive coping, as demonstrated by this adolescent female.

Postoperative Care

Postoperative care includes positioning the infant on the affected side to facilitate expansion of the lung on the unaffected side, observing closely for signs of infection, maintaining respiratory support, managing pain, and carefully monitoring fluid and electrolyte balance. Before discharge, instruct parents in wound care, prevention of infection, and feeding techniques.

Due to the high rate of infant mortality associated with this condition, palliative care may need to be discussed with the parents if the child's condition is deteriorating and unresponsive to treatment. Comfort measures for the infant may become the focus of care. Refer to Chapter 18 🔗 for this discussion.

Evaluation

Expected outcomes for nursing care of the infant with diaphragmatic hernia include:

- The child demonstrates effective breathing patterns following surgical intervention.
- Fluid and electrolyte balance is maintained.
- Parent and infant bonding and attachment are demonstrated.
- The parents demonstrate effective coping with the stress of the child's condition.

Umbilical Hernia

An umbilical hernia results from imperfect closure or weakness of the umbilical ring. Umbilical hernia is a common condition in childhood and occurs more frequently in Black children and low-birthweight infants (Carlo, 2011).

An umbilical hernia presents as a soft swelling covered by skin. Omentum and small intestine herniate or protrude through the opening with coughing, crying, or straining during a bowel movement. It is easily reduced by pushing the bowel back through the fibrous ring. Most defects that appear prior to 6 months of age will resolve spontaneously by 1 year of age. Surgery is indicated in cases of **strangulation** (closure of the muscular ring around a portion of the bowel, preventing it from moving back into the abdomen). Surgery is also recommended if the defect does not resolve by 4 to 5 years of age or if the defect becomes larger after 1 to 2 years of age (Carlo, 2011).

Nursing management is generally supportive. Instruct parents not to apply tape, straps, or coins to reduce the hernia as these methods have not proven to be effective. If surgery is required, it is usually performed in an outpatient surgery unit. Postoperatively, teach parents how to care for the surgical site, to monitor for bleeding, and to recognize signs of infection. Reinforce the importance of returning for follow-up evaluation.

OSTOMIES

An intestinal **ostomy** is an opening, or **stoma,** into the small or large intestine that diverts fecal matter to provide an outlet when a distal surgical anastomosis, obstruction, or nonfunctioning structures prevent normal elimination (Figure 30–13 ■). Depending on the integrity and function of anatomic structures, the ostomy may be temporary or permanent. Infants and small children with imperforate anus, necrotizing enterocolitis, Hirschsprung disease, volvulus, or intussusception may require a temporary or permanent colostomy or ileostomy. Ostomies may also be indicated for children with inflammatory bowel disease, intestinal tumors, or abdominal trauma.

An ostomy may be elective or a surgical emergency. In all cases it affects a child's lifestyle, alters body image, causes anxiety, and increases the risk for alterations in physiologic processes (electrolyte imbalance, increased nutritional requirements). For adolescents, it may also result in dependence at a time when autonomy is a major developmental need (Figure 30–14 ■).

When assessing the family and child approaching ostomy surgery, it is important to determine their ability to understand and accept the physical changes that will occur. Parents may feel guilt and anger about the ostomy surgery when the child has a genetically transmitted disease, has sustained an injury, or has developed an obstruction from necrosis of the bowel. Encourage the parents and child to express their feelings, and correct any misunderstandings. Parents and older children may be referred for counseling and to support groups to help them deal with their feelings. Adolescents often benefit from a visit with an adolescent who has an ostomy and can answer questions about living with an ostomy.

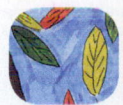

Partnering with Families

Assisting Families to Encourage the Child's Participation in Stoma Care

Assist parents in understanding the child's abilities at various developmental stages when planning the promotion of self-care.

- The preschooler has some manual dexterity and can help with parts of the procedure for changing an ostomy appliance and cleaning the stoma. The child should be taught using a doll or stuffed animal.

- Many school-age children are able to care for their ostomy independently. They should be taught how to avoid leakage around the bag, which could be embarrassing.

- Adolescents are generally independent in their self-care of ostomies; however, they may need support to deal with the fact that they are different from their peers.

Nursing Management

Nursing care focuses on preoperative teaching of the child and family and postoperative care of the child.

Preoperative Care

Preoperative education focuses on educating the child and family and preparing them for postoperative management. Discuss how the appliance, an ostomy pouch, will look, and explain the purpose of the appliance in developmentally appropriate terms. Encourage the parents and child to touch and manipulate all equipment. A younger child can be shown how to place a pouch on a doll, or dolls with ostomies can be used to demonstrate what the ostomy will look like (see Chapter 15, Figure 15–11 ☺). Older children can practice placing a pouch on their skin. These measures help relieve anxiety by providing information and increasing familiarity with the appliance.

In addition to discussion of the appliance, preoperative education includes discussion of pain management (see Chapter 21 ☺) and measures that will be used to prevent postoperative complications. Instructions are geared to the child's developmental level. Encourage parental participation to promote compliance.

Postoperative Care

Postoperative care of a child with an ostomy is similar to that for any child who undergoes abdominal surgery. (See the earlier discussion in this chapter for the child having abdominal surgery and the Nursing Care Plan for the child undergoing surgery in Chapter 15 ☺.) Management of the stoma may be coordinated by an ostomy nurse or other nurses. Major interventions involve ensuring proper function of the stoma, identifying complications, and instituting daily stoma care. Complications include skin breakdown, mucocutaneous separation, necrosis, prolapse, hernia, retraction, and laceration (Coha, 2013; Ratcliff, 2010). Assess the stoma, quality and amount of fecal matter, skin condition, and adherence of the pouch. Evaluate the family's understanding and ability to care for the ostomy.

Clinical Tip

Avoid adhesive enhancers on the skin of newborns and premature infants. Their skin layers are so thin that removal of the appliance can strip off the skin. Remember also that adhesive contains latex, and its frequent use is not advised due to risk of latex allergy development (see Chapter 27 ☺).

Discharge Planning and Home Care Teaching

Identify and address home care needs well in advance of discharge. Instructions include skin and stoma care, appliance removal and application, and frequency of appliance changes.

Begin teaching immediately after surgery with responsibility for care transferred gradually to the parents and child. See Partnering with Families: Assisting Families to Encourage the Child's Participation in Stoma Care. (For information on caring for an ostomy, refer to the Skills Manual ⊂⊃.) Discuss diet, activity level, hygiene, clothing, equipment, and financial considerations. Arrange for home visits to check periodically on the home management program.

Parents and children can be referred to the United Ostomy Association or a local ostomy group for information and support. Referrals should be made to social services, counseling, and a home health agency, if appropriate.

Expected outcomes of nursing care include the child's successful adjustment to the ostomy, thorough evacuation of the bowel, absence of infection and other complications, intact skin, and formation of a positive self-image in the child.

INFLAMMATORY DISORDERS

The gastrointestinal tract may develop an inflammatory disorder in response to trauma caused by injuries, foreign bodies, chemicals, microorganisms, or surgery. These disorders may be acute or chronic and may involve various segments of the gastrointestinal tract. Appendicitis, necrotizing enterocolitis, Meckel diverticulum, recurrent abdominal pain, inflammatory bowel disease (Crohn disease and ulcerative colitis), and peptic ulcer are discussed in this section.

Appendicitis

Appendicitis is an inflammation of the vermiform appendix, the small sac near the end of the cecum, and is the most common cause of emergency surgery in children (Wan, Krahn, Ungar, et al., 2009). Each year in the United States, 70,000 children will develop appendicitis. The condition occurs most often in children and adolescents ages 10 to 19 years. While the overall rate of perforated appendix is 20% to 35%, the rate in children less than 3 years of age is 80% to 100% (Minkes, Bechtel, Billmire, et al., 2011).

Etiology and Pathophysiology

Appendicitis almost always results from an obstruction in the appendiceal lumen. It can be caused by a fecalith (hard fecal mass), parasitic infestations, stenosis, hyperplasia of lymphoid tissue, or a tumor.

Continued secretion of mucus following acute obstruction of the lumen increases pressure, causing ischemia, cellular death, and ulceration. The appendix may perforate or rupture, resulting in fecal and bacterial contamination of the peritoneum. Peritonitis spreads quickly and if untreated can result in small bowel obstruction, electrolyte imbalances, septicemia, hypovolemic shock, and death. Early

Weblink United Ostomy Association

diagnosis and treatment of appendicitis is essential to minimize complications related to rupture (Wan et al., 2009).

Clinical Manifestations

At onset, symptoms include periumbilical cramps, abdominal tenderness, anorexia, nausea, and fever. In adolescent and young adult females, symptoms must be differentiated from those associated with ruptured ectopic pregnancy, ovarian cysts, and pelvic inflammatory disease (Surawicz, 2008).

As the inflammation progresses, pain in the right lower abdomen becomes constant. Pain is often most intense at McBurney point, halfway between the anterior superior iliac crest and the umbilicus (Figure 30–15 ■). Symptoms progress to include guarding, rigidity, nausea, vomiting, onset of pain before vomiting, anorexia, and rebound tenderness following palpation over the right lower quadrant. Diarrhea or constipation may be present (Surawicz, 2008; Watkins, 2010/2011). As appendicitis progresses, the child remains motionless, usually in a side-lying position with knees flexed.

Practice Alert

The most predictive signs and symptoms of acute appendicitis are pain in the right lower quadrant, abdominal rigidity, and migration of pain from the periumbilical region to the right lower quadrant. The nurse assessing these signs or symptoms should immediately report the findings to the primary care provider for urgent interventions.

Sudden relief of abdominal pain usually means that the appendix has ruptured. Notify the physician immediately if the child reports sudden relief of pain.

Assess vital signs for indications of septic shock and peritonitis. Additional signs and symptoms of a ruptured appendix include:

- Fever
- Guarding
- Abdominal distention
- Rapid shallow breathing
- Pallor
- Chills
- Irritability or restlessness

Collaborative Care

The focus of collaborative care includes early identification of appendicitis, pain management, surgical removal of the appendix, and prevention of complications.

Diagnostic Tests

Appendicitis should be suspected in any child with pain in the right lower quadrant. Diagnosis of appendicitis in young children can be difficult because their pain may be less localized and their symptoms more diffuse than in the older child. Continuing evaluations over several hours are often needed to establish diagnosis.

Numerous conditions (e.g., ectopic pregnancy, sickle cell crisis, gastroenteritis, pelvic inflammatory disease) mimic appendicitis and should be considered during the process of diagnosis. The presence of fever and an elevated white blood cell count (above $10,000/mm^3$) generally occur in appendicitis. In the opening scenario, Jenna had a WBC count of $22,000/mm^3$ which was clearly indicative of infection. In addition to these symptoms, a history of midabdominal pain migrating to the right lower quadrant along with rebound tenderness is highly indicative of appendicitis (Surawicz, 2008). Abdominal ultrasound and computed tomography (CT) are both useful in the diagnosis of appendicitis. Ultrasound is preferred by some healthcare providers as the initial screening tool; however, CT scans are more sensitive and should be used in cases where the appendix cannot be seen well on ultrasound or the results are inconclusive (Schwartz, 2008; Zilbert, Stamell, Ezon, et al., 2009).

Clinical Therapy

Treatment involves immediate surgical removal (appendectomy), either through laparoscopic or open method (IPEG, 2008b). Preoperatively the child is kept NPO. Intravenous fluids, electrolytes, and antibiotics are administered. Postoperatively the child has an abdominal incision, and intravenous antibiotics may be administered to prevent infection. The child with uncomplicated appendicitis will generally be discharged the next day.

With ruptured appendix, some surgeons prefer to close the wound, whereas others leave the wound open (delayed primary closure), with or without placement of drains. If the wound is left open, it is packed with sterile saline-soaked gauze. Regardless of whether the wound is left opened or is closed, the child may have a nasogastric tube to decompress the abdomen and will remain NPO until signs of bowel

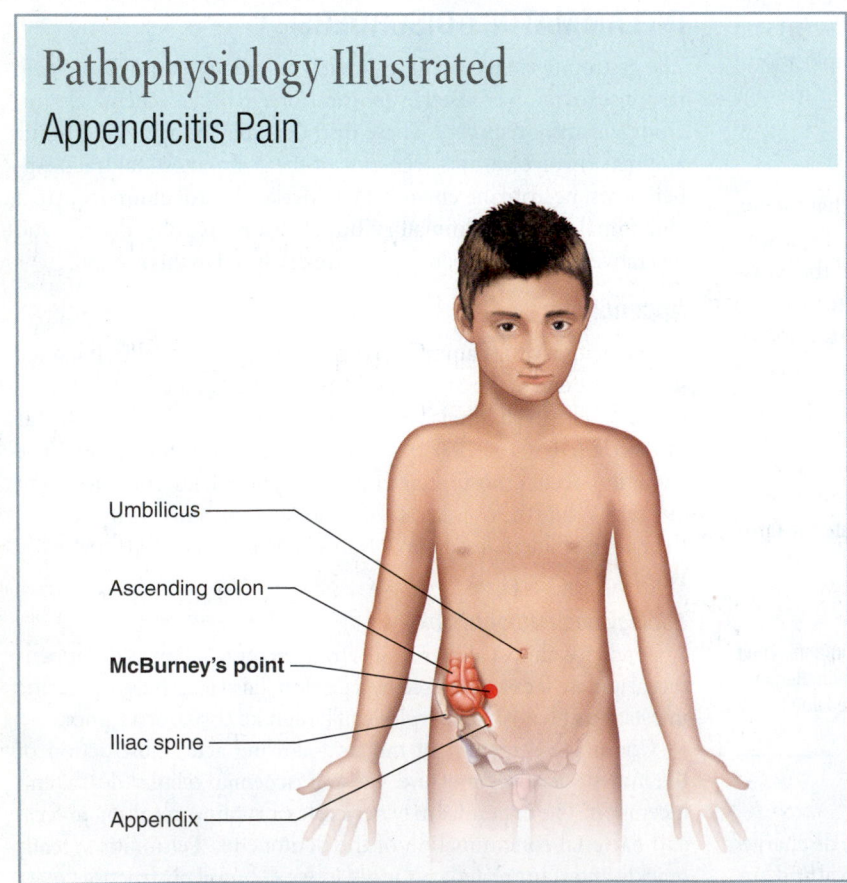

Pathophysiology Illustrated
Appendicitis Pain

Umbilicus

Ascending colon

McBurney's point

Iliac spine

Appendix

FIGURE 30–15 ■ Common location of pain in children and adolescents with appendicitis.

| BOX 30–1 | Research: Antibiotics for Ruptured Appendix |

A prospective randomized trial compared the cost-effectiveness and efficacy of a triple antibiotic regimen of ampicillin, gentamicin, and clindamycin (AGC) to a once-daily dosing of ceftriaxone and metronidazole (CM) for postoperative management of a ruptured appendix. The AGC and CM group each had 100 children with a ruptured appendix. All patients received intravenous antibiotics for at least 5 days. Patients in the AGC group received ampicillin every 6 hours, gentamicin every 8 hours, and clindamycin every 6 hours. Patients in the CM group received one dose of ceftriaxone and one dose of metronidazole daily. Results of the study showed no difference between the two groups in abscess rate, length of hospitalization, or time to oral intake. Significantly higher charges for antibiotics were reported in the AGC group and for the required average of three lab draws to monitor gentamicin levels. The authors concluded that once-daily dosing of ceftriaxone and metronidazole was equal to triple antibiotic therapy in controlling infection in children with a ruptured appendix. Also, CM was more cost-effective and easier for patients and caregivers (St. Peter, Tsao, Spilde, et al., 2008).

function return. Bowel function is best indicated by the passage of flatus or stool. The child will also have a peripheral or temporary central line for administration of intravenous fluids and medications. After surgery for a ruptured appendix, the child will receive antibiotics for several days. The regimen varies among surgeons (Box 30–1). Morphine is generally given for pain. For the child whose wound was left open, the wound will be closed under sedation in about 5 days.

In some cases, where an abscess is formed secondary to rupture of the appendix, the surgeon may choose to place a percutaneous drain, begin broad-spectrum antibiotics, and remove the appendix at a later time. This process is referred to as an interval appendectomy (Santacroce & Ochoa, 2011).

Nursing Management

Nursing management includes collaborative identification of the child with appendicitis, preoperative and postoperative care, and prevention of complications.

Nursing Assessment and Diagnosis

Physiologic Assessment

Preoperatively, a detailed assessment of the child's pain is necessary to differentiate appendicitis from other illnesses (see Chapter 21 🔗). Ask the child to point to the painful area and describe the pain. Recognize that localizing the pain may be difficult for young children. Note onset, location, and intensity of pain; precipitating factors; and relief measures tried. Remember to inspect, auscultate, and then palpate gently to identify distention and areas of pain. Rebound tenderness can also be assessed. Deep palpation of the left side of the abdomen followed by removing the hand quickly can lead to pain in the area of the appendix (rebound tenderness). However, once appendicitis is suspected or verified, avoid abdominal palpation to minimize pain to the child.

Assess vital signs to determine baseline values, and monitor at least every 4 hours thereafter. Ask about the last food and fluid intake and any vomiting that has occurred. Assess history of previous surgeries or abdominal conditions.

Postoperatively, assess fluid volume status every 2 hours. Assess skin turgor, eyes, and mucous membranes for signs of dehydration. Monitor intake and output. Assess for signs of return of bowel function. Assess for pain using the appropriate scale. (See Chapter 21 🔗 for pain assessment and pain management.) Pay careful attention to the wound site for signs of infection such as increased redness or drainage. Vital signs should be monitored at least every 4 hours. Temperature change may be indicative of infection.

Psychosocial Assessment

Because appendicitis usually occurs in school-age children and adolescents, assessment of the child's coping skills is important. Adolescents, because of their preoccupation with body image, may be concerned about the surgical incision scar if open appendectomy is performed. Assess the parents' and child's anxiety about the sudden hospitalization and need for emergency surgery.

Following are nursing diagnoses that may be appropriate for the child with appendicitis:

- Pain, Acute related to inflammation and surgery
- Fluid Volume: Deficient, Risk for related to fluid volume loss and inadequate fluid volume intake
- Anxiety (Parental and Child) related to acute physical condition and need for surgery
- Infection, Risk for related to surgical procedure
- Airway Clearance, Ineffective related to decreased mobility and refusal to cough

NANDA-I © 2012

Planning and Intervention

Nursing care focuses on promoting comfort, maintaining hydration, providing emotional support, supporting respiratory function, providing care of the surgical site, and monitoring for symptoms of infection.

Promote Comfort

Preoperatively, a right side-lying position with knees bent is usually the most comfortable. If the appendix has ruptured, lying on the right side helps the peritoneal cavity drain and facilitates comfort. Allow the child to assume any position that promotes comfort. Ask the family what might be comforting for the child such as music, gently stroking the back, or having family present. Administer analgesics as ordered and note relief from pain.

Postoperatively, the child should be placed in a semi-Fowler or side-lying position on the right side. The child with a ruptured appendix will require intravenous pain medication on a regular basis and prior to scheduled dressing changes if the wound was left open. The child who has an appendectomy for uncomplicated appendicitis will need oral or intravenous pain management for postoperative pain control.

Practice Alert

Be alert to the child who does not complain of pain postoperatively following surgery for a ruptured appendix. This child needs adequate pain medication. While the child may not verbally complain of pain, he or she will cry when approached and will resist or refuse to move in the bed. Proper pain management will facilitate the child's recovery and will help prevent respiratory complications related to immobilization.

Maintain Hydration

An intravenous infusion is initiated preoperatively and continued until bowel function returns after surgery. Once bowel sounds return and after the nasogastric tube has been removed, offer water in small amounts and then other clear fluids. The child should be monitored closely for nausea after beginning to take oral fluids.

Practice Alert

When a child has a nasogastric tube in place, the nurse must keep an accurate measurement of the amount of output from the tube so that adequate fluid replacement can be given. Loss of large amounts of stomach contents without fluid replacement may lead to metabolic alkalosis. Infants are especially at risk for acid–base imbalances. The nurse should be alert to an increase in nasogastric drainage postoperatively, as this drainage should decrease over time. Any concerns should be reported promptly to the physician.

Provide Emotional Support

For many children, appendicitis may be the reason for their first hospitalization and only experience with healthcare personnel other than their primary care provider. The nurse must elicit a history, perform a physical examination, coordinate diagnostic tests, and prepare the child for surgery in a short period of time. Emotional support is essential for both the child and parents. Good preoperative education can reduce anxiety. Answer any questions the child or parents may have.

Support Respiratory Function

General anesthesia during surgery compromises respiratory function. It is important for the child to turn, cough, and breathe deeply to prevent atelectasis. While the child with uncomplicated appendicitis is usually willing to get out of bed and walk soon after surgery, the child with a ruptured appendix is generally hesitant to move and may need to be repositioned by family or staff. The child will need to get out of bed as soon as his or her condition allows and walk two to three times a day to decrease the risk of pulmonary complications and decrease recovery time. Provide adequate analgesia and encourage the child to splint the incision area with a pillow during coughing to decrease pain. Incentive spirometry is frequently ordered for the child. Consider Jenna in the opening scenario. What activities would be appropriate to prevent respiratory complications?

Clinical Tip

Young children may be resistant to incentive spirometry or may be too young to understand the procedure. An effective alternative approach is to give the child bubbles or a pinwheel to blow. Praise and rewards such as stickers each time the child completes the task will likely increase compliance with the procedure and decrease the likelihood of complications.

Recognize Symptoms of Infection

Assess vital signs and observe the abdominal incision every 4 hours for redness, edema, or drainage. If a drain is present, assess drainage for color, consistency, and amount. The amount of drainage from the wound should decrease gradually as the wound heals. If the appendix was ruptured, the child will be hospitalized for several days for intravenous antibiotics. The child with an open wound will require wet to dry dressing changes two to three times a day, depending on physician orders. The wound is generally closed after a few days and prior to discharge.

Discharge Planning and Home Care Teaching

The child with uncomplicated appendicitis is discharged once bowel function returns and he or she has a bowel movement. Give parents instructions on reestablishing a nutritious diet slowly and as tolerated. Teach parents to recognize the signs and symptoms of infection and to seek early treatment.

Normal activities can be resumed fairly quickly, but the child should avoid strenuous activities and contact sports in the immediate postoperative period. Parents should check with the child's physician before allowing the child to resume sports activities. Home tutoring may be needed for a short time so the child can keep up with schoolwork.

Evaluation

Expected outcomes of nursing care include the following:

- The child's pain is effectively managed.
- The child demonstrates effective airway clearance.
- The wound heals without the development of a secondary infection.
- Adequate hydration is achieved and maintained.

Necrotizing Enterocolitis

Necrotizing enterocolitis (NEC) is a potentially life-threatening inflammatory disease of the intestinal tract that occurs primarily in premature infants. NEC is one of the most common gastrointestinal disorders that affects infants in the neonatal intensive care unit (Bradshaw, 2009). While the overall incidence is 1 in 1,000 live births, NEC affects up to 7% of very-low-birth-weight infants and is associated with a mortality rate of 15% to 30% in this population of infants. The disease occurs most often in the ileum (Berman & Moss, 2011).

Early aggressive enteral formula feeding of premature infants is avoided because of the increased incidence of the disease in these cases. Human milk has been shown to protect against the disease; thus, breastfeeding or feeding the mother's expressed milk is the feeding method of choice for premature infants.

Etiology and Pathophysiology

The etiology of NEC is multifactorial. Included are intestinal ischemia, bacterial or viral infection (a result of the premature infant's decreased immune response and greater risk for infection), and immaturity of the gastrointestinal mucosa (Bradshaw, 2009; Morgan, Young, & McGuire, 2011).

Vascular compromise, leading to hypoxia and ischemia, causes a reduced blood flow to the bowel, leading to necrosis of the bowel mucosa. The damaged bowel stops secreting protective enzymes, allowing gas-forming bacteria to invade the necrotic tissue. This bacterial invasion further damages the intestinal mucosa by releasing bacterial toxins and gas, causing abdominal distention. The infant is at risk for intestinal perforation.

Clinical Manifestations

Manifestations generally occur during the second week of life after enteral feedings are started; however, NEC can develop before feedings are started, after several weeks of life, and long after feedings are started (Berman & Moss, 2011). The infant may initially show signs of feeding intolerance (increased gastric residuals, vomiting, irritability, and abdominal distention). These signs are caused by inflammation and dilation of the bowel and accumulation of gas in the intestine. Bloody diarrhea may be present because of the hemorrhagic bowel. The condition progresses to lethargy and then episodes of apnea and bradycardia as the infant develops sepsis (Bradshaw, 2009).

Practice Alert
The infant with NEC is at risk of developing sepsis. Signs of sepsis in the newborn or premature infant include:

- Hypothermia or hyperthermia
- Jaundice
- Respiratory distress
- Hepatomegaly
- Abdominal distention
- Anorexia
- Vomiting
- Lethargy

Report these symptoms to the primary healthcare provider immediately.

Collaborative Care

The goals of collaborative care are to identify and reduce risk factors that lead to necrotizing enterocolitis, to immediately identify and aggressively manage the disorder, and to prevent complications.

Diagnostic Tests

Diagnosis is made on the basis of characteristic clinical findings and the presence of free peritoneal gas, dilated bowel loops, bowel distention, and bowel wall thickening on abdominal radiographs. Stools and emesis are monitored for occult blood. Laboratory data reveal anemia, leukopenia, leukocytosis, thrombocytopenia, electrolyte imbalance, and metabolic or respiratory acidosis. Blood cultures are positive for the organism present.

Clinical Therapy

Necrotizing enterocolitis requires prompt intervention to decrease the morbidity and mortality associated with this illness. Treatment includes bowel rest (NPO status), gastric decompression with nasogastric suction and antibiotic therapy (Gregory et al, 2011; Rapoport & Nishii, 2013: Wright & Miller, 2012). The infant will need central venous access to provide nutrition (Rapoport & Nishii, 2013). Serial radiographs of the abdomen should be performed to detect worsening or resolution of the disease process (Wright & Miller, 2012). Perforation or necrosis of the bowel necessitates surgical resection of the bowel. An ileostomy or colostomy may be performed.

All cases of necrotizing enterocolitis are treated with strict enteric precautions to prevent the spread of infection to other premature infants on the unit.

Long-term complications of necrotizing enterocolitis include short bowel syndrome, strictures, **cholestasis** (disruption of bile flow), impaired nutrition and growth, and delayed developmental performance.

Practice Alert
Cholestasis is a disruption of bile flow, and it is the most common problem in survivors of necrotizing enterocolitis. It is a complication of total parenteral nutrition (TPN) and commonly occurs 2 weeks after TPN therapy has been initiated. It is characterized by hyperbilirubinemia, hepatomegaly, and elevated serum aminotransferase levels (Moyer & Balistreri, 2011).

Nursing Management

Nursing care centers on prevention and early detection of NEC to minimize bowel loss, postoperative care, and family support.

BOX 30–2	Research: Necrotizing Enterocolitis Treatment

Studies continue to demonstrate the effectiveness of supplementation with **probiotics,** live and beneficial microorganisms that promote normal gut flora, in the prevention of necrotizing enterocolitis. *Lactobacillus acidophilus* and *Bifidobacterium infantis* are examples of organisms that can be administered by special formula (Bradshaw, 2009; Martin & Walker, 2008).

Nursing Assessment and Diagnosis

Observe for feeding intolerance by aspirating gastric residual (if the infant is receiving enteral feedings). Measure abdominal circumference and assess bowel sounds in the premature or high-risk infant every 4 to 8 hours. Even minimal changes in circumference can indicate NEC and should be reported to the primary care provider. Careful monitoring of vital signs and intake and output is essential to detect complications.

Nursing diagnoses that apply to the infant with NEC may include:

- Infection, Risk for related to presence of organisms
- Fluid Volume: Deficient, Risk for related to NPO status
- Perfusion: Gastrointestinal, Risk for Ineffective related to vascular compromise
- Nutrition, Imbalanced: Less than Body Requirements related to disease process and NPO status
- Attachment, Risk for Impaired Parent/Infant related to critically ill status of newborn

NANDA-I © 2012

Planning and Implementation

Maintaining fluid and electrolyte balance is essential. Provide comfort by holding and cuddling an infant who is NPO, and offer a pacifier to meet nonnutritive sucking needs. Careful assessment for infection and maintenance of skin integrity are essential. Feedings are gradually reestablished once bowel function returns. Administration of probiotics may be part of therapy (Box 30–2).

Because the symptoms of necrotizing enterocolitis may not appear until several days after feedings begin, parents may not be prepared for the infant's decline. Recovery is slow and can be complicated. Give clear explanations and encourage parents to ask questions and express their fears and concerns. Offer support for the parents of a child with a poor prognosis (see Chapters 17 and 18 ⊘).

Once the child is discharged, frequent follow-up is needed. Parents need specific education related to feedings, medications, and any other treatments prescribed. The infant requires regular and thorough physical assessments to check weight gain, assess development, and identify signs of complications. If the child had to have an ostomy created, the family must be taught ostomy care (see page 1014).

The infant requires regular and thorough physical assessments to identify any complications. Growth of the child is monitored and compared with previous findings. Developmental progress is assessed by regular administration of a developmental test such as the Denver II (see Chapter 8 ⊘).

Evaluation

Expected outcomes of nursing care for the child with necrotizing enterocolitis include:

- The child is free of signs and symptoms of infection.
- Fluid and electrolyte balance is achieved and maintained.
- Tissue perfusion is maintained following surgical removal of necrotic bowel.

- The child consumes adequate nutrition to support growth and development needs.

If surgery is performed, complete healing without infection or other complication is desired. If the infant is not successfully treated, support and comfort for the parents is necessary. When the child survives, desired long-term outcomes include normal developmental progression and nutrition to support growth.

Meckel's Diverticulum

Meckel's diverticulum results when the omphalomesenteric duct, which connects the midgut to the yolk sac during embryonic development, fails to atrophy. Instead, an outpouching of the ileum remains, usually located near the ileocecal valve. The pouch contains gastric or pancreatic tissue, which secretes acid, causing irritation and ulceration. Meckel's diverticulum is one of the most common GI malformations and occurs in 1-4% of the population(Pepper, et al, 2012).

Clinical manifestations usually appear by 2 years of age. Meckel's diverticulum most commonly presents as a gastrointestinal bleeding or obstruction. The child generally presents with bloody stool, irritability, fatigue, abdominal pain and distention, nausea and vomiting (Pepper, et al, 2012).

Collaborative Care

Diagnostic testing for Meckel's diverticulum depends on the presentation and includes laboratory analysis to evaluate for the presence of anemia and dehydration (Pepper, et al, 2012). Imaging studies are also used to assist in the diagnosis and include radiographs, ultrasound, CT scan, and radionuclide scanning (Kotecha, Bellah, Pena, et al, 2012). A Technetium-99m pertechnetate nuclear medicine (also called a Meckel scan) is the current imaging test of choice for a bleeding diverticulum (Pepper, et al, 2012).

Treatment is surgical excision of the diverticulum and removal of any involved bowel. The prognosis is good following surgical excision.

Nursing Management

Preoperatively an intravenous infusion is initiated to correct fluid and electrolyte imbalances. Monitor intake and output. Observe for rectal bleeding and test stools for **occult blood** (blood that is present in small quantities and measurable only by laboratory testing). Keep the child on bed rest. Assess vital signs every 2 hours, and monitor for signs of shock.

Postoperative care is similar to that for an infant or child undergoing abdominal surgery. (See the earlier discussion of postsurgical nursing management of appendicitis and the Nursing Care Plan for the child undergoing surgery in Chapter 15 🔗.)

Recurrent Abdominal Pain

Recurrent abdominal pain (RAP) is a frequent problem among young children and adolescents, particularly school-age girls. The disorder affects approximately 12% of children and adolescents (Wendland, Jackson, & Stokes, 2010). This disorder is associated with the high-stress lifestyles common in contemporary society and has a strong environmental component. However, parents and healthcare professionals should not dismiss the child's pain because the cause is unknown or unidentified.

The pain is generally located in the periumbilical area and occurs on a regular basis. A thorough history and physical examination are necessary to rule out organic causes. The history should explore the pressures and stresses in the child's life, the child's temperament or methods of coping, bowel elimination patterns, and history of sexual abuse.

Laboratory studies such as a complete blood count may be ordered to rule out other illness. Gastrointestinal studies may be performed in an outpatient setting. Children are occasionally hospitalized when their condition is severe and not treatable at home.

When no organic cause can be identified, treatment of recurrent abdominal pain focuses on providing outlets for the release of stress within the family and in other settings in the child's life, enhancing the child's coping methods, and promoting dietary changes that encourage regular bowel movements. Social learning and cognitive behavioral therapies that include relaxation training have proven effective in decreasing parent-reported episodes of pain in the child (Levy, Langer, Walker, et al., 2010).

Nursing Management

Nursing care includes supporting the child during assessment and diagnostic testing. The child can be taught relaxation techniques and methods for coping with stress. Identify what life events are stressors for the child and ask about specific worries. Ask about school and anxiety related to friendships, grades, and activities. Explore methods for giving more independence to the child in the family. Teach the importance of eating a high-fiber diet and maintaining a regular elimination pattern. The child and family may need explanations to understand the pain, which can be compared with neck pain or a headache as an outcome of stress. Children with continuing or recurrent abdominal pain are referred to a mental health professional.

Inflammatory Bowel Disease

Inflammatory bowel disease (IBD) encompasses two distinct chronic disorders, Crohn disease and ulcerative colitis, that have similar symptoms and treatment (see the Clinical Manifestations table). Inflammatory bowel disease differs from irritable bowel syndrome. See Box 30–3.

Etiology and Pathophysiology

Genetic and environmental factors are involved in the development of inflammatory bowel disease. Onset of both of these disorders is most common in adolescence and young adulthood, but either disease can begin in early childhood (Grossman & Baldassano, 2011).

Crohn disease Crohn disease is a chronic, inflammatory process. The disorder can occur randomly throughout the GI tract, with the ileum, colon, and rectum as the most common sites. A distinct feature of Crohn disease is the development of enteric fistulas between loops of bowel or nearby organs. Mucosal ulcers begin in small locations and

---

BOX 30–3	Irritable Bowel Syndrome

Irritable bowel syndrome (IBS) refers to a functional disorder of the gastrointestinal tract that is characterized as chronic and episodic. There is no structural cause, but it seems to be triggered by events such as gastroenteritis or major life events or stressors. Other causative factors may include stress, diet, drugs, and alcohol. IBS is characterized by episodes of abdominal cramping and pain, diarrhea or constipation, bloating, and nausea and vomiting (Holloway, 2010). Management generally focuses on the symptoms. A change in lifestyle and diet might be effective in decreasing the frequency of symptoms. Medications such as antispasmodics, antimotility agents, and laxatives may also be used (Reed, 2010).

Clinical Manifestations Ulcerative Colitis and Crohn Disease

	ULCERATIVE COLITIS	CROHN DISEASE
Type of lesions	Continuous, superficial involvement	Segmental, transmural (through the wall) involvement
Clinical Manifestations		
Anal or perianal lesions	Rare	Common
Anorexia	Mild to moderate	Can be severe
Diarrhea	Often severe	Moderate
Growth retardation	Mild	Significant
Pain	Present	Common
Rectal bleeding	Present	Absent
Weight loss	Moderate	Severe
Risk of cancer	Slightly increased	Greatly increased

then grow in size and depth into the mucosal wall. Submucosal inflammation can be severe. The etiology is unknown. There is strong evidence to support a genetic association. Crohn disease is more common in Whites than in Blacks. It is rare in Asian and Hispanic populations (Grossman & Mamula, 2011). It most often develops in adolescents and young adults. Pediatric Crohn disease has an incidence of approximately 4.56 per 100,000 (Grossman & Baldassano, 2011). Complications associated with Crohn disease include perforation, hemorrhage, strictures, fistulas, liver disease, and toxic megacolon.

Ulcerative colitis Ulcerative colitis is a chronic recurrent disease of the large intestine and rectal mucosa, of unknown etiology. Inflammation is limited to the mucosa, as opposed to Crohn disease, which extends deep into the bowel wall. Ulcerative colitis can involve the entire length of the bowel with varying degrees of inflammation, ulceration, hemorrhage, and edema. Emotional and other psychosocial factors may influence the presentation and course of the disease. It is more prevalent among persons of Jewish heritage. The disease develops before 20 years of age with peak onset at about 12 years. Ulcerative colitis develops in 15 out of 100,000 individuals in the United States (Grossman & Baldassano, 2011).

Complications associated with ulcerative colitis include hemorrhage, sepsis, toxic megacolon, and increased incidence of cancer.

Clinical Manifestations

The onset of *Crohn disease* is subtle. Cramping abdominal pain is usually reported first, followed by diarrhea. Other symptoms include fever, anorexia, growth failure or weight loss, general malaise, and joint pain.

The first symptom of *ulcerative colitis* is usually diarrhea. Lower abdominal pain and cramping are present before and during a bowel movement and are relieved by the passage of stool and flatus. The stool is often mixed with blood and mucus. Weight loss or delayed growth, nutritional deficiencies, and arthralgias often occur as effects of the disease.

Collaborative Care

Collaborative care focuses on promoting remission of the disease, optimal nutritional intake, and optimal growth and development.

Diagnostic Tests

Diagnosis centers on evaluating the cause, identifying the extent of involved bowel, and differentiating an infectious process (organisms such as *Shigella* and *Salmonella*) from inflammatory bowel disease.

Endoscopy with biopsy is helpful to determine the extent and severity of the inflammatory process. Laboratory and bone age studies help to identify related nutritional, electrolyte, and blood abnormalities.

Anemia, an elevated erythrocyte sedimentation rate, hypoalbuminemia, and thrombocytosis are other possible findings. Stools are positive for occult blood (Glick & Carvalho, 2011). Testing for antineutrophil cytoplasmic antibodies (ANCA), anti-*Saccharomyces cerevisiae* antibodies (ASCA), and outer membrane protein of *Escherichia coli* (Anti Omp C) is helpful in differentiating between ulcerative colitis and Crohn disease. A positive ANCA is present in approximately 60% to 80% of children who have ulcerative colitis and in around 18% to 24% of those with Crohn disease. A positive ASCA is present in 40% to 60% of those with Crohn disease as compared to 0% to 7% of those with ulcerative colitis. Anti Omp C is present in 25% of those with Crohn disease as compared to 6% of those with ulcerative colitis (Glick & Carvalho, 2011). Imaging studies assist in the diagnosis of inflammatory bowel disease and in distinguishing ulcerative colitis from Crohn disease. An upper GI series, CT scan, or MRI may be performed. Endoscopy and colonoscopy with biopsy are essential in confirming the diagnosis of IBD (Glick & Carvalho, 2011).

Clinical Therapy

Crohn disease and ulcerative colitis have periods of remission and exacerbation. Treatment for both diseases includes pharmacologic interventions, nutrition therapy, and in severe cases, surgery.

First-line pharmacologic treatment of Crohn disease involves aminosalicylates. Sulfasalazine inhibits prostaglandin synthesis, thereby decreasing inflammation. Corticosteroids and immunosuppressants are used in children with moderate to severe disease. Biological therapies such as infliximab (Remicade) have been effective in patients with Crohn disease and ulcerative colitis who fail to respond to other therapies (Glick & Carvalho, 2011). See the Medications table on page 1022. Some patients with IBD use probiotics as an additional treatment measure.

A nutritionist is part of the team treating the child. The goal of nutrition therapy is to provide adequate caloric intake and nutrients necessary for growth. Vitamin, iron, zinc, and folic acid supplementation is frequently required. Total parenteral nutrition (TPN) is often given to treat nutritional deficiencies and malnutrition, which accompany inflammatory bowel disease. A high-protein, high-carbohydrate, low-fiber diet with normal amounts of fat is recommended.

If other treatment measures fail to reduce inflammation, surgery is generally indicated. Bowel obstruction, perianal disease, abdominal abscess, and strictures are the most common reasons for surgical intervention. A temporary colostomy or ileostomy is performed to allow the bowel to rest. In Crohn disease, however, ulcerations tend to recur elsewhere in the GI tract. In ulcerative colitis, removal of the diseased bowel provides a permanent cure.

Nursing Management

Nursing management occurs mainly in the community and home and focuses on helping the child and family adjust to the emotional impact of a chronic disease, administering medications and diet therapy, monitoring nutritional status, monitoring growth status, and providing appropriate referrals.

Nursing Assessment and Diagnosis

Assess for abdominal distention, tenderness, and pain. Monitor bowel sounds and stool pattern; measure abdominal girth.

Medications Used to Treat Inflammatory Bowel Disease

MEDICATION	INDICATION	NURSING MANAGEMENT
Aminosalicylates	Used for anti-inflammatory effect	Administer after meals.
■ Sulfasalazine ■ Mesalamine	Inhibition of prostaglandins known to cause diarrhea and affect mucosal transport	Do not crush or chew sustained-release tablets. Teach the patient or parents to supplement daily intake of iron. Monitor for side effects: ■ Nausea and vomiting ■ Rash ■ Bloody diarrhea ■ Headache ■ Anorexia
Corticosteroids	Used for anti-inflammatory effect	Administer oral medications with meals to reduce gastric irritation. Teach family to avoid abrupt discontinuation of medication. Teach family to report delayed wound healing. Monitor for side effects:
■ Prednisone ■ Prednisolone ■ Hydrocortisone ■ Budesonide		■ Nausea ■ Growth suppression ■ Vomiting ■ Hypertension ■ Cushingoid appearance ■ Acne ■ Immunosuppression ■ Altered moods
Immunosuppressants	Used for immunosuppressive effect	Monitor for side effects:
■ 6-Mercaptopurine (6-MP) ■ Azathioprine ■ Cyclosporine ■ Methotrexate		■ Nausea ■ Bone marrow suppression ■ Vomiting ■ Infection ■ Anorexia ■ Mucositis ■ Diarrhea Teach family to avoid exposing the child to persons with infection. Teach family the importance of good hygiene for the child to avoid infection.
Biological therapies	Prevents TNF-alpha from binding to its receptors (TNF-alpha has been found in stools of patients with Crohn disease)	Reconstitute IV preparation according to manufacturer directions and administer according to agency protocol. Monitor for side effects: Infusion reactions—fever, chills, chest pain, hypotension, dyspnea, urticaria Discontinue IV infusion if infusion reaction is evident.
■ Infliximab (Remicade) ■ Adalimumab (Humira) ■ Certolizumab (Cimzia)		
Antibiotics	Antibacterial against anaerobic bacteria and some gram-negative bacteria in patients with Crohn disease	Extended-release form should not be chewed or crushed. Administer with food or milk to reduce gastrointestinal distress. Monitor for side effects:
■ Metronidazole ■ Ciprofloxacin		■ Fever ■ Nausea ■ Headache ■ Vomiting ■ Diarrhea ■ Fungal overgrowth

Source: *Data from Baumgart, D. C. (2009). The diagnosis and treatment of Crohn disease and ulcerative colitis.* Deutsches Ärzteblatt International, 106(8), 123–133; Glick, S. R., & Carvalho, R. S. (2011). *Inflammatory bowel disease.* Pediatrics in Review, 32(1), 14–25; Leso, V., Leggio, L., Armuzzi, A., Gasbarrini, G., Gasbarinni, A., & Addolorato, G. (2010). Role of the tumor necrosis factor antagonists in the treatment of inflammatory bowel disease: An update. *European Journal of Gastroenterology and Hepatology, 22(7), 779–786; Peyrin-Biroulet, L. (2011). Why should we define and target early Crohn disease?* Gastroenterology & Hepatology, 7(5), 324–326; Wong, K., & Bressler, B. (2008). *Mild to moderate Crohn disease: An evidence-based treatment algorithm.* Drugs 2008, 68(17), 2419–2425.

Nursing diagnoses that apply to the child with inflammatory bowel disease may include:

- Diarrhea related to disease process
- Nutrition, Imbalanced: Less than Body Requirements related to bowel inflammation and poor nutritional intake
- Pain, Acute or Chronic related to inflammatory disease process
- Fluid Volume, Deficient, Risk for related to loss of fluids through diarrhea
- Body Image, Disturbed related to disease process, presence of stoma, and medication side effects

NANDA-I © 2012

Planning and Implementation

Provide emotional support and counseling to help the child adjust to feeling "different" from peers. Inability to compete with peers and frequent absences from school can affect the child's self-esteem. Collaborate with parents regarding care and assist them in contacting the school district to arrange for tutoring in case extended absences from school become necessary. Encourage the child who is not attending school regularly to maintain contact with friends through telephone calls, texting, e-mail, cards, and visits.

Body image is a major concern for children and adolescents with inflammatory bowel disease. Corticosteroid therapy causes growth

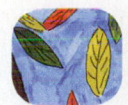

Partnering with Families

Dietary Instructions for Inflammatory Bowel Disease

Families require information regarding dietary accommodations for the child with inflammatory bowel disease. Provide families with the following information:

- Several small feedings are usually better tolerated than three meals daily.
- Limiting fiber intake can help to decrease intestine motility and inflammation. Peel fruits and avoid large quantities of whole grains and nuts.
- If the child is not eating well, offer high-calorie meals. If lactose intolerance is not a problem for the particular child, then cream soups, milkshakes, puddings, and custards can be offered.

- Liquid dietary supplements may be helpful to ensure that protein and caloric requirements are met.
- Watch for foods that cause intestinal problems for the individual child, and avoid them in the future.
- Avoid having mealtime become a reason for family strife. Seek help of nurses and dietitians if needed.

retardation and delayed sexual maturation. Encourage the child to discuss feelings about these side effects. If a permanent colostomy or ileostomy is required, the nurse can assist the child and family to understand the need for surgical treatment. (See the discussion of ostomies earlier in this chapter.) Introduce the child and family to other children who have stomas.

Clinical Tip

Providing adequate stress reduction may be helpful in control of inflammatory bowel disease. Teach young children relaxation techniques, such as deep breathing, progressive tensing and relaxing of muscles, and visualization of favorite places. Encourage busy school-age children and teens to have quiet and restful times each day, in addition to physical activity periods. Meditation might be effective in older children and teens.

Teach parents about medication administration and diet therapy. Reinforce to both the parents and child the importance of adhering to a strict medication regimen. Emphasize that medications should be continued even when the child is asymptomatic. Discuss side effects of the drugs and what to do if any of these symptoms occur. Since immune status may be altered by steroid use, have families avoid contact with infectious diseases when the child is taking steroids. Instruct them to report any diseases and fevers the child experiences, and to report the use of steroids to all healthcare providers. Immunization schedules may need to be altered.

If the child is unable to eat or the intake of calories is insufficient to meet basic nutritional and metabolic needs, TPN will be ordered. Frequent growth measurements and nutritional evaluations must be performed. See Partnering with Families: Dietary Instructions for Inflammatory Bowel Disease.

Parents also will require instructions for TPN and care of a central venous catheter, including dressing changes, sterile and nonsterile techniques, signs of infection, how to handle infusion pumps and tubing, and how to measure the child's intake and output. Assist parents in obtaining equipment and supplies necessary for the child's care. Have parents demonstrate their mastery of care for the central venous catheter and their understanding of TPN techniques during home visits and appointments for health care.

Refer parents to social services, the visiting nurse association, and home healthcare agencies if they are not receiving any of these services. For information about inflammatory bowel disease, refer families to the Crohn's & Colitis Foundation.

Evaluation

Expected outcomes of nursing care for the child with inflammatory bowel disease include the following:

- Normal growth and development is achieved.
- The child demonstrates the ability to cope with episodes of GI distress.
- The child adheres to the medication regimen.
- There is no evidence of central line infection.
- The child has a positive body image.
- The child is able to integrate stress-lowering practices into daily life.

Peptic Ulcer

A peptic ulcer is an erosion of the mucosal tissue in the lower end of the esophagus, in the stomach (usually along the lesser curvature), or in the duodenum (*gastric ulcer* is the term sometimes used when the stomach mucosa is affected).

Etiology and Pathophysiology

Ulcers are classified as primary or secondary, depending on their etiology.

- *Primary peptic ulcers* occur in healthy children.
- *Secondary (stress) ulcers* occur in children with a preexisting illness or injury such as a burn and in children receiving medications such as salicylates, corticosteroids, and nonsteroidal anti-inflammatory drugs.

Diet usually is not a major factor in the development of peptic ulcers in children, although caffeine and alcohol consumption in adolescents may exacerbate the disease. Ulcers in both adults and children are caused by *Helicobacter pylori*, a gram-negative rod. This organism is transmitted by the fecal–oral or oral–oral route (Zagaria, 2010). Infections often occur in several members of a family, especially when the family's water supply is contaminated.

Clinical Manifestations

Clinical manifestations vary according to the age of the child and location of the ulcer. The most common symptom is abdominal pain (burning) associated with an empty stomach, which may awaken the child at night. Vomiting and pain after meals, anemia, occult blood in stools, and abdominal distention may also be present.

Weblink | Crohn's & Colitis Foundation

Collaborative Care

The goals of collaborative care are to relieve discomfort and promote healing.

Diagnostic Tests

Diagnosis is based on the history and radiologic studies. *H. pylori* can be diagnosed by culture of the organism taken via gastroscopy and by measuring urea in the urine and on the breath, since the organism hydrolyzes urea.

Clinical Therapy

When *H. pylori* is the causative agent, treatment regimens may include a proton pump inhibitor such as lansoprazole or omeprazole; two antibiotics such as clarithromycin, amoxicillin, metronidazole, and tetracycline; and a bismuth salt (Zagaria, 2010). Patients should be retested 4 weeks after treatment is completed. If the organism is still present, a regimen using different antibiotics should be implemented (Sherman, 2009). The prognosis is usually good with early intervention.

Nursing Management

Nursing Assessment and Diagnosis

Assess the child for abdominal pain, vomiting, and abdominal distention. Assess for family history of *H. pylori* infection.

Nursing diagnoses that may apply to the child with peptic ulcer include:

- Pain, Acute or Chronic related to erosion of gastric mucosal tissue
- Nutrition, Imbalanced: Less than Body Requirements related to decreased food consumption, vomiting, and nausea
- Coping, Ineffective (Child) related to perceived stressful situations

NANDA-I © 2012

Planning and Implementation

Nursing care centers on interventions to promote adequate nutritional intake, promote healing, and prevent recurrences. A nutritionally sound, age-appropriate diet is provided. Foods should be omitted only if they exacerbate the disorder.

Partner with the family and explain that antibiotics must be administered as scheduled. The family needs encouragement to continue the medications as ordered and to return for follow-up visits. Parents should discuss any additional medications with the primary healthcare provider before administering to the child. Caution parents to avoid ibuprofen, which irritates the gastric mucosa. If an antipyretic or pain medication is needed, acetaminophen should be given. Advise parents to read medication labels if they are unsure of product contents.

Because psychologic stress can contribute to peptic ulcer disease, parents and child should be assisted to identify sources of stress in the child's life. Assess coping mechanisms and provide referral for psychologic counseling, if appropriate. Teach relaxation techniques and recommend community classes on yoga or other stress reduction.

Evaluation

Expected outcomes of nursing care for the child with peptic ulcer include:

- The child demonstrates evidence of pain relief and decreased episodes of pain.
- The child consumes adequate nutrition in order to meet growth and development needs.
- The child participates in stress-reducing activities.

DISORDERS OF MOTILITY

Fluids are an important part of normal gastrointestinal functioning. As food passes through the intestines, fluids are reabsorbed and moderately soft stool is formed and evacuated. In disorders such as diarrhea and constipation, fluid balance is altered, causing either more or less fluid to be reabsorbed. This can severely alter the characteristics of the stool.

Reabsorption of too little water produces diarrhea and can lead to fluid and electrolyte alterations. Reabsorption of too much fluid can cause constipation, which if untreated can lead to bowel obstruction.

Disorders affecting bowel elimination, such as constipation, encopresis, and diarrhea, are discussed in this section. Other disorders that affect bowel elimination, such as Hirschsprung disease, have been previously discussed.

Gastroenteritis (Acute Diarrhea)

Gastroenteritis is an inflammation of the stomach and intestines that may be accompanied by vomiting and diarrhea. Gastroenteritis can affect any part of the gastrointestinal tract. It may be an acute problem, caused by viral, bacterial, or parasitic infections, or a chronic problem. Rotavirus is the leading cause of severe gastroenteritis in infants and young children (Cortese & Parashar, 2009). Children under age 5 years average approximately two episodes of gastroenteritis each year. Infants and small children with gastroenteritis or diarrhea can quickly become dehydrated and are at risk for hypovolemic shock if fluid and electrolyte losses are not replaced (see Chapters 23 and 26 ✍). A significant number of infants and young children are hospitalized each year for dehydration secondary to gastroenteritis.

Etiology and Pathophysiology

Diarrhea in children is related to many different causes (Table 30–5). The specific etiology is not always identified. The common mechanism is a decrease in the absorptive capacity of the bowel through inflammation, decrease in surface area for absorption, or alteration of parasympathetic innervation. Children in childcare centers and those living in substandard housing with improper sanitation are at increased risk.

Clinical Manifestations

Diarrhea may be mild, moderate, or severe.

- In mild diarrhea, stools are slightly increased in number and have a more liquid consistency.
- In moderate diarrhea, the child has several loose or watery stools. Other symptoms include irritability, anorexia, nausea, and vomiting. Moderate diarrhea is usually self-limiting, resolving without treatment within 1 or 2 days.
- In severe diarrhea, watery stools are continuous. The child exhibits symptoms of fluid and electrolyte imbalance (see Chapter 23 ✍), has cramping, and is extremely irritable and difficult to console.

Collaborative Care

Collaborative care focuses on correcting fluid and electrolyte imbalance and restoring normal bowel elimination.

TABLE 30–5	Causes of Diarrhea in Children
ETIOLOGY	**BOWEL MANIFESTATIONS**
Emotional stress (anxiety, fatigue)	Increased motility
Intestinal infection	Inflammation of mucosa
Bacteria	Increased mucous secretion in colon
E. coli	
Salmonella	
Shigella	
Viral	
Human rotavirus	
Enteric	
Adenovirus fungal overgrowth	
Food sensitivity	Decreased digestion of food
Gluten	
Cow milk	
Food intolerance	Increased motility
Lactose	Increased mucous secretion in colon
Introduction of new foods	
Overfeeding	
Medications	Irritation and superinfection
Iron	
Antibiotics	
Colon disease	Inflammation and ulceration of intestinal walls
Colitis	
Necrotizing enterocolitis	Reduced absorption of fluid
Enterocolitis	Increased intestinal motility
Surgical alterations (short bowel syndrome)	Reduced size of colon
	Decreased absorption surface

Diagnostic Tests

Diagnosis is based on the history, physical examination, and laboratory findings. Physical examination provides a guide to the severity of dehydration. Stool cultures or other fecal testing, such as for pus and blood, may be conducted. The stool can be examined for the presence of ova, parasites, infectious organisms, viruses, fat, and undigested sugars. Laboratory evaluation of serum electrolytes and urine helps in identification of electrolyte imbalances and other deficiencies.

Clinical Therapy

Management depends on the severity of the diarrhea and fluid and electrolyte imbalances. The goal of treatment is to correct the fluid and electrolyte imbalances. For mild and moderate dehydration, oral rehydration therapy is the first intervention (see Chapter 23 ●). This may be accomplished at home or in the short-stay observation unit in a hospital.

Clinical Tip

Carbonated beverages and those containing high amounts of sugar should not be given. Fermentation of sugar in the gastrointestinal tract causes increased gas, abdominal distention, and an increased frequency of diarrhea.

For severe dehydration, rehydration is accomplished by intravenous infusion with a solution chosen to correct the specific electrolyte imbalances (see Chapter 23 ● for further information about solutions to correct dehydration). As soon as possible, clear liquids or breast milk are introduced and then the child progresses to a regular diet. Foods generally are not withheld for more than 1 or 2 days. Refer to Chapter 23 ● for discussion of fluid replacement therapy.

If bacteria or parasites cause the diarrhea, antimicrobial therapy may be prescribed. Antiemetics and antidiarrheals are generally not used in young children since they can mask the signs and symptoms of more serious illness.

Nursing Management

The focus of nursing is to prevent complications associated with diarrhea, maintain fluid and electrolyte balance, and promote comfort.

Nursing Assessment and Diagnosis

The nurse may encounter the child and family in the emergency department, urgent care center, clinic, or office. The child may be cared for over several hours at a clinic or urgent care center so that dehydration is treated with intravenous infusion and/or oral rehydration, and then sent home with instructions for parents to care for the child. A thorough history may help in identifying the cause. Ask parents about recent exposure to illnesses, use of antibiotics, travel, food and formula preparation, food sensitivities or allergies, and whether the child attends day care.

If the child is hospitalized it is important to assess onset, frequency, color, amount, and consistency of stools. If the child is also vomiting, monitor the amount and type of vomitus. Initial and ongoing physical assessment of the child focuses on observing for signs and symptoms of dehydration, which reflect underlying fluid and electrolyte status. Evaluate urinary output and specific gravity. An accurate weight must be obtained on admission and daily thereafter. Monitor vital signs every 2 to 4 hours. A febrile child has increased water loss, contributing to the dehydration. Assess skin integrity, especially in the perineal and rectal areas, and note any breakdown or rashes.

The accompanying Nursing Care Plan lists common nursing diagnoses for a child with gastroenteritis. The following diagnoses may also be appropriate:

- Anxiety (Child and Parent) related to change in health status
- Sleep Pattern, Disturbed related to pain
- Nutrition, Imbalanced Less than Body Requirements related to inability to ingest sufficient nutrients

NANDA-I © 2012

Planning and Implementation

Nursing care focuses on providing emotional support, promoting rest and comfort, and ensuring adequate nutrition. The accompanying Nursing Care Plan summarizes nursing care for the child with gastroenteritis.

Practice Alert

When a child has a diaper containing both urine and stool, it is essential that the nurse record the total volume. This will give an accurate measure to the amount of fluid the child is actually losing and lead to appropriate treatment as needed. In addition to amount, color and consistency should also be recorded.

Provide Emotional Support

The child may have been ill for several days or become suddenly ill a short time before seeking health care. The child and parents are

Nursing Care Plan The Child with Gastroenteritis

INTERVENTION	RATIONALE	EXPECTED OUTCOME
1. Nursing Diagnosis: Diarrhea related to infectious process		

INTERVENTION	RATIONALE	EXPECTED OUTCOME
NIC Priority Intervention—*Diarrhea Management:* Prevention and alleviation of diarrhea		**NOC Suggested Outcome**—*Fluid and Electrolyte Balance:* Balance of water and electrolytes in the intracellular and extracellular compartments of the body

GOAL: *The child's bowel function will be restored to normal.*

INTERVENTION	RATIONALE	EXPECTED OUTCOME
■ Obtain baseline vital signs and monitor every 2–4 hours.	■ Fluid and electrolyte imbalances can alter vital body functions.	The child's bowel function returns to normal.
■ Observe stools for amount, color, consistency, odor, and frequency.	■ Observation of stools aids in the diagnosis and in monitoring the child's status.	
■ Test stools for occult blood.	■ Frequent defecation and some infectious organisms can cause bleeding.	
■ Monitor results of the stool culture and sample for ova and parasites.	■ Rapid notification of the physician will facilitate treatment.	
■ Perform hand hygiene before and after contact with the child.	■ Hand washing helps prevent transmission of microorganisms.	
■ Isolate the child until the cause of the diarrhea is determined.	■ Isolation prevents exposure of other patients and staff.	
■ Assist the child with toileting and hygiene.	■ The child may be weak, incontinent, physically impaired, or anxious and require assistance to use the bathroom.	
■ Administer prescribed oral rehydration and intravenous solutions.	■ These solutions provide necessary fluids and nutrients.	
■ Notify the physician if diarrhea persists, stool characteristics change, or other symptoms of dehydration or electrolyte imbalance occur.	■ It is important to ensure early intervention.	

INTERVENTION	RATIONALE	EXPECTED OUTCOME
2. Nursing Diagnosis: Fluid Volume: Deficient related to active fluid volume loss		

INTERVENTION	RATIONALE	EXPECTED OUTCOME
NIC Priority Intervention—*Fluid Monitoring:* Collection and analysis of patient data to regulate fluid balance		**NOC Suggested Outcome**—*Fluid and Electrolyte Balance:* Balance of water and electrolytes in the intracellular and extracellular compartments of the body

GOAL: *The child will become rehydrated and will begin to drink fluids within 24 hours of admission.*

INTERVENTION	RATIONALE	EXPECTED OUTCOME
■ Monitor intake and output. Document time of each voiding. Weigh all diapers.	■ It is important to determine if output exceeds input and to assess renal function.	The child has normal fluid and electrolyte balance as indicated by laboratory evaluation and physical examination.
■ Compare admission weight to preadmission weight. Assess weight daily.	■ The degree of dehydration can be determined by the percentage of weight loss. Daily weights aid in determining progress toward rehydration.	The child should produce 1–2 mL of urine/kg/hr.
■ Assess level of consciousness, skin turgor, mucous membranes, skin color and temperature, capillary refill, eyes, and fontanels every 4 hours.	■ This assessment will determine degree of hydration and adequacy of interventions.	
■ Assess for vomiting.	■ Vomiting frequently accompanies diarrhea and contributes to the child's fluid loss.	
■ Provide oral fluid and electrolyte replacement solution if able to tolerate.	■ Oral fluids are less invasive than IV fluids. This provides for replacement of essential fluids and electrolytes.	
■ Provide and maintain IV replacement therapy, as ordered.	■ Use of IV replacement is based on the degree of dehydration, ongoing losses, insensible water losses, and electrolyte results.	

Nursing Care Plan   The Child with Gastroenteritis, *continued*

INTERVENTION	RATIONALE	EXPECTED OUTCOME
3. Nursing Diagnosis: Skin Integrity, Risk for Impaired related to altered fluid status		
NIC Priority Intervention—*Skin Surveillance*: Collection and analysis of patient data to maintain skin integrity		**NOC Suggested Outcome**—*Tissue Integrity:* Skin and mucous membranes Structural intactness and normal physiologic function of skin and mucous membranes
GOAL: *The child will remain free of skin breakdown and rashes.*		
■ Assess skin of the perineum and rectum for signs of skin breakdown or irritation. ■ Provide prevention or restorative care for infants as follows:	■ Early assessment and intervention can prevent worsening of the condition.	The child's perianal and rectal tissue remains pink and intact.
Preventive Care		
■ Change diapers every 2 hours or as needed. ■ Wash the diaper area with warm water, a cleanser not needing water, or an alcohol-free baby wipe after each soiling. (See Chapter 36 🔗.) ■ Apply A & D ointment, Aquaphor, or another barrier ointment with each diaper change.	■ Frequent diaper changes minimize skin contact with chemical irritants from stool and urine. ■ Washing the diaper area removes traces of stool if present. ■ Ointment provides a barrier and protects intact or reddened skin from becoming excoriated.	
Restorative Care		
■ Leave the buttocks open to air for a few minutes several times daily, placing absorbent pads under the infant. ■ Notify the physician if the skin is severely broken or peeling or if a rash is present. ■ For toddlers and older children: Tub bathe at least daily (if condition allows) in tepid water. Pat the area dry. ■ Discourage the wearing of underwear if possible. ■ Apply barrier ointment with each diaper change or as instructed.	■ Air circulation to the area is promoted. ■ Additional measures such as the use of a barrier cream or paste may be needed to ensure skin healing. ■ Bathing helps loosen any fecal matter without scrubbing, which can cause additional irritation to the skin. ■ Allowing air to circulate will prevent accumulation of moisture. ■ Ointment provides a barrier and protects intact or reddened skin from becoming excoriated.	

NANDA-I © 2012

---

usually anxious, so it is important to allow them to talk and ask questions. The child may require blood tests to help direct rehydration therapy. Most children are cared for at home, although care in a 24-hour monitoring unit may occur. For hospitalization or monitoring units, use therapeutic play techniques, such as allowing the child to manipulate equipment, to reduce anxiety (see Chapter 15 🔗).

Promote Rest and Comfort

Children with gastroenteritis may awaken frequently with periods of vomiting and diarrhea. Provide a quiet, restful environment and cluster nursing care to allow for periods of uninterrupted rest. Darken the room and keep interruptions to a minimum.

To reduce the child's anxiety, encourage parents to room in. Place the child's favorite toys and comfort objects within reach. Keep the child's mouth moistened with a wet washcloth or an occasional ice chip. Provide skin care after each diarrheal episode to maintain skin integrity. Avoid using commercial baby wipes that contain alcohol as these irritate the skin and cause discomfort for the child.

Ensure Adequate Nutrition

Liquids are offered throughout the illness, even if an intravenous infusion is in place. (Follow guidelines for oral rehydration therapy in Chapter 23 🔗.) Small amounts of the normal diet for age are provided. Infants are breastfed or given formula. The child's diet progresses according to protocol or the child's tolerance for feedings.

Clinical Tip

Avoid giving a child with diarrhea foods or fluids containing red dye (Jell-O, Popsicles) as this will turn the stool red and alarm parents who will mistake the red coloring for blood. When in doubt, the stool should be tested for occult blood.

Discharge Planning and Home Care Teaching

Discharge teaching begins on arrival at the healthcare facility. Teach parents about the symptoms of dehydration and what actions to take if diarrhea recurs. Ensure that parents understand the recommended diet progression. Emphasize the necessity of good hygiene practices

TABLE 30–6 Factors Influential in Childhood Constipation		
PHYSICAL FACTORS IN INFANCY	**PHYSICAL FACTORS IN CHILDREN**	**PSYCHOLOGIC FACTORS IN CHILDREN**
Familial stool patterns	Residual stool blockage (fecalith)	Embarrassment/shame related to soiling due to early or coercive toilet training or lack of privacy
High milk and low fiber intake	Overflow fecal soiling around a solid stool	Fear of pain from hard stool
Cow milk allergy	Poor rectal sensation	Being too busy to use the bathroom
Hard stools	Side effects of medications	Refusal to use a public restroom
Dehydration	Diseases that affect the gastrointestinal system such as celiac disease or cystic fibrosis	Parental blame/anger related to soiling and toileting refusal
Group A streptococcal infection of the perianal area	Diseases that affect the neurologic system such as encephalopathy, spina bifida	Teasing and bullying related to incontinence
Medications such as anticonvulsants, narcotics, and antacids	Decreased mobility/activity	
Conditions such as Hirschsprung disease, cystic fibrosis, anorectal malformations, spina bifida		

Source: *Data from Montgomery, D. F., & Navarro, F. (2008). Management of constipation and encopresis in children.* Journal of Pediatric Health Care, 22*(3), 199–204; Pirie, J. (2010). Management of constipation in the emergency department.* Clinical Pediatric Emergency Medicine, 11*(3), 182–188; Dobson, P., & Blannin, J. (2010). Treatment of idiopathic constipation in children and young people.* Primary Health Care, 20*(7), 16–19; Rogers, J. (2011). Functional constipation in childhood.* Nurse Prescribing, 9*(7), 326–331.*

to prevent the spread of microorganisms that can cause gastroenteritis. If the child attends childcare, ask the parent to alert the care center about the gastroenteritis so the staff can monitor for other cases and take steps to prevent the spread of infection.

Practice Alert

Instruct parents in the importance of and techniques for hand hygiene, especially when caring for the child with gastroenteritis. Teach children in childcare centers and schools how to wash their hands effectively to prevent spread of infectious diseases.

Evaluation

Expected outcomes of nursing care are provided on the accompanying Nursing Care Plan.

Constipation

Constipation is a common complaint in the pediatric population and accounts for 3% to 5% of all outpatient visits to the pediatric primary care provider (Pirie, 2010; Tobias, Mason, Lutkenhoff, et al., 2008). The incidence of constipation is 2.9% of children less than 1 year of age and 10.1% of 2-year-olds (Pirie, 2010). Children with functional constipation generally present to the healthcare provider between the ages of 2 and 4 years. Constipation occurs at similar rates in males and females less than 13 years of age (Sood, 2010). Because stool patterns vary among children, identification of an abnormal pattern is sometimes difficult. Infants usually have several bowel movements a day. For a young child, one bowel movement a day may be normal. As the child grows, however, three to four bowel movements in a week may be a normal pattern. The diagnosis of constipation must take into account the child's normal stool patterns.

Etiology and Pathophysiology

Constipation may be caused by an underlying disease, diet, or psychologic factor. Constipation may result from defects in filling, or more commonly emptying, of the rectum. Physiologic and psychologic causes of constipation are listed in Table 30–6.

If the rectum fails to fill, stasis leads to increased water reabsorption and hard, dry stools. Emptying of the rectum depends on the defecation reflex. Lesions of the spinal cord, weakness of the abdominal muscles, local lesions blocking sphincter relaxation, and a desire to avoid painful stools all may impede attempts to defecate.

The three types of constipation are normal-transit constipation, slow-transit constipation, and defecation disorders.

1. **Normal-transit constipation,** also called functional constipation, is the most common form of constipation and accounts for 95% of all cases of constipation in children over 1 year of age. With normal-transit constipation, stool traverses at a normal rate through the colon and the stool frequency is normal, but the individual has a hard time passing a stool, or passes hard stools. Bloating and abdominal pain or discomfort may be experienced (Bisanz, 2007).

2. **Slow-transit constipation** occurs most commonly in young females. With this type of constipation the gastrointestinal time is longer and peristalsis is weaker than it should be. Associated symptoms are bloating and abdominal pain or discomfort (Bisanz, 2007).

3. **Defecation disorders** are commonly due to dysfunction of the pelvic floor or anal sphincter such as in children with anorectal malformations (see discussion in this chapter). A desire to avoid pain associated with passing of a large, hard stool can result in defecation disorders. Symptoms include hard, infrequent stools, bloating, and pain (Bisanz, 2007).

Clinical Manifestations

Constipation is characterized by a decrease in the frequency of stool passage; the formation of hard, dry stools; or the oozing of liquid stool past a collection of hard, dry stool.

Constipation in the newborn should raise the suspicion of an obstructed large bowel such as that due to Hirschsprung disease anal stenosis (Pirie, 2010).

Constipation during infancy is rare and is most often caused by mismanagement of diet. The transition from formula to cow milk may cause a transient constipation, since the bowel must adjust to the increased protein content of cow milk.

Constipation occurs most frequently in the toddler and preschool age groups. This increased incidence is often associated with learning to control body functions. Many children do not like the sensations of a bowel movement and may begin withholding stool, which accumulates in and dilates the rectum until the next urge to defecate. The increasingly hard and painful bowel movement reinforces the child's behavior, and a cycle begins (Montgomery & Navarro, 2008). See the discussion in this chapter on encopresis.

Constipation in the school-age child, older child, and adolescent is generally related to activity, diet, and toileting habits. The child's diet may be lacking in fiber and contain many starchy foods such as bread and cheese (Montgomery & Navarro, 2008). Constipation may occur due to limited time for toileting. The child may not take time during the day to have a bowel movement or may be hesitant to use an unfamiliar bathroom.

Collaborative Care

Collaborative care focuses on determining the underlying pathologic cause of constipation, correcting any structural defect or obstruction, eliminating contributing factors, and assisting the child to establish routine bowel elimination habits.

Diagnostic Tests

Diagnosis is based on a thorough history and physical examination. The presence of stool noted on digital rectal examination is helpful in confirming the diagnosis of constipation (Pirie, 2010). If digital rectal examination is contraindicated or the exam does not yield any findings, abdominal radiographs may be useful in identifying fecal impaction. Refer to the section on Hirschsprung disease on page 1009 for diagnostic tests used to confirm this diagnosis. When constipation occurs along with growth failure, vomiting, or abdominal pain, further investigation is necessary to rule out other disorders. Tests may include thyroid function tests; measurements of calcium, glucose, and electrolytes; a complete blood count; and urinalysis.

Clinical Therapy

Dietary management is the treatment of choice for constipation that has no underlying pathologic cause. Constipation in young infants can usually be corrected by increasing the amount of fluids or adding 2 ounces of pear or apple juice to daily intake. Increasing physical activity and fluid intake may be effective for some children.

Removing constipating foods (e.g., bananas, rice, and cheese) from the child's diet often decreases constipation. Increasing the child's intake of high-fiber foods (e.g., whole grain breads, raw fruits and vegetables) and fluids also promotes bowel elimination. In older infants, increasing the intake of fluids, cereals, fruits, and vegetables in the diet should correct the problem. A single glycerin suppository or enema may be required to remove hard stool.

Encouragement from parents and relaxation of bathroom privileges at school promote regularity and return of usual bowel patterns within a short time for school-age children. Children may need to get up earlier to have breakfast and time for toileting before going to school.

Constipation may follow surgery, especially in children who are immobilized, such as by traction. Stool softeners and a diet high in fiber and fluids are given to prevent and treat constipation.

Pharmacologic management of severe constipation usually occurs in two stages. The first stage involves disimpaction followed by maintenance therapy (Dobson & Blannin, 2010; Rogers, 2011). The evacuation phase is the most difficult for the child and those who are managing the child's constipation.

Consider the most effective means to evacuate the stool while causing the least amount of stress and anxiety to the child. The oral route is less invasive, but if the child experiences nausea and vomiting, the rectal route might be used. Polyethylene glycol solution with or without electrolyte solution has proven successful in relieving impaction (Pirie, 2010). This medication can be administered orally or instilled via a nasogastric tube to promote stool evacuation. Once the stool has been evacuated, a routine stimulant laxative is given to prevent reaccumulation of stool in the bowel. The choice of medication varies among healthcare providers, but mineral oil, polyethylene glycol powder (MiraLax), and lactulose are examples of medications frequently used to maintain a regular stooling pattern (Montgomery & Navarro, 2008; Pirie, 2010).

Behavior management Behavior modification may prove beneficial to managing constipation and may include having the child sit on the toilet for 5 to 10 minutes after meals. Providing rewards for toileting at routinely scheduled times is effective (Montgomery & Navarro, 2008). Rewards can be simple items such as an afternoon spent with the parent playing a game. For children with psychologic issues, child and family psychotherapy may be necessary. In these cases, the family is referred to a child and family counselor.

Nursing Management

Nursing care focuses on teaching parents what constitutes normal bowel patterns in children and the importance of diet in maintaining such patterns.

Nursing Assessment and Diagnosis

Assess the child's diet history and obtain a description of bowel patterns and habits from parents. When was the child toilet trained and have those patterns changed? Has there been incontinence in the toilet-trained child? Ask what the family does to treat constipation. Ask about frequency, consistency, and the presence of blood in the stools. Ask the child or parents about pain upon passing of stool. Assessment of the child's food likes and dislikes may provide a clue to the cause of constipation. Assess fluid intake and level of activity. Assess for previous history of gastrointestinal complications or surgery, as well as present medications. Ask parents when the newborn passed meconium.

Physical Assessment

Palpate and assess the child's abdomen for firmness or tenderness and the presence of a palpable mass (retained stool). Assess for bowel sounds. If a digital rectal examination is performed, assess for the presence of stool in the rectum. Assess for hemorrhoids, anal fissures, or other abnormalities of the abdomen or perineum.

Nursing diagnoses that may apply to the child with constipation include:

- Constipation related to dietary, nutritional, and/or elimination habits
- Bowel Incontinence related to leakage around formed stool

NANDA-I © 2012

Planning and Implementation

Regular bowel habits are encouraged by placing the child on the toilet after a meal or around the time bowel elimination usually occurs. Providing positive reinforcement during toilet training helps to prevent a withholding pattern.

Partner with the family and teach parents dietary measures to promote regularity of bowel movements. Children can be given a high-fiber diet that includes fruits and vegetables. Offer cut fresh fruits, dried fruits, and fruit juice as snacks. A glycerin suppository can be used periodically if needed, as a natural stimulant and lubricant of the bowel.

Complementary Therapy **Herbal Laxatives**

Herbal laxatives are used by some cultures as complementary therapies to treat constipation in children. Examples of herbs and supplements that have been used include psyllium, magnesium, olive oil, glycerol, xanthan gum, guar gum, cascara, senna, and castor oil (Culbert & Banez, 2007). Safety and effectiveness of many of these laxatives have not been established in children. Cascara (*Rhamni purshiana*) and senna (*Sannae folum*) are stimulant laxatives that have been approved by the U.S. Food and Drug Administration for use in children older than 2 years of age to treat constipation (Culbert & Banez, 2007).

Caution parents to avoid frequent use of laxatives, stool softeners, and enemas, because overuse can cause bowel dependency. Herbal stimulant laxatives are discouraged for children less than 12 years, although other intestinal motility aids are not generally harmful. Ask the family about any herbs they may commonly use. See Complementary Therapy: Herbal Laxatives.

Evaluation

Expected outcomes of nursing care for the child with constipation include:

- A routine bowel elimination pattern is established.
- The child demonstrates normal stool patterns with no signs of constipation.

Encopresis

Encopresis is an abnormal elimination pattern characterized by the recurrent soiling or passage of stool at inappropriate times by a child who should have achieved bowel continence. Encopresis is reported to occur in 1% to 3% of children (Montgomery & Navarro, 2008). Children with primary encopresis have never achieved bowel control. Children with secondary encopresis have been continent of stool for several months.

Encopresis is usually associated with voluntary or involuntary retention of stool in the lower bowel and rectum, leading to constipation, dilation of the lower bowel, and incompetence of the inner sphincter. The retention of stool is usually a result of being "too busy"; the child puts off going to the bathroom because of the inconvenience of leaving an activity. The retention of stool leads to constipation that is untreated and chronic. Loose stool leaks around the hard feces, and the child becomes unaware of a need to eliminate. Soiling may occur during the day or night. Bowel movements are irregular, painful, small, and hard. Peers may ridicule the child because of offensive body odor. This rejection leads to withdrawal and behavioral problems, often resulting in altered school performance and attendance. The child continues to hold stool because the passage has become painful. Parents commonly seek health care, believing that the child has diarrhea or constipation.

The underlying constipation that leads to encopresis may be caused by the stress of environmental changes (e.g., birth of a sibling, moving to a new house, attending a new school), issues of anger and control related to bowel training, diet, a full schedule of activities, or a genetic predisposition.

A thorough history, physical examination, and diagnostic studies (possibly including barium or contrast enema) are necessary to rule out organic causes and anatomic abnormalities. Examination of mental health and cognitive functioning may be indicated. Information about the child's toilet-training habits and parents' attitudes concerning those habits is obtained. A dietary history, including eating habits and types of foods eaten, is often helpful. Physical examination sometimes reveals a nontender mass in the lower abdomen.

In addition to dietary management and treatment to evacuate the bowel as discussed in the preceding section, behavior modification techniques and psychotherapy may be used. Behavior modification programs that reward and reinforce appropriate toileting habits can be successful. The child should sit on the toilet for several minutes after morning and evening meals. It takes several months for the bowel to be retrained to respond to sphincter stimulation. Psychologic referral may be needed if the child does not respond to other measures (Montgomery & Navarro, 2008).

Nursing Management

Prevention of encopresis is the nursing goal. Partner with parents to teach toilet-training techniques, emphasizing the child's developmental readiness (see Chapter 5 🔗). Parents are encouraged to praise the child for successes and to avoid punishment and power struggles. Encourage high-fiber diets and regular times for elimination.

Nursing care centers on educating the child and parents about the disorder and its treatment and on providing emotional support. Explain the treatment plan, including dietary changes and use of laxatives or stool softeners. Reassure the child that he or she has a healthy body and, with treatment, will achieve normal functioning. The child is monitored during clinic visits for at least 6 months to be certain new patterns have been established.

INTESTINAL PARASITIC DISORDERS

Intestinal parasitic disorders occur most frequently in tropical regions. Outbreaks take place in areas where water is not treated, food is incorrectly prepared, and people live in crowded conditions with poor sanitation. In the United States, outbreaks of diseases caused by protozoa or helminths (worms) are increasing. Young children, especially those in childcare centers, are most at risk of infection. They often lack good hygiene practices and are more likely to put objects and their hands into their mouths. The most common intestinal parasitic disorders are summarized in the Clinical Manifestations table on pages 1031–1032.

Another common cause of parasitic infection in the young child is related to exposure to pets and wildlife. Pets should be checked regularly for parasites and treated for worms as needed. Sandboxes should be kept covered when not in use, and children should be taught good hand washing after exposure to their pets (Centers for Disease Control and Prevention [CDC], 2011a).

Laboratory examination of stool specimens identifies the causative organism (protozoa, worms, larvae, or ova). Treatment usually involves an anthelmintic.

Nursing Management

Nursing care centers on preventive teaching. Emphasize the importance of good hygiene practices, especially careful hand washing, after toileting and when handling food. Ensure the family understands proper medication administration. Instruct parents to administer prescribed medications as directed even if the child's condition seems to be improved.

Clinical Manifestations Common Intestinal Parasitic Disorders

PARASITIC INFECTION	TRANSMISSION, LIFE CYCLE, PATHOGENESIS	CLINICAL MANIFESTATIONS	CLINICAL THERAPY	COMMENTS
Giardiasis Organism: protozoan *Giardia lamblia* 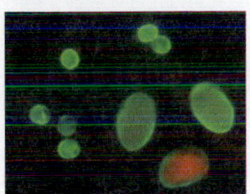	Transmission is through person-to-person contact, unfiltered water, improperly prepared infected food, and contact with animals. Cysts are ingested and passed into the duodenum and proximal jejunum, where they begin actively feeding. They are excreted in the stool.	May be asymptomatic. *Infants:* diarrhea, vomiting, anorexia, failure to thrive *Older children:* abdominal cramps; intermittent loose, foul-smelling, watery, pale, and greasy stools	Medications used to treat giardiasis include metronidazole, tinidazole, and nitazoxanide are the drugs of choice. Quinicrine, furazolidone and paromomycin may be used.	Most common intestinal parasitic organism in the United States. Infection may resolve spontaneously in 4–6 weeks without treatment. Parents or caregivers should wear gloves when handling diapers or stool of an infant or child infected with parasites.
Enterobiasis (Pinworm) Organism: nematode *Enterobius vermicularis* 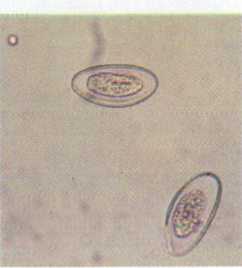 **Source:** *Educational Images Ltd./ Custom Medical Stock Photo.*	Transmission is from discharged eggs inhaled or carried from hand to mouth. Eggs hatch in the upper intestine and mature in 15–28 days. Larvae then migrate to the cecum. After mating, the female migrates out of the anus and lays up to 17,000 eggs. Movement of worms causes intense itching. Scratching deposits eggs on the hands and under the nails.	Intense perianal itching, irritability, restlessness, and short attention span; in females, can migrate to the vagina and urethra to cause infection. Itching intensifies at night when the female comes to the anal opening to lay eggs.	Medications used to treat enterobiasis include mebendazole, pyrantel pamoate, and albendazole. The child and all household members should be treated at the same time. Treatment may be repeated in 2 weeks.	Most common helminthic infection in the United States. Transmission is increased in crowded conditions such as housing developments, schools, and childcare centers.
Ascariasis (Type of Roundworm) Organism: nematode *Ascaris lumbricoides* 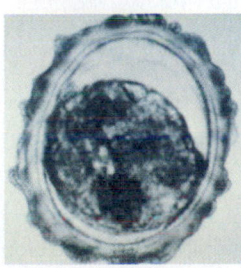 **Source:** *O.J. Staats MD/Custom Medical Stock Photo.*	Transmission is from discharged eggs carried from hand to mouth. The adult lays eggs in the small intestine. Eggs are excreted in stool, where they incubate for 2–3 weeks. Swallowed eggs hatch in the small intestine. Larvae may penetrate intestinal villi, entering the portal vein and liver, then moving to the lung. Larvae that ascend to the upper respiratory tract are swallowed and proceed to the small intestine, where they repeat the cycle.	Mild infection may be asymptomatic. Severe infection may result in intestinal obstruction, peritonitis, obstructive jaundice, and lung involvement.	Medications used to treat ascariasis include ivermectin, mebendazole, albendazole, and nitazoxanide	Most common in warm climates. Primarily affects children 1–4 years of age.
Hookworm Disease Organism: nematode *Necator americanus* 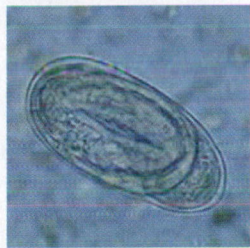	Transmission is through direct contact with infected soil containing larvae. Worms live in the small intestine and feed on villi, causing bleeding. Eggs are deposited in the bowel and excreted in feces. Eggs hatch in damp shaded soil. Larvae attach to and penetrate the skin, then enter the bloodstream, migrating to the lungs. Larvae then migrate to the upper respiratory passages and are swallowed.	In healthy individuals mild infection seldom causes problems. More severe infection may result in anemia and malnutrition. Presence of larvae on the skin may cause burning and itching, followed by redness and papular eruption.	Medications used to treat hookworm disease include mebendazole, albendazole, and pyrantel pamoate. Iron supplements may also be given.	Children should wear shoes when outdoors, although other unprotected areas of the skin may still come in contact with larvae.

(continued)

Clinical Manifestations Common Intestinal Parasitic Disorders (*continued*)

PARASITIC INFECTION	TRANSMISSION, LIFE CYCLE, PATHOGENESIS	CLINICAL MANIFESTATIONS	CLINICAL THERAPY	COMMENTS
Strongyloidiasis (Type of Roundworm) Organism: nematode *Strongyloides stercoralis* 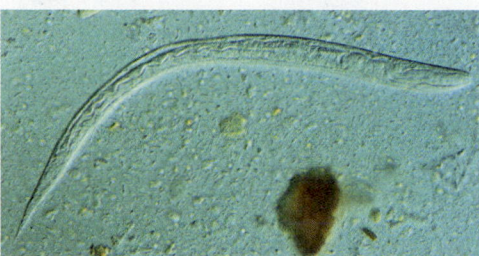	Transmission is from the ingestion of discharged larvae in the soil. Life cycle is similar to that of the hookworm, except this roundworm does not attach to the intestinal mucosa, and feeding larvae (rather than eggs) may be deposited in the soil.	Mild infection may be asymptomatic. Severe infection may result in abdominal pain and distention, nausea, vomiting, and diarrhea. Stools may be large and pale, with mucus. Severe infection may lead to a nutritional deficiency.	Medications used to treat strongyloidiasis include ivermectin, albendazole, and thiabendazole. Treatment may need to be repeated if symptoms recur after treatment.	Most common in older children and adolescents.
Toxocariasis (Type of Roundworm) Organism: nematode *Toxocara canis* or *T. cati*, commonly found in dogs and cats 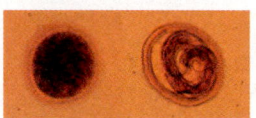	Transmission is through the ingestion of eggs in the soil. Ingested eggs hatch in the intestine. Mobile larvae then migrate to the liver and eventually to all major organs (including the brain). Once migration is complete, they encapsulate in dense fibrous tissue.	Most cases are asymptomatic. Affected children may have a low-grade fever and recurrent upper airway diseases. Severe symptoms include hepatomegaly, pulmonary infiltration, and neurologic disturbances. In all cases there is a hypereosinophilia of the blood.	Medications used to treat toxocariasis include albendazole and mebendazole. Steroids may also be used.	Most common in toddlers. Deworm household pets monthly if indicated. Keep children away from areas contaminated with animal droppings.

Note: Some of the medications listed may not be available in the United States and some of them may not be approved for use in all age groups.

Source: *Data from: American Academy of Pediatrics (2012) Summaries of Infectious Diseases. Red Book 2012. Report of the Committee on Infectious Diseases (29th Ed.). Retrieved online. Elk Grove Village, Illinois; AAP; Centers for Disease Control (2012b). Parasites. Retrieved from www.cdc.gov/parasites/; Gershon, A. A., & Hotez, P. J. (2010). Infectious diseases. In C. D. Rudolph, A. M. Rudolph, G. E. Lister, L. R. First, & A. A. Gershon (Eds.), Rudolph's pediatrics (22nd ed., pp. 878–1247). New York: McGraw-Hill.*

Photos of Giardia lamblia, Strongyloidiasis, Hookworm, and Toxocariasis courtesy of the Centers for Disease Control and Prevention, Atlanta, GA. Ascariasis from O. J. Staats MD/Custom Medical Stock Photo and Enterobiasis from Educational Images Ltd./Custom Medical Stock Photo.

DISORDERS OF MALABSORPTION

Malabsorption occurs when a child cannot digest or absorb nutrients in the diet. Disorders of malabsorption include celiac disease, lactose intolerance, and short bowel syndrome. Celiac disease and lactose intolerance are discussed in Chapter 19 ⊘. Cystic fibrosis, a common cause of malabsorption, is discussed in Chapter 25 ⊘.

Short Bowel Syndrome

Short bowel syndrome is a decreased ability to absorb and digest a regular diet due to a shortened intestine. Loss of intestine may result from extensive bowel resection for treatment of necrotizing enterocolitis or inflammatory disorders or from a congenital bowel anomaly such as intestinal malrotation, gastroschisis, or atresia.

The extent and location of the involved bowel determine severity of the disorder. Because specific types of absorption occur primarily in certain parts of the bowel, the section lost determines the particular vitamins and other nutrients that are inadequate.

During the first 3 months after bowel resection, watery diarrhea is common. In the transition period, the remaining bowel usually increases its absorptive surface area and partially compensates for the absent intestine. At first the infant or young child requires nutritional support to provide sufficient nutrients for adequate growth and development. In the initial period, the child only receives TPN. Once the bowel begins to recover, in addition to TPN, feedings by mouth or by tube may be started in small amounts. Feedings by this method stimulate the bowel and prevent atrophy of the mucosa (Goday, 2009). It is essential that the child receive the appropriate nutritional components regardless of the method in which nutrition is delivered.

Practice Alert

The child with short bowel syndrome will receive TPN via a central line. Aseptic technique in care of the central line is essential to prevent a catheter-associated bloodstream infection and potential sepsis (Gutierrez, Kang, & Jaksic, 2011). Maintaining patency of the central line is also essential as this may be the child's only route for receiving nutrition. It is not uncommon for children with short bowel syndrome to require insertion of multiple central lines over time either due to infection or due to occlusion of the line, especially if they require long-term TPN. This not only places a stress on the child who must undergo yet another surgical procedure, but is a stressor for the family as well.

Nursing Management

Nursing care focuses on meeting the child's nutritional and fluid needs and teaching parents how to care for the child at home. Establishing an adequate nutritional intake and bowel pattern is a lengthy process. TPN is provided initially until a feeding regimen can be established. Oral and enteral feedings are instituted gradually to allow the bowel time to compensate. Refer to Chapter 19 🔗 for nutritional assessment and detailed discussion regarding nutritional needs.

Partner with the family and child to provide support throughout this period. Teach parents how to prepare and administer parenteral feedings and care for the central line (see description in the Skills Manual 🔗). Once enteral or tube feedings are begun, teach management of the feeding pump and care of the feeding tube. Ensure regular bowel function and maintain skin integrity. Arrange home visits to monitor the child's growth and development, care of the central line and tube feeding site, and any side effects such as fluid and electrolyte imbalance and diarrhea.

HEPATIC DISORDERS

The liver is one of the most vital organs in the body. Thus, any inflammatory, obstructive, or degenerative disorder that affects liver function can be life threatening. The following discussion focuses on four common liver disorders in children: hyperbilirubinemia in the newborn, biliary atresia, viral hepatitis, and cirrhosis.

Hyperbilirubinemia of the Newborn

The life span of the red blood cell (RBC) is shorter in newborns than in adults. This increased RBC destruction and the fact that the newborn's liver is immature can lead to delayed clearance of bilirubin, resulting in physiologic jaundice in the newborn. **Hyperbilirubinemia,** an abnormally elevated serum bilirubin level, requires vigilance and frequent assessment of newborns to identify those at risk for central nervous system damage secondary to high bilirubin levels (Moerschel, Cianciaruso, & Tracy, 2008).

Etiology and Pathophysiology

Physiologic jaundice is described as jaundice in the newborn that occurs on the second or third day of life and resolves by the fifth or sixth day and is not associated with any other abnormal laboratory values. The etiology of physiologic jaundice is related to the immaturity of the infant's liver and the inability to effectively conjugate bilirubin (Effron & Piktel, 2008). Jaundice occurs in 60% of term and 80% of preterm infants (less than 37 weeks' gestation). Jaundice is generally noticed when the bilirubin reaches 5 to 6 mg/dL (Brethauer & Carey, 2010).

Practice Alert

In cases of severe and untreated hyperbilirubinemia, bilirubin encephalopathy can cause serious neurologic sequelae. The term *acute bilirubin encephalopathy* describes the acute effects of bilirubin toxicity in the first weeks of life. The term *kernicterus* is used when referring to chronic and permanent brain damage related to bilirubin toxicity (Moerschel et al., 2008).

Clinical Manifestations

Jaundice in the infant is first evident on the face, and then progresses to the trunk and finally to the extremities. While jaundice can usually be detected by blanching the skin with digital pressure in addition to being visible, visual estimates are not reliable. The child whose bilirubin is rising may demonstrate poor feeding and become lethargic (Moerschel et al., 2008).

Collaborative Care

Diagnostic Tests

A blood test, performed by heelstick or venipuncture, measures total serum bilirubin (TSB) in the newborn. A transcutaneous bilirubin (TcB) measurement device is a noninvasive method for estimating serum bilirubin in infants and is equivalent to TSB (Moerschel et al., 2008).

Clinical Therapy

Phototherapy most effectively reduces serum bilirubin in newborns with physiologic jaundice. The point at which phototherapy is implemented depends on whether the infant is full or preterm and how many hours old the infant is at the time the bilirubin rises (Brethauer & Carey, 2010). The goal of phototherapy is to keep the TSB below the exchange transfusion level. The American Academy of Pediatrics provides specific guidelines that clinicians can follow in determining the appropriate treatment (Moerschel et al., 2008).

Phototherapy is thought to reduce the amount of indirect, or unconjugated, bilirubin in the baby's bloodstream by promoting excretion via the intestines and kidneys. Phototherapy exposes the infant's skin to blue light, which changes bilirubin into water-soluble forms that can be excreted. The infant may be placed on fiber-optic pads as the sole means of providing phototherapy when mild jaundice exists or in conjunction with overhead phototherapy when bilirubin levels are higher (Cohen, 2006) (Figure 30–16 ■). The infant will need total serum bilirubin levels checked periodically during treatment to evaluate response to treatment and possibly 24 hours after discharge to see if the bilirubin increases after treatment is discontinued (Moerschel et al., 2008).

Many newborns with hyperbilirubinemia are also mildly dehydrated. When the newborn is breastfed, supplemental breast milk or formula may be given to improve hydration. Supplementation with water or dextrose water is not recommended. If the infant is unable to take adequate fluids and is dehydrated, intravenous fluid should be administered (Moerschel et al., 2008).

Clinical Tip

The infant's eyes are covered during overhead phototherapy to prevent retinal damage (Hansen, 2011). The eye shields can be removed when the lights are off for feeding.

Nursing Management

The nurse in the newborn nursery and in the outpatient setting plays a critical role in identifying the newborn at risk and providing parent education related to hyperbilirubinemia. Although the nurse in the newborn nursery may be providing care to an infant for a few days after birth, many infants are discharged home within 24 hours. The infant may be evaluated for jaundice in the outpatient setting and then admitted to the pediatric unit for treatment. Nurses working in acute care settings must familiarize themselves with the care of very young infants who require treatment for hyperbilirubinemia.

Nursing Assessment and Diagnosis

The newborn should be assessed for jaundice at least every 8 to 12 hours. If the nurse suspects the presence of jaundice, the infant's primary care provider should be notified and TcB (transcutaneous bilirubin) measurement or TSB (total serum bilirubin) level should be obtained (Moerschel et al., 2008).

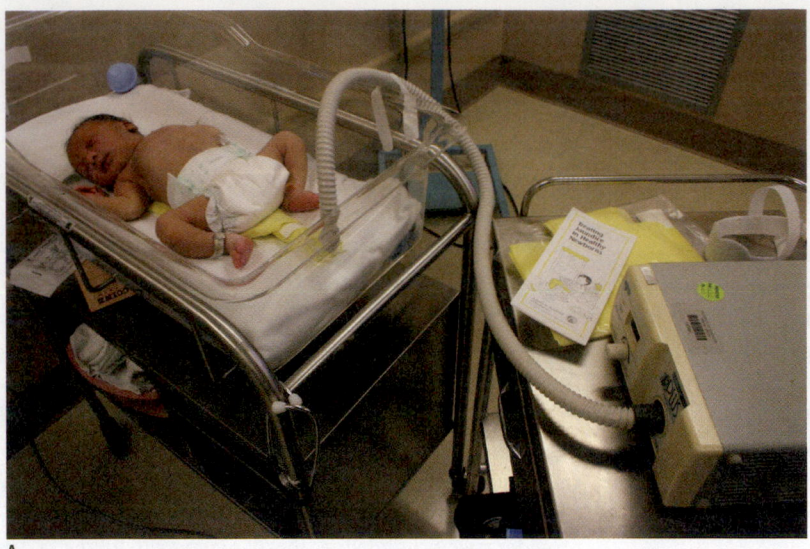
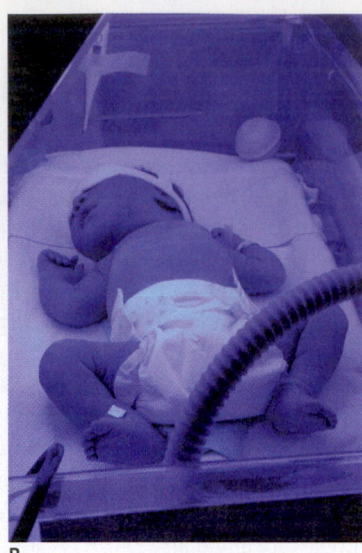

A B

FIGURE 30–16 ■ *A*, Infant receiving phototherapy on a phototherapy blanket. *B*, Infant receiving phototherapy in an incubator with overhead phototherapy lights.

Feeding Assessment

The mother who is breastfeeding should nurse her infant at least 8 to 12 times per day for the first several days (Brethauer & Carey, 2010; Moerschel et al., 2008). The nurse should be alert to mothers and infants who are having difficulty and require lactation support during the hospital stay and following discharge. Adequate hydration is essential for adequate elimination of bilirubin from the body. Newborns that are not well hydrated are at increased risk for hyperbilirubinemia (Brethauer & Carey, 2010). Parents should be educated regarding the number of wet diapers and stools their infant should have each day. Since many mothers and term newborns are discharged within 24 hours after birth, this is important information to teach parents prior to discharge.

Nursing Diagnoses

Nursing diagnoses that may apply to the newborn with hyperbilirubinemia include:

- Fluid Volume, Deficient related to decreased oral intake and ineffective breastfeeding
- Attachment, Risk for Impaired Parent/Newborn related to disruption of parental/newborn interaction due to hospitalization and treatment
- Body Temperature: Imbalanced, Risk for related to phototherapy

NANDA-I © 2012

Planning and Implementation

The role of the nurse is to identify the newborn at risk for hyperbilirubinemia, educate parents about newborn jaundice, and care for the newborn and family undergoing treatment for this condition. For the infant undergoing phototherapy, the nurse should monitor the infant frequently, ensuring that the infant is receiving the phototherapy properly. Vital signs should be assessed every 4 to 8 hours, especially the infant's temperature, which might indicate signs of infection or signs of hypothermia in an infant whose clothing is removed for phototherapy. An accurate measurement of intake and output is essential to make sure the infant is not dehydrated. Assist the family in breastfeeding or bottle-feeding as appropriate.

Discharge Planning and Home Care Teaching

Problems with breastfeeding in the first week of life can contribute to dehydration and subsequent risk of hyperbilirubinemia in the neonate. The nurse assesses adequacy of breastfeeding prior to hospital discharge and coordinates with the newborn's care provider in making appropriate referrals to lactation specialists and support groups in the community when necessary.

For term infants who develop uncomplicated hyperbilirubinemia, home phototherapy may be provided with the use of the fiber-optic pad, also known as a biliblanket (Brethauer & Carey, 2010). Serum bilirubin levels must be monitored regularly at the physician's office, at the neighborhood laboratory, or by the home healthcare worker. A visiting or home healthcare nurse often visits the family to establish the phototherapy and inform parents about the care needed. The nurse partners with other professionals such as staff from a medical supply company to service equipment, a lactation specialist to assist the breastfeeding mother, and a pediatrician to coordinate services.

Evaluation

Expected outcomes of nursing care include:

- Newborns at risk for hyperbilirubinemia are identified prior to discharge, and appropriate and timely follow-up occurs.
- Parents demonstrate an understanding of the basics of newborn jaundice, including who and when to call if they suspect development of hyperbilirubinemia
- Appropriate and timely intervention of hyperbilirubinemia occurs.
- Adequate fluids and nutrition are consumed in order to promote growth and development.

Biliary Atresia

Biliary atresia results when the extrahepatic bile ducts fail to develop or are closed. The disorder leads to cholestasis, cirrhosis, end-stage liver disease, and death by 2 years of age, if left untreated (Flanigan, 2013; Hartley, Davenport, & Kelly, 2009). Biliary atresia occurs in approximately 1 in 14,000 births in the United States (Wadhwani, Turmelle, Nagy, et al., 2008). It is the most common cause of pathologic jaundice in infants and is the leading indication for pediatric liver transplantation (Hartley et al., 2009; Khalil, Thamara, Perera, et al., 2009).

Etiology and Pathophysiology

The cause of biliary atresia is unknown. Absence or blockage of the extrahepatic bile ducts results in blocked bile flow from the liver to the duodenum. This altered bile flow soon causes inflammation and fibrotic changes in the liver. In addition to blockage, the disease can also be caused by hepatocellular dysfunction. Lack of bile acids also interferes with digestion of fat and absorption of fat-soluble vitamins A, D, E, and K, resulting in steatorrhea and nutritional deficiencies. Without treatment the disease is fatal.

Clinical Manifestations

Initially the newborn is asymptomatic. Jaundice may not be detected until 2 or 3 weeks after birth. At that point, bilirubin levels increase, accompanied by abdominal distention and hepatomegaly (see Appendix D 🕭 for bilirubin levels and other liver function tests). As the disease progresses, splenomegaly occurs. The infant experiences easy bruising, prolonged bleeding time, and intense itching. Stools are puttylike in consistency and white or clay colored because of the absence of bile pigments. Excretion of bilirubin and bile salts results in tea-colored urine. Failure to thrive and malnutrition occur as the destructive changes of the disease progress.

Collaborative Care

Collaborative care centers on immediate identification of the infant with biliary atresia, surgical correction of obstruction, and preparation of the child and family for the necessity of liver transplantation.

Diagnostic Tests

Because liver damage develops rapidly in infants with biliary atresia, early diagnosis is essential. Diagnosis is based on the history, physical examination, and laboratory evaluation. Laboratory findings reveal elevated bilirubin levels, elevated serum aminotransferase and alkaline phosphatase values, prolonged prothrombin time, and increased ammonia levels. Percutaneous liver biopsy suggests biliary atresia, and cholangiography and an exploratory laparotomy confirm the diagnosis (Roach & Bruny, 2008).

Clinical Therapy

Treatment involves surgery to attempt correction of the obstruction (hepatoportoenterostomy) and supportive care. In the hepatoportoenterostomy (Kasai procedure), a segment of the intestine is anastomosed to the porta hepatis. The primary purpose of this procedure is to promote bile flow from the liver. Intravenous antibiotics are administered in the postoperative period to prevent cholangitis. Prophylaxis with oral antibiotics is continued for 1 to 2 years after surgery (Flanigan, 2013).

Additional treatment includes administration of intramuscular vitamin K prior to invasive procedures and surgery to decrease the risk of bleeding afterwards and vitamins A, D, E, and K to provide supplementation since absorption of these vitamins is impaired. The infant is breastfed or is given Pregestimil or Nutramigen, formulas that contain medium-chain triglycerides. As the liver disease worsens, the child may need cholestyramine and antihistamines to help decrease itching. Enteral feedings and TPN may be needed as well (Flanigan, 2013). Ursodeoxycholic acid (Actigall) may be given to the child to promote bile flow (Schwarz, 2011).

While bile flow is achieved with the Kasai procedure in many children with biliary atresia, approximately 70% to 80% of children having this surgery will eventually need a liver transplant (Roach & Bruny, 2008). Advances in transplantation surgery now make it possible to perform partial liver transplants from living donor resections. This enables transplantation to be performed before the child develops end-stage liver disease (Flanigan, 2013).

Nursing Management

Nursing care in the initial stages of biliary atresia is the same as that for any healthy newborn. As symptoms develop, the focus of nursing care becomes long-term management and support.

Nursing Assessment and Diagnosis

Assess the abdomen for distention. Monitor stool pattern and assess for clay-colored, puttylike stools and dark urine. Assess skin for jaundice and ecchymosis. Assess comfort.

Nursing diagnoses that apply to the infant with biliary atresia may include:

- Nutrition, Imbalanced: Less than Body Requirements related to altered digestive processes
- Coping: Family, Compromised related to life-threatening illness of infant
- Growth and Development, Delayed related to nutritional deficiencies

NANDA-I © 2012

Planning and Implementation

Nursing care includes providing preoperative and postoperative care, supporting the family, educating the family about home care, and preparing the family for organ transplantation.

Preoperative Nursing Care

Diagnosis of this potentially fatal disorder can be devastating to parents. Provide emotional support and offer frequent explanations of tests during the initial diagnostic evaluation. As the disease progresses, the infant becomes irritable because of intense itching and the accumulation of toxins. Tepid baths may help to relieve itching and provide comfort. Dry the skin by patting rather than rubbing to avoid further skin irritation. Promote rest by grouping nursing activities while the infant is awake. Weigh the infant daily. Administer TPN, intralipids, and fat-soluble vitamins A, D, E, and K as prescribed.

Postoperative Nursing Care

Care following a hepatoportoenterostomy is similar to that for a child undergoing abdominal surgery. (See the earlier discussion of postsurgical nursing management for appendicitis and the Nursing Care Plan for the child undergoing surgery in Chapter 15 🕭.) Posttransplant care includes immunosuppressant drugs and close monitoring for vascular complications.

Discharge Planning and Home Care Teaching

Discharge planning focuses on teaching parents how to care for the child's skin, provide for nutritional needs, administer medications, and monitor for increasing symptoms of liver disease. When the child has received a transplant, teach parents how to identify signs of rejection (nausea, vomiting, fever, and jaundice), as well as the administration and side effects of immunosuppressant medications.

Refer parents to support groups, clergy, or social services if indicated. They will need ongoing visits from a home healthcare nurse to help them manage the child's complex care. Palliative care may need to be discussed with the family if it becomes evident the child will not survive. See Chapter 18 🔗.

Evaluation

Expected outcomes for nursing care of the child with biliary atresia are as follows:

- The child consumes adequate nutrition in order to support growth and development.
- Parents cope effectively with the stress of the child's condition.
- The child achieves growth and developmental milestones expected for age.

Viral Hepatitis

Hepatitis is an inflammation of the liver caused by a viral infection (Figure 30–17 ■). Hepatitis may occur as an acute or chronic disease. Acute hepatitis is rapid in onset and if untreated may develop into chronic hepatitis. The most frequently diagnosed causative organisms are hepatitis A virus (HAV), hepatitis B virus (HBV), and hepatitis C virus (HCV). A lesser known type is hepatitis D virus (HDV), which only occurs in individuals who have HBV infection (CDC, 2009b). Hepatitis E virus (HEV) occurs primarily in developing countries and is rarely seen in the United States (CDC, 2009a). In 2007, the incidence of Hepatitis A declined to only 1 case per 100,000 population reported in the United States. The incidence of hepatitis B has also decreased remarkably over the past several years to a low in 2007 of 1.5 cases per 100,000 in the United States (Daniels, Grytdal, & Wasley, 2009). The decline in both of these illnesses is related to routine vaccine administration, especially in children. (See the following Clinical Therapy section and Chapter 22 🔗 for more information on immunizations for these illnesses.)

Etiology and Pathophysiology

Hepatitis A is highly contagious and traditionally has been called infectious hepatitis. Infection occurs primarily through the fecal–oral route. Transmission is by direct person-to-person spread or through ingestion of contaminated water or food (particularly shellfish). Hepatitis A frequently occurs in children in childcare settings where hygiene practices are poor. Food handlers can spread hepatitis A if not aware of their infection; it is a common cause of foodborne illness. Because the virus is transmitted in the early stages of the disease when individuals are often asymptomatic or only mildly ill, large numbers of people may be exposed before the diagnosis is confirmed (Table 30–7). Most children recover from hepatitis A; however, in rare instances acute liver failure may occur (Yazigi & Balistreri, 2011).

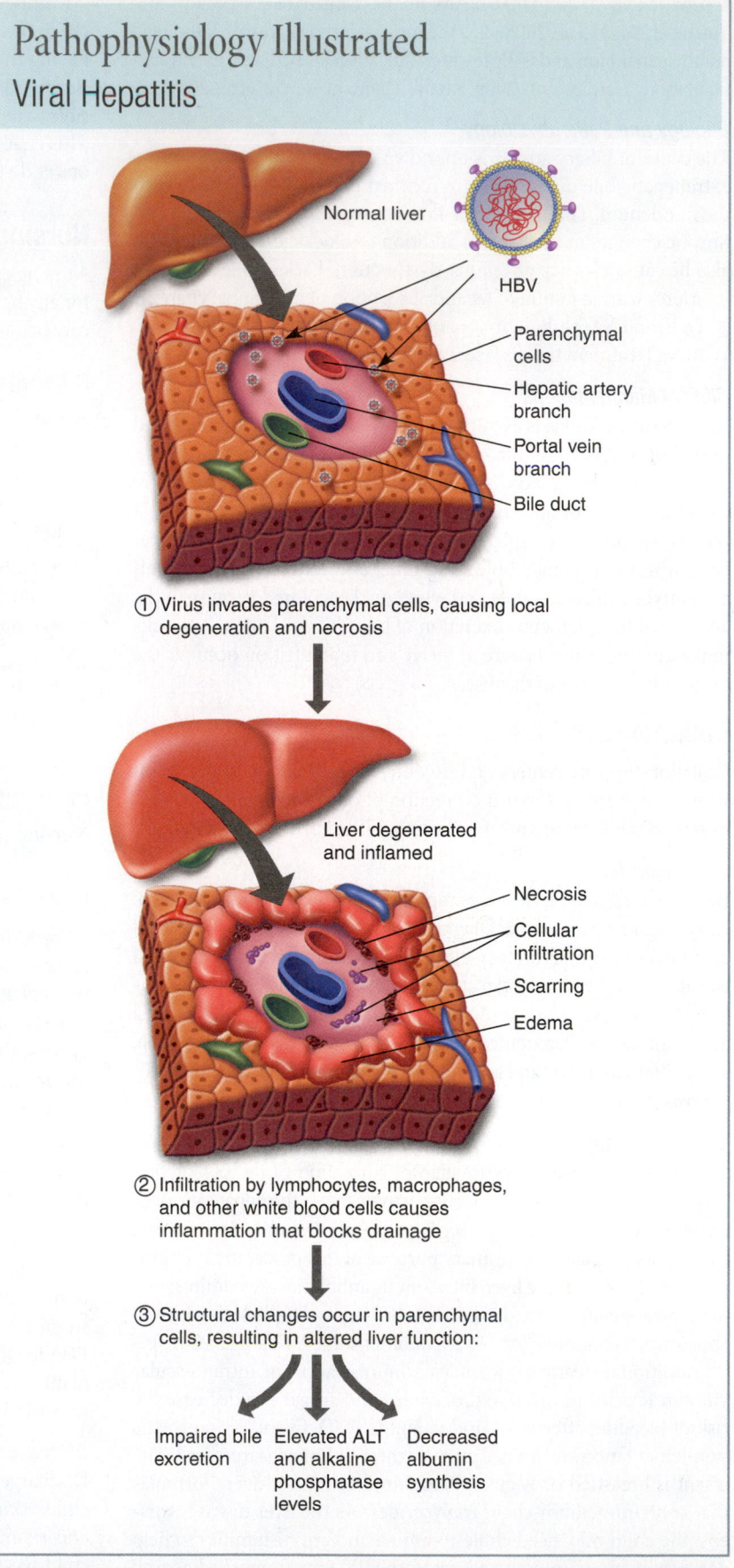

Pathophysiology Illustrated
Viral Hepatitis

Normal liver

HBV

Parenchymal cells

Hepatic artery branch

Portal vein branch

Bile duct

① Virus invades parenchymal cells, causing local degeneration and necrosis

Liver degenerated and inflamed

Necrosis

Cellular infiltration

Scarring

Edema

② Infiltration by lymphocytes, macrophages, and other white blood cells causes inflammation that blocks drainage

③ Structural changes occur in parenchymal cells, resulting in altered liver function:

Impaired bile excretion

Elevated ALT and alkaline phosphatase levels

Decreased albumin synthesis

FIGURE 30–17 ■ The hepatitis virus causes degeneration and necrosis of the liver, which results in abnormal liver function and illness.

TABLE 30–7	Comparison of Hepatitis Types			
TYPE	**IMMUNIZATION AVAILABLE**	**PROPHYLAXIS**	**PRIMARY TRANSMISSION**	**INCUBATION PERIOD**
Hepatitis A	Yes	Immune globulin Hepatitis A vaccine	Fecal–oral	15–19 days
Hepatitis B	Yes	Hepatitis B immune globulin Hepatitis B vaccine	Needlesticks or sharps exposure Intravenous drug use During birth Sexual activity	60–180 days
Hepatitis C	No	None	Needlesticks or sharps exposure Intravenous drug use During birth Sexual activity	14–160 days
Hepatitis D	No	Hepatitis B vaccine	Needlesticks or sharps exposure Intravenous drug use During birth Sexual activity	21–42 days
Hepatitis E	No	None	Fecal–oral	21–63 days

Source: *Data from Centers for Disease Control and Prevention (CDC). (2011b). Hepatitis C information for health professionals. Retrieved from http://www.cdc.gov/hepatitis/HCV/index.htm; Centers for Disease Control and Prevention (CDC). (2009a). Hepatitis E information for health professionals. Retrieved from http://www.cdc.gov/hepatitis/HEV/index.htm; Centers for Disease Control and Prevention (CDC). (2009b). Hepatitis D information for health professionals. Retrieved from http://www.cdc.gov/hepatitis/HDV/index.htm; Centers for Disease Control and Prevention (CDC). (2010a). Hepatitis A information for health professionals. Retrieved from http://www.cdc.gov/hepatitis/HAV/index.htm; Centers for Disease Control and Prevention (CDC). (2010b). Hepatitis B information for health professionals. Retrieved from http://www.cdc.gov/hepatitis/HBV/index.htm; Yazigi, N., & Balistreri, W. F. (2011). Viral hepatitis. In R. M. Kliegman, B. F. Stanton, J. W. St. Geme III, N. F. Schor, & R. E. Behrman, Nelson textbook of pediatrics (19th ed., pp. 1393–1404). Philadelphia, PA: Saunders Elsevier.*

Hepatitis B can result in acute or chronic infection and is transmitted by the parenteral route through the exchange of blood or any body secretion or fluid, sexual activity, and transmission from mother to fetus in utero (Caple, 2011). Adolescents who use intravenous drugs and have unprotected sexual intercourse are at risk for contracting hepatitis B. Major sources for the spread of HBV are healthy chronic carriers. All body fluids of infected individuals are potentially contaminated with the virus.

Hepatitis C is the most common bloodborne infection in the United States (Wasley et al., 2008). The hepatitis C virus is transmitted primarily through blood and blood products, and blood banks now test for this virus. Infected children are commonly individuals who have had repeated transfusions (as in sickle cell disease or hemophilia). Intravenous drug use, body piercing, and multiple sexual partners are also risk factors. Infected mothers may infect their children before birth or during breastfeeding. Chronic infection occurs in 70% to 85% of those individuals infected with hepatitis C (CDC, 2011b).

Hepatitis D (delta virus) is a defective virus that can gain entry to a human only in connection with hepatitis B (CDC, 2009b). Hepatitis E infection is primarily transmitted through contaminated water and is most common in developing countries (Yazigi & Balistreri, 2011).

The liver's response to injury by the viruses that cause hepatitis is similar. Initially, invasion of the parenchymal cells by the virus results in local degeneration and necrosis. Subsequent infiltration of the parenchyma by lymphocytes, macrophages, plasma cells, eosinophils, and neutrophils causes inflammation that blocks biliary drainage into the intestine. Impaired bile excretion causes a buildup of bile in the blood, urine, and skin (jaundice). Structural changes in the parenchymal cells account for other altered liver functions.

Clinical Manifestations

Acute hepatitis infection is characterized by two phases: the anicteric (absence of jaundice) phase and the icteric (jaundice) phase. The anicteric phase usually lasts 5 to 7 days. Signs and symptoms include nausea, vomiting, anorexia, malaise, fatigue, right upper quadrant pain, hepatosplenomegaly, and fever. The child becomes irritable, looks ill, and requires rest. In the icteric phase, signs and symptoms include darkening of urine, clay-colored stools, and the characteristic yellowing of the skin and sclera. However, many children with hepatitis do not have jaundice, leading to difficulty in disease diagnosis and management. As the jaundice worsens, the child begins to feel better. This phase lasts approximately 4 weeks. Complete recovery with return of normal liver function and laboratory values may take 1 to 3 months.

Collaborative Care

The three goals of collaborative care are early detection to prevent complications, support and monitoring during the acute phase of the disease, and prevention of the spread of the disease.

Diagnostic Tests

Diagnosis is often made on the basis of a thorough history and physical examination. A history of exposure to persons with the disease is significant. Physical examination reveals a tender, enlarged liver; abdominal pain; and flulike symptoms. Laboratory evaluation includes serologic testing to detect the presence of antigens and antibodies to HAV, HBV, HCV, or HDV; liver function studies; and a complete blood count to assess for anemia (Caple, 2011).

Clinical Therapy

Early diagnosis is essential to follow the course of the illness and identify potential complications. Management of the illness includes bed rest, hydration, and adequate nutrition during the flulike phase. If prothrombin times are increased, vitamin K is administered.

The spread of viral infections can be interrupted by elimination of the virus from the infected population, institution of proper hygiene, and passive or active immunization. To date, no antiviral agent has been developed to combat the hepatitis viruses. Prevention depends on breaking the cycle of infection.

Active immunization for hepatitis A, a two-dose series, is recommended for all people at increased risk of acquiring infection, for children, and for those who wish to acquire immunity to the illness. The CDC recommends that all children receive the first hepatitis A vaccine at 1 year of age (CDC, 2010a). (Chapter 22 ⊘ provides specific information on immunization schedules.)

Immunization for hepatitis B, a three-dose series, is recommended for all children and at-risk adults. The first dose is given within 12 hours of birth to the infant born to a mother who is infected or to a mother with unknown status (CDC, 2010b).

Individuals who have been exposed to hepatitis A and have not been previously immunized should receive immune globulin within 2 weeks of exposure. Healthy individuals, ages 12 months to 40 years of age, not previously immunized may receive the hepatitis A vaccine instead of immune globulin within 2 weeks of exposure (CDC, 2010a). Passive immunity to HBV can be achieved with hepatitis B immune globulin (HBIG). Used for one-time exposure and for infants of infected mothers, it is given within 12 hours after birth (CDC, 2010b).

Although most children recover from viral hepatitis, some may develop chronic disease. Care is individualized by a pediatric gastroenterologist. Medications are not generally used to treat viral hepatitis; however, some success has been achieved with the use of interferon alfa-2b in children with chronic hepatitis B. Success rates of 25%, similar to those in adults, have been demonstrated. Children who develop liver failure will need to be referred to a transplant center for care (Yazigi & Balistreri, 2011).

Nursing Management

Nursing care focuses on preventing the spread of infection, providing fluid and nutritional support, promoting growth and development, reducing risk of complications, and supporting the parents and child.

Nursing Assessment and Diagnosis

The nurse usually encounters the child and family in an outpatient setting. In addition to being observed for characteristic signs of hepatitis (jaundiced skin and sclera), the child is assessed for the presence of abdominal pain, anorexia, nausea and vomiting, malaise, and arthralgia. A history of the child's contacts over the past 45 days for HAV and up to 180 days for HBV is also obtained. For an infant, the hepatitis history of the mother and other family members is important.

Common nursing diagnoses for the child with acute hepatitis may include the following:

- Nutrition, Imbalanced: Less than Body Requirements related to chronic illness
- Fatigue related to disease state
- Body Image, Disturbed (Older Child) related to jaundice
- Anxiety (Parent and Child) related to threat to health status

NANDA-I © 2012

Planning and Implementation

Nursing care involves home and community considerations, as children with hepatitis are seldom admitted to the hospital. The

hospitalized child is placed in isolation. Prevention of the disease is integrated into all health care by discussion of immunization and universal precautions.

Parents need additional detailed information about health precautions and infection control measures if hepatitis cases have occurred in the family or community. Teach parents the importance of checking with health professionals before administering any medications (even nonprescription medicines). Also teach them to maintain adequate nutrition, promote rest and comfort, and provide diversional activities.

Prevent Spread of Infection

Teach the parents and the child infection control measures to help prevent transmission of the virus. For parents, reinforce good hygiene practices, such as washing hands before and after toileting and proper disposal of soiled diapers. Siblings of a child with hepatitis B who have not already been immunized with the hepatitis B vaccine should be vaccinated immediately. Contacts of the child with hepatitis A should receive immune serum globulin and the first immunization in the hepatitis A series. Rifampin may be given in some cases. All health providers should receive the hepatitis B immunization series and use standard precautions at all times.

Clinical Tip

Nurses in childcare centers can provide assessment of the center's procedures and teaching to prevent hepatitis A transmission. Help the center to set standards about:

- Hand washing after each diaper change
- Proper disposal of diapers
- Cleaning diaper-changing surfaces after each diaper change
- Never having food handlers perform diaper changes
- Instructing parents to keep children at home for at least 2 weeks after a diagnosis of hepatitis A
- Informing parents of other children when there is a case of hepatitis A and teaching them the symptoms of the condition

Maintain Adequate Nutrition

Initially the child is encouraged to eat favorite foods. Once the anorexia and nausea have resolved, a high-protein, high-carbohydrate, low-fat diet is recommended. Increased protein helps to maintain protein stores and prevent muscle wasting. Increased carbohydrates ensure adequate caloric intake and prevent protein depletion. The use of low-fat foods lessens stomach distention. Offer the child small, frequent feedings.

Promote Rest and Comfort

Bed rest is necessary only if the child has severe fatigue and malaise. However, most children voluntarily limit their activities during the initial phase of the disease. Keep the child quiet and comfortable. Offer comfort items such as favorite toys, blankets, and pillows.

Administer Medications

Drug metabolism is altered during hepatitis since the liver cannot detoxify medications readily. As with all liver disorders, medications need to be administered carefully and the child's condition must be monitored for possible drug side effects, especially since so many drugs are metabolized by the liver. Caution parents to check with health professionals before giving any nonprescription medication. For example, acetaminophen is metabolized in the liver, and liver disease can interfere with its breakdown.

Provide Diversional Activities

Hospitalized children with hepatitis are kept in isolation. Nonhospitalized children with hepatitis should be kept at home for 2 weeks following the onset of symptoms. Parents who cannot take time off from work may need to arrange home sitters to stay with the child. Offer suggestions for diversional activities during this period. Young children can be given a new toy or favorite activities. Older children and adolescents can be provided with board games, puzzles, books or magazines, movies, or video games. Phone calls and short visits from friends help school-age children and adolescents maintain contact with peers.

Evaluation

Expected outcomes of nursing care for the child with hepatitis include the following:

- The child demonstrates adequate nutritional intake to meet growth and development needs.
- The child participates in quiet, nonfatiguing activities and self-care.
- Positive body image is achieved.
- Parents demonstrate effective coping with the stress of the child's condition.
- Hepatitis is not spread to the child's contacts.

Cirrhosis

Cirrhosis is a degenerative disease process that results in fibrotic changes and fatty infiltration in the liver. It can occur in children of any age as the end stage of several liver disorders, such as hepatitis and biliary atresia (A-Kader & Balistreri, 2011; Boamah & Balistreri, 2011). The diffuse destruction and regeneration of the hepatic parenchymal cells result in an increase in fibrous connective tissue and disorganization of the liver structure. Progressive scarring that occurs in cirrhosis leads to altered blood flow to the liver which causes further deterioration of liver function (Boamah & Balistreri, 2011).

Clinical manifestations of cirrhosis vary. Hepatomegaly may be evident on exam. Jaundice occurs as the disease progresses and is an indication of hyperbilirubinemia. Jaundice is sometimes the only sign of hepatic dysfunction so its appearance must be investigated. Pruritus is common in children with cirrhosis although it is not related to the degree of hyperbilirubinemia. Other clinical manifestations of cirrhosis in children include ascites, portal hypertension, encephalopathy, and variceal hemorrhage (Boamah & Balistreri, 2011). Severe end-stage complications signaling hepatic failure can occur at any time and with little warning.

Diagnostic evaluation is based on the child's history of infection or disease with liver involvement. Physical examination may reveal jaundice, skin changes, **ascites** (fluid in the peritoneal cavity), and hemodynamic changes. Laboratory evaluation reveals abnormal liver function tests. A liver biopsy may help to determine the extent of the parenchymal damage.

Medical management focuses on treating the child's symptoms and achieving optimal nutritional status and growth. Liver transplantation is the most common treatment for biliary atresia and metabolic disorders and is the only treatment for end-stage liver disease.

Nursing Management

Nursing care focuses on monitoring physiologic and psychosocial changes to identify early signs of end-stage hepatic failure. Monitor vital signs every 2 to 4 hours. Measure weight daily to assess for fluid retention. Close monitoring of electrolytes and liver function test results helps determine the need for fluid replacement therapy.

Careful administration of medications and monitoring for side effects are necessary because drug metabolism is altered in liver disorders. If ascites is present, provide a low-sodium, low-protein diet and restrict fluids. Remove all water pitchers, glasses, and straws to minimize the child's desire to drink.

Parents of a child with cirrhosis are coping with a life-threatening disorder, and their anxiety and stress levels are high. The child may be awaiting a liver transplantation that represents the only hope for recovery. Provide support to parents and encourage them to verbalize their fears and concerns (see Chapter 17). Encourage parents to participate in the child's care. Referral to a support group or counseling may be beneficial.

INJURIES TO THE GASTROINTESTINAL SYSTEM
Abdominal Trauma

Trauma is the leading cause of morbidity and mortality in children. Abdominal injuries in children are caused by blunt trauma in at least 80% of cases. Penetrating injuries account for the remainder (Saxena, 2011).

Etiology and Pathophysiology

Motor vehicle accidents, falls, and intentional injury are the leading causes of abdominal injury in children. Blunt abdominal injury can cause very serious injuries to the spleen, liver, hollow organs, and sometimes the pancreas and kidneys (Karam, Sanchez, Chardot, et al, 2009). Intentional injury that results in abdominal trauma generally involves kicking or punching of the abdomen. While not as common as the unintentional causes listed previously, abdominal trauma related to child abuse carries a mortality rate of 45% to 53% (Pariset, Feldman, & Paris, 2010). Penetrating trauma occurs due to impalement on an object, stabbing, or gunshot wounds (Alterman, Daley, Kennedy, et al., 2011; Mikrogianakis, 2010). Children are more likely to have abdominal injuries because of their small pliable rib cage and less developed abdominal muscles that provide little protection for major solid organs such as the spleen, liver, and kidneys. In addition, the solid organs in children are larger in proportion to their body size compared to adults, so less surface area of the organs is protected by the ribs, making them more exposed and vulnerable to injury (Alterman et al., 2011; Saxena, et al., 2011).

The kind of injury determines the extent of organ damage. High-velocity blunt trauma, which may occur in motor vehicle crashes, usually involves multiple organs. Solid organs such as the liver and spleen can be bruised or lacerated. The sudden increase in abdominal pressure that occurs with a lap belt injury causes hollow organs such as the stomach, intestines, and bladder to burst. Sports-related abdominal trauma is often associated with a direct blow to the abdomen, and a single organ is usually injured. Bicycle accidents account for 5% to 14% of blunt abdominal trauma in children. Serious abdominal injury can result if the handlebars hit the child in the abdomen (Alkan, Iskitt, Soyupak, et al., 2009).

Clinical Manifestations

Clinical manifestations of abdominal injury include pain, abdominal distention, muscle guarding, decreased or absent bowel sounds, nausea and vomiting, hypotension, and shock. The external abdomen and back may have penetrating wounds, abrasions, bruising, or markings (e.g., tire tracks or lap belt marks) that provide a clue to injury beneath the skin surface. Abrasion and contusions in the lower abdominal area are classic visible signs of seat belt trauma (Bansal, Conroy, Tominaga, et al., 2009). See Chapter 7 🔗 for abdominal assessment techniques.

Collaborative Care

Collaborative care focuses on identifying internal organ trauma, replacing blood and fluid loss, and surgical exploration or resection of damaged organs.

Diagnostic Tests

Suspected abdominal trauma in a child necessitates a thorough history and physical examination. The description of the event should be compared with the child's signs and symptoms. Plain abdominal radiographs may reveal air in the abdomen. An ultrasound can reveal free fluid in the abdomen. A CT scan assesses multiple organs for injury and for the presence of free fluid in the abdomen. Urinalysis that shows blood in the urine may be indicative of damage to the urinary tract or kidneys. A CBC is generally obtained every 12 hours for the first 36 hours and then daily to monitor hemodynamic stability. Type and cross match of blood is also necessary in case the child needs a blood transfusion. In addition, liver function tests and pancreatic enzymes are monitored in the case of injury to the liver and pancreas (Saxena, 2011).

Clinical Therapy

In cases of severe trauma, hemorrhage may not be visible. Careful assessment and emergency fluid resuscitation may be needed to prevent or treat hypovolemic shock (see Chapter 26 🔗). The spleen and the liver are the organs most commonly injured in blunt abdominal trauma. Nonsurgical management is preferred. The spleen plays a major role in immune function; therefore, the organ is salvaged whenever possible to help maintain immune function (McKenna & Pieper, 2013; Saxena, 2011). Liver lacerations are treated much like spleen lacerations as long as major vessels have not been injured. Exploratory laparotomy is performed to resect hollow organ injuries or to repair liver or spleen lacerations when bleeding is not controlled.

Treatment of an abdominal, liver, or spleen injury takes place in the pediatric intensive care unit (PICU) and focuses on preventing or managing hemorrhage and monitoring for signs of shock. An intravenous infusion is initiated for fluid maintenance and to provide access for blood products. The child is kept NPO. A nasogastric tube is inserted. Blood transfusions and pharmacologic management are used to treat blood loss.

The child is maintained on strict bed rest until bleeding is controlled and the hemoglobin and hematocrit are stable. The length of time the child is hospitalized ranges from 2 to 5 days depending on the severity of the injury. The length of time for activity restrictions after discharge ranges from 3 to 6 weeks and also depends on the severity of the injury (McKenna & Pieper, 2013).

Nursing Management

Nursing care focuses on promoting hemodynamic stabilization through fluid and blood replacement therapy, providing preoperative and postoperative care, and supporting the child and family.

Nursing Assessment and Diagnosis

Nursing care includes initial and ongoing assessments of the child's condition. Assess the abdomen for pain, guarding, rebound tenderness, distention, and obvious signs of injury such as bruising. See Chapter 7 🔗 for techniques of abdominal assessment.

Nursing care includes initial and ongoing assessments of the child's condition. Monitor hematocrit and vital signs every hour as warranted to detect hypovolemia (see Chapter 26 🔗). Tachycardia and hypotension may indicate hypovolemia or internal bleeding. Strict monitoring of intake and output will give information about the child's fluid status. Monitor the respiratory status as abdominal injuries may also have thoracic involvement. The child with associated thoracic injuries may not take deep breaths if it is painful.

Practice Alert

The child who is restrained in a motor vehicle with only a lap belt is at high risk for abdominal injury in a crash. As the car stops rapidly, the child's body is restrained and flexes around the lap belt. The sudden increase in abdominal pressure causes injury to hollow organs, and sometimes solid organs. Children no longer using car safety seats should sit in a booster seat so that a shoulder restraint is used in addition to the lap belt. A booster seat should be used until the child is 8 years of age or weighs 80 pounds.

Nursing diagnoses for the child with abdominal trauma may include:

- Fluid Volume: Deficient related to loss of blood from trauma
- Pain, Acute related to injury
- Anxiety (Parent and Child) related to trauma and hospitalization
- Infection, Risk for related to release of bacterial organisms from bowel into peritoneum

NANDA-I © 2012

Planning and Implementation

The child and parents are usually fearful and anxious when the child is admitted to the hospital. If the injury was preventable, parents may have feelings of guilt or anger. Provide emotional support and avoid judgmental comments or statements that assign blame. Additional nursing care includes maintenance of the nasogastric tube; administration of antibiotics, intravenous fluids, and blood; and monitoring of lab studies as appropriate. Any concerns should be reported to the physician immediately.

Prepare the child and parents for surgery if necessary. Refer to Chapter 15 🔗 for nursing care of the child undergoing surgery.

Once the child's condition is stabilized, nursing care shifts to preventive teaching. Partner with the child and parents to ensure their understanding of safety measures to prevent future injuries. Provide written materials, when available, to use as a reference when they return home.

Discuss the use of car safety restraint devices for riding in an automobile (see Chapters 10 through 13 🔗). If the child's injury was the result of a bicycle fall or crash, discuss the importance of the proper bicycle size and teach bike safety measures such as use of a helmet and knowledge and proper use of hand signals. Refer to Chapter 20 🔗 for information related to injury to the GI system due to poisoning and ingestion of foreign objects.

Evaluation

Expected outcomes of nursing care for the child with abdominal trauma include:

- Fluid and hemodynamic stability is maintained.
- Parents demonstrate effective coping with stress of the child's injury.
- Wounds heal without signs of infection.

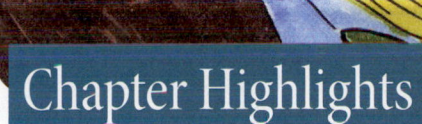

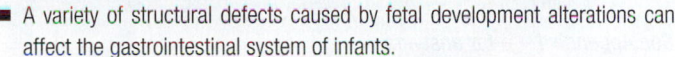

Chapter Highlights

- A variety of structural defects caused by fetal development alterations can affect the gastrointestinal system of infants.
- Cleft lip and palate are structural defects that often involve care by a team of providers such as a plastic surgeon, pediatrician, nurse, audiologist, speech therapist, and orthodontist.
- A variety of defects of the esophagus and trachea can manifest as mild to life-threatening problems in the newborn period.
- Pyloric stenosis is a common cause of projectile vomiting in the newborn period.
- Gastroesophageal reflux is one of the most common gastrointestinal problems in infants and children.
- Abdominal wall defects and anorectal malformations are serious structural defects of infancy.
- Intussusception is one of the most common causes of intestinal obstruction in the pediatric population and primarily occurs in children less than 2 years of age.
- Hirschsprung disease, or aganglionic megacolon, leads to failure to pass normal stools and distention of the abdomen.
- Several of the intestinal problems of childhood necessitate temporary or permanent ostomy placement.

- Hernias can be present in the diaphragmatic area, umbilicus, or inguinal canal.
- The most common inflammatory disorder of the gastrointestinal tract is appendicitis.
- Necrotizing enterocolitis is a potentially life-threatening inflammatory disease of the intestines seen primarily in premature infants after enteral feedings are begun.
- Common inflammatory bowel diseases affecting primarily adolescent and young adult age groups are Crohn disease and ulcerative colitis.
- Peptic ulcer may be primary (often caused by *H. pylori*) or secondary in situations of stress, trauma, or other disease.
- Common disorders of motility include diarrhea, constipation, and encopresis.
- Gastroenteritis and parasitic disorders are common causes of gastrointestinal disturbance and distress in children and may lead to fluid and electrolyte imbalance.
- Short bowel syndrome occurs when surgery is used to treat an intestinal disease and significant sections of the bowel are removed.
- Biliary atresia and hepatitis are the most common liver diseases in young children. Hyperbilirubinemia can occur in newborns.
- Abdominal trauma most often occurs to children involved in motor vehicle accidents.

Clinical Reasoning in Action

INTRODUCTION

Recall Jenna from the chapter-opening scenario, a 4-year-old who has just been admitted to the pediatric unit after surgery for a ruptured appendix.

DESCRIPTION

Jenna is groggy from the anesthesia, but she is scared. Recall that she has a Foley catheter, a nasogastric tube to suction, and a PICC line. She cries as the nurse approaches to perform an initial assessment and states, "My tummy hurts and I want this thing out of my nose!"

DISCUSSION

1. Why was Jenna at increased risk for ruptured appendix compared to a school-age child?
2. Jenna's parents ask why she needs all of the tubes. What information should the nurse include related to the purpose of the nasogastric tube, the Foley catheter, and the PICC line?
3. Considering Jenna's developmental age, how can the nurse help Jenna adapt to the hospitalization experience? (Refer to Chapter 15 🍪 .)
4. What interventions are most appropriate with a 4-year-old to decrease the risk of pulmonary complications associated with surgery?

NCLEX-RN® Review

1. At which developmental stage might a child begin to be capable of assisting an adult with ostomy care?
   1. Preschool age
   2. School age
   3. Toddlerhood
   4. Adolescence

2. The nurse is providing care for a 4-month-old infant who has had reconstructive surgery for an imperforate anus. Which of the following should be included in this child's postoperative care? Select all that apply.
   1. Pain management
   2. Accurate assessment of intake and output
   3. Rectal temperature measurement every 4 hours
   4. Observation of the surgical site for signs of infection
   5. Assessment of cardiac and respiratory status

3. What home care instructions are appropriate for a child who is being discharged following hospitalization for severe diarrhea? (Select all that apply.)
   1. "Have your child drink skim milk instead of 2% milk."
   2. "Call the healthcare provider if your child is unable to keep liquids down."
   3. "Perform hand hygiene frequently, especially after changing diapers."
   4. "Provide small amounts of your child's regular diet."
   5. "Use baby wipes to clean stool and urine at every diaper change."

4. The nurse is performing a home care visit for an infant who was discharged home the previous day following cleft lip repair. The nurse cautions the parents that when the infant cries, they should not attempt to calm her with which item?
   1. A pacifier
   2. Soft music
   3. A mobile
   4. A mirror

See Appendix I 🅔 for answers.

References

A-Kader, H. A., & Balistreri, W. F. (2011). Cholestasis. In R. M. Kliegman, B. F. Stanton, J. W. St. Geme III, N. F. Schor, & R. E. Behrman, *Nelson textbook of pediatrics* (19th ed., pp. 1381–1388). Philadelphia, PA: Saunders Elsevier.

Alkan, M., Iskitt, S. H., Soyupak, S., Tuncer, R., Okur, H., Keskin, E., & Zorludemir, U. (2009). Severe abdominal trauma involving bicycle handlebars in children. *Pediatric Emergency Care, 25*(8), 1–4.

Alterman, D. M., Daley, B. J., Kennedy, A. P., Raju, R., & Lee, S. (2011). *Considerations in pediatric trauma.* Retrieved from http://emedicine.medscape.com/article/435031-overview

American Academy of Pediatrics (2011). *Amount and Schedule of Formula Feedings.* Retrieved http://www.healthychildren.org/English/ages-stages/baby/feeding-nutrition/Pages/default.aspx

Anderson, K. (2010). Gastroesophageal reflux disease. *Radiologic Technology, 81*(3), 251–268.

Applegate, K. E. (2009). Evidence-based diagnosis of malrotation and volvulus. *Pediatric Radiology, 39*(Suppl. 2), S161–S163.

Arikan, D., Alp, H., Gözüm, S., Orbak, Z., & Cifçi, E. K. (2008). Effectiveness of massage, sucrose solution, herbal tea or hydrolysed formula in the treatment of infantile colic. *Journal of Clinical Nursing, 17,* 1754–1761.

Askew, N. (2010). An overview of infantile hypertrophic pyloric stenosis. *Pediatric Nursing, 22*(8), 27–30.

Bansal, V., Conroy, C., Tominaga, G. T., & Coimbra, R. (2009). The utility of seat belt signs to predict intra-abdominal injury following motor vehicle crashes. *Traffic Injury Prevention, 10*(6), 567–572.

Baumgart, D. C. (2009). The diagnosis and treatment of Crohn's disease and ulcerative colitis. *Deutsches Ärzteblatt International, 106*(8), 123–133.

Berman, L., & Moss, R. L. (2011). Necrotizing enterocolitis: An update. *Seminars in Fetal and Neonatal Medicine, 16,* 145–150.

Bisanz, A. (2007). Chronic constipation. *American Journal of Nursing, 107*(4), 72B–72H.

Bischoff, A., Levitt, M. A., Lim, F. Y., Guimarães, C., & Peña, A. (2010). Prenatal diagnosis of cloacal malformations. *Pediatric Surgery International, 26,* 1071–1075.

Blanton, S. H., Henry, R. R., Yuan, Q., Mulliken, J. B., Stal, S., Finnell, R. H., & Hecht, J. T. (2011). Folate pathway and nonsyndromic cleft lip and palate. *Birth Defects Research (Part A): Clinical and Molecular Teratology, 91,* 50–60.

Boamah, L. M., & Balistreri, W. F. (2011). Manifestations of liver disease. In R. M. Kliegman, B. F. Stanton, J. W. St. Geme III, N. F. Schor, & R. E. Behrman, *Nelson textbook of pediatrics* (19th ed., pp. 1374–1381). Philadelphia, PA: Saunders Elsevier.

Bradshaw, W. T. (2009). Necrotizing enterocolitis etiology, presentation, management, and outcomes. *Journal of Perinatal and Neonatal Nursing, 23*(1), 87–94.

Brethauer, M., & Carey, L. (2010). Maternal experience with neonatal jaundice. *American Journal of Maternal Child Nursing, 35*(1), 8–14.

Caple, C. (2011). *Hepatitis B. Cinahl Information Systems.* Retrieved from http://ehis.ebscohost.com.libproxy.uncg.edu/ehost/pdfviewer/pdfviewer?vid=3&hid=20&sid=00a5a37a-1e6e-44fe-ad24-0a32485fa2f7%40sessionmgr15

Carlo, W. A. (2011). The umbilicus. In R. M. Kliegman, B. F. Stanton, J. W. St. Geme III, N. F. Schor, & R. E. Behrman, *Nelson textbook of pediatrics* (19th ed., pp. 622). Philadelphia, PA: Saunders Elsevier.

Cassell, C. H., Daniels, J., & Meyer, R. E. (2009). Timeliness of primary cleft lip/palate surgery. *Cleft Palate-Craniofacial Journal, 46*(6), 588–597.

Centers for Disease Control and Prevention (CDC). (2009a). *Hepatitis E information for health professionals.* Retrieved from http://www.cdc.gov/hepatitis/HEV/index.htm

Centers for Disease Control and Prevention (CDC). (2009b). *Hepatitis D information for health professionals.* Retrieved from http://www.cdc.gov/hepatitis/HDV/index.htm

Centers for Disease Control and Prevention (CDC). (2010a). *Hepatitis A information for health professionals.* Retrieved from http://www.cdc.gov/hepatitis/HAV/index.htm

Centers for Disease Control and Prevention (CDC). (2010b). *Hepatitis B information for health professionals.* Retrieved from http://www.cdc.gov/hepatitis/HBV/index.htm

Centers for Disease Control and Prevention (CDC). (2011a). *Healthy pets, healthy people.* Retrieved from http://www.cdc.gov/Features/HealthyPets/

Centers for Disease Control and Prevention (CDC). (2011b). *Hepatitis C information for health professionals.* Retrieved from http://www.cdc.gov/hepatitis/HCV/index.htm

Chamley, C. A., Carson, P., Randall, D., & Sandwell, M. (2005). *Developmental anatomy and physiology of children.* St. Louis, MO: Elsevier.

Christison-Lagay, E. R., Kelleher, C. M., & Langer, J. C. (2011). Neonatal abdominal wall defects. *Seminars in Fetal & Neonatal Medicine, 16,* 164–172.

Cochran, A. A., Higgins, G. L., & Strout, T. D. (2011). Intussusception in traditional pediatric, nontraditional pediatric, and adult patients. *American Journal of Emergency Medicine, 29,* 523–527.

Coha, T. (2013). Care of the child with an ostomy. In N. T. Browne, L. M. Flanigan, C. A. McComiskey, &

P. Pieper, *Nursing care of the pediatric surgical patient* (2nd ed., pp. 105–129). Boston: Jones & Bartlett.

Cohen, S. M. (2006). Jaundice in the full-term newborn. *Pediatric Nursing, 32*(3), 202–208.

Cohen-Silver, J., & Ratnapalan, S. (2009). Management of infantile colic: A review. *Clinical Pediatrics, 48*(1), 14–17.

Cole, A., Tomlinson, J., Slator, R., & Reading, J. (2009). Understanding cleft lip and palate. 3: Feeding the baby. *Journal of Family Health Care, 19*(5), 157–158.

Collopy, K., & Friese, G. (2010). Pediatric Drug Administration. *Emergency Medical Services Magazine 39,* (6), 52–57.

Cortese, M. M., & Parashar, U. D. (2009). Prevention of rotavirus gastroenteritis among infants and young children. Recommendations of the Advisory Committee on Immunization Practices (ACIP). *Morbidity and Mortality Weekly Report, 58*(RR2), 1–24.

Culbert, T. P., & Banez, G. A. (2007). Integrative approaches to childhood constipation and encopresis. *Pediatric Clinics of North America, 54,* 927–947.

Cuvellier, J., & Lèpine, A. (2010). Childhood periodic syndromes. *Pediatric Neurology, 42,* 1–11.

Daniels, D., Grytdal, S., & Wasley, A.,. (2009). Surveillance for acute viral hepatitis-United States, 2007. *Morbidity and Mortality Weekly Report, 58*(SS03), 1–27.

De Jong, E. M., de Haan, M. A., Gischler, S. J., Hop, W., Cohen-Overbeek, T. E., Bax, N. M. A., . . . Grijseels, E. W. M. (2010). Pre- and postnatal diagnosis and outcome of fetuses and neonates with esophageal atresia and tracheoesophageal fistula. *Prenatal Diagnosis, 30,* 274–279.

Deloach, R., & Farber, L. D. (2013). Intussusception. In N. T. Browne, L. M. Flanigan, C. A. McComiskey, & P. Pieper (Eds.), *Nursing care of the pediatric surgical patient* (3rd ed., pp. 399–406). Burlington, MA: Jones & Bartlett Learning.

Dobson, P., & Blannin, J. (2010). Treatment of idiopathic constipation in children and young people. *Primary Health Care, 20*(7), 16–19.

Effron, D., & Piktel, J. (2008). Photo finish: Acute Dx: What cause of sudden illness? *Consultant for Pediatricians, 7*(5), 217–220.

Fillingham, A., & Rankin (2008). Prevalence, prenatal diagnosis and survival of gastroschisis. *Prenatal Diagnosis, 28,*1232–1237.

Fiorino, K., & Liacouras, C. A. (2011). Congenital aganglionic megacolon (Hirschsprung disease). In R. M. Kliegman, B. F. Stanton, J. W. St. Geme III, N. F. Schor, & R. E. Behrman, *Nelson textbook of pediatrics* (19th ed., pp. 1284–1287). Philadelphia, PA: Saunders Elsevier.

Flanigan, L. M. (2013). Biliary Atresia and Choledochal Cyst. In N. T. Browne, L. M. Flanigan, C. A. McComiskey, & P. Pieper (Eds.). *Nursing care of the pediatric surgical patient* (3rd ed., pp. 435-446). Burlington, MA: Jones & Bartlett Learning.

Forbes, D., & Fairbrother, S. (2008). Cyclic nausea and vomiting in childhood. *Australian Family Physician, 37*(12), 33–36.

Georgeson, K.E. (2010). Hirschsprung's disease. In G.W. Holcomb, III & J. P. *Murphy Ashcraft's Pediatric Surgery* (5th ed., pp. 456-467). Philadelphia: Saunders Elsevier.

Gershon, A. A., & Hotez, P. J. (2010). Infectious diseases. In C. D. Rudolph, A. M. Rudolph, G. E. Lister, L. R. First, & A. A. Gershon (Eds.), *Rudolph's pediatrics* (22nd ed., pp. 1187, 1191). New York, NY: McGraw-Hill.

Glick, S. R., & Carvalho, R. S. (2011). Inflammatory bowel disease. *Pediatrics in Review, 32*(1), 14–25.

Goday, P. S. (2009). Short bowel syndrome: How short is too short? *Clinical Perinatology, 36*, 101–110.

Goldberg, E., Barton, S., Xanthopoulos, M. S., Stettler, N., & Liacouras, C. A. (2010). A descriptive study of complications of gastrostomy tubes in children. *Journal of Pediatric Nursing, 25*(2), 72–80.

Goldson, E., & Reynolds, A. (2011). Child development & behavior. In W. W. Hay, M. J. Levin, J. M. Sondheimer, & R. R. Deterding, *Current diagnosis & treatment: Pediatrics* (20th ed.). Retrieved from http://www.accessmedicine.com.go.libproxy.wfubmc.edu/content.aspx?aID=6576671

Gregory, K.E., DeForge, C.E., Natale, K.M., Phillips, M., VanMarter, L.J. (2011). Necrotizing enterocolitis in the premature infant: Neonatal nursing assessment, disease pathogenesis, and clinical presentation, *Advances in Neonatal Care, 11*(3), 155-164.

Grossman, A. B., & Baldassano, R. N. (2011). Inflammatory bowel disease. In R. M. Kliegman, B. F. Stanton, J. W. St. Geme III, N. F. Schor, & R. E. Behrman, *Nelson textbook of pediatrics* (19th ed., pp. 1294–1295). Philadelphia, PA: Saunders Elsevier.

Grossman, A. B., & Mamula, P. (2011). *Pediatric Crohn disease.* Retrieved from http://emedicine.medscape.com/article/928288-overview

Guardino, K. O., & Pieper, P. (2013). Anorectal malformations in children. In N. T. Browne, L. M. Flanigan, C. A. McComiskey, & P. Pieper (Eds.), *Nursing care of the pediatric surgical patient* (3rd ed., pp. 359–372). Burlington, MA: Jones & Bartlett Learning.

Gutierrez, I. M., Kang, K. H., & Jaksic, T. (2011). Neonatal short bowel syndrome. *Seminars in Fetal & Neonatal Medicine, 16*, 157–163.

Hansen, T. W. R. (2011). *Neonatal jaundice.* Retrieved from http://emedicine.medscape.com/article/974786-overview

Hartley, J. L., Davenport, M., & Kelly, D. A. (2009). Biliary atresia. *Lancet, 374*, 1704–1712.

Holder, M., & Jackson, L. (2013). Hirschsprung's Disease. In N. T. Browne, L. M. Flanigan, C. A. McComiskey, & P. Pieper (Eds.), *Nursing care of the pediatric surgical patient* (3rd ed., pp. 347–358). Burlington, MA: Jones & Bartlett Learning.

Holloway, T. J. (2010). The root of the problem: An irritable bowel or an average American lifestyle? *Gastrointestinal Nursing, 8*(1), 31–37.

Hood, E., & Zimmerman, B. T. (2013). Abdominal wall defects. In N. T. Browne, L. M. Flanigan, C. A.

McComiskey, & P. Pieper (Eds.), *Nursing care of the pediatric surgical patient* (3rd ed., pp. 277–294). Burlington, MA: Jones & Bartlett Learning.

Hunter, A. K., & Liacouras, C. A. (2011). Pyloric stenosis and congenital anomalies of the stomach. In R. M. Kliegman, B. F. Stanton, J. W. St. Geme III, N. F. Schor, & R. E. Behrman, *Nelson textbook of pediatrics* (19th ed., pp. 1274–1275). Philadelphia, PA: Saunders Elsevier.

International Pediatric Endosurgery Group (IPEG). (2008a). IPEG guidelines for the surgical treatment of pediatric gastroesophageal reflux disease (GERD). *Journal of Laparoendoscopic & Advanced Surgical Techniques, 18*(6), x–xiii.

International Pediatric Endosurgery Group (IPEG). (2008b). IPEG guidelines for appendectomy. *Journal of Laparoendoscopic & Advanced Surgical Techniques, 18*(6), vii–ix.

Irving, P. M., & Gibson, P. R. (2007). Infliximab: Getting the most for your money. *Journal of Gastroenterology and Hepatology, 22*, 1557–1565.

Joanna Briggs Institute. (2008). The effectiveness of interventions for colic. *Australian Nursing Journal, 14*(4), 31–34.

Kairam, N., Kaiafis, C., & Shih, R. (2009). Diagnosis of pediatric intussusception by an emergency physician-performed bedside ultrasound. *Pediatric Emergency Care, 25*(3), 177–180.

Karam, O., Sanchez, O., Chardot, C., & La Scala, G. (2009). Blunt abdominal trauma in children: A score to predict the absence of organ injury. *Journal of Pediatrics, 154*(6), 912–917.

Kasten, E. F., Schmidt, S. P., Zickler, C. F., Berner, E., Damian, L. A., Christian, G. M., . . . Hicks, T. L. (2008). Team care of the patient with cleft lip and palate. *Current Problems in Pediatric and Adolescent Health, 38*, 138–158.

Katz, E. R., & DeMaso, D. R. (2011). Rumination, pica, and elimination (enuresis, encopresis) disorders. In R. M. Kliegman, B. F. Stanton, J. W. St. Geme III, N. F. Schor, & R. E. Behrman, *Nelson textbook of pediatrics* (19th ed., pp. 70–75). Philadelphia, PA: Saunders Elsevier.

Kenny, S. E., Tam, P. K. H., & Garcia-Barcelo, M. (2010). Hirschsprung's disease. *Seminars in Pediatric Surgery, 19*, 194–200.

Khalil, B. A., Thamara, M., Perera, P. R., & Mirza, D. F. (2009). Clinical practice: Management of biliary atresia. *European Journal of Pediatrics, 169*(4), 395–402.

Khan, A. N. (2011). *Omphalocele.* Retrieved from http://emedicine.medscape.com/article/404182-overview

Khan, S., & Orenstein, S. R. (2011). Esophageal atresia and tracheoesophageal fistula. In R. M. Kliegman, B. F. Stanton, J. W. St. Geme III, N. F. Schor, & R. E. Behrman, *Nelson textbook of pediatrics* (19th ed., pp. 1262–1263). Philadelphia, PA: Saunders Elsevier.

Kotecha, M., Bellah, R., Pena, A.H., Jaimes, C., & Mattei, P. (2012). Multimodality imaging manifestations of the Meckel diverticulum in children. *Pediatric Radiology, 42*, 95-103.

Leso, V., Leggio, L., Armuzzi, A., Gasbarrini, G., Gasbarrini, A., & Addolorato, G. (2010). Role of the tumor necrosis factor antagonists in the treatment of inflammatory bowel disease: An update. *European Journal of Gastroenterology and Hepatology, 22*(7), 779–786.

Levitt, M. A., & Peña, A. (2010). Imperforate anus and cloacal malformations. In G. W. Holcomb, III & J. P. *Murphy Ashcraft's Pediatric Surgery* (5th ed., pp. 468–490). Philadelphia: Saunders Elsevier.

Levy, R. L., Langer, S. L., Walker, L. S., Romano, J. M., Christie, D. L., Youseff, N., . . . Whitehead, W. E. (2010). Cognitive-behavioral therapy for children with functional abdominal pain and their parents decreases pain and other symptoms. *American Journal of Gastroenterology, 105*, 946–956.

Liacouras, C. A. (2011). Stomach and intestines: Normal development, structure, and function. In R. M. Kliegman, B. F. Stanton, J. W. St. Geme III, N. F. Schor, & R. E. Behrman, *Nelson textbook of pediatrics* (19th ed., pp. 1273). Philadelphia, PA: Saunders Elsevier.

Linton, D. M. (2011). Diagnosing GERD in older children. *Journal for Nurse Practitioners, 7*(4), 328–329.

Lund, C. H., Bauer, K., & Berrios, M. (2007). Gastroschisis: Incidence, complications, and clinical management in the neonatal intensive care unit. *Journal of Perinatal & Neonatal Nursing, 21*(1), 63–68.

Maarse, W., Bergé, S. J., Pistorius, L., van Barneveld, T., Kon, M., Breugem, C., & Mink van der Molen, A. B. (2010). Diagnostic accuracy of transabdominal ultrasound in detecting prenatal cleft lip and palate: A systematic review. *Ultrasound in Obstetrics and Gynecology, 35*(4), 495–502.

Maheshwari, A., & Carlo, W.A. (2011). Congenital Diaphragmatic Hernia. In R. M. Kliegman, B. F. Stanton, J.W. St Geme III, N.F. Schor, & R. E. Behrman, *Nelson textbook of pediatrics* (19th ed., pp. 594–596). Philadelphia: Saunders Elsevier.

Malaty, H. M., O'Malley, K. J., Abudayyeh, S., Graham, D. Y., & Gilger, M. A. (2008). Multidimensional measure for gastroesophageal reflux disease (MM-GERD) symptoms in children: A population-based study. *Acta Pædiatrica, 97*, 1292–1297.

Markowitz, J. E., & Dancel, L. D. (2008). *Volvulus.* Retrieved from http://emedicine.medscape.com/article/932430-overview

Martin, C. R., & Walker, W. A. (2008). Probiotics: Role in pathophysiology and prevention in necrotizing enterocolitis. *Seminars in Perinatology, 32*, 127–137.

McKenna, C., & Pieper, P. (2013). Pediatric trauma. In N. T. Browne, L. M. Flanigan, C. A. McComiskey, & P. Pieper (Eds.), *Nursing care of the pediatric surgical patient* (3rd ed., pp. 513–535). Burlington, MA: Jones & Bartlett Learning.

Miethke, A. G., & Balistreri, W. F. (2011). Morphogenesis of the liver and biliary system. In R. M. Kliegman, B. F. Stanton, J. W. St. Geme III, N. F. Schor, & R. E. Behrman, *Nelson textbook of pediatrics* (19th ed., pp. 1374). Philadelphia, PA: Saunders Elsevier.

Mikrogianakis, A. (2010). Penetrating abdominal trauma in children. *Clinical Pediatric Emergency Medicine, 11*(3), 217–224.

Mills, J. L. A., Lin, Y., MacNab, Y. C., Skarsgard, E. D., & Canadian Pediatric Surgery Network. (2010). Does overnight birth influence treatment or outcome in congenital diaphragmatic hernia? *Journal of Perinatology, 27*(1), 91–95.

Minkes, R. K., Bechtel, K. A., Billmire, D. F., Freitas, M. S., Glick, P., Hennelly, K. A., ... Wolfram, W. (2011). Pediatric Appendicitis. Retrieved from http://emedicine.medscape.com/article/926795-overview

Moerschel, S. K., Cianciaruso, L. B., & Tracy, L. R. (2008). A practical approach to neonatal jaundice. *American Family Physician, 77*(9), 1255–1262.

Montgomery, D. F., & Navarro, F. (2008). Management of constipation and encopresis in children. *Journal of Pediatric Health Care, 22*(3), 199–204.

Mooney, T., & Hogan, P. E. (2011). Pyloric stenosis: Exploring all the options. *Advance for NPs and PAs, 1*(2), 35–37.

Morgan, J. A., Young, L., & McGuire, W. (2011). Pathogenesis and prevention of necrotizing enterocolitis. *Current Opinion in Infectious Disease, 24,* 183–189.

Moules, T., & Ramsay, J. (2008). *The Textbook of Children's and Young People's Nursing.* Maulden, MA.: Blackwell Publishing, Ltd.

Moyer, K. D., & Balistreri, W. F. (2011). Liver disease associated with systemic disorders. In R. M. Kliegman, B. F. Stanton, J. W. St. Geme III, N. F. Schor, & R. E. Behrman, *Nelson textbook of pediatrics* (19th ed., pp. 1405). Philadelphia, PA: Saunders Elsevier.

Nelville, H. L. (2010). *Pediatric Hirschsprung disease.* Retrieved from http://emedicine.medscape.com/article/929733-overview

Nisell, M., Igl, W., Öjmyr-Joelsson, M., Frenckner, B., Rydelius, P., & Christensson, K. (2009). Social issues among children with high or intermediate imperforate anus: A proxy perspective. *Journal of Child and Adolescent Psychiatric Nursing, 22*(3), 132–142.

Nisell, M., Öjmyr-Joelsson, M., Frenckner, B., Rydelius, P., & Christensson, K. (2008). Views on psychosocial functioning: Responses from children with imperforate anus and their parents. *Journal of Pediatric Health Care, 22*(3), 166–174.

Nisell, M., Öjmyr-Joelsson, M., Frenckner, B., Rydelius, P., & Christensson, K. (2009). Psychosocial experiences of parents of a child with imperforate anus. *Journal for Specialists in Pediatric Nursing, 14*(4), 221–229.

Orenstein, S. R., & McGowan, J. D. (2008). Efficacy of conservative therapy as taught in the primary care setting for symptoms suggesting infant gastroesophageal reflux. *Journal of Pediatrics, 152,* 310–314.

Orr, S. (2011). Anal dilatation in children with anorectal malformations. *Gastrointestinal Nursing, 9*(8), 37–40.

Owens, J. (2008). Parents' experiences of feeding a baby with cleft lip and palate. *British Journal of Midwifery, 16*(12), 778–784.

Pakarinen, M. P., & Rintala, R. J. (2010). Management and outcome of low anorectal malformations. *Pediatric Surgery International, 26,* 1057–1063.

Pariset, J. M., Feldman, K. W., & Paris, C. (2010). The pace of signs and symptoms of blunt abdominal trauma to children. *Clinical Pediatrics, 49*(1), 24–28.

Patel, P. K., Ramaswamy, R., Grasseschi, M. F., & Morris, D. E. (2009). *Craniofacial, unilateral cleft lip repair.* Retrieved from http://emedicine.medscape.com/article/1279641-overview

Pepper, V. K., Stanfill, A. B., & Pearl, R. H. (2012). Diagnosis and management of pediatric appendicitis, intussusception, and Meckel's diverticulum. *Surgical Clinics of North America, 92,* 505–526.

Peyrin-Biroulet, L. (2011). Why should we define and target early Crohn's disease? *Gastroenterology & Hepatology, 7*(5), 324–326.

Pirie, J. (2010). Management of constipation in the emergency department. *Clinical Pediatric Emergency Medicine, 11*(3), 182–188.

Rapoport, K., & Nishii, E. K. (2013). Necrotizing enterocolitis. In N. T. Browne, L. M. Flanigan, C. A. McComiskey, & P. Pieper (Eds.), *Nursing care of the pediatric surgical patient* (3rd ed., pp. 295–311). Burlington, MA: Jones & Bartlett Learning.

Ratcliff, C. R. (2010). Early Peristomal Skin Complications Reported by WOC Nurses. *Journal of Wound, Ostomy, Continence Nursing, 37*(5), 505–510.

Razmus, I. S. (2011). Assessment and management of children with abdominal wall defects. *Journal of Wound, Ostomy and Continence Nursing, 38*(1), 22–26.

Reed, L. (2010). Irritable bowel syndrome. *Practice Nurse, 40*(1), 15–20.

Riffe, I., Sayre, J., Waller, T., Brinker, T., & Roberts, P. (2007). Gastroesophageal reflux disease in infants. *Family Practice Recertification, 29*(9), 28–33.

Roach, J. P., & Bruny, J. L. (2008). Advances in the treatment and understanding of biliary atresia. *Current Opinion in Pediatrics, 20,* 315–319.

Rogers, J. (2011). Functional constipation in childhood. *Nurse Prescribing, 9*(7), 326–331.

Rollins, M. D. (2012). Recent advances in the management of congenital diaphragmatic hernia. *Current Opinion in Pediatrics, 24,* (3), 379–385.

Ruano, R., Picone, O., Bernardes, L., Martinovic, J., Dumez, Y., & Benachi, A. (2011). The association of gastroschisis with other congenital anomalies: How important is it? *Prenatal Diagnosis, 31,* 347–350.

Saavedra, H., Losek, J. D., Shanley, L., & Titus, M. O. (2009). Gastrostomy tube related complaints in the pediatric emergency department identifying opportunities for improvement. *Pediatric Emergency Care, 25*(11), 728–732.

Salvadalena, G. (2008). Incidence of complications of the stoma and peristomal skin among individuals with colostomy, ileostomy and urostomy. *Journal of Wound, Ostomy and Continence Nursing, 35*(6), 596–607.

Sandler, A. D. (2010). Repetitive behaviors. In C. D. Rudolph, A. M. Rudolph, G. E. Lister, L. R. First, & A. A. Gershon (Eds.), *Rudolph's pediatrics* (22nd ed., pp. 342–346). New York, NY: McGraw-Hill.

Santacroce, L., & Ochoa, J. B. (2011). *Appendectomy.* Retrieved from http://emedicine.medscape.com/article/195778-overview#a1

Saverino, B. P., Lava, C., Lowe, L. H., & Rivard, D. C. (2010). Radiographic findings in the diagnosis of pediatric ileocolic intussusception: Comparison to a control population. *Pediatric Emergency Care, 26*(4), 281–284.

Saxena, A. K. (2011). Pediatric Abdominal Trauma. Retrieved from http://emedicine.medscape.com/article/1984811-overview

Schwartz, D. (2008). Imaging of suspected appendicitis: Appropriateness of various imaging modalities. *Pediatric Annals, 37*(6), 433–438.

Schwarz, S. M. (2011). Pediatric Biliary Atresia. Retrieved from http://emedicine.medscape.com/article/9300289-overview

Shah, A., & Carroll, M. (2007). *Peptic ulcer disease.* Retrieved from http://emedicine.medscape.com/article/932308-overview

Sherman, C. (2009, August). Managing patients infected with *H. pylori. Clinical Advisor,* 20–24.

Slator, R., Russell, J., Bridges, M., Tomlinson, J., Cole, A., & Morton, J. (2009). Understanding cleft lip and palate. 1: An overview. *Journal of Family Health Care, 19*(3), 101–103.

Slator, R., Russell, J., Cole, A., Tomlinson, J., Bridges, M., Clark, V., . . . Reading, J. (2009). Understanding cleft lip and palate. 2: The first five years. *Journal of Family Health Care, 19*(4), 122–125.

Sluiter, I., van de Ven, C. P., Wijnen, R. M. H., & Tibboel, D. (2011). Congenital diaphragmatic hernia: Still a moving target. *Seminars in Fetal & Neonatal Medicine, 16,* 139–144.

Sood, M. R. (2010). Constipation and fecal incontinence. In C. D. Rudolph, A. M. Rudolph, G. E. Lister, L. R. First, & A. A. Gershon (Eds.), *Rudolph's pediatrics* (22nd ed., pp. 1386–1389). New York, NY: McGraw-Hill.

Srivastava, R., Jackson, W. D., & Barnhart, D. C. (2010). Dysphagia and gastroesophageal reflux disease: Dilemmas in diagnosis and management in children with neurological impairment. *Pediatric Annals, 39*(4), 225–231.

Stafford, S. J., & Klein, M. D. (2011). Anorectal Malformations. In R. M. Kliegman, B. F. Stanton, J. W. St Geme III, N. F. Schor, & R. E. Behrman, *Nelson textbook of pediatrics* (19th ed., pp.1355–1359). Philadelphia: Saunders Elsevier.

St. Peter, S. D., Tsao, K., Spilde, T. L., Holcomb, G. W., III, Sharp, S. W., Murphy, J. P., . . . Ostlie, D. J. (2008). Single daily dosing ceftriaxone and metronidazole vs standard triple antibiotic regimen for perforated appendicitis in children: A prospective randomized trial. *Journal of Pediatric Surgery, 43*(6), 981–985.

Surawicz, C. M. (2008, May). Appendicitis: Toward a better diagnosis. *Clinical Advisor,* 39–41.

Thibodeau, G. A., & Patton, K. T. (2010). *The human body in health & disease* (5th ed.). St. Louis, MO: Mosby.

Tibesar, R. J., Black, A., & Sidman, J. D. (2009). Surgical repair of cleft lip and cleft palate. *Operative Techniques in Otolaryngology, 20,* 245–255.

Tipnis, N. A., & Tipnis, S. M. (2009). Controversies in the treatment of gastroesophageal disease in preterm infants. *Clinical Perinatology, 36,* 153–164.

Tobias, N., Mason, D., Lutkenhoff, M., Stoops, M., & Ferguson, D. (2008). Management principles of organic causes of childhood constipation. *Journal of Pediatric Health Care, 22*(1), 12–23.

Tsao, K., & Lally, K.P (2010). Congenital diaphragmatic hernia and eventration. In In G.W. Holcomb, III & J. P. *Murphy Ashcraft's Pediatric Surgery* (5th ed., pp. 304–321). Philadelphia: Saunders Elsevier.

Upadhyaya, V. D., Gangopadhyay, A., Srivastava, P., Hasan, Z., & Sharma, S. (2008). Evolution of management of anorectal malformation through the ages. *Internet Journal of Surgery, 17*(1). Retrieved from http://www.ispub.com/journal/the_internet_journal_of_surgery/volume_17_number_1/article/evolution_of_management_of_anorectal_malformation_through_the_ages.html

van der Pol, R. J., Smits, M. J., van Wijk, M. P., Omari, T. I., Tabbers, M. M., & Benninga, M. A. (2011). *Pediatrics, 127*(5), 925–935.

Wadhwani, S. L., Turmelle, Y. P., Nagy, R., Lowell, J., Dillion, P., & Shepherd, R. W. (2008). Prolonged neonatal jaundice and the diagnosis of biliary atresia: a single-center analysis of trends in age at diagnosis and outcomes. *Pediatrics, 121*(5), e1438–40.

Wan, M. J., Krahn, M., Ungar, W. J., Edona, C., Sung, L., Medina, L. S., & Doria, A. S. (2009). Acute appendicitis in young children: Cost-effectiveness of US versus CT in diagnosis—A Markov Decision Analytic Model. *Radiology, 250*(2), 378–386.

Wasley, A., Grytdal, S., & Gallagher, K. (2008). Surveillance for acute viral hepatitis—United States, 2006. *Morbidity and Mortality Weekly Report, 57*(SS02), 1–24.

Watkins, J. (2010/2011). Recognizing the signs of acute appendicitis. *British Journal of School Nursing, 5*(10), 488–491.

Wehby, G. L., & Cassell, C. H. (2010). The impact of orofacial clefts on quality of life and healthcare use and costs. *Oral Diseases, 16,* 3–10.

Weill, V. (2008). Gastroesophageal reflux in infancy. *Advance for Nurse Practitioners, 16*(1), 47–50.

Wendland, M., Jackson, Y., & Stokes, L. D. (2010). Functional disability in pediatric patients with recurrent abdominal pain. *Child Care, Health and Development, 36*(4), 516–523.

Werlin, S. L. (2011). Exocrine pancreas. In R. M. Kliegman, B. F. Stanton, J. W. St. Geme III, N. F. Schor, & R. E. Behrman, *Nelson textbook of pediatrics* (19th ed., pp. 1368–1374). Philadelphia, PA: Saunders Elsevier.

Wiet, G. J., Sie, K., Biavati, M. J., & Rocha-Worley, G. (2010). *Reconstructive surgery for cleft palate.* Retrieved from http://emedicine.medscape.com/article/878062-overview#a0102

Wilson, B. E., Etheridge, C. E., Soundappan, V. S. S., & Holland, A. J. A. (2010). Delayed diagnosis of anorectal malformations: Are current guidelines sufficient? *Journal of Paediatrics and Child Health, 46*(5), 268–272.

Wilson, B. A., Shannon, M. T., & Shields, K. M. (2011). *Pearson nurse's drug guide 2011.* New York, NY: Pearson.

Wong, K., & Bressler, B. (2008). Mild to moderate Crohn's disease: An evidence-based treatment algorithm. *Drugs 2008, 68*(17), 2419–2425.

Wright, K., & Miller, H. D. (2012). Evidence-based findings of necrotizing enterocolitis. *Newborn and Infant Nursing Reviews,12,* (1), 17–20.

Yazigi, N., & Balistreri, W. F. (2011). Viral hepatitis. In R. M. Kliegman, B. F. Stanton, J. W. St. Geme III, N. F. Schor, & R. E. Behrman, *Nelson textbook of pediatrics* (19th ed., pp. 1393–1404). Philadelphia, PA: Saunders Elsevier.

Zagaria, M. E. (2010). *Helicobacter pylori:* Recommended eradication regimens. *American Journal for Nurse Practitioners, 14*(1), 30–33.

Zerpa, J. A., & Shapiro, T. J. (2013). Malrotation and Volvulus. In N. T. Browne, L. M. Flanigan, C. A. McComiskey, & P. Pieper (Eds.), *Nursing care of the pediatric surgical patient* (3rd ed., pp. 333–346). Burlington, MA: Jones & Bartlett Learning.

Zilbert, N. R., Stamell, E. F., Ezon, I., Schlager, A., Ginsburg, H. B., & Nadler, E. P. (2009). Management and outcomes for children with acute appendicitis differ by hospital type: Areas for improvement at public hospitals. *Clinical Pediatrics, 48*(5), 499–504.

Pearson Nursing Student Resources
Find additional review materials at
nursing.pearsonhighered.com
Prepare for success with additional NCLEX®-style practice questions, interactive assignments and activities, web links, animations and videos, and more!

Alterations in Genitourinary Function

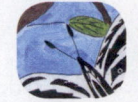
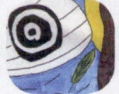
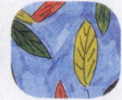

Learning Outcomes

After completing this chapter, you will be able to:

1. Describe the pathophysiologic processes associated with genitourinary disorders in the pediatric population.

2. Develop a nursing care plan for the child with a urinary tract infection.

3. Discuss the collaborative care and nursing management of the child with a structural defect of the genitourinary system.

4. Identify growth and development issues for the child with chronic renal failure.

5. Outline a plan to meet the fluid and dietary restrictions for the child with a renal disorder.

6. Summarize psychosocial issues for the child requiring surgery on the genitourinary tract.

7. Plan nursing care for the child with acute and chronic renal failure.

8. Plan a teaching session for the adolescent with a sexually transmitted infection.

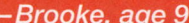

> **"I hope this medicine works! It hurts when I pee and I don't like having to run to the bathroom during class!"**
>
> —*Brooke, age 9*

The school nurse phones Mrs. McIntyre to let her know that her daughter Brooke, 9 years old, was referred by the teacher after she had to run to the bathroom a second time during class. Brooke states that it hurts when she urinates and that she feels very tired. She has a temperature of 100°F orally. The nurse is concerned that Brooke may have a urinary tract infection. Mrs. McIntyre arranges to pick her daughter up at school and take her to the pediatric healthcare facility. Brooke has no prior history of urinary tract infection. History reveals that she recently started taking bubble baths after soccer practice. A urine specimen is obtained by clean catch and the diagnosis of a urinary tract infection is confirmed. Brooke's healthcare provider writes a prescription for oral trimethoprim-sulfamethoxazole for the infection and Pyridium for pain. When Brooke returns to school the following day, she asks the school nurse why she needs to take medicine. The nurse uses an anatomically correct doll to teach Brooke about the infection. What should the clinic nurse teach Brooke and her mother about the antibiotic? In addition to pain medication, what methods can Brooke use to provide pain relief? What information should the school nurse include in the teaching?

Many infections, structural disorders, and disease processes can alter genitourinary function. Given that the kidneys and other urinary system organs perform numerous essential body functions, including removal of waste products and maintenance of fluid and electrolyte balance, disorders that affect these organs pose a significant threat to the health of children.

Although the reproductive system is functionally immature until puberty, disorders involving these organs may also have a significant impact on the health of children. Uncorrected structural defects and sexually transmitted infections can have both psychologic and physiologic implications on the developing child.

ANATOMY AND PHYSIOLOGY

The genitourinary system is made up of the urinary and reproductive organs. The urinary system, composed of the kidneys, ureters, bladder, and urethra, has an important function in excreting wastes and maintaining the acid–base and fluid and electrolyte balance (Figure 31–1 ■). The reproductive system consists of internal and external organs that at maturity promote the conception and healthy development of a fetus. Normal renal function requires the following: unimpaired renal blood flow, adequate glomerular ultrafiltration, normal tubular function, and unobstructed urine flow.

The functional unit of the kidney, the **nephron**, contributes to the formation of urine. The nephron is a tubular structure containing the renal corpuscle, proximal convoluted tubule, loop of Henle, distal convoluted tubule, and collecting duct. The renal corpuscle is composed of the glomerulus (a small group of capillaries) that loops into

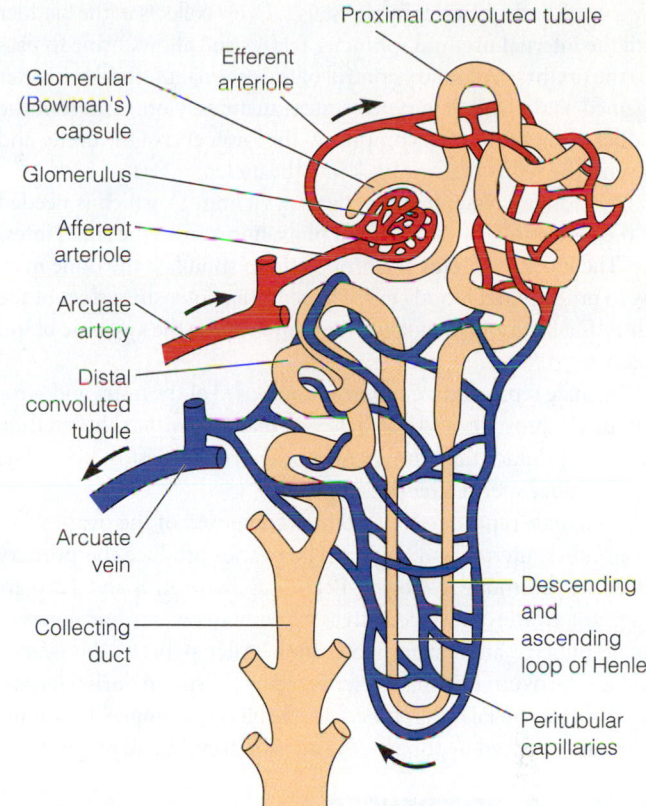

FIGURE 31–2 ■ The nephrons are the structural and functional unit of the kidneys. They filter water and wastes across the glomerular capillaries to maintain the body fluid level, electrolyte composition, and pH.

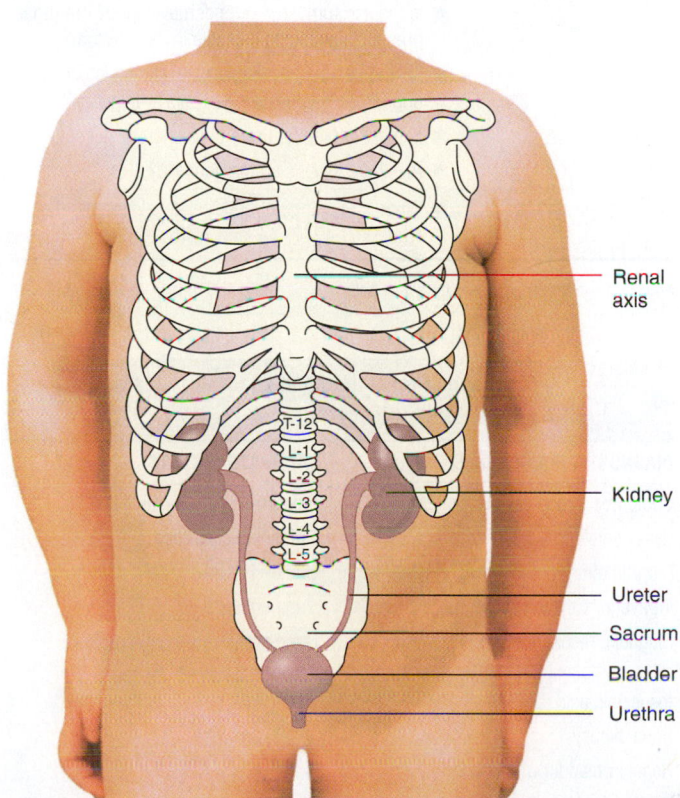

FIGURE 31–1 ■ The urinary system is composed of the kidneys, ureters, bladder, and urethra. The kidneys are located between the twelfth thoracic (T12) and third lumbar (L3) vertebrae.

the Bowman capsule. See Figure 31–2 ■ . The glomerular capillaries serve as the filtration membrane where metabolic wastes and fluids are separated from the blood cells and plasma proteins to form the urine. The kidney maintains the rate of blood flow to keep the **glomerular filtration rate (GFR)** (filtration of plasma) fairly constant. The urine flows through the proximal convoluted tubule, through the loop of Henle, and into the distal convoluted tubule and collecting duct. Water, electrolytes, and other substances are reabsorbed or secreted in the tubules, including the following (Huether, 2010a):

- *Proximal tubule*—Sodium chloride, glucose, potassium, amino acids, bicarbonate, urea, and water are reabsorbed.
- *Loop of Henle*—Water and sodium are reabsorbed, leading to urine concentration and secretion of urea.
- *Distal tubule*—Sodium chloride, bicarbonate, and water are reabsorbed; potassium, urea, hydrogen ions, and ammonia ions are secreted.
- *Collecting tubule*—Water is reabsorbed; sodium, potassium, hydrogen ions, and ammonia ions may be reabsorbed or secreted.

The presence of antidiuretic hormone (ADH) secreted by the posterior pituitary gland causes more water reabsorption leading to urine concentration. Absence of ADH leads to dilute urine. See Chapter 23 🔗 for more information about fluid and electrolyte physiology.

Urine from the nephron flows into the calyces in the renal pelvis and is funneled into the ureters. The lower end of the ureters connect into the posterior aspect of the bladder. The muscle cells of the ureters move urine to the bladder by peristalsis. Urine collects in the bladder until the internal urethral sphincter relaxes and allows urine to pass into the urethra. Voluntary control of the external urethral sphincter is gained as the child's nervous system matures. Contraction of the bladder during urination compresses the lower end of the ureter and prevents the reflux of urine back into the ureter.

The kidney is essential in activating vitamin D, which is needed for the absorption of calcium and phosphorus from the small intestine. The kidney secretes erythropoietin to stimulate the bone marrow to produce red blood cells. The renin-angiotensin system of the kidney is a hormonal regulator that can increase the systemic blood pressure.

The male reproductive system is composed of the testes and scrotum, penis, prostate, and vas deferens that drains into the urethra. The testes produce the primary male sex hormone, testosterone. The testes produce sperm after puberty.

The female reproductive system is composed of the ovaries, fallopian tubes, uterus, and vagina. The ovaries produce the primary female sex hormone, estrogen. Beginning between 8 and 12 years of age, the ovaries produce increasing amounts of sex hormones to initiate puberty and sexual maturation. After puberty, the ovaries produce the ovum that may be fertilized by the sperm during its passage through the fallopian tube into the uterus. Complex hormonal factors are involved in puberty, the menstrual cycle, and pregnancy.

PEDIATRIC DIFFERENCES

Urinary System

All of the nephrons that will make up the mature kidney are present at birth. The kidneys grow and the tubular system matures gradually during childhood, reaching full size by adolescence. Most renal growth occurs during the first 5 years of life. This increase in size is due primarily to enlargement of the nephrons. The kidney's efficiency also increases with age. During the first 2 years of life, the kidneys are less efficient at regulating electrolyte and acid–base balance (see Chapter 23 🔗) and eliminating some drugs from the body. After the age of 2 years, the kidneys' efficiency increases markedly. Urinary output per kilogram of body weight decreases as the child ages because the kidney becomes more efficient at concentrating urine. See Box 31–1 for expected urine output according to age.

Bladder capacity increases with age from 20 to 50 mL at birth to 700 mL in adulthood. A child's bladder capacity (in ounces) can be estimated by adding 2 to the child's age (e.g., a 4-year-old has a bladder capacity of 6 ounces). Stimulation of "stretch receptors" within the bladder wall initiates urination. Simultaneous contraction of the detrusor muscle of the bladder and relaxation of the internal and external sphincters result in emptying of the bladder. Children less than 2 years of age cannot maintain bladder control because of insufficient nerve development (Figure 31–3 ■).

BOX 31–1	Expected Urine Output According to Age

Urinary output per kilogram of body weight decreases as the child ages because the kidney becomes more efficient at concentrating urine. Expected output is:

- Infants, 2 mL/kg/hr
- Children, 0.5–1 mL/kg/hr
- Adolescents, 40–80 mL/hr

Reproductive System

The reproductive system in children is functionally immature until puberty. Throughout childhood the genitalia (with the exception of the clitoris in girls) enlarge gradually. The hormonal changes of puberty accelerate anatomic and functional development (see Chapter 7 🔗 and Figures 7–43, 7–44, and 7–45). In girls, the mons pubis becomes more prominent and hair begins to grow. The vagina lengthens, and the epithelial layers thicken. The uterus and ovaries enlarge, and the musculature and vascularization of the uterus also increase. In boys, downy hair begins to appear at the base of the penis, and the scrotum becomes increasingly pendulous as the testes enlarge. The penis increases in length and width.

See Table 31–1 for guidelines for assessment of the genitourinary system. Table 31–2 lists diagnostic tests and laboratory procedures for the genitourinary system.

TABLE 31–1	Assessment Guidelines for the Child with a Genitourinary Condition*
ASSESSMENT FOCUS	**ASSESSMENT GUIDELINES**
Urine characteristics	■ Does the urine have a strong odor or a dark or unusual color? Does it appear cloudy?
Pain or discomfort	■ Is there pain or burning with urination?
	■ Is there flank or abdominal pain?
	■ Is there scrotal or testicular pain?
Edema	■ Is there generalized edema?
Appearance of genitalia	■ What is the location of the urethra on the glans penis?
	■ Is the scrotum large or underdeveloped? Are rugae present? Are testes palpable in the scrotum?
	■ Do the genitalia have characteristic male or female appearance, or are the genitalia ambiguous?
	■ Is there vaginal or urethral discharge?
	■ Are there lesions on the genitalia?
Sexual development	■ What is the stage of pubertal development? (See Figures 7–43, 7–44, and 7–45 🔗.)

Note: *Refer to Chapter 7 🔗 for the actual techniques of assessment mentioned in this table.

TABLE 31–2	Diagnostic Procedures and Laboratory Tests for the Genitourinary System*
DIAGNOSTIC PROCEDURES	**LABORATORY TESTS**
Computed tomography (CT)	Blood urea nitrogen (BUN)
Cystoscopy	Creatinine clearance
Diuretic renogram (a type of nuclear scan)	Urinalysis (UA)
Intravenous pyelogram	Urine culture
Magnetic resonance imaging (MRI)	Urine protein-to-creatinine ratio
Radionucleotide renal scan with dimercaptosuccinic acid (DMSA)	
Renal biopsy	
Renal or bladder ultrasound	
Voiding Cystourethrogram (Vcug) or Radionuclide Cystography	

Note: *See Appendixes D and E 🔗 for information about these diagnostic procedures and tests.

As They Grow   Development of the Genitourinary System

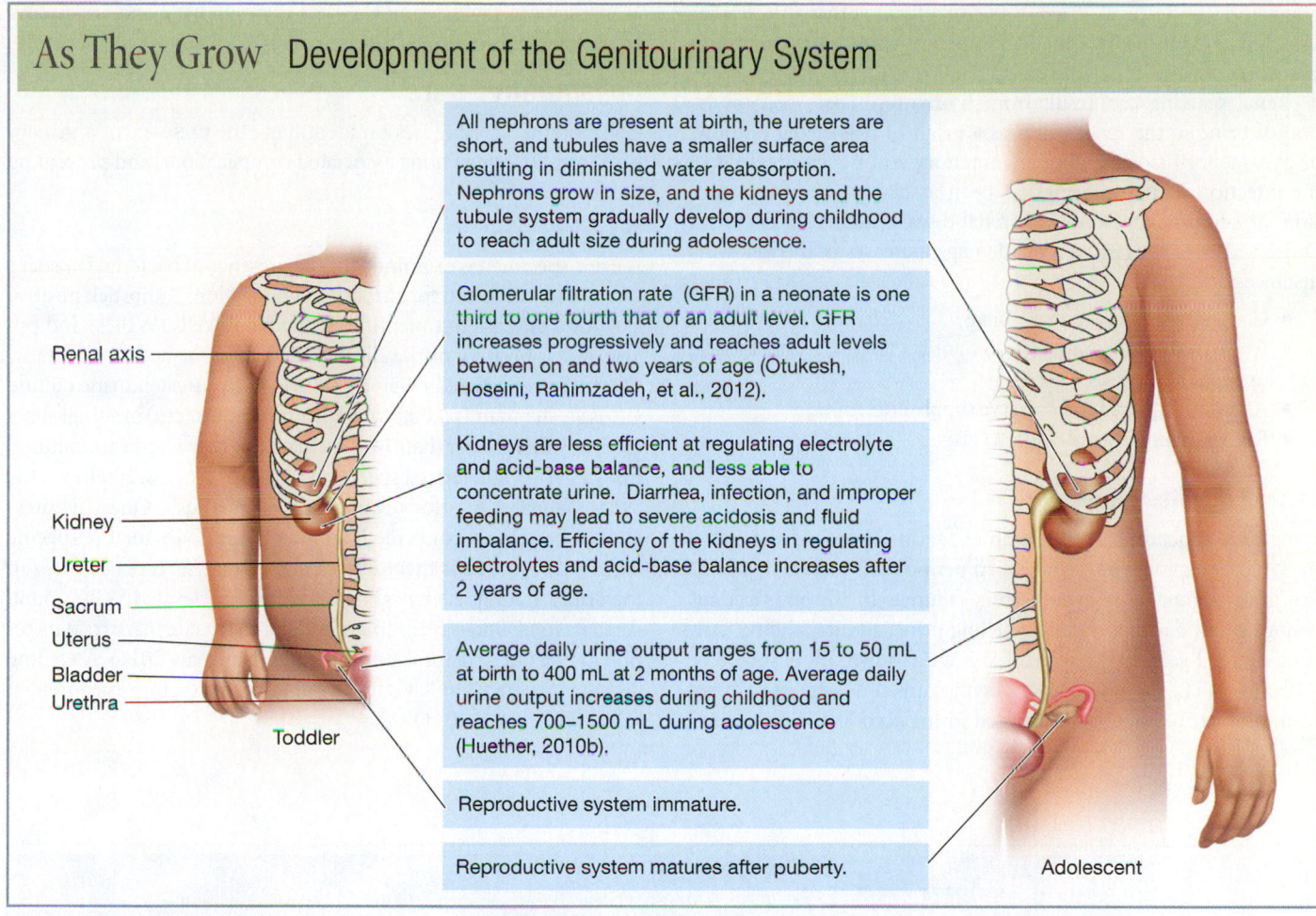

All nephrons are present at birth, the ureters are short, and tubules have a smaller surface area resulting in diminished water reabsorption. Nephrons grow in size, and the kidneys and the tubule system gradually develop during childhood to reach adult size during adolescence.

Glomerular filtration rate (GFR) in a neonate is one third to one fourth that of an adult level. GFR increases progressively and reaches adult levels between on and two years of age (Otukesh, Hoseini, Rahimzadeh, et al., 2012).

Kidneys are less efficient at regulating electrolyte and acid-base balance, and less able to concentrate urine. Diarrhea, infection, and improper feeding may lead to severe acidosis and fluid imbalance. Efficiency of the kidneys in regulating electrolytes and acid-base balance increases after 2 years of age.

Average daily urine output ranges from 15 to 50 mL at birth to 400 mL at 2 months of age. Average daily urine output increases during childhood and reaches 700–1500 mL during adolescence (Huether, 2010b).

Reproductive system immature.

Reproductive system matures after puberty.

Renal axis

Kidney

Ureter

Sacrum

Uterus

Bladder

Urethra

Toddler

Adolescent

FIGURE 31–3 ■ Development of the genitourinary system.

Source: *Data from Huether, S. E. (2010b). Alterations of renal and urinary tract function in children. In K. L. McCance & S. E. Huether,* Pathophysiology: The biologic basis for disease in children and adults *(6th ed., pp. 1402–1419). Maryland Heights, MO: Elsevier Mosby; Otukesh, H. Hoseini, R., Rahimzadeh, N., Hosseini, S. (2012). Glomerular Function in Neonates Iranian.* Journal of Kidney Diseases, 6 *(3), 166–172.*

URINARY TRACT INFECTION

An infection of the urinary tract may be of bacterial, viral, or fungal origin, and can occur in the lower or upper urinary tract. **Cystitis** is a lower urinary tract infection (UTI) that involves the urethra or bladder. **Pyelonephritis** is an upper UTI that involves the ureters, renal pelvis, and renal parenchyma. UTIs can be acute or chronic (the latter either recurrent or persistent).

UTIs are common in children, affecting 8% of females and 2% of males by 7 years of age (Craig, Simpson, Williams, et al., 2009). See Box 31–2.

Etiology and Pathophysiology

The urinary tract is normally sterile. The most common mechanism of infection occurs when an organism enters the genitourinary tract and ascends from the urethra to the bladder and up toward the kidney. Most UTIs in children are caused by *Escherichia coli,* a common gram-negative enteric bacterium (Fisher, Howes, & Thornton 2011).

Urinary stasis enhances the risk of UTI. Stasis may be caused by abnormal anatomic structures or functional abnormalities (e.g., a

BOX 31–2	Growth & Development: Urinary Tract Infections

Urinary tract infections are more common in males than females during the first 6 months of life. Uncircumcised infants in this age group are 10 to 12 times more likely to develop a UTI (Nguyen & Whitehill, 2011). After this age, UTI is much more common in females because the shorter female urethra (2 cm [1 in.] in young girls) has closer proximity to the anus and vagina, increasing the risk of contamination by fecal bacteria.

neurogenic bladder in which an interrupted nerve supply from myelomeningocele or spinal cord trauma impairs bladder voiding function and leads to incomplete bladder emptying). Children normally void five to six times a day. Infrequent voiding, common in school-age children, results in incomplete emptying of the bladder and urinary stasis. Other factors associated with increased risk of UTI include poor hygiene, inadequate cleansing after bowel movements, and an irritated perineum. Uncircumcised males in the first 6 months of life, constipation, and sexual activity in adolescent females also contribute to the incidence of UTI in the pediatric population (Fisher, et al 2011). **Vesicoureteral reflux (VUR),** the backflow of urine from the bladder into the ureters during voiding, is another cause of UTI and is discussed on page 1058.

Renal scarring can result from **hydronephrosis** (accumulation of urine in the renal pelvis as a result of obstructed outflow) or pyelonephritis due to the inflammatory and ischemic effects of the infection. Renal scarring has been associated with hypertension, proteinuria, and end-stage renal disease (Kennedy, Glynn, & Dineen, 2010). The risk of renal damage increases in the following instances:

- UTI in infants under 1 year of age
- Delay in diagnosis and effective antibacterial treatment for an upper UTI
- Anatomic obstruction or nerve supply interruption
- Recurrent episodes of upper UTIs

Clinical Manifestations

Symptoms depend on the location of the infection and the age of the child. Symptoms in the newborn period tend to be nonspecific (e.g., unexplained fever, hypothermia, failure to thrive, poor feeding, vomiting and diarrhea, strong-smelling urine, and irritability). Any child under 2 years of age with a fever of unknown origin should be tested for UTI. The more "classic" symptoms of lower UTI are not seen until the toddler years, as listed in the accompanying Clinical

Manifestations table. Many UTIs are asymptomatic and are discovered incidentally on routine examination.

Collaborative Care

Collaborative care focuses on identifying the presence of a urinary tract infection, preventing associated complications, and preventing reinfection.

Diagnostic Tests

A urine specimen is examined for the presence of bacteria. Dipsticks can be used to screen for urinary tract infection. A dipstick positive leukocyte esterase test identifies white blood cells (WBCs) and pyuria, and a positive nitrite dipstick detects gram-negative bacteria. The UTI is diagnosed when a midstream clean-catch urine culture yields greater than 100,000 colony-forming units (cfu) of a single bacteria, or when greater than 10,000 cfu of a single bacteria are cultured from a sterile catheterized specimen (Robbins & Shew, 2009). See the Skills Manual ⊂⊃ for urine collection methods. Once the presence of bacteria is confirmed, antibiotic sensitivity for the specific organisms cultured is then determined. Urinalysis reveals WBCs in the urine. A complete blood count reveals an elevated WBC count. A renal ultrasound is recommended after the first urinary tract infection to rule out structural abnormalities (Newman, 2011). A voiding cystourethrogram (VCUG) may be obtained to test for vesicoureteral reflux (Fisher, et al 2011).

Clinical Manifestations Urinary Tract Infection

TYPE OF UTI	CLINICAL MANIFESTATIONS	CLINICAL THERAPY
Lower UTI—Cystitis *Neonates*	Poor feeding, vomiting, failure to gain weight, jaundice, abdominal distention, lethargy, fever may be present	- Young infants initially receive parenteral antibiotics until afebrile for 24 hours and then are switched to an oral antibiotic matching organism sensitivity for a complete 10- to 14-day course. - Oral antibiotics are generally prescribed for 10–14 days for children over 2 months of age. - Recommended medications for febrile UTIs include sulfamethoxazole-trimethoprim, a second- or third-generation cephalosporin, or amoxicillin clavulanate. - Length of treatment may vary according to sensitivities, medication used, and age of child. - Encourage fluids. - Analgesics such as acetaminophen or Pyridium may be prescribed. - Review voiding habits if age appropriate and establish a schedule for voiding if needed to increase voiding frequency.
Infants	Fever, diarrhea, vomiting, irritability, lethargy, foul-smelling diapers, poor feeding, failure to gain weight	
Preschoolers	Fever, hematuria, urgency, dysuria, frequency, cloudy urine, foul-smelling urine, dehydration, abdominal pain, enuresis	
School-age children	Dysuria, enuresis, hematuria, strong-smelling urine, diarrhea, frequency or hesitancy, mood changes, abdominal pain, suprapubic or flank pain, dehydration	
Upper UTI—Pyelonephritis	High fever, chills, abdominal pain, nausea, vomiting, flank pain, costovertebral angle tenderness, moderate to severe dehydration	- IV antibiotics are given initially, then transitioned to oral antibiotics matching organism sensitivity once the child has been afebrile for 24–36 hours for a total of 10–14 days of therapy. - Therapy may include rehydration, antipyretics, and analgesics.

Source: *Data from American Academy of Pediatrics: Subcommittee on Urinary Tract Infection, Steering Committee on Quality Improvement and Management. (2011). Urinary tract infection: Clinical practice guideline for the diagnosis and management of the initial UTI in febrile infants and children 2–24 months. Pediatrics, 128(3), 595–610; Fisher, D. J., Howes, D. S., & Thornton, S. L. (2011). Pediatric urinary tract infection: Treatment & management. Retrieved from http://emedicine.medscape.com/article/969643-overview*

Practice Alert

Use of a sterile urine bag to collect urine for culture is likely to yield a contaminated specimen (Karacan, Erkek, Senel, et al., 2010). Confirmation of a UTI should be made with urine collected by catheterization or suprapubic aspiration (American Academy of Pediatrics: Subcommittee on Urinary Tract Infection, Steering Committee on Quality Improvement and Management, 2011).

Urine specimens collected for culture must be delivered to the laboratory within one hour or the specimen must be refrigerated to prevent the growth of organisms that occurs with prolonged room temperature exposure.

Clinical Therapy

Antibiotic therapy is begun as soon as urine samples have been collected. Antibiotics are selected based on the age of the child, sensitivity of the cultured organism, and the child's signs and symptoms. The antibiotic is changed if necessary after culture sensitivity is determined. Children with pyelonephritis should be maintained on antibiotic prophylaxis until radiologic tests are performed to detect any structural defects (Fisher, et al, 2011).

Children who appear ill and cannot tolerate oral antibiotics are often hospitalized because they need rehydration and initiation of parenteral antibiotic treatment until afebrile for 24 hours. Infants may develop permanent kidney damage or generalized sepsis if UTI is not treated aggressively. If a structural defect is identified, surgical correction may be necessary to prevent recurrent infections that could lead to renal damage.

Children treated on an outpatient basis should receive follow-up by phone (or in person if needed) within 24 to 48 hours to validate the child's response to treatment and to make changes to the treatment plan if needed based on urine culture sensitivities. A follow-up visit 7 to 10 days after the initiation of treatment is important to see how the patient responded to treatment (Fisher et al, 2011).

Nursing Management

Goals of nursing care are to collaborate in the identification of the child with a urinary tract infection, to promote adherence to prescribed therapy, and to prevent reinfection.

Nursing Assessment and Diagnosis

Nursing assessment focuses on identifying signs and symptoms of urinary tract infections and related complications.

Physiologic Assessment

Obtain a history of urinary symptoms. Determine if there is a history of recurrent urinary tract infections. Assess the infant for toxic (very ill) appearance, fever, and poor feeding. Evaluate the child's oral fluid intake. Assess for quality, quantity, and frequency of voiding. Assess the infant's or child's vital signs including blood pressure. This is an especially important assessment in infants and toddlers who cannot communicate. Assess for behavioral changes such as bed-wetting and loss of bladder control in older age groups.

Palpate the abdomen and suprapubic and costovertebral areas for masses, tenderness, and distention. Assess for abdominal or flank pain, frequency, urgency, and dysuria. Assess bathing and toileting habits (e.g., determine whether the child takes bubble baths, wipes from front to back, and engages in adequate perineal hygiene). Also be alert for signs of sexual abuse such as bruising or scarring of the perineal region.

Observe the urinary stream if possible and perform a urinalysis, including specific gravity. Proper collection of the urine specimen is essential. Obtain a clean-catch urine specimen if the child is old enough to do this. If not, get a catheterized sample. An early morning urine specimen is preferred because the urine is more concentrated. The early morning specimen may be used for repeat cultures, but in order to facilitate identification of a UTI and initiation of therapy, do not delay in obtaining the urine specimen.

Psychosocial Assessment

Adolescents who are sexually active may deny having symptoms of a UTI because they fear disclosing their sexual activity to their parents. Careful questioning and a visit alone with the adolescent may be necessary to elicit these concerns. Be open and approachable and give the patient and family the chance to address their concerns.

Common nursing diagnoses for the child with a UTI include:

- Urinary Elimination, Impaired related to recurrent urinary tract infections
- Growth and Development, Delayed related to chronic infection and renal damage
- Urinary Retention related to infrequent voiding habits or vesicoureteral reflux
- Fluid Volume: Deficient, Risk for related to fever and inadequate fluid intake
- Pain, Acute related to irritated urethra

NANDA-I © 2012

Planning and Implementation

Nursing care for the hospitalized child with a complicated UTI centers on administering prescribed medications, promoting rehydration, assessing renal function, and partnering with parents and older children to establish methods to minimize the risk of future infection.

Administer antibiotics and antipyretics as prescribed to maintain therapeutic drug levels and reduce fever. Encourage fluid intake according to normal requirements for age to dilute the urine and flush the bladder. Frequent voiding minimizes urinary stasis. Document intake and output. Assess renal function by comparing the child's output to the expected urine output (refer to Box 31–1) and weigh the child daily.

Because bladder training is such an important milestone for young children, any disorder that affects voiding may have developmental implications. A toddler who has been toilet trained may regress and require diapers temporarily due to incontinence related to the pain and frequency associated with the UTI. An older child may develop **enuresis** (repeated involuntary voiding by a child who has reached an age at which bladder control is expected) after a prolonged period of being dry at night. Partner with the family and offer reassurance that regression is normal and emphasize that the child needs support. A preschooler may perceive the infection and any parental disapproval as punishment for an imagined wrong. Reassure the child that he or she has not done anything wrong. (See Chapter 15 .)

Discharge Planning and Home Care Teaching

Children with UTIs such as Brooke from the opening scenario are usually cared for at home. Teach parents that all doses of the antibiotic must be taken as prescribed and that they may be continued even after the infection has cleared to prevent a recurrence. Teach prevention through proper hygiene and avoidance of risk behaviors. See Partnering with Families: Preventive Strategies for Urinary Tract Infections.

Give parents specific guidelines for oral fluid intake. The amount of fluids recommended for a 24-hour period equals the maintenance

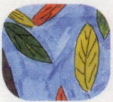

Partnering with Families

Preventive Strategies for Urinary Tract Infections

Provide education to parents about strategies to reduce the risk for future urinary tract infections, including the following:

- Teach proper perineal hygiene. Girls should always wipe the perineum from front to back after voiding.
- Encourage the child to drink plenty of fluids and avoid long periods of "holding urine."
- Caution against tight underwear; children should wear cotton rather than nylon underwear.

- Encourage the child to void more frequently and to fully empty the bladder.
- Discourage bubble baths and hot tubs, which can irritate the urethra.
- Encourage abstinence of sexual activity. However, if girls are sexually active, instruct them to void before and after sexual intercourse to prevent urinary stasis and flush out bacteria introduced during intercourse.

---

fluids for age plus any additional fluids required due to fever and diuresis (refer to Chapter 23 🔗) or as prescribed by the primary healthcare provider. Suggest that the parents avoid giving the child caffeinated and carbonated beverages as these may potentially irritate the bladder mucosa.

The child with a neurogenic bladder (see Chapter 33 🔗) requires a clean intermittent catheterization to be performed several times a day to reduce urinary stasis and the potential for UTI. Although the procedure for inserting the catheter is the same as that for catheterization using sterile technique, families are generally taught to use clean technique. See Partnering with Families: Clean Intermittent Catheterization below for teaching guidelines.

Evaluation

Expected outcomes of nursing care may include:

- The child increases fluid intake and number of times voiding each day.
- Future UTIs are prevented.

STRUCTURAL DEFECTS OF THE URINARY SYSTEM

Structural defects of the urinary system can result in obstructed or reduced urine flow, and may possibly affect reproductive function. Structural defects discussed in this section include bladder exstrophy, hypospadias, epispadias, obstructive uropathy, vesicoureteral reflux, and prune-belly syndrome. (See Chapter 29 🔗 for a discussion of Wilms tumor.)

Bladder Exstrophy

Bladder exstrophy is a rare congenital defect in which the bladder extrudes through the lower abdominal wall (Figure 31–4 ■). The defect occurs in approximately 1 in 35,000 to 40,000 newborns and is twice as common in males than females (Elder, 2011).

Etiology and Pathophysiology

Failure of the abdominal wall to close during fetal development results in eversion and protuberance of the bladder wall, along with a wide separation of the rectus muscles and the symphysis pubis. The upper urinary tract is usually normal.

Clinical Manifestations

The bladder mucosa appears as a mass of bright red tissue, and urine continually leaks from the ureters onto the skin (Huether, 2010b). The defect occurs in varying degrees of severity. Females have a bifid (split) clitoris. Males have a short penis, and the glans is flattened with dorsal **chordee** (a shortage of skin on the ventral side of the penis that causes the penis to curve) and a ventral prepuce. Undescended testicles and inguinal hernias are common in children with bladder exstrophy (Elder, 2011).

Collaborative Care

The goal of collaborative care is to protect the exposed bladder from injury and prevent infection, as well as preserve renal and reproductive function.

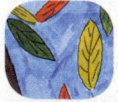

Partnering with Families

Clean Intermittent Catheterization

Clean intermittent catheterization (CIC) is performed to empty the bladder when nerves for bladder control are missing or damaged. Parents must learn to perform this procedure at home since it must be performed every 3 to 4 hours during the day. It is usually not done when the child sleeps at night. The child is ready to learn self-catheterization when he or she really wants to be dry and is learning independence. Until that time, parents usually perform CIC.

- Always have four or five catheters of the needed size and type available.
- Catheters may be used several times until they become hard and brittle or according to the manufacturer's guidelines.

- Use water-soluble lubricant (not petroleum jelly) to lubricate the catheter.
- Wash hands with soap and water or use alcohol-based hand gel prior to beginning the procedure.
- After the procedure, wash the catheter with soap and water and shake out excess water. Store the catheter in a plastic bag, toothbrush holder, or clean container after use.
- Keep a catheter in the car, book bag, fanny pack, or at school.

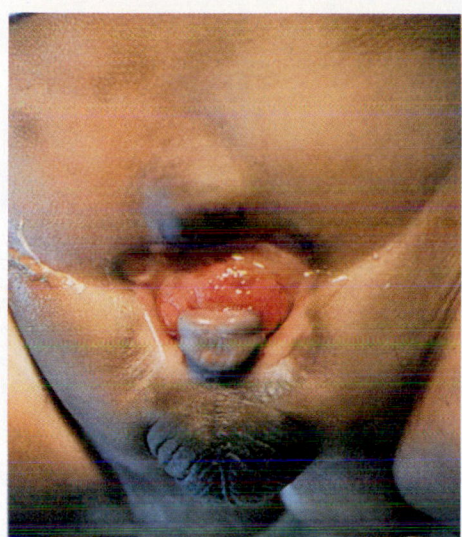

FIGURE 31–4 ■ This child has bladder exstrophy. Note the extrusion of the posterior bladder wall through the lower abdominal wall.

Diagnostic Tests

Prenatal diagnosis may be made with ultrasound. Diagnosis is also made at the time of delivery based on physical appearance of the infant. A renal ultrasound is used to identify hydronephrosis or other renal abnormalities.

Clinical Therapy

The exposed bladder tissue is covered with plastic wrap until surgery is performed to keep the bladder mucosa moist (Elder, 2011). Primary closure of the bladder and abdominal wall is usually completed within 48 to 72 hours after birth (Kozlowski, 2008). The wound and pelvis are immobilized to promote healing. An osteotomy (see Chapter 35 🔗) to rotate the innominate bones of the pelvis to approximate the symphysis pubis reduces tension on the closed bladder and abdominal wall to promote healing. Epispadias repair is often performed between 1 and 2 years of age or at the same time as a surgical procedure to improve continence. Surgery to reconstruct the bladder neck and reimplant the ureters is performed between 3 and 6 years of age when the bladder has achieved capacity of 80 to 90 mL (Elder, 2011). The goals of surgical reconstruction include closure of the bladder wall to provide means for urine storage and voiding and reconstruction of genitalia to creation functional and normal appearing genitalia to allow for sexual and urinary function. Some children require permanent urinary diversion because a functional bladder cannot be reconstructed.

Nursing Management

Goals of nursing management are to protect the exposed bladder until surgery is performed, to prevent complications such as infection, and to provide the family with support.

Nursing Assessment and Diagnosis

Nursing assessment includes immediate newborn assessment (see Chapter 7 🔗) and preoperative and postoperative assessments.

Newborn/Preoperative Assessment

Assess the newborn with exposed bladder tissue on the abdomen for other obvious defects such as epispadias or ambiguous genitalia. Assess the newborn's renal function and hydration status by monitoring the adequacy of urine output and serum and urine chemistries. Measure the newborn's weight daily. Assess family support systems and coping mechanisms when the newborn is diagnosed with the defect.

Postoperative Assessment

Routinely empty and record urine output from each ureteral drainage tube every 2 to 4 hours and note any change in urine output that could indicate an obstruction of the tube. Other signs of obstruction may include urine or blood draining from the urethral meatus or increased intensity of bladder spasms. Monitor for signs of pain (see Chapter 17 🔗). Monitor urine for blood or clots, which are common in the first few days following surgery. Assess incisions to make sure they are intact. Assess peripheral circulation of the lower limbs if a spica cast has been applied (see Chapter 35 🔗).

Family Assessment

Assess the parents for their response to the newborn's defect and the need for immediate surgery. Begin to identify family resources for support and care of an infant requiring long-term care and multiple surgeries.

Nursing diagnoses for the newborn with bladder exstrophy may include:

- Infection, Risk for related to exposed bladder and surgical incision
- Skin Integrity, Impaired related to exposed bladder and surgical incision
- Pain, Acute related to surgical incision
- Attachment, Risk for Impaired Parent/Infant related to newborn with genitourinary structural defect and immediacy of surgery

NANDA-I © 2012

Planning and Implementation
Preoperative Care

Preoperative nursing care centers on preventing infection and trauma to the exposed bladder. The bladder mucosa is covered with plastic wrap to keep the bladder mucosa moist (Elder, 2011). The surrounding area is cleaned daily and protected from leaking urine with a skin sealant.

Practice Alert
At the time of the newborn's delivery, the umbilical cord of the infant with bladder exstrophy should be tied rather than clamped since a clamp could cause trauma to the bladder mucosa (Elmore, Kirsch, Snyder, et al., 2009).

Postoperative Care

After primary closure, the wound and pelvis are immobilized to facilitate healing. Internal and external immobilization techniques are used for pelvic closure (see Chapter 35 🔗). Effective pain management is essential to maintaining immobilization (Kozlowski, 2008). In addition to pain assessment and management, nursing care includes maintaining proper alignment, avoiding abduction of the infant's legs, monitoring peripheral circulation, and providing meticulous wound and skin care. Maintain aseptic technique for wound care and monitor for signs of infection including redness, drainage, and edema.

Monitor renal function by assessing the adequacy of urine output and blood and urine chemistries to detect signs of renal damage. Observe for any signs of obstruction in the drainage tubes such as increased intensity of bladder spasm, decreased urine output, or urine

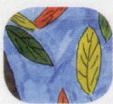

Partnering with Families

Recognizing Signs of Infection Following Surgery

When the child is discharged home following repair of genitourinary structural defects, whether it is shortly after surgery or several days later, ensure that parents understand signs and symptoms of infection and the need to report any complications to the primary healthcare provider. Signs and symptoms of infection include:

- Cloudy and foul-smelling urine
- Increased temperature

- Purulent drainage
- Foul odor from the incision
- Increased fussiness
- Decreased feeding

---

or blood draining from the urethral meatus. Promote comfort and give antibiotics as ordered.

Parents need emotional support to help them cope with the disfiguring nature of the infant's defect and the uncertainty of complete repair. To promote parent–infant bonding, encourage parents to partner with healthcare professionals in all aspects of the infant's care, including bathing, feeding, and wound care. They may also need guidance in the best way to hold the baby. Discharge teaching should include instructions regarding dressing changes and diapering and the need to immediately report any signs of infection or change in renal function. Help parents recognize complications and the need to seek immediate attention for the newborn. (See Partnering with Families: Recognizing Signs of Infection Following Surgery.) Emphasize the need for routine follow-up visits after surgery to assess urinary function and to ensure that the next stages of surgery for continence control are performed at the appropriate time and age in the child's development.

Discharge Planning and Home Care Teaching

Long-term care of the child with bladder exstrophy focuses on establishing continence and addressing social and sexual issues. The family should be aware that achievement of continence is more difficult in children with bladder exstrophy, and urinary diversion to achieve continence may be necessary if surgical procedures are not successful. However, parents should be encouraged to initiate toilet training at the appropriate age for bowel movements. Until urinary continence is achieved, the nurse assists the family in coping with

the child's incontinence and identifying strategies to maintain skin integrity and promote the child's growth and development. Parents may require guidance to promote the child's self-esteem and self-confidence with sexual identity and function. Psychologic counseling may be beneficial to the child during adolescence.

Evaluation

Expected outcomes of nursing care in the immediate postoperative period include:

- The incision heals without signs of infection.
- The child's skin integrity is restored and maintained.
- Pain is managed effectively.
- Parent–infant bonding and attachment is demonstrated.

Hypospadias and Epispadias

Hypospadias and **epispadias** are congenital anomalies involving an abnormal location of the urethral meatus (Figure 31–5 ■). The reported incidence of hypospadias is 1 in 250 male births (Elder, 2011). The incidence of epispadias is 1 in 40,000 to 118,000 births. Epispadias occurs twice as often in males as females (Huether, 2010b).

Etiology and Pathophysiology

Both defects result from failure of the urethral folds to fuse completely over the urethral groove. A familial tendency is recognized, in that about 8% of fathers and 14% of brothers of a boy with hypospadias

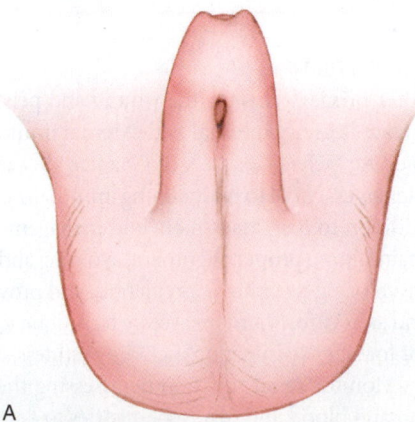 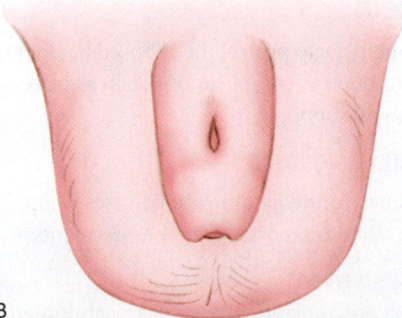

A   B

FIGURE 31–5 ■ Hypospadias and epispadias. *A,* In hypospadias, the urethral canal is open on the ventral surface of the penis. *B,* In epispadias, the urethral canal is open on the dorsal surface.

also have the condition (Pfeil & Lindsay, 2010). Hypospadias often occurs in conjunction with congenital chordee. Associated defects may include inguinal hernia, cryptorchidism (undescended testes), and partial absence of the foreskin (Huether, 2010b). Epispadias and bladder exstrophy are the same condition, but epispadias is the milder expression of the condition (Huether, 2010b). See the section on bladder exstrophy on page 1052. In males with epispadias, the meatal opening is located on the dorsal surface of the penile shaft. The opening may be small or a fissure may extend the entire length of the penis. Females with epispadias have a cleft of the ventral urethra that generally extends to the bladder neck (Huether, 2010b). The remainder of this discussion will focus on hypospadias and males with distal epispadias as the treatment for severe epispadias in males and epispadias in females is similar to the second and third stages of repair of bladder exstrophy (Elder, 2011).

Clinical Manifestations

In hypospadias, the urethral meatus can be located anywhere along the course of the urethra on the ventral surface of the penile shaft, from the perineum to the tip of the glans. Most cases of hypospadias are mild, with the meatus slightly off center from the tip of the penis; in severe cases, the meatus is located on the scrotum.

Collaborative Care

Collaborative care focuses on identification and correction of the defect, prevention of infection, and promotion of urinary elimination and sexual function.

Diagnostic Tests

Diagnosis is made by prenatal ultrasound or by examination at birth. Other diagnostic studies may include urinalysis and urine culture. Refer to the Skills Manual 🔗 for guidelines related to collection of urine specimens. When severe hypospadias occurs in combination with undescended testicle and ambiguous genitalia, a complete endocrine and genetic workup should be performed to rule out intersexuality (Pfeil & Lindsay, 2010).

Clinical Therapy

Surgical correction of the structural defect is the treatment for hypospadias and epispadias. The defects are corrected surgically, usually during infancy to minimize psychologic effects when the child is older. The infant should not be circumcised because the foreskin tissue may be used for surgical repair (Pieretti, Pieretti, & Pieretti-Vanmarcke, 2009). Surgery is generally performed in a single operation and often as an outpatient procedure. Surgery is recommended between 6 and 12 months of age (Pfeil & Lindsay, 2010). For more severe cases, surgical repair may require two stages. Goals of surgical repair are:

- Placement of the urethral meatus at the end of the glans penis with satisfactory caliber and configuration for a urinary stream (enabling the child to void in a standing position)
- Release of chordee to straighten the penis (enabling future sexual function)
- Satisfactory cosmetic appearance of the penis

A caudal nerve block is often used for initial postoperative pain relief. Anticholinergic medications such as oxybutynin may be prescribed to relieve bladder spasms. A urethral stent or catheter is placed to maintain patency of the new urethral canal opening. The stent or catheter may drain directly into the diaper or into a closed drainage collection bag (Pfeil & Lindsay, 2010).

Clinical Tip

A **ureteral stent** is a device used to maintain patency of the ureter, allowing urine flow from the kidney to the bladder. A **urethral stent** is a device used to maintain patency of the urethral canal and allow urine flow from the bladder through the urethra.

Nursing Management

Goals of nursing management are to assist in collaborative identification of the defect, prevent potential complications such as infection and urethral obstruction, promote parental understanding and attachment to the newborn, and promote a normal voiding pattern.

Nursing Assessment and Diagnosis

Perform a thorough newborn assessment to detect the presence of genitourinary defects (see Chapter 7 🔗). Assess the newborn's flow of urine, exit site, and angle of urination. Assess family support systems and coping mechanisms when the newborn is diagnosed with this defect.

Assess the older child's level of understanding of the procedure and need for surgery. Postoperative assessment includes monitoring for penile swelling, dysuria, bleeding at the surgical site, infection, and evidence of pain.

Nursing diagnoses for the child with hypospadias or epispadias may include:

- *Infection, Risk for* related to altered urinary elimination
- *Injury, Risk for* related to dislodged stent or catheter
- *Pain, Acute* related to surgical procedure
- *Anxiety (Parents)* related to genitourinary defect in newborn infant and surgical procedures

NANDA-I © 2012

Planning and Implementation

The nurse addresses the parents' concerns at the time of birth. Preoperative teaching can relieve some of their anxiety about the future appearance and functioning of the penis. For the older child undergoing surgical correction, the use of dolls and pictures to explain the procedure may help the child develop a better understanding. See Chapter 15 🔗 for further discussion on preparing children for surgery.

Postoperative care focuses on protecting the surgical site from injury. The infant or child returns from surgery with the penis wrapped in a simple dressing and a stent or catheter for urinary drainage. Fresh blood may be seen on the dressing and in the stent or catheter during the immediate postoperative period, but the urine should become less bloody over the next few hours. Partner with the family and plan care to ensure that the stent or catheter is not removed. Refer to the hospital's policy for the appropriate use of immobilizers in this situation. (See the Skills Manual 🔗.)

Encourage fluid intake to maintain adequate urinary output and patency of the stent. Accurate and hourly documentation of intake and output is essential to detect postoperative urinary complications. Notify the primary healthcare provider if there is no urine drainage for 1 hour, as this may indicate kinks in the system or obstruction.

Pain may be associated with bladder spasms. Anticholinergic medications such as oxybutynin or hyoscyamine may be prescribed.

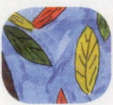

Partnering with Families

Care for the Child After Hypospadias or Epispadias Repair

Guidelines for the care of children at home following hypospadias or epispadias repair include the following:

- Use the double-diapering technique shown in Figure 31–6 ■ to protect the stent (the small tube that drains the urine) or urinary catheter from contamination by stool.
- Do not bathe the child in the tub until the stent or catheter is removed.
- Restrict the infant or toddler from activities that put pressure on the surgical site (e.g., playing on riding toys). Avoid holding the infant or child straddled on the hip. Limit the child's activity for 2 weeks.

- Encourage the infant or toddler to drink fluids to ensure adequate hydration. Provide fluids in a pleasant environment or use a special cup. Offer fruit juice, fruit-flavored ice pops, fruit-flavored juices, flavored ice cubes, and gelatin.
- Administer the *complete course* of prescribed antibiotics to avoid infection.
- Observe for signs of infection: fever, swelling, redness, pain, strong-smelling urine, or change in flow of the urinary stream.
- The urine will be blood tinged for several days. Call the healthcare provider if urine is seen leaking from any area other than the penis.

Once the caudal block wears off, acetaminophen or ibuprofen should be administered for pain as ordered. Antibiotics are usually prescribed until the urinary stent falls out or is removed.

The child is often discharged the day of surgery. Partner with the family to provide instructions regarding care of the reconstructed area, double diapering to protect the stent, fluid intake, medication administration, and signs of infection. (See Partnering with Families: Care for the Child After Hypospadias or Epispadias Repair.)

Evaluation

Expected outcomes of nursing care include:

- The incision heals without signs of infection.
- The catheter or stent remains intact until healing occurs.
- Pain is managed effectively.
- Parents cope with the stress of the child's anomaly and need for surgery.

Obstructive Uropathy

Obstructive uropathy refers to structural or functional abnormalities of the urinary system that interfere with urine flow and result in urine backflow into the kidneys. The uropathy may be bilateral or unilateral

and partial or incomplete. The urinary obstruction may occur anywhere along the urinary tract, including the ureters, renal pelvis, bladder, and urethra. The condition is more common in males than females.

Etiology and Pathophysiology

Obstructive uropathy may be caused by several congenital lesions such as ureteropelvic junction obstruction, posterior urethral valves, and stenosis or hypoplasia of the ureterovesicular junction (Figure 31–7 ■).

- The ureteropelvic junction (UPJ), the tapered point where the renal pelvis transitions to the ureter, is the most frequent site of obstruction of the upper urinary tract in infants and children. UPJ obstruction occurs in 1 out of every 1,000 to 2,000 newborns, making it the most common cause of hydronephrosis in newborns (Han, Rah, & Lee, 2010).
- **Posterior urethral valve (PUV),** abnormal folds of mucosa in the male urethra, is the most common cause of lower urinary tract obstruction in male infants (Hodges, Patel, McLorie, et al., 2009). This condition is also the most common obstructive cause of end-stage renal disease in children and occurs in 1 in 8,000 male births (Uthup, Binitha, Geetha, et al., 2010).
- Stenosis of the distal ureter at the ureterovesicular junction leads to dilation of the entire ureter, renal pelvis, and kidney (Huether, 2010b).
- Other conditions that can lead to hydronephrosis include prune-belly syndrome, myelomeningocele, and neoplasms. See page 1059 for discussion of prune-belly syndrome.

The pressure caused by urine backup compromises kidney function and often causes hydronephrosis. Several physiologic changes may occur as a result of hydronephrosis:

- Cessation of glomerular filtration results when the pressure in the kidney pelvis equals the filtration pressure in the glomerular capillaries. To compensate, the blood pressure increases to increase the glomerular filtration pressure. However, increasing pressure on the glomeruli leads to cell death.
- Metabolic acidosis results when the distal nephron's ability to secrete hydrogen ions is impaired.
- Impairment of the kidney's ability to concentrate urine results in polydipsia and polyuria.
- Obstruction results in urinary stasis, promoting bacterial growth.
- Restriction of urinary outflow causes progressive renal damage and chronic renal failure if untreated.

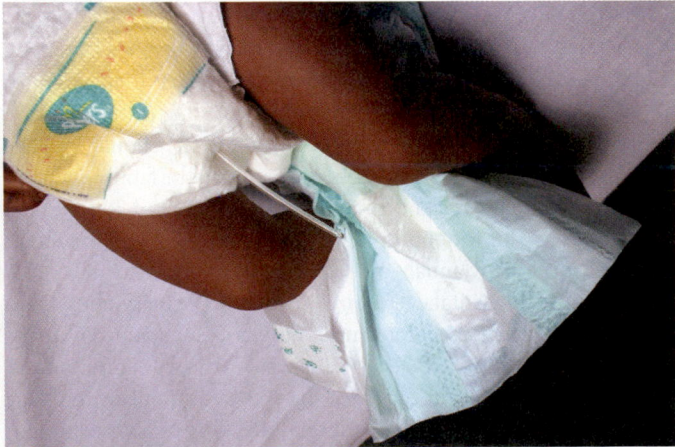

FIGURE 31–6 ■ A double-diapering technique protects the urinary stent after surgery for hypospadias or epispadias repair. The inner diaper collects stool, and the outer diaper collects urine.

Pathophysiology Illustrated
Obstruction Sites

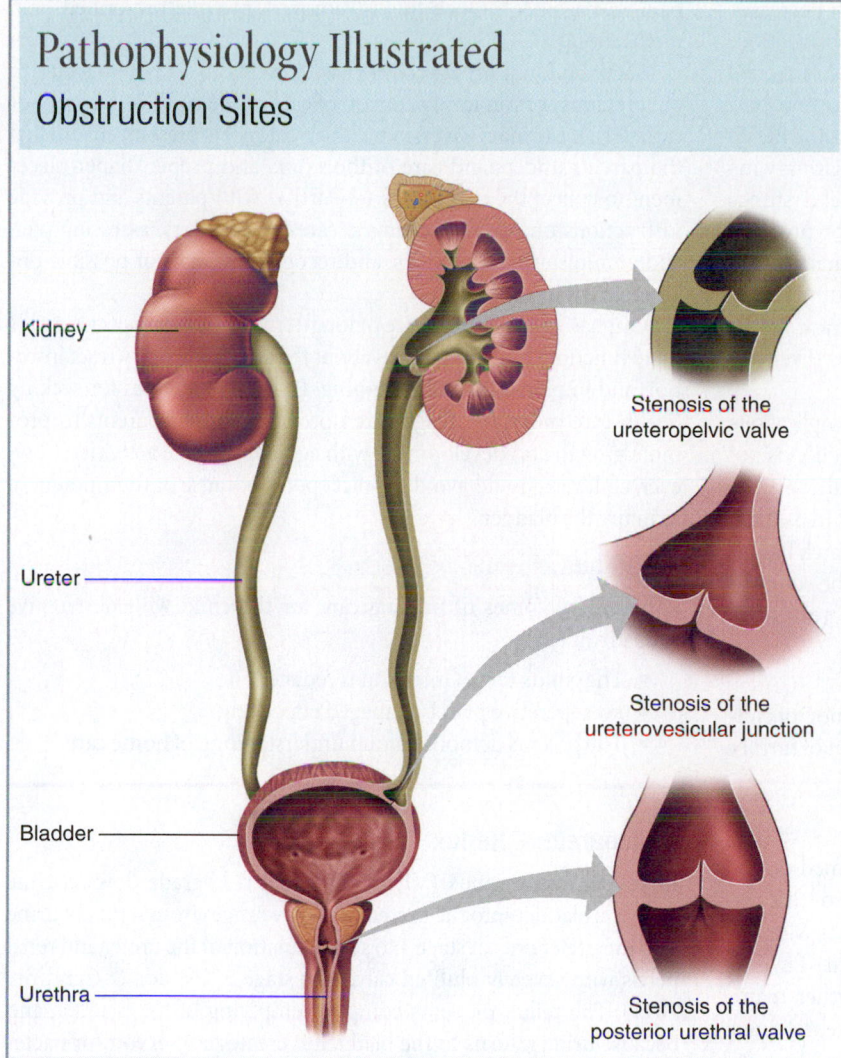

Kidney

Ureter

Bladder

Urethra

Stenosis of the
ureteropelvic valve

Stenosis of the
ureterovesicular junction

Stenosis of the
posterior urethral valve

FIGURE 31–7 ■ Obstruction may occur in either the upper or lower urinary tract. Common sites of obstruction occur at the ureteropelvic valve, the ureterovesicular junction, or the posterior urethral valve. Why would damage from posterior urethral valves potentially be worse than other obstructions? Renal failure is most likely to occur when both kidneys are affected by hydronephrosis.

Clinical Manifestations

Clinical manifestations of obstructive uropathy may include an abdominal mass, palpable bladder, and alternating episodes of increased and decreased urinary output. Some clinical manifestations in infants and children are dependent on the location and severity of the obstructive lesion. See the Clinical Manifestations table.

Collaborative Care

Early diagnosis and treatment is needed to prevent kidney damage and deterioration of renal function. Management of obstructive uropathy focuses on relieving the cause of obstruction.

Diagnostic Tests

Prenatal ultrasound may detect hydronephrosis and PUV. Postnatal assessment reveals a distended bladder and signs and symptoms of **renal insufficiency** (decrease in the kidneys' ability to conserve sodium and concentrate the urine). A diuretic-enhanced radionuclide scan and VCUG is performed when a ureteropelvic or ureterovesicular obstruction is suspected.

A VCUG reveals a dilated posterior urethra, which is diagnostic for PUV. Serial serum creatinine and electrolyte levels are obtained to monitor renal function. Arterial blood gases may reveal metabolic acidosis due to improper renal function.

Clinical Therapy

For acute obstructions, immediate intervention is required. Short-term management includes immediate placement of a urethral catheter in newborns with suspected PUV to promote urine drainage, thereby decreasing pressure in the kidneys (Bomalaski, 2010).

Goals of surgical correction or diversion are to lower the pressure within the collecting system,

Clinical Manifestations Obstructive Lesions of the Urinary System

OBSTRUCTIVE LESION	ETIOLOGY	CLINICAL MANIFESTATIONS
Ureteropelvic junction obstruction	Folds of the upper ureter causing urinary stasis Fibrotic stenosis of the ureteropelvic junction	Infants: Abdominal mass (enlarged kidney), hypertension, urinary tract infection Children: Hematuria, pain, intermittent nausea and vomiting
Posterior urethral valves	Congenital membrane that partially or completely obstructs the posterior urethra	Infants: Abdominal mass (enlarged kidney), distended bladder, poor urinary stream, urinary tract infection, sepsis, low specific gravity, polyuria, increased creatinine level, failure to thrive Older children: Diurnal enuresis, urinary tract infection, dribbling and/or retention of urine, hematuria
Ureterovesical junction obstruction	Maldevelopment of the distal ureteral muscle Ureterocele (dilation of terminal ureter) Ectopic ureter (ureter drains outside of the bladder)	Urinary tract infection (recurrent or chronic), hematuria, pain, abdominal mass (enlarged kidney), enuresis

Source: *Data from Elder, J. S. (2011). Urologic disorders in infants and children. In R. M. Kliegman, B. F. Stanton, J. W. St. Geme III, N. F. Schor, & R. E. Behrman, Nelson textbook of pediatrics (19th ed., pp. 1827–1864). Philadelphia, PA: Saunders Elsevier; Frøkiaer, J., & Zeidel, M. L. (2012). Urinary tract obstruction. In M. W. Taal, G. M. Chertow, P. A. Marsden, K. Skorecki, A. S. L. Yu, & B. M. Brenner, Brenner and Rector's the kidney (9th ed., pp. 1239–1260). Philadelphia, PA: Saunders Elsevier; Hodges, S., Patel, B., McLorie, G., & Atala, A. (2009). Posterior urethral valves. Scientific World Journal, 9, 1119–1126.*

which reduces renal damage, and to prevent stasis, which decreases the risk of infection. Depending on the cause of the obstruction, surgical correction may necessitate **pyeloplasty** (removal of an obstructed segment of the ureter and reimplantation into the renal pelvis), valve repair, or reconstruction. Surgical interventions for PUVs include transurethral ablation or cutaneous vesicostomy. Urinary incontinence resulting from sphincter incompetence, bladder dysfunction, and polyuria related to renal insufficiency is a common problem after surgery, and it can cause hydronephrosis due to urinary retention (Thomas, 2010). Strategies to manage urinary incontinence in some cases include clean intermittent catheterization. In rare cases a urinary diversion with an ostomy may be necessary. This diversion may be either temporary or permanent.

For mild obstructions in the absence of significant complications such as urinary retention or urinary tract infections, correction is not emergent. The child may be observed for a period of time without surgical intervention to see if the obstruction resolves on its own. In the past, children were placed on antibiotic prophylaxis. Recent research has indicated that this is not necessary. Parents should however be educated about signs of urinary tract infection (Islek, Güven, Koyun, et al., 2011).

Nursing Management

The goal of nursing care is to collaborate in the identification of children with obstructive uropathy as well as in the prevention of further renal complications.

Nursing Assessment and Diagnosis

A thorough history and physical examination is performed on the child exhibiting any of the symptoms that are suggestive of this disorder. Palpate the abdomen for a mass or distended bladder. Monitor the urine output and observe the force of the urine stream. If hydronephrosis progresses and urine output diminishes, further manifestations may include peripheral edema and costovertebral angle tenderness.

Parents may be distressed, especially if hydronephrosis was detected on prenatal ultrasound. Assess the parents' coping and ability to hear and understand information presented about the infant's condition.

Nursing diagnoses for the child with obstructive uropathy may include:

- Urinary Elimination, Impaired related to obstructed outflow
- Infection, Risk for related to urinary retention
- Anxiety, (Parent) related to infant's potential for progressive renal failure
- Pain, Acute related to surgical procedure

NANDA-I © 2012

Planning and Implementation

Preoperative nursing care focuses on preparing the parents and child for the procedure and addressing parental concerns about the postsurgical outcome. Provide parents with an opportunity to discuss concerns about the effect of the disorder on the child's long-term renal functioning.

Postoperative care involves monitoring vital signs, as well as intake and output, and observing for signs of urine retention, such as decreased output and bladder distention. Administer medications as prescribed, including antibiotics and antispasmodics such as oxybutynin. An epidural catheter may have been placed for

pain management. Once this is removed, provide prescribed pain medication.

Many children are discharged with stents or catheters (refer to the previous section for discussion of care of the child with a stent or catheter). If a urinary diversion with an ostomy is present, ensure that the parents understand care of the stoma and proper diaper placement to collect the urine outflow. Partner with parents and provide instructions on dressing changes, care for catheters, assessing pain and administering analgesics, and recognizing signs of possible obstruction or infection.

Emphasize the importance of long-term monitoring of the child's renal function. Educate parents about the signs of urinary tract infection and impaired renal functioning. Provide guidelines for seeking health care promptly if signs are noted. Encourage parents to promote growth and development with age-appropriate activities; however, children should avoid contact sports because of their potential to injure the bladder.

Evaluation

Expected outcomes of nursing care for the child with obstructive uropathy include:

- The child's risk of infection is reduced.
- Postoperative pain is managed effectively.
- The parents demonstrate an understanding of home care.

Vesicoureteral Reflux

In vesicoureteral reflux (VUR), there is a retrograde flow of urine from the bladder into the ureters. Severity ranges from reflux of urine into the ureter only at stage 1 to severe dilation of the ureter and renal pelvis with severely blunted calyces at stage 5 (Estrada & Cendron, 2011). The reflux prevents complete emptying of the bladder, and because urine returns to the bladder, it creates a reservoir for bacterial growth (Huether, 2010b; Ključevšek, Ključevšek, Levart, et al., 2010). Bacteria in the urine may be swept up to the kidneys, leading to pyelonephritis.

A renal ultrasound and voiding cystourethrogram reveal the defect and permit grading the severity of reflux (to the ureter and renal pelvis, or causing some dilation of the ureter and renal pelvis). Long-term complications include renal scarring, hypertension, and chronic renal failure (Nelson & Koo, 2008). The goal of treatment is to prevent pyelonephritis and renal scarring. Prophylactic antibiotics may be prescribed to prevent urinary tract infection. See Box 31–3. Surgical intervention, ureteral reimplantation, may be required depending

BOX 31–3	Research: Antibiotic Prophylaxis

A controlled, randomized trial of 338 children, ages 2 months to less than 7 years, who had a first urinary tract infection with fever evaluated the effect of prophylactic antibiotics in preventing recurrence over a 12-month period. These children had pyelonephritis with or without reflux confirmed by scan or clinical pyelonephritis and reflux. The children were randomly assigned to a prophylaxis or no prophylaxis group. Recurrence of a febrile urinary tract infection was not statistically significant between the two groups, with 12 out of 127 or 9.45% in the group not receiving prophylaxis and 15 of 211 or 7.11% in the group receiving prophylaxis. The study concluded that antibiotic prophylaxis is not effective in reducing the recurrence of febrile urinary tract infections in children with or without nonsevere reflux (Montini, Rigon, Zucchetta, et al., 2008).

on the grade of reflux. If a urinary tract infection is present 1 week before surgery, it must be treated to reduce the risk for postoperative complications.

Nursing Management

Following surgery to reimplant the ureters, a urinary catheter will be in place. The urine will be bloody initially and clear within 2 to 3 days. Intravenous fluids will be administered at a rate sufficient to maintain adequate urine output. Monitoring urine output is important as clots may cause an obstruction. If the catheter is not draining adequate urine, notify the healthcare provider, as the catheter may need to be irrigated.

Administer medications as prescribed, including antibiotics and antispasmodics such as oxybutynin. An epidural catheter may have been placed for pain management. Monitor the epidural according to agency protocol. Once this is removed, provide prescribed pain medication.

The child can be discharged when the child has the urinary catheter removed and can void spontaneously. An ultrasound or cystogram may be performed prior to discharge to evaluate the effectiveness of the surgery. Educate the family about the administration of medications including prophylactic antibiotics and antispasmodics if needed. Inform parents of the need for increased fiber in the diet to address the constipating effects of the antispasmodic medication. Guidelines for calling the physician include fever over 38.5°C (101.5°F), abdominal or back pain, or swelling and redness of the incision. The child may take a short shower or tub bath when returning home. The child should avoid active play for 3 weeks following surgery. Provide guidelines for annual follow-up and the potential need to resume prophylactic antibiotics if the child develops recurrent urinary tract infections.

Prune-Belly Syndrome

Prune-belly syndrome, also known as Eagle-Barrett syndrome, is a congenital defect characterized by failure of the abdominal musculature to develop. The skin covering the abdominal wall is thin and resembles a wrinkled prune (Naqvi, Paddack, Kulkarni, et al., 2009). Other characteristics include urinary tract anomalies, poor ureteral peristalsis, enlarged bladder, high risk for recurrent urinary tract infection, vesicoureteral reflux, and bilateral cryptorchidism. Prune-belly syndrome occurs predominantly in males (95%), with an incidence of 1 in 30,000 to 50,000 live births (Papantoniou, Papoutsis, Daskalakis, et al., 2010).

The etiology of prune-belly syndrome is unknown; however, it is thought to be related to a fetal urinary tract obstruction or a specific injury to the mesoderm between 6 and 10 weeks of gestation. In addition to urinary tract anomalies, cardiac, pulmonary, gastrointestinal, and orthopedic anomalies also occur (Papantoniou et al., 2010). See Box 31–4.

Diagnosis is confirmed with abdominal ultrasound. An intravenous pyelogram is useful in assessing structural defects. Abdominal wall reconstruction and correction of genitourinary defects, including orchiopexy, are performed to repair defects. The mortality rate in infants has improved significantly in the past three decades with advances in surgical techniques. Mortality in the neonatal period is related to severe pulmonary hypoplasia. Approximately 30% of children with prune-belly syndrome will develop end-stage renal disease in childhood or adolescence because of inadequate renal function (Elder, 2011).

| BOX 31–4 | Associated Anomalies of Prune-Belly Syndrome |

- **Genitourinary**—cryptorchidism, renal dysplasia, vesicoureteral reflux
- **Respiratory**—pulmonary hypoplasia
- **Cardiovascular**—atrial septal defect, patent ductus arteriosus, tetralogy of Fallot, and ventricular septal defect
- **Gastrointestinal**—gastroschisis, imperforate anus, and malrotation with volvulus
- **Musculoskeletal**—clubfoot, congenital hip dysplasia, pectus excavatum or carinatum

Source: *Data from* Prune Belly Syndrome Network. *(2011). Retrieved from http://www.prunebelly.org*

Nursing Management

Nursing management for the infant with prune-belly syndrome is the same as for other defects of the genitourinary system, including preoperative and postoperative management. Additional management includes psychosocial support for the child and family related to the numerous congenital anomalies, body image concerns, and long-term consequences of the defect.

ENURESIS

Enuresis is repeated involuntary voiding by a child who has reached an age at which bladder control is expected, usually about 5 to 6 years of age. See Table 31–3 for bladder control milestones. Enuresis can occur either at night (**nocturnal enuresis**), during the day (**diurnal enuresis**), or both night and day.

Enuresis is further categorized as primary and secondary.

- **Primary enuresis**—child has never had a dry night; attributed to maturational delay and small functional bladder; not associated with stress or psychiatric cause.
- **Secondary enuresis**—child who has been reliably dry for at least 6 months begins bed-wetting; associated with stress, infections, and sleep disorders.

Primary nocturnal enuresis is the most common type of enuresis and occurs more frequently in males than females (Elder, 2011). Nocturnal enuresis occurs in an estimated 5% to 10% of 7-year-olds (Nevéus, 2011). See Box 31–5.

| TABLE 31–3 | Milestones in the Development of Bladder Control |

AGE	DEVELOPMENTAL MILESTONE
1 1/2 years	Child passes urine at regular intervals.
2 years	Child announces when he or she is voiding.
2 1/2 years	Child makes known need to void; can hold urine.
3 years	Child goes to the bathroom by himself or herself; holds urge if preoccupied with play.
2 1/2–3 1/2 years	Child achieves nighttime control.
4 years	Child shows great interest in going to bathrooms when away from home (shopping centers, movies).
5 years	Child voids approximately seven times a day; prefers privacy; is able to initiate emptying of bladder at any degree of fullness.

| BOX 31–5 | Growth & Development: Wetting Episodes |

Nighttime wetting episodes usually decrease as the child ages. An estimated 21% of children 4.5 years of age and 8% of children 9.5 years of age average less than two episodes of nighttime wetting per week. Wetting episodes occur more than two times per week in 8% of children 4.5 years of age and 1.5% of children 9.5 years of age (Norfolk & Wootton, 2011).

Etiology and Pathophysiology

Primary nocturnal enuresis occurs more often in children who have a positive family history and generally involves more than one causative factor. Factors include reduced or small functional bladder capacity, deep sleep or altered sleep/arousal levels, and nocturnal polyuria (Norfolk & Wootton, 2011; Saldano, Chaviano, & Maizels, 2008). Bowel dysfunction (constipation) may also be a contributing factor (Saldano et al., 2008). Rectal pressure on the posterior bladder wall stimulates the bladder to empty. Nocturnal enuresis is also more prevalent in children with obstructive sleep apnea syndrome (Bascom, Penney, Metcalfe, et al., 2011). Diagnostic tests may be needed to determine the cause of diurnal enuresis (Hoebeke, Bower, Combs, et al., 2010).

Clinical Manifestations

Children with diurnal enuresis may exhibit clinical manifestations of frequency, urgency, constant dribbling, and involuntary loss of control after voiding. Nocturnal enuresis is manifested by bed-wetting.

Collaborative Care

The goal of collaborative care is to identify and treat the cause of enuresis and to establish urinary control. Neurologic defects, structural defects, renal insufficiency, urinary tract infection, and disorders such as diabetes are ruled out.

Diagnostic Tests

Urinalysis on the first voided specimen of the day is performed. Screening for a UTI with a dipstick is performed. A urine culture may reveal that an asymptomatic UTI is present. The specific gravity provides information about the child's ability to concentrate urine. Diabetes mellitus, diabetes insipidus, or renal insufficiency should be ruled out in children with both enuresis and polyuria or **oliguria** (reduced urine volume for age; see Box 31–1 on page 1048). Other diagnostic tests that might be performed include ultrasound of the urinary tract, uroflowmetry, and postvoiding residual urine measurements (Dogan, Akpinar, Gurocak, et al., 2008). A thorough history can help identify potential causes of enuresis (Box 31–6).

The child's lower spine is examined for fistulas, sacral dimples, or tufts of hair that could be signs of spina bifida occulta. (See Chapter 33 .) Prolonged hospitalization, family stressors, and preoccupation with school concerns also have been associated with secondary enuresis.

Clinical Therapy

A multitreatment approach is usually most effective. Fluid restriction, bladder training, and enuresis alarms are common approaches (Table 31–4). Alarms used as the sole management for primary nocturnal enuresis have a 60% success rate, and dryness is generally attained when achieved by this method. The disadvantage is that this method takes a long time to achieve success, and parents discontinue

| BOX 31–6 | Questions to Ask When Taking an Enuresis History |

FAMILY HISTORY
Is there a family history of renal or urinary structural abnormalities?
Is there a family history of bed-wetting? At what age did bed-wetting stop?

FAMILY MANAGEMENT OF ENURESIS
How serious is the problem for the family?
What happens when the child wets? (Who gets up and changes sheets?)
How is the child treated? Is the child punished or blamed for wetting?
What remedies have been tried?

TOILET TRAINING
When was it initiated and what method was used?
Has the child ever been dry during the day or night for an extended period?
How long was the child's longest dry period?
How often does the child void? Have a bowel movement?
Does the child have a history of constipation or encopresis?

STRESSORS
How is the child doing in school?
Are there any new or chronic stressors present in the child's life?
How does the problem interfere with play and social activities?

RISK FACTORS
Diabetes—Are there any signs of polyuria or polydipsia?
Urinary tract infection—Does the child have frequency, urgency, or burning on urination?

due to frustration and the assumption that the method is ineffective (Saldano et al., 2008).

Some children with nocturnal enuresis are treated with medications. Medications are more effective when used in conjunction with other techniques such as alarms because medications alone have low success rates (Saldano et al., 2008).

- Desmopressin is the most common medication used for nocturnal enuresis and has an antidiuretic effect. Desmopressin is

TABLE 31–4	Treatment Approaches for Enuresis
APPROACH	**DESCRIPTION**
Fluid restriction	Fluid intake is limited in the evening and before the child goes to bed.
Bladder exercises	The child drinks a large amount and then holds urine as long as he or she can. The child practices stopping voiding midstream. Exercises should continue for at least 6 months.
Timed voiding	The child with diurnal enuresis is instructed to void every 2 hours and to use a double voiding pattern; this trains the bladder to empty completely and avoid overdistention.
Enuresis alarms	A detector strip is attached to the child's pants. The alarm sounds a buzzer that alerts the child when wetting occurs, so the child can get up and finish voiding in the bathroom. This works best for children over 7 years old, and takes 3 to 4 months for success.
Reward system	Set realistic goals for the child and reinforce dry days or nights with stars and stickers on a chart.
Medications	Imipramine, desmopressin, and oxybutynin are used as per discussion under the Clinical Therapy section.

given at nighttime at the beginning of treatment. Once its effectiveness has been established, it may be used every night or as needed for times when the child is away from home for a short period (e.g., sleepovers or camp) (Nevéus, 2011).

- Imipramine, a tricyclic antidepressant, has anticholinergic and antispasmodic effects and may be used in children who do not respond to other methods. This medication requires close monitoring because of its effects on mood and the associated danger of overdoses (Nevéus, 2011).
- Oxybutynin, an anticholinergic medication, has an antispasmodic effect and is used for children with urgency or an overactive detrusor muscle (Nevéus, 2011).

Relapse often occurs when medications are stopped.

Nursing Management

Goals of nursing include assisting the child and family in achieving the child's urinary control and promoting the child's self-esteem.

Nursing Assessment and Diagnosis

A thorough history can assist in identifying potential causes of enuresis. Review the child's elimination patterns, developmental milestones, toilet-training history, and urinary symptoms. Assess signs of occult spina bifida. Identify any potential stressors that may contribute to enuresis.

Assess the child's and family's feelings and frustrations about the problem of bed-wetting and their motivation to implement therapies.

Nursing diagnoses that apply to the child with enuresis may include:

- Urinary Elimination, Impaired related to inability to control voiding during the day or at night
- Urinary Incontinence, Overflow related to failure to regularly empty bladder
- Knowledge, Readiness for Enhanced related to medication and behavioral interventions for enuresis
- Self-Esteem, Situational Low, Risk for related to embarrassment of lack of bladder control

NANDA-I © 2012

Planning and Implementation

Partner with the child and parents and explain the physiologic development of bladder control and causes and treatment of enuresis. Explore the parents' and child's feelings of guilt or blame. Make sure the parents are aware that the child cannot control the wetting. Psychosocial support is an essential part of care since stress is an important cause of secondary enuresis. Provide emotional support to the parents and child, and encourage the child's participation in the treatment plan. Refer the child for counseling or therapy if appropriate.

Assess the parents' and child's motivation and readiness for interventions. The child needs to be an active participant in the treatment plan for daytime and nighttime wetting. For daytime wetting, the child may need a reminder to go to the bathroom such as a vibrating watch. A discussion with the child's teacher may make it possible for the child to have additional or private bathroom breaks. Before parents purchase an enuresis alarm, suggest that an alarm clock be used in the child's room for several nights to determine if the child will arouse. The child may need the parent's help to arouse initially. Find out if the child shares a room with others who will be disturbed by the alarm. Ask if the child and parents are willing to persist with

---

Complementary Therapy **Biofeedback**

Biofeedback is a complementary therapy that may be used for some cases of enuresis when the child and parents are highly motivated. In the case of bladder sphincter dysfunction, when the pelvic floor muscles contract during voiding, the child may have urgency and frequency associated with daytime or nighttime enuresis. During biofeedback training the child learns to identify the differences in relaxation and contraction of the bladder muscles, as well as straining. The child then learns to sustain and maintain a relaxed pelvic floor and voluntary sphincter opening (Adams & Vohra, 2009).

an enuresis alarm, as it may take months to work. Discuss potential strategies with the family to reduce stressors on the child or to help the child cope with the stressors. See Complementary Therapy: Biofeedback.

Evaluation

Expected outcomes of nursing care include:

- The child has an increased number of dry nights.
- The child and family choose one or more interventions that they prefer and persist in using them.
- The child demonstrates positive self-esteem.

RENAL DISORDERS

The following renal disorders are complex in nature, causing multisystem effects and potentially resulting in loss of kidney function. Renal disorders and therapies discussed in this section include nephrotic syndrome; acute postinfectious glomerulonephritis; renal failure; renal replacement therapy including peritoneal dialysis, hemodialysis, and kidney transplantation; hemolytic uremic syndrome; and polycystic kidney disease.

Nephrotic Syndrome

Nephrotic syndrome (NS) is an alteration in kidney function secondary to increased glomerular basement membrane permeability to plasma protein (Figure 31–8 ■). Nephrotic syndrome refers not to a specific disease, but to a clinical state characterized by edema, massive proteinuria, hypoalbuminemia, hypoproteinemia, hyperlipidemia, and altered immunity. Congenital nephrotic syndrome is generally related to a genetic defect (Jalanko, 2009). Primary nephrotic syndrome results from a disease that affects only the kidney, such as glomerulonephritis. Secondary nephrotic syndrome results from a systemic disease, drugs, or toxins that alter kidney function (Huether, 2010b).

Approximately 85% of children with nephrotic syndrome have a type of primary disease called minimal change nephrotic syndrome (MCNS). It is estimated that more than 95% of these children respond to steroid therapy (Pais & Avner, 2011). MCNS is a common kidney disease in the pediatric population, occurring in 2 to 16 per 100,000 children (Lahdenkari, Suvanto, Kajantie, et al., 2005), and is more common in males than females (Pais & Avner, 2011). MCNS derives its name from the normal or only minimally changed appearance of the glomeruli on light microscopic evaluation. Because MCNS is the most common form of nephrotic syndrome, it is the focus of the following discussion.

Pathophysiology Illustrated Nephrotic Syndrome

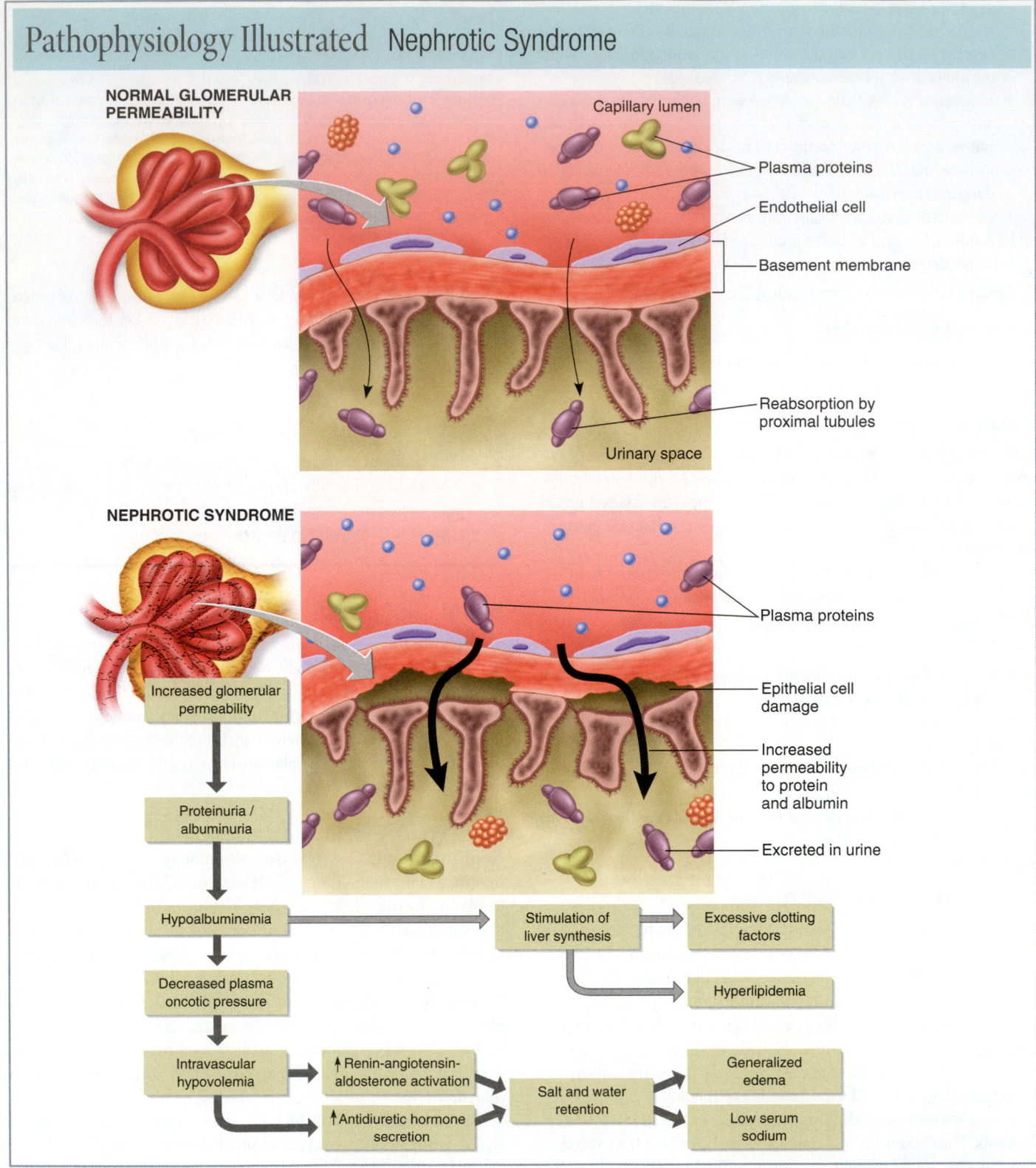

FIGURE 31–8 ■ Note the contrast between the normal glomerular anatomy and the changes that exist in nephrotic syndrome permitting protein to be excreted in the urine. The lower albumin blood level stimulates the liver to generate lipids and excessive clotting factors. Edema results from decreased oncotic plasma pressure, renin-angiotensin-aldosterone activation, and antidiuretic hormone secretion.

Etiology and Pathophysiology

The cause of primary MCNS is unknown, but an immune system role is suspected (Pais & Avner, 2011). The mechanism of increased glomerular permeability is unknown as the glomeruli appear normal, although it may be related to the loss of a negative charge in the glomerular capillary wall (Huether, 2010b). In MCNS, increased permeability of the glomerular membrane permits large negatively charged molecules such as albumin to pass through the membrane and be excreted in the urine. Proteinuria results in decreased oncotic pressure and edema, because fluid remains in the interstitial spaces instead of being pulled back into the vascular compartment (Pais & Avner, 2011). Immunoglobulins are lost, resulting in altered immunity. Loss of protein in the urine, insufficient albumin production by the liver, and a decreased albumin concentration as a result of salt and water retention by the kidney contribute to hypoalbuminemia. Hypercoagulability occurs because of alterations in coagulation factors. The liver, stimulated perhaps by hypoalbuminemia or decreased osmotic pressure, responds by increasing synthesis of lipoprotein, resulting in hyperlipidemia (Huether & Forshee, 2010). Children who develop steroid-resistant nephrotic syndrome are at risk for renal failure (Butani & Ramsamooj, 2009; Hamasaki, Yoshikawa, Hattori, et al., 2009).

Clinical Manifestations

Nephrotic syndrome is characterized by edema, massive proteinuria, and hypoalbuminemia (Akman, Kalay, Akkaya, et al., 2009). In most children, edema develops gradually over several weeks. Children may have a history of periorbital edema on waking that resolves during the day as fluid shifts to the abdomen and lower extremities. Other signs include snug fit of clothing and shoes, pallor, hypertension, irritability, anorexia, hematuria, decreased urine output, and nonspecific malaise. The child's urine may be frothy or foamy. Parents often do not seek medical treatment until generalized edema develops on the child's extremities, abdomen, or genitals (Figure 31–9 ■). Respiratory distress from pleural effusion may occur in some cases.

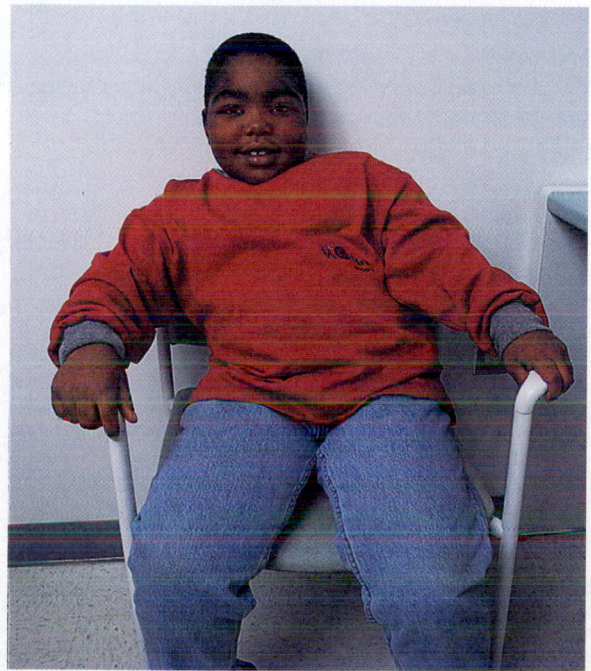

FIGURE 31–9 ■ This boy has generalized edema, a characteristic finding in nephrotic syndrome.

Massive edema resulting in a dramatic weight gain and abdominal pain, with or without vomiting, may occur depending on the amount of albumin lost and the amount of sodium ingested. The child becomes malnourished as a result of protein loss in the urine. The skin is pale and shiny with prominent veins, and the hair becomes more brittle. An increased risk of thrombosis is present.

Collaborative Care

The goal of collaborative care is to induce remission, restore intravascular fluid volume, and avoid complications that may lead to progressive kidney dysfunction.

Diagnostic Tests

Diagnosis is based on the history, characteristic symptoms, and laboratory findings. Urinalysis, serum albumin, sodium, BUN, cholesterol, and electrolytes are ordered. Urinalysis shows 3+ to 4+ protein. Microscopic hematuria may also be present. Other values that confirm the diagnosis include hypoalbuminemia indicated by serum albumin levels of less than 2.5 g/dL, urinary protein excretion of greater than 40 mg/m^2/hr, and a spot urine protein-to-creatinine ratio greater than 2.0 (Pais & Avner, 2011). Renal ultrasound may be performed to detect structural kidney problems. A single-needle kidney biopsy for examination of glomeruli may be performed to assess for renal failure or other disorders.

Diagnostic confirmation of a relapse in children who had at one time achieved remission is the presence of 2+ proteinuria by dipstick testing for 3 consecutive days (Hamasaki et al., 2009).

Clinical Therapy

Children may be hospitalized when severe edema or a major infection is present, but are usually treated as outpatients. Clinical therapy focuses on decreasing proteinuria, relieving edema, managing associated symptoms, improving nutrition, and preventing infection. A corticosteroid (such as prednisone) is prescribed to decrease proteinuria. In most children, urine protein levels fall to trace or negative values within 2 to 3 weeks of the start of therapy. Children who respond successfully to therapy continue to take corticosteroids daily for 6 weeks, followed by at least 4 weeks of alternate-day treatment. The medication is then slowly tapered and discontinued over a 1- to 2-month period of time. Approximately 80% to 90% of children respond to steroid therapy within 3 weeks (Pais & Avner, 2011). Intravenous methylprednisolone may be used in children not responsive to oral steroids (Nachman, Jennette, & Falk, 2012). See Medications Used to Treat Nephrotic Syndrome. Intravenous administration of albumin followed by furosemide may be ordered in the child with massive edema who is unresponsive to fluid restriction and parenteral diuretics (Pais & Avner, 2011). Analgesics may be ordered for pain related to edema or flank pain from a urinary tract infection.

Relapses occur in many children with nephrotic syndrome (Pais & Avner, 2011). Children who have a relapse after drug therapy is discontinued receive repeat therapy. Other medications used include diuretics, antihypertensive agents, and antibiotics. Immunosuppressive or immunomodulator medications, including cyclophosphamide, cyclosporine, tacrolimus, and mycophenolate, may be used to prolong remissions in children with nephrotic syndrome who have frequent relapses (Pais & Avner, 2011). Since diuretics can precipitate hypovolemia, hyponatremia, and hypokalemia, electrolyte levels should be carefully monitored.

Medications Used to Treat Nephrotic Syndrome

MEDICATION	ACTION/IMPLICATION	NURSING MANAGEMENT
Corticosteroid Therapy		
Prednisone Intravenous high-dose methylprednisolone may be used if unresponsive to oral steroids	Stimulates remission Prednisone reduces the excretion of protein in the urine	■ Encourage adherence to prescribed medication. ■ Monitor for infection, changes in blood pressure, and changes in growth and behavior. ■ If long-term courses of corticosteroids are administered, observe for major side effects such as weight gain and moon face, obesity, gastrointestinal bleeding, growth retardation, hyperglycemia, hypertension, adrenal suppression, and bone demineralization. ■ Educate parents about the appetite-stimulating effect of corticosteroids and to limit calorie intake to prevent excessive weight gain. ■ Administration of live vaccines should be delayed until the child is no longer immunosuppressed.
Alkylating/Cytotoxic Agents		
Chlorambucil Cyclophosphamide	Stimulates remission and helps extend the interval between relapses Used when no response to corticosteroids or side effects are a problem	■ Monitor WBC count for leukopenia and neutropenia. Monitor hemoglobin for anemia. Assess for gastrointestinal bleeding, alopecia, and impaired growth. ■ Administer medications 1 hour before breakfast or 2 hours after evening meal. An antiemetic may be prescribed for nausea while taking medication. ■ Encourage adequate hydration to reduce cystitis. ■ Educate the family to report unusual bleeding, bruising, chills, fever, or other signs of infection.
Immunosuppressants		
Cyclosporine Tacrolimus Mycophenolate	Helps to induce and maintain remission in children with corticosteroid refractory nephrotic syndrome by decreasing immunologic responses, decreasing the glomerular filtration rate, and affecting the glomerular basement membrane permeability to albumin	■ Monitor blood pressure for hypertension and other side effects such as nausea, vomiting, anemia, and abdominal discomfort. ■ Monitor electrolytes, cyclosporine serum concentrations, creatinine clearance, and serum creatinine levels to assess renal status. ■ Educate the family to administer medication with meals to reduce nausea, administer the medication at the same time each day, and use a glass rather than plastic container for mixing. May dilute cyclosporine with orange or apple juice and administer immediately. Do not use grapefruit juice.
Diuretics		
Loop diuretics Furosemide Bumetanide	Used for severe edema Prevents reabsorption of water, sodium, and potassium by the renal tubules, thereby reducing massive edema Blocks the sodium-chloride transporter in the distal tubule, thereby reducing massive edema	■ Administer orally or intravenously. ■ Monitor for intravascular volume depletion (hypovolemia). ■ Assess vital signs for tachycardia and hypotension. ■ Monitor for other potential side effects including hyponatremia, hypokalemia, and other electrolyte imbalances.
Angiotensin-Converting Enzyme (ACE) Inhibitor		
Vasotec (enalapril maleate)	Antihypertensive agent Some renal protective effects	■ Monitor blood pressure. Assess for transient hypotension and light-headedness. ■ Monitor serum potassium for side effect of hyperkalemia.

Source: *Data from Butani, L., & Ramsamooj, R. (2009). Experience with tacrolimus in children with steroid-resistant nephrotic syndrome. Pediatric Nephrology, 24, 1517–1523; Hamasaki, Y., Yoshikawa, N., Hattori, S., Sasaki, S., Iijima, K., Nakanishi, K., . . . Honda, M. (2009). Cyclosporine and steroid therapy in children with steroid-resistant nephrotic syndrome. Pediatric Nephrology, 24, 2177–2185; Nachman, P. H., Jennette, J. C., & Falk, R. J. (2012). Primary glomerular disease. In M. W. Taal, G. M. Chertow, P. A. Marsden, K. Skorecki, A. S. L. Yu, & B. M. Brenner, Brenner and Rector's the kidney (9th ed., pp. 987–1046). Philadelphia, PA: Saunders Elsevier; Huether, S. E. (2010b). Alterations of renal and urinary tract function in children. In K. L. McCance & S. E. Huether, Pathophysiology: The biologic basis for disease in adults and children (6th ed., pp. 1402–1419). Maryland Heights, MO: Mosby Elsevier; Pais, P., & Avner, E. D. (2011). Conditions particularly associated with proteinuria. In R. M. Kliegman, B. F. Stanton, J. W. St. Geme III, N. F. Schor, & R. E. Behrman, Nelson textbook of pediatrics (19th ed., pp. 1799–1807). Philadelphia, PA: Saunders Elsevier; Wilson, B. A., Shannon, M. T., & Shields, K. M. (2011). Pearson nurse's drug guide 2011. New York, NY: Pearson.*

Nursing Management

Goals of nursing focus on managing the child's symptoms, including edema, preventing complications such as infection and impaired skin integrity, meeting nutritional needs, and addressing the emotional needs of the child and family.

Nursing Assessment and Diagnosis

Nursing assessment focuses on signs of fluid volume excess, complications related to the disorder, and the psychosocial impact of the condition on the child and family.

Physiologic Assessment

Careful assessment of the child's hydration status and edema is essential. Carefully monitor intake and output. Weigh the child daily using the same scale, and measure abdominal girth to monitor changes in edema and ascites. Refer to Chapter 23 for further information on management of edema.

Monitor vital signs at least every 4 hours and watch for signs of respiratory distress, hypertension, or circulatory overload. Test urine for proteinuria and specific gravity at least once each shift. In addition, assess for:

- Skin breakdown resulting from edema
- Signs of hypovolemia during periods of diuresis
- The child's comfort level and activity tolerance

Psychosocial Assessment

Children and parents are often fearful or anxious on admission. Because edema often develops gradually, parents may feel guilty if they did not seek medical attention immediately. School-age children with generalized edema are often concerned about their appearance. Careful questioning may be necessary to elicit these concerns. The child who is hospitalized for a recurrence of nephrotic syndrome may be frustrated or depressed. Assess individual and family coping mechanisms, support systems, and level of stress.

Following are examples of nursing diagnoses appropriate for the child with MCNS:

- Infection, Risk for related to immunosuppressive therapy
- Fluid Volume: Excess related to renal dysfunction and sodium retention
- Skin Integrity, Risk for Impaired related to edema, lowered resistance to infection, injury, immobility, and malnutrition
- Nutrition, Imbalanced: Less than Body Requirements related to loss of appetite and protein loss in urine
- Fatigue related to fluid and electrolyte imbalance, albumin loss, altered nutrition, and renal failure
- Activity, Deficient Diversional related to fatigue, immobility, and social isolation

NANDA-I © 2012

Planning and Implementation

Nursing care is mainly supportive and focuses on administering medications, preventing infection, preventing skin breakdown, meeting nutritional and fluid needs, promoting rest, and providing emotional support to the parents and child.

Administer Medications

It is important to give prescribed medications at the scheduled time. Monitor closely for side effects of corticosteroids such as moon face, increased appetite, increased hair growth, abdominal distention, and mood swings. Monitor for adverse effects of corticosteroids such as hypertension, nausea, and hyperglycemia. Corticosteroids should be tapered rather than abruptly discontinued. An evaluation of fasting blood sugar may be needed during therapy.

If the child is receiving albumin intravenously, monitor closely for hypertension or signs of volume overload caused by fluid shifts. Severe edema is treated with a loop, thiazide, or potassium-sparing diuretic. Hypovolemia may occur with diuretic administration. Though rarely done because of the associated risk factors, albumin infused simultaneously with diuretics may be required to reduce the

risk of hypovolemic shock. Observe for signs of impending shock (refer to Chapter 26 for discussion of shock).

Prevent Infection

Children with MCNS are at risk for infection because of the loss of immunoglobulins in the urine and corticosteroid therapy. Implement careful hand hygiene and standard precautions. Strict aseptic technique is essential during invasive procedures. Monitor the child's white blood cell count when cytotoxic drugs are given due to the potential for bone marrow suppression as a side effect. Monitor vital signs carefully to detect early signs of infection that may be masked by corticosteroid therapy. Decrease the child's social contacts during immunosuppressive treatment, and caution parents and children to avoid exposure to individuals with respiratory infections and communicable diseases. Educate the family on the importance of avoiding shopping malls, sporting arenas, grocery stores, game stores, and other public areas where the risk of exposure to such infections is increased. Provide instructions to the parents on signs of infection, including fever and changes in behavior. Discuss with parents the need for maintenance of annual recommended influenza immunizations and avoiding those who have recently been vaccinated with live viruses.

> **Practice Alert**
> Children with nephrotic syndrome are on steroids and may be on other medications that suppress the immune system. Care should be taken to limit exposure to infection. Children with nephrotic syndrome who have not been immunized with Varivax or who have not previously had chicken pox should have a varicella zoster titer drawn. If the child is exposed to chicken pox, varicella-zoster immune globulin (VZIG) should be administered within 96 hours of exposure to prevent or lessen the severity of the illness. In addition, the child should receive the polyvalent pneumococcal vaccine if he or she has not already received it. It is best to give the vaccine when the child is in remission and off steroid therapy. Children with nephrotic syndrome should also receive the influenza vaccine annually (Pais & Avner, 2011).

Prevent Skin Breakdown

Meticulous skin care is implemented to prevent skin breakdown and potential infection. Perform repeated skin assessments, turn the child frequently, and use therapeutic mattresses (e.g., egg crate or airflow mattress) to help prevent skin breakdown. Keep the skin clean and dry.

Meet Nutritional and Fluid Needs

Keep the child's food preferences in mind when planning menus. Encourage the child to eat by presenting attractive meals with small portions. Socialization during meals may improve the child's appetite. Fluids are generally not restricted except during severe edema.

> **Practice Alert**
> Traditionally, a high-protein, low-salt diet had been recommended for children with MCNS. Current data, however, suggest that the high-protein diet increases urinary protein loss and may accelerate the development of renal failure. On the other hand, low-protein diets may lead to protein deficiency. For these reasons, a regular-protein, low-salt diet is recommended.

Promote Rest

Provide opportunities for quiet play as tolerated, such as drawing, playing board games, listening to CDs, and watching movies. Adjust the child's daily schedule to allow rest periods after activities. Signs of fatigue may include irritability, mood swings, or withdrawal. Educate the parents and child about the importance of rest. Limiting visitors during the acute phase of the illness may be necessary. Telephone and computer contacts may be encouraged as an alternative to visitors. To provide a sense of control, encourage the child to set his or her own limits on activity.

Provide Emotional Support

Parents and children often require support to cope with this chronic disease. It is important to thoroughly explain the child's disease and treatment regimen to parents. Parental anxiety in combination with the hospitalization may interfere with the child's independence. Assist the parents in promoting the child's independence by allowing the child to select food from the menu or to select the daily activity schedule. Allowing choices when possible provides the child with some sense of control.

Children with MCNS may experience a distorted body image because of sudden weight gain and edema. They may refuse to look in the mirror, refuse to participate in care, and take less interest in their appearance. Encourage children to express their feelings. Help them maintain a normal appearance by promoting normal grooming routines. Encourage them to wear their own pajamas rather than hospital gowns. Scarves or hats may be used to lessen the child's edematous appearance. Adolescents can be encouraged to write their feelings in a journal as a coping mechanism. These children may have a long-term psychosocial adjustment because of having a chronic condition with concerns about potential relapse.

Discharge Planning and Home Care Teaching

Explain the disease process, prognosis, and treatment plan to parents and school-age children. Partner with the family and ensure their understanding of medication administration and their ability to identify potential side effects. Inform parents about fluid restriction until the edema resolves. Instruct parents about the need to monitor urine daily for protein, and have them keep a diary to record results. Monitoring the child's weight each week may help parents identify early stages of fluid retention and signs of relapse before edema occurs.

Care in the Community

Tutoring may be required for a short period after hospital discharge. Partner with the family in establishing a plan for the child to return to school and other normal activities once the acute episode has resolved. In consideration of the child's reduced immunity, emphasize the importance of avoiding contact with individuals who have infectious diseases. Reinforce to parents that as long as the child is receiving corticosteroid therapy or shows signs of MCNS, the no-added-salt diet should be followed. Warn them that steroids stimulate appetite, so they need to control the child's food intake and weight gain. Refer to Chapter 22 🖉 for further discussion of immunizations.

Most children do well with corticosteroid therapy; however, relapses commonly occur. These relapses decrease as the child gets older. Children should have periodic bone density evaluations because of the repeated steroid therapy which can weaken bones and lead to osteoporosis.

Evaluation

Expected outcomes of nursing care may include:

- The child responds to corticosteroid therapy.
- Fluid, electrolyte, and acid–base balance is restored and maintained.
- Skin integrity is maintained.
- The child meets nutritional requirements and follows dietary guidelines.

Acute Postinfectious Glomerulonephritis

Glomerulonephritis is the most common inflammation of the glomeruli of the kidneys. In children, it is most often a response to a group A beta-hemolytic streptococcal infection of the skin or pharynx. It is also caused by other organisms including *Staphylococcus, Pneumococcus,* and *Coxsackie* virus. The incidence of acute postinfectious glomerulonephritis (APIGN), also known as acute poststreptococcal glomerulonephritis (APG), is highest in children between 2 and 6 years of age, and the disorder is more common in boys than in girls (Nachman et al., 2012). Other causes of glomerulonephritis in children and adolescents include immunologic abnormalities, systemic diseases, and viruses (Huether, 2010b). The focus of this discussion is APIGN.

Etiology and Pathophysiology

The child with APIGN usually becomes ill after contracting a nephrogenetic strain of group A beta-hemolytic streptococcal infection of the upper respiratory tract or the skin. Often the child contracts a streptococcal infection (e.g., strep throat), recovers, and then develops signs of APIGN after an interval of 10 to 21 days.

Glomerular damage occurs as a result of an immune complex reaction that localizes on the glomerular capillary wall (Figure 31–10 ■). Antibody–antigen complexes become lodged in the glomeruli, leading to inflammation and obstruction. The glomerular membranes are thickened and capillaries in the glomeruli are obstructed by damaged tissue cells, leading to a decreased glomerular filtration rate. Vascular permeability increases, allowing protein, red blood cells, and red cell casts to be excreted. Sodium and water are retained, expanding the intravascular and interstitial compartments and resulting in the characteristic finding of edema.

Clinical Manifestations

Many children with APIGN are asymptomatic. In other children the onset is usually abrupt with flank or midabdominal pain, irritability, malaise, and fever. Microscopic hematuria is present in nearly all cases, and gross hematuria, resulting in tea-colored urine, is found in up to 50% of cases and may last for 1 to 2 weeks. Mild periorbital edema occurs early along with dependent edema of the feet and ankles. Edema may progress in severity to cause pulmonary congestion or ascites (Nachman et al., 2012). Acute hypertension may cause an encephalopathy that includes headache, nausea, vomiting, irritability, lethargy, and seizures. Oliguria may or may not be present (Huether, 2010b).

Collaborative Care

The goal of collaborative care for the child with APIGN is to preserve renal function and prevent complications associated with the disorder.

Diagnostic Tests

The serum BUN and creatinine concentrations are elevated. Serum protein is decreased (hypoalbuminemia) due to mild to moderate proteinuria. The white blood cell count and erythrocyte sedimentation rate may be elevated. An elevated antistreptolysin O (ASO) titer reflects the presence of antibodies from a recent pharyngeal streptococcal respiratory infection, but the ASO level associated with a recent skin infection is low. The anti-DNAse B titer is helpful for detecting antibodies associated with recent skin infections. Most children have a reduced serum complement (C3) level due to the initial infection (Nachman et al., 2012).

Pathophysiology Illustrated   Acute Postinfectious Glomerulonephritis

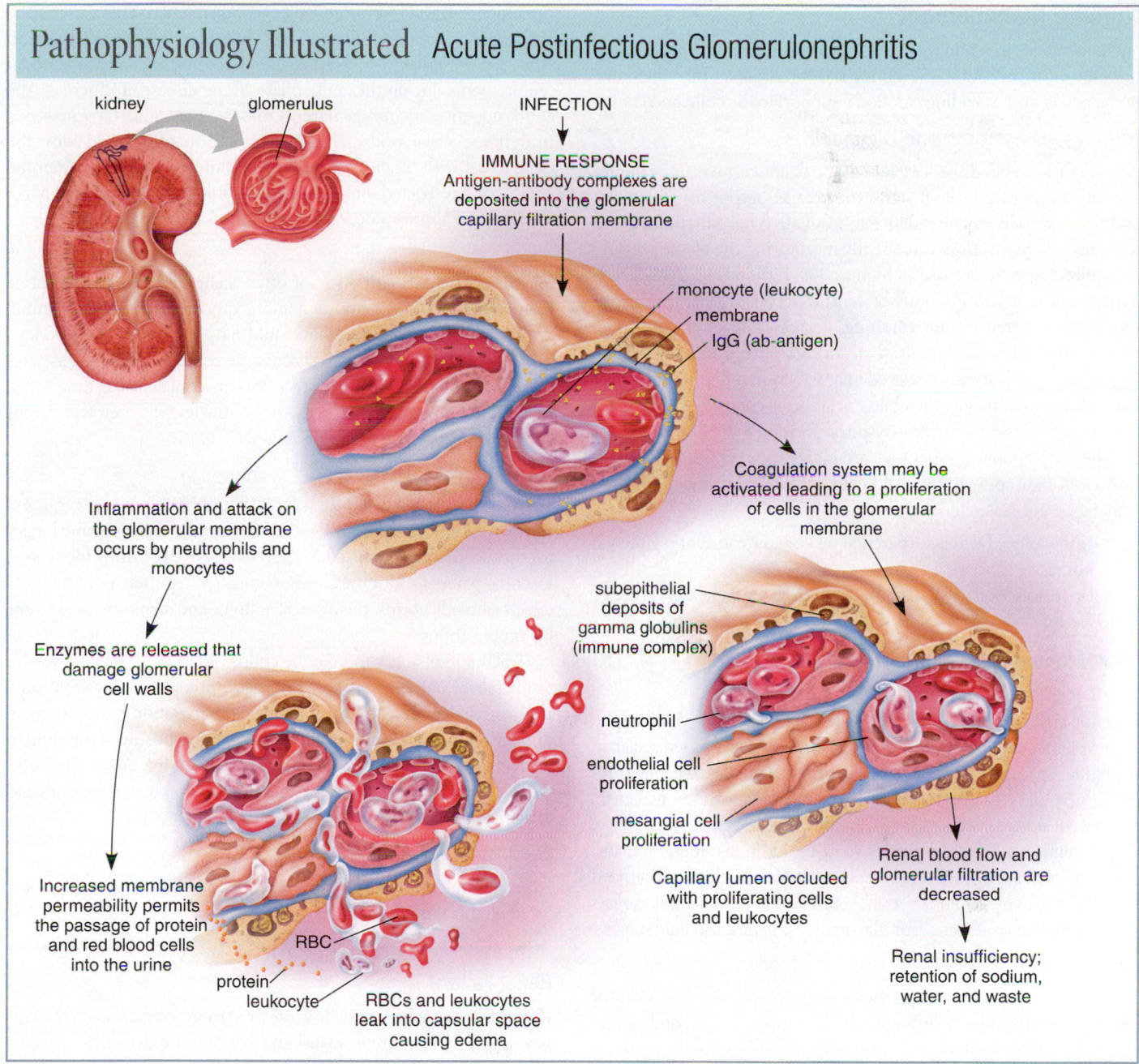

kidney   glomerulus

INFECTION

IMMUNE RESPONSE
Antigen-antibody complexes are
deposited into the glomerular
capillary filtration membrane

monocyte (leukocyte)
membrane
IgG (ab-antigen)

Coagulation system may be
activated leading to a proliferation
of cells in the glomerular
membrane

Inflammation and attack on
the glomerular membrane
occurs by neutrophils and
monocytes

Enzymes are released that
damage glomerular
cell walls

subepithelial
deposits of
gamma globulins
(immune complex)

neutrophil

endothelial cell
proliferation

mesangial cell
proliferation

Increased membrane
permeability permits
the passage of protein
and red blood cells
into the urine

RBC

protein
leukocyte

RBCs and leukocytes
leak into capsular space
causing edema

Capillary lumen occluded
with proliferating cells
and leukocytes

Renal blood flow and
glomerular filtration are
decreased

Renal insufficiency;
retention of sodium,
water, and waste

FIGURE 31–10 ■ Infection from group A beta-hemolytic *Streptococcus* causes an immune response that causes inflammation and damage to the glomeruli. Protein and red blood cells are allowed to pass through the glomeruli. Blood flow to the glomeruli is reduced due to obstruction with damaged cells. Renal insufficiency results, leading to the retention of sodium, water, and waste.

Urinalysis reveals hematuria, proteinuria, and red and white cell casts. Anemia is common in the acute phase, usually because extracellular fluid dilutes the serum. Hemoglobin and hematocrit levels reveal anemia, which is common in the acute phase and is generally caused by dilution of the serum by the extracellular fluid (Bhimma, 2011).

Clinical Therapy

Treatment focuses on relief of symptoms and supportive therapy. Bed rest is a key component of the treatment plan during the acute phase. Edema and mild to moderate hypertension should be treated with sodium restriction and a diuretic such as furosemide (Huether, 2010b; Nachman et al., 2012). Immediate emergency care is needed

for severe hypertension with cerebral dysfunction; medication such as hydralazine or diazoxide is administered intravenously. A course of antibiotics may be given to ensure eradication of the original infectious agent.

Clinical Tip

Antibiotics are *not* a treatment for acute postinfectious glomerulonephritis (APIGN). Instead, antibiotics are prescribed to treat the original infection (such as strep throat).

The prognosis for most children with APIGN is good. Clinical signs, proteinuria, and hematuria resolve within several weeks. Over 95% of children will recover completely (Huether, 2010b).

Nursing Management

Nursing care for the child with APIGN focuses on monitoring fluid status, preventing infection, preventing skin breakdown, meeting nutritional needs, and providing emotional support to the child and family.

Nursing Assessment and Diagnosis

As with other renal disorders, care of the child with APIGN requires careful monitoring of vital signs, intake and output measurement, and fluid and electrolyte balance to evaluate renal functioning and to identify complications. Frequently monitoring the blood pressure is required since it can rise as high as 200/120 mmHg. With severe hypertension, assess for signs of central nervous system problems (headache, blurred vision, vomiting, decreased level of consciousness, confusion, and convulsions). Monitor urine for proteinuria, hematuria, and output. Assess edema, which may be periorbital or dependent and shifts as the child's position is changed. Assess for a pulmonary effusion (crackles, dyspnea, and cough).

The accompanying Nursing Care Plan lists several nursing diagnoses that may apply to the child with APIGN. Additional potential nursing diagnoses include:

- Knowledge, Deficient (parents) related to treatment regimen at home
- Perfusion: Renal, Risk for Ineffective related to disease process

NANDA-I © 2012

Planning and Implementation

Maintain Fluid Status

Monitor vital signs, fluid and electrolyte status, and intake and output. Hypovolemia can occur as a result of fluid shifting from vascular to interstitial spaces despite the outward clinical signs of excess fluid retention. Monitor the degree of ascites by measuring abdominal girth. Document urine specific gravity. Carefully plan the child's fluid intake over the entire day, including meals, so that some fluids are still available at the end of the day. Make sure parents and visitors understand the need to limit fluids to prevent inadvertent excessive intake. Make sure parents understand that gelatin and fruit-flavored ice pops are also fluid sources.

Prevent Infection

Impaired renal function places the child at risk for infection. Monitor for signs of infection including fever, increased malaise, and an elevated white blood cell count. Screen family members for the presence of streptococcal infection and refer for treatment if necessary. Partner with the family to reduce exposure of the child to infection. Instruct the family in good hand hygiene technique. Limit visitors, and screen for upper respiratory infections.

Prevent Skin Breakdown

Bed rest is required during the acute phase. Dependent areas and other pressure areas are vulnerable to skin breakdown. Turn the child frequently. Pad bony prominences or susceptible areas with sheepskin, or protect skin with a transparent dressing. Elevate lower extremities on pillows when in the dependent position or when the child is lying in bed. Make sure the child's bed is free of crumbs or sharp toys. Keep sheets tight and free of wrinkles. Maintain proper hygiene and dry skin.

Meet Nutritional Needs

A team approach (including the nurse, nutritionist, parents, and child) is often needed to meet the child's nutritional needs. In most cases a no-added-salt and low-protein diet is implemented. This diet may be challenging since the child may refuse to eat foods that taste different. Anorexia presents the greatest challenge to meeting daily nutritional requirements during the acute phase of the disease. To increase the child's appetite, encourage parents to bring the child's favorite foods from home, serve foods in age-appropriate quantities, and allow the child to eat with other children or with family members. When the child is on a restricted diet, screen foods brought from home to make sure they are appropriate.

Provide Emotional Support

Parents of a child with APIGN often feel guilty. They may blame themselves for not responding more quickly to the child's initial symptoms or may believe they could have prevented the development of glomerular damage. Discuss the etiology of the disease and the child's treatment, and correct any misconceptions. Emphasize that it is not possible to predict which of the few children with streptococcal infections will develop APIGN.

Discharge Planning and Home Care Teaching

Children are hospitalized for a few days, although it may require 3 weeks for hypertension and gross hematuria to resolve and longer for the disorder to resolve completely. Discharge planning focuses on teaching parents about the child's medication regimen, potential side effects of medications, dietary restrictions, and signs and symptoms of complications.

Teach parents how to take the child's blood pressure and how to test urine for blood or protein, or other routine tasks of patient care. Evaluate the parent's ability by return demonstration of these procedures. Emphasize the importance of avoiding exposure of the child to individuals with upper respiratory tract infections. After discharge, partner with parents to plan the child's return to normal routines and activities, with periods allowed for rest.

Evaluation

Expected outcomes of nursing care for the child with APIGN are listed on the Nursing Care Plan.

Renal Failure

Renal failure, which may be acute or chronic, occurs when the kidney is unable to excrete wastes and concentrate urine. Acute renal failure occurs suddenly (over days or weeks) and may be reversible, whereas in chronic renal failure, kidney function diminishes gradually and permanently over months or years.

Both types of renal failure are characterized by **azotemia** (accumulation of nitrogenous wastes in the blood) and sometimes oliguria, indicating the kidney's inability to excrete metabolic waste products. Chronic renal failure eventually results in **anuria** (absence of urine output). The best indicator of renal function is the glomerular filtration rate (Schwartz & Work, 2009). A glomerular filtration rate calculator is available from the American Kidney Foundation.

Acute Renal Failure

Acute renal failure (ARF) (also called acute renal injury) is a sudden loss of adequate renal function in which the kidneys are unable to clear metabolic wastes and to regulate extracellular fluid volume, sodium balance, and acid–base homeostasis. ARF is seen in 2% to 3% of children cared for in pediatric tertiary care centers and up to 8% of infants cared for in neonatal intensive care units (Sreedharan &

American Kidney Foundation

Weblink

Nursing Care Plan

The Child with Acute Postinfectious Glomerulonephritis

INTERVENTION	RATIONALE	EXPECTED OUTCOME
1. Nursing Diagnosis: Fluid Volume: Excess related to decreased glomerular filtration and increased sodium retention		
NIC Priority Intervention—*Fluid Management:* Promotion of fluid balance and prevention of complications resulting from abnormal and undesired fluid levels		**NOC Suggested Outcome**—*Fluid Balance:* Balance of water in the intracellular and extracellular compartments of the body
GOAL: *The child will regain normal fluid balance.*		
■ Assess for edema (periorbital or dependent areas).	■ Sodium and water retention leads to edema.	The child maintains urine output that is balanced to fluid intake. The child receives the appropriate amount of fluid each day.
■ Calculate fluid intake and plan amounts to offer throughout the day.	■ An intake/output ratio of 1:1 reflects normal hydration and kidney function.	
■ Limit foods with moderate to high sodium content.	■ Further reduction in sodium intake will help balance fluid and sodium retention.	
■ Document intake and output.	■ Documentation is important to prevent excessive fluid intake.	
■ Perform daily weight measurement on the same scale at the same time of day.	■ Changes in weight can indicate fluid retention or improvement in condition.	
■ Administer prescribed medications (diuretics and antihypertensives).	■ Diuretics cause excretion of excess fluid by preventing reabsorption of water and sodium. Antihypertensives increase excretion of water and sodium and cause vasodilation.	
2. Nursing Diagnosis: Skin Integrity, Risk for Impaired related to tissue edema		
NIC Priority Intervention—*Bedrest Care:* Promotion of comfort and safety and prevention of complications for a patient unable to get out of bed		**NOC Suggested Outcome**—*Tissue Integrity: Skin and Mucous Membranes:* Structural intactness and normal physiologic function of skin and mucous membranes
GOAL: *The child's skin integrity will remain intact.*		
■ Assess skin for redness, abrasions, and breakdown secondary to edema, bed rest, and skin rubbing against sheets.	■ Frequent assessment ensures early identification and implementation of preventive measures.	The child develops no areas of redness, abrasions, or skin breakdown over pressure points.
■ Encourage position changes every 1–2 hours. Provide skin care. Use a therapeutic mattress.	■ Prolonged pressure leads to decreased circulation and skin breakdown.	
3. Nursing Diagnosis: Nutrition, Imbalanced: Less than Body Requirements related to loss of appetite		
NIC Priority Intervention—*Nutrition Management:* Assistance with or provision of balanced dietary intake of foods and fluids		**NOC Suggested Outcome**—*Nutritional Status: Nutrient Intake:* Adequacy of nutrients taken into the body
GOAL: *The child will maintain adequate caloric intake.*		
■ Maintain a meal schedule similar to that at home. Serve food in age-appropriate serving sizes.	■ Normal routines and small frequent serving sizes help the child feel less overwhelmed by calories needed.	The child maintains pre-illness body weight and tolerates enough food to meet nutritional requirements.
■ Assess for food likes and dislikes. Provide favorite foods if allowed.	■ Favorite foods with reduced sodium may encourage the child to eat.	
4. Nursing Diagnosis: Activity Intolerance related to fluid and electrolyte imbalance, infectious process, and altered nutrition		
NIC Priority Intervention—*Energy Management:* Regulating energy use to treat and prevent fatigue and optimize function		**NOC Suggested Outcome**—*Energy Conservation:* Extent of active management of energy to initiate and sustain activity
GOAL: *The child will progress in activity tolerance without excessive fatigue as the disease process improves.*		
■ Maintain bed rest during the acute stage. Encourage gradual activity increase as the condition improves.	■ Rest decreases the production of waste materials, which place increased stress on the kidneys.	The child avoids fatigue and exhibits the ability to tolerate activity for a longer period each day.
■ Provide quiet play for the developmental stage of the child (e.g., coloring books, music, videos, television).	■ Quiet activities minimize energy expenditure and stress on the kidneys.	

NANDA-I © 2012

Pathophysiology Illustrated   Acute Renal Failure

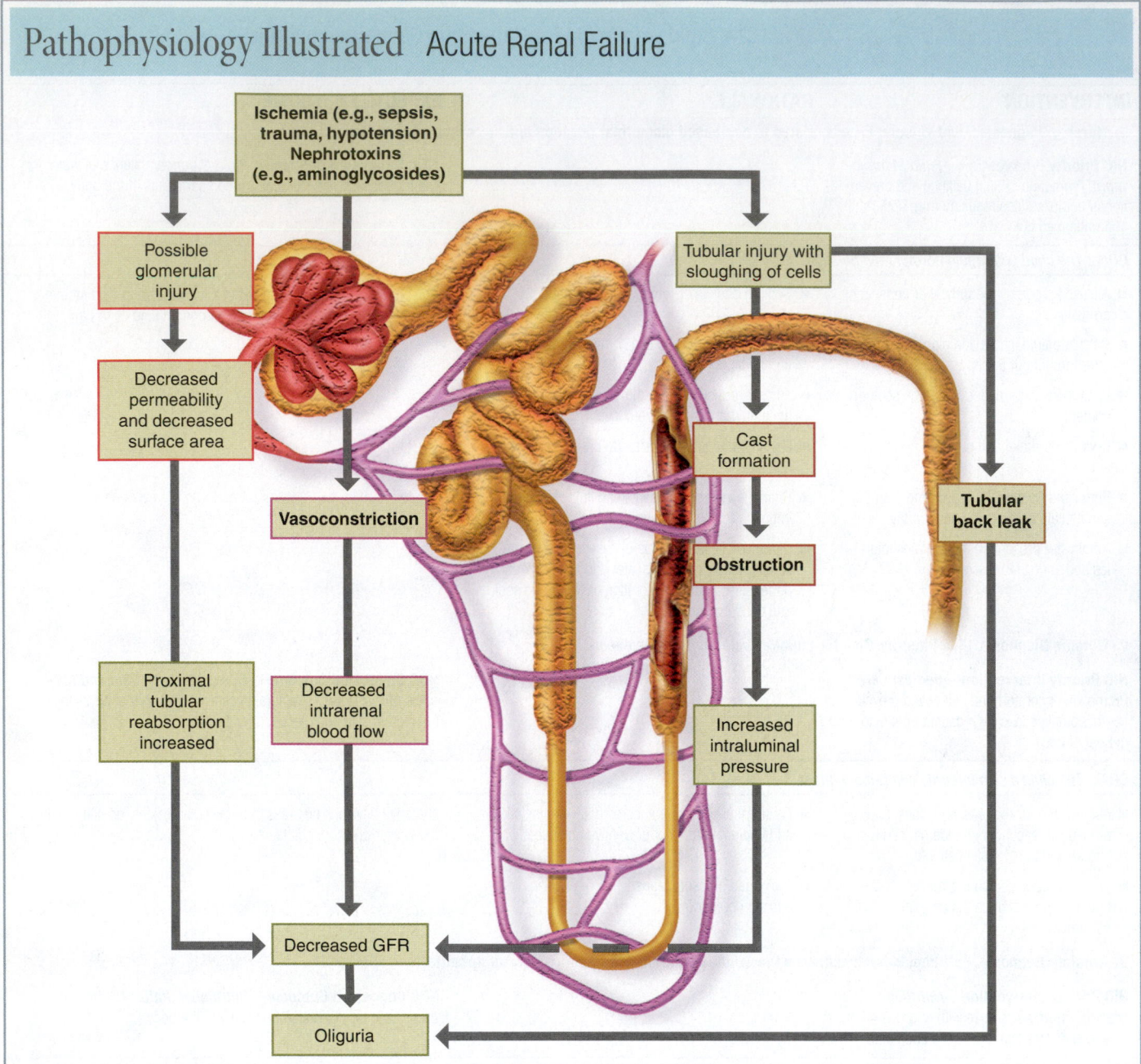

FIGURE 31–11 ■ The initial kidney injury is usually associated with an acute condition such as sepsis, trauma, and hypotension, or the result of treatment for an acute condition with a nephrotoxic medication. Injury to the kidney can occur because of glomerular injury, vasoconstriction of capillaries, or tubular injury. All consequences of injury lead to decreased glomerular filtration and oliguria.

Avner, 2011). Potential causes include hemolytic uremic syndrome, acute glomerulonephritis, sepsis, poisoning, nephrotoxic medications, hypovolemia, obstructive uropathy, and complications of cardiac surgery.

Etiology and pathophysiology ARF may be caused by prerenal or postrenal factors as well as actual kidney damage. See Figure 31–11 ■.

■ Prerenal ARF is a result of decreased perfusion to an otherwise normal kidney in association with a systemic condition. Hypovolemia secondary to dehydration is generally the cause;

however, alterations in renal vasculature or cardiac function may also precipitate prerenal ARF. This is the most common type of ARF in infants and young children (Lum, 2011).

■ Primary kidney damage (intrinsic factors) may result from infection, diseases such as hemolytic uremic syndrome or acute glomerulonephritis, acute interstitial nephritis, and nephrotoxic injury. The structure most susceptible to damage is the kidney tubule. Injury to the tubule resulting in acute tubular necrosis is the most frequent cause of intrinsic renal failure in children (Lum, 2011).

Clinical Manifestations Electrolyte Imbalances in Acute and Chronic Renal Failure

ELECTROLYTE IMBALANCE	CLINICAL MANIFESTATIONS	CLINICAL THERAPY
Hyperkalemia Results from inability to adequately excrete potassium derived from diet and catabolized cells. In metabolic acidosis, there is also movement of potassium from intracellular fluid to extracellular fluid.	■ Peaked T waves, widening of QRS and ECG ■ Dysrhythmias ■ Muscle weakness	Eliminate intake of potassium Kayexalate orally or in retention enema Administration of oral alkalinizing agents Intravenous calcium gluconate or calcium chloride to stabilize the myocardial cell membrane Intravenous sodium bicarbonate, insulin and dextrose, and beta-adrenergic agents such as albuterol may be used to enhance the cellular intake of potassium Dialysis if other methods to reduce the potassium level are ineffective
Hyponatremia In the acute oliguric phase, hyponatremia is related to the accumulation of fluid in excess of solute.	■ Change in level of consciousness ■ Muscle cramps ■ Anorexia ■ Abdominal reflexes, depressed deep tendon reflexes ■ Cheyne-Stokes respirations ■ Seizures	Fluid restriction Electrolyte replacement Hypertonic saline for sodium levels less than 120 mEq/L, seizures Dialysis to correct severe electrolyte disturbance
Hypocalcemia Phosphate retention (hyperphosphatemia) depresses the serum calcium concentration. Calcium is deposited in injured cells. Hyperkalemia and metabolic acidosis may mask the common clinical manifestations of severe hypocalcemia.	■ Muscle tingling ■ Changes in muscle tone ■ Seizures ■ Muscle cramps and twitching ■ Positive Chvostek sign (contraction of facial muscles after tapping facial nerve just anterior to parotid gland)	Low phosphorous diet IV calcium if tetany is present Oral phosphate binders Dialysis to correct severe electrolyte disturbance

Source: *Data from Hines, E. Q. (2012). Fluid and electrolytes. In Johns Hopkins:* The Harriet Lane Handbook *(19th ed., pp. 271–292). Philadelphia, PA: Elsevier; Sreedharan, R., & Avner, E. D. (2011). Renal failure. In R. M. Kliegman, B. F. Stanton, J. W. St. Geme III, N. F. Schor, & R. E. Behrman,* Nelson textbook of pediatrics *(19th ed., pp. 1818–1826). Philadelphia, PA: Saunders Elsevier; Verive, M. J. (2011). Pediatric hyperkalemia. Retrieved from http://emedicine.medscape.com/article/907543-overview*

Note: See Chapter 23 🔗 for more information related to these alterations in electrolytes.

■ Postrenal ARF is generally found in newborns with urologic anatomic anomalies (Lum, 2011). Children may have oliguria, or normal or increased urine output. Renal failure without oliguria usually indicates a less severe renal injury. Children who recover from ARF may have residual kidney damage and compromised renal function.

Clinical manifestations Characteristically, a healthy child suddenly experiences nonspecific symptoms that indicate a significant illness or injury (e.g., nausea, vomiting, edema, gross hematuria, oliguria, and hypertension). These symptoms are a result of electrolyte imbalances, uremia, and fluid overload. The child appears pale and lethargic. See the Clinical Manifestations tables on this page for more information.

Hyperkalemia is the most life-threatening electrolyte disorder associated with ARF. Hyponatremia affects central nervous system function, resulting in symptoms that range from fatigue to seizures. Edema occurs as a result of sodium and water retention. See Chapter 23 🔗 for further discussion of fluid and electrolyte alterations.

Children with ARF are also more susceptible to infection because of depressed immune functioning. Uremia occurs when there is an excess of urea and other nitrogenous waste products in the blood. Neurologic symptoms from accumulating wastes may include headache, seizures, lethargy, and confusion.

Clinical Manifestations Acute Versus Chronic Renal Failure

TYPE OF RENAL FAILURE	CLINICAL MANIFESTATIONS
Acute renal failure	Dark urine or gross hematuria, headache, edema, fatigue, crackles, gallop heart rhythm, hypertension, hematuria, lethargy, nausea and vomiting, oliguria Mass in flank area if a cyst, tumor, or obstructive lesion is present
Chronic renal failure	Fatigue, malaise, poor appetite, nausea and vomiting, failure to thrive or short stature May have oliguria or polyuria Headache, decreased mental alertness or ability to concentrate, chronic anemia, hypertension, edema, fractures with minimal trauma, rickets, valgus deformity

Collaborative Care

The goal of collaborative care is to minimize or prevent permanent kidney damage while maintaining fluid and electrolyte balance and managing complications.

Diagnostic Tests

Diagnosis of renal failure is based primarily on urinalysis and blood chemistry results, including BUN, serum creatinine, sodium, potassium, and calcium levels (Table 31–5). These tests may reveal hematuria, proteinuria, infection, anemia, acidosis, and electrolyte abnormalities. The kidneys are normal in size, and no signs of renal osteodystrophy are found on radiograph. Various imaging studies to assess kidney structures, renal blood flow, and renal perfusion and function may be performed to determine whether the child has ARF or chronic renal failure. A renal biopsy may be required to examine the glomeruli.

Clinical Therapy

Treatment depends on the underlying cause of the renal failure. The goal is to minimize or prevent permanent renal damage while maintaining fluid and electrolyte balance and managing complications. Initial emergency treatment of children with fluid depletion focuses on rapid fluid replacement of saline or lactated Ringer's solution at 20 mL/kg given rapidly or over 5 to 10 minutes and repeated as needed to ensure renal perfusion and stabilize blood pressure. Albumin may also be administered when blood loss is the cause of circulatory depletion. If oliguria persists after restoration of adequate fluid volume, intrinsic renal damage is suspected.

Children with fluid overload, such as those with pulmonary edema, require diuretic therapy and dialysis if they respond poorly to diuretics. Once the child is stabilized, fluid requirements are calculated to maintain zero water balance (intake should equal urine output and insensible fluid loss). All potential sources of potassium should be eliminated until hyperkalemia is controlled. (See Chapter 23 ✏.) Remember that catabolic states or extensive tissue injury may raise potassium levels. Other electrolyte imbalances are treated. Nutrition must be maintained with extra carbohydrate intake during the catabolic state. Antibiotics are prescribed for infection if applicable. Nephrotoxic antibiotics such as aminoglycosides (e.g., gentamicin, vancomycin) should be avoided. Some children whose ARF is unresponsive to management require dialysis to correct severe electrolyte imbalances, manage fluid overload, and cleanse the blood of waste products. The clinical situation and age of the child will determine whether hemodialysis or peritoneal dialysis will be used. Refer to the section on renal replacement therapy on page 1079.

Prognosis depends on the cause of ARF. When renal failure results from drug toxicity or dehydration that is rapidly treated, the prognosis is generally good. However, ARF that results from diseases such as hemolytic uremic syndrome or acute glomerulonephritis may be associated with residual kidney damage.

Nursing Management

Goals of nursing care for the child with acute renal failure are to promote fluid and electrolyte balance, prevent complications such as infection and injury, and support the child and family.

Nursing Assessment and Diagnosis

A complete history and physical examination are necessary to identify progression of symptoms and possible causes for renal failure.

Physiologic Assessment

Assess vital signs, level of consciousness, and other neurologic indicators to help identify signs of electrolyte imbalance (see the Clinical Manifestations table on page 1071). Measure the child's weight on admission to provide a baseline for evaluating changes in fluid status. Monitor urinalysis, urine culture, and blood chemistry studies. Inspect urine for color, specific gravity, intake and output, and odor. Cloudy urine may indicate infection; tea-colored urine suggests hematuria. Assess urine specific gravity and intake and output.

Psychosocial Assessment

The unexpected and acute nature of the child's hospitalization creates anxiety for both parents and child. Assess for feelings of anger, guilt, or fear associated with the hospitalization. Such feelings are likely if ARF developed as a result of dehydration, a preventable injury, or poisoning. Assess coping mechanisms, family support systems, and level of stress.

Several nursing diagnoses may apply to the child with ARF, including:

- Perfusion: Renal, Risk for Ineffective related to hypovolemia, sepsis, or drug toxicity
- Fluid Volume: Excess related to renal dysfunction and sodium retention
- Nutrition, Imbalanced: Less than Body Requirements related to anorexia, nausea, vomiting, and catabolic state
- Infection, Risk for related to invasive procedures and monitoring equipment, and impaired immune functioning
- Coping: Family, Compromised related to sudden hospitalization and uncertain prognosis of child

TABLE 31–5	Diagnostic Tests for Renal Failure
DIAGNOSTIC TESTS	**FINDINGS IN RENAL FAILURE**
Urinalysis	
pH	Acidic urine
Osmolarity	Greater than 500 mOsm/kg: prerenal ARF
	Less than 350 mOsm/kg: intrinsic ARF
Specific Gravity	Greater than 1.020: prerenal ARF
	Less than 1.010: intrinsic ARF
Protein	Positive
Blood	Positive
Serum Chemistry*	
Potassium	Elevated
Sodium	Normal, low, or high, depends solely on the amount of water in the body
Calcium	Low
Phosphorus	High
Urea nitrogen	Increased
Creatinine	Increased
pH	Low acidic

Source: Data from Sreedharan, R., & Avner, E. D. (2011). Renal failure. In R. M. Kliegman, B. F. Stanton, J. W. St. Geme III, N. F. Schor, & R. E. Behrman, Nelson textbook of pediatrics (19th ed., pp. 1818–1826). Philadelphia, PA: Saunders Elsevier; Workeneh, B. T., Agraharkar, M., & Gupta, R. (2012). Acute renal failure. Retrieved from http://emedicine.medscape.com/article/243492-overview

Note: *Refer to Appendix D ✏ for normal values for various ages. ARF = acute renal failure.

NANDA-I © 2012

Planning and Implementation

Nursing care focuses on preventing complications, maintaining fluid balance, administering medications, meeting nutritional needs, preventing infection, and providing emotional support to the child and family.

Prevent Complications

Complications are best prevented by ensuring compliance with the treatment plan. Careful monitoring of vital signs, intake and output, serum electrolytes, and level of consciousness can alert the nurse to changes that indicate potential complications. Nephrotoxic drugs should be avoided.

Practice Alert

Nephrotoxic drugs include the following:

- Antimicrobials: aminoglycosides, cephalosporins, tetracycline, sulfonamides
- Radiographic contrast media with iodine (typically used for CT scans)
- Heavy metals: lead, barium, iron
- Nonsteroidal anti-inflammatory drugs (NSAIDs): indomethacin, aspirin, ibuprofen

Maintain Fluid Balance

Estimate the child's fluid status by monitoring intake and output and blood pressure two or three times daily. Also obtain a weight at least daily on the same scale at the same time of day. Monitor serum chemistry values, especially for sodium and potassium.

Clinical Tip

If serum sodium concentration rises and weight falls, insufficient fluids are being administered. If the serum sodium level falls and the weight increases, excessive fluids are being administered.

If the child has oliguria, limit fluid intake (including parenteral nutrition) to replacement of insensible fluid loss (what is excreted by the lungs, skin, and gastrointestinal tract), which is about one third the daily maintenance requirements in afebrile children. If the child is febrile, fluid administration is increased by 12% for each centigrade degree of temperature elevation.

Clinical Tip

The child with renal insufficiency is at greater risk for fluid loss with illness. In cases of acute gastrointestinal illness, these children are at greater risk for dehydration and ARF.

Administer Medications

Because the kidney's ability to excrete drugs is impaired in ARF, dosages of all medications should be adjusted. The actual dosage of the drug can be reduced, or the time interval between doses may be increased. Check drug levels to monitor for drug toxicity, and know the signs of drug toxicity for each medication the child is receiving.

Meet Nutritional Needs

Children are at risk for malnutrition because of their high metabolic rate during ARF. Parenteral or enteral feeding may be used initially to minimize protein catabolism. The diet is tailored to the individual child's need for calories, carbohydrates, fats, and amino acids or protein hydrolysates. Depending on the degree of renal failure, sodium, potassium, and phosphorus may be restricted. Initiate oral feedings as soon as tolerated. A multidisciplinary team with a nutritionist may be necessary.

Prevent Infection

The child with ARF is extremely susceptible to hospital-acquired infections as a result of altered nutritional status, compromised immunity, and numerous invasive procedures. Thorough hand hygiene and standard precautions are imperative to decrease the risk of infection. Use sterile technique for all invasive procedures and when caring for central lines. Drainage from catheter sites should be cultured to check for the presence of infectious organisms. Assess vital signs and lung sounds frequently.

Provide Emotional Support

The sudden onset of ARF presents parents with an unexpected threat to their child's life. Both the child and the parents experience anxiety related to the unexpected hospitalization and the uncertainty of the prognosis. Parents often feel guilty regardless of the cause of renal failure; guilt is intensified if the parents feel there is something they could have done to prevent the condition. Partner with parents, encourage verbalization of fears, and assist them in working through feelings of guilt. Explain procedures and treatment measures to decrease anxiety. Encouraging parents and older siblings to participate in the child's care can increase their sense of control.

Discharge Planning and Home Care Teaching

Partner with the family to encourage parental involvement early in the child's hospitalization. Be sure parents understand the importance of administering medications correctly. Teach family members proper technique for measuring blood pressure so they can monitor the child's blood pressure for hypertension, if ordered. Ensure the parents can identify signs of progressive renal failure (refer to the chronic renal failure discussion).

Diet counseling is a key component of discharge planning and is usually performed by a nutritionist. Depending on the degree of renal failure, the child's diet may include restrictions on protein, water, sodium, potassium, and phosphorus. Partner with the parents, older child, and dietitian to provide written guidelines identifying appropriate food choices and assist the family in menu planning. Ethnic and cultural preferences, as well as the child's food preferences, are considered in listing menu options. See Developing Cultural Competence: Sodium Intake.

Continued monitoring of kidney function during follow-up examinations is critical as deterioration may occur over time. Referral to support groups can be helpful for parents and children alike. The National Kidney Foundation is a source of numerous publications that are helpful to the child and family.

Weblink | National Kidney Foundation

Developing Cultural Competence
Sodium Intake

Special effort is often needed to reduce the sodium in the diet of a child eating predominantly Asian cuisine. Sauces and seasonings for foods (soy sauce, mustards, monosodium glutamate, and garlic salt) are sodium rich even though the foods seasoned (rice, vegetables, shrimp, and chicken) are low in sodium. A child eating a diet of predominantly Mexican cuisine may also require significant dietary modification, because many of the foods are high in sodium and potassium. Individualized counseling and motivation are needed to encourage families to reduce the child's sodium intake and to use spices low in sodium when preparing meals. A cultural broker may be helpful in assisting the family to understand the need to change dietary habits. (See Chapter 3 .)

Evaluation

Expected outcomes of nursing care may include:

- Kidney function is restored.
- Fluid, electrolyte, and acid–base balance is restored and maintained.
- Nutritional needs are met.
- The parents and child cope effectively with the illness.
- The child does not acquire a secondary infection.

Chronic Renal Failure

Chronic renal failure (CRF) (also called chronic kidney disease) is a progressive, irreversible reduction in kidney function. The prevalence of chronic renal failure in children is approximately 18 per 1 million (Sreedharan & Avner, 2011).

Etiology and pathophysiology In children, CRF usually results from developmental abnormalities of the kidney or urinary tract, obstructed urine flow and reflux, hereditary diseases such as polycystic kidney disease, and infections such as hemolytic uremic syndrome and glomerulonephritis (Lum, 2011).

The gradual, progressive loss of functioning nephrons ultimately results in **end-stage renal disease (ESRD).** In ESRD, the kidneys can no longer maintain homeostasis and the child requires dialysis (Sreedharan & Avner, 2011).

The kidneys excrete excess acid in the body and regulate the body's fluid and electrolyte balance. Renal failure disrupts this fluid and electrolyte balance. As renal failure progresses, metabolic acidosis occurs because the kidneys cannot excrete the acids that build up in the body. Renal osteodystrophy occurs as the kidneys are unable to produce activated vitamin D and to excrete phosphorus, causing phosphorus levels to rise and serum calcium levels to fall. The parathyroid gland responds by drawing calcium and phosphorus from the bones to maintain the adequate serum calcium and phosphorus levels. Hypocalcemia may occur as the parathyroid glands become less responsive to vitamin D and lower serum calcium levels. Osteodystrophy increases the child's risk for spontaneous fractures (Sreedharan & Avner, 2011).

Growth retardation is caused by disturbances in the metabolism of calcium, phosphorus, and vitamin D; decreased caloric intake; and metabolic acidosis. The healthy kidneys also produce erythropoietin (the growth factor responsible for the production and maturation of red cells). Lack of erythropoietin and progressive renal disease are the underlying causes of the anemia of CRF.

Clinical manifestations Children with CRF may not have any symptoms initially. As progression continues, renal insufficiency occurs with polyuria as the kidneys cannot concentrate the urine. Symptoms such as pallor, headache, nausea, and fatigue become more classic. Decreased mental alertness and ability to concentrate may be seen. The child may have anemia leading to tachycardia, tachypnea, and dyspnea on exertion. As the disease progresses, the child experiences a loss of appetite and complications of renal impairment, including hypertension, pulmonary edema, growth retardation, osteodystrophy, delayed fine and gross motor development, and delayed sexual maturation. See the contrast with signs of acute renal failure in the Clinical Manifestations table on page 1071.

In ESRD, the most advanced form of CRF, renal failure adversely affects all body systems. As the severity of the clinical and biochemical disturbances resulting from progressive renal deterioration increases, uremic symptoms develop. Signs and symptoms of uremic syndrome include nausea and vomiting, progressive anemia, anorexia, dyspnea, malaise, **uremic frost** (urea crystals deposited on the skin), unpleasant (uremic) breath odor, headache, progressive confusion, tremors, pulmonary edema, and congestive heart failure.

Collaborative Care

The management goals for the child with chronic renal failure are to preserve remaining kidney function, slow progression to ESRD, maintain fluid and electrolyte balance, prevent associated complications, and promote growth and development.

Diagnostic Tests

Laboratory evaluation, including serum electrolytes, phosphate, BUN, and creatinine levels and pH, is used to confirm the diagnosis of chronic kidney disease and the stage of CRF. An early morning urine sample is collected for culture and to calculate the protein-to-creatinine ratio. The child's GFR is calculated from prediction equations using the serum creatinine level and the patient's height and gender. An online GFR calculator is available through the National Kidney Foundation. Refer to Table 31–5 on page 1072 for diagnostic findings related to renal failure.

Imaging studies are performed to identify renal diseases that could be causing the renal failure. A renal biopsy may sometimes be performed.

Clinical Therapy

Goals of treatment are to slow the progression of kidney disease, prevent complications, and promote growth and development. Conservative treatment includes a combination of dietary, fluid, and electrolyte management, and control of hypertension. If that fails and the child progresses to ESRD, dialysis is initiated.

CRF is irreversible; however, the course of the disease is variable. Some children progress quickly to renal failure, necessitating dialysis. Other children are managed with a combination of medication and diet therapy for some time before significant renal impairment occurs. Frequent modifications in the treatment plan are often necessary to address the child's changing status.

Dietary management focuses on maximizing caloric intake for growth while limiting phosphorus, potassium, and sodium as needed to maintain electrolyte levels in balance (Sreedharan & Avner, 2011). Adequate calcium needs to be part of the meal plan. Enteral or parenteral feedings may be required to achieve optimal protein intake, especially in children under 1 year of age. Complex carbohydrates should be chosen along with vegetables and fruits that are lower in potassium. Vegetable oils, hard candy, sugar, honey, and jelly may be recommended to add calories to the child's diet.

Medications used in the management of chronic renal failure are discussed in the Medications table on page 1075. (See Complementary Therapy: Avoiding Herbal Supplements in Children with CRF.)

Children who progress to ESRD require renal replacement therapy (see page 1079). The timetable for dialysis or renal transplantation is different from that of adults; transplantation is the goal so that the child has an optimal chance for a more normal childhood. Earlier initiation can prevent some complications of ESRD. In addition to the GFR, nonspecific signs such as uremic syndrome, poorly controlled

Medications Used to Treat Children with Chronic Renal Failure

MEDICATION	ACTION OR INDICATION	NURSING MANAGEMENT
Vitamin and mineral supplement (Nephrocaps)	Add vitamins and minerals missing from a heavily restricted diet	Only prescribed vitamins should be used; over-the-counter brands may contain elements that are harmful.
Phosphate binding agents: calcium carbonate (Tums), calcium acetate (PhosLo), or sevelamer hydrochloride (Renagel)	Reduce absorption of phosphorus from the intestines	Ensure that phosphate binding agent is aluminum-free. Take with food.
Calcitriol (Rocaltrol)	Replace the calcitriol that kidneys are no longer producing to keep calcium balance normal	Monitor serum calcium level. Ensure that calcium supplement is provided.
Epoetin alfa (Epogen, Procrit)	Stimulates bone marrow to produce red blood cells, treats anemia due to CRF	Give by IV or subcutaneous injection. Monitor blood pressure as hypertension is an adverse effect. Monitor hematocrit and serum ferritin level according to facility guidelines.
Iron supplementation	Treat iron deficiency when epoetin alfa is prescribed	Give without food or other medications to maximize absorption.
Growth hormone (rhGH)	Used to stimulate growth in children with CRF	Administer daily by subcutaneous injection. Record accurate height measurements at regular intervals.
Antihypertensive agents: Angiotensin-converting enzyme (ACE) inhibitor (enalapril, lisinopril) and angiotensin II blockers (losartan)	Slows the progression to ESRD	Monitor blood pressure. Monitor urine output and electrolyte balance.
Loop diuretics	Used when volume overload is present	

Source: Data from Gulati, S. (2011). Chronic kidney disease in children. Retrieved from http://emedicine.medscape.com/article/984358-overview; Lum, G. M. (2011). Chapter 22. Kidney & urinary tract. In W. W. Hay, M. J. Levin, J. M. Sondheimer, & R. R. Deterding (Eds.), CURRENT diagnosis & treatment: Pediatrics (20th ed.). Retrieved from http://www.accessmedicine.com; Sreedharan, R., & Avner, E. D. (2011). Renal failure. In R. M. Kliegman, B. F. Stanton, J. W. St. Geme III, N. F. Schor, & R. E. Behrman, Nelson textbook of pediatrics (19th ed., pp. 1818–1826). Philadelphia, PA: Saunders Elsevier; Wilson, B. A., Shannon, M. T., & Shields, K. M. (2011). Pearson nurse's drug guide 2011. New York, NY: Pearson.

hypertension, renal osteodystrophy, failure of head circumference measurement to increase normally, developmental delay, and poor growth are used in determining when to initiate renal replacement therapy. Infection is a common complication in children receiving renal replacement therapy in the form of peritoneal dialysis or hemodialysis and often requires hospitalization (Chadha, Schaefer, & Warady, 2010; Stefanidis, 2009).

Nursing Management

Goals of nursing care for the child with chronic renal failure are to promote fluid and electrolyte balance, prevent complications associated with renal dysfunction, and promote growth and development.

Nursing Assessment and Diagnosis

Nursing assessment focuses on identifying signs and symptoms of renal failure and associated complications, as well as assessing the psychosocial effects of renal failure on the child and family.

Physiologic Assessment

The initial and ongoing assessment of the child focuses on identifying complications of renal failure. Observe for signs of edema, poor growth and development, osteodystrophy, and anemia. Assess vital signs, particularly the blood pressure. Observe for signs of electrolyte alterations (see page 1071).

Psychosocial Assessment

As renal disease progresses, the number of stressors on the child and family increases. Denial and disbelief are common first reactions. A

Complementary Therapy Avoiding Herbal Supplements in Children with CRF

Herbal supplements should not be used in children with CRF as they may contain harmful minerals, such as potassium, or they may be toxic to the kidneys. The child with CRF is unable to clear waste products from the body like a healthy child. There is also the risk for interaction between the herbs and other medications taken that could place the child at risk for rejection of a transplanted kidney (National Kidney Foundation, 2011). Parents should discuss with the physician the use of any over-the-counter (OTC) or complementary therapies.

thorough family assessment can help to identify particular needs of the child and family (see Chapter 2). The development of ESRD is particularly challenging during childhood and adolescence because of differences in appearance and social, psychologic, and physical issues. Nonadherence with treatments can endanger the adolescent's life.

Nursing diagnoses for the child with CRF are similar to those previously listed for ARF. Additional diagnoses may include the following:

- Growth and Development, Delayed related to decreased protein and caloric intake and loss of protein in dialysate
- Social Interaction, Impaired related to impaired immunity and dialysis schedule during school hours
- Activity Intolerance related to anemia and fatigue

- Body Image, Disturbed related to short stature and visible external catheter for dialysis
- Therapeutic Regimen Management: Family, Ineffective related to complexity of care plan and economic difficulties

NANDA-I © 2012

Planning and Implementation

Children with CRF are frequently hospitalized for one of the following reasons: initial diagnostic evaluation, dialysis treatment initiation, problems with the treatment plan, or infection. Nursing care for the hospitalized child with CRF focuses on monitoring for side effects of medications, preventing infection, meeting nutritional needs, and providing emotional support and anticipatory teaching.

Monitor for Side Effects of Medications

Assess for signs of electrolyte imbalance such as weakness, muscle cramps, dizziness, headache, and nausea and vomiting in children who are taking diuretics. Supervise the child's activities closely to prevent falls resulting from dizziness, especially at the beginning of diuretic therapy. If antihypertensive medications such as hydralazine are being administered, monitor the child's weight to detect excessive gain resulting from water and sodium retention.

Prevent Infection

The child with CRF is extremely susceptible to infections. Be alert for signs of infection, such as elevated temperature; cloudy, strong-smelling urine; dysuria; changes in respiratory pattern; or productive cough. Cloudy dialysate in the child on peritoneal dialysis is a sign of infection. Emphasize to the child and family the importance of good hand hygiene practices.

Meet Nutritional Needs

Maintaining adequate nutritional intake in a child with CRF who has dietary restrictions is challenging. Provide small, frequent feedings and present meals attractively to encourage the child to eat. A nutritionist partners with the child and family to establish a meal plan with foods that meet the nutritional requirements and acknowledges the child's preferences. See Table 31–6 for foods that children with CRF should avoid.

Maintain Fluid Restrictions

Plan the child's oral intake through the entire 24 hours to ensure that the child has some fluids with meals, to take medications, and when thirsty. Keep in mind that many foods have a high fluid content (gelatin, fruit-flavored ice pops) and must be counted toward the daily fluid allowance. Use medicine cups or small cups for fluids given. Encourage parents and visitors to avoid drinking in the child's presence. Ensure that all visitors know and understand the importance of maintaining the child's fluid restriction.

Provide Emotional Support

Progressive CRF requires a total lifestyle change for the child and family. The parents and child need opportunities to express and work through their feelings related to the disease, prognosis, and treatment restrictions. Help children express their feelings through drawings or therapeutic play.

The need for ongoing dialysis treatments and the wait for a suitable donor kidney are stressful for both parents and the child. Identify effective coping methods and family support systems to promote treatment compliance. The National Kidney Foundation and local support groups for kidney disease can give the family information or additional support.

Discharge Planning and Home Care Teaching

Parents need to understand the necessity of long-term treatments and follow-up care. Partner with the family to develop a schedule for medication administration that fits with their routine. Because of the numerous medications that the child is on, provide or have the hospital pharmacist provide a chart of medications with times to be given. Emphasize the importance of consistency in administration times. Teach parents how to recognize side effects of medications and complications associated with the disease.

Appropriate referrals are made to home care nursing agencies as indicated. Parents of children receiving peritoneal dialysis at home are taught how to perform the treatment and how to identify complications (see the following section on page 1079). Strict aseptic technique is necessary to prevent infection at the catheter site and peritonitis.

Care in the Community

Children with CRF require frequent outpatient visits to monitor the progression of signs and symptoms, and to evaluate the effectiveness of current treatments. The blood pressure is monitored. Blood and urine tests are performed to monitor renal function. Radiographs of the bones are often taken at 6-month intervals to assess changes caused by osteodystrophy. See Health Promotion & Maintenance Overview: The Child with Chronic Renal Failure.

TABLE 31–6	Nutritional Information for the Child with Kidney Disease

Children with kidney disease have restricted diets, which are generally low in sodium, potassium, and phosphorus. The nurse can review this table to help families remember that certain foods must be avoided or eaten in very small quantities.

HIGH-SODIUM CONTENT FOODS	HIGH-POTASSIUM CONTENT FOODS	HIGH-PHOSPHORUS CONTENT FOODS
Soups and sauces: e.g., gravy, spaghetti and tomato sauce, barbeque sauce, steak sauce	*Fruit:* apricots, avocados, bananas, citrus fruits, fresh pears, nectarines, dates, figs, cantaloupe and other melons, prunes, and raisins	*Dairy products:* milk, cheese, yogurt, custard, pudding, ice cream
Processed lunchmeats: e.g., bologna, ham, salami, hot dogs	*Vegetables:* celery, dried beans, lima beans, potatoes, leafy greens, spinach, tomatoes, winter squash	Dried beans, peas
Smoked meat and fish: bacon, chipped beef, corned beef, ham, lox	*Whole grains:* especially those containing bran	Nuts, peanut butter
Sauerkraut, pickles, and other pickled foods	*Dairy products:* milk, ice cream, pudding, yogurt	Chocolate
Seasonings: horseradish, soy sauce, Worcestershire sauce, meat tenderizer, and monosodium glutamate (MSG)	Sardines, clams	Dark cola
	Peanuts	Sausage, hot dogs
	Potassium-containing salt substitutes	

Health Promotion & Maintenance Overview

The Child with Chronic Renal Failure

GROWTH AND DEVELOPMENT SURVEILLANCE

- Compare the child's height, weight, and head circumference to age-specific norms to identify growth retardation and to plot progress.
- Assess developmental progress using the Denver II or another screening tool (refer to Chapter 8).
- Educate parents on normal developmental milestones and measures to promote achieving those milestones.
- Assess the adolescent for signs of delayed sexual maturation and amenorrhea in females.

NUTRITION

- Review the dietary restrictions with the child and parents.
- Partner with the family to assist the child to make food selections and to restrict fluids and sodium as necessary, taking into account the child's preferences and cultural background. Encourage the child and family to take a list of a few favorite foods to the dietitian to see if they can be integrated into the child's meal plan.
- Make mealtime pleasant and make foods taste more appealing with permitted spices.
- Discuss possible behavioral responses by older children and adolescents to dietary restrictions and limitations imposed by the treatment plan. Involve the child and adolescent in discussions about dietary restrictions. When possible, integrate their recommendations for dietary restrictions and fluid management throughout the day.
- Emphasize to the school-age child that dietary and other restrictions are not punishment.
- Use enteral feeding at night to provide the needed calories for growth.

PHYSICAL ACTIVITY

- Encourage the child to participate in developmentally appropriate activities as tolerated.
- Partner with the child to establish a routine plan for physical activity as tolerated that will help promote strong bones.

ORAL HEALTH

- Promote good dentition and oral hygiene.
- Schedule regular dental visits for examination and cleaning to reduce infections.

- Partner with the family to ensure they understand the need for antibiotic prophylaxis before certain invasive procedures, including dental care.

MENTAL AND SPIRITUAL HEALTH

- Ask children how they feel about the need to follow a special diet, take medications, and undergo dialysis treatments. Ask what might make it easier for them to cope with the treatments, and integrate at least one idea into the care plan.
- Encourage parents to promote their child's participation in age-appropriate activities to minimize the psychologic consequences of coping with a chronic disease.
- If available, encourage adolescents to participate in a peer support group to help them cope with dietary restrictions and ongoing dialysis treatments, as they pose a threat to their independence, evolving sense of self, and need for independence. Without support, noncooperation, depression, and hostility are common responses.
- Assist older adolescents to transition to adult health and vocational services.

RELATIONSHIPS

- Attendance at school and contacts with peers promote normal growth and development.
- Work to promote the child's self-worth and a healthy self-esteem.
- Prepare the child for peer conflict.
- Ensure that parents understand the importance of encouraging normal socialization of their child.

DISEASE PREVENTION STRATEGIES

- Partner with the child and family to establish plans to avoid large crowds, people with infections, or other risks that expose the child to infection.
- If possible, provide all immunizations before renal transplantation, as long-term immunosuppressive therapy will then be prescribed.
- Live virus vaccines should not be given to the child taking immunosuppressive agents.
- Encourage the family to maintain scheduled appointments for routine serum and urine diagnostic tests performed to monitor renal function.

Anticipatory Teaching

Provide the child and family with timely information about the disease process, dialysis treatments, and issues related to kidney transplantation as the child's renal failure progresses. Review the child's immunizations on every visit in an effort to have the child fully immunized prior to kidney transplantation. Live virus vaccines cannot be given when the child is immunocompromised following the transplant. Make sure the child receives the 23-valent pneumococcal and the meningococcal vaccine. Some children receive a kidney transplant prior to reaching ESRD (Shapiro & Sarwal, 2010).

Education and Socialization

Parents should be encouraged to register the young child in an early education program to promote development and interaction with other children. The dialysis schedule for school-age children should enable the child to participate in school, or home tutoring should be

provided. Educational progress needs to be assessed in children with ESRD, and additional educational assistance should be provided as needed to promote optimal education attainment. Encourage frequent hand hygiene for all children and adults in the classroom to reduce the spread of infection.

School-age children and adolescents are often embarrassed about being perceived as different from peers. The metabolic abnormalities interfere with the child's height growth and delay pubertal development. Ask the child how he or she feels about the need to follow a special diet, take medications, and undergo dialysis treatments. To minimize the psychologic consequences of coping with a chronic disease, encourage parents to promote the child's participation in age-appropriate activities. Attendance at school and contacts with peers promote normal growth and development. The child with CRF or a kidney transplant may benefit from having a nurse visit the school to talk with the child's peers about the treatments the child requires.

Legal and Ethical Considerations
Kidney Failure and Medicare

In 1972, Congress made children with permanent kidney failure (needing regular dialysis or having a kidney transplant) eligible for Medicare to pay for needed medical care. Additionally, the State Children's Health Insurance Program established by the U.S. Department of Health and Human Services provides assistance to children without health insurance (National Kidney and Urologic Diseases Information Clearinghouse, 2009).

All children have a need for acceptance. Partner with the family to promote the child's self-worth and a healthy self-esteem. Assist the child and family in choosing clothing that can cover the dialysis shunt site and complement and enhance the child's physical appearance. Encourage adolescents to participate in a program that helps them transition to adult health services and job skill training.

Psychosocial Support

The need for ongoing dialysis treatments and the wait for a suitable donor kidney are stressful for parents and child. It is important to identify effective coping methods and family support systems to promote treatment compliance. Partner with the child and family to determine stress factors and strategies for coping. The National Kidney Foundation and local support groups for kidney disease can provide the family with additional information and support. (See Evidence-Based Practice: Living with End-Stage Renal Disease.)

Preparation for Kidney Transplant

Kidney transplantation is the optimal treatment for CRF. While the child is waiting for a transplant, remind the family to keep the transplant center informed of any changes in the child's health status, address, or phone number. This will enable the transplant center to notify the family immediately when a kidney is available for transplant.

Evaluation

Expected outcomes of nursing care include the following:

- The child's fluid status is maintained.
- The child eats foods that meet nutritional needs while adhering to dietary restrictions.
- Growth and developmental milestones are achieved.
- Social needs are met through social interaction.
- The child has a positive body image.

For additional outcomes specific to the child on peritoneal dialysis, see the Nursing Care Plan beginning on page 1080.

Evidence-Based Practice | Living with End-Stage Renal Disease

PROBLEM

End-stage renal disease is a serious chronic condition that requires significant adaptations in lifestyle and complex medical treatments that take a toll on the child and family. What is the impact of end-stage renal disease on children, adolescents, and their families?

EVIDENCE

A cross-sectional study of 81 children and adolescents, ages 10 to 21 years, with end-stage renal disease was conducted to evaluate their health-related quality of life (HRQOL). Of the 81 subjects, 68 had received a kidney transplant and 13 were on dialysis. Results of the study showed that the HRQOL of those patients who had undergone kidney transplant was similar to that of healthy adolescents. However, the patients who remained on dialysis demonstrated a significantly lower HRQOL than kidney recipients or healthy adolescents (Riaño-Galán, Málaga, Rajmil, et al., 2009).

A multicenter study compared quality of life scores between 211 children ages 4 to 18 years who were dialysis patients or kidney transplant recipients and 232 age-matched healthy children. Child-self and parent-proxy scores were also compared with 129 parents of children with kidney disease and 156 parents of healthy children participating in the study. Subscales evaluated included physical well-being, emotional well-being, self-esteem, family, friends, school, and disease perception. Of the children with chronic kidney disease, 139 were renal transplant recipients and 72 were dialysis patients. Children with chronic kidney disease had lower quality of life scores than healthy children in all subscales except for physical well-being. Additionally, dialysis patients had lower scores than transplant recipients in subscales related to physical well-being, friends, and self-esteem, and in the total quality of life score. The study further found that parent-proxy scores and child-self scores were not equivalent, citing the need to evaluate both the child's and parents' perspective (Buyan, Türkmen, Bilge, et al., 2010).

Aldridge's (2008) review of 11 research studies examined how families adjust to having a child with chronic kidney failure. Significant findings from this study demonstrated that families who had children on dialysis reported increased disruption in their family life and increased stress in their marriage. The review also revealed that parents of children with chronic kidney failure have some difficulties in coping and may exhibit high levels of stress, anxiety, and depression. The review established that parents of lower socioeconomic status had more difficulty adjusting to the diagnosis and had decreased rates of adherence to the therapeutic regimen. Lower socioeconomic status was also associated with a higher rate of depression and anxiety among parents of children with chronic kidney failure.

IMPLICATIONS

Effects of chronic illness in children and adolescents can be both physically and psychosocially overwhelming. It is important to evaluate quality of life in children with chronic illness in order to better understand response to the illness and treatment (Heath, MacKinlay, Watson, et al., 2011). Children and adolescents who develop end-stage renal disease are expected to develop skills to cope with the consequences of the illness. Parents must modify lifestyles and their hopes and dreams for their child's future. Strategies for managing the disease differ for every family. These families view their lives and their child as different from other families because of the child's condition. Development of effective coping strategies is essential if the child is to effectively manage living with this illness. Nurses must assess families and determine their level of adjustment to the child's illness and their level of coping because this will impact their adherence to the plan of care. Nurses can facilitate development of these coping strategies by encouraging children and adolescents to express their feelings about the illness and the restraints it places on their lifestyle. Nurses can ensure that distraction techniques, such as music, are utilized when these children are in the hospital or in the dialysis center receiving treatment.

Children who are having difficulty coping with their chronic illness need to be identified early so they may receive counseling and psychiatric help if needed. Nurses can be effective in working with families by listening to the issues and offering suggestions. Often the opportunity to talk through the child's management plan will help the family consider different strategies that may be effective. The nurse may also provide linkages to community resources that may help the family.

CRITICAL THINKING APPLICATION

Initiate a discussion with an older school-age child or adolescent with end-stage renal disease; listen to the child's description of living with the condition. Develop a nursing care plan to help the child take the next steps in self-management.

Renal Replacement Therapy

Renal replacement therapy is the treatment for renal failure and includes both dialysis and kidney transplantation. The preferred method of dialysis is generally dependent on the child's age. Currently 88% of children with renal failure who are 5 years of age and younger are treated with peritoneal dialysis, while 54% of children older than 12 years are treated with hemodialysis (Sreedharan & Avner, 2011).

Peritoneal Dialysis

In peritoneal dialysis, the peritoneum of the abdomen is the membrane through which the body's waste products pass from the blood to the abdominal cavity. A catheter is inserted through the abdominal wall into the peritoneal cavity. In children receiving peritoneal dialysis for ARF, a percutaneously placed catheter can be used for a few weeks. In children with CRF, a catheter is placed surgically for long-term use. The dialysis solution (**dialysate**) that enters the abdomen typically contains dextrose that pulls body wastes and extra fluid into the abdominal cavity. These wastes and extra fluid leave the body with the drained dialysate. This form of dialysis is beneficial to small children since it allows continuous removal of fluids and waste products, decreasing the toxic effects of waste products on the child's developing body. The child can ambulate and interact with the environment. Dietary and fluid restrictions are less severe. The timing of the treatment can be set to minimize the interruption of school, play, or other social events. However, infection or peritonitis is a significant complication.

Two types of peritoneal dialysis are commonly used: continuous ambulatory peritoneal dialysis (CAPD) and automated peritoneal dialysis (APD). Graduated cylinders are used to monitor the volume of fluid exchanged.

- CAPD uses gravity to instill prefilled bags of dialysate into the peritoneal cavity four or five times a day. The fluid remains in the cavity for 4 to 8 hours. The attached bag is folded under the child's clothes, permitting normal activity. After the allotted time, the dialysate is drained by hanging the bag lower than the pelvis. The repeated connections and disconnections with this method are time consuming for the child and family and increase the risk of infection.
- APD is the most commonly used method of dialysis in children (Fischbach & Warady, 2009). APD uses an automatic cycler to instill and drain the dialysate about five times over a 10-hour period, usually overnight. One additional exchange may be needed during the day. With this method, the number of connections and disconnections is minimized, which reduces demands on the family as well as the risk of infection. Infants and young children on peritoneal dialysis generally receive APD while they sleep (Zaritsky & Warady, 2011).

Peritonitis is a common complication of peritoneal dialysis. See Table 31–7. Peritonitis is treated with antibiotics infused in the dialysate (Chadha et al., 2010).

Clinical Judgment

The child on peritoneal dialysis is at high risk of developing peritonitis. What is the nurse's responsibility in assessment and management of the child with peritonitis? What should the nurse teach the family who is performing home dialysis about prevention of peritonitis, recognition of symptoms, and when to notify the healthcare provider?

Nursing Management

Partner with the child and family to assist them in learning appropriate peritoneal dialysis methods and to use sterile technique when performing dialysis and doing catheter care to reduce the risk for peritonitis. Peritoneal dialysis is time consuming, and commitment by family members is required to manage this procedure daily. Assist the family to develop home routines that minimize disruptions to attending school and daily family life. Reinforce the importance of adhering to the prescribed exchanges every day to provide the child with the best clearance and general health status. For additional information, refer to the Nursing Care Plan for the child receiving home peritoneal dialysis.

Hemodialysis

Hemodialysis is a process in which the blood flows from the patient through a machine with a special filter that removes body wastes and extra fluids. Blood is pumped out of the body and through a dialyzer, where waste products and extra fluids diffuse out across a semipermeable membrane, before the blood is returned to the body. Dialysate is pumped in the direction opposite blood flow to promote waste extraction. Differences in osmolarity and concentration between the child's blood and the dialysate alter the intravascular electrolyte concentration and reduce the intravascular volume.

Hemodialysis is used in the critical care setting and for those children with CRF when peritoneal dialysis is not possible for technical reasons, after repeated peritonitis, or when the family is unable to

TABLE 31–7	Complications of Peritoneal Dialysis	
COMPLICATION	**MANIFESTATIONS**	**CAUSE**
Peritonitis	Cloudy dialysate, abdominal pain, tenderness, leukocytosis, nausea or vomiting, fever (neonatal hypothermia), constipation	*Staphylococcus aureus, Staphylococcus epidermidis,* fungal infections, gram-negative rods (risk is proportional to duration of dialysis and inversely proportional to age)
Pain	During inflow	Too rapid a rate of infusion, too large a volume of dialysate, encasement of catheter in a false passage, extremes in temperature of dialysate
	During outflow at end of emptying	Omentum entering catheter at end of outflow
Leakage	Fluid around catheter, edema of penis or scrotum secondary to leakage into abdominal subcutaneous tissue, fluid leakage to pleural spaces through diaphragm	Overfilling of abdomen, catheter that has migrated from peritoneal cavity
Respiratory symptoms	Shortness of breath, decreased breath sounds in lower lobes, inadequate chest expansion	Abdominal fullness that compromises diaphragm movement, hole in diaphragm allowing dialysate into chest cavity

Nursing Care Plan | The Child Receiving Home Peritoneal Dialysis

INTERVENTION	RATIONALE	EXPECTED OUTCOME
1. Nursing Diagnosis: Nutrition, Imbalanced: Less than Body Requirements related to poor appetite, feeling of fullness after a small amount, and loss of protein in dialysate		
NIC Priority Intervention—*Nutrition Management:* Assistance with or provision of a balanced dietary intake of foods and fluids		**NOC Suggested Outcome**—*Nutrition Status: Food and Fluid Intake:* Amount of food and fluid taken into the body over a 24-hour period
GOAL: *The child will obtain adequate nutrients each day.*		
■ Develop a meal plan in collaboration with a nutritionist, to identify the amounts of essential nutrients needed.	■ Parents need concrete guidelines for food preparation.	The child's intake is adequate for an expected growth pattern to be maintained.
■ Provide small, frequent meals of needed nutrients.	■ The child will feel full with smaller amounts of food because of the dialysate.	
■ Make mealtimes pleasant and avoid battles over the child's intake.	■ The child will be more inclined to eat if there is less stress.	
■ Provide supplements by tube feeding if oral intake is inadequate.	■ Adequate nutrition is important for growth and development, and must be supported if oral intake is inadequate.	
2. Nursing Diagnosis: Infection, Risk for related to daily invasive procedure		
NIC Priority Intervention—*Infection Control:* Minimizing the acquisition and transmission of infectious agents		**NOC Suggested Outcome**—*Infection Status:* Presence and extent of infection
GOAL: *The child will not develop peritonitis.*		
■ Wash hands; use sterile gloves and aseptic technique for connection and disconnection of catheters.	■ Aseptic technique reduces the chance of introducing bacteria into the abdomen.	The child does not develop peritonitis.
■ Perform daily catheter site care.	■ Skin around the catheter site will have fewer organisms that could potentially cause infection.	
GOAL: *If peritonitis occurs, it will be treated appropriately.*		
■ Observe for signs of infection (fever, abdominal pain, cloudy dialysate).	■ Early identification of infection will reduce complications.	Hospitalization will not be needed for peritonitis due to early recognition and prompt treatment.
■ Report signs of infection to the physician immediately.	■ Rapid intervention may reduce the need for hospitalization.	
3. Nursing Diagnosis: Caregiver Role Strain related to daily dialysis treatments		
NIC Priority Intervention—*Caregiver Support:* Provision of necessary information, advocacy, and support to facilitate primary patient care by someone other than a healthcare professional		**NOC Suggested Outcome**—*Caregiver Performance: Direct Care:* Provision by family care provider of appropriate personal and health care for a family member or significant other
GOAL: *The family copes with daily demands of the child's dialysis treatments.*		
■ Discuss the importance of daily, consistent dialysis treatments for the child's overall health status.	■ If parents understand the need for consistent dialysis treatments, they are more likely to adhere to guidelines.	The family adheres to daily dialysis treatment guidelines.
■ Collaborate with the family to identify strategies that could reduce the impact of dialysis on the family's life.	■ When the family participates in planning care, compliance is more likely.	
■ Refer the family to local support groups for emotional support, treatment strategies, and respite care.	■ Support groups may help the family develop effective coping strategies.	

Nursing Care Plan | The Child Receiving Home Peritoneal Dialysis, *continued*

INTERVENTION	RATIONALE	EXPECTED OUTCOME
4. Nursing Diagnosis: Body Image, Disturbed related to small size and perception of being and looking different		
NIC Priority Intervention—*Body Image Enhancement:* Improving a patient's conscious and unconscious perceptions and attitudes toward his/her body		**NOC Suggested Outcome**—*Psychosocial Adjustment: Life Change:* Psychosocial adaptation of an individual to a life change
GOAL: *The child will develop a sense of self-worth and self-esteem.*		
■ Identify and emphasize strengths the child has (e.g., interaction style, skills, or cognitive abilities) despite being smaller than peers.	■ Perception of personal strengths should increase self-esteem.	The child effectively interacts with peers and participates in age-appropriate activities.
■ Assist the child and family to identify popular clothing styles that hide the protuberant abdomen, dialysate bag, and catheter.	■ Clothing that conforms to current styles will help the child feel less different from peers.	
■ Increase the child's participation in self-care as appropriate for developmental age.	■ Ability to perform self-care increases the child's sense of control.	
■ Promote participation in safe activities with peers.	■ Social interaction with peers helps reinforce similarities with others.	
■ Encourage the child to participate in support groups with other children receiving dialysis when possible.	■ Interactions with other affected children provide a chance to express feelings and frustrations, and to develop successful coping strategies.	

NANDA-I © 2012

provide peritoneal dialysis safely. Hemodialysis for children is offered in a special dialysis center on an outpatient basis, or it can be performed at bedside during hospitalization. Treatment is usually performed three times a week, with each session lasting approximately 3 to 4 hours.

Children over 20 kg (44 lb) often have an arteriovenous (AV) fistula (connection between an artery and a vein) created for long-term vascular access. Alternatively, a synthetic tube can be implanted under the skin creating a graft between the arterial and venous circulation to provide vascular access. Two needles are inserted into the arteriovenous fistula or the graft—one to carry blood to the dialyzer and one to return cleaned blood to the body. In emergencies and for infants, a double-lumen cannula is inserted into a large vein (e.g., the femoral, jugular, or subclavian vein) for hemodialysis. With current technology, very-low-birth-weight infants can be safely hemodialyzed using a venous catheter for access.

Hemodialysis is more efficient than peritoneal dialysis but requires close monitoring for symptoms related to hypotension or rapid changes in fluid and electrolyte balance. Uncommonly, a **disequilibrium syndrome** (rapid changes in the body's water and electrolyte balance during treatment) may occur during or soon after the dialysis procedure is first initiated. Other complications include access thrombosis and infection. Heparin is used to reduce the risk of thrombosis.

Nursing Management

Nursing management focuses on care of the child during dialysis and teaching the child and family about the administration of heparin and the control of bleeding from minor trauma. Carefully monitor fluid balance in the child undergoing hemodialysis. Check vital signs and blood pressure every half hour. Monitor oral intake and urinary output every half hour when the child is on the dialysis equipment.

Weigh the child before and after the dialysis to determine any fluid imbalances that require adjustment during the next hemodialysis session.

Practice Alert
Monitor the child receiving hemodialysis for complications that can occur suddenly:
- **Hypotension**—sudden nausea and vomiting, abdominal cramping, tachycardia, and dizziness
- **Rapid fluid and electrolyte exchange**—muscle cramping, nausea and vomiting, and dizziness
- **Disequilibrium syndrome**—restlessness, headache, nausea and vomiting, blurred vision, muscle twitching, and altered level of consciousness

Because fluid and dietary limitations (reduced potassium-, sodium-, and phosphorus-containing foods) are needed more often with hemodialysis than with peritoneal dialysis, partner with the family to ensure understanding of how to plan and provide for the child's daily nutritional needs. Review ways to reduce the risk of infection, including daily care of the catheter site. Encourage showering rather than tub baths. Activities such as swimming should be discouraged.

Continuous Renal Replacement Therapy

Continuous renal replacement therapy (CRRT) is a form of continuous hemodialysis treatment, used for children who are hemodynamically unstable in an intensive care setting. CRRT may be indicated in children with inborn errors of metabolism, multisystem organ failure, renal insufficiency, fluid overload, sepsis, electrolyte imbalance, and acid–base imbalance. CRRT allows for gradual therapy without further compromising hemodynamic stability (Eding, Jelsma, Metz, et al., 2011). Disadvantages of CRRT include the need for continual monitoring of hemodynamic and fluid status, continuous anticoagulation, and regular infusion of dialysate (Sarkar, 2009). See Box 31–7.

BOX 31–7	**Research: Complications of Continuous Renal Replacement Therapy (CRRT)**

A prospective observation study of 174 critically ill children treated with CRRT analyzed the incidence of complications of this procedure (Santiago, López-Herce, Urbano, et al., 2009). The study found that the main complications of CRRT in children were hypotension at the time of connection to CRRT (30.4%), clinically significant hemorrhage (10.3%), and problems with venous catheterization (7.4%). Hypotension and hemorrhage were not related to any specific variables; however, problems with venous catheterization were more common in children less than 12 months of age and those weighing less than 10 kilograms. The study also found that electrolyte disturbances occur in children undergoing CRRT and that a decrease in sodium, chloride, and phosphate levels was common. It is very important that children undergoing CRRT are monitored continously for these potential complications.

Nursing Management

Nursing management focuses on monitoring the child's hemodynamic status, cardiac rhythm, mental status, breath sounds, and skin turgor. Admittance to the intensive care unit is required for constant observation, which may include central venous pressure and pulmonary artery pressure monitoring. Intake and output should be monitored hourly. Pharmacologic interventions may include sodium bicarbonate or other electrolytes and vasoactive agents. The nurse should constantly monitor for signs of hemorrhage. The patient needs monitoring for heat loss, which occurs during filtration of the blood (Shingarev, Wille, & Tolwani, 2011).

Kidney Transplantation

Kidney transplantation provides the only alternative to long-term dialysis for children with ESRD and generally yields good outcomes. Good outcomes of kidney transplantation in children are related to improvement in pre- and posttransplant care; surgical techniques; effective immunosuppression; and prevention, diagnosis, and treatment of infection (Shapiro & Sarwal, 2010) (Figure 31–12 ■). The transplanted kidney can normalize physiology and provide a potential for normal growth. Because of the adverse effects on growth and

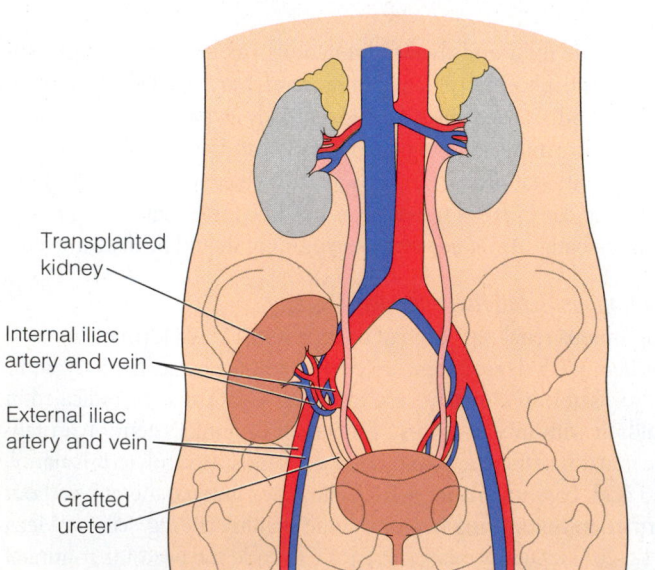

Transplanted kidney

Internal iliac artery and vein

External iliac artery and vein

Grafted ureter

FIGURE 31–12 ■ The transplanted kidney is placed in the iliac fossa with anastomosis to the hypogastric artery, iliac vein, and bladder.

Developing Cultural Competence
Race and the Waiting List

Access to a kidney transplant differs depending on the patient's race. Whites more commonly offer living donor transplants than Blacks, accounting for a higher rate of transplants (Patzer, Amaral, Klein, et al., 2012). Patzer et al. (2012) found that Black children with end-stage renal disease (ESRD) were 12% less likely to be put on a waiting list for a transplant compared to White children with ESRD. Once on a waiting list, the average time that all children wait for a kidney is 12 months. White and Black children wait about the same amount of time, with children of other races waiting the longest (Minnick, Boynton, Ndirangu, et al., 2010).

development resulting from the delay of transplantation, children are often given priority over adults awaiting transplantation.

Blood type compatibility between the kidney donor and the recipient is necessary for a successful transplantation. A human leukocyte antigen (HLA) system match also improves survival of the graft. A living relative donor kidney has a higher survival rate than a cadaver kidney (Shapiro & Sarwal, 2010). Children and their families are screened carefully prior to transplant in an effort to identify problems that could lead to rejection of the kidney or infection that could be life threatening if the immune system is suppressed. See Developing Cultural Competence: Race and the Waiting List.

After transplantation, the child must take immunosuppressive medications such as corticosteroids, azathioprine, cyclosporine, tacrolimus, and monoclonal antibodies to suppress rejection. Immunosuppression regimens use various combinations and sequences of these drugs to reduce the incidence of acute and chronic rejection.

Practice Alert

A large adult kidney is frequently transplanted into the child as parents constitute 80% of living donors (Shapiro & Sarwal, 2010). This results in a large renal reserve as compared to body mass. Clinical signs of rejection may be masked (Sarwal & Wong, 2011; Vogler, Wang, Brink, et al., 2007). Signs of rejection include fever, increased BUN and serum creatinine levels, pain and tenderness over the abdomen, irritability, and weight gain.

Complications of immunosuppressive therapy include opportunistic infection, lymphomas and skin cancer, and hypertension. Adherence with therapy is essential for survival of the graft and for optimal medical outcomes after transplant. Nonadherence to the medication regimen in pediatric transplant patients ranges; it may be as high as 70% (Guilfoyle, Goebel, & Pai, 2011; Ingerski, Perrazo, Goebel, et al., 2011). Nonadherence is related to several factors including forgetting to take medication and refusal to take medication due to expected side effects. Family dynamics, functioning, and flexibility also affect adherence (Guilfoyle et al., 2011). Adherence is higher in adolescents when their parents are knowledgeable and supportive, and when they promote the adolescent to become competent in self-care. Some primary kidney diseases, such as glomerulonephritis and hemolytic uremic syndrome, can also recur in the transplanted kidney.

Nursing Management

Nursing management includes partnering with the child and family to ensure understanding of the transplantation process before it occurs to help prepare them for the experience. The child and family experience rigorous protocols related to the complex medical history and the treatments related to the transplant. Discuss all aspects of the child's care that will have an impact on the family's life, including follow-up appointments, medications, and general health promotion. Emphasize that adherence with the treatment regimen including medications is essential for the success of the transplant. Evaluate the child's and parents' understanding of and adherence to the prescribed regimen. Education is ongoing and requires frequent evaluation of child and parental understanding. Monitor adherence to immunosuppressive treatment at each visit in an effort to identify any issues early. Families and children need to understand that nonadherence places them at risk for rejection of the kidney and return to dialysis. Ensure that the parents, and child if older, have the ability to recognize the signs of acute rejection and infection, and understand when and how to notify the child's physician if immediate care is required. The burden of lifelong treatment, which includes changes in family lifestyle, financial obligations, frequent hospitalizations, and dependency on technology, may lead to stress for the child and family.

Hemolytic Uremic Syndrome

Hemolytic uremic syndrome (HUS) is the most common cause of acute renal failure in young children, occurring primarily in those under 4 years of age (Huether, 2010b). HUS has a classic triad of signs: (1) hemolytic anemia, (2) thrombocytopenia, and (3) acute renal failure (Hedden, 2008; Weil, Andreoli, & Billmire, 2010).

Etiology and Pathophysiology

HUS is most often caused by *Escherichia coli* strain 0157:H7, which is found in undercooked meat and unpasteurized milk and juices (Hedden, 2008; Tan & Silverberg, 2009). The bacteria has also been linked to petting zoos at fairs and festivals. Approximately 16% of patients with this infection will develop HUS (Hedden, 2008).

E. coli strain 0157:H7 produces a toxin that attaches to the glomeruli, collecting ducts, and distal tubules. The toxin damages the lining of the glomerular arterioles, causing the endothelial cells to swell and become occluded with platelets and fibrin clots. This partial occlusion damages the red blood cells, resulting in hemolytic anemia. Platelets cluster in areas of vascular endothelial damage, causing thrombocytopenia. Glomerular filtration is decreased resulting in hematuria and proteinuria. Oliguria and acute renal failure develop in nearly 50% of children affected with HUS (Huether, 2010b).

Clinical Manifestations

An episode of gastroenteritis with diarrhea, upper respiratory infection, or urinary tract infection precedes the development of HUS by 1 to 2 weeks followed by 1 to 5 days without symptoms. Signs and symptoms of HUS include hypertension, pallor, bruising, and oliguria. The child may also be irritable and have fever, anorexia, abdominal pain, vomiting, diarrhea, mild jaundice, and edema or ascites (Huether, 2010b). Up to 20% of children with HUS will develop central nervous system involvement which includes irritability, agitation, confusion, lethargy, and seizures (Huether, 2010b; Listernick, 2009).

Collaborative Care

Care for the child with hemolytic uremic syndrome focuses on preservation of kidney function and prevention of complications associated with edema, thrombocytopenia, and gastrointestinal disturbances.

Diagnostic Tests

The urine is tested for hematuria and proteinuria. Serum chemistries often reveal hyperkalemia and metabolic acidosis as a result of renal failure. A peripheral blood smear with fragments of red blood cells, fibrin fragments, and a decreased platelet count confirms the diagnosis. The hemoglobin is usually less than 8 g/dL, and the platelet count is less than 60,000 per mL (Tan & Silverberg, 2009).

Clinical Therapy

Treatment focuses on the complication of acute renal failure (see page 1072) and includes fluid restrictions and a high-calorie, high-carbohydrate diet that is low in protein, sodium, potassium, and phosphorus. Enteral nutrition is sometimes needed. The use of antibiotics is controversial. Medications may include calcium gluconate or calcium chloride to replace calcium levels, aluminum hydroxide gel to bind to phosphorus, Kayexalate to remove excess potassium, and antihypertensive agents. Transfusions of fresh-packed red blood cells may be ordered to treat severe anemia. Platelets are given if the child is bleeding or if surgery is needed.

Transfusions are carefully administered to prevent hypertension caused by hypervolemia. About two thirds of children with HUS need dialysis (Weil et al., 2010). Peritoneal dialysis is preferred unless the child has severe colitis and abdominal tenderness. Some children may develop chronic renal failure; however, most regain normal renal function (Huether, 2010b).

Nursing Management

The focus of nursing for the child with HUS is to promote renal function, maintain fluid and electrolyte balance, promote adequate nutrition, prevent complications such as bleeding, and provide support to the child and family.

Nursing Assessment and Diagnosis

Monitor vital signs, neurologic signs, and laboratory values including electrolytes and blood counts. Monitor daily weights and calculate intake and output to assess fluid status. Observe the child carefully for evidence of progressive kidney impairment such as oliguria, elevated serum potassium, and creatinine. Monitor for signs of bleeding related to thrombocytopenia, including petechiae and ecchymoses. Assess the coping strategies of the child and family and their availability of support. Monitor the child for abdominal discomfort from diarrhea or other gastrointestinal disturbances.

Nursing diagnoses for the child with HUS may include:

- Fluid Volume: Excess related to impaired kidney perfusion and function
- Skin Integrity, Risk for Impaired related to edema
- Coping: Family, Compromised related to child's sudden severe illness

NANDA-I © 2012

Planning and Implementation

Care for the child with HUS is the same as care for the child with acute renal failure (see page 1072). The child may be cared for in an intensive care or intermediate care unit while on dialysis, depending on the hospital setting and the patient's condition. Carefully monitor neurologic signs, laboratory values, and fluid and electrolyte balance during treatment. Avoid invasive procedures when possible to prevent unnecessary bleeding.

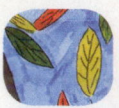

Partnering with Families

Food Preparation

One of the main causes of hemolytic uremic syndrome is the ingestion of undercooked ground beef. The Food Safety and Inspection Service (FSIS) of the U.S. Department of Agriculture (USDA) recommends that ground beef be cooked to an internal temperature of 160°F (USDA, 2011). Teach the family to wash hands carefully when handling raw ground meats and to make sure utensils touching raw meat do not come into contact with cooked meats. Encourage the use of a meat thermometer since the absence of pink in the center of the meat does not ensure that the appropriate temperature has been achieved.

Enteral nutrition may be necessary during the acute illness phase. When able to tolerate oral feeding, promote adequate nutritional intake by offering small feedings that are high calorie, high carbohydrate, and low in sodium, potassium, and phosphorus. Monitor bowel sounds and for vomiting and diarrhea.

Partner with the family and encourage parents to participate in the child's care. Explain the disease process and point out that most children recover completely but some children develop chronic renal failure. Encourage parents to monitor siblings for signs of diarrhea or hemolytic uremic syndrome.

Discharge planning focuses on teaching parents about medications and dietary and fluid restrictions as well as reducing risk of consumption of contaminated beef. See Partnering with Families: Food Preparation.

Clinical Tip

Some cases of hemolytic uremic syndrome have been linked to petting zoos such as those at county and state fairs. Hand hygiene stations should be available for participants. Emphasize to parents the importance of hand hygiene after their child touches the animals.

Evaluation

Expected outcomes of nursing care include:

- The child maintains fluid and electrolyte balance.
- The child has adequate kidney function.
- The parents demonstrate coping and involvement in the child's care.

Polycystic Kidney Disease

Polycystic kidney disease (PKD) is a genetic disorder that has autosomal recessive and dominant forms. Liver abnormalities are associated with both forms of the disease. The incidence of the autosomal recessive form is 1 per 20,000 live births (Salant & Gordon, 2012). The autosomal dominant form is one of the most frequently inherited diseases and is the most common inherited renal disorder in the United States, with a prevalence of 1 in 800 live births (Rizk & Chapman, 2008; Watnick & Dirkx, 2012).

Etiology and Pathophysiology

The autosomal dominant PKD results from mutations on the PKD1 locus on chromosome 16 and PKD2 on chromosome 4. The autosomal recessive gene (PKHD1) is located on chromosome 6 (National Kidney and Urologic Diseases Information Clearinghouse, 2009). In PKD, cellular hyperplasia of the collecting ducts causes dilation of the ducts. Fluid secreted into these ducts enables cyst sacs to form. Initially, cysts are usually less than 2 mm in size and do not obstruct urinary flow. As the child grows, however, the cysts become larger and fibrosis occurs. The cysts slowly replace much of the kidney's mass and reduce kidney function. Tubular atrophy may occur in some children, whereas others have minimal changes in renal function. Polycystic kidney disease is associated with liver abnormalities that progress in severity with age to fibrosis, portal hypertension, and biliary infection.

Newborns with autosomal recessive PKD may have enlarged kidneys, detected at birth. Up to 50% of neonates with this disorder die from pulmonary hypoplasia. This complication is a result of deficient amniotic fluid (*oligohydramnios*) in utero secondary to severe intrauterine kidney disease (Salant & Gordon, 2012).

Clinical Manifestations

Clinical manifestations in infants with autosomal recessive PKD include low-set ears, a small jaw, and a flattened nose. Hypertension develops in early infancy and is often severe. Infants may have expected urine output or oliguria. Respiratory distress and feeding intolerance may develop from the enlarged kidneys (Porter & Avner, 2011). As **uremia** (an excess of urea and other nitrogenous waste products in the blood) develops, infants and children experience **renal osteodystrophy** (a complex bone disease process of chronic kidney disease in which there is increased resorption of bone caused by chronic hyperparathyroidism) and progressive developmental delay and growth failure. While symptoms related to autosomal dominant PKD generally present around 40 to 50 years of age, symptoms including hematuria, hypertension, flank pain, and abdominal masses can be present in infants and children (Porter & Avner, 2011).

Collaborative Care

The goal of management for the child with polycystic kidney disease is to detect the presence of the disorder, maintain fluid and electrolyte balance, prevent associated complications such as hypertension and anemia, and promote growth and development.

Diagnostic Tests

Sonogram or renal biopsy confirms the diagnosis. The disease is often diagnosed on prenatal ultrasound. Liver function tests are usually normal initially. A liver biopsy may also be performed as the condition progresses. If identified, other family members should be screened for subclinical cases of PKD.

Clinical Therapy

Treatment is supportive. Medications such as diuretics are prescribed for hypertension. Fluid and electrolyte abnormalities are managed.

Antibiotics treat urinary tract infection. Growth hormones may be administered to some children to promote growth. Renal osteodystrophy is treated to suppress the parathyroid hormone. Many children with PKD develop end-stage renal disease by 10 years of age. Dialysis or a kidney transplant will prolong survival; however, liver problems may continue to complicate the child's health, even when the kidney condition is well controlled. Up to 20% to 30% of these children die by 15 years of age (Porter & Avner, 2011).

Nursing Management

Nursing care is the same as that for the child with renal insufficiency and chronic renal failure. See discussion on page 1075. Observe the child for signs of progressive renal impairment. Make sure the family schedules and keeps follow-up appointments to assess growth, developmental progress, and the effectiveness of the treatment plan. Partner with the family to establish a home care management plan focusing on medications, diet adequate in protein and calories to support growth, management of acute gastrointestinal illnesses, and care for the child with progressive renal insufficiency and a liver disorder. Since the disease is inherited, the family should be referred for genetic counseling. See Chapter 4 .

STRUCTURAL DEFECTS OF THE REPRODUCTIVE SYSTEM

Structural defects of the reproductive system may interfere with urinary flow or reproductive function. Defects discussed in this section are phimosis, cryptorchidism, inguinal hernia, hydrocele, and testicular torsion.

Phimosis

In **phimosis,** the foreskin over the glans penis cannot be retracted. As a result of natural adhesion, phimosis is a normal finding in uncircumcised infants and young males. Generally the foreskin separates from the glans during childhood, and intermittent erections lead to physiologic foreskin retraction. Obstruction to urine flow may occur when there is narrowing of the preputial opening causing a dribbling stream. **Balanitis** (inflammation or infection of the glans penis) may occur as a result of the obstruction of urine flow.

Paraphimosis, the most serious complication of phimosis, occurs when the foreskin cannot be returned to its normal position over the glans. Blood flow to the penis becomes obstructed with swelling of the glans. Ischemic injury to the glans penis occurs if the constriction is not relieved. Paraphimosis is a medical emergency and requires immediate intervention to preserve the glans penis.

Collaborative Care

Circumcision, surgical removal of the foreskin, has long been a common practice performed in some countries and cultures during the newborn period. It is performed to prevent phimosis, for ease of proper male hygiene, and to prevent urinary tract infections and penile cancer. See Developing Cultural Competence: Circumcision. See Chapter 9 for additional information related to circumcision of the newborn.

The procedure removes the skin covering the end of the penis. Circumcision is considered comparatively safe; however, complications such as damage to the urethra and disfigurement to the penis may occur.

Developing Cultural Competence
Circumcision

Circumcision in male infants is the most common surgical procedure in the United States. Rates of neonatal circumcision in the United States are currently at 56% (Brown-Trask, Sell, Carter, et al., 2009). The Jewish and Islamic faiths practice circumcision for religious reasons (Perera, Bridgewater, Thavaneswaran, et al., 2010). Circumcision is an uncommon practice in other countries except for religious reasons (Wang, Macklin, Tracy, et al., 2010).

Analgesia/anesthesia is provided for neonatal circumcision to prevent pain and physiologic stress on the neonate. EMLA, dorsal penile nerve block, and subcutaneous ring block are methods commonly used (Brown-Trask et al., 2009). Refer to Chapter 21 for further discussion on pain management.

Practice Alert
Circumcision is contraindicated in neonates with hemophilia and those with family history of bleeding disorder. Anomalies such as hypospadias, epispadias, and chordee are also contraindications since the foreskin may be needed for later reconstruction (Brown-Trask et al., 2009).

Nonsurgical treatment of phimosis involves the application of betamethasone cream (0.05%) twice daily for one month or three times a day for 3 weeks to the outer prepuce. It is an effective alternative to surgery for phimosis and has few side effects. Often the child is able to achieve foreskin retraction without surgery (Palmer & Palmer, 2008). Once again, paraphimosis is a medical emergency that must be relieved by surgery.

Nursing Management

Nursing initially focuses on teaching parents how to clean the foreskin and penis of the uncircumcised newborn male. Educate the parents to avoid forcibly retracting the foreskin to prevent complications such as scarring or paraphimosis. Frequent diaper changes help to prevent diaper rash and irritation. When the child is older and the foreskin separates from the penis and easily retracts, teach the parents and child to pull back the foreskin for cleaning and then to return it to its normal position.

If circumcision is requested by parents of the newborn or is the method of treatment for phimosis, nursing care focuses on preoperative preparation of the infant, including the advocacy for and assistance in giving the newborn local anesthesia. Postoperatively the nurse assesses the infant's vital signs and the operative site for bleeding and urination. Partner with the parents to ensure they understand proper care for the surgical site, as infants are discharged within 24 hours of surgery. See Partnering with Families: Care Following Circumcision. If a Plastibell device was used in newborn circumcision, parents should receive specific instructions related to care (Davidson, London, & Ladewig, 2008).

If topical steroids (betamethasone) are prescribed as treatment for phimosis, the nurse partners with the family to ensure the proper application of the medication, including the importance of adherence to the prescribed therapy. Additional instructions include methods of proper hygiene and the signs and symptoms of constriction and infection.

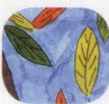

Partnering with Families

Care Following Circumcision

Instruct the family to wash hands well before and after each diaper change and to follow these instructions for care following circumcision:

- Cover the head of the penis with a small amount of petroleum jelly with each diaper change until the redness goes away.
- Pale yellow, sticky drainage may form on the head of the penis and is a normal part of the healing process.
- Squeeze soapy water over the head of the penis once a day, rinse with warm water, and pat dry.

- The diaper should fit appropriately—not too loose as that may cause rubbing with movement and not too tight as that may cause pain.
- Contact the healthcare provider if there is increased redness, bleeding, or swelling of the head of the penis.

Source: *Adapted from Brown-Trask, B., Sell, S. V., Carter, S., & Kindred, C. (2009, February). Circumcision care. RN, 22–28; Davidson, M. R., London, M. L., & Ladewig, P. A. (2008). Old's maternal-newborn nursing and women's health across the lifespan (8th ed.). Upper Saddle River, NJ: Pearson/Prentice Hall.*

Cryptorchidism

Cryptorchidism (undescended testes) occurs when one or both testes fail to descend through the inguinal canal into the scrotum. Normally, the testes descend during the seventh to ninth month of gestation.

Etiology and Pathophysiology

Cryptorchidism may be the result of a testosterone deficiency, an absent or defective testis, or a structural problem such as a narrow inguinal canal, short spermatic cord, or adhesions. This disorder occurs in 3% to 6% of term male infants and in 20% to 30% of preterm infants (Latendresse, McCance, & Morgan, 2010).

The higher temperature in the abdomen than in the scrotum results in morphologic changes to the testis, which begin to occur between 6 and 12 months of age. Complications of cryptorchidism include infertility and malignancy (Cakan & Kamat, 2009). The risk for infertility is much higher when cryptorchidism is bilateral (Chung & Brock, 2011).

Clinical Manifestations

Cryptorchidism is usually detected during the newborn examination when palpation of the scrotum fails to reveal one or both testes. It is not unusual for boys with cryptorchidism to have an inguinal hernia as well. In a majority of cases, the testes descend spontaneously by 3 months of age. An undescended testis may be located in the inguinal canal, abdomen, perineum, or even the thigh.

Collaborative Care

Care for the child with cryptorchidism focuses on identifying the defect, preserving testicular function, maintaining fertility, and maintaining a normal appearance of the scrotum.

Diagnostic Tests

Although diagnosis is made on physical examination, diagnostic studies including ultrasound, CT scan, and MRI are utilized to determine the location of the testes. A diagnostic laparoscope may also be needed to locate the testis. When neither testis can be palpated, hormonal and chromosomal evaluation may be performed to detect an intersex disorder.

Clinical Therapy

If the testes do not descend spontaneously, an orchiopexy is performed around 12 months of age before further testicular damage occurs

(Cakan & Kamat, 2009). The timing for surgery is crucial to preserve fertility and to avoid psychologic effects related to fear of castration and body image issues in older children. With an orchiopexy, an incision is made at the location of the testis, either in the abdomen or in the inguinal area. Blood vessels are disentangled to allow the testis to reach into the lower scrotum. A second incision is made in the scrotum at the point where the testis is stitched to the inside wall to keep it in place. A protective sealant is often put over the incision that peels off in 3 to 5 days. If the testis is defective or undeveloped, it may be removed surgically to decrease the risk of later malignancies, and a prosthesis may be placed in the scrotum. The goals of surgery are to position the testis for future accessibility to palpation, repair any hernia, enhance the possibility of fertility, decrease the potential susceptibility for malignancy, and provide the psychologic benefit of a normal-appearing scrotum. The orchiopexy also makes it easier to examine the testis for tumors. The risk of testicular cancer is 35 to 50 times greater in men with a history of cryptorchidism (Latendresse et al., 2010).

Nursing Management

Nursing care includes assessing the infant for undescended testes; implementing measures to reduce postoperative complications; educating parents on treatment, outcomes, and home care needs; promoting a positive body image in the older child; and teaching testicular self-examination to the adolescent.

Nursing Assessment and Diagnosis

Assess newborns and infants for undescended testes as described in Chapter 7 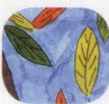. Inspect and then palpate the scrotum. One side or both sides of the scrotum may appear underdeveloped and may feel empty upon palpation. Inspect and palpate the area over the inguinal canal to determine if the testis is in the canal.

Nursing diagnoses that may be appropriate for the child with cryptorchidism include the following:

- Injury, Risk for (Reproductive Function) related to undescended testes
- Infection, Risk for related to surgical procedure
- Knowledge, Deficient (Child) related to understanding of testicular examinations
- Body Image Disturbed (Older Child) related to appearance of scrotum

NANDA-I © 2012

Planning and Implementation

Preoperative nursing care includes preparing the parents and child for the surgical procedure and addressing parents' concerns about the postsurgical outcome. Orchiopexy is often performed as an outpatient procedure. If the child is hospitalized, postoperative nursing care focuses on maintaining comfort and preventing infection. Encourage bed rest and monitor voiding. Apply ice to the surgical area if ordered and administer prescribed analgesics to relieve pain.

Discharge instructions should include demonstration of proper incision care. The diaper area should be cleaned well with each diaper change to decrease chances of infection. Sponge bathe the child for 2 days after surgery, and then a tub bath may be given. No medicine or ointment should be placed over the incision. Teach parents to identify signs of infection such as redness, warmth, swelling, and discharge and to notify the physician if present. Ibuprofen or acetaminophen may be given for pain. Instruct parents to avoid straddling the infant across the hip and to permit no strenuous activity or straddle toy riding for 2 weeks after surgery to promote healing and to prevent injury.

Care in the Community

Because the risk of testicular malignancy is greatly increased with cryptorchidism, long-term planning includes teaching the child to perform monthly testicular examinations after puberty to assist in the early detection of tumors. (See Chapter 13 🔗.) A discussion with the adolescent patient regarding fertility and the possible need for future fertility testing is important since cryptorchidism increases the risk of infertility.

Evaluation

Expected outcomes of nursing care include the following:

- The wound heals without signs of infection.
- Pain is effectively managed.
- Parents verbalize an understanding of postoperative care.
- Understanding of the need for regular testicular self-examinations upon the onset of puberty is verbalized.

Inguinal Hernia and Hydrocele

An **inguinal hernia** is a painless inguinal or scrotal swelling of variable size that occurs when abdominal tissue, such as bowel, extends into the inguinal canal. An inguinal hernia is found in 3.5% to 5% of full-term infants and 9% to 11% of preterm infants and occurs more often in boys than girls by a 6:1 ratio (Aiken & Oldham, 2011).

A hydrocele is a fluid-filled mass in the scrotum. The condition is found in 1% to 2% of male neonates. Most hydroceles resolve spontaneously by reabsorption by 1 year of age (Elder, 2011).

Etiology and Pathophysiology

During fetal development, a peritoneal sac precedes the testicle's descent to the scrotum. The lower sac enfolds the testis to become the tunica vaginalis, and the upper sac atrophies before birth. Fluid may become trapped in the tunica vaginalis and cause the hydrocele. When the tunica vaginalis does not atrophy, an abdominal structure may move into it. Inguinal hernias are often associated with abdominal wall defects such as bladder exstrophy and prune-belly syndrome, and are a common occurrence with undescended testes.

Clinical Manifestations

Diagnosis is made by physical examination at birth or in early infancy. Palpation of the scrotum reveals a round, smooth, nontender mass which is noted with either a hernia or hydrocele. Parents may report an intermittent bulge in the groin or swelling in the scrotum. Swelling associated with a hernia may become more apparent with straining and reduced in size when quiet or asleep.

Collaborative Care

Care for the child with inguinal hernia and hydrocele focuses on identifying and correcting the defect, preventing complications, and promoting growth and development.

Diagnostic Tests

When the hernia appears intermittently, having the older child cough, cry, strain, or engage in vigorous movement increases the intra-abdominal pressure and potentially enhances the ability to palpate a hernia. Transillumination may help determine whether the mass is a hernia or hydrocele. See Chapter 7 🔗.

Clinical Therapy

Outpatient surgery for repair of inguinal hernia is performed as an elective procedure at an early age (usually after 3 months of age to reduce anesthesia risks) to avoid **incarceration** (hernia cannot be reduced and circulation to trapped tissue is impaired), which is a medical emergency. A nerve block may be given in the operating room to reduce postoperative pain. The prognosis is generally excellent. Most hydroceles without inguinal hernia resolve spontaneously as the fluid reabsorbs by the time an infant is 1 to 2 years of age.

Practice Alert

Inguinal hernias can become incarcerated when a bit of bowel becomes trapped in the inguinal opening and the blood supply is constricted. The child has an acute onset of colicky pain, abdominal distention, and vomiting. Other findings may include an edematous, erythematosus scrotum accompanied by fever, and bloody stools (Aiken & Oldham, 2011). The surgeon attempts to reduce the hernia before surgery by sedating the child and applying firm manual pressure on the affected side. If the hernia is reduced, surgery is often performed several days later. If the hernia cannot be reduced, emergency surgery is performed (Hartmann, 2008).

Nursing Management

Nursing care for hydrocele and inguinal hernia includes assessment, explaining the disorder and its treatment, and providing preoperative and postoperative teaching, care, and support.

Nursing Assessment and Diagnosis

Preoperative nursing assessment for the child with an inguinal hernia or hydrocele includes routine newborn assessment and monitoring for signs and symptoms of incarceration.

Postoperative care includes monitoring of vital signs and inspection of the incision for swelling, bleeding, or drainage. Assess the circulation in the leg on the side of the surgical repair to detect any potential blood flow obstruction resulting from edema of the groin. Assess for pain.

Nursing diagnoses for the child with an inguinal hernia or hydrocele may include the following:

- Pain, Acute related to surgical incision (and possibly incarceration)
- Infection, Risk for related to surgical incision in inguinal area

NANDA-I © 2012

Planning and Implementation

The incision is covered with a protective sealant rather than a dressing, and routine wound care is provided. Depending on the type of anesthesia utilized, pain medication requirements may be minimal, especially if a spinal or regional block was used; however, provide pain medication as prescribed. For incarcerated hernias, postoperative care may include management of nasogastric tubes and intravenous antibiotics.

Educate the parents to provide proper care of the incision and reduce the risk of infection to the surgical site, as well as to recognize signs and symptoms of infection. Encourage frequent diaper changes and careful cleaning of the diaper area to reduce the risk of infection. Inform parents that the scrotum may be edematous and may appear bruised after surgery. Encourage the parents to hold the infant normally.

Evaluation

Expected outcomes for nursing care include:

- The wound heals without signs of infection.
- Pain is managed effectively.

Testicular Torsion

Testicular torsion is an emergency condition in which the testis suddenly rotates on its spermatic cord, cutting off its blood supply. The arteries and veins in the spermatic cord become twisted and interrupt the blood supply, leading to vascular engorgement and ischemia. Testicular torsion occurs in an estimated 1 in 4,000 males before 25 years of age (Bradway & Rodgers, 2009; DuFour, 2008). Approximately two thirds of cases occur in boys between the ages of 12 and 18 (DuFour, 2008).

Etiology and Pathophysiology

Testicular torsion most often occurs as a result from trauma to the scrotum but can occur during sporting activities, exercise, and sexual activity. Often the testicles are positioned transversely in the scrotum, secondary to a congenital anomaly known as a bell clapper deformity. In this deformity, the tunica vaginalis has an inappropriately high attachment to the testes, allowing them to rotate freely and twist spontaneously on the spermatic cord. Approximately 12% of males have this deformity (Datta, Dhillon, & Voci, 2011; Rupp & Zwanger, 2010).

Clinical Manifestations

Manifestations include severe pain and erythema in the scrotum, nausea and vomiting, abdominal pain, and scrotal swelling that is not relieved by rest or scrotal support. The testes are tender to palpation and become edematous. The cremasteric reflex is absent. Symptoms generally start when the child is sleeping or inactive, but they can occur after trauma, sexual activity, or exercise.

Collaborative Care

Care for the child focuses on rapid diagnosis so that immediate interventions can be initiated to restore circulation to the testis and save the testicular function.

Diagnostic Tests

Color Doppler ultrasonography is frequently used to confirm the diagnosis. Urinalysis is useful in differentiating testicular torsion from epididymitis. Males with testicular torsion will generally have a normal urinalysis (Bradway & Rodgers, 2009; DuFour, 2008).

Clinical Therapy

Testicular torsion is a surgical emergency. Treatment must be implemented within 6 hours to prevent ischemia and necrosis (Bradway & Rodgers, 2009). During surgery (orchiopexy), the testis is untwisted and stitched to the side of the scrotum in the correct position. The procedure is usually performed bilaterally to prevent future torsion in the other testis. If the testicle does not regain blood flow or is already necrotic, it is removed via orchiectomy (Bradway & Rodgers, 2009; Leung & Kao, 2008).

Nursing Management

The goal of nursing management is to recognize the urgency of the child's condition and to provide the necessary care and advocacy to obtain the emergency intervention.

Nursing Assessment and Diagnosis

Assess the child's symptoms and recognize that pain and swelling in the scrotum is a true emergency. Because the highest incidence of testicular torsion occurs in the adolescent and during sporting activities and trauma, the school nurse should be alert to the possibility of testicular torsion.

Nursing diagnoses that may be appropriate for the child with this condition include:

- Pain, Acute related to swelling and constricted blood flow to the testis
- Anxiety related to urgent onset and fear of mutilation
- Tissue Perfusion, Ineffective (Testis) related to testicular rotation and twisting of blood vessels

NANDA-I © 2012

Planning and Implementation

Provide analgesics as ordered and prepare the child for surgery. The adolescent may be especially anxious about the location of surgery and potential for mutilation. Answer questions the child and family have regarding the surgical procedure and need for rapid intervention.

Nursing management involves psychologic support for the child and family related to the need for emergency surgery and concern about the child's future fertility. Reassure parents that as only one testis is usually affected, fertility should not be affected.

The child often goes home within a few hours following surgery; thus, the child and family require instructions regarding proper care of the incision and pain management. Partner with the family to ensure that the child does not lift heavy objects for 4 weeks or participate in strenuous activity for 2 weeks after surgery to promote healing. Educate the adolescent about the importance of testicular self-examination.

Evaluation

Expected outcomes for nursing care include:

- Pain is managed effectively.
- The incision heals without signs of infection.
- Fear and anxiety in the child are reduced after family support and explanations about care.

SEXUALLY TRANSMITTED INFECTIONS

Sexually transmitted infections (STIs) are a major national public health concern. The Centers for Disease Control and Prevention (CDC) reports that approximately 19 million new cases of STIs occur each year, with young people ages 15 to 24 years accounting for almost half the infections (CDC, 2009). HIV is discussed in Chapter 27 🔗, and hepatitis B, another infection that can be transmitted sexually, is discussed in Chapter 30 🔗.

Children and adolescents can become infected with sexually transmitted organisms through sexual experimentation, sexual play, molestation, sexual abuse, and sexual intercourse.

Practice Alert

When a child younger than 10 years is found to have gonorrhea or other sexually transmitted infection, consider the possibility of sexual abuse. When anorectal symptoms or disease or trauma are found, suspect molestation (see Chapter 20 🔗 for a discussion of child abuse).

Results from the 2009 Youth Risk Behavior Surveillance revealed that among high school students in the United States, 34.2% were currently sexually active and 38.9% of currently sexually active students had not used a condom at last sexual intercourse (CDC, 2010). Adolescents are considered an at-risk population related to their inexperience and lack of knowledge about STIs. Factors contributing to STI risk to the child and adolescent include the avoidance of protective barriers, multiple sexual partners, engaging in sex frequently, and failure to seek medical treatment until symptoms are well advanced.

Frequently diagnosed STIs are chlamydia, genital herpes (herpes simplex type 2), gonorrhea, genital warts (human papillomavirus), trichomoniasis, and syphilis. Human papillomavirus (HPV) is the most common STI in the United States (CDC, 2011), while chlamydia is the most frequently reported infectious disease in the United States (CDC, 2010). Refer to the Clinical Manifestations table for information related to clinical manifestations, complications, clinical therapy, and patient education regarding STIs.

State and local health departments are responsible for controlling the spread of STIs through health promotion programs, staff training, reporting systems, diagnosis, treatment, patient counseling, and the notification of sex partners. To reduce all sexually transmitted infections, the CDC recommends abstinence from sexual contact, or a long-term mutually monogamous relationship with a partner who has been tested for STIs and is known to be uninfected (CDC, 2010). A vaccine is recommended for adolescents to prevent human papillomavirus. See Chapter 22 🔗.

Nursing Management

The goal of nursing is to reduce the transmission of STIs to the child and adolescent. Nursing care focuses on education, prevention, and collaborative treatment of sexually transmitted infections through partnership with the child or adolescent and family.

Nursing Assessment and Diagnosis

Nursing assessment focuses on identifying signs and symptoms indicative of sexually transmitted infections, assessing for the potential of an asymptomatic STI, and assessing the psychosocial impact on the child or adolescent with an STI.

The nurse usually encounters the child or adolescent and family in the emergency department, outpatient clinic, or nursing unit.

Since adolescents are often afraid of the consequences of reporting symptoms, good assessment and communication skills are important considerations for the nurse, particularly when asking questions about sexual activity, partners, and the possibility of abuse. Essential to communication is maintaining a warm, encouraging, nonjudgmental approach and conveying acceptance when discussing sexual health issues with the child or adolescent. In order to achieve the adolescent's cooperation, confidentiality must be ensured. Offer support to the adolescent and encourage the seeking of parental guidance and involvement.

Clinical Tip

Key areas to discuss when obtaining a sexual history include information related to partners, pregnancy prevention, protection from sexually transmitted infections, sexual practices, and past history of STIs (CDC, 2010). Carefully inquire about the potential for date rape or sexual abuse.

During the physical examination, assess the child or adolescent for manifestations as described in the table on pages 1090–1091. When a child or adolescent is diagnosed with one STI, it is essential to screen for the presence of other STIs, as more than one disease may co-exist. Adolescents who are symptomatic may postpone care due to feeling uncomfortable about genital examination. Given that many adolescents have subclinical cases or are asymptomatic, routine screening of adolescents who are sexually active is recommended.

Nursing diagnoses that may apply to the child or adolescent with an STI include:

- Anxiety related to presence of sexually transmitted infection
- Pain, Acute related to genital irritation
- Knowledge, Deficient (Sexually Transmitted Infections) related to cause, transmission, treatments, and prevention
- Body Image, Disturbed related to genital lesions, presence of genital infection

NANDA-I © 2012

Planning and Implementation

The nurse focuses on identifying adolescents at risk for STIs, providing appropriate education, and preventing transmission and complications. Encourage adolescents to seek parental guidance and involvement. Abstinence from sexual contact is the best method to prevent an STI. However, methods to reduce the risk for STIs also include a long-term mutually monogamous relationship with a partner who has been tested for STIs and is known to be uninfected, and the proper use of condoms.

When the adolescent has a confirmed STI, provide information about the specific infection diagnosed, its treatment, potential adverse effects, and recommended follow-up. Encourage the adolescent to complete all prescribed medications if more than a single-dose treatment is used. Provide psychologic support as the adolescent may be upset, ashamed, embarrassed, or angry about having the infection.

When counseling the adolescent, reinforce the importance of treating all sexual partners involved. Partner notification is essential in order to provide treatment if the partner is infected, and to reduce the risk of reinfection. Encourage sexually active adolescents to receive hepatitis B and HPV immunization if not already obtained.

Refer the child with signs of an STI for evaluation of sexual assault by a facility or healthcare provider specializing in collecting evidence and providing specialized care. Similarly refer any adolescent who has been sexually assaulted to a sexual assault nurse examiner

Clinical Manifestations Common Sexually Transmitted Infections

SEXUALLY TRANSMITTED INFECTION	CLINICAL MANIFESTATIONS AND COMPLICATIONS	CLINICAL THERAPY AND PATIENT EDUCATION
Chlamydia *Chlamydia trachomatis*	■ Adolescent females: yellow mucopurulent endocervical discharge, dysuria, pelvic pain, mild abdominal pain, vaginal spotting, cervicitis, salpingitis, pelvic inflammatory disease (PID); asymptomatic infections are common. ■ Adolescent males: **urethritis** (an infection of the urethra), mucoid gray or clear discharge, dysuria, proctitis, epididymitis; may be asymptomatic. ■ Complications associated with chlamydia in females include PID and infertility. ■ Chlamydia is a leading cause of early pneumonia and conjunctivitis in newborns.	■ Diagnosis is by culture or a nucleic acid-amplified test on the urine. ■ Recommended medication therapy includes oral erythromycin twice a day for 7 days, or a single dose of oral azithromycin. ■ Persons who are HIV positive with chlamydia receive the same treatment as those who are HIV negative. ■ All sexual partners should be evaluated, tested, and treated. ■ Infected persons should abstain from sexual intercourse until they and their sex partners have completed treatment to prevent reinfection. ■ Encourage use of condoms. ■ All sexually active female adolescents should be screened at least annually for chlamydia.
Genital herpes *Herpes simplex virus 1* (HSV-1) or *2* (HSV-2)	■ Most individuals infected with HSV-2 are not aware of their infection. ■ Presentation can be variable and ranges from no symptoms to systemic involvement. ■ Common symptoms include dull pain, itching, and small lesions or pimples on genitalia, buttocks, or thighs. ■ Two types of lesions develop, either fluid-filled blisters on an erythematous base or more commonly, painful papules and ulcers. ■ Ulcers can appear between vaginal folds, in posterior cervix, on glans penis, on shaft of penis, in rectum, or in anus. ■ Ulcers heal within 2–4 weeks. ■ Lymph nodes closest to lesions are frequently enlarged. ■ Disease frequently recurs four to five times a year with episodes lasting 5–10 days. ■ Triggers include stress, menses, or trauma.	■ Diagnosis is confirmed by virology and type-specific serologic tests. ■ There is no permanent cure. ■ Recommended drug therapy is acyclovir given for 7–10 days. ■ Antiviral medications can shorten and prevent outbreaks during the period of time the person takes the medication. ■ Daily suppressive therapy for herpes can reduce transmission to partners. ■ A cesarean delivery is usually performed for pregnant women who are infected. ■ Discourage oral sex if ulcers are present in mouth, on lips, in vagina, or on penis. ■ Discourage anal sex when lesions are active. ■ Encourage use of condoms, although they may not prevent transmission. ■ Emphasize that the patient remains contagious, even after lesions are healed.
Gonorrhea *Neisseria gonorrhoeae*	■ Symptoms and severity vary from mild to severe and are different for males and females. ■ In females, areas that can be infected include urethra, cervix, fallopian tubes, and Bartholin and Skene glands. ■ In males, areas include urethra, prostate, seminal vesicles, epididymis, and Littre and Cowper glands. ■ Of females, up to 50% are asymptomatic. ■ The classic sign is discharge from the vagina and urethra; however, infections involving the conjunctiva, pharynx, and rectum are also seen. ■ Lower abdominal pain may be present. ■ Prepubescent girls: heavy, thick green or creamy vaginal discharge, vulvovaginitis. ■ Pubescent girls: purulent vaginal discharge, cervicitis, fallopian tube and PID involvement can lead to sterility. ■ Prepubescent and adolescent boys: yellow purulent urethral discharge, erythematous meatus, frequency, dysuria, and painful or swollen testicles. ■ Although many men with gonorrhea may have no symptoms at all, some men have signs or symptoms that appear 2–5 days after infection; symptoms can take as long as 30 days to appear. ■ Signs and symptoms of rectal infection in both genders include discharge, anal itching, soreness, bleeding, or painful bowel movements. However, they may be asymptomatic. ■ Infections in the throat may cause a sore throat but are usually asymptomatic. ■ Transmission to the neonate during vaginal delivery can cause blindness, joint infection, or sepsis. ■ Gonorrhea is a common cause of PID.	■ Diagnosed by culture of vaginal or urethral discharge or nucleic acid-amplified test on the urine. ■ Recommended drug therapy includes a single dose of ceftriaxone IM or cefixime orally in one dose. ■ Sexual partners should be treated if the adolescent has had sexual contact within 60 days of onset of symptoms. ■ Encourage use of condoms or abstinence. ■ Emphasize the importance of taking all of the medication prescribed to cure gonorrhea. ■ The individual and all sex partners must avoid sex until they have completed their treatment for gonorrhea.

Clinical Manifestations Common Sexually Transmitted Infections (*continued*)

SEXUALLY TRANSMITTED INFECTION	CLINICAL MANIFESTATIONS AND COMPLICATIONS	CLINICAL THERAPY AND PATIENT EDUCATION
Human papillomavirus (HPV)	▪ The most common STI in adolescents in the United States. ▪ Warts are small, flat, and fleshy-colored with a cauliflower appearance. ▪ Adolescent females: warts clustered or alone on the vulva, perineal area, vagina, or cervix; itching, bleeding, burning, irritation. ▪ A subclinical infection may be detected through a Pap smear. ▪ HPV can lead to cervical cancer. ▪ Adolescent males: may be asymptomatic; warts on the penis, near base of penis on scrotal skin, or near anus.	▪ Diagnosis is based upon physical findings or biopsy. The Pap smear may be abnormal. ▪ No cure exists. ▪ Treatment for external genital warts may include cryotherapy, topical podophyllin resin, imiquimod 5% cream, podofilox 0.5% solution or gel, or sinecatechins 15% ointment. ▪ Encourage abstinence or condom use, but condoms are not sufficient to prevent contact transmission. The disorder is transmissible even after treatment. ▪ Encourage adolescent males and females to receive the HPV vaccine (see Chapter 22 🔗).
Trichomoniasis *Trichomonas vaginalis*	▪ Adolescent females: pale yellow to gray-green discharge that may be frothy or have a fishy odor, dysuria, vulvar pruritus, occasional abdominal pain; symptoms worsen during menses, more commonly have symptoms than males. ▪ Adolescent males: most common site is the urethra; mucoid or purulent urethral discharge, pruritus, dysuria; however, males are usually asymptomatic.	▪ Diagnosis is by culture. ▪ Treatment includes metronidazole or tinidazole orally as a single dose or metronidazole orally twice a day for 7 days. ▪ Both partners should be treated at the same time to eliminate the parasite. ▪ Avoid drinking alcohol during and for several days after treatment if a single dose is used. ▪ Sexual contact should be avoided until both partners are cured. ▪ No follow-up test is needed if symptoms resolve after treatment.
Syphilis *Treponema pallidum*	▪ Appearance of classic signs and symptoms of syphilis depends on stage of disease. ▪ *Primary stage:* manifests as an ulcer on labia, within vagina, on penis, in anus, or on lips or tongue that appears at invasion site approximately 2 weeks to 3 months after infection. ▪ Ulcer has an indurated border and smooth base (chancre), and it is painless. ▪ Lymphadenopathy is usually present. ▪ Ulcer spontaneously heals within 5 weeks. ▪ *Secondary stage:* appears up to 10 weeks after initial infection with fever, malaise, lymphadenopathy, patchy alopecia, and diffuse rash. ▪ Rash can be macular, papular, papulosquamous, or bullous, and appearance on the palms and soles is classic. ▪ Flat mucous patches called condylomata latum appear on genitals. ▪ *Latent stage:* asymptomatic, follows the second stage by about 6 weeks. It can last for several years or be lifelong. ▪ *Tertiary stage:* occurs more than 2 years after onset and manifests as changes to the cardiovascular system, bone, skin, or viscera. ▪ *Neurosyphilis:* an infection of the central nervous system, can occur during any stage.	▪ Diagnosis is by serologic tests or direct fluorescent antibody tests of lesion exudates. ▪ Due to the risk of fetal death, every pregnant woman should have a blood test for syphilis. ▪ Syphilis is easy to cure in its early stages. ▪ Recommended drug therapy includes single IM injection of benzathine penicillin G. ▪ Saline compresses and a topical antibiotic are often used to treat lesions on the skin. ▪ Treat all sexual contacts within the past 90 days to 1 year of diagnosis, depending on stage when diagnosed. ▪ During syphilis treatment, abstain from sexual contact with new partners until the syphilis sores are completely healed. ▪ Encourage abstinence or the use of condoms plus spermicidal foams, cream, or jelly to prevent infection.

Source: *Data from American Academy of Pediatrics. (2009). Red book: Report of the Committee on Infectious Disease (28th ed.). Elk Grove Village, IL: Author; Centers for Disease Control and Prevention (CDC). (2011). Genital HPV infection—Fact sheet. Retrieved from http://www.cdc.gov/std/HPV/STDFact-HPV.htm; Centers for Disease Control and Prevention (CDC). (2010). Sexually transmitted diseases treatment guidelines, 2010. Morbidity and Mortality Weekly Report, 59(RR-12), 1–110; de Souza-Thomas, L. (2010). Gonorrhoea: Prevention, diagnosis and treatment. British Journal of School Nursing, 5(3), 116–121; Forhan, S. E., Gottlieb, S. L., Sternberg, M. R., Xu, F., Datta, S. D., McQuillan, G. M., . . . Markowitz, L. E. (2009). Prevalence of sexually transmitted infections among female adolescents aged 14 to 19 in the United States. Pediatrics, 124(6), 1505–1512.*

or other healthcare provider who can collect evidence, coordinate medical treatment, and coordinate mental health support.

Care in the Community

Education includes promoting abstinence, which means avoiding *any* type of sexual contact with a partner. (See Partnering with Families: Preventing STIs and Their Consequences.) The nurse, in partnership with schools and community organizations, should promote sexual health through schools, health clinics, community services, and groups or organizations.

Additional teaching includes dispelling myths of how STIs are spread. Instruct the child or adolescent that STIs are not contracted from sharing bath towels, clothing, and drinking glasses, or from sitting on toilet seats. Inform the adolescent female taking

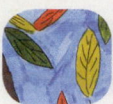

Partnering with Families

Preventing STIs and Their Consequences

It is important when talking with adolescents to give them information about the risks of STIs and strategies to protect themselves. One important strategy is to encourage the adolescent to talk with his or her partner about STI protection, even when the partner is perceived to be at no or little risk of having an STI. Important information to share includes the following:

- Abstinence is the best method to prevent STIs.
- Limit the number of sexual contacts; practice mutual monogamy.
- Always use condoms and spermicidal gels or foams for vaginal and anal intercourse.

- Refrain from oral sex if the partner has active sores in the mouth, vagina, or anus or on the penis.
- Reduce high-risk sexual behaviors. Use of recreational drugs and alcohol can increase sexual risk taking.
- Seek care as soon as symptoms are noticed, make sure the partner gets treatment, and avoid sexual intercourse until the STI is cured.
- Seek annual screening for STIs as some can be present without symptoms.

---

contraceptives (e.g., oral, IM, patch) that this form of birth control offers no protection against STIs. Additional protection is necessary to prevent transmission.

Partner with the adolescent who is sexually active to identify methods of reducing the risk of contracting STIs. Suggestions include the use of latex condoms (though the possibility of STI transmission still exists even with the use of latex condoms), voiding immediately after sexual intercourse, and appropriate genital hygiene with soap and water. Encourage adolescents to discuss the choice of sexual partners and assist them to avoid those partners who are at higher risk for STIs, such as intravenous drug users and those who have multiple sexual partners. Emphasize to the adolescent that even with applying these measures, there is no guaranteed protection with the exception of abstinence. Explain to the adolescent that some STIs, such as chlamydia, are asymptomatic, and it is not possible to tell if a partner is "clean."

Evaluation

Expected outcomes for the child or adolescent with a sexually transmitted infection include:

- The child or adolescent remains free from pain.
- The adolescent demonstrates an understanding of the transmission, prevention, and treatment of sexually transmitted infections.
- The adolescent has a positive body image.
- The child or adolescent displays reduced anxiety.

Pelvic Inflammatory Disease

Pelvic inflammatory disease (PID) is an infection of the upper genital tract caused by the ascending spread of organisms in the cervix and vagina.

Etiology and Pathophysiology

The majority of cases of PID are caused by *Chlamydia trachomatis* or *Neisseria gonorrhoeae*. Approximately 85% of cases of PID are caused by STIs. Other cases are caused by procedures that break the cervical mucus barrier (Abatangelo, Okereke, Parham-Foster, et al., 2010). The infection ascends into the uterus and fallopian tubes during the menses

when the cervix mucosal plug is open and retrograde menstrual blood can flow into the fallopian tubes. A significant complication is a tubo-ovarian abscess, an inflammatory mass that involves the fallopian tube, ovary, and in some cases surrounding structures (Abatangelo et al., 2010).

Clinical Manifestations

Signs and symptoms of PID may include mild or dull bilateral lower abdominal pain, dysmenorrhea that is worse or longer lasting than usual, dysuria, vaginal discharge, pain with sexual activity, prolonged or increased menstrual bleeding, nausea, vomiting, and fever. Most cases are mild.

Collaborative Care

The goal of collaborative care is to diagnose and provide treatment for PID in an effort to reduce the potential consequences of infertility, ectopic pregnancy, and chronic pelvic pain.

Diagnostic Tests

No specific laboratory test exists for PID. During a pelvic examination, uterine or adnexal tenderness or tenderness with cervical motion is present. Other criteria that help support the diagnosis of PID include an elevated erythrocyte sedimentation rate, elevated C-reactive protein level, white blood cells seen on microscopic examination of vaginal secretions, and documented cervical infection with gonorrhea or chlamydia (CDC, 2010). A transvaginal sonogram may reveal thickened and fluid-filled fallopian tubes with or without free pelvic fluid. A pregnancy test, HIV test, and cultures for STIs should be performed.

Clinical Therapy

Parenteral antibiotic therapy is often used for the first 24 hours before converting to oral antibiotics for the remaining 14 days of treatment. Common intravenous antibiotics used include a combination of cefotetan or cefoxitin plus doxycycline. An alternative parenteral regimen combines clindamycin and gentamicin. Oral regimens include ceftriaxone or cefoxitin, plus doxycycline with or without metronidazole (CDC, 2010). Follow-up physical examination is performed in 72 hours to ensure treatment adherence and to detect improvement in symptoms and reduced tenderness of the uterus, adnexae, and cervix. Rehospitalization and IV antibiotics are initiated if no improvement is noted.

Nursing Management

Goals of nursing management are to identify the adolescent at risk for PID, provide medications for treatment, and provide education to reduce the risk for reinfection.

Nursing Assessment and Diagnosis

A sexual history should be obtained from all adolescent females to identify the risk for sexually transmitted infection and PID. Risk factors for adolescents include those who have an STI, multiple sexual partners, lack of consistent condom use, use of douching, smoking, alcohol use, and the exchange of sex for money or drugs (Abatangelo et al., 2010; Reyes, Kumar, & Abbuhl, 2009).

Nursing diagnoses that may be applicable for the adolescent with PID include the following:

- Pain, Acute related to inflammation and swelling of uterus and fallopian tubes
- Self Health Management, Readiness for Enhanced related to requested information on methods to reduce risk for sexually transmitted infections

NANDA-I © 2012

Planning and Implementation

Administer medications intravenously for the first 24 hours, making arrangements for the adolescent to return for a second dose 12 hours after the first. Provide education for the ongoing treatment with oral antibiotics, ensuring that the adolescent understands the importance of taking all medications on schedule for the full 14 days. Provide signs of adverse effects and actions to take if they occur.

Determine if the adolescent's parents have been informed about the illness, and assist the adolescent to discuss the health problem with them. If the parents are unaware of the health problem, discuss the importance of telling the parents so that they can help identify any problems that develop during treatment. Refer to Chapter 1 for information related to confidentiality issues.

Provide counseling about methods to reduce the risk for reinfection with a sexually transmitted infection. Provide information about the potential consequences of infertility, ectopic pregnancy, and chronic abdominal pain for this infection and the increased risk for these consequences with subsequent infections. Encourage regular health visits with screening for sexually transmitted infections in the future. Chlamydia and gonorrhea infections may be asymptomatic.

Evaluation

Expected outcomes for the child or adolescent with PID are as follows:

- The infection and pain resolve through adherence to the treatment plan.
- The adolescent demonstrates an understanding of methods to reduce the risk for future episodes of sexually transmitted infections and PID.

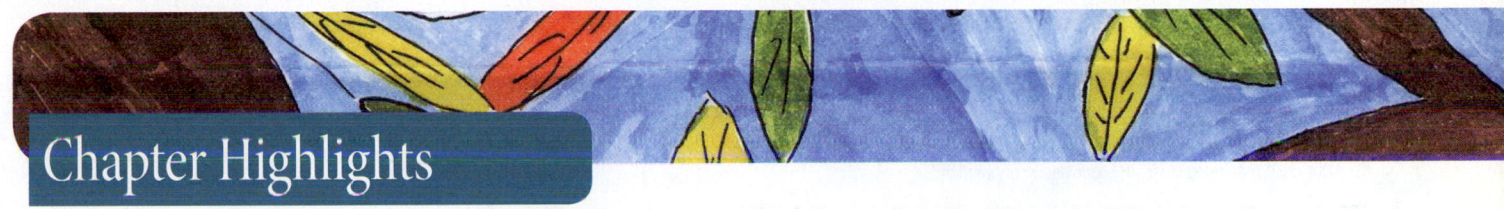

Chapter Highlights

- Functions of the urinary system include excretion of wastes, maintenance of acid–base and fluid and electrolyte balance, regulation of blood pressure, production of erythropoietin, and regulation of calcium metabolism.
- Bladder capacity increases with growth, from 20 to 50 mL in newborns to 700 mL in adults.
- Urinary tract infections are common infections in children. Factors placing the child at risk for a UTI include urinary stasis, infrequent voiding, irritated perineum, constipation, masturbation, sexual abuse, and sexual activity in adolescent females.
- Structural defects of the urinary system—including bladder exstrophy, hypospadias and epispadias, obstructive uropathy, vesicoureteral reflux, and posterior ureteral valves—generally require surgical treatment.
- Bladder exstrophy is a congenital defect in which the abdominal wall does not fuse during fetal development, leading to exposure of the bladder wall, a separation of the rectus muscles, and widening of the symphysis pubis.
- Surgical correction of hypospadias and epispadias generally occurs during the first year of life to minimize psychologic effects on the child.
- Obstruction of the urinary tract interferes with urine flow and results in hydronephrosis or urine backflow into the kidneys. This results in significant damage to the kidney and is a common cause of renal failure in children.
- Vesicoureteral reflux may result from a structural anomaly in which the ureters insert in an abnormal position into the bladder. Urinary tract infections are often a complication of this disorder.

- Prune-belly (Eagle-Barrett) syndrome is a rare congenital disorder in which the skin covering the abdominal wall is thin and resembles a wrinkled prune. Anomalies associated with this syndrome include urinary tract anomalies, enlarged bladder, vesicoureteral reflux, and bilateral cryptorchidism.
- Nocturnal enuresis often occurs in children whose parents have a history of enuresis. Very few children have a structural or neurologic cause. Higher rates of enuresis have been noted in children with obstructive sleep apnea.
- Minimal change nephrotic syndrome is characterized by edema that develops over several weeks, weight gain, hypertension, irritability, hematuria, malaise, anorexia, and foamy or frothy urine.
- Acute postinfectious glomerulonephritis results from a beta-hemolytic group A streptococcal infection of the respiratory tract or skin. Most children have a complete recovery of kidney function.
- Hemolytic uremic syndrome is often associated with ingestion of *E. coli* strain 0157:H7, which produces a toxin that attacks the kidneys. The child develops hemolytic anemia, thrombocytopenia, and acute renal failure that can progress to chronic renal failure.
- Polycystic kidney disease is a genetic disorder with both autosomal recessive and autosomal dominant forms that lead to chronic renal failure. It may be detected prenatally or in young children by ultrasound.
- Acute renal failure occurs when kidney function diminishes abruptly and is often reversible. It may occur as a complication of trauma, sepsis, cardiac

surgery, or drug toxicity. It is also seen in critically ill neonates with asphyxia, sepsis, or shock.

■ Chronic renal failure is progressive and irreversible reduced function of the kidneys, eventually resulting in end-stage renal disease. It often results from developmental abnormalities of the kidneys or urinary tract.

■ Children with end-stage renal disease are treated with renal replacement therapy, including hemodialysis, peritoneal dialysis, or kidney transplant.

■ Structural defects of the male reproductive system include phimosis, cryptorchidism, inguinal hernia and hydrocele, and testicular torsion.

■ Nursing care of sexually transmitted infections includes identifying the cause and organism, providing appropriate treatment, preventing transmission and complications, and educating the child, adolescent, and family.

■ Pelvic inflammatory disease (PID) is an infection of the upper genital tract (uterus and fallopian tubes) caused by the ascending spread of organisms (usually chlamydia or gonorrhea) in the cervix and vagina.

Clinical Reasoning in Action

INTRODUCTION
Recall Brooke from the opening scenario who has a urinary tract infection. She was given a prescription for oral antibiotics. Her recent UTI forced her to leave class to run to the bathroom.

DESCRIPTION
Brooke is an active 9-year-old who is involved in many activities at school. Brooke commonly wears nylon panties and tights under her school uniform.

DISCUSSION
1. What developmental factors should the nurse take into consideration when teaching Brooke about prevention of future UTIs?
2. What desired outcomes should the nurse include in the teaching plan?
3. What are the potential problems that Brooke could encounter if she does not take the medication as prescribed?
4. If Brooke has another urinary tract infection in the next few months, what diagnostic procedures might be used to rule out other potential causes?

NCLEX-RN® Review

1. A nurse is providing discharge teaching to the parents of a child who has a urinary tract infection (UTI). Which statement would demonstrate to the nurse that the parents need more extensive teaching?
   1. "Urinary tract infections always cause renal scarring."
   2. "Urine can cause bacterial growth when the bladder is not emptied completely."
   3. "A fever could be a sign of a UTI."
   4. "Our child may need to be on prophylactic antibiotics."

2. The nurse is helping a 10-year-old child with chronic renal failure select menu items for lunch. Which menu is the best choice?
   1. Pasta with tomato sauce, lettuce salad, and vanilla ice cream
   2. Peanut butter and jelly sandwich, chocolate pudding, and a fresh pear
   3. Hot dog on a bun with ketchup, french fries, and blueberry yogurt
   4. Broiled chicken, broccoli, and noodles with low-salt butter

3. When planning care for a child on dialysis due to renal failure, which of the following nursing diagnoses is priority?
   1. Caregiver Role Strain
   2. Disturbed Body Image
   3. Risk for Infection
   4. Imbalanced Nutrition

4. A 3-year-old female with nephrotic syndrome is being admitted to the general pediatric floor. Who is the most appropriate roommate for this child?
   1. A 2-year-old female recovering from varicella
   2. A 4-year-old female with a fractured femur
   3. A 6-year-old male postoperative appendectomy
   4. A 3-year-old female with cystic fibrosis

See Appendix I 🏮 for answers.

References

Abatangelo, L., Okereke, L., Parham-Foster, C., Parrish, C., Scaglione, L., Zotte, D., & Taub, L. M. (2010). If pelvic inflammatory disease is suspected empiric treatment should be initiated. *Journal of the American Academy of Nurse Practitioners, 22*(2), 117–122.

Adams, D., & Vohra, S. (2009). Complementary, holistic, and integrative medicine: Nocturnal enuresis. *Pediatrics in Review, 30*(10), 396–400.

Akman, S., Kalay, S., Akkaya, B., Koyun, M., Akbas, H., Baysal, Y. E., & Guven, A. G. (2009). Beneficial effect of triple treatment plus immunoglobulin in experimental nephrotic syndrome. *Pediatric Nephrology, 24,* 1173–1180.

Aiken, J. J., & Oldham, K. T. (2011). Inguinal hernias. In R. M. Kliegman, B. F. Stanton, J. W. St. Geme III, N. F. Schor, & R. E. Behrman, *Nelson textbook of pediatrics* (19th ed., pp. 1362–1368). Philadelphia, PA: Saunders Elsevier.

Aldridge, M. D. (2008). How do families adjust to having a child with chronic kidney failure? A systematic review. *Nephrology Nursing Journal, 35*(2), 157–162.

American Academy of Pediatrics. (2009). *Red book: Report of the Committee on Infectious Disease* (28th ed.). Elk Grove Village, IL: Author.

American Academy of Pediatrics: Subcommittee on Urinary Tract Infection, Steering Committee on Quality

Improvement and Management. (2011). Urinary tract infection: Clinical practice guideline for the diagnosis and management of the initial UTI in febrile infants and children 2–24 months. *Pediatrics, 128*(3), 595–610.

Bascom, A., Penney, T., Metcalfe, M., Knox, A., Witmans, M., Uweira, T., & Metcalfe, P. D. (2011). High risk of sleep disordered breathing in the enuresis population. *Journal of Urology, 184*(4), 1710–1714.

Bhimma, R. (2011). *Acute poststreptococcal glomerulonephritis.* Retrieved from http://emedicine.medscape.com/article/980685-overview

Bomalaski, M. D. (2010). *Posterior urethral valves, treatment and management.* Retrieved from http://emedicine.medscape.com/article/1016086-overview

Bradway, C., & Rodgers, J. (2009). Evaluation and management of genitourinary emergencies. *Nurse Practitioner, 34*(5), 37–43.

Brown-Trask, B., Sell, S. V., Carter, S., & Kindred, C. (2009, February). Circumcision care. *RN,* 22–28.

Butani, L., & Ramsamooj, R. (2009). Experience with tacrolimus in children with steroid-resistant nephrotic syndrome. *Pediatric Nephrology, 24,* 1517–1523.

Buyan, N., Türkmen, M. A., Bilge, I., Baskin, E., Haberal, M., Bilginer, Y., . . . Dogrucan, N. (2010). Quality of life in children with chronic kidney disease (with child and parents assessments). *Pediatric Nephrology, 25,* 1487–1496.

Cakan, N., & Kamat, D. (2009). Cryptorchidism: Primary care evaluation and management. *Consultant for Pediatricians, 8*(2), 46–50.

Centers for Disease Control and Prevention (CDC). (2009). *Trends in reportable sexually transmitted diseases in the United States, 2007: National surveillance data for chlamydia, gonorrhea, and syphilis.* Retrieved from http://www.cdc.gov/STD/stats07/trends.htm

Centers for Disease Control and Prevention (CDC). (2010). Sexually transmitted diseases treatment guidelines, 2010. *Morbidity and Mortality Weekly Report, 59*(RR-12), 1–110.

Centers for Disease Control and Prevention (CDC). (2011). *Genital HPV infection—Fact sheet.* Retrieved from http://www.cdc.gov/std/HPV/STDFact-HPV.htm

Chadha, V., Schaefer, F. S., & Warady, B. A. (2010). Dialysis-associated peritonitis in children. *Pediatric Nephrology, 25,* 425–440.

Chung, E., & Brock, G. B. (2011). Cryptorchidism and its impact on male fertility: A state of art review of current literature. *Canadian Urological Association Journal, 5*(3), 210–214.

Craig, J., Simpson, J., Williams, G. J., Lowe, A., Reynolds, G. J., McTaggart, S. J., . . . Roy, L. P. (2009). Antibiotic prophylaxis and recurrent urinary tract infection in children. *New England Journal of Medicine, 361*(18), 1748–1759.

Datta, V., Dhillon, G., & Voci, S. (2011). Testicular torsion/detorsion. *Ultrasound Quarterly, 27*(2), 127–128.

Davidson, M. R., London, M. L., & Ladewig, P. A. (2008). *Olds' maternal-newborn nursing and women's health across the lifespan* (8th ed.). Upper Saddle River, NJ: Pearson/Prentice Hall.

de Souza-Thomas, L. (2010). Gonorrhoea: Prevention, diagnosis and treatment. *British Journal of School Nursing, 5*(3),116–121.

Dogan, H. S., Akpinar, B., Gurocak, S., Akata, D., Bakkaloglu, M., & Tekgul, S. (2008). Non-invasive evaluation of voiding function in asymptomatic primary school children. *Pediatric Nephrology, 23,* 1115–1122.

DuFour, J. L. (2008). Testicular torsion: Respond quickly to urologic emergency. *Advance for Nurse Practitioners, 16*(6), 65–66.

Eding, D. M., Jelsma, L. R., Metz, C. J., Steen, V. S., & Wincek, J. M. (2011). Innovative techniques to decrease blood exposure and minimize interruptions in pediatric continuous renal replacement therapy. *Critical Care Nurse, 31*(1), 64–71.

Elder, J. S. (2011). Urologic disorders in infants and children. In R. M. Kliegman, B. F. Stanton, J. W. St. Geme III, N. F. Schor, & R. E. Behrman, *Nelson textbook of pediatrics* (19th ed., pp. 1827–1864). Philadelphia, PA: Saunders Elsevier.

Elmore, J. M., Kirsch, A. J., Snyder, H. M., & Cooper, C. S. (2009). *Pediatric urologic gynecology.*

Retrieved from http://emedicine.medscape.com/article/1017296-overview#a1

Estrada, C. R., & Cendron, M. (2011). *Vesicoureteral reflux.* Retrieved from http://emedicine.medscape.com/article/439403-overview

Fischbach, M., & Warady, B. A. (2009). Peritoneal dialysis prescription in children: Bedside principles for optimal practice. *Pediatric Nephrology, 24,* 1633–1642.

Fisher, D. J., Howes, D. S., & Thornton, S. L. (2011). *Pediatric urinary tract infection: Treatment & management.* Retrieved from http://emedicine.medscape.com/article/969643-overview

Forhan, S. E., Gottlieb, S. L., Sternberg, M. R., Xu, F., Datta, S. D., McQuillan, G. M., . . . Markowitz, L. E. (2009). Prevalence of sexually transmitted infections among female adolescents aged 14 to 19 in the United States. *Pediatrics, 124*(6), 1505–1512.

Frøkiaer, J., & Zeidel, M. L. (2012). Urinary tract obstruction. In M. W. Taal, G. M. Chertow, P. A. Marsden, K. Skorecki, A. S. L. Yu, & B. M. Brenner, *Brenner and Rector's the kidney* (9th ed., pp. 1239–1260). Philadelphia, PA: Saunders Elsevier.

Guilfoyle, S. M., Goebel, J. W., & Pai, A. L. (2011). Efficacy and flexibility impact perceived adherence barriers in pediatric kidney post-transplantation. *Families, Systems, & Health, 29*(1), 44–54.

Gulati, S. (2011). *Chronic kidney disease in children.* Retrieved from http://emedicine.medscape.com/article/984358-overview

Hamasaki, Y., Yoshikawa, N., Hattori, S., Sasaki, S., Iijima, K., Nakanishi, K., . . . Honda, M. (2009). Cyclosporine and steroid therapy in children with steroid-resistant nephrotic syndrome. *Pediatric Nephrology, 24,* 2177–2185.

Han, S. W., Rah, K. H., & Lee, H. (2010). *Pediatric ureteropelvic junction obstruction.* Retrieved from http://emedicine.medscape.com/article/1016988-overview

Hartmann, R. W. (2008). Congenital complete inguinal-scrotal hernia. *Consultant for Pediatricians, 7*(12), 526–527.

Heath, J., MacKinlay, D., Watson, A. R., Hames, A., Wirz, L., Scott, S., . . . McHugh, K. (2011). Self-reported quality of life in children and young people with chronic kidney disease. *Pediatric Nephrology, 26,* 767–773.

Hedden, A. Z. (2008). *E. coli* 0157:H7 infection. *Advance for Nurse Practitioners, 16*(10), 69–72.

Hines, E. Q. (2012). Fluid and electrolytes. In Johns Hopkins: *The Harriet Lane handbook* (19th ed., pp. 271–292). Philadelphia, PA: Elsevier.

Hodges, S., Patel, B., McLorie, G., & Atala, A. (2009). Posterior urethral valves. *Scientific World Journal, 9,* 1119–1126.

Hoebeke, P., Bower, W., Combs, A., DeJong, T., & Yang, S. (2010). Diagnostic evaluation of children with daytime incontinence. *Journal of Urology, 183,* 699–703.

Huether, S. E. (2010a). Structure and function of the renal and urologic systems. In K. L. McCance & S. E. Huether, *Pathophysiology: The biologic basis for disease in adults and children* (6th ed., pp. 1344–1364). Maryland Heights, MO: Mosby Elsevier.

Huether, S. E. (2010b). Alterations of renal and urinary tract function in children. In K. L. McCance & S. E. Huether, *Pathophysiology: The biologic basis for disease in adults and children* (6th ed., pp. 1402–1419). Maryland Heights, MO: Mosby Elsevier.

Huether, S. E., & Forshee, B. A. (2010). Alterations of renal and urinary tract function. In K. L. McCance & S. E. Huether, *Pathophysiology: The biologic basis for*

disease in adults and children (6th ed., pp. 1365–1401). Maryland Heights, MO: Mosby Elsevier.

Ingerski, L., Perrazo, L., Goebel, J., & Pai, A. L. H. (2011). Family strategies for achieving medication adherence in pediatric kidney transplantation. *Nursing Research, 60*(3), 190–196.

Islek, A., Güven, A. G., Koyun, M., Akman, S., & Alimoglu, E. (2011). Probability of urinary tract infection in infants with ureteropelvic junction obstruction: Is antibacterial prophylaxis really needed? *Pediatric Nephrology, 26,* 1837–1841.

Jalanko, H. (2009). Congenital nephrotic syndrome. *Pediatric Nephrology, 24,* 2121–2128.

Karacan, C., Erkek, N., Senel, S., Gunduz, S., Catli, G., & Tavil, B. (2010). Evaluation of urine collection methods for the diagnosis of urinary tract infection in children. *Medical Principles and Practice, 19,* 188–191.

Kennedy, K. M., Glynn, L. G., & Dineen, B. (2010). A survey of the management of urinary tract infection in children in primary care and comparison with the NICE guidelines. *BMC Family Practice, 11*(6), 1–6.

Ključevšek, D., Ključevšek, T., Levart, T. K., Novljan, G., & Kenda, R. B. (2010). Catheter-free methods for vesicoureteric reflux detection: Our experience and a critical appraisal of existing data. *Pediatric Nephrology, 25*(7), 1201–1206.

Kozlowski, L. J. (2008). The acute pain service nurse practitioner: A case study in the postoperative care of the child with bladder exstrophy. *Journal of Pediatric Health Care, 22,* 351–359.

Lahdenkari, A., Suvanto, M., Kajantie, E., Koskimies, O., Kestila, M., & Jalanko, H. (2005). Clinical features and outcome of childhood minimal change nephrotic syndrome: Is genetics involved? *Pediatric Nephrology, 20,* 1073–1080.

Latendresse, G. A., McCance, K. L., & Morgan, K. (2010). Alterations of the reproductive systems. In K. L. McCance & S. E. Huether, *Pathophysiology: The biologic basis for disease in adults and children* (6th ed., pp. 816–922). Maryland Heights, MO: Mosby Elsevier.

Leung, A. K. C., & Kao, C. P. (2008). A collage of genital lesions, Part 2. *Consultant for Pediatricians, 7*(9), 369–370.

Listernick, R. (2009). An 8-year-old girl with kidney failure. *Pediatric Annals, 38*(7), 355–358.

Lum, G. (2011). Kidney & urinary tract. In W. W. Hay, M. J. Levin, J. M. Sondheimer, & R. R. Deterding, *CURRENT diagnosis and treatment: Pediatrics* (20th ed.). New York, NY: McGraw-Hill. Retrieved from http://accessmedicine.com

Minnick, M. L., Boynton, S., Ndirangu, J., & Furth, S. (2010). Sex, race, and socioeconomic disparities in kidney disease in children. *Seminars in Nephrology, 30*(1), 26–32.

Montini, G., Rigon, L., Zucchetta, P., Fregonese, G., Toffolo, A., Gobber, D., . . . Dall'Amico, R. (2008). Prophylaxis after first febrile urinary tract infection in children? A multicenter, randomized, controlled, noninferiority trial. *Pediatrics, 122*(5), 1064–1071.

Nachman, P. H., Jennette, J. C., & Falk, R. J. (2012). Primary glomerular disease. In M. W. Taal, G. M. Chertow, P. A. Marsden, K. Skorecki, A. S. L. Yu, & B. M. Brenner, *Brenner and Rector's the kidney* (9th ed., pp. 987–1046). Philadelphia, PA: Saunders Elsevier.

Naqvi, M., Paddack, J., Kulkarni, A., Akangire, G., & Subhani, M. (2009). What's your diagnosis? Sharpen your physical diagnostic skills. *Consultant for Pediatricians, 8*(9), 333–335.

National Kidney Foundation. (2011). *Use of herbal supplements in chronic kidney disease.* Retrieved from http://www.kidney.org/atoz/content/herbalsupp.cfm

National Kidney and Urologic Diseases Information Clearinghouse. (2009). *Financial help for treatment of kidney failure.* NIH Publication No. 09–4765. Retrieved from http://kidney.niddk.nih.gov/kudiseases/pubs/pdf/Financial-Help-Kidney.pdf

Nelson, C. P., & Koo, H. P. (2008). *Vesicoureteral reflux.* Retrieved from http://emedicine.medscape.com/article/1016439-overview

Nevéus, T. (2011). Nocturnal enuresis-theoretic background and practical guidelines. *Pediatric Nephrology, 26,* 1207–1214.

Newman, T. B. (2011). The new American Academy of Pediatrics urinary tract infection guidelines. *Pediatrics, 128*(3), 572–575.

Nguyen, S., & Whitehill, J. (2011). *Treatment of urinary tract infections in children.* Retrieved from http://www.medscape.com/viewarticle/740362

Norfolk, S., & Wootton, J. (2011). Supporting children with nocturnal enuresis. *British Journal of School Nursing, 6*(5), 225–228.

Otukesh, H. Hoseini, R., Rahimzadeh, N., Hosseini, S. (2012). Glomerular Function in Neonates Iranian. *Journal of Kidney Diseases, 6*(3), 166–172.

Pais, P., & Avner, E. D. (2011). Nephrotic syndrome. In R. M. Kliegman, B. F. Stanton, J. W. St. Geme III, N. F. Schor, & R. E. Behrman, *Nelson textbook of pediatrics* (19th ed., pp. 1799–1807). Philadelphia, PA: Saunders Elsevier.

Palmer, L. S., & Palmer, J. S. (2008). The efficacy of topical betamethasone for treating phimosis: A comparison of two treatment regimens. *Urology, 72,* 68–71.

Papantoniou, N., Papoutsis, D., Daskalakis, G., Chatzipapas, I., Sindos, M., Papaspyrou, I., . . . Antsaklis, A. (2010). Prenatal diagnosis of prune-belly syndrome at 13 weeks of gestation: Case report and review of literature. *Journal of Maternal-Fetal and Neonatal Medicine, 23*(10), 1263–1267.

Patzer, R. E., Amaral, S., Klein, M., Kutner, N., Perryman, J. P., Gazmararian, J. A., & McClellan, W. M. (2012). Racial disparities in pediatric access to kidney transplantation: Does socioeconomic status play a role? *American Journal of Transplantation, 12*(2), 369–378.

Perera, C. L., Bridgewater, F. H., Thavaneswaran, P., & Maddern, G. J. (2010). Safety and efficacy of nontherapeutic male circumcision: A systematic review. *Annals of Family Medicine, 8*(1), 64–72.

Pfeil, M., & Lindsay, B. (2010). Hypospadias repair: An overview. *Urological Nursing, 4*(1), 4–12.

Pieretti, R. V., Pieretti, A., & Pieretti-Vanmarcke, R. (2009). Circumcised hypospadias. *Pediatric Surgery International, 25,* 53–55.

Porter, C. C., & Avner, E. D. (2011). Anatomic abnormalities associated with hematuria. In R. M. Kliegman, B. F. Stanton, J. W. St. Geme III, N. F. Schor, & R. E. Behrman, *Nelson textbook of pediatrics* (19th ed., pp. 1796–1799). Philadelphia, PA: Saunders Elsevier.

Prune Belly Syndrome Network. (2011). Retrieved from http://www.prunebelly.org

Reyes, I., Kumar, R., & Abbuhl, S. (2009). *Pelvic inflammatory disease.* Retrieved from http://emedicine.medscape.com/article/796092-overview

Riaño-Galán, I., Málaga, S., Rajmil, L., Ariceta, G., Navarro, M., Loris, C., & Vallo, A. (2009). Quality of life of adolescents with end-stage renal disease and kidney transplant. *Pediatric Nephrology, 24,* 1561–1568.

Rizk, D., & Chapman, A. (2008). Treatment of autosomal dominant polycystic kidney disease (ADPKD): The new horizon for children with ADPKD. *Pediatric Nephrology, 23,* 1029–1036.

Robbins, C., & Shew, M. L. (2009). UTIs in adolescents: Common infections, uncommon challenges. *Contemporary Pediatrics, 26*(7), 48–54.

Rupp, T. J., & Zwanger, M. (2010). *Testicular torsion.* Retrieved from http://emedicine.medscape.com/article/778086-overview

Salant, D. J., & Gordon, C. E. (2012). Polycystic kidney disease and other inherited tubular disorders. In D. L. Longo, A. S. Fauci, D. L. Kasper, S. L. Hauser, J. L. Jameson, & J. Loscalzo, *Harrison's principles of internal medicine* (18th ed., pp. 1797–1806). New York, NY: McGraw-Hill.

Saldano, D. D., Chaviano, A. H., & Maizels, M. (2008). Sustainability of remission of pediatric primary nocturnal enuresis—Comparison of remission using try for dry vs. non-try for dry treatment plans. *Urologic Nursing, 28*(4), 263–266.

Santiago, M. J., López-Herce, J., Urbano, J., Solana, M. J., del Castillo, J., Ballestero, Y., . . . Bellón, J. M. (2009). Complications of continuous renal replacement therapy in critically ill children: A prospective observational evaluation study. *Critical Care, 13*(6). Retrieved from http://ccforum.com/content/13/6/R184

Sarkar, S. (2009). Continuous renal replacement therapy (CRRT). *Internet Journal of Anesthesiology, 21*(1). Retrieved from http://www.ispub.com/journal/the-internet-journal-of-anesthesiology/volume-21-number-1/continuous-renal-replacement-therapy-crrt.html

Sarwal, M. M., & Wong, C. J. (2011). Renal transplantation. In R. M. Kliegman, B. F. Stanton, J. W. St. Geme III, N. F. Schor, & R. E. Behrman, *Nelson textbook of pediatrics* (19th ed., p. 1826). Philadelphia, PA: Saunders Elsevier.

Schwartz, G. J., & Work, D. F. (2009). Measurement and estimation of GFR in children and adolescents. *Clinical Journal of the American Society of Nephrology, 4,* 1832–1843.

Shapiro, R., & Sarwal, M. M. (2010). Pediatric kidney transplantation. *Pediatric Kidney Transplantation, 57*(2), 393–400.

Shingarev, R., Wille, K., & Tolwani, A. (2011). Management of complications in renal replacement therapy. *Seminars in Dialysis, 24*(2), 164–168.

Sreedharan, R., & Avner, E. D. (2011). Renal failure. In R. M. Kliegman, B. F. Stanton, J. W. St. Geme III, N. F. Schor, & R. E. Behrman, *Nelson textbook of pediatrics* (19th ed., pp. 1818–1826). Philadelphia, PA: Saunders Elsevier.

Stefanidis, C. J. (2009). Prevention of catheter-related bacteremia in children on hemodialysis: Time for action. *Pediatric Nephrology, 24,* 2087–2095.

Tan, A. J., & Silverberg, M. A. (2009). *Hemolytic uremic syndrome.* Retrieved from http://emedicine.medscape.com/article/779218-overview

Thomas, J. (2010). Etiopathogenesis and management of bladder dysfunction in patients with posterior urethral valves. *Indian Journal of Urology, 26*(4), 480–489.

United States Department of Agriculture (USDA). (2011). *Meat preparation: Color of cooked ground beef as it relates to doneness.* Retrieved from http://www.fsis.usda.gov/Factsheets/Color_of_Cooked_Ground_Beef/index.asp

Uthup, S., Binitha, R., Geetha, S., Hema, R., & Kailas, L. (2010). A follow-up study of children with posterior urethral valve. *Indian Journal of Nephrology, 20*(2), 72–75.

Verive, M. J. (2011). *Pediatric hyperkalemia.* Retrieved from http://emedicine.medscape.com/article/907543-overview

Vogler, C., Wang, Y., Brink, D., Wood, E., Belsha, C., & Walker, P. D. (2007). Renal pathology in the pediatric transplant patient. *Advances in Anatomic Pathology, 14*(3), 202–216.

Wang, M. L., Macklin, E. A., Tracy, E., Nadel, H., & Catlin, E. A. (2010). Updated parental viewpoints on male neonatal circumcision in the United States. *Clinical Pediatrics, 49*(2), 130–136.

Watnick, S., & Dirkx, T. (2012). Kidney disease. In S. J. McPhee, M. A. Papadakis, & M. W. Rabow, *Current medical diagnosis and treatment 2012* (51st ed.). New York, NY: McGraw-Hill.

Weil, B. R., Andreoli, S. P., & Billmire, D. F. (2010). Bleeding risk for surgical dialysis procedures in children with hemolytic uremic syndrome. *Pediatric Nephrology, 25*(9), 1693–1698.

Wilson, B. A., Shannon, M. T., & Shields, K. M. (2011). *Pearson nurse's drug guide 2011.* New York, NY: Pearson.

Workeneh, B. T., Agraharkar, M., & Gupta, R. (2012). *Acute renal failure.* Retrieved from http://emedicine.medscape.com/article/243492-overview

Zaritsky, J., & Warady, B. A. (2011). Peritoneal dialysis in infants and young children. *Seminars in Nephrology, 31*(2), 213–224.

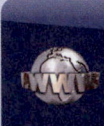

Pearson Nursing Student Resources
Find additional review materials at
nursing.pearsonhighered.com
Prepare for success with additional NCLEX®-style practice questions, interactive assignments and activities, web links, animations and videos, and more!

Alterations in Endocrine and Metabolic Function

CHAPTER 32

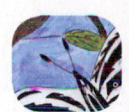 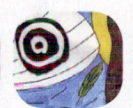 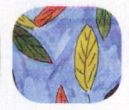

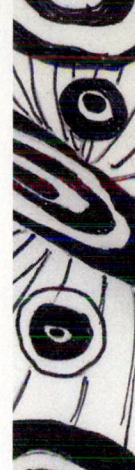

KEY TERMS

Learning Outcomes

After completing this chapter, you will be able to:

1. Describe the general function of the endocrine system.

2. Identify the function of important hormones of the endocrine system.

3. Summarize signs and symptoms that may indicate a disorder of the endocrine system.

4. Identify all conditions for which short stature is a sign.

5. Prioritize nursing care for each type of acquired metabolic disorder.

6. Develop a family education plan for the child who needs lifelong cortisol replacement.

7. Distinguish between the nursing care of the child with type 1 and type 2 diabetes.

8. Outline collaborative management for the child with type 1 and type 2 diabetes.

9. Plan care for the child with an inherited metabolic disorder.

"I don't like this at all—I know I have to check my glucose levels and eat the right foods—but I still don't like it. Why doesn't my body make insulin like it's supposed to?"

—*Anthony, 12 years old*

Anthony Maxwell, 12 years old, has just been diagnosed with type 1 diabetes. His parents sought medical attention from their family physician after Anthony complained of being constantly thirsty and hungry for over a week. Despite his vigorous appetite, he has lost 5 pounds since his last recorded weight. The family recalls that Anthony had a viral illness 3 months ago but recovered from the illness without difficulty. His mother says that Anthony has seemed lethargic for the last several days.

Anthony and his family must now learn to manage his diabetes using a combination of diet, exercise, and insulin therapy. Monitoring his serum glucose level is important in determining how much insulin he will require every day. Anthony's meals and activities will be coordinated with his insulin doses. During his short hospitalization and follow-up sessions, the nurse partners with Anthony and his family in educating them regarding the cause, management, and long-term implications of diabetes. What are the key components of the teaching plan for Anthony and his family related to management of type 1 diabetes? How can Anthony be involved in his care while hospitalized?

The endocrine system controls the cellular activity that regulates growth and body metabolism through the release of hormones. **Hormones** are chemical messengers secreted by various glands that exert controlling effects on the cells of the body. Overlapping with all body systems, the general functions of the endocrine system include the following:

- Differentiation of the reproductive and central nervous systems in the fetus
- Regulation of the pace of growth and development in concert with the central nervous system throughout childhood and adolescence
- Coordination of the male and female reproductive systems, enabling sexual reproduction
- Maintenance of an optimal level of hormones for body functioning
- Maintenance of homeostasis, a healthy internal environment, in the presence of a constantly changing external environment

The endocrine and nervous systems interact to regulate responses within the body and with the external environment.

ANATOMY AND PHYSIOLOGY

The hypothalamic-pituitary axis (or system) produces a number of releasing and inhibiting hormones that regulate the function of many endocrine glands, including the thyroid, adrenal, and male and female reproductive glands. The hypothalamus synthesizes many hormones, and the pituitary gland works by stimulating or inhibiting the release of these hormones. The pituitary gland also secretes certain hormones. Hormones originating from this axis regulate growth. Other endocrine glands include the parathyroid glands and the islets of Langerhans in the pancreas (Figure 32–1 ■). All of these glands secrete hormones into the bloodstream, which carries them to target organs or tissues. Most hormones exert their influence through interaction with receptors in the target cells of specific tissues (Table 32–1).

Hormone secretion regulation occurs through a **negative feedback** mechanism that maintains an optimal internal body environment (Figure 32–2 ■). Negative feedback occurs when an endocrine gland or secretory tissue receives a message that the target cells have received an adequate amount of hormone. In response, further secretion is inhibited. Secretion is resumed only when the secretory tissue receives another message indicating that levels of the hormone are low.

PEDIATRIC DIFFERENCES

The endocrine system is responsible for sexual differentiation during fetal development. As the embryo develops, the initial reproductive structures are the same (a pair of gonads, two pairs of ducts, and the genital tubercle). Beginning at 7 to 8 weeks of gestation, the male embryo begins secreting testosterone, which causes the gonads to differentiate into testes. The pairs of ducts develop into the vas deferens. The female embryo begins secreting estrogen, causing the gonads to differentiate into ovaries, while the ducts develop into the uterus and the fallopian tubes. The genital tubercle also differentiates and develops the male and female external genitalia.

During childhood, the production of sex hormones (estrogen, progesterone, and testosterone) is low. **Puberty** (sexual maturation,

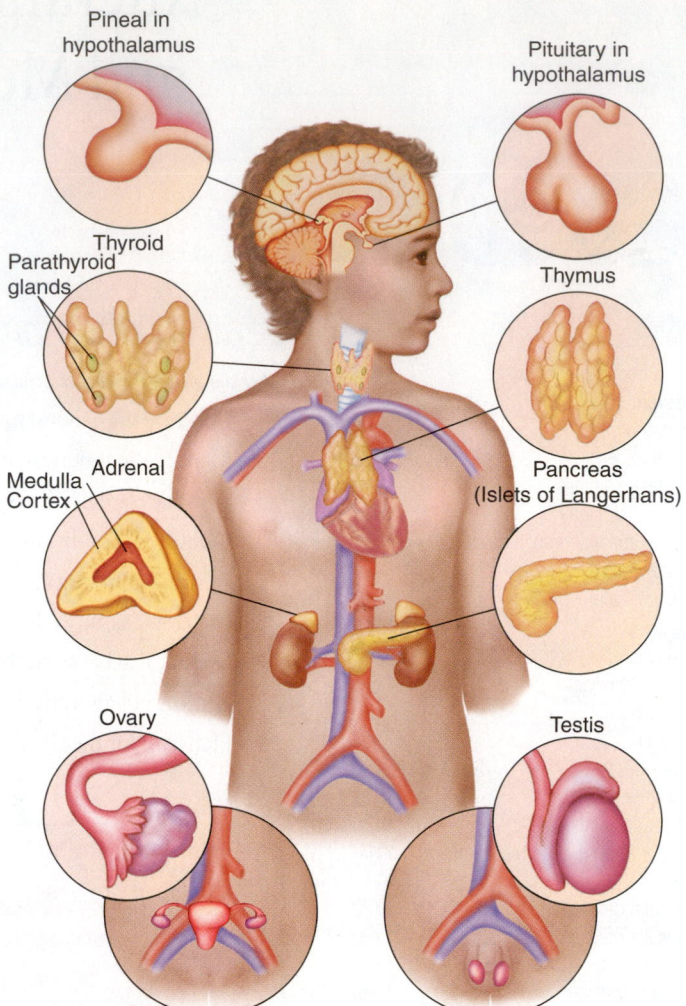

FIGURE 32–1 ■ Major organs and glands of the endocrine system.

lasting an average of 4.5 years) occurs when the gonads begin to secrete increased amounts of the sex hormones estrogen and androgens. At the average age of 9 years in girls and 11 years in boys, the hypothalamus produces increased amounts of gonadotropin-releasing hormone (GnRH). This hormone stimulates the anterior pituitary gland to secrete luteinizing hormone (LH) and follicle-stimulating hormone (FSH). In boys, LH stimulates testosterone production, and FSH stimulates sperm production. In girls, LH and FSH stimulate development and maturation of the ova and ovulation. These hormones in turn stimulate the gonads to secrete more sex hormones, resulting in the development of primary and secondary sex characteristics. They also stimulate the genitalia to grow to adult proportions. **Adrenarche** refers to the onset of adrenal androgen production. These adrenal hormones lead to the development of acne, pubic hair, and adult body odor (Bordini & Rosenfield, 2011a). Pubertal development usually follows a specific sequence (breast development, pubic hair growth, and menarche in females; testicular enlargement, pubic hair growth, appearance of spermatozoa in seminal fluid, facial hair, and voice change in males) (Bordini & Rosenfield, 2011b). See Figures 7–43, 7–44, and 7–45 in Chapter 7 🔗 for the development of secondary sexual characteristics in males and females. See Box 32–1.

TABLE 32–1	Endocrine Glands and Their Functions

GLAND/HORMONE	FUNCTION
Anterior Pituitary	
Growth hormone (somatotropin)	Regulates metabolic process related to growth
Thyroid-stimulating hormone (TSH)	Stimulates thyroid hormone secretion which regulates body metabolism and is essential for normal growth
Adrenocorticotropic hormone (ACTH) (corticotropin)	Stimulates adrenal glands to produce cortisol (stress hormone) and other hormones that enable the body to respond to stress
Follicle-stimulating hormone (FSH) (a gonadotropin)	Stimulates secretion of estrogen; stimulates follicle maturation in ovaries; also critical for sperm production in males
Luteinizing hormone (LH) and interstitial cell-stimulating hormone (ICSH) (male analog) (a gonadotropin)	Stimulates secretion of androgens in males and progesterone in females
Prolactin-releasing hormone	Stimulates secretion of prolactin which stimulates the secretion of milk during lactation
Melanocyte-stimulating hormone (MSH)	Stimulates skin pigmentation
Posterior Pituitary	
Antidiuretic hormone (ADH)	Promotes water reabsorption back into blood, decreasing urine output
Oxytocin	Stimulates uterine contractions and breast milk letdown reflex
Beta endorphins	May regulate body temperature, food and water intake
Thyroid	
Thyroxine (T_4) and triiodothyronine (T_3)	Regulates metabolic rate of all cells, body heat production; protein, fat, and carbohydrate catabolism in all cells
Thyrocalcitonin	Stimulates bone ossification and development
Parathyroid	
Parathyroid hormone	Regulates serum calcium levels and excretion of phosphorus
Adrenal	
Aldosterone	Increases sodium ion reabsorption, and increases potassium and hydrogen ion excretion in the kidneys
Androgens	Stimulates bone development and secondary sexual characteristics
Cortisol	Stimulates anti-inflammatory reactions, protects from stress
Epinephrine	Activates sympathetic nervous system; stimulates increase in blood pressure and blood glucose levels
Pancreas (islets of Langerhans)	
Insulin	Facilitates cellular glucose utilization
Glucagon	Increases blood glucose when low by stimulating glycogenolysis
Somatostatin	Inhibits insulin and glucagon secretion; may prevent excess insulin secretion
Ovaries	
Estrogen	Stimulates development of breasts and ova
Progesterone	Stimulates breast glandular development; acts to maintain pregnancy
Testes	
Testosterone	Stimulates production of sperm, development of secondary sexual characteristics, and closure of epiphysis

BOX 32–1	Growth & Development: Puberty and Weight

Delayed puberty or slow progression through puberty in females may be related to excessive exercise without adequate caloric intake and is most often associated with participation in gymnastics, competitive swimming, and ballet dancing. Delayed puberty may also occur in the presence of anorexia nervosa (Kaplowitz, 2010).

Menarche, the onset of menstruation, occurs at an average age of 12.1 years in African American girls and 12.6 years in White girls (Bordini & Rosenfield, 2011b). Menstruation is controlled by several hormones (FSH, LH, estrogen, and progesterone). For 1 to 2 years, cycles are anovulatory of variable duration. In contrast, males begin producing sperm once testicular and penile growth has occurred, during genital stages 3 and 4 (Bordini & Rosenfield, 2011b).

Use the guidelines in Table 32–2 to perform a nursing assessment of the endocrine system. Table 32–3 lists some common diagnostic procedures and laboratory procedures for the endocrine system. See Appendixes D and E 🔗 for examples of diagnostic and laboratory tests used to evaluate endocrine conditions. Additional tests are discussed in this chapter.

Endocrine disturbances result in alterations in metabolism, growth and development, and behavior that may have significant implications for children. If not diagnosed and treated early, these conditions can result in delays in growth and development, intellectual disability, and, occasionally, death. However, treatment, which usually consists of supplementation of missing hormones, adjustment of hormone levels, or dietary measures, allows most children to live a normal life.

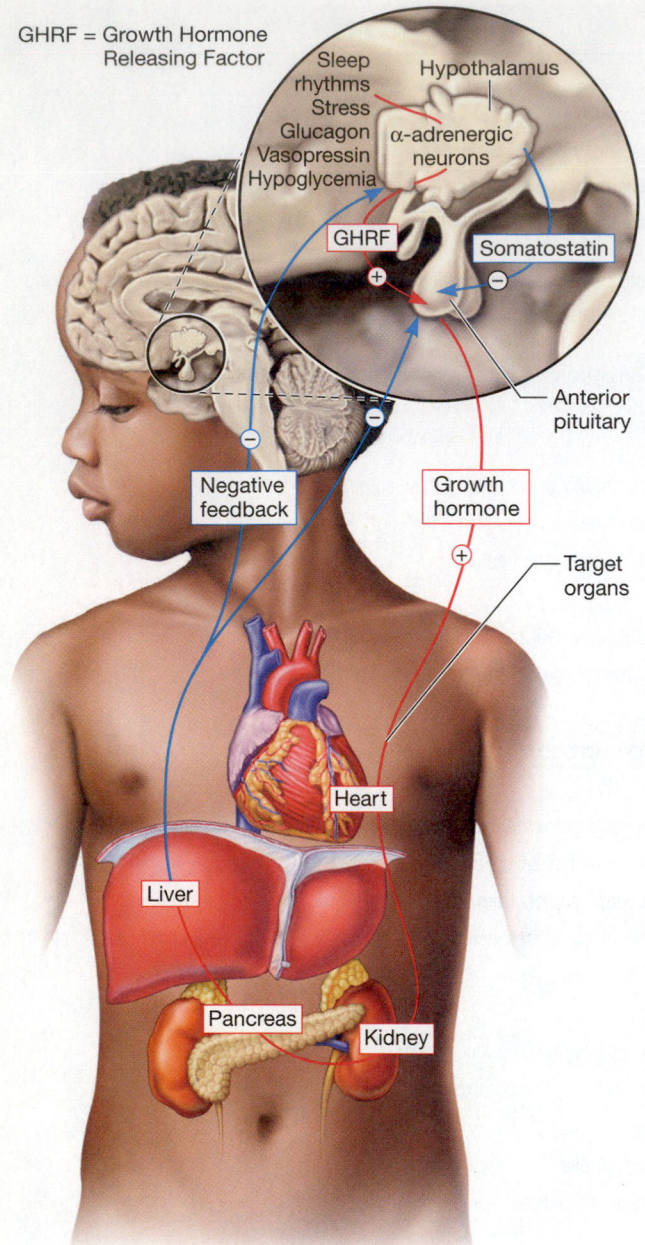

GHRF = Growth Hormone
Releasing Factor

Sleep rhythms
Stress
Glucagon
Vasopressin
Hypoglycemia

Hypothalamus

α-adrenergic neurons

GHRF

Somatostatin

Anterior pituitary

Negative feedback

Growth hormone

Target organs

Heart

Liver

Pancreas

Kidney

FIGURE 32–2 ■ Feedback mechanism in hormonal stimulation of the gonads during puberty.

TABLE 32–2	Assessment Guidelines for the Child with an Endocrine Condition*
ASSESSMENT FOCUS	**ASSESSMENT GUIDELINE**
Growth	■ Carefully measure weight, length, or height and plot on a growth curve.
	■ Compare measurements at different ages to assess the growth pattern over time and to assess the growth velocity.
Blood pressure/pulse	■ Assess blood pressure and compare to expected norms for age. See Appendix B 🖉.
Facial characteristics	■ Inspect the face for unusual features such as a protuberant tongue, protuberant eyes, or moon face.
Neck	■ Palpate the neck for an enlarged thyroid or goiter.
Muscles	■ Assess strength and muscle tone.
Genitalia and secondary sexual characteristics	■ Assess external genitalia for signs of ambiguous genitalia, or inappropriate size for age.
	■ Determine the child's stage of development for each characteristic (breast and pubic hair for girls, genital and pubic hair for boys) by comparing to the images in Figures 7–43, 7–44, and 7–45 🖉.
	■ Assess the sexual maturity rating with information in Figure 7–46 🖉. Compare the stage of development to the age of the boy or girl to determine early or delayed onset of puberty.
Body odor	■ Assess body odor for unusual smell (e.g., sweet, musty, cheesy, sweaty feet).
Skin	■ Assess skin color, noting areas of unusual pigmentation.
Mental status	■ Note affect. Assess for anxiety, irritability, or lethargy.
Family history	■ Assess for family history of metabolic or endocrine disorders.

Note: *Refer to Chapter 7 🖉 for the actual techniques of assessment mentioned in this table.

The anterior pituitary gland is considered to be the "master gland" of the body. The major function of the anterior pituitary gland is the production and release of thyroid-stimulating hormone (TSH), adrenocorticotropic hormone (ACTH), luteinizing hormone (LH), follicle-stimulating hormone (FSH), growth hormone (GH), and

TABLE 32–3	Diagnostic Procedures and Laboratory Tests for the Endocrine System*	
DIAGNOSTIC PROCEDURES	**LABORATORY TESTS**	
ACTH stimulation test	Fasting plasma glucose	
Adrenal (ACTH) suppression test	Hemoglobin A$_{1c}$	
Bone age	Hormone levels	
Computed tomography (CT)	Insulin-like growth factor (IGF-1) and Insulin-like growth factor-binding protein 3 IGFBP-3	
Fluid deprivation test		
Karyotype		
Magnetic resonance imaging (MRI)	Newborn metabolic screening	
Thyroid radioactive iodine uptake (RAIU) scan	Provocative growth hormone testing	
	Thyroid antibodies	

Note: *See Appendixes D and E 🖉 for information about these diagnostic procedures and for expected laboratory tests values.

Inborn errors of metabolism (inherited biochemical abnormalities of the urea cycle and amino acid and organic acid metabolism) often have a significant impact on the endocrine system's ability to support growth and development. Some chromosomal abnormalities also result in disturbances in growth and sexual development. These disorders are discussed on page 1141.

DISORDERS OF PITUITARY FUNCTION

The pituitary gland consists of two lobes, an anterior lobe and a posterior lobe. The functions of the posterior pituitary gland include regulation of fluid balance through release of antidiuretic hormone (ADH), which is stored in the hypothalamus; and production of oxytocin, which is also stored in the hypothalamus.

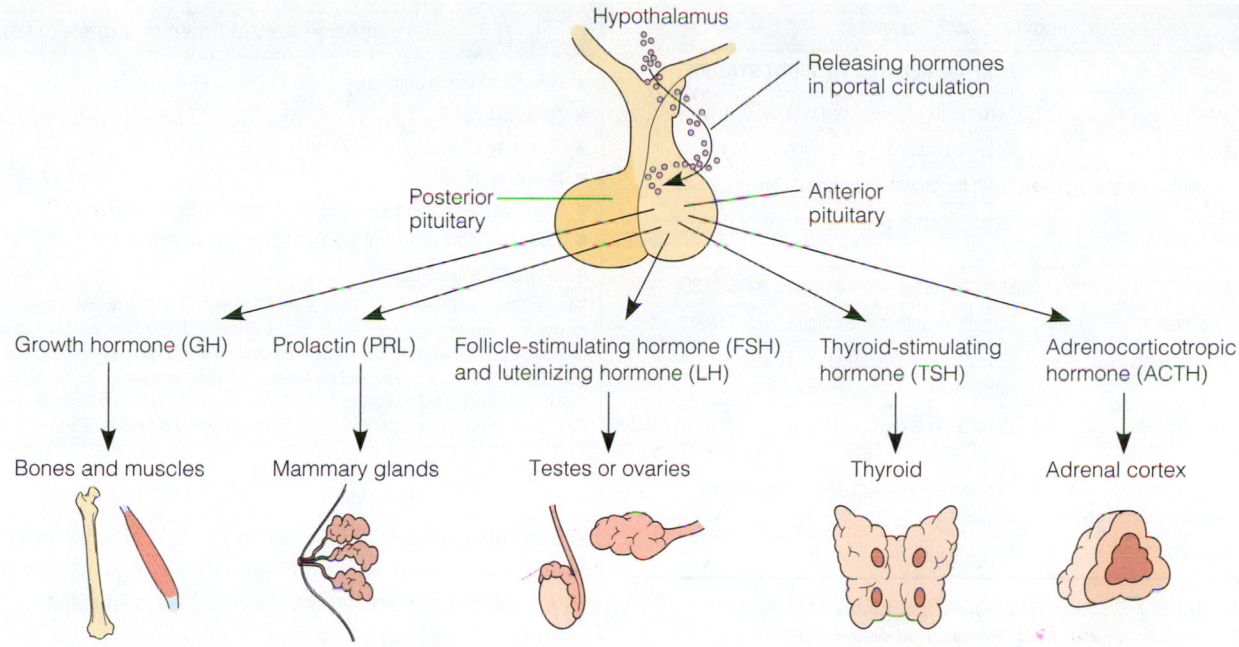

FIGURE 32–3 ■ Actions of the major hormones of the anterior pituitary.

prolactin (PRL). Most of these hormones regulate the secretion of other hormones. See Table 32–1.

Pituitary disorders such as growth hormone deficiency, hyperpituitarism, and precocious puberty directly affect the child's growth, while diabetes insipidus is a disorder affecting fluid balance. These disorders are discussed in the following section.

Growth Hormone Deficiency

Growth hormone deficiency (GHD) is a disorder caused by decreased activity of the pituitary gland. Because most children with this disorder secrete inadequate amounts of growth hormone, the term *growth hormone deficiency* is often preferred to *hypopituitarism*. The disorder is diagnosed earlier in males than females because males are referred sooner for evaluation of short stature (Grimberg, Stewart, & Wajnrajch, 2008).

Etiology and Pathophysiology

The release of growth hormone from the anterior pituitary gland is controlled by the hypothalamus, which secretes releasing and inhibitory factors (somatostatin) (Figure 32–3 ■). Growth hormone stimulates linear growth and bone mineral density, as well as the growth of all body tissues. Growth hormone also stimulates the synthesis of proteins in the liver, among them the somatomedins or insulin-like growth factors (IGFs), which promote glucose utilization by the cells and cell proliferation.

Growth hormone deficiency can be caused by several conditions that interfere with the production or release of growth hormone. These conditions include infarction of the pituitary gland (such as that related to sickle cell disease), central nervous system disease, tumors of the pituitary gland or hypothalamus (primarily craniopharyngiomas and gliomas), other brain tumors, cranial irradiation, brain trauma, chemotherapy, and psychosocial deprivation. Other major causes of short stature include familial short stature, hypothyroidism, Turner syndrome, **constitutional growth delay** (a late pubertal growth spurt caused by delayed pubertal hormone secretion), chronic renal failure, malnutrition, Cushing syndrome, Down

syndrome, inborn error of metabolism, and severe cardiac, pulmonary, immunologic, or gastrointestinal disease. Psychosocial dwarfism is a syndrome of emotional deprivation that causes transient growth hormone deficiency that is reversed by placing the child in a nurturing environment (Sirotnak, 2008).

Clinical Manifestations

Children with growth hormone deficiency have normal birth weights and lengths. By the age of 1 year, however, they are below the 3rd percentile on the growth chart. The child characteristically grows at a rate of less than 5 cm (2 in.) per year. Other characteristic findings in infants include hypoglycemic seizures, hyponatremia, neonatal jaundice, pale optic discs, micropenis, and undescended testes. Children with growth hormone deficiency tend to appear "cherubic" and exhibit youthful facial features, higher pitched voices, delayed dentition, "ripply" abdominal fat, decreased muscle mass, delayed skeletal maturation, and delayed sexual maturation.

Collaborative Care

The goal of collaborative care is attainment of maximum adult height potential.

Diagnostic Tests

Any child whose height is 2 to 3 standard deviations below the mean height for age or whose measurement is falling off the normal growth chart should be evaluated for short stature (Table 32–4). A child whose screening tests reveal low levels of insulin-like growth factors (IGF-1) requires further evaluation by a pediatric endocrinologist. A careful history, physical examination, assessment of pubertal development and unusual facies, and radiologic studies are necessary to rule out familial short stature and constitutional growth delay, which are normal variants, and skeletal dysplasias or psychosocial short stature, which requires further evaluation.

In some cases, the onset of puberty is delayed with GnRH analogs to provide more time for growth hormone therapy to stimulate growth. Provocative growth hormone testing, in which various

TABLE 32–4	Diagnostic Tests for Short Stature
TEST	**PURPOSE RELATED TO SHORT STATURE**
IGF-1 and IGFBP-3	Screens for growth hormone deficiency
MRI of the pituitary gland	Detects pituitary malformation or tumor
Provocative growth hormone testing	Tests for growth hormone deficiency
Bone age	Identifies other potential causes of delayed growth
Karyotype (girls)	Detects Turner syndrome (see page 1139)
Thyroid function studies	Detects hypothyroidism (see page 1108)
ACTH and cortisol levels	Detects other pituitary hormonal deficiencies
Urine creatinine, pH, specific gravity, urea nitrogen, electrolytes	Detects chronic renal failure (see Chapter 31 🔗)
Complete blood count and erythrocyte sedimentation rate	Screens for inflammatory bowel disease with anemia
Antigliadin antibodies	Screens for celiac disease

Source: Data from Parks, J. S., & Felner, E. I. (2011). Hypopituitarism. In R. M. Kliegman, B. F. Stanton, J. W. St. Geme III, N. F. Schor, & R. E. Behrman, Nelson textbook of pediatrics (19th ed., pp. 1876–1881). Philadelphia, PA: Saunders Elsevier; Cooke, D. W., Divall, S. A., & Radovick, S. (2011). Normal and aberrant growth. In S. Melmed, K. S. Polonsky, P. R. Larsen, & H. M. Kronenberg, Williams textbook of endocrinology (12th ed., pp. 935–1053). Philadelphia, PA: Saunders Elsevier.

BOX 32–2	FDA-Approved Uses of Growth Hormone in Children

- Growth hormone deficiency
- Renal failure
- Turner syndrome
- Noonan syndrome
- Short stature from Prader-Willi syndrome (PWS)
- Children with a history of intrauterine growth retardation
- Idiopathic short stature

Source: Data from Cooke, D. W., Divall, S. A., & Radovick, S. (2011). Normal and aberrant growth. In S. Melmed, K. S. Polonsky, P. R. Larsen, & H. M. Kronenberg, Williams textbook of endocrinology (12th ed., pp. 935–1053). Philadelphia, PA: Saunders Elsevier; Ferguson, L. A. (2011). Growth hormone use in children: Necessary or designer therapy? Journal of Pediatric Health Care, 25(1), 24–30; Sperling, M. A. (2010). Treatment of short children with GH plus IGF-1: Are two hormones better than one? Infectious Diseases in Children, 23(1), 46–48.

medications (arginine, clonidine, glucagon, insulin, L-dopa) are administered to stimulate release of growth hormone, may be used to confirm growth hormone deficiency. Confirmation of the disorder is based on failure to demonstrate a growth hormone response (with a GH level greater than 10 ng/mL) after presentation of two provocative stimuli as previously mentioned. However, some endocrinologists believe this test is less reliable than other tests, such as low IGF-1 levels. Growth hormone deficiency may occur alone or with one or more other pituitary hormone deficiencies. It may be total deficiency (no growth hormone produced) or partial deficiency (some growth hormone produced, but not enough to support normal growth).

Early diagnosis and treatment are important to ensure attainment of maximum adult height potential. **Bone age** (an estimation of skeletal maturity) is used to evaluate the child with a growth problem and can be used to predict final height. Radiographic imaging of the hand or wrist bone is used to evaluate the stage of bone ossification and thus the bone age of the child. Using standardized norms for bone ossification, radiologists can determine if the child's chronologic and bone ages match. Significantly delayed (less than the child's age) or advanced (greater than the child's age) bone age may be indicative of a systemic chronic disease or hormone abnormality requiring investigation (Figure 32–4 ■).

Clinical Therapy

For growth hormone deficiency, replacement therapy with GH is administered to promote growth and development. Growth hormone replacement requires subcutaneous injections 6 to 7 times per week and generally continues for several years until growth is complete. The pediatric endocrinologist adjusts the dosage based on response to treatment (Ferguson, 2011). See Box 32–2.

The child usually experiences increased growth velocity for the first year of treatment, followed by a gradual decrease in growth for subsequent months or years. Growth should progress at least at the normal growth rate for age while the child is continued on growth hormone treatment. If growth is slower than anticipated, compliance to therapy must be considered before the dosage is increased. Replacement therapy is continued until either the child achieves an acceptable height or growth velocity drops to less than 2 cm (1 in.)

As They Grow   Bone Age

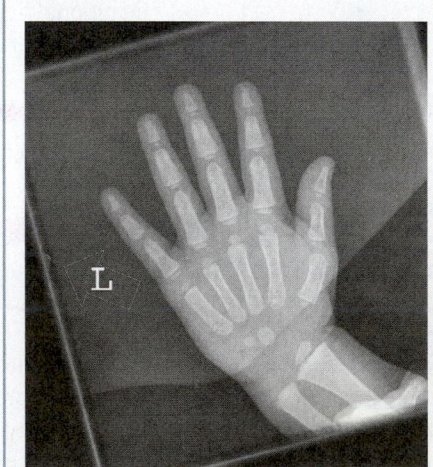
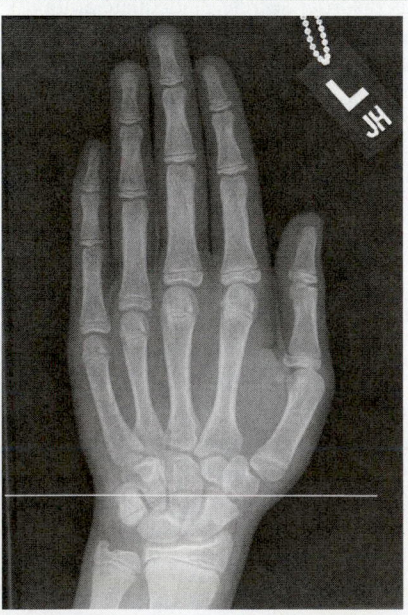

FIGURE 32–4 ■ The radiograph of the hand and wrist of a 3-year-old and 13-year-old girl reveal significant differences in skeletal maturation that are closely tied to physiologic maturation. The 3-year-old has many bones in the hand and wrist that have not fully developed. The secretion of estrogen during puberty has resulted in the development and calcification of secondary ossification centers of most of the bones in the hand and wrist of the 13-year-old.

Source: *Courtesy of Dorothy Bulas, M.D., Children's National Medical Center.*

per year. Additionally, a bone age of greater than 14 years in girls and 16 years in boys is criteria to stop treatment. In some cases, the onset of puberty is delayed with GnRH analogs to provide more time for growth hormone therapy to stimulate growth (Parks & Felner, 2011).

Side effects of growth hormone therapy are rare and include headache, progression of scoliosis, slipped capital femoral epiphysis, hypothyroidism, hyperglycemia, and intracranial hypertension (Cooke, Divall, & Radovick, 2011; Ferguson, 2011). Though rare, lipoatrophy may occur at growth hormone injection sites if sites are not rotated.

Practice Alert

Slipped capital femoral epiphysis has been associated with growth hormone therapy (Ferguson, 2011). Any child receiving growth hormone treatment who complains of hip pain or knee pain, or who manifests a limp, must be evaluated for this disorder (Cooke et al., 2011). See Chapter 35 for further information on this condition.

Nursing Management

Nursing care consists of monitoring growth, teaching the child and family about the disorder and its treatment, and providing emotional support.

Nursing Assessment and Diagnosis

The child's height and weight are carefully measured and plotted on a growth chart (refer to Appendix A) to monitor growth changes over time. Assess the child's psychosocial adaptation to short stature. Assess parents for coping with the child's short stature and treatment regimen.

Nursing diagnoses that apply to the child with growth hormone deficiency may include the following:

- Growth: Disproportionate, Risk for related to poor adherence to daily injection regimen
- Body Image, Disturbed related to short stature
- Self-Esteem, Chronic Low, Risk for related to physical appearance
- Knowledge, Deficient (Parent) related to growth hormone administration

NANDA-I © 2012

Planning and Implementation

Partner with the child and family in providing instructions regarding growth hormone replacement therapy and injection. Injections are given subcutaneously, and parents must understand site selection, safe administration, and the importance of site rotation. Some growth hormone preparations are available in injection pen form, which improves ease of preparation and delivery. Daily injections of growth hormone may be a source of major stress to the child. Assist the family in establishing techniques to minimize the trauma to the child who is receiving regular injections. Some growth hormone may require dilution before administration. Ensure parents utilize proper diluent techniques. Educate the family about potential side effects and actions to take if noticed.

Direct family members to educational resources such as the Magic Foundation and Human Growth Foundation. Replacement therapy is expensive, costing more than $52,000, and may not be covered by insurance (Ferguson, 2011).

Children with growth hormone deficiency, especially those due to tumors and trauma from radiation or surgery, may experience academic problems resulting from acquired learning disabilities. Before the child enters or returns to school, a comprehensive evaluation is performed to identify potential problems. Partner with the family and school officials to ensure that the child is appropriately screened.

Encourage parents and teachers to treat the child in an age-appropriate manner. The child should dress in clothing that reflects his or her chronologic age. Encourage parents to emphasize the child's strengths, support independence, and promote participation in age-appropriate activities to assist in the development of a positive self-image. Suggest that the child take part in sports in which ability does not depend on size (e.g., swimming, gymnastics, wrestling, ice skating, and martial arts). Identifying positive role models, people of short stature who accomplish their goals, also promotes a positive image. Refer the child for counseling if appropriate.

The best results occur when treatment is initiated at an early age, before psychologic effects of short stature become apparent and when attainment of near normal height can be reached. People often treat children who are short on the basis of their size rather than their age, and such children experience social prejudice about height. Teasing is a common problem. The teenage years may be particularly stressful because of adolescents' characteristic preoccupation with body image. Partner with the adolescent and family to promote positive coping mechanisms.

Evaluation

Outcomes of nursing care for the child with growth hormone deficiency may include the following:

- The child achieves linear growth that is near normal for adult height.
- The parents and child adhere to the treatment regimen, being able to identify side effects and appropriately administer growth hormone.
- The child demonstrates a positive body image.
- The child demonstrates positive self-esteem.

Growth Hormone Excess (Hyperpituitarism)

Hyperpituitarism, a disorder in which excessive secretion of growth hormone increases the growth rate, is rare in children. If combined with precocious puberty, a tumor of the hypothalamus may be present. Affected children can grow to 7 or 8 feet in height when oversecretion occurs before closure of the epiphyseal plates. If the disorder occurs after closure of the epiphyseal plates, **acromegaly** occurs. In acromegaly, abnormal growth of the hands and feet occurs as well as a protruding brow and lower jaw; the nasal bone enlarges, and spacing of the teeth increases.

Because tall stature is valued in our society, assessment of children, particularly males, with accelerated growth is often delayed. Any child whose predicted height exceeds that consistent with parental height should be evaluated for possible growth problems and underlying pathologic conditions.

A complete history is obtained, and physical examination and laboratory testing are performed. Increased levels of insulin-like growth factor (IGF-1) establish the diagnosis of hyperpituitarism. Radiologic examination for bone age is obtained to determine if the epiphyseal plates have begun to fuse. Radiologic studies are used to detect a tumor. Thorough evaluation is required to differentiate growth hormone excess from familial tall stature.

Treatment depends on the cause of the excessive growth and may involve surgical removal of a tumor or pituitary gland

Weblink | Growth Hormone Deficiency Resources

(hypophysectomy), radiation therapy, or radioactive implants. High doses of sex steroids are given to close the epiphyseal plates. The child may need lifelong pituitary hormone replacement following surgery.

Nursing Management

Early identification of the child with excessive growth rate is essential. Monitor growth trends and refer children whose height growth rate exceeds expected development for further evaluation and treatment to retard the accelerated growth rate. Nursing care focuses on educating the parents and child about the disorder and its treatment, providing emotional support, and, if surgery is required, providing preoperative and postoperative teaching and care (refer to Chapter 15 🔗).

Tall stature, like short stature, can be stressful for children. Tall children are often treated as if they are older than their chronologic age. Tall adolescents may have problems with self-image, and girls in particular may worry about their appearance. Partner with the child and family to promote a positive body image and self-esteem. Provide the child opportunities to express concerns regarding body image.

Diabetes Insipidus

Diabetes insipidus is a disorder of the posterior pituitary gland and is defined as an inability of the kidneys to concentrate urine. Two forms of diabetes insipidus occur, central (neurogenic) and nephrogenic diabetes insipidus. Central diabetes insipidus results from inadequate production of vasopressin (antidiuretic hormone), and nephrogenic diabetes insipidus results from ineffective action of vasopressin in the kidneys (McHugo & Harden, 2011).

Etiology and Pathophysiology

Normally, fluid balance is maintained by actions of the hypothalamus, kidney, and pituitary gland by the following mechanisms:

- The antidiuretic hormone (ADH) is produced by the hypothalamus and is stored in the posterior pituitary gland.
- The hypothalamus detects dehydration and sends a message to the pituitary, which in turn releases antidiuretic hormone into the blood and carries it to the kidney.
- In the kidney, antidiuretic hormone acts on the collecting and distal tubules to reabsorb water—promoting concentration of urine and *retention* of fluids (decreased urine output) to restore fluid balance.
- When excess fluid volume occurs, the hypothalamus sends a message to the pituitary to inhibit secretion of antidiuretic

hormone, promoting *excretion* of fluids to restore fluid balance.

Plasma osmolarity, or the concentration of solutes in the blood, is an important factor in ADH secretion. Osmolarity is sensed in the hypothalamus by osmoreceptor neurons, and those neurons provide feedback to the posterior pituitary gland to produce appropriate antidiuretic hormone.

- A low serum osmolality causes a reduction in antidiuretic hormone production, which leads to increased urine output and increased serum sodium (from hemoconcentration).
- An elevated serum osmolality causes an increase in antidiuretic hormone production, which leads to water retention and decreased urine output.

ADH facilitates concentration of the urine by stimulating reabsorption of water from the distal tubule of the kidney. When ADH is inadequate, the tubules do not resorb water, leading to **polyuria** (passage of a large volume of urine in a given period). Therefore, the body is unable to conserve water, resulting in severe dehydration.

Causes of central diabetes insipidus include brain tumors, brain trauma, central nervous system infection, and neurosurgery (McHugo & Harden, 2011). Genetic nephrogenic diabetes insipidus is not as common as the acquired type, but its presentation is more severe. Acquired nephrogenic diabetes insipidus may be caused by drug toxicity, an adverse drug reaction, or illnesses that impair the ability of the kidneys to concentrate urine (Breault & Majzoub, 2011).

Clinical Manifestations

Polyuria and **polydipsia** (excessive thirst) are the cardinal signs of diabetes insipidus. Enuresis is common in children. Polydipsia is the body's attempt to preserve fluid balance. Additional manifestations observed in children with diabetes insipidus include hypernatremia, dilute urine, and dehydration. See the Clinical Manifestations table for signs and symptoms associated with the cause.

Although the onset of symptoms is often sudden, the diagnosis is often delayed. Children who can quench their thirst may not complain to parents about symptoms. In infants, symptoms may include irritability, lethargy, vomiting, poor feeding, failure to thrive, and constipation (Buckley & Walsh, 2011; McHugo & Harden, 2011). Their diapers are typically saturated. Dehydration in the infant is manifested by sunken fontanels, sunken eyes, and mottled skin. Older children exhibit excessive fluid intake, nocturia, poor appetite, and delayed growth. Seizures may occur in response to extreme

Clinical Manifestations   Diabetes Insipidus

ETIOLOGY	CLINICAL MANIFESTATIONS	CLINICAL THERAPY
Central diabetes insipidus ADH (vasopressin) deficiency Familial or idiopathic	Polyuria, polydipsia Nocturia, enuresis Thirsty at night Irritable if fluids withheld Constipation, fever, dehydration	Desmopressin acetate
Nephrogenic diabetes insipidus Inherited or acquired Decreased responsiveness of kidneys to ADH (vasopressin)	Polyuria, polydipsia Hypernatremia in neonatal period Dehydration, fever, vomiting Mental status changes	Diuretics High fluid intake Salt and protein restricted diet

electrolyte imbalances. Hypotension, tachycardia, and poor perfusion due to dehydration may also occur.

In all forms of diabetes insipidus, the urine cannot be concentrated, no matter how dehydrated the child becomes. A dehydration episode usually leads to the diagnosis. The serum sodium concentration and osmolality increase rapidly to pathologic levels. Often an unconscious child is admitted to the emergency department with dehydration and hypernatremia.

Collaborative Care

The goals of collaborative care include restoration and maintenance of fluid and electrolyte balance using fluid and pharmacologic management, identifying and correcting the underlying pathology, and preventing complications associated with the disorder. Early recognition and treatment are essential to prevent complications, such as secondary neurologic impairment associated with hypernatremic dehydration (see Chapter 23).

Diagnostic Tests

Initial testing involves serum electrolyte concentrations and a urinalysis including specific gravity and osmolality. Serum osmolality is increased (greater than 300 mOsm/kg), and urine osmolality is decreased (less than 300 mOsm/kg) (Breault & Majzoub, 2011). Urine specific gravity is decreased (less than 1.005), and serum sodium is elevated (greater than 145 mEq/L) (Buckley & Walsh, 2011). An MRI may be ordered to visualize the pituitary gland to detect a tumor. Diagnosis is confirmed by a water deprivation test, which is usually conducted in the inpatient setting.

Clinical Tip
During the water deprivation test, advise parents that the child will be frustrated and irritable from thirst. No one should drink in front of the child during the testing period. Monitor the child's vital signs, intake, output, and weight carefully (McHugo & Harden, 2011).

Clinical Therapy

Children who can access water and who have an intact thirst mechanism can maintain serum sodium and osmolality status; however, medications decrease polyuria and polydipsia. Fluid management may be the safest and preferred treatment in infants (Breault & Majzoub, 2011).

Practice Alert
When the child with diabetes insipidus has an acute illness, the child's physician should be notified immediately. Dehydration and hypernatremia may develop rapidly, and hypernatremia can cause intellectual disability, seizures, and cerebral calcification. Intravenous fluids will be needed to prevent or treat dehydration. See Chapter 23 . Serum sodium and serum osmolality must be carefully monitored.

Pharmacologic treatment for neurogenic diabetes insipidus Central ADH deficiency is treated by intranasal or oral desmopressin acetate (DDAVP). The medication reduces urinary output, enabling the child to live a more normal life with a decrease in thirst and nocturia. The dose of DDAVP is based on route of administration, age, and response to therapy (McHugo & Harden, 2011).

Pharmacologic treatment for nephrogenic diabetes insipidus Nephrogenic diabetes insipidus is treated with thiazide diuretics, which promote sodium excretion and stimulate the proximal

tubule to reabsorb water. Indomethacin and amiloride may also be prescribed to have an additive effect on decreased water excretion (Breault & Majzoub, 2011). The child's sodium and potassium levels must be carefully monitored to prevent hypernatremia and hypokalemia (see Chapter 23) (McHugo & Harden, 2011).

Nursing Management

Nursing care centers on administering medications and teaching parents how to manage the condition and recognize signs of altered fluid status.

Nursing Assessment and Diagnosis

Assess for signs of fluid volume deficit. Weigh the child and compare to previous weight when healthy to detect fluid volume loss. Assess skin integrity and mucous membranes. Assess fontanels in infants. Monitor intake and output and assess thirst or water craving. Monitor vital signs to detect changes in blood pressure and heart rate. Assess level of consciousness or responsiveness as the child is usually irritable or lethargic as a result of hypernatremia and dehydration. Observe the cardiac monitor for rhythm disturbances associated with electrolyte imbalances. Assess the child's sleeping pattern.

Clinical Tip
A weight loss of 2 pounds indicates a loss of 1 liter of fluid.

Nursing diagnoses that apply to the child with diabetes insipidus may include the following:

- Urinary Elimination, Impaired related to polyuria
- Fluid Volume, Deficient related to polyuria
- Sleep Pattern, Disturbed related to nocturia and enuresis
- Skin Integrity, Risk for Impaired related to incontinence
- Therapeutic Regimen Management: Family, Ineffective related to dietary and medication plan adherence

NANDA-I © 2012

Planning and Implementation

Care in the hospital includes fluid replacement either orally or intravenously. Monitor urine specific gravity as indicated and report decreasing values. Monitor serum osmolality and sodium for increasing values. Keep fluids within the child's reach at all times, with the exception of testing restrictions. Implement preventive measures for skin integrity if the child is incontinent.

Care in the Community

Educate parents about making fluids available to the child as needed, administering DDAVP, obtaining and recording daily weights, measuring intake and output, and recognizing signs of dehydration (see Chapter 23). Parents may need to weigh diapers to monitor urine output in infants. Cold fluids are often preferred and help relieve thirst. The child's fluid intake will need to be adjusted to prevent dehydration during an illness. Children often wake to drink fluids at night, but infants will need to have fluids provided. Many infants have co-existing brain damage and need nasogastric or gastrostomy feeding to maintain adequate hydration and nutrition. However, care should be taken to avoid the intake of excessive fluid as the child will not be able to excrete the excess water load with DDAVP treatment.

The child with chronic diabetes insipidus should always wear a medical identification alert (tag, bracelet, or necklace) to indicate the presence of the disorder. Partner with the parents and school officials to make arrangements to provide the child unrestricted access to toilet facilities and water.

Parents may require assistance to manage the child's care. Arrangements for a visiting nurse, a home health nurse, or respite care may be required. Assist the family in obtaining the appropriate support needed.

Evaluation

Outcomes of nursing care for the child with diabetes insipidus may include the following:

- The child's frequency of urination is decreased; fluid balance is restored.
- The child obtains adequate rest and sleep for optimal growth and development.
- The parents and child demonstrate an understanding of disease management, administer medication correctly, and monitor and record intake, output, and weight.
- The child's skin integrity remains intact.

Syndrome of Inappropriate Antidiuretic Hormone

Syndrome of inappropriate antidiuretic hormone (SIADH) results from an excessive amount of serum ADH. It is seen in children with central nervous system infections, brain tumors, and brain trauma; in children with pulmonary disorders such as pneumonia, asthma, or cystic fibrosis; and in children receiving positive-pressure ventilation. Some medications, including diuretics and chemotherapy, have been associated with SIADH.

Etiology and Pathophysiology

Failure of normal feedback mechanisms from the hypothalamus, pituitary gland, and kidney results in excessive secretion of ADH, leading to water reabsorption despite the presence of low serum osmolality. ADH secretion causes increased permeability of the distal renal tubules and collecting ducts, resulting in water reabsorption, increased intravascular volume, and decreased urine output (Ferry & Pascual-y-Baralt, 2010). Elevated ADH can also cause suppression of the renin-angiotensin mechanism and sodium excretion. The outcome is **water intoxication** (an abnormal proportion of water to sodium in the extracellular fluid), hyponatremia, and cellular edema.

Clinical Manifestations

Manifestations of SIADH are related to water intoxication and hyponatremia, and include elevated blood pressure, distended jugular veins, crackles in lung fields, weight gain without edema, fluid and electrolyte imbalance, and concentrated urine with decreased urine output. As serum sodium levels continue to fall, lethargy, confusion, headache, an altered level of consciousness, seizures, and coma occur due to cerebral edema.

Collaborative Care

The goal of collaborative care is to restore fluid volume and electrolyte balance, and identify and correct the underlying cause of the disorder.

Diagnostic Tests

Laboratory findings include a high urine osmolality, elevated specific gravity, low serum osmolality, low serum sodium, and decreased blood urea nitrogen (Ferry & Pascual-y-Baralt, 2010).

Clinical Therapy

Treatment includes fluid management, medications, and treatment of the underlying condition when possible. Fluids are restricted to prevent further dilution of the blood. Medications include diuretics, demeclocycline to block action of ADH at the renal collecting tubules, and hypertonic saline IV fluids. Oral urea has recently been evaluated for treatment with promising results (Robinson & Verbalis, 2011). After the acute phase, a daily fluid allowance is calculated to two-thirds maintenance to prevent excess water intake and potential complications such as congestive heart failure or pulmonary edema. See Chapter 23 for calculation of the maintenance fluid amount for the child.

Nursing Management

The goal of nursing care is to promote maintenance of fluid and electrolyte balance and prevent complications associated with the disorder.

Nursing Assessment and Diagnosis

Assess for changes in level of consciousness, mentation, and cognition, including headache and seizure activity. Monitor vital signs, and intake and output. Weigh the child daily to assess for weight gain, which may indicate a sign of water intoxication. Assess nutritional intake status and appetite.

Nursing diagnoses that apply to the child with SIADH may include the following:

- Fluid Volume: Excess related to water retention
- Knowledge, Deficient related to disease process and treatment regimen
- Injury, Risk for related to the potential for seizures

NANDA-I © 2012

Planning and Implementation

Nursing care focuses on preventing injury and monitoring fluid balance, administering medications, and managing nutritional intake. Monitor intake and output, serum sodium, urine osmolality, and specific gravity. Educate the parents about the child's fluid restrictions and the hidden sources of water and fluids in foods to help avoid excessive fluid intake.

Care in the Community

Partner with the family to ensure understanding of home care instructions. Teach the importance of checking weight daily and reporting weight gain, which may indicate fluid retention. Refer the family to a nutritionist to assist in identifying hidden sources of water and fluids, such as fruit-flavored ice pops, gelatin, watermelon, and citrus fruit, to prevent excessive fluid intake.

Depending on the cause of the disorder, lifelong medication may be required. If the child is prescribed demeclocycline, emphasize to the family the importance of follow-up care since the drug has nephrotoxic side effects. The child should wear a medical identification alert tag, bracelet, or necklace identifying the disorder and treatment.

Evaluation

Outcomes of nursing care for the child with syndrome of inappropriate antidiuretic hormone may include the following:

- The child's fluid balance is restored.
- The child has adequate nutritional intake to promote growth and development.

- The child and family demonstrate understanding of the disorder, treatment regimen including fluid restriction and sources of sodium and water, and medication administration.
- The child is free from injury.

Precocious Puberty

Precocious puberty is defined as the appearance of any secondary sexual characteristics before 8 years of age in girls (breast development or pubic hair) and 9 years of age in boys (pubic hair or genital development) (Bordini & Rosenfield, 2011b). (See Developing Cultural Competence: Onset of Puberty.) Precocious puberty is 5 times more common in females than males. While 90% of cases of precocious puberty are idiopathic in females, only 50% of cases are idiopathic in males. Precocious puberty in males is likely related to an organic central nervous system disorder (Bordini & Rosenfield, 2011b).

Etiology and Pathophysiology

Earlier than expected secretion of the normal hormones responsible for pubertal changes is not usually associated with an endocrine system abnormality (an idiopathic problem). External sources of hormones such as anabolic steroids or estrogen may be identified. Central precocious puberty or true precocious puberty occurs when the hypothalamus is activated to secrete GnRH. Other potential causes include tumors of the ovary, adrenal gland, and pituitary gland, and a rare genetic condition known as McCune-Albright syndrome (Carel & Léger, 2008).

Clinical Manifestations

Isolated signs of premature sexual development such as **thelarche** (breast development), menarche (vaginal bleeding without other signs of sexual development), and adrenarche (development of pubic and axillary sexual hair) before 8 years of age in girls and 9 years of age in boys often need no treatment.

Children with central precocious puberty have an advanced bone age (premature skeletal maturation) and may appear unusually tall for their age. Their growth ceases prematurely, however, as the hormones stimulate early closure of the epiphyseal plates, resulting in short stature. Behavior changes may include mood swings and emotional lability.

Collaborative Care

The goal of collaborative care is to determine the cause of precocious puberty, decrease the growth rate, stabilize development of secondary sexual characteristics, and promote optimal growth and development.

Diagnostic Tests

Serum diagnostic studies include LH, FSH, testosterone, or estradiol. Provocative testing includes GnRH stimulation to confirm the

> ### Developing Cultural Competence
> **Onset of Puberty**
>
> Differences exist by race in the onset of thelarche in girls of normal weight. Non-Hispanic African American girls and Mexican American girls normally undergo breast development during the seventh year, about one year earlier than non-Hispanic White girls (Bordini & Rosenfield, 2011b).

diagnosis. Radiologic imaging of the brain, as well as a bone age, may be performed.

Clinical Tip

Hormone levels vary throughout the day, making it difficult to get a measurement of the child's peak hormone level. Provocative testing is used to measure hormone levels when an endocrine condition is suspected. A medication known to stimulate the secretion of the hormone being tested is administered and serial blood samples are collected to measure the child's response.

Clinical Therapy

Central nervous system (CNS) tumors require surgery, radiation, and/or chemotherapy. Treatment may be initiated immediately to slow or stop the progression of sexual development in children below the expected age of puberty. A GnRH agonist is administered (Carel & Léger, 2008). Treatment often continues until a more normal age for puberty is reached (e.g., 11 years in girls and 12 years in boys). Simple monitoring of growth patterns may be the only intervention for children closer to the lower expected age for puberty to begin.

Nursing Management

Nursing care focuses on educating the child and parents about the condition and its treatment, promoting growth and development, and providing emotional support.

Nursing Assessment and Diagnosis

A thorough history and physical examination are performed, including assessment of the child's secondary sexual characteristic development and sexual maturity rating using Tanner staging (see Chapter 7). Measure the child's height and weight and plot on a growth curve to detect changes in the growth rate from prior measurements. Assess the child's psychosocial adaptation to changes in body image. Assess for parental anxiety related to the child's physical changes.

Nursing diagnoses that apply to the child with precocious puberty may include the following:

- Body Image, Disturbed related to premature development of secondary sexual characteristics and rapid growth in height
- Growth: Disproportionate, Risk for related to accelerated growth and advanced bone age at an early age
- Coping: Family, Compromised related to early sexual maturation changes

NANDA-I © 2012

Planning and Implementation

Promoting Positive Body Image

The goal of nursing care is to promote a positive body image in the child and to ensure proper medication administration. Partner with the child and family to explain to the child in age-appropriate terms that physiologic changes are normal but occurring at an earlier than usual age. Reassure the child that friends will experience the same stages of development eventually. Emphasize to the family that the child's social, cognitive, and emotional development corresponds with his or her age, even though the physical development is advanced.

Children with precocious puberty become self-conscious as body changes occur. Provide the child opportunities to express concerns and discuss issues related to body changes. The child may need to practice role-playing as a coping mechanism to manage teasing by other children. Partner with the family to encourage dressing the child in a manner appropriate to his or her chronologic age, even though the child may look older. Provide privacy during physical examinations. Advise parents that they may need to discuss issues of sexuality with the child at an earlier age than normal. Refer the child and family for counseling if appropriate.

Medication Administration

Teach the family proper medication administration and adherence to the treatment regimen. Determine the family's ability to financially manage the cost of treatment. Assistance in covering the cost of therapy may be available through pharmaceutical companies and third-party payers. Refer the family to organizations that can assist them in obtaining support.

Evaluation

Expected outcomes of care for the child with precocious puberty include the following:

- The child demonstrates a positive body image.
- The child achieves growth stabilization and cessation of developing secondary sexual characteristics.
- The family and child demonstrate an understanding of the disorder and the treatment regimen.

DISORDERS OF THYROID FUNCTION

TSH = 0.5–40mU/m (handwritten)

The function of the thyroid gland is to regulate the rate of cellular metabolism. In children, the hormones are responsible for normal development of the muscular, skeletal, and nervous systems.

Thyroxine, triiodothyronine, and calcitonin are hormones secreted by the thyroid. Thyroxine (tetraiodothyronine or T_4) and triiodothyronine (T_3) maintain metabolism and regulate growth and development. T_4 is a **precursor**—a substance that precedes another substance or from which another substance is synthesized—to T_3. Calcitonin targets kidney and bone cells to regulate serum calcium ion concentrations. TSH controls T_3 and T_4 production; therefore, thyroid-stimulating hormone function is evaluated in all thyroid disorders.

The two major disorders of the thyroid gland—hypothyroidism and hyperthyroidism—are discussed in this section.

Hypothyroidism

Hypothyroidism, a disorder in which levels of active thyroid hormones (TH) are decreased, may be congenital or acquired. Congenital hypothyroidism occurs in approximately 1 in 3,000 live births and is twice as common among females as it is among males. In comparison to White infants, it is less prevalent among Black infants but more prevalent in Hispanic infants (LaFranchi, 2011).

Etiology and Pathophysiology

Thyroid hormones are important for growth and development and for the metabolism of nutrients and energy. When these hormones are not available for stimulation of other hormones or specific target cells, growth is delayed and intellectual disability develops.

Congenital hypothyroidism Congenital hypothyroidism is usually caused by a spontaneous gene mutation, an autosomal recessive genetic transmission of an enzyme deficiency, hypoplasia or aplasia of the thyroid gland, failure of the central nervous system–thyroid

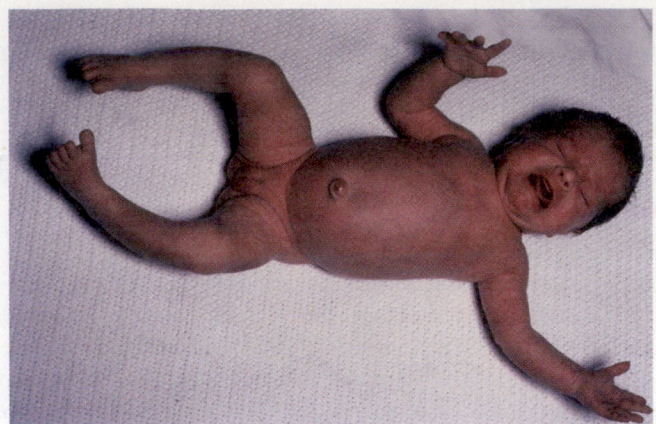

FIGURE 32–5 ■ Child with congenital hypothyroidism.
Source: © 2012 Wellcome Trust Library—Custom Medical Stock Photo, All Rights Reserved.

feedback mechanism to develop, or iodine deficiency. Intellectual disability is irreversible if the disorder is not treated. A small percentage of these cases are caused by hypothalamic-pituitary hypothyroidism and have TSH resistance. Some children have a transient form of congenital hypothyroidism due to transplacental transfer of maternal thyroid-blocking antibodies or antithyroid medications (LaFranchi, 2011).

Acquired hypothyroidism Acquired hypothyroidism can be idiopathic or result from autoimmune thyroiditis (Hashimoto thyroiditis), late-onset thyroid dysfunction, isolated TSH deficiency due to pituitary or hypothalamic dysfunction, or exposure to drugs or substances such as lithium that interfere with thyroid hormone synthesis. In the case of Hashimoto thyroiditis, the thyroid is infiltrated by lymphocytes that cause an autoimmune reaction and an enlarged thyroid. A genetic predisposition to autoimmune thyroiditis and an autosomal dominant inheritance of thyroid antibodies has been identified (LaFranchi, 2011).

Clinical Manifestations

Congenital hypothyroidism Infants with congenital hypothyroidism have few clinical signs of the disorder in the first weeks of life. In untreated infants, characteristic cretinoid features (thickened protuberant tongue, thick lips, and dull appearance) appear during the first few months of life (Figure 32–5 ■). Other signs include prolonged hypotonia, cool extremities, mottling, umbilical hernia, difficulty feeding, lethargy, constipation, and a hoarse cry (Péter & Muzsnai, 2009).

Acquired hypothyroidism Children with acquired hypothyroidism have many of the same signs as adults: decreased appetite, dry cool skin, thinning hair or hair loss, depressed deep tendon reflexes, bradycardia, constipation, sensitivity to cold temperatures, abnormal menses, and a **goiter** (a nontender enlarged thyroid gland). Manifestations unique to children include changes in past normal growth patterns with a weight increase, decreased height velocity, delayed bone and dental age, muscle hypertrophy with muscle weakness, and delayed or precocious puberty. However, children with acquired hypothyroidism may not exhibit the typical symptoms. The disorder should be suspected in the presence of a family history or other conditions—for example, another autoimmune disease such as diabetes—that predispose the child to acquired hypothyroidism.

TABLE 32–5	Diagnostic Laboratory Values for Testing Thyroid Function	
DIAGNOSTIC STUDY	**HYPOTHYROIDISM**	**HYPERTHYROIDISM**
Serum T_4 (tests level of thyroxine)	Decreased	Markedly elevated
Serum T_3 (tests level of triiodothyronine)	Normal	Markedly elevated
Serum TSH (tests level of thyroid-stimulating hormone)	Elevated	Decreased

Note: *Normal values vary based on infant/child age.*

A major complication associated with hypothyroidism is **myxedema,** a life-threatening crisis of hypothyroidism. Myxedema occurs when levels of thyroid hormone are extremely low. The disorder is characterized by nonpitting edema, puffy face and tongue, severe metabolic disorders, and hypothermia, with progression to hypoglycemia, hypotension, cardiovascular collapse, and coma (called myxedema coma) (Brent & Davies, 2011; Ganie & Kalra, 2010). This complication is rare in children.

Collaborative Care

Goals of collaborative care include early identification of the disorder, treatment with thyroid hormone for restoration of normalized thyroid function, and promotion of optimal growth and development.

Diagnostic Tests

Congenital hypothyroidism is usually detected during newborn screening, which is mandatory in all 50 states. Newborn screening has greatly reduced the incidence of intellectual disability associated with this disorder (Péter & Muzsnai, 2009). Most newborn screening programs screen for thyroxine (T_4) as the initial screening test and utilize TSH levels for confirmation. Some programs use both tests for initial screening (Pass & Neto, 2009). A decreased T_4 and elevated TSH level indicate hypothyroidism. TSH levels are often above 100 mU/L in congenital hypothyroidism (LaFranchi, 2011) (Table 32–5). An elevated TSH level indicates that the disease originated in the thyroid, not the pituitary. The screening is generally performed between 2 and 5 days of life. Rapid response from the laboratory that is testing the samples is important to reduce the time to diagnosis and the effects of hypothyroidism on the infant's development. Once there is notification of an abnormal screen, the infant should be evaluated for symptoms. A thyroid scan or ultrasound of thyroid to confirm presence and position of the thyroid gland and radiologic examinations of bone growth may also be performed.

Antithyroid antibodies are measured in children with a goiter and suspected Hashimoto thyroiditis, as increased titers of antithyroglobulin and antimicrosomal antibodies are often found.

Clinical Therapy

Oral levothyroxine (Synthroid) is the treatment of choice. The recommended starting dose for newborns with congenital hypothyroidism is 10 to 15 mcg/kg per day (Counts & Varma, 2009). The dose is increased gradually as the child grows to ensure a **euthyroid** (thyroid hormones in appropriate balance) state. A pediatric endocrinologist monitors treatment. Periodic evaluation of T_4 and TSH serum levels is necessary to assess for signs of excess or inadequate

thyroid hormone. A trial without medication may be attempted when the child is about 3 years of age if the child has not required increasing doses of levothyroxine to maintain the TSH level. If the TSH level is elevated and the T_4 level is low off therapy, permanent hypothyroidism is confirmed and treatment is resumed (Counts & Varma, 2009).

Practice Alert

Soy formulas should not be used in children who are being treated for hypothyroidism as they reduce the absorption of T_4 (Counts & Varma, 2009).

To ensure an adequate growth rate and prevent intellectual disability, the hormone must be taken throughout life. Children with congenital hypothyroidism that is diagnosed before 3 months of age have the best prognosis for optimal cognitive development. Children with acquired hypothyroidism usually have normal growth following a period of catch-up growth. Many adolescents with Hashimoto thyroiditis have a spontaneous remission.

Nursing Management

Nursing care focuses on educating the parents and child about the disorder and its treatment, monitoring the child's growth rate, and promoting optimal growth and development.

Nursing Assessment and Diagnosis

Routine neonatal screening is performed before discharge from the hospital and is often repeated at the infant's first health visit to evaluate levels of circulating thyroid hormones. If the nurse is making a home visit several days after discharge to assess the health of the mother and infant, the neonatal screening may be performed at that visit. Neonatal screening must be ensured for all infants, whether they are born in the hospital or at home.

Serial measurements and recording of height and weight are performed at each follow-up visit with growth parameters plotted on a growth curve. Assess the child for signs of inadequate growth to determine if the dose of thyroid hormone requires adjustment and to monitor adherence with medication. Conduct developmental screenings to detect delays in achievement of developmental milestones.

Nursing diagnoses appropriate for the child with hypothyroidism may include the following:

- Development, Delayed, Risk for related to late initiation of thyroid replacement therapy
- Growth: Disproportionate, Risk for related to poor adherence to thyroid hormone therapy
- Body Image, Disturbed related to physical changes associated with condition
- Fatigue related to inadequate dose of thyroid medication

NANDA-I © 2012

Planning and Implementation

Nursing care focuses on teaching the parents and child about the disorder and its treatment and monitoring the child's growth rate. Explain how to administer thyroid hormone, which is only available in tablet form (e.g., tablets can be crushed and mixed in a small amount of formula or applesauce, as long as it can be ensured that the child gets all of the medication). Advise parents that the child may experience temporary sleep disturbances or behavioral changes in response to therapy. Teach the parents how to assess for an increased pulse rate, which could indicate the presence of too much thyroid hormone, and advise them to report problems such as fatigue, which could indicate an improper drug dose that needs to be adjusted.

Caution parents to dress the child appropriately for the season to prevent hypothermia. Modify the child's diet by increasing the amount of fruits and bulk if constipation is a problem.

Reassure the family that the child has the best chance of normal development when the hormone replacement therapy is given as prescribed. Reinforce the importance of follow-up visits to assess growth rate and response to therapy and to regulate drug dosages as the child grows. Periodic assessments of educational achievement are needed. Even with good control, adolescents may have persistent visual-spatial deficits, and memory and attention problems. Parents should be informed that in most cases therapy will be lifelong and it is needed to promote the child's cognitive development. When the cause is genetic, make a referral for genetic counseling. See Chapter 4 🔗.

Evaluation

Expected outcomes of nursing care for the child with hypothyroidism include the following:

- The child maintains adequate growth of height and weight, following a percentile curve throughout childhood.
- The child's cognitive development is appropriate for age.
- The child demonstrates a positive body image.
- The child participates in activities of daily living and other activities appropriate for age without experiencing fatigue.
- The parents (and child if older) demonstrate an understanding of the disorder and treatment regimen.
- Medications are administered properly and assessment for complications is ongoing.

Hyperthyroidism

Hyperthyroidism occurs when thyroid hormone levels are increased, resulting in excessive levels of circulating thyroid hormones. This leads to increased basal metabolic rate, cardiovascular function, gastrointestinal function, neuromuscular function, weight loss, and heat intolerance. It also leads to increased metabolism of fats, proteins, and carbohydrates. Hyperthyroidism is rare in children and adolescents. It occurs in only 0.02% of children, primarily in adolescents ages 11 to 15. The disorder is almost always due to Graves disease and occurs 5 times more often in females than in males (LaFranchi, 2011).

Etiology and Pathophysiology

Graves disease is an autoimmune disorder. Immunoglobulins produced by the B lymphocytes stimulate oversecretion of thyroid hormones, resulting in the clinical symptoms. It has a high familial incidence.

Other less common causes of hyperthyroidism result from thyroiditis and thyroid hormone-producing tumors, including thyroid adenomas and carcinomas, and pituitary adenomas. Congenital hyperthyroidism can occur in infants of mothers with Graves disease as a result of transplacental transfer of immunoglobulins. This condition generally resolves by 6 to 12 weeks of age but can last longer (LaFranchi, 2011).

Clinical Manifestations

Signs and symptoms are caused by hyperactivity of the sympathetic nervous system. Characteristic findings include an enlarged,

Clinical Manifestations (Graves Disease)	Hyperthyroidism
SYSTEM	**CLINICAL MANIFESTATIONS**
Cardiovascular	Palpitations Tachycardia Hypertension
Neuromuscular	Eyelid lag Fatigue Irritability Muscle weakness Nervousness, restlessness Pruritus Tremors
Endocrine	Diaphoresis Heat intolerance Increased growth rate Goiter Exophthalmos
Gastrointestinal	Frequent bowel movements Increased appetite Nausea Thirst Weight loss
Genitourinary	Urinary frequency, nocturia
Psychosocial	Anxiety Behavioral problems Declining school performance Emotional lability Inability to concentrate Insomnia

Source: *Data from Bahn, R. S., Burch, H. B., Cooper, D. S., Garber, J. R., Greenlee, C., Klein, I., . . . Stan, M. N. (2011). Hyperthyroidism and other causes of thyrotoxicosis: Management guidelines of the American Thyroid Association and American Association of Clinical Endocrinologists. Thyroid, 21(6), 593–646; Bauer, A. J. (2011). Approach to the pediatric patient with Graves' disease: When is definitive therapy warranted? Journal of Clinical Endocrinology and Metabolism, 96(3), 580–588; Fitzgerald, P. A. (2012). Endocrine disorders. CURRENT medical diagnosis & treatment 2012. New York, NY: McGraw-Hill.*

nontender thyroid gland (goiter), prominent or bulging eyes (**exophthalmos**) (Figure 32–6 ■), eyelid lag, tachycardia, nervousness, restlessness or irritability, increased appetite with weight loss,

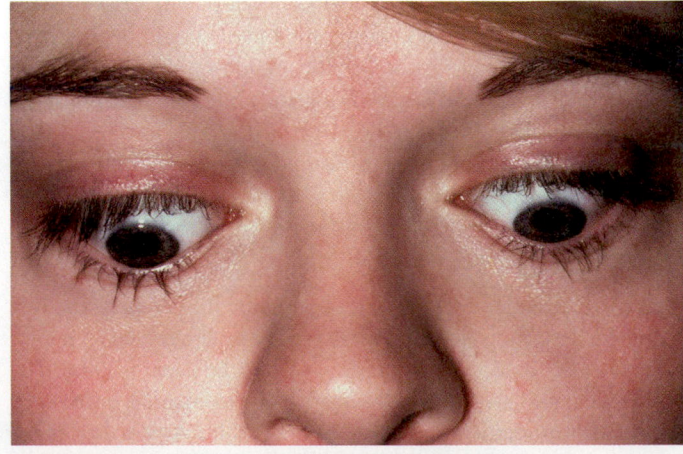

FIGURE 32–6 ■ Exophthalmos in an adolescent with Graves disease.
Source: *Wellcome Images/Custom Medical Stock Photography.*

Medications Used in Management of Hyperthyroidism

MEDICATION	ACTION OR INDICATION	NURSING MANAGEMENT
Antithyroid medications Methimazole (Tapazole) Propylthiouracil (PTU)	Inhibits thyroid hormone secretion	Monitor for side effects including fever, rash, mild leukopenia, nausea, arthralgia, pruritus, hives, and mild increase in liver enzymes; more serious side effects include liver and bone marrow failure. Emphasize the importance of taking medications as prescribed and to take them at the same time each day. Monitor for symptoms of hypothyroidism.
Propranolol Atenolol Metroprolol	Beta-blocking agent Decreases beta-adrenergic activity to relieve tremors, tachycardia, anxiety, heat intolerance, and restlessness	Monitor for side effects including hypotension and bradycardia. Emphasize the importance of taking the medication as prescribed.
Radioiodine Oral, in solution or capsule	Produces radiation thyroiditis and fibrosis, resulting in euthyroid state	Assess for allergy to iodine. Antithyroid medications should be discontinued 5–7 days prior to treatment. Ensure adolescent is not pregnant before beginning treatment. Partner with family to ensure avoidance of physical contact with secretions (urine, stool, saliva, sweat) for several days following the treatment. Emphasize the importance of keeping follow-up appointments to monitor thyroid function. Hypothyroidism is a potential complication.

Source: *Data from LaFranchi, S. (2011). Disorders of the thyroid gland. In R. M. Kliegman, B. F. Stanton, J. W. St. Geme III, N. F. Schor, & R. E. Behrman,* Nelson textbook of pediatrics *(19th ed., pp. 1894–1923). Philadelphia, PA: Saunders Elsevier; Rivkees, S. A. (2010). Pediatric Graves' disease: Controversies in management.* Hormone Research in Pediatrics, 74, *305–311; Wilson, B. A., Shannon, M. T., & Shields, K. M. (2011).* Pearson nurse's drug guide 2011. *New York, NY: Pearson.*

emotional lability, heat intolerance, diaphoresis, insomnia, tremor, and muscle weakness. The thyroid gland may be slightly enlarged or grow to three to four times its normal size; feel warm, soft, and fleshy; and have an auditory bruit on auscultation. See the table for clinical manifestations of hyperthyroidism. Onset is subtle, and the condition often remains unrecognized for 1 to 2 years.

Children with Graves disease usually have difficulty concentrating, behavioral problems, and declining performance in school. They become easily frustrated in the classroom and overheated and fatigued during physical education class. Children with this disorder find it difficult to relax or sleep. These symptoms usually prompt parents to seek medical treatment for the child.

Collaborative Care

Management includes identifying hyperthyroidism, inhibiting excessive secretion of thyroid hormones, and promoting normal growth and development.

Diagnostic Tests

Diagnostic studies include laboratory evaluation of serum TSH, T_3 and T_4 levels, and a thyroid scan. T_3 and T_4 levels are markedly elevated while the TSH level is decreased. Serum studies are also performed to detect thyroid autoantibodies anti-TG (anti-thyroglobulin) and anti-TPO (anti-peroxidase), usually present in Graves disease and Hashimoto thyroiditis. In addition, a thyroid scan is performed to identify nodules or to confirm the high uptake of radioactive iodine associated with Graves disease.

Clinical Therapy

The goal of clinical therapy is to inhibit excessive secretion of thyroid hormones. Treatment may include medication therapy, radiation therapy, or surgery (Glaser & Styne, 2008).

Medication therapy Medication therapy is most often the initial treatment, but compliance is often a problem because of side effects. Methimazole (Tapazole) and propylthiouracil (PTU) are antithyroid drugs that are used in children with hyperthyroidism (Rivkees, 2010). Due to the concern for severe liver disease with the administration of PTU, current recommendations are that children with hyperthyroidism receive methimazole instead (Bauer, 2011; LaFranchi, 2011; Rivkees, 2010). See the Medications table on this page.

It is estimated that 20% to 30% of children achieve remission after a 1- to 2-year course of treatment with medication (Leger, Gelwane, Kaguelidou, et al., 2012; Rivkees, 2010). Symptoms usually improve within weeks of starting treatment. Adjunct therapy with beta-adrenergic blocking agents such as propranolol, atenolol, or metoprolol may be administered to relieve symptoms of tremors, tachycardia, lid lag, and excessive sweating (Bahn, Burch, Cooper, et al., 2011; LaFranchi, 2011).

Radiation therapy If medication therapy is ineffective, radiation therapy using oral radioactive iodine (RAI) is the next treatment choice. Current data do not indicate a relationship between radioactive iodine used to treat Graves disease in children and the development of thyroid cancer (Rivkees, 2010).

Surgical removal of thyroid Thyroidectomy (removal of most of the thyroid) provides an immediate cure and avoids radiation along with possible long-term complications of radioactive iodine. However, destruction or removal of the thyroid gland often results in permanent hypothyroidism, necessitating lifelong hormone replacement therapy (Kaguelidou, Carel, & Leger, 2009).

Manipulation of the parathyroid gland during surgery can result in excess release of parathyroid hormone, leading to hypercalcemia. Monitoring of serum calcium levels following a thyroidectomy is essential.

Nursing Management

Nursing care focuses on educating the child and parents about the disorder and its treatment, promoting rest, providing emotional support, and, if the child requires surgery, providing preoperative and postoperative teaching and care.

Nursing Assessment and Diagnosis

Assess the child's vital signs, as blood pressure and pulse may be elevated. Keep a record of food intake. Accurate measurement and recording of height and weight are important to establish a baseline and identify patterns of growth. Observe the child's behavior, activity, and level of fatigue.

If surgery is performed, assess the vital signs and monitor the child's surgical site. Assess the site postoperatively for bleeding, hoarseness, swelling, and difficulty breathing. Assess serum calcium levels. Monitor for signs of hypocalcemia by assessing Chvostek and Trousseau signs (see Chapter 23 🔗) for numbness and tingling of extremities or lips, and assessing for muscle twitching. Assess for thyrotoxicosis, as it can be life-threatening.

Practice Alert

The most serious complication of hyperthyroidism is severe thyrotoxicosis, also called thyroid crisis or thyroid storm. It is a life-threatening emergency resulting from extreme hyperthyroidism, in which elevated circulating levels of thyroid hormone result in a hypermetabolic state. Symptoms include muscle weakness, diaphoresis, tachycardia, tremor, palpitations, diarrhea, irritability, nervousness, and anxiety (Bahn et al., 2011; Bauer, 2011; Fitzgerald, 2012).

Assess the family's response to the chronic condition, as well as the family's response to the child's disturbing symptoms (e.g., irritability, heat intolerance, and muscle weakness). Common nursing diagnoses for the child with hyperthyroidism may include the following:

- Thermoregulation, Ineffective related to illness and excessive activity of the sympathetic nervous system
- Nutrition, Imbalanced: Less than Body Requirements related to high metabolic needs
- Body Image, Disturbed related to physical changes caused by illness (prominent eyes, excessive perspiration, and tremors)
- Fatigue related to hypermetabolic state and sleep deprivation

NANDA-I © 2012

Planning and Implementation

Promote increased caloric intake by providing five or six moderate meals per day. Encourage the child and family to express their feelings and concerns about the disorder, especially when deciding among the three treatment options or during the period when medication dosage adjustments are frequently needed. Pointing out even slight improvements in the child's condition may increase the child's adherence with therapy.

Promote Symptom Management

Children with hyperthyroidism are easily fatigued. Partner with the family and school officials to plan scheduled rest periods at school and to develop an education plan tailored to the child's needs during the state of hyperthyroidism. Emphasize to the family and teachers that home and physical activities should be kept to a minimum until symptoms resolve. Encourage parents to provide a cool environment and allow the child to wear fewer clothes until symptoms subside.

If exophthalmos is present, teach the family about measures to protect the eye. Encourage regular eye examinations and eye protection

measures such as safety tinted glasses, artificial tears as necessary, sleeping with the head of the bed elevated to minimize pressure on the optic nerve, and patching eyes at bedtime if the eyelid does not completely cover the eye. Report changes in vision or appearance of the eye.

Preoperative and Postoperative Care

Children who have partial or total removal of the thyroid gland receive antithyroid medications, such as iodine, for approximately 2 weeks before surgery to reduce the vascularity and size of the thyroid gland and to decrease the risk of thyroid storm.

Instruct parents to observe for side effects of antithyroid medications, including fever, urticaria, and lymphadenopathy. Ensure the child and family understand the medication therapy. Provide routine preoperative teaching (refer to Chapter 15 🔗). Explain the procedure to the child using developmentally appropriate terms. Young children in particular may be fearful about having their throat "cut."

Postoperatively, elevate the head of the bed to 30 degrees to promote patent airway. An endotracheal tube, oxygen, suction supplies, and IV calcium gluconate should be immediately available for emergency treatment of hypocalcemia and respiratory distress. If thyroidectomy is performed and thyrotoxicosis develops, it does not immediately resolve because the half-life of T_4 is 7 to 8 days. Antithyroid medications should be slowly tapered (Sharma & Barr, 2010).

Discharge Planning and Home Care Teaching

Emphasize to the child and family the need for lifelong thyroid hormone replacement if radiation or surgery is performed. Encourage the family to adjust food intake to prevent obesity because the child's metabolic rate declines and weight gain may occur. The child should wear a medical alert identification. Explain to the parents the importance of the child's scheduled follow-up visits for evaluation to ensure that the T_4 level is adequate to sustain growth and development.

Evaluation

Expected outcomes of nursing care for the child with hyperthyroidism may include the following:

- The child achieves balanced thermoregulation.
- The child maintains adequate nutritional intake to meet growth and development needs.
- The child participates in activities of daily living without experiencing fatigue.
- The child demonstrates a positive body image.

DISORDERS OF THE PARATHYROID

Children usually have four parathyroid glands located posterior to the thyroid gland. Their primary function is to work in conjunction with vitamin D to regulate total body calcium. Ionized calcium influences release of parathyroid hormone, which acts on both bone and the kidney to maintain normal serum levels. The hormone also acts on the kidney to increase vitamin D synthesis, which assists in calcium balance. It is related also to magnesium and phosphorus balance. Low magnesium levels stimulate parathyroid hormone release, and the hormone leads to lowered phosphate serum levels.

Hyperparathyroidism

Primary hyperparathyroidism, rare during childhood, may result from a tumor (adenoma) or hyperplasia (Doyle, 2011). Secondary hyperparathyroidism is due to disease outside of the parathyroid gland, leading to excessive secretion of parathyroid hormone. This is commonly seen in chronic renal failure when the kidneys are unable to reabsorb calcium, causing low serum calcium levels and stimulating continual secretion of parathyroid hormone to maintain normal serum calcium levels (Molina, 2010). See Chapter 31 🖉 for further discussion of renal failure. Secondary hyperparathyroidism can also result from malabsorption syndromes or diets deficient in calcium or vitamin D, or which contain excessive phosphorus. Transient neonatal hyperparathyroidism has been reported in a small number of infants whose mothers had hypoparathyroidism or pseudohyperthyroidism that was untreated or inadequately treated. The bones are the primary area of involvement and generally heal between 4 and 7 months of age (Doyle, 2011).

At any age, symptoms of primary hyperparathyroidism may include bone pain, nephrolithiasis (kidney stones), and pathologic bone fractures. Hypercalcemia may cause symptoms of muscle weakness, peptic ulcer disease, fatigue, volume depletion, and subtle mental disturbance. Abdominal pain may be present and may indicate pancreatitis (Potts & Jüppner, 2012).

Collaborative Care

There is often a delay between development of symptoms and diagnosis. Elevated serum calcium and parathyroid hormone (PTH) levels are diagnostic. Radiographic images may reveal signs of rickets. For primary hyperparathyroidism, unilateral surgical parathyroid exploration is performed to remove the affected gland and biopsy the other gland on the same side (George, Acharya, Bandgar, et al., 2010). Treatment of secondary hyperparathyroidism focuses on prevention of hypercalcemia utilizing vitamin D replacement and phosphorus binders.

Nursing Management

Nursing care centers on fluid management and electrolyte monitoring. In children who require surgery, assess for respiratory distress and a potential airway obstruction due to edema and a potential hematoma around the tracheal space. Monitor for signs of infection.

Following surgery, educate the child and parents to recognize signs of hypocalcemia and appropriate calcium supplementation. After diagnosis or after surgical intervention, follow-up is important to monitor serum calcium and phosphorus levels to detect persistence of hyperparathyroidism.

Hypoparathyroidism

Primary hypoparathyroidism is rare but may result from congenital disorders (e.g., parathyroid aplasia, DiGeorge syndrome), surgical removal of the parathyroid glands (e.g., parathyroid adenoma, thyroidectomy), disease processes that destroy the parathyroid glands (Wilson disease, hemochromatosis), or medications (e.g., aluminum, asparagine, doxorubicin, cytosine, and arabinoside). Hypoparathyroidism can also be idiopathic. The primary result is hypocalcemia and hyperphosphatemia in the blood.

Infants may display hyperirritability, muscle rigidity, seizures, vomiting, abdominal distention, apneic episodes, intermittent cyanosis, or twitching. Muscle pain and cramps may progress to numbness, stiffness, and tingling of the hands and feet. A positive **Chvostek sign** (spasm of facial muscles after tapping facial nerve) may be present. Tetany and convulsions may occur with severe hypocalcemia (Doyle, 2011).

Collaborative Care

Serum calcium and PTH levels are low and serum phosphorus is elevated. Radiographs often demonstrate increased bone density. A 12-lead electrocardiogram (ECG) may demonstrate a prolonged QT interval.

In emergencies, intravenous calcium and calcitriol are administered to treat seizures, tetany, life-threatening hypotension, and cardiac arrhythmias. Oral calcitriol and calcium are prescribed. Foods with high phosphorus content (dairy products and eggs) are limited (Doyle, 2011).

Practice Alert

Dilute intravenous calcium per hospital protocol. Infiltration of IV calcium can cause extravasation and tissue sloughing. Always check the patency of the IV prior to administration. Monitor ECG during administration. Evaluate for hypocalcemia and hypercalcemia after administration.

Nursing Management

Assess and stabilize the airway, breathing, and circulation. In the acute care setting, children should be placed on a cardiorespiratory monitor. Maintain seizure precautions until normal serum calcium levels are attained. Obtain intravenous access and administer calcium supplementation as ordered.

Partner with the family to ensure their understanding of the need for calcium supplementation and reduced intake of phosphorus. Teach the family that periodic monitoring of calcium levels is important. Inform the family that hypoparathyroidism may require lifelong therapy.

DISORDERS OF ADRENAL FUNCTION

The adrenal glands are composed of the inner cortex and the outer medulla. The adrenal medulla secretes the **catecholamines** epinephrine and norepinephrine, which affect the nervous system, cardiovascular system, metabolic rate, temperature, and smooth muscles. The adrenal cortex produces the steroid hormones **glucocorticoids** (affect protein and carbohydrate metabolism and protect against stress) and **mineralocorticoids** (involved in regulation of fluid and electrolytes). Cortisol, the main glucocorticoid, affects the metabolism of proteins, glucose, and fats; stress responses; and inhibition of inflammation. The most important mineralocorticoid, aldosterone, maintains extracellular fluid volume and blood pressure by conserving sodium, chloride, water, and excretion of potassium by the kidneys.

Disorders of adrenal function discussed in this section are Cushing syndrome, congenital adrenal hyperplasia, adrenal insufficiency (Addison disease), and pheochromocytoma.

Cushing Syndrome and Cushing Disease

Cushing syndrome, also called adrenocortical hyperfunction, is characterized by a group of symptoms resulting from excess blood levels of glucocorticoids (especially cortisol) (Moriarty & Hoe, 2009; White, 2011). Cushing disease is a type of Cushing syndrome and is caused by a pituitary tumor.

Etiology and Pathophysiology

The most common cause of Cushing syndrome is the prolonged administration of glucocorticoid hormones (Fraser & Van Uum, 2010;

BOX 32–3	Cushing Syndrome and Corticosteroids

Cushingoid features occur most often in children receiving high doses of corticosteroids or corticosteroids over a prolonged period of time. Cushingoid features may develop in a shorter time than occurs with Cushing disease (see Figure 29–8B in Chapter 29). Corticosteroids suppress adrenal function when administered long term. These children have exogenous Cushing syndrome and are at increased risk of hypertension, hyperglycemia, weight gain, linear growth retardation, and fractures (White, 2011). These children may also exhibit mood swings and are at increased risk of infection (Wilson, Shannon, & Shields, 2011).

White, 2011). During infancy, most cases of endogenous Cushing syndrome are due to an adrenocortical tumor. The most common cause of endogenous Cushing syndrome in children older than 7 years of age is Cushing disease in which a pituitary tumor (adenoma) secretes excess ACTH. This leads to bilateral adrenal hyperplasia (White, 2011). The remainder of this discussion will focus on the child with Cushing syndrome caused by a pituitary tumor (Cushing disease). See Box 32–3 for a discussion of Cushing syndrome caused by corticosteroid administration.

Clinical Manifestations

Obesity is common in children with Cushing syndrome. Excessive weight gain is followed by slowed linear growth (Moriarty & Hoe, 2009). The child develops the characteristic cushingoid features that include a rounded (moon) face with prominent cheeks. Additional manifestations include hirsutism, acne, deepening of the voice, and hypertension (White, 2011). Older children may also experience delayed puberty, irregular menstrual periods, headaches, weakness, pathologic fractures, emotional problems, and hyperglycemia (Pluta, Burke, & Golub, 2011; White, 2011).

Collaborative Care

The goals of collaborative care for Cushing syndrome caused by a pituitary tumor (Cushing disease) are the surgical removal of the tumor, replacement of cortisol, restoration of normal physical appearance, and promotion of growth and development.

Diagnostic Tests

Diagnosis is based on characteristic physical findings and laboratory values, including increased 24-hour urinary levels of free cortisol and elevated nighttime salivary cortisol levels. The child will also have an abnormal glucose tolerance test (White, 2011). See Appendix D for usual laboratory values.

The adrenal suppression test with an 11 p.m. dose of dexamethasone reveals that adrenal cortisol output is not suppressed overnight as would occur normally in children. Computed tomography (CT) and magnetic resonance imaging (MRI) are used to detect the specific location of tumors in the adrenal and pituitary glands (Pluta et al., 2011; White, 2011).

Clinical Therapy

Surgical removal of the pituitary adenoma is the current treatment of choice when this is the cause of Cushing syndrome. Irradiation of the pituitary is performed when surgical removal of the adenoma does not substantially reduce cortisol levels. Bilateral removal of the adrenal glands may be necessary in some cases to stop the excessive secretion of cortisol. Lifelong hormone replacement is required when both adrenal glands are removed (Pluta et al., 2011; White, 2011).

Nursing Management

The nurse usually encounters a child with Cushing syndrome when the child has a pituitary tumor (Cushing disease) and is hospitalized for diagnostic evaluation or surgery. Nursing care focuses on assessment, management of symptoms, educating the family, and providing support.

Nursing Assessment and Diagnosis

Nursing assessment includes monitoring the child's vital signs, fluid status, nutritional status, and weight. Additional assessment includes monitoring muscle strength and endurance during hospital play activities.

Nursing diagnoses that apply to the child with Cushing syndrome caused by a pituitary tumor (Cushing disease) may include the following:

- Fluid Volume: Excess related to elevated serum sodium and fluid retention
- Infection, Risk for related to surgical incision
- Body Image, Disturbed related to body changes
- Anxiety (Child and Parent) related to surgical procedure and serious disorder

NANDA-I © 2012

Planning and Implementation

Partner with the child and family to ensure understanding of the disorder and its treatment. For children undergoing surgery, provide preoperative and postoperative teaching and care. Answer any questions the child and family may have and explain all laboratory and diagnostic tests. Explain to the parents and child that the cushingoid appearance is reversible with treatment. Provide nutritional guidance or refer the child and parents to a nutritionist to promote maintenance of an appropriate weight. Encourage the child to discuss feelings regarding changes in physical appearance. Assist the child and family to identify effective coping strategies.

Preoperative and postoperative teaching and care are similar to those for the child undergoing surgery (see Chapter 15). Refer to Chapter 29 for general nursing care of the child with cancer. Postoperatively, elevate the head of the bed 30 degrees to promote effective breathing. Take care to prevent tension on the incision line during repositioning.

For children who need cortisol replacement therapy following the surgical removal of both adrenal glands, administering the medication early in the morning or every other day causes fewer symptoms and mimics the normal diurnal pattern of cortisol secretion. Cortisol replacement in the postoperative period must be explained carefully to the parents. Hydrocortisone (Cortef, Solu-Cortef, cortisone acetate) is available in liquid, tablet, or injectable form. Parents may need to crush the tablet and mix with a small amount of applesauce, but the entire dose of medication must be taken. The oral preparations of cortisone have a bitter taste and can cause gastric irritation. Giving the dose at mealtimes and using antacids between meals helps reduce these side effects. Teach parents how and when to administer the injectable form—usually when the child is vomiting, has diarrhea, or cannot take the oral medication. Failure to give medication when the child is ill may lead to severe illness and cardiovascular collapse. See Partnering with Families: Hydrocortisone Administration on page 1115.

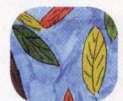

Partnering with Families

Hydrocortisone Administration

Teach the family the following tips regarding hydrocortisone administration:

- Always give the medication at times prescribed since the schedule follows the body's normal cortisol release pattern.
- Never abruptly discontinue the medication.
- The child should wear a medical identification alert.
- If the child has vomiting or diarrhea and is unable to take the medication by mouth, administer the injections to replace oral doses as instructed

and notify the physician immediately. Higher doses of hydrocortisone are needed when the child is ill.

- Always have injectable hydrocortisone available at home, at school, and everywhere the child travels. An emergency kit should be available at all times to supply cortisol to the child during acute illnesses and stressful situations. Check expiration dates frequently and maintain current medications in the emergency kit.

Evaluation

Examples of outcomes of care for the child with Cushing syndrome caused by a tumor include the following:

- The child achieves fluid volume balance.
- The child is free from infection.
- The child's appearance returns to a normalized state and the child exhibits positive body image.
- The family and child demonstrate understanding of the disease and treatment.
- The child and family are free from anxiety.

Congenital Adrenal Hyperplasia

Congenital adrenal hyperplasia (CAH), sometimes called adrenogenital syndrome, adrenocortical hyperplasia, or congenital adrenogenital hyperplasia, results from a deficiency of one of the enzymes necessary for the synthesis of cortisol and aldosterone. CAH is considered to be an inborn error of metabolism.

Etiology and Pathophysiology

Approximately 95% of children with congenital adrenal hyperplasia have a deficiency in 21-hydroxylase, which results in inadequate production of aldosterone and cortisol. This disorder occurs in 1 in 15,000 live births. This form has an autosomal recessive inheritance pattern, and the defective gene CYP21A2 is located on chromosome 6p21.3 (Ryzin, 2009).

Of the two classic forms of the disorder, 75% are salt-losing, caused by aldosterone deficiency and overproduction of androgen, and 25% are non-salt-losing with **virilization** (the production of masculine secondary sexual characteristics in females). In all forms, increased secretion of ACTH occurs in response to diminished cortisol levels (Kwon & Tsai, 2007).

During fetal development, the lack of cortisol triggers the pituitary to continue secretion of ACTH. This in turn stimulates overproduction of the adrenal androgens. Virilization of the female external genitalia begins in week 10 of gestation. If untreated after birth, the overproduction of androgens results in accelerated height, early closure of the epiphyseal plates, and premature sexual development with both pubic and axillary hair.

Clinical Manifestations

Congenital adrenal hyperplasia is the most common cause of **pseudohermaphroditism** (ambiguous genitalia) in newborn girls. The female infant is born with an enlarged clitoris and partial or complete

labial fusion. The vagina usually has a common opening with the urethra (Figure 32–7 ■). Females who are severely virilized may be mistaken for males with cryptorchidism, hypospadias, or micropenis. The uterus, ovaries, and fallopian tubes are normal. The male infant may look normal at birth or may have a slightly enlarged penis and hyperpigmented scrotum. The boy may have tall stature and an adult-sized penis by school age, but the testes are appropriately sized for age. Partial enzyme deficiency produces less obvious symptoms. Precocious puberty, tall stature for age, acne, and excessive muscle development may be noted in both males and females as the child grows. Due to early epiphyseal fusion, adult stature is shorter.

Signs of adrenal insufficiency may be the first indication of the disorder. Recurrent vomiting, dehydration, metabolic acidosis, hypotension, and hypoglycemia are characteristic signs of the salt-wasting form of the disorder. Hypertension with hypokalemic alkalosis is alternately found in children with 11-hydroxylase deficiency.

Collaborative Care

The goals of collaborative care are to identify the newborn with congenital adrenal hyperplasia, suppress adrenal secretion of androgens, maintain homeostasis, and correct ambiguous genitalia.

Diagnostic Tests

Diagnosis in infants and children is usually confirmed by laboratory evaluation of serum 17-alpha-hydroxyl progesterone (17-OHP)

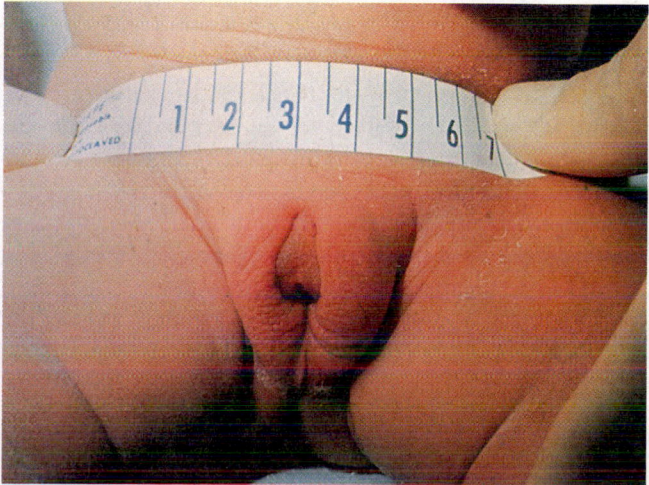

FIGURE 32–7 ■ Newborn girl with ambiguous genitalia.
Source: Courtesy of Patrick C. Walsh, MD.

level. Routine newborn screening for congenital adrenal hyperplasia is performed in all 50 states (National Newborn Screening and Genetics Resource Center, 2011). Prenatal diagnosis is available. In instances of ambiguous genitalia, a karyotype determines the infant's gender. (See Chapter 4 🔗.) Ultrasonography may be used to visualize pelvic structures.

In the salt-wasting form of the disorder, the child may have hyponatremia, hyperkalemia, acidosis, hypoglycemia, a high urine sodium level, and low serum and urinary aldosterone levels. Serum concentrations of testosterone in girls and androstenedione in boys and girls are elevated in affected infants. Measurement of ACTH and 17-hydroxyprogesterone levels reveals high readings, while serum cortisol is inappropriately low in comparison to ACTH (White, 2011). Diagnosis may be delayed in the non-salt-losing form until 3 to 7 years.

Clinical Therapy

The goal of treatment is to suppress adrenal secretion of androgens by replacing deficient hormones. Antenatal steroids (dexamethasone) have been shown to reduce the severity of genital masculinization in females with congenital adrenal hyperplasia. Continued use of dexamethasone in the postnatal period has been shown to be effective as well (Kulshreshtha, Khadgawat, Eunice, et al., 2010). Treatment of affected children is accomplished by the lifelong use of oral administration of glucocorticoids (dexamethasone, prednisone, or hydrocortisone). The glucocorticoid replacement reduces secretion of ACTH, which had overstimulated the adrenal cortex. As a result, excessive adrenal androgen production is suppressed. The dose is individualized by monitoring growth parameters, bone age, and hormone levels. If the infant has the salt-wasting form of the disorder, salt is added to the infant's formula and a mineralocorticoid (Florinef) is given to replace the missing hormone. Hormone dosage must be doubled or tripled during acute illnesses or injury and for surgery. Injectable hydrocortisone is administered for severe stress. Generally there are no side effects to the hormone; however, elevated doses can result in hypertension and growth impairment. Adrenalectomy is recommended only in cases in which medical therapy is ineffective (White, 2011).

Reconstructive surgery of the enlarged clitoris is often performed on girls during the first year of life; however, some centers support waiting until adolescence, allowing the patient to participate in the decision for surgery.

Nursing Management

Nursing care of the newborn with congenital adrenal hyperplasia focuses on teaching parents about the disorder and its treatment, providing emotional support, and preoperative and postoperative teaching for parents of infants undergoing reconstructive surgery.

Nursing Assessment and Diagnosis

Assess the infant and child for signs of dehydration, electrolyte imbalance, and hypovolemic shock in the salt-wasting form of the disease. See Chapter 26 🔗 for information on hypovolemic shock. Monitor airway, breathing, circulation, and responsiveness. Assess vital signs and assess peripheral perfusion (capillary refill, distal pulses, color and temperature of the extremities) frequently to detect early changes in condition, such as hypovolemia.

Assess the parents' emotional response to a newborn with ambiguous genitalia and a chronic condition. Explore their values

and beliefs regarding gender roles and sexuality while awaiting results of the karyotype.

Nursing diagnoses for the child with congenital adrenal hyperplasia may include the following:

- *Parenting, Impaired* related to a child with undetermined gender identity
- *Fluid Volume: Deficient, Risk for* related to failure of regulatory mechanisms and excess excretion of salt by the kidneys
- *Growth: Disproportionate, Risk for* related to accelerated growth and premature closure of epiphyseal plates
- *Caregiver Role Strain* related to care of a child with a chronic, potentially life-threatening condition

NANDA-I © 2012

Planning and Implementation

It is often difficult for parents to accept that their infant, whose genitalia look male, is really female. Reassure parents that with medication and surgery, the genitalia can assume a female appearance and all organs necessary for future childbearing are usually functional. Several surgeries may be performed before 2 years of age and then during adolescence to dilate the vagina. Because of the risk for adrenal insufficiency, the child will most likely be hospitalized for surgery rather than having outpatient surgery.

Nurses can assist parents in educating the child's siblings, grandparents, other family members, and childcare workers about the condition. In the newborn nursery, the infant should be referred to as "your beautiful infant," not "your son" or "your daughter," until gender identity is confirmed.

Inform parents that genetic counseling should be provided for the child during adolescence. Inform parents considering a future pregnancy that prenatal testing may detect congenital adrenal hyperplasia in the fetus. Refer the family for supportive counseling if indicated.

Care in the Community

The child will need frequent follow-up to monitor growth and appropriate dosage of glucocorticoids. Teach parents about the special problems that develop in the salt-wasting form of the disease during acute illness. Explain the medication regimen and help the family develop an emergency care plan. The child should wear a medical identification alert. Teach parents how to administer intramuscular injections of hydrocortisone. (See Partnering with Families: Hydrocortisone Administration on page 1115.) Ensure that parents have an emergency kit of injectable hydrocortisone at home and at school to be used when the child is vomiting or has diarrhea. Emphasize that the emergency kit should be carried wherever the child goes. If injectable hydrocortisone is not available, the child requires treatment in an emergency department. The child may become dehydrated quickly and require intravenous fluid and electrolyte replacement in addition to higher doses of hydrocortisone. An individualized health plan should be developed to inform the school nurse and teachers about the special care needed if the child becomes ill at school.

Evaluation

Expected outcomes of nursing care for the child with congenital adrenal hyperplasia may include:

- Parent/newborn attachment is achieved.
- The child maintains fluid volume balance.

- The child achieves age-appropriate growth and developmental milestones.
- The parents demonstrate understanding of treatment and respond appropriately when injectable medication is needed.

Adrenal Insufficiency (Addison Disease)

Adrenal insufficiency, also known as Addison disease, is a rare disorder in childhood characterized by a deficiency of glucocorticoids (cortisone) and mineralocorticoids (aldosterone). The lack of glucocorticoids affects the body's ability to handle stress.

Etiology and Pathophysiology

The majority of cases of Addison disease are caused by an autoimmune process, but it may also be acquired after infection, metabolic disease, and metastatic disease (Antal & Zhou, 2009). Worldwide, infectious diseases such as fungal infections, cytomegalovirus, and tuberculosis are still important causes of Addison disease. Acute hemorrhage related to meningococcal septicemia is also a cause of adrenal insufficiency in some children, although this is not very common (O'Connell & Siafarikas, 2010).

Clinical Manifestations

Adrenal insufficiency usually develops slowly as the adrenal glands deteriorate. The early signs may not be noticed initially but include weakness with fatigue, lethargy and emotional lability, anorexia and salt craving, and poor weight gain or weight loss. Skin changes include hyperpigmentation at pressure points, lip borders and gingival margins, nipples, palms and soles, body creases, and scarred areas of the body; and generalized bronzing of the skin or freckling without tan lines even in winter months. Additional signs include abdominal pain, nausea, vomiting and diarrhea, and symptomatic hypoglycemia.

Adrenal crisis can be caused by dehydration, stress, sepsis, or trauma. Nonadherence to therapy, inappropriate reduction of the cortisol dose, and failure to adjust the cortisol dose in the presence of stress can also lead to adrenal crisis in children previously diagnosed with adrenal insufficiency (O'Connell & Siafarikas, 2010).

Practice Alert

Signs of adrenal crisis include altered consciousness, severe hypotension, weakness, fever, abdominal pain, hypoglycemia, hyponatremia, hyperkalemia, seizures, circulatory collapse, shock, and coma. Monitor the child for these symptoms as immediate interventions are required (O'Connell & Siafarikas, 2010).

Collaborative Care

The goal of collaborative care is to maintain fluid and electrolyte balance and establish normal levels of corticosteroids and mineralocorticoids.

Diagnostic Tests

Serum cortisol and urinary 17-hydroxycorticoid levels are measured in the early morning. Low levels of serum cortisol are associated with adrenal insufficiency. The ACTH stimulation test is used to detect adrenal gland reserve. See Appendix E 🔗. Electrolyte values generally reveal low serum sodium, elevated serum potassium, and low fasting blood glucose levels. CT may be used to visualize the adrenal glands.

Clinical Therapy

Treatment involves replacement of the deficient hormones. Oral hydrocortisone is given in the lowest therapeutic dose to control symptoms and promote normal growth. Fludrocortisone acetate (Florinef) replaces the missing mineralocorticoid in children with aldosterone deficiency.

Adrenal crisis is treated by aggressive fluid resuscitation, intravenous glucose, and intravenous hydrocortisone. The precipitating illness or injury is then treated along with adequate doses of glucocorticoid and maintenance doses of mineralocorticoid. Children will also need increased doses of steroids during periods of increased physiologic stress, such as surgical procedures, illnesses, and injuries. In these cases, the dose of hydrocortisone should be at least tripled and given three times a day for 24 to 48 hours or for as long as the stress lasts before resuming the maintenance dose. Injectable hydrocortisone should always be available in case the child is vomiting or unable to take oral fluids (Antal & Zhou, 2009).

Nursing Management

Nursing management focuses on restoring hemodynamic homeostasis in the child with Addison disease who is acutely ill. Educating the child and parents about the disorder, providing emotional support, and caring for the child during acute episodes are other aspects of nursing management.

Nursing Assessment and Diagnosis

Assess vital signs for changes in heart rate and blood pressure. Assess weight, skin turgor, and mucous membranes to determine the presence of dehydration. Monitor nutritional intake, elimination patterns, muscle strength, and level of consciousness. Monitor laboratory values, intake and output, and daily weight.

Nursing diagnoses that apply to the child with adrenal insufficiency may include the following:

- Fluid Volume: Deficient related to dehydration
- Knowledge, Deficient related to disease process and treatment regimen
- Body Image, Disturbed related to changes in skin pigmentation

NANDA-I © 2012

Planning and Implementation

Encourage fluid intake as prescribed. Administer intravenous fluids as indicated. Monitor serum electrolytes as ordered. Partner with the family to ensure that proper medication and fluid administration is added to family routines. Educate the family and child to promote an understanding that the treatment for this disorder is lifelong replacement therapy.

If the child vomits within 1 hour of taking the medication, the dose is repeated. Parents may be instructed to double or triple medication in anticipation of stressful events and to increase the medication in the event of illness. Since stress increases the body's need for cortisol, Solu-Cortef hydrocortisone injections should be available at home and in the school setting for emergencies. If the child is unable to take the medications orally or is unconscious, hydrocortisone injections are indicated (O'Connell & Siafarikas, 2010).

Discuss skin pigment changes with older children and adolescents. Encourage the child to identify clothing colors that are complementary despite skin color changes. Help the child identify personal strengths and abilities to promote self-esteem.

Ensure the family recognizes symptoms that require reporting, including bleeding, dizziness, lethargy, weakness, changes in blood pressure or pulse, and weight gain. The child should wear a medical alert identifying the disorder and medications for treatment. As the child assumes independence, encourage the adolescent to share information about the disorder with at least one close friend who can provide assistance in an emergency. See Chapter 16 🔗.

Refer to the earlier discussion of congenital adrenal hyperplasia for further information on nursing care.

Evaluation

Expected outcomes of care for the child with adrenal insufficiency include the following:

- The child maintains hemodynamic stability.
- The child achieves fluid balance.
- The child and family demonstrate understanding of the disease and treatment regimen.
- The child demonstrates a positive body image.

Pheochromocytoma

Pheochromocytoma is a tumor of the adrenal gland, but it may be extra-adrenal with no anatomic connection. In most cases, these tumors are benign and curable. They can occur in a familial pattern. Most tumors diagnosed in children are identified between the ages of 6 and 14 years; however, this only accounts for 10% of these tumors as most are identified during the adult years. Pheochromocytomas may also be associated with neurofibromatosis (White, 2011). See Chapter 33 🔗.

The tumor results in excessive release of the catecholamines epinephrine and norepinephrine, leading to hypertension. Clinical manifestations include episodes of severe hypertension, palpitations, profuse sweating, and headache. Because release of catecholamines (norepinephrine and epinephrine) from the tumor is not continuous, these symptoms occur intermittently (Cook, 2009).

Collaborative Care

Diagnosis is based on 24-hour urine studies to detect the presence of increased urinary catecholamines and vanillylmandelic (VMA) levels. Radiologic imaging with CT or MRI is used to provide the location of the tumor. Most are located on the adrenal gland, but they may also be located on the thorax, mediastinum, and pelvis (Cook, 2009).

The treatment of choice is curative surgical removal of all identified tumors. However, the procedure is dangerous and may result in pheochromocytoma crisis.

Practice Alert

Pheochromocytoma crisis manifests with profound hypertension, seizures, shock, altered level of consciousness, disseminated intravascular coagulation, rhabdomyolysis (skeletal muscle destruction), and acute renal failure. This crisis can result in death. Monitor blood pressure frequently in patients with pheochromocytoma to detect changes.

Alpha- and beta-adrenergic blocking agents to control hypertension, tachycardia, and catecholamine release are administered for 7 to 14 days before surgery (Cook, 2009). Plasma catecholamines are used to measure the effectiveness of the preoperative adrenergic blockade. Postoperatively for several days, a 24-hour urine collection is measured for catecholamines to determine if all tumor sites were removed. With successful removal of all tumor sites, the prognosis is generally good, and catecholamine secretion should return to normal within 1 week. Follow-up is important to assess for recurrence of tumor.

Nursing Management

Nursing care is mainly supportive. Provide preoperative and postoperative teaching and care (refer to Chapter 15 🔗). Preoperatively, monitor vital signs and observe for signs of complications associated with pheochromocytoma crisis. Administer antihypertensives and observe for any signs of hyperglycemia (refer to page 1134).

Postoperatively, the child may be managed initially in an intensive care unit. Monitor blood pressure and glucose levels. Hypoglycemia and hypotension may occur following the withdrawal of excessive amounts of catecholamines. Observe for changes in neurologic status, respiratory distress, and signs of shock. Lifelong follow-up care with screening for hypertension and increased urinary catecholamine levels is required because symptoms recur if the child has other tumors not yet detected that activate at a later age (White, 2011).

DISORDERS OF PANCREATIC FUNCTION

The primary function of the pancreas is to regulate blood glucose metabolism. The islets of Langerhans of the pancreas consist of alpha, beta, and delta cells.

- Alpha cells secrete the hormone **glucagon,** which accelerates liver **glycogenolysis** (conversion of glycogen to glucose) to increase blood glucose. Glucagon acts as an antagonist to the hormone **insulin,** the hormone responsible for glucose metabolism.
- Beta cells produce insulin, which promotes glucose, protein, and fatty acid transport into the cells. Insulin also accelerates the movement of potassium and phosphate ions through the cell membranes with glucose, which reduces blood glucose levels and increases glucose metabolism.
- Delta cells produce somatostatin, the hormone that inhibits secretion of insulin and glucagons.

The pancreas normally secretes approximately 40 to 50 units of insulin per day. Normal blood glucose range in the child is 60 to 100 mg/dL (Tschudy & Arcara, 2012). Normally, after consumption of food, insulin secretion increases to move glucose from the blood into the liver, muscle, and fat cells for energy. When glucose is unavailable, as in lack of insulin, lipolysis (breakdown of fat), which results in the production of ketones, and proteolysis (breakdown of protein) occur to meet the body's energy demands.

Other hormones that increase blood glucose levels are epinephrine, norepinephrine, cortisol, and growth hormone.

The major disorders of pancreatic function are diabetes mellitus types 1 and 2, which are discussed in the following section. Associated complications of diabetes, such as hypoglycemia and diabetic ketoacidosis, are also discussed.

Diabetes Mellitus

Diabetes mellitus is a disorder of hyperglycemia resulting from defects in insulin secretion, insulin action, or both, leading to abnormalities in carbohydrate, protein, and fat metabolism (American Diabetes Association, 2011a) (Figure 32–8 ■). There are two main types of diabetes mellitus. Most children with diabetes mellitus have immune-mediated type 1 diabetes, formerly called insulin-dependent diabetes

Pathophysiology Illustrated Mechanism of Diabetes Mellitus

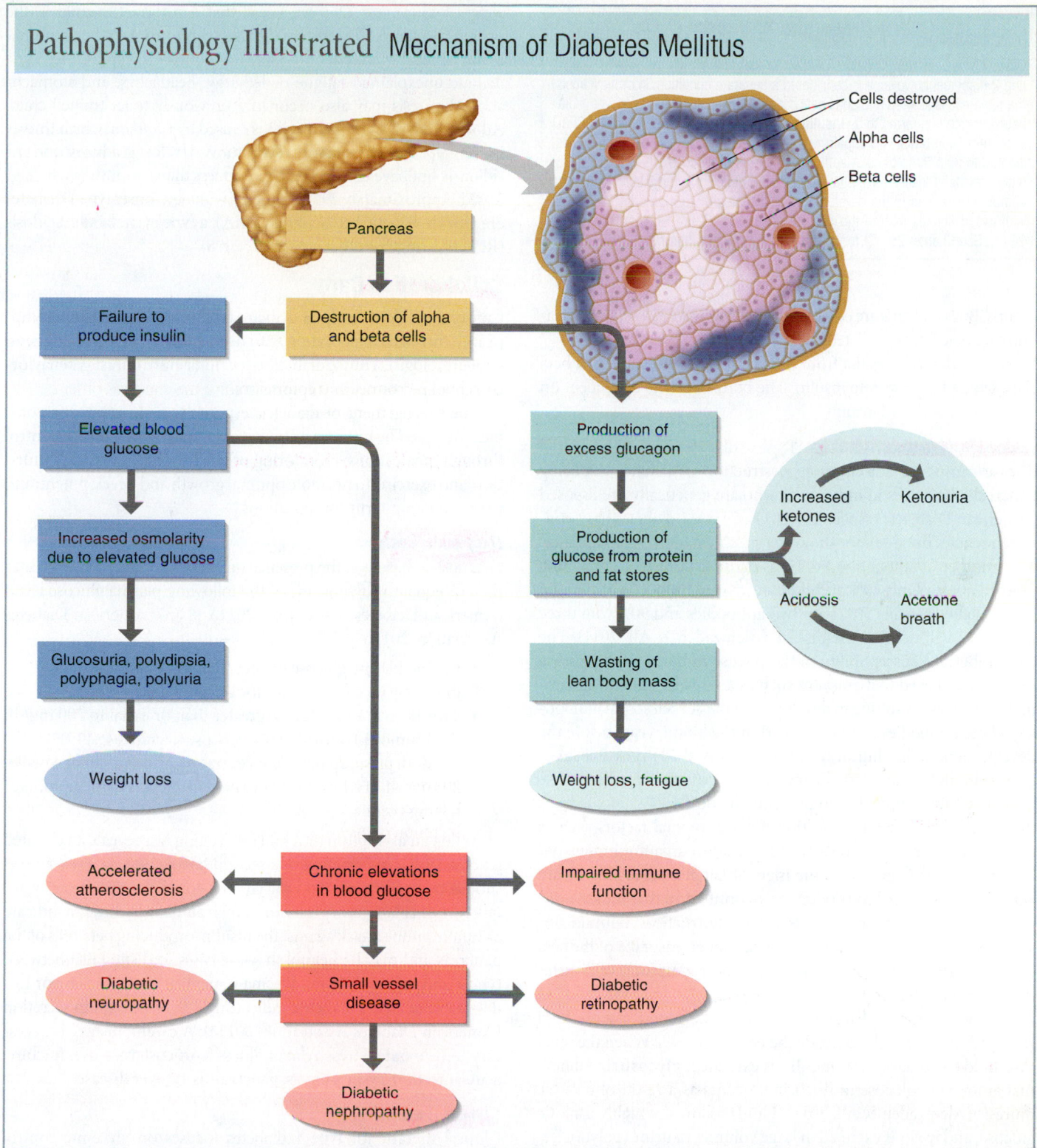

FIGURE 32–8 ■ Destruction of the alpha and beta cells in the islets of Langerhans produces multiple metabolic changes. Acute signs and symptoms are followed by short-term and long-term complications if the disease is not well managed. See Figure 32–9.

mellitus or juvenile diabetes. However, up to 30% of new cases of diabetes in children are classified as type 2 (Alemzadeh & Ali, 2011).

Type 1 Diabetes

In the United States, approximately 1 in every 400 to 600 children and adolescents have type 1 diabetes (Bachman & Hsueh, 2008). Each year more than 13,000 children under age 18 are diagnosed with type 1 diabetes (Centers for Disease Control and Prevention, 2011). Peak incidence in childhood is between 7 and 15 years of age; however, type 1 diabetes can present at any age (Alemzadeh & Ali, 2011). Caucasians experience a higher incidence of type 1 diabetes than other racial

---

BOX 32–4 **Cystic Fibrosis–Related Diabetes (CFRD)**

Cystic fibrosis–related diabetes (CFRD) has features similar to those of types 1 and 2 diabetes; however, it is considered a separate condition. In cystic fibrosis, the pancreas is scarred and does not produce sufficient insulin (as in type 1 diabetes), which is referred to as **insulin deficiency**. Another mechanism of CFRD is **insulin resistance**, an impairment in insulin receptors on cell membranes, leading to inability to transfer sufficient amounts of glucose into cells, requiring higher levels of insulin for metabolism. Insulin deficiency and insulin resistance combined can lead to the development of diabetes more frequently in patients with cystic fibrosis than in the general population (Cystic Fibrosis Foundation, 2011). See Chapter 25 🅔 for information about cystic fibrosis.

---

groups. Boys and girls are equally affected. (See Box 32–4 for information on cystic fibrosis–related diabetes.)

Type 1 diabetes results from destruction of pancreatic islet beta cells, which fail to secrete insulin. The body becomes dependent on exogenous sources of insulin.

Etiology and pathophysiology Type 1 diabetes is a multifactorial disease caused by autoimmune destruction of insulin-producing pancreatic beta cells in individuals who are genetically predisposed (American Diabetes Association, 2011a). Type 1 diabetes has familial tendencies but does not show any specific pattern of inheritance. The number of autoantibodies helps predict the risk of developing type 1 diabetes. Only 30% of children with one antibody will develop type 1 diabetes, while 70% with two antibodies and 90% with three antibodies will develop the disease (Alemzadeh & Ali, 2011). The child inherits a susceptibility to the disease rather than the disease itself. It is believed that an event such as a virus triggers the inflammatory process, resulting in development of islet cell serum antibodies. These antibodies can be detected in the blood, years before the development of the clinical symptoms (Cooke & Plotnick, 2008a).

Insulin helps transport glucose into the cells so the body can use it as an energy source. It also prevents the outflow of glucose from the liver to the general circulation. Environmental factors such as enteroviruses or toxins are believed to lead to an autoimmune destruction of the beta cells in the islets of Langerhans. Antigens are generated which lead to production of antibodies that indicate ongoing destruction of the islet cells. As the destruction continues, insulin secretion decreases. It is estimated that at least 80% of the beta cells are destroyed before the onset of clinical symptoms of diabetes (Cooke & Plotnick, 2008a).

As the secretion of insulin decreases, the blood glucose level rises and the glucose level inside the cells decreases. When the renal threshold for glucose (180 mg/dL) is exceeded, **glycosuria** (abnormal amount of glucose in the urine) occurs as a result of osmotic diuresis (Alemzadeh & Ali, 2011). Fluids follow the highly osmotic glucose, and water is excreted in large volumes of urine (polyuria).

When glucose is unavailable to the cells for metabolism, free fatty acids provide an alternative source of energy. The liver metabolizes fatty acids at an increased rate, producing acetyl coenzyme A (CoA). The by-products of acetyl CoA metabolism (ketone bodies) accumulate in the body, resulting in a state of metabolic acidosis, or ketoacidosis. (See Chapter 23 🅔 for discussion of metabolic acidosis; see page 1132 for discussion of ketoacidosis.)

Clinical manifestations The classic signs of type 1 diabetes are polyuria, polydipsia, and **polyphagia** (excessive appetite) with significant

weight loss (Figure 32–9 ■). Recall that Anthony, the child in the opening scenario, demonstrated these symptoms. See the accompanying Clinical Manifestations table for diabetes by type. Other signs include unexplained fatigue or lethargy, headaches, and stomachaches. Enuresis may also occur in a previously toilet-trained child. Adolescent girls may have vaginitis caused by *Candida*, which thrives in the hyperglycemic tissues. Symptoms develop gradually and insidiously but have usually been present less than a month when diagnosed. Approximately 29% of patients with new-onset type 1 diabetes are ill with diabetic ketoacidosis (DKA), a type of metabolic acidosis (Rewers, Klingensmith, Davis, et al., 2008).

Collaborative Care

Care of the child with type 1 diabetes requires a multidisciplinary approach through collaboration with primary healthcare providers, an endocrinologist, a nurse diabetic educator, a nutritionist, a behaviorist, school personnel, and counselors.

The management of diabetes, especially in children, is a complex process. The goals are to achieve optimal blood glucose control through medications, monitoring of glucose levels, adequate nutrition, and exercise; to promote optimal growth and development; and to prevent long-term complications.

Diagnostic Tests

Diagnosis is based on the presence of a hemoglobin A_{1c} level greater than or equal to 6.5% or one of the following plasma glucose levels (American Diabetes Association, 2011a, p. S67; American Diabetes Association, 2011b, p. S4):

- Fasting plasma glucose greater than or equal to 126 mg/dL (7 mmol/L), no caloric intake for at least 8 hours
- Two-hour plasma glucose greater than or equal to 200 mg/dL (11.1 mmol/L) during an oral glucose tolerance test
- Random plasma glucose concentration greater than or equal to 200 mg/dL (11.1 mmol/L) in a patient with classic symptoms of hyperglycemia

When an asymptomatic child's screening test reveals an elevated glucose level, confirmation of a second fasting plasma glucose level should be performed. An oral glucose tolerance test is rarely required. Other laboratory tests for known autoantibodies can indicate an autoimmune attack against the insulin-producing beta cells of the pancreas and may be helpful in some cases to distinguish between type 1 and type 2 diabetes. Plasma C-peptide levels are low or undetectable in type 1 diabetes, indicating little or no insulin secretion (American Diabetes Association, 2011a). A careful history is necessary to rule out a stress-related illness, corticosteroid use, fracture, acute infection, cystic fibrosis, pancreatitis, or liver disease.

Clinical Therapy

Clinical therapy for type 1 diabetes focuses on glycemic control by combining insulin therapy, nutrition management to support growth and to maintain blood glucose at near normal levels, an exercise regimen, and psychosocial support.

Insulin therapy Multiple approaches to insulin therapy for children and adolescents are available, and an approach that works for the child and family should be selected. Children often need several daily injections of insulin before meals and at bedtime to maintain an optimal blood glucose level. Several forms of insulin are available as identified in the accompanying Medications table.

Pathophysiology Illustrated Multisystem Effects of Diabetes

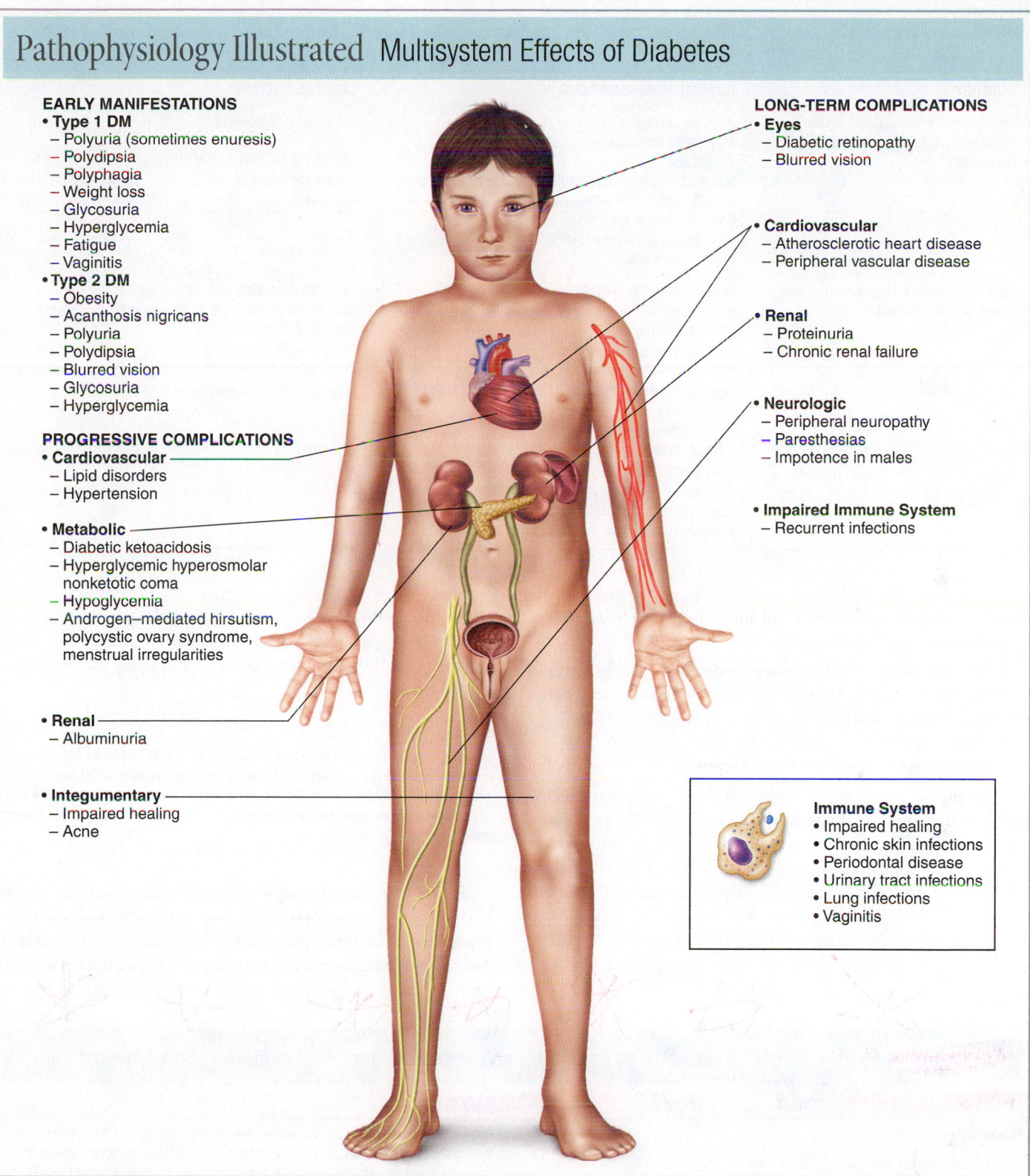

EARLY MANIFESTATIONS
- **Type 1 DM**
  - Polyuria (sometimes enuresis)
  - Polydipsia
  - Polyphagia
  - Weight loss
  - Glycosuria
  - Hyperglycemia
  - Fatigue
  - Vaginitis
- **Type 2 DM**
  - Obesity
  - Acanthosis nigricans
  - Polyuria
  - Polydipsia
  - Blurred vision
  - Glycosuria
  - Hyperglycemia

PROGRESSIVE COMPLICATIONS
- **Cardiovascular**
  - Lipid disorders
  - Hypertension

- **Metabolic**
  - Diabetic ketoacidosis
  - Hyperglycemic hyperosmolar nonketotic coma
  - Hypoglycemia
  - Androgen–mediated hirsutism, polycystic ovary syndrome, menstrual irregularities

- **Renal**
  - Albuminuria

- **Integumentary**
  - Impaired healing
  - Acne

LONG-TERM COMPLICATIONS
- **Eyes**
  - Diabetic retinopathy
  - Blurred vision

- **Cardiovascular**
  - Atherosclerotic heart disease
  - Peripheral vascular disease

- **Renal**
  - Proteinuria
  - Chronic renal failure

- **Neurologic**
  - Peripheral neuropathy
  - Paresthesias
  - Impotence in males

- **Impaired Immune System**
  - Recurrent infections

Immune System
- Impaired healing
- Chronic skin infections
- Periodontal disease
- Urinary tract infections
- Lung infections
- Vaginitis

FIGURE 32–9 ■ Multiple body systems are affected by metabolic changes resulting from diabetes.

A basal-bolus insulin regimen has resulted in improved glycemic control in the pediatric population (American Diabetes Association, 2011b). Insulin can be administered by an insulin pump or by multiple daily injections. When multiple injections are used, basal insulin is administered once a day using a very long-acting insulin. A bolus of rapid-acting insulin is administered with each meal and snack based on the carbohydrate grams consumed and the blood glucose level. This means that a child may get six to seven injections a day. Stress, infection, and illness may either increase or decrease insulin needs. If basal-bolus therapy for type 1

Clinical Manifestations Diabetes by Type

ETIOLOGY	CLINICAL MANIFESTATIONS	CLINICAL THERAPY
Type 1—immune mediated, insulin deficiency due to pancreatic beta cell destruction	Polyuria, polydipsia May have polyphagia Weight loss Ketoacidosis on initial presentation in 30–40% of cases, at continued risk for ketoacidosis Short duration of symptoms Initial period of decreased insulin requirement, then need insulin for survival	Blood glucose monitoring Insulin Dietary management, balancing carbohydrate intake to insulin and exercise Exercise
Type 2—Insulin resistance with relative insulin secretory defect	Obese, little or no weight loss, or may have significant weight loss Acanthosis nigricans Long duration of symptoms Polyuria, polydipsia may be mild or absent Glycosuria without ketonuria in 33% of cases on initial presentation Ketoacidosis may be present Lipid disorders Hypertension Androgen-mediated problems such as acne, hirsutism, menstrual disturbances, polycystic ovary disease Excessive weight gain and fatigue due to insulin resistance	Diet with decreased calories and low-fat foods Decrease sedentary activity time or increase routine physical activity Blood glucose monitoring Oral medication (metformin) to improve insulin sensitivity May need insulin initially

diabetes is to be effective, the child and family need to do each of the following:

- Monitor the blood glucose appropriately to establish insulin requirements. For example, test glucose before and 2 hours after meals, as well as once a week at midnight and 3 a.m.
- Count carbohydrates consumed.
- Incorporate exercise in to the daily routine.

Continuous subcutaneous insulin infusion (CSII) pump therapy is increasingly used by children and adolescents as the technology makes it possible to more closely match plasma insulin levels to levels found in children who do not have diabetes. CSII pump therapy has been used successfully in children of all ages and has been found to improve glycemic control with less hypoglycemia. Pump therapy requires the willingness of the patient or parent (with young children) to monitor blood glucose frequently, practice advanced insulin management skills, learn how to troubleshoot the pump, and be technology capable (Carchidi, Holland, Minnock, et al., 2011). Advantages and disadvantages of an insulin pump are outlined in Table 32–6.

Clinical Tip
Insulin is usually provided in prepackaged doses of 100 units/mL. Diluted insulin prepared by a pharmacist may be used for infants and toddlers who require a small insulin dosage. Insulin cartridges, disposable pens, and other devices are available, making insulin easy to carry by older children and adolescents for frequent insulin injections during the day.

The goal of insulin therapy is to maintain a range of blood glucose levels as near normal as possible, while avoiding episodes of severe hypoglycemia. Glycemic goals for children younger than 6 years are generally not as tight since this age group is at higher risk for severe or

Medications Used in Management of Diabetes Mellitus and Average Insulin Action Times (Subcutaneous Route)

TYPE	ONSET	PEAK	DURATION	ACTION
Rapid Acting				Insulin is an endogenous hormone, secreted by the beta cells of the pancreas. It lowers the blood glucose level by stimulating glucose passage across cell membranes and uptake into the cells. It also promotes the conversion of glucose to glycogen and inhibits hepatic glucose production from glycogen.
Insulin lispro, insulin glulisine, or insulin aspart	10–30 min	0.5–1.5 hr	3–5 hr	
Short Acting				
Regular	0.5–1 hr	2–5 hr	5–8 hr	
Very Long Acting				
Glargine or detemir	1–2 hr	None	Up to 24 hr	

Source: *Data from Fleury-Milfort, E. (2008). Insulin replacement therapy: Minimizing complications and side effects. Advance for Nurse Practitioners, 16(11), 32–39; Wright, E. E. (2009). Overview of insulin replacement therapy. Journal of Family Practice, 58(8), S3–S9; Miles, H. L., & Acerini, C. L. (2008). Insulin analog preparations and their use in children and adolescents with type 1 diabetes mellitus. Pediatric Drugs, 10(3), 163–176.*

TABLE 32–6 Advantages and Disadvantages of an External Insulin Infusion Pump

ADVANTAGES	DISADVANTAGES
■ Delivers a continuous infusion of insulin to match the basal rate needed plus an insulin bolus at mealtime to more closely simulate normal pancreatic function	■ Requires highly motivated child and supportive parents and healthcare professionals
■ Helps maintain blood glucose control between meals	■ Requires willingness to live connected to a device (can be disconnected for short periods by removing or clamping the catheter; however, DKA can occur within hours of interruption of insulin flow)
■ Decreases HbA$_{1c}$ level	■ Requires the site to be changed every 2–3 days
■ Improves glycemic control	■ Overuse of catheter-site locations
■ Improves growth in children	■ Must still monitor blood glucose levels and carbohydrates consumed
■ Reduces number of injections, reduces number of injection sites, so variation in absorption decreases	■ Risk of infections at the injection site
■ New pumps calculate bolus insulin dose to carbohydrates consumed	■ Possible weight gain when blood sugar control improves
■ Allows child to eat with less adherence to a schedule and have a more flexible lifestyle	■ Increased cost
■ Fewer incidents of diabetic ketoacidosis	■ Risk of DKA secondary to pump failure or dislodgment of catheter
■ Decreases frequency of hypoglycemia	
■ Improves quality of life	
■ Stores Information	

Source: *Data from Bangstad, H., Danne, T., Deeb, L. C., Jarosz-Chobot, P., Urakami, T., & Hanas, R. (2009). Insulin treatment in children and adolescents with diabetes. Pediatric Diabetes, 10(Suppl. 12), 82–99; Campbell, F. (2008). The pros and cons of continuous subcutaneous insulin infusion (CSII) therapy in the pediatric population and practical considerations when choosing and initiating CSII in children. British Journal of Diabetes and Vascular Disease, 8(Suppl. 1), S6–10; Carchidi, C., Holland, C., Minnock, P., & Boyle, D. (2011). New technologies in pediatric diabetes care. MCN, 36(1), 32–39; Ho, J., Loh, C. T. F., Pacaud, D., & Leung, A. K. C. (2010). Type 1 diabetes mellitus in children and adolescents: Part 2, Management. Consultant for Pediatricians, 9(2), 69–77.*

unrecognized hypoglycemia (Carchidi et al., 2011; Ho, Loh, Pacaud, et al., 2010).

Evaluation of insulin therapy Insulin therapy is evaluated every 3 months with a hemoglobin A$_{1c}$ (HbA$_{1c}$) level, an objective measurement of glycemic control. It represents the amount of glucose that binds to the hemoglobin molecule, predicting average glucose concentration over the prior 2 months (Cooke & Plotnick, 2008a). See Table 32–7 for the HbA$_{1c}$ goals for children of different ages. It is also important to determine if the HbA$_{1c}$ matches recorded blood sugars.

Nutrition therapy The goal of nutrition therapy is to provide adequate calories for the child's normal growth and development. An evaluation of the child's food intake, metabolic status, and lifestyle is necessary before establishing a nutrition plan. Daily caloric requirements are individualized for each child according to need. To facilitate adherence to the nutritional plan, an individualized approach with considerations of the child and family's culture, lifestyle, and financial means should be incorporated. Careful instruction by a nutritionist is essential in the management of diabetes.

Carbohydrate counting provides flexibility in meal planning and is simple for children and adolescents to use. One carbohydrate choice equals 15 grams of carbohydrates. The number of carbohydrate choices needed at meals and snacks vary depending on the child's individualized nutrition plan. Generally, one unit of insulin covers 15 grams of carbohydrates, making insulin dosage calculation for meal coverage relatively easy; however, a different ratio of insulin to carbohydrates may be calculated for individual children. If additional carbohydrates are eaten at a meal or snack, the number of insulin units can also be adjusted, providing further flexibility. A high-fiber diet is also recommended for improved control of blood glucose.

Practice Alert
Avoid use of sorbitol and xylitol as artificial sweeteners because they are carbohydrates and have been associated with some diabetes complications (Alemzadeh & Ali, 2011).

Exercise program Physical activity is associated with increased insulin sensitivity. Regular exercise and fitness improves blood glucose control, reduces cardiovascular risk factors, contributes to weight loss, and improves overall well-being. Blood lipid levels are also positively affected. However, the child must have an adequate caloric

TABLE 32–7 Goals for Blood Glucose and Hemoglobin A$_{1c}$ by Age of the Child

PRACTICE ALERT			CLINICAL TIP
Blood glucose goals for younger children are not as tight since they cannot verbalize symptoms of hypoglycemia. Overnight goals are higher in all age groups to decrease the risk of hypoglycemia during the night. Guidelines are as follows:			Hemoglobin A$_{1c}$ goals vary by age and are higher for younger children. Guidelines are as follows:

AGE	BEFORE MEALS	BEDTIME/ OVERNIGHT	HEMOGLOBIN A$_{1c}$
Less than 6 years of age	100–180 mg/dL	110–200 mg/dL	7.5–8.5%
6–12 years of age	90–180 mg/dL	100–180 mg/dL	Less than 8%
13–19 years of age	90–130 mg/dL	90–150 mg/dL	Less than 7.5%

TABLE 32–8	Complications Associated with Diabetes Mellitus	
ACUTE COMPLICATIONS	**CHRONIC COMPLICATIONS**	**COMPLICATIONS RELATED TO GROWTH AND DEVELOPMENT**
Diabetic ketoacidosis	Retinopathy	Delay in growth
Hypoglycemia	Nephropathy	Delay in puberty
	Neuropathy	Emotional disturbances
	Peripheral vascular disease	Menstrual disturbances

BOX 32–5	Questions to Ask When Planning Diabetes Education

1. Do both parents work or does the single parent work? What hours?
2. Who else is involved in the child's care?
3. What is the child's usual daily schedule? Does the schedule vary on the weekend or any other days of the week?
4. Does the child have health insurance? What coverage exists for diabetes education, treatment, and home management?
5. Does the child have any cognitive, behavioral, motor, or visual problems co-existing with this condition?
6. What other family stressors co-exist with the diagnosis?

intake to prevent hypoglycemia. Excessive exercise associated with sports requires careful planning and management.

Complications Complications of type 1 diabetes (retinopathy, heart disease, renal failure, and peripheral vascular disease) result from long-term hyperglycemic effects on the blood vessels. Without careful management, children with diabetes may develop renal failure and loss of vision in adulthood. Intensive therapy is expected to reduce the risk for or delay the development of these complications. Risk may be further reduced if the adolescent does not begin smoking and if the blood pressure is controlled. See Table 32–8.

Nursing Management

Nursing care focuses on teaching the child and parents about the disease and its management—managing dietary intake, promoting growth and developmental milestones, providing emotional support, and planning strategies for daily management in the community.

Nursing Assessment and Diagnosis

Nursing assessment focuses on a physiologic assessment of the child and also on collecting the environmental, developmental, and psychosocial information that is needed to develop a nursing care plan for the family's management of a chronic illness.

Physiologic Assessment

Children with type 1 diabetes are frequently admitted to the hospital at the time of diagnosis. Assess the child's physiologic status, focusing on vital signs and level of consciousness. Assess hydration by checking mucous membranes, skin turgor, and urine output. Blood is initially collected to monitor blood gases, glucose, and electrolytes. The frequency of blood collections will depend on whether the child is in diabetic ketoacidosis. Once the child is stable, assess dietary and caloric intake and the ability of the child or family to manage care.

Psychosocial Assessment

Parents may feel guilty at the time of diagnosis if they waited to seek care until the child began to experience symptoms of diabetic ketoacidosis. Assess coping mechanisms, family strengths and resources, ability to manage the disease, and educational needs of both the child and parents. Assess the child's understanding and ability to cope with the diagnosis of diabetes. Assess the child's previous experience with diabetes, for example, a relative with diabetes who experienced complications such as amputation or blindness. Examples of questions to ask in assessing the family's strengths and limitations in the child's disease management are provided in Box 32–5. Assess the child's or adolescent's willingness and motivation to adhere to the treatment regimen. See Evidence-Based Practice: Adolescent Diabetes, Quality of Life, and Self-Efficacy.

Developmental Assessment

Assess the child's developmental level, particularly fine motor skills, and cognitive level. The child will need to learn how to obtain and read a blood glucose sample and to inject insulin. Children can usually perform some of these tasks with supervision by 6 to 8 years of age.

Adolescents often perceive type 1 diabetes as a disability and may deny having the disease so they can be like their peers when eating and exercising. Talk with adolescents and assess problem-solving skills associated with daily condition management, and their ability to manage special circumstances such as illness or changes in exercise. Self-management is the eventual goal, and the child's responsibilities are gradually increased. See Box 32–6.

Several nursing diagnoses that may apply to the child newly diagnosed with type 1 diabetes are provided in the accompanying Nursing Care Plans. Additional diagnoses that may be appropriate are as follows:

- Fluid Volume, Deficient, Risk for related to active fluid loss associated with hyperglycemia
- Breathing Pattern, Ineffective related to neuromuscular dysfunction associated with metabolic acidosis
- Coping, Ineffective related to inability to admit impact of disease on lifestyle

NANDA-I © 2012

Planning and Implementation

Nursing care focuses on teaching the child and parents about the disease and its management, planning dietary intake, providing emotional support, and planning strategies for daily management in the community. Refer to the accompanying Nursing Care Plans, which summarize nursing care for the child who is hospitalized with newly diagnosed type 1 diabetes, and the child who is receiving care in the community.

Provide Education

The nurse is an important member of the management team (physician, nurse, nutritionist, and social worker) and is usually responsible for educating the child and family. The majority of teaching may be performed by an advanced practice nurse or a certified diabetes nurse educator in the clinic setting, since children may be hospitalized only briefly following diagnosis.

The timing and amount of information provided are especially important in the first days following diagnosis. Both the child and parents are very tired, and they are often in a state of shock and disbelief. Information presented during this period needs to be repeated. This time should be used to assess learning needs and to answer the family's questions. Initial teaching focuses on the survival skills

Evidence-Based Practice

Adolescent Diabetes, Quality of Life, and Self-Efficacy

PROBLEM

Adolescents with type 1 diabetes not only experience the normal psychologic and physiologic changes that occur during the adolescent growth period, but they must also cope with the responsibility of increasing self-management of their disease including insulin administration, exercise, nutrition, and self-esteem issues associated with a chronic illness. How can self-efficacy and quality of life be maximized in adolescents with type 1 diabetes?

EVIDENCE

A randomized controlled trial measured how monitoring and discussing health-related quality of life (HRQoL) improved psychosocial well-being in adolescents with type 1 diabetes. Ninety-one adolescents between the ages of 13 and 17 with type 1 diabetes participated in the study and were randomly assigned to the HRQoL intervention group or the control group. During a 12-month period, all participants had 3 scheduled visits for routine diabetes care at 3-month intervals. The intervention group completed the Pediatric Quality of Life Inventory on a computer at each visit prior to being seen by the healthcare provider. The results were discussed with the adolescent during the visit. Over the 12-month period, mean scores for psychosocial health, behavior, mental health, and family activities improved in the intervention group except for those adolescents with the highest hemoglobin A_{1c} values. Adolescents in the intervention group demonstrated higher self-esteem at follow-up visits and were more satisfied with care than those in the control group (de Wit, Delemarre-van de Waal, Bokma, et al., 2008).

A cross-sectional design was utilized to determine the impact of family support and environment on quality of life, adherence to treatment, and metabolic control in 157 adolescents ages 10 to 18 with type 1 diabetes. Four instruments were used in the study: a self-report questionnaire on adherence, Diabetes Family Behavior Scale, Family Environment Scale, and Diabetes Quality of Life. Results of the study indicated that increased family support predicted a better quality of life in both males and females, and higher family conflict predicted a lower quality of life. Increased family support also predicted an increase in adherence in females. Additionally, the study found that the longer the teen had been diagnosed with diabetes, the less likely he or she was to be adherent to a management plan and to have good metabolic control. Results

of the study also indicated that participants from a lower socioeconomic level were less likely to be adherent to the treatment plan and had a poorer quality of life when compared to participants from a higher socioeconomic level (Pereira, Berg-Cross, Almeida, et al., 2008).

A descriptive comparative pilot study explored the concepts of self-efficacy and resilience in 81 adolescents ages 10 to 16 years who attended a diabetes camp. The Self-Efficacy for Diabetes Scale was used. Results showed that both self-efficacy and resilience scores were moderately high in this population. African Americans scored significantly higher than Caucasians on both measures. Participants who lived in single-parent homes had poorer diabetic control, as indicated by a higher hemoglobin A_{1c}, but had higher scores in resilience (Winsett, Stender, Gower, et al., 2010).

IMPLICATIONS

Developmental tasks of adolescents focus on development of self-concept and self-esteem. Adolescents with type 1 diabetes must also cope with the increasing responsibility for complex self-management, including insulin administration, blood glucose testing, exercise, and nutrition. Self-esteem and self-concept often become linked with the disease as peers react to the differences noted. Life satisfaction, perceived control, and worries associated with having diabetes are important considerations when counseling the teenager and family about the management of diabetes. Additionally, it is important to know that adolescents value parental involvement and care rather than perceiving it as a reason for conflict. Parental involvement and supervision is important in helping adolescents transition successfully to self-management of their disease. Peers are also very important to adolescents with diabetes. Continued involvement in school activities and summer camps provide excellent avenues for friendship and promote a positive quality of life.

CRITICAL THINKING APPLICATION

What questions can be used to explore an adolescent's perceptions of family involvement, care, and control? How can you address quality of life issues in adolescents with diabetes? What questions can be asked to determine the adolescent's self-efficacy and resilience?

---

necessary for home management, including insulin administration, blood glucose testing, meal planning, and the recognition and treatment of both hypoglycemia and hyperglycemia. Partner with the child and family to identify barriers to management.

Explain the goals of insulin therapy. Teach the parents and child (if age appropriate) how to draw up and administer insulin or how to use an insulin pen. Insulin pens might be accepted more readily than the traditional syringe and vial method; they are easier to transport, they provide more accurate dosing, and they decrease

anxiety associated with needles and insulin administration in public (Hanas, de Beaufort, Hoey, et al., 2011). Rotating the injection sites is important to decrease the chances of **lipoatrophy,** loss of subcutaneous tissue, or hypertrophy, in which collagen is replaced by fat cells (Figure 32–10 ■). The absorption rate of insulin varies by the site used. Insulin is usually absorbed most rapidly from the abdomen; however, insulin absorption is increased in the extremities with exercise. An understanding of the different types of insulin and their actions is essential.

BOX 32–6 Research: Communication Between Adolescents with Type 1 Diabetes and Their Parents

Transcripts of interactions between adolescents ages 11 to 15 years with type 1 diabetes and their parents were analyzed. Participation in the study required that the adolescent had been diagnosed with type 1 diabetes for at least a year and have no other chronic illness, psychologic problems, or learning disability. Transcripts were based on a 10-minute interaction between the adolescent and his or her parents in which a diabetes management task, identified by the teen as a source of disagreement, was discussed.

Five themes were identified from the transcripts: fear, frustration, discounting, normalizing, and trusting. Parents demonstrated frustration, fear, and difficulty in trusting the child with the daily management of diabetes. Parents were also fearful of long-term complications. Adolescents demonstrated frustration because they did

not feel their parents recognized their successes in their diabetes management. Discounting was noted in statements by parents that showed a lack of respect for the adolescents' opinions and failure to include the adolescents in decisions related to their care. These statements further added to the child's frustration. The theme of normalizing was noted in only a few families and included statements indicating that the family was attempting to view diabetes as a normal aspect of the adolescent's life. The other themes of fear, frustration, trust, and discounting were cited as barriers to achieving the goal of normalcy.

The study concluded that effective communication between parents and adolescents with type 1 diabetes is essential and that nurses should work with families to facilitate communication related to diabetes management (Ivey, Wright, & Dashiff, 2009).

Nursing Care Plan   The Child Hospitalized with Newly Diagnosed Type 1 Diabetes Mellitus

INTERVENTION	RATIONALE	EXPECTED OUTCOME
1. Nursing Diagnosis: Knowledge, Deficient (Survival Skills) related to lack of exposure to diabetic management in the newly diagnosed child		
NIC Priority Intervention—*Teaching, Individual:* Planning, implementing, and evaluating a teaching program designed to address a patient's particular needs		**NOC Suggested Outcome**—*Knowledge:* Extent of understanding conveyed about diabetic treatment regimen
GOAL: *The child and parents will acquire survival skills for home management.*		
■ Assess the child's developmental level and select an educational approach and self-care activities to match.	■ Learning goals for the child must match knowledge and skill expectations appropriate for developmental level.	The child and parents demonstrate proper technique for blood glucose monitoring, urine testing for ketones, drawing up and injecting insulin doses, survival food guidelines, and record keeping.
■ Teach blood glucose monitoring, drawing up and injecting insulin, urine testing for ketones, record keeping, survival food guidelines, and when to call the healthcare provider.	■ Diabetic management survival skills are needed for initial home management until more extensive education can be completed that permits more independent management.	
■ Use demonstration/return demonstration until the child and family are comfortable with procedures.	■ Return demonstration permits evaluation, positive reinforcement, and guidance for modification of techniques.	
GOAL: *The child and parents will recognize signs and symptoms of hypoglycemia and hyperglycemia.*		
■ Teach signs and symptoms of hypoglycemic and hyperglycemic reactions.	■ Recognition and treatment of poor glucose control will prevent progression of symptoms.	The child and family can describe symptoms of hypoglycemia and hyperglycemia.
■ Teach the child to test blood glucose when feeling different than usual, and record the reading and symptoms felt.	■ The child learns his or her specific symptoms of hyper- and hypoglycemia.	
2. Nursing Diagnosis: Injury, Risk for (Complication) related to potential episodes of hypoglycemia and diabetic ketoacidosis		
NIC Priority Intervention—*Risk Identification:* Analysis of potential risk factors, determination of health risks, and prioritization of risk reduction strategies for an individual or group		**NOC Suggested Outcome**—*Risk Control:* Actions to eliminate or reduce actual, personal, and modifiable health threats
GOAL: *The child will experience few episodes of hypoglycemia during hospitalization.*		
■ Assess the child at least every 2 hours for signs of hypoglycemia. if signs are present, check blood glucose to verify and administer the source of quick sugar.	■ Hypoglycemia commonly occurs during hospitalization because of change in diet, lack of food intake, or illness.	The child and staff manage episodes of hypoglycemia without a crisis developing.
■ When the child is NPO for a special procedure, verify with the physician when food, fluids, and insulin are to be given, or if an intravenous infusion with dextrose is to be given.	■ Giving insulin without calorie intake can lead to hypoglycemia. Intravenous dextrose and insulin can be used when the child must be NPO.	
■ Have glucose paste or 50% dextrose solution readily available.	■ Dextrose is used for emergency iv treatment of severe hypoglycemia. Glucose paste is used for oral treatment.	
GOAL: *The child's condition is treated slowly to gradually reverse hyperglycemia and ketoacidosis and to prevent cerebral edema.*		
■ Assess the child's mental status for improvement or deterioration.	■ Improvement in mental status may indicate successful treatment. Deterioration may indicate onset of cerebral edema.	The child's hyperglycemia and ketoacidosis resolve without additional complications.
■ Check blood glucose and urine ketones frequently to confirm reduction in blood glucose level and ketosis, and to identify the insulin dose for administration.	■ Frequent blood glucose and ketone level determination helps assess progress in treating ketoacidosis.	
■ Monitor and control IV fluid intake. Measure output.	■ The child with ketoacidosis will be dehydrated. IV fluid intake needs to be carefully controlled to prevent cerebral edema.	
■ Have insulin doses checked by a second nurse.	■ Doses are frequently small, and the possibility of error is great.	

Nursing Care Plan   The Child Hospitalized with Newly Diagnosed Type 1 Diabetes Mellitus, *continued*

INTERVENTION	RATIONALE	EXPECTED OUTCOME
GOAL: *The child and parents will demonstrate emergency management of hypoglycemia.*		
■ Identify sources of glucose to give in case of hypoglycemic reaction. Tell the child and parent to carry glucose tablets or paste with them at all times.	■ Access to sources of glucose and its rapid administration are important for emergency care.	The child and family can identify several glucose sources for emergencies. The child and family have a source of glucose with them at each visit.
GOAL: *The child and parents will demonstrate management of sick days.*		
■ Teach the child and family to test blood glucose and urine for ketones with acute symptoms and to notify the healthcare provider.	■ When the child is ill, hyperglycemia needs special management to prevent progression to ketoacidosis.	The child's hyperglycemic episodes do not progress to ketoacidosis.
3. Nursing Diagnosis: Nutrition, Imbalanced: Less than Body Requirements related to glycosuria		
NIC Priority Intervention—*Nutrition Management:* Assistance with or provision of a balanced dietary intake of foods and fluids		**NOC Suggested Outcome—***Nutritional Status:* Extent to which nutrients are available to meet metabolic needs
GOAL: *The child will eat a well-balanced diet and maintain normal height and weight proportions.*		
■ Encourage and serve meals and snacks with a consistent number of carbohydrates at the same time each day.	■ A consistent food plan keeps blood glucose levels stable during the initial disease management stages.	The child regains weight lost and demonstrates normal growth and stable blood glucose levels.
■ Provide a calorie-nonrestricted diet food plan.	■ This enables weight lost during the onset of diabetes to be regained.	
GOAL: *The child and parents will state understanding of dietary management of type 1 diabetes.*		
■ Make an appointment with a nutritionist who can assess the child's favorite foods and promote their integration into the child's meal plan. reinforce the dietary information taught.	■ The nutritionist can develop dietary recommendations that fit the specific growth needs of the child and include favorite foods, thereby increasing compliance with the meal plan.	The child and parents describe nutritional needs of the child and select the dietary management best suited to the family's and child's eating habits.
■ Provide sample menus and teach the use of carbohydrate counting.	■ This information assists the family and adolescent with meal planning.	

NANDA-I © 2012

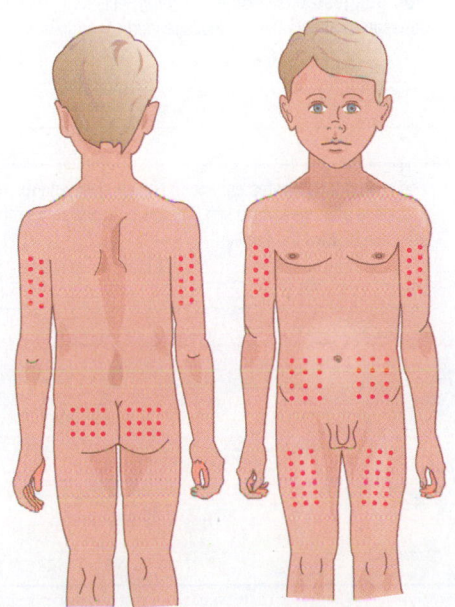

FIGURE 32–10 ■ Insulin injection sites. Give all morning insulin in one site (e.g., arms) and all evening insulin in another (e.g., legs) because of different rates of absorption from these sites. Space injections about 1.25 cm (0.5 in.) apart.

Once the child and parents demonstrate understanding of this information, teach guidelines for recognizing and managing episodes of hyperglycemia during acute illness and using an insulin correction scale. A correction scale indicates specific insulin dosages appropriate for a particular blood glucose level. The family also needs to learn "sick day" care guidelines to prevent diabetic ketoacidosis. (See Partnering with Families: Teaching About Sick Day Guidelines.)

Clinical Tip

Caution parents to check the blood glucose level of a toddler who is extremely sleepy or irritable, as these can be signs of either hypoglycemia or hyperglycemia.

Manage Food Intake

While no specific meal plan is recommended for children with diabetes, 50% of their calories should be carbohydrates, 10% to 20% of their calories should be protein, and 30% of their calories should be fat (American Academy of Pediatrics, 2009). The child needs adequate calories to reach or maintain a desirable body weight. The MyPlate Food Guide (see Chapter 19 ⬟) may be used to teach the child and family the correct portions and which foods are considered carbohydrates, fats, and proteins. A variety of simple and complex carbohydrates should be eaten. Poly- and monounsaturated fats are preferred for meeting fat needs with avoidance of saturated and trans fats.

Nursing Care Plan | The Child with Previously Diagnosed Type 1 Diabetes Being Cared for at Home

INTERVENTION	RATIONALE	EXPECTED OUTCOME
1. Nursing Diagnosis: Nutrition, Imbalanced: Less than Body Requirements related to chronic illness (type 1 diabetes)		
NIC Priority Intervention—_Nutrition Management:_ Assistance with or provision of a balanced dietary intake of foods and fluids		**NOC Suggested Outcome—**_Nutritional Status:_ Nutrient Intake: Adequacy of nutrients taken into body
GOAL: _The child will eat a well-balanced diet that maintains weight proportional to height._		
■ Assess height and weight regularly and plot on a growth chart.	■ A change in body mass index may indicate a potential weight problem.	Diet records indicate meals and snacks have the appropriate distribution of carbohydrates, protein, and fats, and daily caloric intake goals are met.
■ Review the child's 24-hour intake on a weekday and a weekend day to assess adequacy of calories and proportion of carbohydrates, protein, and fats in foods consumed. Obtain information about usual exercise.	■ Dietary recall provides information to help guide recommendations for changes in food plans to match growth needs and usual exercise routines.	Food intake is adequate for growth and exercise.
■ Make an appointment with a nutritionist who can assess the child's favorite foods and integrate them into a food plan that controls caloric intake. Encourage the child to keep a food diary.	■ Inclusion of the child's favorite foods helps the child adapt to changes in the food plan.	
2. Nursing Diagnosis: Family Processes, Readiness for Enhanced related to management of a chronic disease		
NIC Priority Intervention—_Family Process Maintenance:_ Minimization of family process disruption effects		**NOC Suggested Outcome—**_Family Functioning:_ Ability of family to meet the needs of its members through developmental transitions
GOAL: _The child and family will manage the food plan, exercise, blood glucose monitoring, and medications regimen._		
■ Assess the family's lifestyle and attempt to fit the child's care needs into the family's schedule.	■ Fitting the care to the family's lifestyle promotes adherence with the regimen.	The child and family make minimal changes in their usual lifestyle while managing the type 1 diabetes.
■ Discuss the family's routines for special occasions and vacations. Identify ways to modify the child's management for these occasions.	■ It is important for the child to participate in special events with the family and peers to promote psychologic development.	
3. Nursing Diagnosis: Coping, Ineffective (Individual) related to inadequate level of confidence in ability to cope		
NIC Priority Intervention—_Coping Enhancement:_ Assisting a patient to adapt to perceived stressors, changes, or threats which interfere with meeting life demands and roles		**NOC Suggested Outcome—**_Coping:_ Actions to manage stressors that tax an individual's resources
GOAL: _The child will demonstrate enhanced coping skills._		
■ Ask how the child has solved problems in the past. Review possible problems the child may encounter. Together evaluate the effectiveness of solutions. Suggest other solutions to consider.	■ Children's success in mastering maturational conflicts and daily psychosocial problems will influence their pattern of coping.	The child demonstrates enhanced coping skills and expresses a positive attitude toward self. The child displays warmth and affection toward the family.
GOAL: _The child will develop positive self-esteem._		
■ Role-play ways to talk about diabetes with friends and teachers. Encourage the child to express feelings about diabetes to those he or she trusts.	■ Sharing information about the condition helps others understand changes in lifestyle needed by the child. Expressing feelings decreases anxiety.	
■ Encourage the child to attend diabetes camp.	■ Learning and support networks experienced at camp can promote development of self-esteem.	
■ Encourage the child to continue previous social activities and hobbies.	■ Increased social interaction, especially in group sessions, improves self-esteem.	

NANDA-I © 2012

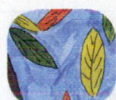

Partnering with Families

Teaching About Sick Day Guidelines

When the child with diabetes is sick, parents need to be extra attentive to the child's glycemic control. The following recommendations should be followed (Doyle & Grey, 2010):

- Seek medical attention for fever or other signs of infection.
- Monitor the blood glucose levels more often than routine (every 1 to 4 hours or as instructed by the healthcare provider).
- Test urine ketones when the blood glucose level is greater than 200 mg/dL or as instructed by the healthcare provider.

- The usual dose of insulin may be increased for high blood glucose levels.
- Do not skip doses of insulin.
- Maintain hydration. A large fluid intake is essential if the child cannot eat as usual. Fluids should have carbohydrates to maintain the child's usual caloric intake. If the child cannot consume adequate amounts of fluids, seek medical attention.

Eating at consistent intervals is important for glycemic control, whether counting carbohydrates or following a conventional meal plan (three meals a day and three snacks a day). Although the child with diabetes is not restricted from eating any food, the child and parents need to learn about the relationship between foods eaten and insulin needed. Meal plans also need to be adjusted for exercise. Nonnutritive sweeteners such as aspartame and saccharin may be used in moderation. The child and family should learn how to read food labels. The meal plan should be customized, with the assistance of a nutritionist, to the child's age, cultural and family food preferences, and activity level.

Clinical Tip

Children with type 1 diabetes need a balanced diet for growth. Assist them to understand their meal plan and that they will need to count carbohydrates for the rest of their lives.

Provide Emotional Support

The diagnosis of type 1 diabetes often comes as a shock to the family. If there is a familial history, parents may feel guilty about having caused the disease. The diagnosis of a chronic disease that requires daily management can be difficult to accept. Provide the family with information about diabetes education programs, refer them to support groups with other parents of children with diabetes, and assist them in learning the role of disease management. It is important to help the family develop the practices and routines needed to adhere to the regimen of care.

Support for the child depends on age and developmental stage. Encourage the child to express feelings about the disease and its management. The adolescent may benefit from contact with other adolescents who have diabetes. Refer the family to organizations that focus on support for children with diabetes and their families.

Discharge Planning and Home Care Teaching

Home care needs should be addressed before discharge. Initial survival skills as described in the Nursing Care Plan on page 1126 are taught with the plans for ongoing outpatient education, often beginning the day after discharge.

Partner with the family to incorporate the diabetic regimen (insulin administration, food plan, blood glucose monitoring, and exercise) into the present lifestyle. Demonstrate and ensure return demonstration of injection administration. The fewer changes the

---

BOX 32–7	The Honeymoon Phase

The family and child newly diagnosed with diabetes should be made aware of the "honeymoon phase." This is a period during new-onset diabetes when the child has some residual β-cell function, which reduces exogenous insulin requirements. The child and family may assume this is an indication that the diabetes "is better." However, the insulin requirement does eventually return. The duration of the honeymoon phase varies among individuals.

---

family has to make, the greater the chance of adherence. Assist the family with the transition of the child with diabetes going to school. Attending school can be a source of fear and concern for parents of young children with diabetes as they experience concerns regarding insulin injections, glucose monitoring, nutrition, safety, and other associated issues. For adolescents, common fears include being perceived as different, the inconvenience of injections, self-monitoring of glucose, and dietary issues. The nurse can assist the family in collaboration with school personnel to establish a routine and plan. See Box 32–7.

Provide written materials and refer parents to books and other materials they can use in teaching the child about diabetes. The Juvenile Diabetes Research Foundation and the American Diabetes Association are excellent sources of information.

Care in the Community

During follow-up visits, ask the child or parents about signs indicating problems with diabetic control (see Box 32–8). Maintain a record of the child's growth measurements and vital signs. Review the child's typical dietary intake and exercise regimens. Assess the child's secondary sexual characteristics development using Tanner staging guidelines (refer to Chapter 7). Puberty may be delayed if diabetic control is inadequate.

Evaluation for the potential complications of diabetes should be performed annually, including blood for lipid levels, blood pressure, liver and renal function, urine for albumin, an ophthalmologic examination for retinopathy, and a neurologic examination of the extremities for neuropathies. Partner with the child and family to ensure an ongoing shared responsibility of the child's care. The child's developmental stage and cognitive level influence his or her readiness to assume responsibility for some aspects of self-care (Figure 32–11 ■).

Weblink | Diabetes Resources

| BOX 32–8 | Questions to Ask to Identify Problems with Diabetic Control |

- Is the child hungry at meals? Between meals?
- How much fluid is the child drinking?
- Has the child been going to the bathroom frequently or had episodes of bed-wetting?
- Does the child have dry skin?
- Are there sores on the feet? Do scratches or scrapes take a long time to heal?
- Has the child had any skin infections?
- Does the child have changes in mood (depression, unexplained sadness, irritability) or energy level from day to day or throughout the day?
- Have there been any changes in vision?

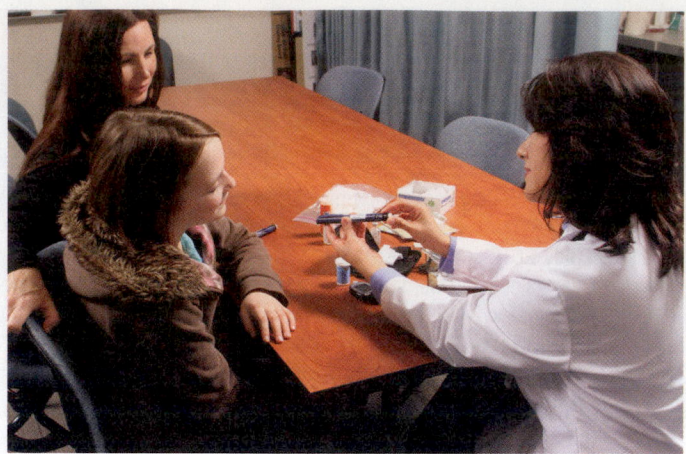

FIGURE 32–12 ■ This mother and child are being taught how to use an insulin pen.

Learning Self-Management

Education is ongoing, especially for children who develop diabetes at a young age. As they grow and assume more responsibility for their care, they need to learn more about the pathophysiology of the disease and the rationale for its management. New advances in diabetes care need to be integrated into the ongoing education.

The child with diabetes should be treated as any other child without a chronic condition, including limit setting and consistent discipline for unacceptable behavior. Children with type 1 diabetes may learn maladaptive behaviors, using their disease to obtain something they want. Teach parents to be alert to signs of maladaptation, such as helpless, demanding, or whining behaviors, and any evidence of poor coping. Additional behaviors may include skipping blood glucose testing and losing or damaging equipment. Food may become a battleground for toddlers who are picky eaters but must eat enough for the insulin dose. Referral for counseling may be appropriate for some families.

Continually work with the child to help him or her assume responsibility for self-care, and with parents to promote the child's self-care (Figure 32–12 ■). Summer camps for children with diabetes are often helpful in providing education and support. See the Photo Story on the next page. Children can learn more about their care, learn from others with diabetes, have normal activities, and add to their knowledge base.

The preschool child's need for autonomy and control can be met by allowing the child to choose snacks or to pick which finger to stick for glucose testing and by helping parents to gather necessary supplies. School-age children can learn to test blood glucose, administer insulin, and keep records. They should be taught how to select foods and portion sizes appropriate for dietary management and how to plan food intake for an exercise program. School-age children need to learn to recognize the signs of hypoglycemia and hyperglycemia, and understand the importance of carrying a rapidly absorbed sugar product.

Although adolescents understand explanations about the potential complications of diabetes, they are present-time oriented and may rebel against the daily regimen of insulin injections, the food plan, and the exercise plan. Successful self-care depends in part on the adolescent's adjustment to the chronic nature of the disease and feelings of being different from peers. Although adolescents are able to manage self-care, the desire to be like peers may interfere with treatment adherence. Talk with adolescents to assess their mood and to evaluate their motivation to manage the meal plan, exercise regimen, blood glucose monitoring, and insulin therapy. Discuss how carbohydrate counting and insulin dose adjustment may provide the flexibility to participate in activities with peers. Collaborate with the adolescent in preparation to assume care, and assist parents in accepting the growing independence from adult supervision. A discussion of the hazards associated with having diabetes and the use of alcohol, drugs, and tobacco should occur. At every subsequent healthcare visit, the adolescent should be asked about alcohol intake.

The child with type 1 diabetes may develop circulatory and neurologic changes over time. Emphasize the importance of good foot care from an early age—for example, wearing clean cotton socks, changing socks and shoes when they are damp, carrying an extra pair of socks, washing and drying feet, and keeping toenails short. Adolescents getting pedicures should inform the person performing them that they have diabetes.

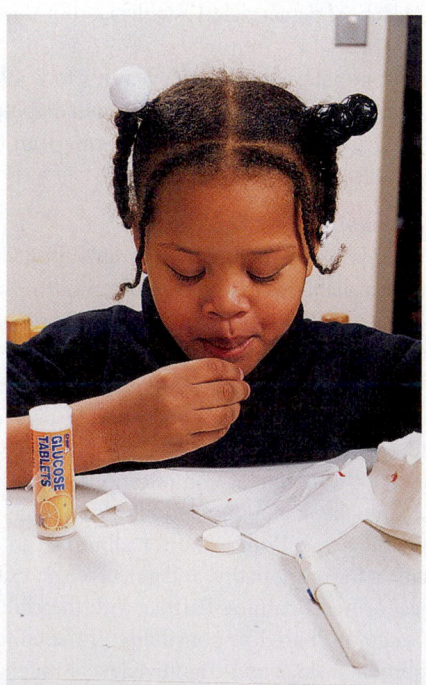

FIGURE 32–11 ■ This girl is old enough to understand the need to take glucose tablets or another form of a rapidly absorbed sugar when her serum glucose level is low.

PHOTO STORY...

MANAGING TYPE 1 DIABETES

Anna is now able to participate in her disease management, learning about monitoring serum glucose levels and eating well-balanced meals.

Anna is a 5-year-old girl with type 1 diabetes. Following Anna's diagnosis of diabetes at age 2, her parents, Cathy and Tom Deaver, have been able to successfully manage her diabetes with an insulin pump and frequent glucose monitoring. Her mother also has type 1 diabetes and uses an insulin pump. Anna is now able to participate in her disease management, learning about monitoring serum glucose levels and eating well-balanced meals.

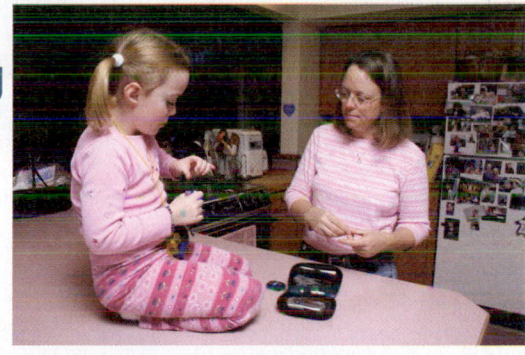

Anna prepares her equipment to perform self-glucose monitoring as her mother observes.

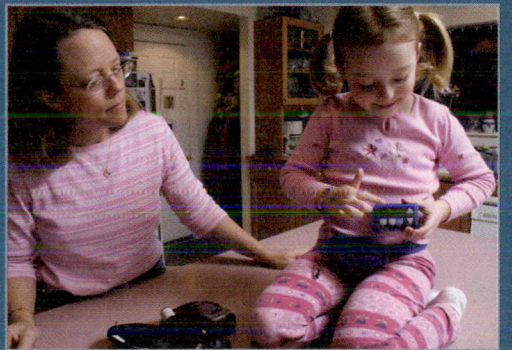

Anna checks her insulin pump. Note the waist pack on Anna. This is where she keeps her insulin pump.

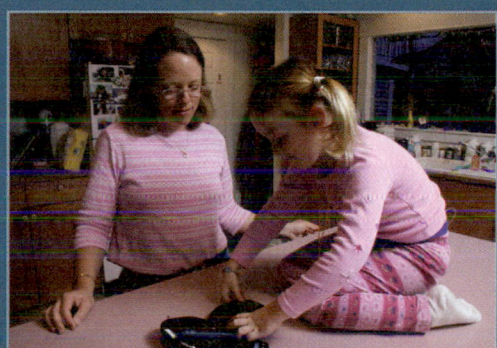

Anna and Cathy check the test results.

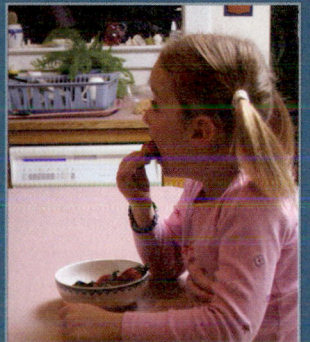

Cathy ensures nutritious snacks are always available.

Cathy started working with the diabetes nurse educator a few months ago to identify developmentally appropriate skills for Anna to learn. Cathy began by talking to Anna about each step while performing a serum glucose test on herself. Then she had Anna gather all the needed supplies. Now Anna is able to perform the fingerstick and put the drop of blood on the test strip. As Anna grows older, she will learn to interpret the serum glucose reading. Anna is also learning about foods that are good for her to eat and foods she should ask about first.

Management of Anna's diabetes takes a considerable amount of time and supervision. However, Cathy and Tom ensure that Anna participates in activities typical for a 5-year-old to promote her growth and development. In addition to ballet and gymnastics, Anna attends a childcare center. Transitioning Anna into day care required adaptations by both the family and the childcare center, but her parents emphasize that Anna's condition is manageable and should not interfere with her ability to engage in developmentally appropriate activities.

To ensure Anna's diabetes is managed at the childcare center, Anna, her parents, a community health nurse, and a nutritionist met with the staff to discuss Anna's goals and needs. Although Anna is learning how to monitor her serum glucose levels, staff members are also trained, and Cathy and Tom provide the childcare center with phone numbers so that they can be reached anytime that the serum glucose level indicates additional treatment is needed.

Foods Anna can eat are sent with her each day to help keep her diabetes controlled. The childcare center staff have also been told to contact her parents if there is a planned party so that Anna's meal plan is modified for the day and she can eat some party foods.

Health Promotion & Maintenance Overview

The Child with Diabetes Mellitus

GROWTH AND DEVELOPMENT SURVEILLANCE
- Compare the child's height, weight, and head circumference to age-specific norms to determine if growth is meeting expectations for age. Monitor body mass index (BMI) percentile at each healthcare visit.
- Assess developmental progress using the Denver II or another screening tool (refer to Chapter 8 ✪). Assess school performance.
- Assess for delays in development of sexual secondary characteristics and pubertal changes.

NUTRITION
- Promote adherence to nutrition guidelines by including the child's personal preferences in the food plan.

PHYSICAL ACTIVITY
- Encourage regular physical activity, and educate the child how to modify insulin dosage or food intake for extra physical activity periods.
- Encourage the child to participate in sports, and help the child and family learn to balance exercise, food intake, and insulin dosage.

ORAL HEALTH
- Promote good dentition and oral hygiene.
- Regular dental visits are important to reduce risk of infections.
- The child with poorly controlled diabetes is at risk of gingivitis and cavities.

MENTAL AND SPIRITUAL HEALTH
- Provide the child and adolescent an opportunity to discuss feelings regarding diabetes.
  - Assess the adolescent periodically for self-concept, and conduct screening for depression.

RELATIONSHIPS
- The child should attend school or childcare as any other child. Parents may need support to find facilities able to monitor the child as needed and to provide the teaching required for facility employees.
- Encourage the development of special friends who can be informed about the child's disorder and who will seek help when the child has signs of hypoglycemia or hyperglycemia.

DISEASE PREVENTION STRATEGIES
- Encourage the family to ensure that the child receives all recommended immunizations, including an annual influenza vaccine.
- Refer the child for an annual ophthalmologic examination.
- Maintain appointments for regular evaluation of HbA$_{1c}$ to monitor glycemic control.

INJURY PREVENTION STRATEGIES
- Encourage the child to wear a medical identification alert.
- Encourage daily inspection of feet and foot care.
- Provide the family with strategies for safe disposal of needles and syringes.

Explain to parents that the child should wear some type of medical alert identification. Help them have an individualized health plan developed (see Chapter 16 ✪) to ensure that school administrators and teachers can identify the signs of hypoglycemia or hyperglycemia and provide emergency management.

Emphasize to the parents the importance of the child receiving annual or more frequent evaluations for potential complications of diabetes. Continued education about long-term complications and prevention measures should be included at each visit. See the Health Promotion & Maintenance Overview above.

Clinical Tip

The child with diabetes needs an individualized health plan (IHP) for management of diabetes while in school or childcare. Information that should be in the IHP includes when blood glucose testing should be performed, insulin administration and storage, meals and snacks needed, and symptoms and management of hypoglycemia and hyperglycemia. Parents need to ensure that the school or childcare provider has all essential equipment and supplies for the child's management as well as phone numbers for the parents and the child's healthcare provider for diabetes (American Diabetes Association, 2011c). When the child transitions to a new childcare facility, school, or even college, IHPs should be shared, evaluated, and revised.

Evaluation

Expected outcomes of nursing care for children with type 1 diabetes can be found on the Nursing Care Plans.

Diabetic Ketoacidosis

Diabetic ketoacidosis (DKA) is a common and potentially life-threatening condition that occurs primarily in children with type 1 diabetes.

Etiology and pathophysiology Potential causes of DKA include incorrect or missed insulin doses or incorrect administration of insulin, an illness, trauma, or surgery. DKA may be present in children with new-onset diabetes.

Insulin deficiency is accompanied by a compensatory increase in hormones (epinephrine, norepinephrine, cortisol, growth hormone, and glucagon) that are released when inadequate glucose is delivered to the cells. The muscle cells break down protein into amino acids that are then converted to glucose by the liver, leading to hyperglycemia. The adipose tissue releases fatty acids that are transformed by the liver into ketone bodies. Their accumulation leads to ketoacidosis. The hyperglycemia causes an osmotic diuresis resulting in dehydration, acidosis, and hyperosmolarity. The rising ketones lead to metabolic acidosis. DKA is associated with severe metabolic, electrolyte, and fluid imbalances (see Chapter 23 ✪).

Clinical manifestations Characteristic signs of DKA include polyuria, polydipsia, weight loss, abdominal pain, nausea, and vomiting, tachycardia, signs of dehydration, flushed ears and cheeks, Kussmaul respirations, acetone breath (fruity smell), altered level of consciousness, and hypotension. Hyperglycemia, glycosuria, and ketonuria are also present. In response to metabolic acidosis, children complain of abdominal or chest pain, nausea, and vomiting. The disorder may progress to electrolyte disturbances, arrhythmias, altered consciousness, pupillary changes, irregular respirations, inappropriate slowing of the heart rate, and widening pulse pressure. See the table on page 1134 for clinical manifestations of hypoglycemia and hyperglycemia.

TABLE 32–9	Laboratory Findings in the Child with Diabetic Ketoacidosis
LABORATORY STUDY	**RESULTS**
Serum glucose	Greater than 200 mg/dL
Serum ketones	Positive
Arterial blood gas pH	Acidotic—pH less than 7.3 and bicarbonate less than 15 mEq/L
Urine	Positive for ketones (ketonuria)
Serum potassium	Elevated, decreased, or normal
Serum chloride	Elevated
Serum sodium	Decreased
Serum phosphate	Decreased
Serum osmolality	Elevated

Source: Data from Cooke, D. W., & Plotnick, L. (2008b). Management of diabetic ketoacidosis in children and adolescents. Pediatrics in Review, 29, 431–436; Jerreat, L. (2010). Managing diabetic ketoacidosis. Nursing Standard, 24(34), 49–55; McFarlane, K. (2011). An overview of diabetic ketoacidosis in children. Paediatric Nursing, 23(1), 14–19.

Collaborative Care

The immediate goal of collaborative care is to normalize the pH level, restore blood glucose to target level, and correct fluid and electrolyte imbalance. The long-term goal of management includes preventive education to reduce the risk of further diabetic ketoacidosis episodes.

Diagnostic Tests

See Table 32–9 for laboratory findings in diabetic ketoacidosis. CT scan of the brain and possible intubation and implementation of intracranial pressure (ICP) lowering strategies will be required.

Clinical Therapy

The child with ketoacidosis is hospitalized. Medical management includes isotonic intravenous fluids and electrolytes for dehydration and acidosis. Short-acting insulin (0.1 unit/kg per hour) is administered by continuous intravenous infusion pump to decrease the serum glucose level at a rate not to exceed 100 mg/dL/hr. Faster reduction of hyperglycemia and serum osmolality increases the risk for cerebral edema. When glucose is lowered too rapidly, water is freed and attracted to the glucose, which has accumulated in large quantities in the brain. Bicarbonate is not routinely used for treatment of DKA as it places the child at increased risk for hypokalemia, acidosis, and cerebral edema (Cooke & Plotnick, 2008b). As insulin is administered, potassium shifts to the cells, resulting in hypokalemia. Potassium supplementation is given only after confirmation of renal function.

Cerebral edema is the most common cause of DKA-related deaths. Mannitol is kept on standby for treatment of neurologic symptoms secondary to cerebral edema (Cooke & Plotnik, 2008b). See Chapter 33 🔗 for information about cerebral edema.

Nursing Management

Nursing care focuses on administering insulin, fluids, and electrolytes, and monitoring the child for signs and symptoms of associated complications. Once the child is stabilized, the focus of care shifts to educating the child and family on methods to prevent further episodes of diabetic ketoacidosis.

Nursing Assessment and Diagnosis

Continuously monitor the child's vital signs, respiratory status, perfusion, and mental status. Assess for changes in neurologic status, respiratory pattern, blood pressure, and heart rate. Monitor for cardiac arrhythmias associated with hypokalemia. Assess for signs of dehydration, including dry skin and mucous membranes, and depressed fontanels in infants.

Nursing diagnoses that apply to the child with diabetic ketoacidosis may include:

- Injury, Risk for related to altered cerebral function
- Fluid Volume: Deficient related to osmotic diuresis
- Nutrition, Imbalanced: Less than Body Requirements related to catabolism of protein and fat for fuel
- Knowledge, Deficient related to recognition, treatment, and prevention of diabetic ketoacidosis

NANDA-I © 2012

Planning and Implementation

Intravenous fluids are given in boluses of 10 to 20 mL/kg rapidly over 5 minutes if the child is in hypovolemic shock. Adequate fluids are given to reverse the fluid deficit. The insulin infusion must be carefully titrated to control the gradual reduction in hyperglycemia. Monitor blood glucose levels hourly or as indicated. Frequently monitor the electrolytes and acid–base status, as well as urine glucose and ketone levels as indicated. Intake and output are monitored hourly. Assess for signs of hypoglycemia which may occur during insulin infusion.

Practice Alert

Only regular insulin is administered intravenously for treatment of hyperglycemia or diabetic ketoacidosis. Do not use other insulin types as they may lower the blood glucose too rapidly or too slowly.

The child is tapered off intravenous insulin and transitioned to subcutaneous insulin when clinically stable. Oral feedings are reintroduced when the child is alert enough and the glucose level is stabilized. This plan varies according to the primary healthcare provider or endocrinologist.

Clinical Tip

Insulin binds to IV tubing. Run 50 to 100 mL of insulin through the new IV tubing to saturate all the binding sites. This ensures that the full dose of insulin reaches the child from the outset.

Electrolytes are replaced as needed. Potassium is not administered until the child has voided to confirm renal function. Monitor for signs and symptoms of hypokalemia, including hypotension, weak pulse, shallow respirations, and muscle weakness. Continuous cardiac monitoring is performed to detect cardiac conduction changes related to hypokalemia. Weigh the child daily. Provide emotional care and support to the child and family.

Care in the Community

The prevention of future episodes of diabetic ketoacidosis is important. Partner with the child and family to ensure they learn strategies to keep hyperglycemic episodes from progressing to diabetic ketoacidosis. (See Partnering with Families: Preventing DKA.) Parents should have specific instructions on how often to check the blood glucose and when to check the urine for ketones when the child is

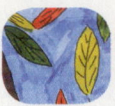

Partnering with Families

Preventing DKA

WHEN TO MONITOR FOR DKA:
- Abdominal pain
- Nausea and vomiting that persists for over 6 hours
- More than five diarrheal stools in 1 day
- A 1- or 2-day history of polyuria and polydipsia
- Has illness (e.g., viral or other) and is unable to eat

RECOGNIZING SIGNS OF DKA:
- Change in mental status
- Temperature over 102°F (38.9°C) for 12 hours
- Blood glucose 400 mg/dL on two separate readings

- Moderate to large ketones present in urine
- Fruity breath odor
- Evidence of a bacterial infection (e.g., fever, drainage, dysuria, or other evidence of a urinary tract infection)
- Difficulty breathing
- Decreased urine output

Source: *Data from Doyle, E. A., & Grey, M. (2010). Diabetes mellitus (types 1 and 2). In P. J. Allen, J. A. Vessey, & N. A. Schapiro (Eds.), Primary care of the child with a chronic condition (5th ed., pp. 427–446). St. Louis, MO: Mosby; Masharani, U. (2011). Chapter 27. Diabetes mellitus & hypoglycemia. In S. J. McPhee, M. A. Papadakis, & M. W. Rabow (Eds.), CURRENT medical diagnosis & treatment 2012. New York, NY: McGraw-Hill.*

sick. If the child has an elevated blood glucose and moderate or large amounts of ketones, treatment with extra insulin and fluids can be initiated. Increased attention to blood glucose and urine ketone monitoring is especially important when the child has significant stressors such as an illness. It is important for the child and family to understand that insulin is required even when the child is not eating to counter the hormones secreted in response to the stressor.

Evaluation

Expected outcomes of care for the child with diabetic ketoacidosis include:

- The child is free from neurologic impairment.
- The child achieves fluid volume balance.
- The child's nutritional intake is adequate to support growth and development and is balanced to insulin administration.
- The child is free from infection.
- The child and family identify measures to prevent or reduce the risk of DKA.

- The child and family recognize symptoms that require notification of a healthcare provider.
- The child experiences a reduced number of DKA episodes.

Hypoglycemia in the Child with Diabetes

Hypoglycemia can develop within minutes in children with type 1 diabetes mellitus. The symptoms outlined in the Clinical Manifestations table below may occur when blood glucose levels suddenly drop or fall below 70 mg/dL. Children are at risk of hypoglycemia due to their rapid growth rates, unpredictable eating habits, and physical activity. Severe hypoglycemia episodes may occur at night in children who are treated with two to three injections per day. Other common causes include an error in insulin dosage, errors in injection technique, inadequate calories because of missed meals, or exercise without a corresponding increase in caloric intake. Severe hypoglycemia can cause seizures.

Clinical Manifestations   Hypoglycemia and Hyperglycemia

ETIOLOGY	CLINICAL MANIFESTATIONS	CLINICAL THERAPY
Hypoglycemia - Insulin dose too high for food eaten - Insulin injection into muscle - Too much exercise for insulin dose - Too long between meals/snacks - Too few carbohydrates eaten - Illness, stress	*Rapid onset* Irritability, nervousness, tremors, shaky feeling, difficulty concentrating or speaking, behavior change, confusion, repeating something over and over Unconsciousness, seizure, shallow breathing, tachycardia Pallor, sweating Moist mucous membranes, hunger Headache, dizziness, blurred vision, double vision, photophobia Numb lips or mouth	If conscious, give 15 g of carbohydrate. Wait 15 minutes and recheck blood glucose level. Give another 15 g of carbohydrate if 70 mg/dL or below. Recheck the blood glucose level in 15 minutes. If unconscious, give glucagon by injection.
Hyperglycemia - Insulin dose too low for food eaten - Illness or injury, stress - Too many carbohydrates eaten - Meals/snacks too close together - Insulin injected just under skin or into hypertrophied areas - Decreased activity	*Gradual onset* Lethargy, sleepiness, slowed responses, or confusion Deep, rapid breathing Flushed skin, dry skin Dry mucous membranes, thirst, hunger, dehydration Weakness, fatigue Headache, abdominal pain, nausea, vomiting Blurred vision Shock	Give additional insulin at usual injection time. Give correction scale insulin doses for specific blood glucose levels when ill or injured. Give extra injections if hyperglycemic and moderate to large ketones. Increase fluids.

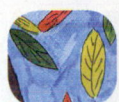

Partnering with Families

Treating Hypoglycemic Episodes

The nurse collaborates with the family to ensure that they can recognize symptoms indicating hypoglycemic episodes and the appropriate interventions.

- If the child shows signs of hypoglycemia (pallor, sweating, tremors, dizziness, numb lips or mouth, confusion, irritability, altered mental status), test the blood glucose level.
- Assist the child to perform the test. Skills needed to get an accurate reading deteriorate with the child's altered mental status.
- If the blood glucose reading is less than or equal to 70 mg/dL, give glucose rapidly. Use one of the following to give 15 grams of rapid-acting glucose to raise the blood sugar level:
  - 1/2 cup fruit juice
  - 1/2 cup of regular cola or soda

- 1 small box raisins
- 3–4 glucose tablets
- Wait 15 minutes and recheck the blood glucose level. Repeat the 15 grams of rapid-acting glucose if it is still less than or equal to 70 mg/dL. Recheck the blood glucose level in another 15 minutes.
- Once blood glucose has returned to at least 80 mg/dL, give a more substantial snack such as cheese and crackers if the next meal will be more than 30 minutes later or an activity or exercise is planned.
- If the child is unconscious, spread glucose paste on the gums or administer intramuscular subcutaneous glucagon.

Hypoglycemia can be diagnosed on the basis of the sudden onset of signs and symptoms. A blood glucose reading should be taken to confirm the diagnosis, since signs of hyperglycemia and hypoglycemia may be difficult to distinguish. Give glucose immediately in the form of a low-fat carbohydrate-containing snack or drink, sugar gel, glucose tablets, or glucose paste.

If the child becomes unconscious, administer glucagon or, if unavailable, administer sugar gel or glucose paste squeezed onto the gums. In the hospital setting, administer an intravenous infusion of dextrose to prevent progression of symptoms. Since the effects of dextrose and glucagon are temporary, additional snacks or a meal is provided. The child should be continually observed for several hours after treatment.

Clinical Tip

Do not use cake frosting or candy bars for treatment of hypoglycemia. The fat in the frosting and candy prevents the sugar from absorbing quickly. Hard candy takes too long to dissolve to provide rapid treatment for hypoglycemia.

Clinical Judgment

Symptoms such as confusion and behavior changes can be present with both hyperglycemia and hypoglycemia. When blood glucose monitoring equipment is immediately available, the nurse should check the child's blood glucose level prior to initiating treatment. What action should the nurse take if blood glucose monitoring equipment is not readily available?

Nursing Management

Recognition of hypoglycemia is essential to quickly manage symptoms and prevent further reduction of glucose. Partner with the child and family to ensure they are able to recognize the signs of hypoglycemia and take appropriate action. (See Partnering with Families: Treating Hypoglycemic Episodes.) Parents are taught to give an intramuscular or subcutaneous dose of glucagon (a hormone produced by the pancreas that helps release stored glucose from the liver) for cases of severe hypoglycemia and to activate the emergency medical system (911).

Reinforce the importance of achieving a daily balance between food intake, insulin administration, and exercise. Partner with the family to educate school personnel about the signs and symptoms of

hypoglycemia and appropriate interventions. The child should wear a medical alert identification indicating the disease and treatment. Expected outcomes include maintenance of optimal blood glucose level and a reduced number of episodes of hypoglycemia.

Neonatal hypoglycemia The neonate's serum glucose declines after a normal delivery (without complications) to a serum glucose concentration of 50 mg/dL by 2 hours of age, and then stabilizes at approximately 70 mg/dL at approximately 72 hours after birth.

Neonatal hypoglycemia occurs as a result of increased metabolic requirements during the initial newborn period. Causes of neonatal hypoglycemia are identified in Box 32–9. Signs and symptoms of neonatal hypoglycemia include apnea, tachypnea, cyanosis, hypotonia, jitteriness, poor feeding, lethargy, hypothermia, and seizures (DePuy, Coassolo, Som, et al., 2009). Serum glucose less than 30 mg/dL in the first day of life and less than 45 mg/dL after that point is considered hypoglycemia in the neonate and should be evaluated and treated to avoid permanent brain damage (Cranmer, 2011). Treatment includes administration of breast milk or formula, or parenteral glucose if the neonate refuses oral fluids.

BOX 32–9	Causes of Neonatal Hypoglycemia

- Intrauterine growth retardation
- Hyperinsulinism
- Prematurity
- Growth hormone deficiency
- Polycythemia
- Sepsis
- Hypoxia
- Hyperthermia
- Inborn errors of metabolism
- Infant of mother with diabetes
- Adrenal insufficiency

Source: *Data from Cranmer, H. (2011). Pediatrics, hypoglycemia. Emedicine. Retrieved from http://emedicine.medscape.com/article/802334-overview; Sperling, M. A. (2011). Hypoglycemia. In R. M. Kliegman, B. F. Stanton, J. W. St. Geme III, N. F. Schor, & R. E. Behrman,* Nelson textbook of pediatrics *(19th ed., pp. 517–531). Philadelphia, PA: Saunders Elsevier.*

Type 2 Diabetes

Type 2 diabetes is a disease associated with insulin resistance. Significant risk factors for type 2 diabetes include obesity, low levels of physical activity, intake of high-energy foods, low socioeconomic status, race, and family history of diabetes (Alemzadeh & Ali, 2011; Cox & Polvado, 2008; Dea, 2011). (See Developing Cultural Competence: Type 2 Diabetes Risk.) Over 75% of children with type 2 diabetes have a first- or second-degree relative with diabetes (Dea, 2011). Most children diagnosed with type 2 diabetes are over 10 years of age (Beckwith, 2010).

The increasing number of children being diagnosed with type 2 diabetes has caused significant concern in the healthcare community. An estimated 8% to 45% of children older than 10 years of age with a new diagnosis of diabetes have type 2 (Dea, 2011). The true incidence in children is unknown as many children are undiagnosed.

Etiology and pathophysiology Type 2 diabetes is a complex metabolic disorder with insulin resistance as the central abnormality. In response to increased body weight, the visceral fat produces a cytokine hormone (tumor necrosis factor) that desensitizes cellular insulin receptors to insulin. The pancreatic cells produce more insulin in an attempt to overcome insulin resistance and facilitate glucose transfer. This results in **hyperinsulinemia** (elevated insulin levels in the blood). The child maintains a balance between hyperinsulinemia and insulin resistance and a normal glycemic state. As insulin resistance worsens, the islet of Langerhans beta cells fail in their ability to hypersecrete insulin. This leads to impaired glucose tolerance and develops overt diabetes. The onset of puberty and increased secretion of the growth hormone is believed to be a contributing factor in the development of insulin resistance (Beckwith, 2010; Dea, 2011).

Clinical manifestations Signs and symptoms of type 2 diabetes vary upon initial presentation from those for type 1. See the Clinical Manifestations table on page 1122. Onset is more insidious, and diagnosis is frequently made at a routine screening appointment or after presentation of mild polydipsia or polyuria (Beckwith, 2010). **Acanthosis nigricans** (Figure 32–13 ■)—hyperpigmentation and thickening of the skin with velvety irregularities in the skinfolds of the back of the neck and medial aspect of the thighs and axillae—is a common finding and is associated with insulin resistance. The finding is present in up to 90% of children with type 2 diabetes (Beckwith, 2010). The child is usually obese with a high waist circumference. Approximately 5% to 25% of children with type 2 diabetes present with diabetic ketoacidosis at the time of diagnosis (Dea, 2011). Children with type 2 diabetes often come from home environments with a poor understanding of healthy eating habits. Behaviors frequently observed in these children include heavy snacking on calorie-dense foods, skipping meals, and sedentary activities such as using the computer, watching television excessively, and playing video games (Dea, 2011).

Collaborative Care

The goals of management are to reduce risk factors associated with type 2 diabetes, promote normal physical and emotional development, maintain target glucose, reduce hypoglycemic and hyperglycemic episodes, and minimize long-term complications.

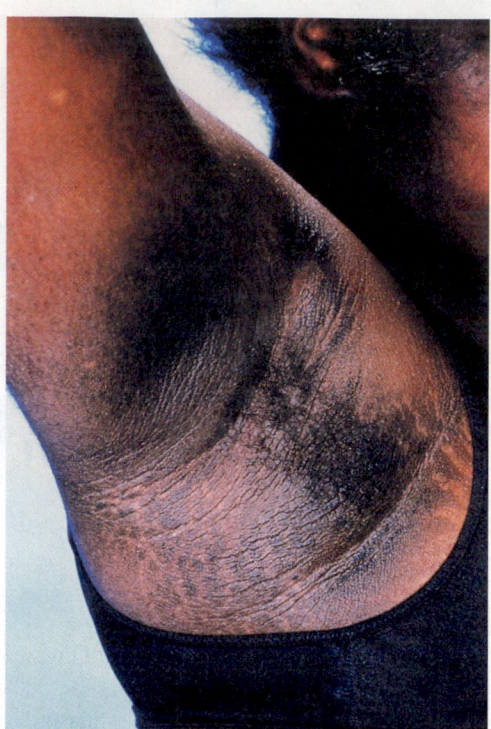

FIGURE 32–13 ■ Acanthosis nigricans.

Source: *Courtesy of Audrey Austin, MD, Children's National Medical Center, Washington, DC.*

Clinical Tip

Both the American Diabetes Association and the American Academy of Pediatrics recommend diabetes screening for children over 10 years of age when the child has a BMI greater than the 85th percentile for age and gender and at least two additional risk factors (Cox & Polvado, 2008; Dea, 2011):

- Family history of type 2 diabetes in a first- or second-degree relative
- Member of a high-risk racial or ethnic group, such as Native American, African American, Latino, Asian American, or Pacific Islander
- Signs of insulin resistance or an associated condition such as acanthosis nigricans, hypertension, dyslipidemia, or polycystic ovary syndrome

Diagnostic Tests

Blood glucose levels of 200 mg/dL or greater without fasting, or a fasting glucose of 126 mg/dL or greater, are diagnostic of diabetes. Hemoglobin A_{1c} provides an indicator of average glucose concentration over the prior 2 months (Cooke & Plotnick, 2008a). Islet cell autoantibodies, fasting insulin levels, and C-peptide levels are used to help differentiate between type 1 and type 2 diabetes but are not definitive. Islet cell autoantibodies (GAD-65, islet cell antibodies, insulin) are suggestive for type 1 diabetes; however, autoantibodies specific to a certain antigen are not present in approximately 15% of children with type 1 diabetes. Additionally, some children with type

---

Developing Cultural Competence
Type 2 Diabetes Risk

Children of African American, Native American, Latino, Asian American, and Pacific Islander origins are at greater risk for developing type 2 diabetes. Pima Indians have the highest incidence of type 2 diabetes in children, with 51 per 1,000 affected (Cox & Polvado, 2008).

2 diabetes will have detectable autoantibodies. While insulin and C-peptide levels are usually low in children with type 1 diabetes, there is some overlap with type 2, so these values are not helpful with the initial classification (Cohee, 2012). A fasting lipid profile is obtained since dyslipidemia (primarily elevated triglycerides and LDL cholesterol) is usually present (Alemzadeh & Ali, 2011). High blood pressure for age, gender, and height percentile is also seen.

Clinical Tip

The American Diabetes Association considers a fasting glucose level of 100 to 125 mg/dL (5.6 to 6.9 mmol/L) to be an *impaired fasting glucose (IFG)*, and a 2-hour postload glucose level of 140 to 199 mg/dL (7.8 to 11.0 mmol/L) to be an *impaired glucose tolerance (IGT)*. Individuals with IFG or IGT are considered at increased risk for developing diabetes. A hemoglobin A_{1c} value of 5.7% to 6.4% is an additional risk factor for the development of diabetes (American Diabetes Association, 2011b).

Clinical Therapy

The multiple goals for managing the child with type 2 diabetes include the following: normalizing the blood glucose and HbA_{1c} levels, decreasing weight, increasing exercise, normalizing lipid profile and blood pressure, and preventing complications. Nutrition education and weight loss is the major therapy. The child needs to have gradual sustained weight loss, metabolic control of blood glucose levels, exercise, and emotional support.

If the child or adolescent presents with severe hyperglycemia or diabetic ketoacidosis, insulin will be required to gain initial glycemic control. Once metabolic control is achieved, oral medication (metformin) is initiated as the child is weaned off insulin. Metformin is used when diet and exercise efforts are inadequate to control hyperglycemia. Metformin improves the sensitivity of target cells to insulin, slows the gastrointestinal absorption of glucose, and reduces the hepatic and renal glucose production. It can be used when there is normal liver and kidney function and no ketosis. The dosage may be gradually increased to improve metabolic control. If additional medication is needed, sulfonylureas may be used if metformin alone is not adequate or is contraindicated, but their use in pediatrics is limited. Thiazolidinediones are not approved for use in children but may be used if metformin is contraindicated. Insulin may only be needed for periods of increased stress, but the adolescent may ultimately require insulin for glycemic control if weight and exercise goals are not met (Alemzadeh & Ali, 2011).

Nursing Management

Nursing care focuses on promoting the child's blood glucose levels within target range if hospitalization is required and providing emotional support to the child and family. Assess growth and dietary intake, evaluate goals for weight loss and exercise programs, and review the child's knowledge about diabetes and strategies for management at home.

Nursing Assessment and Diagnosis

Because the child with type 2 diabetes often does not have an acute onset, assess any child with a BMI greater than the 85th percentile for age and gender for signs of insulin resistance (acanthosis nigricans, hypertension, and dyslipidemia). Family history of diabetes in a child who is overweight is a reason to begin screening for the condition. Once the child has been diagnosed with the disorder, monitor serum glucose levels and blood pressure. Assess the child's diet and activity

patterns to determine appropriate changes for disease management. Consider evaluating the siblings for diabetes.

Nursing diagnoses that may apply to the child with type 2 diabetes include the following:

- Nutrition, Imbalanced: More than Body Requirements related to obesity and ethnic or cultural norms
- Activity Intolerance related to sedentary lifestyle and disease state (insulin resistance)
- Therapeutic Regimen Management: Family, Ineffective related to family conflict over changing eating patterns
- Self-Esteem, Situational Low related to situational crisis associated with diagnosis of new-onset chronic illness

NANDA-I © 2012

Planning and Implementation

The child with type 2 diabetes may be hospitalized at the time of diagnosis because of ketoacidosis. However, the nurse in an inpatient setting is more likely to encounter this child when hospitalized for another condition or during visits for health care in clinics or schools. Nursing care focuses on managing the child's blood glucose levels and hypertension during the hospitalization, assessing growth and dietary intake, evaluating goals for weight loss and exercise programs, and reviewing the child's knowledge about diabetes and strategies for management at home.

Care in the Community

Since the child is usually diagnosed with type 2 diabetes and managed on an outpatient basis, nursing care focuses on teaching the child and parents about the disease and its management, managing dietary intake, providing emotional support, and planning strategies for daily management in the community.

Partner with the child and family to provide education about the disease and its management. Assist the child and family to establish lifestyle changes required for effective management of the condition. Focus on the need to increase activity with routine exercise of at least 30 to 60 minutes daily and to decrease sedentary activity time, such as computer, texting, gaming, and television viewing, to no more than 2 hours daily. Customize the activity strategy for each child with motivation to develop a regular routine.

Clinical Tip

Early intervention is needed to reduce the incidence of type 2 diabetes in a child who is at risk as well as potential complications such as hypertension. *Metabolic syndrome* is a precursor for type 2 diabetes and is characterized by elevated triglycerides, dyslipidemia, hypertension, elevated waist circumference, and high blood glucose (Steinberger, Daniels, Eckel, et al., 2009). Monitor children at risk for these associated conditions.

Work with the family to substitute alternatives to high-calorie and high-fat foods with a meal plan sensitive to the family's resources and ethnic preferences. Suggestions include limiting fast foods and using fruits and vegetables as snacks rather than foods high in fat and sugar. Assess the child's height, weight, and BMI on each visit, and plot them on the appropriate growth curve for age and gender. A gradual sustained weight loss or decrease in BMI is the goal. If the child is experiencing a height growth spurt, maintenance of weight rather than weight loss is the goal. Encourage the entire family to make dietary changes, especially since other family members are also at risk for the condition. The nutritional patterns in the family are a key part of treatment.

Partner with the child and family to ensure their ability to perform home serum glucose testing to monitor glycemic control. This will let the child and family know that efforts to manage the disease are successful. Take HbA$_{1c}$ levels at each visit to determine the average blood glucose level for the past 2 months. When dietary control and exercise are not successful in reducing blood glucose levels, teach the child and family about the prescribed oral medication.

Give the child and family opportunities to talk about the impact of the disease on their lives. Identify resources for information about strategies that have worked for other families. Identify local support groups and peer groups for the family and child. Suggest weekly activities, summer camps, and other ongoing programs to provide necessary support and motivation.

Make sure the child gets annual evaluations for potential complications of diabetes. The tests to be performed include blood for lipid levels and lipoproteins, blood pressure, liver and renal function, urine for albumin, an eye exam for retinopathy, and a neurologic exam of the extremities for neuropathies. The child with type 2 diabetes has the same risk for developing long-term vascular complications as the child with type 1 diabetes when hyperglycemia is poorly controlled.

Evaluation

Examples of expected outcomes of nursing care include:

- The child decreases sedentary activity time to less than 2 hours a day.
- The child's daily intake of fruits and vegetables increases to 5 to 8 servings daily, and total fat intake decreases to less than 30% of total calories.
- The child's body mass index slowly and consistently decreases.

DISORDERS OF GONADAL FUNCTION

The female gonads, or ovaries, regulate secondary sexual characteristics and reproduction in females. Estrogens are responsible for stimulating cells to develop secondary sexual characteristics, follicle maturation, and growth of the uterine lining. The male gonads, or testes, regulate secondary sexual characteristics and reproduction in males. Androgens, primarily testosterone, are responsible for maturation of sperm, secondary sexual characteristics, and stimulation of cells for protein synthesis.

Gynecomastia, amenorrhea, and dysmenorrhea are the disorders of gonadal function presented in this section.

Gynecomastia

Gynecomastia is a proliferation of glandular breast tissue in males occurring in approximately 50% to 60% of adolescent boys (Johnson & Murad, 2009). It is sometimes confused with subcutaneous fat pads in obese males. Gynecomastia occurs when the ratio of estrogen to testosterone is greater than the usual male ratio. It is also associated with Klinefelter syndrome and many drugs including marijuana, amphetamines, tricyclic antidepressants, calcium channel blockers, anabolic steroids, methadone, some anti-ulcer medications, cardiovascular drugs, and chemotherapy agents. Herbal supplements, especially those containing phytoestrogen, may also cause gynecomastia. The condition generally disappears in less than a year. If gynecomastia persists and is causing pain or distress to the

adolescent, a referral to a surgeon for possible reduction is indicated (Johnson & Murad, 2009).

Nursing Management

Nursing care focuses on reassuring the child and his parents that gynecomastia is common and transient. Because of the body image concerns common during adolescence, embarrassment is a frequent problem. Recommend clothing styles and other methods to camouflage the enlarged breasts.

Amenorrhea

Amenorrhea, or lack of menstruation, may be primary or secondary. Criteria for primary amenorrhea include absence of menarche by age 14.5 years in association with no growth or development of secondary sexual characteristics or absence of menses by age 16 when secondary sexual characteristics and growth are present.

Secondary amenorrhea is the cessation of menstrual periods 6 months or three cycles after menstruation has begun; it is characterized by an absence of spontaneous bleeding for at least 120 days. Pregnancy is the most common cause of secondary amenorrhea in adolescents. It is common for adolescents to have irregular menstrual cycles and duration of the menstrual period for 1 to 2 years after menarche. A large number of cycles are anovulatory for the first 2 years after menarche.

Primary amenorrhea is most often caused by structural defects of the reproductive system, chromosomal abnormalities (such as Turner syndrome, hypothalamic), pituitary tumors, thyroid dysfunction, or polycystic ovary disease. No underlying pathologic condition is identified in some adolescents.

Primary or secondary amenorrhea may be identified in competitive athletes, particularly those who are pressured to be strong competitors. Girls competing in sports such as gymnastics, ballet, and long-distance running feel the need to maintain a low weight and specific body type. Reduced adipose tissue leads to a reduction in leptin and subsequently a reduction in gonadotropin-releasing hormone and low serum estrogen levels. Amenorrhea or oligomenorrhea may result when exercise leads to excessive weight loss. Bone demineralization or osteopenia may also occur. Low levels of estrogen that occur in the presence of amenorrhea increase the female's chances of osteoporosis and fractures (Landry, 2011) (see Chapter 35).

Collaborative Care

A thorough history (including sexual activity), physical examination, and laboratory evaluation are required to determine the cause of amenorrhea. The history focuses on asking questions about recent excessive weight loss or gain; excessive physical activity or sports training; chronic illness; use of illegal drugs, birth control pills, or phenothiazines; emotional problems; and age of the mother at menarche. A family history helps to identify other female family members with similar issues.

The physical examination focuses on evaluating the adolescent's stage of sexual development and assessing for hirsutism (refer to Chapter 7). A vaginal exam is performed to determine vaginal patency and if the vaginal mucosa is estrogenized. A pregnancy test is performed. Bone age and hormone levels are evaluated (estrogen, LH, FSH, and prolactin).

Treatment of amenorrhea depends on the specific cause. The most common approach is to administer birth control pills containing both estrogen and progesterone. Athletic teenagers are encouraged to eat a well-balanced, high-calorie diet. Calcium supplements may be ordered. Estrogen with progesterone in low doses may be prescribed for athletes to reduce the risk for osteoporosis.

Nursing Management

Nursing management for the adolescent with amenorrhea centers on education and providing emotional support. The goal is to promote normal growth and development.

The nurse teaches the adolescent that it is common to have irregular menstrual cycles and variable duration in menstrual periods for 1 to 2 years after menarche. A large number of cycles are anovulatory for the first 2 years after menarche. If the adolescent female is or is considering becoming sexually active, the nurse should provide education about safe sex practices and birth control. Refer to obstetric or women's health textbooks for more information about birth control.

Dysmenorrhea

Dysmenorrhea (menstrual pain or cramping) is the most common gynecologic problem in adolescent females. Primary dysmenorrhea is usually caused by an increased secretion of prostaglandins that are produced during the ovulatory cycle. Prostaglandin causes smooth muscle contraction in the uterus, leading to ischemia and pain. Primary dysmenorrhea affects 40% to 50% of adolescent females, with an overall incidence of 40% to 90% in women. Pain may be mild or severe, with 1 out of 13 females who experience dysmenorrhea being incapacitated 1 to 3 days each month. Dysmenorrhea is the leading cause of school absence in the adolescent female population (Woo & McEneaney, 2010).

Dysmenorrhea usually occurs prior to the beginning of the menstrual period and ends on the second day of the period. The cramping pain in the lower abdomen and pelvic region ranges from mild to severe and varies with the individual. Pain may also radiate to the back or thighs. Other symptoms may include dizziness, syncope, nausea, vomiting, diarrhea, headache, and fatigue (Woo & McEneaney, 2010).

The treatment of choice for primary dysmenorrhea is nonsteroidal anti-inflammatory drugs (NSAIDs), such as ibuprofen and naproxen sodium. These drugs inhibit prostaglandin synthesis, which leads to a reduction in uterine activity and pain. Oral contraceptives may be prescribed to prevent ovulation and to decrease prostaglandin production. A gynecologic examination may be conducted to rule out any structural abnormalities.

Secondary dysmenorrhea is defined as painful menstruation associated with pelvic abnormalities. Common causes of secondary dysmenorrhea include endometriosis, fibroids, and pelvic inflammatory disease (Holder, 2011). Vaginal and cervical cultures are taken when a sexually transmitted infection is possible. See Chapter 31 🔗.

Nursing Management

Nursing care centers on providing patient education and emotional support. Instruct the adolescent with chronic dysmenorrhea to keep a calendar and begin taking NSAIDs 1 day before the onset of the menstrual period. The medications should be taken with food to minimize side effects. See Complementary Therapy: Dysmenorrhea for nonpharmacologic interventions.

Complementary Therapy   Dysmenorrhea

Nonpharmacologic methods that may be useful in the treatment of dysmenorrhea include heat, acupuncture, and exercise. Intake of vitamin B_1, vitamin E, vitamin B_6, magnesium, and omega-3 fatty acids may also help relieve symptoms of dysmenorrhea (Woo & McEneaney, 2010).

DISORDERS RELATED TO SEX CHROMOSOME ABNORMALITIES

Sex chromosome abnormalities are gender specific. Males inherit an X and a Y chromosome, whereas females inherit two X chromosomes. Male abnormalities are the result of irregular numbers of either the X or the Y chromosome or both. Female abnormalities are the result of variations in the number of X chromosomes.

The two most common sex chromosome abnormalities, Turner syndrome in females and Klinefelter syndrome in males, are discussed in this section.

Turner Syndrome

Turner syndrome is the most common sex chromosome abnormality in females. Affected girls have a missing or partial absence of one X chromosome. It occurs in approximately 1 in 2,000 live female births (Simpson, 2009). Only an estimated 1% of fetuses with this disorder survive to term (Malaisamy, Cakan, & Kamat, 2008).

Clinical Manifestations

In the absence of one X chromosome, the oocytes in the ovaries disappear and are nearly all gone by age 2 years. Other specific clinical manifestations are related to specific missing genes.

Characteristic clinical findings in the newborn include lymphedema of the hands and feet, a webbed neck, a low hairline, low-set ears, cubitus valgus (increased angle at the elbow), and widely separated nipples. Other characteristic signs include high arched palates, small mandibles, and short fourth metacarpals. During childhood, short stature becomes apparent (less than the 5th percentile). During adolescence, there is a lack of breast development, pubertal delay, and amenorrhea (Malaisamy et al., 2008; Simpson, 2009) (Figure 32–14 ■).

Growth usually proceeds at a normal rate for the first 2 to 3 years of life and then slows. Breast tissue, which begins to bud at about 10 to 12 years, fails to develop fully. Only in rare instances does a

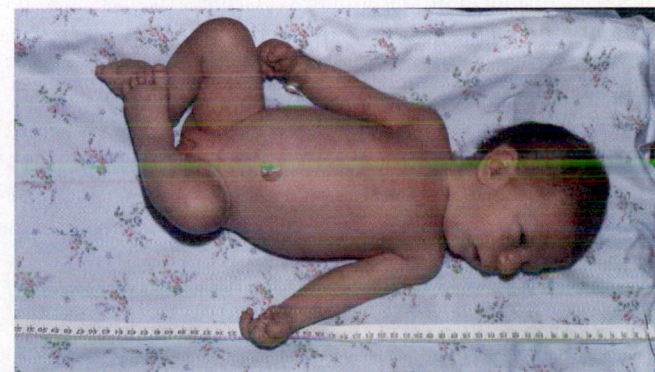

FIGURE 32–14 ■ What characteristic physical manifestation of Turner syndrome can you identify in this girl?

Source: © 2012 Wellcome Trust Library—Custom Medical Stock Photo, All Rights Reserved.

girl with Turner syndrome menstruate spontaneously or become able to conceive. Without treatment, final height is approximately 20 cm (7.8 in.) lower than the expected mean adult female height (Malaisamy et al., 2008).

Among the conditions that may be associated with Turner syndrome are congenital heart defects such as coarctation of aorta or bicuspid aortic valve, hearing loss, structural abnormalities of the kidney, ophthalmic abnormalities such as strabismus, ptosis, amblyopia, myopia, and musculoskeletal disorders such as congenital hip dysplasia and scoliosis (Scales & Weber, 2010).

Collaborative Care

The condition is diagnosed definitively by a karyotype. The most common and most severe phenotype is 45,XO, indicating an absent X chromosome, which occurs in 50% of girls with Turner syndrome. Partial X deletion occurs in 30% of girls with Turner syndrome. In this case, both X chromosomes are present, but one arm of one of the X chromosomes is either malformed or missing. In a third type, mosaicism, the child generally has a less severe type of Turner syndrome. Diagnosis of Turner syndrome may be determined prenatally by amniocentesis and should be confirmed after birth (Scales & Weber, 2010). If the diagnosis is not made prenatally, it may be made based on clinical features in infancy or in childhood as the child fails to achieve physical developmental milestones such as breast development, menarche, and height (Kansra & Donohoue, 2011).

Because of the incidence of certain disorders associated with Turner syndrome, additional diagnostic testing should be performed at the time of diagnosis. For example, cardiac abnormalities occur in approximately 50% of females with Turner syndrome. Echocardiogram is used to detect the presence of these abnormalities (Mortensen, Hjerrild, Andersen, et al., 2010). Renal ultrasound may be performed to detect kidney malformations, which occur in 30% to 60% of individuals with Turner syndrome (Styne & Grumbach, 2011).

The goal of collaborative care is to promote growth and development of the child. Treatment involves careful monitoring of the child's growth. A growth chart specifically for assessing the child with Turner syndrome is available from the Turner Syndrome Society. Growth hormone therapy may be prescribed to promote growth during childhood (Kansra & Donohoue, 2011). Anabolic steroids, preferably oxandrolone, may be used in combination with growth hormone therapy to augment growth (Malaisamy et al., 2008). Supplemental estrogen therapy is usually begun during the preteen years. This treatment produces pubertal changes such as breast development and pubic hair. Estrogen therapy also helps to preserve bone mineral density (Kansra & Donohoue, 2011).

Nursing Management

Nursing assessment is focused on monitoring growth rates and observing for signs of cardiac, renal, gastrointestinal, vision, hearing, musculoskeletal, or thyroid dysfunction. Carefully measure the child's height and plot on the growth curve. Teach the family the correct administration of growth hormone and potential side effects.

The lack of growth and sexual development associated with Turner syndrome presents problems not only for physical growth but also for psychosocial development. The girl's perception of her body and how she differs from peers affects self-image, self-consciousness, and self-esteem. In the United States, cultural values place importance on attaining normal to tall stature. Children who are short tend

to be treated according to their size rather than their age. Emphasis is also placed on sexual maturity. Encourage parents to treat the child by her chronologic age rather than size. Even though intelligence is generally normal, learning disabilities are common (Tsai, Manchester, & Elias, 2011).

The nurse can help the child adapt to the condition and gain self-esteem. Be an active listener and reinforce abilities and skills that the girl exhibits. Encourage parents to provide support.

Partner with the child and family to promote adaptive skills and positive self-esteem. Active listening and reinforcement of abilities and skills that the child exhibits promote self-esteem. Encourage parents to partner with the healthcare team to provide the child or adolescent with ongoing support. The Turner Syndrome Society can provide additional information about the disorder for parents and adolescents.

Klinefelter Syndrome

Klinefelter syndrome is a common genetic condition that occurs in boys who have an extra X chromosome (usually 47,XXY). It occurs in approximately 1 in 650 males. Klinefelter syndrome is associated with hypogonadism (decreased secretory activity of the gonad), infertility in males, and tall stature (Boada, Janusz, Hutaff-Lee, et al., 2009).

Clinical Manifestations

Klinefelter syndrome is frequently diagnosed when the onset of puberty is delayed or an abnormal progression is evident. Testicular size is decreased at all ages. Less facial and body hair may develop. Gynecomastia is a characteristic finding. Other physical features include fifth-finger *clinodactyly* (bending or curving), hypotonia, and *hypertelorism* (increased distance between the eyes) (Zeger, Zinn, Lahlou, et al., 2008).

Klinefelter syndrome may also be diagnosed during the school-age years when the child is having difficulty at school. Speech and reading delays are common (Zeger et al., 2008). Boys with Klinefelter syndrome have normal to borderline IQs, and a small percentage demonstrates cognitive disabilities (Tsai et al., 2011).

Collaborative Care

Chromosomal analysis revealing one or more extra X chromosomes confirms the diagnosis. The goal of treatment is to stimulate masculinization and the development of secondary sex characteristics when adolescence is delayed. Testosterone replacement is begun at puberty, when the male is 11 or 12 years of age. A testosterone preparation is given by intramuscular injection every 3 to 4 weeks to maintain serum testosterone levels within the normal range. The dose is increased gradually every 6 to 9 months until a maintenance dose is achieved in adults (Ali & Donohoue, 2011).

Nursing Management

Assess secondary sexual characteristics, history, and height and weight. Nursing care consists of educating the parents and child about the syndrome, evaluating the child's and family's coping mechanisms, assisting with school problems, and reinforcing the child's strengths.

Partner with the family and school officials to encourage an education environment tailored to the child's needs. The family may require assistance in coordinating an individualized developmental and educational program for their son. Language therapy to promote communication skills may be required. Refer the family to speech and communication specialists as indicated.

Encourage parents to channel their son's energy into areas that will provide opportunities for success and productive experiences. Emphasize the importance of rewarding the child's successes in school, sports, or hobbies. Encourage the child to express concerns related to body image. Genetic counseling should be made available to adolescents, if indicated, given that sexual functioning and fertility may be impaired.

INBORN ERRORS OF METABOLISM

Inborn errors of metabolism are inherited biochemical abnormalities of the urea cycle, amino acid, and organic acid metabolism. Therefore, protein, carbohydrate, fat, electrolyte, blood, and respiratory metabolism can be affected. Individually they are rare disorders; however, as a group they are a significant health problem in infancy.

The biochemical defect usually causes an abnormal chemical by-product to accumulate in the blood, urine, or tissues or results in a decreased amount of normal enzymes. Most disorders are associated with protein intolerance, with symptoms developing shortly after formula or breast milk feedings are begun.

Clinical manifestations usually occur within days or weeks of birth. Signs and symptoms may include lethargy and poor feeding, persistent vomiting, abnormal muscle tone and seizures, apnea and tachycardia, and an unusual urine or body odor (musty, sweet odor of maple syrup or burnt sugar, cheesy, or sweaty feet).

Newborn screening has been demonstrated to save lives and to prevent serious disability. The March of Dimes recommends that newborn screening tests for 30 disorders that have effective treatment be made available to all newborns (March of Dimes, 2010). In most states, newborn screening programs lead to the detection of several conditions before symptoms develop. See Chapters 4 and 9 🔵.

In some cases, disorders associated with inborn errors of metabolism are not detected until signs and symptoms are present. Initial laboratory tests include measurement of serum glucose, electrolytes, blood gases, and serum ammonia. Test results make it possible to classify the disorder by the presence of hypoglycemia, metabolic acidosis, hyperammonemia, or liver dysfunction. Further diagnostic laboratory tests are then performed on newborns with positive results.

Treatment, when available, focuses on replacing or reducing the amount of the substance causing the biochemical abnormality.

Four of the more common inborn errors of metabolism—phenylketonuria, galactosemia, fatty acid oxidation defects, and maple syrup urine disease—are presented in this section. Congenital hypothyroidism and congenital adrenal hyperplasia, which are also considered inborn errors of metabolism, were discussed earlier in this chapter.

Phenylketonuria

Phenylketonuria (PKU) is an autosomal recessive inherited disorder of amino acid metabolism that affects the body's utilization of protein. It is caused by a mutation of the phenylalanine hydroxylase gene. The incidence is greater than 1 in 15,000 live births per year in the U.S. population (Arnold, 2009). The defect results in an accumulation of phenylalanine in the blood or phenylalanine metabolites in the urine. If untreated, this disease leads to irreversible brain damage and severe intellectual disability. Phenylalanine levels above 20 mg/dL are indicative of classic PKU (Widaman, 2009).

Etiology and Pathophysiology

Children with PKU have a deficiency of the liver enzyme phenylalanine hydroxylase that normally breaks down the essential amino acid phenylalanine into tyrosine. As a result, phenylalanine accumulates in the blood, causing a musty or mousy body and urine odor, irritability, vomiting, hyperactivity, hypertonic or hyperreflexive deep tendon reflexes, seizures, and an eczema-like rash (Rezvani & Melvin, 2011). Persistence of elevated phenylalanine leads to disruption of cellular processes of myelination and protein synthesis and results in a seizure disorder and untreatable intellectual disability.

Clinical Manifestations

Infants appear normal at birth except for a lighter skin complexion than their nonaffected siblings. If diagnosis is delayed, a mousy or musty body odor is noticed and intellectual disability may be severe. Microcephaly, prominent maxilla and widely spaced teeth, enamel hypoplasia, and growth retardation commonly occur in untreated children (Rezvani & Melvin, 2011).

Collaborative Care

The goal of collaborative care is to diagnose the condition as soon as possible, before the toxic effect of phenylalanine has a chance to cause extensive harm to the body, and to begin treatment with medical formula and foods as soon as the diagnosis is made.

Screening for phenylketonuria is required by law in all 50 states (see Legal and Ethical Considerations: Neonatal Screening). For best results, the newborn should have begun formula or breast milk feeding before specimen collection. Early hospital discharge places newborns at risk for false-negative screening tests if screened within 24 hours of birth. Screening must occur no sooner than 48 hours after birth, or the test should be repeated at 1 to 2 weeks of age. If the test shows elevated levels of plasma phenylalanine, a repeat quantitative test is performed. If the second test is positive, the family is referred to an outpatient treatment center. Serum levels of phenylalanine should be measured periodically throughout life. Levels greater than 15 mg/dL are considered dangerous.

Clinical Therapy

Phenylketonuria is treated using special formulas and a diet low in phenylalanine to keep plasma phenylalanine levels between 2 and 6 mg/dL (Arnold, 2009). The diet must also meet the child's needs for optimal growth. Breastfeeding is possible if phenylalanine levels are monitored. High-protein foods (meats and dairy products) and aspartame are avoided since they contain large amounts of phenylalanine. Elemental medical foods (modified protein hydrolysates in which the phenylalanine has been removed) are used instead.

Legal and Ethical Considerations
Neonatal Screening

Neonatal screening for many conditions, including congenital hypothyroidism, sickle cell disease, sickle C disease, sickle beta thalassemia, galactosemia, phenylketonuria, and cystic fibrosis, is required by state law in all 50 states. A complete list of conditions for which all 50 states require screening is available from the National Newborn Screening and Genetics Resource Center (National Newborn Screening and Genetics Resource Center, 2011).

The low-phenylalanine diet should be maintained for life to avoid declines in IQ and neuropsychologic abilities (White, Waisbren, & van Spronsen, 2010). The low-phenylalanine diet is especially important for adolescent females and women prior to conception and during pregnancy to prevent congenital anomalies (low birth weight, microcephaly, intellectual disability, and congenital heart defects) in the fetus (March of Dimes, 2008; Widaman, 2009).

Nursing Management

Nursing care is mainly supportive and focuses on teaching parents about the disorder and its management.

Nursing Assessment and Diagnosis

Assess the infant and child for consequences of PKU, including neurologic findings such as tremor and hyperactive deep tendon reflexes, cognitive and behavioral problems, and atopic dermatitis (related to toxic effects of phenylalanine and its metabolites) (Clements, 2010). The severity of findings may provide a clue as to how well the dietary control is maintained.

Nursing diagnoses that may be applicable to a child with PKU include the following:

- Development: Delayed, Risk for related to effects of disorder and less than optimal dietary control
- Noncompliance (PKU diet) related to desire to eat same foods as peers
- Parenting, Risk for Impaired related to child with inherited disorder and need for lifelong special formula and foods

NANDA-I © 2012

Planning and Implementation

The low-phenylalanine diet is a rigid, strict diet that excludes many foods. Educate the family about sources of phenylalanine, and refer the family to a nutritionist to establish an appropriate meal plan. Parents and children need a great deal of support to promote compliance. The formula and elemental medical food costs are relatively expensive. The formula is usually reimbursed by insurance, but negotiations with health plans may help parents to obtain support for medical foods. The current recommendation is that all individuals with PKU remain on the phenylalanine restricted diet for life (Rezvani & Melvin, 2011).

Like children with diabetes mellitus, children with PKU may rebel against the dietary limitations in an effort to be like their peers. Reinforcement of the need for dietary control is important during this time. Educate the child's teacher and school nurse about the child's special meal plan in an effort to encourage compliance while the child is at school. Parents of an affected child who are considering a future pregnancy, and adolescents with the disorder should be referred for genetic counseling. See Chapter 4 🔗.

Evaluation

Examples of expected outcomes of nursing care for the child with PKU include the following:

- The child demonstrates age-appropriate development.
- The child adheres to special dietary requirements at school.
- The parents adapt by integrating the child's special care needs into the family's routines.

Galactosemia

Galactosemia is a disorder of carbohydrate metabolism that has an autosomal recessive inheritance pattern. It occurs in greater than 1 in 50,000 live births (March of Dimes, 2010). Galactosemia results from a deficiency of the liver enzyme galactose-1-phosphate uridyltransferase (GALT), one of three enzymes needed to convert galactose to glucose. The lack of enzyme leads to an accumulation of galactose metabolites in the eyes, liver, kidney, and brain, rapidly damaging the organs and causing life-threatening problems. Children become susceptible to gram-negative sepsis.

Early signs include poor sucking, failure to gain weight due to vomiting followed by diarrhea, hypoglycemia, and an enlarged liver. Later signs include intellectual disability, jaundice, ascites, sepsis, lethargy, seizures, hypotonia, cataracts, and coma. Babies may die within 1 month without treatment, usually due to sepsis. If the infant is not diagnosed with galactosemia at birth, cirrhosis of the liver and intellectual disability progress and become irreversible (Kishnani & Chen, 2011).

Collaborative Care

Routine newborn screening for galactosemia is performed in all U.S. newborn screening programs (March of Dimes, 2008). Infants who are not screened at birth are identified once they become symptomatic. The diagnosis is based on history, physical examination, and laboratory tests (galactose, alanine aminotranferease (ALT) and aspartate aminotransferase (AST) are abnormally high). Urine specimens are checked for reducing substances (the Clinitest is positive and the Clinistix is negative) in several specimens while the patient is receiving human milk or formula with lactose.

Treatment involves placing infants on a lactose- or galactose-free formula. Improvement in the infant's condition is generally observed within 24 hours. A galactose-free diet (no milk or cheese products, including foods with dry milk products) is prescribed when the infant is ready for solid foods. These dietary restrictions are lifelong (March of Dimes, 2010). Despite compliance with the diet, complications (learning disabilities, speech defects, ovarian failure, and neurologic syndromes) develop in many children (Kishnani & Chen, 2011).

Nursing Management

Nursing management focuses on educating the parents and child about the disorder and required diet, assessing coping abilities, and providing emotional support. Refer the family to a nutritionist for diet counseling. Families must learn to screen foods for added milk solids and to avoid medications, such as antibiotics, that have lactose fillers. Calcium supplementation may be needed. Advise parents that several galactose-free cheeses are sold commercially. Because the disorder is inherited, refer the family for genetic counseling.

Defects in Fatty Acid Oxidation

Mitochondrial oxidation of fatty acids is an energy-producing pathway that becomes essential during periods of starvation when the body fuel converts from carbohydrate to fat. Gene defects can occur in nearly every stage in the fatty acid oxidation pathway, resulting in many subclasses of fatty acid oxidation defects. All of these defects are autosomal recessive traits that occur in both males and females (Stanley & Bennett, 2011).

Fatty acid oxidation disorders are among the most common inborn errors of metabolism. These defects include medium-chain acyl-CoA dehydrogenase (MCAD) deficiency (most common), very long-chain acyl-CoA dehydrogenase deficiency, long-chain 3-OH acyl-CoA dehydrogenase deficiency, trifunctional protein deficiency, and carnitine uptake defect. If undiagnosed, these disorders can lead to serious complications affecting the brain and other organs. Symptoms can progress to coma and then death (March of Dimes, 2010).

The most common presentation is an acute-onset life-threatening coma and hypoglycemia induced by a period of fasting. Other manifestations often include cardiomyopathy, hepatomegaly, and muscle weakness. Infants and children can be asymptomatic except for times during fasting or stress.

Diagnosis can occur during routine newborn screening when laboratories use mass spectrometry. Most cases are identified during an acute presentation of symptoms. Laboratory evaluation may include blood gases, electrolytes, hepatic profile, plasma lactate, plasma amino acids, urine organic acids, acylcarnitine profile, quantitative carnitine levels, and urine for ketones. Hypoglycemia is usually present and ketone levels are unusually low (Thomas & Van Hove, 2011). Liver function tests demonstrate elevated transaminases, urea, and ammonia. Plasma and tissue concentrations of total carnitine are reduced. Skin biopsies are often obtained for fibroblast analysis. Physical examination may reveal hepatomegaly due to fatty infiltration.

Treatment includes the prevention of hypoglycemia by avoiding fasting, ensuring that no more than 8 to 12 hours passes before food is eaten. Carnitine supplementation may be required in some disorders as it is useful in preventing low blood sugar and assists in removing metabolic waste from cells (Thomas & Van Hove, 2011).

Nursing Management

Nurses can educate parents about the importance of frequent feedings and avoidance of fasting. Teach parents that these children should go no longer than 8 to 12 hours without food. Infants should be fed around the clock every 2 to 4 hours. If the infant or child is unable to sustain oral intake during an acute illness, he or she must be referred to the hospital for intravenous dextrose supplementation. Even simple infections such as an ear infection or influenza can become life threatening for these children. Several snacks and meals of low-fat and high-carbohydrate foods (e.g., cereal, pasta) are recommended throughout the day. Genetic counseling should be offered to the family. If one child in the family is diagnosed with the disorder, the siblings should also be tested, even if they are asymptomatic.

Maple Syrup Urine Disease

Maple syrup urine disease (MSUD) is a disorder of amino acid metabolism that has an autosomal recessive inheritance pattern. It is rare, occurring in approximately 1 in 180,000 newborns, but occurs as often as 1 in 176 newborns among some Pennsylvania Mennonites (Bodamer & Lee, 2008).

In MSUD, leucine, isoleucine, and valine cannot be metabolized due to an enzyme defect in the branched chain of these three essential amino acids (Bodamer & Lee, 2008). All three amino acids are essential to form normal structures such as the hair, skin, and muscle. Accumulation of these three amino acids leads to encephalopathy and progressive neurologic impairment if left untreated (Bodamer & Lee, 2008).

Within 4 to 7 days of life, the newborn develops symptoms of poor feeding, lethargy, vomiting, poor weight gain, variable muscle tone, irritability, seizures, high-pitched cry, severe ketoacidosis, and a sweet odor of maple syrup in urine. The symptoms may quickly progress to coma and death if not treated (Bodamer & Lee, 2008; March of Dimes, 2010).

Collaborative Care

Most but not all states require newborn screening for MSUD. Diagnosis is made with laboratory tests of the urine for positive ketones and blood tests for elevated leucine, isoleucine, alloisoleucine, and valine. Treatment during the acute stage involves removal of the branch-chained amino acids and their metabolites from the tissues and body fluids. Some critically ill infants may require dialysis to remove these compounds because renal clearance is poor.

Lifelong treatment includes specially designed medical formulas and foods rich in amino acids, calories, vitamins, minerals, and other nutrients as prescribed; these special medical foods have the three amino acids removed. The child needs special low-protein foods that are adequate for growth with enough calories to support twice the child's basal metabolic rate. Daily urine testing is required to determine if ketones are being excreted, an indication that the body is in a catabolic state. Liver transplants have been performed in a few affected children who were subsequently able to tolerate a normal diet. The long-term prognosis of children with MSUD is guarded (Rezvani & Rosenblatt, 2011).

Nursing Management

Nursing care includes educating the family about the disorder and special dietary requirements. Partner with the family to ensure their understanding of how to mix the child's special formula with a natural protein source, amino acid supplements, and water. The child requires formula even when ill. Parents should have a sick day plan to prevent ketoacidosis. The child should be permitted moderate exercise only to prevent increases in leucine levels. Help families identify sources of information or support groups who can share recipes and tips for managing the child's condition.

Chapter Highlights

- Puberty is the process of sexual maturation that occurs when the gonads secrete increased amounts of the sex hormones estrogen and testosterone, resulting in the development of primary and secondary sexual characteristics.

- The anterior pituitary gland is considered to be the "master gland" of the body because of its role in the production of hormones that regulate the secretion of other hormones.

- Children with hypopituitarism have short stature as a result of growth hormone deficiency. Treatment with growth hormone early in life enables these children to have near normal heights.

- An excessive secretion of growth hormone or hyperpituitarism may cause children to have tall stature, growing up to 7 or 8 feet in height if no intervention is provided before the epiphyseal plates close.

- In diabetes insipidus, the urine cannot be concentrated, no matter how dehydrated the child becomes. Diagnosis rarely occurs until the child experiences hypernatremic dehydration.

- Syndrome of inappropriate antidiuretic hormone (SIADH) results from an excessive amount of serum antidiuretic hormone (ADH) leading to water intoxication and hyponatremia.

- Precocious puberty is defined as the appearance of any secondary sexual characteristics before 8 years in girls and 9 years in boys. If no treatment is provided, the hormones will stimulate closure of the epiphyseal plates and the child will have short stature as an adult.

- Untreated or ineffectively treated congenital hypothyroidism results in impaired growth and intellectual disability.

- Signs of hyperthyroidism include an enlarged, nontender thyroid gland (goiter), prominent eyes, eyelid lag, tachycardia, nervousness, restlessness or irritability, increased appetite with weight loss, emotional lability, heat intolerance, increased sweating, insomnia, tremor, and muscle weakness.

- During infancy and childhood, most cases of Cushing disease are due to a malignant adrenal tumor. It generally takes up to 5 years for the child to develop the characteristic cushingoid appearance.

- Congenital adrenal hyperplasia has two forms, salt-losing or non-salt-losing with virilization. The salt-losing form accounts for 75% of cases and is caused by aldosterone deficiency and overproduction of androgen. The non-salt-losing form accounts for the other 25% of cases.

- Adrenal insufficiency, though rare in children, is characterized by weakness with fatigue, anorexia and salt craving, poor weight gain or weight loss, hyperpigmentation at pressure points, generalized bronzing of the skin, abdominal pain, nausea and vomiting, and diarrhea.

- Congenital adrenal hyperplasia is the most common cause of pseudohermaphroditism (ambiguous genitalia) in newborn girls.

- Pheochromocytoma is a rare benign tumor of the adrenal gland which causes labile hypertension and intermittent signs associated with epinephrine and norepinephrine secretion.

- Diabetes mellitus type 1 is the most common metabolic disease in children and one of the most common chronic diseases in school-age children. It is a disorder of carbohydrate, protein, and fat metabolism.

- Treatment of the child with diabetic ketoacidosis includes intravenous fluids and electrolytes for dehydration and acidosis. Insulin is given by continuous infusion pump to decrease the serum glucose level at a slow but steady rate to prevent the development of cerebral edema.

- Common causes of hypoglycemia in children with type 1 diabetes include an error in insulin dosage, inadequate calories because of missed meals, or exercise without a corresponding increase in caloric intake.

- Type 2 diabetes mellitus is a condition that results from insulin resistance and affects 8% to 45% of children over 10 years of age. The true incidence in children is unknown as many children are undiagnosed. Children most commonly affected are obese, and many have family members with the same type of diabetes.

- Secondary amenorrhea is the cessation of spontaneous menstrual periods for at least 120 days and occurs 6 months or three cycles after menarche.

- Turner syndrome is diagnosed definitively by a karyotype, which reveals the classic 45,X chromosome pattern or 46,XX pattern with one misshapen X chromosome.

- Signs of Klinefelter syndrome include gynecomastia, delayed onset of puberty with an abnormal progression, decreased testicular size, and less facial and body hair than normal.

- Inborn errors of metabolism—inherited biochemical abnormalities of the urea cycle and amino acid and organic acid metabolism—often have a significant impact on the endocrine system's ability to support growth and development. These disorders include phenylketonuria, galactosemia, defects in fatty acid oxygenation, and maple syrup urine disease.

- Children with phenylketonuria (PKU) have a deficiency of the liver enzyme phenylalanine hydroxylase that normally breaks down the essential amino acid phenylalanine into tyrosine. It is treated with special formula and engineered foods.

- Galactosemia results from a deficiency of a liver enzyme needed to convert galactose to glucose. This leads to an accumulation of galactose metabolites in the eyes, liver, kidney, and brain, rapidly damaging the organs and causing life-threatening problems.

- In the inborn error of metabolism involving a defect in fatty acid oxygenation, the most common presentation is an acute-onset life-threatening coma and hypoglycemia induced by a period of fasting.

- Maple syrup urine disease is a rare inherited enzyme deficiency that results in ketoacidosis unless special formula, engineered foods, and extra calories are eaten.

Clinical Reasoning in Action

INTRODUCTION

Recall Anthony, the 12-year-old in the opening scenario, who is newly diagnosed with type 1 diabetes. His glucose is now stabilized and he is receiving basal-bolus insulin therapy.

DESCRIPTION

Anthony is learning to check his own serum glucose and demonstrates the correct technique. He states that he is afraid of giving himself a "shot" and becomes anxious when he receives injections. Anthony will soon be discharged from the hospital and will receive further diabetes education on an outpatient basis. Anthony's parents are eager to learn about caring for him but express concerns now that he will not be able to participate in sports activities as he has in the past.

DISCUSSION

1. Considering Anthony's age and developmental level, how will the nurse explain type 1 diabetes to Anthony?
2. How will the nurse address Anthony's reluctance to self-administer his insulin? What are some potential causes of Anthony's reluctance?
3. What skills must Anthony's parents demonstrate prior to his discharge from the hospital?
4. What will the nurse explain to Anthony and his parents regarding activity, exercise, and participation in sports?

NCLEX-RN® Review

1. When a child with type 1 diabetes is sick, which is the most appropriate recommendation?
   1. The usual dose of insulin may need to be decreased or omitted.
   2. Test blood glucose if the urine ketones are positive.
   3. Urine ketones are tested when the glucose level is greater than 200 mg/dL.
   4. Maintain fluid intake, avoiding fluids that contain carbohydrates.

2. Identify the priority nursing diagnosis for an adolescent with hyperthyroidism.
   1. Disturbed Body Image related to changes in appearance caused by process of metabolic disorder
   2. Imbalanced Nutrition: More than Body Requirements related to decreased metabolic needs
   3. Risk for Decreased Fluid Volume related to excess salt excretion
   4. Constipation related to thyroid medication side effects

3. A 4-year-old child with congenital renal hyperplasia is being admitted for an elective surgical procedure. Which indicates effective teaching has taken place?
   1. The hormone dosage is held for 24 hours prior to surgery.
   2. Injectable hydrocortisone is on hand for stressful situations such as surgery.
   3. Surgery is avoided unless absolutely necessary.
   4. The hydrocortisone dose is decreased prior to the surgery.

4. The nurse is caring for a newborn in the nursery. The child has lymphedema of the hands and feet, a webbed neck, and a low hairline. Which disorder does the nurse suspect?
   1. Turner syndrome
   2. Klinefelter syndrome
   3. Phenylkeytonuria
   4. Galactosemia

See Appendix I ⊘ for answers.

References

Alemzadeh, R., & Ali, O. (2011). Diabetes mellitus. In R. M. Kliegman, B. F. Stanton, J. W. St. Geme III, N. F. Schor, & R. E. Behrman, *Nelson textbook of pediatrics* (19th ed., pp. 1968–1997). Philadelphia, PA: Saunders Elsevier.

Ali, O., & Donohoue, P. A. (2011). Hypofunction of the testes. In R. M. Kliegman, B. F. Stanton, J. W. St. Geme III, N. F. Schor, & R. E. Behrman, *Nelson textbook of pediatrics* (19th ed., pp. 1943–1950). Philadelphia, PA: Saunders Elsevier.

American Academy of Pediatrics. (2009). *Pediatric nutrition handbook* (6th ed., pp. 673–699). Elk Grove Village, IL: Author.

American Diabetes Association. (2011a). Diagnosis and classification of diabetes mellitus. *Diabetes Care, 34*(Suppl. 1), S62–S69.

American Diabetes Association. (2011b). Standards of medical care in diabetes—2011. *Diabetes Care, 34*(Suppl. 1), S11–S61.

American Diabetes Association. (2011c). Diabetes care in the school and day care setting. *Diabetes Care, 34*(Suppl. 1), S70–S74.

Antal, Z., & Zhou, P. (2009). Addison disease. *Pediatrics in Review, 30*(12), 491–493.

Arnold, G. L. (2009). *Genetics of phenylketonuria.* Retrieved from http://emedicine.medscape.com/article/947781-overview

Bachman, J. A., & Hsueh, K. (2008). Evaluation of online education about diabetes management in the school setting. *Journal of School Nursing, 24*(3), 151–157.

Bahn, R. S., Burch, H. B., Cooper, D. S., Garber, J. R., Greenlee, C., Klein, I., . . . Stan, M. N. (2011). Hyperthyroidism and other causes of thyrotoxicosis: Management guidelines of the American Thyroid Association and American Association of Clinical Endocrinologists. *Thyroid, 21*(6), 593–646.

Bangstad, H., Danne, T., Deeb, L. C., Jarosz-Chobot, P., Urakami, T., & Hanas, R. (2009). Insulin treatment in children and adolescents with diabetes. *Pediatric Diabetes, 10*(Suppl. 12), 82–99.

Bauer, A. J. (2011). Approach to the pediatric patient with Graves' disease: When is definitive therapy warranted? *Journal of Clinical Endocrinology and Metabolism, 96*(3), 580–588.

Beckwith, S. (2010). Diagnosing type 2 diabetes in children and young people. *British Journal of School Nursing, 5*(1), 15–19.

Boada, R., Janusz, J., Hutaff-Lee, C., & Tartaglia, N. (2009). The cognitive phenotype in Klinefelter syndrome: A review of the literature including genetic and hormonal factors. *Developmental Disabilities Research Reviews, 15*, 284–294.

Bodamer, O. A., & Lee, B. (2008). *Maple syrup urine disease*. Retrieved from http://emedicine.medscape.com/article/946234-overview

Bordini, B., & Rosenfield, R. L. (2011a). Normal pubertal development: Part I: The endocrine basis of puberty. *Pediatrics in Review, 32*(6), 223–229.

Bordini, B., & Rosenfield, R. L. (2011b). Normal pubertal development: Part II: Clinical aspects of puberty. *Pediatrics in Review, 32*(7), 281–292.

Breault, D. T., & Majzoub, J. A. (2011). Diabetes insipidus. In R. M. Kliegman, B. F. Stanton, J. W. St. Geme III, N. F. Schor, & R. E. Behrman, *Nelson textbook of pediatrics* (19th ed., pp. 1881–1884). Philadelphia, PA: Saunders Elsevier.

Brent, G. A., & Davies, T. F. (2011). Hypothyroidism and thyroiditis. In S. Melmed, K. S. Polonsky, P. R. Larsen, & H. M. Kronenberg, *Williams textbook of endocrinology* (12th ed., pp. 406–439). Philadelphia, PA: Saunders Elsevier.

Buckley, L. L., & Walsh, K. (2011, July). Diabetes insipidus. *CINAHL Information Systems.*

Campbell, F. (2008). The pros and cons of continuous subcutaneous insulin infusion (CSII) therapy in the paediatric population and practical considerations when choosing and initiating CSII in children. *British Journal of Diabetes and Vascular Disease, 8*(Suppl. 1), S6–10.

Carchidi, C., Holland, C., Minnock, P., & Boyle, D. (2011). New technologies in pediatric diabetes care. *MCN, 36*(1), 32–39.

Carel, J., & Léger, J. (2008). Precocious puberty. *New England Journal of Medicine, 358*, 2366–2377.

Centers for Disease Control and Prevention. (2011). *SEARCH for diabetes in youth*. Retrieved from http://www.cdc.gov/diabetes/pubs/factsheets/search.htm

Clements, A. L. (2010). Phenylketonuria. In P. J. Allen & J. A. Vessey (Eds.), *Primary care of the child with a chronic condition* (5th ed., pp. 739–755). St. Louis, MO: Mosby.

Cohee, L. (2012). Endocrinology. In *Johns Hopkins: The Harriet Lane handbook* (19th ed., pp. xxxx). Philadelphia, PA: Elsevier.

Cook, L. K. (2009). Pheochromocytoma. *American Journal of Nursing, 109*(2), 50–53.

Cooke, D. W., Divall, S. A., & Radovick, S. (2011). Normal and aberrant growth. In S. Melmed, K. S. Polonsky, P. R. Larsen, & H. M. Kronenberg, *Williams textbook of endocrinology* (12th ed., pp. 935–1053). Philadelphia, PA: Saunders Elsevier.

Cooke, D. W., & Plotnick, L. (2008a). Type 1 diabetes mellitus in pediatrics. *Pediatrics in Review, 29*, 374–385.

Cooke, D. W., & Plotnick, L. (2008b). Management of diabetic ketoacidosis in children and adolescents. *Pediatrics in Review, 29*, 431–436.

Counts, D., & Varma, S. K. (2009). Hypothyroidism in children. *Pediatrics in Review, 30*, 251–258.

Cox, D., & Polvado, K. (2008). Type 2 diabetes in children and adolescents. *Advance for Nurse Practitioners, 16*(11), 43–45.

Cranmer, H. (2011). Pediatrics, hypoglycemia. *Emedicine*. Retrieved from http://emedicine.medscape.com/article/802334-overview

Cystic Fibrosis Foundation. (2011). *Cystic fibrosis-related diabetes*. Retrieved from http://www.cff.org/LivingWithCF/StayingHealthy/Diet/Diabetes/

Dea, T. L. (2011). Pediatric obesity & type 2 diabetes. *MCN, 36*(1), 42–48.

DePuy, A. M., Coassolo, K. M., Som, D. A., & Smulian, J. C. (2009). Neonatal hypoglycemia in term, nondiabetic pregnancies. *American Journal of Obstetrics & Gynecology, 200*(5), e45–51.

de Wit, M., Delemarre-van de Waal, H. A., Bokma, J. A., & Hass, K. (2008). Monitoring and discussing health-related quality of life in adolescents with type 1 diabetes improve psychosocial well-being. *Diabetes Care, 31*(8), 1521–1526.

Doyle, D. A. (2011). Disorders of the parathyroid gland. In R. M. Kliegman, B. F. Stanton, J. W. St. Geme III, N. F. Schor, & R. E. Behrman, *Nelson textbook of pediatrics* (19th ed., pp. 1916–1923). Philadelphia, PA: Saunders Elsevier.

Doyle, E. A., & Grey, M. (2010). Diabetes mellitus (Types 1 and 2). In P. J. Allen, J. A. Vessey, & N. A. Schapiro (Eds.), *Primary care of the child with a chronic condition* (5th ed., pp. 427–446). St. Louis, MO: Mosby.

Ferguson, L. A. (2011). Growth hormone use in children: Necessary or designer therapy? *Journal of Pediatric Health Care, 25*(1), 24–30.

Ferry, R. J., & Pascual-y-Baralt, J. F. (2010). *Pediatric syndrome of inappropriate antidiuretic hormone secretion*. Retrieved from http://emedicine.medscape.com/article/924829-overview

Fitzgerald, P. A. (2012). Endocrine disorders. *CURRENT Medical Diagnosis & Treatment 2012*. New York, NY: McGraw-Hill.

Fleury-Milfort, E. (2008). Insulin replacement therapy: Minimizing complications and side effects. *Advance for Nurse Practitioners, 16*(11), 32–39.

Fraser, L., & Van Uum, S. (2010). Work-up for Cushing syndrome. *Canadian Medical Association Journal, 182*(6), 584–587.

Ganie, A. M., & Kalra, S. (2010). Hypothyroidism: Clinical features. *Internet Journal of Family Practice, 8*(2), 9p.

George, J., Acharya, S. V., Bandgar, T. R., Menon, P. S., & Shah, N. S. (2010). Primary hyperparathyroidism in children and adolescents. *Indian Journal of Pediatrics, 77*(2), 175–178.

Glaser, N. S., & Styne, D. M. (2008). Predicting the likelihood of remission in children with Graves' disease: A prospective multicenter study. *Pediatrics, 121*(3), e481–e488.

Grimberg, A., Stewart, E., & Wajnrajch, M. P. (2008). Gender of pediatric recombinant human growth hormone recipients in the United States and globally. *Journal of Clinical Endocrinology and Metabolism, 93*(6), 2050–2056.

Hanas, R., de Beaufort, C., Hoey, H., & Anderson, B. (2011). Insulin delivery by injection in children and adolescents. *Pediatric Diabetes, 12*, 518–526.

Ho, J., Loh, C. T. F., Pacaud, D., & Leung, A. K. C. (2010). Type 1 diabetes mellitus in children and adolescents: Part 2, Management. *Consultant for Pediatricians, 9*(2), 69–77.

Holder, A. (2011). *Dysmenorrhea in emergency medicine*. Retrieved from http://emedicine.medscape.com/article/795677-overview#a0104

Ivey, J. B., Wright, A., & Dashiff, C. J. (2009). Finding the balance: Adolescents with type 1 diabetes and their parents. *Journal of Pediatric Health Care, 23*(1), 10–18.

Jerreat, L. (2010). Managing diabetic ketoacidosis. *Nursing Standard, 24*(34), 49–55.

Johnson, R. E., & Murad, M. H. (2009). Gynecomastia: Pathophysiology, evaluation, and management. *Mayo Clinic Proceedings, 84*(11), 1010–1015.

Kaguelidou, F., Carel, J. C., & Leger, J. (2009). Graves' disease in childhood: Advances in management with antithyroid drug therapy. *Hormone Research, 71*, 310–317.

Kansra, A. R., & Donohoue, P. A. (2011). Hypergonadotropic hypogonadism in the female (primary hypogonadism). In R. M. Kliegman, B. F. Stanton, J. W. St. Geme III, N. F. Schor, & R. E. Behrman, *Nelson textbook of pediatrics* (19th ed., pp. 1951–1957). Philadelphia, PA: Saunders Elsevier.

Kaplowitz, P. B. (2010). Delayed purberty. *Pediatrics in Review, 31*(5), 189–195.

Kishnani, P. S., & Chen, Y. (2011). Defects in galactose metabolism. In R. M. Kliegman, B. F. Stanton, J. W. St. Geme III, N. F. Schor, & R. E. Behrman, *Nelson textbook of pediatrics* (19th ed., pp. 502–503). Philadelphia, PA: Saunders Elsevier.

Kulshreshtha, B., Khadgawat, R., Eunice, M., & Ammini, A. C. (2010). Congenital adrenal hyperplasia: Results of medical therapy on appearance of external genitalia. *Journal of Pediatric Urology, 6*(6), 555–559.

Kwon, K. T., & Tsai, V. W. (2007). Metabolic emergencies. *Emergency Medicine Clinics of North America, 25*(4), 1041–1060.

LaFranchi, S. (2011). Disorders of the thyroid gland. In R. M. Kliegman, B. F. Stanton, J. W. St. Geme III, N. F. Schor, & R. E. Behrman, *Nelson textbook of pediatrics* (19th ed., pp. 1894–1923). Philadelphia, PA: Saunders Elsevier.

Landry, G. L. (2011). Female athletes: Menstrual problems and the risk of osteopenia. In R. M. Kliegman, B. F. Stanton, J. W. St. Geme III, N. F. Schor, & R. E. Behrman, *Nelson textbook of pediatrics* (19th ed., pp. 2421–2422). Philadelphia, PA: Saunders Elsevier.

Leger, J., Gelwane, G., Kaguelidou, F., Benmerad, M., Alberti, C., and the French Childhood Graves' Disease Study Group. (2012). Positive impact of long-term antithyroid drug treatment on the outcome of children with Graves' disease: National long-term cohort study. *Journal of Clinical Endocrinology and Metabolism. 97*(1), 1–10.

Malaisamy, A., Cakan, N., & Kamat, D. M. (2008). Genetic disorders: What is this disorder—And what is the prognosis? Two girls with short stature. *Consultant for Pediatricians, 7*(7), 277–284.

March of Dimes. (2008). *Phenylketonuria*. Retrieved from http://www.marchofdimes.com/baby/birthdefects_pku.html

March of Dimes. (2010). *Recommended newborn screening tests*. Retrieved from http://www.marchofdimes.com/baby/bringinghome_recommendedtests.html

Masharani, U. (2011). Chapter 27. Diabetes mellitus & hypoglycemia. In S. J. McPhee, M. A. Papadakis, M. W. Rabow (Eds.), *CURRENT medical diagnosis & treatment 2012*. New York, NY: McGraw-Hill.

McFarlane, K. (2011). An overview of diabetic ketoacidosis in children. *Paediatric Nursing, 23*(1), 14–19.

McHugo, J., & Harden, A. (2011). Diabetes insipidus: Navigating troubled waters. *Advance for NPs and PAs, 2*(4), 20–24.

Miles, H. L., & Acerini, C. L. (2008). Insulin analog preparations and their use in children and adolescents with type 1 diabetes mellitus. *Pediatric Drugs, 10*(3), 163–176.

Molina, P. E. (2010). Parathyroid gland & Ca^{2+} & Po_4^- regulation. In *Endocrine physiology* (3rd ed.). New York, NY: McGraw-Hill.

Moriarty, M., & Hoe, F. (2009). Cushing disease in a toddler: Not all obese children are just fat. *Current Opinion in Pediatrics, 21*, 548–552.

Mortensen, K. V., Hjerrild, B. E., Andersen, N. H., Sørensen, K. E., Hørlyck, A., Pedersen, E. M., . . . Gravholt, C. H. (2010). Abnormalities of the major intrathoracic arteries in Turner syndrome as revealed by magnetic resonance imaging. *Cardiology in the Young, 20,* 191–200.

National Newborn Screening and Genetics Resource Center. (2011). *National newborn screening status report.* Retrieved from http://genes-r-us.uthscsa.edu/nbsdisorders.pdf

O'Connell, S., & Siafarikas, A. (2010). Addison disease: Diagnosis and initial management. *Australian Family Physician, 39*(11), 834–837.

Parks, J. S., & Felner, E. I. (2011). Hypopituitarism. In R. M. Kliegman, B. F. Stanton, J. W. St. Geme III, N. F. Schor, & R. E. Behrman, *Nelson textbook of pediatrics* (19th ed., pp. 1876–1881). Philadelphia, PA: Saunders Elsevier.

Pass, K. A., & Neto, E. C. (2009). Update: Newborn screening for endocrinopathies. *Endocrinology Metabolic Clinics of North America, 38,* 827–837.

Pereira, M. G., Berg-Cross, L., Almeida, P., & Machado, J. C. (2008). Impact of family environment and support on adherence, metabolic control, and quality of life in adolescents with diabetes. *International Journal of Behavioral Medicine, 15,* 187–193.

Péter, F., & Muzsnai, O. (2009). Congenital disorders of the thyroid: Hypo/hyper. *Endocrinology Metabolism Clinics of North America, 38,* 491–507.

Pluta, R. M., Burke, A. E., & Golub, R. M. (2011). Cushing syndrome and Cushing disease. *Journal of the American Medical Association, 306*(24), 2742.

Potts, J. T., & Jüppner, H. (2012). Disorders of the parathyroid gland and calcium homeostasis. In D. L. Longo, A. S. Fauci, D. L. Kasper, S. L. Hauser, J. L. Jameson, & J. Loscalzo (Eds.), *Harrison's principles of internal medicine* (18th ed.). New York, NY: McGraw-Hill.

Rewers, A., Klingensmith, G., Davis, C., Petitti, D. B., Pihoker, C., Rodriquez, B., . . . Dabelea, D. (2008). Presence of diabetic ketoacidosis at diagnosis of diabetes mellitus in youth: The search for diabetes in youth study. *Pediatrics, 121*(5), e1258–e1266.

Rezvani, I., & Melvin, J. J. (2011). Phenylalanine. In R. M. Kliegman, B. F. Stanton, J. W. St. Geme III, N. F. Schor, & R. E. Behrman, *Nelson textbook of pediatrics* (19th ed., pp. 418–421). Philadelphia, PA: Saunders Elsevier.

Rezvani, I., & Rosenblatt, D. S. (2011). Valine, leucine, isoleucine and related organic acidemias. In R. M.

Kliegman, B. F. Stanton, J. W. St. Geme III, N. F. Schor, & R. E. Behrman, *Nelson textbook of pediatrics* (19th ed., pp. 430–438). Philadelphia, PA: Saunders Elsevier.

Rivkees, S. A. (2010). Pediatric Graves' disease: Controversies in management. *Hormone Research in Pediatrics, 74,* 305–311.

Robinson, A. G., & Verbalis, J. G. (2011). Posterior pituitary. In S. Melmed, K. S. Polonsky, P. R. Larsen, & H. M. Kronenberg, *Williams textbook of endocrinology* (12th ed., pp. 292–323). Philadelphia, PA: Saunders Elsevier.

Ryzin, C. V. (2009). Nonclassic congenital adrenal hyperplasia: An overview. *Journal of Pediatric Nursing, 24*(6), 535–537.

Scales, R., & Weber, C. (2010). Turner syndrome: Do not miss this diagnosis. *Journal of Pediatric Nursing, 25,* 66–68.

Sharma, P. K., & Barr, L. J. (2010). *Complications of thyroid surgery.* Retrieved from http://emedicine.medscape.com/article/852184-overview#a1

Simpson, T. (2009). Short stature in a 6-year-old female. *Pediatric Nursing, 35*(1), 64, 68.

Sirotnak, A. P. (2008). *Child abuse and neglect: Psychosocial dwarfism.* Retrieved from http://emedicine.medscape.com/article/913843-overview

Sperling, M. A. (2010). Treatment of short children with GH plus IGF-1: Are two hormones better than one? *Infectious Diseases in Children, 23*(1), 46–48.

Sperling, M. A. (2011). Hypoglycemia. In R. M. Kliegman, B. F. Stanton, J. W. St. Geme III, N. F. Schor, & R. E. Behrman, *Nelson textbook of pediatrics* (19th ed., pp. 517–531). Philadelphia, PA: Saunders Elsevier.

Stanley, C. A., & Bennett, M. J. (2011). Disorders of mitochondrial fatty acid b-oxidation. In R. M. Kliegman, B. F. Stanton, J. W. St. Geme III, N. F. Schor, & R. E. Behrman, *Nelson textbook of pediatrics* (19th ed., pp. 456–462). Philadelphia, PA: Saunders Elsevier.

Steinberger, J., Daniels, S. R., Eckel, R. H., Hayman, L., Lustig, R. H., McCrindle, B., & Mietus-Snyder, M. L. (2009). Progress and challenges in metabolic syndrome in children and adolescents. A scientific statement from the American Heart Association Atherosclerosis, Hypertension, and Obesity in the Young Committee of the Council on Cardiovascular Disease in the Young; Council on Cardiovascular Nursing; and Council on Nutrition, Physical Activity, and Metabolism. *Circulation. 119,* 628–647.

Styne, D. M., & Grumbach, M. M. (2011). Puberty: Ontogeny, neuroendocrinology, physiology, and disorders. In S. Melmed, K. S. Polonsky, P. R. Larsen, & H. M. Kronenberg, *Williams textbook of endocrinology* (12th ed., pp. 1054–1201). Philadelphia, PA: Saunders Elsevier.

Thomas, J. A., & Van Hove, J. L. K. (2011). Inborn errors of metabolism. In W. W. Hay, M. J. Levin, J. M. Sondheimer, & R. R. Deterding, *CURRENT diagnosis and treatment: Pediatrics* (20th ed.). New York, NY: McGraw-Hill.

Tsai, A. C., Manchester, D. K., & Elias, E. R. (2011). Genetics & dysmorphology. In W. W. Hay, M. J. Levin, J. M. Sondheimer, & R. R. Deterding, *CURRENT diagnosis and treatment: Pediatrics* (20th ed.). New York, NY: McGraw-Hill.

Tschudy, M. M., & Arcara, K. M. (2012). Blood chemistries and body fluids. In *Johns Hopkins: The Harriet Lane handbook* (19th ed., p. 643). Philadelphia, PA: Elsevier.

White, D. A., Waisbren, S., & van Spronsen, F. J. (2010). The psychology and neuropathology of phenylketonuria. *Molecular Genetics and Metabolism, 99,* s1–s2.

White, P. C. (2011). Disorders of the adrenal gland. In R. M. Kliegman, B. F. Stanton, J. W. St. Geme III, N. F. Schor, & R. E. Behrman, *Nelson textbook of pediatrics* (19th ed., pp. 1923–1943). Philadelphia, PA: Saunders Elsevier.

Widaman, K. F. (2009). Phenylketonuria in children and mothers: Genes, environments, behavior. *Current Directions in Psychological Science, 18*(1), 48–52.

Wilson, B. A., Shannon, M. T., & Shields, K. M. (2011). *Pearson nurse's drug guide 2011.* New York, NY: Pearson.

Winsett, R. P., Stender, S. R., Gower, G., & Burghen, G. A. (2010). Adolescent self-efficacy and resilience in participants attending a diabetes camp. *Pediatric Nursing, 36*(6), 293–296.

Woo, P., & McEneaney, M. J. (2010). New strategies to treat primary dysmenorrhea. *Clinical Advisor for Nurse Practitioners, 13*(11), 43–49.

Wright, E. E. (2009). Overview of insulin replacement therapy. *Journal of Family Practice, 58*(80), S3–S9.

Zeger, M. P. D., Zinn, A. R., Lahlou, N., Ramos, P., Kowal, K., Samango-Sprouse, C., & Ross, J. L. (2008). Effect of ascertainment and genetic features on the phenotype of Klinefelter syndrome. *Journal of Pediatrics, 152,* 716–722.

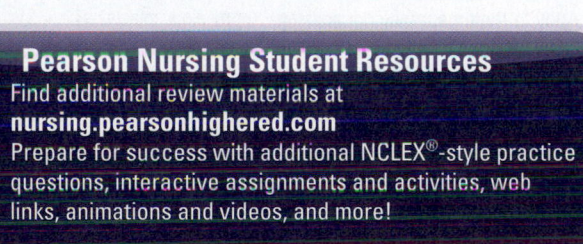

Pearson Nursing Student Resources

Find additional review materials at
nursing.pearsonhighered.com
Prepare for success with additional NCLEX®-style practice questions, interactive assignments and activities, web links, animations and videos, and more!

33 Alterations in Neurologic Function

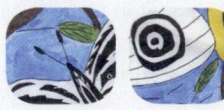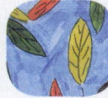

Learning Outcomes

After completing this chapter, you will be able to:

1. Describe the anatomy and physiology of the neurologic system.

2. Choose the appropriate assessment guidelines and tools to examine infants and children with altered levels of consciousness and other neurologic conditions.

3. Differentiate between the signs of a seizure and status epilepticus in infants and children, and plan appropriate nursing management for each condition.

4. Differentiate between signs of bacterial meningitis, viral meningitis, encephalitis, and Guillain-Barré syndrome in infants and children.

5. Plan family-centered nursing care for the child with myelodysplasia and hydrocephalus.

6. Plan family-centered nursing care for the child with cerebral palsy in a community setting.

7. Contrast the initial nursing management for the child with mild traumatic brain injury and severe traumatic brain injury.

8. Discuss initiatives to prevent drowning in children.

> "I am so glad I finally got to visit Andy. Even though Mom and Dad told me he would be okay, I could tell they were really worried. Even though he had all those tubes hooked up to him, I was so glad he could play with me."
>
> —*Timmy, age 6*

Andy Davis, 8 years old, was admitted to the hospital after being diagnosed with meningitis. Andy's mother took him to see his primary care physician after he complained of a severe headache and discovered that he had a fever. The physician immediately sent Andy to the emergency department to be evaluated for meningitis. Andy had a lumbar puncture in the emergency department that revealed white blood cells in his spinal fluid. The spinal fluid was sent to the lab for culture and sensitivities. An intravenous line was inserted and antibiotics were initiated as soon as the culture was obtained.

On admission, Andy was lethargic and irritable, and he complained of a severe headache. Both Kernig and Brudzinski signs were positive. No petechial lesions or signs of increased intracranial pressure were identified. A fever of 40.0°C (104°F) was present. Andy reported a pain level of 8 in his head and neck. An opioid pain medication and acetaminophen were prescribed.

Andy's antibiotic was changed to match the culture sensitivities when the results became available 2 days later, and after 24 hours on the appropriate antibiotic he was no longer considered infectious. Four days have passed, and Andy is beginning to feel like getting up for short periods to visit the playroom.

What is the nurse's role in the acute care of the child with meningitis? What support does the family need to cope with this serious infection and provide supportive care for the child? What are some potential long-term consequences of this condition?

Why do certain neurologic disorders occur more often in children than in adults? What effect do these disorders have on a child's growth and development? Why are some neurologic injuries more likely to be seen in children? What role do nurses play in ensuring early diagnosis and treatment of neurologic disorders? This chapter will answer these questions by examining some of the more common disorders of neurologic function in children.

ANATOMY AND PHYSIOLOGY

Knowledge of the anatomy of the nervous system makes neurologic symptoms easier to understand. The brain, spinal cord, and nerves are the major structures of the nervous system. The brain is protected by the skull and covered by three layers of tissue called the meninges—the dura mater, arachnoid, and pia mater (Figure 33–1 ■). Cerebrospinal fluid circulates within the ventricles of the brain and around the brain and spinal cord.

The brain is a complex organ that controls, regulates, or coordinates many body functions, including cognition, behaviors, the senses, and motor ability. Stimuli are received from the environment, and the brain enables response for adaptation, survival, and maintenance of body functions. See Table 33–1 for the primary functions of the brain's structures, including the cerebrum, the cerebellum, and the brainstem. The brainstem connects the cerebral hemispheres, the cerebellum, and the spinal cord. The 12 cranial nerves arise from the brainstem and have many important sensory and motor functions (Table 33–2).

TABLE 33–1 | **The Brain Structures and Their Primary Functions**

BRAIN STRUCTURE	FUNCTIONS AND CONTROL
Cerebrum	Higher mental functions, general movement, perception, and integration of all functions in lobes listed below
Frontal lobe	Voluntary skeletal muscle movement, fine repetitive motion, eye movements, motor aspects of speech
Parietal lobe	Interpretation of sensations (taste, vision, smell, hearing, temperature, pressure, touch, pain, texture, two-point discrimination); recognition of body parts, proprioception
Occipital lobe	Vision center and interpretation of vision
Temporal lobe	Hearing or the perception, reception, and comprehension of speech, long-term memory
Insula (corpus callosum)	Coordination of activities between the two hemispheres of the cerebrum
Limbic system	Mediation of certain primitive behavior responses, visceral emotional responses, feeding behaviors, biological rhythms, and the sense of smell
Thalamus	Interpretation of most sensations except smell, relay center for sensory motor information
Hypothalamus	Maintenance of temperature, autonomic nervous system function, endocrine function, wakefulness; regulation of emotional expression
Cerebellum	Conscious and reflexive control of muscle tone and voluntary muscle activity, maintenance of balance and posture
Brainstem	Location of the descending and ascending motor and sensory pathways; connects the cerebrum, cerebellum, and spinal cord; origin of the 12 cranial nerves

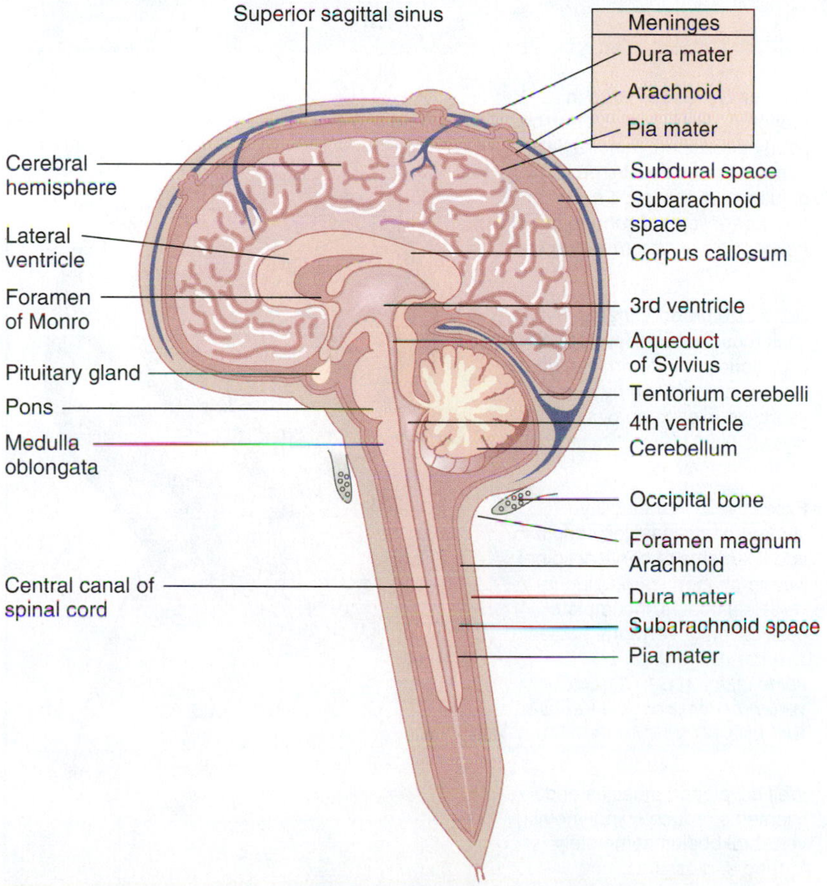

FIGURE 33–1 ■ Transverse section of the brain and spinal cord. Knowledge of brain and spinal cord anatomy is helpful in understanding the symptoms of neurologic dysfunction.

The spinal cord, covered by the vertebrae, transmits impulses to and from the brain, conveying sensory information and relaying impulses that stimulate motor responses. Spinal nerves have sensory and motor components that send and receive information to specific body locations. Nerve impulses are transmitted by chemical substances (e.g., norepinephrine, acetylcholine, dopamine, histamine, and serotonin) and electrical conduction, enabling the impulse to travel through the synapses from neuron to neuron.

The peripheral nerves permit transmission of impulses from the nerve pathways to the cerebral cortex through simple spinal reflex arcs. The upper motor neurons consist of fibers originating in the anterior horn of the spinal cord that travel to the brainstem and the nerve cells in the cerebral cortex. The lower motor neurons consist of the peripheral nerves and branches that transmit impulses from the body to the anterior horn of the spinal cord.

The autonomic nervous system maintains a steady state of the internal body organs' and glands' involuntary functions. It is divided into the *sympathetic nervous system*, which mobilizes the body to respond in times of need or stress, and the *parasympathetic nervous system*, which works to conserve and restore energy.

PEDIATRIC DIFFERENCES

The brain and spinal cord are formed early in gestation from the neural plate which evolves into the neural groove and neural folds. By the fourth week of

TABLE 33–2   The Cranial Nerves and Their Functions*

CRANIAL NERVES	FUNCTION
Olfactory (I)	Reception and interpretation of smell
Optic (II)	Visual acuity, visual fields
Oculomotor (III)	Many eye movements, raise the eyelids, pupil constriction
Trochlear (IV)	Inward and downward eye movement
Trigeminal (V)	Opening and closing the jaw, chewing; eyelid and corneal eye sensation; sensation of the face, mouth and nose mucosa, tongue, and ear
Abducens (VI)	Lateral eye movement
Facial (VII)	Facial expression, eye closure, and lip speech sounds; taste sensation on anterior two thirds of tongue; and pharyngeal sensation
Acoustic (VIII)	Sense of hearing and equilibrium
Glossopharyngeal (IX)	Muscles for swallowing and guttural speech; gag reflex; taste sensation of posterior one third of tongue, nasopharyngeal sensation
Vagus (X)	Sensation behind ear and in a portion of the external ear canal; involuntary control of the heart and lungs
Spinal accessory (XI)	Shrug the shoulders and turn the head
Hypoglossal (XII)	Tongue movement; swallowing, speech sounds involving the tongue

*See Chapter 7 🔗 for assessment guidelines.

gestation, the neural folds close to form the **neural tube,** the embryonic origin of the central nervous system (CNS). The neural folds close first in the cervical region. Closure then progresses in both the cranial and caudal directions. The brain develops from the cranial end of the neural tube, and the spinal cord develops in the remainder of the neural tube (Boss & Huether, 2010). Any insult (such as inadequate folic acid) or critical event (teratogen, infection, substance abuse, or trauma) during this early period of gestation can result in a neural tube defect such as spina bifida.

The anatomic and physiologic differences between the nervous systems of children and adults help explain why children and adults have different neurologic problems (Figure 33–2 ■). For example, the brain and spinal cord are protected by the skeletal structures of the skull and vertebrae. In infants, however, the cranial bones and vertebrae are not completely ossified. The infant's brain and spinal cord are thus at greater risk for injury resulting from trauma. The bones of the skull are separated but held together with bands of connective tissue to allow for normal brain growth. **Fontanels** are spaces of connective tissue covering the brain at the junction of skull bones, which gradually close and ossify. The posterior fontanel closes at 3 months of age, and the anterior fontanel closes at about 18 to 24 months of age. See Figure 7–12 in Chapter 7 🔗. The suture lines between the skull bones interlock as early as 6 months of age, and by 8 years of age the sutures are completely ossified (Boss & Huether, 2010).

As They Grow   Anatomic Differences in the Structures of the Nervous System Between Children and Adults

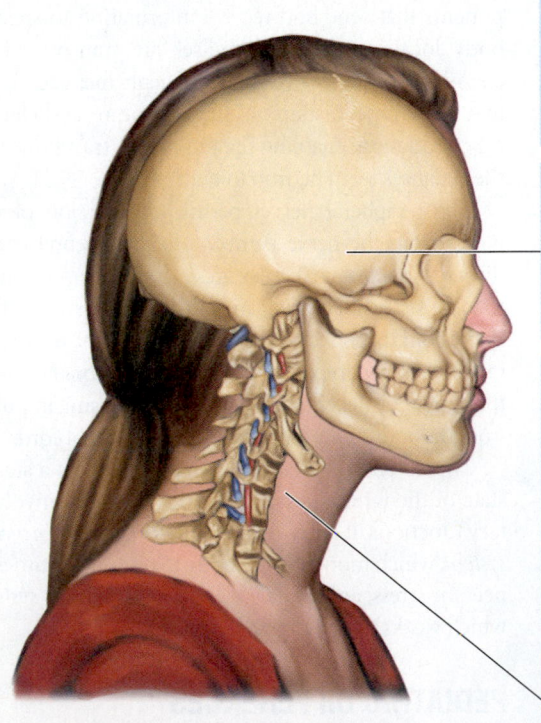
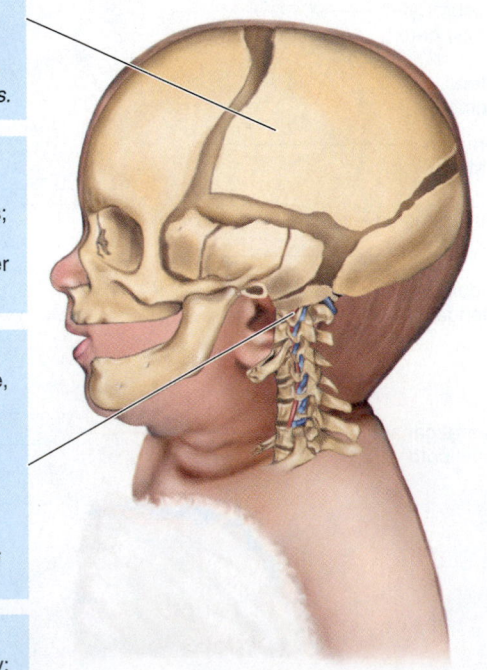

Top heavy, head is large in proportion to body; neck muscles poorly developed; thin cranial bones not well developed; unfused sutures; skull expands until age 2 years. *Prone to brain injury and skull fracture with falls.*

Head size proportional to body; neck muscles well developed, can reduce risk for brain injuries; sutures are ossified by age 12 years; no expansion of skull after 5 years.

Excessive spinal mobility; immature muscles, joint capsule, and ligaments of cervical spine; wedge-shaped, cartilaginous vertebral bodies; incomplete ossification of vertebral bodies. *Greater risk for high cervical spine injury at C1-C2 level or vertebral compression fractures with falls.*

Well developed muscles and ligaments reduce spinal mobility; vertebral bodies completely formed and ossified.

FIGURE 33–2 ■ The skull and brain grow and develop rapidly during early childhood. Infants and young children are at higher risk for injury to the brain and spinal cord because of developing anatomic structures.

The full-term newborn has a complete but immature nervous system at birth. The infant is born with all of the nerve cells that will exist throughout life, but maturation of these nerve cells continues after birth. The number of glial cells and dendrites, which enable receipt of nerve impulses, continues to increase until approximately 4 years of age. Brain growth results in the increasing head circumference in infants and toddlers. Brain growth continues until the child is 12 to 15 years of age.

Myelination, the progressive covering of axons with layers of myelin or a lipid protein sheath, is also incomplete at birth. Lack of myelination is associated with the presence of primitive reflexes. As the myelination progresses, the primitive reflexes disappear. See Table 7–19 🔗 for the expected appearance and disappearance of primitive reflexes during early infancy. This process continues throughout childhood, proceeding in a cephalocaudal direction. The myelination process accounts for the progressive acquisition of fine and gross motor skills and coordination during early childhood, and it is ultimately responsible for the speed and accuracy of nerve impulses.

In infants and young children the vertebral bodies are wedge shaped, the ligaments permit more movement, and the articulating facets at C1 and C2 permit more sliding in cases of injury. The child's spinal cord attains adult characteristics after 10 years of age when the vertebral body loses its wedge shape and the facets become more vertically aligned (Mathison, Kadom, & Krug, 2008).

The brain depends on a continuous blood flow to meet its high demands for oxygen. Through an autoregulatory process, the cerebral blood vessels dilate to maintain the cerebral blood flow in response to physiologic changes such as fluctuating cerebral perfusion pressure from decreased cardiac output, increased intracranial pressure, or constriction of the neck's blood vessels due to positioning. When blood flow and oxygenation are not maintained, the brain cells become damaged in a very short time. Because the nervous system helps to control and coordinate many body functions, alterations in neurologic function can have widespread effects on the body's metabolism.

NEUROLOGIC ASSESSMENT

Performing a nursing assessment of the child with a potential or actual neurologic condition involves a careful review of the signs and symptoms in many body systems and analysis of their relationship to neurologic functioning. Use the guidelines in Table 33–3 to perform a comprehensive assessment of a child with a neurologic condition. Numerous diagnostic procedures and laboratory tests are used for the diagnosis of neurologic conditions (Table 33–4). Additional information about these diagnostic procedures and laboratory tests can be found in Appendixes D and E 🔗.

ALTERED STATES OF CONSCIOUSNESS

Level of consciousness (LOC) is perhaps the most important indicator of neurologic dysfunction. **Consciousness,** the responsiveness or awareness of the mind to sensory stimuli, has two components: (1) Alertness, or arousal, the ability to react to stimuli, is controlled

---

TABLE 33–3	**Assessment Guidelines for the Child with a Neurologic Condition**
ASSESSMENT FOCUS	**ASSESSMENT GUIDELINES**
Level of consciousness	■ Is the infant or child difficult to arouse? ■ Is the infant or child irritable or difficult to calm or console? ■ Is the child oriented? Can the child tell the examiner his or her name and age? ■ What is the child's ability to concentrate? Can the young child name pictures of animals? Can the older child answer simple math questions or spell words? ■ The Glasgow Coma Scale provides a numeric score for future comparison. See Table 33–5.
Cranial nerves	■ Assess the cranial nerves. See Table 7–18 🔗. See Table 33–6 for methods to indirectly assess cranial nerves in the unconscious child.
Fontanels and sutures	■ Palpate fontanels and suture lines on the infant's scalp.
Cognitive function	■ Are the child's verbal skills developmentally appropriate for age? ■ Does the child follow directions and respond appropriately?
Pupils	■ Check the pupils for size and reaction to light and accommodation. See Figure 33–4 on page 1154.
Vital signs	■ Assess heart rate, respiratory rate, and blood pressure. ■ Monitor for an increased systolic blood pressure, a widened pulse pressure, bradycardia, and irregular respirations (late signs of increased intracranial pressure).
Posture and movement	■ Inspect the infant's posture and movement by using the primitive reflexes. See Table 7–19 🔗. ■ Observe the child's play or other spontaneous activity to assess strength as well as symmetry and smoothness of movements. ■ Are the child's motor skills developmentally appropriate for age? Were motor skills acquired at the appropriate age? Has the child lost a previously acquired skill? ■ Evaluate muscle strength and tone, comparing side to side. Is any weakness present? ■ Test the child's coordination for smoothness and symmetry of response. ■ Assess deep tendon reflexes for smoothness and symmetry of response. See Table 7–20 🔗.
Neck stiffness	■ Assess for neck stiffness (nuchal rigidity).
Pain	■ Assess level of pain when present.
Family history	■ Is there a family history of headaches, seizures, neurofibromatosis, or other neurologic condition?

TABLE 33–4	Diagnostic Procedures and Laboratory Tests Used to Evaluate Neurologic Conditions*	
DIAGNOSTIC PROCEDURES	**LABORATORY TESTS**	
Radiograph	Arterial blood gases	
Computed tomography (CT)	Complete blood cell count	
Magnetic resonance imaging (MRI)	Serum electrolytes and osmolality	
Positron emission tomography (PET) scan	Cerebrospinal fluid analysis	
Single-photon emission computed tomography (SPECT)	Clotting factors	
Electroencephalogram (EEG)	Blood culture	
Intracranial pressure (ICP) monitoring	Toxicology screens (blood, urine, hair)	
Lumbar puncture	Enzyme-linked immunosorbent assay (ELISA)	
Ultrasonography		
Myelography		

*See Appendixes D and E 🔗 for more information about these diagnostic procedures and laboratory tests.

by the reticular activating system. (2) **Cognitive power,** the ability to process the data and respond either verbally or physically, is controlled by cerebral function. Consciousness is dependent upon an intact brainstem and functioning cerebral hemispheres. **Unconsciousness,** on the other hand, is depressed cerebral function, or the inability of the brain to respond to stimuli. Altered levels of consciousness can be further categorized as follows:

- *Confused*—disorientation to time, place, or person. The child has loss of clear thinking. Answers to simple questions may be correct, but responses to complex ones may be inaccurate.
- *Delirious*—a state characterized by disorientation, fear, irritability or agitation, and mental or motor excitement.
- *Obtunded*—mild or moderate reduction in level of alertness. The child has a decreased interest in the environment and slower than usual response to stimuli.
- *Lethargic*—profound slumber in which speech and movement are limited. The child can be aroused with moderate stimulation but falls asleep easily once stimulation is removed.
- **Stuporous**—deep sleep or unresponsiveness in which the child can be aroused only with repeated vigorous stimulation,

such as pain. The child returns to the unresponsive state when the stimulus is removed.
- **Comatose**—unconsciousness from which the child cannot be aroused even by painful stimuli.
- **Persistent vegetative state**—permanent loss of function of the cerebral cortex retaining only reflexive responses (e.g., eyes may open briefly and spontaneously).

Etiology and Pathophysiology

Many conditions may alter the level of consciousness, including the following: obstructed airway, trauma, hypoxia, infection, poisoning, seizures, alcohol or substance abuse, endocrine or metabolic disturbances (e.g., diabetic ketoacidosis), electrolyte or acid–base imbalance, intracranial space-occupying lesion, stroke, and a congenital structural defect. Infection of the brain and/or meninges is a common cause of altered consciousness in children. Any of these pathologic processes can also cause increased **intracranial pressure** (force exerted by brain tissue, cerebrospinal fluid, and blood within the cranial vault). Decreased **cerebral perfusion pressure,** the amount of pressure needed to ensure that adequate oxygen and nutrients will be delivered to the brain, often results when the arterial blood flow to the brain is reduced due to the increase in intracranial pressure. Discovering the cause of an altered level of consciousness is essential so that immediate treatment can begin, to prevent possible secondary effects of the illness or injury.

Clinical Manifestations

Decline in a child's level of consciousness often follows a sequential pattern of deterioration. Initial changes may be subtle such as a slight disorientation to time and place. The child may become restless or fussy, and actions that normally calm or soothe the child only increase irritability. As responsiveness decreases, the child may become drowsy but still respond to loud verbal commands and withdraw from painful stimuli. Keeping the child awake is sometimes difficult. The response to pain progresses from purposeful to nonpurposeful. The child may exhibit flexor or extensor **posturing,** the abnormal positions assumed after severe injury or damage to the brain (Figure 33–3 ■). In some cases, the decline will be rapid and stages may be skipped, such as when the child has a serious brain injury. Other conditions such as poisoning may cause a slower decline.

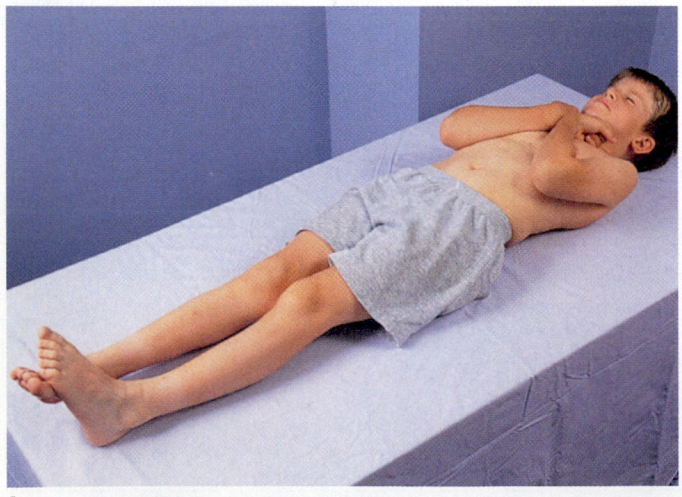

A

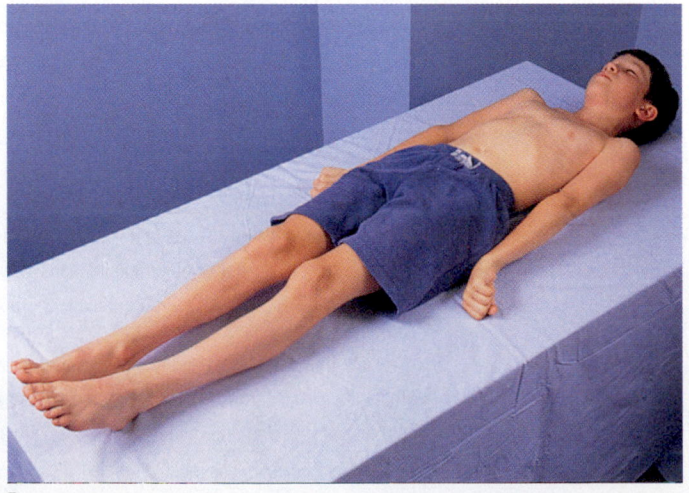

B

FIGURE 33–3 ■ *A,* Flexor or decorticate posturing, characterized by rigid flexion, is associated with lesions above the brainstem in the corticospinal tracts. *B,* Extensor or decerebrate posturing, distinguished by rigid extension, is associated with lesions of the brainstem.

Detection of an altered level of consciousness in newborns is more difficult due to the time they spend sleeping. Newborns may have lethargy, irritability, or hyperalertness as key findings of altered consciousness.

See the Clinical Manifestations table on increased intracranial pressure, which may occur in association with various causes of altered mental status.

Clinical Manifestations   Increased Intracranial Pressure

TIMING OF SIGNS	SIGNS
Early signs	Headache Visual disturbances, diplopia Nausea and vomiting Dizziness or vertigo Slight change in vital signs Pupils not as reactive or equal **Sunsetting eyes** (sclera visible above the iris), cranial nerve VI palsy Slight change in level of consciousness, restlessness
Additional signs in infants	Bulging fontanel Wide sutures, increased head circumference Dilated scalp veins Irritability High-pitched, catlike cry
Late signs	Significant decrease in level of consciousness Seizures **Cushing triad** ■ Increased systolic blood pressure and widened pulse pressure ■ Bradycardia ■ Irregular respirations Fixed and dilated pupils, papilledema

Collaborative Care

The goal of collaborative care is to rapidly identify the cause of an altered level of consciousness and to provide therapy to prevent further insult to the central nervous system.

Diagnostic Tests

The Glasgow Coma Scale (GCS) is used to quantify the level of consciousness, most commonly for acute brain injury. Pediatric criteria for preverbal children have integrated the child's developmental age for each category of the scale. See Table 33–5.

Laboratory tests and diagnostic procedures selected depend on the suspected condition based upon clinical manifestations (Lehman & Mink, 2008). Laboratory tests may include a complete blood cell count, blood chemistry, clotting factors, and blood culture; toxicology assessments of both blood and urine; and urinalysis with culture. A lumbar puncture may be performed if infection is suspected to assess the cerebrospinal fluid (CSF) for protein, glucose, or blood cells as well as CSF pressure level. An electroencephalogram (EEG) identifies damaged or nonfunctioning areas of the brain. Computed tomography (CT) or magnetic resonance imaging (MRI) is used to detect any lesions, structural abnormalities, vascular malformations, hemorrhage, or edema. Skull radiograph studies are used to detect fractures or bony malformations. Intracranial pressure monitoring is discussed on page 1199. See Appendix E 🔗 for more information about these procedures.

Practice Alert

The lumbar puncture should be postponed if any signs of increased intracranial pressure are present, which would place the child at risk for brain **herniation** (protrusion of brain contents into the brainstem area). Part of that assessment should include the ophthalmoscopic examination to determine if papilledema, or pressure on the optic nerve, is present.

TABLE 33–5	**Glasgow Coma Scale for Assessment of Coma in Infants and Children**		
CATEGORY	**SCORE***	**PREVERBAL CHILD CRITERIA**	**OLDER CHILD AND ADULT CRITERIA**
Eye opening	4	Spontaneous opening	Spontaneous opening
	3	To voice or sound	To voice or command
	2	To pain	To pain
	1	No response	No response
Verbal response	5	Smiles, coos, babbles, cries to appropriate stimuli, words, or sentences normal for age	Oriented to time, place, and person; uses appropriate words and phrases
	4	Irritable; cries	Confused
	3	Cries to pain	Inappropriate words or verbal response
	2	Moans to pain	Incomprehensible words
	1	No response	No response
Motor response	6	Spontaneous movement	Obeys commands
	5	Purposeful, localizes pain	Localizes pain
	4	Withdraws to pain	Withdraws to pain
	3	Flexor posturing to pain	Flexor posturing
	2	Extensor posturing to pain	Extensor posturing
	1	No response/flaccid	No response/flaccid

*Add the score from each category to get the total. The maximum score is 15, indicating the best level of neurologic functioning. The minimum is 3, indicating total neurologic unresponsiveness. A score of 5 is strongly correlated with the critical outcome of death or severe disability with pediatric brain injury.

Source: Data Kirkham, F. J., Newton, C. R., & Whitehouse, W. (2008). Pediatric coma scales. Developmental Medicine and Child Neurology, 50(4), 267–274. Copyright 2008. Reproduced with permission of John Wiley & Sons Ltd.

Clinical Therapy

Clinical therapy focuses on any lifesaving care needed, and then on an early diagnosis of the cause of altered level of consciousness. Initial care involves ensuring that the child's airway is open. Then, the child is treated with oxygen, and assisted ventilation is provided when gas exchange is inadequate. Any metabolic, acid–base, or electrolyte imbalances are corrected. Antibiotics are initiated for suspected infection.

Efforts are made to maintain the cerebral perfusion pressure so that oxygen and nutrients are supplied to the brain. In cases of hypovolemia, intravenous fluids are given. In cases of poor perfusion and fluid overload, a vasopressor medication such as dopamine is administered to increase cardiac output and perfusion of the brain. If the intracranial pressure is markedly increased and is caused by an obstruction leading to the accumulation of cerebrospinal fluid, a ventricular catheter can be inserted to drain cerebrospinal fluid and to decrease the intracranial pressure, temporarily relieving a life-threatening condition. See Skills Manual ⬭. See page 1199 for care specific to increased intracranial pressure and traumatic brain injury.

Nursing Management

Nursing care is focused on assessing potential causes of altered consciousness, monitoring the child's condition, and providing support to the child and family.

Nursing Assessment and Diagnosis

Take a thorough history to identify a potential cause of altered consciousness. Assess whether the child had a recent head trauma, has an infection, has ingested toxins, or has a shunt, tumor, or other condition that could affect the level of consciousness.

Initially assess the child's physiologic status, focusing on the child's responsiveness to the environment or stimuli, ability to maintain the airway, head circumference, and breathing patterns. Assess the child's airway. The presence of a cough or gag reflex indicates that the child is able to protect the airway from aspiration. Assess the child's respiratory effort and color, as well as other vital signs. Monitor pulse oximetry and arterial blood gas measurements. Adequate air exchange to keep oxygen and carbon dioxide levels within normal ranges and maintaining acid–base balance are critical to reduce the risk of hypoxemia and increased intracranial pressure. If the child cannot maintain adequate respiratory effort, mechanical ventilation will be necessary.

Practice Alert

Assess vital sign readings and detect important changes. An increased systolic blood pressure, a wide pulse pressure, and bradycardia indicate increased intracranial pressure.

A baseline neurologic assessment should be performed, including assessment of the pupils (pupil size, reaction to light, and consensual response to light), eye movements, and motor function (Figure 33–4 ■). Repeated assessments should be performed and compared to baseline findings. The Glasgow Coma Scale may be used to assess the child at specified intervals. Observe for other physiologic signs of increased intracranial pressure listed in the Clinical Manifestations table on page 1153.

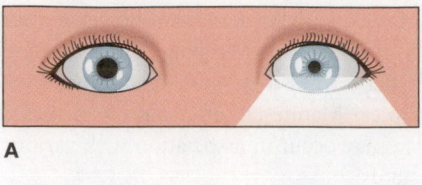

A

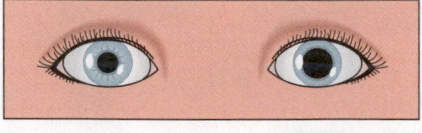

B

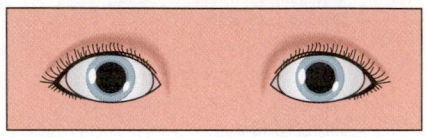

C

FIGURE 33–4 ■ Pupil findings in various neurologic conditions with altered consciousness. *A,* A unilateral dilated and reactive pupil is associated with an intracranial mass. *B,* A fixed and dilated pupil may be a sign of impending brainstem herniation. *C,* Bilateral fixed and dilated pupils are associated with brainstem herniation from increased intracranial pressure.

Clinical Tip

The Glasgow Coma Scale assessment of infants and young children is performed by noting the following:

- **Eye opening**—Note if the eye opening is spontaneous or occurs in response to stimuli.
- **Verbal response**—Crying in an infant is a positive response. The 2-year-old who says *no* to each command is also responding in an age-appropriate way.
- **Motor response**—Motor score is probably the most critical aspect of this test, since the child cannot control reflexes. A fearful toddler may refuse to open the eyes or talk to strangers, but the child's reflexes should automatically respond to appropriate stimuli. To help the toddler feel less threatened when assessing motor skills, ask the child to reach for a finger puppet or doll rather than your hand. The toy can serve as a reward.

See Box 33–1 and Chapter 7 ⬭ for additional tips in assessing the responsiveness of an infant.

Assess the child's cranial nerves (see Table 7–18 ⬭). The child's responses may differ significantly when stress and anxiety are reduced. Encourage the parents to take part in the examination to reduce the child's anxiety. In the unconscious child, cranial nerve assessment and interpretation are more challenging. See Table 33–6 for cranial nerve assessment guidelines in the unconscious child.

BOX 33–1	Assessment of Infant Responsiveness

When initially checking the responsiveness of infants, the acronym AVPU provides a method for rapid assessment.

Alert, responsive to parents, cuddles, coos or babbles, smiles

Verbal, responsive to verbal stimulation

Pain, responsive to painful stimulation only

Unresponsive to painful stimulation

Additionally assess the infant for a loud energetic quality to the cry, feeding for a strong suck and suck-swallowing coordination, and the presence of appropriate primitive reflexes for age. These signs all indicate intact mental status.

TABLE 33–6	Assessment of Cranial Nerves in the Unconscious Child
CRANIAL NERVES AND REFLEX	**REFLEX ASSESSMENT PROCEDURE AND *NORMAL FINDINGS***
II, III Pupillary	Shine a light source in the eye.
	Rapid, concentrically constricting pupils indicate intact cranial nerves II, III.
II, IV, VI Oculocephalic	Perform with eyes held open (doll's eyes) and head moved horizontally or vertically.
	When head is turned suddenly to the right, the eyes of an infant or comatose patient look to the left, and similarly look to the right when the head is turned to the left. Absence of this reflex suggests brainstem dysfunction in comatose patients.
	Precaution: Cervical spine injury must be ruled out before this assessment is performed.
III, VIII Oculovestibular	Place the head in a midline and slightly elevated position. Inject ice water into the ear canal.
	Eyes deviating toward the irrigated ear indicate intact cranial nerves III, VIII.
	Precaution: Ensure that the tympanic membrane is intact to keep fluid from entering the middle ear.
	Note: A physician usually performs this assessment.
V, VII Corneal	Gently touch the cornea with a sterile cotton swab.
	A blink indicates intact cranial nerves V, VII.
IX, X Gag	Irritate the pharynx with a tongue depressor or cotton swab.
	A gagging response indicates intact cranial nerves IX, X.

Clinical Judgment

Some signs of the intact neurologic status of an infant (newborn to 2 months of age) are a cry with a loud and energetic quality, a strong suck, and suck-swallowing coordination. What is one additional sign?

Following are nursing diagnoses that may be appropriate for the child with an altered level of consciousness:

- Breathing Pattern, Ineffective related to neuromuscular dysfunction associated with increased intracranial pressure
- Aspiration, Risk for related to poor control of secretions with decreased level of consciousness
- Skin Integrity, Risk for Impaired related to agitation and skin rubbing against bedding
- Communication: Verbal, Impaired related to physiologic condition of decreased level of consciousness
- Family Processes, Interrupted related to care of a child with an acquired disability

NANDA-I © 2012

Planning and Implementation

Nursing care of the child with altered consciousness or increased intracranial pressure focuses on maintaining airway patency, monitoring neurologic status, performing routine care, providing sensory stimulation, and providing emotional support to parents. Nursing care for the child with increased intracranial pressure is described beginning on page 1199.

Maintain Airway Patency

Make sure the child's airway is clear at all times. If the child does not have a gag reflex or has difficulty swallowing secretions, endotracheal intubation is performed. A tracheostomy may be performed for long-term airway management. Frequent suctioning may be required. Keep suction apparatus with catheters at the bedside along with oxygen, resuscitation bag and mask, and extra endotracheal or tracheostomy tubes (if applicable). Pulse oximetry or arterial blood gas analysis is performed at regular intervals to ensure that gas exchange is adequate. Assisted ventilation may be required (refer to the Skills Manual ⬤▭).

Anticipate that seizures may occur. Pad the side rails to protect the child from injury.

Perform Routine Nursing Care

If the corneal reflex is absent, place artificial tears in the eyes and cover with gauze, taping over so they remain closed. Perform routine mouth care by brushing the teeth and using swabs with water. Gently clean the oral mucosa in newborns and keep secretions from accumulating.

Provide adequate nutrition. Initially, nutrients may be supplied intravenously. A nasogastric or transpyloric tube may be inserted if the infant or child remains unconscious or is not alert enough to take food by mouth. A gastrostomy tube may be inserted if it is anticipated that enteral feeds will be needed for longer than 3 months. (See the Skills Manual ⬤▭.)

Prevent complications associated with immobility (muscle atrophy, contractures, and skin breakdown) as described in Box 33–2. Nurses support physical therapy efforts with extra passive range of motion exercises.

Provide Sensory Stimulation

Because the child with a severely altered level of consciousness may still be able to hear, talking to him or her may be beneficial. Listening to music or tapes of family members talking or reading can soothe a child when family members cannot be present. Explain all procedures and actions to the parents and child. Encourage the parents to stroke and touch the child in a soothing manner.

When the child becomes more alert, gradually and repeatedly orient the child to time, place, and person, depending on his or her age and level of understanding. Encourage parents to bring objects or toys from home to make the environment more familiar and promote a feeling of security.

Provide Emotional Support

Explain the child's condition to the family in simple terms. Encourage parents to take part in the child's care and therapy as much as possible.

BOX 33–2	Care of the Child Who Is Immobile

- Help keep the body in proper alignment with splints or rolls made of towels or blankets.
- Perform passive or gentle range of motion exercises three to four times per day according to physician's orders.
- Assess the child's skin frequently and maintain skin integrity:
  - Change position every 2 hours.
  - Place the child on a special mattress or bed designed to relieve pressure points, or use sheepskin under the child when special beds are not available.
  - Massage the child gently using lotion.
  - Place transparent dressings over skin surfaces exposed to rubbing or friction.
- Sequential compression devices may be used for some children to prevent deep vein thrombosis.

If the child's normal functioning has been permanently impaired, re-fer the family to the appropriate psychologic and social services for emotional support. (See Chapter 17 🥏 for more information about helping families cope with a child's life-threatening illness.) Provide family members with opportunities to express their feelings.

Discharge Planning and Home Care Teaching

The child's transition from the hospital to home, a long-term care facility, or an inpatient rehabilitation center must be planned well in advance of discharge. A case manager or social worker should be identified who can help plan the child's long-term care needs, includ-ing home health nursing, adaptation of the home, and the purchase of special equipment.

Care in the Community

Home care nurses play a vital role in the care of children with an acquired neurologic dysfunction and prolonged altered consciousness. Teach the family how to care for the child with severe neurologic dysfunction and to perform routine procedures such as suctioning and maintaining the airway, skin care, feeding, positioning, performing range of motion ex-ercises, and offering stimulation. Regular follow-up visits are needed to assess the child's progress and to modify the treatment plan.

The child also needs to be linked with community rehabilitation services through an early intervention program or school-based pro-gram. The home health nurse or case manager should assist the fam-ily to have an individualized education plan developed for the child (see Chapter 16 🥏).

Evaluation

Expected outcomes of nursing care include the following:

- The child's airway and cerebral perfusion pressure are main-tained to oxygenate the brain.
- Complications of immobility are prevented.
- The risk for long-term disabilities is reduced through the provi-sion of appropriate care.

SEIZURE DISORDERS

Seizures are periods of abnormal electrical discharges (excessive concurrent firing) in the brain that cause involuntary movement, and behavior and sensory alterations. They are a common neurologic dis-order in children. Approximately 120,000 children and youth under 18 years of age will experience a first seizure each year, with the great-est incidence in children under 2 years of age (Epilepsy Foundation, 2010a).

Epilepsy is a chronic disorder characterized by recurrent, unpro-voked seizures secondary to an underlying brain abnormality. In the United States, approximately 45,000 children under age 15 years develop epilepsy each year, and 326,000 children live with epilepsy (Epilepsy Foundation, 2010a). Approximately 30% of epilepsy cases occur by age 4 years (Boss & Huether, 2010). See Developing Cultural Competence: Seizures.

Etiology and Pathophysiology

A seizure is a clinical event in which abnormal discharges of electrical activity occur within the brain. When an excessive number of the neu-rons become overexcited, they discharge abnormally. Seizures may result from a central nervous system (CSN) disorder, a CNS structural defect,

---

Developing Cultural Competence
Seizures

Seizures may have a special meaning to different cultural groups. For example, the Hmong believe the child is experiencing *quag dab peg*, or "the spirit catches you and you fall down." Traditional Hmong view the condition as serious, but they take pride in children who have the condition as they have a link to the spirit world. In 1997, Anne Fadiman wrote a compelling story about the cultural conflict between a Hmong family and healthcare providers over the treatment of their daughter's seizures, *The Spirit Catches You and You Fall Down* (Fadiman, 1997; Spector, 2009).

---

or a disorder that affects CNS functioning, such as brain injury, infection, electrolyte disturbance such as hypoglycemia, endocrine dysfunction, toxins, and brain tumor. Genetic factors or familial predisposition may lead to seizures. Some seizures have no known cause. See the Clinical Manifestations table for the etiology of various types of seizures.

Partial or **focal** seizures are caused by abnormal electrical activity in one hemisphere or a specific area of the cerebral cortex, most often the temporal, frontal, or parietal lobes. The symptoms displayed de-pend on the region of the cerebral cortex affected.

In contrast, generalized seizures are the result of diffuse electrical activity that begins in both hemispheres of the brain simultaneously and spreads throughout the cortex into the brainstem. As a result, movements and spasms displayed by the child are bilateral and sym-metric, and consciousness is impaired.

Febrile seizures occur in approximately 2% to 5% of infants and children in connection with a temperature greater than 39°C (102.2°F) during the first 24 hours of an acute respiratory or ear in-fection. No evidence of intracranial infection or systemic metabolic disorder is found. A familial predisposition may be present. These sei-zures are usually seen in children between 9 months and 5 years, with a peak age of 14 to 18 months (Boss & Huether, 2010). Simple febrile seizures last less than 15 minutes and do not recur within 24 hours. Complex febrile seizures occur in some children with a 15-minute or longer duration and recurrence within 24 hours. Children with com-plex febrile seizures may have a greater risk for developing epilepsy.

Newborn seizures usually occur because of primary CNS disease (intraventricular or other hemorrhage), CNS infection, inborn errors of metabolism, asphyxia, electrolyte disorder, drug withdrawal or toxicity, kernicterus, or other underlying disease.

Status epilepticus is a prolonged continuous seizure of 20 min-utes or two or more seizures without full return to baseline between episodes (Goldstein, 2008). Fever, infection, and a recent medical change are the most common risk factors in children (Shearer & Riviello, 2011). Status epilepticus has an incidence of 20 per 100,000 children per year, with the highest incidence in infants under age 1 year. Approximately 10% of children with epilepsy will have at least one episode of status epilepticus (Goldstein, 2008). The length of a seizure episode is important because the airway may be compro-mised, leading to cerebral hypoxia and the death of some neurons. The basal metabolic rate rises during the peak of seizure activity. This change, in turn, increases the demand for oxygen and glucose.

Clinical Manifestations

The symptoms of a seizure depend on its type and duration. Seizures are classified into two types: partial (focal) seizures and generalized seizures of nonfocal origin. The specific characteristics of the various types of partial and generalized seizures are presented in the Clinical Manifestations table. Seizure characteristics and patterns may change as the child's nervous system grows and matures. Seizures in infants may be subtle. As neurons and their connections throughout the cortex develop, neurons can fire in repetitive high-frequency bursts, leading to more sustained and organized seizures (Boss & Huether, 2010).

Clinical Manifestations Seizures

TYPE OF SEIZURE AND ETIOLOGY	CLINICAL MANIFESTATIONS

Partial seizures
 	
 Simple partial seizures
 	
 (focal seizures)
   Focal damage (e.g., with cerebral palsy)
   Tumors or lesions
   Arteriovenous malformation
   Brain abscess
	Onset: any age
	 No loss of consciousness, lasts less than 30 seconds, no postseizure confusion, may occur many times a day
	 No **aura** (a sensation preceding the onset of a seizure, such as taste, visual, auditory, dizziness, or numbness)
	 Motor responses may involve one extremity, part of extremity, or ipsilateral extremities with eyes and head turning in opposite direction
	 Sensory responses involve **paresthesia** (decreased sensation or tingling); auditory, olfactory, or visual sensations; autonomic (e.g., sweating, pupil dilation) or psychic symptoms
	 Motor and sensory involvement may be combined and progress to a generalized seizure
	 Jacksonian march (rare in children): tonic contractions of either fingers of one hand, toes of one foot, or one side of face become clonic or tonic-clonic movements that spread to adjacent muscles of the affected extremity or same side of body

Complex partial seizures
 	
 (psychomotor seizures)
   Lesions, cysts, or tumors
   Perinatal trauma
   Focal sclerosis (e.g., scarring of the mediotemporal lobe from prolonged febrile seizures)
   Vascular anomalies (e.g., arteriovenous malformations, a congenital tangling of blood vessels in the brain)
   Brain trauma
	Onset: 3 years of age to adolescence
	 Consciousness is impaired immediately; lasts 30 seconds to 5 minutes; postseizure amnesia or confusion
	 May have abnormal motor activity, twitching, loss of tone
	 May have sensory changes such as tingling or numbness
	 May progress to a generalized seizure
	 Aura frequently occurs, such as an unusual taste or odor
	 Abdominal pain
	 Posturing
	 Feelings of anxiety, fear, or déjà vu (sensation that event occurred before)
	 Automatisms (unusual body movements without purpose) such as lip smacking, lip chewing, or sucking

Generalized seizures
 	
 Tonic-clonic seizures
 	
 (grand mal seizures)
   Cerebral damage from perinatal trauma, brain trauma, tumors, structural lesions, metabolic and neuromuscular degenerative disorders
   Genetic link
   Many are idiopathic
	Onset: any age, rare before 6 months of age, strong familial incidence
	 Abrupt-onset seizure, 1- to 2-minute loss of consciousness, postseizure confusion (few minutes to hours)
	 May or may not have aura
	 Body becomes stiff and rigid when all muscles contract (tonic phase), followed by rhythmic jerking motions (clonic phase)
	 Eyes roll upward or deviate to one side; pupils dilate
	 Drooling or foaming at mouth as secretions are not swallowed
	 Abdominal or chest wall rigidity with leg, head, and neck extended, and arms flexed or contracted
	 Cry or grunt as air is forced out when diaphragm and chest muscles contract
	 Urinary or bowel incontinence as muscles become flaccid during clonic phase
	 Characterized by sleepiness, difficulty in arousal; hypertension; diaphoresis; headache, nausea, vomiting; poor coordination, decreased muscle tone; confusion, amnesia; slurred speech; visual disturbances; combativeness

Absence seizures
 	
 (petit mal, or lapse seizures)
   Hyperventilation
   Genetic predisposition
	Onset: age 3–12 years with remission in adolescence
	 More prevalent in females
	 May go on to develop other generalized seizures
	 May be triggered by hyperventilation or flashing lights
	 No aura
	 Brief loss of consciousness, usually lasts 5–10 seconds, rarely exceeds 30 seconds, no postseizure confusion, lethargy, or sleepiness; has amnesia regarding the seizure
	 Frequent attacks (50–100 or more per day), may cluster, interfere with learning; episodes may be confused with daydreaming or inattentiveness
	 Eye blinking or fluttering of eyelids, staring, usually a glazed eye appearance
	 Child may continue simple movements such as walking or looking; ceases activities such as reading
	 Slight decrease or loss of muscle tone (head may droop, handheld objects may be dropped)
	 Cannot be interrupted by verbal or touch stimulation

Juvenile myoclonic ***Epilepsy*** Genetic disorder with locus on chromosome 6p11, 15q14, 6q24, and 10q35 (Boss & Huether, 2010)	*Onset:* more prevalent in adolescents, peak age of 12–15 years No loss of consciousness, child recovers in seconds, no postictal period Attacks occur most often upon falling asleep or awakening Quick involuntary muscle jerks of the neck, shoulders, and arms; injury is possible if thrown to ground Child usually has normal intelligence

(continued)

Clinical Manifestations Seizures (continued)

TYPE OF SEIZURE AND ETIOLOGY	CLINICAL MANIFESTATIONS
Infantile spasms (West syndrome, salaam seizures) ARX and CDKL5 gene mutations (Boss & Huether, 2010) Tuberous sclerosis Hypoxic-ischemic injury Congenital infections, diseases Inborn errors of metabolism CNS malformations	*Onset:* begin between ages 4 and 18 months; more common in males Severe form of epilepsy; may occur with altered consciousness as part of a complex partial seizure Spasms with abrupt flexion and extension of muscle groups in the neck, trunk, and extremities, involving head nods or jackknife body contractions; episodes are worse when the infant is waking up or falling asleep Child may cry during episodes Occur in clusters, 5–150 per day Seizure activity increases in intensity and severity over time Developmental delays and disability occur High risk for developing other types of epilepsy or intractable seizures
Lennox-Gastaut syndrome (akinetic or atonic seizures) Gray matter degenerative diseases and subacute seizures Sclerosing panencephalitis Many are idiopathic	*Onset:* first seen in early childhood, between 3 and 5 years, predominantly in males Combination of tonic, absence, and myoclonic seizure activity; drop attack (falls to ground with sudden loss of postural tone, inability to break fall, is limp for period of time) Associated cognitive impairment, delayed psychomotor development, and severe behavioral problems

Partial seizures often start with an aura or abrupt unprovoked alteration in behavior. When the child recognizes the pattern of an aura, he or she may have time to avoid injury by getting to the floor. Generalized seizures often begin with a **tonic** phase characterized by unconsciousness, continuous muscular contraction, and sustained stiffness. The tonic phase is followed by the **clonic** phase, characterized by alternating muscular contraction and relaxation as a rhythmic repetitive jerking. The **postictal period** following seizure activity is a phase during which the level of consciousness is decreased. The length of the postictal period varies among children. Children may have a partial seizure and progress to a generalized seizure.

Simple febrile seizures are generalized seizures that involve generalized tonic-clonic movements and rolling back of the eyes lasting a few seconds to less than 15 minutes. The seizure is followed by a brief postictal period. Complex febrile seizures look like a simple febrile seizure but additionally have focal signs and last longer than 10 to 15 minutes.

Clinical Tip
The only evidence of seizures in a neonate may be roving eye movements, repetitive blinking, sucking, lip smacking, tongue thrusting, pedaling movements, and sustained posturing (Kothare, Khurana, Madsen, et al., 2009).

Collaborative Care

The goal of collaborative care is to identify the underlying cause of the seizure and identify the appropriate clinical therapy to interrupt a prolonged seizure and to prevent future seizures.

Diagnostic Tests

After the child's first seizure, it is essential that a thorough history be taken from the parent, primary caretaker, or witnesses to the event. Details such as the description and length of the seizure, presence or absence of an aura, and if the child lost consciousness should be noted. This information is used to identify the type of seizure according to the International Classification of Epileptic Seizures descriptions in the Clinical Manifestations table on pages 1157–1158.

Based on the physical findings and history, diagnostic tests ordered may include a complete blood cell count, blood chemistry, and urine toxicology. A urine culture, blood culture, and lumbar puncture are performed if the child is febrile and meningitis is suspected. A lead level and tests for inborn errors of metabolism may be considered. Radiologic tests such as a CT scan or an MRI and angiography may be performed to identify a cerebral lesion or to identify a metabolic disorder of the brain. An EEG is often performed at a follow-up visit between seizures. If the child is taking any anticonvulsants, the serum drug level is checked and monitored over time.

Clinical Therapy

Many seizures are self-limiting and require no emergency intervention. If the child is still having a seizure upon arrival at the healthcare facility, therapy should be initiated. Emergency therapy includes maintaining the airway, supplemental oxygen, intravenous benzodiazepines, and careful monitoring of vital signs. Serum electrolytes, glucose, blood gases, and vital signs may be monitored. Continued motor activity, if present, may be less intense after benzodiazepines are given, but it must be monitored because of the potential for status epilepticus. The postictal period ranges from 30 minutes to 2 hours. When the child's seizure does not stop as expected, management of the child with status epilepticus should be performed as described in Table 33–7.

Febrile seizures Children with febrile seizures are generally not treated with an anticonvulsant at the time of a seizure because the seizure has usually ended before the child arrives at the emergency care or health center. Acetaminophen is administered to reduce the fever and to make the child more comfortable. Long-term anticonvulsants are not recommended for prevention of future simple febrile seizures because of the adverse effects of the three medications effective against febrile seizures (phenobarbital, primidone, and valproic acid). Diazepam may be ordered for rectal or oral administration at the onset of a child's febrile illness when the parents are severely anxious about a subsequent febrile seizure (American Academy of Pediatrics, 2008).

Medications Most seizure disorders are treated with antiepileptic drugs (AEDs). A single medication (monotherapy) is preferred for seizure control to minimize side effects that can be significant (sleepiness, decreased attention and memory, difficulty with speech, ataxia, and diplopia). Monotherapy works for approximately 60% of children with new-onset epilepsy (Stafstrom, 2009). If seizure control is not

TABLE 33–7	Collaborative Care for Status Epilepticus
TYPE OF CARE	**COLLABORATIVE CARE**
Emergency assessment and interventions	■ Maintain a patent airway. Muscle rigidity may compromise the airway. Keep suction equipment at the bedside to clear secretions. ■ Give oxygen by mask, as increased metabolic demands deplete oxygen stores. ■ Monitor vital signs and circulation with pulse oximeter and cardiorespiratory monitor. ■ Perform neurologic assessments, every 5 to 10 minutes.
Ongoing urgent management	■ Establish an intravenous line to administer fluids or medications. ■ Assess blood glucose level and administer glucose if the child is hypoglycemic; the physical stress of the seizure may result in declining glucose levels. ■ Insert a nasogastric tube to reduce risk of aspiration due to vomiting. ■ Protect the child from injury. ■ Manage thermoregulation.
Medications	■ Administer benzodiazepines such as diazepam, lorazepam, or midazolam. If there is no response, the dose may be repeated. Fosphenytoin or phenobarbital may be necessary if seizure activity continues. ■ Cumulative doses of benzodiazepines, including the rectal diazepam (Diastat) that parents may have given, may produce apnea, so be prepared to assist with ventilatory support and endotracheal intubation if needed.
EEG	■ If status epilepticus is persistent despite treatment, an EEG may be ordered to ensure that seizure activity has stopped.

Source: *Data from Shearer, P., & Riviello, J. (2011). Generalized convulsive status epilepticus in adults and children: Treatment guidelines and protocols.* Emergency Care Clinics of North America, 29, 51–64.

initially achieved with the first antiepileptic medication, the dosage is increased to a high therapeutic level or until toxicity is noted. Only at that time is an alternate medication used. The first medication may be continued or tapered as the second medication is initiated. Only when monotherapy is unsuccessful with two different medications will multiple medications be prescribed (Raspall-Chaure, Neville, & Scott, 2008). The side effects are often cumulative with multiple medications. Some medications have been found most effective for certain types of seizures. No seizure medication should be stopped abruptly to prevent status epilepticus. See the Medications table for a listing of antiepileptic medications.

Serum drug levels (for each AED if multiple drugs are prescribed) may be obtained to assess the achievement of therapeutic levels or to identify toxicity; however, the tests are expensive. Medication dosage adjustments are often needed as the child grows. See Complementary Therapy: Herbs and Antiepileptic Drugs.

The child is monitored for medication adverse effects and toxicity, especially those related to the hepatic and hematologic systems, and for hypersensitivity reactions. Many of the AEDs potentially cause lethargy, sedation, and dizziness or other problems that interfere with the child's learning. Children treated with single and multiple antiepileptic medications should have regular blood testing performed to identify any developing hematologic or liver problems.

Complementary Therapy Herbs and Antiepileptic Drugs

Families should be educated that herbal preparations with ginkgo may increase the risk of seizures in individuals with a history of seizures. Ginkgo has been found to decrease the effectiveness of anticonvulsants including phenytoin, valproic acid, ethosuximide, carbamazepine, gabapentin, topiramate, felbamate, and oxcarbazepine.

Kava and valerian may increase the sedative effects of primidone and phenobarbital (Wilson, Shannon, & Shields, 2011). Parents should make the healthcare provider aware of all herbal preparations used.

A trial of medication withdrawal is often attempted for children who have been seizure-free for 2 years or longer. Medications are tapered slowly, over a few months (Clore, 2010). Approximately 70% of children remain seizure-free for 2 years without medications, and if seizures recur, in most cases they will happen within the first year after AED withdrawal. Up to 20% of children with seizure recurrence do not regain seizure control (Raspall-Chaure et al., 2008).

Some children have refractory or **intractable seizures,** which continue to occur even when treated with three or more medications. These children should be referred to an epilepsy center for other potential treatments such as the ketogenic diet, vagal nerve stimulation, or evaluation for surgical treatment.

Invasive procedures Surgery may occasionally be performed to remove a tumor, lesion, or portion of the brain with a localized seizure focus, particularly when the seizures are not responsive to multiple antiepileptic medications. In some cases, the precise area of seizure focus can be determined for surgical resection. Types of surgery include a temporal lobectomy, nontemporal resection, corpus callosotomy (disconnecting the two cerebral hemispheres), and hemispherectomy. Surgery performed at earlier ages is believed to lead to a better neurodevelopmental outcome (Stafstrom, 2009).

A vagus nerve stimulator is another option for some children with intractable epilepsy when no focal lesion can be identified and the child is not a candidate for surgery. A pulse generator is implanted in the chest, and leads are threaded under the skin and wrapped around the left vagus nerve. The pulse generator is programmed to stimulate the vagus nerve. The patient can activate the device after experiencing an aura and reduce the spread of the seizure.

Ketogenic diet A ketogenic diet is occasionally used for children with intractable seizures. This high-fat (up to 80% of calories), adequate protein for growth, and very-low-carbohydrate diet is customized to help the child maintain ideal body weight, maximize ketosis, and achieve optimal seizure control (Figure 33–5 ■). The child usually begins the diet in the hospital with a fast for 24 hours. The very-low-carbohydrate intake forces the child to burn fat for fuel, leading to ketosis. While the actual mechanism of action is unknown, the ketosis is believed to produce an anticonvulsant and antiepileptic effect. All foods and liquids given to the child must be carefully weighed and measured, and they are usually planned by a nutritionist specially trained to help families develop the daily meal plan. Each meal typically has about four times as much fat as protein or carbohydrate (Epilepsy Foundation, 2010b). Family motivation must be high to maintain the rigid diet for 1 or more years because improved seizure control is directly related to diet compliance.

Medications Used to Treat Seizures

MEDICATION	ACTION	NURSING MANAGEMENT
Benzodiazepines IV Diazepam (Valium) Lorazepam (Ativan) Rectal diazepam (Diastat) Intranasal midazolam Used for status epilepticus	Produces CNS depression by acting on the limbic, thalamic, and hypothalamic regions of the brain	■ IV push medication is administered into the IV entry site closest to the child's body. Administer very slowly. Monitor vital signs for hypotension, tachycardia, and respiratory depression. ■ The rectal or nasal preparation may be prescribed for home administration to treat prolonged seizures.
Phenobarbital PO, IV, IM Used for generalized tonic-clonic, simple partial and complex partial seizures, and status epilepticus	Enhances GABAergic (gamma-aminobutyric acid) neurotransmitter inhibition by prolonging the time that chloride channels are open in response to GABA	■ IV medication must be administered into the IV entry site closest to the child's body. Administer very slowly. ■ Monitor the child's vital signs frequently when given IV, and monitor the child for excessive sedation. ■ Tablets may be crushed and mixed with food or fluid. ■ The medication may be associated with hyperactivity, learning difficulties, irritability, and sleep disturbance. ■ Ensure extra intake of foods with vitamin D and folate, or provide vitamin D and folic acid supplementation when drug is used long term.
Phenytoin (Dilantin) PO, IV **Fosphenytoin** (Cerebyx) IV Used for generalized tonic-clonic, partial, and tonic seizures	Inhibits seizure activity by blocking the neuronal sodium channels; reduces voltage, frequency, and spread of electrical discharges within motor cortex	■ Monitor the child's vital signs frequently after IV dosage for respiratory depression. ■ Educate the family to ensure adequate intake of foods with vitamin D, folate, and calcium. ■ Promote frequent dental care for gingival hyperplasia. ■ Urine may turn pink, red, or red-brown.
Carbamazepine (Tegretol) PO Used for partial and generalized tonic-clonic seizures	Inhibits sustained repetitive impulses and reduces synaptic transmission to the spinal cord, limiting the spread of seizure activity	■ Give with food to enhance absorption. Grapefruit may increase drug levels. ■ Ensure that chewable tablets are fully chewed and that sustained-release capsules are not chewed. ■ Do not administer suspension simultaneously with another liquid medication to prevent formation of a precipitate. ■ Erythromycin may increase carbamazepine toxicity. ■ Be aware that it causes photosensitivity reactions.
Valproic acid (Depacon, Depakote) PO Used for absence, partial and generalized tonic-clonic, and myoclonic seizures	Enhances GABAergic neurotransmitter inhibition and suppresses repetitive neuronal firing by inhibiting sodium channels	■ Do not use carbonated beverage to dilute syrup. ■ Tablets and capsules should not be chewed. Sprinkles within special capsules should be placed on a teaspoon of soft food and swallowed without chewing. ■ Give with food to decrease gastrointestinal upset. ■ Monitor platelet count and bleeding times. ■ Teratogenic effects, such as neural tube defects, atrial septal defect, cleft palate, hypospadias, polydactyly, and craniosynostosis, may occur (Jentink, Loane, Dolk, et al., 2010). Encourage adolescent females to plan pregnancy so that medication may be changed prior to conception.
Ethosuximide (Zarontin) PO Used for absence seizures	Blocks calcium channels, interrupting the thalamocortical feedback loop associated with seizure activity	■ Monitor for weight loss or anorexia. ■ Give with food if gastrointestinal upset occurs. ■ Do not expose medication to light. Do not freeze.
Primidone (Mysoline) PO Used for generalized tonic-clonic and partial seizures	Raises the seizure threshold and changes seizure patterns; may control seizures unresponsive to phenobarbital	■ Give with food if gastrointestinal upset occurs. ■ Ensure adequate intake of foods with folate, or provide folic acid supplementation.
Felbamate (Felbatol) PO Used for partial seizures and generalized seizures of Lennox-Gastaut syndrome	Blocks repetitive firing of neurons and increases seizure threshold	■ Monitor weight for gain or loss. ■ The child needs regular monitoring for hematologic and liver problems. ■ Use as a monotherapy.
Gabapentin (Neurontin) PO Used for partial seizures	Related to inhibitory GABA neurotransmitter analog; actual mechanism of action is unknown	■ Vision and concentration may be impaired by the medication. ■ Do not take medication within 2 hours of an antacid.
Lamotrigine (Lamictal) PO Used for Lennox-Gastaut syndrome and partial and generalized seizures	Inhibits release of glutamate and aspartate (excitory neurotransmitters) in sodium channels, decreasing seizure activity	■ Drug increases photosensitivity. ■ Serious skin rashes occur in 10% of children; Stevens-Johnson syndrome occurs in 0.8% of children with epilepsy (see Chapter 36 🔗). ■ Monitor for adverse effects if used with valproic acid, which inhibits the drug's metabolism.

Medications Used to Treat Seizures (*continued*)

MEDICATION	ACTION	NURSING MANAGEMENT
Tiagabine (Gabitril filmtabs) PO Used for partial seizures	Prevents reuptake of released GABA back into the presynaptic terminal and prolongs the time GABA is available for synaptic inhibition	■ Give with food. ■ Monitor for signs of central nervous system depression. ■ Avoid using with over-the-counter (OTC) medications that cause drowsiness.
Topiramate (Topamax) PO Used for partial and generalized seizures, Lennox-Gastaut syndrome, and infantile spasms	Complex mechanism of action involving the sodium and calcium channels and glutamate receptors; GABA enhancer	■ Increase fluid intake to reduce risk of kidney stones. ■ Psychomotor slowing as well as speech and language problems may develop with use of medication. ■ Monitor weight as weight loss may occur.
Levetiracetam (Keppra) PO Used for simple and complex partial seizures in adolescents	Mechanism of action is unknown	■ The child and adolescent should not engage in hazardous activities such as driving an all-terrain vehicle (ATV) or car until effect of the drug is known. ■ Monitor for gait and coordination problems.
Oxcarbazepine (Trileptal) PO Used for partial and generalized seizures in children over age 4 years	Similar mechanism of action to carbamazepine	■ Monitor for hyponatremia. ■ Monitor for excess drowsiness, dizziness, lack of coordination, and frequent headaches.
Vigabatrin (Sabril) PO Used for refractory partial and generalized seizures, and infantile spasms	Inhibitor of GABA transaminase; decreases GABA breakdown in the brain	■ Vision should be monitored because vigabatrin can cause visual field constriction. ■ Vigabatrin is not available in the U.S. as of 2011.
Zonisamide (Zonegran) PO Used for partial seizures in adults but may have broader action for other seizures	Mechanism of action is unknown	■ Zonisamide is contraindicated if hypersensitivity to sulfonamides. ■ Increase fluid intake to reduce risk of kidney stones. ■ Report dizziness, excess drowsiness, lack of coordination, or double vision.
Rufinamide PO Used for Lennox-Gastaut syndrome in children age 4 years and older	Modulation of sodium channels results in limiting the firing of sodium-dependent action potentials in neurons	■ Give medication with a meal because fats increase drug absorption.

Source: *Data from Wilson, B. A., Shannon, M. T., & Shield, K. M. (2011). Nurse's drug guide 2011. Upper Saddle River, NJ: Pearson; Stafstrom, C. E. (2009). The epilepsies. In R. B. David (Ed.), Clinical Pediatric Neurology (pp. 151–188). New York, NY: Demos Medical Publishing; Ferrie, C. D. (2010). Rufinamide: A new antiepileptic drug treatment for Lennox–Gastaut syndrome. Expert Review of Neurotherapeutics, 10(6), 851–860.*

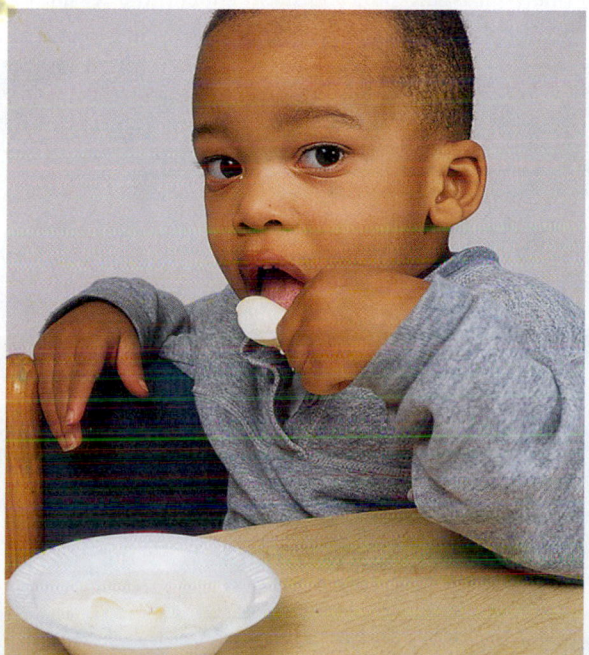

FIGURE 33–5 ■ The family must make an effort to make the high-fat diet appealing to the child on a ketogenic diet, despite their personal feelings about eating large amounts of food such as mayonnaise, as this child is doing.

Kidney stones occur in 5% of children on the ketogenic diet, and they are treated with increased fluid intake and alkalinization of the urine. Height and weight may decrease during treatment (Neal, Chaffe, Edwards, et al., 2008). Constipation sometimes occurs and can be treated with medium-chain triglycerides (MCT oil) and increased fluids. Effectiveness of the diet is determined by lack of seizures or significant reduction in frequency. A recent randomized control trial found the ketogenic diet to be effective in reducing seizure frequency after 3 months among children who averaged seven or more seizures a week and failed to respond to two or more AEDs (Neal, Chaffe, Schwartz, et al., 2008).

Long-term effects Epilepsy is associated with high rates of learning disabilities; developmental delay; and psychosocial, psychiatric, and behavioral problems in up to 50% of children affected. Common behavioral problems include depression, anxiety, attention deficit hyperactivity disorder, conduct problems, and aggression; these might be present in up to half of children and adolescents with epilepsy (Spencer & Huh, 2008).

Nursing Management

Nursing care at the time of a seizure focuses on maintaining airway patency, ensuring safety, administering medications, and providing emotional support. The nurse also assists the family to manage the condition long term.

Nursing Assessment and Diagnosis

Nursing assessment first focuses on assessing the child with a seizure to identify immediate care needed. For the child with known seizures, assessment focuses on adaptation of the child and family to the seizure disorder.

Assess and monitor the child's physiologic status. Observe the specific seizure activity, level of consciousness, vital signs, and signs of hypoxia. During the postictal period, monitor the child's vital signs, perform neurologic checks, and keep the environment safe. Once the child is stable, a more definitive assessment can be made. Level of consciousness is a vital indicator of neurologic function. Remember that the child's lack of response may be the result of the postictal state or cumulative medication dosages.

Collect and analyze historical information about the seizure activity, clustering, aura, description of motor activity or changes in muscle tone, automatisms, and any changes in development or school performance to help determine the type of seizures the child experiences. See Box 33–3.

Assess the family's adaptation to the seizure disorder because epilepsy is a disorder with a stigma associated with it. Identify how well the family is coping with the uncertainty of when the next seizure will occur. Identify how well the child is coping with a visible condition, such as when a seizure happens at school. Inquire about any behavioral, social, or emotional problems.

Common nursing diagnoses for the child with a seizure disorder include the following:

- Breathing Pattern, Ineffective, related to neuromuscular dysfunction during the tonic phase of a seizure
- Airway Clearance, Ineffective, related to inability to manage secretions during seizure
- Trauma, Risk for, related to fall with onset of seizure activity
- Self-Esteem, Chronic Low, related to loss of bowel and bladder control during seizure activity
- Anxiety related to unpredictable nature of seizure disorder
- Therapeutic Regimen Management: Family, Ineffective, related to poor adherence to medications prescribed for seizures
- Family Processes, Readiness for Enhanced, related to care of a child with a chronic disorder

NANDA-I © 2012

| BOX 33–3 | Questions to Ask About Seizures |

- What was the child doing just before the seizure?
- Did the child complain of not feeling well or feeling "funny" just before the seizure? Was the child sick or feverish before the seizure? Did the child complain of headache, nausea, or muscle pain? Did the child vomit?
- Did the child suffer any trauma before the seizure?
- Did the child get into any medications or poisons before the seizure?
- What movements of the arms and legs were seen? Were the movements on one or both sides of the body or in one extremity only? Did the child exhibit any chewing or other type of automatic behavior? If the parent struggles with a description, ask the parent to demonstrate movements and behaviors.
- Was the child's vision normal? Were the pupils dilated or the eyes deviated to one side?
- Was the child aware of surroundings? Could the child respond to questions?
- Was the child incontinent of urine or stool?
- How long did the episode last? When did the child begin to wake up? Was the child lethargic, weak, or uncoordinated upon arousal? Did the child have amnesia, loss of memory, or confusion after the event?
- Was the child injured during the convulsion?
- Did the child's color change (pale, red, blue)?

Planning and Implementation

Children may be hospitalized for a rapid (over several days) taper of the antiepileptic medication for a presurgical evaluation to provoke a seizure. Other children may be hospitalized for another condition but also have a seizure disorder. Nursing care focuses on maintaining airway patency, ensuring safety, administering medications, and providing emotional support.

Maintain Airway Patency

Be sure that nothing is placed in the child's mouth during a seizure to avoid knocking out loose teeth that could be aspirated. Position the child on his or her side so secretions can drain out of the mouth. Monitor the child to ensure adequate oxygenation. The child's color should be pink, the heart rate at a normal or slightly elevated rate for age, and the pulse oximetry reading greater than 95%. Oxygen is usually administered when the pulse oximetry reading (SpO_2) falls below 95% (refer to the Skills Manual ⬭).

Ensure Safety

Protect the child from self-harm during violent seizures (Figure 33–6 ■). If the child is in bed, the side rails should be padded to prevent injury. The child who has frequent, recurrent seizures should wear a helmet to protect the head during falls. All children with seizure disorders should wear a form of medical alert identification. Children with seizures that cause respiratory compromise or loss of consciousness should have seizure precaution supplies and equipment at the bedside (bag-valve mask, suction source and catheter, cardiorespiratory monitor and pulse oximetry) (Clore, 2010).

Administer Medications

Take special precautions when administering intravenous medications (benzodiapezines) for the acute management of seizures. These medications should be given very slowly to minimize the risk of respiratory or circulatory collapse.

Medications for the ongoing management of seizures are given orally. Crushing pills and mixing them in a teaspoonful of

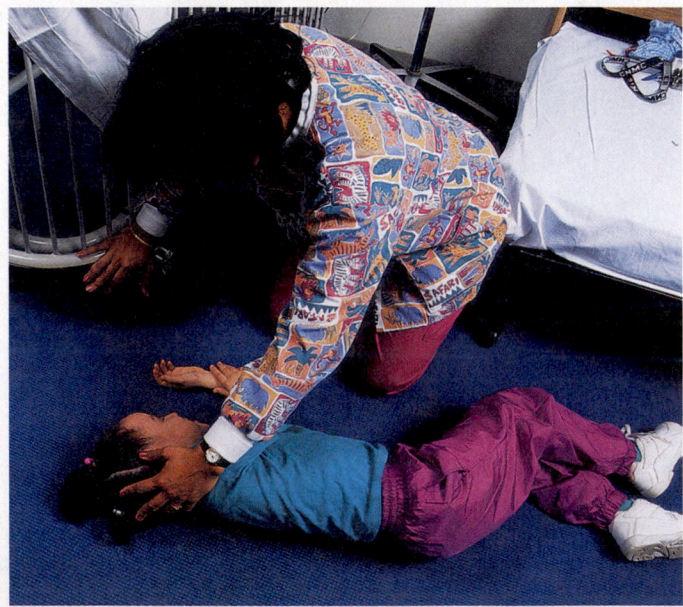

FIGURE 33–6 ■ A child who has a seizure when standing should be gently assisted to the floor and placed in a side-lying position. Clear the area of any objects that might cause harm to the child.

applesauce, pudding, or other soft food make them more palatable and easier for the child to swallow. For some medications, elixirs and flavored chewables are available. If the child has a sustained-release medication prescribed, this medication should not be chewed or crushed.

When a child is NPO (nothing by mouth) due to illness or on the day of surgery, seizure medications are usually given with a swallow of water. Obtain medication orders for these cases.

Practice Alert

When the child on a ketogenic diet is hospitalized, it is important to limit glucose and dextrose from all sources. Normal saline intravenous fluid should be used. Medications in elixirs, suspensions, and syrups cannot be used. Alternatively obtain medications in pill form, crush them, and mix with an allowable food approved by the pharmacy for medication mixing.

Provide Emotional Support

The loss of control of body movements and possible loss of consciousness make seizures frightening and difficult to accept for the child, parents, and other family members. Make sure that parents are informed about the cause of the seizures when possible to allay concerns about a potential brain tumor and prognosis. Parents may also be concerned about the effect of epilepsy on the child's development and relationships, and this stress and worry can affect their mental health (Duffy, 2011).

Parents often feel guilty about the child's seizure disorder and compensate by not disciplining or restricting the child appropriately. Stress the need to treat the child as normally as possible. Refer the child and family to support groups and counseling services if indicated. See Evidence-Based Practice: Supporting Children with Epilepsy and Their Parents.

Discharge Planning and Home Care Teaching

Encourage parents to express their fears and anxieties. Answer their questions honestly, and refer them to organizations, such as the Epilepsy Foundation of America, where they can obtain more information about the child's disorder. Be sure parents know how to administer medications and provide for the child's safety. Discuss with them whom to call with questions and when to return for follow-up. See Box 33–4 for books that may be useful to families and children.

Care in the Community

Parents and children should be regularly informed about new seizure management, be encouraged to ask questions about their concerns, and receive important information about injury prevention strategies. See Partnering with Families: Safety for the Child with a Seizure Disorder.

BOX 33–4	Epilepsy Resources for Families

- *Seizures and Epilepsy in Childhood: A Guide for Parents*, John M. Freeman, Johns Hopkins University Press, 2003.
- *Epilepsy on Our Terms: Stories by Children with Seizures and Their Parents (The Brainstorms Series)*, Stephen C. Schactner, Georgia Montouris, & John M. Pellock, Oxford University Press, 2008.
- *Epilepsy in Children* (2nd ed.), Sheila J. Wallace & Kevin Farrell (Eds.), Arnold Publications, 2004.
- *Keto Kid: Helping Your Child Succeed on the Ketogenic Diet*, Deborah Snyder, Demos Medical Publishing, 2007.
- *Children with Seizures: A Guide for Parents, Teachers, and Other Professionals*, Martin Kutscher & M. D. Kutscher, Jessica Kingsley Publishers, 2006.
- *Mommy I Feel Funny: A Child's Experience with Epilepsy*, Danielle M. Rocheford, 2009.

Evidence-Based Practice | Supporting Children with Epilepsy and Their Parents

PROBLEM

Epilepsy is a chronic neurologic condition that causes concern due to its unpredictable nature and potential for injury during a seizure. What is the nature of the stress that parents and children experience related to epilepsy? Is the parent's stress related to the child's psychologic adaptation to the disorder?

EVIDENCE

A study involving 49 parents of children with epilepsy and 54 parents of children with asthma, each with children between 8 and 13 years old, investigated differences in parental stress associated with each condition. The parents of children with epilepsy had a significantly higher stress level than the parents of children with asthma on four of seven domains of Abidin's Parenting Stress Index: restrictions of role, depression, relationship to spouse, and parental health. Parents also rated their children with epilepsy as having statistically significant differences in three of seven domains: adaptability, demanding, and hyperactivity/distractibility. These child characteristics likely contribute to problems with behavior, peer relationships, and self-esteem (Chiou & Hsieh, 2008).

The parenting stress of parents of 32 children (2 to 12 years old) with new-onset epilepsy was investigated and contrasted with the stress of parents of 29 healthy control children using the Abidin Parenting Stress Index, a life stress score, and the seizure-specific version of the family stress scale. No significant differences existed between the parent groups on any of the Parenting Stress Index composite scales and the life stress score. Stresses were higher in parents whose children experienced a seizure within a month of diagnosis. Parents of children with new-onset

epilepsy did identify more stress with finances, disciplining the child with epilepsy, concerns about education, and their marital relationship (Modi, 2009).

A study with 9 youth (10 to 15 years old) investigated a pilot intervention project that focused on enhancing coping skills, self-efficacy, and self-management to promote resilience in the youth and parents. Parents reported improved coping skills in their children. Children had improved knowledge of epilepsy and self-efficacy. The sample size was inadequate to investigate the effectiveness of the program on parental stress (Wagner, Smith, Ferguson, et al., 2010).

IMPLICATIONS

Parents often have no prior experience with epilepsy, and they may not have their concerns and needs well addressed by healthcare providers. Soon after diagnosis, parents do not yet demonstrate stress associated with the child's epilepsy condition; however, after some time, parents experience much greater stress. This could potentially be related to the stigma associated with epilepsy, the unpredictable nature of when and where seizures may occur, and loss of control. Intervention programs may help provide support for parents and children that improves the family's healthy adaptation to epilepsy.

CRITICAL THINKING APPLICATION

When caring for a child with epilepsy, what questions may help reveal the stressors that the parents and child are experiencing? Once stressors are identified, investigate resources with regard to parenting strategies, management of epilepsy, and support groups.

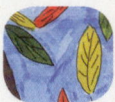

Partnering with Families

Safety for the Child with a Seizure Disorder

Children with epilepsy may potentially have more injuries of all sorts, including burns, falls, and drowning. Children are at increased risk for death due to drowning. Planning for safety includes the following:

- Children who bathe alone should use the shower. The child should not be left alone in the bathtub.
- A buddy and lifeguard should always be present when the child swims.
- A life vest should always be worn when boating.

- The child with frequent seizures should wear a helmet to protect the head in case of a fall.
- The child should not play or stand around open flames or outdoor grills.
- The child should avoid areas where fall risks are increased.
- A form of medical identification should be worn (e.g., medical alert bracelet).

Medication Education

Educate the child and parents about antiepileptic medication (AED) regimens. Explain the purpose of each drug, its schedule for administration, and the importance of giving all doses. As the child grows older, ensure that information is shared directly with the child so that the child can begin to take more responsibility for condition management. Teaching the older child to take medications without parental intervention provides a sense of self-control. Child and adolescent growth should be monitored; rapid changes in weight may lead to loss of seizure control if medication dosage is not appropriately adjusted. Ask questions at each visit that may reveal actual medication adherence, such as questions that can verify remaining doses or difficulties paying for medications. See Box 33–5 for research on medication adherence. Serum medication level may also be monitored to maintain drug levels within the therapeutic range.

Clinical Tip
The blood for serum drug levels is ideally obtained just prior to a dose so that it can be representative of the child's lowest serum level for that day.

Provide information about the side effects of medications ordered, and alert parents to the signs of toxic reactions or undermedication. Ensure that adolescents understand that alcohol intake is contraindicated and may result in medication toxicity. Regular dental care is important because some AEDs cause gingival hyperplasia. Explain the importance of follow-up visits to healthcare providers so the effectiveness of the child's medications can be monitored. Ensure that the family knows that dosage adjustments will be needed as the child grows, particularly during the time of growth spurts. Children at risk for continuous seizures or status epilepticus should have an emergency care plan developed so families know appropriate actions to take (see Chapter 14 ⊘).

Adolescent females need to be educated about the potential teratogenicity of some AEDs, such as valproic acid. Contraception should

be used when the adolescent is sexually active. When pregnancy is desired, an AED with a lower risk for birth defects may be prescribed. Refer the adolescent to a healthcare provider who can help select an effective contraceptive, or collaborate with the adolescent's primary care provider to manage epilepsy and reduce the risk of birth defects when pregnancy is desired.

Clinical Tip
Some AEDs, such as phenobarbital, primidone, phenytoin, carbamazepine, and oxcarbazepine, cause a drug interaction with low-estrogen oral contraceptives that can lead to contraceptive failure. Other more effective contraception should be prescribed.

Parents of children with febrile seizures should be taught how to properly administer acetaminophen or ibuprofen and to keep the child cool with light clothing. Parents need to know, however, that antipyretics may not prevent a future febrile seizure associated with an acute illness. The potential toxicity of an AED in a child with febrile seizures is often considered greater than the risk of having a seizure, and parents can be reassured that complications from febrile seizures are rare. If a rectal or intranasal benzodiazepine is prescribed, make sure the parents know when and how to administer it.

Care When a Seizure Occurs
Parents should learn how to care for the child having a seizure that is typical for the child rather than calling the healthcare provider each time. See Partnering with Families: Care When a Seizure Occurs.

Ketogenic Diet
When families choose to follow the ketogenic diet, help coordinate their care with a dietitian who can customize the diet to the child's growth and activity needs. Ensure that vitamins and other medications used are carbohydrate-free so ketosis is maintained. Alert parents that sunscreen lotions and shampoos with sorbitol should not be used; sorbitol is a carbohydrate that can be absorbed through the skin. When it is time to discontinue the ketogenic diet, it should be tapered by slowly decreasing the ratio of fats to protein and carbohydrates.

Family and Child Support
Assist the family to develop an individualized health plan so the child can receive medications during school hours, if necessary. If the child could potentially have a seizure while at school, it may be desirable to provide students with information about seizures, what happens, and how they can help the child. Parents may also want to provide a towel and change of clothing for the child to use if incontinence occurs with

BOX 33–5	Research: Medication Adherence

A study explored nonadherence to AEDs in 124 newly diagnosed children ages 2 to 12 years. Researchers discovered that 58% of children had persistent nonadherence and 42% had near perfect adherence during the first 6 months of therapy. The pattern of adherence was established within the first month of therapy. Socioeconomic status was the only factor associated with adherence, and lower socioeconomic status was associated with higher nonadherence (Modi, Rausch, & Glauser, 2011).

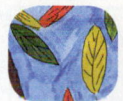
Partnering with Families

Care When a Seizure Occurs

First aid techniques to care for the child who has a seizure include the following:

- Place the child on the floor or bed, lying on one side so that saliva or vomit can drain out of the mouth.
- Loosen the clothing around the neck.
- Move objects away from the child so they are not close enough to cause injury.
- Put no objects into the child's mouth or between the teeth. Loose teeth may be knocked out and aspirated.

- Administer rectal diazepam (Diastat) or intranasal midazolam if it has been prescribed.
- Stay with the child until he or she is fully awake.
- Call 911 or your emergency number if the child's seizure lasts longer than 5 to 10 minutes, if a second seizure occurs, or if the child does not become conscious immediately after the seizure. Have a completed and current emergency medical information form available for the emergency care personnel.

---

the seizures. Teachers and school administrators should know what actions to take if the child has a seizure and what information to report about the seizure.

Physical activity and exercise are important for all children. Encourage participation in sports when supervision is provided. Some activities are potentially more dangerous for children, especially when seizures are not completely controlled, such as rope climbing, rock or mountain climbing, tree climbing, snow skiing, scuba diving, and skydiving. Swimming and water sports require one-to-one supervision.

The child may be afraid of having a seizure in front of friends. Reassure the child and family that taking medications regularly should control seizures. Children should explain to peers what a seizure is and what to do if they are present when one occurs. Summer camps for children with seizures can be a safe and comfortable place for the child to enjoy outdoor activities. Tell parents to boost the child's self-image by emphasizing what the child can do, rather than focusing on contraindicated activities. Depending on state laws, most adolescents can drive after they have been seizure-free for at least 2 years.

Evaluation

Expected outcomes of nursing management for the child and family include the following:

- The child achieves good seizure control with medication, ketogenic diet, or surgical intervention.
- The use of effective safety measures prevents injuries during seizures.
- The adolescent successfully manages seizures and maintains a healthy life.
- The child or adolescent gains enhanced self-esteem through participation in well-supervised sports and activities.

INFECTIOUS DISEASES

Bacterial Meningitis

Meningitis, an inflammation of the meninges, can be caused by either bacterial or viral agents. Bacterial meningitis is more serious than viral meningitis and is sometimes fatal. Newborns and infants are at greatest risk for bacterial meningitis. Infants and children who develop meningitis have the potential for acute complications and long-term morbidity.

Etiology and Pathophysiology

Meningitis may occur secondary to other infections such as otitis media, sinusitis, pharyngitis, cellulitis, pneumonia, tuberculosis, or septic arthritis; brain trauma; or a neurosurgical procedure. Two organisms, *Neisseria meningitidis* and *Streptococcus pneumoniae*, cause the majority of meningitis cases in children in the United States. *Haemophilus influenzae* type b remains a common causative organism in developing countries. *Group B streptococcus*, *Escherichia coli*, and *Listeria monocytogenes* are most likely to cause meningitis in newborns (Malhotra, Bell, & Henderson, 2009). (See Chapter 22 for more information about these infectious organisms.) Risk factors for meningitis include immunosuppression, a ventriculoperitoneal shunt, cochlear implant, CNS trauma, or a recent sinus or ear infection (Mann & Jackson, 2008).

In many cases, bacteremia in the blood spreads to the CNS where it enters the subarachnoid space, leading to an inflammatory response (Figure 33–7 ■). Bacterial endotoxins cause the brain to become inflamed and edematous, leading to **cerebral edema** (the increase in intracellular and extracellular fluid in the brain that results from anoxia, vasodilation, or vascular stasis) and increased intracranial pressure. If the infection spreads to the ventricles, they can become obstructed and impede the flow of cerebrospinal fluid, causing hydrocephalus as an acute complication. The infection may trigger the syndrome of inappropriate antidiuretic hormone (SIADH).

Clinical Tip

Haemophilus influenzae type b was the leading cause of bacterial meningitis in children prior to the use of the Hib conjugate vaccine. Immunization of infants with the pneumococcal vaccine is reducing the incidence of meningitis caused by specific serotypes of *Streptococcus pneumoniae* included in the vaccine (Mann & Jackson, 2008).

Clinical Manifestations

Symptoms are variable and depend on the child's age, the pathogen, and the length of the illness before diagnosis. Onset may be sudden or may develop over 1 to 2 days.

Symptoms in the young infant may include fever or hypothermia, change in feeding pattern, vomiting, or diarrhea. The anterior fontanel may be bulging or flat. The infant may be alert, restless, lethargic, or irritable. Rocking or cuddling, which normally calms a fussy infant, only irritates the infant with meningitis.

Older children are usually febrile, have altered consciousness (confusion, delirium, lethargy, or irritability), and may have vomiting and

Pathophysiology Illustrated   Central Nervous System Infection

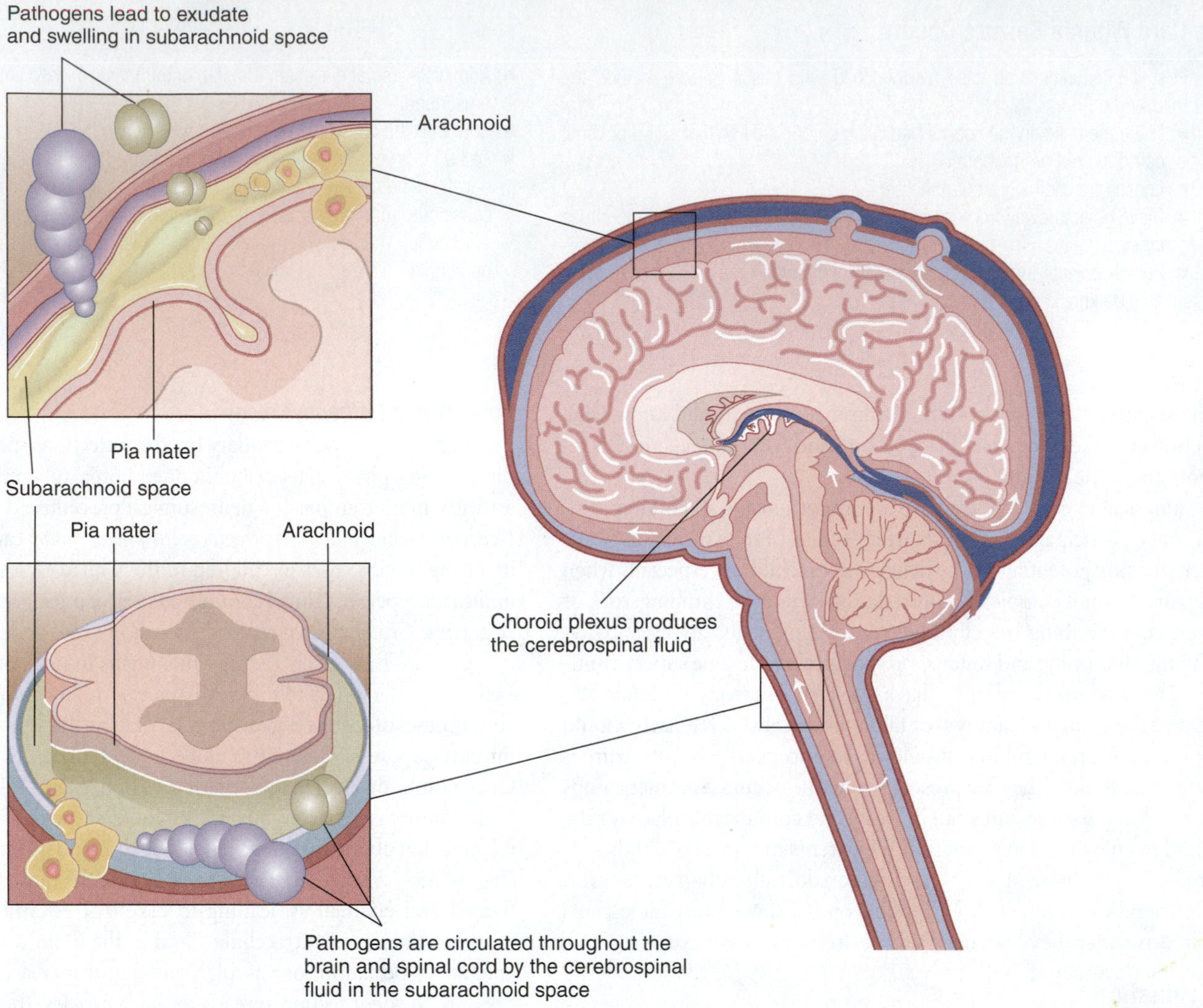

Pathogens lead to exudate
and swelling in subarachnoid space

Arachnoid

Pia mater

Subarachnoid space

Pia mater

Arachnoid

Choroid plexus produces
the cerebrospinal fluid

Pathogens are circulated throughout the
brain and spinal cord by the cerebrospinal
fluid in the subarachnoid space

FIGURE 33–7 ■ After bacteria reach the central nervous system, the pia mater, the arachnoid, and the cerebrospinal fluid–filled subarachnoid space become infected. The cerebrospinal fluid then circulates the pathogens throughout the brain and spinal cord.

complaints of muscle or joint pain. A hemorrhagic rash, first appearing as petechiae and changing to purpura or large necrotic patches, may be seen in meningococcal meningitis (see Chapter 22 ⊘). The child also displays other symptoms consistent with meningeal irritation: headache (most often frontal), back pain, photophobia, esotropia (inward eye deviation), and **nuchal rigidity** (resistance to neck flexion). The child is often comfortable only in an **opisthotonic position** in which the head and neck are hyperextended to relieve discomfort (Figure 33–8 ■). The child may have a positive Kernig or Brudzinski sign, or both, on examination (Figure 33–9 ■).

Collaborative Care

The goal of collaborative care is to identify the causative organism and rapidly begin clinical therapy in an effort to reduce the risk for complications.

Diagnostic Tests

Diagnosis is based on the history, clinical presentation, and laboratory findings. Laboratory tests include a complete blood count, blood

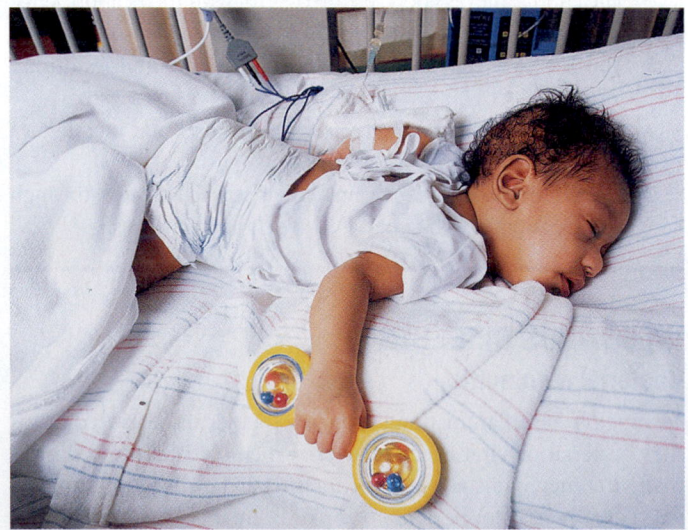

FIGURE 33–8 ■ The child with bacterial meningitis assumes an opisthotonic position, with the neck and head hyperextended, to relieve discomfort.

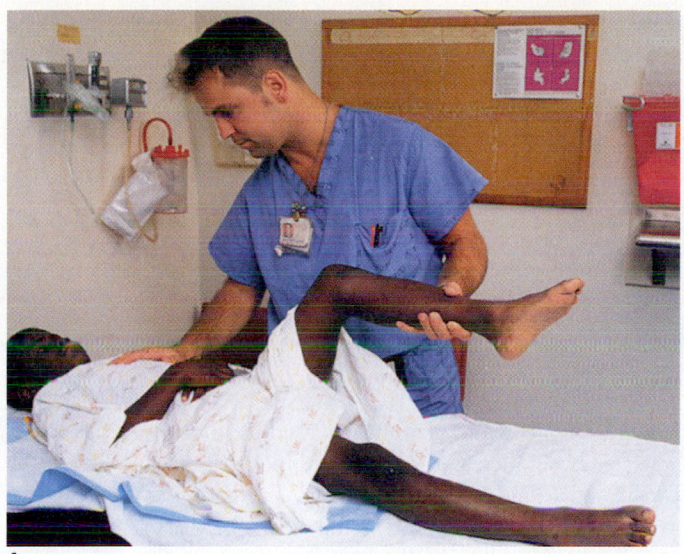
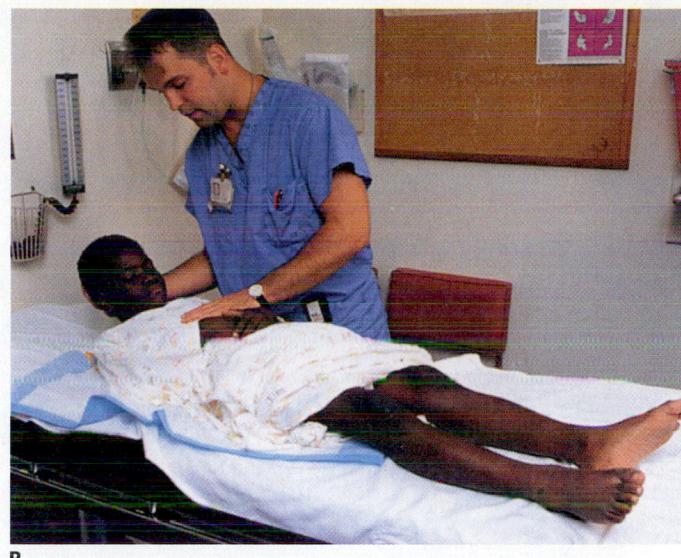

A   **B**

FIGURE 33–9 ■ *A*, To test for **Kernig sign,** raise the child's leg with the knee flexed. Then extend the child's leg at the knee. If any resistance is noted or pain is felt, the result is a positive Kernig sign. This is a common finding in meningitis. *B*, To test **Brudzinski sign,** flex the child's head while in a supine position. If this action makes the knees or hips flex involuntarily, a positive Brudzinski sign is present. This is a common sign in meningitis.

cultures, serum electrolytes and osmolality, and clotting factors. Blood cultures usually identify the responsible bacteria causing meningitis. A lumbar puncture, performed to culture the cerebrospinal fluid (CSF), measure the CSF pressure, and assess the fluid for the number of white blood cells and protein and glucose levels, confirms the diagnosis. The CSF glucose level is low in bacterial meningitis, and the protein level may be elevated. A gram stain of the CSF will usually show bacteria. CT scanning may be performed when increased intracranial pressure or a brain abscess is suspected. Repeat assessment of cerebrospinal fluid analysis may be performed to evaluate response to treatment (refer to the Skills Manual ⬭). See Box 33–6.

Clinical Therapy

Antibiotics must be able to cross the blood-brain barrier into the cerebrospinal fluid. In the majority of cases, antibiotics are administered as soon as diagnostic tests are obtained. Those commonly used to treat bacterial meningitis include ampicillin, aminoglycosides, cefotaxime, ceftriaxone, penicillin G, and vancomycin. Antibiotics are often changed once culture and sensitivity results are known, since many organisms have resistance to certain antibiotics. These medications are administered intravenously at the highest recommended therapeutic dose for 7 to 21 days, depending on the organism and the child's clinical response. Dexamethasone is given as an adjunct to children over 6 weeks of age and is initiated at the same time antibiotics are started to reduce the risk of severe neurologic sequelae such as sensorineural hearing loss in cases of *Haemophilus influenzae*

type b meningitis. The effectiveness of dexamethasone in meningitis caused by other organisms is not confirmed by research (Kim, 2010). Additional treatments include control of fever and seizures, management of increased intracranial pressure (ICP) if present, and fluid and electrolyte management.

Infants and children receive nothing by mouth and are started on IV fluids. The IV fluids are managed to maintain cerebral perfusion pressure, but the fluid volume administered may be less than maintenance dosage when the child is adequately hydrated to treat cerebral edema (Malhotra et al., 2009). The child is carefully monitored for increased intracranial pressure and SIADH (see Chapter 32 ⬤). Many child survivors have significant disabilities. Hearing impairment is reported in 30% to 50% of survivors of pneumococcal meningitis, 10% to 30% of *Haemophilus influenzae* meningitis, and 5% to 25% of meningococcal meningitis (Peltola, Roine, Fernandez, et al., 2010). See Box 33–7 for research on meningitis consequences.

Nursing Management

The goals of nursing care are to carefully monitor the child for signs of illness progression or development of complications, to support the family, to administer medications, and to manage pain.

Nursing Assessment and Diagnosis

Frequently assess the child's physiologic status, including vital signs and level of consciousness, and compare to the baseline neurologic assessment to identify changes in the child's condition. Measure head circumference frequently in infants during hospitalization and compare to previous measurements because of the potential for hydrocephalus to develop. Be alert for signs of a change in the child's

BOX 33–6	Research: Clinical Criteria for Bacterial Meningitis Diagnosis

A study that conducted a systematic review of prospective data identified several historical and clinical criteria related to a higher likelihood of bacterial meningitis. The potential for meningitis was higher if the parent reported neck stiffness, bulging fontanel, nonfebrile seizures, or reduced feeding in the child. Clinical signs with a higher likelihood for bacterial meningitis included jaundice, toxic appearance, neck stiffness, bulging fontanel, Kernig or Brudzinski sign, increased tone, and fever greater than 40°C (104°F) (Curtis, Stobart, Vandermeer, et al., 2010).

BOX 33–7	Research: Meningitis Consequences

A recent study of 1,433 infant and child survivors of bacterial meningitis revealed that 49% had at least one long-term consequence. Hearing loss was in 6.7% of children, gross neurologic deficits in 14.3%, and behavior and intellectual disorders in 45% of children (Chandran, Herbert, Misurski, et al., 2011).

condition and response to treatment. Monitor the child's ability to control secretions and to drink sufficient fluids. Monitor intake and output. Assess for any sensory deficits. Identify parents' concerns related to this potentially life-threatening condition.

Several nursing diagnoses that may apply to the child with bacterial meningitis are given in the accompanying Nursing Care Plan. Additional nursing diagnoses may include the following:

- Aspiration, Risk for, related to altered level of consciousness and poor secretion control
- Fluid Volume: Deficient, Risk For related to poor oral fluid intake
- Grieving (Parent) related to the child's potentially life-threatening condition
- Family Processes, Interrupted, related to serious illness and hospitalization of the child
- Caregiver Role Strain related to a hospitalized child and other family responsibilities

NANDA-I © 2012

Planning and Implementation

The Nursing Care Plan summarizes care for the child with bacterial meningitis. Nursing care begins with emergency treatment and continues as the child's condition stabilizes. Monitor respiratory and neurologic status, maintain hydration, administer medications, and prevent complications. Promote the child's comfort with reduced stimulation (dim lights, quiet room) and by placing the child in a side-lying position. Isolate the child according to hospital protocol until the causative organism is identified and at least 24 hours of effective treatment has occurred.

Practice Alert
Monitor the serum sodium concentration and urine specific gravity because these children are at risk for SIADH (see Chapter 32 🕜). Maintenance and replacement fluids are usually given to children with bacterial meningitis. If SIADH occurs, moderate fluid restriction with an isotonic solution is ordered until serum sodium levels return to normal.

Monitor the child's response to antibiotic therapy. Observe for signs of gastrointestinal bleeding (e.g., intestinal discomfort and blood in the stools), which is a potential complication of corticosteroid use.

Respond to parents' concerns about their child's condition, explaining all measures to reduce the child's discomfort and provide adequate treatment. Identify ways parents can participate in meeting the child's comfort needs. Parents may also need assistance in identifying the best strategies for meeting the needs of other children at home while spending time with the hospitalized child.

A major role of nurses is prevention. Encourage the parents to get their infants and children fully immunized, especially the Haemophilus influenzae type b, pneumococcal, and meningococcal vaccines (see Chapter 22 🕜).

Discharge Planning and Home Care Teaching
Home care needs should be identified and addressed well in advance of discharge. Follow-up visits are important to monitor for complications and sequelae. Help parents deal with any physical requirements resulting from the child's illness and any emotional, social, and financial repercussions of the child's condition. Teach parents what to do if the child has a seizure.

Infants and toddlers with neurologic sequelae should be referred to an early intervention program. If the child has had a hearing loss, referral to an otolaryngologist and speech and language specialist

should be made. Encourage early identification of other neurologic sequelae, such as learning problems. Children with hearing, learning, or other neurologic sequelae need to have an individualized education plan (see Chapter 16 🕜), and parents may need assistance in planning for the child's special education needs. Refer parents to appropriate social service agencies for support and assistance.

Evaluation

Expected outcomes of nursing care are provided in the Nursing Care Plan.

Viral (Aseptic) Meningitis

Viral meningitis is an inflammatory response of the meninges characterized by an increased number of blood cells and protein in the cerebrospinal fluid. In the United States, an enterovirus is the cause of a majority of cases (Irani, 2008). Viral meningitis due to enteroviruses occurs more frequently in the summer and fall.

Generally, the child with aseptic meningitis does not appear as ill as the child with bacterial meningitis. The child may have an abrupt onset of fever of 38°C to 40°C (100.4°F to 104°F) and have meningeal signs (headache, photophobia, stiff neck, and back pain), myalgia, irritability, and lethargy. Other symptoms include general malaise, vomiting, diarrhea, upper respiratory symptoms, and rash. The infant may have a tense anterior fontanel. Seizures are rare. Symptoms usually resolve spontaneously within 3 to 10 days.

The child with fever and meningeal signs is hospitalized. Blood, urine, and cerebrospinal fluid analyses are performed. A polymerase chain reaction test of the cerebrospinal fluid is performed for diagnosis of viral meningitis and is often available within 24 hours. Until the diagnosis of aseptic meningitis is confirmed, the child is treated aggressively, as if he or she has bacterial meningitis. Other treatment is supportive of symptoms. Children usually make a full recovery.

Nursing Management

Initial nursing care focuses on providing supportive care as described for the child with bacterial meningitis. Give acetaminophen as ordered to reduce fever, headache, and muscle or joint pain. Keep the room dark and quiet (to decrease stimuli and meningeal irritation), give fluids either intravenously or orally, and promote comfort with proper positioning.

The child and family need information about the disease. Explain medical and nursing procedures in terms that the child and family can understand. Keep parents informed about the child's progress. Once the diagnosis of viral meningitis is made, discharge planning and teaching for home care must begin immediately. Explain that recovery may take several weeks but that complete recovery is expected.

Encephalitis

Encephalitis is an acute inflammation of the brain often caused by a virus that is transmitted by a mosquito, such as West Nile virus and western equine virus. Inflammation of the meninges is also common. Epidemics occur most commonly in warm weather seasons. The incidence is estimated to be 10 per 100,000 child-years (Fowler, Stödberg, Eriksson, et al., 2010).

The encephalitis may occur as a direct or primary infection by an organism (virus, bacteria, fungi, or parasite) that successfully passes through the blood-brain barrier, such as herpes viruses or

Nursing Care Plan
The Child with Bacterial Meningitis

INTERVENTION	RATIONALE	EXPECTED OUTCOME
1. Nursing Diagnosis: Gas Exchange, Impaired, related to decreased level of consciousness		
NIC Priority Intervention—*Respiratory Monitoring:* Collection and analysis of patient data to ensure airway patency and adequate gas exchange		**NOC Suggested Outcome**—*Ventilation:* Movement of air in and out of the lungs
GOAL: *The child's respiratory failure does not progress to respiratory arrest.*		
■ Place the child on a cardiorespiratory monitor with a 20-second alarm.	■ The alarm on the monitor alerts staff if the child has bradycardia or an apneic spell.	The child's respiratory failure is managed with assessment and prompt treatment.
■ Have resuscitation equipment, including oxygen, resuscitation bag with mask, and suction apparatus, at the bedside.	■ Equipment is readily available in case of respiratory arrest.	
■ Stimulate the child if apneic; if no response, begin assisted ventilations and call for the resuscitation team.	■ Stimulation may encourage spontaneous respirations; if not, ventilation is necessary. The resuscitation team can help manage the child's condition.	
■ Monitor heart rate and perform compressions if necessary.	■ The apneic child may have bradycardia resulting from cardiac hypoxia.	
2. Nursing Diagnosis: Injury, Risk for, related to infection of cerebrospinal fluid and potential sequelae		
NIC Priority Intervention—*Health Screening:* Detecting health risks or problems by means of history, examination, and other procedures		**NOC Suggested Outcome**—*Immune Status:* Adequacy of natural and acquired appropriately targeted resistance to internal and external antigens
GOAL: *The child will suffer minimal CNS injury secondary to infection.*		
■ Administer antibiotics and corticosteroids (if prescribed).	■ Antibiotics help eradicate the pathogen and prevent cerebral edema. Corticosteroids may reduce the risk for neurologic **sequelae** (abnormal conditions resulting from a disease, treatment, or injury).	The child's condition improves significantly within 48–72 hours (fever decreases and no signs of neurologic sequelae are detected).
■ Note return of fever, nuchal rigidity, or irritability. Monitor vital signs, assess for signs of increased ICP, and measure head circumference once or twice daily. Note changes in responsiveness. Notify the physician immediately if any signs are detected.	■ Watching for common sequelae, such as subdural effusion or hydrocephalus, ensures prompt treatment.	
GOAL: *The child will not develop cerebral edema as a result of water retention.*		
■ Monitor serum sodium for development of SIADH and watch for signs of increased ICP.	■ SIADH can be either avoided or quickly managed if recognized early.	Cerebral edema does not develop. If SIADH or increased ICP occurs, the condition is treated promptly so effects are minimized.
■ Perform strict intake and output measurements. Determine urine specific gravity. Check electrolytes and osmolality of both serum and urine. Weigh the child daily. Restrict fluids and give sodium chloride as prescribed.	■ Low urine output with a high specific gravity is a sign of fluid retention and SIADH. The child is maintained with restricted fluids and is provided sodium supplements to reduce the possibility for cerebral edema.	
GOAL: *The child will be free of injury resulting from disseminated intravascular coagulation (DIC).*		
■ Be aware of needlesticks that continue to bleed and lesions that continue to ooze. Monitor clotting times.	■ Prompt recognition leads to management of the coagulopathy.	The child does not sustain injury from DIC.
■ Administer blood products, vitamin K, or heparin as ordered.	■ Prompt recognition allows for early initial treatment of DIC. The child may bleed to death if treatment is delayed.	
GOAL: *The child with any degree of hearing loss will be identified.*		
■ Arrange for hearing assessment prior to discharge.	■ Hearing loss is a common complication. Early intervention is needed to promote growth and development.	The child with identified hearing loss is referred to an appropriate specialist or program for intervention.

(continued)

Nursing Care Plan | The Child with Bacterial Meningitis, *continued*

INTERVENTION	RATIONALE	EXPECTED OUTCOME
3. Nursing Diagnosis: Pain, Acute, related to meningeal irritation		
NIC Priority Intervention—*Pain Management:* Alleviation of pain or reduction in pain to a level of comfort acceptable to patient		**NOC Suggested Outcome**—*Comfort Level:* Feelings of physical and psychological ease
GOAL: *The child will be as comfortable as possible.*		
■ Assess pain with an age-appropriate pain scale.	■ Pain scales provide the ability to quantify pain for future comparison.	The child is calm and expresses increased comfort.
■ Minimize tactile stimulation.	■ Sensory stimulation increases discomfort.	
■ Allow the child to assume a comfortable position.	■ The child determines the most comfortable position. The opisthotonic position may be the most comfortable.	
■ Keep the lights dim and maintain a quiet environment.	■ Dim lights reduce the discomfort from photophobia. Noise can disturb the child.	
■ Provide pain medication as prescribed.	■ Pain medication is appropriate for acute discomfort associated with illness.	
4. Nursing Diagnosis: Infection, Risk for (Family and Close Contacts) related to pathogens in the cerebrospinal fluid		
NIC Priority Intervention—*Infection Control:* Minimizing the acquisition and transmission of infectious agents		**NOC Suggested Outcome**—*Infection Status:* Presence and extent of infection
GOAL: *Caretakers or family members will have no apparent evidence of infection.*		
■ Explain rationale and dose schedule for taking rifampin or ciprofloxacin.	■ Rifampin and ciprofloxacin provide prophylaxis for many bacterial pathogens responsible for meningitis.	Family members and other close contacts verbalize the schedule for rifampin or ciprofloxacin therapy.

NANDA-I © 2012

rabies. Arboviruses (viruses causing eastern equine, western equine, St. Louis, and La Crosse encephalitis, and Colorado tick fever), enteroviruses, and Epstein-Barr virus are other potential organisms causing encephalitis.

Some children only have symptoms of a flulike illness after being infected and never develop encephalitis. Signs and symptoms include fever, irritability, severe headache, and bulging fontanel, followed by altered mental status. The child may have flaccid or spastic paralysis. Meningeal irritation signs such as nuchal rigidity, photophobia, and positive Kernig or Brudzinski signs are common. Focal or generalized seizures may occur. Altered mental status may progress to coma over hours or days.

Diagnosis is based on history and laboratory findings. Information about recent immunizations, insect bites, and residing in or travel to areas where cases of encephalitis are present should be obtained (e.g., cases of West Nile virus or eastern equine encephalitis). CSF culture and analysis, blood serologic tests, and nasopharyngeal and stool specimens are evaluated to identify viral pathogens. Testing for virus-specific immunoglobulin M antibodies with an enzyme-linked immunosorbent assay (ELISA) is performed after 5 days of the acute illness. A polymerase chain reaction test is used to assay for herpes DNA in the spinal fluid. A CT scan, MRI, and EEG may also be performed. An EEG may help assess seizure activity and help localize the area of the brain affected.

The child with encephalitis at risk for seizures, respiratory failure, and increased intracranial pressure receives supportive treatment in an intensive care unit. Physical therapy, occupational therapy, and speech therapy may be prescribed for these children. Children admitted to the intensive care unit with serious symptoms are more likely to have persistent symptoms that last up to 6 months. Those who survive often have significant neurologic sequelae, such as personality changes, memory changes, noise sensitivity, and poor concentration (Fowler et al., 2010).

Nursing Management

Nursing care focuses on monitoring cardiorespiratory function, preventing complications resulting from immobility, reorienting the child, and teaching the parents about the child's condition.

The child is usually admitted to the intensive care unit during acute stages. Monitor the child's cardiorespiratory function. Check the child's airway and ability to handle secretions. Monitor respiratory status by observing color, respiratory rate, use of accessory muscles, pulse oximetry readings, and arterial blood gas values. Provide seizure precautions, and have appropriate equipment for managing seizures at bedside (refer to the Skills Manual 🔗). Provide support to parents as they cope with the serious nature of this condition.

Prevent complications resulting from immobility as described in Box 33–2 on page 1155. Maintain skin integrity. Proper positioning with frequent turning is important. When indicated by the physician, perform chest physiotherapy to prevent pneumonia.

As the level of consciousness begins to improve, the child may at first be confused and disoriented and have residual effects of the disease. Orient the child to the hospital environment. Encourage parents to take an active role in the child's physical and emotional care during recovery. They can, for example, bring favorite stuffed animals or music from home. Engage in therapeutic play (refer to Chapter 15 🔗 for techniques). Give the child age-appropriate toys to encourage a return to normal behavior.

Provide parents with instructions for home care. Plan follow-up visits so the child can be evaluated for neurologic sequelae. Ensure that children are referred for physical or speech therapy as needed. Refer parents to home care, social services, family counseling, and support groups as needed.

Reye Syndrome

Reye syndrome is an acute **encephalopathy,** a cerebral dysfunction caused by a toxic, inflammatory, or anoxic insult or injury that may result in permanent tissue damage and hepatic dysfunction. In the 1980s, an association was reported between the use of aspirin for influenza or varicella and the subsequent development of Reye syndrome. The condition is now rare (approximately 35 cases a year) since most parents now give children acetaminophen or ibuprofen rather than aspirin for viral illnesses and flulike symptoms (Carey & Balistreri, 2011). The mortality rate for children who develop Reye syndrome is high.

Reye syndrome is classified as a secondary mitochondrial hepatopathy, caused by a drug toxic to the liver, toxin, metal, or metabolite from a poorly functioning organ. In the case of Reye syndrome an interaction between a viral illness and aspirin occurs in a susceptible individual (Carey & Balistreri, 2011). The disorder is characterized by cerebral edema, hypoglycemia, and an enlarged, fatty, poorly functioning liver (due to an elevation of short-chain fatty acid levels and hyperammonemia).

Reye syndrome begins with a preceding viral illness that seems to be resolving, followed by an acute onset of vomiting, mental status changes, seizures, and progressive unresponsiveness. The condition has five stages that demonstrate increasing signs of cerebral edema and neurologic dysfunction. See the Clinical Manifestations table for the signs associated with each stage.

The diagnosis of Reye syndrome is based on an abrupt change in the child's level of consciousness and diagnostic laboratory tests that reveal liver dysfunction and no other identifiable cause. CSF analysis usually reveals white blood cells, while radiographic imaging reveals cerebral edema. Liver enzyme and ammonia levels are elevated, blood glucose levels are below normal, and prothrombin time is prolonged. Serum bilirubin levels are normal. A liver biopsy is sometimes performed to confirm the diagnosis. Death occurs due to increased intracranial pressure and herniation of the brainstem. If the child survives, full liver function occurs, but these children should be screened for a fatty-acid oxidation metabolic disorder (Carey & Balistreri, 2011).

The child with Reye syndrome is cared for in a pediatric intensive care unit. The goal of medical management is to provide supportive treatment and to prevent the secondary effects of cerebral edema and metabolic injury associated with the elevation of short-chain fatty acid levels and hyperammonemia. Mechanical ventilation is often needed once the child is comatose. Arterial and venous pressure monitoring are performed. The child is carefully monitored for signs of increased intracranial pressure, which can be secondary to cerebral edema. Hypoglycemia is treated with intravenous glucose; and electrolytes, blood chemistry, and blood pH are monitored (refer to the Skills Manual 🔗).

Nursing Management

Nursing care focuses on monitoring the child's physical status, providing emotional support, and teaching parents about disease prevention.

Clinical Manifestations   Reye Syndrome by Stages

STAGE	CLINICAL MANIFESTATIONS
I	Vomiting, lethargy and sleepiness, usually quiet, laboratory evidence of liver dysfunction
II	Deep lethargy, confusion, delirium, combativeness, hyperventilation, hyperactive reflexes
III	Obtunded, light coma, seizures may or may not be present, decorticate rigidity, pupillary light reflex is intact
IV	Seizures, deepening coma, decerebrate rigidity and posturing, absent oculocephalic reflex, fixed pupils
V	Coma, loss of deep tendon reflexes, respiratory arrest, fixed dilated pupils, intermittent flaccidity and decerebrate posturing

Source: *Data from Carey, R. G., & Balistreri, W. F. (2011). Mitochondrial hepatopathies. In R. M. Kliegman, B. F. Stanton, J. W. St. Geme, N. F. Schor, & R. E. Behrman, Nelson textbook of pediatrics (19th ed., pp. 1405–1408). Philadelphia, PA: Elsevier Saunders.*

Clinical Tip

Make sure all parents know to use acetaminophen or ibuprofen when the child has a viral illness, such as influenza, to prevent the development of Reye syndrome. Most over-the counter-medications for children are now made with acetaminophen or ibuprofen rather than aspirin or salicylate compounds, but parents should be encouraged to verify this. Emphasize the importance of obtaining health care whenever a child's condition worsens at the end of a viral illness.

Check the child's respiratory and neurologic status frequently, and note any signs of improvement or deterioration. Refer to the discussion of nursing management of altered states of consciousness on page 1154 for specific nursing interventions. Monitor laboratory tests for acidosis, elevation of ammonia levels, or hypoglycemia. Carefully monitor the child's intake and output. Correct imbalances by administering fluids, electrolytes, or medications as ordered. Prevent complications associated with immobility.

Provide emotional support to the parents, who are dealing with a sudden life-threatening condition. Keep them informed about the child's condition, and prepare them for potential deterioration in the course of the disease. Explanations of treatments can help reduce anxiety. Encourage the parents to participate in the child's care when possible.

If the child survives and is discharged, monitoring is needed to observe for sequelae of the illness. Developmental and neurologic deficits may occur and are more severe in children under 2 years of age. Arrange for home nursing visits or frequent office visits during the recovery period so that developmental and neurologic status can be assessed. Be sure the parents are informed about resources in the community that can assist them in dealing with the child's recovery.

Guillain-Barré Syndrome (Postinfectious Polyneuritis)

Guillain-Barré syndrome is a peripheral neuropathy with an acute onset of rapidly developing symmetric motor weakness. This disorder affects children at an estimated rate of 0.6 per 100,000 per year. The disorder occurs in all seasons, and males are reported to be affected more than females (McGrogan, Madle, Seaman, et al., 2009).

Guillain-Barré syndrome is thought to be caused by an immune response to an infectious organism rather than an autoimmune or systemic disorder. Children usually have a respiratory or gastrointestinal infection within 3 weeks of weakness development.

Campylobacter jejuni is the most commonly reported antecedent infection, but other organisms associated with Guillain-Barré syndrome include cytomegalovirus, Epstein-Barr virus, *Mycoplasma pneumoniae*, and *Haemophilus influenzae*. An association between some immunizations, such as for influenza, and development of the disorder has not been confirmed. Some research evidence suggests that the disorder is caused by an infection-induced aberrant immune response that damages the peripheral nerves (van Doorn, Ruts, & Jacobs, 2008). The damaged peripheral nerves then begin to atrophy.

Infants have an onset of rapidly progressive severe **hypotonia** (reduced muscle tone), possible respiratory distress, irritability, and feeding difficulties. Older children initially have pain, numbness, paresthesia, or weakness in all limbs. Weakness progresses bilaterally over days up to 4 weeks. Maximum weakness is often reached in 2 to 4 weeks. Deep tendon reflexes are diminished or absent. The child may develop acute ataxia or an inability to walk. Respiratory muscles and cranial nerves may not be affected, but difficulty swallowing and bilateral facial nerve weakness are signs of impending respiratory failure. A dysfunctional autonomic nervous system may cause such symptoms as blood pressure fluctuations, cardiac arrhythmias, sweating abnormalities, pupillary abnormalities, and bladder and bowel dysfunction (van Doorn et al., 2008).

Collaborative Care

Diagnostic criteria of Guillain-Barré syndrome include progressive motor weakness (minimal weakness of the legs to total paralysis of all extremities) and varying degrees of **areflexia** (no reflex response to stimulation). Cerebrospinal fluid analysis usually reveals a protein that may be normal in the first week but nearly twice the upper limit of normal after the second week (van Doorn et al., 2008). Bacterial and viral cultures are usually negative. Electroconduction tests such as electromyography show acute muscle denervation. Muscle biopsy is usually not required for diagnosis.

The preferred clinical therapy for Guillain-Barré syndrome is intravenous immune globulin (IVIG) at a dose of 0.4 g/kg/day for 5 days when the child is unable to ambulate (van Doorn et al., 2008). Guidelines for administration of IVIG can be found in Chapter 27 🔗. Responses to intravenous immune globulin are dramatic, often within days. Plasma exchange to remove autoantibodies has also been documented as an effective therapy (Cirillo, 2008). Oral and intravenous corticosteroids are not effective. Pain management is important. Physical therapy and supportive care are initiated early to promote ambulation. Rehabilitation begins as soon as improvement is noted. The condition is rarely fatal. Children may report severe fatigue during recovery.

Nursing Management

Nursing care focuses on monitoring respiratory status, meeting nutritional needs, managing autonomic nervous system dysfunction, preventing complications associated with immobility, providing emotional support, and teaching the parents how to care for the child after discharge.

Monitor Cardiorespiratory Status

Place the child on a cardiorespiratory monitor to continuously assess the child's cardiorespiratory status, especially in the early phase of illness. Look for such signs as dyspnea, inability to handle secretions, inadequate respiratory effort, and color changes that may indicate the need for endotracheal intubation and mechanical ventilation.

Manage Autonomic Nervous System Dysfunction

Monitor the child's vital signs closely for episodes of tachycardia, bradycardia, blood pressure fluctuations, sweating, and bowel and bladder dysfunction. Observe frequently for decreased responsiveness. Promptly report the occurrence of these signs of autonomic nervous system dysfunction to the child's physician.

Meet Nutritional Needs

Assess whether the child is having difficulty swallowing. If the child has no gag reflex, nutritional needs are maintained with intravenous supplements or nasogastric tube feedings.

Prevent Complications

Prevent complications associated with immobility (see Box 33–2 on page 1155). Ensure good postural alignment, and turn the child every 2 hours. Interventions to prevent deep vein thrombosis may be prescribed. Maintaining skin integrity is also important.

Evaluate the child's muscle tone, strength, and symmetry. When the child's condition begins to improve, recovery of lost strength is the priority. Active exercise is emphasized in physical therapy. Encourage family members to participate in the child's care, especially during the recovery phase. They can help with the activities of daily living and reinforce what the child has learned in physical therapy.

Provide Emotional Support

Explain the progression of Guillain-Barré syndrome to the parents during the initial stages. Witnessing a rapid deterioration in their child's physical status can be frightening; therefore, informing parents that deterioration may continue until the treatment becomes effective is essential to reduce their anxieties. Be honest when discussing recovery and prognosis for the child.

Have parents bring in favorite toys, dolls, or books to make the child feel more secure. Playing with or reading to the child can be comforting.

Discharge Planning and Home Care Teaching

Home care needs should be identified and addressed well in advance of discharge. Support the parents as they prepare for the child's return home, especially when return to full strength is expected to be slow. Outpatient physical sessions may be needed several times a week in the early recovery stages. Frequent follow-up visits to the health center are essential to monitor the child's recovery. Refer the parents to social workers who can help with financial arrangements as needed.

Care in the Community

Help the child adjust to any residual effects of Guillain-Barré syndrome. Help the child practice exercises learned in physical therapy sessions, and encourage the child to perform activities of daily living, such as brushing the teeth or combing the hair.

To promote a positive self-image, praise any effort the child makes to be self-sufficient. The child may have feelings of frustration and anger. Allow the child to express these feelings in an appropriate way, either during play or in conversation. Home schooling may be needed until the child has strength to walk and participate in a full school day.

HEADACHES

Children commonly experience headaches. They may be the cause of school absence, decreased extracurricular activity, and poor academic achievement. Up to 82% of children experience a headache

Clinical Manifestations Headaches

TYPE OF HEADACHE AND ETIOLOGY	CLINICAL MANIFESTATIONS	CLINICAL THERAPY
Migraine—vascular Acute Recurrent	■ Prodrome may include a visual or motor aura less than 30 minutes before headache; child without aura may have mood changes, food cravings, or anorexia hours before the attack ■ Unilateral, bifrontal, or bitemporal pain, gradual but rapid onset, pulsatile throbbing, moderate to severe pain intensity aggravated by physical activity ■ Headache lasts 2 to 3 hours, often relieved by sleep; may last 48 to 72 hours if untreated ■ Nausea and/or vomiting ■ Photophobia and/or phonophobia ■ Preschool-age children may have irritability, malaise, head banging, head holding, and behaviors indicating sensitivity to light and sound	■ Medications to abort migraine (e.g., sumatriptan nasal spray) for adolescents ■ Noise and light avoidance during acute headache ■ Ibuprofen or acetaminophen at onset of aura or headache ■ Relaxation techniques, biofeedback, and cognitive behavioral therapies ■ Regular patterns of eating, sleep, and exercise; adequate fluid intake ■ Food elimination trial to identify food triggers (e.g., caffeine, chocolate, cheese, lunch meats, food coloring, monosodium glutamate) ■ May prescribe prophylactic daily administration of topiramate or valproic acid for children with frequent disabling migraines
Tension—muscular contraction Acute recurrent (less than 15 days a month) Chronic nonprogressive (more than 15 days a month)	■ Pressure or tightening (nonpulsatile) pain of mild to moderate intensity, may last for 30 minutes to 7 days ■ Intermittent or constant pain with fluctuations in degree of pain ■ Unlikely to have nausea and vomiting, sensitivity to light and sound, abdominal pain, or visual disturbances ■ Dizziness and fatigue may be present ■ Pain not aggravated by walking or climbing stairs	■ Relaxation techniques, biofeedback therapy ■ Ibuprofen or acetaminophen ■ Ice pack ■ Rest, adequate hydration, regular meals and exercise, regular sleep pattern ■ Minimize intake of caffeine ■ Review schedule to ensure some relaxation time daily
Medication Overuse	■ Pain may be bandlike, over entire head, or crushing; may be bad enough to interfere with academic performance ■ Occurs more than 15 times a month or more; lasts longer than 3 to 4 hours daily ■ Usually increases in frequency and severity over time, paralleling the increase in medication use ■ Recurs with the abortive therapy or when medication wears off	■ Withdrawal of all medications for headaches (e.g., acetaminophen, NSAIDs, opioids, ergotamines, and triptans) for a 2- to 4-week period; may permit use of one of the medications up to twice a week after withdrawal period ■ Prophylactic daily amitriptyline, calcium channel blocker, or antiepileptic drug may be prescribed ■ Adequate hydration, three meals a day, daily exercise, and 8 hours uninterrupted sleep ■ Avoid foods, beverages, and medications with caffeine
Inflammatory—sinusitis or dental abscess Acute Localized	■ Facial pain or tenderness over affected sinus, gum area, or periorbital, may be associated with nasal congestion ■ Dull, constant pressure ■ Severity of pain varies with position of head ■ Fever may be present ■ No nausea, visual changes, light or sound sensitivity	■ Analgesic, antipyretic, and anti-inflammatory medications ■ Antibiotic medications ■ Cold or heat application
Structural—space-occupying lesion, hemorrhage, increased intracranial pressure Chronic progressive	■ Severe pain, increases in frequency and severity, often in occipital or frontal location ■ Pain awakens child or occurs in morning ■ Pain increases with coughing, sneezing, or straining ■ Vomiting that is persistent or preceded by recurrent headache ■ Abnormal neurologic signs (e.g., double vision, papilledema, strabismus, weakness, ataxia)	■ Surgery (see Chapter 29 🔗 for brain tumors) ■ Analgesic medications

Source: *Data from Dooley, J. M., & Pearlman, E. M. (2010). The clinical spectrum of migraine in children. Pediatric Annals, 39(7), 408–415; Hershey, A. D., Kabbouche, M. A., & Powers, S. W. (2010). Treatment of pediatric and adolescent migraines. Pediatric Annals, 39(7), 416–423; Pakalnis, A., & Yonker, M. (2010). "Other" headache syndromes in children. Pediatric Annals, 39(7), 440–446; Partap, S., & Fisher, P. G. (2010). Managing chronic daily headaches. Contemporary Pediatrics, 27(4), 30–41; Blume, H. K., & Szperka, C. L. (2010). Secondary causes of headaches in children: When it isn't a migraine. Pediatric Annals, 39(7), 431–439.*

by age 15 years, and the prevalence increases between preschool age and adolescence. Migraine headache 1 year prevalence in children between ages 12 and 17 years was 5% in boys and 7.7% in girls, and the prevalence is higher in Caucasian compared to African American children (Bigal & Arruda, 2010).

Headaches have both benign (migraine, inflammatory, and tension) and structural causes (e.g., tumors or increased intracranial pressure). Signs and symptoms of headaches in children and adolescents vary by cause. Classifications and clinical manifestations for various headaches can be found in the Clinical Manifestations table above.

■ Migraines may be triggered by stress; foods containing nitrates, glutamate, caffeine, tyramine, and salt; menses; oral contraceptives; fatigue; and hunger. Another family member often has similar headaches, so genetic predisposition may also be a factor. Some children with migraines have previously experienced cyclic vomiting syndrome or abdominal migraine episodes (Dooley & Pearlman, 2010).

- Tension headaches may be triggered by stresses associated with school, anxiety, demanding schedules, fasting, and inadequate sleep. Tension headaches are more common than migraines.
- Medication overuse (rebound) headaches are associated with the frequent use of headache medications more than two to three times a week. They occur in more than 50% of children with chronic headaches. A higher risk of chronic headaches occurs in the child or adolescent who is obese (Partap & Fisher, 2010). Medications associated with this disorder include acetaminophen, nonsteroidal anti-inflammatory drugs (NSAIDs), decongestants, triptans, opioids, benzodiazepines, and ergotamines.

Clinical Tip
Some children with migraine headaches experience an aura or warning of an impending migraine headache less than 30 minutes prior to the pain. Ask the young child to draw the visual aura, or show pictures of common patterns (zigzag lines, holes in central vision, sparkles or stars, or kaleidoscope patterns with multiple colors) to help him or her describe the experience. Other children experience numbness, weakness, confusion, or motor auras (Dooley & Pearlman, 2010).

Collaborative Care

The goal of collaborative care is to differentiate a serious structural cause of headache from the benign headache classifications and to select appropriate clinical therapy to promote the child's ability to function and participate in school and daily living.

Diagnostic Tests

Diagnosis is usually made by obtaining a detailed history of the following headache characteristics: onset; warning signs; duration; time of day; pain severity, impact on activity, quality, and location; change in symptoms over time; treatment or medications used; and associated symptoms such as abdominal pain, nausea, vomiting, blurred vision, and photophobia. Laboratory tests are not useful for diagnosing the most common headaches. The child is assessed for neurologic signs such as altered consciousness, abnormal cranial nerves, papilledema, and motor or sensory deficits. Headache characteristics such as explosive headache with straining, steadily worsening headache awakening the child from sleep, and abnormal neurologic signs are indications for radiologic studies (CT scan, MRI, or magnetic resonance arteriography or venography). A lumbar puncture is performed if an infection (e.g., meningitis) or inflammatory process (e.g., Guillain-Barré syndrome) is suspected.

Clinical Therapy

Treatment includes relaxation techniques, analgesics, and anti-inflammatory medications. A behavior management program to reduce common headache triggers (inadequate sleep, stress, missed meals, caffeine, chocolate, excessive extracurricular activities) may be implemented (Kemper & Breuner, 2010). Medications to abort migraines (e.g., sumatriptan by mouth or nasal spray) are used in adolescents old enough to identify an aura, or signs of an impending headache. Children and adolescents with headaches that significantly interfere with school or social activities may have prophylactic medications prescribed (e.g., amitriptyline, valproic acid, topiramate, and gabapentin). More specific therapies are provided in the Clinical Manifestations table.

Nursing Management

Nursing management involves assessing the child for potential neurologic signs associated with headaches and assisting the child and family to identify strategies for relieving the headaches. Encourage

---

Complementary Therapy
Treating Headaches

Numerous behavioral cognitive therapies have been evaluated and found effective in reducing the frequency and severity of headaches in children, including biofeedback, guided imagery, relaxation, and hypnosis. Magnesium is often deficient in the adolescent's diet, and supplementation with magnesium L-lactate dehydrate may reduce the frequency of migraines in adolescents. Butterbur and feverfew are herbal preparations that have been found to reduce migraines in pediatric patients (Kemper & Breuner, 2010).

---

the child to keep a calendar or diary of headaches, including the events and stresses occurring at the time, foods eaten, and hours of sleep. Assist the child to see patterns of stress that appear in the headache diary, and discuss strategies that may help reduce that stress.

Encourage the family to implement behavior changes to reduce headache triggers, including the following: develop a consistent bedtime and wake-up time that includes weekends, eat on a regular schedule and avoid hunger, participate in regular physical activity for 30 to 45 minutes at least 5 days a week, limit or avoid identified food triggers, avoid smoke and other strong odors, and avoid excessive use of over-the-counter analgesics. See Complementary Therapy: Treating Headaches.

Make sure the child learns to take prescribed medications appropriately at the first sign of a migraine headache. An individualized health plan may be needed to ensure that the child gets access to medications rapidly when at school. Analgesic medications should not be taken in any combination for more than 2 to 3 days a week to reduce the risk for medication overuse chronic headaches.

STRUCTURAL DEFECTS
Microcephaly

Microcephaly is a small brain with a head circumference greater than 3 standard deviations below the mean for age and sex, or below the 3rd percentile on growth curves (Gaitanis & Mandelbaum, 2009). It may be caused by a genetic disorder or destructive insult during infancy, such as infection, metabolic disorder, or hypoxia-ischemia. Intellectual disability is common. See Chapter 34 for care of the child with intellectual disability.

Hydrocephalus

Hydrocephalus is the body's response to an imbalance between the production and absorption of cerebrospinal fluid, leading to an increase in the CSF volume and widening of the ventricles. The condition is often congenital or associated with other central nervous system malformations. Other causes may include an intraventricular hemorrhage in a preterm newborn, meningitis, traumatic brain injury, and tumors. The overall incidence is estimated to be 1 per 500 children (National Institute of Neurological Disorders and Stroke, 2008). It occurs in 90% of children with a lumbar **myelomeningocele** (meningomyelocele), a spinal fluid–filled meningeal sac that contains a portion of the spinal cord and nerves protruding through a vertebral defect (Gaitanis & Mandelbaum, 2009). See page 1178 for care of the child with myelomeningocele.

Etiology and Pathophysiology

CSF is produced by the choroid plexus within the lateral, third, and fourth ventricles at a consistent rate of 500 mL per day (Duffy, 2010).

Pathophysiology Illustrated   Hydrocephalus

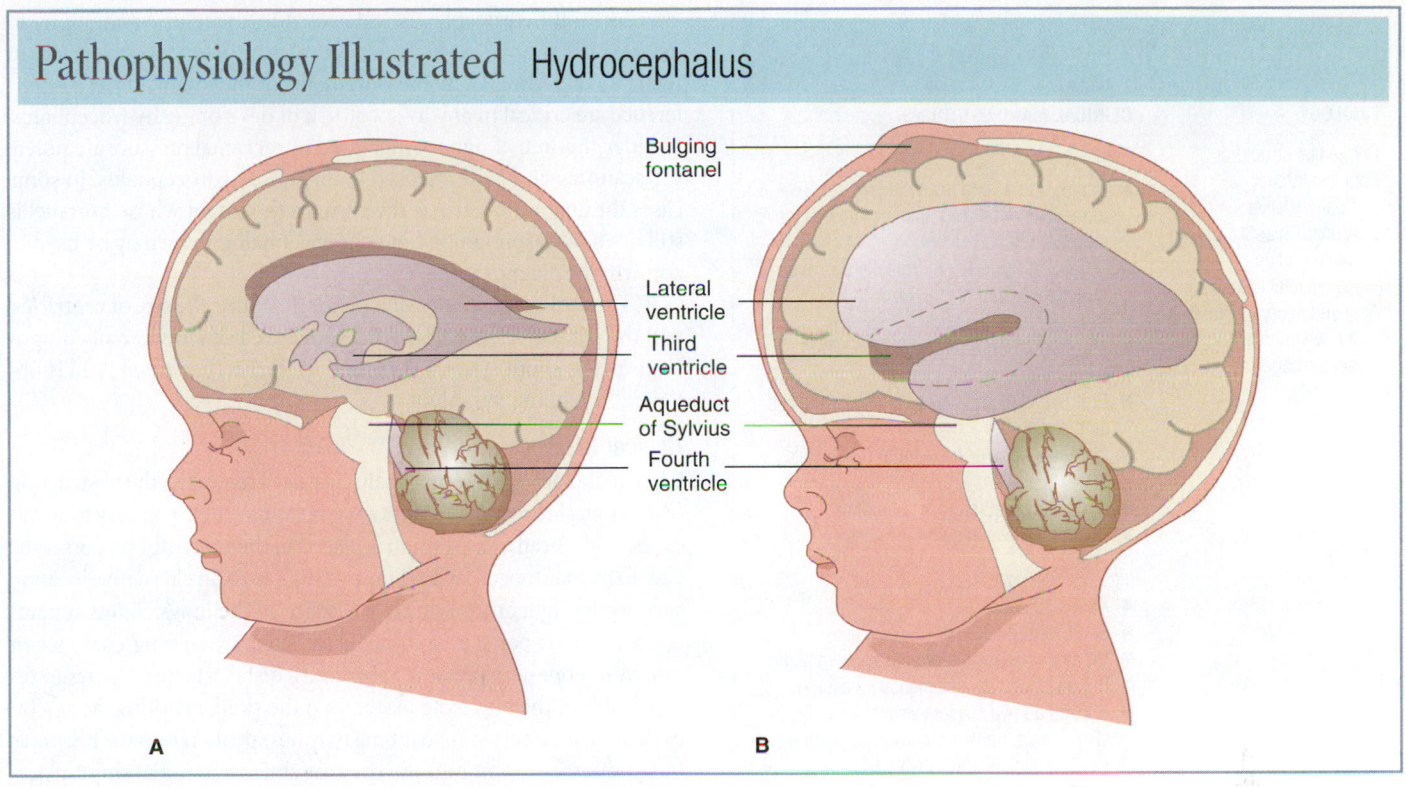

Bulging fontanel

Lateral ventricle

Third ventricle

Aqueduct of Sylvius

Fourth ventricle

A   B

FIGURE 33–10 ■ *A*, Normal size of ventricle. *B*, Enlarged ventricles, characteristic of hydrocephalus.

In usual circumstances, the same amount of CSF is absorbed by the subarachnoid space into the venous circulation. Cerebrospinal fluid must pass through a number of channels and pathways between the ventricles, around the brainstem and spinal cord, and to the surface of the brain until it reaches the subarachnoid space. When the amount of CSF absorbed is less than the amount produced, the ventricles enlarge. Hydrocephalus may be either communicating or noncommunicating, and congenital or acquired.

In communicating hydrocephalus the CSF flows freely between ventricles, normal channels, and pathways, but absorption of CSF in the subarachnoid space and the arachnoid villi is impaired. This form of hydrocephalus is often acquired from postinfectious meningitis, intraventricular hemorrhage in a preterm infant, or a congenital malformation of the subarachnoid spaces.

Noncommunicating hydrocephalus is responsible for the majority of cases in children. It results from a blockage in the ventricular system that prevents CSF from entering the subarachnoid space, resulting in enlargement of one or more ventricles (Figure 33–10 ■). This obstruction can be caused by infection, hemorrhage, tumor, surgery, or structural deformity. Congenital structural defects causing noncommunicating hydrocephalus include the Chiari II malformation (found in most children with myelomeningocele), aqueduct of Sylvius stenosis (a recessive X-linked cause of hydrocephalus), and the Dandy-Walker syndrome (includes hydrocephalus, a posterior fossa cyst, and hypoplasia of the cerebellum).

The Arnold-Chiari malformation (Chiari type II) occurs when myelomeningocele and hydrocephalus exist together along with an inferior placement of the medulla and lower cerebellum through the foramen magnum. Bony defects of the foramen magnum, occiput, and upper cervical vertebrae are seen. This defect has a mortality rate ranging from 21% to 60%, and significant morbidity also

occurs, including cognitive disability and epilepsy (Gaitanis & Mandelbaum, 2009).

Practice Alert

With the Chiari II malformation there is progressive hydrocephalus along with the myelomeningocele. Symptoms may begin during infancy and consist of stridor, a weak cry, and apnea. An older child may have an extremity weakness, difficulty swallowing, choking, hoarseness, vocal cord paralysis, and breath-holding episodes. Because the structures herniating through the foramen magnum control respiration and the protective reflexes, the child may also have apnea episodes, aspiration, and disordered breathing during sleep.

Clinical Manifestations

The signs and symptoms of hydrocephalus, which vary depending on the age of the child, are listed in the Clinical Manifestations table on page 1176. The predominant sign of the condition in infants is a rapidly increasing head circumference. Once the skull sutures have closed, children develop signs of increased intracranial pressure.

Signs of shunt malfunction are often related to increased intracranial pressure. In the child under age 1 year, signs are nonspecific and include irritability, vomiting, poor appetite, disordered sleep, and fever. Older children may have a headache, nausea, vomiting, and decreased level of consciousness.

Collaborative Care

The goal of collaborative care is to rapidly diagnose the hydrocephalus and perform surgery to reduce the consequences of excessive CSF on the child's developing cognitive and motor function.

Diagnostic Tests

The diagnosis of hydrocephalus may be made prenatally by ultrasound or based on clinical manifestations and neuroimaging studies

Clinical Manifestations Hydrocephalus

ETIOLOGY	CLINICAL MANIFESTATIONS

Congenital structural defect in infancy
  Dandy-Walker syndrome
  Arnold-Chiari II malformation
  Aqueductal stenosis
Acquired injury in infancy
  Intraventricular hemorrhage
	Early signs
	■ Rapidly increasing head circumference; tense, full, or bulging anterior fontanel; split sutures
	■ Bossing (protrusion) of frontal area, face disproportionate to skull size
	■ Difficulty holding head up
	■ Macewen or "cracked-pot" sign with percussion
	■ Prominent, distended scalp veins, translucent scalp skin
	■ Increased tone or hyperreflexia, Babinski sign
	■ Irritability or lethargy, poor feeding
	■ Decline in level of consciousness
	
	Late signs
	■ Apnea episodes
	■ Shrill, high-pitched cry
	■ Difficulty swallowing or feeding; vomiting
	■ Regression in developmental milestones
	■ Sunsetting eyes (sclera visible above iris), sixth cranial nerve palsy causing paralysis of upward gaze (Figure 33–11 ■)
	■ Cardiopulmonary depression (severe cases)

Acquired hydrocephalus in older child after closure of sutures
  Postinfectious
  Tumor
  Hemorrhage
	■ Signs of increased intracranial pressure
	■ Headache upon arising with nausea and vomiting
	■ Fussiness, sleepiness, confusion, apathy, or altered level of consciousness
	■ No head enlargement
	■ Irritability, lethargy, poor appetite
	■ Personality change, loss of interest in daily activities
	■ Poor judgment or verbal incoherence, worsening school performance, memory loss
	■ Ataxia, spasticity, or other alterations in motor development
	■ Visual problems due to pressure on the sixth cranial nerve (strabismus, double vision)

after birth. If hydrocephalus is detected in the fetus, sonography to detect other anomalies, such as a neural tube defect, is performed. In the hospital setting, daily measurements of the infant's head circumference are critical in any infant at risk of developing hydrocephalus. In older children, if signs of increased intracranial pressure are noted, CT scanning and MRI are used to diagnose hydrocephalus. In some cases the anatomic cause is revealed. In the infant whose fontanel is still open, ultrasonography or echoencephalography may be used to confirm the diagnosis.

CT scanning is used to evaluate shunt failure, the size of ventricles, and the parts of the shunt. Radiographs are used to view all components of the shunt system. A culture of the cerebrospinal fluid is obtained by tapping the shunt.

Clinical Therapy

Clinical therapy for hydrocephalus involves removing the obstruction (e.g., surgical removal of a tumor) or creating a new pathway to divert excess CSF. A catheter or shunt is placed in the ventricle and passes the CSF to the peritoneal cavity (Figure 33–12 ■) or an alternative location such as the right atrium or pleural space of the lungs. Shunt systems consist of four parts: a ventricular catheter, a pumping chamber or reservoir, a one-way pressure valve, and a distal catheter. The reservoir is palpable at the burr hole placed into the skull, providing access for evaluation of function. The tubing may be palpated from the burr hole to the insertion point into the chest or abdomen. Initial shunt placement is usually performed early in infancy. Tubing of adequate length

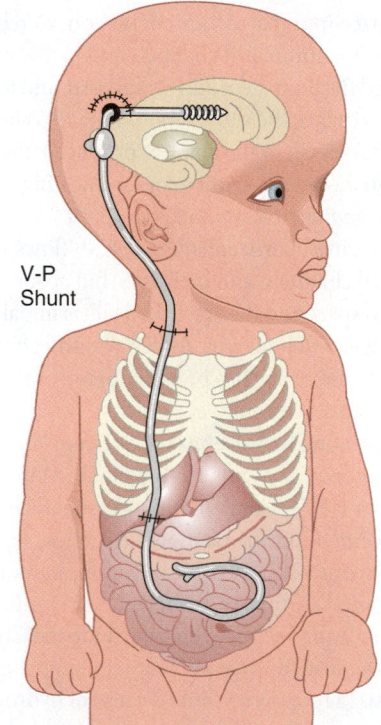

V-P Shunt

FIGURE 33–12 ■ A ventriculoperitoneal shunt, commonly used to treat children with hydrocephalus, is often placed at about 3 to 4 months of age; however, it may be placed at any age as needed to treat secondary hydrocephalus from conditions such as meningitis or tumors. The shunt system consists of four parts: a ventricular catheter, a pumping chamber or reservoir, a one-way pressure valve, and a distal catheter. The tubing drains the excess cerebrospinal fluid from the ventricles to the abdomen. The main goal of treatment is to reduce the intracranial pressure and to preserve central nervous system function.

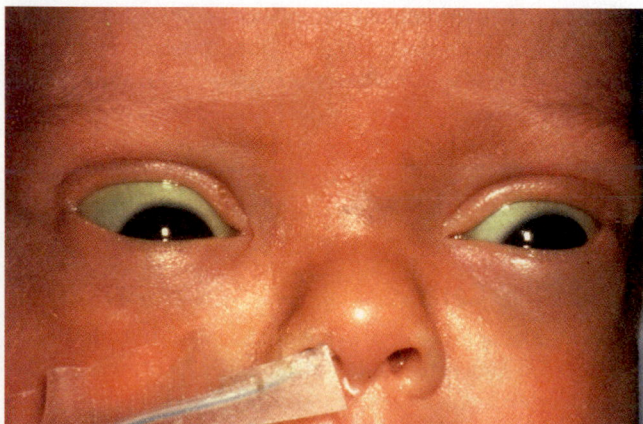

FIGURE 33–11 ■ Sunsetting eyes or sunsetting sign. Notice the sinking of the iris below the lower eyelid and the white above the iris caused by paresis of cranial nerve VI.

Source: Copyright 2012 NMSB—Custom Medical Stock Photo, All Rights Reserved.

is inserted to accommodate the child's growth and reduce the need for future surgery. CSF drainage is regulated by the one-way valve. Children often need shunt revisions four times before 10 years of age (Jea & Kulkarni, 2009). Children with ventriculoatrial shunts may receive perioperative intravenous antibiotics to reduce the risk for reinfection.

Practice Alert

Technology advances have resulted in programmable shunts that enable adjustment of pressure, resulting in a reduction in the number of shunt revisions. These shunts are sensitive to magnets, so they must be checked and reprogrammed to the correct pressure level after an MRI diagnostic procedure (Duffy, 2010).

Mechanical complications may include blockage at either the proximal or the distal end of the catheter, kinking of the tubing, or valve breakdown. Infants or children with shunt failure show signs and symptoms of recurrent hydrocephalus and increased intracranial pressure. Shunt materials and systems continue to be refined in an attempt to reduce mechanical problems.

The most serious complication is shunt infection, which may occur at any time, but most often occurs within 6 months after placement in approximately 8% of cases (Jea & Kulkarni, 2009). The infection may present as meningitis, peritonitis, shunt obstruction, wound infection, or some combination. The infection may be confirmed by culture of the CSF obtained from the shunt reservoir. The shunt is surgically removed and an external ventricular drainage device is placed. Intravenous antibiotics are prescribed until the CSF is sterile, after which a new shunt is inserted.

An alternative to the placement of a CSF shunt is an endoscopic third ventriculostomy in children who have a mechanical obstruction, such as aqueductal stenosis. A small hole is placed in the floor of the third ventricle which allows CSF to drain directly into the subarachnoid space and bypass the obstruction. The surgery can cause complications by disturbing hypothalamic function and causing endocrine deficiency (e.g., diabetes insipidus). Lifelong follow-up is required because late failure can occur (Jea & Kulkarni, 2009).

Children with the Arnold-Chiari malformation may have an upper cervical laminectomy performed within the first few weeks of life to prevent an emergency. Alternative treatment includes symptomatic care while maintaining the airway and preventing aspiration. Rapid surgical decompression may be needed to reduce brainstem compression and to prevent death.

Children often have cognitive impairment with poor math skills and problems with reading comprehension and inference skills (Jea & Kulkarni, 2009). Children may also have lower fine motor skills than healthy children.

Nursing Management

The goals of nursing management are to monitor infants for signs of unexpected increases in head circumference and increased intracranial pressure and to provide nursing care during the recuperation from surgery and community follow-up.

Nursing Assessment and Diagnosis

It is important for nurses to become familiar with the clinical manifestations of hydrocephalus to ensure prompt identification and treatment of children with this condition. Measure the head circumference of all infants at each well-child visit and plot on a growth curve to detect the condition at an early stage (refer to the Skills Manual 🔗).

Following surgery to place a shunt, the child's vital signs and levels of responsiveness and irritability are assessed frequently to monitor signs and symptoms of shunt failure and infection. Measure the infant's head circumference daily when shunt failure is suspected. Report any abnormalities to the physician immediately. Surgical sites are evaluated for signs of drainage and infection as well as redness and swelling of the shunt tract. Carefully assess respiratory status. Assess intake and output in the immediate postoperative period. Assess pain in the postoperative period.

Practice Alert

In infants under age 1 year, important signs and symptoms of shunt failure include unusual irritability, bulging fontanel, separation of sutures, increasing head circumference, vomiting, diminished appetite, sleep pattern disturbance, and fever. In older children, observe for signs of increased intracranial pressure, such as a headache, nausea and vomiting, and decreased level of consciousness. The symptoms may be subtle, and symptom-free periods may occur (Lee & DiPatri, 2008).

Nursing diagnoses that may be appropriate for the child with hydrocephalus include the following:

- Infection, Risk for related to surgical procedure
- Mobility: Physical, Impaired (Level 2), related to decreased neck muscle mass from lifting the increased weight of head
- Caregiver Role Strain, Risk for, related to care of a child with a chronic condition or life-threatening illness
- Growth and Development, Delayed, related to repeated shunt infections and hospitalizations
- Injury, Risk for, related to potential shunt failure

NANDA-I © 2012

Planning and Implementation

Nursing care in the hospital setting focuses on providing postoperative care and providing emotional support.

Provide Preoperative Care

Position the child carefully; do not stretch or strain neck muscles, since they must support a large head. Holding the child may be difficult because of the additional weight of the head. Provide good skin care. Reduce the chances for skin breakdown by placing sheepskin or a lamb's wool blanket under the head. Prevent any other complications associated with immobility (see Box 33–2). Attend to the child's special nutritional needs. Because the infant is prone to vomiting, frequent small feedings with frequent burping are beneficial.

Provide Postoperative Care

After surgery, the child is usually placed in a flat position to prevent rapid CSF drainage. The head of the bed is elevated gradually over a day or two. Take vital signs every 2 to 4 hours. Maintain aseptic technique when performing incision care. Monitor the child carefully for any signs of shunt malfunction, increased intracranial pressure, or infection.

Provide Emotional Support

Provide parents with explanations about the child's condition and all procedures to be performed. Encourage parents and family to help with the child's care in the hospital when appropriate. Be sympathetic and understanding, and allow parents to express their concerns. If hydrocephalus occurs during early infancy, the parents will be anxious about the impact of the chronic condition and subsequent surgical procedures. If hydrocephalus is secondary to neoplasm, however, the parents' anxieties are compounded by their child's life-threatening illness.

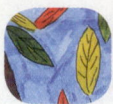

Partnering with Families

Signs of Shunt Malfunction or Infection

Parents should seek immediate medical attention if the infant or child experiences any of the following signs of shunt malfunction or infection:
- Headache, progressive or worsening
- Drowsiness, irritability, or inappropriate sleepiness during the day

- Nausea or vomiting
- Personality changes or changes in school performance
- Fever
- Redness or swelling along the shunt tract

Assure parents that most children with shunts attend school and interact with family members and peers as other children do.

Discharge Planning and Home Care Teaching

Address home care needs well in advance of discharge. Parents must learn how to care for the surgical site until healed. Educate parents and other family members about important signs and symptoms of both shunt failure and infection. See Partnering with Families: Signs of Shunt Malfunction or Infection. Provide telephone numbers of the pediatrician and the neurosurgeon, and instruct parents to contact a physician immediately if the child develops seizures (or a change in the characteristics of seizures in a child with a seizure disorder) or if a problem with the shunt is suspected. Refer families to the appropriate home care, social services, and support groups such as the Hydrocephalus Association.

Care in the Community

Infants and children need frequent monitoring to ensure proper functioning of the shunt. Head circumference is measured at each visit and compared to expected growth curves to monitor growth. Assess the child for visual problems and cognitive, speech, and motor developmental delays that are often associated problems. The child and family should be referred to an early intervention program to promote developmental progress. School-age children may need to have an individualized education plan developed (see Chapter 16 🔗).

Clinical Tip
After the shunt placement, the head circumference may decrease by 1 to 2 cm as the pressure is relieved. Head growth due to brain development may then be noted in 2 to 4 months. If head growth resumes sooner than that, shunt failure may be present (Duffy, 2010).

Teach parents to protect the infant from injury by using a rear-facing car safety seat. These infants have poor head control due to an enlarged head, and the forward-facing position increases the risk of cervical spine injury and death in a car crash. Support the child's head and body position with towel rolls to maintain proper positioning in the seat. For older children, participation in contact sports with high potential for head and abdominal impact should be discouraged; however, sports like tennis and swimming should be encouraged. A helmet should be worn for skiing, skateboarding, and bicycle riding.

Parents should be encouraged to promote optimal health status by promoting good nutrition and reducing exposure to infections. Teach parents alternate positions for burping infants with an enlarged head and to use an infant seat for positioning after feeding to reduce regurgitation. Constipation that increases abdominal pressure may interfere with drainage of CSF through the ventriculoperitoneal shunt.

Teach parents to provide foods with fiber to promote regular bowel movements.

Parents seeking childcare for the child under age 2 years should be encouraged to use a setting with fewer children, such as family or home-based childcare, to decrease exposure to infection. Encourage the use of good hand hygiene by all caregivers to reduce the spread of infections.

Evaluation

Expected outcomes of nursing care for the child include the following:
- The child develops adequate neck-muscle control to interact with the environment.
- The parents identify signs of shunt infections and malfunctions and promptly seek medical attention.
- The child's growth and development is maximized with care and a stimulating environment.

Neural Tube Defects

The neural tube is the tissue that ultimately develops into the central nervous system, including the brain and spinal cord. Neural tube defects occur in about 3,000 pregnancies each year in the United States (Boss & Huether, 2010). See Box 33–8 for types of neural tube defects.

Myelodysplasia or Spina Bifida

Myelodysplasia (sometimes called myelomeningocele) refers to a malformation of the spinal cord and spinal canal. **Spina bifida** refers to a defect in one or more vertebrae through which spinal cord contents can protrude. It is often associated with a protrusion of a meningeal sac filled with a portion of the spinal cord. The malformation can occur anywhere along the vertebral column, but is most common at the lumbar or sacral portion of the spine. This is the most common developmental disorder of the central nervous system.

BOX 33–8	Types of Neural Tube Defects

Anencephaly—no development of the brain above the brainstem

Encephalocele—protrusion of meningeal tissue or meningeal-covered brain through a defect in the skull

Spina bifida occulta—a vertebral defect in which the posterior vertebral arches fail to fuse (usually the fifth lumbar or first sacral vertebrae)

Meningocele—protrusion of a meningeal sac filled with CSF through a vertebral defect, associated with no abnormalities of the spinal cord

Meningomyelocele—protrusion of a meningeal sac that contains CSF, a portion of the spinal cord, and nerves through a vertebral defect

Each year, approximately 1,500 infants are born with spina bifida. Hispanic women (4.17 per 10,000) are at greater risk having of a newborn with a neural tube defect than non-Hispanic White women (3.22 per 10,000) or non-Hispanic Black women (2.64 per 10,000) (Centers for Disease Control and Prevention, 2011). The infant mortality rate associated with spina bifida is 10% (Adzick, Thom, Spong, et al., 2011).

Etiology and pathophysiology The cause of spina bifida is unknown, although environmental factors such as chemicals (excessive use of alcohol), medications (e.g., valproic acid and carbamazepine used for seizures and isotretinoin for acne), genetic factors, and maternal health conditions (diabetes mellitus, gestational diabetes, folic acid deficiency, and maternal obesity) have been implicated. The increased incidence within families indicates a possible genetic influence.

Clinical Tip

Mandatory fortification of all enriched grain products with folate was initiated in 1998, leading to a decrease in the number of infants born with myelodysplasia. Prior to folic acid food supplementation in 1996, the prevalence of spina bifida was 5.04 per 10,000 children, decreasing 31% to 3.04 per 10,000 children in 2006 (Centers for Disease Control and Prevention, 2011).

Several other problems develop in children with spinal bifida. Bowel and bladder control is affected in children with defects in the thoracic and lumbar regions. Renal damage may result from neurologic impairment and urinary retention. Hydrocephalus is present in 85% of children with spina bifida. Seizures and visual-perceptual problems may also occur. The Arnold-Chiari II malformation commonly occurs with spina bifida. See page 1175. Tethering of the spinal cord to scar tissue in the spinal canal may prevent the spinal cord from its normal ascent between birth and puberty, often leading to clinical signs between 6 and 12 years of age (Sandler, 2010).

Clinical manifestations There are several different types of spina bifida (Figure 33–13 ■). A saclike protrusion on the infant's back indicates meningocele or myelomeningocele. The clinical manifestations seen depend on the location of the defect: the higher the defect, the greater the neuromotor dysfunction as described here:

- **Thoracic**—paralysis of the legs, weakness and sensory loss in the trunk and lower body region; may eventually stand upright with hip, knee, and ankle braces; bowel and bladder incontinence
- **Lumbar 1–2 level**—have some hip flexion and adduction, cannot extend knees; may eventually stand upright with hip, knee, and ankle braces; bowel and bladder incontinence
- **Lumbar 3**—can flex hips and extend knees; paralysis of the ankles and toes; need knee and ankle braces and forearm crutches to mobilize; bowel and bladder incontinence

Pathophysiology Illustrated
Types of Spina Bifida

Spina bifida occulta	Failure of posterior vertebral arches to fuse, most commonly at fifth lumbar or first sacral vertebrae; spinal cord and meninges entirely within vertebral canal; condition usually not visible externally; tuft of hair, a dermoid cyst, or hemangioma may be found over the site; mildest form.
Spina bifida cystica	Defect in closure of posterior vertebral arch with protrusion through bony spine, including meningocele and myelomeningocele lesions.
Meningocele	Saclike protrusion through bony defect containing meninges and cerebrospinal fluid; sac covering defect may be translucent or membranous; spinal cord and spinal root in normal position.
Myelomeningocele	Saclike herniation through bony defect holding meninges, cerebrospinal fluid, and a portion of spinal cord or nerve roots; fluid leakage may also occur; lesion poorly covered with imperfect tissue; mobility impairment 99% of time; more common than meningocele.

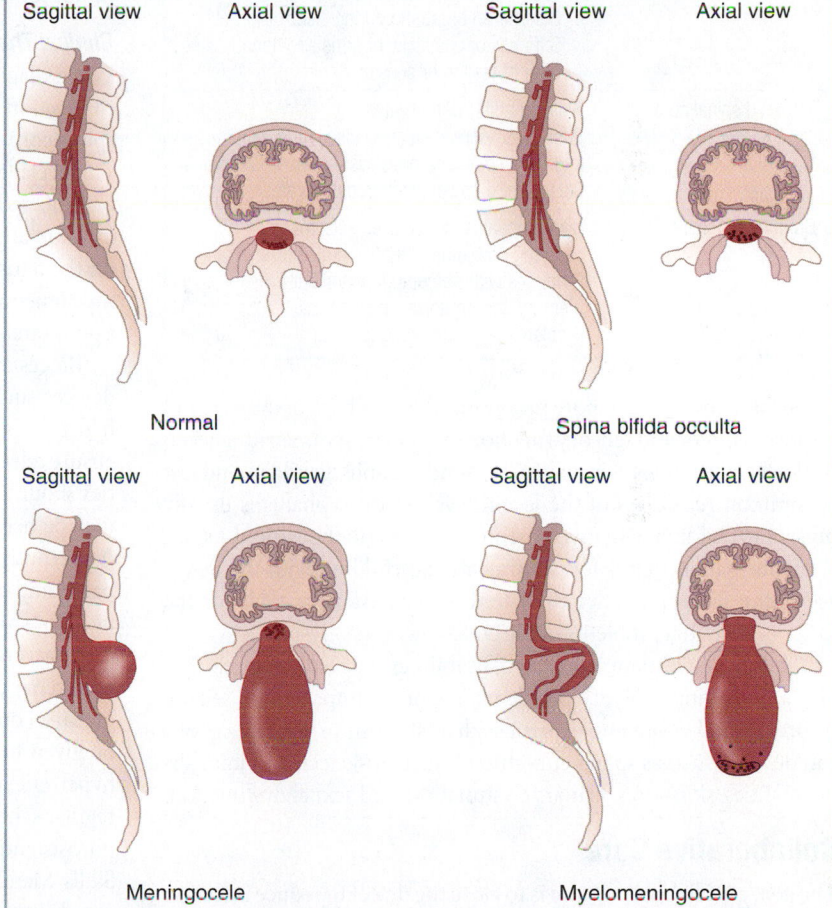

FIGURE 33–13 ■ Note the different conditions that result from a vertebral bony defect.

- **Lumbar 4–5 level**—can flex hips and extend knees; weak or absent ankle extension, toe flexion, and hip extension; bowel and bladder incontinence
- **Sacral level**—mild weakness in ankles and toes; walk by 2 to 3 years, may need ankle braces; bladder and bowel function may be affected

Clinical Manifestations Myelodysplasia

CAUSE	CLINICAL MANIFESTATIONS
Interruption of the spinal cord at site of the spinal defect	Loss of motor and sensory function of the abdomen and lower extremities, dependent on defect level Scoliosis or kyphosis Incontinence of urine or urinary retention Incontinence of feces or constipation Sensory loss around genitalia
Muscle imbalance	Hip abnormalities, hip dysplasia Foot deformities, e.g., clubfoot

Chiari II malformation	Hydrocephalus
	Infants:
	    Difficulty swallowing
	    Apnea, respiratory difficulty, inspiratory stridor
	    Weak or poor cry
	    Sustained backward arching of the head (opisthotonos)
	Older children:
	    Choking, hoarseness, vocal cord paralysis
	    Disordered breathing during sleep
	    Stiffness or spasticity of arms and hands
	    Loss of feeling or sensation

Tethered spinal cord	Walking ability deteriorates Back pain, increasing scoliosis Leg pain, spasticity, progressive foot deformity Bladder and bowel function deteriorates
Brain Abnormalities	Hydrocephalus, generalized seizures Learning problems, attention deficit disorder Problems with perceptual motor skills Memory and organization problems Problems with numeric reasoning

Sensory loss is often more pronounced on the back of the legs, and the loss of motor and sensory function may not be symmetric between the lower extremities. Sensory loss around the anus, genitalia, and feet is common regardless of the lesion level. Hydrocephalus is usually present in children with myelomeningocele due to the Arnold-Chiari II malformation that is found in nearly all children with the defect above the sacral level. See the Clinical Manifestations table for the range of potential problems in the child with myelodysplasia.

Children have many associated disabilities as a result of myelodysplasia, including mobility problems, cognitive impairment, seizure disorders, and visual impairment such as strabismus. Complications can develop such as spinal curvatures, musculoskeletal and joint abnormalities, skin sores, urinary dysfunction, and sexual dysfunction.

Collaborative Care

The goal of collaborative care is to close the defect to reduce infection and evaluate the neurologic complications resulting from the defect. Clinical therapy is then focused on managing the complications of the disorder while promoting the child's growth and development.

Diagnostic Tests

Diagnosis is often made prenatally by an elevated maternal serum alpha-fetoprotein level, which increases suspicion that the newborn will have a neural tube defect, followed by a high-resolution fetal ultrasound. After birth a multidisciplinary team examines the lesion and evaluates neurologic status. Radiographic imaging by ultrasonography, CT scan, MRI, and flat films of the spinal column can

---

BOX 33–9   Research: Fetal Surgery for Myelomeningocele

A randomized controlled trial investigated two outcomes of fetal surgery to correct myelomeningocele. Infants were evaluated at 12 months of age to identify the number that needed a shunt for hydrocephalus, and infants were evaluated again at 30 months to assess motor and functional development. The research was stopped early because of findings that revealed a significant reduction in shunt placement for infants with fetal surgery (40%) compared to postnatal surgery (82%). Infants with fetal surgery also had an improved composite score for mental development and motor function at 30 months of age. Fetal surgery was associated with a higher risk for preterm delivery and uterine dehiscence at the time of delivery (Adzick et al., 2011). Neurodevelopmental evaluation of 30 children at 5 years of age who had fetal repair of myelomeningocele revealed that mean verbal and performance intelligence quotient (IQ) scores fell within the normal population range. Mean full IQ scores were higher in children who did not have a shunt placed (Danzer, Gerdes, Bebbington, et al., 2010).

---

pinpoint the bony defect and nerve involvement. Subsequent testing is performed to evaluate bladder and bowel function, neurologic and motor function, and cognitive function.

Clinical Therapy

When diagnosed prenatally, the newborn is often delivered by cesarean section to minimize trauma to the spinal lesion or traction on the spinal cord. Surgery to close and repair the meningocele or myelomeningocele lesion usually occurs within 24 to 48 hours of the infant's birth to reduce infection. Depending on the size of the defect, the excision area may be extensive. In some cases, a repair is performed on the fetus in utero. See Box 33–9 for research on fetal surgery for myelomeningocele. In cases of spina bifida occulta, surgical intervention is rarely needed.

Braces are used to support joint position and mobility. Assistive devices such as walkers, crutches, and wheelchairs are used to enhance mobility. To minimize the risk for osteoporosis, the diet should ensure adequate calcium and vitamin D, and weight-bearing activities should be encouraged. Surgery to release a tethered spinal cord may be needed to relieve pain and reduce neurologic deterioration. An orthotic jacket may correct spinal deformities that affect lung capacity and interfere with mobility and sitting, potentially delaying the need for spinal fusion or stabilization with rods.

Interventions for a neurogenic bladder are initiated early to prevent renal damage, to maintain bladder function, and to promote urinary continence. Anticholinergic medication (oxybutynin) may be given to lower urinary storage pressures and manage sphincter hyperreflexia. Clean intermittent catheterization is performed on a regular schedule (every 3 to 4 hours) to reduce the risk for hydronephrosis and renal damage, as well as promote continence. (See the Skills Manual ⊂▭.) Clean intermittent catheterization does not greatly increase the risk for febrile urinary tract infections when compared to sterile urinary catheterization (Mourtzinos & Stoffel, 2010). Various surgical strategies may be used to promote urinary continence, such as a Mitrofanoff procedure that creates a reservoir for urine and a stoma for catheterization, an artificial urinary sphincter, or bladder neck reconstruction (Figure 33–14 ■). Botulinum toxin type A injection into the external bladder sphincter may improve continence, but more research is needed to determine best practices (Mourtzinos & Stoffel, 2010).

Dietary fiber supplements, stool softeners, and glycerin or bisacodyl suppositories are often prescribed for bowel evacuation and to

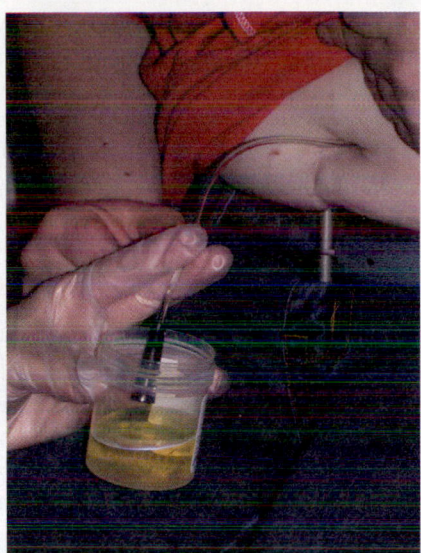

FIGURE 33–14 ■ This child has had a Mitrofanoff procedure to make it easier to perform self-catheterization and maintain modesty. Clean intermittent self-catheterization is performed, and the catheters can be reused until they become brittle. Catheters should be washed with soap and water, rinsed, and stored in a plastic bag.

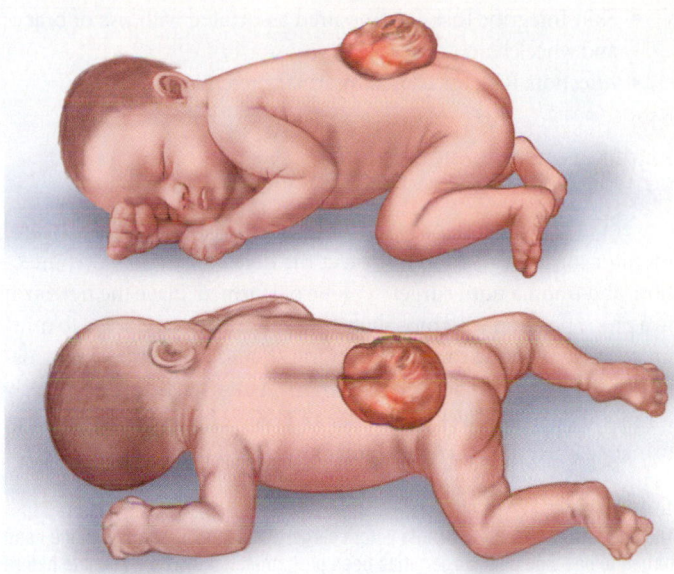

FIGURE 33–15 ■ Lumbosacral myelomeningocele is caused by a neural tube defect that results in incomplete closure of the vertebral column. As shown here, the meninges (and sometimes the spinal cord) protrude as a saclike structure. Observe for leakage of cerebrospinal fluid.

promote bowel continence. Surgery to create a channel between the skin and bowel using the appendix (Malone antegrade continence enema) is often performed in children with fecal incontinence or severe constipation. This procedure enables a child or adolescent to have delivery of an enema to the ascending and transverse colon to promote bowel evacuation (Sandler, 2010).

Prognosis depends on the type of defect, the level of the lesion, and the presence of other complicating factors, such as renal damage. Children need multiple surgeries and invasive procedures. A team of physicians, nurses, and therapists from the neurosurgery, orthopedic, urology, and physical medicine departments will work with the child and family to form a comprehensive care plan. Pediatric referral centers often establish a clinic for children with myelodysplasia in which services by all disciplines are coordinated in a single visit. Parents and their children often need to travel to these centers to obtain needed care. With the improved care of these children, the majority survive into adulthood. Transition to adult healthcare services is essential to ensure that the individual continues to receive urology and other specialized services.

Nursing Management

Nursing care of the infant or child in the hospital focuses on assessing the child for infection, signs of hydrocephalus, and wound healing, as well as providing preoperative and postoperative care, promoting mobility, and providing emotional support.

Nursing Assessment and Diagnosis

Newborn

The newborn should be monitored for integrity of the sac and leakage of CSF (Figure 33–15 ■). Assess the extremities for deformities. Frequently assess the vital signs and stay alert for signs of infection. Following surgery, observe the wound healing. Note any signs of infection and CSF leakage. Measure the head circumference daily after surgery to assess for potential hydrocephalus. Assess intake and output.

Child

During healthcare visits, assess the child's vital signs, growth, and head circumference. Assess neurologic status for any deterioration in function that could be associated with shunt failure or a tethered spinal cord. Assess the range of motion of joints, mobility status, and urinary function.

The child with spina bifida may be hospitalized for surgery to correct deformities or for other health conditions. After surgery, assess the child's vital signs, responsiveness, and level of pain. As the child may have decreased pain sensation in the lower extremities, careful assessment is needed. Assess dressing sites for bleeding and draining. Monitor the distal extremities for swelling and circulation. Assess intake and output.

Practice Alert

It is estimated that 73% of children and adolescents with spina bifida have sensitivity to latex, based on an allergic reaction or blood test (Spina Bifida Association, 2011). See Chapter 27 🔗. Anaphylaxis caused by latex exposure in children has been reported. All children with latex allergy need to carry a kit with premeasured epinephrine for emergency treatment of anaphylaxis. Non-latex materials should be used when providing care to the child in the hospital, in the outpatient setting, or at home. The Spina Bifida Association maintains an updated list of products containing latex and potential substitutes (see Table 27–12 🔗).

Examples of nursing diagnoses for the child with myelodysplasia include:

- Mobility: Physical, Impaired related to neuromuscular impairment
- Urinary Incontinence, Overflow related to hyperactive sphincter
- Allergy Response, Latex, Risk for related to multiple surgical procedures
- Growth: Disproportionate, Risk for related to excessive caloric intake and limited mobility

- Skin Integrity, Risk for Impaired associated with use of braces and wheelchair
- Infection, Risk for related to urinary retention

NANDA-I © 2012

Planning and Implementation

Newborn

Cover the sac with a sterile saline dressing to protect its integrity, and monitor for leakage of CSF. Protect the defect from pressure, infection, and trauma until surgery can be performed. Place the newborn in a prone position with hips slightly flexed and legs abducted to minimize tension on the sac. This position should be maintained by using towel rolls placed between the knees. Assess the neonate regularly for motor deficits as well as bladder and bowel involvement. Perform urinary catheterization on a regular schedule if needed.

Clinical Tip

The newborn is difficult to handle before surgery. Feed the newborn with the head turned to one side until surgery has been performed. Comfort the neonate before surgery with tactile stimulation such as touching, patting, and cuddling.

Monitor the infant's vital signs and assess for pain during the postoperative period. Watch closely for symptoms of infection, especially meningitis, and increasing head circumference. Inspect the surgical site for CSF leakage. The infant should be placed in the prone or side-lying position for sleep until healing has occurred (despite guidelines to put infants to sleep on their backs), and then a supine position for sleep may be used. Keep stool and the diaper away from the incision site which may be difficult if the repair is in the lower lumbar or sacral area.

Promote Mobility

Begin gentle range of motion exercises as soon as possible to prevent muscle contractures and atrophy. Extreme caution should be used because these children have brittle bones and are subject to idiopathic fractures. Splints may be used to maintain extremity alignment.

Provide Emotional Support

Keep the parents informed about their infant's status. Allow them to express their frustrations and anger. As soon as parents are able to cope with the infant's condition, encourage them to become involved in the infant's care in the hospital.

Discharge Planning and Home Care Teaching

Home care needs should be identified and addressed well in advance of discharge. Make sure family members understand how to care for the infant or child at home. Help them obtain special devices such as splints, wedges, and rolls, if indicated, to prevent complications. Instruct parents how to position, handle, and feed the infant, and to perform range of motion exercises. Parents need to learn to perform intermittent catheterization prior to discharge and establish a schedule to perform catheterization every 3 to 4 hours.

Teach parents the signs and symptoms of increased intracranial pressure, hydrocephalus, shunt infection or malfunction, and urinary tract infection. Home care nursing may be needed for the initial transition to reinforce skills learned in the hospital setting. A case manager should be identified to coordinate the numerous healthcare professionals who will be working with the child and family. Refer parents to resource groups such as the Spina Bifida Association of America.

Care in the Community

To reduce complications and promote optimal development, children with spina bifida require comprehensive care that is planned and coordinated by a knowledgeable team of healthcare professionals at a pediatric referral center. This care may be provided in partnership with the primary care physician. Parents are faced with the long-term financial issues of caring for the child who needs regular new adaptive equipment to match growth, as well as other medical supplies. The nurse has an important role in ensuring that families with limited financial resources are linked with social services for assistance with transportation, housing, and other care needs. See the Photo Story.

Parents need to learn how to catheterize the child and then at an appropriate age teach the child intermittent self-catheterization to prevent urinary tract infections and other renal complications (see Chapter 31 🔗). If urinary incontinence occurs after having urinary control, this should be reported to the physician. When the child begins school, an individualized health plan should be developed to ensure that the child has access to the restroom and assistance as needed for toileting, as well as accommodations for mobility challenges.

Clinical Tip

The child who has clean intermittent catheterization performed usually has bacteria in the urine, but this is not treated unless the child becomes symptomatic. Symptoms indicating a urinary tract infection that should be treated include fever, dysuria, or new-onset incontinence.

Good nutrition planning is important to prevent obesity and to reduce constipation and complications such as fecal impaction. Bowel training is initiated to control bowel evacuation at appropriate times and places. A diet high in fiber and fiber supplementation helps ensure adequate stool. At a convenient time, either morning or night, a glycerin or bisacodyl suppository can be given. The child should have a bowel movement at least every 1 to 2 days to avoid impaction. Consistency in time of day for bowel evacuation is important to promote continence. Children must learn to assume greater responsibility for self-care as they get older. See Box 33–10 for research on challenges with bowel management.

Promote safety and independent mobility with proper use of braces, walkers, crutches, canes, and in some cases custom-designed wheelchairs and car safety seats (Figure 33–16 ■). Promote good skin care to reduce the risk for skin injury. Encourage daily inspection of all skin areas under braces and splints. For other safety guidelines see Partnering with Families: Safety for the Child with Myelodysplasia and Chapter 36 🔗.

Treat older children according to their intellectual level, not their motor development. Encourage them to take responsibility for self-care, and recognize their need to control their body functions. Promote interaction with peers in the hospital and participation in community activities.

> **BOX 33–10   Research: Bowel Management Challenges**
>
> A qualitative descriptive study involving seven parents of children with spina bifida focused on bowel management. Parents described their frustration with finding a bowel management program that was effective for their child to prevent embarrassment when accidents occurred. They were concerned with the child's self-image because of incontinence, malodor, and fecal soiling. Additionally, parents felt that healthcare providers did not view bowel management with the same priority that parents did (Sawin & Thompson, 2009).

Spina Bifida Association of America

Weblink

PHOTO STORY...

MANAGING MYELODYSPLASIA

Daily exercise using crutches is important for Sam to maintain the strength to continue bearing weight and walking independently.

Sam is a 7-year-old child with myelodysplasia. Sam and his parents are seen every few months in the multidisciplinary spina bifida clinic located in the university medical center about 100 miles from his home. The health professionals in this clinic help the family coordinate care for Sam with his local pediatrician and physical therapy center. An important part of the health visit is to measure his height and weight and to determine that growth is occurring as expected. In particular, it is important to monitor for signs of excessive weight gain as this would potentially reduce his mobility.

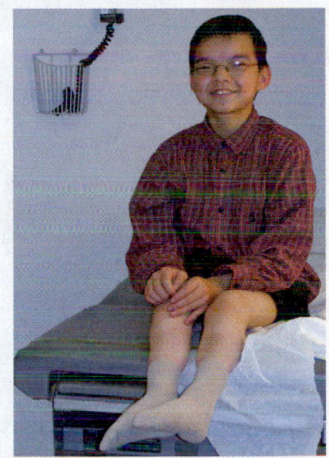

Sam has been placed on the examining table so his lower extremities can be evaluated. Next his socks will be removed so his feet can be inspected.

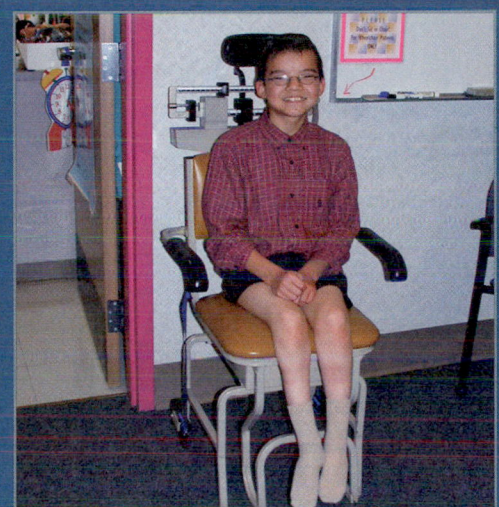

A scale with a chair attached is often used to measure the weight of children with an inability to stand without support.

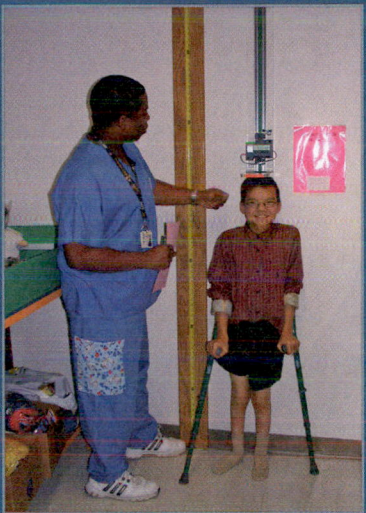

Assessing height is also important to contrast with weight and to calculate a body mass index. In this case Sam is using crutches to stand erect.

Sam's lesion is at the L4 to L5 level, so he can flex his hips and extend his knees, but he has weak ankle extension, toe flexion, and hip extension. He has minimal sensation in his lower legs and feet. His bladder and bowel sphincters are also affected. Sam and his parents have worked hard to establish bowel control with a high-fiber diet and to establish a specific time of day for bowel evacuation. Sam has learned to perform intermittent self-catheterization for bladder control to reduce the risk for kidney damage.

During the health visit, Sam's general health is reviewed, along with changes in muscle tone, joint range of motion, and any signs of damage to

his skin. As this visit is completed, his socks will be removed to check for signs of redness or lesions on his feet and lower extremities, especially where braces may rub.

The health professionals at the spina bifida clinic are encouraging Sam to be as mobile as possible. Daily exercise using crutches is important for him to maintain the strength to continue bearing weight and walking independently. This enables Sam to interact with his environment and other children in school. As the visit is finishing, Sam's mobility is evaluated by watching him walk down the hall with his crutches.

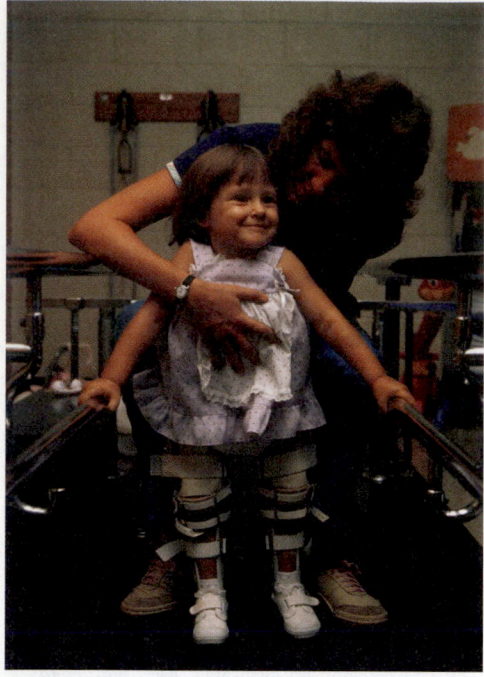
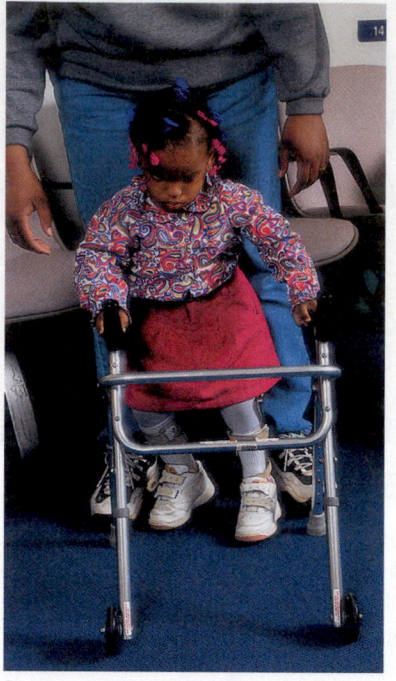
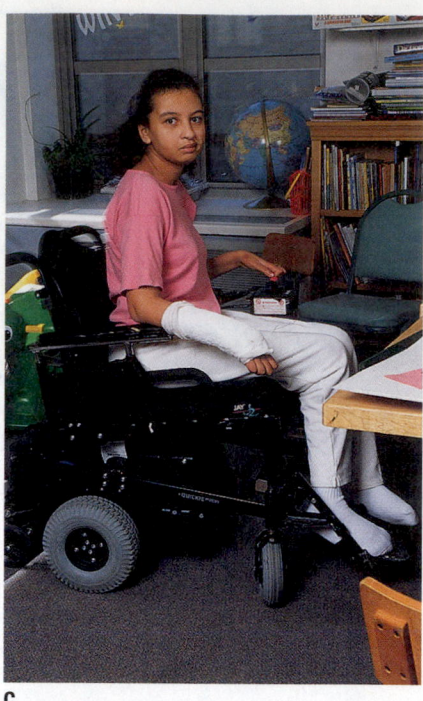

A   B   C

FIGURE 33–16 ■ Help determine the best assistive device for the child to gain the most independence for mobilizing and to promote development. The child may change devices in different settings to promote optimal independence. *A* and *B,* Braces and walkers may be best for young children to promote an upright posture that encourages a normal interaction with the environment. *C,* A motorized wheelchair can assist the child with a significant neurologic impairment to achieve independence and mobility.

Source: *A, Copyright 2012. K. Glaser & Associates—Custom Medical Stock Photo, All Rights Reserved.*

Educational services must be coordinated. An individualized education plan needs to be developed that addresses learning needs and mobility. Adaptive equipment may be needed in the school setting. Planning for vocational and transition services is important for the adolescent. Monitor the adolescent for depression and need for counseling services, particularly at the time when differences and challenges in lifestyle become of more concern.

Evaluation

Expected outcomes of nursing care for the child and family include the following:

- The child maintains weight bearing and mobility as much as possible using a walker and crutches.
- The family promptly identifies signs of neurologic impairment and immediately seeks care.

- Pressure ulcers are prevented through daily skin inspection and skin care.
- The child gains urinary continence and minimizes the risk for kidney damage.
- The child is integrated into peer groups and social activities resulting in the development of self-esteem.

Craniosynostosis

Craniosynostosis is the premature closing of the cranial sutures in utero or during the first 18 to 20 months of life. This condition occurs in up to 1 in 1,800 to 2,200 live births, and boys are affected twice as often as girls. Craniosynostosis not associated with a syndrome may affect one or more sutures, and the cause is often unknown. Syndromes of chromosome abnormalities and autosomal dominant

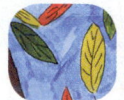

Partnering with Families

Safety for the Child with Myelodysplasia

Due to the loss of sensation in the lower extremities, injuries to the skin may not be immediately noticed by the child. Several actions routinely taken by the child and family will reduce the risk for injury.

- Perform a daily check of all skin surfaces and pressure points associated with sitting, braces, and shoes to identify abrasions, scrapes, reddened areas, and other lesions. Stop using the braces or shoes until the skin heals or redness disappears.
- Keep all skin surfaces clean and dry. Wear socks under braces.

- Use a gel-filled cushion and teach the child to shift his or her position hourly when in the wheelchair to avoid pressure sores.
- Avoid burns to the lower extremities by checking the temperature of bath water and car safety seats during hot weather.
- Take latex precautions as the child is at high risk for latex allergy. Avoid latex whenever a nonlatex substitute is available. Inform all healthcare providers about the child's latex allergy.
- Use safe ambulation techniques with walkers, canes, and crutches.

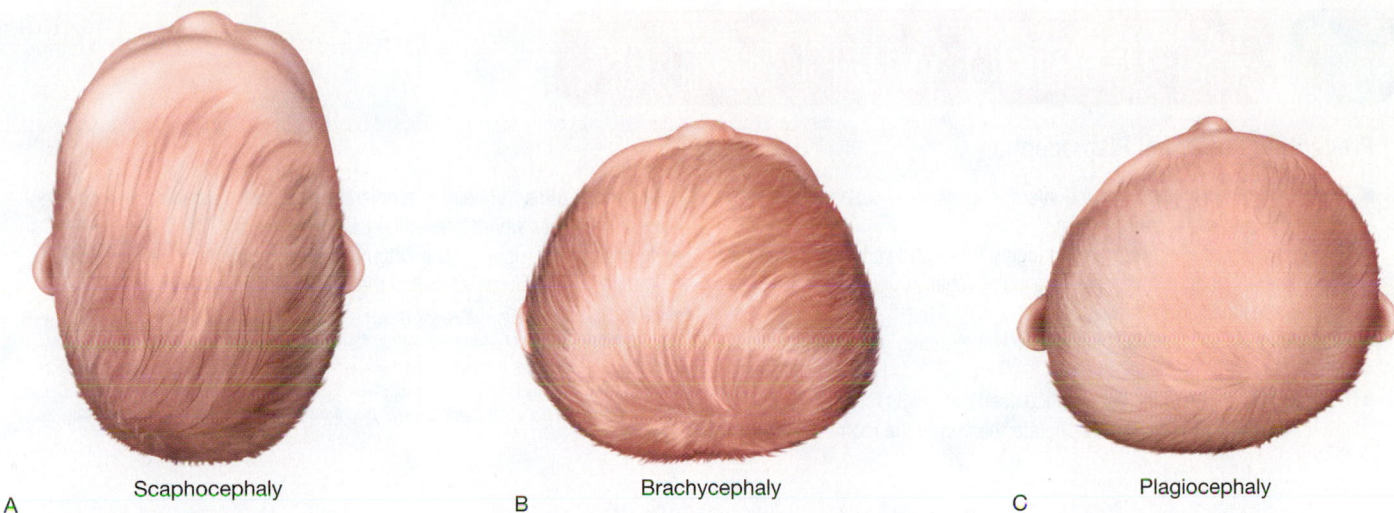

A   Scaphocephaly   B   Brachycephaly   C   Plagiocephaly

FIGURE 33–17 ■ In craniosynostosis, the head shape is dependent on which sutures are involved. *A,* Scaphocephaly accounts for more than 50% of cases (Boss & Huether, 2010). Premature closure of the sagittal suture causes a long, narrow skull and flattened parietal bones with a prominent occiput, a broad forehead, and small or absent anterior fontanel. The infant typically has an elongated head and bilateral bossing on the frontal and occipital areas. The parietal bones appear flattened. A ridge over the sagittal suture is palpable, and facial symmetry is apparent. *B,* Brachycephaly or bicoronal synostosis is associated with Apert syndrome or Crouzon syndrome. The head shape is shortened anterior to posterior, and the occiput is flattened. The infant may have hypertelorism and underdeveloped eye orbits with prominent eyes. *C,* Positional plagiocephaly is often asymmetric flattening of the occiput due to preferred position when supine or torticollis.

conditions such as Apert syndrome and Crouzon syndrome are responsible for up to 40% of cases (Boss & Huether, 2010).

Closure of the sutures usually takes place at predetermined times during the infant's development. Problems arise if one or more sutures close early. Bone growth continues in a direction parallel to the suture line rather than perpendicular as the brain pushes the sutures apart while it grows. Compensatory overgrowth at normal suture lines and the classic skull deformities associated with craniosynostosis occur with early suture closures. Sagittal synostosis (scaphocephaly), occurring more commonly in males, is the most common form of craniosynostosis (Brown & Proctor, 2011). See Figure 33–17A ■. When one coronal suture is involved, facial and skull asymmetry is apparent with eyes and ears out of alignment. Bicoronal synostosis, more common in females, is associated with Apert or Crouzon syndrome (Figure 33–17B ■). Palpation of the skull is used to detect bony ridges along suture lines and absence of an open anterior fontanel prior to 12 months of age; these are signs associated with craniosynostosis. Uncorrected craniosynostosis leads to increased intracranial pressure and delayed cognitive and psychosocial development (Brown & Proctor, 2011).

Diagnosis is often made at birth by clinical appearance and palpation of a bony ridge along a skull suture line. Skull measurements, radiographs, and a CT scan confirm the diagnosis. Surgery is performed when closure of multiple sutures causes chronic increased intracranial pressure, or for cosmetic reasons. One surgical approach is reconstructive skull remodeling, which removes the fused suture and cuts out parts of bone to reposition the bone and modify the skull shape. An alternative surgical technique, the endoscopically assisted strip craniectomy, is performed at about 3 months of age to remove the fused suture, and then a custom orthotic helmet is used for 3 to 9 months to promote optimal skull reshaping (Brown & Proctor, 2011). Children having surgery before 1 year of age have a better outcome. After surgery, it is important for the incision to remain dry and intact. The nurse should monitor intake and output, manage patient

positioning, protect skin integrity, monitor for infection, and observe the child for symptoms of increased intracranial pressure (see the Clinical Manifestations table on page 1153). Explain to parents that surgery will improve the child's appearance. Assure them that most children with corrected craniosynostosis are healthy and that their brains develop normally.

Positional Plagiocephaly

Positional plagiocephaly (a flattening of the occipital area of the skull) is seen increasingly in healthy infants put to sleep on their backs to prevent sudden infant death syndrome (Taub & Pierce, 2010). See Figure 33–17C ■. The sutures do not close prematurely. However, when the infant's sleep position does not change and the newborn is unable to control or lift the head, this leads to constant pressure on one side of the skull. The weight of the head flattens the skull, potentially making the skull asymmetric. Congenital torticollis, or shortening of the sternocleidomastoid muscle, and too little tummy time is believed to be associated with development of this disorder (Taub & Pierce, 2011). See Partnering with Families: Preventing Positional Plagiocephaly.

A helmet device to correct severe cases of positional plagiocephaly or brachycephaly is most effective in infants under 12 months of age and when treatment is initiated at 6 months of age when the skull bones are most malleable. The helmet, worn 23 hours a day for 3 months, relieves pressure on the flattened areas, allowing outward growth to occur. Remolding of the head shape continues after that treatment period because the infant spends more hours awake and sitting upright.

Neurofibromatosis

Neurofibromatosis 1 (NF1), or von Recklinghausen disease, is an autosomal dominant genetic disorder in which tumors grow along nerves. Skin pigmentation changes and bone deformities also occur. The incidence of the disorder is 1 per 3,500 individuals (Black &

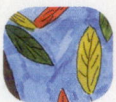

Partnering with Families

Preventing Positional Plagiocephaly

- Encourage tummy time when the infant is awake and supervised to promote neck and motor development.
- Encourage use of a baby carrier or snuggly. Reduce the amount of time the infant spends in an infant carrier, car safety seat, or infant swing, where the head rests against a firm surface.
- Hold the child for feeding, cuddling, and interaction. Alternate positions used.
- Change the position of the infant's face used each night for sleep to reduce the chance of a side preference. Rotate the crib in the room each day so

the infant turns the head in a different direction to look at the door. Alternate crib sides where interesting toys are placed.

- In children developing skull flattening, physical therapy exercises may be taught to the parents to stretch the sternocleidomastoid muscle.

Source: Data from Taub, P. J., & Pierce, P. (2011). Positional plagiocephaly, part 2: Prevention and treatment. Consultant for Pediatricians, 10(1), 13–15; Lennartsson, F. (2011). Developing guidelines for child health care nurses to prevent nonsynostotic plagiocephaly: Search for the evidence. Journal of Pediatric Nursing, 26, 348–358; Miller, L. C., Johnson, A., Duggan, L., & Behm, M. (2011). Consequences of the "back to sleep" program in infants. Journal of Pediatric Nursing, 26, 364–368.

Wilson, 2009). The NF1 gene (a tumor suppressor gene) is located on chromosome 17. Approximately 30% to 50% of cases result from a new mutation (National Institute of Neurological Disorders and Stroke, 2011). The condition varies in severity with most individuals having the milder form of the disease, but it can be debilitating when the severe form of the disease is present.

Etiology and Pathophysiology

Neurofibromas develop from cells of the nerve sheath, usually at some point along the peripheral nerves or at nerve endings. The neurofibroma may be an isolated growth, or extend along the length of a nerve and include nerve branches (plexiform neurofibromas). Plexiform neurofibromas are congenital and found in 25% of individuals (Hersh & the Committee on Genetics, 2008). Dermal neurofibromas, which usually begin to appear around the time of puberty, may reside in the skin or project above the skin surface. Tumors may also develop in the brain, along a cranial nerve, or along spinal nerve roots. Children with NF1 may be at higher risk for malignancies, such as peripheral nerve sheath tumors, leukemia, rhabdomyosarcoma, and pheochromocytoma (Hersh & the Committee on Genetics, 2008).

Clinical Manifestations

Signs and symptoms may be present at birth and progress over time. The disorder is characterized by multiple, light tan-colored café-au-lait spots 5 mm or larger seen at birth or by 2 years of age. In darker skinned children, the spots are darker than surrounding skin. The spots grow to 15 mm or larger in diameter by adulthood. Multiple neurofibromas or benign tumors, composed of nervous system tissue and fibrous tissue, grow on or under the skin beginning during puberty. Other findings include plexiform neurofibromas, and freckling in the axillary or inguinal areas (Figure 33–18 ■). See the Clinical Manifestations table. The expression of the disorder is variable, from mild to severe. Pain may occur when tumors grow around and compress a nerve or when a tumor grows in the spinal cord. Most children and adults with mild symptoms can live a normal, productive life.

Collaborative Care

The goal of collaborative care is to accurately diagnose the condition and monitor for complications that arise from the development of neurofibromas in different body sites.

Diagnostic Tests

Diagnosis is made in infancy or early childhood by the presence of two or more clinical signs of the disorder (see Box 33–11). Radiologic

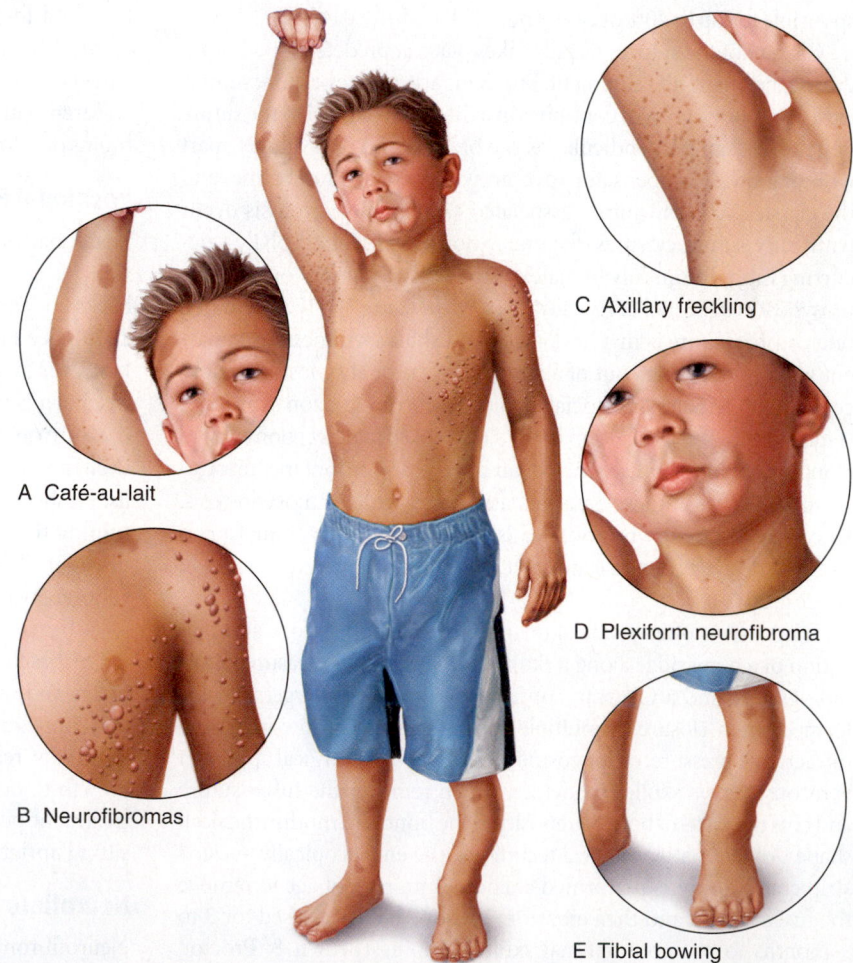

A Café-au-lait
B Neurofibromas
C Axillary freckling
D Plexiform neurofibroma
E Tibial bowing

FIGURE 33–18 ■ Physical signs of neurofibromatosis 1 become more apparent during adolescence. Café-au-lait spots enlarge, axillary freckling appears, and multiple neurofibromas develop. Some children develop plexiform neurofibromas.

Clinical Manifestations Neurofibromatosis Type 1

SYSTEM INVOLVED	CLINICAL MANIFESTATION
Skin	Six or more café-au-lait spots, dark macules that range in size from 5 mm to several centimeters Dermal neurofibromas, benign tumors that grow around nerves under the skin Plexiform neurofibromas, tumors involving multiple nerves that can be disfiguring Freckling in the axillary and inguinal areas
Eye	Lisch nodules, tan or brown benign tumors on the iris of the eye
Bones	Thinning or bowing of the tibia resulting in fractures that fail to heal properly Scoliosis
Cardiovascular	Hypertension due to renal vascular stenosis or pheochromocytoma
Central nervous system	Optic glioma, tumor along the optic pathway, found in 15% of children, causing vision loss, proptosis Learning disabilities, hyperactivity, and speech abnormalities Seizures Pain due to growing tumor
Endocrine	Precocious puberty or delayed puberty if optic glioma tumor invades the hypothalamus

imaging (MRI of brain and radiographs of the spine and other bones) is performed when problems are detected. Vision examinations are performed annually to detect vision loss and optic tumors. Prenatal diagnosis using amniocentesis or chorionic villus sampling procedures is possible. Genetic testing is available in families with documented cases.

Clinical Therapy

Clinical therapy focuses on monitoring the child for signs of developing problems associated with the condition. Regular health visits focusing on growth, developmental screening, blood pressure monitoring, scoliosis screening, inspection for limb abnormalities,

---

BOX 33–11	Diagnostic Criteria for Neurofibromatosis 1

Diagnostic criteria for neurofibromatosis 1 include the presence of two or more of the following characteristics (National Institute of Neurologic Disorders and Stroke, 2011):

- Six or more café-au-lait spots over 5 mm in diameter in prepubertal children and over 15 mm in diameter in postpubertal individuals
- Two or more neurofibromas of any type or one plexiform neurofibroma (grow diffusely under the skin or in deeper areas of the body)
- Freckling in the axillary or inguinal regions
- Optic glioma (a tumor of the optic nerve)
- Two or more Lisch nodules, usually in children over 5 years of age
- A distinctive osseous lesion such as sphenoid dysplasia or thinning of the long bone cortex with or without incomplete healing associated with fractures
- A first-degree relative (parent, sibling, offspring) with neurofibromatosis 1 by the above criteria

---

ophthalmic evaluation, timing of sexual development, and development of neurofibromas are encouraged.

When neurofibromas are disfiguring or cause problems because of their location, surgery may be performed to remove the tumor. Surgical removal of plexiform neurofibromas is more often attempted when tumors are painful, are disfiguring, or cause paralysis, or when life-threatening problems develop.

Nursing Management

The goals of nursing management are to assess the child and identify emerging problems with the disorder and to provide support to the child and family living with the condition.

Nurses assess the child to identify signs of neurofibromatosis, including café-au-lait spots, axillary and inguinal freckling, and small tumors on the body. Assess growth, including head circumference, as infants may have a large head or tumor development in the brain. Vital signs and blood pressure are monitored to detect hypertension. Vision screening to detect any vision impairment and proptosis is performed. Monitor growth and development to detect any unusual patterns, identifying signs of early or late pubertal development. Perform scoliosis screening on a frequent basis. Note any evidence of tibial bowing or other skeletal abnormalities. School performance should be monitored as learning disabilities and hyperactivity may occur. Pay attention to any mass that is rapidly enlarging or causing new pain.

Provide psychologic support to the child and family. Children with NF1 have more challenges with social development, especially if attention deficit hyperactivity disorder is present. As tumor development increases during adolescence, problems with self-image and self-esteem are common. The adolescent may have a difficult adjustment to the disorder. Identify peers or refer the adolescent to a support group. Assist children and adolescents to learn to live with the disorder. Focus on the child's strengths and encourage continuing development of those strengths. Refer families and adolescents to resources and support groups.

CEREBRAL PALSY

Cerebral palsy (CP) describes a group of permanent disorders of movement and posture development causing activity limitation, which is attributed to nonprogressive disturbances that occurred in the developing fetal or infant brain. The child with CP may also have disturbances in sensation, perception, cognition, communication, and behavior (Nehring, 2010). It is the major physical disability affecting functional development in children. The overall prevalence of CP is 2 to 3 cases per 1,000 live births (Lie, Gröholt, & Eskild, 2010). The four types of motor dysfunction seen with cerebral palsy—spastic, dystonia, athetosis, and ataxic—are related to the location of brain insult. A mix of motor dysfunctions may also be found. Dystonia and athetosis are sometimes categorized together as dyskinesia.

Etiology and Pathophysiology

It is estimated that 70% of cases of CP occur during the prenatal period, 20% during the perinatal period, and 10% during the first 2 years of life (Nehring, 2010). Most cases of CP are caused by brain insult (complications of prematurity, prenatal and genetic factors, teratogens, and viral infection of the fetus). Problems during labor and delivery, such as fetal heart rate decompression, asphyxia, and preeclampsia, may be factors in the development of CP. See Box 33–12.

| BOX 33–12 | Research: Apgar Score and Cerebral Palsy |

A recent study reviewed Apgar scores of all newborns in Norway between 1986 and 1995 to identify children diagnosed with CP. Findings revealed that 10% to 17% of children born with an Apgar score of 3 at birth, regardless of birth weight group (less than 1500 g, 1500 to 2499 g, and 2500 g or greater) developed CP. Only 0.1% of children having an Apgar score of 10 were diagnosed with CP. The child in the birth weight group of 2500 g or greater with an Apgar score of 3 had significantly greater odds of developing CP than children in lower birth weight groups. The Apgar score is a measure of the neonate's vitality at birth, so factors that affect a neonate's vitality could be associated with the neurologic insult causing CP (Lie et al., 2010).

Postnatal factors include neonatal sepsis, hyperbilirubinemia, intraventricular hemorrhage, meningitis or encephalitis, toxins, traumatic brain injury, infections, and stroke.

Spasticity of muscles inhibits muscle growth, so the muscle may not grow in coordination with bone growth. This can lead to a contracture that limits joint movement or deformities such as scoliosis or hip displacement (Blair, 2010). Spasticity is also associated with muscle weakness that interferes with gross motor activities.

Clinical Manifestations

Cerebral palsy is characterized by abnormal muscle tone and lack of coordination with spasticity found in the majority of cases. Children have a variety of symptoms depending on their ages, and the pattern or extremities involved may vary:

- **Diplegia** —both legs are affected.
- **Hemiplegia** —one side of the body is involved, the arm is usually more severely affected than the leg.
- **Quadriplegia** —all four extremities are affected.

All children with CP have motor impairment, with spasticity present in more than 75% of cases, ataxia in 2% to 8% of cases, and athetosis and dystonia in 2% to 15% (Blair, 2010). Even if both sides of the body are affected, the impairment is usually more severe on one side. See the table for clinical manifestations by type of CNS injury. A wide variability in symptoms for this lifelong disability occur depending on the area of the brain involved and the extent of brain injury.

Children with cerebral palsy usually are delayed in meeting developmental milestones (Figure 33–19 ■). For example, after 6 months of age, they may be unable to sit up, have persistent back arching, and have little spontaneous movement. Motor deficits become more obvious as the child grows, and the functional consequences progress even though the brain injury is nonprogressive. These children frequently have other complications, including intellectual disabilities, vision impairments, hearing loss, speech and language impairments, and seizures. Feeding may be difficult because of oral motor involvement, including hypotonia, with poor sucking and swallowing coordination.

Collaborative Care

The goal of collaborative care is to cautiously diagnose cerebral palsy and then to promote motor function and provide specific therapies that enable the child to develop the greatest amount of independence possible.

Diagnostic Tests

Diagnosis is usually based on clinical findings, including delayed development and increased or decreased muscle tone. CP is difficult to

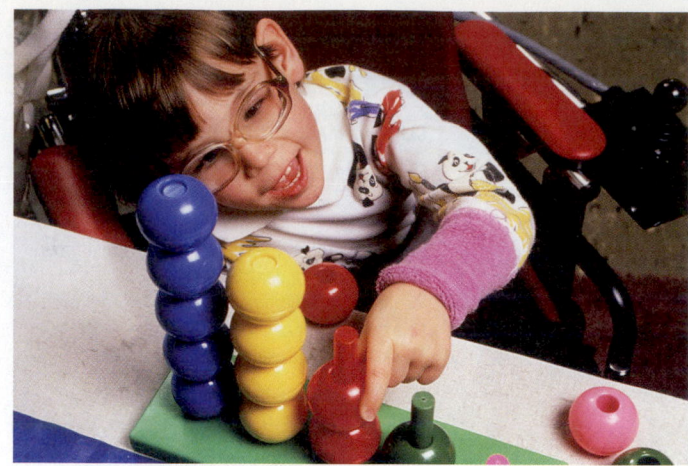

FIGURE 33–19 ■ A child with cerebral palsy has abnormal muscle tone and lack of physical coordination.
Source: *Will & Deni McIntyre/Science Source.*

diagnose in the early months of life because it must be distinguished from other neurologic conditions and signs may be subtle. Suspicious historical findings include risk factors described in the section on etiology and pathophysiology.

Ultrasonography can be used to detect fetal and neonatal abnormalities of the brain, such as intraventricular hemorrhage. Neuromotor tests that evaluate the presence of normal movement patterns and the absence of primitive reflexes and abnormal tone in young infants have been developed. Once CP is suspected, CT scans and MRI provide information about anatomic structures and help to define the cause of CP. Genetic and metabolic tests should be performed if congenital anomalies are present. Hearing and vision should be evaluated.

Functional mobility and manual ability of children are often categorized using a standardized scale, such as the Gross Motor Function Classification System, Functional Mobility Scale, and Manual Ability Classification System. For example, a child's mobility may be classified as Level 1—walks without limitations, Level 2—walks with limitations, Level 3—walks using a handheld mobility device, Level 4—self-mobility with limitations and may use powered mobility, and Level 5—transported in a manual wheelchair (Rethlefsen, Ryan, & Kay, 2010).

Clinical Therapy

It is not uncommon for children who are delayed in meeting developmental milestones or have neuromuscular abnormalities at 1 year of age to show gradual improvement in function. Half of the infants suspected to be at risk for CP at age 1 year are unimpaired neurologically by age 2 years (Nehring, 2010). Careful monitoring and early referral for evaluation is important to promote the child's development.

Clinical therapy focuses on helping the child develop to his or her maximum level of independence and to perform activities of daily living. This involves promoting mobility, an optimal range of motion, muscle control, balance, and communication. Referrals are made for physical, occupational, and speech therapy, as well as special education to improve motor function and ability. Braces and splints, serial casting, and positioning devices (prone wedges, standers, and side-lyers) are used to promote range of motion, skeletal alignment, stability, and control of involuntary movements, and to prevent contractures. Mobility devices such as scooters, tricycles, and wheelchairs help the child to move independently and explore the environment.

Clinical Manifestations Cerebral Palsy by Type of Insult

CLASSIFICATION AND TYPE OF INSULT	CLINICAL MANIFESTATIONS	CLINICAL THERAPY
Spastic Cerebral cortex or pyramidal tract injury 75% of cases	Increased muscle tone through a joint's range of motion Positive Babinski reflex Exaggerated deep tendon reflexes, clonus Persistence of primitive reflexes Leads to contractures and abnormal curvature of the spine	▪ Braces and splints to prevent contractures, braces to manage scoliosis ▪ Tone-reducing casts to keep spastic muscles in stretched position ▪ Static positioning devices to promote skeletal alignment
Dyskinetic—Athetosis Extrapyramidal, basal ganglia injury 10%–15% of cases	Slow involuntary writhing motions that interfere with ability to maintain a stable posture Abnormalities of muscle tone that affect the entire body Difficulty with fine and purposeful movements or coordinating the timing of movement; tremors	▪ Adaptive equipment for mobility and positioning ▪ Diazepam, baclofen, dantrolene to control spasticity ▪ Nerve blocks
Dyskinetic—Dystonia Basal ganglia, extrapyramidal injury	Involuntary sustained muscle contractions that lead to sustained or intermittent exaggerated and distorted posturing, twisting, or repetitive movements Develops around 5–10 years after myelination Rigid muscles when awake; normal or decreased muscle tone when asleep	▪ Botulinum toxin injections into the nerve-muscle junction to control spasticity ▪ Physical and occupational therapy to promote improved muscle tone and better motor control for function ▪ Speech therapy to address oral motor problems ▪ Surgery to lengthen tendons
Ataxic Cerebellar (extrapyramidal) injury 5%–10% of cases	Irregularity in muscle coordination, tone, and balance Abnormalities of voluntary movement involving balance and position of the trunk and limbs; have difficulty maintaining a posture Difficulty controlling hand and arm movements during reaching (overshooting or past-pointing) Increased or decreased muscle tone Hypotonia in first couple of years Muscle instability and wide-based unsteady gait Intellectual disability	▪ Carefully designed seating to promote function and to reduce contractures and joint deformities ▪ Mobility options—tricycle, walker, wheelchair ▪ Early intervention program ▪ Individualized education plan ▪ Assistive technology such as a computer ▪ Therapies to match specific symptoms
Mixed Injuries to multiple areas	No dominant motor pattern; may have mild spasticity, dystonia, and/or athetoid movement	

Orthopedic surgery interventions may be required to improve function by balancing muscle power and stabilizing uncontrollable joints (e.g., lengthening the Achilles tendon to increase the ankle's range of motion or releasing the hamstrings to correct knee flexion contractures). Other procedures may be performed to improve hip adduction, to correct spinal deformities, or to reduce spasticity by muscle lengthening and tendon transfers. Dorsal rhizotomy, cutting the afferent fibers that contribute to spasticity, may be performed in some children.

Medications are given to control seizures, to control spasms (skeletal muscle relaxants, baclofen, and benzodiazepines), and to minimize gastrointestinal side effects (cimetidine or ranitidine). See the Medications table. Baclofen is administered orally or by intrathecal pump to decrease muscle spasticity. See Figure 33–20 ▪. Botulinum toxin injections into specific muscles is a new therapy that helps to temporarily control spasticity.

The prognosis for infants and children with cerebral palsy depends on the level of physical disability and on the presence of intellectual, visual, or hearing deficits. Early intervention programs can significantly improve performance and can help the transition to the school setting. Some children are able to ambulate, but many others will need assistance with mobility and activities of daily living. Many of these children have difficulty with swallowing and aspiration, making feeding a challenge for families. A gastrostomy tube may ultimately be needed to ensure that the child has adequate nutrition and to prevent aspiration. These children are usually cared for in their homes, but in some cases receive care in long-term care facilities.

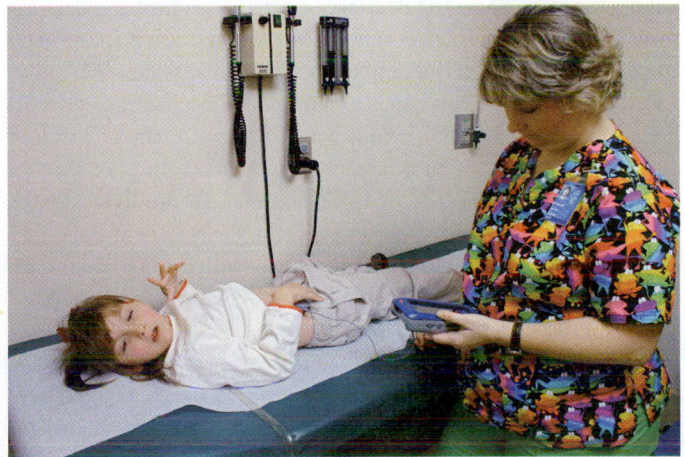

FIGURE 33–20 ▪ Child having baclofen pump filled.

Nursing Management

The goal of nursing care is to support the early identification of children with cerebral palsy and then to provide supportive care to promote cognitive, motor, and social functioning.

Nursing Assessment and Diagnosis

Be alert for children whose histories indicate an increased risk for CP. Assess all children at each healthcare visit for developmental delays (see Chapters 9, 10, and 11 🔗). Any orthopedic, visual, auditory, or intellectual deficits should be noted. Assess for the presence

Medications Used to Treat Cerebral Palsy

MEDICATION	ACTION	NURSING MANAGEMENT
Diazepam, lorazepam, clonazepam *Oral*	Affect brain control of muscle tone to help control spasticity and rigidity	Can cause drowsiness and excessive drooling. May interfere with feeding and speech. Physiologic dependence can develop, so taper drug when discontinued.
Dantrolene *Oral*	Calcium channel blocker that inhibits muscle contraction; skeletal muscle relaxant	Can cause drowsiness, muscle weakness, and increased drooling. Perform liver function testing periodically. Educate parents to report signs of jaundice. Supervise ambulation until effects are known.
Baclofen *Intrathecal* *Oral*	Inhibits motor nerve conduction at the level of the spinal cord Delivered intrathecally to the cerebrospinal fluid by a pump placed in the abdomen	Side effects with oral drug include drowsiness, nausea, headache, and low blood pressure. Lower continuous dosing is possible with intrathecal route, reducing side effects which may include hypotonia, increased seizures in children with known epilepsy, sleepiness, and nausea and vomiting. Monitor for pump failure and signs of infection.
Botulinum toxin type A *Injection*	When injected into the muscles of the trunk and limbs, inhibits the release of acetylcholine and a reversible chemically induced denervation. This weakens the spastic muscle and prevents a contracture (Berker & Yalçin, 2008); reduces spasticity for 3–6 months	Used to improve walking in children with equinus gait, may be used in hip adductors and hamstrings to improve positioning. Manage the pain associated with injections. May have stumbling, leg cramps, leg weakness, and calf atrophy. Repeated injections are needed to continue effect.

Source: *Data from Pellegrino, L. (2007). Cerebral palsy. In M. L. Batshaw, L. Pellegrino, & N. J. Roizen (Eds.), Children with disabilities (6th ed., pp. 387–408). Baltimore, MD: Paul H. Brooks; Wilson, B. A., Shannon, M. T., & Shields, K. M. (2011). Nurse's drug guide 2011. Upper Saddle River, NJ: Pearson.*

of newborn primitive reflexes, which may persist beyond the normal age in a child with CP (see Chapter 7 ⬦). Identify infants who appear to have an abnormal muscle tone or abnormal posture (head lag beyond 6 months of age, arched back, poor trunk control and balance, toe walking or scissoring). A simple screening test can be performed by placing a clean light piece of cloth on the infant's face. The unaffected infant will use two hands to remove it. Be concerned if the infant over 6 months of age uses one hand or does not remove the cloth at all. Asymmetric or abnormal crawling by using three extremities may indicate a motor problem. Hand dominance prior to 18 months of age is another sign of a motor problem. Determine if the infant has any problems sucking and swallowing or with feeding. Record dietary intake and height and weight percentiles for children suspected to have or diagnosed with the condition.

The child has many potential sources of pain, so care must be taken to identify a potential cause. For example, the child could have dental caries or abscesses, headaches, constipation, muscle spasms, bladder spasms, or decubitus ulcers. Take a careful history to identify potential causes of pain (e.g., time of day, association with aspects of care), especially in a child who is nonverbal, is irritable, and cries with pain (Dodge, 2008).

Nursing diagnoses for the child with CP depend on the type of CP, the child's symptoms and age, and the family situation. See the Nursing Care Plan for several diagnoses that may be appropriate for the child with CP. Additional nursing diagnoses may include the following:

- Constipation, Risk for, related to low intake of fiber and fluids and insufficient physical activity
- Tissue Integrity, Impaired, related to decreased physical mobility and limited self-care ability
- Communication: Verbal, Impaired, related to hearing and/or speech impairment
- Home Maintenance, Impaired, related to child's developmental disability and inadequate support system
- Pain, Chronic, related to spasticity and stretching exercises to prevent contractures
- Growth and Development, Delayed, related to lack of muscle strength or limited social interaction

NANDA-I © 2012

Planning and Implementation

The accompanying Nursing Care Plan summarizes care for the child with CP. Because the condition can range from mild to severe and involve numerous manifestations, interventions need to be adapted to the child and family. Nursing care focuses on providing adequate nutrition, maintaining skin integrity, promoting physical mobility, promoting safety, promoting growth and development, teaching parents how to care for the child, and providing emotional support.

Provide Adequate Nutrition

Children with CP require high-calorie diets or supplements to the diet because of feeding difficulties associated with spasticity or hypotonia. Many children have difficulty chewing and swallowing, and they are at risk for aspiration. Give the child small amounts of soft foods at a time. Feeding utensils with large, padded handles and adaptive cups may be easier for the child to use. Make sure the child gets adequate fluids as the child may not be able to communicate thirst. Children with severe CP may require a gastrostomy tube to obtain adequate nutrition.

Constipation is a common issue in children with CP because of dietary intake, lack of exercise, and difficulty sitting on the toilet. Adequate dietary fiber and fluid is needed to prevent constipation, and

Nursing Care Plan   The Child with Cerebral Palsy

INTERVENTION	RATIONALE	EXPECTED OUTCOME
1. Nursing Diagnosis: Mobility: Physical, Impaired, related to increased muscle tone and spasticity		
NIC Priority Intervention—*Exercise Therapy, Joint Mobility:* Use of active and passive body movement to maintain joint flexibility		**NOC Suggested Outcome**—*Joint Movement–Active:* Range of motion of joints with self-initiated movement
GOAL: *The child will attain maximum physical abilities possible.*		
■ Perform developmental assessment and record age when milestones are achieved (e.g., reaching for objects, sitting).	■ Delayed developmental milestones are characteristic of CP. Interventions are revised as each milestone is achieved, to focus on the next.	The child reaches maximum physical mobility and all developmental milestones.
■ Plan activities to use gross and fine motor skills (e.g., holding eating utensils, toys positioned to encourage reaching). Allow time for the child to complete activities.	■ Many activities of daily living and play activities promote physical development. The child may perform tasks more slowly than most children.	
■ Perform range of motion exercises every 4 hours for the child unable to move body parts. Position the child to promote tendon stretching (e.g., foot plantar flexion instead of dorsiflexion, legs extended rather than flexed at the knees and hips).	■ Exercises and positioning promote mobility and increased circulation, and decrease the risk of contractures.	
■ Arrange for and encourage parents to keep appointments with a rehabilitation therapist.	■ A regularly reevaluated and revised rehabilitation program helps to promote development.	
■ Teach the family to use braces and other positioning devices.	■ Adaptive devices are often necessary to prevent contractures and to maximize physical mobility.	
2. Nursing Diagnosis: Nutrition: Imbalanced, Less than Body Requirements related to chewing and swallowing difficulty and high metabolic needs		
NIC Priority Intervention—*Nutrition Management:* Assistance with or provision of a balanced dietary intake of foods and fluids		**NOC Suggested Outcome**—*Nutritional Status: Nutrient Intake:* Adequacy of nutrients taken into body
GOAL: *The child will receive nutrients needed for normal growth.*		
■ Monitor height and weight and plot on a growth grid. Perform hydration status assessment.	■ Insufficient intake can lead to impaired growth and dehydration.	The child shows normal growth patterns for height, weight, and other physical parameters.
■ Teach the family techniques to promote swallowing and caloric and nutrient intake:	■ Special techniques can facilitate food intake. Adaptive handles may help the child better manage feeding self.	
■ Position the child upright for feedings.		
■ Place foods far back in the mouth to overcome tongue thrust.		
■ Use soft and blended foods. Allow extra time for chewing and swallowing.		
■ Obtain adaptive handles for utensils and encourage self-feeding skills.		
■ Perform frequent respiratory assessment. Teach the family to prevent aspiration. Teach gastrostomy tube care and tube-feeding technique as appropriate.	■ Aspiration pneumonia is a risk for the child with poor swallowing. Special feeding techniques may be needed.	
3. Nursing Diagnosis: Therapeutic Regimen Management: Family, Ineffective, related to excessive demands made on family with child's complex care needs		
NIC Priority Intervention—*Family Mobilization:* Utilization of family strengths to influence patient's health in a positive direction		**NOC Suggested Outcome**—*Family Functioning:* Ability of the family to meet the needs of its members through developmental transitions
GOAL: *The family will adapt to growth and development needs of the child with CP.*		
■ Allow opportunities for parents to verbalize the impact of CP on the family. Refer them to other parents and support groups.	■ The family needs to explore the emotional and social impact of the child's care so they can integrate and grow from the experience.	The child demonstrates appropriate growth and developmental progress.

(continued)

Nursing Care Plan   The Child with Cerebral Palsy, *continued*

INTERVENTION	RATIONALE	EXPECTED OUTCOME
▪ Explore community services for rehabilitation, respite care, childcare, and early intervention programs, and refer the family as appropriate.	▪ Diverse services may be available and will be needed due to the multiple impacts of CP on the child.	
▪ During home and office visits, recognize the child's achievements, and praise the family for care provided.	▪ The child's achievements are positive reinforcement of the family's efforts.	
▪ Teach the family skills needed to manage the child's care (e.g., medication administration, muscle stretching, seizure management).	▪ Complex skills must be learned before they can be performed efficiently.	
▪ Teach case management techniques.	▪ The child requires care by many specialists, and many parents become case managers to coordinate care.	
▪ Involve siblings in the care of the child with CP. Review with parents the needs of all children in the family.	▪ Siblings of the child with CP may feel left out because of the care provided. Special efforts help to meet the developmental needs of all family members.	The family successfully supports all of its members.

4. Nursing Diagnosis: Activity, Deficient Diversional, (Child) related to poor social skills

NIC Priority Intervention—*Recreation Therapy:* Purposeful use of recreation to promote relaxation and enhancement of social skills		**NOC Suggested Outcome—*Play Participation:*** Use of activities as needed for enjoyment, entertainment, and development by children

GOAL: *The child will engage in activities that maximize growth and development.*

▪ Refer the family to an early intervention program. Encourage contact with other children.	▪ The child needs a variety of activities and contact with other children and adults to maximize development.	The child engages in activities to maximize development.
▪ Work with the school to develop an individualized education plan that encourages interaction with peers and a variety of activities that support development.	▪ The education system is obligated to work with families to provide methods to enhance learning, including social interactions.	
▪ Investigate recreational programs for children with disabilities and share information with the parents.	▪ Recreational programs for children with disabilities may provide social experiences and physical activity.	

NANDA-I © 2012

some children need a bowel management program to treat chronic constipation.

Maintain Skin Integrity

Take special care to protect the bony prominences from friction injury and pressure sores. Monitor splints and braces for proper fit, and the skin under them for redness. If the skin is red, the braces or splints should be removed and not worn until the redness is gone. See Partnering with Families: Safety for the Child with Myelodysplasia on page 1184.

Promote Physical Mobility

Proper body alignment should be maintained at all times. Support the child with pillows, towels, and bolsters whether the child is in bed or in a chair. Use splints and braces to help support joints in extension or functional position and to reduce the risk for contractures. Support the head and body of a floppy infant. A child with spasticity and scissored, extended legs, or a child with athetosis who writhes constantly may be difficult to carry and transport.

Range of motion exercises are essential to maintain joint flexibility and to prevent contractures. Consult with the physical therapists who work with the child and assist with recommended exercises. Teach

parents to position the child to foster flexion rather than extension so that interaction with the environment can be enhanced (e.g., the child can bring objects closer to the face). Encourage parents to bring the child's adaptive appliances (e.g., customized wheelchairs, braces, positioning devices) for use in the hospital; however, secure the child's appliances as it may be difficult for the family to get them replaced if lost. Refer parents to the appropriate resources for help with the acquisition of adaptive devices. Massage may be helpful when performing stretching exercises. See Complementary Therapy: Hippotherapy.

Complementary Therapy
Hippotherapy

A few studies have investigated the benefit of hippotherapy (therapeutic horseback riding) for children with CP. Although the studies have small sample sizes, children are believed to benefit by improved balance and postural control from the muscular effort of adjusting to the gait of the horse. It is believed that this movement and the warmth of the horse help hypertonicity and promote relaxation in the child (Zadnikar & Kastrin, 2011).

Weblink | Cerebral Palsy Resources

Promote Safety

Teach parents the importance of using safety belts with children in strollers and wheelchairs. Determine if an adaptive car safety seat is needed so the child can be safely transported. A helmet should be worn by the child with chronic seizures to protect from further injury during seizures.

Promote Growth and Development

Remember that some children with CP are physically but not intellectually disabled. Use terminology appropriate for the child's developmental level. Help the child develop a positive self-image to ensure emotional health and social growth. Children with a hearing impairment may need referral to learn American Sign Language or other communication methods. Provide audio and visual activities for the child who is unable to mobilize independently.

Adaptive and assistive technology may be needed to promote mobility and communication. **Assistive technology** is any item, piece of equipment, or product customized for use to promote the functional capabilities of individuals with disabilities so that they are as independent as possible. Examples include computers, communication devices, adaptive utensils, and customized wheelchairs.

Foster Parental Knowledge

Teach parents about the disorder and arrange sessions to teach them about all of the child's special needs. Teach administration, desired effects, and side effects of medications prescribed for seizures. Make sure parents are aware of the need for dental care because enamel defects and malocclusion commonly occur in children with CP, and gingival hyperplasia occurs when anticonvulsants are prescribed.

Provide Emotional Support

Refer parents to individual and family counseling if appropriate. Listen to the parents' concerns and encourage them to express their feelings and ask questions. Explain what they can expect regarding future treatment. Work with other healthcare professionals to help families adjust to this chronic disease.

Care in the Community

Children with CP need continuous support in the community. A case manager such as the parent or nurse is often needed to coordinate care. Parents may need financial assistance to provide for the child's needs and to obtain appliances such as braces or a customized wheelchair. Children need new adaptive devices, ongoing developmental assessment and care planning, and possibly surgery as they grow. Although the brain lesion does not change, it manifests differently as the child grows. For example, once the child begins to walk, the extensor tone may cause Achilles cord tightening. Braces may decrease deformities, but surgery may eventually be needed. Technology offers many new strategies to promote communication and self-care by these children.

Monitor the child's growth. If the child is unable to ambulate, a scale that accommodates a wheelchair should be used. Standing height measurements may be inaccurate, and tools to assess ulnar length or tibial length may be more accurate for a height measurement (Dodge, 2008). Schedule regular appointments for vision and hearing screening as many children with CP have vision and sensorineural hearing deficits. Children need regular dental visits to assess for malocclusion and gingivitis, and for dental cleaning. Give immunizations according to the recommended schedule, even though the pertussis, measles, mumps, and rubella vaccines may increase the risk of seizures in children with a seizure disorder. Educate parents about the possible risk for a seizure associated with the vaccines.

Early intervention programs can help parents learn how to meet their child's special needs, including physical, occupational, and speech therapy, as well as educational needs. The nurse can help parents meet the needs of the child with CP in preschool, school, and healthcare settings. The child often needs an individualized education plan (IEP) to maximize learning potential and mobility. See Chapter 16 . Many children with CP have a normal IQ, but problems with behavior, perception, and speech create challenges for learning. In addition, the nurse makes referrals as appropriate to support groups and organizations such as the United Cerebral Palsy Association and Shriners Hospitals. Recreational activities may be identified through the National Association of Sports for Cerebral Palsy.

An individualized transition plan developed during adolescence assists the family and adolescent with CP to plan for adult living. Vocational training options can be explored. The young adult, age 18 to 21 years, may be able to move into a group home or live independently, if desired. Both the special mobility needs and educational support needed by the child must be addressed (see Chapter 16). Nurses in hospital programs may coordinate transition into smaller communities and settings and assist the family in gaining access to available resources.

Evaluation

Expected outcomes of nursing care for the child with cerebral palsy are provided in the Nursing Care Plan. Some additional outcomes include:

- The child's constipation is effectively managed.
- Successful communication techniques are identified for the child.
- The child is integrated into school, recreation, and social activities.

NEONATAL ABSTINENCE SYNDROME

Illicit substances that may cause neonatal abstinence syndrome when used by the mother during pregnancy include opioids (heroin, meperidine, methadone), CNS stimulants (cocaine, propoxyphene, amphetamines), and CNS depressants (barbiturates, alcohol, and marijuana). It is estimated that 4.4% of women 15 to 44 years of age use illicit drugs during pregnancy, but the rates vary by age: women 15 to 17 years (16.2%), women 18 to 25 years (7.4%), and women 26 to 44 years (1.9%). Among pregnant women 15 to 44 years of age, 10.8% report current alcohol use, 3.7% report binge drinking, and 1% report heavy drinking. Regular or binge alcohol use is reported by 4.1% of pregnant women (Substance Abuse and Mental Health Services Administration, 2011). See Chapter 34 for information about fetal alcohol syndrome.

Etiology and Pathophysiology

Illicit substances readily cross the placenta, enter the fetal circulation, and have the same effects on the fetus that they do on the mother. For example, cocaine acts on the developing fetus by decreasing placental blood flow, which deprives the fetus of essential oxygen and nutrients while elevating the fetal blood pressure and heart rate. The mother's repeated use of narcotics and illicit substances leads to fetal tolerance

Clinical Manifestations Neonatal Abstinence Syndrome

SYSTEM INVOLVED	CLINICAL MANIFESTATIONS	CLINICAL THERAPY
Central nervous system	Irritability, restlessness, tremors, seizures, high-pitched cry, abnormal sleep patterns, drowsiness, yawning, and hypertonicity	Phenobarbital, diazepam, methadone, clonidine, or paregoric may be prescribed to relieve symptoms of drug withdrawal. Provide skin care to protect skin surfaces that rub against sheets.
Autonomic nervous system	Sneezing, stuffy nose, sweating, tachycardia, and tachypnea	Keep the newborn's nasal passages clear. Bathe skin with warm water. Swaddle the newborn to reduce stimuli.
Gastrointestinal system	Diarrhea, vomiting, and poor feeding	Provide small frequent feedings. Monitor weight gain.

and physical dependence. When the mother stops taking drugs during pregnancy, both she and the fetus have withdrawal symptoms. If the infant is born to a mother who is still actively using drugs, the neonate has signs of abrupt withdrawal from the illicit substance shortly after birth. See Chapter 21 ℰ for information about opioid withdrawal.

Clinical Manifestations

Withdrawal symptoms for opioids usually appear 24 to 48 hours after birth, barbiturate withdrawal symptoms occur between 4 and 14 days afer birth, and cocaine or amphetamine withdrawal symptoms appear up to 7 days after birth. The onset of symptoms may be attributed to the type and amount of drug taken by the mother and how soon before birth it was taken. Mothers, however, may use multiple substances which makes it difficult to determine which substance was used.

Signs of opioid withdrawal include hypertonia, irritability, excitability, jitteriness, tremors, tachypnea, sneezing, stuffy nose, high-pitched cry, diarrhea, regurgitation, poor feeding, apnea, and seizures (Sweeney, 2009). These newborns may have excoriated skin, especially on the heels, toes, hands, elbows, nose, or chin, as a result of continuous movement against bed linens. Fetal cocaine exposure increases the risk for prematurity, low birth weight, and small for gestational age (Wallman, Smith, & Moore, 2011). See the Clinical Manifestations table for neonatal abstinence syndrome.

The neonate exposed to methamphetamine is often small for gestational age, similar to the effects of cocaine. However, neonates are often sleepy and lethargic in the initial weeks, making them difficult to feed. After a couple of weeks they become jittery, startle easily, and have a shrill cry, similar to characteristics of neonates exposed to cocaine (Wells, 2009).

Collaborative Care

The goal of collaborative care is to identify the newborn with neonatal abstinence syndrome and to initiate supportive care during the withdrawal process.

Diagnostic Tests

Diagnosis is based on the history of maternal substance abuse and physical signs in the newborn. EEG abnormalities may be noted. Urine testing provides information on drug use immediately prior to labor, and meconium screening provides information of drug use by the mother for the last half of the pregnancy. If urine is positive, compare results with medications used during labor and delivery. The

newborn's hair may also be tested. Chain of custody for specimens may be needed. CordStat, a test of a portion of the umbilical cord for drugs of abuse, is being adopted by many hospitals.

Behavioral and neurologic functioning may also be assessed with diagnostic tools such as the Brazelton Neonatal Behavioral Assessment Scale. This tool evaluates infants on four developmental abilities: (1) ability to control their breathing, temperature, and autonomic nervous system, (2) inhibiting random movement and controlling activity level, (3) ability to control states from quiet sleep to crying and the ability to tune out irritating stimuli, and (4) social interaction (Brazelton Institute, 2008).

Clinical Therapy

Treatment is generally supportive. Infants with cocaine exposure need to have reduced environmental stimuli and swaddling. Medications such as phenobarbital, diazepam, methadone, clonidine, and paregoric may be prescribed to alleviate symptoms of drug withdrawal. If the mother is still using illicit drugs, breastfeeding is discouraged as the drugs cross over into milk.

The most serious and prevalent complication for the neonate whose mother used illicit drugs is congenital infection, such as with human immunodeficiency virus (HIV), hepatitis B, hepatitis C, or syphilis. Assessment and treatment for these conditions is implemented. See Chapters 27, 30, and 31 ℰ for treatment of these infections. Another important consideration for the infant with methamphetamine exposure is whether the newborn will be living in a setting where a clandestine laboratory exists, which would increase the infant's exposure to toxic chemicals used in methamphetamine production. Infants living with a parent who uses illicit drugs are also at greater risk for child abuse (Wells, 2009). The long-term effects of this condition on cognitive function continue to be studied. Children with prenatal cocaine exposure are reported to have problems with behavior and executive functioning (Salisbury, Ponder, Padbury, et al., 2009).

Nursing Management

Nursing care focuses on monitoring withdrawal symptoms, administering prescribed medications, and meeting the infant's emotional needs.

Nursing Assessment and Diagnosis

Prevention and early identification of the infant with neonatal abstinence syndrome is an important nursing role. Providing information for all parents about the risks and effects of various abused substances increases the chance that they will avoid these substances in future pregnancies.

Crying and poor feeding should increase the nurse's suspicion of neonatal abstinence syndrome. Observe the newborn carefully for poor sucking, seizures, vomiting, diarrhea, dehydration, and an increased metabolic rate. Many withdrawal symptoms are identical to symptoms of infection, bowel obstruction, electrolyte disorder, hydrocephalus, and intracranial anomaly, so consider the possibility that the infant could have both neonatal abstinence syndrome and another condition. Monitor the condition of the skin to identify abrasions associated with rubbing against sheets.

Assess the strengths, safety, and competence of the mother and other potential caregivers. Determine if the mother is still using illicit drugs, and identify other family supports that may help provide the care and safety needed by the newborn.

Examples of nursing diagnoses may include:

- Infant Feeding Pattern, Ineffective related to prematurity and oral hypersensitivity
- Infant Behavior: Disorganized related to prenatal cocaine exposure
- Development: Delayed, Risk for related to intrauterine exposure to illicit substances
- Parenting, Impaired to mother who continues to use illicit substances

NANDA-I © 2012

Planning and Implementation

Provide Supportive Care

Provide frequent, small, high-calorie feedings, which are more readily tolerated by these infants. Infants suffering from withdrawal need increased calories; a formula with 24 calories per ounce may be recommended. Breastfeeding is not recommended for mothers continuing to use cocaine and other illicit drugs, as the substance is excreted in the breast milk. Patience is needed when feeding these infants because their sucking and swallowing is poorly coordinated. Teach parents to use a calm approach and soothing voice when feeding. Newborns may initially feed better in a side-lying position while swaddled. Hold the infant with the spine flexed to decrease extensor tone.

Administer prescribed medications, if ordered, for drug withdrawal and monitor the infant's response. Keep in mind that many infants are managed without drugs. Protect the newborn's skin because jitteriness may lead to greater skin surface rubbing against sheets and cause scratches and abrasions.

Clinical Tip

Several techniques are used to calm and soothe the newborn with neonatal abstinence syndrome:

- Keep the infant in a quiet environment, away from monitors that beep and paging speakers.
- Keep the lighting subdued, and minimize stimulation to promote rest and sleep.
- Comfort and pacify the infant with swaddling and a pacifier for sucking needs. Rocking and soothing music may also be calming. Infant massage may be beneficial for some neonates.

Begin working with the mother and other family members to demonstrate strategies for promoting parent–infant interaction, minimizing stimulation, and promoting feeding. Make plans for careful follow-up by health professionals (social services, physicians, and nurses) so that the infant's safety is ensured and growth and development are monitored and promoted.

Care in the Community

Long-term follow-up care of the child should be planned to ensure regular developmental testing and assessment for catch-up growth, neurobehavioral problems, and fetal alcohol syndrome (as multiple substances could have been used by the mother). Care of the infant with neonatal abstinence syndrome and the substance-abusing mother often presents complex family situations, and support from social services is often needed. The infant is at risk for neurobehavioral problems that a substance-abusing parent has difficulty meeting. Family resources, child protective services, and foster care may be needed if the infant does not have adequate growth. See the Health Promotion & Maintenance Overview to identify key areas for attention during follow-up visits.

Evaluation

Expected outcomes of nursing management for the infant and family include:

- The infant is receptive to interaction at periods during the day.
- Parent and infant bonding is observed.
- Assessment of growth and development occurs during regular healthcare visits.

INJURIES OF THE NEUROLOGIC SYSTEM

Traumatic Brain Injury

Traumatic brain injury (TBI) is defined as a blunt force to the head or penetrating injury that disrupts normal brain functioning, such as a change in level of consciousness. Traumatic brain injuries are the most common injuries in childhood, and they are the leading cause of death and disability during childhood. Among children from birth to 19 years of age in 2007, traumatic brain injury caused 5,500 deaths. The highest rate of death (16.4 per 100,000) occurred in adolescents 15 to 19 years of age, followed by children from birth to 4 years of age (4.7 per 100,000) (Coronado, Xu, Basavaraju, et al., 2011). Annually in the United States in children younger than 15 years, approximately 515,000 experience a TBI, 474,000 require an emergency department visit, 35,000 require hospitalization, and 2,100 die from their TBI (Faul, Xu, Wald, et al., 2010). Young children are at risk for long-term cognitive deficits following a traumatic brain injury (Podell, Gifford, Bougakov, et al., 2010).

Etiology and Pathophysiology

TBI may be caused by blunt (head struck by an object or shaking) or penetrating (e.g., bullet) mechanisms, and children more commonly have a blunt injury mechanism. Motor vehicle crashes are the major mechanism of injury causing TBI deaths in all children and adolescents, closely followed by firearms in adolescents 15 to 19 years of age (Coronado et al., 2011). Leading TBI mechanisms of injury resulting in emergency department visits or hospitalization vary by age (Faul et al., 2010):

- **Children 0 to 4 years**—falls, struck by or against an object (e.g., shaken baby syndrome and child abuse) (see Chapter 20 for more information), and motor vehicle crashes
- **Children 5 to 9 years**—falls, struck by or against an object, and motor vehicle-related injury as passengers or pedestrians
- **Children 10 to 14 years**—falls, struck by or against an object, assault, and motor vehicle-related injury as passengers or pedestrians
- **Adolescents 15 to 19 years**—motor vehicle crashes, struck by or against an object, falls, and assault

Health Promotion & Maintenance Overview

The Infant with Prenatal Exposure to Illicit Substances

GROWTH AND DEVELOPMENT SURVEILLANCE
- Monitor the child's motor, psychosocial, and language development, and refer the infant for a complete assessment if a developmental delay or other problem is suspected.
- Enroll the infant in an early intervention program to assist the parents or caregivers to promote the infant's development.
- Encourage enrollment in Head Start programs when the child is old enough as this may help later school performance.

NUTRITION
- Assess the parent's techniques for feeding the infant and the amount of formula ingested. Breastfeeding is not encouraged if the mother is still using illicit substances. Assess the number of calories ingested, and determine if calories are adequate for growth.
- Provide guidance about introduction of solid foods as the infant may have a strong tongue thrust and oral hypersensitivity. Refer to an occupational therapy feeding specialist if the parent continues to have difficulty feeding the infant.

SLEEP AND REST
- Encourage parents or caregivers to establish a regular sleeping pattern. Use swaddling, low lighting, low noise, infant massage, rocking the infant in a flexed position, and a pacifier to relax the infant and promote sleep.

- Place the infant on its back to sleep because these infants are at higher risk for sudden infant death syndrome.

RELATIONSHIPS
- Assess the patience and ability of the parents or caregivers to care for an infant having behaviors such as irritability, excessive crying, and hyperactivity. Provide support to the parents or caregivers with education, support groups, or respite care to enable them to continue effective parenting of the infant.
- Monitor the parent for continued use of drugs to determine the infant's safety and the ongoing ability of the parents to provide care. Monitor for potential signs of child abuse or neglect.
- Conduct home visits if ongoing use of drugs is suspected. Coordinate care with social services as necessary to determine the infant's need for foster care placement.

DISEASE PREVENTION STRATEGIES
- Work with the parents to ensure that the infant receives all immunizations according to the recommended schedule. Hepatitis B vaccine is especially important because of the mother's potential to acquire the infection through needle sharing or as a sexually transmitted disease.
- Perform all recommended screening tests to identify health problems.
- Weigh and measure the infant regularly to monitor catch-up growth. Monitor head circumference.

The injury impact transfers energy through the skull and meninges to the brain. The primary injury occurs on impact, when the initial cellular damage occurs. The injury may result from a direct blow to the head (**coup injury**) or from movement of the brain within the skull (**contrecoup injury**), such as from shaken baby syndrome (Figure 33–21 ■). At the time of impact, scalp injuries, skull fractures, contusions, and hematomas of brain tissue may occur. Movement of the head, such as from shaking, causes the brain tissues within the skull to keep moving, causing bruising and tearing of nerves, fibers, and blood vessels.

The secondary injury is the biochemical and cellular response to the primary injury. Brain swelling begins to occur immediately after the TBI, impairing cerebral blood flow that can lead to ischemia and brain damage. Brain cells are further damaged by the release of amino acids and an inflammatory response that increase the permeability of the blood-brain barrier. Cerebral edema results in increased ICP. The brain injury is further compounded by decreased cerebral perfusion pressure, limiting the blood flow that delivers oxygen and nutrients and removes accumulated toxins from cell death.

Clinical Manifestations

The signs and symptoms of brain injuries in children depend on the pathologic features and severity of the injury. The child with a mild brain injury may remain conscious or have a brief loss of consciousness (seconds to a few minutes) or amnesia. The child with a moderate brain injury loses consciousness for 5 to 10 minutes. Following mild and moderate brain injuries, children may have amnesia about the event, headache, nausea, and vomiting. The child with a severe brain injury is usually unconscious for more than 10 minutes and may rapidly show signs of increased ICP. See the Clinical Manifestations table on page 1153.

Unconsciousness may result from increased ICP, cerebral edema, intracranial hemorrhage, or parenchymal damage to the cortex in both cerebral hemispheres or the brainstem. The presence of retinal hemorrhages, rib fractures, and apnea with TBI, especially in an infant less than 6 months of age, should raise the suspicion of child abuse (Maguire, Pickerd, Farewell, et al., 2009).

Vital signs are important indicators of brain injury. Changes in respiratory effort or periods of apnea may result from shock, injury to the spinal cord above C4, or damage to or pressure on the medulla. Heart rate and blood pressure are indices of brainstem function. Tachycardia can be a sign of blood loss, shock, hypoxia, anxiety, or pain. Cushing triad (increased systolic blood pressure with a wide pulse pressure, bradycardia, and irregular respirations) is associated with significantly increased ICP, impending herniation, or compromised blood flow to the brainstem. Refer to the earlier discussion of altered states of consciousness for more information about increased ICP. Reflexes may be hyporesponsive, hyperresponsive, or nonexistent. The child may assume a flexor, extensor, or flaccid posture (see Figure 33–3). See the Clinical Manifestations table for specific traumatic brain injuries.

Collaborative Care

The goal of collaborative care is to rapidly identify the brain injuries that may lead to serious morbidity or mortality if untreated and to initiate aggressive interventions to reduce increased ICP and minimize complications.

Pathophysiology Illustrated Brain Injury

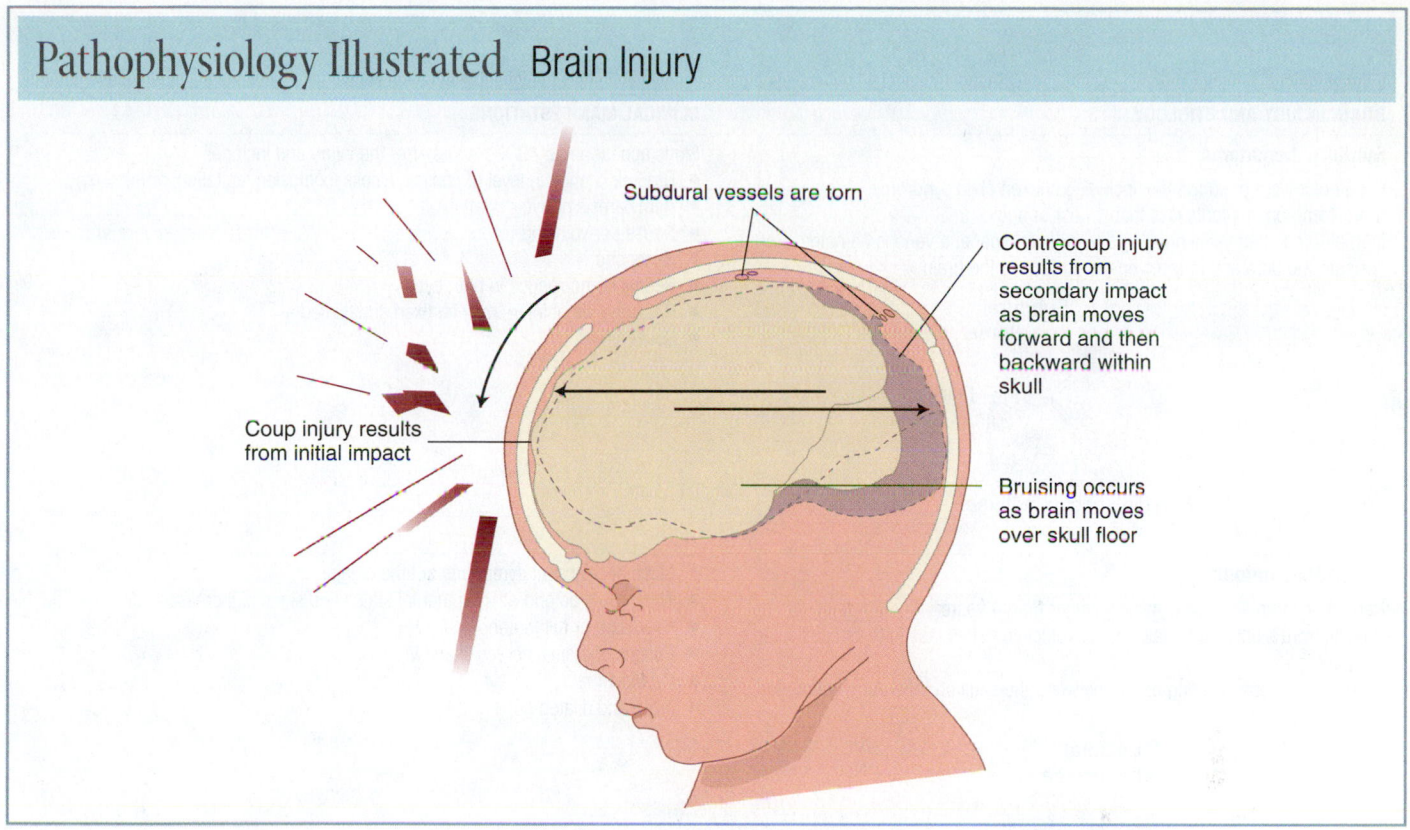

Subdural vessels are torn

Contrecoup injury results from secondary impact as brain moves forward and then backward within skull

Coup injury results from initial impact

Bruising occurs as brain moves over skull floor

FIGURE 33–21 ■ Brain injury can result from a direct blow to the head just under the skull where the initial impact occurs (coup injury). The acceleration-deceleration movement of the brain within the skull also results in an injury where the brain strikes the skull (contrecoup injury).

Clinical Manifestations Traumatic Brain Injury by Severity

TYPE OF BRAIN INJURY	CLINICAL MANIFESTATIONS
Concussion or mild brain injury	Low-grade headache that will not go away Slowness in thinking, acting, speaking, reading Memory problems Loss of balance, unsteady walking Poor concentration, change in performance at school, lack of motivation, or lack of interest in favorite toys Feeling tired all the time, change in sleeping pattern Change in eating patterns Increased sensitivity to lights, sounds, distractions Easily irritated
Moderate brain injury	Glasgow Coma Scale score of 9–12 Posttraumatic amnesia for 1–24 hours Loss of consciousness
Severe brain injury	Glasgow Coma Scale score of 8 or less Posttraumatic amnesia lasting longer than 24 hours Coma or unconsciousness Increased intracranial pressure Posttraumatic seizures

Diagnostic Tests

Identifying the severity of a brain injury involves history, observation, neurologic examination, and diagnostic testing. Ask questions about how the injury occurred, the child's initial responses and current responses, any loss of consciousness or confused behavior, and the child's memory of the event. Important elements of the history include the following:

- If the injury resulted from a fall: What was the distance fallen? What surface did the head strike? Where on the head was the primary impact?
- Did the child lose consciousness (for how long), or did the child act confused or dazed after the injury?
- Did the child have a seizure or vomit?

Practice Alert

Any infant who arrives in the emergency department with seizures, failure to thrive, vomiting, lethargy, respiratory irregularities, or coma should be evaluated for child abuse, particularly shaken baby syndrome or shaken impact syndrome. The infant has a relatively large head with relatively weak neck muscles. A frustrated adult can shake an infant and cause inertial injuries (acceleration and deceleration) to the head that tear nerve fibers as the brain moves back and forth in the skull. Throwing the infant down onto a solid surface further increases the forces with which the brain hits the back of the skull (Dubowitz & Lane, 2011). See Chapter 20 for more information about nursing management of child abuse.

Neurologic evaluation with the pediatric Glasgow Coma Scale is performed frequently to describe the level of consciousness, to determine severity of the brain injury, and to detect changes in consciousness over time (see Table 33–5). Review the discussion of altered

Clinical Manifestations Specific Brain Injuries

BRAIN INJURY AND ETIOLOGY	CLINICAL MANIFESTATIONS
Subdural hematoma Result of severe brain trauma, including shaken child syndrome More common in infants less than 1 year of age Inertial forces tear veins bridging the subdural space; a venous hematoma forms beneath the dura and presses on the surface of the brain 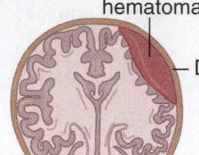 Bleeding occurs between dura and brain	Signs appear about 48–72 hours after the injury and include: ■ Gradual change in level of consciousness (confusion, agitation, or lethargy) ■ Hemiparesis or eye deviation ■ Nausea or vomiting ■ Headache ■ Retinal hemorrhages in both eyes ■ Pupil on side of injury may be fixed and dilated ■ Seizures
Epidural hematoma Rare in children, especially those younger than 4 years Results from blunt trauma falls, motor vehicle crashes, assaults, or baseball to temporal area Arterial or venous bleeding occurs between the skull and the dura; associated with skull fracture 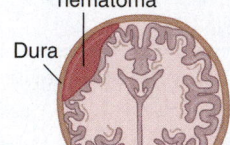 Bleeding occurs between dura and skull	■ Minimal or absent symptoms at time of injury ■ Then, rapid deterioration in mental status and signs of increased ICP ■ Headache or full fontanel ■ Paresis of cranial nerves III and VI ■ Papilledema ■ Fixed and dilated pupil
Cerebral contusion Bruising on surface of brain from hitting the skull associated with coup and contrecoup injuries, including the base of the brain as it moves across the bony prominences in the base of the skull Common on frontal and temporal lobes Most common TBI	■ Altered levels of consciousness ranging from confusion and disorientation to being obtunded ■ Focal symptoms depending on the area of injury
Diffuse axonal injury Results from rapid acceleration-deceleration injuries, such as with motor vehicle crash or shaken child syndrome Nerve fibers torn in both hemispheres of the cerebrum and other brain areas Frequent accompanying trauma to other organ systems or to the spine	■ Immediate loss of consciousness ■ Unconsciousness lasting longer than 6 hours ■ Abnormal movements or posturing ■ Seizures ■ Increased intracranial pressure ■ Difficulty regulating blood pressure and breathing
Subarachnoid hemorrhage Associated with severe head injuries such as intracranial hematomas or contusions, result from tearing of arteries or veins in the subarachnoid space	■ Progressive decrease in level of consciousness ■ Severe headache, nausea, and vomiting ■ Ipsilateral pupil dilation ■ Diplopia ■ Hemiparesis ■ Nuchal rigidity
Intracerebral hematoma Often result of acceleration-deceleration injury or secondary to impalement with hemorrhage to frontal or temporal lobe 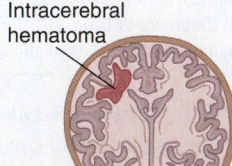 Bleeding occurs within cerebrum	■ Focal symptoms depend on size and location of hematoma, such as epilepsy

states of consciousness at the beginning of the chapter for further details. Cranial nerves are assessed, including pupils (see Table 7–18 and Table 33–6). The skull is palpated for any depressions. Deep tendon reflexes and signs of extremity weakness are assessed.

Laboratory tests include a complete blood cell count, blood chemistry, coagulation tests, toxicology screening, and urinalysis. Radiographs detect fractures of the skull and cervical vertebrae. A CT scan detects fractures, intracranial bleeding, swelling, and diffuse axonal injury. An MRI is used during recovery to determine the extent of brain damage. PET scans measure blood flow in the brain. Many children with head injuries have other injuries. A fracture indicates a more severe injury. Even though cervical spine injuries are rare, children with moderate and severe brain injury should have a cervical spine injury ruled out by radiologic examination.

Clinical Therapy

The initial management of a child with a severe brain injury is based on the child's physiologic status. When the child has altered consciousness, the airway must be stable and patent. Oxygen is administered to prevent hypoxemia. If indicated, the child is intubated (and in some cases chemically paralyzed) to protect the airway and prevent aspiration. Mechanical ventilation with supplemental oxygen at the child's normal respiratory rate is used to maintain the oxygenation level. Hyperventilation is not used unless the child has signs of herniation (Huh & Raghupathi, 2009). Cerebral perfusion pressure (difference between the mean arterial pressure minus the ICP or central venous pressure) must be maintained to ensure that the blood flow to the brain delivers oxygen and nutrients and removes accumulated neurotoxins. Surgery to remove hematomas may be performed as an emergency.

Invasive procedures may be necessary to reduce increased intracranial pressure. Burr holes may be made or more extensive surgery performed as a method of evacuating a lesion or hematoma. A ventriculostomy catheter may be placed to drain cerebrospinal fluid and to monitor pressure when brain swelling reaches dangerous heights (refer to the Skills Manual ⬭). Decompressive craniectomy may be considered as a last resort when ICP cannot be otherwise controlled. Therapeutic hypothermia is being investigated as a treatment to protect the brain.

Practice Alert

In the child with moderate head injury, the oxygen saturation should remain over 95%. For the severely injured child who is intubated, monitor arterial blood gas results. The Pao_2 of 70 to 100 mmHg indicates satisfactory management of oxygenation.

Hypovolemic shock therapy Shock is treated aggressively with fluid boluses using isotonic IV solutions (0.9% normal saline or lactated Ringer's) until the blood pressure can sustain the appropriate cerebral perfusion pressure. Keep the head of the bed flat until adequate cerebral perfusion pressure is ensured and maintained at greater than 40 mmHg or higher as appropriate for age (Huh & Raghupathi, 2009). Inotropic medications may be used to maintain the blood pressure and ensure perfusion if cerebral edema is present. Ongoing fluid administration is focused on maintaining the blood pressure level within a normal range for age.

Increased intracranial pressure management The goal is to maintain ICP to 20 mmHg or less (Huh & Raghupathi, 2009). If increased ICP occurs and is not relieved, brain shifting in the cranium begins, which may be a precursor of herniation. Hypoxia and hypercapnia

---

BOX 33–13	Research: Hypothermia

A randomized controlled trial involving 225 children studied the use of hypothermia to treat severe TBI. Children in the experimental group were cooled to 32.5°C for 24 hours within 8 hours of injury. Children in the control group were maintained at 37°C. No improvement in outcomes was found for the hypothermia group, and it is possible that hypothermia increases mortality (Hutchison, Ward, Lacroix, et al., 2008).

---

have disastrous effects on cerebral function, as they can cause vasodilation and increased ICP. Continuous capnography is essential to monitor for hypercarbia. Mechanical ventilation with 100% oxygen at the child's normal respiratory rate is used in the first 24 hours after injury to maintain oxygenation levels. Sedation, analgesia, and paralytic agents may be administered to eliminate the child's resistance to mechanical ventilation, relieve pain, and lower the ICP (Huh & Raghupathi, 2009). Hyperthermia is avoided because it increases cell death in severe TBI. See Box 33–13 for research on hypothermia.

In children with severe brain injury and increased ICP, invasive ICP monitoring and CSF drainage may be initiated, particularly if the child is sedated and cannot be evaluated by physical signs. Treatment for increased ICP is started when the intracranial pressure is greater than or equal to 20 mmHg. Mannitol or hypertonic saline (3%) may be administered to decrease the intracranial pressure. The child may be placed in a chemically induced coma to reduce brain activity during this acute care phase. See the Medications table on page 1200.

If there is no cervical spine injury, the head of the bed is elevated up to 30 degrees. The child's head is kept in the midline to promote venous (jugular) drainage. Hip flexion is avoided. The child's body temperature is kept within normal limits. The environment is kept as quiet as possible. A urinary catheter is inserted to monitor output, and electrolytes should be checked frequently to ensure that glucose and sodium levels stay within targeted ranges. Nutritional support should be started early with enteral nutrition using a postpyloric feeding tube to decrease risk of aspiration.

Rehabilitation care Initial stages of rehabilitation are made during the acute phase of management to prevent complications from immobilization, disuse, and neurologic dysfunction. Physical therapists, occupational therapists, speech-language specialists, and social workers all play vital roles in the rehabilitation process. When long-term rehabilitation is needed, the primary goals are to improve mobility, to perform basic self-care skills (bathing, grooming, dressing, and feeding), and to regain language skills. Moderate and severe TBI may result in permanent disability, such as epilepsy, motor and cognitive impairments, learning problems, hearing and vision impairments, communication problems, and behavioral or emotional problems. Difficulties with learning skills are common, such as with short-term memory, attention span, goal setting, problem solving, and sequencing multistep actions (Catroppa & Anderson, 2009).

Reliable predictions of outcome following a severe TBI cannot be made until 6 to 12 months postinjury. Sometimes despite all efforts, the child dies due to the consequences of the TBI. (See Table 18–1 for brain death criteria.)

Nursing Management

The child with a moderate or severe TBI is hospitalized. A severe TBI can be life threatening, so care is provided in a critical care unit. Nursing

Medications Used for Increased Intracranial Pressure

MEDICATION	ACTION	NURSING MANAGEMENT
Analgesics and sedatives Benzodiazepines Opioids Barbiturates	Sedation and reduction of pain and anxiety help prevent increases in ICP. These medications reduce the ICP by decreasing the cerebral metabolic rate. The combined effects of these medications are more likely to cause respiratory depression and the need for assisted ventilation.	■ ICP monitoring is needed to accurately monitor neurologic status. ■ Monitor respiratory status with pulse oximetry and blood gases. ■ Monitor blood pressure. Maintain the systolic pressure at 80 mmHg or higher to ensure an adequate cerebral blood flow rate. ■ Monitor physiologic responses (heart rate, blood pressure, and ICP) to assess adequacy of pain management. ■ When mechanical ventilation is needed, suction airway secretions to maintain airway patency.
Mannitol	The ICP is lowered for about 75 minutes by reducing blood viscosity, leading to reflex vasoconstriction of the arterioles and decreased cerebral blood volume. In addition, serum osmolality increases, pulling fluid out of the brain cells into the intravascular space and decreasing cellular edema, an effect lasting about 6 hours.	■ Carefully monitor ICP as well as intake and output. Rebound increased ICP may occur 12 hours after dose. ■ Monitor serum osmolality so it is maintained at less than 320 mOsm/L to prevent renal toxicity and hypotension. ■ Monitor serum and urine electrolytes to detect syndrome of inappropriate antidiuretic hormone secretion.
Hypertonic saline (3%) continuous IV infusion	Has an osmotic effect similar to mannitol. Used in children when signs of herniation are present. It is believed to preserve the intravascular volume.	■ Administered in a continuous infusion. Carefully monitor the IV site for extravasation. ■ Monitor serum osmolality and keep at less than 320 mOsm/L to prevent renal toxicity and hypotension. ■ Serum sodium levels should be gradually returned to normal when hypertonic saline is discontinued.
Anticonvulsants	Anticonvulsants may be used prophylactically to prevent seizures in the first 7 days following injury. Seizures may cause hyperthermia and increased ICP.	■ Monitor the child for seizures. ■ Immediate medications are needed to stop seizure activity.

Source: *Data from Huh, J. W., & Raghupathi, R. (2009). New concepts in treatment of pediatric traumatic brain injury. Anesthesiology Clinics of North America, 27, 213–240; Little, R. D. (2008). Increased intracranial pressure. Clinical Pediatric Emergency Medicine, 9, 83–87; Mansfield, R. T. (2007). Severe traumatic brain injury. Clinical Pediatric Emergency Medicine, 8, 156–164.*

management of the child with a severe TBI focuses on assessment of changes in neurologic status and vital signs, management of clinical therapies, prevention of complications, and support for the family.

Nursing Assessment and Diagnosis

Assess the child's ability to maintain an open airway and regulate breathing. Assess circulation. As level of consciousness drops, protective gag and cough reflexes are lost, and the tongue obstructs the airway. If the child is intubated, assess the CO_2 monitor on the endotracheal tube to confirm tube placement in the trachea.

Neurologic Assessment

Assess the child's neurologic status frequently using the guidelines in Table 33–3, and compare the child's status to baseline findings, noting improvement, stability, or deterioration. Evaluate the child's level of consciousness using the pediatric Glasgow Coma Scale (see Table 33–5). Assess the pupils for size and reactivity. Check the cranial nerves for impaired functioning. Note flexor or extensor posturing. The cause of any deterioration must be quickly identified and appropriate interventions taken.

Clinical Tip

A child who has a decreased level of consciousness shortly after a brain injury may have had a posttraumatic seizure and may still be in the postictal state.

Monitor vital signs closely. Stay alert for changes in vital signs and behavior that indicate increased ICP and potential progression to Cushing triad (bradycardia, irregular respirations, and increased systolic blood pressure with a widening pulse pressure). See the Clinical Manifestations table on page 1153. Changes in vital signs may indicate hypoxia, decreased perfusion, shock, or increased ICP. If a ventricular catheter or bolt is inserted, monitor the actual ICP readings.

Suspect that the child with increased ICP is in pain, even when unresponsive. Observe for physiologic and behavioral signs of pain. See Chapter 21 🔗.

Psychologic Assessment

Assess the family's coping with the uncertainty of the child's severe injury and the support systems available to them. Assess their ability to understand the information about the child's status. They may feel guilty if the child was in their care when the life-threatening injury occurred. Refer to Chapter 17 🔗.

The following nursing diagnoses may be appropriate for the child with a serious traumatic brain injury:

- Tissue Perfusion: Cerebral, Risk for Ineffective, related to hypoventilation, hypovolemia, and/or reduction of arterial blood flow to the brain due to increased ICP
- Aspiration, Risk for, related to decreased level of consciousness and loss of protective reflexes
- Skin Integrity, Risk for Impaired, related to bed rest and immobility
- Fluid Volume: Imbalanced, Risk for related to therapies for reducing ICP
- Coping: Family, Compromised related to life-threatening injury to child

NANDA-I © 2012

Planning and Implementation

Critical Care

Nursing care focuses on maintaining cardiopulmonary function and cerebral perfusion, preventing complications, promoting recovery, and providing emotional support. The goal of nursing management is to prevent secondary injury and to promote return to an optimal level of function.

Maintain Cerebral Perfusion

In the child who is severely injured, measures are taken to reduce or minimize increases in the ICP. Maintain oxygenation and ventilation to prevent hypoxemia. Keep the airway clear and cautiously suction the airway only when excessive secretions are present, as suctioning can increase the ICP. Administer intravenous fluids at the rate that maintains hydration and blood pressure thus ensuring an adequate cerebral perfusion pressure. Monitor the effects of medications on hydration status. Report any sign of decreased oxygenation, bradycardia, and lowered blood pressure to the physician immediately.

When an intraventricular catheter or bolt is inserted, stabilize and protect the catheter or bolt to keep it from becoming displaced. Position the child with head at midline position either on a flat surface or with the bed elevated 15 to 30 degrees to prevent compression of the neck blood vessels. Elevating the head may help promote venous drainage from the cerebral circulation; however, elevation should only be used if the cerebral perfusion pressure is maintained. Avoid excessive flexion of the hips and neck that could slow venous circulation. The child may also be placed in a side-lying position with the head in neutral position (not flexed or extended). Logroll the child for turning to prevent intra-abdominal and intrathoracic pressure that could cause an increase in ICP.

Reduce Intracranial Pressure

Reduce physiologic stresses on the body that can increase ICP. Provide careful thermoregulation and keep the environment quiet. Minimize unpleasant stimuli when possible, such as jarring the bed. Minimize pain associated with painful procedures, and control pain associated with increased ICP. Monitor the effect of nursing procedures on the level of ICP and determine if clustering procedures is better than spreading procedures over time. Administer medications as ordered. Mannitol or hypertonic saline may be administered to reduce ICP. Sedatives may be given to decrease the metabolic demands on the brain. Pain medication is provided to promote comfort.

Promote Nutrition

Nutrition is implemented as soon as possible to promote wound healing. Enteral feeding may be used initially, slowly progressing to oral foods as tolerated. Fluids are given to meet daily fluid requirements or to maintain the child's blood pressure within normal ranges for age.

Provide Routine Care

Provide oral care to keep mucous membranes moist and intact, but use care when the gag reflex is absent. Pad and cushion bony prominences, provide skin care, and change the child's position frequently. The eyes should be protected from corneal irritation with ophthalmic ointment and patching. Prevent constipation with stool softeners and suppositories as needed. The bed side rails should be padded to protect the child if a seizure occurs.

Promote Recovery and Prevent Physical Deformities

Physical, occupational, and speech therapy should begin in the hospital, and often in the intensive care unit. Perform passive range of

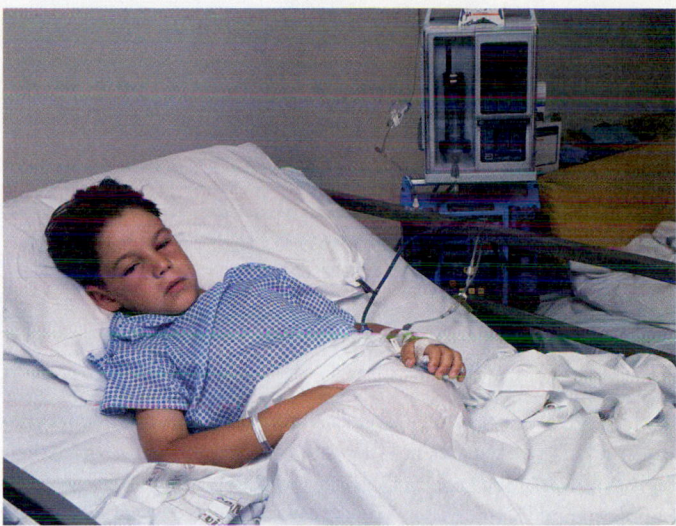

FIGURE 33–22 ■ This child experienced a severe traumatic brain injury, and he is just beginning to regain consciousness after 2 weeks. His intracranial pressure has stabilized after aggressive care in the pediatric intensive care unit. He is fed through a gastrostomy tube. Plans for his transfer to an inpatient rehabilitation program are proceeding.

motion exercises to prevent contractures. Splints may be used to position extremities in functional positions. Work with therapists to reinforce exercises and help teach parents the techniques so they can work with the child in the hospital and at home. The nurse can reinforce what has been done during these sessions, noting positive changes.

After the child survives the critical injury and is moved to the pediatric care unit, begin promoting general awareness when the child is ready by using toys, books, music, or games based on the child's age and ability. Encourage parents to bring in favorite toys, stuffed animals, and recordings of the child's favorite music or family members talking. Assist the family to provide stimulation but to also provide quiet when the child displays agitation (Figure 33–22 ■).

Provide Emotional Support

Nurses, social workers, physicians, psychologists, rehabilitation therapists, and members of the clergy can support and help parents adjust to having a child with a new disability. Encourage parents to participate in the child's care.

Despite all care, the child with a serious brain injury may die. See Table 18–1 🔗 for brain death criteria. Provide support to the family while testing for brain death criteria is performed. Allow the family to have time with the child to make important decisions regarding termination of life support and potential organ donation. See Chapter 18 🔗.

Discharge Planning and Home Care Teaching

Children with serious TBIs may be transferred to an inpatient rehabilitation center to promote optimal achievement of function. Other children may have outpatient rehabilitation prescribed, and thus home care needs should be identified and addressed well in advance of discharge. If the child's condition qualifies for inpatient rehabilitation, encourage the family to visit the rehabilitation center to learn more about the care that will be provided and the family's role in the child's care. Rehabilitation focuses on augmenting abilities regained during recovery and teaches adaptive compensation for lost function. For children with disabilities, determine what adaptations and assistive technology are needed in the home, such as a wheelchair, walker,

Legal and Ethical Considerations
Social Security Supplemental Income

A child with a TBI that results in severe functional limitations may qualify for Social Security's Supplemental Security Income (SSI). The child must have a physical or mental condition that seriously limits his or her activities and that is expected to last at least one year or result in death (Social Security Online, 2011). The child may become eligible when the parents' or child's income meets federal poverty guidelines, which might occur if a parent needs to stop working to provide full-time care for the child.

braces, or special bed. A case manager is often needed to coordinate services and resources during rehabilitation. Social services intervention may be needed when TBI results from child abuse or shaken baby syndrome. See Legal and Ethical Considerations: Social Security Supplemental Income.

Give parents information about home care for children with mild and moderate TBIs and possible behaviors to expect from the child. See the discussion on concussion below.

Care in the Community

Home care nursing may be important for the child with an acquired neurologic dysfunction and prolonged altered consciousness. The home care nurse can assume the role of case manager for the child and make sure the environment is safe. The nurse can also teach the family how to care for the child's needs, monitor intake of fluids and nutrition, as well as position the child and protect the skin over pressure areas from skin breakdown. See Chapter 36 🖉 for information on pressure ulcers. During the acute rehabilitation phase, physical therapy may be provided in the home to help educate the parents to appropriately position the child and exercise the muscles to reduce contractures and to promote improved functioning. Regular follow-up visits are needed to assess the child's progress and to modify the treatment plan. The family of a child with a significant brain injury will need continuing psychologic support, case management, and linkage to rehabilitation services that may help promote improvements in the child's functioning. See Legal and Ethical Considerations: Traumatic Brain Injury Act.

Children with moderate or severe traumatic brain injuries may require academic accommodations. Children with moderate injuries commonly have problems with attention, problem solving, and speed of information processing that compromise their school performance, as well as behavioral problems (e.g., impulsivity, irritability, frustration, apathy, aggression, and social withdrawal). Neuropsychologic testing is needed to identify the subtle learning disabilities that are not usually revealed on standardized school achievement tests. Educational accommodations needed are usually different from

Legal and Ethical Considerations
Traumatic Brain Injury Act

Public Law 104-166, the Traumatic Brain Injury Act, was enacted by Congress in 1996 to prevent brain injuries and to minimize the severity of dysfunction as a result of brain injury by providing funding to states to identify mechanisms to improve access to services. States apply for funding to develop services to promote rehabilitation and recovery for individuals with TBI and to educate families of victims about resources available.

those made for children with other learning disabilities. The severity of deficits and functional capabilities may influence whether the best resources for the child are in a mainstreamed or separate classroom. Future neuropsychologic testing is often needed as the child progresses to different developmental stages or when educational demands increase, such as deductive reasoning and organizational abilities needed in middle school and high school. The brain injury impairs new learning more than the retention of prior learning. Children who experience a brain injury at a young age may be at a special disadvantage because they have not had the time to store knowledge and develop learning strategies.

The child or adolescent who is facing long-term rehabilitation requires support to adjust to the disability and to find the strength to maximize his or her abilities. Identify recreational opportunities for the child with disabilities to promote exercise and self-esteem. The adolescent may need to gain vocational skills and learn to live independently. Refer parents to the Brain Injury Association for further information.

Prevention of brain injury is another important role of the nurse. Encourage parents to require children to use protective helmets for bicycling, skateboarding, in-line skating, and other sports. Parents should be encouraged to wear a helmet themselves as role models. Encourage parents to monitor playgrounds for appropriate use of wood chips or cushioning tiles to reduce severity of injuries associated with falls.

Evaluation

Examples of expected outcomes of nursing care for the family and child with TBI include the following:

- The child's cerebral perfusion pressure is maintained at a rate that sustains oxygenation of the brain.
- The child regains consciousness allowing rehabilitation to begin.
- Prevention of physical deformities through range of motion exercises to maintain muscle function and splinting occurs during the acute recovery stages.
- The parents are educated to provide appropriate care for the child at home.
- The child receives appropriate educational resources to promote learning.

Concussion or Mild Brain Injury

A concussion is a mild TBI that usually results from a direct blow to the head, face, neck, or other part of the body. The blow causes an impulsive force to be transmitted to the head, with a rapid onset of short-term functional impairment that may or may not involve loss of consciousness, but signs resolve spontaneously (Halstead, Walter, & the Council on Sports Medicine and Fitness, 2010). The signs are primarily caused by acceleration-deceleration and rotational forces that may cause stretching, compression, or shearing of nerve fibers as the brain moves within the skull, as well as disruption of brain chemicals responsible for brain functioning. No structural abnormality is seen on radiographic imaging.

Concussions account for 144,000 emergency department visits each year in children and adolescents less than 20 years of age (Meehan & Mannix, 2010). Children between 8 and 13 years of age account for 35% of these visits, potentially because of increased participation in organized sports (Bakhoa, Lockhart, Myers, et al., 2010). Sports-related concussions represent 8.9% of all high school athletic injuries (Halstead et al., 2010). Sports associated with higher rates of concussion in children and adolescents include football, soccer, basketball, ice hockey, and lacrosse (Halstead et al., 2010). Other common activities associated with concussion include falls from bicycles, snow skiing, skateboarding, and horseback riding (Bakhoa et al., 2010).

Clinical manifestations of concussions include disturbances in physical, cognitive, emotional, and sleep-related domains (Halstead et al., 2010; McGuire & McCambridge, 2011):

- *Physical*—headache, sensitivity to light or noise, dazed, visual problems, balance problems, fatigue, and nausea and vomiting
- *Cognitive*—feeling foggy or sluggish, difficulty concentrating and remembering, confused about recent events, answers slowly
- *Emotional*—irritable, sad, nervous, more emotional than usual
- *Sleep*—drowsy, sleeps more or less than normal, difficulty falling asleep

Pediatric concussive syndrome, believed to be caused by an injury to the brainstem, is seen in children who are under 3 years of age. Toddlers seem stunned at the time of injury but do not lose consciousness. Later, however, these children become pale, clammy, and lethargic, and they may vomit.

Initial evaluation of the child injured in an organized sport should occur on the sideline by asking questions that detect subtle problems with orientation, memory, and concentration. Amnesia is an important sign of a more serious injury, so questions about events before and after the injury should be asked. In the health center or emergency department, the child should have a complete physical examination and history that identifies any prior mild brain injuries. Brain imaging studies are usually normal and are usually ordered only when an intracranial structural injury may be present (Halstead et al., 2010). Computerized neuropsychologic tests are available to test a high school athlete's baseline performance for comparison after concussion to monitor recovery.

Treatment is supportive. Children are observed in the emergency department for several hours before being sent home with instructions to the parents to watch the child closely for decreased responsiveness. Any child who is unconscious for more than 5 minutes or has amnesia of the event may be admitted to the hospital or observed in a short-stay unit to rule out other injury. All cognitive activities, including cell phone texting, television and computer use, and loud music, should be limited in the first few days after injury. Physical activities are gradually increased, particularly before permitting the child to return to organized sports. Before returning to play, the child should be symptom-free and off all analgesia for headache, and have no symptoms with graduated increases in physical activity. The child may start with light aerobic activity, and progress to running drills, to noncontact training, to full practice, and then return to play if the child remains asymptomatic at each stage (McGuire & McCambridge, 2011). Symptoms usually disappear within several weeks but may last up to 6 months.

Young athletes suffering a second concussion before complete recovery from the first may develop *second impact syndrome*. This injury results in acute brain swelling, neurologic or cognitive deficits, and sometimes death from the cumulative effect of these concussions.

BOX 33–14	**Community Care: Mild TBI and School Return**

Strategies to assist the child or adolescent with a mild TBI to return to school over the first few weeks include the following (Halstead et al., 2010):

- The child may need to stay home for a few days and return with shortened school days.
- Recognize that the child may look well, but be aware that the student will have difficulty with concentration.
- After return to school, give extra time to complete make-up assignments, and reduce assignments as possible.
- Reduce the homework and class workload, and allow more time to complete work.
- Do not give standardized tests during the recovery period as scores will likely not be reflective of the student's capability.
- Physical activity should be limited and gradually increased.

Recommendations should be followed for the management of sports-related concussions to reduce the risk of disability and death.

Even though the child looks normal within days of a mild or moderate TBI, the parents and teachers need to be aware that brain healing takes up to 6 weeks. Typical behavior during this period may include any of the following: tiring easily, memory loss or forgetfulness, easy distractibility, difficulty concentrating, difficulty following directions, irritability or short temper, and needing help starting and finishing tasks (Box 33–14). The child should not return to a full school schedule too quickly to prevent fatigue and frustration.

Prevention of brain injuries is an important nursing role. Encourage the use of appropriate helmets for the activity or sport.

Specific Head Injuries

Scalp Injuries

Injuries to the scalp, which can be caused by falls, blunt trauma, or penetration of a foreign body, are usually benign. Although bleeding may be extensive, hypovolemia or shock is uncommon unless the patient is an infant.

Lacerations should be irrigated with copious amounts of sterile normal saline solution and inspected for bony fragments or depressions, cerebrospinal fluid leakage with a tear of the dura mater, or debris. If the injury is simple, the laceration can be sutured and the child discharged from the emergency department. If not, a neurosurgeon should be consulted.

Skull Fractures

A fracture to any of the eight cranial bones is caused by a considerable force to the head. The types of skull fracture include the following:

- **Linear fracture**—most common type of fracture, can potentially be caused by child abuse; may have overlying hematoma or soft tissue swelling; usually no symptoms
- **Depressed skull fracture**—break in skull itself or an area shattered into many fragments; pieces of bone may be depressed into brain tissue with hematoma forming on top
- **Basilar fracture**—fracture at the base of the skull; may involve the frontal, ethmoid, sphenoid, temporal, or occipital bones; a dural tear may be present; increases risk for meningitis

The skull fracture of a newborn in association with a traumatic birth is often a linear fracture or a depressed "ping-pong" fracture (Doumouchtsis & Arulkumaran, 2008).

Diagnosis is made by visual inspection, palpation, and a plain radiograph or CT scan. Any area of the skull with swelling or a hematoma should be evaluated for possible fracture. Diagnosis of a basilar skull fracture is confirmed by signs of blood behind the tympanic membranes, CSF leakage from the nose or ears, periorbital ecchymosis (raccoon eyes), or bruising of the mastoid (Battle sign).

Treatment should always include neurosurgical consultation. Surgery may be required for debridement or to elevate bone fragments of a depressed skull fracture. Tetanus prophylaxis and antibiotic therapy may be prescribed in some cases. Some of these injuries may be associated with intracranial bleeding, cranial nerve injuries, and post-traumatic epilepsy.

Penetrating Injuries

Gunshot wounds to the head can damage tissue, bone, and vessels. Low-velocity bullets enter but do not exit the skull; instead they ricochet within the cranial vault, destroying brain tissue and vessels. Although the child may be conscious just after the injury, the level of consciousness quickly deteriorates due to the edema surrounding the penetration tract. High-velocity bullets, on the other hand, cause immediate, severe damage on impact. (See Chapter 20 🔴 for a discussion of violence in childhood.)

CT is used to evaluate gunshot trauma and to pinpoint the location of bullet and bone fragments as well as parenchymal damage. Treatment involves surgical debridement of the bullet tract, evacuation of any hematomas, and removal of accessible bone or bullet particles. A high percentage of children with gunshot wounds to the head die. Those who survive may suffer multiple focal deficits and seizures.

Impalement injuries may occur in children in association with projectiles or dog bites. All objects must be left in place and removed in the operating room by a neurosurgeon. The child with an impalement injury is at high risk for focal injury and infection. After surgery, children with this type of injury are managed as with other postoperative head injuries, with attention focused on level of consciousness, increased ICP, and infection control.

Spinal Cord Injury

Spinal cord injury occurs at a rate of 1.99 per 100,000 children, and only 10% of these injuries occur in children under age 10 years (Parent, 2010). Motor vehicle crashes (passenger and pedestrian) account for nearly 55% of cases, while the remainder are associated with sports such as football, ice hockey, bicycling, trampoline injuries, and driving an all-terrain vehicle (Mathison et al., 2008). Child abuse and penetrating injuries such as stabbing and gunshot wounds are other potential causes of spinal cord injury.

Etiology and Pathophysiology

The mechanism of injury and the direction of forces determine the type of lesion that occurs (Figure 33–23 ■). The increased elasticity of the pediatric spine predisposes it to injury. Hyperflexion injuries (e.g., extreme bending as occurs with whiplash or around a safety seat belt) produce tears or avulsions and fractures of vertebral bodies, as well as subluxation and dislocation. Rotation may cause joint dislocations or unstable spinal fractures. Hyperextension may result in the so-called hangman's fracture, ligament tears, avulsion fractures of vertebral bodies, and central or posterior spinal cord syndrome (damage to the center of the cord only). Compression fractures may occur when the child falls from a height.

Children are prone to specific kinds of spinal cord injuries due to the extreme mobility and flexibility of their spinal column. The upper cervical region (C1 to C3) is the most mobile section of the spine in children less than age 8 years. The vertebrae are also incompletely ossified in children under 9 years. The facet joints of the vertebrae are more shallow and horizontal, allowing them to slide over each other more easily. The young child's head is relatively large compared with the strength of the neck muscles. The ligaments supporting the neck and spinal column are more elastic and allow for more stretching between the vertebrae, but the spinal cord does not stretch. Thus, injuries are more likely to occur at the C1–C3 level in children under age 9 years, but injuries are more likely at the C4–C6 level in children 9 to 15 years.

Injuries can be caused by penetration (e.g., by a bullet), a significant force bending the vertebral column, compression of the vertebrae (a direct blow to the top of the head, e.g., football or diving injury), or dislocation of the vertebrae. The spinal cord can have tears, contusions, and even transection without bony damage. Table 33–8 on page 1206 describes the spinal cord injuries most common in children.

Clinical Manifestations

Spinal cord injuries are classified as complete or incomplete. Complete lesions are irreversible and involve a loss of sensory, motor, and autonomic function below the level of the injury. Incomplete lesions involve varying degrees of sensory, motor, and autonomic function below the level of injury. Hypotension, loss of bladder and bowel control, and loss of environmental thermoregulatory function are associated with autonomic dysfunction. The higher the level of spinal cord injury, the more severe the neurologic damage.

At the time of injury, the child may be flaccid and lose reflexes below the lesion due to **spinal shock,** spinal cord concussion resulting in a transient suppression of nerve function below the level of the acute injury. Some return of function occurs within the first 72 hours of injury. As neurologic recovery begins, spinal reflex activity returns and increasing spasticity below the level of the lesion is seen.

Children can experience neurogenic shock in which there is loss of vasomotor tone and sympathetic innervation of the heart, resulting in hypotension, bradycardia, and peripheral vasodilation (a form of distributive shock). See Chapter 26 🔴. Priapism may be seen. Respiratory compromise may be present due to paralysis of the diaphragm.

The child with a spinal cord injury is often a victim of multiple trauma and may display signs of hypovolemic shock resulting from other injuries, increased ICP, or respiratory depression.

Collaborative Care

The goal of collaborative care is to determine the extent of spinal cord injury and to aggressively treat the injury to reduce the potential for permanent disability.

Diagnostic Tests

Diagnosis is made by a detailed neurologic examination of motor, reflex, and sensory function, as well as radiographic studies. Radiographic studies include lateral cervical spine and anteroposterior and lateral views of the thoracic and lumbosacral spine to determine if a vertebral fracture or compression on the spinal cord is present. The child's immobilized position is unchanged until radiographs are read by a radiologist and the spine is declared uninjured. In addition, CT scanning, MRI, fluoroscopy, or myelography may be performed. See Box 33–15.

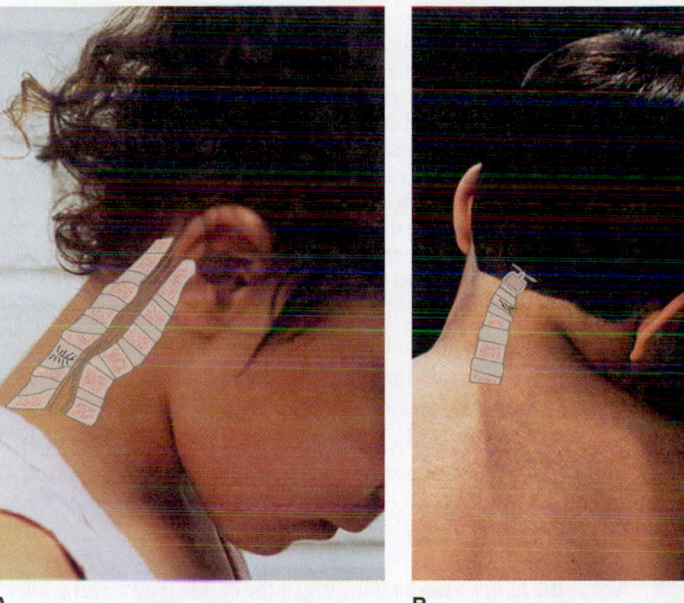
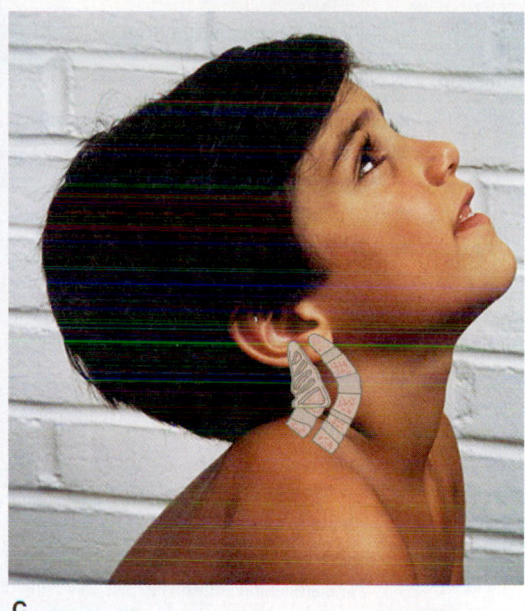

A   **B**   **C**

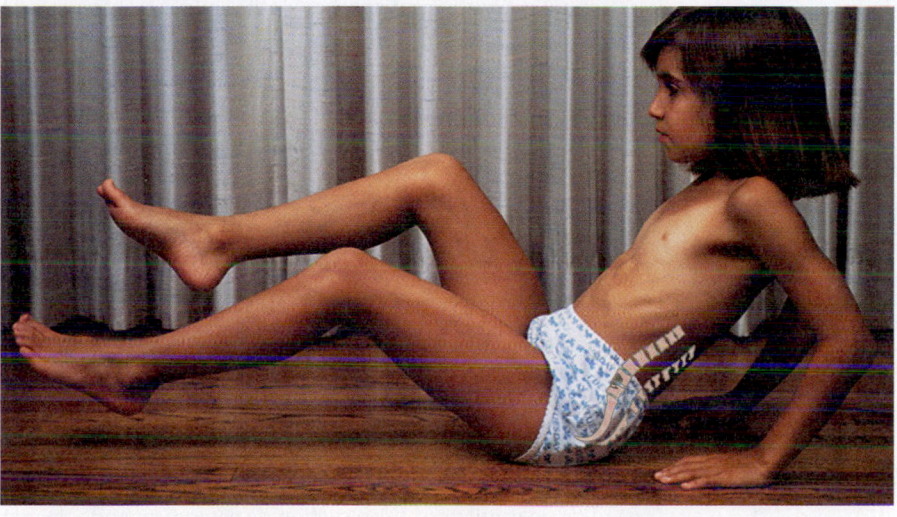
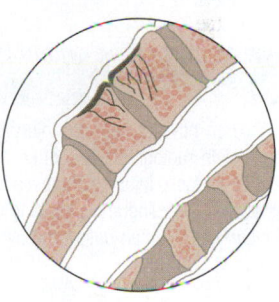

D

FIGURE 33–23 ■ Mechanics of injury to the spinal cord: *A,* hyperflexion often due to diving and frontal motor vehicle crashes; *B,* rotation in which the head and neck are twisted; *C,* hyperextension often due to rear-end motor vehicle crashes and falls; *D,* compression due to falls that put vertical pressure on the spinal column. Infants and young children are at higher risk for injury to the brain and spinal cord because of developing bones and muscles.

Clinical Therapy

Immediate stabilization and immobilization of the child with a suspected spinal injury from the scene of the injury is essential until radiographic evidence of spinal cord injury is confirmed or cleared. The child with a confirmed spinal cord injury may be placed in external immobilization with a halo device. Surgery to reduce and internally fixate the fracture may be performed for unstable fractures, dislocations, and progressive deformity. Decompression of the spinal cord and nerve roots may also be performed if transection is not complete or if compression by a clot, herniated disk, or other lesion is present and can be relieved.

To decrease neurologic sequelae in children with motor deficits, a high-dose methylprednisolone continuous infusion may be administered over 48 hours when the infusion is started within 3 to 8 hours of the injury (Mathison et al., 2008). Gastrointestinal prophylaxis is provided to reduce the risk for an ulcer. Other medications such as atropine and norepinephrine may be given to manage spinal shock. Intravenous fluid resuscitation is also performed if the child could have hypovolemic shock from other injuries. Complications of spinal cord injury include the following:

- Impaired respiratory function due to a paralyzed diaphragm or diminished vital capacity
- Scoliosis if injury occurs before the skeleton is mature
- Hip instability due to poor acetabular development
- Pathologic fractures of the long bones due to immobilization hypercalcemia
- Pressure sores
- Deep vein thrombosis
- Autonomic dysreflexia

TABLE 33–8	Spinal Cord Injuries in Children
SPINE REGION	**INJURY CHARACTERISTICS**
Cervical	▪ Site of a majority of spinal injuries in children under 10 years
	▪ Injury above C3 segment causes respiratory arrest and death without ventilatory support; many of these injuries are fatal
	▪ Diaphragm function present when injury is at C5 level
	▪ Quadriplegia, some function of upper extremities when injury is at C6–C7 level
	▪ Loss of sphincter function
	▪ Sensory level lost below the sternum
Thoracic	▪ Site of spinal injuries more common between 8 and 14 years
	▪ Full control of upper extremities including hands
	▪ Poor trunk balance
Thoracolumbar	▪ Full control of muscles in abdomen and upper back
	▪ Good trunk balance
Lumbar	▪ Most injuries at the L1–L3 level occur when children 4 to 8 years are restrained with lap belt only rather than child safety or booster seats during a motor vehicle crash (Mathison et al., 2008)
	▪ Below L3 may have functioning of muscles in upper leg
	▪ Loss of ankle and foot control

BOX 33–15	SCIWORA

Some young children have spinal cord injury without radiographic abnormality (SCIWORA) on a plain radiograph. It is often associated with a rear-end motor vehicle crash or direct facial injury that causes hyperextension of the cervical vertebrae. Unless additional radiographic imaging is performed, the child is believed to be free of injury. An MRI can detect the injury to ligaments and soft tissues (Looby & Flanders, 2011).

Spasticity, muscle atrophy, increased risk of respiratory problems, weight gain, osteoporosis, and other skeletal problems are long-term issues for many children. An interdisciplinary approach is required to manage the rehabilitation and long-term care needs of the child and family. The goal of rehabilitation is to promote independence in daily activities, as well as mobility, strength, power, and endurance.

Nursing Management

Nursing care focuses on monitoring vital signs, meeting nutritional needs, maintaining skin integrity, promoting independent functioning, encouraging therapeutic play, providing emotional support, and promoting rehabilitation.

Nursing Assessment and Diagnosis

Monitor Physiologic Status

Be alert for any changes in vital signs, especially those that may signify neurogenic shock (hypotension, bradycardia, and peripheral vasodilation), increased ICP (see the Clinical Manifestations table on page 1153), or autonomic dysreflexia. Monitor the child's respiratory status and vital capacity to determine the functioning of the diaphragm. Notify the physician immediately if autonomic dysreflexia occurs. Monitor intake and output. Monitor for bladder function and constipation. Assess the skin for integrity.

Practice Alert

Autonomic dysreflexia is a condition associated with injuries above the level of T6 that can be caused by constipation, a full bladder, sexual activity, pain, and diseases of the gastrointestinal tract (Schottler, Vogel, Chafetz, et al., 2009). It can become a medical emergency in which overactivity of the autonomic nervous system causes an abrupt onset of hypertension, cardiac arrhythmia, severe headaches, flushing above the level of the spinal cord lesion, and sweating. Treatment involves positioning the patient upright, loosening tight clothing, emptying the bladder, and eliminating any precipitating stimulus. The child's blood pressure and heart rate should be assessed every 2 to 5 minutes. Antihypertensive medications are given if hypertension is sustained. Prevention of autonomic dysreflexia involves an effective bowel and bladder program (Somani, 2009).

Monitor Neurologic Functioning

With higher cervical injuries, assess the cranial nerves as they may be affected by swelling around the cord. Assess for the return of segmental reflex function and change from flaccid tone to spasticity. Note any changes in level of sensation and motor function. Carefully check the immobilizing devices to ensure that the spine remains stable.

Family Coping

Assess the family's understanding of the child's injury and coping. Begin identifying family resources and needs for future home management of the child.

Examples of nursing diagnoses for the child with a spinal cord injury include:

- Breathing Pattern, Ineffective, related to lack of spinal nerve innervation of diaphragm
- Constipation, Risk for, related to immobility and loss of sphincter innervation
- Thermoregulation, Ineffective, related to spinal shock
- Skin Integrity, Risk for Impaired, related to inability to change positions independently
- Urinary Elimination, Impaired, related to loss of sphincter innervation

NANDA-I © 2012

Planning and Implementation

Some children with cervical lesions have tracheostomies performed to help maintain airway patency; others with very high lesions are dependent on ventilators. Keep suctioning equipment and other emergency equipment at bedside at all times.

Meet Nutritional Needs

Ensure adequate nutrition. A child with complete paralysis may require a gastrostomy tube. When the child is able to begin eating, feed soft foods slowly as the child may have some swallowing problems. Encourage the family to work with occupational therapists to learn strategies to feed the child and promote self-feeding.

Maintain Skin Integrity

Provide skin care to prevent skin breakdown and pressure sores. See Chapter 36 ⊘. Observe surgical sites and traction pin sites for signs of infection or inflammation. Perform regular traction pin site skin care according to facility guidelines.

Promote Independent Functioning

Reinforce the exercises and skills learned in physical and occupational therapy. Use supports, boots, footboards, splints, and braces as recommended by therapists to prevent contractures (Figure 33–24 ■). If hand mobility is limited, explore options for independence. Encourage the child to be as independent as possible while using a wheelchair. An important mobility goal is to achieve wheelchair transfer and to

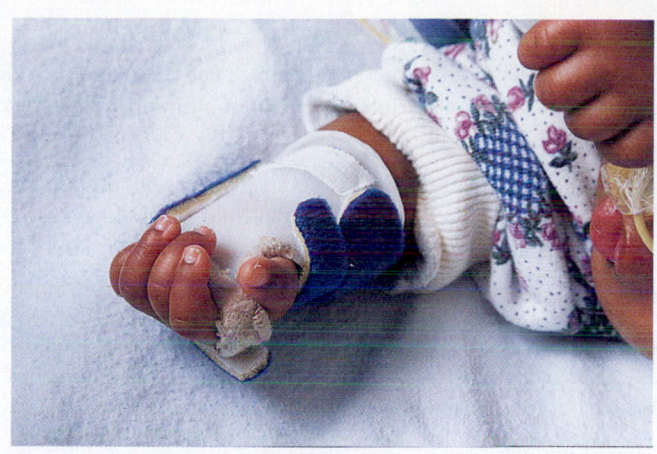

FIGURE 33–24 ■ Splints are often used to prevent contractures, thus maintaining optimal functioning of the child's hands or feet.

perform self-care. Identify adaptive equipment that makes it possible to achieve those goals.

When bladder and bowel sphincter control is impaired, bowel and bladder control may be hard to achieve. When urinary retention occurs, perform intermittent catheterizations on a regular schedule to prevent hydronephrosis, urinary tract infection, and kidney damage (see Chapter 31 🔗). Anticipate that constipation will occur and initiate bowel training with a diet high in fiber and the use of stool softeners.

Encourage Therapeutic Play

Therapeutic play appropriate for the child's developmental level is an important part of the healing process. Provide as many normal activities for the child as possible, but do not assign tasks that the child will have difficulty completing. Child life teachers or tutors can help the child keep up with schoolwork once the child is beyond the acute stage.

Television, DVDs, computer games, Internet connections, and music can offer diversion for prolonged hospitalization. Children with paraplegia can learn to use their arms and hands to play interactive games. Devices can also be adapted so the child can use the computer, play computer games, and manipulate the television or music devices. Assistive devices to provide recreation for the child with quadriplegia should also be identified.

Provide Emotional Support

Support the child or adolescent emotionally. Encourage the child to meet small, short-term goals, including those that involve self-care. Encourage the child to express fears and frustrations.

Be compassionate and understanding. Encourage siblings to visit, answer their questions honestly, and help them to discuss their feelings. Involve the parents and siblings in the care of the child as much as possible. When appropriate, encourage them to help with activities of daily living.

Discharge Planning and Home Care Teaching

Many children and adolescents with spinal cord injury are discharged to inpatient rehabilitation facilities. Assist with arrangements for the child's transfer from the hospital to the rehabilitation facility. Work closely with the child, parents, and other members of the healthcare team concerning placement. Home care needs, reintegration into educational programs, and safety issues should be identified and addressed well in advance of discharge from the rehabilitation facility. Refer families to social services, family counseling, and support groups if indicated.

Evaluation

Expected outcomes of nursing care include the following:

- Complications such as pressure ulcers and contractures are prevented.
- The child receives adequate nutrition to support growth.
- Bowel and bladder control are established.
- The child and family adapt to the child's disability.

Hypoxic-Ischemic Brain Injury (Drowning)

Drowning is defined as the process resulting in primary respiratory impairment from submersion/immersion in a liquid medium resulting in death (Figure 33–25 ■). *Submersion injury* is the term used when the child survives. This new definition replaces other commonly used terms such as near drowning, wet drowning, and dry drowning, and is the term used for children who do and do not survive. Drowning is a leading cause of injury death for children between 1 and 19 years of age, accounting for 1,093 deaths in 2008. Children between birth and 4 years and adolescents 15 to 19 years had the highest number of drowning deaths in 2008 (National Center for Health Statistics, National Vital Statistics System, 2011). In 2008, 3,800 children visited an emergency department after a submersion injury, and 60% of these children were hospitalized (Weiss & the

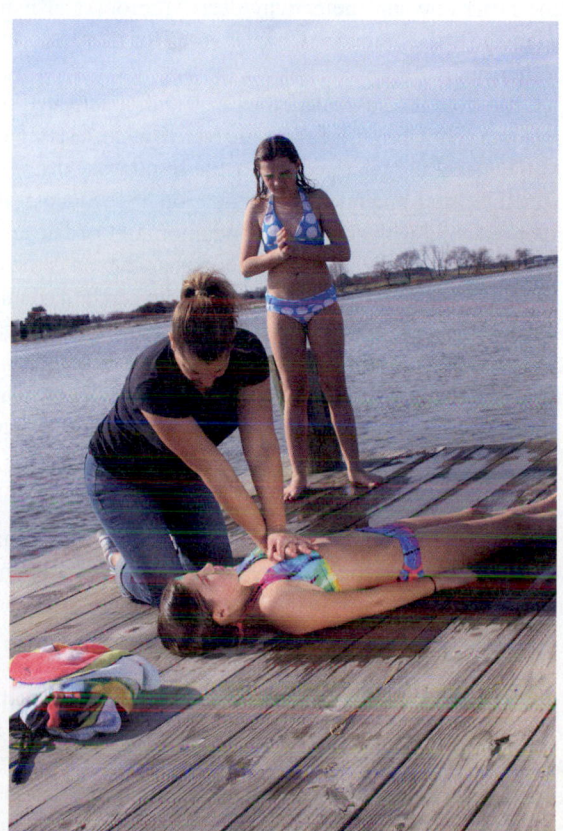

FIGURE 33–25 ■ The best chance of survival after a submersion injury is immediate CPR. Another bystander ran to call 911.

Committee on Injury, Violence, and Poison Prevention, 2010). Boys are more commonly affected than girls.

In children and adolescents less than age 20 years, 47% of drownings occur in fresh bodies of water, 32% occur in artificial pools, 9% occur in the home (e.g., bathtub or large buckets), and 4% occur in salt water. The bathtub is the most frequent location (78%) for infant drowning (Weiss & the Committee on Injury, Violence, and Poison Prevention, 2010). Adolescent drowning may be associated with risk-taking behaviors and alcohol or illicit substance use. Children with seizure disorders may experience a sudden and uncontrollable loss of body position that places them at a significantly higher risk for drowning.

Etiology and Pathophysiology

A child can drown in as little water as it takes to cover the nose and mouth. Infants and young children do not have the physical or cognitive ability to rescue themselves. The events preceding drowning follow a sequential pattern. The child trapped in water panics, struggles, attempts to move using swimming motions, and holds his or her breath. Then the child aspirates a small amount of water from the oropharynx, which triggers an involuntary laryngospasm lasting no longer than 2 minutes, leading to hypoxia. Because of the increasing panic and hypoxia, the child swallows more liquid. As the laryngospasm passes, the child breathes water into the lungs. The child may vomit and aspirate stomach contents as well. Aspirated water damages the surfactant in the lungs and impairs the capillary gas exchange in the alveoli, leading to hypoxemia. Hypothermia may result because the child's body cools more quickly in water than in air, and systemic perfusion decreases as a result. Hypothermia may be protective in young children as it decreases the tissue oxygen needs, slows the heart rate, and potentially delays the onset of hypoxia-related damage to the brain. See Chapter 36 for more information on hypothermia.

When the child is resuscitated, the lungs with inactivated surfactant develop a ventilation/perfusion mismatch, atelectasis, and poor lung compliance. Pulmonary edema, acute respiratory distress syndrome (ARDS), and pneumonia may develop. (See Chapter 25 for care of the child with ARDS and pneumonia.) Cardiac arrhythmias may result from hypothermia or hypoxia. Anoxia is the major insult associated with drowning. Anoxia leads to cerebral edema and increased ICP, leading to secondary cerebral injuries. Little can be done to resuscitate the brain, but with aggressive treatment, children may survive but with brain injury. Approximately 20% of surviving drowning victims have neurologic impairment that limits recovery (Wagner, 2009).

Clinical Manifestations

The child who has been immersed exhibits a wide variety of signs and symptoms depending on the length of time underwater, the temperature of the water, the response to the episode, and the initial treatment performed at the scene. The child may be pulseless and apneic. Children who are submerged for short periods (less than 5 to 10 minutes who are resuscitated at the scene) have few symptoms, and often fully recover without neurologic impairment. Signs and symptoms in the rescued child may be decreased level of consciousness ranging from stupor to total unresponsiveness, apnea or irregular respirations, gastric distention, and seizures. The child who waits for basic life support to be started for more than 10 minutes or is pulseless for more than 25 minutes is most likely to have a poor prognosis (Wagner, 2009).

Collaborative Care

The goal of collaborative care is to begin resuscitation and provide supportive diagnostic and clinical care to promote the child's recovery.

Diagnostic Tests

Initial diagnosis is made from physical assessment signs of spontaneous breathing and a heart rate. Once the child arrives in the emergency department, monitoring equipment is applied to assess for arrhythmias and oxygen saturation. Pupils are assessed for reactivity. The Glasgow Coma Scale is used to quantify and monitor the level of consciousness. Arterial blood gases are obtained to detect changes in gas exchange and pH. A chest radiograph may be ordered to establish baseline information about lung expansion and pulmonary integrity.

Clinical Therapy

Initial care of the child at the scene involves clearing the mouth of foreign matter and initiating cardiopulmonary resuscitation (CPR) as soon as the child is removed from the water. Immediate CPR at the scene is associated with the best outcomes. It is hoped that spontaneous respiratory effort by the child will begin within 5 minutes after removal from the water. Emergency personnel with a defibrillator should assess the heart rhythm and defibrillate if ventricular fibrillation is present. Emergency transport to a hospital emergency department should occur as soon as possible, even if spontaneous breathing is initiated.

Practice Alert

All submersion injury victims should be observed in a short-stay observation unit for 6 to 8 hours, even when initially asymptomatic. Most life-threatening complications, including respiratory distress and cerebral edema, usually develop within 7 hours after the incident. If the child remains asymptomatic, emergency department discharge may occur (Wagner, 2009).

In the emergency department, CPR is continued if necessary. Supplemental 100% oxygen is provided. If the child is unconscious, an airway is secured with an endotracheal tube. Mechanical ventilation may be used to keep the alveoli open, to promote adequate oxygenation, and to prevent hypercarbia. If the child is severely hypothermic (less than 30°C), active and passive rewarming actions are used during resuscitation. Intravenous fluids are administered to address hypovolemia. Once hypovolemia is corrected, fluids may be restricted, and diuretics may be used to help reduce the risk of cerebral edema. Vasopressor medications may be used to maintain a normal blood pressure.

Nursing Management

Nursing care of the child who survives a submersion incident focuses on monitoring the child's neurologic and cardiopulmonary status, providing emotional support to the family, and implementing needed therapies.

Nursing Assessment and Diagnosis

Assess the child's responsiveness, spontaneous respiratory efforts, and pulse. As resuscitation proceeds, monitor the child's respiratory status, oxygenation, cardiopulmonary function, and neurologic status. Frequent neurologic monitoring with the Glasgow Coma Scale, pupil checks for reactivity, and assessment of vital signs are performed.

Attach a cardiorespiratory monitor and pulse oximetry to provide continuous assessment information about the child's oxygenation status. Once the child has been resuscitated, the child is monitored frequently for signs of potential complications such as respiratory distress and worsening mental status indicating potential cerebral edema. Assess intake and output.

Parents and family members are assessed for their response and need for support associated with the child's life-threatening injury.

Examples of nursing diagnoses that may be appropriate for the child with drowning include:

- Tissue Perfusion: Cerebral, Risk for Ineffective, related to interruption of arterial blood flow
- Infection, Risk for, related to aspiration and trauma to the respiratory system
- Gas Exchange, Impaired, related to damage to the alveolar-capillary membranes of the lungs
- Decisional Conflict (continue or terminate life support for child) related to divergent sources of information
- Family Processes, Interrupted, related to situational crisis of child with life-threatening injury

NANDA-I © 2012

Planning and Implementation

Nursing management focuses on observation and support of cardiopulmonary and central nervous system function. The child with seriously compromised respiratory and neurologic status will be cared for in the intensive care unit. Oxygen and positive end-expiratory pressure or mechanical ventilation will be needed if acute respiratory distress develops. Position the child properly to promote respiratory function and venous drainage from the head. Note any change in respiratory status and blood gases, and notify the physician promptly.

Implement other nursing interventions for the child with altered states of consciousness as described on page 1154. If cerebral edema develops, implement nursing interventions as described on page 1199.

Family Support

Provide emotional support to the family. Be nonjudgmental and provide a forum for parents to express their feelings. Reassure parents who exhibit guilt reactions that their child is receiving all possible medical treatment. Parents may be faced with an unknown prognosis. See Chapter 18 🔗. Encourage parents to seek assistance from social workers, clergy, close friends, and relatives. Arrange for appropriate referrals. The child and family need support to work through the feelings surrounding the drowning incident, the unexpected

hospitalization, and an uncertain prognosis that may mean the child will not return to normal functioning. If the child's prognosis is poor, an ethical consult may be offered to educate the family about options for decision making regarding terminating life support.

Prevention

Another significant nursing role is prevention. Drowning can be prevented through education, legislation, and changes in the environment. Infants and toddlers should never be left unattended in a bathtub. Pool owners should erect climb-proof 5-foot fences around all four sides of the pool to reduce access to the pool by young children living in or visiting the home. If fencing is on three sides, the door to the pool area should be kept locked and have an alarm. Local ordinances may require such fences. Pool owners should learn CPR so that immediate resuscitation can begin if a child is found submerged. Hot tubs and pools should all have drain covers or other safety devices that prevent a child from having a limb or hair entrapped in a drain. Adolescents should learn the dangers of mixing alcohol and swimming. Five- and 10-gallon buckets should be kept empty when not used. Personal flotation devices should be used for recreational boating. Emphasize the importance of closely supervising children when near or in the water, whether in pools, at the beach or water park, or in the bathtub.

Discharge Planning

Home care needs should be identified and addressed well in advance of discharge when the child has neurologic impairment. Assign a case manager to the child with significant neurologic impairments so that long-term care options can be explored. Inpatient or outpatient rehabilitation services should be matched to the child's needs and family resources.

Evaluation

Expected outcomes of nursing care for the family and child with a drowning episode include the following:

- Consciousness is regained following rapid response cardiopulmonary resuscitation.
- Any change in mental status or respiratory distress is rapidly detected and managed.
- All family members learn and use drowning prevention strategies.

Chapter Highlights

- The nervous system is complete with all nerve cells at birth, but the number of glial cells and dendrites continues to increase until 4 years of age. Myelination continues throughout childhood.
- Altered level of consciousness may be caused by trauma, hypoxia, infection, poisoning, seizures, alcohol or substance abuse, endocrine or metabolic disturbances (e.g., diabetic ketoacidosis), electrolyte or acid–base imbalance, intracranial space-occupying lesion, stroke, and congenital structural defects.
- Monitor any child with a prolonged generalized seizure for electrolyte levels, glucose, blood gases, increasing fever, and abnormal blood pressure to identify any conditions that can be treated and reduce the risk of significant CNS injury. Carefully document the duration of the seizure or series of seizures to detect status epilepticus.
- Neurologic damage from bacterial meningitis often occurs in infants and young children despite early, aggressive management. The most common sequelae involve cranial nerves, especially the eighth, resulting in hearing loss, as well as seizures, developmental delay, and learning problems.
- Viral (aseptic) meningitis in most cases is not as virulent as bacterial meningitis, and the child with aseptic meningitis appears less ill than the child with bacterial meningitis.
- Encephalitis is usually caused by a virus, such as West Nile virus or herpes simplex 1, and has a high mortality rate. Presenting signs include a severe headache, fever, altered level of consciousness, and vomiting.
- Reye syndrome is an encephalopathy with a high mortality rate that is associated with aspirin use for a mild viral illness. Because most parents give children acetaminophen or ibuprofen rather than aspirin for flulike symptoms and varicella, Reye syndrome has become rare.
- Guillain-Barré syndrome is a peripheral neuropathy with an acute onset of rapidly developing symmetric motor weakness. It is caused by an immune response to an infectious organism, usually from a gastrointestinal or respiratory illness 1 to 3 weeks prior to onset.
- More than 80% of children experience a headache by late adolescence, and migraine is the most common type of benign headache in children. Other benign headache types are inflammatory (sinusitis) and tension.
- Microcephaly is a small brain that may be caused by chromosomal abnormalities, fetal insult, maternal infection, or destructive insult during infancy, such as infection, metabolic disorder, or anoxia.
- Hydrocephalus is caused by blockage of cerebrospinal fluid flow through normal channels and pathways or the impaired absorption of cerebrospinal fluid in the subarachnoid space and the arachnoid villi. It can be associated with a congenital condition or acquired from meningitis or intraventricular hemorrhage, tumor, or structural deformity.
- The more common types of neural tube defects include anencephaly (no development of the brain above the brainstem), encephalocele (protrusion of meningeal or skin-covered brain through the skull), and myelodysplasia or spina bifida.
- Myelodysplasia or spina bifida is a malformation of the spinal cord and spinal canal that may be associated with a protrusion of a meningeal sac filled with a portion of the spinal cord. It is the most common developmental disorder of the CNS. Its prevalence is decreasing due to the fortification of all enriched grain products with folate.
- Positional plagiocephaly, a flattened area of the occiput, occurs when infants placed on their backs to prevent sudden infant death syndrome do not change the position of the head during sleep. The weight of the infant head sometimes flattens the skull. It may be treated with a helmet device to help reshape the skull.
- Neurofibromatosis 1 is characterized by multiple café-au-lait spots, darker than the surrounding skin, that are 5 mm or larger in infants but grow to 15 mm in diameter during adolescence. Multiple benign tumors grow on or under the skin beginning during puberty.
- Most cases of cerebral palsy are characterized by spasticity and a lack of coordination. The risk for cerebral palsy is increased when an intrauterine infection is documented. Neonatal sepsis and hyperbilirubinemia also increase the child's risk of developing cerebral palsy.
- Irritability, jitteriness, high-pitched cry, and excessive sucking may be seen in infants having withdrawal from illicit substances. The infant may also have excoriated skin, especially on the heels, toes, hands, elbows, nose, or chin, because of continuous rubbing against the crib sheets.
- Traumatic brain injuries are the most common injuries during childhood. They result from falls, motor vehicle crashes, sports injuries, and child abuse. Traumatic brain injuries are responsible for a majority of injury-related deaths and disability in children.
- Concussions are associated with a transient impairment of consciousness resulting from the stretching, compression, and shearing of nerve fibers after an impact injury to the head. Impairment in consciousness may include amnesia, dizziness, memory or orientation impairment, and unsteady gait.
- Spinal cord injuries, although relatively rare in children, often result from significant forces such as from motor vehicle crashes. Because of the child's larger and heavier head, undeveloped vertebrae, and weaker neck muscles, cervical spine injuries are more common.
- Children who have the best outcomes following submersion injury include those submerged less than 5 minutes and those who need cardiopulmonary resuscitation for less than 10 minutes.

Clinical Reasoning in Action

INTRODUCTION

Return to the beginning of the chapter to review the case of 8-year-old Andy Davis, who has meningitis. Andy has a cochlear implant that increases his risk for development of meningitis; however, this is the first time he has developed it. He lives with his mother, a stepfather, and two brothers, 6-year-old Timmy and 2-year-old Zach. Both of Andy's parents work and have limited time that can be taken away from their jobs. Andy's father lives in another state, but he has called to stay informed about his progress. Andy's grandmother lives close by, so she helps the family by spending time with him in the hospital while the parents work.

DESCRIPTION

During the first days of Andy's hospital stay, he is irritable and resists moving because his head and neck hurt. His IV fluid is carefully managed for the first few days while determining if any complications such as SIADH will develop. Intravenous pain medication is provided around the clock during the first few days, and it is administered orally after he begins to eat. Although he remains responsive throughout the early days of hospitalization, he spends a lot of time napping. On the second day, Andy has a generalized seizure that is effectively treated with diazepam. Although it is uncertain whether Andy will have a seizure disorder resulting from meningitis, seizure precautions are taken in the hospital. As the infection begins to resolve, Andy begins feeling better and seeks opportunities for diversion.

DISCUSSION

Andy's family is adapting to the sudden serious infection that has some potential long-term consequences.

1. Using the tools described in Chapter 2 🖉, identify the strengths and coping strategies in this family. Identify those factors that will be most helpful as the nursing care plan is developed.
2. Describe the pathophysiology that could account for Andy's infection.
3. Develop a nursing care plan for Andy that takes into account his treatment, pain, and lethargy. Be sure to address hydration, seizure precautions, and diversion.
4. Develop an education program to prepare the parents to manage a seizure if Andy has another seizure after discharge.
5. Identify the follow-up care assessments that should occur to assess Andy for complications of bacterial meningitis.

NCLEX-RN® Review

1. Along with medication, a 5-year-old child with myoclonic seizures uses a ketogenic diet for seizure control. Which choices should the nurse suggest for the child's lunch?
   1. Tuna with mayonnaise, potato chips, and broccoli
   2. Hot dog on a bun with orange Jell-O
   3. Grilled cheese on white bread, bacon, and apple juice
   4. Macaroni and cheese, pear, and skim milk

2. The parent of a child recently diagnosed with viral meningitis is concerned about permanent effects from the disease. Her neighbor's child had viral encephalitis with learning and mobility sequelae as a result. How should the nurse respond to her concerns?
   1. "Let's wait and see if this disease becomes viral encephalitis."
   2. "Have they been playing together?"
   3. "Most children with viral meningitis have future learning problems. You'll need to make plans for a special school."
   4. "Children who have viral meningitis usually have a complete recovery without permanent effects."

3. A nurse is providing discharge teaching to the family of a 5-year-old child who just had a ventriculoperitoneal shunt surgically placed. Which statement indicates the parents understand the teaching?
   1. "There is no chance my child will have a seizure as long as the shunt is functioning correctly."
   2. "We should let our doctor know if the child complains of a worsening headache."
   3. "Our child does not need to be followed by any early intervention programs, unless a problem develops."
   4. "We will observe for symptoms of shunt malfunction until our child has had the shunt for 6 months."

4. An infant is brought to the emergency department with assessment findings of failure to thrive, vomiting, and a decreased level of consciousness. Which should the nurse suspect?
   1. Influenza
   2. Reaction to the DTaP immunization
   3. Shaken baby syndrome
   4. A malabsorption syndrome

See Appendix I 🖉 for answers.

References

Adzick, N. S., Thom, E. A., Spong, C. Y., Brock, J. W., Burrows, P. K., Johnson, M. P., . . . Farmer, D. L. (2011). A randomized trial of prenatal versus postnatal repair of myelomeningocele. *New England Journal of Medicine, 364*, 993–1004.

American Academy of Pediatrics, Steering Committee on Quality Improvement and Management & Subcommittee on Febrile Seizures. (2008). Febrile seizures: Clinical practice guideline for the long-term management of the child with simple febrile seizures. *Pediatrics, 121*(6), 1281–1286.

Bakhoa, L. L., Lockhart, G. R., Myers, R., & Linakis, J. G. (2010). Emergency department visits for concussion in young child athletes. *Pediatrics, 126*(3), e550–e556.

Berker, A. N., & Yalçin, M. C. (2008). Cerebral palsy: Orthopedic aspects and rehabilitation. *Pediatric Clinics of North America, 55*, 1209–1255.

Bigal, M. E., & Arruda, M. A. (2010). Migraine in the pediatric population—Evolving concepts. *Headache, 50*(7), 1130–1143.

Black, J. S., & Wilson, B. (2009). Neurofibromatosis type 1. *Consultant for Pediatricians, 8*(12), 433.

Blair, E. (2010). Epidemiology of the cerebral palsies. *Orthopedic Clinics of North America, 41*, 441–455.

Blume, H. K., & Szperka, C. L. (2010). Secondary causes of headaches in children: When it isn't a migraine. *Pediatric Annals, 39*(7), 431–439.

Boss, B. J., & Huether, S. E. (2010). Alterations in neurologic function in children. In K. L. McCance, S. E. Huether, V. L. Brashers, & N. S. Rote, *Pathophysiology: The biologic basis for disease in adults and children* (6th ed., pp. 665–695). St. Louis, MO: Mosby Elsevier.

Brazelton Institute. (2008). *Understanding the baby's language.* Retrieved from http://www.brazelton-institute.com/intro.html

Brown, L., & Proctor, M. R. (2011). Endoscopically assisted correction of sagittal craniosynostosis. *AORN Journal, 93*(5), 566–579.

Carey, R. G., & Balistreri, W. F. (2011). Mitochondrial hepatopathies. In R. M. Kliegman, B. F. Stanton, J. W. St. Geme, N. F. Schor, & R. E. Behrman, *Nelson textbook of pediatrics* (19th ed., pp. 1405–1408). Philadelphia, PA: Elsevier Saunders.

Catroppa, C., & Anderson, V. (2009). Neurodevelopmental outcome in pediatric traumatic brain injury. *Future Neurology, 4*(6), 811–821.

Centers for Disease Control and Prevention. (2011). *Spina bifida: Data and statistics in the United States.*

Retrieved from http://www.cdc.gov/ncbddd/spinabifida/data.html

Chandran, A., Herbert, H., Misurski, D., & Santosham, M. (2011). Long-term sequelae of childhood bacterial meningitis: An underappreciated problem. *Pediatric Infectious Disease Journal, 30*(1), 3–6.

Chiou, H., & Hsieh, L. (2008). Parenting stress in parents of children with epilepsy and asthma. *Journal of Child Neurology, 23*(3), 301–306.

Cirillo, M. L. (2008). Neuromuscular emergencies. *Clinical Pediatric Emergency Medicine, 9,* 88–95.

Clore, E. T. (2010). Seizure precautions for pediatric bedside nurses. *Pediatric Nursing, 36*(4), 191–194.

Coronado, V. G., Xu, L., Basavaraju, S. V., McGuire, L. C., Wald, M. M., Faul, M. D., . . . Hemphill, J. D. (2011). Surveillance for traumatic brain injury-related deaths—United States, 1997–2007. *Morbidity and Mortality Weekly Report, 60*(5), 1–32.

Curtis, S., Stobart, K., Vandermeer, B., Simel, D. L., & Klassen, T. (2010). Clinical features suggestive of meningitis in children: A systematic review of prospective data. *Pediatrics, 126*(5), 952–960.

Danzer, E., Gerdes, M., Bebbington, M. W., Zarnow, D. M., Adzick, N. S., & Johnson, M. P. (2010). Preschool neurodevelopmental outcome of children following fetal myelomeningocele closure. *American Journal of Obstetrics and Gynecology, 202*(5):450, e1–e9.

Dodge, N. N. (2008). Cerebral palsy: Medical aspects. *Orthopedic Clinics of North America, 41,* 1189–1207.

Dooley, J. M., & Pearlman, E. M. (2010). The clinical spectrum of migraine in children. *Pediatric Annals, 39*(7), 408–415.

Doumouchtsis, S. K., & Arulkumaran, S. (2008). Head trauma after instrumental births. *Clinics in Perinatology, 35,* 69–83.

Dubowitz, H., & Lane, W. G. (2011). Abused and neglected children. In R. M. Kliegman, B. F. Stanton, J. W. St. Geme, N. F. Schor, & R. E. Behrman, *Nelson textbook of pediatrics* (19th ed., pp. 135–142). Philadelphia, PA: Elsevier Saunders.

Duffy, L. V. (2010). Hydrocephalus. In P. J. Allen, J. A. Vessey, & N. A. Shapiro (Eds.), *Primary care of the child with a chronic condition* (5th ed., pp. 546–561). St. Louis, MO: Elsevier Mosby.

Duffy, L. V. (2011). Parental coping and childhood epilepsy: The need for future research. *Journal of Neuroscience Nursing, 43*(1), 29–35.

Epilepsy Foundation. (2010a). *Incidence and prevalence.* Retrieved from http://www.epilepsyfoundation.org/aboutepilepsy/whatisepilepsy/statistics.cfm

Epilepsy Foundation. (2010b). *Ketogenic diet.* Retrieved from http://www.epilepsyfoundation.org/aboutepilepsy/treatment/ketogenicdiet/

Fadiman, A. (1997). *The spirit catches you and you fall down.* New York, NY: Farrar, Strauss, Giroux.

Faul, M. D., Xu, L., Wald, M. M., & Coronado, V. G. (2010). *Traumatic brain injury in the United States: Emergency department visits, hospitalizations, and deaths 2002–2006.* Retrieved from http://www.cdc.gov/traumaticbraininjury/pdf/tbi_blue_book_age.pdf

Ferrie, C. D. (2010). Rufinamide: A new antiepileptic drug treatment for Lennox–Gastaut syndrome. *Expert Review of Neurotherapeutics, 10*(6), 851–860.

Fowler, A., Stödberg, T., Eriksson, M., & Wickström, R. (2010). Long-term outcomes of acute encephalitis in childhood. *Pediatrics, 126*(4), e828–e835.

Gaitanis, J. N., & Mandelbaum, D. E. (2009). Disorders of nervous system development: Cellular and molecular mechanisms. In R. B. David (Ed.), *Clinical pediatric neurology* (pp. 415–432). New York, NY: Demos Medical Publishing.

Goldstein, J. (2008). Status epilepticus in the pediatric emergency department. *Clinical Pediatric Emergency Medicine, 9,* 96–100.

Halstead, M. E., Walter, K. D., & the Council on Sports Medicine and Fitness. (2010). Clinical report—Sports-related concussion in children and adolescents. *Pediatrics, 126*(3), 597–615.

Hersh, J. H., & the Committee on Genetics. (2008). Health supervision for children with neurofibromatosis. *Pediatrics, 121*(3), 633–642.

Hershey, A. D., Kabbouche, M. A., & Powers, S. W. (2010). Treatment of pediatric and adolescent migraines. *Pediatric Annals, 39*(7), 416–423.

Huh, J. W., & Raghupathi, R. (2009). New concepts in treatment of pediatric traumatic brain injury. *Anesthesiology Clinics of North America, 27,* 213–240.

Hutchison, J. S., Ward, R. E., Lacroix, J., Hébert, P. C., Barnes, M. A., Bohn, D. J., . . . Skippen, P. W. (2008). Hypothermia therapy after traumatic brain injury in children. *New England Journal of Medicine, 358*(23), 2447–2456.

Irani, D. N. (2008). Aseptic meningitis and viral myelitis. *Neurologic Clinics, 26,* 635–655.

Jea, A., & Kulkarni, A. V. (2009). Hydrocephalus. In J. Legido & J. H. Piatt, *Clinical pediatric neurosciences for primary care* (pp. 459–478). Elk Grove Village, IL: American Academy of Pediatrics.

Jentink, J., Loane, M. A., Dolk, H., Barisic, I., Garne, E., Morris, J. K., . . . EUROCAT Antiepileptic Study Working Group. (2010). Valproic acid monotherapy in pregnancy and major congenital malformations. *New England Journal of Medicine, 362*(23), 2185–2193.

Kemper, K. J., & Breuner, C. C. (2010). Complementary, holistic, and integrative medicine: Headaches. *Pediatrics in Review, 31*(2), e17–e23.

Kim, K. S. (2010). Acute bacterial meningitis in children. *Lancet Infectious Diseases, 10*(1), 32–42.

Kinsman, S. L., & Johnston, M. V. (2011). Craniosynostosis. In R. M. Kliegman, B. F. Stanton, J. W. St. Geme, N. F. Schor, & R. E. Behrman, *Nelson textbook of pediatrics* (19th ed., pp. 2011–2013). Philadelphia, PA: Elsevier Saunders.

Kirkham, F. J., Newton, C. R., & Whitehouse, W. (2008). Pediatric coma scales. *Developmental Medicine and Child Neurology, 50*(4), 267–274.

Kothare, S. V., Khurana, D. S., Madsen, J., & Papanastassiou, A. (2009). Epilepsy. In J. Legido & J. H. Piatt, *Clinical pediatric neurosciences for primary care* (pp. 267–301). Elk Grove Village, IL: American Academy of Pediatrics.

Lee, P., & DiPatri, A. J. (2008). Evaluation of suspected cerebrospinal fluid shunt complications in children. *Clinical Pediatric Emergency Medicine, 9,* 76–82.

Lehman, R. K., & Mink, J. (2008). Altered mental status. *Clinical Pediatric Emergency Medicine, 9,* 68–75.

Lennartsson, F. (2011). Developing guidelines for child health care nurses to prevent nonsynostotic plagiocephaly: Search for the evidence. *Journal of Pediatric Nursing, 26,* 348–358.

Lie, K. K., Gröholt, E. K., & Eskild, A. (2010). Association of cerebral palsy with Apgar score in low and normal birthweight infants: Population based cohort study.

British Medical Journal, 341, c4990. Retrieved from http://www.bmj.come/content/341/bmj.c4990.full.pdf+html

Little, R. D. (2008). Increased intracranial pressure. *Clinical Pediatric Emergency Medicine, 9,* 83–87.

Looby, S., & Flanders, A. (2011). Spine trauma. *Radiologic Clinics of North America, 49,* 129–163.

Maguire, S., Pickerd, N., Farewell, D., Mann, M., Tempest, V., & Kemp, A. M. (2009). Which clinical features distinguish inflicted from noninflicted brain injury? A systematic review. *Archives of Diseases in Childhood, 94,* 860–867.

Malhotra, A., Bell, W. E., & Henderson, F. W. (2009). Infections of the central nervous system. In R. B. David (Ed.), *Clinical pediatric neurology* (pp. 151–188). New York, NY: Demos Medical Publishing.

Mann, K., & Jackson, A. (2008). Meningitis. *Pediatrics in Review, 29*(12), 417–429.

Mansfield, R. T. (2007). Severe traumatic brain injury. *Clinical Pediatric Emergency Medicine, 8,* 156–164.

Mathison, D. J., Kadom, N., & Krug, S. E. (2008). Spinal cord injury in the pediatric patient. *Clinical Pediatric Emergency Medicine, 9,* 106–123.

McGrogan, A., Madle, G. C., Seaman, H. E., & deVries, C. S. (2009). The epidemiology of Guillain-Barré syndrome worldwide. *Neuroepidemiology, 32,* 150–163.

McGuire, C. S., & McCambridge, T. M. (2011). Concussion in the young athlete: Diagnosis, management, and prevention. *Contemporary Pediatrics, 28*(5), 30–46.

Meehan, W. P., & Mannix, R. (2010). Pediatric concussions in United States emergency departments in the years 2002 to 2006. *Journal of Pediatrics, 157*(6), 889–893.

Miller, L. C., Johnson, A., Duggan, L., & Behm, M. (2011). Consequences of the "back to sleep" program in infants. *Journal of Pediatric Nursing, 26,* 364–368.

Modi, A. C. (2009). The impact of new pediatric epilepsy diagnosis on parents: Parenting stress and activity patterns. *Epilepsy and Behavior, 14,* 237–242.

Modi, A. C., Rausch, J. R., & Glauser, T. A. (2011). Patterns of nonadherence to antiepileptic drug therapy in children with newly diagnosed epilepsy. *Journal of the American Medical Association, 305*(16), 1669–1679.

Mourtzinos, A., & Stoffel, J. T. (2010). Management goals for the spina bifida neurogenic bladder: A review from infancy to adulthood. *Urology Clinics of North America, 37,* 527–535.

National Center for Health Statistics, National Vital Statistics System. (2011). *2008, United States drowning deaths and rates per 100,000, all races, both sexes, ages 0 to 19.* Retrieved from http://webappa.cdc.gov/cgi-bin/broker.exe

National Institute of Neurological Disorders and Stroke. (2008). *Hydrocephalus fact sheet.* Retrieved from http://www.ninds.nih.gov/disorders/hydrocephalus/detail_hydrocephalus.htm

National Institute of Neurological Disorders and Stroke. (2011). *Neurofibromatosis fact sheet.* Retrieved from http://www.ninds.nih.gov/disorders/neurofibromatosis/detail_neurofibromatosis.htm#192803162

Neal, E. G., Chaffe, H. M., Edwards, N., Lawson, M. S., Schwartz, R. H., & Cross, J. H. (2008). Growth of children on classical and medium-chain triglyceride ketogenic diets. *Pediatrics, 122*(2), e334–e340.

Neal, E. G., Chaffe, H., Schwartz, R. H., Lawson, M. S., Edwards, N., Fitzsimmons, G., . . . Cross, J. H. (2008). The ketogenic diet for the treatment of childhood epilepsy: A randomised controlled trial. *Lancet Neurology, 7*(6), 500–506.

Nehring, W. M. (2010). Cerebral palsy. In P. J. Allen, J. A. Vessey, & N. A. Shapiro, *Primary care of the child with a chronic condition* (5th ed., pp. 326–346). St. Louis, MO: Elsevier Mosby.

Pakalnis, A., & Yonker, M. (2010). "Other" headache syndromes in children. *Pediatric Annals, 39*(7), 440–446.

Parent, S. (2010). Unique features of pediatric spinal cord injury. *Spine, 35*(Suppl. 21): S202–S208.

Partap, S., & Fisher, P. G. (2010). Managing chronic daily headaches. *Contemporary Pediatrics, 27*(4), 30–41.

Peltola, H., Roine, I., Fernández, J., González Mata, A., Zavala, I., Gonzalez, A. S., … Jauhiainen, T. (2010). Hearing impairment in childhood bacterial meningitis is little relieved by dexamethasone or glycerol. *Pediatrics, 125*(1), e1–e8.

Podell, K., Gifford, K., Bougakov, D., & Goldberg, E. (2010). Neuropsychological assessment in traumatic brain injury. *Psychiatric Clinics of North America, 33*, 855–876.

Raspall-Chaure, M., Neville, B. G., & Scott, R. C. (2008). The medical management of the epilepsies in children: Conceptual and practical considerations. *Lancet Neurology, 7*(1), 57–69.

Rethlefsen, S. A., Ryan, D. D., & Kay, R. M. (2010). Classification systems in cerebral palsy. *Orthopedic Clinics of North America, 41*, 457–467.

Salisbury, A. L., Ponder, K. L., Padbury, J. F., & Lester, B. M. (2009). Fetal effects of psychoactive drugs. *Clinics in Perinatology, 36*, 595–619.

Sandler, A. D. (2010). Children with spina bifida: Key clinical issues. *Pediatric Clinics of North America, 57*, 879–892.

Sawin, K. J., & Thompson, N. M. (2009). The experience of finding an effective bowel management program for children with spina bifida: The parent's perspective. *Journal of Pediatric Nursing, 24*(4), 280–291.

Schottler, J., Vogel, L., Chafetz, R., & Mulcahey, M. J. (2009). Parent and caregiver knowledge of autonomic dysreflexia among youth with spinal cord injury. *Spinal Cord, 47*, 681–686.

Shearer, P., & Riviello, J. (2011). Generalized convulsive status epilepticus in adults and children: Treatment guidelines and protocols. *Emergency Medical Clinics of North America, 29*, 51–64.

Social Security Online. (2011). *Disability programs.* Retrieved from http://www.ssa.gov/disability/child_factsheet.htm#disability

Somani, B. K. (2009). Autonomic dysreflexia: A medical emergency with spinal cord injury. *International Journal of Clinical Practice, 63*(3), 350–352.

Spector, R. E. (2009). *Cultural diversity in health and illness* (7th ed., pp. 3–4). Upper Saddle River, NJ: Pearson.

Spencer, S., & Huh, L. (2008). Outcomes of epilepsy surgery in adults and children. *Lancet Neurology, 7*(6), 525–537.

Spina Bifida Association. (2011). *Latex (natural rubber) allergy in spina bifida.* Retrieved from http://www.spinabifidaassociation.org/site/c.liKWL7PLLrF/b.2700271/k.1779/Latex_Natural_Rubber_Allergy_in_Spina_Bifida.htm

Stafstrom, C. E. (2009). The epilepsies. In R. B. David (Ed.), *Clinical pediatric neurology* (pp. 151–188). New York, NY: Demos Medical Publishing.

Substance Abuse and Mental Health Services Administration. (2011). *Results from the 2010 National Survey on Drug Use and Health: Summary of national findings.* Retrieved from http://oas.samhsa.gov/NSDUH/2k10NSDUH/2k10Results.htm#2.6

Sweeney, N. M. F. (2009). Neonatology. In J. W. Custer & R. E. Rau (Eds.), *The Harriet Lane handbook* (18th ed., pp. 481–505). Philadelphia, PA: Elsevier Mosby.

Taub, P. J., & Pierce, P. (2010). Positional plagiocephaly, Part 1: A practical guide to evaluation. *Consultant for Pediatricians, 9*(12), 421–428.

Taub, P. J., & Pierce, P. (2011). Positional plagiocephaly, Part 2: Prevention and treatment. *Consultant for Pediatricians, 10*(1), 13–15.

van Doorn, P. A., Ruts, L., & Jacobs, B. C. (2008). Clinical features, pathogenesis, and treatment of Guillain-Barré syndrome. *Lancet Neurology, 7*, 939–950.

Wagner, C. (2009). Pediatric submersion injuries. *Air Medical Journal, 28*(3), 116–119.

Wagner, J. L., Smith, G., Ferguson, P., van Bakergem, K., & Hrisko, S. (2010). Pilot study of an integrated cognitive-behavioral and self-management intervention for youth with epilepsy and caregivers: Coping openly and personally with epilepsy (COPE). *Epilepsy and Behavior, 18*, 280–285.

Wallman, C. M., Smith, P. B., & Moore, K. (2011). Implementing a perinatal substance abuse screening tool. *Advances in Neonatal Care, 11*(4), 255–267.

Weiss, J., & the Committee on Injury, Violence, and Poison Prevention. (2010). Technical report—Prevention of drowning. *Pediatrics, 126*(1), e253–e262.

Wells, K. (2009). Substance abuse and child maltreatment. *Pediatric Clinics of North America, 56*, 345–362.

Wilson, B. A., Shannon, M. T., & Shields, K. M. (2011). *Nurse's drug guide 2011.* Upper Saddle River, NJ: Pearson.

Zadnikar, M., & Kastrin, A. J. (2011). Effects of hippotherapy and therapeutic horseback riding on postural control and balance in children with cerebral palsy: A meta-analysis. *Developmental Medicine and Child Neurology, 53*(8), 684–691.

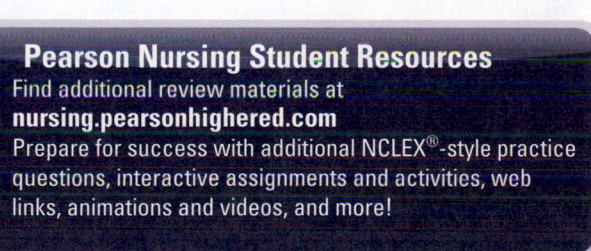

Pearson Nursing Student Resources

Find additional review materials at
nursing.pearsonhighered.com
Prepare for success with additional NCLEX®-style practice questions, interactive assignments and activities, web links, animations and videos, and more!

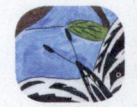 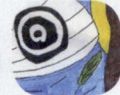 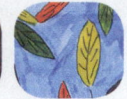

Learning Outcomes

After completing this chapter, you will be able to:

1. Define mental health and describe major mental health alterations in childhood.
2. Contrast pediatric differences and issues related to mental health and cognition.
3. Discuss the clinical manifestations of the major mental health alterations of childhood and adolescence.
4. Plan for the nursing management of children and adolescents with mental health alterations in the hospital and community settings.
5. Describe characteristics of common cognitive alterations of childhood.
6. Use evidence-based practice to plan nursing management for children with cognitive alterations.
7. Establish and evaluate expected outcomes of care for the child with a cognitive alteration.

> "We love Jeremiah. He's cool, and our friends like him to come with us when we're hanging out."
>
> —*Jeffrey, Jeremiah's brother, age 19 years*

Jeremiah, a 7-year-old boy with Down syndrome, enjoys attending his special education classroom. Jeremiah is the youngest of four children and was born after an unplanned pregnancy to a mother and father in their 40s. Their youngest child at that time was 12 years of age. Although they accepted that they would have another child, Jeremiah's parents learned after an amniocentesis during the pregnancy that their son had Down syndrome. His parents progressed through stages of shock, denial, anger, and sadness. Thanks to a strong support system, they soon learned more about Down syndrome, resolved their grief, and grew to love their infant son. The siblings loved their new brother and seemed to have little trouble accepting the fact that he was different from their original expectations.

During infancy, Jeremiah developed gastroesophageal reflux and frequent otitis media. Since his parents had adequate health care, they were able to seek assistance as needed. When Jeremiah was almost a year of age, the family enrolled him in an early intervention program. He was about 4 months behind in developmental milestone achievement, but through the intervention program he quickly gained fine and gross motor skills. He eventually progressed from the early intervention program to preschool, and recently began attending a special education classroom. The school nurse has worked with the family to review Jeremiah's transport to school, provide information about obtaining and wearing medical alert identification, and monitor his health status in school.

How can the school nurse partner with the teachers and family to assist in establishing an educational plan for Jeremiah? How can the strengths and protective factors of the family be used to maximize Jeremiah's developmental skills?

Much of the care for mental health disruptions is provided by psychiatric–mental health specialists, so the nurse partners with these specialists to identify problems, support and carry out the therapy, provide education to the family, and refer the family to appropriate resources. Cognitive conditions are commonly managed by the family and school personnel. The nurse forms partnerships with families and school personnel to plan and evaluate care for the child with cognitive conditions such as intellectual disability, as in the case of Jeremiah. A thorough knowledge of development is a prerequisite to understanding mental health disruptions and cognitive conditions since developmental status is often altered in both. A number of conditions are discussed in this chapter, and related issues may be found in other chapters. For example, see Chapter 20 🖉 for a discussion of many of the environmentally related mental health conditions such as violence and substance use. Eating disorders are discussed in Chapter 19 and mental health needs of children with chronic disease are examined in Chapter 16 🖉.

This chapter provides the knowledge and tools to help you plan and implement care for children with alterations in mental health or cognition. Most mental health and cognitive conditions are treated in community settings, and nurses in these settings play an active role in the treatment and support of the child and family. Nurses may function as case managers, assisting a family to deal with all areas of the child's care. Occasionally a child is hospitalized for treatment of a significant mental health disruption, or is hospitalized for treatment of another health problem and requires continued mental health services. Cognitive and developmental characteristics must be considered and integrated into care for all children. In this chapter, mental health disruptions will be discussed first, with cognitive conditions following. Children can manifest both mental health and cognitive alterations, necessitating integration of concepts from both areas to plan care.

MENTAL HEALTH AND COGNITION

Mental health is foundational to a sense of personal well-being, physical health, relationships, and learning (Simpson, Cohen, Pastor, et al., 2008). It involves successful engagement in activities and relationships and the ability to adapt to and cope with change. **Cognition** refers to the change in thought, intelligence, and language that occurs over time as brain maturation and life experiences interact to mutually influence child performance (Santrock, 2011). Disruptions in mental health and cognition are common in children; specifics about these alterations are described throughout the chapter.

Nurses have been leaders in the field of pediatric mental health care. An initiative known as KySS (Keep your children/yourself Safe and Secure) was launched by nurses with goals of identification of assessment, implementation, and dissemination strategies for promoting the mental health of children and teens in primary care and alternative care settings, and review of evidence-based practice to make recommendations for interventions and needed research areas (DiMarco & Melnyk, 2009). Recommendations regarding screening for specific mental health conditions will be found throughout this chapter.

PEDIATRIC DIFFERENCES

The brain develops from the fetal neural tube early in development, with much critical embryology occurring in the fourth to sixth weeks of gestation at which time many women do not even know they are pregnant. During this time, the brain is not protected by the blood-brain barrier and is at risk for injury from the fetal environment. Environmental conditions such as maternal alcohol ingestion, intake of certain medications, and exposure to environmental toxins can influence the developing fetus's brain. Most of the brain structure is present at birth, but during the first 5 years of life the brain continues to develop and mature as the young child gains fine and gross motor, social, and language skills. Development and differentiation occur during childhood spurts with fine motor skills improvement and during adolescent years when perception, motor function, and advanced thinking processes further develop (Santrock, 2011). The child remains vulnerable to external forces during periods of brain growth and development. The influence of drugs, poor nutrition, traumatic brain injury, and absence of emotional nurturance are all examples of factors that can interfere with healthy brain and cognitive development.

Mental health and cognition in children is different from adults because developmental progression and abilities influence perceptions and reactions. The brain matures and life experiences become more complex, while the interactions among these factors create a unique mental health state. Childhood is a crucial period for development of mental health that provides for the social skills, emotional health, developmental progression, and cognitive abilities that prepare youth for mental health and achieving maximum potential in adulthood.

Children differ from adults both in mental healthcare needs and in the types and progression of mental health disruptions. During childhood, the necessity for bonding and attachment to significant adults forms the cornerstone of the child's healthy mental development. Therefore, young children rely on adults for establishment of mental health. The child's unique genetic makeup couples with environmental factors such as bonding with adults and physical factors such as chemical exposure (see Chapter 20 🖉 for a description of the effects of environment on children) to influence mental health status. Cognitive disorders are also a result of a unique interplay of genetic and environmental causes.

In addition, children with mental health disruptions sometimes display different clinical manifestations for mental illness than adults; therefore, diagnosis is difficult and challenging. For example, a child with a tic syndrome may be mistakenly diagnosed as hyperactive, and the treatment would not be appropriate to the underlying condition. More than one mental health disruption may occur in the same child, leading to difficulty in diagnosis and treatment.

Use the guidelines in Table 34–1 to perform a nursing assessment of the child with a mental health or cognitive alteration.

MENTAL HEALTH ALTERATIONS

Approximately 15 million children in the United States have a mental illness that is severe enough to impair functioning at home or school. Overall, about one in five children and adolescents has a mental health disorder, and 1 in 10 has a disorder that profoundly interferes with daily functioning (National Center for Children in Poverty, 2010). Even more striking is that less than 35% of children with mental health alterations receive mental health services to treat their impairment (Storch & Elder, 2009). Further, some of the services received are not comprehensive or multidisciplinary, leading to

TABLE 34–1	Assessment Guidelines for the Child with an Alteration in Mental Health or Cognition
ASSESSMENT FOCUS	**ASSESSMENT GUIDELINES**
History	■ Describe prenatal care and problems. Was there any trauma at birth? ■ Is there a diagnosed mental health disorder in the child or other family members? ■ Is there a history of any neurologic injuries or diseases such as cancer? ■ What medications is the child taking? What medications has the child taken in the past? ■ Has there been exposure to environmental pesticides or other chemicals?
Growth	■ Is growth progressing along the same channel or growth percentile? ■ Is head circumference within normal limits?
Development	■ Perform regular developmental screening to identify any variations from expected developmental milestones. Further testing is required if screening suggests any abnormalities. ■ What is the progression of skills reported by the family? ■ Are there any unusual capabilities or deficits? ■ Inquire about progression in school and extracurricular activities.
Social skills	■ Describe the relationship between the child and significant adults. Is close attachment evident? Are there signs of attachment disorders such as lack of eye contact, smiles, or response to others in the environment? ■ Describe the school-age child's daily schedule, including family and peer activities. Does the child have friends and engage in several activities with them on a regular basis? Does the child generally interact well with others? Has the child recently had a change in school performance? ■ Have the school-age child or teen describe daily activities and friends. Is there a combination of peer and family influence on personal decision making?
Affect	■ Describe the child's facial expression and response to the nurse. ■ Observe body size, position, and posture. ■ Are interaction behaviors typical for the setting and age of the child? ■ Does the child display interest in surroundings? ■ Is the child dressed in an appropriate manner? Does the child establish eye contact?
Appearance	■ Is the child's clothing appropriate for age, setting, and developmental level?
Behaviors	■ Describe level of consciousness and interaction with surroundings. ■ Inquire about recent reported changes in behavior (e.g., sleep, eating patterns, communication with others, school performance, friendships, risky activities). ■ Are problem behaviors identified by the child or parent? ■ Are there particular events that were associated with problem behaviors?
Life events	■ Has the child or family experienced recent stress or trauma? ■ Have there been any changes in family structure? ■ Evaluate chronic health conditions in family members.

unmet mental health needs. In other cases, the interventions used are not established on evidence-based practice.

Certain population groups are at increased risk for mental disorders. Children from homes with low income are twice as likely to have mental health disruptions. Approximately 50% of children in the child welfare system and 70% of youth in the juvenile justice system have mental disorders (National Center for Children in Poverty, 2010). Children with special healthcare needs and those living in military families have particular barriers to accessing mental health services (Sogomonyan & Cooper, 2010).

Etiology and Pathophysiology

Some mental health and cognitive alterations in children originate from a genetic or physiologic cause. Examples include intellectual disability and childhood schizophrenia. Often the family and surrounding environments in which children live influence their characteristics and contribute to dysfunctions such as anxiety, depression, and posttraumatic stress disorder. A unique interplay of genetics and the environment influences mental health and cognitive conditions, making prevention, diagnosis, and treatment challenging.

Clinical Manifestations

The manifestations of mental health alterations in children are varied, but most can be identified through careful developmental and behavioral screening. Children with mental health conditions often do not display usual developmental milestones at the times predicted. They may have social interaction problems with family members or other people, or they may have demonstrated a change in performance from former developmental achievement. Functional patterns of living such as the ability to feed and care for self, regulation of sleep and nutritional intake, and the ability to self-regulate during activities may be lacking. Repetitive actions, behavioral instability

TABLE 34–2	Diagnostic Procedures and Laboratory Tests for Mental Health and Cognition*	
DIAGNOSTIC PROCEDURES	**LABORATORY TESTS**	
Magnetic resonance imaging (MRI)	Toxicology screening	
Radiograph (x-ray)		
Electroencephalogram		

Note: *See Appendixes D and E 🔗 for information about these diagnostic procedures and for expected laboratory test values.

and outbursts, and withdrawal are other important signs of mental health disruption.

Collaborative Care

Many professionals work in the field of mental health, and the nurse establishes partnerships with them in caring for children. In the following sections, general assessments, treatments, and nursing care for mental health alterations are discussed. Later sections in this chapter address specific alterations and related care.

Diagnostic Tests

Teachers or parents may notice changes in behavior and refer a child to the school nurse or other health professional. The nurse may identify developmental or behavioral problems during clinic, school, or home visits, and refer the child to a physician, psychiatric mental health nurse practitioner, or psychologist for further assessment. Evaluation commonly includes observing behavior, asking family and teachers to complete behavioral questionnaires, and examining the past history about pregnancy, birth, developmental milestone achievement, family health conditions, and recent changes in the child's behavior. Serum toxicology screen, radiographs, and other diagnostic tests may be performed (Table 34–2).

Clinical Therapy

From the ages of 10 to 21 years, mental health issues are among the top two leading causes of hospitalization in all age groups (see Chapter 1 🔗). This high rate of hospitalization suggests that children are not receiving clinical therapy early, when outpatient care is appropriate and prognosis is best. Indeed, 75% to 80% of children with mental health needs do not receive necessary services, and quality of care is often insufficient (National Center for Children in Poverty, 2010). Application of evidence-based care concepts in curricula for students can best prepare care providers to provide comprehensive interventions to promote child mental health (Melnyk, Hawkins-Walsh, Beauchesne, et al., 2010).

The primary treatment goal in the management of children and adolescents with mental health disorders is to assist the child and family to achieve and maintain an optimal level of functioning through interventions designed to reduce the impact of stressors. Therapeutic interventions and communication are based on the principle that feelings motivate behaviors. Parents and others who are close to the child often fall into the habit of reacting to the child's behaviors rather than trying to find out what feelings may be precipitating the undesirable actions. Although behaviors may be considered in treatment, feelings and life experiences are often explored to provide insight and to lead to behavior change. Medication may be used to enhance and support other therapy, or may be the major therapeutic measure.

Treatment modes **Evidence-based practice** (EBP) refers to a body of scientific knowledge and its relationship to healthcare services (see further discussion in Chapter 1 🔗). Although the research basis for care in all areas of pediatric health is generally scant, there is even less scientific basis to support interventions in mental health services. Nurses must seek to apply evidence-based practice to enhance mental health care when possible, and to participate in research and outcomes measurement so that additional strong evidence can be gathered on the best approaches to care.

Three basic treatment modes based on evidence-based practice are used: individual, family, and group therapy. The choice of treatment mode must take into account the child's age and developmental stage, as well as the family situation and access to care. Most therapists incorporate several intervention strategies simultaneously within these modes. Different strategies are more or less effective and appropriate for children and adolescents in various stages of development. A thorough understanding of developmental needs, expectations, and abilities is therefore essential for mental health professionals. Treatment modes and therapeutic strategies commonly used with children and adolescents are described in the following text.

Individual therapy Individual therapy involves only the child and the therapist. Treatment of specific emotional problems or disorders may involve various techniques such as play therapy, psychodrama, art therapy, and **cognitive therapy** (a technique used to help a person recognize automatic negative thinking). Individual therapy may be short term (four to six sessions) or long term (lasting for several years).

Family therapy Family therapy involves the exploration of a particular emotional problem and its manifestations among the family members. Family therapy is based on the idea that an individual's emotional symptoms or problems are an expression of emotional symptoms or problems in the family. The focus is on the relationships among the family members, rather than the psychologic conflict within each individual member.

Group therapy Group therapy involves an ongoing or limited number of sessions in which several individuals participate. The emphasis is on the interpersonal styles of relating to one another in the group. Group therapy is particularly effective with adolescents because of the importance of the peer group at this age. An advantage of group therapy is that stimuli and feedback come from multiple sources (the group members) instead of just one person (the therapist).

Therapeutic strategies

Play therapy Play is often called the language or work of the child. From a developmental perspective, children progressively learn to express feelings and needs through action, fantasy, and finally language. The special quality of play buffers children against the pressures and demands of daily life. Play facilitates mastery of developmental stages by strengthening physical and neurologic processes. Play also assists in cognitive learning, setting the stage for problem solving and creativity.

Play therapy is a technique that reveals problems using fantasy through the use of toys, dolls, clay, art, and other creative objects. It is often used with preschool and school-age children who are experiencing anxiety, stress, and other specific nonpsychotic mental disorders. Play therapy encourages the child to act out feelings such as anger, hostility, sadness, and fear. It also provides the opportunity for the therapist to help the child understand, on a conscious or unconscious level, personal responses and behavior in a safe, supportive environment.

Clinical Tip

Play therapy, a technique used with children who have psychosocial disorders, is different from therapeutic play, which may be used with many hospitalized children (see Chapter 15 ⊘). Although some techniques overlap, only a specialist is qualified to provide play therapy. However, anyone with a basic knowledge of development can plan therapeutic play approaches.

Art therapy   Children who may be apprehensive about playing can sometimes be encouraged to participate in art therapy, using brief drawing exercises. This technique is appropriate for children of all ages, including adolescents. The drawings can help the therapist gain information about the child, the family, and the interactions between the child and family. However, children's drawings should never be used solely to form a definitive diagnosis.

When used in conjunction with a thorough history and appropriate psychologic testing information, art therapy can guide the child's treatment. These drawing exercises provide an opportunity to help in the healing process. The therapist can assist the child to release feelings of anger, pain, or fear onto paper, where they can be examined objectively. Figures 34–1 to 34–4 ■ present examples of this technique (Box 34–1).

Cognitive and behavioral therapy (CBT)   A combination of cognitive and behavioral therapy is useful in treating many mental health conditions in children. Cognitive therapy teaches thinking patterns to change reactions to situations that cause anxiety or other undesirable conditions. Children are taught how their brain and body are working; this understanding assists them in having control over the experience and responding with appropriate behaviors (Mayo Clinic, 2010).

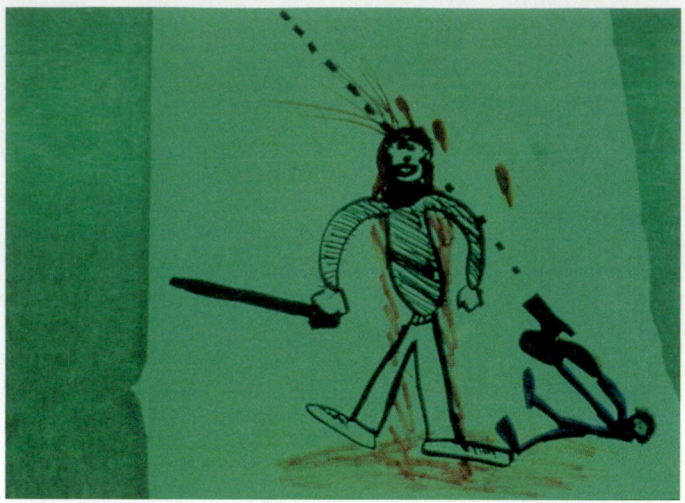

FIGURE 34–2 ■ "Self-Portrait." Drawn by a 15-year-old boy who was admitted through the emergency department after a failed suicide attempt by hanging. He had a psychiatric diagnosis of depression and polysubstance abuse (including inhalants and alcohol) and insisted that he was a member of a satanic cult in his hometown. Most of his drawings depicted a preoccupation with violence and suicide. The boy said he always felt a "darkness" like a shadow that followed him around and wanted him dead. His family history was significant for depression and suicide on both his mother's and his father's side. His father also had a lengthy history of polysubstance abuse and alcoholism. The boy was discharged to a long-term residential treatment facility for adolescents.

Behavior modification is a therapeutic technique that uses stimulus and response conditioning to alter inappropriate behaviors. It is used to reinforce desirable behaviors by helping the child to replace maladaptive behaviors with more appropriate ones. This technique is based on the assumption that any learned behavior can be unlearned. Thus, if parents, nurses, teachers, and other adults

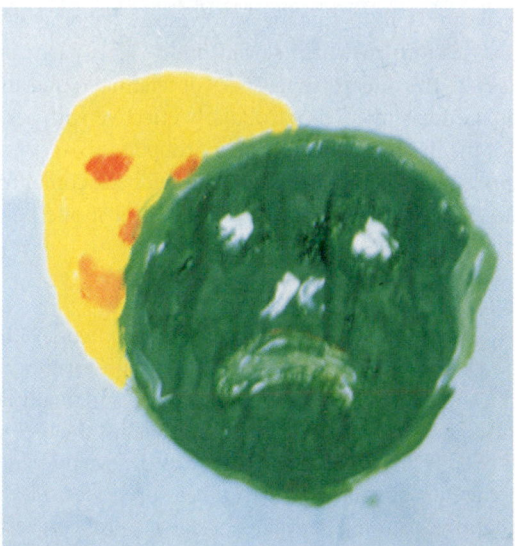

FIGURE 34–1 ■ "Me." Drawn by a 14-year-old girl with major depression, anxiety, and school phobia who had experienced multiple losses over several years. Her mother had severe chronic lung problems and diabetes, and the girl had stopped attending school for fear that something would happen to her mother. This drawing represents the girl's obvious feelings of sadness and depression but also indicates a glimmer of hope (represented by the yellow mask coming from behind the dark mask of depression).

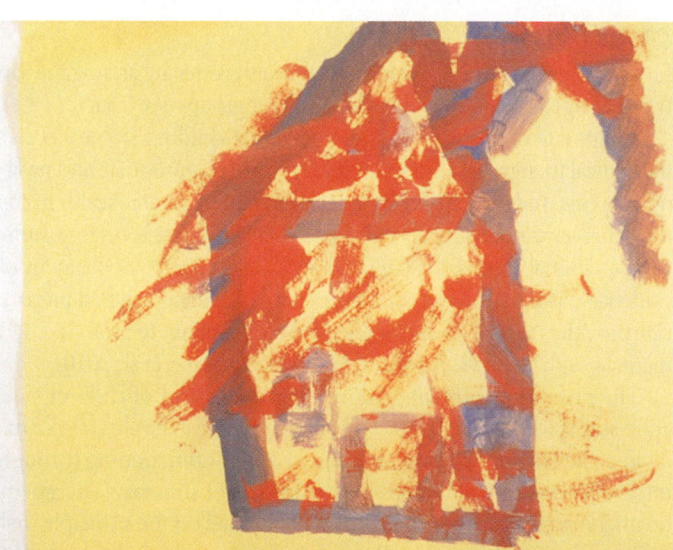

FIGURE 34–3 ■ "An Activity." Drawn by an 8-year-old boy who was initially admitted to the medical-surgical floor of a pediatric hospital for dehydration resulting from vomiting and diarrhea. Psychiatric evaluation was ordered for extreme anxiety. These drawings, completed during the initial interview, led to further investigation, which revealed that the child had started a house fire in which his grandmother was killed. The family's home and all their belongings were lost. No one knew that the child had set the fire. Further sessions indicated that he had been setting neighborhood garage fires and watching them burn from a distance.

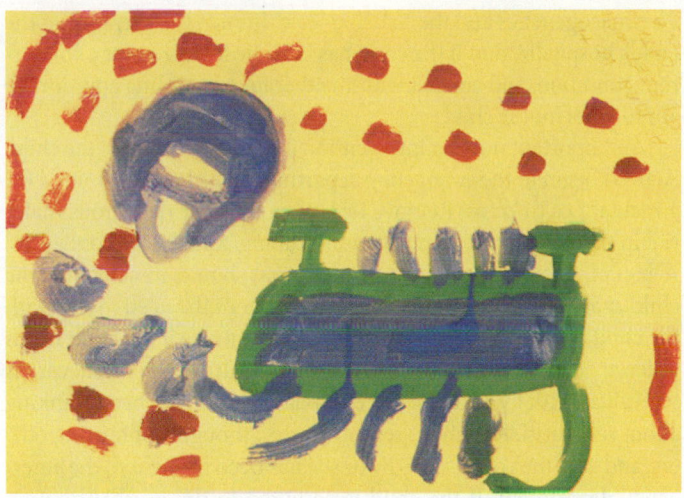

FIGURE 34–4 ■ "A Family Activity." By the same boy who drew Figure 34–3. This drawing depicts a recurring incident of physical and emotional abuse by his mother's live-in boyfriend. It shows the family bathtub with feces and blood smeared on the floor and walls. The boy reported that when either he or his 3-year-old brother had a toileting accident the boyfriend would make them go into the bathroom and stand in the bathtub while he smeared the feces on the walls. He would then hit the children and make them clean up the mess. The boy had previously been removed from the mother's custody for neglect. He was transferred from the medical-surgical area to the inpatient children's psychiatric unit, where he received a diagnosis of depression, anxiety disorder, and child abuse (physical and emotional). Charges were filed against the mother's boyfriend, and custody of both children was temporarily revoked.

consistently reinforce desirable behaviors, the child will eventually alter or discontinue undesirable behaviors.

Behavior modification may include (1) removing the child from the home to a more structured environment, such as a hospital, for a brief time; and (2) instructing the parents, teachers, and other appropriate adults to be agents of behavioral change. Several ongoing sessions may be required with the adults involved, using role-play and other techniques. Consistency is the most important principle in the successful use of behavior modification.

Visualization and guided imagery The techniques of visualization and guided imagery begin with specific directions for progressive relaxation according to the child's ability. These forms of therapy use the child's own imagination and positive thinking to reduce stress and anxiety, decrease the experience of pain or discomfort, and promote healing. The techniques are especially useful in the management of

| BOX 34–1 | Research: Art Therapy |

Drawing as a means for communication with children has been used for many years. Art can be viewed as a window or doorway through which a child's emotions and experiences can be viewed (Kortesluoma, Punamaki, & Nikkonen, 2008). Art is also versatile and can be accomplished in practically any setting. This makes it an effective assessment technique with children too young to express certain situations verbally (Massimo & Wiley, 2008). In addition, it allows them expression of feelings and thus becomes an intervention. Following a drawing session with a discussion in which the child explains a piece of art is especially helpful. Children can also be shown drawings by children with similar experiences and asked to tell a story about the drawings (Wilson, Megel, Enenback, et al., 2010).

Nurses who work with children in various settings should consider the use of drawings. Provide a table and drawing materials for children waiting for a healthcare examination, bring art materials to the child in the hospital, and consider the activity with children who have experienced trauma.

anxiety disorders and chronic pain. It is not easy for every child to use his or her imagination in this way, so the technique may not work or be appropriate for every child.

Hypnosis Hypnosis involves varying degrees of suggestibility and deep relaxation effects. This technique is useful for children and adolescents because they can usually be hypnotized more easily than adults. Hypnosis is especially helpful in treating physical symptoms with a psychologic component, anxiety, and phobias, as well as managing severe physical symptoms or discomfort (pain or nausea) associated with a physiologic disorder or its treatment (e.g., cancer or juvenile rheumatoid arthritis).

Nursing Management

Nursing Assessment and Diagnosis

Mental health conditions often escalate to a level of crisis for families because they are not identified early. To avoid serious mental health problems, ongoing assessment of all children for risks is imperative. During all health visits, mental health screening should be integrated into care so that teaching can focus on promotion of mental health and so that disruptions can be identified. See Chapters 8 to 13 🔗 for specific questions to ask during health promotion and health maintenance visits. When a potential mental health condition exists, the child should receive further assessment from a mental health specialist. A resource commonly used is the *Diagnostic and Statistical Manual of Mental Disorders,* which lists diagnostic criteria for known mental health conditions. The current edition is the *DSM-IV-TR* (American Psychiatric Association, 2000), and its criteria for several conditions are listed throughout this chapter and other chapters in this book. The *DSM-V* is scheduled for publication in May 2013.

Once a mental health problem is identified, the nurse assesses the child for related issues and conditions. Mental health is linked to development, so developmental screening tests are administered. Mental health status can influence activity level, physiologic parameters, and risk for certain conditions. Therefore, height and weight, review of systems, vital signs, physical activity levels, dietary intake, and medication/substance use history are important to assess. Family interactions, stressors, and methods of coping are also assessed (see Chapter 2 🔗 for further detail on family assessment). Consider cultural variations to definitions and components of mental health (see Developing Cultural Competence: Mental Health Definition and Treatments). See Table 34–1 for pertinent assessment topics.

Many nursing diagnoses can be formulated based on particular mental health conditions and child situations. Examples include:

- Powerlessness related to multiple stressors
- Anxiety related to situational or maturational crises
- Coping, Ineffective related to inadequate social support
- Grieving, Complicated related to difficulty expressing loss of significant other
- Role Performance, Ineffective related to inadequate support system and inadequate linkage with healthcare system

NANDA-I © 2012

Planning and Implementation

The primary treatment goal in the management of children and adolescents with mental health disruptions is to assist the child and family to achieve and maintain an optimal level of functioning through

Developing Cultural Competence
Mental Health Definition and Treatments

Mental health is defined in different ways by various cultural groups. For most it is a sense of well-being, peace, and productive use of the mind. In many cultures, care of the "spirit" is believed necessary to promote mental health. An identity with one's community and spiritual wholeness is promoted by storytelling, singing, and rites of passage. An array of therapies is used to support and restore mental health. Use of certain objects such as bags of herbs may be considered important to preserve mental health. Other therapies may include healers, family and community support, relaxation or meditation, teas and other herbal products, and exorcism. Find out how individuals and groups define mental health and how they believe health is maintained. Be alert to learn if mental disorders are viewed as a negative stigma or are openly accepted and discussed within the culture. Ask about what the family believes will help to enhance the child's mental health and integrate these practices into the plan of care whenever it is safe to do so.

interventions designed to reduce the impact of risk factors and to enhance protective factors such as coping ability.

Care in the Hospital

Although most mental health disorders are managed effectively with therapy and/or medication on an outpatient basis, some necessitate admission to an inpatient psychiatric setting. In addition, you may encounter the child with a mental health disorder during hospitalization for a concurrent physiologic problem. If hospitalized for a concurrent problem, the child's current level of mental health functioning needs to be assessed in addition to the admitting diagnosis in order to plan appropriate interventions.

Nursing care includes carrying out the prescribed treatment plan and administering psychotropic medications. The child's medication regimen should be evaluated for administration schedule, dosage, side effects, and effectiveness. See Evidence-Based Practice:

Pharmacogenetics and the Nursing Role. Inform the therapist of the child's hospitalization if the child has been hospitalized for a concurrent condition, and consult with the therapist regarding appropriate approaches for the child.

An important nursing intervention is to ensure safety of the child. Actions begin in the emergency department if a child is admitted for a mental health crisis. Remove or lock potentially dangerous material in the room such as medications, tubing, and sharps containers. A parent, guardian, or health professional should remain with the child at all times. Inform the family member of the need to stay with the child and how to immediately notify the nurse if the adult needs to leave or if the child's condition changes. Part of the initial care is to evaluate risk by asking if the child has tried or has been thinking about self-harm. Ask about recent stresses, thoughts of hurting others, and why the child thinks he or she has been brought to the emergency department. If the child is admitted to the psychiatric unit, follow unit policies for ensuring safety for children who are at risk of hurting themselves or others.

Psychiatric hospitalization is a stressful event for all families, and both the family and child need supportive care. Continuation of family involvement is critical. The nurse frequently is the liaison between the family and the therapist in making follow-up arrangements at the time of discharge. The nurse must be aware of the meaning of mental illness in various cultural groups and the treatments that may be commonly used. These complementary therapies should be integrated within the care plan when considered safe, and families must feel that their responses and approaches to the child with a mental disorder are not judged by health professionals.

Care in the Community

The nurse in the community assesses how a child with a mental health disorder is functioning in each part of the microsystem, such as home, childcare, school, and with friends. Risks and protective factors of the

Evidence-Based Practice — Pharmacogenetics and the Nursing Role

PROBLEM
Great variability is seen in the response to psychotropic medicines used to treat mental health disorders such as depression. Children and adolescents show even more variability than adults, related to developmental variation in absorption, distribution, metabolism, and elimination; therefore, close monitoring is essential (Van den Anker, 2010). New technologies provide information about individual responses to medications, but nurses may be unaware of the applications.

EVIDENCE
The fields of genetics and genomics are growing rapidly (see Chapter 4 🔗). Currently, pharmacogenetic testing is being used so that clinicians can select the best psychotropic medications for particular patients. For example, a genetic test for a gene that codes for high manufacture of a body enzyme that metabolizes a particular medication predicts the patient will not respond well to that medication. Another psychotropic can be chosen to enhance response. On the other hand, if the patient is a slow metabolizer of the medication, an increased risk of toxicity results (Prows & Saldana, 2009). Depression is inadequately treated in about one third of patients because of genetically determined enzymes that influence drug availability. Genetic testing and serum blood levels of medication assist in effective drug treatment (Krauter & Cook, 2011). Recent research suggests that treatment for attention deficit hyperactivity disorder may influence drug variability and effectiveness of treatment with common medications (Froehlich et al., 2011).

IMPLICATIONS
The nurse in a setting where children and adolescents are treated for psychiatric disorders has an important role in applying new knowledge related to pharmacogenetics. First, the nurse needs to take a careful history of other medications, over-the-counter products, and herbal remedies because many of these substances compete with psychotropic medications for metabolism in the body. When a DNA test is recommended prior to beginning medication, families need to understand the reason for the test. They will also need explanations about the test results and how they relate to the specific medication that has been prescribed. It is important that all children and adolescents receiving psychotropic medications be closely monitored for responses and side effects. The nurse is integral to the ongoing evaluation of the prescribed therapy (Theoktisto, 2009).

CRITICAL THINKING APPLICATION
What is the nursing role in history taking and monitoring for the child or adolescent on psychotropic medication? What questions do you think a family is likely to ask when they learn that a genetic test is recommended before prescribing medication to an adolescent experiencing a mental health disruption such as severe depression? Where will you find the information about pharmacogenetics and pharmacogenomics that will provide necessary background for you and the family? How can pharmacogenetic testing enhance the treatment of individuals by both leading to a therapeutic response in a short time and avoiding serious side effects?

child and family are assessed (see Chapter 5 🔗). The nurse conducts therapy sessions and performs ongoing evaluation and updates of the child's level of functioning. Changes in the child and family stressors and coping mechanisms are evaluated. Explore the family's access to, use of, and acceptance of complementary therapy, such as yoga, relaxation, music, and pet therapy. Such techniques can provide stress relief and assist in the child's mental health treatment. See Chapter 3 🔗 for further description of complementary therapies.

Since many children do not receive adequate mental health services, nurses need to be knowledgeable about resources for mental health care and facilitate their use by the child and family. The nurse in the community often acts as a partner to inform other health professionals such as psychiatrists, psychologists, psychiatric nurse practitioners, school counselors, teachers, and hospital nurses about the child's mental health status.

Evaluation

Desired outcomes for mental health care depend on the particular condition and the child's situation. Examples are:

- The child demonstrates the ability to self-restrain compulsive or impulsive behaviors.
- The child who experiences a change in family structure manifests healthy psychosocial adaptation.
- The youth verbalizes feelings of productivity and self-worth.
- The family identifies and uses available social support.
- Family members demonstrate the ability to draw on spiritual beliefs for comfort.

DEVELOPMENTAL AND BEHAVIORAL DISORDERS

Autism Spectrum Disorders (Pervasive Developmental Disorders)

It is estimated that 12% to 16% of children have a developmental or behavioral disorder. One of the most common types of disorders is pervasive developmental disorder. **Autism spectrum disorders (ASDs),** also called **pervasive developmental disorders (PDDs),** begin in early childhood and are characterized by impaired social interactions and communication, with restricted interests, activities, and behaviors (Centers for Disease Control and Prevention [CDC], 2009a). The disorders are classified into five types:

- Autistic disorder
- Asperger syndrome
- Rett disorder
- Childhood disintegrative disorder
- Pervasive developmental disorder not otherwise specified

About 1% of children or 1 in 100 to 150 have autism spectrum disorder, with about half of the cases composed of autistic disorder (commonly called *autism*). This incidence represents an increase from formerly described levels. Before 1985, less than 1 child in 1,000 was diagnosed with autistic disorder; it is unclear whether there is a true increase in cases or simply improved techniques in making the diagnosis, as well as an enlarged diagnostic category that includes more children (Inglese & Elder, 2009). The disorder is 4 to 5 times more common in males than females (CDC, 2009a). Peak age at diagnosis is 6 to 11 years, but symptoms often begin

by 18 to 24 months of age. A rare subtype of autism is the *autistic savant*, or a person capable of performing at an extraordinarily high level of skill in one area, such as arithmetical computation, calendar calculation, music performance, art, or memory feats (Hughes, 2010).

Etiology and Pathophysiology

The etiology of autism spectrum disorders is unknown although they are biologically based with multiple and complex phenotypes. Genetics plays a role because monozygotic twins have an affected twin 60% to 90% of the time, whereas dizygotic twins have a 1% to 24% chance of the condition if a twin is affected. Immune responses, environmental exposures, certain drugs during pregnancy, and neuroanatomy are being investigated as influences that interact with genetics to cause ASDs (CDC, 2010a). Neurotransmitters such as dopamine, serotonin, and opioids are abnormal in some children and are also a focus of research. Fetal alcohol syndrome, fragile X syndrome, phenylketonuria, Down syndrome, and tuberous sclerosis are all associated with a higher than normal incidence of autism (CDC, 2010a). Despite concern expressed in earlier medical and lay press, there has been no demonstrated relationship between measles-mumps-rubella vaccine or thimerosal (mercury-containing vaccines) and the incidence of ASDs (see Chapter 22 🔗 for further information on immunizations and this issue) (American Academy of Pediatrics, 2010).

Clinical Manifestations

The essential features typically become apparent by the time a child is 3 years of age. They involve impairments in socialization, communication, and behavior (CDC, 2009a).

A primary finding is impairment in social interactions. Social interactions are always complex and involve perceptions of the other person as well as social behaviors. The infant has limited eye contact, rarely smiles, and does not babble or point to objects (Inglese, 2009). The child with autism does not learn the common characteristics of social interchanges. The child may be unable to converse normally, fail to initiate conversations, and have impaired observations of nonverbal behavior.

Communication difficulties or delays in speech and language are common and are often the first symptoms that lead to diagnosis. Absence of babbling and other communication by 1 year, absence of two-word phrases by 2 years, and deterioration of previous language skills are characteristic. Some children manifest beginning language skills and then regress between 15 and 24 months of age, losing previously acquired communication skills. Abnormal communication patterns include both verbal and nonverbal communication. Children with autism may eventually learn to talk, in some cases well, but their speech is likely to show certain abnormalities: use of "you" in place of "I"; **echolalia** (a compulsive parroting of what is heard); repeating questions rather than answering them; and fascination with rhythmic, repetitive songs and verses.

Children with autism are often unable to relate to people or to respond to social and emotional cues. In addition, they may engage in **stereotypy,** or rigid and obsessive behavior. Characteristically these repetitive behaviors in affected children include head banging, twirling in circles, biting themselves, and flapping their hands or arms. Frequently a child's behavior is self-stimulating or self-destructive. Responses to sensory stimuli are frequently abnormal and include an extreme aversion to touch, loud noises, and bright lights. Emotional lability is common (Figure 34–5 ■).

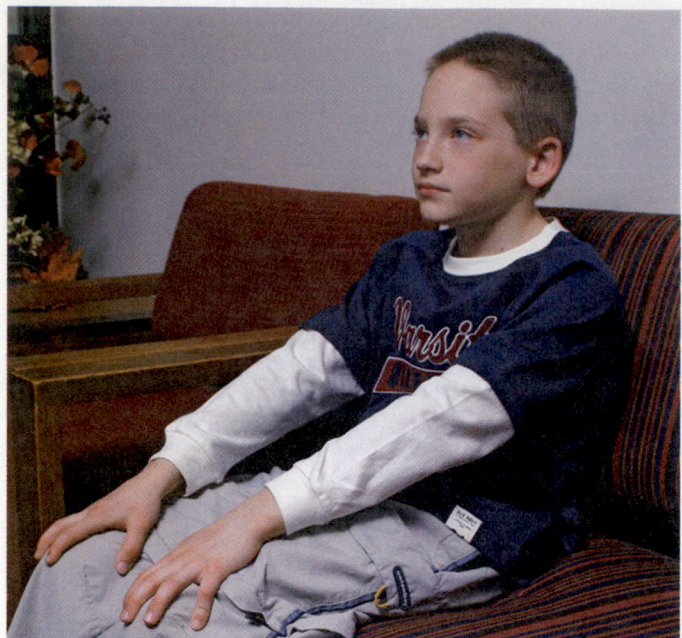

FIGURE 34–5 ■ This child with autism sits stiffly in the chair and engages in rhythmic rocking behavior. He has a disengaged look and does not readily interact with other children or adults who are in his environment.

Behaviors of affected children show several differences from others. They do not commonly explore objects during early childhood, but have stereotyped behaviors. They may line up objects, play with the same objects over and over, and have certain rituals that must be performed. They often become upset if these normal routines are disrupted. In fact, the child often has a great deal of difficulty dealing with new situations, and shows agitation and withdrawal when routines are changed. Rituals may involve eating only certain types or colors of foods or eating in specific patterns.

Children with ASD may manifest disturbances in the rate or sequence of development. They are frequently cognitively impaired but can demonstrate a wide range of intellectual ability and functioning. Cognitive impairment may become manifested early in life by slow developmental progression, particularly in social skills. Some children are impaired in particular areas of development, whereas others are above normal.

The specific differences in clinical manifestations of the types of autism spectrum disorder are listed in the Clinical Manifestations table.

Collaborative Care

Nurses partner with families and other health professionals to identify children with autism spectrum disorders. Care involves collaborative efforts of many resources, including speech therapists, psychologists, teachers, and mental health therapists.

Diagnostic Tests

The first step in identification of children at risk of ASD is surveillance at each healthcare visit. Since diagnosis and treatment have often been delayed, the American Academy of Pediatrics has now identified a multistage process for surveillance and screening:

1. Perform surveillance at early healthcare visits to identify if a sibling has ASD, if parents or other caregivers are concerned about the developmental progression of the child, or if the provider notes abnormalities in the child's behavior.

Clinical Manifestations	Autism Spectrum Disorders (Pervasive Developmental Disorders)	
DISORDER	**CLINICAL MANIFESTATIONS**	**CLINICAL THERAPY**
Autistic disorder	Impaired social, communicative, and behavioral development, usually noted in the first year of life.	Early intervention is key to maximal performance. Interventions focus on improving behaviors and communication skills, providing physical and occupational therapy, structuring play interactions with other children, and educating parents about the child's needs.
Asperger syndrome	Impaired social interactions with normal language development for age; pitch, tone, and other speech characteristics may be abnormal. Verbal skills involving spelling and vocabulary are high, but concept formation, language flexibility, and comprehension are low. Intellectual functioning may be at a very high level, particularly in certain areas, while social skills are limited.	Social interactions are the focus of therapy.
Rett disorder	Early development appears normal and symptoms emerge at 6–18 months. Ataxia, hand-wringing, intermittent hyperventilation, dementia, and growth retardation show progressive increase. Appears only in females as an X-linked dominant disorder; mutations occur in the gene MeCP2, affecting methyl-CpG-binding protein 2, which is important in brain development.	Early intervention focuses on areas of abnormal behaviors.
Childhood disintegrative disorder	First 2–5 years of development appear normal, followed by deterioration in many areas of functioning. Behaviors finally stabilize at some point without further deterioration.	Focus on areas of developmental function that show abnormality. Individualized education plans are needed in school to deal with communication, play, physical therapy, and teaching management skills to parents. Regression in toileting and other skills may occur.
Pervasive developmental disorder not otherwise specified	Severe social impairment without meeting *DSM* criteria for other types of autism spectrum disorder.	Behavioral therapy focuses on building social skills.

TABLE 34–3	Screening Tests for Autism
TEST	**SOURCE**
Clinical Practice Guidelines—Early Intervention Program of the New York State Department of Health	http://www.health.ny.gov/community/infants_children/early_intervention/disorders/autism/
Checklist for Autism in Toddlers (CHAT) or Modified Checklist for Autism in Toddlers (MCHAT)	http://www.aheadwithautism.com/chat_screening.htmlhttp://www.firstsigns.org/downloads/m-chat.PDF
Autism Diagnostic Interview—Revised	http://portal.wpspublish.com/portal/page?_pageid=53,70436&_dad=portal&_schema=PORTAL
Communication and Symbolic Behavior Scales Developmental Profile (CSBS DP)	http://www.brookespublishing.com/store/books/wetherby-csbsdp/checklist.htm
Screening Tool for Autism in Two-Year-Olds	http://kc.vanderbilt.edu/triad/training/page.aspx?id=821
Autism Diagnostic Observation Schedule—Generic (ADOS-G)	http://www.ehow.com/how_2095042_use-adosg.html
Childhood Autism Rating Scale (CARS)	http://oreilly.com/medical/autism/news/diag_tools.html
Developmental Behaviour Checklist—Early Screen (DBC-ES)	http://www.med.monash.edu.au/spppm/research/devpsych/download/dbc-info-package.pdf
Childhood Asperger Syndrome Test (CAST)	http://www.anst.uu.se/abduahma/Saxlemxane/Instruments/CAST/CAST.pdf

2. Determine if the child appears to be at risk for ASD.

3. Evaluate the risks. If risk exists, administer an age-appropriate and ASD-specific screening tool.

4. If no risk exists, an ASD-specific tool is administered at the 18- and 24-month visits.

5. Select the appropriate screening tool for age and risk profile of the child.

6. If screening is negative for a child with some risk, provide information to parents and evaluate again in 1 month. If screening is positive, refer for comprehensive ASD evaluation, including audiology, and begin early intervention programs (Johnson et al., 2007; reaffirmed 2010).

Several screening tests are available for use in health maintenance visits if autistic disorder is suspected (Table 34–3). Because of a rising number of cases, researchers have developed and are testing the reliability of many measures for use at different ages and with siblings. Additional testing is performed to rule out other causes of the child's behavior. Tests may include neuroimaging (CT scan or MRI), lead screening, metabolic studies, DNA analysis, and electroencephalogram. See Chapters 7 and 33 🔗 for further descriptions related to neurologic system assessment.

Diagnosis is based on the presence of specific criteria, as described in the American Psychiatric Association's *Diagnostic and Statistical Manual of Mental Disorders*, 4th edition (*DSM-IV-TR*), and the results of the examination. See the specific criteria for autistic disorder (autism) in Box 34–2; consult *DSM-IV-TR*, which lists similar criteria for other autistic syndrome disorders. Symptoms may emerge as early as 6 months for some disorders, or later for others.

Clinical Therapy

Early intervention assists in maximizing the child's potential by improving developmental skills and behaviors, as well as establishing helpful support for parents (Myers, 2009; Rogers & Vismara, 2008). Treatment focuses on behavior management to reward appropriate behaviors (known as applied behavior analysis or ABA), foster positive or adaptive coping skills, and facilitate effective communication. The goals of treatment are to reduce rigidity or stereotypy

(repetitive, obsessive, machinelike movements) and other maladaptive behaviors. Often the child must be physically restrained from aggressive or self-destructive behaviors. Speech therapy is an essential part of treatment. Instruction in social skills and occupational therapy to improve fine motor dexterity and sensory integration are provided (Myers, 2009). Some parents choose to use complementary therapies such as vitamin supplements and dimethylglycine or trimethylglycine. Foods such as sugar, aspartame, milk products, and wheat are sometimes eliminated from the diet. See Complementary Therapy: Autism.

Medications are used with some children to treat associated disorders but are not effective in treatment of autistic syndrome itself. Medications used for associated conditions include stimulants, selective serotonin reuptake inhibitors (SSRIs), and mood stabilizers.

The overall prognosis for children with autism to become functioning members of society is guarded. The extent to which adequate adjustment is achieved varies greatly. Successful adjustment is more likely for children with higher IQs, adequate speech, and access to specialized programs.

Nursing Management

Nursing Assessment and Diagnosis

The nurse may encounter the child with autism during routine well-child visits or when parents seek care for a suspected hearing impairment, speech difficulty, or developmental delay. Early and frequent developmental screening of all children can help in referral for thorough assessment and identification of cases. Parents may report abnormal interaction such as lack of eye contact, disinterest in cuddling, minimal facial responsiveness, and failure to talk. Be alert to parental observations that the baby or young child does not look at them or provides other developmental or behavioral cues of aversion to contact. Become familiar with the "red flags" of the American Academy of Neurology and Child Neurology Society that require immediate evaluation:

- No babbling or communication gestures by 12 months
- No single word by 16 months

BOX 34–2   *DSM-IV-TR* **Diagnostic Criteria for Autistic Disorder**

A. A total of six or more items from 1, 2, and 3, with at least two from 1, and one each from 2 and 3:

1. Qualitative impairment in social interaction, as manifested by at least two of the following:

   a. Marked impairment in the use of multiple nonverbal behaviors such as eye-to-eye gaze, facial expression, body posture, and gestures to regulate social interaction

   b. Failure to develop peer relationships appropriate to developmental level

   c. Lack of spontaneous seeking to share enjoyment, interests, or achievements with other people

   d. Lack of social or emotional reciprocity

2. Qualitative impairments in communication as manifested by at least one of the following:

   a. Delay in, or total lack of, the development of spoken language (not accompanied by an attempt to compensate through alternative modes of communication such as gesture or mime)

   b. In individuals with adequate speech, marked impairment in the ability to initiate or sustain a conversation with others

   c. Stereotyped and repetitive use of language or idiosyncratic language

   d. Lack of varied, spontaneous make-believe play or social imitative play appropriate to developmental level

3. Restricted repetitive and stereotyped patterns of behavior, interests, and activities, as manifested by at least one of the following:

   a. Encompassing preoccupation with one or more stereotyped and restricted patterns of interest that is abnormal either in intensity or in focus

   b. Apparently inflexible adherence to specific, nonfunctional routines or rituals

   c. Stereotyped and repetitive motor mannerisms (e.g., hand or finger flapping or twisting, or complex whole-body movements)

   d. Persistent preoccupation with parts of objects

B. Delays or abnormal functioning in at least one of the following areas, with onset prior to age 3 years: (1) social interaction, (2) language as used in social communication, or (3) symbolic or imaginative play.

C. The disturbance is not better accounted for by Rett's Disorder or Childhood Disintegrative Disorder.

Source: *Reprinted with permission from the* Diagnostic and Statistical Manual of Mental Disorders, *fourth edition, text revision. Copyright © 2000 American Psychiatric Association.*

Complementary Therapy   **Autism**

Some parents who have a child with autism choose to use complementary therapy in an attempt to help the child. A popular treatment approach includes dietary therapy with vitamin A, vitamin C, vitamin B$_6$, magnesium, omega-3 fatty acids, zinc, or use of gluten-free or casein-free diets. Probiotics such as those in yogurt, kefir, and tempeh may be taken. Complementary drug therapy includes secretin, a pancreatic gastrointestinal peptide, and Pepcid or other antacids. Some parents believe that detoxification by limiting intake of certain dietary components or using Epsom salt baths can be helpful. Music therapy has been used to improve social interaction, and massage has been used to enhance response to touch and communication. Additional therapies include homeopathy, craniosacral therapy, Reiki, hyperbaric chambers, and biofeedback. Chelation therapy is not approved but has been used by some physicians and families as a treatment for autism. The rationale is that autism is related to collection of heavy metals such as mercury in the body. Chelation is a treatment with serious potential side effects (see Chapter 20 🔗 for further information about chelation for treatment of lead poisoning). The report of a death of a young boy being treated for autism with chelation reinforces the danger of using untested therapies (CDC, 2010a, 2010b; Golnik & Maccabee-Ryaboy, 2010).

Nurses can help parents to evaluate studies on complementary and alternative therapy and encourage them to initiate only one treatment at a time to measure effectiveness. Ask about therapies being used, and discuss safeguards to avoid any undesired side effects. Read about new studies on complementary therapies, and evaluate the rationale, efficacy, side effects, and other pertinent findings to bring current information to families.

---

patterns. Perform hearing and vision screening to rule out sensory problems. Integrate within child health care in all settings at least one screening tool for autism appropriate for the age groups served.

Clinical Judgment

The infant or toddler often displays signs of autism at an early age. Since communication abnormalities are red flags for autism, what speech would you normally expect in a 12-month-old, 16-month-old, or 24-month-old?

When a child with a diagnosis of autistic disorder is hospitalized for a concurrent problem, obtain a history from the parents regarding the child's routines, rituals, and likes and dislikes, as well as ways to promote interaction and cooperation. Children with autism may carry a special toy or object that they play with during times of stress. Ask parents about these objects and their use.

Ask about the child's behaviors as well as observing them on admission. Observe interactions with parents, other adults, and children. Obtain a history of acute and chronic illnesses and injuries. Ask about eating patterns and food restrictions. Inquire about complementary therapies used in a nonjudgmental and supportive manner.

Nursing diagnoses must be tailored to fit the individual needs of the child. Examples of diagnoses that may be appropriate for children with autism or other pervasive developmental disorders include the following:

- Communication: Verbal, Impaired related to psychological condition
- Social Interaction, Impaired related to developmental disability
- Confusion, Chronic related to mental disorder
- Injury, Risk for related to cognitive impairment
- Caregiver Role Strain, Risk for related to chronicity and demands of child's condition
- Coping: Family, Disabled Compromised related to having a child with prolonged disability

NANDA-I © 2012

- No spontaneous two-word phrases by 24 months
- Loss of language or social skills previously achieved

Johnson et al., 2007, 2010.

Assessment at every healthcare visit focuses on language development, response to others, and hearing acuity (see Chapters 7 and 24 🔗). Carefully evaluate the child for history of developmental milestones and refer for abnormalities. Perform developmental screening that considers several areas of development including motor activity, social skills, and language. Recall that the child with autism may have normal performance in one area such as motor skills and delayed development in another area such as language skills. Likewise, language may be normal for age but social interactions may be delayed. Include questioning about adaptive skills such as toilet training and feeding patterns. Inquire about school performance since some areas of achievement may be normal while others are delayed. Observe the child in play situations, and evaluate the use of creative and exploratory play versus more repetitive

Planning and Implementation

Nursing care focuses on stabilizing environmental stimuli, providing supportive care, enhancing communication, maintaining a safe environment, and offering the parents anticipatory guidance.

Stabilize Environmental Stimuli

Children with autism interpret and respond to the environment differently from other individuals. Sounds that are not distressing to the average person may be interpreted by children with autism as louder, more frightening, and overwhelming. The child needs to be oriented to new settings such as a classroom or the hospital room and may adjust best to a small classroom or a hospital room with only one other child. Encourage parents to bring the child's favorite objects from home, and try to keep these objects in the same places, because the child often does not cope well with changes in the environment.

Provide Supportive Care

Developing a trusting relationship with the child who has autism is often difficult. Adjust communication techniques and teaching to the child's developmental level. Ask parents about the child's usual home routines, and maintain these routines as much as possible if the child is not in the home setting. Because self-care abilities are often limited, the child may need assistance to meet basic needs. When possible, schedule daily care and routine procedures at consistent times to maintain predictability. Encourage parents to remain with the hospitalized child and to participate in daily care planning. Parents are integral parts of the treatment team when the child's learning goals are established in early intervention or school programs. Identify rituals for naptime and bedtime, and maintain them to promote rest and sleep. Integrate patterns that facilitate intake of nutritious foods at mealtimes.

School programs, behavioral therapy, and individualized education plans (see Chapter 14 🔗) can help the child to learn self-care skills within community settings. See additional suggestions for family support in the community care section.

Enhance Communication

Because children with autism have impaired communication, nursing care focuses on utilizing and improving communication with the child. Speech is used when possible; short, direct sentences are usually most effective. If the child responds well to visual cues, then pictures, computers, and other visual aids may form an important part of interaction. Sign language is used with some children.

Maintain a Safe Environment

Monitor children with autism at all times, including bath time and bedtime. Close supervision is needed to ensure that the child does not obtain any harmful objects or engage in dangerous behaviors. For the child who engages in head banging or other abusive behaviors, bicycle helmets and hand mitts can be the least restrictive method to provide safety. They enable the child to participate in activities and engage in a social environment to the degree possible.

Provide Anticipatory Guidance

Approximately half of all children with autistic disorder require lifelong supervision and support, especially if the disorder is accompanied by intellectual disability. Some children may grow up to lead independent lives, although they will have social limitations with impaired interpersonal relationships. Encourage parents to promote the child's development through behavior modification and specialized educational programs. The overall goal is to provide the child with the guidance, education, and support necessary for optimal functioning. Parents need support over a long period and may benefit from contact with other families in similar situations. They may be vulnerable to "quick cures" offered on the Internet and other sources, and need reliable materials and opportunities to discuss what they have read or heard.

Care in the Community

Families of children with autism need a great deal of support. The diagnosis may trigger feelings of grief and shock (Elder & D'Alessandro, 2009). Then, the challenges of families who have a child with a chronic disorder emerge (see Chapter 16 🔗). Participating in parent support groups and learning how to reframe the condition to view its positive aspects are helpful strategies. Help families to identify resources for childcare, such as special toddler programs and preschools. They may need specialized transportation services for the child or other social supports. The child will need an individualized education plan. The parent or primary caretaker often has difficulty obtaining respite care and may need assistance to find suitable resources. Siblings of the child with autism may need help to explain the disorder to their friends or teachers. The nurse can be instrumental in assisting these siblings to understand and explain autism. School nurses partner with health professionals in other settings to implement communication plans and other strategies for the child with autism. Individualized education and health plans are needed, and the school nurse is instrumental in team management to achieve these plans (Lobar, Fritts, Arbide, et al., 2008).

Genetic counseling should be offered to the family. Information on immunizations is necessary, because parents may have heard about a potential connection between immunization and the disorder. They should be encouraged to have the child immunized on the recommended schedule. Parents may have questions about where to find information on complementary and alternative therapies.

Local support groups for parents of children with autism are available in most areas. Parents can also be referred to the Autism Society of America, the American Academy of Pediatrics, and the Centers for Disease Control and Prevention for information on autism.

Evaluation

Expected outcomes of nursing care for the child with autism are as follows:

- Behavioral symptoms are effectively managed.
- The child performs elements of self-care.
- The child remains free from injury.
- Consistent developmental progression is observed.
- The child develops successful communication strategies.

Attention Deficit Disorder and Attention Deficit Hyperactivity Disorder

Attention deficit disorder (ADD) is a variation in central nervous system processing characterized by developmentally inappropriate behaviors involving inattention. When hyperactivity and impulsivity accompany inattention, the disorder is called attention deficit hyperactivity disorder (ADHD). The latter is the most common mental health alteration of childhood, affecting about 8.4% of all school-age children (CDC, 2012). Boys are affected almost four times more commonly than girls. It is now known to affect adolescents and adults; those with the disorder often continue to manifest at least some of the symptoms as they grow into adulthood. Hyperactivity and impulsivity may improve as the child nears adulthood, with inattentiveness the most persistent characteristic. The adolescent may have difficulty due to the increasing cognitive demands of school.

Etiology and Pathophysiology

Although a variety of physical and neurologic disorders are associated with ADHD, children with identifiable causes represent a small proportion of this population. Examples of known associations include exposure to high levels of lead or mercury in childhood and prenatal exposure to alcohol or tobacco smoke. Other prenatal factors associated with a higher incidence of ADHD include preterm labor, impaired placenta functioning, and impaired oxygenation. Seizures and serious head injury are other potential associations. Genetic factors may be important, as well as family dynamics and environmental characteristics. Although ADHD occurs more commonly within families (25% have a first-degree relative with the disorder), a single gene has not been located and a specific mechanism of genetic transmission is not known. It is believed that a genetic predisposition interacts with the child's environment, so that both factors contribute to the appearance of the condition. Family stress, poverty, and poor nutrition may also be contributing factors. Although daily television exposure at ages 1 to 3 years has been associated with attentional symptoms of the condition later in childhood, not all studies verify this finding (Cheng, Maeda, Yoichi, et al., 2010; Ferguson, 2011; Swing, Gentile, Anderson, et al., 2010). It is likely that there are many types of attention deficit, resulting from several different mechanisms that involve interaction of genetic, biological, and environmental risk factors.

The pathophysiology of ADD/ADHD is unclear, but certain brain characteristics provide clues. Some children may exhibit a deficit in the catecholamines dopamine and norepinephrine, lowering the threshold for stimuli input. The disorder is marked by brain maturation delay in the area of self-regulation. Increased input from stimuli and decreased self-regulation cause the hallmark inability to inhibit stimuli and motor activity. Slow brain maturity, as much as 3 years, has been demonstrated on imaging studies. The cortex is particularly affected and may explain the school and concentration difficulty associated with the disorder (National Institutes of Health, 2011).

Clinical Manifestations

Children with ADD and ADHD have problems related to decreased attention span, impulsiveness, and/or increased motor activity (Figure 34–6 ■). Symptoms can range from mild to severe. The disorders often co-exist with various developmental learning disabilities, motor disorders, and aggressive behaviors. The child has difficulty completing tasks, fidgets constantly, is frequently loud, and interrupts others. Sleep disturbances are common. Because of these behaviors, the child often has difficulty developing and maintaining social relationships and may be shunned or teased by other children. This only increases the anxiety of the already compromised child, whose behavior is set on a downward spiraling course.

Typically, girls with ADHD show less aggression and impulsiveness than boys, but far more anxiety, mood swings, social withdrawal, rejection, and cognitive and language problems. Girls tend to be older

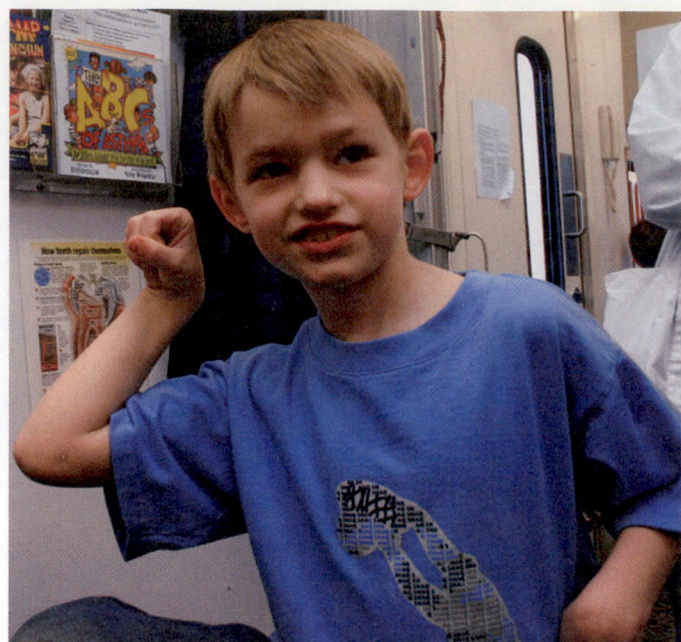

FIGURE 34–6 ■ This child with ADHD is challenged by a visit to a healthcare facility for dental care. He found it difficult to remain in the chair for the examination, and once it was over, he rapidly ran from one piece of equipment to another in the facility. He asked what things were for but did not wait for answers. His engaging personality can be seen as he poses briefly for a picture. Such behaviors can be exhausting for parents to manage and may create safety hazards in the healthcare setting.

at the time of diagnosis. Children are frequently diagnosed with the disorder soon after beginning school, when demands increase for attentive behavior. See Box 34–3 for the *DSM-IV-TR* diagnostic criteria for attention deficit hyperactivity disorder.

Collaborative Care

Families and professionals collaborate to make the diagnosis and ensure adequate treatment for the child with ADHD. Parents often seek a pediatrician or other primary care provider. A specialist in the disorder should then be consulted for the diagnosis. School personnel will be asked for their observations in order to meet diagnostic criteria. Parents and professionals in health care and school partner to plan and provide care for the child.

Diagnostic Tests

Children are usually brought for evaluation when behaviors escalate to the point of interfering with the daily functioning of teachers or parents. Any child from 4 through 18 years who has academic problems, behavior difficulties, inattention, hyperactivity, or impulsivity should be evaluated for ADHD (Subcommittee on Attention-Deficit/Hyperactivity Disorder, 2011). When children have learning disabilities or anxiety disorders, the problem is commonly misdiagnosed as ADHD if full and accurate evaluation of the child's symptoms is not performed. Obtaining an accurate diagnosis after comprehensive testing by a pediatric mental health specialist is vital (Becker, Goobie, & Thomas, 2009). Specific diagnostic criteria must be applied to all children with the potential diagnosis (see *DSM-IV-TR* criteria in Box 34–3). The diagnosis of ADD is often difficult due to the absence of hyperactivity behaviors. Behaviors both at home and school or childcare must be evaluated, because abnormal patterns in two

BOX 34–3 | *DSM-IV-TR* Diagnostic Criteria for Attention Deficit Hyperactivity Disorder

A. Either 1 or 2:

1. Inattention: Six (or more) of the following symptoms of inattention have persisted for at least 6 months to a degree that is maladaptive and inconsistent with developmental level:

   a. Often fails to give close attention to details or makes careless mistakes in schoolwork, work, and other activities

   b. Often has difficulty sustaining attention in tasks or play activities

   c. Often does not seem to listen when spoken to directly

   d. Often does not follow through on instructions and fails to finish schoolwork, chores, or duties in the workplace (not due to oppositional behavior or failure to understand instructions)

   e. Often has difficulty organizing tasks and activities

   f. Often avoids, dislikes, or is reluctant to engage in tasks that require sustained mental effort (such as schoolwork or homework)

   g. Often loses things necessary for tasks or activities (e.g., toys, school assignments, pencils, books, or tools)

   h. Is often easily distracted by extraneous stimuli

   i. Is often forgetful in daily activities

2. Hyperactivity-impulsivity: Six (or more) of the following symptoms of hyperactivity-impulsivity have persisted for at least 6 months to a degree that is maladaptive and inconsistent with developmental level:

   Hyperactivity

   a. Often fidgets with hands or feet or squirms in seat

   b. Often leaves seat in classroom or in other situations in which remaining seated is expected

   c. Often runs about or climbs excessively in situations in which it is inappropriate (in adolescents or adults, may be limited to subjective feelings of restlessness)

   d. Often has difficulty playing or engaging in leisure activities quietly

   e. Is often "on the go" or often acts as if "driven by a motor"

   f. Often talks excessively

   Impulsivity

   a. Often blurts out answers before questions have been completed

   b. Often has difficulty awaiting turn

   c. Often interrupts or intrudes on others (e.g., butts into conversations or games)

B. Some hyperactive-impulsive or inattentive symptoms that caused impairment were present before age 7 years.

C. Some impairment from the symptoms is present in two or more settings (e.g., at school [or work] and at home).

D. There must be clear evidence of clinically significant impairment in social, academic, or occupational functioning.

E. The symptoms do not occur exclusively during the course of a Pervasive Developmental Disorder, Schizophrenia, or other Psychotic Disorder and are not better accounted for by another mental disorder (e.g., Mood Disorder, Anxiety Disorder, Dissociative Disorder, or a Personality Disorder).

Source: *Reprinted with permission from the* Diagnostic and Statistical Manual of Mental Disorders, *fourth edition, text revision. Copyright © 2000 American Psychiatric Association.*

and teachers, and any other emotional and behavioral conditions (Subcommittee on Attention-Deficit/Hyperactivity Disorder, 2011). A physical examination should be performed to rule out neurologic diseases and other health problems. The mental health specialist then performs testing of the child and administers questionnaires to the parent and teacher. See Table 34–4 for examples of comprehensive testing resources. It is important to identify other conditions that may either mimic ADD/ADHD or co-exist with the disorders. These might include depression, anxiety, learning disorder, conduct disorder, or oppositional defiant disorder.

Clinical Therapy

Based on the findings, desired outcomes are established for the child's performance. Treatment is established to meet the desired behavioral outcomes, and includes a combination of approaches, such as environmental changes, behavior therapy, and pharmacotherapy (Vierhile, Robb, & Ryan-Krause, 2009). The condition is chronic, so treatment will continue over time.

Children often benefit from environmental changes. Decreasing stimulation—for example, by turning off television, keeping the environment quiet, and maintaining an orderly and clutter-free desk or study area without distractions—may help the child to stay focused on the task at hand. Another relatively simple change is appropriate classroom placement, preferably in a small class with a teacher who can provide close supervision and a structured daily routine. Consistent limits and expectations should be set for the child. Children living in chaotic homes and communities may function better if the environment can be simplified. When aggressive behaviors occur, therapeutic approaches such as play and group therapy may be useful.

Behavior therapy involves rewarding the child for desired behaviors and applying consequences for undesirable behaviors. Children may be rewarded by praise or earn points toward a movie or other desired outing for staying seated during meals or quietly listening in a classroom. Cues are established so the child can subtly be reminded when impulsive or hyperactive behaviors are escalating. All adults who are in close contact with the child, such as parents and teachers, must be educated to carry out the behavioral program (Subcommittee on Attention-Deficit/Hyperactivity Disorder, 2011).

Children with moderate to severe ADD/ADHD are treated with pharmacotherapy. Methylphenidate (Ritalin, Concerta) is most often prescribed with dextroamphetamine (Dexedrine or Adderall) and the nonstimulant medication atomoxetine as alternatives. A skin patch that releases medication over a 9-hour period is available, facilitating ease of administration (May & Kratochvil, 2010). Usually a favorable response (a decrease in impulsive behaviors and an increase in the ability to sit still and attend to an activity for at least 15 minutes) is seen in the first 10 days of treatment and frequently with the first few doses. New guidelines have been issued to recommend thorough evaluation of children before a stimulant or other medication is prescribed, in order to rule out any cardiac condition that could be affected by medication use. Guidelines include:

- Patient and family history of conditions associated with sudden cardiac death
- All medications and health supplements
- Physical examination, especially of the cardiovascular system
- Electrocardiogram
- Pediatric cardiology consult if any abnormalities are identified

Hammerness, Traum, Becker, et al., 2009; Vetter, Elia, Erickson, et al., 2008.

settings are needed for diagnosis. A variety of tests are available for use by the trained professional in establishing the diagnosis.

Diagnosis begins with a careful history of the child, including family history, birth history, growth and developmental milestones, behaviors such as sleep and eating patterns, progression and patterns in school, social and environmental conditions, reports from parents

TABLE 34–4	Screening Tests for ADD/ADHD
TEST	**SOURCE**
Vanderbilt Parent and Teacher Scales	http://www.brightfutures.org/mentalhealth/pdf/professionals/bridges/adhd.pdfhttp://www.childrenshospital.vanderbilt.org/uploads/documents/DIAGNOSTIC_PARENT_RATING_SCALE(1).pdf
Connors' Parent and Teacher Rating Scales—Revised—Long Form	http://psychcorp.pearsonassessments.com/HAIWEB/Cultures/en-us/Productdetail.htm?Pid=PAg116
Swanson, Nolan and Pelham Questionnaire II Teacher and Parent Rating Scale (SNAP-IV)	http://www.ourgirlwednesday.com/downloads/snap-iv-instructions.pdf
Disruptive Behavior Disorder Scale	http://vinst.umdnj.edu/VAID/TestReport.asp?Code=DBRSF
ADHD Rating Scale	http://www.fmpe.org/en/documents/appendix/Appendix%201%20-%20ADHD%20Rating%20Scale.pdf
Revised Behavioral Problems Checklist	http://vinst.umdnj.edu/VAID/TestReport.asp?Code=RBPC
Child Behavior Checklist	http://vinst.umdnj.edu/VAID/TestReport.asp?Code=CBCA

Source: *Data from Vierhile, A., Robb, A., & Ryan-Krause, P. (2009). Attention-deficit/hyperactivity disorder in children and adolescents: Closing diagnostic, communication, and treatment gaps.* Journal of Pediatric Health Care, 23, S5–S21.

See the Medications table below for a listing of common pharmacologic treatments.

A variety of other treatments have been attempted for ADHD and are used by families. Chiropractic manipulation, biofeedback, and dietary interventions (both elimination diets and supplement use) are examples of common complementary or alternative therapies.

Although ADHD was once thought to be a disorder of childhood that gradually improved with age, it is now known that ADHD is a chronic condition requiring ongoing management; for many individuals, symptoms continue into adulthood.

Nursing Management

Nursing management consists of referring children with possible ADHD for appropriate screening, monitoring the child's growth and development, following progress in behavioral manifestations, and partnering with parents and other professionals in the treatment of the disorder.

Nursing Assessment and Diagnosis

The nurse often encounters the family who is concerned about the child's behavior before a diagnosis has been made. Ask about

Medications Used to Treat ADHD

MEDICATION	ACTION AND INDICATION	NURSING MANAGEMENT
Methylphenidate	A derivative of piperidine that acts like amphetamine. May work in ADHD treatment by inhibiting reuptake of dopamine and norepinephrine, thereby enhancing catecholamine effects in the nervous system, improving attention span and task performance. Schedule II drug in Schedule of Controlled Substances.	Available in short-acting forms as Ritalin, Methylin, and Focalin. Also in intermediate-acting forms of Ritalin SR, Metadate ER, and Methylin ER. Available in long-acting forms of Concerta, Daytrana, Focalin XR, Methylin ER, Metadate CD, and Ritalin LA. Transdermal 9-hour patches are available. The variety of available forms makes it important to read labels carefully and inform families about proper administration of the child's specific type of drug. The most common side effects are headache, insomnia, and anorexia. Periodic growth measurements and cardiac assessments are needed. Behavior and school performance are monitored.
Amphetamine preparations	Synthetic sympathomimetic amine with stimulant effect on central nervous system. Increases release of norepinephrine and dopamine by blocking their reuptake. Schedule II drug in Schedule of Controlled Substances.	Available in short-acting forms of Dexedrine, DextroStat, Adderall, and Procentra. Intermediate-acting forms include Adderall and Dexedrine Spansules. Long-acting forms include Adderall-XR and Vyvanse. Read labels and instruct in proper administration. Anorexia, weight loss, insomnia, and headache are common side effects. Monitor vital signs, cardiac status, and growth measurements periodically.
Atomoxetine	This is the first nonstimulant drug for treatment of ADHD. It inhibits norepinephrine reuptake, decreases hyperactivity and impulsivity of ADHD, and may assist with improving mood and decreasing anxiety.	Available as Strattera in a variety of dosages. Recommended starting dose for children is 0.5 mg/kg/day. Has been shown to have long-lasting effect of 1 day or longer. Side effects are uncommon and transient, with dyspepsia or vomiting, fatigue, decreased appetite, and dizziness most common. Have the child change position slowly if dizziness occurs; caution the teen not to drive until effects of the drug are clear. Perform periodic growth measurements. Monitor for increased irritability and agitation. The drug must be labeled with the caution that it has been associated with increased suicide ideation in some youth.

Source: *Ganem, J. A. (2008). Treating children with ADHD. Retrieved from http://www.jobsoneducation.com/cliniciansCME.index.asp?page= courses/105821/disclaimer.htm&lsn_id= 105821; Ryan-Krause, P. (2011). Attention deficit hyperactivity disorder: Part III.* Journal of Pediatric Health Care, 25, 48–54.

family and birth history, and have the parents describe the child's behaviors. Perform developmental testing and look specifically for attention span and physical activity. Refer the family to their pediatric healthcare home for further assessment and then to a mental healthcare specialist who is experienced in diagnosing ADD/ADHD. Schedule a visit for a complete patient and family history, physical examination, and electrocardiogram before medication is begun (Vetter et al., 2008).

The nurse may encounter the child with known ADHD in the hospital when parents bring the child for treatment of an injury (e.g., fracture) or other problem. Explore the parents' report of the child's attention span in detail. Usually within a few minutes in an unstructured setting or waiting area, the child with ADHD becomes restless and searches for distraction. Gather information about the child's activity level and impulsiveness. Be alert for information that reveals a serious problem, such as hurting animals or other children. Obtain information about distractibility, attention deficit in activities of daily living, characteristic ways of reacting, and the extent of impulsiveness when the child is receiving medication. Find out how the family manages at home and what treatment is being used.

Examples of nursing diagnoses that may be appropriate for a child with ADD/ADHD include the following:

- Communication: Verbal, Impaired related to altered perceptions
- Social Interaction, Impaired related to chronic episodes of impulsive behavior
- Self-Esteem, Chronic Low related to behaviors associated with ADD/ADHD
- Injury, Risk for related to high level of impulsiveness and excitability
- Caregiver Role Strain, Risk for related to management of child with unpredictable moods and high energy

NANDA-I © 2012

Planning and Implementation

Nursing care of the hospitalized child with ADD/ADHD focuses on administering medications, managing the child's environment, implementing behavioral management plans, providing emotional support to the child and family, promoting self-esteem, and ensuring ongoing care. Care in the community includes the same components along with guiding parents to appropriate resources when needed. Prevention can focus on discouraging regular television exposure for young children from 1 to 3 years and encouraging daily vigorous physical activity for all children.

Administer Medications

Stimulant and nonstimulant medications increase the child's attention span and decrease distractibility. Be alert for the common side effects of these medications, including anorexia, insomnia, and tachycardia. Administering medication early in the day helps to alleviate insomnia. Anorexia can be managed by giving medication at mealtimes. Baseline cardiac examinations are needed, as well as periodic reevaluation. Careful periodic monitoring of weight, height, and blood pressure is necessary. Instruct families about the abuse potential of stimulant drugs; they should be kept locked and administered only as directed. Youth going to college or camps with the medication should be provided with a locked container in which to store the drug. Inquire about camp and school policies and procedures for medication use and storage. See Box 34–4.

BOX 34–4	**Research: Diversion of Stimulants Prescribed for ADHD**

Most of the drugs that are used to treat ADHD can be abused when used by others. One study of 2,744 secondary school students found that about one in seven had diverted their prescribed controlled substances by selling, trading, or giving them away (McCabe, West, Teter, et al., 2011). A large systematic review of 21 studies on diversion of prescribed ADHD stimulants with 113,104 subjects found that 16% to 29% of students had diverted controlled drugs at some time (Wilens, Adler, Adams, et al., 2008). College students are the most frequent abusers of these prescription drugs. Nurses should screen all youth for substance use (see Chapter 20 🔗) and should perform teaching with youth and their families about safe storage of ADHD drugs to avoid inadvertent use by others. Secondary and college students should be asked if they have ever diverted their prescribed medications to others, and clear education on misuse and dangers of diversion should be provided.

Minimize Environmental Distractions

The child may need to be placed in an environment with minimal distractions. When hospitalized, this may mean a room with only one other child. Potentially harmful equipment should be kept out of reach. Television and video game time needs to be monitored and limited. Use shades to darken the room during naps or at bedtime and minimize noise. Teach parents to minimize distractions at home during periods when the child needs to concentrate, for example, when doing schoolwork (Figure 34–7 ■). Visits to areas such as shopping malls and playgrounds may need to be limited. Plenty of daily physical activity assists the child in the ability to focus on school and other tasks.

Implement Behavioral Management Plans

Behavior modification programs can help to reduce specific impulsive behaviors. An example is setting up a reward program for the child who has taken medication as ordered or completed a homework

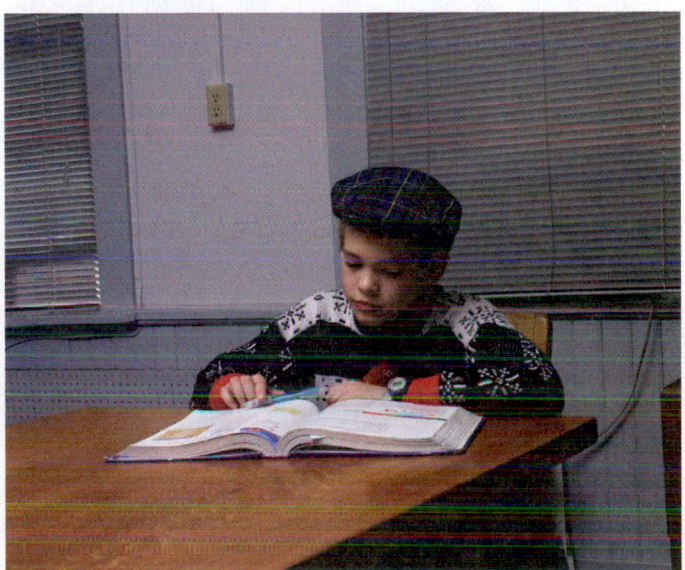

FIGURE 34–7 ■ Managing the environment to provide quiet places with minimal distractions is often necessary for the child with ADHD. This boy reads and does homework in a room with few pictures, no music, and only the book with homework on the table. He is also assisted by structure such as a scheduled time for homework, with short breaks to walk around every 10 to 15 minutes.

assignment. The rewards may be daily as well as weekly or monthly, depending on the child's age. For example, one completed homework assignment might be rewarded with 30 minutes of basketball or a bike ride; assignments completed for a week might be rewarded with participation in an activity of the child's choice on the weekend. Find out what behavioral rewards are being used at school and home, and integrate them as much as possible into hospital routines.

If punishment is necessary, the behavior should be corrected while simultaneously supporting the child as a person. Punishment is generally withdrawal of a privilege, and should follow the offense quickly as the child may not otherwise connect the punishment with the behavior.

Provide Emotional Support

Children with ADD or ADHD offer a special challenge to parents, teachers, and healthcare providers. Parents must cope simultaneously with managing the difficult needs and demands of a child who is hard to handle, obtaining appropriate evaluation and treatment, and understanding and accepting the diagnosis, even when the child exhibits different behaviors with different people. Family support is essential. Educate both the parents and the child about the importance of appropriate expectations and consequences of behaviors. Teach skills that will help as the child grows older: making lists of tasks to accomplish; implementing routines for eating, sleeping, recreation, and schoolwork; minimizing stimuli in the environment when completing work; and asking teachers and friends to identify when behavior is inappropriate. When the child is hospitalized for another condition, the time may provide a brief respite from constant care by the parent. The activity, impulsivity, and general high energy of children with ADHD can fatigue parents. They may wish to spend a few hours each day at home or a nearby residence for families when the child is hospitalized. Ask them how they manage at home, and offer ideas for respite care.

Promote Self-Esteem

As the child grows, ask about school and friends in order to assess self-concept and self-esteem. Help the child to understand the disorder at an appropriate developmental level, and facilitate a trusting relationship with healthcare providers. Assist the child with social skills through the use of role-play, small-group play, and modeling. Promote the child's self-esteem by emphasizing the positive aspects of behavior and treating instances of negative behavior as learning opportunities. Help the child to develop ego strengths (the conscious ability to screen outside stimuli and to control internal demands), which will result in better impulse control and thus increase self-esteem over time (Houck, Kendall, Miller, et al., 2011). Praise the child for remaining still for a procedure, taking a medication on time, or helping a staff member in the playroom.

Care in the Community

Most children with ADD or ADHD are only hospitalized when needing care for another condition. Parents need support to understand the diagnosis and to learn how to manage the child. This will usually be accomplished in the pediatric healthcare home or in the office of a mental health specialist. Explain the diagnosis and what is known about attention deficit disorders. Provide written materials and Internet sites, and an opportunity to ask questions. See Developing Cultural Competence: ADHD and Family Response.

Developing Cultural Competence
ADHD and Family Response

Many families who have a child with ADHD or another mental health disorder are embarrassed and feel shame because of the diagnosis, especially in certain cultures such as some Asian groups and in very structured and highly achieving families. When taking histories from family members, it is best to be sensitive to the stigma they may feel. Ask questions in a private setting, and ask about the family's feelings regarding a mental health disorder. Is there someone in their family who they can talk to about the diagnosis? Provide information in a nonjudgmental manner, and offer support if appropriate from other families with similar experiences.

Emphasize the importance of a stable environment, at home as well as at school. At home, the child may have difficulty staying on task. Parents need to consider the child's age and the developmental appropriateness of tasks, give clear and simple instructions, and provide frequent reminders to ensure completion. Routines in the evening can promote good sleep patterns.

The nurse can serve as a liaison to teachers and school personnel, or as the case manager for the child. An individualized education plan may be needed (see Chapter 14 🔴), with clear expected outcomes stated for the child's behaviors. Special classrooms or periods of instruction free from the distractions of the entire class may enable the child to improve school performance. Parents may have difficulty understanding the need for these approaches because the child often tests with above-average intelligence. Reinforce the importance of providing a structured environment free from unnecessary external stimuli. Be sure that parents understand behavioral approaches that will help the child, how to administer prescribed medications, and the importance of returning for healthcare visits to monitor for side effects. (See Partnering with Families: School Suggestions for Children with ADD/ADHD.) Ensure that medication is safely stored.

Children with ADD or ADHD may have few friends due to their impulsivity, lack of connectedness with other children, and other behaviors. Ask about social interactions and recommend participation in school and community sports and clubs where the rules of working with others can be learned.

Parents may have heard about attention deficit disorder in the media and may have many questions about its cause and management. Providing information about complementary and alternative treatments is a nursing role (see Complementary Therapy: ADD/ADHD). The National Institutes of Health sponsors the National Center for Complementary and Alternative Medicine (NCCAM) and is a reliable source for parents and professionals.

As the child grows older, provide explanations about the disorder and information about techniques that will assist in dealing with problems. Emphasize the importance of doing homework or other tasks requiring concentration in a quiet environment without background noise from a television or radio. Encourage children with ADD/ADHD to keep assignment notebooks and use checklists to help them accomplish specific tasks. Such interventions lead to establishment of a positive self-image and confidence in the ability to manage the condition successfully.

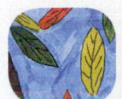

Partnering with Families

School Suggestions for Children with ADD/ADHD

Parents can work with teachers to provide for a school environment that fosters attention and learning. Ideas that may be helpful include:

- Have the child sit near the front of the class.
- Plan a reminder that is apparent to the teacher and student but not to other children when the child needs to concentrate on attention. This might be an object placed on the student's desk or a hand placed gently on the shoulder or arm.
- Give instructions verbally and in written form and repeat them more than once.
- Provide opportunities to take notes and make lists of assignments and mark them off when accomplished. Have a planned time for the parent to go through the child's backpack daily so notices are seen and homework is completed and in a uniform location.

- Use computers to make lists and take notes. The child may need to listen in class, record the teacher, and take notes later from the recording.
- If the child has well-developed fine or gross motor skills, integrate motor movement into learning situations when possible.
- Provide quiet places with minimal distraction for examinations. Offer additional time.
- Allow time for organizing clothing, the desk, and other areas.
- Go over assignments and tests with the child to explain areas that are understood and those that need attention.
- Find the child's areas of excellence and allow for performance in these ways. Some children are talented in dance, others in art or extemporaneous speech.
- Never call the child names, make fun of behavior or performance, or call the child "hyperactive" in front of other children, teachers, or parents.

Complementary Therapy ADD/ADHD

A variety of complementary approaches, in addition to or instead of traditional behavioral therapy and medication, have been tried in children with ADD or ADHD. Chiropractic manipulation, biofeedback, yoga, massage, visual or auditory therapy, and dietary interventions have been used. Dietary therapies include elimination of dietary components such as highly processed foods, sugar, aspartame, or yeast; use of supplements such as omega-3 fatty acids, iron, magnesium, zinc, and vitamin B_6; and herbs such as Pycnogenol, melatonin, *Echinacea*, St. John's wort, and *Ginkgo biloba*. Ask parents about alternative therapies used, and investigate what is known about them in order to share this information with parents (Brulotte, Bukutu, & Vohra, 2009; Rucklidge, Johnstone, & Kaplan, 2009).

Evaluation

Expected outcomes of nursing care for the child with ADD or ADHD include the following:

- The parents and child demonstrate an understanding of the condition.
- Medications are administered and managed safely and as prescribed.
- The child demonstrates increased attentiveness and decreased hyperactivity, impulsivity, and sleep disturbance.
- The child forms a positive self-image.
- The child forms healthy social interactions with peers and family.
- Educational performance is achieved to maximum potential.

MOOD DISORDERS

The major mood disorders in children are depression and bipolar disease, both of which are discussed in this chapter. A third disorder, dysthymia, is less common in children. It has similar but milder symptoms than depression; however, it lasts longer with a mean duration of 3 years.

Depression

Depression is psychologic distress that can range from mild to severe. Only in recent years has depression in children been recognized as a clinical condition. Many children referred to child guidance centers and mental health professionals due to behavioral difficulties or poor achievement actually suffer from depression. The incidence of major depression is estimated to be about 3% in childhood and 14% in adolescence (Hamrin & Magorno, 2010). A history of substance abuse and anxiety disorder increases risk, and cultural variations in rates exist (Hamrin & Magorno, 2010). (See Developing Cultural Competence: Depression Rates.)

Etiology and Pathophysiology

Theories have been proposed to explain the cause of depression in children and adolescents. Depression may be biological in origin or a result of learned helplessness, cognitive distortion, social skills deficit, or family dysfunction. The physiologic theory focuses on monoamine neurotransmission. These amines include indolamine, serotonin, norepinephrine, and dopamine, and decreases are sometimes found in depression. Magnetic resonance imaging has identified brain changes in individuals who are depressed, suggesting a biological basis (National Institute of Mental Health, 2009).

Developing Cultural Competence
Depression Rates

Ethnic and racial differences in depression rates exist. The highest rates of depression are observed in Hispanic and Native American youth. Although there is scant data with Asian American youth, their rates of depression appear to be less. Data do not provide a clear picture of depression in Black youth as compared to White youth; in some studies rates are higher and in others rates are lower. However, Black males report more depressive symptoms than Black females, whereas the reverse trend is usually reported in White youth (Anderson & Mayes, 2010). It is likely that genetics, environment, and culture interact to influence the differences in prevalence of depression.

BOX 34–5	Growth & Development: Symptoms of Depression

Symptoms of depression can vary among age groups, although sadness and **anhedonia** (inability to experience pleasure) are common at all ages. Differences include the following:

- Infants experiencing depression may fail to eat and grow.
- Toddlers can show regressive behaviors in toileting and other activities.
- Preschoolers have less symbolic and other play activities, and demonstrate self-destructive play themes. They may whine and show irritability, disinterest, and lack of confidence.
- School-age children may show a decrease in academic performance, increased or decreased physical activity, somatic complaints, and loss of friends. The older school-age child may talk of running away or show signs of boredom and low self-esteem.
- The adolescent can have a wide array of symptoms such as anxiety, decreased social contact, poor school performance, lack of involvement in typical activities, poor self-care, difficulty with parents and teachers, or focus on violence.

Source: *National Institute of Mental Health. (2010). Depression in children and adolescents. Retrieved from http://www.nimh.nih.gov/health/topics/depression/depression-in-children-and-adolescents.shtml*

Parental depression is a strong predictor of childhood depression. Abuse and neglect, family conflict, parental death, and low socioeconomic status predispose children to depression. Other psychiatric diagnoses are common in children with depression; these include conditions such as ADHD, anxiety disorder, bipolar disease, or substance abuse (Lack & Green, 2009).

Clinical Manifestations

Characteristic findings of major depression in children and adolescents include declining school performance, withdrawal from social activities, sleep disturbance (either too much or too little), appetite disturbance (too much or too little), multiple somatic complaints (especially headaches and stomachaches), decreased energy, difficulty concentrating and making decisions, low self-esteem, and feelings of hopelessness. There is much variation among children in the symptoms displayed, and they often have some but not all of the major criteria.

Symptoms of depression in children vary according to their developmental levels (Box 34–5).

Collaborative Care

Nurses partner with families and other health professionals to ensure adequate treatment of the child with depression. They may include parents, school nurses and teachers, pediatricians, and mental health specialists.

Diagnostic Tests

All youth should be screened for depression (U.S. Preventive Services Task Force, 2009). Once depression or major depressive disorder is diagnosed, comprehensive assessment of the child should occur to rule out physical illness that can be linked to depressive symptoms, such as diabetes, cancer, and obesity (U.S. Preventive Services Task Force, 2009). The child is tested for various mental health problems since comorbidities (combination with other disorders) are common (Bukstein, 2009). A history of bullying and substance abuse are examples of these comorbidities.

A child psychologist or child psychiatrist performs the initial psychiatric assessment. A variety of scales and techniques are used;

however, very little guidance is available relating to evaluation of children under 6 years of age. Examples of useful tools are:

- Children's Depression Inventory Revised (CDI-R)
- Revised Children's Manifest Anxiety Scale
- Beck Depression Inventory
- Preschool Feelings Checklist
- Reynolds Child Depression Scale
- Reynolds Adolescent Depression Scale
- Patient Health Questionnaire for Adolescents (PHQ-A)
- Guideline for Adolescent Preventative Services Questionnaire
- Hopelessness Scale for Children
- Center of Epidemiologic Studies Depression Scale of Children (CES-DC)

Hamrin & Magorno, 2010.

Clinical Therapy

Treatment may include psychotherapy with psychotropic medication, a combination that is more effective than either approach alone. Often a combination of individual, family, and group therapy provides the greatest benefit for young children and adolescents. Involving parents, other family members, school personnel, and friends in the treatment plan is essential. Group therapy is an effective treatment measure for adolescents because of the importance of peer group relationships during the teenage years. Cognitive behavioral therapy (CBT) may be used with adolescents, and play therapy may be used with younger children. CBT focuses on thoughts and behaviors, leading to understanding of negative thoughts, and increasing activities that provide pleasure. Supportive interactions with healthcare providers and active problem solving are approaches that improve outcomes in adolescents. Healthcare providers should educate families about depression and counsel as needed. Confidentiality should be ensured. Refer to community resources as needed. Ensure a plan for the adolescent's safety.

Antidepressant medications, most commonly the SSRIs and the tricyclic antidepressants (TCAs) such as imipramine (Tofranil), desipramine (Norpramin), and amitriptyline (Elavil), may be prescribed. The only antidepressant approved to treat major depressive disorders in pediatric patients is fluoxetine HCl (Prozac), but clinicians use others when the child does not respond to Prozac.

Practice Alert

Sudden cardiac death has occurred in several children on tricyclic antidepressants (TCAs). Due to this risk, serum levels should be monitored and electrocardiograms (ECGs) performed. Specific ECG changes along with a resting heart rate above 100, systolic blood pressure above 130 mmHg, and diastolic blood pressure above 85 mmHg necessitate immediate report to the prescriber. A narrow margin exists between the therapeutic and lethal dose in children (Zemrak & Kenna, 2008).

The SSRIs act to block reuptake of serotonin in the synapse, so that serotonin levels (which influence mood) increase. Although the SSRIs are generally considered safer than some other types of antidepressants, their use in children has been limited, so side effects must be monitored. Generally the child is started with a low dose, which is increased slowly to minimize the chance of side effects. Because of some reports of increased suicidal ideation and the lack of efficacy evidence, children and adolescents taking SSRIs must be closely monitored by a psychiatric mental health specialist (U.S. Preventive Services Task Force, 2009). A patient medication guide with the risks and precautions, as well as drug label information, must be provided for every patient.

A major serious side effect of SSRIs is serotonin syndrome, a condition characterized by agitation, muscle twitching, gastric upset, chills, fever, confusion, and dizziness (Arora & Kannikeswaran, 2010; Evans, Tepper, Shapiro, et al., 2010; Lovrin, 2009). This life-threatening side effect of SSRIs is caused by overstimulation

TABLE 34–5	Risk Factors for Child and Adolescent Depression	
CHILD	**FAMILY**	**SCHOOL AND SOCIAL SITUATIONS**
■ Frequent feelings of sadness, sleep problems, loss of interest in activities ■ Increase in risk taking and impulsivity ■ Previous suicide attempt ■ Alcohol or substance abuse ■ Diagnosed psychotic disorder ■ Chronic illness and frequent hospitalization	■ Parental neglect, abuse, or loss ■ Dysfunctional family relationships ■ Family history of depression, suicide, substance abuse, alcoholism, other psychopathology	■ Academic pressures and underachievement ■ Stressful social relationships ■ Declining participation in social events

of serotonin receptors. It is more likely to develop when the child or adolescent is also taking St. John's wort, other antidepressants, alcohol, or diet pills, or abusing drugs such as Ecstasy and LSD. Be certain to ask questions in a nonjudgmental way about intake of any alternative therapies, other medications, or substance use to identify those most at risk.

Nursing Management

Nursing management focuses on encouraging the child and family to participate in therapy and to report side effects of drugs and any changes in condition.

Nursing Assessment and Diagnosis

A thorough history and physical examination, including observation of behavior, are obtained at the time of admission. Assess the child for common risk factors for depression (Table 34–5).

Several nursing diagnoses that may be appropriate for the child or adolescent hospitalized with depression are included in the accompanying Nursing Care Plan. Other diagnoses may include the following:

- Nutrition, Imbalanced: More than Body Requirements related to eating in response to internal cues other than hunger
- Powerlessness related to sense of helplessness
- Self-Esteem, Chronic Low related to negative self-evaluation

NANDA-I © 2012

Planning and Implementation

Becoming hospitalized for depression may be difficult and indicate failure to both the youth and the family. Information about the condition and need for hospitalization should be provided. Nursing care of the child or adolescent hospitalized for depression includes administering medications and other therapy, and providing supportive care. Monitor vital signs of youth receiving antidepressant medications. Watch for common side effects of the agents used. Carefully monitor for serious side effects of TCAs or SSRIs, and be aware that lower doses are used at initiation with doses increasing slowly to the desired level. Frequent face-to-face follow-up visits are needed. When dosages are altered, all behavior and ideation changes must be closely monitored. Monitor cardiovascular status, including hypertension and tachycardia, observe motor movement, and record dietary intake. Help parents to evaluate inpatient settings to be certain the care provided will best meet the needs of the child or adolescent. See Partnering with Families: Selecting Residential and Inpatient Care for the Child with Mental Illness. Refer to the Nursing Care Plan for specific nursing interventions for the child or adolescent hospitalized with depression.

Discharge Planning and Home Care Teaching

When the child has been hospitalized and is returning home, teach parents to recognize signs and symptoms of worsening depression. Parents should also be taught dosages and side effects of any prescribed medications. Review data in the patient medication guide for any medications with the family. Caution not to alter the dose or discontinue the drug without guidance and monitoring of the prescriber. Instruct the family to remove guns, ammunition, and other potentially harmful items from the home. Have the family immediately seek emergency care if they are concerned about the child's safety or worsening condition. Refer the family to appropriate healthcare professionals and to support groups for family members dealing with depression.

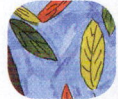

Partnering with Families

Selecting Residential and Inpatient Care for the Child with Mental Illness

Families need guidelines to assist them in evaluating inpatient facilities when a child with a mental disorder must be placed in an institution. They can be referred to the National Alliance for the Mentally Ill website. Nurses can provide questions for the families to ask:

- What is the staff-to-youth ratio?
- What are the guidelines for chemical and physical restraint?
- Are children isolated when behaviors are inappropriate?
- Are children constantly monitored visually when in restraint or when potentially dangerous to self or others?

- Does the child have a full physical and psychologic evaluation by a specialist within 24 hours of entry to the facility?
- What professionals review the plan of care and how often?
- To whom can the family speak for regular updates on the child?
- How often can the family visit?
- What services will be covered by insurance?
- What subjective feelings does the family member have when visiting the unit and facility?
- What services will be offered on an ongoing basis upon discharge?

Care in the Community

Most children with depression are cared for in the community. Maintain regular contact with family members through their healthcare visits to outpatient agencies and by making home visits. Monitor the child's affect, activity, and food intake. School teachers and counselors often are aware of the child's ability to perform in the school setting. Have the family schedule after-school care so young children with depression are not left at home alone for extended periods. Assist the family in finding support for financial and emotional needs related to managing the child's depression.

Evaluation

Expected outcomes of nursing care for the child with depression are found in the accompanying Nursing Care Plan.

Bipolar Disorder (Manic Depression)

Bipolar disorder is a mental illness in which extreme changes in affect and energy are manifested. Moods most often alter between mania (high energy and euphoria) and depression. Children often present with irritability or hyperactivity. About 1% of children and adults have bipolar illness, with a high rate of onset from 15 to 19 years, although onset as young as preschool age can occur. There is a high rate of attempted suicide in those with bipolar disease, as well as co-occurrence with other disorders such as ADHD, anxiety, and substance abuse, all of which complicates diagnosis (Apps, Winkler, & Jandrisevits, 2008; Lack & Green, 2009).

Bipolar disorder is classified into four types:

- *Bipolar I*—includes a severe manic episode that requires hospitalization or causes functional impairment in life
- *Bipolar II*—at least one episode of mild to moderate mania (hypomania) and one of depression
- *Cyclothymic disorder*—manifests as multiple mild manic and depressive episodes
- *Bipolar not otherwise specified*—rapid mood fluctuations, mania without depressive episodes, or chronic depression with hypomania episodes

National Institute of Mental Health, 2009.

When parents or close relatives are affected, the child is more likely to have the disorder. Thus, a genetic etiology is probable. It is believed that genetics and environment interact to create the condition in youth. Brain imaging shows abnormalities of the frontal and prefrontal cortex, the hippocampus, the basal ganglia, and the left amygdala, which is the center for experiencing fear (National Institute of Mental Health, 2009).

The manic phase of bipolar illness is characterized by hyperactivity and high energy, irritability, aggression, and sometimes hallucinations. In the depressive phase, the child is sad, has alterations in sleep and eating patterns, feels worthless, is lacking in energy, and is socially withdrawn, similar to any depressive illness. Mania may be the persistent symptom in children, or rapid cycles of mania and depression can occur throughout the day (Lack & Green, 2009).

Collaborative Care

Collaborative care focuses on early identification of bipolar illness so that treatment can begin when it is most effective.

Diagnostic Tests

Diagnosis and treatment of bipolar disorder should be performed by mental health specialists. Use of alcohol or illegal drugs should be ruled out as a cause of symptoms, even in children. Since the manic phase is often manifested by hyperactivity, the child may be incorrectly treated with stimulants (see discussion of ADHD earlier in this chapter), and the disease can be worsened. Although there are criteria for diagnosis of the disorder in adults, the presentation in children differs so diagnosis can be difficult. Labile moods and sleep disturbance in children are associated with the condition; irritability and elation may occur in children (Apps et al., 2008; Lack & Green, 2009).

Clinical Therapy

The treatment of bipolar disease involves a variety of drugs used to stabilize mood. Lithium, valproate, divalproex, carbamazepine, olanzapine, oxcarbazepine, lamotrigine, quetiapine, and risperidone are examples of drugs used. Only lithium is approved by the U.S. Food and Drug Administration (FDA) for use in those from 12 to 18 years (Apps et al., 2008). However, clinicians prescribe other drugs with careful monitoring performed. Early treatment is key to preventing chronic, serious mental illness. Individual and family education and therapy can be helpful. Once initial therapy is successful, co-existing conditions such as ADHD or alcohol use are treated as well.

Nursing Management

Nurses are instrumental in identifying children with the disorder, providing information to families, and monitoring the drugs and psychotherapy for the child.

Nursing Assessment and Diagnosis

The nurse is aware of children with symptoms of bipolar disorder when they appear in any setting. Be alert for the child described as having wide mood swings and irritability. A low tolerance for frustration and overactive stress and startle response may occur. Ask about response to stressful situations and change in behavior over time. Be alert for substance abuse and other mental health disorders. Based on the assessment, several diagnoses may be established, including:

- Injury, Risk for related to behaviors in manic phase and potential suicide in depressive phase
- Social Interaction, Impaired related to irritability and frustration
- Powerlessness related to mood instability

NANDA-I © 2012

Planning and Implementation

The child with bipolar disorder needs ongoing care to ensure implementation of therapy and return to function. The nurse administers medications in some settings and instructs parents, the child, and other family members in other settings. Observe for side effects specific to the drug regimen used. Assist parents to find resources for health care since medications and other treatments may be costly. Parents and children need information about the disorder as it may recur several times throughout the child's life and affects family functioning. Once successful treatment occurs, the child may need developmental intervention to catch up on skills that were lost or not developed during the bipolar episode. Assist the family to plan for developmentally appropriate activities. Assist the child to find social events and groups that build a sense of self-esteem.

Nursing Care Plan

The Child or Adolescent Hospitalized with Depression

INTERVENTION	RATIONALE	EXPECTED OUTCOME
1. Nursing Diagnosis: Hopelessness related to long-term stress		
NIC Priority Intervention—*Hope Instillation*: Facilitation of the development of a positive outlook		**NOC Suggested Outcome**—*Hope*: Presence of internal state of optimism that is personally satisfying and life supporting
GOAL: *The child or adolescent will discuss feelings of hopelessness.*		
■ Encourage open expression of feelings. Explore hopeless, sad, or lonely feelings. Point out the connection between feelings and behavior. Assess the child or adolescent to identify the precipitating event when feelings of sadness arose. Maintain an accepting and nonjudgmental attitude regarding any feelings expressed by the child.	■ Expressing feelings may help to relieve sadness, loneliness, despair, and hopelessness.	By discharge, the child or adolescent expresses an interest in the future.
■ Encourage the child or adolescent to take part in self-care and unit activities. Use routines to establish feelings of control.	■ An active role in self-care and treatment helps the child or adolescent to feel more in control.	
■ Medicate as ordered and document results.	■ Antidepressants modify mood to a more hopeful outlook.	
2. Nursing Diagnosis: Coping, Ineffective related to inadequate social support or disturbance in pattern of appraisal of threat		
NIC Priority Intervention—*Coping Enhancement*: Assisting a patient to adapt to perceived stressors, changes, or threats which interfere with meeting life demands and roles		**NOC Suggested Outcome**—*Coping:* Actions to manage stressors that tax an individual's resources
GOAL: *The child or adolescent will use effective coping skills.*		
■ Teach positive, effective coping strategies such as guided imagery and relaxation. Assist the child or adolescent to focus on strengths rather than weaknesses.	■ Therapeutic techniques can help the child or adolescent to replace negative thoughts and images with more positive and effective beliefs and images. These interventions foster resilience.	The child or adolescent verbalizes and demonstrates the ability to cope appropriately for his or her age.
■ Assist the child or adolescent to identify friends, family members, and others who are positive and supportive.	■ The child or adolescent becomes aware that people can be caring and supportive (thus validating self-esteem).	
3. Nursing Diagnosis: Social Interaction, Impaired related to self-concept disturbance		
NIC Intervention—*SOcialization Enhancement*: Facilitation of ability to interact with others		**NOC Outcome**—*Social Interaction Skills*: An individual's use of effective interaction behaviors
GOAL: *The child or adolescent will participate in and initiate activities and conversation.*		
■ Assist the child or adolescent to identify topics and activities of interest.	■ The more the child or adolescent focuses on areas of interest, the less he or she will focus on internal anxiety and depression.	By discharge, the child or adolescent initiates conversation and activities with staff and peers.
■ Encourage interaction with peers and staff.	■ Each positive interaction reinforces feelings of success. Each success reinforces the desire for future social interaction.	
■ Facilitate visits from family and friends.	■ Visits from family and friends reinforce positive and rewarding relationships.	
■ Provide guidance to family regarding interaction that promotes self-esteem.	■ The family's existing interaction style is often negative.	

(continued)

Nursing Care Plan	The Child or Adolescent Hospitalized with Depression, *continued*

INTERVENTION	RATIONALE	EXPECTED OUTCOME
4. Nursing Diagnosis: Nutrition, Imbalanced, Less than Body Requirements related to loss of appetite secondary to depression		
NIC Intervention—*Nutrition Management*: Assistance with or provision of a balanced dietary intake of foods and fluids		**NOC Outcome**—*Nutritional Status:* Amount of food and fluid taken into the body over a 24-hour period
GOAL: *The child or adolescent's daily intake will be adequate to maintain optimal nutritional status.*		
■ Offer nutritious finger foods, sandwiches, and high-calorie liquid supplements frequently throughout the day.	■ Convenient easy-to-eat foods encourage the child or adolescent to eat and maintain nutritional status.	The child or adolescent's daily intake will be adequate to maintain optimal nutritional status by discharge.
■ Offer easy-to-carry drinks that are high in vitamins, minerals, and calories.	■ These are a convenient method for meeting hydration and electrolyte needs.	
■ Encourage daily vigorous physical activity of at least 30 minutes.	■ Physical activity stimulates appetite.	

NANDA-I © 2012

Evaluation

The desired outcomes for a child with bipolar disorder include:

■ The child manifests interest in school, family, and other life events.

■ The family successfully manages stressors that challenge resources.

■ The child is confident in ability to manage life and its stresses.

■ The child manifests congruence with expected role behaviors for developmental age.

ANXIETY AND RELATED DISORDERS

A large group of anxiety disorders can affect youth as well as adults. Some of the more common types seen in children and adolescents are described in this section, with detailed nursing management described for posttraumatic stress disorder.

Generalized Anxiety Disorder

Anxiety is a subjective feeling of uncertainty, worry, and helplessness, usually accompanied by central nervous system (CNS) signs, including restlessness, trembling, perspiration, and rapid pulse. The disorder is often manifested in children with restlessness, excessive fatigue, poor concentration, irritability, muscle tension, and sleep disturbance. Anxiety is second only to substance abuse (see Chapter 20 🔗) in incidence for mental disorders, and it is a common mental disorder of childhood. From 20% to 28% of youth experience some type of anxiety disorder. Although all children experience anxiety at certain times, those with anxiety disorder are excessively worried about many things, are difficult to reassure, and are not able to distract themselves from worry. Many youth have accompanying physical complaints, such as headache or stomachache, and comorbid diagnoses such as depression and substance use are common (Keeley & Storch, 2009).

Anxiety disorders are strongly linked to familial and genetic factors. Diagnosis is performed by a mental health specialist. Treatment is usually cognitive behavioral therapy (CBT) and may involve medication. CBT can include child or family interventions that focus on relaxation, recognition of feelings, and self-talking (learned words or phrases said to oneself to aid in management of distress). Medications

that have been reported to be successful in children include SSRIs and benzodiazepines (Keeley & Storch, 2009).

Separation Anxiety Disorder

Separation anxiety disorder is characterized by an extreme state of uneasiness when in unfamiliar surroundings and often by refusal to visit friends' homes or attend school for at least 2 weeks. It is a common type of anxiety disorder manifested by children (Beesdo, Knappe, & Pine, 2009; Kendall, Compton, Walkup, et al., 2010). Approximately 75% of children with separation anxiety disorder refuse to attend school (see the discussion of school phobia or social phobia to follow). This disorder occurs in approximately 4% to 5% of children and in twice as many girls as boys. The peak age for occurrence is 7 to 9 years. It may be recurrent and become worse at certain times. The condition may be acute in onset (preceded by a traumatic event) or slow in developing over time (Keeley & Storch, 2009).

Children with separation anxiety disorder tend to be perfectionistic, overly compliant, and eager to please. They appear to cling to the parent or caretaker. They may use physical complaints such as headaches, abdominal pain, nausea, and vomiting in an attempt to avoid being away from the parent. Depression frequently accompanies separation anxiety disorder. The resulting avoidant behaviors can interfere with personal growth and development, academic achievement, and social functioning.

Clinical Tip

The separation anxiety experienced by a toddler differs from the psychiatric disorder in age appropriateness, duration, and severity. Separation anxiety disorder affects children of preschool age or older, lasts for at least 2 weeks, and is characterized by excessive anxiety. In contrast, the separation anxiety experienced by the toddler directly follows a separation from a familiar caretaker, lasts only for a short time after the separation, and is a normal developmental response in toddlers.

A mental health specialist makes the diagnosis. Treatment includes CBT with both the child and parents. Parents learn about the disorder and how to structure the setting so that the child is expected to attend school. Consistency in expectations is necessary; if the child is permitted to stay home some days or has missed school and other activities for longer periods, treatment is more difficult. The child learns what situations cause anxiety and how to manage for situations and feelings. Both parents and child work out the expectations for behavior for the child with the mental health therapist. School personnel and those from other settings where the child spends time need to be included in the treatment plan. Medication has occasionally been used if CBT is not effective.

Panic Disorder

Panic disorder is the presence of recurrent, unexpected panic attacks. These attacks are periods of intense fear and discomfort in the absence of real danger. The lifetime risk of panic disorder is from 1% to 5% (Keeley & Storch, 2009). Predictive factors for panic attacks in adolescence include a history of separation anxiety or other anxiety disorders earlier in life and a history of parental panic attacks.

Examples of the physical symptoms experienced are palpitations, sweating, chills, hot flashes, shaking, shortness of breath, choking, chest pain, nausea, and dizziness. The person describes feelings of danger or doom. There may be accompanying agoraphobia in some people. **Agoraphobia** is an anxiety of being in places or situations from which escape may be difficult or embarrassing, or in which help may not be available. The attacks may be continuous or episodic but generally are chronic in nature.

Diagnosis is made by a mental health specialist. Similar to anxiety, treatment may involve individual and family interventions using CBT, and the use of medication (SSRIs) in some cases.

Obsessive-Compulsive Disorder

Individuals with obsessive-compulsive disorder (OCD) may be mildly or severely affected. From 1% to 4% of children are affected, and about 80% of adults with OCD had the condition in childhood (Keeley & Storch, 2009). Affected children have recurrent obsessive thoughts, commonly about contamination, harm, sex, or moral concerns. These obsessions are handled through a series of compulsive behaviors that interfere with daily life. Examples of behaviors and concerns are excessive hand washing, counting objects, and hoarding substances. These practices may take 1 or more hours each day. Children with OCD differ from adults in several ways. Children have more aggressive obsessions, such as fears of catastrophe, more commonly hoard objects, and are more likely to have religious obsessions. Comorbidity with other mental health disorders is common.

The basal ganglia of the brain are affected and a genetic link is observed. A neurochemical cause may be related to abnormal serotonin metabolism. MRI changes in the globus pallidus and anterior cingulated gyrus of the brain have been noted. Poststreptococcal autoimmune disorder may be a cause in some cases (D'Alessandro, 2009) (Box 34–6).

Diagnosis is made by a mental health specialist. The disorder may have been present for some time before diagnosis since parents tend to overlook or deny the symptoms, and children may hide the behaviors. Treatment may involve CBT, where the feared occurrence is presented and the person learns that no harm will occur. Involvement of the family in treatment is important so that members learn how to handle the child's ritualistic behaviors. Medications, such as clomipramine and the SSRIs, are effective in most children and adolescents.

School Phobia (Social Phobia)

School phobia (also known as social phobia, school avoidance, or school refusal) is a persistent, irrational, or excessive fear of negative evaluation or embarrassment in social situations and therefore of attending school.

BOX 34–6	Research: PANDAS

Pediatric autoimmune neuropsychiatric disorders associated with streptococcal infections (PANDAS) are characterized by obsessive-compulsive and/or tic disorder in childhood or adolescence with worsening of symptoms after group A beta-hemolytic streptococcal infection. Exact prevalence is unknown due to inadequate application of all diagnostic criteria (Gabbay, Coffey, Babb, et al., 2008; National Institute of Mental Health, 2012). It is believed that in certain children, the strep infection leads to a neural autoimmune response, resulting in the psychiatric disorder. Research continues to identify possible mechanisms, results, and treatments for this cause of OCD (D'Allesandro, 2009; Gabbay et al., 2008). Pediatric acute-onset neuropsychiatric syndrome (PANS) is a recent term that describes all cases of abrupt onset of obsessive-compulsive disorder (OCD). In addition to the rapid onset of OCD, PANS is characterized by two additional symptoms: (1) anxiety, mood swings, depression, aggression, behavioral regression, or somatization, and (2) no other explanation for the behaviors. Separation anxiety, hyperactivity, sensory abnormalities, difficulty concentrating, and urinary frequency are other common symptoms (National Institute of Mental Health, 2012). Sudden behavior changes in children should be referred for further evaluation.

The child may fear being harmed or losing control. Social and school phobia can occur in children as young as 5 years of age, often presents at 11 or 12 years, but can occur in children up to 16 years; about 7% of children manifest the phobia (Keeley & Storch, 2009).

Children with social phobia may fear asking for directions, ordering food at a restaurant, and speaking in the classroom. They commonly report that teachers and peers "pick on" them. Somatic complaints are similar to those in children with separation anxiety disorder. Characteristically, symptoms are present only on school days and not on weekends or holidays. The social withdrawal that occurs in this disorder further impairs the child since social interactions are needed for normal developmental progression.

A mental health specialist makes the diagnosis. Treatment includes the family and child, and establishes firm limits for behavioral expectations and consequences. CBT is used, including education of the youth about the condition, body awareness of symptoms, and methods of changing feelings. SSRI medications may sometimes be needed to lessen anxiety in social situations so the child can experience success in these interactions.

Conversion Reaction

Conversion reaction is a disorder in which a disturbance or loss of sensory, motor, or other physical functions suggests neurologic or other somatic disease. The disturbance or loss cannot be explained by any known pathophysiologic mechanism. Instead, psychologic factors are involved. About 3% of the population experiences conversion reactions at some time. Adolescence and early adulthood are common times for the onset to occur, with onset rare before 10 years or after 35 years (Kozlowska, Scher, & Williams, 2011).

Conversion reactions develop in response to a catastrophic event such as threat, loss, or harm. Clinical manifestations include altered sensations such as blindness or deafness; paralysis or ataxia, including inability to stand or walk and loss of ability to speak (aphonia); involuntary movements, such as pseudoepileptic convulsions; and constant complaints of pain with no physical basis (psychogenic pain). Children under 10 years may present with gait abnormalities or seizures. The onset of conversion symptoms is usually dramatic and sudden. Symptoms often appear to be neurologic, but on careful examination obvious discrepancies are found. The person is usually calm about the symptoms even though they are serious. Often the child or family members appear indifferent or unconcerned over what healthcare providers consider an overwhelming physical disability. Children suspected of having a conversion reaction require a complete physical and neurologic evaluation to rule out any possible physiologic basis for the symptoms. Individual and family therapy is usually necessary to identify the source of the psychologic conflict, pain, or need resulting in the conversion symptoms. Pharmacologic approaches may also be used.

Posttraumatic Stress Disorder

Acute stress disorder can occur after any life-threatening event and is manifested in the first month after exposure to the event. Symptoms include repeatedly reliving the traumatic experience, anxiety, and increased arousal. Similarly, individuals with *posttraumatic stress disorder* (PTSD) have experienced or witnessed a life-threatening event; however, the symptoms of distress continue for more than 1 month and cause impairment in functioning. Estimates of the incidence of PTSD are hard to obtain. It is assumed that about 40% of youth have an episode of trauma that could lead to PTSD and that 6% have symptoms of the disorder. While 20% of children may experience PTSD after traumatic events, the prevalence rises to 90% when the trauma is severe (Hamblen, Norris, Pietruszkiewicz, et al., 2009; Kassam-Adams, Marsac, & Cirilli, 2010).

Etiology and Pathophysiology

Examples of traumatic events that are associated with posttraumatic stress include sexual or other child abuse, rape, car crash, fire, witnessing violence, and having an experience in war. The treatment of PTSD is discussed in this section; consult Chapter 20 🕮 for further examples of the types of violence that affect children, as well as methods for reducing youth exposure to violent, traumatic events.

The disorder involves both a traumatic event and the child's reaction to this event. It is believed that brain changes occur in trauma, leading to neurobiological alterations that cause dysfunction of memory. Overreactivity of the amygdala, underreactivity of the prefrontal cortex, and increased dopamine in the medial prefrontal cortex are observed. Children with other psychiatric disorders, a family history of psychiatric illness, and severe or lengthy trauma all possess risk factors.

Clinical Manifestations

The very young child with PTSD may show regression in behavior, sleep disturbance, or demonstration of anxiety. Children may be unable to remember the truesequence of the traumatic event and reenact the event in play and drawings. Adolescents commonly exhibit impulsive or aggressive behaviors. Children of any age have feelings of fear, terror, and helplessness, and may relive the event frequently in thought and nightmares. There is a state of hypervigilance and exaggerated startle response, such as to touch or loud noises. The child feels detached from others and alone. Even if the child appears to have adapted and functions normally immediately after the traumatic event, several weeks or even months later, the symptoms of PTSD can begin to appear (National Center for PTSD, 2008).

Collaborative Care

Collaborative care for children with PTSD involves identification of the condition and treatment so that long-term consequences can be avoided.

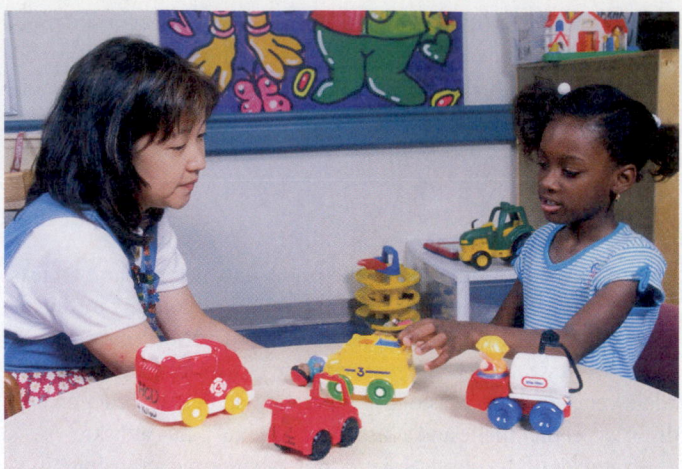

FIGURE 34–8 ■ A psychologist uses play therapy to help Cassandra, a young girl who is experiencing PTSD. The child was in a car crash and physically recovered but has had nightmares about the event. She also developed a fear of leaving home. The therapist allows Cassandra to play with cars and talk about the event. She uses cognitive behavioral therapy to suggest ways of handling the thoughts and fears. This helps Cassandra to gain control over the event so it is not so frightening and does not interfere with her functioning in daily life.

Diagnostic Tests

The diagnosis is made by a mental health specialist. A history of a traumatic event with normal childhood developmental behaviors before the event is characteristic. A variety of instruments are available to screen for symptoms characteristic of the disorder. Examples include the Screening Tool for Early Predictors of PTSD (STEPP) that asks questions of both parent and child (Center for Injury Research and Prevention, 2011).

Clinical Therapy

Counseling by a mental health specialist is the main therapy for PTSD (Figure 34–8 ■). CBT is the treatment of choice, with both the child and family members included. Young children show significant improvement in symptoms after a course of CBT (Legerstee, Tulen, Dierckx, et al., 2010). A variety of antidepressants and SSRIs can be used for pharmacologic treatment, with medication tailored to the specific symptoms that are most distressing and have been resistant to CBT.

Nursing Management

Nursing management for PTSD and other anxiety disorders focuses on partnering with other health professionals and families to relieve the child's anxiety and return the child to a normal, developmentally appropriate level of functioning.

Nursing Assessment and Diagnosis

Nurses often help to identify PTSD patients and others with anxiety disorders so that care can be obtained. Ask about traumatic events in the past and how the child reacted. Inquire about recent changes in the child's behavior. Include school attendance, complaints of physical illness, sleep patterns, and rituals in behavior. A family history of mental disorders may be useful. Youth who run away from home and present at homeless shelters are often suffering from PTSD; assessment for the condition should be part of initial history and evaluation. Based on the data gathered, the child's symptoms, and the

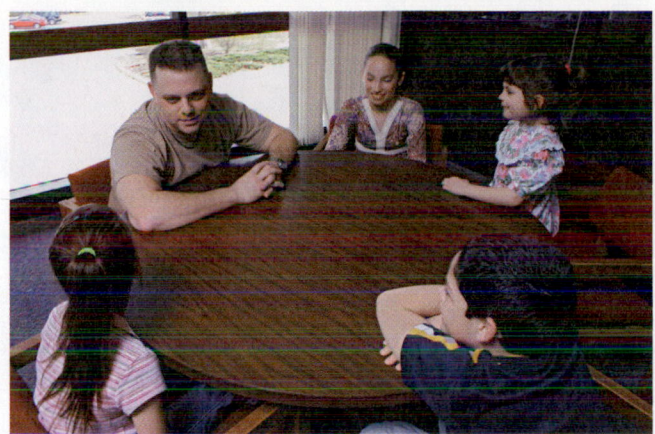 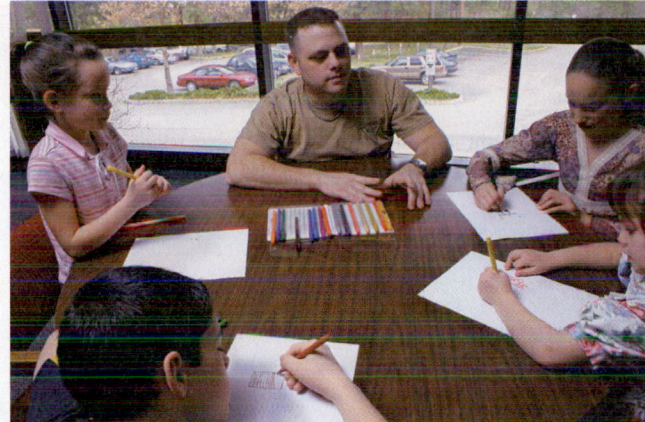

FIGURE 34–9 ■ This nurse conducts a group therapy session for children who have experienced traumatic events and have resulting anxiety disorders. He is clearly engaged, has a positive rapport, and fosters exchanges among the children. Games and drawing are frequent techniques used in the group.

mental health diagnosis, the nurse determines nursing diagnoses. Examples include:

- Anxiety related to unconscious conflict
- Coping, Ineffective related to perceived high degree of threat
- Powerlessness related to chronic mental illness
- Sleep Pattern, Disturbed related to anxiety
- Post-Trauma Syndrome related to motor vehicle crash or other traumatic events

NANDA-I © 2012

Planning and Implementation

Nursing care for anxiety disorders focuses on behavioral and cognitive therapies to enhance coping skills. Mental health nurses may conduct group therapy sessions both in inpatient and community settings (Figure 34–9 ■). Group sessions for children often provide a forum for discussion of fears, an opportunity to enhance skills of working together, and an opportunity to learn coping skills. Being a member of a group with other children experiencing anxiety or trauma can remove the stigma and allow the child the freedom to explore feelings, behaviors, and their causes. Several of the techniques described earlier in the chapter, such as drawing pictures and discussing them or telling stories, are used by mental health nurses in child therapy groups.

Children need to learn relaxation techniques, and nurses may teach such techniques or recommend that the child consider participation in yoga or guided imagery classes. Inquire about alternative therapies that the child and family are using or have an interest in beginning, and refer as needed. See Complementary Therapy: Selected Methods for Anxiety Disorders.

Parents or other significant people should be included in the treatment program. Nurses often teach them basic information about the child's diagnosis and therapy. They should be in at least some therapy sessions with the child. Provide resources that they need for relief from worry about the child, guilt about causing an accident that triggered the child's symptoms, or other feelings related to the diagnosis. See Partnering with Families: Talking with Children About Traumatic Events.

Insurance companies may provide limited payment for mental health services. Help the family to see the importance of recommended therapy, and assist them to find resources for care if needed.

School personnel may need to know about the child's treatment. Partner with the families to provide needed information. Some

---

Complementary Therapy Selected Methods for Anxiety Disorders

- Herbal therapy—e.g., St. John's wort, kava, ginseng, ginkgo biloba, lemon balm
- Diet—e.g., omega-3 fatty acids, vitamin and mineral supplements, removal of food dyes
- Self-hypnotic relaxation—to reduce pain and anxiety
- Acupuncture—for anxiety, depression
- Massage therapy—for anxiety, anger, grief
- Reflexology (manual stimulation of specific points on the foot)—for anxiety
- Guided imagery—to relieve anxiety
- Biofeedback (use of machines to watch muscle or skin responses)—for anxiety

Source: *Soh, J. L., & Walter, G. (2008). Complementary and alternative medicine (CAM) treatments and pediatric psychopharmacology. Journal of the American Academy of Child and Adolescent Psychiatry, 47, 364–368.*

---

schools have counselors who can be instrumental in carrying out treatment plans at school and acting as a resource in that setting. School personnel may be asked to provide feedback about the child's attendance, performance, and social skills as a measure of the success of therapy, and the community or school nurse can relay this information.

Nurses often administer medications to children being treated for anxiety. Be alert for side effects, and ensure the family knows how to safely administer the drugs. They should be kept locked securely. Have the child return for follow-up as needed since some medications may take several weeks to achieve effects, and close monitoring is essential. The child should have a medication alert tag for drugs being taken.

Evaluation

The outcomes of nursing care for the child with anxiety disorder center on return to normal developmental activities, engagement in social relationships, learned coping skills for dealing with stress, and maintenance of safety.

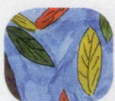

Partnering with Families

Talking with Children About Traumatic Events

Whether a child or adolescent experiences trauma from a car crash, abuse, or environmental event, parents can help to decrease the effects of the stress and prevent the appearance of posttraumatic stress disorder by doing the following:

- Be sure children feel comfortable asking parents, teachers, or others about the events and their feelings.
- Assure children that their feelings are normal and may return over time.
- Be honest and open in responses, without overloading children with more details than they need.
- Be prepared to repeat answers and discuss the same topics many times.
- Get help from counselors who can suggest how to talk with children.

- Use communication methods appropriate at various ages, such as reading books, doing art projects, or drawing.
- Show children that they are loved by spending time and planning activities with them.
- Limit the television and other media time where children are exposed to violence and traumatic events. Do not have television on so often that children repeatedly view a traumatic event.
- Restore a sense of normal routines into children's lives.
- Be alert for increasing signs of distress, and seek care from a professional if they occur.

SUICIDE

Suicide is the third leading cause of death in adolescents between 15 and 19 years of age. About 4,400 youth commit suicide annually, and an additional 149,000 receive care after attempted suicide. In any one year, about 15% of youth admit to contemplating suicide (CDC, 2009b). The prevalence of suicide is about 7.32 per 100,000, with 86% of the deaths among males. Firearms, suffocation, and poisoning are the most common means of suicide (CDC, 2009c). See Developing Cultural Competence: Suicide and Ethnicity.

It is not unusual for healthcare professionals and parents to label suicide attempts by children and adolescents as accidents. Up to half of childhood suicides may be recorded as accidents; suicide data for children under age 10 years are not maintained. Adults may have difficulty believing that young children, in particular, would have any reason to want to end their lives. For this reason, many children who are brought to the emergency department with indications of a suicide attempt are often classified as unintentional injury victims and released without arrangements for appropriate follow-up care. Accurate identification and treatment are needed for youth at risk of suicide.

Many risk factors for suicide exist in children and adolescents, and there are also known protective factors (Table 34–6). The most common precursor to adolescent suicide is depression (see previous discussion). Common signs or symptoms of an underlying depression that could lead to suicide include boredom, restlessness, problems with concentration, irritability, lethargy, intentional misbehavior, preoccupation with one's own body or health, and excessive

dependence on or isolation from others (especially adults or caregivers). The depression may be exacerbated by a recent psychosocial stress such as loss or perceived rejection or ridicule. Youth who are gay or lesbian may feel stigmatized, and have a higher risk of suicide. A previous attempt is also a common risk factor.

The child or adolescent found to be at high risk for suicide may be admitted to a mental health unit or may be cared for in a community mental health facility. When a suicide attempt is made, the child or adolescent may be hospitalized for 24 hours, kept in a short-term monitoring unit, or sent home under close observation to ensure adequate assessment and monitoring. It is important to provide crisis

TABLE 34–6   Risk and Protective Factors for Suicide in Children and Adolescents

RISK FACTORS	PROTECTIVE FACTORS
History of previous attempted suicide	Emotional well-being
Friend committed or attempted suicide	Satisfactory school performance
School problems or changes in grades	Participation in sports or other group events
Pregnancy	
Drug use or abuse	Weight satisfaction
Problems with a romantic relationship	Parent/family connectedness
Gay or lesbian sexual practice	Frequent discussions of important issues with family
Loneliness, withdrawal	
Feelings of anxiety	School connectedness
History of chronic family problems	Safe school
Chronic illness	Safe neighborhood
Physical, emotional, or sexual abuse	Caring adult presence at school or elsewhere
History of suicide in a family member	
History of depression	Availability of school counseling
Chronic low self-esteem	School policies to limit and cope with fighting, bullying
Change in behavior	
Change in weight	
Giving away special possessions	
Access to firearms and ammunition	

Developing Cultural Competence
Suicide and Ethnicity

Some ethnic groups have a high rate of suicide. For example, Native Americans and Alaska Natives have a suicide rate of 27.72 per 100,000 males and 8.5 per 100,000 females. The historic pain experienced by this ethnic group and lack of opportunities for many youth may be some of the reasons for a high suicide rate. White males also have a high rate of suicide at about 13 per 100,000 (CDC, 2009c). *Healthy People 2020* goals focus on eliminating such health disparities by finding the causes, decreasing rates of suicide, educating about risk factors, and establishing prevention programs (U.S. Department of Health and Human Services, 2010).

intervention at the time of the suicide attempt to minimize the opportunity for repeat attempts and to begin a therapeutic treatment plan.

Treatment may include individual, group, or family therapy. Negotiating a no-suicide contract is an important first step in therapy. In the contract, the child agrees not to attempt suicide during a specified period. The presence of a contract is not a guarantee of child safety, so vigilant monitoring of the youth's condition continues. Comorbidities such as depression or substance abuse must also be addressed for treatment to be successful.

Nursing Management
Nursing Assessment and Diagnosis

The major nursing role is in prevention of suicide. All children and adolescents in health promotion visits and emergency departments should be evaluated for risk. Health promotion visits are an opportunity to be alert for children with depression (see previous discussion), substance abuse, recent stresses, and changes in behavior. Inquire about sleep patterns, feelings of sadness, and use of alcohol and other substances. Gather a family history of mental health disorders, suicide attempts, and stresses. Ask about how often the youth talks with or has meals with the family. Be aware of the risk of self-inflicted strangulation.

Practice Alert

A tragic cause of unintentional suicide in children is the choking "game." About 25 children annually die in the United States from this practice with a mean age of 13 years. When the blood supply to the brain is interrupted and then rushes back, some people report a feeling of euphoria or a "high." Children and adolescents may seek the experience for the feelings it creates and may even become addicted to it. Unfortunately, some children become unintentionally strangled and die from the experience. Methods that children use to cut off oxygen include using their hands to apply pressure to the carotids in the neck, or tying belts, cords, towels, and other items to the neck and then around doorways or other solid objects. Some children perform these rituals with others who then rescue them so that they begin breathing; many of the injuries occur when children are alone since there is no one to perform a rescue. Teachers, parents, and other adults typically have not heard of or are unaware that children are performing these rituals. Adults can watch for signs such as conjunctival hemorrhage, headaches, bruising in the neck area, periods of disorientation, hoarseness, and finding items tied to doors and other solid objects. Parents can also be alert if the history of a family computer has shown the child's entry to a website that describes the practice. Nurses in schools and other settings should educate children about the dangers of strangulation and should provide materials for parents to inform them of the risk (CDC, 2008b, 2010c).

Recall that all youth who receive medications for treatment of depression should be carefully monitored, especially in the first several weeks, to identify those who may develop suicide ideation and risk. Although antidepressants have demonstrated efficacy for treating depression in youth, there is an increased risk of suicidal ideation or behaviors in children and adolescents treated with these drugs.

Most suicides are committed with firearms that are usually obtained from the home. Determine at each healthcare visit if the family has firearms. Teach them to keep the guns unloaded, with ammunition and firearms locked in separate locations. Be sure that children and adolescents do not have access to the keys for the locked firearms.

Possible nursing diagnoses for the child at risk of suicide are:

- Suicide, Risk for related to hopelessness and substance abuse
- Violence: Self-Directed, Risk for related to history of suicide attempts, present suicidal ideation, and recent failure in school
- Coping: Family, Readiness for Enhanced related to recent teen attempted suicide

NANDA-I © 2012

Planning and Implementation
Care in the Hospital

Many children at risk for suicide or who have made a suicide attempt will be admitted to the hospital for a period of monitoring. Therapy is initiated and medications can be given under close supervision.

Nursing care centers on taking appropriate precautions to ensure the safety of a child or adolescent at risk of suicide. The child and the environment of the hospital or other setting are monitored for any object that could be used for self-harm. All potentially harmful objects, such as shoestrings, belts, pantyhose, and hair ribbons, are removed. All personal care items (including toothbrush and shampoo) are kept locked at the nursing station and monitored constantly when used by the child.

Children or adolescents who are considered at high risk for suicidal behaviors are attended by a nursing staff member at all times, including while using the bathroom and sleeping. It may be necessary for the child to dress in a plain hospital gown, be kept in a visually monitored seclusion room, or (if seriously impaired and self-abusive) be medicated for restraint for a period of time. Restraints are used only when ordered by the physician and interdisciplinary team caring for the youth. Physical restraint is only a short-term approach to provide immediate safety if necessary. Chemical restraint (medication) may be needed to prevent self-injury by the suicidal person. See page 1233 for information for families to consider when choosing residential care for their child who is suicidal.

Hospitalization continues as long as the child's behavior is self-destructive. Children are referred for intensive individual and family therapy to begin in the hospital and continue after discharge.

Care in the Community

Encourage parents to keep follow-up clinic appointments, to watch for self-destructive behaviors, and to administer any prescribed medications according to the treatment schedule. Arrange home visits and other community resources for families. Fewer than one half of adolescents who attempt suicide are referred for mental health evaluation and follow-up, so nurses are instrumental in referrals and in encouraging the care that youth need.

Education in all school settings is appropriate to assist children in awareness of resources for help when needed and in identifying peers at risk. Mental health services of all types should be available and embedded in schools since that is the setting where youth spend much of their time (U.S. Department of Health and Human Services, 2010). Be alert for children and adolescents at risk for suicide in any setting. Assess children and adolescents in schools, outpatient settings, and emergency departments for the possibility of suicidal behavior. Report threats of suicide and depressive behavior. Recognize that when one suicide has occurred, there may be an increased risk for friends of the victim. Teach students to report to teachers, nurses, or counselors about friends who have threatened suicide or seem depressed or display behaviors different than usual. Nurses often plan with mental health specialists to implement suicide prevention programs in schools and communities (U.S. Department of Health and Human Services, 2010). Provide supportive services to family and friends when suicide occurs. Consult websites and refer parents as appropriate. The Suicide Prevention Resource Center has helpful regional offices to facilitate networks at national, state, territorial, community, and tribal levels.

Weblink Suicide Prevention Resource Center

Evaluation

Desired outcomes related to suicide risk include:

- The family develops coping strategies to support a suicidal member.
- The child or adolescent takes actions to decrease sadness and increase interest in life events.
- The child or adolescent remains safe with no further suicide attempts or ideation.

TIC DISORDERS AND TOURETTE SYNDROME

Tics are sudden, rapid, recurrent, nonrhythmic, and brief motor movements or vocalizations. They may involve movement of the head or upper body, blinking of eyes, or a variety of verbal noises. They may be worse during periods of stress or tiredness. Many children have mild motor tics at some time that gradually disappear with no intervention. Midadolescence is the most common age for tics to appear. When the tics are severe or last over 1 year, they are considered chronic and may require attention from a mental health provider.

Severe motor tics accompanied by verbal utterances are known as Tourette syndrome. The syndrome is seen in 3 out of 1,000 children and is often accompanied by other diagnoses such as attention deficit and learning disabilities. Children with Tourette syndrome may exhibit **coprolalia,** the involuntary utterance of obscenities, profanities, and racial slurs, or **copropraxia,** the involuntary use of obscene gestures.

It is believed that there is an underlying genetic cause for tic disorders since about 75% have a family history. Boys are more affected than girls, suggesting an autosomal dominant transfer. The direct pathophysiology of the disorder is unknown, but dopamine, serotonin, and other neurotransmitter and neuropeptide levels are disrupted. Comorbidity commonly involves obsessive-compulsive disorder and ADHD (National Institute of Neurological Disorders and Stroke, 2010).

Clinical Tip
Children with Tourette syndrome may initially be diagnosed with ADHD due to their increased activity. If they are medicated with a drug such as methylphenidate (Ritalin, Concerta), their activity will worsen. Monitor symptoms carefully after the child begins taking medication, and be sure the child is seen regularly for ongoing care.

Diagnosis and identification of the disruptive effects of tics are the first steps. Education and reassurance may assist some children. Relaxation and management of stresses in school and other settings may be helpful. Tic disorders have been treated with medications in some cases (National Institute of Neurological Disorders and Stroke, 2010).

Nursing care involves supporting parents and encouraging normal developmental progression for the child. Stress should be minimized and relaxation techniques taught. Administer medications and teach families about desired outcomes and side effects. If the child's verbal utterances are disruptive in the classroom, partner with the family and school to arrange for home tutors for a while if needed. The nurse can teach school personnel and other children about the disorder so that they understand the child's behaviors.

TRICHOTILLOMANIA

Trichotillomania, or chronic hair pulling, can affect children and adolescents. Head hair is most commonly pulled, leaving patches of baldness, but eyebrows, eyelashes, pubic hair, and other body hair may be involved. Incidence is greatest in middle childhood, but it can occur earlier or later. Hair pulling may occur in brief periods of stress or over longer periods during sedentary activities. Gastrointestinal distress can occur when the person swallows the hair that is pulled out.

Trichotillomania is classified as an impulse control disorder. It has similarities to both obsessive-compulsive disorder and Tourette syndrome, described earlier in the chapter (Guynn & Gulley, 2009). Behavioral therapy, hypnosis, and SSRI medication therapy are generally used in treatment. Group therapy may be an effective support mechanism that helps to decrease guilt and feelings of isolation about the disorder.

People affected by the disorder usually feel shame and guilt. They try to hide the disorder and may not seek help for an extended period. The nurse should be alert for the disorder when head or body hair is missing, someone is wearing a wig, or eyebrows are heavily penciled. An appropriate way to question is to say, "Some people pull out their hair. I notice that you have no eyebrows or eyelashes. Is pulling them out something you do?"

Refer the child or adolescent to a healthcare professional. Try to establish a trusting atmosphere that fosters communication about the disorder. Encourage participation in the treatment plan. Ensure follow-up for care so effectiveness of treatment can be measured.

SCHIZOPHRENIA

Schizophrenia, a psychotic disorder that is relatively rare in young children, occurs in 1 in 10,000 children. The condition can manifest in childhood but is more common in adolescence (Addington & Rapoport, 2009; Mayo Clinic, 2009).

The cause of schizophrenia is unknown, but genetic predisposition and neurointegration deficits are suspected causes (Mayo Clinic, 2009). The brain is altered in the disease, with progressively enlarged ventricles and nervous system arousal. Impaired glucose metabolism is often present. Onset is usually slow with increasing intensity over time. Most often the child demonstrates restlessness, poor appetite, and social withdrawal over several weeks to months. Behavioral problems, slowed development, and minor neurologic symptoms may occur.

The clinical manifestations of schizophrenia are the same in children as in adults. Characteristic behaviors of the individual with schizophrenia include social withdrawal, impaired social relationships, flat **affect** (outward appearance of feeling or emotion), regression, loose associations (thought characterized by speech in which ideas shift from one subject to another that is unrelated), poor judgment and problem solving, anxiety, delusions, and hallucinations. Motor abnormalities may include rocking and arm flapping.

During adolescence, acute schizophrenia can occur suddenly while the teenager is making plans to leave home to attend college, marry, or work in another area. Onset of symptoms may be triggered by an important loss (death of a significant other, parent, child, or friend).

Prompt diagnosis can lead to early treatment and more positive outcomes. Clinical therapy for childhood schizophrenia is multifaceted, including individual psychotherapy, family therapy, and various psychotropic medications (antipsychotics such as haloperidol [Haldol], clozapine, olanzapine, and risperidone; antianxiety agents such as lorazepam [Ativan]; and antidepressants such as imipramine [Tofranil]). Drugs are only moderately effective at controlling hallucinations and delusions, responses vary considerably among individuals, and children may have different responses than adults. Side effects will determine what drugs are used and their duration. Antipsychotic medication is continued for at least 4 to 6 weeks before effectiveness can be determined. Medications often must be continued for several months or years after recovery from an acute schizophrenic episode, although medication-free trials may be attempted in children who have shown an absence of symptoms for 6 to 12 months.

Episodes of acute schizophrenia often require inpatient hospitalization on a psychiatric unit for thorough diagnosis and beginning management. Treatment may include an intensive school-based program in a structured, supervised setting with specially trained professionals. The goal of initial treatment is to reduce or control psychotic episodes and provide a safe, structured environment for the child or adolescent, enabling the child to live each day at an optimal level of functioning. Outpatient care is provided following initial diagnosis and establishment of the treatment regimen.

Most children require long-term treatment, including intermittent periods of hospitalization. Children or adolescents whose symptoms are difficult to control and who present a safety risk to themselves or others may require long-term residential treatment. Earlier age at diagnosis and delay in treatment lead to a poorer prognosis.

Nursing Management

The nurse may encounter the child or adolescent with schizophrenia during hospitalization for an acute episode, during treatment of another problem, or while working with the individual in the community. Nursing care centers on providing for physical safety and psychologic care, and normal growth and development for the child.

Family education and involvement in the treatment plan are essential. The family is taught to monitor the child's symptoms and progression. Educating the child and parents about the risk of recurrence and methods to alleviate side effects of prescribed medications may increase compliance with the treatment plan. The nurse performs assessments of the child for common medication side effects. For example, when excess weight is a potential side effect, frequent growth measurements are made. Neurologic assessment and laboratory studies may be needed with some medications.

The family is assisted in establishing educational plans for the child and for integration within the school system. The nurse communicates with school personnel to ensure understanding of the child's condition and ongoing management of the individualized education plan (IEP).

Desired outcomes of nursing care for the child with schizophrenia include physical and psychologic security, normal growth and development, and decrease in psychotic symptoms.

COGNITIVE DISORDERS

A wide array of cognitive conditions occur in childhood. Some are mild and not diagnosed until a child has difficulty in school, whereas others may be associated with physical signs that are visible at birth.

Learning Disabilities

Learning disabilities are a common problem of young children, affecting about 5% to 10% of school-age children (Boyle, Boulet, Schieve, et al., 2011; CDC, 2008a). They involve neurologic conditions in which the brain cannot receive or process information in the normal manner. Often the impairment is only in one or two types of learning, making diagnosis difficult. Common types of learning

Clinical Manifestations Various Learning Disabilities	
DISORDER	**CLINICAL MANIFESTATIONS**
Dyslexia	Difficulty with writing, reading, spelling
Dyscalculia	Mathematics and computation problems
Dysgraphia	Difficulty with writing, spelling, and composition
Dyspraxia	Problems with manual dexterity and coordination

disorders are listed in the Clinical Manifestations table. Children may have difficulty in processing visual information, which may be manifested in reading, writing, and mathematics performance. Others may have more difficulty with oral information, leading to problems in language development and reading.

The causes of learning disorders are complex. Sometimes they are related to low birth weight or problems during the perinatal period. There may be a genetic component since their occurrence is more common when other family members are affected. Learning disabilities are manifested in diverse ways. The disabilities should be diagnosed by a learning specialist such as a psychologist with specialty training. A series of cognitive and developmental tests are most commonly used. Brain scanning with MRI is showing promise for diagnostic clues in the future. Treatments involve learning how to compensate for the difficulties by using capabilities that are intact. Some children need to have all material written for them, and others need verbal presentations. Specific learning goals are established with the assistance of learning specialists. Children with learning disabilities should have IEPs established with realistic goals for school performance (see Chapter 14 ⊘ for further information about IEPs).

Nurses play a major role in identification of children with learning disabilities. You may be in contact with families during health promotion visits or in other settings when parents relay concern about the child's performance or difficulty in some aspect of school. Ask about a family history of learning problems, and evaluate the child's history for prematurity, low birth weight, head injury, seizure activity, and other chronic health conditions. Assess the child for delay in the following developmental milestones, which can indicate learning disability:

- Tasks such as tying shoes, buttoning, or hopping
- Expressive and receptive speech
- Naming objects or reading
- Fine and gross motor milestones
- Following simple instructions

National Joint Committee on Learning Disabilities, 2010.

When a child may have a learning disability, refer the family to the school or other testing resource. Partner with the family to plan for the child's learning needs. Help the family to work closely with the child, provide a setting at home to maximize potential for learning, and build healthy self-esteem in the child. Assist the family to work with the school to establish annual goals for the child. A multidisciplinary team commonly works within the school, and includes teachers, therapists, and the family to plan for the child's learning needs. Most children with learning disabilities can learn to perform well in

TABLE 34–7   Common Conditions Associated with Intellectual Disability

PRENATAL CONDITIONS	BIOLOGICAL ENVIRONMENT	EXTERNAL FORCES
Down syndrome	Inborn errors of metabolism (e.g., phenylketonuria, hypothyroidism)	Traumatic brain injury
Fragile X syndrome		Poison ingestion (acute or chronic)
Fetal alcohol syndrome		Hypoxia/anoxic insult
Maternal Infection (e.g., rubella, cytomegalovirus)		Infection (e.g., meningitis)
		Environmental deprivation

their areas of strength and compensate for areas of difficulty. Early intervention is key to success and building positive self-image regarding abilities.

Intellectual Disability (Mental Retardation)

Intellectual disability is now the preferred term for what was previously called mental retardation. **Intellectual disability** is defined as significant limitation in intellectual functioning and adaptive behavior. It is manifested in differences in conceptual, social, and practical life skills, and begins before the age of 18 years (American Association on Intellectual and Developmental Disabilities, 2012). Later events that lead to limitations in function are generally referred to as brain injury. Intellectual disability is generally characterized by an IQ below 70 to 75, with significant impairments in **adaptive functioning** (the ability of an individual to meet the standards expected for his or her cultural group). The child with intellectual disability has adaptive deficits in at least two areas such as communication, self-care, home living, social and interpersonal skills, use of community resources, self-direction, functional academic skills, work, leisure, health, or safety. A low IQ score by itself does not necessarily correlate with impairment in the ability to carry out adaptive skills. The child should be evaluated within the contexts of the individual cultural and community environment. The IQ score and the level of adaptive skills together determine the degree of severity of intellectual disability.

Intellectual disability is one type of **developmental disability,** any of a variety of chronic conditions that are characterized by mental or physical impairments. Other examples include pervasive developmental disorder, cerebral palsy (see Chapter 33), and sensory loss (see Chapter 24). A developmental disability begins by the age of 21 years and lasts throughout the lifetime.

Etiology and Pathophysiology

Intellectual disability occurs in 12 per 1,000 children (CDC, n.d.). The causes of intellectual disability can be grouped into three general categories: prenatal errors in the development of the CNS, prenatal or postnatal changes in the biological environment of the person, and external forces leading to CNS damage. In each instance, the precipitating factor causes a change in the form, function, and adaptation of the CNS. Table 34–7 provides examples of common causes of intellectual disability for each category.

Three conditions associated with intellectual disability from prenatal conditions are Down syndrome, fragile X syndrome, and fetal alcohol syndrome. They will be discussed in greater detail in this section. See Table 34–8 for physical characteristics of children with each of these conditions.

In the United States, about 1 in 800 to 1,000 infants, or 5,500 infants each year, are born with *Down syndrome* (American Academy

of Pediatrics, 2009). See Figure 34–10 ■. The condition is caused by an extra chromosome; the child has 47 rather than 46 chromosomes (see discussion of genetic transmission in Chapter 4). The most common chromosome affected is 21, so that the child often has trisomy 21, or three instead of two copies of chromosome 21. In addition to intellectual disability and physical signs, the child with Down syndrome is at higher risk of developing other conditions such as cardiac defects, hearing loss, strabismus, gastrointestinal problems, orthodontic conditions, thyroid disease, dermatologic conditions, and leukemia (Fonatsch, 2010). Jeremiah, who was described in the opening scenario, was born with Down syndrome. He had gastroesophageal reflux and otitis media frequently as a young child.

Fragile X syndrome is caused by a single recessive gene abnormality on the X chromosome. A permutation to the X chromosome may occur in males or females. When a father or mother passes the faulty X chromosome to a daughter, it may remain as a permutation or may change into a true mutation. The daughter has two X chromosomes

TABLE 34–8   Characteristics of Three Common Conditions Associated with Intellectual Disability

DOWN SYNDROME	FRAGILE X SYNDROME	FETAL ALCOHOL SYNDROME
Small head (microcephaly)	Long face	Flat midface
Flattened forehead	Prominent jaw	Low nasal bridge
Wide, short neck	Large ears	Long philtrum with narrow upper lip
Epicanthal eye folds	Frequent otitis media	Short upturned nose
White spots on eye iris (Brushfield spots)	Large testicles	Poor coordination
Congenital cataracts	Epicanthal eye folds	Failure to thrive
Flat nose	Strabismus	Skeletal and joint abnormalities
Small, low-set ears	High-arched palate	Hearing loss
Protruding tongue	Scoliosis	
Short broad hands	Pliable joints	
Single transverse crease that crosses the entire palm of the hand		
Wide space between first and second toes		
Hearing loss		
Increased incidence of diabetes, congenital heart defect, and leukemia		
Hypotonia		

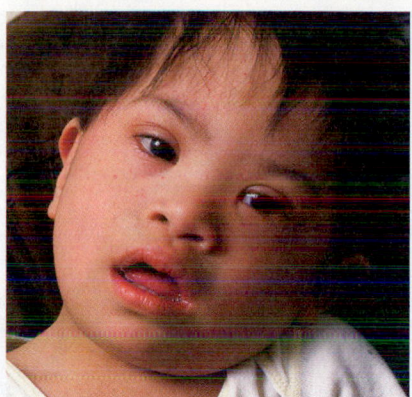

FIGURE 34–10 ■ A child with Down syndrome.

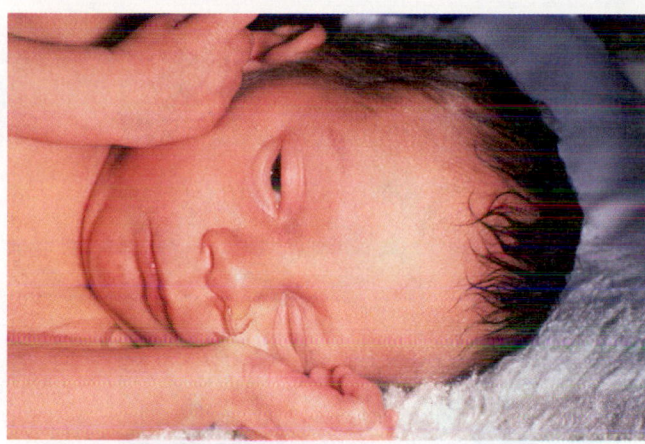

FIGURE 34–11 ■ A child with fetal alcohol syndrome.
Source: © 2012--Custom Medical Stock Photo, All Rights Reserved.

and therefore does not manifest this recessive disorder; however, she can give the mutated X chromosome to her son who becomes affected with fragile X. The mutation of fragile X is on gene FMRP-1, which instructs cells to make a protein necessary for normal brain development. The faulty gene creates a deficiency in the FMR1 protein that leads to brain changes. The condition is often associated with other conditions such as ADHD, anxiety, and autism (Hay, 2008; Roberts, Mankowski, Sideris, et al., 2009).

Fetal alcohol syndrome (FAS) is caused by the effect of ethyl alcohol on the developing fetus. The term *fetal alcohol spectrum disorder* (FASD) describes the wide range of effects from the condition, which can range from FAS to a milder condition called *fetal alcohol effects* (FAE) (Ismail, Buckley, Budacki, et al., 2010). Alcohol ingestion by the pregnant woman can influence development of many body organs, and effects can range from mild to severe. Despite many years of education, alcohol use remains a leading cause of intellectual disability, affecting 0.3 to 1.5 in 1,000 births in the United States, or 8,000 to 12,000 infants annually (CDC, 2010d). (See Chapter 33 ✪ for treatment of the drug-addicted newborn.) Chapter 32 ✪ discusses phenylketonuria and hypothyroidism, two common biochemical causes of intellectual disability. Other causes involve traumatic brain injury and infections of the CNS (see Chapter 33).

Clinical Manifestations

Mild intellectual disability was originally described as an IQ between 50 and 70, moderate intellectual disability as an IQ of 35 to 50, severe intellectual disability as an IQ of 20 to 35, and profound intellectual disability as an IQ below 20. Although an IQ below 70 is generally considered indicative of intellectual disability, the functional assessment of the child is now considered to be a more accurate identification of the child's performance and needs. Children who have intellectual disability manifest delays in several areas of development, including motor movement, language, and adaptive behavior. They usually achieve developmental milestones more slowly than the average child. These developmental delays may be the first indication to parents and care providers of the child's condition.

Intellectual disability is sometimes accompanied by sensory impairment, speech problems, motor and orthopedic disabilities, and seizure disorders. Of children with intellectual disability, 10% to 30% manifest one such disorder. See Table 34–8 for several physical characteristics associated with Down syndrome, fragile X syndrome, and fetal alcohol syndrome (Figure 34–11 ■).

Collaborative Care

Many professionals, family members, and community partners work together to provide a nurturing environment for children with intellectual disability.

Diagnostic Tests

Intellectual disability is diagnosed and initial treatment is planned in a multistep process involving a multidisciplinary team. Members of the team are commonly a developmental specialist, physician, geneticist, nurse, teacher, language therapist, occupational therapist, and physical rehabilitation specialist. See Box 34–7 for the *DSM-IV-TR* criteria for intellectual disability.

First, a comprehensive history and evaluation of the child's physical characteristics, developmental level, and intellectual and adaptive functioning is carried out. Laboratory tests such as chromosome analysis, blood enzyme levels, lead levels, or cranial imaging provide valuable information in some circumstances. A three-generation family history is performed.

Developmental screening using a test such as the Denver II (see Chapter 8 ✪) can help to identify children who may be at risk. Tests of intellectual and adaptive functioning are performed when

BOX 34–7	*DSM-IV-TR* Diagnostic Criteria for Intellectual Disability (Mental Retardation)

Criteria A, B, and C are present:

A. Significantly subaverage intellectual functioning: an IQ of approximately 70 or below on an individually administered IQ test (for infants, a clinical judgment of significantly subaverage intellectual functioning)

B. Concurrent deficits or impairments in present adaptive functioning (i.e., the person's effectiveness in meeting the standards expected for his or her age by his or her cultural group) in at least two of the following areas: communication, self-care, home living, social/interpersonal skills, use of community resources, self-direction, functional academic skills, work, leisure, health, and safety

C. The onset is before age 18 years

Source: Reprinted with permission from the Diagnostic and Statistical Manual of Mental Disorders, *fourth edition, text revision.* Copyright © 2000 American Psychiatric Association.

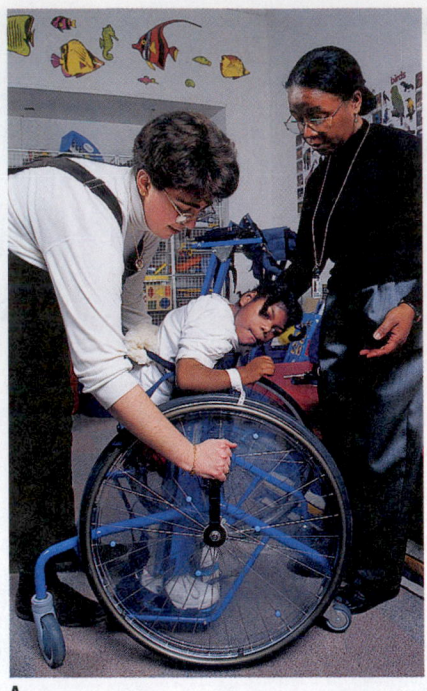

A

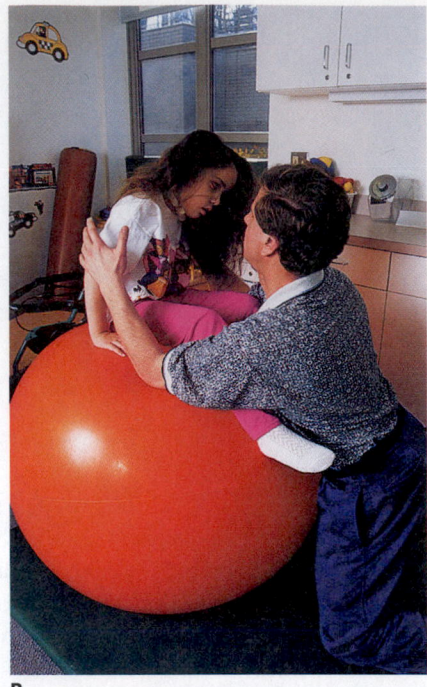

B

FIGURE 34–12 ■ Physical therapy is an important component of medical management for many children who have intellectual disabilities. *A,* This girl with severe intellectual disability uses a wheelchair. She is being positioned in a mobile prone stander, which enables her to interact in a different manner with her therapists and the environment. *B,* Physical therapists also provide outpatient care in the community to children with varying degrees of disability.

intellectual disability is suspected. A neurologic examination may indicate asymmetry of movement or strength, irritability or lethargy, or abnormal pitch to an infant's cry. Because intellectual disability may be accompanied by physical abnormalities, it is important to observe the child for facial symmetry, distance between the eyes, level of the ears, hair growth, and palmar creases. These abnormalities may be cues to other health problems.

Clinical Therapy

Based on results of the evaluation, the multidisciplinary team plans the support needed to maximize the child's potential for development. Management focuses on early intervention to improve the degree of adaptive functioning. Simultaneous treatment of associated physical, emotional, and behavioral problems is provided. Depending on the child's condition, special education programs and physical or occupational therapy may be necessary (Figure 34–12 ■). The Education for All Handicapped Children Act, PL 94-142, provides free appropriate education to all children with disabilities, between 2 and 21 years of age. Amendments to this act in 1986 (PL 99-457) encouraged states to provide early intervention services for infants and toddlers with developmental delay conditions through federal funding.

The child may require supportive care and assistance with activities of daily living. The plans for intervention change as the child grows and family situations evolve. Respite services for parents and other family members may be required periodically.

Nursing Management

Nursing management of the child with intellectual disability focuses on prevention when possible, and support of the child and family to enhance development throughout the life span.

Nursing Assessment and Diagnosis

Nurses can help to identify children with intellectual disability through history taking, observation, and developmental screening during early childhood. The history should provide information about the mental and adaptive functioning of birth parents and other family members. Intellectual disability may cluster in some families, and conditions such as fragile X syndrome are genetic in origin. The pregnancy and birth history can provide important information relating to alcohol and drug use by the mother during pregnancy. Be alert for a history of difficult pregnancy and problems during delivery. Prematurity places the child at risk of displaying below normal cognitive development. Premature infants are expected to reach developmental milestones at approximately the same age they would reach them if they were born at normal gestational age. For example, an infant born 2 months prematurely should be evaluated on milestones of an infant 2 months younger than the infant's current chronologic age. The infant gradually catches up and reaches the chronologic age milestones by about 2 years of age.

Clinical Tip

The premature infant needs frequent, thorough neurologic and developmental examinations, particularly in the first 2 years of life. Encourage parents to keep health promotion appointments, and be sure the child receives developmental screening at each visit.

When genetic conditions in the family predispose family members to intellectual disability, careful assessment of the child is needed. Children from deprived environments or those at risk because of environmental factors such as lead poisoning (see Chapter 30 ∂) are more likely to manifest intellectual disability.

Many children with intellectual disability are not diagnosed with the condition until they reach school age, particularly if the condition is mild. Early intervention, however, can help to enhance the child's functioning later. During home visits and clinic appointments, in childcare centers, and during hospitalization, be alert for signs of developmental delays, multiple (more than three) physical anomalies associated with a specific condition, or neurologic alterations. Developmental assessment should be part of each health promotion and health maintenance visit to aid in early identification.

Once the diagnosis of intellectual disability has been made, assess the adaptive functioning of the child and family. A functional assessment of the child should be performed, including toileting, dressing, and feeding skills. Assess the child's language, sensory, and psychomotor functioning. Assess the home and community for safety hazards. Observe how the family is managing with the child. To determine the impact of the child with intellectual disability on the family, ask parents to describe (1) family activities that include the child, (2) strategies that parents and siblings use to deal with community attitudes about the child, and (3) in the case of a child with other disabilities, methods of managing the child's care and planning for future care needs.

Assess the availability of services such as support groups for parents and special education opportunities for children. Evaluate the coping skills of family members.

Several nursing diagnoses may be appropriate for the child with intellectual disability, depending on the degree, cause, and outcome of the condition. Diagnoses that relate to impairments in adaptive functioning and family impact include the following:

- Growth and Development, Delayed related to neonatal disease or condition
- Nutrition, Imbalanced, Less than Body Requirements related to inability to ingest sufficient food
- Self-care Deficit: Bathing, Dressing, Toileting related to developmental disability
- Communication: Verbal, Impaired related to developmental disability
- Injury, Risk for related to lack of understanding of environmental hazards
- Coping: Family, Compromised related to the child's developmental variations

NANDA-I © 2012

Planning and Implementation

Prevention is important for some types of intellectual disability. All pregnant women or those who may become pregnant should stop ingestion of alcohol and nonprescription drugs (Box 34–8). Encourage regular prenatal visits; this helps to prevent premature births, which have a higher association with intellectual disability than birth at term.

BOX 34–8	Community Care: Fetal Alcohol Syndrome

Fetal alcohol syndrome (FAS) is a preventable cause of intellectual disability. About 12% to 15% of women consume alcohol while pregnant, and 2% engage in frequent or binge drinking (CDC, 2010d). This indicates that all women must receive clear messages about the dangers of drinking while pregnant. Teach all pregnant women that total abstention from alcohol for the entire length of pregnancy is the only completely effective method of preventing FAS. Include this in teaching to all adolescent girls, so they are aware of the potentially harmful effects of alcohol on their infant if they become pregnant. Emphasize that the most dangerous time may be early in pregnancy before women know they are pregnant (Monsen, 2009).

Nearly all children who are intellectually disabled are cared for in the community; however, they may have conditions that require periodic hospitalization or frequent healthcare visits. When needed, nursing care focuses on providing emotional support and information to family members, assisting the child with adaptive functioning, and fostering parental management of the child's activities.

Provide Emotional Support and Information

Family members need empathy and support both at the time of diagnosis and in the ensuing years. Parents may be in an acute or chronic state of grief over the loss of the "perfect" child. Encourage them to verbalize their feelings. Introducing them to parents of other children with intellectual disabilities may provide assistance and support as they learn how to manage the child's needs. Emphasize the child's strengths and capabilities. Discuss the availability of respite care to provide parents with a break from caretaking. Other family members such as grandparents and siblings may also be experiencing grief or guilt and should be given an opportunity to talk about their feelings.

Parents need honest information and answers to their questions about the child's condition. Reinforce information provided by genetic counselors and other healthcare professionals. Parents need to be informed about community resources designed to assist children with intellectual disability. Such resources include the Zero to Three Project, special education preschools and schools, county health services, and respite care. Ask parents if they have questions about individualized education plans. Refer parents to Internet sources, and help them to interpret information received and analyze its strengths and limitations. See Legal and Ethical Considerations: Laws to Provide Services for Persons with Disabilities.

Maintain a Safe Environment

Children with intellectual disability require close supervision because they may lack an understanding of common hazards. Ensure safety in the hospital environment. Assist parents to provide safety at home and school and to teach their child necessary skills such as pedestrian safety. Consider both physical and emotional safety. The child with intellectual disability may be trusting of others and sometimes is at risk for physical or sexual abuse.

Legal and Ethical Considerations
Laws to Provide Services for Persons with Disabilities

Federal and state laws and services provide for persons with intellectual disability. Public Laws 94-142, 99-457, and the Individuals with Disabilities Education Amendment mandate public education for those with disabilities (see Chapter 16 ⚙). Additional examples of pertinent laws and organizations are as follows:

- Public Law (PL) 101-336 of 1990 is known as the Americans with Disabilities Act (ADA). It prohibits discrimination and ensures equal opportunity for persons with disabilities in employment, state and local government services, public accommodations, commercial facilities, and transportation.
- The Administration on Developmental Disabilities (ADD) is the U.S. organization that ensures that the Developmental Disabilities (DD) Act goals are met. The DD Act implemented the Developmental Disabilities and Bill of Rights Act of 2000 and seeks to enhance life through training activities, community education, eliminating barriers, and influencing policy (Administration for Children and Families, 2010).
- A State Council on Developmental Disabilities (SCDD) is present in each state to increase integration of children with developmental disabilities into their communities.

Provide Assistance with Adaptive Functioning

Encourage parents' efforts to maximize the child's areas of strength and identify needs related to adaptive behaviors. Refer them to resources to assist in the areas of adaptive functioning in which the child has impairment, such as communication, self-care activities, or social skills. During hospitalization, support parents' efforts to maintain the child's skills in toileting, dressing, and self-care by planning interventions to use the skills being taught at home.

Care in the Community

The child with intellectual disability needs ongoing care throughout childhood, and adaptation of interventions as development occurs and the family's needs evolve. Parents often act as case managers for the child's care. Partner with parents as necessary to acquire the skills required to coordinate the child's plan of care. Evaluate the child's needs regularly and assist parents with the treatment plan as necessary. Provision of education is a primary goal for children who have intellectual disability. Collaborate with the family and other healthcare professionals to provide for education and for services such as physical or speech therapy. Most children with intellectual disability have an IEP designed to meet their specific learning needs (see Chapter 14 🔗 for further information). Parents, nurses, and others such as teachers and language therapists are part of the team that establishes this plan. Promote optimal development and socialization. As the child reaches adolescence, education is directed toward a vocation, issues of sexuality, and the goal of independent living, when appropriate (Box 34–9).

Specific guidelines for care are available for the child with Down syndrome (Bull & the Committee on Genetics, 2011). These guidelines suggest specific times for evaluation of hearing, growth, cardiac function, and other areas designed for early identification and treatment of associated disorders. Specific growth grids for children with Down syndrome are available, and relevant topics to suggest for anticipatory guidance during health care are recommended.

Evaluation

The expected outcomes of nursing care depend on the child's needs and developmental level. Early in the diagnostic phase, desired outcomes may involve the family's understanding of the diagnosis and the child's special needs. Later outcomes may focus on the child's communication or self-help skills. Outcomes related to cognitive performance and adaptive skills may be developed during childhood.

BOX 34–9	Community Care: Planning for the Future

Some schools and community agencies offer transitional classes when children who are intellectually disabled reach adolescence and young adulthood. These services help to teach self-care skills that may enable some youth to live in group homes or other community settings. Families receive help in planning for the child's future as parents look toward retirement. Information is provided on living options, health insurance, work opportunities, and other needs.

Clinical Judgment

Jeremiah, described in the opening scenario, has recently been enrolled in a school program. Think ahead to his needs as an adolescent with Down syndrome. What information will his family need to provide a healthy and safe experience for him regarding alcohol, sexuality, and other adolescent issues? Where will you find information to assist Jeremiah and his family when he reaches adolescence?

Chapter Highlights

- Major treatment modes for children with mental health disorders include individual therapy, family therapy, and group therapy.
- Therapeutic strategies for treatment of children and adolescents with mental health disorders include play therapy, art therapy, cognitive behavioral therapy (CBT), visualization, and hypnosis.
- Families often attempt to treat mental health conditions with use of alternative and complementary therapy; nurses can provide information to assist families in evaluating the results of these therapies.
- Nurses are involved in conducting mental health assessments, preventing disorders when possible, participating in intervention to treat disorders, and evaluating success of treatments.
- Autism spectrum disorder is the major type of pervasive developmental disorder and is manifested by abnormal behavior, social interaction, and communication.
- Attention deficit disorder (ADD) and attention deficit hyperactivity disorder (ADHD) are characterized by developmentally inappropriate behaviors involving inattention, and sometimes hyperactivity.

- ADD and ADHD must be diagnosed using recommended criteria and are commonly treated with a combination of behavioral, environmental, and medication therapies.
- Schizophrenia is a psychotic disorder manifested by social withdrawal, delusions, and hallucinations.
- Mood disorders in childhood and adolescence are commonly manifested as depression or manic depression (bipolar disorder).
- Several anxiety disorders occur in children and adolescents, most notably generalized anxiety, separation anxiety, panic, obsessive-compulsive disorder, school phobia, conversion reaction, and posttraumatic stress disorder.
- Behavioral therapy and selective serotonin reuptake inhibitors (SSRIs) are used in treatment of anxiety disorders; their use in children must be closely monitored.
- Posttraumatic stress disorder may occur as children relive the terror of traumatic events.
- Suicide is a preventable and significant cause of death among youth.

- Nurses are key health professionals in identifying youth at risk of suicide, instituting suicide prevention programs, and counseling family and friends of suicide victims.
- Children may experience tic disorders that impair development and social interactions; medications are helpful in treatment of these disorders.
- Childhood schizophrenia presents a crisis for families and may require inpatient hospitalization for youth affected.
- Nurses play a role in identifying children with potential learning disabilities, referring for diagnosis, and partnering with the family to provide a positive learning environment for the child.

- Intellectual disability is defined as subaverage intellectual and adaptive functioning, and is caused by chromosomal, genetic, or environmental factors.
- Nurses identify children with possible intellectual disability by careful evaluation of development.
- A multidisciplinary team plans the care for children with intellectual disability and periodically evaluates the child's progress and the family's needs.
- Nurses play a vital role in maintaining the mental health of children, preventing mental health problems, identifying children at risk of mental health disorders, and providing care or referring families for mental health services.

Clinical Reasoning in Action

INTRODUCTION

Recall the opening scenario. Jeremiah is a 7-year-old child who has Down syndrome. He has been relatively healthy after some ear infections in early childhood. His early intervention programs and now his entrance into school have provided a strong and nurturing environment for learning.

DESCRIPTION

It appears that Jeremiah is in a warm and nurturing environment. He has a supportive family and school environment. The school nurse and classroom teacher recently invited the parents to a meeting to establish Jeremiah's learning goals and individualized education program. During the meeting, Jeremiah's mother and father expressed concern because they would both like to retire in about 5 years but are concerned about health care, education, and other resources for Jeremiah. They expressed that they feel fortunate that their older children can often care for Jeremiah for several hours or even a couple of days at a time, thereby freeing the parents for short trips and respite from the care their son needs.

DISCUSSION

1. How will you decide if the physical growth and psychologic development that Jeremiah is demonstrating are what would be expected for a child with his diagnosis? What regular physical assessments are needed, due to some common accompanying health problems seen in children with Down syndrome?

2. Based on his history of frequent otitis media, what assessments will you perform now? See Chapter 24 🔗 for ideas.

3. What is the genetic basis for Down syndrome? Why are older parents more at risk for having a child with the syndrome?

4. Plan some physical activities that Jeremiah is likely to enjoy. How will you integrate them into his family and school life?

5. Jeremiah's parents are requesting information about what plans they should make for his care when they start planning for retirement. How can you assist them in locating resources to assist with the future care that Jeremiah will need as he grows into teen years and young adulthood?

NCLEX-RN® Review

1. A 14-year-old child experiences sudden alternating sweating and chills, shortness of breath, and dizziness when on a bus for a school field trip. She believes all on the bus are in danger. What is the priority action for this teen?
   1. Get the child off the bus for a while.
   2. Offer the child a caffeinated sports drink.
   3. Encourage others on the bus to distract the teen.
   4. Offer her some crackers with peanut butter.

2. A nurse is making a home visit for a 6-year-old child with intellectual disability. Which assessment finding indicates the need for further discussion with the family?
   1. The nurse notices household cleaners stored under the kitchen sink.
   2. The parents state they are comfortable caring for the child's toileting needs.
   3. The family has support from a grandparent who watches the child.
   4. The child has an individualized education plan (IEP).

3. A school nurse is planning care for the child with auditory learning disabilities. What are appropriate school interventions to aid the child's school success?
   1. Place the child in a special classroom.
   2. Homeschool the child.
   3. Wait until the child asks for help.
   4. Develop an individualized education plan (IEP).

4. A 6-year-old child is enrolled in kindergarten. What developmental milestone indicates a potential learning disability?
   1. Inability to write cursive
   2. Inability to hop
   3. Inability to ride a skateboard
   4. Having difficulty composing a short story

See Appendix I 🔗 for answers.

References

Addington, A. M., & Rapoport, J. L. (2009). The genetics of childhood onset schizophrenia: When madness strikes the prepubescent. *Current Psychiatric Reports, 11*, 156–161.

Administration for Children and Families. (2010). *Administration on developmental disabilities*. Retrieved from http://www.acf.hhs.gov/opa/fact_sheets/add_factsheet.html

American Academy of Pediatrics. (2009). *Down syndrome*. Retrieved from http://www.healthychildren.org

American Academy of Pediatrics. (2010). *Vaccines and side effects: The facts*. Retrieved from http://www.healthychildren.org

American Association on Intellectual and Developmental Disabilities. (2012). *FAQ on the AAIDD definition of intellectual disability*. Retrieved from http://www.aaidd.org/IntellectualDisabilityBook/content_7473.cfm?navID=366

American Psychiatric Association. (2000). *Diagnostic and statistical manual of mental disorders* (4th ed., text revision). Washington, DC: Author.

Anderson, E. R., & Mayes, L. C. (2010). Race/ethnicity and internalizing disorders in youth: A review. *Clinical Psychology Review, 30*, 338–348.

Apps, J., Winkler, J., & Jandrisevits, M. D. (2008). Bipolar disorders: Symptoms and treatment in children and adolescents. *Pediatric Nursing, 34*, 84–88.

Arora, B., & Kannikeswaran, N. (2010). The serotonin syndrome—The need for physician's awareness. *International Journal of Emergency Medicine, 3*, 373–377.

Becker, L., Goobie, K., & Thomas, S. (2009). Advising families on AD/HD: A multimodal approach. *Pediatric Nursing 35*, 47–52.

Beesdo, K., Knappe, S., & Pine, D. S. (2009). Anxiety and anxiety disorders in children and adolescents: Developmental issues and implications for DSM-V. *Psychiatric Clinics of North America, 32*, 483–524.

Boyle, C. A., Boulet, S., Schieve, L. A., Cohen, R. A., Blumberg, S. J., Yeargin-Allsop, M., . . . Kogan, M. D. (2011). Trends in the prevalence of developmental disabilities in US children, 1997–2008. *Pediatrics*. doi:10.1542/peds.2010-2989

Brulotte, J., Bukutu, C., & Vohra, S. (2009). Complementary, holistic, and integrative medicine: Fish oils and neurodevelopmental disorders. *Pediatrics in Review, 30*(4), e29–e33.

Bukstein, O. G. (2009). Long-term effectiveness of ADHD treatments. *Consultant for Pediatricians, 8*(8), S19–S24.

Bull, M. J., & the Committee on Genetics. (2011). Clinical report—Health supervision for children with Down syndrome. *Pediatrics, 128*, 393–406.

Center for Injury Research and Prevention. (2011). *PTSD in children and parents*. Retrieved from http://injury.research.chop.edu/our_research/carit_research.php

Centers for Disease Control and Prevention (CDC). (2008a). QuickStats: Percentage of children ages 6–17 years with learning disability (LD) and attention deficit hyperactivity disorder (ADHD) by birthweight—National Health Interview Survey, United States, 2004–2006. *Morbidity and Mortality Weekly Report, 57*, 947.

Centers for Disease Control and Prevention (CDC). (2008b). Unintentional strangulation deaths from the "choking game" among youths ages 6–19 years—United States, 1995–2007. *Morbidity and Mortality Weekly Report, 57*, 141–146.

Centers for Disease Control and Prevention (CDC). (2009a). Prevention of autism spectrum disorders—Autism and developmental disease monitoring network, United States, 2006. *Morbidity and Mortality Weekly Report, 58*(SS-10), 1–28.

Centers for Disease Control and Prevention (CDC). (2009b). *Youth suicide*. Retrieved from http://www.cdc.gov/violenceprevention/pub/youth_suicide.html

Centers for Disease Control and Prevention (CDC). (2009c). *National suicide statistics*. Retrieved from http://www.cdc.gov/ViolencePrevention/suicide/statistics/rates03.html

Centers for Disease Control and Prevention (CDC). (2010a). *Autistic syndrome disorders treatment*. Retrieved from http://www.cdc.gov/ncbddd/autism/treatment.html

Centers for Disease Control and Prevention (CDC). (2010b). *Autistic spectrum disorders research*. Retrieved from http://www.cdc.gov/ncbddd/autism

Centers for Disease Control and Prevention (CDC). (2010c). The choking game: Risky youth behavior. Retrieved from http://www.cdc.gov

Centers for Disease Control and Prevention (CDC). (2010d). *Fetal alcohol spectrum disorders (FASDs)*. Retrieved from http://www.cdc.gov

Centers for Disease Control and Prevention (CDC). (2012) *Attention deficit hyperactivity disorder (ADHD)*. Retrieved from http://www.cdc.gov/nchs/fastats/adhd.htm

Centers for Disease Control and Prevention (CDC). (n.d.). *Intellectual disabilities among children*. Retrieved from http://www.cdc.gov

Cheng, S., Maeda, T., Yoichi, S., Yamagata, Z., Tomiwa, K., & Japan Children's Study Group. (2010). Early television exposure and children's behavioral and social outcomes at age 30 months. *Journal of Epidemiology, 20*(Suppl. 2), S482–S489.

D'Alessandro, T. M. (2009). Factors influencing the onset of childhood obsessive compulsive disorder. *Pediatric Nursing, 35*, 43–46.

DiMarco, M. A., & Melnyk, B. (2009). The mental health needs of children and adolescents. *Archives of Psychiatric Nursing, 23*, 334–336.

Elder, J. H., & D'Alessandro, T. (2009). Supporting families of children with autism spectrum disorders: Questions parents ask and what nurses need to know. *Pediatric Nursing, 35*, 240–253.

Evans, R. W., Tepper, S. J., Shapiro, R. E., Sun-Edelskin, C., & Tiethen, G. E. (2010). The FDA alert on serotonin syndrome with use of triptans combined with serotonin reuptake inhibitors or selective serotonin-norepinephrine reuptake inhibitors. *Headache, 50*, 1089–1099.

Ferguson, C. J. (2011). The influence of television and video game use on attention and school problems: A multivariate analysis with other risk factors controlled. *Journal of Psychiatric Research, 45*, 808–813.

Fonatsch, C. (2010). The role of chromosome 21 in hematology and oncology. *Genes and Chromosomes in Cancer, 49*, 497–508.

Froehlich, T. E., Epstein, J. N., Nick, T. G., Melguizo Castro, M. S., Stein, M. A., Brinkman, W. B., . . . Kahn, R. S. (2011). Pharmacogenetic predictors of methylphenidate dose-response in attention-deficit/hyperactivity disorder. *Journal of the American Academy of Child and Adolescent Psychiatry, 50*, 1129–1139.

Gabbay, V., Coffey, B. J., Babb, J. S., Meyer, L., Wachtel, C., Anam, S., & Rabinovitz, B. (2008). Pediatric autoimmune neuropsychiatric disorders associated with streptococcus: Comparison of diagnosis and treatment in the community and at a specialty unit. *Pediatrics, 122*, 273–278.

Ganem, J. A. (2008). *Treating children with ADHD*. Retrieved from http://www.jobsoneducation.com/cliniciansCME.index.asp?page=courses/105821/disclaimer.htm&lsn_id=105821

Golnik, A., & Maccabee-Ryaboy, N. (2010, November). Autism: Clinical pearls for primary care. *Contemporary Pediatrics*, 42–60.

Guynn, C., & Gulley, T. (2009, November). Trichotillomania. *Consultant for Pediatricians, 408*.

Hamblen, J. L., Norris, F. H., Pietruszkiewicz, S., Gibson, L. E., Naturale, A., & Louis, C. (2009). Cognitive behavioral therapy for postdisaster distress: A community based treatment program for survivors of Hurricane Katrina. *Administration and Policy in Mental Health, 36*, 206–214.

Hammerness, P., Traum, A. Z., Becker, J., & Deshpande, A. (2009). Cardiovascular risk in ADHD pharmacotherapy. *Contemporary Pediatrics, 26*(11), 34–45.

Hamrin, V., & Magorno, M. (2010). Assessment of adolescents for depression in the pediatric primary care setting. *Pediatric Nursing, 36*, 103–111.

Hay, D. A. (2008). Fragile X—A challenge to models of the mind and to best clinical practice. *Cortex, 44*, 626–627.

Houck, G., Kendall, J., Miller, A., Mirrell, P., & Wiebe, G. (2011). Self-concept in children and adolescents with attention deficit hyperactivity disorder. *Journal of Pediatric Nursing, 26*, 239–247.

Hughes, J. R. (2010). A review of Savant syndrome and its possible relationship to epilepsy. *Epilepsy Behavior, 17*, 147–152.

Inglese, M. D. (2009). Caring for children with autism spectrum disorder, Part II: Screening diagnosis, and management. *Journal of Pediatric Nursing, 24*, 49–59.

Inglese, M. D., & Elder, H. (2009). Caring for children with autism spectrum disorder, Part I: Prevalence, etiology, and core features. *Journal of Pediatric Nursing, 24*, 41–47.

Ismail, S., Buckley, S., Budacki, R., Jabbar, A., & Gallicano, G. I. (2010). Screening, diagnosing and prevention of fetal alcohol syndrome: Is this syndrome treatable? *Developmental Neuroscience, 32*, 91–100.

Johnson, C. P., Myers, S. M., & the Council on Children with Disabilties (2007, reaffirmed 2010). Identification and evaluation of children with autism spectrum disorders. *Pediatrics 120*, 1183–1215.

Kassam-Adams, N., Marsac, M. L., & Cirilli, C. (2010). Posttraumatic stress disorder symptom structure in injured children: Functional impairment and depression symptoms in a confirmatory factor analysis. *Journal of the American Academy of Child and Adolescent Psychiatry, 49*, 616–625.

Keeley, M. L., & Storch, E. A. (2009). Anxiety disorders in youth. *Journal of Pediatric Nursing, 24,* 26–40.

Kendall, P. C., Compton, S. N., Walkup, J. T., Birmaher, B., Albano, A. M., Sherill, J., … Piacentini, J. (2010). Clinical characteristics of anxiety disordered youth. *Journal of Anxiety Disorders, 24,* 360–365.

Kortesluoma, R. L., Punamaki, R. L., & Nikkonen, J. (2008). Hospitalized children drawing their pain: The contents and cognitive and emotional characteristics of pain drawings. *Journal of Child Health Care, 12,* 284–300.

Kozlowska, K., Scher, S., & Williams, L. M. (2011). Patterns of emotional-cognitive functioning in pediatric conversion patients: Implications for the conceptualization of conversion disorders. *Psychosomatic Medicine, 73*(9), 775–788.

Krauter, R. R., & Cook, S. S. (2011). Pharmacogenetics and the pharmacological management of depression. *Nurse Practitioner, 36*(10), 15–21.

Lack, C. W., & Green, A. L. (2009). Mood disorders in children and adolescents. *Journal of Pediatric Nursing, 24,* 13–25.

Legerstee, J. S., Tulen, J. H., Dierckx, B., Treffers, P. D., Verhulst, F. C., & Utens, E. M. (2010). CBT for childhood anxiety disorders: Differential changes in selective attention between treatment responders and non-responders. *Journal of Child Psychology and Psychiatry, 51,* 162–172.

Lobar, S. L., Fritts, M. K., Arbide, Z., & Russell, D. (2008). The role of the nurse practitioner in an individualized education plan and coordination of care for the child with Asperger's syndrome. *Journal of Pediatric Health Care, 22,* 111–119.

Lovrin, M. (2009). Treatment of major depression in adolescents: Weighing the evidence of risk and benefit in light of black box warnings. *Journal of Child and Adolescent Psychiatric Nursing, 22*(2), 63–68.

Massimo, L. M., & Wiley, T. J. (2008). Young siblings of children with cancer deserve care and a personalized approach. *Pediatrics and Blood Cancer, 50,* 708–710.

May, D. E., & Kratochvil, C. J. (2010). Attention-deficit hyperactivity disorder: Recent advances in pediatric pharmacotherapy. *Drugs, 70,* 15–40.

Mayo Clinic. (2009). *Childhood schizophrenia.* Retrieved from http://www.mayoclinic.com/health/childhood-schizophrenia/DS00868

Mayo Clinic. (2010). *Cognitive behavioral therapy.* Retrieved from http://www.mayoclinic.com/health/cognitive-behavioral-therapy/MY00194

McCabe, W. E., West, B. T., Teter, C. J., Ross-Durow, P., Young, A., & Boyd, C. J. (2011). Characteristics associated with the diversion of controlled medications among adolescents. *Drug and Alcohol Dependence, 118,* 452–458.

Melnyk, B. M., Hawkins-Walsh, E., Beauchesne, M., Brandt, P., Crowley, A., Choi, M., & Greenburg, E. (2010). Strengthening PNP curricula in mental/behavioral health and evidence-based practice. *Journal of Pediatric Health Care, 24,* 81–94.

Monsen, R. B. (2009). Prevention is best for fetal alcohol syndrome. *Journal of Pediatric Nursing, 24,* 60–61.

Myers, S. M. (2009). Management of autism spectrum disorders in primary care. *Pediatric Annals, 38,* 42–49.

National Center for Children in Poverty. (2010). *Children's mental health.* Retrieved from http://www.nccp.org/publications/pub_929.html

National Center for PTSD. (2008). *PTSD in children and adolescents.* Retrieved from http://ncptsd.va.gov/ncmain/ncdocs/fact_shts/fs_children.html

National Institutes of Health (2011). *Attention deficit hyperactivity disorder (ADHD).* Retrieved from http://report.nih.gov/nihfactsheets/viewfactsheet.aspx?csid=25&key=a

National Institute of Mental Health. (2009). *Bipolar disorder.* Retrieved from http://www.nimh.nih.gov/health/publications/bipolar-disorder/how-is-bipolar-disorder-diagnosed.shtml

National Institute of Mental Health. (2010). *Depression in children and adolescents.* Retrieved from http://www.nimh.nih.gov/health/topics/depression/depression-in-children-and-adolescents.shtml

National Institute of Mental Health (2012). *A PANDAS study.* Retrieved from http://intramural.nimh.nih.gov/pdn/web.htm

National Institute of Neurological Disorders and Stroke. (2010). *Tourette syndrome fact sheet.* Retrieved from http://www.ninds.nih.gov/disorders/tourette.detail_tourette.htm

National Joint Committee on Learning Disabilities. (2010). *Learning disabilities and young children.* Retrieved from http://www.ldonline.org/article/11511/

Prows, C. A., & Saldana, S. N. (2009). Nurses' genetic/genomics competencies when medication therapy is guided by pharmacogenetic testing: Children with mental health disorders as an exemplar. *Journal of Pediatric Nursing, 24,* 179–188.

Roberts, J. E., Mankowski, J. B., Sideris, J., Goldman, B. D., Hatton, D. D., Mirrett, P. L., … Bailey, B. D. (2009). Trajectories and predictors of the development of very young boys with fragile X syndrome. *Journal of Pediatric Psychology, 34,* 827–836.

Rogers, S. J., & Vismara, L. A. (2008). Evidence-based comprehensive treatments for early autism. *Journal of Clinical Child and Adolescent Psychology, 37,* 8–38.

Rucklidge, J. J., Johnstone, J., & Kaplan, B. J. (2009). Nutrient supplementation approaches in the treatment of ADHD. *Expert Review of Neurotherapeutics, 9,* 461–476.

Ryan-Krause, P. (2011). Attention deficit hyperactivity disorder: Part III. *Journal of Pediatric Health Care, 25*(1), 50–56.

Santrock, J. W. (2011). *Child development* (13th ed.). Boston, MA: McGraw-Hill.

Simpson, G. A., Cohen, R. A., Pastor, P. N., & Reuben, C. A. (2008). *Use of mental health services in the past 12 months by children ages 4–17 years: United States 2005–2006 (NCHS Data Brief No. 8).* Hyattsville, MD: National Center for Health Statistics.

Sogomonyan, F., & Cooper, J. L. (2010). *Trauma faced by children of military families.* New York, NY: National Center for Children in Poverty.

Soh, J. L., & Walter, G. (2008). Complementary and alternative medicine (CAM) treatments and pediatric psychopharmacology. *Journal of the American Academy of Child and Adolescent Psychiatry, 47,* 364–368.

Storch, E. A., & Elder, J. H. (2009). Introduction to the special series on child and adolescent mental health. *Journal of Pediatric Nursing, 24,* 1–2.

Subcommittee on Attention-Deficit/Hyperactivity Disorder, Steering Committee on Quality Improvement and Management. (2011). ADHD: Clinical practice guideline for the diagnosis, evaluation, and treatment of attention-deficit/hyperactivity disorder in children and adolescents. *Pediatrics.* doi:10.1542/peds.2011-2654

Swing, E. L., Gentile, D. A., Anderson, C. A., & Walsh, D. A. (2010). Television and video game exposure and the development of attention problems. *Pediatrics, 126,* 214–221.

Theoktisto, K. M. (2009). Pharmacokinetic considerations in the treatment of pediatric behavioral issues. *Pediatric Nursing, 35,* 369–375.

U.S. Department of Health and Human Services. (2010). *Healthy People 2020.* Retrieved from http://www.healthypeople.gov/hp2020/

U.S. Preventive Services Task Force (2009). *Screening and treatment for major depressive disorder in children and adolescents: Recommendation statement* (AHRQ Publication No. 09-05130-EF-2). Rockville, MD: Association for Healthcare Research and Quality.

Van den Anker, J. N. (2010). Developmental pharmacology. *Developmental Disabilities Research Reviews, 16,* 233–238.

Vetter, V. L., Elia, J., Erickson, C., Berger, S., Blum, N., Uzark, K., & Webb, C. L. (2008). Cardiovascular monitoring of children and adolescents with heart disease receiving stimulant drugs: A scientific statement from the American Heart Association Council on Cardiovascular Disease in the Young Congenital Cardiac Defects Committee and the Council on Cardiovascular Nursing. *Circulation, 117,* 2407–2423.

Vierhile, A., Robb, A., & Ryan-Krause, P. (2009). Attention-deficit/hyperactivity disorder in children and adolescents: Closing diagnostic, communication, and treatment gaps. *Journal of Pediatric Health Care, 23,* S5–S21.

Wilens, T. E., Adler, L. A., Adams, J., Sgambati, S., Rotrosen, J., Sawtelle, R., … Fusillo, S. (2008). Misuse and diversion of stimulants prescribed for ADHD: A systematic review of the literature. *Journal of the American Academy of Child and Adolescent Psychiatry, 47,* 21–31.

Wilson, M. E., Megel, M. E., Enenback, L., & Carlson, K. L. (2010). The voices of children: Stories about hospitalization. *Journal of Pediatric Health Care, 24,* 95–102.

Zemrak, W. R., & Kenna, G. A. (2008). Association of antipsychotic and antidepressant drugs with QT-interval prolongation. *American Journal of Health-System Pharmacy 65,* 1029–1038.

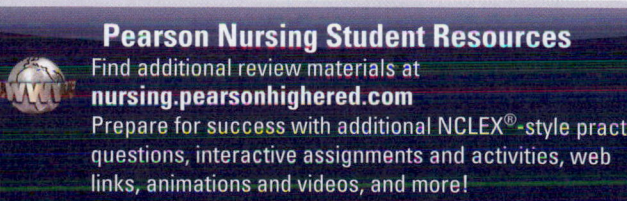

Pearson Nursing Student Resources
Find additional review materials at
nursing.pearsonhighered.com
Prepare for success with additional NCLEX®-style practice questions, interactive assignments and activities, web links, animations and videos, and more!

35 Alterations in Musculoskeletal Function

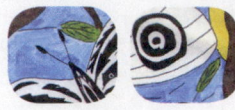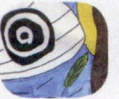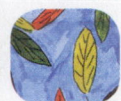

Learning Outcomes

After completing this chapter, you will be able to:

1. Describe pediatric variations in the musculoskeletal system.

2. Plan nursing care for children with structural deformities of the foot, hip, and spine.

3. Recognize signs and symptoms of infectious musculoskeletal disorders and refer for appropriate care.

4. Partner with families to plan care for children with musculoskeletal conditions that are chronic or require long-term care.

5. Plan nursing interventions to promote safety and developmental progression in children who require braces, casts, traction, and surgery.

6. Recommend nursing care for fractures, including teaching for injury prevention and nursing implementations for the child who has sustained a fracture.

> "How am I going to go back to school? There are stairs and you wouldn't believe all the kids in the hallways between classes."
>
> *—Douglass, age 12*

Douglass Langlois was admitted to the clinic today for application of a short leg cast. He broke his left lower fibula nearly a week ago when he was on a trampoline with three friends, trying to see who could jump the highest. Douglass slipped and his lateral leg hit the frame on the side. His friends helped him off the trampoline and called his mother, who transported Douglass to the emergency room.

His mother states that Douglass is 12 years old and in middle school. He has been going to a friend's house nearly every day after school and spending time on activities such as the trampoline and in-line skating, as well as watching television and playing video games. She felt this was safer than him being at home alone during her work hours, but is now starting to wonder whether to allow Douglass to engage in activities with his friend. In the emergency room after the accident, a splint was used to provide support for a few days and allow the swelling to decrease before today's cast application. Douglass has been non–weight bearing on his leg and has been using crutches.

What teaching does Douglass need to keep the cast intact and to ensure his safety? What special adaptations will be needed in his home and school? How can the clinic nurse partner with the school nurse to provide for Douglass's transition back to school? Is there any way his injury could have been avoided? The information in this chapter will discuss issues such as these and help you to provide effective care for children like Douglass who have musculoskeletal disorders.

he musculoskeletal system helps the body to protect its vital organs, support weight, control motion, store minerals, and supply red blood cells. *Bones* provide a rigid framework for the body, and *joints* are the articulations or places where adjoining bones meet. *Muscles* are fibrous tissue that provide for movement. *Ligaments* are bands of connective tissue holding bones together, and *tendons* are connective tissue that connects bones and muscles. Bones, muscles, and supporting structures are needed for gross and fine motor development. Therefore, alterations in musculoskeletal functioning can have a significant impact on a child's growth and development.

ANATOMY AND PHYSIOLOGY

The musculoskeletal system is composed of the bones and muscles; joints, the supporting structures that facilitate movement; and tendons and ligaments that connect parts of the system. Cartilage is the connective tissue precursor to bone, and remains in some structures such as ears and ribs throughout life. Bone formation is a dynamic system at any age, but particularly so in children and adolescents. Children depend on a functioning musculoskeletal system to enable support and movement, which in turn ensures that exposure to various stimuli and normal development can occur.

Bones are composed of osseous or dense connective tissue. They contain an exterior shell or cortex, and an inner, primarily protein, matrix (Figure 35–1 ■). The cells covering the cortex are called lining cells or compact bone. They protect the bone from penetration by circulating blood cells and other components of circulation; this covering is called the **periosteum.** The inner matrix is composed of a series of interconnected plates called cancellous, trabecular, or spongy bone. Spaces between these plates are called bone marrow,

and this is the area where **hematopoiesis** (production and development of blood cells) occurs. In addition to the lining cells found on the bone exterior, other types of cells include **osteoblasts,** which synthesize and lay down bone and then attract calcium and phosphates to strengthen the bone; **osteoclasts,** which resorb bone in the constant process of bone formation and breakdown; and **osteocytes,** which are special osteoblasts that sense and respond to bone pressure and bending to direct the process of bone remodeling. The process of bone growth and remodeling is influenced by factors such as pressure (via physical activity), hormones (parathyroid hormone, glucocorticoids, insulin-like growth factor, calcitonin), and external factors (dietary intake of calcium and phosphorus, bisphosphonate drugs, gallium, and so on).

The 206 bones of the human body are composed of several types. They include:

- *Long bones* such as the fibula, tibia, femur, humerus, and ulna; most childhood growth occurs in these bones
- *Short bones* such as those in the wrist and ankle
- *Flat bones* such as the skull, sternum, and ribs; the ribs retain large components of cartilage even when mature
- *Irregular bones* which have a variety of shapes and sizes, such as vertebrae, pelvis bones, and scapulae

Muscles are collections of cells that can contract, causing the accompanying skeleton to move. Muscle fibers require a supply of blood and nerves, and vary from small to quite large in size. Muscle cells develop in response to the stimulation of activity. Types of muscle cells include:

- *Skeletal* (striated) or *voluntary* muscles that involve the biceps, triceps, deltoid, gluteus maximus, and others
- *Smooth* (short-fibered) or *involuntary* muscles such as those in the gastrointestinal tract, lungs, and pupils of the eye
- *Cardiac* (striated, special-function) muscles that ensure the heart's constant contraction and relaxation

Muscles enable parts of the body to flex and extend, abduct and adduct, and carry out other motions (see Figure 35–2 ■ for terms used to describe the positions of limbs and the motions possible in the body extremities). As one muscle flexes, the opposing muscle must extend to allow the movement.

Several other structures enable the musculoskeletal system to function. The **joints** are articulations or connections between bones. Fibrous joints provide for little movement (those in the skull are an example), cartilaginous joints allow for slight movement (vertebral joints are a good example), while synovial joints are movable within certain limits (knee, hip, elbow, and shoulder are examples). Joints are complex in structure and function, containing the fibrous end of the bone, synovial membrane and fluid, other sacs called bursae, and ligaments. **Ligaments** are tough fibers that bind the ends of bones together. **Tendons** are fibrous bands that connect bone to its accompanying muscles, allowing the bone to move when a muscle contracts or relaxes.

PEDIATRIC DIFFERENCES

Bones

Several differences exist between the bones of children and those of adults. Although primary centers of **ossification** (bone formation) are nearly complete at birth, a fibrous membrane still exists between the cranial bones (fontanels). The posterior fontanel closes between

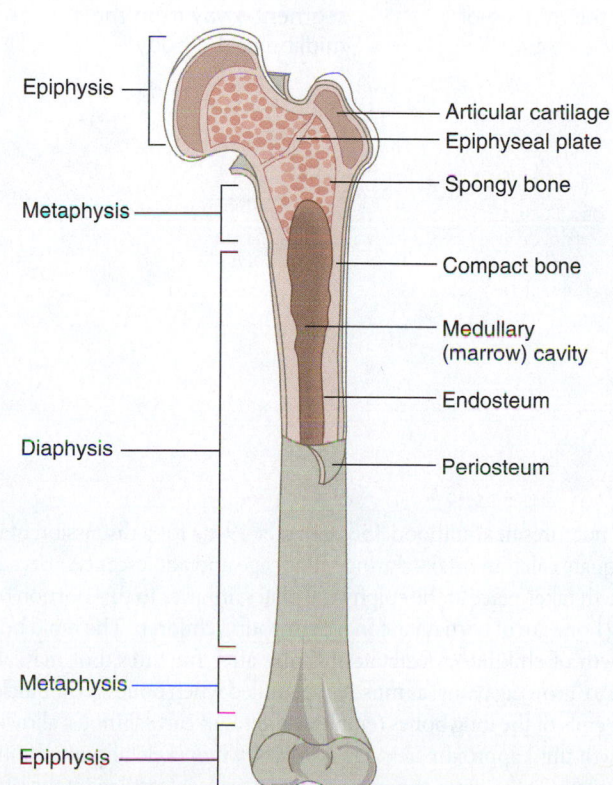

Epiphysis

Metaphysis

Diaphysis

Metaphysis

Epiphysis

Articular cartilage
Epiphyseal plate
Spongy bone
Compact bone
Medullary (marrow) cavity
Endosteum
Periosteum

FIGURE 35–1 ■ The parts of long bones.

Varus
An abnormal position of limb that involves bending inward toward the midline of the body

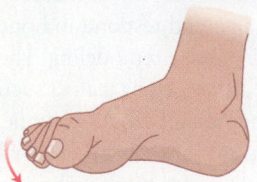

Valgus
An abnormal position of a limb that involves bending outward away from the midline of the body

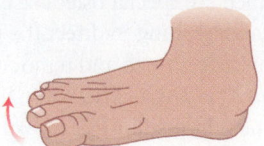

Supination
Lying on the back or placing the hand so that palm faces upward

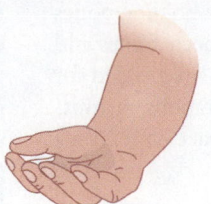

Pronation
Lying on the stomach or placing the hand so the palm faces downward

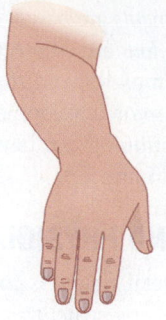

Adduction
Lateral movement of limbs toward the midline of the body

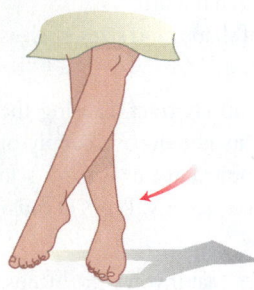

Abduction
Lateral movement of limbs away from the midline of the body

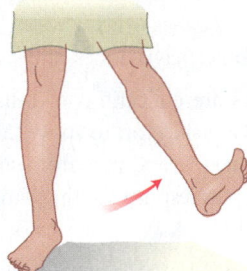

Flexion
A decrease in angle between bones forming a joint

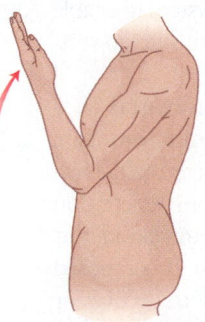

Extension
A movement that brings a limb into a straight position

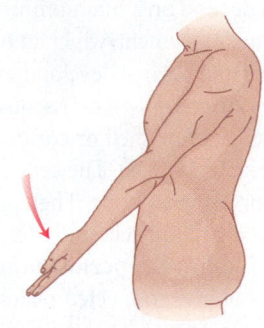

Inversion
Turning inward, usually more than normal

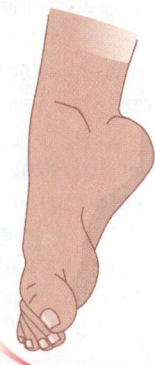

Eversion
Turning outward

Internal rotation
Rotation of a body part towards the midline of the body

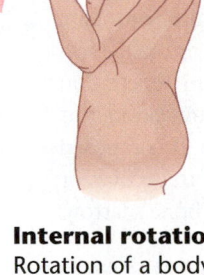

External rotation
Rotation of a body segment away from the midline of the body

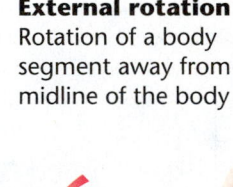

FIGURE 35–2 ■ Musculoskeletal positions and joint motions.

2 and 3 months of age. The anterior fontanel does not close until approximately 7-19 months of age, allowing for growth of the brain and skull. Most growth of the skull occurs by 2 years of age, with the skull reaching full size by 16 years (National Institutes of Health, 2012).

Secondary ossification occurs as the long bones grow. Cartilage cells at the epiphyses (an area enriched with blood cells) are replaced by osteoblasts (immature bone cells), which push the end of the bone away from the shaft and engineer the deposition of calcium within the newly formed bone. Calcium intake during childhood and adolescence is essential to provide adequate bone density that will prevent osteoporosis

and fractures in adulthood. (See Chapter 19 🖉 for a discussion of inadequate calcium intake during school age and adolescence.) Because growth takes place at the epiphyseal plates, injuries to this portion of a long bone are of particular concern in young children. The rapid bone growth of childhood facilitates healing after fractures, but may also lead to "growing pains" as muscles are pulled when bones grow quickly. The ends of the long bones (epiphyses) remain cartilaginous, allowing growth until approximately age 20 years, when skeletal maturation is complete. At this time, the epiphyseal plate closes, cartilage at the site is replaced by bone, and only an epiphyseal line remains (Figure 35–3 ■).

Children and adolescents may suffer injury to the musculoskeletal system from falls, car crashes, and sports. Fractures are one type of common injury. The long bones of children are porous and less dense than those of adults. For this reason, children's bones can bend, buckle, or break as a result of a simple fall. In addition to the structural differences between the bones of children and adults, there are functional differences in the skeletal system of children. Before birth, the thoracic and sacral regions of the spine are convex curves. As the infant learns to hold up the head, the cervical region becomes concave. When the child learns to stand, the lumbar region also becomes concave. Failure of the spine to assume these final curves results in an abnormal curvature of the spine (kyphosis or lordosis).

Muscles, Tendons, and Ligaments

The muscular system, unlike the skeletal system, is almost completely formed at birth, with any remaining increase achieved in the first year of life. As a child grows, muscles do not increase in number, but rather in length and circumference. Muscle fibers reach maximum diameter in girls at about 10 years of age, and in boys at 14 years. Muscle strength continues to increase until about 25 to 30 years of age (Chamley et al., 2005).

Until puberty, both ligaments and tendons are stronger than bone. When these structural differences are not recognized, a childhood fracture is sometimes mistaken for a sprain. A **sprain** is a tearing of ligaments, the structural support connecting bones, usually caused when a joint is twisted or otherwise traumatized. Tendons, which connect bones to muscles, grow in length and fibrous tissue as mechanical pressure is placed on them. Fractures are breakages in bones and are common injuries during the childhood years.

Use the guidelines in Table 35–1 to perform a nursing assessment of the musculoskeletal system. Examples of diagnostic and laboratory tests used for the musculoskeletal system are provided in Table 35–2.

Musculoskeletal disorders may be congenital, such as clubfoot, or acquired, such as osteomyelitis. They may require short- or long-term management, and may be treated on an outpatient basis or require hospitalization. Many musculoskeletal disorders require surgical correction, casting, or braces.

DISORDERS OF THE FEET AND LEGS
Metatarsus Adductus

Metatarsus adductus, the most common congenital foot deformity, is characterized by an inward turning of the forefoot at the tarsometatarsal joints (Figure 35–4 ■). The forefoot is adducted, leading to a convex or curved lateral border and concave medial border. Often referred to as "intoeing," metatarsus adductus affects male and female infants equally and occurs in approximately 1 in 1,000 births, with more common incidence among siblings, twins, and multiple births. This condition is most likely caused by both intrauterine positioning and genetic factors. It occurs more often in certain neurologic conditions such as cerebral palsy (see Chapter 33) (Hagmann, Dreher, & Wenz, 2009; Hutchinson, 2010; Sankar, Weiss, & Skaggs, 2009).

Practice Alert
Metatarsus adductus is one cause of intoeing. There are other potential causes that should be considered; some are more likely at certain ages in development. If intoeing is first observed when the child walks (12 to 18 months), internal tibial torsion may be the cause. This generally improves with walking. Intoeing that persists until 2 to 4 years may be related to femoral anteversion. Stretching exercises, ballet, and ice skating may help to decrease intoeing.

TABLE 35–1	Assessment Guidelines for the Child with a Musculoskeletal System Alteration*
ASSESSMENT FOCUS	**ASSESSMENT GUIDELINES**
Muscles	▪ Is muscle mass symmetric? ▪ Do fine and gross motor movements correspond to developmental expectations? ▪ Can you identify any abnormal signs such as asymmetry of movement, tenderness, masses, weakness, hypotonia, or hypertonia? ▪ Can the school-age child get up from a lying or sitting position in the usual manner? ▪ Can you describe the child's usual daily physical activity? ▪ Has there been a loss of ability to perform developmental milestones?
Joints	▪ Are movements smooth and symmetric? ▪ Are there any signs of tenderness, decreased range of motion, inflammation, crepitus/grinding, or masses? ▪ Do the hips of newborns and infants manifest symmetric full range of motion? ▪ Were there recent events of trauma such as in sports or a fall?
Bones	▪ Are any masses noted? ▪ Are arms and legs the same length? ▪ Is there a recent decrease or change in mobility, such as limping? ▪ Are bones in alignment, or are abnormalities noted such as bowlegs or knock-knees? ▪ Upon spinal screening, is the spine properly aligned? (See screening procedure within this chapter.) ▪ In what sports does the child participate? Is recommended protective gear worn?
Tendons and ligaments	▪ Do all joints move through full range of motion? ▪ Is there any pain upon joint motion or palpation? ▪ Are there feelings of grinding or crepitus as the joint moves? ▪ Has there been a recent sports or other injury? ▪ In what sports does the child participate?
Family history	▪ Is there a family history of disorders of the muscular or skeletal systems?

*Refer to Chapter 7 for the actual techniques of assessment mentioned in this table.

TABLE 35–2	Diagnostic Procedures and Laboratory Tests for the Musculoskeletal System*	
DIAGNOSTIC PROCEDURES		**LABORATORY TESTS**
Arthrogram		Alkaline phosphatase (ALP)
Bone scan		C-reactive protein (CRP)
Computed tomography (CT)		Erythrocyte sedimentation rate (ESR or sed rate)
Dual energy x-ray absorptiometry (DEXA)		Rheumatoid factor (RF)
Electromyelogram		
Evoked potential		
Magnetic resonance imaging (MRI)		
Radiograph (x-ray)		
Ultrasound		

*See Appendixes D and E for information about these diagnostic procedures and for expected laboratory tests values.

As They Grow Musculoskeletal System

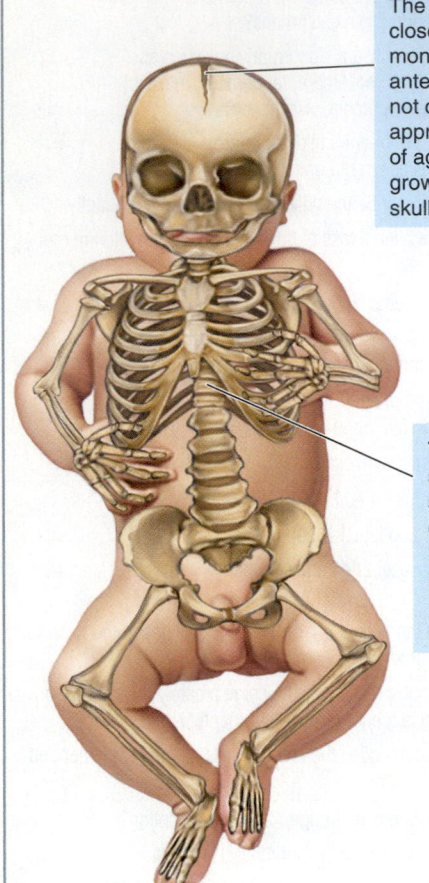

A fibrous membrane still exists between the cranial bones (fontanels). The posterior fontanel closes between 2 and 3 months of age. The anterior fontanel does not close until approximately 18 months of age, allowing for growth of the brain and skull.

The thoracic and sacral regions of the spine are convex curves. As the infant learns to hold up the head, the cervical region becomes concave.

Most growth of the skull occurs by 2 years of age, with the skull reaching full size by 16 years.

The long bones of children are porous and less dense than those of adults, leading to higher rates of fracture.

When the child learns to stand, the lumbar region becomes concave in shape.

As a child grows, muscles do not increase in number, but rather in length and circumference. Muscle fibers reach maximum diameter in girls at about 10 years of age, and in boys at 14 years.

During childhood, cartilage cells at the epiphyses (an area enriched with blood cells) are replaced by osteoblasts (immature bone cells), which push the end of the bone away from the shaft and engineer the deposition of calcium within the newly formed bone.

The rapid bone growth of childhood facilitates healing after fractures, but may also lead to "growing pains" as muscles are pulled when bones grow quickly.

FIGURE 35–3 ■ Skeletal and muscle development throughout childhood.

Foot radiographs may be taken and physical assessment of the foot is performed. Treatment depends on the degree of foot flexibility and age of the child. If the foot can be readily maneuvered past the neutral position, simple exercises may correct the problem. (See Partnering with Families: Stretching Exercises for Metatarsus Adductus.) The exercise protocol of several weeks may be followed by use of a Denis Browne splint to maintain the adducted position. Although most cases will resolve spontaneously by the time the infant is about 3 months of age, therapy is recommended since the condition is most treatable during early infancy when the bones and cartilage are soft.

Passive stretching with serial casting to follow is the treatment of choice for curvature angles greater than 15 degrees, or in cases that

are rigid. The infant's feet are placed in a position as close to neutral as possible and are held secure with casts. Casts are changed weekly until the desired correction is achieved. Braces and orthopedic shoes may also be used to maintain correction after casting. Rarely, surgery is required to correct the condition.

Nursing Management

Reassure parents that the child's condition can be corrected. If the deformity is mild, teach parents simple stretching exercises that can be performed at each diaper change. Emphasize that performing the stretching as instructed is important to ensure treatment success for metatarsus adductus. Have the parent demonstrate techniques used

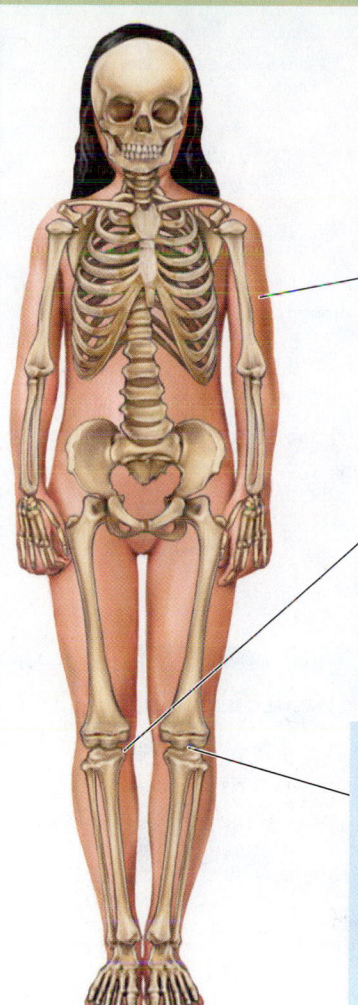

Muscle strength continues to increase until about 25–30 years of age.

The ends of long bones (epiphyses) remain cartilaginous, allowing growth, until approximately age 20 years, when skeletal maturation is complete. At this time the epiphyseal plate closes, cartilage at the site is replaced by bone, and only an epiphyseal line remains.

Until puberty, both ligaments and tendons are stronger than bone. As the child ages and cartilage is replaced by bone, the resulting bone is stronger than ligaments or tendons. Rates of fractures decrease while injuries to ligaments and tendons increase.

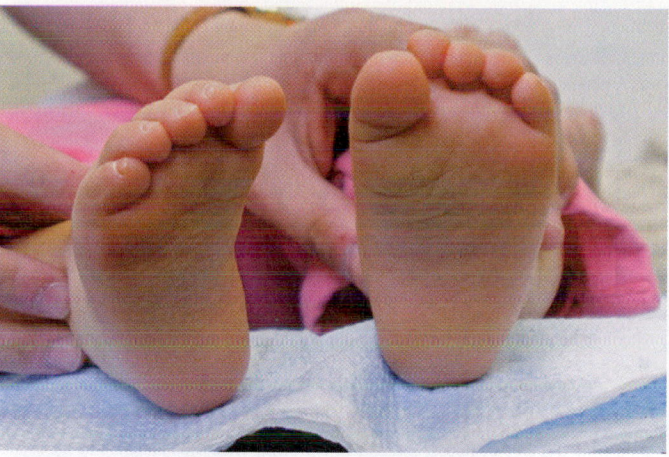

FIGURE 35–4 ■ Metatarsus adductus is characterized by convexity (curvature) of the lateral border of the foot. The child's right foot demonstrates the disorder. Note that the forefoot turns inward and appears out of alignment with the remainder of the foot.

at each healthcare visit so corrections can be made if needed. If casting is necessary, provide cast care and teach parents how to care for the child in a cast at home (Box 35–1). See Partnering with Families: Care of the Child with a Cast on page 1259. If metatarsus adductus persists into childhood without correction, skewfoot (forefoot adduction, plantar flexion, and hindfoot valgus) can result, providing a challenge to find shoes that accommodate the unusual shape of the foot. Surgery may be needed in these cases.

Clubfoot

Clubfoot is a congenital abnormality in which the foot is twisted out of its normal position. It occurs in approximately 1 to 2 in 1,000 births, affects boys nearly twice as often as girls, and is bilateral in about half of affected infants (Gurnett, Boehm, Connolly, et al., 2008). It is more common in families with a history of the condition, and occurs in conjunction with several syndromes and in conditions such as myelomeningocele (see Chapter 33 🔗).

Etiology and Pathophysiology

The exact cause of clubfoot is unknown; however, several possible etiologies have been proposed. Neuromuscular or vascular problems are suspected as causes by some experts. Yet other experts believe there is a genetic component, either at the chromosomal level or by the arrest of normal fetal development. Uterine positioning and biochemical causes are also cited as possibilities. A positive family history is present in 15% of cases (Paton, Fox, Foster, et al., 2010).

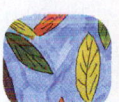

Partnering with Families

Stretching Exercises for Metatarsus Adductus

- Hold the infant's foot securely with the heel in your palm and your index finger on the Achilles tendon. Maintain the back of the foot in this position.
- Move the forefoot outward away from the body with the other hand.

- Hold the foot in this position for the time recommended by your health professional. Time varies based on the treatment method and the infant's foot.
- Treatment will usually continue for 3 to 4 weeks.

BOX 35–1	Nursing Care of the Child in a Cast

- A plaster cast takes anywhere from 24 to 48 hours to dry. When handling the cast, be gentle and use the palms of your hands, as fingertips can indent plaster and create pressure areas.
- After the cast is applied, elevate the extremity on a pillow above the level of the heart. Elevation helps to reduce swelling and increases venous return.
- If the cast is applied after surgery, there may be drainage or bleeding through the cast material. Circle the stain and note the date and time on the cast to provide a means of assessing the amount of fluid lost. Once a cast is dry a "window" or opening is sometimes cut so that a wound can be viewed or to allow the stomach to expand more comfortably.
- Assess the distal pulses, and check the fingers and toes for color, warmth, capillary refill, and edema. Assess sensation as well as movement. Any deviation from normal may indicate nerve damage or decreased blood supply.
- During the first 24 hours, the casted extremity should be checked every 15 to 30 minutes for 2 hours, then every 1 to 2 hours thereafter. The skin should be warm. It should blanch when slight pressure is applied and then return to its normal color within 3 seconds (**A**). For the next 2 days, the casted extremity should be assessed at least every 4 hours.

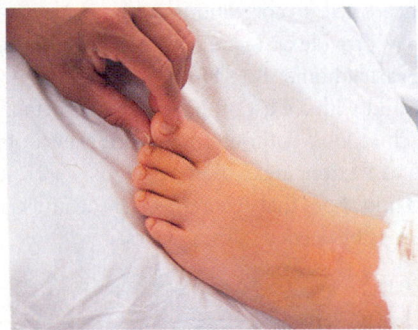

A

- Check the edges of the cast for roughness or crumbling. If necessary, pull the inner stockinette over the edge of the cast and tape.
- The rough edges of the cast may also be alleviated by "petaling." This is done by securing tape or padding to the inside of the cast and pulling it over the edge, covering the jagged or broken pieces of plaster, and securing it to the outer surface of the cast (**B, C, D**). Moleskin may be used on the cast as well. Petal the opening around a window in the cast if one is present.
- Keep the cast as clean and dry as possible. Cover the cast with a plastic bag or plastic wrap when the child bathes or showers.

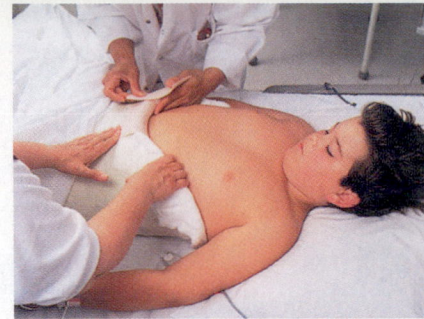

B

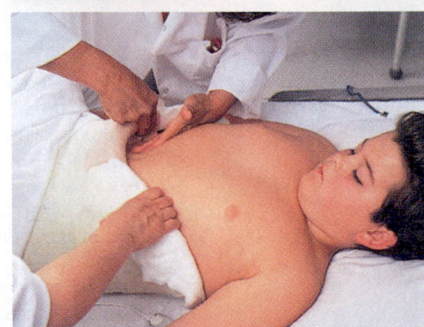

C

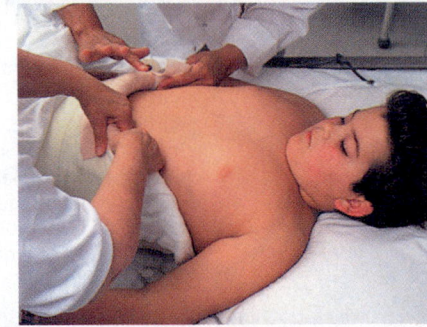

D

- The skin under the cast may itch; however, do not use powders or lotions near the edges or under the cast as they can cause skin irritation.
- Be sure that children do not put small objects between the casts and their extremities; these actions can cause skin irritation as well as neurovascular compromise.

Clinical Manifestations

A clubfoot (talipes equinovarus) involves three areas of deformity: the midfoot is directed downward (**equinus**), the hindfoot turns inward (**varus**), and the forefoot curls toward the heel (adduction) and turns upward in partial supination. (*Talipes* refers to foot and ankle.) Most children with clubfoot have this combination of findings, with muscles, tendons, and bones involved. The condition may range from mild to severe involvement, with the latter often associated with additional malformations in the newborn such as meningomyelocele. The foot is small with a shortened Achilles tendon. Muscles in the lower leg are atrophied, but leg lengths are generally normal (Figure 35–5 ■).

Collaborative Care

The goal of collaborative care for the child with clubfoot is successful treatment to facilitate normal ambulation.

Diagnostic Tests

Diagnosis is made at birth on the basis of visual inspection. Radiographs after birth are used to confirm the severity of the condition.

Clinical Therapy

Early treatment is essential to achieve successful correction and reduce the chance of complications. Serial casting is the treatment of choice. Casting should begin as soon as possible after birth. Timing is critical, because the short bones of the foot, which are primarily cartilaginous at birth, begin to ossify shortly thereafter. The foot is manipulated to achieve maximum correction first of the varus deformity and then of the equinus deformity. A long leg cast is applied to hold the foot in the desired position. The cast is changed every 1 to 2 weeks. This regimen of manipulation and casting continues for approximately 8 to 12 weeks until maximum correction is achieved. If the deformity has been corrected, the child may begin wearing a splint with a crossbar between shoes (most commonly called a Denis Browne splint) or reverse last corrective shoes (shoes with the toes pointing outward rather than inward) to maintain the correction (Gurnett et al., 2008). If the deformity has not been corrected, surgical intervention is required. Casting is maintained to hold the foot in position until surgery is performed (Figure 35–6 ■).

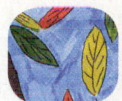

Partnering with Families

Care of the Child with a Cast

SKIN CARE
- Check the skin around the cast edges for irritation, rubbing, or blistering. The skin should be clean and dry.
- Cleanse the skin just under the cast edges and between the toes or fingers with a cotton-tipped applicator and rubbing alcohol. Avoid using lotions, oils, and powders near the cast as they may collect on and irritate the skin.
- Avoid poking sharp objects down inside the cast as this may result in sores.

CAST CARE
- Keep the cast dry. Protect plaster with a cast shoe, thick sock, or sling.
- Raise the casted arm or leg above heart level and rest it on pillows to prevent or reduce any swelling.
- Allow a new, wet cast to air-dry for 24 hours.
- Begin walking on a leg cast only when the physician gives permission.

BE ALERT FOR POSSIBLE COMPLICATIONS
- Toes or fingers should be pink, not blue or white.
- Skin should be warm and the tips of the toes should blanch when pinched.

NOTIFY THE HEALTHCARE PROVIDER IF ANY OF THE FOLLOWING OCCUR
- Unusual odor beneath the cast
- Burning, tingling, or numbness in the casted arm or leg
- Drainage through the cast
- Swelling or inability to move the fingers or toes
- Slippage of the cast
- Cast cracked, soft, or loose
- Sudden, unexplained fever
- Unusual fussiness or irritability in an infant or child
- Fingers or toes that are blue or white
- Pain that is not relieved by any comfort measures (e.g., repositioning or pain medication)

Source: *Courtesy of Shriners Hospital for Children, Spokane, WA.*

The age at which a child undergoes clubfoot surgery varies among surgeons. However, most children have surgery between 3 and 12 months of age. The one-stage posteromedial release procedure, which involves realignment of the bones of the foot and release of the constricting soft tissue, is most commonly performed. The foot is held in the proper position by one or more stainless steel pins. A cast is then applied with the knee flexed to prevent damage to the pin and to discourage weight bearing. Casting continues for 6 to 12 weeks. The child may then need to wear a brace or corrective shoes, depending on the severity of the deformity and the surgeon's preference. Alternatively, the Ponseti technique uses a simple Achilles tenotomy (incision of the Achilles tendon) after serial manipulation

Pathophysiology Illustrated
Bilateral Clubfoot Deformity

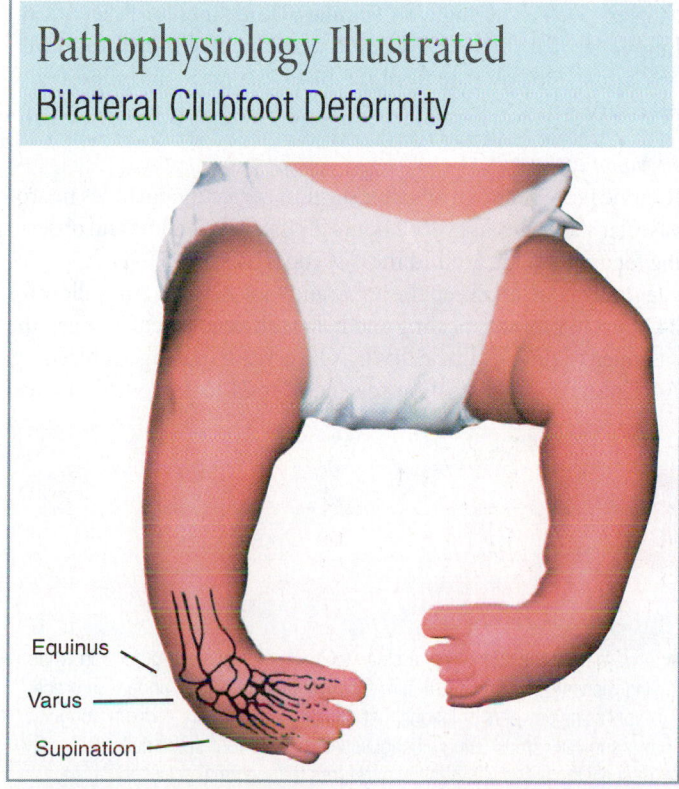

Equinus
Varus
Supination

FIGURE 35–5 ■ Parents of a child with clubfoot will have many questions. Can the condition be treated? Will the child be able to walk normally after surgery? Will they need help caring for the infant? How much will surgery and other care cost? Will any subsequent children have a clubfoot?

Source: *Modified from Staheli, L. T. (1992). Fundamentals of pediatric orthopedics (p. 5.10). New York, NY: Raven Press.*

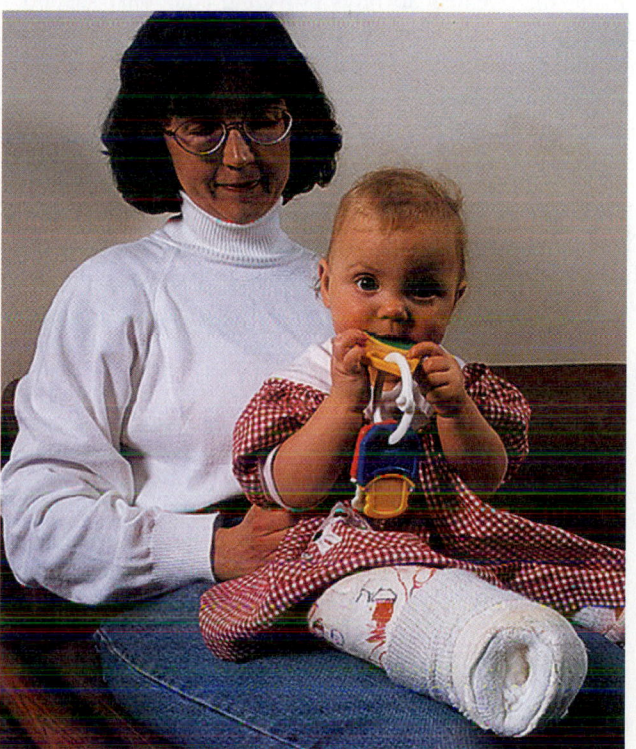

FIGURE 35–6 ■ This girl has a long leg cast, which was applied after surgery to correct her clubfoot.

and casting, and is followed by use of a foot-abduction brace (Gott-schalk, Karol, & Jeans, 2010). This technique is less invasive, does not cause scar tissue that can impair later mobility, and shows success in treatment. More severe cases or those not corrected in infancy may require more than one surgery to correct the foot.

Nursing Management

The goals of nursing care for the child with a clubfoot are to provide necessary information to parents and ensure adequate healing during the treatment process.

Nursing Assessment and Diagnosis

Nursing assessment, which begins at birth and continues throughout the child's subsequent outpatient casting visits and hospitalization for surgery, includes taking a genetic and birth history, performing a physical examination (including position and appearance of the foot), and assessing the child's motor development and family's coping mechanisms. Because parents will need to bring the child for frequent cast changes, assess the family's access to transportation and other arrangements that are necessary to facilitate these visits.

Nursing diagnoses that may apply to the child with a clubfoot deformity are as follows:

- Mobility: Physical, Impaired related to restricted movement due to cast
- Skin Integrity, Risk for Impaired related to pressure from cast
- Parenting, Risk for Impaired related to birth of a child with a physical defect
- Knowledge, Deficient related to lack of information about deformity, treatment, and home care

NANDA-I © 2012

Planning and Implementation

Nursing management involves providing emotional support and educating the family about the treatment plan as well as home care of the child in a cast or brace. The importance of keeping appointments at the outpatient facility for cast changes is emphasized. The family is prepared for the child's hospitalization if surgery is to occur, and for providing postsurgical care.

Provide Emotional Support

Clubfoot is a condition that affects both the child and the family. The child's foot deformity may be upsetting to parents, and they need emotional support to allay their fears. Helping parents understand the condition and its treatment is essential.

Encourage parents to hold and cuddle the child and to take an active role in the child's care to help promote bonding. Explain that, with treatment, the child will grow and develop normally.

Provide Cast and Brace Care

Routine cast care is important to ensure skin and neurovascular integrity (see Box 35–1). Teach parents how to safely bathe, carry, and care for the child in a cast. Discomfort after application of a new cast or after tenotomy may require analgesics; be sure parents know the recommended dosage and administration techniques.

Clinical Tip

When an infant is receiving serial casting for clubfoot, the physician often recommends that the parent soak the cast off the night before a scheduled cast change. Teach the parents how to remove the plaster cast. The infant can be placed in a warm bath, and the cast will start to disintegrate and can be unrolled. This avoids exposure of the infant to the loud sound of the cast cutter and allows for the infant's leg to be washed and out of the cast overnight. Parents can also be encouraged to bring a bottle to the clinic. If the infant is hungry and feeding, the foot is more easily kept still for the cast application.

Provide information about the treatment to parents during the casting process. After serial casting is complete, or following surgery, the child may progress to wearing a brace or special shoe for 6 to 12 months. Braces should fit snugly but should not interfere with neurovascular function. Before the child begins to wear a brace, check the skin for any areas of redness or breakdown. Provide parents with guidelines for brace wear as outlined later in the chapter. (See Partnering with Families: Guidelines for Brace Wear.) Emphasize that proper skin care is essential. If skin redness develops, arrange to have the fit of the brace evaluated and modified if necessary.

Provide Postsurgical Care

Routine postoperative care after surgical correction includes neurovascular status checks every 2 hours for the first 24 hours and observing for any swelling around the cast edges (see Box 35–1). Apply ice bags to the foot, and keep the ankle and foot elevated on a pillow for 24 hours to promote healing and help with venous return. Keep the cast open to air to facilitate drying. Observe for drainage or bleeding. Administer pain medication routinely for 24 to 48 hours. Popliteal

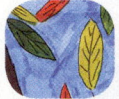

Partnering with Families

Guidelines for Brace Wear

- Braces should be as comfortable as possible, and the child should have adequate mobility while wearing the brace.
- Begin wearing the brace for periods of 1 to 2 hours and then progress to 2 to 4 hours.
- Check the skin every 1 to 2 hours initially, then lengthening to every 4 hours once the skin has been clear for several days. If redness is apparent, leave the brace off and allow the skin to clear. If breakdown has occurred, the brace cannot be replaced until healing is complete. (See Chapter 36 🔗 for a discussion of pressure ulcers.)

- Always have the child wear a clean white sock, T-shirt, or other thin white liner beneath the brace. Be sure the liner is wrinkle-free under the brace. Avoid using powders or lotions that can cause skin to break down. Toughen any sensitive areas using alcohol wipes three to four times daily.
- Reapply the brace when the skin returns to its normal color.
- Return to the physician or orthotic specialist if discomfort or red areas persist or if the brace needs adjustment or repair or is outgrown.
- Check the brace daily for rough edges.

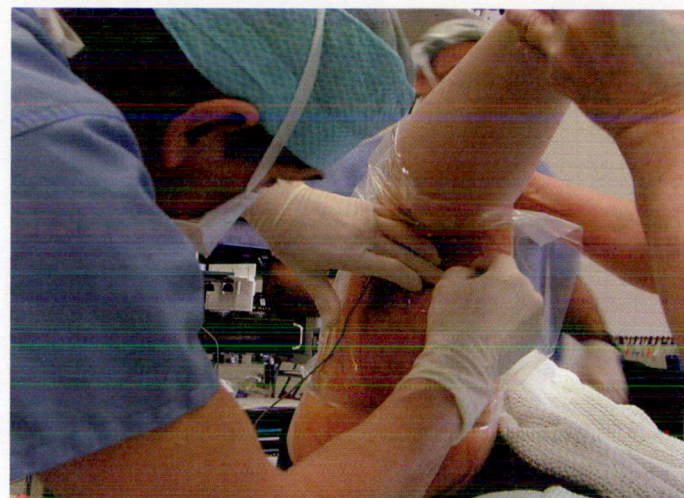

FIGURE 35–7 ■ The insertion of a popliteal block during surgery. The site will be wrapped and the tubing connected to an infusion pump. The nurse will monitor the infusion and pain control after surgery.

Source: *Courtesy of Shriners Hospital for Children, Spokane, WA.*

or epidural blocks may be placed during surgery and used in the immediate postsurgical period for pain control (Figure 35–7 ■). The nurse monitors these blocks for effectiveness and any undesired effects (see Chapter 21 🔗 for detailed instructions on pain management). See the Skills Manual 🔗 for detail on monitoring nerve blocks.

Discharge Planning and Home Care Teaching

Parents should be given written instructions for care of the child with a cast (see page 1259). In addition, assist them in the following ways:

- Demonstrate the use of a sponge bath to protect the cast from water breakdown. Have parents contact the healthcare provider if the cast gets wet with water or urine.
- Discuss several options for clothing that accommodate a cast, for example, one-piece snap suits or sweatpants.
- Discuss potential safety hazards that may result from awkward positioning. Be sure the child is properly situated in a car safety seat for the trip home.
- Suggest that parents make an effort to place toys within the child's reach, because movements of a child in a cast may be slowed.
- Provide safety teaching to avoid slippage of the cast. Have parents report slippage immediately.

Practice Alert

Advise parents that "umbrella" strollers are not sturdy enough to support an infant's casted leg. Some infant swings do not provide a foot rest; its absence can contribute to cast slippage or breakdown. Observe the child in the family's car seat to be sure the casted leg is adequately supported. A pillow may be needed under the leg to provide adequate support for the casted leg.

Evaluation

Expected outcomes of nursing care include maintenance of skin integrity, recovery without complications after surgery, normal developmental progression of the child, and demonstrated knowledge by parents for care of braces or casts, as needed.

Genu Varum and Genu Valgum

Genu varum (bowlegs) is a deformity in which the knees are widely separated while the ankles are close together and the lower legs are turned inward (varus). In genu valgum (knock-knees), the knees are close together while the ankles are widely spaced so that the lower legs are directed outward (**valgus**) (Figure 35–8 ■). Chapter 7 🔗 discusses the assessment for genu varum and genu valgum in children.

At certain stages of a child's development, the appearance of bowlegs or knock-knees is normal. Until 2 to 3 years, the knees are normally bowed, showing varus alignment, and by 4 to 5 years, some knock-knee or valgus alignment commonly emerges (see Figure 7–53 🔗). Persistent genu varum or genu valgum should be evaluated by an orthopedist. Two pathologic causes of genu varum are Blount disease and rickets. **Blount disease** is characterized by abnormal growth on the medial side of the proximal tibia which causes an increasing varus deformity. It is believed to be due to increasing compression forces across the medial knee. It is more common in overweight, Black, and female children, and has been associated with low serum vitamin D levels (Montgomery, Young, Austen, et al., 2010; Sabharwal, 2009). **Rickets** is a result of inadequate bone mineralization, usually caused by a deficiency of calcium and/or vitamin D. (See Chapter 19 🔗 for a description of the association between rickets and diet.) Since the bones are decalcified or softened, long bones such as those in the legs may bend into a bowed position. Occasionally rickets is congenital and is caused by an X-linked autosomal dominant or recessive gene with the chromosomal location Xp22.31-p21.3. It results in an enzyme deficiency of alkaline phosphatase which in turn leads to excessive inhibitors of bone mineralization. This type of rickets is rare and is called familial hypophosphatemic rickets (FHR).

Excessive or continued genu valgum should also be evaluated by an orthopedist although, unlike genu varum, the condition has no pathologic causes.

Measurements, radiographic studies, arthrography (joint radiographs), MRI, and CT imaging are used for accurate diagnosis of varus and valgus conditions.

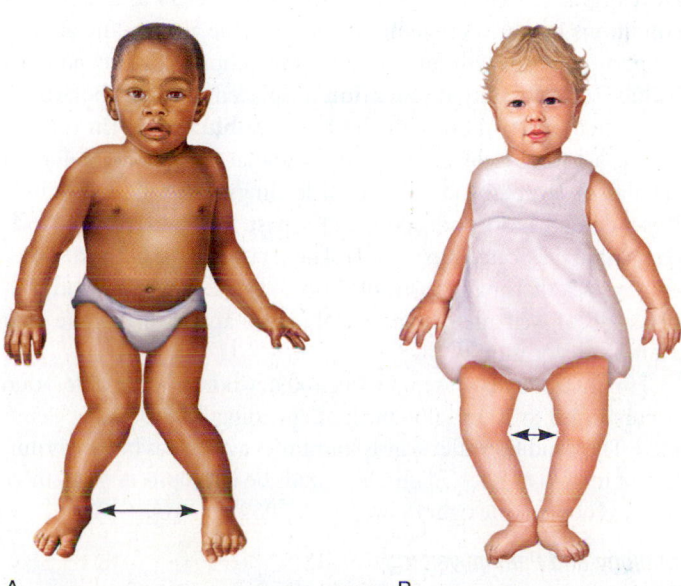

A   B

FIGURE 35–8 ■ *A,* Genu valgum, or knock-knees. Note that the ankles are far apart when the knees are together. *B,* Genu varum, or bowlegs. The legs are bowed so that the knees are far apart as the child stands.

Braces are often used to correct mild varus and valgus deformities that could worsen as the child grows. Braces for varus deformities (bowlegs) are worn at night; those for valgus deformities (knock-knees) are worn both day and night. Duration of brace wear is determined by the severity of the deformity. If the deformity continues to worsen, surgical intervention is necessary. Surgery may be needed, particularly in treatment of Blount disease. An **osteotomy** (cutting of the bone) is performed and the tibiofemoral angle surgically corrected. The child is then placed in a cast for approximately 6 to 10 weeks, or until full healing has occurred.

When dietary rickets is the cause of varus deformity, supplementation with calcium and vitamin D is needed. FHR is treated with calcium and phosphorus in five to six daily doses.

Nursing Management

Reassure parents that bowlegs and knock-knees are usually a normal part of a child's growth and development. These conditions often resolve spontaneously and require no treatment other than monitoring. Encourage them to ask for evaluation at each health promotion visit to be sure the condition is not worsening. Ask about familial bone diseases.

Nursing care focuses on educating the parents and child about the conditions and their treatment. Provide the child and family with guidelines for brace wear and maintenance if this therapy is used (see page 1260). Instruct about intake of calcium and vitamin D when there is a deficiency, and partner with parents to plan for dietary supplements in children with dietary rickets or FHR. Provide postoperative care and cast care as needed for the child who undergoes surgery.

Desired outcomes for nursing care include establishment of normal gait patterns and activities for the child, maintenance of intact skin and neurovascular status during treatment, and understanding by the parent of assessment and intervention when needed.

DISORDERS OF THE HIP
Developmental Dysplasia of the Hip

Developmental dysplasia of the hip (DDH) refers to a variety of conditions in which the femoral head and the acetabulum are improperly aligned with an unstable connection. These conditions include hip instability, **dislocation** (displacement of the bone from its normal articulation with the joint), **subluxation** (in this instance, a partial dislocation), and acetabular **dysplasia** (abnormal cellular or structural development leading to instability) (Sewell, Rosendahl, & Eastwood, 2009). In the past, DDH was referred to as congenital dislocated hip (CDH). The revised name of the disorder emphasizes that many cases of dislocation, subluxation, and dysplasia occur well after the neonatal period and involve more than a simple dislocation.

Hip instability is present in 1 in 100 newborns, while dislocation occurs in 1.5 to 20 in 1,000 births, depending on the studies examined. The condition affects girls four times as often as boys. It is unilateral in 80% of affected children, and the left hip is affected three times as often as the right (Sewell et al., 2009).

Etiology and Pathophysiology

Although the exact cause of DDH is unknown, genetic factors appear to play a role. DDH is 20 to 50 times more common in first-degree relatives of an infant with the condition than in the general population. If one child of a set of identical twins has DDH, the other twin is affected 30% to 40% of the time. Some types of DDH are linked to early gestational events at 12 and 18 weeks' gestation, as the lower limbs rotate and surrounding muscles develop. However, milder cases may be influenced by mechanical forces in the last month of pregnancy such as breech position, oligohydramnios, or fetal size, and some cases develop after birth as the hip assumes an extended rather than flexed posture (Kleposki, Abel, & Sehgal, 2010; Sewell et al., 2009).

The left hip is involved more often than the right hip as a result of intrauterine positioning of the left side of the fetus against the mother's sacrum. Maternal estrogen may cause laxity of the hip joint and capsule, leading to joint instability, especially in females who respond more than males to these estrogen levels. Cultural factors may also be associated with DDH with the condition occurring less commonly in infants carried on the mothers' hips since the infants' legs are maintained in the abducted position.

Clinical Manifestations

Common signs and symptoms of DDH include limited abduction of the affected hip, asymmetry of the gluteal and thigh fat folds, and telescoping or pistoning of the thigh (Figure 35–9 ■). The older child with untreated DDH walks with a significant limp, which results from telescoping of the femoral head into the pelvis. The longer the disorder goes untreated, the more pronounced the clinical manifestations become, and the worse the prognosis.

Collaborative Care

The purpose of care is to identify all children with DDH early in infancy, when treatment is most successful. Partnership between many health professionals is needed to provide care and ensure normal mobility.

Diagnostic Tests

From 60% to 80% of hip abnormalities noted in infants resolve by 2 months of age, so practitioners use care and caution in diagnosing DDH. However, only 15% to 25% of infants have known risk factors for the disorder. Therefore, the American Academy of Pediatrics and the Pediatric Orthopaedic Society of North America recommend that all infants and young children should be screened for DDH until

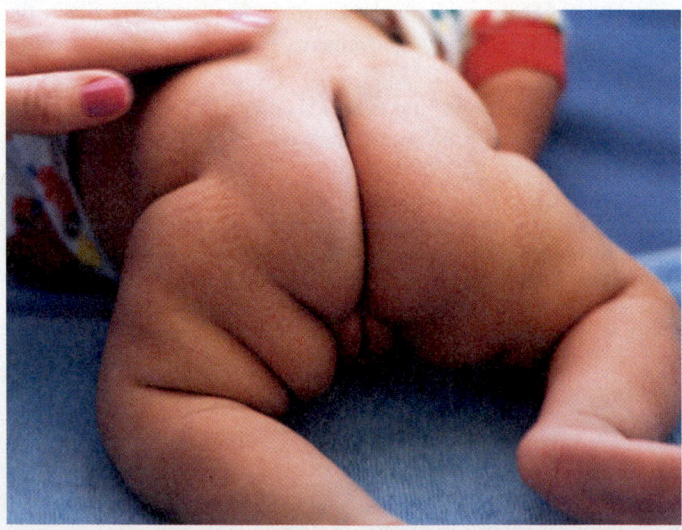

FIGURE 35–9 ■ The asymmetry of the gluteal and thigh fat folds is easy to see in this child with developmental dysplasia of the hip.

walking is well established at about 1 year of age (American Academy of Orthopaedic Surgeons, 2009). Physical examination reveals Allis sign (one knee lower than the other when the knees are flexed) and positive Ortolani-Barlow maneuver. Refer to Chapter 7 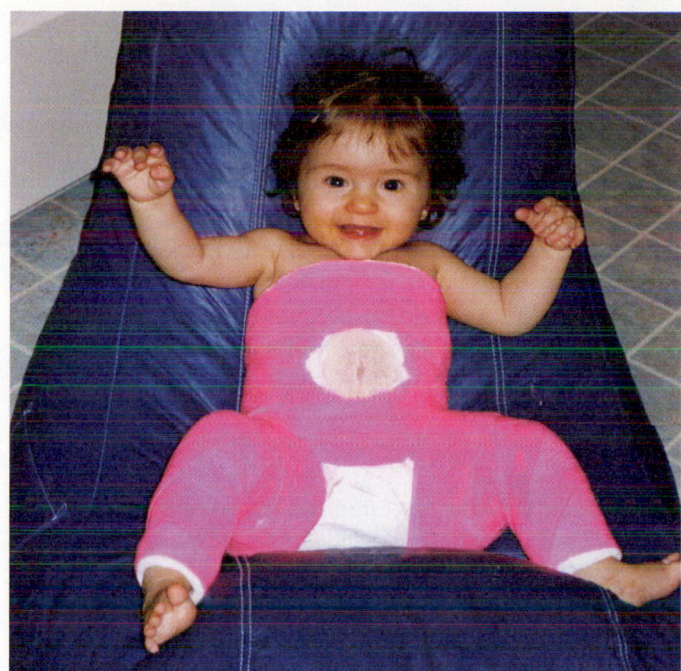 for a discussion of the assessment of hip dysplasia in newborns and infants. Radiographs are generally not reliable until approximately 4 months of age, because the pelvis in a newborn is still primarily cartilaginous. Before 4 months, ultrasonography may be useful for diagnosis. After that age, radiographs are used for diagnosis. Radiographs or ultrasound should be considered for the female infant born in the breech position because of the increased risk of DDH in these infants. A family history may also suggest the need for these studies (Mahan, Katz, & Kim, 2009).

Clinical Therapy

Treatment plans vary according to the child's age. For infants younger than 6 months, the Pavlik harness is the most commonly used method for hip reduction (Figure 35–10 ■). The Pavlik harness is a dynamic splint, that is, a splint that allows movement. It ensures hip flexion and abduction but does not allow hip extension or adduction. For infants older than 6 months, surgery with closed reduction is generally performed (positioning the head of the femur into the acetabulum without an incision of the skin) followed by the application of a spica cast (Figure 35–11 ■). Surgery may be preceded by a course of Bryant traction to facilitate stretching of the tissues that will promote positive surgical outcomes. In children over 18 months of age, open or closed reduction surgery and casting are necessary and bracing may also be required. Outcomes of treatment are monitored by physical examination and ultrasound.

Early screening, detection, and treatment enable the majority of affected children to attain normal hip function.

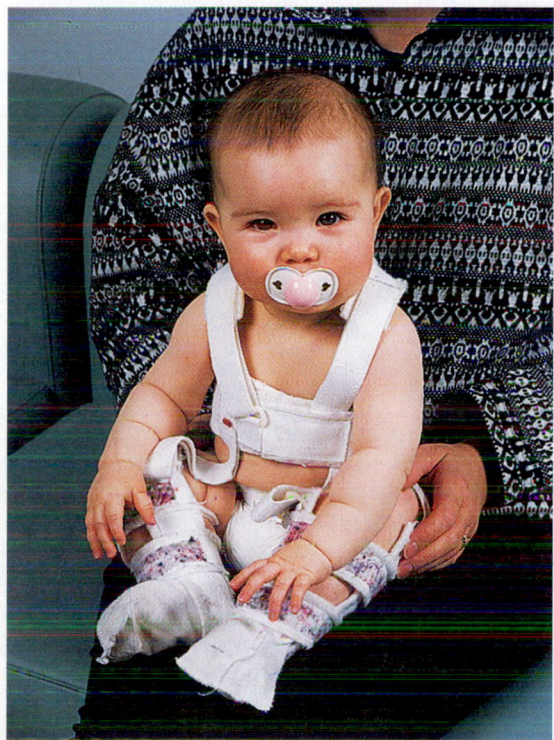

FIGURE 35–10 ■ The most common treatment for DDH in a child under 3 months of age is a Pavlik harness. A shirt should be worn under the harness to prevent skin irritation (it was omitted for clarity in this photograph).

FIGURE 35–11 ■ The infant treated for DDH is often in a hip spica cast after surgery.
Source: *MarylandWebdesigners.com*

Nursing Management

The goal of nursing management is to promote early identification of DDH and to provide safe care for the child using a brace or traction, requiring surgery, or wearing corrective shoes.

Nursing Assessment and Diagnosis

Assessment for DDH begins at delivery and continues through all health promotion visits during the first 2 years of life. The specific family history or birth data may indicate a high-risk infant, as does oligohydramnios, large-for-gestational-age infant, or breech birth. Instructions for performing the physical examination to assess the infant for DDH are given in Chapter 7 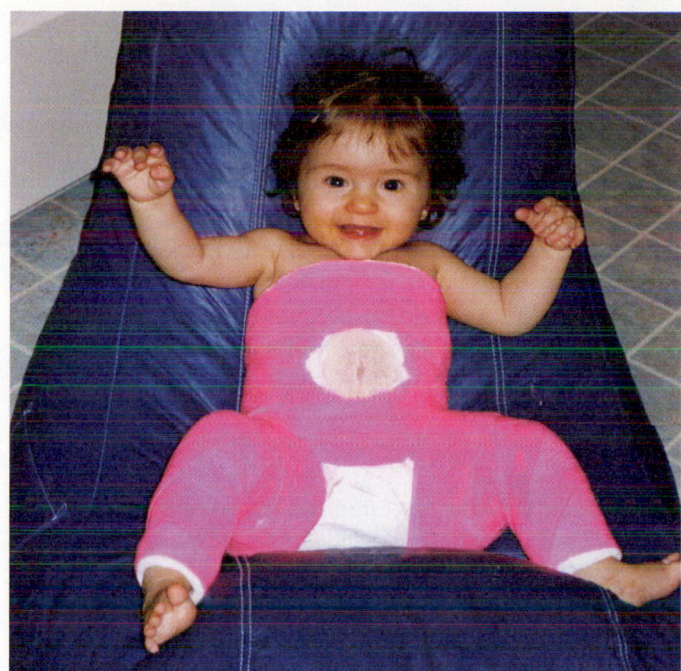. Further assessments are determined by the treatment provided. Skin assessments are performed on the child in a cast, every few minutes in the immediate postoperative period and progressing to once or twice daily at home. Respiratory and circulatory assessments are included when the child is immobilized. Ongoing assessments of the child's growth and development are needed when mobility is impaired. Weigh the casted child once the cast is dry so a baseline casted weight can be used for comparison during the weeks and months while the cast remains in place.

The following nursing diagnoses may apply to the child with DDH:

- Mobility: Physical, Impaired related to prescribed movement restriction (Pavlik harness, traction, spica cast, brace)
- Skin Integrity, Risk for Impaired related to irritation from harness straps
- Urinary Elimination, Impaired or Constipation related to immobility caused by treatment
- Nutrition, Imbalanced: Less than Body Requirements related to decreased appetite
- Growth and Development, Delayed related to limited mobility and potential decreased exposure to stimulation
- Knowledge, Deficient related to lack of information about disease process and treatment

NANDA-I © 2012

Planning and Implementation

The infant with DDH is often cared for at home and in outpatient facilities. If surgery is performed, the child is hospitalized for surgery and the immediate postoperative period. Nursing care varies according to the medical treatment and the child's age. Management includes ensuring follow-up visits are scheduled and kept, providing cast care, preventing complications resulting from immobility, promoting normal growth and development, and counseling parents about the condition and care (e.g., management of a cast or a Pavlik harness) (Causon, 2010). Because treatment may interfere with the child's normal movement, the treatment plan should take into consideration the age and developmental stage of the child.

Provide Cast Care and Correct Harness Alignment

The principles of routine cast care presented in Box 35–1 apply to the care of hip spica casts. Special techniques should be used to help keep the cast clean and dry in children who are not toilet trained. Female and male urinals can be used for older children. Use a plastic lining to protect the cast edges during elimination for older children, and use a small disposable diaper to cover the perineum in babies, tucking edges beneath the cast. Be sure to change the diaper frequently to prevent soiling of the cast.

The child in a Pavlik harness has the harness applied in the healthcare facility. Parents need instructions on maintaining the child in the harness at all times. Return visits are scheduled to ensure proper fit, maintenance of hip position, and skin condition (Box 35–2).

Control Pain

If the child has surgery to correct DDH, pain control in the immediate postoperative period is needed. Assess the child's pain frequently in a method appropriate for age (see Chapter 21 🔗). Administer intravenous and then oral pain medications as ordered. Use methods such as holding, rocking, and gentle music to calm the child. An ice bag placed on top of the cast at the operative site may be helpful. Encourage parents to be present and provide care when possible.

BOX 35–2 **Guidelines for Pavlik Harness Application and Fitting**

1. Position the chest halter at the nipple line and fasten with Velcro.
2. Position the legs and feet in the stirrups, being sure the hips are flexed and abducted. Fasten with Velcro.
3. Connect the chest halter and leg straps in front.
4. Connect the chest halter and leg straps in back.

The harness is usually worn constantly, with removal only for bathing. Clinic visits every 1 to 2 weeks check for proper fit and skin condition.

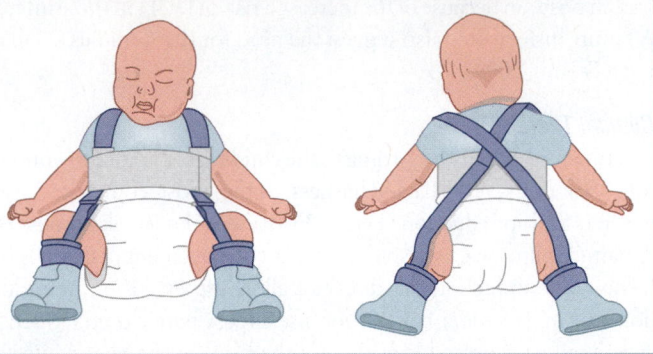

Clinical Tip

If pain is not controlled or if it increases over time, compression at the surgical site may be occurring; promptly report this to the physician. Pain in the infant may be manifested by a combination of physiologic and behavioral changes (see Chapter 21 🔗 for a description of pain in infancy).

Prevent Complications Resulting from Immobility

Immobilization from a cast can cause alterations in physiologic functioning. Take the following actions to prevent complications:

- Assess breathing patterns and lung sounds frequently for congestion or respiratory compromise.
- Perform skin and neurovascular assessments approximately every 2 hours.
- Use adequate padding and skin wrapping to avoid placing pressure on the popliteal space. Such pressure could lead to nerve damage.

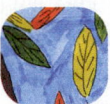

Partnering with Families

Transporting the Child with an Orthopedic Device

The American Academy of Pediatrics and the National Center for the Safe Transportation of Children with Special Health Care Needs have established guidelines for transporting children with special healthcare needs.

- Placement in the rear seat is preferable.
- If the front seat must be used, the front passenger air bag should be disconnected. The National Highway and Traffic Safety Administration provides information and assistance (1-888-327-4236).
- Use only car seat transport systems approved for use with children with special needs.
- Install and use seats as instructed. Never alter a car safety seat to transport a child.
- When reasonable, a child should be moved from a wheelchair or other special device to be placed in the vehicle safety seat.

- Pieces of medical equipment required during transportation (such as monitors or oxygen) or that are being transported with the child (such as wheelchair or walker) should be secured to the floor of the vehicle.
- If the child is transported by school bus, state and federal recommendations for school bus transportation of children with special needs should be followed.
- Keep a cellular phone and emergency equipment in the vehicle.

Source: *Data adapted from American Academy of Pediatrics, Committee on Injury and Poison Prevention. (1999, affirmed 2006). Children with special health care needs. Retrieved from* http://www.aap.org/healthtopics/specialneeds.cfm; *Parenting corner: Questions and answers: Transporting children with special health care needs. Retrieved from* http://www.aap.org/publiced/BR_SpNeedsCarSeats.htm; *Special needs transportation. Retrieved from* http://www.preventinjury.org/NationalCenter.asp

- Change the position of the child in a cast every 2 to 3 hours while awake to help avoid areas of pressure and promote increased circulation. The child can be placed either prone or supine or positioned on the floor and supported with pillows.

- Help prevent skin irritation and breakdown in the child with a cast. Use moleskin to provide protection from rough edges. Place tape around the perineal opening of the cast to prevent soiling.

- Increase fluids and fiber in the child's diet, as a change in bowel or bladder status is commonly associated with immobility.

Clinical Tip

Neurovascular assessment involves evaluation of temperature, movement, color, capillary refill, and sensation. Even if the child is not old enough to respond to questions about feeling, usually brushing the hands or sheets along the toes elicits a movement from the child indicating sensation. Report any abnormalities immediately. Keep limbs aligned as prescribed. For the child in a hip spica, immediately after surgery elevate the lower body on pillows to decrease edema under the cast at the operative site.

Promote Normal Growth and Development

Engage the child in activities that stimulate the upper extremities and all five senses. Provide stimulating toys such as stacking blocks, brightly colored mobiles, Koosh balls, or musical toys. Position toys within the child's reach and interact with the child as much as possible (Box 35–3).

Discharge Planning and Home Care Teaching

Parents must learn how to care for a child in a hip spica cast at home. The active participation of family members in the daily care of the child while hospitalized gradually increases confidence in their ability to provide care at home. Home care needs should be identified and addressed early in hospitalization. Before discharge, be sure the parents have the following information:

- Instruct about general cast care (see page 1259), positioning, bathing, toileting, and age-appropriate diversional activities.
- Emphasize the importance of performing neurovascular checks and reporting any abnormalities immediately.
- Be sure that parents understand that the bar between the legs on the cast is not to be used for holding or turning the child. The bar is used to position the legs at the proper distance; using it to lift can cause the cast to fracture, weaken, or disintegrate.
- Make appropriate referrals for periodic assessment by a visiting nurse or home health nurse.
- Provide the family with resources to care for the child.

Before discharge, have parents demonstrate how to dress and feed a child in a hip spica cast. Ensure that safe travel arrangements have been made for the day of discharge (see Partnering with Families: Transporting the Child with an Orthopedic Device). Help parents to obtain an appropriate car safety seat in advance of discharge. Some agencies have loaner programs for families. Encourage parents to let the child interact with other children at home, and to provide the child in a cast opportunities for play and social activities.

Care in the Community

Have parents of an infant in a Pavlik harness demonstrate care of the infant while in the harness. Teach family members about daily care (bathing, dressing, and feeding) of the infant. The harness is worn full time; instructions generally include sponge bathing while it is in place although some physicians may allow it to be removed briefly each day for bathing. One shoulder strap is removed at a time to change a T-shirt while the legs are held in proper position. The hips and buttocks should be supported carefully in the abducted position at all times. Demonstrate how to feed the infant in an upright position to maintain abduction and how to change a diaper without removing the harness.

Instruct the parents of an infant with a harness to look for any reddened or irritated areas near the harness or cast edges and to check toes frequently for proper circulation. Frequent repositioning reduces the risk of pressure sores or circulatory compromise. The infant should wear an undershirt and socks under the harness to prevent rubbing of the skin.

Safety precautions are important as the child will not have normal mobility. Parents will need to use a specially designed car seat that accommodates the child with abducted hips. Strollers and cribs should provide sufficient room to protect the legs from injury and to prevent hip adduction.

Evaluation

Expected outcomes of nursing care for the child with developmental dysplasia of the hip include the following:

- The skin remains intact.
- The child has no complications related to immobility.
- Parents demonstrate adequate knowledge regarding the condition, treatment, and necessary home care.
- A safe environment is maintained for the child.
- The child regains normal mobility.

Legg-Calvé-Perthes Disease

Legg-Calvé-Perthes disease (often called *Perthes disease*) is a self-limiting condition in which there is avascular necrosis of the femoral head. The disease occurs in approximately 1 in 12,000 children and affects boys four to five times more often than girls. It usually occurs between the ages of 2 and 12 years, with an average age of 7 years at onset. The disease can be unilateral or bilateral (Perry & Hall, 2011).

Etiology and Pathophysiology

The necrosis associated with Legg-Calvé-Perthes disease results from an interruption of the blood supply to the femoral epiphysis. How and why this occurs is not completely understood, but several predisposing factors have been identified. A coagulation system disorder causes repeated vascular interruptions to the proximal femur. Disturbed blood supply to the epiphyseal plate of the femoral bone is noted, leading to necrosis of the femoral head (Kleposki et al., 2010). The incidence of this condition is increased in families with a history of the disease, which suggests that genetic factors may play a role. In 17% of the cases, onset of the disease is preceded by a mild traumatic injury, and 10% of children affected have a history of breech birth

---

BOX 35–3	Growth & Development: Cast Precautions

Use caution in selecting toys appropriate for the child's developmental age. If the child is in a cast, be sure that toys or parts cannot be swallowed or inserted under the edges of the cast. Place a T-shirt over the cast so that the edges are securely covered and it is difficult for the child to place something under them. Provide toys that are large and soft. Use diversion such as play and music to occupy the child's attention, and assess the child frequently.

Developing Cultural Competence
Legg-Calvé-Perthes Disease

Legg-Calvé-Perthes disease is most common among White, Chinese, and Japanese children. It is less common among Blacks and Native Americans. This suggests a genetic link to the disease. However, Legg-Calvé-Perthes disease is most common in children from low socioeconomic backgrounds, suggesting an environmental or intrauterine connection (Perry & Hall, 2011).

(Burns, Dunn, Brady, et al., 2009). Trauma may cause a subchondral fracture and resultant synovitis, which in turn causes pressure that occludes the blood supply. Children with Legg-Calvé-Perthes disease often have delayed skeletal maturation, increased thyroid levels, and low somatomedin C (insulin-like growth factor). It is more common in those with low birth weight, increased parental age, and exposure to environmental tobacco smoke. Some cultural variations occur. (See Developing Cultural Competence: Legg-Calvé-Perthes Disease.)

Clinical Manifestations

Legg-Calvé-Perthes disease progresses through four distinct stages after the original insult (usually unidentified) occurs, over a period of 1 to 4 years. Early symptoms of the disease include a mild pain in the knee, hip, or anterior thigh and a limp, which are aggravated by increased activity and relieved by rest. The child favors the affected hip and limits hip movement to avoid discomfort. See the Clinical Manifestations table.

As the disease progresses, range of motion becomes limited, walking becomes more difficult, and weakness and muscle wasting develop. The affected thigh is 2 to 3 cm smaller than the unaffected thigh. Prolonged hip irritability may produce muscle spasms and pain increases. This period of the disease varies from 1 to 4 years. Gradually, revascularization begins and pain decreases.

Collaborative Care

Medical management and prognosis depend on the degree of femoral involvement. Early detection is important to the success of treatment.

Diagnostic Tests

Because the child's initial symptoms are so mild, parents often do not seek medical attention until symptoms have been present for several months. Diagnosis is made using standard anteroposterior and frog-leg radiographs. As noted, radiographs taken early in the course of the disease may be normal or show vague widening of the cartilage space. Bone scans, MRI, and arthrogram may be used in diagnosis. Laboratory studies of the blood, such as white blood cell count, help to rule out inflammatory synovitis of the hip. Protein C, protein S, and APC-R (resistance to activated protein C) may sometimes be performed to evaluate if a coagulation abnormality is present (Burns et al., 2009; De Sanctis, 2011; Milani & Dobashi, 2011).

Clinical Therapy

Medical management and prognosis depend on the degree of femoral involvement and the clinician's decision. Early detection is important to the success of therapy. The desired outcome is a pain-free hip that functions properly. To promote healing and prevent deformity, the femoral head must be contained within the acetabulum to maintain its sphericity. Observation and examination over time are most commonly used with physical rehabilitation, and occasionally traction, casting, or bracing. Toronto (Figure 35–12 ■) and Scottish-Rite braces are most commonly used. Anti-inflammatory medications are used to treat the pain and discomfort. Severe disease may be treated by surgery to release adductor muscles (adductor tenotomy), treat the acetabulum or femur, and restore range of motion.

Prognosis is good if the child is young (under 8 years) and has a mild form of the disease (Fabry, 2010). Children with untreated disease or those diagnosed late in the disease process may develop osteoarthritis, hip dysfunction, or leg-length discrepancy later in life.

Nursing Management

Goals of nursing management include early identification of Perthes disease and ensuring maintenance of the treatment regimen in active children.

Clinical Manifestations Legg-Calvé-Perthes Disease

STAGE	CLINICAL MANIFESTATIONS
Prenecrosis	An insult or coagulation disorder causes loss of blood supply to the femoral head.
I—Necrosis	Avascular stage (3–6 months); the child is asymptomatic, bone radiographs are normal, and the head of the femur is structurally intact but avascular.
II—Revascularization	Period of 1–4 years characterized by pain and limitation of movement. Bone radiographs show new bone deposition and dead bone resorption. Fracture and deformity of the head of the femur can occur.
III—Bone healing	Reossification takes place; pain decreases.
IV—Remodeling	The disease process is over, pain is absent, and improvement in joint function occurs.

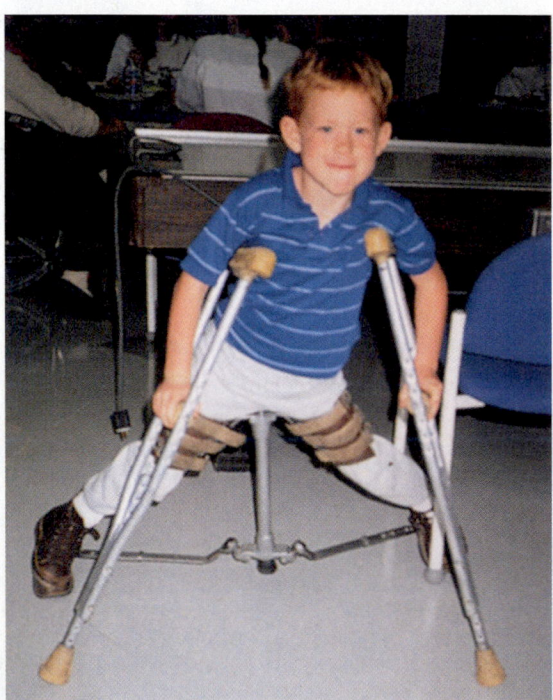

FIGURE 35–12 ■ Although the Toronto brace used for treatment of Legg-Calvé-Perthes disease may seem formidable for a child to wear, you can see by this photograph that, as usual, children adapt quite well to it.

Nursing Assessment and Diagnosis

Legg-Calvé-Perthes disease should be suspected in any child, especially a boy age 2 to 12 years, who complains of hip discomfort accompanied by a limp. The school nurse may be the first health professional to observe the child with symptoms of the disease. The child may complain of pain and have to rest during physical education classes. Immediate referral should be made to the healthcare provider. Question the child who has an apparent limp about pain, and assess the child's range of motion. Ask if the child previously injured the hip.

Nursing diagnoses for the child with diagnosed Legg-Calvé-Perthes disease center on altered activities and compliance, and may include the following:

- Mobility: Physical, Impaired related to restriction of brace or cast
- Injury, Risk for related to potential complications resulting from noncompliance with the treatment regimen
- Stress Overload related to duration of treatment and nonadherence to recommended therapy
- Coping, Ineffective related to inactivity
- Body Image, Disturbed, related to brace

NANDA-I © 2012

Planning and Implementation

Children with Legg-Calvé-Perthes disease often receive all of their treatment at home. Helping the child and family adhere to the prescribed treatment plan may be challenging, because children develop the disease at an age when they are usually very active. The child, who may have little pain, often finds immobilization and physical rehabilitation recommendations difficult.

Promote Normal Growth and Development

Parents should be given suggestions to help redirect the child's energy within the limitations in mobility imposed by treatment. A return to school promotes a feeling of normalcy. Coordinate the return to school by facilitating the child's use of an elevator or ramp as needed in that setting. An individualized health plan may be needed. Partner with the family to provide instruction for school personnel and other children to foster understanding of the child's condition and treatment. Activities that involve peers also help the child achieve developmental milestones. Help the child adjust to wearing a brace.

Clinical Judgment

Legg-Calvé-Perthes disease primarily affects boys with an average age of 7 years. These school-age children are industrious and independent. What suggestions will you offer for physical activities that redirect energy, allow for hip adduction, and promote normal development?

Care in the Community

Both the child and the family should be aware that treatment generally takes approximately 2 years. Emphasize the importance of following the treatment plan to ensure adequate hip containment and proper healing. Teach the family how to care for a child in traction and how to check the child's skin for breakdown. Follow-up visits should be arranged at regular intervals, and home visits may be helpful for some families. Provide suggestions to alter the home environment to facilitate treatment recommendations.

Evaluation

Expected outcomes of nursing care are elimination of hip pain and discomfort, normal development during the period of immobilization, parent and child knowledge of treatment regimen, and eventual normal proximal femur function without joint deformity.

Slipped Capital Femoral Epiphysis

Slipped capital femoral epiphysis (SCFE) occurs when the femoral head is displaced from the femoral neck. This condition is seen in 10 per 100,000 adolescents, commonly during the adolescent growth spurt, between the ages of 12 and 15 years in boys and 10 and 13 years in girls. Boys are more often affected than girls. Black children are affected more often than other ethnic groups, as are children with certain predisposing factors described below (Gholve, Cameron, & Millis, 2009; Shank, Thiel, & Klingele, 2010).

Etiology and Pathophysiology

The cause of SCFE is unknown. Predisposing factors include obesity, a recent growth spurt, sports injuries or other trauma, history of radiation therapy, and endocrine disorders such as hypothyroidism, hypopituitarism, and hypogonadism (Box 35–4).

Slippage of the femoral head occurs at the proximal epiphyseal plate, and the femur displaces from the epiphysis (Figure 35–13 ■). Slippage is usually gradual (chronic), but may also result from acute trauma. The synovial membrane becomes inflamed, edematous, and painful. If untreated, callous formation occurs, resulting in a deformed hip with limited range of motion.

Clinical Manifestations

Symptoms include a limp; knee, thigh, groin, or hip pain; and loss of hip motion. Out-toeing, decreased internal rotation, and external rotation with flexion of the leg are suggestive of the condition (Kleposki et al., 2010). The condition is categorized as acute, chronic, or acute-on-chronic. *Acute* SCFE has a sudden onset of less than 3 weeks' duration. The child with an acute slip has sudden, severe pain and cannot bear weight. An acute slip may be associated with traumatic injury.

Chronic SCFE has a duration of longer than 3 weeks. It involves persistent hip pain, which is generally aching or mild and can be referred to the thigh, knee, or both. A limp and decreased range of motion may also occur.

Acute-on-chronic SCFE is an additional slippage in a child with a chronic condition. The child with a chronic slip sustains a traumatic incident that causes further slippage of the femoral head, causing sudden, severe pain.

BOX 35–4	Research: Obesity and SCFE

Obesity is a known risk factor for SCFE. Increasing rates of obesity among children contribute to an increasing risk for the disorder. Research continues to demonstrate a relationship between body mass index (BMI) and SCFE. In one study of over 100 youth with SCFE from 8 to 18 years, over 81% had a BMI above the 95th percentile for their age and gender (Chan & Chen, 2009). Another study examined factors associated with bilateral SCFE; about 20% of children with SCFE eventually develop the condition in both hips. This study also identified that in the last 25 years the incidence of SCFE has risen from 3.78 per 100,000 to 9.66 per 100,000, and the average age at diagnosis has fallen from 13.4 to 12.6 years. High rates of elevated BMI likely play a role in both bilateral SCFE occurrence and increased incidence of the condition (Murray & Wilson, 2008). Nurses are well positioned to work with children and families to teach weight reduction strategies and to share information about the numerous health risks associated with elevated BMI.

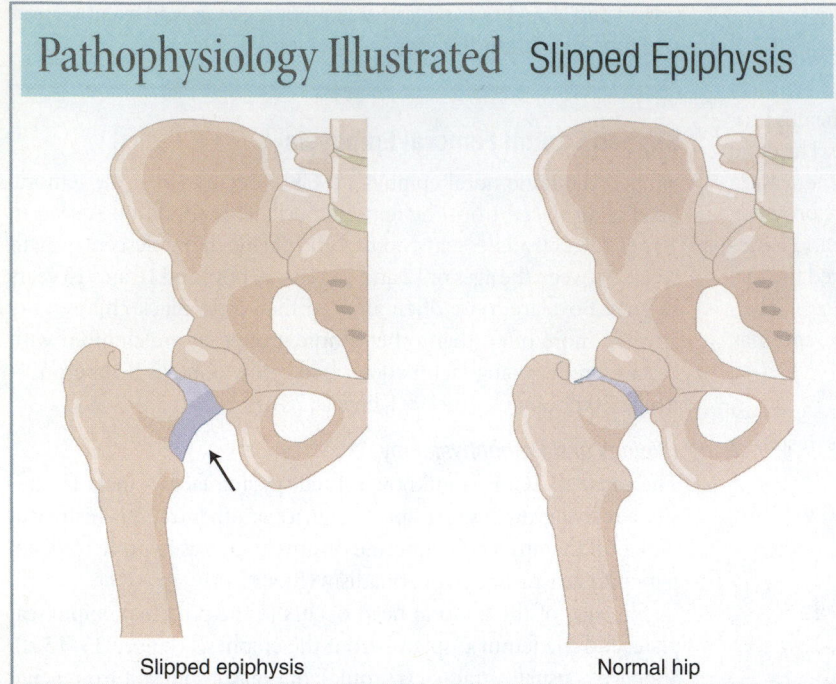

Pathophysiology Illustrated Slipped Epiphysis

Slipped epiphysis   Normal hip

FIGURE 35–13 ■ In slipped capital femoral epiphysis, the femoral head is displaced from the femoral neck at the proximal epiphyseal plate.

The condition is further classified as stable if the youth can walk on it, or unstable when walking is not possible.

Collaborative Care

The goal of medical management is to stabilize the femoral head while keeping displacement to a minimum and retaining as much hip function as possible.

Diagnostic Tests

A complete history provides information about risk factors and the development of the condition. Radiographs are used to confirm the diagnosis; lateral radiographs display the slippage most clearly. A bone scan, ultrasound, CT, and MRI are sometimes performed to verify the extent of injury.

Clinical Therapy

Surgical treatment is usually necessary; this involves fixation of the epiphysis with screws or pins. If the condition is stable, a single screw into the hip in an outpatient procedure may be sufficient for stabilization; if unstable, surgery becomes more complicated and may include both traction and surgery (Peck, 2010).

Prognosis is related to the severity of the deformity and the occurrence of complications, such as avascular necrosis of the femoral head or **chondrolysis** (the breaking down and absorption of cartilage).

Nursing Management

The goals of nursing management are early detection and referral of potential slipped epiphysis and provision of care for the adolescent who is surgically treated.

Nursing Assessment and Diagnosis

The child usually presents with hip pain or referred pain to the groin, thigh, or knee, and limited mobility. A thorough history is used to assess for injury as a cause. Assess the child's range of motion, pain,

and limp, if apparent. Refer the child for treatment immediately if SCFE is suspected. This condition is considered to be an emergency, and it is essential that the child be treated immediately to keep weight off the affected joint (Kleposki et al., 2010; Plante, Wallace, & Busconi, 2011).

Nursing diagnoses that may apply to the child with SCFE are as follows:

- Mobility, Physical, Impaired related to treatment
- Pain related to hip injury
- Body Image, Disturbed related to treatment
- Growth and Development, Delayed related to mobility restrictions
- Nutrition, Imbalanced: More than Body Requirements related to immobility
- Tissue Perfusion: Peripheral, Ineffective related to traction, casting, and other treatments
- Knowledge, Deficient related to disease process and treatment

NANDA-I © 2012

Planning and Implementation

Nursing management involves caring for the child in traction or after surgery, administering medications and other pain control interventions, maintaining mobility within the limits imposed by treatment, providing adequate nutrition, educating the child and family about the disorder, providing emotional support, and promoting compliance with the treatment plan.

Encourage Appropriate Nutritional Intake and Physical Activity

A growing adolescent needs increased amounts of proteins, carbohydrates, and calcium to promote skeletal healing. Provide written instructions about nutritional requirements necessary to promote bone healing and maintain an ideal body weight. If a child is overweight, encourage weight loss by decreasing percent of fat and carbohydrate in the diet and by increasing physical activity as appropriate. This decreases pressure on the femoral epiphysis and can also lead to a more positive self-image. Incorporate upper body exercises into treatment, both to assist in weight control and to build muscle. A few visits to physical therapy may facilitate a program of upper body exercise and teach safe ways of increasing total amount of physical activity.

Provide Emotional Support

Because the onset of SCFE is usually unexpected, the child and family may find themselves facing surgery with little warning. Explain the treatment plan simply and thoroughly. Reassure the child and family that with proper compliance, treatment should be successful.

Discharge Planning and Home Care Teaching

Partner with the family to help them plan for the child's return to school. If attendance is not possible for a period of time due to traction or surgery, suggest tutors and computer communication with the school as needed. Assist the family and school in establishment of an individualized education plan. Follow-up visits are necessary until the child's epiphyseal plates close. Make sure the child and family are aware of symptoms such as decreased range of motion or pain that could indicate onset of the disorder in the other hip. Tell parents to contact their healthcare provider immediately if these symptoms occur.

Evaluation

Expected outcomes of nursing care for the child with SCFE include maintenance of normal weight and recommended nutritional intake, absence of complications of immobility, successful adaptation to school following treatment, and family recognition of the need for ongoing monitoring for complications.

DISORDERS OF THE SPINE

Scoliosis

Scoliosis is a lateral S- or C-shaped curvature of the spine that is often associated with a rotational deformity of the spine and ribs. Many individuals exhibit some degree of spinal curvature, but curvatures of more than 10 degrees are considered abnormal. Curves are either idiopathic or compensatory, the latter occurring as the spine curves to compensate for a structural deformity such as leg length discrepancy. Idiopathic scoliosis occurs most often in girls, especially during the growth spurt between the ages of 10 and 13 years. From 1% to 3% of adolescents manifest with idiopathic scoliosis of greater than 10 degrees. A smaller number of children manifest infantile scoliosis before 3 years of age or juvenile scoliosis from 3 to 10 years (Lombardi, Akoume, Colombini, et al., 2011).

Etiology and Pathophysiology

The cause of scoliosis is complex. Structural scoliosis may be congenital, idiopathic, or acquired (associated with neuromuscular disorders such as muscular dystrophy or myelodysplasia, or secondary to spinal cord injuries).

In idiopathic scoliosis (the most common type), the spine for unknown reasons begins to curve laterally, with vertebral rotation. The most common curve is a right thoracic and left lumbar deformity. As the curve progresses, structural changes occur. The ribs on the concave side (inside the curve) are forced closer together, while the ribs on the convex side separate widely, causing narrowing of the thoracic cage and formation of the rib hump. The lateral curvature affects the vertebral structure. Disk spaces are narrowed on the concave side and spread wider on the convex side, resulting in an asymmetric vertebral canal (Figure 35–14 ■).

Scoliosis can also occur in congenital diseases involving the spinal structure and in the musculoskeletal changes seen in conditions such as myelomeningocele, cerebral palsy (see Chapter 33 🔗), or muscular dystrophy. Disturbances in platelet function, melatonin levels, and bone-related trace substances are sometimes evident (Lombardi et al., 2011). Scoliosis can also be acquired after injury to the spinal cord. The child in Figure 35–15 ■ acquired scoliosis after chemotherapy and radiation to the chest during treatment for cancer.

Clinical Manifestations

The classic signs of scoliosis include truncal asymmetry, uneven shoulder and hip height, a one-sided rib hump, and a prominent scapula. The child does not complain of pain or discomfort. If diagnosis does not occur before the curvature reaches about 40 degrees, some compensatory problems may develop. Hip and back pain can result, and lung compromise can lead to fatigue or dyspnea with exertion.

Collaborative Care

The goal of medical management is to limit or stop progression of the curvature. School and office nurses often screen children for scoliosis and refer abnormalities for further evaluation. Many professionals

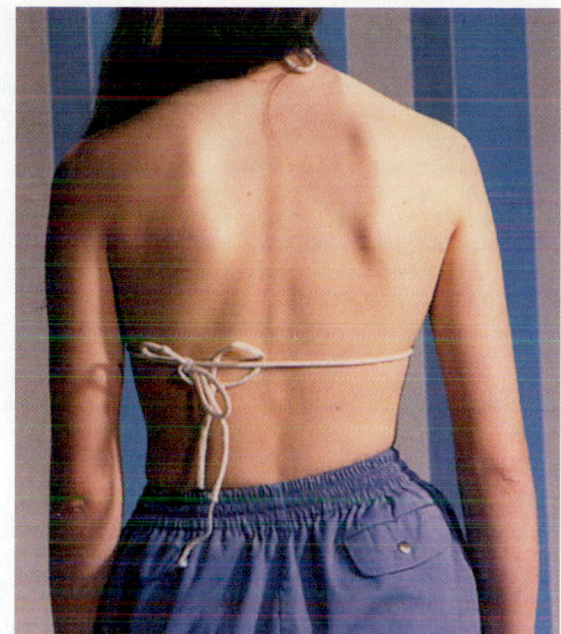

FIGURE 35–14 ■ A child may have varying degrees of scoliosis. For mild forms, treatment will focus on strengthening and stretching. Moderate forms will require bracing. Severe forms may necessitate surgery and fusion. Clothes that fit at an angle, such as this teenage girl's shorts, and anatomic asymmetry of the back provide clues for early detection.

such as physical therapists, physicians, and nurses partner with families to treat the adolescent with scoliosis.

Diagnostic Tests

Generally, observation and radiographic examination are used to diagnose scoliosis. An inclinometer (Scoliometer) can be placed on the spine with the child bent forward; a variation from one side to the other of greater than 7 degrees warrants referral for further evaluation (Scottish Rite Hospital, 2011). Additional diagnostic studies include MRI, CT scan, and bone scan, which are used occasionally to assess the degree of curvature.

Clinical Therapy

Early detection is essential to successful treatment. Adequate treatment and follow-up maximize the child's chances for proper spinal alignment. The treatment regimen chosen depends on the degree

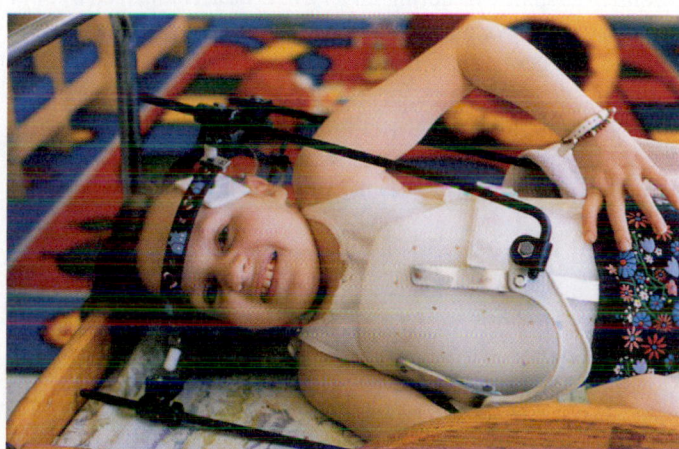

FIGURE 35–15 ■ In severe scoliosis, the child may wear a halo brace, shown here, to hold the body in position after surgery.

BOX 35–5   **Research: Adolescent Quality of Life and Braces**

We know that adolescents are concerned about body image and that wearing a brace can be challenging. Research suggests that the quality of the adolescent's life can influence acceptance of and adaptation to brace wearing. Adolescents who were noncompliant with brace wear rated themselves lower in a quality-of-life questionnaire, and had poor physical, emotional, and social characteristics (Rivett, Rothberg, Stewart, et al., 2009). Health professionals may need to address psychosocial coping issues in order to ensure compliance with brace therapy. What assessments can assist you in learning the activity level, social interactions, and well-being of adolescents beginning scoliosis treatment?

and progression of the curvature and the response of the child and family to medical management.

Treatment of children with mild scoliosis (curvatures of 10 to 20 degrees upon radiographic study) consists of exercises to improve posture and muscle tone and to maintain, or possibly increase, flexibility of the spine. Emphasis is placed on building strength toward the outside of the curve while stretching the inside of the curve. These exercises are not a cure, however, and the child should be evaluated by a physician at 3-month intervals, with radiographic evaluation every 6 months.

Medical management of moderate scoliosis (curvatures of 20 to 40 degrees) includes bracing, most commonly with a Boston brace. The goal of wearing a brace is to maintain the existing spinal curvature with no increase. Brace wear begins immediately after diagnosis. To achieve maximum effectiveness, the brace should be worn 23 hours per day. Brace treatment is lengthy and requires a high degree of compliance, which can be difficult for adolescents who view body image or sports involvement as important (Box 35–5).

Electrical stimulation is used occasionally as an alternative treatment. An electric current stimulates the back muscles to contract, thus helping to correct the spinal curvature. This treatment, which is performed at night, eliminates the need for bracing.

Children with severe scoliosis (curvatures of 40 to 50 degrees or more) generally require surgery, which involves spinal fusion. The majority of spinal fusions are performed using segmental instrumentation of the spinal cord with hooks, wires, rods, and screws (Lubicky, Hanson, Riley, et al., 2011). Examples of surgical approaches include Luque wires, Cotrel-Dubousset (CD) instrumentation, Texas Scottish Rite Hospital system, and Moss-Miami system. These treatments stabilize the spine well during surgery, may be accompanied by bone grafting to the spine, and require no long-term therapy or postoperative casting; they permanently remain in the back. Following surgery with wires or instrumentation, the child is on bed rest during a recovery period and then is generally fitted with anteroposterior plastic shells (also called thoracolumbar sacral orthotics) that are worn for several months to provide stability for the spine.

Nursing Management

Nursing management focuses on screening and early detection, teaching about brace wear, caring for the adolescent having surgery for scoliosis, and partnering with the adolescent and family to provide support during all treatments.

Nursing Assessment and Diagnosis

School nurses often screen children for scoliosis, generally in the fifth and seventh grades. This screening is mandated by law in several states, but not universally recommended (U.S. Preventive Services Task Force, 2011). When abnormalities are noted, the child is referred to an orthopedic center for further evaluation. Children should be examined every 6 to 9 months thereafter. If scoliosis is detected, the child's brothers and sisters should be examined and observed closely. See Chapter 7 🔗 for photographs of scoliosis screening, Figures 7–48 and 7–49.

Scoliosis screening involves visual observation of the following:

From the Front

- Is the head midline?
- Are the shoulders at the same height?
- Is there the same amount of space between the arms and body on each side?

From the Back

- Is the head midline?
- Are the shoulders at the same height?
- Are the scapulae equally prominent and at the same height?
- Is the spine straight?
- Is there the same amount of space between the arms and body on each side?
- Are the hips at the same height?

With the Adolescent Holding Hands Together and Bent Over Slightly

- Are the scapular humps even?

With the Adolescent Holding Hands Together and Bent Over Toward the Floor

- Are the flank humps even?
- Is the spine straight?
- Is there a marked roundness when viewed from the side (evidence of kyphosis)?

Once scoliosis has been identified, the nurse's focus becomes education and follow-up. Any child with scoliosis should have a comprehensive neurologic, cardiac, and respiratory examination, since the rib cage deformity can influence the functioning of these systems.

The following nursing diagnoses may apply to the child with scoliosis who is not undergoing surgery:

- Coping, Ineffective related to duration and intensity of exercise
- Mobility: Physical, Impaired related to brace
- Skin Integrity, Impaired related to brace
- Ineffective Breathing Pattern related to rib cage deformity
- Health Maintenance, Impaired related to unfamiliarity with disease process
- Body Image, Disturbed related to deformity and brace wear

NANDA-I © 2012

Common nursing diagnoses for the child who is having surgery can be found in the accompanying Nursing Care Plan.

Planning and Implementation

An important aspect of nursing care is patient education. Patient adherence with prescribed measures is critical to the success of treatment. Children and their families need to understand the condition and the stages of treatment, particularly adolescents who are undergoing treatment for scoliosis. Adherence to exercise programs and bracing can be challenging for adolescents and their families. Nurses can institute follow-up contacts to encourage treatments as

Nursing Care Plan — The Child Undergoing Surgery for Scoliosis

INTERVENTION	RATIONALE	EXPECTED OUTCOME
1. Knowledge, Deficient (Child and Parents) related to lack of information about surgery and home care		
NIC Priority Intervention—*Teaching, Disease Process and Preoperative:* Assisting the patient to understand information and mentally prepare for surgery and postoperative recovery; *Teaching: Prescribed Teaching:* Preparing family to understand and perform prescribed treatment		**NOC Suggested Outcome**—*Knowledge:* Extent of understanding conveyed about scoliosis treatment and follow-up care

GOAL: *The child and parents will verbalize understanding of the disease, the surgical procedure, and home care treatment.*

■ Teach the child and family about the course of the disease, its signs and symptoms, and treatment. Provide appropriate handouts. Encourage the child and parents to ask questions.	■ Understanding and involvement increase motivation and compliance while reducing fear.	The child and family accurately verbalize knowledge about the disease and its treatment. The child and family ask appropriate questions about postoperative care.
■ Begin preoperative teaching at the time of admission. Orient the child to hospital and postoperative procedures. Before surgery, have the child demonstrate logrolling, range of motion exercises, and the use of an incentive spirometer. Discuss pain management.	■ Preoperative teaching and familiarity with hospital procedures reduces the stress related to surgery and postoperative complications.	
■ Teach cast or brace care before discharge. Provide oral and written instructions and a list of activity limitations.	■ Providing education decreases anxiety and increases adherence to the treatment plan.	
■ Provide resources for questions or concerns. Schedule follow-up visits.	■ Follow-up visits assist the physician, nurse, and family in evaluating the effectiveness of the treatment plan.	

2. Breathing Pattern, Ineffective related to hypoventilation syndrome		
NIC Priority Intervention—*Airway Management and Respiratory Monitoring:* Facilitation of patency of air passages and analysis of patient data		**NOC Suggested Outcome**—*Respiratory Status: Ventilation:* Movement of air in and out of the lungs

GOAL: *The child will show no signs of respiratory compromise.*

■ Monitor respiratory status, especially after the administration of analgesics. Apply a pulse oximeter.	■ Evaluation of the child's respiratory condition anticipates and avoids complications. Analgesics such as morphine may increase or potentiate respiratory compromise.	The child has no respiratory complications.
■ Administer oxygen if ordered.	■ Oxygen increases peripheral oxygen saturation to 95–100%.	
■ Have the child use an incentive spirometer.	■ Spirometry increases lung expansion and aeration of the alveoli.	
■ Monitor intake and output.	■ Good hydration promotes loose secretions and helps prevent infection.	
■ Reposition the child at least every 2 hours.	■ Repositioning ensures inflation of the lung fields.	

3. Injury, Risk for related to neurovascular deficit secondary to instrumentation		
NIC Priority Intervention—*Injury Prevention:* Instituting special precautions with patient at risk		**NOC Suggested Outcome**—*Risk Control:* Actions to eliminate or reduce modifiable health risks

GOAL: *The child's neurovascular system will remain intact as evidenced by circulation, sensation, and motor checks. The child will feel no numbness or tingling.*

■ Monitor the child's color, circulation, capillary refill, warmth, sensation, and motion in all extremities. Perform neurovascular checks every 2 hours for the first 24 hours and then every 4 hours for the next 48 hours. Record presence of pedal and distal tibial pulses every hour for 48 hours. Report changes and abnormal findings immediately.	■ When the spinal column is manipulated during surgery, altered neurovascular status, thrombus formation, and paralysis are possible complications. Postoperative risks include loss of bowel or bladder control, weakness or paralysis, and impaired vision or sensation.	The child exhibits only temporary alteration (pale skin, faint pulse, and edema occur, but then resolve within the initial postoperative phase). The child returns to the preoperative baseline state by discharge.

(continued)

Nursing Care Plan

The Child Undergoing Surgery for Scoliosis, *continued*

INTERVENTION	RATIONALE	EXPECTED OUTCOME
▪ Have the child wear antiembolism stockings until ambulatory. The stockings may be removed for 1 hour 2–3 times daily.	▪ Antiembolism stockings prevent blood clots and promote venous return. Thrombus formation is a postoperative risk.	
▪ Check for any pain, swelling, or a positive Homans sign (pain in the calf of the leg when the toes are dorsiflexed). Record any evidence of edema.	▪ Swelling may indicate a tight dressing and tissue damage. A positive Homans sign and pain may indicate thrombus formation.	
▪ Monitor input and output.	▪ Abnormalities may indicate a fluid shift problem.	
▪ Encourage and assist the child with range of motion exercises, both passive and active.	▪ Activity promotes mobility and reduces risk of thrombus formation.	

4. Nursing Diagnosis: Pain related to spinal fusion with instrumentation

NIC Priority Intervention—*Pain Management:* Alleviation of pain or a reduction of pain to a level of comfort acceptable to the patient		**NOC Suggested Outcome**—*Pain Level:* Amount of reported or demonstrated pain

GOAL: *The child will verbalize an adequate level of comfort or show absence of pain behavior within 1 hour of a specific nursing intervention.*

▪ Assess the level of pain and initiate pain management strategies as soon as possible. Use patient-controlled analgesics if ordered.	▪ Adequate pain management allows for faster healing and a more cooperative patient. Patient-controlled analgesics may be effective.	The child experiences pain relief early in the postoperative period.
▪ Administer pain medication around the clock to help ensure pain relief, especially during the first 48 hours. Monitor epidural blocks and patient-controlled analgesia or other methods used for pain control.	▪ Medicating around the clock helps to maintain comfort. Monitoring ensures patient safety.	
▪ Use nonpharmacologic pain management techniques, such as imagery, relaxation, touch, music, application of heat and cold, and reduced environmental stimulation to supplement medications (see Chapter 21 🔗).	▪ Alternative treatments also interrupt the pain stimulus and provide relief. Nonpharmacologic methods can be an effective adjunct to pain management.	
▪ Document pain assessment, interventions, and the child's reactions.	▪ Proper documentation guides the selection of the most effective means of pain control.	
▪ Reassure the child that some discomfort is expected and that a variety of measures can be tried to reduce discomfort.	▪ Realistic expectations decrease anxiety and give the child a sense of control.	

5. Mobility: Physical, Impaired related to movement restrictions and pain

NIC Priority Intervention—*Positioning and Ambulation:* Moving the patient to provide comfort and promote healing, assist with walking		**NOC Suggested Outcome**—*Ambulation:* Ability to walk from place to place

GOAL: *The child will maintain proper body alignment and progress with activity as ordered by the physician. If no anteroposterior shell bracing is required, the child will have active mobility by the third to fifth postoperative day.*

▪ Reposition the child every 2 hours using the logroll technique. Support the back, feet, and knees with pillows.	▪ Proper positioning prevents twisting or turning the spine.	The child is as mobile as appropriate for condition within 3–5 days after surgery.
▪ Have the child perform passive and active range of motion exercises every 2 hours for 48 hours and then every 4 hours while awake. Have the child dangle his or her legs at bedside by the second to fourth postoperative day or as ordered by the surgeon. Begin ambulation generally by the third to fifth postoperative day. Note any complaints of dizziness or pallor. Proceed slowly.	▪ Exercises help maintain strength, circulation, and muscle tone. If the spine is stable and the physician has ordered no external support, the child may progress to full ambulation as tolerated. If the spine is not stable, great care must be taken until external supportive devices are used.	

NANDA-I © 2012

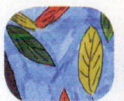

Partnering with Families

Postoperative Activities After Spinal Surgery

RECOMMENDED
- Lying
- Sitting
- Standing
- Walking (including normal stair climbing)
- Swimming, gentle (except if in a cast); diving is not permitted

NOT RECOMMENDED
- Bending or twisting at the waist
- Lifting more than 10 pounds
- Household chores such as vacuuming, unloading groceries, mowing the lawn, taking out the garbage
- Sports such as bicycle riding, horseback riding, skiing, in-line skating
- Physical education classes

prescribed and assist the youth and family to problem-solve issues that lead to decreased treatment adherence. Establish baseline exercise levels and use them for comparison during subsequent visits.

Children or adolescents facing surgery require education, reassurance, and support. Teach about pain control and the patient-controlled analgesia (PCA) pump, and general postoperative care routines. Often the child donates some of his or her own blood prior to surgery, and the family may also donate so blood transfused in surgery is the child's or a family member's. Explain to the child the safety that this ensures. The adolescent will benefit from learning about deep breathing, positioning, surgical incision, and all other aspects of postoperative care. The accompanying Nursing Care Plan summarizes nursing care for the child undergoing surgery for scoliosis.

Promote Understanding and Acceptance of the Treatment Plan

Provide instructions about exercises that will help to decrease the severity of the spinal curvature. Demonstrate the exercises, and explain their purpose (e.g., to strengthen back muscles). Help the child adjust to wearing a brace. Adolescents, in particular, may be reluctant to wear an external device such as a brace. To promote a sense of control, allow the adolescent to choose when to exercise and when to be out of the brace, within the treatment guidelines. Provide reassurance and encouragement and promote interaction with peers. Consider suggesting that the adolescent work with a peer support person who is being treated for scoliosis or has had the condition in the past. Provide information about fashionable clothing that can be worn with the brace.

Discharge Planning and Home Care Teaching

Home care needs should be identified and addressed well in advance of discharge after spinal surgery. The child must learn to adapt to a new set of body mechanics. Show the child how to perform simple tasks without bending or twisting the torso. Have the child demonstrate the ability to perform activities of daily living before discharge from the hospital. Partner with physical therapy/rehabilitation to plan for the youth's needs related to safe and effective movement with the brace.

Activities for the child who has had spinal surgery are commonly limited for a period of time. Restrictions usually should be followed for 6 to 8 months, depending on the type of surgery and the surgeon's choice. Emphasize to both the child and the family the importance of adhering to therapy, and give them written discharge instructions. Follow-up visits are important. The child should be examined 4 to 6 weeks after discharge, then every 3 to 4 months for 1 year, and every 1 to 2 years thereafter (see Partnering with Families: Postoperative Activities After Spinal Surgery).

Clinical Tip

Youth with metal hardware in their back after scoliosis surgery need to carry an explanation from the physician on airplane flights as they will set off metal detectors in airports. Have families call airlines before flights to be certain what documentation will be needed. Encourage families to arrive early for flights in order to facilitate transportation security screening.

Several organizations provide information and assistance to families of children with scoliosis. Referrals can be made as appropriate.

Evaluation

Expected outcomes of nursing care for the child with scoliosis treated by brace are maintenance of intact skin and compliance with prescribed therapy. Expected outcomes after surgical correction are listed on the accompanying Nursing Care Plan.

Torticollis, Kyphosis, and Lordosis

Torticollis is tilt of the head caused by rotation of the cervical spine. The cause is generally an injury sustained to the sternocleidomastoid muscle at the time of birth or to a cervical spine abnormality. Stretching exercises or surgical lengthening of the sternocleidomastoid muscle are usual treatments. Occasionally the cause of torticollis is visual impairment, leading to constant turning in one direction to see with the better eye.

Kyphosis (hunchback) and lordosis (swayback) are two other types of spinal curvature that may occur in children. The type of kyphosis in adolescence is most commonly Scheuermann kyphosis, an abnormality in ossification of anterior vertebral bodies; it differs from the degenerative kyphosis sometimes seen in the elderly. Postural lordosis is a characteristic finding in toddlers, but it should disappear by the school-age years.

Nurses perform thorough musculoskeletal assessments of children (see Chapter 7) and refer any children with abnormalities for further evaluation. Clinical therapy depends on the cause and degree of the curvature, and the age of the child at onset. Refer to the Clinical Manifestations table for clinical manifestations, treatment, and nursing management of kyphosis and lordosis.

ADDITIONAL DISORDERS OF THE BONES AND JOINTS

Osteoporosis and Osteopenia

Osteoporosis, a condition in which there is decreased density and mass of bone, promotes the risk of fractures and is commonly

Clinical Manifestations Kyphosis and Lordosis

CONDITION	CLINICAL MANIFESTATIONS	CLINICAL THERAPY
Kyphosis Excessive convex curvature of the cervical thoracic spine. (Scheuermann kyphosis is a common type.)	*Clinical manifestations:* Visible hunchback or rounded shoulders; shortness of breath or fatigue; pain; abdominal creases and tight hamstrings in severe cases. *Diagnostic tests:* Spinal curvature is assessed by having the child bend 90 degrees at the waist and noting roundness at the scapular area from the side. Sharp angulation is visible. Diagnosis is confirmed by radiograph.	*Medical therapy:* Exercises are prescribed for mild conditions; bracing is commonly used; spinal fusion surgery is performed in severe cases. *Nursing management:* Provide support. Encourage exercises and diligent brace wear. Help the child to deal with the psychologic stress of altered body image.
Lordosis Excessive concave curvature of the lumbar spine with an angle of more than 60 degrees; most common in prepubescent girls and Blacks.	*Clinical manifestations:* Presence of swayback; prominent buttocks; hip flexion contractures; tight hamstrings. *Diagnostic tests:* Spinal curvature is assessed by looking at the standing child from the side. Lumbar lordosis is confirmed by visualizing the spine on standing, and by lateral radiograph.	*Medical therapy:* Treatment focuses on exercises and postural awareness. Bracing and surgery are rarely prescribed. *Nursing management:* Provide support. Reassure the child and family that the condition is often outgrown as the child matures. Encourage physical conditioning exercises and follow-up examinations on a yearly basis.

associated with aging. However, children can have **osteoporosis** (also known as metabolic bone disease or a bone mineral density more than 2.5 standard deviations below the norm) related to imbalanced nutrition or other pathologic conditions. Osteoporosis is preceded by **osteopenia** or low bone mass which is between 1 and 2.5 standard deviations below the norm (National Institute of Arthritis and Musculoskeletal and Skin Diseases, 2009).

Etiology and Pathophysiology

Very-low-birth-weight infants who are premature often have osteopenia of prematurity because much of their bone mass is usually acquired in the latter weeks of pregnancy. In addition, they may have other health problems after birth and be unable to ingest enough nutrients to meet metabolic needs for bone growth. Prematures are often less active than other infants which decreases the amount of mechanical loading on their bones, a factor known to increase bone resorption and decrease bone mass (Harrison, Johnson, & McKechnie, 2008).

A group of children who may show signs of osteoporosis are those who have decreased mechanical loading. Children with spina bifida or cerebral palsy, conditions that interfere with ambulation, have limited pressure on bones and lowered bone mass in affected extremities and the spine. Other conditions associated with lower bone mass include Turner syndrome, growth hormone deficiency, osteogenesis imperfecta, juvenile rheumatoid arthritis, and diabetes. Children treated for some types of cancer have increased rates of osteoporosis. Children who are treated for disorders or injuries with casting and bracing are also at high risk of osteoporosis due to immobilization. See Figure 35–16 ■ for other effects of immobility on body systems.

Lastly, adolescence is a period when adequate intakes of calcium and vitamin D are needed to maximize bone formation and prevent osteoporosis later in life. Adolescents, particularly females, often do not meet the Recommended Dietary Allowance (RDA) for these nutrients and are at risk for osteoporosis even though it may not be manifested for years. Other lifestyle patterns of youth that decrease bone formation are smoking, alcohol use, and keeping weight at a very low level. Those with anorexia nervosa are at risk for osteoporosis and have an increased lifetime risk for fractures (Mehler, Cleary, & Gaudiani, 2011).

Clinical Manifestations

Osteoporosis is a silent disease, as is its precursor osteopenia; those who have the disorders are often without signs or symptoms for

years. The problem may become apparent when a baby or child has a fracture and radiologic studies make the problem evident.

Collaborative Care

All health professionals should partner with parents and children to increase awareness of the silent and insidious disease of osteoporosis. The goal of care is to prevent the disease in all youth and to direct special attention to those conditions that may contribute to its occurrence.

Diagnostic Tests

Bone mineral content and density are measured by single-photon absorptiometry (SPA), dual-photon absorptiometry (DPA), or DEXA; ultrasound may be used to assess preterm infants (Rack, Lochmuller, Janni, et al., 2011). Although uncommonly used, serum studies such as bone-specific alkaline phosphatase, phosphorus, and type I collagen can be used to measure osteoblastic and osteoclastic activity. Recall that over 90% of the body's calcium is stored in bone, so serum calcium is not reflective of bone density.

Clinical Therapy

Premature newborns at risk of osteopenia of prematurity need collaborative management by neonatologists, neonatal nutritionists, and neonatal nurses. Breast milk is enhanced by adding special fortifiers; premature formula should be used rather than regular baby formula. When infants need enteral or parenteral feedings, calcium to phosphorus ratios are carefully balanced to enhance osteoblastic activity. Extremity range of motion for very-low-birth-weight newborns may decrease bone loss in the period after birth. Assisted range of motion exercise decreases loss of bone strength and enhances bone health in low-birth-weight premature infants (Chen, Lee, Tseng, et al., 2010).

For older children at risk of developing osteoporosis, calcium and vitamin D intake is encouraged and oral supplements may be given. Standing therapy for those who are nonambulatory can provide mechanical weight and enhance bone density. Bisphosphonates, calcitonin, fluoride, and parathyroid hormone may be used to treat children and adolescents with osteoporosis (Cheung, 2009). When a cast or other immobilizing device is removed from a child, a program of gradually increasing exercise in collaboration with physical rehabilitation professionals promotes bone strengthening and lowers the risk for fractures or related sequelae.

Pathophysiology Illustrated   Effects of Immobility

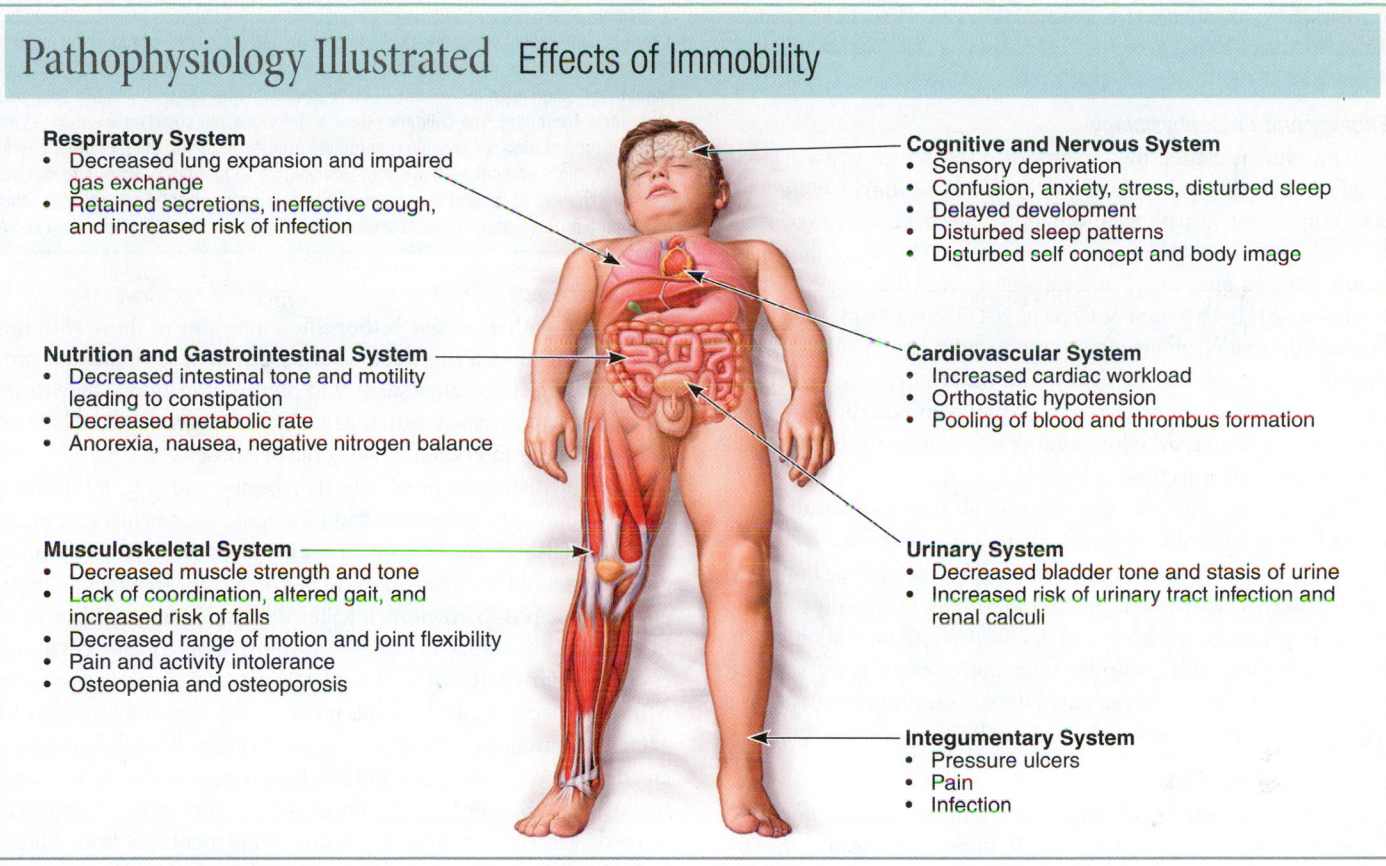

Respiratory System
- Decreased lung expansion and impaired gas exchange
- Retained secretions, ineffective cough, and increased risk of infection

Nutrition and Gastrointestinal System
- Decreased intestinal tone and motility leading to constipation
- Decreased metabolic rate
- Anorexia, nausea, negative nitrogen balance

Musculoskeletal System
- Decreased muscle strength and tone
- Lack of coordination, altered gait, and increased risk of falls
- Decreased range of motion and joint flexibility
- Pain and activity intolerance
- Osteopenia and osteoporosis

Cognitive and Nervous System
- Sensory deprivation
- Confusion, anxiety, stress, disturbed sleep
- Delayed development
- Disturbed sleep patterns
- Disturbed self concept and body image

Cardiovascular System
- Increased cardiac workload
- Orthostatic hypotension
- Pooling of blood and thrombus formation

Urinary System
- Decreased bladder tone and stasis of urine
- Increased risk of urinary tract infection and renal calculi

Integumentary System
- Pressure ulcers
- Pain
- Infection

FIGURE 35–16 ■ The effects of immobility on the body involve all systems.

Nursing Management

The goal of nursing care is to prevent osteopenia, osteoporosis, and resultant fractures in all children, from newborns through adolescence and on into adulthood.

Nursing Assessment and Diagnosis

Nurses identify newborns, children, and adolescents at risk of developing low bone mass and density. This is accomplished by identifying diseases putting the child at risk. Ask about exercise and activity patterns, and physical therapy for children who are nonambulatory. Dietary intake is measured periodically for all youth at health promotion visits, and RDAs for calcium, phosphorus, and vitamin D are compared to the child's intake.

Nursing diagnoses that may apply to the child with osteoporosis include the following:

- Nutrition, Imbalanced: Less than Body Requirements related to inability to consume essential nutrients
- Injury, Risk for related to decreased bone mass and density
- Health Maintenance, Ineffective related to inadequate dietary intake

NANDA-I © 2012

Planning and Implementation

Perform dietary analysis of children at risk (see Chapter 19 🖱 for detailed methods for diet assessment). Refer children at risk to nutritionists and physicians for further education and diagnosis. Suggest referrals to physical rehabilitation to recommend weight-bearing exercise. Administer nutritional supplements when prescribed and teach families how to give these medications. Partner with families to provide therapy that stimulates weight bearing for children who are nonambulatory. Teach parents how to recognize fractures in children who may not have normal sensation and are unable to report them. Edema, unusual shape of a limb, fussiness of the child, and falls should be reported promptly.

Effects of Immobility

When osteoporosis is due to immobility, many other symptoms occur as well. Be alert for these problems, and integrate physical activity in care as much as possible to minimize their effects. All organ systems, such as respiratory, gastrointestinal, cardiovascular, urinary, and integumentary, are affected by immobility. Including range of motion as tolerated and allowed, changing body position frequently, and providing diversionary activities are examples of nursing care strategies used to minimize effects of immobility.

Evaluation

Expected outcomes for the child with a potential for osteoporosis include adequate intake of recommended amounts of nutrients, absence of fractures, and normal findings on studies of bone mineral content and density.

Osteomyelitis

Osteomyelitis is an infection of the bone, most often one of the long bones of the lower extremity. It may be acute or chronic and may spread into surrounding tissues. Although osteomyelitis may occur at any age, it is most common in children between the ages of 1 and

12 years. Boys are affected two to three times as often as girls, primarily because they have a greater incidence of trauma. Overall incidence is 5 in 10,000 youth (Thomsen & Creech, 2011).

Etiology and Pathophysiology

Osteomyelitis is caused by a microorganism, which is usually bacterial but can be viral or fungal. *Staphylococcus aureus* is the most common causative pathogen; others include *Escherichia coli*, *Neisseria meningitidis*, *Streptococcus pneumoniae*, *Mycobacterium tuberculosis*, *Borrelia burgdorferi*, and *Kingella kingae* (Bautista, Gholve, & Dormans, 2011; Thomsen & Creech, 2011). See Chapter 22 🔗 for further information about community-acquired methicillin-resistant *Staphylococcus aureus* (CA-MRSA) and other infections. Trauma to the bone or surgical interventions are other common causes of infection. Osteomyelitis may follow another infection in the body, such as upper respiratory infection.

The infecting organism spreads through the bloodstream or via a penetrating injury to the bone, where it becomes established. Infections in children often begin in the metaphysis of long bones (see Figure 35–1), which has a sluggish blood supply. Eventually the infection may penetrate the bone cortex and periosteum. Inflammation and abscess formation can lead to interruption of the blood supply to the underlying bone, involvement of the surrounding soft tissue, and, if the infection is left untreated, necrosis (Box 35–6).

Clinical Manifestations

Symptoms include constant bone pain, edema, decreased mobility of the infected joint or bone, and fever. Redness over the area may occur. The child may refuse to walk or may limp. Because the onset of acute osteomyelitis is generally rapid, it is sometimes misdiagnosed as a sports injury.

Collaborative Care

The goal of treatment is eradication of the causative organism and prevention of any complications or long-term sequelae from the infection.

Diagnostic Tests

A history suggestive of osteomyelitis includes an upper respiratory infection or blunt trauma followed by pain at the area of a growth plate. Laboratory evaluation shows leukocytosis and an elevated erythrocyte sedimentation rate (ESR) and C-reactive protein. Radiographs, MRI, and bone scans may identify the area of involvement. A needle aspiration of the site or a blood culture can confirm the diagnosis and provide a culture of the causative organism. Other studies may be carried out depending on the history. Examples include enzyme-linked immunosorbent assay (ELISA) for Lyme antibody titer, antistreptolysin-O for recent streptococcus infections, or purified protein derivative (PPD) for exposure to tuberculosis (Thomsen & Creech, 2011).

BOX 35–6	**Growth & Development: Osteomyelitis and Newborns**

Osteomyelitis in a newborn is of great concern because the blood vessels cross the growth plates before 18 months of age. This creates a higher risk of epiphyseal involvement with resultant limb length discrepancy and other problems. Be alert for the newborn who exhibits poor feeding, fussiness when moved, or refusal to move a limb. Fever and other signs of infection are less often seen in newborns.

Clinical Tip

Children can present with elevated temperature and bone pain due to many causes. Nurses are instrumental in performing ongoing history and assessments that augment those taken upon admission. Such "detective" work can assist in the diagnosis and proper treatment. The child may have an infection, but could have cancer, Lyme disease, tuberculosis, or juvenile rheumatoid arthritis. Can you think of other conditions that might present as bone pain? Investigate all laboratory work and discuss the combination of laboratory abnormalities and assessment findings with other healthcare professionals. What assessments will provide clues to proper diagnosis?

Clinical Therapy

In children with extensive orthopedic surgery, or in those with immunosuppression, a short course of prophylactic antibiotic is commonly administered after surgery to prevent infection. Three doses are generally prescribed, with the first before surgery and the last two at 8- to 12-hour intervals following the first dose.

Medical management of infection begins with the intravenous administration of a broad-spectrum antibiotic, even before culture results are available. Because *S. aureus* is a common cause of infection, the antibiotic should be effective against this organism. Treatment is influenced by the possibility of methicillin-resistant *S. aureus* (MRSA), so intravenous antibiotics are usually vancomycin or clindamycin, drugs effective against MRSA. (See Chapter 22 🔗 for further discussion of MRSA.) Once the culture results are obtained, the antibiotic may be altered. Intravenous antibiotics may be changed to oral forms once an adequate response has occurred. However, extended intravenous home therapy may be used. Antibiotic therapy continues for about 3 to 6 weeks. The cause of infection is not always identified from culture so ESR and C-reactive protein are followed carefully in these cases to identify if treatment is successful. When an adequate response to antibiotic is not obtained within 2 to 3 days, the area may be aspirated again, or surgical drainage may be performed. Intravenous fluids may be administered to ensure adequate hydration. Prompt diagnosis and treatment usually result in complete resolution of the infection. The prognosis is related to the initiation of therapy—the earlier treatment begins, the better the outcome. Long-term unfavorable outcomes include disruption of the growth plate, which can interrupt growth, damage the joints from septic arthritis, and cause recurrent infection.

Nursing Management

The goals of nursing management include early identification of osteomyelitis and careful monitoring for outcomes of treatment.

Nursing Assessment and Diagnosis

A thorough history, including information about the onset of symptoms and a history of recent infections or trauma, is essential. Ask about immunization status, especially tetanus. Assess the affected area for signs of redness, swelling, pain, and decreased range of motion. Measure vital signs; increased temperature and pulse in particular may provide clues about worsening infection.

Nursing diagnoses that may apply to the child with osteomyelitis are as follows:

- **Pain, Acute** related to biologic injury
- **Mobility: Physical, Impaired** related to discomfort
- **Infection, Risk for** related to spread of infection throughout the body
- **Nutrition, Imbalanced: Less than Body Requirements** related to anorexia
- **Knowledge, Deficient** related to long-term intravenous therapy

NANDA-I © 2012

Planning and Implementation

Nursing management focuses on performing cultures and obtaining blood samples, administering antibiotics, protecting the child from spread of the infection, and encouraging generous amounts of fluid and a well-balanced diet. Standard precautions should be used, with transmission-based precautions for any drainage from the site of infection.

Obtain Cultures and Blood Work

Blood cultures and cultures of any open wound must be performed before the first dose of antibiotic when osteomyelitis is suspected. Treatment may then begin, even before the results of the cultures are available. Obtain continuing blood samples as needed to monitor ESR and C-reactive protein.

Administer Fluids and Medications

Administer intravenous fluids as ordered to maintain the hydration status of the child. Offer oral fluids that will encourage oral intake by affected young children. Antibiotics are administered intravenously at first, then orally. Monitor the intravenous site and provide care for the central line, if used (refer to the Skills Manual ⬭). In the early stages of the infection, analgesics are prescribed to relieve the associated pain and joint tenderness.

Protect from the Spread of Infection

Strict aseptic technique and transmission-based precautions should be used during all dressing changes. Children and family members should avoid direct contact with any dressings or drainage. Teach good hygiene practices, including hand washing, to maintain infection control. Take vital signs and evaluate the child frequently for symptoms indicating the spread of infection (e.g., increasing pain, difficulty breathing, increased pulse rate, or fever).

Encourage a Well-Balanced Diet

Educate both the child and the parents about healthy dietary choices that promote the healing process. Providing a high-protein diet and extra vitamin C will contribute to this process. Encourage increased fluid intake to provide adequate hydration and circulation.

Discharge Planning and Home Care Teaching

Emphasize the importance of completing the full course of antibiotic therapy, especially for children who have undergone surgical drainage of an abscess or lesion. Some children may be discharged on intravenous antibiotics if the family is willing to learn the procedure for medication administration and care of the central line. Several sessions of demonstration and return demonstration are needed to ensure safe administration. If the family is unable to perform antibiotic therapy, a home infusion company may be available to come to the home and administer the medication. Explain that failure to follow the prescribed antibiotic therapy may result in chronic infection. Emphasize the importance of returning for blood analysis to monitor progression of healing.

Consider the child's age and developmental level, and partner with the family to plan quiet activities and access to schoolwork if the child will be immobilized at home. If the child is homebound during treatment, assist the family in planning for completion of school tasks.

- Contact the school and ask that work be sent home.
- Arrange for a tutor if needed.
- Facilitate computer communication between the child, teacher, and other students.
- Help family members to plan for help at home, to monitor the child when they are at work or to perform other tasks.
- Refer to financial resources as appropriate for the services the child needs.
- Suggest activities that the child can do at home to foster developmental progression.

Evaluation

Expected outcomes of nursing care for the child with osteomyelitis include the following:

- There are no signs of infection or sepsis.
- The child completes the prescribed course of antibiotics.
- Intake of fluids and nutrients is adequate for good health.
- The child's pain is effectively managed.
- The child is able to return to normal activities of daily living.

Skeletal Tuberculosis and Septic Arthritis

Skeletal tuberculosis (Figure 35–17 ■) and septic arthritis are two infections that, although infrequent, may affect children and adolescents. See the Clinical Manifestations table for diagnostic tests and medical and nursing management for these infections.

Osgood-Schlatter Disease

Osgood-Schlatter disease is an inflammation of the proximal tibial physis as it inserts into the patellar tendon. The condition is painful and is associated with repeated stress on the site resulting from sports such as hockey, gymnastics, or basketball. The child presents with knee pain centered at the tibial tubercle, particularly during sporting

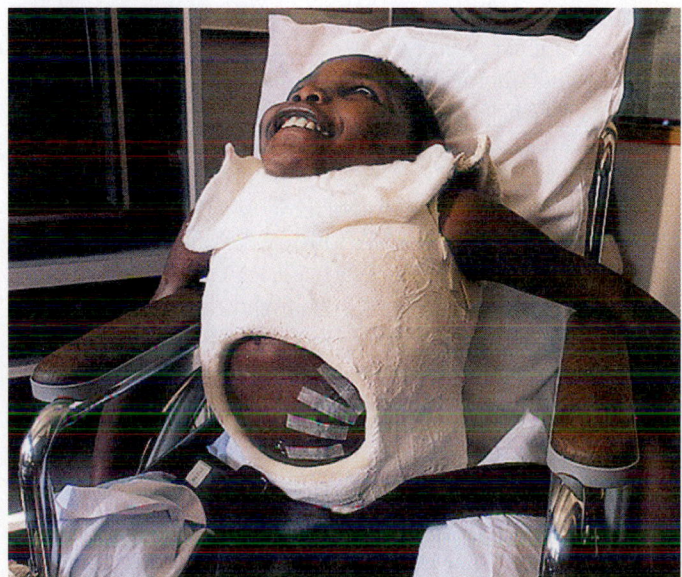

FIGURE 35–17 ■ This boy from Kenya had surgery to correct severe kyphosis and scoliosis, caused by tuberculosis of the spine. A Risser cast has been applied to maintain stability of the spine and thoracic cage during healing. Notice the area cut out of the cast to allow for auscultation of the abdomen, as well as to facilitate the child's comfort and adequate intake of food.

Clinical Manifestations Treatment of Skeletal Tuberculosis and Septic Arthritis

CONDITION	CLINICAL MANIFESTATIONS	DIAGNOSTIC TESTS AND CLINICAL THERAPY	NURSING MANAGEMENT
Skeletal Tuberculosis Rare mycobacterial infection that can be destructive. The spine is the most frequent site of infection (Pott disease), with joints and other sites sometimes affected.	Depending on the site, pain, limp, severe muscle spasms, kyphosis, muscle atrophy, "doughy" swelling of joints, decreased joint motion, changes in reflexes, low-grade fever.	*Diagnostic tests:* Diagnostic studies include tuberculosis skin test, complete blood count (CBC), synovial fluid analysis, and radiographs of affected limb or joint. *Clinical Therapy:* Antibiotic therapy (using a combination of drugs) for 6–9 months is the treatment of choice. The affected site is immobilized. Disease may become resistant to these drugs, and additional drug therapy may be necessary.	Educate the child and family about the disorder, and stress the importance of complying with long-term antibiotic therapy. Test all members of the family for tuberculosis. Report the disease to the local health department. Facilitate the immobilization and physical therapy of the child at home.
Septic Arthritis Joint infection of the synovial space most often caused by *Haemophilus influenzae, Staphylococcus,* and *Streptococcus.* The most common site of infection is the knee, followed by the hip, ankle, and elbow. Most common in children less than 3 years of age.	Fever, pain and local inflammation, joint tenderness, swelling, loss of spontaneous movement. Infant may be irritable, cries when handled, refuses food.	*Diagnostic tests:* CBC with differential, ESR, blood cultures. Diagnosis is made based on joint aspiration findings. Results are commonly 100,000 white blood cells (WBCs) and 75% neutrophils, ESR greater than 44 mm/hr. Radiographic changes may not be evident until later in the disease process. *Clinical Therapy:* This is a medical emergency requiring prompt treatment to avoid permanent disability. Treatment involves joint aspiration, open drainage, and irrigation, followed by intravenous antibiotic therapy for 3–4 weeks and then oral antibiotics. If the full course of antibiotic treatment is not completed, the child risks recurrent infection and further degeneration of the infected joint.	Educate the child and family about the disorder and emphasize the importance of proper antibiotic therapy. Carefully position the painful joint. Administer antibiotics as prescribed. Use transmission-based precautions. Encourage fluids to ensure adequate hydration. Support and rest the joint; provide activities that do not require joint movement.

activities (Weiler, Ingram & Wolman, 2011). Swelling or prominence of the tubercle may be present. The condition is observed in preadolescents and adolescents. The condition is diagnosed by its history, localization of pain, and radiographs.

Osgood-Schlatter disease is treated conservatively by resting the limb from vigorous activity for several weeks. Anti-inflammatory medications may provide comfort. Exercises to stretch and strengthen the quadriceps may be helpful. Wrapping the knee during activities and application of ice after can be recommended. If the condition does not improve, a brace to immobilize the knee or physical therapy may be helpful. After several weeks the condition generally improves. It may recur while growth continues but disappears after full growth has occurred.

Nursing management consists of recognizing recurrent knee pain and referring for diagnosis so that Osgood-Schlatter can be differentiated from other abnormalities such as Legg-Calvé-Perthes disease, slipped capital femoral epiphysis, osteomyelitis, and arthritis. Explain to the family the chronic nature of Osgood-Schlatter during the growth period and the need to rest the limb for several weeks to decrease the inflammation. Teach the child to wrap the knee and apply ice after activities resume.

Achondroplasia

Dwarfism is a genetic condition usually resulting in an adult height of 58 inches or less. The most common cause of dwarfism is achondroplasia which causes short arms and legs. The torso and head are approximately normal size, but decreased growth of long bones causes short stature. This is known as disproportionate short stature. Achondroplasia is caused by an abnormal gene of chromosome 4 and occurs in 1 in 10,000 to 30,000 births (Baujat, Legeai-Mallet, Finidori,

et al., 2008). The gene is coded to produce proteins called fibroblast growth factor receptors. When fewer receptors are produced the cells cannot respond normally to signals from growth factors. Achondroplasia occurs as a new genetic mutation with no previous family history (80% of cases), or can occur when one or both parents are also dwarfs. There are other less common forms of dwarfism, with about 200 identified types. Most children with the disorder inherit the gene from one parent. Since only one affected gene must be present for manifestation of the disorder, it is a dominant characteristic (review as needed the genetic transfer described in Chapter 4 ☞). When a child inherits two copies of the gene from two affected parents, a fatal form of achondroplasia occurs which is characterized by a small thorax, respiratory failure, and death in infancy.

Children with achondroplasia have short legs and arms, short fingers with a separation between the middle and ring fingers, and a large, prominent forehead. Hydrocephalus sometimes occurs in children with achondroplasia (see Chapter 33 ☞ for a description of hydrocephalus).

Children with the disorder are diagnosed prenatally, at birth, or shortly after. When there is a family history, genetic testing before or after birth identifies the presence of the fibroblast growth factor receptor 3 (FGFR3) gene on chromosome 4. Characteristics common in the growth disorder during childhood include short fingers, frequent otitis media, dental malocclusion, bowing of legs, sleep apnea, and marked lordosis. The child may be slow at meeting gross motor developmental milestones. Low back and leg pain are common as the child grows into adulthood. Usually adult males are about 4 feet tall. Perhaps the greatest challenge for families is helping the child to establish a positive self-image in a society that values tall height.

There is no treatment for the disorder at this time. Gene therapy and growth plate targeting are being explored as possible treatments for the future (Laederich & Horton, 2010). Some children and adults with dwarfism have undergone limb-lengthening procedures, described later in this chapter. Other orthopedic interventions may be needed to treat back pain or bone problems. For those children who develop hydrocephalus, insertion of a shunt to divert excess fluid may be needed. Treatment of conditions such as otitis media and malocclusion of teeth is provided.

Nursing Management

Nurses play an important role in helping families when a child is diagnosed with achondroplasia. If a parent is a dwarf or a family has a positive history of dwarfism, genetic counseling should be offered prenatally. Explain findings of testing and provide assistance with decision making about pregnancy if needed. Nurses assist parents who have a child with achondroplasia to adjust to the diagnosis, particularly if the parents have had no previous experience with the condition. They may feel guilt and anxiety; contact with other families who have children with achondroplasia can be a supportive intervention.

Nurses help the child with achondroplasia to develop a positive self-concept during childhood. Many resources are available that provide suggestions about how to foster a positive self-concept, adjust the home to facilitate the child with dwarfism, and assist the child with adjustments in school settings. Partner with school nurses to ensure the child's successful inclusion in all school facilities. An individualized education plan (IEP) will likely be needed. Frequent otitis media and related disorders may create a need for adaptation in communication methods. While some families decide to explore limb-lengthening procedures, most organizations encourage a focus placed on development of a healthy self-image rather than limb lengthening.

Nurses provide careful assessments of children throughout childhood. Head circumference is especially important in early childhood to identify hydrocephalus if it should occur. Carefully evaluate growth with specialized growth grids for achondroplasia, evaluate dental health at each visit, and perform developmental assessment with special emphasis on gross motor skills. Refer for care for otitis media and provide postoperative care if tympanostomy tubes are inserted (see Chapter 24 ⊘). Refer to dentists and orthodontists and encourage regular dental care. Assess nutritional intake and engage teaching to improve diet if needed.

Assist the family by providing resources to help with planning for car safety seats. As the child grows older, focus on methods of adjusting the home (light switches, counters, toileting, etc.) and partnering with the school to provide a supportive atmosphere for the child. Helpful organizations include Little People of America, Dwarf Athletic Association of America, Human Growth Foundation, Magic Foundation for Children's Growth and Related Adult Disorders, and March of Dimes. Review at each visit the support groups the family is using, and make additional suggestions as needed.

As the child grows, suggest activities that foster physical and social development. Swimming and biking provide activity with little stress on bones. Investigate the physical education program in the school and suggest appropriate activities for integration in which the child with achondroplasia can participate. As the youth grows into adolescence, assist the family with plans for transition to independent living. Driving will require adaptations to a car. Attending college, moving to an apartment, or taking a job will all require adaptations.

Marfan Syndrome

Marfan syndrome is another example of a condition inherited in an autosomal dominant manner. About 1 in 5,000 to 10,000 children are affected with the syndrome which manifests with several conditions of connective tissue (Gonzales, 2009). The most common problems are cardiac (mitral valve prolapse, aortic regurgitation, aortic aneurysm, abnormal aortic root dimensions), skeletal (pectus excavatum, long arms and digits, scoliosis, elongated head, high arched palate), ocular (lens subluxation or dislocation), and respiratory (pneumothorax). The woman with Marfan syndrome has an increased risk of complications during pregnancy, primarily due to the extra requirements placed on the heart.

The average age for diagnosis is 3 years, with a heart murmur the usual finding. Careful assessment identifies additional characteristics of the condition along with a positive family history. Diagnosis is made after a complete family history, a detailed physical examination, an eye examination, a thorough heart examination, radiographs of the chest, and MRI or CT.

There is no treatment for the syndrome, which causes abnormal formation of fibrillin matrix in connective tissue. Early diagnosis can be successful in treating the cardiac abnormalities with medication or surgery to prevent dissection of the aorta, the major cause of death. However, diagnosis in children is often difficult because many features of Marfan syndrome are not apparent until adolescence. Surgery may be needed to correct scoliosis, pectus excavatum, or pneumothorax. Careful monitoring throughout life is needed to prevent and treat abnormalities associated with the disorder.

Nursing management of Marfan syndrome begins with identification of infants and children with symptoms of the disorder. Once diagnosed, collaboration with a cardiologist, ophthalmologist, and orthopedist is needed throughout life. The child may require surgery for one or more conditions, can require antibiotics during elective procedures or dental care if the mitral valve is affected, and needs echocardiogram and other cardiac studies regularly. The nurse may need to explain the disorder to the family and provide referrals for genetic counseling. The child needs support during childhood to learn about the disorder and to manage the medication and monitoring required.

Osteogenesis Imperfecta

Osteogenesis imperfecta, also known as brittle bone disease, is a connective tissue disorder that primarily affects the bones. Children with this condition have fragile bones that are more likely to fracture. Osteogenesis imperfecta (OI) occurs in 1 in 10,000 to 15,000 live births and affects boys and girls equally. Prognosis depends on the type of disease, as described in this section.

Etiology and Pathophysiology

The underlying disorder is a biochemical defect in the production of collagen. The disease is genetically transmitted, generally in an autosomal dominant inheritance pattern, although some types are transmitted in a recessive pattern. The most common types are caused by mutations on the COL1A1 or COL1A2 genes on chromosomes 17 and 7, respectively (Online Mendelian Inheritance in Man, 2008).

Clinical Manifestations

Clinical manifestations include multiple and frequent fractures; blue sclerae; thin, soft skin; increased joint flexibility; enlargement of the anterior fontanel; weak muscles; soft, pliable, brittle bones; and short stature. Most children with OI are short in stature and may have

Weblink · Achondroplasia Resources

decreased range of motion in several joints. Conductive hearing loss can occur by adolescence or young adulthood due to changes in the bones of the inner ear.

The disease is classified into four major phenotypes, with several other minor types recently identified (Starr, Roberts, & Fischer, 2010). In type I disease, the most common form, children have fragile bones, blue sclerae, weakened tooth dentin, and hearing loss that manifests in adolescence. In type II disease, the ribs and skeleton are extensively involved; most children with this form of the disease die in utero or shortly after birth. Type III disease is identified in the newborn period or in infancy when the child sustains numerous fractures and manifests blue sclerae. Severe bone fragility and kyphoscoliosis are observed. Most children with type III disease die in childhood as a result of cardiorespiratory failure. Type IV disease is characterized by fractures without other symptoms of the disease. Bowing of the legs and other structural deformities can occur; however, the incidence of fractures decreases beginning in puberty.

Collaborative Care

There are many goals for the child and family with osteogenesis imperfecta. Genetic counselors work with the family to explain the transmission. Physicians perform surgery and ongoing management. Nurses and physical rehabilitation unite to plan for health promotion, physical activity, and developmental stimulation. Nurses partner with the school for an individualized education plan.

Diagnostic Tests

Improved knowledge about the genetic transmission of this disease means that some cases of osteogenesis imperfecta can be identified before birth using ultrasound, collagen analysis of chorionic villus cells, or genetic testing. In many cases, however, diagnosis of osteogenesis imperfecta is made only when the child has a delay in walking or sustains a fracture. Radiographic evaluation may detect both old and new fractures.

Clinical Tip

Multiple fractures in various stages of healing may be seen in infants or young children with both child abuse and osteogenesis imperfecta. Collect data to assist in determining the cause. Ask about family history of diseases, stress to the family, and other pertinent factors.

Tests such as DEXA can be used to measure bone density. Serum alkaline phosphatase may be elevated; other measures of bone metabolism such as serum osteocalcin, procollagen 1 C-terminal peptide, collagen 1 teleopeptide, and urine deoxypyridinoline may be performed to measure effects of experimental medication.

Clinical Therapy

There is no cure for osteogenesis imperfecta. Medical management consists primarily of fracture care and prevention of deformities. The goal is to maximize the child's independence and mobility while minimizing the risk of fractures. Treatment includes physical therapy; casting, bracing, or splinting; surgical stabilization; nutritional management with high vitamin D and calcium; and bisphosphonate medication such as pamidronate. Health supervision that includes dental examinations and hearing screening is important. Surgery to insert telescoping rods in long bones may be helpful to stabilize bones. Hematologic stem cell transplant has been used successfully in some children with severe osteogenesis imperfecta

---

BOX 35–7	Research: Pamidronate

Pamidronate is a bone resorption inhibitor that absorbs calcium phosphate crystals in bone and is used in adults to treat hypercalcemia of cancer and Paget disease. It is now being used and studied in children with osteogenesis imperfecta. Low-dose medication is given intravenously or orally. Density of lumbar bones has improved in children receiving the medication, and fractures and pain are lessened in some studies (Bishop, 2010; Castillo & Samson-Fang, 2009).

and is under further investigation (Jethva, Otsuru, Dominici, et al., 2009) (Box 35–7).

Nursing Management

Nursing care is primarily supportive and focuses on educating the parents and child about the disease and its treatment.

Nursing Assessment and Diagnosis

The child with OI is assessed carefully and frequently for signs of fractures. Ask about the child's favorite activities since these will need to be integrated into plans for physical activity and developmental progression. Perform careful growth measures and developmental screening.

Nursing diagnoses that may apply to the child with OI include the following:

- Injury, Risk for related to learning to walk and other developmental tasks
- Nutrition, Imbalanced: Less than Body Requirements related to increased needs to heal from fractures
- Walking, Impaired related to frequent immobility and bone changes

NANDA-I © 2012

Planning and Implementation

Nursing care focuses on fostering safety and minimizing the chance of fractures; encouraging healing of fractures; reducing pain; supporting the family during the management of this chronic condition; providing care when surgery is required, along with rehabilitation after surgical interventions; ensuring health promotion visits, including dental and hearing screenings; and fostering normal growth and development.

Foster Safety

To prevent fractures, children with osteogenesis imperfecta must be handled gently. The trunk and extremities should be supported when the child is moved. Tasks such as bathing and diapering may cause fractures and should be performed carefully. Newborns and infants are at particular risk. Use a blanket or pillow under the child for additional support when lifting and moving the child. Do not pull the legs upward when changing a diaper as this can cause a fracture. Instead, slip a hand under the hips to raise the child, sliding the diaper carefully in, and then bringing it up as the legs are slightly abducted.

Partner with families to provide safe activities for the child. Discourage contact sports and other activities that are likely to lead to fractures.

Encourage Healing

Children commonly have several fractures during childhood. The period of immobility and casting causes further bone breakdown due to decreased mechanical loading, further increasing the chance of fracture. The child should eat a well-balanced diet with additional vitamin C, vitamin D, and calcium to encourage healing and bone growth. Calories should be limited to maintain weight at recommended levels since immobility can lead to overweight and the child is generally short for age. Partner with parents if the child is receiving experimental bisphosphonate medication, so that doses are properly administered and serum/urine samples are obtained for monitoring.

Family Support

The family may have been suspected of child abuse before the disease was diagnosed, and they should be given an explanation about the similar presenting symptoms if this occurred. Parents should be offered access to genetic counseling.

Parents may initially feel guilt or anger about the diagnosis. As time progresses and they focus on care of the child, they must deal with the disappointment that occurs with each fracture, and a rehabilitation period after. The Osteogenesis Imperfecta Foundation provides information about the disease and can put families in touch with others who have the disease.

For parents who have a child with type II or III OI, the terminal nature of the condition necessitates psychologic support, linkage to potential resources, and assistance with managing other tasks of family life (see Chapters 16, 17, and 18 🔗 for management of chronic conditions and end-of-life care). The siblings and extended family will need support to understand the disease and deal with their feelings and the affected child.

Surgical Care and Rehabilitation

When the child needs a fracture stabilized in surgery, or is having rods inserted to strengthen bones, surgical care management is important. Assess the child's vital signs and growth measurements. Obtain accurate weight before surgery and again after with the cast in place. Administer fluids and use pain control techniques such as medication and other comfort measures. Be alert for signs of infection such as osteomyelitis, or respiratory or urinary tract infection. Begin fluids and perform dietary teaching before discharge to promote intake that fosters healing. Follow activity orders precisely to minimize safety hazards for the child. Partner with physical and occupational therapists to plan rehabilitation for the child's return to home and school, and to ensure the family can perform range of motion exercises and other therapies. Ensure that the family has an approved car safety seat to transport the child.

Foster Normal Growth and Development

Ensure health promotion visits with special emphasis on growth measurement, nutrition, immunizations, and screening for dental or hearing problems. Emphasize the importance of maintaining normal patterns of growth and development. Toddlers should be helped to explore and interact safely in their environment. Socialization is essential during the school-age and adolescent years. Encourage exercise, such as swimming, to improve muscle tone and prevent obesity. Independent functioning is promoted by the use of adaptive equipment and motorized wheelchairs. Maintenance of function can depend on proper rehabilitation services. The nurse can arrange and manage such services for the family. If the child is hospitalized or must remain out of school for a period of time, partner with the family to provide for continuing learning at home and for safe transition back to the school setting.

Evaluation

Expected outcomes for the child with osteogenesis imperfecta include the following:

- The child experiences minimal fractures with optimal healing.
- The child maintains normal range of motion and activity levels.
- A normal weight and a diet rich in vitamins and calcium is maintained.
- The child meets expected developmental milestones.
- The family receives adequate information, resources, and support.

MUSCULAR DYSTROPHIES

The muscular dystrophies are a group of inherited diseases characterized by muscle fiber degeneration and muscle wasting. These disorders can begin early or late in life, and onset can be at birth or gradual. They are all terminal disorders, but the progression can vary from a few to many years.

Etiology and Pathophysiology

Many types of muscular dystrophies affect children and adults. The most common form of childhood muscular dystrophy is Duchenne muscular dystrophy (pseudohypertrophic), which occurs in 1 per 3,500 live male births (Wagner, 2008). **Pseudohypertrophy** refers to enlargement of the muscles as a result of their infiltration with fatty tissue. The gene for Duchenne muscular dystrophy was identified in 1987; it is carried in the Xp21.2 region of the chromosome and is either absent or deleted in affected children. This area codes for a protein called dystrophin which is needed as a muscle membrane stabilizer. In the absence of dystrophin, a cascade of cellular events occurs, leading to necrosis in the fibers and their replacement by connective tissue. Since this is an X-linked disorder, it is seen only in males. There is similar incidence in various ethnic groups.

Becker muscular dystrophy is also X-linked and affects 1 in 30,000 males (Becker Muscular Dystrophy, n.d.). Although the gene mutation is similar to Duchenne, it is milder in form. Other rare muscular dystrophies manifest in infancy, later childhood, or adolescence. There are a variety of genetic mutations ranging from X-linked to autosomal.

Clinical Manifestations

Clinical manifestations vary with type of disease. With Duchenne muscular dystrophy, muscle weakness begins in the lower extremities in early childhood. Children compensate for weak lower extremities by using the upper extremity muscles to raise themselves to a standing position (Gowers maneuver) (Figure 35–18 ■). The parents may notice the child tripping, toe walking, and displaying enlargement of the calf muscles. In fact, the calf is not enlarged but muscle is replaced by connective tissue. By the middle teen years, the child's condition has usually progressed so that walking is not possible. The disease progresses up the body, potentially causing conditions such as scoliosis, other musculoskeletal conditions, cardiomyopathy, difficulty ingesting foods, and respiratory distress. Fractures may occur when the child falls due to weakness. Becker dystrophy is similar but emerges later and more slowly.

The dystrophies of infancy are manifested by generalized weakness and hypotonia. The infant may have difficulty with sucking and

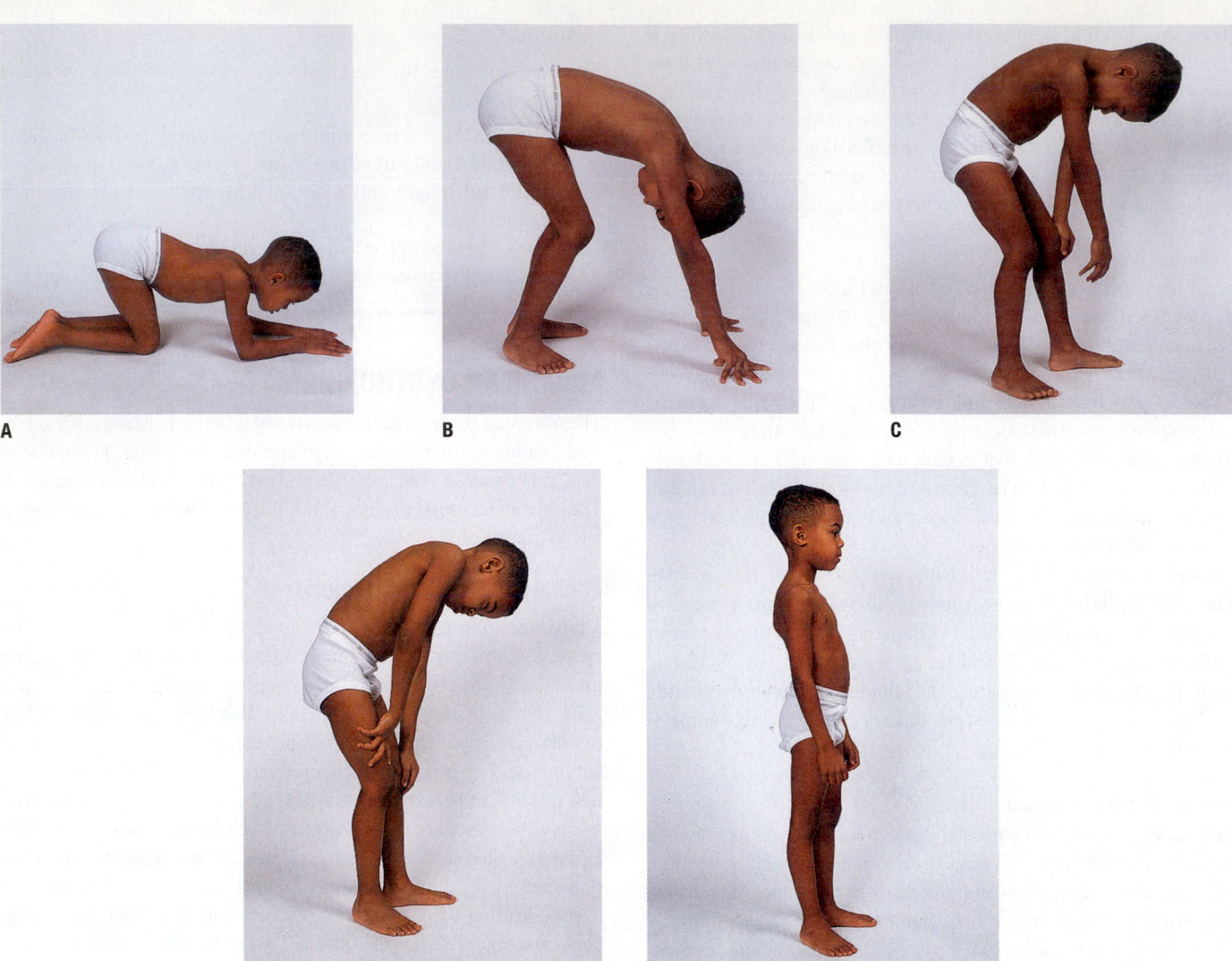

FIGURE 35–18 ■ Because the leg muscles of children with muscular dystrophy are weak, they must perform the Gowers maneuver to raise to a standing position. *A* and *B,* The child first maneuvers to a position supported by arms and legs. *C,* The child next pushes off the floor and rests one hand on the knee. *D* and *E,* The child then pushes himself upright.

swallowing; ocular problems may be present. Adolescent-onset disease is generally milder and slower to progress. Some individuals may live into middle adulthood. See the Clinical Manifestations table for some of the more common muscular dystrophies of childhood.

Collaborative Care

The goal of medical management is to provide support and prevent complications such as infection or spinal deformities.

Diagnostic Tests

Diagnosis and classification are most often based on clinical signs and the pattern of muscle involvement. Biochemical examinations such as serum enzyme assay, muscle biopsy, and electromyography confirm the diagnosis. Serum creatine kinase (CK) is elevated early in the disease. Dystrophin, the muscle protein that is deficient in muscular dystrophy, can be measured by muscle biopsy. Genetic testing establishes the specific abnormality and type of disease present. Testing of newborns may be offered to families who have one child with the disease since this helps some families to adapt and prepare for the care the child will need. Respiratory function is measured periodically with pulmonary function tests and overnight pulse oximetry.

Clinical Therapy

There is no effective treatment for childhood muscular dystrophy. At the present time, research is directed at several techniques to repair mutations by gene therapy, override the genetic error to produce dystrophin, and apply stem cell therapy (Goyenvaile, Seto, Davies, et al., 2011). The steroids prednisone and deflazacort may preserve muscle function, preserving walking and pulmonary function for a longer period (Wagner, 2008).

Progressive weakness and muscle deformity result in chronic disability (Figure 35–19 ■). Respiratory infections are vigorously treated with deep breathing, coughing, nebulizer treatments, and antibiotics. Comprehensive and regular cardiac evaluations are recommended. Surgery may be used to correct scoliosis developing from the disease in order to facilitate lung expansion. Rehabilitative therapy is needed to maximize independence and physical activity, and to decrease hazards of immobility (see Figure 35–16).

Children and families can benefit from mental health support due to the progressive and terminal nature of the disease. The team approach to managing the child with muscular dystrophy ensures collaborative partnering of parents with all health professionals

Clinical Manifestations Muscular Dystrophies of Childhood

TYPE OF DYSTROPHY	CLINICAL MANIFESTATIONS	CLINICAL THERAPY
Duchenne muscular dystrophy X-linked recessive disorder seen in boys (on Xp21 gene); however, 30–50% of affected children have no family history. Onset: within the first 3–4 years of life.	Delayed walking; frequent falls; easily tired when walking, running, or climbing stairs; toe walking, hypertrophied calves; waddling gait; lordosis; positive Gowers maneuver; intellectual disability frequently seen.	Supportive care; physical therapy and braces to help maintain mobility and prevent contractures. Most children are wheelchair bound by 12 years of age; death commonly occurs during young adulthood from respiratory or cardiac failure.
Becker muscular dystrophy X-linked recessive disorder. Onset: usually after 5 years.	Symptoms are similar to those of Duchenne muscular dystrophy, but milder and delayed; child is mobile until late teens; normal intelligence; congestive heart failure; contractures.	Supportive care, same as for Duchenne muscular dystrophy. Slow progression; death usually occurs by 30–50 years of age.
Facioscapulohumeral muscular dystrophy Autosomal dominant disorder (on 4q35 chromosome). Onset: later childhood and adolescence.	Face, shoulder girdle, lower limbs affected; unable to raise arms over head; lordosis; cannot close eyes, whistle, smile, or drink from a straw because of inability to move face; characteristic appearance includes facial weakness, winging of the scapulae, thin arms, well-developed forearms.	Physical therapy. Slow progression; confined to wheelchair as older adult, but usually attains normal life span.
Emery-Dreifuss muscular dystrophy X-linked recessive disorder (on Xq28 gene). Onset: childhood.	Early onset of contractures followed by weakness; Achilles tendon, elbow, and spine affected; muscle weakness in upper body follows, with lower body weakness occurring later; cardiac conduction defect may occur.	Physical therapy; surgery; pacemaker insertion.
Congenital muscular dystrophies Autosomal recessive group of disorders. Onset: present at birth.	Muscle weaknesses present at birth; motor development delay; contractures and joint deformities; hypotonia.	Correction of skeletal deformity (orthosis or surgery). Usually nonprogressive.

and a comprehensive management plan. Team members should include parents, the child when able, physicians (pediatrician, orthopedic surgeon, neurologist), nurses, physical and occupational therapists, a nutritionist, a psychologist or mental health therapist, and a social worker.

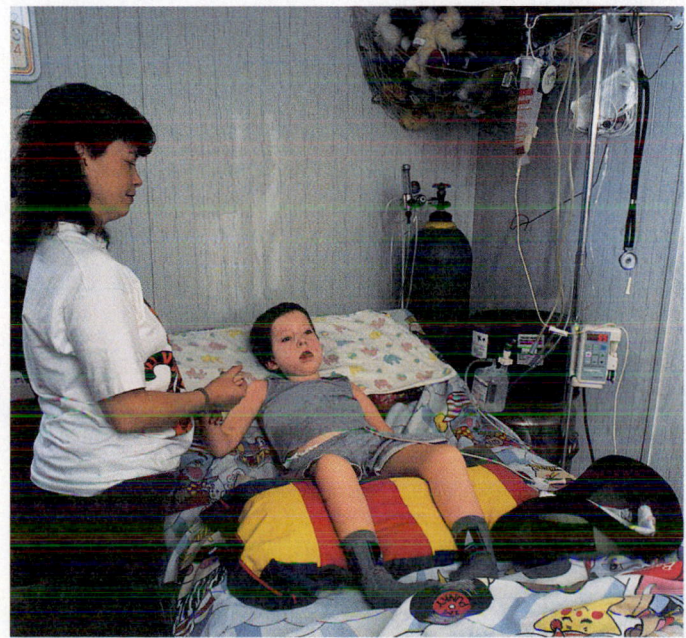

FIGURE 35–19 ■ This young boy with muscular dystrophy needs to receive tube feedings and home nursing care. He attends school when possible and is able to use an adapted computer.

Nursing Management

Nursing care focuses on promoting independence and mobility and providing psychosocial support that helps the child and family deal with this progressive, incapacitating disease. Nearly all body systems become involved in the care required, and emotional care is important for the child and family.

Nursing Assessment and Diagnosis

Monitor all vital signs as well as cardiac and respiratory functioning. Assess urinary function and frequency of bowel movements. Periodically measure strength and range of motion. Assess mobility via ambulation or assisted device. Perform periodic developmental and nutritional assessments. Meet with teachers to evaluate the child's learning needs and functional level in the classroom. Evaluate the family's risk and protective factors for dealing with this chronic and fatal disorder.

Nursing diagnoses that may apply to the child and family with muscular dystrophy include the following:

- Caregiver Role Strain due to increasing dependence of child on care
- Activity Intolerance related to weakness
- Anxiety, Hopelessness, and Powerlessness (Child and Family) related to diagnosis of terminal disease
- Coping: Family, Compromised related to a family member with chronic disease and worsening condition
- Infection, Risk for related to impaired respiratory system and stasis in urinary system
- Constipation, Risk for related to immobility

- Nutrition, Imbalanced: Less than Body Requirements related to inability to ingest adequate nutrients
- Grieving (Child and Family) related to terminal illness

NANDA-I © 2012

Planning and Implementation

Care for the child with muscular dystrophy is usually long term and offers challenges to maintain both physical and emotional health of the entire family. Periods of crisis occur when the child is diagnosed and at any time the condition worsens. Nurses often provide home healthcare services to such children, work with them in school nursing positions, and partner with parents in clinics and other facilities to provide health promotion and maintenance as the child grows; this is often a close and meaningful relationship for the child, family, and nurse. See the Health Promotion & Maintenance Overview for detailed nursing activities. Provide other therapies to maintain function of body systems and support the family as needed (see Legal and Ethical Considerations: Muscular Dystrophy Care).

Maintenance of Body Systems

Ensure that regular cardiac and respiratory evaluations are performed by specialists in those fields. Administer oxygen or respiratory therapy as ordered. Soft foods or enteral tube feedings may be needed to promote nutrition. The infant with dystrophy of infancy may need gavage feedings. Maintain bowel function with fluids, high-fiber foods, and medications as needed. Monitor and ensure adequate fluid output. Watch for signs of infection. Perform range of motion and provide for physical activity to level of ability. Physical therapy helps the child ambulate and prevents joint contractures. It is important to provide good back support and posture by keeping the child's body in alignment when confined to a wheelchair. Splints may be needed to maintain extremities in the proper position.

Child and Family Support

Perform periodic developmental assessments and provide parents with suggestions for encouraging the child's development. Arrange a conference with family members and teachers to evaluate the child's cognitive performance and learning needs and to determine educational goals. An individualized education plan should be established. Partner with the school to provide tutors or home computers if needed. Young children should be enrolled in early intervention programs before they are old enough for school.

Encourage the child to be independent for as long as possible. Concentrate on what the child can accomplish, and do not ask the child to complete tasks that may prove frustrating. Reading books to the child, listening to tapes, and watching television offer the child stimulation during hospitalization. Exercise as tolerated contributes to muscle strength and a general sense of well-being.

Families may be challenged by the care the child needs. Surgery, hospitalization for respiratory infection, transportation of the child in a wheelchair, visits to physical therapy, and constant daily care are examples of the challenges faced. Managing this care, providing a nurturing environment for other children and family members, and obtaining necessary financial resources over many years creates a need for assistance from various resources. Refer the family to respite care, assist them in finding resources, and be certain that either a family member or health professional acts as case manager to coordinate various services needed. Refer family members to resource and support groups such as the Muscular Dystrophy Association. Ask what treatments they are using and what is helpful to the child and family (see Complementary Therapy: Muscular Dystrophy).

Weblink | Muscular Dystrophy Association

Legal and Ethical Considerations
Muscular Dystrophy Care

The child with muscular dystrophy has a shortened life span. Parents provide comprehensive care and require support both physically and emotionally as the child's condition progresses. The child continues to develop in many ways, especially cognitively, as the years pass. Therefore, the needs for explanation and ability to understand the diagnosis change for the child over time. Parents may have difficulty initiating discussions with the growing child about desire for end-of-life care (Penner, Cantor, & Siegel, 2010). An ethical approach to care demands that such a complex chronic disease be managed by an interdisciplinary team that collaborates on a regular basis. The child, family, and a variety of health, social, and educational professionals should all be part of the team. The plan of care will include physical, emotional, cognitive, and palliative care; it will evolve and change as the child grows older. Nurses are essential members of the team and may work with families as team managers.

Parents may exhibit feelings of guilt and hopelessness. The mother who learns she has carried the gene that affects her son can be devastated. Encourage parents to express their feelings. Genetic counseling is recommended for the entire family, and it is especially important to identify women who are carriers of one of the X-linked disorders. Siblings may feel neglected because their brother or sister is receiving so much attention. They may be concerned that they will develop the disease. Sometimes multiple children in a family are affected with the condition and as one child worsens, the effect on siblings is profound. On the other hand, siblings without the disease may feel guilty for their good health. Encourage the parents to involve siblings in the affected child's care to reassure them of their importance. (See Chapter 16 ⚓ for ideas about involvement of siblings in care.)

As the child's condition weakens, the family again needs additional support. They experience grieving, each person in their own way. They have lived with chronic sorrow and now need to prepare for the child's death. The child is usually old enough to recognize the deteriorating condition. See Chapter 18 ⚓ for further discussion of bereavement and end-of-life care.

Evaluation

Expected outcomes of nursing care for the child with muscular dystrophy include maintenance of optimal mobility and development, positive self-image for the affected child, and positive management of the emotional challenges by all family members.

Complementary Therapy
Muscular Dystrophy

Many families who have a child with muscular dystrophy use different types of complementary care. The nurse always assesses for such approaches, provides information as needed by the family, makes recommendations for complementary therapies that may be helpful, and cautions against those that could be harmful due to interactions with medications or other problems. Common complementary care used in muscular dystrophy includes dietary enhancement. This enhancement includes vitamins A, C, E, D, and B-complex; minerals such as calcium, magnesium, zinc, and selenium; probiotic supplement; omega-3 fatty acids; herbal remedies such as green and rhodiola rosea teas; muscular and immunologic enzymes such as coenzyme Q10, N-acetyl cysteine, acetyl-L-carnitine, creatine, and L-theanine; melatonin to promote sleep; and massage to assist with reduction of muscle spasms (University of Maryland Medical Center, 2011).

Health Promotion & Maintenance Overview

The Child with Muscular Dystrophy

The child with muscular dystrophy needs close monitoring and intervention to foster growth and development in spite of a chronic and terminal disease. The nurse in health promotion can assist the child and family in many ways.

GROWTH AND DEVELOPMENT SURVEILLANCE

- Perform developmental screening of the young child.
- Refer to early intervention programs that establish educational plans to foster development.
- Provide resources and ideas for the parents based on the child's status rather than expected age norms.
- Measure growth at each healthcare visit and plot on growth grids. Be alert for the child who is gaining weight due to decreased activity in order to avoid overweight.
- Ensure visits with specialists in respiratory medicine and cardiology as recommended.

NUTRITION

- Perform 24-hour analysis and evaluate for all essential nutrients. Base the analysis on the child's height and weight rather than chronologic age.
- Ask about appetite and food likes and dislikes.
- Encourage adequate fluid, whole grains, fruits, and vegetables to maintain bowel function.
- For the infant with muscular dystrophy, evaluate intake carefully; gavage feeding or nutritional supplementation such as with high-calorie formula may be needed.

PHYSICAL ACTIVITY

- Carefully monitor physical ability at each visit. Observe for decreases in movement, difficulty ambulating, or a history of falls.
- Partner with physical therapists to ensure range of motion and proper positioning of extremities.
- Explore activities that the child can do as mobility decreases. Swimming and upper body exercise may be good options.
- If the child is using a wheelchair, evaluate fit, safety, and ability to move the chair by arm controls.
- Physical activity should be regular and daily. Ensure that the family has resources to accomplish this need.

ACTIVITIES OF DAILY LIVING

- Partner with occupational therapy to evaluate the child's ability to feed, bathe, dress, and provide own oral care. Provide adaptive devices as needed.
- Encourage the family to provide time for the child to perform self-care as much as possible.
- Make a home visit or discuss with the family adaptations that could make it easier for the child to be independent in activities of daily living. Low drawers for clothing, or open shelves that do not require pulling out to get items are examples of important adaptations.

MENTAL AND SPIRITUAL HEALTH

- Inquire about the child's general mood.
- Ask the parents what is best and worst about their lives at this time. Use the information to establish a list of their meaningful activities and to identify the areas most in need of support.

- Ask about sources of support such as a group for parents of a child with muscular dystrophy, family participation in faith-based activity, and extended family or neighbors.
    - Be alert for signs of depression in the child or family (see Chapter 34).
    - Assist the family to establish activities to increase self-esteem in the youth. The youth should be able to make choices appropriate for developmental age.
    - If the child was diagnosed at a younger age, ask what the parents have told him or her about the disease. Provide support and role-playing opportunities for parents who wish to tell the child about the terminal nature of the disorder.
- Refer for services such as genetic counseling, grief counseling, or other supportive interventions.

RELATIONSHIPS

- Ask about siblings and their relationship with the child with muscular dystrophy.
- Inquire about the child's participation in early intervention or school programs and community groups. Refer the family to resources that encourage the child's interactions with peers. This is particularly important for teens.
- Ask the parents if and how often they are able to spend time with other adults.

DISEASE PREVENTION STRATEGIES

- Immunize the child at recommended times. If the child is ill and immunization is delayed, be sure to call the family back promptly to reschedule administration of vaccines so that infectious diseases can be avoided. Annual influenza vaccine is needed. If the child is treated with steroids for the disease, follow recommendations for immunization of children on steroids.
- Teach the family to avoid crowds and known infectious persons. The child may need to be out of school for a few days or weeks if there is an influenza or other disease outbreak in the school population.
- Teach the family signs of infection, especially of the respiratory tract. Have them report these symptoms promptly.
- Monitor effects of antibiotics when administered for infection.
- Encourage daily activities that encourage deep breathing. Swimming, blowing into an incentive spirometer, or playing with a pinwheel are examples.

INJURY PREVENTION STRATEGIES

- Inquire about whether the family has an emergency evacuation plan for the child in case of house fire or other emergency. Assist them to develop a plan.
- If the child is using oxygen, teach about fire safety.
- When mechanical ventilation is used at home, help the family establish emergency backup systems for power outage, such as portable generators.
- Assist the family to learn proper body mechanics to safely transfer and provide care for the child.

Clinical Manifestations Strains, Sprains, and Dislocations

CONDITION	CLINICAL MANIFESTATIONS	CLINICAL THERAPY
Strain ■ Stretching or tearing of either a muscle or a tendon, usually from overuse (e.g., back strain resulting from improper or overly heavy lifting, shoulder and elbow tears from baseball).	■ Vary according to the type and severity of the strain. Pain can be acute or chronic.	■ Rest and support of the injured part until the muscle or tendon heals and normal activity can occur.
Sprain ■ Stretching or tearing of a ligament, usually caused by a fall, sports injury, or motor vehicle crash (e.g., anterior cruciate ligament [ACL] tear is a severe sprain requiring reconstruction).	■ Edema, joint immobility, and pain.	■ For the first 24–36 hours: Rest Ice Compression Elevation ■ After the first 24–36 hours, mobility is gradually increased.
Dislocation ■ Complete displacement of an articular joint surface, usually associated with a fall, sports injury, or motor vehicle crash. Although almost any joint may be dislocated, most dislocations occur in the shoulder, knee, and hip.	■ Pain and tenderness, swelling and obvious deformity, and instability of the joint.	■ Varies according to the site and severity of the injury, and consists of: Shoulder: Open or closed reduction followed by the application of a sling. Knee: Closed reduction with gentle traction, then immobilization with a splint. Hip (posterior): Immediate closed reduction or possibly open reduction, traction, or hip spica cast. Hip (anterior): Immediate closed reduction, extension traction, and hip spica cast.

INJURIES TO THE MUSCULOSKELETAL SYSTEM

Musculoskeletal injuries are classified according to the mechanism, location, and force of the injury. Strains, sprains, dislocations, and fractures are the most common musculoskeletal injuries in children. Distinguishing among these injuries is often difficult. Athletic participation and injuries in car crashes are frequent causes of strains, sprains, dislocations, and fractures. (See Evidence-Based Practice: Backpacks and Pain.) Serious injuries affecting the brain and spinal cord are discussed in Chapter 33. See the Clinical Manifestations table for descriptions of strains, sprains, and dislocations. A detailed discussion of fractures follows.

Fractures

A fracture is a break in a bone that occurs when more stress is placed on the bone than the bone can withstand. Fractures, which may occur

Evidence-Based Practice   Backpacks and Pain

PROBLEM

Many children wear backpacks that are heavy and carry them for large parts of the day. Low back, neck, and shoulder pain are prevalent in children, and a possible connection with backpacks has been suggested (Talbott, Bhattacharya, Davis, et al., 2009).

EVIDENCE

Several studies have investigated the relationships between backpack use and complaints of pain. One study found that carrying a backpack over one shoulder, having heavier backpacks, and carrying the pack lower rather than higher were associated with greater back and shoulder pressure (Macias, Murthy, Chanbers, et al., 2008). Postural angle and lumbar curvature are altered by heavy backpacks (Neuschwander, Cutrone, Macias, et al., 2010; Ramprasad, Alias, Raghuveer, 2010). Another study found that younger students and females were more prone to injury from heavy backpacks. No more than 10% of body weight should be carried in a backpack (Bauer & Freivalds, 2009).

IMPLICATIONS

An association between backpack use and weight and complaints of pain appears to be evident, especially among females. Therefore, nurses should ask about backpack use at health promotion visits and advise on how to wear them. The American Academy of Pediatrics and North American Spine Society list recommendations for backpack use:

■ Have wide, padded shoulder straps and wear the pack on both shoulders, close to the body.
■ Use a padded back and waist strap.
■ Be sure the backpack is lightweight (no more than 10% to 15% of the youth's weight) or consider a rolling pack if it is heavy.
■ Practice back-strengthening exercises and learn to bend at the knees when lifting objects.

CRITICAL THINKING APPLICATION

How will you partner with youth who are in sports after school to plan how to carry school items and sports gear safely? What exercises can you plan to help strengthen the back and thighs for carrying a pack? What children are most at risk for back pain from heavy backpacks (consider gender and weight)?

at any age, occur frequently in children because their bones are less dense and more porous than those of adults.

Etiology and Pathophysiology

Fractures in children may result from direct trauma to a bone (falls, sports injuries, abuse, motor vehicle crashes) or bone diseases (osteogenesis imperfecta) that cause weakening of the bone. Children with osteoporosis or osteopenia are more prone to fractures (see description of these conditions earlier in the chapter). Trauma may be caused by an acute injury, direct and forceful impact, or overuse such as in chronic and repetitive activities. Due to their porous nature, the bones of children may bow, leading to more common greenstick or spiral fractures (Table 35–3). Child abuse is a cause of fracture and should be suspected when the type of fracture is uncommon for a given age. For example, femur fractures are most common at 2 to 3 years and in adolescence; a femur fracture in an infant is suggestive of the possibility of abuse. In the opening scenario of this chapter, Douglass experienced an acute injury when his leg forcefully hit the trampoline frame, suffering a closed fracture of the fibula (Box 35–8).

Clinical Manifestations

Signs and symptoms of fractures vary depending on the location, type, and nature of the causative injury. Fractures are generally characterized by pain, abnormal positioning, edema, immobility or decreased range of motion, ecchymosis, guarding, and crepitus. Childhood fractures most often involve the clavicle, tibia, ulna, and femur, with distal forearm fractures of the radius or ulna the most common type. Fractures to the pelvis are often associated with motor vehicle crashes. Stress fractures are most common in the tibia, fibula, metatarsals, and calcaneus (Custer & Rau, 2009). Epiphyseal (growth plate) injuries are dangerous in children as they can interfere with future growth at the site. Types of fractures are described using the Salter-Harris classification system (Figure 35–20 ■).

Collaborative Care

Emergency care focuses on accurate diagnosis, pain management, and establishment of a treatment plan. Medical management consists of two basic steps: reduction to realign displaced or fragmented bones, and immobilization so that healing can take place. Some fractures have sides that are properly aligned and no reduction is needed.

Diagnostic Tests

Radiographs are useful for determining the exact location and type of fracture. However, in very young children the higher amounts of collagen and cartilage make diagnosis by radiograph challenging at times. Examination and palpation of the area by a skilled clinician is essential.

Clinical Therapy

Immobilization is essential for the bone healing process to take place. A closed reduction aligns the bone by manual manipulation or traction. Sedation and additional pain management techniques are used during closed reduction. An open reduction requires surgical alignment of the bone, often using pins, plates, wires, or screws. For open

TABLE 35–3	Common Fractures	
FRACTURE TYPE	**DESCRIPTION**	**COMMENTS**
Closed	Bone breaks cleanly but does not penetrate the skin.	Also called a simple fracture.
Open	Broken ends of bone protrude through soft tissues and skin.	Serious; may result in osteomyelitis. Also called a compound fracture.
Comminuted	Bone fragments into many pieces.	Common in those with conditions causing brittle bones, such as osteogenesis imperfecta.
Compression	Bone is crushed.	Common in patients with osteoporosis.
Impacted	Broken ends of bone are forced into each other.	Commonly results from falls; also common in hip fracture.
Depressed	Broken bone is pressed inward.	Common in skull fractures.
Spiral	Jagged break due to twisting force applied to bone.	Common fracture due to sports injuries.
Greenstick	Bone breaks incompletely, much in the way a green twig breaks.	Common in children, whose bones have proportionally more organic matrix and are more flexible than those of adults.

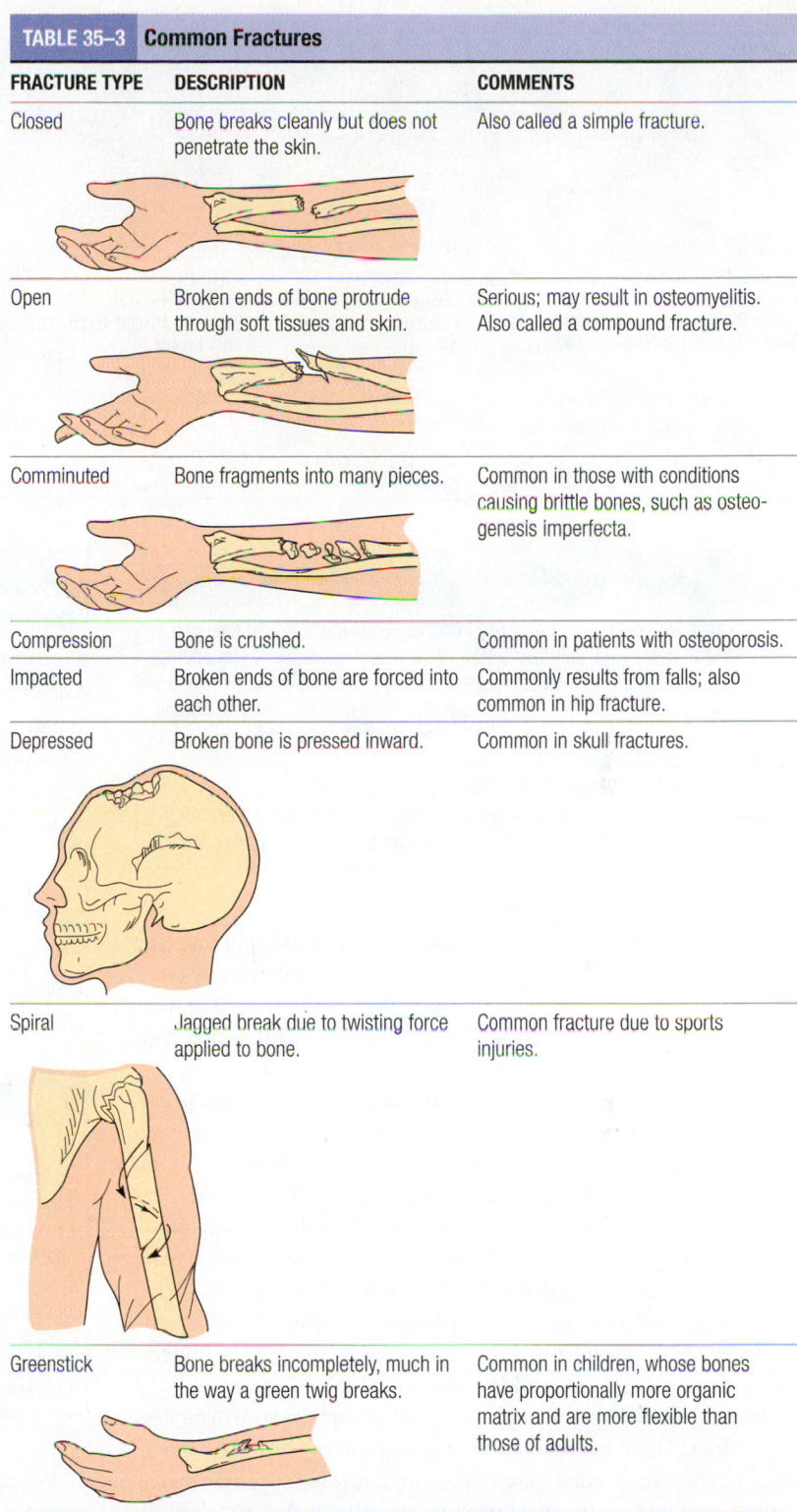

Source: *Drawings adapted from Marieb, E. N. (1998). Human anatomy and physiology (4th ed., p. 180). Menlo Park, CA: Benjamin Cummings.*

fractures, surgery must also be performed for debridement, to remove dead tissue and clean the wound. Casting is the most common external method of immobilization. Casts may be placed on extremities (short or long leg or arm cast) or the upper body to immobilize the spine, or may be applied from chest to legs to stabilize the pelvis or hips (hip spica cast). Leg casts may be walking or nonwalking casts. Cast material is either plaster or a synthetic fabric. Other

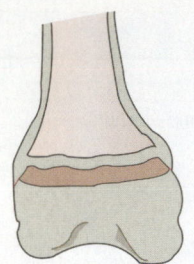

Type I
Common
Growth plate undisturbed
Growth disturbances rare

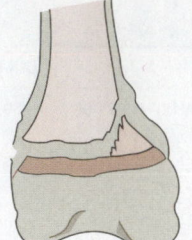

Type II
Most common
Growth disturbances rare

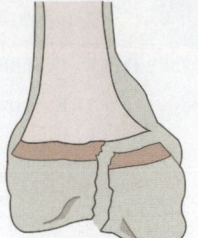

Type III
Less common
Serious threat to growth
and joint

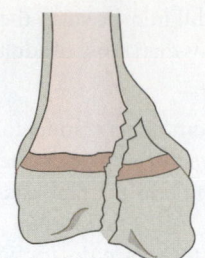

Type IV
Serious threat to growth

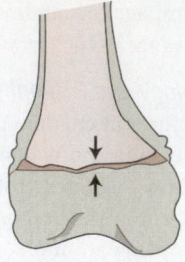

Type V
Rare
Crush injury causes cell death in
  growth plate, resulting in
  arrested growth and limited
  bone length
If growth plate is partially
  destroyed, angular deformities
  may result

FIGURE 35–20 ■ The Salter-Harris classification system is based on the angle of the fracture in relation to the epiphysis.

BOX 35–8	Growth & Development: Stress Fractures

Stress fractures occur more frequently in adolescents and are most common in females and those who limit their intake of calories and calcium in an attempt to remain lean for sports such as distance running, cheerleading, or gymnastics (Field, Gordon, Pierce, et al., 2011). These fractures may present with chronic pain that changes in intensity. Be alert to this possibility when teenagers' diets and athletic activities place them at risk.

The risk of bone fractures is increased with high cola consumption and television viewing time and with lower levels of physical activity and lower milk intake. Assess for these health risks and teach preventive diet and activity patterns.

---

external methods of stabilization include traction and splinting (see Table 35–5 on page 1292 for types of traction). Pins may be inserted to stabilize the fracture, and can be used with or without casts or traction. A combination of treatments may be needed in the child with multiple fractures following a car crash or other trauma.

Healing of fractures is influenced by factors including age, size of the involved bone, and fracture site. The healing process progresses from cartilaginous callous formation to bone remodeling and bony callous formation (Figure 35–21 ■ on page 1290). Fractures heal more quickly in children than in adults, because the periosteum or vascular outer layer of bone is thicker and remains intact even during a fracture (American Academy of Orthopaedic Surgeons, 2010). This blood supply enhances the healing process. Immobilization is essential for the bone healing process to take place. If a fracture is properly reduced, complications should be minimal (Table 35–4).

Fractures involving the epiphyseal plate disrupt the growth process in children. These injuries require ongoing care to evaluate for outcomes such as limb length discrepancy, joint incongruity, and angular deformities. Further surgery or treatment may be needed in such cases.

Nursing Management

The goals of nursing management are early identification and immobilization of fractures, and providing care to promote safety during the healing process.

Nursing Assessment and Diagnosis

Assess the diets of all youth who might be at risk for fractures, and insert dietary teaching in health promotion visits. Ask about sports and other activities that might lead to injury (Box 35–9).

TABLE 35–4	Complications of Fracture Reduction
COMPLICATION	**CLINICAL THERAPY**
Infection Acute (may occur with open fractures) Chronic (osteomyelitis)	Debridement, drainage, culture, and treatment with antibiotics
Neurovascular injury resulting from physical nerve damage	Nerve repair
Vascular injury	Vascular repair, amputation, tendon lengthening
Malunion (undesired healed alignment of bone) or delayed union	Corrective osteotomy; prolonged immobilization
Nonunion	Surgical intervention; internal fixation
Leg length discrepancy	Shoe lift

BOX 35–9	Research: Heelys, Wheelies, and Street Gliders

Children generally love to move fast and explore new shoe technology. A trend currently popular among youth is wheeled shoes. These shoes alter normal gait and may lead to injury; fractures of the radius are the most common injury. Protective gear, though recommended, is usually not worn by injured children. Teaching is needed so that children who get the shoes wear protective gear (helmet, wrist guards, knee pads, and elbow pads) and practice in safe areas before wearing the shoes to other environmental settings (Beach, Garcia Pena, & Linares, 2009; Norem, Feuerstein, Traverso, et al., 2009; Thing, Wade, & Clark, 2008). Do you see children in your clinical practice area using wheeled shoes? Design a program to provide needed information to children and their parents.

When dealing with an injured child, be alert to the signs and symptoms of fractures before moving the child. Try to identify the cause of the injury by asking the child, parents, or other family members what happened.

Clinical Tip

When in doubt about the nature of an injury, apply a splint. Splinting immobilizes the site, prevents further damage, and decreases pain. Be sure to immobilize both the joints directly above and directly below the injury.

Evaluate pain, swelling, and any abnormal positioning of the injured area. When a child is admitted to the emergency department or hospital, nursing assessment includes the extent of the injury, the degree of pain, and the child's vital signs (respiratory status, pulse, blood pressure).

The following nursing diagnoses may apply to the child with a fracture:

- Pain related to injury
- Skin Integrity, Risk for Impaired related to treatment
- Infection, Risk for related to open fracture or trauma
- Mobility: Physical, Impaired related to treatment
- Knowledge, Deficient related to lack of information about treatment and expected outcome

NANDA-I © 2012

Planning and Implementation

Nurses may be in community settings when children experience a fracture, and need to provide emergency care and arrange for transport. Emergency personnel are informed of the assessment data to provide for safe care. In addition, nurses are aware that repeated fractures in the same child can be a sign of other healthcare conditions.

Practice Alert

It is uncommon for children to have repeated fractures. If they occur, make further assessments for their cause. The child may have osteogenesis imperfecta. If attention deficit hyperactivity disorder (ADHD) is present or if the child has a mental health problem, excessive risky behavior may be the cause of fractures. When children are found on radiograph to have several old and healing fractures, or multiple fractures of the same or different bones, they may be victims of physical abuse, particularly if the caretaker explanation of fracture does not match the clinical picture. An example could be the parent who claims the child fell from a chair, but there is a severe arm fracture and skull fracture. See Chapter 20 for a description of child abuse and Chapter 34 for a discussion of ADHD.

Nursing care focuses on care of the child before and after fracture reduction, encouraging mobility as ordered, maintaining skin integrity, preventing infection, and teaching the parents and child how to care for the fracture. If sedation or pain blocks are used, nursing care for these procedures is needed. When caring for a child who has undergone fracture reduction, it is important to be aware of the signs of complications (see Table 35–4). Notify the physician immediately if these signs occur. The major serious complication is **compartment syndrome,** or a condition of increased pressure in a limited space such as the soft tissue of an extremity, which compromises circulation and nervous innervation (Wright, 2009). See the Clinical Manifestations table. Compartment syndrome is a medical emergency and needs to be reported immediately to the primary healthcare provider or medical personnel on hand. Have a cast cutter available so the cast can be removed if needed.

Maintain Proper Alignment

Immobilization is used to maintain proper alignment of the fracture. Casts and traction are methods used for immobilizing an injured child. Cast care guidelines are included on page 1258.

Different types of traction are used, depending on the location and type of fracture (Table 35–5). Nursing care for the child in traction is described in Box 35–10.

Monitor Neurovascular Status

Neurovascular assessment is used for early detection of compartment syndrome, which may occur with a crush injury or when a fracture is reduced. Swelling associated with inflammation reduces blood flow to the affected area, and casting causes further constriction of blood

Clinical Manifestations	Compartment Syndrome
CLINICAL MANIFESTATIONS	**ASSESSMENT**
Clinical manifestations begin about 30 minutes after tissue ischemia starts. Major manifestations are: - Paresthesia (tingling, burning, loss of two-point discrimination) - Pain (unrelieved by medication, characterized by crying in the young child) - Pressure (skin is tense, cast appears tight) - Pallor (pale, gray, or white skin tone) - Paralysis (weakness or inability to move extremity) - Pulselessness (weak or absent pulse)	Check extremities for: - Color - Temperature - Capillary refill - Peripheral pulses (can be checked with Doppler when available) - Edema - Sensation - Motor ability - Pain

Document results and report changes or abnormal results immediately.

Source: Data from Custer, J. W., & Rau, R. E. (Eds.). (2009). The Harriet Lane handbook. Philadelphia, PA: Mosby Elsevier; Wright, E. (2009). Neurovascular impairment and compartment syndrome. Paediatric Nursing, 21(3), 26–29.

flow. Douglass, in the opening scenario, had a splint applied for several days, with casting later, to allow swelling to decrease and to minimize risk for compartment syndrome. Monitor the child's sensation to touch, temperature, movement, strength of the pulse, and capillary refill time in the extremity distal to the injury. Monitor every 15 minutes after the cast is applied for at least 2 hours and then every 1 to 2 hours, depending on the care facility's policy and the child's condition. Keep the cast elevated above heart level to minimize edema.

Promote Mobility

The amount of mobility the child is allowed is ordered by the physician. Restrictions depend on the extent and site of the fracture. Fractures of the hip or pelvis may involve body casts, and providing wheeled carts makes mobility possible. Children with leg fractures can sometimes bear weight on the cast. If they cannot bear weight, they move around with crutches, walkers, or wheelchairs. See the Skills Manual for information on crutch walking.

Discharge Planning and Home Care Teaching

Most fractures can be easily managed at home. Activities are generally limited for approximately 8 weeks. Teach the parents and child cast care, activity restrictions, and how to identify problems that should be reported (see page 1259). Help parents to identify any modifications that may be needed at home and school. The child who has to manage steps at home or school may need special training with crutches or a temporary ramp. Refer parents to home health nurses or home teaching services if indicated. Provide pertinent teaching to prevent future injuries.

While every healthcare encounter is a time to promote safe activity practices for youth, an injury provides a special opportunity to share safety information with the family. The American Academy of Pediatrics has a number of policy statements such as *Boxing Participation by Children and Adolescents, Baseball and Softball, Bicycle Helmets,* and *In-Line Skating Injuries in Children and Adolescents.* Similarly, the American Academy of Orthopaedic Surgeons has policy statements on topics such as *Trampolines and Trampoline Safety* and *The Risks of Shoulder and Elbow Injury from Participation in Youth Baseball.* The

Weblink | American Academy of Pediatrics

Pathophysiology Illustrated Process of Bone Healing

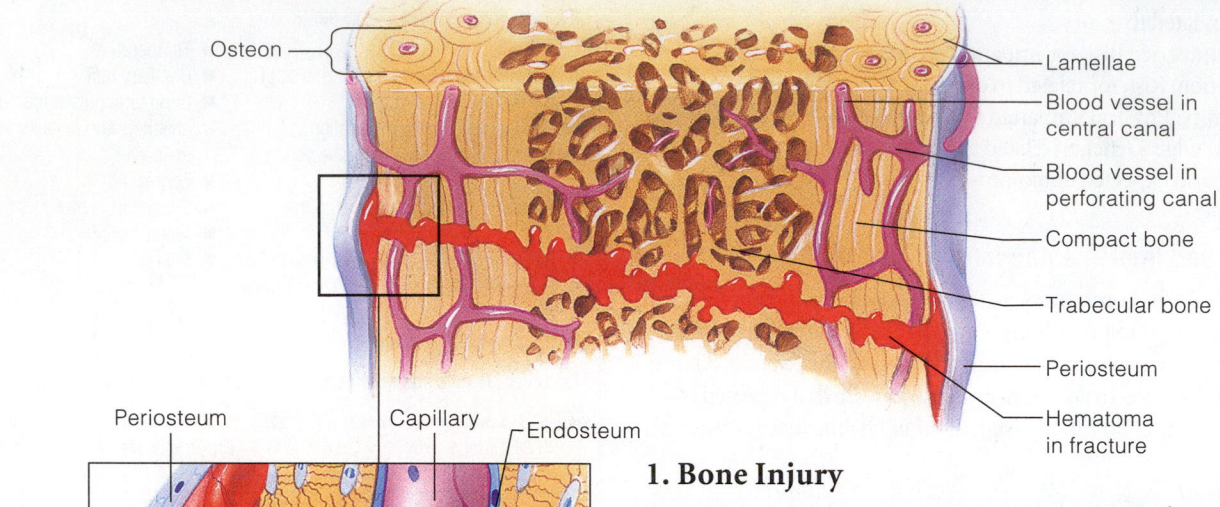

Osteon

Lamellae

Blood vessel in central canal

Blood vessel in perforating canal

Compact bone

Trabecular bone

Periosteum

Hematoma in fracture

Periosteum   Capillary   Endosteum

Fibrin

Bone fragment

Osteocyte

1. Bone Injury

When a bone fractures, blood vessels within the bone and surrounding soft tissues tear and begin to bleed, forming a hematoma. Necrotic bone tissue adjacent to the fracture causes an intense inflammatory response characterized by vasodilation, exudate formation, and white cell migration to the fracture site.

2. Fibrocartilaginous Callus Formation

Clotting factors within the hematoma form a fibrin meshwork. Within 48 hours, fibroblasts and new capillaries growing into the fracture form granulation tissue that gradually replaces the hematoma. Phagocytes begin to remove cell debris.

Osteoblasts, bone-forming cells, proliferate and migrate into the fracture site, forming a fibrocartilaginous callus. The osteoblasts build a web of collagen fibers from both sides of the fracture site that eventually unites to connect bone fragments, thus splinting the bone. Chondroblasts lay down patches of cartilage that provide a base for bone growth.

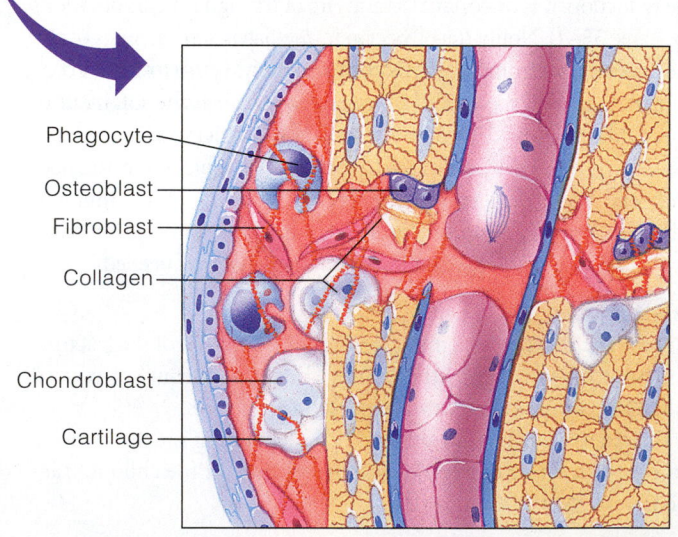

Phagocyte

Osteoblast

Fibroblast

Collagen

Chondroblast

Cartilage

FIGURE 35–21 ■ Any injury to the bone brings about a multistep process of bone formation that lasts about 3 months.

Pathophysiology Illustrated Process of Bone Healing

4. Bone Remodeling

Osteoblasts continue to form new woven bone, which is in turn organized into the lamellar structures of compact bone. Osteoclasts resorb excess callus as it is replaced by mature bone.

As the bone heals and is subjected to the mechanical stress of everyday use, osteoblasts and osteoclasts respond by remodeling the repair site along the lines of force. This ensures that the repaired section of bone eventually resembles the structure of the uninjured part.

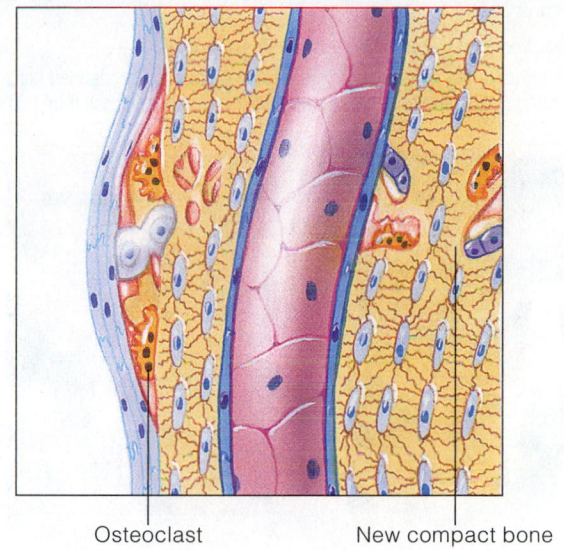

Osteoclast   New compact bone

3. Bony Callus Formation

Osteoblasts continue to proliferate and synthesize collagen fibers and bone matrix, which are gradually mineralized with calcium and mineral salts to form a spongey mass of woven bone. The trabeculae of woven bone bridge the fracture. Osteoclasts migrate to the repair site and begin removing excess bone in the callus. Bony callus formation usually continues for 2 to 3 months.

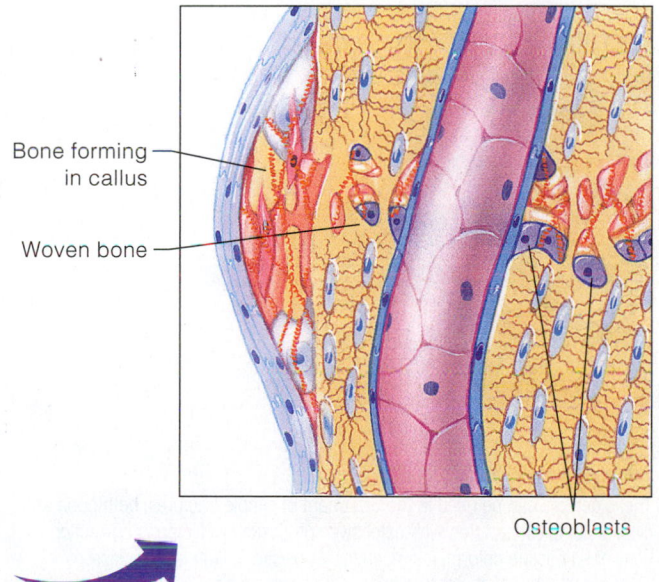

Bone forming in callus

Woven bone

Osteoblasts

FIGURE 35–21 ■ (continued)

TABLE 35–5	Types of Traction

Skin Traction

Pull is applied to the skin surface, which puts traction directly on the bones and muscles. Traction is attached to the skin with adhesive materials or straps, or foam boots, belts, or halters.

Dunlop Traction (can be either skeletal or skin)

Used for fracture of the humerus. The arm, which is flexed, is suspended horizontally with straps placed on both the upper and lower portions for pull from both sides.

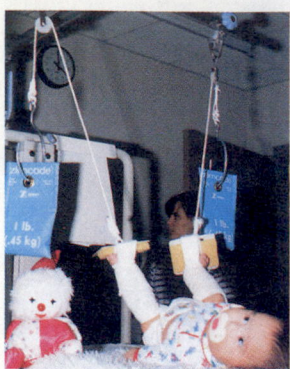 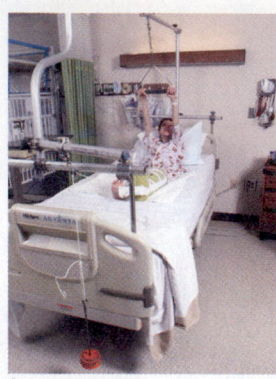

1   2

Bryant Traction (1)

Used specifically for the child under 3 years of age and weighing less than 17.5 kg (35 lb), who has developmental dysplasia of the hip or a fractured femur. This bilateral traction is applied to the child's legs and kept in place by wrapping the legs from foot to thigh with elastic bandages. The hips are flexed at a 90-degree angle, with knees extended. This position is maintained by attaching the traction appliance to weights and pulleys, which are suspended above the crib. The buttocks do not rest on the mattress, but are slightly elevated off the bed.

Buck Traction (2)

Used for knee immobilization; to correct contractures or deformities; or for short-term immobilization of a fracture. It keeps the leg in an extended position, without hip flexion. Traction is applied to the extremity in one direction (straight line) with a single pulley system.

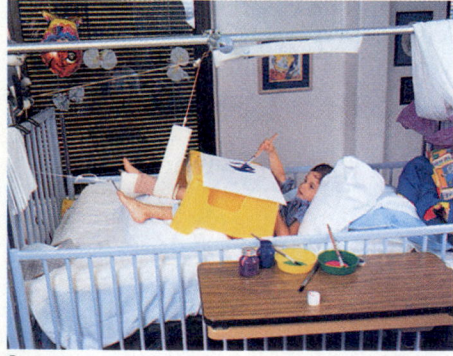

3

Russell Traction (3)

Used for fractures of the femur and lower leg. Traction is placed on the lower leg while the knee is suspended in a padded sling. The hips and knees, which are slightly flexed, are immobilized. One force is applied by a double pulley to the foot, and another force is applied upward using a sling under the knee and an overhead pulley.

Skeletal Traction

Pull is directly applied to the bone by pins, wires, tongs, or other apparatus that have been surgically placed through the distal end of the bone.

Skeletal Cervical Traction

Used for cervical spine injuries to reduce fractures and dislocations. Crutchfield, Gardner-Wells, or Vinke tongs are placed in the skull with burr holes. Weights are attached to the apparatus with a rope and pulley system to the hyperextended head.

Halo Traction

Used to immobilize the head and neck after cervical injury or dislocation. Also used for positioning and immobilization after cervical injury.

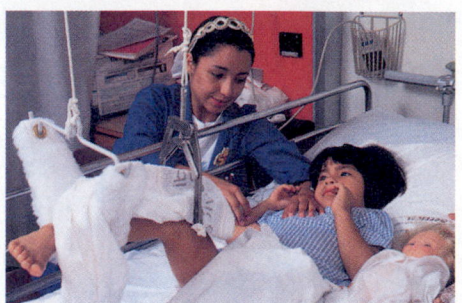

4

90-90 Traction (4)

Used for fractures of the femur or tibia. A skeletal pin or wire is surgically placed through the distal part of the femur, while the lower part of the extremity is in a boot cast. Traction ropes and pulleys are applied at the pin site and on the boot cast to maintain the flexion of both the hip and knee at 90 degrees. This traction can also be used for treatment of an upper extremity fracture.

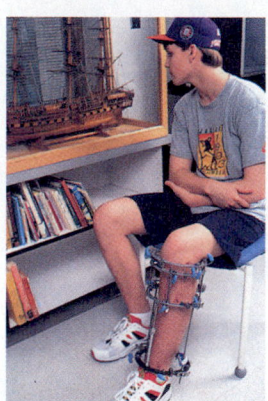

5

External Fixators (5)

These devices can be used in the treatment of simple fractures, both open and closed; complex fractures with extensive soft tissue involvement; correction of bony or soft tissue deformities; pseudoarthrosis; and limb length discrepancy. They are attached to the extremity by percutaneous transfixing of pins or wires to the bone.

---

pediatric nurse should be familiar with and share information from such policy statements.

Practice Alert

When a child has a fracture from sports or other activities, ask details about how the injury occurred. If protective gear is recommended and was not worn, reinforce the need for protection. Suggest financial resources as necessary.

Sports Injuries

Sports injuries are the most common type of injury in youth from 13 to 19 years. Football, soccer, cycling, and basketball are the sports commonly associated with injury (Halstead, 2010). Fractures, as described, are common sports injuries of young athletes, and many severe fractures that require hospitalization are related to sports and

BOX 35–10	Nursing Care of the Child with Traction or External Fixator

1. Assess the child in traction by first checking the equipment. Make sure that the equipment is in the proper position. Observe both the body appliance and the attached weights and pulleys. Make certain that the child's body is in proper alignment.

2. Assess the skin under the straps and pin insertion sites for any signs of redness, edema, or skin breakdown.

3. Assess the extremity by checking neurovascular status frequently (check warmth, color, distal pulses, capillary refill time, movement, sensation).

4. Provide pin care when ordered using sterile technique. Clean the area surrounding the pin with cotton-tipped applicators saturated with normal saline or half-strength hydrogen peroxide. Clean the area again with sterile water or more saline. Apply an antibacterial ointment, if ordered, using another cotton-tipped applicator.

5. With skin traction, skin care should be performed every 4 hours when the traction device is removed.

6. Place a sheepskin pad under the child's extremity if prescriptions permit.

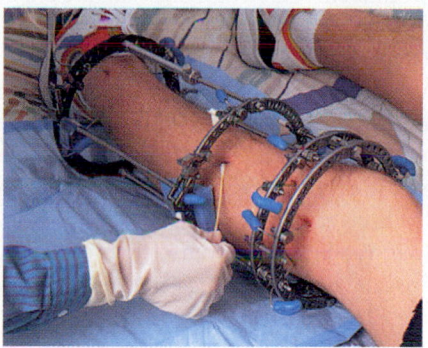

BOX 35–11	Research: Overuse Syndrome

The National Athletic Trainers' Association has investigated overuse injuries in youth and designed a position statement on prevention of pediatric overuse injuries. They recommend physical examinations that review risk factors for injury such as pain, fatigue, and decreased performance. Youth athletes should have no more than 16 to 20 hours per week of vigorous sports activity, and overhead throwing should be limited. Training programs that focus on balance, coordination, strength, and flexibility should be planned, and 1 to 2 days off a week should be part of an athletic program (Valovich McLeod, Decoster, Loud, et al., 2011). Nurses can take careful histories of youth athletes, become involved in coach training programs, and refer families to knowledgeable coaches.

coach and supervise children. Encourage youth to gradually increase time and intensity at a sport, rather than immediately playing a new sport for long periods of time. Have parents inquire about the coach's experience and also verify that the coaching staff is prepared in emergency care.

The nurse should be alert for sports injuries during contacts with children and adolescents in health promotion visits. Ask about sports participation for all youth, but especially when there are complaints of sore muscles, edema of body parts, and bruises. Perform neurovascular assessment of extremities, including color, temperature, capillary refill time, edema, pulses, sensation, and pain. Phrase questions so that you identify sports such as skateboarding or snowboarding which may not be performed under supervision or in organized sports programs. Youth may not consider these "sports."

Teach the importance of warming up for 10 to 15 minutes before participation, and to cool down for a corresponding period at the end of activity. Encourage wearing recommended safety gear for the sport such as a well-fitted protective helmet, face mask, eye protection, mouth guard, elbow and wrist guards, gloves, knee pads, and shin pads. Parents may need assistance to learn recommended equipment

activity injuries. Douglass, in the opening scenario, is an example of a child with this type of injury. He had a tibial fracture, common in sports; distal radial fractures are also frequent. However, a variety of other injuries that affect the musculoskeletal system are common in sports; strains and sprains are examples. Overuse injuries can occur when tendons, muscles, or bones are stressed excessively without adequate rest periods (Luke, Lazaro, Bergeron, et al., 2011) (Box 35–11). Children and adolescents have characteristics that put them at risk for injury. These include:

- Vulnerability of growth plates to injury, especially distal tibia and fibula
- Increased joint mobility from lax tendons and ligaments, leading to injury of knee, ankle, and hip
- More porous bones that lead to fractures and more common injury to underlying organs
- Lack of experience in the sport and inadequate training
- Lack of acceptance of protective gear
- Impatience with taking the time to heal after injury

Common sports injuries are listed in Table 35–6. Treatments for sprains, strains, dislocations, and fractures are described in the previous sections. Head and neck injuries are discussed in Chapter 33 and dental emergencies in Chapter 24. General approaches to minimize and treat injuries for youth athletes follow.

Athletes can benefit from teaching that enhances performance of their sports and also minimizes the chance of injury. They should receive instruction in correct techniques from a person qualified to

TABLE 35–6	Common Sports Injuries

SPORT	TYPE OF INJURIES
Baseball/basketball	■ Hand and finger fractures and sprains
	■ Contusions and sprains of upper or lower extremities; wrists, elbows, knees, and ankles are common sites
	■ Injury to body parts when hit by a ball, e.g., broken teeth; face, head, eye, and chest injuries
Football	■ Head and neck injury such as skull or cervical vertebrae fracture
	■ Pulled muscles or dislocations in shoulders and legs
Gymnastics	■ Wrist and elbow fractures and strains
	■ Tendonitis in elbows and ankles/legs
Hockey (ice and in-line)	■ Dental injury
	■ Leg fractures
	■ Head and neck injury
Soccer	■ Head and neck injury
	■ Strains and fractures of legs
Wrestling	■ Fractures and dislocations of upper and lower extremities

and resources for purchase. Frequent updates are needed as the child grows. Teach the child not to ignore pain.

Clinical Tip

Nurses are instrumental in checking on helmet use and application for risky sports. The helmet should sit low on the forehead (parallel plane to the ground when child looks ahead), there should be no more than two fingers of space between the chin strap and the chin, and it should move minimally when the child shakes the head vigorously (American Academy of Orthopaedic Surgeons, 2011). Helmets should be used only for the sport for which they were designed and should be replaced every 5 years to ensure product integrity and good fit. Plan to insert teaching and demonstrations of helmets in healthcare, school, and home settings with youth and their parents.

Injuries such as muscle strains should be treated promptly. Treatment involves several steps:

- Resting the injury for 24 to 48 hours; applying ice for 20 minutes four times daily; compression with an elastic wrap to provide comfort and decrease edema; elevating the part affected above heart level
- Gradually increasing motion to the part
- Adding flexibility and resistance or strengthening exercises
- Returning gradually to the sport, usually in 2 to 3 weeks after injury

Partner with the child, family, and other health professionals to plan for activity when an injury has occurred. Praise the family and youth for physical activity, an important part of a healthy lifestyle. Provide community resources to foster sports participation.

Amputations

Amputation—the complete absence of a body extremity—can be either congenital or acquired. Approximately two thirds of amputations in children are congenital and one third are acquired. Congenital amputations can be caused by constrictive amniotic bands, drugs, or irradiation. Acquired amputations are generally associated with trauma or the result of a disease or disorder. Children are prone to such injuries because of small extremities and limited skeletal mass. Lawn mower injury, exercise equipment, and car crashes are common causes. Most traumatic amputations involve fingers or toes, but hands and limbs are also at risk.

The child with an absent hand or limb should be fitted with a prosthesis as soon as feasible and encouraged to use it several hours daily to foster a positive body image, independence, activity, and self-confidence and to ensure that the child's motor skills develop as normally as possible (Ulger & Sener, 2011). The prosthetic device should be reevaluated as the child progresses physically and developmentally. A variety of devices are now available for persons with amputations, including blades for running, devices that connect with skis, and others. Periodic stump reconstructions may be necessary in children with traumatic amputations, because as children grow, so do their bones, and the skin tends to adhere to the bone. Bone may need to be cut and soft tissue added to keep the stump rounded. Joint fusions or stump lengthenings may also be needed to allow for the effective use of a prosthesis. Several prosthetic revisions will be needed as the child grows and develops.

Nursing Management

Nursing care focuses on providing emotional support regarding altered body image, managing pain, maintaining skin integrity, and encouraging maximal independent functioning.

Recovering from the loss of a limb is one of the most difficult challenges facing a child. Emphasize what the child can do rather than what he or she cannot do. Good listening skills are important.

The child who has had surgery or a traumatic injury experiences pain. Many of the techniques discussed in Chapter 21 🔗 are useful interventions. After surgery, an epidural may be the treatment of choice. Oral analgesics are used during the period of adaptation to a prosthesis if tenderness is present. Children can experience "phantom" limb pain in the lost extremity, although this phenomenon decreases significantly in the first year after amputation (Burgoyne, Billups, Jiron, et al., 2012; Wolff, Vanduynhoven, van Kleef, et al., 2011).

The child usually begins wearing the prosthetic device for 1 to 2 hours at a time. Check the skin for any redness or breakdown. If such conditions develop, leave the prosthesis off and allow the skin to clear before reapplying. Have the prosthesis adjusted if necessary, and increase wearing time as tolerated by the child.

Children with amputated limbs quickly learn how to accommodate to the prosthetic device. Make use of physical therapy programs that are specifically designed to help the child perform activities of daily living.

Answer any questions the family has about how to care for the prosthetic device and how to perform skin checks. Encourage parents to allow the child to participate in peer activities that are physically and emotionally challenging. Sporting activities that enable the child to participate using modified equipment are a good way to build self-confidence and motivation. For example, ski centers may offer programs that teach children with physical disabilities how to ski, and Special Olympics is a motivating option for some children. Assess the need for counseling and offer referrals as appropriate.

Weblink | Special Olympics

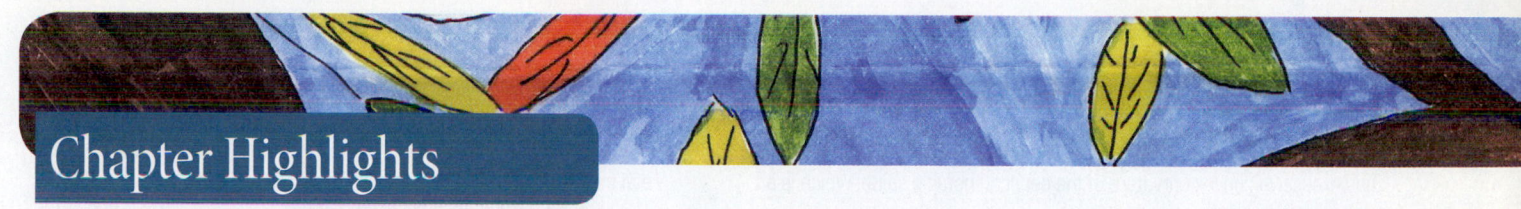

Chapter Highlights

- Children may develop musculoskeletal conditions as a result of congenital conditions, developmental variations, or trauma.
- Talipes equinovarus (clubfoot) is a common unilateral or bilateral variation in newborns that is treated by casting, traction, or surgery.
- Genu varum and genu valgum are normal variations at certain times in development that may need treatment if they persist.
- The nurse may identify developmental dysplasia of the hip (DDH) during newborn assessments and must refer the child for care to a specialist.
- Mild DDH may be treated by a harness, but more severe cases may require surgery for the child to walk normally.
- Legg-Calvé-Perthes is a reversible disease most commonly seen in school-age boys, and causes necrosis of the femoral head.
- Slipped capital femoral epiphysis is treated by casting, traction, or more commonly surgery with pinning, to stabilize the epiphysis.
- Scoliosis is a lateral curvature of the spine, and nurses commonly screen adolescents to identify the disorder.
- Scoliosis may require exercises, bracing, or surgery with instrumentation and spinal fusion.

- Osteoporosis can occur in premature infants, in children with conditions that lead to immobility and decreased weight bearing, and in youth with inadequate calcium or vitamin D intake.
- Osteomyelitis most commonly follows another infection and requires prompt treatment to prevent sepsis and serious injury to the bone.
- The child with osteogenesis imperfecta (brittle bone disease) requires careful handling by the nurse and parents to prevent fractures while fostering developmental progression.
- Muscular dystrophies are inherited diseases characterized by muscle wasting and degeneration.
- Children can experience a variety of fractures due to sports, car crashes, and other injuries.
- Many sports injuries experienced by youth can be avoided with proper equipment and training.
- Casts, braces, and traction are common interventions for musculoskeletal disorders; nursing interventions minimize development of problems related to these treatments.

Clinical Reasoning in Action

INTRODUCTION

Recall the opening scenario. Douglass, 12 years old, has a fractured fibula from a fall while jumping on a trampoline. He talks openly in the office about how much fun he has at his friend's house after school and shares that he hopes his mother will still let him go there. He is also nervous about returning to his busy school with a cast and crutches.

DESCRIPTION

Douglass has normal vital signs and neurovascular checks of the lower extremities. He ambulates well with crutches but appears slow and careful. Douglass admits that he has been pretty "crazy" at his friend's house and takes chances on the trampoline that he should not take. He is worried that his friends at school will make fun of him now that he has a cast and crutches.

DISCUSSION

1. Douglass's fracture did not disrupt the growth plate. What is the type of his fracture according to the Salter-Harris classification? If his growth plate had been disturbed, what would be some possible long-term outcomes?

2. What is Douglass's developmental stage according to Erikson? Can that explain his risk-taking behaviors at his friend's house?

3. Douglass's mother is worried about whether she should allow her son to continue going to his friend's house. What questions can you help her to ask the friend's parents about supervision, activities allowed, and plans for emergencies?

4. What are some of the microsystems you can identify in Douglass's life? How are these supportive or offering challenges to him?

5. List two nursing diagnoses dealing with the physical systems and two focusing on psychosocial systems for Douglass.

6. What nursing interventions can you establish for each nursing diagnosis?

NCLEX-RN® Review

1. The nurse is screening eighth-grade students for scoliosis and notes one has excessive convex curvature of the cervical thoracic spine. Which is an appropriate action for the nurse?
1. Refer the child for further evaluation of scoliosis.
2. Refer the child for further evaluation of lordosis.
3. Refer the child for further evaluation for kyphosis.
4. The nurse should take no action, as this is developmentally appropriate for a child of this age.

2. Which statement indicates the parents of a child with Duchenne muscular dystrophy have an accurate understanding of the genetics of the disease?
1. "Because our first son has muscular dystrophy, our next child will have a 50% chance of having the disease."
2. "All of our sons will have a 50% chance of having the disease."
3. "All of our daughters will have a 50% chance of having the disease."
4. "Because our first child has muscular dystrophy, our next child will be normal."

3. Which intervention is appropriate when providing care for a child in skeletal traction?
1. Ensure the weights are in the proper position.
2. Weights are supported on a table.
3. Nuts and bolts should be movable.
4. The line of pull has some slack for adjustment.

4. The nurse is working with a child who has just had a fracture reduction and casting. The nurse knows that the child is at risk for compartment syndrome. What objective assessment items will the nurse monitor for while completing the nursing assessment? (Select all that apply).
1. Weak pulse
2. Pale grey extremity
3. Tingling
4. Burning
5. Fever

See Appendix I 🔴 *for answers.*

References

American Academy of Orthopaedic Surgeons. (2009). *Developmental disease (dysplasia) of the hip (DDH)*. Retrieved from http://orthoinfo.aaos.org/topic.cfm?

American Academy of Orthopaedic Surgeons. (2010). *Forearm fractures in children*. Retrieved from http://orthoinfo.aaos.org/topic.cfm?topic=A00039&return_link=0

American Academy of Orthopaedic Surgeons. (2011). *Helmet safety*. Retrieved from http://www.orthoinfo.aaos.org/topic.cfm?topic=a00425

American Academy of Pediatrics. (1999, reaffirmed 2006). *Children with special health care needs*. Retrieved from http://www.aap.org/healthtopics/specialneeds.cfm

Bauer, D. H., & Freivalds, A. (2009). Backpack load limit recommendation for middle school students based on physiological and psychophysical measurements. *Work, 32,* 339–350.

Baujat, G., Legeai-Mallet, L., Finidori, G., Cormier-Daire, V., & LeMerrer, M. (2008). Achondroplasia. *Best Practices & Research in Clinical Rheumatology, 22,* 3–18.

Bautista, S. R., Gholve, P., & Dormans, J. P. (2011). Pediatric musculoskeletal infections: Managing the significant organisms. *Consultant for Pediatricians, 10*(2), 41–45.

Beach, H., Garcia Pena, B. M., & Linares, M. Y. (2009). Heelys injuries: A review of the National Electronic Injury Surveillance System data. *Pediatric Emergency Care, 25,* 642–644.

Becker Muscular Dystrophy. (n.d.). *Becker muscular dystrophy*. Retrieved from http//www.beckermuscular-dystrophy.org

Bishop, N. (2010). Characterizing and treating osteogenesis imperfecta. *Early Human Development, 86,* 743–746.

Burgoyne, L. L., Billups, C. A., Jiron, J. L., Dakkoum, R. N., Wright, B. B., Bikhazi, G. B., . . . Pereiras, L. A. (2012). Phantom limb pain in young cancer-related amputees: Recent experience at St Jude Children's Research Hospital. *Clinical Journal of Pain, 28,* 222–225

Burns, C. E., Dunn, A. M., Brady, M. A., Starr, N. B., & Blosser, C. G. (2009). *Pediatric primary care* (4th ed.). Philadelphia, PA: Elsevier Saunders.

Castillo, H., & Samson-Fang, L. (2009). Effects of bisphosphonates in children with osteogenesis imperfecta: An AACPDM systematic review. *Developmental Medicine and Child Neurology, 51,* 17–29.

Causon, E. (2010). The nurse's role in educating, counseling and preparing parents to care for a child with developmental dysplasia of the hip (DDH). *International Journal of Orthopaedic & Trauma Nursing, 14,* 40–47.

Chamley, C. A., Carson, P., Randall, D., & Sandwell, M. (2005). *Developmental anatomy and physiology of children*. St. Louis, MO: Elsevier.

Chan, G., & Chen, C. T. (2009). Musculoskeletal effects of obesity. *Current Opinion in Pediatrics, 21,* 65–70.

Chen, H. L., Lee, C. L., Tseng, H. I., Yang, S. N., Yang, R. C., & Jao, H. C. (2010). Assisted exercise improves bone strength in very low birthweight infants by bone quantitative ultrasound. *Journal of Pediatric and Child Health, 46,* 653–659.

Cheung, M. (2009). Drugs used in pediatric bone and calcium disorders. *Endocrine Development, 16,* 218–232.

Custer, J. W., & Rau, R. E. (Eds.). (2009). *The Harriet Lane handbook*. Philadelphia, PA: Mosby Elsevier.

De Sanctis, N. (2011). Magnetic resonance imaging in Legg-Calvé-Perthes disease: Review of literature. *Journal of Pediatric Orthopaedics, 31*(Suppl. 2), S163–S167.

Fabry, G. (2010). The hip from birth to adolescence. *European Journal of Pediatrics, 169,* 143–148.

Field, A. E., Gordon, C. M., Pierce, L. M., Ramappa, A., & Kocher, M. S. (2011). Prospective study of physical activity and risk of developing a stress fracture among preadolescent and adolescent girls. *Archives of Pediatrics and Adolescent Medicine, 165,* 723–728.

Gholve, P. A., Cameron, D. B., & Millis, M. B. (2009). Slipped capital femoral epiphysis update. *Current Opinion in Pediatrics, 21,* 39–45.

Gonzales, E. A. (2009). Marfan syndrome. *Journal of the American Academy of Nurse Practitioners, 21,* 663–670.

Gottschalk, H. P., Karol, L. A., & Jeans, K. A. (2010). Gait analysis of children treated for moderate clubfoot with physical therapy versus the Ponseti cast technique. *Journal of Pediatric Orthopaedics, 30,* 235–239.

Goyenvaile, A., Seto, J. T., Davies, K. E., & Chamberlain, J. (2011). Therapeutic approaches to muscular dystrophy. *Human Molecular Genetics, 20*(Review Issue I), R69–R78.

Gurnett, C. A., Boehm, S., Connolly, A., Reimschisel, T., & Dobbs, M. B. (2008). Impact of congenital talipes equinovarus etiology on treatment outcomes. *Developmental Medicine & Child Neurology, 50,* 498–502.

Hagmann, S., Dreher, T., & Wenz, W. (2009). Skewfoot. *Foot and Ankle Clinics, 14,* 409–434.

Halstead, M. E. (2010). Contact sports for young athletes: Keys to safety. *Pediatric Annals, 39,* 275–278.

Harrison, C. M., Johnson, K., & McKechnie, E. (2008). Osteopenia of prematurity: A national survey and review of practice. *Acta Paediatrica, 97,* 407–413.

Hutchinson, B. (2010). Pediatric metatarsus adductus and skewfoot deformity. *Clinics in Podiatric Medicine and Surgery, 27,* 93–104.

Jethva, R., Otsuru, S., Dominici, M., & Horwitz, E. M. (2009). Cell therapy for disorders of bone. *Cytotherapy, 11,* 3–17.

Kleposki, R. W., Abel, K., & Sehgal, K. (2010, June). Common pediatric hip diseases in primary care. *Clinical Advisor,* 21–26.

Laederich, M. B., & Horton, W. A. (2010). Achondroplasia: Pathogenesis and implications for future treatment. *Current Opinion in Pediatrics, 22,* 516–523.

Lombardi, G., Akoume, M. Y., Colombini, A., Moreau, A., & Banfi, G. (2011). Biochemistry of adolescent idiopathic scoliosis. *Advances in Clinical Chemistry, 54,* 165–182.

Lubicky, J. P., Hanson, J. E., Riley, E., & Spinal Deformity Study Group. (2011). Instrumentation constructs in pediatric patients undergoing deformity correction correlated with Scoliosis Research Society scores. *Spine, 36,* 1692–1700.

Luke, A., Lazaro, R. M., Bergeron, M. F., Keyser, L., Benjamin, H., Brenner, J., . . . Smith, A. (2011). Sports-related injuries in youth athletes: Is overscheduling a risk factor? *Clinical Journal of Sports Medicine, 21,* 307–314.

Macias, B. R., Murthy, G., Chanbers, H., & Hargens, A. R. (2008). Asymmetric loads and pain associated with backpack carrying by children. *Journal of Pediatric Orthopaedics, 28,* 512–517.

Mahan, S. T., Katz, J. N., & Kim, N. (2009). To screen or not to screen? A decision analysis of the utility of screening for DDH. *Journal of Bone and Joint Surgery of America, 91,* 1705–1719.

Mehler, P. S., Cleary, B. S., & Gaudiani, J. L. (2011). Osteoporosis in anorexia nervosa. *Eating Disorders, 19,* 194–202.

Milani, C., & Dobashi, E. T. (2011). Arthrogram in Legg-Calve-Perthes disease. *Journal of Pediatric Orthopaedics, 31*(Suppl. 2), S156–S162.

Montgomery, C. O., Young, K. L., Austen, M., Jo, C. H., Blasier, R. D., & Ilyas, M. (2010). Increased risk of Blount disease in obese children and adolescents with vitamin D deficiency. *Journal of Pediatric Orthopaedics, 30,* 879–882.

Murray, A. W., & Wilson, N. I. (2008). Changing incidence of slipped capital femoral epiphysis: A relationship with obesity. *Journal of Bone and Joint Surgery, 90,* 92–94.

National Center for the Safe Transportation of Children with Special Health Care Needs. (2010). *Special needs transportation.* Retrieved from http://www.preventinjury .org/NationalCenter.asp

National Institute of Arthritis and Musculoskeletal and Skin Diseases. (2009). *Osteoporosis: The diagnosis.* Retrieved from http://www.niams.nih.gov/Health_Info/ Bone/Osteoporosis/diagnosis.asp

National Institutes of Health (2012). Fontanelles. Retrieved from http://www.nlm.nih.gov/medlineplus/ ency/article/003310.htm

Neuschwander, T. B., Cutrone, J., Macias, B. R., Cutrone, S., Murthy, G., Changers, H., & Hargens, A. R. (2010). The effect of backpacks on the lumbar spine in children: A standing magnetic resonance imaging study. *Spine, 35,* 83–88.

Norem, N., Feuerstein, C., Traverso, V., Zomaya, N., Crews, R., & Wrobel, J. S. (2009). Gait changes with the use of Heelys: A case study. *Journal of the American Podiatric Medicine Association, 99,* 247–250.

Online Mendelian Inheritance in Man. (2008). *Osteogenesis imperfecta.* Retrieved from http://www.ncbi.nlm .nih.gov/entrez/dispomin/cgi?id=166200

Paton, R. W., Fox, A. E., Foster, P., & Hehily, M. (2010). Incidence and etiology of equino-varus with recent population changes. *Acta Orthopaedica Belgium, 76,* 86–89.

Peck, D. (2010). Slipped capital femoral epiphysis: Diagnosis and management. *American Family Physician, 82,* 258–262.

Penner, L., Cantor, M., & Siegel, L. (2010). Joseph's wishes: Ethical decision-making in Duchenne muscular dystrophy. *Mount Sinai Journal of Medicine, 77,* 394–397.

Perry, D. C., & Hall, A. J. (2011). The epidemiology and etiology of Perthes disease. *Orthopedic Clinics of North America, 42,* 279–283.

Plante, M., Wallace, R., & Busconi, B. D. (2011). Clinical diagnosis of hip pain. *Clinical Sports Medicine, 30,* 225–238.

Rack, B., Lochmuller, E. M., Janni, W., Lipowsky, G., Engelsberger, I., Friese, K., & Kuster, H. (2011). Ultrasound for the assessment of bone quality in preterm and term infants. *Journal of Perinatology.* doi: 10.1038/jp.2011.82

Ramprasad, M., Alias, J., & Raghuveer, A. K. (2010). Effect of backpack weight on postural angles in preadolescent children. *Indian Pediatrics, 47,* 575–580.

Rivett, L., Rothberg, A., Stewart, A., & Berkowitz, R. (2009, January 14). The relationship between quality of life and compliance to a brace protocol in adolescents with idiopathic scoliosis: A comparative study. *BMC Musculoskeletal Disorders,* 10–15.

Sabharwal, S. (2009). Blount disease. *Journal of Bone and Joint Surgery of America, 91,* 1758–1776.

Sankar, W. N., Weiss, J., & Skaggs, D. C. (2009). Orthopaedic conditions in the newborn. *Journal of the American Academy of Orthopaedic Surgeons, 17,* 112–122.

Scottish Rite Hospital. (2011). *Scoliosis and spine.* Retrieved from http://www.tsrhc.org/scoliosis-scoliometer.htm

Sewell, M. D., Rosendahl, K., & Eastwood, D. M. (2009). Developmental dysplasia of the hip. *British Medical Journal, 339,* b4464. doi: 10.1136/bmj.b4454

Shank, C. E., Thiel, E. J., & Klingele, K. E. (2010). Valgus slipped capital femoral epiphysis: Prevalence, presentation, and treatment options. *Journal of Pediatric Orthopaedics, 30,* 140–146.

Starr, S. R., Roberts, T. T., & Fischer, P. R. (2010). Osteogenesis imperfecta: Primary care. *Pediatrics in Review, 31,* e54–e64.

Talbott, N. R., Bhattacharya, A., Davis, K. G., Shukla, R., & Levin, L. (2009). School backpacks: It's more than just a weight problem. *Work, 34,* 481–494.

Thing, J., Wade, D., & Clark, H. (2008). "Heely"-related injuries in children. *Emergency Medicine Journal, 25,* 572–574.

Thomsen, K., & Creech, C. B. (2011). Advances in the diagnosis and management of pediatric osteomyelitis. *Current Infectious Disease Reports, 13,* 451–460.

Ulger, O., & Sener, G. (2011). Functional outcome after prosthetic rehabilitation of children with acquired and congenital lower limb loss. *Journal of Pediatric Orthopaedics, 20,* 178–183.

University of Maryland Medical Center. (2011). *Muscular dystrophy.* Retrieved from http://www.wmm.edu/ altmed/articles/musculardystrophy-000113.htm

U.S. Preventive Services Task Force. (2011). *Screening for idiopathic scoliosis in adolescents.* Retrieved from http:// www.uspreventiveservicestaskforce.org/3rduspstf/ scoliosis/scoliors.htm

Valovich McLeod, T. C., Decoster, L.C., Loud, K. J., Micheli, L. J., Parker, J. T., Sandrey, M. A., & White, C. (2011). National Athletic Trainers' Association position statement: Prevention of pediatric overuse injuries. *Journal of Athletic Training, 46,* 206–220.

Wagner, K. R. (2008). Approaching a new age in Duchenne muscular dystrophy treatment. *Journal of the American Society for Experimental NeuroTherapeutics, 5,* 583–591.

Weiler, R., Ingram, M., & Wolman, R. (2011). Osgood-Schlatter disease. *British Medical Journal, 343.* doi:10.1136/bmj.d4534

Wolff, A., Vanduynhoven, E., van Kleef, M., Huygen, F., Pope, J. E., & Mehhail, N. (2011). Phantom pain. *Pain Practice, 11,* 403–413.

Wright, E. (2009). Neurovascular impairment and compartment syndrome. *Paediatric Nursing, 21*(3), 26–29.

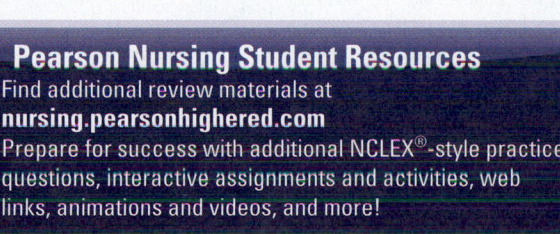

Pearson Nursing Student Resources

Find additional review materials at
nursing.pearsonhighered.com
Prepare for success with additional NCLEX®-style practice questions, interactive assignments and activities, web links, animations and videos, and more!

36 Alterations in Skin Integrity

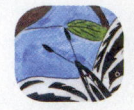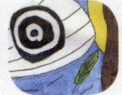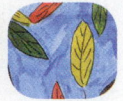

Learning Outcomes

After completing this chapter, you will be able to:

1. Describe important pediatric differences in the anatomy and physiology of the child's skin.

2. Classify the characteristics of skin lesions caused by irritants, drug reactions, mites, infection, and injury.

3. Differentiate between the stages of wound healing.

4. Compare the skin conditions that have a hereditary cause or predisposition.

5. Prepare an education plan for adolescents with acne to promote self-care.

6. Plan the nursing care for the child with alterations in skin integrity, including dermatitis, infectious disorders, and infestations.

7. Summarize the process to measure the extent of burns and burn severity in children.

8. Develop a nursing care plan for the child with a full-thickness burn injury.

9. Evaluate preventive strategies to reduce the risk of injury from burns, bites, and stings.

> "Why can't I go back to school? I really miss my friends and the fun we have together."
> —*Joshua, 6 years old*

Joshua Needham, 6 years old, was admitted to the hospital with a burn to his lower leg. He was playing with matches, and his pant leg caught on fire. Fortunately his father heard his cries and quickly put out the flames. Joshua received emergency care to stop the burning process and then went to the operating room for wound debridement. His pain was initially managed with IV morphine. By Joshua's second day of hospitalization, it was determined that most of his burn injury was deep partial thickness. It was not known at that time if a skin graft would be needed. A burn dressing and a vacuum-assisted closure device were applied to his leg to promote healing. Joshua was discharged home with the vacuum-assisted closure device after 4 days.

Three days later, Joshua has returned to the hospital's burn clinic for the first of his twice-weekly burn dressing changes. It is performed in the sedation suite, in case additional debridement is needed. Joshua's mother stays with him while the sedation is administered and then goes to the waiting room. Joshua's dressing change and sedation experience are uneventful. When the dressing is removed, granulation tissue is seen and no odor or purulent drainage that might indicate infection is present. The dressing and vacuum-assisted closure device are reapplied.

After the dressing change, some time is spent talking with Joshua's mother. She reports that Joshua has been eating the recommended high-protein, high-calorie diet to promote wound healing. She admits that it has been challenging to keep Joshua occupied so that he does not move more than recommended, especially since he is such an active child. Joshua's mother wonders how long it will take to determine if a skin graft will be needed.

What is the nurse's role in providing care to the child with a burn injury? What strategies will help the child cope with dressing changes when sedation is not provided? What other members of the healthcare team are important to promote an optimal recovery?

Skin disorders are seen frequently by nurses who work in outpatient clinics, schools, emergency departments, and pediatric units of hospitals. Many of these disorders are not unique to children, but children are at greater risk for some skin conditions for a variety of reasons discussed in this chapter.

ANATOMY AND PHYSIOLOGY
Function of the Skin

The skin is the largest organ in the body. It performs several essential functions. The skin protects underlying tissues from invasion by microorganisms and from trauma. The nerves in the skin enable the perception of touch, pain, pressure, heat, and cold. The skin also assists the body to conserve heat by constricting blood vessels. Dilation of blood vessels and the secretion of sweat by the eccrine sweat glands enable the body to release excess heat. The sweat glands, secreting a solution of water, electrolytes, and urea, also help to rid the body of toxins. The skin supplements the body's intake of vitamin D by synthesizing this vitamin from ultraviolet light.

The skin consists of three distinct layers: the epidermis, dermis, and subcutaneous fatty layer that separates the skin from the underlying tissue (Figure 36–1 ■). The epidermis is the thin, rapidly growing, outermost layer of skin. Skin is continually shed by the **stratum corneum,** the superficial layer of the epidermis, composed of flat keratinized, nonnucleated cells. The thickness of the epidermis varies by location on the body (e.g., 0.3 mm on the eyelids and 1.5 mm on the soles of the feet) (Nicol & Huether, 2010b). The epidermis contains the melanocytes that synthesize and secrete melanin when the skin is exposed to ultraviolet light. The Langerhans cells within the epidermis initiate the skin's immune response when exposed to environmental antigens.

The dermis, the middle layer of the skin, is mostly composed of connective tissue which allows the skin to stretch and contract with movement. Nerves, muscles, hair follicles, sebaceous and sweat glands, lymph channels, and blood vessels are all contained in the dermis. Mast cells located within the dermis play a role in the skin's hypersensitivity reactions.

The third skin layer, the subcutaneous layer, connects the dermis to the muscle below. This layer of fat cells helps insulate the body from cold temperatures. The sebaceous glands appear all over the body, except the palms of the hands and soles of the feet, and are connected with hair follicles in most cases. Sebum, a lipid substance produced and secreted into the hair follicle or directly onto the skin, lubricates the skin and hair.

Eccrine sweat glands, located in the dermis, open onto the skin's surface. They secrete sweat, an odorless, watery fluid containing sodium, chloride, urea, and other body wastes. As the body temperature increases, the glands increase their production of sweat; its evaporation cools the body.

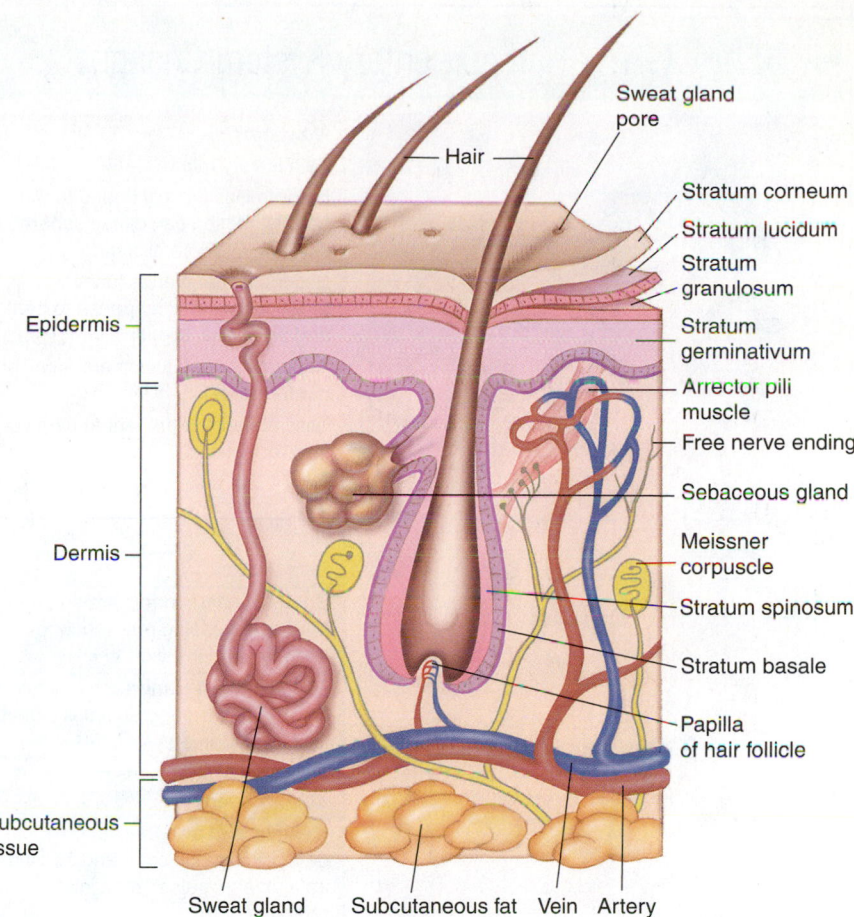

FIGURE 36–1 ■ Layers of the skin with accessory structures.

Apocrine sweat glands are primarily located in the axillary and genital areas, and their secretions contain more lipids and proteins. Decomposition of the fluid secreted by these glands leads to body odor.

Nails are protective keratinized plates that appear at the ends of fingers and toes. They grow at a rate of 1 mm or less a day.

PEDIATRIC DIFFERENCES

The newborn's skin is the largest organ of the body, but it is 40% to 60% thinner than adult skin (Lund & Kuller, 2007). The infant's skin is thin, about 1 mm thick at birth, with little underlying subcutaneous fat. The skin grows to 2 mm thick by adulthood. With thinner skin and less subcutaneous fat, the infant loses heat more rapidly, has greater difficulty regulating body temperature, and becomes more easily chilled than an older child or an adult. The thinner skin also increases the potential absorption of topical medications. The infant's skin contains more water than an adult's and has loosely attached cells. As the infant grows, the skin toughens and becomes less hydrated, making it less susceptible to bacteria (Figure 36–2 ■).

Melanin, a peptide synthesized by an enzyme in melanocytes, influences skin color. Melanin production is low at birth and during the newborn period, accounting for the lighter skin in newborns of all races. Newborns and young infants are therefore more susceptible to the harmful effects of the sun.

As They Grow Integumentary System Changes

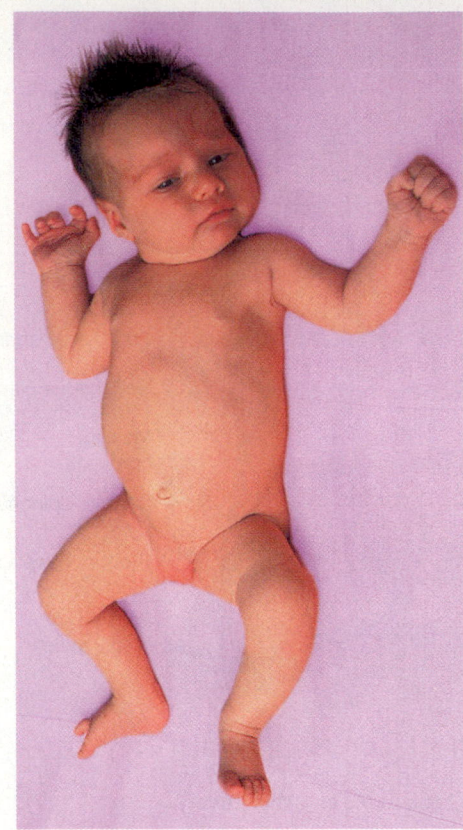

Newborns

Skin is very thin
Epidermis is loosely bound to the dermis, friction can cause separation of the layers with blistering
Eccrine sweat glands function, produce sweat in response to heat and emotional stimuli
Apocrine sweat glands are small and nonfunctional
Less melanin is present at birth so skin is lighter colored

Adolescents

Skin thickens
Epidermis and dermis are tightly bound, increasing resistance to infection and irritation
Eccrine sweat glands achieve full function, after puberty males sweat more than females
Apocrine sweat glands mature during puberty
Melanin is at adult levels, determining skin color and serving as a shield against ultraviolet radiation

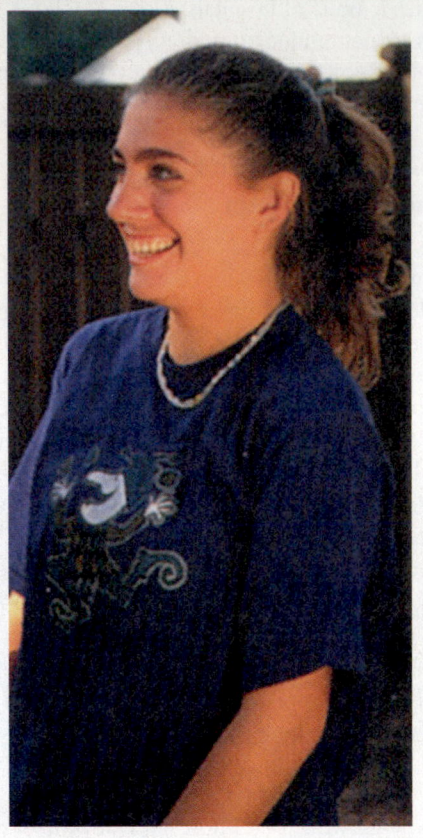

FIGURE 36–2 ■ The structures of the skin mature during childhood, reaching adult function at puberty.

Sebaceous glands and eccrine sweat glands are functional at birth in a term infant, although somewhat immaturely. The apocrine glands do not function until puberty.

Guidelines for performing a nursing assessment of the integumentary system are provided in Table 36–1. Examples of diagnostic and laboratory tests used to evaluate skin disorders are provided in Table 36–2. A description of these diagnostic procedures and nursing considerations are provided in Appendix E; values for laboratory tests are provided in Appendix D 🌐.

SKIN LESIONS

Skin lesions vary in size, shape, color, and texture characteristics. The two major types of skin lesions are primary lesions and secondary lesions. Primary lesions arise from previously healthy skin and include macules, patches, papules, nodules, tumors, vesicles, pustules, bullae, and wheals (see Figure 7–11 🌐). Secondary lesions result from changes in primary lesions. They include crusts, scales, **lichenification** (thickening of the skin with increased visibility of normal skin furrows), scars, keloids, excoriation, fissures, erosion, and ulcers (Table 36–3). It is important for the nurse to be able to identify and describe the primary and secondary skin lesions and understand their underlying cause and treatment. Some families may use complementary therapies to treat skin lesions. See Complementary Therapy: Oils and Gels.

TABLE 36–1	Assessment Guidelines for the Child with a Skin Condition*
ASSESSMENT FOCUS	**ASSESSMENT GUIDELINES**
Skin characteristics	■ Inspect the skin for color, elevations, and imperfections.
	■ Palpate the skin for texture, moisture, temperature, turgor, and edema.
Hair	■ Inspect the scalp hair for color, distribution, and cleanliness. Inspect for nits (lice eggs) that adhere to the hair.
	■ Inspect for areas of hair loss, bald spots, or broken hairs.
Lesions	■ Describe skin lesions according to characteristics listed in Figure 7–11 🌐 and Table 36–3. Note erythema, signs of scratching (excoriation), or secondary infection.
	■ Identify the location or distribution of lesions on the body (e.g., generalized, diaper area, flexor surfaces).
	■ Palpate lesions for induration and temperature.
	■ Measure the size of lesions (length, width, and height when appropriate).
Pain	■ Assess level of pain when present.
Temperature	■ Assess the body temperature.
Family history	■ Identify any family members with allergies or chronic skin conditions.

Note: *See Chapter 7 🌐 for examination techniques.

TABLE 36–2	Diagnostic Procedures and Laboratory Tests for Skin Disorders*
DIAGNOSTIC PROCEDURES	**LABORATORY TESTS**
Culture of wound or skin drainage	Complete blood count
Tissue biopsy	Immunoglobulin E
Computed tomography (CT)	Potassium hydroxide on skin scrapings
Radiograph	
Ultrasound	

Note: *See Appendixes D and E 🔴 for more information about these procedures and tests.

Wound Healing

Wound healing occurs in three overlapping phases: inflammation, reconstruction, and maturation; the wound fills in, seals, and finally shrinks (Rote & Huether, 2010). See Figure 36–3 ■.

The initial healing begins within a few hours. Hemostasis and inflammation, the initial response at the injury site, lasts approximately 3 to 5 days after injury (Bookout, 2008). This phase prepares the injury site for the repair process. Vasodilation allows leukocytes and neutrophils to travel to the injury site where they ingest bacteria and debris. Plasma leaks from the blood vessels due to capillary permeability and the increased blood flow. The wound is sealed with a clot to prevent bacterial invasion and join the wound edges. Bacteria, dead cells, and other inflammatory products are drained by lymphatic vessels.

Tissue formation or **epithelialization** (the process by which epithelial cells grow into the wound from surrounding healthy tissue), the second phase, may last from 3 to 21 days (Bookout, 2008). Capillary budding to reestablish the blood flow and **natural debridement** (enzyme action by macrophages and neutrophils to clean the lesion and dissolve the clot or scab) occur. The wound contracts as fibroblasts multiply, producing **collagen** (a protein that is the material of tissue repair) and granulation tissue to fill the wound to skin level. A fine layer of epithelial cells forms over the site.

Maturation or remodeling, the third phase, involves continued collagen production for scar production. The scar gradually strengthens and devascularizes, eventually achieving about 80% of the tissue's preinjury strength (Rote & Huether, 2010). Maturation can take months to years, depending on the extent of the injury. Formation of a **keloid,** a scar that extends beyond the original boundaries of the wound, is caused by an imbalance between collagen synthesis and collagen breakdown. The cause is unknown, but there is a familial tendency. A **hypertrophic scar** is one that is raised but stays within the original boundaries of the wound.

Wounds that heal well with minimal tissue loss are those that heal by *primary intention*. An example is the wound healing after an incision in which there is little tissue loss, wound edges are joined together, and little epithelialization and contraction are needed. Wounds that are open and require much tissue regeneration heal by *secondary intention*. See Box 36–1.

Complementary Therapy Oils and Gels

Some skin conditions have complementary therapies for which scientific studies have demonstrated a benefit. Evening primrose oil given orally is used for atopic dermatitis. Aloe vera gel used topically is effective for superficial burns and abrasions (National Center for Complementary and Alternative Medicine, 2011).

BOX 36–1 Causes of Dysfunctional Wound Repair and Healing

- **Predisposing chronic condition**—e.g., diabetes
- **Hypoxemia**—insufficient oxygen in the tissues, making them susceptible to infection
- **Hypovolemia**—inflammation is inhibited because of low circulating blood volume
- **Prolonged infection**—can cause excessive scarring
- **Corticosteroid treatment**—macrophages are prevented from migrating to the site of injury and epithelialization is suppressed
- **Poor nutrition**—inadequate caloric, protein, and vitamin intake to meet metabolic needs for healing prolongs inflammation

Source: *Data from Rote, N. S., & Huether, S. E. (2010). Innate immunity: Inflammation. In K. L. McCance & S. E. Huether (Eds.),* Pathophysiology: The basis for disease in adults and children *(5th ed., pp. 183–216). St. Louis, MO: Elsevier Mosby.*

TABLE 36–3	Common Secondary Skin Lesions and Associated Conditions	
LESION NAME	**DESCRIPTION**	**EXAMPLE**
Burrow	A narrow, raised irregular channel caused by a parasite	Scabies
Comedones	Plugs of sebaceous and keratin material in hair follicles	Acne
Crust	Dried residue of serum, pus, or blood	Impetigo
Erosion	Loss of superficial epidermis; moist but does not bleed	Ruptured chicken pox vesicle
Excoriation	Abrasion or scratch mark	Scratched insect bite
Fissure	Linear crack in skin	Tinea pedis (athlete's foot)
Keloid	Overdevelopment or hypertrophy of scar that extends beyond wound edges and above skin line due to excess collagen	Healed skin area following traumatic injury
Lichenification	Thickening of skin with increased visibility of normal skin furrows	Atopic dermatitis (eczema)
Scale	Thin flake of exfoliated epidermis	Dandruff, psoriasis
Scar	Replacement of destroyed tissue with fibrous tissue	Healed surgical incision
Telangiectasia	Dilated, superficial blood vessels	Birthmark
Ulcer	Deeper loss of skin surface; bleeding or scarring may ensue	Pressure ulcer

Pathophysiology Illustrated Phases of Wound Healing

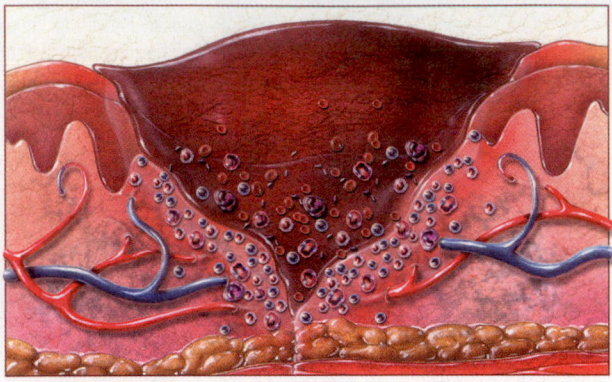

Hemostasis and Inflammation (3–5 days)

Platelets flow to site and form a clot to stop bleeding

Platelets release inflammatory mediators (cytokines, chemokines, and growth factors

Increased blood flow to site delivers leukocytes, phagocytes, and lymphocytes

Increased capillary permeability causes swelling

Bacteria are destroyed and cellular debris and foreign particles are removed

Clot formation seals the wound with fibrin, trapped cells, and platelets

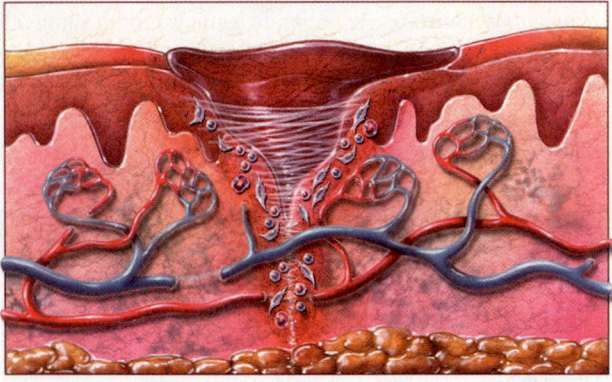

Tissue Formation (4 days to 2 weeks)

Fibrinolytic enzymes dissolve the fibrin clots

Fibroblasts and endothelial cells in surrounding tissue direct the migration of cells to the newly developed fibrin matrix (replacing the clot) so remodeling can begin

Granulation tissue forms and the wound is closed

Capillary budding occurs for development of new blood vessels

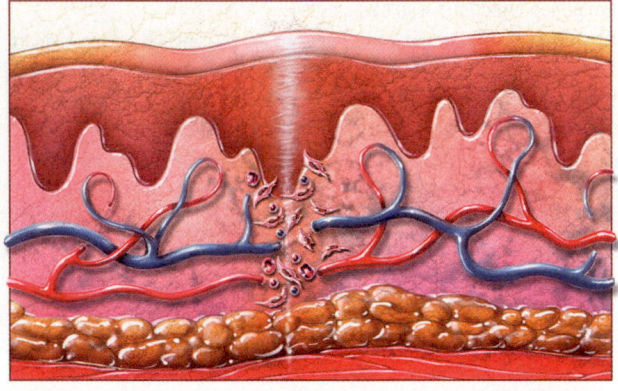

Maturation (Months to 2 Years)

Wound contraction occurs

Epithelial cells migrate from the peripheral areas

Collagen development leads to scar formation and strengthening

Capillaries disappearance from the scar tissue

FIGURE 36–3 ■ Wound healing occurs in three overlapping phases: hemostasis and inflammation, tissue formation, and maturation.

Source: Data from: *Rizzi, S. C., Upton, Z., Bott, K., & Dargaville, T. R. (2010). Recent advances in dermal wound healing: Biomedical device approaches. Expert Reviews of Medical Devices, 7(1), 143–154; Brown, T. S., Safford, S., Caramanica, J., & Elster, E. A. (2010). Biomarker use in tailored combat casualty care. Biomarkers Medicine, 4(3), 465-473; and Rote, N. S., & Huether, S. E. (2010). Innate immunity: Inflammation. In K. L. McCance, S. E. Huether, V. L. Brashers, & N. S. Rote. Pathophysiology: The biologic basis for disease in adults and children (6th ed., pp. 183–216). St. Louis, MO: Elsevier Mosby; © 2012 K. Somerville—Custome Medical Stock Photo, All Rights Reserved..*

DERMATITIS

Many skin inflammations occur in early childhood. Most are easily treated and have no long-term consequences. *Dermatitis* is a broad term describing changes that occur in the skin in response to external stimuli. The three most common types of acute dermatitis in infants, children, and adolescents are contact dermatitis, diaper dermatitis, and seborrheic dermatitis. (Atopic dermatitis or eczema is discussed on page 1312.) These skin disorders can cause an emotional response in the child and family. Be supportive and reassure them that the child is not infectious.

Contact Dermatitis

Contact dermatitis is an inflammation of the skin that occurs in response to direct contact with an allergen or irritant. Irritant contact dermatitis is more common.

Etiology and Pathophysiology

In the case of contact dermatitis caused by external irritants, an inflammatory reaction occurs without an immune response. Common irritants include soaps, detergents, fabric softeners, bleaches, lotions, urine, and stool. An irritant can affect the skin any time there is

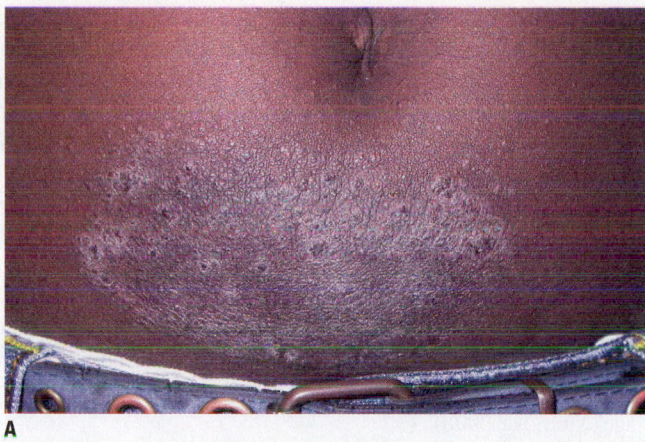

A

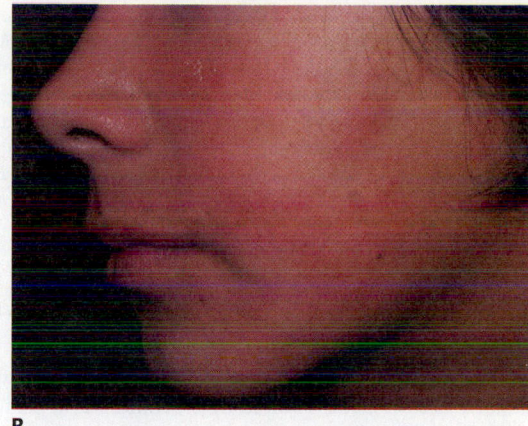

B

FIGURE 36–4 ■ *A,* Contact dermatitis caused by nickel often affects the lower abdomen as the result of exposure to belt buckles or clothing snaps. This results in a chronic dermatitis characterized by hyperpigmented scaling papules and patches. *B,* Contact dermatitis caused by poison ivy. There are clustered tiny erythematous papules involving the face and neck. In some areas (particularly the neck), lesions are distributed in a linear fashion.

Source: *A, B, Courtesy of Daniel P. Krowchuk, MD, Professor of Pediatrics and Dermatology, Department of Pediatrics, Wake Forest School of Medicine, Medical Center Blvd., Winston-Salem, NC.*

adequate concentration and contact duration. Sweating and friction enhance the skin damage caused by the irritant. For example, shin guards or gloves used for sports are potential sources of irritation.

Clinical Tip
Phytodermatitis can result when the child has contact with a chemical (furocoumarin) found in plants and vegetables such as citrus fruits, celery, fennel, parsley, fig leaves, or St. John's wort that sensitizes the skin to radioviolet (sun) light. Phytodermatitis commonly occurs in the mid to late summer when the chemical concentration is higher in the plants. Following sun exposure, the child develops erythema and blistering at the site of the exposure that then becomes hyperpigmented. Wet skin, heat, and sweating increase the response. The hyperpigmentation fades over several months (Krakowski, 2011).

Allergic contact dermatitis is a delayed hypersensitivity reaction. See Chapter 27 🔗 for a complete explanation of the immune response to allergens. An antigen is absorbed from the skin surface during the initial sensitization phase, and an immune memory is created. A repeated exposure or a long-term exposure is required to cause the immune response and the resulting dermatitis. Common allergens include nickel, poison ivy, poison oak, lanolin, neomycin or bacitracin, rubber, chemicals in shoe leather, fragrances, and latex. Children may have both an irritant and allergic reaction to latex, often found in hospital equipment and supplies, as well as in products in the home and community (see Chapter 27 🔗 for a list of products and potential substitutes).

Clinical Manifestations
Irritant contact dermatitis is a discrete area of redness that corresponds to the exposure location. The rash usually develops within a few hours of contact, peaks within 24 hours, and quickly resolves with removal of the irritant, unless the irritant is used frequently. With frequent exposure, reactions may include painful erythema, edema, vesicles, and exudation.

Allergic contact dermatitis is characterized by erythema, edema, pruritus, vesicles, or bullae that rupture, ooze, and crust (Figure 36–4 ■). The rash is usually limited to the area of contact, for example, the rash may be linear where a poison ivy leaf brushes against the skin. Symptoms develop several hours after exposure, after the immunologic response has been activated. Symptoms can last up to 3 to 4 weeks without treatment.

Collaborative Care
The goal of collaborative care is to remove the irritant or allergen causing the skin reaction and to promote reduced itching and healing.

Diagnostic Tests
The patient history and distribution of the lesions provide clues about the source and identity of the allergen or irritant. See Table 36–4. Patch testing, placing an adhesive patch with common allergens on the back between the scapulae, may be used to identify the allergen, but this test is not useful for irritant contact dermatitis.

Clinical Therapy
Treatment involves removal and future avoidance of the offending agent (e.g., clothes, plant, soap). The American Contact Dermatitis Society has a database of replacement products for individuals with allergies that can be accessed by organization members.

Calamine lotion can be applied to the affected skin. Cool compresses with aluminum acetate (Burow's solution) promote drying and relieve itching. Oatmeal or Aveeno may be added to the bathwater to relieve itching. Antihistamines may be given to reduce itching or for a sedative effect when the child is too irritable to sleep.

TABLE 36–4	Distribution of Lesions by Type of Allergen
DISTRIBUTION OF LESION	**ALLERGEN**
Face, eyelids	Cosmetics, hair and skin care products, nail cosmetics, eyeglasses with nickel, cleansers
Earlobes, neck	Nickel, fragrances
Lips, mouth	Oral hygiene products, bubblegum, lipstick
Feet	Rubber or leather chemical in shoes, metal buckles on sandals
Trunk	Snaps, buckles, moisturizers, cleansers, sunscreen products, detergents

Source: *Data from Nijhawan, R. I., Matiz, C., & Jacobs, S. E. (2009). Contact dermatitis: From basics to allergodromes. Pediatric Annals, 38(2), 99–108; and Nichols, K. M., & Cook-Bolden, F. E. (2009). Allergic skin disease: Major highlights and recent advances. Medical Clinics of North America, 93, 1211–1224.*

Practice Alert

Products containing formaldehyde or formaldehyde-releasing preservatives are not recommended for children, especially those with allergies. Common products that contain formaldehyde include shampoo, conditioner, hair gels, baby wipes, and vitamins. Foods that have formaldehyde-releasing preservatives may include aspartame, coffee, smoked ham, shitake mushrooms, and maple syrup (Nelson & Yiannias, 2009). Some medications are made with aspartame, so parents should remind healthcare providers about the child's formaldehyde sensitivity to avoid a systemic response.

Acute allergic contact dermatitis is managed with medium-potency topical corticosteroids when less than 10% of the body surface area is affected; however, the topical medication should not be applied to open lesions. The topical corticosteroids limit the production of cytokines, stop lymphocyte proliferation, and limit the inflammatory response to the allergens. The topical corticosteroid is applied to the affected area twice a day for 2 to 3 weeks. Stopping the treatment too soon can cause rebound dermatitis. Reactions to poison ivy or other allergens covering more than 10% of the body surface area require treatment with oral corticosteroids for 7 to 10 days and a tapered dose over another 7 to 10 days.

Nursing Management

Patient education for home care management focuses on care of the skin and on prevention of future exposures. Teach parents how to apply topical corticosteroids and to keep using the ointment for 2 to 3 weeks, even when the skin shows signs of healing. When oatmeal soaks are used, caution parents that the tub will be slippery. Place the oatmeal in a sock that is tied to prevent the oatmeal from clogging pipes. Instruct them to pat the child dry to leave the oatmeal film in place. Wet dressings may be soothing, and they help to loosen crusts. Burow's solution as a soak helps dry lesions. Familiarize parents with the symptoms of infection in the affected area (e.g., increased redness, oozing, fever), and tell them when to return for follow-up care.

Teaching the child and family how to avoid exposure to the allergen or irritant is an important nursing role. See Partnering with Families: Exposure to Poison Ivy or Poison Oak.

- Advise parents to wash all clothes before the first wearing and to rinse clothes an extra time to remove all soap. Mild soap should be used to clean the skin.
- Place a barrier between the allergen and the skin. For example, cover all metal snaps on clothing with cloth, and wear socks to avoid exposure to tanning chemicals left on shoe leather. If barriers do not reduce the dermatitis, then efforts to find clothing without nickel or shoes with specific tanning chemicals may be necessary.
- Make sure nickel jewelry and belt buckles are not used if a nickel allergy exists.
- Children should remove clothing worn after outside activities and take a shower. Clean clothes should then be worn.

Diaper Dermatitis

Diaper dermatitis, one of the most common causes of irritant contact dermatitis, occurs in approximately one third of young children, usually in a mild form. It is most common in infants from 9 to 12 months of age (Montoya, 2008).

Etiology and Pathophysiology

Diaper dermatitis is a primary reaction to urine, feces, moisture, or friction. Urine and feces interact with the skin to cause dermatitis. Urine increases the wetness and pH of the skin, increasing abrasion and its permeability to irritants and microbes. Urine also metabolizes to ammonia, producing another irritant. Fecal organisms provide more irritants.

Secondary infection with *Candida albicans* is a common complication of diaper dermatitis or antibiotic therapy for another condition. It is frequently the underlying cause of severe diaper rash. Diaper candidiasis often occurs simultaneously with oral candidiasis (see page 1310).

Clinical Manifestations

The primary irritant diaper rash is characterized by raw, moist, or weeping macules and papules of the skin in direct contact with the diaper. Usually the perineum, genitals, and buttocks are affected, and the skinfolds are spared. In severe cases, the infant develops a rash that is fiery red, raised, and confluent. Pustules with tenderness can also be present.

When a secondary infection with *Candida albicans* occurs, the rash has bright red beefy plaques with sharp margins that may rupture and leave scales. Small papules and pustules may be seen, along with satellite lesions (Figure 36–5 ■). Skinfolds may be involved.

Collaborative Care

The goal of collaborative care is to correctly distinguish between types of diaper dermatitis, and provide appropriate ointments to promote healing and improve the infant's comfort.

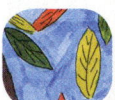

Partnering with Families

Exposure to Poison Ivy or Poison Oak

- The rash is caused by contact with urushiol, a resin of the plants, either from the plants directly or indirectly, such as transfer from animal fur or clothing.
- React quickly after contact. Wash the exposed skin with soap and water, and scrub under the nails as soon as possible. Zanfel Poison Ivy Wash, an over-the-counter cleanser, removes poison ivy resin and reduces the extent of redness and blisters if used promptly (Boelman, 2010).
- Do not rub hands exposed to poison ivy or poison oak urushiol against other body areas or in the eyes, as the resin will transfer to other areas.
- Avoid hugging a pet exposed to poison ivy until after it has been bathed.

- Launder clothing worn during exposure, and wash hands after handling exposed clothing.
- Wear vinyl gloves to handle plants (cloth and rubber gloves allow the resin to penetrate).
- Search the yard and remove all plants. Do not burn the plants. An individual with sensitivity may inhale the urushiol particles in the smoke and develop airway inflammation or severe dermatitis.
- For children with sensitivity to poison ivy or poison oak, some over-the-counter barrier creams such as IvyBlock can help prevent skin penetration by the plant oil.

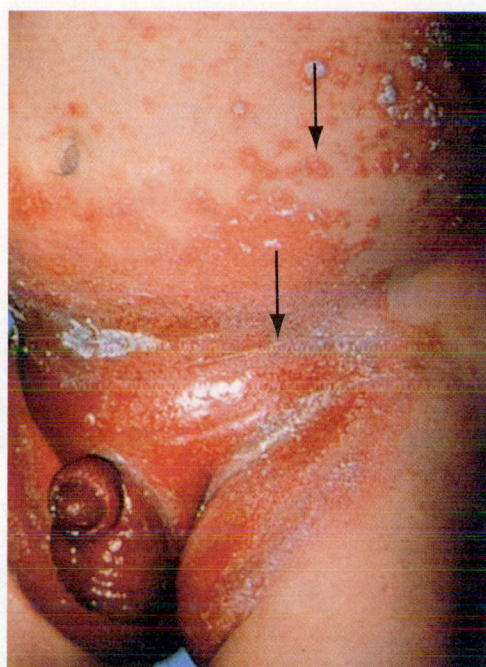

FIGURE 36–5 ■ Diaper dermatitis with *Candida albicans* secondary infection. Note the inflammation in the skinfold and satellite lesions above the diaper area.

Source: *Courtesy of the Centers for Disease Control and Prevention, Atlanta, GA.*

Diagnostic Procedures

When *Candida albicans* is suspected as a cause of the diaper rash, a skin scraping is sometimes taken for microscopic examination with potassium hydroxide (KOH).

Clinical Therapy

Mild diaper dermatitis is treated with a water-impermeable barrier or protective sealant such as zinc oxide, Aquaphor, Desitin, or Balmex after every diaper change. In some cases a combination product, containing a diaper ointment or cream plus a protective powder (e.g., karaya powder, Stomahesive protective powder), may be effective. An antifungal topical medication (e.g., nystatin) is applied to the skin before the barrier product when *Candida albicans* is present, and continued until 3 days after the rash has cleared. Topical corticosteroids are not recommended for diaper dermatitis because occlusion in the diaper area increases corticosteroid systemic absorption (Montoya, 2008).

Nursing Management

Severe diaper dermatitis can be a major source of stress for parents who must deal with a child in constant discomfort. Instruct parents to change the diaper as soon as the infant is wet or has a bowel movement, or minimally every 2 hours during the day and once during the night to limit prolonged skin contact with the urine and fecal irritants. Topical barriers (ointments or pastes such as Desitin, Triple Paste, A & D ointment, Balmex, white petrolatum, or zinc oxide ointment or paste) should be applied with each diaper change. If the diaper sticks to the skin due to these barriers, apply white petrolatum over the topical barrier. Mineral oil on a soft cloth may be helpful in removing pastes from the skin once or twice a day so that fresh medication may be applied, but more frequent removal of pastes is not necessary. Allowing the child to spend part of each day without a diaper so the skin is exposed to the air may also help healing.

Observe for signs of infection since the skin is damaged and can allow infectious organisms to grow. If significant improvement in the infant's skin is not seen within a week, encourage the parents to return for further assessment and care.

Provide parents with advice about preventing diaper dermatitis. Encourage parents to use superabsorbent disposable diapers, which tend to reduce the frequency and severity of diaper dermatitis. When wet, these diapers form a gel that keeps the skin drier than cloth diapers; however, diapers should still be changed every 2 to 3 hours. Tell parents to avoid using tight diapers and waterproof pants.

Advise parents to wash the perianal area with warm water or a cleanser not needing water (Aquanil HC lotion or Cetaphil) after a bowel movement. Advise parents to use soft cloths or paper towels with warm tap water or to use baby wipes without alcohol if baby wipes are preferred. The skin should be patted dry to reduce friction and skin injury. Powders or corn starch are not recommended because they may increase friction.

Seborrheic Dermatitis

Seborrheic dermatitis is a recurrent inflammatory skin condition thought to be caused by an overgrowth of a yeast *Malassezia furfur* (previously known as *Pityrosporum ovale*). The condition is also thought to be influenced by hormones. The rash is found over the areas of the body where the sebaceous glands are most plentiful: scalp (cradle cap), forehead, and postauricular and periorbital areas. It may also occur on the skin of the eyelids, inguinal area, or nasolabial folds. The condition is frequently seen in infants up to 3 months of age and in adolescents.

Common symptoms are pruritus and a mildly erythematous, adherent waxy scaling of the scalp (or "dandruff"). Yellow-red patches with greasy scaling may be present, typically on the scalp and nasolabial folds on the face, behind the ears, on the upper chest, and sometimes on the **intertriginous areas** (skinfolds of the neck, axillae, antecubital fossa) (Figure 36–6 ■). Itching with this rash is less intense than in atopic dermatitis.

Treatment of young infants for seborrheic dermatitis consists of daily shampooing with baby shampoo. An **emollient,** a topical

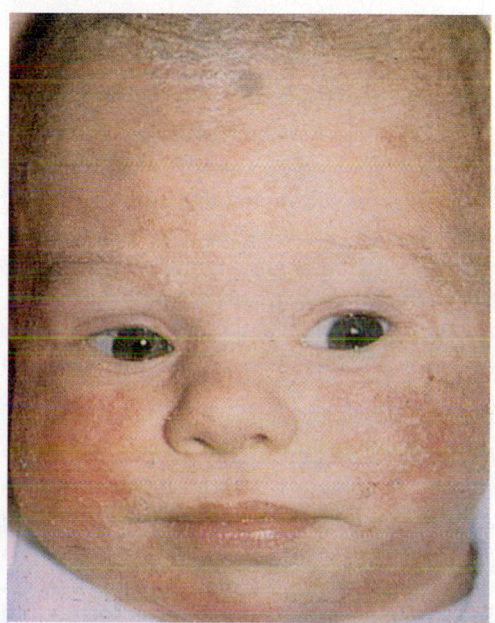

FIGURE 36–6 ■ Seborrheic dermatitis.

product that soothes and softens the skin (e.g., white petrolatum or baby oil), is left on the scalp of infants for about 20 minutes to soften the crusts. The scales are removed by brushing with the fingertips, a baby hairbrush, or a soft toothbrush. The hair is then rinsed thoroughly. A tar-containing shampoo may be used in infants if baby shampoo is not effective (O'Connor, McLaughlin, & Ham, 2008).

Lesions on the body of adolescents can be treated with shampoos containing selenium sulfide (Selsun or Head and Shoulders) or salicylic acid. Use baby shampoo to wash lesions on the eyelids and eyelashes. Treatments are continued for several days after the lesions disappear. Topical corticosteroids are often used to treat seborrhea, but they should not be used around the eyes. Topical calcineurin inhibitors (e.g., tacrolimus and pimecrolimus) are also effective for adolescents with seborrhea (Poindexter, Burkhart, & Morrell, 2009).

Nursing Management

Teach new parents that the young infant's hair should be washed daily with each bath to reduce the risk for seborrheic dermatitis. Reassure parents that gentle cleansing will not harm the infant's "soft spot." Provide a bath demonstration to show them the proper technique, if necessary. Follow-up is seldom necessary, as the condition resolves with treatment.

Educate adolescents about the daily use of shampoo and topical corticosteroid ointment or cream application. Advise adolescents that emotional distress may trigger future **flares** (exacerbations of symptoms) and to initiate treatment promptly when symptoms begin.

BACTERIAL INFECTIONS

Bacterial infections commonly occur in children due to minor skin injuries. The most common superficial infections include impetigo and folliculitis. Cellulitis is a more serious and deeper bacterial skin infection (see page 1308).

Impetigo

Impetigo, the most common bacterial skin infection, is highly contagious and superficial (involving the epidermis). The most common sites are the face and around the mouth, the hands, the neck, and the extremities.

Etiology and Pathophysiology

Minor skin injuries, insect bites, and dermatitis provide the portal for the infectious agent commonly present in the environment. For these reasons, impetigo is more common in the summer months. Either *Staphylococcus aureus*, group A beta-hemolytic streptococcus, or both together are usually responsible for the infection. *Streptococcus pyogenes* may be responsible in some cases. *Staphylococcus aureus* is the more common pathogen in the United States as it colonizes on the skin and mucous membranes, particularly in the nose and throat. Children may touch or pick their nose and spread the organism to a break in the skin. Streptococcal organisms tend to colonize on the epidermis after an injury. Impetigo occurs more commonly in children who are in close physical contact with others, such as in childcare settings, or who have poor hygiene. Bullous impetigo results from *Staphylococcus aureus* that produces an exfoliative toxin that blisters the epidermis. It most commonly occurs in infants and young children and may be a localized form of staphylococcal scalded skin syndrome (Morelli, 2011a).

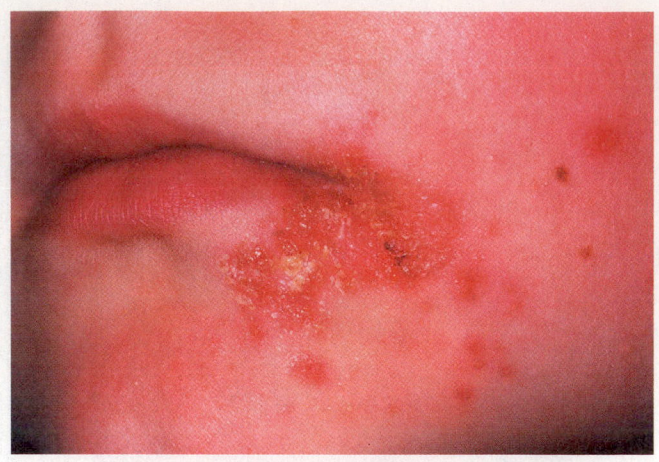

A

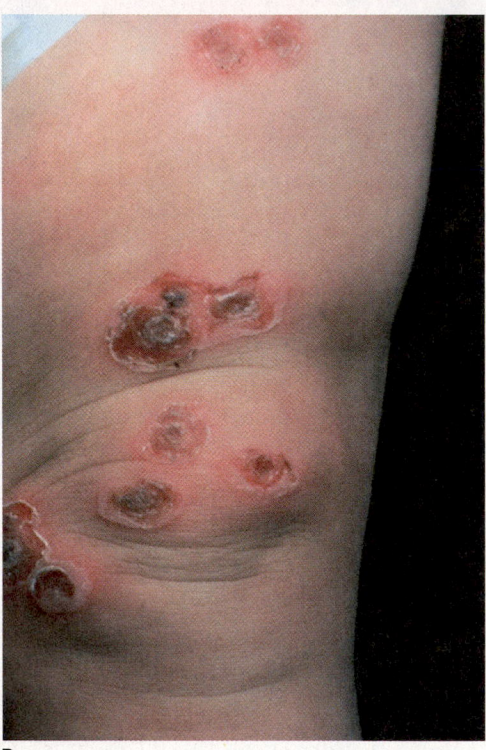

B

FIGURE 36–7 ■ Characteristic lesions of *A*, honey-colored crusts of impetigo on the face, and *B*, bullous impetigo.

Source: *A*, Images and Text Copyright © 2012 Photo Researchers, Inc. Alll Rights Reserved; *B*, © 2012 Wellcome Image Library / Custom Medical Stock Photo, All Rights Reserved.

In staphylococcal scalded skin syndrome, known as Ritter syndrome in the newborn, the exfoliative endotoxins, produced by a strain of *Staphylococcus aureus*, spread systemically, causing the skin to separate at the level of the superficial epidermis. Newborns are at the highest risk as they have no antibodies, but the condition also occurs in children up to age 5 years (Berk & Bayliss, 2010; Morelli, 2011a).

Clinical Manifestations

Impetigo lesions begin as a papule that turns into a vesicle at the site of an injury or insect bite. The vesicle ruptures and forms an erosion, and the serous fluid forms the characteristic honey-colored crusts (Figure 36–7A ■). Pruritus and regional lymphadenopathy may be present. The child may develop multiple lesions through self-inoculation.

In bullous impetigo, vesicles stimulated by the bacterial toxin enlarge and coalesce to form the bullae with sharp margins and no surrounding erythema (Figure 36–7B ■). A thin, honey-colored crust forms when the bullae rupture. When the crust is removed, a moist, erythematous lesion with a collar of skin around the shining, superficial erosion is seen. Lesions seem to occur more frequently in moist skinfold areas.

In staphylococcal scalded skin syndrome, the newborn or child may have fever; malaise; irritability; and painful, widespread erythema that is more pronounced at the flexor areas of the body and around the mouth. The erythematous skin may have a wrinkled appearance as the bullae form, enlarge, and rupture, exposing moist red skin that has a scaled appearance. Extension of blistering may occur with gentle pressure on the side of a bulla (Nikolsky sign).

Collaborative Care

The goal of collaborative care is to diagnose the organism causing the infection and to implement effective antibiotic therapy.

Diagnostic Tests

Impetigo is usually diagnosed by appearance of the lesions, but in some cases a Gram stain and bacterial culture are performed. For staphylococcal scalded skin syndrome, bacterial culture, histology, and exfoliated skin cytology testing are performed to distinguish the condition from toxic epidermal necrolysis (see the Clinical Manifestations table on page 1323).

Clinical Therapy

Local treatment involves removal of the crusts and application of a topical antibiotic. Crusts are soaked in warm water and gently scrubbed off with an antiseptic soap. A topical bactericidal ointment is applied, such as mupirocin 2% (three times a day for 5 to 7 days), retapamulin 1% (twice a day for 5 days), or fusidic acid (Morelli, 2011a). Oral antibiotics are prescribed if lesions are extensive or when lesions are on the mouth and the topical ointment may be licked off. Skin generally heals without scars. As methicillin-resistant *Staphylococcus aureus* (MRSA) has become more common, a culture and sensitivity should be performed if lesions do not clear within 7 days to identify an appropriate antibiotic for treatment. The infection continues to be communicable for 24 hours after antibiotic ointment treatment is begun.

Some cases of postinfectious streptococcal glomerulonephritis have been noted following impetigo caused by specific strains of group A beta-hemolytic streptococcus (see Chapter 31 ⊙). Cellulitis is another potential complication.

Practice Alert

If the child has a history of recurrent impetigo, determine if a caregiver or family member is a nasal carrier of *Staphylococcus aureus*. The carrier can be effectively treated with topical mupirocin ointment applied to the nares two times daily for 5 days (Zajac & Jacobson, 2009).

Staphylococcal scalded skin syndrome in infants and children with extensive skin involvement is treated with intravenous (IV) antibiotics, pain management, gentle handling, and a pressure-relieving mattress. The skin is moistened and cleaned, followed by an application of emollient to lubricate the skin and decrease discomfort. Dehydration, fluid and electrolyte imbalances, problems with temperature regulation, and secondary infections (pneumonia, septicemia, or cellulitis) may occur. Pain management is important. Healing generally occurs without scarring.

Nursing Management

Teach parents how to clean the lesions and apply topical ointment or give the oral antibiotic.

Advise parents that topical or oral medications must be continued for the full number of days prescribed. Caution parents that a child who is infected should not share towels or toiletries with others and that all linens and clothing used by the child should be washed separately with detergent in hot water. Fingernails should be kept short and clean to prevent the spread of infection from scratching. Frequent hand hygiene by the child and caregivers is important to prevent the spread of infection. Tell the parents to observe all close contacts and family members for the development of lesions. Inform the childcare center about the child's infection, so toys and surfaces can be sanitized. If the child's lesions do not improve within a couple of days of described care, have the parent contact the healthcare provider. A culture of the lesions may be needed. The child can return to childcare after 24 hours of treatment.

Discourage athletes from sharing towels and clothing. Wounds should be covered to reduce exposure to other athletes. Teach adolescents and coaches signs and symptoms of MRSA. Skin infections that worsen rather than heal with regular topical antibiotics should be seen by a healthcare provider. Athletes should not return to practice or compete until treatment is determined to be effective.

Community-Acquired Methicillin-Resistant *Staphylococcus aureus*

Community-acquired methicillin-resistant *Staphylococcus aureus* (CA-MRSA) is an organism that causes an aggressive skin and soft tissue infection in healthy children. Severe skin infections were the seventh most common reason for hospitalization in children in 2009, largely attributable to CA-MRSA (Friedman, Berdahl, Simpson, et al., 2011).

CA-MRSA is colonized on the skin, the mucous membranes, and nares of healthy individuals who are carriers. Transmission may occur by droplet during respiratory infection or contact with contaminated surfaces or hands. Athletes are at high risk because of their potential for frequent skin-to-skin contact, cuts or abrasions, and wound contact. Additional risk factors include poor hygiene, crowded living conditions, childcare center attendance, and recurrent skin infections (Hinckley & Allen, 2008).

Clinical manifestations include furuncles or abscesses. Localized swelling, redness, warmth, purulent drainage, fever, and pain may be present. The lesion may invade deeper tissues.

Diagnosis is made by culturing the drainage from an incised abscess. Treatment involves incision and drainage and wound care for simple abscesses. Systemic antibiotics are often prescribed for CA-MRSA after determining sensitivities, such as clindamycin, trimethoprim-sulfamethoxazole, doxycycline, or linezolid (Liu, Bayer, Cosgrove, et al., 2011). Children with repeated CA-MRSA infections may be encouraged to bathe in a tub with diluted bleach solution (one-half cup to a tub one-quarter full) (Neville-Swensen & Clayton, 2011).

Nursing Management

Make sure parents and adolescents understand the importance of taking the full course of the prescribed antibiotic. Educate parents about meticulous wound care to prevent the spread of CA-MRSA.

Ensure that the wound and drainage are completely covered all the time. The dressing should be changed twice a day using vinyl gloves. Dispose of the used dressing in a plastic bag that is tightly closed and placed in the trash. Good hand hygiene is important before and after dressing changes. Encourage parents to disinfect surfaces that come into contact with the wound or wound drainage using a bleach solution. Use hot water to wash linens and clothing used by the child, and dry clothes in a hot dryer.

Nurses have a major role in prevention of CA-MRSA infections. Teach adolescents the signs of a skin infection that needs treatment. Encourage good hand hygiene and a shower with soap and hot water after each practice and competition. Towels and personal items should not be shared. Shared athletic equipment should be cleaned regularly. Encourage athletes to cover and care for wounds and report those that are potentially infected.

Folliculitis

Folliculitis is a superficial inflammation of the pilosebaceous follicle caused by infection, trauma, or irritation. The causative organism is usually *Staphylococcus aureus*. The condition is common in children and teenagers because of increased sweat production. Folliculitis may be associated with *Pseudomonas aeruginosa* from an inadequately chlorinated pool or hot tub in which lesions develop 8 to 48 hours after exposure (Morelli, 2011a).

Symptoms include pain or pruritus, localized swelling, and the formation of tiny dome-shaped, yellowish pustules and red papules at follicular openings with surrounding erythema. Individual lesions may become deeper and form an abscess (furuncle). Lesions are usually seen in clusters on the face, scalp, trunk, and extremities. Some children have fever, aching, and flulike symptoms. If associated with *Pseudomonas* exposure in a pool or hot tub, lesions may develop on areas covered by bathing suits.

Treatment of inflamed follicles consists of washing the affected area with a topical antibacterial cleanser (e.g., chlorhexidine) and water. A benzoyl peroxide gel or wash or another drying agent will also help clear the infection. The lesions usually resolve within 1 to 2 weeks. Ruptured lesions heal with hyperpigmentation and no scarring. Complications are rare. If the child or adolescent has systemic symptoms, oral antibiotics (e.g., ciprofloxacin) may be prescribed. A **furuncle,** a deep infection of a hair follicle, may develop in some cases and need incision and drainage. Children who are immunocompromised should not use hot tubs because of the potential for complications from *Pseudomonas*.

Nursing Management

Nursing management focuses on educating the parents and child about prevention. Advise children to shower daily and shortly after exercise, to cleanse with an antibacterial soap, and to wear loose cotton clothing. Talk with parents about the importance of maintaining the correct pH level and chlorine concentration in swimming pools, whirlpools, and hot tubs. Bathing suits of affected children should be laundered and well dried before the next use.

Cellulitis

Cellulitis is an acute inflammation of the loose connective tissue with some limited involvement of the dermis. The child with diabetes mellitus or immunosuppression is at higher risk for cellulitis.

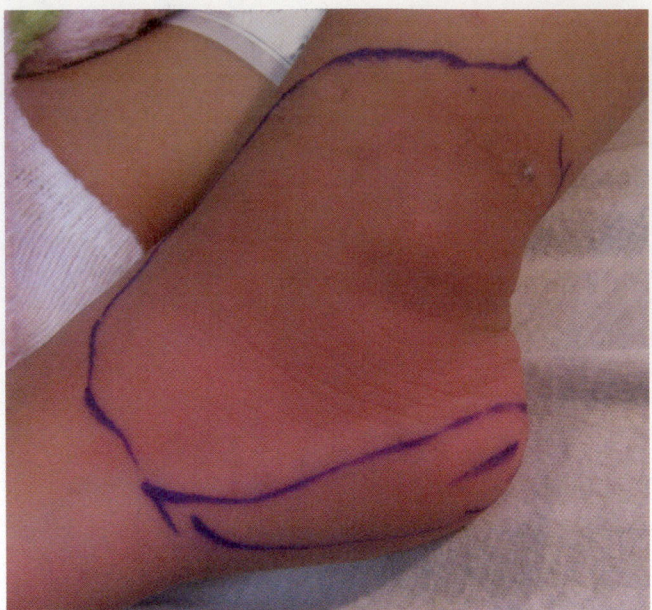

FIGURE 36–8 ■ Characteristic appearance of cellulitis.

Source: *Daniel P. Krowchuk, MD, Professor of Pediatrics and Dermatology, Department of Pediatrics, Wake Forest School of Medicine, Medical Center Blvd., Winston-Salem, NC.*

The condition usually occurs on the face and extremities as a result of trauma or a compromised skin barrier.

Etiology and Pathophysiology

Children with cellulitis often have a history of trauma, surgery, or a skin lesion. Common causative organisms are *Staphylococcus aureus* and *Streptococcus pyogenes*. The condition may also result from a nearby abscess or sinusitis.

Clinical Manifestations

Classic signs and symptoms include red or lilac, tender, warm, edematous skin around the infected site (Figure 36–8 ■). The border is often indistinct because the infection is deep in the tissue. The onset may be rapid and children may appear ill. Other symptoms include fever, chills, malaise, and enlarged, tender regional lymph nodes. **Lymphangitis,** inflammation of the lymphatic system draining the site of infection seen as tender, erythematous streaks extending in a proximal direction from the infection, may be present.

Collaborative Care

The goal of collaborative care is to initiate rapid effective antibiotic treatment of the infection to prevent progression of the infection into deeper tissues or to septicemia.

Diagnostic Tests

A complete blood count with differential often reveals an increased white blood cell count. Cultures may be taken by needle aspiration to identify the causative organisms. Blood cultures and a lumbar puncture are performed for an infant or child who has a toxic (very ill) appearance.

Clinical Therapy

Children with severe cases or a large affected surface area are hospitalized and treated with systemic antibiotics and analgesics to prevent sepsis. If the face is involved, intravenous antibiotic therapy is administered to avoid serious complications. Children with cellulitis on the trunk, limbs, or perianal area may be treated on an outpatient basis with oral antibiotics. Recovery begins within 48 hours, but therapy should continue for at least 10 days (Morelli, 2011a). See Chapter 24 🔗 for treatment of periorbital cellulitis. In some cases, a rapidly progressive lesion may result in bacteremia, abscess, septic arthritis, and thrombophlebitis.

Nursing Management

The goal of nursing management is to recognize the severity of the infection and to provide support and education to the family for effective home care and recognition of complications.

Assessment centers on recognition of infection, documentation of location and related symptoms, and monitoring of vital signs and response to therapy. Administer prescribed oral or IV antibiotics as scheduled. Supportive care includes warm compresses to the affected area four times daily, elevation of the affected limb, and bed rest. Outpatient follow-up is crucial to ensure appropriate response to therapy.

Advise parents about possible complications, such as abscess formation. Instruct parents of children who are treated at home to contact their healthcare provider if the child displays any of the following:

- Spread of the infected area in the 24- to 48-hour period after the start of treatment
- Temperature over 38.3°C (101°F)
- Increased lethargy

Reinforce to parents the importance of adherence to the treatment regimen and the seriousness of potential complications.

VIRAL INFECTIONS
Molluscum Contagiosum

Molluscum contagiosum is a viral infection of the skin caused by the poxvirus. It is transmitted by direct contact; sexual contact; or contact with contaminated clothing, towels, or other objects. Spread occurs by autoinoculation. The incubation period is 2 to 7 weeks (American Academy of Pediatrics, 2012, p. 512). Children 2 to 11 years of age are most commonly affected, but risk is increased in children with atopic dermatitis and immunodeficiency.

Multiple pearl-like, flesh-colored smooth papules (usually less than 30) are about 1 to 5 mm in diameter. Lesions are often noted on the trunk, axillae, and antecubital and popliteal fossa but may be found on the mucous membranes and conjunctiva. If found on the genitals in children, consider possible sexual abuse. The lesion develops a central depression as it enlarges, and it is filled with a plug of cheesy material that can be expressed when punctured. Pruritus may be present and disturb the child's sleep.

In mild cases the lesions resolve spontaneously within 6 months, but new lesions may appear over 2 to 4 years. In other cases, treatment may involve destruction of the lesions, using curettage, **cryotherapy** (freezing each lesion with liquid nitrogen), or cantharidin. Topical anesthesia is needed for curettage. Cantharidin, a vesicant or blistering agent, may be the treatment of choice because it is painless and effective (Mathes & Frieden, 2010). Application to the lesion causes a small blister, leading to extrusion of the lesion core with the blister rupture. Scarring or hypopigmentation change may result from any of the clinical therapies. Pruritus may be managed with emollients, topical corticosteroids, or oral antihistamines. Secondary infections are a potential complication. Oral antibiotics, warm compresses, and drainage are prescribed if the child develops an abscess in a lesion.

Nursing Management

Nursing education focuses on reducing disease transmission. Children who are infected should not use public swimming pools or hot tubs, and they should not share a bathtub with other children because the virus is transmitted more easily when the skin is wet. Transmission of the virus among household members is high. Towels, sponges, and clothing should not be shared.

The parents or child should wash the skin daily with gentle fragrance-free cleansers. A hypoallergenic moisturizer or emollient is then applied to the entire skin surface. Educate parents to recognize potential secondary infections.

When intervention such as curettage, cryotherapy, or cantharidin is performed, provide information to help the child understand what will happen, and then provide distraction during the procedure to reduce anxiety. Ensure that the child has adequate topical anesthetic to minimize any pain from the intervention. If the child has discomfort after any of the interventions, acetaminophen or ibuprofen may be used as an analgesic.

Warts (Papillomavirus)

Several types of human papillomavirus infect epithelial cells and cause warts. Various types of warts are found in children; common warts appear on any skin surface, and plantar warts are found on the feet. The human papillomavirus is commonly transmitted by direct skin-to-skin contact or mucous membrane contact, and then autoinoculation. The virus also survives on various surfaces, and transmission can occur with contact, such as plantar warts from locker room floors. The incubation period may be 2 to 6 months; however, a latency period may exist in some cases. Children with immune compromise are more susceptible to the human papillomavirus and often have numerous warts.

Common warts appear as skin-colored, rough, scaly papules and nodules on exposed skin surfaces. Individual and multiple warts may be seen, but large plaques may form if autoinoculation occurs. Warts usually cause no pain or itching unless on skin surface areas or creases that become irritated. Plantar warts appear as papules and plaques on the bottom of feet that grow inward and cause pain. Small black dots result from thrombosed vessels on the surface of the warts caused by weight bearing.

No intervention may be recommended because warts often resolve spontaneously over a couple of years, and clinical therapy may be traumatic for children. Warts do not produce scarring unless treated surgically or in an aggressive manner. Clinical therapy may be provided when warts have a social stigma or cause pain, as in the case of plantar warts. Therapy usually involves some form of destruction, such as liquid nitrogen or pulsed dye laser. Salicylic acid plasters may be applied over 5 days followed by a 2-day rest. The extremity with the warts is soaked in hot water, and debris from the wart can be removed with an emery board or pumice stone. A keratolytic agent (imiquimod) is used to treat external genital and perianal warts, as well as nongenital warts (Morelli, 2011c). Immunotherapy may also be used.

Nursing Management

Educate the parents and child about how warts may spread by picking at the wart or by sucking or chewing it. If the child will not stop sucking or chewing on the wart, bitter apple or a pepper solution may discourage the child. Teach the parents about the application of peeling agents and caustic substances when prescribed for home use. If the reaction to the substance is painful, encourage the parents to reduce the frequency of the treatment until the pain subsides and then to resume the original treatment schedule. Successful treatment may take several months, and parents may need encouragement to continue the therapy and remain optimistic. Other viral skin conditions are described in Chapter 22 🔗.

FUNGAL INFECTIONS
Oral Candidiasis (Thrush)

Oral candidiasis (moniliasis or thrush) is a fungal infection that occurs as an acute condition in newborns. Children who regularly use a corticosteroid inhaler or have received antibiotics disturbing normal flora are also at risk. Candidiasis may become a chronic condition when the child has an immune disorder.

Candida albicans causes most of the infections, as it is commonly present on the skin and mucous membranes, including the intestines and vagina. Newborns may become infected in utero, during passage through the vagina, or postnatally. Transmission rarely occurs from person to person. Children at risk for invasive *Candida* infection have an impaired immune status (immunodeficiency), have a central venous catheter, are receiving hyperalimentation long term, or are receiving broad-spectrum antibiotics (American Academy of Pediatrics, 2012, pp. 265).

Oral thrush is characterized by white patches that resemble coagulated milk on the oral mucosa, which may bleed when removed (Figure 36–9 ■). Milk residue can be removed from the oral mucosa with gentle swabbing, but with thrush, attempts to remove lesions may cause bleeding and are unsuccessful. The infant may refuse to nurse or feed because of discomfort and pain. Fever is usually not present. *Candida* lesions may also be seen in the diaper area or various skinfolds of the neck, groin, axillae, and **paronychia** (infection in the tissue surrounding the nail). (See page 1304 for the discussion on candidal diaper rash.)

Diagnosis is made by clinical appearance or by microscopic examination of a skin scraping suspended in potassium hydroxide. The appearance of yeast cells and threadlike structures of the fungus is diagnostic. A fungal culture may also be taken.

Treatment involves oral nystatin suspension or clotrimazole, which is applied to the mouth and tongue after feedings. Fluconazole or itraconazole may be beneficial for immunocompromised patients with oropharyngeal candidiasis. Intravenous amphotericin B may be used for invasive and systemic *Candida* infections. Duration of treatment depends on severity of illness, the age of the child, and the extent of compromise to the immune status.

Nursing Management

Educate the family to give oral nystatin to infants and children, using a swab to apply the suspension to the buccal mucosa and tongue surfaces. Then allow the infant to swallow the remaining suspension. Instruct older children to swish the solution around in the mouth before swallowing.

A significant nursing role is prevention of *Candida* infections, especially in infants and children at risk. Educate parents about the appropriate sterilization technique for bottle nipples and pacifiers. Good hand hygiene is important to reduce the transmission of the fungus. Breastfeeding mothers should be treated with nystatin cream applied to the nipples, as the breasts may have become infected from contact with lesions in the infant's mouth. A commercial antiseptic spray may be used on toys the infant or child puts in the mouth that cannot be autoclaved, but follow directions carefully so the child does not ingest any harmful residue.

Teach parents and older children with asthma to rinse the mouth well with water after using a corticosteroid inhaler to prevent candidiasis. If the child uses a spacer, that should also be rinsed with water after use. Meticulous nursing care for central or intravascular lines in children with impaired immune status or in those receiving prolonged hyperalimentation is critical in reducing the risk of invasive *Candida* infections.

Dermatophytoses (Ringworm)

Dermatophytoses are fungal infections that affect the skin, hair, or nails. Children of all ages may be affected. The most common infections are as follows:

- Tinea capitis, involving the hair of the scalp, usually seen in prepubertal children
- Tinea corporis, involving the skin of the body, excluding the scalp, groin, hands, or feet; seen in children and adolescents
- Tinea cruris, jock itch or involving the inner thighs, inguinal creases, or perianal area; rare before adolescence
- Tinea pedis, athlete's foot or involving the plantar surface or interdigital webbed areas of the toes and feet

Etiology and Pathophysiology

Many species of dermatophytoses may be spread from person to person or from animal to person, or by contact with an inanimate object such as the clothing, furniture, and bed linen of another infected individual. An asymptomatic carrier may exist in the family and reinfect the child and other family members. See Developing Cultural Competence: Tinea Capitis.

Clinical Manifestations

The Clinical Manifestations table compares and contrasts the dermatophyte infections.

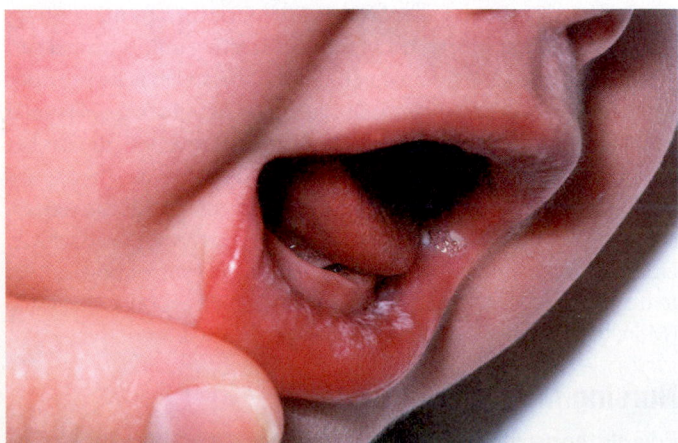

FIGURE 36–9 ■ Thrush, an acute pseudomembranous form of oral candidiasis, is a common fungal infection in infants and children.

Source: © Medical-on-Line / Alamy.

Clinical Manifestations Tinea Infections

SITE AND COMMON DERMATOPHYTE	CLINICAL MANIFESTATIONS	CLINICAL THERAPY
Tinea capitis (scalp) *Trichophyton tonsurans* in 90% of cases (American Academy of Pediatrics, 2012, p. 712) *Trichophyton mentagrophytes* *Microsporum canis* in animal-human transmission *Microsporum audouinii* Usually prepubertal children between 1 and 10 years 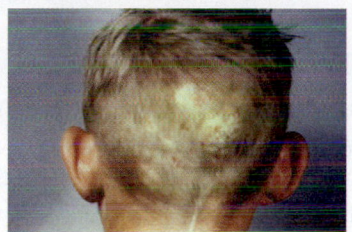	■ Circumscribed hair loss; broken hairs; dotted stubbed appearance where weakened hair has broken off ■ Many scaly pustular bald areas with indistinct margins; may appear as seborrhea, with yellow, greasy scales; erythema or lesion lighter than skin color ■ Mild itching ■ **Kerion**—large purulent tender boggy mass on scalp with drainage ■ Suboccipital or posterior cervical nodes	■ Give griseofulvin orally for 8–12 weeks, or for 2–4 weeks after symptoms disappear OR terbinafine orally once a day for 6 weeks in children older than 4 years. ■ Use selenium sulfide shampoo 2 times weekly in addition to oral medication. Leave the shampoo on the scalp for 10 minutes before rinsing to help eliminate scalp spores. Family members should also use the shampoo 2 times a week to reduce the number of spores in the household. ■ Alternative antifungal agents, e.g., fluconazole and itraconazole, are not FDA approved in children less than 12 years of age. ■ Oral corticosteroid therapy in addition to griseofulvin may be used to treat a kerion.
Tinea corporis (trunk) *Trichophyton tonsurans* *Trichophyton rubrum* *Trichophyton mentagrophytes* *Microsporum canis* *Epidermophyton floccosum* Children and adolescents 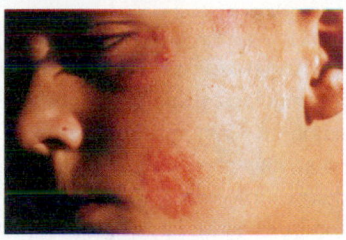	■ Pink, scaly circular patch with an expanding border, may be scaly or erythematous throughout ■ Slightly raised borders with a clearing center ■ Usually acquired from contact with infected human, animal, or contaminated object	■ Use a topical cream (e.g., clotrimazole, miconazole, ketoconazole, and terbinafine approved for ages 12 years and older; tolnaftate, naftifine, or ciclopirox approved for ages 10 years and older) twice a day for 4–6 weeks, even if the rash clears sooner. ■ Topical corticosteroids are not used to reduce the risk for a persistent or recurrent infection. ■ Selenium sulfide shampoo should be used 2 times a week on the child's body in addition to topical cream. The shampoo helps to reduce the number of spores. Family members may also use the shampoo. ■ An oral antifungal agent may be needed when there is no response to topical therapy.
Tinea cruris ("jock itch") *Epidermophyton floccosum* *Trichophyton rubrum* *Trichophyton mentagrophytes* Rare before adolescence	■ Scaly, erythematous annular lesions on groin and upper thighs; may spread to abdomen and buttocks, usually spare the penis and scrotum ■ May have elevated lesions, papules, or vesicles ■ Tinea pedis may have been spread by hand to groin area	■ Use a topical antifungal agent (e.g., clotrimazole, miconazole, and terbinafine for ages 12 years and older, tolnaftate or ciclopirox for 10 years and older) for 4–6 weeks. ■ Topical corticosteroids are not used to reduce the risk for a persistent or recurrent infection. ■ Decrease moisture and occlusion in area.
Tinea pedis ("athlete's foot") *Trichophyton rubrum* *Trichophyton mentagrophytes* *Epidermophyton floccosum* Older children and adolescents	■ Vesicles or erosions on instep or between toes (fissures, red scaly); dry scaly patches or plaques with mild erythema on plantar and lateral surfaces of foot ■ Peeling maceration and fissures in lateral toe web spaces (indicate a secondary bacterial involvement) ■ Pruritus	■ Use a broad-spectrum topical antifungal agent with antibacterial properties, such as econazole, clotrimazole, or miconazole. ■ Keep feet dry with absorbent antifungal foot powder. ■ Allow feet to air-dry frequently. ■ Use 100% cotton socks, change twice daily. ■ Put socks on before other clothing to reduce transmission of fungus to groin.

Source: *Data from American Academy of Pediatrics. (2012).* Red book: Report of the Committee on Infectious Diseases *(29th ed., pp. 712–719). Elk Grove Village, IL: Author.*
Photos courtesy of the Centers for Disease Control and Prevention, Atlanta, GA.

Developing Cultural Competence
Tinea Capitis

Although tinea capitis can occur in any racial or ethnic group, infection with *Trichophyton tonsurans* is most prevalent in African American children. It is not known if this is due to hair type or ethnicity. For this reason, all African American children with scaling in the scalp should be screened for tinea capitis (Meadows-Oliver, 2009).

Collaborative Care

The goal of collaborative care is the accurate diagnosis of the lesions and effective therapy to treat the condition.

Diagnostic Tests

Diagnosis may be confirmed through microscopic examination of the hair and scalp scrapings using a KOH wet mount to reveal rows and chains of spores within the hair shaft. A fungal culture can also be taken by rubbing a cotton-tipped applicator across a moistened area of the scalp and placing it in a throat culture tube. A Wood's lamp may help identify some forms of tinea such as *Microsporum* infection, which fluoresces a brilliant green with ultraviolet light. However, the most common forms of tinea (e.g., *Trichophyton tonsurans*) do not fluoresce (American Academy of Pediatrics, 2012, p. 713).

Clinical Therapy

An oral antifungal agent (e.g., griseofulvin and terbinafine) is usually prescribed for tinea capitis. Resistance is developing to griseofulvin, and high doses for 8 to 12 weeks are needed; however, it has the best safety record. Treatment continues for 2 to 4 weeks after clinical resolution to help prevent a recurrence. Terbinafine, given once per day for 6 weeks, was recently approved for children 4 years of age and older. The medication comes in granules that can be sprinkled on food as well as tablets. Antifungal shampoo may reduce the risk of transmission. The child should not be excluded from school as asymptomatic carriers are probably present. Kerions are treated with oral antifungal agents, and often oral corticosteroid therapy is prescribed for 2 weeks with tapering doses toward the end of therapy (American Academy of Pediatrics, 2012, p. 714).

Practice Alert

A large number of children treated for tinea capitis and tinea pedis will develop an extensive, itchy papulovesicular rash on the trunk, extremities, and face similar to atopic dermatitis. This is called the "id" reaction. It is a hypersensitivity reaction to the fungal antigen, not an allergic reaction to the oral medication (Morelli, 2011b). Continuing therapy with the antifungal agent is critical to resolving the fungal infection.

Topical antifungal agents are used for tinea corporis, tinea cruris, and tinea pedis, and medication should be applied at least 2 cm beyond the border of the lesion. Oral therapy is required if the response to topical agents is poor after the recommended length of treatment. Treatment should continue for 1 to 2 weeks after the skin lesions have cleared to ensure that the infection is fully treated. Topical medications with corticosteroids should not be used as first-line agents. Resolution of the inflammation may confuse families who think the infection is cleared earlier than expected. They may discontinue treatment too soon, resulting in a recurrence of the infection.

Nursing Management

All members of the family and household pets should be assessed for fungal lesions after the child's diagnosis. In many cases, a family member is an asymptomatic carrier, so treatment of all family members with selenium sulfide shampoo may be encouraged. Because person-to-person transmission is common, personal contact with hair and the sharing of hair accessories, brushes, and hats should be avoided. Ensure that the child's brush and comb are cleaned. Teach parents and children that fungi are found in soil and animals and are transmitted through direct contact.

Advise parents to give oral griseofulvin with fatty foods such as whole milk or peanut butter to enhance absorption. The medications must be used for the entire prescribed period, even if the lesions are gone, to prevent recurrence of the infection. Alert parents to the possibility of the "id" reaction rash so they do not stop the medication.

For children with tinea cruris, encourage the use of cotton underwear and loose-fitting undergarments to promote dryness. An antifungal powder may help promote dryness and serve as a prophylaxis.

With tinea pedis, feet should be kept clean and dry and nails clipped short. Use of 100% cotton socks that wick moisture away from the skin is helpful in reducing the maceration and potential for secondary infection. Socks should be changed frequently. To help prevent tinea pedis, encourage children to wear shower shoes in public showers and the locker room.

Parents of children with tinea capitis should be told that hair regrowth is slow and may take 6 to 12 months. In rare cases hair loss is permanent, which can be particularly stressful for older children or adolescents. Provide emotional support and suggestions for hairstyles.

CHRONIC SKIN CONDITIONS

Atopic Dermatitis (Eczema)

Atopic dermatitis, also called eczema, is a chronic, relapsing, superficial inflammatory skin disorder characterized by intense pruritus (Figure 36–10 ■). The condition affects approximately 20% of infants, children, and adolescents (Shaw, Burkhart, & Morrell, 2009). Up to 60% of children who develop the condition do so during the first year of life (Gonzalez, Unwala, & Connelly, 2008). Some children have recurrent symptoms that continue into adulthood, and some children may have or develop other allergic conditions such as asthma or food allergy.

Etiology and Pathophysiology

The etiology of atopic dermatitis is unknown; a complex interaction of genetic predisposition, environmental exposure, infectious agents, defects in the skin barrier, and immunologic responses contributes to its development. A genetic mutation involving filaggrin, a protein essential for the skin barrier function, may play a role in the increased loss of water through the epidermis, infections, and inflammation (Ong & Boguniewicz, 2008). Atopic dermatitis has two forms, nonallergic and allergic (associated with high levels of IgE). The nonallergic

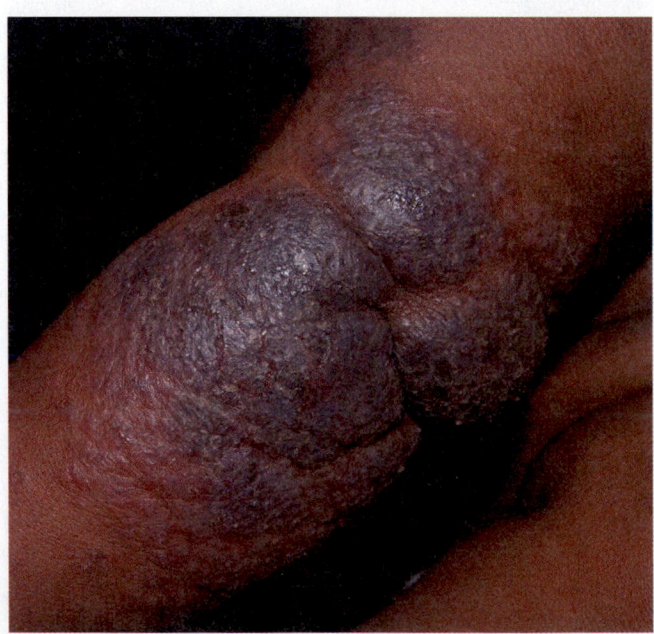

FIGURE 36–10 ■ Severe atopic dermatitis in an infant. Note the thick (i.e., lichenified), hyperpigmented plaque on the extensor surface of the elbow.

Source: *Courtesy of Daniel P. Krowchuk, MD, Professor of Pediatrics and Dermatology, Department of Pediatrics, Wake Forest School of Medicine, Winston-Salem, NC.*

(not IgE-mediated) form is more common in preschool children and in adults (Caubet & Eigenmann, 2010). Allergens, especially food allergens, are believed to play a significant role in atopic dermatitis. The impaired skin barrier also makes the child more responsive to allergens in the environment. Both the IgE-mediated immediate immune response and T-cell-mediated delayed immune response are involved. Inhalant allergens become more common after age 3 years and include pollen, mold, cockroaches, dust mites, and animal dander, as well as bacterial and fungal organisms (Caubet & Eigenmann, 2010).

Due to the increased loss of water through the epidermis, the child has **xerosis,** generally dry skin that is more likely to crack and fissure. Chronically dry skin allows irritants to penetrate and makes the child more susceptible to infection. Children with atopic dermatitis have been found to have a deficiency of a skin lipid that has anti-*Staphylococcus aureus* properties and a decrease in antimicrobial peptide, likely resulting in the recurrent infections. Approximately 90% of children with atopic dermatitis have *Staphylococcus aureus* colonized on their skin compared to 10% of healthy children (Ong & Leung, 2010). Exotoxins secreted by *Staphylococcus aureus* stimulate the immune system, leading to the persistence of inflammation (Epps, 2010). These children are also susceptible to other bacterial, viral, and fungal infectious organisms.

Clinical Manifestations

Acute atopic dermatitis is characterized by erythematous papulovesicular lesions with exudates, crusts, and pruritus. Excoriation from scratching is common. Some patches may weep. Chronic atopic dermatitis characteristics include darkened, thickened skin with prominent skin lines (lichenification), excoriation, dryness, and scaling. Inflammation usually occurs on the face, neck, and extensor surfaces in infants, but lesions on flexor surfaces (antecubital and popliteal areas) often occur in children over age 2 years. The diaper area is usually spared in infants because the skin is damp, and the diaper protects the area from scratching. Adolescents may have the following areas affected: the eyelids, where the earlobe touches the face, fingertips, toes, nipple, and the vulva, plus sites affected in the childhood phase.

The itching interferes with sleep and causes irritability. The child may wiggle to scratch so much that a perception of hyperactivity may occur. Areas with erythema and warmth may indicate a secondary bacterial skin infection. Some children have repeated flares or chronic atopic dermatitis that persists into adulthood. Other children may have skin resolution when respiratory symptoms such as asthma develop.

Collaborative Care

The goals of collaborative care are to identify potential triggers for atopic dermatitis, to keep the skin hydrated and lubricated, and to treat flare-ups aggressively so the risk for infection is reduced.

Diagnostic Tests

Atopic dermatitis is distinguished from other forms of dermatitis by the child's history and clinical manifestations. Diagnostic criteria for atopic dermatitis include an itching skin condition and three of the following signs (Ong & Boguniewicz, 2008):

- History of flexural dermatitis (e.g., popliteal or antecubital area)
- History of respiratory allergic condition (asthma or allergic rhinitis) in a first-degree relative
- History of dry skin in past year
- Skin rash occurring before 2 years of age
- Visible flexural dermatitis; dermatitis on cheeks, forehead, or extensor surfaces in an infant

No laboratory tests are diagnostic. Skin prick tests or radioallergosorbent tests (RAST) may be used to identify food allergies, and children may not use antihistamines or corticosteroids for several days before these tests to ensure effective evaluation of the child's response (Epps, 2010). See Chapter 27 🔗. Cultures of the skin may be used when a secondary infection is suspected.

Clinical Therapy

As there is no cure, the goals of treatment are to hydrate and lubricate the skin, reduce pruritus, minimize inflammatory changes, and try to determine what triggers flare-ups for future avoidance. The skin is lubricated by applying an occlusive topical emollient cream or ointment within 3 minutes of leaving the water after bathing. This traps moisture in the skin and promotes flexibility of the skin without cracking. Moisturizing ointments and creams should be applied three to four times a day or whenever the skin feels dry. Numerous types of medications are used to treat atopic dermatitis. See the Medications table on page 1314.

Clinical Tip
Emollients selected should have a cream or ointment base and be fragrance-free. Lotions contain alcohol which will further dry the skin. Examples of emollients include Eucerin cream, Aveeno cream, Vanicream, Cetaphil cream, SBR-Lipocream, and white petroleum. White petroleum (e.g., Vaseline) has the benefit of lower cost, especially since so much of the emollient must be used.

Topical corticosteroids are used to reduce inflammation and help control the flare. Ointments are preferred over creams because of their occlusive effect, which ensures a stronger barrier and absorption into the skin. Many different preparations and seven categories of corticosteroid strength exist to treat acute flares. Midstrength corticosteroids are applied twice daily for 2 weeks under the emollient. Lower strength corticosteroids are used for thinner skin areas, such as the face, diaper area, and skinfolds. When the inflammation resolves, topical corticosteroids are tapered in frequency of application and strength, and then discontinued. Topical steroids are not used on healthy skin to reduce the risk of adrenal suppression and other side effects. Oral corticosteroids may be used for a severe acute exacerbation; however, a consequence is a rebound effect after the medication is discontinued, in which the rash is even more severe than when oral corticosteroids were started (Epps, 2010).

Practice Alert
The potency or strength of a topical corticosteroid is based on whether it is fluorinated and contains other ingredients. Do not rely on the percentage listed on the medication label to inform you about the medication's potency. Avoid the use of fluorinated corticosteroids on the face, genitalia, and intertriginous (skinfold) areas where absorption of the medication may be increased because of the thinness of the stratum corneum.

Children with atopic dermatitis often have *Staphylococcus aureus* colonization, which can trigger an immune cascade that increases pruritus. Topical antibiotics are not effective for atopic dermatitis. Oral antibiotics, such as a cephalosporin for 5 to 7 days, are prescribed to treat an infection associated with a flare. Consider antibacterial resistance patterns in the community when selecting the

Medications Used to Treat Atopic Dermatitis

MEDICATIONS	ACTION	NURSING MANAGEMENT
Antihistamines (e.g., diphenhydramine, hydroxyzine) Oral	Provides sedation to control nighttime itching.	■ Encourage nighttime use when acute flares interfere with sleep. If given during the day, sleepiness will interfere with learning.
Antibiotics Topical or oral	Treats cutaneous skin superinfections.	■ Educate parents about potential for a hypersensitivity reaction.
Corticosteroids Topical or oral	Helps control skin inflammation.	■ Apply topical product to all lesions immediately after bathing, and then apply emollients. ■ Educate parents to avoid using topical product around the eyes to reduce the potential for development of glaucoma or cataracts. ■ Do not use topical product on healthy skin. ■ Do not use topical product under occlusive dressings that can increase absorption.
Calcineurin inhibitors (second-line drug) Tacrolimus ointment (Protopic) Pimecrolimus (Elidel, SDZ-ASM-981) Topical	Inhibits T-lymphocyte activation and the release of cytokines and inflammatory mediators from anti-IgE-activated skin mast cells and basophils. Approved for children over 2 years of age. May increase the risk for viral skin infections (Epps, 2010).	■ Inform the child and parents to expect a sensation of burning, redness, and itching for the first few days of therapy; symptoms generally decrease over a few days. ■ Apply to clean and dry skin for treatment between skin flares; can be used on the face and other thin skin areas (Epps, 2010). ■ Do not apply under an occlusive dressing. ■ Educate the child and parents to use sunscreens because of potential increased risk for skin cancer with sun exposure.

appropriate antibiotic. If the child has a fever and is not responsive to treatment, a culture and sensitivity test is needed to identify an appropriate antibiotic (Epps, 2010). Children may be encouraged to soak in a tub with dilute chlorine bleach (one-quarter to one-half cup of bleach to a tub filled 4 to 6 inches) to help reduce the number of *Staphylococcus aureus* infections, especially if lesions improve after swimming in a chlorinated pool (Epps, 2010). See Box 36–2. Superinfections with herpes simplex may be treated with oral or intravenous acyclovir, depending upon the severity of the infection.

Immunomodulator ointments such as tacrolimus (Protopic) and pimecrolimus (Elidel) are increasingly used as a second-line treatment for some children; however, the expense of the medication may be prohibitive for some families. The medication has been approved by the U.S. Food and Drug Administration (FDA) for children over 2 years of age for short-term or intermittent treatment who are not responsive to conventional therapy. The FDA has placed a black box warning on both drugs indicating that long-term safety has not been established (Epps, 2010). However, topical corticosteroids also have

significant potential adverse effects such as skin atrophy, hypopigmentation, and suppression of the hypothalamic-pituitary axis when used long term, so all treatments for atopic dermatitis have risks.

Oral immunomodulating agents (e.g., azathioprine, cyclosporine, mycophenolate, or methotrexate) or phototherapy may be used when atopic dermatitis does not respond to other therapies; however, these are not generally FDA-approved treatments for atopic dermatitis. Experience with these agents is limited, especially in children, and adverse effects of long-term use may include carcinogenesis (Shaw et al., 2009).

Antihistamine agents such as diphenhydramine (Benadryl) or hydroxyzine (Vistaril and Atarax) have a limited effect on itching, but the sedative effect is beneficial for promoting sleep for several nights during a flare. Tolerance to the sedating effects of these medications occurs, so limit their use for 2 to 7 nights. The tricyclic antidepressant doxepin may also be prescribed to manage pruritus. Topical antihistamines are not recommended because of the potential for hypersensitivity reactions and contact dermatitis. See Complementary Therapy: Probiotics and Atopic Dermatitis.

BOX 36–2   Research: Bleach Baths

A recent study investigated the effectiveness of soaking in a bath with dilute chlorine bleach (one-half cup in a 40-gallon bathtub) for 5 to 10 minutes twice a week on atopic dermatitis severity. A total of 31 children 6 months to 17 years of age were randomly assigned to either soak in dilute bleach baths and have intranasal application of mupirocin ointment (to treat *Staphylococcus aureus* colonization) or soak in a tub with plain bathwater and have white petrolatum nasal treatment. The atopic dermatitis severity scores decreased significantly for all body sites except the unexposed head and neck in children assigned to dilute bleach baths and nasal mupirocin treatment (Huang, Abrams, Tlougan, et al., 2009).

Complementary Therapy Probiotics and Atopic Dermatitis

Probiotics were found in one randomized controlled study to reduce the incidence of atopic dermatitis. Mothers (n=159) with a first-degree relative with atopic dermatitis were prescribed a probiotic or placebo to take during pregnancy, and the infants were also prescribed a probiotic or placebo after birth. During the next 2 years, infants taking probiotics had a lower incidence of atopic dermatitis than infants treated with a placebo (Morelli, Calmet, & Jhingade, 2010).

Methods to reduce pruritus include aggressively treating flares and other environmental controls, such as humidification in the winter and air conditioning in the summer. The humidifier counteracts dryness of the surrounding air, minimizing loss of skin moisture. Air conditioning limits unnecessary sweating that can exacerbate inflamed areas.

Food allergies may be a significant factor for up to 40% of children with atopic dermatitis (Epps, 2010). Food triggers are more common in children under age 3 years and include cow milk, eggs, soy, wheat, peanuts, tree nuts, fish, and shellfish. A food elimination test may be suggested for these children to see if improvements in the skin condition occur. Cow milk, wheat, eggs, soy products, citrus, and peanuts are the foods most often withheld for 2 or more weeks to determine if any change in skin condition occurs. Foods withheld are then introduced one at a time to determine which ones are the allergens. See Chapter 19 for more information on food allergies.

Nursing Management

The goal of nursing management is to provide support and education to the family to manage the child's skin condition and reduce the number of flares requiring medical intervention.

Nursing Assessment and Diagnosis

A thorough history, including any family history of allergy, environmental factors, and past exacerbations of skin problems, is necessary. Note the distribution and type of lesions. Attempt to identify what makes the skin condition flare (e.g., sweating, detergent use, food). Note the presence of weeping lesions or signs of infection.

Clinical Judgment
What are the signs and symptoms that help distinguish between chronic atopic dermatitis and an acute flare?

Identify the potential impact that the skin disorder is having on the child and family. How does the family describe living with a child having atopic dermatitis? How is the family managing the daily care routine? Do the child, sibling, or other family members have disturbed sleep because of scratching? What stresses have been imposed on the family? What concerns does the child have about his or her appearance? How is the child's appearance affecting the family's social relationships? What are the family's concerns about medication use?

Common nursing diagnoses that may be appropriate for the child with atopic dermatitis include the following:

- Tissue Integrity, Impaired, related to dry skin, chemical irritants, and mechanical factors (abrasive clothing)
- Sleep Pattern, Disturbed, related to prolonged physical discomfort (itching)
- Infection, Risk for, related to breaks in the skin barrier
- Self-Esteem, Chronic Low, related to chronic illness and peer reaction to visible skin lesions
- Therapeutic Regimen Management: Family, Ineffective, related to excessive demands made on the family to keep the condition under control

NANDA-I © 2012

Planning and Implementation

Nursing management focuses on education and emotional support. Atopic dermatitis can be controlled, but there is no cure. Advise parents that the lesions are not contagious and will not usually result in scarring. Help parents and children of all ages deal with the frustration of the acute condition flares by reinforcing that remissions do occur with good home care.

Skin Care
Bathing and cleaning the skin once a day is important to hydrate the skin and to allow topical corticosteroids to penetrate the skin. A brief warm soak in the bathtub or shower should be followed with patting excess water from the skin and application of adequate emollient to the entire body within 3 minutes to trap moisture in the skin. If soap is used, select an unscented product such as Dove or Cetaphil liquid cleanser. If water stings the child's open lesions, salt or baking soda can be added to the bathwater to make the water more like the child's physiologic fluids. See recommended emollients in the Clinical Tip on page 1313. Emollients should be reapplied several times a day. When the child has a flare, the child may be bathed twice a day followed by the application of topical medications on affected areas and emollients on unaffected skin, unless the child has too much discomfort from the bathwater. If the child has increased dryness associated with bathing, less frequent bathing is recommended.

Teach parents and children appropriate application of topical ointments or creams. Depending on the topical corticosteroid or calcineurin inhibitor prescribed, it should be spread in a thin layer over all lesions once or twice daily. The medication should be rubbed in gently and completely. As the skin clears, the topical corticosteroid is changed to a lower strength product as a tapering dose before discontinuing its use. Medications should be applied first, with emollients applied on top. Emollients should be continued after topical corticosteroids and calcineurin inhibitors are discontinued. See Partnering with Families: Skin Care for Atopic Dermatitis for additional tips for skin care.

Emotional Support
Allow parents to discuss their feelings about having a child with visible skin lesions, and the types of comments they hear from family, friends, and strangers. Reassure parents that the condition does improve with age in most cases and with consistent skin care.

Atopic dermatitis produces visible changes that can affect a child's self-confidence and self-esteem. Identify activities that the child can participate in to improve self-esteem. Even though humidity and sweating can make the condition worse, encourage the child to participate in sports. However, the child should shower as soon as possible after a sporting event or strenuous activity to clean the skin, and then apply emollients.

The child, parents, and siblings may be tired because of lost sleep when the child scratches at night during a flare. This may affect school performance if the child has sleep deprivation or if the child has physical discomfort that interferes with learning. If an oral antihistamine has been ordered, make sure the parents understand when to give the medication to maximize its effectiveness to produce a full night of sleep.

Parents may feel guilty or embarrassed because of their inability to clear the child's skin and to keep it clear. Make an effort to have the child return for follow-up visits about 2 weeks after a flare to monitor progress in controlling the skin inflammation. Provide encouragement and positive reinforcement for improvements in the child's skin. See Health Promotion & Maintenance Overview: The Child with Atopic Dermatitis.

Food Allergy Management
Food allergies may be identified as a trigger for atopic dermatitis. Educate parents that increased itching within hours of eating a food may be

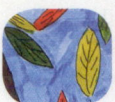

Partnering with Families

Skin Care for Atopic Dermatitis

- Help select an appropriate emollient ointment or cream for the family to use; the child may respond to one better than another. Avoid ointments and creams with a fragrance because these may irritate the skin.
- Consider the cost of emollient ointments and creams and make sure it fits into the family's budget as this is an out-of-pocket cost. Large quantities are needed to cover the body at least twice a day. White petroleum is inexpensive, safe, and easily applied.
- Help ensure that parents receive adequate amounts of topical corticosteroids for effective treatment. It takes about 6 g to cover the entire body of a 6-month-old infant, so a 12-g tube of corticosteroid ointment is enough for only 1 day and 84 g are needed for an entire week. Similarly, it takes 10 g to cover the entire body of a 2-year-old, 13 g for a 5-year-old, and 18 g for a 10-year-old (Findlay, 2007). Corticosteroids should be applied

no more than twice a day. Fortunately, most children do not have atopic dermatitis over the entire body, and the ointment is used only where there is inflammation.
- For immunomodulators, a pea-size amount should cover a 2-inch circle.
- In areas where the humidity is low, more frequent application of emollients to the skin is needed.
- Encourage the child to wear loose cotton clothing rather than wool or other materials that can irritate the skin. Keep the child's fingernails trimmed, and place clean cotton gloves or socks over the hands of an infant or child to decrease scratching and the risk for secondary infection.
- Educate children about the disorder and skin care. Emphasize the importance of following the treatment plan to promote healing of existing lesions and to reduce the number of flares and secondary infections.

---

associated with an atopic dermatitis flare. Teach parents how to control the skin inflammation that results, as described. Once a specific food allergy has been identified, such as eggs, refer the parents to a nutritionist for counseling related to alternative food options that will fulfill daily nutritional requirements. Caution parents that food allergies can change, so foods connected with atopic dermatitis can sometimes be safely eaten at a later age. Different food sensitivities may also develop. See Chapter 19 . Refer the family to the Food Allergy Network.

Evaluation

Expected outcomes of nursing care include the following:

- The child has longer periods of remission as skin care improves and fewer atopic dermatitis flares.

- Atopic dermatitis triggers are identified and avoided.
- The child's sleep is minimally disturbed due to itching.

Psoriasis

Psoriasis is a chronic, relapsing, pruritic, papulosquamous skin condition that has its onset during childhood and adolescence in about a third of cases (Bard, Torchia, & Schachner, 2010). An estimated 20,000 children under age 10 years are thought to have the disorder (Hanson, Thompson, Langemo, et al., 2008). Psoriasis is a T-cell-mediated autoimmune disease. Inflammatory cytokines from activated T cells, B cells, and macrophages are responsible for the skin

---

Health Promotion & Maintenance Overview

The Child with Atopic Dermatitis

GROWTH AND DEVELOPMENT SURVEILLANCE
- Assess growth measurements and plot on a growth chart. Identify any changes in weight and height that could be related to an altered meal plan due to food allergies.
- Perform a Denver II to assess developmental progress for age.

NUTRITION
- Identify any patterns of skin flares associated with newly introduced foods. If food allergies are identified, ensure that the parents receive nutritional counseling to provide all essential nutrients to the child.
- If atopic dermatitis develops early in infancy, postponing the introduction of eggs into the diet may be beneficial. Ensure that alternative sources of protein and iron are provided in the diet.

PHYSICAL ACTIVITY
- Encourage physical activity, but bathing and application of emollients should occur as soon as possible.
- If swimming is a preferred activity, rinse chlorine immediately after leaving the pool and apply emollients immediately after rinsing off chlorine.
- Between physical activities, keep the child in a cool environment to reduce itching and sweating that further irritates the skin.

FAMILY INTERACTIONS
- Identify how frequently the child's sleep is disturbed by scratching. Are other family members disturbed, such as a child sharing the room?

MENTAL AND SPIRITUAL HEALTH
- Determine the child's level of frustration with skin flares and desire for clear skin.
- Assess the child's self-esteem and impact of skin lesions on relationships with peers.
- Identify how disturbed sleep affects behavior and learning. Encourage the use of an antihistamine to promote sleep when a skin flare occurs.

DISEASE PREVENTION STRATEGIES
- Provide all immunizations on schedule.
- Perform all recommended screening tests for age.
- Teach the family that good hand hygiene is essential to reduce the risk of infection.
- Educate the child and parents to provide skin care as described in Partnering with Families in an effort to minimize skin inflammation and to reduce the risk for secondary infection.

changes (Nicol & Huether, 2010b). A family history of psoriasis is often present, but a multifactorial inheritance is suspected. The dermis and epidermis become thickened along with excessive proliferation of keratinocytes, abnormal differentiation of keratinocytes, and inflammation. Because cells proliferate so rapidly, the keratinocytes do not mature. The epidermis thickens and plaques form with a silvery, scaly appearance.

The typical psoriatic lesion is a thick, silvery scaly erythematous plaque with an irregular border, surrounded by normal skin. Pruritus is often present. These lesions commonly are found on the scalp, elbows, knees, umbilicus, and genitals. Nails may also be involved. Lesions also often appear at the site of trauma. Small points of bleeding may be noted when a scale is removed. Triggers may be infection, skin injury, and stress. One of the most common infectious triggers of psoriasis in children, particularly guttate type, is group A beta-hemolytic streptococcus (Mukherjee, 2011). Guttate psoriasis is characterized by an eruption of small round or oval papules on the trunk, face, and extremities. The child may have remissions and exacerbations that occur throughout life.

Diagnosis is based on observation of skin lesions, but microscopic examination of skin lesions is sometimes performed. Treatment includes midstrength or stronger topical corticosteroids twice a day and topical vitamin D. A topical retinoid may also be prescribed. A tar shampoo may be used to clear scales in the scalp prior to topical steroid application. Ultraviolet B phototherapy is used for children who do not respond to topical therapy. Systemic therapy with drugs such as methotrexate, oral retinoids, and cyclosporine is reserved for children with severe psoriasis. The condition cannot be cured, and lifelong relapses and remissions occur.

Nursing Management

The child's skin should be assessed for extent of lesions and response to therapy. Spend time talking with the child and family to learn how the condition affects them. Educate them about the condition and reasonable expectations related to treatment. Families need to understand that lesions are not contagious and that there will be periods of remissions and flares. Make sure that the family and child are actively involved in decision making regarding the treatment plan. Parents and adolescents need education to appropriately apply topical medications. The child should be encouraged to avoid situations in which chemical and physical trauma to the skin could occur.

Children and adolescents may have feelings of embarrassment, anger, and frustration related to their visible skin lesions. The impact on their daily lives may involve problems with school, personal relationships, and social acceptance. Children may anticipate rejection and withdraw from social interactions. Children and adolescents may withdraw from physical activities that require them to expose affected skin areas, such as swimming. The mental health of adolescents should be monitored to identify psychologic distress, depression, or substance abuse. The National Psoriasis Foundation provides supportive information and local or Internet support group contacts. Peers may help the child learn how to handle social situations.

Acne

Acne is a chronic inflammatory disorder of the pilosebaceous hair follicles located on the face and trunk. It is the most common skin disorder in the pediatric population. It affects 85% of the population between 12 and 25 years of age (Nicol & Huether, 2010a). Acne is found in all ethnic groups and is present equally in males and females, but severe acne is more common in males.

Etiology and Pathophysiology

Keratin and sebum usually flow to the skin surface. Androgens released as puberty begins trigger the sebaceous glands to increase the production of sebum. When the extra sebum mixes with the keratinocytes and causes them to clump together, the pilosebaceous hair follicle canal becomes obstructed by comedones (whitehead and blackheads). The sebum behind the comedones is an ideal environment for the anaerobic *Propionibacterium acnes*, allowing it to proliferate. This bacterium metabolizes the sebum, causing an inflammatory rather than infectious reaction (Clayton & Tom, 2010). When the inflammatory reaction is close to the surface, a papule or pustule develops. If the hair follicle ruptures, the inflammatory reaction is deeper, and a larger papule or nodule develops. Extensive rupture and inflammation leads to cysts that can result in scars. Familial trends have been recognized, particularly in cases of severe acne, but a pattern of inheritance has not been identified.

Acne may also occur in 20% of neonates in response to maternal androgen hormones. This form of acne may develop in the first month of life and resolves spontaneously in a few months. Drugs such as anabolic steroids, systemic corticosteroids, phenytoin, phenobarbital, lithium, trimethadione, and isoniazid are reported to cause acne (Morelli, 2011d). Other factors that can help trigger acne include friction of the skin from hairbands, helmets, and hats, as well as oil-based cosmetics. Females may have an exacerbation of acne with hormonal changes associated with the menstrual cycle.

Clinical Manifestations

Lesions most often occur on the face, upper chest, shoulders, and back. Initial skin lesions are closed and open comedones without signs of inflammation. Closed comedones are whiteheads or flesh-colored papules with tiny follicular openings. Open comedones are blackheads in which the follicular plug has enlarged and dilated the follicular opening. As inflammation occurs, papules and pustules develop (Figure 36–11 ■). Nodules are larger areas of inflammation that may involve more than one hair follicle. Cysts are compressible nodules without overlying inflammation. Scars form when the surrounding dermis is damaged and may be pitted, atrophic, hypertrophic, or keloid. Severity of acne may be graded as mild, moderate, moderately severe, or severe (Habif, 2010):

- Mild—non-inflammatory comedones
- Moderate—inflammatory, papules, pustules, and comedones; may have mild disease on chest and back
- Moderately severe—inflammatory, numerous papules, localized cysts or nodules; face, chest, and back widely involved
- Severe—nodular and cystic acne on face, back and chest; numerous cystic lesions that may connect, pustules may be present

Collaborative Care

The goal of collaborative care is to identify the therapy to match the severity of the adolescent's acne and to provide guidelines for safe and effective use of these treatments.

Diagnostic Tests

Diagnosis is based on examination of the skin. The most predominant type of lesion present is identified, and the severity of skin lesions is graded. A young child who develops acne that persists despite treatment should be evaluated for potential causes of increased androgen, such as a virilizing tumor or congenital adrenal hyperplasia (Morelli, 2011d). See Chapter 32 🖉 for a discussion of congenital adrenal hyperplasia.

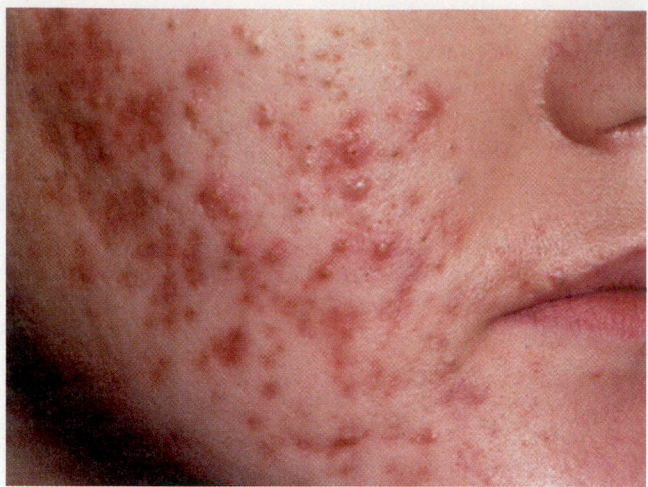

FIGURE 36–11 ■ Severe acne can have a significant effect on an adolescent's self-esteem.

Source: © 2012 National Medical Slide Bank—Custom Medical Stock Photo, All Rights Reserved.

Clinical Therapy

Treatment is customized to the predominant type of lesion present and severity of lesions. The goal of treatment is to suppress lesions until the condition is outgrown, thus preventing infection and scarring, and minimizing psychologic distress. A variety of topical and oral medications and therapies are prescribed. Topical corticosteroids are not used because they thin the skin and promote acne. See the accompanying Medications table. Once inflammatory lesions are under control, oral and topical antibiotics are discontinued. Acne will recur gradually if treatment is stopped, so maintenance therapy with topical retinoids continues once acne is controlled. See Complementary Therapy: Light Treatment.

Skin irritation related to topical preparations may occur in adolescents with sensitive skin. Using a lower concentration product and removing it after a few hours may reduce the initial irritation. With continued use the skin adapts, permitting the product concentration to be changed. Creams are used for adolescents with more sensitive skin whereas adolescents with more oily skin or those who live in a hot and humid climate should use gels. See Developing Cultural Competence: Acne Lesions in Individuals with Dark Skin.

Isotretinoin (Accutane) is reserved for severe acne that is not responsive to other therapies. A 4- to 6-month course of treatment is given, often resulting in a dramatic improvement in up to 85% of patients (Merritt, Burkhart, & Morrell, 2009). Serious birth defects are associated with isotretinoin, so the FDA program iPLEDGE, a mandatory Internet-based registry for prescribers, patients, and pharmacies, was developed to prevent fetal exposure. A one-month supply of the medication is provided to ensure compliance with the program. See the Medications Used to Treat Acne table for important guidelines. Because of the potential association of isotretinoin with depression and suicide, a history regarding past depression and suicide attempts is essential.

Nursing Management

The goal of nursing management is to support the adolescent with the psychologic impact of acne, and provide education about potential triggers, appropriate medication use, and skin care for optimal treatment outcomes.

Nursing Assessment and Diagnosis

Physical assessment should include documentation regarding distribution, type, and severity of acne lesions. Assess the adolescent's and parents' knowledge about the cause and treatment of acne, and identify the home therapies used.

Explore the amount of emotional distress the acne causes the adolescent. Studies have identified that acne has a significant impact on quality of life, self-esteem, and social functioning (Groff, Tromberg, & Wilson, 2009).

Common nursing diagnoses are presented in the accompanying Nursing Care Plan on page 1320.

Planning and Implementation

Nursing management focuses on educating the child and parents about acne and its treatment. Inform the child and parents that daily treatment must be consistently performed for 4 to 8 weeks before improvement is noticed. Advise adolescents to wash their hands before touching affected areas and to avoid picking or squeezing lesions. Provide guidance about skin and hair care. Adolescents should be warned to expect flare-ups despite treatment. For example, increased sweating, heat, and humidity may exacerbate acne, and emotional stress may increase adrenal androgen production, sebum production, and acne flares. Correct any misconceptions adolescents and their families have about dietary causes of acne. Although no food has been found to cause acne or to increase the severity of lesions, good nutrition is important to help the skin heal. See Partnering with Families: Caring for Acne on page 1321.

Topical medication should be spread in a thin film over the skin, according to directions. Avoid getting the topical medications near the eyes, lips, and mucous membranes. Inform the adolescent that acne may seem to worsen with treatment as the comedones are being pushed out, but this is a sign that the treatment is working. While some improvement is seen at 4 to 8 weeks, significant improvement

---

Complementary Therapy Light Treatment

Daily treatment with mixed blue and red light for several weeks is an alternative treatment for mild to moderate acne on the face. The bacteria *P. acnes* has porphyrins that fluoresce, and these porphyrins become excited by the wavelength of the blue light and kill the bacteria. Red light has an anti-inflammatory effect. Studies have reported improvement for many patients with acne with light therapy, as well as laser therapy, and most recently with photodynamic therapy preceded by application of methyl aminolevulinic acid (Shamban & Narurkar, 2009). Unfortunately, these treatments are currently expensive, may not be covered by insurance, and require daily visits to the healthcare provider, so they are not practical for most patients.

Developing Cultural Competence
Acne Lesions in Individuals with Dark Skin

Inflammatory acne in adolescents with darker skin color is commonly associated with a brown or black discoloration, as extra pigment gets deposited in the areas of inflammation. If protected from sun exposure, this darker coloration fades over 3 to 18 months. Additional therapies for the darker pigmentation are chemical peels, bleaching agents, and laser therapy (Shamban & Narurkar, 2009). Encourage adolescents with dark skin to use noncomedonic sunscreen (SPF 30 or higher) whenever sun exposure is likely.

Medications Used to Treat Acne Based on Severity

MEDICATION	ACTION	NURSING MANAGEMENT
Topical retinoids Tretinoin (Retin-A), adapalene, tazarotene For mild and moderate comedonal and papulopustular acne	Prevents the formation of new lesions by regulating the follicular keratinocyte shedding Has anti-inflammatory properties Enhances the penetration of topical antibiotics and benzoyl peroxide	■ Skin irritation is common, and lower concentrations may be used initially. ■ Divide and spread a pea-sized amount over the entire face. Do not use as spot therapy. ■ Apply at night to help reduce the photosensitivity effect. Encourage use of a sunscreen.
Benzoyl peroxide (BPO) For mild or moderate papulopustular acne	Topical antimicrobial with bactericidal action	■ A lower strength may be used initially if skin irritation occurs. ■ A water-based product is used for dry skin; an alcohol-based product is used for oily skin. ■ Use a pea-size amount for the entire face. ■ Treat chest and back lesions with a BPO wash in the shower. Allow it to penetrate the skin for 20–30 seconds before rinsing. ■ Apply in the morning.
Antibiotics Topical for mild inflammatory acne (erythromycin, clindamycin) Oral for moderate to severe inflammatory acne (tetracycline, doxycycline, minocycline)	Antimicrobial action, reduces skin bacterial colonization	■ Inform the adolescent it will take 6–8 weeks to see improvement. ■ Give tetracycline and minocycline on an empty stomach. Give doxycycline with food. ■ Use in combination with topical retinoid or benzoyl peroxide to increase response and reduce bacterial resistance. ■ Use of oral antibiotics is evaluated after 3 months to determine need for longer treatment.
Azelaic acid Mild to moderate acne	Has keratolytic and anti-inflammatory properties	■ Use with patients who cannot tolerate topical retinoids.
Oral contraceptives For persistent inflammatory papules and nodules	Suppress gonadotropin secretion and reduce ovarian androgen production	■ Use as an adjunct for other treatments. ■ Teach the adolescent female about the correct administration schedule.
Spironolactone Severe acne	Blocks the androgen receptor on the sebaceous gland	■ This is not FDA approved for use in treating acne but is commonly prescribed for that purpose. ■ Prescribe for 1–3 months along with an antibiotic.
Isotretinoin For severe nodular acne, especially when resistant to other treatment Drug of last resort	Causes sebaceous gland atrophy and decreases sebum production Reverses effect of androgens on sebaceous glands Represses inflammatory response and comedone production	■ Requires informed consent, commitment for the 4- to 6-month treatment period, and enrollment in the iPLEDGE program. ■ Females must use contraception due to teratogenic effects on skull and limb development. ■ Requires monthly pregnancy tests and monthly blood tests for blood counts, lipid levels, and liver enzymes. ■ A lower dose may be used initially to reduce the initial flare. ■ Take medication with food to increase oral absorption. ■ Encourage the use of sunscreen and protective clothing to prevent sunburn.

Source: *Data from Ramanathan, S., & Hebert, A. A. (2011). Management of acne vulgaris. Journal of Pediatric Health Care, 25(5), 332–337; Webster, G. F. (2009). Acne: Tips and tricks for the pediatrician. Pediatric Annals, 38(2), 80–83; Merritt, B., Burkhart, C. N., & Morrell, D. S. (2009). Use of isotretinoin for acne vulgaris. Pediatric Annals, 28(6), 311–320.*

may not be seen until at least 6 to 12 weeks after the start of treatment. Emphasize that treatment is often long term, including maintenance therapy after the acute acne is controlled.

Teach correct procedures for taking other prescribed drugs, such as tetracycline, doxycycline, minocycline, and isotretinoin (Accutane), to reduce potential side effects. Emphasize the importance of return visits to the adolescent's healthcare provider to monitor treatment progress and for side effects of medications.

Psychologic support is an important aspect of care. Because adolescents are preoccupied with their body image and peer relationships, they often find having acne embarrassing. Encourage them to express their feelings, and refer for counseling if necessary.

Evaluation

Expected outcomes of nursing care can be found in the accompanying Nursing Care Plan on page 1320.

VESICULOBULLOUS SKIN DISORDERS

Several serious skin disorders are characterized by vesiculobullous lesions, vesicles that become blisters and bullae as the condition develops. Examples include epidermolysis bullosa and some serious drug reactions such as Stevens-Johnson syndrome and toxic epidermal necrolysis.

Nursing Care Plan — The Adolescent with Acne

INTERVENTION	RATIONALE	EXPECTED OUTCOME
1. Nursing Diagnosis: Health Maintenance, Ineffective, related to daily hygiene and skin care		
NIC Priority Intervention—*Health Education:* Developing and providing instruction and learning experiences to facilitate voluntary adaptation of behavior conducive to health in individuals, families, groups, or communities		**NOC Suggested Outcome**—*Health-Promoting Behavior:* Personal actions to sustain or increase wellness

GOAL: *The adolescent will verbalize proper hygiene, nutrition, and treatment of acne.*

INTERVENTION	RATIONALE	EXPECTED OUTCOME
■ Teach good skin care: ■ Wash skin with mild soap and water twice a day. Do not scrub the skin. ■ Wash hands frequently, especially after eating greasy foods. ■ Do not use astringents or abrasive cleansers. ■ Apply topical retinoid 20 minutes after washing and drying the face.	■ Good hygiene and appropriate skin care reduce irritation, surface oils, and bacteria, which intensify inflammatory reactions. Scrubbing irritates the skin and increases inflammation. Astringents and after-shave may contain alcohol and further dry the skin.	The adolescent exhibits good hygiene habits and adheres to the daily skin care regimen.
■ Praise good habits related to prescribed skin care and frequent hand washing.	■ Positive reinforcement encourages continued effort.	
■ Advise the adolescent to wash hair with antiseborrheic shampoo and avoid oil-based cosmetics, pomades, or petroleum-based hair products.	■ Seborrhea frequently accompanies acne. Oil-based products can obstruct sebaceous glands, exacerbating acne.	
■ Encourage a balanced diet, adequate fluids, exercise, and adequate rest.	■ Adequate nutrients, water, and exercise promote healthy skin.	A 24-hour recall of food and fluid intake and daily activities reveals adequate nutrient and water intake, exercise, and rest.
■ Encourage the adolescent to keep a diary of skin health and diet habits.	■ A record may help identify associations with flares that can be avoided in the future.	

GOAL: *The adolescent will verbalize understanding of the treatment regimen.*

INTERVENTION	RATIONALE	EXPECTED OUTCOME
■ Educate the adolescent about medications (action, side effects, dosage, and application technique).	■ Proper application of medication enhances healing of lesions.	The adolescent implements the treatment regimen as outlined, resulting in a noticeable reduction in lesions after 3 months.
■ Encourage application of tretinoin at night. Encourage use of noncomedonic sunscreens of at least SPF 30 during the day.	■ Nighttime application helps reduce sensitivity to sun, and sunscreen helps to prevent sunburn.	
■ Educate the adolescent about the time needed for a therapeutic response and the importance of adhering to the daily regimen.	■ Up to 3 months may be needed for significant improvement. The adolescent needs a reason to continue with the care plan.	
■ Encourage continuation of daily therapies even when acne has improved significantly.	■ Acne will return if treatment stops.	

INTERVENTION	RATIONALE	EXPECTED OUTCOME
2. Nursing Diagnosis: Body Image, Disturbed, related to biophysical factors (visible facial lesions)		
NIC Priority Intervention—*Self-Esteem Enhancement:* Assisting a patient to increase his or her personal judgment of self-worth		**NOC Suggested Outcome**—*Self-Esteem:* Personal judgment of self-worth

GOAL: *The adolescent will demonstrate increased self-confidence and self-esteem.*

INTERVENTION	RATIONALE	EXPECTED OUTCOME
■ Establish a rapport with the adolescent.	■ A trusting relationship promotes verbalization of concerns and fears.	The adolescent freely discusses concerns and fears.
■ Provide education about the condition and therapy modalities.	■ Providing information better enables the adolescent to take control of the condition.	
■ Encourage the adolescent to be responsible for treatment and follow-up, and give positive reinforcement.	■ Responsibility reinforces a sense of self-esteem.	The adolescent demonstrates active involvement in own care.
■ Encourage the adolescent to become involved with school activities and peers	■ Involvement in activities helps enhance self-esteem and allows the adolescent to explore new experiences and friendships.	The adolescent shows increased confidence, as demonstrated by involvement in extracurricular activities.

NANDA-I © 2012

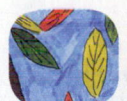

Partnering with Families

Caring for Acne

- Wash hands often and avoid touching the face to reduce the transfer of oils (e.g., greasy foods) and bacteria to the face.
- Use gentle cleansers (without an oil base) to wash the face twice a day. Do not use abrasive sponges or cloths. Wait 20 minutes until the skin is thoroughly dry before applying topical retinoid. Hair should be shampooed regularly, and the seborrhea that can accompany acne should be treated.
- Avoid picking and squeezing pimples as this may rupture lesions beneath the skin and cause more inflammation.
- Avoid the use of astringents and aftershaves that contain alcohol. They may further dry the skin and make it difficult to tolerate the prescribed treatments.

- Limit the use of pomades or petroleum-based hair products. Keep hair spray and other hair products away from the face.
- Use noncomedonic or water-based skin care products (e.g., moisturizers, makeup, sunscreen).
- Avoid hats or headgear that can cause friction and occlusion of the skin.
- Wear protective clothing even on cloudy days as acne medications make the skin more sensitive to sun exposure. Protect the face from cold, windy weather.
- Continue daily topical therapies, even when acne has improved significantly, so that acne does not return.

Epidermolysis Bullosa

Epidermolysis bullosa (EB) is a rare and severe chronic skin disorder that is associated with blistering of the skin and mucous membranes with minor trauma. The most common variants are inherited in an autosomal dominant pattern whereas other variants are inherited in an autosomal recessive pattern. (See Chapter 4 .) The incidence in the United States is estimated to be 10.7 per 1 million live births (Arbuckle, 2010). Depending upon the variant, the condition may either be mild, cause functional impairment, or be life threatening.

The condition is thought to be caused by defective keratin function (Sprecher, 2010). Three general classifications are simplex, junctional, and dystrophic. Autosomal dominant epidermolysis bullosa simplex (EBS) is the most common form of the disease (Sprecher, 2010). With localized EBS, blistering is limited to the hands and feet and is often diagnosed when the child begins to walk or during puberty. This form can become incapacitating during exacerbations. In generalized EBS, blistering is apparent at birth and occurs with minor trauma to any skin surface area. Blistering often lessens in severity with age in this form. Scarring occurs in some forms but not in epidermolysis bullosa simplex. In the most severe forms of epidermolysis bullosa, blistering and skin erosions occur on all parts of the body and ulcerations can occur in the respiratory, gastrointestinal, and urologic systems. These children lose protein and have electrolyte and fluid imbalances, malnutrition, and anemia. The severe forms have a high mortality rate because of secondary infection.

Children with this condition have extremely fragile skin, and blisters form with minor trauma, friction, or heat applied to the skin. In severe forms, blisters and skin erosions occur on all parts of the body and involve the nails, and healing is delayed. Fingers and toes may fuse and webbing may occur, leading to malformations. Children experience pain with blisters and may have difficulty walking when feet are affected.

In newborns, the severe forms of the condition must be distinguished from staphylococcal scalded skin syndrome (see page 1306). Diagnosis can be made by biopsy of the skin lesions and examination under an electron microscope. Prenatal diagnosis can be made by amniocentesis or chorionic villus sampling (Sprecher, 2010).

The condition is managed by prevention of new blisters, wound care, good nutrition, and minimizing the risk for infection. Open

wounds increase the risk of infection so wound care is important. In EBS, blisters are pricked on two sides with a sterile needle each day and drained so that they do not extend. The blister roof is not removed because it acts as a natural biologic dressing. Antibiotic ointments are applied to wounds, and the antibiotic is rotated monthly to reduce the risk for bacterial resistance. Wounds are covered, and care is taken to avoid placing adhesives directly on the skin. Biologic dressings may be used to cover larger wounds in some cases (see page 1330). These infants need additional protein and calories, similar to children with burns, because of the chronic wound healing. Pain management must be customized to the child's condition severity and pain with wound care.

Nursing Management

Teach the family to provide wound care at home; it can be quite time consuming. In newborns, dressing changes need to be performed at a time that is good for the parents and the infant. The process needs to become a daily part of the care routine. Give new parents tips on aspects of dressing changes, such as gathering all supplies together first and using soft music and distraction to help calm the infant. Use other complementary pain management strategies when performing dressing changes on older children (see Chapter 21).

Parents must learn to inspect the skin each day, to lance the blisters with a sterile needle, and to drain the fluid. A second person is needed to assist the parent by carefully preventing movement of an extremity during blister lancing and dressing changes. Holding or grabbing the extremity too tightly can cause friction injury. Dressings that are stuck to the skin cause pain and anxiety for the child, so they should be soaked off. Encourage parents to remove dressings from one location at a time as exposure to the air will be painful for the child. Nonadherent dressings that can absorb the fluid from blisters are helpful in preventing dressings from sticking to the skin. A bulky cover over the dressing (roller gauze or elastic tube dressings) is often used to protect the skin and promote healing. Fingers and toes must be wrapped separately so they do not fuse together with healing.

Provide information to parents about the signs of infection that should be monitored daily. Determine if financial support is needed to ensure that parents have the dressing supplies needed to effectively manage the child's wounds.

Help the parents to identify ways to prevent or reduce blistering of the skin but still permit the child to interact with other children and have opportunities for development. Soft cotton clothing that covers the skin should be worn, with rough seams that can irritate the skin on the outside. Foam padding can be sewn into clothing over the knees and elbows for the infant who is crawling or walking. Shoes without seams on the inside should be worn with seamless cotton socks. Cotton socks can be used to mitten the infant's hands during sleep. The child should also avoid sun exposure and stay where temperatures are cool, as heat and sweating may cause blistering.

Promote good nutrition with adequate calories to meet growth needs. Protein is lost with blisters, and chronic wound healing requires extra calories, so ensure that high-protein meals are provided. In infants, blistering in the mouth may interfere with feeding. A soft nipple with a larger hole may be easier for the infant to use. Vaseline on the lips may help reduce trauma to the mouth. Food temperature should be cool or room temperature and nonacidic to prevent injury to the gastrointestinal tract. In some cases a gastrostomy tube is inserted for nutritional supplementation. Regularly measure height and weight and plot measurements on a growth curve to monitor growth and to identify growth deficiencies early.

Help parents and the child manage the psychologic impact of this disfiguring disorder and the inability to fully participate in all activities. An individualized health plan with educational accommodations will be necessary. Because the hands and feet are often involved, writing and test taking may be challenging. Mobility and walking throughout the school may also be a problem. Help parents inform classroom teachers and classmates about the need to minimize injury.

Drug Reactions

Adverse reactions to over-the-counter or prescription medications are relatively common. Children with drug allergies usually have reactions after ingestion (e.g., aspirin, antibiotics, sedatives), injection (e.g., penicillin), or direct skin contact with medications. Drug sensitivities may result from variations in an individual's ability to tolerate a particular drug or drug concentration, or from allergic responses. (See Chapter 27 for a description of allergic reactions.)

Sensitivity reactions may occur after a dose or two when the child has been previously sensitized, but the reaction may take up to 7 days to develop when no previous exposure to the drug has occurred. The most common reactions in children are the development of erythematous macules and papules or urticaria, which may be pruritic. Drugs that may cause sensitivity reactions include sulfonamides, anticonvulsants, antibiotics (penicillins, cephalosporins, erythromycin, vancomycin), and nonsteroidal anti-inflammatory drugs (NSAIDs). Be alert to the possibility of serious drug reactions that may become a medical emergency. See the Clinical Manifestations table for signs associated with drug reactions of varying severity.

The treatment of choice for most drug sensitivity reactions is discontinuation of the causative drug. In rare cases, a drug may be continued with careful monitoring when the child has a sensitivity reaction because it is the best treatment choice. Supportive measures should be taken to decrease the intensity of the reaction. An antihistamine may be used to block the release of histamine, which causes the rash. Topical corticosteroids, cool compresses, and baths may also be prescribed for pruritus. For some severe drug reactions the child must be hospitalized and treated on a burn unit. Therapies for differing types of drug reactions are identified in the Clinical Manifestations table.

Practice Alert

Children with a true drug allergy (having a serious systemic reaction) should not be treated with that drug again. Prominently mark the child's health records so that all allergies are easily identified. The child should wear medical alert identification.

Nursing Management

Nurses can play an important role by teaching parents to be alert for the signs of drug sensitivity reactions. Obtain a careful history of the child's past reactions to medications before starting new therapies. If a reaction occurs, discontinue the medication until the physician is notified. See the information on nursing care for the child with a burn injury on page 1336 for additional nursing interventions for the care of damaged skin due to severe drug reactions.

INFESTATIONS

Pediculosis Capitis (Lice)

Pediculosis capitis is a lice infestation of the hair and scalp. Infestation occurs among children of all socioeconomic levels, and it is most common in children between 3 and 12 years of age (Diamantis, Morrell, & Burkhart, 2009). The presence of lice may be noted by parents or teachers or by healthcare providers during routine examination of the child (see Chapter 7). Outbreaks occur periodically among preschool and school-age children, particularly those in childcare and elementary school. Head lice rarely infest African American children for some unknown reason (Morelli, 2011f).

Etiology and Pathophysiology

Head lice live and reproduce only on humans and are transmitted by direct hair-to-hair contact or by indirect contact such as sharing hair accessories, brushes, hats, towels, and bedding. Lice do not fly or jump, but they can crawl quickly. The female louse can lay up to 10 eggs (nits) per day on the hair shaft, close to the scalp for food, moisture, and warmth. The eggs hatch 8 to 9 days later. Lice inject a small amount of saliva and anticoagulant into the scalp as they feed on human blood several times a day. Sensitization from the saliva leads to pruritus.

Clinical Manifestations

Classic signs include intense pruritus and complaints of "dandruff" that sticks to the hair (actually the nits) and "bugs" in the hair. Nits look like silvery-white, yellow, or darker 1 mm teardrops adhering to one side of the hair shaft. See Figure 36–12 ■. Nits are found most commonly behind the ears and near the scalp. Lice are wingless insects about the size of sesame seeds (2 to 3 mm long). They move quickly away from light and are not easily seen. Secondary effects of scratching include inflammation, pustules, and bacterial infection. Occipital and posterior cervical nodes are frequently palpable.

Collaborative Care

Diagnosis is based on physical findings. Treatment involves the use of a pediculicide shampoo, such as pyrethrin with an enzymatic lice egg remover, or an ovicidal rinse, such as permethrin (Nix). Permethrin cream rinse is applied to dry hair for 10 minutes before rinsing it off. The hair is then towel dried and the nits are removed with a fine-tooth comb. A second treatment is needed in 7 to 10 days after eggs have hatched because the pediculicide neurotoxin is not effective on nits. If live lice still persist after two treatments, a prescription pediculicide such as malathion may be ordered. See the Medications

Clinical Manifestations Drug Reactions

TYPE OF REACTION AND OFFENDING DRUGS	CLINICAL MANIFESTATIONS	CLINICAL THERAPY
Allergic drug reaction Most common offending drugs include sulfon-amides, tetracyclines, NSAIDs, oral contraceptives, barbiturates, phenytoin, carbamazepine, benzodiazepines, and morphine.	Erythematous, pruritic macules and papules; urticaria, begins on the trunk and extends in a symmetric fashion, often sparing mucous membranes. Some children have urticarial reaction with wheals of various shapes and sizes. The child may have fever and pruritus. The affected area darkens over 1–2 weeks, and skin peeling may occur. May heal with pigment changes.	Discontinue offending drug. Administer oral antihistamines. Use emollients for pruritus. Use mild topical corticosteroids to improve the child's comfort. Avoid sun exposure to allow pigment changes to resolve.
Drug hypersensitivity syndrome Has been documented to occur with antibiotics, antifungals, anticonvulsants, dapsone, NSAIDs, and allopurinol.	Fever and malaise followed by facial edema with erythematous macules on the face and upper body. These lesions become confluent and change to deep red papular lesions that eventually peel. Mucous membranes are usually spared. Pruritus.	Stop the offending drug. Use systemic corticosteroids to treat internal organ involvement. Use topical corticosteroids and give oral antihistamines for pruritus. Monitor the blood count and function of all vital organs. Anticipate potential relapse after corticosteroids are tapered.
Erythema multiforme minor Hypersensitivity reaction to anticonvulsants, penicillins, salicylates, sulfa antibiotics, barbiturates, and phenytoin; infectious agents. Herpes simplex virus infection or reactivation may trigger the disorder, often in association with sun exposure.	Skin lesions may be preceded by fever, malaise, and upper respiratory symptoms. Widespread pruritic macules progress to target lesions with dusky centers (papules, vesicles, or bullae in a pale ring with an erythematous border), and then to plaques. May progress to blisters and bullous lesions. Lesions may itch or burn. Lesions on the mucosa are minimal. Lesions are common on palms and soles, elbows, extensor surface of forearms, and legs.	Remove offending drug and treat infection with alternative medication. Apply emollients or topical antipruritics. Administer oral antihistamines. Administer analgesics. Use cool compresses or baths. Apply or administer topical or oral corticosteroids if prescribed.
Stevens-Johnson syndrome (SJS) and toxic epidermal necrolysis (TEN) Potential life-threatening hypersensitivity reaction to penicillins, sulfonamides, fluoroquinolones, cephalosporins, anticonvulsants, or NSAIDs, or reaction to an infectious disease such as *Mycoplasma pneumonia*. Believed to be a form of the same disease and the most severe form of erythema multiforme.	Prodrome of an upper respiratory infection for 1–7 days with low-grade fever, sore throat, or malaise. Headache, muscle aches, joint pain, and vomiting and diarrhea may be seen. Initial target lesions are on the face and trunk with dusky purple areas or blisters in the center. The dusky areas and blisters are necrotic skin. The lesions may rapidly progress to blistering, sloughing, and erosions. SJS has mucosal involvement appearing 2 days before the rash. Mucous membranes (oral, conjunctival, and anogenital) have blisters, erosions, ulcerations, and hemorrhagic crusting. Painful crusting and sloughing of the lips and oral membranes occurs. Respiratory and gastrointestinal mucosa may also be affected. Erosions (similar to partial-thickness burns) may spread to cover up to 10% of the skin surface in SJS, 10–30% in overlapping SJS and TEN, and more than 30% in TEN. Corneal blistering can lead to scarring and blindness.	Discontinue offending drug. Admit to a burn center and carefully monitor fluid and electrolyte balance, see page 1333. Debride blisters and necrotic epidermis. Clean gently with saline or Burow's solution (aluminum acetate) compresses. Ensure pain and fever management. Apply sterile nonadherent dressings. Wounds may be covered with biosynthetic dressing or human allografts to reduce infection and pain. Provide intensive nutritional support. Obtain ophthalmic consultation and provide eye care. Administer IV immune globulin over 2–4 days. Apply topical antibiotics around the mouth and areas at high risk of secondary infection. Provide oral care. Systemic corticosteroids are not used to reduce the risk for sepsis.

Source: *Data from Nicol, N. H., & Huether, S. E. (2010). Structure, function, and disorders of the integument. In K. L. McCance, S. E. Huether, V. L. Brashers, & N. S. Rote,* Pathophysiology: The biologic basis for disease in adults and children *(6th ed., pp. 1644–1679). St. Louis, MO: Elsevier Mosby; Juhas, E., & Gehris, R. P. (2010). Drug eruptions: The benign—and the life threatening. Consultant for Pediatricians, 9(Suppl. 6), S2–S9; Morelli, J. G. (2011e). Vesiculobullous disorders. In R. M. Kliegman, B. F. Stanton, J. W. St. Geme, N. F. Schor, & R. E. Behrman,* Nelson textbook of pediatrics *(19th ed., pp. 2241–2249). St. Louis, MO: Elsevier Mosby; Treat, J. (2010). Stevens-Johnson syndrome and toxic epidermal necrolysis. Pediatric Annals, 39(1), 667–674.*

table for products used to treat lice. See Box 36–3. None of the treatments remove nits. Various chemical-free shampoos and rinses are available to help with nit removal. See Complementary Therapy: Hot Air Treatment for Lice for one new therapy being investigated.

Practice Alert

Lindane is a second-line treatment for head lice, and it must be used with caution in any child weighing less than 50 kg (110 lb) because of neurotoxicity and potential to cause seizures. High levels of resistance by lice have been documented. Lindane is no longer recommended for treatment of head lice (American Academy of Pediatrics, 2012, p. 545).

Nursing Management

The goal of nursing management is to educate parents about how to shampoo and comb the hair to eradicate lice and nits, and ways to prevent infestation among other family members.

Nursing Assessment and Diagnoses

Carefully assess children who have been exposed to head lice. Use a bright light and magnifying glass to see the lice and nits along the hair shaft close to the scalp. Make sure to distinguish lice and nits from dandruff flakes. To avoid potential infestation of other children,

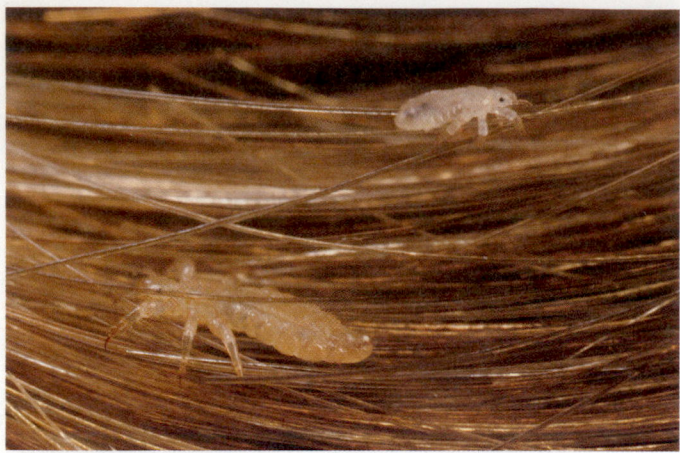

FIGURE 36–12 ■ Note the presence of lice (highly magnified) crawling through the hair.
Source: *Darlyne A. Marawski/National Geographic Image Collection.*

BOX 36–3	Research: Lice

A recent study was conducted at multiple centers with 812 children with live lice. All children had been unsuccessfully treated for lice with topical insecticides in the prior 2 to 6 weeks. Children in the study were randomly assigned to treatment for lice at the study site with either malathion application to the hair or oral ivermectin on days 1 and 8. Of the children receiving ivermectin, 95.2% were lice-free on day 15 versus 85% receiving malathion treatment. Oral ivermectin was significantly superior to malathion in these difficult-to-treat lice infestations and could be an alternative therapy to malathion (Chosidow, Giraudeau, Cottrell, et al., 2010).

change gloves frequently when assessing several children in a classroom setting.

Examples of nursing diagnoses that might apply with the child who has a lice infestation include:

- Skin Integrity, Risk for Impaired, related to scratching
- Therapeutic Regimen Management: Family, Ineffective, related to proper use of pediculicide and removal of nits
- Social Isolation related to exclusion from school until all nits associated with lice infestation are removed

NANDA-I © 2012

Planning and Implementation

Infestation with lice can be upsetting for both the child and family. Emphasize to the family that anyone can get lice. All family members and contacts of the child should be examined for infestation and should be treated as necessary. Teach the child not to share clothing, headwear, or combs. Parents of children exposed to an infested child should be notified so they can watch for signs of lice.

Correct use of pediculicides is essential for effective treatment. Explain to parents that the shampoo and rinses prescribed are pesticides and must be used for the time specified and as directed. Parents should not use a crème rinse, combination shampoo/conditioner, or conditioner before using the lice shampoo or lotion as it may reduce the ovicide activity and cause treatment failure. An extra bottle of the pediculicide may be needed if the child has extra long hair. The hair should not be washed again for 1 to 2 days after the lice medication is removed.

To remove the nits, use a fine-tooth comb, tweezers, and a basin filled with water or isopropyl alcohol to dip and clean the comb and

Medications and Preparations for Head Lice

NAME OF MEDICATION/ PREPARATION	NURSING MANAGEMENT
First-line pesticide treatment	
Permethrin 1% Creme Rinse—Nix	Apply to the hair after shampooing and towel drying the hair. Leave on 10 minutes and rinse. Repeat in 7–10 days.
Pyrethrin shampoo (0.17–0.33%) or piperonyl butoxide (2–4%)—Rid, A-200, R&C, TripleX, Pronto, Tisit, Licide	Apply to *dry hair and scalp.* Lather, leave on 10 minutes, and rinse with cool water. Repeat 7–10 days later. Wet hair dilutes the product and may contribute to treatment failure.
Benyzl alcohol 5% (Ulesfia), FDA-approved nonneurotoxic treatment for children age 6 months and older. Lice die by suffocation.	Apply to *dry hair,* saturating the hair and scalp. Rinse after 10 minutes. Repeat in 7 days. Protect eyes during use. Available by prescription.
Second-line pesticide treatment	
Malathion 0.5% lotion or gel Organophosphate that causes paralysis and death of lice. Approved for children over age 6 years.	Apply to *dry hair.* Leave on 4 minutes and rinse. No retreatment is needed. Treatment is flammable; do not expose the child to electric heat sources.
Non-FDA approved	
Trimethoprim/sulfamethoxazole Ivermectin—anthelmintic agent	Drug in bloodstream is ingested by louse and destroys bacterial flora in louse intestine. One oral dose is repeated 7 days later. May cause adverse drug reaction in young children.

Source: *Data from Diamantis, S. A., Morrell, D. S., & Burkhart, C. N. (2009). Pediatric infestations. Pediatric Annals, 38(6), 326–332; Frankowski, B. L., Bocchini, J. A., & the Council on School Health and Committee on Infectious Disease. (2010). Clinical report—Head lice. Pediatrics, 126(2), 392–403; U.S. Food and Drug Administration Center for Drug Evaluation and Research. (2009). Ulesfia. Retrieved from http://www.accessdata.fda.gov/scripts/cder/drugsatfda/index.cfm?fuseaction=Search.DrugDetails*

Complementary Therapy
Hot Air Treatment for Lice

The LouseBuster is a commercial machine with a hose and comb on the end that uses hot air to kill lice and nits. While the hot air is blowing, the hair is slowly combed, taking about 30 minutes to treat the entire scalp. One study reported a mortality rate for eggs and lice of nearly 100% without the use of any medications. The specially developed device could potentially be available for use in a healthcare setting by an individual trained in its use (Frankowski, Bocchini, & the Council on School Health and Committee on Infectious Disease, 2010).

tweezers. Comb 1-inch sections from the scalp outward and pin these out of the way when done. Nits adhere to the hair shaft and must be manually pulled down the hair shaft with the comb, tweezers, or fingernails. Have blunt-nosed scissors available to cut the hair shaft below the level of the nit when it cannot be easily removed. All nits must be removed. Make sure the parents know that it may take hours for all the lice and nits to be removed because they are firmly cemented to the hair shaft. Put the child under a bright light and use distraction techniques such as a video to keep the child cooperative during the procedure. Check the hair every 2 to 3 days and remove any lice or nits seen. An alternative therapy for boys is to cut off the hair in a close buzz cut or shave the head. A shorter haircut for girls may also help with nit removal.

Although lice can survive for only about 3 days away from a human host, nits may hatch 8 to 10 days later. For this reason, bedding, clothing, and bath towels used by the child should be changed daily, laundered in hot water with detergent, and dried in a hot dryer for 20 minutes. Nonessential bedding and clothing can be stored in a tightly sealed bag for 2 to 3 weeks and then washed. Hair accessories, brushes, and combs should be discarded or soaked in hot soapy water (54.4°C [130°F]) for 10 minutes. Furniture and carpets should be vacuumed (remember to change the bag after vacuuming) and treated with a hot iron when possible. It is not recommended that the family use an insecticide in the home to kill lice on carpets, furniture, and other items, especially if young children and pets will come into contact with them. Seal toys and other personal items that cannot be washed or dry-cleaned in a plastic bag for 2 weeks.

Clinical Tip

Teachers with one or more children who have lice should be educated to take preventive measures to stop the spread of lice. Children with lice can be temporarily moved to prevent close head contact with other students. If the classroom is carpeted and children play on the floor, the carpet should be vacuumed daily. Sleeping mats should be assigned. Discourage children from sharing hats, helmets, earphones, and other items that could enable lice transfer to another child.

There is no evidence that lice continue to be transmitted after the treatment, even if the parents have not yet been able to remove all nits. Both the American Academy of Pediatrics and the National Association of School Nurses have policies that allow the child to stay in school even if all nits have not been removed. Some schools and childcare centers still have a "no nit" policy, meaning the child cannot return until all nits have been removed.

If treatment failure is found, discuss the following issues with the parents to determine a strategy for improved outcomes:

- Review the application and use of selected products with the parents to ensure proper use.
- Review any potential sources for continued infestation.
- Make sure lice is the proper diagnosis.
- Actual resistance to pediculicides may be present, and an alternative pediculicide treatment may be needed.

Evaluation

Expected outcomes of nursing care include:

- The child receives effective pediculicide treatment and nit removal.
- Reinfestation is prevented.

Scabies

Scabies is a highly contagious infestation caused by the mite *Sarcoptes scabiei*. It is spread by close skin-to-skin contact, sexual contact, or contact with shared objects such as sheets and towels. Transmission within a household, especially when crowding is present, and in childcare facilities is common. The mites are so tiny a microscope is needed to see them. Children of all ages and both sexes are affected.

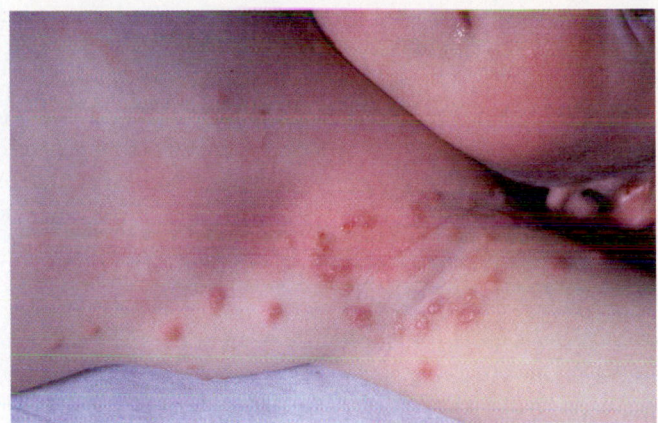

FIGURE 36–13 ■ Diffuse scabies in an infant. The lesions are most numerous around the axillae, chest, and abdomen.

Source: © 2012—Custom Medical Stock Photo, All Rights Reserved.

It takes the pregnant female mite about 30 minutes to burrow into the outer layer of the epidermis (stratum corneum) to lay her eggs, leaving a trail of debris and feces. The larvae hatch in approximately 3 to 4 days and proceed toward the surface of the skin. The cycle is repeated 14 to 17 days later. A delayed type IV hypersensitivity reaction to the mites, debris, and feces occurs within 2 to 4 weeks of the infestation; however, response to a reinfestation can occur within 24 hours (Orrico & Krause-Parello, 2010).

Symptoms include a rash with various types of lesions (papules, burrows, and pustules), severe pruritus that worsens at night, and restlessness. Lesions are usually located in the webs of the fingers, in the intergluteal folds, around the axillae, or on the palms, wrists, elbows, inner thighs, and waist (Figure 36–13 ■). In children under 2 years, insteps of the feet, as well as the head, neck, face, palms, and soles, can be affected. The burrow lesions appear as linear, threadlike, grayish burrows 1 to 10 cm in length, which may end in a pinpoint vesicle. Burrows are often more easily seen on the hands and feet. The lesions may look like widespread atopic dermatitis. The child's scratching and secondary infection may obliterate the burrow lesions. Nodules 2 to 20 mm in size occasionally develop as a granulomatous response to the dead mite antigens and feces and can persist for weeks after effective treatment.

Diagnosis is confirmed by physical examination for intact burrows and by skin scrapings from the end of the burrow that is examined under the microscope. Actively moving mites, fecal pellets, and eggs or nits may be seen. An enzyme-linked immunosorbent assay to identify a specific antigen or antibody to *S. scabiei* is available in Europe and potentially soon in the United States (Orrico & Krause-Parello, 2010).

Treatment involves application of a scabicide, such as 5% permethrin lotion, over the entire body with special attention to the hands, fingers, feet, and toes, and under the nails. The scabicide should also be applied to the face, neck, ears, and scalp, but avoid getting the solution in the eyes and mucous membranes. Application of 5% permethrin lotion is preceded by a warm soap and water bath. The skin must be cool and dry before the lotion is applied. The lotion is left in place for 8 to 12 hours (overnight) before washing it off. A second treatment is used 1 week later. All close contacts, members of the household, and childcare contacts should be treated at the same time, even if not symptomatic. An oral antihistamine (e.g., Benadryl, Atarax) may be prescribed to help relieve itching. Antibiotics may be needed when a secondary infection occurs. If symptoms, including itching, persist for more than 2 weeks after treatment, the possibility of treatment failure is considered (Orrico & Krause-Parello, 2010). Treatment failure is usually due to inadequate treatment or reinfestation by an untreated contact. Oral ivermectin is a new antiparasitic product with FDA approval for children weighing more than 15 kg, but it is a second-line therapy, used when other treatments are unsuccessful.

Nursing Management

Educate parents about the proper application of the scabicide. Make sure parents understand the importance of keeping the medication on the skin for the full 8 to 12 hours. The child should have the scabicide reapplied to the hands if hands are washed or if the child sucks the fingers or thumb. Mitts or socks over the hands of young children who suck the fingers or thumb may reduce the chance of ingesting the scabicide.

Advise parents that scabies is easily transmitted by close contact. All clothing, bedding, and pillowcases used by the child should be changed daily, washed with hot water, and dried in a hot dryer. Nonwashable toys and other items should be sealed in plastic bags for 5 to 7 days.

All household family members should be treated simultaneously. Individuals who are not infected should avoid touching the affected child until after treatment is completed. If contact is made, hands should be washed well. Inform the parents about signs of secondary infections and that itching and nodules may persist for weeks after effective treatment. Encourage the use of emollients as the treatment dries the skin.

Scabies, like pediculosis, can be embarrassing or upsetting for the child and family. Educate them about the condition, its spread, and treatment measures to prevent recurrence.

MISCELLANEOUS SKIN CONDITIONS

Birthmarks

Children are born with a variety of birthmarks or congenital problems that affect the integumentary system. Congenital nevi and vascular birthmarks are among the more common conditions. See the accompanying table for clinical manifestations and clinical therapy.

Parents are very distressed by the presence of birthmarks on their newborn, especially when it is on the face and is viewed as disfiguring. Encourage parents to discuss their concerns and feelings. Provide education about the birthmark, expected changes, and when intervention might be appropriate. Since some birthmarks spontaneously improve, parents should be encouraged to be patient. Help them identify ways to discuss the birthmark with other family members and friends to gain support rather than be pressured to treat the skin lesion.

Vascular Tumors (Hemangiomas)

A vascular tumor, or **hemangioma,** occurs in 1% to 2% of all newborns but up to 10% of White infants within a year of birth (Morelli, 2011h, p. 2227). An increased incidence has been noted in females, low-birth-weight infants, White infants, and infants of multiple births. A familial tendency has also been noted (Holland & Drolet, 2010).

Clinical Manifestations   Common Birthmarks

CONDITION	CLINICAL MANIFESTATIONS	CLINICAL THERAPY
Salmon patch (stork bite or nevus simplex) Occurs in 44% of neonates	Pink to scarlet colored patch that blanches on the forehead or neck; may also appear on nose, upper eyelids, or upper lip. Deepens in color with vigorous activity.	Usually disappears within 2 years without therapy, few if any cosmetic problems.
Vascular formations (port-wine stain or nevus flammeus) Occurs in 0.3% of neonates	Red plaques or patches that progressively darken with age, becoming dark purple red during adolescence; flat at birth, but become thicker or nodular with age; most common site is one side of the face, but may be found any place on the body. When the patch involves the upper face and eyelid (in distribution of the ophthalmic branch of the fifth cranial nerve), the child may have Sturge-Weber syndrome with associated cerebral atrophy, seizures, developmental delay, hemiplegia, vision loss, or glaucoma.	Pulsed dye laser therapy on the small blood vessels of the patch to destroy the vasculature and lighten the discoloration. Early treatment is encouraged and may be more effective when young. In cases of Sturge-Weber syndrome: ■ Regular ophthalmic assessments for glaucoma begin at birth. ■ Magnetic resonance imaging is performed to detect central nervous system vascular problems or atrophic changes.
Congenital melanocytic nevus Occurs in about 1% of neonates.	Lesions are flat, elevated, or nodular in various shades of brown, blue, or black. Vary in size from less than 2 cm to greater than 20 cm in diameter. Giant congenital nevi, covering more than 20 cm or more skin surface area, are rare.	Because of the risk of melanoma, regular examination (inspection and palpation) and comparison to photographs should occur at 6-month intervals for 5 years and yearly thereafter. Excision is considered in some cases.
Café-au-lait spots	Macules or patches darker than surrounding skin that may have smooth or irregular borders. May vary from a few mm to 10 cm in size. May be an indication of neurofibromatosis or McCune-Albright disease.	Monitor child for increase in size and number of café-au-lait spots and development of skin tumors indicative of neurofibromatosis (see Chapter 33 🥖).

Source: *Data from Leung, A. K. C. (2011). Port-wine stain versus salmon patch: How to tell the difference.* Consultant for Pediatricians, 10(2), 33; Huang, J. T., & Liang, M. G. (2010). Vascular malformations. Pediatric Clinics of North America, 57, 1091–1110; Morelli, J. G. (2011g). Cutaneous nevi. In R. M. Kliegman, B. F. Stanton, J. W. St. Geme, N. F. Schor, & R. E. Behrman, Nelson textbook of pediatrics (19th ed., pp. 2317–2322). St. Louis, MO: Elsevier Mosby; Black, J. S., & Wilson, B. (2009). Neurofibromatosis type 1. Consultant for Pediatricians, 8(12), 433.

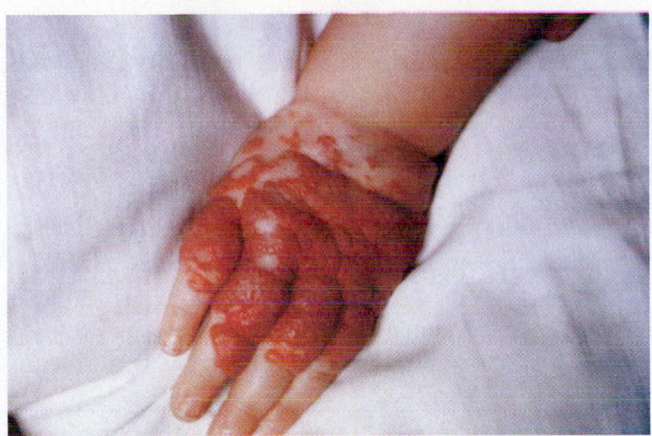

FIGURE 36–14 ■ Superficial hemangioma on the hand.

Source: *Custom Medical Stock Photo, Inc.*

Etiology and Pathophysiology

Hemangiomas are vascular tumors believed to arise initially from embolized fetal placental cells followed by a proliferation of mast cells that promote the development of a vascular network of small blood vessels. These tumors undergo rapid growth and proliferation during the first 6 to 10 months during infancy and may undergo ulceration. This phase is followed by a slow **involution** (process of decreasing in size) phase that may take years. Hemangiomas may be superficial (located in the epidermis), deep (located in the dermis or subcutaneous tissue), or mixed superficial and deep. When multiple hemangiomas are found, some may be in major organs such as the liver. Complications are caused by the rapid growth and pressure against or obstruction of vital structures, such as the airway, eye, or ear canal. A large facial hemangioma may be associated with PHACE syndrome (**p**osterior fossa or other structural brain anomaly, a large **h**emangioma that is usually on the face, **a**rterial anomalies, **c**ardiac defects, and **e**ye anomalies) (Metry, Siegel, Cordisco, et al., 2008).

Clinical Manifestations

Infantile hemangiomas begin as barely visible telangiectasias or red macules that begin to grow rapidly and become bright red and compressible. Some lesions ulcerate with rapid growth. Most growth occurs during the first 5 months, attaining 80% of the full size (Holland & Drolet, 2010). Some hemangiomas are localized, superficial, and discrete; they are usually oval or round and bright red, resembling a strawberry. See Figure 36–14 ■ . Deep hemangiomas appear as bluish tumors covered with normal-appearing epidermis. Mixed hemangiomas have features of both superficial and deep tumors. Some lesions are segmental, having a geographic shape over a broad anatomic region, and these lesions are often at greater risk for complications and associated anomalies (Holland & Drolet, 2010). They have no bruit or thrill. Some children have multiple lesions. The lesions, appearing any place on the body, are minimally compressible during rapid growth and become more compressible with involution. As the vascular tumors involute, signs of tissue atrophy, wrinkles, telangiectasias, and hypopigmentation may be noted.

Collaborative Care

The goal of collaborative care is focused on identifying the hemangioma early, evaluating the infant for potential complications, and providing clinical therapy that will result in the best cosmetic appearance.

Diagnostic Tests

Initial diagnosis is by physical examination and monitoring the growth of the vascular tumor. When a vital organ could be obstructed, or either Sturge-Weber or PHACE syndrome is suspected, ultrasound, computed tomography scanning, or magnetic resonance imaging may be performed.

Clinical Therapy

Some hemangiomas are monitored and receive no treatment. Hemangiomas in problem areas or at risk for ulceration, bleeding, permanent disfigurement, or pressure on a vital organ are usually referred to a dermatology specialist for treatment. Treatment with high doses of oral systemic corticosteroids may be initiated in the first weeks of life during the proliferation phase to slow growth. Injections of corticosteroids into small localized hemangiomas are sometimes performed (Stier, Glick, & Hirsch, 2008). Vincristine may be used for infants resistant to or unable to tolerate systemic corticosteroids; however, there are serious adverse effects and a central line must be inserted for drug administration (Holland & Drolet, 2010). See Box 36–4 for research on using propranolol hydrochloride as a treatment for hemangiomas.

Pulsed dye laser treatment may be used for hemangiomas after involution when residual telangiectasia remains. Pulses of light energy are targeted to the lesion's oxyhemoglobin, which absorbs the wavelength of light and heats it. Topical anesthesia and eye protection should be provided. The lesion may darken for 1 to 2 weeks, as purpura result from extravasation of the red blood cells when blood vessels rupture. The darkness fades to red, and the treated skin surface eventually lightens. Surgical removal of an ulcerated hemangioma tissue may be considered if a poor cosmetic outcome is expected (Holland & Drolet, 2010).

Nursing Management

The goal of nursing care is to support families through the period of rapid hemangioma growth and treatment, helping them to deal with emotional responses to the infant's appearance and potential complications.

Nursing Assessment and Diagnoses

Assess the distribution of the hemangioma, and consider the potential for complications as it goes through a rapid growth stage. Monitor the child during regular visits for development of any complications, such as ulceration or stridor that could be associated with compression on the airway.

Assess the parents' response to the infant's appearance and how they are managing interactions with friends and family about the

BOX 36–4	Research: Treatment of Vascular Hemangiomas

A recent study with 40 infants less than 6 months old evaluated the effectiveness of propranolol hydrochloride versus placebo for the treatment of vascular hemangiomas over 24 weeks. The size of the hemangioma was measured every 4 weeks. Infants receiving propranolol had significantly better outcomes. Among the infants receiving propranolol, most of the hemangiomas stopped growing within 1 month and involution occurred at a much younger age than usual (Hogeling, Adams, & Wargon, 2011). Infants did need to be monitored in an observation unit for 4 hours after the initial dose and subsequent dose increase for bradycardia and hypotension before continuing the medication.

infant's changing appearance. Take photos of the infant at each visit so that parents have a record of improvements once therapy is initiated.

Examples of nursing diagnoses that might apply with the infant who has a hemangioma include:

- Parenting, Risk for Impaired, related to infant with an extensive vascular lesion on the face
- Skin Integrity, Impaired, related to presence of rapidly growing vascular lesion
- Infection, Risk for, related to potential ulceration of hemangioma

NANDA-I © 2012

Planning and Implementation

Provide education to parents about the type of vascular lesion and potential treatment options. When corticosteroids are prescribed, teach the parents about administration and the need to take the full course as prescribed. Inform the parents about potential side effects, including gastrointestinal upset, sleep disturbance, temporary growth retardation, decreased appetite, and transient facial edema. Reassure parents that growth catch-up will occur once corticosteroid treatment ends. Inform parents about the possibility of ulceration as the hemangioma grows rapidly and what signs to expect. Provide guidelines for covering and protecting the ulcerated skin from infection until the infant can be seen by the healthcare provider.

Listen to parents as they describe challenges with family and friends who comment about the infant's appearance. Role-play possible responses that parents can make to these individuals. To promote attachment, help parents see positive characteristics in the infant, such as responsiveness to interaction and smiling. Show parents photos of other children with similar lesions who have completed therapy. Demonstrating that improvements in appearance are gradual, but possible, is encouraging to parents overwhelmed with the infant's current appearance. Take photos of the child at intervals during treatment to show parents when improvements have occurred.

Prepare parents for changes to the child's appearance with pulsed dye laser therapy. Explain that the initial appearance will be darkening of the hemangioma for 1 to 2 weeks, and then the darkness will fade to red and eventual lightening of the treated skin surface. Some swelling may occur after the treatment, so the application of ice packs for 10 minutes every hour during the first day may help. Teach parents to protect the treated skin surface from trauma and keep the infant's nails short to prevent scratching. Cleanse the area treated with water and pat it dry. Instruct parents to avoid sun exposure for 6 weeks following the treatments and to use SPF 30 sunscreen on the area in the future.

Evaluation

Expected outcomes of nursing care for the child and family include:

- The parents form a close attachment with the infant.
- The parents cope with comments about the infant's appearance.
- Hemangioma treatment is effective without causing additional injury to the treated skin.

INJURIES TO THE SKIN

Pressure Ulcers

An increasing number of children with disabilities are cared for in hospital, community, and home care settings. Many of these children are at risk for skin breakdown and pressure ulcer formation.

| BOX 36–5 | Research: Pressure Ulcer Prevalence |

The Braden Scale was used to identify the prevalence of pressure ulcers in 155 children ages newborn to 17 years in four German pediatric hospitals. A total of 43 children (27%) were found to have one or more pressure ulcers, most being grade or stage 1. However, 7 children (4.5%) had pressure ulcers of grade or stage 2 or higher. Many of the pressure ulcers were associated with splints, cables, and tubes used in the child's care (Schlüer, Cignacco, Müller, et al., 2009).

Prevalence rates range from 0.5% to 13%, but have been reported as high as 27% in neonatal and pediatric intensive care units (Mukherjee, Coha, & Torres, 2010). See Box 36–5.

Etiology and Pathophysiology

Soft tissues and capillary beds can be compressed for a prolonged period between a bony prominence and another surface (see Table 36–5). Tissue ischemia occurs when arterial and venous blood flow is impeded to the skin and deeper tissues. The cells are deprived of oxygen and nutrients, and metabolic waste products accumulate, resulting in tissue hypoxia and soft tissue injury. Without appropriate intervention, the injury becomes rapidly progressive and a pressure ulcer forms. Skin damage can also occur when adhesive products are removed from the skin of infants and children with fragile skin.

Clinical Manifestations

Pressure ulcer severity is defined in four stages (Figure 36–15 ■). The earliest sign of skin damage (stage 1) is an area of redness in intact skin that does not blanch and remains 30 minutes after removing the pressure or skin irritant. Children with dark skin may have persistent red, blue, or purple discoloration. As the injury progresses, the skin looks rubbed or raw like an abrasion or blister (stage 2). If intervention does not occur, the skin damage extends through the epidermis and dermis (full-thickness injury), forming an ulcer (stage 3). The ulcer then deepens to underlying muscles, bone, or connective tissue unless treated (stage 4).

Clinical Tip

The site of greatest pressure in infants and young children is the occiput. Older children have increased pressure on the sacral and occipital areas.

Collaborative Care

Diagnostic Tests

No laboratory diagnostic tests are needed. Several tools have been developed to assess the risk for development of pressure ulcers in

TABLE 36–5	Sites and Potential Causes of Pressure Ulcers
SITES	**POTENTIAL CAUSES**
Occipital region of scalp, earlobes	Inability to lift or reposition head, common in infants
Sacrum and buttocks	Confinement to bed or wheelchair
Legs and feet	Orthotics, leg braces, casts
Spine and neck	Scoliosis brace
Knees, elbows, and heels of feet	Rubbing against bed sheet
Sternum, iliac crest	Prone positioning for mechanical ventilation

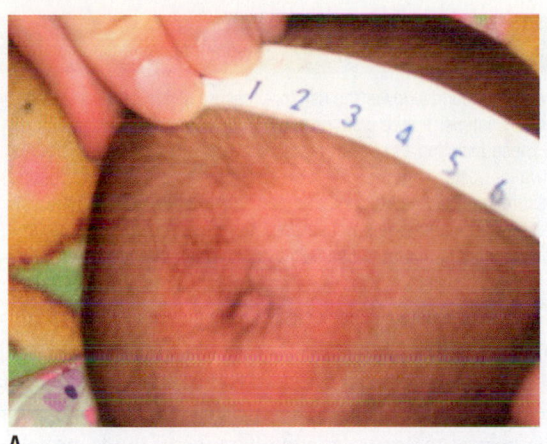

A

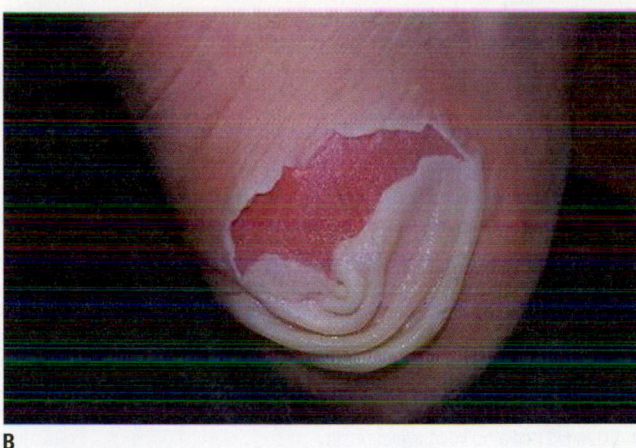

B

FIGURE 36–15 ■ The two (out of four) most common stages of ulcer formation seen in children as described by the National Pressure Ulcer Advisory Panel. *A,* Stage 1, nonblanchable erythematous area of intact skin, usually over a bony prominence that does not resolve within 30 minutes of pressure relief. This stage may be difficult to detect in children with darker skin tones. *B,* Stage 2, a partial-thickness injury (blister or abrasion) in which a shallow open ulcer with a reddened wound area is noted.

Source: *Courtesy of Sandra Quigley, Children's Hospital, Boston, MA.*

infants and children, such as the Braden Q Scale for children under age 5 years. The Braden Scale can be used for older children. These scales assess risk associated with mobility, activity, sensory perception, moisture, friction-shear, nutrition, and tissue perfusion/oxygenation.

Clinical Therapy

Initial treatment for early stages of skin damage involves removing pressure from the affected site until the skin has healed. Children who use leg braces for alignment and mobility are often put in wheelchairs. Children who use wheelchairs are often put on bed rest on a pressure-reducing surface. Frequent repositioning is needed. A transparent film may be applied to affected red skin to minimize friction. Pressure ulcers are treated with various dressings, such as hydrocolloids, gels or hydrogels, and calcium alginates that do not adhere to the wound.

Nursing Management

The goal of nursing care is the prevention of pressure ulcers by regular assessment of children at higher risk, skin care, and position change.

Nursing Assessment and Diagnosis

Carefully inspect the dependent skin surfaces of all infants and children confined to bed at least three times in each 24-hour period using an appropriate scale for the child's age. Additionally, monitor the skin around all tubing and cables that can be pressed against the skin. See Evidence-Based Practice: Pressure Ulcers in Children. Evaluate the risk for skin damage based on factors that can contribute to skin breakdown. See Box 36–6 for risk factors.

Identify and record the size (measuring the length, width, and depth) and character of the skin lesion. Note any signs of infection,

Evidence-Based Practice | Pressure Ulcers in Children

PROBLEM
Pressure ulcers have a prevalence rate of up to 27% in hospital and intensive care unit (neonatal and pediatric) settings. What tools exist to identify infants and children at risk for pressure ulcers?

EVIDENCE
Investigators reviewed patient data to identify specific factors associated with pressure ulcers in children as a foundation for development of the Glamorgan Pediatric Pressure Ulcer Assessment Scale. Findings led to a scale that weighs two factors contributing to the development of pressure ulcers, the extent of immobility and the presence of equipment pressing on the skin, while adding other variables to the scale. The resulting scale had high sensitivity (98.4%) and lower specificity (67.4%) for predicting a pressure ulcer when the total score was 15 (Willock, Baharestani, & Anthony, 2009). The Glamorgan Scale was further evaluated and found to have validity and interrater reliability (Willock, Anthony, & Richardson, 2008). A systematic review investigated the validity and reliability of 12 pressure ulcer risk assessment scales. All studies related to validity and reliability of these scales had limitations, and some were developed for specific populations (e.g., neonates and children with burns). The study concluded that no scale was superior to the other, and diagnostic accuracy was unclear in some of the scales (Kottner, Hauss, Schlüer, et al., 2011).

IMPLICATIONS
Many pressure ulcer risk scales exist such as the Braden, Braden Q for children ages 5 years and younger, Star Kids, Norton, Glamorgan, and others. Most pressure ulcer assessment scales are designed to identify the risk for pressure ulcers; however, a child needs to have a full skin assessment to see if pressure ulcers exist or may be developing. Many infants and children are at risk for development of pressure ulcers, but nurses may choose to intervene when a child has specific risk factors rather than performing a risk assessment routinely. Perhaps having a risk assessment tool would encourage nurses to pay closer attention to a child's risk factors for pressure ulcers. Knowledge of these risk factors is important when developing guidelines to prevent pressure ulcers, such as a turning or repositioning schedule, careful inspection of skin under braces and orthotics, frequently moving pulse oximetry sensors, and taping endotracheal, tracheostomy, and nasogastric tubes to avoid their pressure against the skin.

CRITICAL THINKING APPLICATION
Use the Braden Scale, the Braden Q Scale (for children under 5 years), or the Glamorgan Scale to assess the pressure ulcer risk of one child with an acute illness and one with a chronic illness. Then perform a complete assessment of these children to identify any skin breakdown. Plan the appropriate nursing intervention for the prevention and treatment of pediatric skin breakdown.

BOX 36–6	Factors That Place the Child at Greater Risk for Skin Breakdown

- Prolonged pressure over a bony prominence
- Compression of the skin by cables, tubes, or other medical devices
- Decreased mobility and activity
- Decreased sensory perception of pressure-related discomfort or injury
- Prolonged exposure to moisture; incontinence of urine or feces inappropriate for age
- Excessive movement that can lead to friction injury
- Edema
- Poor nutritional status or anemia
- Use of orthotics, braces, or prosthetics
- Extended pediatric intensive care stay
- Conditions causing vasoconstriction, such as low cardiac output, in which blood is shunted away from nonvital organs like the skin
- Impaired tissue perfusion and oxygenation requiring ventilator support

BOX 36–7	Research: Preventing Pressure Ulcers

Nursing interventions found to lower the risk for pressure ulcers in children cared for in nine pediatric intensive care units revealed that basic nursing interventions are valuable. These included turning the patient every 2 hours, use of blanket rolls and pillows for positioning, use of a draw sheet to reposition the child, and use of a pressure-reduction surface. Other valuable nursing interventions included a nutrition consultation, dry weave diapers, disposable underpads, and application of moisturizer (Schindler, Mikhailov, Kuhn, et al., 2011).

the appearance of wound edges, and the type of tissue at the wound base. Describe drainage amount, color, and type.

Examples of nursing diagnoses that may be appropriate for the child at risk for pressure ulcers are as follows:

- Skin Integrity, Risk for Impaired, related to infant's heavy head and inability to shift position
- Injury, Risk for, related to sensory/perceptual alterations
- Mobility: Physical, Impaired, related to decreased muscle strength and control

NANDA-I © 2012

Planning and Implementation

Develop protocols for pressure ulcer prevention so that children at high risk are identified. Initiate appropriate interventions such as

increased ambulation, frequent position changes, pressure-reducing surfaces, and moisture barriers. If the child is incontinent, change the diaper frequently to keep the skin clean and dry. A nutrition consultation may be helpful to ensure adequate intake of fluids, proteins, and vitamins to keep the skin healthy or to promote wound healing. See Box 36–7 for research on preventing pressure ulcers.

Moist wounds heal more rapidly than dry wounds because granulation and cell migration across the wound bed fight infection and remove cellular debris; such cell migration occurs more readily in a moist environment. A **primary dressing** comes directly in contact with the wound, and a **secondary dressing** is used to cover the primary dressing when further protection from contamination is needed. An **occlusive dressing** protects the wound from the outside environment and keeps all moisture at the wound site. A semiocclusive dressing allows some oxygen and moisture to evaporate from the wound environment. Dressings should be selected based on the amount of exudate that needs to be absorbed (see Table 36–6). Provide wound care and dressing changes according to agency guidelines. These guidelines may include irrigating the site with saline, debridement, and the application of a dressing appropriate for the wound condition. Gauze wraps may be used to hold the dressing in place to prevent skin damage caused by adhesives (refer to the Skills Manual 🔗).

TABLE 36–6   Characteristics of Wound Dressings

DRESSING	TYPE	PROPERTIES	NURSING MANAGEMENT
Hydrocolloid	Primary, semiocclusive	Reacts with wound exudate to form a gel-like covering to protect the wound bed and maintain a moist environment. Is occlusive and adhesive. Promotes autolytic debridement.	Use for granulating and epithelializing wounds with low or moderate amounts of exudates. Use with caution in infected wounds. Cover at least 1 inch of intact skin around the wound.
Hydrogel	Primary, semiocclusive	Increases and maintains the moisture content. Helps to clean and debride necrotic tissue. Does not adhere to the wound, so removal is pain-free.	Use with minimal or moderate exudate. Cover at least 1 inch of intact skin around the wound.
Foam	Primary, semiocclusive	Keeps the exudates off the wound to decrease the maceration of surrounding tissue. Can be left in place 3–4 days, but is often changed daily.	Use for wounds with heavy exudates and for packing deep wounds. Use during the inflammatory phase following debridement, when drainage is at its peak.
Calcium alginates	Primary, semiocclusive	Alginate fibers absorb exudate and convert it to a gel that provides a moist healing environment.	Use for moderate to heavy exudate. A secondary dressing may be needed to absorb excess drainage.
Film dressing	Primary or secondary, occlusive	Helps to protect a wound from bacterial contamination. Is permeable to oxygen, but waterproof. Helps maintain a moist environment. Provides visible wound evaluation.	Use on wounds with little or no drainage, on skin tears, or on areas of friction.

Source: *Data from Wound Care Information Network. (2010). Wound care product and category index. Retrieved from http://medicaledu.com/prodindx.htm; Mukherjee, S., Coha, T., & Torres, Z. (2010). Common skin problems in children with special healthcare needs. Pediatric Annals, 39*(4), 206–215; Butler, C. T. (2006). Pediatric skin care: Guidelines for assessment, prevention, and treatment. Pediatric Nursing, 32*(5), 448.

Care in the Community

Teach parents of children with impaired mobility and diminished pain sensation to inspect the brace fit and skin under the braces daily for signs of irritation (redness or blisters). Take the braces off once or more daily and help the child to use a mirror with a long handle to inspect skin on the bottom and sides of the feet, behind the knees, and on the lower legs. Check all edges of the braces for roughness or breakage that can pinch or scrape the skin. If any sign of skin irritation is seen and redness does not diminish within 30 minutes, do not wear the brace until the skin heals. Inform the child's healthcare provider so that an appropriate treatment regimen can be started immediately. To prevent braces from rubbing on bare skin, have the child wear cotton socks under the braces. To avoid irritation of the foot, shoes should be purchased that are large enough to accommodate the brace and the foot in the shoe. Advise parents to return to a prosthetist regularly for refitting as the child grows. See Chapter 35 🖉 and the Skills Manual ⊂⊃ for further information on the care of the child with braces.

Children who use a wheelchair are at risk for skin breakdown on the buttocks and lower back because of the pressure from sitting for hours. A wheelchair cushion can distribute and shift the child's weight when sitting in the chair. Frequent position changes are needed to relieve the pressure on the skin. Teach the child to do wheelchair push-ups or to shift the weight by leaning to the side or forward for several minutes every 10 to 15 minutes. Make sure the child wears a safety belt when sitting in the wheelchair. Teach school personnel about the child's recommended protocol so they can provide opportunities in school to change positions and reinforce the routine.

Evaluation

The expected outcomes of nursing care for the child and family include:

- Routine skin assessment is performed in children at high risk to identify early signs of pressure ulcer development.
- Effective treatment is provided to treat pressure ulcers.
- Pressure ulcers are prevented by repositioning and good skin care.

Burns

Burns are among the top five leading causes of injury deaths in children between 1 and 14 years of age (National Center for Health Statistics, National Vital Statistics System, 2011). See Table 1–1 in Chapter 1 🖉. An average of 120,856 children and adolescents under age 21 years are treated for burns in emergency departments each year. Children less than age 6 years, particularly boys, experience the most burn injuries. The majority of burn injuries occur in the home (D'Souza, Nelson, & McKenzie, 2009).

The four main types of burns are thermal, chemical, electrical, and radioactive. Thermal burns, the most common burns in children, may occur through exposure to flames or scalds (such as hot coffee or grease), or contact with a hot object (such as a woodstove or curling iron). Joshua, described in the opening vignette, sustained a thermal burn from flames when playing with matches. Chemical burns occur when children touch or ingest caustic agents. Electrical burns occur from exposure to direct or alternating current (in electrical wires, appliances, or high-voltage wires) that passes through muscles, organs,

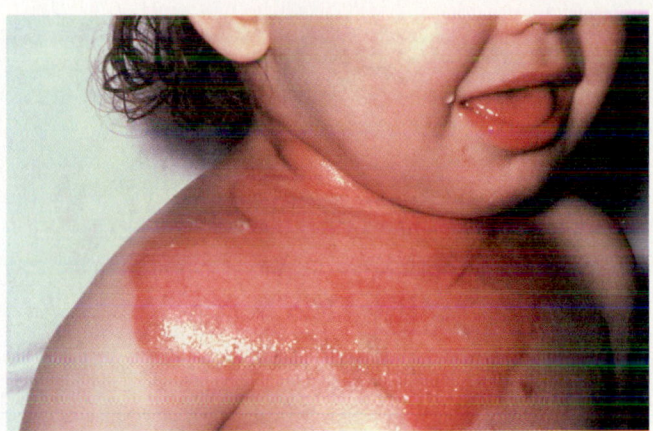

FIGURE 36–16 ■ Thermal (scald) burns are the most common burn injury in infancy. Notice the distribution of the burned skin, a wide area on the upper chest and arm where the hottest liquid fell, with a narrower area indicating the liquid cooled as it traveled down the chest.
Source: © 2012—NMSB—Custom Medical Stock Photo, All Rights Reserved.

and nerve and vascular pathways. Radiation burns result from exposure to radioactive substances or sunlight. Burns are a common form of child abuse, accounting for up to 25% of all cases (Mahindra, Guillen, & Glick, 2009). See Chapter 20 🖉 for a description of burns related to child abuse.

Etiology and Pathophysiology

Children at different developmental stages are at risk for different types of burns:

- Infants are most often injured by thermal burns (scalding liquids, house fires) (Figure 36–16 ■).
- Toddlers are at risk for thermal burns (pulling hot liquids or grease onto themselves), electrical burns (biting electrical cords or chewing through the insulation of electrical cords) (Figure 36–17 ■), contact burns, and chemical burns (ingesting cleaning agents and other substances) associated with exploring the environment.
- Preschool-age children are most often injured by scalding or contact with hot appliances (curling irons, ovens).

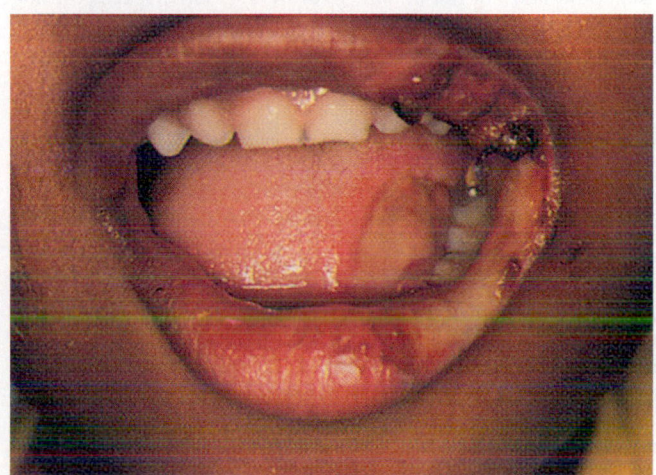

FIGURE 36–17 ■ Electrical burn caused by biting an electric cord. The burn is caused when the current arcs through the lips, often causing a full-thickness injury through the mucosa, submucosa, muscle, nerves, and blood vessels. The labial artery may be injured and cause significant bleeding once the eschar falls off after 2 to 3 weeks.
Source: Courtesy of Dr. Lezley McIlveen, Department of Dentistry, Children's National Medical Center, Washington, DC.

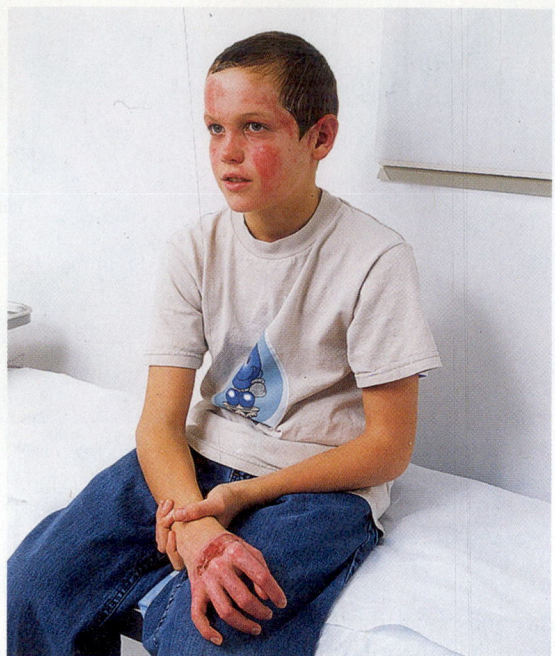

FIGURE 36–18 ■ The burns on the face and hands of this school-age boy were the result of a flash burn caused by igniting gasoline.

- School-age children are at risk for thermal burns (playing with matches, fireworks), electrical burns (climbing high-voltage towers, climbing trees, and contact with electrical wires), and chemical burns (combustion experiments) associated with their curiosity and interest in experimentation (Figure 36–18 ■).
- Adolescents also experience thermal, chemical, and electrical burns, as well as radiation burns associated with sunbathing (see page 1342).

Immediately after the burn, intense vasoconstriction occurs in response to substances released by the injured cells. Ischemia due to vasoconstriction may increase the depth of the burn injury. Vasoactive hormones are then released that increase capillary permeability. This permits fluid and plasma to shift into the interstitial spaces causing edema and decreased circulating volume in the vascular beds. Capillary integrity is not restored for 18 to 36 hours after the burn injury. The child loses increased water and heat through the injured epidermis. The child's metabolic rate and need for calories increases as the child tries to maintain body temperature and begin healing. The depth of the burn injury depends upon the temperature and duration of the heat application, and on the ability of tissues to dissipate the transferred energy.

Practice Alert

A full-thickness burn can occur in an infant or young child after immersion for only 5 seconds in water with a temperature of 60°C (140°F) and after 15 seconds if the temperature is 56°C (133°F). Coffee and other hot beverages are served at temperatures high enough to cause a serious scald burn injury (Burn Foundation, 2010). Set hot water heaters to 48°C (120°F) to help prevent scald burns. Do not hold young children in the lap when drinking hot beverages.

Clinical Manifestations

Burns are classified by depth, and different depths have specific clinical manifestations. Burn depth may be defined as partial thickness or full thickness. Partial-thickness burns, in which the injured tissue

can regenerate and heal, encompass first- and second-degree burns. Full-thickness burns, in which the injured tissue cannot regenerate, are also known as third-degree burns. See Figure 36–19 ■.

When the child places an electric plug in the mouth, a deep burn occurs at the corner of the mouth, causing necrosis of tissues and cosmetic problems. A central blackened area is surrounded by a gray-white ring and then an erythematous ring. The **eschar** (the tough leathery scab that forms over severely burned areas) forms and then separates about 1 to 2 weeks after injury, potentially causing serious bleeding.

Other clinical manifestations are included in the Clinical Manifestations table on page 1334. Signs of infection include purulent drainage, swelling, erythema, discoloration of wound margins, and pain in the uninjured skin around the wound.

Collaborative Care

The goal of therapy is to promote healing with optimal functioning, minimal scarring, and minimal psychologic impact. A team of healthcare providers is important in caring for the child with severe burns. Physical therapy and occupational therapy are important in promoting joint and muscle function with passive and active range of motion, as well as self-care skills. Splints may be needed to prevent contractures and to reduce scarring. Child life specialists can help the child cope with the stress and anxiety of the hospitalization through therapeutic play activities.

Diagnostic Tests

Burn severity is determined by the depth of the burn injury, percentage of body surface area (BSA) affected, and involvement of specific body parts. A Lund and Browder Chart with BSA distributions for various body parts at different ages is used to calculate the area affected by the burn injury (Figure 36–20 ■). Alternatively the palm of a child's hand can be used to assess the BSA to make a quick estimate of the burn size. The palmar surface (without fingers and thumb) is equal to 1% BSA.

Reassessment of the extent of thermal injury is performed 24 to 48 hours after the injury when the true extent of the injury can be identified. Criteria for major burns that should be cared for in a specialized burn center include (American College of Surgeons, 2012, p. 240):

- A partial-thickness burn greater than 10% BSA in a child under 10 years
- Burns involving the hands, face, eyes, ears, feet, genitalia, perineum, and skin over major joints
- Full-thickness burns of any size
- Chemical burns
- Electrical burns, including lightning injury
- Inhalation injury
- Local facility does not have qualified personnel and equipment to care for children who are burned
- Child requires special social and emotional or long-term rehabilitation support, including cases of suspected child maltreatment

Clinical Therapy

Initial treatment The first step is to ensure that the child has an airway, is breathing, and has a pulse. Then stop the burning process by removing any jewelry and all clothing. Moist soaks or ice (if small surface area is affected) are used to stop the burning process and

Pathophysiology Illustrated   Classification of Burns

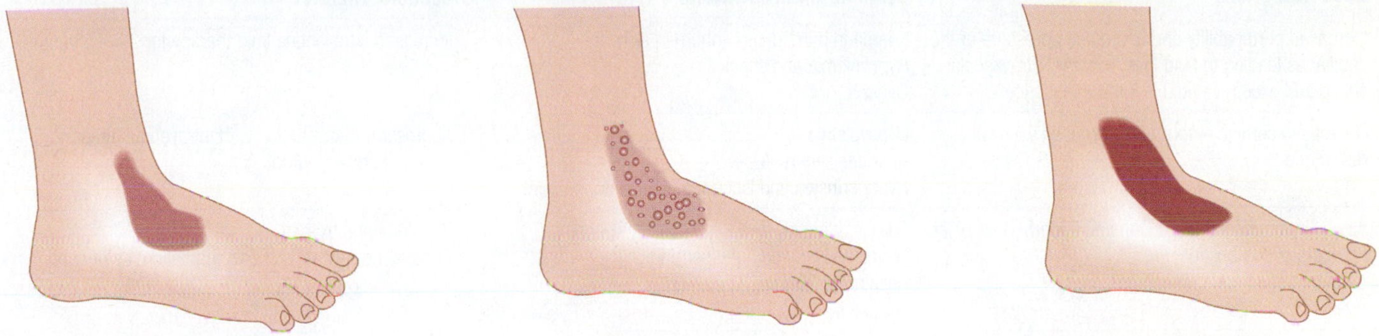

Superficial Partial Thickness (first degree)

Damages only outer layer of skin; burn is painful and red; heals in a few days (e.g., sunburn)

Partial Thickness (second degree)

Involves epidermis and upper layers of dermis; may have sparing of sweat glands and sebaceous glands; heals in 10–14 days

Full Thickness (third degree)

Involves all of epidermis and dermis; may also involve underlying tissue; nerve endings usually destroyed; requires skin grafting

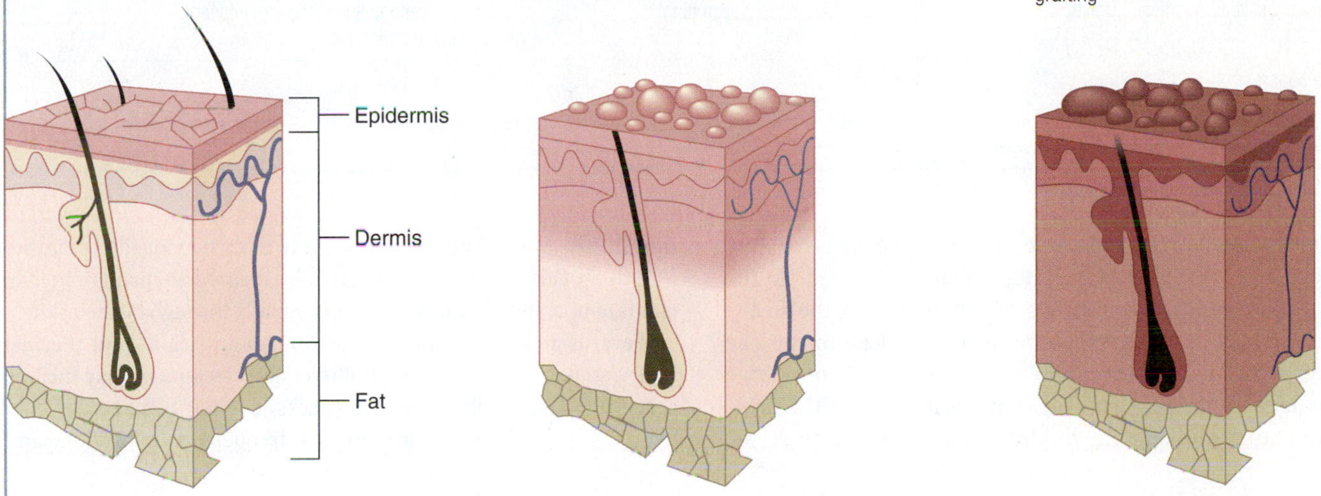

- Epidermis
- Dermis
- Fat

Erythema, blanches on pressure, no bullae, peeling after a few days due to premature cell death

Blisters or bullae, erythema, blanches on pressure, pain and sensitivity to cold air, minimal scar formation

Skin may appear brown, black, deep cherry red, white to gray, waxy or translucent, usually no pain, injured area may appear sunken

FIGURE 36–19 ■ Characteristics of burns by depth of thermal injury.

to relieve pain. If a chemical causes the burns, remove the clothing and wash with large amounts of water or an appropriate neutralizing agent.

If the child has been struck by lightning, immediate resuscitation is initiated even if the child is not breathing and has no pulse. Begin cardiopulmonary resuscitation (CPR) and give oxygen as soon as possible as the effect of the electric shock may be reversible. Once the child has been resuscitated, then entrance and exit injuries associated with the electrical burn can be identified and cared for.

A tetanus vaccine booster is given if more than 5 years have passed since the last vaccine, or when the child has not completed the full vaccine series.

Treatment of major burns Treatment focuses on decreasing burn fluid losses, preventing infection, controlling pain, promoting nutrition, and salvaging all viable burned tissue.

Fluid replacement is necessary to maintain the cardiovascular and renal systems and to prevent hypovolemic shock in cases of major burn injury. Fluid shifts from the vasculature to the interstitial spaces (third spacing) occur soon after the burn and can result in hypovolemic shock. Fluid replacement for the first 24 hours after the injury is based on a fluid volume formula calculated from the child's body weight, affected BSA, and normal maintenance needs. The Parkland and Galveston formulas are two examples used to calculate the amount of fluid needed.

- Parkland Formula: 4 mL × body weight (kg) × percentage of total body surface area burned = total 24-hour fluid requirement in mL. Maintenance fluids must be added to the amount of fluid calculated with this formula.
- Shriners Burn Hospitals–Galveston Formula: 5000 mL/m^2 burned area + 2000 mL/m^2 of total BSA = total 24-hour fluid requirement in mL.

Clinical Manifestations Moderate to Severe Burn Injury

BODY RESPONSES	CLINICAL MANIFESTATIONS	CLINICAL THERAPY
Increased permeability and hydrostatic pressure of the capillaries leading to fluid loss from the intravascular space and excessive fluid in interstitial space	Edema in burned and unburned skin Hypovolemia and shock Oliguria	Increased intravenous fluid therapy for 24–48 hours
Decreased cardiac output and increased vascular resistance	Hypovolemia Poor capillary refill Hypoperfusion and ischemia of tissues	Aggressive resuscitation with intravenous fluids to maintain urinary output
Airway inflammation due to inhaled superheated air or products of combustion	Edema of airway and airway tissue sloughing Hoarseness, stridor, or wheezing Respiratory distress Hypoxemia	Supplemental oxygen Endotracheal intubation and ventilation, as needed
Hematologic response from bone marrow suppression	Anemia	Transfusion of packed red cells
Hypermetabolic state and depletion of protein stores, increased catecholamines, glucocorticoids, and glucagon	Loss of weight and lean body mass Hyperglycemia	High-protein diet by enteral feeding until oral feeding is adequate Insulin therapy
Changed digestive absorption, paralytic ileus	Food aversion, nausea, vomiting	Intravenous fluids and electrolytes Nasogastric tube
Immune suppression	Infection	Antibiotics

Source: *Data from Hazinski, M. F., Mondozzi, M. A., & Baker, R. A. U. (2010). Shock, multiple organ dysfunction syndrome, and burns in children. In K. L. McCance, S. E. Huether, V. L. Brashers, & N. S. Rote,* Pathophysiology: The biologic basis for disease in adults and children *(6th ed., pp. 1727–1754). St. Louis, MO: Elsevier Mosby.*

Lactated Ringer's or normal saline solution is the preferred fluid (see Chapter 23 🅔). Half of the total volume calculated for the 24-hour period is infused over the first 8 hours, starting at the time of the burn, not the time of arrival in the emergency department. The remainder is then distributed evenly over the next 16 hours. Urine output is used to monitor end-organ perfusion. When the urine output reaches 1 mL/kg/hr in children weighing less than 30 kg,

fluid resuscitation ends, and the fluid rate is reduced (Hazinski, Mondozzi, & Baker, 2010). Efforts are also focused on maintaining the child's temperature because heat is lost rapidly through burned skin.

Fever is a normal, expected outcome of any significant thermal injury, so it is not always a sign of infection. Treatment may include acetaminophen or ibuprofen, ice packs, cooling blankets, or cool hydrotherapy sessions. Infection is a frequent complication, and

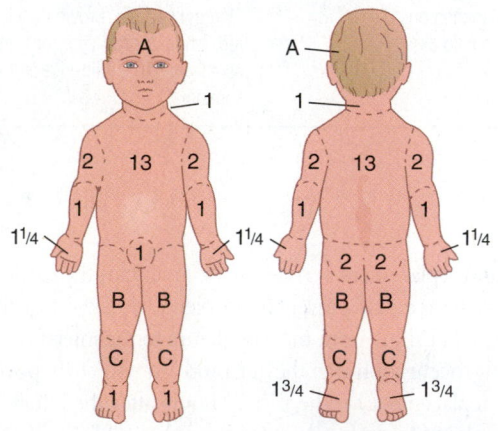

Relative Percentages of Areas Affected by Growth

Area	0	1	5	10	11	Adult
A = 1/2 of head	9 1/2	8 1/2	6 1/2	5 1/2	4 1/2	3 1/2
B = 1/2 of one thigh	2 3/4	3 1/4	4	4 1/2	4 1/2	4 3/4
C = 1/2 of one lower leg	2 1/2	2 1/2	2 3/4	3	3 1/4	3 1/2

Age in years

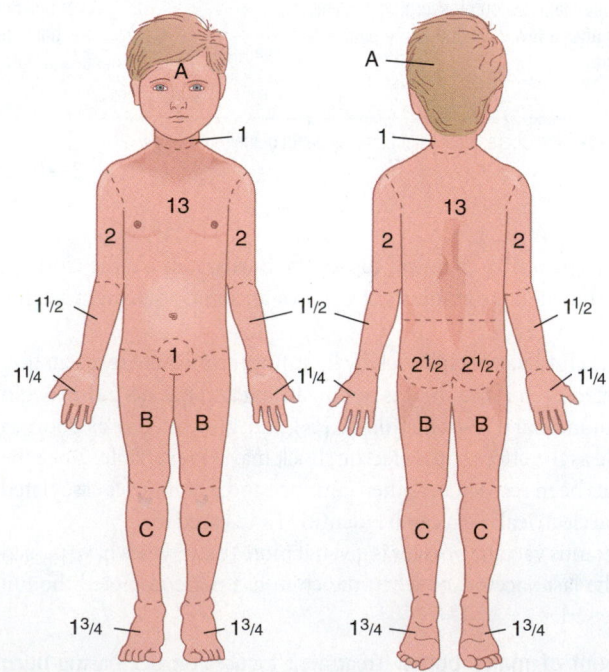

FIGURE 36–20 ■ Lund and Browder Chart for determining percentage of body surface areas in pediatric burn injuries.

Source: *Adapted from Artz, C. P., & Moncrief, J. A. (1969). The treatment of burns (2nd ed.). Philadelphia, PA: Saunders.*

wounds are cultured to identify specific organisms and sensitivities before prescribing antibiotic therapy.

A serious burn injury causes a hypermetabolic state. Continuous enteral feedings are often initiated within 6 hours of the burn injury to support the child's nutritional requirements for increased calories and additional protein. Such enteral feedings support wound healing and the body's stress response to injury. Supplemental vitamins C and E, zinc, copper, iron, and selenium are given to promote wound healing (Gauglitz, Herndon, & Jeschke, 2008).

Aggressive pain management with intravenous opioids is needed around the clock and for all procedures. The burns cause a significant emotional overlay that increases the perception of pain. See Chapter 21 🔗 for a discussion of pain management. Cimetidine or other H_2 blockers may be prescribed to prevent a burn stress ulcer.

Special consideration is needed when burns involve certain areas of the body:

- Deep partial-thickness and full-thickness burns develop eschar with no elasticity. When the burn is **circumferential,** completely around the chest or extremity, blood flow can become restricted due to edema and the scab, leading to impaired circulation and tissue hypoxia. An **escharotomy** (incision into the leathery eschar that is limiting circulation or ventilation) may be necessary to restore peripheral circulation.
- Facial burns usually cause significant edema. Care must be taken to ensure airway patency. An ophthalmologist should be consulted for burns to the eyes to assess damage and prescribe treatment. If the lips are burned, an infant may be unable to suck.
- Burns of the hands require careful management to maintain function. Special splinting and physical therapy are usually necessary.
- Perineal burns are at higher risk for infection because of frequent contamination with urine and stool. Frequent dressing changes are required. A urinary catheter is usually inserted but is removed once hydration status is stable to minimize the risk of urinary tract infection.

Wound management Burn wound care has several goals: (1) to remove necrotic tissue and speed wound debridement, (2) to maintain moist wound conditions and adequate circulation, (3) to conserve body heat and fluids, (4) to protect the wound from infection, and (5) to control scarring and prevent scar contracture. Several treatment regimens are used to achieve these goals.

When the child has an extensive burn, the entire body is bathed to initiate **debridement** (removal of dead tissue to speed the healing process). Sedation, pain management, and anesthesiology support are often used during debridement sessions. Intact blisters provide a natural, pain-free, sterile dressing; however, some healthcare providers believe the fluid provides a medium for bacterial infection. Some burn centers keep blisters intact, whereas others break blisters open. In either case the tissues should be carefully cut away when the wound is being prepared for skin grafting.

Clinical Tip
Be sure to follow all agency guidelines for assessment and monitoring of a child when sedation is used during the debridement process (see Chapter 21 🔗).

Various options are used for wound management after debridement. Traditional burn care for a partial-thickness injury involves the application of antibacterial agents, such as silver sulfadiazine

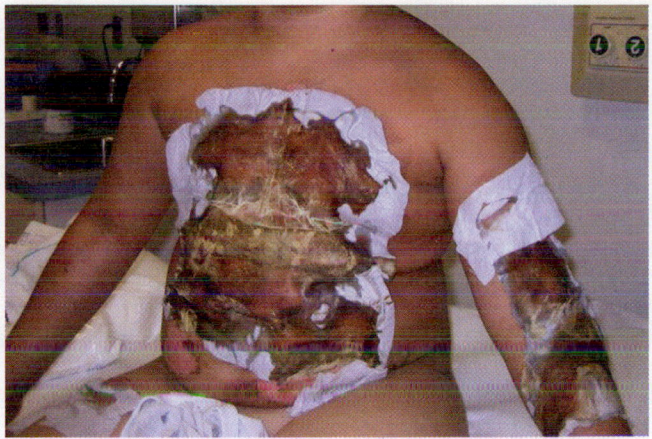

FIGURE 36–21 ■ Child with a scald burn treated with an Aquacel AG dressing, one of the newer silver-embedded dressings. Note the absorbed exudate that is visible through the burn dressing.

Source: *Courtesy of Martin Eichelberger, MD, and Lisa Ring, RN, PNP, Children's National Medical Center, Washington, DC.*

(Silvadene), mafenide acetate (Sulfamylon), or bacitracin after initial cleansing. Dressings are added to cover the burned area and are changed once or twice daily.

Newer silver-based antimicrobial dressings (e.g., Aquacel, Acticoat) have been developed that provide a sustained-release delivery of silver, valued for its antimicrobial activity. As these dressings also absorb exudates from the wound, they can be left in place for several days (Figure 36–21 ■). When the dressing is removed, a layer of eschar may also be debrided. These dressing changes are often painful, so pain management is needed. See Chapter 21 🔗.

Hydrotherapy (whirlpool) baths may be used to cleanse extensive wounds before debridement, to increase vasodilation and circulation, and to speed healing. Hydrotherapy and debridement may be performed with the child in a shower rather than a tub to reduce the risk of infection. The water loosens exudates, topical medications, and dead tissue. In addition, the dressings that adhere to the skin may be soaked to help loosen them. Tap water and an antimicrobial soap are often used for cleansing. Gentle washing is necessary to protect new epithelial cells. Granulation tissue forms as a result of daily debridement. Superficial partial-thickness burns reepithelialize within 3 weeks.

Skin grafting is necessary with any deep partial-thickness and full-thickness burn. Often a biologic dressing (e.g., Integra or Biobrane) or **allograft** (cadaver skin from a skin bank) is used to cover deep burns until an **autograft** (use of healthy skin taken from a non-burned area of the child's body) can be placed. The biologic dressing or allograft is effective in decreasing infection risk and pain, protecting against fluid loss, and promoting revascularization. The autograft is placed after the wound is debrided in the operating room to reveal healthy, bleeding tissue. The donor site (where the autograft was harvested) is a new wound, causing pain and requiring close monitoring for signs of infection.

Vacuum-assisted wound closure (negative pressure wound therapy) is sometimes used for management of partial-thickness burns, graft sites, and other complex wounds. Vacuum-assisted wound closure consists of a pump that generates a vacuum, dressing materials used to pack the wound and seal it, tubing for fluid removal from the wound area, and a container/canister to collect waste materials that are removed from the wound area by suction. Once the burn site is debrided, a foam dressing is applied and sealed

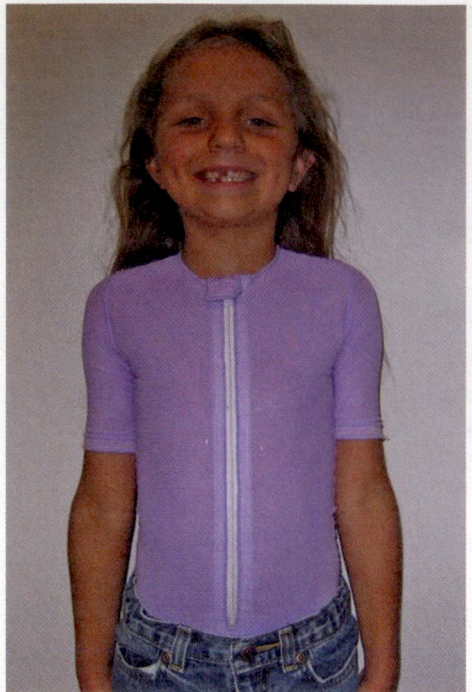

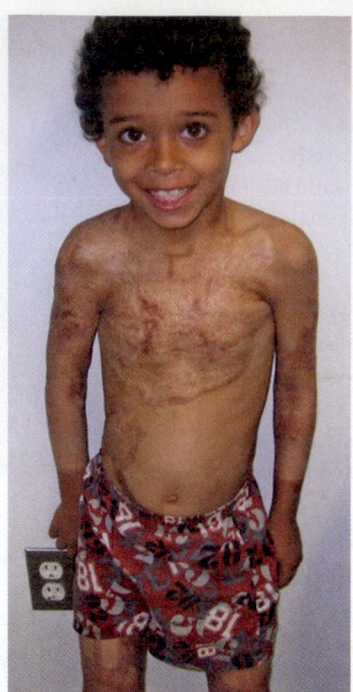

A   **B**

FIGURE 36–22 ■ *A*, Pressure garment used to reduce hypertrophic scarring from a burn to the chest and upper arms. *B*, Hypertrophic scar on the chest.

Source: *Courtesy of Martin R. Eichelberger, MD, and Lisa Ring, RN, PNP, Children's National Medical Center, Washington, DC.*

with adhesive before the device is attached. The vacuum over the surface of the wound draws out fluids, increases blood perfusion, decreases bacterial colonization, and draws wound edges together to speed healing.

Practice Alert
Vacuum-assisted wound closure devices are not approved by the FDA for use in infants and children. The FDA issued a warning about rare and serious side effects of these devices, such as life-threatening bleeding and serious infection. Patients should be carefully monitored for these problems, and parents should be taught how to identify problems and seek help when these devices are used at home (U.S. Food and Drug Administration, 2011).

During the rehabilitation stage, pressure garments (e.g., Jobst) are used to reduce development of hypertrophic scarring and contractures (Figure 36–22A ■). Such garments are worn 23 hours a day for 6 to 8 months to shorten the time of scar maturation and to reduce the thickness of the scars (Figure 36–22B ■).

Severe morbidity is likely to occur with major burns. Significant scarring may occur despite the use of autografts and pressure garments. Contractures and loss of function are also possible. Children with major burns require comprehensive follow-up, sometimes involving repeated hospitalizations for surgery to release burn contractures and perform new grafting or cosmetic surgery for scar revision.

Nursing Management

The goals of nursing care include prevention of burns, careful assessment and monitoring of the child's condition and burn injury, pain management, psychosocial support of the child and family, treatment of the burn injury, and prevention of complications.

Nursing Assessment and Diagnosis
Emergency Assessment

Nursing assessment first focuses on the potential for life-threatening injuries that need immediate care. Assessment of the airway is necessary, especially when signs of smoke inhalation or burns to the face and neck are present. It is important to identify other potential injuries when the mechanism of injury also includes a fall or explosion which compounds the severity of the burn injury. Identify signs of respiratory distress and any potential bleeding source. A weak, thready pulse, tachycardia, and pallor are important signs of early shock that may provide clues to an internal injury.

History

Obtain information about the type of burn (e.g., thermal, electrical, chemical) and a complete history. When taking a burn history, carefully document the type and time of injury, people present at the time of the injury, first aid administered, and history of other unusual injuries or emergency department visits. If a burn injury was preventable, parents may be emotionally stressed by feelings of guilt. Take care to avoid sounding accusatory when questioning parents about the injury. Be alert to signs of child abuse when the history does not match the burn injury. Child neglect can be a factor in the burn of a child who was not adequately supervised.

Practice Alert
Signs of child abuse include glove and stocking burns, burns that spare flexor surfaces (e.g., perineum or popliteal area), contact burns from cigarettes or an iron, or zebra burn lines from contact with a hot grate (Figure 36–23 ■). Photographs are often taken to document these burn injuries.

Physical Assessment

Assess the extent of burn injury (depth and BSA affected). Frequently monitor the vital signs and pain level. Monitor the child's circulatory and respiratory status to identify signs of hypovolemia in the first 24 hours or fluid overload as capillary integrity is restored.

Perform a head-to-toe assessment at the beginning of every shift followed by system-specific assessments, depending on clinical findings and changes in the child's status. For example, frequently assess edema, eschar, and distal pulses in a burned extremity to monitor peripheral circulation. Monitor electrolytes as well as the child's intake and output carefully. A urinary catheter may be inserted to monitor urine output. Be alert to signs of infection such as purulent drainage and edematous, red, or discolored wound margins.

Practice Alert
If a burn is circumferential, assess for an increase in cyanosis, deep-tissue pain, and capillary refill time, and a decreased pulse distal to the circumferential burn. If you detect these signs, notify the physician immediately.

Psychosocial Assessment

Assess the child's concerns over appearance and the stress of hospitalization. Determine if the child has memories or nightmares about the

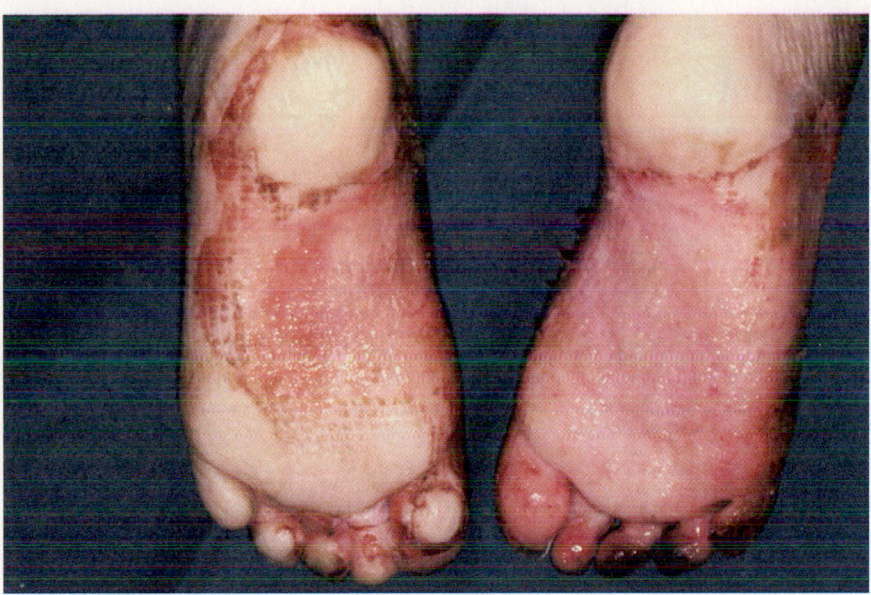

FIGURE 36–23 ■ Burn injuries associated with child abuse. Burns of the hands or feet that are distributed like gloves or stockings that often have a clear demarcation matching the depth of hot water and few splash marks. Note the skin protected that was in contact with the cooler tub surface.

Source: *© 2012—Custom Medical Stock Photo, All Rights Reserved.*

burn so psychologic support can be provided as needed. Identify any family stressors that might need to be addressed during the child's care.

Common nursing diagnoses for the child with a major burn injury are included in the accompanying Nursing Care Plan. Additional nursing diagnoses for the child with a major burn may include the following:

- Hyperthermia related to increased metabolic rate and trauma
- Tissue Perfusion: Peripheral, Ineffective related to mechanical reduction in blood flow (edema) to an extremity with a circumferential burn
- Body Image, Disturbed related to burn injury and scars
- Anxiety related to situational crisis and threat of death or disfigurement

NANDA-I © 2012

Planning and Implementation

Nursing care focuses on performing burn care, promoting healing, preventing complications, and providing emotional support. Care includes dressing changes, hydrotherapy, antibiotic therapy, fluid and nutrition management, analgesic support, physical therapy, play therapy, and possibly skin grafting. See the Nursing Care Plan for some important aspects of burn care.

Promote Comfort

Assess the child's pain frequently and provide pain management day and night (see Chapter 21 🔗 for pain management guidelines). Begin pain and sedation management as soon as possible for the initial debridement to reduce the stress on the child. Perception of procedural pain may be intensified if the child has ongoing background pain from the injury (Connor-Ballard, 2009). Provide diversion to help the child focus on a pleasant activity rather than pain.

Promote the child's comfort during periods of elevated temperature while keeping burns covered to reduce pain. Keep room

temperature at a comfortable level. Change bed linens as needed when the child perspires heavily.

Fluid and Nutritional Support

Fluids should be administered at the rate prescribed for resuscitation for the first 24 hours, and then adjusted as prescribed. Enteral feeding may be needed initially by the child with extensive burns until the child is able to eat adequate amounts. Once the child is able to eat, provide a diet high in protein and calories. Identify food items that the child likes, and encourage the family to bring food in that the child may prefer to eat. Provide small frequent feedings to increase the number of calories consumed each day.

Wound Care

The burned area is debrided and cleaned, often with a chemical enzyme. Then an antibacterial/antimicrobial medication or dressing is applied. Topical medications are often covered with dressings. At each dressing change, the wound needs to be assessed for appearance, exudate, odor, appearance of surrounding tissue, and presence of granulation tissue.

A semipermeable wound membrane may be applied to a debrided superficial partial-thickness burn. These membranes protect the burned tissue from trauma, prevent fluid loss, create a moist environment for healing, and provide a physical barrier to bacteria. Monitor the burn under the transparent membrane carefully for infection which could deepen the burn wound. When the burn heals, the wound membrane loosens, permitting it to be trimmed.

Allografts or autografts may be placed in the operating room after debridement to prepare the burned tissue for the graft. Following the grafting procedure, wet dressings with antibiotic solution are used for several days, commonly followed by other dry dressings with antibiotics. Splints may be required to promote healing when the skin over a joint is burned. The child may be on bed rest for several

Nursing Care Plan

The Child with a Major Burn Injury

INTERVENTION	RATIONALE	EXPECTED OUTCOME
1. Nursing Diagnosis: Pain, Acute related to physical injury agents		
NIC Priority Intervention—_Pain Management:_ Alleviation of pain or a reduction in pain to a level of comfort that is acceptable to the patient		**NOC Suggested Outcome—**_Comfort Level:_ Extent of positive perception of physical and psychologic ease
GOAL: _The child will verbalize adequate relief from pain and will be able to perform activities of daily living (ADLs)._		
■ Assess the level of pain frequently using pain scales (see Chapter 21 🔗).	■ Pain scales provide objective measurement. Pain is always present, but changes in location and intensity may indicate complications.	The child verbalizes adequate relief from pain and is able to perform ADLs.
■ Cover burns with dressings as much as possible.	■ Temperature changes or movement of air causes pain.	
■ Change the child's position every 2–4 hours. Perform range of motion exercises at least twice a day.	■ Position changes and exercises reduce joint stiffness and increase comfort.	
■ Encourage verbalization about pain by asking questions.	■ This provides an outlet for emotions and helps the child cope.	
■ Provide diversion activities such as videos, games, or other activities that the child can participate in.	■ Activities help lessen the focus on pain.	
■ Promote uninterrupted sleep with use of a quiet environment, medications, and other comfort measures.	■ Sleep deprivation can increase pain perception.	
■ Use analgesics before all dressing changes and burn care. Use sedation when appropriate for major debridement.	■ Analgesics and sedatives help to reduce pain and decrease anxiety for subsequent dressing changes.	
2. Nursing Diagnosis: Infection, Risk for related to trauma and destruction of skin barrier		
NIC Priority Intervention—_Infection Protection:_ Prevention and early detection of infection in a patient at risk		**NOC Suggested Outcome—**_Risk Control:_ Actions to eliminate or reduce actual, personal, and modifiable health threats
GOAL: _The child will be free of infection during the healing process._		
■ Take vital signs frequently.	■ Increased temperature is an early sign of infection, but it is also a common response to burn injury.	The child either stays free of secondary infection or has infection diagnosed and treated early.
■ Use standard precautions (gown, gloves, mask) when wounds of a major burn are exposed. Do not allow visitors who have an infectious disease.	■ These measures reduce the risk of wound contamination.	
■ Clip hair around burns.	■ Hair harbors bacteria and can irritate the wound.	
■ Keep the burn dressing clean and intact.	■ A clean dressing helps reduce the number of bacteria introduced to the burned site.	
■ Do not place the IV in any burned area.	■ This reduces the risk of wound contamination.	
■ Administer oral or IV antibiotics for diagnosed infections as prescribed.	■ Antibiotics administered as prescribed help to clear the infection quickly.	
3. Nursing Diagnosis: Fluid Volume: Imbalanced, Risk for related to loss of fluids through wounds and to subsequent excess fluid intake		
NIC Priority Intervention—_Fluid Management:_ Promotion of fluid balance and prevention of complications resulting from abnormal or undesired fluid levels		**NOC Suggested Outcome—**_Fluid Balance:_ Balance of water in the intracellular and extracellular compartments of the body
GOAL: _The child will maintain adequate urine output._		
■ Monitor vital signs, central venous pressure, capillary refill time, and pulses.	■ The child is initially at risk for hypovolemic shock and needs fluid resuscitation (see Chapter 26 🔗).	The child maintains normal urine output, and burn site edema is not excessive.
■ Administer IV and oral fluids as ordered.	■ Careful calculation of fluid needs and ensuring proper intake helps keep the child properly hydrated and reduces the risk for renal damage.	

Nursing Care Plan   The Child with a Major Burn Injury, *continued*

INTERVENTION	RATIONALE	EXPECTED OUTCOME
■ Monitor intake and output.	■ The child is at risk for fluid overload during hydration, and for edema in the burned tissues.	
■ Weigh the child daily using the same scale and amount of clothing.	■ Significant weight loss or gain can help determine fluid imbalances.	
■ Insert a urinary catheter if prescribed.	■ A catheter helps maintain accurate output measurement during the critical care stage.	
■ Monitor for hyponatremia and hyperkalemia (see Chapter 23 🔗).	■ Sodium is lost with burn fluid and potassium is lost from damaged cells, causing electrolyte imbalances.	

4. Nursing Diagnosis: Mobility: Physical, Impaired related to joint stiffness due to burns

NIC Priority Intervention—*Exercise Therapy, Joint Mobility:* Use of active or passive body movement to maintain or restore joint flexibility		**NOC Suggested Outcome**—*Joint Movement (Active):* Range of motion of joints with self-initiated movement

GOAL: *The child will maintain maximum range of motion.*

■ Arrange physical and occupational therapy twice daily for stretching and range of motion exercises. Splint as ordered. Encourage independent activities of daily living.	■ Positioning in alignment and range of motion exercises help to prevent contractures. Self-care encourages developmental progression and enhances self-concept.	The child maintains maximum range of motion without contractures.
■ Encourage activities to promote range of motion (toss a beanbag, mimic animal movements).	■ Fun activities help the child with diversion and provide movement.	

5. Nursing Diagnosis: Nutrition: Imbalanced, Less than Body Requirements related to high metabolic needs

NIC Priority Intervention—*Nutrition Management:* Assistance with or provision of balanced dietary intake of foods and fluids		**NOC Suggested Outcome**—*Nutritional Status:* Extent to which nutrients are available to meet metabolic needs

GOAL: *The child will maintain weight and demonstrate adequate serum albumin and hydration.*

■ Provide an opportunity to choose meals. Offer a variety of high-protein and high-calorie foods. Provide snacks.	■ A variety of food choices encourages intake. General malaise and anorexia lead to poor healing.	The child maintains weight, adequate hydration, and normal serum albumin.
■ Encourage the child to have meals with other children.	■ Socialization improves intake.	
■ Provide a multivitamin supplement.	■ Vitamin C aids zinc absorption; zinc aids in healing.	
■ Provide enteral feedings as needed.	■ A child with a burn greater than 10% of BSA needs assistance to meet nutrition requirements.	
■ Weigh the child daily.	■ Daily weights provide an objective evaluation.	

6. Nursing Diagnosis: Anxiety (Child) related to threat to or change in health status

NIC Priority Intervention—*Anxiety Reduction:* Minimizing apprehension, dread, foreboding, or uneasiness related to an unidentified source of anticipated danger		**NOC Suggested Outcome**—*Coping:* Actions to manage stressors that tax an individual's resources

GOAL: *The child will verbalize reduced anxiety.*

■ Provide continuity of care providers.	■ Continuity of care helps to build a trusting relationship.	The child expresses and shows signs of reduced anxiety.
■ Encourage parents to stay with the child; calls from home; and pictures from classmates.	■ Familiar surroundings, people, and items encourage relaxation.	
■ Group tasks and activities.	■ Grouping activities helps to reduce overstimulation and encourage rest.	

(continued)

Nursing Care Plan   The Child with a Major Burn Injury, *continued*

INTERVENTION	RATIONALE	EXPECTED OUTCOME
7. Nursing Diagnosis: Anxiety (Parent) related to situational crisis		
NIC Priority Intervention—*Coping Enhancement:* Assisting a patient to adapt to perceived stressors, changes, or threats that interfere with meeting life demands and roles		**NOC Suggested Outcome**—*Anxiety Control:* Ability to eliminate or reduce feelings of apprehension and tension from an unidentified source
GOAL: *Parents will verbalize decreased anxiety.*		
■ Provide educational materials about healing, grafting, dressing changes, and course of action.	■ Knowledge reduces anxiety.	Parents state decreased anxiety, and they describe plans and solve problems related to care of the child at home.
■ Be flexible when teaching parents about wound care.	■ Adults learn in many different ways.	
■ Allow parents to talk about their feelings, concerns, and frustrations. Provide referral to social services or a parent support group.	■ It is important to allow for venting of fears and guilt feelings, and to provide exchange of ideas on dealing with hospitalization and long-term care.	
■ Encourage parents to participate in the child's care and development of the care plan.	■ An actual role in planning the child's care helps them gain some control and comfort in the setting.	

NANDA-I © 2012

days following an autograft to protect the graft until it has a vascular supply. Donor sites are treated as separate wounds.

Provide Emotional Support

Children with burns have received a profound insult to their body and their self-image. Fear and anxiety related to disfigurement and scarring are common, especially among adolescents. The shock and pain of the injury cause increased stress, as do the unfamiliar surroundings and presence of healthcare providers.

An attitude of genuine interest and concern on the part of the nurse is essential. The child should be oriented to his or her surroundings frequently and given ample preparation for procedures, when possible. Continuity of care providers is important in developing a trusting relationship and partnership with the child and family. Make appropriate referrals to social workers, chaplains, and child life specialists to ensure that the child and family receive necessary services.

Therapeutic play is encouraged for children, even if they can only observe initially. It serves several purposes for the child with a major burn:

- It provides an outlet for frustration, independence, and creativity.
- It promotes activities that challenge range of motion.
- It normalizes the child's daily routine.
- It encourages the child, who sees the progress that other children make day by day.

Families are at risk for emotional stress. The family needs information and frequent updates. This promotes trust between the family and the healthcare team. Warn them to expect edema and changes in the child's body with the injury response. Parents often feel guilty and responsible for the child's injury. It is important to help parents focus on recovery rather than on past actions. Anxiety usually results from lack of knowledge about the severity of the burn and the child's status, especially in the early stages of burn care and admission to the intensive care unit. Involve parents in their child's care, learning how to change dressings, assessing for infection and dehydration, and performing range of motion exercises to aid in the child's recovery.

Prevent Complications

The healthcare team works to prevent complications such as infections, sepsis, pneumonia, and renal failure, as well as possible irreversible loss of function of the burned area. Standard precautions are often used to reduce the child's risk for infection. Identified infections need to be treated early to reduce the risk for sepsis and pneumonia.

Significant scarring may occur regardless of autografting. Contractures and loss of function are also possible.

Discharge Planning and Home Care Teaching

Home care needs should be identified and addressed well in advance of discharge. Thorough assessment is necessary to identify the family's needs related to the child's discharge home or to a rehabilitation facility. Discharge planning may include instructing parents in nutrition and diet needs, safety in the home, protection of the burned area, wound care, signs of infection and actions to take, use of pressure garments, and range of motion exercises to prevent contractures.

Provide support and encouragement to parents when they are learning how to care for the child with a burn injury. Many burn centers use burn dressings (e.g., silver-embedded dressings) that reduce the frequency of burn dressing changes needed. As with Joshua, dressing changes are often performed in a clinic setting or sedation suite to reduce the risk for infection and to provide effective pain management for the procedure. If parents provide dressing changes, provide pain medication and give guidelines about how soon before the dressing change to give the pain medication. Specific guidelines for dressing changes should be outlined so that parents and healthcare team members will have the same focus. Parents should first observe care being performed and then provide repeat demonstrations until competent.

Care in the Community

Care of the child with a burn requires long-term therapy and rehabilitation. Nurses in the clinic and home care settings continue the care provided in the hospital. Long-term care commonly occurs in the home, with frequent visits to healthcare professionals. Children with extensive burns or with burns in locations where scarring may limit function must often wear a pressure garment (see Figure 36–22A), and sometimes a face mask if the face is burned. The garment is removed only for bathing and laundry of the garment. The pressure garment may present a threat to the child's self-image, but it is an important way to decrease scarring. Help families understand the need for the special garments and masks, and how to clean and care for them.

Clinical Tip

Moisturizing creams can be used after burns heal to relieve residual drying. The healed skin is highly sensitive to sunburn, so cover the area or use a sunscreen. Use of a sunscreen will also help prevent hyperpigmentation after burn healing.

Continued physical therapy and occupational therapy are often needed to increase strength and dexterity in performing self-care skills and to prevent contractures. Emphasis is placed on returning to normal activities of daily living as soon as possible, such as returning to school as soon as health permits. Some children have home tutors and are provided with computer connections to school activities for a time to ensure opportunities to continue learning while decreasing their exposure to infection.

School reentry can be a traumatic experience, especially for older children and adolescents, because of the fear of rejection, decreased self-esteem, and impaired body image. The child's primary nurse, social worker, child life specialist, and parent may visit the school of a child with a burn injury before the child returns to school—bringing photographs of the child, pressure garments, or other items—to inform the classmates and allow them to explore their emotions relating to the child's burn injury. Several communities offer support groups for families and children with burn injuries. Referral to these groups may be beneficial.

A major role of nurses in the community is prevention. Provide burn prevention information to parents at each health promotion visit. Become involved with a Safe Kids coalition or local firefighters to help educate families and caregivers about ways to prevent scald burns and house fires. Examples of prevention messages include the following:

- Appropriate temperature settings for hot water heaters
- Keeping the handles of pots on the stove turned toward the wall and dishes with hot liquids out of the toddler's reach
- Keeping infants and toddlers off the lap when drinking hot beverages or eating soup

- Keeping matches, lighters, and flammable materials away from children
- Installing smoke detectors and replacing the batteries annually

Encourage families to develop and practice escape plans from the home in case of a house fire. See Chapter 14 🔗. Look for burn hazards when making home visits. Provide adolescents and parents with first aid training so they can provide appropriate care when a child or other family member becomes injured.

Evaluation

Examples of expected outcomes of nursing management are included in the Nursing Care Plan. Some additional outcomes include:

- The child has effective pain management for the injury and dressing changes.
- Hypovolemia and later fluid overload due to intravenous fluid management is prevented in the child with burns.
- The child has appropriate wound management that prevents infection.

Management of Minor Burns

Many children with minor burns are cared for at home after an initial visit to the emergency department or urgent care clinic. Discuss home remedies for minor burn care. See Partnering with Families: Caring for Minor Burns. For superficial burns covering a small area, use moist soaks or ice to stop the burning process and to relieve pain. Any open blisters are debrided, and a thin layer of an antibiotic medication (e.g., silver sulfadiazine) is applied over the burn. Do not place this medication close to the eyes or mouth. Bacitracin is often used for burns on the face. The burn is then covered with one or two layers of gauze. Acetaminophen with codeine may be prescribed for burn dressing changes at home. Burn dressings should be changed once or twice daily. This involves cleaning the burn and reapplying antibiotic medication. See the Skills Manual 🔗.

Educate the parents about increasing the child's fluid intake to compensate for loss of fluid through damaged skin. A high-calorie, high-protein diet is necessary to meet the increased nutritional requirement of healing. Infection is a common complication. Educate the parents to observe for signs of infection (inflammation extending under the dressing, bad odor, excessive exudates, and fever), and notify the physician immediately if noticed. The child should be seen

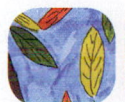 # Partnering with Families

Caring for Minor Burns

- Place the burn under cool, running water to stop the burning process and to help reduce pain. Do not use ice as it can cause more damage to the injured skin.
- Do not use butter or margarine on the burn as it may introduce bacteria into the wound.
- Remove all clothing and jewelry from the burned area.
- Topical application of gel from the leaf of an aloe vera plant may help promote healing (National Center for Complementary and Alternative Medicine, 2011).

- Apply a topical antibiotic such as bacitracin to the burned area, and cover the area with a couple of layers of gauze. Keep the area clean and dry.
- Clean and change the dressing twice daily. The pain medication should be given about an hour before the dressing change is planned. The dressing may be saturated with sterile normal saline and gently removed if it adheres to the burn area.

BOX 36–8	Community Care: Assessing UV Exposure Risk

Harmful exposure to UV rays is more intense in the summer, at higher altitudes, and closer to the equator. Surfaces like sand, snow, and water reflect UV rays, in some cases making intensity higher than expected. The UV index, published in most newspapers and on the Internet, provides daily information about the strength or intensity of the sun's rays in any given community. Encourage parents to monitor the UV index and use it as a guide for dressing children with protective covering when playing outside, and the use of sunscreen.

BOX 36–9	*Healthy People 2020* Skin Cancer Prevention Objectives

- Increase the proportion of persons who participate in behaviors that reduce their exposure to harmful ultraviolet (UV) irradiation and avoid sunburn.
- Reduce the proportion of adolescents in grades 9 through 12 who report sunburn.
- Reduce the proportion of adolescents in grades 9 through 12 who report using artificial sources of ultraviolet light for tanning.
- Increase the proportion of adolescents in grades 9 through 12 who follow protective measures that may reduce the risk of skin cancer.

Source: From U.S. Department of Health and Human Services. (2011). Healthy People 2020. Washington, DC. Retrieved from http://healthypeople.gov/2020/topicsobjectives2020/objectiveslist.aspx?topicId=5

within 48 hours of initial treatment to monitor progress. Reinforce to parents the importance of follow-up appointments.

Sunburn

Sunburn is a burn injury to the outer layer of skin caused by excess ultraviolet (UV) light exposure, or sun exposure after taking **phototoxic** drugs (acne medication, sulfonamides, tetracycline, NSAIDs, and birth control pills). Young children have less melanin to protect their skin against harmful UV rays. More than half of a person's lifetime sun exposure occurs before 20 years of age (Land & Small, 2008). An estimated 83% of children are sunburned during the summer, and approximately 36% of adolescents have repeated sunburns during the summer (Koshy, Sharabi, Jerkins, et al., 2010). See Box 36–8. A childhood sun exposure history that includes intense repeated sunburns and chronic overexposure to UV radiation for the purpose of tanning is strongly associated with the development of skin cancer in future years (Koshy et al., 2010). Avoiding sunburn during childhood is believed to be more important than protecting the skin during adulthood.

Practice Alert

Melanoma is the most common form of cancer in adolescents and young adults. Behaviors and skin characteristics that increase the risk for pediatric melanoma include light-colored eyes, freckling, fair skin, blond or red hair, family history of melanoma, intermittent large blasts of UV radiation causing blistering sunburns before 20 years of age, frequent sun exposure without the use of sunscreen, melanocytic nevi, and immunosuppression (Berwick, Erdei, & Hay, 2009; Muhrer, 2009).

Erythema, pain, skin tenderness, swelling, blistering, and itching usually develop between 3 and 5 hours after exposure to ultraviolet B (UVB) rays. UVA rays cause deeper skin damage (Bell, 2008). Increased vasodilation and vascular permeability result in the extravasation of fluid to the tissues and white blood cell migration to the damaged skin. The erythema peaks at 12 to 24 hours and subsides after 72 hours. Systemic complaints include malaise, insomnia (because of skin tenderness), fatigue, headaches, and chilling (because of rapid heat loss).

Treatment is generally supportive. Pain can be relieved by cool water compresses, ice packs, local anesthetic sprays or creams, and emollients. Extra fluids should be provided. Some healthcare providers prescribe the application of a low-potency topical corticosteroid (on unblistered skin) and NSAIDs for pain relief and to reduce inflammation (Land & Small, 2008). See Chapter 21 🔗 for information on NSAIDs.

Nursing Management

Educate parents and children about ways to prevent sunburn. See Box 36–9 for the *Healthy People 2020* objectives for the reduction of sun exposure and skin cancer in children and adolescents. Advise that repeated sunburns may lead to permanent skin damage, skin cancer, cataracts, and premature aging of the skin. Be alert for medications that a child is taking that have side effects of increased reaction to sun exposure. Advise the family of increased risk. See Partnering with Families: Preventing Sunburn.

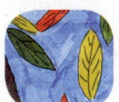

Partnering with Families

Preventing Sunburn

- Keep children out of direct sunlight as much as possible, especially the midday sun. Avoid scheduling outdoor activities during the hours of maximum exposure (10 a.m. to 3 p.m.), or have children play in the shade.
- When outdoors, minimize sun exposure by wearing hats with a 3-inch brim, and closely woven cotton long-sleeved shirts and pants. Wear T-shirts while swimming. Special sun protection clothing is now available from some manufacturers.
- Obtain sunglasses with 99% UV blockage for children to wear.
- Be aware that water, concrete, and sand reflect sunlight and increase exposure up to 90% by reflecting up to 85% of the UV rays.
- Use sunscreen with at least 15 SPF. For optimal protection, apply thickly to all exposed areas at least 30 minutes before sun exposure. Remember to apply it behind the knees and on the ears, eye areas, and neck. Reapply 15 to 20 minutes after first sun exposure, and then again

every 2 hours as needed. Reapply sooner if swimming, toweling off, or perspiring heavily.
- Use a waterproof sunscreen when swimming; this provides protection in water for approximately 60 to 80 minutes. Then reapply. Avoid placing waterproof sunscreen near the eyes as it causes severe pain and a chemical burn. Call the poison control center immediately for guidance if the eyes are exposed.
- Use UV blocking agents such as zinc oxide or titanium oxide for infants under age 6 months as they may absorb sunscreen chemicals through their skin.
- Remember that a child can be burned even on a cloudy day. Up to 80% of UV rays can penetrate the cloud cover.
- If the child is taking any medications, check with the healthcare provider before exposure (some medications cause hypersensitivity to sunlight).
- Adolescents should avoid indoor tanning facilities and artificial tanning devices because the rays are as damaging to the skin as the sun.

Participate in educating students about sun safety, and promote policy changes to reduce sun exposure in school settings, such as hats worn for play or physical education when outside during peak sun hours. Teach adolescents how to monitor for changes in moles that could signal the development of skin cancer and to seek care immediately. Characteristics of moles that indicate a need for evaluation include those that are asymmetric and have an irregular border.

Hypothermia

Hypothermia is a condition in which the core body temperature falls below 35°C (95°F). This occurs when the heat produced by the body is less than the body heat lost. Hypothermia is a life-threatening emergency that can occur in any season and any geographic location. Infants and young children are at risk because of immature thermoregulatory mechanisms, thinner skin, limited subcutaneous fat, and high surface area to body mass ratio. Adolescents are at risk due to risk-taking behaviors such as drug and alcohol use, and engaging in remote outdoor activities without proper equipment.

Etiology and Pathophysiology

Primary hypothermia results from environmental exposure. Heat is lost through four primary mechanisms:

- **Radiation**—heat transfers from the body to cooler surfaces not in direct contact with the skin, such as moving through a cool hallway. Most heat is lost from uncovered parts of the body.
- **Convection**—loss of heat to cooler air currents. The rate of heat loss can be increased dependent on wind speeds or the wind chill factor.
- **Conduction**—transfer of heat from the body to a cooler surface in direct contact with the skin. This mechanism of heat loss is increased when the child is submerged in water.
- **Evaporation**—loss of heat when water or sweat is converted to a vapor.

As the core temperature falls, the body tries to conserve body heat and to rewarm blood by vasoconstriction to shunt blood to the body core and increasing muscle tone and shivering. An increased metabolic rate occurs. Hypothermia leads to increased blood viscosity, slows blood through the capillaries, and facilitates blood coagulation.

Hypothermia is associated with drowning episodes, because body heat is lost quickly in water, as compared with air. Other causes of hypothermia include prolonged exposure to cold environments, ingestion of alcohol or barbiturates, trauma or a brain disorder that interferes with temperature regulation, and overwhelming sepsis.

Clinical Manifestations

Symptoms of hypothermia are associated with severity.

- Mild hypothermia (32°C to 35°C) signs include fatigue, slurred speech, poor coordination, confusion, poor judgment and inappropriate behavior, shivering, and muscle stiffness. Exposed skin may be pale or bluish. Tachycardia and peripheral vasoconstriction maintain the cardiac output and blood pressure. Tachypnea with increased secretions and bronchospasm are also present. The kidneys respond with increased urine production.
- Moderate hypothermia (29°C to 32°C) signs include depressed respirations, bradycardia, low blood pressure, pale or cyanotic color, shivering, and dilated pupils. Lethargy, mental

impairment, irrational thinking, hallucinations, and coma develop as the central nervous system becomes depressed. Atrial and ventricular arrhythmias may occur. As the child becomes colder, the gag and cough reflexes are lost, breathing is hard to detect, shivering stops, and muscle rigidity occurs.
- Profound hypothermia (body temperature below 28°C) is characterized by coma, dilated and unresponsive pupils, apnea, no shivering, reduced cardiac output and blood pressure, ventricular fibrillation, and asystole. It may be impossible to distinguish between severe hypothermia and death.

Collaborative Care

Diagnostic testing involves measuring the core body temperature using a rectal probe inserted about 15 cm.

Clinical therapy focuses on resuscitation, if necessary, and gradual core body rewarming. If the child was immersed or submerged in water, remove the wet clothing and wrap the child in a blanket. The child who has profound hypothermia should receive CPR until the body temperature returns to normal because the hypothermia may have preserved vital organs. Volume expanders are needed to promote cardiac output. Aggressive techniques for rewarming in the emergency department include humidified, warm oxygen; warmed intravenous fluids; and warm packs to the core circulation areas (axillae, groin, and posterior neck). Peritoneal lavage or hemodialysis (and in some cases extracorporeal membranous oxygenation) may be used for profound hypothermia. Hypoglycemia is a common complication and should be treated with IV glucose.

For mild hypothermia (temperature above 35°C [95°F]), external heat lamps, immersion in warm water, and an electric blanket may be all that are necessary.

If a child becomes hypothermic during an outing such as a camping trip, a warm person should get into a sleeping bag (or under the blankets) next to the child. This action will warm the child and prevent further heat loss.

Nursing Management

Prevention of hypothermia is an important nursing education role. Educate parents to properly dress the child for cold weather by layering, and putting on a warm hat, gloves, socks, and insulated boots. Parents and adolescents should learn to recognize signs of hypothermia, decrease time of exposure to cold, and be aware of actions to take for mild hypothermia. Teach school-age children and adolescents who go on camping and hunting trips how to recognize and manage hypothermia in themselves and others. First aid for hypothermia includes moving the child to a dry area and removing any wet clothing. Replace with warm, dry clothing, and encourage the child to drink a warm, high-calorie liquid, if able. Teach all children and adolescents not to ride a snowmobile or walk on ice that is not known to be thick enough to support the weight.

The child with moderate or profound hypothermia will be treated in the emergency department and critical care unit as efforts are made to stabilize the child's temperature and manage potential complications. Monitor vital signs, including the core body temperature, and urine output during rewarming. Avoid excessive manipulation and stress on the child as arrhythmias can be triggered. Care must be taken in administering medications that may not be metabolized during the rewarming period. Once the circulation is reestablished, potential toxicity is possible if extra medication doses were administered during resuscitation.

Frostbite

Frostbite is a cold injury that results from the overexposure of skin cells, which have high concentrations of water, to temperatures low enough to cause crystal formation. Frostbite develops in tissues exposed to temperatures below freezing for more than 1 hour when environmental protection is inadequate. Wind velocity, altitude, wetness of tissue, the child's vascular status, and previous exposure to cold injury are factors in the severity of the cold injury. Areas of the body at high risk for frostbite include the hands, feet, cheeks, nose, and ears. Ice crystallizes in the tissues, resulting in cellular dehydration and ischemic damage.

With cold exposure, the skin initially responds with vasoconstriction and lost sensation. As ice crystals develop in the extracellular fluid, water moves out of and dehydrates the cells. When the cold injury progresses, circulation to the area is impaired, and cell death results from ischemia. Vascular stasis leads to thrombosis. In severe cases, gangrene may develop (Nicol & Huether, 2010b).

Clinical manifestations depend on the severity and depth of the cellular damage (Nicol & Huether, 2010b):

- **Superficial skin affected.** Numb, central white area surrounded by redness and edema, no blistering.
- **Full-thickness skin affected.** Erythema, vesicle formation with clear or pink fluid, surrounded by edema and redness.
- **Full-thickness and subcutaneous skin affected.** Local edema, grayish blue color, hemorrhagic vesicles, tissue necrosis.
- **Deeper cold injury.** Deep cyanosis, no vesicles or local edema, necrosis of subcutaneous tissue or lower, possibly involving the muscles and tendons. Gangrene develops.

With superficial injury, the skin at first appears pale and is numb. Rapid rewarming causes a flush and the sensation of tingling, burning, or prickling in the affected area. With deeper injury, the skin may appear mottled and cyanotic followed by erythema, swelling, and burning pain with rewarming. Vesicles and bullae develop in 24 to 48 hours, which slowly heal. The extent of injury is not initially apparent.

If frostbite is suspected, get the child to a warmer environment for rewarming and remove any wet clothes. Because the frostbitten area is numb, extreme caution is needed to protect it from any trauma. Do not rub or massage the area. Slowly rewarm the affected area to decrease the risk of cellular damage. Immerse the affected part in water warmed to between 40°C and 42°C (104°F and 107.6°F) until it is thawed. Analgesics are needed because thawing causes severe pain. Gently clean the affected skin with saline. Cover the exposed skin with sterile dressings and elevate the affected extremity. As the extent of the cold injury is gradually revealed, the ruptured vesicles and eschar are debrided. Wound care may be similar to that provided to a child with burns. Physical therapy treatment may be important to improve circulation and maintain function.

Nursing Management

As with hypothermia, the goal of management is prevention. Teach parents to layer children's clothing for warmth and to pack extra blankets and clothing if cold temperatures are expected during outdoor activities. Hats covering the ears and gloves should be worn. Teach adolescents how to avoid frostbite during hunting and other cold weather expeditions. Wet clothing should be changed quickly.

Practice Alert

Frostbite can also occur if a chemical ice pack (such as a freezer pack used in coolers) is left in contact with the skin for an extended period. Avoid using these chemical ice packs with children if possible. When one is used, cover it with a few layers of clothing or a towel and monitor the skin under the pack frequently. Remove the chemical ice pack if the skin starts to look white or has decreased sensation. Remove the ice pack periodically to allow the skin to rewarm.

Early care is instrumental in minimizing permanent injury. Severe frostbite will require hospitalization, with fluid management, dressing changes, and careful attention to diet. Provide emotional support to the child and family while they wait to learn the full extent of injury and disability.

Animal Bites

Dog and cat bites account for approximately 1% of all emergency department visits in the United States and about 19% of all bites (Gilchrest, 2008; Oehler, Velez, Mizrachi, et al., 2009). Children ages 5 to 9 years have the highest rate of dog bites (Centers for Disease Control and Prevention, 2009). In many cases the dog is known to the child, and most bites occur in the home or a familiar place. Bites are often associated with the child's inappropriate behavior, such as teasing, rough play, or interfering with feeding or the care of puppies. Other animals that may bite include birds, turtles, and wild animals such as bats, squirrels, and raccoons.

Collaborative Care

Immediate care includes assessment of the location and number of puncture wounds, abrasions, lacerations, and crushing injuries; redness or swelling at entry sites; redness extending from the site (possible cellulitis); and any drainage related to the bite. Examination for damage to nerves, muscles, tendons, and blood vessels is also performed. Dog bites tend to be crushing, rather than clean, sharp lacerations. Cat bites tend to be puncture wounds, 50% of which become infected (American Academy of Pediatrics, 2012, p. 203). Head and neck bites require radiographic examination to rule out any associated injury, such as trauma to the airway or breathing structures or a depressed skull fracture.

Initial treatment includes irrigation of the wound, removal of devitalized tissue, and a clean dressing. Povidone iodine solution (a virucidal agent) may be used to irrigate the wound if rabies exposure is suspected (Michos, 2011). Sedation and pain management may be needed for some children. Puncture wounds may be debrided in the operating room. Prophylactic antibiotics may be prescribed to treat organisms that commonly are found in the mouths of dogs or cats (Oehler et al., 2009).

Small or deep wounds may be closed with adhesive strips rather than suturing because of the potential for infection. Severe bites sometimes require surgical closure or reconstruction. Facial wounds require repair by a plastic surgeon. Wounds over joints should be immobilized and elevated. Children who acquire an abscess or infection (cellulitis, septic arthritis, or osteomyelitis) may be admitted to the hospital for treatment. Bites on the hands are common and may become infected, resulting in limitations in function if not properly treated. Cultures from deep in the wound should be obtained before antibiotics are prescribed for infection.

Dog bites should be reported, and the dog should be confined and observed for 10 days for signs of rabies. Cat bites are also dangerous because cats less often have rabies vaccinations. If the animal develops rabies during that interval, human rabies immune globulin (HRIG) is administered immediately, followed by a rabies vaccine injection on days 3, 7, 14, and 28 following the first injection. There should be no delay in administering HRIG and human diploid cell rabies vaccine (HDCV) to any child bitten by wild animals in which rabies cannot be excluded. See Chapter 22 for a description of rabies treatment.

Nursing Management

If a child sustains an animal bite, a complete and accurate history is essential. Document the extent of injury, circumstances surrounding the attack, present location of the animal, and attempts to assess the animal's health.

Wound care is an important nursing intervention. To decrease infection, the wound should be gently washed with antibacterial soap and water, followed by high-pressure wound irrigation with large quantities of sterile saline or lactated Ringer's solution if not a puncture wound. One method of high-pressure irrigation involves the use of an 18-gauge needle on a 60-mL syringe filled with saline. A clean dressing is applied, and the affected part is elevated to reduce bleeding. Instruct parents about how to care for the wound, the expected healing process, and signs of infection that indicate a need to return for care.

Review the child's immunization record to determine if a tetanus booster is necessary. Refer to Chapter 22 for immunization information.

Children who receive traumatic animal bites often experience significant psychologic trauma, such as posttraumatic stress disorder (Dendle & Looke, 2009). See Chapter 34 for information on posttraumatic stress disorder. They may develop a fear of strange animals and a decreased capacity to enjoy the presence of household pets. Give parents information about the symptoms and potential for posttraumatic stress syndrome following a serious dog bite. Counseling and follow-up may be necessary.

Prevention of animal bites is another important nursing role. See education recommendations in Partnering with Families: Preventing Animal Bites.

Human Bites

Human bites are more common than most people realize. They usually occur in toddlers and young children, and adolescents may also receive human bites in association with an altercation. The majority of bites occur on the upper extremities. The skin may be broken with erythema, an abrasion, bruising, or laceration. Because the mouth harbors many bacteria, infection is fairly common. Assess the risk for hepatitis B and HIV infection. Initial treatment includes irrigating with sterile saline and debridement. Antibiotics may be prescribed to prevent systemic complications. Instruct parents about how to care for the wound. Follow-up is important to watch for infection.

Nursing Management

Educate parents about ways to prevent human bites and the importance of teaching young children appropriate behavior around other children. When these bites occur in a childcare or school setting, inform parents about the human bite so they can discuss potential risks and follow-up with a healthcare provider.

As these children are often cared for at home, teach the parents about the normal healing process, proper wound care, and the signs and symptoms of infection. Assist childcare centers and schools to set up policies related to care of and reporting human bites. Parents should be informed when their child has been bitten by another child, and recommendations for care should be provided.

Insect Bites and Stings

Insect bites and stings occur frequently in children and usually are not a cause for concern. Exceptions include bites or stings by insects that carry parasites or communicable diseases (ticks, mosquitoes), those of venomous nature (spiders), and those that produce an allergic reaction. About 3% of the population are sensitized to Hymenoptera (bees, wasps, fire ants) stings and have a generalized response, but the response is lower in children (Järvinen, 2009). For a discussion of communicable diseases carried by ticks and mosquitoes (e.g., Lyme disease, Rocky Mountain spotted fever, malaria, and West Nile virus), see Chapter 22.

See the Clinical Manifestations table for information about signs, symptoms, and clinical therapy for various insect and spider bites. See Chapter 27 for information on immune reactions and anaphylaxis.

Nursing Management

The goal of nursing care is prevention. Become familiar with the harmful insects in your geographic area so you can identify them and recognize their effects. Children should be taught to avoid spiders

---

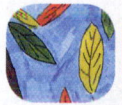

Partnering with Families

Preventing Animal Bites

GENERAL GUIDELINES FOR PETS IN THE HOME
- Never leave a young child alone with an animal.
- Do not buy or adopt a pet unless you are confident of your child's ability to respect it.
- Spay or neuter the pet to reduce aggression.

TEACH CHILDREN THE FOLLOWING RULES
- Avoid all unfamiliar animals and report them to a parent.
- Avoid contact with all wild animals. If an animal (wild or unknown) is sick or acting strangely, notify the health department.

- Do not touch an animal when it is eating, sleeping, or nursing its young.
- Never overexcite an animal, even in play. Do not roughhouse or play games that stimulate aggressive behavior. Do not tease or throw objects at an animal.
- Never put your face close to an animal. Seek permission before hugging or petting an animal.
- If approached by a dog, stay calm, stand still, talk softly, and back away slowly until the dog loses interest; do not run or scream.
- If attacked, pretend to be a tree or a log and protect the face. If knocked down, curl into a ball and protect the face and neck.

TYPE	CLINICAL MANIFESTATION	CLINICAL THERAPY
Mosquitoes and fleas Local inflammation results from sensitization to mosquito salivary proteins. 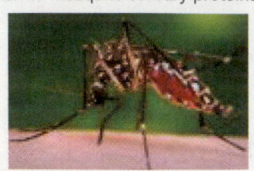	Local reactions: - Discrete, red papules and edema at the bite site with itching; minimal discomfort. - Pruritic wheals and bullae tend to develop with repeat exposure. Rare systemic reactions with generalized urticaria, angioedema, nausea, vomiting, wheezing, and other signs of anaphylaxis.	- Treatment is supportive for local reactions. - Apply cold compresses or ice to the site. - Antihistamine medication may be given. - Systemic reactions need emergency medical treatment.
Bed bugs Local inflammation results from injected saliva, an anesthetic and anticoagulant during feeding. 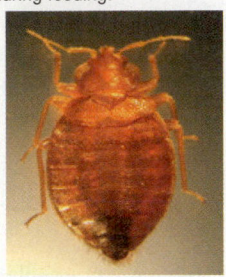 *Photo courtesy of Dr. Harold Harlan, Armed Forces Pest Management Board Image Library.*	- Numerous pruritic papules, often in pattern of three papules. - Child often wakes up with numerous lesions that were not present the night before. - Rare severe allergic reaction.	- Keep skin clean. - Topical corticosteroids may be applied. - Antihistamines may be prescribed. - Oral corticosteroids may be prescribed for severe allergic reaction. - Treat infested areas, and discard infested bedding.

Bee or wasp sting
 	
Hymenoptera
Venoms contain enzymes that affect vascular tone and permeability.
 	
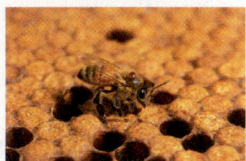
U.S. Department of Agriculture.
	Local reactions:
	- Mild, local pain
	- Erythema and edema
	Systemic reactions:
	- Cutaneous—generalized urticaria, flushing, angioedema, hives, pruritus
	- Respiratory—wheezing, throat tightening, dysphagia, hoarseness, cough
	- Circulatory—dizziness, hypotension, loss of consciousness
	- Gastrointestinal—abdominal pain, vomiting, diarrhea
		- Remove stinger as soon as possible, if present. Scrape the stinger off with a sharp edge and avoid squeezing the venom sac if present.
		- Apply ice or cold compresses and elevate the extremity.
		- Massage a dash of meat tenderizer (papain powder) with a drop of water into the skin for 5 minutes to relieve the pain.
		- Antihistamine medication may be given.
		- For systemic reactions:
		  - Administer glucocorticoids and antihistamines or epinephrine as prescribed.
		  - Have the child carry an epinephrine auto-injector.
		  - Venom immunotherapy is used for severe reactions.

Fire ants Venom is hemolytic and neurotoxic, causing a histamine-like response. 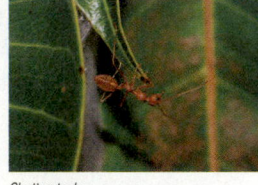 *Shutterstock.*	Local reactions: - A black center at the point of the bite, or a trail of lesions across the skin. - Initial wheal becomes a vesicle in a few hours; in 24 hours the fluid is cloudy and the vesicle has a red halo. - Pruritus, erythema, edema, and induration. - Systemic and anaphylactic reactions can occur.	- Apply ice or cold compresses. - Antihistamine medication may be prescribed. - Elevate the extremity. - Provide the same therapy as for systemic reactions for bee stings.
Black widow spider Venom is neurotoxic. The black widow spider can be recognized by the red and orange hourglass-shape markings on its underside; usually bites in self-defense and avoids light areas. 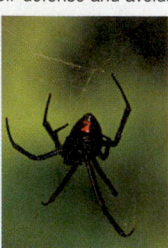 *John Cancalosi/Alamy.*	- Stinging sensation at time of bite - Localized edema and erythema, two fang marks, petechiae branching from site Systemic reaction in 1–3 hours; symptoms peak in 3–12 hours and diminish within 72 hours: - Muscle rigidity of chest and abdomen - Severe muscle cramping, sweating, nausea, vomiting, dizziness, restlessness, insomnia, and diaphoresis - Hypertension and arrhythmias - Oliguria	- Apply ice to site. - Benzodiazepines may be prescribed for muscle spasms. - Opioids may be prescribed for pain management. - Antihistamine medication may be given. - Hydrocortisone may decrease the inflammatory response. - Antivenom IV is used in severe reactions; however, the child should be monitored for an allergic reaction to horse serum.

Clinical Manifestations Insect Bites and Stings (*continued*)

TYPE	CLINICAL MANIFESTATION	CLINICAL THERAPY
Brown recluse spider Venom contains proteolytic enzymes and sphingomyelinase D, a cytotoxic factor. The brown recluse spider is recognized by the fiddle-shape marking on its head; usually not aggressive and bites only when provoked. 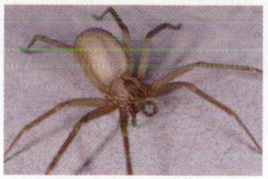 *Reprinted with permission of the University of California, Riverside.*	■ Within 2 hours, sinking blue macule with a halo of inflammation at the bite site; pain. ■ Systemic symptoms include fever, chills, nausea and vomiting, and hemolysis. ■ A hemorrhagic blister forms in 1–2 days with a necrotic ulcer seen when it breaks. Most ulcers are 1–2 cm in diameter, but some progress to 15 cm in diameter with full-thickness injury.	■ Apply ice or cold compresses. ■ Clean the wound and provide good wound care. ■ Analgesics are prescribed for pain management. ■ An oral anti-inflammatory agent may be prescribed. ■ Antibiotics are prescribed for a secondary infection. ■ Excision and skin grafting are performed in cases of severe necrosis.

Source: *Data from Jarvinen, K. M. (2009). Allergic reactions in stinging and biting insects and arachnids. Pediatric Annals, 38(4), 199–209; Holve, S. (2009). Venomous spiders, snakes, and scorpions in the United States. Pediatric Annals, 38(4), 210–217; and Wilson, K. M. (2011). They only come out at night: Bed bugs and their alarming resurgence. Nursing 2011, 41(11), 54–58.*

and other biting or stinging insects. Teach children to stay calm when a bee or wasp approaches and to slowly walk away without swatting.

Many commercial repellents (OFF, Cutter's, Deep Woods OFF) are available. Most products contain DEET (diethyltoluamide), picaridin, or oil of lemon eucalyptus and are effective against many insects including mosquitoes, fleas, ticks, and chiggers. The insect repellent produces a vapor layer that is malodorous and distasteful to insects. However, DEET does not repel stinging insects. The repellent should be reapplied if washed off by sweating or getting wet. Wash DEET off the skin with soap and water once the child is back indoors. Caution parents to avoid overuse of products containing DEET, especially with infants and small children. Do not apply it to young children's hands, as they may rub it into the eyes and mouth.

Warn parents against using heavily perfumed shampoos, powders, soaps, or lotions, or dressing children in bright-colored or floral-print clothing when outdoors, as these may attract insects. Light-colored and smooth-textured clothing is less attractive to bees and wasps. Long sleeves and pants, and wearing shoes rather than sandals, reduce the risk for stings and bites. Wear gloves for working in the garden and around shrubs.

Avoid eating sweet foods and beverages outdoors as these will attract bees and wasps. Bees and wasps may crawl into a canned beverage and not be seen. Pour beverages into a cup rather than drinking them from the can to prevent stings to the mouth and lips.

Household pets may be a source of fleas or ticks. Encourage frequent inspection of pets and preventive treatments against fleas and ticks before pets are allowed prolonged contact with children. See the Clinical Manifestations table for interventions appropriate for the treatment of local reactions. See Complementary Therapy: Garlic.

Complementary Therapy Garlic

Garlic is a plant that has a long history as a therapeutic agent for many health problems, such as insect bites, parasites, fatigue, and respiratory complaints. Chemical burns are a potential adverse effect when raw garlic is crushed and applied to the skin to treat insect bites, especially if the skin is sensitive.

When a systemic reaction to Hymenoptera has occurred, the child should wear a medical alert identification and carry an emergency kit with epinephrine (EpiPen). See Chapter 27 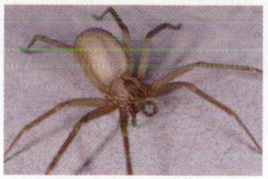. Educate parents to monitor the expiration date and check the medication weekly for discoloration or a precipitate, indicating a need for replacement. Teach the child and parents how to administer the epinephrine. Make sure the school nurse receives the written order for the epinephrine injector so it can be administered if necessary. If the epinephrine is administered, call 911 for emergency transport for the child as the epinephrine's effectiveness lasts only about 20 minutes. Desensitization injections may be given to children with an anaphylactic reaction or severe systemic reaction.

Snakebites

Venomous snakes are found in most areas of the country. During warm months of the year, snakes are active and likely to bite if disturbed. Fortunately many bites are dry, delivering no venom. A cell phone photo of the snake is useful in identifying whether the snake is venomous.

Rattlesnake, copperhead, and cottonmouth venom is composed of proteolytic enzymes, glycoproteins, and vasoactive substances that are hemotoxic and neurotoxic, and cause other systemic symptoms. Coral snake venom causes neuromuscular paralysis (Holve, 2009). The amount and toxicity of the venom injected have an impact on the consequences of the snakebite. Because children usually receive a higher amount of venom relative to body mass, their response may be greater than that of an adult.

Puncture marks, white wheal, and burning sensation appear at the site of the bite. If the bite is dry, minimal swelling and signs will develop. With envenomation, pain, erythema, petechiae, bruising, and edema rapidly develop and extend from the site for up to 24 hours. The swelling may progress without treatment to involve the entire extremity. Swelling may put the child at risk for compartment syndrome. Systemic signs include dizziness, tachycardia, nausea, vomiting, diarrhea, diaphoresis, chills, and muscle fasciculation. A severe response may include hypotension, altered consciousness, bleeding from multiple sites (disseminated intravascular coagulation), pulmonary edema, and renal failure. Bites from the coral snake are accompanied by numbness and mild soft tissue swelling. Neurologic signs include diplopia and ptosis, difficulty speaking and swallowing, hypersalivation, and altered mental status (lethargy, drowsiness, or euphoria). If untreated, signs progress to pharyngeal spasm, cyanosis, hypotension, and tachycardia, heralding the onset of respiratory failure.

Collaborative Care

Clinical therapy involves immobilization of the extremity and a cold compress to slow the spread of the venom. Laboratory studies include complete blood count, platelet count, coagulation studies, electrolytes, creatine phosphokinase, and renal function. The poison control center is contacted to provide guidelines for treatment. Specific antivenom is usually administered within 4 to 6 hours. CroFab, a newer antivenom used for cottonmouth, copperhead, and rattlesnake bites, is available and has a lower rate of severe hypersensitivity reactions than antivenoms made from horse serum (Holve, 2009). Children at risk for a severe hypersensitivity reaction are pretreated with IV antihistamines and corticosteroids (Holve, 2009). Children receiving CroFab must be monitored for thrombocytopenia and bleeding related to the development of coagulopathy 2 to 14 days after envenomation (Smollin, 2010). The use of NSAIDs is avoided because of coagulopathies (Reuter-Rice, 2008). Acetaminophen and codeine may be prescribed for pain management. The child's immunization record is reviewed to determine if a tetanus toxoid booster is needed. Antibiotics are not administered unless an infection develops.

Practice Alert

First aid for a snakebite no longer involves a tourniquet or excision of the bite. Instead, remove constrictive clothing and jewelry, minimize movement of the injured extremity, and keep it below the level of the heart. Keep the child calm to slow the spread of the venom. Call 911 or transport the child to the nearest medical facility (Kumar, Kimura, & Kamat, 2009).

Nursing Management

Nursing care involves assessing the child for initial and progressive signs of the venom's effect. Monitor the child's vital signs and the distal extremity's neurovascular status. Manage the child's pain. Measure, mark, and record the circumference of the affected extremity above and below the site, and reassess every 15 to 30 minutes to monitor the progression of edema. Clean the wound with germicidal soap and water. Keep the child quiet and calm to slow the circulation. If a photo is unavailable, help the child identify the snake from pictures of snakes common to the area; however, keep in mind that other venomous snakes may be kept as exotic pets.

The antivenom is diluted in saline and slowly administered intravenously as ordered. Help locate additional antivenom if the hospital does not have an adequate supply. Carefully and frequently monitor the child for progressive signs of venom effect and for antivenom hypersensitivity. Provide skin care for the swollen and tense skin to prevent abrasions and additional injury. Monitor the site for necrosis and secondary infection. Provide emotional support to the child and family.

As children with bites are often cared for at home after the emergency management, teach the parents about the normal healing process, proper wound care, and the signs and symptoms of infection. Teach children and their families how to avoid future snakebites. When in areas where snakes may live, the child should wear protective clothing such as leather boots, avoid reaching into areas where snakes may hide, and avoid any actions that may provoke a snake.

Scorpion Bites

Scorpions are an arthropod with a stinger on the tail. One species of scorpion, found in the Southwest, is potentially dangerous to humans. Scorpions are not aggressive, and they sting in self-defense. Stings cause intense pain that worsens with light pressure on the sting site. Swelling, redness, itching, and burning are common. Neurologic signs may include neuromuscular excitation, paresthesias, tachycardia, and hypertension. Pain usually resolves in 4 hours and symptoms resolve in 24 hours. Stings rarely result in death, except in small children who may experience respiratory failure.

No diagnostic procedures are performed. Efforts to capture the scorpion for identification should be attempted. Treatment involves supportive measures such as intravenous access, oxygen, pulse oximetry, and cardiac monitoring. Sedation may be required for neuromuscular symptoms. Narcotics are not used as they may worsen the neurotoxicity. Antivenom is available for some species and is sometimes used.

Nursing Management

Nursing care involves supportive care during the day after the bite. Carefully monitor vital signs, oxygen saturation, and cardiac rhythm. Clean the sting site with warm soap and water. Apply ice to the sting site and keep the extremity elevated. Monitor intake and output. If antivenom is used, provide care as described for snakebite antivenom. Provide reassurance to the child and family that the pain and reaction will be gone within 24 hours.

MINOR SKIN INJURIES
Contusions

Contusions are soft tissue injuries that result from a variety of causes. Often it is difficult to assess whether an injury has caused underlying tissue damage. An injury does not have to break the skin to result in internal damage. Radiographic examination may be necessary to rule out broken bones or further tissue damage. Signs and symptoms that indicate a need for treatment include swelling that does not subside within 72 hours, intense pain, inability to move the injured part, and infection. Elevate the injured extremity and apply ice as soon as possible after injury to reduce inflammation and swelling in the area.

Foreign Bodies

Many skin injuries result from penetration of foreign particles. Common substances include gravel in abrasions, bee stingers, and splinters. Treatment of a superficial foreign body involves irrigating the wound to try to forcibly dislodge the debris. A deeply embedded foreign body is best removed under medical supervision to avoid permanent injury or scarring.

Lacerations

Lacerations are caused by cuts or tears to the skin. In many cases the cut is minor and can be managed at home with gentle cleansing, antibiotic ointment, and a bandage. More extensive lacerations, and those on the face or over joints, often need closing to promote healing and reduce scarring. Laceration repair is performed after wound cleansing and appropriate local analgesia to control pain. Sutures or dermal adhesive may be used. Sutures are usually removed about 7 days later.

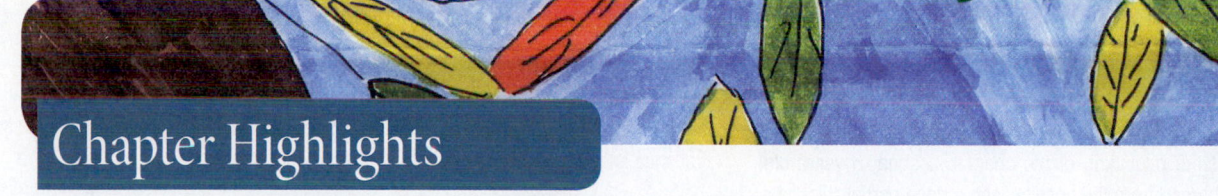

Chapter Highlights

- Functions of the skin include perception of pain, heat, and cold; serving as a protective barrier against microorganisms, ultraviolet radiation, and loss of body fluids; temperature regulation; vitamin D synthesis; and excretion.

- Wound healing has three overlapping phases: inflammation, proliferation (reconstruction), and remodeling (maturation).

- Contact dermatitis is an inflammation of the skin that occurs in response to direct contact with either an allergen, causing an immune response, or an irritant, resulting in no immune response.

- Superabsorbent disposable diapers reduce the frequency and severity of diaper dermatitis because, when wet, a gel forms inside the diaper keeping moisture from contacting the skin. The skin stays drier than when cloth diapers are used.

- Seborrheic dermatitis is an inflammatory skin condition due to an overgrowth of *Malassezia furfur* yeast in areas of sebaceous gland activity. It is commonly found on the scalp, forehead, and postauricular and periorbital areas.

- The classic impetigo lesion begins as a vesicle surrounded by edema and redness. The vesicle fluid turns cloudy and ruptures, leaving a honey-colored crust on an ulcerated base.

- Folliculitis, a superficial inflammation of the pilosebaceous follicle, may be associated with *Pseudomonas* exposure in a poorly chlorinated pool or hot tub.

- Children with cellulitis appear ill with fever, chills, malaise, and enlarged lymph nodes. The infected site is red or lilac in color, warm, edematous, and tender. The lesion border is often indistinct.

- Viral skin infections include molluscum contagiosum and warts (papillomavirus).

- Oral thrush (candidiasis) is characterized by white patches that resemble coagulated milk on the oral mucosa and may bleed when removed.

- Treatment for tinea capitis involves griseofulvin orally for 8 to 12 weeks, or for 2 to 4 weeks after symptoms disappear. Children being treated may develop an "id" hypersensitivity reaction rash to the fungal antigen, not an allergic reaction to the medication.

- Treatment of atopic dermatitis involves hydration and lubrication of the skin by bathing followed by emollients to trap in skin moisture. Topical corticosteroids are used to treat flares and then tapered and stopped.

- Psoriasis is a T-cell-mediated autoimmune disease that causes pruritic, thick, silvery, scaly erythematous plaques with irregular borders surrounded by normal skin.

- Acne medications, tretinoin or isotretinoin, are phototoxic, resulting in sunburn with even minimal exposure. Protection with sunscreen and protective clothing is important to prevent significant sunburn.

- Epidermolysis bullosa is a rare and severe chronic blistering skin disorder that is associated with minor trauma, friction, or heat to the skin.

- Drug reactions vary in severity from a simple allergic reaction and erythema multiforme minor to drug hypersensitivity reaction to potential life-threatening responses such as erythema multiforme major (Stevens-Johnson syndrome and toxic epidermal necrolysis).

- Treatment for lice includes a pediculicide applied to the hair, and combing the hair with a fine-tooth comb to remove all the nits. A second treatment is needed in 7 days to treat lice emerging from eggs.

- Scabies is an infestation caused by direct contact in which the female mite burrows under the skin to lay eggs. The eggs, feces, and debris left behind cause irritation and intense itching. Often the child's scratching and secondary infection result in lesions with no distinct appearance.

- Birthmarks or skin lesions that can indicate an underlying condition include a port-wine stain (Sturge-Weber syndrome) and café-au-lait spots (neurofibromatosis).

- Hemangiomas undergo a period of rapid growth during infancy before involuting. The rapid growth may cause significant complications, such as pressure on the airway, eye, or ear canal if near those body areas.

- Children at greatest risk for pressure ulcers are those with limited mobility, sensory deficits, or the inability to change positions. Tissue ischemia occurs when the soft tissues and capillary beds are compressed between a bony prominence and another surface.

- Of the four main types of burns (thermal, chemical, electrical, and radioactive), thermal burns are most common in children. Infants, toddlers, and preschool-age children most commonly suffer scald burns. Other types of thermal burns include flames and contact with a hot object.

- Initial treatment for a child with a significant burn injury includes emergency assessment of the airway, breathing, and circulation; and stopping the burning process by removing jewelry and clothing, and applying moist soaks or ice.

- More than half of a person's lifetime exposure to the sun occurs before 20 years of age. Repeated blistering sunburns during childhood increase the risk for development of malignant melanoma in adolescence and early adulthood.

- Children are at greater risk for hypothermia because of their thinner skin, limited subcutaneous fat, and high surface area to body mass ratio. Body heat is lost more quickly in water or when clothing is wet.

- Frostbite occurs when ice crystallizes in the tissues, causing cellular dehydration and ischemic damage.

- Children at highest risk for dog bites are those 5 to 9 years old. Most children know the dog that bites them, and most bites are associated with the child's inappropriate behavior, such as teasing, rough play, or interfering with feeding or the dog's care of puppies.

- Insects and spiders with venomous bites include bees, fire ants, black widow spiders, and brown recluse spiders.

- Venomous snakes living in the wild in the United States include rattlesnakes, copperheads, water moccasins, and coral snakes. Initial treatment includes immobilization of the extremity and cold compresses to slow the spread of the venom.

- Minor skin injuries that may need clinical therapy include contusions, foreign bodies, and lacerations.

Clinical Reasoning in Action

INTRODUCTION

Return to the scenario at the beginning of the chapter. Joshua, 6 years old, was admitted to and discharged from the hospital with a deep partial-thickness burn caused by flames associated with playing with matches. He is making his second visit to the burn clinic for a burn dressing change 5 days after discharge. He will continue visits to the burn clinic twice a week until the burn is healed.

DESCRIPTION

Because no debridement is expected on this visit, he will not go to the sedation suite. Joshua is given pain medication in the burn clinic to help cover the discomfort of the burn dressing change. He is anxious about the dressing change and worries that it will hurt. Joshua's burn is showing granulation tissue and no signs of infection at this visit. It is now possible to determine that skin grafting will not be needed.

Finding activities to keep Joshua occupied is already becoming a challenge to his mother. She is concerned about how to keep Joshua occupied now that he is feeling better. She and Joshua's father are worried about how they will prevent future injuries since Joshua is so energetic and curious. Joshua's mother has had no difficulty identifying high-calorie foods for him to eat, but she is not sure if Joshua is getting enough extra protein to promote the wound healing.

DISCUSSION

1. What are potential appropriate pain medications to give Joshua for a dressing change? How far in advance of the dressing change should the pain medication be administered?

2. Describe complementary interventions that could further reduce Joshua's pain and anxiety.

3. What are signs of wound infection that you must observe for?

4. What nursing support may help Joshua deal with a painful and disfiguring injury?

5. Discuss injury prevention strategies that the family can implement to protect Joshua from future injuries.

6. What are some foods or strategies that Joshua's mother can use at home to provide the high-protein and high-calorie diet needed for healing?

NCLEX-RN® Review

1. When assessing the history of a child recently diagnosed with atopic dermatitis, which question is important to ask the parents?
   1. "Does your child have any allergies to foods or other substances?"
   2. "Has your child ever had these symptoms before?"
   3. "Has your child had any cystic lesions?"
   4. "Are your child's immunizations up to date?"

2. The nurse is planning care for a 3-month-old infant with eczema. Which intervention will take the highest priority?
   1. Maintaining adequate hydration
   2. Keeping the baby content
   3. Preventing infection of lesions
   4. Applying antibiotics to lesions

3. In order to increase compliance with the acne treatment regimen for a teenager, the nurse should include what information in the education plan?
   1. Teenagers must be responsible for their own treatment and must be trusted to follow through and be compliant.
   2. It often takes up to 12 weeks to see an improvement and a response to treatment.
   3. Apply sunscreen every morning and anti-acne medication every night.
   4. Teach parents to praise the good habits of their teenager.

4. A 6-year-old child is having burn care following premedication for pain. The child is not cooperative for dressing changes and begins screaming and kicking. What is the best action by the nurse?
   1. Inform the child that cooperation is necessary for proper healing and will shorten the hospital stay.
   2. Allow the parents to change the dressings with coaching from the nurse.
   3. Allow the child to participate in the dressing change process as much as possible.
   4. Inform the child that restraints will be used if there is no cooperation.

See Appendix I ⬚ *for answers.*

References

American Academy of Pediatrics, Committee on Infectious Disease. (2012). *Red book: 2012 report of the Committee on Infectious Disease* (29th ed.). Elk Grove Village, IL: Author.

American College of Surgeons Committee on Trauma. (2012). *Advanced trauma life support* (9th ed). Chicago, IL: Author.

Arbuckle, H. A. (2010). Epidermolysis bullosa care in the United States. *Dermatology Clinics, 28,* 387–389.

Bard, S., Torchia, D., & Schachner, L. A. (2010). Managing pediatric patients with psoriasis. *American Journal of Clinical Dermatology, 11*(Suppl. 1), 15–17.

Bell, E. A. (2008). An update on sunscreen. *Infectious Diseases in Children, 21*(6), 14–15.

Berk, D. R., & Bayliss, S. J. (2010). MRSA, staphylococcal scalded skin syndrome, and other cutaneous bacterial emergencies. *Pediatric Annals, 39*(10), 627–633.

Berwick, M., Erdei, E., & Hay, J. (2009). Melanoma epidemiology and public health. *Dermatology Clinics, 27,* 205–214.

Black, J. S., & Wilson, B. (2009). Neurofibromatosis type 1. *Consultant for Pediatricians, 8*(12), 433.

Boelman, D. J. (2010). Treating poison ivy, oak, and sumac. *American Journal of Nursing, 110*(6), 49–52.

Bookout, K. (2008). Wound care product primer for the nurse practitioner: Part 1. *Journal of Pediatric Health Care, 22*(1), 60–63.

Brown, T. S., Safford, S., Caramanica, J., & Elster, E. A. (2010). Biomarker use in tailored combat casualty care. *Biomarkers Medicine, 4*(3), 465–473.

Burn Foundation. (2010). Safety facts on scald burns. Retrieved from http://burnfoundation.org/programs/resource.cfm?c=18a=3

Butler, C. T. (2006). Pediatric skin care: Guidelines for assessment, prevention, and treatment. *Pediatric Nursing, 32*(5), 443–450.

Caubet, J. C., & Eigenmann, P. A. (2010). Allergic triggers in atopic dermatitis. *Immunology and Allergy Clinics of North America, 30*, 289–307.

Centers for Disease Control and Prevention. (2009). *Dog bite prevention.* Retrieved from http://www.cdc.gov/HomeandRecreationalSafety/Dog-Bites/biteprevention.html

Chosidow, O., Giraudeau, B., Cottrell, J., Izri, A., Hofmann, R., Mann, S. G., & Burgess, I. (2010). Oral ivermectin versus malathion lotion for difficult-to-treat head lice. *New England Journal of Medicine, 362*(10), 896–905.

Clayton, L. A., & Tom, W. L. (2010). Individualizing treatment for adolescent acne to achieve optimal outcomes. *Journal of Pediatric Health Care, 24*(2), 127–132.

Connor-Ballard, P. A. (2009). Understanding and managing burn pain: Part 1. *American Journal of Nursing, 109*(4), 48–56.

Dendle, C., & Looke, D. (2009). Management of mammalian bites. *Australian Family Physician, 38*(11), 868–874.

Diamantis, S. A., Morrell, D. S., & Burkhart, C. N. (2009). Pediatric infestations. *Pediatric Annals, 38*(9), 326–332.

D'Souza, A. L., Nelson, N. G., & McKenzie, L. B. (2009). Pediatric burn injuries treated in US emergency departments between 1990 and 2006. *Pediatrics, 124*(5), 1424–1430.

Epps, R. (2010). Atopic dermatitis and ichthyosis. *Pediatrics in Review, 31*(7), 278–285.

Findlay, J. (2007). Treating atopic dermatitis. *Contemporary Pediatrics, 24*(Suppl. 6), 4–12.

Frankowski, B. L., Bocchini, J. A., & the Council on School Health and Committee on Infectious Disease. (2010). Clinical report—Head lice. *Pediatrics, 126*(2), 392–403.

Friedman, B., Berdahl, T., Simpson, L. A., McCormick, M. C., Owens, P. L., Andrews, R., & Romano, P. S. (2011). Annual report on health care for children and youth in the United States: Focus on trends in hospital use and quality. *Academic Pediatrics, 11*(4), 263–279.

Gauglitz, G. G., Herndon, D. N., & Jeschke, M. G. (2008). Emergency treatment of severely burned pediatric patients: Current therapeutic strategies. *Pediatric Health, 2*(6), 761–775.

Gilchrest, J. (2008). Dog bites: Still a problem? *Injury Prevention, 14*(5), 296–301.

Gonzalez, M. E., Unwala, R., & Connelly, E. A. (2008). A red scaly baby. *Contemporary Pediatrics, 25*(6), 28–33.

Groff, B. M., Tromberg, J. S., & Wilson, B. B. (2009). Adolescent acne: Effective therapy for a serious condition. *Consultant for Pediatricians, 8*(6, suppl.), S5–S14.

Habif, T. P. (2010). *Clinical Dermatology: A Color Guide to Diagnosis and Therapy,* (5th ed, pp. 217–247), Philadelphia, PA: Elsevier Mosby.

Hanson, D., Thompson, P. A., Langemo, D., Hunter, S., Tinkler, J., & Anderson, J. W. (2008). What you should know about psoriasis. *Nursing, 38*(6), 58–59.

Hazinski, M. F., Mondozzi, M. A., & Baker, R. A. U. (2010). Shock, multiple organ dysfunction syndrome, and burns in children. In K. L. McCance, S. E. Huether, V. L. Brashers, & N. S. Rote, *Pathophysiology: The biologic basis for disease in adults and children* (6th ed., pp. 1727–1754). St. Louis, MO: Elsevier Mosby.

Hinckley, J., & Allen, P. J. (2008). Community-associated MRSA in the pediatric primary care setting. *Pediatric Nursing, 34*(1), 64–71.

Hogeling, M., Adams, S., & Wargon, O. (2011). A randomized controlled trial of propranolol for infantile hemangiomas. *Pediatrics, 128*(2), e259–e266.

Holland, K. E., & Drolet, B. A. (2010). Infantile hemangioma. *Pediatric Clinics of North America, 57*, 1069–1083.

Holve, S. (2009). Venomous spiders, snakes, and scorpions in the United States. *Pediatric Annals, 38*(4), 210–217.

Huang, J. T., Abrams, M., Tlougan, B., Rademaker, A., & Paller, A. S. (2009). Treatment of *Staphylococcus aureus* colonization in atopic dermatitis decreases disease severity. *Pediatrics, 123*(5), e808–e814.

Huang, J. T., & Liang, M. G. (2010). Vascular malformations. *Pediatric Clinics of North America, 57*, 1091–1110.

Järvinen, K. M. (2009). Allergic reactions in stinging and biting insects and arachnids. *Pediatric Annals, 38*(4), 199–209.

Juhas, E., & Gehris, R. P. (2010). Drug eruptions: The benign—and the life threatening. *Consultant for Pediatricians, 9*(Suppl. 6), S2–S9.

Koshy, J. C., Sharabi, S. E., Jerkins, D., Cox, J., Cronin, S. P., & Hollier, L. H. (2010). Sunscreens: Evolving aspects of sun protection. *Journal of Pediatric Health Care, 24*(5), 343–346.

Kottner, J., Hauss, A., Schlüer, A. B., & Dassen, T. (2011). Validation and clinical impact of paediatric pressure ulcer risk assessment scales: A systematic review. *International Journal of Nursing Studies.* doi:10.1016/j.ijnurstu.2011.04.014.

Krakowski, A. C. (2011). Teenage girl, young boy present with edema, erythema and bullae in bizarre streaking pattern. *Infectious Diseases in Children, 24*(9), 24–25.

Kumar, J., Kimura, L., & Kamat, R. (2009). Snakebite envenomation. *Consultant for Pediatricians, 8*(9), 340–343.

Land, V., & Small, L. (2008). The evidence on how to best treat sunburn in children: A common treatment dilemma. *Pediatric Nursing, 34*(4), 343–348.

Leung, A. K. C. (2011). Port-wine stain versus salmon patch: How to tell the difference. *Consultant for Pediatricians, 10*(2), 33.

Liu, C., Bayer, A., Cosgrove, S. E., Daum, R. S., Fridkin, S. M., Gorwitz, R. J., . . . Chambers, H. F. (2011). Clinical practice guidelines by the Infectious Diseases Society of America for the treatment of methicillin-resistant *Staphylococcus aureus* infections in adults and children. *Clinical Infectious Diseases, 52*(1), 1–38.

Lund, C. H., & Kuller, J. M. (2007). Integumentary system. In C. Kenner & J. W. Lott, *Comprehensive neonatal care: An interdisciplinary approach* (4th ed., pp. 65–91). Philadelphia, PA: Saunders Elsevier.

Mahindra, P., Guillen, C., & Glick, S. A. (2009). A 5-year old girl with scarring. *Pediatric Annals, 38*(7), 359–364.

Mathes, E. F. D., & Frieden, I. J. (2010). Treatment of molluscum contagiosum with cantharidin: A practical approach. *Pediatric Annals, 39*(3), 124–130.

Meadows-Oliver, M. (2009). Tinea capitis: Diagnostic criteria and treatment options. *Pediatric Nursing, 35*(1), 53–57.

Merritt, B., Burkhart, C. N., & Morrell, D. S. (2009). Use of isotretinoin for acne vulgaris. *Pediatric Annals, 28*(6), 311–320.

Metry, D. W., Siegel, D. H., Cordisco, M. R., Pope, E., Prendiville, J., Drolet, B. A., . . . Frieden, I. J. (2008). A comparison of disease severity among affected male versus female patients with PHACE syndrome. *Journal of the American Academy of Dermatology, 58*(1), 81–87.

Michos, Z. (2011). Bats and rabies. *Contemporary Pediatrics, 28*(10), 46–55.

Montoya, C. (2008). Diaper dermatitis: Smart and effective management. *American Journal for Nurse Practitioners, 12*(9), 11–20.

Morelli, J. G. (2011a). Cutaneous bacterial infections. In R. M. Kliegman, B. F. Stanton, J. W. St. Geme, N. F. Schor, & R. E. Behrman, *Nelson textbook of pediatrics* (19th ed., pp. 2299–2308). Philadelphia, PA: Elsevier Saunders.

Morelli, J. G. (2011b). Cutaneous fungal infections. In R. M. Kliegman, B. F. Stanton, J. W. St. Geme, N. F. Schor, & R. E. Behrman, *Nelson textbook of pediatrics* (19th ed., pp. 2309–2314). Philadelphia, PA: Elsevier Saunders.

Morelli, J. G. (2011c). Cutaneous viral infections. In R. M. Kliegman, B. F. Stanton, J. W. St. Geme, N. F. Schor, & R. E. Behrman, *Nelson textbook of pediatrics* (19th ed., pp. 2315–2317). Philadelphia, PA: Elsevier Saunders.

Morelli, J. G. (2011d). Acne. In R. M. Kliegman, B. F. Stanton, J. W. St. Geme, N. F. Schor, & R. E. Behrman, *Nelson textbook of pediatrics* (19th ed., pp. 2322–2328). Philadelphia, PA: Elsevier Saunders.

Morelli, J. G. (2011e). Vesiculobullous disorders. In R. M. Kliegman, B. F. Stanton, J. W. St. Geme, N. F. Schor, & R. E. Behrman, *Nelson textbook of pediatrics* (19th ed., pp. 2241–2249). St. Louis, MO: Elsevier Mosby.

Morelli, J. G. (2011f). Arthropod bites and infestations. In R. M. Kliegman, B. F. Stanton, J. W. St. Geme, N. F. Schor, & R. E. Behrman, *Nelson textbook of pediatrics* (19th ed., pp. 2317–2322). St. Louis, MO: Elsevier Mosby.

Morelli, J. G. (2011g). Cutaneous nevi. In R. M. Kliegman, B. F. Stanton, J. W. St. Geme, N. F. Schor, & R. E. Behrman, *Nelson textbook of pediatrics* (19th ed., pp. 2231–2236). St. Louis, MO: Elsevier Mosby.

Morelli, J. G. (2011h). Vascular disorders. In R. M. Kliegman, B. F. Stanton, J. W. St. Geme, N. F. Schor, & R. E. Behrman, *Nelson textbook of pediatrics* (19th ed., pp. 2223–2231). St. Louis, MO: Elsevier Mosby.

Morelli, V., Calmet, E., & Jhingade, V. (2010). Alternative therapies for common dermatologic disorders: Part 2. *Primary Care Clinics in Office Practice, 37*, 285–296.

Muhrer, J. C. (2009). Melanoma: Current incidence, diagnosis, and preventive strategies. *Journal for Nurse Practitioners, 5*(1), 35–46.

Mukherjee, S. K. (2011). Streptococcal infection as a trigger for psoriasis. *Contemporary Pediatrics, 28*(3), 27–36.

Mukherjee, S., Coha, T., & Torres, Z. (2010). Common skin problems in children with special health care needs. *Pediatric Annals, 39*(4), 206–215.

National Center for Complementary and Alternative Medicine. (2011). *Aloe vera*. Retrieved from http://nccam.nih.gov/health/aloevera/

National Center for Health Statistics, National Vital Statistics System. (2011). *Ten leading causes of injury deaths, United States, 2008, all races, both sexes*. Retrieved from http://webappa.cdc.gov/cgi-bin/broker.exe

Nelson, S. A., & Yiannias, J. A. (2009). Product allergens: Pearls and pitfalls. *Dermatology Clinics, 27*, 329–336.

Neville-Swensen, M., & Clayton, M. (2011). Outpatient management of community-associated methicillin-resistant *Staphylococcus aureus* skin and soft tissue infection. *Journal of Pediatric Health Care, 25*(5), 308–315.

Nicol, N. H., & Huether, S. E. (2010a). Alterations of the integument in children. In K. L. McCance, S. E. Huether, V. L. Brashers, & N. S. Rote, *Pathophysiology: The biologic basis for disease in adults and children* (6th ed., pp. 1680–1695). St. Louis, MO: Elsevier Mosby.

Nicol, N. H., & Huether, S. E. (2010b). Structure, function, and disorders of the integument. In K. L. McCance, S. E. Huether, V. L. Brashers, & N. S. Rote, *Pathophysiology: The biologic basis for disease in adults and children* (6th ed., pp. 1644–1679). St. Louis, MO: Elsevier Mosby.

Nichols, K. M., & Cook-Bolden, F. E. (2009). Allergic skin disease: Major highlights and recent advances. *Medical Clinics of North America, 93*, 1211–1224.

Nijhawan, R. I., Matiz, C., & Jacobs, S. E. (2009). Contact dermatitis: From basics to allergodromes. *Pediatric Annals, 38*(2), 99–108.

O'Connor, N. R., McLaughlin, M. R., & Ham, P. (2008). Newborn skin: Part 1. Common rashes. *American Family Physician, 77*(1), 47–52.

Oehler, R. L., Velez, A. P., Mizrachi, M., Lamarche, J., & Gompf, S. (2009). Bite-related and septic syndromes caused by cats and dogs. *Lancet Infectious Diseases, 9*, 439–447.

Ong, P. Y., & Boguniewicz, M. (2008). Atopic dermatitis. *Primary Care Clinics in Office Practice, 35*, 105–117.

Ong, P. Y., & Leung, D. Y. M. (2010). The infectious aspects of atopic dermatitis. *Immunology and Allergy Clinics of North America, 30*, 309–321.

Orrico, J. A., & Krause-Parello, C. A. (2010). Facts, fiction, and figures of the *Sarcoptes scabiei* infection. *Journal of School Nursing, 26*(4), 260–266.

Poindexter, G. B., Burkhart, C. N., & Morrell, D. S. (2009). Therapies for pediatric seborrheic dermatitis. *Pediatric Annals, 38*(6), 333–338.

Ramanathan, S., & Hebert, A. A. (2011). Management of acne vulgaris. *Journal of Pediatric Health Care, 25*(5), 332–337.

Reuter-Rice, K. (2008). Bites that bleed: Crotalid envenomation. *Journal of Pediatric Health Care, 22*(4), 258–261.

Rizzi, S. C., Upton, Z., Bott, K., & Dargaville, T. R. (2010). Recent advances in dermal wound healing: Biomedical device approaches. *Expert Reviews of Medical Devices, 7*(1), 143–154.

Rote, N. S., & Huether, S. E. (2010). Innate immunity: Inflammation. In K. L. McCance, S. E. Huether, V. L. Brashers, & N. S. Rote, *Pathophysiology: The biologic basis for disease in adults and children* (6th ed., pp. 183–216). St. Louis, MO: Elsevier Mosby.

Schindler, C. A., Mikhailov, T. A., Kuhn, E. M., Christopher, J., Conway, P., Riding, D., . . . Simpson, V. S. (2011). Protecting fragile skin: Nursing interventions to decrease development of pressure ulcers in pediatric intensive care. *American Journal of Critical Care, 20*(1), 26–34.

Schlüer, A. B., Cignacco, E., Müller, M., & Halfes, R. J. (2009). The prevalence of pressure ulcers in four pediatric institutions. *Journal of Clinical Nursing, 18*, 3244–3252.

Shamban, A. T., & Narurkar, V. A. (2009). Multimodal treatment of acne, acne scars, and pigmentation. *Dermatology Clinics, 27*, 459–471.

Shaw, M. G., Burkhart, C. N., & Morrell, D. S. (2009). Systemic therapies for pediatric atopic dermatitis. *American Journal for Nurse Practitioners, 11*(4), 28–35.

Smollin, C. G. (2010). Toxicology: Pearls and pitfalls in the use of antidotes. *Emergency Medical Clinics of North America, 28*, 149–161.

Sprecher, E. (2010). Epidermolysis bullosa simplex. *Dermatology Clinics, 28*, 23–32.

Stier, M. F., Glick, S. A., & Hirsch, R. J. (2008). Laser treatment of pediatric vascular lesions: Port wine stains and hemangiomas. *Journal of American Academy of Dermatology, 58*(2), 261–285.

Treat, J. (2010). Stevens-Johnson syndrome and toxic epidermal necrolysis. *Pediatric Annals, 39*(1), 667–674.

U.S. Department of Health and Human Services. (2011). *Healthy People 2020*. Retrieved from http://healthypeople.gov/2020/topicsobjectives2020/objectiveslist.aspx?topicId=5

U.S. Food and Drug Administration (FDA). (2011). *FDA safety communication: Update on serious complications associated with negative pressure wound therapy systems*. Retrieved from http://www.fda.gov/MedicalDevices/Safety/AlertsandNotices/ucm244211.htm

U.S. Food and Drug Administration Center for Drug Evaluation and Research. (2009). *Ulesfia*. Retrieved from http://www.accessdata.fda.gov/scripts/cder/drugsatfda/index.cfm?fuseaction=Search.DrugDetails

Webster, G. F. (2009). Acne: Tips and tricks for the pediatrician. *Pediatric Annals, 38*(2), 80–83.

Willock, J., Anthony, D., & Richardson, J. (2008). Interrater reliability of the Glamorgan pediatric pressure ulcer risk assessment scale. *Pediatric Nursing, 20*(7), 14–19.

Willock, J., Baharestani, M. M., & Anthony, D. (2009). The development of the Glamorgan pediatric pressure ulcer assessment scale. *Journal of Wound Care, 18*(1), 17–21.

Wilson, K. M. (2011). They only come out at night: Bed bugs and their alarming resurgence. *Nursing 2011, 41*(11), 54–58.

Wound Care Information Network. (2010). *Wound product and category index*. Retrieved from http://medicaledu.com/prodindex.htm

Zajac, L., & Jacobson, A. (2009). Impetigo: Taking on a common skin infection. *Clinical Advisor, 12*(7), 30–34.

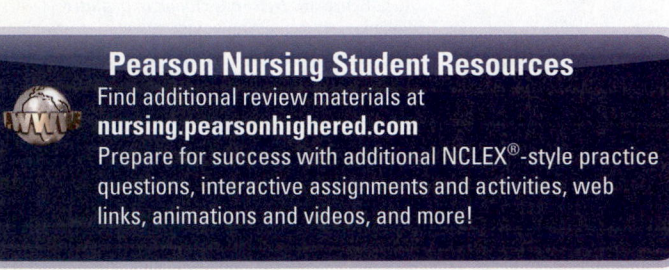

Pearson Nursing Student Resources

Find additional review materials at **nursing.pearsonhighered.com**
Prepare for success with additional NCLEX®-style practice questions, interactive assignments and activities, web links, animations and videos, and more!

APPENDICES

Appendix A
Physical Growth Charts

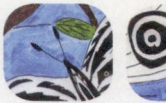 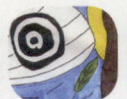 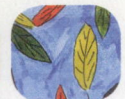

FIGURE A–1 ■ Classification of newborns based on maturity and intrauterine growth.

Source: *Adapted from Lubchenco, L. O., Hansman, C., & Boyd, E. (1966). Intrauterine growth in length and head circumference as estimated from live births at gestational ages from 26 to 42 weeks. Pediatrics, 37, 403–408; Battaglia, F. C., & Lubchenco, L. D. (1967). A practical classification of newborn infants by weight and gestational age. Journal of Pediatrics, 71, 159.*

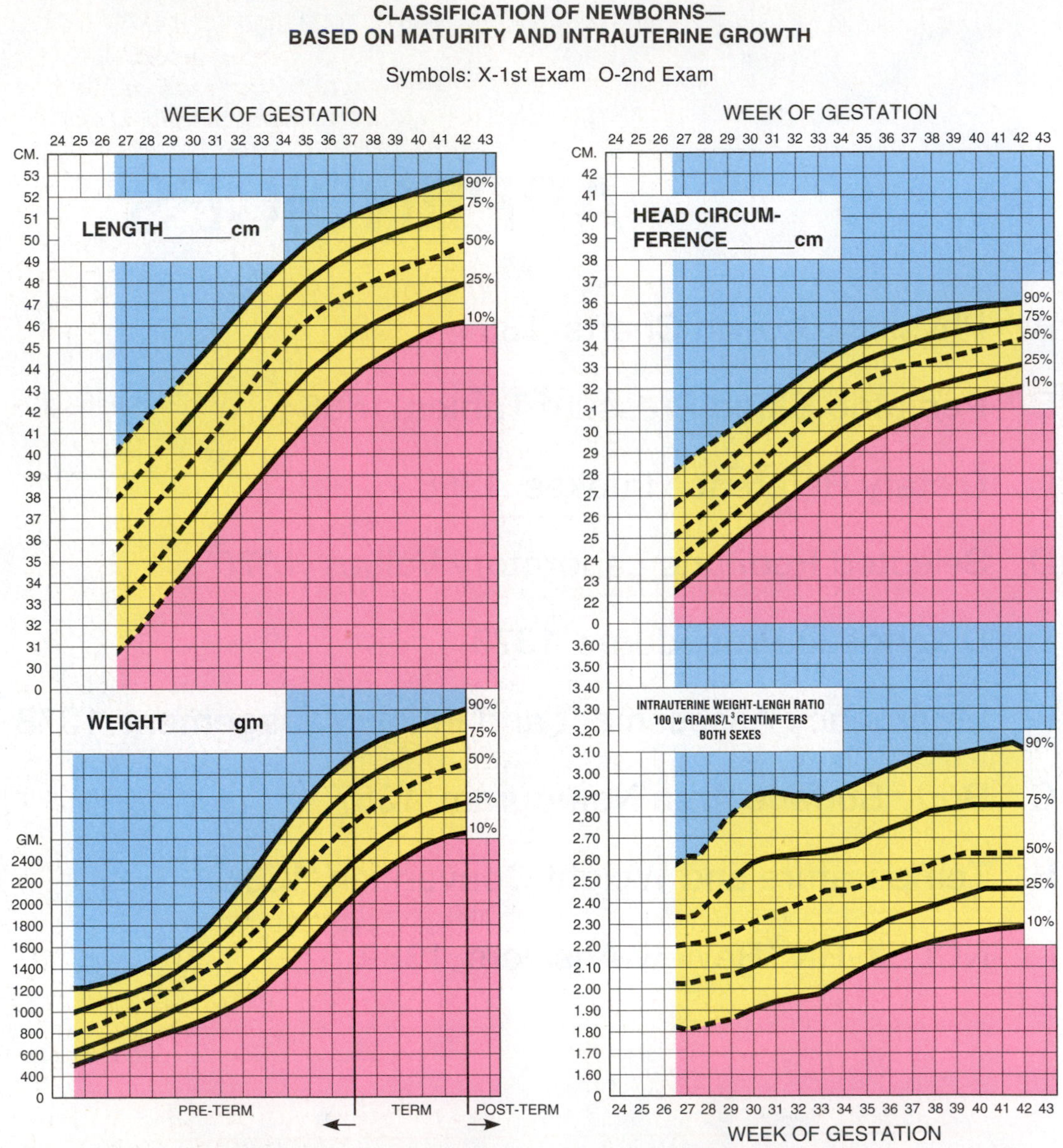

CLASSIFICATION OF NEWBORNS— BASED ON MATURITY AND INTRAUTERINE GROWTH

Symbols: X-1st Exam O-2nd Exam

WEEK OF GESTATION

LENGTH_____cm

WEIGHT_____gm

PRE-TERM   TERM   POST-TERM

HEAD CIRCUM-FERENCE_____cm

INTRAUTERINE WEIGHT-LENGH RATIO
100 w GRAMS/L³ CENTIMETERS
BOTH SEXES

WEEK OF GESTATION

	1st Exam (X)	2nd Exam (O)
LARGE FOR GESTATIONAL AGE **(LGA)**		
APPROPRIATE FOR GESTATIONAL AGE **(AGA)**		
SMALL FOR GESTATIONAL AGE **(SGA)**		
Age at Exam	hrs	hrs
Signature of Examiner	M.D.	M.D.

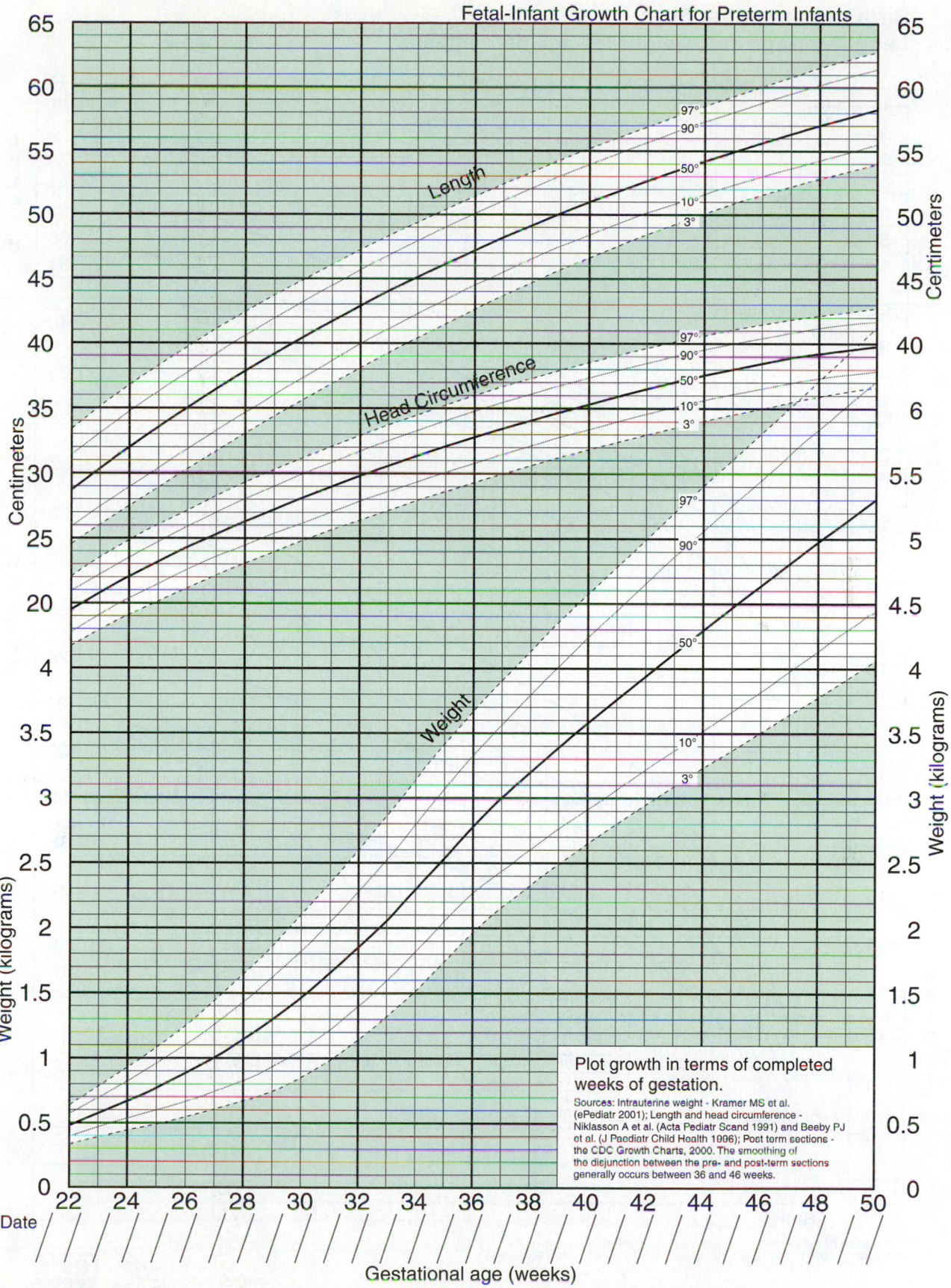

Fetal-Infant Growth Chart for Preterm Infants

Plot growth in terms of completed weeks of gestation.

Sources: Intrauterine weight - Kramer MS et al. (ePediatr 2001); Length and head circumference - Niklasson A et al. (Acta Pediatr Scand 1991) and Beeby PJ et al. (J Paediatr Child Health 1996); Post term sections - the CDC Growth Charts, 2000. The smoothing of the disjunction between the pre- and post-term sections generally occurs between 36 and 46 weeks.

Gestational age (weeks)

Date

FIGURE A–2 ■ Fetal-infant growth chart for preterm infants.

Source: *Fenton, T. R. A new growth chart for preterm babies: Babson and Benda's chart updated with recent data and new format. BMC Pediatrics, 3(1), 13.*

Birth to 24 months: Boys
Length-for-age and Weight-for-age percentiles

NAME _____

RECORD # _____

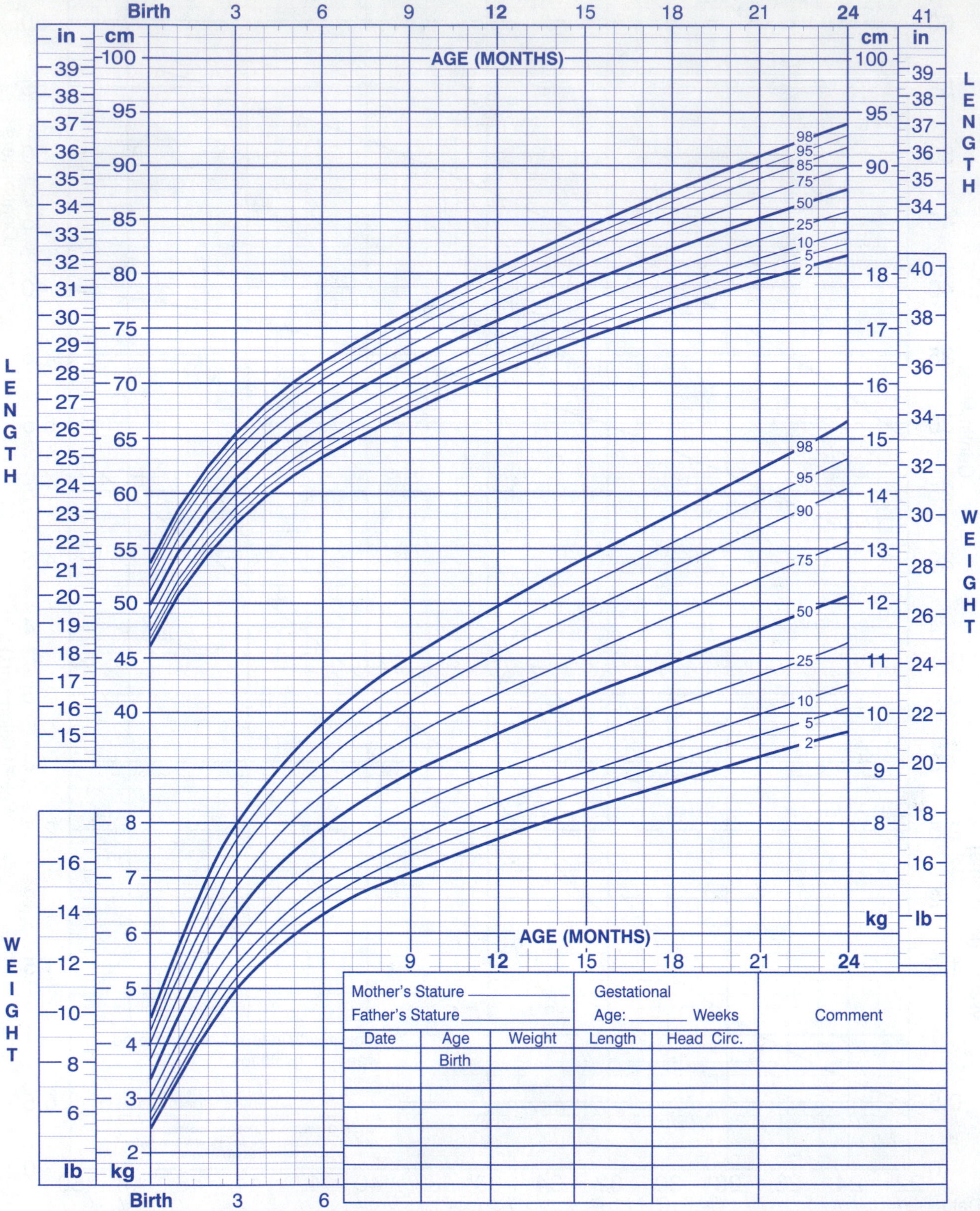

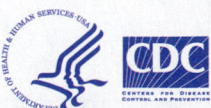

Published by the Centers for Disease Control and Prevention, November 1, 2009
SOURCE: WHO Child Growth Standards (http://www.who.int/childgrowth/en)

FIGURE A–3 ■ Physical growth percentiles for length and weight—boys: birth to 24 months.

Source: WHO Child Growth Standards: http://www.who.int/childgrowth/en

Birth to 24 months: Boys
Head circumference-for-age and Weight-for-length percentiles

NAME ______________________

RECORD # ______________

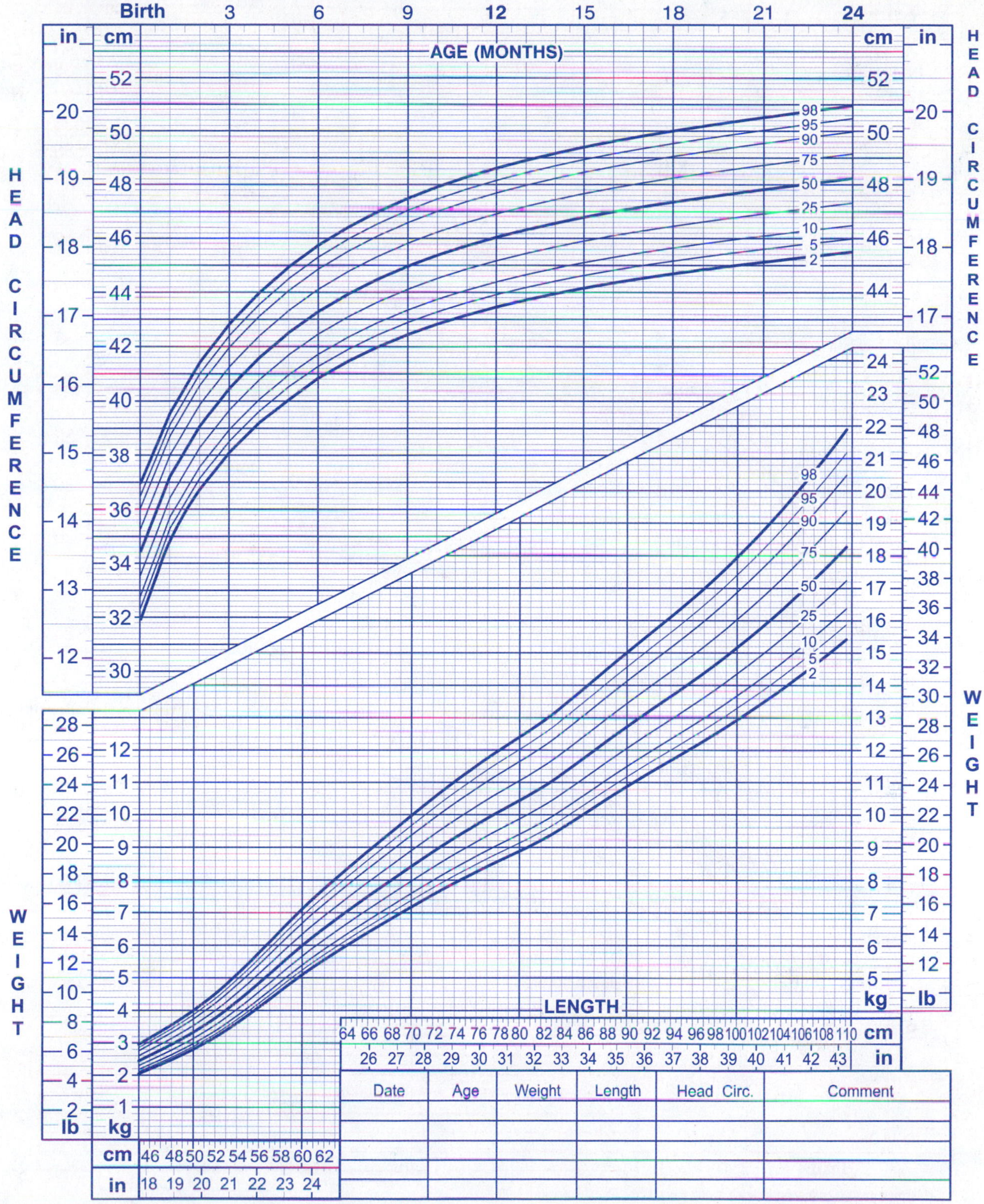
Birth 3 6 9 12 15 18 21 24
AGE (MONTHS)
HEAD CIRCUMFERENCE
in
cm
52 50 48 46 44 42 40 38 36 34 32 30
20 19 18 17 16 15 14 13 12
98 95 90 75 50 25 10 5 2
WEIGHT
lb
kg
LENGTH
cm 46 48 50 52 54 56 58 60 62
in 18 19 20 21 22 23 24
64 66 68 70 72 74 76 78 80 82 84 86 88 90 92 94 96 98 100 102 104 106 108 110 cm
26 27 28 29 30 31 32 33 34 35 36 37 38 39 40 41 42 43 in

Date	Age	Weight	Length	Head Circ.	Comment

Published by the Centers for Disease Control and Prevention, November 1, 2009
SOURCE: WHO Child Growth Standards (http://www.who.int/childgrowth/en)

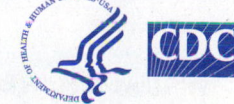

FIGURE A–4 ■ Physical growth percentiles for head circumference, weight for length—boys: birth to 24 months.

Source: WHO Child Growth Standards: http://www.who.int/childgrowth/en

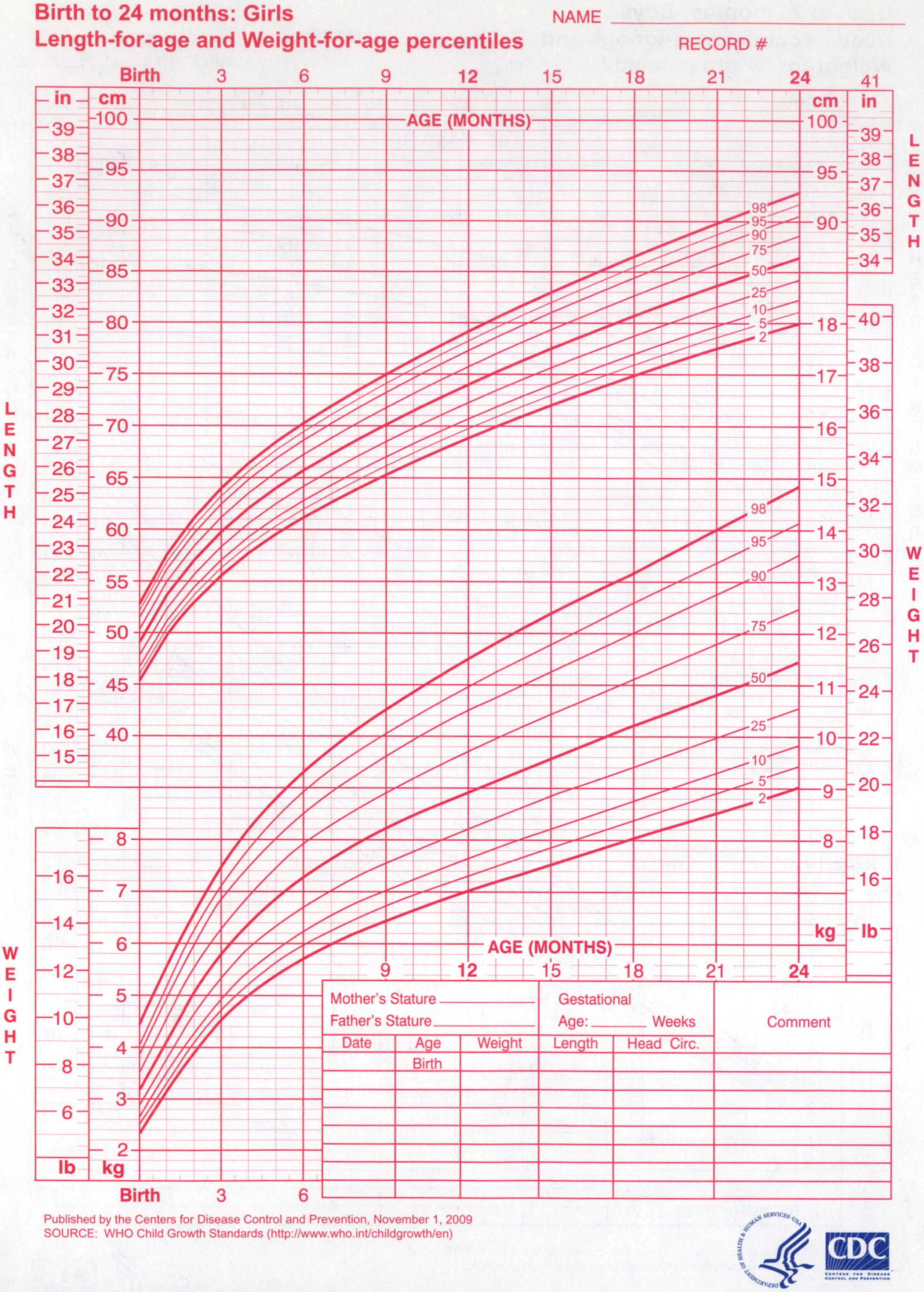

Birth to 24 months: Girls
Length-for-age and Weight-for-age percentiles

NAME _____

RECORD # _____

Published by the Centers for Disease Control and Prevention, November 1, 2009
SOURCE: WHO Child Growth Standards (http://www.who.int/childgrowth/en)

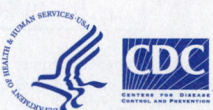

FIGURE A–5 ■ Physical growth percentiles for length and weight—girls: birth to 24 months.

Source: WHO Child Growth Standards: http://www.who.int/childgrowth/en

**Birth to 24 months: Girls
Head circumference-for-age and
Weight-for-length percentiles**

NAME _____

RECORD # _____

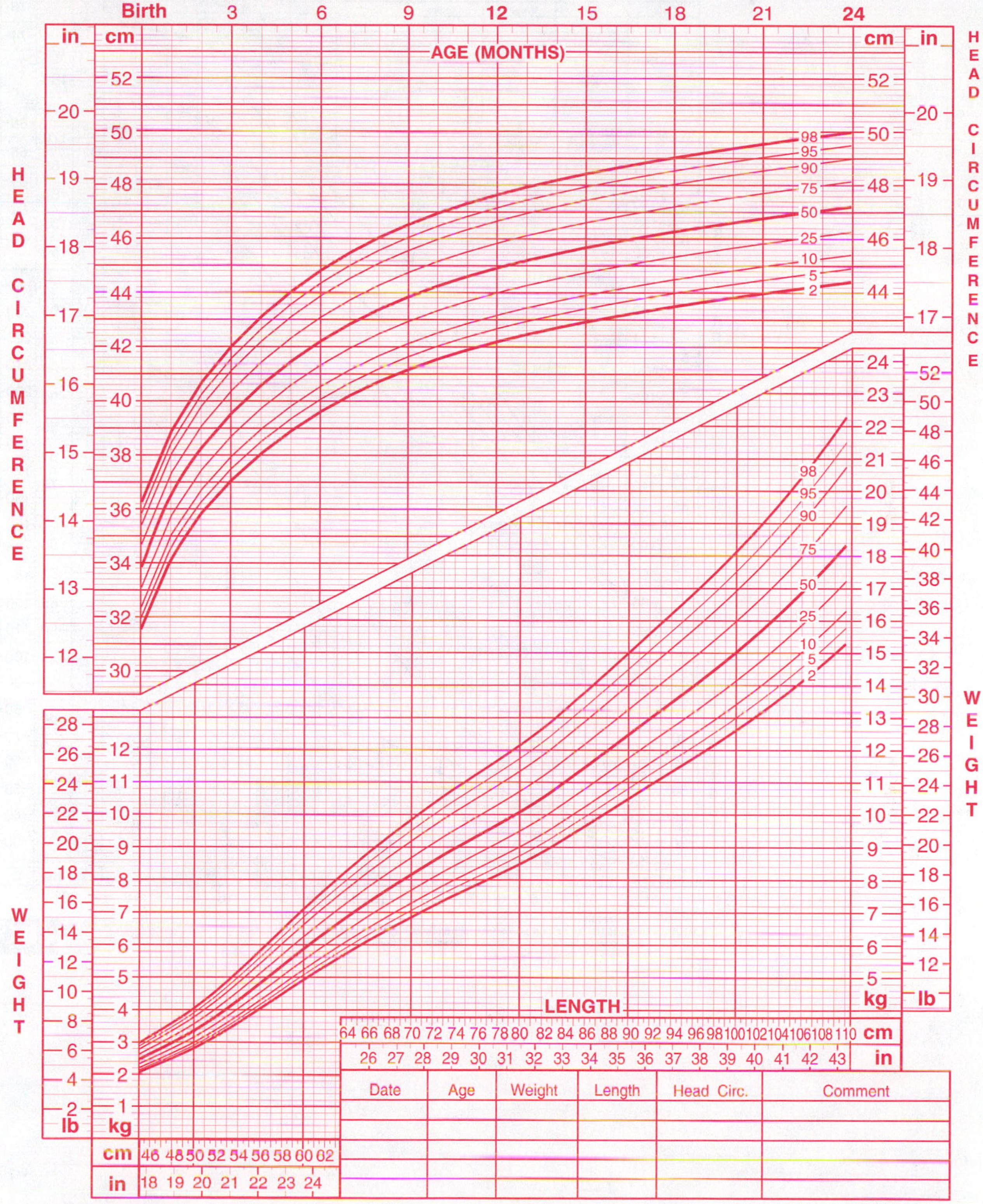

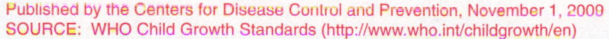

FIGURE A–6 ■ Physical growth percentiles for head circumference, weight for length—girls: birth to 24 months.

Source: WHO Child Growth Standards: http://www.who.int/childgrowth/en

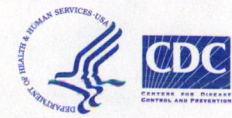

FIGURE A–7 ■ Physical growth percentiles for stature and weight according to age—boys: 2 to 20 years.

Source: From CDC, 2001. www.cdc.gov/growthcharts

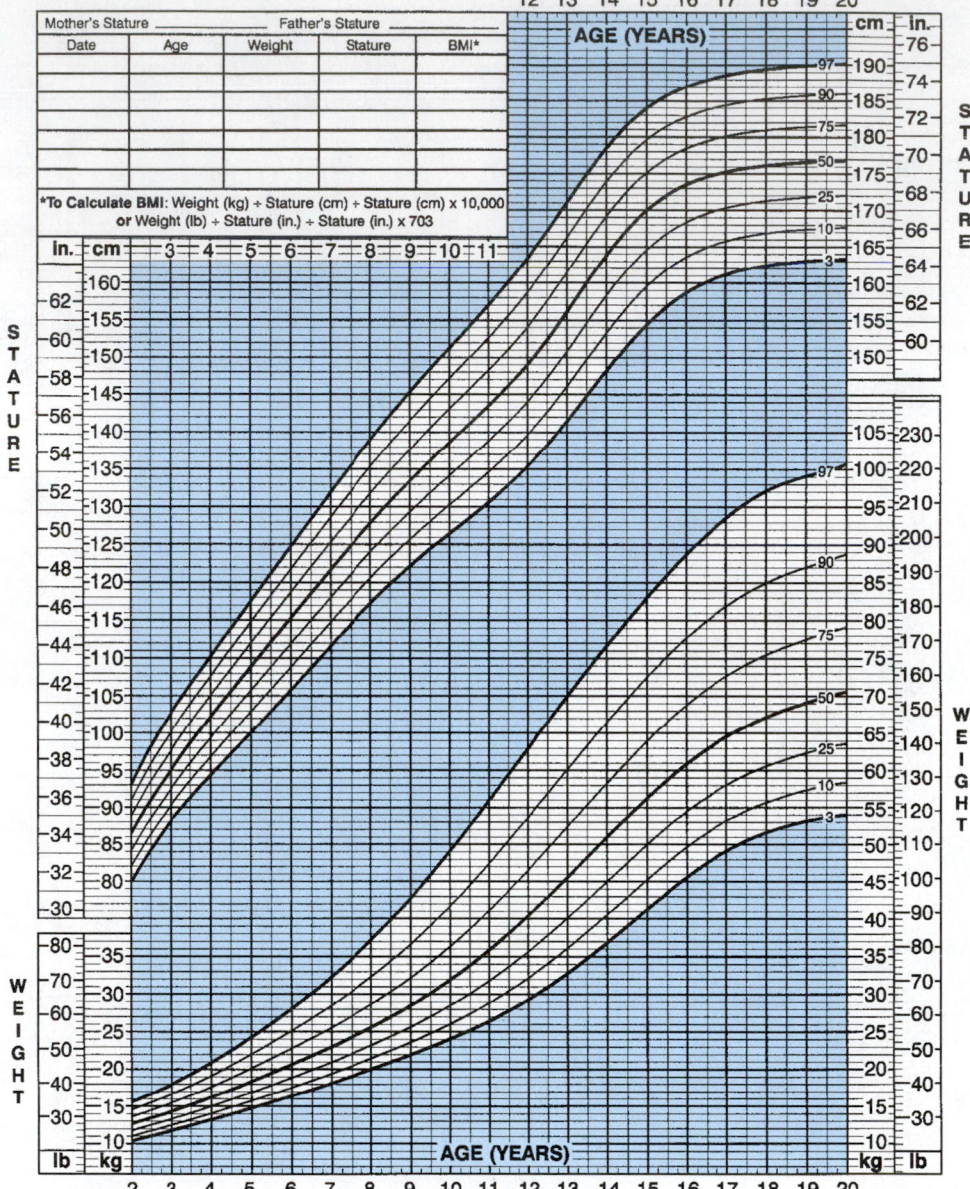

2 to 20 years: Boys
Stature-for-age and Weight-for-age percentiles

NAME _____

RECORD # _____

Revised and corrected November 21, 2000.
SOURCE: Developed by the National Center for Health Statistics in collaboration with
the National Center for Chronic Disease Prevention and Health Promotion (2000).
http://www.cdc.gov/growthcharts

2 to 20 years: Boys
Body Mass Index-for-age percentiles

NAME _____

RECORD # _____

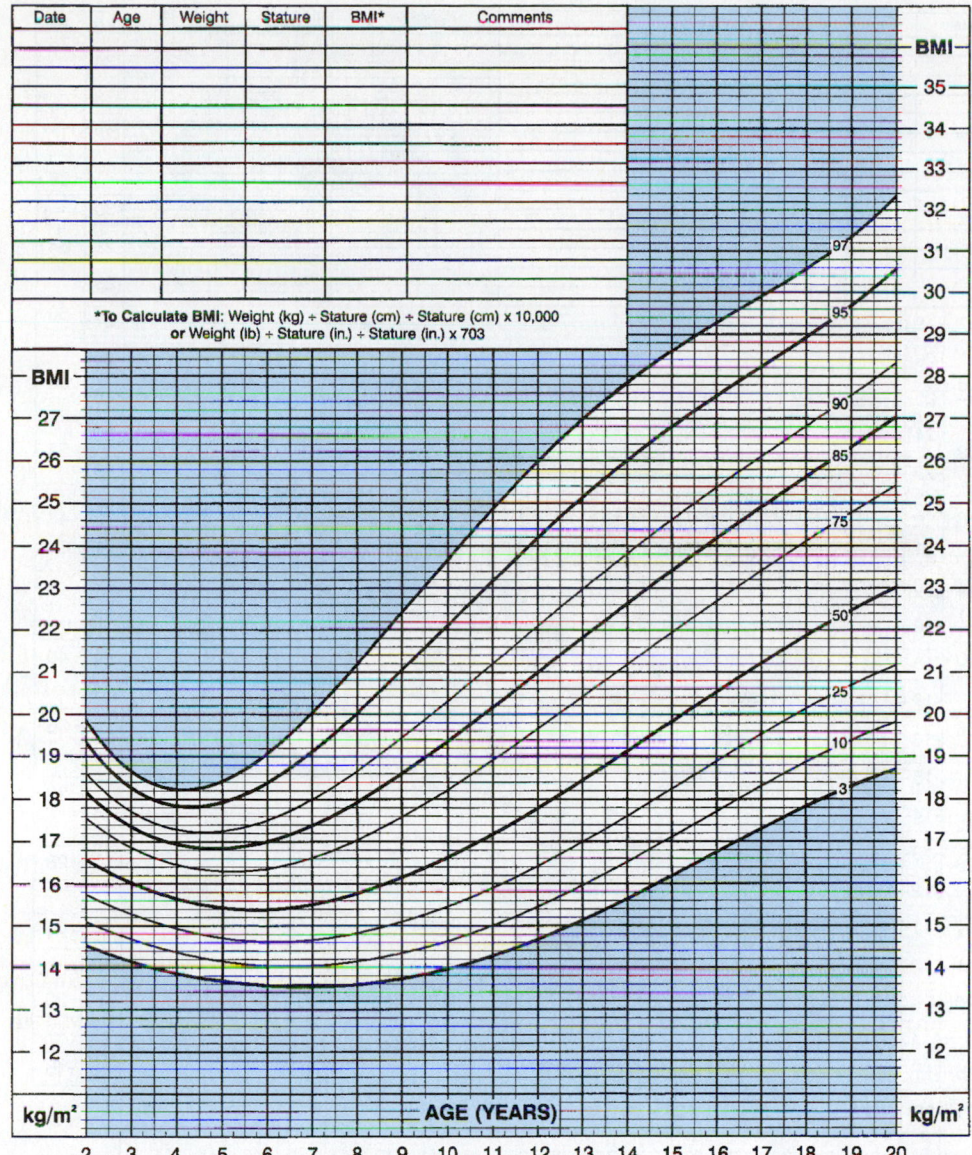

Date	Age	Weight	Stature	BMI*	Comments

*To Calculate BMI: Weight (kg) ÷ Stature (cm) ÷ Stature (cm) x 10,000
or Weight (lb) ÷ Stature (in.) ÷ Stature (in.) x 703

FIGURE A–8 ■ Physical growth percentiles for body mass index according to age—boys: 2 to 20 years.

Source: From CDC, 2001. www.cdc.gov/growthcharts

SOURCE: Developed by the National Center for Health Statistics in collaboration with
the National Center for Chronic Disease Prevention and Health Promotion (2000).
http://www.cdc.gov/growthcharts

FIGURE A–9 ■ Physical growth percentiles for weight for stature—boys: 2 to 20 years.
Source: From CDC, 2001. www.cdc.gov/growthcharts

NAME _____

RECORD # _____

Weight-for-stature percentiles: Boys

Date	Age	Weight	Stature	Comments

STATURE

cm   80   85   90   95   100   105   110   115   120

in.   31 32 33 34 35 36 37 38 39 40 41 42 43 44 45 46 47

SOURCE: Developed by the National Center for Health Statistics in collaboration with
the National Center for Chronic Disease Prevention and Health Promotion (2000).
http://www.cdc.gov/growthcharts

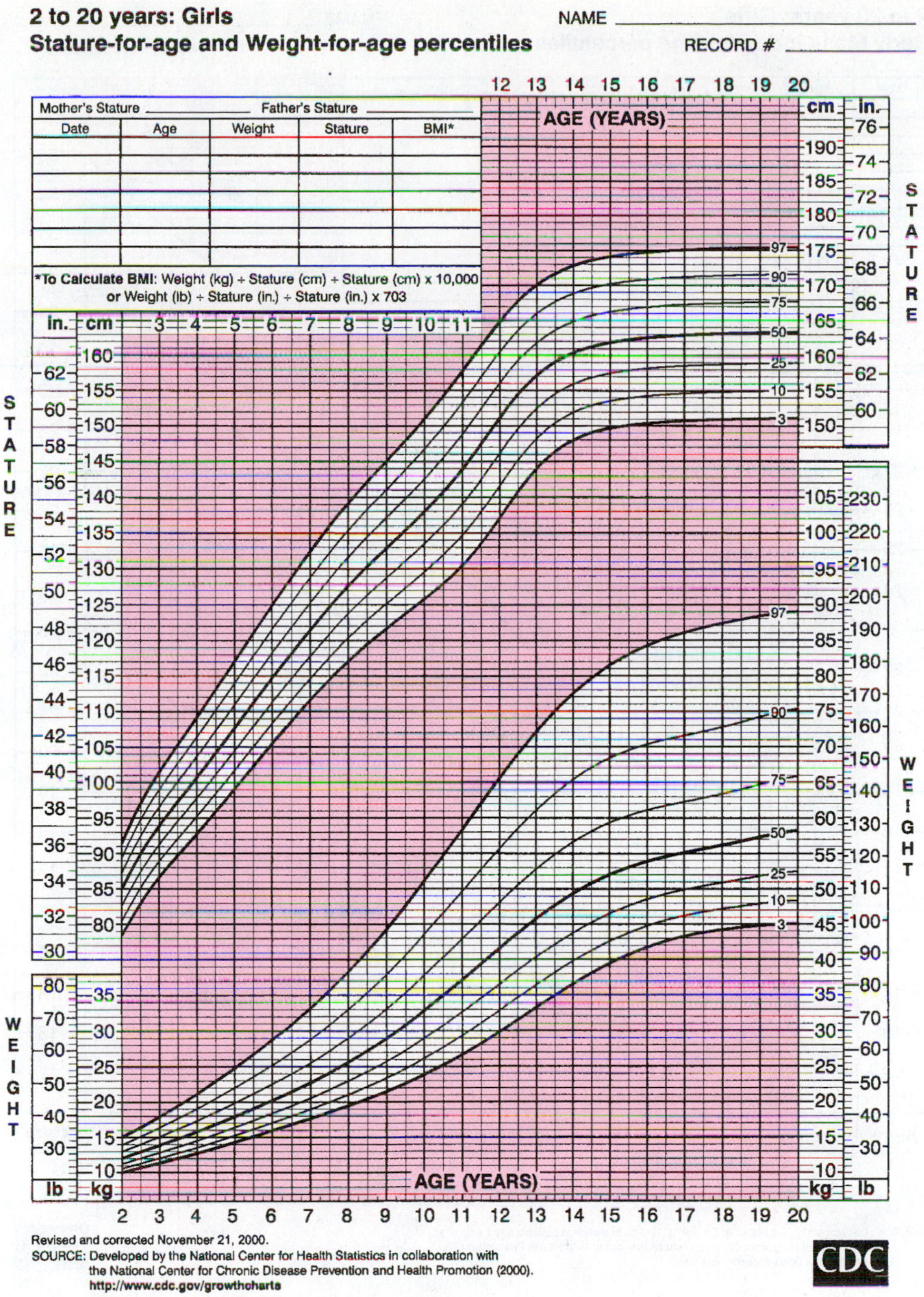

2 to 20 years: Girls
Stature-for-age and Weight-for-age percentiles

NAME _____

RECORD # _____

Mother's Stature		Father's Stature		
Date	Age	Weight	Stature	BMI*

*To Calculate BMI: Weight (kg) ÷ Stature (cm) ÷ Stature (cm) x 10,000
or Weight (lb) ÷ Stature (in.) ÷ Stature (in.) x 703

AGE (YEARS)

STATURE

WEIGHT

AGE (YEARS)

Revised and corrected November 21, 2000.
SOURCE: Developed by the National Center for Health Statistics in collaboration with
the National Center for Chronic Disease Prevention and Health Promotion (2000).
http://www.cdc.gov/growthcharts

CDC

FIGURE A–10 ■ Physical growth percentiles for stature and weight according to age—girls: 2 to 20 years.

Source: From CDC, 2001. www.cdc.gov/growthcharts

FIGURE A–11 ■ Physical growth percentiles for body mass index according to age—girls: 2 to 20 years.

Source: From CDC, 2001. www.cdc.gov/growthcharts

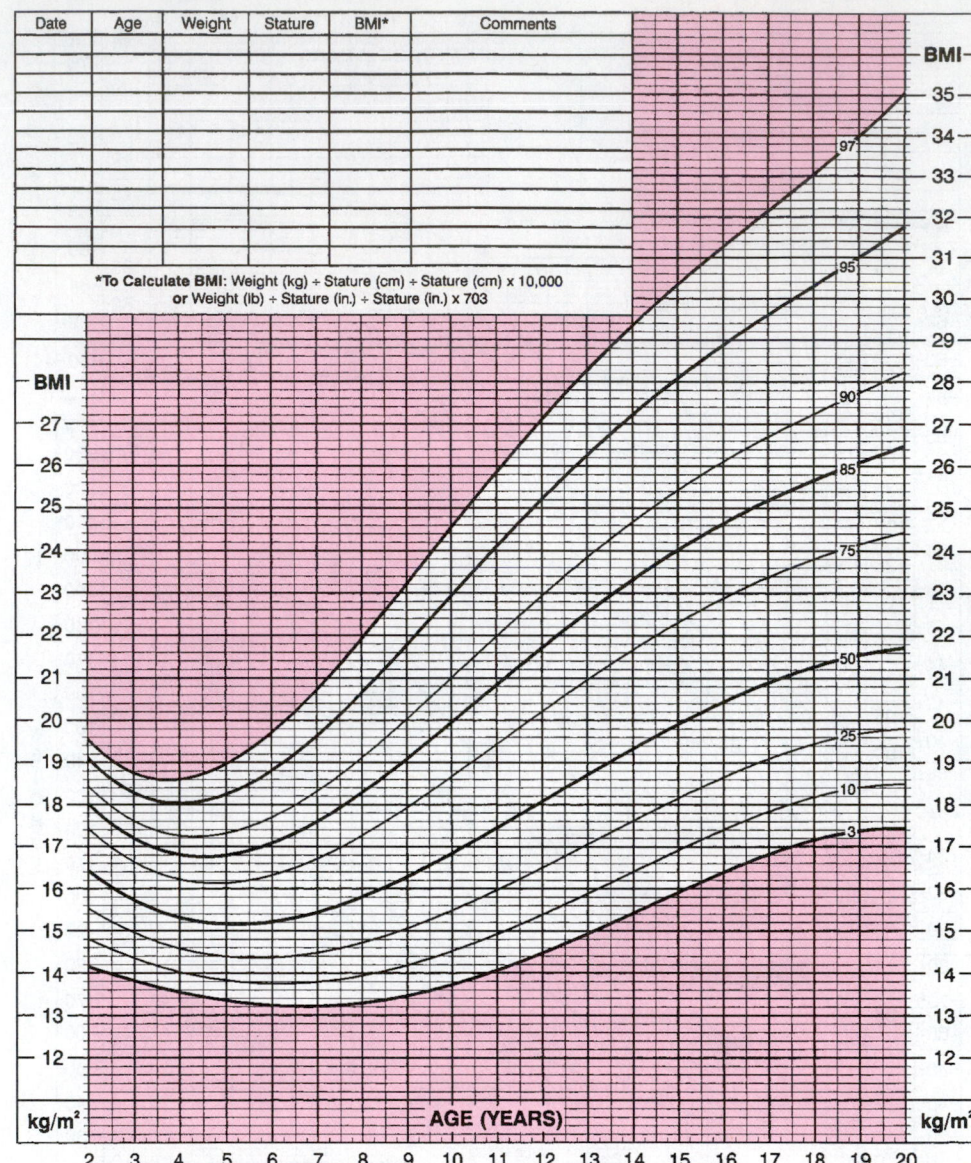

2 to 20 years: Girls
Body Mass Index-for-age percentiles

NAME _____

RECORD # _____

Date	Age	Weight	Stature	BMI*	Comments

*To Calculate BMI: Weight (kg) ÷ Stature (cm) ÷ Stature (cm) x 10,000
or Weight (lb) ÷ Stature (in.) ÷ Stature (in.) x 703

AGE (YEARS)

SOURCE: Developed by the National Center for Health Statistics in collaboration with
the National Center for Chronic Disease Prevention and Health Promotion (2000).
http://www.cdc.gov/growthcharts

FIGURE A–12 ■ Physical growth percentiles for weight for stature—girls: 2 to 20 years.

Source: From CDC, 2001. www.cdc.gov/growthcharts

Weight-for-stature percentiles: Girls

NAME _____

RECORD # _____

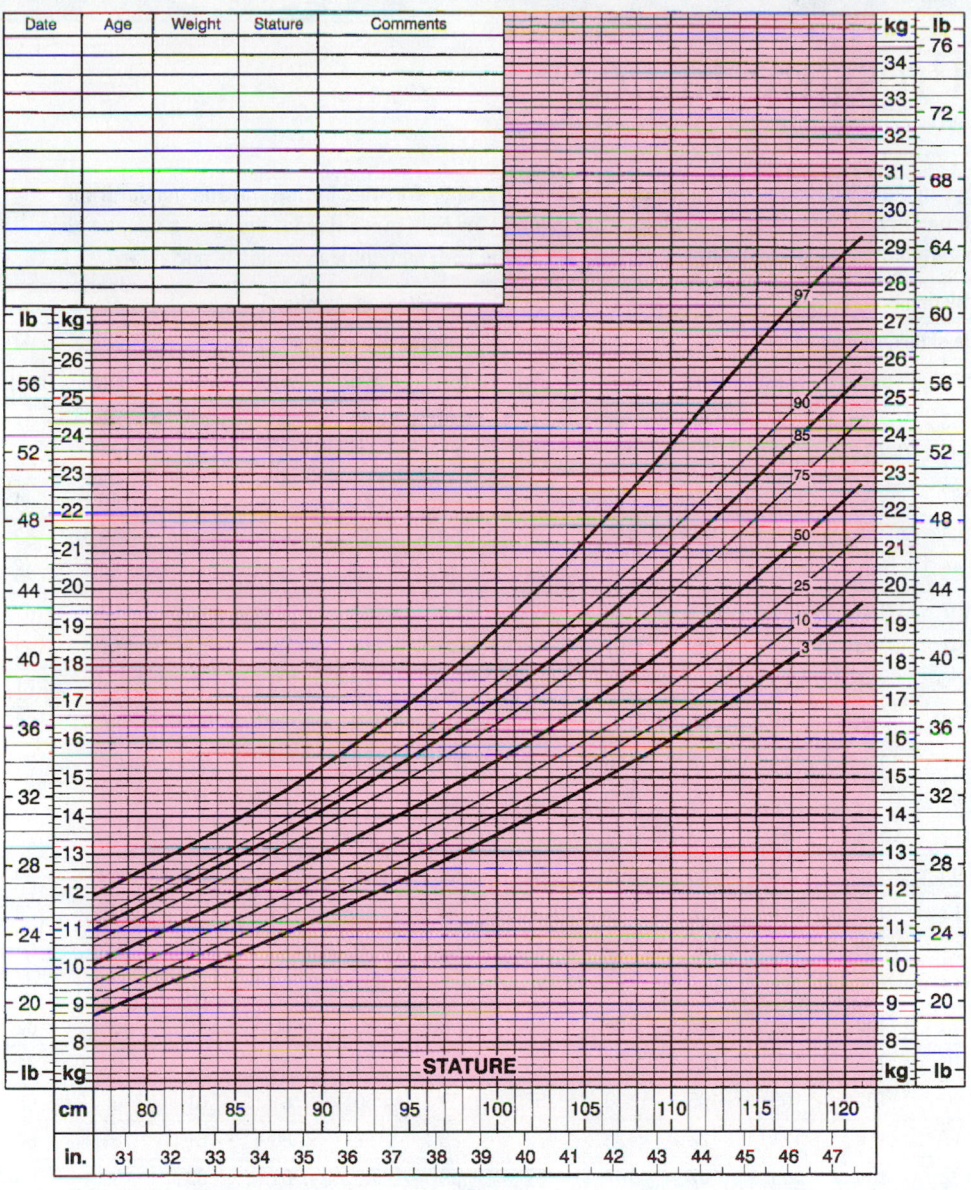

STATURE

SOURCE: Developed by the National Center for Health Statistics in collaboration with
the National Center for Chronic Disease Prevention and Health Promotion (2000).
http://www.cdc.gov/growthcharts

CDC

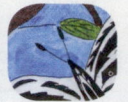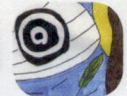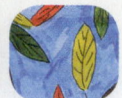
Pediatric Blood Pressure Tables

TABLE B–1 **Blood Pressure Levels for Boys by Age and Height Percentile.** Use the child's height percentile for the age and gender from the standard growth charts found in Appendix A 🔗. A blood pressure value at the 50th percentile for the child's age, gender, and height is considered the midpoint of the normal range. A reading above the 95th percentile indicates hypertension.*

AGE (YEAR)	BP PERCENTILE	Systolic BP (mmHg) Percentile of Height							Diastolic BP (mmHg) Percentile of Height						
		5TH	10TH	25TH	50TH	75TH	90TH	95TH	5TH	10TH	25TH	50TH	75TH	90TH	95TH
1	50th	80	81	83	85	87	88	89	34	35	36	37	38	39	39
	95th	98	99	101	103	104	106	106	54	54	55	56	57	58	58
2	50th	84	85	87	88	90	92	92	39	40	41	42	43	44	44
	95th	101	102	104	106	108	109	110	59	59	60	61	62	63	63
3	50th	86	87	89	91	93	94	95	44	44	45	46	47	48	48
	95th	104	105	107	109	110	112	113	63	63	64	65	66	67	67
4	50th	88	89	91	93	95	96	97	47	48	49	50	51	51	52
	95th	106	107	109	111	112	114	115	66	67	68	69	70	71	71
5	50th	90	91	93	95	96	98	98	50	51	52	53	54	55	55
	95th	108	109	110	112	114	115	116	69	70	71	72	73	74	74
6	50th	91	92	94	96	98	99	100	53	53	54	55	56	57	57
	95th	109	110	112	114	115	117	117	72	72	73	74	75	76	76
7	50th	92	94	95	97	99	100	101	55	55	56	57	58	59	59
	95th	110	111	113	115	117	118	119	74	74	75	76	77	78	78
8	50th	94	95	97	99	100	102	102	56	57	58	59	60	60	61
	95th	111	112	114	116	118	119	120	75	76	77	78	79	79	80
9	50th	95	96	98	100	102	103	104	57	58	59	60	61	61	62
	95th	113	114	116	118	119	121	121	76	77	78	79	80	81	81
10	50th	97	98	100	102	103	105	106	58	59	60	61	61	62	63
	95th	115	116	117	119	121	122	123	77	78	79	80	81	81	82
11	50th	99	100	102	104	105	107	107	59	59	60	61	62	63	63
	95th	117	118	119	121	123	124	125	78	78	79	80	81	82	82
12	50th	101	102	104	106	108	109	110	59	60	61	62	63	63	64
	95th	119	120	122	123	125	127	127	78	79	80	81	82	82	83
13	50th	104	105	106	108	110	111	112	60	60	61	62	63	64	64
	95th	121	122	124	126	128	129	130	79	79	80	81	82	83	83
14	50th	106	107	109	111	113	114	115	60	61	62	63	64	65	65
	95th	124	125	127	128	130	132	132	80	80	81	82	83	84	84
15	50th	109	110	112	113	115	117	117	61	62	63	64	65	66	66
	95th	126	127	129	131	133	134	135	81	81	82	83	84	85	85
16	50th	111	112	114	116	118	119	120	63	63	64	65	66	67	67
	95th	129	130	132	134	135	137	137	82	83	83	84	85	86	87
17	50th	114	115	116	118	120	121	122	65	66	66	67	68	69	70
	95th	131	132	134	136	138	139	140	84	85	86	87	87	88	89

BP, blood pressure

*The 90th percentile is 1.28 SD, the 95th percentile is 1.645 SD, and the 99th percentile is 2.326 SD over the mean.

Source: From National Heart, Lung, and Blood Institute. (2004). Blood pressure tables for children and adolescents from the fourth report on the diagnosis, evaluation, and treatment of high blood pressure in children and adolescents. Retrieved from http://www.nhlbi.nih.gov/guidelines/hypertension/child_tbl.htm

TABLE B–2	Blood Pressure Levels for Girls by Age and Height Percentile. Use the child's height percentile for the age and gender from the standard growth charts found in Appendix A 🔗. A blood pressure value at the 50th percentile for the child's age, gender, and height is considered the midpoint of the normal range. A reading above the 95th percentile indicates hypertension.

AGE (YEAR)	BP PERCENTILE	Systolic BP (mmHg) Percentile of Height							Diastolic BP (mmHg) Percentile of Height						
		5TH	10TH	25TH	50TH	75TH	90TH	95TH	5TH	10TH	25TH	50TH	75TH	90TH	95TH
1	50th	83	84	85	86	88	89	90	38	39	39	40	41	41	42
	95th	100	101	102	104	105	106	107	56	57	57	58	59	59	60
2	50th	85	85	87	88	89	91	91	43	44	44	45	46	46	47
	95th	102	103	104	105	107	108	109	61	62	62	63	64	65	65
3	50th	86	87	88	89	91	92	93	47	48	48	49	50	50	51
	95th	104	104	105	107	108	109	110	65	66	66	67	68	68	69
4	50th	88	88	90	91	92	94	94	50	50	51	52	52	53	54
	95th	105	106	107	108	110	111	112	68	68	69	70	71	71	72
5	50th	89	90	91	93	94	95	96	52	53	53	54	55	55	56
	95th	107	107	108	110	111	112	113	70	71	71	72	73	73	74
6	50th	91	92	93	94	96	97	98	54	54	55	56	56	57	58
	95th	108	109	110	111	113	114	115	72	72	73	74	74	75	76
7	50th	93	93	95	96	97	99	99	55	56	56	57	58	58	59
	95th	110	111	112	113	115	116	116	73	74	74	75	76	76	77
8	50th	95	95	96	98	99	100	101	57	57	57	58	59	60	60
	95th	112	112	114	115	116	118	118	75	75	75	76	77	78	78
9	50th	96	97	98	100	101	102	103	58	58	58	59	60	61	61
	95th	114	114	115	117	118	119	120	76	76	76	77	78	79	79
10	50th	98	99	100	102	103	104	105	59	59	59	60	61	62	62
	95th	116	116	117	119	120	121	122	77	77	77	78	79	80	80
11	50th	100	101	102	103	105	106	107	60	60	60	61	62	63	63
	95th	118	118	119	121	122	123	124	78	78	78	79	80	81	81
12	50th	102	103	104	105	107	108	109	61	61	61	62	63	64	64
	95th	119	120	121	123	124	125	126	79	79	79	80	81	82	82
13	50th	104	105	106	107	109	110	110	62	62	62	63	64	65	65
	95th	121	122	123	124	126	127	128	80	80	80	81	82	83	83
14	50th	106	106	107	109	110	111	112	63	63	63	64	65	66	66
	95th	123	123	125	126	127	129	129	81	81	81	82	83	84	84
15	50th	107	108	109	110	111	113	113	64	64	64	65	66	67	67
	95th	124	125	126	127	129	130	131	82	82	82	83	84	85	85
16	50th	108	108	110	111	112	114	114	64	64	65	66	66	67	68
	95th	125	126	127	128	130	131	132	82	82	83	84	85	85	86
17	50th	108	109	110	111	113	114	115	64	65	65	66	67	67	68
	95th	125	126	127	129	130	131	132	82	83	83	84	85	85	86

BP, blood pressure

Appendix C

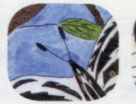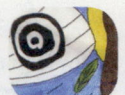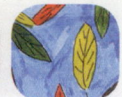

Dietary Reference Intakes

TABLE C–1	Dietary Reference Intakes for Infants, Children, and Adolescents

	AGE	VITAMIN A (MCG/D)	VITAMIN D (MCG/D)	VITAMIN E (MG/D α-TOCOPHEROL)	VITAMIN K (MCG/D)	VITAMIN C (MG/D)	THIAMIN (MG/D)	RIBOFLAVIN (MG/D)	NIACIN (MG/D)	VITAMIN B₆ (MG/D)
Infants	0–6 months	400*	10*	4*	2.0*	40*	0.2*	0.3*	~0.2*	0.1*
	7–12 months	500*	10*	5*	2.5*	50*	0.3*	0.4*	~0.4*	0.3*
Children	1–3 years	300	15	6	30*	15	0.5	0.5	6	0.5
	4–8 years	400	15	7	55*	25	0.6	0.6	8	0.6
Males	9–13 years	600	15	11	60*	45	0.9	0.9	12	1.0
	14–18 years	900	15	15	75*	75	1.2	1.3	16	1.3
Females	9–13 years	600	15	11	60*	45	0.9	0.9	12	1.0
	14–18 years	700	15	15	75*	65	1.0	1.0	14	1.2

*Values are Adequate Intakes (AIs) rather than Recommended Dietary Allowances (RDAs). All other values on chart are RDAs. See Chapter 19 for a discussion of nutrient requirements.

TABLE C–2	Recommended Dietary Allowances

	AGE	PROTEIN	CARBOHYDRATE	POLYUNSATURATED FATTY ACIDS n-6	POLYUNSATURATED FATTY ACIDS n-3	TOTAL FAT	FIBER
Infants	0–6 months	9.1 g/d or 1.52 g/kg/d*	60 g/d*	4.4 g/d	0.5 g/d	31 g/d	NE
	7–12 months	1.5 g/kg/d	95 g/d*	4.6 g/d	0.5 g/d	30 g/d	NE
Children	1–3 years	1.1 g/kg/d or 13 g/d	130 g/d	7 g/d (linoleic)	0.7 g/d (α-linolenic)	NE	19 g/d
	4–8 years	0.95 g/kg/d or 19 g/d	130 g/d	10 g/d (linoleic)	0.9 g/d (α-linolenic)	NE	25 g/d
Males	9–13 years	0.95 g/kg/d or 34 g/d	130 g/d	12 g/d (linoleic)	1.2 g/d (α-linolenic)	NE	31 g/d
	14–18 years	0.85 g/kg/d or 52 g/d	130 g/d	16 g/d (linoleic)	1.6 g/d (α-linolenic)	NE	38 g/d
Females	9–13 years	0.95 g/kg/d or 34 g/d	130 g/d	10 g/d (linoleic)	1.0 g/d (α-linolenic)	NE	26 g/d
	14–18 years	0.85 g/kg/d or 46 g/d	130 g/d	11 g/d (linoleic)	1.1 g/d (α-linolenic)	NE	26 g/d

*Values are Adequate Intakes (AIs) rather than Recommended Dietary Allowances (RDAs). All other values on charts are RDAs.

NE = not established

Source: *Data from Institute of Medicine. (2002). Dietary Reference Intakes.Washington, DC: National Academy Press; Otten, J. J., Hellwig, J. P., & Meyers, L. D. (Eds.). (2006). Dietary Reference Intakes: The essential guide to nutrient requirements. Washington, DC: National Academies Press; Wagner, C. L., Greer, F. R., & Section on Breastfeeding and Committee on Nutrition. (2008). Prevention of rickets and vitamin D deficiency in infants, children, and adolescents. Pediatrics, 122(5), 1142–1152; Ross, A. C., Taylor, C. L., Yaktine, A. L., & Del Valle, H.B. (Eds.). (2011). Dietary Reference Intakes for calcium and vitamin D. Washington, DC: Institute of Medicine.* (www.nap.edu/iom)

FOLATE (MCG/D)	VITAMIN B$_{12}$ (MCG/D)	CALCIUM (MG/D)	PHOSPHORUS (MG/D)	MAGNESIUM (MG/D)	IRON (MG/D)	ZINC (MG/D)	IODINE (MCG/D)	SELENIUM (MCG/D)
65*	0.4*	200*	100*	30*	0.27*	2.0*	110*	15*
80*	0.5*	260*	275*	75*	11	3	130*	20*
150	0.9	700	460	80	7	3	90	20
200	1.2	1000	500	130	10	5	90	30
300	1.8	1300	1250	240	8	8	120	40
400	2.4	1300	1250	240	11	11	150	55
300	1.8	1300	1250	410	8	8	120	40
400	2.4	1300	1250	360	15	9	150	55

Appendix D

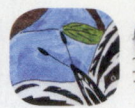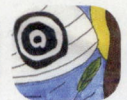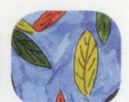

Selected Pediatric Laboratory Values

All laboratory value intervals listed are approximate. Consult your local laboratory for guidelines as to normal values for the specific testing procedures used.

NORMAL HEMATOLOGY VALUE INTERVALS (B)

Values for children 2 to 12 years

Hematocrit (HCT)[1]

31.7–39.8%

Hemoglobin (Hb)[1]

10.2–13.4 g/dL

Mean Corpuscular Hemoglobin (MCH)[1]

23.7–29.5 picograms

Mean Corpuscular Hemoglobin Concentration (MCHC)[1]

31.8–34.9%

Mean Corpuscular Volume (MCV)[1]

71.3–87.6 micrometer[3]

Red Blood Cell (RBC)[1]

$3.89–5.03 \times 10^{12}$/L

White Blood Cell (WBC)[1]

$4.86–11.4 \times 10^{9}$/L

Differential[1]

Neutrophils	22.4–74.7%
Eosinophils	0–4.7%
Basophils	0.1–0.6%
Lymphocytes	18.1–57.8%
Atypical lymphocytes	2–4%
Monocytes	4.1–12.3%

Platelet Count[3]

$202–367 \times 10^{9}$/L

Reticulocyte Count[1]

0.82–1.49%

NORMAL BLOOD CHEMISTRY VALUE INTERVALS

Albumin (S)[1]

1 month–1 year:	2.8–4.8 g/dL
1–18 years:	3.2–4.7 g/dL

KEY for Type of Specimen: S = serum; B = whole blood; P = plasma

Alkaline Phosphatase (S)[1]

AGE	MALE UNITS/L	FEMALE UNITS/L
1–30 days	75–316	48–406
1–3 years	104–345	108–317
4–6 years	93–309	96–297
7–9 years	86–315	69–325
10–12 years	42–362	51–332
13–15 years	74–390	50–162
16–18 years	52–171	47–119

Alpha-fetoprotein (AFP) (S)[1]

Newborn:	50–100,000 ng/mL
1–3 months:	40–1000 ng/mL
4 months–18 years:	0–12 ng/mL

Bilirubin (S)[1]

Conjugated	Newborn:	Less than 0.6 mg/dL
Total	Birth–5 days:	Less than 11.7 mg/dL

Blood Gases

Carbon Dioxide, Partial Pressure (Pco_2) (B)[1]

Infant:	27–41 mmHg (3.6–5.5 kPa)
Children:	32–48 mmHg (4.3–6.4 kPa)

Oxygen, Partial Pressure (Po_2) (B)[1]

Greater than 1 day: 83–108 mmHg (11–14.4 kPa)

Bicarbonate, Actual (P)[3]

22–29 mmol/L

pH (B)[1]

0–6 months:	7.18–7.50
6–12 months:	7.27–7.49

Base Excess (B)[1]

Infant:	–7 to –1 mmol/L
Child:	–4 to +2 mmol/L
Thereafter:	–3 to +3 mmol/L

Oxygen Saturation (B)[1]

Newborns:	85–90%
Thereafter:	95–99%

BUN—see Urea Nitrogen

Cholesterol (S)[2]

Total Cholesterol
    Borderline: 170–199 mg/dL
    Elevated: Greater than 200 mg/dL

High-Density Lipoprotein
    Greater than 35 mg/dL

Low-Density Lipoprotein
    Borderline: 110–129 mg/dL
    Elevated: 130 mg/dL and higher

Triglycerides
    Less than 150 mg/dL

Coagulation Values[4]

Fibrinogen 175–400 mg/dL
International normalized ratio (INR) 2–3
Partial thromboplastin time, activated (aPTT) 22–34 seconds
Prothrombin time (PT) 11–15 seconds

C-Peptide (S)[5]

0.8–1.8 ng/mL or 0.27–0.63 nmol/L

C-Reactive Protein (CRP) (P, S)[1]

0.068–8.2 mg/L

Creatinine (S, P)[1]

1–7 days:	0.7–1.2 mg/dL
7 days–1 year:	0.2–0.5 mg/dL
1–9 years:	0.2–0.8 mg/dL
10–18 years:	0.5–1.1 mg/dL

Electrolytes[1]

Calcium (S, P)

Newborn:	7.9–10.7 mg/dL
Thereafter:	8.7–10.7 mg/dL

Chloride (S, P)
102–112 mmol/L

Glucose, Fasting (S, P)[6]

Newborn over 1 day old:	50–90 mg/dL (2.8–5.0 mmol/L)
Child:	60–100 mg/dL (3.3–5.5 mmol/L)
16 years and older:	70–105 mg/dL (3.9–5.8 mmol/L)

Magnesium (P, S)
1.6–2.4 mg/dL (0.66–0.99 mmol/L)

Phosphorus, Inorganic (S, P)
2.8–5.6 mg/dL (0.91–1.8 mmol)

Potassium (S, P)
3.7–5 mmol/L

Sodium (P, S)
134–143 mmol/L

Urea Nitrogen (S, P)

1–13 years:	5–17 mg/dL (1.8–6 mmol/L)
14–19 years:	8–21 mg/dL (2.9–7.5 mmol/L)

Erythrocyte Sedimentation Rate (Micro)[4]

1–13 mm/hr

Hemoglobin A$_{1c}$ (B)[1]

Normal:	4–6%

Hemoglobin, Fetal (B)[1]

Birth:	77–97.9%
6 weeks–3 months:	23.9–67.2%
3–9 months:	4.4–27.8%
9–15 months:	0.4–8.4%
15 months–6 years:	0.1–4.9%
6–17 years:	0–2%

Growth Hormone (P, S)[1]

0–6.9 years:	Less than 13.7 mcg/L
7–10.9 years:	Less than 16.5 mcg/L
11–14.9 years:	Less than 14.5 mcg/L
15–18.9 years:	Less than 13.5 mcg/L

Iron-Related Values

Ferritin (P, S)[1]

1–5 years:	6–24 ng/mL
6–9 years:	10–55 ng/mL
10–19 years:	Males 23–70 ng/mL
	Females 6–40 ng/mL

Iron (S, P)[1]

1–5 years:	22–136 mcg/dL (4–25 micromol/L)
6–9 years:	39–136 mcg/dL (7–25 micromol/L)
10–14 years:	28–134 mcg/dL (5–24 micromol/L)
14–19 years:	34–162 mcg/dL (6–29 micromol/L)

Iron-Binding Capacity (S, P)[1]

1–5 years:	268–441 mcg/dL (48–79 micromol/L)
6–9 years:	240–508 mcg/dL (43–91 micromol/L)
10–19 years:	290–570 mcg/dL (52–102 micromol/L)

Lead (B)[3]

Less than 10 mcg/dL (0.48 mmol/L)

Osmolality (S)

280–300 mOsm/kg

Thyroid Hormones

Thyroid-Stimulating Hormone (TSH) (P, S)[1]

AGE	MALES	FEMALES
0–12 months	0.9–5.4 milli International Unit/L (mIU/L)	
1–5 years	0.7–4.5 mIU/L	0.7–4.8 mIU/L
11–14 years	0.6–3.6 mIU/L	0.5–4.1 mIU/L

Thyroxine (T₄) (S, P)[1]

1–5 years:	5–14.45 mcg/dL
6–20 years:	4.4–12.1 mcg/dL

Thyroxine, "Free" (Free T₄) (S, P)[1]

Under 1 year:	1.3–2.8 ng/dL (16.8–36.1 picomol/L)
1–18 years:	1.3–2.42 ng/mL (16.8–31 picomol/L)

Thyroxine-Binding Globulin (TBG) (P)[1]

AGE	MALES	FEMALES
Cord blood	19–39 mg/L	19–39 mg/L
1–11 months	16–36 mg/L	17–37 mg/L
1–9 years	12–28 mg/L	15–27 mg/L
10–19 years	14–26 mg/L	14–30 mg/L

Triiodothyronine (T₃) (S)[1]

1–5 years:	106–203 ng/dL
6–10 years:	104–183 ng/dL
11–14 years:	68–186 ng/dL
15–20 years:	71–175 ng/dL

NORMAL VALUE RANGES: URINE

Albumin[4]

Less than 1 mg/dL

Catecholamines (Norepinephrine, Epinephrine)[1]

Values in mmol/mol creatinine

AGE	NOREPINEPHRINE	EPINEPHRINE
0–24 months	0–0.28	0–0.46
2–4 years	0–0.8	0–0.035
5–9 years	0–0.059	0–0.022
10–19 years	0–0.055	0–0.021

Creatinine[1]

3–8 years:	0.11–0.68 g/24 hr
9–12 years:	0.17–1.41 g/24 hr
13–17 years:	0.29–1.87 g/24 hr
Adults:	0.63–2.5 g/24 hr

Osmolality[4]

500–800 mOsm/kg water

Should be higher than serum osmolality

Protein[4]

Less than 150 mg/24 hr

Specific Gravity

1.01–1.03

NORMAL VALUE RANGES: SWEAT

Electrolytes[1]

Sodium and chloride: under 40 mmol/L

NORMAL VALUE RANGES: CEREBROSPINAL FLUID

Protein[1]

Under 1 month:	15–153 mg/dL
Over 1 month:	15–48 mg/dL

Glucose[1]

All ages: 41–84 mg/dL (60–80% of blood glucose)

REFERENCES

[1]Adapted from Soldin, S. J., Wong, E. C., Brugnara, C., & Soldin, O. P. (2011). *Pediatric reference ranges* (7th ed.). Washington, DC: AACC Press.

[2]Data from Daniels, S. R., Greer, F. R., & the Committee on Nutrition. (2008). Lipid screening and cardiovascular health in childhood. *Pediatrics, 122*(1), 198–208.

[3]Data from Kliegman, R. M., Stanton, B. F., St. Geme, J. W., Schor, N. F., & Behrman, R. E. (2011). *Nelson textbook of pediatrics* (19th ed., Table 708.6). Philadelphia, PA: Elsevier Saunders.

[4]Data from Corbett, J. V. (2008). *Laboratory tests and diagnostic procedures with nursing diagnoses* (7th ed.). Upper Saddle River, NJ: Pearson Prentice Hall.

[5]Data from Kee, J. L. (2010). *Laboratory and diagnostic tests* (8th ed.). Upper Saddle River, NJ: Pearson.

[6]Tschudy, M. M., & Arcara, K. M. (2012). Blood chemistries and body fluids. *The Harriet Lane handbook* (19th ed., p. 643). St. Louis, MO: Elsevier Mosby.

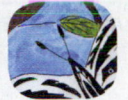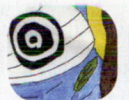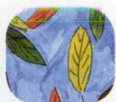

Diagnostic Procedures

Consider the growth and developmental level of the child when preparing the child for a procedure, and supporting the child during and after the procedure. See Chapter 15 🔊. Parents need to complete a signed consent with an understanding of the procedure, results, and risk factors. When possible, allow the parent to remain with the child during the procedure.

PROCEDURE, DESCRIPTION, AND PURPOSE	NURSING MANAGEMENT
ACTH stimulation test A drug, metyrapone, is administered to block the production of cortisol. In persons with pituitary insufficiency, the ACTH level does not increase as expected.	▪ Phenytoin and estrogen compounds interfere with the test results. ▪ Contact the laboratory for timing of the blood specimens to be collected.
Adrenal suppression test Dexamethasone, a potent corticosteroid, is administered to suppress the pituitary and ACTH production. In cases of Cushing syndrome, high levels of serum cortisol continue to be produced.	▪ Administer dexamethasone as prescribed. ▪ Contact the laboratory for timing of the blood specimens to be collected. A plastic tube is used rather than glass.
Arteriography/angiogram A contrast dye is injected to allow visualization of blood vessels. It is useful in evaluating patency of blood vessels and blood flow to parts of the body and in identifying abnormal vasculature.	▪ Obtain history of hypersensitivity to iodine, seafood, or radiographic contrast dye. Antihistamines and/or steroids may be ordered if allergy is suspected. ▪ Tell the child to expect a warm, flushing feeling that could last a few minutes. ▪ Ensure the child remains still during procedures so that pictures are clear. ▪ During and after the test, monitor vital signs; assess for vasovagal and allergic reactions.
Arthrogram After a local anesthetic, a needle is inserted into a joint (e.g., knee or shoulder). Samples of joint fluid may be aspirated, and then dye is injected into the joint cavity. The joint is moved to spread the dye. Radiographs are taken with the joint in various positions to detect joint damage.	▪ Prepare the child and family for the procedure. ▪ Local anesthesia is often used with general anesthesia for very young children. Support the child when the local anesthetic is inserted. ▪ Rest, ice on the joint, elevation, and an analgesic may be needed for discomfort after the procedure.
Barium or contrast enema Barium or barium and air are administered via a tube through the rectum to the colon. The large intestine is visualized to detect any abnormalities. Fluoroscopy is used to monitor the process and radiographs are taken.	▪ Give parents preprocedure instructions regarding diet, laxatives, and/or enemas. ▪ Prepare the child and parents for the procedure and to expect the sensation of fluid entering the rectum. Tell the child of the need to not have a bowel movement until told it is okay to do so. ▪ Ensure that the child holds still while the radiographs are taken.
Biopsy Biopsy is removal and examination of tissue from the body organs or skin to detect malignancies or the presence of disease. Biopsies can be obtained in several ways: ▪ Surgical excision at tissue site ▪ Needle aspiration at tissue site, with or without ultrasound ▪ Needle insertion into skin ▪ Brush method, scraping cells and tissue with stiff bristles as is done with a Pap smear ▪ Punch, using an instrument to excise a small area of tissue	▪ Prepare necessary instruments and specimen containers. Assist with preparation of the biopsy site. ▪ Monitor the child receiving sedation and analgesia according to protocol. ▪ Ensure that the child remains still during the procedure. ▪ Apply a dressing if appropriate to the site after the procedure. ▪ Label specimens accurately and arrange for specimen transport as recommended. ▪ Teach the family to care for the wound and to monitor the site for infection.
Bone marrow aspiration Marrow is removed from pelvic or iliac crest bones through a needle with a syringe used for aspiration. The test is diagnostic for leukemia, metastatic tumors, and some anemias. Marrow may also be harvested for transplant.	▪ The child is usually given anesthesia, or sedation and analgesia. Follow monitoring guidelines during and after the procedure. ▪ The site is prepped with a cleansing agent according to agency protocol. ▪ Positioning is determined by the site used, e.g., side-lying for the iliac crest. ▪ After the procedure, maintain the child on bed rest for at least 1 hour. ▪ Mild analgesics are provided for pain at the harvest site.
Bronchoscopy A flexible, fiber-optic bronchoscope is used to visualize the trachea and bronchi to identify and extract foreign objects in the airway, or for a biopsy.	▪ Maintain NPO status preprocedure according to agency guidelines. ▪ The child will often be sedated for the procedure, so monitor the child according to agency guidelines. ▪ Monitor vital signs per protocol postprocedure. Resume oral feedings as prescribed.

(continued)

PROCEDURE, DESCRIPTION, AND PURPOSE	NURSING MANAGEMENT
Cardiac catheterization A radiopaque catheter is passed through a large vein or artery in an arm or leg to the heart. It is then threaded to the heart chambers or coronary arteries, or both, guided by fluoroscopy. The procedure enables precise measurement of oxygen saturation within the heart's chambers and great arteries and pressure gradients in the pulmonary vessels or heart chambers. This helps assess for: ■ Congenital heart defects ■ Cardiac valvular disease ■ Coronary artery disease ■ Evaluation of artificial valves Other purposes of cardiac catheterization include heart muscle biopsy, tissue sampling for heart transplant rejection, or radiofrequency ablation for a heart rhythm disturbance.	■ Preparation includes discontinuation of anticoagulant therapy a week prior to the test and no food or fluid 6–8 hours preprocedure. Have the child void. ■ Prepare the child for the equipment to be used and sensations that will be felt. ■ Obtain a history of hypersensitivity to iodine, seafood, or radiographic contrast dye. Antihistamines and/or steroids may be ordered if allergy is suspected. Assess for allergic reaction during the procedure. ■ An IV is started for sedation administration, and to provide access for emergency drugs if needed. ■ ECG leads are applied to the chest to monitor heart activity. Vital signs and heart rhythm are monitored according to agency protocol. ■ See Chapter 26 🔗 for nursing management after the procedure.
Computed tomography (CT) The CT scan is a radiographic procedure that examines body sections from different angles, producing a three-dimensional cross section of any body structure. It may be performed with or without contrast dye. CT is used to screen for head, liver, abdominal, and renal lesions; tumors; edema; abscesses; bone destruction; and to locate foreign objects in soft tissue, such as the eye.	■ Depending upon the body system evaluated the infant or child may be NPO and require bowel evacuation prior to study. ■ If contrast dye is to be used, obtain a history about any hypersensitivity to iodine, seafood, or radiographic contrast dye. If allergy is suspected, antihistamines and/or steroids may be ordered prior to the procedure. Assess for allergic reaction during the procedure. ■ Prepare the child for the procedure by describing the equipment, noises, and other expected sensations, and how the child can help during the procedure. ■ If sedation is ordered for infants and small children to keep them still, monitor them according to protocol. ■ If contrast dye is used, encourage fluids after the procedure.
Cultures Cultures are taken to isolate and identify microorganisms causing infection, and often to identify the specific antibiotics to which the organisms are sensitive. Cultures commonly used with children include blood, throat, sputum, stool, wound, urine, and cerebrospinal fluid.	■ Collect culture specimens before administering new antimicrobials to prevent false results. List any antimicrobials given on the laboratory slip. ■ Send all specimens immediately to the laboratory, or refrigerate the specimen. ■ Use strict aseptic technique to handle the specimen. Keep lids on sterile specimen containers.
Cystoscopy A flexible fiber-optic scope is inserted through the urethra into the bladder to inspect the interior urethra and bladder for inflammation, tumors, stones, or structural abnormalities. The procedure may be done simultaneously with a voiding cystourethrogram (see page 1377).	■ Keep infants and children NPO prior to the study if sedation will be used. ■ Administer sedation as prescribed and monitor the child according to protocol. ■ Encourage fluids after the procedure to detect problems with voiding. ■ Inform the child and parents that dysuria and frequency may occur for a short time following the procedure.
Dual energy x-ray absorptiometry (DEXA) DEXA is a radiographic procedure emitting two photon energy beams used to measure bone mineral density in children at risk for glucocorticoid-induced osteoporosis.	■ Identify factors increasing a child's risk for osteoporosis or skeletal problems. ■ Explain the procedure and equipment to be used to the child and parents. ■ Inform the child of the need to not move, and let the child know the test does not cause pain.
Echocardiography An ultrasound study of the heart is used to identify the heart size, structure, pattern of movement, hemodynamics, blood flow, and blood flow disturbances. The ultrasound probe (transducer) is held over the chest (transthoracic) or inserted through the esophagus (transesophageal) to send an ultrasound beam to the tissues. The reflected sound waves are then transformed into scans, graphs, or sounds (Doppler).	■ Explain the procedure to the parents and child. Inform the child of the need to hold still for the procedure. ■ Inform the child that a gel will be applied to the skin and a transducer will move over the area, but that the test causes no pain.
Electrocardiography (ECG or EKG) and ambulatory electrocardiography An ECG records the electrical impulses of the heart via electrodes and a galvanometer (ECG machine). Eight electrodes are placed on the chest, and an electrode is placed on each extremity. The lead selector is turned to read the 12 standard leads. A Holter monitor may be attached to capture ambulatory ECG readings over a 24-hour period. An ECG is used to detect cardiac arrhythmias, identify electrolyte imbalances, or monitor ECG changes during an exercise or stress test.	■ Obtain a list of current medications and when they were last taken. ■ Inform the child that patches will be applied to the skin and wires will be attached, and that the test causes no pain. ■ Ask the child to hold still for a brief time. A pacifier or bottle may help the infant be still. ■ Encourage the child with a Holter monitor to engage in usual activities, but no swimming or bathing in a tub or shower is allowed until the electrodes are removed. ■ Ask the parents of the child wearing a Holter monitor to keep a diary of any events or emotional stress that causes symptoms. A daily schedule of sleep, eating, exercise, and other activities may be requested.

PROCEDURE, DESCRIPTION, AND PURPOSE	NURSING MANAGEMENT
Electroencephalogram (EEG) Approximately 20 electrodes are applied to the scalp to record cerebral cortex electrical activity over 1–2 hours. In some cases an EEG is performed when the child is asleep. An EEG is used to identify the potential for seizures, to determine brain death, and to detect other abnormalities such as a tumor, abscess, or intracranial hemorrhage.	■ Inform the parents and child about all medications and other substances (e.g., cola, tea, or coffee) to withhold for 24–48 hours. ■ Ensure that the hair is clean and dry, and that no hair products (oil, gel, spray, etc.) have been applied. ■ Do not permit infants or children to nap before the test. ■ Explain that the procedure is not painful as electrodes are applied. ■ Explain that washing the child's hair will remove electrode gel.
Electromyography (EMG) Needle electrodes are inserted into skeletal muscles, and muscle activity is measured during rest, voluntary activity, and electrical stimulation. The test is useful in assisting with diagnosis of muscular dystrophy and to differentiate muscle diseases and lower motor neuron neuropathies such as those caused by hypothyroidism or diabetes.	■ Be alert to medications that could affect EMG results. ■ Inform the child that there may be slight pain when the needle electrodes are inserted. Support the child with age-appropriate relaxation techniques or distraction techniques. If pain persists, inform the technician. ■ Administer analgesic as needed for pain.
Endoscopy A flexible, fiber-optic endoscope is used to visualize the internal structures of the esophagus, stomach, and duodenum. This procedure is also used to collect cytology specimens and to confirm gastrointestinal pathology.	■ Keep the child NPO prior to the procedure. ■ Administer sedation as prescribed and monitor the child during and post procedure according to protocol. ■ Inform the child that some pressure will be felt when the endoscope is inserted. ■ Resume oral feedings as prescribed.
Evoked potential A child who is awake is monitored by electrodes measuring brain and muscle activity. The baseline of electrical activity obtained is then used during later surgery, such as a spinal fusion for scoliosis, in order to monitor innervation to muscle groups and avoid injury to the spinal cord during the surgical procedure.	■ Prepare the child for the procedure, including the size of equipment, sounds, and time it will take. ■ Assist the child to relax with quiet music during the test.
Exercise testing A test is performed with a treadmill or stationary bicycle to evaluate exercise tolerance. ECG leads, a blood pressure cuff, and sometimes an oxygen consumption monitor are attached. Acceleration and pitch of the treadmill or bicycle are increased at intervals until the patient is fatigued, symptomatic, or a predetermined endpoint is reached. An ECG recording with a controlled activity increase helps to identify significant cardiac compensation or inadequate cardiac output.	■ Inform the adolescent about the test, what to expect, and that the test can be stopped at any time. ■ Instruct the adolescent to report vertigo, extreme shortness of breath, chest pain, and excessive fatigue. ■ Ensure that the adolescent understands that the test is of greater value when the exercise continues until the predetermined stopping level is reached. ■ Take baseline vital sign measurements prior to the exercise and throughout per agency protocol.
GI series Upper GI and small bowel series are fluoroscopic and radiographic examinations of the esophagus, stomach, and small intestine as ingested oral barium or water-soluble contrast agent passes through the digestive tract. This series identifies ulcers; gastroesophageal reflux; polyps, tumors, or hiatal hernias in the GI tract; pyloric stenosis; or foreign bodies, varices, or strictures.	■ Keep the child NPO before the procedure. A low-residue diet may be ordered for the night before the test. ■ Withhold medications as ordered. ■ Record vital signs; note epigastric pain or discomfort. ■ Inform the child that all of the liquid must be swallowed, but that the test will not cause pain or discomfort. ■ Inform parents that the stool will be light colored after the test.
Hyperoxitest Arterial blood is collected before and at least 10 minutes after giving the infant 100% oxygen. Differences between the arterial blood gas levels when an infant has central cyanosis help to distinguish between cardiac disease and pulmonary disease (Park, 2008).	■ Follow guidelines for arterial blood collection from the upper right side of the body. ■ Administer oxygen through a plastic hood for at least 10 minutes to replace all alveolar air with oxygen.
Intraesophageal pH probe monitoring A probe is placed in the distal esophagus for 24 hours to detect pH changes below 4. The pH is measured and recorded every 4–8 seconds. The test is used to diagnose gastroesophageal reflux disease and for evaluating atypical symptoms such as apnea, stridor, or cough.	■ Prevent the infant or child from inadvertent removal of the probe. Use soft mittens on the child's hands if necessary. ■ Monitor and record pH measurements per protocol. ■ Instruct parents to keep a diary of the child's activities while the probe is in place, e.g., feeding or sleeping.
Intravenous pyelogram A contrast dye is administered IV and excreted by the urinary system. A series of radiographs are taken at various intervals over an hour to evaluate the kidney cortex, kidney pelvis, ureters, and bladder. A postvoid radiograph is taken to see how well the bladder empties. The test is used to diagnose structural defects and tumors in the urinary system.	■ Assess for potential allergy to the contrast dye. An antihistamine or corticosteroid may be given to children with a potential allergy. Monitor the child carefully for an allergic reaction. ■ Obtain a serum creatinine and BUN prior to the test to assess renal function. ■ Follow orders for an NPO or clear liquid diet prior to the study. ■ Encourage fluids after the procedure to flush out the contrast media.

(continued)

PROCEDURE, DESCRIPTION, AND PURPOSE	NURSING MANAGEMENT
Lumbar puncture A lumbar puncture is performed at the L3-4 or L4-5 level to obtain a specimen of cerebrospinal fluid (CSF) and to measure the CSF pressure. CSF is cultured and analyzed for glucose and protein content, and the number of lymphocytes present.	■ Obtain a blood glucose level prior to the test for comparison with the CSF glucose level. ■ Hold the infant or child in knee-chest position and keep the child still during the procedure. ■ Label the tubes of CSF by numeric sequence obtained. ■ Assess breathing and any changes in neurologic function during the test. ■ Administer analgesics as ordered for headache.
Magnetic resonance imaging (MRI) A radiographic examination uses a large magnet to produce a magnetic field and radio waves to produce detailed images without ionizing radiation. The MRI scanner is a large, doughnut-shaped cylinder and the child lies on a table in the cylinder. An intravenous contrast dye is often used. An MRI provides images of the internal organ structure, blood flow patterns, and abnormalities in soft tissues.	■ Prepare the child for the loud sounds, size of equipment, and tunnel. Cardiorespiratory leads are often placed on the chest when contrast dye is used. ■ Assess the child for potential allergy to the contrast dye. An antihistamine or corticosteroid may be ordered if the child is at risk for allergy. Monitor the child for allergy during the procedure. ■ Remove all metal objects from the body. Only preapproved medical equipment can be in the room. ■ Sedation may be needed to keep the infant or child still. Monitor the child according to protocol. Commonly the examiner can talk with the child via a speaker system to provide information and reassurance.
Nuclear scan or radionuclide imaging A radioactive isotope (an unstable isotope that decays or disintegrates, emitting radiation) is given by mouth or IV which concentrates in certain parts of the body. Scintillation (gamma) camera detectors are used to create a two-dimensional image in gray tones or color. The scans may be taken in several minutes, hours, or 24 hours later. The test may identify a functional (rather than a structural) problem in the bone, brain, gastrointestinal tract, kidney, or thyroid scan, such as hyperthyroidism or hypothyroidism may be diagnosed.	■ Explain the procedure to the parents and child. Inform them that the amount of radiation received from radionuclide imaging is usually less than that received from a radiograph, and that there will be no discomfort. ■ Inform the child and family that radionuclide is excreted from the body in 6–24 hours. ■ The child may be NPO for several hours before the initial scan. ■ The nurse should wear two pairs of disposable gloves when in direct contact with the child's wastes for several hours. Follow agency guidelines for handling waste products.
Polysomnography (sleep study) Electrodes are attached to the head and chest. Recordings of brain activity, eye movement, apnea episodes, oxygen desaturation, and sleep disturbances are taken during sleep over an 8-hour period. The test is used to identify apnea during sleep and to determine the cause of sleep disorders.	■ Instruct the family to keep a sleep log 1–2 weeks prior to sleep studies, including notes about snoring and sleepiness during the day. Review the sleep log. ■ Instruct the patient/family to avoid caffeine products, sedatives, and naps 1–2 days prior to testing. ■ Obtain a history related to medications, head injury, headache, and seizures. ■ Explain the procedure to the parents and child. ■ Monitor vital signs and observe for respiratory distress during the test.
Positron emission tomography (PET) scan and single-photon emission computed tomography (SPECT) PET alone or in combination with CT uses an intravenous radioisotope to measure emission of positive electrons in body organs, such as the brain or heart, or to detect tumors and metastases. PET is effective in evaluating and measuring cerebral blood flow and myocardial perfusion as well as detecting recurrent cancer. SPECT is used to measure blood perfusion in the brain.	■ Monitor vital signs. ■ Start two IVs, one for the radioisotope and the other for serial blood gases. ■ Assess for potential allergies to the radioisotope medium. ■ Prepare the child for the procedure in order to reduce anxiety.
Pulmonary function tests (spirometry) The patient breathes into a spirometer connected to a computer, and the results are analyzed. The vital capacity (maximum amount of air that can be expired after a normal inspiration) and forced expiratory volume (FEV), the percentage of air expired at 1, 2, and 3 seconds, can be calculated. Pulmonary function tests are used to identify the severity of obstructive airway disease.	■ Obtain a list of any bronchodilators and steroids the child is taking. ■ Record the child's age, height, weight, and vital signs. ■ Assess for signs and symptoms of respiratory distress. ■ Explain the purpose of tests and procedures. ■ Help the child to practice breathing patterns required for the test. ■ Take two readings and average the values.
Pulse oximetry Pulse oximetry provides an estimate of the hemoglobin saturated by oxygen, measured percutaneously (SpO_2). It serves as an alternate to the direct measurement of PaO_2 (SaO_2) through arterial blood gas analysis.	■ Explain that the sensor needs to be over a finger or nail bed. ■ Monitor the skin for breakdown under the sensor if it is kept in place for a constant measurement.
Radiograph (x-ray) The most common form of imaging, radiographs use electromagnetic radiation to obtain images of body structures on film for diagnostic purposes. Radiographs are commonly used to detect abnormalities in size, structure, and shape of bone and body structures, or to detect abnormalities of the chest such as air trapping in the alveoli (hyperinflation), consolidation of lung tissue (pneumonia), or lung collapse.	■ Determine if any other radiographic procedures have been performed recently, as the contrast dye used may distort radiograph images. ■ Explain the procedure to the parents and child and the need for a lead apron. Explain that one or more films will be taken in about 5–10 minutes. Explain that modern equipment decreases radiation exposure. ■ Prepare the child. Have the child practice holding still and holding a breath in preparation for the test.

PROCEDURE, DESCRIPTION, AND PURPOSE	NURSING MANAGEMENT
Sweat chloride test Gel pads containing pilocarpine are placed on the child's arms. A small generator attached to the pads stimulates sweating until enough sweat is collected. The arms are covered with plastic. Sweat is analyzed for the concentration of chloride and osmolality. The test is used to diagnose cystic fibrosis.	■ Explain the purpose of the test ■ Explain the need for the child to keep the plastic covering over the lower arms in place for the duration of the test (about 30 minutes).
Tympanogram The procedure provides an estimate of middle ear pressure and an indirect measure of tympanic membrane movement. This helps identify the presence of fluid accumulation in the middle ear.	■ Explain the procedure to the parents and child. The young child should be held still by the parent. ■ Insert the earpiece with the probe into the auditory canal until the canal is sealed tightly. ■ Use the machine according to the manufacturer's instructions. ■ Repeat the test in the other ear.
Ultrasound An ultrasound probe (transducer) is held over the skin or body cavity to transmit ultrasound waves to the tissues and receives deflected sound waves as they bounce off various body structures. The computer transforms the deflected sound waves into two-dimensional scans or audible sounds (Doppler). Ultrasound is a noninvasive procedure used to detect tissue abnormalities.	■ Explain the procedure to the parents and child. Inform them that the procedure is painless, and there is no exposure to radiation. ■ Maintain NPO status preprocedure for abdominal studies. ■ Confirm the child has not received any tests that will interfere with results, e.g., upper GI series. ■ Instruct the child to remain still during the procedure.
Voiding cystourethrogram or radionuclide cystography A cystoscopy procedure is combined with a radionucleotide scan to examine bladder structure and function, urethral anatomy, and bladder masses. The test may detect vesicoureteral reflux.	■ Assess for potential allergies to the radioisotope medium. ■ Explain catheterization to the child and that the bladder will be filled. ■ Provide coaching strategies for parents accompanying the child to help the child cooperate and cope during the test. ■ Encourage fluids after the procedure to flush out the contrast media.

Data from Corbett, J. V. (2008). Laboratory tests and diagnostic procedures with nursing diagnosis (7th ed.). Upper Saddle River, NJ: Pearson Prentice Hall; Kee, J. L. (2010). Laboratory and diagnostic tests with nursing implications (8th ed.). Upper Saddle River, NJ: Pearson; Park, M. (2008). Pediatric cardiology for practitioners (5th ed., pp. 374–375). St. Louis, MO: Mosby; Bindler, R. C., & Ball, J. W. (2012). Clinical skills manual for principles of pediatric nursing: Caring for children (5th ed.). Upper Saddle River, NJ: Pearson.

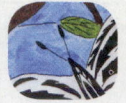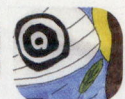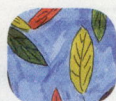

Emergency Assessment and Initial Management

EMERGENCY ASSESSMENT OF THE CHILD
Initial Assessment

An initial assessment begins as soon as the child comes in to view. It is important to gain an initial impression of the severity of the child's condition. Experienced healthcare providers use visual and auditory clues (based on appearance, breathing effort, and circulation of the skin) to make a rapid judgment about the urgency of the child's condition. This may take only 5 to 10 seconds to perform. It is not necessary to touch or disturb the child to make these assessments.

Appearance

Before touching the child, quickly look at the following characteristics and behavior of the infant or child:

- Observe for alertness, eye contact and interaction with parent or caregiver, and interest in toys or objects.
- Observe for spontaneous movement and good muscle tone.
- Observe consolability.
- Note quality of speech or cry.

Be concerned when the infant or child does not make eye contact with the parent or caregiver, is uninterested in toys or objects, is limp or flaccid, is inconsolable, or has a weak, hoarse, or muffled cry.

Breathing Effort

Increased effort associated with breathing indicates an attempt by the child to overcome hypoxia, especially when some airway obstruction or problem with ventilation exists.

- Observe for nasal flaring, retractions, and head bobbing.
- Listen for abnormal airway sounds such as stridor, wheezing, grunting, snoring, or muffled or hoarse speech.
- Observe for tripod positioning, sitting with the head and neck extended, or refusal to lie down.

Presence of any of the signs may be associated with respiratory distress.

Practice Alert

If the infant or child is not responsive and not breathing (gasping is not breathing), check the pulse for 10 seconds. If no pulse is detected, begin cardiopulmonary resuscitation. See page 1383.

Circulation of the Skin

Constriction of the blood vessels occurs when the child has reduced circulating blood volume due to hemorrhage or dehydration. This action shifts blood flow to the vital organs to keep them oxygenated.

- Observe the color of the skin and mucous membranes.
- Inspecting the mucous membranes is especially important in children of darker skin because the mucous membranes are usually pink, regardless of skin color.

Pallor is an early sign of poor tissue perfusion. Mottling, caused by constriction of the blood vessels to the skin, indicates poor tissue perfusion (Figure F–1 ■). Cyanosis, a blue discoloration of the skin and mucous membranes, indicates severely impaired tissue perfusion.

Forming an Initial Impression

To make a judgment about the child's physiologic stability, consider all the findings from the child's appearance, breathing effort, and circulation of the skin. The child's condition is more serious when a larger number of abnormal findings are present. See Figure F–2 ■ for an example of an infant with poor physiologic stability that is characterized by an insecure airway, respiratory distress, impaired circulation, or unresponsiveness.

When the initial impression of a child's condition indicates an emergency due to an injury or acute medical condition, the sequence of assessment is changed to quickly identify the presence of a life-threatening condition. This sequence is focused on recognizing physiologic changes that require immediate care to save the child's life. The physiologic body functions that are most critical for survival are assessed first:

- *A*irway (for example, if the child's airway is obstructed, no oxygen can enter the child's system)
- *B*reathing (for example, if there is damage to the child's lungs or the bronchioles are constricted, the child may be unable to ventilate and support gas exchange)

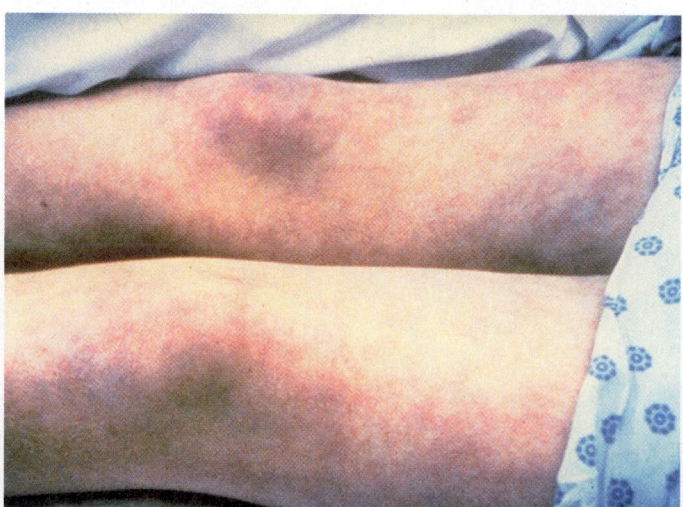

FIGURE F–1 ■ Mottling of the skin indicates vasoconstriction and poor tissue perfusion.
Source: *Courtesy of Health Resources and Services Administration, Maternal and Child Health Bureau, EMSC Program.*

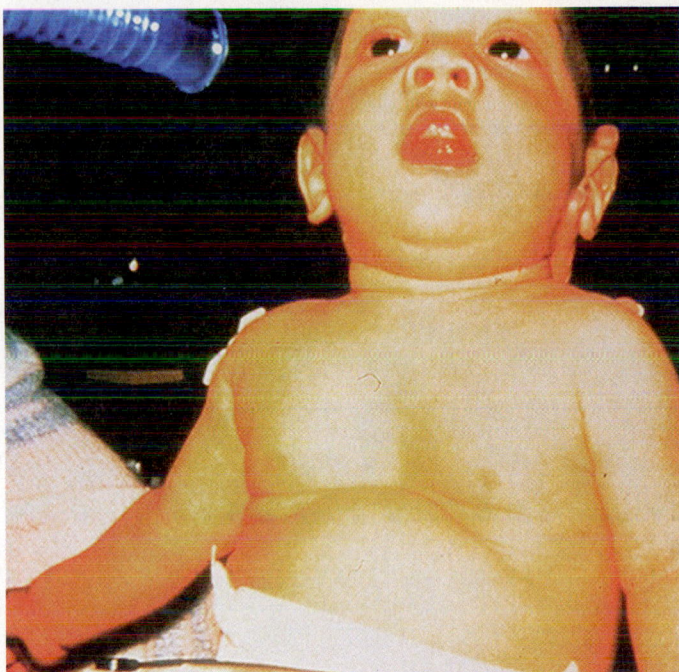

FIGURE F–2 ■ Using the initial assessment of appearance, breathing effort, and circulation of the skin, this infant is determined to have an emergency condition. *What are the visual clues that resulted in that assessment?*
Source: *Courtesy of Health Resources and Services Administration, Maternal and Child Health Bureau, EMSC Program.*

■ Circulation (for example, hemorrhage may reduce blood volume to the extent that it is inadequate to circulate oxygen to the brain and other vital organs)

As soon as a potential life-threatening physiologic condition is identified, the assessment is interrupted to provide the needed lifesaving care. Only when the physiologic condition is stabilized does the nurse continue on to the next physiologic assessment, or on to assessment of other body systems. When a child has an emergency condition, the physiologic status of the airway, breathing, and circulation are assessed frequently (every 5 minutes) because the child's condition can change and deteriorate rapidly.

ASSESSING THE ABCs

Airway Assessment

Is the infant or child crying or talking?	Crying or talking indicates an open airway at that point in time.
Are any airway sounds heard?	Airway sounds may indicate an upper or lower airway obstruction due to a foreign body, inflammation, secretions, or blood.
Could the tongue be blocking the airway?	When a child is unresponsive and lying supine, the tongue can fall back into the pharynx and obstruct the airway.
Is there rhythmic chest rise and abdominal movement?	Periodic and synchronized chest and abdominal rise indicate movement of air within the airway.

Airway Management

Take immediate actions to open the airway if the child is not breathing or if the airway is obstructed.

■ Perform a head tilt–chin lift maneuver to lift the tongue out of the pharynx. Use a jaw thrust maneuver only if the child has a head or neck injury. See Figure F–3 ■ for guidance in performing those maneuvers.

■ An oropharyngeal or nasopharyngeal airway may be inserted to maintain the airway in an unconscious child. Secretions and blood should be gently suctioned to clear the airway.

■ If the chest does not rise and fall, perform rescue breathing (using a mouth-to-mouth and nose barrier device) and give two slow breaths. A bag-valve mask can be used by trained health professionals.

If the chest does not rise, check the child's head position with the chin lift or jaw thrust. Give two slow breaths again. If the chest does not rise, initiate procedures for removing a foreign body obstruction.

Clinical Tip

An endotracheal tube may be inserted by trained healthcare providers to maintain and secure the airway. Capnography or end-tidal CO_2 monitoring may be used to confirm endotracheal tube placement. See the Skills Manual 🔗. Once placement is confirmed, the tube is secured and the level of the tube at the teeth is recorded. The nurse monitors endotracheal tube placement to make sure it does not become dislodged from the trachea.

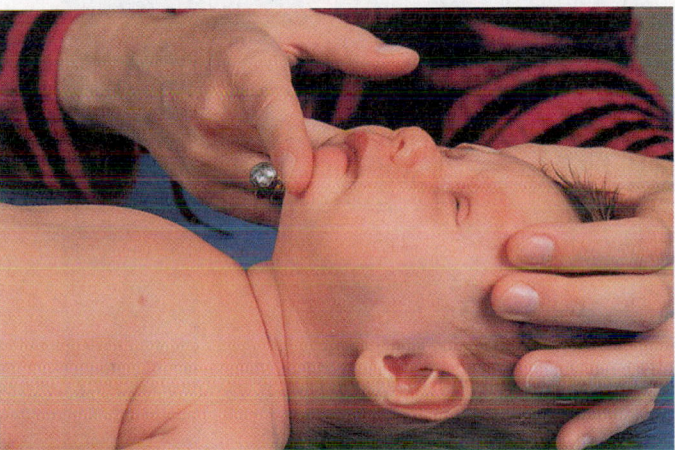

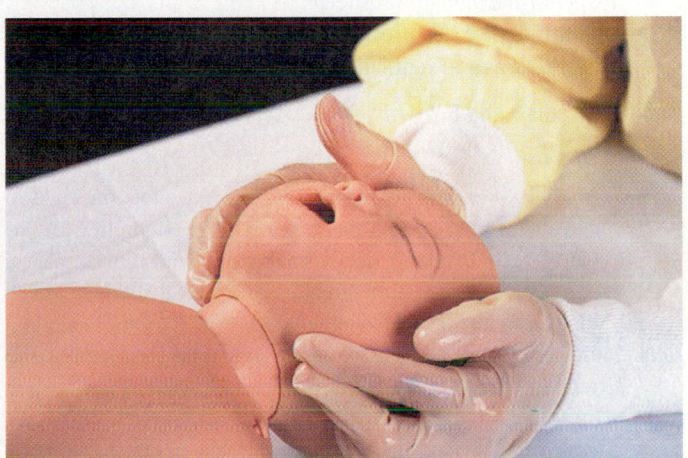

FIGURE F–3 ■ Opening the airway of an infant. For both techniques place the child's head in sniffing position (as if to move your head forward slightly to smell a flower). Avoid hyperextending the neck. Place a small towel under the shoulders of an infant and young child to maintain the head position. This helps offset the child's large occiput. *A,* Perform the chin lift by tilting the head back (as described) and lifting the chin up and out. *B,* Perform the jaw thrust by placing two fingers under each side of the jaw at its angle and lifting the jaw upward and outward.

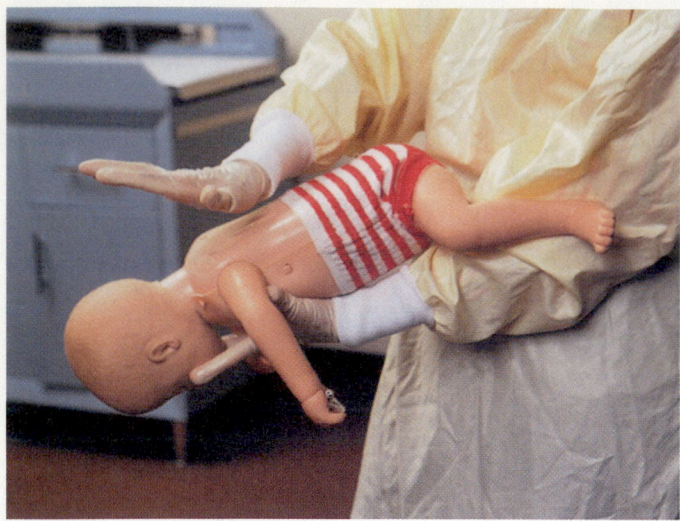

A

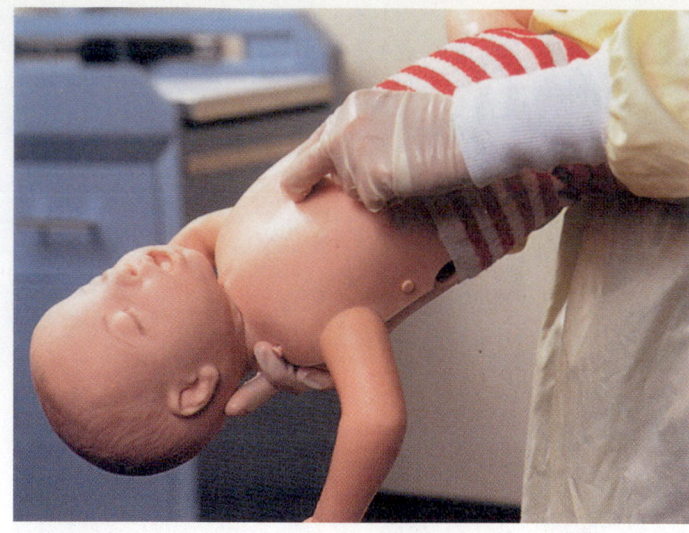

B

FIGURE F–4 ■ *A,* Position for back blows (slaps); *B,* Hand position for chest compressions in an infant with a foreign body airway obstruction or for cardiopulmonary resuscitation.

Removing a Foreign Body Obstruction

Follow the most current guidelines for severe foreign body obstruction and cardiopulmonary resuscitation (CPR) from the American Heart Association (Berg, Schexnayder, Chameides, et al., 2010).

Infant

- Position the infant face down on your arm supporting the head.
- Perform five back blows (slaps) with the heel of the hand between the infant's shoulder blades. Then rotate the infant to be face up on your forearm.
- Give five chest compressions, placing the fingers in the same position used for CPR (Figure F–4 ■).
- Repeat this sequence until the object is expelled or the infant becomes unresponsive. If the infant becomes unresponsive, start CPR (do not perform a pulse check).
- After 30 compressions, place your index finger on the bony prominence of the infant's chin and your thumb in the mouth on the tongue. Pull up and out to open the mouth. Look in the infant's mouth for the foreign body and remove it if seen. *Do not perform a blind finger sweep.*
- Attempt to give two breaths and continue with cycles of chest compressions and ventilations until the object is expelled.

Child Between 1 and 8 Years

Conscious Child

- When the child's airway obstruction is mild, allow the child to cough and assume a position of comfort while attempting to clear the airway. If the obstruction is severe (the child cannot make a sound), perform subdiaphragmatic abdominal thrusts (Heimlich maneuver) with the child in either a sitting or standing position.
- Stand behind the child, with your arms under the child's axillae and around the chest. Place the thumb of one fist against the abdomen in the midline, under the xiphoid process and above the umbilicus.
- Grasp your fist with the other hand. Deliver up to five quick upward thrusts against the abdomen (Figure F–5 ■). Each thrust should be a distinct effort to remove the obstruction.
- After the thrusts, assess the ability of the child to breathe. Repeat the series of five thrusts until the obstruction is cleared.

Unconscious Child

- If the child becomes unconscious, move the child to the floor to begin CPR with chest compressions (do not perform a pulse check). See page 1383.

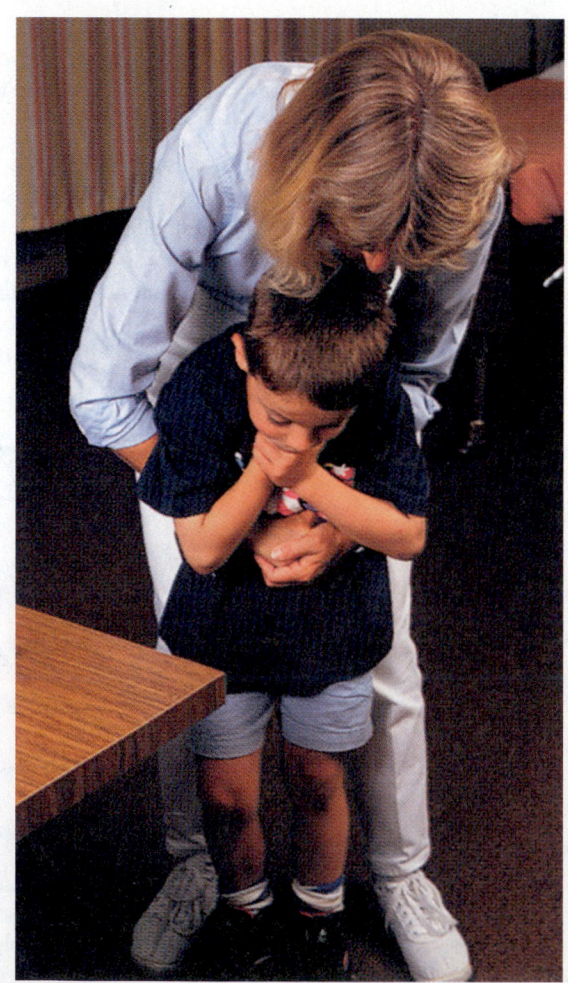

FIGURE F–5 ■ Hand positioning for abdominal thrusts when the child is standing.

- After 30 compressions open the mouth to look for an object in the pharynx. Remove the object if seen, but do not perform a blind finger sweep.
- Attempt to give two breaths and continue the cycles of chest compressions and ventilations until the object is expelled.

Additional information about management of the child with a foreign body airway obstruction, croup, or asthma can be found in Chapter 25 🔗.

Breathing Assessment

What is the effort associated with breathing?	The presence of retractions, nasal flaring, stridor, wheezing, or grunting is a sign of respiratory distress. Periodic gasping is not breathing.
What is the respiratory rate and how does it compare with the expected rate by age?	See Table F–1 for expected respiratory rates by age. A rate higher than expected may be a sign of respiratory distress, especially when accompanied by increased breathing effort. A rate that is consistently higher than 60 breaths per minute is abnormal. An inadequate or decreasing respiratory rate accompanied by altered level of consciousness is a sign of respiratory failure (Kleinman, Chameides, Schexnayder, et al., 2010).
What sounds are heard when auscultating the chest?	Absent or decreased breath sounds with respiratory effort are associated with an airway obstruction such as asthma or a foreign body. Identify any adventitious sounds such as wheezes, crackles, grunting, and rhonchi. Adventitious sounds may indicate an injury, aspiration, or inflammatory process.
Is there a penetrating chest injury? Are marks on the chest present that indicate an injury? Are there any rib fractures?	Any obvious openings on the anterior and posterior chest wall, and sounds that could be air sucked into or escaping from the chest, are indications of a penetrating chest injury. An open chest wound can develop into a life-threatening tension pneumothorax (see Chapter 25 🔗). Bruises on the chest wall may indicate a deeper injury to the lung tissue such as a pulmonary contusion or pneumothorax. Rib fractures are uncommon in children, but if present interfere with the ability to adequately ventilate the child.

Breathing Management

High-concentration oxygen is provided to most infants and children with emergency conditions. A nonrebreather mask has a face mask and a reservoir bag that enables delivery of up to 95% oxygen at a flow rate of 10 to 15 L/min when the mask maintains a tight seal on the face (Berg et al., 2010). High-concentration oxygen can also be

TABLE F–1   Normal Respiratory Rate Ranges by Age

AGE	RESPIRATORY RATE PER MINUTE
Newborn	30–55
1 year	25–40
3 years	20–30
6 years	16–22
10 years	16–20
17 years	12–18

delivered through a bag-valve mask (used to assist ventilations). In some cases, low-concentration oxygen is provided to the infant or child using a simple face mask, nasal cannula, or blow-by tubing. See the Skills Manual 🔗 for additional information.

Assisted Ventilation

When the child has minimal or no respiratory effort, assisted ventilation is initiated with a bag-valve mask.

- Select the appropriate size mask for the child, one that extends from the bridge of the nose to the cleft of the chin.
- Select the appropriate size resuscitation bag to ensure that adequate tidal volume is delivered. A pediatric bag has a volume of 450 to 500 mL, while an adult bag has a volume of 1000 mL.
- Connect the bag to the oxygen tubing and set the flow rate at 15 mL/min.
- Apply the mask to the face and get an airtight seal. Hold the mask securely to the face to maintain the seal. Form a C with the thumb and index finger to hold the mask securely over the face to cause an airtight seal. Place the remaining fingers of the hand against the mandible to secure the mask to the face (Figure F–6 ■).
- When assisting ventilation with the resuscitation bag, give the breath slowly over one second using only enough force to make

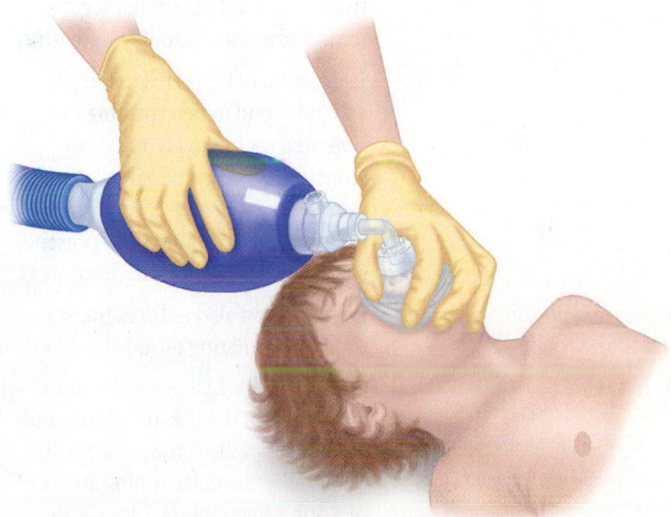

FIGURE F–6 ■ Proper placement of the hand to hold the mask of a resuscitation bag. Note the C formed by the thumb and index finger and the three fingers forming an E on the mandible to become the E-C clamp. This helps promote a tight seal with the face and prevents the remaining fingers from occluding the airway by pressing on the soft tissue of the neck.

the chest rise. If the chest does not rise, reopen the airway and make sure the seal is tight between the face and the mask. Then attempt ventilation again.

- Avoid hyperventilation; ventilate at a rate of 12 to 20 breaths per minute when the infant or child has a heart rate that is greater than or equal to 60 beats per minute. During CPR, the assisted ventilation rate is approximately 8 to 10 breaths per minute (Berg et al., 2010).

Excessive assisted ventilation often causes gastric distention because more air is forced into the airway than is needed to inflate the lungs. The extra air enters the stomach, and over a short period of time the stomach becomes distended and presses against the diaphragm. A nasogastric or orogastric tube may be inserted to keep the stomach deflated and improve ventilation. The nasogastric tube also reduces the risk for vomiting which can compromise the airway.

Managing a Chest Injury

An open chest wound is immediately covered with an occlusive dressing and taped on three sides. This prevents air from entering the chest while permitting an outlet for air escaping from the chest. A chest tube is inserted when a pneumothorax is present to reduce the elevated pressure in the chest and to help reinflate the lung. See the Skills Manual ⊂⊃ for information on assisting with chest tube insertion. Additional information for the management of respiratory conditions and injuries, such as croup, asthma, and pneumothorax, can be found in Chapter 25 ℰ.

Circulatory Assessment

What is the circulation to the skin?	When the skin is warm and the child's color is pink, tissue perfusion is good. Cool extremities accompanied by pallor, mottling, or cyanosis is associated with poor tissue perfusion.
What is the capillary refill time?	Delayed capillary refill, greater than 2 seconds, is associated with poor tissue perfusion. See Chapter 7 ℰ for assessment of capillay refill time.
Is there any bleeding or potential internal bleeding? How much blood has been lost?	Estimation of blood loss from all sites is helpful in determining the potential for hypovolemic shock. Consider if there could be bleeding into the chest or abdomen from the type of injury sustained and presence of bruises or abrasions in those areas.
Is the child possibly dehydrated?	Dehydration also reduces the volume of circulating blood.
What is the heart rate?	Check the brachial pulse in infants and the carotid pulse in children and adolescents. Check the pulse for 10 seconds before determining absence of a pulse. See Table F–2 for the expected heart rates by age. A sustained and increasing heart rate greater than 130 beats per minute in a child is associated with continuing blood loss and hypovolemia.

Are the peripheral pulses palpable?	Weak peripheral pulses compared to central pulses may be an indication of early hypovolemic shock. When the peripheral pulses cannot be palpated and the central pulses are weak, the child is in uncompensated hypovolemic shock.
What is the child's skin temperature and color?	Cool, cold, or pale skin is an indicator of poor tissue perfusion, and an early sign of hypovolemic shock.
What is the child's mental status?	Deteriorating mental status is an indication that the brain is not being perfused, and hypoxia and uncompensated shock are present.
What is the child's blood pressure?	See Appendix B ℰ for expected blood pressure by age, height percentiles, and gender. Children are able to maintain their blood pressure by constricting blood vessels, until blood volume loss exceeds their ability to compensate. A falling systolic blood pressure or hypotension is a significant sign of uncompensated shock. Hypotension is described as the following (Kleinman et al., 2010):

- Less than 60 mmHg in newborns up to 28 days
- Less than 70 mmHg in infants (1 to 12 months)
- Less than 70 mmHg 1 (2 × age in years) for children (1 to 10 years)
- Less than 90 mmHg for children 10 years and older

Circulation Management

When bradycardia (a heart rate of 60 beats per minute or less) and poor perfusion of the tissues (e.g., pallor, mottling, or cyanosis) are present, provide oxygen and assist ventilations as described under the breathing management section.

- Attach a cardiorespiratory monitor to the child and monitor the heart rate during interventions to see if the heart rate increases and stabilizes.
- An intravenous line is established to provide medications that stimulate and support myocardial function, as well as to treat arrhythmias and to correct metabolic acidosis. See the

TABLE F–2	Normal Heart Rate Ranges by Age
AGE	**HEART RATE RANGE (BEATS/MIN)**
Newborn	100–150
Infant to 2 years	80–120
2–6 years	70–110
6–10 years	60–95
10–16 years	60–85

commonly used resuscitation drugs in the Medications table on page 1384. Monitor the blood pressure, heart rate, and ECG continuously during drug interventions.

- If an IV line cannot be started, but an endotracheal tube is in place, small amounts of medication can be administered down the endotracheal tube.

If no response to oxygen and ventilation is noted, begin chest compressions as cardiac arrest is imminent (Berg et al., 2010).

Cardiopulmonary Resuscitation

If no pulse can be palpated within 10 seconds or the pulse rate is less than 60 beats per minute in an infant or child with poor tissue perfusion, cardiac compressions are initiated using American Heart Association guidelines (Berg et al., 2010).

Infants

- Place the child on a firm surface. Give 30 rapid chest compressions (rate of 100 compressions a minute) before initiating ventilations (if a single rescuer). Two rescuers should initiate 15 compressions before ventilations.
  - For newborns and small infants, place the two thumbs over the lower sternum and encircle the hands around the chest when two rescuers are present. The thumbs compress the sternum and the fingers squeeze the thorax. A single rescuer should use two fingers on the lower sternum, one finger's width below the nipple line. Avoid pressure over the xiphoid process.
  - For children, position the heel of one or two hands (one hand over the other) at about the nipple line for compressions.
- Perform chest compressions pushing with enough pressure to depress the chest by one third of its anterior-posterior diameter (1½ inches [4 cm] in infants and 2 inches [5 cm] in children). Allow the chest to fully recoil after each compression by lifting the fingers or heel of the hand slightly. Minimize interruptions during compressions.
- Open the airway and have the second rescuer maintain the open airway position while providing rescue breaths.
  - Position the infant or child on its back while supporting the head and neck. Open the airway by performing a chin lift—tilt the head back and lift the chin up and out.
  - If the child is suspected of having a cervical spine injury, open the airway by performing a jaw thrust—from a position behind the infant's head, place two or three fingers under each side of the jaw at its angle and lift the jaw upward and outward.
  - A visible chest rise should be seen with each ventilation. If the chest does not rise with ventilation, reposition the head and try again. If the chest still does not rise, perform the procedure for choking (see page 1380).
- Initiate ventilations after 30 compressions for a single rescuer or 15 compressions for two rescuers. When one rescuer is present, the compression to ventilation ratio is 30:2 for infants and children. For two rescuers the ratio is 15:2.
  - Give rescue breaths, about 1 second each, making the chest rise visibly. Seal your lips or mouth to the barrier device around the child's mouth or around the infant's mouth and nose.

- Compressions should be paused for rescue breaths, but interruptions should be minimal.
- When an advanced airway (endotracheal tube or tracheostomy tube) has been inserted, give 8 to 10 ventilations a minute without interrupting compressions.
- Begin using a bag-mask resuscitator hooked up to oxygen (flow rate of 10 to 15 L/min) as soon as possible. Ensure that the mask is the correct size, extending from the bridge of the nose to the cleft of the chin, and tightly sealed. Avoid excessive ventilations. Give each breath slowly over 1 second using only enough force to make the chest rise.
- Continue coordination of compressions and ventilations. Rescuers should rotate the compression role every 2 minutes, making the switch in about 5 seconds.
- Use an automated external defibrillator or manual defibrillator as soon as available for the patient with a sudden witnessed collapse. The shock causes a sudden depolarization of the myocardial cells and terminates the ventricular fibrillation rhythm long enough for a more organized myocardial rhythm to start.
  - Minimize interruption of chest compressions by continuing them until the defibrillator is ready to deliver the shock.
  - Apply child-size pads or child paddles as directed by the equipment manual for any child between 1 and 8 years. Apply adult pads or paddles for any child over age 8 years as directed by the equipment manual (Figure F–7 ■).
  - For the first shock, apply 2 joules/kg, and immediately follow with chest compressions and ventilations. The rhythm is then rechecked. A second shock of 4 joules/kg is given if needed.
  - After each shock has been given, immediately resume CPR. Resuscitation medications are also given.
- If the infant or child has a return of both pulse and respirations and is not a trauma patient, place the child in the side-lying position to protect the airway in case of vomiting. See the Medications table on page 1385 for drugs used in the postresuscitation and stabilization period.

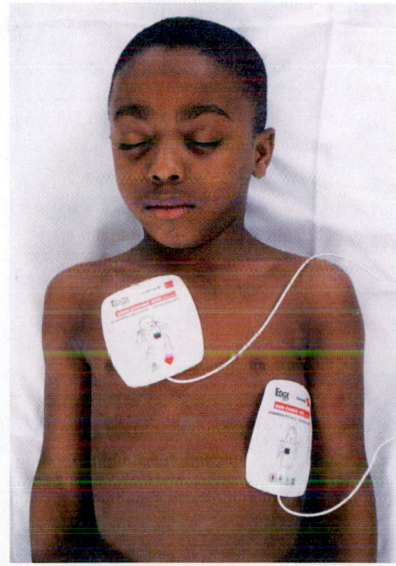

FIGURE F–7 ■ Proper placement of pads for defibrillation on the child. One pad is on the right chest under the clavicle. The pad on the left chest is below the nipple line on the ribs so that the heart is positioned between the two pads.

Medications Used for Cardiac Arrest and Symptomatic Arrhythmias

DRUG	DOSAGE (PEDIATRIC)	NURSING MANAGEMENT
Adenosine	0.1 mg/kg (maximum dose: 6 mg) Repeat dose: 0.2 mg/kg (maximum dose: 12 mg)	■ Rapid IV/IO bolus followed by normal saline flush to push drug to central circulation. ■ May cause hypotension, transient bradycardia, or asystole, so monitor the ECG.
Amiodarone	5 mg/kg IV/IO push bolus for VF and pulseless VT; may repeat twice up to 15 mg/kg maximum dose Maximum single dose: 300 mg	■ Rapid IV bolus if the patient has VF or pulseless VT. ■ Should not be used in combination with another drug that prolongs the QT interval. ■ Monitor ECG continuously and blood pressure frequently, hypotension is a common side effect.
Atropine sulfate	0.02 mg/kg, IV/IO 0.04–0.06 mg/kg, ET Minimum dose: 0.1 mg Maximum single dose: 0.5 mg Higher dose may be used for organophosphate poisoning.	■ Use for symptomatic bradycardia and rapid sequence intubation. ■ Tachycardia, hypotension, and pupil dilation may occur. Distorts pupil exam in children with a brain injury.
Calcium chloride 10% (100 mg/mL)	20 mg/kg (0.2 mL/kg) IV/IO Maximum dose: 2 g	■ Give slowly IV push preferably using a central vein. ■ Use during cardiac arrest only when hypocalcemia, calcium channel blocker overdose, hypermagnesemia, or hyperkalemia is documented. ■ Hypotension and bradycardia may occur.
Dextrose (glucose) (10% or 25% or 50%)	0.5–1 g/kg IV/IO ■ 5–10 mL/kg 10% dextrose for newborns ■ 2–4 mL/kg 25% dextrose for infants and children ■ 1–2 mL/kg 50% dextrose for adolescents	■ Hypoglycemia may result due to high glucose needs and low glycogen stores. ■ Use during cardiac arrest only if hypoglycemia is documented by a rapid glucose test.
Epinephrine (1:10,000 and 1:1000)	0.01 mg/kg (0.1 mL/kg with 1:10,000), IV/IO, repeat every 3–5 minutes 0.1 mg/kg (0.1 mL/kg with 1:1000), ET Maximum dose is 1 mg IV/IO; 2.5 mg ET	■ At doses used during resuscitation, causes vasoconstriction that increases coronary artery perfusion and tachycardia. ■ For endotracheal administration, dilute medication with 5 mL of normal saline and follow with five positive-pressure ventilations. ■ May cause tachyarrhythmias, hypertension.
Lidocaine	Bolus loading dose is 1 mg/kg IV/IO followed by infusion of 20–50 mcg/kg per minute	■ Suppresses ventricular arrhythmias. May be used for VF and pulseless VT and rapid sequence intubation.
Magnesium sulfate	25–50 mg/kg IV/IO in infusion over 10–20 minutes Maximum dose: 2 g	■ Rapid IV infusion for pulseless VT with *torsades de pointes* (a VT rhythm with a long QT interval). ■ Also used with documented hypomagnesemia. ■ May cause hypotension if administered rapidly.
Procainamide	15 mg/kg IV/IO, infuse slowly over 30–60 minutes	■ Monitor the blood pressure and ECG as drug may prolong the QT interval or heart block. ■ Used for perfusing tachyarrhythmias. ■ Do not use in combination with amiodarone (or other drugs prolonging QT interval).
Sodium bicarbonate	1 mEq/kg per dose IV/IO, infuse slowly.	■ Not used routinely during resuscitation, but may be used for some toxicologic emergencies. ■ Ensure adequate ventilation. ■ Irrigate IV/IO tubing with normal saline before and after infusion.

IV, intravenous; IO, intraosseous; ECG, electrocardiogram; ET, endotracheal; SQ, subcutaneous; VT, ventricular tachycardia; VF, ventricular fibrillation; SVT, supraventricular tachycardia

Source: *Adapted from Kleinman, M. E., Chameides, L., Schexnayder, S. M., Samson, R. A., Hazinski, M. F., . . . Zaritsky, A. L. (2010). Pediatric advanced life support. Circulation, 122(Suppl. 3), S876–S908.*

Medications Used to Maintain Cardiac Output and for Postresuscitation Stabilization

MEDICATION	DOSE RANGE	COMMENT
Dobutamine	2–20 mcg/kg per minute IV/IO, titrated to desired effect	Used to improve cardiac output and blood pressure due to poor myocardial function. Do not mix with sodium bicarbonate.
Dopamine	2–20 mcg/kg per minute, IV/IO	Used to treat shock that is not responsive to fluids and when systemic vascular resistance is low. Higher doses than recommended may cause too much vasoconstriction. Do not mix with sodium bicarbonate.
Epinephrine	0.1–1 mcg/kg per minute, IV/IO	This drug needs to be titrated for the desired response, either tachycardia and decreased systemic vascular resistance at lower doses or vasoconstriction at higher doses.
Inamrinone	0.75–1 mg/kg, IV/IO given as a slow loading dose bolus over 5 minutes; may be repeated twice; then given as an infusion at 5–10 mcg/kg per minute	Used to augment cardiac output. Fluids must be infused to manage vasodilation effects to prevent hypotension.
Milrinone	IV/IO loading dose: 50 mcg/kg, IV/IO, given as a slow loading dose bolus over 10–60 minutes; then given as an infusion: 0.25–0.75 mcg/kg per minute	Used to augment cardiac output. Fluids must be infused to manage vasodilation effects to prevent hypotension.
Norepinephrine	0.1–2 mcg/kg per minute infusion, IV/IO; titrated to desired effect	Used to treat shock when low vascular resistance exists that is unresponsive to fluids. Do not mix with sodium bicarbonate.
Sodium nitroprusside	0.5–1 mcg/kg per minute infusion, IV/IO; then titrate to desired effect up to 8 mcg/kg per minute	Increases cardiac output by decreasing vascular resistance. Fluid administration may be needed when vasodilation causes hypotension. Prepare only in D5W. Wrap container with opaque cover to protect drug from exposure to sunlight during administration.

IV indicates intravenous; IO, intraosseous.

Source: *Adapted from Kleinman, M. E., Chameides, L., Schexnayder, S. M., Samson, R. A., Hazinski, M. F., . . . Zaritsky, A. L. (2010). Pediatric advanced life support.* Circulation, 122*(Suppl. 3), S876–S908.*

Hypovolemic Shock

See the Clinical Manifestations table on page 857 for signs of hypovolemic shock.

Control bleeding with direct pressure using a gloved hand and elevate the body part if it is safe to do so. In the case of hemorrhage, apply pressure to an arterial pressure point proximal to the injury to slow the flow of bleeding.

Two intravenous lines are usually established when the child has signs of severe or *uncompensated shock* (signs of shock plus a drop in the systolic blood pressure). An intraosseous or central venous line may be used if peripheral lines cannot be obtained easily. A bolus (20 mL/kg) of crystalloid fluids (lactated Ringer's or normal saline) is administered quickly (over 5 to 20 minutes) to increase the volume of circulating blood so that remaining blood can get to and oxygenate the vital organs. The heart rate, capillary refill, and responsiveness are reassessed frequently over the next 5 to 15 minutes to determine the child's response to the extra fluid volume and to determine the need for additional crystalloid IV fluid, albumin, or blood. Additional fluids or blood are given until the circulatory system is stabilized. See Chapter 28 🔗 for blood administration guidelines. Drugs used to support the child in shock are listed in the Medications table above. Additional information for the management of the child with dehydration and hypovolemic shock can be found in Chapters 23 and 26 🔗.

Disability (Neurologic) Assessment

What is the infant's or child's level of responsiveness using AVPU? What is the Glasgow Coma Scale score?	See Box F–1 and Table 33–5 🔗 for assessment guidelines. When the child is alert or responsive to verbal stimuli, a mild injury or condition may be present. When the child is responsive only to pain or unresponsive, a severe injury or condition is usually present.
Check the pupils for size, symmetry, and reactivity to light.	Dilated or asymmetric pupils that do not react to light may indicate the development of increased intracranial pressure. Pupillary response may also be abnormal in the presence of drugs, seizures, or hypoxia.
Has the child had a seizure?	Seizures may happen when the infant or child has had a brain injury or a hypoxic event. Seizures may also be due to hypoglycemia or a metabolic disorder.

Is the child moving spontaneously? Is the child flaccid? Is any abnormal posturing present? Spontaneous movement of the extremities is a positive sign of neurologic integrity. Limpness accompanied by decreased responsiveness may indicate hypoxia or a brain injury. Total loss of flexor and extensor tone may indicate a spinal cord injury. Flexor or extensor posturing indicates a significant brain injury.

Disability Management

Initial management of the child with a severe brain injury is to provide supplemental oxygen with assisted ventilation at the normal respiratory rate for the infant or child for the first 24 hours. See Chapter 33 🔗 for management of the child with a brain injury.

When a seizure occurs following a brain injury or other hypoxic event, a benzodiazepine medication is usually administered. See Chapter 33 🔗 for management of the child with a seizure.

If spinal cord injury is suspected, immobilize the head in neutral position and prevent movement of other parts of the body. This helps protect the child from additional injury. Radiographs and often CT scanning are required to determine if a spinal cord injury is present.

Exposure

Full Body Inspection

When the child's condition is stabilized, a rapid inspection of the entire body is conducted to identify any additional injuries such as fractures of the extremities or soft tissue injuries. Check for the presence of pulses in extremities distal to the injury. Any object impaling a part of the body is stabilized in place until it can be surgically removed. Assess the child's pain level.

Temperature Management

Temperature control is important in children who have experienced an emergency. Remember that infants and children have a larger body surface area and lose body heat quickly if skin surface is exposed. Often the clothes have been removed to assess and provide treatment. Keep the child warm with heat lamps and warmed IV fluids. Maintaining a neutral temperature is beneficial for management of the child's emergency condition.

HISTORY

An abbreviated history of the event leading to the emergency is collected from the parent, caregiver, or witness by another healthcare provider while the emergency assessment and resuscitation is occurring. The acronym for the key elements of this history is SAMPLE:

- *Signs and symptoms*—onset and nature of the symptoms
- *Allergies*—any known allergies

BOX F–1	Assessment of Responsiveness

When initially checking the responsiveness of infants, the acronym AVPU provides a method for rapid assessment:

Alert, responds to parents, cuddles, coos or babbles, smiles
Verbal, responds to verbal stimulation
Pain, responds to painful stimulation only
Unresponsive to painful stimulation

- *Medications*—names and doses of prescribed and over-the-counter medications, including aerosol medications and complementary therapies
- *Past medical problems*—any significant health conditions, past hospitalizations, immunizations
- *Last food or liquid*—when the infant or child last ate or had liquids, including breast or bottle feeding
- *Events leading to the injury or illness*—progression of illness over time, activities contributing to injury

QUICK REVIEW

- Use the initial assessment guidelines to quickly identify the need for emergency intervention.
- Always start by ensuring that the child has a patent airway.
- Assess breathing and provide assisted ventilation as needed.
- Check the circulation and intervene as needed with chest compressions or IV fluids.
- Repeat the assessment of ABCs every 5 minutes and intervene immediately if any deterioration in status is noted.
- Continue with other parts of the physical examination only when the infant's or child's condition is stabilized.

REFERENCES

Berg, M. D., Schexnayder, S. M., Chameides, L., Terry, M., Donoghue, A., . . . Hazinski, M. F. (2010). Pediatric basic life support. *Circulation, 122*(Suppl. 3), S862–S875.

Kleinman, M. E., Chameides, L., Schexnayder, S. M., Samson, R. A., Hazinsky, M. F., . . . Zaritsky, A. L. (2010). Pediatric advanced life support. *Circulation, 122*(Suppl. 3), S876–S908.

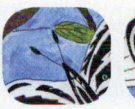
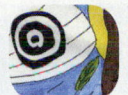
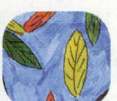

Body Surface Area Nomogram

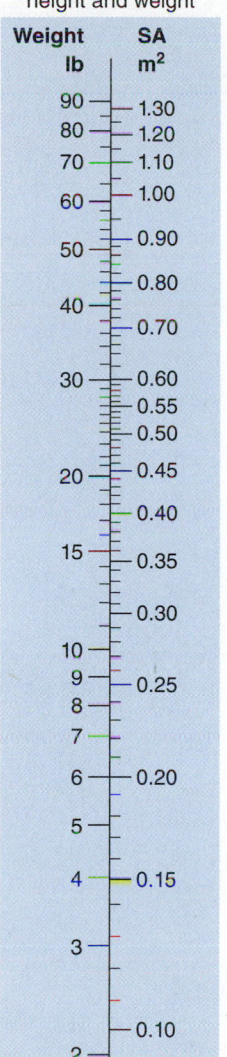

Nomogram
for child with proportional
height and weight

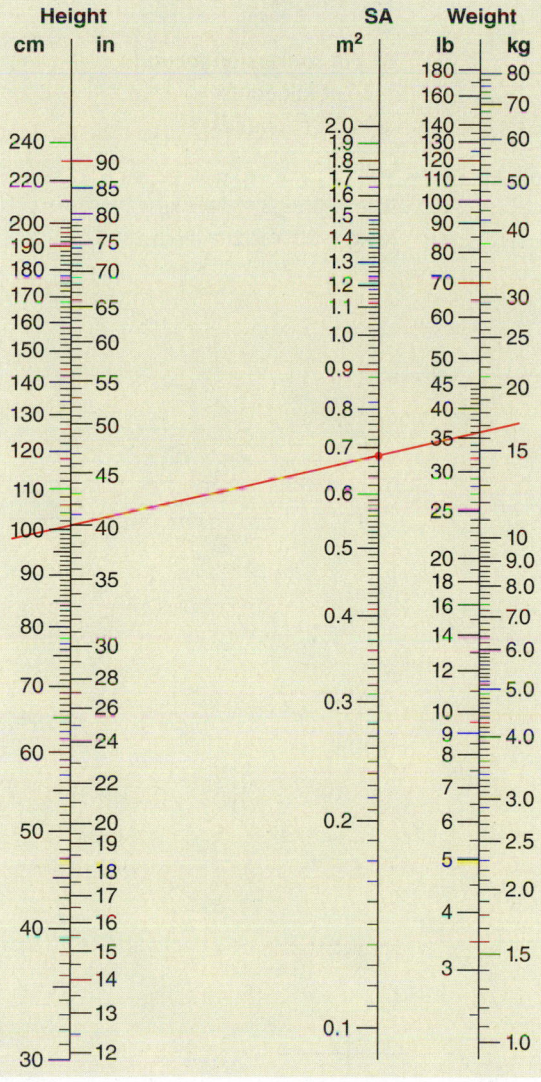

Nomogram
for child with varied
height and weight percentiles

The proportion between height and weight in children is different from the proportion in adults. These differences are most manifest in newborns, infants, and young children. Therefore, dosages of drugs that have been established for adults cannot simply be reduced and correspondingly be safe for young children. Weight is used as a better method of calculating drug dosage in children and is used when medications have a dose of drug recommended in mg/kg.

However, weight alone is not always accurate as a method of calculating a drug dosage for a child. Another more accurate method is that of body surface area (BSA). BSA is a relationship of height to weight and is measured in square meters. BSA increases about 7 times from birth to adulthood, and is a good reflection of many physiologic processes significant in metabolizing, transporting, and eliminating drugs, such as metabolic rate, extracellular fluid and total fluid volumes, cardiac output, and glomerular filtration rate. BSA is calculated by the formula:

$$\text{Surface area}(m^2) = \sqrt{\frac{\text{height (cm)} \times \text{weight (kg)}}{3600}}$$

A nomogram or graph has been developed to calculate BSA quickly and accurately. The nomogram on the left can be used when a child has height and weight in proportion, or in the same percentile range. (See Chapter 19 for description of growth and percentiles.) When the percentiles for height and weight differ, the nomogram on the right can be used. To calculate the BSA, draw a straight line from the height to the weight. The point at which this line intersects the surface area (SA) column is the BSA in square meters. Medications that are prescribed using the BSA are dosed in mg/m².

Appendix H

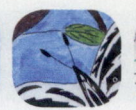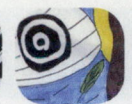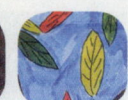

Temperature and Weight Conversion

°C	°F
35	95
35.2	95.4
35.3	95.7
35.6	96.1
35.8	96.4
36	96.8
36.2	97.2
36.4	97.5
36.6	97.9
36.8	98.2
37	98.6
37.2	99
37.4	99.3
37.6	99.7
37.8	100
38	100.4
38.2	100.8
38.4	101.1
38.6	101.5
38.8	101.8
39	102.2
39.2	102.6
39.4	102.9
39.6	103.3
39.8	103.6
40	104
40.2	104.4
40.4	104.7
40.6	105.1
40.8	105.4
41	105.8

Temperature conversion formula
°F = (°C × 9/5) – 32 or (°C × 1.8) + 32
°C = (°F – 32) × 5/9 or (°F – 32) × 0.55

Weight conversion formula
lb/2.2 = kilograms
kg × 2.2 = pounds
Example:
40 lb = 40/2.2 = 18.2 kg
20 kg = 20 × 2.2 = 44 lb

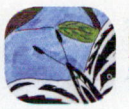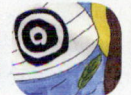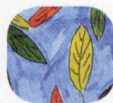

NCLEX-RN® Review Answers

CHAPTER 1

1. **Correct answer:** 4; Prescription of medication

   Rationale: All nurses are able to act as patient advocates, educators, and case managers. The new RN can administer medication but is not able to prescribe medication. A nurse with an advanced practice degree, such as a pediatric nurse practitioner, is able to prescribe medication. Cognitive Level: Application; Client Need: Safe, Effective Care Environment; Nursing Process: Implementation; Learning Outcome: Differentiate between the general nurse and advanced practice nurse roles in child health nursing.

2. **Correct answers:** 1, 3, 4, 5

   Rationale: In all but one of these situations, there is the possibility of the child getting hurt. The infant may put small parts of the toys in his or her mouth; the toddler may fall while on the playground; the school-age child may not physically be capable of safely doing the same movements as her older sibling; and adolescents are more likely to do activities as a result of peer pressure, when other adolescents are around. The safe babysitter class poses no immediate threat to the adolescent's safety. Cognitive Level: Comprehension; Client Need: Physiologic Integrity; Nursing Process: Assessment; Learning Outcome: Analyze the current causes of child morbidity and mortality and identify opportunities for nursing intervention.

3. **Correct answer:** 1; Unintentional injury prevention

   Rationale: Toddlers ages 1 to 4 are most likely to be hospitalized or killed from unintentional injury. Therefore, the nurse should concentrate on this topic for these parents. Seizure management is not primary prevention, and although child abuse can occur in this age group, injuries occur more frequently. SIDS does not occur in this age group. Cognitive Level: Analysis; Client Need: Physiological Integrity; Nursing Process: Planning; Learning Outcome: Analyze the current causes of child morbidity and mortality and identify opportunities for nursing intervention.

4. **Correct answer:** 1; Obtain the custodial parent's telephone number for permission.

   Rationale: No indication is given regarding the nature of the injuries for either the grandfather or the child. Therefore, permission to treat should be obtained from the custodial parent. Implied consent only applies in life or death situations and there is no indication of this in the stem. Registration can occur while permission to treat is obtained, and transferring cannot occur until the child has a medical screening exam. Cognitive Level: Application; Client Need: Physiological Integrity; Nursing Process: Implementation; Learning Outcome: Contrast the policies for obtaining informed consent of minors with policies for adults.

CHAPTER 2

1. **Correct answer:** 2; Authoritative

   Rationale: The authoritative parent sets limits while establishing an atmosphere of open discussion, thus promoting developmental integrity and trust. Permissive and indifferent parents do not set limits whereas authoritarian parents use stricter methods of discipline than do authoritative parents. Cognitive Level: Application; Client Need: Health Promotion and Maintenance; Nursing Process: Assessment; Learning Outcome: Analyze the impact of each of the four different parenting styles on child personality development.

2. **Correct answer:** 3; Identity versus role confusion

   Rationale: Identity versus role confusion is the developmental task of adolescence. Given the history of adoption, the behavioral changes may be even more pronounced. Industry versus inferiority is the developmental task of the school-age child, trust versus mistrust is the developmental task of the infant, and intimacy versus isolation is the developmental task of the young adult. Cognitive Level: Analysis; Client Need: Psychosocial Integrity; Nursing Process: Assessment; Learning Outcome: Explain the effect of major family changes on children, including divorce, gaining a stepparent, being placed in foster care, and adoption.

3. **Correct answer:** 3; Head Start or Early Head Start

   Rationale: The parents are looking to save money by decreasing the use of a private babysitter. Both parents work but are having financial difficulty. This family may qualify for Head Start or Early Head Start. These programs provide an all-day preschool for children who financially qualify. School-based counseling services are not appropriate as the child is not school age. Although a play group may help the child to socialize, it does not save the family money on a babysitter. There is no indication that the child is high-risk and would require a home visiting program. Cognitive Level: Application; Client Need: Safe, Effective Care Environment; Nursing Process: Evaluation; Learning Outcome: Assemble a list of family support services that might be available in the community.

4. **Correct answer:** 3; "I will place the order for a Kosher diet. I will check with you when his meal comes to make sure he received the appropriate foods."

   Rationale: The hospital should be able to provide foods appropriate for a Kosher diet. The nurse is demonstrating cultural sensitivity when she assures the father that she will order this diet and make sure this diet is delivered. A child who has an order for a regular diet can have Kosher foods. Cognitive

Level: Application; Client Need: Health Promotion and Maintenance; Nursing Process: Evaluation; Learning Outcome: Design a nursing care plan for the child and family that integrates key concepts of family-centered care.

CHAPTER 3

1. **Correct answer:** 1; Listen to the family's preferences.

   Rationale: The quickest and most accurate method for learning how to care for this child and family is to ask questions and then listen to their answers about preferences that may differ from traditional Western medicine. Cognitive Level: Application; Client Need: Safe, Effective Care Environment; Nursing Process: Assessment; Learning Outcome: Apply strategies for nurses to achieve cultural competence when providing care to the child and family.

2. **Correct answer:** 1, 2, 3, 4, and 5

   Rationale: Religious beliefs and the healing practices that can accompany them vary widely from culture to culture. The use of and belief in different alternative therapies can also differ widely. Time orientation and nutritional preferences are also areas for vast differences. In addition, the use of hands in talking or hand gestures may also differ from culture to culture. Cognitive Level: Application; Client Need: Safe, Effective Care Environment; Nursing Process: Implementation; Learning Outcome: Apply strategies for nurses to achieve cultural competence when providing care to the child and family.

3. **Correct answer:** 3; "How do you know when your child is sick?"

   Rationale: Although asking how a person knows a child is sick is an assessment, it is not particular to a cultural assessment. The other options ask about healthcare practices, childrearing responsibilities, and spiritual practices. Cognitive Level: Application; Client Need: Health Promotion and Maintenance; Nursing Process: Evaluation; Learning Outcome: Apply strategies for nurses to achieve cultural competence when providing care to the child and family.

4. **Correct answer:** 1; "I don't know of any other way that is better than mine."

   Rationale: Stating that one way is better than others represents ethnocentrism, which believes one cultural perspective and thinking is better than all others. The others are just opinions or thoughts about cultural differences in general. Cognitive Level: Application; Client Need: Health Promotion and Maintenance; Nursing Process: Planning; Learning Outcome: Apply strategies for nurses to achieve cultural competence when providing care to the child and family.

CHAPTER 4

1. **Correct answer:** 4; Affect males and females equally.

   Rationale: In autosomal recessive disorders, males and females are affected equally. Each gender has a 25% chance of being affected with each birth. An affected child will have an unaffected parent, but may have affected siblings. An affected male who can only have carrier daughters is a characteristic of X-linked recessive disorders. Cognitive Level: Analysis; Client Need: Health Promotion and Maintenance; Nursing Process: Evaluation;

Learning Outcome: Integrate basic genetic concepts into child and family education and the reinforcement of information provided to clients by genetic professionals.

2. **Correct answer:** 1, 2, 3, 4; A family medical history for the three previous generations, relationships between any affected family members, the birth history for any siblings of the baby, and the medical history for both mother and father.

   Rationale: A family pedigree contains information about medical history for three previous generations; the relationships between any affected family members; the medical history for mother, father, and any siblings of the baby; and the birth history of any siblings. The estimated date of birth is not necessary information to obtain for genetic counseling. Cognitive Level: Application; Client Need: Safe, Effective Care Environment; Nursing Process: Implementation; Learning Outcome: Incorporate genetic physical assessment and a family history pedigree into the delivery of nursing care.

3. **Correct answer:** 2; Speech problems

   Rationale: A speech problem is a developmental indicator that would support the need for genetic testing of this child. Deafness, a short stature, and skin lesions are all physical indicators for genetic testing. Cognitive Level: Application; Client Need: Safe, Effective Care Environment; Learning Outcome: Identify children or families with actual or potential genetic conditions and initiate referrals to a genetics professional.

4. **Correct answer:** 1: Implement developmentally appropriate assessment skills.

   Rationale: Developmentally appropriate assessment skills are useful with any age child. Asking the adults to leave the room may only be appropriate for adolescents, and allowing the parent to answer may only be appropriate for young children. Detailed explanations would not be helpful for some children since some can be easily overwhelmed with such details. Cognitive Level: Application; Client Need: Safe, Effective Care Environment; Nursing Process: Implementation; Learning Outcome: Prepare children and their families for a genetic evaluation.

CHAPTER 5

1. **Correct answer:** 3; Chart the assessment.

   Rationale: The baby's weight should be just about double the birth weight by 6 months. The other options treat the weight as if it is either too high or too low. Cognitive Level: Analysis; Client Need: Health Promotion and Maintenance; Nursing Process: Evaluation; Learning Outcome: Synthesize information from several theoretic approaches to plan assessments of the child's growth and developmental milestones.

2. **Correct answer:** 1; Encourage the child to continue schoolwork.

   Rationale: The developmental task of a 9-year-old is industry according to Erikson; thus, the nurse should encourage the continuation of schoolwork. The separate recreation room is appropriate for adolescents, toddlers need reminders to brush, and playing with medical toys is appropriate for preschool-age children. Cognitive Level: Analysis; Client Need: Health Promotion and Maintenance; Nursing Process: Planning; Learning

Outcome: Plan nursing interventions that are appropriate for the child's developmental state and that apply developmental theories and frameworks.

3. **Correct answer:** 3; Knocking on the door before entering the room

   Rationale: The most appropriate intervention for the school-age child is knocking on the door prior to entering. According to Freud this child is experiencing the latency stage where the child places importance on privacy and understanding the body. Using toys for distraction of a painful medical procedure is appropriate for an infant in Piaget's sensorimotor stage. Offering medical equipment to decrease anxiety is appropriate for the preschooler who is experiencing Erikson's initiative versus guilt stage. Providing information on sexuality is appropriate for the adolescent patient experiencing Freud's genital stage. Cognitive Level: Application; Client Need: Health Promotion and Maintenance; Nursing Process: Evaluation; Learning Outcome: Plan nursing interventions that are appropriate for the child's developmental state and that apply developmental theories and frameworks.

4. **Correct answer:** 2; "Do not expect the child to adapt quickly to new situations."

   Rationale: Toddlers are not flexible and do not adapt to anything quickly. Associative play does not occur until preschool age, and spanking should not be encouraged. Cognitive Level: Analysis; Client Need: Health Promotion and Maintenance; Nursing Process: Planning; Learning Outcome: Use data collected during developmental assessments to plan appropriate nursing interventions that promote development of children and adolescents.

CHAPTER 6

1. **Correct answer:** 1; "I need to discuss your medical history with you. Should your dad leave or stay?"

   Rationale: Adolescents should be offered privacy and choices whenever possible. Words that suggest disapproval are not helpful when communicating with an adolescent and should be avoided. Lastly, nurses should make adolescents aware they only have to discuss what they are ready to. Cognitive Level: Application; Client Need: Psychosocial Integrity; Nursing Process: Implementation; Learning Outcome: Apply concepts of communication to the developmental levels of childhood.

2. **Correct answer:** 1; Accepting

   Rationale: The nurse is conveying acceptance by respecting the child's emotions by allowing the child to cry in pain and letting the child know that crying is OK. Collaborating would be portrayed by assisting the child and family through problem solving. Giving recognition occurs when the nurse identifies observed behaviors or cues of the child, which indicates an interest. Offering self occurs when the nurse is available to listen and be with the child. Cognitive Level: Application; Client Need: Psychosocial Integrity; Nursing Process: Implementation; Learning Outcome: Apply concepts of communication to the developmental levels of childhood.

3. **Correct answer:** 3; Listens and observes the family interactions.

   Rationale: Getting the family whatever they want is not therapeutic even though the student should keep promises. False reassurances and avoiding difficult topics are also not helpful for the family. Listening attentively and observing nonverbal communications can assist in understanding family dynamics, which can lead to more effective communication. Cognitive Level: Application; Client Need: Psychosocial Integrity; Nursing Process: Evaluation; Learning Outcome: Integrate the nursing process to promote effective communication and establish a therapeutic nurse–child–family relationship.

4. **Correct answer:** 2; Encourage the child to engage in play with dolls, puppets, or safe medical equipment.

   Rationale: Play with dolls, puppets, or safe medical equipment is a developmentally appropriate means by which preschool children are able to express themselves. Detailed explanations and writing a story are not developmentally appropriate for a preschool-age child. Visitors are important to children this age. Parents should be allowed to stay at all times. Cognitive Level: Application; Client Need: Psychosocial Integrity; Nursing Process: Implementation; Learning Outcome: Integrate the nursing process to promote effective communication and establish a therapeutic nurse–child–family relationship.

CHAPTER 7

1. **Correct answer:** 1; Position the child on the parent's lap with his or her legs apart.

   Rationale: This will help to alleviate stress from having privacy invaded. Positioning the child on the exam table will increase stress as most preschool-age children are taught strangers are not allowed to look at their "private parts." Examining the genital area last is appropriate for adolescents, and examining the area first is not appropriate in any age group. Cognitive Level: Analysis; Client Need: Health Promotion and Maintenance; Nursing Process: Planning; Learning Outcome: Modify physical assessment techniques according to the age and developmental stage of the child.

2. **Correct answer:** 2; At the apices and midaxillary areas

   Rationale: The apices and midaxillary sites offer the greatest distance between the two lungs, which assists in identifying absent or diminished breath sounds in each lung separately. Cognitive Level: Analysis; Client Need: Health Promotion and Maintenance; Nursing Process: Assessment; Learning Outcome: Modify physical assessment techniques according to the age and developmental stage of the child.

3. **Correct answer:** 3; Normal finding in a child at this age

   Rationale: Firm, nontender, movable lymph nodes up to 1 cm in diameter are common in young children, and therefore do not require antibiotics. Cognitive Level: Analysis; Client Need: Health Promotion and Maintenance; Nursing Process: Assessment; Learning Outcome: Analyze findings from the assessment of multiple systems and identify signs indicating the presence of a health condition.

4. **Correct answer:** 2; Report the blood pressure to the physician.

   Rationale: All of the vital signs listed are normal for a 2-year-old child except for the blood pressure. This reading is greater than the 99th percentile for a 2-year-old child, and should be reported promptly to the physician. Cognitive Level: Application; Client Need: Psychosocial Integrity; Nursing Process: Implementation; Learning Outcome: Analyze findings from the assessment of multiple systems and identify signs indicating the presence of a health condition.

CHAPTER 8

1. **Correct answer:** 4; The family does not have health insurance.

   Rationale: Children with parents who are poor, have low educational level, or lack health insurance are more likely to have unmet dental needs. The other options do not place the child at risk for poor dental care. Cognitive Level: Application; Client Need: Health Promotion and Maintenance; Nursing Process: Planning; Learning Outcome: Apply the nursing process to assess, diagnose, establish goals, intervene, and evaluate care related to health promotion and health maintenance of children and adolescents in a variety of settings.

2. **Correct answer:** 1; Knowledge, Deficient related to inexperience as a parent

   Rationale: Implementing a teaching plan can inform parents of both primary prevention activities and anticipatory guidance activities which can prevent health problems before they begin. Thus, this is the best option. Cognitive Level: Analysis; Client Need: Health Promotion and Maintenance; Nursing Process: Diagnosis; Learning Outcome: Apply the nursing process to assess, diagnose, establish goals, intervene, and evaluate care related to health promotion and health maintenance of children and adolescents in a variety of settings.

3. **Correct answer:** 1; It can take place in any healthcare setting.

   Rationale: Health maintenance and promotion should be implemented in all settings in which children and adolescents are served. Cognitive Level: Comprehension; Client Need: Health Promotion and Maintenance; Nursing Process: Implementation; Learning Outcome: Apply the nursing process to assess, diagnose, establish goals, intervene, and evaluate care related to health promotion and health maintenance of children and adolescents in a variety of settings.

4. **Correct answer:** 2; Explore with the teen ways to forge new friendships.

   Rationale: Suggesting ways to begin new friendships is the priority as it is a health maintenance activity focusing on preventing social interaction problems. The other options do not address the specific concern or present a "don't worry" attitude which is nontherapeutic. Cognitive Level: Application; Client Need: Health Promotion and Maintenance; Nursing Process: Implementation; Learning Outcome: Apply the nursing process to assess, diagnose, establish goals, intervene, and evaluate care related to health promotion and health maintenance of children and adolescents in a variety of settings.

CHAPTER 9

1. **Correct answer:** 3; The parent touches, massages, and gently rubs the infant in an attempt to soothe.

   Rationale: Attempts to soothe the infant are expected behaviors of healthy parent–infant attachment. The nurse would expect both parents to be involved by comforting, asking questions, and expressing an interest in the care of the infant. Cognitive Level: Analysis; Client Need: Health Promotion and Maintenance; Nursing Process: Assessment; Learning Outcome: Apply assessment skills to gather data regarding nutrition, physical activity, mental health status, and growth and development of newborns.

2. **Correct answer:** 1, 2, 3; Developmental progressions, Newborn sleep patterns, Dietary needs

   Rationale: It is important to address health promotion and health maintenance needs for your patients and their families. Topics include developmental progression, sleep, nutrition, social interactions, physical activity, and other areas that are pertinent to the family and the age of the child. Establishing a plan of action for further care and clarifying information are both important but these will build effective partnerships with the family and they do not promote health and health maintenance needs for the patient and family. Cognitive Level: Analysis; Client Need: Health Promotion and Maintenance; Nursing Process: Planning; Learning Outcome: Diagnose and plan interventions with newborns and their families to integrate health promotion and maintenance behaviors.

3. **Correct answer:** 2; Ask to hold the baby while discussing safer holding techniques.

   Rationale: Asking to hold the baby while discussing safer holding techniques will not only allow the mother to see a demonstration but also conveys respect for the mother. It is too important just to document and discuss later. The nurse must take advantage of "teachable moments" when they occur. The others are disrespectful and may offend the mother. Cognitive Level: Application; Client Need: Health Promotion and Maintenance; Nursing Process: Implementation; Learning Outcome: Diagnose and plan interventions with newborns and their families to integrate health promotion and maintenance behaviors.

4. **Correct answer:** 2; Place the infant in a crib with a tight fitting, firm mattress.

   Rationale: Placing the infant in a crib with a tight fitting, firm mattress will keep the infant's mouth free of obstructions. Quilts, blankets, and other soft items should not be used in baby beds. Put the infant in a blanket sleeper instead. Finally, research has shown that supine is the safest sleeping position for infants. "Back to Sleep" and "Face Up to Wake Up" campaigns are designed to educate the public that infants should be placed on their backs for sleeping. Cognitive Level: Analysis; Client Need: Health Promotion and Maintenance; Nursing Process: Planning; Learning Outcome: Synthesize data from history and examination of the newborn and family to plan approaches useful with the family during health supervision encounters.

CHAPTER 10

1. **Correct answer:** 3; A 9-month-old is able to sit with support from pillows on each side.

   Rationale: The child should sit independently without support by 9 months. Thus, the 9-month-old sitting only with support indicates the need for more extensive developmental assessment. Cognitive Level: Application; Client Need: Health Promotion and Maintenance; Nursing Process: Assessment; Learning Outcome: Assess nutrition, physical activity, mental health status, and growth and development of infants.

2. **Correct answer:** 4; A 9-month-old avoids eye contact with the parents and the nurse.

   Rationale: The nurse should expect the 9-month-old to have eye contact with the parents and the nurse. If no eye contact is made, the nurse should implement a more detailed assessment of the infant's mental health. The other options are normal behavior for each respective age of the child. Cognitive Level: Analysis; Client Need: Health Promotion and Maintenance; Nursing Process: Assessment; Learning Outcome: Apply therapeutic communication skills with infant and family during health supervision visits in infancy.

3. **Correct answer:** 2; Ask the parents how close together the crib slats are.

   Rationale: If the crib slats are too far apart, the infant may get the head stuck in between and essentially get hanged in the crib. Crib slats should therefore be no more than 6 cm (2 3/8 inches) apart. The mattress should be firm and tight fitting. Cognitive Level: Analysis; Client Need: Safe, Effective Care Environment; Nursing Process: Assessment; Learning Outcome: Prioritize interventions for infants and their families to integrate activities to promote health and prevent disease and injury.

4. **Correct answer:** 1; A 6-month-old infant whose birth weight was at the 50th percentile and current weight is just above the 25th percentile.

   Rationale: A 6-month-old infant whose birth weight was at the 50th percentile and current weight is just above the 25th percentile has dropped several percentiles. This is abnormal. The other options contain measurements a nurse would consider normal growth. Cognitive Level: Analysis; Client Need: Health Promotion and Maintenance; Nursing Process: Assessment; Learning Outcome: Synthesize data from history and examination of the infant and family with knowledge of infant development to plan approaches useful with the family during health supervision encounters.

CHAPTER 11

1. **Correct answer:** 4; The need for a complete developmental evaluation.

   Rationale: These findings are not the expected findings for a 4-year-old child. Further testing is needed. While these findings are below the level expected for a 4-year-old child, a screening assessment is not diagnostic, so further testing is needed. Cognitive Level: Application; Client Need: Health Promotion and Maintenance; Nursing Process: Assessment; Learning Outcome: Apply assessment skills to gather data regarding nutrition, physical activity, mental health status, and growth and development of toddlers and preschoolers.

2. **Correct answer:** 1; "Now that our child is 4 years old we will still need to use a car seat with a harness until she reaches the top height or weight limit that is allowed by the car seat's manufacturer."

   Rationale: The child can be in a forward-facing car seat with a harness until she reaches the top height or weight limit that is allowed by the car seat's manufacturer. The child should continue to use a belt positioning booster seat until her knees extend to the edge of the seat and the shoulder belt fits appropriately. Children should not be in the front seat of the vehicle with passenger side air bags. Cognitive Level: Application; Client Need: Safe, Effective Care Environment; Nursing Process: Evaluation; Learning Outcome: Apply therapeutic communication skills with the toddler/preschooler and family during health supervision visits in toddlerhood/preschool.

3. **Correct answer:** 1; "I think you should start using time-outs when he throws a temper tantrum."

   Rationale: A time-out lets the child know there are limits and also removes him from the stimulus causing the tantrum. Rewards are not the best option as they will be interpreted as a reward for the behavior, which may be repeated to get more rewards. Temper tantrums are common at this age. They do not indicate emotional disturbance. Tantrums should decrease as the child ages. With age a child is better able to maintain control and to feel in control of situations. Cognitive Level: Analysis; Client Need: Safe, Effective Care Environment; Nursing Process: Implementation; Learning Outcome: Prioritize interventions to promote health and to prevent disease and injury for toddlers/preschoolers and their families.

4. **Correct answer:** 4; The child should eat five servings of fruits and vegetables each day.

   Rationale: One of the most important nutrition recommendations is an intake of five fruits and vegetables each day. They provide for a wide variety of vitamins and minerals, as well as adding fiber and water to the diet. A national initiative to encourage intake of produce has been used to teach families about the importance of integrating fruits and vegetables into the daily diet. Nurses should apply this teaching tool when working with families of young children. Cognitive Level: Synthesis; Client Need: Health Promotion and Maintenance; Nursing Process: Planning and Implementation; Learning Outcome: Synthesize data from history and examination of toddler/preschooler and family with knowledge of toddler/preschooler development to plan approaches useful with the family during health supervision encounters.

CHAPTER 12

1. **Correct answer:** 4; 12–14 years

   Rationale: At 12–14 years old the self-concept is developing. The child is beginning to associate with peers, and associates with same-sex groups. It becomes increasingly important to look like their peer group. This becomes even more important during adolescence. Hair loss will have little effect on the 3- and 4-year-old child. The 6-year-old child is still very egocentric and does not compare self to others. It is not yet important to look like peers, or dress like peers. Cognitive Level: Application; Client Need: Health Promotion and Maintenance; Nursing Process: Assessment; Learning Outcome: Assess nutrition, physical activity, oral health, mental health status, and growth and development of school-age children.

2. **Correct answer:** 1; Use a special black light solution to show the children how effectively they washed their hands.

   Rationale: Active participation in a concrete learning activity will be best received by this age group. This is the only active participation option. Cognitive Level: Application; Client Need: Safe, Effective Care Environment; Nursing Process: Planning; Learning Outcome: Apply therapeutic communication skills with the school-age child and family during health supervision visits.

3. **Correct answer:** 1; Before announcing the program, discuss the content with the parents.

   Rationale: The topic may be sensitive and contain new information for most children. Involving the parents initially would enable them to give permission and have discussions with their child before, during, and after the presentation. Some children might not be comfortable having their parents present, in front of their friends, during a program of such sensitive content. Having boys and girls together might be stressful and uncomfortable for the school-age child. Many students would not be able to attend. More students would be exposed to the information if it were presented during routine school hours. Cognitive Level: Analysis; Client Need: Health Promotion and Maintenance; Nursing Process: Planning; Learning Outcome: Intervene with school-age children and their families to integrate activities to promote health and to prevent disease and injury.

4. **Correct answer:** 4; Limit all screen viewing time to a maximum of 2 hours per day.

   Rationale: Two hours of all screen viewing per day, including video games, television, computers, and handheld video games, is sufficient for children of this age. The remainder of their free time should be spent in active play. At this age, milk should be nonfat. Access to play equipment may be increased, but access to screen viewing will need to be decreased in order to encourage use of the equipment. Finally, increasing contact time with other children will not necessarily decrease his weight. Cognitive Level: Synthesis; Client Need: Health Promotion and Maintenance; Nursing Process: Planning; Learning Outcome: Plan developmentally appropriate approaches for the school-age child and family during health supervision encounters.

CHAPTER 13

1. **Correct answer:** 1; Anthropometric measurements, 24-hour dietary recall, and activity information

   Rationale: Early adolescence is a time of rapid growth. Complete assessment is essential to positive outcomes, and this includes anthropometric measurements, 24-hour dietary recall, and activity information. Although blood pressure is an important part of a health maintenance visit, it does not provide for a comprehensive nutritional assessment. Lipid screening may be

indicated for those with a family history of early heart disease, but it is not the priority in assessing the nutritional status of an early adolescent. Scoliosis screening is not part of a nutritional assessment. Cognitive Level: Application; Client Need: Health Promotion and Maintenance; Nursing Process: Assessment; Learning Outcome: Apply assessment skills to gather data regarding nutrition, physical activity, mental health status, and growth and development of adolescents.

2. **Correct answer:** 4; Suggest to the mother that she can join her daughter after the exam to discuss findings and have all questions answered.

   Rationale: The nurse has suggested the girl be alone for the questions and exam. The girl has the option to allow her mother to come with her. This is easier than asking the mother to leave partway through the exam. The initial assessment questions are the responsibility of the nurse, not the physician. The girl might not answer truthfully if asked about sexuality in front of her mother. Cognitive Level: Application; Client Need: Safe, Effective Care Environment; Nursing Process: Implementation; Learning Outcome: Demonstrate therapeutic communication skills with the adolescent and family during health supervision visits.

3. **Correct answer:** 4; Driving and substance abuse

   Rationale: School dances, social gatherings, and dating increase during high school along with drug and alcohol experimentation. Cognitive impairment related to alcohol and drug consumption can cause motor vehicle crashes leading to injuries. Although learning CPR, avoiding sports injuries, and fire prevention are important, they are not the priority in this age group. Cognitive Level: Analysis; Client Need: Health Promotion and Maintenance; Nursing Process: Planning; Learning Outcome: Intervene with adolescents and their families to integrate activities to promote health and to prevent disease and injury.

4. **Correct answer:** 3; "I have the knowledge, support and strength to achieve my goal to quit smoking."

   Rationale: Self-efficacy indicates that the individual feels confident that behavior can be changed. The necessary support and resources are available so that the person believes lifestyle alterations will be successful. Cognitive Level: Application; Client Need: Psychosocial Integrity; Nursing Process: Evaluation; Learning Outcome: Synthesize data from history and examination of the adolescent and family.

CHAPTER 14

1. **Correct answer:** 3; Provide training for teachers and health aides to provide appropriate care for the child.

   Rationale: Public Law 94-142 and Public Law 99-457 ensure all children with disabilities ages 3 to 21 receive a free education. Accommodations need to be made for this child. Therefore since the 8-year-old child has an established tracheostomy and is at risk for aspiration, teachers should be instructed on the care needs of the child and how to recognize symptoms if needed. It is not necessary for a registered nurse to be assigned to the child while at school. While it is desirable for a school nurse to have only one school, it is unlikely to happen just for this child. Cognitive Level: Application; Client Need: Safe, Effective Care Environment; Nursing Process: Planning; Learning Outcome:

Compare the roles of the nurse in each identified community healthcare setting.

2. **Correct answer:** 1; Whether or not the children were actively exposed to any chemical agents

   Rationale: Exposure to chemical agents can cause skin, respiratory, and other organ complications. Therefore, this assessment must take priority. Although posttraumatic stress syndrome is important, it is not an initial priority. Diversion activities are important for children, but are secondary to physical safety in this situation. Finally, the nurse would be concerned about reassuring the children, but their physical well-being must take priority. Cognitive Level: Application; Client Need: Physiological Integrity; Nursing Process: Assessment; Learning Outcome: Summarize the potential roles of the pediatric nurse or school nurse in supporting a community assessment process.

3. **Correct answer:** 2; The child and family need to have a definite evacuation plan in place.

   Rationale: Evacuation education is priority. The child should be instructed to evacuate if indicated, not to find parents and other family members. As each fire situation is different, the child may be required to evacuate the building for the outdoors. Finally, while drinking the water after fire exposure is important, it is not the priority in fire prevention and evacuation planning. Cognitive Level: Application; Client Need: Safe, Effective Care Environment; Nursing Process: Planning; Learning Outcome: Examine the special needs of children that should be considered in disaster preparedness.

4. **Correct answer:** 4; A portable automatic external defibrillator

   Rationale: An automatic external defibrillator is not indicated in this population, as it is unusual for children to present with ventricular fibrillation. The blueprint, portable radios, and list of staff and students are important to include. Cognitive Level: Application; Client Need: Safe, Effective Care Environment; Nursing Process: Implementation; Learning Outcome: Examine the special needs of children that should be considered in disaster preparedness.

CHAPTER 15

1. **Correct answer:** 4; "Yes, it is OK to bring your child's siblings for a visit as long as we educate them on what to expect when they visit."

   Rationale: The child's siblings should be allowed to visit as long as the child and the siblings all wish to see each other and the siblings are educated on what to expect during the visit. Seeing siblings would not necessarily make the child feel worse. Although it may be upsetting for the child's siblings to see the patient, proper education on what to expect is required prior to the visit. The parents would not be required to bring someone to watch their other children during the visit. Cognitive Level: Analysis; Client Need: Health Promotion and Maintenance; Nursing Process: Assessment; Learning Outcome: Apply family-centered care principles to the hospital setting.

2. **Correct answer:** 4; Encourage parental involvement in the child's care and suggest rooming-in if possible.

   Rationale: Parents should be encouraged to room-in with and hold their child and to participate in the child's care as much as possible. The child's anxiety will increase when the parent leaves or the child is left alone. Cognitive Level: Analysis; Client Need: Health Promotion and Maintenance; Nursing Process: Assessment; Learning Outcome: Apply family-centered care principles to the hospital setting.

3. **Correct answer:** 2; The parents give the medication to the child using the appropriate technique in the nurse's presence.

   Rationale: While all four options indicate understanding, watching the parents correctly administer the medication provides the most information about their understanding. Cognitive Level: Analysis; Client Need: Physiological Integrity; Nursing Process: Evaluation; Learning Outcome: Evaluate the effectiveness of teaching strategies used with the hospitalized child and his or her family.

4. **Correct answer:** 3; Use dolls to teach the child about the procedure.

   Rationale: A 5-year-old child should be taught about a surgical procedure through the use of pictures, books, dolls, and safe medical equipment in order to clarify misconception and teach about the upcoming procedure. Although providing the mother with a brochure may be appropriate, this does not teach the child. Sitting with the child while he watches a video or allowing the child to talk to other children who have had the procedure is not appropriate for this age group. Cognitive Level: Analysis; Client Need: Safe, Effective Care Environment; Nursing Process: Evaluation; Learning Outcome: Evaluate the effectiveness of teaching strategies used with the hospitalized child and his or her family.

CHAPTER 16

1. **Correct answer:** 1; Encourage the child to use a peak flow meter and record results every day.

   Rationale: Only encouraging the child to use the flow meter and record results every day is directed toward independent self-care. The other nursing interventions are all important, but they do not address the child's independent management of symptoms. Cognitive Level: Application; Client Need: Physiological Integrity; Nursing Process: Implementation; Learning Outcome: Assess the child with a chronic condition and identify specific nursing interventions for the child at different ages.

2. **Correct answer:** 1; "I can call respite caregivers to give me a break from her daily requirements."

   Rationale: Respite care is a short-term skilled care that helps a family take a break from the daily routine and stress. The family needs respite care more than other assistance due to the child's skilled care needs. The other options may provide support but cannot provide skilled care for the child. Cognitive Level: Analysis; Client Need: Health Promotion and Maintenance; Nursing Process: Planning; Learning Outcome: Assess the child with a chronic condition and apply specific nursing interventions for the child at different ages.

3. **Correct answer:** 4; Assess the family's understanding of leukemia.

Rationale: A child with leukemia has a life-threatening chronic condition that requires ongoing nursing and medical care. The nurse first must assess if the family understands the gravity of the child's condition and required treatment. Assessment of the situation must take precedence over evaluation of wheelchair accessibility. Although the physician needs to know of this request, it is more important to assess the situation first so the physician can be aware of the family's exact situation. Demonstrating respect is important, but the nurse must first ensure the family understands their child's diagnosis and possible outcomes. Cognitive Level: Analysis; Client Need: Psychosocial Integrity; Nursing Process: Implementation; Learning Outcome: Assess the family of a child with a chronic condition and discuss the impact of the child's condition on the family.

4. **Correct answer:** 3; The family provides appropriate home care for the child while maintaining family routines.

Rationale: Maintenance of family routines while successfully caring for the ill child is the only answer that addresses the hospital-to-home transition. The child is too young to do self-care. Suctioning the child's tracheostomy and taking vital signs are skills required of the parents before discharge, but performance of skills does not indicate that the parents will successfully navigate the transition to home care. Cognitive Level: Analysis; Client Need: Psychosocial Integrity; Nursing Process: Evaluation; Learning Outcome: Assess the family of a child with a chronic condition and discuss the impact of the child's condition on the family.

CHAPTER 17

1. **Correct answer:** 1; The child will appear more relaxed with fewer indications of anxiety.

Rationale: The expected outcome in this situation is that the child will be able to eliminate or reduce feelings of apprehension. The expected outcome would be for the child to not only verbalize the source of the fear, but also better control the feelings. The focus of this situation is on the child, not the parents. Cognitive Level: Application; Client Need: Psychosocial Integrity; Nursing Process: Evaluation; Learning Outcome: Develop a plan of care for the child with a life-threatening illness and the family.

2. **Correct answer:** 4; Involve the adolescent in planning care goals.

Rationale: Adolescents prefer to be in control. Involving them in planning care will facilitate this. Touching and talking to the adolescent are not a priority. Consistent caregivers are important, but more so with younger children who experience stranger anxiety. Many pediatric facilities allow open visitation. It is important for siblings and friends to be allowed to visit in addition to parents. Cognitive Level: Application; Client Need: Psychosocial Integrity; Nursing Process: Implementation; Learning Outcome: Develop a plan of care for the child with a life-threatening illness and the family.

3. **Correct answer:** 2; Empowering the child

Rationale: It is the child's life and possible death, and he or she should be empowered to have control over it as much as developmentally possible. Pain medications should be given on a schedule and not on an as-needed basis. The child may not be able to communicate pain to the nurse. Open visitation or a quiet room may or may not be something the child or family wants. It is more important to let the child/family make the decisions that work best for them. Cognitive Level: Analysis; Client Need: Physiological Integrity; Nursing Process: Planning; Learning Outcome: Develop a plan of care for the child with a life-threatening illness and the family.

4. **Correct answer:** 4; Explain the child's condition and what is being done at this time for the child.

Rationale: Nurses must be nonjudgmental and not punitive to facilitate trust from families. Now is not an appropriate time to teach the mother about safety or iron poisoning; this will only reinforce her guilt. The parents' most important identified need is for information about their child's condition and the child's medical and nursing interventions. The visiting policy is secondary. Cognitive Level: Analysis; Client Need: Psychosocial Integrity; Nursing Process: Implementation; Learning Outcome: Develop a plan of care for the child with a life-threatening illness and the family.

CHAPTER 18

1. **Correct answer:** 1, 2, 3, 4; Determining whether the family's and child's goals are curative, comfort, or not yet decided, Helping the family make decisions about medical interventions that are desired, Identifying the decision makers for the child's health care, Evaluating the family's understanding of the child's illness and prognosis.

Rationale: Planning palliative care includes determining the family's and child's goals: curative, comfort, or not yet decided; helping the family make decisions about medical interventions that are desired; identifying the decision makers for the child's health care; and assessing the family's understanding of the child's illness and prognosis. Assisting the family in making funeral arrangements is not part of palliative care. Cognitive Level: Application; Client Need: Psychosocial Integrity; Nursing Process: Planning; Learning Outcome: Devise a nursing care plan to provide family-centered care for the child who is dying and his or her family.

2. **Correct answer:** 1, 3, 4, 5; Cultural traditions, Beliefs related to loss, Coping skills, Spiritual rituals

Rationale: Cultural traditions should be identified and accommodated in the plan of care. Income and other financial factors are not part of a family-centered plan of care for a child who is dying. Beliefs related to loss should be identified and respected. The family's coping skills should be assessed and assistance and resources offered as necessary. Spiritual rituals are an important part of family life and should be identified and respected. Cognitive Level: Application; Client Need: Psychosocial Integrity; Nursing Process: Planning; Learning Outcome: Devise a nursing care plan to provide family-centered care for the child who is dying and his or her family.

3. **Correct answer:** 1; Anticipatory Grieving related to terminal illness

Rationale: Families need to be prepared for the impending death, and nurses should provide this support by discussing the events forthcoming. In a situation involving a dying child, preparing the family for death is the priority. Preparing the family for the impending death takes precedence over the change in family processes. This is not a concern as the child is dying. It is more important to prepare the family for the death. Cognitive Level: Analysis; Client Need: Psychosocial Integrity; Nursing Process: Diagnosis; Learning Outcome: Devise a nursing care plan to provide family-centered care for the child who is dying and his or her family.

4. **Correct answer:** 2; Allow the family to ask questions about the recent events and future expectations.

   Rationale: Making the visit personal is important to share memories of the child as a way to help provide support. The priority support would be for the nurse to let the family lead the conversation, not to ask them questions. Cognitive Level: Analysis; Client Need: Psychosocial Integrity; Nursing Process: Implementation; Learning Outcome: Plan bereavement support for the parents and siblings after the death of a child.

CHAPTER 19

1. **Correct answer:** 2; "My infant will only eat from a bottle or breast for 4 to 6 months."

   Rationale: Infants do not begin eating with a spoon at 2 weeks of age. Sucking is the only method of feeding for infants for the first 4 to 6 months of life. Infants must use their tongue in a different way when learning to eat from a spoon. This is often confused with food dislike. Infants will not consume anything other than formula or breastmilk for the first 4 to 6 months of life. Cognitive Level: Application; Client Need: Health Promotion and Maintenance; Nursing Process: Assessment; Learning Outcome: Describe and plan nursing interventions to meet nutritional needs for all age groups from preterm infants through adolescents.

2. **Correct answer:** 1, 2, 3, 4; The child's diet, Food content, Food preferences, Parent feeding practices

   Rationale: The child's diet, food content, and food preferences must be assessed with the diagnosis of a feeding disorder. The feeding practices that the parent uses must also be assessed with a diagnosis of a feeding disorder. The dietary habits of the parent do not need to be assessed with the diagnosis of a feeding disorder. Cognitive Level: Analysis; Client Need: Safe, Effective Care Environment; Nursing Process: Evaluation; Learning Outcome: Apply the nursing process to care for children and adolescents with feeding and eating disorders.

3. **Correct answer:** 4; The child demonstrates sufficient intake of all nutrients while achieving or maintaining optimal weight for height.

   Rationale: The desired outcome is that the child takes in nutrients sufficient to meet metabolic needs, but without taking in excess. The child may need to lose weight or to maintain weight while height grows in proportion to weight. Plans to achieve this outcome would likely include an increase in activity, healthy food choices, and appropriate serving sizes. Cognitive Level: Analysis; Client Need: Psychosocial Integrity; Nursing Process:

Planning; Learning Outcome: Apply the nursing process to care for children or adolescents with feeding and eating disorders.

4. **Correct answer:** 1; "I will start my infant on rice cereal since it is iron fortified and has little chance of causing allergy."

   Rationale: Rice cereal is the recommended first food for infants since it has a low risk of causing allergy, and it is iron fortified. Infants should not have egg whites as they can cause severe allergies. Foods should be introduced one at a time, and the infant should progress to other single-ingredient cereals, followed by fruits and vegetables. Cognitive Level: Application; Client Need: Health Promotion and Maintenance; Nursing Process: Evaluation; Learning Outcome: Describe and plan nursing interventions to meet nutritional needs for all age groups from preterm infants through adolescents.

CHAPTER 20

1. **Correct answer:** 3; Encourage the parents to set consistent limits and be involved in their children's lives.

   Rationale: Children who are given consistent limits and have involved parents are less likely to abuse drugs. When a teen is unsupervised, it can lead to risk-taking behaviors. Teens need intensive therapy if they are using drugs. Methamphetamine is a risk, especially for youth, with the recent increase in the amount of people using this drug. Cognitive Level: Analysis; Client Need: Physiological Integrity; Nursing Process: Implementation; Learning Outcome: Examine the effects of substance use, physical activity, and other lifestyle patterns on health.

2. **Correct answer:** 4; The parents state they will examine each room of their house to assess for safety risks for their child.

   Rationale: Prevention of ingestions is the key and the priority when teaching about risk potential. Examining for safety risks in the house is the most important step in prevention of unintentional ingestions in children. While every home with small children should have quick access to this number, it is more important that parents focus on prevention of unintentional ingestions. It is not necessary to throw all medications away. However, parents should keep them locked up and away from children. Inducing vomiting with syrup of ipecac is no longer recommended for home treatment of poisonings. Cognitive Level: Analysis; Client Need: Safe, Effective Care Environment; Nursing Process: Evaluation; Learning Outcome: Evaluate the environment for hazards to children, such as exposure to substances and potential for poisoning.

3. **Correct answer:** 1; Report suspected child abuse to the appropriate authority.

   Rationale: The multiple bruising on the buttocks and the looped cord mark are symptoms highly suspicious of physical abuse and must be reported to legal authorities. In addition, bruises in different stages of healing might also be indicative of intentional trauma. If the parents are informed of the nurse's suspicion, they might leave before further evaluation can be performed. Detailed charting of the findings is essential and required, not just charting the main findings. A child who is learning to walk might have multiple bruises on the front of the legs but should not have multiple bruises on the buttocks or looped cord marks. Cognitive Level: Analysis; Client Need: Psychosocial Integrity; Nursing Process: Implementation; Learning Outcome: Explore the nursing role in prevention and treatment of child abuse and neglect, and other forms of violence.

4. **Correct answer:** 2; Accept delayed reactions in the child.

   Rationale: When a disaster or act of war or terrorism has occurred, the preschool-age child might have difficulty coping. The amount of television the child watches should be limited, since repeated showing of the event by the media might cause this age child to think the event is occurring over and over again. Parents should take cues from the child regarding how much to discuss about the event. It is normal for delayed reactions to occur. The parents should spend time with the child and continue with planned events as much as possible. Maintain the child and family's routine as much as possible. Cognitive Level: Analysis; Client Need: Psychosocial Integrity; Nursing Process: Planning; Learning Outcome: Plan nursing interventions for children related to social and environmental situations.

CHAPTER 21

1. **Correct answer:** 3; The infant has a heart rate of 180.

   Rationale: Tachycardia is a physiologic consequence of pain and stress and is one that infants exhibit frequently. The other options suggest controlled pain. Cognitive Level: Analysis; Client Need: Physiological Integrity; Nursing Process: Assessment; Learning Outcome: Summarize the physiologic and behavioral consequences of pain in infants and children.

2. **Correct answer:** 4; Teach progressive muscle relaxation

   Rationale: Progressive muscle relaxation is a complementary therapy for pain management that is appropriate for a child 6 years of age or older. Wrapping in a blanket is appropriate for newborns and infants but not for a 12-year-old. Offering bubbles would be appropriate for a child who is 2 to 6 years of age. Cognitive Level: Analysis; Client Need: Physiological Integrity; Nursing Process: Implementation; Learning Outcome: Plan the nursing care for an infant or child that integrates pharmacologic interventions, and developmentally appropriate nonpharmacologic (complementary) therapies.

3. **Correct answer:** 1; Ensure the child has pain medication for uncontrolled pain.

   Rationale: The assessment indicates that the child is experiencing pain. Uncontrolled pain can cause decreased bowel function as exhibited by hypoactive bowel sounds upon auscultation. The most appropriate intervention is to ensure the child has pain medication for uncontrolled pain. Cognitive Level: Analysis; Client Need: Physiological Integrity; Nursing Process: Implementation; Learning Outcome: Distinguish between the clinical therapies used for acute and chronic pain.

4. **Correct answer:** 3; Obtain a prescription for EMLA from the healthcare provider or L-M-X4 from the pharmacy and instruct the parents how to use it.

   Rationale: EMLA and L-M-X4 are topical anesthetics that are appropriate to use to prevent or decrease pain associated with minor medical procedures. Venipuncture is a painful procedure and intervention prior to the procedure is indicated. Although distraction is helpful, it is not as effective as topical anesthesia. Therapeutic play can be a useful method to teach the child briefly about the procedure and to help relieve anxiety following the procedure, but it will not actually decrease the discomfort that a child of this age will experience from a needle stick. Cognitive Level: Application; Client Need: Physiological Integrity; Nursing Process: Implementation; Learning Outcome: Compare the effectiveness of pain management strategies for procedures such as venipuncture and immunizations.

CHAPTER 22

1. **Correct answer:** 3; Infection, Risk for related to inadequate acquired immunity

   Rationale: If children do not receive immunizations as scheduled, they are at risk for infection from many infectious diseases. If children do not receive immunizations as scheduled, there is no effective therapy management or risk for injury related to immunization reaction. Children who receive immunizations will always have anxiety. However, the risk for infection is the priority should they not receive them. Cognitive Level: Application; Client Need: Health Promotion and Maintenance; Nursing Process: Diagnosis; Learning Outcome: Plan the nursing care for children of all ages needing immunizations.

2. **Correct answer:** 4; A medication refrigerator is necessary for vaccine storage.

   Rationale: The Joint Commission requires medications and food items to be stored separately. Most vaccines require refrigeration to maintain safety and potency. Thus, medication refrigeration is the priority consideration. Although educating staff on proper vaccine administration is important, it is not the priority and it not related to equipment needs. Cognitive Level: Analysis; Client Need: Safe, Effective Care Environment; Nursing Process: Planning; Learning Outcome: Design a plan to maintain the potency of vaccines.

3. **Correct answer:** 2; Malaria

   Rationale: Based on the patient's presenting symptoms and the history of travel to South America the nurse suspects the child may have contracted malaria. The child is not exhibiting symptoms of Lyme disease, tetanus, or rubella. Cognitive Level: Analysis; Client Need: Health Promotion and Maintenance; Nursing Process: Evaluation; Learning Outcome: Differentiate between common communicable diseases and vector-borne diseases.

4. **Correct answer:** 2; Rubella

   Rationale: The child's pattern of rash eruption is characteristic of rubella. Hand, foot, and mouth lesions are papulovesicular and last 7 to 10 days. The child with scarlet fever has a fine, red, sandpaper rash that spares the face and appears on the neck and trunk. The toes and fingers can peel, and a strawberry tongue is seen on day 4 or 5. The child with meningococcus is very ill, and has a red-to-purple urticarial, maculopapular, or petechial rash that can progress to purpura. Chickenpox or varicella would have lesions all over that crust over as they age. Cognitive Level:

Analysis; Client Need: Physiological Integrity; Nursing Process: Assessment; Learning Outcome: Differentiate between common communicable diseases and vector-borne diseases.

CHAPTER 23

1. **Correct answer:** 1; The infant is having a seizure.

   Rationale: Seizure activity is usually not noted until the child is severely dehydrated. Slight elevation of pulse rate can be seen in moderate dehydration. Dry mucous membranes are seen in moderate dehydration. Normal skin turgor indicates no signs of mild dehydration. Cognitive Level: Analysis; Client Need: Physiological Integrity; Nursing Process: Assessment; Learning Outcome: Analyze assessment findings to recognize fluid-electrolyte problems and acid–base imbalance in children.

2. **Correct answer:** 1 and 2; "Your child may be placed on medication to strengthen the heart."; "Your child may be given a diuretic."

   Rationale: The child may be placed on a medication to strengthen the heart in this instance. The child may be given a diuretic to remove excess fluid from the body. Children with extracellular fluid volume excess are not started on an IV drip of lactated Ringer's. This is appropriate for a child with dehydration. An oral rehydration solution is given to treat dehydration, not extracellular fluid volume excess. Bronchodilators are not used to treat extracellular fluid volume excess. Cognitive Level: Analysis; Client Need: Physiological Integrity; Nursing Process: Assessment: Learning Outcome: Analyze assessment findings to recognize fluid-electrolyte problems and acid-base imbalance in children.

3. **Correct answer:** 4; Poor fluid intake

   Rationale: Poor fluid intake correlates with hypernatremia. Although poor fluid intake can indicate child abuse, the nurse would not expect to find it immediately. Children with developmental delays may not be able to recognize thirst or communicate that thirst to caregivers. However, this was not a primary expectation. Cognitive Level: Analysis; Client Need: Physiological Integrity; Nursing Process: Assessment; Learning Outcome: Analyze assessment findings to recognize fluid-electrolyte problems and acid–base imbalance in children.

4. **Correct answer:** 3; An ABG with a pH of 7.2, an HCO_3 of 35, and a CO_2 of 50

   Rationale: The ABG indicates respiratory acidosis which can occur in status asthmaticus. The CBC, potassium, and BUN are not indicative of respiratory issues. Cognitive Level: Analysis; Client Need: Physiological Integrity; Nursing Process: Assessment; Learning Outcome: Analyze assessment findings to recognize fluid-electrolyte problems and acid-base imbalance in children.

CHAPTER 24

1. **Correct answer:** 1; Encourage the child to use all five senses.

   Rationale: It is important to encourage children with vision impairment to use all five senses, including vision as much as possible, to allow development to progress as normally as possible. While teaching parents to read body language is an appropriate intervention, the priority intervention focuses on the child. Teaching parents about special safety measures is an appropriate intervention, but the priority intervention focuses on the child. It has already been determined that the child has a visual impairment, so screening is not the priority. Cognitive Level: Application; Client Need: Health Promotion and Maintenance; Nursing Process: Evaluation; Learning Outcome: Plan for screening programs and identification of children with vision and hearing abnormalities.

2. **Correct answer:** 1; "Prevention is the key."

   Rationale: Primary prevention, or avoiding or decreasing risk factors, is key to decreasing the frequency of ear disorders in children. Antibiotics for otitis media are not automatically prescribed; it is recommended that the child be observed for 48 to 72 hours first. There is insufficient evidence either way, but the literature suggests that herbal medications might be as effective for ear pain in children as anesthetic eardrops. Regularly listening to loud music or using earphones at high volume are causes of hearing loss. Cognitive Level: Analysis; Client Need: Physiological Integrity; Nursing Process: Implementation; Learning Outcome: Apply current recommendations when implementing care and teaching for children with abnormalities of the eyes, ears, nose, throat, and mouth.

3. **Correct answer:** 1; Facilitating communication.

   Rationale: Nursing care focuses on facilitating the child's ability to receive spoken language and send information. Not all children with hearing impairment want or will receive a cochlear implant. The priority focus is on the child, not the parents. The first priority focuses on the child's ability to communicate, not on preparing an IEP. Cognitive Level: Application; Client Need: Physiological Integrity; Nursing Process: Implementation; Learning Outcome: Apply current recommendations when implementing care and teaching for children with abnormalities of the eyes, ears, nose, throat, and mouth.

4. **Correct answer:** 2; The child is having increased swallowing.

   Rationale: The child having increased swallowing could be a sign of increased bleeding from the surgical site. White crusts on the back of the throat, eating only Popsicles, and complaining of throat pain are all normal following a tonsillectomy. Cognitive Level: Application; Client Need: Physiological Integrity; Nursing Process: Assessment; Learning Outcome: Prioritize preventive and treatment principles when implementing care for children related to the eyes, ears, nose, and throat.

CHAPTER 25

1. **Correct answer:** 3; Decreased pulse oximeter saturations

   Rationale: Signs of increased respiratory distress including decreased pulse oximeter saturations should be reported immediately to the health care provider. Increased temperature, increased heart rate, and decreased bowel sounds are significant but would not require immediate notification. Cognitive Level: Analysis; Client Need: Safe, Effective Care Environment; Nursing Process: Assessment; Learning Outcome: Distinguish between mild, moderate, and severe respiratory distress and plan the appropriate nursing care for each level of respiratory distress severity.

2. **Correct answer:** 2; "I can expect my baby to be on oxygen therapy for the rest of his life."

   Rationale: Although most babies will initially be placed on oxygen, every attempt is made to discontinue oxygen as soon as possible. Babies with BPD will require at least one treatment of corticosteroid and/or a bronchodilator daily due to permanent damage to the lung tissue. Diuretics are required to reduce excess fluid in the lungs as well as decrease pulmonary resistance. Some babies can be weaned from them after they grow. Since babies with BPD are at high risk for respiratory syncytial virus, they should receive palivizumab (Synagis) during winter months at least through age 1. Cognitive Level: Analysis; Client Need: Physiological Integrity; Nursing Process: Evaluation; Learning Outcome: Contrast respiratory conditions and injuries that can cause respiratory distress in infants and children.

3. **Correct answer:** 4; "Antibiotics are not effective for viral pneumonia. Bacteria can grow later in the duration of the illness, making antibiotics necessary later."

   Rationale: The nurse responds with the most informative, accurate response. The decision not to use antibiotics for viral pneumonia was based on sound rationale about the etiology of the illness, and not to save money. This situation does not indicate the viral pneumonia was misdiagnosed. The nurse should not diagnose the illness since it is outside a nurse's scope of practice. Only a nurse practitioner or physician should diagnose. Cognitive Level: Application; Client Need: Safe, Effective Care Environment; Nursing Process: Implementation; Learning Outcome: Create a nursing care plan for a child with a common acute respiratory condition.

4. **Correct answer:** 3, 4, 5; "Does your child have any signs of hyperactivity?"; "Does your child have difficulty with school-work?"; "Does your child wet the bed?"

   Rationale: Asking about hyperactivity, school work difficulty, and wetting the bed are appropriate assessment questions. Children with obstructive sleep apnea often assume unusual sleep positions and have morning headaches, not evening headaches. Cognitive Level: Analysis; Client Need: Physiological Integrity; Nursing Process: Evaluation; Learning Outcome: Plan the nursing care for a child with a chronic respiratory condition.

CHAPTER 26

1. **Correct answer:** 1; A heart rate of 90

   Rationale: A heart rate under 100 beats per minute indicates bradycardia. The medication should be held and the healthcare provider should be notified. The normal serum digoxin level has therapeutic levels ranging from 1.0 to 2.0 ng/mL. A potassium level of 4 mEq/L is normal. Withholding the digoxin is not indicated. Cognitive Level: Analysis; Client Need: Physiological Integrity; Nursing Process: Assessment; Learning Outcome: Recognize the signs and symptoms of congestive heart failure in an infant and child.

2. **Correct answer:** 3; Feed the infant prior to other interventions.

   Rationale: Providing calories is imperative and will aid in providing more energy for other activities. Although psychosocial support is important, physical care needs are always considered first. Providing familiar toys is beneficial, but this intervention is not priority, especially since the child is an infant. Bathing the infant before feeding will cause expenditure of energy during the bath and may interfere with successful feeding. Cognitive Level: Analysis; Client Need: Physiological Integrity; Nursing Process: Planning; Learning Outcome: Recognize the signs and symptoms of congestive heart failure in an infant and child.

3. **Correct answer:** 4; Encourage the infant to take a small amount of formula by mouth each day.

   Rationale: Even taking a small amount of formula each day will provide positive oral stimulation. The infant is using a naso-gastric tube because he or she is having difficulty maintaining caloric intake. Weaning an older infant from a bottle should be done after surgery, when more energy is available to the infant. Exposure to other children at this time could cause infection and a delay in surgery. Cognitive Level: Analysis; Client Need: Health Promotion and Maintenance; Nursing Process: Implementation; Learning Outcome: Create a nursing care plan for the child with a congenital heart defect cared for at home prior to corrective surgery.

4. **Correct answer:** 2; Capillary refill

   Rationale: Although cardiopulmonary monitoring may be necessary, this is not the best assessment for hypovolemia. Capillary refill is an appropriate assessment parameter to monitor for hypovolemia. Although monitoring the pulse is necessary, this is not the best assessment for hypovolemia. Although assessing the history of the injury is important, this is not the best way to assess for hypovolemia. Cognitive Level: Analysis; Client Need: Physiological Integrity; Nursing Process: Assessment; Learning Outcome: Plan the nursing care for the child undergoing open heart surgery.

CHAPTER 27

1. **Correct answer:** 1; Give epinephrine through an EpiPen.

   Rationale: The nurse's first action will be to administer epinephrine through an EpiPen. Giving prednisone and oxygen would be done after the epinephrine. Diphenhydramine would be given if epinephrine is not available. Cognitive Level: Analysis; Client Need: Physiological Integrity; Nursing Process: Implementation; Learning Outcome: Apply nursing interventions and prevention measures for the child experiencing hypersensitivity reactions.

2. **Correct answer:** 2; "The temperature should be taken rectally every day."

   Rationale: Rectal temperature should be avoided as this will increase the risk of infection. All other statements are appropriate. Cognitive Level: Application; Client Need: Safe, Effective Care Environment; Nursing Process: Evaluation; Learning Outcome: Develop a nursing care plan in partnership with the family for a child with human immunodeficiency virus (HIV) infection.

3. **Correct answer:** 4; Cleaning frequently with moist cloths

   Rationale: The family should be taught to clean frequently with moist cloths and mops to remove dust. Pets should be kept outside of the child's room. Plastic covers should be used on mattresses and pillows. Carpeting, not hardwood floors, should be avoided. Cognitive Level: Application; Client Need: Safe, Effective Care Environment; Nursing Process: Evaluation; Learning Outcome: Apply nursing interventions and prevention measures for the child experiencing hypersensitivity reactions.

4. **Correct answer:** 3; Kiwi fruit, bananas, and avocados

   Rationale: Some of the proteins present in latex are also present in kiwi fruit, bananas, and avocados. Oranges, broccoli, and carrots should be encouraged in the diet due to vitamin enrichment. Cognitive Level: Application; Client Need: Safe, Effective Care Environment; Nursing Process: Implementation; Learning Outcome: Describe exposure prevention measures for the child with latex allergy.

CHAPTER 28

1. **Correct answer:** 2; Preventing infection

   Rationale: Preventing infection is a priority goal of the child with neutropenia. Preventing bruising is a concern when the platelet count is decreased. Although developmental issues are always a concern in pediatric care, it is not priority in the care of a child with neutropenia. Cognitive Level: Application; Client Need: Physiological Integrity; Nursing Process: Planning; Learning Outcome: Develop a family-centered nursing care plan for the management of a child with a hematologic disorder.

2. **Correct answer:** 1; Erythrocytes

   Rationale: Erythrocytes are responsible for transporting oxygen to the tissues. Leukocytes are responsible for specific and nonspecific immune response. Thrombocytes are responsible for coagulation. Granulocytes are a type of leukocyte, and they are responsible for fighting infection. Cognitive Level: Analysis; Client Need: Physiological Integrity; Nursing Process: Assessment; Learning Outcome: Develop a family-centered nursing care plan for the management of a child with hematologic disorder.

3. **Correct answer:** 4; "I will make sure my child has a rectal temperature every 4 hours."

   Rationale: Perforation of the anus or rectum can cause bleeding and infection. Taking a rectal temperature is an incorrect intervention in this population. If frequent blood draws are anticipated, inserting a saline lock is a safe intervention. Frequent mouth care promotes improved gum integrity and decreases the chance of bleeding. Using paper tape prevents shearing of the skin and subsequent bleeding. Cognitive Level: Application; Client Need: Safe, Effective Care Environment; Nursing Process: Evaluation; Learning Outcome: Develop a family-centered nursing care plan for the management of a child with a hematologic disorder.

4. **Correct answer:** 2; "Flying at high altitudes causes decreased oxygen, causing increased sickling."

   Rationale: High altitude increases the demand for O_2, which is impaired in the child with sickle cell anemia. The child with sickle cell anemia is at no higher risk for infection than a child without the disease. Water and other fluids for oral consumption are available on flights. Cognitive Level: Analysis; Client Need: Health Promotion and Maintenance; Nursing Process: Implementation; Learning Outcome: Develop a family-centered nursing care plan for the management of a child with a hematologic disorder.

CHAPTER 29

1. **Correct answer:** 1; Weight gain

   Rationale: Administration of steroids causes weight gain. Steroids cause an elevation of blood pressure, an increase in appetite, and mood instability and irritability. Cognitive Level: Application; Client Need: Physiological Integrity; Nursing Process: Assessment; Learning Outcome: Synthesize information about diagnostic tests and clinical therapy for cancer to plan comprehensive care for children undergoing these procedures.

2. **Correct answer:** 4; Administer intravenous fluids.

   Rationale: Intravenous fluids aid in the removal of the contents of malignant cells into the bloodstream or lysis syndrome. Daily (and sometimes twice daily) weights are imperative for assessment of fluid balance. Urine specific gravity should be at or below 1.010, as it reflects dilute urine or adequate hydration. Antiemetics must be administered at least 30 minutes before the start of chemotherapy and need to be administered as frequently as possible if the patient is nauseated, especially during the administration of chemotherapy. Cognitive Level: Application; Client Need: Physiological Integrity; Nursing Process: Planning; Learning Outcome: Integrate information about oncologic emergencies into plans for monitoring all children with cancer.

3. **Correct answer:** 3; Hemorrhage

   Rationale: The platelet count is decreased, thus putting the child at risk for hemorrhage. The white blood cell count is normal; however, a differential should be analyzed. The red blood cell count is within normal limits. Anemia is not a priority; however, hemoglobin and hematocrit levels should be monitored. Pain should always be considered, but it is not the focus in this situation. Cognitive Level: Analysis; Client Need: Physiological Integrity; Nursing Process: Planning; Learning Outcome: Plan care for children and adolescents of all ages who have a diagnosis of leukemia.

4. **Correct answer:** 1; Create an individualized health plan (IHP) and organize a meeting with the child's teachers.

   Rationale: Communicating an individualized health plan to all teachers is essential for readjustment to the school environment. Reintroduction to the classroom and socialization with friends adds to the feeling of normalcy. Pressure to make up schoolwork may lead to feelings of being overwhelmed and depression. Homeschooling may be necessary for an extended period of time, to aid in readjustment to the classroom and the grasping of concepts for present and future schoolwork. Cognitive Level: Analysis; Client Need: Psychosocial Integrity; Nursing Process: Planning; Learning Outcome: Recommend methods for an oncology team including nurses, social workers, psychologists, and child life specialists to partner with school personnel, children and adolescents, families, and others to meet the needs of children with cancer.

CHAPTER 30

1. **Correct answer:** 1; Preschool age

   Rationale: Preschool-age children have the manual dexterity to assist in caring for an ostomy. School-age children should be able to do most, if not all, of the ostomy care independently. Toddlers do not have the dexterity to assist with ostomy care. Adolescents are able to care for an ostomy independently. Cognitive Level: Application; Client Need: Health Promotion and Maintenance; Nursing Process: Assessment; Learning Outcome: Analyze developmentally appropriate approaches for nursing management of gastrointestinal disorders in the pediatric population.

2. **Correct answer:** 1, 2, 4, 5; Pain management; Accurate assessment of intake and output; Observation of the surgical site for signs of infection; Assessment of cardiac and respiratory status

   Rationale: The child who has had reconstructive surgery for an imperforate anus should not have anything inserted into the rectum in the postoperative period. A sign should be placed over the bed that reads "Nothing per rectum." All of the other choices are important aspects of this child's care. Cognitive Level: Application; Client Need: Physiological Integrity; Nursing Process: Implementation; Learning Outcome: Contrast nursing management and plan care for disorders of the gastrointestinal system for the child needing surgery versus the child needing nonoperative management.

3. **Correct answer:** 2, 3, 4; "Call the health care provider if your child is unable to keep liquids down."; "Perform hand hygiene frequently, especially after changing diapers."; "Provide small amounts of your child's regular diet."

   Rationale: The child's eating patterns may not have returned to normal, raising the risk of dehydration. Liquids should be encouraged; if the child cannot tolerate liquids, the health care provider should be notified. The child may still shed virus in the stool; parents need to use good hand hygiene techniques to prevent the spread of disease. Although appetite may be diminished, the child should be offered smaller, more frequent meals consistent with the normal diet. Liquids should include clear fluids with electrolyte replacement. Parents should be instructed to cleanse the diaper area with warm water and a clean washcloth rather than baby wipes that contain alcohol and may further irritate the skin. Cognitive Level: Analysis; Client Need: Physiological Integrity; Nursing Process: Implementation; Learning Outcome: Analyze developmentally appropriate approaches for nursing management of gastrointestinal disorders in the pediatric population.

4. **Correct answer:** 1; A pacifier

   Rationale: Sucking on a pacifier can disrupt the suture line and should not be used to calm an infant following cleft lip repair. Playing soft music, providing a mobile, and providing a mirror are appropriate ways to soothe and keep the infant calm.

Cognitive Level: Analysis; Client Need: Health Promotion and Maintenance; Nursing Process: Implementation; Learning Outcome: Analyze developmentally appropriate approaches for nursing management of gastrointestinal disorders in the pediatric population.

CHAPTER 31

1. **Correct answer:** 1; "Urinary tract infections always cause renal scarring."

   Rationale: Urinary infections do not always cause renal scarring. It is noted most often in hydronephrosis. Urine returned to the bladder, mostly due to vesicoureteral reflux, creates a reservoir for bacterial growth. It is true that fever can be a sign of a UTI. Prophylactic antibiotics may be ordered until all radiologic tests are completed and a specific diagnosis is made. Cognitive Level: Analysis; Client Need: Physiological Integrity; Nursing Process: Evaluation; Learning Outcome: Develop a nursing care plan for the child with a urinary tract infection.

2. **Correct answer:** 4; Broiled chicken, broccoli, and noodles with low-salt butter

   Rationale: Broiled chicken, broccoli, and noodles with low-salt butter are low in sodium, potassium, and phosphorus, which are compatible with the restrictions for children with kidney disease. Tomatoes and leafy greens are high in potassium. Ice cream is high in phosphorus. All are limited in children with chronic renal failure. Peanuts and fresh pears are high in potassium. Chocolate pudding is high in phosphorus. Both must be limited in children with chronic renal failure. Hot dogs and ketchup are high in sodium. Yogurt is high in phosphorus. Both are limited in the child with kidney disease. Cognitive Level: Analysis; Client Need: Physiological Integrity; Nursing Process: Planning; Learning Outcome: Outline a plan to meet the dietary restrictions of a child with a renal disorder.

3. **Correct answer:** 3; Infection, Risk for

   Rationale: Acquiring an infection due to the daily invasive procedure is an ongoing problem and is priority. Caregiver role strain is important but diagnoses directly involving the child's safety are priority. A disturbed body image is psychosocial and the physical risk for infection has higher priority. Imbalanced nutrition is important but the child's physical safety takes priority. Cognitive Level: Analysis; Client Need: Safe, Effective Care Environment; Nursing Process: Planning; Learning Outcome: Plan nursing care for the child with acute and chronic renal failure.

4. **Correct answer:** 2; A 4-year-old female with a fractured femur

   Rationale: A 4-year-old child with a fractured femur is a developmentally appropriate roommate for the 3-year-old female. Exposure to this child will not promote infection. The patients with varicella and cystic fibrosis are not appropriate roommates due to the risk of infection for the patient on hemodialysis. The child who is postoperative appendectomy is a male and thus is not the most appropriate choice. Cognitive Level: Analysis; Client Need: Safe, Effective Care Environment; Nursing Process: Evaluation; Learning Outcome: Plan nursing care for the child with acute and chronic renal failure.

CHAPTER 32

1. **Correct answer:** 3; Urine ketones are tested when the glucose level is greater than 200 mg/dL.

   Rationale: Urine ketones are tested when the blood glucose level is greater than 200 mg/dL. Blood glucose levels may need to be monitored more frequently than is routine. The usual dose of insulin may actually need to be increased. Higher blood glucose levels may necessitate increases in insulin doses. The child will need increased fluid intake, greater than normal demands. If the child cannot eat to maintain food intake, fluids should have carbohydrates to maintain the usual caloric intake. Cognitive Level: Synthesis; Client Need: Physiological Integrity; Nursing Process: Implementation; Learning Outcome: Prioritize nursing care for each type of acquired metabolic disorder.

2. **Correct answer:** 1; Disturbed Body Image related to changes in appearance caused by process of metabolic disorder

   Rationale: A teenager is most affected by changes in body image. Teenagers who are different from their peers or have a change in appearance may have a difficult time adjusting and need emotional and psychosocial support. Metabolic needs are higher than usual in hyperthyroidism, leading to a potential inability to meet the body's requirements. Fluid volume deficit is not associated with hyperthyroidism. The child may have increased appetite, weight loss, diaphoresis, and weakness. Cognitive Level: Analysis; Client Need: Psychosocial Integrity; Nursing Process: Assessment; Learning Outcome: Prioritize nursing care for each type of acquired metabolic disorder.

3. **Correct answer:** 2; Injectable hydrocortisone is on hand for stressful situations such as surgery.

   Rationale: Injectable hydrocortisone will be given prior to surgery or any other stressful event. Parents should be educated to have injectable hydrocortisone on hand at home in the event of an emergency. The dosage should not be held prior to surgery. The stress of surgery may necessitate an increase in dosage prior to surgery and for a short time after surgery. The child will need more intensive care before, during, and after surgery than the average child. Careful monitoring of hormone and drug levels is vital. Cognitive Level: Analysis; Client Need: Physiological Integrity; Nursing Process: Evaluation; Learning Outcome: Develop a family education plan for the child who needs lifelong cortisol replacement.

4. **Correct answer:** 1; Turner Syndrome

   Rationale: Turner syndrome presents with lymphedema of hands and feet, a webbed neck, and a low hairline. Klinefelter syndrome typically does not manifest until the school-age years. PKU infants will appear lighter than nonaffected siblings. Galactosemia does not present in this fashion. Cognitive Level: Analysis; Client Need: Physiological Integrity; Nursing Process: Implementation; Learning Outcome: Plan care for the child with an inherited metabolic disorder.

CHAPTER 33

1. **Correct answer:** 1; Tuna with mayonnaise, potato chips, and broccoli

   Rationale: Acceptable foods on the ketogenic diet are low in sugars. The other choices include foods high in sugar and should not be offered on the ketogenic diet. Cognitive Level: Analysis; Client Need: Physiological Integrity; Nursing Process: Planning; Learning Outcome: Differentiate between the signs of a seizure and status epilepticus in infants and children, and plan appropriate nursing management for each condition.

2. **Correct answer:** 4; "Children who have viral meningitis usually have a complete recovery without permanent effects."

   Rationale: Prognosis for viral meningitis is excellent. Some children with viral encephalitis may also have complete recoveries but many have intellectual, visual, auditory, or motor deficits. Viral meningitis is a different disease than viral encephalitis. There is no connection. Viral encephalitis is not contagious. It occurs as a response to a virus, specifically herpes simplex type 1. Cognitive Level: Analysis; Client Need: Physiological Integrity; Nursing Process: Implementation; Learning Outcome: Differentiate between signs of bacterial meningitis, viral meningitis, encephalitis, and Guillain-Barré syndrome in infants and children.

3. **Correct answer:** 2; "We should let our doctor know if the child complains of a worsening headache."

   Rationale: Signs of shunt malfunction include a worsening headache. The parents should be taught that there is a risk of the child developing seizures, even if the shunt is functioning properly. All children with this condition should be referred to early intervention programs for tracking developmental milestones and appropriate therapy. Usually a shunt malfunction or infection will occur within the 6-month time frame; however, it can occur at any time. Cognitive Level: Application; Client Need: Physiological Integrity; Nursing Process: Evaluation; Learning Outcome: Plan family-centered nursing care for the child with myelodysplasia and hydrocephalus.

4. **Correct answer:** 3; Shaken baby syndrome

   Rationale: Clinical manifestations of shaken baby syndrome include seizure, lethargy, failure to thrive, and vomiting. It is caused by the tearing of the nerve fibers as the brain moves back and forth. Influenza is an acute illness and should not have accompanying signs of failure to thrive or a decreased level of consciousness. Response to the DTaP immunization includes fever and irritability. A malabsorption syndrome can cause failure to thrive but not a decreased level of consciousness. Cognitive Level: Application; Client Need: Physiological Integrity; Nursing Process: Assessment; Learning Outcome: Contrast the initial nursing management for the child with mild traumatic brain injury and severe traumatic brain injury.

CHAPTER 34

1. **Correct answer:** 1; Get the child off the bus for a while.

   Rationale: The teen needs to get off the bus since she is experiencing panic because of agoraphobia; she does not need to eat. Caffeinated drinks may actually exacerbate a panic disorder. Promoting attention can exacerbate the symptoms. Cognitive Level: Application; Client Need: Psychosocial Integrity; Nursing Process: Implementation; Learning Outcome: Plan for the nursing management of children and adolescents with mental health alterations in the hospital and community settings.

2. Correct answer: 1; The nurse notices household cleaners stored under the kitchen sink.

Rationale: Children with intellectual disability might lack an understanding of household hazards, so placing all chemicals out of reach is an important issue to discuss with the parents. Families with children who have intellectual disability often have to aid with more physical tasks due to the child's inability to provide self-care. Families with special needs children need help and support. All children with intellectual disability should have an IEP through the school. Cognitive Level: Application; Client Need: Safe, Effective Care Environment; Nursing Process: Evaluation; Learning Outcome: Establish and evaluate expected outcomes for children with cognitive alterations.

3. Correct answer: 4; Develop an individualized education plan (IEP).

Rationale: The IEP provides learning accommodations for the child with a learning disability. Most children with an auditory learning disability do not have intellectual disability and can attend a regular classroom. A child with learning disabilities can be an integral part of the classroom. By planning ahead and acting quickly, the child with learning disabilities can receive learning accommodations and build healthy self-esteem. Cognitive Level: Application; Client Need: Psychosocial Integrity; Nursing Process: Planning; Learning Outcome: Use evidence-based practice to plan nursing management for children with cognitive alterations.

4. Correct answer: 2; Inability to hop

Rationale: A 6-year-old child should have the ability to hop. Cursive writing occurs in the second grade, at approximately 7 to 8 years of age. Riding a skateboard is not an expectation for a 6-year-old child and does not indicate developmental delay. Composing a short story is not an expectation for a 6-year-old child. Cognitive Level: Analysis; Client Need: Health Promotion and Maintenance; Nursing Process: Assessment; Learning Outcome: Establish and evaluate expected outcomes of care for the child with a cognitive alteration.

CHAPTER 35

1. Correct answer: 3; Refer the child for further evaluation for kyphosis.

Rationale: The child fits the description of having kyphosis, a convex curvature of the spine that results in a bulging appearance at the upper back. Further evaluation is necessary. Scoliosis is a lateral C or S curve in the spine. Lordosis is a concave curvature of the lumbar spine, resulting in a swayback appearance. Cognitive Level: Analysis; Client Need: Physiological Integrity; Nursing Process: Assessment; Learning Outcome: Plan nursing care for children with structural deformities of foot, hip, and spine.

2. Correct answer: 2; "All of our sons will have a 50% chance of having the disease."

Rationale: Duchenne muscular dystrophy is an X-linked disorder, so only males are affected. There is a 25% chance the next child will be affected. If he is male, there is a 50% chance. For each pregnancy, the following outcomes are possible for this X-linked disorder (where Xd is the affected gene):

	X	Xd
X	XX	XXd
Y	XY	XdY

With each pregnancy the risk is the same, regardless of previous pregnancy outcomes. Cognitive Level: Analysis; Client Need: Psychosocial Integrity; Nursing Process: Evaluation; Learning Outcome: Partner with families to plan care for children with musculoskeletal conditions that are chronic or require long-term care.

3. Correct answer: 1; Ensure the weights are in the proper position.

Rationale: Proper positioning is essential for proper functioning of traction. Weights should be in proper position on a tight line and hanging free. Nuts and bolts should be tight to prevent movement. If weights are supported on a table, they cannot be pulling traction. Slack in the line means that the traction is not being applied. Cognitive Level: Analysis; Client Need: Physiological Integrity; Nursing Process: Implementation; Learning Outcome: Plan nursing interventions to promote safety and developmental progression in children who require braces, casts, traction, and surgery.

4. Correct answer: 1 and 2; Weak pulse; Pale grey extremity

Rationale: Objective symptoms of compartment syndrome include a weak pulse and a pale grey extremity. Tingling and burning are subjective symptoms of compartment syndrome. A fever is not associated with compartment syndrome. Cognitive Level: Analysis; Client Need: Physiological Integrity; Nursing Process: Assessment; Learning Outcome: Recommend nursing care for fractures, including teaching for injury prevention and nursing implementations for the child who has sustained a fracture.

CHAPTER 36

1. Correct answer: 1; "Does your child have any allergies to foods or other substances?"

Rationale: The majority of children with atopic dermatitis, which has a hereditary disposition, also have a history of food allergy or allergy to other substances. Questions about the recurrence of symptoms and the presence of dry skin will not provide useful information as the child may have had symptoms of atopic dermatitis for an extended time. Although the nurse will need information about immunizations, it is not directly related to the chief complaint. Cognitive Level: Analysis; Client Need: Physiological Integrity; Nursing Process: Assessment; Learning Outcome: Plan the nursing care for the child with alterations in skin integrity, including dermatitis, infectious disorders, and infestations.

2. Correct answer: 3; Preventing infection of lesions

Rationale: Although nutrition may be important for a child with atopic dermatitis it is not the highest priority. Keeping the infant content is not the top priority. Nursing care should focus on preventing infection of lesions. Due to impaired skin barrier function and cutaneous immunity, an infant with atopic dermatitis is at greater risk for the development of skin infections by organisms. Antibiotics are not routinely applied to the lesions, since the lesions are not related to infection. Cognitive Level: Analysis; Client Need: Physiological Integrity; Nursing Process: Implementation; Learning Outcome: Plan the nursing care for the child with alterations in skin integrity, including dermatitis, infectious disorders, and infestations.

3. **Correct answer:** 2; It often takes up to 12 weeks to see an improvement and a response to treatment.

Rationale: The teenager should know that the treatment often takes 6 to 12 weeks before a response is noted. Knowing that they may not see results for up to 3 months may encourage them to continue their treatment plan and maintain compliance. Although teenagers must take responsibility for their own treatment, they need to know that results will not be immediate. Sunscreen and acne medication can be applied as directed by a healthcare provider. There is no contraindication to applying them at the same time of day. Encouragement from parents is probably not enough to maintain compliance with the treatment if the teenager perceives that it is not effective. Cognitive

Level: Analysis; Client Need: Psychosocial Integrity; Nursing Process: Implementation; Learning Outcome: Prepare an education plan for adolescents with acne to promote self-care.

4. **Correct answer:** 3; Allow the child to participate in the dressing change process as much as possible.

Rationale: The school-age child is striving for feelings of achievement and control. Giving the child the opportunity to help with the procedure will provide a sense of control and accomplishment. Effective pain management improves the chance the child will participate. A shortened hospital stay is no guarantee with or without cooperation and should never be used as leverage with a child. The parents may not be able to tolerate the procedure and may not wish to participate. The school-age child will not respond well to threats and further loss of control. Cognitive Level: Analysis; Client Need: Health Promotion and Maintenance; Nursing Process: Planning; Learning Outcome: Develop a nursing care plan for the child with a full-thickness burn injury.

Glossary

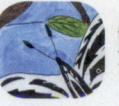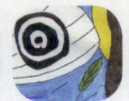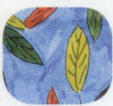

A

Abstract communication Communication displayed through play, visual images, and even clothing.

Acanthosis nigricans Hyperpigmentation and thickening of the skin associated with chronic hyperinsulinemia.

Accommodation The process of changing an individual's cognitive structures to include data from recent experiences.

Accommodations Services or special assistance provided in the school setting to ensure that a student with a physical or mental impairment has access to an appropriate education.

Acculturation An involuntary process in which people adapt to or borrow traits from another culture.

Acellular pertussis vaccine A vaccine that uses proteins from the microorganism rather than the whole cell to stimulate the process of active immunity.

Acidemia Decreased blood pH.

Acidosis Condition caused by excess acid in the blood.

Acquired immunity Humoral and cell-mediated immunity that is not fully developed until a child is about 6 years of age.

Acromegaly Abnormal growth of the hands and feet as well as a protruding brow and lower jaw; the nasal bone enlarges, and spacing of the teeth increases.

Active immunity Antibody development for specific infections through immunization or exposure to the natural disease.

Active transport A process of moving electrolytes against the concentration gradient, from lower to higher areas of concentration, requiring metabolic energy.

Acute pain Sudden pain of short duration, associated with a tissue-damaging stimulus.

Adaptive functioning The ability of an individual to meet the standards expected for his or her age by his or her cultural group.

Addiction A patient's loss of control over the use of a substance with a compulsive use of the substance despite harm.

Adherence The extent to which a patient or parent acts consistently with regard to recommended care.

Adoption A legal relationship between the child and parents who are not related by birth in which the adoptive parents assume all legal and financial responsibility for the child; all ties with the birth family are legally severed.

Adrenarche Stage at which adrenal glands begin increased secretion of hormones.

Advance directives A patient's living will or appointed durable power of attorney for healthcare decisions.

Adventitious sounds Breath sounds that are not normally heard, such as crackles and rhonchi.

Advocacy Acting to safeguard and advance the interests of another.

Affect Outward manifestation of feeling or emotion; the tone of a person's reaction or response to people or events.

Afterload Resistance to the ventricular ejection of blood.

Agoraphobia Anxiety of being in places or situations from which escape may be difficult or embarrassing, or in which help may not be available.

Air hunger The most severe form of dyspnea.

Airway remodeling Irreversible thickening of the subepithelial basement membrane and proliferation of smooth muscle cells in size and number as the result of asthma.

Airway resistance The effort or force needed to move oxygen through the trachea to the lungs.

Alkalemia Increased blood pH.

Alkalosis Condition caused by too little acid in the blood.

Alleles Different forms of a gene or DNA occupying the same place on a pair of chromosomes; an allele for each gene is inherited from each parent.

Allergen An antigen capable of inducing hypersensitivity.

Allergy An abnormal immune response (hypersensitivity) to a substance (allergen).

Allodynia A normally nonpainful sensation, such as touch, is felt as pain.

Allogeneic transplantation Hematopoietic stem cell transplant in which the donor, often a sibling (related), has a compatible human leukocyte antigen (HLA).

Allograft A temporary skin replacement, often with cadaver skin.

Allow natural death Continuing ongoing care and choosing not to initiate CPR if the child stops breathing or the heart stops beating.

Alternative medicine A type of nontraditional medicine used in place of conventional medicine.

Alveolar hypoventilation The condition in which the volume of air entering the alveoli during gas exchange is inadequate to meet the body's metabolic needs.

Amblyopia Reduced vision of the eye.

Anabolism The synthesis or building up of body tissues.

Anemia A reduction in the number of red blood cells to below normal levels.

Anemia of prematurity Insufficient iron stores at birth, resulting in anemia at 2 to 3 months of age.

Anencephaly No development of the brain above the brainstem, most severe congenital malformation of the central nervous system.

Anhedonia Inability to experience pleasure.

Animal-assisted activity (or pet therapy**)** Use of a specially trained animal to provide comfort, companionship, and distraction during an illness; often used in hospitals.

Animism The process of attributing lifelike qualities to nonliving things; common in thoughts of young children.

Anion Negatively charged particle.

Anthropometric measurement The growth assessment of various body parts.

Antibodies Proteins capable of responding to specific infections.

Anticipation The tendency for certain genetic disorders to display earlier onset and increased severity in successive generations of a family.

Anticipatory guidance The process of understanding upcoming developmental needs and then teaching caretakers to meet those needs.

Anticipatory loss The anticipation of loss experienced before the loss actually transpires.

Anticipatory mourning Grief occurring before an expected loss in anticipation of that loss.

Antigen A foreign substance that triggers an immune system response.

Anuria Complete cessation of urine production by the kidneys.

Apical impulse Point of maximum intensity, where the left ventricle taps the anterior chest during systole.

Apnea Cessation of respiration lasting longer than 20 seconds.

Apoptosis Programmed or physiologic cell death caused by the cell itself when its growth becomes abnormal.

Appropriate for gestational age An infant whose weight, length, and head circumference falls between the tenth and ninetieth percentiles when plotted on a standard intrauterine growth/gestational age chart. An AGA newborn can be term, preterm, or postterm. For example, a baby born at 33 weeks' gestation who weighs 1800 grams (4 pounds) is preterm and AGA.

Areflexia No reflex response to verbal, sensory, or pain stimulation.

Arrhythmias Abnormal rhythms or dysrhythmias.

Ascites Fluid in the peritoneal cavity.

Assent Voluntary agreement to participate in a research project or to accept treatment.

Assimilation Adopting and incorporating characteristics of a new culture within one's practices.

Assistive technology A piece of equipment or system modified or customized to improve or maintain functional capabilities of individuals with disabilities.

Association in dysmorphology A group of abnormalities of unknown cause that is seen together more often than would be expected by chance.

Associative play A type of play that emerges in preschool years when children interact with one another, engaging in similar activities and participating in groups.

Asthma flare Sudden appearance of breathing difficulty (cough, wheeze, or breathlessness), often called an asthma attack.

Atelectasis Incomplete expansion of the lungs at birth, or collapse of the lungs or a section of the lungs.

Atresia Absence or closure of a normal body orifice.

Attachment A strong emotional bond between people.

Attachment behaviors Behavior of infant toward caregiver, and caregiver toward infant that demonstrates an emotional connection; eye contact, sounds, and touches between a parent and newborn that build the core emotions a parent feels for a child, such as protectiveness and amazement. This initial process helps lay the foundation for attachment, which develops over time as the caregiver and infant build their relationship.

Audiography A test used to assess hearing in which sounds of various pitches and intensity are presented to children through earphones.

Audiometry A hearing screening using air conduction that measures hearing for pure-tone frequencies and loudness.

Aura A sensation preceding the onset of a seizure, such as taste, visual, auditory, dizziness, or numbness.

Auscultation Listening to sounds produced by the airway, lungs, stomach, heart, and blood vessels to identify their characteristics; usually performed with the stethoscope to enhance the sounds heard.

Autism spectrum disorder (ASD) or pervasive developmental disorder (PDD) A condition that begins in early childhood and is characterized by impaired social interactions and communication, with restricted interests, activities, and behaviors.

Autografting Use of healthy skin taken from a nonburned area of the patient's body.

Autoimmune disease When the immune system produces antibodies against cells of the body.

Autologous transplantation When the child's own marrow is taken, treated, stored, and reinfused after the child has received chemotherapy.

Automatism Unusual or typical body movements without purpose such as lip smacking, lip chewing, or sucking in association with a seizure.

Autonomic dysreflexia Condition in which hypertension, bradycardia, severe headaches, pallor below and flushing above the level of the spinal cord lesion, and seizures occur due to an impaired autonomic nervous system, triggered by simultaneous sympathetic and parasympathetic activity.

Autonomy Right for self-determination in decision making or to protect the informed choices of patients who are capable of decision making.

Autosome A single chromosome from any one of the 22 pairs of chromosomes not involved in sex determination (X or Y); humans have 22 pairs of autosomes.

Azotemia Accumulation of nitrogenous wastes in the blood.

B

Balanitis Inflammation or infection of the glans penis.

Behavior modification A technique used to reinforce desirable behaviors, helping the child to replace maladaptive behaviors with more appropriate ones.

Beneficence An obligation to act or make a decision to benefit the patient.

Benign A growth that does not endanger life or health.

Bereavement The situation of having experienced loss through the death of a loved one.

Bias Preference for a certain set of ideas.

Bibliotherapy The use of books related to topics and events the child is experiencing or will experience.

Binge eating A compulsion to consume large quantities of food in a short period.

Binocularity Ability of the eyes to function together.

Biotherapy Use of biologic response modifiers to treat cancer.

Bladder exstrophy A rare congenital defect in which the posterior bladder wall extrudes through the lower abdominal wall.

Blount disease A disorder characterized by abnormal growth on the medial side of the proximal tibia

which causes an increasing varus deformity, leading to bowlegs.

Body fluid Body water that has substances (solutes) dissolved in it.

Body image The idea that one forms about one's body.

Body language Movement of body parts, including gestures and posture, used during communication.

Body mass index (BMI) A calculation (kilograms of weight/m^2 of height) used to determine the proportion between a child's height and weight.

Body surface area (BSA) Measurement of the relationship between height and weight, measured in squared meters (m^2).

Bone age An estimation of skeletal maturity.

Bones Osseous or dense connective tissue that contains an exterior shell or cortex, and an inner, primarily protein, matrix that forms the skeleton.

Brain death The irreversible cessation of all functions of the brain, including the cerebral cortex and brainstem.

Branding Burning of skin to create a scar, usually in a desired design (scarification).

Breakthrough pain Pain that emerges as the pain medication wears off.

Bronchiolitis obliterans Chronic rejection of transplanted lungs that is unresponsive to immunologic medication management.

Broncophony Change in vocal resonance in the presence of a lung consolidation, in which there is increased intensity and clarity of sounds while the words remain indistinct.

Brudzinski sign If flexing the child's head while in a supine position makes the knees or hips flex involuntarily, a positive Brudzinski sign is present; this is a common sign in meningitis.

Buffer Related acid-base pair that gives up or takes up hydrogen ions as needed to prevent large changes in the pH of a solution.

Bullying Repeatedly aggressive behavior intended to cause physical or emotional harm that exists in a relationship with an imbalance of power.

C

Cachexia A syndrome characterized by anorexia, weight loss, anemia, asthenia (weakness), and early satiety (feeling of being full).

Caput succedaneum An edematous swelling and ecchymosis over the presenting part of the head due to birth trauma.

Carbohydrate Macronutrients composed of carbon, hydrogen, and oxygen that are arranged in various configurations to form saccharides (sugar molecules).

Carcinogens Chemicals or processes that, when combined with genetic traits and in interaction with one another, cause cancer.

Cardiac output Volume of blood ejected from the left ventricle each minute.

Cardiomegaly Enlargement of the heart by hypertrophy of its muscles.

Caregiver burden The burden family or caregivers feel when caring for the child with a chronic condition.

Caring Emotional investment in the child and family by the nurse or other healthcare providers.

Carrier Any individual who carries a single copy of an altered gene or mutation for a recessive condition on one chromosome of a chromosome pair and an unaltered form of that gene on the other chromosome; a carrier generally is not affected by

the gene alteration; on the average, each person in the general population is a carrier of five or six gene mutations for recessive disorders.

Case management A process of coordinating the delivery of healthcare services in a manner that focuses on both quality and cost outcomes.

Case manager Person who coordinates health care to prevent gaps or overlaps.

Catabolism The destruction or breaking down of body tissues.

Cataract Condition that occurs when all or part of the lens of the eye becomes opaque, which prevents refraction of light rays onto the retina.

Catecholamine (epinephrine and norepinephrine) Affects the nervous system, cardiovascular system, metabolic rate, temperature, and smooth muscles.

Cation Positively charged particle.

Cell The basic unit of life, and the working unit of all living systems.

Cellulitis An acute inflammation of the dermis and underlying connective tissue characterized by red or lilac colored, tender, warm, edematous skin.

Centration Focus on only one particular aspect of a situation; common in thoughts of preschoolers.

Cephalhematoma A subperiosteal hemorrhage that results from birth trauma.

Cephalocaudal development The process by which development proceeds from the head downward through the body and toward the feet.

Cerebral edema The increase in intracellular and extracellular fluid in the brain that results from anoxia, vasodilation, or vascular stasis.

Cerebral perfusion pressure Amount of pressure needed to ensure that adequate oxygen and nutrients are delivered to the brain.

Channel The medium through which the message is transmitted.

Chelation A reaction in which an organic compound, containing carbonyl (CO) and hydroxyl (OH) groups, coordinates with a metal to form a firmly bound ringlike structure.

Chemotherapy Treatment to combat cancer that involves drugs taken orally, intravenously, intrathecally, or by injection, which kill both normal and cancerous cells.

Cheyne-Stokes respirations Periods of shallow breathing alternating with apnea, a sign of imminent death.

Child life specialist Trained professional who plans therapeutic activities for hospitalized children.

Child sex abuse The exploitation of a child for the sexual gratification of an adult.

Children with special healthcare needs (CSHCN) Children who have or are at increased risk for a chronic physical, developmental, behavioral, or emotional condition and who also require services beyond those usually required by children.

Cholestasis Disruption of bile flow.

Cholesterol A steroid or sterol compound found only in animal cells that is essential to cell membranes; may be ingested from foods as well as manufactured in the body.

Chondrolysis The breaking down and absorption of cartilage.

Chordee A fibrous line of tissue that results in ventral curvature of the penile shaft.

Chronic condition A health or medical condition that lasts or is expected to last 3 months or more.

Chronic pain Persistent pain lasting longer than 3 months, generally associated with a prolonged disease process.

Chronic sorrow A coping mechanism of periodic grieving.

Chronic vomiting Low-grade nearly daily emesis.

Circumcision Surgical removal of the foreskin.

Circumferential Injury completely surrounding the thorax or an extremity.

Clinical practice guidelines Comprehensive evidence-based interdisciplinary care statements to assist healthcare provider decision making about the appropriate care for a specific condition.

Clinical reasoning The process by which nurses collect cues, process the information, come to an understanding of a patient problem or situation, plan and implement interventions, evaluate outcomes, and reflect on and learn from the process.

Clonic Alternating muscular contraction and relaxation; rhythmic repetitive jerking, often used to describe seizure activity.

Clubbing Widening of the nail bed with an increased angle between the proximal nail fold and nail.

Cognition The change in thought, intelligence, and language that occurs from the mutual interaction of brain maturation with life experiences.

Cognitive power The ability to process the data and respond either verbally or physically.

Cognitive therapy A therapeutic approach that attempts to help the person recognize automatic thought patterns that lead to unpleasant feelings.

Collagen A protein that is the material of skin repair.

Collective monologue Speaking in separate conversations even though each person waits for the other to speak; common in speech of preschoolers.

Coloboma A keyhole-shaped pupil caused by a notch in the iris.

Coma State of unconsciousness in which the patient cannot be aroused, even with powerful stimuli.

Comdones Whiteheads and blackheads.

Comfort care Continuation of ongoing care, managing pain, and choosing not to initiate CPR if the child stops breathing or if the heart stops beating.

Communicable disease An illness that is transmitted directly or indirectly from one person to another.

Communication The exchange of information, thoughts, and feelings.

Community assessment A process of compiling data about a community's health status and resources for the purpose of program planning to address health needs.

Compartment syndrome A condition of increased pressure in a limited space such as in soft tissue of an extremity, which compromises circulation and nervous innervation.

Compassion fatigue An emotion that comes from knowing about the traumatizing events experienced by families and the stress from helping or wanting to help that family.

Competence An ability to be involved in healthcare decisions requiring a certain degree of intellect, an ability to communicate, and an ability to remember.

Complementary medicine Nontraditional medicine that is used in combination with conventional medicine.

Complementary therapy Nontraditional medicine that is used in combination with conventional medicine.

Compliance Ability of the lungs and chest wall to expand during inspiration and recoil with expiration; amount of distention or expansion the ventricles can achieve to increase stroke volume.

Complicated grief An unhealthy grief that is not resolved; the grief is intensified to the level that the individual is so overwhelmed that it interferes with ability to function.

Conductive hearing loss Hearing loss caused by inadequate conduction of sound from the outer to the middle ear.

Confidentiality An agreement between a patient and a provider that information discussed during the healthcare encounter will not be shared without the patient's permission.

Congenital Present at birth.

Conjugate vaccine A vaccine in which an altered organism is joined with another substance to increase the immune response, such as the pneumococcal conjugate vaccine, meningococcal polysaccharide conjugate vaccine, and *Haemophilus influenzae* type b (Hib) vaccine.

Consanguinity Related by having a common ancestor; close blood relationship.

Consciousness The responsiveness of the mind to sensory stimuli, consciousness has two components: alertness and cognitive power.

Conservation The knowledge that matter is not changed when its form is altered.

Constipation Difficult and infrequent defecation with passage of hard, dry stool.

Constitutional growth delay A late pubertal growth spurt caused by delayed pubertal hormone secretion.

Continuity of care An interdisciplinary process of facilitating a patient's transition between and among settings based on changing needs and available resources.

Continuum of care The ongoing relationship between the healthcare provider and family, providing a "seamless continuum of care" so that the patient perceives no interruption of services as a variety of healthcare needs are provided.

Contractility The ability of the heart muscle fibers to contract forcefully.

Contrecoup injury Brain injury resulting from inertial forces, the acceleration-deceleration movement of the brain within the skull.

Cooperative play A type of play that emerges in school years when children join into groups to achieve a goal or play a game.

Coping Use of behavioral and cognitive strategies to manage or relieve perceived stress.

Coprolalia The involuntary utterance of obscenities, profanities, and racial slurs.

Copropraxia The involuntary use of obscene gestures.

Cor pulmonale Obstruction of pulmonary blood flow that leads to right ventricular hypertrophy and heart failure.

Corrected age Number of weeks or months after a baby's birth, minus the number of weeks or months the baby was born prematurely. For example, a 12-week-old baby born at 32 weeks' gestation (8 weeks before its due date) would have a corrected age of 4 weeks. A preterm infant is assessed according to his or her corrected age, not age since birth.

Coup injury Brain injury resulting from a direct blow to the head.

Crepitus A crinkly sensation palpated on the chest surface caused by air escaping into the subcutaneous tissues.

Critical thinking An individualized, creative thinking or reasoning process that the nurse uses to solve problems.

Crossing over A process that occurs during meiosis in which homologous maternal and paternal chromosomes break and exchange corresponding sections of DNA and then rejoin; this process can cause an exchange of alleles between chromosomes and provides human diversity.

Cryosurgery Freezing a lesion with liquid nitrogen.

Cryptorchidism Undescended testes.

Cues An action or behavior that indicates a baby's readiness for and reaction to stimulation, which indicates an important method of infant communication, for example, a baby making eye contact with the caregiver. Disengagement cues include looking away, arching, and crying.

Cultural broker One who serves as a go-between or advocate for people from different cultural backgrounds.

Cultural competence The ability of the nurse to understand and effectively respond to the needs of patients and families from different cultural backgrounds.

Culture "The combination of a body of knowledge, a body of belief and a body of behavior. It involves a number of elements, including personal identification, language, thoughts, communications, actions, customs, beliefs, values, and institutions that are often specific to ethnic, racial, religious, geographic, or social groups" (U.S. Department of Health and Human Services, National Institutes of Health, 2010).

Culture shock The experience that a person has in attempting to understand or adapt to a culture that is fundamentally different from his or her own culture.

Curandero A highly respected shaman in the Hispanic and other Mexican American cultures who uses white magic and herbs to bring about cures.

Cushing triad Reflex response associated with increased intracranial pressure or compromised blood flow to the brainstem, characterized by hypertension, increased systolic pressure with wide pulse pressure, bradycardia, and irregular respirations.

Customs Common practices of a culture.

Cutting Creating a break in the skin to result in a scar, usually in a desired design.

Cyberbullying Socially aggressive and often anonymous targeting of a child or adolescent via Internet posting or other digital technology; the youth victim is threatened, tormented, harassed, humiliated, embarrassed, or excluded from communication; personal information may be disclosed or fabricated; offensive messages may be sent, or harmful messages sent out under the target person's name.

Cyclic vomiting Repeated severe vomiting of an episodic nature.

Cystitis Infection of the bladder.

Cytogenetics The study of chromosomes and alterations to health caused by abnormalities in the number or structure of chromosomes.

Cytokines Proteins that carry messages for immune system function.

D

Deamination Removal of amino group from amino compound.

Death anxiety A feeling of apprehension or fear of death.

Death imagery Any reference to death or death-related topics, such as going away, separation, funerals, and dying, given in response to a picture or story that would not usually stimulate a child to discuss death-related topics.

Debridement Enzyme action to clean a lesion and dissolve fibrin clots or scabs; or removal of dead tissue to speed the healing process.

Debulk To reduce the size of a solid tumor.

Decibels Units used to measure the loudness of sounds.

Deciduous teeth Primary set of 20 teeth that are complete by about 2 years of age and will be lost during childhood, beginning at about 6 years.

Decode To translate the meaning of the message.

Decontamination The removal of chemicals and nerve agents from the skin.

Deep sedation A controlled state of depressed consciousness or unconsciousness in which the child may experience partial or complete loss of protective reflexes.

Defensive mechanism Technique used by the ego to unconsciously change reality, thereby protecting the individual from excessive anxiety.

Dehydration The state of body water deficit.

Deletion Loss of all or part of a chromosome resulting in missing chromosomal material.

Dental caries Cavities, tooth decay, decalcification of enamel and dentin.

Dental home A specialized primary dental care provider who manages and facilitates all aspects of oral health care for infants and young children 6 months after the first tooth erupts or by 12 months of age and who provides preventive dental health care.

Dermatophytoses Fungal infections that affect primarily the skin but may affect the hair and nails.

Desaturated blood Blood with a lower than normal oxygen level resulting when a heart defect causes oxygenated and unoxygenated blood to mix.

Development An increase in capability or function.

Developmental delay Failure to achieve anticipated developmental milestones during specific developmental stages.

Developmental disability A variety of chronic conditions characterized by mental and/or physical impairments.

Developmental surveillance A flexible, continuous process of skilled observations of children's fine and gross motor skills, language, and psychosocial behavior milestones during child health visits.

Dialysate The solution used in dialysis.

Diarrhea Frequent passage of abnormally watery stool.

Dietary Reference Intakes (DRIs) A set of nutrient values that can be used to assess and plan intake for individuals of different ages.

Diffusion Movement of molecules across a membrane from an area of higher concentration to lower concentration.

Digitalization Process of giving a higher than normal dose of digoxin initially to speed response to the drug and achieve therapeutic blood levels faster.

Direct transmission Illness passed from one person or animal to another by contact with body fluids.

Disability A limitation that interferes with a child's ability to fully participate in society.

Disaster preparedness Planning and coordinated response readiness by a community to meet the personal safety, healthcare, emotional, and environmental needs of children and their families in the event of a natural or man-made disaster.

Disasters Monumental occurrences involving serious and massive events that impact many people and are beyond the community's ability to manage.

Discipline A method for teaching the rules that govern behavior or conduct or the action taken to enforce the rules when the child misbehaves.

Disease surveillance Continuous monitoring and tracking of the incidence and patterns of infections.

Disequilibrium syndrome Occurs during or soon after dialysis and results from cerebral edema caused by a drop in plasma osmolality during dialysis.

Dislocation Displacement of a bone from its normal articulation with a joint.

Distraction The ability to focus attention on something other than pain, such as an activity, music, or a story.

Diurnal enuresis Enuresis occurring during the day.

Do-not-intubate (DNI) order An order written by a physician at the family's request not to intubate a child who stops breathing.

Do-not-resuscitate (DNR) order An order written by a physician at the family's request not to resuscitate or take other lifesaving interventions for a child who stops breathing.

Domains Categories or foci of developmental progression, including fine motor skills, gross motor skills, language, self-help skills, social skills, and reading.

Domestic violence A pattern of violent and coercive behavior that includes physical, sexual, and psychologic attacks, as well as economic coercion that adults or adolescents use against their intimate partners to gain or maintain power and control.

Dominant A characteristic or gene that is apparent even when the relevant gene is present in only one copy; a person with a dominant gene usually expresses that gene trait.

Dramatic play A type of play in which a child acts out the drama of daily life.

Drowning Death from suffocation in the first 24 hours after submersion in a liquid.

Ductus arteriosus The fetal vascular channel between the pulmonary artery and the descending aorta.

Ductus venosus The fetal vascular channel between the umbilical vein and the inferior vena cava.

Dwarfism A genetic condition usually resulting in an adult height of 58 inches or less.

Dysfluency A disruption in the smooth transition between sounds, syllables, and words.

Dysmorphology The study of human congenital defects or abnormalities of body structure that begin before birth.

Dysphagia Difficulty in swallowing.

Dysphonia Muffled, hoarse, or absent voice sounds.

Dysplasia Abnormal development resulting in altered size, shape, and cell organization.

Dyspnea Shortness of breath; difficulty in breathing.

E

Early childhood caries The presence of one or more decayed, lost, or filled tooth surfaces in primary teeth from birth to 6 years of age; frequently caused by drinking from a bottle or nursing for prolonged periods, especially when sleeping; previously referred to as nursing bottle mouth syndrome and baby bottle tooth decay.

Early intervention Special services for infants and toddlers up to age 3 years who have developmental delay or are at risk for developmental delay.

Ecchymosis Bruising.

Echolalia A compulsive parroting of what is heard.

Ecological theory A theory of development that emphasizes the importance of interactions between the developing child and the settings in which the child lives.

Ecomap An illustration of the family's relationships and interactions with the community, describing the family's social network.

Edema An accumulation of excess fluid in the interstitial spaces.

Ego The realistic part of the person, which develops during infancy and searches for acceptable methods of meeting impulses.

Egocentrism The inability to consider the perspective of another; seeing things only from one's own point of view.

Egophony A change in vocal resonance in the presence of a lung consolidation condition in which the transmission of the "eee" sound becomes a nasal "ay" sound.

Electroanalgesia A method of delivering electrical stimulation to the skin, to compete with pain stimuli for transmission to the spinal cord; also known as transcutaneous electrical nerve stimulation (TENS).

Electrolytes Charged particles (ions) dissolved in body fluid.

Emancipated minors Self-supporting adolescents under 18 years of age not subject to parental control.

Emergency preparedness Readiness to manage a healthcare emergency that involves planning, equipment and supplies for responses, and provider training and guidelines for action when an emergency occurs.

Emollient A topical product that soothes and softens the skin.

Emotional abuse Shaming, ridiculing, embarrassing, or insulting a child.

Emotional neglect A caretaker's inability to meet the psychosocial needs of a child.

Empathy The ability to perceive another individual's experience and to understand the perception of that individual's view of the situation.

Empyema A collection of pus in the pleural space.

Encephalocele Protrusion of meningeal tissue or meningeal-covered brain through a defect in the skull.

Encephalopathy Cerebral dysfunction resulting from an insult (toxin, injury, inflammation, or anoxic event) of limited duration; the tissue damage is often permanent, but the dysfunction may improve over time.

Encopresis Abnormal elimination pattern characterized by the recurrent soiling or passage of stool at inappropriate times by a child who should have achieved bowel continence.

Endocardial cushions Fetal growth centers for mitral and tricuspid valves and the atrial and ventricular septum.

Endocardium The tissue lining the heart chambers.

Endogenous pyrogens Pyrogens that are released in response to an invasive organism and travel through the circulatory system to the hypothalamus, where they trigger the production of prostaglandins.

Endorphins Endogenous opioids produced by the brain in response to painful stimuli that help inhibit pain impulses in the spinal cord and the brain.

End-stage renal disease Irreversible kidney failure.

Enteral Nutrition introduced through the intestinal tract, including oral or tube feedings.

Enterocolitis Inflammation of the intestines.

Enuresis Involuntary micturition by a child who has reached the age at which bladder control is expected.

Epicanthal fold An extra layer of skin covering all or part of the medial canthus of the eye.

Epigenetic Describes any factor that can affect gene function (usually by changing gene expression, or translation) without changing the DNA sequence.

Epispadias A congenital anomaly involving an abnormal location of the urethral meatus in males; the meatal opening is located on the dorsal surface of the penile shaft.

Epithelialization The process by which epithelial cells grow into the wound from surrounding healthy tissue.

Equianalgesic dose The amount of a drug, whether administered orally or parenterally, needed to produce the same analgesic effect.

Equinus A condition that limits dorsiflexion to less than normal; usually associated with clubfoot.

Ergogenic aids Products that enhance physical performance.

Erythrocytes Red blood cells.

Erythropoiesis Formation of red blood cells.

Erythropoietin A hormone produced by the kidney that stimulates red blood cell production.

Eschar Slough or layer of dead skin or tissue.

Escharotomy Incision into constricting dead tissue of a burn injury to restore peripheral circulation.

Esotropia Momentary turning inward of eyes.

Espiritista A healer who communicates with spirits for the physical and emotional development of the patient.

Essential amino acid Amino acid that cannot be manufactured by humans but must be ingested in the diet.

Ethics The philosophic study of morality, and the analysis of moral problems and moral judgments.

Ethnicity Cultural group's sense of identification associated with the group's common social and cultural heritage.

Ethnocentrism The belief that an individual's own culture is superior to all others.

Euthanasia The action taken with the sole intent of ending a patient's life.

Euthyroid Normal thyroid state.

Evidence-based practice Integration of the best research evidence with an individual's clinical expertise and the patient's values or preferences.

Exercise-induced asthma Bronchospasm caused by hyperventilation of air that is cooler and dryer than the respiratory tree.

Exophthalmos Prominent or bulging eyes.

Exotropia Outward deviation of eyes ("wall-eyes").

Expressive jargon Use of unintelligible words with normal speech intonations as if truly communicating in words; common in toddlerhood.

Expressive speech Words a young child can speak; usually less than the child is able to understand (receptive speech).

Extracellular fluid The fluid in the body that is outside the cells, including interstitial and intravascular fluid.

Extravasation Damage that occurs when a chemotherapeutic drug leaks into the soft tissue surrounding the infusion site.

F

Faith-based belief An organized system of shared beliefs regarding the significance of the nature, cause, and purpose of life and the universe.

Family Individuals who are joined together by marriage, blood, adoption, or residence in the same household; a living social system, consisting of a small group of individuals who are closely interrelated and interdependent and who collaborate to attain family functions and goals.

Family APGAR A quick five-item questionnaire that may be used as an initial screening tool for family assessment.

Family-centered care A partnership between families, the nurse, and other health professionals in which the priorities and needs of the family are addressed when the family seeks health care; a dynamic, deliberate approach to building collaborative relationships between health professionals and families that are respectful of diversity and beliefs about the nature of the child's condition and ways to manage it.

Family crisis An event occurring when a family encounters problems that seem insurmountable and with which the family is unable to cope in its usual ways.

Family strengths Relationships and processes that support and protect families and family members during times of adversity and change.

Fats Macronutrients also known as lipids; complex molecules of several types, consisting of carbon, hydrogen, and oxygen, arranged so that glycerol and fatty acids are the structural subcomponents.

Fatty acids The major components of fats; may be referred to as saturated (no additional hydrogen atoms could be absorbed by the structure) or unsaturated (some additional bonds with hydrogen are possible). Unsaturated fatty acids are further designated as monounsaturated (only one potential bond with hydrogen possible) or polyunsaturated (two or more potential bonds). Trans-fatty acids are formed when food manufacturers partially hydrogenate unsaturated fatty acids.

Febrile seizure A seizure associated with a fever and acute illness but with no evidence of intracranial infection or other defined cause.

Fiber Indigestible carbohydrate components that ensure healthy movement of fecal contents through the bowel.

Filtration Movement into or out of capillaries as the net result of several opposing forces.

Flares Exacerbations of symptoms associated with a condition.

Focal Located in one hemisphere or a specific area of the cerebral cortex.

Folk healers Members of a community who conduct healing in their home or home of the patient; specific to certain cultures.

Fontanels Spaces of connective tissue covering the brain at the junction of skull bones that gradually close and ossify.

Food allergy An IgE-mediated reaction that is potentially systemic, characteristically rapid in onset, and may be manifested as swelling of the lips, mouth, uvula, or glottis, generalized urticaria, and, in severe reactions, anaphylaxis.

Food insecurity An inability or uncertainty that an individual will be able to acquire or consume adequate quality or quantity of foods in socially acceptable ways.

Food intolerance (sensitivity) An abnormal physiologic response to a food that is not IgE-mediated.

Food jags Eating only a few foods for several days or weeks.

Food security Access at all times to enough nourishment for an active, healthy life.

Foramen ovale The opening between the right and left atria in the fetal heart.

Foster care The provision of protection and shelter for a child in an approved living situation away from the family of origin.

Frostbite A cold injury that results from the overexposure of skin cells to temperatures low enough to cause crystal formation.

Furuncle A deep infection around a hair follicle.

Futility A situation in which treatments do not provide a clear clinical benefit.

G

Gallop A third heart sound that produces a rhythm like the gait of a horse.

Gamete A reproductive cell (i.e., an ovum or sperm) containing a single copy of each of the 23 chromosomes that make up the human genome.

Gastroesophageal reflux (GER) The return of gastric contents into the esophagus, the result of relaxation of the lower esophageal sphincter.

Gastroesophageal reflux disease (GERD) A more serious manifestation of GER; a pathologic process in infants manifested by poor weight gain, recurrent vomiting, generalized irritability, refusal to feed, arching, and respiratory symptoms such as wheezing.

Gastroschisis A congenital defect of the ventral abdominal wall, characterized by herniation of abdominal viscera outside the abdominal cavity through a defect in the abdominal wall to the side (most often to the right) of the umbilicus.

Gene A sequence of DNA on a chromosome that represents a fundamental unit of heredity; occupies a specific spot on a chromosome (gene locus).

Gene expression When the protein product of a gene is visible (presence of a body structure or identifiable through biochemical tests such as insulin or phenylalanine levels).

Genetic disease Any disease associated with gene dysfunction. While genetics diseases have traditionally been thought of as relatively rare inherited diseases, it is now known that nearly all diseases have a genetic component.

Genogram An illustration that incorporates information about significant life events and health and illness status of family members over at least three generations.

Genome The entire DNA sequence that makes up the complete genetic information of a gamete, an individual, a population, or a species.

Genomics The study of all the genes in the human genome together, including their interactions with each other, the environment, and the influence of other psychosocial and cultural factors.

Genotype The genes and the variations therein that a person inherits from his or her parents.

Glaucoma Condition resulting from increased intraocular pressure.

Glomerular filtration rate Refers to the filtration of plasma and is mainly influenced by hydrostatic pressure in the glomerular capillaries.

Glomerulonephritis Inflammation of the glomeruli of the kidneys.

Glucagon A hormone produced by the pancreas that helps release stored glucose from the liver.

Glucocorticoid Affects protein and carbohydrate metabolism and is active in protecting against stress.

Gluconeogenesis Formation of glycogen from noncarbohydrate sources such as protein or fat.

Glycemic index The blood glucose response to 50 grams of carbohydrate from any specific food, as compared to the glucose level after ingestion of white bread.

Glycogen Stored form of carbohydrate that can be returned to glucose for use when the body requires energy and food is not being ingested.

Glycogenolysis Conversion of glycogen to glucose.

Glycosuria Abnormal amount of glucose in the urine.

Goiter Enlargement of the thyroid gland.

Graft-versus-host disease A series of immunologic responses mounted by the host of a transplanted organ with the purpose of destroying the transplant cells.

Grief An individual's feelings and behaviors in response to death.

Growth An increase in physical size.

Growth channel Another term for percentile range.

Grunting A sound produced by the rapid breath release at the end of expiration after the newborn has used the vocal cords to hold the expiratory breath in the lungs to prevent alveolar collapse.

Gynecomastia The presence of unilateral or bilateral enlarged breast tissue in males.

H

Hazing An activity that is forced upon an individual, causes humiliation, and is required for membership in an organization or group.

Health A state of complete physical, mental, and social well-being and not merely the absence of disease and infirmity.

Health literacy The degree to which individuals have the capacity to obtain and understand basic health information needed to make appropriate health decisions.

Health maintenance (health protection) Activities that preserve an individual's present state of health and prevent disease or injury occurrence.

Health promotion Activities that increase wellbeing, enhance wellness or health, and lead to actualization of positive health potential; strategies that seek to foster conditions to allow populations to be healthy and to make healthy choices.

Health supervision Services that focus on disease and injury prevention (health maintenance), growth and developmental surveillance, and health promotion at key intervals during the child's life.

Heave Lifting of the chest wall during contraction.

Hemangioma Benign vascular tumor or malformation.

Hemarthrosis Bleeding into joint spaces.

Hematopoiesis Blood cell production.

Hemodynamics Pressures generated by blood and passage of blood through the heart and pulmonary system.

Hemoglobinopathy Disease characterized by abnormal hemoglobin.

Hemoptysis Coughing up blood from the respiratory tract.

Hemosiderin Iron containing pigment accumulated from hemoglobin as the red blood cells are destroyed.

Hemosiderosis Increased storage of iron in body tissues and associated with diseases involving the destruction of red blood cells.

Hepatitis An inflammation of the liver caused by a viral infection.

Herd immunity Protection provided by persons with immunity to an infection to others who are susceptible or not protected.

Hernia Protrusion or projection of a body part or structure through the muscle wall of the cavity that normally contains it.

Herniation Protrusion of brain contents through the cranial vault at the base of the skull.

Heterozygous Nonidentical copies of a particular gene (different alleles) on the paired chromosomes.

Holistic health paradigm Belief that the forces of nature must be maintained in balance or harmony, and that human life is one aspect of nature that must be in harmony with the rest of nature. Illness results when the natural balance or harmony is disturbed; also called naturalistic health belief.

Holosystolic Heart murmur heard during the entire phase of systole.

Homologous chromosomes Chromosomes that are members of the same pair and normally have the same number and arrangement of genes; usually one copy is from the mother and the other copy is from the father.

Homosexuality Sexual attraction to people of the same sex.

Homozygous Identical copies of a particular gene (same alleles) on both paired chromosomes.

Hormone A chemical substance produced by a gland or organ and carried in the bloodstream to another part of the body where it has a regulatory effect on particular cells.

Hospice A philosophy of care for a terminally ill child that is focused exclusively on comfort and making sure the remaining time for the child is lived as comfortably and fully as possible.

Human genome The total amount of the DNA (genes) in an individual's cells.

Hydronephrosis Collection of urine in the renal pelvis as a result of obstructed outflow.

Hyperalgesia Increased response to a pain stimulus because of peripheral sensitization.

Hyperbilirubinemia An excessive amount of bilirubin in the blood.

Hypercapnia Greater than normal amounts of carbon dioxide in the blood.

Hypercyanotic episode An abrupt decrease in systemic vascular resistance and pulmonary blood flow triggered by activity that occurs in children with heart defects with decreased pulmonary blood flow.

Hypergastrinemia Too much gastrin in the blood.

Hyperinsulinemia Elevated insulin levels in the blood.

Hypersensitivity response An overreaction of the immune system, responsible for allergic reactions.

Hypersplenism A syndrome characterized by splenomegaly and blood cell deficiencies.

Hypertelorism Widely spaced eyes.

Hypertonic dehydration (or hypernatremic dehydration) Sodium loss that is proportionately greater than water loss.

Hypertonic fluid Fluid that is more concentrated than normal body fluid.

Hypertrophic scar A scar that is raised but stays within the original boundaries of the wound.

Hypoplastic Small and nonfunctional.

Hypospadias A congenital anomaly involving an abnormal location of the urethral meatus in males; the urethral meatus may be located anywhere along the course of the anterior urethra on the ventral surface of the penile shaft, from the perineum to the tip of the glans.

Hypotonia Floppiness, increased joint range of motion, and diminished reflex response.

Hypotonic dehydration (or hyponatremic dehydration) Fluid loss characterized by a proportionately greater loss of sodium than water.

Hypotonic fluid Fluid that is more dilute than normal body fluid.

Hypoxemia Lower than normal amounts of oxygen in the blood.

Hypoxia Lower than normal amounts of oxygen in the tissues.

I

Id The basic sexual energy that is present at birth and drives the individual to seek pleasure.

Immigrants Individuals who are foreign-born and migrate to the United States to live and work.

Immunodeficiency A state of the immune system in which it cannot cope effectively with foreign antigens.

Immunoglobulin A protein that functions as an antibody, responsible for humoral immunity.

Inborn errors of metabolism Inherited biochemical abnormalities of the urea cycle, amino acid, and organic acid metabolism.

Incarceration Occurs when the presence of intestine in the groin causes constriction of the blood supply to the scrotal sac, leading to intestinal strangulation and testicular ischemia.

Incest Sexual activity between close family members so that marriage between them would be legally or culturally prohibited.

Independent assortment The random distribution of different combinations of parental genes to gametes.

Indirect transmission The passage of an infectious disease involving survival of pathogens outside humans before they invade a new host.

Individualized approach Health assessment and intervention performed with a particular child.

Individualized education plan (IEP) Formulation of a specific learning approach for a child with a physical or mental disability, following thorough assessment of the child's capabilities and areas of need.

Individualized family service plan (IFSP) Developed for the early intervention process for infants with special healthcare needs and their families, the IFSP contains information about the services required to support a child's development and enhance the family's capacity to facilitate the child's development.

Individualized health plan (IHP) A formal mechanism to ensure that the child's health needs are managed in the school setting.

Individualized transition plan (ITP) A plan that focuses on assisting the individual in moving successfully from school and home into other community settings.

Induration Skin area of extra firmness with a distinct border.

Infant state Characteristics that regularly occur together: body activity, eye movements, facial movements, breathing pattern, and level of response to external stimuli such as handling and internal stimuli such as hunger. Newborns demonstrate six states: quiet sleep, active sleep, drowsy, quiet alert, active alert, and crying.

Infectious disease Illness caused by a microorganism that is commonly communicated from one host (human or otherwise) to another.

Informed consent A formal preauthorization for an invasive procedure or participation in research.

Inguinal hernia A painless inguinal or scrotal swelling of variable size that results when a portion of an abdominal organ or tissue protrudes into the groin.

Inotropic medications Agents that improve the velocity of heart contractility.

Insensible fluid loss Water loss not directly measurable or observable, such as through skin and respirations.

Inspection Purposeful observation by carefully looking at the characteristics of the child's physical features and behaviors, including size, shape, color, movement, position, and location.

Insulin The hormone responsible for glucose metabolism.

Insulin deficiency Insulin resistance; pancreas does not produce sufficient insulin.

Insulin resistance Insulin resistance where the body fails to utilize insulin normally.

Intellectual disability Significant limitation in intellectual functioning and adaptive behavior.

Interstitial fluid Extracellular fluid that is between the cells and outside the blood and lymphatic vessels.

Intertriginous areas Skinfolds of the neck, axillae, and antecubital fossa.

Intimate partner violence Physical, sexual, or emotional abuse or threat from a spouse, partner, or other person in an intimate relationship.

Intracellular fluid The fluid in the body that is inside the cells.

Intracranial pressure Force exerted by brain tissue, cerebrospinal fluid, and blood within the cranial vault.

Intractable seizure Seizures that continue to occur even with optimal medical management.

Intravascular fluid That portion of the extracellular fluid that is in the blood vessels.

Intussusception A condition that occurs when one portion of the intestine prolapses and then invaginates or telescopes into another.

Inversion A chromosomal alteration in which a gene or DNA sequence in a segment of a chromosome has been reversed.

Involution Process of decreasing in size.

Iontophoresis Use of a small machine that generates electric current to transport anesthetic into the skin.

Isotonic dehydration (or isonatremic dehydration) Fluid loss that is not balanced by intake; the loss of water and sodium are in proportion.

Isotonic fluid Fluid that has the same osmolality as normal body fluid.

J

Joint custody A legal situation in which both parents have equal responsibility and legal rights for a child, regardless of where the child lives.

Joints Articulations or connections between bones.

Justice Fairness in the use of resources.

K

Karyotype The arrangement of chromosome pairs by number according to length, centromere position, and banding patterns.

Keloid A scar that extends beyond the original boundaries of the wound.

Kerion A large tender boggy mass on the scalp with drainage associated with tinea capitis.

Kernig sign Resistance or pain when a child's leg is raised with the knee flexed and then extended at the knee is a positive Kernig sign, a common finding in meningitis.

Killed virus vaccine A vaccine that contains a killed microorganism that is still capable of inducing the human body to produce antibodies to the disease.

Kinesthesia The sense of one's body position and movement.

Kussmaul respirations Increased rate and depth of respirations (hyperventilation).

Kwashiorkor A deficiency disease that occurs when insufficient protein is ingested.

L

Lacto-ovovegetarians Vegetarians that eat eggs and dairy products.

Lactovegetarians Vegetarians that eat dairy products.

Lanugo The fine, soft hair covering the fetus during intrauterine development.

Large for gestational age (LGA) A newborn whose weight (and possibly length and head circumference) falls above the ninetieth percentile when plotted on a standard intrauterine growth/gestational age chart. An LGA newborn is larger than expected for the amount of time spent in the uterus. An LGA baby can be preterm, term, or postterm. For example, a baby born at 36 weeks' gestation that weighs 3630 grams (8 pounds) is preterm and LGA.

Laryngospasm Spasmodic vibrations of the larynx, which create sudden, violent, unpredictable, involuntary contractions of airway muscles.

Latchkey children Children who come home to an empty house after school.

Learning disabilities Neurologic conditions in which the brain cannot receive or process information in the normal manner.

Legal guardianship An alternative permanent arrangement for the child, often with kin, in which the child retains legal connections with the birth family and relationships with the extended family, and the guardian assumes limited financial liability for the child's care.

Lethal gene When this gene is expressed, it results in death.

Leukocytes White blood cells.

Leukocytosis A higher than normal leukocyte count.

Leukopenia A lower than normal white blood cell count.

Level of consciousness (LOC) General description of cognitive, sensory, and motor response to stimuli.

LGBQ Lesbian, gay, bisexual, or questioning.

LGBT Lesbian, gay, bisexual, or transgendered.

Lichenification Thickening of the skin with increased visibility of normal skin furrows.

Life-threatening condition One in which there is a considerable likelihood of death even though treatment may prolong the child's life or the child may have a complete recovery from the illness or injury.

Ligaments Tough fibers that bind the ends of bones together.

Limit setting Established rules or guidelines for behavior.

Lipoatrophy Loss of subcutaneous tissue.

Lipoproteins Combinations of fat and protein that transport fats in the blood.

Live virus vaccine A vaccine that contains the microorganism in a live but attenuated, or weakened, form.

Loss When something of value is changed, is no longer available, or can no longer be experienced.

Lymphangitis Inflammation of the lymphatic system draining the site of infection seen as tender, erythematous streaks extending in a proximal direction from the infection.

M

Macronutrients The major building blocks of the body, including carbohydrates, protein, and fat.

Macro-religious belief view The belief that health and illness are dominated by supernatural forces.

Magical thinking The belief of young children that events occur because of their thoughts or wishes.

Major anomaly A serious structural defect present at birth that may have severe medical or cosmetic consequences, interfere with normal functioning of body systems, lead to a lifelong disability, or even cause early death.

Malignant The progressive growth of a tumor that will, if not checked by treatment, result in death.

Managed care A health delivery system that combines financing and delivery of specified healthcare services with the following elements in place: clinicians are contracted to provide services for a preset fee, clinicians are selected according to specific standards, formal programs of quality assurance and utilization review are in place, and members of the health program have incentives to use selected clinicians.

Marasmus A deficiency disease that occurs when insufficient carbohydrates are ingested.

Mastoiditis An infection of the mastoid process of the temporal bone of the skull.

Mature minors Adolescents of 14 and 15 years of age who are able to understand treatment risks and who, in some states, can consent to or refuse treatment.

Medical futility The treatment of an irreversibly dying patient that provides no physiologic benefit to the patient.

Medical home A continuous, comprehensive, family-centered, and compassionate source of health care.

Medical jargon The technical language associated with health care.

Medically fragile Children who need skilled nursing care with or without medical equipment to support vital functions.

Meiosis Cell division that produces reproductive cells (egg or sperm); meiosis results in daughter cells, which contain half of the chromosome complement (23).

Melanin A peptide present in the skin and synthesized by an enzyme in melanocytes that influences skin color.

Menarche The onset of menstruation.

Meningocele A spinal fluid-filled meningeal sac protruding through a vertebral defect, associated with no abnormalities of the spinal cord.

Menorrhagia Increased menstrual bleeding.

Mental health Successful engagement in activities and relationships and the ability to adapt to and cope with change.

Newborn screening Blood test conducted on the newborn, usually taken by heelstick sample, to identify those newborns who require further diagnostic testing for an array of genetic diseases and metabolic disorders such as phenylketonuria. The department of health in each state regulates newborn metabolic screening, including which tests are included in the screen.

Metastasis The spread of cancer cells to other sites in the body.

Microarray analysis A laboratory method in which labeled RNA from a specimen is added to a glass slide or other platform upon which DNA fragments are arranged. Useful for identifying and quantifying mRNA and indicating which genes are actively expressed in a tissue.

Microcephaly A small brain with a head circumference greater than 3 standard deviations below the mean for age and sex.

Micronutrients Substances like vitamins and minerals that are needed in small quantities for healthy body functioning.

Mineralocorticoids Hormones involved in regulation of fluid and electrolytes.

Minor anomaly An unusual morphologic feature that is of no serious medical or cosmetic concern.

Mitosis Cell division that results in new (daughter) cells that are genetically identical to each other and to the parent cell.

Mixed hearing loss Hearing loss having a combination of conductive and sensorineural causes.

Modeling Exhibiting appropriate behavior for someone else.

Moderate sedation Sedation level when the child maintains protective reflexes, retains the ability to independently and continuously maintain a patent airway, and retains the ability to make an appropriate response to physical stimuli or verbal command, formerly called conscious sedation.

Molding An overriding of the cranial bones to accommodate the head's passage through the vaginal canal.

Monosomic (monosomy) When one member of the chromosome pair is missing, for example, Turner syndrome (45, XO).

Moral dilemma A conflict of social values and ethical principles that support different courses of action.

Morbidity An illness or injury that limits activity, requires medical attention or hospitalization, or results in a chronic condition.

Mosaicism A chromosome variation or abnormality that occurs after fertilization during mitosis at an early cell stage so not all cells are affected with the variation; for example, a child who is mosaic for Down syndrome will have some cells with two copies of chromosome 21 and some that have an extra chromosome 21.

Mottled Patchy pink, pale, and cyanotic variations in skin color associated with hypoxia.

Mourning The behavioral and psychologic process of adapting to the loss.

Multifactorial Health conditions determined by multiple factors, including genetic and environmental factors, each having an additive effect.

Muscles Collections of cells that can contract, causing the accompanying skeleton to move.

Mutagenesis Permanent changes in the fetus's genetic material.

Myelination The progressive covering of axons with layers of myelin or a lipid protein sheath.

Myelinization Establishment of the myelin or fatty sheath on nerve fibers.

Myelodysplasia Any malformation of the spinal cord and spinal canal.

Myelomeningocele (meningomyelocele) A spinal fluid-filled meningeal sac that contains a portion of the spinal cord and nerves protruding through a vertebral defect.

Myelosuppression A decreased production of blood cells in the bone marrow.

Myringotomy A procedure whereby an incision is made in the tympanic membrane to drain fluid.

Myxedema A life-threatening crisis of hypothyroidism.

N

Nasal flaring Widening of the nares with breathing that is a sign of respiratory distress.

Natural debridement Enzyme action by macrophages and neutrophils to clean the lesion and dissolve the clot or scab.

Natural immunity Natural antibodies passed from mother to the newborn.

Nature The genetic or hereditary capability of an individual.

Negative feedback Mechanism for regulation of hormone concentration.

Neonatal intensive care unit (NICU) A highly specialized care unit for neonates with critical conditions.

Neoplasms Cancerous growths.

Nephron The functional unit of the kidney that contributes to the formation of urine.

Nephrotic syndrome (NS) An alternation in kidney function secondary to increased glomerular basement membrane permeability to plasma protein.

Neural tube The embryonic origin of the central nervous system.

Neurogenic bladder The result of urinary tract obstruction related to an interrupted nerve supply to the bladder.

Neuropathic pain An abnormal processing of pain stimuli by the peripheral or central nervous system; may be initiated or caused by a primary lesion or dysfunction of the nervous system.

Neutropenia A decreased number of neutrophils.

Nightmares Frightening dreams that awaken a child.

Night terrors In contrast to nightmares, the child having a night terror is not fully awake and may appear disoriented.

Nitrogen balance Protein balance. Positive nitrogen balance is when more nitrogen is taken into the body than excreted and occurs during periods of growth during childhood, when additional body tissues are being manufactured, and when the body is replenished after illness or surgery. Negative nitrogen balance indicates that the body excretes more nitrogen than it ingests and occurs when dietary intake is limited.

Nociceptive pain The normal processing of pain stimuli caused by tissue injury or damage.

Nociception Transmission of pain impulses.

Nociceptors Free nerve endings at the site of tissue damage that detect pain stimuli.

Nocturnal enuresis Enuresis that occurs at night.

Nondisjunction An error in cell division where a pair of homologous chromosomes do not separate as expected, resulting in monosomy or trisomy in gametes.

Nonessential amino acid Amino acid that humans can manufacture when in good health.

Nonmaleficence To prevent harm.

Nonsteroidal anti-inflammatory drugs (NSAIDs) Non-opioid drugs, used for the treatment of pain.

Nonverbal communication The use of body language, facial expressions, touch, and other forms of gestures to express thoughts and feelings.

Normalization The process of family management that involves acknowledging that the child has a chronic health problem but encouraging the family members to make an effort to lead normal lives.

Nosocomial infection An infection acquired in a healthcare agency, not present at the time of entrance to the agency.

Nuchal rigidity Resistance to neck flexion.

Nurture The effects of environment on an individual's performance.

Nutrition Taking in food and assimilating it metabolically for use by the body.

Nystagmus Involuntary rapid eye movement.

O

Object permanence The knowledge that an object or person continues to exist when not seen, heard, or felt.

Obstructive uropathy Structural or functional abnormalities of the urinary system that interfere with urine flow and can result in kidney damage and underdevelopment of the lungs.

Occlusive dressing A wound covering that protects the wound from the outside environment and keeps all moisture at the wound site.

Occult blood Blood that is present in minute quantities and can be seen only on microscopic examination or through chemical testing.

Oliguria Diminished urine output (less than 0.5 to 1 mL/kg/hr).

Omphalocele A congenital malformation in which intra-abdominal contents herniate through the umbilical cord.

Oncogene A portion of the DNA that is altered and, when duplicated, causes uncontrolled cellular division.

Oncotic pressure The part of the blood osmotic pressure that is due to plasma proteins; also called blood colloid osmotic pressure.

Opioids Synthetic narcotic drugs used for the treatment of pain.

Opisthotonos/opisthotonic position Rigid hyperextension of the entire body; hyperextension of the head and neck to relieve discomfort.

Opportunistic infection An infection that is often caused by normally nonpathogenic organisms in persons who lack normal immunity.

Organelle A small cellular structure such as a ribosome or mitochondria that performs specific cellular functions.

Osmolality The amount of concentration of a fluid; technically, the number of moles of particles per kilogram of water in the solution.

Osmosis Movement of water across a semipermeable membrane into an area of higher particle concentration.

Ossification Formation of bone from fibrous tissue or cartilage.

Osteoblasts Cells that synthesize and lay down bone and then attract calcium and phosphates to strengthen the bone.

Osteoclasts Cells that resorb bone in the constant process of bone formation and breakdown.

Osteocytes Special osteoblasts that sense and respond to bone pressure and bending to direct the process of bone remodeling.

Osteomalacia Softening of bones.

Osteopenia Decreased mineralization and bone mass; bone mass between 1 and 2.5 standard deviations below norm.

Osteoporosis Softening of bone due to marked decrease in mineralization and bone mass; bone mass is more than 2.5 standard deviations below norm; also known as metabolic bone disease.

Osteotomy Surgical cutting of bone.

Ostomy An artificial abdominal opening into the urinary or gastrointestinal canal that provides an outlet for the diversion of urine or fecal matter.

Outcome expectancy What the person expects to get from performing a certain behavior.

Oxygen saturation The amount of oxygen that can potentially be delivered to the tissues.

P

Pain A highly personal and subjective unpleasant sensory and emotional experience associated with actual or potential tissue damage. Pain exists when the patient says it does.

Pain threshold The point at which the transmission of pain stimulus begins.

Pain tolerance Duration of time or intensity of pain a child will endure before demonstrating pain responses.

Palliative care A multidisciplinary care approach to prevent and relieve suffering and to enhance quality of life for patients and their families, regardless of the stage of the disease or the need for other therapies.

Palliative procedure Surgical procedure that does not create normal anatomic or hemodynamic results that are used for children with a potentially fatal or lethal condition. Examples include shunts that are lifesaving, pulmonary artery banding, and final surgeries that do not produce normal blood flow, such as the Fontan procedure.

Palpation The technique of touch to identify characteristics of the skin, internal organs, and masses, including texture, moistness, tenderness, temperature, position, shape, consistency, mobility of masses, and organs.

Pancytopenia A decreased number of blood cell components.

Pandemic The emergency and worldwide spread of an influenza or other viral or bacterial pathogen that causes significantly increased morbidity and mortality.

Paradoxical breathing Severe respiratory distress in which the chest falls and the abdomen rises on inspiration.

Paralanguage The tone and pitch of the voice; speed, pace, volume, and inflection of the conversation, as well as other vocalizations.

Parallel play A type of play that emerges in toddlerhood when children play side by side but demonstrate little or no social interaction.

Paraphimosis When the foreskin cannot be returned to its normal position over the glans, causing constriction of the penis and resulting in swelling of the glans and obstruction of penile blood flow.

Parenteral Nutrition introduced outside the intestinal tract, usually by the intravenous route.

Parenting A leadership role in the family in which children are guided in learning acceptable behaviors, beliefs, morals, and rituals of the family and become socially responsible, contributing members of society.

Paresthesia Decreased sensation or tingling.

Paronychia Infection in the tissue surrounding the nail.

Partnership A relationship in which participants join together to ensure healthcare delivery in a way that recognizes the critical role and contribution of each partner in promoting health, preventing illness, and managing healthcare conditions.

Passive immunity Placental transfer of antibodies, or antibodies are produced in another human or animal host and injected into the recipient.

Patient-controlled analgesia (PCA) A method for administering an intravenous analgesic, such as morphine, using a computerized pump that the patient controls.

Patient safety The freedom from unintentional injury caused by medical care, including harm or death related to adverse drug events, misidentification of the patient, and healthcare-associated infections.

Pco₂ The partial pressure of carbon dioxide in arterial blood.

Pediatric healthcare home (or medical home) Site of comprehensive health care by a pediatric healthcare professional.

Pediatric intensive care unit (PICU) A highly specialized care unit for children with critical illness or injuries.

Pedigree A pictorial family history diagram that traces genetic characteristics and disorders in a family.

Penetrance The percentage or likelihood that an individual who has inherited a gene mutation will actually express the disease signs and symptoms in his or her lifetime.

Percussion Striking the surface of the body, either directly or indirectly, to set up vibrations that reveal the density of underlying tissues and borders of internal organs.

Perfusion Oxygenated blood flow to all portions of the lungs.

Periodic breathing Pauses in respiration lasting less than 20 seconds; a normal breathing pattern in infancy and childhood.

Periosteum The fibrous membrane that covers the bones.

Peristalsis A progressive, wavelike muscular movement that occurs involuntarily throughout the gastrointestinal tract.

Persistent vegetative state Permanent loss of function of the cerebral cortex retaining only reflexive responses.

Pet therapy Use of a specially trained animal to provide comfort, companionship, and distraction during an illness.

Petechiae Pinpoint red lesions.

pH Negative logarithm of the hydrogen ion concentration; used to monitor the acidity of body fluid.

Phagocytosis The engulfment and destruction of microorganisms, dead cells, and foreign particles.

Phantom pain Pain that feels as if it is in an amputated extremity and is caused by trauma to the nerves in the area of the amputation.

Pharmacogenomics The study of how an individual's genotype affects his or her response to medications.

Phenotype The expression of a person's entire physical, biochemical, and physiologic makeup, as determined by the individual's genotype and environmental factors.

Phimosis When the foreskin over the glans penis cannot be retracted.

Phototoxic A rapid nonimmunologic reaction of the skin when exposed to sunlight.

Physical abuse The deliberate maltreatment of another individual that inflicts pain or injury and may result in temporary or permanent disfigurement or even death.

Physical dependence The physiologic adaptation to an analgesic or sedative drug at the peripheral and central neurons.

Physical neglect The deliberate withholding of or failure to provide the necessary and available resources to a child.

Physiologic anemia of infancy A normal occurrence after the first few weeks of life in which the hemoglobin reaches a low level of 9 to 11 g/dL in term infants and 7 to 9 g/dL in premature infants.

Physiologic anorexia A decrease in appetite manifested when the extremely high metabolic demands of infancy slow down to keep pace with the more moderate growth rate of toddlerhood.

Pica An eating disorder characterized by ingestion of nonfood items or food items consumed in abnormal quantities or forms.

Pitting edema A "pit" or concave indentation that remains after an edematous area is pressed downward by the examiner's fingers.

Play therapy A therapeutic intervention often used with preschool and school-age children, in which the child reveals conflicts, wishes, and fears on an unconscious level while playing with dolls, toys, clay, and other objects.

Pneumonitis A chemical lung injury and resulting inflammatory response.

Pneumothorax Condition that occurs when air enters the pleural space because of tears in the tracheobronchial tree, the esophagus, or the chest wall.

Po₂ The partial pressure of oxygen in arterial blood.

Polycythemia An excess production of red blood cells by the bone marrow in response to chronic hypoxemia to increase the amount of hemoglobin available to carry oxygen to the tissues.

Polydipsia Excessive thirst.

Polymorphism One of two or more variants of a particular DNA sequence. Polymorphisms most commonly involve substitution of a single base pair (called a single nucleotide polymorphism or SNP) but can represent variation in longer DNA sequences.

Polyphagia Excessive or voracious eating.

Polypharmacy The use of many drugs at one time to treat multiple health conditions.

Polysomnography A sleep study that simultaneously records the brain activity, eye movement, and respiration.

Polyuria Passage of a large volume of urine in a given period.

Population The collection of individuals that make up a community.

Population-based approach Health assessment and intervention performed with a group of children.

Posterior urethral valves Abnormal folds of mucosa in the male urethra.

Postictal period Period after seizure activity during which the level of consciousness is decreased.

Postpartum Taking place after giving birth.

Postpartum blues Mild and self-limited depression, thought to be caused by hormonal shifts in the mother during the postpartum period, evidenced by predominantly positive moods marked by labile and intense episodes of tearfulness, irritability, and sadness.

Postpartum depression A serious form of depression requiring medical intervention, usually starting within 2 to 3 months postpartum; marked by symptoms of depression lasting longer than 2 weeks, such as consistently depressed mood, poor concentration or indecisiveness, recurrent thoughts of death, fatigue or loss of energy, significant decrease or increase in appetite, and insomnia or hypersomnia.

Postpartum mood disorders A group of disorders affecting women in the postpartum period, including postpartum blues, postpartum depression, and postpartum psychosis.

Postpartum psychosis A psychiatric emergency in the postpartum period, usually presenting within 2 to 4 weeks postpartum but can start as early as 2 to 3 days after delivery. Signs include restlessness, irritability, and a rapidly evolving or shifting depressed or elated mood with increasingly disorganized, confused, or disoriented behavior. Hallucinations or delusions, frequently focused on the baby, can present life-threatening scenarios.

Postterm Born after 42 weeks' gestation.

Posturing Abnormal position assumed after injury or damage to the brain that may be seen as extreme flexion or extension of the limbs.

Prebiotic A nondigestible food ingredient that can stimulate growth or activity of probiotic bacteria.

Precursor A substance that precedes another substance or from which another substance is synthesized.

Prejudice A negative feeling about someone who is perceived as being different.

Preload Volume of blood in the ventricle at the end of diastole that stretches the heart muscle before contraction.

Prenatal care Healthcare supervision during pregnancy.

Preterm Born prior to 37 weeks' gestation.

Prevalence The percentage of the population that has a condition at a specific point in time.

Priapism Sustained and painful penile erection.

Primary dressing The layer of dressing that comes directly in contact with the wound.

Primary immune response The process in which B lymphocytes produce antibodies specific to a particular antigen on first exposure.

Primary immune deficiency Congenital immunodeficiency.

Primary prevention Activities that decrease opportunity for illness or injury.

Privacy Ability of an individual to relate information in a protected manner.

Proband The family member around whom a family history is collected.

Probiotic A food supplement containing a live microorganism that alters the balance of gut microflora, thereby providing a health benefit.

Projectile vomiting Vomiting in which the stomach contents are ejected with great force.

Prostration Extreme exhaustion, unable to make any effort.

Protective factors Characteristics of a child and family that provide strength and assistance in dealing with a crisis.

Protein A molecule composed of amino acids linked together in a particular order specified by a gene's DNA sequence; proteins perform a wide variety of functions in the cell, including serving as enzymes, structural components, or signaling molecules.

Proteomics The study of the interactions of expressed proteins in a cell.

Protocol A plan of action for chemotherapy that is based on the type of cancer, its stage, and the particular cell type.

Proto-oncogene A gene that regulates cellular growth and development but can become an oncogene, capable of causing cancerous growth.

Proximodistal development The process by which development proceeds from the center of the body outward to the extremities.

Pseudohermaphroditism Ambiguous development of the external genitalia.

Pseudohypertrophy Enlargement of the muscles as a result of infiltration by fatty tissue.

Ptosis Drooping of the eyelid over the pupil.

Puberty Period of life when the ability to reproduce sexually begins, characterized by maturation of the genital organs, development of the secondary sex characteristics, and the onset of menstruation in females.

Pulse oximeter A transcutaneous assessment method to detect the amount of hemoglobin saturated with oxygen.

Pulsus paradoxus The decrease in arterial blood pressure during inspiration by 10 mmHg that may be present in severe asthma episodes.

Punishment The action taken to enforce the rules when the child misbehaves.

Purpura Irregular bluish purple areas of bleeding into the tissues.

Pyelonephritis Upper urinary tract infection involving the ureters, renal pelvis, and renal parenchyma.

Pyeloplasty Removal of an obstructed segment of the ureter and reimplantation into the renal pelvis.

Pyrogens Substances that stimulate fever.

Q

Quality improvement The continuous study and improvement of the processes and outcomes of providing healthcare services to meet the needs of patients by examining the system and processes of care and service delivery.

R

Race A group of people who share biological similarities such as skin color, bone structure, and genetic traits.

Radiation Cancer treatment using unstable isotopes that release varying levels of energy to cause breaks in the DNA molecule and thereby destroy cells.

Radioallergosorbent test (RAST) A technique in which radioimmunoassay is used to measure the presence of IgE antibodies to certain antigens in the blood.

Radiofrequency ablation The use of radio energy to destroy a very small section of the myocardium through which an accessory conduction pathway passes.

Receptive language The words a young child is able to understand; usually greater than the number of words spoken (expressive speech).

Recessive A characteristic that is apparent only when two copies of the gene encoding it are present, one from the mother and one from the father.

Recombinant vaccine A vaccine in which an organism has been genetically altered.

Red reflex The orange-red glow of the vascular retina as light travels through the cornea, aqueous humor, lens, and vitreous humor to the retina.

Refugee A person who is unable or unwilling to return to his or her country because of persecution or a well-founded fear of persecution based on race, religion, nationality, membership in a particular social group, or political opinion.

Regression Return to an earlier behavior (a common reaction to stress).

Rehabilitation Assisting a child with physical or mental challenges to reach his or her fullest potential through therapy and education that considers the physiologic, psychologic, and environmental strengths and limitations of the child.

Reliability The extent to which the same score is obtained when an instrument or scale is used either by different persons or by the same person at different times.

Religion An organized system of shared beliefs regarding the significance of the nature, cause, and purpose of life and of the universe.

Renal failure An acute or chronic condition that occurs when the kidney is unable to excrete wastes and concentrate urine.

Renal insufficiency Decrease in the kidneys' ability to conserve sodium and concentrate the urine.

Renal osteodystrophy A complex bone disease process of chronic kidney disease in which there is increased resorption of bone caused by chronic hyperparathyroidism.

Renal replacement therapy The treatment for kidney failure, including dialysis and kidney transplantation.

Repression Involuntary forgetting of uncomfortable situations.

Resilience The ability to function with healthy responses, even during significant stress and adversity.

Respiratory effort The work of breathing.

Respite care A family support service that provides periodic breaks from the constant stress of caring for the child.

Reticulocytes Immature erythrocytes.

Retinoblastoma Tumor of the retina.

Retractions Visible depressions of tissue between the ribs of the chest wall with each inspiration.

Rickets Deossification of bones due to calcium and/or vitamin D deficiency, resulting in bending of long bones and bowlegs.

Risk factors Characteristics of a child or family that promote or contribute to health system challenges.

Risk management A process established by a healthcare institution to identify, evaluate, and reduce the risk of injury to patients, staff, and visitors, and thereby reduce the institution's liability.

Rooming in Practice in which parents stay in the child's hospital room and care for the child.

S

Saline A mixture of salt and water; normal saline refers to the mixture of salt and water in equal concentration in body fluids.

Scientific or biomedical health belief The belief that life and life processes are controlled by physical and biochemical processes that can be manipulated by humans.

Screening A procedure used to detect the possible presence of a health condition before symptoms are apparent, usually conducted on large groups of individuals at risk for a condition.

Secondary cancers Also called second malignant neoplasm (SMN) and most commonly solid tumors, these occur after the primary cancer and treatment but are of a different histologic type.

Secondary dressing A cover for the primary dressing when further protection from contamination is needed.

Secondary immune response The body's response to an antigen at any time other than the initial exposure.

Secondary immune deficiency Acquired immunodeficiency.

Secondary prevention Early diagnosis and treatment of a condition to lessen its severity.

Sedation A medically controlled state of depressed consciousness (light to deep) used for painful diagnostic and therapeutic procedures and analgesia.

Seizures Periods of abnormal electrical discharges (excessive concurrent firing) of the cortical neuronal network of cells on the surface of the brain that cause involuntary movement and behavior and sensory alterations.

Self-concept Evaluations of the self in certain specific areas, such as those related to academic achievement, athletic ability, physical appearance, and social interactions.

Self-efficacy A person's belief that he or she can change behavior to produce a desired outcome.

Self-esteem The feelings and beliefs of children about their competence and worth as individuals, their ability to meet challenges, and their ability to learn lessons from success and failure.

Self-regulation The infant's ability to maintain state and self-console, for example by sucking his or her fingers to stay calm instead of crying.

Sensible fluid loss Water loss that is measurable and observable, such as urine and drainage from tubes.

Sensitivity The ability of a test to accurately identify those with a condition being tested; a high-sensitivity test is able to detect the condition when only a small amount of the indicator is present or early in the disease process.

Sensitization An increased reaction to pain over time, or a reduced threshold for reaction to painful stimuli.

Sensorineural hearing loss Hearing loss caused by damage to the inner ear structures or the auditory nerve.

Separation anxiety Inconsolable crying and other signs of distress in an infant when parents are not present, commonly beginning in the second half of the first year of life.

Sex chromosome One of the chromosomes (X or Y) involved in sex determination. Normal human females have two X chromosomes in each cell, while normal males have one X and one Y.

Sexual maturity rating An average of the breast and pubic hair Tanner stages in females and of the genital and pubic hair Tanner stages in boys.

Sexuality A person's view of self as a sexual being.

Shaman A man or woman who enters an altered state of consciousness, at will, to contact and utilize another type of reality to acquire knowledge and power and to help other people.

Shock An acute, complex state of circulatory dysfunction resulting in failure to deliver sufficient oxygen and other nutrients to meet cell and tissue demands. It can be caused by a variety of conditions such as hemorrhage, dehydration, sepsis, obstruction of blood flow, and cardiac pump failure.

Shunt Movement of blood between the systemic and pulmonary circulation through an abnormal anatomic or surgically created opening. Left to right shunting is systemic to pulmonary circulation, and right to left shunting is pulmonary to systemic circulation.

Single nucleotide polymorphism (SNP) A variation in DNA sequence in which a single nucleotide base (A, T, C, or G) is substituted for another.

Sleep hygiene Behaviors that foster a regular and sufficient sleep pattern, as well as daytime alertness

Small for gestational age (SGA) A newborn whose weight (and possibly length and head circumference) falls below the tenth percentile when plotted on a standard intrauterine growth/gestational age chart. An SGA newborn is a small size for the amount of time spent in the uterus. An SGA baby can be preterm, term, or postterm.

Sobadores Individuals that use massage and manipulation to treat patients with joint and muscle problems.

Solitary play Playing alone, with one's self.

Specificity The ability of a test to exclude those who do not have the condition being tested.

Spina bifida A defect in one or more vertebrae through which spinal cord contents can protrude.

Spina bifida occulta A vertebral defect without visible protrusion of the meninges or spinal cord tissue.

Spinal shock Spinal cord concussion resulting in a transient suppression of nerve function below the level of the acute injury.

Spiritual dimension Belief in a connection with a greater power that guides a person to strive for inspiration, respect, meaning, and purpose in life.

Spiritual health The ability to develop a spiritual nature, including awareness of a life purpose and fulfillment.

Spirituality The individual's experience and interpretation of his or her relationship with a Supreme Being.

Sprain A tearing of ligaments usually caused when a joint is twisted or otherwise traumatized.

Stadiometer Height-measuring device attached to the wall.

Stakeholders All residents, policy makers, health providers, and funders concerned with the outcome of the assessment.

Status epilepticus A continuous seizure that lasts for more than 30 minutes, or two or more seizures without full recovery of consciousness between episodes.

Stenosis/stenotic Narrowing of a valve or below the valve, or in the blood vessel.

Stereotyping The assumption that all members of a culture, ethnic, or racial group are alike and share the same attitudes and beliefs.

Stereotypy Repetitive, obsessive, machine-like movements, commonly seen in children with autism or schizophrenia.

Stoma An opening, commonly in the abdominal wall, to provide for drainage from the intestinal or urinary systems.

Strabismus An abnormal turning of the eye, usually inward or outward, due to a weak eye muscle.

Stranger anxiety Wariness of strange people and places, often shown by infants between 6 and 18 months of age.

Strangulation Closure of the muscular ring around a portion of the bowel, preventing it from moving back into the abdomen.

Stratum corneum The superficial layer of the epidermis.

Stridor An audible crowlike inspiratory and expiratory breath sound.

Stroke volume The amount of blood ejected from the heart with each contraction.

Stupor Deep sleep or unresponsiveness with arousal only to repeated vigorous stimulation.

Subcutaneous emphysema Air leakage in the tissue.

Subluxation Partial or incomplete dislocation of a joint.

Sudden infant death syndrome (SIDS) The sudden unexpected death of an infant less than 1 year of age, occurring during sleep that is unexplained after autopsy and clinical investigation.

Sunsetting eyes A condition in which the sclera is visible above the iris.

Superego A moral and ethical system that develops in childhood and contains a set of values and conscience.

Supernumerary nipples Extra small, undeveloped nipples and areolae found along the mammary line between the neck and pubic area that may be mistaken for moles.

Support systems The extended network of family, friends, and religious and community contacts that provide nurturance, emotional support, and direct assistance to parents.

Surfactant A lipid-protein secreted in the lungs that lowers the surface tension of the alveoli.

Surveillance A continuous process in which skilled observations are carried out in collaboration with families, specialists, childcare providers, and other professionals.

Synchronized cardioversion The timed administration of a calibrated electrical charge by a defibrillator in an effort to convert the arrhythmia to a sinus rhythm.

Syncope Transient loss of consciousness and muscle tone.

Syndrome A collection of anomalies that occur in a consistent pattern and have a common cause.

Syngeneic Hematopoietic stem cell transplant from an identical twin.

Systemic vascular resistance The force or resistance of the blood in the body's blood vessels that helps return blood to the heart.

T

Tachypnea An elevated respiratory rate.

Tactile fremitus Vibrations that can be palpated on the chest when the child cries or talks.

Technology-assisted Special services for infants and toddlers up to age 3 years who have developmental delay or are at risk for developmental delay.

Telangiectasia Permanent dilation of superficial capillaries and venules.

Telephone triage Talking with a family member by telephone to address concerns about the child, analyze the child's symptoms, and determine if or how quickly the child needs to be seen by the healthcare provider.

Temperament The unique characteristic style of activity, mood, and reaction of an infant, made up of genetically derived characteristics that evolve and develop over time and often underlie interaction and behavior.

Tendons Fibrous bands that connect bone to its accompanying muscles, allowing the bone to move when a muscle contracts or relaxes.

Teratogenesis Abnormal development of the fetus.

Term Born between 37 and 42 weeks gestation.

Tertiary prevention Activities designed to rehabilitate or restore optimum function.

Testicular torsion An emergency condition in which the testis suddenly rotates on its spermatic cord, obstructing its blood supply.

Thelarche Breast development.

Therapeutic play Planned play techniques that provide an opportunity for children to deal with fears and concerns related to illness or hospitalization.

Therapeutic recreation Using recreational therapy interventions to improve functioning of individuals with illness or disabling conditions.

Third-spacing Loss or pooling of fluid in a body space.

Thrombocytes Platelets.

Thrombocytopenia A low platelet count.

Thyrotoxicosis (thyroid storm) When thyroid hormone is suddenly released into the bloodstream during surgery; the child experiences fever, diaphoresis, and tachycardia, progressing to shock and, if untreated, death.

Tidal volume The amount of air inhaled and exhaled during a normal breath.

Tinnitus Ringing in the ears.

Tolerance An altered state of response to an opioid or other pain agent in which increasing amounts of the drug are needed to produce or maintain the same level of pain relief or sedation effect.

Tonic Continuous muscular contraction; sustained stiffening, often used to describe seizure activity.

Torsades de pointes A distinct form of ventricular tachycardia in patients with marked QT prolongation on the ECG, appearing as "twisting of the points."

Toxic appearance Lethargy, poor perfusion, hypoventilation or hyperventilation, and cyanosis.

Toxicants Natural or synthetic chemicals not metabolically produced by an organism.

Toxins Damaging or poisonous chemicals produced by metabolism or an organism.

Toxoid A toxin that has been treated (by heat or chemical) to weaken its toxic effects but retain its antigenicity.

Tracheostomy The creation of a surgical opening into the trachea through the anterior neck at the cricoid cartilage, often performed if long-term airway management is needed.

Transcultural Across cultures.

Transductive reasoning Connecting two events in a cause-and-effect relationship simply because they occur together in time; common in thoughts of preschoolers.

Translocation The joining of a part of or a whole chromosome to another separate chromosome.

Transplacental immunity Passive immunity that is transferred from mother to infant.

Treatment interference The self-removal of technologic devices in hospitalized patients.

Treatment room A special room used for the pediatric population for procedures such as intravenous starts, lumbar punctures, and blood drawing. The treatment room is used so that the child always has a "safe" environment and comfort zone by knowing that no unpleasant or painful procedures will occur in his or her own hospital room.

Triage Rapid assessment to sort injured children by the urgency of their condition.

Trigger A stimulus that initiates an asthmatic episode; a substance or condition, including exercise, infection, allergy, irritants, weather, or emotions.

Triglycerides The major fats consumed by humans, consisting of three fatty acids connected to a glycerol base.

Tripod position Sitting forward with arms on knees for support and extending the neck.

Trisomy Having three chromosomes instead of the usual two as in trisomy 21 or Down syndrome.

Tumor suppressor genes Genetic material that controls the growth of cells, decreasing the effects of oncogenes.

Tympanogram A graph showing the ability of the middle ear to transmit sound energy; measured by inserting an airtight probe into the external ear entrance and emitting a tone.

Tympanometry A test to estimate the pressure in the middle ear and an indirect measure of tympanic membrane movement.

Tympanostomy tubes Small Teflon tubes inserted surgically into the tympanic membrane to equalize pressure, promote fluid drainage, and ventilate the middle ear.

U

Unconsciousness Depressed cerebral function, or the inability of the brain to respond to stimuli.

Uremia Toxicity resulting from the buildup of urea and nitrogenous waste in the blood.

Uremic frost Urea crystals deposited on the skin.

Ureteral stent A device used to maintain patency of the ureter allowing urine flow from the kidney to the bladder.

Urethral stent A device used to maintain patency of the ureteral canal and allow urine to flow from the bladder through the urethra.

Urethritis Infection of the urethra.

Uveitis Inflammation of the middle layer of the eye.

V

Vacuum-assisted wound closure Negative-pressure wound therapy.

Valgus Bending inward of a limb toward the midline of the body.

Validity A test's ability to accurately measure the characteristics it is established to measure.

Valsalva maneuver A forced expiratory effort against a closed airway (e.g., holding the breath and bearing down as if to have a bowel movement, inducing the gag reflex, or blowing forcefully on the thumb), which increases intrathoracic and venous pressures and thus slows the heart rate.

Valvuloplasty Dilating a stenotic pulmonic or aortic valve.

Varus A condition in which the hindfoot turns inward, usually associated with clubfoot.

Vasculitis Inflammation of the blood vessels.

Vaso-occlusion Blockage of a blood vessel.

Vectors Insects or animals that transmit infectious organisms by biting humans.

Vegan Strict vegetarian who eats no animal products.

Vegetarian Individual who eats no poultry, meat, or fish.

Ventilation The movement of oxygen into the lungs and carbon dioxide out of the lungs.

Verbal communication The use of language, spoken or written or vocalizations, such as laughter or crying to convey messages.

Vertical transmission The passage of disease from the mother to the fetus during the period of pregnancy.

Vesicoureteral reflux (VUR) The backflow of urine from the bladder into the ureters during voiding.

Violence Threatened or actual use of physical force that leads to potential or actual physical or emotional trauma.

Virilization Production of masculine secondary sex characteristics in females.

Vision A complex process of acquiring meaning from what is seen, involving the eye, brain, and related neurologic and physiologic structures.

Visual acuity Measurement of the ability to discriminate a letter or other object to test sight.

Volvulus A twisting of the intestine.

W

Water intoxication Intake of excessive water without sodium.

Weaning The process of a baby giving up breastfeeding or a bottle to drink from a cup.

Wheezing A noise resulting from the passage of air through mucus or fluids in a narrowed lower airway; is associated with asthma.

Whispered pectoriloquy Change in vocal resonance when syllables are heard distinctly as a whisper.

Wild type gene The most common type of gene; designated as normal.

Windshield survey A walking or driving tour around a neighborhood or community for the purpose of identifying resources and characteristics of the community.

Withdrawal The physical signs and symptoms that occur when a sedative or pain drug is stopped suddenly in a patient who is physically tolerant.

X

Xerosis Generally dry skin that is more likely to crack and fissure.

X-linked Any gene found on the X chromosome, or traits determined by such genes; also refers to the specific mode of inheritance of such genes; one altered gene on an X chromosome in a male can produce disease, such as hemophilia.

Z

Zoonosis Infectious disease transmitted to humans from an insect or animal host.

Zygote A fertilized ovum.

Index

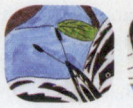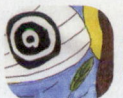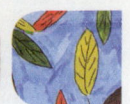

Page numbers followed by *f* indicate figures and those followed by *t* indicate tables, boxes, or special features. The titles of special features (e.g., Clinical Reasoning in Action, Developing Cultural Competence, Partnering with Families) are also capitalized.

Evidence-Based Practice

Health Promotion & Maintenance Overview

Legal and Ethical Considerations

Medications

Nursing Care Plan

Partnering with Families